DISEASES/CONDITIONS AND ICD-9-CM CODES

Abruptio placentae 641.2**
Acne vulgaris 706.1
Acromegaly 253.0
Actinic keratosis 702.0
Acute bronchitis 466.0
Acute and chronic viral hepatitis 070.9
Acute diarrhea (NOS) 787.91
Acute leukemia (plain leukemia) 208.0**
Acute myocardial infarction 410.9**
Acute otitis media 382.9
Acute pancreatitis 577.0
Acute peripheral facial paralysis (Bell's palsy) ...351.0
Acute renal failure 584.9
Acute respiratory failure 518.81
Acute stress disorder 308.9
Adrenocortical insufficiency 255.4
Adverse reactions to blood transfusions ...999
Alcoholism 303.9**
Allergic reactions to drugs 995.2
Allergic reactions to insect stings 989.5
Allergic rhinitis 477.8
Alopecia areata 704.01
Alzheimer's disease 331.0
Amebiasis 006.9
Amenorrhea 626.0
Anal fissure, ...565.0
Anaphylaxis, NOS 995.0
Angina pectoris 413.9
Angioedema 995.1
Ankle fracture 824.8
Ankylosing spondylitis 720.0
Anorectal abscess ....566.
Anorexia nervosa 307.1
Aortic aneurysm and dissection 441.00
Aplastic anemia 284.9
Asthma 493.9**
Atelectasis 518.0
Atopic dermatitis 691.8
Atopic fibrillation 427.31
Attention deficit/hyperactivity disorder ...314.01
Autoimmune hemolytic anemia 283.0
Bacterial meningitis ....320.
Bacterial pneumonia 482.9
Bacterial vaginitis 616.1
Benign prostatic hyperplasia ....600.
Blastomycosis 116.0
Bleeding esophageal varices 456.0
Brain abscess ....324.
Brain tumors 239.6
Breast cancer 174
Brucellosis 023
Bulimia nervosa 307.51
Bullous diseases 694
Burns 940-949
Bursitis 726-727
Cancer of the endometrium 182.0
Cancer of the skin 172-173
Cancer of the uterine cervix 180
Cardiac arrest, sudden cardiac death ...427.5
Care after myocardial infarction 414.8
Cellulitis ....682.
Chancroid 099.3
Chlamydia trachomatis infection 079.88
Cholelithiasis and cholecystitis 574.1-574.9
Cholera 001
Chronic fatigue syndrome 780.71
Chronic leukemia 208.1**
Chronic obstructive pulmonary disease ...491.2**
Chronic pancreatitis 577.1
Chronic renal failure 585
Chronic serous otitis media 381.1**
Coccidioidomycosis 114*
Colorectal cancer 153
Concussion 850
Congenital heart disease 745-747
Congenital rubella 771.0
Congestive heart failure 428.0
Conjunctivitis, acute 372.0**
Connective tissue disease 710*
Constipation 564.0
Contact dermatitis 692
Cough 786.2
Cushing's syndrome 255.0
Delirium 780.0
Dementia, multi-infarct, uncomplicated ...294.8
Depression psychosis 298.0
Depression with anxiety 300.4

Diabetes insipidus 253.5
Diabetes mellitus, I 250.01
Diabetes mellitus, II 250.02
Diabetic ketoacidosis 276.2**
Diphtheria 032*
Diseases of the mouth 528*
Disseminated intravascular coagulation ...286.6
Diverticulitis 562.11
Drug abuse (nondependent) 305.9**
Dysfunctional uterine bleeding 626.6
Dysmenorrhea 635.5
Dysphagia and esophageal obstruction ...530.3
Ectopic pregnancy 633*
Elbow dislocation 832.0**
Encephalitis 323*
Endometriosis 617*
Enuresis 786.30
Epididymitis 604**
Episodic vertigo 386.11
Erythema multiforme 695.1
Fetal lung immaturity 770.4
Fever 780.6
Fibrocystic diseases of the breast 610.1
Fibromyositis 729.1
Fifth disease 057.0
Finger dislocation, closed 834.0**
Finger fracture 816.0**
Fistula (anal) 565.1
Fitting of diaphragm V25.02
Folliculitis 704.8
Food allergy 693.1
Food poisoning 005*
Foot fracture 825.2**
Frostbite 991*
Gangrene 785.4
Gastritis ....535.
Gastroesophageal reflux disease (GERD) ...530.81
Generalized anxiety disorder 300.02
Generalized epilepsy 345.1**
Genital warts (condylomata acuminata) ...078.11
Giant cell arteritis 446.5
Giardiasis 7.1
Gilles de la Tourette syndrome 307.23
Glaucoma 365**
Gonorrhea 098.0
Gout 274.9
Granuloma inguinale (donovanosis) 099.2
Guillain-Barré syndrome 357.0
Headache. 784.0
Heart block 426.1**
Heat exhaustion 992.3
Heat stroke 992.0
Hemochromatosis 285.0
Hemolytic disease of the fetus and newborn ...773.2
Hemophilia and related conditions 286.0
Hemorrhoids 455.6
Herpes gestationis 646.8**
Herpes simplex 054*
Herpes zoster 053*
Hiccups 786.8
High-altitude sickness 993.2
Histoplasmosis 115**
HIV-associated infections 042.0
HIV infection, asymptomatic V08
HIV infection, early symptomatic 042
HIV infection, late symptomatic 042
Hyperlipoproteinemias 272*
Hyperparathyroidism 252.0
Hyperprolactinemia 253.1
Hypersensitivity pneumonitis 495
Hypertension (essential) 401*
Hyperthyroidism 242**
Hypertrophic cardiomyopathy 425.4
Hypoparathyroidism 252.1
Hypothyroidism 244*
Immunization practices V03, VO4, VO5, VO6**
Impetigo 684
Impotence 302.72
Indigestion 536.8
Infectious diarrhea 009.2
Infectious mononucleosis 075
Infective endocarditis 424.9**
Influenza 487.2
Ingrowing nail 703.0
Insect and spider bite 989.5
Insertion of intrauterine device V25.1
Insomnia (NOS) 780.52

DISEASES/CONDITIONS AND ICD-9-CM CODES *(Continued)*

Intracerebral hemorrhage 431
Iron deficiency anemia.....280.0-280.9
Irritable bowel syndrome 564.1
Jellyfish sting.....989.5
Juvenile rheumatoid arthritis 714.3**
Keloids 701.4
Laryngitis 464.00
Lead poisoning 984*
Legionnaires' disease 482.84
Leishmaniasis 085*
Leprosy 030*
Lichen planus 697.0
Low back pain 724.2
Lyme disease 088.81
Lymphogranuloma venereum 099.1
Malabsorption 579*
Malaria 084.6
Measles (rubeola) 055.9
Meconium aspiration 770.1
Melanoma, malignant 172*
Ménière's disease 386.0**
Meningitis 320-322
Menopausal.....627.2
Migraine headache 346**
Mitral valve prolapse 424.0
Monilial vulvovaginitis 121.1
Multiple myeloma 203.0**
Multiple sclerosis 340
Mumps 072.9
Myasthenia gravis 358.0**
Mycoplasmal pneumonias 483.0
Mycosis fungoides 202.1**
Nausea and vomiting 787.01
Neoplasm of the vulva 239.5
Neutropenia 288.0
Nevi 216*
Newborn physiologic jaundice 774.6
Nongonococcal urethritis.....099.4**
Non-Hodgkin's lymphomas 202.8**
Non-autoimmune hemolytic anemia 283.1**
Normal delivery 650
Obesity.....278.0**
Obsessive-compulsive disorders 300.3
Onychomycosis 110.1
Optic neuritis 377.3**
Osteoarthritis 715**
Osteomyelitis 730**
Osteoporosis 733.00
Otitis externa 380.10
Paget's disease of bone 731.0
Panic disorder 300.01
Pap smear V72.3
Parkinsonism 332.0
Paronychia 681.0**
Partial epilepsy 345.4**
Patent ductus arteriosus 747.0
Pediculosis 132*
Pelvic inflammatory disease 614*
Peptic ulcer disease 533*
Pericarditis 432.9
Peripheral arterial disease 443.9
Peripheral neuropathies 356*
Pernicious anemia 281.0
Personality disorder 301**
Pheochromocytoma 227.0
Phobia 300.2**
Pigmentary disorders—vitiligo 709.01
Pinworms 127.4
Pityriasis rosea 696.3
Placenta previa 641**
Plague 020*
Platelet-mediated bleeding disorders 287.1
Pleural effusion 511.9
Polycythemia vera 238.4
Polymyalgia rheumatica 725
Porphyria 277.1
Postpartum hemorrhage 666.1**
Post-traumatic stress disorder 309.81
Pregnancy V22.2
Pregnancy-induced hypertension 642**
Premature beats 427.6**
Premenstrual tension syndrome (PMS) 625.4
Prescribed oral contraceptive.....V25.01
Pressure ulcers 707.0
Preterm labor 644.2**
Primary glomerular disease 581-583
Primary lung abscess.....513.0
Primary lung cancer 162.9
Prostate cancer.....185

Prostatitis 601*
Pruritus.....698.9
Pruritus ani.....698.0
Pruritus vulvae 698.1
Psittacosis (ornithosis) 073*
Psoriasis 696.1
Pulmonary embolism 415.1
Pyelonephritis 590*
Q fever 083.0
Rabies 071
Rat-bite fever 026*
Relapsing fever 087*
Renal calculi 592
Reye syndrome 331.81
Rheumatic fever 390
Rheumatoid arthritis 714.0
Rib fracture 807.0**
Rocky Mountain spotted fever 082.0
Rosacea 695.3
Roseola 057.8
Rubella 056*
Salmonellosis 003.0
Sarcoidosis 135
Scabies.....133.0
Schizophrenia 295**
Seborrheic dermatitis.....690.1**
Septicemia 038*
Sézary's syndrome 202.2**
Shoulder dislocation 831.0**
Sickle cell anemia 282.6**
Silicosis 502
Sinusitis, chronic 473*
Skull fracture 800, 801, 803
Sleep apnea 780.57
Sleep disorders 780.50
Snakebite 989.5
Stasis ulcers 454.0
Status epilepticus 345.3
Stomach cancer 151*
Streptococcal pharyngitis.....034.0
Stroke 436
Strongyloides infection 127.2
Subdural or subarachnoid hemorrhage.....852**
Sunburn 692.71
Syphilis 090-097
Tachycardias.....785.0
Tapeworm infections 123*
Telogen effluvium 704.02
Temporomandibular joint syndrome 524.6**
Tendonitis 726.90
Tetanus 037
Thalassemia 282.4**
Therapeutic use of blood components V59.0**
Thrombotic thrombocytopenic purpura 446.6
Thyroid cancer 193
Thyroiditis 245*
Tinea capitis 110.0
Tinnitus.....388.3**
Toe fracture 826.0
Toxic shock syndrome 040.82
Toxoplasmosis 130*
Transient cerebral ischemia 435*
Trauma to the genitourinary tract 958,959
Trichinellosis 124
Trichomonal vaginitis 131.01
Trigeminal neuralgia 350.1
Tuberculosis, pulmonary 011**
Tularemia 021*
Typhoid fever 002.0
Typhus fevers 080, 081
Ulcerative colitis 556*
Urethral stricture 598*
Urinary incontinence 788.30
Urticaria.....708*
Uterine inertia 661.0**
Uterine leiomyoma 218*
Varicella 052*
Venous thrombosis 453.8
Viral pneumonia 480.9
Viral respiratory infections 465.9
Vitamin deficiency 264-269
Vitamin K deficiency 269.0
Warts (verrucae) 078.10
Wegener's granulomatosis 446.4
Whooping cough (pertussis) 033*
Wrist fracture 814.0**

*4th digit needed
**5th (or 4th and 5th) digit needed

CONN'S
Current Therapy 2006

More Volumes in the Current Therapy Series

Upcoming

Current Surgical Therapy, 9th Edition
CAMERON, 2007

Gellis & Kagan's Current Pediatric Therapy, 18th Edition
BURG, INGELFINGER, POLIN, GERSHON, 2006

Current Therapy in Vascular Surgery, 5th Edition
STANLEY, VEITH, WAKEFIELD, 2007

Current Therapy in Trauma and Surgical Critical Care
ASENSIO, TRUNKEY, 2007

Published

Current Therapy in Plastic Surgery
MCCARTHY, GALIANO, ABD BOUTROS, 2006

Current Therapy in Colon and Rectal Surgery, 2nd Edition
FAZIO, CHURCH, AND DELANEY, 2005

Current Surgical Therapy, 8th Edition
CAMERON, 2004

Current Therapy in Thoracic and Cardiovascular Surgery
YANG AND CAMERON, 2004

Current Therapy in Allergy, Immunology and Rheumatology, 6th Edition
LICHTENSTEIN, BUSSE, AND GEHA, 2003

Gellis and Kagan's Current Pediatric Therapy, 17th Edition
BURG, INGELFINGER, POLIN, AND GERSHON, 2002

Current Therapy in Neurologic Disease, 7th Edition
JOHNSON, GRIFFIN, AND MCARTHUR, 2006

Current Therapy of Infectious Disease, 2nd Edition
SCHLOSSBERG, 2001

Current Therapy in Vascular Surgery, 4th Edition
ERNST AND STANLEY, 2001

Current Ocular Therapy, 5th Edition
FRAUNFELDER AND ROY, 2000

Current Therapy in Obstetrics and Gynecology, 5th Edition
QUILLIGAN AND ZUSPAN, 2000

CONN'S
Current
Therapy
2006

Robert E. Rakel, MD

Professor, Department of Family and
    Community Medicine
Baylor College of Medicine
Houston, Texas

Edward T. Bope, MD

Family Practice Residency Director
Riverside Family Practice Residency Program
Clinical Professor
Department of Family Medicine
The Ohio State University
Columbus, Ohio

LATEST APPROVED METHODS
OF TREATMENT FOR
THE PRACTICING PHYSICIAN

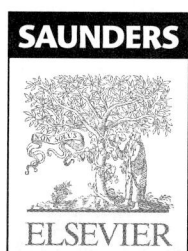

SAUNDERS

ELSEVIER

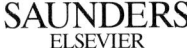

SAUNDERS
ELSEVIER

1600 John F. Kennedy Blvd.
Ste 1800
Philadelphia, PA 19103-2899

ISBN-13: 978-1-4160-2376-0
ISBN-10: 1-4160-2376-3

CONN'S CURRENT THERAPY 2006

Library of Congress Cataloging-in-Publication Data
Current therapy; latest approved methods of treatment for the practicing physician.
Editors: H. F. Conn and others
    v. 28 cm. annual
        ISBN 1-4160-2376-3
    1. Therapeutics.   2. Therapeutics, Surgical.   3. Medicine—Practice.
        I. Conn, Howard Franklin, 1908–1982 ed.

    RM101.C87   616.058   49–8328 rev*

Acquisitions Editor: Joanne Husovski
Publishing Services Manager: Frank Polizzano
Senior Project Managers: Pete Faber and Natalie Ware
Design Direction: Karen O'Keefe-Owens

Printed in the United States of America.

Last digit is the print number: 9 8 7 6 5 4 3 2 1

Contributors

Ali F. AbuRahma, MD
Professor of Surgery, West Virginia University School of
Medicine; Chief, Vascular Surgery; Medical Director,
Vascular Laboratory; Co-Medical Director, Vascular Center
of Excellence, Department of Surgery, Robert C. Byrd
Health Sciences Center of West Virginia University,
Charleston, West Virginia
Venous Thrombosis

Harold Pomeroy Adams, Jr., MD
Professor, Department of Neurology, The University of
Iowa Roy J. and Lucille A. Carver College of Medicine,
Iowa City, Iowa
Ischemic Cerebrovascular Disease

Paul C. Adams, MD
Professor of Medicine, The University of Western Ontario
Faculty of Medicine, London, Ontario, Canada
Hemochromatosis

Tod C. Aeby, MD
Residency Program Director, Department of Obstetrics,
Gynecology, and Women's Health, University of Hawaii
John A. Burns School of Medicine, Honolulu, Hawaii
Uterine Leiomyomas

Marc E. Agronin, MD
Director of Mental Health Services, Miami Jewish Home and
Hospital for the Aged; Assistant Professor of Psychiatry,
University of Miami School of Medicine, Miami, Florida
Delirium

Bandar Al Ghamdi, MD
Electrophysiology Fellow, University of British Columbia
Faculty of Medicine, Vancouver, British Columbia, Canada
Premature Beats

Carl M. Allen, DDS, MSD
Professor, Department of Oral Pathology, The Ohio State
University College of Dentistry; Director, Oral &
Maxillofacial Surgery and Pathology, University Hospital;
Professor, Department of Pathology, The Ohio State
University College of Medicine and Public Health,
Columbus, Ohio
Diseases of the Mouth

Emine Alp, MD
Assistant Professor, Department of Infectious Disease,
Erciyes University Faculty of Medicine, Kayseri, Turkey
Brucellosis

Navin M. Amin, MD
Professor and Chairman, Department of Family
Medicine/Pediatrics, University of California, Irvine,
School of Medicine, Irvine; Associate Professor of Medicine,
David Geffen School of Medicine at UCLA, Los Angeles;
Associate Professor of Family Medicine, Stanford University
School of Medicine, Bakersfield, California
Infective Endocarditis

Robert J. Anderson, MD
Chief, Section of Endocrinology, VA Medical Center;
Professor of Medicine, Creighton University School of
Medicine, Omaha, Nebraska
Hypopituitarism

Aydin Arici, MD
Professor, Department of Reproductive Endocrinology and
Infertility, Yale University School of Medicine, New Haven,
Connecticut
Dysfunctional Uterine Bleeding

David C. Aron, MD, MS
Professor of Medicine and Epidemiology and Biostatistics,
Division of Clinical and Molecular Endocrinology, Case
Western Reserve University School of Medicine; Director,
VA-HSR&D Center for Quality Improvement Research,
Louis Stokes Cleveland Department of Veterans Affairs
Medical Center, Cleveland, Ohio
Adrenal Insufficiency

Gopal H. Badlani, MD
Vice Chairman, Department of Urology, Long Island Jewish
Medical Center, New Hyde Park, New York
Benign Prostatic Hyperplasia

David A. Baker, MD
Professor, Department of Obstetrics, Gynecology, and
Reproductive Medicine, State University of New York at
Stony Brook Health Sciences Center School of Medicine,
Stony Brook, New York
Vulvovaginitis

Robert A. Balk, MD
Director, Division of Pulmonary and Critical Care Medicine,
Rush University Medical Center; Rush Medical College,
Chicago, Illinois
Severe Sepsis and Septic Shock

Robert Baran, MD
Former Head, Department of Dermatology, Cannes General
Hospital, Nail Disease Center, Cannes, France
Diseases of the Nails

Uriel S. Barzel, MD
Professor, Department of Medicine (Endocrinology), Albert
Einstein College of Medicine of Yeshiva University; Primary
Care Physician/Specialist, Montefiore Medical Center, Bronx,
New York
Osteoporosis

Heidi M. Bauer, MD, MS, MPH
Chief, Office of Medical and Scientific Affairs, STD Control
Branch, California Department of Health Services, Oakland,
California
Nongonococcal Urethritis

Joel S. Bennett, MD
Professor of Medicine, University of Pennsylvania School of
Medicine, Philadelphia, Pennsylvania
Platelet-Mediated Bleeding Disorders

Karl R. Beutner, MD, PhD
Associate Clinical Professor of Dermatology, University of
California, San Francisco, School of Medicine, San Francisco,
California
Condyloma Accuminata (Genital Warts)

Zulfiqar A. Bhutta, MB, BS, PhD
Husein Lalji Dewraj Professor of Pediatrics, Aga Khan
University and Medical Center, Karachi, Pakistan
Typhoid Fever

Emil Bisaccia, MD
Professor of Clinical Dermatology, Columbia University
College of Physicians and Surgeons, New York, New York
Diseases of the Hair

Peter B. Bloland, DVM, MPVM
Chief, Case Management Unit, Malaria Branch, Division of
Parasitic Diseases, National Center for Infectious Diseases,
Centers for Disease Control and Prevention, Atlanta, Georgia
Malaria

Brian A. Boehlecke, MD, MSPH
Professor of Medicine, University of North Carolina School of
Medicine, Chapel Hill, North Carolina
Obstructive Sleep Apnea

Jonathan Bond, MB, MRCPI
Specialist Registrar in Hematology, The Adelaide and Meath
Hospitals, Tallaght, Dublin, Ireland
Chronic Leukemias

Stephen Boorjian, MD
Chief Resident, Joan and Sanford I. Weill Medical College of
Cornell University; New York–Presbyterian Hospital, New
York, New York
Urethral Stricture

Valia Boosalis, MD
Assistant Professor, Department of Medicine, Boston
University School of Medicine; Staff
Hematologist/Oncologist, Jamaica Plain Boston Veterans
Medical Center, Boston, Massachusetts
Thalassemia

William Z. Borer, MD
Professor, Department of Pathology, Jefferson Medical
College at Thomas Jefferson University, Philadelphia,
Pennsylvania
Reference Intervals for the Interpretation of Laboratory Tests

Patrick Borgen, MD
Chief, Breast Service, Department of Surgery, Memorial
Sloan-Kettering Cancer Center, New York, New York
Diseases of the Breast

Phillipe Bossi, MD, PhD
Department of Infectious Diseases, Pitié-Salpêtrière
Hospital, Paris, France
Plague

Louis-Philippe Boulet, MD
Pneumologist, Laval Hospital, and Professor of Medicine,
Laval University, Quebec City, Canada
Asthma in Adolescents and Adults

Maxime Breban, MD, PhD
Professor of Rheumatology, University Versailles-Saint-
Quentin en Yvelines; Division of Rheumatology, Hospital
Ambroise Paré, Boulogne-Billancourt, France
Ankylosing Spondylitis

François Bricaire, MD
Plague

Sylvia L. Brice, MD
Associate Professor of Dermatology, University of Colorado
Health Sciences Center School of Medicine, Aurora,
Colorado
Viral Diseases of the Skin

Kenneth R. Bridges, MD
Founder, Joint Center for Sickle Cell and Thalassemic
Disorders, Brigham and Women's Hospital; Associate
Professor of Medicine, Partners in HealthCare, Harvard
Medical School, Cambridge, Massachussetts
Management Issues in Sickle Cell Disease

Charles K. Brown, MD
Professor and Vice Chair for Education, Department of
Emergency Medicine, The Brody School of Medicine at East
Carolina University, Greenville, North Carolina
Marine Trauma, Envenomations, and Intoxications

Deborah Brown, MD
Assistant Professor, Department of Pediatrics, The
University of Texas Medical School at Houston and M.D.
Anderson Cancer Center, Houston, Texas
Disseminated Intravascular Coagulation

Forrest C. Brown, MD
Clinical Professor, Department of Dermatology,
University of Texas, Southwestern Medical School;
Chief, Division of Dermatology, Medical City Hospital,
Dallas, Texas
Premalignant Lesions

Richard L. Brown, MD, MPH
Associate Professor, Department of Family Medicine,
University of Wisconsin Medical School, Madison,
Wisconsin
Alcohol Use Disorders

Philip Alfred Brunell, MS, MD
Professor Emeritus of Pediatrics, David Geffen School of
Medicine at University of California—Los Angeles,
Los Angeles, California
Varicella

Paul C. Bryson, MD
Resident, University of North Carolina Voice Center, Chapel Hill, North Carolina
Hoarseness and Laryngitis

Robert Buckmire, MD
Associate Professor, Department of Otolaryngology–Head and Neck Surgery, University of North Carolina School of Medicine; Director, University of North Carolina Voice Center, Chapel Hill, North Carolina
Hoarseness and Laryngitis

James J. Burke II, MD
Assistant Professor, Department of Obstetrics and Gynecology, Mercer University School of Medicine, Macon; Attending Physician, Memorial Health University Medical Center, Savannah, Georgia
Endometrial Cancer

Michael J. Burke, MD, PhD
Director of Medical Student Education and Associate Professor, Department of Psychiatry and Behavioral Medicine; Director of Inpatient Services and Director of Electroconvulsive Therapy (ECT) Services, Patient Care Clinic, University of Kansas School of Medicine–Wichita; Director of Psychiatry Education, Department of Medicine, Via Christi Regional Medical Center, Wichita, Kansas
Mood Disorders

Kenneth D. Burman, MD
Chief, Endocrine Section, Washington Hospital Center, Washington DC, Professor, Department of Medicine, Georgetown University, Washington DC
Hyperthyroidism

Ruth L. Bush, MD
Assistant Professor, Division of Vascular Surgery and Endovascular Therapy, Michael E. DeBakey Department of Surgery, Baylor College of Medicine, Houston, Texas
Acquired Diseases of the Aorta

Thomas M. Bush, MD
Clinical Associate Professor, Stanford University School of Medicine, Stanford; Chief of Rheumatology, Santa Clara Valley Medical Center, San Jose, California
Cutaneous Vasculitis

Kevin A. Bybee, MD
Assistant Professor of Medicine, Mayo Clinic College of Medicine, Rochester, Minnesota
Acute Myocardial Infarction

Alexander Bystritsky, MD, PhD
Professor, Department of Psychiatry and Biobehavioral Sciences, David Geffen School of Medicine at University of California—Los Angeles, Director, Anxiety Disorders Program, Neuropsychiatric Institute and Hospital, Los Angeles, California
Panic Disorder

Sally A. Campbell-Lee, MD
Associate Medical, Director, Division of Transfusion Medicine; Assistant Professor, Department of Pathology, Johns Hopkins Medical Institutions, Baltimore, Maryland
Therapeutic Use of Blood Components

Thomas R. Caraccio, PharmD
Associate Professor of Emergency Medicine, State University of New York at Stony Brook Health Sciences Center School of Medicine, Stony Brook; Assistant Professor of Pharmacology and Toxicology, New York College of Osteopathic Medicine, Old Westbury, New York
Medical Toxicology: Ingestions, Inhalations, and Dermal and Ocular Absorptions

Brett S. Carver, MD
Urologic Oncology Fellow, Memorial Sloan-Kettering Cancer Center; Department of Urology, Sidney Kimmel Center for Prostate and Urologic Cancers, New York, New York
Malignant Tumors of the Urogenital Tract

F. Xavier Castellanos, MD
Brooke and Daniel Neidich Professor of Child and Adolescent Psychiatry, New York University School of Medicine; Director, Institute for Pediatric Neuroscience; Director of Research, New York University Child Study Center, New York, New York
Attention Deficit Hyperactivity Disorder (ADHD)

Daniel Cattran, MD
Senior Scientist, Division of Clinical Investigation and Human Physiology, Toronto General Research Institute, Toronto, Ontario, Canada
Primary Glomerular Diseases

Frank R. Cerniglia, Jr., MD
Director of Pediatric Urology, Urologic Institute of New Orleans, New Orleans, Louisiana
Childhood Enuresis

Miriam M. Chan, RPh, PharmD
Director of Pharmacy Education, Riverside Family Practice Residency Program, Columbus, Ohio
Some Popular Herbs and Nutritional Supplements; New Drugs in 2004 and Agents Pending FDA Approval

Ying Chan, MD
Attending Perinatologist, Englewood Hospital and Medical Center, Englewood, New Jersey
Antepartum Care

Aruna Chandran, MD, MPH
General Preventive Medicine Resident, Johns Hopkins University Hospital, Baltimore, Maryland
Acute Infectious Diarrhea

Eugene Chang, MD
Martin Boyer Professor of Medicine, Department of Medicine, University of Chicago Pritzker School of Medicine, Chicago, Illinois
Malabsorption

Darren Chapman, MD
Resident, Urology, The Ohio State University School of Medicine and Public Health, Columbus, Ohio
Epididymitis

John P. Cheatham, MD
Director, Cardiac Catheterization and Interventional Therapy, The Heart Center, Columbus Children's Hospital; Professor of Pediatrics and Internal Medicine–Cardiology, The Ohio State University College of Medicine and Public Health, Columbus, Ohio
Congenital Heart Disease

Rahul K. Chhablani, MD
Resident, Department of Medicine, Hospital of the University of Pennsylvania, Philadelphia, Pennsylvania
Inflammatory Bowel Disease

Deborah Chirnomas, MD
Fellow in Pediatric Hematology/Oncology, Dana-Farber Cancer Institute, Children's Hospital Boston, Boston, Massachusetts
Aplastic Anemia

Hester H. Choi, MD
Gastroenterology Fellow, Department of Medicine, Division of Gastroenterology and Hepatology, University of Virginia Health System, Charlottesville, Virginia
Tumors of the Stomach

James Christensen, MS, MD
Emeritus Professor, Internal Medicine, The University of Iowa Roy J. and Lucille A. Carver College of Medicine, Iowa City, Iowa
Irritable Bowel Syndrome

George W. Christopher, MD
Chief, Infectious Diseases Service, Wilford Hall Medical Center, Lackland Air Force Base, Texas
Anthrax

Julie J. Chuan, MD
Sports Medicine Fellow, University of California, San Diego, School of Medicine; Family Practice, La Jolla, California
Common Sports Injuries

Bart L. Clarke, MD
Assistant Professor of Medicine, Mayo Clinic College of Medicine; Consultant, Division of Endocrinology, Diabetes, Metabolism, Nutrition and Internal Medicine, Mayo Clinic, Rochester, Minnesota
Paget's Disease of Bone

Bruce A. Cohen, MD
Professor, Davee Department of Neurology, Northwestern University Feinberg School of Medicine, Chicago, Illinois
Viral Meningitis and Encephalitis

Keith K. Colburn, MD
Chief, Division of Rheumatology, Loma Linda University Medical Center, Loma Linda, California
Bursitis, Tendonitis, Myofascial Pain, and Fibromyalgia

Robert R. Conley, MD
Professor of Psychiatry and Pharmacy Science, University of Maryland, Baltimore, Chief, Inpatient Research Program, Maryland Psychiatric Research Center, Baltimore, Maryland
Schizophrenia

Michael P. Conroy, MD, MS
Fellow in Dermatology, Mayo School of Graduate Medical Education, Mayo Clinic, and Mayo Clinic College of Medicine, Rochester, Minnesota
Pruritus

Stephen C. Cook, MD
Fellow, Pediatric Cardiology & Adult Cardiovascular Medicine, Division of Cardiology, Columbus Children's Hospital, Columbus, Ohio
Congenital Heart Disease

Laura Cooling, MD, MS
Associate Medical Director, Transfusion Medicine, University Hospital, University of Michigan Hospitals and Health Centers, Ann Arbor, Michigan
Thrombotic Thrombocytopenia Purpura

Jody P. Corey-Bloom, MD, PhD
Clinical Chief, Neurosciences Clinical Center, Perlman Ambulatory Care Center, La Jolla, California
Alzheimer's Disease

Yvon Cormier, MD
Professor, Department of Medicine, Laval University Faculty of Medicine, Ste Foy, Québec, Canada
Hypersensitivity Pneumonitis

John F. Coyle II, MD
Clinical Professor, Department of Medicine, University of Oklahoma College of Medicine–Tulsa, Tulsa, Oklahoma
Disturbances Caused by Heat

Gail Cresci, MS, RD
Assistant Clinical Professor, Department of Surgery, Medical College of Georgia, Augusta, Georgia
Total Parenteral Nutrition in Adults

Burke A. Cunha, MD
Chief, Infectious Disease Division, Winthrop-University Hospital, Mineola; Professor of Medicine, State University of New York at Stony Brook Health Sciences Center School of Medicine, Stony Brook, New York
Psittacosis (Ornithosis); Streptococcal Pharyngitis; Urinary Tract Infections in Women

Dennis Cunningham, MD
Assistant Professor of Clinical Pediatrics, The Ohio State University College of Medicine and Public Health, Columbus, Ohio
Rubella and Congenital Rubella Syndrome

Guido Dalbagni, MD
Associate Professor of Urology, New York University School of Medicine/Joan and Sanford I. Weill Medical College of Cornell University; Attending Physician, Department of Urology, Sidney Kimmel Center for Prostate and Urologic Cancers, New York, New York
Malignant Tumors of the Urogenital Tract

Stella Dantas, MD
Physician, Department of Obstetrics & Gynecology, Beaverton Medical Office, Northwest Permanente PC, Physicians and Surgeons, Beaverton, Oregon
Uterine Leiomyomas

Daniel F. Danzl, MD
Professor and Chair, Department of Emergency Medicine, University of Louisville School of Medicine, Louisville, Kentucky
Disturbances Due to Cold

Kenneth R. Dardick, MD
Clinical Assistant Professor, University of Connecticut School of Medicine, Farmington; Attending Physician, Windham Community Memorial Hospital, Storrs, Connecticut
Travel Medicine

Susan A. Davidson, MD
Associate Professor, University of Colorado Health Sciences Center School of Medicine; Chief, Gynecologic Oncology, University of Colorado Hospital, Denver, Colorado
Neoplasms of the Vulva

Terence M. Davidson, MD
Professor of Surgery–Head and Neck, University of California, San Diego, School of Medicine; Staff Physician, VA San Diego Health Care System, San Diego, California
Snake Venom Poisoning

Harold H. Davis, MD
Polycythemia Vera

Kepler A. Davis, MD
Fellow Infectious Diseases Service, Brooke Army Medical Center, Fort Sam Houston, Texas
Anthrax

Phillip J. DeChristopher, MD, PhD
Medical Director, Blood Bank/Transfusion Medicine, University of Illinois—Chicago Medical Center, Chicago, Illinois
Adverse Effects of Blood Transfusions

Jean-Pierre Dedet, MD, BSc
Head, Laboratoire de Parasitologie, Centre Hospitalier Universitaire de Montpellier, Montpellier, France
Leishmaniasis

Alfred DeMaria, Jr., MD
Director, Bureau of Communicable Disease Control; State Epidemiologist, Massachusetts Department of Public Health, Boston, Massachusetts
Giardiasis

David T. Dennis, MD, MPH
Guest Researcher, Division Vector-Borne Infectious Diseases, National Center for Infectious Diseases, Centers for Disease Control and Prevention; Faculty Affiliate, Department of Microbiology, Immunology and Pathology, Colorado State University, Fort Collins, Colorado
Relapsing Fever

Stephen R. Deputy, MD
Assistant Professor of Neurology, Louisiana State University Health Sciences Center, Children's Hospital, New Orleans, Louisiana
Acute Brain Injury in Children

Robert L. Deresiewicz, MD
Assistant Professor of Medicine, Harvard Medical School; Associate Physician, Channing Laboratory and Infectious Disease Division, Brigham and Women's Hospital, Boston, Massachusetts
Toxic Shock Syndrome

Kenneth R. DeVault, MD
Professor of Medicine, Mayo Clinic College of Medicine, Jacksonville, Florida
Dysphagia and Esophageal Obstruction

Ronald K. de Venecia, MD, PhD
Department of Otology and Laryngology, Massachusetts Eye and Ear Infirmary, Boston, Massachusetts
Ménière's Disease

Richard B. Devereaux, MD
Professor of Medicine, Joan and Sanford I. Weill Medical College of Cornell University; Director, Laboratory of Echocardiography, New York–Presbyterian Hospital, New York, New York
Mitral Valve Prolapse

Jack A. DiPalma, MD
Professor of Medicine, University of South Alabama College of Medicine; Director, USA Digestive Health Center; Director, Division of Gastroenterology, USA Medical Center, Mobile, Alabama
Constipation

Alice N. Do, DO
Research Fellow, Solano Clinical Research, Division Dow Pharmaceutical Sciences, Vallejo, California
Condyloma Accuminata (Genital Warts)

Mehmet Doganay, MD
Professor, Department of Infectious Disease, Erciyes University Faculty of Medicine, Kayseri, Turkey
Brucellosis

Pere Domingo, MD, PhD
Chairman, Department of Internal Medicine, Hospital de la Santa Creu i Sant Pau; University of Barcelona School of Medicine, Barcelona, Spain
Q Fever

James F. Donohue, MD
Professor, Department of Medicine, Division of Pulmonary and Critical Care Medicine, University of North Carolina School of Medicine, Chapel Hill, North Carolina
Acute Respiratory Failure

Anne Hamilton Dougherty, MD
Professor of Medicine, Division of Cardiology–Cardiac Electrophysiology, The University of Texas Medical School at Houston, Houston, Texas
Heart Block

Alan B. Douglass, MD
Assistant Director, Family Practice Residency Program, Middlesex Hospital, Middletown, Connecticut
Pain; Low Back Pain

Katharine A. Downes, MD
Assistant Professor of Pathology, Case Western Reserve
School of Medicine; Associate Director of Blood
Banking/Transfusion Medicine, University Hospitals of
Cleveland, Cleveland, Ohio
Autoimmune Hemolytic Anemia

Andjela Drincic, MD
Assistant Professor of Medicine, Division of Endocrinology,
Creighton University School of Medicine, Omaha, Nebraska
Hypopituitarism

Mark S. Dykewicz, MD
Professor of Internal Medicine, Saint Louis University School
of Medicine, St. Louis, Missouri
Allergic Reactions to Insect Stings

Lynne A. Eaton, MD, MS
Assistant Professor, Department of Obstetrics and
Gynecology, Division of Gynecologic Oncology, The Ohio
State University College of Medicine and Public Health; Staff
Physician, James Cancer Hospital and Solove Research
Institute, Columbus, Ohio
Ovarian Cancer

Kamryn T. Eddy, MA
Boston University; Center for Anxiety and Related Disorders,
Boston, Massachusetts
Bulimia Nervosa

Libby Edwards, MD
Southeast Vulvar Clinic; Associate Clinical Professor of
Dermatology, Wake Forest University School of Medicine,
Winston-Salem; Private Practice, Charlotte, North Carolina
Pruritus Ani and Vulvae

Eric Eggenberger, DO
Professor, Department of Neurology, Michigan State University
College of Human Medicine, East Lansing, Michigan
Optic Neuritis

George E. Ehrlich, MD
Adjunct Professor, Department of Medicine, University of
Pennsylvania School of Medicine, Philadelphia, Pennsylvania;
Adjunct Professor of Clinical Medicine, New York University
School of Medicine, New York, New York
Osteoarthritis

Lawrence F. Eichenfield, MD
Clinical Professor of Pediatrics and Medicine (Dermatology),
University of California, San Diego, School of Medicine;
Chief, Pediatric and Adolescent Dermatology; Medical
Director of Research, Children's Hospital and Health Center,
San Diego, California
Atopic Dermatitis

Millicent Eidson, MA, DVM
State Public Health Veterinarian and Director, Zoonoses
Program, Bureau of Communicable Disease Control,
New York State Department of Health, Albany, New York
Rabies

Magda Elkabani, MD
Hematology/Oncology Fellow, Department of Medicine,
Division of Infectious and Tropical Diseases, University of
South Florida College of Medicine; H. Lee Moffitt Cancer
Center & Research Institute, Tampa, Florida
Polycythemia Vera

Sean P. Elliott, MD
Clinical Instructor, Department of Urology, University of
California, San Francisco, School of Medicine; Staff
Physician, San Francisco General Hospital, San Francisco,
California
Trauma to the Genitourinary Tract

Craig A. Elmets, MD
Professor and Chairman, Department of Dermatology,
University of Alabama at Birmingham School of Medicine,
Birmingham, Alabama
Sunburn

Helen Enright, MD
Department of Haematology, Adelaide and Meath Hospitals,
Tallaght, Dublin, Ireland
Chronic Leukemias

Per-Olaf Eriksson, DDS, PhD
Professor, Department of Odontology, Clinical Oral
Physiology, Umeå University Faculty of Medicine, Umeå;
Center for Musculoskeletal Research, Gävle University,
Gävle and Umeå, Sweden
Temporomandibular Disorders

Tommaso Falcone, MD
Professor and Chairman, Department of Obstetrics and
Gynecology, Cleveland Clinic Foundation, Cleveland, Ohio
Endometriosis

Adel G. Fam, MD
Professor Emeritus of Medicine, Division of Rheumatology,
Sunnybrook Health Science Center, Toronto, Ontario,
Canada
Gout and Hyperuricemia

Vahab Fatourechi, MD
Professor of Medicine, Mayo Clinic College of Medicine,
Rochester, Minnesota
Thyroiditis

Eve S. Ferdman, BA
Managing Editor, *Brachytherapy*, Memorial Sloan-Kettering
Cancer Center, New York, New York
Brain Tumors

Jonathan F. Finks, MD
Instructor of Surgery, Oregon Health & Science University
School of Medicine, Portland, Oregon
Gastroesophageal Reflux Disease

Juan M. Flores-Cordero, MD, PhD
Intensive Care Medicine Specialist, Critical Care and
Emergency Department, University Hospital Virgen del
Rocío, Seville, Spain
Bacterial Meningitis

Matthew I. Fogg, MD
Fellow, Department of Allergy and Immunology, University
of Pennsylvania School of Medicine, Philadelphia,
Pennsylvania
Asthma in Children

K. Wade Foster, MD, PhD
Staff Physician, Department of Dermatology, University of
Alabama at Birmingham School of Medicine, Birmingham,
Alabama
Sunburn

Nathan B. Fountain, MD
Associate Professor and Director, Comprehensive Epilepsy Program, Department of Neurology, University of Virginia School of Medicine, Charlottesville, Virginia
Seizures and Epilepsy in Adolescents and Adults

Roger D. Freeman, MD
Clinical Professor Emeritus of Psychiatry and Associate Professor, Department of Pediatrics, University of British Columbia Faculty of Medicine, Vancouver, British Columbia, Canada
Gilles de la Tourette Syndrome

Michael P. Frenneaux, MB, BS, MD
British Heart Foundation, Chair of Cardiology, University of Birmingham, Birmingham, United Kingdom
Hypertrophic Cardiomyopathy

Faith Joy Frieden, MD
Director, Maternal-Fetal Medicine, Englewood Hospital and Medical Center, Englewood, New Jersey; Clinical Assistant Professor, Mount Sinai School of Medicine, New York, New York
Antepartum Care

John J. Friedewald, MD
Assistant Professor of Medicine, Division of Nephrology and Organ Transplant, Northwestern University Feinberg School of Medicine, Baltimore, Maryland
Acute Renal Failure

R. Michael Gallagher, DO
Director, University Headache Center; Professor and Dean, University of Medicine and Dentistry of New Jersey School of Osteopathic Medicine, Stratford, New Jersey
Headache

Niall T. M. Galloway, MD
Associate Professor of Urology, Emory University School of Medicine; Director, Emory Continence Center, Atlanta, Georgia
Urinary Incontinence

Donald G. Gallup, MD
Professor and Chairperson, Department of Obstetrics and Gynecology, Mercer University School of Medicine, Macon; Attending Physician, Memorial Health University Medical Center, Savannah, Georgia
Endometrial Cancer

Michael Thomas Gambla, MD
Urology Surgeon, Riverside Methodist Hospital; Urology Surgeons, Inc., Columbus, Ohio
Epididymitis

Ramasamy Ganapati, BSc, MBBS
Director, Bombay Leprosy Project, Mumbai, Maharashtra, India
Leprosy (Hansen's Disease)

Vani Gandhi, MD
Attending Physician, St. Luke's–Roosevelt Hospital Center; Clinical Instructor, Columbia University College of Physicians and Surgeons, New York, New York
Management of the Patient with HIV Disease

Bruce J. Gantz, MD
Professor of Otolaryngology, The University of Iowa Roy J. and Lucille A. Carver College of Medicine; Head, Department of Otolaryngology–Head and Neck Surgery, University of Iowa Hospitals and Clinics, Iowa City, Iowa
Acute Facial Paralysis (Bell's Palsy)

Juan Armando Garcia, MD
Assistant Professor of Medicine, Pulmonary and Critical Care Division, University of Texas Health Science Center at San Antonio, Audie Murphy VA Medical Center, San Antonio, Texas
Management of Chronic Obstructive Pulmonary Disease

James M. Gebel, Jr., MD
Medical Director, Jewish Hospital Emergency Stroke Center, Louisville Kentucky
Intracerebral Hemorrhage

Luciano Z. Goldani, MD, PhD
Associate Professor of Internal Medicine, Universidade Federal do Rio Grande do Sul; Staff Physician, Infectious Diseases Unit, Hospital de Clinicas de Porto Alegre, Porto Alegre, Brazil
Infectious Mononucleosis

Nora Goldschlager, MD
Professor of Clinical Medicine, University of California, San Francisco, California, Co-Director, Division of Cardiology, San Francisco General Hospital, San Francisco, California, Director, Coronary Care Unit, ECG Laboratory and Pacemaker Clinic, San Francisco General Hospital, San Francisco, California
Tachycardias

Eduardo Gotuzzo-Herencia, MD
Insituto de Medicina Tropical "Alexander von Humboldt," Universidad Peruana, Cayetano Heredia; Departamento de Enfermedades Infecciosas, Tropicales y Dermatológicas, Hospital Nacional Cayetano Heredia, Lima, Peru
Cholera

Marina Grandis, MD
Neurologist, Department of Neurosciences, Ophthalmology, and Genetics, University of Genova, Genova, Italy
Peripheral Neuropathies

William Kevin Green, MD
Assistant Professor, Department of Medicine, University of South Alabama College of Medicine, Mobile, Alabama
Bacterial Pneumonia

Stephen B. Greenberg, MD
Professor and Chair, Department of Medicine, Baylor College of Medicine, Houston, Texas
Viral and Mycoplasmal Pneumonia

Joseph Greensher, MD
Professor of Pediatrics, State University of New York at Stony Brook Health Sciences Center School of Medicine, Stony Brook; Medical Director and Associate Chair, Department of Pediatrics, Long Island Regional Poison and Drug Information Center, Winthrop-University Hospital, Mineola, New York
Medical Toxicology: Ingestions, Inhalations, and Dermal and Ocular Absorptions

Hans W. Grünwald, MD
Associate Professor of Medicine, Division of Hematology-Oncology, Mount Sinai School of Medicine; Staff Physician, Queens Hospital Center, Jamaica, New York
Acute Leukemia in Adults

Eva C. Guinan, MD
Director, Hematopoietic Stem Cell Transplantation, Children's Hospital Boston; Pediatric Oncologist, Dana Farber Cancer Institute; Harvard Medical School, Boston, Massachusetts
Aplastic Anemia

Joan Guitart, MD
Professor of Dermatology, Northwestern University Feinberg School of Medicine, Chicago, Illinois
Nevi

Vivek Gumaste, MD
Associate Professor of Medicine, Mount Sinai School of Medicine; Chief, Division of Gastroenterology, Mount Sinai Services, Elmhurst, New York
Acute Pancreatitis; Chronic Pancreatitis

Hiroyuki Hara, MD, PhD
Associate Professor, Department of Dermatology, Nihon University School of Medicine, Tokyo, Japan
Pigmentary Disorders

Laura Harrell, MD
Gastroenterology Fellow, Department of Medicine, University of Chicago Pritzker School of Medicine, Chicago, Illinois
Malabsorption

Thomas M. Harvey, MD
Vision Correction Procedures

David S. Haynes, MD
Assistant Professor of Otolaryngology, Vanderbilt School of Medicine; Director of Otology/Neurotology, Vanderbilt Bill Wilkerson Center for Otolaryngology and Communication Sciences; Medical Director, Vanderbilt Hearing and Balance Center, Nashville, Tennessee
Otitis Externa

Adelaide A. Hebert, MD
Professor, Department of Dermatology, The University of Texas Medical School at Houston, Houston, Texas
Fungal Diseases of the Skin

Nicholas J. Hegarty, MD
Endourology Research Fellow, Glickman Urological Institute, The Cleveland Clinic Foundation, Cleveland, Ohio
Renal Calculi

Sharon M. Henry, MD
Associate Professor of Surgery, University of Maryland School of Medicine; Chief, Section of Wound Healing and Metabolism, R. Adams Cowley Shock Trauma Center, University of Maryland Medical System, Baltimore, Maryland
Necrotizing Skin and Soft Tissue Infections

David B. Herzog, MD
President, Harvard Eating Disorders Center at Massachusetts General Hospital; Professor of Psychiatry (Pediatrics), Harvard Medical School; Pediatrician, Massachusetts General Hospital; Psychiatrist, Massachusetts General Hospital; and Associate Psychiatrist, Massachusetts General Hospital, Boston, Massachusetts
Bulimia Nervosa

David G. Hill, MD
Waterbury Pulmonary Associates, Waterbury, Connecticut; Yale University School of Medicine, New Haven, Connecticut
Cough

Richard H. Hongo, MD
Cardiac Electrophysiologist, California Pacific Medical Center, Cardiology Division, San Francisco, California
Tachycardias

A. A. Hoosen, MD
Professor and Head of Department, Department of Microbiological Pathology, University of Limpopo Faculty of Medicine, Medunsa Campus, Pretoria, South Africa
Granuloma Inguinale/Donovanosis and Lymphogranuloma Venereum

William K. Hoots, MD
Professor, Department of Pediatrics, The University of Texas School of Medicine at Houston and M.D. Anderson Cancer Center, Houston, Texas
Disseminated Intravascular Coagulation

Michael P. Hopkins, MD, MEd
Professor, Department of Obstetrics and Gynecology, Northeastern Ohio Universities College of Medicine; Atending Physician, Aultman Hospital, Canton, Ohio
Cancer of the Uterine Cervix

Mark Horowitz, MD
Assistant Professor, Department of Urology, Joan and Sanford I. Weill Medical College of Cornell University; Staff Physician, New York–Presbyterian Hospital, New York, New York
Urethral Stricture

John W. House, MD
Clinical Professor, Department of Otolaryngology–Head and Neck Surgery, Keck School of Medicine of the University of Southern California, Private Practice, House Ear Clinic, Los Angeles, California
Tinnitus

Tamara Salam Housman, MD
Resident, Department of Dermatology, Wake Forest University Health Sciences Center, Winston-Salem, North Carolina
Warts (Verrucae)

Shirley H. Huang, MD
Pediatric Nutrition Fellow, Division of Gastroenterology and Nutrition, The Children's Hospital of Philadelphia, Philadelphia, Pennsylvania
Normal Infant Feeding

John G. Hunter, MD
Professor and Chairman, Department of Surgery, Oregon Health & Science University School of Medicine, Portland, Oregon
Gastroesophageal Reflux Disease

Raymond J. Hutchinson, MS, MD
Professor of Pediatrics, University of Michigan Medical
School; Staff Physician, Division of Pediatric Hematology/
Oncology, University of Michigan Comprehensive Cancer
Center, Ann Arbor, Michigan
Acute Leukemia in Childhood

Jeffrey A. Jackson, MD
Associate Professor, Department of Dermatology, University
of Texas—Dallas, Southwestern Medical School; Director,
Phototherapy Clinic, The University of Texas Southwestern
Medical Center at Dallas, Dallas, Texas
Hyperparathyroidism and Hypoparathyroidism

James J. James, MD, DrPH, MHA
Director, Center for Disaster Preparedness and Emergency
Response, American Medical Association, Chicago, Illinois
*Toxic Chemical Agents Reference Chart: Symptoms and Treatments;
Biologic Agents Reference Chart: Symptoms, Tests, and Treatment*

Stephen G. Jenkinson, MD
Chief, Pulmonary Diseases Section, Audie Murphy VA
Medical Center, San Antonio, Texas
Management of Chronic Obstructive Pulmonary Disease

Kowichi Jimbow, MD, PhD
Professor and Chair, Department of Dermatology, Sapporo
Medical University School of Medicine, Sapporo, Hokkaido,
Japan
Pigmentary Disorders

Candice E. Johnson, MD, PhD
Professor of Pediatrics, University of Colorado Health
Sciences Center School of Medicine; Staff Physician,
The Children's Hospital, Denver, Colorado
Bacterial Infections of the Urinary Tract in Girls

David R. Jones, MD
Associate Professor of Surgery, University of Virginia School
of Medicine; Chief, General Thoracic Surgery, University of
Virginia Hospital, Charlottesville, Virginia
Atelectasis

Marc A. Judson, MD
Professor of Medicine, Division of Pulmonary and Critical
Care Medicine, Medical University of South Carolina,
Charleston, South Carolina
Sarcoidosis

Matthew H. Kanzler, MD
Clinical Professor, Stanford University School of Medicine,
Stanford; Chief of Dermatology, Santa Clara Valley Medical
Center, San Jose, California
Cutaneous Vasculitis

Matthew E. Karlovsky, MD
Fellow, Neurourology & Prosthetics, Department of Urology,
Long Island Jewish Medical Center, New Hyde Park,
New York
Benign Prostatic Hyperplasia

David E. Katz, MD
Epidemic Intelligence Service Officer, Centers for Disease
Control and Prevention, Atlanta, Georgia; Epidemic
Intelligence Service Officer, Massachusetts Department of
Public Health, Jamaica Plain, Massachusetts
Giardiasis

Steven E. Katz, MD
Associate Professor of Ophthalmology, The Ohio State
University College of Medicine and Public Health; William H.
Havener Eye Center, Columbus, Ohio
Conjunctivitis

Andrew M. Kaunitz, MD
Professor, Department of Obstetrics and Gynecology,
University of Florida College of Medicine, Jacksonville,
Florida
Contraception

Deanna L. Kelly, PharmD
Assistant Professor, University of Maryland School of
Medicine–Maryland Psychiatric Research Center, Baltimore,
Maryland
Schizophrenia

James W. Kendig, MD
Professor of Pediatrics, Pennsylvania State University School
of Medicine; Staff Pediatrician, Division of Newborn
Medicine, Penn State Children's Hospital, Hershey,
Pennsylvania
Hemolytic Disease of the Newborn

Azim J. Khan, MD
Assistant Professor of Clinical Dermatology, State University
of New York at Stony Brook Health Sciences Center School
of Medicine, Stony Brook, New York
Diseases of the Hair

Ramesh K. Khurana, MD
Chief of Neurology, Union Memorial Hospital, Baltimore,
Maryland
Tetanus

Jeremy A. King, MD
Reproductive Endocrinology Fellow, Division of Reproductive
Endocrinology, Department of Gynecology and Obstetrics,
Johns Hopkins School of Medicine and Johns Hopkins
Hospital, Baltimore, Maryland
Hyperprolactinemia

Abbas E. Kitabchi, PhD, MD
Professor of Medicine and Molecular Sciences, The
University of Tennessee Health Science Center College of
Medicine; Director, Division of Endocrinology, Diabetes and
Metabolism, The University of Tennessee Health Science
Center, Memphis, Tennessee
Diabetic Ketoacidosis

Douglas D. Koch, MD
Professor and The Allen, Mosbacher, and Law Chair in
Ophthalmology, Cullen Eye Institute, Baylor College of
Medicine, Houston, Texas
Vision Correction Procedures

Luciano Kolodny, MD
Endocrinologist, HealthPartners Medical Group, Woodbury,
Minnesota
Erectile Dysfunction

Stephen L. Kopecky, MD
Associate Professor of Medicine, Mayo Clinic College of
Medicine, Mayo Clinic, Rochester, Minnesota
Acute Myocardial Infarction

Amy M. Kopp, MD
Ophthalmology Resident, The Ohio State University;
William H. Havener Eye Center, Columbus, Ohio
Conjunctivitis

David S. Kotlyar, BS
Medical Student, University of Pennsylvania School of
Medicine, Philadelphia, Pennsylvania
Cirrhosis

Peter R. Kowey, MD
Professor, Department of Medicine, Jefferson Medical
College at Thomas Jefferson University, Philadelphia,
Pennsylvania
Atrial Fibrillation

Carl A. Krantz, Jr., MD
Associate Program Director, Riverside Methodist Hospital;
Clinical Assistant Professor, The Ohio State University
College of Medicine and Public Health, Worthington, Ohio
Amenorrhea

Jeffrey A. Kraut, MD
Chief of Dialysis, Veterans Affairs Greater Los Angeles
Healthcare System; Professor of Medicine, David Geffen
School of Medicine at University of California—Los Angeles,
Los Angeles, California
Chronic Renal Failure

John N. Krieger, MD
Professor, Department of Urology, University of Washington
School of Medicine, Seattle, Washington
Bacterial Infections of the Urinary Tract in Males

John G. Kuldau, MD
Director of Advanced Endoscopy, Scripps Clinic, La Jolla,
California
Diverticula of the Alimentary Tract

Roshni Kulkarni, MD
Professor and Division Chief, Pediatric and Adolescent
Hematology/Oncology, Michigan State University College of
Human Medicine; Director (Pediatric), Michigan State
University Center for Bleeding and Clotting Disorders,
East Lansing, Michigan
Hemophilia and Related Conditions

Robert F. Kushner, MD
Professor of Medicine, Northwestern University Feinberg
School of Medicine, Chicago, Illinois
Obesity

Timothy M. Kuzel, MD
Associate Professor of Medicine, Department of Medicine,
Division of Hematology/Oncology, Northwestern University
Feinberg School of Medicine; Staff Physician, Robert H. Lurie
Comprehensive Cancer Center, Chicago, Illinois
Cutaneous T-Cell Lymphomas (Mycosis Fungoides and Sézary Syndrome)

Robert A. Kyle, MD
Consultant, Division of Hematology and Internal Medicine,
Mayo Clinic; Professor of Medicine and of Laboratory
Medicine, Mayo Clinic College of Medicine, Rochester,
Minnesota
Multiple Myeloma

Christopher J. Lahart, MD
Associate Medical Director, Hepatitis and Oncology, Gilead
Sciences, Inc., Foster City, California
Tuberculosis and Other Mycobacterial Diseases

Gabriella Lakos, MD, PhD
Connective Tissue Disorders

Charles R. Lambert, MD, PhD
Professor of Medicine, Division of Cardiovascular Medicine,
Interventional Cardiology Section, University of Florida
College of Medicine, Gainesville, Florida
Angina Pectoris

Corey J. Langer, MD
Medical Director, Thoracic Oncology, Fox Chase Cancer
Center, Philadelphia, Pennsylvania
Lung Cancer

Barbara A. Latenser, MD
Associate Professor of Surgery, The University of Iowa Roy J.
and Lucille A. Carver College of Medicine; Director, Burn
Treatment Center, University of Iowa Hospitals and Clinics,
Iowa City, Iowa
Burn Treatment Guidelines

Luca Lazzarini, MD
Department of Infectious Diseases and Tropical Medicine,
San Bortolo Hospital, Vicenza, Italy
Osteomyelitis

Miguel Sabria Leal, MD, PhD
Chief, Infectious Diseases Section, Hospital Universitario
Germans Trias i Pujol; Professor of Medicine, University of
Barcelona School of Medicine, Barcelona, Spain
Legionellosis (Legionnaires' Disease and Pontiac Fever)

Mark G. Lebwohl, MD
Professor and Chair, Department of Dermatology, The
Mount Sinai School of Medicine, New York, New York
Papulosquamous Eruptions

Clifford L. S. Leen, MB ChB, MD
Consultant Physician & part time Senior Lecturer
(Edinburgh University), Regional Infectious Diseases Unit,
Western General Hospital, Edinburgh
Salmonellosis

Enrique C. Leira, MD
Assistant Professor, The University of Iowa Roy J. and
Lucille A. Carver College of Medicine, Iowa City, Iowa
Ischemic Cerebrovascular Disease

Anthony Lembo, MD
Instructor of Medicine, Division of Gastroenterology,
Harvard Medical School; Director of Gastrointestinal
Motility, Beth Israel Deaconess Medical Center, Boston,
Massachusetts
Gaseousness and Indigestion

J. Keith Lemmon, MD
Fellow in Allergy and Immunology, Division of Allergy
and Immunology, St. Louis University School of Medicine,
St. Louis, Missouri
Allergic Reactions to Insect Stings

Matthew E. Levison, MD
Professor of Medicine and Public Health, Drexel University College of Medicine, Philadelphia, Pennsylvania
Primary Lung Abscess

Robert Libke, MD
Chief of Infectious Diseases and Clinical Professor of Medicine, University of California, San Francisco, School of Medicine, San Francisco; University of California, Fresno, School of Medicine, Fresno, California
Coccidioidomycosis

Gary R. Lichtenstein, MD
Professor of Medicine, University of Pennsylvania School of Medicine; Director, Center for Inflammatory Bowel Diseases, Division of Gastroenterology, Hospital of the University of Pennsylvania, Philadelphia, Pennsylvania
Inflammatory Bowel Disease

Phillip L. Lieberman, MD
Clinical Professor of Medicine and Pediatrics, Departments of Internal Medicine and Pediatrics (Divisions of Allergy and Immunology), University of Tennessee, College of Medicine, University of Tennessee, Allergy and Asthma Care, Memphis, Tennessee
Nonallergic Rhinitis

Marcia Torres Lima, MD
Visiting Scientist, Division of Allergy and Clinical Immunology, Department of Internal Medicine, The University of Texas Medical School at Houston, Houston, Texas
Anaphylaxis and Serum Sickness

Markéta Limová, MD
Assistant Clinical Professor, Department of Dermatology, University of California, San Francisco, School of Medicine, Fresno, California
Venous Ulcers

Jana Lincoln, MD
Mood Disorders

Jeffrey A. Linder, MD
Associate Physician, Division of General Medicine and Primary Care, Brigham and Women's Hospital; Instructor in Medicine, Harvard Medical School, Boston, Massachusetts
Acute Bronchitis

Gary H. Lipscomb, MD
Professor and Vice Chairman, The University of Tennessee Health Science Center College of Medicine; Director, Division of Gynecologic Specialties, The University of Tennessee Health Science Center, Memphis, Tennessee
Ectopic Pregnancy

James A. Litch, MD
Clinical Assistant Professor, University of Washington School of Medicine and School of Public Health, Seattle, Washington
High Altitude Illness

Dan L. Longo, MD
Scientific Director, National Institute on Aging, National Institutes of Health, Baltimore, Maryland
Pernicious Anemia and Other Megaloblastic Anemias

Kirk A. Ludwig, MD
Assistant Professor of Surgery, Duke University School of Medicine; Chief of Gastrointestinal Surgery, Duke University Medical Center, Durham, North Carolina
Tumors of the Colon and Rectum

Jeanne Lusher, MD
Marion Barnhart Hemostasis Research Professor, Wayne State University School of Medicine; Co-Director, Pediatric Hematology/Oncology, Children's Hospital of Michigan, Detroit, Michigan
Hemophilia and Related Conditions

Garrett Lynch, MD
Professor of Medicine, Baylor College of Medicine, Houston, Texas
Non-Hodgkin's Lymphomas

James M. Lyznicki, MS, MPH
Senior Scientist, Center for Disaster Preparedness and Emergency Response, American Medical Association, Chicago, Illinois
Toxic Chemical Agents Reference Chart: Symptoms and Treatments; Biologic Agents Reference Chart: Symptoms, Tests, and Treatment

Scott C. Manning, MD
Professor, Department of Otolaryngology, University of Washington School of Medicine; Staff Physician, Children's Hospital and Regional Medical Center, Seattle, Washington
Sinusitis

Woraphong Manuskiatti, MD
Associate Professor, Mahidol University School of Medicine; Laser and Cutaneous Surgery Division, Department of Dermatology, Siriraj Hospital, Bangkok, Thailand
Keloids

Susan M. Manzi, MD, MPH
Associate Professor of Medicine, University of Pittsburgh School of Medicine, Pittsburgh, Pennsylvania
Connective Tissue Disorders

Barry J. Marshall, MD
Clinical Professor of Microbiology, University of Western Australia Faculty of Medicine, Nedlands, Western Australia, Australia
Gastritis and Peptic Ulcer Disease

Gailen D. Marshall, Jr., MD, PhD
Professor of Medicine and Pediatrics and Vice Chair, Department of Medicine, University of Mississippi School of Medicine; Director, Division of Clinical Immunology and Allergy, University of Mississippi Medical Center, Jackson, Mississippi
Anaphylaxis and Serum Sickness

Jose Martagon-Villamil, MD
House Officer, Department of Internal Medicine, Baystate Medical Center, Westfield, Massachusetts
Histoplasmosis

Robert Martindale, MD
Chief, Gastrointestinal Surgery, Medical College of Georgia Medical Center; Professor of Surgery, Medical College of Georgia, Augusta, Georgia
Parenteral Nutrition in Adults

Alexander Mauskop, MD
Director, New York Headache Center, New York, New York,
Associate Professor of Clinical Neurology, State University of
New York - Downstate Medical Center, New York, New York
Trigeminal Neuralgia

Martin J. McCaffrey, MD
Director, Neonatal Intensive Care Unit, Naval Medical
Center; Specialty Advisor to the Navy Surgeon General for
Neonatology, San Diego, California
Resuscitation of the Newborn

Carol F. McCammon, MD
Assistant Professor, Department of Emergency Medicine,
Eastern Virginia Medical School, Virginia Beach, Virginia
Acute Pyelonephritis

Kurt A. McCammon, MD
Assistant Professor of Urology, Eastern Virginia Medical
School, Virginia Beach, Virginia
Acute Pyelonephritis

Jacqueline Carinhas McGregor, MD
Director, Baylor Child Psychiatry Clinic; Associate Professor,
Menninger Department of Psychiatry and Behavioral
Sciences, Baylor College of Medicine, Houston, Texas
Anxiety Disorders

Michael McGuigan, MD
Medical Director, Long Island Regional Poison and Drug
Information Center, Winthrop-University Hospital, Mineola,
New York
*Medical Toxicology: Ingestions, Inhalations, and Dermal and Ocular
Absorptions*

Christopher R. McHenry, MD
Professor and Vice-Chairman, Department of Surgery
(General, Neck and Endocrine Surgery), Case Western
Reserve School of Medicine; Director, Division of General
Surgery, MetroHealth Medical Center, Cleveland, Ohio
Thyroid Cancer

Terrance P. McHugh, MD
Attending Physician, Palmetto Richland Memorial Hospital,
Columbia, South Carolina
Rat-Bite Fever

Dilcia McLenan, MD
Assistant Professor of Pediatrics, Baylor College of Medicine,
Pearland, Texas
Care of the High-Risk Neonate

Donald McNeil, MD
Associate Professor of Clinical Medicine, Department of
Immunology, Ohio State University College of Medicine and
Public Health, Columbus, Ohio
Allergic Reactions to Drugs

Jennifer Meddings, MD
Resident Physician, Internal Medicine and Pediatrics, The
Ohio State University & Columbus Children's Hospital,
Columbus, Ohio
Rubella and Congenital Rubella Syndrome

Bella Mehta, PharmD
Assistant Professor of Clinical Pharmacy and Director,
Clinical Partners Program, The Ohio State University
College of Pharmacy, Columbus, Ohio
New Drugs in 2004 and Agents Pending FDA Approval

Ted A. Meyer, MD, PhD
Fellow, Department of Otolaryngology–Head and Neck
Surgery, The University of Iowa Roy J. and Lucille A. Carver
College of Medicine, and University of Iowa Hospitals and
Clinics, Iowa City, Iowa
Acute Facial Paralysis (Bell's Palsy)

Shirwan A. Mirza, MD
Consultant Endocrinologist, Auburn Memorial Hospital,
Auburn; Clinical Assistant Professor of Medicine, State
University of New York Upstate Medical University College
of Medicine, Syracuse; Adjunct Clinical Assistant Professor of
Medicine, New York College of Osteopathic Medicine,
Auburn, New York
Diabetes Mellitus in Adults

William F. Miser, MD, MA
Associate Professor, Department of Family Medicine, Ohio
State University College of Medicine and Public Health,
Columbus, Ohio
Nausea and Vomiting

Candace L. Mitchell, MD
Assistant Professor, Louisiana State University Health
Sciences Center School of Medicine, Shreveport, Louisiana
Blastomycosis

Howard C. Mofenson, MD
Professor of Pediatrics and Emergency Medicine, State
University of New York at Stony Brook Health Sciences
Center School of Medicine, Stony Brook; Professor of
Pharmacology and Toxicology, New York College of
Osteopathic Medicine, Old Westbury, New York
*Medical Toxicology: Ingestions, Inhalations, and Dermal and Ocular
Absorptions*

Imran T. Mohiuddin, MD
Vascular Surgery Fellow, Division of Vascular Surgery and
Endovascular Therapy, Michael E. DeBakey Department of
Surgery, Baylor College of Medicine, Houston, Texas
Acquired Diseases of the Aorta

Mark E. Molitch, MD
Professor of Medicine, Northwestern University Feinberg
School of Medicine, Chicago, Illinois
Acromegaly

Eugene W. Monroe, MD
Assistant Clinical Professor of Dermatology, Medical College
of Wisconsin; Advanced Healthcare, Milwaukee, Wisconsin
Urticaria and Angioedema

James E. Moon, MD, CPT, MC, USA
Infectious Diseases Service, Brooke Army Medical Center,
Fort Sam Houston, Texas
Anthrax

Dilip Moonka, MD
Medical Director of Liver Transplantation, Gastroenterology
Division, Henry Ford Health System, Detroit, Michigan
Acute and Chronic Viral Hepatitis

Sherif B. Mossad, MD
Staff Member, Department of Infectious Disease, Cleveland
Clinic Foundation, Cleveland, Ohio
Histoplasmosis

Patrick J. Mulrow, MD
Professor Emeritus, Department of Medicine, Medical
College of Ohio, Toledo, Ohio
Hypertension

Diya F. Mutasim, M.D.
Professor and Chairman, Department of Dermatology,
University of Cincinnati College of Medicine, Cincinnati, Ohio
Bullous Diseases

Joseph B. Nadol, Jr., MD
Walter Augustus LeCompte Professor and Chairman,
Department of Otology and Laryngology, Harvard Medical
School; Chief, Department of Otolaryngology, Massachusetts
Eye and Ear Infirmary, Boston, Massachusetts
Ménière's Disease

Ashwatha Narayana, MD
Assistant Professor, Department of Radiation Oncology,
Memorial Sloan-Kettering Cancer Center, New York,
New York
Brain Tumors

Lisa R. Nash, DO
Assistant Professor, Department of Family Medicine,
The University of Texas Medical Branch School of Medicine,
Galveston, Texas
Postpartum Care

Paul M. Ness, MD
Director, Blood Bank, Division of Transfusion Medicine,
Department of Pathology, Johns Hopkins Medical
Institutions, Baltimore, Maryland
Therapeutic Use of Blood Components

Peter E. Newburger, MD
Professor and Vice Chair, Department of Pediatrics,
University of Massachusetts Medical School, Worcester,
Massachusetts
Neutropenia

Courtney A. Noble, MD
Clinical Instructor of Medicine, Department of Medicine,
Northwestern University Feinberg School of Medicine,
Chicago, Illinois
Obesity

R. Craig Nodurft, MD
Scripps Clinic, La Jolla, California
Diverticula of the Alimentary Tract

Robert L. Norris, MD
Associate Professor of Surgery, Stanford University School of
Medicine, Stanford; Chief, Division of Emergency Medicine,
Stanford Hospital and Clinics, Palo Alto, California
Spider Bites and Scorpion Stings

Joyce Olutade, MD
Assistant Professor, Division of Rheumatology, Allergy, and
Immunology, The Ohio State University College of Medicine
and Public Health; Midwest Allergy and Asthma Associates,
Columbus, Ohio
Dysmenorrhea

Mary B. O'Malley, MD, PhD
Fellowship Director, Norwalk Hospital Sleep Disorders
Center, Norwalk, Connecticut
Sleep Disorders Except Insomnia and Sleep Apnea

Brian J. O'Neil, MD
Wayne State University School of Medicine, Detroit; Staff
Physician, Department of Emergency Medicine, Saint John
Hospital and Medical Center, Detroit; William Beaumont
Hospital, Royal Oak, Michigan
Sudden Cardiac Death

Vivek V. Pai, MBBS, DVD
Additional Director, Bombay Leprosy Project, Mumbai,
Maharashtra, India
Leprosy (Hansen's Disease)

Biff F. Palmer, MD
Professor of Internal Medicine, Department of Internal
Medicine, Division of Nephrology, Universtiy of Texas,
Southwestern Medical School, Dallas, Texas
Hyponatremia

John E. Parker, MD
Professor of Medicine and Chief, Section of Pulmonary and
Critical Care Medicine, West Virginia University School of
Medicine, Morgantown, West Virginia
Silicosis and Asbestosis

Lorne S. Parnes, MD
Professor and Chairman, Department of Otolaryngology,
The University of Western Ontario Faculty of Medicine,
London, Ontario, Canada
Episodic Vertigo

Robert M. Pascuzzi, MD
Professor and Interim Chair, Department of Neurology,
Indiana University School of Medicine, Indianapolis,
Indiana
Myasthenia Gravis and Related Disorders

Sonal M. Patel, MD
Fellow, Division of Gastroenterology, Beth Israel Deaconess
Medical Center, Boston, Massachusetts
Gaseousness and Indigestion

Susan P. Perrine, MD
Associate Professor, Departments of Medicine, Pediatrics,
and Pharmacology and Experimental Therapeutics;
Director, Hemoglobinopathy-Thalassemia Research Unit,
Boston University School of Medicine, Boston,
Massachusetts
Thalassemia

William A. Petri, Jr., MD, PhD
Wade Hampton Frost Professor of Epidemiology and
Professor of Medicine, Microbiology, and Pathology,
University of Virginia School of Medicine; Chief, Division of
Infectious Diseases and International Health, University of
Virginia Health Systems, Charlottesville, Virginia
Amebiasis

Claus A. Pierach, MD
Professor of Medicine and Professor of History of Medicine,
Department of Medicine, University of Minnesota Medical
School, Minneapolis, Minnesota
The Porphyrias

Germania A. Pinheiro, MD, MSc, PhD
Epidemic Intelligence Service Officer, Centers for Disease
Control and Prevention, National Institute for Occupational
Safety and Health, Division of Respiratory Disease Studies,
Morgantown, West Virginia
Silicosis and Asbestosis

Michael A. Polis, MD, MPH
Office of Clinical Research, National Institutes of Allergy and
Infectious Diseases, National Institutes of Health, Bethesda,
Maryland
Food-Borne Illness

Michel A. Pontari, MD
Associate Professor, Department of Urology, Temple
University School of Medicine, Philadelphia, Pennsylvania
Prostatitis

Steven M. Powell, MD
Associate Professor of Medicine, Department of Medicine,
Division of Gastroenterology and Hepatology, University of
Virginia School of Medicine, Charlottesville, Virginia
Tumors of the Stomach

Richard P. Propp, MD
Medical Director, Patient Safety Center, New York State
Department of Health, Delmar, New York
Otitis Media

Christiane Querfeld, MD
Postdoctoral Fellow, Department of Medicine, Division of
Hematology/Oncology, Northwestern University Feinberg
School of Medicine and Robert H. Lurie Comprehensive
Cancer Center, Chicago, Illinois
Cutaneous T-Cell Lymphomas (Mycosis Fungoides and Sézary Syndrome)

Hamid Rabb, MD
Physician Director, Kidney Transplant Program, Johns
Hopkins Hospital; Associate Professor, Division of Nephrology,
Johns Hopkins School of Medicine, Baltimore, Maryland
Acute Renal Failure

Beth W. Rackow, MD
Instructor, Department of Reproductive Endocrinology and
Infertility, Yale University School of Medicine, New Haven,
Connecticut
Dysfunctional Uterine Bleeding

S. Vincent Rajkumar, MD
Consultant, Division of Hematology and Internal Medicine,
Mayo Clinic; Associate Professor of Medicine, Mayo Clinic
College of Medicine, Rochester, Minnesota
Multiple Myeloma

Annemarei Ranta, MD
Epilepsy and EEG Fellow, Department of Neurology,
University of Virginia School of Medicine, Charlottesville,
Virginia
Seizures and Epilepsy in Adolescents and Adults

K. Rajender Reddy, MD
Professor of Medicine and Surgery, University of Pennsylvania
School of Medicine; Director of Hepatology and Medical
Director of Liver Transplantation, Department of Medicine,
Gastroenterology Division, University of Pennsylvania
Health Systems, Philadelphia, Pennsylvania
Cirrhosis

Steven Reid, MD, PhD
Consultant Liaison Psychiatrist, St Mary's Hospital London,
United Kingdom; Senior Lecturer, Imperial College School of
Medicine, London, United Kingdom
Chronic Fatigue Syndrome

Andreas Otto Reiff, MD
Associate Professor of Pediatrics, Keck School of Medicine
of the University of Southern California; Staff Physician,
Children's Hospital Los Angeles, Los Angeles, California
Juvenile Arthritis

Martin Reite, MD
Professor of Psychiatry, University of Colorado Health
Sciences Center School of Medicine; Director, Insomnia and
Sleep Disorders Clinic, University of Colorado Hospital,
Denver, Colorado
Treatment of Insomnia

Jeffrey Rentz, MD
Resident in Thoracic Surgery, Beth Israel Deaconess Medical
Center, Boston, Massachusetts
Pleural Effusion and Empyema Thoracis

James P. Richardson, MD, MPH
Chief, Geriatric Medicine, Union Memorial Hospital,
Baltimore, Maryland, Clinical Professor of Family Medicine,
University of Maryland School of Medicine, Baltimore,
Maryland
Tetanus

Alan G. Robinson, MD
Executive Associate Dean and Associate Vice Chancellor,
Medical Sciences, David Geffen School of Medicine at
University of California—Los Angeles, Los Angeles,
California
Diabetes Insipidus

Steven T. Rosen, MD
Geneviève Teuton Professor, Department of Medicine,
Division of Hematology/Oncology, Northwestern University
Feinberg School of Medicine; Staff Physician, Robert H. Lurie
Comprehensive Cancer Center, Chicago, Illinois
Cutaneous T-Cell Lymphomas (Mycosis Fungoides and Sézary Syndrome)

Richard M. Rosenfeld, MD, MPH
Professor of Otolaryngology, State University of New York,
Downstate Medical Center College of Medicine, Delmar,
New York
Otitis Media

Oscar Ruiz, MD
Program Director, General Surgery Residency, Riverside
Methodist Hospital, Columbus, Ohio
Cholelithiasis and Cholecystitis

Brian K. Rundall, DO
Senior Thoracic Surgery Research Fellow, Division of
Thoracic and Cardiovascular Surgery, University of Virginia
School of Medicine, Charlottesville, Virginia
Atelectasis

Asad Salim, MD
Clinical Pediatric Fellow, Children's Hospital and Health
Center, San Diego, California
Atopic Dermatitis

Karl J. Sandin, MD
Central Coast Physical Medicine and Rehabilitation Medical
Group, Santa Barbara, California
Rehabilitation of the Stroke Patient

Mathuram Santosham, MD, MPH
Director and Professor, Department of International Health,
Johns Hopkins Bloomberg School of Public Health;
Baltimore, Maryland
Acute Infectious Diarrhea

Denis Sasseville, MD
Director, Division of Dermatology, McGill University
Health Centre; Associate Professor of Dermatology,
McGill University Faculty of Medicine, Montreal,
Quebec, Canada
Contact Dermatitis

Wilson Sawa, MD
Professor, Department of Obstetrics and Gynecology,
Northeastern Ohio Universities College of Medicine; Staff
Physician, Aultman Hospital, Canton, Ohio
Cancer of the Uterine Cervix

Thomas M. Scalea, MD
Francis X. Kelly/MBNA Professor of Trauma Surgery;
Director, Program in Trauma, University of Maryland School
of Medicine; Physician-in-Chief, R. Adams Cowley Shock
Trauma Center, Baltimore, Maryland
Necrotizing Skin and Soft Tissue Infection

Dwight Scarborough, MD
Adjunct Assistant Professor of Dermatology, Columbia
University College of Physicians and Surgeons, New York,
New York
Diseases of the Hair

Randall T. Schapiro, MD
Director, The Schapiro Center for Multiple Sclerosis and
The Minneapolis Clinic of Neurology, Minneapolis,
Minnesota
Multiple Sclerosis

Anouk Scheres, PhD
Associate Research Scientist, Institute for Pediatric
Neuroscience, New York University Child Study Center,
New York, New York
Attention Deficit Hyperactivity Disorder (ADHD)

Isaac Schiff, MD
Joe Vincent Meigs Professor of Gynecology, Harvard Medical
School; Chief, Vincent Memorial Obstetrics and Gynecology
Service, Massachusetts General Hospital, Boston,
Massachusetts
Menopause

George P. Schmid, MD, MSc
Department of HIV & AIDS/Evidence and Information
for Policy, World Health Organization, Geneva,
Switzerland
Chancroid; Gonorrhea

Robert T. Schoen, MD
Clinical Professor of Medicine, Yale University School of
Medicine, New Haven, Connecticut
Lyme Disease

Kathryn G. Schuff, MD
Associate Professor of Endocrinology and General Clinical
Research Center, Clinical Research Compliance Manager,
Oregon Health and Science University School of Medicine,
Portland, Oregon
Cushing's Syndrome

Carlos Seas, MD
Insituto de Medicina Tropical "Alexander von Humboldt,"
Universidad Peruana Cayetano Heredia, Lima, Peru;
Departamento de Enfermedades Infecciosas, Tropicales y
Dermatológicas, Hospital Nacional Cayetano Heredia,
Lima, Peru
Cholera

Hilliard Seigler, MD
Professor of Surgery and Immunology, Duke University
School of Medicine, Durham, North Carolina
Malignant Melanoma

Ralph Shabetai, MD
Professor of Medicine Emeritus, University of California,
San Diego, School of Medicine, La Jolla, California
Acute Pericarditis

Mrunal Shah, MD
Clinical Assistant Professor of Family Medicine, The Ohio
State University College of Medicine and Public Health;
Assistant Program Director, Riverside Family Practice
Residency Program, Columbus, Ohio
Syphilis

Samir S. Shah, MD
Instructor, Department of Pediatrics, University of
Pennsylvania School of Medicine; Division of Infectious
Diseases and General Pediatrics, The Children's Hospital of
Philadelphia, Philadelphia, Pennsylvania
Cat-Scratch Disease

Snehal N. Shah, MD
Epidemic Intelligence Service Officer, Malaria Branch,
Division of Parasitic Diseases, National Center for Infectious
Diseases, Centers for Disease Control and Prevention,
Atlanta, Georgia
Malaria

Joseph C. Shanahan, MD
Assistant Professor of Medicine, Division of Rheumatology
and Immunology, Duke University School of Medicine,
Durham, North Carolina
Rheumatoid Arthritis

Joel Sheinfeld, MD
Vice-Chairman, Department of Urology, Memorial-Sloan
Kettering Cancer Center, Professor of Urology, Weill Medical
School, Cornell University
Malignant Tumors of the Urogenital Tract

Philip D. Shenefelt, MD, MS
Associate Professor, Division of Dermatology, University of
South Florida, Tampa, Florida
Parasitic Diseases of the Skin

Raj D. Sheth, MD
Director, Comprehensive Epilepsy Program; Professor,
University of Wisconsin–Madison School of Medicine,
Madison, Wisconsin
Epilepsy in Infancy and Childhood

Jan L. Shifren, MD
Assistant Professor of Obstetrics, Gynecology, and
Reproductive Biology, Harvard Medical School; Director,
Menopause Program, Vincent Memorial Obstetrics and
Gynecology Service, Massachusetts General Hospital,
Boston, Massachusetts
Menopause

Lydia A. Shrier, MD, MPH
Assistant Professor of Pediatrics, Harvard Medical School;
Assistant in Medicine, Children's Hospital Boston, Boston,
Massachusetts
Pelvic Inflammatory Disease

Ira A. Shulman, MD
Professor and Vice Chair, Department of Pathology, Keck
School of Medicine of University of Southern California;
Director of Transfusion Medicine, Los Angeles County–
University of Southern California, Medical Center, Los
Angeles, California
Autoimmune Hemolytic Anemia

Michael E. Shy, MD
Professor of Neurology, Professor of Molecular Medicine and
Genetics, Wayne State University School of Medicine,
Detroit, Michigan
Peripheral Neuropathies

Dee E. Silver, MD
Head, Section of Neurology, Scripps Memorial Hospital,
La Jolla; Medical Director, Parkinson's Disease Association,
San Diego, California
Parkinsonism

Marc A. Silver, MD
Clinical Professor of Medicine, University of Illinois at
Chicago College of Medicine, Chicago; Adjunct Professor,
Department of Biomedical Engineering, Illinois Institute of
Technology, Chicago; Chairman, Department of Medicine,
and Director, Heart Failure Institute, Advocate Christ
Medical Center, Oak Lawn, Illinois
Heart Failure

A. Larry Simmons, MD
Assistant Professor, Department of Pediatrics–General
Pediatrics, University of Arkansas for Medical Sciences: Staff
Physician, Arkansas Children's Hospital, Little Rock,
Arkansas
Whooping Cough (Pertussis)

Peter A. Singer, MD
Professor of Clinical Medicine, Department of
Medicine, Keck School of Medicine of University of Southern
California, Los Angeles, California
Hypothyroidism

James E. Skinner, MD
Director of Research and Development, Vicor Technologies,
Inc., Bangor, Pennsylvania
Sudden Cardiac Death

Kenneth J. Smith, MD
Assistant Professor of Medicine, University of Pittsburgh
School of Medicine, Pittsburgh, Pennsylvania
Influenza

Jonathan M. Spergel, MD, PhD
Assistant Professor of Pediatrics, University of Pennsylvania
School of Medicine; Staff Physician, The Children's Hospital
of Philadelphia, Philadelphia, Pennsylvania
Asthma in Children

Peter C. Spittell, MD
Assistant Professor of Medicine, Mayo Medical School;
Consultant, Division of Internal Medicine and
Cardiovascular Disease, Mayo Clinic and Mayo Foundation,
Rochester, Minnesota
Peripheral Arterial Disease

Katherine Spooner, MD
Deputy Director for Clinical Interventions, U.S. Military HIV
Research Program/HJF, Infectious Diseases Division, Walter
Reed Army Medical Center, Washington, DC
Food-Borne Illness

E. William St. Clair, MD
Professor of Medicine and Immunology, Division of
Rheumatology and Immunology, Duke University School of
Medicine, Durham, North Carolina
Rheumatoid Arthritis

Virginia A. Stallings, MD
Director, Nutrition Center, The Children's Hospital of
Philadelphia, Philadelphia, Pennsylvania
Normal Infant Feeding

Andrew P. Steenhoff, MD, MBBCh
Fellow, Division of Infectious Diseases, The Children's
Hospital of Philadelphia, Philadelphia, Pennsylvania
Cat-Scratch Disease

John R. Stephenson, MD
Honorary Senior Lecturer, Department of Infectious and
Tropical Diseases, London School of Hygiene and Tropical
Medicine, London, England
Measles (Rubeola)

Dana Kazlow Stern, MD
Resident, Mount Sinai Medical Center, New York, New York
Papulosquamous Eruptions

Tasha Stevens, BS
Resident, Baylor College of Medicine, Houston, Texas
Non-Hodgkin's Lymphomas

Catherine Stevens-Simon, MD
Associate Professor of Pediatrics, Division of Adolescent
Medicine, University of Colorado Health Sciences Center
School of Medicine; Staff Physician, Children's Hospital,
Denver, Colorado
Chlamydia trachomatis

Greg V. Stiegmann, MD
Professor and Head, Gastrointestinal, Tumor, and Endocrine
Surgery, Department of Surgery, University of Colorado
Health Sciences Center School of Medicine; Staff Physician,
Denver Veterans Affairs Hospitals, Denver, Colorado
Bleeding Esophageal Varices

Mathias L. Stoenescu, MD
Fellow, Department of Electrophysiology, Lankenau
Hospital, Wynnewood, Pennsylvania
Atrial Fibrillation

John H. Stone, MD, MPH
Associate Professor of Medicine, Division of Rheumatology, Johns Hopkins School of Medicine; Director, The Johns Hopkins Vasculitis Center, Johns Hopkins Bayview Medical Center, Baltimore, Maryland
Giant Cell Arteritis and Polymyalgia Rheumatica

Patrick A. Stone, MD
Chief Surgical Resident, Department of Surgery, Robert C. Byrd Health Sciences Center of West Virginia University, Charleston, West Virginia
Venous Thrombosis

David J. Straus, MD
Attending Physician, Department of Medicine, Memorial Sloan-Kettering Cancer Center; Professor of Clinical Medicine, Joan and Sanford I. Weill Medical College of Cornell University, New York, New York
Hodgkin's Disease: Chemotherapy

Stevan B. Streem, MD
Head, Section of Endourology and Stone Disease, Glickman Urological Institute, The Cleveland Clinic Foundation; Professor of Surgery, Cleveland Clinic Lerner College of Medicine/Case Western University School of Medicine, Cleveland, Ohio
Renal Calculi

Jin S. Suh, MD
Associate Medical Director, Center for Comprehensive Care, St. Luke's–Roosevelt Hospital Center; Assistant Clinical Professor of Medicine, Columbia University College of Physicians and Surgeons, New York, New York
Management of the Patient with HIV Disease

Paniti Sukumvanich
Fellow, Breast Service, Department of Surgery, Memorial Sloan-Kettering Cancer Center, New York, New York
Diseases of the Breast

Britta M. Svoren, MD
Fellow, Pediatric Endocrinology, Division of Endocrinology, Children's Hospital Boston, Boston, Massachusetts
Diabetes Mellitus in Children and Adolescents

Mehmet Tanyuksel, MD
Professor of Medical Parasitology; Chief of Medical Parasitology, Gulhane Military Medical Academy, Ankara, Turkey
Amebiasis

Victor F. Tapson, MD
Associate Professor of Medicine, Division of Pulmonary and Critical Care, Duke University School of Medicine, Durham, North Carolina
Pulmonary Embolism

Kenneth S. Taylor, MD
Director University of California-San Diego Sports Medicine Fellowship, Associate Professor, Department of Family and Preventive Medicine
Common Sports Injuries

David R. Thomas, MD
Professor of Medicine, Division of Gerontology and Geriatric Medicine, Saint Louis University School of Medicine, St. Louis, Missouri
Pressure Ulcers

Robert L. Thurer, MD
Associate Professor of Surgery, Harvard Medical School; Associate Chief of Thoracic Surgery, Beth Israel Deaconess Medical Center, Boston, Massachusetts
Pleural Effusion and Empyema Thoracis

Susan Thys-Jacobs, MD
Assistant Professor, Department of Medicine, Columbia University College of Physicians and Surgeons, New York, New York
Premenstral Syndrome

Joyce A. Tinsley, MD
Associate Professor, Department of Psychiatry; Director of Psychiatric Residency Training and Director of Addiction Psychiatry Training, University of Connecticut School of Medicine, Farmington, Connecticut
Drug Abuse

Lama L. Tolaymat, MD, MPH
Assistant Professor, Department of Obstetrics and Gynecology, University of Florida College of Medicine, Jacksonville, Florida
Contraception

Marcia G. Tonnesen, MD
Associate Professor of Dermatology and Medicine, State University of New York at Stony Brook Health Sciences Center School of Medicine, Stony Brook; Chief of Dermatology, Veterans Affairs Medical Center, Northport, New York
Erythema Multiforme, Stevens-Johnson Syndrome, and Toxic Epidermal Necrolysis

Peter P. Toth, MD, PhD
Chief of Medicine, CGH Medical Center; Visiting Clinical Associate Professor, University of Illinois at Chicago School of Medicine, Chicago; Director of Preventive Cardiology, Sterling Rock Falls Clinic, Sterling, Illinois
Dyslipoproteinemias

Charles V. Trimarchi, MD
Chief, Laboratory of Zoonotic Disease and Clinical, Griffin Laboratory, Slingerlands, New York
Rabies

Penny Turner, MD
Assistant Clinical Professor, Department of Medicine, University of Alberta, Edmonton, Alberta, Canada
Primary Glomerular Diseases

Ronald B. Turner, MD
Professor, Department of Pediatric Infectious Diseases, University of Virginia School of Medicine, Charlottesville, Virginia
Viral Respiratory Infections

Douglas Tyler, MD
Associate Professor of Surgery, Duke University School of Medicine; Chief, Surgical Oncology; Vice Chairman, Department of Surgery, Duke University Medical Center, Durham North Carolina
Malignant Melanoma

Jay Umbreit, MTS, MD, PhD
Professor of Hematology/Oncology, Emory University School of Medicine; Winship Cancer Institute, Atlanta, Georgia
Iron Deficiency

Varsha Vaidya, MD
Assistant Professor of Psychiatry and General Internal
Medicine, Johns Hopkins School of Medicine, Silver Spring,
Maryland
Hiccups

John A. Vande Waa, PhD, DO
Associate Professor, Department of Medicine, University of
South Alabama College of Medicine, Mobile, Alabama
Bacterial Pneumonia

John Varga, MD
Professor of Medicine, Division of Rheumatology,
Northwestern University School of Medicine, Chicago,
Illinois
Connective Tissue Disorders

Ronald K. de Vencecia, MD, PhD
Otology-Neurology Fellow, Department of Otology and
Laryngology, Massachusetts Eye and Ear Infirmary, Boston,
Massachusetts
Ménière's Disease

Todd W. Vitaz, MD
Director of Neurosurgical Oncology; Co-Director of
Neurosciences ICU; Assistant Professor of Neurological
Surgery, University of Louisville School of Medicine,
Louisville, Kentucky
Management of Head Injuries

Fritz-Henry Volmar, MD
Fellow, Gastroenterology Division, Henry Ford Health
System, Detroit, Michigan
Acute and Chronic Viral Hepatitis

Matthew D. Vrees, MD
Colorectal Surgery Resident, Cleveland Clinic Foundation,
Weston, Florida
Hemorrhoids, Anal Fissure, Anorectal Abscess and Fistula

Richard F. Wagner, Jr., MD
Professor, Department of Dermatology, The University of
Texas Medical Branch School of Medicine, Galveston, Texas
Cancer of the Skin

Laura Waikart, MD
Fellow (Allergy), University of Tennessee, Knoxville,
Tennessee
Nonallergic Rhinitis

David H. Walker, MD
Professor and Chairman, Department of Pathology,
The University of Texas Medical Branch School of Medicine,
Galveston, Texas
Rickettsial and Ehrlichial Infections

Philip D. Walson, MD
Professor of Pediatrics and Pharmacology, University of
Cincinnati College of Medicine; Director, Clinical
Pharmacology Division, Clinical Trials Office, Cincinnati
Children's Hospital Medical Center, Cincinnati, Ohio
Fever

Thomas T. Ward, MD
Associate Professor of Medicine, Oregon Health and Science
University School of Medicine; Chief, Infectious Diseases,
Portland Veterans Affairs Medical Center, Portland, Oregon
Toxoplasmosis

Peter C. Weber, MD
Professor and Program Director; Director of Implantable
Hearing Devices, Head and Neck Institute, Cleveland Clinic,
Cleveland, Ohio
Acute Facial Paralysis (Bell's Palsy)

Guy F. Webster, MD, PhD
Professor and Vice Chair, Department of Dermatology,
Jefferson Medical College at Thomas Jefferson University,
Philadelphia, Pennsylvania
Acne Rosacea

Max M. Weder, MD
Department of Medicine, Division of Pulmonary and Critical
Care Medicine, University of North Carolina School of
Medicine, Chapel Hill, North Carolina
Acute Respiratory Failure

Michael Wein, MD
President, Florida Allergy, Asthma, and Immunology Society;
Chief of Allergy, Indian River Memorial Hospital, Vero
Beach, Florida
Allergic Rhinitis

Robert N. Weinreb, MD
Hamilton Glaucoma Center; Department of Ophthalmology,
University of California, San Diego, School of Medicine,
La Jolla, California
Glaucoma

David G. Weismiller, MD, ScM
Associate Professor and Vice Chair, Department of Family
Medicine, The Brody School of Medicine at East Carolina
University, Greenville, North Carolina
Hypertensive Disorders of Pregnancy

Eric G. Weiss, MD
Residency Program Director and Director of Surgical
Endoscopy, Cleveland Clinic Foundation, Weston, Florida
Hemorrhoids, Anal Fissure, Anorectal Abscess and Fistula

Thomas R. Welch, MD
Professor and Chair, Department of Pediatrics, State
University of New York Upstate Medical University College
of Medicine, Syracuse, New York
Parenteral Fluid Therapy for Infants and Children

Simon Wessely, MD, PhD
Professor of Epidemiology and Liaison Psychiatry, Institute
of Psychiatry, King's College London, London, United
Kingdom
Chronic Fatigue Syndrome

Derek S. Wheeler, MD
Assistant Professor of Clinical Pediatrics, Division of Critical
Care Medicine, Cincinnati College of Medicine; Staff
Physician, Cincinnati Children's Hospital Medical Center,
Cincinnati, Ohio
Resuscitation of the Newborn

J. Gary Wheeler, MD
Professor of Pediatrics, Department of Pediatrics, Infectious
Diseases, University of Arkansas for Medical Sciences; Staff
Physician, Arkansas Children's Hospital, Little Rock,
Arkansas
Whooping Cough (Pertussis)

A. Clinton White, Jr., MD
Department of Medicine, Infectious Disease Section, Baylor
College of Medicine, Houston, Texas
Intestinal Parasites

Richard J. Whitley, MD
Professor of Pediatrics, Microbiology, Medicine, and
Neurosurgery, University of Alabama at Birmingham School
of Medicine, Birmingham, Alabama
Smallpox: A Twenty-First Century View

Scott C. Wickless, DO
Dermatologist/Dermatopathologist, Northwestern
University, Chicago, Illinois
Nevi

Michael G. Wilkerson, MD
Clinical Assistant Professor of Dermatology, University of
Oklahoma College of Medicine–Tulsa, Tulsa, Oklahoma
Bacterial Diseases of the Skin

Kira Williams, MD
Chief Resident in Psychiatry, Anxiety Disorders Clinic,
Department of Psychiatry and Biobehavioral Sciences,
Neuropsychiatric Institute and Hospital, Los Angeles,
California
Panic Disorder

Lynne K. Williams, MB, BCh
Research Fellow, Specialist Registrar in Cardiology,
University of Birmingham, Birmingham, United Kingdom
Hypertrophic Cardiomyopathy

Steven R. Williams, MD
Clinical Assistant Professor, Department of Obstetrics and
Gynecology, The Ohio State University, Columbus, Ohio
Infertility

Phillip M. Williford, MD
Associate Professor, Department of Dermatology, Wake
Forest University School of Medicine, Winston-Salem,
North Carolina
Warts (Verrucae)

Joseph I. Wolfsdorf, MB, BCh
Director, Diabetes Program; Associate Chief, Division of
Endocrinology, Children's Hospital; Associate Professor of
Pediatrics, Harvard Medical School, Boston, Massachusetts
Diabetes Mellitus in Children and Adolescents

Kimberly Workowski, MD
Associate Professor of Medicine, Division of Infectious
Diseases, Emory University School of Medicine; Division of
STD Prevention, Centers for Disease Control and
Prevention, Atlanta, Georgia
Nongonococcal Urethritis

Ted Wun, MD
Professor of Medicine, University of California, Davis, School
of Medicine; Associate Chief and Fellowship Program
Director, Division of Hematology-Oncology; Chief, Section of
Hematology and Oncology, VA Northern California Health
Care System, Davis, California
Nonimmune Hemolytic Anemia

Joachim Yahalom, MD
Member, Department of Radiation Oncology, Memorial
Sloan-Kettering Cancer Center; Professor of Radiation
Oncology in Medicine, Joan and Sanford I. Weill Medical
College of Cornell University, New York, New York
Hodgkin's Lymphoma: Role of Radiation Therapy

Terry Yamauchi, MD
Professor and Vice Chairman, Department of Pediatrics,
University of Arkansas for Medical Sciences; Staff Physician,
Arkansas Children's Hospital, Little Rock, Arkansas
Mumps

Linda Yancey, MD
Fellow, Infectious Diseases, Ben Taub General Hospital and
Baylor College of Medicine, Houston, Texas
Intestinal Parasites

Barbara P. Yawn, MD, MSc, FAAFP
Adjunct Professor of Family and Community Health,
University of Minnesota Medical School, Minneapolis;
Director of Research, Department of Research, Olmsted
Medical Center, Rochester, Minnesota
Office-Based Immunization Practices

John A. Yeung-Lai-Wah, MB, ChB
Clinical Associate Professor, University of British Columbia
Faculty of Medicine; Director of Electrophysiology
Laboratory, St. Paul's Hospital, Vancouver, British
Columbia, Canada
Premature Beats

James A. Yiannias, MD
Consultant, Department of Dermatology, Mayo Clinic,
Scottsdale, Arizona; Associate Professor of Dermatology,
Mayo Clinic College of Medicine, Rochester, Minnesota
Pruritus

William F. Young, Jr., MD
Professor of Medicine, Mayo Clinic College of Medicine;
Consultant, Divisions of Endocrinology, Diabetes,
Metabolism, and Nutrition and Internal Medicine, Mayo
Clinic and Mayo Foundation, Rochester, Minnesota
Primary Aldosteronism; Pheochromocytoma

Howard A. Zacur, MD, PhD
Director, Division of Reproductive Endocrinology,
Department of Gynecology and Obstetrics, Johns Hopkins
School of Medicine, Baltimore, Maryland
Hyperprolactinemia

Hamayun Zafar, PT, PhD
Assistant Professor, Department of Odontology–Clinical Oral
Physiology, Umeå University Faculty of Medicine, Umeå;
Center for Musculoskeletal Research, Gävle University,
Gävle and Umeå, Sweden
Temporomandibular Disorders

Robert L. Zanni, MD
Director, Pediatric Pulmonary Medicine; Director, Cystic
Fibrosis Center, Saint Barnabas Health Care System,
Monmouth Medical Center, Long Branch, New Jersey
Cystic Fibrosis

Jami Star Zeltzer, MD
Associate Professor, Department of Obstetrics and
Gynecology, Division of Maternal-Fetal Medicine, University
of Massachusetts Medical School, Worcester, Massachusetts
Vaginal Bleeding in Late Pregnancy

Steven Zgliniec, MD
Fellow, Division of Pulmonary and Critical Care Medicine,
Rush Medical College; Rush University Medical Center,
Chicago, Illinois
Severe Sepsis and Septic Shock

Kenneth S. Zuckerman, MD
Harold H. Davis Professor of Cancer Research and Professor
of Oncology, Internal Medicine, and Biochemistry/Molecular
Biology, University of South Florida School of Medicine,
Tampa, Florida
Polycythemia Vera

Preface

This is the 58th edition, the first having been published by Howard Conn, M.D. in 1949. In 2006, the goal remains exactly the same, that is, to provide a concise and up-to-date reference of the most recent advances in therapy for conditions most commonly encountered in practice. Also included are several less common problems that could have serious consequences if not diagnosed and managed properly.

Each year we turn to new authorities to assure that the information remains current. The presentation by different experts often provides the health care professional a different approach to managing the problem than was presented the previous year.

Although most of our authors are from the United States, we often turn to authors in other countries. An outstanding example this year is the Australian, Barry Marshall, MD, who was awarded the Nobel Prize for his discovery of *H. pylori* as the cause of peptic ulcer disease. Presentations by authors from other countries provides readers the benefit of their extensive experience with diseases seen less frequently in the United States. For example, this year there are 25 authors from countries such as Turkey (Amebiasis, Brucellosis), Peru (Cholera), India (Leprosy), South Africa (Granuloma Inguinale, Lymphogranuloma Venereum), France (Leishmaniasis, Plague, Ankylosing Spondylitis), Pakistan (Typhoid Fever), Japan (Pigmentary Disorders), Italy (Osteomyelitis), Thailand (Legionellosis), Brazil (Infectious Mononucleosis), Switzerland (Gonorrhea, Chancroid), Spain (Bacterial Meningitis), Sweden (Temporomandibular Disorders), and many from Canada and the United Kingdom.

New topics added this year are Heparin-Induced Thrombocytopenia, Hyponatremia, Sleep Disorders, Infertility, and Ovarian Cancer.

A major change has been made in the format of this edition to make essential information even more visible and easy to retrieve by including Key Points shown as Key Diagnostic and Key Treatment boxes. These provide the reader immediate access to the most useful and important features of diagnosis and treatment.

The 2006 edition also provides a website containing the entire book with some additional features of calculators and a drug reference. Any of the content on the web can be downloaded to a handheld device.

Also new this year are approximately ten references for each chapter that list the most important studies regarding management of that problem.

Every manuscript is reviewed by a pharmacist, physician, and multiple copy editors to ensure accuracy and easy readability. We are indebted to the excellent editorial staff at Elsevier, to our pharmacist reviewers Miriam Chan RPH, PharmD, and Bella Mehta, PharmD, and especially to Raegan Thompson, our editorial assistant who handles all correspondence and ensures that the tight deadlines required for an annual publication are met.

Robert E. Rakel, M.D.

Edward T. Bope, M.D.

Contents

SECTION 3
Diseases of the Head and Neck

SECTION 4
The Respiratory System

SECTION **7**
The Digestive System

SECTION **8**
Metabolic Disease

SECTION 11
Sexually Transmitted Diseases

SECTION 12
Diseases of Allergy

SECTION 13
Diseases of the Skin

SECTION **19**
Appendices and Index

Symptomatic Care Pending Diagnosis

Pain

Method of
Alan B. Douglass, MD

Pain, an almost ubiquitous human condition, is a common reason for seeking medical care. Ninety percent of patients with advanced cancer, 45% to 80% of nursing home patients, and 25% to 50% of community adults report daily pain. Pain is a major cause of lost productivity, with United States (U.S.) annual costs of more than $60 billion in lost work alone. Improving pain assessment and management is currently a U.S. national priority.

The literature clearly documents that 90% of pain can be adequately controlled using standard techniques such as the World Health Organization (WHO) pain ladder and the Agency for Healthcare Policy and Research (AHCPR) (now known as the Agency for Healthcare Research and Quality [AHRQ]) guidelines. However, undertreatment is rife. More than 50% of patients, even those at the end of life, do not receive adequate analgesia.

Pain is defined by the International Association for the Study of Pain as "an unpleasant sensory and emotional experience associated with actual or potential tissue damage, or described in terms of such damage." Pain is a complex and subjective sensory, emotional, and cognitive phenomenon. The degree of pain experienced by a patient does not always correlate well with identifiable tissue injury, making assessment challenging.

Acute pain often follows an injury but may also arise de novo as the result of structural degeneration, infection, or metabolic changes. Acute pain tends to abate as tissues heal, and it generally responds well to analgesics and other therapies. Chronic pain persists over time and is generally defined as either lasting longer than 3 to 6 months or lasting 1 month longer than the usual time required for an injury to heal. The management of chronic pain is often complex.

Pain is generally divided into two broad categories: nociceptive and neuropathic. Nociceptive pain is induced when nociceptive receptors are stimulated by a tissue injury process and is further divided into visceral and somatic pain. Visceral pain originates in internal organs. It is often poorly localized and described as cramping, squeezing, or colicky, if originating from a hollow viscus, or aching and dull, if originating from a solid organ. Somatic pain is more easily localized and usually described as achy, throbbing, or dull.

Neuropathic pain is induced by pathophysiologic changes to the central and peripheral nervous systems. It is typically described as a sharp, tingling, burning, or electric sensation that often radiates. Pain of neuropathic origin may be associated with dysesthesias (unpleasant abnormal sensations), hyperalgesia (mildly painful stimuli perceived as very painful), or allodynia (nonpainful stimuli perceived as painful). Neuropathic pain usually requires a multimodal approach to therapy and tends to be more refractory to treatment than nociceptive pain.

Patient Assessment

Pain is a subjective, complex, multidimensional experience perceived only by the patient. Patient response to pain involves physical, psychologic, and cognitive facets. Pain assessment is always challenging for clinicians because no single objective measurement is available. Consequently, the patient's assessment of the severity and quality of the pain should be considered the best available assessment tool.

Pain reporting by patients can be subject to exaggeration, minimization, and misinterpretation. Many factors can influence the pain perception of others. Generally speaking, family members tend to overestimate, whereas health care professionals tend to underestimate. Reduced cognitive ability, reduced level of consciousness, and stoicism can result in under-reporting. Cultural, ethnic, and gender factors on the part of both patients and caregivers all can affect pain interpretation and communication.

Effective pain management begins with comprehensive patient assessment. A number of validated pain assessment tools of varying length and complexity are available. Simple examples include the numeric rating scale (1 to 10) and visual analogue scale. Special instruments, such as the faces scale, are available when language barriers are present and for rating discomfort in young children and the cognitively impaired. Frequent reevaluation is an essential part of effective pain management.

Pharmacologic Management

Medication is the mainstay of pain management. The pharmacologic management of pain is based on the WHO analgesic ladder, where the selection of agent depends on the severity and type of pain experienced. Patients with mild pain are treated with step 1 nonopioid agents such as acetaminophen or nonsteroidal anti-inflammatory drugs (NSAIDs), with or without the addition of adjuvant medications. Pain that is moderate in intensity is treated with step 2 weak opioids in addition to step 1 medications. Severe pain is treated with step 3 strong opioids, such as morphine, in addition to adjuvants and appropriate adjuvants. Some authors recommend a fourth step in the ladder, representing interventional pain management techniques. If pain is initially severe, the treating physician does not have to proceed up the ladder sequentially but may begin with either step 2 or step 3.

ACETAMINOPHEN OF PHARMACOLOGIC MANAGEMENT

Full-dose acetaminophen (Tylenol) is an effective, well-tolerated analgesic in a variety of pain scenarios. Although 4 g per day are listed as the maximal safe dosage, many experts advocate maximum dosages of 2 to 3 g per day. Furthermore, in alcoholism, fasting states, hepatic disease, the presence of certain medications (especially anticonvulsants), or in the frail elderly, liver toxicity can occur at recommended doses. Toxicity increases when acetaminophen is taken in conjunction with an NSAID. Particular care should be taken that daily dose limits are not exceeded inadvertently when patients are taking combination analgesics containing acetaminophen.

NONSTEROIDAL ANTI-INFLAMMATORY DRUGS OF PHARMACOLOGIC MANAGEMENT

Strong evidence indicates the efficacy of NSAIDs in acute and chronic pain. The efficacy of all NSAIDs appears roughly equivalent, but patient response to any particular agent is highly idiosyncratic.

Nonacetylated salicylates (choline magnesium trisalicylate [Trilisate], salsalate [Disalcid]), and cyclooxygenase (COX)-2-specific inhibitors are effective and may have fewer gastrointestinal side effects than traditional NSAIDs. Salicylates have the additional advantage of low cost. If traditional NSAIDs are chosen, gastric cytoprotection should be considered based on the patient's risk profile. Clinicians should also be aware of potential nephrotoxicity in the elderly and in patients with renal disease. Recent research suggests that at least some NSAIDs may increase the risk of cardiovascular events. Care should be taken in prescribing to at-risk patients. NSAIDs should be particularly considered when inflammation is playing a substantial role in the production of the pain process.

OPIOIDS OF PHARMACOLOGIC MANAGEMENT

Opioids are an effective option in the management of moderate to severe pain. They are often the drug of choice in acute and chronic cancer pain. Opioids recently became more accepted in the long-term management of severe chronic noncancer pain, although concerns are raised about the safety and efficacy of prolonged high-dose opioid therapy.

Traditionally, opioids were thought superior to other agents because of the absence of a ceiling effect. Recent research suggests a ceiling may exist, but it is variable and often determined by side effects such as myoclonus. Doses can be escalated by 50% to 100% in a 24-hour period for severe uncontrolled pain. Increases of less than 25% are usually ineffective in this situation, but smaller increases may be effective for moderate pain.

Immediate-release opioids commonly prescribed orally in the ambulatory setting include codeine, hydrocodone, and oxycodone (Roxicodone). Codeine tends to be very constipating and should be used with care in the elderly. Propoxyphene (Darvon) has a limited analgesic effect and active metabolites accumulate over time. Its use should be limited to the short term. Partial agonists such as butorphanol (Stadol) are strongly discouraged as first-line agents. They should not be given to patients taking pure opioid agonists because they may precipitate withdrawal.

Morphine, the prototypical opioid, is available in a variety of dosage forms and widely used. Fentanyl (Duragesic) and hydromorphone (Dilaudid) are also commonly used. Hydromorphone is particularly useful because of its high potency but is available only in short-acting preparations. Methadone (Dolophine) is increasingly used in the management of chronic pain because of its low cost and beneficial side-effect profile. Because of its peculiar pharmacokinetics that can lead to drug accumulation and toxicity, however, it should be prescribed only after careful consideration and only by physicians experienced in its use. Meperidine (Demerol) is not recommended because of accumulation of active metabolites that can trigger neurotoxicity and seizures. In patients with renal failure fentanyl and methadone carry the least risk.

In patients with chronic pain, the use of sustained-release morphine and oxycodone should be considered. Once at steady state, sustained-release opioids are more convenient and prevent the peaks and valleys associated with short-acting agents. However, many patients, particularly those with cancer pain, require an additional short-acting agent to manage breakthrough pain.

The diversity of opioid receptors allows the transition from one opioid agonist to another when one agent ceases to be effective or side effects limit dose escalation. Opioid rotation must be done with care. Doses of different agents are not equivalent, so a conversion table (Table 1) should be used to calculate the equianalgesic doses.

TABLE 1 Single-Dose Opioid Equianalgesic

Drug	Doses in milligrams	
	Oral dose	Parenteral dose
Morphine	15	5
Meperidine (Demerol)	150	50
Hydromorphone (Dilaudid)	3.75	0.75
Oxycodone (Roxicodone)	10	NA
Hydrocodone	15	NA
Codeine	90	NA

Alternatively, the dose of the original agent can be converted to oral morphine equivalents (Table 2) and then converted to the correct dosage of the new agent. To account for the phenomenon of incomplete cross-tolerance, the equianalgesic dose of the new agent should be decreased by 25% to 50%.

Opioids can be delivered by a variety of routes, including orally, rectally, intravenously, and subcutaneously. The intramuscular route is not recommended because of the pain associated with injections and wide fluctuations in blood levels. Fentanyl (Duragesic) is highly lipophilic and can be delivered transdermally through a 72-hour patch. Butorphanol (Stadol NS), a mixed agonist-antagonist, can be delivered intranasally. Interventional delivery of a variety of agents through the intrathecal or epidural route is also possible. Patient-controlled analgesia through the intravenous or epidural route can be very effective. When changing from one route to another, doses must be recalculated even if the same agent is used (see Table 1).

The most common side effect of opioid therapy is constipation, which, once established, can be severe and difficult to treat. All patients started on an opioid should receive a prophylactic bowel regimen with a stimulant laxative. Use of a stool softener alone is rarely effective. Nausea and vomiting are common but usually transient. Sedation and impaired psychomotor function occur in a dose-dependent fashion and are most common when initiating therapy. Symptoms typically dissipate over time, and patients on long-term opioid therapy are often capable of carrying out their usual daily activities, including working and driving.

The long-term use of opioids in the management of chronic noncancer pain is currently being debated. Some patients clearly can benefit from this approach.

TABLE 2 Oral Morphine Equivalents (OME)

Drug	OME
Morphine	1
Codeine, 30 mg	1-2
Hydrocodone, 5 mg	2
Oxycodone, 5 mg	5
Hydromorphone, 4 mg	15

Rakel and Bope: *Conn's Current Therapy 2006.*

Recent research on prolonged high-dose opioid therapy raises concerns of opioid-induced abnormal pain sensitivity, hormonal changes, including changes in libido and fertility, and immune suppression. Daily doses of more than 180 mg of daily morphine equivalent are not validated as effective in clinical trials and may present an increased risk of toxicity. The decision on an appropriate dose in a given patient should be individualized, with a focus on efficacy, avoiding potential toxicities, and functional improvement.

Both physicians and patients are often leery about using opioids because of fears of addiction and abuse. The nature of addiction and its risk in the use of opioids for pain management is frequently misunderstood, and confusion over definitions worsens the problem. The result often is undertreatment of pain.

Addiction is a primary, chronic, neurobiologic disease with genetic, psychosocial, and environmental risk factors. It is characterized by behaviors such as impaired control over drug use, cravings and excessive or compulsive drug use, and persistent use despite adverse consequences. Addiction occurs very infrequently in patients receiving opioid analgesia, and the risk is generally overrated. *Pseudoaddiction* is the manifestation of opioid-seeking behaviors that superficially appear similar to addiction but in reality are driven by undertreatment of pain. Unlike addiction, symptoms of pseudoaddiction disappear when pain is treated effectively.

Two terms describe the physiologic adaptation to chronic opioid therapy. Both are universal and predictable. *Dependence* is adaptation to a medication that results in a class-specific withdrawal syndrome if that medication is discontinued abruptly. This abstinence syndrome should not be confused with addiction. *Tolerance* is the development of diminution of drug effect over time, resulting in the need for increasing dosages to achieve the same analgesic effect. Tolerance occurs most commonly early in the course of opioid therapy. In cancer patients, an increasing need for opioid therapy usually reflects disease progression rather than tolerance.

ADJUVANT ANALGESICS OF PHARMACOLOGIC MANAGEMENT

Anticonvulsants are effective treatments for all types of neuropathic pain. Responses can be complete and dramatic in some patients. They are often used in combination with analgesics. All require gradual dose titration to maximize response while minimizing side effects. Gabapentin (Neurontin)[1] is commonly prescribed and has few drug interactions, although sedation and ataxia can be problematic at higher doses. Topiramate (Topamax),[1] because of its several mechanisms of action, may be more effective than existing anticonvulsants but is not as well studied. Older anticonvulsants, such as carbamazepine (Tegretol), are as effective as and less expensive than newer agents but associated with more side effects and adverse reactions.

Tricyclic antidepressants can be effective adjuvants in the management of headache and neuropathic pain,

[1]Not FDA approved for this indication.

although it is unusual for responses to be complete. Amitriptyline (Elavil)[1] has been studied extensively. Secondary amines, such as nortriptyline (Pamelor)[1] and desipramine (Norpramin),[1] are also effective, however, and they have less anticholinergic side effects. Small doses (10 to 25 mg at bedtime) can be effective in some patients, but the response is generally dose dependent and greatest in the 100 to 150 mg per day range. Dose-limiting side effects include dry mouth, sedation, weight gain, constipation, and urinary retention. Serious side effects, including cardiac rhythm disturbances, are reported, so patients should be evaluated for cardiac abnormalities prior to initiating therapy.

Serotonin reuptake inhibitors do not have a demonstrably independent analgesic effect beyond their antidepressant action, although research is ongoing. Venlafaxine (Effexor),[1] an atypical antidepressant, is effective in reducing pain but not yet studied in nondepressed patients.

Corticosteroids are highly useful agents in the management of a variety of painful cancer syndromes, including bone, visceral, and neuropathic pain, as well as headaches caused by increased intracranial pressure and soft tissue infiltration by tumor. In addition to their analgesic actions, they have a number of beneficial secondary effects, such as antiemetic activity, improved mood, energy, and sense of well-being, and appetite stimulation. Choice of agent is empirical. There is no therapeutic dose ceiling, but toxicities are related to dose and duration of therapy. To minimize problems, including hyperglycemia, immunosuppression, myopathy, osteoporosis, and gastrointestinal toxicity, short-term use at the lowest effective dose is recommended.

Topical anesthetics such as transdermal lidocaine (Lidoderm) are effective in neuropathic pain with minimal side effects.

Muscle relaxants can sometimes be helpful in acute musculoskeletal pain. Side effects, such as sedation and the potential for abuse of some agents, limit their use. They have a limited role in long-term pain management.

In addition to their role in the management of hypercalcemia, bisphosphonates can substantially reduce cancer-related bone pain caused by osteolytic metastases either alone or in combination with radiation therapy. Pamidronate (Aredia)[1] and zoledronic acid (Zometa)[1] are available only in intravenous form.

Nonpharmacologic Management

Although pharmacologic therapies are clearly a mainstay of pain management, optimal care often also involves the use of nonpharmacologic strategies that complement and supplement medications.

PHYSICAL MODALITIES OF PHARMACOLOGIC MANAGEMENT

Substantial high-quality evidence indicates that a variety of physical modalities can be effective in managing both acute and chronic pain. Physical rehabilitation,

---

[1]Not FDA approved for this indication.

 CURRENT DIAGNOSIS

- Pain, an almost ubiquitous human condition, is commonly underdiagnosed and undertreated.
- Acute, chronic, somatic, visceral, and neuropathic pain should be distinguished.
- Comprehensive patient assessment is critical.
- Pain is subjective and perceived only by the patient. The patient's perception should be considered the best available assessment tool.
- Factors that can affect symptom interpretation and communication should be carefully explored.
- Clinicians must differentiate addiction, pseudoaddiction, dependence, and tolerance.

such as stretching, exercise, and ergonomic attention, is of benefit in many pain situations and can prevent maladaptive deconditioning. Thermotherapy and neurostimulatory approaches can have independent analgesic effects. In certain musculoskeletal problems, massage, mobilization, and manipulation can be helpful.

PSYCHOLOGIC METHODS OF PHARMACOLOGIC MANAGEMENT

In appropriate clinical settings, individual counseling, group therapy, relaxation training, biofeedback, and support groups all can be useful adjuncts. Treatment of coincident depression and anxiety is clearly shown to improve pain control, quality of life, and functionality.

 CURRENT THERAPY

- Most pain can be adequately controlled using standard techniques, such as the WHO pain ladder.
- Acetaminophen and nonsteroidal anti-inflammatory drugs (NSAIDs) are effective analgesics, but clinicians should be mindful of their potential toxicities.
- Opioids in a variety of forms are an effective option in the management of moderate to severe pain. Constipation is common with opioid use and should be managed proactively. Other side effects, such as nausea and sedation, typically dissipate over time.
- For neuropathic pain, adjunctive agents, such as tricyclic antidepressants and anticonvulsants, should always be considered.
- Nonpharmacologic measures, such as physical modalities, psychologic methods, and alternative approaches supported by evidence of benefit, should be used whenever feasible.
- Referral for an interventional procedure should be considered if a structural lesion is likely and a potentially beneficial procedure is available.

ALTERNATIVE MODALITIES OF PHARMACOLOGIC MANAGEMENT

Americans are turning to alternative therapies in ever-increasing numbers. Studies of the treatment efficacy of a variety of alternative modalities are ongoing, but strong evidence currently supports only a limited number of therapies. Physicians should discuss alternative therapies openly with patients and be knowledgeable about evidence of efficacy, side effects, and the potential for interactions with other conventional therapies.

INTERVENTIONAL APPROACHES OF PHARMACOLOGIC MANAGEMENT

Interventional pain specialists offer a variety of diagnostic and therapeutic techniques that can be helpful in the care of some patients. These include diagnostic facet and nerve blocks, therapeutic rhizotomies and nerve ablations, and selective joint and epidural injections. Referral to an interventionalist is appropriate if a structural defect is likely and a potentially beneficial procedure is available. Good communication between treating physicians is critical for overall treatment success.

REFERENCES

American Geriatrics Society Panel on Persistent Pain in Older Persons: The management of persistent pain in older persons. J Am Geriatr Soc 2002;50:S205-S224.
American Pain Society: Principles of Analgesic Use in the Treatment of Acute Pain and Cancer Pain, 5th ed. Glenview, IL: American Pain Society, 2003.
Ballantyne JC, Mao J: Opioid therapy for chronic pain. New Engl J Med 2003;349(20):1943-1953.
Dean M: Opioids in renal failure and dialysis patients. J Pain Symptom Management 2004;28(5):497-504.
Dworkin RH, Backonja M, Rowbotham MC, et al: Advances in neuropathic pain: Diagnosis, mechanisms, and treatment recommendations. Arch Neurol 2003;60(11):1524-1534.
Graham AW, Schultz TK, Mayo-Smith MF, et al: Principles of Addiction Medicine, 3rd ed. Chery Chase, MD, American Society of Addiction Medicine, 2003.
Levy MH: Pharmacologic treatment of cancer pain. N Engl J Med 1996;335(15):1124-1132.
Loeser JD, Butler SH, Chapman CR, Turk DC: Bonica's Management of Pain, 3rd ed. Philadelphia, Lippincott, Williams, & Wilkins, 2001.

Nausea and Vomiting

Method of
William F. Miser, MD, MA

Nausea and vomiting are common, anxiety-provoking symptoms that often prompt patients to seek medical attention. The causes are myriad and range from benign, self-limiting conditions to chronic, potentially life-threatening disorders. The challenge for clinicians is to determine, in a cost-effective and orderly manner, the most likely causes and to decide whether or not further intervention is required. However, current

evidence suggests there is a lack of consistency in the management of these symptoms in clinical practice.

Definitions

The sensation of *nausea* is purely subjective, the degree of which can only be judged by the individual. It is a vague, unpleasant feeling described as being "sick to the stomach" or "queasy," and is often associated with a flushed feeling, fatigue, and an urge to vomit. *Vomiting* (emesis) is a physical event that results in a quick and forceful expulsion of the stomach's contents in a retrograde fashion up to and out of the mouth. This emptying can either be voluntary or involuntary. *Retching* is repetitive, spasmodic contractions of the diaphragm and abdominal wall muscles that may or may not result in the evacuation of gastric contents. In contrast, *regurgitation* is a passive, retrograde flow of gastric and esophageal contents into the mouth, with water that has a brash or acidic taste, most often the results of gastroesophageal reflux. Some individuals may experience *rumination*, which, likewise, is an effortless regurgitation of recently ingested food into the mouth, followed by either a spitting out or a rechewing and reswallowing. Although nausea and vomiting may be associated symptoms, *dyspepsia* is marked by chronic or recurrent epigastric discomfort with early satiety. Most instances of nausea and vomiting are acute with rapid resolution. *Chronic nausea and vomiting*, defined as the persistence of these symptoms for more than 1 month, present a diagnostic challenge to clinicians.

Differential Diagnosis

The causes for nausea and vomiting are numerous (Box 1). The key organs involved are the brain (chemoreceptor trigger zone, cerebral cortex, vestibular apparatus, and vomiting center), and the gastrointestinal tract. Neurotransmitter receptors that mediate nausea include dopamine, serotonin, acetylcholine, and histamine.

A common cause of nausea is an adverse reaction to a recently prescribed medication. Patients will often complain about their new medicine making them "sick." Almost any medication can cause nausea, but nonsteroidal anti-inflammatory drugs (NSAIDs), opioids, aspirin, and alcohol are probably the best known causes because of concomitant local gastric irritation. The most "notorious" drugs that cause nausea and vomiting are chemotherapeutic agents, particularly cisplatin (Platinol-AQ), cyclophosphamide (Cytoxan), dacarbazine (DTIC-Dome), and nitrogen mustard. Postchemotherapy nausea and vomiting (PCNV) can be acute (within 24 hours of administration), delayed (beyond 1 day of administration), or anticipatory; the latter is most common if the nausea and vomiting were not well controlled during previous courses of therapy.

Nausea and vomiting caused by viral infections (e.g., Norwalk virus, reoviruses, and adenoviruses) are of an acute onset, usually occurring in the autumn and winter. Bacterial infections (e.g., *Staphylococcus aureus*,

---

BOX 1   Differential Diagnosis of Nausea and Vomiting

Medications

Analgesics—acetaminophen, aspirin, nonsteroidal anti-inflammatory drugs (NSAIDs), rheumatologic and antigout drugs, opioids (codeine, morphine, oxycodone [Roxicodone])

Anesthetic agents—halothane, fentanyl (Sublimaze)

Antiasthmatics—theophylline

Anticonvulsants—phenobarbital, phenytoin (Dilantin)

Antidepressants—selective serotonin reuptake inhibitors (SSRIs)

Antimicrobials—acyclovir (Zovirax), erythromycin, itraconazole (Sporanox), metronidazole (Flagyl), sulfonamides, tetracycline

Antiparkinsonian drugs—levodopa (Dopar), carbidopa (Lodosyn)

Cancer chemotherapy—cisplatin (Platinol-AQ), cyclophosphamide (Cytoxan), dacarbazine (DTIC-Dome), nitrogen mustard

Cardiovascular agents—antiarrhythmics, antihypertensives, β-blockers, calcium channel antagonists, digoxin, diuretics

Corticosteroids—prednisone

Diabetic drugs—sulfonylureas, metformin (Glucophage)

Ergot alkaloids—dihydroergotamine (Migranal), ergotamine (Ergomar), methysergide (Sansert)[1]

Gastrointestinal agents—azathioprine (Imuran), sulfasalazine (Azulfidine)

Hormonal agents—estrogen, progesterone, oral contraceptives

Iron replacement—ferrous sulfate

Substance abuse—alcohol, nicotine

Infectious Causes

Gastroenteritis—viral, bacterial, parasitic

Other—otitis media, systemic sepsis

Gastrointestinal Disorders

Functional disorders—chronic intestinal pseudo-obstruction, gastroparesis, irritable bowel syndrome, nonulcer dyspepsia

Mechanical obstruction—gastric outlet obstruction, small-bowel obstruction

Organic gastrointestinal disorders

Appendicitis

Hepatobiliary disease—biliary colic, cholecystitis, hepatitis, neoplasia

Inflammatory bowel disease—Crohn's disease

Mesenteric ischemia

Peptic diseases—esophagitis, gastritis, *Helicobacter pylori,* nonulcer dyspepsia, peptic ulcer disease

Pancreatic disease—pancreatitis, pancreatic adenocarcinoma

Paralytic ileus

Peritoneal irritation—peritonitis, metastases

Postoperative gastric surgery

Retroperitoneal fibrosis

Central Nervous System (CNS) Disorders

Increased intracranial pressure—abscess, hemorrhage, hydrocephalus, infarction, malignancy, meningitis, pseudotumor cerebri

Demyelinating disorders

Labyrinthine disorders—labyrinthitis, Ménière's disease, motion sickness

Migraine headaches

Parkinsonian disorders

Seizures—complex partial

Psychologic/Psychiatric Disorders

Anxiety

Depression

Eating disorders—anorexia nervosa, bulimia nervosa

Pain

Psychogenic vomiting

Medical Conditions

Cardiac—acute myocardial infarction, congestive heart failure

Genitourinary—acute nephritis, nephrolithiasis, ovarian torsion, pyelonephritis, testicular torsion

Endocrinologic and metabolic conditions—acute intermittent porphyria, Addison's disease, diabetic ketoacidosis, hypercalcemia, hyperparathyroidism, hyperthyroidism, hypoparathyroidism, uremia

Pregnancy—hyperemesis gravidarum, morning sickness

Postoperative Nausea and Vomiting

Radiation Therapy

Idiopathic Conditions

Cyclic vomiting syndrome

Gastric dysrhythmias

[1]Not FDA approved for this indication.

Salmonella species., *Bacillus aureus,* and *Clostridium perfringens*) are associated with contaminated water or food, and accompanied by abdominal cramping, fever, and profuse diarrhea. Other infectious agents, such as cytomegalovirus and herpes simplex virus, can cause nausea and vomiting in those who are immunocompromised.

Small-bowel obstruction can also be acute and is associated with intermittent abdominal pain. Mesenteric ischemia can result in unexplained nausea. Gastroparesis, which is frequently seen in those with uncontrolled diabetes mellitus, scleroderma, amyloidosis, and systemic lupus erythematosus, causes nausea because of an inability to clear secretions and retained food. Lesions within the central nervous system, especially those involving the brainstem where the structures mediating vomiting (vomiting center) are located, can be a cause of nongastrointestinal vomiting. Psychogenic vomiting is usually associated with a previous history of psychiatric illness or social stressors and is often suspected when an

individual maintains adequate nutrition despite a reported prolonged course of vomiting.

Pregnancy is another common cause of nausea and vomiting, particularly in the first trimester. Typically, younger, primigravida women are the most prone to "morning sickness," which often resolves by the end of the first trimester. Hyperemesis gravidarum, marked by intractable vomiting, weight loss, and ketosis, occurs in up to 5% of pregnancies. Postoperative nausea and vomiting (PONV) complicates up to half of all surgeries and is associated with several risk factors, including type of inhalation anesthetic used (particularly nitrous oxide), female gender, and younger patients. Concomitant use of opiate medication postoperatively can worsen this condition.

A rare condition causing nausea and vomiting is cyclic vomiting, also known as "abdominal migraine" or "abdominal epilepsy." Individuals with this condition typically have discrete, acute episodes of vomiting lasting up to 20 hours, with frequent attacks during the year.

Rakel and Bope: *Conn's Current Therapy 2006.*

This condition usually starts early in life and is more common in girls. Associated conditions include migraine headaches and motion sickness.

Clinical Approach to Patients With Nausea and Vomiting

Because the differential diagnosis for the causes of nausea and vomiting is so great, the clinician must arrive at the diagnosis in an orderly and careful fashion. Several questions that need to be addressed as one evaluates the patient include: Is this an emergency situation (e.g., mechanical obstruction, perforation, peritonitis) that requires immediate attention? Does the patient need to be hospitalized to correct electrolyte abnormalities or dehydration or to treat intractable, incapacitating symptoms? Are there any clues clinically that would suggest a self-limited condition (e.g., viral gastroenteritis)? Was a medication recently started that could be the source of symptoms, and, if so, can it be safely discontinued? Is there a need to empirically prescribe an antiemetic? A comprehensive history and physical examination will often answer these questions, and help pinpoint the cause of the nausea and vomiting.

INITIAL HISTORY

The first step in making a proper diagnosis is to obtain a clear description of the patient's symptoms. The clinician should obtain a history of the duration, frequency, and severity of the nausea and vomiting, and the nature of any other associated symptoms. An acute onset of symptoms suggests conditions such as viral gastroenteritis, pancreatitis, biliary tract disease, or an adverse reaction to a medication. The nausea and vomiting caused by acute viral gastroenteritis are often accompanied by low-grade fever, malaise, headache, and diarrhea. Typically, the symptoms are self-limited and will resolve within 5 days. A more insidious onset of nausea and vomiting is seen in conditions such as gastroparesis, gastroesophageal reflux disease (GERD), metabolic disorders, and pregnancy.

The timing and characteristics of the vomiting can also provide clues as to the potential diagnosis. Early morning vomiting, especially before breakfast, can be seen with pregnancy, alcohol ingestion, uremia, and increased intracranial pressure. Projectile vomiting characterizes this latter condition. If fever accompanies the vomiting, one must consider acute gastroenteritis, appendicitis, hepatitis, or cholecystitis. Vomiting consisting of partially digested food or chyme caused by mechanical outlet obstruction or gastroparesis is usually delayed 1 hour or longer after eating, while the vomiting caused by psychiatric conditions such as bulimia or anorexia usually occurs during or right after eating. Bilious vomiting suggests small-bowel obstruction, while hematemesis (coffee-ground or black emesis) can be a result of peptic ulcer disease or esophageal varices. Sometimes the pressure generated by vomiting can be so great that it results in linear tears of the esophageal mucosa in the region of the gastroesophageal junction (Mallory-Weiss syndrome) or, rarely, rupture of the esophagus (Boerhaave's syndrome); these conditions will also result in hematemesis.

While taking the patient's history, the clinician should also ask about other associated symptoms. If abdominal pain is present, a precise description of the location may help to isolate the more serious causes. An organic cause, such as from an obstruction, usually causes abdominal pain, which precedes the vomiting. Significant weight loss may be associated with malignancy or chronic peptic ulcer disease with gastric outlet obstruction. A history of recent travel or similar symptoms found in family or friends point toward an infectious cause. Vertigo suggests Ménière's disease, benign positional labyrinthitis, or motion sickness. A headache with fever, stiff neck, or focal neurologic symptoms indicates a central nervous system disorder.

PHYSICAL EXAMINATION

After obtaining a detailed history, the clinician next must search for physical examination clues that indicate consequences or complications from the vomiting, and for signs that help to identify the potential cause of the symptoms. Dry mucus membranes with normal vital signs are a result of mild dehydration. In contrast, orthostatic changes in the vital signs, with a postural lowering of the blood pressure with increased heart rate, suggest significant dehydration. Other physical examination clues can include jaundice, lymphadenopathy, abdominal masses, and occult blood in the stool.

A careful abdominal examination can detect distension or hernias. Specific areas of abdominal tenderness provide clues as to potential causes. Midepigastric pain is seen with peptic ulcer disease, right upper quadrant pain occurs with hepatobiliary disease, and right lower quadrant tenderness suggests the possibility of appendicitis. Auscultation of the abdomen may detect the increased bowel sounds seen with obstruction, or absent bowel sounds that occur with an ileus. Examining the fingernails and teeth may disclose findings suggestive of self-induced vomiting. A thorough neurologic examination should also be done, including an examination of the cranial nerves, looking for nystagmus, a funduscopic examination to rule out increased intracranial pressure, and observation of the patient's gait to evaluate cerebellar function.

LABORATORY AND OTHER DIAGNOSTIC EVALUATIONS

Findings from the history and physical examination will help guide what further laboratory and diagnostic studies are required. Basic laboratory studies, if done, should include a complete blood count, looking for anemia or an elevated white blood count suggesting infection, and electrolytes, which may detect hypokalemia, hyponatremia, metabolic alkalosis, or uremia. A pregnancy test should be done in women of childbearing age who are still menstruating. Further laboratory tests might include screening for hyperthyroidism and drug toxicity (e.g., salicylates, digoxin, and theophylline).

Rakel and Bope: *Conn's Current Therapy 2006.*

The clinical picture should direct other diagnostic testing. If the symptoms suggest a mechanical obstruction, radiographic studies, such as upright and supine abdominal radiographs, should be obtained. However, the results of these films may be nonspecific or normal with intermittent small-bowel obstruction. Esophagogastroduodenoscopy (EGD) can detect abnormalities in the esophageal, gastric, or duodenal mucosa suggestive of esophagitis or peptic ulcer disease. Further gastrointestinal studies, such as an upper gastrointestinal barium study, small bowel follow-through, and

enteroclysis, may sometimes be needed to detect underlying disorders such as gastroparesis or small-bowel obstruction. Other diagnostic studies that might help in making the diagnosis include an abdominal ultrasound of the right upper quadrant or an abdominal CT scan. Tests of gastric motility function include gastric emptying scintigraphy, antroduodenal manometry, and electrogastrography.

If a gastrointestinal disorder is not found, the clinician should consider systemic illness, central nervous system disorders, or psychologic conditions. The clinician should

TABLE 1 Commonly Used Medications for Nausea and Vomiting

Class/medication	Usual dosage	Route(s)	Adverse effects
Anticholinergic			
Scopolamine (Transderm Scop)	1 patch every 3 d	Transdermal	Dry mouth, drowsiness, impaired eye accommodation; rare: disorientation, memory disturbance, dizziness, hallucinations
Antihistamines			
Diphenhyhramine (Benadryl)	25-50 mg q 4-6 h	IM, IV, PO	Sedation, dry mouth, constipation, confusion, blurred vision, urinary retention
Hydroxyzine (Atarax, Vistaril)	25-100 mg q 6 h	IM, PO1	
Meclizine (Antivert)	25-50 mg q 6 h	PO	
Promethazine (Phenergan)	12.5-25 mg q 4-6 h	IM, IV, PO, PR	
Benzamides			
Metoclopramide (Reglan)	5-15 mg q 6 h	IM, IV, PO	Sedation, restlessness, diarrhea, agitation, central nervous depression, extrapyramidal effects, hypotension, neuroleptic syndrome, supraventricular tachycardia
Trimethobenzamide (Tigan)	250 mg q 6-8 h	IM, PO, PR	
Benzodiazepines			
Lorazepam (Ativan)[1]	0.5-2.5 mg q 8-12 h	IM, IV, PO	Sedation, amnesia, respiratory depression, ataxia, blurred vision, hallucinations, emotional reactions
Butyrophenones			
Droperidol (Inapsine)	0.625-1.25 mg q 3-4 h[3]	IM, IV	Sedation, hypotension, tachycardia, extrapyramidal effects, dizziness, blood pressure increase, hallucinations, chills, QT prolongation, torsades de pointes
Haloperidol (Haldol)[1]	0.5-5 mg q 8 h	IM, IV, PO	
Cannabinoids			
Dronabinol (Marinol)	2.5-5 mg q 8 h	PO	Drowsiness, euphoria, vision difficulties, somnolence, vasodilation, abnormal thinking, dysphoria, diarrhea, flushing, tremor, myalgias
Corticosteroids			
Dexamethasone (Decadron)[1]	4 mg q 6 h	IM, IV, PO	Gastrointestinal upset, anxiety, insomnia, hyperglycemia, facial flushing, euphoria, perineal itching
Phenothiazines			
Chlorpromazine (Thorazine)	10-25 mg q 4-6 h	IM, PO, PR	Sedation, lethargy, skin irritation, cardiovascular effects, extrapyramidal effects, cholestatic jaundice, hyperprolactinemia, neuroleptic malignant syndrome, blood abnormalities
Prochlorperazine (Compazine)	5-10 (25PR) mg q 6 h	IM, IV, PO, PR	
Thiethylperazine (Torecan)	10-20 mg q 6 h[3]	IM, IV, PO	
5-HT3 Serotonin Antagonists			
Ondansetron (Zofran)	8 mg q 8 h	IV, PO	Headache, constipation, fever, asthenia, arrhythmias, diarrhea, dizziness, ataxia, tremor, somnolence, thirst, nervousness, elevated hepatic transaminases
Granisetron (Kytril)	2 mg per 24 h	IV, PO	
Dolasetron (Anzemet)	100 mg per 24 h	IV, PO	

[1]Not FDA approved for this indication.
[3]Exceeds dosage recommended by manufacturer.
Abbreviations: IM = intramuscular; IV = intravenous; PO = orally; PR = per rectum; q = every.

obtain a head imaging study in those cases in which the nausea and vomiting are severe, unexplained, and chronic. Magnetic resonance imaging (MRI) of the brain is superior to computed tomographic (CT) scanning to detect lesions in the posterior fossa. In those patients with chronic, unexplained nausea and vomiting, a psychologic evaluation should be performed. Rarely, some causes of nausea and vomiting remain undiagnosed despite this thorough evaluation, in which case, consultation with a gastroenterologist is warranted.

Management of Nausea and Vomiting

Goals in managing nausea and vomiting include:

• Identifying and correcting any fluid, electrolyte, acid-base, and/or nutritional deficiencies that are a result of the nausea and vomiting
• Identifying and eliminating, if possible, the underlying cause of the symptoms
• Suppressing or eliminating the symptoms if the underlying cause cannot be quickly identified

If oral rehydration is not possible, the individual may need intravenous hydration with normal saline solution and appropriate potassium replacement.

Initially in acute nausea and vomiting, the best treatment is often nutritional discretion. When nauseated, individuals should slowly drink small amounts of clear, cool liquids that contain some caloric content, preferably 30 to 60 minutes before and after meals. If vomiting occurs, solid foods should be avoided. To avoid dehydration, salty rehydration solutions such as Gatorade or bullion are good choices, while sweetened and acidic juices (e.g., orange or grapefruit juices) should be avoided. The goal is to consume 1 to 2 L of fluid during the day in multiple, small (1-4 oz) amounts.

If liquids are well tolerated, individuals may cautiously advance their diet to include a variety of easily digested foods such as crackers, dry toast, broth-based soups with rice or noodles, and hard candy. The goal is to ingest approximately 1500 calories daily. Creamy, milk-based liquids should be avoided at this time. Once this is tolerated, individuals may try other mild-flavored, low-fat foods such as plain pasta, baked potatoes, chicken, fish, vegetables, and fruit. They should eat the food slowly and stop once satisfied. Also, they should rest, either sitting or lying down slightly propped up, after eating, because activity may increase the nausea and lead to vomiting.

Typically, if the nausea is mild, dietary changes may be all that is needed because the symptoms are usually short-lived and resolve spontaneously. However, if symptoms persist despite dietary changes, or if the nausea and vomiting are severe, the individual may require treatment empirically with an antiemetic while the cause of the symptoms is sought.

There are a wide variety of antiemetic agents available (Table 1). Many of these drugs act primarily within the central nervous system (CNS) to suppress the nausea and prevent vomiting. This mechanism of action also explains the potential CNS side effects that can occur

 CURRENT DIAGNOSIS

• Medications are a common cause of nausea, especially chemotherapeutic agents, NSAIDs, opioids, and alcohol.
• Postoperative N&V occurs in up to half of all surgeries and is made worse by the use of opioids.
• Morning sickness occurs in the first trimester and is most common in young, primigravida women.
• An accurate diagnosis requires evaluation of the timing, duration, frequency, and severity of the N&V.

with these medicines. As such, one must weigh the potential benefit of relieving the symptoms against the potential risk of developing other intolerant symptoms.

Except in the cases of PCNV and PONV, there are relatively few randomized trials that provide insight into which are the antiemetics of choice. One of the most widely used drugs for moderate to severe nausea and vomiting is prochlorperazine (Compazine). It is available in oral, rectal, and parenteral forms. However, side effects are common and include sedation, extrapyramidal symptoms, including dystonic and tardive dyskinesias. Metoclopramide (Reglan), provides both antiemetic and prokinetic activities and is useful in GERD and gastroparesis. However, it, too, has associated significant side effects which include fatigue and extrapyramidal symptoms such as oculogyric crisis, opisthotonos, akathisia, dyskinesia, and dystonia.

Normally, antiemetics should be avoided in the nausea and vomiting of pregnancy, especially during the first trimester. Pyridoxine (vitamin B$_6$)[1] has been used with some success. In severe cases of hyperemesis gravidarum marked by weight loss, ketosis, and dehydration, the patient should be hospitalized and given intravenous fluids. In severe cases, meclizine (Antivert)[1] or promethazine (Phenergan)[1] may be used.

---

[1]Not FDA approved for this condition.

 CURRENT THERAPY

• For nausea I recommend small amounts of cool, clear liquids, such as Gatorade or bullion, 30 to 60 minutes before and after meals.
• Avoid sweetened and acidic juices, and creamy, milk-based liquids.
• Chlorpromazine (Thorazine) and prochlorperazine (Compazine) are available in oral, rectal, and parenteral forms, but run the risk of extrapyramidal side effects.
• Ondansetron (Zofran) and granisetron (Kytril) are especially effective in postchemotherapy N&V, are well tolerated, and have few side effects.
• Antiemetics should be avoided in N&V of pregnancy, especially during the first trimester, although pyridoxine (vitamin B6) may be helpful.

The 5-HT$_3$ serotonin antagonists ondansetron (Zofran), granisetron (Kytril), and dolasetron (Anzemet) have both central and peripheral activities, and are usually very well tolerated with few adverse effects. These drugs, along with corticosteroids, are highly effective in PCNV. At equivalent doses, each of these drugs has equivalent safety and efficacy and can be interchanged based on availability, cost and convenience. Single doses are effective, and their oral forms are equally effective and are as safe as their intravenous forms.

Nonpharmacologic options for nausea and vomiting exist. Studies of acupressure, using the P6 (Neiguan) point, located 5 cm proximal to the palmar aspect of the wrist between the flexor carpi radialis and the palmaris longus tendons, show favorable results. In addition, some studies suggest that ginger (Zingiber officinale Roscoe)[1] may help.

---

[1]Not FDA approved for this indication.

Gaseousness and Indigestion

Method of
Sonal M. Patel, MD, and
Anthony Lembo, MD

Gaseousness

Excessive "gas" can cause significant discomfort and embarrassment. The symptoms of gaseousness can refer to excessive belching (or eructation), flatus, or even abdominal bloating. These symptoms are especially prominent in patients with irritable bowel syndrome (IBS). In most cases, gaseousness is not caused by an increased volume of gas within the gastrointestinal tract. Recent studies in patients with IBS demonstrate that it is not increased gas production but rather the altered transit of gas or the location of trapping of gas within the gastrointestinal (GI) tract that creates symptoms of gaseousness. Most patients who complain of excessive gas actually have symptoms that fall within range of normal and can be reassured. However, the patient's perception that his or her symptoms are abnormal can make successful treatment of gaseousness difficult.

EXCESSIVE BELCHING (ERUCTATION)

Symptoms and Physiology

Occasional belching is a normal physiologic process, which allows for swallowed air to be removed from the stomach. The normal frequency of belching has not been well documented but patients who complain of it usually have repetitive and uncontrollable episodes of belching.

Involuntary belching usually occurs after meals and is the release of swallowed air after gastric distension. The most common cause of excessive, repetitive belching is excessive air swallowing (aerophagia). Swallowing food, or even saliva, can result in some air entering the upper gastrointestinal tract. Air can also be swallowed by itself consciously and unconsciously. Factors that can result in increased aerophagia include stress, gastroesophageal reflux, increased salivary production from excessive sucking on hard candy or chewing gum, and cigarette smoking. Rarely, other upper gastrointestinal diseases such as peptic ulcer disease (PUD), gastroesophageal reflux disease (GERD), and cholecystitis can present with excessive belching.

Patient Treatment

Although belching is usually the result of excessive air swallowing, a complete history and physical examination are important to exclude the rare causes of upper gastrointestinal disorders that may produce these symptoms (e.g., GERD, PUD, or cholecystitis). If other associated gastrointestinal symptoms are present, appropriate diagnostic tests should follow. In most patients, no other diagnostic testing is necessary. Rather, the patient should be reassured that the symptom is not associated with an organic disorder. In this group of patients, treatment is focused on techniques that reduce air swallowing. Dietary modifications, such as avoiding sucking on hard candies or chewing gum, eating slowly with small swallows, and avoiding carbonated beverages, can be suggested, although they have not been sufficiently tested and are usually disappointing in practice. Another technique is to hold an object (such as a pencil) between one's teeth. Simethicone (Mylicon) and activated charcoal preparations (Charcoal Plus) are ineffective. Stress management may be helpful in those patients whose excessive air swallowing seems exacerbated by underlying stress. Other forms of psychotherapy (e.g., cognitive behavioral therapy) should be considered in patients who remain symptomatic.

EXCESSIVE FLATUS

Symptoms and Physiology

The range of normal volume and frequency of flatus varies widely. Adults pass flatus on average 10 to 14 times per day for a total volume of 400 to 2500 mL per day. Because flatus volume is difficult to measure, clinicians rely on the frequency of flatulence to estimate volume. To do this, patients record the number of flatulence "episodes" per day over the course of one week (normal is less than 22 per day). Most individuals can evacuate relatively large volumes of gas without any difficulty. Recent evidence demonstrates that when gas is infused into the proximal small bowel there are a minority of patients who are "gas retainers." These patients develop symptoms such as bloating, pressure, or cramping in response to gas in their small bowel. Furthermore, the location of gas retention may be important. Specifically, gas trapped in the jejunum seems to create a worsening of symptoms in gas retainers. Although helpful in understanding the physiology, impaired transit alone does not explain gas-related symptoms. Visceral hypersensitivity, as seen in IBS, may also help explain why some patients perceive that they have excessive flatus.

Rectal gas comes from either swallowed air or from bacterial fermentation. Malabsorption of carbohydrates, which can occur in patients with celiac sprue, pancreatic insufficiency, and short-bowel syndrome, can result in increased flatus production. Lactose and fructose are simple sugars commonly found in many foods that are commonly malabsorbed. Likewise, many common starches found in various fruits, vegetables, and flours are not fully absorbed by healthy patients.

Patient Management

The first step is to determine if excessive flatulence is present by having the patient record the frequency of rectal gas passage for 2 weeks. Patients who pass flatus more than 22 times per day without signs of malabsorption should undergo dietary modification. Specifically, patients should be advised to restrict lactose- and fructose-containing foods. It is virtually impossible to restrict all carbohydrates, but certain carbohydrates that may be malabsorbed include fructose (soft drinks), lactose (dairy), trehalose (mushrooms), raffinose and stachyose (legumes), and resistant starches (fruits, flours, vegetables).

A patient diary of foods associated with concomitant symptoms may be instrumental in determining any salient offending carbohydrates. Hydrogen breath testing can be helpful in the diagnosis of lactose and fructose intolerances. Patients not responding to dietary modifications should be advised to reduce behaviors associated with excessive air swallowing, including stress, smoking, chewing gum, or sucking on candy. α-D-Galactosidase enzyme (Beano), which facilitates oligosaccharide digestion and is available over the counter, can be a helpful treatment. Pharmacologic treatments for noxious flatus odor are zinc acetate,[1] bismuth subsalicylate (Pepto-Bismol),[1] and carbohydrate laxatives.[1] The charcoal cushion, which decreases flatus odor immediately after passage, is another treatment option for noxious flatus.

Indigestion (Dyspepsia)

DEFINITION AND EPIDEMIOLOGY

Indigestion, or dyspepsia, is defined as a persistent or recurrent pain or discomfort centered in the upper abdomen. Other associated characteristics include postprandial fullness, upper abdominal bloating, early satiety, anorexia, nausea, and vomiting. Its prevalence in the United States is estimated to be as high as 40%. Dyspepsia is responsible for substantial health care costs and considerable time loss from work. Dyspepsia has a

number of possible etiologies. Symptoms and causes can overlap, which can make the initial diagnosis difficult. The most common cause of dyspepsia encountered in primary care practice is functional dyspepsia; however, more serious conditions should always be considered in the initial evaluation.

DIFFERENTIAL DIAGNOSIS

PUD accounts for 15% to 25% of patients with dyspepsia; 30% to 60% of these patients will be positive for *Helicobacter pylori* if tested. Nonsteroidal anti-inflammatory drug (NSAID) use accounts for the majority of the remaining patients.

GERD is defined as epigastric burning that radiates substernally. Heartburn and regurgitation are the most common symptoms. The symptom of substernal radiation is somewhat specific for GERD; however, many patients with GERD may not have the classic radiation, but solely complain of epigastric pain or discomfort.

Functional or nonulcer dyspepsia (NUD) accounts for up to 60% of patients who present with dyspepsia. This syndrome is a diagnosis of exclusion when other organic etiologies have been excluded. Although up to 40% of patients with IBS can also have dyspeptic symptoms, isolated functional dyspepsia appears to be a separate syndrome. Various theories or factors that have not been conclusively implicated include *H. pylori* infection, visceral hypersensitivity, and abnormal motility.

Biliary or pancreatic disease can be mistaken for dyspepsia, but a proper history and physical examination should point to these disease processes with further diagnostic tests such as blood work and imaging.

Although gastric and esophageal malignancies are rare (<2%) in patients presenting with dyspepsia, the risk increases with age.

PATIENT MANAGEMENT

Patients who present with dyspepsia who are older than age 45 years should undergo an upper endoscopy to rule out serious processes such as malignancy. Also, any patient who has any alarming features, such as unexplained weight loss, anemia, GI bleeding (hematemesis or melena), or significant examination (tenderness, lymphadenopathy or jaundice), also should undergo an upper endoscopy.

For patients who are younger than age 45 years and without alarming symptoms, empiric testing for *H. pylori* infection, either by serology or a breath test, is a reasonable first step. However, this strategy may not suit all patients or physicians. Alternatively, upper endoscopy with biopsies for *H. pylori* may provide the patient added reassurance if the study is negative. If the patient is positive for *H. pylori* infection, the patient should be treated with eradication therapy.

Treatment of functional dyspepsia can be challenging. Important aspects of the therapy include explanation and reassurance. Acid suppression with either an H_2 blocker or proton pump inhibitor should be the first-line of therapy. If these do not provide any relief, a promotility

---

[1]Not FDA approved for this indication.

agent such as metoclopramide (Reglan)[1] or erythromycin (E-Mycin)[1] can be considered. Tricyclic antidepressants such as amitriptyline (Elavil)[1] have also been used with some anecdotal success. Other behavioral therapies, such as biofeedback or hypnosis, have not been studied, but may be reserved for severely refractory patients.

---

[1]Not FDA approved for this indication.

Hiccups

Method of
Varsha Vaidya, MD

Hiccups usually occur in brief episodes, causing embarrassment and annoyance in the patient and sometimes amusement in the observer. They can become a more serious phenomenon associated with significant morbidity and even death. The medical term "singultus" comes from "singulut," the act of catching one's breath when sobbing. The term *hiccup* derives from the sound of the event. It is also called *hiccough*, which erroneously implies an association with the respiratory reflexes. Hiccups are defined as a sudden contraction of the inspiratory muscles, terminated by abrupt contraction of the glottis to produce the characteristic sound. A bout of hiccups usually lasts a few minutes. The term *persistent hiccups* is used when the episodes last for more than 8 hours, often implying a serious organic etiology, which can be central or peripheral. *Intractable* defines duration of more than 1 month. The longest recorded attack is 6 decades. There was a report of familial intractable hiccup in which seven members of a patient's family suffered from the same affliction.

Pathophysiology

Hiccups do not appear to be protective or purposeful in humans or other mammals. Although the entire diaphragm can be affected, the left hemidiaphragm alone is affected in 80% of cases. In women, hiccups tend to occur most frequently in the first half of the menstrual cycle and decrease markedly during pregnancy. The frequency is relatively constant for a given individual and varies inversely with arterial P_{CO_2}.

The exact cause has been a source of much speculation for centuries. It was associated with liver inflammation and other conditions according to Hippocrates and Celsus. Galen thought hiccups occurred because of violent emotions arousing the stomach.

An Edinburgh physician, Shortt, in 1833 first made the association between hiccups and the phrenic nerve.

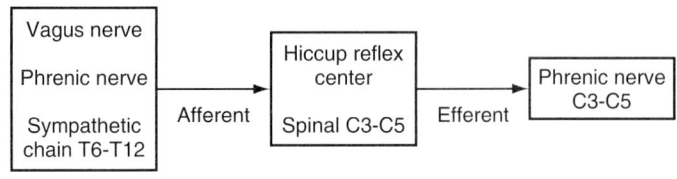

FIGURE 1. Hiccup-Phrenic Nerve connection.

The credit of first delineating the reflex arc goes to Bailey, who proposed it in 1943. The reflex arc consists of the following:

- The afferent limb, the vagus and phrenic nerves, and a sympathetic chain arising from T6-12.
- The hiccup center has been established in the upper cervical region C3 and C5 in addition to connections with the central nervous system [CNS] respiratory center, phrenic nerve nuclei, medullary reticular formation, and hypothalamus, (Figure 1).
- The efferent limb is the phrenic nerve C3-5, anterior scalene muscles (C5-7), external intercostals (T1-11), and glottis (recurrent laryngeal component of the vagus nerve, inhibitory autonomic processes, decreasing esophageal tone).

Diagnosis

Hiccups occur equally in men and women; however, intractable hiccups occur more frequently in men (82% of cases); 90% of men and only 8% of women have an organic cause for their hiccups.

They occur in all ages, as well as in utero; preterm infants tend to spend 2.5% of their time hiccupping.

BOX 1   Etiology of Hiccups

Begin/self-limited
1. Gastrointestinal distension, e.g., overeating aerophagia
2. Sudden change in temperature, e.g., too hot or cold food/drink
3. Alcohol ingestion, excessive smoking
4. Psychogenic causes: anxiety, sudden stress, or excitement.

Organic/Intractable
5. Medical: CNS, peripheral damage to the vagus nerve, diaphragm trauma or inflammation or vascular lesions. Toxic: uremia, diabetes mellitus, gout, hypokalemia, alcoholism, hyponatremia.
   Tumors or metastasis involving reflex arc
   Degenerative disorders: multiple sclerosis.
6. Surgical: general anesthesia and complications thereof and manipulation of structures during surgery causing stretch on the vagus or phrenic nerve and diaphragm.
7. Drug induced, e.g., analeptic agents, benzodiazepines, dexamethasone (Decadron), chlordizepoxide (Librium), methyldopa, short-acting barbiturates.

Abbreviation: CNS = central nervous system

Rakel and Bope: *Conn's Current Therapy 2006.*

Hiccups that are brief and episodic need no further investigations. Intractable or persistent hiccups are frequently associated with an underlying pathologic process, which may result in significant morbidity and need careful investigation.

History should include onset, duration, and progress of the episodes. This should include aggravating and relieving factors as well as remedies already tried. A full surgical and drug history and substance abuse, especially alcohol, history is important to rule out potential differentials.

LABORATORY STUDIES

Include the following laboratory studies:

- Electrolytes: hyponatremia can be the cause and effect of hiccups. Other causes include hypokalemia, hypocalcemia, and hyperglycemia.
- Renal function: look for uremia.
- Liver function: rule out hepatitis.
- Amylase and lipase: look for pancreatitis.
- White blood count.
- Urine, sputum, and cerebral spinal fluid (CSF) exam: rule out infectious etiology.

IMAGING STUDIES

Include the following imaging studies:

- Chest radiograph checks for tumors, infection, thoracic aorta.
- Fluoroscopy of diaphragmatic movement confirms diagnosis if malingering is suspected, as well as determines if there is unilateral or bilateral involvement of the diaphragm.
- Computed tomography (CT) scan of the head, thorax, and abdomen rules out tumors, infection, and structural lesions.

BOX 2   Treatment of Hiccups

Non-drug therapies

- Forcible change in respiration such as breath holding, Valsalva maneuver, and rebreathing into paper bags.
- Irritation of the uvula or nasopharynx such as gargling, drinking water rapidly, sipping ice water, and biting a lemon.
- Counter irritation of the vagus nerve such as pressure on eyeballs, carotid sinus compression and digital rectal massage.
- Disruption of the phrenic nerve such as phrenic nerve block, and galvanic sinusoidal current.
- Counter irritation of the diaphragm by applying pressure to points of diaphragmatic insertion.
- Relieve gastric distension by gastric lavage, emetic induced vomiting, nasogastric aspiration.
- C3-5 dermatome stimulation such as tapping or rubbing of the back of the neck, coolant sprays, and acupuncture.
- Prayer has been known to cure at least one patient with intractable hiccups that lasted for 8 years.
- Phrenic nerve ablation is a very drastic measure. Fluoroscopic examination may reveal unilateral involvement thereby allowing limited measures.
- Psychotherapy/relaxation techniques, and hypnosis can work for patients with anxiety related hiccups.

Drug therapies

- Baclofen (Lioresal)[1] is a GABA analogue that contains phenylethylamine moiety. It is thought to activate inhibitory neurotransmitters that lead to the blockade of the hiccup stimulus. Adult dose is 10 mg orally twice or four times daily.
- Chlorpromazine (Thorazine) is thought to act by dopamine blockade in the hypothalamus, the central component of the reflex arc. (It is the only drug with an FDA approved indication for hiccups). The adult dose is 25 to 30 mg orally three or four times daily or slow IV infusion with patient lying flat. When symptoms persist give 25 to 50 mg IM for 2 to 3 d.
- Metoclopramide (Reglan)[1] acts by inhibiting the intensity of esophageal contractions, relaxes the proximal stomach, and reduces gastric secretion. It blocks dopamine receptors in the chemoreceptor trigger zone.

The adult dose is 10 to 20 mg orally three or four times daily for 7 days; pediatric dose is 1 to 2 mg/kg three or four times daily for 7 d.
- Valproic acid (Depakene)[1] is thought to act by enhancing transmission of GABA centrally, thereby inhibiting the hiccup stimulus. The adult dose is 10 to 15 mg/kg orally daily in one to three divided doses.
- Nifedipine (Procardia) is a calcium-channel blocker. It is theorized that the hiccup reflex arc contains the abnormal depolarized elements of dendrites. Nifedipine reverses this abnormal depolarization.
- Phenytoin (Dilantin) inhibits the spread of motor activity by its effect in the motor cortex. The adult dose is 15 to 20 mg/kg IV loading dose, followed by a maintenance dose of 2 to 3 mg/kg twice daily.
- Carbamazepine (Tegretol) may block post-tetanic potentiation by reducing summation of temporal stimulation. The adult dose is 200 mg orally twice daily.
- Ketamine (Ketalar) acts on the cortex and limbic system, decreasing muscle spasms. The adult dose is 0.4 mg/kg IV; supplemental dose of 1/3 to 1/2 initial dose for maintenance.
- Lidocaine (Xylocane) inhibits depolarization of type C sensory neurons by blocking sodium channels. The adult dose is 1 mg/kg loading, followed by an infusion of 2 mg/min.
- Orphenadrine (Norflex) mode of action is not known, however, it is clinically effective. The adult dose is 100 mg orally twice daily as needed or 60 mg IM every 12 hours as needed.
- Haloperidol (Haldol) is useful in treatment of spasmodic muscle movements. The adult dose is 2 to 5 mg orally every 4 to 8 h.
- Amitriptyline (Elavil) inhibits reuptake of 5HT and norepinephrine in the CNS and reduces GI motility. The adult dose is 10 to 40 mg orally.
- Sertraline (Zoloft) is reported to help the proposed mechanism because of effects on the GI system. The adult dose is 50 to 100 mg daily.

[1]Not FDA approved for this indication.
Abbreviations: FDA = Food and Drug Administration; GABA = γ-amino butyric acid; GI = gastrointestinal; IM = intramuscular; IV = intravenous

---

- Magnetic resonance imaging (MRI) rules out multiple sclerosis and checks vascular relations to vagus and phrenic nerve.
- Electrocardiogram (ECG): Sometimes a myocardial infarction presents with hiccups, as well as pericarditis and arrhythmias.
- Nerve conduction studies prior to invasive therapy confirm the presence of unilateral or bilateral involvement.
- Endoscopy, bronchoscopy, or gastrointestinal (GI) radiography.

Etiology

There are more than 100 causes of hiccups described; in many cases, however, the cause remains idiopathic. Usual causes include gastric distension (food, alcohol, air), sudden changes in ambient or gastric temperature, and use of alcohol and/or tobacco in excess. Sudden excitement and stress can precipitate hiccups in some.

Persistent or intractable hiccups are usually precipitated by direct injury or an underlying disease resulting in irritation or inflammation of one of the components of the hiccup reflex arc. The list of possible causes is extensive (Box 1).

Treatment

Once an etiology is established, it is usually helpful to treat the cause, and the hiccups abate. However, relief is not commonly immediate, and frequently the etiology remains a mystery. Most treatment recommendations are based on case reports purporting their success. The Mayo Clinic accurately described the situation in treating hiccups: "The amount of knowledge on any subject such as this can be considered as being in inverse proportion to the number of treatments suggested and tried."

Many traditional remedies have a sound physiological basis affecting components of the hiccup reflex arc, which include the following:

- Stimulation of the nasopharynx
- C3-5 dermatome stimulation

CURRENT DIAGNOSIS

- Brief episodes of hiccups require no investigation, however, persistent (lasting for more than 8 hours) or intractable (lasting for more than 1 month) hiccups need full investigation to rule out the broad differential and outline specific treatment. A full history and physical along with laboratory results, chest radiographs and MRIs help rule out potentially dangerous and/or treatable causes. Often the etiology remains a mystery.

Abbreviations: IM = intramuscular injection; MRI = magnetic resonance imaging

CURRENT THERAPY

- Use nondrug therapy or pharmacotherapy. Nondrug therapies are more traditional remedies with some physiological basis, affecting various components of the hiccup reflex arc.
- Medication that can be used is chlorpromazine (Thorazine) at 25 to 30 mg orally three times daily or as a slow intravenous infusion. Baclofen (Lioresal)[1] 5 to 60 mg daily, Haloperidol (Haldol)[1] 2 mg IM or 5 to 10 mg daily orally.

- Direct pharyngeal stimulation
- Direct uvular stimulation
- Removal of gastric contents
- Vagal stimulation
- Behavioral conditioning:
- Phrenic nerve block surgery
- Prayer: a patient suffered from intractable hiccups for 8 years. After more than 60,000 suggested treatments, what cured him was a prayer to St. Jude, patron Saint of lost causes!
- Medication: a list of medications tried with some success appears in Box 2. The first line medications often are chlorpromazine (Thorazine) 25 to 50 mg intravenous (IV) or intramuscular (IM). Other agents like baclofen (Liaresal)[1] or ketamine (Ketalar)[1] have been tried with success.

REFERENCES

Burke AM: Baclofen for intractabe hiccups. N Engl J Med 1998; 319:1354.
Grant JA, Steiner EM: Treatment of persistent hiccups (letter). J Neurol Neurosurg Psychiatry 1991;54:468.
Lauds S, Psizec JL: Hiccups in adults: An overivew. Eur Respir J 1993;6(4):563-575.
Lewis J: Hiccups: Causes and cures. J Clin Gastroenterol 7(6): 539-552.
Peabody CA, Dewitt J: Intractable hiccups treated with Amitriptyline. Am J Psychiatry 1988;145:1036.
Vaidya V: Sertraline in the treatment of hiccups. Psychosomatics 2000;41:353-355.
Williamson BWA: Management of intractable hiccups. Br Med J 1977; 2:501-503.

---

[1]Not FDA approved for this indication.

Acute Infectious Diarrhea

Method of
*Mathuram Santosham, MD, MPH, and
Aruna Chandran, MD, MPH*

Infectious diarrhea is a leading cause of mortality worldwide. The World Health Organization (WHO) reported nearly 1.8 million deaths caused by diarrheal diseases in 2002. Even in the United States acute diarrhea represents a significant disease burden, with an estimated 211 million to 375 million episodes per year. Among children, acute diarrhea accounts for more than 1.5 million outpatient visits, 200,000 hospitalizations, and approximately 300 deaths per year.

Diagnosis

Acute diarrhea is defined by most experts as the passage of three or more loose or watery stools per day, for fewer than 14 days. Evaluation of a patient with diarrhea requires a detailed history and physical examination. The physical examination should include documentation of signs and symptoms of dehydration, as this will determine the volume of fluid required to rehydrate the individual. Table 1 gives the recommendations made by the Centers for Disease Control and Prevention (CDC) and the WHO regarding criteria for determining levels of dehydration in children.

Laboratory tests are unnecessary to manage uncomplicated diarrhea. The presence of fecal leukocytes increases the chances of identifying a pathogenic bacterium by stool culture. The diagnostic yield of stool culture is only between 1.5% and 5.6%. Thus, the estimated cost of each positive culture is more than $1000. If there is visible blood in the stool, a stool sample should be sent for bacterial cultures to test for organisms that may require antibiotic therapy.

Further testing may be necessary in specific circumstances, such as recent travel. In such cases, testing for organisms such as *Entamoeba histolytica* or *Vibrio cholerae* should be considered. Immunocompromised individuals may require testing for *Cryptosporidium parvum* or opportunistic infections.

Common Causative Organisms

There is limited information regarding the etiology of diarrheal illnesses in the United States, even for those illnesses resulting in hospitalization. One study showed that in children younger than 4 years of age, the etiology of 64% of diarrhea-related hospitalizations was unknown. Viruses were reported as the causative agent for 33%, with rotavirus being the most common. Bacterial causes accounted for 4%, whereas parasites accounted for less than 1% of hospitalizations because of diarrhea. The highest rates of hospitalization occur in the winter months. Most of the excess cases of diarrhea in the winter are caused by rotavirus.

BACTERIA

Salmonella

Salmonella are gram-negative organisms in the Enterobacteriaceae family with more than 2600 serotypes, most of which can cause human disease. *Salmonella* are broadly grouped into two classifications: typhoidal and nontyphoidal. The typhoidal species *Salmonella typhi*

TABLE 1 Signs and Symptoms Associated With Dehydration in Children

Sign/symptom	Minimal or no dehydration (<3% loss of body weight)	Mild to moderate dehydration (3%-9% loss of body weight)	Severe dehydration (>9% loss of body weight)
Mental Status	Well; alert	Normal, fatigued or restless, irritable	Apathetic, lethargic, unconscious
Thirst	Drinks normally; might refuse liquids	Thirsty; eager to drink	Drinks poorly; unable to drink
Heart rate	Normal	Normal to increased	Tachycardia, with bradycardia in most severe cases
Quality of pulse	Normal	Normal to decreased	Weak, thready, or impalpable
Breathing	Normal	Normal; fast	Deep
Eyes	Normal	Slightly sunken	Deeply sunken
Tears	Present	Decreased	Absent
Mouth and tongue	Moist	Dry	Parched
Skin fold	Instant recoil	Recoil in <2 seconds	Recoil in >2 seconds
Capillary refill	Normal	Prolonged	Prolonged; minimal
Extremities	Warm	Cool	Cold; mottled; cyanotic
Urine output	Normal to decreased	Decreased	Minimal

From King, CK, et al: Managing acute gastroenteritis among children. MMWR 2003;52(No. RR-16).

and *Salmonella paratyphi* cause typhoid fever, which is endemic in many parts of the developing world.

Nontyphoidal *Salmonella* typically cause an acute self-limited illness lasting 5 to 7 days. The incubation period is 6 to 48 hours. The diarrhea can be watery or bloody, and associated symptoms include fever, abdominal pain, and vomiting. The attack rate is highest in children younger than 4 years. The major reservoirs are animals, including poultry, cattle, reptiles, and rodents. Infection is acquired through contact with or ingestion of contaminated animals, eggs, or dairy products. Several large-scale, food-borne epidemics of *Salmonella* have been described in the literature.

Children younger than 3 months of age, as well as patients with immunodeficiencies, HIV, malignancy, or hemoglobinopathies, are at higher risk for more severe illness. Manifestations of severe disease include bacteremia, constitutional symptoms, hepatosplenomegaly, or meningitis.

Antimicrobial therapy is not indicated in patients with uncomplicated nonbacteremic illness caused by nontyphoidal *Salmonella*; in fact, antibiotics may prolong fecal excretion of the organism. For high-risk patients, individuals with bacteremic illness, and those with typhoid fever, appropriate therapy should be based on the antimicrobial susceptibility of the organism.

There are two licensed vaccines against *S. typhi*, one parenteral capsular antigen (Typhim Vi) and one oral live-attenuated immunogen (Vivotif Berna). Both are recommended for and used by travelers from industrialized countries going to developing regions. Neither vaccine is effective in children younger than 2 years of age.

Shigella

Shigella is a gram-negative organism, with humans as the primary natural host. This is a highly virulent and contagious microbe, with as few as 10 organisms necessary to cause disease in a healthy adult. The most common species is *Salmonella sonnei*, which caused 78% of infections in the United States in 2000. *Salmonella flexneri*, *Salmonella boydii*, and *Salmonella dysenteriae* also cause human disease. Transmission occurs through the fecal–oral route. The typical incubation period is 1 to 3 days.

Clinical symptoms include diarrhea or dysentery and may include fever, abdominal cramps, and tenesmus. The presentation can vary by species of infection. *S. sonnei* usually results in watery diarrhea, whereas *S. flexneri*, *S. boydii*, and *S. dysenteriae* typically cause severe systemic illness with dysentery. Children under age 5, their caregivers, and those living in crowded conditions are at higher risk for disease. Severe infection with high fever may be associated with seizures in patients younger than 2 years of age.

Most cases of *Shigella* are self-limited, and even without treatment, the carrier state usually ceases in approximately 4 weeks. However, antimicrobial therapy is effective in shortening the duration of illness and eradicating the organisms from feces. Documenting stool culture with antibiotic sensitivities is recommended in all cases because of widespread antimicrobial resistance.

Campylobacter

The majority of human *Campylobacter* disease is caused by only one species, *Campylobacter jejuni*. Poultry is the major reservoir, but infection can also occur by ingestion of unpasteurized milk and untreated water. The incubation period is 2 to 7 days.

Symptoms include bloody diarrhea, cramping, abdominal pain, fever, nausea, and vomiting. The illness typically lasts 1 week, and in the majority of patients, recovery is spontaneous. However, immunoreactive complications such as reactive arthritis, Reiter syndrome, and Guillain-Barré syndrome have been reported during convalescence. Immunocompromised individuals are at risk for prolonged, relapsing, or extraintestinal infections, particularly with the less common *Campylobacter* species.

Antimicrobial therapy should be used only in cases of severe illness or for immunocompromised hosts. There is some evidence that macrolides, if given early in the course of infection, can shorten the duration of illness and prevent relapse.

Escherichia coli

Escherichia coli is a gram-negative organism with at least five diarrhea-causing types, each with distinct virulence characteristics and clinical manifestations. Table 2 summarizes the types of diarrhea-causing *E. coli*. It is transmitted by contaminated food and water with an incubation period of 3 to 4 days. Shiga toxin–producing *E. coli* has been documented to be transmitted via undercooked ground beef and unpasteurized milk.

The most virulent is Shiga toxin–producing *E. coli* (STEC), formerly known as enterohemorrhagic *E. coli*, with the most common serotype being *E. coli* 0157:H7. Sequelae associated with infection are hemolytic uremic syndrome (HUS), postdiarrheal thrombotic thrombocytopenic purpura (TTP), and hemorrhagic colitis. *E. coli* 0157:H7 can be specifically serotyped, and positive results should be reported to public health authorities. Some studies have suggested an increased association with HUS if patients are treated with antimicrobial agents, but this has not been confirmed.

Cholera

Vibrio cholerae is a gram-negative rod that characteristically causes copious watery diarrhea. The organism is highly contagious, with an incubation period of 1 to 3 days. Epidemics have been caused by serotypes 01 and 0139, although many other serotypes exist. The vast majority of illness occurs in developing countries; however, there is an endemic focus in the Gulf Coast of the United States of a unique strain of serotype 01. The usual sources of infection are contaminated water or undercooked shellfish.

Symptoms include severe watery diarrhea that is often described as having the consistency of "rice water." Without treatment, severe dehydration, electrolyte imbalances, and hypovolemic shock can occur in 4 to 12 hours. Metabolic acidosis and potassium deficiency can cause

TABLE 2 *Escherichia coli* Pathotypes Associated With Diarrhea

Organism	Susceptible populations	Clinical syndrome	Duration of illness	Antimicrobial therapy
Enterohemorrhagic (STEC/EHEC)	All	Watery diarrhea progressing to bloody, severe abdominal pain	5–10 days	Not recommended
Enteropathogenic (EPEC)	Children younger than 2, developing countries	Severe watery diarrhea, fever	Persistent	Trimethoprim-sulfamethoxazole (Bactrim)[1]
Enterotoxigenic (ETEC)	Travelers to developing nations	Watery stools, abdominal cramps	1–5 days	Fluoroquinolones, Trimethoprim-sulfamethoxazole
Enteroinvasive (EIEC)	All	Watery stools, fever, crampy abdominal pain	7 days	Trimethoprim-sulfamethoxazole (Bactrim)[1], Fluoroquinolones
Enteroaggregative (EAEC)	Young children, developing countries	Watery diarrhea, low-grade fever	Persistent	No Specific Recommendations

[1]Not FDA approved for this indication.
Abbreviations: EAEC = enteroadherent *Escherichia coli*; EHEC = enterohemorrhagic *Escherichia coli*; EIEC = enteroinvasive *Escherichia coli*; EPEC = enteropathogenic *Escherichia coli*; ETEC = enterotoxigenic *Escherichia coli*; STEC = Shiga toxin–producing *Escherichia coli*.

severe muscle cramps. Without treatment, the case-fatality rate is approximately 50%.

Isolated organisms should be sent to the local public health department for serotyping. Treatment with rapid rehydration and electrolyte repletion should be initiated as soon as the diagnosis is suspected. Oral rehydration should be used in patients with mild to moderate dehydration. Patients presenting with severe dehydration will require initial fluid therapy intravenously with solutions such as normal saline or lactated Ringer's.

Antimicrobial therapy eradicates the organism, as well as decreases the duration and severity of illness. Giving antibiotics to household contacts within 24 hours of identification of the organism may help prevent coprimary cases. However, antibiotic prophylaxis is not recommended for routine cholera control, particularly in the United States.

Although unavailable in the United States, two oral cholera vaccines are commercially available in some countries. One of these, a killed oral vaccine (Dukoral),[1] has been recommended by the WHO for use in refugee populations at immediate risk for cholera. There are numerous live and killed oral vaccines currently in field trials that may become available in the near future.

Clostridium difficile

Clostridium difficile is a gram-positive anaerobe that is the leading cause of nosocomial infectious diarrhea. Disease usually results as a complication of antibiotic therapy, most commonly the cephalosporins, penicillins, and clindamycin (Cleocin), although colitis has been associated with nearly every antimicrobial agent. Antibiotics disrupt the normal intestinal flora, which allows colonization and growth of the pathogen. The toxins produced by the organism result in colitis and diarrhea.

The illness varies in severity, and can cause pseudomembranous colitis or toxic megacolon, particularly in the elderly and immunocompromised hosts. Of note, neonates have high rates of asymptomatic colonization. Diagnosis can be made by detection of the toxin in stool specimens. Treatment begins with discontinuation of the causative antibiotic. If symptoms persist, alternate antibiotic therapy should be considered.

VIRUSES

Rotavirus

The CDC estimates that rotavirus causes more than 2 million hospitalizations and 440,000 deaths annually in children younger than 5 years of age. Children from the poorest countries account for 82% of deaths. In the United States, approximately 55,000 children are hospitalized each year from the disease. It is the most common cause of severe diarrhea in children under 2 years of age in all countries.

Children ages 6 to 24 months are most commonly affected. The disease is characterized by vomiting and watery diarrhea, with associated fever and abdominal pain. In temperate climates, the peak incidence of rotavirus occurs in winter. Transmission occurs by fecal–oral contact. The incubation period is 1 to 3 days. The illness is usually self-limited, lasting 3 to 8 days; however, persistent infection can develop in immunocompromised hosts. Diagnosis can be confirmed by rapid antigen detection in stool specimens.

Treatment is entirely supportive. There are no available antimicrobial agents for rotavirus. Nearly every infant is affected with rotavirus by 3 years of age. Although immunity is incomplete, subsequent episodes are less severe.

Rotavirus serotypes are determined by two capsid protein gene segments, the glycoprotein (G protein) and the protease-cleaved (P) protein. The main serotypes

[1]Not FDA approved for this indication.

Rakel and Bope: *Conn's Current Therapy 2006.*

that cause human disease in the United States are G1, G2, G3, G4, and G9 combined with P1a, P1b, or P2. Several candidate rotavirus vaccines have been evaluated in the past 20 years. One quadrivalent reassortant candidate vaccine containing serotypes G1 to G4 was derived from the rhesus monkey strain of rotavirus. The vaccine (RotaShield) was licensed in the United States in 1998 but was subsequently withdrawn because of reports of association with intussusception. There is a monovalent lamb rotavirus vaccine licensed in China. No rotavirus vaccine is currently licensed in the United States, although several clinical trials are underway for products under development. One pentavalent reassortant vaccine and one monovalent human strain are in the late stages of clinical development and may be available in the near future.

Norovirus

The noroviruses, also known as Norwalk-like viruses, are of the *Caliciviridae* family. According to the CDC, noroviruses are the cause of at least 50% of food-borne outbreaks in the United States. Transmission occurs via the fecal–oral route, or through contaminated food or water. Virus excretion lasts for more than a week. Most sporadic cases occur in children under 4 years of age, although outbreaks have occurred in all age groups.

The incubation period is less than 2 days. The most common symptoms are vomiting, diarrhea, and abdominal cramps, with associated fever and malaise. The illness is usually self-limited, lasting 1 to 3 days. There are no known long-term sequelae.

Outbreaks in the United States have been linked to raw shellfish, water, eggs, and salad ingredients. The CDC found that 96% of nonbacterial gastroenteritis outbreaks reported from January of 1996 through June of 1997 were caused by noroviruses. In 2002 there was a marked increase in norovirus outbreaks on cruise ships. In that year, out of 21 gastrointestinal illness outbreaks on 17 ships, 9 were confirmed to be caused by norovirus. In that same year, there were 26 land-based gastroenteritis outbreaks associated with norovirus. Since then, several waterborne outbreaks have been associated with private wells, small water systems, and recreational pools and lakes. One outbreak in February of 2004 at a swimming pool resulted in 53 cases of norovirus diarrhea and was attributed to lapses in pool maintenance and management.

Treatment for this illness is supportive. Commercial diagnostic assays are not routinely available. However, local public health department laboratories can test for norovirus in the event of a suspected outbreak. No antiviral medications or vaccines are available for norovirus.

PARASITES

Giardia lamblia

Giardiasis is caused by a protozoan that infects the small intestine and biliary tract. Humans are the primary reservoir, but dogs, cats, and beavers can be infected as well. Transmission occurs through fecal–oral contact,

and community outbreaks have occurred from contaminated water.

The incubation period is 1 to 4 weeks, and many people remain asymptomatic. Disease symptoms vary widely, from occasional acute watery diarrhea to protracted passage of foul-smelling stools associated with flatulence, abdominal distension, and anorexia. Symptoms may last 2 to 6 weeks, and may recur several times if untreated.

Diagnosis is made by antibody testing or direct smear examination of stool specimens. Treatment consists of rehydration and oral antimicrobials. Immunocompromised patients may require prolonged treatment because relapse is common.

Amebiasis

Entamoeba histolytica is a protozoan that causes intestinal infections and liver abscesses. Prevalence is highest in people of low socioeconomic status living in developing countries. In industrialized countries, persons at highest risk include recent immigrants, travelers, and institutionalized populations.

The incubation period is 1 to 4 weeks on average but can be highly variable. Approximately 10% of individuals infected with the organism manifest clinically. The clinical syndrome usually consists of 1 to 3 weeks of increasingly severe diarrhea that progresses to dysentery, lower abdominal pain, and tenesmus. Rarely, progressive involvement of the colon can result in toxic megacolon, fulminant colitis, or perforation.

Diagnosis can be made by identification of cysts in the stool specimen. However, this may not distinguish the organism from the nonpathogenic *Entamoeba dispar*. Therefore, antibody-based antigen detection assays or polymerase chain reaction (PCR) are recommended if available. Treatment is with oral amebicides.

Unique Populations

THE ELDERLY

Infectious diarrhea is an underappreciated problem in the elderly. According to a CDC survey, individuals older than age 65 years in the United States report 0.66 episodes of diarrhea per person each year. Mortality and case-fatality rates are higher in the elderly than in younger adults for nearly all types of diarrhea. Studies have shown that in the United States, the elderly represent between 51% and 85% of all deaths because of diarrhea. One study showed that individuals aged 80 years and older have a 3% case fatality rate from gastroenteritis requiring hospitalization.

The elderly are at higher risk for diarrheal infections because of diminished immune function, as well as decreased intestinal motility associated with medications, frequent use of antibiotics, and history of prior surgeries. The elderly are more likely than the general population to have chronic medical conditions and are less able to adapt to fluid and electrolyte shifts. Finally, associated medical conditions frequently predispose the elderly to serious sequelae of infectious diarrhea such as ischemic colitis.

Outbreaks are common, particularly in nursing homes or skilled nursing facilities. Nursing home outbreaks of *E. coli* 0157:H7 have resulted in three times the morbidity and mortality seen in younger persons. Spread occurs through common caregivers and food handlers. Etiologic agents include norovirus, *E. coli*, rotavirus, and *C. difficile*.

Recommendations for treatment are the same in the elderly as for younger adults. However, symptomatic dehydration requires closer monitoring during fluid and electrolyte replacement.

TRAVELERS

Traveler's diarrhea refers to an enteric illness acquired by a person from an industrialized country while traveling to a developing country or within 10 days of return. Currently, 20% to 50% of more than 50 million travelers annually report having diarrhea. Despite efforts by the tourism and health care industries, there has been no significant decrease in the incidence of traveler's diarrhea since the 1970s.

The following organisms cause more than 80% of cases: *E. coli*, *Shigella*, *C. jejuni*, *Salmonella*, *Aeromonas*, *V. cholerae*, rotavirus, *G. lamblia*, *E. histolytica*, *Cryptosporidium parvum*, and *Cyclospora*. Etiology and severity vary by geographic region and a variety of host factors.

There are several approaches for prevention. Dietary recommendations include eating only cooked foods and drinking water that has been boiled or treated with water purification tablets. Unfortunately, travelers' compliance with these measures is poor.

Routine administration of chemoprophylaxis is not recommended. Fluoroquinolones, including ciprofloxacin (Cipro), are frequently used; however, there is now emerging resistance of both *C. jejuni* and *E. coli* to these medicines.

Most cases are self-limited, lasting 3 to 5 days. Treatment involves replacement of fluid losses with appropriate oral rehydration. Bismuth subsalicylate is somewhat effective for traveler's diarrhea; it may, however, be impractical for the traveler to carry the large quantities of medicine that would be needed. If the diarrhea is moderate or severe, or is associated with fever or bloody stools, empiric antibiotic therapy may be used but should be continued for no more than 3 days.

CHILD-CARE CENTERS

Children in group care settings are at high risk for diarrheal diseases. One study showed between 2 and 3 diarrheal episodes per child each year among children attending daycare centers compared to less than 1 episode per child each year in children who did not attend daycare. Important preventive measures include caregivers' practice of hygiene, environmental sanitation, and careful food handling procedures.

Children with diarrhea or with bloody stools should be excluded from daycare settings. The principal organisms implicated in child-care center associated outbreaks are *Shigella*, STEC, *Cryptosporidium parvum*, hepatitis A, rotavirus, and *G. lamblia*. In contrast, nontyphoidal *Salmonella* and *Campylobacter* are rarely associated with such outbreaks.

If *S. typhi*, *Shigella*, STEC, or *G. lamblia* is documented in a child or staff member, all symptomatic children, staff, and family members should be tested and treated. Reports should be made to local health departments as appropriate. Children should remain excluded until symptoms resolve. Furthermore, *Shigella* and *E. coli* require two subsequent negative stool cultures prior to return. For *S. typhi*, children younger than 5 years of age must have three subsequent negative stool specimens.

IMMUNOCOMPROMISED INDIVIDUALS

Organisms that cause mild self-limited illness in immunocompetent hosts can cause severe, persistent, and even life-threatening conditions in immunocompromised individuals. Symptomatic intestinal infections can occur in immunocompromised hosts from organisms that commonly do not cause disease in otherwise healthy individuals, including illness caused by the following organisms: *Cryptosporidium parvum*, microsporidia, *Isospora belli*, *Cyclospora cayetanensis*, Cytomegalovirus, *Mycobacterium avium-intracellulare* and *Histoplasma capsulatum*. Treatment is often complex. Courses of antibiotics are usually longer, and relapses can occur. In addition, antimicrobial therapy may be needed against organisms that do not require treatment in otherwise healthy individuals.

Treatment

REHYDRATION

Because most diarrheal illnesses are self-limited, the main strategy for treatment is the replacement of fluids along with appropriate feeding. In the late 1970s, the WHO recommended an oral rehydration solution (ORS) containing 90 mmol/L of sodium and 111 mmol/L of glucose, with an osmolarity of 311 mOsm/L. The extensive use of this solution worldwide is credited with saving millions of lives in the last three decades. Recently, the WHO has recommended a reduced osmolarity ORS that contains 75 mmol/L of sodium and 75 mmol/L of glucose, with an osmolarity of 245 mOsm/L. The reduced osmolarity ORS has been demonstrated to reduce the need for unscheduled intravenous therapy among children with noncholera diarrhea. Table 3 shows the commercially available ORS formulations commonly used in the United States. Although ORS can be prepared from home ingredients, errors in mixing can occur and may result in serious electrolyte imbalances. Therefore, commercially prepared ORS should be recommended whenever possible.

In cases of severe dehydration in which a patient may be obtunded and unable to drink, IV or intraosseous (IO) fluids should be used in the initial management. ORS should then be instituted as soon as the patient is able to drink oral fluids. In addition to delivering the

TABLE 3 Composition of Commercial Oral Rehydration Solutions

Solution	Sodium (mmol/L)	Potassium (mmol/L)	Carbohydrate (gm/L)	Osmolarity (mOsm/L)
Pedialyte® (Ross)	45	20	25	250
Enfalyte® (Mead- Johnson)	50	25	30	200
Rehydralyte® (Ross)	75	20	25	305
CeraLyte® (Cera Products)	50–90	20	40	220

From King, CK, et al: Managing acute gastroenteritis among children. MMWR 2003;52(No. RR-16).

appropriate quantity of ORS to replace the calculated fluid deficit, ongoing fluid losses should be replaced. Table 4 summarizes the recommended quantities of fluid for different levels of dehydration.

The individual's usual diet should be continued. Breast-fed infants should continue breastfeeding, and formula-fed infants should continue their usual formula. Commercial carbonated beverages and undiluted fruit juices should be avoided because the high carbohydrate content can aggravate diarrhea.

ZINC SUPPLEMENTATION

Based on recent evidence that zinc[1] supplementation during a diarrheal illness reduces the severity of diarrhea, the WHO recommends the use of daily supplementation for 10 to 14 days with 20 mg of oral zinc sulfate for children older than 6 months of age and 10 mg

[1]Not FDA approved for this indication.

for infants younger than 6 months of age in developing countries.

ANTIMICROBIALS

Antimicrobial therapy should be used only in specific cases of acute infectious diarrhea when the etiologic agent has been identified. Table 5 summarizes the common diarrhea-causing organisms for which therapy is indicated in immunocompetent, otherwise healthy individuals. Whenever possible, therapeutic decisions should be based on the antibiotic susceptibility of the organism. Immunocompromised hosts or patients with severe concomitant illnesses may require additional specific therapy.

Widespread and continually emerging antibiotic resistance in pathogenic bacteria has led to the dissemination of numerous policies regarding the judicious use of antibiotics in ill patients. However, of antimicrobial agents used annually in the United States, between

TABLE 4 Summary of Treatment Based on Degree of Dehydration

Degree of dehydration	Rehydration therapy	Replacement of losses	Nutrition
Minimal or no dehydration	Not applicable.	<10 kg body weight: 60–120 mL ORS for each diarrheal stool or vomiting episode. >10 kg body weight: 120–240 mL ORS for each diarrheal stool or vomiting episode.	Continue breast-feeding or resume age-appropriate normal diet after initial hydration, including adequate caloric intake for maintenance.
Mild to moderate dehydration	ORS, 50–100 mL/kg body weight over 3–4 hours.	Same.	Same.
Severe dehydration	Lactated Ringer's solution or normal saline in 20 mL/kg body weight intravenous boluses until perfusion and mental status improve. Then administer 100 mL/kg body weight ORS over 4 hours or 5% dextrose ½ normal saline intravenously at twice maintenance fluid rates.	Same. If unable to drink, administer through nasogastric tube or administer 5% dextrose ¼ normal saline* with 20 mEq/L potassium chloride intravenously.	Same.

*Some experts recommend the use of ½ normal saline instead of ¼ normal saline.
Abbreviations: ORS = oral rehydration solution.
From King, CK et al: Managing acute gastroenteritis among children. MMWR 2003;52(No. RR-16).

TABLE 5 Antimicrobial Recommendations for Infectious Diarrhea Caused by Specific Pathogens

Organism	Antimicrobial regimen
Salmonella typhi	Ampicillin[1] or trimethoprim-sulfamethoxazole (Bactrim)[1] (14 days); ceftriaxone (Rocephin)[1] (7–10 days); or ciprofloxacin (Cipro) (adults, 5–7 days)
Shigella	Ampicillin or trimethoprim-sulfamethoxazole (5 days); ciprofloxacin (adults, 5 days); or ceftriaxone (Rocephin)[1] (5 days)
Enteropathogenic *Escherichia coli*	Ciprofloxacin (Cipro)[1] (adults, 5 days) or trimethoprim-sulfamethoxazole (Bactrim)[1] (5 days)
Enterotoxigenic *Escherichia coli*	Ciprofloxacin (Cipro) (adults, 5 days) or trimethoprim-sulfamethoxazole (Bactrim) (5 days)
Vibrio cholerae	Doxycycline (Vibramycin) (adults, 3 days); trimethoprim-sulfamethoxazole (Bactrim)[1] (3 days); or erythromycin (Ery-Tab)[1] (3 days)
Clostridium difficile	Metronidazole (Flagyl)[1] or oral vancomycin (Vancocin) (7–10 days)
Giardia lamblia	Metronidazole (Flagyl)[1] (5–7 days); tinidazole (Tindamax) (adults, single dose); or furazolidone (Furoxone) (children, 7–10 days)
Entamoeba histolytica	Metronidazole (Flagyl) (7–10 days); or tinidazole (Tindamax) (3 days) followed by Iodoquinol (Yodoxin) (20 days); or paromomycin (Humatin) (7 days)

[1]Not FDA approved for this indication.

40% and 80% are used in food animals, mostly in healthy animals to promote growth or prevent disease. Evidence shows that this results in the selection and dissemination of resistant organisms. For example, one study showed that of the grocery store chicken that was contaminated with *Campylobacter* species, 24% were resistant to fluoroquinolones. Further studies showed that patients with fluoroquinolone resistant *Campylobacter* infection had a longer duration of diarrhea. Similar patterns are emerging with *Salmonella* and *Enterococcus* species.

PROBIOTICS

Probiotics are microbial cell preparations or components of microbial cells that have a beneficial effect on the health and well-being of the host. They grow in fermented foods, and are thought to facilitate an improved balance in the intestinal microflora.

For more than a century, researchers have hypothesized that live bacterial cultures could be used to prevent or treat diarrhea. The proposed mechanisms of action include competition with pathogenic bacteria for intraluminal nutrients, making the intestinal contents acidic, production of antibiotic substances, or enhancement of the host immune system. No serious adverse effects have been associated with probiotic use by healthy individuals; however, infections have been reported in immunocompromised hosts.

The most widely used products are lactobacilli,[1] which are found in normal human intestinal and perineal flora. Some studies suggest differential effects, modified by disease etiology or species of *Lactobacillus*. For example, *L. GG* has been shown in several placebo-controlled studies to reduce the duration and severity of rotavirus diarrhea accompanied by decreased viral shedding, although the same effect was not demonstrated with *Lactobacillus rhamnosis*, *Lactobacillus delbrueckii*, or *Lactobacillus acidophilus*.

Several placebo-controlled studies have demonstrated decreased diarrheal incidence and severity in patients treated with probiotics concomitantly with antibiotics. The probiotics most often used in these studies were *L. GG*, *L. acidophilus*, and the nonpathogenic yeast *Saccharomyces boulardii*. However, studies using probiotics for the treatment of antibiotic associated diarrhea have not been as convincing. The use of probiotics in traveler's diarrhea has been extensively studied. Efficacy seems to vary by strain of probiotic and travel destination.

Additional well-designed controlled trials are needed to elucidate the role of probiotics in acute infectious diarrhea, particularly to establish dosing schedules and specificity of treatment for different pathogens. Furthermore, U.S. experts warn that because the FDA does not regulate dietary supplements, the potential exists for variance in product safety and efficacy.

NONANTIMICROBIAL DRUG THERAPY

There are several over-the-counter and prescription antimotility (e.g., loperamide [Imodium]), antisecretory

---

 CURRENT DIAGNOSIS

For all Patients
- History, including duration of diarrhea and vomiting, fever, and number of water stools in past 24 hours
- Physical examination, including assessment of level of dehydration

If Indicated
- Stool examination and culture: for patients with bloody stools, history of recent travel, immunocompromised hosts

---

[1]Not FDA approved for this indication.

Rakel and Bope: *Conn's Current Therapy 2006.*

CURRENT THERAPY

Rehydration

- ORS: Use commercially prepared solutions when possible; initiate early in the course of illness.
- Intravenous fluid therapy: For patients who are unable to drink, initiate ORS as soon as possible.

Medicinal Therapy

- Zinc[1] is recommended, particularly for children in developing countries.
- Probiotics:[1] Further testing is required for specific recommendations.
- Antimicrobial drugs: When indicated for particular pathogens, obtain stool culture for identification and antibiotic sensitivities.

[1]Not FDA approved for this indication.
Abbreviations: ORS = Oral rehydration solution.

(e.g., racecadotril [Tiorfan][2]), and toxin-binding agents (e.g., cholestyramine [Questran][1]) available for treatment of diarrhea but few have demonstrated efficacy in randomized clinical trials. Because of the limited evidence and uncertain side-effect profiles, most experts do not recommend the use of any of these agents, particularly for pediatric patients. In fact, most experts believe that the use of these medications could be harmful especially in children. For example, antimotility agents have been implicated in prolonged fever in shigellosis and toxic megacolon in *C. difficile* colitis. Also, reliance on pharmaceutic management may shift emphasis away from proven therapeutic methods such as ORS.

REFERENCES

Allan SJ, Okoko B, Martinez E, Gregorio G, Dans LF: Probiotics for treating infectious diarrhoea. The Cochrane Database of Systematic Reviews 2003, Issue 4. Art. No; CD003048.pub2. DOI: 10.1002/14651858.CD003048.pub2.
Casburn-Jones AC, Farthing MJG: Traveler's diarrhea. J Gastroenterol Hepatol 2004;19:610-618.
Centers for Disease Control and Prevention: Outbreaks of gastroenteritis associated with norovirus on cruise ships–United States, 2002. MMWR 2002;51(49):1112-1115.
Imhoff B, et al: Burden of self-reported acute diarrheal illness in FoodNet surveillance areas, 1998-1999. Clin Infect Dis 2004; 38(Suppl 3):S219-S226.
King CK, et al: Managing acute gastroenteritis among children: Oral rehydration, maintenance, and nutritional therapy. MMWR 2003; 52(No. RR-16):1-16.
Parashar UD, et al: Hospitalizations associated with rotavirus diarrhea in the United States, 1993-1995: Surveillance based on the new ICD-9-CM rotavirus-specific diagnostic code. J Infect Dis 1998; 177:13-17.
Pickering LK (ed.): Red book: 2003 report of the Committee on Infectious Diseases. 26th ed. Elk Grove Village, IL, American Academy of Pediatrics, 2003.
Roberts L, et al: Effect of infection control measures on the frequency of diarrheal episodes in child care: A randomized controlled trial. Pediatrics 2000;105(4):743-746.
Sack DA, et al: Cholera. Lancet 2004;363:223-233.
Shea KM, et al: Nontherapeutic use of antimicrobial agents in animal agriculture: Implications for pediatrics. Pediatrics 2004;114(3): 862-868.
Slotwiner-Nie PK, Brandt LJ: Infectious diarrhea in the elderly. Gastroenterology Clinics of North America 2001;30(3):625-635.
Svennerholm AM, Steele D: Progress in enteric vaccine development. Best Pract Res Clin Gastroenterol 2004;18(2):421-445.
Thielman NM, Guerrant RL: Acute infectious diarrhea. N Engl J Med 2004;350(1):38-47.
WHO/UNICEF Joint Statement: Clinical management of acute diarrhoea. The United Nations Children's Fund/World Health Organization, May 2004.

Constipation

Method of
Jack A. Di Palma, MD

Between 15% and 20% of the U.S. population report that they are constipated or take laxatives. The aisles of any drugstore attest to the frequency of constipation and related symptoms. Constipation is more frequent in the elderly, and in children it accounts for 3% of office visits and 25% of referrals to pediatric gastroenterologists. Despite approximately 2.6 million annual visits, only a minority of patients seem to seek care. Many "suffer in silence" and self-medicate.

What is Constipation?

Regularity varies. The *Federal Register* defines normal bowel frequency as three times a day to three times a week. The frequency definition alone, however, ignores the commonly associated symptoms that patients consider as constipation. When patients report constipation they may mean straining, hard stools, inability to defecate on demand, infrequent defecation, feelings of pain or bloating, or the sensation of incomplete defecation. Some describe anal blockage or report the need for manual digital disimpaction. The International Congress of Gastroenterology committees convened in Rome have described and revised criteria to devise a uniform standard (Box 1). Some authors have shown inconsistency of these criteria, but criteria-based symptom evaluations encourage clinicians to focus on frequency and the associated symptoms of consistency, stool passage, and discomfort.

Objectives of the Clinical Evaluation

Gastroenterologists focus on detecting pelvic floor dysfunction syndromes, but the majority of patients that seek care for constipation will have normal- or

[1]Not FDA approved for this indication.
[2]Not available in the United States.

BOX 1	Rome II Diagnostic Criteria for Constipation

At least 12 weeks, which need not be consecutive, in the preceding 12 months of two or more of:
- Straining with >25% defecations
- Lumpy or hard stools with >25% defecations
- Sensation of incomplete evacuation with >25% defecations
- Sensation of anorectal obstruction/blockage with >25% defecations
- Manual maneuvers to facilitate >25% defecations
- More than three defecations per week
- Loose stools are not present, and insufficient criteria for IBS

Abbreviations: IBS = irritable bowel syndrome.

BOX 2	Medications Associated With Constipation

- Analgesics
   Nonsteroidal anti-inflammatory agents, opiates
- Anticholinergics
   Atropine agents, antidepressants, neuroleptics, antiparkinsonian drugs
- Anticonvulsants
- Antihistamines
- Antihypertensives
   Calcium channel antagonists, clonidine (Catapres), hydralazine (Apresoline), MAO inhibitors, methyldopa (Aldomet)
- Chemotherapeutic agents
   Vinca derivatives
- Diuretics
- Metal ions
   Aluminum (antacids, sucralfate [Carafate]), barium sulfate, bismuth (Pepto-Bismol), calcium, iron, heavy metals (arsenic, lead, mercury)
- Resins
   Cholestyramine (Questran), polystyrene (Kayexalate)

slow-transit constipation. The clinical evaluation should be directed first toward a specific diagnosis of constipation using defined clinical criteria, and then detecting the presence of irritable bowel syndrome because the management approach may be different. Medications need to be carefully reviewed with attention to over-the-counter, herbal, and other self-medicating regimens. Endocrinopathies and neuromuscular conditions should be considered to determine whether colonic inertia or obstructed defecation is present. Structural evaluation is important to exclude stricture or obstructing diverticular disease; however, colon cancer screening may be the most important objective of the clinical evaluation.

MEDICATION CONSTIPATION

The Physician's Desk Reference (PDR) lists more than 900 drugs that are reported to cause constipation. More than 100 drugs noted constipation as an adverse experience that occurs in more than 3% of patients using the product. In a survey of patients who considered themselves constipated, more than 40% were using medications known to cause constipation. Box 2 lists medications that commonly cause constipation. Many over-the-counter and herbal products also cause it. Clinicians should anticipate constipation from medicines known to cause constipation and use preemptive treatment. Some have said that "one should write a laxative with one hand when prescribing narcotics with the other."

DIAGNOSTIC EVALUATION

Physical examination should give careful attention to the perineum and anus. In the left lateral position, with the buttocks separated, perineal descent and elevation is observed during simulated defecation and retention squeeze, and the skin is examined for fecal soiling. The anal verge is observed for any patulous opening. The digital exam should evaluate resting tone and squeezing effort. The puborectalis should be palpated and expulsionary forces tested by having the patient try to expel the finger. An examination should be made to look for rectocele.

Testing should include a metabolic profile and thyroid-stimulating hormone (TSH). The structural evaluation should be based on symptoms, age, and colon cancer screening indications. The preferred screening strategy is colonoscopy. Some use radiopaque colon transit markers (sitz markers) to assess transit and to screen for disorders of obstructed defecation. These patients may benefit from specialty center referral for more detailed testing with balloon expulsion, defecography, anorectal manometry or electromyelogram (EMG).

OBSTRUCTED DEFECATION

Constipated patients usually have normal or slow transit or a disorder of obstructed defecation. Outlet obstruction can be excluded by a careful examination by sigmoidoscopy, colonoscopy, or barium enema radiograph. Patients should be carefully examined for cystocele and rectocele, which might require radiologic evaluation or gynecologic examination. Intussusception and prolapse are other considerations.

Pelvic floor dyssynergia also may be present. These patients have normal or slightly delayed colon transit. There is storage of fecal residue for prolonged periods in the rectum and they have the inability to adequately defecate. Often, patients report that the stool is in the position to defecate and they feel the need to defecate, but they are unable to expel the rectal contents. This syndrome has several names and is referred to as *outlet obstruction, obstructed defecation, dyschezia, anismus, or dyssynergia*. They may represent different disorders of dysfunction with muscular hypertonicity and spasm, failure to relax the pelvic floor, incomplete relaxation, or paradoxical contractions. There may be muscular hypotonicity with megarectum and excessive pelvic floor descent.

Treatment

EDUCATION

"Normal" expectations for bowel habits should be reviewed, educating patients on typical frequency. They should be encouraged to recognize and respond to the "call to defecate." Modest exercise is advised and patients should observe the situations such as travel that disrupt their usual routines. Patients can monitor their bowel habits by using a diary to record movements, stool characteristics, and associated discomfort.

LAXATIVES

Laxatives are drugs that induce defecation. Box 3 lists a useful classification. When diet and lifestyle interventions fail, the choice of initial laxative is subject to personal opinion and consensus. There are few well-designed and well-conducted trials comparing laxative classes, but most have not been evaluated head to head. There are also conflicting opinions about the initial approach to diagnosis before treatment.

BOX 3   Laxatives

- Bulk Laxatives
    Dietary fiber, psyllium (Metamucil), polycarbophil (Mitrolan), methylcellulose (Citrucel), carboxymethylcellulose[2]
- Lubricating Agent
    Mineral oil
- Stimulant Laxatives
    Surface acting agents: Docusate (Colace), bile salts*
    Diphenylmethane derivatives: Phenolphthalein,[2] bisacodyl (Dulcolax), sodium picosulfate
    Ricinoleic acid: Castor oil
    Anthraquinones: Senna, cascara sagrada,* aloe,* rhubarb*
- Osmotic Agents
    Saline laxatives: Magnesium hydroxide (Milk of Magnesia), magnesium sulfate (Epsom Salt), sodium and phosphate salts (Fleet Phospho-Soda)
    Poorly absorbed sugars: Lactulose (Chronulac), sorbitol, mannitol, lactose, glycerine suppositories
    Polyethylene glycol (MiraLax)
- Neuromuscular Agents
    5HT4 Agonists: Cisapride (Propulsid),[2] norcisapride,[2] prucalopride,[†] tegaserod (Zelnorm)
    Colchicine[1]
    Prostaglandin agent: Misoprostol (Cytotec)[1]
    Cholinergic agents: Bethanechol (Urecholine),[1] neostigmine (Prostigmin)[1]
    Opiate antagonists: Naloxone (Norcan),[1] naltrexone (ReVia)[1]
- Investigational Agents
    Recombinant brain-derived neurotropic factor (r-metHuBDNF), Neurotropin-3

[1]Not FDA approved for this indication.
[2]Not available in the United States.
*Not FDA approved for this indication but available as herbal supplement.
[†]Investigational drug in the United States.

CURRENT DIAGNOSIS

- The diagnosis of constipation is made by a careful history addressing bowel frequency and associated symptoms of stool passage, consistency, and discomfort.
- The physical exam is directed at a careful anal and perineal inspection.
- Lab testing includes metabolic profile and TSH.
- Colon cancer screening indications are addressed based on age and risks related to underlying medical conditions and family history.

Abbreviations: TSH = thyroid-stimulating hormone.

Some recommend initially addressing the contribution of pelvic floor dysfunction and algorithmic treatment approaches have been developed based on whether constipation *is slow transit* or *normal transit*. Others advise that a dietary fiber trial be conducted before technical investigations. Because the response to biofeedback for pelvic floor dysfunction is inconsistent and typical initial algorithms are similar regardless of transit status, laxative therapy could be initiated based on symptoms before additional diagnostic evaluation. Most empiric regimens begin with fiber.

Most patients do not seek care for constipation and try to treat themselves, mostly with drugstore-shelf remedies and with alternative and complementary medicine agents. It is thus important to carefully ask about prior treatment before making new recommendations. An appropriate trial of fiber should increase dietary fiber or use medicinal bulk agents such as psyllium (Metamucil), polycarbophil (Mitrolan), or methylcellulose (Citrucel). These are dosed as 1 to 2 heaping tablespoons daily. For severe infrequency or acute constipation, PEG 3350 (MiraLax 17 g daily), saline laxatives (Milk of Magnesia), senna or bisacodyl (Dulcolax, 5 mg, 1 to -4 tablets when needed) are reasonable choices and can also be used as *rescue* treatment if patients need relief while adjusting to a new regimen. If initial therapy fails, larger doses of saline (Milk of Magnesia), PEG laxative (MiraLax, 34 g to 68 g), or lactulose can be used. Neuromuscular agents such as tegaserod (Zelnorm 6 mg twice a day) (see Box 3) or combination therapy are other options for severe constipation. For outlet obstruction, surgery should be avoided. Osmotic laxatives (Milk of Magnesia or MiraLax)

CURRENT THERAPY

- Patient education reviews normal expectations and situations like travel which tend toward causing constipation.
- Dietary fiber or laxatives are initial treatments.
- Use preemptive laxative treatment when prescribing medicines with a high likelihood of causing constipation.

can be used to liquefy the stool and improve passage of stool.

REFERENCES

DiPalma JA: Current treatment options for chronic constipation. Rev Gastroenterol Disord 2004;4;S34-S42.
Jones MP, Talley NJ, Nuyts G, Dubois D: Lack of objective evidence of efficacy of laxatives in chronic constipation. Dig Dis Sci 2002; 47:2222-2230.
Locke GR, Pemberton JH, Phillips SF: AGA technical review on constipation. Gastroenterology 2000;119:1766-1778.
Schiller LR: Review article: The therapy of constipation. Aliment Pharmacol Ther 2001;15:749-763.
Talley NJ: Definitions, epidemiology, and impact of chronic constipation. Rev Gastroenterol Disord 2004;4;S3-S10.

Fever

Method of
Philip D. Walson, MD

Fever is the single most common symptom treated by primary care physicians. In the majority of visits, patients receive medications. Numerous studies have increased our knowledge about the pathophysiology of fever, as well as of the risks and benefits of treating it. Unfortunately, as many as 91% of parents and caregivers, as well as many health providers, harbor misconceptions about the dangers of, and the need to treat, fever. The unrealistic concerns of parents was termed *fever phobia* by Barton Schmitt in 1980. This phobia can result in many unnecessary diagnostic and therapeutic interventions.

Fever is a common manifestation of many medical conditions, both trivial and serious. Only in rare situations, and only when extremely high (i.e., above 41.1°C [106.1°F]), can elevated body temperature cause harm, and it may even be protective. Treatment of fever can cause delay in seeking needed, disease-specific treatment or prolong recovery from disease. However, fever treatment can also have benefits, providing comfort, improving oral intake, and allowing for sleep, as well as discouraging unnecessary diagnostic evaluation or dangerous therapeutic interventions.

Pathophysiology of Fever

Both the decision whether to treat fever and the choice of methods used to lower body temperature require an appreciation of the pathophysiology of fever. There are multiple causes of elevated body temperature. Infectious causes of fever are the most common and are the only causes associated with an altered *setpoint* of the central *thermostat* located in the preoptic anterior hypothalamic region. It is important clinically to distinguish these infectious causes of fever from hyperthermia.

Hyperthermia results from excessive heat production, altered heat dissipation, or pharmacologic or physiologic alterations in homeostatic temperature regulatory mechanisms. A risk-to-benefit analysis of lowering temperature depends on the underlying cause(s) of temperature elevation. True hyperthermia should be treated only by external cooling, whether it was caused by, for example, chemicals (e.g., salicylates, nitrophenol, anticholinergics, stimulants, anesthetics), dehydration, elevated environmental temperature or wrapping, excessive exercise, head trauma, or neurosurgery. Other noninfectious causes of fever, such as malignancy, hyperthyroidism, autoimmune diseases, and so forth, should receive disease-specific treatment.

This discussion deals with the symptomatic treatment of infection-associated fever caused by increases in inflammatory mediators (i.e., cytokines such as interleukin [IL]-1, IL-8, and tumor necrosis factor [TNF]) that are released from cells, especially white blood cells (WBCs), in response to infection. These mediators act on the central thermostat to reset the body temperature by causing production of prostaglandin E_2. There are many patient-specific factors that alter the response to these mediators. For example, patients who are very young or very old, malnourished, treated with certain drugs (i.e., steroids or nonsteroidal anti-inflammatory drugs [NSAIDs]), or have renal diseases all can have altered fever responses.

Definition of Fever

The definition of fever is arbitrary, in part because temperature variability, both between and within individuals, is rather large. *Normal* baseline temperatures differ between individuals. They also vary during the day from 36°C (96.8°F) to 37.8°C (100°F), in the same individual, with the higher temperatures at night. Some temperature variabilities result from differences in measurement techniques, patient age, environmental temperature, dress, body composition, exercise, and metabolic state. In older children (over age 12) and adults, an oral temperature above 37.5°C (99.5°F), a rectal temperature above 38°C (100.4°F), or an axillary temperature above 37.2°C (99°F) is generally accepted to constitute a fever.

Tympanic membrane temperature measurements are capable of predicting core, or rectal, temperatures, but not all studies have validated the accuracy of tympanic measurements, especially in inexperienced hands. Accurate measurement of body temperature is not trivial, especially in ill or uncooperative patients. The site of measurement, the equipment used, the ambient temperature, the skill of the observer, and the cooperation of the subject all can have major effects on the accuracy of temperature measurements. For example, consumption of liquids, location and duration of the thermometer in the mouth, and mouth breathing all alter oral temperature measurements, especially if electronic temperature devices are used without disabling their automatic timing devices. Electronic temperature probes that are ingested orally and transmit core temperatures to a radio receiver device have even been used experimentally to obtain accurate measurements. Fortunately, there is seldom any need to obtain accurate temperatures in the vast majority of clinical situations.

Risks and Benefits of Fever

Fever is associated with some harmful clinical effects such as fetal damage from fever in pregnancy, increased metabolic needs in malnutrition, and increased cardiac demand with borderline cardiac function. However, most of the misconceptions concerning fever are the result of other weak, noncausal associations. There is a sound evolutionary theory that fever is beneficial, and despite some contrary opinions, there are also some data to support this theory. Fever has been shown in animal studies to enhance the immune response to many infectious agents and to some malignancies. Use of antipyretic drugs to lower fever increases both morbidity and mortality in infected laboratory animals and prolongs *varicella* infection in humans. Much of the fear of fever is the result of concern that high fever can cause *brain damage*. There are simply no data to support these fears, which appear to be perpetuated by the common association between fever and conditions such as brain trauma, central nervous system (CNS) infections, neurosurgery, hyperthermia, and febrile convulsions. Febrile convulsions are a special cause of fear. Yet in previously normal children, almost all simple febrile convulsions are associated with neither recurrence of seizures (febrile or otherwise) nor with any brain damage. Most, if not all, children who are found to have brain damage after a high fever, with or without convulsions, were either suffering from a disease known to cause damage (e.g., meningitis) or had abnormal brain development prior to the onset of fever and convulsions. It is the presence of abnormal development preceding the seizure, not the recurrence of high fever or the clinical characteristics of the febrile seizures themselves, which is most predictive of seizure recurrence or brain damage. There is also no evidence that parents can prevent recurrent febrile convulsions with the use of antipyretic drugs. Prescribing or using such therapy can lead to failure, frustration, and parental guilt.

Clinical Aspects of Treatment Decisions

In addition to the risks of symptomatic therapies (described later in this article), the major risk of fever treatment involves delays in diagnosis and initiation of specific treatment. The physician must always first attempt to diagnose the cause of the fever and determine what benefit, if any, would come from specific or nonspecific therapy.

Treatment of hyperthermia requires cooling and specific therapy as mentioned previously. Fevers from drugs or toxins require specific toxicologic management. Malignancies and autoimmune diseases need specific drug therapy. Symptomatic therapy also can be used but can be dangerous. For example, shock can occur in

Hodgkin's lymphoma patients given antipyretics. In infectious causes of fever, treatment decisions involve the type and seriousness of the infection, and which, if any, specific and nonspecific therapy is needed. The assessment of the febrile patient is a critically important, complicated, clinical process that is often transparent to the patient or parent. The need for therapy depends on a clinical assessment of how ill the patient is rather than how high the temperature is. This is especially true in patients who have any decreased ability to generate a febrile response or to tolerate delay in specific treatment (e.g., elderly, malnourished, immunocompromised, newborn, or renal patients). In all patients, the decision to treat and what to use are based on the patient's history, physical findings, and occasionally on laboratory test results.

There is a general misconception that trivial causes of fever respond more readily to antipyretic medication than do serious infections. In fact, there is no difference in the response of fever to symptomatic therapy between children with serious as opposed to trivial illnesses. Whether symptomatic therapy is given or not, the physician must continually assess the patient's overall clinical condition and not just whether the temperature decreases.

Nonpharmacologic Therapy

A number of nondrug therapies are available. If used, they should make the patient more comfortable rather than just lower the reading on a thermometer. Overwrapped patients should have extra clothing removed. Activities that raise the body temperature, such as shivering, crying, and excessive motor activity, should be minimized. Excessive environmental temperature (i.e., above 25°C [77°F]) should be avoided, but the child should not become chilled enough to shiver. Extra fluids should be encouraged to prevent dehydration. Sponge bathing is controversial. If attempted, only water at a comfortable temperature should be used and only small portions of the body exposed to the water. The sponging should be stopped if the child becomes too upset or inconsolable, and the child should be held and comforted by a competent adult at all times. Ice water and alcohol bathing must *not* be used. Alcohol is absorbed through the skin and lungs and can cause a chemical pneumonitis or ketosis; both ice water and alcohol can cause shivering, discomfort, and increased motor activity.

Antipyretics/analgesics are commonly used for the symptomatic treatment of fever. Their major advantage is their ability to control pain. They may make patients more comfortable even when the fever is not controlled. Studies in adults demonstrate that there is only a modest correlation between improvement in subjective feelings of wellness and temperature decrease. Parents and patients should be encouraged to think of these drugs as pain killers rather than as fever reducers. The goal of therapy with antipyretic/analgesics is to make patients more comfortable. If this were understood, caretakers would be less likely to treat thermometer readings and less likely to awaken quietly sleeping patients to dose them again or to continue to dose comfortable, awake patients with minimally elevated temperatures.

There are two general classes of antipyretics/analgesics: acetaminophen (Tylenol) and NSAIDs (e.g., salicylates, ibuprofen [Advil], and the newer relatively selective cyclooxygenase-2 [COX-2] inhibitors). The choice of drug is based on a number of things, including the clinical situation, cost, availability, dosage forms, patient age, drug allergies, and other patient characteristics that influence the relative safety of the individual agents.

There are a number of prescription and over-the-counter NSAIDs that are effective antipyretics/analgesics; some have specific benefits such as parenteral dosage forms (e.g., ketorolac [Toradol]) or prolonged durations of action (e.g., naproxen [Naprosyn]). Although the drugs are useful in selected clinical situations, the relative safety and efficacy of these alternatives have not yet been sufficiently studied to recommend them for routine symptomatic fever therapy. This includes the many parenteral antipyretics that are marketed in other countries (e.g., antipyrine, propacetamol), but are not available in the United States.

Pharmacotherapeutic Agents

ACETAMINOPHEN

Acetaminophen (Tylenol) can be inexpensive and is available in a wide variety of brands and dosage forms. Although it does have the ability to inhibit certain peripheral prostaglandin synthetic enzymes, it is not generally classified as an NSAID. It has been available chemically for more than a century and used clinically for almost 60 years. It is rapidly and well absorbed orally and rectally. Parenteral dosage forms are available in some European, but not North American, countries. It is an effective antipyretic and analgesic, but its anti-inflammatory activity is weak. There is a 1- to 3-hour delay between the attainment of maximal plasma concentrations and therapeutic effects. Clearance is largely by hepatic metabolism to inactive and nontoxic metabolites. However, in overdose, its usual metabolic pathways can be saturated and a toxic quinone produced. This metabolite can be detoxified by endogenous glutathione. However, when production of the toxic metabolite exceeds glutathione stores, such as in overdosed patients or patients whose hepatic metabolizing enzymes are induced (by cigarettes, anticonvulsants, etc.), these detoxification mechanisms can be overwhelmed, leading to hepatic or even renal toxicity. Except for rare, poorly substantiated reports of hepatotoxicity in alcoholic patients who took therapeutic doses chronically, the drug appears to be very safe in patients taking usual therapeutic doses. Even in overdose, if diagnosed and treated (especially if within 12 to 24 hours), the use of acetylcysteine (Mucomyst) (as a glutathione substitute) is remarkably effective in preventing serious morbidity or mortality. However, if the diagnosis of overdose is delayed, especially in patients taking enzyme-inducing drugs, pregnant women, and malnourished patients, serious or even fatal hepatic or renal

toxicity can occur. Despite its potential to produce toxicity in overdose, acetaminophen (Tylenol) is by far the safest analgesic/antipyretic drug to use therapeutically, especially in patients with gastrointestinal (GI) ulcers, bleeding problems, allergies, asthma, or renal diseases, and in pregnant or elderly patients. Therapeutic acetaminophen (Tylenol) use can be problematic only in patients at risk for chronic, accidental, or intentional overdose or who are pregnant. Dosing is generally 10 to 15 mg/kg every 4 to 6 hours for 3 to 4 days. There is good theoretical and clinical evidence that at least 15 mg/kg, and probably 20 to 30 mg/kg,[3] can be given safely, especially as a *loading dose,* and be effective for up to 8 hours (therefore not changing the total daily mg/kg exposure). Doses in adults are from 325 to 650 mg every 3 to 4 hours. There are multiple dosage forms available, including drops, elixirs, syrups, tablets, capsules, caplets, chewable tablets, and suppositories, and even prolonged-release preparations that allow for less frequent dosing. It is not known whether double-dosing of a rapid-release preparation would be more effective or less safe than use of these less frequent, higher dose, prolonged-release products.

IBUPROFEN

Ibuprofen (Advil) is a classic NSAID that works as a reversible inhibitor of prostaglandin synthesis. Of note, it is available as a racemic mixture of two optical (R and S) isomers, which differ in pharmacokinetics, as well as in therapeutic and toxic effects. The R isomer is converted enzymatically in the body to the more active and less toxic S isomer. It is unclear whether the use of pure S isomer would improve the therapeutic ratio, and this could increase costs significantly. Although used for decades as an anti-inflammatory and analgesic, ibuprofen (Advil) has more recently been widely used as an antipyretic. It is rapidly absorbed, but the percentage absorbed can differ between preparations and can be decreased by food. Ibuprofen (Advil) at the doses used for antipyresis produces a more rapid temperature fall and longer duration of action (usually 5 to 6 and up to 8 hours) than acetaminophen (Tylenol) after the first dose, especially in children with higher (i.e., above 39.2°C [102.5°F]) temperatures. This advantage may not be maintained with repeated dosing.

The toxicity of ibuprofen (Advil) is similar to that of all NSAIDs. GI upset is much more common than with acetaminophen (Tylenol) but is usually minor, especially in children. Serious GI, renal, pulmonary, allergic, and bone marrow toxicity occurs rarely. Patients with hypovolemia or renal disease can develop renal failure after taking ibuprofen (Advil). Asthmatic patients can develop bronchospasm. If taken by a pregnant woman in the third trimester, fetal toxicity can occur (e.g., closure of the ductus arteriosus, delayed labor, decreased fetal urine output, oligohydramnios, bleeding, etc.). Sudden, previously silent, life-threatening GI hemorrhage (especially in the elderly), GI ulcers, hepatic damage, platelet

---

[3]Exceeds dosage recommended by the manufacturer.

dysfunction, hypertension, rashes (even fatal), worsening of psoriasis, bone marrow suppression, headaches, confusion, and even aseptic meningitis all can occur. Toxicity after single therapeutic doses is much more common than with acetaminophen (Tylenol), but it is less common than with other NSAIDs including salicylates or naproxen (Naprosyn). The risk of Reye syndrome is unknown. The major advantage of ibuprofen (Advil), in addition to its longer duration of action and excellent efficacy, is its safety in overdose. Although ibuprofen (Advil) can produce life-threatening toxicity in certain susceptible populations (e.g., ulcer or renal patients, pregnant women, or asthmatics), it appears to be extremely safe when taken in overdose by most of the general population. Except for mild acidosis and some CNS changes, there are few reports of serious, nonidiosyncratic, acute, or long-term toxicity after even massive overdoses.

Ibuprofen (Advil) is available both by prescription and over the counter in a number of liquid and solid dosage forms from a number of manufacturers at a variety of prices. Over-the-counter dosing recommendations result in approximately 5 to 10 mg/kg per dose, which is given every 6 to 8 hours. Higher temperatures may respond better to the higher dosages, but after the first dose, repeat doses as little as 2.5 mg/kg[*] may be equally effective. The adult over-the-counter dose is 200 to 400 mg given every 4 to 6 hours.

SALICYLATES

Aspirin (acetylated salicylic acid) is the classic NSAID. Although still important analgesic and antiplatelet drugs, the salicylates are seldom used as only antipyretics because of safety concerns. Use is especially rare in children. Fear of drug-induced Reye syndrome has stopped salicylate use in all but rare childhood diseases (e.g., for Kawasaki disease, arthritis, or inflammatory bowel diseases) or as components of various preparations (e.g., topical methylsalicylate and bismuth subsalicylate preparations).

All salicylates are rapidly and well absorbed and both metabolized and excreted renally as both metabolites and unchanged drugs. The metabolism and distribution of salicylates are saturable, as well as time, dose, duration, and pH-dependent processes. This is part of the reason that toxicity is so problematic. The onset of different effects is variable. Noncompetitive antiplatelet effects occur very rapidly; platelet prostaglandin synthetase is irreversibly acetylated when aspirin is rapidly deacetylated (the half-life is approximately 15 minutes). This results in inhibition of platelet function that persists for the life of the affected platelet, because platelets cannot resynthesize the prostaglandin synthetase. The antipyretic and additional antiplatelet effects of salicylates are reversible, last only approximately 3 to 4 hours, and are slower in onset.

Aspirin and other salicylates are inexpensive and effective antipyretics, analgesics, and anti-inflammatory drugs. They are probably the standard in terms of efficacy against which other drugs (at least in adults)

should be compared. Toxicity, rather than cost or efficacy, limits their more widespread use. Adverse effects from salicylates are common and can be serious after both therapeutic use and with accidental and intentional overdose. They produce the same GI, hepatic, renal, allergic, platelet, fetal, and pulmonary toxicity as ibuprofen (Advil). Asthmatic patients with nasal polyps are especially prone to aspirin-induced bronchospasm. Unique to aspirin as an NSAID is its ability to produce irreversible (in addition to reversible) platelet dysfunction. This has been used to prevent conditions associated with platelet adhesion such as myocardial dysfunction and intracardiac valve replacement. Salicylate toxicity from therapeutic, accidental, or suicidal overdose is common and often life-threatening. Because there are safer, inexpensive, equally effective drugs available, the use of salicylates for symptomatic antipyresis cannot be recommended, especially in children.

COMBINATIONS

Use of combinations of two antipyretics for fever, although a common clinical practice, is mentioned only to seriously question this approach. The combination of aspirin and acetaminophen (Tylenol) was historically shown to be more effective at lowering temperature

CURRENT DIAGNOSIS

- Fever is the most commonly treated symptom.
- Misconceptions about fever, especially unrealistic fear, are pervasive.
- Fever can be a manifestation of both serious and trivial illness.
- One must distinguish fever from hyperthermia.
- Fever's definition is arbitrary and depends on patient characteristics and measurement technique.

CURRENT THERAPY

- The risk/benefit of any treatment depends on the cause.
- Treat the underlying cause first whenever possible.
- This article discusses only infection-associated fever.
- Fever can be protective, and lowering it can be harmful.
- Seriousness of infection is *not* related to antipyretic effectiveness.
- Antipyretics/analgesics should be used for comfort; not to lower temperature.
- Therapy is not without risks; be careful with dose, duration, and combinations.
- Proper therapy can be inexpensive and comforting.
- Improper therapy is dangerous and causes irrational *fever phobia*.

---

[*]Less than dosage recommended by the manufacturer.

than either drug alone. Similar data are unavailable for acetaminophen (Tylenol) plus ibuprofen (Advil). However, more than 50% of pediatricians use this approach, many of whom cite as the source of this unproven practice recommendations from the American Academy of Pediatrics that simply do not exist. There is no reason to believe that it is necessary to lower temperature more than can be done with adequate doses of a single drug. Combinations have not been proven to produce quicker or longer-lasting responses, and studies show that lowering of temperature does not correlate well with comfort provided. It is also unknown whether the current practice of alternating usual therapeutic doses of acetaminophen (Tylenol) with ibuprofen (Advil) is either more effective than or as safe as the use of a single drug alone at usual or increased doses. Combining drugs is more expensive, adds toxicity, could delay proper diagnosis or therapy, and contributes to the impression that lowering temperature, rather than controlling symptoms, is the primary goal of therapy. This practice perpetuates unnecessary *fever phobia.*

Proper treatment of fever can be inexpensive and effective and can relieve discomfort and anxiety. However, much needs to be done to educate patients, parents, and health providers about rational fever evaluation and treatment.

REFERENCES

Aronoff DM, Nielson EG: Antipyretics: Mechanisms of action and clinical use in fever suppression. Am J Med 2001;111(4):304-315.

Arons MM, Wheeler AP, Benard GR, et al: Effects of ibuprofen on the physiology and survival of hypothermic sepsis. Ibuprofen in Sepsis Study Group. Crit Care Med 1999;27(4) 699-707.

Baker RC, Tiller T, Bausher JC, et al: Severity of disease correlated with fever reduction in febrile infants. Pediatrics 1989;83(6):1016-1019.

Crocetti M, Moghbeli N, Serwint J, et al: Fever phobia revisited: Have parental misconceptions about fever changed in 20 years? Pediatrics 2001;107(6):1241-1246.

Eskerud JR, Andrew M, Stromnes B, Toverud EL: Pharmacy personnel and fever: A study on perception, self-care and information to customers. Pharm World Sci 1993;15(4):156-160.

Greisman LA, Mackowiak PA: Fever: Beneficial and detrimental effects of antipyretics. Curr Opin Infect Dis 2002;15(3):241-245.

Hasday JD, Garrison A: Antipyretic therapy in patients with sepsis. Clin Infect Dis 2000;31(Suppl 5):S234-S41.

Mackowiak PA, Plaisance KI: Benefits and risks of antipyretic therapy. Ann N Y Acad Sci 1998;856:214-223.

Acknowledgment

This work was supported by a cooperative agreement from the Agency for Healthcare Research and Quality for the UNC Center for Education and Research on Therapeutics (award number U18 HS 10397).

Cough

Method of
David G. Hill, MD

Cough is among the most common presenting complaints of outpatients in the United States. It serves as a protective reflex against foreign material and as a method to clear secretions from the airway. The cough center is located in the medulla, and the cough reflex is mediated by way of multiple nervous system pathways including the trigeminal, glossopharyngeal, vagus, and phrenic nerves. Cough is mediated by separate neural pathways from bronchoconstriction. When cough occurs there is a synchronized activation of muscles, the glottis opens, and the lungs expand. At the peak of inspiration the glottis closes and expiratory muscles contract. This results in increased intrathoracic pressure; when the glottis opens airflow can reach 500 miles per hour. The cough reflex varies in different patient populations. Women have a more sensitive cough reflex than men. Smokers' cough reflexes are depressed despite the increased frequency of cough in this population. Patients who have a decreased cough sensitivity following cerebral vascular accidents have an increased incidence of pneumonia. Angiotensin-converting enzyme (ACE) inhibitors increase cough reflex sensitivity and have been shown to decrease the risk of pneumonia in patients with cerebrovascular accidents. The evaluation of cough as a patient complaint may best be pursued by examining the duration of the symptoms. Cough can be subcategorized into acute and chronic cough. Cough that occurs following an acute respiratory infection may narrow the differential diagnosis and is addressed separately.

Acute Cough

Acute cough may be defined as cough that has been present for less than 8 weeks. Because all causes of chronic coughs initially cause acute symptoms, patients with acute cough may actually have cough caused by one of the etiologies discussed later in this section; however, acute cough more commonly is the result of a less indolent process (Box 1). Infectious etiologies are a frequent cause of acute cough. Most acute cough is the result of viral infections, specifically the common cold. Most cough resulting from the common cold is self-limited

---

BOX 1 Causes of Acute Cough

- Viral upper respiratory infections (the common cold)
- Acute sinusitis (usually viral, occasionally bacterial)
- Exacerbation of chronic obstructive pulmonary disease
- Allergic rhinitis
- *Bordetella pertussis* infection

---

and lasts less than 3 weeks. Most episodes of sinusitis are of viral etiology; however, bacterial sinusitis can also result in acute cough. The presence of a significant smoking history raises the possibility of an acute exacerbation of chronic obstructive pulmonary disease (COPD) as the cause of acute cough, especially in patients with previously documented COPD. *Bordetella pertussis* infection may also be the etiology of an acute episode of cough. Noninfectious processes that lead to acute cough include allergic rhinitis, congestive heart failure, asthma, and aspiration. The clinical history, physical exam, and diagnostic testing are of particular importance in differentiating these disease states and often point to the diagnosis.

Postinfectious Cough

Postinfectious cough begins with an acute upper respiratory tract infection but persists following the resolution of the other acute symptoms (Box 2). Postnasal drip syndrome may present following the common cold or sinusitis. Bronchospasm may lead to postinfectious cough either as a result of a single episode of postinfectious wheezing or an exacerbation of underlying asthma. Postinfectious cough may be the initial presentation of asthma. Recurrent episodes of airflow obstruction are required to confirm the diagnosis of this chronic illness. Because *B. pertussis* can present with an indolent course, this infection can be confused with a postinfectious cough. Similarly, bacterial sinusitis can be confused with postinfectious cough. Both of these etiologies of cough are the result of ongoing infection rather than true postinfectious cough. *Mycoplasma pneumoniae* and *Chlamydia pneumoniae* infections may also result in postinfectious cough likely because of persistent airway inflammation and increases in cough reflex sensitivity.

Chronic Cough

Chronic cough presents the most difficult diagnostic dilemma for the health care practitioner. Cough of greater than 8 weeks, duration can be considered chronic. Lesser duration of symptoms may still be indicative of one of the etiologies discussed in this section, but such cough is more likely the result of one of the infectious or postinfectious etiologies described previously. In patients who have never smoked, chronic cough is most likely the result of asthma, postnasal drip syndrome, or gastroesophageal reflux. These three etiologies are the most common cause of chronic cough regardless of

patient age. In nonsmokers with a normal chest radiograph who are not taking an ACE inhibitor, these three etiologies alone or in combination are the cause of more than 85% of chronic cough (Box 3). Postnasal drip syndrome is the most common of these etiologies. Cough may be the sole presenting symptom of any of these conditions; they are not mutually exclusive and may coexist, particularly in the patient with troublesome, persistent symptoms. Most patients with problematic, persistent cough have multiple etiologies contributing to their symptoms. COPD must be considered in current smokers and in those patients with a significant smoking history. Smokers can have a cough of any etiology, however, and it should not be assumed that their cough is the result of smoking or COPD. Although smokers frequently admit to cough when a history is taken, they infrequently seek medical attention for this symptom. Cough resulting from the use of ACE inhibitors must be considered in all patients being treated with these medications. Less common, yet frequent causes of cough include chronic bronchitis from irritants other than tobacco smoke and eosinophilic bronchitis. Occasionally, chronic cough may be the result of:

- Bronchogenic carcinoma
- Metastatic carcinoma
- Bronchiectasis
- Sarcoidosis
- Pulmonary fibrosis
- Pneumoconiosis
- Hypersensitivity pneumonitis
- Congestive heart failure
- Chronic infection, such as tuberculosis or *mycobacterium avium* complex
- Recurrent aspiration because of pharyngeal or esophageal abnormalities

Key Diagnostic Points

The evaluation of acute cough should focus on the history and physical exam. Most acute cough will be the result of self-limited viral upper respiratory infections. More thorough evaluation is necessary in the workup of cough of longer duration particularly if the cough has been present for more than 2 months. The history of onset of the cough and whether it was associated with an acute infectious episode should be elicited. Exposure to sick contacts particularly to a known case of *B. pertussis* are important historic considerations. The timing and nature of the cough and any associated sputum

---

BOX 2   Causes of Postinfectious Cough
• Postnasal drip syndrome • Bronchospasm • *Bordetella pertussis* infection • Bacterial sinusitis • *Mycoplasma pneumoniae/Chlamydia pneumoniae* infection

BOX 3   Causes of Chronic Cough
• Postnasal drip syndrome • Asthma • Gastroesophageal reflux disease (GERD) • Eosinophilic bronchitis • Angiotensin converting enzyme inhibitors

must be described. Factors that mitigate or worsen the cough should be examined, and prior history of episodic cough, allergies, wheezing, asthma, and gastroesophageal reflux should be questioned. A thorough medication history particularly regarding use of ACE inhibitors must be obtained. Environmental factors both at home and in the work place should be reviewed. Although smoking history is important, it is again noted that smoking-related cough is an infrequent reason for a patient to seek medical attention. The physical exam should focus most on the head, neck, and thorax with a thorough examination of the upper respiratory tract including the auditory canal, nose, and oropharynx. The cardiopulmonary exam should also be thorough to elicit signs of less common illnesses.

Acute cough associated with an acute respiratory illness and prominent upper airway symptoms can be assumed to be secondary to the common cold. Diagnostic testing is not indicated in such patients; a chest radiograph would be normal and is thus not recommended. Patients who have abnormal sinus transillumination, purulent nasal secretions, sinus pain or tenderness, or maxillary toothache could possibly have bacterial sinusitis. Again, a viral etiology of sinusitis is more likely than bacterial sinusitis, and antibiotic therapy should be initiated only in patients with persistent symptoms despite symptomatic therapy. Patients with documented COPD who present with acute cough, purulent sputum, dyspnea, and wheezing have an exacerbation of their underlying COPD and should be treated appropriately. Allergic rhinitis usually presents with a clear clinical history of episodic nasal and other allergy symptoms, and allergen avoidance can be initiated. It is important to note that allergic rhinitis can present with perennial symptoms.

Postinfectious cough should be evaluated with thorough history and physical exams followed by limited diagnostic evaluation and empiric therapies. Patients should be treated for postnasal drip syndrome, particularly in the setting of described rhinitis, postnasal drip, or frequent throat clearing. The presence of nasal inflammation and congestion, cobblestoning of the pharyngeal mucosa, or mucus in the oropharynx should also lead to empiric therapy for postnasal drip syndrome. If cough persists in the patients with suspected postnasal drip syndrome, evaluation of the sinuses with imaging and treatment of those patients with evidence of bacterial sinusitis should be pursued. Computed tomography (CT) imaging of the sinuses is the gold standard for diagnosing bacterial sinusitis. Patients with postinfectious cough and an abnormal respiratory exam should have a chest radiograph. Patients with a normal radiograph and evidence of bronchospasm can be empirically treated for airway hyperreactivity. Again the diagnosis of asthma requires recurrent airflow obstruction and cannot be made on the basis of a single episode of postinfectious wheezing or airway hyperreactivity. In subjects with cough and vomiting, known exposure to a case of *B. pertussis*, or in the presence of a *B. pertussis* epidemic in the community, empiric therapy for this illness should be pursued.

Before the vaccine era, *B. pertussis* was an endemic disease, which occurred in cyclic epidemics. It has been documented that *B. pertussis* continues to circulate in the adult population despite control of the disease in the pediatric population by vaccination. Immunity to *B. pertussis,* whether as a result of primary infection or immunization, is shortlived. The longer the elapsed interval since prior infection or immunization and repeat infection, the more likely repeat infection will be symptomatic. Perhaps repeat adolescent and adult booster immunization programs should be implemented to effectively control or eliminate this infection.

History and physical exam remain paramount in the patient presenting with chronic cough. The majority of patients should have a chest radiograph obtained as part of their evaluation. If the history and physical exam suggest that postnasal drip, asthma, or gastroesophageal reflux is the etiology of a patient's symptoms, empiric therapy for these conditions should be initiated. Cough triggered by environmental factors or changes may be secondary to rhinitis and postnasal drip or airway hyperreactivity and asthma. Substernal burning or a sour taste in the mouth, particularly when triggered by supine positioning or bending, should increase the suspicion of gastroesophageal reflux.

If asthma is suspected, spirometry should be performed to document whether airflow obstruction is present. Response to inhaled bronchodilator with normal spirometry is indicative of airway hyperreactivity. Improvement in symptoms and spirometry with empiric asthma therapy even in the setting of normal baseline flow rates also confirms an asthmatic etiology. A methacholine challenge can be performed to confirm airway hyperreactivity. If cough in the setting of a positive methacholine challenge shows absolutely no response to empiric asthma therapy with inhaled corticosteroids and bronchodilators, consider a trial of systemic steroids. If the cough does not respond to aggressive asthma therapy, the methacholine challenge test results were probably false positive; asthma therapy can be discontinued and diagnostic efforts focused elsewhere.

Cough patients being treated with ACE inhibitors should cease these medications. Up to 30% of patients treated with ACE inhibitors will develop a persistent cough, more commonly in women, nonsmokers, and patients of Chinese ancestry. It may take 4 weeks or more for cough caused by ACE inhibitors to resolve following cessation of these medications. In the presence of ACE inhibitor use, further evaluation of dry cough should not be pursued until the patient has been withdrawn from these medications for 1 month.

An abnormal chest radiograph can direct further diagnostic studies and therapies, whereas a normal chest radiograph makes less common etiologies of chronic cough such as carcinoma, congestive heart failure, sarcoidosis, or interstitial lung disease unlikely. Evidence of basilar infiltrates or fibrosis may suggest interstitial lung disease or chronic aspiration. Severe gastroesophageal reflux must be considered in those patients with radiographic evidence of chronic aspiration.

Chronic cough without a definitive etiology can be troubling to both patient and health care provider. A systematic approach can simplify both diagnosis and treatment (Figure 1). It is again stressed that such a

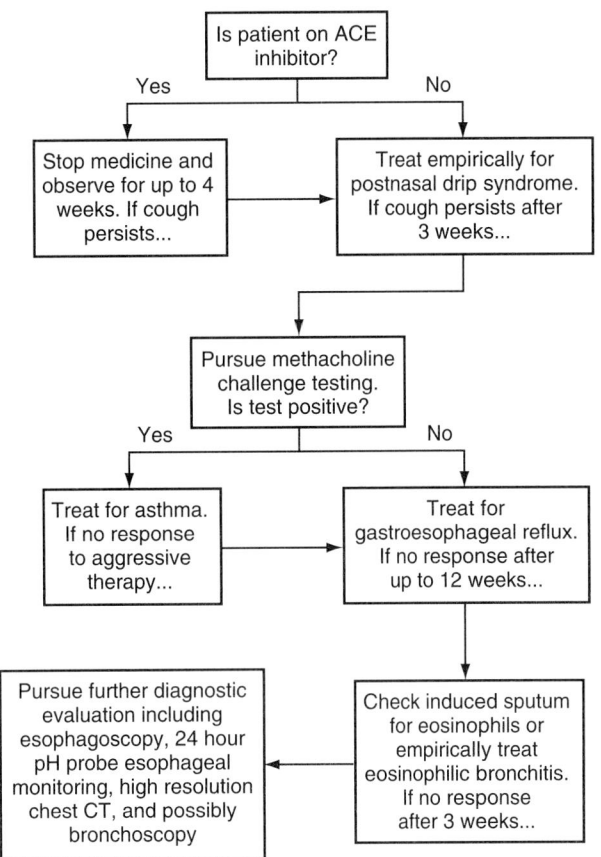

FIGURE 1. Approach to chronic cough of uncertain origin.
ACE = angiotensin-converting enzyme; CT = computed tomography.

cough may be the result of multiple etiologic factors. In the absence of specific factors that help to point to an etiology of chronic cough, empiric treatment for post-nasal drip syndrome should be pursued. Methacholine challenge testing will rule out asthma if it is negative and should also be performed early in the evaluation of chronic cough. Cough may be the sole manifestation of asthma in nearly 60% of patients presenting with chronic cough. A positive methacholine challenge does not have 100% predictive value but should lead to empiric asthma therapy.

Empiric therapy for silent gastroesophageal reflux should be initiated in those who do not respond to treatment for postnasal drip syndrome and do not have evidence of or respond to treatment for asthma. Cough may be the only manifestation of gastroesophageal reflux up to 30% of the time. Definitive diagnosis of gastroesophageal reflux requires invasive testing and may require more than one testing modality. Therefore it is recommended that empiric therapy for reflux be pursued before diagnostic testing. Reflux therapy should include conservative approaches such as dietary and lifestyle changes, bed positioning, and pharmacologic treatment. Gastroesophageal reflux–related cough can be particularly troublesome and persistent and may take weeks or months to respond to appropriate and intensive antireflux therapy. This may include higher-than-normal

doses of proton pump inhibitors and promotility agents. Surgical treatment of reflux may be necessary to effectively treat reflux related cough in some patients. In patients with persistent cough, the common etiologies of cough often coexist and exacerbate one another. Therapy should often be additive, for instance treating both asthma and reflux, rather than mutually exclusive. Persistent cough should result in further diagnostic evaluation including sputum studies, esophagoscopy, 24-hour pH probe esophageal monitoring, high-resolution chest CT, and possibly bronchoscopy. In the presence of normal chest imaging, bronchoscopy is unlikely to yield beneficial diagnostic information in the patient with chronic cough.

Eosinophilic bronchitis in the absence of asthma is also a frequent cause (up to 13% of cases) of chronic cough. Patients with eosinophilic bronchitis will have normal spirometry and a negative methacholine challenge. The disease may be diagnosed by appropriate induced sputum analysis showing at least 3% eosinophils. Alternatively it can be empirically treated with a course of inhaled corticosteroids. Most patients appear to respond to inhaled corticosteroids within 3 weeks. Systemic corticosteroids may be required to improve the symptoms in some cases. There may be an association of gastroesophageal reflux with eosinophilic bronchitis. Patients with gastroesophageal reflux have been found to have increased sputum eosinophilia.

Bronchiectasis may infrequently result in chronic cough. Bronchiectasis is characterized by the abnormal

 CURRENT DIAGNOSIS

All Patients Presenting With Cough

- Perform thorough history and physical examination.
- Review timing and nature of cough along with exacerbating or mitigating factors.
- Review prior history of cough, allergies, asthma, or gastroesophageal reflux.
- Take medication history, particularly use of ACE inhibitors.
- Focus physical exam on head, neck, and thorax.

Patients With Postinfectious or Chronic Cough

- Obtain chest radiograph, particularly in patients with an abnormal respiratory exam.
- Evaluate airflow obstruction with spirometry.
- Stop ACE inhibitors and assess for improvement.
- Administer empiric therapy for postnasal drip, asthma, or gastroesophageal reflux.
- Consider methacholine challenge testing to evaluate for airway hyperreactivity.
- Induce sputum for eosinophils or empiric trial of corticosteroids for eosinophilic bronchitis.
- If cough persists, consider esophagoscopy, 24-hour pH probe monitoring, high-resolution chest CT, or bronchoscopy.

Abbreviations: ACE = angiotensin-converting enzyme; CT = computed tomography.

Rakel and Bope: *Conn's Current Therapy 2006.*

CURRENT THERAPY

Treatment of Acute Cough

- Common cold: Supportive care with dexbrompheniramine, 6 mg, and pseudoephedrine, 120 mg (Drixoral Cold and Allergy tablets); or ipratropium nasal spray (Atrovent, 0.06%), two 42-mcg sprays in each nostril 3 times daily for 4 to 7 days depending on duration of symptoms.
- Acute sinusitis: Treat as a common cold. Add oxymetazoline (Afrin), two sprays twice daily for three days. If symptoms persist, consider antibiotic therapy directed against *Haemophilus influenzae* and *Streptococcus pneumoniae* such as azithromycin (Zithromax), 500 mg daily for 3 days.
- Exacerbation of chronic obstructive pulmonary disease: Antibiotics directed against *H. influenzae* and *S. pneumoniae* for 3 to 7 days such as clarithromycin (Biaxin), 500 mg twice daily for 7 days; systemic corticosteroids such as prednisone (Deltasone), 40 mg tapered over 10 days; inhaled anticholinergics such as tiotropium (Spiriva), one inhalation daily; and short-acting beta agonists such as albuterol (Proventil), two inhalations every 4 hours as needed; smoking cessation.
- Allergic rhinitis: Nasal corticosteroids such as mometasone (Nasonex), two sprays in each nostril daily; nonsedating antihistamines such as fexofenadine (Allegra), 180 mg daily; allergen avoidance if possible.
- *Bordetella pertussis*: Erythromycin 500 mg four times daily for 14 days or trimethoprim 160 mg/sulfamethoxazole (Bactrim DS),[1] 800 mg twice daily for 14 days. Other macrolide antibiotics such as azithromycin (Zithromax)[1] or clarithromycin (Biaxin)[1] are likely effective and may be better tolerated.

Treatment of Postinfectious Cough

- Postnasal drip syndrome: Dexbrompheniramine, 6 mg, and pseudoephedrine (Drixoral Cold and Allergy Tablets), 120 mg for up to 3 weeks; ipratropium (Atrovent), 0.06% nasal spray for up to 3 weeks; azelastine (Astelin) nasal spray (137 mcg), two sprays each nostril twice daily for up to 3 weeks.
- Bronchospasm: Inhaled corticosteroid such as budesonide (Pulmicort),[1] two inhalations daily with or without inhaled long-acting beta agonist

such as formoterol (Foradil), two inhalations twice daily; short-acting beta agonist such as albuterol (Ventolin), two puffs every 4 hours as needed. Oral steroids such as prednisone (Deltasone), 40 mg tapered over 10 days.
- *Bordetella pertussis*: Erythromycin, 500 mg four times daily for 14 days, or trimethoprim 160 mg/sulfamethoxazole, 800 mg (Bactrim DS)[1] twice daily for 14 days. Other macrolide antibiotics such as azithromycin (Zithromax)[1] or clarithromycin (Biaxin)[1] are likely effective and may be better tolerated.
- Bacterial sinusitis: Dexbrompheniramine, 6 mg, and pseudoephedrine (Drixoral Cold and Allergy Tablets), 120 mg for up to 3 weeks; oxymetazoline (Afrin), two sprays twice daily for 3 days; azithromycin (Zithromax), 500 mg daily for 3 days.
- Chlamydia/mycoplasma: Clarithromycin (Biaxin), 500 mg twice daily for 14 days.

Treatment of Chronic Cough

- Postnasal drip syndrome
  Nonallergic: Dexbrompheniramine, 6 mg, and pseudoephedrine (Drixoral Cold and Allergy Tablets), 120 mg for up to 3 weeks; ipratropium (Atrovent), 0.06% nasal spray for up to 3 weeks; azelastine (Astelin) nasal spray (137 mcg), two sprays each nostril twice daily for up to 3 weeks.
  Allergic: Fluticasone (Flonase) (50 mcg), two sprays each nostril daily; fexofenadine (Allegra), 180 mg daily; allergen avoidance.
- Asthma: Albuterol (Proventil), two puffs every 4 hours as needed; inhaled corticosteroid such as budesonide (Pulmicort), two inhalations daily with or without inhaled long-acting beta agonist such as formoterol (Foradil), two inhalations twice daily; combination of long-acting beta agonist and inhaled steroid such as fluticasone/salmeterol (Advair) (100/50 mcg), inhaled twice daily; montelukast (Singulair), 10 mg daily; prednisone (Deltasone), 40 mg daily with tapering dose over 10 days.
- Gastroesophageal reflux: Dietary and lifestyle modifications, lansoprazole (Prevacid), 30 mg daily for up to 3 months; metoclopramide (Reglan), 10 mg before meals and sleep.
- Eosinophilic bronchitis: Fluticasone (Flovent)[1] (110 mcg), two inhalations twice daily; prednisone (Deltasone), 30 mg daily for 3 weeks.
- ACE inhibitor: Discontinue medication.

[1]Not FDA approved for this indication.

dilatation of one or more branches of the bronchial tree. It can effectively be diagnosed by high resolution CT scan of the thorax. Bronchiectasis may occur following a severe infection, distal to an area of airway obstruction, congenitally, from chronic inflammatory processes, and as a result of chronic parenchymal scarring and traction. Patients with bronchiectasis may present with productive or nonproductive coughs. They may have recurrent episodes of infection resulting from persistent colonization of the abnormal bronchial segment. Infectious agents may include routine bacterial organisms and typical or atypical mycobacterium. Bronchiectasis may be seen in a variety of chronic illnesses. The presence of bronchiectasis in a patient without a known predisposing cause should prompt the clinician to look for appropriate clinical states. such as:

- Primary or acquired immunodeficiencies
- Abnormalities of ciliary function, such as ciliary dyskinesia or cystic fibrosis
- Postinfectious inflammatory processes, such as allergic bronchopulmonary aspergillosis
- Collagen vascular diseases
- Inflammatory bowel disease
- Sarcoidosis
- Yellow nail syndrome

The presence of localized bronchiectasis may be an indication to pursue flexible fiberoptic bronchoscopy to rule out an obstructing lesion and to obtain appropriate culture specimens. Treatment of bronchiectasis is aimed at the underlying disease state if one can be identified. Infections should be treated with appropriate antibiotics. Clearance of bronchial secretions can be aided with mucolytics and chest physiotherapy including use of percussive devices. In some cases surgical therapy to remove the bronchiectatic segment can be considered.

Treatment

The key treatments for cough are best described based on the suspected etiology. Acute cough therapy should focus on supportive treatment of the underlying suspected etiology, which will likely be a viral upper respiratory infection. Therapy for exacerbation of chronic obstructive pulmonary disease, allergic rhinitis, bacterial sinusitis, or *B. pertussis* infection is more specific. Postinfectious cough should focus on therapy for postnasal drip syndrome or airways reactivity if suspected. In chronic cough of uncertain etiology (see Figure 1), cough therapy should begin with empiric treatment of postnasal drip syndrome, evaluation and treatment of asthma, empiric treatment of gastroesophageal reflux syndrome, and finally evaluation or empiric therapy for eosinophilic bronchitis.

Cough is a frequent and troublesome symptom for both patient and health care provider. Acute cough although at times troubling is usually self-limiting. Postinfectious cough and chronic cough are more problematic, but can effectively be evaluated and treated by performing a thorough history and physical exam and pursuing a systematic approach to diagnostic evaluation and both empiric and guided therapies. The resolution of chronic troubling cough is a therapeutic relief for the patient and a gratifying experience for the caregiver.

REFERENCES

Barnes TW, Afessa B, Swanson KL, Lim KG: The clinical utility of flexible bronchoscopy in the evaluation of chronic cough. Chest 2004;126:268-272.
Breitling CE, Ward R, Goh KL: Eosinophilic bronchitis is an important cause of chronic cough. Am J Respir Crit Care Med 1999; 160:406-410.
Cherry JD: Epidemiological, clinical, and laboratory aspects of pertussis in adults. Clin Infect Dis 1999;28(suppl2):S112-S117.
Cohen M, Sahn SA: Bronchiectasis in systemic diseases. Chest 1999; 116:1063-1074.
Irwin RS, Madison JM: Symptom research on chronic cough: A historical perspective. Ann Intern Med 2001;134:809-814.
Irwin RS, Madison JM: The diagnosis and treatment of cough. N Engl J Med 2000;343:1715-1721.
Irwin RS, Madison JM: The persistently troublesome cough. Am J Respir Crit Care Med 2002;165:1469-1474.
Kiljander TO: The role of proton pump inhibitors in the management of gastroesophageal reflux disease-related asthma and chronic cough. Am J Med 2003;115(3A):S65-S71.

Treatment of Insomnia

Method of
Martin Reite, MD

Three things should be remembered when considering treatment of an insomnia complaint. First, insomnia is more often a symptom, than a specific disorder. Second, it is important to perform a systematic differential diagnosis, keeping in mind the possibility that there will be very likely more than one cause of an insomnia complaint. Finally, the cause of the complaint usually can be determined, and most patients complaining of insomnia can be helped. Also, insomnia must not be trivialized.

Insomnia is among the most frequent complaints in the population; untreated insomnia is associated with increases in new-onset anxiety and depression, increased daytime sleepiness, and increased health-related concerns.

Insomnia can include difficulty in getting to sleep (sleep-onset insomnia), difficulty staying asleep (sleep-maintenance insomnia), or early morning awakening (terminal insomnia). Because such subtypes are not stable over time, this method of subtyping may have little clinical usefulness. As a rule, insomnia complaints are more frequent in women, elderly persons, and patients of lower socioeconomic status.

Screening for Sleep Complaints

Three routine questions, illustrated in Box 1, will detect most significant sleep problems. A positive answer to any of these questions merits consideration of a more detailed sleep history to determine whether in fact a

---

BOX 1   Detection of Specific Sleep Disorders

Are you content with your sleep? (identifies most insomnia complaints)
Are you excessively sleepy during the day? (identifies most disorders of excessive sleepiness)
Does your bed partner complain about your sleep? (identifies most parasomnia disorders)

---

sleep disorder is present. Box 2 outlines the items to be covered in a sleep history.

Sources of diagnostic information should include the bed partner whenever possible because many sleep-related symptoms are apparent only to the bed partner. A several-week daily sleep diary also can be useful at this stage of the evaluation because it can provide a detailed daily description of sleep/wake activity patterns.

Transient and Short-Term Insomnia

Transient (1 to several days) and short-term (up to 3 weeks) insomnias are typically stress related, and respond well to pharmacologic (short-term hypnotic) intervention. They should be considered for active treatment, because untreated short-term insomnia can lead to a state of "conditioned arousal" resulting in a chronic insomnia.

Differential Diagnosis of the Chronic Insomnia Complaint

The differential diagnosis of a chronic insomnia complaint can represent a more challenging task and requires a thorough differential diagnostic evaluation, which includes systematically considering the conditions or combinations of conditions that are most likely to result in insomnia complaints. General practice parameters for the evaluation of chronic insomnia complaints can be found at: http://www.aasmnet.org/PDF/ChronicParameter.pdf. Box 3 lists the common causes of insomnia (not necessarily listed in order of frequency). Each cause is briefly discussed.

MEDICAL CONDITIONS AND TREATMENT

Medical conditions, and in susceptible patients, many pharmacologic treatments of medical conditions, can result in insomnia complaints. The endocrinopathies are notorious for being associated with sleep-related complaints, as are conditions associated with chronic pain, breathing difficulties, cardiac arrhythmias, arthritis, renal failure, and central nervous system (CNS) disorders. Box 4 lists the more commonly used medications that can result in insomnia complaints.

BOX 2 Sleep History Questionnaire

When did the symptoms start, and what was going on at the time?
What has been the symptom pattern across time?
Are symptoms stress or situationally related?
What is your typical daily schedule, hour by hour?
What medications and treatments have been and are currently being used to date?
Is there a presence of familial sleep-related symptoms?

BOX 3 Common Causes of Insomnia

Medical conditions and/or pharmacologic treatment of medical conditions
Psychiatric disorders (especially depression, anxiety, and post-traumatic stress disorder [PTSD])
Substance abuse disorders
Circadian rhythm disorders presenting as insomnia
Periodic limb movements in sleep (PLMS)
Central sleep apnea
The primary insomnia, conditioned insomnia, and sleep-state misperception group

---

The treatment of insomnia associated with medical conditions is first to isolate and appropriately treat the medical condition and the symptoms (e.g., pain) causing the insomnia. If the insomnia complaint persists, evaluate the possibility of an additional cause for the sleep complaint. Supplementary use of a short half-life hypnotic agent [e.g., zolpidem (Ambien), 5-10 mg at bedtime] may be helpful. Insomnia associated with fibromyalgia and chronic fatigue syndrome is frequently resistant to treatment, although small doses of amitriptyline (Elavil)[1] (10-50 mg at bedtime) or cyclobenzaprine (Flexeril)[1] (10 mg three times a day) have been reported to be helpful; occasionally, zolpidem (5-10 mg) will help with the associated insomnia complaints.

Dementing illnesses are often associated with severe insomnia complaints that are quite disruptive to patients and families and often are the factors precipitating institutional care. Sleep is often disturbed in such disorders on the basis of disease-associated CNS lesions, and different specific pathophysiologies (not yet well understood) may respond to different treatments. Until such specific treatments can be based on specific pathophysiology, we should adhere to optimal environmental circadian principles (quiet, dark nocturnal environment; bright, socially stimulating daytime environment). Appropriate use of hypnotics may be helpful, although responses may be variable.

---

[1]Not FDA approved for this indication.

BOX 4 Medications Often Associated with Insomnia

Anticholinergics
Antidepressants
Antihypertensives
Antineoplastic agents
Bronchodilators
CNS stimulants
Corticosteroids
Decongestants
Diuretics
Histamine-2 (H2) blockers
Smoking cessation aids

Rakel and Bope: *Conn's Current Therapy 2006.*

PSYCHIATRIC DISORDERS

Psychiatric disorders, especially those associated with anxiety or depression, frequently include insomnia (delayed sleep onset, frequent awakening, or early morning awakening) as an associated symptom. Effective treatment of the psychiatric condition will often relieve the insomnia complaint, although a supplemental hypnotic might be indicated early in treatment. Different antidepressant agents have quite different effects on sleep as illustrated in Table 1, and the initial choice of an antidepressant might profitably take such effects into account.

If, for a patient already complaining of insomnia, an antidepressant with a known high incidence of insomnia side effects is chosen, it may be useful to augment it with a hypnotic agent early in the course of treatment.

SUBSTANCE USE SLEEP DISORDERS

Alcohol abuse remains a significant problem in the etiology of sleep complaints, as do stimulants and other drugs of abuse. Treatment includes withdrawal of the offending substance, with long-term abstinence as the goal. Treatment of substance abuse-related insomnia should emphasize behavioral treatment strategies to the fullest extent possible, because psychoactive agents have already proved to be a problem.

CIRCADIAN RHYTHM DISORDERS

Disturbances in the regulation of the circadian system frequently present as sleep-related complaints, although the source of the problem lies in the circadian system rather than sleep pathology. Sleep per se may be adequate, but it occurs at the wrong time. Delayed sleep-phase syndrome (DSPS) is the most common, and is likely a genetically based disorder with frequent onset in adolescence or early adulthood. These individuals cannot get to sleep (because of phase delay in the body temperature rhythm) until 3 to 4 a.m., and if allowed to sleep, 8 to 9 hours may do well. If they have to arise at 7 a.m. for school or work, they will be sleep deprived and complain of insomnia.

Early morning bright-light exposure, with restriction of light exposure in the evening, has been found to be effective for phase-advancing the circadian system in DSPS. Evening bright-light treatment is effective in treating advanced sleep-phase syndrome. Low-dose (1-3 mg) melatonin[1,*] at bedtime may help regulate circadian rhythms in some individuals.

Jet lag and shift-work–related sleep problems also fall in the category of circadian rhythm problems. A detailed discussion of these problem areas is beyond

[1]Not FDA approved for this indication.
*Available as a dietary supplement.

TABLE 1 Effect of Antidepressants on Sleep Scale*

Effects on EEG Sleep

Drug	Trade Name	Continuity	SWS	REM	Sedation Effects
TCAs					
Amitriptyline	Elavil	I (3)	I (1)	D (3)	4
Doxepin	Sinequan	I (3)	I (2)	D (2)	4
Imipramine	Tofranil	I (0-1)	I (1)	D (2)	2
Nortriptyline	Pamelor	I (1)	I (1)	D (2)	2
Desipramine	Norpramin	(0)	I (1)	D (2)	1
Clomipramine	Anafranil	I (0-1)	I (1)	D (4)	0
MAOIs					
Phenelzine	Nardil	D (1)	(0)	D (4)	0
Tranylcypromine	Parnate	D (2)	(0)	D (4)	0
SSRIs					
Fluoxetine	Prozac	D (1)	D (0-1)	D (0-1)	0
Paroxetine	Paxil	D (1)	D (0-1)	D (2)	0
Sertraline	Zoloft	(0)	(0)	D (2)	0
Citalopram	Celexa	D (1)	(0)	D (1)	ND
Fluvoxamine	Luvox	D (1)	(0)	D (1)	ND
Escitalopram	Lexapro	(0)	(0)	D (2)	0
Other					
Bupropion	Wellbutrin	D (0-1)	(0)	I (1)	0
Venlafaxine	Effexor	D (1)	D (1)	D (3)	2
Trazodone	Desyrel	I (3)	I (0-1)	D (1)	4
Mirtazapine	Remeron	I (3)	I (2)	(0)	3
Nefazodone	Serzone	I (1)	(0)	I (1)	1

Abbreviations: EEG = electroencephalogram; MAOIs = monoamine oxidase inhibitors; REM = rapid eye movement; SSRIs = selective serotonin reuptake inhibitors; SWS = slow-wave sleep; TCAs = tricyclic antidepressants.
*Scale 0-4: 0 = no significant effect; I = increase and D = decrease.

Rakel and Bope: *Conn's Current Therapy 2006.*

the scope of this article, but recently emerging data suggest that properly timed bright-light exposure, supplemented with melatonin[1],[*] administration and appropriate hypnotic use, can significantly reduce associated symptoms.

PERIODIC LIMB MOVEMENTS OF SLEEP AND RESTLESS LEGS SYNDROME

Both restless legs syndrome (RLS) and periodic limb movements of sleep (PLMS) are associated with a variety of medical conditions, including iron deficiency, but they may occur in otherwise healthy individuals (especially the elderly). A polysomnogram (PSG) is usually required for accurate diagnosis of a PLMS disorder, quantifying both the number of events and their association with awakenings or arousals. Table 2 lists the drugs currently used in the treatment of PLMS and RLS.

CENTRAL SLEEP APNEA

Central sleep apnea with frequent arousals is a relatively rare cause of chronic insomnia except at higher altitudes, and may require a PSG for accurate diagnosis. Both oxygen and continuous positive airway pressure (CPAP) can be used in the treatment of central apnea in patients with medical disorders. The efficacy of pharmacologic agents in the treatment of central sleep apnea has yet to be clearly established in well-controlled studies. Acetazolamide (Diamox)[1] (250 mg twice a day) may be effective for the prevention of high altitude-induced central apnea.

---

[1]Not FDA approved for this indication.
[*]Available as a dietary supplement.

THE PRIMARY INSOMNIA, CONDITIONED INSOMNIA, AND SLEEP-STATE MISPERCEPTION SYNDROME GROUP

Although there are several more rare causes of a chronic insomnia complaint, most often it is generally safe to assume that once the aforementioned specific causes have been systematically excluded or appropriately treated (and the insomnia complaints remain), we are in all probability left with either a primary insomnia disorder (DSM-IV 307.42), a conditioned insomnia, a sleep-state misperception syndrome (SSMS), or some combination thereof.

A treatment approach that combines both behavioral and pharmacologic approaches is generally recommended. Such a combined treatment approach offers the advantage of a pharmacologic agent that can produce rapid relief of the sleep complaint, along with behavioral strategies, which take longer to become effective but provide long-term results that are under a patient's control. Active and continued involvement of the patient is important for any chronic insomnia treatment.

Sleep Laboratory Studies

All night PSGs, which monitor multiple physiologic variables during sleep, are rarely needed in the evaluation of insomnia complaints, except for symptoms associated with PLMS or for a sleep-related breathing disorder, where a PSG is usually required for accurate diagnosis. A recent review of the use of PSGs in the insomnia complaints can be found at: http://www.aasmnet.org/PDF/260616.pdf

The 24-hour recording of activity (Actigraphy) can also be useful in the diagnosis of circadian rhythm-based

---

TABLE 2 Beginning Dose Schedules for PMLS and RLS

Drug	Dose (mg)	Administration
Dopa Agonists		
Carbidopa/Levodopa	25/100-50/200	Bedtime/(Sinemet)[1] symptom onset
Controlled-release	25/100-50/200	Bedtime/Carbidopa/Levodopa symptom onset (Sinemet CR)[1]
Bromocriptine (Parlodel)[1]	2.5-5	Bedtime
Baclofen (Lioresal)[1]	20-40	Bedtime
Pergolide (Permax)[1]	0.05	Bedtime/symptom onset
Pramipexole (Mirapex)[1]	0.125	Bedtime
Ropinirole (Requip)[1]	0.25	Bedtime
Other Agents		
Oxycodone (Roxicodone)[1]	5-15	Bedtime
Codeine[1]	10-60	Bedtime
Triazolam (Halcion)[1]	0.125-0.25	Bedtime
Temazepam (Restoril)[1]	15-30	Bedtime
Clonazepam (Klonopin)[1]	0.5-1.5	Bedtime
Gabapentin (Neurontin)[1]	100-300	Bedtime

[1]Not FDA approved for this indication.

sleep complaints (e.g., see: http://www.aasmnet.org/PDF/260315.pdf

Treatment

After completing the evaluation of a chronic insomnia complaint and arriving at a diagnostic formulation, a treatment plan should be developed addressing all likely contributing causes. The treatment plan will likely include both behavioral and pharmacologic components, and should be discussed in detail with the patient. Patients might be encouraged to visit the web pages of the American Sleep Disorders Association (www.asda.org) and the National Sleep Foundation (www.nsf.org) to learn more about factors influencing sleep. Patient education facilitates effective treatment.

BEHAVIORAL TREATMENTS

Behavioral treatment strategies are aimed at (a) breaking bad sleep habits and replacing them with sleep-promoting habits; (b) directly decreasing physiologic arousal levels using cognitively based or learned strategies; and (c) providing the patient with several types of cognitive strategies to deal with sleep difficulties, thus promoting a sense of competence and diminishing anxiety about sleep. First and foremost among the behavioral strategies is good sleep hygiene—the behaviors and habits that foster good sleep. Box 5 highlights the principles of good sleep hygiene. It is helpful to prepare a handout for patients summarizing good sleep hygiene practices that they can take with them. Box 6 lists additional behavioral strategies.

PHARMACOLOGIC TREATMENTS

Benzodiazepine (BZ) compounds and newer nonbenzodiazepine agents active at the level of the BZ receptor are the most commonly used hypnotic agents. Older hypnotic agents (chloral hydrate, paraldehyde [Paral], barbiturates) may have limited usefulness for very short-term use in specific patients, but they cannot be recommended for the treatment of chronic insomnia.

BOX 5   Good Sleep Hygiene

Establish a regular sleep schedule that does not vary by more than 1 hour.
Maintain a state of good aerobic fitness with regular exercise (but not within 3 hours of sleep onset).
Do not use caffeine or alcohol to excess.
Ensure a quiet, dark, cool bedroom.
Provide a time to wind down in the evening before sleeping.
Consider a high-tryptophan snack (milk, cookies, banana) before bed.
Use the bedroom for sleep and sex but not for reviewing or thinking about the affairs of the day.
Minimize exposure to late evening bright light to avoid phase-delaying the circadian system.

BOX 6   Other Behavioral Strategies for the Treatment of Insomnia

Biofeedback (EMG and EEG): teaches subjects to decrease autonomic arousal
Progressive relaxation: training in systematic total body relaxation
Sleep restriction: good for subjects spending excessive time in bed with poorly consolidated sleep
Yoga, transcendental meditation (TM): self-control strategies
Cognitive behavioral therapy (several types): improved self-confidence and self-control

---

BZ agents activate all BZ receptors (hypnotic, anxiolytic, muscle relaxant, anticonvulsant), and different agents demonstrate relatively little receptor specificity.

The BZ compounds differ substantially in terms of half-life and are illustrated in Table 3. The clinician can choose the agent with a half-life most appropriate for the clinical situation.

Long half-life BZ agents may be associated with residual daytime sedation and impairments in psychomotor performance. All BZ agents interfere with memory consolidation, the more potent agents (e.g., triazolam [Halcion]) most prominently. All BZ agents are prone to the development of tolerance, dependence, and rebound insomnia in response to rapid withdrawal. BZ agents also tend to decrease stages 3 to 4 sleep, and increase fast activity in the waking and sleeping electroencephalogram (EEG). These results may continue after drug discontinuation. Clearly useful for the treatment of insomnia associated with anxiety, the use of long-term BZ treatment of primary insomnia is problematic, especially in light of the research and development of new, apparently safe and effective nonbenzodiazepine agents designed to be selectively more active on the hypnotic receptor.

Newer non-BZ agents selectively active at the omega$_1$ (primarily hypnotic) BZ receptor include the imidazopyridine zolpidem (Ambien), and the cyclopyralone zaleplon (Sonata) that are effective and relatively safe hypnotics that do not alter sleep architecture, and do not appear to induce significant tolerance, dependence, or withdrawal. Both agents have a rapid onset of action, but differ in half-life and duration of action. Zolpidem (5-10 mg) can be taken if the patient has 6 to 7 hours to sleep. Zaleplon can be taken if the patient has 4 hours available for sleep.

Antidepressant agents, especially sedative tricyclics, are frequently used at low doses to manage chronic insomnia despite the relative lack of well-controlled double-blind studies demonstrating efficacy. These agents are clearly indicated in insomnia that accompanies depressive disorders, where their effectiveness is clear. These agents are normally taken about one hour before bedtime so their sedative effects have time to emerge. This effectively teaches the patient to take a pill to sleep, which is counterproductive for treating insomnia. The new non-BZ hypnotics with their rapid onset of action

TABLE 3 Benzodiazepines

Name		Dose (mg)			
Generic	Trade Name	Adult	Elderly	Onset	Half-Life (Hours)
Triazolam	Halcion	0.125-0.25	0.125-0.25	Rapid	1.5-5.5
Estazolam	ProSom	1-2	0.5-1	Rapid	20-30
Temazepam	Restoril	15-30	7.5-15	Intermediate	8-20
Quazepam	Doral	7.5-15	7.5	Intermediate	15-120
Flurazepam	Dalmane	15-30	7.5	Intermediate	36-250

can be placed at the bedside and are taken if the patient has not fallen asleep within 30 minutes.

Several agents more directly involved in modulating γ-aminobutyric acid (GABA) activity, such as tiagabine (Gabitril)[1] and sodium oxybate (Xyrem),[1] have been used in limited studies to promote slow-wave sleep, but there are insufficient published data to make specific recommendations as to their potential usefulness in insomnia at this time.

LONG-TERM USE OF HYPNOTIC AGENTS

Current thinking suggests we might best conceptualize primary insomnia as a chronic disorder that will likely require long-term treatment. Considering the known adverse effects of chronic sleep loss, in the context of the present availability of relatively safe and effective hypnotic agents, there would appear to be no reason to withhold or severely limit pharmacologic treatment in those responsible patients for whom a comprehensive and thorough diagnostic evaluation has established the presence of a primary insomnia disorder. It should go without saying, however, that behavioral treatment also should be actively implemented in those patients who are being considered for long-term pharmacologic management.

---

[1]Not FDA approved for this indication.

Pruritus

Method of
James A. Yiannias, MD, and
Michael P. Conroy, MD, MS

Pruritus is a subjective sensation of itch with a host of causes and treatment options. The sensation is most often a clinical finding associated with a purely dermatologic disorder, but it may also be a presenting symptom of an underlying systemic condition.

In dermatology practices, pruritus is commonly associated with numerous entities labeled *dermatitis*. Contact dermatitis, particularly allergic contact dermatitis (ACD),

is observed in virtually all medical specialties. Although seeking the cause of *the itch* can be daunting, it is manageable when approached systematically. Likewise, pruritus often can be treated appropriately with a logically ordered therapeutic algorithm. In most cases, successful treatment lies in aggressive lubrication, whereas more involved cases may require mitigation of systemic disease.

Pathophysiology

Mediators of itch are unique to the skin, mucous membranes, and cornea. This article is limited to a discussion of cutaneous itch. Although the origin of itch has not been fully elucidated, it likely emanates from the free nerve endings. These unencapsulated structures are localized within the dermis and possibly around the dermoepidermal junction. After stimulation, the impulse is transmitted along C fibers to the dorsal roots of the spine, producing a scratch reflex.

A heterogeneous group of mechanisms can induce itching, including the release of histamine (in urticaria and allergic reactions) or serotonin, peripheral neuropathies, immune mechanisms (atopic dermatitis, ACD), and drugs (opioids). Pruritus can be heightened by xerosis (dry skin). Hydration of the skin therefore increases the patient's level of comfort, regardless of the cause.

Key Diagnostic Points

The treatment approach to patients with pruritus necessitates a systematic, logical, and thorough workup. Simply stated, the causes can be classified as dermatologic (Table 1) or systemic (Table 2). Dermatologic causes, such as urticaria, xerosis, ACD, or atopic dermatitis, account for most physician visits associated with pruritus.

Urticaria is a common cutaneous condition associated with transient pink or red edematous plaques and marked pruritus mediated by histamine. This condition can be frustrating to patient and clinician alike, because it may be controlled but not cured and its cause typically remains elusive. Xerosis is common in older adults and patients living in cold or dry environments. ACD may be caused by numerous potential allergens, such as urushiol (the allergen in poison ivy), which are obvious by history and physical examination.

Other less-apparent allergens (e.g., nickel, rubber, neomycin, and the preservatives and fragrances used in

TABLE 1 Common Dermatologic Causes of Pruritus

Cause	Feature
Urticaria	Urticarial papules or plaques Transient (>24 h; if lesions persist, question diagnosis) Variants (caused by cold, exercise, vibration, or pressure)
Allergic contact dermatitis	History (particularly important) Acute: vesicles or bullae Subacute: juicy papules Chronic: lichenification
Atopic dermatitis	Morphologic characteristics as above in contact dermatitis Asthma, hay fever (often in association) Common involvement with flexural skin (antecubital or popliteal fossae)
Psoriasis	Red plaques with silvery scales (well marginated and often involving elbows, knees, and intergluteal cleft)
Lichen planus	5 Ps (purple, polygonal, planar, pruritic, papules)
Scabies	Burrows (finger webs, waistband area, genitals) Contagiousness (treat intimate contacts)
Bullous pemphigoid	Tense bullae (evolves classically with pruritus as presenting symptom) Age (affects adults older than age 55 years)
Dermatitis herpetiformis	Microvesicles, often localized to lumbar back, elbows, and knees Celiac sprue (often in close association)

TABLE 2 Common Systemic Causes of Pruritus

Cause	Feature
Medication Opioids (common offenders)	Stimulation of μ receptors in central nervous system
Thyroid disease Hyperthyroidism	Moist skin, heat intolerance, weight loss, infrequently pretibial myxedema
Hypothyroidism	Dry skin, cold intolerance, weight gain
Infection Human immunodeficiency virus Parasitic (schistosomiasis, filariasis)	Itchiness
Uremia	*Uremic frost* (uncommon) Intermittent itching (more common)
Liver disease	Itchiness (possibly stimulated by bile salts in skin)
Malignancy Hodgkin lymphoma Multiple myeloma	Itchiness frequently precedes diagnosis Bone pain, anemia, renal failure (may be more common in patients 60 years old or older)

skin-care and cleaning products) may necessitate patch testing. The pruritus of atopic dermatitis is in patients of virtually any age group and may not demonstrate a profound rash. Other dermatologic conditions with an often substantial component of pruritus include scabies, psoriasis, lichen planus, bullous pemphigoid, dermatitis herpetiformis, and mycosis fungoides (cutaneous T-cell lymphoma).

Of patients who present with generalized pruritus, 10% to 50% have an underlying systemic cause, so further workup is warranted for refractory itching. In general, any failure to improve after several weeks of symptomatic therapy should trigger a more extensive evaluation. Diagnostic considerations of systemic causes include medications, uremia, liver disease, thyroid disease (hyperthyroidism or hypothyroidism), malignancy (Hodgkin's lymphoma or multiple myeloma), infection (HIV or parasitic infection), peripheral neuropathy, and cutaneous mastocytosis.

The typical approach to the diagnosis of pruritus follows an algorithm that begins with a thorough history and physical examination (Figure 1). The history should identify the location of lesions and their onset, duration, and evolution. It should also include a detailed medication history (prescription and over-the-counter; oral and topical), any occupational exposures, a travel history, and affected persons with whom the patient came in contact. Lest they omit them, patients should be asked specifically about over-the-counter and as-needed medications.

When the patient history and physical examination do not indicate a prominent or worrisome systemic illness, symptomatic treatment may be implemented. If there is no improvement after several weeks of compliance, then a first-tier laboratory evaluation should include a complete blood cell count (CBC) and measurements of thyroid-stimulating hormone (TSH), liver function enzymes (aspartate transaminase, alanine transaminase, alkaline phosphatase), and renal function (blood urea nitrogen [BUN], creatinine clearance).

If the initial laboratory workup provides no clinically significant findings, then second-tier laboratory tests should be considered. These tests should be directed at age-appropriate diagnostic considerations, such as serum protein electrophoresis (SPEP), to rule out multiple myeloma in patients older than 50 years of age.

An age- and sex-appropriate malignancy workup is of particular importance. Thus, the further evaluation of middle-aged or elderly women with refractory pruritus should include mammography and pelvic ultrasonography. Men older than age 50 should have prostate evaluations. Both men and women should have chest radiography and a colonoscopy. Indeed, both hematologic and solid tumors may demonstrate itch as an initial manifestation, sometimes years before an established diagnosis. Nevertheless, *total-body* computed tomography (CT) should be reserved for patients with a negative initial screening or other suggestive features, such as unexplained fatigue or weight loss.

Patients with smoldering immunobullous diseases, such as pemphigus or pemphigoid, can present with the

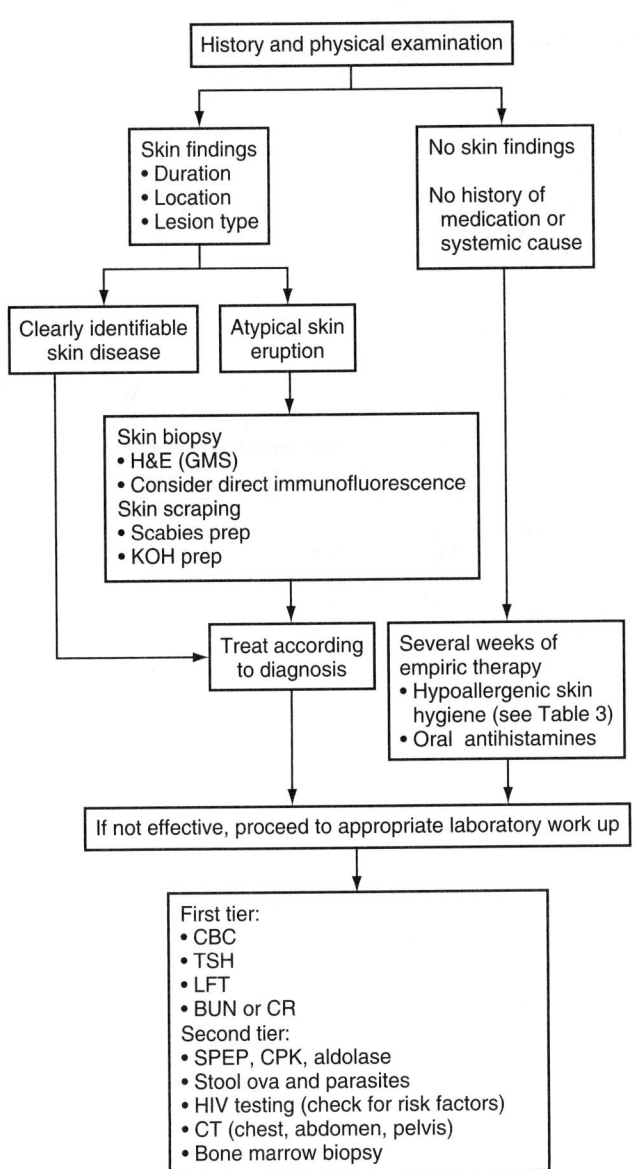

FIGURE 1. A useful diagnostic algorithm for patients with pruritus proceeds from the history and physical examination through first- and second-tier laboratory tests, if necessary. BUN = blood urea nitrogen; CBC = complete blood cell count; CPK = creatine phosphokinase; CR = creatinine ratio; CT = computed tomography; GMS = Gomori methenamine silver stain; H&E = hematoxylin and eosin; HIV = human immunodeficiency virus; KOH = potassium hydroxide; LFT = liver function test; SPEP = serum protein electrophoresis; TSH = thyroid-stimulating hormone.

Key Treatment

Treatment should aim to eliminate triggers and, when applicable, to correct underlying causes. Simplification of basic skin care is an essential but often overlooked component of management. It is also important to educate the patient about the *dos and don'ts* of skin care, such as the sensibility of using truly fragrance-free soaps and detergents, frequently lubricating (particularly after bathing), bathing in lukewarm water to which unscented moisturizing oil has been added, and using household humidification in cold or dry environments (Table 3). In addition, patients with excoriations should be encouraged to trim their nails short. These general therapies usually provide substantial relief, moderating the itch-and-scratch cycle.

Oral antihistamines are often the medication mainstay of pruritus treatment. They are the preferred drug for any histamine-mediated process of itch, producing a local antipruritic effect, but they also have overall beneficial or central antipruritic effects on the central nervous system (CNS), irrespective of cause. Maximal therapy is usually attained with first-generation H_1 antihistamines (i.e., diphenhydramine hydrochloride [Benadryl], doxepin hydrochloride [Sinequan],[1] hydroxyzine hydrochloride [Atarax], or cyproheptadine hydrochloride [Periactin]).

Doxepin hydrochloride (Sinequan)[1] often is prescribed for several reasons. First, it demonstrates much greater affinity for the histamine receptor than other antihistamines. Second, it provides modest anxiolytic action and sedation, which can be of particular benefit in attenuating emotional states and perceptions of itch. Doxepin hydrochloride (Sinequan)[1] should be taken in 10-mg doses approximately 2 hours before bedtime. The dose can be advanced as tolerated to 300 mg per day,[2] with sedation the typical dose-limiting adverse effect. Given its long half-life, doxepin hydrochloride (Sinequan)[1] can be administered as a single evening dose. If more than 100 mg per day are prescribed, a baseline electrocardiogram should be obtained, because this medication may prolong the QT interval. It is metabolized by the cytochrome P450 system, so patients with hepatic disease in particular should be started with a low dose slowly titrated upward.

Second-generation H_1 antihistamines (fexofenadine hydrochloride [Allegra], cetirizine hydrochloride [Zyrtec], loratadine [Claritin], desloratadine [Clarinex]) may also benefit patients with pruritus. These medications can be used alone or with first-generation H_1 antihistamines. They are typically more helpful with less anxious patients, because they do not cross the blood-brain barrier. However, they cost substantially more than first-generation antihistamines. Also of note is that both first- and second-generation agents can be found in combination with pseudoephedrine. This combination[1] can be particularly effective for urticaria because the vasoconstrictive effect of pseudoephedrine complements their histamine-inhibitory effect.

solitary finding of pruritus. In such cases, serum studies for causative circulating autoantibodies (indirect immunofluorescence) may be diagnostic.

Patch testing can help unmask causes of ACD by identifying sensitizing allergens. To obtain a higher yield, individualized patch-testing panels can be tailored to specific patients such as hairdressers. However, such expanded testing is typically performed only at referral centers.

---

[1]Not FDA approved for this indication.
[2]Exceeds dosage recommended by the manufacturer.

Rakel and Bope: *Conn's Current Therapy 2006.*

TABLE 3 Skin Care "Dos and Don'ts" for Patients With Eczema* or Dermatitis*

Yes	No

Soap
    Vanicream Cleansing Bar, Free and Clear Liquid
    Cleanser, Aveeno Dry Skin Soap (bar or liquid),
    Oilatum Unscented Soap, Neutrogena Original
    Formula Fragrance-Free (bar or liquid)
Shave gel
    Aveeno or Edge unscented
	No hot water (lukewarm only)
	Avoid hot tubs
	No creams, lotions, oils, or powders other
	    than those recommended on this handout
	    No neosporin
	No rubbing alcohol
	No perfumes, colognes, aftershave, or preshave on
	    any part of body or clothing

Moisturizer
    Over-the-counter plain moisturizers to be used twice
    daily (even on face)
Vanicream or Vanicream Lite, Aveeno Dry Skin,
    DML Unscented, or plain Vaseline
Shampoo and conditioner
    Free & Clear Shampoo and Conditioner,
    DHS Clear or DHS Sal Shampoo, DHS Conditioner,
    Neutrogena T/Sal Shampoo (not T-Gel)
        Use shampoo as body or liquid hand soap
        (especially in public bathrooms)
        Conditioners can be left on and used as hair gel
Bath Oil
    Robathol Bath Oil
Hair spray
    Free & Clear Hair Spray or other fragrance-free (not unscented)
	No fabric softener in washer
	No fabric softener sheets in dryer
	No washing machine water softener, such as Calgon
	    (in-house water softeners are acceptable)
	White vinegar in rinse cycle helps remove soap and
	    may be used as a general household cleaner
	No scented deodorants (use plain cornstarch or a
	    fragrance-free antiperspirant such as Certain Dri
	    or Almay unscented antiperspirants)
	
	No wetting of hands more than 5 times per day
	
	No tight-fitting clothes
	No scrubbing

Unscented laundry detergent
    Tide Free, Cheer Free, All Free & Clear, Arm &
    Hammer, Wisk Free, or Purex (not Dreft)
Sunscreen
    Vanicream Sunscreen no. 15 or Solbar Zinc
        Use every morning and at lunchtime, 365 days
        a year, rain or shine
    Apply in only one direction to avoid white discoloration
Miscellaneous
    Wash all new clothes and linens 5 times before using
    Old clothes and fabrics are preferred
    Wear white cotton gloves under rubber or vinyl gloves for
    any activities where hand wetting is expected
    Trim nails short (nails are dangerous to skin, especially
    while sleeping)
Cream schedule:
    Generously apply over-the-counter plain moisturizer
    (eg, Vanicream) to all skin twice daily and anytime skin is dry
Apply prescription creams twice daily, as needed for
    rash or itch:
        Hydrocortisone Prescription Cream to face, ears,
        neck, underarms, and groin
    Triamcinolone Prescription Cream to arms, legs, chest,
    and back
    To ease cream application after showering, don't use
    a towel to dry off. Just wipe off water with hands,
    then apply cream
    With improvement, decrease use of prescription creams
    but continue to apply plain moisturizer generously
    at least twice daily to all skin
	No loofah
	No pumice stone
	No washcloth
	Do not pull off dead skin (snip off with scissors)

*Inflammation of the skin, usually caused by dryness, irritation, or possible external allergy.

CURRENT DIAGNOSIS

- Pruritus is the most common presenting complaint to dermatologists.
- Objective cutaneous physical examination findings may not be present despite complaints of pruritus.
- Diagnosis can be challenging considering the breadth of potential dermatologic and systemic etiologies of pruritus (dermatitis, medication reactions, and malignancies).

REFERENCES

Charlesworth EN, Beltrani VS: Pruritic dermatoses: Overview of etiology and therapy. Am J Med 2002;113(Suppl 9A):25S-33S.
Koblenzer CS: Itching and the atopic skin. J Allergy Clin Immunol 1999;104(3 Pt 2):S109-S113.
Moses S: Pruritus. Am Fam Physician 2003;68:1135-1142.
Twycross R, Greaves MW, Handwerker H, et al: Itch: Scratching more than the surface. QJM 2003;96:7-26.
Yosipovitch G, Fleischer A: Itch associated with skin disease: Advances in pathophysiology and emerging therapies. Am J Clin Dermatol 2003;4:617-622.
Zirwas MJ, Seraly MP: Pruritus of unknown origin: A retrospective study. J Am Acad Dermatol 2001;45:892-896.

Although oral antihistamines typically provide beneficial antipruritic action independent of diagnosis, the effectiveness of topical therapies depends more on the diagnosis. For example, in cases of ACD, topical corticosteroids are the primary treatment. Yet, topical corticosteroids are not typically effective for urticaria or many systemic causes of itch. As demonstrated in cases of atopic dermatitis and oral lichen planus, the newer steroid-sparing topical agents, such as pimecrolimus (Elidel) and tacrolimus (Protopic), certainly have a role in managing dermatologic causes of pruritus.

For patients with recalcitrant pruritus, especially inflammatory cutaneous disease such as a drug eruption or dermatitis, short courses of systemic steroids (prednisone 10 to 40 mg/day) can be used. However, using systemic steroids without a parallel effort to identify and treat the underlying cause invites a return of pruritus when the steroid is tapered.

Determining whether to refer patients with pruritus to a dermatologist depends on the comfort level of the primary care physician in treating itch. With an unclear history or a nondiagnostic physical examination, a dermatologist will follow the diagnostic and therapeutic regimens described above. A dermatologist may also facilitate the interpretation of complex skin biopsy specimens, which are often encountered in inflammatory skin disorders. Additionally, treatments such as phototherapy or systemic immunosuppression may be used for recalcitrant cases of pruritus.

 CURRENT THERAPY

- Management ultimately should be tailored to addressing the etiology as directed by a thorough workup.
- Effective moisturization and avoidance of potential allergens or irritants are fundamental components of pruritus management.
- Topical steroids and oral antihistamines typically are the mainstay of symptomatic therapy.

Tinnitus

Method of
John W. House, MD

Tinnitus is a symptom, not a disease. Many patients, under the misimpression they have a disease, are concerned about how their ailment may progress. In fact, 80% of patients with hearing loss have associated tinnitus. Approximately 20 to 30 million people in the United States experience it. Most of these patients learn to live with tinnitus and are unaware of it much of the time. Perhaps only 5% of patients are disturbed and require some form of therapy. When dealing with patients who have tinnitus, it is important to determine the etiology of the symptom.

Tinnitus is defined as one or more sounds perceived by the patient in the absence of an external source of the sound. It may be perceived in one ear, both ears, or in the head. Tinnitus usually is benign, but it may represent a serious underlying pathology. The tinnitus may be constant, intermittent, steady state, or pulsatile. Its frequency is variable from one patient to another and may vary within the same patient. At times, it may be barely perceptible or it may be described as quite loud. When tinnitus-matching tests are performed, the average relative loudness, regardless of patients' perception, is only 5 decibels above their hearing threshold. The two types of tinnitus are objective and subjective.

Objective Tinnitus

Objective tinnitus, which is uncommon, can be heard by an observer and may be of vascular or muscular origin. Vascular tinnitus may arise from either arterial or venous causes or from vascular tumors, such as glomus tympanicum and glomus jugulare. The arterial causes include conditions that cause turbulent flow, such as arterial sclerosis associated with aging, aberrant carotid artery, arterial-venous fistula, or an arterial-venous malformation. It also may be associated with conditions that cause an increase in blood flow around the ears, such as anemia, hyperthyroidism, or Paget's disease. The venous causes include a large or exposed jugular bulb on one side and benign intracranial hypertension. The venous type of tinnitus is easily differentiated from the arterial type. The sound typically stops or is reduced when light pressure is applied over the internal jugular vein on the involved side. In addition, patients may report the sound is reduced when they turn their head toward the involved ear and increased when they turn their head away from it. Evaluation includes radiographic and ultrasound studies as indicated. High-resolution computed tomography (CT) scanning with contrast and bone program is helpful in identifying erosive lesions or tumors. Magnetic resonance angiography (MRA) and magnetic resonance venography (MRV) are helpful in defining vascular lesions or aberrant vessels. Standard angiography is performed less often because of the effectiveness of MRA, MRV, and ultrasound studies. This type of tinnitus responds well to treatment aimed at the vascular lesion or correction of the anemia or hyperthyroidism.

The three causes of muscular tinnitus are myoclonic activity of the stapedial muscle, the tensor tympani muscle, or the palatal muscle. These types of tinnitus are characterized by brief periods of clicking, popping, or banging sounds in the ear. Palatal myoclonus can be differentiated from the other causes by observing rhythmic contractions of the soft palate that are synchronized with the patient's sounds. While observing the palate, the patient should not open the mouth widely because this action usually stops the myoclonus. It may be possible to observe movement of the tympanic membrane either with the microscope or the tympanometer. Treatment often is successful and aimed at the offending muscle. By cutting the tendon to the stapedial or tensor tympani muscle, the symptoms are relieved. If the cause is the palatal muscle, treatment is more difficult and palliative. Placing the patient on muscle relaxants or performing a myringotomy with tubes may help. Botulinum toxin (Botox)[1] injections into the levator palatini muscle help relieve the sound in some patients.

Subjective Tinnitus

The vast majority of tinnitus is subjective, and only the patient is able to hear the sound. It usually is associated with some type of hearing loss. Approximately 90% of tinnitus patients have a sensorineural hearing loss, 5% have a conductive loss, and 5% have normal hearing.

Because tinnitus is a symptom, the underlying cause must be determined by a history, physical examination, audiogram, and any additional tests that are indicated. The physical examination includes otoscopy and, at times, auscultation and palpation around the ear and neck. The remainder of the head and neck examination is performed. Tuning fork tests (Rinne's test or Weber's test for hearing) are routinely performed to determine if the hearing loss is conductive or sensorineural. The possible

causes of a conductive hearing loss with tinnitus are cerumen impaction, otitis externa, otitis media (acute and chronic), chronic otitis media with effusion (serous otitis), and otosclerosis. Some of the causes of sensorineural hearing loss associated with tinnitus include presbycusis (age-related hearing loss), noise-induced hearing loss, ototoxic medications, sudden hearing loss as a result of either vascular or viral causes, Ménière's disease, and cerebellopontine angle tumors (acoustic neuromas or meningiomas). The latter are usually associated with unilateral symptoms (hearing loss with or without tinnitus). Patients having unilateral complaints must have a neurotologic evaluation that includes an MRI with gadolinium to rule out a tumor. Blood tests may be indicated if there is a fluctuating or rapidly progressive hearing loss associated with the tinnitus. This would include a complete blood cell count (CBC) with sedimentation rate, a fluorescent treponemal antibody (FTA), and possibly an antinuclear antibody (ANA) test. These tests are performed to rule out syphilitic or autoimmune hearing loss.

Treatment

Because tinnitus is a symptom and not a disease, no one treatment is effective for all. Victor Goodhill, MD, in 1950, put it very well: "Any management which is based upon a single panacea for the treatment of a symptom and not a disease will result in failure." The important steps in the management of the patient with tinnitus are the evaluation, the examination, and the explanation. The explanation is very helpful when it is accompanied by reassurance that the tinnitus does not represent serious pathology and the patient is not going deaf. Approximately 95% of the patients seen in my office who have tinnitus are not particularly bothered by it, but 5% are driven to distraction.

If the tinnitus is associated with a hearing loss, amplification with a hearing aid usually helps. The normal environmental sounds mask out the tinnitus and at the same time improve the patient's hearing. At night, a noise generator, fan, air conditioner, or a radio tuned to an FM station can help mask the tinnitus. Tinnitus maskers are wearable devices that generate sound to help mask the tinnitus. These have limited success in helping reduce the annoyance of the tinnitus. For those patients with tinnitus and a hearing loss who find a masker or hearing aid alone are not helpful, a tinnitus instrument (combined hearing aid and masker) may help both mask the tinnitus and provide amplification. A new promising tinnitus treatment is auditory habituation as proposed and developed by Pawel Jastreboff. This therapy involves retraining the auditory system to ignore the tinnitus sounds. Therapeutic noise devices emit stable broadband noise that is softer than the patient's tinnitus. The theory is not to cover up the tinnitus but to help the patient learn to ignore it. This training takes time (as long as 1 year) and requires the therapist to spend a great deal of time counseling the patient.

---

[1]Not FDA approved for this indication.

For approximately 80% of a selected group of patients, biofeedback training helps reduce the tinnitus by teaching the patient relaxation techniques. Muscle tension and stress worsen the perceived tinnitus. The biofeedback consists of monitoring muscle tension and skin temperature. When patients are able to learn to relax the muscles and increase circulation in the skin, their tinnitus is reduced. In addition, patients recognize the relationship between their stress level and the perceived loudness of the tinnitus.

Over the years many medications have been tried for the treatment of tinnitus. No single medication works uniformly in reducing tinnitus. Antidepressants are effective in some patients. Most severe tinnitus sufferers have sleep problems and are anxious and depressed. Small doses of either amitriptyline (Elavil)[1] or nortriptyline (Pamelor)[1] given at bedtime seem to help the patient get through the night and reduce the aggravation of the tinnitus during the day.

Other medications that might be helpful include antianxiety agents such as alprazolam (Xanax),[1] clonazepam (Klonopin),[1] and diazepam (Valium).[1] Schulman reports some success recently in relieving severe tinnitus by combining clonazepam and gabapentin (Neurontin).[1] Because of the potential for abuse and dependence, this category of medication is rarely prescribed, however.

Box 1 lists additional medications that are cited as possibly helping tinnitus. In a recently completed double-blind study using a combination of ginkgo biloba,[1] magnesium,[1] and vitamin B_{12},[1] the active treatment group did no better than the placebo group.

In conclusion, no sure cure for tinnitus is available. Many patients have tinnitus, but most learn to ignore it and live with it after an evaluation and a reassuring explanation. No magical cure exists, but many avenues of treatment are available to help a patient cope with and overcome the problem of tinnitus.

REFERENCES

House JW: Treatment of severe tinnitus with biofeedback training. Laryngoscope 1978;88(3):406-412.
Jastreboff PJ, Gray WC, Gold SL: Neurophysiological approach to the tinnitus patient. Am J Otol 1996;17(2):236-240.
Jastreboff PJ, Jastreboff MM: Tinnitus retraining therapy for patients with tinnitus and decreased sound tolerance. Otolaryngol Clin North Am 2003;36(2):321.
Sullivan M, Katon W, Russo J, et al: A randomized trial of nortriptyline for severe chronic tinnitus. Effects on depression, disability, and tinnitus symptoms. Arch Intern Med 1993;153(19):2251.
Sullivan M, Katon W, Russo J, et al: Coping and marital support as correlates of tinnitus disability. Gen Hosp Psychiatry 1994;16(4):259-266.

BOX 1   Medications Proposed to Help Tinnitus*

Anesthetics
- Lidocaine[1] (Intravenous provides temporary relief in approximately 80% of patients.)
- Procaine (Novocain)[1]
- Tocainide (Tonocard)[1] (oral lidocaine analogue)
- Flecainide (Tambocor)[1]
- Mexiletine (Mexitil)[1] (oral lidocaine analogue)

Antianxiety
- Alprazolam (Xanax)[1]
- Diazepam (Valium)[1]
- Clonazepam (Klonopin)[1]

Anticonvulsants
- Carbamazepine (Tegretol)[1]
- Phenytoin (Dilantin)[1]
- Primidone (Mysoline)[1]
- Gabapentin (Neurontin)[1]

Antidepressants
- Amitriptyline (Elavil)[1]
- Nortriptyline (Pamelor)[1]
- Diuretics (in Ménière's disease)
- Triamterene/hydrochlorothiazide (HCTZ) (Dyazide)[1]
- Vitamins and herbs
- Niacin
- Misoprostol (Cytotec)[1] (synthetic prostaglandin)
- Magnesium
- Vitamin B_{12}
- Ginkgo biloba

*Results are inconsistent.
[1]Not FDA approved for this indication.

Low Back Pain

Method of
Alan B. Douglass, MD, FAAFP

Definitions

Low back pain is defined as pain, muscle tension, and/or stiffness located below the costal margin and above the inferior gluteal folds. Sciatica is sharp, burning, lancinating, or electric-like pain radiating down the posterior or lateral aspect of the leg often associated with numbness or paresthesias. It is caused by compression of an inflamed, sensitized nerve root and occurs in 1% to 3% of patients. Neurologic compromise in the context of low back pain is defined as motor, sensory, or reflex dysfunction in the lower extremities, or bladder or bowel dysfunction.

Epidemiology

Low back pain is experienced by 90% of adults at some point in their lives, and 50% of working adults experience it each year. Back pain is second only to upper respiratory infection as a reason for physician office visits in the United States. It is the leading cause of work-related disability. Typically 70% of patients recover within 6 weeks and 85% by 12 weeks, but progress thereafter is slow. Chronic back pain develops in 2% to 7% of patients with lifetime recurrence rates up to 85%.

In North America, back disorders generate more than $100 billion in annual direct and indirect costs. Psychosocial factors such as depression, previous back trouble, substance abuse, pursuit of disability compensation, and ongoing litigation all increase the risk of recurrent and chronic symptoms.

Etiology

The majority of patients with isolated low back pain cannot be given a precise anatomic diagnosis. Potential pain generators include the myofascial tissues, ligaments, facet joints, intervertebral discs, spinal nerve roots, and bony structures. The vast majority of back pain seen in primary care practice is caused by mechanical factors such as musculoligamentous injuries (70%) and age-related degenerative changes of the discs and facet joints (10%). Disc herniation (4%), spinal stenosis (3%), compression fractures (4%), and spondylolisthesis (3%) are also relatively common. Uncommon but potentially serious etiologies include tumor (0.7%), inflammatory arthritis (0.3%), and spinal infection (0.01%). Occasionally low back pain can be secondary to visceral disease such as abdominal aortic aneurysm or renal, pelvic, or gastrointestinal disease (2%). As patients age neoplasms, compression fractures, spinal stenosis, and aortic aneurysms become more common.

Diagnostic Evaluation

A basic principle of diagnosis is to attempt to specifically define the anatomic source of a patient's pain. However, in the majority of cases of low back pain this is not possible. In these circumstances the most important thing is for the physician to exclude the relatively rare *red-flag* disorders that require early, aggressive intervention before proceeding with symptom-directed therapy. These disorders include fractures, systemic disease such as infection, neoplasm, or inflammatory arthritis, and evidence of neurologic compromise. Psychosocial factors that may affect symptoms and recovery should be carefully explored.

HISTORY

Take history carefully and consistently, with attention to current symptoms; underlying medical conditions; prior back injuries and treatment; and lifestyle, social, legal, and disability issues. Particularly, focus on identifying red-flag symptoms suggestive of serious pathology including age older than 50, a history of high-impact trauma or osteoporosis (fractures), progressive motor or sensory deficit (nerve-root impingement), fever, night sweats, weight loss, or a personal history of malignancy (infection or neoplasm), rest pain, unremitting pain or night pain (bony pathology), or loss of bladder or bowel function with or without saddle anesthesia (cauda equina syndrome). The presence of sciatic symptoms is both sensitive (0.95) and specific (0.88) for lumbar disc herniation.

PHYSICAL EXAMINATION

Physical examination should focus on identifying patterns of findings suggestive of a diagnosis. Key examination components that should be consistently performed on every patient with back pain include inspection of the back and posture; palpation of bony and muscular structures; spinal range of motion assessment; and neurologic examination of motor, sensory, and reflex function in the lower extremities. Sciatic tension signs such as straight leg raises have a sensitivity of 0.8 but a specificity of only 0.4 for nerve root impingement. Crossed straight leg raises have poor sensitivity but a specificity of 0.9. Rectal examination should be performed in any patient when the possibility of cauda equina syndrome is being entertained.

IMAGING

Most patients with low back pain do not require diagnostic imaging. Further, there is a high incidence of radiographic abnormalities in asymptomatic individuals. In one study, 64% of asymptomatic subjects had disc abnormalities on magnetic resonance imaging (MRI). Therefore, unnecessary imaging should be minimized to avoid identifying potentially misleading findings. Plain radiographs should be ordered in patients with a history of osteoporosis, significant trauma, advanced age, or a suspicion of serious underlying red-flag disease such as infection or a malignancy. However, a normal plain film does not in and of itself exclude underlying disease. More advanced imaging studies such as MRI, computed tomography (CT), or myelography should be reserved for patients with symptoms of nerve root compression, neurogenic claudication, or other neurologic compromise severe enough to consider surgery, or when there is a clinical suspicion of serious spinal pathology.

Treatment

MEDICATIONS

Acetaminophen is an effective, well-tolerated analgesic. Many experts advocate maximum dosages of 2 to 3 g per day. In alcoholism, fasting states, hepatic disease, the presence of certain medications (especially anticonvulsants), or in the frail elderly, liver toxicity can occur at recommended doses. Toxicity increases when acetaminophen is taken in conjunction with a nonsteroidal anti-inflammatory drug (NSAID). Particular care should be taken when patients are taking combination analgesics containing acetaminophen; daily dose limits must not be inadvertently exceeded.

There is strong evidence of efficacy for NSAIDS in acute and chronic back pain. The efficacy of all NSAIDs appears roughly equivalent, but patient response to any particular agent is highly idiosyncratic. Nonacetylated salicylates (choline magnesium trisalicylate [Trilisate], salsalate [Disalcid]) and cyclooxygenase-2 (COX-2) specific inhibitors are effective and may have fewer gastrointestinal side effects than traditional NSAIDs.

CURRENT DIAGNOSIS

- Most adults experience low back pain, and recurrence is common.
- Most symptoms are caused by biomechanical causes, but a precise anatomic diagnosis often cannot be made.
- History and physical exam should focus on early identification of those relatively rare red-flag etiologies such as fracture, infection, malignancy, and major neurologic compromise that require prompt, aggressive therapy.
- Imaging should be reserved for patients with a history of trauma or a suspicion of underlying systemic disease because of the high incidence of radiographic abnormalities in asymptomatic individuals.
- Psychosocial factors that may affect symptoms and recovery should be carefully explored.

CURRENT THERAPY

- Most patients improve promptly in the absence of an underlying serious etiology, and most treatment is symptom-directed.
- Acetaminophen and NSAIDs are effective analgesics, but physicians should be mindful of their potential toxicities.
- Tricyclic antidepressants are effective in depressed patients and in conjunction with anticonvulsants if pain has a neuropathic component.
- Epidural steroid injections can be helpful in patients with sciatic symptoms that have not responded to conservative therapy.
- Bed rest is not recommended. Physicians should advise a rapid return to normal activity.
- Physical modalities with evidence of benefit should be used.
- Surgery should be reserved for the small group of patients with progressive neurologic deficit, cauda equina syndrome, or sciatic symptoms caused by nerve root compression that have not improved with conservative therapy.

Abbreviations: NSAIDs = nonsteroidal anti-inflammatory drugs.

Salicylates have the additional advantage of low cost. If traditional NSAIDs are chosen, gastric cytoprotection should be considered in patients at elevated risk for gastric toxicity. Clinicians also should be aware of potential nephrotoxicity in the elderly and patients with renal disease, the potential of NSAIDs to exacerbate hypertension and heart failure, and linkages between COX-2 specific inhibitors and cardiovascular events.

Opioids are an effective option in the management of severe acute low back pain and are slowly becoming more accepted in the long-term management of severe chronic pain. Little evidence of long-term benefit is available, however, and concerns have been raised about the safety and efficacy of prolonged, high-dose therapy.

Some muscle relaxants are more effective than placebo in the management of low back pain. However, effects are modest, greatest in the first 4 days of therapy, and come at the price of greater adverse effects. Sedative hypnotics are effective in relieving spasm but are ineffective analgesics.

If a patient with low back pain is depressed, antidepressants clearly are of benefit. Evidence is conflicting in the absence of depression. Tricyclic antidepressants appear most consistently effective, whereas serotonin reuptake inhibitors do not appear to be of benefit. Anticonvulsants and tricyclic antidepressants are supported by evidence of benefit in patients with a neuropathic component to their pain.

Epidural injection of steroids can provide short-term sciatic symptom reduction in patients that have not responded to conservative therapy, but current evidence of efficacy remains mixed. There is no clear rationale for epidural steroid injection in patients with nonradicular pain. Small trials of the efficacy of systemic steroids have been inconclusive, and clinical trials comparing oral with epidural steroids have not been performed.

Rakel and Bope: *Conn's Current Therapy 2006.*

PHYSICAL MODALITIES

Once back pain has been deemed to be uncomplicated, physical modalities should be emphasized. Bed rest should be avoided and patients encouraged to return to their usual activities as soon as possible. Stretching, ice, heat, and low-stress aerobic exercise are all effective. There is limited evidence of short-term effectiveness for spinal manipulation. Back exercises, lumbar supports, massage, acupuncture, transcutaneous electrical nerve stimulator (TENS) units, magnet therapy, and traction are not supported by strong evidence of benefit.

SURGERY

Only 2% of all patients with low back pain will ever require surgery. Most patients, and 90% of patients with sciatic symptoms and nerve compression on imaging, recover with conservative treatment. However, referral to a back surgeon is indicated in patients with progressive neurologic deficit, cauda equina syndrome, and those with a lesion seen on imaging that correlates with symptoms and clinical findings of nerve compression and have failed to respond to four to six weeks of conservative management.

REFERENCES

American Pain Society: Principles of analgesic use in the treatment of acute pain and cancer pain. 5th ed. (2003) Glenview IL: American Pain Society.

Ballantyne JC, Mao J: Opioid therapy for chronic pain. N Engl J Med 2003;349(20):1943-1953.

Carette S, Leclaire R, Marcoux S, et al: Epidural corticosteroid injections for sciatica due to herniated nucleus pulposus. N Engl J Med 1997;336:1634-1640.

Deyo RA: Drug therapy for back pain: which drugs help which patients? Spine J 1996;24:2840-2850.

Deyo RA, Rainville J, Kent DL: What can the history and physical examination tell us about low back pain? JAMA 1992;268:760-765.

Deyo RA, Weinstein JN: Low back pain. N Engl J Med 2001;344: 363-370.

Hagen KB, Hilde G, Jamtvedt G, Winnem M: Bed rest for acute low-back pain and sciatica. Cochrane Database Syst Rev 2004; 3:CD001254.

Jarvik JG, Deyo RA: Diagnostic evaluation of low back pain with emphasis on imaging. Ann Intern Med 2002;137:586.

Jensen MC, Brant-Zawadzki MN, Obuchowski N, et al: Magnetic resonance imaging of the lumbar spine in people without back pain. N Engl J Med 1994;331:69-73.

Nelemans PJ, de Bie RA, de Vet HCW, Sturmans F: Injection therapy for subacute and chronic benign low-back pain. Cochrane Database Syst Rev 1999;4:CD001824.

Staiger TO, Gaster B, Sullivan MD, Deyo RA: Systematic review of antidepressants in the treatment of low back pain. Spine J 2003; 28:2540.

Van Tilder M, Koes B: Low back pain and sciatica. Clinical Evidence 2003;286-291.

The Infectious Diseases

Management of the Patient with HIV Disease

Method of
Jin S. Suh, MD, and Vani Gandhi, MD

Epidemiology

HIV disease is a global public health problem affecting millions of individuals worldwide. As of July 2004, the pandemic had claimed more than 20 million lives, and another 38 million people are estimated to be living with HIV/AIDS. The virus has spread to all continents of the world. Sub-Saharan Africa is most severely affected, with an estimated 25 million infected. Other affected regions include South/Southeast Asia with 6.5 million, Latin America with 1.6 million, Eastern Europe with 1.3 million, and North America with 1.0 million. HIV/AIDS is now the leading cause of death worldwide among persons 15 to 59 years of age. Moreover, the epidemic is considered a threat to the economic well-being and sociopolitical stability of many nations. In the United States, the estimated number of people living with HIV/AIDS as of 2003 was 950,000. The exposure category was as follows: male-to-male sexual contact (48%), injection drug use (27%), heterosexual contact (16%), male-to-male sexual contact combined with intravenous drug use (IDU) (7%), and others, including hemophilia, blood transfusion, perinatal, and risk not reported or not identified (2%). Perinatally acquired AIDS has decreased significantly, primarily because of the use of zidovudine (AZT, Retrovir) to prevent HIV transmission. Racial/ethnic disparities among people with HIV and AIDS continue to be worrisome. African Americans represent 45% and Hispanics 20% of reported AIDS cases, far out of proportion to their respective representation in the U.S. population. HIV infection occurs at any age at which individuals are sexually active or may have shared needles. In 2002 the age group 25 to 34 years represented 28% of all new diagnoses of HIV/AIDS. The use of highly active antiretroviral therapy (HAART) became widespread during 1996, and the estimated number of deaths among persons with AIDS in 2002 represented a 14% decline since 1998. The declining rates of morbidity and mortality, as well as improvement in quality of life, are well documented among HIV-infected individuals who have access to diagnostic monitoring and antiretroviral (ARV) medications. But patients are still dying from HIV and associated opportunistic infections, especially in yet undiagnosed patients not receiving ARV therapy, patients who cannot adhere to regimens, and those who fail therapy.

The Virus

HIV-1 is established as the principal cause of AIDS. HIV-2 is less prevalent, isolated primarily in West African patients. Both viruses belong to the family of human retroviruses (Retroviridae) and the subfamily of lentiviruses. The HIV virion is an icosahedral structure containing spikes formed by envelope proteins. It is an RNA virus and noted for reverse transcription of its genomic RNA to DNA by the enzyme *reverse transcriptase*. The two viruses are only 60% homologous, and significant differences in the envelope of glycoprotein exist. The hallmark of HIV infection is the progressive destruction of $CD4^+$ T lymphocytes (helper cells), leading to decreased cell-mediated immunity and memory responses. As a person's $CD4^+$ cell count falls below $200/mm^3$, the likelihood of developing opportunistic infection increases. HIV-1 is accountable for causing more than 90% of the HIV infections in the world. HIV-1 is divided into three groups: M, O, and N. Group M accounts for as much as 95% of the world's HIV-1 infection and is further subdivided into *clades,* or subtypes, designated A to K. More than 98% of HIV-1 infections in the United States are caused by subtype B; most non-B subtypes in the United States were acquired in other countries. In Africa, more than 75% of strains are subtypes A, C, and D, with C predominating. In Asia, subtypes E, C, and B are most common; in India, subtype C is most prevalent. The newest group, N, which was reported in 1998, and group O are found primarily in West Africa. HIV-2 is less transmissible, associated with lower viral load and a slower rate of disease progression. HIV-2 is not susceptible to non-nucleoside reverse transcriptase inhibitors (NNRTIs) and may have multiple protease inhibitor (PI)–associated substitutions, suggesting possible PI resistance.

Natural History of HIV Infection

The natural history of untreated infection is divided into several stages. Viral transmission is followed by the symptoms of the acute retroviral syndrome within 2 to 6 weeks. This syndrome is seen in 50% to 70% of individuals. Symptoms may include fever, fatigue, pharyngitis, weight loss, night sweats, lymphadenopathy, myalgias, headaches, nausea, and diarrhea. Neurologic presentations such as aseptic meningitis, seventh nerve palsy, and radiculopathy may occur. Symptoms can last approximately 14 days but may be up to 10 weeks in duration. Early viremia is noted at 4 to 11 days when a peak of several million copies per milliliter is reached. When HIV-1 specific cytotoxic T lymphocytes (CTLs) are activated, it is associated with a decrease in HIV viral load. The CTL response determines the set point, which predicts the rate of long-term progression. Recent seroconversion could be diagnosed by the so-called detuned enzyme-linked immunoabsorbent assay (ELISA), which generally becomes positive at a mean of 129 days after transmission and suggests infection within the past 18 weeks. If treatment is not initiated, viral load decreases along with seroconversion and development of an immune response. With continued untreated infection, HIV RNA replication increases. Symptomatic HIV infection or late-stage disease is characterized by a CD4$^+$ count of less than 200 cells/mm^3 and the development of opportunistic infections, selected tumors, wasting, and neurologic complications. Median survival after the CD4$^+$ count falls to less than 200 cells/mm^3 is 3.7 years, and the median survival after an AIDS-defining complication is 1.3 years.

Modes of Transmission

There are three recognized ways to become HIV infected: sexual contact, parenteral exposure, and perinatal transmission. Heterosexual contact with an infected person is the predominant mode of transmission worldwide. Men who have sex with men (MSM) and bisexual men account for the majority of cases in the United States. HIV infection can occur when the potential host's mucous membranes or blood comes into contact with infected body fluids, especially blood, semen, and vaginal secretions. Available data indicate certain sexual practices pose higher risk than others; higher rates of transmission are observed with receptive anal intercourse compared to receptive vaginal intercourse, and oral sex carries a lower risk than does anal or vaginal sex. There is a close association between genital ulcerations and transmission. History of sexually transmitted disease, multiple sex partners, and users of illicit substances also appear to be major risk factors. Alcohol consumption and illicit drug use are associated with unsafe sexual behavior, which leads to increased risk of sexual transmission of HIV. The chief predictor of heterosexual transmission of virus in some studies is the level of plasma viremia. Hence decrease in viral load by treatment decreases transmission risk. Condoms decrease the risk of infection but do not eliminate it.

Circumcision may decrease acquisition risk in heterosexual men. Exposure to nonbloody oral secretions, feces, urine, tears, and other nongenital fluids is very low risk, even when the exposure is via mucous membranes. No evidence indicates that HIV is transmitted through casual contact: sharing utensils or toilet facilities or spread by insects such as by a mosquito bite, or via respiratory droplets. Transmission of HIV through receipt of blood and blood products can still occur, especially in parts of the world where blood is screened improperly. Parenteral transmission of HIV during injection drug use can occur because of contamination through intravenous puncture or by subcutaneous ("skin popping") or intramuscular ("muscling") injections. Perinatal HIV prophylaxis has significantly decreased rates of vertical (mother-to-child) transmission. But higher risks are associated with vaginal versus cesarean delivery, mothers with higher viral loads, and those who breastfeed their children.

Initial Evaluation

The history and physical should be a comprehensive assessment of the patient. Relevant HIV-related history should include sexual behavior and any sexually transmitted diseases. Prior laboratory information (if available) should include viral load, CD4$^+$ count, nadir CD4$^+$, and peak viral load. Current and previous ARV regimens, including adverse drug reactions, HIV-related illness, opportunistic infections, and psychiatric and substance use history should also be discussed. Physical examination should include vital signs and pain assessment, and complete evaluation targeting HIV-related conditions such as seborrheic dermatitis, Kaposi's sarcoma (KS), molluscum contagiosum, onychomycosis, oral candidiasis, hairy leukoplakia, oral herpes simplex, and fat maldistribution changes. Genital examination should be done for venereal warts (human papillomavirus [HPV]), classic and atypical herpes simplex virus (HSV) lesions, and ulcerative genital disease, and pelvic examination in women. Rectal examination is necessary, and if perianal lesions exist, an anal Pap smear should be considered. Ophthalmologic and ear, nose, throat examinations to evaluate funduscopic findings, as well as evidence for sinus infection, odynophagia, dysphagia, and hearing loss, are necessary. A complete neurologic assessment including mental status examination should be done along with a screen for depression and anxiety; appetite and sleep habits should also be discussed.

Diagnostic and Other Laboratory Testing

Detection of antibody against viral antigens is the standard method of HIV diagnosis. HIV enzyme immunoassay (EIA) provides a highly sensitive screening test. False-positive EIAs occur at approximately less than 1% in the overall population. Serum samples that are reactive by EIAs should be retested; if repeatedly positive, samples must be confirmed by Western blot (WB) test.

CURRENT DIAGNOSIS

- CD4$^+$ count and viral load should be monitored every 3 months.
- Resistance testing should be performed in patients failing therapy and before starting therapy in patients with acute infection.
- Laboratory monitoring should be done to monitor for complications.
- *Pneumocystis* pneumonia is the most common opportunistic infection associated with HIV.
- Candidiasis is the most common fungal condition seen in HIV-positive persons.
- Pseudomembranous candidiasis, or thrush, appears as removable white plaques on any oral mucosal surface.
- HIV infection has emerged as by far the most important predisposing factor for the development of tuberculosis (TB).
- *Mycobacterium avium* complex (MAC) disease continues to be the most common systemic bacterial infection in AIDS and is responsible for significant morbidity.
- Cytomegalovirus (CMV) infection is the most common intraocular infection in patients with AIDS, accounting for at least 90% of HIV-related infectious retinopathies.

The two tests when combined provide a specificity of more than 99.99%. WBs that meet the standard Centers for Disease Control and Prevention (CDC) criteria of detecting antibodies to at least two of the p24, gp41, or gp120/160 viral antigens rarely give false positives. False-negative results occur during the window period prior to seroconversion and less commonly in patients with prolonged immune reconstitution because of HAART, agammaglobulinemia, and persons infected with type N or O strains of HIV-2. False-positive results can occur with autoimmune diseases and occasionally with immunizations. Indeterminate results occur with early HIV infection, HIV-2 infection, pregnancy, cross-reacting nonspecific antibodies, and HIV vaccines.

RAPID HIV TESTING

There are three FDA-approved rapid serologic tests: OraQuick Rapid HIV-1 test, Reveal Rapid HIV-1 Antibody Test, and Uni-Gold Recombigen HIV Test. A negative test is definitive unless tested in the window period of 3 months postexposure. Positive tests are considered preliminary positive results and should be confirmed by WB or EIA. Indeterminate tests should be repeated in 1 month. Sensitivity and specificity of these tests are consistently higher than 99%.

QUANTITATIVE PLASMA HIV VIRAL LOAD

Currently available techniques include branched chain DNA (bDNA), HIV RNA PCR (polymerase chain

reaction), and the NucliSens HIV-1 QT (quick test). Following initiation of therapy, there is a rapid initial decline in HIV RNA level over 1 to 4 weeks, reflecting activity against free-plasma HIV virions in acutely infected CD4$^+$ cells. This is followed by a second decline that is longer in duration (months) and more modest in degree, which reflects activity against HIV-infected macrophages and HIV released from other compartments, especially those trapped in follicular dendritic cells of lymph follicles. Maximum antiviral effect is expected by 4 to 6 months. Viral load should be measured at baseline and later at 3- to 4-month intervals, or earlier as indicated clinically. An expected response to therapy is a decrease of 0.75 to 1.0 log$_{10}$ cells/mL at 1 week, a decrease of 1.5 to 2.0 log$_{10}$ to more than 5000 cells/mL at 4 weeks, less than 500 cells/mL at 8 to 16 weeks, and undetectable at 16 to 24 weeks.

CD4$^+$ T LYMPHOCYTES

The CD4$^+$ T lymphocyte count is the standard test to assess prognosis for progression to AIDS, to make therapeutic decisions regarding antiviral treatment, to provide prophylaxis against opportunistic pathogens, and to formulate the differential diagnosis in symptomatic patients. Normal values, depending on laboratory used, range between 500 to 1400 cells/mm^3. The CD4$^+$ count should be repeated every 3 to 6 months in untreated patients and at 2- to 4-month intervals in patients on ARV therapy. The CD4$^+$ cell count is affected by seasons, diurnal variations, and corticosteroid administration. Deceptively high CD4$^+$ counts may occur with HTLV-1 (human T-lymphotropic virus type 1) co-infection or after splenectomy. The CD4$^+$ count typically increases to 50 cells/mm^3 or more at 4 to 8 weeks after viral suppression with HAART and then increases an additional 50 to 100 cells/mm^3 per year thereafter.

Drug Resistance Testing

Testing for HIV resistance to ARV drugs is a useful tool for guiding antiviral therapy. There are different types of resistance testing: genotypic assays and phenotypic assays. When combined with a detailed drug history and efforts to maximize drug adherence, these assays improve the short-term virologic response to ARV therapy. In general, resistance testing is recommended in the setting of virologic failure and considered in persons with acute HIV infections, incomplete viral suppression, and in the chronically infected patient with high suspicion for viral resistance.

Genotyping assays detect drug resistance mutations that are present in the relevant viral genes (e.g., reverse transcriptase, protease). Genotyping can be performed rapidly, and results reported within 1 to 2 weeks of sample collection. Interpretation of test results requires knowledge of the mutations that are selected for by different ARV drugs and of the potential for cross-resistance to other drugs conferred by certain mutations.

Phenotyping assays measure the virus's ability to grow in different concentrations of ARV drugs.

Phenotyping assays are more costly to perform than genotyping assays. Drug concentrations that inhibit 50% and 90% of viral replication (i.e., the median inhibitory concentration [IC] IC_{50} and IC_{90}) are calculated, and the ratio of the IC_{50} of test and reference viruses is reported as the fold increase in IC_{50} (i.e., fold resistance). Interpretation of phenotyping assay results is complicated by the paucity of data regarding the specific resistance level (i.e., fold increase in IC_{50}) associated with drug failure, although clinically significant fold increase cutoffs are now available for some drugs.

Further limitations of both genotyping and phenotyping assays include the lack of uniform quality assurance for all available assays, relatively high cost, and insensitivity for minor viral species. If drug-resistant viruses constitute less than 10% to 20% of the circulating virus population, they may not be detected by available assays. If drug resistance had developed to a drug that was subsequently discontinued, the drug-resistant virus can become a minor species because its growth advantage is lost. Hence resistance assays should be performed while the patient is taking his or her ARV regimen, and resistance testing should be interpreted cautiously in relation to the previous treatment history.

Antiretroviral Therapy

All symptomatic patients and individuals with AIDS-defining illness need treatment. The U.S. Department of Health and Human Services (DHHS) in 2004 revised the guidelines, with $CD4^+$ count the most important criterion and an increased viral load threshold for initiation of treatment (Table 1). Considerations in choosing an initial regimen include potency, convenience, tolerability, pharmacokinetics, drug interactions, toxicity, and sequencing potential (i.e., options for subsequent therapy in the event of treatment failure). Table 2 shows current preferred and alternative regimens. Resistance testing is generally recommended in treatment-naïve patients, especially when there is a high prevalence of resistance in the community or when infection is believed to have occurred within the last 2 years. Currently, there are four classes of ARV agents: the nucleoside reverse transcriptase inhibitors (NRTIs), PIs, NNRTIs, and fusion inhibitors (FIs) (Table 3).

NUCLEOSIDE REVERSE TRANSCRIPTASE INHIBITORS

The NRTI class of drugs serves an important role as a backbone component of HAART, or as part of triple or quadruple NRTI-based therapy. Zidovudine/lamivudine/abacavir (Trizivir) in combined formulation is effective and convenient, although perhaps less effective in advanced patients with plasma HIV-1 RNA more than 100,000 copies/mL. Recent studies show higher rates of virologic failure in triple-nucleoside regimens when compared to PI-containing arms. The current guidelines list several potential dual-NRTI combinations for use in initial three-drug or four-drug regimens. These include zidovudine/lamivudine (Combivir) and bacavir-lamivudine

CURRENT THERAPY

- Preferred HAART regimens are two NRTIs with one PI or NNRTI.
- Failure of HAART therapy is most commonly caused by poor adherence.
- Substance use is not a contraindication to antiretroviral therapy.
- Certain complications may necessitate change of HAART therapy.
- For patients who have $CD4^+$ T lymphocyte count responses, primary and/or secondary prophylaxis for certain opportunistic infections can be discontinued.
- Trimethoprim-sulfamethoxazole (Bactrim, Septra) is always the drug of choice for PCP unless the patient has a history of life-threatening intolerance.
- There are no proven alternative therapies to penicillin for treatment of neurosyphilis in HIV patients; penicillin desensitization is recommended.
- Presentation of malignancy in patients infected with HIV is often different from that seen in immunocompetent hosts.
- In general, patients with controlled HIV and moderate $CD4^+$ counts are equally capable of tolerating full-dose chemotherapy and radiotherapy for treatment of malignancies.

Abbreviations: HAART = highly active antiretroviral therapy; NNRTI = non-nucleoside reverse transcriptase inhibitor; NRTI = nucleoside reverse transcriptase inhibitor; PCP = *Pneumocystis carinii* pneumonia; PI = protease inhibitor.

(Epzicom), and tenofovir-emtricitabine (Truvada), which can be used with a PI or NNRTI. The newer co-formulated options provide low pill burden and once-daily dosing. Stavudine (Zerit) has greater long-term toxicity including mitochondrial toxicity, neuropathy, lipoatrophy, and lactic acidosis. The abacavir (Ziagen) hypersensitivity reaction can occur in approximately 5% of patients who initiate therapy with the drug. Tenofovir (Viread) is the only nucleotide analogue. Similar to lamivudine, it is also active against hepatitis B.

PROTEASE INHIBITORS

The discovery and subsequent use of PIs in combination with at least two other NRTIs marked the beginning of the HAART era. Currently, the following PIs are approved by the Food and Drug Administration (FDA): saquinavir (Fortovase, Invirase), ritonavir (Norvir), indinavir (Crixivan), nelfinavir (Viracept), amprenavir (Agenerase), lopinavir/ritonavir (Kaletra), atazanavir (Reyataz), and fosamprenavir (Lexiva). Ritonavir is an inhibitor of the cytochrome P-450 pathway. Thus when co-administered with other PIs, it increases their bioavailability (called boosting) and lessens the pill burden. Most PIs are now used in this boosted fashion. PIs as a whole are considered a potent and durable component of a HAART regimen, but drug-drug interactions

TABLE 1 Department of Health and Human Services (DHHS) and International AIDS Society-USA (IAS-USA) Guidelines for Initiating Antiretroviral Therapy*

Disease Type	DHHS Recommendations	IAS-USA Recommendations
Symptomatic HIV disease	Treatment recommended.	Treatment recommended.
Asymptomatic HIV disease, CD4$^+$ count <200 cells/mm^3	Treatment recommended.	Treatment recommended.
Asymptomatic HIV disease, CD4$^+$ count >201-350 cells/mm^3	Treatment should be offered following full discussion of pros and cons with each patient.	Physicians and patients must weigh risks and benefits of treatment thoroughly and make individualized informed decisions.
Asymptomatic HIV disease, CD4$^+$ count >350 cells/mm^3	For patients with HIV RNA <100,000 copies/mL, defer therapy. For patients with HIV RNA >100,000 copies/mL, most clinicians recommend deferring therapy, but some clinicians would treat.	For patients with HIV RNA >50,000-100,000 copies/mL or a rapidly declining CD4$^+$ count (loss of >100 cells/mm^3/y), initiation of therapy may be considered.

*This table provides general guidance rather than absolute recommendations for an individual patient. All decisions regarding initiating therapy should be made on the basis of prognosis as determined by CD4$^+$T cell count and level of plasma HIV RNA, the potential benefits and risks of therapy, and the willingness of the patient to accept therapy.
[3]Exceeds dosage recommended by the manufacturer.
Adapted from recommendations of Department of Health and Human Services (Guidelines for the use of antiretroviral agents in HIV-1-infected adults and adolescents, October 29, 2004) and the International AIDS Society-USA (IAS-USA) Panel.

and both short- and long-term side effects can occur (see Table 3). Potential toxicities should be discussed with patients before initiation of any new therapy.

NON-NUCLEOSIDE REVERSE TRANSCRIPTASE INHIBITORS

Many consider NNRTI-based regimens better tolerated and easier to take than PI-based regimens. They have less long-term metabolic toxicity than PIs. The most commonly used NNRTIs are efavirenz (Sustiva) and nevirapine (Viramune). Efavirenz-based regimens demonstrate excellent potency and durability in clinical trials. Efavirenz can cause neuropsychiatric side effects during the first few days or weeks of therapy, whereas nevirapine is associated with higher rates of hepatotoxicity and skin rash. Risk of hepatotoxicity is higher in women with CD4$^+$ counts above 250 cells/mm^3 or in men with counts above 400 cells/mm^3 and in the first 6 weeks of therapy. Delavirdine (Rescriptor) is considered less potent and now used infrequently.

FUSION INHIBITORS

Enfuvirtide (Fuzeon) is currently the only injectable ARV drug. This drug should be carefully chosen for treatment-experienced patients. Major disadvantages include high cost, inconvenient route of administration, and occurrence of injection-site reactions.

Adherence to Antiretroviral Therapy

Nonadherence among patients on HAART was the strongest predictor for failure to achieve viral suppression below the level of detection. Studies have reported that 90% to 95% of doses must be taken for optimal suppression. Suboptimal adherence is common and leads to decreased virologic control, increased morbidity and mortality, and drug resistance. Patients should be asked about all missed doses, especially in the last 3 days, with reasons for missing doses. Patients may be advised to bring their medications and medication diaries to clinic visits. The patient's literacy and readiness to take medication should be assessed over several visits. Patient education should include the goals of therapy, possible side effects of treatment, and information about the treatment for side effects. A multidisciplinary approach using family, friends, community-based case managers, peer educators, and adherence support groups should be used if available.

Complications of Antiretroviral Therapy

BONE MARROW SUPPRESSION

Zidovudine (AZT, Retrovir) is the most common cause of bone marrow toxicity; anemia may occur within 4 to 6 weeks; neutropenia usually occurs later, after 12 to 24 weeks. Complete blood counts should be measured at baseline and every 3 to 4 months following initiation of therapy. Patients at higher risk for bone marrow suppression may need monitoring more frequently. Significant drug-induced cytopenias become more common in the later stages of symptomatic HIV infection but occasionally develop abruptly in patients at earlier stages. Severe anemia or neutropenia may require discontinuation of azidothymidine (AZT) and support with erythropoietin (Epogen, Procrit) and/or filgrastim[1] (Neupogen).

_____

[1]Not FDA approved for this indication.

TABLE 2 Antiretroviral Regimens Recommended for Treatment of HIV-1 Infection in Antiretroviral-Naïve Patients

	Preferred Regimens	Number of Pills per Day
NNRTI based	Efavirenz (Sustiva) + (lamivudine [Epivir] or emtricitabine [Emtriva]) + (zidovudine [Retrovir] or tenofovir DF [Viread]) (Note: Efavirenz is not recommended for use in first trimester of pregnancy or in women with high pregnancy potential.[†])	2-3
PI based	Lopinavir/ritonavir (co-formulation) (Kaletra) + (lamivudine or emtricitabine) + zidovudine	8-9

	Alternative Regimens	Number of Pills per Day
NNRTI based	Efavirenz + (lamivudine or emtricitabine) + (abacavir [Ziagen] or didanosine [Videx] or stavudine [Zerit]) (Note: Efavirenz is not recommended for use in first trimester of pregnancy or in women with high pregnancy potential.[†])	2-4
	Nevirapine (Viramune) + (lamivudine or emtricitabine) + (zidovudine or stavudine or didanosine or abacavir or tenofovir) (Note: High incidence (11%) of symptomatic hepatic events observed in women with pre-nevirapine CD4[+] T cell count >250 cells/mm^3 and men with CD4[+] >400 cells/mm^3 [6.3%]. Use with caution in these patients, with close clinical and laboratory monitoring, especially during the first 18 weeks of therapy.)	3-6
PI based	Atazanavir (Reyataz) + (lamivudine or emtricitabine) + (zidovudine or stavudine or abacavir or didanosine) or (tenofovir or ritonavir [Norvir] 100 mg/d)	3-6
	Fosamprenavir (Lexiva)+ (lamivudine or emtricitabine) + (zidovudine or stavudine or abacavir or tenofovir or didanosine)	5-8
	Fosamprenavir/ritonavir[‡] + (lamivudine or emtricitabine) + (zidovudine or stavudine or abacavir or tenofovir or didanosine)	5-8
	Indinavir/ritonavir[‡] + (lamivudine or emtricitabine) + (zidovudine or stavudine or abacavir or tenofovir or didanosine)	7-12
	Lopinavir/ritonavir (Kaletra) + (lamivudine or emtricitabine) + (stavudine or abacavir or tenofovir or didanosine)	7-10
	Nelfinavir (Viracept) + (lamivudine or emtricitabine) + (zidovudine or stavudine or abacavir or tenofovir or didanosine)	5-8
	Saquinavir (sgc [Fortovase] or hgc [Invirase])/ritonavir[‡] + (lamivudine or emtricitabine) + (zidovudine or stavudine or abacavir or tenofovir or didanosine)	13-16
Triple-NRTI based	Abacavir + zidovudine + lamivudine: only when an NNRTI- or a PI-based regimen cannot or should not be used as first-line therapy.	2

*The generic and brand names for all the drugs listed are: abacavir (Ziagen), amprenavir (Agenerase), atazanavir (Reyataz), didanosine (Videx), efavirenz (Sustiva), emtricitabine (Entriva), fosamprenavir (Lexiva), lopinavir/ritonavir (Kalentra), nelfinavir (Viracept), nevirapine (Viramune), ritanovir (Norvir), saquinavir HGC (Invirase). saquinavir SGC (Fortovase), stavudine (Zerit), tenofovir (Viread), zidovudine (Retrovir).
†Women with childbearing potential implies women who want to conceive or those who are not using effective contraception.
‡Low-dose (100-200 mg) ritonavir.
Abbreviations: hgc = hard gel capsule; NNRTI = non-nucleoside reverse transcriptase inhibitor; PI = protease inhibitor; sgc = soft gel capsule.
From Department of Health and Human Services. Guidelines for the use of antiretroviral agents in HIV-1-infected adults and adolescents, October 29, 2004.

DISTAL SYMMETRIC POLYNEUROPATHY

The dideoxynucleoside class of ARV agents (didanosine [ddl, Videx], zalcitabine[ddc, Hivid], stavudine [d4T, Zerit]) may cause polyneuropathy. Paresthesias, pain and numbness occurring in the extremities, can be severely debilitating in many cases. Deep tendon reflexes are reduced or absent; pinprick, temperature, and vibration sensation may also be diminished in a stocking-and-glove distribution. Nerve conduction studies (NCSs) and electromyography (EMG) and nerve biopsy may be necessary with atypical presentations. Treatment consists of pain control with analgesics; in some cases, adjunctive agents such as tricyclic antidepressants (amitriptyline [Elavil], desipramine[1] [Norpramin]) and

anticonvulsants (gabapentin[1] [Neurantin], lamotrigine[1] [Lamictal]) may decrease symptoms. The decision to discontinue the offending ARV drug must consider the risks and benefits of virologic control versus neuropathic symptom control.

PANCREATITIS

Didanosine (ddI, Videx) is the agent most often associated with the complication of pancreatitis. Frequency is dose related and the fatality rate reported as 6%. Risk factors for ddI-associated pancreatitis include alcohol abuse, renal failure, morbid obesity, and hypertriglyceridemia. Dosage adjustment is required when the drug is used concurrently with tenofovirm (TDF, Viread), which increases levels of ddI. Asymptomatic patients with modest elevations in amylase and lipase levels (≤3-fold) may be monitored closely without change in therapy.

___
[1]Not FDA approved for this indication.

5 Management of the Patient with HIV Disease **55**

The Infectious Diseases

TABLE 3 Antiretroviral Medications: Dose and Adverse Events

Generic Name/ Trade Name	NRTIs	
	Dosing Recommendations	**Adverse Events**
Abacavir (ABC)/ Ziagen	300 mg bid or with ZDV and 3TC as Trizivir, one dose bid	Hypersensitivity reaction that can be fatal
Didanosine (ddI)/ Videx, Videx EC	Body weight ≥60 kg: 400 mg once daily (buffered tablets or enteric-coated capsule); or 200 mg bid (buffered tablets); body weight <60 kg: 250 mg daily (buffered tablets or enteric-coated capsule); or 125 mg bid (buffered tablets)	Pancreatitis; peripheral neuropathy; nausea; diarrhea Lactic acidosis with hepatic steatosis; rare but potentially life-threatening toxicity
Emtricitabine (FTC)/ Emtriva	200 mg once daily	Minimal toxicity; lactic acidosis with hepatic steatosis
Lamivudine (3TC)/ Epivir	150 mg bid; or 300 mg daily with ZDV as Combivir, or with ZDV and abacavir as Trizivir, one dose bid	Minimal toxicity; lactic acidosis with hepatic steatosis
Stavudine (d4T)/ Zerit, Zerit XR	Zerit: Body weight ≥60 kg: 40 mg bid; body weight <60 kg: 30 mg bid Zerit-XR: Body weight ≥60 kg: 100 mg once daily; body weight <60 kg: 75 mg once daily	Peripheral neuropathy; lipodystrophy; rapidly progressive ascending neuromuscular weakness (rare); pancreatitis; lactic acidosis with hepatic steatosis;
Tenofovir Disoproxil/ Fumarate Viread	300 mg daily for patients with creatinine clearance ≥60 mL/min	Asthenia, headache, diarrhea, nausea, vomiting, and flatulence; lactic acidosis with hepatic steatosis—not yet reported with tenofovir use; rare reports of renal insufficiency
Zalcitabine (ddC)/ Hivid	0.75 mg tid	Peripheral neuropathy; stomatitis; lactic acidosis with hepatic steatosis; pancreatitis
Zidovudine (AZT, ZDV)/ Retrovir	300 mg bid or 200 mg tid with lamivudine as Combivir, one dose bid or, with abacavir and lamivudine as Trizivir, one dose bid	Bone marrow suppression: anemia or neutropenia; subjective complaints: GI intolerance, headache, insomnia, asthenia; lactic acidosis with hepatic steatosis
	NNRTIs	
Delavirdine/Rescriptor	400 mg by mouth tid; four 100-mg tablets can be dispersed in ≥3 oz. of water to produce slurry; 200-mg tablets should be taken as intact tablets	Rash; increased transaminase levels; headaches
Efavirenz/Sustiva	600 mg by mouth daily on an empty stomach, preferably at bedtime	Rash; central nervous system symptoms; increased transaminase levels; false-positive cannabinoid test; teratogenic in monkeys
Nevirapine/Viramune	200 mg by mouth daily for 14 d; thereafter, 200 mg by mouth bid	Rash; hepatitis, including hepatic necrosis, is reported
	PIs	
Amprenavir/Agenerase	Body weight >50 kg: 1200 mg bid (capsules) or 1400 mg bid (oral solution) Body weight <50 kg: 20 mg/kg bid (capsules) to maximum 2400 mg daily total; 1.5 mL/kg bid (oral solution) to maximum 2800 mg daily total	GI intolerance: nausea, vomiting, diarrhea; rash; oral paresthesias; transaminase elevation; lipid abnormalities; noted with all PIs are hyperglycemia, fat redistribution
Atazanavir/Reyataz	400 mg once daily If taken with efavirenz (or tenofovir): Ritonavir 100 mg + atazanavir 300 mg once daily	Indirect hyperbilirubinemia; prolonged PR interval; some patients experience asymptomatic first-degree AV block; use with caution in patients with underlying conduction defects or on concomitant medications that can cause PR prolongation No lipid abnormalities
Fosamprenavir (f-APV)/Lexiva	700-mg tablet	Skin rash (19%), diarrhea, nausea, vomiting, headache, transaminase elevation

Continued

Rakel and Bope: *Conn's Current Therapy 2006*

TABLE 3 Antiretroviral Medications: Dose and Adverse Events—cont'd

Generic Name/ Trade Name	NRTIs	
Trade Name	Dosing Recommendations	Adverse Events
Indinavir/Crixivan	800 mg every 8 hours; recommendation without food, but with 1.5 L water per day	Nephrolithiasis; GI intolerance: nausea; lab: Increased indirect bilirubinemia (inconsequential); miscellaneous: headache, asthenia, blurred vision, dizziness, rash, metallic taste, thrombocytopenia, alopecia, and hemolytic anemia; lipid abnormalities
Lopinavir + Ritonavir/Kaletra	400 mg lopinavir + 100 mg ritonavir (three capsules) bid	GI intolerance: nausea, vomiting, diarrhea; Asthenia; elevated transaminase enzymes; lipid abnormalities Oral solution contains 42% alcohol
Nelfinavir/Viracept	750 mg tid or 1250 mg bid	Diarrhea; lipid abnormalities; serum transaminase elevation
Ritonavir/Norvir	600 mg every 12 hours (when ritonavir is used as sole PI)	GI intolerance: nausea, vomiting, diarrhea; paresthesias: circumoral and extremities; hepatitis; pancreatitis; asthenia; taste perversion; lab: triglycerides increase >200%, transaminase elevation, elevated CK and uric acid; lipid abnormalities
Saquinavir hard gel capsule/Invirase	Invirase is not recommended to be used as sole PI *With ritonavir:* ritonavir 100 mg + Invirase 1000 mg bid ritonavir 400 mg + Invirase 400 mg bid	GI intolerance: nausea and diarrhea; Headache; elevated transaminase enzymes; lipid abnormalities
Saquinavir soft gel capsule/Fortovase	1200 mg tid *With ritonavir:* ritonavir 100 mg + Fortovase 1000 mg bid ritonavir 400 mg + Fortovase 400 mg bid	As above
Fusion Inhibitors		
Enfuvirtide/Fuzeon	90 mg (1 mL) subcutaneously bid	Local injection site reactions (pain, erythema, induration, nodules and cysts, pruritus, ecchymosis); increased rate of bacterial pneumonia; hypersensitivity reaction (<1%): symptoms may include rash, fever, nausea, vomiting, chills, rigors, hypotension, or elevated serum transaminases; may recur on rechallenge

Abbreviations: AV = atrioventricular; bid = two times per day; CK = creatine kinase; GI = gastrointestinal; NNRTI = non-nucleoside reverse transcriptase inhibitor; NRTI = nucleoside reverse transcriptase inhibitor; PI = protease inhibitor; tid = three times per day.
From Department of Health and Human Services. Guidelines for the use of antiretroviral agents in HIV-1-infected adults and adolescents, October 29, 2004.

LACTIC ACIDOSIS/HEPATIC STEATOSIS

Severe decompensated lactic acidosis with hepatomegaly and steatosis is now considered rare but is potentially fatal when it occurs. Risk factors include pregnancy, obesity, being female, and prolonged use of NRTIs. NRTI-associated mitochondrial dysfunction is postulated as a cause of cellular injury, although the exact mechanism of action remains unclear. Signs and symptoms include nausea, abdominal pain, vomiting, diarrhea, anorexia, dyspnea, generalized weakness, myalgias, paresthesias, and hepatomegaly. Laboratory evaluation reveals an increased anion gap, elevated aminotransferases, creatine kinase, lactate dehydrogenase, lipase, and amylase. Computed tomography (CT) scans may indicate an enlarged fatty liver, and microvesicular steatosis may be noted on histologic exam. Treatment includes discontinuation of ARV treatment and supportive care, which may include hydration, mechanical ventilation, and/or dialysis. Anecdotal case reports show possible benefit with thiamine,[1] riboflavin,[1] and antioxidants.[1]

[1]Not FDA approved for this indication.

Rakel and Bope: *Conn's Current Therapy 2006*

HEPATOTOXICITY

Hepatotoxicity may occur with any NNRTIs and PIs. The majority of patients are asymptomatic. Among the NNRTIs, nevirapine (NVP, Viramune) has the greatest potential for causing clinical hepatitis. Similarly, PI-associated liver enzyme abnormalities can occur any time during the treatment course. Severe hepatotoxicity is noted more often among patients receiving regimens containing ritonavir (RTV, Norvir) or ritonavir/saquinavir (SQV, Fortovase, Invirase) compared to those receiving indinavir (IDN, Crixivan), nelfinavir (NFV, Viracept), or saquinavir. HAART-induced immune reconstitution may be the cause of liver decompensation in hepatitis B or C co-infected patients. Other risk factors include alcohol abuse, stavudine (d4T, Zerit) use, and concomitant use of other hepatotoxic agents.

RENAL TOXICITY

Indinavir (IDV, Crixivan) may cause renal abnormalities, especially when used with ritonavir (RTV, Norvir). Nephrolithiasis is most common, reported in 15% of patients on indinavir. Patients taking this drug are instructed to drink at least 48 oz of fluid per day to avoid renal complications. Tenofovir (TDF, Viread) may cause a Fanconi-like syndrome, especially in persons with low estimated glomerular filtration rates (GFRs). The incidence rate has yet to be determined.

HYPERGLYCEMIA

Hyperglycemia, new-onset diabetes mellitus, diabetic ketoacidosis, and exacerbation of preexisting diabetes mellitus may be observed, most notably with PI use. The pathogenesis is believed to be multifactorial, involving peripheral and hepatic resistance, insulin deficiency, and duration of exposure to ARV medications. Symptoms of hyperglycemia were reported at a median of 60 days after initiation of PI therapy. Hyperglycemia resolves in certain cases when PI therapy is discontinued. In other patients, oral hypoglycemics and/or insulin are added to their PI regimen. Data are lacking regarding what is the better option. Most experts recommend continuation of HAART in the absence of severe diabetes.

FAT MALDISTRIBUTION

Localized fat accumulations are reported with NRTI monotherapy. Fat maldistribution syndromes are more common with use of highly active ARV therapy. Fat maldistribution with insulin resistance and hyperlipidemia is referred to as lipodystrophy syndrome. Multifactorial causation is suggested. Prevalence increases with duration of ARV therapy and with use of protease inhibitors. Loss of subcutaneous fat in the face and extremities (lipoatrophy) is most commonly attributed to long-term NRTI exposure, especially with stavudine (d4T, Zerit). Discontinuation of ARV medications or class switching does not result in substantial benefit.

HYPERLIPIDEMIA

ARV therapy is associated with the elevation of total serum cholesterol, low-density lipoprotein (LDL), and fasting triglycerides (TGs). Dyslipidemias primarily occur with PIs and might be associated with accelerated atherosclerosis and cardiovascular complications among HIV-infected patients. Treatment includes dietary interventions, regular exercise, control of blood pressure, and smoking cessation. Addition of lipid-controlling agents, such as 3β-hydroxy-3β-methylglutaryl-CoA reductase inhibitors (statins), may be necessary. Interactions of certain statins with PIs can result in increased statin levels. Pravastatin (Pravachel) and atorvastatin (Lipitor) are less affected by the inhibitory effect of PIs via the cytochrome P-450 system and can be used with PIs. Fibrates can be added to statin therapy with additional monitoring for rhabdomyolysis and hepatotoxicity. For severe lipid elevations, modifications might be required in the HAART regimen. Certain PIs (atazanavir [Reyataz]) and NNRTIs (nevirapine [Viramune]) are considered less dyslipidemic.

CARDIOVASCULAR DISEASE

Etiology of cardiovascular disease is multifactorial, including traditional risk factors, HIV disease–related factors, and ARV-related issues. Potential risk factors include dyslipidemia, insulin resistance, endothelial dysfunction, hypercoagulability, elevated C-reactive protein, hypertension, and elevated homocysteine. Most PIs increase very-low-density lipoprotein (VLDLP)/TGs, and increase LDL, but have little effect on high-density lipoprotein (HDL). NNRTIs increase HDL; NRTIs, especially stavudine (d4T, Zerit) increases LDL and TGs. Data suggest increased risk of myocardial infarction in association with ARV use; many HIV-infected patients are at increased long-term risk of atherosclerosis. The management of cardiac risk plays an increasing role in the treatment of HIV/AIDS.

OSTEONECROSIS

Also known as avascular necrosis (AVN), osteonecrosis results from direct or indirect damage to the affected bone's vascular supply. AVN involving the hips is described among HIV-infected adults and more recently among HIV-infected children. Chief complaint is pain in an affected bone; most common sites are the femoral head, followed by the humoral head, and less frequently the wrist, knee, and ankle. Diagnosis usually made by CT scan or magnetic resonance imaging (MRI). Although a causal relationship between AVN and HAART is proposed, recent epidemiologic data suggest other recognized risk factors are involved. These factors include alcohol abuse, hemoglobinopathies, corticosteroid treatment, hyperlipidemia, and hypercoagulability states. Surgery may be necessary to treat disabling symptoms.

SKIN RASH

Skin rash occurs with the NNRTI class of drugs, especially with nevirapine (NVP, Viramune). The majority of cases occur within the first weeks of therapy. Serious cutaneous manifestations (e.g., Stevens-Johnson syndrome [SJS] and toxic epidermal necrolysis [TEN]) are rare, and the drug should be discontinued. Using a 2-week lead-in dose escalation schedule when initiating nevirapine therapy might reduce the incidence of rash. Corticosteroid or antihistamine therapy may worsen the condition and should be discouraged. Skin rash may be one of the symptoms of abacavir (ABC, Ziagen)-associated systemic hypersensitivity reaction and therapy should be discontinued. Among PIs, skin rash occurs most frequently with amprenavir (APV, Agenerase).

IMMUNE RECONSTITUTION INFLAMMATORY SYNDROME

Immune reconstitution inflammatory syndrome (IRIS) has symptoms and/or signs consistent with an infectious/inflammatory condition and temporally related to initiation of ARV therapy and can not be explained by a newly acquired infection, the expected clinical course of a previously recognized infectious agent, or the side effects of ARV therapy itself. Symptoms and signs are significant for paradoxical worsening or atypical manifestations of the subclinical disease present prior to starting ARV therapy. Various infections are described, including *Mycobacterium avium* infection, tuberculosis, cytomegalovirus (CMV) retinitis, progressive multifocal leukoencephalopathy, rarely *Pneumocystis jiroveci* pneumonia, cryptococcal meningitis, herpes simplex infection, and hepatitis B or hepatitis C infection. In patients who are ARV naïve and who have an opportunistic infection, the underlying infection should be treated and ARV therapy should be considered after 2 to 4 weeks at least, but there are no clear guidelines.

OPPORTUNISTIC INFECTIONS

The incidence of nearly all AIDS-defining opportunistic infections (OIs) decreased significantly in the United States after HAART was introduced. The success of HAART in reducing the incidence of AIDS-related OIs led to a reassessment of the role of prophylaxis against these infections in HIV-infected patients who have sustained antiviral responses (Table 4). There is now sufficient data to recommend that for patients who have CD4$^+$ T lymphocyte count responses, primary and/or secondary prophylaxis for some OIs can be discontinued. But despite the encouraging trends in incidence of OI, patients are still dying from HIV and associated OIs. These occurrences are most notable among individuals who are unaware of their HIV seropositivity, adhere poorly to prophylaxis, or have poor access to adequate health care. These three groups pose an important challenge in management, especially in light of recent studies indicating that the best treatment for many OIs remains effective ARV therapy.

Pneumocystis Pneumonia

The report of *Pneumocystis jiroveci* pneumonia (formerly *Pneumocystis carinii* pneumonia [PCP]) in previously healthy men in 1981 heralded the onset of the current AIDS epidemic. In the following two decades, PCP gained notoriety as the most common opportunistic infection associated with HIV and the most common infection to have occurred among persons who died with AIDS. The best predictor of PCP is the CD4$^+$ lymphocyte blood count. The majority of AIDS patients have CD4$^+$ cell counts in the range of 50 to 70/mm^3 at the time of their first episode of PCP; more than 90% of episodes occur when counts are below 200/mm^3. Clinical presentation includes exertional dyspnea, nonproductive cough, fever, and hypoxemia. Symptoms may persist for weeks and be accompanied by weight loss and malaise. Lung examination is usually normal, although fine basilar inspiratory rales may be heard on auscultation. Laboratory findings often include an elevated serum lactate dehydrogenase (LDH), although this abnormality is neither sensitive nor specific for PCP. The best indicator of prognosis is the alveolar-arterial gradient at the time specific therapy is initiated. Chest radiograph classically reveals a diffuse bilateral, interstitial, and then alveolointerstitial infiltrate progressing from perihilar to peripheral regions. Apical disease, often confused with tuberculosis, is associated with use of aerosol pentamidine (NebuPent) prophylaxis. Pleural effusions and intrathoracic adenopathy are rare, whereas spontaneous pneumothoraces are more common in PCP. Normal chest radiographs are reported in the range of 0% to 40%. Extrapulmonary disease is rarely encountered in patients receiving systemic chemoprophylaxis. Reported sites of disseminated *P. jiroveci* infection include the lymph nodes, liver, spleen, bone marrow, intestine, peritoneum, adrenal gland, pancreas, skin, eye, ear, and meninges.

Diagnosis of PCP is established with identification of *P. jiroveci* on microscopic examination with Gomori's methenamine silver stain or toluidine blue O. Expectorated sputum is rarely suitable for microscopic evaluation. Similarly, purulent sputum, even when induced, may be inadequate for examination because of presence of cellular debris and artifact. Bronchoscopy with bronchoalveolar lavage (BAL) is the diagnostic procedure of choice for obtaining adequate pulmonary secretions. Gallium citrate scanning is a highly sensitive (90%) but nonspecific test (50%) for PCP but seldom used in routine cases because of high cost and time delay for results (3 days).

Empirical treatment prior to confirmation of diagnosis may be appropriate for patients who are clinically stable or individuals who do not have prompt access to diagnostic facilities. Trimethoprim-sulfamethoxazole (Bactrim, Septra) for at least 21 days is always the drug of choice unless the patient has a history of life-threatening intolerance. No other agent demonstrates higher efficacy for PCP; it is well absorbed orally and can be used for outpatient therapy for mild disease (room air P$_{O2}$ more than 80 mm Hg) in patients with no major gastrointestinal dysfunction. Table 5 outlines dosing and alternative options. In patients receiving HAART, primary and secondary prophylaxis against PCP can be safely discontinued after the CD4$^+$ cell count has increased to 200/mm^3 or more for longer than 3 months (Table 6).

TABLE 4 Prophylaxis against Common Opportunistic Disease in Adults and Adolescents Infected with Human Immunodeficiency Virus

Pathogen	Indication	Preventive Regimens	
		First Choice	**Alternatives**
Pneumocystis jiroveci	CD4$^+$ count <200/μL or oropharyngeal candidiasis	Trimethoprim-sulfamethoxazole (TMP-SMZ [Bactrim]), 1 DS PO qd TMP-SMZ, 1 SS PO qd	Dapsone,[1] 50 mg PO bid *or* 100 mg PO qd; dapsone, 50 mg PO qd, *plus* pyrimethamine, 50 mg PO qw, *plus* leucovorin, 25 mg PO qw; dapsone, 200 mg PO, *plus* pyrimethamine (Daraprim), 75 mg PO, *plus* leucovorin, 25 mg PO qw; aerosolized pentamidine (NebuPent), 300 mg qm via Respirgard II nebulizer; atovaquone (Mepron), 1500 mg PO qd; TMP-SMZ, 1 DS PO tiw
Toxoplasma gondii	IgG antibody to *Toxoplasma* and CD4$^+$ count <100/μL	TMP-SMZ,[1] 1 DS PO qd	TMP-SMZ, 1 SS PO qd: dapsone,[1] 50 mg PO qd, *plus* pyrimethamine, 50 mg PO qw, *plus* leucovorin, 25 mg PO qw; dapsone, 200 mg PO, plus pyrimethamine, 75 mg PO, *plus* leucovorin, 25 mg PO qw; atovaquone,[1] 1500 mg PO qd with or without pyrimethamine, 25 mg PO qd, *plus* leucovorin, 10 mg PO qd
Mycobacterium avium complex	CD4$^+$ count <50/μL	Azithromycin (Zithromax), 1200 mg PO qw, or clarithromycin (Biaxin), 500 mg PO bid	Rifabutin (Mycobutin), 300 mg PO qd; azithromycin, 1200 mg PO qw *plus* rifabutin, 300 mg PO qd

[1]Not FDA approved for this indication.
Notes: Prophylaxis should also be considered for persons with a CD4$^+$ percentage of <14%, for persons with a history of an AIDS-defining illness, and possibly for those with CD4$^+$ counts >200 but <250 cells/μL. TMP-SMZ also reduces the frequency of toxoplasmosis and some bacterial infections. Patients receiving dapsone should be tested for glucose-6 phosphate dehydrogenase deficiency. The efficacy of parenteral pentamidine (e.g., 4 mg/kg/mo) is uncertain. Patients who are administered therapy for toxoplasmosis with sulfadiazine-pyrimethamine are protected against *Pneumocystis jiroveci* pneumonia and do not need additional prophylaxis against PCP.
Abbreviations: DS = double-strength tablet; PCP = *Pneumocystis carinii* pneumonia; PO = by mouth; qd = daily; qm = monthly; qw = weekly; SS= single-strength tablet; tiw = three times a week; TMP-SMZ = trimethoprim-sulfamethoxazole.
From Masur H, Kaplan JE, Homes KK, and the USPHS/IDSA Prevention of Opportunistic Infections Working Group: 2001 USPHS/IDSA guidelines for the prevention of opportunistic infections in persons infected with human immunodeficiency virus.

Candidiasis

Candidiasis is the most common fungal condition seen in HIV-positive persons. Progression of HIV infection to AIDS is associated with development of oropharyngeal candidiasis. *Candida albicans* causes most disease; however, other species, including *Candida tropicalis, Candida krusei,* and *Candida dubliniensis,* are also reported, although much less frequently. *Candida glabrata* and *Candida parapsilosis* infections tend to occur in patients with very advanced disease who had previous exposure to antifungals. Chronic courses of azole therapy (e.g., in prophylaxis) may result in selecting out of more azole-resistant species.

Presentation is generally limited to oral, vaginal, or esophageal mucosa. Systemic disease is extremely rare and should not be included in the differential diagnosis of unexplained fever. Symptoms of oropharyngeal candidiasis include burning, pain, and altered taste sensation, although many patients are asymptomatic. Pseudomembranous candidiasis, or thrush, appears as removable white plaques on any oral mucosal surface. The erythematous form is seen as smooth red patches and often missed on routine examination. Candidiasis can also cause angular cheilitis, producing erythema,

cracks, and fissures at the corner of the mouth. Vaginal candidiasis presents as a creamy white vaginal discharge and often is the first evidence of immune dysfunction in women because it can precede the development of oral infection. Recurrent infection is common, and chronic suppressive therapy may be necessary. Esophageal involvement may present with severe dysphagia or odynophagia in patients with or without evidence of oral infection. Diagnosis of oral or vaginal disease often is made on clinical appearance alone. In patients who fail to respond to standard therapy, potassium hydroxide (KOH) preparation and fungal cultures are indicated. Esophageal disease is diagnosed by endoscopic examination and culture, although response to empirical antifungal therapy is often used as an indirect means of establishing the diagnosis.

Patients with localized oral or vulvovaginal candidiasis respond well to topical therapy: clotrimazole (Mycelex) oral troches, 10 mg five times per day, or nystatin oral pastilles (Mycostatin) (200,000 U) or oral suspension (500,000 U/5 mL), five times per day. For patients who do not respond to standard therapy or who have esophageal disease, the antifungal azole compounds are effective. Treatment of esophageal candidiasis

TABLE 5 Treatment of *Pneumocystis jiroveci* Pneumonia (PCP)

Regimens	Side Effects
First Choice	
Trimethoprim/sulfamethoxazole (Bactrim), 15 mg/kg/d IV or PO trimethoprim and 75 mg/kg/d of sulfamethoxazole divided q6-8h × 21 d	Neutropenia, rash, GI upset, increased creatinine and potassium
Alternatives	
Trimethoprim,[1] 15 mg/kg/d, *plus* dapsone,[1] 100 mg PO/d × 21 d	Rash, neutropenia, GI upset, methemoglobinemia, hemolytic anemia (dapsone)
Intravenous pentamidine (Pentam), 4 mg/kg/d IV × 21 d	Pancreatitis, hypoglycemia, hyperglycemia, rash, hypotension, cardiac arrhythmias
Clindamycin (Cleocin)[1], 600 mg IV q8h/300-450 mg PO q6h *plus* primaquine,[1] 30 mg PO qd × 21 d	GI upset, neutropenia, diarrhea, *Clostridium difficile* infection
Atovaquone (Mepron), 750 mg suspension PO bid × 21 d	Rash, GI upset
Trimetrexate (Neutrexin), 45 mg/m² IV qd *plus* folinic acid (leucovorin), 20 mg mg/m² PO IV q6h ± dapsone, 100 mg PO qd × 21 d	Neutropenia, rash, fever

[1]Not FDA approved for this indication.
Note: Tapering doses of corticosteroids is recommended in patients with severe disease (PO₂ <70 mm Hg or A-a gradient >35 mm Hg): prednisone 40 mg PO bid on days 1 through 5, followed by prednisone 40 mg PO qd on days 6 through 10, then prednisone 20 mg PO qd on days 11 through 21.
Abbreviations: A-a = arterial-alveolar; bid = twice per day; GI = gastrointestinal; IV = intravenous; PO = by mouth; q = every; qd = every day.

requires systemic therapy. Options include fluconazole (Diflucan), 100 to 200 mg per day, by mouth or intravenous for 14 to 21 days, and itraconazole (Sporanox), 200 mg per day (tablets) or 100 mg twice per day (oral suspension). Maintenance suppressive therapy may be necessary in cases of recurrent esophagitis; fluconazole up to 800 mg per day[3] may be successful despite in vitro resistance. Drug resistance, particularly azole-resistant candidiasis, is increasingly common. Some patients respond to increased doses of the drug, and some respond to a switch from one azole to another (e.g., fluconazole to itraconazole or voriconazole). However, low-dose therapy with intravenous amphotericin B or caspofungin may be required.

Mycobacterial Infection

Mycobacterium tuberculosis infection continues to be a devastating disease worldwide. HIV infection is by far the most important predisposing factor for the development of tuberculosis (TB). The risk of death in HIV-infected patients with TB is reported to be twice that in HIV-infected patients without TB, independent of CD4⁺ cell count. Resistant tuberculosis is seen with increasing frequency, especially in urban areas. This disease is particularly difficult to treat in the HIV-infected patient. HIV-infected persons latently infected with tuberculosis develop reactivation tuberculosis at a rate of 8% to 10% per year, rather than 5% to 10% per lifetime. HIV-infected persons exposed to an infectious index case develop acute tuberculosis at a rate as high as 40% over 6 to 12 months rather than 2% to 5% over 2 years, as seen in normal hosts. Finally, tuberculosis may accelerate the progression of HIV infection by activating expression of HIV from macrophages. Three principles for treatment of TB in HIV-infected patients are emphasized. First, ARV therapy should be administered when indicated, regardless of anti-TB therapy. Second, a short-course regimen (6 to 9 months, depending on the regimen used) should be administered as directly observed therapy to enhance compliance. Third, rifabutin[1] (Mycobutin) at a lower dosage (150 mg) is preferred over rifampin (Rifadin) because of significant drug interactions of rifampin (RIF) with PIs and NNRTIs.

Mycobacterium Avium Complex Disease

The prevalence of diagnosed disseminated *Mycobacterium avium* complex (MAC) for patients with CD4⁺ cell counts of fewer than 100/mm³ is approximately 10% at autopsy. Prior to HAART and routine use of prophylaxis, the rate was approximately 50%. Despite declining incidence, MAC continues to be the most common systemic bacterial infection in AIDS and is responsible for significant morbidity. Clinical presentation of disseminated MAC includes fever, night sweats, severe weight loss, and, less often, diarrhea. High spiking temperatures and a toxic appearance may be seen. Hepatosplenomegaly may be present, but the examination often is quite nonspecific and unrevealing. Common laboratory abnormalities include anemia, neutropenia, and elevated alkaline phosphatase. Diagnosis depends on culturing the organism from blood and/or bone marrow. The utility of cultures from other sites, including lymph node and liver, is less well established. Blood cultures using special culture media (i.e., BACTEC system and Dupont Isolator system) yield the highest results. Whereas a single blood culture is diagnostic for MAC infection, a negative culture does not rule disseminated infection because patients can have low levels of mycobacteremia.

Treatment of MAC continues to improve. Many drugs have activity, including the macrolides (azithromycin [Zithromax] and clarithromycin [Biaxin]), the rifamycins

---

[3]Exceeds dosage recommended by the manufacturer.

[1]Not FDA approved for this indication.

TABLE 6 Criteria for Starting, Discontinuing, and Restarting Opportunistic Infection Prophylaxis for Adults With Human Immunodeficiency Virus Infection

	Criteria for initiating primary prophylaxis	Criteria for discontinuing primary prophylaxis	Criteria for restarting primary prophylaxis	Criteria for initiating secondary prophylaxis	Criteria for discontinuing secondary prophylaxis	Criteria for restarting secondary prophylaxis
Opportunistic Illness						
Pneumocystis jiroveci pneumonia	$CD4^+$ <200 cells/μL or oropharyngeal candidiasis	$CD4^+$ >200 cells/μL for ≥3 mo	$CD4^+$ <200 cells/μL	Prior PCP	$CD4^+$ >200 cells/μL for ≥3 mo	$CD4^+$ <200 cells/μL
Toxoplasmosis	IgG antibody to toxoplasma and $CD4^+$ <100 cells/μL	$CD4^+$ >200 cells/μL for ≥3 mo	$CD4^+$ <100-200 cells/μL	Prior toxoplasmic encephalitis	$CD4^+$ >200 cells/μL sustained (e.g., ≥6 mo) and completed initial therapy and asymptomatic for toxo	$CD4^+$ <200 cells/μL
Disseminated Mycobacterium avium complex	$CD4^+$ <50 cells/μL	$CD4^+$ >100 cells/μL for ≥3 mo	$CD4^+$ <50-100 cells/μL	Documented disseminated disease	$CD4^+$ >100 cells/μL sustained (e.g., ≥6 mo) and completed 12 mo of MAC therapy and asymptomatic for MAC	$CD4^+$ <100 cells/μL
Cryptococcosis	None	Not applicable	Not applicable	Documented disease	$CD4^+$ >100-200 cells/μL sustained (e.g., ≥6 mo) and completed initial therapy and asymptomatic for cryptococcosis	$CD4^+$ <100-200 cells/μL
Histoplasmosis	None	Not applicable	Not applicable	Documented disease	No criteria recommended for stopping	Not applicable
Coccidioidomycosis	None	Not applicable	Not applicable	Documented disease	No criteria recommended for stopping	Not applicable
Cytomegalovirus retinitis	None	Not applicable	Not applicable	Documented end-organ disease	$CD4^+$ >100-150 cells/μL sustained (e.g., ≥6 mo) and no evidence of active disease Regular ophthalmic examination	$CD4^+$ <100-150 cells/μL

From Masur H, Kaplan JE, Homes KK, and the USPHS/IDSA Prevention of Opportunistic Infections Working Group: 2001 USPHS/IDSA guidelines for the prevention of opportunistic infections in persons infected with human immunodeficiency virus.

(rifabutin [Mycobutin] and rifampin[1] [Rifadin]), ciprofloxacin[1] (Cipro), ethambutol[1] (Myambutol), and amikacin[1] (Amikin). Therapy initially should include a macrolide and ethambutol. A third agent, such as rifamycin or ciprofloxacin, can be either included in the initial regimen or added if there is a slow response. The addition of amikacin as a fourth agent may be needed in some patients who fail to respond or who relapse. In patients who are very ill with MAC disease, some experts recommend using a multidrug regimen initially (e.g., clarithromycin, ethambutol, rifamycin, and amikacin) to try to diminish rapidly the bacteremic load of organisms.

Rakel and Bope: *Conn's Current Therapy 2006*

Once the patient clinically responds, switching to at least two oral agents (e.g., ethambutol and clarithromycin) simplifies an outpatient regimen. Clofazimine[1] (Lamprene) is no longer recommended because of an association with increased mortality. Prophylaxis for MAC disease is recommended for patients with CD4+ cell counts of less than 50/mm³ (see Table 6). Patients with prior history of opportunistic infections or colonization with MAC in the respiratory or gastrointestinal tract should also be considered for chemoprophylaxis. Studies support the discontinuation of prophylaxis in patients who respond to HAART with sustained increases in CD4+ cell counts to greater than 100/mm³ for 3 to 6 months.

Cytomegalovirus (CMV) Infection

Prior to HAART, CMV infection was diagnosed in up to 40% of AIDS patients. Virtually all patients with disease because of CMV have CD4+ counts less than 100/mm³. Linking detection of CMV to disease may be difficult because the presence of CMV in culture does not necessarily indicate invasive disease. Therefore, clinical presentation, physical examination, histopathologic findings, and viral culture all must be considered. Chorioretinitis is now seldom the presenting manifestation but occurs when the CD4+ count is less than 50/mm³. It remains the most common intraocular infection in patients with AIDS, accounting for at least 90% of HIV-related infectious retinopathies. Symptoms include decreasing visual acuity, the presence of so-called floaters, and visual field cut defects. Blindness results if CMV infection is left untreated. Diagnosis is made clinically by ophthalmologic examination. Typical findings include creamy or yellow-white granular areas with perivascular exudates and hemorrhages. These lesions are found initially in the periphery of the fundus but can progress to involve the macula and optic disc. Antigenemia testing and nucleic acid amplification testing are used to identify at-risk patients for prophylaxis and to predict CMV end-organ disease. Extraocular CMV manifestations include esophagitis, pneumonitis, enteritis, colitis, adrenalitis, and encephalitis. Four drugs that act to inhibit viral DNA polymerase are currently available for therapy: ganciclovir (Cytovene), valganciclovir (Valcyte), foscarnet (Foscavir), and cidofovir (Vistide). Induction therapy includes 2 weeks or more of high-dose drug. When retinitis is stable, patients are placed on lifelong maintenance therapy until evidence of immune recovery is apparent. Alternative therapies include intraocular ganciclovir (Vitrasert) implants and fomivirsen intravitreal (Vitravene) injection. Some experts feel the implants are superior to systemic therapy in time to relapse, but there is increased risk of involvement of the other eye and increased risk of extraocular disease. So any local therapy should be accompanied by systemic anti-CMV therapy such as oral ganciclovir or valganciclovir. Current data suggest that secondary prophylaxis can be safely discontinued after resolution of lesions, if the CD4+ cell count is

above 100 to 150/mm³ for at least 3 to 6 months, if the lesions are not life-threatening, and if regular follow-up with an ophthalmologist can be ensured. Discontinuation of secondary prophylaxis for extraocular CMV disease is not supported by the literature.

Toxoplasmosis

Toxoplasmosis gondii is the most common cause of focal encephalitis in AIDS patients. Disease is usually caused by recrudescence of latent infection, and therefore all patients with antibodies to *T. gondii* are at risk. Approximately 25% to 40% of seropositive patients eventually develop disease unless given prophylaxis. In patients with HIV infection, the risk of reactivation of toxoplasma infection increases with a decreasing CD4+ cell count; especially when the CD4+ count falls below 100/mm³. In the United States, toxoplasmic encephalitis (TE) is reported in 1% to 5% of patients with AIDS. Clinical presentation ranges from focal neurologic findings to generalized symptoms, including weakness, confusion, seizures, and coma. Constitutional symptoms such as fever and malaise are variable, but meningism is rare. The cerebrospinal fluid (CSF) may show a mononuclear pleocytosis and elevated protein or may be normal. Disseminated toxoplasmosis, involving heart, lung, colon, skeletal muscles, and other organs, is described. Septic shock is also seen, with presentation of prolonged fever, dyspnea, thrombocytopenia, and high lactate dehydrogenase levels.

Diagnosis is made definitively by demonstration of the tachyzoite form of *T. gondii* in brain biopsy specimens; however, histologic diagnosis can be difficult because changes can resemble other infectious processes and the organism may be difficult to find. Most often, diagnosis is made presumptively based on positive serology, radiographic findings, and response to specific therapy. Radiographic evaluation of the central nervous system (CNS) reveals single or multiple lesions with ring or nodular enhancement. Lesions are most frequently found in the basal ganglia or corticomedullary junction. The MRI scan is the best diagnostic imaging technique and may detect lesions not seen in CT scanning. The presence of edema, a mass effect, and hemorrhage may help distinguish TE from CNS lymphoma. Thalllium-201 single-photon emission computed tomography (SPECT) scans are used with greater frequency to distinguish these two entities: A negative scan is unlikely to represent lymphoma. Serologic diagnosis is highly reliable but not specific for active disease. Almost all patients with toxoplasmosis have IgG antibody. Seronegative toxoplasmosis is rare, accounting for 0% to 3% of cases. The level of antibody does not predict the likelihood of reactivation or severity of disease. The use of PCR enables detection of *T. gondii* DNA in brain tissue, CSF, BAL fluid, sputum, and blood in patients with AIDS. Response to empirical treatment is the most practical means of making the diagnosis. In some series, 50% of patients with toxoplasmosis respond clinically to therapy by day 3 and 90% by day 14 and radiographically within 2 weeks. Administration of corticosteroids results in radiologic

---

[1] Not FDA approved for this indication.

improvement if the disease is either lymphoma or toxoplasmosis and should therefore not routinely be given unless the diagnosis is already secured. The mainstay of treatment is combination chemotherapy. Most agents act synergistically to block folic acid metabolism (see article "Toxoplasmosis" for treatment options). Primary prophylaxis should be offered to all patients with positive IgG antibody and CD4$^+$ more than 100 cells/mm^3. Secondary prophylaxis or lifelong suppressive therapy should be given following primary treatment (see Table 6). The role of immune reconstitution in modifying this rule is still unclear; discontinuation should be considered when CD4$^+$ count is more than 200 cells /mm^3 for longer than 3 months and viral load more than 5000 copies/mm^3.

Cryptococcosis

Cryptococcus neoformans most often causes meningitis or disseminated disease. Approximately 6% to 10% of patients with AIDS develop cryptococcal infection; it is the most common systemic fungal infection in HIV-infected patients. It is the third most common AIDS CNS disorder, behind toxoplasmosis and CNS lymphoma. Cryptococcal meningitis is usually an indolent disease. Symptoms, including headache, fever, and malaise, typically are present for weeks prior to diagnosis. Classic meningism and focal neurologic signs are uncommon, occurring less than 10% of the time. Lethargy, mental status changes, and forgetfulness are common. CSF analysis reveals a poor inflammatory response. Protein and glucose may be normal, with little pleocytosis. Poor prognostic factors include impaired mental status at presentation, fewer than 20 white blood cells (WBCs) in CSF, raised opening pressure (more than 200 mm H$_2$O), and a CSF cryptococcal antigen titer of greater than 1:1054. Positive CSF culture for *C. neoformans* is the standard for diagnosis of meningitis. The latex agglutination test for the cryptococcal polysaccharide antigen is highly sensitive and specific. In general, any serum titer in excess of 1:4 should be repeated and consideration given to a full evaluation; any titer in excess of 1:32 should be considered diagnostic. All patients with a positive serum cryptococcal antigen titer should undergo a spinal tap. CSF India ink stains are positive approximately 75% of the time. Routine screening of patients with the serum cryptococcal antigen test, however, is not recommended.

Therapy for cryptococcosis in AIDS patients is lifelong. Amphotericin B (Fungizane) (0.7 to 1.0 mg/kg per day intravenously) for a total dose of 2.5 g, with concurrent flucytosine (Ancoban) (25 mg/kg by mouth every 6 hours for 14 days), is the treatment of choice, followed by fluconazole (Diflucan), 400 mg daily, to complete an 8- to 10-week course. Lifelong maintenance with fluconazole, 200 mg daily, is recommended. Weekly amphotericin B prophylaxis produces a higher relapse rate compared to fluconazole. Increased intracranial pressure greater than 250 mm H$_2$O requires urgent CSF drainage. In absence of obstructive hydrocephalus, serial lumbar punctures are recommended for complications of increased intracranial pressure. In addition, corticosteroids may ameliorate the sequelae of increased intracranial pressure. If cerebral edema occurs in any patient with cryptococcosis, high-dose steroids may offer temporary benefit. Limited studies support the use of antifungal prophylaxis in preventing cryptococcosis. Although the incidence of cryptococcal meningitis decreases with the use of either fluconazole[1] or itraconazole[1] (Sparanox) prophylaxis, no survival benefit is noted. Because of concerns regarding potential development of antifungal resistance, relative infrequency of cryptococcal disease, the possibility of drug interactions, and costs, guidelines do not recommend routine prophylaxis.

ENDEMIC FUNGAL INFECTIONS

Histoplasmosis occurs in at least 5% of HIV-infected patients residing within endemic regions (central and south central) of the United States. For these HIV-infected patients, it often is the first opportunistic infection (more than 70%), and nearly all cases are disseminated at the time of diagnosis. Disseminated infection may result either from direct contact with *Histoplasma capsulatum* or from reactivation of latent foci. More than 95% of patients present with fever and weight loss, and more often 50% have pulmonary complaints. The chest roentgenogram may show streaky infiltrates but can be normal in half of the cases. An elevated lactate dehydrogenase level, often higher than 1000 U/L, may be another clue to diagnosis. With disseminated disease, HIV-infected patients can present with sepsis-like syndrome characterized by hypotension, respiratory and liver failure, and disseminated intravascular coagulopathy. Diagnosis of active disease is made by isolation of *H. capsulatum* from appropriate sites, including blood, bone marrow, lung tissue, or lymph node. Therapy with amphotericin B (Fungizone) is effective in most patients. Failures are seen in patients who are severely ill at diagnosis. Itraconazole (Sparanox) can be used for less severe, nonmeningeal, nonsepticemic cases. Lifetime maintenance therapy is required to prevent relapse. Coccidioidomycosis is a systemic fungal disease endemic to areas of the southwestern United States. Rates and severity of illness are higher in HIV-infected persons. Presentation depends on the immunologic status of the patient. For patients with CD4$^+$ cell counts of less than 250/mm^3, pneumonia and meningitis are more common. The disease may present as an fever of unknown origin (FUO) with diffuse lymphadenopathy and pancytopenia. Diagnosis is by culture of blood, bone marrow, CSF, or pulmonary specimen and serologic tests. Treatment of systemic disease is with amphotericin B (1 mg/kg per day) for a total dose of as much as 2.5 g. The oral azoles, including itraconazole[1] (200 mg twice daily) and fluconazole[1] (Diflucan) (400 mg per day), are also used with success as initial therapy. Maintenance therapy with either intermittent amphotericin B or oral azoles is recommended because relapse rates are high. Blastomycosis is a systemic fungal disease endemic to areas of the midwestern and south-central United States.

---

[1] Not FDA approved for this indication.

It rarely causes disease in HIV-infected persons even in endemic regions.

Herpesvirus Infection

Herpes simplex virus (HSV) types 1 and 2 commonly cause disease in HIV-infected persons; 95% of homosexual men with AIDS have positive serology for HSV, as does up to 77% of the HIV-infected population in general. Reactivation occurs frequently, resulting in chronic, persistent mucocutaneous disease in many patients with AIDS. Direct contact with oral secretions (HSV-1) or genital secretions (HSV-2) is the primary mode of transmission. Clinical manifestations of HSV infection include large, painful, grouped vesicles with an erythematous base that can involve any areas of the body but occur most frequently in the orolabial, genital, and anorectal regions. Diagnosis of HSV infection is made by clinical presentation or by viral culture. HSV should be considered a cause of any chronic nonhealing ulcer or indistinct erosion. For initial therapy, oral acyclovir (Zovirax) (200 to 400 mg five times daily) is the treatment of choice for routine lesions. Bioavailability of oral acyclovir is approximately 10% to 20%. Topical acyclovir* is not highly effective in patients with HIV infection and should not be used. Famciclovir (Famvir), 250 mg by mouth three times per day,* and valacyclovir (Valtrex), 1.0 g by mouth two times per day, both given for 7 to 10 days, are equally effective. Both have excellent bioavailability after oral administration. Suppressive therapy is recommended for patients with recurrent infection or relapses after the discontinuation of therapy. Many patients can be controlled with acyclovir, 400 to 800 mg per day in divided doses; famciclovir, 125 to 250 mg by mouth two times per day; or valacyclovir, 500 mg by mouth two times per day or 1 g by mouth every day. Doses should be individualized because different patients require different doses. Acyclovir-resistant HSV infection is increasingly common. Patients at risk usually have an extensive prior history of acyclovir use. Foscarnet (Foscavir) (40 to 60 mg/kg per day intravenously) is the treatment of choice for acyclovir-resistant strains despite its potential toxicity and added costs.

Human Herpesvirus 8 Infection

The most common neoplasm in AIDS is KS. Approximately 30% to 40% of homosexual men infected with HIV are seropositive for human herpesvirus 8 (HHV-8). More than half of patients with cutaneous KS have oral involvement. In AIDS patients, KS is usually aggressive. It is a multicentric tumor that initially presents as purplish nodules on the skin or mucous membranes. In the early stage, lesions are irregular reddish blue or purple to violaceous macules. The macules may become papular or nodular or coalesce to form large patches, plaques, and fusiform or ovoid tumors. KS frequently spreads to lymph nodes and visceral organs and is seen in any organ in the body. In advanced disease, lymph node involvement may result in edema, particularly of the legs and scrotum. Diagnosis is confirmed by biopsy, which shows vascular proliferation. Any patient with presumed KS should have a confirmatory biopsy because other conditions, such as bacillary angiomatosis, may mimic the disease. Therapy for KS can be local or systemic. Local therapies include surgical excision, cryotherapy, laser, intralesional injections, and radiation therapy. Recombinant interferon-α (Roferon-A) therapy is used for extensive cutaneous lesions. Systemic treatments involve chemotherapy regimens with various combinations of vinblastine (Velban), etoposide[1] (VePesid), bleomycin[1] (Blenoxane), and doxorubicin (Adriamycin). Paclitaxel (Taxol) is generally well tolerated and the treatment of choice for refractory KS. Remission of cutaneous and pulmonary disease is noted in patients receiving HAART.

Progressive Multifocal Leukoencephalopathy

Progressive multifocal leukoencephalopathy (PML) is a progressive demyelinating disease caused by the JC virus (JCV). Clinical presentation varies depending on the area involved and ranges from diffuse encephalopathy to focal deficits such as ataxia, hemiparesis, or speech difficulties. Symptoms tend to progress rapidly over several months, although rare patients have a waxing and waning clinical course extending for years. The typical finding is progressive dementia concurrent with a stroke syndrome. Definitive diagnosis requires a brain biopsy–positive direct fluorescent antibody (DFA) stain for JCV and typical inclusions in oligodendrocytes. CSF PCR detection of JCV has a diagnostic sensitivity of 70% to 80% and specificity of virtually 100%. Suggestive CT findings include multiple nonenhancing lesions scattered throughout the white matter without mass effect. MRI may also be suggestive: Lesions are hypodense in T1 images and hyperdense on T2 lesions. There is no proven treatment for PML. Treatment with prednisone[1], acyclovir (Zovirax),[1] vidarabine (Vira-A),[1] HLA (human leukocyte antibody)-matched platelets, amantadine (Symmetrel)[1], interferon alfa (Roferon-B)[1], and cytarabine (Cytasor)[1] have been disappointing in patients with PML. Response to HAART is also inconsistent.

Syphilis

Syphilis and HIV infection are uniquely associated. Epidemiologic studies show that a history of sexually transmitted disease (STD) such as syphilis is associated with an increased risk of HIV infection, and the genital ulcerations caused by *Treponema pallidum* may facilitate transmission of the virus. Coexistent HIV infection may alter the clinical course of syphilis, especially latent and tertiary disease. Screening test for syphilis should be performed annually in HIV-infected patients because of high rates of co-infection. Most HIV-infected patients with early syphilis have clinical manifestations

---

*Not FDA approved for initial episode.

[1]Not FDA approved for this indication.

comparable to those observed in HIV-uninfected persons. A higher incidence of neurosyphilis may be seen, which may develop rapidly or years after therapy. Serologic tests, patient history, clinical examination, and dark-field examination of tissue all are used. Serologic testing, however, remains a cornerstone of diagnosis when the clinical manifestations are not readily apparent. The Venereal Disease Research Laboratory (VDRL) test and the rapid plasma reagin (RPR) test are nontreponemal tests used for screening. Unfortunately, up to 6% of HIV-infected patients have biologic false-positive tests. False-negative tests also occur but are rare. The fluorescent treponemal antibody absorption test (FTA-ABS) and the microhemagglutination assay for *T. pallidum* (MHA-TP) detect antibodies directed against *T. pallidum* antigens. The treponemal tests are used to confirm reactive nontreponemal tests. Once positive, treponemal test assays usually stay positive for life. Current recommendations include lumbar puncture for all patients with latent syphilis regardless of the apparent duration of infection. Diagnosis of neurosyphilis is made by a positive CSF serology, high protein, or pleocytosis; however, there are many false-negative tests. Treatment with penicillin is currently recommended by the CDC whenever possible for all stages of syphilis in HIV-infected patients. Furthermore, there are no proven alternative therapies to penicillin for treatment of congenital syphilis, neurosyphilis, or syphilis in pregnancy. Penicillin desensitization is recommended for these situations. Benzathine penicillin G (Bicillin-LA), 2.4 million U intramuscularly, is recommended for primary or secondary syphilis in patients who have no evidence of neurosyphilis in CSF. A total of 7.2 million U (administered as 2.4 U intramuscularly weekly for 3 weeks) is advised for treatment of non-neurologic latent syphilis regardless of apparent duration of infection. Follow-up nontreponemal serologies should be obtained at 3, 6, 9, and 12 months. In HIV-positive patients, a slower decrease in serologic response may be seen, but clinical failures are rare. Recurrence is more often caused by reinfection than relapse. Treatment of neurosyphilis is with high-dose aqueous crystalline penicillin G, 18 to 24 million U per day, administered as 3 to 4 million U intravenously every 4 hours for 10 to 14 days.

Hepatitis C Virus (HCV) Infection

The hepatitis C virus (HCV) has emerged as a major pathogen in HIV-infected patients, reflecting shared epidemiologic risk factors. HCV is transmitted chiefly by percutaneous exposure to blood; injection drug use is the leading route of HCV transmission in the United States. Sexual transmission occurs less commonly. All HIV-infected patients should be screened for HCV because approximately 30% to 50% are co-infected. HIV is an important cofactor for HCV disease progression. The majority of these patients develop chronic hepatitis; others may progress to cirrhosis, hepatic decompensation, and even hepatocellular carcinoma. Awareness of HCV status is also important so liver function abnormalities can be properly evaluated in patients on HAART. Patients may complain of lethargy,

inability to concentrate, or abdominal pain. Jaundice, encephalopathy, ascites, splenomegaly, or gastrointestinal bleed secondary to portal hypertension may be seen with decompensated cirrhosis. Laboratory values may reveal hypoalbuminemia, thrombocytopenia, coagulopathy, and elevated hepatic transaminases. Hepatocellular carcinoma should be suspected in patients with sudden decompensation in previously stable chronic liver disease and elevated α-fetoprotein. Diagnosis is made by detection of antibody to HCV in blood by EIA. EIA-positive patients should undergo confirmation testing with recombinant immunoblot assay (RIBA) or reverse transcriptase polymerase chain reaction (RT-PCR) for HCV RNA. Liver biopsy provides information about degree of inflammation and the stage of fibrosis. Despite advancements in treatment of HCV, the data regarding safety and efficacy in HIV co-infected persons are limited. Interferon-α (Intron A) was the first licensed treatment for HCV infection. Results of therapy in HIV–co-infected patients are limited and mostly disappointing. Ribavirin (Rebetol) is an oral nucleoside analogue that is active in vitro against many RNA and DNA viruses. The major toxic effect of ribavirin appears to be reversible dose-dependent hemolytic anemia. Therapy with interferon alpha-2a (Roferon-A) and ribavirin, used together, appears to have a synergistic effect with increased sustained-response rates to approximately 50%. Adverse events commonly associated with interferon therapy include self-limited, dose-dependent, flu-like illness. Symptoms include mild fever, chills, headache, lethargy, arthralgias, and myalgias. These early symptoms may progress to depression, irritability, anorexia, rash, and alopecia. Patients need to be warned about these and other potential adverse events. Pegylated interferon alpha-2a (PEG-IFN) (Pegasys) has a longer half-life, may be administered once weekly, and appears to be better tolerated.

ASSOCIATED BACTERIAL INFECTIONS

Pulmonary infections continue to cause significant morbidity and mortality in HIV-infected patients. Recurrent bacterial pneumonia as an AIDS-defining disease is defined as two or more episodes of bacterial pneumonia within 1 year. In contrast to PCP, bacterial pneumonia can occur at any CD4+ cell level. *Streptococcus pneumoniae* is the most common identifiable bacterium causing pneumonia in HIV-infected patients. Pneumococcal bacteremia occurs with an estimated 100 times greater frequency in the HIV population. Injection drug use is an independent risk factor for both bacterial pneumonia and pneumococcal bacteremia. Other pathogens causing bacterial pneumonia in HIV-infected patients include *Staphylococcus aureus*, *Haemophilus influenzae*, and gram-negative organisms, most notably *Klebsiella* and *Pseudomonas*. A lobar infiltrate generally suggests bacterial pneumonia, but radiographic findings alone do not identify the causative agent. HIV patients with pneumonia have higher rates of positive blood cultures compared to HIV-negative individuals with pneumonia. It is essential to identify the pathogen to treat the pneumonia appropriately and improve the outcome.

More invasive procedures such as bronchoscopy may be necessary in patients with poor response to the initial antibiotic therapy or when PCP is suspected. Selection of the best agent should be based on local patterns of drug resistance. Once the pathogen(s) are identified, appropriate adjustments in antibiotic therapy should be made.

Salmonella infections, particularly bacteremia, are seen in higher frequency in HIV-infected patients and often present without intestinal symptoms. Nontyphoid *Salmonella* species, especially *Salmonella enteritidis* and *Salmonella typhimurium*, are isolated most often. Enteric infections are seen in traveler's diarrhea, often producing a more severe diarrheal illness that may be more resistant to therapy in HIV-infected patients. Diagnosis is made by bacterial culture of blood, stool, or urine. Treatment with ampicillin[1], quinolones, third-generation cephalosporins, or trimethoprim-sulfamethoxazole[1] (Septra Bactrim) is effective. Therapy should extend for at least 7 to 10 days after defervescence. Some experts place all patients with salmonellosis on chronic suppressive therapy; others give suppressive therapy only to those with recurrent disease (see also article "Salmonellosis").

Associated Malignancies

The association between certain malignancies and HIV infection was recognized early in the AIDS epidemic. KS was noted in homosexual men at a 20,000-fold increased rate compared to the pre-AIDS era. Increased incidence of other cancers, such as squamous cell neoplasia, in particular cervical and anal intraepithelial neoplasia (CIN, AIN), non-Hodgkin's lymphoma (NHL), Hodgkin's disease (HD), and primary CNS lymphoma, is also well documented. A correlation with viral co-infections appears to exist with several of these malignancies. HHV 8 promotes the development of KS. Certain types of HPV, often associated with more advanced CIN lesions (CIN II and CIN III), are found in a majority of cases of invasive carcinoma. The presence of Epstein-Barr virus (EBV) is reported in approximately 40% of systemic HIV-associated lymphomas and in a majority of primary CNS lymphomas. Although some AIDS-related malignancies have declined in frequency because of HAART, lymphomas other than primary CNS lymphoma have not changed dramatically. Similarly, available but limited data indicate no significant impact of HAART on CIN or AIN. Although the presentation of malignancy in patients infected with HIV is often different from that seen in immunocompetent hosts, patients with controlled HIV and moderate CD4+ counts are generally equally capable of tolerating full-dose chemotherapy and radiotherapy.

REFERENCES

Aberg JA, Gallant JE, Anderson J, et al: Primary care guidelines for the management of persons infected with human immunodeficiency virus: Recommendations of the HIV Medicine Association of the Infectious Diseases Society of America. Clin Infect Dis 2004;39(5):609-629.
Bartlett, JG, Gallant JE: Medical management of HIV infection. Baltimore, Johns Hopkins Medicine Health Publishing Business Group, 2004.
Department of Health and Human Services: Guidelines for the use of antiretroviral agents in HIV-1-infected adults and adolescents, October 29, 2004. Available online at http://aidsinfo.nih.gov (accessed November 2, 2004).
Hirsch MS, Brun-Vezinet F, Clotet B, et al: Antiretroviral drug resistance testing in adults infected with human immunodeficiency virus type 1: 2003 recommendations of an International AIDS Society-USA Panel. Clin Infect Dis 2003;37(1):113-128.
Recommendations of the 2002 United States Public Health Service/Infectious Disease Society of America: Guidelines for the Prevention of Opportunistic Infections in Persons Infected with Human Immunodeficiency Virus. Morb Mortal Wkly Rep (MMWR) 2002;51[RR-8]:1.
Suh JS, Sepkowitz KA: Treatment of HIV-related opportunistic infections. In RE Reese and RF Betts (eds): A Practical Approach to Infectious Diseases, 5th ed. Philadelphia, Lippincott Williams & Wilkins, 2003.
UNAIDS 2004: Report on the global AIDS epidemic 2004. Available online at http://www.unaids.org/bangkok2004 (accessed November 2, 2004).

Amebiasis

Method of
Mehmet Tanyuksel, MD, and
William A. Petri, Jr., MD, PhD

Amebiasis is a common disease caused by the protozoan *Entamoeba histolytica*. It is estimated that approximately 10% of the world's population is infected by the closely related parasites *E. histolytica*, *Entamoeba dispar*, and *Entamoeba moshkovskii*. Each year, more than 50 million individuals are infected, resulting in more than 100,000 deaths worldwide. Generally, infection caused by nonpathogens *E. dispar* and *E. moshkovskii* are approximately 10 times more frequent than infection caused by invasive *E. histolytica*. The indistinguishable morphology of *E. histolytica*, *E. dispar*, and *E. moshkovskii* makes it important to diagnose amebiasis using an *E. histolytica*–specific test such as the TechLab antigen detection test (*E. histolytica* II test) or polymerase chain reaction (PCR) assay.

Amebiasis is a worldwide infection and is commonly found in tropical and subtropical countries. It is endemic to poor areas in developing countries. The majority of the morbidity and mortality is in Central and South Americas, Africa, and the Indian subcontinent. *E. histolytica* is found only in human hosts, and amebiasis is commonly transmitted by a fecal–oral route through food and water contamination with fecal matter. Transmission also occurs by sexual practice (through oral-anal contact).

The life cycle of *E. histolytica* is simple. The enteric protozoan parasite can exist as either a cyst or a motile, vegetative trophozoite form. The cyst is responsible for the transmission of infection. It is a metabolically reduced

---
[1] Not FDA approved for this indication.

tetra-nucleated cell and resistant to desiccation as well as other environmental factors. The infection is attributable to contamination of food or drinking water by the cyst form. Once a cyst is ingested by a new host, it lives in the ileum and transforms to the trophozoite form of the organism yielding four and then eight trophozoites. The trophozoite can colonize colonic epithelial cells of the bowel lumen and invades into the intestinal epithelium of the host. Adherence of *E. histolytica* trophozoites to host surfaces—colonic mucin, epithelium, and other target cells, as well as a variety of cell lines—is mediated by the amebic galactose (Gal) and *N*-acetyl D-galactosamine (GalNAc), a specific lectin. After adherence the parasite kills the epithelial cells, causing dysentery with blood and mucus in the stool. Immunologic and antigenic differences are distinguishable between *E. histolytica* and the nonpathogenic *Entamoeba* with the use of monoclonal antibodies; significant systemic humoral immune responses occur only with *E. histolytica*—not with *E. dispar* or *E. moshkovskii* infection.

E. histolytica also secretes proteases that degrade the extracellular matrix and permit invasion of the bowel wall. Furthermore, *E. histolytica* can spread through the portal circulation and cause amebic liver abscesses. The infection may spread further by direct extension from the liver or through the bloodstream to the lungs, brain, and other organs.

The Gal/GalNAc lectin is a logical vaccine candidate because of its critical role in pathogenicity. Genetic conservation of the Gal/GalNAc lectin between isolates may reveal that the lectin is under well-built, well-designed assortment or that *E. histolytica* is a clonal population. The high sequence conservation of the lectin heavy subunit reveals that immune responses against it could be broadly cross protective.

Clinical Manifestations

Basically, the clinical classifications of the disease caused by *E. histolytica* are asymptomatic colonization and symptomatic disease (intestinal and extra-intestinal). The wide spectrum of the clinical intestinal disease ranges from asymptomatic carrier state to a fulminant colitis with an array of manifestations that may include toxic megacolon, perianal ulcer, peritonitis, and cutaneous amebiasis.

Most infections are in the form of asymptomatic (up to 90%) colonization, which is commonly caused by the nonpathogen protozoa *E. dispar* and *E. moshkovskii*; *E. histolytica* also frequently causes asymptomatic infection. In the United States and Europe, most isolates from homosexual men are *E. dispar*. In the case of asymptomatic colonization with *E. histolytica*, all subjects should be treated at least by luminal agents. If these individuals are not treated, they may be hazardous environmentally or may develop amebic colitis within months. Intestinal amebiasis can masquerade or simply be confused with bacillary dysentery, intestinal schistosomiasis, ulcerative colitis, acute fulminant dysentery, inflammatory bowel disease, ischemic colitis, diverticulitis and carcinoma of the colon.

Symptoms of amebic colitis/dysentery are:

- Abdominal pain or tenderness
- Diarrhea (watery/bloody/mucous)
- Tenesmus
- Flatulence
- Decrease of appetite
- Loss of weight
- Dehydration

Fever is uncommon. In the colon, inflammation and lesions may display as thickening of the mucosal wall, flask-shaped ulcerations or necrosis of the intestinal wall depending on the grade of invasion (Figure 1). Amebic liver abscess (ALA) is the most common manifestation of extra-intestinal amebiasis. The clinical presentation of ALA commonly includes fever, cough, abdominal pain or tenderness in right upper quadrant (in acute stage), enlarged liver, weight loss, fever, and abdominal pain (in subacute stage). Although patients with ALA may report a history of dysentery within the last year, in most patients it is impossible to identify the organism in stool (Figure 2).

ALA is a disease predominantly of young men, whereas pyogenic liver abscess (PLA) is commonly seen in older population of patients between ages 50 and 70 years, in equal ratios of men to women. Both ALA and PLA are

2

KEY INTESTINAL AMEBIASIS DIAGNOSTIC POINTS

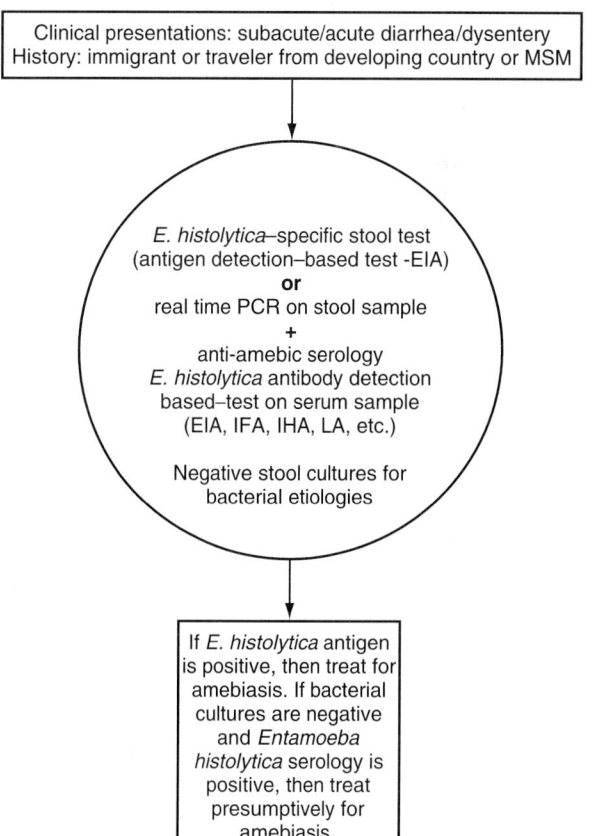

FIGURE 1. Practical diagnostic points for patients with intestinal amebiasis. *Abbreviations:* EIA = enzyme immuno assay; IFA = immunofluorescence assay; IHA = indirect hemagglutination assay; MSM = men who have sex with men

KEY AMEBIC LIVER ABSCESS (ALA) DIAGNOSTIC POINTS

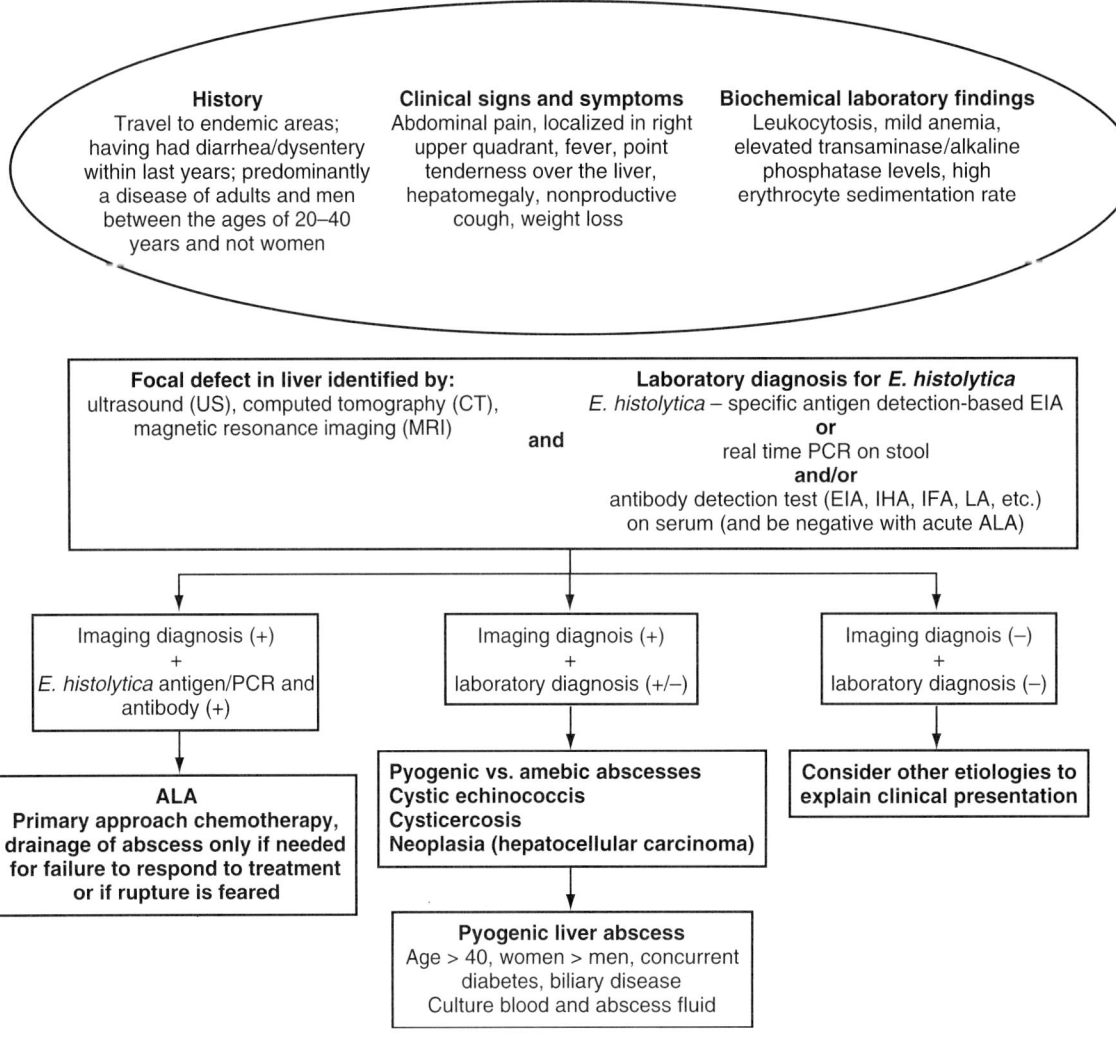

FIGURE 2. Practical diagnostic points for patients with amebic liver abscess. *Abbreviation:* EIA = enzyme immunoassay; IFA = immunofluorescence assay; IHA = indirect hemagglutination assay; PCR = polymerase chain reaction.

usually located in the right lobe of the liver, and both ALA and PLA are multiple in approximately 50% of all cases. Patients with PLA have a tendency to present with symptoms ranging in a period anywhere from 2 weeks to 1 or more months. Other clinical manifestations more common in patients with PLA include concurrent diabetes mellitus (DM)—in approximately 27% of patients—and biliary disease, jaundice, pruritus, elevated bilirubin and alkaline phosphatase levels, sepsis, and positive bacterial cultures of blood or abscess fluid.

DIAGNOSIS

There are several methods used for amebiasis diagnosis and monitoring of *E. histolytica* infection. Microscopy is a relatively nonspecific and insensitive but widely available diagnostic test for *E. histolytica*, *E. dispar*, and *E. moshkovskii*. Enzyme-linked immunoassays (ELISAs) to detect *E. histolytica* antigen in the stool, where available, have replaced the traditional microscopy for diagnosis of *E. histolytica*.

Serologic tests are useful for diagnosis of infection. The traditional but time-consuming immunofluorescence, counterimmunoelectrophoresis, indirect hemagglutination assays (IHAs) have been supplanted in most laboratories by tests based on enzyme-linked immunosorbent assay or *E. histolytica*–specific antigen (ELISA). However, serologic techniques are not entirely satisfactory because of inadequate sensitivity and specificity in the detection of early infections and the fact that serologic assays remain positive for months to years after exposure to the parasite.

Several newer molecular diagnostic tests that facilitate accurate monitoring of amebiasis have become available. The ELISA/DNA detection-based test (PCR) and culture remain the principal means of diagnosis of infection in individuals. Rapid diagnosis and the early treatment of clinical cases are important in reducing the morbidity and mortality in amebiasis. Several PCR-based assays for the detection of the *E. histolytica* infecting humans have been described, and the results of evaluating these molecular tests have been encouraging, indicating

CURRENT DIAGNOSIS

Intestinal Amebiasis

- Ask about a clinical presentation such as diarrhea/dysentery (remember many infections are asymptomatic).
- Remember conventional microscopic examination is insensitive and cannot distinguish invasive *Entamoeba histolytica* from the nonpathogen *Entamoeba dispar*.
- Test the stool sample with the *E. histolytica*–specific EIA or real-time PCR, and also perform a serology (*E. histolytica* antibody detection based–test on serum sample EIA, IFA, IHA, LA, etc.).

Amebic Liver Abscess (ALA)

- Obtain travel history to endemic areas/residence immigrant from developing country for amebiasis, age (20-40 years), history of alcohol abuse, and gender (male/female 9:1).
- Ask history of having had dysentery within the last year.
- Ask clinical manifestations (i.e., abdominal pain localized in right upper quadrant, fever, point tenderness over the liver, hepatomegaly).
- Obtain biochemical laboratory findings (i.e., leukocytosis, mild anemia, elevated transaminase/ alkaline phosphatase levels).
- Screen for presence of abscess with imaging analyses and obtain the *E. histolytica*–specific EIA or real-time PCR testing on stool sample, and/or serology (*E. histolytica* antibody detection–based test on serum sample EIA, IFA, IHA, LA, etc.).
- Differentiate pyogenic liver abscess with some findings (i.e., age older than 40, women more than men, concurrent diabetes mellitus, and biliary disease) and positive cultivation for bacteria in the blood and abscess fluid.

Abbreviations: EIA = enzyme immunoassay; IFA = immunofluorescence assay; IHA = indirect hemagglutination; LA = latex agglutination assay; PCR = polymerase chain reaction.

sensitivities and specificities higher than those achievable by routine microscopy. Newer molecular diagnostic tests provide important insights into the state and level of activity of *E. histolytica* infection and will continue to be used more widely, especially among patients with severe infection or in case of require to interpretation in immunocompromised patients. Now the antigen-detection ELISAs offer the capability of identifying and distinguishing *E. histolytica* from *E. dispar* and *E. moshkovskii* infections. Table 1 summarizes sensitivities and specificities of diagnostic assays for diagnosis of amebiasis in patients with colitis and amebic liver abscess.

Several studies indicate that early detection of amebiasis based on genomic amplification (as is done with PCR) may provide an adjunct and may be a more sensitive method than conventional methods. Because of the development of molecular biology–based diagnostic tests such as the PCR, it is possible to detect low numbers of cyst and trophozoites of *E. histolytica* in clinical specimens; these tests also enormously powerful tools for genetically typing different amoebic strains. Particularly, real-time PCR is a rapid and sensitive method.

Treatment

There are a number of drugs available that are effective in treating amebiasis. Figure 3 summarizes the recommended therapy for amebiasis in adults. The major drugs used to treat asymptomatic cyst passers are paromomycin (Humatin), iodoquinol (Yodoxin), and diloxanide furoate (Furamide).[2] Paromomycin (Humatin), a nonabsorbable aminoglycoside, has the advantage of being poorly absorbed, making it possible to use in pregnancy, and well tolerated in children. Iodoquinol (Yodoxin) is a highly effective luminal agent but has some gastrointestinal side effects and may interfere with thyroid function tests caused by a high iodine content. Diloxanide furoate (Furamide)[2] is relatively nontoxic and is used as a luminal agent worldwide (available only from the Centers for Disease Control and Prevention in the United States).

---

[2]Not available in the United States.

TABLE 1 Evaluation of Sensitivity and Specificity of Tests of Diagnosis for Amebiasis

Assay	Amebic Colitis		ALA
	Sensitivity	Specificity	Sensitivity
Microscopy (stool)	Moderate	Poor	Poor
Stool antigen detection (ELISA)	Excellent	Excellent	NA
Real-time PCR (stool)*	Excellent	Excellent	Excellent
Microscopy (abscess fluid)	NA	NA	Poor
Serum antigen detection (ELISA)*	Moderate (early)	Excellent	Excellent (first 3 days), poor (late)
Abscess antigen detection (ELISA)*	NA	NA	Excellent (before treatment)
Serum antibody detection (ELISA)	Good	Good	Good (acute), excellent (recovery)
Serum antibody detection (IHA)	Excellent	-	Excellent (recovery)

*Investigational; not in routine clinical use.
Abbreviations: ALA = amebic liver abscess; ELISA = *Entamoeba histolytica*–specific antigen; IHA = indirect hemagglutination assay; NA = not available; PCR = polymerase chain reaction.

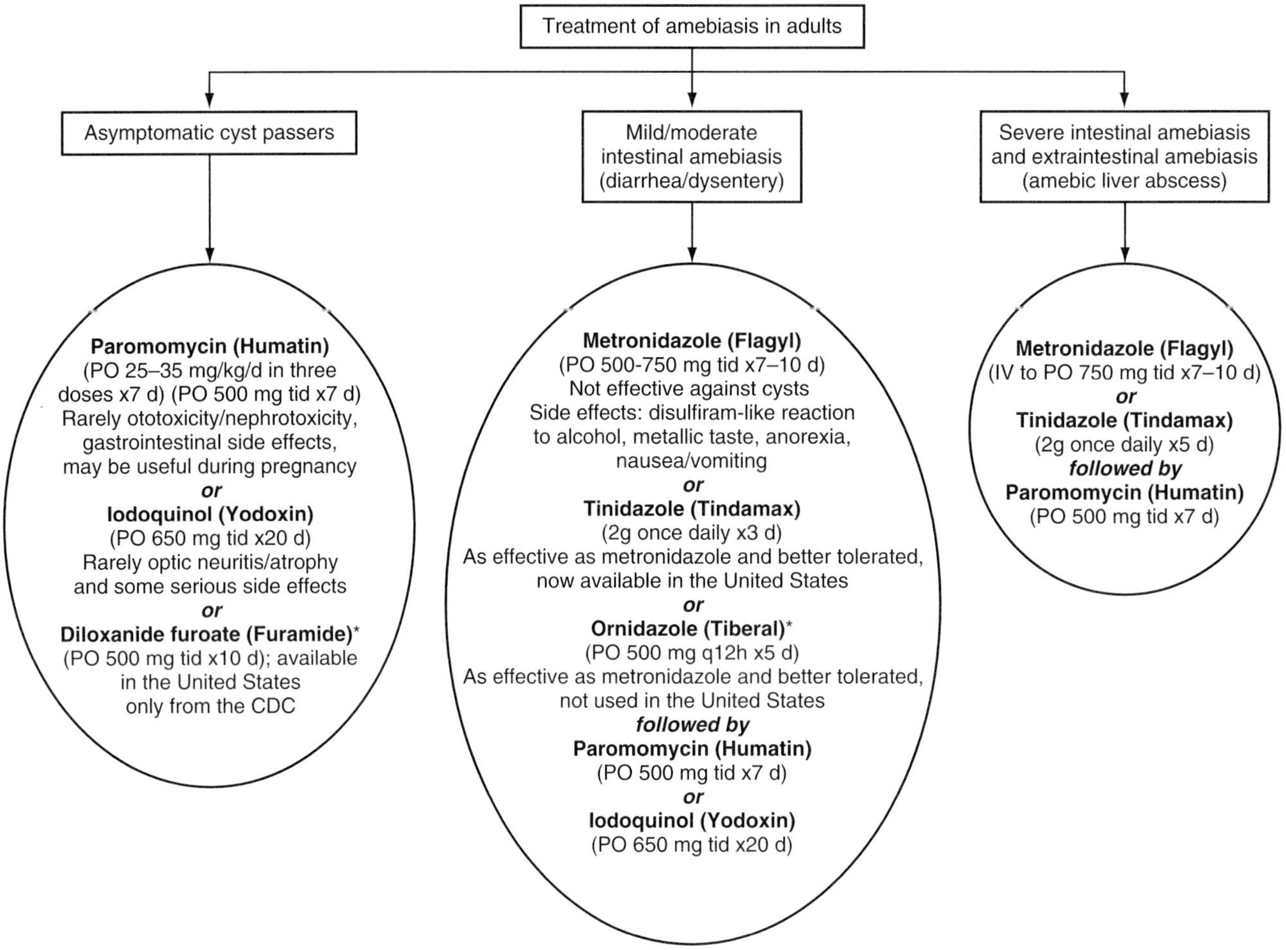

Treatment of amebiasis in adults

Asymptomatic cyst passers

Mild/moderate
intestinal amebiasis
(diarrhea/dysentery)

Severe intestinal amebiasis
and extraintestinal amebiasis
(amebic liver abscess)

Paromomycin (Humatin)
(PO 25–35 mg/kg/d in three
doses x7 d) (PO 500 mg tid x7 d)
Rarely ototoxicity/nephrotoxicity,
gastrointestinal side effects,
may be useful during pregnancy
or
Iodoquinol (Yodoxin)
(PO 650 mg tid x20 d)
Rarely optic neuritis/atrophy
and some serious side effects
or
Diloxanide furoate (Furamide)*
(PO 500 mg tid x10 d); available
in the United States
only from the CDC

Metronidazole (Flagyl)
(PO 500-750 mg tid x7–10 d)
Not effective against cysts
Side effects: disulfiram-like reaction
to alcohol, metallic taste, anorexia,
nausea/vomiting
or
Tinidazole (Tindamax)
(2g once daily x3 d)
As effective as metronidazole and better tolerated,
now available in the United States
or
Ornidazole (Tiberal)*
(PO 500 mg q12h x5 d)
As effective as metronidazole and better tolerated,
not used in the United States
followed by
Paromomycin (Humatin)
(PO 500 mg tid x7 d)
or
Iodoquinol (Yodoxin)
(PO 650 mg tid x20 d)

Metronidazole (Flagyl)
(IV to PO 750 mg tid x7–10 d)
or
Tinidazole (Tindamax)
(2g once daily x5 d)
followed by
Paromomycin (Humatin)
(PO 500 mg tid x7 d)

*Not available in the United States

FIGURE 3. Practical key treatment algorithm for patients with amebiasis.

CURRENT THERAPY

Intestinal Amebiasis

■ Consider medical therapy for asymptomatic
cyst passers: paromomycin or iodoquinol
or diloxanide furoate (available in the
United States only from the CDC).

■ Remember paromomycin may be useful during
pregnancy.

■ For mild to moderate intestinal amebiasis
(diarrhea/dysentery), consider metronidazole
or tinidazole or ornidazole followed by
paromomycin.

■ For severe intestinal amebiasis, metronidazole or
tinidazole followed by paromomycin is
recommended.

Amebic Liver Abscess (ALA)

Metronidazole or tinidazole followed by
paromomycin is recommended.

The drug of choice for the therapy of invasive intestinal
amebiasis and amebic liver abscess is metronidazole
(Flagyl) or the related (and now available in the United
States) drug tinidazole (Tindamax). Metronidazole
(Flagyl), a nitroimidazole, is given in divided doses for
7 days, with an efficacy of more than 90%. It has a high
gastrointestinal absorption and is tolerated well in
infants and children. Metronidazole (Flagyl) may also
be associated with a disulfiram-like reaction to alcohol
when consumed with the drug. The most effective available therapeutic regimen is the combination of metronidazole followed by (not given concurrently) a luminal
agent such as paromomycin (or iodoquinol) in intestinal
amebiasis. Because the teratogenic effect of metronidazole seems greatest during the first trimester,
it can possibly be used safely in the last two trimesters
of pregnancy in severe amebiasis. Tinidazole, another
nitroimidazole, has shown tremendous efficacy when
given in doses of 2 g orally once daily for 3 days; as
mentioned above, this drug is now available in the
United States. Response to drug therapy depends on

the cyst size, location, and host immunity and also is the best monitored by serial imaging and serology. Indications for therapeutic draining of ALA are:

- Clinically a lack of response to drug therapy over 3 to 7 days. Normally patients with ALA regularly respond up to 5 days to metronidazole therapy with a decline in fever and right-upper quadrant pain.
- High possibility of ruptured abscess (large) as characterized by cavity size larger than 5 cm.
- A left-lobe abscess that appears to be ruptured into pericardium.
- A differential diagnosis still including pyogenic abscess.

REFERENCES

Anonymous: Amoebiasis. Wkly Epidemiol Rec 1997;72:97-99.
Beck DL, Tanyuksel M, Mackey AJ, et al: *Entamoeba histolytica*: Sequence conservation of the GalNAc lectin from clinical isolates. Exp Parasitol 2002;101:157-163.
Dunzendorfer T, Kasznica J: Amebic and/or ulcerative colitis? (Letter). Gastrointest Endosc 1998;48:450-451.
Gathiram V, Jackson TF: A longitudinal study of asymptomatic carriers of pathogenic zymodemes of *Entamoeba histolytica*. S Afr Med J 1987;72:669-672.
Gilbert DN, Moellering RC, Eliopoulos GM, Sande MA: The Sanford guide to antimicrobial therapy, 34th ed. Hyde Park, Vt, Antimicrobial Therapy, 2004.
Haque R, Faruque ASG, Hahn P, et al: *Entamoeba histolytica* and *Entamoeba dispar* infection in children in Bangladesh. J Infect Dis 1997;175:734-736.
Irusen EM, Jackson TFHG, Simjee, AE: Asymptomatic intestinal colonization by pathogenic *Entamoeba histolytica* in amebic liver abscess—prevalence, response to therapy, and pathogenic potential. Clin Infect Dis 1992;14:889-893.
Petri WA Jr, Jackson TFHG, Gathiram V, et al: Pathogenic and non-pathogenic strains of *Entamoeba histolytica* can be differentiated by monoclonal antibodies to the galactose-specific adherence lectin. Infect Immun 1990;58:1802-1806.
Ravdin JI, Guerrant RL: Role of adherence in cytopathogenic mechanisms of *Entamoeba histolytica*. Study with mammalian tissue culture cells and human erythrocytes. J Clin Invest 1981;68:1305-1313.
Tanyuksel M, Petri WA Jr: Laboratory diagnosis of amebiasis. Clin Microbiol Rev 2003;16: 713-729.
Weinke T, Friedrich-Janicke B, Hopp P, Janitschke K: Prevalence and clinical importance of *Entamoeba histolytica* in two high-risk groups: Travelers returning from the tropics and male homosexuals. J Infect Dis 1989;161:1029-1031.

Giardiasis

Method of
*David E. Katz, MD, and
Alfred DeMaria, Jr., MD*

Background/Organism

Giardiasis is an intestinal infection caused by the protozoan parasite *Giardia lamblia* (also known as *Giardia intestinalis* and *Giardia duodenalis*). Giardiasis is the most common protozoal infection in humans. *Giardia* exists in two forms: The trophozoite is responsible for

the clinical illness, and the environmentally resistant cyst is responsible for transmission of infection. Trophozoites are pear shaped, flagellated, and binucleate and contain a ventral disc thought to aid in attachment of the organism to small intestine villi. Trophozoites measure 9 μm to 15 μm long, 5 μm to 15 μm wide, and 2 μm to 4 μm thick. Cysts are oval, contain four nuclei, and are approximately 10 μm to 12 μm long.

Pathogenesis

Giardia cysts persist in the environment. After ingestion, excystation in the proximal small intestine is thought to be triggered by exposure to gastric acid in the stomach and/or the alkaline, protease-rich environment of the proximal duodenum. Excystation releases two mobile trophozoites, which replicate by binary fission. *Giardia* is not invasive but causes mucosal damage in the proximal small bowel, which leads to malabsorption and diarrhea. Trophozoites encyst in the jejunum, triggered by biliary secretions. Trophozoites and cysts are then passed intermittently in the stool.

Epidemiology

Giardiasis occurs worldwide. The prevalence of *Giardia* in stool ranges from 2% to 5% in industrialized countries to 20% to 30% in developing countries. However, patients are often asymptomatic or have nonspecific symptoms. In 1997 the incidence of reported disease in the United States was 9.5 cases per 100,000 population. It is estimated that nearly 5000 people are hospitalized annually in the United States with severe giardiasis. Reservoir hosts include human beings as well as farm, wild, and domesticated animals. Two major groups of *G. lamblia* organisms have been recognized as infecting humans worldwide. Although no consensus exists as to nomenclature, the term *assemblages* has been widely used. Current research endeavors to understand how genetic variability of the parasite is correlated with pathogenicity. Studies have shown that *G. lamblia* from certain animals can potentially infect humans. Although isolates of *G. lamblia* from humans and various animals are morphologically similar, the existence of distinct host-adapted genotypes has been demonstrated.

Transmission is via fecal–oral spread and can be person-to-person, food-borne, or waterborne. Waterborne transmission is the major source for epidemic spread. Because cysts are killed by cooking, food-borne spread is uncommon. The age distribution is bimodal, with peaks at ages 0 to 5 years as well as 31 to 40 years. The incidence of giardiasis is similar among men and women. Seasonal variation exists with most cases occurring in the summer. High-risk groups include:

- Diaper-age children
- Children in daycare settings
- Child-care workers
- Immunocompromised persons
- Institutionalized persons

- Foreign travelers
- Persons who drink untreated water from lakes, streams, and swimming pools
- Men who have sex with men
- Patients with intestinal metaplasia and/or hypochlorhydria

Studies of giardiasis in poorly nourished children in developing regions have demonstrated growth retardation, cognitive impairment, and delayed psychomotor development. Repeated or chronic low-level exposure to *Giardia* likely stimulates some protection from symptomatic infection. Children born to nonimmune mothers are significantly more likely to acquire *Giardia* infection and develop giardiasis with more severe symptoms compared with children of immune mothers. Antibodies in mother's milk may protect children against giardiasis.

Clinical Presentation

Clinical presentation can vary greatly and may depend on variations among strains of *Giardia*. Ingestion of as few as 10 to 25 cysts can lead to giardiasis. After an incubation period of 1 to 2 weeks, signs and symptoms may develop such as nausea, vomiting (less common), malaise, flatulence, cramping, diarrhea, steatorrhea, and weight loss. A history of gradual onset of diarrhea is characteristic. Symptoms lasting 2 to 4 weeks with weight loss are typical. Chronic giardiasis may follow an acute syndrome or present without severe antecedent symptoms. Chronic signs and symptoms such as loose stool, steatorrhea (with frothy, foul-smelling stools), a 10% to 20% weight loss, malabsorption (of fats, vitamin B_{12}, and D-xylose [D-XYL]), malaise, fatigue, and depression may wax and wane over many months in untreated individuals. Rash and urticaria may be present in a hypersensitivity reaction. Giardiasis may rarely be associated with reactive arthritis or asymmetric synovitis, usually of the lower extremities.

Approximately 60% of infected individuals may be asymptomatic. Even asymptomatic infection may lead to vitamin deficiencies (A, B_{12}, and folate) and hypoalbuminemia. Acquired lactose intolerance occurs in up to 20% to 40% of cases because of a transient lactase deficiency, which can take many weeks to normalize.

Diagnosis

Diagnosis is based on detection of trophozoites, or more commonly, cysts in the stool and is difficult because the number of cysts excreted varies from day to day. In addition, shedding occurs intermittently. Eosinophilia and fecal leukocytosis do not occur. Radiographic imaging is not useful. Stool microscopy (ova and parasite examination) may require three separate stool specimens collected on nonconsecutive days for maximum yield. The sensitivity of parasite identification is 50% to 70% with a single specimen and 90% after three specimens. Several commercial antigen detection immunoassays for stool exist, including counterimmunoelectrophoresis (CIE),

CURRENT DIAGNOSIS

- Clinical presentation can vary greatly.
- More than half of infected individuals may be asymptomatic.
- Chronic infection can last for months and result in significant weight loss.
- Lactose intolerance may persist after symptoms resolve.
- Cyst excretion occurs intermittently.
- Diagnosis is optimized with three separate specimens for stool microscopy.
- Assays that detect soluble antigen may give false positives in individuals recently cured of infection.

enzyme-linked immunosorbent assay (ELISA), enzyme immunoassay (EIA; detects soluble antigens), direct fluorescent antibody (DFA; detects intact organisms), and the immunochromatographic lateral-flow immunoassay (rapid assay). Many of these tests have demonstrated sensitivities and specificities greater than 95%. However, sensitivity and specificity of diagnostic methods based upon *Giardia* antigen detection may be affected by genetic variability of *Giardia* isolates present in a given geographic area. Antigen assays are quick and are similar in cost to ova and parasite exam. Assays that detect *Giardia* antigen should be carefully interpreted because they might be positive even after a person stops shedding intact organisms, giving false-positive results in individuals who might actually be cured but still symptomatic because of disaccharidase deficiency. Serology is of limited value because IgG and IgM antibodies both persist after infection. Secretory antibodies found in saliva may be used for diagnosis in the future. Duodenal aspirates, biopsies, brush cytology, and the string test are invasive and/or costly procedures. Although biopsy is most sensitive, it should be reserved for confusing or refractory cases. Culture and polymerase chain reaction (PCR) tests are available only as research tools.

Treatment

Table 1 provides the current therapy for giardiasis. Metronidazole (Flagyl)[1] is the first-line agent for treatment of giardiasis in the United States, despite not being approved by the U.S. Food and Drug Administration (FDA). Reported cure rates range from 80% to 95%. Side effects are uncommon but include gastrointestinal upset, headache, nausea, leukopenia, a metallic taste in the mouth, and a possible disulfiram-like reaction with alcohol ingestion. Because metronidazole (Flagyl)[1] is reported to be carcinogenic, teratogenic, and mutagenic, it is contraindicated in pregnant women during the first trimester. Seizures, peripheral neuropathy, depression, irritability, restlessness, and insomnia are

---

[1]Not FDA approved for this indication.

TABLE 1 Common Current Therapies for Treating Giardiasis

Drug	Dose	Comment
Metronidazole (Flagyl)[1]	Adult: 250 mg PO tid for 5d or 2 g qhs for 3d[3] Pediatric: 15 mg/kg/d PO tid for 5d	Cost effective.
Albendazole (Albenza)[1]	Adult: 400 mg PO for 5d Pediatric: 10 mg/kg/d PO for 5d	Recommended dosages vary.
Paromomycin (Humatin)[1]	Adult: 500 mg PO qid for 7d Pediatric: 25–35 mg/kg/d PO tid for 7d	Useful in pregnancy.
Tinidazole (Tindamax)	Adult: 2.0 g PO for 1d Pediatric: 50 mg/kg PO for 1d (2 g max)	Tindamax FDA approved May 2004. For use in children ages >3 years.
Nitazoxanide (Alinia)	12–47 months: 100 mg (5mL) PO bid for 3d 4–11 years: 200 mg (10 mL) PO bid for 3d ≥12 years: 500 mg (25 mL) PO bid for 3d	Available in liquid and tablet form. Approved for children 1 year of age or older.

[1]Not FDA approved for this indication.
[3]Exceeds dosage recommended by the manufacturer.
Abbreviations: bid = twice daily; d = days; PO = by mouth; qhs = at bedtime; qid = four times daily; tid = three times daily.

rarely reported. Drug resistance is not yet widespread but has been reported.

ALBENDAZOLE (ALBENZA)

Albendazole (Albenza)[1] is an antihelminthic used as an alternative treatment for giardiasis. It is a benzimidazole derivative comparable in efficacy to metronidazole (Flagyl).[1] Cure rates are reported as 62% to 95%. It is becoming a first-line drug for giardiasis and a variety of other parasitic gastrointestinal diseases. Side effects include gastrointestinal upset, abdominal pain, nausea, vomiting, diarrhea, dizziness, vertigo, fever, increased intracranial pressure, and variable increases in transaminases (seen in approximately 15% of patients and reversible). Discontinuation of the drug is usually not required for abnormal liver function tests. In vitro resistance has been reported.

[1]Not FDA approved for this indication.

 CURRENT THERAPY

- Metronidazole (Flagyl)[1] is the current first-line agent but cannot be used in the first trimester of pregnancy.
- Patients taking metronidazole (Flagyl)[1] should abstain from alcohol.
- Paromomycin (Humatin)[1] can be used in pregnancy.
- Nitazoxanide (Alinia) is available in suspension and tablet form and is approved for children greater that 1 year of age.
- Diet modification may reduce acute symptoms and promote host defenses.
- Asymptomatic carriers may need to receive treatment during an outbreak.

[1]Not FDA approved for this indication.

Rakel and Bope: *Conn's Current Therapy 2006*

PAROMOMYCIN (HUMATIN)

Paromomycin (Humatin)[1] is considered investigational for giardiasis by the FDA. It is a poorly absorbed aminoglycoside and, therefore, is one of the only antigiardial medications recommended for symptomatic pregnant patients. Reported efficacy against giardiasis is 60% to 70%. Side effects include nausea, increased gastrointestinal motility, abdominal pain, and diarrhea.

FURAZOLIDONE (FUROXONE), QUINACRINE (ATABRINE), AND NITROIMIDAZOLE DERIVATIVES

Furazolidone (Furoxone)[2] and quinacrine (Atabrine)[2] have been used in the past but are no longer readily available in the United States and have been supplanted by other agents. Nitroimidazole derivatives include tinidazole (Tindamax), now available in the United States, and ornidazole (Tiberal).[2] Ornidazole (Tiberal)[2] is not approved in the United States, but it is used as a frontline agent in other countries. Advantages are a reported cure rate of 90% and less frequent dosing. Side effects include gastrointestinal upset, vertigo, and bitter taste.

NITAZOXANIDE (ALINIA)

Nitazoxanide (Alinia), a 5-nitrothiazole derivative, has activity against protozoans, helminths, and some aerobic and anaerobic bacteria. It is available in liquid or tablet form and is approved for the treatment of giardiasis in immunocompetent children (>1 year of age) and adults. Nitazoxanide (Alinia) has the advantages over metronidazole (Flagyl)[1] of a liquid formulation and shorter duration of treatment. Trials show nitazoxanide (Alinia) to be 83% to 100% effective. Side effects include abdominal pain, diarrhea, nausea, vomiting,

[1]Not FDA approved for this indication.
[2]Not available in the United States.

and headache similar to those for placebo; yellow sclera caused by drug deposition occurs rarely and resolves after discontinuation. Nitazoxanide (Alinia) should be taken with food. Caution is needed when adding nitazoxanide (Alinia) to regimens consisting of other highly plasma protein-bound medication (warfarin, valproic acid, carbamazepine, and aspirin). Metronidazole (Flagyl)[1]-refractory cases should be treated with nitazoxanide (Alinia), higher doses of metronidazole (Flagyl), or combination therapy (e.g., quinacrine [Atabrine][2] and metronidazole [Flagyl][1]).

ALTERNATIVE AND COMPLEMENTARY THERAPIES

Alternative and complementary therapies are used by many patients and include nutritional interventions and phytotherapeutics. This approach advocates a whole-food, high-fiber, low-fat, low simple–carbohydrate diet. Ingestion of wheat germ and probiotics might possibly aid in parasite clearance. The phytotherapeutic agents with most potential benefit appear to be the berberine-containing herbs, garlic, and the Ayurvedic combination pippali rasayana.[†] These modalities demonstrate some efficacy, without significant side effects. Seirogan, a herbal medicine containing wood creosote (45 to 135 mg/dose), has been marketed in Asia for the treatment of acute diarrhea, with minimal reported side effects.

Immunocompromised patients might experience relapses and require prolonged treatment or combination therapy. Patients with persistent symptoms after treatment, or for whom repeated treatment has failed, should be evaluated for lactose intolerance, underlying common variable immunodeficiency, and functional irritable bowel disease.

Prevention and Control Measures

Centers for Disease Control and Prevention (CDC) publishes recommendations for the prevention and control of giardiasis (http://www.cdc.gov/ncidod/dpd/parasites/giardiasis/factsht_giardia.htm). Prevention of giardiasis is accomplished through proper sewage disposal, water treatment, and hygiene. Water should be treated by flocculation, sedimentation, filtration, or chlorination. *Giardia* cysts can be inactivated by boiling water for at least 1 minute using filters (pore size less than 1 μm). Halogens, including chlorine and iodine, may not be effective in all circumstances. When traveling overseas, bottled beverages (preferably carbonated) are the safest. Raw food should be washed with uncontaminated water. Fecal exposure should be avoided during sexual activity. In daycare centers, strict hand washing and separate diaper-changing areas should be implemented. Symptomatic children, teachers, and family members should be treated. People with diarrhea should be excluded from child care. Individuals diagnosed with giardiasis should not swim in recreational water for at least 2 weeks after diarrhea stops.

Treatment of asymptomatic carriers is generally not recommended. Possible exceptions are carriers in households of patients with hypogammaglobulinemia or cystic fibrosis, diaper-age children in households with pregnant women, and food handlers, or in the presence of an outbreak. If a child does not have diarrhea but is experiencing nausea, fatigue, weight loss, or a poor appetite, treatment should be considered. If an outbreak is continuing to occur at a daycare center despite control efforts, screening and treating asymptomatic children should be considered.

REFERENCES

Adam RD: Biology of *Giardia lamblia*. Clin Microbiol Rev 2001;14:447-475.
Anonymous: Nitazoxanide (Alinia)—a new antiprotozoal agent. Med Lett Drugs Ther 2003;45(1154):29-31.
Bailey JM, Erramouspe J: Nitazoxanide treatment for giardiasis and cryptosporidiosis in children. Ann Pharmacother 2004;38:634-640.
Caccio SM, De Giacomo M, Pozio E: Sequence analysis of the β-giardin gene and development of a polymerase chain reaction-restriction fragment length polymorphism assay to genotype *Giardia duodenalis* cysts from human faecal samples. Int J Parasitol 2002;32:1023-1030.
Faubert G: Immune response to *Giardia duodenalis*. Clin Microbiol Rev. 2000;13:35-54.
Furness BW, Beach MJ, Roberts JM. Giardiasis surveillance—United States, 1992-1997. MMWR 2000;49(7):1-13.
Gardner TB, Hill DR: Treatment of giardiasis. Clin Microbiol Rev 2001;14:114-128.
Johnston SP, Ballard MM, Beach MJ, et al: Evaluation or three commercial assays for detection of *Giardia* and *Cryptosporidium* organisms in fecal specimens. J Clin Microbiol 2003;41:623-626.
Mineno T, Avery MA: Giardiasis: Recent progress in chemotherapy and drug development. Curr Pharm Des 2003;9:841-855.
Petri WA Jr: Therapy of intestinal protozoa. Trends Parasitol 2003;19(11):523-526.
Sulaiman IM, Fayer R, Bern C, et al: Triosephosphate isomerase gene characterization and potential zoonotic transmission of *Giardia duodenalis*. Emerg Infect Dis 2003;9(11):1444-1452.

Severe Sepsis and Septic Shock

Method of
Steven Zgliniec, MD, and *Robert A. Balk, MD*

Sepsis has been defined as the systemic inflammatory response to an infection. The true incidence of sepsis is unknown, in part related to the lack of a uniformly accepted definition. The Centers for Disease Control and Prevention (CDC) had previously reported a dramatic 139% increase in the septicemia discharge diagnosis over a decade of monitoring. Using discharge-coding data from seven states, it has been recently suggested that there are more than 750,000 episodes of severe

---

[1]Not FDA approved for this indication.
[2]Not available in the United States.
[†]This herbal supplement is not FDA approved for this indication.

sepsis each year in the United States. Severe sepsis accounts for 1 out of every 10 intensive care unit (ICU) admissions and represents 2% to 3% of all hospital admissions. Furthermore, incidence of sepsis in the United States is projected to rise at a rate of 1.5% per year. Factors responsible for this increase include the continued growth in the number of elderly patients, an increased number of immunocompromised patients, the increased use of invasive procedures and devices to care for patients, the growing problem with resistant micro-organisms, and a greater awareness and recognition of this disorder.

Sepsis is now reported to be the tenth most common cause of death in the United States and is one of the two most common causes of death in the noncoronary ICU. Using the extrapolated annual incidence of 750,000 episodes of sepsis in the United States and a relatively conservative mortality estimate of 28%, there would be an annual mortality of greater than 220,000. This surprisingly high mortality rate has been projected despite our enhanced understanding of the pathophysiologic alterations that occur in sepsis, technologic improvements in monitoring and support of the critically ill patient, and use of more potent antibiotic therapy. There have also been multiple attempts to improve the outcome of the septic patient using innovative therapeutic strategies that are designed to target selected aspects of the pathophysiologic response to the causative microorganism(s).

A recent epidemiologic review of sepsis in the United States reported that sepsis is more common in males and in the nonwhite population. Over the past 22 years, gram-positive organisms have become the predominant cause of sepsis, but there has also been a dramatic increase in the number of episodes of fungal sepsis. During this observation period, the incidence and number of sepsis-related deaths have increased, whereas the actual sepsis mortality rate has improved.

Definitions of Systemic Inflammatory Response Syndrome and Sepsis

The approach to management of patients with severe sepsis and septic shock begins with prompt recognition of the septic process (Current Diagnosis box). As mentioned, in the past there has been difficulty in identifying septic patients, in part related to the lack of a uniformly accepted definition. In 1991 the American College of Chest Physicians and the Society of Critical Care Medicine convened a consensus conference to develop a set of definitions that would assist the medical community in communication about sepsis and provide for the early recognition of the septic patient. The definition would incorporate predominantly readily available clinical criteria that would facilitate patient identification and enrollment in investigational trials of innovative therapeutic agents. The consensus conference recognized that some patients with presumed sepsis based on their clinical presentation lacked a positive culture or other evidence of a documented infection.

CURRENT DIAGNOSIS

Infection (documented or suspected) and some of the following:

General Variables

- Fever (core temperature >38.3°C [101°F]
- Hypothermia (core temperature <36°C [96.8°F]
- Heart rate >90/min or >2 SD above the normal value for age
- Tachypnea
- Altered mental status
- Significant edema or positive fluid balance (>20 mL/kg more than 24 h)
- Hyperglycemia (plasma glucose >120 mg/dL, or 7.7 mmol/L in the absence of diabetes)

Inflammatory Variables

- Leukocytosis (WBC count >12,000/μL)
- Leukopenia (WBC count <4000/μL)
- Normal WBC count with >10% immature forms (bands)
- Plasma C-reactive protein >2 SD above the normal value
- Plasma procalcitonin >2 SD above the normal value

Hemodynamic Variables

- Arterial hypotension (systolic BP <90 mm Hg, MAP <70, or a systolic BP decrease >40 mm Hg in adults or <2 SD below normal for age)
- SvO_2 >70%
- Cardiac index >3.5 L/min/m^2
- Organ Dysfunction Variables
- Arterial hypoxemia (PaO_2/FiO_2 <300)
- Acute oliguria (urine output <0.5 mL/kg/h or 45 mmol/L for at least 2 h)
- Creatinine increase >0.5 mg/dL
- Coagulation abnormalities (INR >1.5 or aPTT >60s)
- Ileus (absent bowel sounds)
- Thrombocytopenia (platelet count <100,000/μL)
- Hyperbilirubinemia (plasma total bilirubin >4 mg/dL or 70 mmol/L)

Tissue Perfusion Variables

- Hyperlactatemia (>1 mmol/L)
- Decreased capillary refill or mottling

Abbreviations: aPTT = activated partial thromboplastin time; BP = blood pressure; INR = international normalized ratio; MAP = mean arterial pressure; SD = standard deviation; WBC = white blood cell.
From Levy MM, Fink MP, Marshall JC, et al: 2001 SCCM/ESICM/ACCP/ATS/SIS International sepsis definitions conference. Crit Care Med 2003;31:1250-1256.

These individuals were classified as having the systemic inflammatory response syndrome (SIRS). SIRS can result from a diverse group of insults, such as trauma, burns, pancreatitis, and so forth. Sepsis was defined as the SIRS response to a documented infection.

Defined as a widespread systemic inflammatory response to a variety of insults, SIRS includes but is not limited to infection. SIRS was operationally defined by the presence of two or more of the following:

- Temperature greater than 38°C (100.4°F) or less than 36°C (96.8°F)
- Heart rate more than 90 beats per minute (bpm)
- Respiratory rate greater than 20 breaths per minute or $PaCO_2$ less than 32 mm Hg

- White blood cell (WBC) more than 12,000 cells/mm^3, fewer than 4000 cells/mm^3, or greater than 10% immature band forms

Sepsis is the systemic inflammatory response to a documented infection. The diagnosis of sepsis requires the presence of at least two of the above SIRS criteria as a response to an infection. Signs of infection include an inflammatory response to the presence of microorganisms and the invasion of normally sterile host tissue by those organisms. There is a continuum of injury severity in SIRS and sepsis. Severe SIRS and severe sepsis are defined by the presence of organ dysfunction or hypoperfusion as a result of the inflammatory response. Hypoperfusion and perfusion abnormalities may include, but are not limited to, lactic acidosis, oliguria, or an acute alteration in mental status. Sepsis-induced hypotension occurs when systolic blood pressure (BP) falls to less than 90 mm Hg or there is a reduction of at least 40 mm Hg from baseline systolic pressure in the absence of other causes for hypotension.

Septic shock is a subset of severe sepsis with hypotension despite adequate fluid resuscitation, along with the presence of perfusion abnormalities. Patients receiving inotropic or vasopressor agents may no longer be hypotensive by the time they manifest hypoperfusion abnormalities or organ dysfunction, yet they would still be considered to have septic shock. Multiple organ dysfunction syndrome (MODS) is the alteration of organ function such that normal homeostasis cannot be maintained without intervention. Unfortunately, there is no consensus on how to define the dysfunction or failure of specific organ systems. However, most would agree that the need for organ support or replacement therapy signifies the presence of specific organ failure.

Validation of these conference definitions came from a prospective evaluation of University of Iowa patients who met the SIRS criteria, as well as sepsis, severe sepsis, and septic shock definitions. These patients demonstrated an increase in mortality as they moved down this continuum of injury severity.

In 2001 the International Sepsis Definitions Conference convened to revisit the American College of Chest Physicians/Society of Critical Care Medicine (ACCP/SCCM) Consensus Conference Definitions. Representatives from the SCCM, ACCP, European Society of Intensive Care Medicine, American Thoracic Society, and the Surgical Infection Society reaffirmed the basic validity of the 1991 definitions. To enhance the clinician's ability to recognize severe sepsis and to possibly enhance the specificity of the clinical diagnosis of sepsis, the conference provided a listing of common signs and symptoms of sepsis (see Current Diagnosis box). In addition, the International Sepsis Definitions Conference developed a classification scheme for sepsis modeled after the TNM system used in cancer staging (Table 1). The PIRO classification system to hoped to aid in stratifying septic patients on the basis of the predisposing condition(s), the nature of the insult, the nature and magnitude of the host's response, and the degree of concomitant organ dysfunction. The potential utility of the proposed staging systems is the ability to

TABLE 1   PIRO Staging of Sepsis

Predisposition: Premorbid conditions that influence likelihood of infection, sepsis, morbidity, survival (i.e., age, sex, hormonal state, genetic polymorphisms for TNF, IL-10, IL-6, IL-1ra, TLR)

Insult/Infection: Insult or organism associated with the sepsis response (i.e., type of organism, sensitivity pattern, community, or nosocomial acquisition)

Response: Clinical manifestations of the SIRS response (procalcitonin, IL-6, HLA-DR, TNF, PAF, CRP, etc.)

Organ dysfunction: Type and number of dysfunctional organs (reversible versus irreversible dysfunction) Severity of dysfunction (judged by scoring systems, e.g., MODS, LODS, SOFA)

Abbreviations: CRP = C-reactive protein; HLA-DR = human leukocyte antigen-D region–related; IL = interleukin; LODS = logistic organ dysfunction system; MODS = multiple organ dysfunction syndrome; PAF = platelet-activating factor; SOFA = sepsis-related organ failure assessment; TNF = tumor necrosis factor.
From Levy MM, Fink MP, Marshall JC, et al: 2001 SCCM/ESICM/ACCP/ATS/SIS International sepsis definitions conference. Crit Care Med 2003;31:1250-1256.

discriminate the morbidity associated with the infection from the morbidity arising from the response to infection.

Pathogenesis of Sepsis

The septic response begins as a normal physiologic response to an infection that attempts to wall off and eliminate the offending microbiologic organism(s). The pathologic process clinically recognized as sepsis results from an excessive and uncontrolled physiologic response that may culminate in endothelial cell injury, MODS, or death. The normal response to infection involves a process that serves to localize and contain an invading organism, usually resulting in the initiation of repair of injured host tissue. When this inflammatory response to infection becomes generalized and extends to healthy host tissue, it becomes the SIRS. With the onset of SIRS, normal host tissue whether infected or not, becomes damaged. This results in the release of proinflammatory and anti-inflammatory molecules and mediators capable of producing injury and/or altering the host's immune response. These contrasting elements help facilitate host tissue repair and healing. When there is an imbalance in the complex and intricate septic cascade, however, either a SIRS or a compensatory anti-inflammatory response syndrome (CARS) can predominate. If the SIRS response predominates, there is a predisposition for an exaggerated proinflammatory response that can culminate in the production of MODS. In contrast, when the CARS response predominates, there is a state of immune suppression that can result in secondary or nosocomial infections. These additional inflammatory insults may supply additional *hits* to the immune system; this pathomechanism has been termed the *multiple hits hypothesis* for the production of multiple organ dysfunction (MOD) or failure. The sepsis cascade has been categorized into five stages by Bone and colleagues (Table 2).

TABLE 2 The Five Stages of Sepsis

The infectious insult
Preliminary systemic response
Overwhelming systemic response
The compensatory anti-inflammatory reaction
Immunomodulatory failure

TABLE 3 Potential Molecules Involved in the Pathogenesis of Systemic Inflammatory Response Syndrome and Sepsis

Pro-inflammatory Molecules and Cells

PMNLs
Tissue macrophages and monocytes
Platelets
Arachidonic acid metabolites
Prostaglandins, prostacyclin, thromboxane, leukotrienes
Cytokines (interleukins 1, 2, 6, 8, 15, TNF, G-CSF)
Soluble adhesion molecules
PAF
Complement and activation of the complement cascade
Various kinins (e.g., bradykinin)
Endorphins
Histamine and serotonin
Proteolytic enzymes
Elastase and lysosomal enzymes
Protein kinase, tyrosine kinase
Toxic oxygen metabolites
Superoxide, hydroxyl radical, hydrogen peroxide, peroxynitrite, etc.
Endotoxin and other bacterial and microbial toxins
Activation of the coagulation cascade
Neopterin
PAI-1
CD14
Toll-like receptors 2 & 4
NF-κB
Vasoactive neuropeptides
MCP-1 and -2

Potential Anti-inflammatory Molecules

IL-1ra
Type II IL-1 receptor
IL-4, IL-10, IL-13
Transforming growth factor-β (TGF-β)
IκB
Glucocorticoid receptors
Epinephrine
sTNFr
Leukotriene B$_4$ receptor antagonist
Soluble CD14
LPS binding protein

Abbreviations: G-CSF = granulocyte colony-stimulating factor; IL = interleukin; IL-1ra = interleukin-1 receptor antagonist; LPS = lipopolysaccharide; MCP = monocyte chemoattractant protein; NF-κB = nuclear factor-kappa B; PAF = platelet-activating factor; PAI1 = plasminogen activator inhibitor-1; PMNL = polymorphonuclear leukocyte; sTNFr = soluble TNF receptor; TNF = tumor necrosis factor.

Host factors responsible for important first line of defense against the infectious insult include epithelial barriers, mucociliary flow, pH of body fluids, urine volume, and secretory immunoglobulins. Overall immune function of the host is also a key consideration. Chronic diseases such as diabetes mellitus, HIV infection, and chronic alcoholism commonly predispose the host to an infectious insult. The adaptive and innate immunity of the host also provide key defenses against infectious insults. The adaptive arm of host immunity is composed of specialized B cells and T cells. Receptors unique to each of these cell lines results in a proliferation of immune response when stimulated. The innate arm of the immune response uses receptors that recognize highly conserved antigenic regions in large groups of microorganisms. A group of cell surface receptors that have become of particular interest are the toll-like receptors (TLR). For example, activation of TLR-4 by circulating endotoxin from the gram-negative bacterial cell wall induces the transcription of a number of inflammatory and immune response genes. Gram-negative organisms contain a component of endotoxin within the cell wall that is responsible for many of the manifestations of sepsis. Gram-positive organisms produce exotoxins that may function as superantigens. The result is a massive activation of mononuclear cells and macrophages with an overproduction of cytokines and an out of control immune response.

Mediators of the host inflammatory response are initially found in high concentrations locally, at the nidus of infection. In severe infections proinflammatory cytokines will produce systemic symptoms. This usually becomes the telltale sign that the infection is unable to be contained locally. Some of the more common primary pro- and anti-inflammatory molecules and mediators are listed in Table 3. Included in the list of pro-inflammatory cytokines are tumor necrosis factor (TNF)-α, interleukin (IL)-1, IL-6, and interferon-γ.

An overwhelming systemic inflammatory response results when the host is unable to contain the pro-inflammatory response locally. The massive, uncontrolled production of pro-inflammatory molecules and cytokines produce the SIRS. Endothelial dysfunction typically ensues from the inflammatory response coupled with the activation of the coagulation syndrome. The result is microvascular thrombi as well as upregulation of endothelial adhesion molecules causing increased microvascular permeability, vasodilatation, organ dysfunction, and shock.

The overwhelming pro-inflammatory response is then followed by CARS, which down-regulates the pro-inflammatory cascade. The balance that ensues during the mixed antagonistic response syndrome (MARS) will determine the clinical manifestations and outcome of the response to the infection. The principal mediators of the CARS response include IL-4, IL-10, and transforming growth factor (TGF)-β. In some cases the compensatory reaction can lead to excessive production of counterregulatory cytokines leading to immune suppression. This can be recognized by a decreased production of IL-6 and TNF-α by monocytes. The final result may be immunomodulatory failure, progression of infection, or superinfection along with coagulation activation or abnormalities of fibrinolysis leading to MODS and death.

Management of Severe Sepsis and Septic Shock

In 2003 critical care and infectious disease experts representing 11 international organizations developed management guidelines for severe sepsis and septic shock entitled the "Surviving Sepsis Campaign." These were published in 2004 in both *Critical Care Medicine* and *Intensive Care Medicine* journals. Management of sepsis and septic shock begins with prompt recognition of the process. Along with recognition and determination of a probable site and cause of the infection, the initial management begins with an assessment of the physiologic derangements. In critically ill patients the general management involves source control, restoration and maintenance of normal hemodynamic function, adequate oxygenation, ventilation, tissue oxygen delivery, and prevention of complications. The assessment of adrenal function and detection of occult adrenal insufficiency in vasopressor-dependent patients with septic shock is important for defining a role for physiologic adrenal replacement therapy. It is also imperative to evaluate for the presence of complications of critical illness and to administer preventive strategies where appropriate. The Current Therapy box outlines the general management principles.

SOURCE CONTROL

Prompt, effective management of the source of the infection is the cornerstone of sepsis management. Early initiation of appropriate, effective antimicrobial therapy is essential for a favorable outcome in the septic patient. Necessary specimens should be sent for culture and sensitivity testing as early as possible, because this information will guide subsequent antimicrobial therapy and allow for good antimicrobial stewardship. The initial antimicrobial therapy is empirical and should be directed toward the organisms likely to cause the infection giving rise to the septic response. A review of nosocomial infections suggests that the urinary tract (UT), respiratory system (RS), and bloodstream are the three most common sources of hospital-acquired infections.

Clinical trials of new agents for the treatment of sepsis have observed that the respiratory tract and the abdomen are the most common sources of infection. After identification of the likely site and cause of the infection, the initial antibiotic selection should be made taking into account the antibiogram of the institution or specific unit where the infection was acquired. When the results of the various cultures and their sensitivity pattern are available, the antimicrobial therapy should then be appropriately tailored. It has been well documented that the use of early effective antimicrobial therapy will decrease mortality, particularly in patients with gram-negative bacteremia, elderly patients with *Streptococcus pneumoniae* pulmonary infection, and critically ill patients with bloodstream infections and/or hospital-acquired

 CURRENT THERAPY

Identify the Cause and Source of Infection
Obtain suitable material for needed cultures, Gram stains, and diagnostic studies.
Implement surgical drainage where appropriate.

Initiate Appropriate Antibiotic Therapy
Initial therapy will be empirical, but tailored therapy may be started when more data are available.
Survival is improved when the initial antibiotic therapy is effective against the isolated organism(s) and started early.

Restore and Maintain Hemodynamic Function
Implement an early goal-directed therapeutic approach.
Fluids are the initial choice for volume resuscitation and may include crystalloids, colloids, volume expanders, or blood products.
If hypotension and poor perfusion persist, then vasoactive agents should be used as necessary to ensure adequate hemodynamic function.
Hemodynamic monitoring is frequently used to ensure the adequacy and effectiveness of therapy (i.e., arterial line, CVP, PA catheter).
Physiologic dose corticosteroid replacement therapy may be beneficial for vasopressor-dependent patients with inadequate cortisol response.

Support Oxygenation and Ventilation
Supplemental oxygen as needed to ensure the patient has adequate arterial oxygen saturation.
Ensure adequate tissue oxygen delivery.
Implement mechanical ventilation as necessary.
Use lung protective ventilator support.
Implement protocol-derived weaning.

Antithrombotic, Profibrinolytic, Anti-inflammatory Therapy
Use drotrecogin alfa (activated) (Xigris) as per package insert recommendations.

Metabolic Support
Maintain early nutritional support.
Maintain intestinal mucosa barrier function by enteral route, the preferred method.
Control hyperglycemia to decrease infectious complications, may need IV insulin therapy.

Prevent Complications of Critical Illness
Prevent DVT prophylaxis.
Prevent stress-related gastrointestinal bleeding.
Prevent organ system dysfunction.
Prevent nosocomial and secondary infections.
Recognize critical illness polyneuropathy/myopathy.
Anticipate anemia of critical illness.

Abbreviations: CVP = central venous pressure; DVT = deep vein thrombosis; IV = intravenous; PA = pulmonary artery.
Adapted from Balk RA: Optimum treatment of patients with severe sepsis and septic shock: Evidence in support of the recommendations. Dis Mon 2004;50:168-213.

pneumonia. The use of early effective antibiotic therapy in critically ill patients is associated with significant reductions in infection-related and all-cause mortality rates. This benefit was present despite the addition of effective antibiotics once the culture and sensitivity data was available. This observation underscores the importance of initiating the correct initial empirical therapy. Correct antibiotic decisions are crucial in this era of increasing antibiotic resistance. It is important to know the ecology of organisms in your institution along with the antibiogram for the institution. Several recent reviews have been published to assist with the initial empirical antibiotic selection.

HEMODYNAMIC MANAGEMENT

Sepsis is characterized by vasodilatory or distributive shock, and there is an increase in vascular capacitance along with the decrease in the systemic vascular resistance. Septic patients are typically intravascularly volume depleted related to the presence of increased permeability as a result of endothelial cell injury and an increase in fluid loss coupled with a decrease in fluid replacement. Early recognition of significant hemodynamic derangements and restoration of normal organ perfusion are vital in preventing organ dysfunction and failure. The goal of hemodynamic resuscitation should be either to raise the mean arterial pressure above 60 to 65 mm Hg or to achieve a systolic BP of at least 90 mm Hg. The resuscitative efforts and the adequacy of tissue perfusion can be assessed at the bedside by monitoring heart rate, BP, orthostatic BP changes, mental status, hourly urine output, and skin perfusion.

The initial hemodynamic resuscitation should take the form of fluid for volume replacement. The fluid resuscitation can be accomplished with a variety of fluids including crystalloid, colloid, blood, synthetic starches, and hypertonic saline. Most clinicians accomplish the fluid resuscitation with intravenous (IV) infusion of either crystalloid or colloid. Bolus infusions are typically administered using the clinical response and/or measurements of central venous pressure (CVP) or pulmonary capillary wedge pressure (PCWP) as a guide. In many instances adequate volume resuscitation may be sufficient to restore normal perfusion pressure. The choice of crystalloids versus colloids for fluid resuscitation has been the subject of numerous studies and reviews. The Saline versus Albumin Fluid Evaluation (SAFE) trial, a large multicenter, prospective, randomized trial conducted by the Australia-New Zealand Critical Care Trials Group found that saline and 5% albumin (Albuminar-5) were equally effective for fluid resuscitation of the patient with shock. Currently there is no clear benefit of one fluid over the other. Crystalloids tend to be cheaper and more readily available, but a larger volume is required. Generally it may take significant liters of fluid to adequately resuscitate patients with severe septic shock. Colloids are typically more expensive and may be associated with coagulation abnormalities, but smaller volumes are needed.

Invasive vascular monitoring may be used to aid in the determination of adequate hemodynamic resuscitation.

If a central venous catheter is present, the CVP can be measured to assess the adequacy of the intravascular volume status. In selected patients with hemodynamic insufficiency, the insertion of pulmonary artery catheters to measure the left-sided (and right-sided) filling pressures and the various hemodynamic parameters may be beneficial. A sphygmomanometer may be unreliable for BP measurement in hypotensive septic patients. Insertion of an arterial line may be required, especially if the patient is unresponsive to volume resuscitation and requires the addition of vasopressor therapy for hemodynamic resuscitation.

VASOPRESSOR MANAGEMENT

If adequate fluid resuscitation is insufficient to restore adequate hemodynamic function, then vasopressor and/or inotropic therapy will be necessary. There are a wide variety of vasoactive medications that are useful in the hemodynamic resuscitation of septic shock. Table 4 lists some of the more commonly used agents. Despite a wide range of possible agents, dopamine (Intropin) and norepinephrine (Levophed) are typically used in most clinical units. Some centers prefer to use phenylephrine (Neo-Synephrine) in patients with tachycardia or a history of arrhythmias because this pure alpha agent will cause less tachycardia and arrhythmias.

Unfortunately, there is a lack of large, prospective, randomized, protocol-controlled clinical trials that have compared dopamine (Intropin) to norepinephrine (Levophed) for the management of patients with septic shock. Therefore, until such data are available to guide the decision process, there is no clear benefit of one vasopressor strategy over the other, so either agent is acceptable in the management of hypotensive patients. Dopamine (Intropin) has been the preferred agent in many units, in part related to its ease of use, the concept that it improves splanchnic and renal perfusion, and its safety record. Recent clinical trial results have revealed that there is no specific beneficial effect of so called renal dose dopamine (Intropin) in preventing the development of renal failure or in decreasing the need for renal replacement therapy. In addition, the use of dopamine (Intropin) has been associated with an increase in the incidences of arrhythmias and a decrease in the gastric intramucosal pH (an indicator of splanchnic oxygen delivery and use). Norepinephrine (Levophed) is a potent vasoconstrictor that also has some increased inotropic and chronotropic effect on the heart. There is no decrease in renal or splanchnic perfusion as was once thought, and in fact there is an increase in the perfusion of these vascular beds as a result of the increased cardiac output and vasoconstriction. A large observational study of French septic shock patients who required high doses of vasopressor therapy, demonstrated a significant improvement in survival with the use of norepinephrine (Levophed) as compared to high doses of dopamine (Intropin) with or without the addition of epinephrine.

There has been renewed interest in the use of vasopressin in patients with vasodilatory shock. The initial release of stored vasopressin (Pitressin)[1] from the posterior pituitary during hypotension depletes the body's

TABLE 4 Vasoactive Agents Commonly Used in the Management of Severe Sepsis[1]

Drug	Receptor Activity	Dose	Effect	Notes
Norepinephrine (Levophed)	α_1: 3+, α_2: 2+, β_1: 2+	0.03-1.5 µg/kg/min	Vasoconstriction	Little change in heart rate or CI. May decrease lactate.
Epinephrine	α_1: 3+, α_2: 3+, β_1: 3+, β_2: 2+	0.1-0.5 µg/kg/min	Increase stroke volume and CI	Unpredictable dose-response. Decrease splanchnic blood flow. Increase oxygen consumption and delivery.
Dopamine (Intropin)	α_1: 3+, α_2: 3+, β_1: 3+, β_2: 2+	<5 µg/kg/min	Vasodilation	Dopaminergic effects predominate. Dilation of renal, mesenteric, and coronary arteries. Increased GFR. Sodium excretion.
Dopamine (Intropin)	α_1: 3+, α_2: 3+, β_1: 3+, β_2: 2+	5-10 µg/kg/min	↑ Inotropy and chronotropy	β-adrenergic effects predominate. Increased CI primarily caused by increased stroke volume.
Dopamine (Intropin)	α_1: 3+, α_2: 3+, β_1: 3+, β_2: 2+	>10 µg/kg/min	Vasoconstriction	α-Adrenergic effects predominate.
Dobutamine (Dobutrex)	α_1: 1+, v_2: 1+, β_1: 3+, β_2: 2+	2-20 µg/kg/min	↑ Inotropy and chronotropy	25%-50% increase in CI. Decreases PAOP.
Phenylephrine (Neo-Synephrine)	α_1: 3v	0.5-8 µg/kg/min	Vasoconstriction	Increases MAP without change in heart rate. CI may decrease.
Vasopressin (Pitressin)[1]	V_1	0.01-0.04 U/min IV	Vasoconstriction	Hormone replacement therapy may potentiate the vasoconstrictor effect of endogenous catecholamines or act directly on a V_1 receptor.

[1]Not FDA approved for this indication.
Abbreviations: CI = cardiac index; GFR = glomerular filtration rate; IV = intravenous; MAP = mean aortic pressure; PAOP = pulmonary artery occluded pressure.
Modified from Steel A, Bihari D: Choice of catecholamine: Does it matter? Curr Opin Crit Care 2000;6:347-353.

store of the hormone. As the shock state persists, there is a state of vasopressin deficiency, which some view as a hormone-deficiency state that is amenable to replacement therapy. Some centers are now infusing vasopressin (Pitressin)[1] as a hormone replacement therapy in a constant, nonescalating dose to augment dopamine (Intropin) or the pressor effects of norepinephrine (Levophed). The importance of early goal-oriented hemodynamic resuscitation was emphasized in a recent trial comparing this technique with more traditional resuscitation efforts. The early goal-oriented protocol was associated with significant improvement in ICU and hospital survival and significantly fewer deaths from sudden hemodynamic collapse.

Some patients with severe sepsis and septic shock have a reversible biventricular myocardial dysfunction, which has been attributed to circulating TNF-α, IL-1, and/or nitric oxide that are elaborated as part of the SIRS response. Ventricular dilatation and a reduced ejection fraction comprise this myocardial depression. Inotropic agents such as dobutamine (Dobutrex) or epinephrine can improve the myocardial contractility and hemodynamic function in these patients. By increasing stroke volume and heart rate, dobutamine (Dobutrex) increases the cardiac index. Although epinephrine can also increase the cardiac index, its use should be limited in the septic patient because it can impair splanchnic blood flow and increase systemic and regional lactate concentrations.

[1]Not FDA approved for this indication.

SUPPORT OXYGENATION AND VENTILATION

Abnormalities of the respiratory system are some of the most common evidence of organ systems involvement in sepsis. Septic patients should be assessed for adequacy of oxygenation, oxygen delivery, ventilation, and the ability to protect the airway. Septic patients commonly have abnormalities of oxygenation and increased work of breathing. Patients who are hypoxemic should be given supplemental oxygen with a goal of achieving arterial oxygen saturation of at least 90%.

Another decision to make in caring for the septic patient is the need and timing for endotracheal intubation and ventilatory support. Acute lung injury (ALI) and ARDS are relatively common manifestations of pulmonary dysfunction in the patient with severe sepsis and septic shock. Up to 35% of septic patients may manifest ARDS. The goal of mechanical ventilation is to maintain the PaO_2 in the 55 to 70 mm Hg range while keeping the FiO_2 below 60% (0.6). The traditional approach to mechanically ventilating patients with ALI and ARDS has been to employ tidal volumes in the 10 to 15 mL/kg range. The Acute Respiratory Distress Syndrome Network (ARDSNet) trial of low tidal volume ventilation of 6 mL/kg ideal body weight, coupled with maintaining an end-inspiratory plateau pressure up to 30 cm H_2O and a nomogram for positive end-expiratory pressure (PEEP) titration based on FiO_2, and oxygenation goals demonstrated an overall decrease in hospital mortality along with an increase in ventilator-free and organ failure–free days.

The risk of infection and ventilator-associated complications increases with the duration of ventilatory support. Patients should be removed from the ventilator as soon as they no longer need mechanical ventilatory support. The use of weaning protocols implemented by trained ICU support staff have been shown to speed the weaning process and improve the overall process of extubating the critically ill patient. It is also important to use sedation and analgesia appropriately in this critically ill population. Excessive sedation and analgesia have been linked to prolonged stays on mechanical ventilatory support and increased complications.

In a large, multicenter, controlled trial conducted in critically ill patients without ischemic cardiac disease or acute blood loss, the restrictive practice of packed red blood cell (RBC) transfusions in the management of anemia and low hemoglobin (Hb) levels (between 7.0 and 9.0 g/dL) was shown to provide adequate oxygen delivery to the tissues and in a subgroup of younger patients and less ill patients was found to be associated with a lower mortality rate compared to a more liberal transfusion policy with Hb levels maintained between 10.0 and 12.0 g/dL. The use of weekly recombinant erythropoietin (Epogen)[1] has also been shown to reduce the need for transfusions in critically ill patients. Aggressive use of packed RBC transfusions in an effort to achieve supernormal oxygen delivery states should be discouraged.

SUPPORTIVE CARE FOR THE CRITICALLY ILL PATIENT

Patients with severe sepsis and septic shock are critically ill and susceptible to the multiple complications common in the critically ill population. These complications include deep vein thrombosis and pulmonary emboli, stress-related gastrointestinal (GI) bleeding, nosocomial infections, MODS, and critical illness polyneuropathy/myopathy. Patients in the ICU with sepsis or septic shock should receive prophylaxis for deep vein thrombosis with unfractionated heparin or low-molecular-weight heparin, unless they have contraindications for their use. Pneumatic compression devices can be used if they have a coagulopathy or increased risk of bleeding. Prophylaxis for stress-related GI bleeding may be accomplished with H_2-receptor blockers, proton pump inhibitors,[1] sucralfate (Carafate)[1] or early enteral feeding.

Nutritional support of the patient with severe sepsis is important from multiple standpoints. Proper nutrition is important to maintain the necessary immune function during the catabolic septic metabolic process. Enteral administration of nutrition may prevent stress-related GI bleeding and may prevent the translocation of bowel organisms and/or endotoxin by maintaining the integrity of the GI tract's mucosal barrier function. Nutritional requirements during severe sepsis and septic shock have been addressed by numerous organizations and

medical societies. Adequate nutrition is responsible for improved wound healing, decreasing susceptibility of critically ill patients to infection and optimizing immune function. The following nutritional guidelines have been recommended for patients with sepsis:

- Daily caloric intake: 25 to 30 kcal/kg per usual body weight per day
- Protein: 1.3 to 2.0 g/kg per day
- Glucose: 30% to 70% of total nonprotein calories to maintain serum glucose fewer than 150 mg/dL
- Lipids: 15% to 30% of total nonprotein calories
- Omega-6 polyunsaturated fatty acids: reduce in septic patients, maintaining that level, which avoids deficiency of essential fatty acids (7% of total calories—generally 1 g/kg per day)

Metabolic management also includes correction of electrolyte abnormalities as well as tight control of blood sugar, which may require constant insulin infusion. In a report of postsurgical predominantly ventilated patients, tight glucose control aimed at keeping the blood sugar between 80 and 110 mg/dL was associated with a significant improvement in ICU and hospital survival. There were four times more deaths from multiple organ failure secondary to a proven septic focus in the group that did not receive the tight glucose control.

Innovative Therapies in Severe Sepsis and Septic Shock

Severe sepsis and septic shock have continued to be associated with significant mortality despite the improvements in our understanding of the septic process, the use of powerful antibiotic agents, and the provision of basic sepsis management. Advances in technology have also brought forward antibodies, receptor blockers, and other innovative agents designed to interrupt or block aspects of the septic cascade. The majority of innovative experimental strategies were directed at various components of the proinflammatory response evident during the initial phases of SIRS and sepsis. Because most of these trials were unsuccessful, there has been a shift in the target for interruption toward a later stage aspect of the septic cascade. A number of these recent strategies have taken aim at the coagulation system to inhibit the generation of thrombin and fibrin, which may be instrumental in the disorder of the microcirculation that may be at least partially responsible for the organ system dysfunction and MODS seen in severe sepsis and SIRS.

CORTICOSTEROID THERAPY

Experimental studies in animal models of sepsis and septic shock have demonstrated improved survival with the pretreatment or early treatment with high doses of corticosteroids. Such doses in humans with severe sepsis and septic shock have not been associated with significant improvements in survival except for one study. As a result of multiple trials of high-dose steroids in patients

---

[1]Not FDA approved for this indication.

with severe sepsis showing no benefit and potentially harm this practice has been abandoned. Recently, the observation that basal cortisol levels and the cortisol response to the administration of adrenocorticotropic hormone (ACTH) (Corticotropin)[1] could predict survival in patients with severe sepsis, and septic shock has drawn attention back to the use of steroid therapy. A French study of patients with septic shock demonstrated that a basal cortisol level of up to 34 µg/dL along with the ability to increase the cortisol level by at least 9 µg/dL was associated with a 74% survival rate. In comparison, patients who had a basal cortisol level of more than 34 µg/dL and were unable to increase their cortisol level by at least 9 µg/dL had an 18% survival rate. The investigators proposed that some patients with septic shock have a state of relative adrenal insufficiency or problems with their glucocorticoid receptors that can be improved with the use of more physiologic corticosteroid replacement therapy. A recent multicenter, prospective, randomized, controlled trial of 300 patients with vasopressor-dependent septic shock who were all receiving mechanical ventilatory support and were resuscitated according to a defined protocol demonstrated an improved survival rate in patients who failed to increased their basal cortisol level by more than 9 µg/dL and were given physiologic corticosteroid replacement therapy. For this trial the physiologic corticosteroid replacement therapy consisted of 50 mg of IV hydrocortisone (Solu-Cortef)[1] every 6 hours for 7 days combined with once-daily fludrocortisone (Florinef)[1] given enterally at 50 µg per day. The authors of this trial concluded that physiologic corticosteroid therapy is beneficial and should be administered to vasopressor-dependent patients in septic shock who manifest relative adrenal insufficiency as defined by the failure to increase the cortisol level by more than 9 µg/dL after ACTH stimulation.

HIGH-VOLUME CONTINUOUS VENOVENOUS HEMOFILTRATION THERAPY

The use of high-volume, continuous hemofiltration (either continuous arteriovenous or venovenous) benefits the hemodynamic course and outcome in patients with intractable circulatory failure resulting from septic shock. The use of this form of management is expensive, requires defined expertise, and may be associated with metabolic and coagulation abnormalities. Further studies are needed to determine if this mode of therapy improves outcome in septic patients. Its use should probably be limited to patients with renal indications for hemofiltration.

ANTITHROMBOTIC THERAPY

Newer therapies have been directed toward inhibitors of the coagulation system as a potential therapeutic strategy for patients with severe sepsis and septic shock. Earlier therapies targeting the pro-inflammatory stage have shown little benefit in reducing mortality.

Among the therapies that have been used are Antithrombin, tissue factor pathway inhibitor (TFPI),* and activated protein C replacement therapy.

Antithrombin (AT)* is an endogenous serine protease that has antithrombotic and anti-inflammatory properties. In an early trial in a small number of patients, the administration of AT to patients with septic shock and disseminated intravascular coagulation demonstrated a trend toward improved survival. Subsequently a large multicenter, prospective, randomized, double-blind, placebo-controlled trial was conducted, which unfortunately showed no difference in mortality compared to placebo at 30, 60, and 90 days.

TFPI* inhibits factor VIIa within the factor VIIa/tissue factor complex, after first binding and inactivating factor Xa. Recently, a phase 3 multicenter, prospective, randomized, double-blind, placebo-controlled trial has been completed and failed to demonstrate a significant benefit in the primary endpoint, which was 28-day all-cause mortality.

As with antithrombin, the protein C system is one of the endogenous antithrombotic agents. Drotrecogin alfa (activated) (Xigris) is recombinant human activated protein C. A recent phase 3 trial was stopped after the second interim analysis demonstrated a significant survival benefit associated with the use of activated protein C versus placebo in 1690 patients with severe sepsis and septic shock. Treatment with a 96-hour infusion of drotrecogin alfa (activated) (Xigris) produced a 6.1% absolute risk reduction and a 19.4% relative risk reduction in the 28-day all-cause mortality in patients with severe sepsis ($P = 0.005$) The drotrecogin alfa (activated) (Xigris)-treated population experienced more serious bleeding complications (3.5%) compared to the placebo group (2.0%), and this difference trended toward significance. These results suggest that for every 66 patients treated with drotrecogin alfa (activated) (Xigris), 1 additional serious bleeding event would occur. The number needed to treat to save an additional life was 16.

The Food and Drug Administration (FDA) and 19 other regulatory bodies in other countries (including the European Union) have approved the use of drotrecogin alfa (activated) (Xigris) for the treatment of severe sepsis in adult patients with a high risk of mortality. The FDA gives the example of using the Acute Physiology and Chronic Health Evaluation (APACHE) II to estimate the risk of death (APACHE II score ≥25) and other means such as the number of dysfunctional organs to determine the target population of patients. Currently, the safety and efficacy of drotrecogin alfa (activated) (Xigris) in pediatric patients has not been determined. Contraindications to the use of drotrecogin alfa (activated) (Xigris) include patients with known sensitivity to drotrecogin alfa (activated) (Xigris) and patients with a high risk of death from or significant morbidity associated with bleeding. This group would include patients with active internal bleeding, recent (within 3 months) hemorrhagic stroke, recent (within 2 months) intracranial or intraspinal surgery or severe head trauma, trauma with increased risk

---

[1]Not FDA approved for this indication.

*Investigational drug in the United States.

of life-threatening bleeding, the presence of an epidural catheter, an intracranial neoplasm, or mass lesion or evidence of cerebral herniation. Septic patients who have undergone surgery within the prior month were also found to have a higher mortality rate when given activated protein C and clinicians are warned about using this agent in this group of patients.

Prognosis

Despite the tremendous advances in our appreciation of the pathophysiologic processes that comprise the septic response coupled with improved antibiotics and technologic support of the critically ill, the mortality rate for patients with severe sepsis and septic shock remains high. Clinical trials have reported placebo-group mortality rates attributable to severe sepsis and septic shock of 20% to 50%, with mortality rates up to 80% to 85% with septic shock and multiple organ failure. This high rate of morbidity and mortality demands an aggressive approach for early diagnosis and treatment in an attempt to improve the outcome of these critically ill patients. A number of factors have been found to impact survival including, age, co-morbid condition, site and type of infection, severity of illness, the number, and specific organ system failures. In addition, a patient's genetic makeup and/or gender may have a dramatic impact on whether they develop sepsis, as well as the severity, clinical manifestations, and outcome of the sepsis. Also, survivors of sepsis have increased 6- and 12-month mortality rates compared to nonseptic critically ill patients. There is a reduced quality of life and more health-related issues in patients who have survived an episode of sepsis. These observations underscore the importance of early aggressive management of the septic patient and suggest that our future focus should also be directed toward prevention of sepsis.

REFERENCES

Angus DC, Linde-Zwirble WT, Lidicker J, et al: Epidemiology of severe sepsis in the United States: Analysis of incidence, outcome, and associated costs of care. Crit Care Med 2001;29: 1303-1310.

Annane D, Sebille V, Charpentier C, et al: Effect of treatment with low doses of hydrocortisone and fludrocortisone on mortality in patients with septic shock. JAMA 2002;288:862-871.

Balk RA: Optimum treatment of patients with severe sepsis and septic shock: Evidence in support of the recommendations. Dis Mon 2004; 50:168-213.

Bernard GR, Vincent J-L, Laterre P-F, et al: Efficacy and safety of recombinant human activated protein C for severe sepsis. N Engl J Med 2001;344:699-709.

Dellinger RP, Carlet JM, Masur H, et al: Surviving Sepsis Campaign guidelines for management of severe sepsis and septic shock. Crit Care Med 2004;32(3):858-873.

Levy MM, Fink MP, Marshall JC, et al: 2001 SCCM/ESICM/ACCP/ ATS/SIS International sepsis definitions conference. Crit Care Med 2003;31:1250-1256.

Martin GS, Mannino DM, Eaton S, et al: The epidemiology of sepsis in the United States from 1979 through 2000. N Engl J Med 2003;348:1546-1554.

Rivers E, Nguyen B, Havstad S, et al: Early goal-directed therapy in the treatment of severe sepsis and septic shock. N Engl J Med 2001;345:1368-1377.

Steel A, Bihari D: Choice of catecholamine: Does it matter? Curr Opin Crit Care 2000;6:347-353.

The Acute Respiratory Distress Syndrome Network: Ventilation with lower tidal volumes as compared with traditional tidal volumes for acute lung injury and the acute respiratory distress syndrome. N Engl J Med 2000;342:1301-1308.

The SAFE Study Investigators: A comparison of albumin and saline for fluid resuscitation in the intensive care unit. N Engl J Med 2004; 350:2247-2256.

Van den Berghe G, Wouters P, Weekers F, et al: Intensive insulin therapy in critically ill patients. N Engl J Med 2001;345:1359-1367.

Brucellosis

Method of
Mehmet Doganay MD, and Emine Alp, MD

Brucella species are gram-negative coccobacillary, non-motile, aerobic microorganisms. The six known species of *Brucella* are *Brucella melitensis*, *Brucella abortus*, *Brucella suis*, *Brucella canis*, *Brucella ovis*, and *Brucella neotomae*, and recently *Brucella maris* was isolated. Brucellosis remains a major public health problem in many parts of the world. It affects mainly domestic animals and transmitted from animals to humans. Table 1 shows the animal reservoirs of *Brucella* species.

Epidemiology

Humans are usually infected in one of three ways: ingestion of infected food products, direct contact with an infected animal, or inhalation of aerosols. The most common way is eating or drinking contaminated milk products (milk, cream, butter, fresh cheese, ice cream). Human-to-human transmission is rare, but the organism can be transmitted through blood transfusion, bone marrow transplantation, breast-feeding, placenta, and sexual transmission.

According to the World Health Organization (WHO) reports, approximately 500,000 cases of brucellosis have been reported each year. It is a common disease in the Mediterranean Basin (Portugal, Spain, Southern France, Italy, Greece, Turkey, North Africa), South and Central America, Eastern Europe, Asia, Africa, the Caribbean, and the Middle East.

Pathogenesis and Immunity

Brucella species are facultative intracellular pathogens, surviving and multiplying within the cells of the reticuloendothelial system. Virulent *Brucella* organisms can infect both nonphagocytic and phagocytic cells. The intracellular environment of host cells sustains extensive reproduction, allowing bacterial expansion and subsequent transmission to new host cells. No classical virulence factors have been described in *Brucella* organisms.

TABLE 1 Species of *Brucella* and Animal Reservoirs

Species	Reservoir	Other Hosts	Human Cases (Worldwide)
Brucella melitensis	Goat, sheep, camel	Cattle, antelope	(70% cases)
Brucella abortus	Cattle, buffalo, yaks, bison	Horse	(25% of cases)
Brucella suis	Swine	Cattle, caribou	(5% of cases)
Brucella ovis	Sheep	—	No
Brucella canis	Dog	—	Few
Brucella neotomae	Desert wood rat	—	No
Brucella maris	Marine mammals	—	Few*

*Two cases reported.
Adapted from Doganay M, Aygen M: Human brucellosis: An overview. Int J Infect Dis 2003;7:173-182.

Some molecular determinants are described for *Brucella* species as virulence elements.

In humans, *Brucella* species infection results in the formation of granulomas consisting of epithelioid cells, polymorphonuclear leukocytes, lymphocytes, and some giant cells. The granulomatous response is characteristic of *Brucella abortus* infections. *Brucella melitensis* is the most virulent species.

Although humoral and cellular immunity play roles in the immunity to *Brucella*, cell-mediated immunity appears to be the principal mechanism of recovery. Serum IgM antibodies raise within the first week of infection, followed later by IgG and IgA antibodies. After treatment, IgG antibodies decline faster than IgM antibodies. The failed decrease of the IgG titers points out relapse or chronic infection.

Clinical Manifestations

Brucellosis is a systemic disease and any organ or body system can be involved. The incubation period varies between 1 and 5 weeks but may be as long as several months. Asymptomatic or symptomatic forms of the brucellosis can be seen. According to the length and severity of symptoms, the disease is classified as acute (less than 8 weeks), subacute (from 8 to 52 weeks), or chronic (more than 1 year).

The symptoms of brucellosis are generally nonspecific, including fever, sweats, malaise, anorexia, headache, arthralgia, and back pain (Table 2). The subclinical or asymptomatic form is diagnosed by positive serology, usually seen in farmers and veterinarians. Any organ involvement is often referred to as localized disease. If the localized infection occurs as a result of systemic infection, it is named as a complication and can be seen in 27.7% of cases. The identification of any organ involvement is very important for the choice of regimen and its duration and the prognosis.

Diagnosis

The diagnosis is based on the isolation of *Brucella* species from blood or body tissues, or the combination of suggestive clinical presentations and positive serology.

The patient's history that includes ingestion of high-risk foods (e.g., unpasteurized dairy products), exposure to animals, occupation, and travel to enzootic areas is important. The isolation rate of *Brucella* species from blood cultures ranges from 15% to 80%. The bone marrow cultures are significantly more sensitive than cultures of blood, and the time to detection is shorter for bone marrow cultures than for blood cultures. The culture material should be taken from the affected places (liver, lymph node, abscess, synovial fluid, prostatic fluid, or cerebrospinal fluid) in the case of focal complications. Amplification of DNA by polymerase chain reaction (PCR) is the diagnostic test used in recent years, with high sensitivity (100%) and specificity (93%).

TABLE 2 Symptoms and Clinical Findings in Brucellosis

Symptoms	%
Malaise	90.0
Sweating	84.4
Arthralgia	81.9
Fever	79.8
Back pain	58.5
Myalgia	49.2
Weight loss	44.4
Anorexia	41.3
Nausea	32.3
Vomiting	21.7
Abdominal pain	21.0
Headache	19.0

Findings	%
Fever	39.0
Hepatomegaly	21.3
Osteoarticular involvement	19.0
Splenomegaly	14.2
Neurologic involvement	6.5
Genitourinary involvement	1.0
Endocarditis	0.4
Peritonitis	0.4
Cutaneous involvement	0.4
Pneumonia	0.2

Adapted from Aygen B, Doganay M, Sümerkan B, et al: Clinical manifestations, complications and treatment of brucellosis: An evaluation of 480 patients. Med Mal Infect 2002;32:485-493.

CURRENT DIAGNOSIS

- The symptoms of brucellosis are generally nonspecific, including fever, sweats, malaise, anorexia, headache, arthralgia, and back pain.
- Any organ or body system can be involved.
- The diagnosis is based on the isolation of *Brucella* species from blood or body tissues, or the combination of suggestive clinical presentations and positive serology.

CURRENT THERAPY

- Tetracycline, doxycycline (Vibramycin), rifampin,[1] streptomycin, trimethoprim-sulfamethoxazole (Bactrim), some third-generation cephalosporins and quinolones are active against *B. melitensis*.
- Combination antibiotic therapy should be used.
- A combination of doxycycline (100 mg twice daily for 6 weeks) and streptomycin (1 g per day for 2 weeks) has been used widely and successfully.
- Doxycycline and rifampin combination is generally suggested to patients following in outpatient clinics.
- The therapy for any organ involvement or complications is the same as for brucellosis without focal disease, only the duration of the therapy should be longer (8–12 weeks or longer).

[1]Not FDA approved for this indication.

In the absence of bacterial isolation, the serologic tests (the tube agglutination test, the rose Bengal test, the anti-Brucella Coombs test, enzyme-linked immunosorbent assay [ELISA]) can be used for the diagnosis. The tube agglutination test is widely used, and a single titer of greater than or equal to160 or a fourfold rise in titer is significant.

Treatment

Appropriate antibiotics should have in vitro activity against *Brucella* species and adequate intracellular concentrations. *Brucella* species are extremely sensitive to many antibiotics; however, the results of in vitro susceptibility tests do not always expect clinical efficacy. Previous studies have shown that tetracycline, doxycycline (Vibramycin), rifampicin (Rifadin),[1] streptomycin, trimethoprim-sulfamethoxazole (TMP-SMZ) (Bactrim),[1] some third-generation cephalosporins,[1] and quinolones[1] are active against *B. melitensis* (Table 3).

Currently monotherapy is unacceptable because of high rate of failure and relapse and the potential development of resistance. The tetracyclines are, at present,

the antibiotics of choice in brucellosis. A combination of doxycycline (Vibramycin) (100 mg twice daily for 6 weeks) and streptomycin (1 g per day for 2 weeks) has been used widely and successfully, with an associated relapse rate of 5%. Combinations of gentamicin (Garamycin)[1] or netilmicin (Netromycin)[1] with doxycycline (Vibramycin) have also proved to be effective, and could cause fewer adverse reactions. The second suggesting combination is doxycycline (Vibramycin) (200 mg daily) and rifampicin (Rifadin)[1] (600 to 900 mg daily) for 6 weeks. The combination of ofloxacin (Floxin)[1] or ciprofloxacin (Cipro)[1] with rifampicin (Rifadin)[1] is also an alternative regimen. The combination of TMP-SMZ (Bactrim)[1] and rifampicin (Rifadin)[1] can be used in pregnancy and children (younger than 7 years). Older children should receive the same antibiotics as adults.

[1]Not FDA approved for this indication.

[1]Not FDA approved for this indication.

TABLE 3 Drugs Used in the Treatment of Brucellosis

Generic Name	Trade Name	Adult Dosage	Pediatric Dosage
Doxycycline	Doryx, Vibramycin, Monodox	100 mg, PO, bid	5 mg/kg qd, PO <8y not suggested
Rifampin[1]	Rifadin, Rimactane	600–900 mg, PO/IV, qd	10–20 mg/kg qd, PO/IV, not to exceed 600 mg qd
Sulfamethoxazole and trimethoprim[1] (TMP/SMZ)	Bactrim, Septra	1 double strength tab, PO, bid (160 mg TMP; 800 mg SMZ) 8–10 mg/kg IV based on TMP divided q6h, q8h, or q12h	5 mL/10 kg, PO, bid; 5 mL:40 mg TMP; 200 mg SMZ
Gentamicin[1]	Garamycin, Jenamicin	5 mg/kg, IV/IM, qd	5 mg/kg/d, IM for 5 d
Streptomycin sulfate	Streptomycin	15 mg/kg, not to exceed 1 g qd, IM, qd	20–40 mg/kg qd IM, not to exceed 1 g qd
Ciprofloxacin[1]	Cipro	500–750 mg, PO, bid or tid	Not suggested
Ofloxacin[1]	Floxin	400 mg, PO, bid	Not suggested

[1]Not FDA approved for this indication.
Abbreviations: bid = twice daily; d = days; h = hours; IM = intramuscular injection; IV = intravenous; PO = by mouth; q = each; qd = daily; qid = four times daily; SMZ = sulfamethoxazole; tid = three times daily; TMP = trimethoprim.

The therapy for any organ involvement or complications is the same as for brucellosis without focal disease with a longer duration of the therapy. In recent studies patients with osteoarticular involvement had better results in doxycycline-streptomycin regimen than doxycycline-rifampicin (Vibramycin-Rifadin). In neurobrucellosis, an addition of a third-generation cephalosporin (ceftriaxone [Rocephin][1] for 2 to 3 weeks) to doxycycline-rifampicin (Vibramycin-Rifadin) combination have shown low therapeutic failure. In osteoarticular involvement and neurobrucellosis, surgery may be required under rare circumstances. Endocarditis and myocarditis are rare but serious complications of *Brucella* species, and a combination of medical and surgical therapy is required for the successful management of *Brucella* infective endocarditis. The duration of therapy in the localized forms should be at least 8 to 12 weeks or longer.

Prevention

There is no safe effective vaccine available for humans. Unpasteurized milk and milk products should not be consumed. Hunters and animal herdsman should use rubber gloves when handling viscera of animals.

REFERENCES

Ariza J, Gudiol F, Pallares R, et al: Treatment of human brucellosis with doxycycline plus rifampin or doxycycline plus streptomycin. Ann Intern Med 1992;117:25-30.

Aygen B, Doganay M, Sümerkan B, et al: Clinical manifestations, complications and treatment of brucellosis: An evaluation of 480 patients. Med Mal Infect 2002;32:485-493.

Aygen B, Sümerkan B, Mirza M, et al: Treatment of neurobrucellosis with a combination of ceftriaxone, rifampicin and doxycycline. Med Mal Infect (Elsevier) 1996;26:1199-1201.

Black FT: Brucellosis. In Cohen J, Powderly WG (eds): Infectious Diseases, 2nd ed. Edinburgh, Mosby, 2004, pp 1665-1669.

Doganay M, Aygen B, Esel D: Brucellosis due to blood transfusion. J Hosp Infect 2001;49:151-152.

Doganay M, Aygen M: Human brucellosis: An overview. Int J Infect Dis 2003;7:173-182.

Sümerkan B, Doganay M, Bakiskan V, et al: Antimicrobial susceptibility of clinical isolates of *Brucella melitensis*. Turkish J Med Sci 1993;18:17-22.

Young EJ: *Brucella* species. In Mandell GL, Bennett JE, Dolin R (eds): Principles and Practice of Infectious Disease, 5th ed. Philadelphia, Churchill Livingstone, 2000, pp 2387-2393.

Varicella (Chickenpox)

Method of
Philip Alfred Brunell, MS, MD

Varicella (chickenpox) is a highly contagious infection that is caused by a herpesvirus, varicella-zoster virus (VZV). Both active and passive immunizations are available. It is characterized by a vesicular rash, which is generalized in distribution tending to be more evident on the trunk and head than the extremities. Systemic symptoms in normal children are mild and complications infrequent. It is more severe in adults and in the immunocompromised. Varicella can be treated with antiviral drugs.

Etiology and Epidemiology

The etiologic agent of varicella is a herpes DNA virus that contains approximately 125,000 base pairs with approximately 70 open reading frames. Although significant polymorphism can be demonstrated, there is only one human genotype. Vaccine and wild-type viruses are distinguishable by laboratory testing.

Initial VZV infection results in varicella, which usually occurs in childhood. Approximately half of all children were infected prior to school entry before the introduction of routine immunization in 1995. Less than 2% of reported cases occurred after the second decade, which attests to the infectiousness of the disease. It is reported that 87% of children with a negative history are infected within an incubation period after introduction of a case into a household and 96% after two incubation periods. The attack rate is much lower in other settings. The most contagious period is probably the day prior to rash. Transmission of cases after the fourth day of rash is unlikely. Breakthrough cases in vaccinees with fewer than 50 lesions are less contagious than natural varicella. The incubation period is approximately 14 days; 99% of cases occur between 10 and 20 days following exposure. Passive immunization may lengthen the incubation period.

After the clinical illness resolves, this herpes virus continues to remain latent in dorsal root ganglion cells. In persons older than 50 years of age, the rate of activation of this herpes virus increases progressively. By 75 years of age there is a 1% chance per year of developing the manifestation of activation, zoster.

Zoster is common in infants whose mothers have chickenpox during pregnancy and in the immunocompromised.

Clinical Course

NORMAL UNIMMUNIZED CHILDREN

Varicella usually produces little or no prodrome or significant systemic symptoms other than pruritus. Often the appearance of vesicular lesions is the first sign of illness.

---

[1]Not FDA approved for this indication.

Fever below 39°C (102°F) is the rule. High fever raises suspicion of complication or misdiagnosis. The first lesions often appear in the scalp and may be appreciated by palpation of raised vesicular lesion before the appearance of lesions on the face and trunk. The extremities are last to be affected. Different stages of lesions, erythematous macules, papules, vesicles and crusted lesions may be seen simultaneously in the same site. Vesicles continue to appear for a few days and soon crust. Itching may cause considerable discomfort.

NORMAL IMMUNIZED CHILDREN

Breakthrough cases in vaccinated children are becoming more common as a greater proportion of children receive live varicella vaccine (LVV). These children usually have fewer than 50 lesions, many of which do not vesiculate. They are mainly on the trunk. Systemic symptoms are uncommon. Occasionally, immunized children may have more extensive rashes. These may represent children who did not have a successful immunization.

IMMUNOCOMPROMISED PATIENTS

Patients with cellular immune deficiencies, malignant diseases, and receiving immunosuppressive therapy including high doses of corticosteroids, can develop progressive varicella. These patients can have high fever with extensive vesicular rashes that continue to erupt for more than 1 week if untreated. Visceral involvement with pneumonia is the most common complication and can result in the demise of untreated patients. The course of these patients is very variable, however; some respond in similar manner as normal patients, and others contract fatal illnesses. The illness is modified by antiviral treatment or by active or passive immunization.

NORMAL ADULTS

Varicella is much more severe in adults and in some adolescents. There often is a prodrome with malaise, muscle aches, and fever. The rash distribution is similar to children but usually is more extensive and prolonged. Often there is an erythematous base around the vesicular lesions. Pneumonia is seen more frequently on roentgenographic exam than is clinically apparent. It is more common during pregnancy.

VARICELLA OF THE NEWBORN AND FETAL VARICELLA SYNDROME

Maternal infection during pregnancy rarely affects the fetus. During the first half of pregnancy approximately 1% of mothers will have babies with malformations. The hallmark of the syndrome is an atrophic limb, often with scars suggesting intrauterine zoster had occurred. Ophthalmologic involvement includes cataracts, retinopathy, and microphthalmia.

Microcephaly also is found. Maternal infections within 1 week prior to delivery and perhaps 1 or 2 days after may result in infants developing varicella shortly after birth. Some of these babies, if untreated in the absence

of maternal passive immunization, will develop generalized visceral disease with pneumonia.

Complications

The most common complication in the normal host is secondary bacterial infection. Some infections, caused by group A streptococci, may progress to necrotizing fasciitis and the "toxic strep syndrome," which is similar to staphylococcal toxic shock syndrome. Staphylococcal super infection also is common. Hemorrhagic complication can occur including purpura fulminans or thrombocytopenia. The neurologic complications include cerebellitis, which usually is self-limited, or encephalitis, which can end fatally. Less common complications include nephritis, optic neuritis, and transverse myelitis.

Diagnosis

In past years, varicella stood out as a distinctive illness, which rarely needed to be differentiated from others. However, with the threat of smallpox and the introduction of LVV resulting in "breakthrough disease," this is no longer the case. Smallpox usually has a more marked prodrome, and the rash is peripheral rather than centripetal. It is more deeply seeded and usually is in the same stage in a given skin area. Progressive varicella can resemble smallpox because of an underlying immune problem in patients. Both can have hemorrhagic manifestations. Disseminated zoster usually has a localized segmental rash from which the rash becomes generalized, but in severely immunocompromised patients, this is not always the case. Insect bites can be confused with breakthrough disease, but the lesions of this entity are usually on exposed areas rather than truncal. Herpetic lesions are usually localized in normal individuals but may pose a problem in the immunocompromised or when herpetic zosteriform lesions appear. Direct fluorescent antibody testing or polymerase chain reaction (PCR) are most useful in differentiating the two. PCR also can be useful in distinguishing vaccine from wild-type virus. The latter can cause disease in a recently immunized individual who was exposed to chickenpox.

 CURRENT DIAGNOSIS

- Generalized vesicular rash
- Centripetal distribution
- Erythematous macules, papules, vesicles, and crusts at the same time at one skin site
- Few systemic symptoms in normal children
- Rare mucous membrane lesions
- Prominent itching
- Approximately 2-week incubation period
- Modified disease occurs in previous vaccines

Prevention

PASSIVE IMMUNIZATION

Varicella-zoster immune globulin (VZIG) is useful in protecting susceptible individuals at high risk of severe disease who have had an intimate exposure, which is likely to result in transmission. It is used in immunocompromised persons and susceptible pregnant women. It should be given as soon as possible following exposure. It also is given at birth to newborns whose mothers had onset of varicella within 5 days prior to or 2 days following delivery and certain exposed young infants who had been born prematurely.

ACTIVE IMMUNIZATION

LVV (Varivax) is recommended now for all children older than 1 year of age. It also is recommended for children younger than 13 years of age if they have not had varicella. One dose is required prior to 13 years of age and two doses, separated by 4 to 8 weeks for older individuals. It can be given a few days following exposure. It also is recommended for susceptible adults who work in health care environments, are in contact with people at high risk, are international travelers, work with children or in environments where transmission is likely (e. g., day care), and nonpregnant women of child-bearing age. Note that false-negative history of varicella in adults is common. In our studies of health care workers, less than 9% of those who said they had not had the disease were found to be seropositive. The most reliable test for immunity is latex agglutination and is highly recommended over other commercially available tests. The vaccine can be given at the same time as other vaccines, and simultaneous immunization is encouraged. Significant complications are rare, but a few vesicular lesions can appear at the site of immunization or in a more generalized distribution in a very small number of patients. Documented spread from these vaccinees is rare, but because of the potential for dissemination to contacts, immunization of those likely to expose high-risk patients or pregnant women probably should be avoided if possible. LVV should not be given to pregnant women or to those who are immunocompromised or are receiving drugs that impair immune response. However, some HIV-infected individuals receive the vaccine, and the manufacturer (Merck) provides the vaccine for some patients with leukemia. The vaccine should not be given to patients receiving salicylates for fear of precipitating Reye's syndrome.

ANTIVIRAL DRUGS

Although not approved for this use, acyclovir (Zovirax) given to normal children in a dose of 20 mg/kg four times daily starting on day 7 following exposure and continuing for 7 days has been found to prevent varicella. However, it will not be apparent which individuals had subclinical infection, and thus will be protected against future exposure, or were completely protected from infection and will be susceptible if exposed subsequently.

Treatment

ANTIVIRAL THERAPY

Acyclovir (Zovirax) can be used to treat adults or adolescents who develop varicella. The drug is most effective if given within the first 24 hours after onset of lesions. Delay beyond this time will have a relatively small impact on the course of the disease. The drug is not usually used in children, as the effect on the course of illness is minimal. It should be given parenterally to immunocompromised patients or newborns. Acyclovir is very safe, and resistance in normal individuals is rare. A registry of pregnant women who have received the drug has not revealed any untoward effects on the fetus.

Acyclovir is usually given orally to adults and adolescents four times daily in doses of 800 mg for 5 days. Parenterally, the dose is 30 mg/kg daily for infants younger than 1 year of age and 1500 mg/m^2 daily for immunocompromised children older than 1 year of age given every 8 hours for 7 to 10 days. Contact a pediatric infectious disease consultant for use in the newborn as much higher doses are used for neonatal herpes. The parenteral dose for adults is 30 mg/kg daily given every 8 hours for 7 days. Valacyclovir (Valtrex)[1] and famciclovir (Famvir)[1] are better absorbed orally administered drugs and can be given less frequently. Although these drugs have been found to be at least as effective as acyclovir in the treatment of zoster, there is no approval for their use for varicella.

OTHER MEASURES

Although bathing persons with chickenpox is avoided by many for fear that it might spread the lesions, this is not the case. Although there is no evidence to support the use of bathing with antibacterial soap to decrease the risk of bacterial superinfection, it probably is a good idea. Colloidal baths (Aveeno) have been recommended by some to relieve itching, but there is little evidence that this or other antipruritic preparations are effective. I have used trimeprazine (Temaril)[2] in a dose of 2.5 mg three times daily in children older than 3 years, and 1.25 mg three times daily in those 6 months to 3 years of age. Calamine lotion containing some menthol, again, may be useful, but there is no proof that this is the case.

---

[1]Not FDA approved for this indication.
[2]Not available in the United States for human use.

 CURRENT THERAPY

- Normal children are not treated.
- Therapy is indicated for adults and some adolescents.
- Therapy must be started within 24 hours of onset.
- Immunocompromised individuals should receive parental therapy.

REFERENCES

Asano Y, et al: Post exposure prophylaxis of varicella in family contacts by oral acyclovir. Pediatrics 1993;92:219-222.

Brunell PA, Wood D: Varicella serologic status of health care workers as a guide to who to test immunize. Infect Control Hosp Epidemiol 1999;50(5):355-357.

Cohen JI, Brunell PA, Straus SE, et al: Varicella-zoster virus infection: New advances in an ancient disease. Ann Intern Med 1999;130: 922-932.

Peterson C, Mascola L, Chao SM, et al: Children hospitalized for varicella: A prevaccine review. J Pediatr 1996;129:529-536.

Prevention of varicella: Recommendations of the advisory committee on immunization practices (ACIP). MMWR 1996;45(RR11):1-25.

Prevention of varicella updated recommendations of the advisory committee on immunization practices (ACIP). MMWR 1999; 48(RR06):1-5.

Report of the Committee of Infectious Diseases 2003, 26th ed. Evanston, IL, American Academy of Pediatrics, 2003.

Ross AH: Modification of chickenpox in family contacts by administration of gamma globulin. N Engl J Med 1962;267:369-376.

Varicella vaccine update. Pediatrics 2000; 105(1):136-141.

Cholera

Method of
Carlos Seas, MD, and
Eduardo Gotuzzo, MD, FACP

Cholera is the most feared of all diarrheal diseases in history. Epidemics of cholera have been reported since the time of Hippocrates, but the modern time began approximately in 1817. Since then, cholera has caused seven pandemics, affecting all continents and remaining endemic in almost all affected areas. Recent examples of severe epidemics are the Latin American extension of the seventh pandemic by way of Peru in 1991, explosive epidemics among refugees in Africa, and unexpected epidemics of cholera caused by a new serogroup in Asia since 1992. We can conclude from these epidemics that it is very difficult to predict when a new epidemic will start, appropriate treatment reduces the mortality to values below 1%, and the pathogen continues to evolve in the environment despite interventions to control its spread.

Organism and Pathophysiology

Cholera is caused by a curved gram-negative bacillus that belongs to the family Vibrionaceae. Two serogroups are associated with clinical cholera, O1 and O139; both cause the same clinical entity. These serogroups spread not only locally but regionally and among continents. *Vibrio cholerae* is a natural inhabitant of certain aquatic environments, where it lives attached to copepods, algae, and crustacean shells in a symbiotic association. If conditions are not favorable for growth, *V. cholerae* adopts a dormant state. In this state it remains metabolically inactive for long periods of time. The switch to a metabolically

CURRENT DIAGNOSIS

- History of travel to an endemic area.
- Acute voluminous watery diarrhea with rice watery appearance, leading to severe dehydration in a matter of hours.
- Muscle cramps, vomiting, and signs of severe dehydration such as loss of skin elasticity (slow skin pinch retraction), hoarse voice, sunken eyes, and wrinkled hands and feet (*washerwoman hands*).
- Fever is absent in the majority of patients.
- Milder forms of dehydration cannot be distinguished from other common causes of acute diarrhea.
- Stool culture using proper media is positive for *Vibrio cholerae* O1 or O139; darkfield microscopy of a fresh stool sample may detect the presence of vibrios, specific antiserum confirms the serogroup.

active state occurs when conditions are suitable again for division. Humans are infected by drinking or eating contaminated water, beverages, or food. During epidemics a single source can be identified, but usually multiple routes of transmission play a role simultaneously. Epidemics tend to occur during the warmest months of the year, and association with climate variability and El Niño southern oscillation has been recently documented.

V. cholerae O1 and O139 secrete a number of potent exotoxins that induce the characteristic isotonic dehydration of cholera. The cholera toxin, which has subunits A and B, is better studied. The B subunit allows the toxin to attach to a specific receptor present along the small intestine of humans, and the A subunit activates the adenylate cyclase enzyme. The chain of events that follows this enzymatic activation are mediated by cyclic adenosine monophosphate (cAMP) and include blocking sodium and chloride absorption by the microvillus and promoting secretion of chloride and water by crypt cells. Table 1 illustrates the resulting massive liberation of water and electrolytes into the intestinal lumen.

Treatment

The objectives of therapy are to replace the fluid and electrolyte losses caused by diarrhea and vomiting, maintain hydration, and reduce the volume of diarrhea and excretion of vibrios to the environment. The treatment is divided into two phases, rehydration and maintenance. The rehydration phase has the objective to replace the losses that ensued before admitting the patient. This phase begins with a thorough evaluation of the degree of dehydration. Table 2 shows the clinical signs according to the degree of dehydration. Patients with severe dehydration present a constellation of signs that reflect a deficit of at least 10% of body weight. The pulse is feeble and rapid, blood pressure is not recordable, skin

TABLE 1 Electrolyte Concentration of Cholera Stools and Rehydration Solutions Recommended for Treatment
Electrolyte and Glucose Concentration (mmol/L)

	Sodium	Chloride	Potassium	Bicarbonate	Osmolality
Cholera stool					
Adults	130	100	20	44	
Children	100	90	33	30	
Intravenous solutions					
Lactated Ringer's*	130	109	4	28	271
Normal saline	154	154	0	0	308
WHO ORS (reduced osmolality)†	75	65	20	10	245
Rice-based ORS	75	65	20	10	180

*Lactated Ringer's does not contain HCO_3 but instead lactate.
†Bicarbonate is replaced with trisodium citrate which persists longer than bicarbonate in sachets.
Abbreviations: ORS = oral rehydration solution; WHO = World Health Organization.

elasticity is lost, eyes are sunken, and the voice is not audible or hoarse. The intravenous route is recommended for all patients with severe dehydration. The rate and speed of the infusion are recommended at 50 to 100 mL/kg per hour for the first 2 to 4 hours. After this time, the

CURRENT THERAPY

- Identify the degree of dehydration on admission.
- Register the intake and output regularly in predesigned charts.
- Rehydrate the patients in two phases. The rehydration phase lasts 2 to 4 hours. The maintenance phase lasts until diarrhea abates.
- Use the intravenous route for patients with severe dehydration during the rehydration phase, who purge more than 10 to 20 mL/kg/hour, and who do not tolerate the oral route during the maintenance phase. The amount and speed of the intravenous infusion varies between 50 and 100 mL/kg/hour.
- Use the preferred intravenous solution, lactated Ringer's solution. Normal saline can be used, but recovery from acidosis is less efficient.
- Use the oral rehydration solution advised by the World Health Organization (WHO) during the maintenance phase for severely dehydrated patients and for milder forms of dehydration. The amount of oral fluids advised is 500 to 1000 mL/hour.
- Start antibiotics once the patient can tolerate the oral route. Single-dose, 300 mg of doxycycline (Vibramycin) is the preferred regimen, given with a light food.
- Start normal diet as soon as the patient tolerates the oral route.
- Discharge patients when all the following criteria are fulfilled: oral tolerance more than 600 to 800 mL/hour, stool output more than 400 mL/hour, urine output more than 30 to 40 mL/hour.

patient has to be fully rehydrated to begin the maintenance phase. The preferred intravenous solution is lactated Ringer's solution. If this solution is not available, normal saline may be used, but the recovery from metabolic acidosis is less efficient. An oral rehydration solution (ORS) should be started as soon a possible in these patients. Milder forms of dehydration caused by cholera can not be clinically distinguished from other common causes of acute diarrhea. Symptoms caused by some degree of dehydration are seen when water deficit is higher than 5% of body weight. The intravenous route may be used in these patients if the stool output is high (more than 10 to 20 mL/kg per hour) or if the patient does not tolerate the oral method. The great majority of patients with milder forms of dehydration can be rehydrated by the oral route. Laboratory abnormalities in patients with severe cholera reflect hemoconcentration and include a high hematocrit, increased white blood cell count, azotemia, and elevation in the specific gravity and total proteins. These laboratory parameters are good indicators of the degree of dehydration on admission but are not useful to follow the rehydration status. Metabolic acidosis with a high anion gap is typical in patients with severe cholera. Hypokalemia or normal values caused by acidosis, and normal- or low-serum sodium and chloride are also observed in these patients. Hyperglycemia results of high levels of epinephrine, glucagon, and cortisol stimulated by hypovolemia. Hypoglycemia is rare but carries a poor prognosis, particularly in children.

The maintenance phase begins when the patient has been fully rehydrated. A good indicator of the recovery of the normal hydration status is not only the absence of clinical signs of dehydration, but also the urine output. Urine output more than 0.5 mL/kg per hour is expected in a fully hydrated patient. The maintenance phase has the objective of keeping the normal hydration status and lasts until diarrhea abates. The oral route is advised for this phase, with an ORS recommended by the World Health Organization (WHO) as the preferred oral solution. More recently WHO has promoted the use of ORS with lower osmolality (75 mmol/L of sodium and total osmolality of 245 mOsm/L versus former presentation containing 90 mmol/L of sodium and total

TABLE 2 Clinical Findings According to Degree of Dehydration

	Some Dehydration	Severe Dehydration
Loss of fluid (% of body weight)	5%-10%	More than 10%
Mentation	Restless	Drowsy or comatose
Radial pulse		
Rate	Rapid	Very rapid
Intensity	Weak	Feeble or impalpable
Respirations	Normal or deep	Deep and rapid
Systolic blood pressure	Low	Very low or unrecordable
Skin elasticity	Retracts slowly	Retracts very slowly
Eyes	Sunken	Very sunken
Voice	Hoarse	Not audible
Urine production	Scant	Oliguria

osmolality of 311 mOsm/L) to treat all kinds of acute diarrheal diseases. Caution about observing hyponatremia in adults should be made with this reduced osmolality ORS. An ORS uses the principle of common transportation of solutes, electrolytes and water not affected by cholera in the intestine. An ORS containing rice instead of glucose is also preferred, because the purging rate is lower with a solution containing rice than with a glucose-based solution. If an ORS in packets is unavailable, a home preparation adding 2.6 g of sodium chloride, 2.9 g of sodium citrate, 1.5 g of potassium chloride, and 13.5 g of glucose or 50 g of rice powder to 1 L of boiled water can be made. The amount of oral fluids should match the ongoing losses to avoid dehydration during this phase. Periodic review of the patient's chart is advised for this purpose. Predesigned forms to register intake and output and vital signs should be available to monitor the hydration status regularly. Cholera cots or cholera chairs facilitate the collection and measurement of stools and urine during treatment. Discharging patients from the hospital is a critical issue, particularly when health centers are overloaded with patients with various degrees of dehydration. Patients can be safely discharged if all the following criteria are met:

- Oral intake between 600 and 800 mL per hour
- Urine output between 30 to 40 mL per hour
- Stool output lower than 400 mL per hour

Case fatality rates in centers with experience in the treatment of cholera are extremely low-approximately 0.14%.

An oral antibiotic is advised to reduce the volume of diarrhea, the requirement of intravenous fluids, and hospital stay. Antibiotics are not lifesaving and should not be offered if the patient cannot tolerate the oral route. A reduction in almost 50% of the volume and duration of diarrhea, and a reduction in the excretion of vibrios to 1 to 2 days have been documented with the use of effective antimicrobials. Single-dose regimens are preferred over multiple-dose regimens. A single 300-mg dose of doxycycline (Vibramycin), given with light food is the preferred regimen. Table 3 lists alternative regimens. More recently the quinolones have emerged as the best alternatives for resistant *V. cholerae* strains prevalent in Asia and Africa. Norfloxacin (Noroxin)[1] or ciprofloxacin (Cipro)[1] are the most extensively studied to date. Quinolones should not be used in children and pregnant women. Chemoprophylaxis with antimicrobials to prevent transmission of cholera is not recommended.

The most severe complication of cholera is acute renal failure. A careful evaluation of the medical charts of these patients disclosed improper replacement of fluids during the rehydration or maintenance phases. The nonoliguric form predominates. All age groups are affected, and the mortality rate is very high. The presentation of cholera in children is similar to adults. Certain features

---

[1]Not FDA approved for this indication.

TABLE 3 Antimicrobial Regimens for the Treatment of Cholera

Drug	Dose	
	Adult	Children
Tetracycline	500 mg qid × 3d	50 mg/kg of body weight qid × 3d
Doxycycline (Vibramycin)	300 mg as a single dose	Not evaluated
Erythromycin[1]	250 mg qid × 3d	30 mg/kg in 3 divided doses × 3d
Furazolidone (Furoxone)	100 mg qid × 3d	5 mg/kg of body weight per day qid × 3d, or 7 mg/kg, single dose
Cotrimoxazole (Bactrim)[1]	160 mg of trimethoprim/800 mg of sulfamethoxazole bid × 3d	8 mg of trimethoprim + 40 mg of sulfamethoxazole/kg divided in two doses × 3d
Norfloxacin (Noroxin)[1]	400 mg bid × 3d	Not recommended
Ciprofloxacin (Cipro)[1]	1 g single dose	Not recommended
	250 mg qd × 3d	Not recommended
	500 mg bid × 3d	Not recommended

[1]Not FDA approved for this indication.
Abbreviations: bid = twice daily; d = days; qd = daily; qid = four times daily; tid = three times daily.

are distinctive in children, however, such as the presence of fever, seizures, mental alteration, and hypoglycemia. Cholera in the elderly carries a bad prognosis. The common presence of co-morbid conditions, difficulties in evaluating the hydration status properly, and higher incidence of acute renal failure and pulmonary edema account for the higher mortality observed in this population. Cholera in pregnant women is associated with more severe illness and fetal losses.

REFERENCES

Carpenter CJ: The treatment of cholera: Clinical science at the bedside. J Infect Dis 1992;166:2-14.

Colwell RR: Global climate and infectious diseases: The cholera paradigm. Science 1996;274:2025-2031.

Khan WA, Bennish ML, Seas C, et al: Randomized controlled comparison of single-dose ciprofloxacin and doxycycline for cholera caused by *Vibrio cholerae* O1 or O139. Lancet 1996;348:296-300.

Rodó X, Pascual M, Fuchs G, Faruque ASG: ENSO and cholera: A nonstationary link related to climate change? Proc Natl Acad Sci USA 2002;99:12901-12906.

Sack DA, Sack RB, Nair GB, Siddique AK: Cholera. Lancet 2004;363: 223-233.

Seas C, Gotuzzo E: Cholera. In Mandell GL, Bennett JE, Dolin R (eds): Principles and Practice of Infectious Diseases. Philadelphia, Churchill Livingstone, 2000, pp 2266-2272.

Food-Borne Illness

Method of
Katherine Spooner, MD, and
Michael A. Polis, MD, MPH

Food-borne illness remains a significant cause of morbidity and mortality worldwide. More than 200 known diseases are transmitted through food, and the disease agents include bacteria, viruses, parasites, toxins, metals, and prions. These agents cause syndromes commonly manifested by the acute onset of gastrointestinal symptoms with or without systemic complications. In recent years, the impact of food-borne illness has gone beyond being a public health problem and become a broad perception of an unsafe food supply with economic repercussions. A notable economic impact of food safety was seen in the beef industry between the emergences of *Escherichia coli* O157:H7 and "mad cow disease" in the United Kingdom in the 1990s. The recent terrorist attacks and fear of bioterrorism have contributed to heightened concerns about food safety. This article reviews the syndromes and microbial pathogens commonly encountered.

The true incidence of food-borne syndromes is not known, because reported outbreaks greatly underestimate the impact of the problem. The Centers for Disease Control and Prevention (CDC) estimates that food-borne illness leads to approximately 75 million cases of diarrhea, up to 325,000 hospitalizations, and 5000 deaths annually.

In 1996 the CDC established an active surveillance program known as FoodNet, that monitors the prevalence of specific pathogens, including those recognized as recently emerging, such as *Cyclospora cayetanensis, Crytosporidium parvum, Campylobacter jejuni, E. coli* O157:H7, and *Listeria monocytogenes*. From this research, the estimated frequency of a variety of microbes has been reported (Table 1). It is thought that changes in the epidemiology and incidence of food-borne illness result from several factors, including increased travel, global distribution of foods, expansion of commercial food services, and an increased market for convenience foods.

In the evaluation of suspected food-borne illness, the following general guidelines should be used to establish an etiologic diagnosis and treatment plan:

• Define the clinical features of the illness, including incubation time, type of symptoms, and severity of disease.
• Define the epidemiology of the disease, including recent travel, the type of food ingested (including origin and method of preparation), the time of year, and the presence of similar symptoms in the patient's recent contacts.
• Attempt, when possible, to document the etiology by means of laboratory confirmation. This can be done by collecting appropriate specimens and performing cultures as well as assays for the presence of toxins.

The diagnosis of food-related illness should be entertained when a patient develops an acute gastrointestinal or neurologic illness and should be suspected strongly when two or more persons develop an acute illness after ingesting food from the same source within the previous 72 hours. The presentation and time course of the illness provide important clues about the pathogenesis and etiology. A summary of the common microbial agents that cause food-borne illness, their sources, and appropriate therapy appears in Table 2; and Table 3 provides a summary of common chemical agents that cause food poisoning.

Pathogenesis and Clinical Presentation

BACTERIAL AGENTS AND THEIR TOXINS

In a patient who develops nausea and vomiting within 1 to 6 hours of ingesting a food item, the major etiologic considerations are *Staphylococcus aureus* and *Bacillus cereus*. These are examples of enterotoxigenic organisms, a term referring to bacteria that cause disease by producing a toxin. The short incubation time for *S. aureus* and *B. cereus* food poisoning is a reflection of a preformed toxin that is present in the food before consumption. *S. aureus* contamination usually is caused by improper handling of food during preparation, whereas *B. cereus* most often is associated with reheating fried rice. Both toxins cause an acute, self-limited illness that generally lasts less than 12 hours.

In a patient who develops abdominal cramps and diarrhea within 8 to 16 hours after the ingestion of food,

TABLE 1 Incidence of Selected Common Infectious Causes of Food-Borne Illness

Disease or Agent in Order of Frequency	Estimated Total Cases Annually	Percentage of Food-Borne Transmission	Percentage of Hospitalizations*	Percentage of Deaths*
Norwalk-like virus (noroviruses)	23,000,000	40	33.0	7.0
Campylobacter species	2,453,926	80	17.0	5.0
Giardia lamblia	2,000,000	10	1.0	0.1
Salmonella, nontyphoidal	1,412,498	95	26.0	31.0
Shigella	448,240	20	2.0	0.8
Cryptosporidium parvum	300,000	10	0.3	0.4
Clostridium perfringens	248,000	100	0.1	0.4
Staphylococcal food poisoning	185,060	100	2.9	0.1
Yersinia enterolitica	96,368	90	1.8	0.1
Escherichia coli O157:H7	73,480	85	3.0	2.9
E. coli, non-O157 STEC	36,740	85	1.5	1.4
Bacillus cereus	27,360	100	0.0	0.0
Cyclospora cayetanensis	16,264	90	0.0	0.0
Listeria monocytogenes	2,518	99	3.8	27.6

*Expressed as a percentage of the number of hospitalizations and deaths caused by food-borne pathogens.
Abbreviation: STEC = Shiga toxin–producing *E. coli.*
Modified from Mead PS, Slutsker L, Dietz V, et al. Food related illness and death in the United States. Emerg Infect Dis 1999;5:607

2

the likely agent is also an enterotoxin. In this setting, the toxin probably is formed in vivo, as opposed to the preformed toxins produced by *S. aureus* and *B. cereus.* The most common pathogens are *Clostridium perfringens* and *B. cereus* (which produces both types of toxins), causing illness that tends to last longer than does illness related to preformed toxin. This type of illness occasionally is associated with nausea, vomiting, and, rarely, fever. The illness is self-limited, resolving within 24 hours, and treatment is solely supportive.

In a patient who presents with fever, abdominal cramps, and diarrhea 16 to 48 hours after the ingestion of contaminated food, the likely etiology is an enteroinvasive bacteria: microbial infection with tissue invasion. The major organisms to be considered in acute infectious colitis are *Salmonella, Shigella, C. jejuni, Vibrio parahaemolyticus,* and invasive *E. coli.* Fever and fecal leukocytes provide evidence of tissue invasion; bloody diarrhea is common with *Shigella, E. coli* O157:H7, and Shiga toxin–producing *E. coli* serogroups other than O157 (STEC); such invasion also may occur with *Salmonella, V. parahaemolyticus,* and *Yersinia enterocolitica. C. perfringens* type C has been associated with a severe hemorrhagic jejunitis and ileitis, a syndrome known as enteritis necroticans or pigbel. Symptoms from these invasive diarrheal illnesses generally last less than a week, but severe complications occasionally occur, including seizures and meningism associated with shigellosis and those discussed later in reference to *Campylobacter* and *E. coli* O157:H7.

Salmonella, which is discussed extensively in a separate article, *Salmonellosis,* generally is considered a disease associated with undercooked poultry and eggs. However, it recently has been implicated in an outbreak involving imported mangoes, underscoring the impact of increased reliance on imported foods. A multistate

outbreak involving 78 individuals from 13 states who developed salmonellosis from *Salmonella* serotype Newport (SN) was reported, and the outbreak involved 15 hospitalizations and two deaths. The source was traced to a single Brazilian farm where a hot water treatment to prevent importation of the Mediterranean fruit fly was the possible point of contamination.

Campylobacter recently has been appreciated as the most common bacterial cause of acute infectious colitis in adults and adolescents, although historically *Salmonella* has received more attention. *Campylobacter* is associated with meat and raw poultry, and in fact more poultry is contaminated with *Campylobacter* than with *Salmonella. Campylobacter* also can be identified in unpasteurized milk, and waterborne outbreaks have been reported. Guillain-Barré syndrome (GBS) is an acute flaccid paralysis associated with *Campylobacter,* with up to 30% of GBS patients demonstrating evidence of recent *Campylobacter* infection. An increasing concern with *Campylobacter* infections is the development of fluoroquinolone resistance, with a recent survey of retail poultry demonstrating resistance in up to 20% of isolates.

Outbreaks of *E. coli* O157:H7 have been associated with ground beef, contaminated water, unpasteurized milk and apple cider, sprouts, and lettuce. In 1997, 25 million pounds of ground beef was recalled by the U.S. Department of Agriculture (USDA) after an outbreak of *E. coli* O157:H7 in Colorado was associated with contaminated frozen hamburger patties. The U.S. Food and Drug Administration (FDA) published warnings about uncooked sprouts after outbreaks caused by radish sprouts occurred in Japan and the United States. Severe complications include the hemolytic uremic syndrome (HUS), which occurs in up to 4% of reported cases. *E. coli.* STEC causes a similar illness, including a propensity to cause HUS, but cases are not reported

TABLE 2 Microbial Causes of Food-Borne Illness: Common Syndromes and Therapy

Etiologic Agent	Associated Foods and Transmission	Clinical Syndrome	Therapy (Adult Dosages)
Viral Agents			
Norwalk-like viruses	Shellfish, fecally contaminated foods, airborne, contact with vomitus	Nausea, vomiting, watery diarrhea	Fluids, supportive care
Rotavirus, astrovirus	Same	Same	Same
Hepatitis A	Same	Flulike illness, vomiting, jaundice	Same
Bacterial Agents			
Campylobacter jejuni	Undercooked poultry, meat contaminated water	Vomiting, diarrhea (may be bloody), abdominal cramps, fever	Fluids, ciprofloxacin (Cipro) 500 mg PO bid × 3d or azithromycin (Zithromax)[1] 500 mg qd × 3d
Salmonella (nontyphoidal)	Undercooked poultry, eggs, contaminated fruits and vegetables, mangoes	Diarrhea (occasionally bloody), cramps, vomiting, fever; sometimes sepsis	Fluids, antibiotics not usually indicated. If sepsis or immunocompromised host, ciprofloxacin[1] 500 mg PO bid × 3d
Shigella	Fecally contaminated food	Fever, cramps, diarrhea	Fluids, ciprofloxacin 500 mg PO bid × 3d or TMP-SMZ (Septra) DS PO bid × 3d
Escherichia coli O157:H7 and STEC	Undercooked beef, unpasteurized milk/juice, raw fruits, vegetables (sprouts)	Diarrhea (often bloody), cramps, vomiting; rarely, fever	Fluids Antibiotics contraindicated
Yersinia enterolitica	Undercooked pork, unpasteurized milk	Fever, vomiting, cramps, diarrhea; sometimes pseudoappendicitis	Fluids, antibiotics if invasive disease; ciprofloxacin[1] 500 mg PO bid × 3d, TMP-SMZ DS[1] PO bid × 3d
Clostridium perfringens	Precooked meats, poultry, gravy	Nausea, cramps, watery diarrhea; rarely, fever	Fluids, supportive care
Staphylococci (food poisoning)	Improperly refrigerated meat or egg/mayonnaise products	Acute onset nausea and vomiting	Fluids, supportive care
Food-borne Streptococcus	Food contamination by infected handlers	Pharyngitis	PEN VK 500 mg PO BID × 10d, or azithromycin 500 mg PO × 5d
Bacillus cereus	Emetic toxin: Improperly refrigerated rice	Acute-onset nausea, vomiting	Fluids, supportive care
	Diarrheal toxin: Precooked meats, stews	Nausea, watery diarrhea, cramps	
Vibrio cholerae (non-O1/O139), Vibrio parahaemolyticus	Raw shellfish, seafood	Watery diarrhea	Fluids, severe cases: doxycycline (Vibramycin) 100 mg PO bid × 3d
E. coli, enterotoxigenic	Fecally contaminated food	Watery diarrhea, cramps, vomiting	Fluids, severe cases: ciprofloxacin 500 mg PO bid × 3d; TMP/SMZ DS PO bid × 3d
Vibrio vulnificus	Raw, undercooked shellfish	Sepsis in patients with liver disease	Doxycycline[1] 100 mg bid plus ceftazidime (Fortaz) 2 g q8h
Listeria monocytogenes	Unpasteurized milk, ready-to-eat meats, hot dogs, cheese	Fever, myalgias, nausea, diarrhea	
		Severe disease in immunosuppressed, elderly, and pregnant women	Fluids, ampicillin[1] 2 g IV q4-6h, or TMP-SMZ DS PO bid × 3d
Botulism (Clostridium botulinum)	Home-canned foods	Nausea, vomiting, diarrhea,	Supportive care Notification to state health department/CDC

TABLE 2 Microbial Causes of Food-Borne Illness: Common Syndromes and Therapy—cont'd

Etiologic Agent	Associated Foods and Transmission	Clinical Syndrome	Therapy (Adult Dosages)
Parasitic Agents			
Cryptosporidium parvum	Contaminated water, vegetables, fruits, unpasteurized milk	Cramping, watery diarrhea	Supportive care
Cyclospora cayetanensis	Imported berries, basil, lettuce, contaminated water	Prolonged diarrhea, fatigue, weight loss	TMP-SMZ DS[1] PO bid × 7d
Giardia lamblia	Contaminated water	Acute or chronic diarrhea, bloating, and flatulence	Metronidazole (Flagyl)[1] 250 mg PO tid × 5d
Toxoplasma gondii	Undercooked meats (pork, lamb), contact with cat feces	Generally asymptomatic except in pregnant women and immunocompromised persons	No treatment for asymptomatic disease; pyrimethamine (Daraprim) and sulfadiazine in immunocompromised persons

[1]Not FDA approved for this indication.
Abbreviations: bid = twice daily; d = days; h = hours; PO = by mouth; q = every; tid = three times per day; TMP-SMZ = trimethoprim-sulfamethoxazole; DS = double strength.
Adapted from Diagnosis and management of food-borne illnesses: A primer for physicians. MMWR Morb Mortal Wkly Rep 2001;50(RR02):1-69.

routinely because many clinical laboratories are unable to identify it. The incidence of STEC has been estimated to be between 20% and 50% of that of *E. coli* O157:H7.

The presentation of abdominal cramps and watery diarrhea within 16 to 72 hours after exposure to contaminated food suggests an enterotoxin-producing agent. This includes enterotoxigenic strains of *E. coli* (ETEC), *V. parahaemolyticus*, *Vibrio cholerae* (either non-O1/O139 or O1 in endemic locales), and occasionally *C. jejuni*, *Salmonella*, and *Shigella*. Occasionally vomiting and fever may occur, and in the majority of cases these illnesses resolve within 72 to 96 hours. Cholera has been described in outbreaks from contaminated Gulf Coast waters and contaminated imported coconut milk in Maryland, but up to 96% of cases are acquired abroad. The cornerstone to treating cholera and, in the developing world, reducing mortality is aggressive fluid replacement.

The appearance of nausea, vomiting, diarrhea, and progressive paralysis within 18 to 36 hours of food ingestion strongly suggests the diagnosis of food-borne botulism. Botulism is a syndrome that is caused by a neurotoxin produced by *Clostridium botulinum*. Although the current focus on botulism is that of a potential agent of bioterrorism, it is a rare but reported illness in the United States. In 2001, 169 cases of botulism were reported to the CDC. Among them, 33 were food-borne, 112 were infant botulism, and 23 were cases of wound botulism. Botulism is manifested by progressive neurologic symptoms of dry mouth, diplopia, dysphagia, and progressive weakness, with respiratory failure in severe cases. Nausea, vomiting, and diarrhea can occur in the initial stages of the illness, but once the neurologic symptoms predominate, constipation is a common feature. The incubation period of this illness usually ranges from 12 to 36 hours but can be as long as 8 days. Typically, the disease results from the ingestion of any of three distinct neurotoxins A, B, and E produced by

C. botulinum spores. The source is usually inadequately prepared home-processed or canned foods. In Alaska, for example, home-processed fish prepared in oils and spices and allowed to ferment in plastic bags has been associated with botulism. Infant botulism is a similar illness, but in these cases the toxin is produced in vivo after ingestion of the spores, with honey being the usual source. Botulism is a potentially fatal illness, with fatality rates estimated to be as high as 25%. Death usually is caused by rapidly progressive neuromuscular paralysis. All patients with suspected botulism should be hospitalized and should be considered for treatment with a trivalent antiserum available from the CDC. Medical care providers who suspect a diagnosis of botulism in a patient should call the state health department's emergency 24-hour telephone number immediately. State health departments should call 770-488-7100, the CDC Emergency Operations Center. Apart from the intravenous (IV) antiserum (botulism Ig [BIG-IV]), treatment is primarily supportive, including mechanical ventilation as indicated. Penicillin[1] has been used to eradicate *C. botulinum* in the gastrointestinal tract, but the clinical benefit is not known.

Several infectious diseases are transmitted by foods and present with symptoms that are not gastrointestinal or neurologic. Listeriosis, which is of increasing concern in the United States, can be caused by the ingestion of improperly pasteurized milk and cheese products, undercooked chicken, and non-reheated hot dogs containing *L. monocytogenes*. In late 2002, a multistate outbreak of 53 cases of listeriosis occurred in the northeastern United States, leading to eight deaths and three stillbirths or miscarriages. After the outbreak was traced to sliced turkey delicatessen meat, approximately 27 million pounds of fresh and frozen ready-to-eat turkey

[1]Not FDA approved for this indication.

TABLE 3 Chemical/Natural Toxin Causes of Food-Borne Illness: Common Syndromes and Therapy

Etiologic Agent	Associated Sources	Clinical Syndrome	Therapy
Seafood Toxins			
Ciguatera toxin	Large reef fish: barracuda, grouper, red snapper, amberjack, seabass	2-6h: nausea, vomiting abdominal pain; 3h: Paresthesias, pain, weakness, rare death; 2-5d: bradycardia, hypotension, T wave changes	Supportive care, atropine IV, mannitol in severe cases
Scombroid	Tuna, skipjack, mackerel, mahimahi, marlin	Histamine toxicity; flushing, rash, burning sensation in mouth and throat, urticaria	Antihistamines, supportive care
Paralytic shellfish poisoning	Scallops, mussels, clams cockles (Alaska, Pacific northwest, California, Maine)	Paresthesias, ataxia, dysphagia, weakness; respiratory paralysis in severe cases	Supportive care
Tetrodotoxin	Puffer fish	Paresthesias, vomiting, diarrhea, ascending paralysis, respiratory failure	Supportive care; possibly respiratory support
Heavy Metals			
Antimony	Metallic container	Vomiting, metallic taste	Supportive care
Arsenic	Contaminated food	Vomiting, colic, diarrhea	Gastric lavage
Cadmium	Seafood, grains, peanuts	Nausea, vomiting, myalgia, increased salivation	Supportive care
Copper	Metallic container	Nausea, blue or green vomitus	Supportive care
Mercury	Fish exposed to organic mercury; tuna	Numbness, weakness, spastic paralysis, impaired vision, blindness, coma; pregnant woman/fetus vulnerable	Supportive care
Thallium	Contaminated food	Nausea, vomiting, diarrhea, paresthesias, hair loss	Supportive care
Tin	Metallic container	Nausea, vomiting, diarrhea	Supportive care
Mushroom Poisoning			
Short incubation	Amanita, Inocybe, Clitocybe, Psilocybe, Coprinus, Panaeolus species	Vomiting, confusion, visual disturbance, salivation; Disulfiram-like reaction with Coprinus	Supportive case
Long incubation	Amanita phalloides	4-8h: diarrhea, abdominal cramps; 24-48h: hepatic and renal failure	Supportive care; possibly life support
	Gyromitra species	Nausea, vomiting, hemolysis, hepatic failure, seizures	Supportive care
	Corinarius species	Nausea, headache, renal failure	Supportive care

Abbreviations: d = days; h = hours; IV = intravenously.
Adapted from Diagnosis and management of food-borne illnesses: A primer for physicians. MMWR Morb Mortal Wkly Rep 2001;50(RR02):1-69.

and chicken products were recalled by the implicated processing plant in Pennsylvania. The disease occurs most often in the elderly, immunocompromised persons, and pregnant women. Listeriosis is a severe illness; the mortality rate is 20%, and recent FoodNet data suggest that 90% of reported patients are hospitalized.

Other illnesses that present with systemic syndromes include brucellosis (from *Brucella abortus* found in goat's milk cheese), anthrax (from *Bacillis anthracis* found in contaminated undercooked meat), a sepsis-like syndrome in patients with liver diseases caused by *Vibrio vulnificus* (raw oysters), hepatitis A (seafood, improperly prepared salads, imported green onions), trichinosis (from *Trichinella spiralis* found in contaminated pork), tularemia (from *Francisella tularensis* found in contaminated water from streams and wells and in contaminated meat), and Q fever (from *Coxiella burnetii* found in contaminated raw milk). Anthrax, tularemia, and Q fever are all considered potential agents of bioterrorism.

VIRAL AGENTS

If a patient presents with vomiting as a major symptom, viral agents must be considered. The Norwalk-like viruses, small round structured caliciviruses, are the most common causes of acute gastroenteritis in the

United States, with more than 9 million estimated cases per year. The incubation period is 24 to 48 hours, and recent outbreaks were identified readily when large numbers of individuals were infected from a common food source. The most renowned examples have been the recent outbreaks on cruise ships. Shellfish may harbor the noroviruses, but those viruses are readily transmitted by food handlers (either by the fecal-oral route or by vomitus) and also may be transmitted by an aerosol route. The illness, consisting primarily of vomiting but also including watery diarrhea and low-grade fever, lasts 48 to 72 hours and requires supportive care only. In outbreak settings, polymerase chain reaction (PCR) assay and electron microscopy have been useful in the identification of these viruses. Other enteric viruses associated with vomiting and watery diarrhea are rotavirus (causing up to 40,000 infections annually), astrovirus, and enteric adenovirus. Hepatitis A also causes vomiting but usually is associated with systemic symptoms, including jaundice. A recent outbreak of hepatitis A was reported in association with contaminated green onions.

PROTOZOAL AGENTS

In patients who present with chronic watery diarrhea, protozoal pathogens must be considered. *C. parvum* gained notoriety in the early 1990s after the water supply in Milwaukee was found to be contaminated and more than 400,000 individuals were affected. The organism is endemic in cattle, but outbreaks have been associated with water, fresh produce, unpasteurized milk, and person-to-person spread. The incubation period is 2 to 28 days. Cryptosporidiosis is associated with persistent chronic diarrhea in immunocompromised hosts, particularly HIV-infected individuals. There is no reliably effective therapy for this illness. Healthy individuals are susceptible as well; however, they tend to develop a self-limited disease. *C. cayetanensis* has been recognized as a pathogen in the United States only since 1996 after a well-publicized outbreak caused by contaminated raspberries from Guatemala; this is another emerging disease that highlights the impact of imported food supplies. More recently it has been associated with contaminated basil products. *Cyclospora* infection also results in a chronic watery diarrheal illness after an incubation period of 1 to 11 days but responds well to therapy with trimethoprim-sulfamethoxazole (Bactrim).[1]

Other parasitic agents that lead to food-borne illness include *Giardia lamblia* and *Toxoplasma gondii*. Giardiasis is associated with contaminated water and often results in significant watery diarrhea, bloating, and flatulence. Toxoplasmosis is associated with undercooked meats (pork, lamb) and is generally asymptomatic, although a mononucleosis-like syndrome can develop in up to 20% of individuals. Central nervous system (CNS) disease is seen in immunocompromised hosts, particularly those with AIDS, and fetal CNS disease can develop if a pregnant woman is infected.

SEAFOOD-RELATED TOXINS

Seafood ingestion also is associated with several types of food poisoning related to toxin ingestion. Ciguatera poisoning has a worldwide incidence that has been reported to be as high as 50,000 cases per year and is believed to be caused by a neurotoxin produced by marine dinoflagellates and algae. This neurotoxin is concentrated up the food chain in grouper, snapper, barracuda, jack, surgeon fish, and sea bass. The largest concentrations of contaminated fish are found in the Pacific, Caribbean, and Indian oceans during the spring and summer months. The onset of illness usually occurs a few hours after consumption of the implicated fish and presents with nausea, vomiting, abdominal pain, pruritus, perioral paresthesias, dizziness, and blurred vision. Rarely, it can lead to temporary blindness, paralysis, and death. The toxin can be present in affected fish without any apparent indication of contamination. The heat-stable toxins are not affected by cooking and processing and can persist for weeks. Treatment is supportive, although one can consider cholinesterase-reactivating drugs because the toxin appears to inhibit cholinesterase activity in red blood cells.

Scombroid poisoning is also toxin-mediated and is frequently misdiagnosed as a seafood allergy. Although it is recognized worldwide, most incidents are reported in the United States, Japan, and Great Britain. Illness is caused by eating fish that contain high levels of histamine, which is produced as a result of the decarboxylation of histidine. Although it initially was reported in association with fish of the Scombridae and Scomberesocidae families (tuna, mackerel, and bonito), other species, such as mahi-mahi, have been implicated. Flushing, pruritus, urticaria, headache, nausea, and, rarely, bronchospasm develop within 10 minutes to 2 hours of the ingestion of contaminated fish. This self-limited process typically resolves within 4 hours, although antihistamines and bronchodilators can be used for symptomatic relief.

Other seafood-related, toxin-mediated illnesses include paralytic and neurotoxic shellfish poisoning and puffer fish poisoning. Paralytic shellfish poisoning is caused by the ingestion of shellfish contaminated with marine dinoflagellates (the cause of "red tide") that contain saxitoxin. Mollusks feed on dinoflagellates, and contaminated species are in ambient waters at latitudes higher than 30 degrees. Most patients present with the onset of symptoms within 1 hour of food ingestion and develop paresthesias of the mouth, lips and face, and extremities. Rarely, patients develop severe complications, including dyspnea, dysphagia, weakness or paralysis, and respiratory failure. Treatment involves removal of remaining toxin from the gastrointestinal tract (cathartics, enemas), supportive care, and, rarely, mechanical ventilation.

Neurotoxic shellfish poisoning is similar to paralytic shellfish poisoning, but paralysis does not occur. Outbreaks in North America have been reported in association with the ingestion of oysters, clams, and mollusks. Puffer fish poisoning is seen primarily in Japan and is caused by tetrodotoxin. This toxin is found in puffer fish, porcupine fish, and ocean sunfish as well as

---

[1]Not FDA approved for this indication.

Rakel and Bope: *Conn's Current Therapy 2006*

some newts and salamanders and is associated with improper cleaning of fish. Tetrodotoxin is similar to saxitoxin and can cause a severe neuromuscular paralysis, including respiratory failure; it is associated with a mortality of up to 60%.

MUSHROOM POISONING

Ingestion of toxic mushrooms can lead to clinically distinct syndromes that vary with the type of mushroom ingested. At least six species of toxic mushrooms lead to illness within 2 hours of ingestion, and three species lead to an illness with an incubation up to 24 hours (see Table 3). Clinicians can contact the local poison control center for assistance in the identification and treatment of mushroom toxicity. Types of illnesses seen in the early presentations of poisoning include confusion, delirium (similar to alcohol intoxication), parasympathetic hyperactivity, acute psychotic behavior and hallucinations, a disulfiram-like reaction if alcohol is ingested, and gastrointestinal manifestations (nausea, vomiting, and abdominal cramps). With the exception of the illness associated with parasympathetic hypersensitivity, the symptoms are self-limited and require only supportive treatment. Mushrooms of the muscarine-containing varieties (*Clitocybe* and *Inocybe* species) produce an anticholinergic syndrome that presents as sweating, salivation, and bradycardia as well as other indications of parasympathetic hyperactivity. Rarely, this syndrome is fatal, and thus it should be treated with atropine sulfate, 1 to 2 mg every 2 to 6 hours, until the symptoms resolve (typically within 24 hours).

A patient who develops abdominal cramps and diarrhea within 6 to 24 hours of mushroom ingestion suggests a more serious mushroom intoxication that can lead to hepatorenal failure. The etiology is most commonly ingestion of amatoxin or phallotoxin, which produces a biphasic illness that accounts for 95% of cases of fatal mushroom poisoning. Initially, the patient presents with gastrointestinal symptoms (nausea, vomiting, abdominal cramps, and diarrhea) as well as fever in the first 6 to 12 hours after ingestion. These symptoms resolve within 24 hours, and then, after remaining well for up to 2 days, the patient becomes severely ill with renal and hepatic failure. Treatment consists of supportive intensive care, but mortality approaches 50% even with that care.

A similar syndrome also develops with the ingestion of *Gyromitra* species of mushrooms containing gyromitrin, which, after metabolism to methylhydrazine, inhibits pyridoxal phosphate. Initially the patient experiences gastrointestinal symptoms, which are followed by hepatic failure, hemolysis, methemoglobinuria, convulsions, and coma.

MISCELLANEOUS FOOD-RELATED ILLNESS

Ingestion of heavy metals, often through contaminated food or metallic containers, can cause a variety of syndromes, most often a self-limited gastrointestinal disease (see Table 3). Of particular interest recently has been the ingestion of mercury, which is found in some large fish species, including tuna. The primary concern with mercury toxicity involves pregnant women and the potential effect on a developing fetus's CNS and kidneys; thus, the FDA has recommended limiting the consumption of certain fish by pregnant women and young children.

Ingestion of alkaloids found in fungi that contaminate wheat and rye can lead to ergotism, which is characterized by severe vasoconstriction that can progress to ischemic necrosis of muscle. Ingestion of the mycotoxin aflatoxin, which is found in peanut butter, can lead to gastrointestinal bleeding and hepatic complications. Other mycotoxins known as trichothecenes can be found as contaminants of grains and can lead to gastrointestinal symptoms as well as anemia and leukopenia. Ingestion of the Italian fava bean can cause hemolytic anemia in patients with glucose-6-phosphate dehydrogenase deficiency. Ingestion of solanine, which is found in jimsonweed and in the milk of cows that ingest that weed, can cause a syndrome similar to atropine poisoning, with headache, confusion, abdominal pain, and diarrhea. Other toxin-related illnesses caused by ingestion of food items include oxalic acid poisoning (rhubarb leaves, beets, spinach, houseplants), lathyrism (progressive spastic paraplegia caused by ingestion of sweet peas of *Lathyrus* species), digitalis poisoning (home-brewed foxglove or oleander tea), and cyanide poisoning (seen, rarely, after ingestion of large amounts of seeds from apples, cherries, pears, peaches, cassava, and lima beans).

The "Chinese restaurant syndrome," which is caused by the ingestion of monosodium L-glutamate (MSG), causes a flushing and burning sensation of the face and chest, headache, and diaphoresis. Most commonly, this occurs after a person eats wonton soup as a first course, as the MSG is absorbed more rapidly on an empty stomach. The syndrome is self-limited and rarely requires treatment.

Prion disease has been of international interest in the last decade with the emergence of mad cow disease, or bovine spongiform encephalopathy (variant Creutzfeldt-Jakob disease [vCJD]). A discussion of vCJD is beyond the scope of this article, but it is an example of a rare pathogen that has had a profound economic and social impact and at one time led to the slaughter of more than 35 million cattle in the United Kingdom and heightened public fear about the safety of the food supply.

Diagnosis

Although the history and clinical presentation can lead to a presumptive diagnosis of food-related illness, confirmation requires laboratory evaluation. Appropriate specimens to evaluate include blood, stool, vomitus, and the suspected contaminated food. Most often, however, no diagnosis is made because of the rapid resolution of symptoms with appropriate supportive care.

Stool cultures are helpful for the diagnosis of *Salmonella, Shigella, Campylobacter, Yersinia, V. cholerae* (types O1, O139 and non-O1), and *V. parahaemolyticus*. Gram stain of the stool is rarely helpful, but the presence of fecal leukocytes on stool examination is useful in establishing the diagnosis of an invasive organism

CURRENT DIAGNOSIS

- Evaluate blood, stool, vomitus, and the suspected contaminated food.
- Stool cultures help diagnose *Salmonella, Shigella, Campylobacter, Yersinia, Vibrio cholerae* (types O1/O139 and non-O1), and *Vibrio parahaemolyticus.*
- Toxin assays can identify several etiologies of food poisoning (e.g., *Clostridium botulinum, Escherichia coli* O15:H7, *Staphylococcus aureus*), fish and shellfish poisoning, and mushroom poisoning.

(*Salmonella, Shigella*, invasive *E. coli*). In outbreaks of staphylococcal poisoning, the organism can be isolated from stool and vomitus, as well as the suspected food item. *B. cereus* also can be isolated from feces but has been reported on occasion as flora in healthy patients, and so confirmation by serotyping may be useful. *C. perfringens* is seen frequently in the normal flora of healthy patients, and so stool culture is helpful only if a colony count of more than 10^6 *C. perfringens* spores per gram of feces is found. Confirmation of this illness can be made by isolating the organism in the suspected food.

C. parvum can be identified by acid-fast staining of the stool as well as by stool antigen immunoassay. *C. cayetanensis* is identified by a modified acid-fast stain of the stool. Electron microscopy of the stool plays a role in identifying some viruses (e.g., Norwalk agent) but is not routinely available. PCR is also useful in outbreaks of viral agents. Serology is used to identify hepatitis A and toxoplasmosis.

Toxin assays are important for identifying several etiologies of food poisoning. These assays are most helpful for *C. botulinum, E. coli* O15:H7, *S. aureus*, fish and shellfish poisoning, and mushroom poisoning. Most of these assays require the use of a reference laboratory. Scombroid poisoning can be documented by the presence of histamine in the suspected fish (100 mg of histamine in 100 g of fish confirms the diagnosis). Ciguatera usually is diagnosed on the clinical picture alone. Assays demonstrating the toxin in suspected fish have been developed but are not commonly available. The clinician can contact local public health authorities for more specialized assays. Despite an extensive evaluation, one can expect to find the etiology of food-related illness in less than 50% of cases.

Treatment

Although specific therapy occasionally is indicated, the mainstay of treatment of food-borne illness is supportive. Most of the syndromes discussed here are self-limited in nature but may require extensive fluid replacement. In severe cases of toxin-mediated disease, the patients also should be monitored closely for changes in vital signs and neurologic symptoms. As was noted previously,

local health departments and poison control centers should be contacted for severe toxin-mediated illnesses, and the CDC should be contacted in cases of suspected botulism.

Fluid replacement can be either oral or parenteral, depending on the patient's clinical status. The degree of dehydration can be assessed by the patient's vital signs as well as examination of mucous membranes and skin turgor. If oral hydration is chosen as the route of replacement, the patient must be advised to take a fluid with adequate sodium and carbohydrate content. Acceptable fluids include Rehydrate, Ricelyte, and the World Health Organization (WHO) oral rehydration formula or another replacement formula containing 3.5 g NaCl, 1.5 g KCl, 2.5 g NaHCO$_3$, and 20 g glucose in 1 L of boiled water. Clear liquids such as Gatorade are less appropriate because the sodium content is lower. In severe cases, rapid infusion of intravenous fluids such as normal saline is necessary.

Symptomatically the patient can be treated for nausea and vomiting with antiemetics such as prochlorperazine (Compazine), 5 to 10 mg orally or 25 mg by rectal suppository. Symptomatic relief of diarrhea should be used in patients with mild, nondysentery gastroenteritis but should be avoided in those with toxin-related illness and severe invasive diarrhea. An appropriate agent is loperamide hydrochloride (Imodium), 4 mg followed by 2 mg after each episode of diarrhea, to a maximum of 16 mg daily.

The role of antibiotics has not been clarified in the treatment of most causes of invasive diarrhea, but antibiotics should be included in the treatment of shigellosis, cholera, and typhoid. Studies have shown that antibiotics may decrease the duration of microbial carriage but generally do not affect the clinical course. Antimicrobials are of no known benefit in the treatment of illness caused by staphylococcal, *C. perfringens*, or *B. cereus* food poisoning and are likely to have minimal to no benefit in the treatment of food poisoning caused by *V. parahaemolyticus*,

CURRENT THERAPY

- Treat dehydration with either oral or parenteral fluid replacement, depending on the patient's clinical status.
- In severe cases, rapid infusion of IV fluids is necessary.
- Treat nausea and vomiting with antiemetics.
- For patients with mild, nondysentery gastroenteritis, symptomatic relief of diarrhea can be used; avoid in toxin-related illness and severe invasive diarrhea.
- Use antibiotics to treat shigellosis, cholera, and typhoid.
- Contact local health departments and poison control centers for severe toxin-mediated illnesses; contact the CDC for cases of suspected botulism.

E. coli, and *Y. enterolitica*. Of note, antibiotics are contraindicated in patients with *E. coli* O157:H7 disease.

Treatment for traveler's diarrhea should start with counseling before travel, and clinicians can refer to the CDC Web site under Traveler's Health for guidance (www.cdc.gov/travel/). Recommendations from the CDC include ways to avoid contaminated food and water and location-specific vaccination requirements. The issue of chemoprophylaxis for travelers is controversial; the use of antimicrobial agents will decrease the incidence of diarrhea but is associated with a significant incidence of side effects and potentially increased microbial resistance. Antidiarrheal agents such as loperamide hydrochloride (Imodium) are useful in decreasing the symptoms of traveler's diarrhea (defined as >3 loose stools daily) but are contraindicated in patients with evidence of invasive disease (fever and bloody stools). In the setting of invasive disease, effective antibiotics are indicated and may shorten the course of illness from the typical 3 to 5 days to 1 to 1.5 days. The antibiotic regimen most likely to be effective is ciprofloxacin (Cipro) (500 mg twice daily for three days); ofloxacin (Floxin)[1] and levofloxacin (Levaquin)[1] are considered equally effective. The effectiveness of antibiotic therapy depends on the etiologic agent and its antibiotic sensitivity, and clinicians should keep in mind the global increase in antibacterial resistance. The most prominent example of this is the fluoroquinolone resistance of *Campylobacter* in Southeast Asia, and travelers to that region should be provided with azithromycin (Zithromax)[1] (500 mg daily for 3 days). Travelers should be advised to consult a physician rather than attempt self-medication if the diarrhea is severe or does not resolve within several days, if fever occurs with shaking chills, or if there is dehydration with persistent diarrhea.

REFERENCES

Diagnosis and management of foodborne illness: A primer for physicians. MMWR Morb Mortal Wkly Rep 2004;53(RR04):1-33.

Guerrant RL, Van Gilder T, Steiner TS, et al. Practice guidelines for the management of infectious diarrhea. Clin Infect Dis 2001;32: 331-351.

Kaferstein FK, Motarjemi Y, Bettcher DW. Foodborne disease control: A transnational challenge. Emerg Infect Dis 1997;3(4):503-510.

Lasky T. Foodborne illness-old problem, new relevance. Epidemiology 2002;13(5):593-598.

Mead PS, Slutsker L, Dietz V, et al. Food-related illness and death in the United States. Emerg Infect Dis 1999;5(5):607-625.

Olsen SJ, MacKinnon LC, Goulding JS, et al. Surveillance for foodborne-disease outbreaks—United States, 1993-1997. MMWR Surveill Summ 2000;49(1):1-62.

_____

[1]Not FDA approved for this indication.

Necrotizing Skin and Soft Tissue Infections

Method of
Sharon M. Henry, MD, FACS, and
Thomas M. Scalea, MD, FACS

Although uncommon, necrotizing soft tissue infections are not rare. Initial symptoms are often nonspecific and may be confused with less invasive soft tissue infection. Undertreated, non-necrotizing infection can develop into necrotizing infection.

Table 1 lists the many synonyms used to describe necrotizing soft tissue infection. The term *necrotizing fasciitis,* coined by Wilson in 1952 to describe infection that involved subcutaneous fat and superficial fascia, is used here to simplify the discussion. Regardless of the name used, treatment principles remain the same. Early diagnosis is paramount. Treatment involves wide surgical débridement, antibiotics, and other adjunctive measures. Mortality rates vary but are quite significant, ranging from 6% to 76%.

Pathophysiology

Necrotizing fasciitis is a deep soft tissue infection that typically involves the subcutaneous fat and superficial and/or deep fascia. Usually there is necrosis of the subcutaneous fat and superficial fascia accompanied by inflammation of the dermis. Muscle may also be involved, although it is usually spared. Typically, there is intense polymorphonuclear infiltration in the subcutaneous tissue and fascia. Microabscess formation and vascular thrombosis in the subcutaneous tissue layer often occurs.

TABLE 1 Terms to Describe Necrotizing Soft Tissue Infections

Hospital gangrene	Described by Joseph Jowes, a Confederate Army surgeon, rapidly progressive fascial necrosis caused by bacteria
Necrotizing erysipelas	
Hemolytic streptococcal gangrene	
Necrotizing fasciitis	Described by Wilson, 1952
Acute dermal gangrene	Described by Brewer and Meleney, 1926
Synergistic gangrene	Occurs after injury presenting with erythema, swelling, violaceous zone, and central necrotic zone
Clostridial gangrene	
Synergistic necrotizing cellulitis	

CURRENT DIAGNOSIS

- Possible diagnosis in patients with cellulitis and shock
- Physical examination:
    Tense edema
    Severe erythema
    Purple skin discoloration or necrosis
    Bullae
    Crepitus
- Co-morbid conditions:
    Diabetes mellitus
    Intravenous drug abuse
    Alcohol abuse
    Immunosuppression
- Cellulitis not responding to appropriate antibiotics within appropriate time frame
- Rapid progression

A loss of tissue plane integrity may be the most significant finding in cases that are treated earliest. The bacteria produce enzymes that allow spread along fascial planes.

Clinical Findings

Erythema, warmth, and swelling are the earliest signs of necrotizing fasciitis. These symptoms are woefully non-specific (Box 1). Initially, there is often induration of the subcutaneous tissue and skin with exquisite tenderness. As the process progresses, blisters and bullae develop. Later, discoloration of the skin occurs and crepitus may appear.

Physical findings most specific for necrotizing fasciitis are tense edema, crepitus, bullae, and necrosis. Initially, these findings are absent 20% of the time. The overlying skin, in fact, may be relatively normal. In patients at risk, clinicians must maintain a high level of suspicion.

Any anatomic location may be involved (Table 2). This infection can be rapidly progressive. These patients are often toxic and develop hypotension and respiratory failure early. They often progress to multiple organ failure and death. Early diagnosis is mandatory, but the nonspecific signs and symptoms can make differentiation from less invasive infections difficult (Box 2).

TABLE 2 Sites, Sources, and Signs of Necrotizing Fasciitis

Sites	%
Lower extremity	32%
Upper extremity	24%
Perineum	16%
Trunk	16%
Head and neck	10%

Etiological Source
Insect bites
Skin ulcers
Tooth abscess
Abrasions
Gunshot wounds
Blunt trauma

Bacteriology	
Single pathogen	29%
Polymicrobial	71%
Cultures +	73%

Signs of Deep Infection — any 3 of the following
Confusion
Shock
Marked local pain
Pitting edema
Cyanosis of skin
Necrosis

Laboratory values may be nonspecific. A small series evaluated basic laboratory data to determine if a value could distinguish non-necrotizing from necrotizing infection. Hyponatremia and leukocytosis were present more commonly in patients with necrotizing infections. Specifically, a serum sodium of less than 135 mmol/L or white blood cell count (WBC) greater than 15,400, or both, identified patients with necrotizing infections with sensitivity of 90% and specificity of 76%.

The group from Singapore Hospital designed a laboratory risk score for necrotizing fasciitis to aid in early detection (Table 3). The score is based on C-reactive protein, WBC, hemoglobin level, sodium, creatinine, and glucose. A score less than 5 has a negative predictive value of 96%. A score of more than 8 has a positive predictive value of 93%. The study is based on a retrospective analysis and requires prospective validation.

An inciting event can often be identified. Insect bites, minor traumatic wounds, surgical wounds, injection sites (illicit or medicinal), hematomas, tooth abscesses, and pharyngitis may be the portal of entry for bacteria.

BOX 1 Clinical Signs and Symptoms of Necrotizing Fasciitis

- Pain
- Erythema
- Skin necrosis and hemorrhage bullae
- Edema
- Crepitus
- Systemic toxicity
- Decreased sensation
- Crepitus, blistering, and radiographic air: 85%
- Sensitivity

BOX 2 Differential Diagnosis of Necrotizing Fasciitis

- Cellulitis
- Deep-seated abscess
- Compartment syndrome
- Rhabdomyolysis
- Deep vein thrombosis
- Myositis

TABLE 3 Laboratory Risk Indicator for Necrotizing Fasciitis Score

Variable (U)	Score
C-reactive protein (mg/dL)	
<15	0
>15	4
White blood cell count (cells/mm^3)	
<15	0
15-25	1
>25	2
Hemoglobin (g/dL)	
>13.5	0
11-13.5	1
<11	2
Creatinine (mg/dL)	
<1.59	0
>1.59	2
Glucose (mg/dL)	
<180	0
>180	1

BOX 3 Medical Diseases Associated with Necrotizing Fasciitis

- Diabetes mellitus
- Preexisting skin lesion
  - Dermatitis
  - Decubitus ulcers
  - Diabetic ulcers
  - Vascular ulcers
  - Injection sites
  - Simple abscess
  - Traumatic wounds
  - Insect bites
- Hepatic cirrhosis
- Alcoholism
- Illicit drug use
- Immune compromise
- Obesity
- Malnutrition
- Peripheral vascular disease
- Surgical sites

An inciting event cannot be identified in as many as 20% of patients, however. In addition, an undertreated non-necrotizing infection can develop into necrotizing fasciitis. Patient factors may influence the development. Diabetics seem to be quite susceptible. Many other risk factors are associated (Box 3).

Radiography

Radiographic studies can support the diagnosis, but no study can exclude the diagnosis. Identifying fluid collections or areas of air helps verify the diagnosis when doubt exists. Studies that fail to demonstrate these findings should not override clinical suspicion. Subcutaneous gas on plain films virtually assures the diagnosis, but its absence does not exclude the diagnosis. Ultrasonography is more sensitive in diagnosing subcutaneous air and fluid collections. Often, only diffuse edema is seen, which neither confirms nor refutes the diagnosis. Computerized tomography and magnetic resonance imaging can delineate the extent of disease and more sensitively identify air and fluid, but radiographic findings should not supersede clinical judgment.

Bacteriology

Necrotizing fasciitis is often polymicrobial. Two types exist. Type I is associated with culture of multiple organisms, occurring in approximately 85% of patients with positive cultures. Gram-negative bacteria commonly cultured include *Escherichia coli*, *Proteus mirabilis*, *Klebsiella pneumoniae*, and *Pseudomonas*. Anaerobes are often present in polymicrobial infections (*Bacteroides* and clostridia), as well as non–group A streptococcal species. *Staphylococcus aureus* may be seen alone or in combination with other organisms. Enterococcus is frequently isolated. Type II necrotizing fasciitis is seen when group A streptococcus is isolated as a single organism or in combination with staphylococcus.

Given this wide spectrum of potential pathogens, initial antibiotic therapy must be broad spectrum and should cover anaerobes as well as gram-negative and gram-positive organisms. Antibiotic therapy can be tailored once culture results are available. Particular suspicion for group A streptococcus mandates the addition of clindamycin (Cleocin), 600 to 900 mg every 6 to 8 hours. Clindamycin neutralizes exotoxin and is administered in addition to penicillin; extended-spectrum penicillins are also an excellent initial choice.

Patients with community-acquired infections can usually be managed with ampicillin/clavulanic acid (Unasyn), 3 g every 6 hours. Patients exposed to antibiotics or who may have more resistant organisms should receive piperacillin/tazobactam (Zosyn), 3.375 to 4.5 g every 6 hours. Individuals with a penicillin allergy should receive a combination of clindamycin and a fluoroquinolone or aminoglycoside. Vancomycin (1 g every 8 hours) should be started in patients who are known to have methicillin S. *aureus* and have normal renal function.

If the clinical history includes saltwater exposure, *Vibrio vulnificus* (photobacterium) infection should be considered. This organism can be especially virulent in diabetics and cirrhotics. Fourth-generation cephalosporins, Ceftazidime, 1 to 3 g intravenously every 8 to 12 hours, or Cefepime, 0.5 to 2.0 g intravenously every 12 hours, combined with doxycycline, should be used. In the case of freshwater exposure, *Aeromonas hydrophila* should be considered. Piperacillin/tazobactam, Cefepime, and fluoroquinolones can be used.

Surgical Therapy

Surgical treatment should begin as soon as the patient is adequately resuscitated. No other therapy should take precedence. Outcome is directly related to the timeliness and adequacy of the surgical intervention.

CURRENT THERAPY

- Timely operative intervention is the cornerstone of therapy.
- Broad-spectrum antibiotics should cover gram-negative, gram-positive, and anaerobic bacteria tailored to cultures later.
- Hyperbaric oxygen is adjunctive.

In many patients, a definitive diagnosis cannot be made despite multiple diagnostic tests. In this instance, surgical exploration is performed. The diagnosis may be obvious when the soft tissue, fascia, or muscle is directly visualized. Tissue biopsy may be obtained to help make the diagnosis when the diagnosis is not clear.

Dèbridement may result in loss of significant amounts of skin and soft tissues. These large defects often cannot be closed primarily and require grafting or healing by secondary intention. With extremity involvement, amputation may be required when muscle and soft tissue are extensively involved or when the patient is in a dire clinical condition. This is more likely to be required with infections because of clostridia or group A streptococcus. Repeat exploration is usually required to assure adequate dèbridement is accomplished.

Hyperbaric Oxygen

Hyperbaric oxygen is an adjunctive therapy. Its role is best supported in necrotizing infection because of clostridia. Bacterial killing is improved, and toxins are neutralized with hyperbaric oxygen. The role in the treatment of necrotizing fasciitis of other etiologies is less supported. Data suggest there may be a survival advantage when used for these indications as well. Hyperbaric oxygen has some role in modulating cytokine response to infection. It decreases tumor necrosis factor expression. If it is available and can be administered safely, it should be used.

Necrotizing fasciitis is a serious infection that requires prompt identification. Once the diagnosis is established and resuscitation accomplished, surgical exploration and wide dèbridement should be performed. The patient should receive empirical antibiotic therapy. Antibiotics are then tailored to operative culture findings once available. Repeated operative treatments may be required. If available, hyperbaric oxygen therapy should be offered.

REFERENCES

Andreasen TJ, Green SD, Childers BJ: Massive infectious soft-tissue injury: Diagnosis and management of necrotizing fasciitis and purpura fulminans. Plast Reconstr Surg 2001;107(4):1025-1034.
Chapnick EK, Abter EI: Necrotizing soft tissue infections. Infect Dis Clin North Am 1996;10(4):835-855.
Elliott DC, Kufera JA, Myers RA: Necrotizing soft tissue infections: Risk factors for mortality and strategies for management. Ann Surg 1996;224(5):672-683.
File T: Necrotizing soft tissue infections. Curr Infect Dis Reports 2003;5:407-415.
McHenry CR, Piotrowski JJ, Petrinic D, Malangoni MA: Determinants of mortality for necrotizing soft tissue infections. Ann Surg 1995;221(5):558-563.
Morgan MS, Lytle J, Bryson PJV: The place of hyperbaric oxygen in the treatment of gas gangrene. Br J Hospital Med 1995;53:424-426.
Stevens DL: Necrotizing soft tissue infections. Curr Treat Options Infect Dis 2000;2:359-368.
Wall DB, Klein SR, Black S, de Virgilio C: A simple model to help distinguish necrotizing fasciitis from nonnecrotizing soft tissue infection. J Am Coll Surg 2000;191(3):227-231.
Wilson B: Necrotizing fasciitis. Am Surg 1952;18:416.
Wong CH, Khin LW, Heng KS, et al: The LRINEC (Laboratory Risk Indicator for Necrotizing Fasciitis) score: A tool for distinguishing necrotizing fasciitis from other soft tissue infections. Crit Care Med 2004; 32(7):1535-1541.
Wu WC, Scannell C, Lieber M, Huang M: Hyperbaric oxygen therapy: Current status in the management of severe non-clostridial necrotizing soft tissue infections. Curr Opin Infect Dis 2001;3:217-225.

Toxic Shock Syndrome

Method of
Robert L. Deresiewicz, MD

Staphylococcal toxic shock syndrome (TSS) is an acute, severe, febrile illness characterized by fever, hypotension, rash, multiorgan dysfunction, and convalescent-stage desquamation. It results from intoxication by any of several related *Staphylococcus aureus* exotoxins, most commonly TSS toxin type-1 (TSST-1). A related and clinically indistinguishable illness, toxic shock–like syndrome (TSLS), may follow infection by toxigenic strains of *Streptococcus pyogenes*.

TSS was first described in a pediatric population but became widely known in 1980 following a large outbreak among young, menstruating women, the overwhelming majority of whom were tampon users. Menstrual cases presently account for about half of TSS cases reported in the United States. The remainder are attributable to staphylococcal colonization or infection of diverse body sites, and occur in patients of either gender and at any age. With prompt recognition and proper management the outcome is usually good; the principal challenge, as with many rare and severe diseases, is to recognize the illness and promptly intervene.

Etiology and Pathogenesis

Virtually all menstrual TSS cases and about 60% of nonmenstrual cases are caused by TSST-1. Most of the remainder are caused by staphylococcal enterotoxin B (SEB) and a small fraction by enterotoxin C. Coagulase-negative staphylococci do not produce TSS toxins and, therefore, cannot cause TSS. The TSS toxins are encoded by variable genetic elements, meaning that the genetic capability to produce one or more of the toxins is present in only a subset of strains. Approximately 10% to 20% of human *S. aureus* isolates produce TSST-1 and 7% to 14% produce SEB.

Necessary steps in the pathogenesis of TSS are colonization of a nonimmune host by a toxigenic strain, toxin production, toxin absorption, and intoxication. Approximately 4% to 10% of people harbor toxigenic staphylococci at any site at any given time, including approximately 1% to 4% of postmenarcheal women who carry TSST-1–producing staphylococci in the vagina. Most people acquire protective levels of antibodies to TSST-1 and SEB during youth and adolescence, presumably consequent to benign staphylococcal colonization or trivial infection. By adulthood, more than 90% of people are immune to each toxin.

Toxigenic staphylococci that have the genetic capability to produce a TSS toxin actually do so only at limited times. The risk of TSS associated with the use of tampons or certain surgical dressings likely results from changes that these products cause to the local microenvironment, and the stimulus to toxin production resulting therefrom. For example, tampon use introduces oxygen into the normally anaerobic vagina; oxygen is required for TSST-1 synthesis, at least in vitro. Once produced, TSST-1 is rapidly transported across the vaginal mucosa.

The TSS toxins are superantigens—V{ΣB}β{/ΣB}-restricted T-cell mitogens—whose toxicity to humans is thought to derive from their ability to stimulate certain immune cells and thereby provoke exuberant, dysregulated cytokine release. How cytokine release culminates in the various manifestations of TSS remains uncertain. An important sequela, however, is the development of capillary leak syndrome, which may be principally responsible for the hypotension and end-organ damage that occurs in TSS.

Epidemiology

TSS is principally a disease of the first three decades of life. As noted, cases may be classified as menstrual or nonmenstrual. Menstrual cases peak in incidence between the third and fifth days of menses. The vast majority are in tampon users. Nonmenstrual cases include those related to colonization or infection of the female genitourinary tract (e.g., puerperal cases and cases associated with barrier contraceptive use, septic abortion, and nonobstetric gynecologic surgery); those associated with skin or soft-tissue infections (including both primary staphylococcal infections such as folliculitis, cellulitis, and furunculosis, and secondary infections such as of burns, bites, varicella lesions, or surgical wounds); and those related to infections of the respiratory tract (e.g., staphylococcal pharyngitis, tracheitis, sinusitis, or pneumonia) the musculoskeletal system (e.g., osteomyelitis, septic arthritis), or, rarely, the bloodstream. In postoperative cases, the illness may manifest within hours of the surgical procedure or may be delayed for days or weeks.

The number of TSS cases reported annually to the Centers for Disease Control and Prevention (CDC) has dropped considerably since the early 1980s. The drop is partly attributable to the development of safer tampons and tampon usage practices, but likely also reflects substantial under-reporting. The true frequency of menstrual TSS is probably at least 1 per 100,000 women per year, and is likely higher among women in their teens and early twenties. According to a recent study, the incidence of postoperative (nonmenstrual) TSS is 3 cases per 100,000 women.

Mortality also appears to have diminished over time. For the 10 years ended in 1996, the minimum case fatality rate for definite or probable menstrual cases reported to the CDC was 1.8%; for nonmenstrual cases the minimum rate was 5.5%.

Clinical Manifestations

Mild prodromal, flu-like symptoms occur in a minority of patients. The acute illness begins precipitously, with high fever, chills, headache, severe myalgias, muscle tenderness, abdominal pain, nausea, vomiting, and profuse watery diarrhea. Oral, conjunctival, and vaginal mucosal irritation also typically occurs. Orthostasis or hypotension and the characteristic macular erythroderma develop during the next 2 days. The erythroderma is usually generalized, often intense, and blanches with pressure. However, it may be locally distributed, mild, or fleeting; and it may be subtle, particularly in the presence of severe hypotension. On admission patients appear toxic, with hypotension, tachycardia, and oliguria. Examination may reveal conjunctival suffusion; tender, beefy-red oral or vaginal mucosa; and a strawberry tongue. Peripheral cyanosis and edema are common, as is diffuse abdominal tenderness. Rales may be present. The liver, spleen, and lymph nodes are usually unremarkable. Encephalopathy as evidenced by confusion, disorientation, agitation, or somnolence is also common, but the neurologic examination is typically nonfocal. The site of staphylococcal toxin production may be purulent or erythematous, or it may appear entirely benign. Laboratory studies reflect multiorgan dysfunction. Frequent findings include leukocytosis, thrombocytopenia, coagulopathy, azotemia, transaminitis, hypoalbuminemia, hypocalcemia, hypophosphatemia, and pyuria. Disseminated intravascular coagulation is not a common feature of TSS.

Like many other toxin-mediated diseases, TSS follows a fairly predictable course. The early manifestations of fever, erythroderma, gastrointestinal distress, and blood chemistry abnormalities resolve within the first few days of illness. In severe cases, hypotension may persist and may be complicated by myocardial dysfunction, pulmonary edema, rhabdomyolysis, hepatic damage, renal failure, or peripheral gangrene.

Desquamation is a late event in TSS. Superficial flaking of the skin on the trunk and extremities begins about a week into the illness. The characteristic full-thickness desquamation of the palms, soles, and digits follows in the second week and may continue for up to 1 month. Late sequelae of TSS include postfebrile telogen effluvium (reversible loss of the hair and nails), prolonged weakness or fatigue, memory loss, emotional changes, and impaired ability to concentrate. Fatalities typically occur within the first few days of illness, most commonly from refractory shock, respiratory failure, or cardiac arrhythmia.

Rakel and Bope: *Conn's Current Therapy 2006*

Although not included in the case definition of TSS, mild systemic intoxications by the TSS toxins probably occur. Such cases lack two or more criteria for TSS but have certain clinical or epidemiologic features suggestive of the diagnosis (e.g., erythroderma, severe gastrointestinal disturbance, and/or convalescent desquamation). The occurrence of such an illness during menses in a young tampon user should prompt a search for evidence of TSST-1 involvement, particularly if the illness is recurrent. Compatible findings include the isolation of TSST-1-producing *S. aureus* from the vagina, and the demonstration of a nonprotective titer of serum anti-TSST-1 antibodies. Although such findings do not prove that an illness was TSST-1-related (certainly most perimenstrual flu-like illness is not attributable to TSST-1), they should, nevertheless, prompt discontinuation of tampon use until seroconversion has been documented. An attempt to eradicate vaginal staphylococcal carriage in such circumstances is also reasonable.

Diagnosis

The diagnosis of TSS is made exclusively on clinical grounds (Table 1). A host of possibilities other than TSS should be considered in the patient acutely ill with fever, rash, and hypotension. These include severe group A streptococcal infections (scarlet fever, necrotizing fasciitis, streptococcal TSLS), Kawasaki disease (particularly in children younger than 4 years of age), staphylococcal scalded skin syndrome, Rocky Mountain spotted fever, leptospirosis, meningococcemia, exanthematous viral syndromes, and severe allergic drug reactions.

In menstrual TSS cases, particularly when a purulent vaginal discharge is present, the diagnosis may be readily apparent. The challenge is to recognize subtle cases including nonmenstrual cases and cases in which the rash is evanescent. A careful history with attention to past health, possible infectious exposures, travel, vocation, avocation, vaccination status, menstrual status, and medication usage often considerably narrows the diagnostic possibilities. Backdrops particularly suggestive of TSS include the menstruating or postpartum female, the female who uses barrier contraceptive methods, the postoperative patient, the patient with varicella-zoster infection, and the patient with chemical or thermal burns.

Laboratory evaluation should include a complete blood count and differential, serum electrolytes, calcium, phosphate, albumin levels, liver and renal function tests, creatine phosphokinase level, coagulation studies, and urinalysis. A chest radiograph and an electrocardiogram should also be obtained. In females, vaginal culture should be performed. Blood, urine, and respiratory tract cultures should also be obtained, as should cultures of all wounds, regardless of how benign they might appear. The laboratory should be instructed to speciate any staphylococci isolated from mucosal sites. *S. aureus* isolates (mucosal or otherwise) should be referred for TSST-1 testing, if possible.

Acute and convalescent sera should be tested for antibody to TSST-1, particularly in suspected menstrual cases. The absence initially of a protective titer to TSST-1

TABLE 1 Staphylococcal Toxic Shock Syndrome: Case Definition

Criteria	Definition
1. Fever	Temperature ≥38.9°C (102°F)
2. Rash	Diffuse macular erythroderma (sunburn rash)
3. Hypotension	Systolic blood pressure ≤90 mm Hg (adults) or <5th percentile for age (children younger than 16 years of age) Orthostatic hypotension (orthostatic drop in diastolic blood pressure ≥15 mm Hg, orthostatic dizziness, or orthostatic syncope)
4. Organ involvement (at least 3 of the defined organ systems)	**GI** (vomiting or diarrhea at onset of illness) **Muscular** (severe myalgias or serum creatine phosphokinase level at least twice the upper limit of normal) **Mucous membranes** (vaginal, oropharyngeal, or conjunctival hyperemia) **Renal** (blood urea nitrogen or creatinine at least twice the upper limit of normal, or pyuria [≥5 leukocytes per high-power field] in the absence of urinary tract infection) **Hepatic** (total serum bilirubin or transaminase level [alanine aminotransferase or aspartate aminotransferase] at least twice the upper limit of normal) **Hematologic** (thrombocytopenia [platelets ≤100,000 per μL]) **CNS** (disorientation or alteration in consciousness in the absence of focal neurologic signs at a time when fever and hypotension are absent)
5. Desquamation	1 to 2 weeks after onset of illness (typically of palms and soles)
6. Evidence against alternative diagnosis	If obtained, negative cultures of blood, throat, or cerebrospinal fluid*; absence of a rise in antibody titers to the agents of Rocky Mountain spotted fever, leptospirosis, or rubeola

*Blood cultures may be positive for *Staphylococcus aureus*.
Abbreviations: CNS = central nervous system; GI = gastrointestinal.
Adapted from Reingold AL, Hargrett NY, Shands KN, et al: Toxic shock syndrome surveillance in the United States, 1980 to 1981. Ann Intern Med 1982; 96(Part 2):875-880.

supports the clinical diagnosis of TSS, and seroconversion, if it occurs, confirms it. The majority of patients, however, do not seroconvert following TSS; such patients, particularly those whose illness occurred in the perimenstrual period, are at risk for recurrent disease.

Treatment

With prompt treatment, the serious consequences of TSS (organ failure, limb loss, death) can often be avoided. Treatment involves four components:

1. Decontamination of the site of toxin production
2. Administration of antistaphylococcal antibiotics
3. Fluid resuscitation
4. General supportive care

The nidus of toxin production should be carefully sought. If present, vaginal tampons or other types of foreign bodies should be removed. Purulent foci should be drained and débrided and cutaneous lesions copiously irrigated. Thorough lavage lowers the burden of organisms and potentially slows toxin accretion. For TSS occurring in the postoperative period, the surgical wound must be explored, even if it appears uninfected.

Antibiotic administration offers a second opportunity to interrupt intoxication. While β-lactamase-resistant semisynthetic penicillins or first-generation cephalosporins have historically been given for TSS, growing evidence suggests that clindamycin (Cleocin) is superior. Under conditions of saturating (stationary phase) growth, staphylococci produce only low levels of penicillin-binding proteins. Penicillin-binding proteins are the molecular targets of β-lactam antibiotics. beta lactams are, therefore, relatively ineffective against such cells. On the other hand, TSST-1 is essentially only produced under those saturating conditions. Organisms producing TSST-1 are likely to be relatively resistant to β lactams. In addition, β-lactam levels fluctuate widely during dosing, and may fall below the minimum inhibitory concentration for *S. aureus* toward the end of each dosing interval. Subinhibitory concentrations of β lactams may actually enhance TSST-1 production.

Clindamycin, on the other hand, is a protein synthesis inhibitor; its antistaphylococcal activity is independent of growth phase. Moreover, clindamycin potentially suppresses TSST-1 production in vitro, even at concentrations insufficient to inhibit staphylococcal growth. The great majority of *S. aureus* strains causing TSS, particularly menstrual TSS, remain susceptible to clindamycin (and to methicillin). I suggest clindamycin 900 mg intravenously every 8 hours for suspected cases of TSS. In the critically ill patient in whom clindamycin- or methicillin-resistant infection may be a concern, it is reasonable to co-administer vancomycin (Vancocin) 1 g intravenously every 12 hours until microbiologic data are available. If the diagnosis of TSS is initially uncertain, broader empiric coverage is prudent. Antibiotics should be administered for at least 10 days but can be given orally once the patient has stabilized.

Aggressive fluid resuscitation should be initiated to reverse hypotension and forestall end-organ damage.

Adult patients may require up to 10 liters of crystalloid for the first 24 hours to maintain adequate cardiac filling. The principal mechanism of hypotension in TSS is capillary leak syndrome. Fluid therapy is, therefore, typically complicated by massive weight gain and peripheral edema. Pressors and central hemodynamic monitoring may be useful in cases of refractory hypotension, particularly if oxygenation is impaired.

In addition to the specific interventions outlined above, intensive care should be provided. Metabolic abnormalities should be corrected, and potential complications should be diligently sought. A final therapeutic option, especially for refractory cases or cases associated with an undrainable purulent focus, is pooled human immunoglobulin.[1] All commercial preparations contain anti-TSST-1 at concentrations sufficient to generate protective titers after a single intravenous dose of 400 mg/kg. Evidence supporting this therapy in humans is strictly anecdotal, but the approach makes sense on theoretical grounds.

---

[1] Not FDA approved for this indication.

Influenza

Method of
Kenneth J. Smith, MD, FACP

Influenza occurs annually during winter months, producing an upper respiratory infection that can lead to complications with significant morbidity and mortality and causing an average of 36,000 deaths per year in the United States. Two viruses, influenza A and B, cause the typical influenza syndrome in humans. Changes in two viral surface glycoproteins, hemagglutinin (H) and neuraminidase (N), the main sites of immunologic recognition, lead to changes in population susceptibility to infection over time. Influenza A is prone to minor or major changes in either glycoprotein, whereas influenza B has only had minor changes in hemagglutinin described. Minor changes are termed *antigenic drift* and occur as often as yearly, leading to localized outbreaks of influenza. Major glycoprotein changes are called *antigenic shift* and occur at irregular intervals (9 to 50 years), leading to worldwide influenza outbreaks or pandemics.

Traditionally, influenza control effects have centered on illness prevention by vaccinating persons most susceptible to influenza complications in addition to health care workers. Antiviral medication use for prophylaxis and treatment had a relatively minor role, and tests were unavailable to assist clinicians in diagnosing influenza. More recently, vaccination is being recommended for lower risk groups, nasal vaccination and newer antiviral agents are available, and rapid influenza tests can now potentially assist decision making.

The Infectious Diseases

Clinical Manifestations

Clinical features of influenza are nonspecific but mainly respiratory. Onset is often abrupt—with fever, myalgia, and cough—but often resembles other upper or lower respiratory infections with nasal congestion, sore throat, fatigue, and malaise. In uncomplicated cases, fever and other symptoms are classically described as lasting approximately 3 days or longer with a convalescent period of 1 to 2 weeks. Recent antiviral trials show illness of 4 to 5 days median duration in placebo recipients, with 70% reaching full recovery within 9 days after illness onset. The most common physical findings besides fever are hyperemic, nonexudative nasal and pharyngeal mucosa and small, tender cervical nodes; chest findings are typically absent.

Influenza complications can occur in up to 10% or more of otherwise healthy persons and more frequently in high-risk groups (patients with cardiac, renal, or pulmonary disease, or with diabetes, hemoglobinopathy, or immunosuppression; nursing home or chronic care–facility residents; and person older than age 65 years). Common complications are sinusitis, otitis media, bronchitis, and pneumonia. Pneumonia causes most of influenza's morbidity and mortality and can be caused by the influenza virus itself, a bacterial superinfection (most commonly), or a mix of viral and bacterial pathogens. Primary influenza pneumonia is fortunately rare, because it is often fatal. As a viral illness, it does not respond to antibiotics and response to antiviral agents is unknown. Secondary bacterial pneumonia often presents as recurrent fever and systemic symptoms after improvement in acute influenza symptoms has occurred. *Streptococcus pneumoniae*, *Staphylococcus aureus*, and *Haemophilus influenzae* are often cited as the leading causes based on a 1971 study; more recent data are unavailable. Other complications include exacerbations of chronic obstructive pulmonary disease (COPD) and asthma, myositis, and central nervous system involvement. Reye's syndrome—characterized by nausea, vomiting, and mental status changes caused by liver dysfunction—can be seen in children with influenza (most often influenza B) and is associated with aspirin use.

Diagnosis

Because its clinical manifestations can resemble many other respiratory infections, influenza is typically a clinical diagnosis based on the presence of fever, nasal congestion, cough, and myalgia when influenza is active in the community. In this situation, the diagnosis is correct in 60% to 70% of patients. Previously, if confirmation of the diagnosis was desired, viral culture or other research-based techniques (immunofluorescence or polymerase chain reaction assays) were needed, or acute and convalescent serologies could be performed. Unfortunately, there was not time enough for the test results to become available to help.

Now there are enzyme immunoassay tests that can be performed in physician's offices with test procedures that take less than 30 minutes. Tests are available to

CURRENT DIAGNOSIS

- Influenza is mainly diagnosed when fever, nasal congestion, cough, and myalgia are present during known influenza activity in the community.
- Available rapid influenza tests have low sensitivity, leading to many false-negative tests when influenza is prevalent. Testing is more reasonable in situations when influenza likelihood is lower.

detect either influenza A or B with no differentiation between the two (Flu OIA, QuickVue Influenza Test, and ZstatFlu), or detect either one with the ability to tell which virus is present (BD Directigen Flu A+B). Test specificity is generally high at 90% or greater; however when influenza prevalence is high, test sensitivity is low (65% to 86%), which leads to many false-negative tests when influenza prevalence is high.

Decision analyses and cost-effectiveness analyses have shown that rapid testing for influenza is reasonable when influenza is relatively uncommon, such as early or late in the typical influenza season or during influenza seasons where prevalence is low. When influenza prevalence is high, however, testing before treatment is not recommended because high rates of false-negative tests can lead to patients with influenza going untreated. Hence this strategy is not worth the expense of testing ($15 to $20).

Prevention and Treatment

VACCINE

Influenza vaccination prevents influenza illness, complications, and death in high-risk groups, with cost-effectiveness analyses showing that vaccination is cost saving compared to no vaccination. Based on worldwide surveillance data, vaccine composition is modified to match that year's predictions of circulating influenza viruses. The Centers for Disease Control and Prevention (CDC) recommends intramuscular administration of inactivated influenza virus vaccine to the following groups at increased risk for influenza complications:

- Persons older than 65 years of age
- Residents of nursing homes and other chronic care facilities
- Adults and children with chronic cardiac or pulmonary disorders or with chronic metabolic diseases (including diabetes), renal dysfunction, hemoglobinopathy, or immunosuppression (including AIDS)
- Children and adolescents on chronic aspirin therapy (because of Reye's syndrome risk)
- Women who will be pregnant during the influenza season (influenza complication rates increase during pregnancy)
- Children ages 6 to 23 months

CURRENT THERAPY

- Antiviral agents are an adjunct to, not a replacement for, influenza vaccination.
- Antiviral therapy is clinically and economically reasonable based on clinical features without confirmatory testing when fever and typical symptoms are present during influenza outbreaks.
- Amantadine and rimantadine are relatively inexpensive, but they only cover influenza A and are more prone to side effects and antiviral resistance development. Zanamivir and oseltamivir are reasonable, if more expensive, options.

Intramuscular vaccination is also recommended for persons 50 to 64 years of age, because of greater likelihood of high-risk conditions and proven benefits for persons of this age who are not at high risk. Persons who can transmit influenza to those at high risk should also be vaccinated, including all personnel who have contact with patients in hospitals, outpatient settings, nursing home or chronic care facilities, assisted living or retirement communities; home care personnel; and household contacts of persons in high-risk groups.

Live, attenuated influenza vaccine (LAIV) (FluMist) administered via the nasal passages is also available, but it is more expensive than the inactivated vaccine. It may be given to healthy children and adolescents 5 to 17 years of age and healthy adults 18 to 49 years of age. If LAIV is given to persons who have contact with severely immunosuppressed patients, the CDC recommends refraining from contact for 7 days after vaccination because of virus shedding associated with this vaccine. LAIV is not recommended for persons at high risk for influenza complications, or for patients younger than 5 years or older than 49 years of age. No significant differences in vaccine efficacy have been shown between the two modes of vaccination in adults younger than 50 years old.

Neither vaccine should be administered to persons with anaphylactic reactions to eggs or to other influenza vaccine components. If high risk of influenza complications exists however, allergy evaluation and desensitization followed by vaccination can be considered.

Optimal time of vaccination is October or November, but vaccination can continue into December and beyond. Acute febrile or nonfebrile illnesses are not a contraindication to vaccination according to the CDC, particularly in children with mild upper respiratory infections or allergic rhinitis, but vaccination should usually be delayed until symptoms have diminished.

Vaccine Dosage

Dosage of intramuscular inactivated vaccine is 0.50 mL, except in children 6 to 35 months old, where the dose is 0.25 mL. In children younger than 9 years old who have not previously received influenza vaccination, a second dose should be administered at least 1 month after the first dose, ideally before December. Adults and older children should be vaccinated in the deltoid muscle, infants and younger children in the anterolateral thigh.

The live vaccine dose is 0.5 mL, divided equally between each nostril. Children ages 5 to 8 years, who have not previously received influenza vaccination of either type, should receive two doses separated by 6 to 10 weeks, while persons ages 9 to 49 years should receive one dose.

Vaccine Side Effects

Intramuscular inactivated vaccine causes local pain at the injection site in 10% to 64%, lasting less than 2 days and rarely interfering with daily activities. Systemic reactions with fever, malaise, and myalgia lasting 1 to 2 days can occur, mainly in young children with no prior exposure to antigens contained in the vaccine. Placebo-controlled trials in healthy young adults and the elderly show no difference in systemic symptoms between placebo and influenza vaccine injections. Inactivated vaccine, containing killed virus, cannot cause influenza.

Intranasal vaccination of live, attenuated virus can lead to higher rates of nasal congestion, headache, fever, and other systemic complaints than that seen in placebo recipients, particularly after the first dose. These side effects are largely mild and self-limited. Serious adverse effects are reported in less than 1%, and the incidence of pneumonia or other possible influenza complications were not statistically different from controls.

Guillain-Barré syndrome (GBS) occurred in less than 10 per million persons receiving the 1976 swine influenza vaccination. Since then, no statistically significant association between influenza and GBS has been found. If there is a risk of GBS with vaccination, it is approximately 1 per million vaccinations according to the CDC, much less than the risk of severe influenza complications, particularly in high-risk groups.

ANTIVIRALS

Two of the four available antiviral medications for influenza management, amantadine (Symmetrel) and rimantadine (Flumadine), are active only against influenza A, whereas the neuraminidase inhibitors zanamivir (Relenza) and oseltamivir (Tamiflu) are active against both influenza A and B. When given to patients with illness caused by susceptible virus within 48 hours, all agents decrease illness duration by approximately 1 day. Whether these medications decrease the likelihood of influenza complications is unclear; however, recent studies of zanamivir and oseltamivir strongly suggest that impact on complications is likely, particularly in high-risk adults.

Deciding which drug to use for influenza treatment is complicated (Table 1). Amantadine and rimantadine are less expensive but are only effective for influenza A and more prone to side effects and induction of viral resistance. The likelihood of influenza being caused by influenza A varies greatly and unpredictably from year to year and within single influenza seasons.

TABLE 1 Approved Indications for Influenza Antiviral Medications

	Spectrum	Duration	Age Group (y)					
			1–6	7–9	10–12	13–64	≥65	
Treatment								
Amantadine (Symmetrel)	Influenza A	5d	5 mg/kg/d*	5 mg/kg/d*	100 mg bid	100 mg bid	"100 mg/d	
Rimantadine (Flumadine)	Influenza A	5d	Not approved	Not approved	Not approved	100 mg bid	100 mg/d	
Zanamivir (Relenza)	Influenza A or B	5d	Not approved	10 mg bid	10 mg bid	10 mg bid	10 mg bid	
Oseltamivir (Tamiflu)	Influenza A or B	5d	Varies by weight	Varies by weight	Varies by weight	75 mg bid	75 mg bid	
Prophylaxis								
Amantadine	Influenza A	†	5 mg/kg/d*	5 mg/kg/d*	100 mg bid	100 mg bid	"100 mg/d	
Rimantadine	Influenza A	†	5 mg/kg/d*	5 mg/kg/d*	100 mg bid	100 mg bid	100 mg/d	
Oseltamivir	Influenza A or B	†	Not approved	Not approved	Not approved	75 mg/d	75 mg/d	

*Up to 150 mg per day in two divided doses.
†Duration of influenza activity.
Abbreviations: bid = twice a day; d = days; y = years.

Rakel and Bope: *Conn's Current Therapy 2006*

Central nervous system (CNS) side effects (nervousness, anxiety, insomnia, difficulty concentrating, and lightheadedness) have occurred with amantadine (13%) and rimantadine (6%) and at higher levels in older populations. More severe CNS effects (marked behavioral changes, delirium, agitation, seizures) are rare; gastrointestinal (GI) side effects occur in 1% to 3% of patients. Zanamivir should not be used in patients with asthma or COPD because of reported induction of bronchospasm and worsening pulmonary function after its use; otherwise systemic side effects with zanamivir were similar to placebo. Unlike the oral formulations of the other agents, zanamivir is inhaled nasally and could be difficult to administer for some individuals. Oseltamivir causes nausea or vomiting in approximately 10% of patients; taking the medication with food may decrease this effect. Drug-resistant viruses occur in approximately a third of patients receiving amantadine or rimantadine, appearing within 2 to 3 days of starting therapy. Viral resistance to zanamivir and oseltamivir appears to be infrequent; surveillance for resistant viruses is being conducted. When antiviral therapy of influenza is warranted, cost-effectiveness analyses have shown that treatment with zanamivir or oseltamivir is clinically and economically reasonable, with amantadine or rimantadine as lower cost options when influenza B is uncommon.

Chemoprophylaxis with antiviral agents, as an adjunct to vaccination, should be considered in:

- High-risk patients who are vaccinated during an influenza outbreak
- Persons caring for high-risk patients
- Persons with immunodeficiency and inadequate response to vaccination
- High-risk patients who cannot be vaccinated

Amantadine and rimantadine are approved for influenza A prophylaxis in patients ages 1 year and older (see Table 1). Oseltamivir is approved for influenza A and B prophylaxis in patients ages 13 years or older. Thus, there are no approved drugs for prophylaxis of influenza B in those younger than 13 years old, but studies have shown efficacy for both zanamivir and oseltamivir in children with household influenza contacts. When used with vaccination, antiviral prophylaxis should be given for at least 2 weeks after vaccination is completed. Otherwise, chemoprophylaxis should be continued for the duration of influenza activity in the community, although cost-effectiveness analysis suggests use only during peak influenza activity. When live, attenuated vaccine is used, antiviral agents should not be used for 2 weeks afterward, because antivirals interfere with viral replication and subsequent immunity.

REFERENCES

Centers for Disease Control and Prevention: Prevention and control of influenza: Recommendations of the Advisory Committee on Immunization Practices (ACIP). MMWR 2003;52[No. RR-8]:1-34.

Hayden FG, Osterhaus AD, Treanor JJ, et al: Efficacy and safety of the neuraminidase inhibitor zanamivir in the treatment of influenzavirus infections. N Engl J Med 1997;337(13):874-880.

Jefferson TO, Demicheli V, Deeks JJ, Rivetti D: Amantadine and rimantadine for preventing and treating influenza A in adults. Cochrane Database Syst Rev 2002;(3):CD001169.

Kaiser L, Wat C, Mills T, et al: Impact of oseltamivir treatment on influenza-related lower respiratory tract complications and hospitalizations. Arch Intern Med 2003;163(14):1667-1672.

Muennig PA, Khan K: Cost-effectiveness of vaccination versus treatment of influenza in healthy adolescents and adults. Clin Infect Dis 2001;33(11):1879-1885.

Rothberg MB, Bellantonio S, Rose DN: Management of influenza in adults older than 65 years of age: Cost-effectiveness of rapid testing and antiviral therapy. Ann Intern Med 2003;139(5 Pt 1):321-329.

Smith KJ, Roberts MS. Cost-effectiveness of newer treatment strategies for influenza. Am J Med 2002;113(4):300-7.

Treanor JJ, Hayden FG, Vrooman PS, et al: Efficacy and safety of the oral neuraminidase inhibitor oseltamivir in treating acute influenza: A randomized controlled trial. JAMA 2000;283(8):1016-24.

Leishmaniasis

Method of
Jean-Pierre Dedet, MD, BSc

The leishmaniases are parasitic diseases caused by protozoan flagellates of the genus *Leishmania,* which infect numerous mammals, including humans, and are transmitted through the bite of an insect vector, the phlebotomine sandfly.

Leishmania are protozoa belonging to the order Kinetoplastida and the family Trypanosomatidae. They are dimorphic parasites that present as two principal morphologic stages: the intracellular amastigote, within the mononuclear phagocytic system of the mammalian host, and the flagellated promastigote within the intestinal tract of the insect vector and in culture. The genus *Leishmania* includes around 20 taxa (Table 1), most of which commonly infect humans, in whom they are responsible for various types of disease such as visceral, cutaneous (localized or diffuse), and mucocutaneous leishmaniasis.

The leishmaniases occur in 88 countries, of which 72 are developing and 13 are among the poorest in the world. They range over the intertropical zones of the world, and extend into temperate regions in South America, southern Europe, and Asia. Because of increased risk factors, they remain a major public health problem in numerous developing countries. An estimated 350 million people are at risk of infection, and the world annual incidence of new cases is liable to be between 1.5 and 2 million.

Pathology

Transmission is usually by the bite of an infected sandfly, resulting in the intradermal inoculation of metacyclic promastigotes. Remarkably, establishment in the

TABLE 1 Short, Practical Classification of the Genus *Leishmania* According to Subgenera, the Main Geographical Domains, and the Usual Tropism of the Species*

Subgenus	Subgenus *Leishmania*		Subgenus *Viannia*	
Old word	Leishmania donovani Leishmania infantum	Leishmania major Leishmania tropica Leishmania killicki Leishmania aethiopica		
New word	Leishmania infantum (= Leishmania chagasi)	Leishmania mexicana Leishmania amazonensis Leishmania venezuelensis	Leishmania guyanensis Leishmania panamensis Leishmania shawi Leishmania naiffi Leishmania lainsoni Leishmania peruviana	Leishmania braziliensis
Tropism	Viscerotropic	Dermotropic		Mucosatropic

*This table is limited to the main anthropotropic species.

mammalian host is facilitated by the sandfly saliva delivered at the same time, which enhances the infectivity of the parasites.

Within the dermis of mammalian skin, the metacyclic promastigotes are phagocytosed by dendritic cells and macrophages, within which they transform into amastigotes resistant to intracellular digestion. The localization of the parasite in various organs is directly related to the tropism of the parasite species (Table 2). Clinical expression of the disease depends on the organs infected and the immunologic condition of the patient.

A localized lesion of cutaneous leishmaniasis (CL) develops when the intracellular multiplication of the amastigotes remains restricted to the inoculation site. Alternatively, the parasites spread to the organs of the mononuclear phagocytic system, giving rise to visceral leishmaniasis (VL). Amastigotes may also spread to other cutaneous sites, such as diffuse cutaneous leishmaniasis (DCL), or to mucosae in mucocutaneous leishmaniasis (MCL).

Parasitologic diagnosis (demonstration of parasites in different types of sample according to the clinical form) has been revolutionized by the use of PCR for the detection of specific DNA. Immunologic diagnosis is based on the detection of circulating antibodies (VL) or delayed-type hypersensitivity (CL, MCL).

TABLE 2 Usual Tropism and Clinical Expressions of the Main Anthropophilic Species of *Leishmania*

Usual Tropism	Species	Clinical Expression	
		Usual	Exceptional
Viscerotropic species	Leishmania donovani	VL, PKDL	LCL
	Leishmania infantum	VL	LCL, DCL*
Dermotropic species	Leishmania major	LCL	DCL*
	Leishmania tropica	LCL	VL
	Leishmania killicki	LCL	
	Leishmania aethiopica	LCL	DCL
	Leishmania mexicana	LCL	DCL, VL*
	Leishmania amazonensis	LCL	DCL, VL
	Leishmania venezuelensis	LCL	
	Leishmania guyanensis	LCL	MCL
	Leishmania panamensis	LCL	MCL, DCL*
	Leishmania shawi	LCL	
	Leishmania naiffi	LCL	
	Leishmania lainsoni	LCL	
	Leishmania peruviana	LCL	
Mucosatropic species	Leishmania braziliensis	LCL, MCL	DCL,* VL*

*During immunosuppression.
Abbreviations: DCL = diffuse cutaneous leishmaniasis; LCL = localized cutaneous leishmaniasis; MCL = mucocutaneous leishmaniasis; PKDL = post–kala-azar dermal leishmaniasis; VL = visceral leishmaniasis.

CURRENT DIAGNOSIS

Visceral leishmaniasis

- Immunologic diagnosis
    Detection of circulating antibodies (ELISA, IFAT, Western blot, DAT, etc.)
- Parasitologic diagnosis
    Demonstration of parasites in smears made from bone marrow, spleen, or lymph node aspirates
    Detection of parasite DNA in peripheral blood, bone marrow, spleen, or lymph nodes using PCR
    Culture on blood agar or liquid media (+FCS)

Cutaneous leishmaniasis

- Parasitologic diagnosis
    Demonstration of parasites in smears made from a cutaneous lesion
    Detection of parasite DNA in a cutaneous lesion sample using PCR
- Immunologic diagnosis
    DTH detected by skin test

Mucocutaneous leishmaniasis

- Parasitologic diagnosis
    Demonstration of parasites in smears made from mucosal lesion
    Detection of parasite DNA in biopsy of mucosal lesion, using PCR
- Immunologic diagnosis
    DTH detected by skin test
    Detection of circulating antibodies (ELISA, IFAT, etc.)

Abbreviations: DAT = direct agglutination test; DTH = delayed type hypersensitivity; ELISA = enzyme-linked immunosorbent assay; FCS = fetal calf serum; IFAT = indirect immunofluorescence test; PCR = polymerase chain reaction [assay].

Treatment

For approximately a century, the treatment of leishmaniasis has been based on pentavalent antimonial compounds. Significant changes have, however, been introduced throughout the past two decades. Following the increasing incidence of VL cases in immunocompromised patients and the rise of acquired resistances to antimonials, amphotericin B (AMB) (Fungizone) has joined the antimonials as a first line drug for leishmaniasis. A liposomal formulation (AmBisome) may soon supplant antimonials in several countries. Miltefosine (Miltex),* a new oral compound, has shown promising results, and could completely change the therapy of leishmaniasis in a near future.

*Investigational drug in the United States.

 CURRENT THERAPY

Visceral leishmaniasis

- Pentavalent antimonials (Pentostam):* 20 mg H Sb^v/kg per day, over the course of 28 days
- Lipid-associated AMB (AmBisone): Five daily injections plus 1 on day 10; total dose 15 to 18 mg/kg VL (immunocompetent patients); up to 10 injections (total dose 20-30 mg/kg) (HIV patients)

Cutaneous leishmaniasis

- Therapeutic abstention
- Intralesional pentavalent antimonials: 5 to 10 infiltrations of 1 to 5 mL
- Pentamidine (Pentacarinat):[1] four to five IM injections, 4 mg/kg per injection
- Pentavalent antimonials: 20 mg H Sb^v/kg per day, for 20 days

Mucocutaneous leishmaniasis

- Primary cutaneous lesion
    Pentavalent antimonials: 20 mg H Sb^v/kg per day for 20 days
- Secondary mucosal involvement
    AMB (Fungizone): 0.5 to 1 mg/kg per infusion (in dextrose 5%), 14 to 20 infusions
    Pentavalent antimonials: 20 mg H Sb^v/kg per day, for 28 days

*Available in the United States from the CDC.
[1]Not FDA approved for this indication.
Abbreviations: ABM = amphotericin B; IM = intramuscular; H Sb^v = H pentavalent antimony; VL = visceral leishmaniasis.

CURRENT PRODUCTS

Pentavalent Antimonials

Two closely related antimony (Sb) derivatives are currently used: sodium stibogluconate (Pentostam)* and meglumine antimonate (Glucantime).[2] They have distinct antimony rates of 100 and 85 mg H pentavalent antimony (Sb^v)/mL, respectively. When properly manufactured and stored, they have comparable efficacy and toxicity. A generic antimonial (Albert David) is presently manufactured in India for local use.

Although long-term use has proved antimonials to be efficient in leishmaniasis treatment, their mechanisms of action remain unclear. Possibly, antimonial salts are efficiently concentrated within the macrophage or parasite and are then transformed into active trivalent metabolites highly toxic to both *Leishmania* stages. They seem to inhibit ATP synthesis, but the mechanism is unknown. Antimonials have poor oral absorption, so they are administered by parenteral route. They are rapidly excreted by the kidneys.

Although numerous side effects have been attributed to antimonials, the scarcity of reported accidents

*Available in the United States from the Centers for Disease Control.
[2]Not available in the United States.

and absence of any better alternative justify their continued use. The side effects of pentavalent antimonials can be divided into signs of intolerance (shivers, fever, arthralgias, myalgias, skin rashes, abdominal symptoms, and headache) and toxic effects occurring at the end of treatment. Stibointoxication signs include reversible elevation of hepatocellular enzymes, subclinical pancreatitis, decrease in the hemoglobin level and the platelet count. Cardiac side effects are the most worrisome. Several transient electrocardiogram changes occur, including flattening and/or inversion of T waves, prolongation of the corrected QT interval, concave ST abnormality, and prolongation of PR interval. Exceptionally, sudden deaths have been reported in patients who received more than the recommended dose of SBV.

Sodium stibogluconate and meglumine antimonate are administered on the basis of their H Sb^v content. The recommended dosage is 20 mg H Sb^v/kg per day, for 20 days in CL and 28 days in VL and MCL. They are currently injected intravenously (IV) or intramuscularly (IM). The IV route is preferred for the large volumes of drug required for most adults. In the case of a few localized cutaneous lesions, intralesional injections are used.

Amphotericin B (Fungizone)

AMB (Fungizone) is a polyene antibiotic isolated in 1955 from a strain of *Streptomyces*. It is used in the treatment of systemic fungal infections. The target of AMB (Fungizone) is ergosterol-like sterols, which are the major membrane sterols of *Leishmania* as well as fungi; so it is a powerful antileishmanial used in the treatment of severe leishmaniasis (VL, MCL) or cases resistant to antimonials. Throughout the last 15 years, it has become an alternative first-line drug.

AMB (Fungizone) is only used by IV injection. Effective plasma concentrations are rapidly reached, and even exceeded, from the beginning of the infusion, and persist more than 24 hours. The product has slow renal elimination.

There are two types of side effects to AMB (Fungizone). Intolerance signs occur during infusion and include chills, headache, cramps, hypotension, vertigo, paresthesias, vomiting, and exceptionally anaphylactic or cardiogenic shocks. These manifestations are usually controlled by addition of corticoids in the liquid of suspension, or by slowing down the rate of infusion. Nephrotoxicity is the most important of toxic effect of AMB (Fungizone).

AMB (Fungizone) is administered as a slow (6 to 8 hours) IV infusion (0.5 to 1 mg/kg dissolved in 500 mL dextrose 5%) on alternate days. The common regimens range from 14 to 20 infusions, for a total dose of 1.5 to 2 g. Major advances have recently been in lipid formulations of AMB (Fungizone).

Lipid-Associated Amphotericin B (AmBisome)

When associated with lipids, AMB (Fungizone) is delivered to the site of intracellular infection, which leads to more drug accumulation in infected cells, thereby increasing the therapeutic index.

The three existing formulations are similar in some respects and altogether less toxic than AMB (Fungizone), but they have different tolerability and kinetics. Liposomal AMB (AmBisome) is formed from several phospholipids in a membrane bilayer containing amphotericin B (Fungizone). This compound is licensed for VL treatment in Europe and the United States. The two other formulations, AMB phospholipid complex (Abelcet) and AMB cholesterol dispersion (Amphotec) are not yet licensed for VL.

Liposomal AMB (AmBisome) has been tested in several countries for VL treatment, and it has proved less toxic than conventional AMB (Fungizone) and more efficient in both immunocompetent and immunocompromised patients. Short-course treatment currently consists of five daily injections, plus another injection on day 10 (total dose 15 to 18 mg/kg) with 95% to 100% efficacy. Single-dose liposomal AMB (AmBisome) has been successfully tested in India.

Pentamidine (Pentacarinat)[1]

Pentamidine (Pentacarinat)[1] is an aromatic diamine first synthesized in the late 1930s. It has been used as an alternative drug to treat antimonial-resistant VL in India and Kenya and infantile VL in courses alternating with antimonials in several countries of the Mediterranean basin. At present, the isethionate salt (Pentamidine [Pentacarinat][1]) is the only form available for human use and is restricted to treatment of CL.

Pentamidine (Pentacarinat)[1] inhibits the synthesis of parasitic DNA by blocking thymidine synthase and fixation of the messenger RNA. In the absence of oral absorption, the drug is administered by parenteral route, which provides a transient blood concentration, with rapid subsequent dispersal and high tissue fixation. It is excreted slowly by kidney.

Pentamidine (Pentacarinat)[1] can be responsible for immediate side effects, mainly in case of rapid IV injection (hypotension, tachycardia, nausea, vomiting, facial erythema, pruritus, syncope). Local reactions can also occur (urticaria, abscess formation, phlebitis). Toxic side effects depend on the dose and can affect pancreas, kidney, and blood cell lines. Changes in glucose metabolism are directly linked to the toxicity of the drug to pancreatic cells and can induce diabetes mellitus.

Pentamidine (Pentacarinat)[1] is given in doses of 4 mg/kg per injection. The IM or slow IV injections are made on alternate days, to patients confined to bed and fasting. Short courses (four doses) are currently used for treatment of CL. Long courses lasting several weeks, suggested for treatment of resistant VL, have significant potential side effects.

---

[1]Not FDA approved for this indication.

DRUGS UNDER DEVELOPMENT

Various molecules already used against other infectious agents have been tested during recent decades for leishmaniasis treatment. To date not one of them has been recognized as a genuine antileishmanial. The most promising alternative product seems to be miltefosine (Miltex).*

Miltefosine (Miltex)

Miltefosine (Miltex),* an alkyl phospholipid, is a phosphocholine analogue used as an oral antineoplastic agent, which affects cell-signaling pathways and membrane synthesis. It is effective in the treatment of experimental murine leishmaniasis. Since the beginning of the 1990s, several clinical trials have been carried out in India where a phase-IV study is in progress. Several thousand patients have been successfully treated with side effects limited to digestive troubles. Regulatory approval for adult use in India was obtained in 2002. Miltefosine (Miltex)* is as effective and well tolerated in Indian children with VL as in adults. Clinical trials are planned in other countries and other clinical forms of leishmaniasis.

Aminosidine

Aminosidine (paromomycin)[1] is an aminoglycoside antibiotic. It showed powerful antileishmanial activity in vitro and in animal models. Like other aminoglycosides, paromomycin has renal and eighth cranial nerve toxicity. It is administered by IM injection or IV infusion at the recommended dose of 15 mg/kg per day for 10 days.

Paromomycin[1] has been used efficiently for VL treatment as monotherapy and in combination with pentavalent antimonials, but it is not yet available in parenteral formulation. Paromomycin,[†] used in regular topical applications for 4 to 12 weeks, has good effects in the treatment of certain forms of CL.

Immunomodulation

Because defective macrophage activation is key to the development of leishmanial infection, use of immunomodulation drugs appears to be a relevant strategy. Interferon gamma (IFN-γ) (Actimmune)[1] has been used in combination with pentavalent antimonials in the treatment of VL and MCL. However, despite some efficacy, its use remains limited because of hematologic toxicity and high cost. Clinical trials of imidazoquinoline imiquimod (Aldara)[1] are presently in progress.

Imidazoles

The antifungal azoles inhibit the sterol synthesis pathway of *Leishmania*. Some of them [ketoconazole (Nizoral),[1] itraconazole (Sporanox)[1]] have been tested in the treatment of CL, with contradictory results. In spite of their low toxicity and the comfort of oral administration, these products are of little interest in leishmaniasis treatment. New formulations (fluconazole [Diflucan][1] posaconazole)* are under investigation.

Allopurinol (Zyloprim)

Allopurinol (Zyloprim)[1] is a purine structural analogue that can be incorporated into *Leishmania* RNA, with a lethal effect on the parasite. It is administered orally and rapidly metabolized and eliminated by renal route. Limited clinical trials showed some efficacy in CL, and synergy with pentavalent antimonials. Although not applicable for human leishmaniasis, this product is currently in use for the treatment of canine leishmaniasis.

TREATMENT REGIMENS ACCORDING TO CLINICAL FEATURES

Because of the diversity of clinical forms of leishmaniasis, with different levels of gravity and distinct progression, the drug regimen must be decided on a case-by-case basis. This strategy is all the more relevant because the available antileishmanial drugs are not devoid of toxicity.

Visceral Leishmaniasis

VL may be treated as soon as diagnosis is made. The efficacy of treatment depends on the duration because advanced cases are less responsive to antileishmanial drugs. Treatment requires confirmed first-line products, principally antimonials and AMB (Fungizone).

The conventional treatment is based on a 28-day course of pentavalent antimonial sodium stibogluconate (Pentostam) at 20 mg H Sb^v/kg per day. A single course can be insufficient to obtain a complete cure, and treatment should be repeated after a pause.

Clinical resistance to antimony is increasing, particularly in one geographical focus, the state of Bihar in India, where primary resistance to antimony exceeds 60% of cases. Various alternative treatments have been tested in this situation, including AMB (Fungizone), liposomal AMB (AmBisone), pentamidine (Pentacarinat),[1] aminosidine (paromomycin),[1] and more recently, miltefosine (Miltex).

Because of its excellent results, liposomal AMB (AmBisome) tends to be the drug of choice. Treatment begins with five daily injections (3 mg/kg/injection).

A final injection on day 10 brings the total dosage to 18 mg/kg. In poor countries its use is limited by cost.

Management of VL cases includes correction of nutritional deficiencies in severely wasted patients, blood transfusion in case of dramatic anemia, and treatment of any secondary bacterial infection with appropriate antibiotics.

VL in HIV-infected patients appears generally nonresponsive to the classical antileishmanial drugs, with incomplete cure and frequent relapses. Side effects of antileishmanial drugs are more frequent and serious than in immunocompetent patients. Liposomal AMB (AmBisome) can be used in these cases, and at higher doses, the total injections reaching 10 (total dose: 30 mg/kg).

VL following organ transplantation poses therapeutic problems resulting from the toxicity of the main antileishmanial drugs for transplanted organs. However, these cases do need to be treated because they are fatal in the absence of specific treatment. Antimonials and AMB (Fungizone) are equally efficient; the best results are obtained by treating patients successively by both drugs.

Once the antileishmanial treatment has been concluded, the problem with immunocompromised patients is that of secondary prophylaxis to prevent relapses. Numerous schemes have been proposed—such as monthly injections of antimonial, twice-monthly injections of liposomal AMB (AmBisome) or of pentamidine (Pentacarinat)[1]—but available data are insufficient for evaluating their respective efficiency. All these protocols need to be evaluated.

Localized Cutaneous Leishmaniasis

Management of patients with LCL depends on the type and characters of the lesion(s), the *Leishmania* species involved, the risk of expansion or dissemination, and the opinion of the patient. Briefly, three options are possible: therapeutic abstention, local treatment, or general treatment.

Mild, rapidly self-healing forms of CL, such as those because of *Leishmania major* or *Leishmania peruviana*, can probably remain untreated. It is well known that patients in the placebo group can cure more rapidly than those receiving antileishmanial drugs.

Various local treatments have been proposed, including diverse physical means (diathermy, cryotherapy, radiotherapy, laser), surgical excision or local applications of ointments. Trials have generally been limited, without control groups, and the results have been inconclusive. These procedures cannot generally be recommended.

Local infiltration of pentavalent antimonials is recommended for the treatment of small numbers of lesions. Various protocols have been proposed consisting of a course of 5 to 10 infiltrations of 1 to 5 mL of antimonial, often accompanied by local anesthetic to prevent pain,

and associated with cryotherapy or not. Infiltration is repeated two or three times per week.

Systemic treatment is recommended for CL with large and/or multiple lesions, with lymphangitic dissemination, of the recidivans type or with a risk of mucosal involvement. CL of immunocompromised patients should also be treated systemically. The currently used systemic treatment is a course of 20 days of pentavalent antimonial, at a dose of 20 mg H Sb^v/kg per day. A course of 4 to 5 IM injections of pentamidine (Pentacarinat)[1] (4 mg/kg/injection) on alternate days is used with good results in *L. guyanensis* lesions. Oral fluconazole (Diflucan)[1] can be proposed as an alternative.

Diffuse Cutaneous Leishmaniasis

Once established, DCL is resistant to treatment. Systematic pentavalent antimonials can temporarily improve the clinical condition. Pentamidine (Pentacarinat)[1] showed some efficacy, but high doses were close to toxicity. Tests of various new molecules or formulations (liposomal AMB [AmBisome], immunomodulators) are needed. However, the scarcity of cases precludes clinical trials with control groups.

Mucocutaneous Leishmaniasis

Systemic treatment of the primary cutaneous lesion is recommended with the hope of preventing the spread of the parasites to facial mucosae. The treatment currently used in endemic areas is pentavalent antimonial, 20-day course of IM injections, 20 mg H Sb^v/kg per day. However, it has been shown that correct treatment does not consistently prevent the development of secondary mucosal lesions.

Mucosal lesions should be treated as early as possible to prevent the expansion of lesions and subsequent mutilation. The antimonials, at standard doses, are injected daily over the course of 28 days. The rate of cure varies in different countries and according to the stage of development of the lesions. AMB (Fungizone) has been used for late cases or those responding poorly to antimonials. Cure has sometimes been obtained from 1 g, but higher doses (2 to 3 g) were often necessary. Cases of resistance seem to occur, but few observations are documented. Liposomal AMB (AmBisome) and combined paromomycin and antimonials need to be investigated.

REFERENCES

Bhattacharya SK, Jha TK, Sundar S, et al: Efficacy and tolerability of miltefosine for childhood visceral leishmaniasis in India. Clin Infect Dis 2004;38: 217-221.
Dedet JP, Pratlong F: Leishmaniasis. In Cook GC, Zumla A (eds): Manson's Tropical Diseases. Philadelphia, WB Saunders, 2003, pp 1339-1371.
Desjeux P: Leishmaniasis: Current situation and new perspectives. Comp Immunol Microbiol Infect Dis 2004;27:305-318.

[1]Not FDA approved for this indication.

[1]Not FDA approved for this indication.

Herwaldt BL, Berman JD: Recommendations for treating leishmaniasis with sodium stibogluconate (Pentostam) and review or pertinent clinical studies. Am J Trop Med Hyg 1992;46:296-306.

Laguna F: Treatment of leishmaniasis in HIV-positive patients. Ann Trop Med Parasitol 2003;97(suppl):135-142.

Sundar S, Jha TK, Thakur CP, et al: Oral miltefosine for Indian visceral leishmaniasis. N Engl J Med 2002;347:1739-1746.

Sundar S, Mehta H, Suresh AV, et al: Amphotericin B treatment for Indian visceral leishmaniasis: Conventional versus lipid formulations. Clin Infect Dis 2004;38:377-383.

Titus RG, Ribeiro JMC: Salivary gland lysates from the sand fly *Lutzomyia longipalpis* enhance *Leishmania* infectivity. Science 1988;239:1306-1308.

Zilberstein D, Ephros M: Clinical and laboratory aspects of *Leishmania* chemotherapy in the era of drug resistance. In Farrell JP (ed): World Class Parasites, vol 4: *Leishmania*. Boston, Kluwer Academic Publishers, 2002, pp 115-136.

Leprosy (Hansen's Disease)

Method of
*Ramaswamy Ganapati, BSc, MBBS, DDV and
Vivek V. Pai, MBBS, DVD, FCGP*

Definition

Leprosy is one of the oldest diseases of humankind. Leprosy bacilli are also known as Hansen's bacilli after the name of their discoverer. The onset of the disease is usually slow, after a long and variable incubation period (latent period). The disease is mainly characterized by lesions in the skin and/or polyneuritic changes caused by involvement of and damage to the peripheral nerves. Jopling (1984) has defined it as "a chronic mycobacterial disease (infectious in some cases) primarily affecting the peripheral nervous system and secondarily involving skin and certain other tissues."

Causative Agent

As far back as 1873, Norwegian scientist Gerhard Armauer Hansen demonstrated bacilli (later called *Mycobacterium leprae*) in leprosy lesions. Stained by the Ziehl-Neelsen method, they appear as pink rods, which may be arranged in groups (globi) or may occur singly. They are less toxic and less pathogenic in nature than many other organisms, with a generation time of 13 to 14 days. Because of these properties, as well as host factors, 2 to 5 years may elapse before clinically detectable disease is apparent.

Transmission

An untreated patient with multibacillary leprosy is the only source of infection, discharging as many as 100 million bacilli from nasal secretions every day. The inhalation of bacilli-laden droplets is the most likely mode of entry of leprosy bacilli. Only susceptible persons develop the disease. Any person who has specific deficiency in cell-mediated immunity (CMI) toward *M. leprae* is susceptible. Research on genetic factors determining susceptibility is inconclusive. The possible role of indirect transmission through insects, mosquitoes, and bedbugs is also reported, as are extrahuman reservoirs such as soil, water, and animals.

Pathogenesis

According to Khanolkar (1964) the distal endoneurial involvement with *M. leprae* ascending along axons is generally believed to be the method of infection. Scollard (2000) showed that in infected armadillos the endothelial cells of peripheral nerve vasculature may be the "gatekeepers" by which *M. leprae* infect nerves. It is generally accepted that Schwann cells are the target for *M. leprae* and multiply gradually, depending upon host resistance, for example, cell-mediated immunity (CMI) determined by T lymphocytes. Subclinical infection in leprosy is reported. Advance in knowledge is limited because the bacillus is not cultivable in laboratory media, but it can be grown in mouse footpads and armadillos.

Clinical Features

The spectral concept of Ridley and Jopling (1966) for classifying the disease into five groups has led to a better understanding of the clinicopathologic events in leprosy. However, this classification does not refer to macular lesions of "indeterminate" leprosy and "pure neuritic" without skin lesions. The World Health Organization (WHO) (1994) has offered a simple field classification as multibacillary (MB), which is more than five skin lesions and/or more than two nerve trunks, or paucibacillary (PB), which is less than five skin lesions or one nerve trunk.

INDETERMINATE LEPROSY (I)

Indeterminate leprosy (I) features hypopigmented lesions, 2 cm to 5 cm in diameter with ill-defined margins, which may be seen on trunk, thighs, buttocks, and arms. There may be only blunting of pain sensation and impairment of sweat function because autonomic nerves may be involved. Thickening nerves are not found and skin smears are negative for acid-fast bacillus (AFB). Indeterminate lesions may heal spontaneously or may evolve into determinate forms with an increase in the number and progress to severe forms. Response to lepromin test (discussed later) is variable, and a positive response indicates a favorable course.

TUBERCULOID LEPROSY (TT)

In tuberculoid leprosy (TT), skin lesions are well circumscribed, raised (infiltrated), or macular of varying sizes. The surface of the lesion is dry because of anhidrosis with or without hair loss. Thickening of cutaneous nerves in relation to lesion is common. If the lesion is over the distribution of a major nerve trunk, it may be enlarged. The routine skin smear examination is negative for AFB, and the lepromin test is strongly positive. The lesion may continue for a long time without any change, even under treatment.

BORDERLINE-TUBERCULOID LEPROSY (BT)

Skin lesions in borderline-tuberculoid leprosy (BT) present a morphologic resemblance of the lesions to TT leprosy. The number of skin lesions is more than four, sometimes numerous with bilateral distribution. Small satellite lesions may be seen around lesions. Patches may occupy large parts of the trunk or limbs but seldom the entire face. Lesions are rarely encountered in unusual sites like the penis, scrotum, scalp, palms, and soles. The edge is abrupt and well demarcated and may present as plaques and annular lesions with a band of infiltration at the periphery with a normal looking center.

MIDBORDERLINE LEPROSY (BB)

Midborderline leprosy (BB) has multiple lesions that tend to be symmetrical with varying sizes. Papules, plaques, and circinate lesions are evident. In the circinate lesions, the inner edge is abrupt, whereas the outer edge slopes toward the normal skin. Concentric or geographic patterns of lesions are also encountered. Patches may have an abrupt edge, whereas another part might be sloping. Rough or smooth surfaces may be seen in different lesions. Nerve damage depends on the BT element present in the individual case. Skin smears are moderately positive in many of the lesions and a there is a weak lepromin response.

BORDERLINE-LEPROMATOUS LEPROSY (BL)

Midborderline leprosy may evolve into borderline-lepromatous leprosy (BL). Lesions, soft in consistency, are always numerous, with symmetrical distribution and sloping margins; plaques may be small or medium sized. The face may show diffuse infiltration, which may be topped by occasional nodules over the pinna or chin. The patient may present with deformities of hands and feet because of damage to the nerves. Lesions may be seen on the eyelids, scrotum, penis, palms, soles, and scalp. The lepromin response is negative.

LEPROMATOUS LEPROSY (LL)

Lepromatous leprosy (LL) patients are anergic to *M. leprae*, and their tissues are ideal for multiplication of *M. leprae*. In early stages it presents as shiny, oily skin with diffuse infiltration. Papulonodular lesions gradually appear. Lepromata are also found in lymph nodes, spleen, liver, bone marrow, adrenal glands, smooth and striated muscles, and testes. The nose and eyes are frequently affected in LL. Saddle nose, blindness, madarosis, and gynecomastia form the late manifestations.

SPECIAL FORMS OF LEPROMATOUS LEPROSY

Lucio's Leprosy

Lucio's leprosy, only found in Mexico and Central America, is a special form of LL first described in 1852 by Lucio & Alvarado in Mexico. It is characterized by a diffuse, widespread infiltration of the skin with loss of sensation, hair, and eyebrows.

Histoid Leprosy

Histoid leprosy, described by Wade (1963), is characterized by the formation of firm, pedunculated nodules and/or plaques in the skin and subcutis of MB patients. A biopsy shows elongated or spindle-shaped histiocytes containing bacilli in a whorled arrangement.

Primary Neuritic Leprosy

Wade first recognized polyneuritic cases as a separate subgroup in the histoid leprosy classification. The Indian classification and the revised version have placed primary neuritic leprosy (PNL) as a distinct group in the classification. In an epidemiologic study of intensive long-term follow-up of a population of 8000 in a rural part of South India, Noordeen (1972) found the prevalence rate of pure polyneuritic leprosy to be 8.2 per 1000, and it formed 18% of the area's new cases. According to Browne, this variety is unknown in Africa. However, it is relatively common in India (Dongre, 1966; Bhushan and colleagues, 2004). Diagnosis is made on complaints of paresthesia, finding nerve thickening and sensory impairment in area of distribution of the nerve. A spectrum from TT to BL leprosy has been observed in the histopathology of polyneuritic leprosy. A positive lepromin response strongly indicates TT or BT leprosy. Ulnar, median, and lateral popliteal nerves are commonly involved. Cutaneous nerves like the sural, musculocutaneous, superficial radial, and great auricular are also included. Early diagnosis of pure neuritic leprosy is critical to prevent disabilities from developing.

Diagnosis

Leprosy mimics a variety of dermatologic and neurologic conditions, so it is imperative to rule out the area's other common, prevalent diseases. A doubtful case should be kept under observation until the cardinal signs are demonstrated. In diagnosing leprosy it is advisable to consider the information in the following sections.

HISTORY

Any hypopigmented skin patch that has been present for a considerable time, is not scaly, does not itch, increases in size gradually, and does not respond to topical drugs could be ascribed to leprosy. There may be diagnostic problems, especially in children, when lesions are on the cheeks. Generally these types of lesions are associated with helminthiasis, infection by

CURRENT DIAGNOSIS

Leprosy can be diagnosed by the presence of any one of the following cardinal signs:

- Hypopigmented or erythematous skin lesions with sensory impairment
- Enlargement of peripheral nerves associated with signs of sensory loss or muscle paralysis and pain in some stages of the disease
- Demonstration of acid-fast bacilli in skin smears

tinea versicolor, malnutrition, avitaminosis, and chronic rhinorrhea.

Family history is important because the contacts of cases of lepromatous leprosy are at higher risk than those of borderline or tuberculoid cases. A negative family history does not rule out leprosy, however, because in hyperendemic areas the disease may not necessarily be contracted from intrafamilial sources. Assessing sensory loss in adults is far easier than in children.

CLINICAL EXAMINATION

A thorough clinical examination includes the following:

- Examination should be from head to toe because solitary lesions have been observed, albeit rarely, even on scalp and the plantar surface of the foot. Involvement of external genital organs is not unusual.
- All the nerve trunks, including cutaneous nerves, must be examined carefully for thickening and tenderness irrespective of the presence or absence of skin lesions. Any beaded thickening or abscesses of nerves should be recorded carefully.
- Sensory testing is very important because anesthesia is one of the cardinal signs of leprosy. Depending on the types of nerve fiber involved, either all three sensory modalities (temperature, pain, and touch) or any one of them may be lost. It is generally observed that thermal sensation is lost first and touch sensation is the last to be affected. Touch and pain sensations are tested with a pointed pin, whereas thermal sensation is tested with a test tube containing hot and cold water. The WHO has developed a battery-operated thermal tester, a simple and handy instrument to test the sensation in the field.
- In pure neuritic leprosy, the peripheral loss of sensation (including loss of sweating) is directly proportional to the degree of nerve thickening in most cases. However, it has been observed that one or more nerve trunk may be grossly thickened, yet the loss of sensation in the related area may be minimal. Contrariwise, sensory loss and muscle wasting may be marked, although the nerve is not greatly thickened. This may be either because of treatment or to gradual fibrosis of the nerve.

LABORATORY DIAGNOSIS

The laboratory tests for leprosy are:

- **Skin smears:** Demonstration of AFB in the skin smears is a definite sign of leprosy. Diagnosis of leprosy by this technique is limited to approximately 20% of MB cases. The rest are negative for AFB. A negative skin smear, therefore, does not rule out leprosy.
- **Biopsy:** A good biopsy specimen of a skin lesion or of a nerve may be helpful in diagnosis and in accurate typing. In the very early stages of leprosy, however, a biopsy may not show any definite evidence and any changes may be nonspecific.
- **Serologic tests (uncommon):** Serologic tests involve the demonstration of circulating anti–PGL-IgM antibodies using a particle agglutination assay or enzyme-linked immunoabsorbent assay (ELISA) techniques but are low in sensitivity in PB leprosy and hence are unlikely to contribute to early diagnosis. Additionally antibodies to 35-kDa protein of *M. leprae* have been similarly tested for its value in early diagnosis with same results.
- **Polymerase chain reaction (PCR):** Procedures employing the PCR are extremely sensitive and are applicable on a variety of clinical specimens. Recently specific DNA probes have been developed that improve leprosy diagnosis. High sensitivity of the test makes it very vulnerable to cross reactivity leading to nonspecificity. However the technology has to be made very simple and cost effective for application under field conditions.
- **Electromyography:** This may be necessary in exceptional instances.
- **Lepromin test:** This is not a diagnostic test, but it is useful to find the level of CMI in any individual against leprosy infection. It contains suspension of autoclaved *M. leprae* obtained from leprosy patients and 0.1 mL is injected intradermally into the forearm. The reading after 48 to 72 hours (Fernandez reaction) and 3 to 4 weeks (Mitsuda reaction) are recorded. A Mitsuda reaction measuring less than 3 mm is negative, 3 mm to 5 mm is doubtful or weak, and greater than 5 mm is positive.

Chemotherapy

Concepts on chemotherapy in the management of leprosy have undergone a phenomenal change over the last two decades. Although the current multidrug therapy (MDT) advocated by WHO has been quite successful, a search for newer drugs continues.

WORLD HEALTH ORGANIZATION MULTIDRUG THERAPY: DOSE AND DURATION

Extensive data now available indicate the efficacy of fixed duration treatment (FDT) in terms of bacterial killing and relapses. There is no reason to continue the drugs until smear negativity is reached (Ganapati, 1987). Even persistence of clinical signs and symptoms in such

CURRENT THERAPY

- The MDT as recommended by the WHO is the standard and accepted treatment of all categories of untreated leprosy patients.
- All leprosy patients with active disease must be treated for 6 months in PB leprosy (two drugs) and 12 months in MB leprosy (three drugs) in full dosages without interruption.
- The success of MDT largely depends on effective drug delivery system and patients' compliance.
- Episodes of reactions are treated with anti-inflammatory drugs.

Abbreviations: MDT = multidrug therapy; MB = multibacillary PB = paucibacillary; WHO = World Health Organization.

patients may not be interpreted as an indication for continuation of chemotherapy (Ganapati, 1992). The success of MDT is evident from its efficacy to bring down prevalence rates. Almost negligible relapse rates have been reported in both PB and MB patients. WHO has recommended a standard regimen for the treatment of leprosy (Table 1).

UNIFORM MULTIDRUG THERAPY (U-MDT)

WHO (2002) has proposed a large-scale field trial of MB-MDT regimen for 6 months as uniform regimen for both PB and MB patients. Trials are in progress.

ACCOMPANIED MULTIDRUG THERAPY (A-MDT)

Accompanied MDT (A-MDT) is designed by WHO to address frequent problems in the field programs by providing only certain patients with a full course of treatment on their first visit to the leprosy clinic after diagnosis. WHO feels that A-MDT is user friendly and suitable to mobile populations, patients living in remote areas, and in the areas of civil strife.

NEWER CHEMOTHERAPEUTIC AGENTS

A review by Ganapati (1996) on newer drugs shows a lot of promise with several of them, as discussed in the following sections.

Fluoroquinolones

Ofloxacin (Floxin)[1] as a single dose has significant bactericidal activity but less than that of rifampicin (Rimactane).[1] This forms the basis of short-term clinical trials. A combination of ofloxacin (Floxin),[1] 400 mg, and rifampicin (Rimactane),[1] 600 mg, administered daily for 28 days is being tested, and results on relapses will be known shortly.

Tetracyclines

Minocycline (Minocin, Arestin)[1] is the only member of tetracycline group that has significant action against *M. leprae,* but much less than rifampin. This in a dose of 100 mg once a month forms a component of rifampin, ofloxacin, and minocycline (ROM) therapy.

Macrolides

Clarithromycin (Biaxin, Claribid),[1] the drug of choice in this group of compounds, has appreciable bactericidal activity. The adult dose is 500 mg daily. Although no specific recommendation is made on the combination and duration, clarithromycin (Biaxin, Claribid),[1] is advocated along with clofazimine (Lamprene, Hansepran), ofloxacin (Floxin),[1] and minocycline (Minocin, Arestin) in leprosy patients with proven rifampicin resistance or toxicity.[1]

---

[1]Not FDA approved for this indication.

TABLE 1 Standard World Health Organization Multidrug Therapy for Leprosy

		Less than 10 years	10–14 years	More than 14 years	Duration
PB Leprosy					
Monthly dose*	Rifampin (Rifadin)	300 mg	450 mg	600 mg	6m
Daily dose†	Dapsone	25 mg	50 mg	100 mg	
MB Leprosy					
Monthly dose*	Rifampicin (Rifadin)	300 mg	450 mg	600mg	12m
	Clofazimine (Lamprene)[1]	100 mg	150 mg	300 mg	
Daily dose†	Dapsone	25 mg	50 mg	100 mg	
	Clofazimine (Lamprene)[1]	50 mg biw	50 mg Alt. Day	50 mg	

*Monthly dose is always supervised.
†Daily dose is self-administered.
[1]Not FDA approved for this indication.
Abbreviations: biw = twice a week; m = months; MB = multibacillary; PB = paucibacillary.

Monthly Administered Compound for Multibacillary and Paucibacillary Leprosies

Efficacy of once-a-month ROM in both MB (for 12 months) and PB (for 6 months) leprosy patients is currently being conducted in Myanmar, Guinea, and Senegal. The final results will be available in mid-2007.

Newer Drug Combinations

Moxifloxacin (Avelox),[1] a new broad-spectrum fluoroquinolone, with minocycline and Rifapentine (Priftin)[1] is believed to be the most powerful bactericidal combination. Reports on human trials are anticipated.

WORLD HEALTH ORGANIZATION– RECOMMENDED COMBINATIONS (ROUTINE AND RESEARCH): A SUMMARY

Table 2 portrays how concepts on duration of treatment for MB and PB leprosies have changed over the years.

Reactions and Management

Uneventful response to chemotherapy, which occurs in most patients, may be intercepted in approximately 20% to 30% of patients by a phenomenon called *reactions*. Reactions may occur spontaneously or may be precipitated by other immunocompromised disorders.

---

[1]Not FDA approved for this indication.

---

[1]Not FDA approved for this indication.

TABLE 2 Evolution of Treatment Regimens for Leprosy

Regimen	Duration
DDS Mono-therapy*	Life-long (continuous)
WHO-MDT (21 days intensive therapy)*	24m or until skin smear negativity
WHO-MDT (Modified)*	24m or until skin smear negativity
WHO-MDT (FDT-24)*	24m (continuous)
WHO-MDT (FDT-12)†	12m (continuous)
WHO-MDT (FDT-6)†	6m (continuous)
ROM-12‡	12m (intermittent)
ROM-6‡	6m (intermittent)
RO‡	28 days (continuous)
ROM§-1	1 day (single dose)
P*MM*-1‡	1 day (single dose)

*Not in vogue.
†Universally recommended by WHO.
‡Trials in progress.
§In vogue for some time, now given up.
Abbreviations: m = months; M = minocycline (Minocin)[1]; *M* = moxifloxacin (Avelox)[1]; MDT = multidrug therapy; O = ofloxacin (Floxin)[1]; P = rifapentine (Priftin)[1]; R = rifampin (Rifadin)[1]; WHO = World Health Organization.[1]
[1]Not FDA approved for this indication.

TYPE I REACTIONS

Type I reactions are hypersensitivity reactions following an increase in the CMI. Neuritis is a common feature and may be associated with sudden muscle paralysis. The mainstay for treatment of type I reactions continues to be corticosteroids. Although type I, or reversal, reactions (RRs) are started on 30 mg to 40 mg of prednisolone (Prelone), once daily, Naafs (1979) observed that 15 mg to 20 mg was the critical dose of prednisolone to control a RR after the initial high dose of corticosteroids. The WHO recommends using a standard course of prednisolone (Prelone) for a total duration of 12 weeks, which is now available in blister calendar packs known as Prednipac.[2] The long-term, low-dose steroid therapy was observed to be more useful than high dose-short term steroid therapy in prevention of nerve damage. The newer and alternative drugs with promise like cyclosporine (Neoral) and azathioprine (Imuran) are under research.

TYPE II REACTION

The type II reaction is a humoral hypersensitivity reaction (erythema nodosum leprosum) and is not associated with alteration in CMI. In patients who are not responding to corticosteroid therapy, clofazimine, up to 300 mg per day, may be added or even thalidomide (Thalomid) can be considered under supervision and with precautions. The newer and alternative drugs with promise are pentoxifylline (Trental)[1] alone or in combination with clofazimine and/or prednisolone.

THALIDOMIDE ANALOGUES

The associated adverse effects of thalidomide analogues, such as teratogenicity, peripheral neuropathy, and drowsiness among others, may limit the use of thalidomide in clinical settings. Hence the thalidomide analogues like lenalidomide Revimid (CC-5013)* and Actimid (CC-4047),* which are chemically similar to thalidomide but appear to lack its side effects are being pursued.

Prevention of Disability

Approximately 25% of the patients who go undetected and untreated at an early stage of the disease develop deformities of hands, feet, and eyes. As a single disease entity, leprosy is one of the foremost causes of deformities leading to handicap. Deformities in leprosy are of two main types, primary and secondary. They may also be of the mixed variety with loss of sensation in their distribution, muscle weakness or paralysis, and lack of sweat and sebum causing physical damage to the affected limbs and eyes. Other deformities such as sagging face, loss of eyebrows, depressed nose, and gynecomastia mostly occur in LL. Most of the paralytic

---

[1]Not FDA approved for this indication.
[2]Not available in the United States.
*Investigational drug in the United States.

deformities can be partially or fully corrected by simple physiotherapy and with the use of aids and appliances. Every effort should be made to educate the patient to practice self-care measures to prevent worsening of deformities. Reconstructive surgery also plays an important role in restoring functional and cosmetic benefits. Rehabilitation measures should be considered as a means of reintegrating the needy individuals affected by leprosy into the community.

Epidemiology

A report published by the WHO (2003), states that the leprosy load in the world was reduced by approximately 90% in more than 100 countries by the end of the year 2002. Currently there are 523,605 registered cases in the world with a prevalence rate (PR) of 0.84 per 10,000 people. The total number of new cases detected during 2002 was 612,110, giving an annual new case detection rate of 0.98 per 10,000 people. As of the end of 2003, there are still 17 countries with a PR of more than 1 per 10,000 people and another 8 countries with a large number of leprosy cases. India reports 65.8% of the global leprosy cases.

REFERENCES

Bhushan K, Kaur I, Dogra S, Kumaran: Pure neuritic leprosy in India: An appraisal. Int J Lepr Other Mycobact Dis 2004;72(3)284-290.
Dongre VV, Ganapati R, Chulawala RG: A study of mononeuritic lesions in a leprosy clinic. Indian J Lepr 1966;48(2)132-137.
Ganapati R, Pai VV: Newer chemotherapeutic agents in leprosy, Editorial. Indian Journal of Dermatology 1996;41(l):1-4.
Ganapati R, Shroff HJ, Gandewar KL, et al: Five-year follow-up of multibacillary leprosy after fixed duration chemotherapy. Quaderni di cooperazione sanitaria—Health cooperation papers, Proceedings of the VI Symposium on Leprosy Research, Genoa, Italy, 1992;12,223-229.
Ganapati R, Revankar CR, Pai RR: Three years assessment of multibacillary leprosy cases. Indian J Lepr 1987;59(1)44-49.
Jopling WH: In Handbook of Leprosy, 3rd ed. London: William Heinemann Medical Books, 1984, pp 1-7.
Khanolkar VR: Pathology of leprosy. In Leprosy in Theory and Practice, 2nd ed. Bristol, UK, John Wright & Sons Limited, 1964, pp 125-151.
Naafs B, Pearson JMH, Wheate HW: Reversal reactions: The prevention of permanent nerve damage. Comparison of short and long term steroid treatment. Int J Lepr Other Mycobact Dis 1979; 47(1)7-12.
Noordeen, SK: Epidemiology of (poly)neuritic type of leprosy. Indian J Lepr 1972;44,90-96.
Ridley DS, Jopling WH: Classification of leprosy according to immunity. A five group system. Int J Lepr Other Mycobact Dis 1966; 34(3)255-277.
Scollard DM: Endothelial cells and the pathogenesis of lepromatous neuritis: Insights from the armadillo model. Microbes Infect 2000; 2(15)1835-1843.
Wade, HW: The histoid variety of lepromatous leprosy. Int J Lepr Other Mycobact Dis 1963;31,129
World Health Organization: Chemotherapy of Leprosy. Report of a WHO study group. Geneva, WHO Technical Report Series, No 847, 1994.
World Health Organization: Report on the third meeting of the WHO Technical Advisory group on elimination of leprosy. Brasilia, February 2002.
World Health Organization: Bulletin of the Leprosy Elimination Alliance, Jan-Jun, 2003. See also http://www.who.int/lep.

Malaria

Method of
Snehal N. Shah, MD, and
Peter B. Bloland, DVM, MPVM*

Malaria is caused by infection with one or more of the four species of human *Plasmodium: Plasmodium falciparum, Plasmodium vivax, Plasmodium ovale,* and *Plasmodium malariae.* Malaria is transmitted by the bite of an infected female *Anopheles* mosquito, which serves as the vector and definitive host for plasmodia. Rarely, malaria can be transmitted through exposure to infected blood and blood products, injection equipment, or organ transplantation (induced malaria); vertical transmission (congenital malaria); or an unidentified mechanism (cryptic malaria). *P. falciparum* and *P. vivax* are more common causes of malaria than are *P. ovale* and *P. malariae. P. falciparum* is the species responsible for most of the morbidity and mortality associated with malaria infection.

Despite significant progress in malaria control over the last two decades, malaria remains one of the most prevalent infectious diseases in the world. There are 300 million to 500 million cases every year, and more than 1 million deaths, mostly of children younger than 5 years of age, are attributable to this disease. The majority of those at risk for malaria, which includes more than 40% of the world's population, live in countries that lack the resources to combat the disease. The burden of malaria is greatest in the developing world, where it is not only a leading cause of morbidity and mortality but a major barrier to economic development.

In nonendemic countries, imported malaria (malaria acquired while traveling in an endemic area) remains a concern. Each year in the United States, more than 21 million people travel to malaria-endemic countries. The Centers for Disease Control and Prevention (CDC) reported more than 1300 cases of imported malaria and 8 malaria deaths in the United States in 2002. There were five cases of malaria in individuals who did not have a travel history: one case of congenitally acquired *P. vivax* infection, one case of transfusion-transmitted *P. malariae* infection, one case of cryptic *P. falciparum* infection, and two cases of probable locally acquired mosquito-borne *P. vivax* infection.

In areas where malaria is not endemic, such as the United States, locally acquired mosquito-borne transmission of malaria (introduced malaria) can occur when a local mosquito acquires the parasite by biting an infected individual and then transmits that infection to another individual. There have been 11 outbreaks of locally acquired mosquito-borne malaria transmission in the United States since 1992, with the most recent

*The use of trade names is for identification purposes only and does not imply endorsement by USPHS or the U.S. Department of Health and Human Services.

one involving eight cases of *P. vivax* infection in Florida in 2003. Although the United States was officially recognized as being malaria-free in 1970, competent malaria vectors continue to exist in the 48 continental states. Local transmission can occur whenever gametocytemic individuals, competent vectors, conducive environmental conditions, and opportunities for exposure of susceptible individuals to mosquitoes come together.

Etiology

Infection with protozoa of the genus *Plasmodium* causes malaria. Only four species of *Plasmodium* typically cause clinical disease in humans: *P. falciparum, P. vivax, P. ovale,* and *P. malariae.* Transmission occurs with the inoculation of sporozoites into humans from the salivary glands of a female *Anopheles* mosquito during a blood meal. The sporozoites pass rapidly into the liver, infecting hepatocytes. Within the hepatocytes, the sporozoites undergo asexual multiplication and development in a process called exoerythrocytic schizogony. After 6 to 14 days, each infected hepatocyte contains a tissue schizont that releases thousands of merozoites, which in turn infect susceptible red blood cells. In the erythrocyte, the merozoite develops into a trophozoite. After a period of growth, the trophozoite undergoes asexual reproduction, or erythrocytic schizogony, to produce a blood schizont that contains merozoites. The merozoites, when released from the erythrocyte, invade new red blood cells to continue the cycle. Some merozoites develop into sexual forms: the microgametocytes (male) and macrogametocytes (female). Both male and female gametocytes must be ingested during a blood meal by a female *Anopheles* mosquito for the sexual life cycle to occur in the mosquito's gut. In a process involving several steps, sporozoites are produced in the wall of the mosquito's gut and migrate to the salivary glands; they are transmitted to humans when the mosquito takes its next blood meal, completing the life cycle.

In *P. vivax* and *P. ovale* infections, some sporozoites may not enter exoerythrocytic schizogony but instead develop into latent forms, or hypnozoites. These forms may reactivate later to complete exoerythrocytic schizogony and cause acute illness. The resulting infection, which is termed a relapse, can occur months to years after the initial infection. Persons with *P. vivax* or *P. ovale* infection can have multiple relapses for up to 4 years and occasionally longer after the primary infection. However, if *P. vivax* or *P. ovale* infections are acquired congenitally or through exposure to blood or blood products, no liver phase occurs and therefore relapses cannot occur. Neither *P. falciparum* nor *P. malariae* has a hypnozoite form. However, if *P. malariae* infection is not treated, symptomatic recrudescences, often associated with splenectomy or immunosuppression, can occur decades after the primary infection.

The incubation period, or the period from infection to the appearance of symptoms, is species-dependent. The incubation period is 9 to 14 days for *P. falciparum*, 12 to 17 days (or up to 6 to 12 months after initial infection with some strains) for *P. vivax*, 16 to 18 days for

P. ovale, and 18 to 40 days (or longer) for *P. malariae.* Individuals taking chemoprophylaxis and those who have acquired partial immunity from repeated exposure to malaria infection may experience a prolonged incubation period.

Epidemiology

Malaria is endemic to Africa, South Asia, Southeast Asia, parts of Central Asia and the Caucasus, Oceania, Central America, parts of South America, Haiti and the Dominican Republic, and parts of Turkey and the Middle East. The species-specific geographic distribution is presented in Table 1. *P. falciparum* is the most common species in the tropics and subtropics. *P. vivax* is prevalent in many temperate zones as well as in the tropics and subtropics, making it the species with the widest geographic distribution. Together, *P. falciparum* and *P. vivax* account for more than 90% of clinical malaria infections worldwide.

The development of resistance to antimalarial drugs has complicated malaria prophylaxis and treatment. Species-specific resistance patterns are presented in Table 1. Knowledge of species-specific resistance patterns is essential to making appropriate decisions about chemoprophylaxis and treatment.

Clinical Manifestations

The clinical presentation of malaria is nonspecific; therefore, clinicians must maintain a high index of suspicion of malaria and routinely elicit a travel history from febrile patients. The clinical presentation of malaria can vary substantially, depending on the infecting species, the level of parasitemia, and the immune status of the patient. The initial clinical symptoms usually include a flulike prodrome with headache, malaise, and myalgias that is followed by fever. In travelers with these symptoms, the differential diagnosis should include meningitis, typhoid fever, dengue fever and other arboviral infections, leptospirosis, typhus, hepatitis, and influenza.

Malaria paroxysms are produced when infected red blood cells rupture and release merozoites. After a number of cycles of erythrocytic schizogony, the release of merozoites may become synchronized, resulting in classic cyclic fevers. With *P. falciparum, P. vivax,* and *P. ovale* infections (tertian malaria), the paroxysm may occur in 48-hour cycles, whereas with *P. malariae* infections (quartan malaria), the cycles are 72 hours. However, patients, particularly those with *P. falciparum*, may not develop cyclic paroxysms at all, and so a lack of cyclic fevers should not rule out a diagnosis of malaria. Other symptoms include headache, chills, rigors, myalgias and arthralgias, and abdominal pain. Patients also may complain of diarrhea, vomiting, chest pain, and cough. The presence of gastrointestinal and respiratory symptoms should not lead the physician to exclude malaria as a potential diagnosis. On physical examination, a patient may have jaundice, tachycardia, hypotension (usually secondary to dehydration), and splenomegaly.

TABLE 1 Species Distribution and Drug Resistance Pattern

Species	Known Geographic Distribution	Drug Resistance Pattern
Plasmodium falciparum	Most malaria-endemic areas except Republic of Korea, China north of Yunnan province, and some areas of Central Asia and the Caucasus	• Chloroquine (Aralen) resistance in nearly all endemic countries with the exception of Haiti, the Dominican Republic, Central America west of the Panama Canal, and parts of the Middle East (resistance identified in Iran, Oman, Saudi Arabia, and Yemen) • Sulfadoxine pyrimethamine (Fansidar) resistance widespread in South America, Southeast Asia, and Africa • Mefloquine (Lariam) resistance in parts of Southeast Asia • Reduced susceptibility to quinine in Southeast Asia; longer course of therapy required
Plasmodium vivax	• Central and South America, South Asia, Southeast Asia, Oceania, parts of Middle East, Mexico, North Africa, and Horn of Africa • Not common to absent in sub-Saharan Africa, Haiti, and Dominican Republic	Chloroquine resistance in Papua New Guinea, Indonesia, and East Timor; sporadically reported elsewhere
Plasmodium ovale	• Sub-Saharan Africa • Reported sporadically in southern China, Burma, and Southeast Asia	Chloroquine resistance not documented
Plasmodium malariae	As for P. falciparum	Chloroquine resistance not documented

Laboratory abnormalities in cases of uncomplicated malaria may include mild anemia, an elevated reticulocyte count, thrombocytopenia, lymphopenia, hyperbilirubinemia, and mildly elevated transaminases.

An uncomplicated malaria infection can progress to severe disease or death within hours. Risk factors for severe malaria include delays in treatment, inadequate or inappropriate treatment, a high parasite burden, and lack of acquired immunity. P. falciparum, more than any other species of Plasmodium, is responsible for the severe disease and death associated with malaria. This tendency has been linked to several features of this species. The tissue and blood schizonts in P. falciparum release a larger number of merozoites when they rupture, resulting in a more rapid rise in parasitemia. P. falciparum, unlike the other species, can infect both reticulocytes and mature erythrocytes. In addition, P. falciparum–infected erythrocytes adhere to the vascular endothelium of postcapillary venules. It is believed that cytoadherence and severe anemia contribute to tissue hypoxia and end-organ dysfunction.

Severe malaria is associated with a 15% to 20% mortality rate. Signs and symptoms of severe malaria include impaired consciousness, unarousable coma (cerebral malaria), generalized convulsions, severe normocytic anemia, acute renal failure, pulmonary edema, acute respiratory distress syndrome, hypotension and circulatory collapse, disseminated intravascular coagulation, spontaneous bleeding, metabolic acidosis, hypoglycemia, hemoglobinuria, jaundice, and/or a parasitemia greater than 5%.

Cerebral malaria entails an unarousable coma that is not attributable to any other cause in a patient infected with P. falciparum. It is a life-threatening complication with an estimated 10% to 40% mortality rate. Coma or impaired mental status caused by malaria has to be distinguished from other causes of neurologic symptoms, including hyperpyrexia, hypoglycemia, and concurrent infections. Signs of cerebral malaria may range from disorientation to focal neurologic signs to unarousable coma with extensor posturing (including decorticate or decerebrate rigidity) or opisthotonos.

Complications with other species are rare. Splenic rupture has been described in patients who, because of long-standing untreated P. vivax infection, have developed massive splenomegaly. With effective chemotherapy, this complication is unusual. Nephritis is a rare complication of persistent P. malariae infection but occurs more commonly in children.

Diagnosis

To provide appropriate therapy, it is essential to identify the infecting malaria species, determine where the infection was acquired, and determine the parasite density. Initial evaluation of individuals with slide-confirmed malaria ideally also should include glucose, a complete blood count, electrolytes, creatinine, urea, and liver function tests. In patients with severe disease or respiratory symptoms, lactate level and arterial blood gas to determine acid-base status also should be obtained.

Malaria should be considered in any febrile patient with a history of travel to an area of malaria transmission regardless of whether the patient gives a history of taking prophylaxis. Information on the location and duration of the trip, the date of return, the history of prophylaxis, and the date of symptom onset enables the physician to assess the risk of malaria and, if necessary, choose an appropriate course of treatment. Rapid diagnosis and institution of antimalarial treatment can prevent the development of severe morbidity and mortality. A list of key diagnostic points, including risk factors for malaria, clinical presentation, and useful laboratory investigations, is presented in the Current Diagnosis box.

A thick and a thin blood smear should be obtained from any patient suspected of having malaria. Blood smears can be used to detect the presence of parasites, identify the species, and determine the parasite density. Initial blood smears may be negative, particularly in symptomatic semi-immunes and those taking prophylaxis. Consequently, a diagnosis of malaria cannot be dismissed on the basis of a single negative smear. Blood smears should be repeated every 12 to 24 hours for a total of 48 to 72 hours before the diagnosis of malaria is excluded. Most patients with clinical symptoms caused by malaria will have detectable parasites on well-stained thick blood smears within 48 hours.

Blood smears should be prepared with Giemsa stain and examined under light microscopy. Thick blood smears are more sensitive in detecting malaria parasites, and thin smears are more reliable for identifying species.

CURRENT DIAGNOSIS

Risk factors for malaria:

- Travel to malaria-endemic areas (including duration of journey and date of return)
- Malaria prophylaxis
- Compliance with malaria prophylaxis
- History of blood transfusion, organ transplant, intravenous drug use
- History of malaria
- Exposure to mosquitoes
- Visitors from endemic areas

Clinical presentation (can be very nonspecific):

- Prodrome with headaches, myalgias, malaise,
- Fever (cyclic?)
- Chills
- Rigors
- Abdominal pain, nausea, vomiting, diarrhea
- Respiratory distress
- Splenomegaly
- Tachycardia
- Hypotension
- Jaundice
- Seizures
- Altered consciousness/coma

Initial laboratory investigations:

- Thick and thin blood smear required for diagnosis
  Thick smear used for parasite detection
  Thin smear used for species identification and determination of parasite density
- Complete blood count
- Electrolytes
- Blood urea nitrogen
- Creatinine
- Liver function tests

Both thick and thin smears should be scanned at low magnification and then examined using the 100× oil immersion lens. To determine the percent parasitemia using the thin smear, one should count the parasitized erythrocytes among 500 to 2000 erythrocytes and divide the number of parasitized erythrocytes by the total number of erythrocytes counted and multiply by 100. An alternative method that is used less commonly calculates the parasite density by using the thick smear. To avoid missing low-density infections, at least 300 high-power fields should be examined before a slide is considered negative. Further details about preparation and interpretation of smears can be found at the CDC's Division of Parasitic Diseases diagnostic Internet site: http://www.dpd.cdc.gov/dpdx.

The severity of malaria may vary with the percent parasitemia. Persons with parasitemia lower than 1% usually have mild disease. Individuals with 1% to 5% parasitemia can have manifestations of more moderate disease. Although severe malaria can occur even with apparently low parasitemia, persons with greater than 5% parasitemia are at high risk for severe malaria.

If malaria parasites are detected, blood smears should be repeated every 12 to 24 hours, depending on the severity of illness, until the smears are negative. Sequential smears are useful for monitoring the response to treatment and detecting potential drug failure. Although gametocytes may persist much longer, blood smears should be negative for asexual parasites within 48 to 72 hours after the completion of therapy or sooner when more rapidly acting drugs or longer-duration treatment (such as quinine) is used.

Alternative methods for diagnosis are available. Rapid diagnostic tests (RDTs) detect the presence of parasite antigens by measuring either histidine-rich protein-2 (HRP-2) or parasite lactate dehydrogenase (pLDH). Determination of parasite density is not possible with these methods. These assays are not approved by the U.S. Food and Drug Administration (FDA) and are not available in the United States. The polymerase chain reaction (PCR) method may be more sensitive for detecting parasites than is microscopy. PCR is particularly valuable for identifying a the species of a parasite when that cannot be determined by morphology alone. Currently, PCR is used mostly as a research tool and is available only in reference laboratories . Malaria serology detects antibodies to all four species but cannot be used to diagnose current infections. However, it may be useful for identifying an infective donor in cases of transfusion-related malaria, investigating congenital malaria, confirming malaria diagnosis in empirically treated nonimmunes, and diagnosing tropical splenomegaly syndrome.

Antimalarial Drugs

Because of the emergence and spread of drug-resistant strains, the slow rate of development of new antimalarial drugs, and the infrequency with which new drugs that are developed are submitted for FDA approval, relatively few drugs are available for the prophylaxis and treatment of malaria infections in the United States. The choice of antimalarial therapy should be guided by several factors: the infecting species, where it was acquired (or at least a travel history), drug resistance patterns, and percent parasitemia. Details about the specific drugs are given later in this article. Treatment options are discussed in the next section.

Quinine sulfate (oral) and its dextroisomer, quinidine gluconate (intravenous and oral[1]), are blood schizonticides that are effective against the erythrocytic stages of all four species of plasmodia and are also active against the gametocytes of *P. vivax, P. ovale,* and *P. malariae.* Common side effects include cinchonism, a syndrome of tinnitus, deafness, headache, nausea, and visual disturbance, as well as hyperinsulinemic hypoglycemia. The longer the duration of therapy, the higher the risk of adverse events. To shorten the course of therapy, quinine and intravenous quinidine often can be combined with doxycycline (Vibramycin),[1] tetracycline,[1] or clindamycin (Cleocin)[1] (see the treatment section for details).

Mefloquine (Lariam*) is a long-acting blood schizonticide that is effective against the erythrocytic stages of all four species. Mefloquine is used most commonly for prophylaxis but will not prevent *P. vivax* and *P. ovale* relapses. Side effects include nausea, vomiting, diarrhea, abdominal pain, mild neuropsychiatric complaints (dizziness, headache, somnolence, sleep disorders), myalgia, a mild skin rash, and fatigue. Mefloquine has been associated with rare serious adverse reactions such as seizures and psychoses at prophylactic doses. Although mefloquine can be used to treat chloroquine-resistant *P. falciparum,* adverse reactions are more common at the higher doses used for treatment. Because other options that have fewer adverse events are available for treatment, mefloquine normally is not recommended. Mefloquine is contraindicated for use in patients with known hypersensitivity to the drug and persons with a history of psychiatric disease. Mefloquine also is contraindicated in persons with a history of seizures (not including febrile seizures in childhood). It should be avoided in patients with cardiac conduction disorders because it prolongs the QTc interval and should be used with caution in persons taking β-blockers. Concomitant administration of mefloquine and quinine or quinidine may produce arrhythmias and increase the risk of convulsions. Mefloquine prophylaxis in the second and third trimesters is not associated with an adverse fetal or pregnancy outcome. More limited data suggest that it is probably safe in the first trimester.

Atovaquone-proguanil (Malarone*), a fixed combination antimalarial drug that is active against both blood and tissue schizonts, can be used for prophylaxis and treatment of chloroquine-resistant *P. falciparum.* The most common side effects are abdominal pain, nausea, vomiting, and headache. Atovaquone-proguanil should not be used for prophylaxis in children who weigh less than 11 kg or for treatment in children who weigh less than 5 kg. It is contraindicated in pregnant women, women who are breast-feeding infants who weigh less than 11 kg, and persons with severe renal impairment.

Chloroquine phosphate (Aralen phosphate) and chloroquine sulfate (Nivaquine)[2] are blood schizonticides that are active against the erythrocytic stages of all four *Plasmodium* species. Chloroquine also has gametocytocidal activity against *P. vivax, P. ovale,* and *P. malariae.* Chloroquine is the treatment of choice for susceptible strains of *P. falciparum* and *P. vivax* as well as for the treatment of *P. ovale* or *P. malariae* infections. Chloroquine can be taken safely by pregnant women and children. Side effects include gastrointestinal disturbance, dizziness, blurred vision, insomnia, headache, and pruritis. Overdose (ingestion of more than 25 mg of base per kilogram at one time) can lead to acute toxic effects. The toxic effects are predominantly cardiac, leading to cardiac arrest and respiratory failure, usually within 1 to 3 hours after an overdose. For adults, 2.5 to 3 g base may be a fatal dose; for children, 30 to 50 mg base per kg may be fatal.

Tetracyclines are blood schizonticides that are effective against the erythrocytic stages of all four species of *Plasmodium.* They have some activity against liver schizonts, but not enough to prevent relapses. Tetracyclines[1] should never be used alone for treatment. Combined with quinine or quinidine, they are effective against chloroquine-resistant *P. falciparum* and *P. vivax.* Doxycycline (Vibramycin) alone is effective as prophylaxis against chloroquine-resistant and mefloquine-resistant *P. falciparum.* Side effects include gastrointestinal symptoms, *Candida* vaginitis or stomatitis, and idiosyncratic photosensitivity reactions. Tetracyclines should not be used in pregnant women or in children younger than 8 years old.

Clindamycin (Cleocin)[1] is active against blood schizonts of all four species of *Plasmodium.* Clindamycin can be used in combination with quinine to treat chloroquine-resistant *P. falciparum* infections in people who are not able to take doxycycline. Side effects include diarrhea, nausea, and skin rashes. Bloody diarrhea secondary to *Clostridium difficile* has been reported.

Derivatives of artemisinin (such as artesunate,[2] artemether,[2] and dihyroartemisinin[2]) are compounds derived from the Chinese medicinal plant quinghaosu (*Artemisia annua*) that are active against blood schizonts and gametocytes. Artemisinin and its derivatives are short-acting, highly effective antimalarial drugs for the treatment of uncomplicated multidrug-resistant *P. falciparum* and severe *P. falciparum* infection. These drugs are available in oral, rectal, and intravenous formulations. Although they can be used alone for 5 to 7 days, combining them with other antimalarial drugs

---

[1]Not FDA approved for this indication.
*Use of trade names is for identification purposes only and does not imply endorsement by the United States Public Health Service or the United States Department of Health and Human Services.

---

[1]Not FDA approved for this indication.
[2]Not available in the United States.

can treat malaria infection effectively and decrease the length of treatment to as little as 3 days. Therefore, using these drugs as a component of combination therapy is recommended. Commonly used artemisinin-based combination therapies (ACTs) include artesunate combined with mefloquine, sulfadoxine-pyrimethamine (Fansidar), or amodiaquine.[2] Artemether plus lumefantrine (Coartem or Riamet)[2] is currently the only coformulated ACT available. Artemisinin and its derivatives are not available in the United States.

Primaquine phosphate, a tissue schizonticide with gametocytocidal properties, is the only drug available to prevent relapse of *P. vivax* and *P. ovale* infections. Primaquine may be used for primary prophylaxis when other prophylactic agents are contraindicated or unavailable. Primaquine can cause hemolysis and methemoglobinemia in glucose-6-phosophate dehydrogenase (G6PD)-deficient persons. Before primaquine is used, G6PD deficiency must be ruled out by appropriate laboratory testing. The most common side effect is abdominal pain. Primaquine is contraindicated in pregnant and breast-feeding women.

Treatment

GENERAL INFORMATION

Ideally, treatment for malaria should not be initiated until the diagnosis has been confirmed by laboratory investigations. Empirical treatment should be reserved for extreme situations (e.g., an individual has severe illness and the clinician has a strong clinical suspicion but is unable to obtain prompt laboratory diagnosis). Once the diagnosis is confirmed, appropriate antimalarial therapy must be initiated immediately. The choice of treatment should be guided by the degree of parasitemia and the species of *Plasmodium* found, the clinical status of the patient, and the likely drug susceptibility of the infecting species as determined by where the infection was acquired. Although all four species require treatment with a rapidly acting blood schizonticide, patients with *P. vivax* or *P. ovale* also require treatment with primaquine phosphate to decrease the likelihood of a relapse.

Species identification is necessary to distinguish falciparum malaria from nonfalciparum malaria. *P. falciparum* can cause rapid progression of disease and death. Patients with *P. falciparum*, mixed infections with *P. falciparum*, or infections in which the species cannot be identified immediately should be hospitalized and monitored closely. If the infecting species or probable origin of infection cannot be determined, patients should be treated for multidrug-resistant *P. falciparum* until otherwise identified.

Using available clinical and laboratory data, physicians must determine whether a patient has uncomplicated or severe malaria. Individuals with uncomplicated malaria typically can be treated with oral therapy but may need parenteral therapy if they are unable to take oral medication because of nausea, vomiting, or other reasons. Individuals with severe malaria should be treated at least initially with parenteral malaria therapy.

For detailed treatment information, including doses and frequency of therapy, refer to the Current Therapy box.

DRUG-RESISTANT *P. FALCIPARUM*

For *P. falciparum* infections acquired in chloroquine-resistant areas, there are three treatment options: quinine sulfate plus doxycycline (Vibramycin),[1] tetracycline,[1] or clindamycin (Cleocin)[1]; atovaquone-proguanil (Malarone[1]) alone; and mefloquine alone. Because mefloquine has a higher rate of severe neuropsychiatric reactions at treatment doses, it is not recommended unless the other two options are not available. Also, mefloquine is not recommended for the treatment of falciparum malaria in persons who acquired the infection in Burma, Thailand, or Cambodia because of the potential for mefloquine-resistant strains.

CHLOROQUINE-SENSITIVE *P. FALCIPARUM*, *P. VIVAX*, *P. OVALE*, AND *P. MALARIAE*

For *P. malariae*, *P. ovale*, chloroquine-sensitive *P. vivax*, and chloroquine-sensitive *P. falciparum* infection, prompt treatment with oral chloroquine phosphate (Aralen) is recommended. In addition, infections with *P. vivax* and *P. ovale* require primaquine to reduce the likelihood of a relapse. Before starting primaquine treatment, patients must be screened for G6PD deficiency.

DRUG-RESISTANT *P. VIVAX*

Chloroquine-resistant *P. vivax* should be treated with either quinine sulfate plus doxycycline (Vibramycin)[1] or tetracycline[1] or with mefloquine alone. After screening for G6PD deficiency, chloroquine-resistant *P. vivax* should be treated with primaquine phosphate. Some *P. vivax* infections acquired in Southeast Asia or Oceania can be poorly responsive to normal doses of primaquine.

SEVERE MALARIA

Patients diagnosed with severe malaria and those who are unable to take oral medications because of depressed sensorium, vomiting, or other reasons should be treated with parenteral antimalarial therapy. Severe malaria is a medical emergency, and treatment with intravenous (IV) quinidine should be initiated immediately (see Current Therapy box). If possible, the patient should be admitted to an intensive care unit. Continuous blood pressure and cardiac monitoring (to follow the QT interval) and regular assessments of blood glucose are strongly recommended for patients who receive quinidine therapy. In addition to antimalarial therapy, patients should receive the necessary supportive care. The airway should be secured, and breathing and circulation assessed.

---

[2]Not available in the United States.

[1]Not FDA approved for this indication.

CURRENT THERAPY

Diagnosis	Recommended Drug	Adult Dose	Pediatric Dose
Chloroquine-sensitive uncomplicated *Plasmodium falciparum*	Chloroquine phosphate (Aralen)	600 mg base (= 1 g salt) PO, then 300 mg base (500 mg salt) at 6, 24, 48h.	10 mg base/kg PO, then 5 mg base/kg at 6, 24, 48h.
Chloroquine-resistant uncomplicated *P. falciparum* OR resistance unknown OR species unknown	Quinine sulfate* *plus* one of the following: Doxycycline (Vibramycin),[†1] Tetracycline,[†] or Clindamycin (Cleocin)[†]	Quinine sulfate: 650 mg salt (= 542 mg base) PO tid × 3–7d, *PLUS EITHER:* Doxycycline: 100 mg PO bid × 7d, OR Tetracycline: 250 mg PO qid × 7d, OR Clindamycin: 20 mg (base)/kg/d PO divided tid × 7d.	Quinine sulfate: 10 mg salt/kg (8.3 mg base/kg) PO tid × 3–7d, *PLUS EITHER:* Doxycycline: 4 mg/kg/d PO divided bid × 7d, OR Tetracycline: 25 mg/kg/d PO divided qid × 7d, OR Clindamycin: 20 mg (base)/kg/d PO divided tid × 7d.
	Atovaquone-proguanil (Malarone)	4 adult tabs PO qd × 3d Adult tab = 250 mg atovaquone/100 mg proguanil.	5–8 kg: 2 peds tabs PO qd × 3d, 9–10 kg: 3 peds tabs PO qd × 3d, 11–20 kg: 1 adult tab PO qd × 3d, 21–30 kg: 2 adult tabs PO qd × 3d, 31–40 kg: 3 adult tabs PO qd × 3d, >40 kg: 4 adult tabs PO qd × 3d, Peds tab = 62.5mg atovaquone/25 mg proguanil.
	Mefloquine[‡] (Lariam)	750 mg salt (= 684 mg base) PO as initial dose, followed by 500 mg salt (= 456 mg base) PO given 6–12h after initial dose.	15 mg salt/kg (= 13.7 mg base/kg) PO as initial dose, followed by 10 mg salt/kg (= 9.1 mg base/kg) PO given 6–12h after initial dose.
Uncomplicated *Plasmodium malariae*	Chloroquine phosphate	600 mg base (= 1 g salt) PO, then 300 mg base (500 mg salt) at 6, 24, 48h.	10 mg base/kg PO, then 5 mg base/kg at 6, 24, 48h.
Uncomplicated *Plasmodium vivax* or *Plasmodium ovale* except chloroquine-resistant *P. vivax*	Chloroquine phosphate *plus* Primaquine phosphate	Chloroquine phosphate: 600 mg base (= 1g salt) PO, then 300 mg base (500 mg salt) at 6, 24, 48h. Primaquine phosphate: 30 mg (base)[3] PO qd × 14 days.	Chloroquine phosphate:10 mg base/kg PO, then 5 mg base/kg at 6, 24, 48h. Primaquine phosphate: 0.6 mg (base)/kg[2] PO qd × 14d.
Chloroquine-resistant *P. vivax*	Quinine sulfate[1] *plus* one of the following: Doxycycline,[1,†] Tetracycline,[1,†] or Clindamycin[1]	Quinine sulfate: 650 mg salt (= 542 mg base/kg) PO tid × 3–7d, *plus either*: Doxycycline: 100 mg PO bid × 7d, OR Tetracycline: 250 mg PO qid × 7d, OR Clindamycin: 20 mg (base)/kg/d PO divided tid × 7d.	Quinine sulfate: 10 mg salt/kg (8.3 mg base/kg) PO tid × 3–7d, *plus either*: Doxycycline: 4 mg/kg/day PO divided bid × 7d, OR Tetracycline: 25 mg/kg/day PO divided qid × 7d, OR Clindamycin: 20 mg (base)/kg/day PO divided tid × 7d.
	Mefloquine *plus* primaquine phosphate	Mefloquine: 750 mg salt (= 684 mg base) PO as initial dose, followed by 500 mg salt (= 456 mg base) PO given 6–12h after initial dose. Primaquine phosphate: 30 mg (base)[2] PO qd × 14d.	Mefloquine: 15 mg salt/kg (= 13.7 mg base/kg) PO as initial dose, followed by 10 mg salt/kg (= 9.1 mg base/kg) PO given 6–12h after initial dose. Primaquine phosphate: 0.6 mg (base)/kg[2] PO qd × 14d.

Continued

CURRENT THERAPY—cont'd

Diagnosis	Recommended Drug	Adult Dose	Pediatric Dose
Chloroquine-sensitive infection during pregnancy[§]	Chloroquine phosphate	600 mg base (= 1 g salt) PO, then 300 mg base (500 mg salt) at 6, 24, 48h.	Not applicable.
Chloroquine-resistant *P. talciparum* infection during pregnancy	Quinine sulfate* plus clindamycin[1]	Quinine sulfate: 650 mg salt (= 542 mg base) PO tid × 3–7d, *plus* Clindamycin: 20 mg (base)/kg/day PO divided tid × 7d.	Not applicable.
Chloroquine-resistant *P. vivax* infection during pregnancy	Quinine sulfate	Quinine sulfate: 650 mg salt (= 542 mg base) PO tid × 7d.	Not applicable.
Severe malaria	Quinidine gluconate[(ParaMarks)] *plus* one of the following: Doxycycline,[1,†] Tetracycline,[1,†] or Clindamycin[1]	Quinidine gluconate: 6.25 mg/kg base (= 10 mg salt/kg) loading dose IV over 1–2h, then 0.0125 mg/kg/min base (= 0.02 mg salt/kg/min) continuous infusion for at least 24h; once parasite density <1% and patient can take oral medication, complete treatment with oral quinine, dose as above. Quinidine/quinine course = 7 days in multidrug-resistant areas; = 3 days in non–multidrug-resistant areas. *plus either:* Doxycycline: 100 mg PO bid × 7d; If patient not able to take oral medication, may start IV dose at 100 mg q 12h and then switch to oral doxycycline (as above) as soon as patient is able. For IV use, avoid rapid administration. OR Tetracycline: 250 mg PO qid × 7d OR Clindamycin: 20 mg (base)/kg/d PO divided tid × 7d. If patient not able to take oral medication, give IV loading dose of 10 mg (base)/kg followed by 5 mg (base)/kg IV every 8h. Switch to oral clindamycin (oral dose as above) as soon as patient is able. For IV use, avoid rapid administration.	Quinidine gluconate: Same mg/kg dosing and recommendations as for adults, *plus either:* Doxycycline: 4 mg/kg/d PO divided bid × 7d; If patient not able to take oral medication, may start IV dose. For children <45 kg, give 4 mg/kg IV q12h and then switch to oral doxycycline (dose as above) as soon as patient is able. For children >45 kg, use same dosing as for adults. For IV use, avoid rapid administration. OR Tetracycline: 25 mg/kg/d PO divided qid × 7d, OR Clindamycin: 20 mg (base)/kg/d PO divided tid × 7d. If patient not able to take oral medication, give IV loading dose of 10 mg. (base)/kg followed by 5 mg (base)/kg IV q8h. Switch to oral clindamycin (oral dose as above) as soon as patient is able. For IV use, avoid rapid administration. Treatment course = 7d.

[1]Not FDA approved for this indication.
[2]Exceeds dosage recommended by the manufacturer.
*Quinine course = 3 days if infection was acquired in South America and Africa. Quinine course = 7 days if infection was acquired in Southeast Asia.
[†]Doxycycline and tetracycline are not indicated for use in children younger than 8 years of age.
[‡]Because of resistant strains, treatment with mefloquine is not recommended in persons who have acquired infections from the Southeast Asian region of Burma, Thailand, and Cambodia.
[§]All pregnant women with *P. vivax* and *P. ovale* infection should be given chloroquine prophylaxis for the duration of the pregnancy to avoid relapses and can be treated with primaquine after delivery.
[(ParaMarks)] Patients should be given a loading dose of quinidine unless they have received more than 40 mg/kg of quinine in the preceding 48 hours or if they received mefloquine treatment within the preceding 12 hours.
Abbreviations: bid = twice a day; IV = intravenous; PO = orally; qd = every day; tid = three times a day.

Fluid status, level of consciousness, and vital signs including blood pressure, temperature, and respiratory rate should be monitored closely. Because these patients are at risk for hypoglycemia, severe anemia, renal failure, and acidosis, regular assessment of blood glucose, hemoglobin/hematocrit, creatinine, urea, electrolytes, and acid-base status also is required. Patients are potentially at risk for septicemia and may require parenteral antibiotics. Severe anemia requires blood transfusion with packed red blood cells. Dialysis is usually necessary in patients with acute renal failure. Oxygen and other respiratory support may be required in individuals with noncardiogenic pulmonary edema. Corticosteroids should not be used because they have not been shown to provide benefit and have been associated with increased mortality in this setting. One should consider exchange transfusion if parasitemia is greater than 10% or if the patient has altered mental status, noncardiogenic pulmonary edema, or renal complications. Blood smears should be repeated every 8 to 12 hours to monitor the therapeutic response. Once parasite density is lower than 1% and the patient can take oral medication, treatment can be completed with oral quinine.

MALARIA IN PREGNANCY

Malaria in pregnancy affects both the mother and her fetus. Infection with *P. falciparum* during pregnancy can increase the mother's risk of developing severe disease and anemia as well as increase the risk of stillbirth, prematurity, and low birth weight. Chloroquine and quinine or quinidine alone or in combination with clindamycin[1] have been used successfully and safely in the treatment of malaria during pregnancy. Babies born to nonimmune mothers with acute malaria are at risk for congenital malaria. If a mother is parasitemic at the time of delivery, blood smears should be performed on the infant. If the blood smears demonstrate malaria parasite, the infant should be treated according to the species present (there is no need to treat the liver stage in *P. vivax* or *P. ovale* congenital malaria). Even if the infant's blood smear is negative at the time of delivery, it is often most prudent to treat the infant empirically, although close clinical follow-up is also an option. Congenital malaria often presents as fever, anemia, or failure to thrive at 1 to 2 months of age and can be difficult for an unsuspecting clinician to detect.

For pregnant women diagnosed with uncomplicated malaria caused by *P. malariae*, *P. ovale*, chloroquine-sensitive *P. vivax*, or chloroquine-sensitive *P. falciparum*, prompt treatment with chloroquine is recommended. For pregnant women diagnosed with chloroquine-resistant *P. vivax*, treatment with quinine for 7 days is recommended. After treatment, all pregnant women with *P. vivax* and *P. ovale* should be given chloroquine prophylaxis for the duration of the pregnancy to avoid relapses; women can be treated with primaquine after delivery if they have a normal G6PD screening test. Primaquine treatment of infants is unnecessary because there is no liver phase with congenital infections. For pregnant women diagnosed with uncomplicated chloroquine-resistant *P. falciparum* malaria, prompt treatment with quinine and clindamycin is recommended.

MALARIA IN CHILDREN

For pediatric patients, the treatment options are the same as those for adults except that the drug dose is adjusted by patient weight. The pediatric dose should not exceed the recommended adult dose. For treatment of chloroquine-resistant *P. falciparum* in children younger than 8 years old, doxycycline and tetracycline

---

TABLE 2 Malaria Prophylaxis Regimens*

Drug	Duration	Adult Dose	Pediatric Dose
Chloroquine-Resistant Areas			
Atovaquone-proguanil (Malarone)	Start 1–2d before travel and continue for 7d after leaving endemic area	1 adult tablet orally, daily	11–20 kg: 1 pediatric tablet 21–30 kg: 2 pediatric tablets 31–40 kg: 3 pediatric tablets > 40 kg: 1 **adult tablet daily
Doxycycline (Vibramycin)	Start 1–2d before travel and continue for 4 weeks after leaving endemic area	100 mg orally, daily	≥ 8 years of age: 2 mg/kg up to adult dose of 100 mg/d
Mefloquine (Lariam)	Start 1–2 weeks before travel and continue for 4 weeks after leaving endemic area	228 mg base (250 mg salt) orally, once/week	**5–10 kg: 1/8 tablet orally, once/week **10–20 kg: 1/4 tablet once/week 20–30 kg: 1/2 tablet, once/week : 30–45 kg 3/4 tablet once/week >45 kg: 1 tablet, once/week **The recommended dose of mefloquine is 5 mg/kg body weight once weekly
Chloroquine-Sensitive Areas			
Chloroquine phosphate (Aralen)	Start 1–2 weeks before travel and continue for 4 weeks after leaving endemic area	300 mg base (500 mg salt) orally, once/week	5 mg/kg base (8.3 mg/kg salt) orally, once/week, up to maximum adult dose of 300 mg base

*Prophylaxis choices are not presented in any particular order.

TABLE 3 Travel Risk, Diagnosis, and Treatment Resources

Type of Information	Source	Telephone Number, Internet Address or e-mail Address
Travel risk data	CDC Traveler's Health Internet site (includes online access to *The Yellow Book*)	http://www.cdc.gov/travel
Travel risk data, diagnosis, and treatment	CDC Malaria Branch	http://www.cdc.gov/malaria
Travel risk data	World Health Organization	http://www.who.int/ith/preface.html
Diagnosis	CDC's Division of Parasitic Diseases diagnostic internet site	http://www.dpd.cdc.gov/dpdx

Abbreviation: CDC = Centers for Disease Control and Prevention.

should not be used; quinine sulfate given in combination with clindamycin[1] and atovaquone-proguanil alone are the recommended treatment options. Mefloquine can be considered if these options are not available. In rare instances, doxycycline[1] or tetracycline[1] can be used in combination with quinine in children younger than 8 years old if other treatment options are not available or are not tolerated and the benefit of adding doxycycline or tetracycline is judged to outweigh the risk.

Prevention

A combination of personal protective measures and chemoprophylaxis can be highly effective in preventing malaria. Travelers should avoid being outdoors during the peak *Anopheles* biting period between dusk and dawn. When outdoors, travelers should wear clothing that minimizes the amount of exposed skin and apply insect repellents that contain DEET (diethylmethyltoluamide). DEET may be used on adults and children and infants older than 2 months of age. Higher concentrations of DEET may have a longer repellent effect; however, concentrations over 50% provide no added protection. Travelers who are not staying in well-screened or air-conditioned rooms should sleep under insecticide-treated bed nets.

The choice of prophylactic medication should be made in light of the traveler's destination, length of stay, type of exposure, and accommodation; the presence of resistant strains; and the traveler's age, drug allergies, other medications, and medical history. Detailed prophylaxis recommendations are presented in Table 2.

Malaria infection in pregnant women can be more severe than it is in nonpregnant women. Women who are pregnant or likely to become pregnant should be advised to avoid travel to malaria-risk areas. However, pregnant women who choose to travel to these areas should take appropriate antimalarial prophylaxis and use personal protective measures.

Travelers should be advised that they can contract malaria despite the use of prophylaxis and personal protective measures. Travelers should be aware of the signs

and symptoms of malaria and should seek medical care if they develop fever or experience flulike symptoms.

A list of Internet-based malaria travel risk, diagnosis, and treatment resources is provided in Table 3.

REFERENCES

CDC Guidelines for Treatment of Malaria in the United States. Available at http://www.cdc.gov/malaria/pdf/treatmenttable.pdf (accessed January 3, 2005).
Congenital malaria as a result of Plasmodium malaria–North Carolina, 2000. MMWR Morb Mortal Wkly Rep 2002;51(8):164-165.
Hulbert TV. Congenital malaria in the United States: Report of a case and review. Clin Infect Dis 1992;14(4):922-926.
Management of Severe Malaria: A Practical Handbook, 2nd ed. Geneva: World Health Organization, 2000.
Multifocal autochthonous transmission of malaria–Florida, 2003. MMWR Morb Mortal Wkly Rep 2004;53(19):412-413.
Probable transfusion-transmitted malaria–Houston Texas, 2003. MMWR Morb Mortal Wkly Rep 2003;52(44):1075-1076.
White NJ. The treatment of malaria. N Engl J Med 1996;335(11):800-806.
World Health Organization Expert Committee on Malaria. World Health Organ Tech Rep Ser 2000;892:1-74.
World Health Report 2004. Geneva: World Health Organization, 2004.
Zucker JR, Campbell CC. Malaria: Principles of prevention and treatment. Infect Dis Clin North Am 1993;7(3):547-567.

Bacterial Meningitis

Method of
Juan M. Flores-Cordero, MD, PhD

Bacterial meningitis is the infection of the leptomeninges (pia mater and arachnoid) and the subarachnoid space, which is occupied by the cerebrospinal fluid (CSF). The term *meningitis* always means a cerebrospinal involvement. Bacterial meningitis must be considered a medical emergency because inappropriate or delayed treatment may increase the risk of death or neurologic

_____
[1]Not FDA approved for this indication.

sequelae between survivors. It tends to be a common disease in the extreme ages of life, but it may occur at any age.

Etiology

Haemophilus influenzae, Neisseria meningitidis, and *Streptococcus pneumoniae* are the responsible pathogens in 70% to 85% of episodes of acute community-acquired bacterial meningitis. Each of them predominates in a different population according to the age and the underlying conditions of the host.

H. influenzae type B has been the most common origin of meningitis in infants and toddlers, but the introduction of conjugate vaccines (HibTITER) for this pathogen has reduced its incidence dramatically. Predisposing factors such as acquired breach of normal anatomic barriers (basilar skull fractures or cerebrospinal fluid [CSF] leakage) or impaired humoral immunity are present in most adult patients with *H. influenzae* meningitis.

N. meningitidis and *S. pneumoniae* are now the most common pathogens from childhood through adulthood. *N. meningitidis* is the leading cause of bacterial meningitis in children and young adults but is rare after age 45 years. *S. pneumoniae* is the most common causative agent of bacterial meningitis in adults, but pneumococcal meningitis may occur at any age. This pathogen is especially common either in patients who have sustained a previous head injury or in presence of CSF leakage. Approximately 50% of pneumococcal meningitis episodes are associated with pneumonia, otitis, or sinusitis. The emergence of penicillin resistance among pneumococcal isolates in various part of the world has resulted in increased incidence of meningitis caused by *S. pneumoniae* resistant to penicillin and other β-lactam antibiotics.

Meningitis caused by other different bacteria is usually associated with specific clinical conditions of the host. The principal pathogens of neonatal meningitis are group B streptococcus (*Streptococcus agalactiae*), gram-negative bacilli, and *Listeria monocytogenes*. Among adults, predisposing factors for gram-negative bacillary meningitis include neurosurgical procedures, head trauma, malignancy, and alcoholic liver disease. Risk factors for meningitis caused by *L. monocytogenes* include advanced age, organ transplantation, and immunosuppressive conditions. *Staphylococcus aureus* may cause meningitis following trauma or neurosurgery, and community-acquired cases are usually in conjunction with endocarditis or soft-tissue infections. Skin flora as staphylococcal species, gram-negative bacilli, and *Propionibacterium acnes* may cause meningitis in patients with CSF shunts.

Mortality and Neurologic Morbidity

Since the beginning of the antibiotic era, the fatality rate from acute bacterial meningitis has declined but remains high for a disease in which rapid microbiologic

cure might be the rule. Mortality rates of meningitis caused by *H. influenzae* and *N. meningitidis* have declined below 10%, whereas mortality caused by pneumococcal meningitis is still between 20% and 30%. Equally, long-term neurologic morbidity (Box 1) is quite variable in those who survive after an episode of acute bacterial meningitis. Mortality and neurologic morbidity are influenced by specific bacterial etiology, patient age, overall severity of the disease, and development of systemic complications.

Pathogenesis and Pathophysiology

Most cases of bacterial meningitis are caused by hematogenous dissemination. The mechanisms of neuroinvasion are related to several virulence factors that allow bacteria to overcome specific host defense mechanisms, effectively colonize and invade mucosal epithelium, survive within the bloodstream, and successfully cross the blood–brain barrier (BBB) into the CSF.

Once the bacteria reach the CSF, the subcapsular surface components, such as the bacteria cell wall, seem to serve as the critical components in stimulating host-mediated meningeal inflammation. This inflammatory activity seems to play a major role in the pathophysiologic events of bacterial meningitis: (a) increased permeability in the BBB results in vasogenic cerebral edema; (b) increased resistance to cerebrospinal outflow impedes reabsorption of CSF and thus increased CSF volume; and (c) cerebrovascular involvement, one of the major determinants of long-term outcome of patients.

Clinical Presentation

Meningitis should be considered in patients who are febrile and have an altered mental status. The clinical presentation of meningitis is similar in adults and older children with an acute onset. At least two of the classic signs—fever, neck stiffness, headache, and altered mental status—occur in more than 90% of adults presenting with meningitis. However, the sensitivity of the classic

---

BOX 1 Neurologic Morbidity of Bacterial Meningitis

- Seizures
- Cranial nerve palsies
- Hearing impairment
- Focal neurologic deficits
- Hydrocephalus
- CNS hemorrhage
- Herniation
- Mental retardation
- Behavior disturbances
- Epilepsy

Abbreviation: CNS = central nervous system.

triad of fever, neck stiffness, and a change in mental status is low, presenting only in 44% of adult patients. Other symptoms include nausea, vomiting, and photophobia. In children younger than age 2 years, meningeal signs are not reliably present, but almost all present with abnormal thermoregulation and altered state of consciousness. Elderly patients may only present with alterations of mentation and consciousness.

Approximately 50% of patients have symptoms for less than 24 hours, but meningitis may also present a subacute progression over 1 to 7 days with fever, malaise, nausea, vomiting, and other nonspecific signs and symptoms. Predisposing factors for meningitis such as infected contiguous site (otitis, sinusitis), alcoholism, altered immune state, head trauma, and CSF leakage should be considered during the hospital admission.

The signs of meningeal irritation, stiff neck, and Kernig and Brudzinski signs must be explored during the physical exam, but they may be absent in young, old, or severely obtunded patients. Fullness or bulging of the anterior fontanelle may be detected in neonates and infants and is evidence of intracranial hypertension. There are certain special clinical features that correlate with particular types of meningitis. Meningococcal meningitis should always be suspected when a petechial or purpuric rash is present. The petechiae correlate with the degree of thrombocytopenia and are important as an indicator in the evolution of bleeding complications secondary to ensuing disseminated, intravascular coagulopathies.

Seizures were encountered most often in children with *H. influenzae* meningitis. They occur in approximately 5% to 12% of adult patients and may be focal or generalized. Focal neurologic deficits may be present on admission from 9% to 33% of episodes. When meningitis progress rapidly, clinical signs of acute intracranial hypertension may be present and include depressed consciousness, sluggishly reactive or dilated pupils, ophthalmoplegia, impaired respiratory function, posturing, hyperreflexia, and spasticity. Systemic signs may also be present in meningitis. Arterial hypotension may indicate the presence of severe sepsis or septic shock accompanying the meningitis.

Diagnosis

The diagnosis of bacterial meningitis requires the examination and the culture of CSF. Blood samples must also be obtained for culture because bacteremia is usually detected in more than 50% of episodes. Once there is suspicion of acute bacterial meningitis, a lumbar puncture must be performed immediately to determine whether the CSF formula is consistent with the clinical diagnosis. Nevertheless, in adult patients, computed tomography (CT) of the head is routinely ordered prior to the performance of the lumbar puncture to identify intracranial abnormalities and thus avoid the risk of brain herniation resulting from the removal of CSF. A series of clinical findings at baseline has been associated with an abnormal finding on CT. These clinical findings are the following: an age of at least 60 years;

 CURRENT DIAGNOSIS

- Obtain medical, weight, and family/social histories.
- Measure BMI and waist circumference to risk stratify.
- Screen for common obesity-related, co-morbid conditions (i.e., check blood pressure, fasting glucose, lipid risk panel).
- Assess patient's readiness to make lifestyle changes.

immunocompromise; prior central nervous system (CNS) disease; and recent history of seizure, an abnormal level of consciousness, abnormal visual fields, limb drift, and aphasia. Among the patients investigated who lacked these findings, fully 97% of the scans have been normal, emphasizing that clinical features can be used to identify patients who do not need to undergo CT before lumbar puncture.

The CSF samples obtained by lumbar puncture must be analyzed for cell count and differential, protein, and glucose measurement and microbiologic examination. Concomitant with the lumbar puncture, blood glucose level should be recorded.

Typical CSF findings in bacterial meningitis are polymorphonuclear pleocytosis and low glucose concentration (Table 1). CSF normally contains fewer than 5 white blood cells (WBC)/mm^3 in adults and children and fewer than 30 WBC/mm^3 in infants younger than 1 month of age. Polymorphonuclear pleocytosis ranges usually from several hundred to several thousand WBC/mm^3. Approximately 70% of patients have greater than 1000 WBC/mm^3. Normal CSF glucose concentration is greater than 40 mg/dL in adults and children, and concentration below this value is common in bacterial meningitis. The CSF to blood glucose ratio is also decreased in meningitis and is usually less than 0.4.

The CSF protein concentration in adults and children is less than 45 to 50 mg/dL; normally in newborns it is

TABLE 1 Characteristic Cerebrospinal Fluid Findings in Bacterial Meningitis

	Normal	Bacterial Meningitis
Cell count	<5 WBC/mm^3 (15% neutrophils)	100-10,000 WBC/mm^3 (>50% neutrophils)
CSF glucose	45-80 mg/dL	<40 mg/dL
CSF:blood glucose ratio	>0.5	≤0.4
Protein	15-50 mg/dL	50-500 mg/dL
Lactate	<2 mmol/L	>3 mmol/L

Abbreviations: CSF = cerebrospinal fluid; WBC = white blood cells.

between 80 and 150 mg/dL. The majority of adults and children with meningitis have an increased CSF protein concentration, with values ranging from 50 to 500 mg/dL. Elevated CSF lactate (normal <2 mmol/L) may be seen in patients with bacterial meningitis and it may be a useful test, if available, for distinguishing bacterial from nonbacterial meningitis.

Gram stain examination of CSF permits a rapid, accurate identification of the causative pathogen in 60% to 90% of patients with bacterial meningitis, and it has a specificity of up to 97%. The likelihood of having a positive Gram stain result depends on the CSF concentration of bacteria and the specific pathogen-causing meningitis; *S. pneumoniae* is most often identified.

Several rapid diagnostic tests have been developed to aid in the etiologic diagnosis of bacterial meningitis. Latex particle agglutination tests are available for detecting the antigens of common meningeal pathogens: *S. pneumoniae*, *N. meningitidis*, *H. influenzae*, and *S. agalactiae*. These tests may be most useful for the patient who has received antibiotics before the lumbar puncture and whose Gram stain and CSF culture results are negative.

Neuroimaging Studies

The role of neuroimaging studies in community-acquired meningitis has not been clearly established. In more seriously affected patients, however, CT and magnetic resonance imaging (MRI) scans have demonstrated significant abnormalities, including ventricular dilatation, cerebral edema, subdural effusions, and cerebral infarction. The incidence of these abnormalities varies among the reported series. In a series of 64 adults with acute community-acquired bacterial meningitis admitted to the intensive care unit (ICU), CT findings associated with meningitis were observed in 27.5% of episodes; ventriculomegaly was the most common abnormality.

Ventricular dilatation and enlargement of the subarachnoid spaces are early findings in patients with bacterial meningitis. Resolution of this increase in CSF volume occurs within several days to a week in the majority of patients. Cerebral edema is determined primarily by changes in brain water content, and severe diffuse edema may correlate with death early in the course of the disease.

Cranial CT may be a useful technique in the early management of patients with acute bacterial meningitis because it may show the presence of abnormalities that may require adjunctive therapy. Cranial CT may also be useful both in detecting a parameningeal infection that may require surgical drainage and in ruling out subsequent complications in patients with normal initial CT and poor clinical evolution.

Cerebral Hemodynamics

Changes in global and regional cerebral blood flow (CBF) have been reported in patients with acute bacterial meningitis. CBF autoregulation may also be impaired

in these patients. Currently, transcranial Doppler (TCD) sonography is a noninvasive technique for monitoring the cerebral hemodynamics in a variety of pathologic conditions and can be used to guide medical strategies in the neurocritical patient. TCD sonography of patients with bacterial meningitis has revealed cerebral hemodynamic alterations, both in the anterior and posterior circulation. TCD recordings suggesting transient stenoses of the intracranial arteries have been reported between days 3 and 5 in bacterial meningitis and have been associated with a complicated course of the disease. Increase in pulsatility index (PI) of TCD recording has also been found in adult patients with acute community-acquired bacterial meningitis. This finding may indicate an increased intracranial pressure (ICP). Compliance in the distal vascular tree is first affected by small increases in ICP and this leads to a pattern of increased resistance with larger PI. The normalization of PI values is accompanied by an improvement in level of consciousness.

Treatment

The initial management approach to the patient with acute bacterial meningitis depends on early recognition of the disease, rapid diagnostic evaluation, and appropriate antibiotic and adjunctive therapy (Figure 1).

ANTIBIOTIC THERAPY

Currently, antibiotic therapy remains the cornerstone in the treatment of this disease, and a delay in the onset of treatment has usually been associated with an adverse clinical outcome. Bacterial meningitis is a medical emergency, and appropriate antibiotic therapy should be initiated as soon as possible after the diagnosis is deemed likely.

Empirical antibiotic therapy is initiated either when the diagnosis is strongly suspected based on history and physical exam findings and lumbar puncture must be delayed, or for patients with purulent meningitis (cloudy or purulent CSF) and a negative CSF Gram stain result. The choice of antimicrobial agents for empirical therapy is based on the age of the patient, the current knowledge of bacterial resistance patterns in a given

---

 CURRENT THERAPY

- Remember dietary recommentations (i.e., well-balanced, calorie-restricted diet containing 45-65% carbohydrates, 10-35% protein, and 20-35% fat, as well as a daily fiber intake of at least 25 g per day).
- Accumulate at least 30 minutes per day of moderate physical activity.
- Consider pharmacotherapy for patients with BMI >30 or >27 and co-morbid conditions.
- Consider surgical therapy for patients with BMI >40 or >35 and co-morbid conditions.

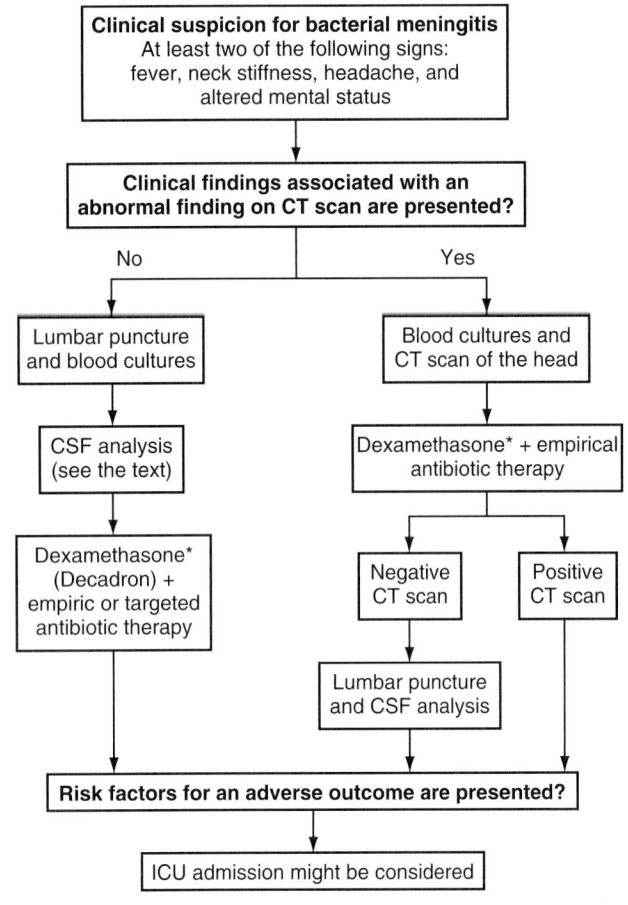

Clinical suspicion for bacterial meningitis
At least two of the following signs:
fever, neck stiffness, headache, and
altered mental status

**Clinical findings associated with an
abnormal finding on CT scan are presented?**

No — Lumbar puncture and blood cultures

Yes — Blood cultures and CT scan of the head

CSF analysis (see the text)

Dexamethasone* + empirical antibiotic therapy

Dexamethasone* (Decadron) + empiric or targeted antibiotic therapy

Negative CT scan | Positive CT scan

Lumbar puncture and CSF analysis

Risk factors for an adverse outcome are presented?

ICU admission might be considered

*Not FDA approved for this indication.

FIGURE 1. Algorithm showing the key management points for bacterial meningitis.

area, and specific predisposing factors for the patient (Table 2). Because of the emergence of penicillin- and cephalosporin-resistant pneumococci, empiric regimens for meningitis treatment should include vancomycin (Vancocin), at least until the results of identification and susceptibility testing is available.

Targeted antibiotic therapy may be based on either presumptive pathogen identification by CSF Gram stain or once the bacterial pathogen isolation and in vitro susceptibility testing have been performed. Decision on the choice of a specific antibiotic must be based on knowledge of in vitro susceptibility and relative penetration into CSF in the presence of meningeal inflammation (Table 3). Table 4 outlines antibiotic recommended dosages.

The duration of antibiotic therapy in patients with bacterial meningitis is not standardized, and it may need to be individualized on the basis oh the patient's clinical response. Most patients need antibiotic therapy for 10 to 14 days. However, treatment for uncomplicated *N. meningitidis* and *H. influenzae* meningitis should be for 7 days. Treatment of gram-negative bacillary meningitis should be for 21 days. In patients who respond

appropriately to antibiotic therapy, repeated lumbar puncture to document CSF sterilization is not routinely indicated. Repeated CSF analysis should be performed for any patient who has not responded clinically after 48 hours of appropriate antibiotic therapy.

ADJUNCTIVE DEXAMETHASONE (DECADRON) THERAPY

The role of adjunctive therapy with corticosteroids has been widely debated. Numerous clinical trials have been undertaken to assess the efficacy of dexamethasone (Decadron) as adjunctive therapy in meningitis. In children with meningitis caused by *H. influenzae* type B, the use of dexamethasone (Decadron) as adjunctive therapy demonstrated reduction of hearing impairment. Current recommendations for adjunctive use of dexamethasone (Decadron) in children are to initiate it 10 to 20 minutes before or concomitant with the first antibiotic dose, at 0.15 mg/Kg every 6 hours for 2 to 4 days. In children who have already received antibiotic therapy, dexamethasone (Decadron) should not be given because is unlikely to improve patient outcome.

A prospective, randomized, double-blind, multicenter trial of dexamethasone (Decadron) in adults with bacterial meningitis showed reduction in death and neurologic impairment in patients who received dexamethasone (Decadron). This was particularly remarkable in adult patients with pneumococcal meningitis. On the basis of this available evidence, dexamethasone (Decadron) is recommended at 10 mg given every 6 hours intravenously (IV) for 4 days. Dexamethasone (Decadron) administration should be initiated 10 to 20 minutes before or concomitant with the first antibiotic dose.

SUPPORTIVE CARE

Bacterial meningitis remains a serious disease that carries high mortality and morbidity rates. Appropriate general supportive care for patients with meningitis is critical. Different studies have found that some baseline clinical features are associated with adverse outcome. Reported clinical risk factors for an adverse outcome are an advanced age, a low level of consciousness, the presence of seizures and/or focal neurologic findings, and signs indicative of systemic compromise, such as hypotension and tachycardia. Other prognostic factors include a positive blood culture, an elevated erythrocyte sedimentation rate, thrombocytopenia, and a low CSF WBC count. Patients with these baseline features might best be admitted to the ICU early to adjust their medical care to the severity of the disease, monitor clinical response to antibiotic therapy closely, and detect possible complications.

Adult patients with acute bacterial meningitis admitted to the ICU may require several adjunctive or support therapies. In the series of 64 episodes of acute community-acquired bacterial meningitis admitted to the ICU, nearly 30% of patients required treatment with mannitol and/or phenytoin, 25% necessitated mechanical ventilation, and 6% required an external ventricular drainage.

Rakel and Bope: *Conn's Current Therapy 2006*

TABLE 2 Antibiotic Therapy in Bacterial Meningitis
Empiric Therapy Based on Patient Age and Predisposing Factors

Age and Predisposing Factor	Recommended Antibiotics	Common Bacteria
Neonates (<1 mo)	Ampicillin + Cefotaxime (Claforan)* or Gentamicin	Enterobacteriaceae Group B streptococcus *Listeria monocytogenes*
1-3 mo	Ampicillin + Cefotaxime (Claforan)* or Cefotaxime (Claforan)+ Vancomycin (Vancocin)	*Neisseria meningitidis* *Haemophilus influenzae*
3 mo-2 y	Cefotaxime (Claforan)* or Cefotaxime (Claforan)*+ Vancomycin (Vancocin)	*N. meningitidis* *H. influenzae* *Streptococcus pneumoniae*
>2 y and adults	Cefotaxime (Claforan)* or Cefotaxime (Claforan)* + Vancomycin (Vancocin)	*N. meningitidis* *S. pneumoniae*
Elderly	Cefotaxime (Claforan)* + Vancomycin (Vancocin) + Ampicillin	*S. pneumoniae* Gram-negative bacilli *L. monocytogenes*
Skull fracture CSF leakage	Cefotaxime (Claforan)* + Vancomycin (Vancocin)	*S. pneumoniae* Group A β-hemolytic streptococci *H. influenzae*
Neurosurgery	Vancomycin (Vancocin) + Ceftazidime or Vancomycin (Vancocin) + Meropenem or Vancomycin (Vancocin) + Cefepime	Enterobacteriaceae *Pseudomonas aeruginosa* *Streptococcus aureus* *Streptococcus epidermidis*
Altered immune state	Cefotaxime (Claforan)* + Vancomycin (Vancocin) + Ampicillin	*N. meningitidis* *S. pneumoniae* Enterobacteriaceae

*Ceftriaxone (Rocephin) could be used, too.

Prevention

Close contacts of patients who have meningococcal disease have a significant risk of developing meningococcal infection after exposure to an index case. Antibiotic chemoprophylaxis is recommended for these close contacts (family members, daycare, and school contacts). Rifampin (Rifadin) is the drug of choice and is administered twice daily for 2 days (600 mg every 12 hours for adults, 10 mg/Kg every 12 hours for children older than 1 month, and 5 mg/Kg every 12 hours for infants younger than 1 month). Ciprofloxacin (Cipro) is also effective in chemoprophylaxis for adults and a single 750 mg oral dose may be given as an alternative to rifampin (Rifadin). Ceftriaxone administered in a single intramuscular dose is an alternative for pregnant

TABLE 3 Antibiotic Therapy in Bacterial Meningitis
Antibiotic Choices Based on Suspected or Documented Organism

Pathogen	Antibiotics
Streptococcus pneumoniae	Cefotaxime (Claforan),* vancomycin (Vancocin), penicillin G, fluoroquinolone[†]
Neisseria meningitidis	Cefotaxime (Claforan),* penicillin G, ampicillin, chloramphenicol, fluoroquinolone,[†] aztreonam.
Haemophilus influenzae	Cefotaxime (Claforan),* ampicillin, cefepime, chloramphenicol, fluoroquinolone[†]
Listeria monocytogenes	Ampicillin, penicillin G, TMP-SMZ, meropenem
Streptococcus agalactiae	Ampicillin , penicillin G, cefotaxime (Claforan)*

Streptococcus aureus
  (methicillin-sensitive)
  (methicillin-resistant)
	
	Nafcillin, oxacillin, vancomycin (Vancocin)
	Vancomycin (Vancocin), TMP-SMZ, linezolid

Streptococcus epidermidis	Vancomycin, linezolid
Gram-negative bacilli	
Enterobacteriaceae	Cefotaxime (Claforan),* meropenem, aztreonam, fluoroquinolone,[†] TMP-SMZ
Pseudomonas aeruginosa	Ceftazidime (Fortaz), cefepime, aztreonam, meropenem

*Ceftriaxone (Rocephin) could be used, too.
[†]Gatifloxacin, moxifloxacin.
Abbreviation: TMP-SMZ = trimethoprim-sulfamethoxazole.

TABLE 4 Antibiotic Therapy in Bacterial Meningitis: Recommended Dosages

Antibiotic	Children Total Daily Dose (Schedule)	Adults Total Daily Dose (Schedule)
Ampicillin	300 mg/kg (q6h)	12 g (q4h)
Aztreonam	—	6-8 g (q6-8h)
Cefepime	—	6-8 g (q6-8h)
Cefotaxime (Claforan)	200 mg/kg (q8h)	8-12 g (q4–6h)
Ceftriaxone	100 mg/kg (q12h)	4 g (q12h)
Ceftazidime (Fortaz)	150 mg/kg (q8h)	6 g (q8h)
Chloramphenicol	50-100 mg/kg (q6h)	4-6 g (q6h)
Gatifloxacin	—	400 mg (q24h)
Gentamicin	5-7.5 mg/kg (q8h)	5 mg/kg (q8h)
Meropenem	120 mg/kg (q8h)	6 g (q8h)
Moxifloxacin	—	400 mg (q24h)
Nafcillin	200 mg/kg (q6h)	9-12 g (q4h)
Oxacillin	200 mg/kg (q6h)	9-12 g (q4h)
Penicillin G	200,000 U/kg (q4-6h)	24 mU (q4h)
TMP-SMZ	20 mg/kg (q6-12h)	20 mg/kg (q6-12h)
Vancomycin (Vancocin)	60 mg/kg (q6h)	2 g (q12h)

Abbreviation: TMP-SMZ = trimethoprim-sulfamethoxazole.

women (250 mg intramuscular [IM]) and children (125 mg IM <12 years of age, 250 mg IM >12 years of age).

Conjugate vaccines against *H. influenzae* type B have declined the incidence of meningitis in children. Similarly, the introduction of heptavalent conjugate vaccine for *S. pneumoniae* and the development of tetravalent conjugate vaccine against meningococcal disease may contribute to reduce the incidence of meningitis in the future.

REFERENCES

Auburtin M, Porcher R, Bruneel F, et al: Pneumococcal meningitis in the intensive care unit. Prognostic factors of clinical outcome in a series of 80 cases. Am J Respir Crit Care Med 2002;165:713-717.

Aronin SI, Peduzzi P, Quagliarello VJ: Community-acquired bacterial meningitis: Risk stratification for adverse clinical outcome and effect of antibiotic timing. Ann Intern Med 1998;129:862-869.

de Gans J, van de Beek D: Dexamethasone in adults with bacterial meningitis. N Engl J Med 2002; 347:1549-1556.

Flores-Cordero JM, Amaya-Villar R, Rincón-Ferrari MD, et al: Acute community-acquired bacterial meningitis in adults admitted to the intensive care unit: Clinical manifestations, management and prognostic factors. Intensive Care Med 2003;29:1967-1973.

Hasbun R, Abrahams J, Jekel J, Quagliarello VJ: Computed tomography of the head before lumbar puncture in adults with suspected meningitis. N Engl J Med 2001;345:1727-1733.

McIntyre PB, Berkey CS, King SM, et al: Dexamethasone as adjunctive therapy in bacterial meningitis. A meta-analysis of randomized clinical trials since 1988. JAMA 1997;278:925-931.

Schuchat A, Robinson K, Wenger JD, et al: Bacterial meningitis in the United States in 1995. N Engl J Med 1997;337:970-976.

Tunkel AR, Hartman BJ, Kaplan SL, et al: Practice guidelines for the management of bacterial meningitis. Clin Infect Dis 2004;39: 1267-1284.

van de Beek D, de Gans J, Spanjaard L, et al: Clinical features and prognostic factors in adults with bacterial meningitis. N Engl J Med 2004;351:1849-1859.

Infectious Mononucleosis

Method of
Luciano Z. Goldani, MD, PhD

Epstein-Barr virus (EBV) is the cause of heterophile-positive infectious mononuceosis and atypical lymphocytosis. The virus is a ubiquitous human herpesvirus spread by contact with oral secretions and frequently transmitted from asymptomatic adults to infants and among young adults by transfer of saliva during kissing. More than 90% of asymptomatic seropositive individuals shed the virus in oropharyngeal secretions.

Infectious mononucleosis is usually a disease of young adults. In lower socioeconomic groups and in areas of the world with lower standards of hygiene, EBV tends to infect children at an early age, and symptomatic infectious mononucleosis is uncommon. In areas with higher standards of hygiene, infection with EBV is often delayed until adulthood, and infectious mononucleosis is more prevalent. The incidence of infectious mononucleosis in a large epidemiologic study in the United States was 45.2 cases per 100,000 per year.

Clinical Manifestations

EBV induces a broad spectrum of illness in humans. The incubation period in young adults is approximately 4 to 6 weeks. A prodrome of fatigue, malaise, retro-orbital headaches, and myalgias may last for 1 to 2 weeks before the onset of fever, sore throat, and lymphadenopathy. Fever is low-grade, and it may persist for more than a month. Lymphadenopathy most often involving the posterior cervical nodes and pharyngitis are most prominent during the first 2 weeks of illness, whereas splenomegaly is more prominent during the second and third weeks. Pharyngitis can be accompanied by enlargement of the tonsils with an exudate resembling that of streptococcal pharyngitis. A morbilliform or papular rash on the arms and trunk develops in approximately 5% of cases. Most patients treated with ampicillin develop a macular rash. Most patients have symptoms for 2 to 4 weeks, but malaise and difficulty concentrating can persist for months. Symptomatic infectious mononucleosis is uncommon in infants and young children. In elderly, infectious mononucleosis presents relatively often as nonspecific symptoms, including prolonged fever, fatigue, myalgia, and malaise. In contrast, pharyngitis, lymphadenopathy, splenomegaly, and atypical lymphocytes are relatively rare in elderly patients.

Most patients with infectious mononucleosis recover uneventfully over a 2- to 3-week period. Deaths are very rare and most often are a result of central nervous system complications, splenic rupture, upper airway obstruction, or bacterial superinfection. Splenic rupture is a rare but dramatic complication of infectious mononucleosis. Meningitis and encephalitis are the most common neurologic abnormalities. Acute EBV infection is also associated with cranial nerve palsies, Guillain-Barré syndrome, acute transverse myelitis, and peripheral neuritis. Autoimmune hemolytic anemia occurs in approximately 2% of cases during the first 2 weeks. Most patients with hemolysis have mild anemia that lasts for 1 to 2 months. Infectious mononucleosis has been associated with red-cell aplasia, severe granulocytopenia, thrombocytopenia, pancytopenia, and hemophagocytic syndrome. Splenic rupture occurs in fewer than 0.5% of cases. Splenic rupture is more common among males than females and may manifest as abdominal pain or hemodynamic compromise.

Hypertrophy of lymphoid tissue in the tonsils or adenoids can result in upper airway obstruction. Patient may develop streptococcal pharyngitis after the initial sore throat resolves. Other rare complications associated with infectious mononucleosis include hepatitis, myocarditis or pericarditis, pneumonia with pleural effusion, interstitial nephritis, genital ulcerations, and vasculitis.

during the first week of illness and in 80% to 90% during the third week. Tests usually remain positive for 3 months after the onset of illness, but heterophile antibodies can persist for up to 1 year. The antibodies are not detectable in children less than 5 years of age, in the elderly, or in patients presenting with symptoms not typical of infectious mononucleosis. The commercially available monospot test for heterophile antibodies is more sensitive than the classic heterophile test. False-positive monospot occurs in patients with connective tissue disease, lymphoma, viral hepatitis, and malaria.

In most cases, the diagnosis of infectious mononucleosis is straightforward. Difficulties arise, however, when the clinical manifestations are less striking, particularly when the heterophile test is negative. Differential diagnosis of infectious mononucleosis and atypical lymphocytosis includes acute infection with cytomegalovirus, Toxoplasma, HIV, human herpesvirus 6, and hepatitis A, B, and C virus. Other diseases with some features of infectious mononucleosis include rubella, lymphoma, and leukemia. A streptococcal sore throat may also mimic infectious mononucleosis clinically. Adenopathy is generally submandibular and anterior cervical, and splenomegaly is absent.

EBV-specific antibody testing as measured by immunofluorescence is used for patients, especially young children with infectious mononucleosis who lack heterophile antibodies. IgM and IgG antibodies to viral capsid antigen are elevated in the serum of more than 90% of patients at the onset of the disease. IgM antibody to viral capsid is useful for the diagnosis of acute infection. In contrast, IgG antibody to viral capsid is usually not useful for diagnosis of infectious mononucleosis but is often used to assess exposure to EBV in the past because it persists for life. Antibodies to Epstein-Barr virus nuclear antigen (EBNA) are detectable 3 to 6 weeks after the onset of symptoms in nearly all case of acute infectious mononucleosis and persist for lifetime. Antibodies to early antigens are detectable 3 to 4 weeks after the onset of symptoms in patients with infectious mononucleosis. Early antigens restricted to the cytoplasm and nucleus (EA-D) are especially likely in those with relatively severe disease. EA-D antibodies are also elevated in patients with nasopharyngeal carcinoma or

Laboratory Diagnosis

Laboratory findings include an elevated white count from to 10,000 to 20,000/μL with lymphocytosis (10% > atypical lymphocytes). Low-grade neutropenia and thrombocytopenia are common during the first month of illness. Liver function is abnormal in more than 90% of cases. Microscopic hematuria and proteinuria are the most frequently noted renal abnormalities. The heterophile test is used for the specific diagnosis. A titer of 40-fold or greater is diagnostic of infectious mononucleosis in a patient who has symptoms compatible with infectious mononucleosis and atypical lymphocytes. Heterophile antibodies are positive in 40% of patients

 CURRENT DIAGNOSIS

- Fever, sore throat, lymphadenopathy, malaise, splenomegaly
- Lymphocytosis (more than 10% atypical lymphocytes)
- Thrombocytopenia (50% of the cases)
- Heterophile antibodies—Paul-Bunell test (90% of the cases)
- IgM antibodies to viral capsid antigen (VCA) (highly sensitive and specific and useful in patients with no detectable heterophile antibodies)

Rakel and Bope: *Conn's Current Therapy 2006*

chronic active EBV infection. Early antigens restricted to the cytoplasm are only occasionally found in patients with African Burkitt's lymphoma or chronic active EBV infection. EBV may be cultured from oropharyngeal washings or from circulating lymphocytes of patients with infectious mononucleosis. Cultivation of the virus is, however, not routinely available in most diagnostic laboratories.

Treatment/Management

Therapy for infectious mononucleosis includes supportive measures such as rest and analgesia. Excessive physical therapy should be avoided in patients with splenomegaly to avoid splenic rupture. Corticosteroids should not generally be used in uncomplicated infectious mononucleosis. Prednisone (40 to 60 mg/day) has been used to prevent airway obstruction in patients with severe tonsillar hypertrophy, for autoimmune hemolytic anemia, and for severe thrombocytopenia. The response is usually rapid, and dosage can be tapered over a 1- to 2-week period.

Acyclovir (Zovirax)[1] has had no significant clinical impact on infectious mononucleosis in controlled trials. These trials included patients with mild, moderate, and severe mononucleosis. Because EBV infection is predominantly latent, it is not surprising that this agent is ineffective in the treatment of infectious mononucleosis. The isolation of patients with infectious mononucleosis is unnecessary.

---

[1]Not FDA approved for this indication.

CURRENT THERAPY

- Supportive
  Low level of physical activity
  Avoid trauma, if splenomegaly
  Acetaminophen or nonsteroid anti-
    inflammatory agents

- Antiviral agents
  Not significant benefit of acyclovir (Zovirax)[1]
    (meta-analysis)

- Corticosteroids
  Helpful in complicated cases (hemolytic
    anemia, severe thrombocytopenia, airway
    compromise)
  Avoid in uncomplicated cases (risk for
    encephalitis and myocarditis)
  Decrease the period of febrility
  Hasten the resolution of tonsil-pharyngeal
    symptoms
  No effect on lymphadenopathy or liver and
    spleen involvement

[1]Not FDA approved for this indication.

REFERENCES

Cohen JI: Epstein-Barr virus infection. N Engl J Med 2000;343-481.
Macsweenn KF, Crawford DH: Epstein-Barr virus: Recent advances. Lancet Infect Dis 2003;3:131.
Okano M, Thiele GM, Davis JR, et al: Epstein-Barr virus and human diseases: Recent advances in diagnosis. Clin Microbiol Rev 1988;1:300.
Tynell E, Aurelius E, Brandella A, et al: Acyclovir and prednisolone treatment of acute infectious mononucleosis: A multicenter, double-blind, place-controlled study. J Infect Dis 1996;174;324.

Chronic Fatigue Syndrome

Method of
*Steven Reid, MB, PhD and
Simon Wessely, MD, PhD*

Chronic fatigue syndrome (CFS) denotes an illness of uncertain etiology characterized by severe, disabling physical and mental fatigue made worse by minimal activity and not relieved by rest. In recent years it has attracted a resurgence of interest, at the same time becoming the subject of controversy regarding its cause and management. Along with fatigue, CFS is typically associated with other symptoms, including musculoskeletal pain, sleep disturbance, impaired concentration, and headaches. Together, these form the basis of the widely used case definition developed by the Centers for Disease Control and Prevention (CDC) (Current Diagnosis box). The severity and duration of CFS varies considerably from patient to patient, but many experience a substantial decline in physical and cognitive functioning. Those who do not meet the fatigue severity or symptom criteria are given a diagnosis of idiopathic chronic fatigue.

Epidemiology

Fatigue is a common medical complaint, reported on one in five primary care visits. A smaller number suffer from idiopathic chronic fatigue, and studies based on community and primary care report the prevalence of CFS as 0.007% to 2.8%, depending on the definition and exclusion criteria used. Most studies show an increased prevalence of CFS in women, with a relative risk of 1.3 to 1.7. In contrast to those patients attending specialist clinics, community samples show an association with lower socioeconomic status and certain ethnic groups: Latinos, African Americans, and Native Americans are at increased risk. Most of those who fulfill the criteria do not use the term *chronic fatigue syndrome* to describe their illness, however.

CURRENT DIAGNOSIS

International Consensus Definition of Chronic Fatigue Syndrome

1. Clinically evaluated, unexplained, persistent or relapsing chronic fatigue (lasting more than 6 months) that is of new or definite onset (has not been lifelong); is not the result of ongoing exertion; is not substantially alleviated by rest; and results in substantial reduction in previous levels of occupational, educational, social, or personal activities.
2. Four or more of the following symptoms are concurrently present for more than 6 months:
   - Impaired memory or concentration
   - Sore throat
   - Tender cervical or axillary lymph nodes
   - Muscle pain
   - Multijoint pain
   - New headaches
   - Unrefreshing sleep
   - Postexertion malaise
3. Exclusionary clinical diagnoses:
   - Any active medical condition that could explain the chronic fatigue
   - Any previously diagnosed medical condition whose resolution has not been documented beyond reasonable clinical doubt and whose continued activity may explain the chronic fatiguing illness
   - Psychotic major depression; bipolar affective disorder; schizophrenia; delusional disorders; dementias; anorexia nervosa; bulimia nervosa
   - Alcohol or other substance abuse within 2 years prior to the onset of the chronic fatigue and at any time afterward

Adapted from Fukuda K, Straus SE, Hickie I, et al: The chronic fatigue syndrome: A comprehensive approach to its definition and study. Ann Intern Med 1994;121:953-959.

Etiology

Despite considerable research effort and several hypotheses, the cause of chronic fatigue syndrome remains elusive. Hypocortisolism and a blunted adrenal response to stress are found in many patients, leading to a disturbance of the hypothalamic-pituitary-adrenal (HPA) axis posited as a cause of CFS symptoms. These abnormalities of HPA function are the most consistent and reproducible to date, but whether they are causal or epiphenomenal is yet to be established. Alterations in immune function are found in some patients, but many of the findings are inconsistent and nonspecific. One replicated finding is that of chronic low-level immune system activation, with increased expression of activation markers on the surface of T cells. Again, the significance of this abnormality in the development of CFS remains unclear.

Chronic fatigue syndrome is frequently attributed to viral infection, but epidemiologic studies do not demonstrate any association with common infective agents. Certain infections, such as Epstein-Barr virus, toxoplasmosis, cytomegalovirus, and Q fever, can precipitate prolonged periods of fatigue, however. Clinical and laboratory evidence suggests a single infectious agent is unlikely to be responsible for CFS. Rather, a number of infections may act as triggers in predisposed individuals and perpetuate CFS symptoms.

The relationship between depression and CFS is complex. Many depressed patients complain of prolonged fatigue, and depression is very common in CFS populations. As well as similarities, significant differences exist between the two illnesses. Patients with CFS often do not show the cognitions typically associated with depression—low self-esteem, hopelessness, suicidal ideation—and studies of neurotransmitter and neuroendocrine function in the two conditions emphasize a distinction. Depression is an indicator of poorer outcome in CFS.

CFS shares many similarities with other medically unexplained syndromes, such as fibromyalgia, irritable bowel syndrome, and multiple chemical sensitivity. Of particular importance in all of these illnesses are patients' health beliefs and attributions. Evidence suggests these factors have a significant role in influencing outcome. What is less clear is their role in symptom development.

Assessment

The management of CFS is by necessity collaborative, and establishment of a positive relationship with the patient, beginning at the assessment, is key. Unfortunately, many patients with chronic fatigue are confronted with disbelief when they consult medical practitioners, or they may be reassured nothing is physically wrong and their symptoms are "all in the mind." This interpretation understandably leads to resentment and a distrust of the medical profession, with the patient seeking alternatives either within the general medical sphere or in more unorthodox circles. So an important first step in management is to validate the patients' symptoms and allow them to ventilate the difficulties they may have experienced with previous medical encounters.

Fatigue is a common feature of a wide range of medical disorders, but most can be excluded on clinical grounds and with the use of simple screening tests. The need to rule out an organic disorder must also be balanced with the potential adverse consequences of continued investigation. The importance of an adequate history cannot be overemphasized. As well as detailing the nature and development of the presenting complaint, the history should include a comprehensive account of the patient's background, including family history, past medical and psychiatric history, employment, and financial situation. The mental state and physical examinations are both of central importance to making a diagnosis. The aim of the mental state examination, as well as excluding clearly distinguishable diagnoses such as psychotic illness, is to identify disorders such as anxiety and depression, which have significant implications for treatment. It is also important to identify potential obstacles to recovery by exploring the patient's illness beliefs, coping strategies, and prior experience of medical care, as well as the attitude of caregivers or family members. A thorough physical examination is essential, and abnormal findings such as pyrexia or persistent lymphadenopathy merit further investigation and should not be ascribed to CFS. There may be evidence on examination of prolonged physical inactivity, such as muscle wasting and postural hypotension, which indicate the severity of the illness.

A careful history and examination should be linked with appropriate use of investigations in patients presenting with chronic fatigue (Box 1). No diagnostic test is available for CFS, and laboratory tests are generally unremarkable. More detailed investigations should also be considered in the following circumstances: extremes of age, recent foreign travel, or absence of mental fatigue. Weight loss in particular is unusual in CFS and needs careful inquiry. Likewise, absence of any evidence of mental fatigue should increase suspicion of a primary neuromuscular disorder because the fatigue in CFS is of central origin and associated with both physical and mental fatigability.

A diagnosis of chronic fatigue syndrome should be made pragmatically (i.e., the patient complains of chronic physical and mental fatigue; fatigability manifests substantial disability in the absence of identifiable organic disease). A diagnosis provides patients with a coherent (although simply descriptive) label for their illness. It should be given in the context of understanding that the cause of the illness is poorly understood but treatment is available and recovery possible. The acronyms ME (myalgic encephalomyelitis) and CFIDS (chronic fatigue and immune function syndrome) should be avoided because *myalgic encephalomyelitis* is a misleading term that implies a known disease process, and no consistent evidence justifies the addition of "immune dysfunction" to the diagnosis. There will also be patients with idiopathic chronic fatigue (not quite meeting the case definition for CFS) who may still benefit from this approach to treatment.

Treatment

The principal aim of treatment is a reduction in functional disability, and the emphasis should be on rehabilitation rather than cure. Management follows a few basic principles, but the CFS population includes many people with differing needs. Treatments should be broadly divided into general and specific areas (Current Therapy) and tailored to the individual patient.

General education about chronic fatigue syndrome is necessary for most patients, and for some may be all that is required. The reality of the illness and its associated symptoms should be firmly acknowledged while emphasizing there is no specific underlying, ongoing disease process (i.e., it is not like HIV). The next step is to agree on a model for thinking about the illness that encompasses the many factors, both physical and psychological, involved in its development, but especially its persistence. Thus patients learn how they can influence the outcome of their illness by modifying these factors. A helpful analogy is being involved in a hit-and-run accident, emphasizing the futility of searching for a cause but the importance of rehabilitation. Patients may also be reassured that CFS is not associated with mortality and people can improve and recover, but they have a significant role to play. For most patients, this involvement includes a gradual and monitored increase in activity levels, linked to overcoming previous and present avoidance behavior where relevant. Advice also needs to be offered on the importance of reducing stressors from employment or lifestyle that may be contributing to symptoms and hindering recovery.

PHARMACOLOGIC TREATMENTS

Patients who have a co-morbid depressive illness, whether it is considered a primary or secondary problem, should be offered treatment with antidepressants. For patients who are not depressed, the evidence for the use of antidepressants is unclear. Tricyclic antidepressants do have

---

BOX 1   Recommended Investigations for the Fatigued Patient

Routine investigations
- Full blood count
- Erythrocyte sedimentation rate or C-reactive protein
- Urea and electrolytes
- Thyroid function tests
- Urine protein and glucose

Special investigations
- Epstein-Barr virus serology
- Toxoplasmosis serology
- Cytomegalovirus serology
- HIV serology
- Celiac disease serology
- Chest radiograph
- Creatine kinase
- Rheumatoid factor
- Cerebral magnetic resonance imaging (MRI) (for demyelination)

 CURRENT THERAPY

General
- Help patient accept illness.
- Educate patient about the illness.
- Encourage self-help and normal activity.
- Treat co-morbid psychiatric illness.

Pharmacologic
- Consider antidepressant medication.
- Avoid untested treatments.

Nonpharmacologic
- Set goals.
- Explain sleep hygiene.
- Suggest graded activity schedule.
- Refer for cognitive behavior therapy.
- Refer for other psychotherapies if indicated.

analgesic properties, however, and they may also be beneficial in patients complaining of insomnia. To minimize side effects (commonly dry mouth, constipation, postural hypotension), the patient should be started at the lowest possible dose, such as 10 mg of amitriptyline (Elavil) or imipramine (Tofronil), which may be increased incrementally. For depressed patients, the ideal dosage is 150 to 300 mg daily (divided if necessary). In nondepressed patients complaining of myalgia or insomnia, lower dosages are often effective. Selective serotonin reuptake inhibitors and other more recently developed antidepressants are more easily tolerated and may also have an alerting effect, but their analgesic properties are less clear. Although many other drug treatments are being evaluated in the management of chronic fatigue syndrome, there is as yet insufficient evidence to recommend their use.

NONPHARMACOLOGIC TREATMENTS

Nonpharmacologic treatments consist of a combination of educational and behavioral interventions, which can be used without recourse to a special clinic. Graded activity is central to the treatment of chronic fatigue syndrome. As part of the assessment, patients should record levels of activity in a diary. Many patients with CFS initially overdo attempts to exercise, become severely fatigued, and develop a pattern of over- and underactivity—"boom and bust," as it is sometimes called. Other patients avoid all levels of exercise and may develop features of deconditioning. So before any exercise plan is advised, current activity levels should be stabilized, which may even mean an overall reduction at the start of treatment. The aim is to produce consistency in activity before embarking on any program of gradually increasing activity. Activities should be set at an attainable level, and the patient should be made aware that initially symptoms may worsen but will subsequently improve. The first steps may involve simple tasks such as getting out of bed or going to the toilet unaided, and at this stage involvement of a partner or caregiver in supervising management can be helpful. Periods of adequate rest should also be included in the activity schedule. This treatment approach benefits children and adolescents as well as adults.

Sleep disturbance occurs commonly in chronic fatigue syndrome and may have a considerable impact on the patient's ability to participate in daily activities. A number of measures can be taken to correct abnormal sleep patterns. Daytime naps should be avoided; so should stimulants such as caffeine or nicotine in the evening. The bedroom should be used only for sleep and intimacy and not for other activities such as eating or watching television. Time spent in bed should be curtailed to the actual time spent sleeping, with the goal to build up a mild sleep debt that increases the patient's ability to stay asleep. Should these measures not prove sufficient, it may be necessary to consider a sedative antidepressant.

For some patients, their interpersonal problems and psychosocial difficulties may make progress with treatment difficult. In such cases, supportive therapy

BOX 2 Perpetuating Factors in Chronic Fatigue Syndrome

- Depression and anxiety
- Lack of physical fitness
- Sleep disorder
- Chronic life stresses and difficulties
- Inaccurate or unhelpful illness beliefs
- Avoidance of activities

and graded activity may be insufficient, and referral to a specialist is required. Considerable research now backs the effectiveness of cognitive behavioral therapy, which include the principles of treatment already discussed and also places an emphasis on the reappraisal of illness beliefs. Other psychotherapies, such as family therapy and psychodynamic therapy, may have a role in the management of some patients, if specifically indicated.

In patients with a long history of severely impaired functioning or who prove consistently resistant to treatment, management is essentially supportive with infrequent but regular contact. This approach provides emotional support, reduces further deterioration, and assists in mobilizing social support.

Prognosis

Most studies of prognosis in CFS focus on people attending special clinics, who are likely to have a poorer prognosis. Outcome appears to be influenced by the presence of psychiatric disorders and beliefs about causation and treatment (Box 2). Approximately 20% to 50% of adults with the disorder show some improvement in the medium term, but few return to their previous level of functioning. Conversely, children and adolescents appear to have a better outlook, with the majority showing definite improvement when followed up in the longer term.

Mumps

Method of
Terry Yamauchi, MD

Mumps is an acute, generalized infection caused by a paramyxovirus. The disease is usually self-limiting with very low mortality. The most frequently observed manifestation is painful enlargement of the parotid gland. Unilateral parotitis is sometimes seen; however, the opposite side usually becomes involved 2 to 3 days later. Submandibular glands may also have swelling and tenderness. Mumps infection of other endocrine tissues is rare, but does occur. Pancreatitis should be considered in patients with severe abdominal pain, chills, fever, and vomiting. Oophoritis, mastitis, arthritis, and hematologic complications are unusual.

Epidemiology

The association of mumps virus infection of the pancreas and the development of diabetes mellitus (DM) remains speculative. Pancreatic involvement and transient diabetes has been well documented; however, cause and effect remain to be more clearly delineated.

Mumps parotitis during pregnancy has been temporally associated with various congenital abnormalities, but no specific syndromes have been identified. The finding of subendocardial fibroelastosis in infants born to mumps-infected mothers remains speculative.

Central nervous system (CNS) infection can occur from 1 week before to 3 weeks after onset of parotitis and is probably underdiagnosed. Mumps meningitis/encephalitis may be present without parotid swelling. Meningitis usually starts shortly after parotid swelling, whereas encephalitis begins during the second week. Other neurologic complications include neuritis and myelitis. Deafness, unrelated to central nervous system involvement has been reported. The deafness is usually unilateral and temporary.

Eating acidic foods is reported to cause discomfort in some infected individuals. Likewise, inflammation of Stensen's duct has been an inconsistent finding. Anorexia is a frequent complaint, but vomiting is not often seen unless the patient is severely ill.

Diagnosis

Mumps is a clinical diagnosis and laboratory tests are unnecessary. If needed, confirmation can be established by viral isolation and/or serologic testing.

The differential diagnoses of parotid swelling and pain include infection with parainfluenza virus types 1 and 3, influenza A virus, cytomegalovirus, coxsackieviruses, enteroviruses, lymphocytic choriomeningitis virus, Epstein-Barr virus, and HIV. Bacterial infections such as from *Staphylococcus aureus*, pneumococcus, gram-negative bacilli, and nontuberculosis mycobacteria can also cause parotitis. Metabolic disorders (cirrhosis, diabetes mellitus, and malnutrition) and drug reactions (iodides, thiouracil, and phenylbutazone) are rare causes of parotid gland inflammation.

Treatment

There is no specific therapy and no antibody-specific gamma globulin or antiviral agent available for mumps infection. The treatment of mumps infection is symptomatic relief and supportive measures. Analgesics for fever and pain control may be necessary. Warm or cold compresses sometimes offer local, but brief, relief. Adequate hydration and bed rest should be provided as needed.

Prevention

Considerations for preventing the spread of mumps include use of standard precautions for the hospitalized patient; however, isolation in the home or community setting is not practical because patients are infectious before parotid swelling is evident. Daycare children should be excluded from the time of onset of parotid gland swelling for 9 days, or until they have been immunized.

In the United States, attenuated live mumps virus vaccine (Mumpsvax) is routinely given to children, usually in combination with measles and rubella vaccine as the measles-mumps-rubella vaccine (MMR). The vaccine provides long-lasting immunity and appears to have no adverse effects. Although the attenuated mumps vaccine strain has been recovered from placental tissue, no fetal involvement has been demonstrated.

Persons with a history of immediate reactions (anaphylactic or anaphylactoid) following egg ingestion may be at an increased risk for reactions after immunization.

REFERENCES

American Academy of Pediatrics: Mumps. In Pickering LK (ed): Red Book: 2003 Report of the Committee on Infectious Diseases, 26th ed. Elk Grove Village, IL, American Academy of Pediatrics, 2003, pp 439-443.

Henle W, Enders JF: Mumps virus. In Horsfall FL, Tamm I (eds): Viral and Rickettsial Infections of Man, 4th ed. Philadelphia, JB Lippincott, 1965, pp 755-768.

Kanra G, Kara A, Cengiz AB, et al: Mumps meningoencephalitis effect on hearing. Pediatr Infect Dis J 2002;21(12):1167-1169.

Schwartz HA: Mumps in pregnancy. Am J Obstet Gynecol 1950; 60(4):875-876.

CURRENT DIAGNOSIS

- Unilateral painful parotid gland enlargement usually progresses to opposite-side involvement.
- Low-grade fever and sometimes discomfort in the parotid gland occurs when ingesting acidic foods.
- Occasionally, inflammation of Stensen's duct occurs.
- Anorexia is sometimes associated with mumps.
- Laboratory confirmation is established by viral isolation and/or serology.

CURRENT THERAPY

- Symptomatic relief and supportive measures are the only treatments.
- Analgesics may be given for fever and pain.
- Warm or cold compresses may offer relief.
- Adequate hydration and bed rest are recommended.

St Geme JW Jr, Noren GR, Adams P Jr: Proposed embryopathic relation between mumps virus and primary endocardial fibroelastosis. N Engl J Med 1966;275(7):339-347.

Yamauchi T, Wilson C, St Geme JW Jr: Transmission of live, attenuated mumps virus to the human placenta. N Engl J Med 1974; 290(13):710-712.

Plague

Method of
Philippe Bossi, MD, PhD, and
François Bricaire, MD

Plague is an acute bacterial infection caused by the organism *Yersinia pestis*. Historically, three plague pandemics have killed more than 200 million people, including the Black Death epidemics in the 14th century in Europe. This disease, primarily the bubonic form, is still reported in several countries in Africa, Asia, South America, and rural southwestern United States There is currently no plague in Europe; the last reported cases occurred shortly after World War II. Worldwide, it is estimated that 1000 to 6000 cases occur each year. It remains an enzootic infection of rats and other rodents. Plague occurs in sylvatic rats and then may spread among more domestic rat species and finally among humans. Bacteria are usually passed to humans through the bite of a flea that has previously fed on an infected rat. In nature, at least 200 mammal species and 80 species of fleas serve as reservoirs. Contamination may also occur by direct contact with infected tissues or fluids from handling a sick or dead plague-infected animal, by respiratory droplets of animals to humans (especially cats with plague pneumonia), by laboratory exposure to plague bacteria, or by human-to-human transmission through infectious respiratory droplets in cases of plague pneumonia. Bubonic and other forms of plague in humans, without secondary pneumonia, are not considered to be contagious.

Plague and Bioterrorism

Y. pestis appears to be a good candidate for a bioterrorist attack agent. The use of an aerosolized form of this agent could be associated with an explosive outbreak of primary plague pneumonia in the exposed population. Moreover, secondary infection via the rodent population could be expected. Intentional aerosol release should be suspected in patients presenting with plague pneumonia in nonendemic areas or in patients without risk factors. As few as 1 to 10 bacteria are sufficient to infect rodents via the oral, intradermal, subcutaneous, and intravenous routes. Estimates of infectivity by the respiratory route vary from 100 to 20,000 organisms.

In 1347, Tartars were the first to use plague as a biological weapon. During a siege on the Genoese-controlled Black Sea port of Caffa, they hurled the bodies of their plague victims over the city walls. In World War II, it was reported that the Japanese army dropped plague-infected fleas in China. In 1970, it was reported that if 50 kg of *Y. pestis* were released over a city of 5 million people, plague pneumonia could occur in as many as 150,000 persons, resulting in 36,000 deaths. In May 2000, during the virtual exercise called TOPOFF (for top officials) in the United States, an aerosol of *Y. pestis* was released covertly at the Denver Performing Arts Center. The estimated result was that 4000 cases of plague pneumonia would have occurred, including 950 deaths.

Clinical Features

The three typical clinical presentations of plague are bubonic, primary septicemic, and pneumonic disease.

BUBONIC PLAGUE

Bubonic plague is the most common clinical form of naturally occurring plague (75% to 97% of all cases). After an incubation period of 2 to 8 days, there is a sudden onset of fever (38.5°C to 40° [101.3°F to 104°F]), chills, headache, nausea, vomiting, malaise or prostration, and weakness; and 6 to 8 hours after the onset of symptoms, a bubo develops. The bubo is characterized by severe pain, swelling, and marked tenderness. It develops in the area of an infected bite, becoming visible after 24 hours, and its size varies from 1 to 10 cm in diameter. There is surrounding edema, and the overlying skin is warm, erythematous, and adherent. Pustules, vesicles, eschars, papules, or skin ulcerations may occur at the site of the fleabite. Rarely, the bubo may become fluctuant and suppurate. Other manifestations include apathy, confusion, fright, anxiety, oliguria or anuria, tachycardia, and hypotension. Without specific treatment, complications are common and include primary (without discernible bubo) or secondary septicemia, secondary pneumonia, and meningitis. The mortality rate or case-fatality rate for untreated bubonic plague is 60%, which becomes less than 5% with antibiotic treatment. This form is unlikely to occur in a bioterrorist attack unless fleas were used as the contaminated vector.

PNEUMONIC PLAGUE

Pneumonic plague may be caused by a primary respiratory infection, or be a complication of the bubonic and septicemic forms of the disease (secondary pneumonia). Plague pneumonia is highly contagious to other humans by airborne transmission.

Primary pneumonia would be the most frequent clinical form in a bioterrorist attack. In this case, the incubation period is 1 to 6 days. It begins abruptly with intense headache and malaise, high fever, vomiting, abdominal pain, diarrhea, and marked prostration. Chest pain, cough, dyspnea, and hemoptysis develop thereafter.

Chest radiographs show evidence of multilobar consolidation, cavities, or bronchopneumonia. Laboratory findings are consistent with a bacterial infection with disseminated intravascular coagulation. Respiratory failure develops quickly with septic shock, and mortality is high. Without antibiotics, the disease is fatal in almost all patients within 2 or 3 days. With the use of antibiotics, the fatality rate decreases below 10%.

SEPTICEMIC PLAGUE

Septicemic plague may occur as a complication of untreated bubonic plague or pneumonic plague (secondary septicemic plague), and may develop in the absence of obvious signs of primary disease (primary septicemic plague). It includes septic shock and disseminated intravascular coagulation with vasculitis, livid cyanotic petechiae, purpura, and large ecchymoses that can mimic lesions of meningococcemia. Gangrene of acral regions, caused by small artery thrombosis, may appear in advanced disease. If the disease is left untreated, the mortality rate approaches 100%.

PLAGUE MENINGITIS

Plague meningitis is rare but may occur as a complication of inadequately treated infection elsewhere.

PHARYNGEAL PLAGUE

Pharyngeal plague is very rare and possibly results from ingestion or inhalation of the organism. The tonsils are swollen and inflamed with anterior cervical lymphadenopathy and swelling of the parotid area.

Diagnosis

Case definitions of possible, probable, and confirmed cases are reported in the Current Diagnosis box. Smears from blood, sputum, bubo aspirate, and cerebrospinal fluid (CSF) may be stained with Gram, Giemsa, or Wayson stain to demonstrate bipolar-staining coccobacilli. The diagnosis of plague is then confirmed by culture. *Y. pestis* grows aerobically on most culture media.

Antimicrobial susceptibility tests must be set up as early as possible. Serologic diagnosis is possible, but antibodies may not be detectable when the patient first presents. Detection of anticapsular antibodies with either a more than fourfold rise in titers from acute to convalescent serum or a single titer of more than 1:128 in patients not previously vaccinated confirms the diagnosis. Other tests include direct immunofluorescence for F1 antigen, specific phage lysis, and polymerase chain reaction (PCR) assay for the plasminogen activator gene.

Treatment

Treatment should be initiated as soon as the diagnosis is suspected. Many antibiotics are active against *Y. pestis*. Most of the therapeutic guidelines suggest using gentamicin (Garamycin) or streptomycin as first-line therapy, with ciprofloxacin (Cipro)[1] as an optional treatment. Persons in contact with patients who present with pneumonic plague should receive antibiotic prophylaxis with doxycycline (Vibramycin) or ciprofloxacin (Cipro)[1] for 7 days.

Prevention of human-to-human transmission from patients with plague pneumonia can be achieved by implementing standard isolation procedures until they have received at least 4 days of antibiotic treatment. For the other clinical types of the disease, patients should be isolated for the first 48 hours after the initiation of treatment.

A killed whole cell plague vaccine that was efficacious against bubonic disease was available until 1999 in the United States. This vaccine was associated with poor protection against pneumonic disease. It was recommended for persons working with *Y. pestis* in a laboratory, in plague-affected areas, or with potentially infected animals. A live attenuated vaccine[2] is also available in the United States, but it retains some virulence and is therefore not considered suitable for human use in most countries. Recent vaccine research in Europe is focused on the development of a subunit vaccine containing F1 antigens and recombinant V antigens, which proved to be efficacious against pneumonic plague in mice.

---

[1]Not FDA approved for this indication.
[2]Not commercially available in the United States.

 CURRENT DIAGNOSIS: CASE DEFINITIONS OF POSSIBLE, PROBABLE, AND CONFIRMED CASES

Possible cases
- Sudden onset of severe, unexplained febrile respiratory illness
- Unexplained death following a short febrile illness
- Sepsis with gram-negative coccobacilli identified from clinical specimens

Probable case
- A case that clinically fits the criteria for suspected plague, and in addition, positive results are obtained on one or more specimens

Definitive diagnosis
- A clinically compatible case with confirmatory laboratory results
- Culture of *Y. pestis* from a clinical specimen and confirmation of identification by phage lysis
- A significant (4-fold) change in antibody titer to F1 antigen in paired serum samples
- A definitive diagnosis, by positive PCR or detection of F1 antigen on suspect isolates, will be available within one working day

CURRENT THERAPY: RECOMMENDATIONS FOR TREATMENT AND POSTEXPOSURE PROPHYLAXIS OF PLAGUE

		Treatment of suspected or confirmed clinical cases* (10 days)	Postexposure prophylaxis* (7 days)
Adults Pregnant women It is recommended in all cases, when possible, to cease breast-feeding.	First-line treatment	▪ Gentamicin (Garamycin)[1]: 5 mg/kg IV in 1 or 2 doses qd ▪ - Streptomycin: 1 g IM bid	
	Second-line treatment; first-line prophylaxis	▪ Ciprofloxacin (Cipro)[1]: 400 mg IV bid followed by 500 mg PO bid ▪ Ofloxacin (Floxin)[1]: 400 mg IV bid followed by 400 mg PO bid ▪ - Levofloxacin (Levaquin)[1]: 500 mg IV once qd, followed by 500 mg PO once qd	▪ Ciprofloxacin (Cipro)[1]: 500 mg PO bid ▪ Ofloxacin (Floxin)[1]: 400 mg PO bid ▪ Levofloxacin (Levaquin)[1]: 500 mg PO once qd
	Third-line treatment; second-line prophylaxis	▪ Doxycycline (Vibramycin): 100 mg IV bid followed by 100 mg bid PO	▪ Doxycycline (Vibramycin): 100 mg bid PO
Children	First-line treatment	▪ Gentamicin (Garamycin)[1]: 2.5 mg/kg IV in 3 doses daily ▪ Streptomycin: 15 mg/kg IM twice daily (max 2 g)	
	Second-line treatment; first-line prophylaxis	▪ Ciprofloxacin (Cipro)[1]: 10-15 mg/kg IV bid followed by 10-15 mg/kg PO bid	▪ Ciprofloxacin (Cipro)[1]: 10-15mg/kg PO bid
	Third-line treatment; second-line prophylaxis	▪ Doxycycline (Vibramycin): • >8 years and >45 kg: adult dose • >8 years and <45 kg or <8 years[1]: 2.2 mg/kg IV bid followed by 2.2 mg/kg PO bid (max 200 mg/d)	▪ Doxycycline (Vibramycin): • >8 years and >45 kg: adult dose • >8 years and <45 kg or <8 years[1]: 2.2 mg/kg PO bid (max 200 mg/d)

*In cases where multiple treatments are listed, choose only one.
[1]Not FDA approved for this indication.
Abbreviations: bid = twice daily; IM = intramuscular; IV = intravenous; PO = by mouth; qd = daily.
Adapted from The European Agency for the Evaluation of Medicinal Products/CPMP guidance document on use of medicinal products for treatment and prophylaxis of biological agents that might be used as weapons of bioterrorism. July 2002. Available online at http://www.emea.eu.int/pdfs/human/bioterror/404801.pdf

REFERENCES

Brubaker R: Factors promoting acute and chronic diseases caused by *Yersinia*. Clin Microbiol Rev 1991;4:309-324.

Du Y, Rosqvist R, Forsberg A: Role of fraction 1 antigen of *Yersinia pestis* in inhibition of phagocytosis. Infect Immun 2002;70: 1453-1460.

Franz D, Jahrling P, Friedlander A, et al: Clinical recognition and management of patients exposed to biological warfare agents. JAMA 1997;278:399-411.

Health Aspects of Chemical and Biological Weapons. Geneva, Switzerland: World Health Organization; 1970:98-109.

Inglesby T, Grossman R, O'Toole T: A plague on your city: Observations from TOPOFF. Clin Infect Dis 2001;32:436-445.

Inglesby TV, Dennis DT, Henderson DA, et al: Plague as a biological weapon: Medical and public health management. JAMA 2000; 283:2281-2290.

Jefferson T, Demicheli V, Pratt M: Vaccines for preventing plague. Cochrane Database Syst Rev 2000;2:CD000976.

Levison M: Lessons learned from history on mode of transmission for control of pneumonic plague. Curr Infect Dis Rep 2000;2:269-271.

McGovern T, Christopher G, Eitzen E: Cutaneous manifestations of biological warfare and related threat agents. Arch Dermatol 1999; 135:311-322.

McGovern T, Friedlander A: Plague. In Textbook of Military Medicine, Medical Aspects of Chemical and Biological Warfare. Office of the Surgeon General. 1997;23:479-502.

The European Agency for the Evaluation of Medicinal Products/ CPMP guidance document on use of medicinal products for treatment and prophylaxis of biological agents that might be used as weapons of bioterrorism. July 2002. Available online at http://www.emea.eu.int/pdfs/human/bioterror/404801.pdf

Tiball R, Williamson E: Vaccination against bubonic and pneumonic plague. Vaccine 2001;19:4175-4184.

Anthrax

Method of
Kepler A. Davis, MD, James E. Moon, MD,
and George Christopher, MD

Anthrax was brought to the forefront of American consciousness by the bioterrorism (BT) attacks during the autumn of 2001. Letters containing spores of *Bacillus anthracis* in a highly concentrated powder resulted in 22 cases and 5 deaths among people who had either handled contaminated mail or who had been exposed to aerosols generated from contaminated mail or mail-processing equipment.

Historically, anthrax has been a disease of livestock and wild animals, especially herbivores that ingest spores of *B. anthracis* while grazing. Naturally occurring (zoonotic) anthrax in humans derives from contact with infected animals or contaminated animal products. Between 20,000 and 100,000 cases of anthrax occur worldwide annually. Until 2001 the incidence in the United States was less than one case per year, with the last case of inhalational anthrax occurring in 1979.

The vast majority of zoonotic cases are cutaneous (95%), followed distantly by other forms including inhalational, gastrointestinal (GI), oropharyngeal, and meningeal disease. In contrast, cases from the 2001 BT epidemic were evenly divided between cutaneous and inhalational disease (11 each), with 1 inhalational case complicated by meningoencephalitis.

Cutaneous Anthrax

Cutaneous anthrax results from the introduction of spores through abrasions, cuts, and possibly insect bites and unapparent skin lesions. After an incubation of 1 to 5 days, a small pruritic macule or papule forms at the site of entry, and develops into a vesicular lesion containing clear or serosanguineous fluid. The vesicles undergo ulceration and central necrosis, resulting in a characteristic black eschar, often surrounded by significant local edema. Eschar is painless and aids in differentiating anthrax from other diseases that cause eschars such as scrub typhus, brown recluse spider bites, rickettsial spotted fevers, tularemia, and ecthyma gangrenosum. Although cutaneous anthrax can be self-limited, untreated cutaneous anthrax carries a mortality rate of approximately 20%, caused by bacteremia and disseminated infection. Antimicrobial therapy reduces

---

*Disclaimer: The views expressed herein are those of the authors and do not reflect the official policy or position of the Department of the Army, Department of the Air Force, Department of Defense, or the U.S. government. The authors are employees of the U.S. government. This work was prepared as part of their official duties and, as such, there is no copyright to be transferred. Use of trade names and commercial sources is for identification only and does not imply endorsement by the authors or the U.S. Department of Defense.

the mortality rate to less than 1%. All of the 11 patients with BT-associated cutaneous anthrax cases of 2001 survived with treatment.

Inhalational Anthrax

Before the 2001 BT attacks, experience with inhalational anthrax during the antibiotic era was rare—cases primarily occurred among textile workers (i.e., *woolsorter's disease*), and an outbreak followed an accidental release of spores from a Soviet laboratory in Yekaterinburg (Sverdlovsk), Russia, in 1979.

The inoculum of inhaled spores required to cause disease in humans is not clearly defined, but the median lethal dose (lethal for 50% of test subjects) (LD_{50}) for nonhuman primates based on challenge studies is estimated at 4100 to 8000 spores. Incubation is typically 1 to 6 days but has been reported as long as 43 days. Nonhuman primate models have confirmed the persistence of spores in lung tissue up to 100 days after exposure; these observations lead to the prolonged (60-day) courses recommended for postexposure prophylaxis and therapy following BT exposures.

Inhaled spores are phagocytized by alveolar macrophages and transported to mediastinal and pleura-based lymph nodes, where they germinate and give rise to vegetative bacteria. Edema toxin and lethal toxin lead to the characteristic features of inhalational anthrax including hemorrhagic thoracic lymphadenitis and mediastinitis and hemorrhagic pleural effusions. Bacteremia results in metastatic infection, sepsis, and death.

Inhalational anthrax begins with nonspecific symptoms—including fever, chills, profuse sweating, nausea, vomiting, diarrhea, nonproductive cough, headache, and chest pain—followed by dyspnea and shock. Features that may discriminate between inhalational anthrax and influenza-like illness include non-headache neurologic symptoms (confusion or dizziness), dyspnea, nausea or vomiting, and the features of rhinorrhea or sore throat (Table 1). The diagnosis is supported by findings of hypoxia, hemorrhagic pleural fluid, elevated serum transaminase levels, and abnormal chest radiograph findings, and confirmed by culture, direct fluorescent assay (DFA), polymerase chain reaction (PCR) assay, or serology. In contrast to the historically estimated mortality rate of 85 to 100%, 6 of the 11 (55%) cases during the 2001 BT epidemic survived, possibly because of modern intensive care and combination antimicrobial therapy.

Oropharyngeal and Gastrointestinal Anthrax

The consumption of meat that contains spores can lead to two similar but distinct clinical syndromes. Following an incubation of 1 to 6 days, lesions similar to those of cutaneous disease develop in the oropharynx or GI tract accompanied by high fever. These lesions necrose, ulcerate, and can result in substantial local edema. The extent and location of these lesions result in symptoms specific

TABLE 1 Differentiating Inhalational Anthrax from Influenza or Influenza-Like Illnesses

Symptom/Sign on Initial Presentation*	Inhalational Anthrax (n = 11)	Laboratory-Confirmed Influenza	Influenza-Like Illnesses
Fever or chills	100	68-77	40-73
Fatigue/malaise	100	83-90	75-89
Cough (minimal/nonproductive)	91	84-93	72-80
Abdominal pain	27	22	22
Chest discomfort	55	35	23
Shortness of breath†	73	6	6
Nausea or vomiting†	73	12	12
Sore throat†	18	64-84	64-84
Rhinorrhea†	9	79	68
Hypoxemia/increased arteriolar-alveolar gradient† (7 cases)	86	N/A	N/A
Elevated transaminase levels+ (9 cases)	78	N/A	N/A
Abnormal chest radiograph*	91	N/A	N/A
Hemorrhagic pleural fluid* (6 cases)	100	N/A	N/A

*Findings reported for 11 cases unless noted otherwise.
†Potential discriminators: Inhalational anthrax versus uncomplicated influenza or influenza-like illness.
Abbreviation: N/A = data not available.
From Morb Mortal Wkly Rep 2001;50:984-986 and Morb Mortal Wkly Rep 2001;50:1049-1051.

to each syndrome. In oropharyngeal disease, lesions predominate in the upper aerodigestive tract, leading to sore throat, dysphagia, and possibly life-threatening oropharyngeal edema. Ulcerations in the oropharynx are often covered by white pseudomembranes. Cervical lymphadenopathy (often unilateral) is frequently present. In GI disease, lesions occur in the stomach and lower GI tract and may lead to bowel edema and hemorrhage, ileus, mesenteric adenitis, and massive ascites. Symptoms include nausea, vomiting, anorexia, severe abdominal pain, and diarrhea.

Aggressive antimicrobial therapy reduces mortality from more than 50% to approximately 30%. At least one study suggests that oropharyngeal is the milder of the two conditions, with 13% mortality in treated patients.

Anthrax Meningoencephalitis

Meningoencephalitis was the clinical presentation of the index case of the 2001 BT epidemic. This complication historically occurred in approximately 50% of inhalational anthrax cases and may also complicate cutaneous and GI anthrax. Cerebrospinal fluid (CSF) findings are typical of bacterial meningitis because of other organisms, with the exception that the CSF is usually hemorrhagic, and large gram-positive bacilli may be seen on a Gram stain. Unfortunately, even if promptly treated, anthrax meningoencephalitis is fatal in more than 95% of cases within 1 to 6 days.

Key Diagnostic Points

Guidance for obtaining, handling, and shipping specimens to the Centers for Disease Control and Prevention

(CDC) Laboratory Response Network is available by calling (888) 246-2675 or accessing http://www.bt.cdc.gov/agent/anthrax/faq/labtesting.asp/.

Cutaneous anthrax is confirmed by punch biopsy at the edge of the lesion, with silver staining, tissue culture, DFA for *B. anthracis* polysaccharide cell wall capsular antigen, and PCR.

Leukocyte counts were normal or only modestly elevated (ranging from 7500 to 13,300) at the initial presentation of the BT inhalational anthrax cases in 2001, but marked leukocytosis (ranging from 11,900 to 46,900) subsequently developed. Transaminase levels were elevated in seven of nine cases for which results were reported. Pleural fluid was hemorrhagic with relatively low leukocyte counts.

Blood cultures were positive within 12 to 24 hours in all BT-related inhalational anthrax patients cultured before antibiotics were started, but were negative when obtained after the start of therapy. A nasal swab yielded growth on a culture obtained on the fifth day of antibiotic therapy in a suspected case, caused by persistent spores on nasal hair or epithelium. Other confirmatory tests for inhalational, meningeal, or oropharyngeal or GI anthrax include Gram stain and culture, PCR, and DFA of clinically relevant specimens (e.g., pleural fluid cytology preparations, pleural, transbronchial or other directed tissue biopsy specimens, cerebrospinal fluid, or stool). Serologic testing may be useful in all forms of anthrax; IgG antibody to *B. anthracis*–protective antigen may be detectable within 10 to 40 days after the onset of symptoms.

Of the 11 patients with inhalational anthrax in the 2001 BT outbreak, 10 had abnormal chest radiographs at initial presentation. Pleural effusions were present in 9, and infiltrates were found in 8 of the cases. However, the classically described widened mediastinum was observed only in 7, and was occasionally subtle.

CURRENT DIAGNOSIS

- Cutaneous anthrax: Skin lesion evolves from a small papule/macule to a vesicle to a painless eschar. Biopsy at the edge of the lesion with silver stain, tissue culture, DFA, or PCR confirms the diagnosis.
- Inhalational anthrax: Presents with an abnormal chest radiograph (pleural effusion, infiltrate, widened mediastinum) preceded by nonspecific influenza-type symptoms, followed by dyspnea and shock. Concomitant nonheadache neurologic symptoms and hypoxia frequently occur. Diagnosis is confirmed by blood culture, or Gram stain and culture of pleural fluid that is typically hemorrhagic.

Abbreviations: DFA = direct fluorescent assay; PCR = polymerase chain reaction.

Computed tomography may be more sensitive than plain radiography for the detection of mediastinal adenopathy; this key finding was observed in 7 of the 8 patients scanned.

Key Treatment

Early empirical antimicrobial therapy should be started without waiting for diagnostic confirmation. Table 2 lists the treatment guidelines issued by the U.S. Department of Health and Human Services (DHHS) for BT-associated anthrax

The duration of therapy for BT-associated cutaneous anthrax (60 days) differs from that of naturally acquired

CURRENT THERAPY

The following are recommendation for adults (see Table 2).
- Cutaneous anthrax: Ciprofloxacin (Cipro) 500 mg orally every 12 hours or doxycycline (Vibramycin) 100 mg orally every 12 hours for 60 days.
- Inhalational anthrax: Either ciprofloxacin (Cipro) 400 mg IV every 12 hours or doxycycline (Vibramycin) 100 mg IV every 12 hours, along with one or two additional antimicrobials (see Table 2 footnote). Continue parenteral therapy until clinical improvement; then convert to oral therapy to complete a total of 60 days; duration of therapy.
- Any confirmed case of anthrax (cutaneous or inhalational) needs to be evaluated as a possible BT event, and all cases should be reported to local health departments, the CDC, and local/national law enforcement agencies.

Abbreviations: BT = bioterrorism; CDC = Centers for Disease Control and Prevention (CDC); IV = intravenously.

zoonotic disease (7 to 10 days) because of the potential that in the BT context, the patient may have inhaled a large inoculum of spores at the time of cutaneous exposure; antibiotic therapy is extended to provide postexposure prophylaxis for inhalational anthrax.

Therapy of inhalational anthrax includes intensive supportive care, drainage of effusions, and parenteral antimicrobials. The DHHS recommendations combine either ciprofloxacin (Cipro) or doxycycline (Vibramycin) with one or two additional agents with activity against *B. anthracis* (see Table 2). Combination parenteral therapy is recommended until the patient is stable, followed by oral therapy for a total of 60 days. Therapy should be based on susceptibility testing. Penicillin has been FDA approved for use in anthrax but may be inappropriate because many strains of *B. anthracis* produce an inducible β-lactamase that confers penicillin resistance.

Antibiotic therapy of meningoencephalitis, oropharyngeal, and GI anthrax is similar to the treatment of inhalational anthrax summarized in Table 2, with the caveats that doxycycline (Vibramycin) is not recommended for meningoencephalitis because of its relatively low central nervous system (CNS) bioavailability, and the duration of therapy for non-BT related cases is not well defined. Adjunctive measures for GI anthrax may include aggressive fluid and electrolyte resuscitation, drainage of ascites, and wide surgical resection of diseased bowel segments for patients failing medical therapy.

Adjunctive corticosteroid therapy has been suggested for meningoencephalitis (based on experience with bacterial meningitis because of other organisms), cutaneous anthrax complicated by severe edema (especially head and neck lesions), oropharyngeal anthrax (potential upper airway obstruction), and inhalational anthrax with severe mediastinal edema. There is only limited clinical experience using corticosteroids in the treatment of anthrax.

Pre-exposure Prophylaxis

The currently licensed anthrax vaccine, adsorbed (AVA) (BioThrax),* has been licensed since 1970. It is indicated for use in individuals between 18 and 65 years of age who are at high risk of occupational exposure to *B. anthracis*. These include veterinarians, laboratory workers, and goat hair and woolen mill workers. A similar vaccine was proved effective in preventing cutaneous anthrax in textile workers. Although no cases of inhalation anthrax occurred among vaccine recipients, the incidence among the unimmunized was too low to demonstrate statistical significance. Proof of efficacy in preventing inhalational anthrax is derived from nonhuman primate models; the vaccine has protected animals exposed to more than 950 LD_{50}s of aerosolized spores. The U.S. Department of Defense (DOD) directed an anthrax vaccination program in 1997 as a countermeasure to the potential use of aerosolized anthrax spores as a biological weapon by adversaries.

---

*Currently not available for the general public.

TABLE 2 Treatment of Bioterrorism-Associated Anthrax*

	Initial Therapy	Duration of Therapy
Inhalational		
Adults[†]	Ciprofloxacin (Cipro) 400 mg IV q12h or doxycycline (Vibramycin) 100 mg IV q12h *plus* one or two additional antimicrobials[‡§]	IV initially until clinically improved, then convert to ciprofloxacin (Cipro) 500 mg PO q12h or doxycycline (Vibramycin) 100 mg PO q12h. Complete duration: 60 days
Children	Ciprofloxacin (Cipro) 10-15 mg/kg IV q12h or Doxycycline (Vibramycin): >8y and >45 kg: adult dose >8y and ≤45 kg: 2.2 mg/kg IV q12h ≤8y: 2.2 mg/kg IV q12h *plus* one or two additional antimicrobials[§]	IV initially until clinically improved, then convert tociprofloxacin (Cipro) 10-15 mg/kg PO q12h or Doxycycline (Vibramycin): >8y and >45 kg: adult dose >8y and ≤45 kg: 2.2 mg/kg IV q12h ≤8y: 2.2 mg/kg IV q12h Complete duration 60 days.
Cutaneous		
Adults[†]	Ciprofloxacin (Cipro) 500 mg PO q12h or Doxycycline (Vibramycin) 100 mg PO q12h Amoxicillin (Amoxil)[1] 500 mg PO tid may be considered after initial clinical improvement in cases because of susceptible strains	60 days
Children	Ciprofloxacin (Cipro) 10-15 mg/kg PO q12h or Doxycycline (Vibramycin): >8y and >45 kg: adult dose >8y and ≤45 kg: 2.2 mg/kg IV q12h ≤8y: 2.2 mg/kg IV q12h Amoxicillin[1] 500 mg/kg/daily divided in three doses may be considered after initial clinical improvement in cases because of susceptible strains	60 days

*Use of trade names and commercial sources is for identification only and does not imply endorsement by the U.S. Department of Defense.
[†]Therapy for pregnant women same as for nonpregnant adults; therapy for immunocompromised persons same as for nonimmunocompromised persons
[‡]Doxycycline (Vibramycin) is not recommended for cases complicated by meningoencephalitis (see text).
[§]Other antimicrobials with in vitro activity include rifampin (Rifadin),[1] vancomycin (Vancocin),[1] chloramphenicol (Chloromycetin),[1] imipenem (Primaxin),[1] clindamycin (Cleocin),[1] and clarithromycin (Biaxin).[1]
[1]Not FDA approved for this indication.
From Investigation of bioterrorism-related anthrax and interim guidelines for exposure management and antimicrobial therapy. Morb Mortal Wkly Rep 2001;50:909-919.

By October 2002 more than 2 million doses had been administered to more than 500,000 individuals, with only 11 reports of serious adverse events. The program was interrupted pending further FDA review in October 2004. Further information is available on the Internet at http://www.vaccines.army.mil/.

Postexposure Prophylaxis

Postexposure prophylaxis is generally not indicated following exposure to an animal with enzootic anthrax or contaminated animal products in a typical agricultural or industrial setting. However, exposure to an aerosol of highly concentrated spores in a BT context represents a special case. Given the prolonged persistence of spores in lung tissue demonstrated by animal models and a reported incubation of up to 43 days during the Sverdlovsk epidemic, the DHHS has recommended either ciprofloxacin (Cipro), 500 mg orally twice daily, or doxycycline (Vibramycin), 100 mg orally twice daily for 60 days (Table 3). Pediatric recommendations are similar because the potential benefit for children at risk

outweighs potential toxicity. Options offered by the DHHS are the extension of prophylaxis for 100 days with or without the addition of three doses of anthrax vaccine. Vaccine administered as postexposure prophylaxis is given as an investigational new drug under an informed consent protocol.

Case Reporting

Anthrax should be reported to local health departments; suspected BT attacks should be reported to local health departments, the CDC, local law enforcement agencies, and the Federal Bureau of Investigation (FBI).

Hospital Infection Control

Anthrax is not transmitted person to person; standard precautions are appropriate. Transmission risk is associated with spores present during clinical infection, not vegetative bacteria. However, sporulation and infectious aerosols may be generated during the handling of

TABLE 3 Postexposure Prophylaxis for Bioterrorism-Associated Anthrax[†]*

	Primary Therapeutic Option	Alternative Therapeutic Option
Adults[‡]	Ciprofloxacin (Cipro) 500 mg PO tid	Doxycycline (Vibramycin) 100 mg PO tid or Amoxicillin[1] 500 mg PO tid[§]
Pregnant women	Ciprofloxacin (Cipro) 500 mg tid	Amoxicillin 500 mg PO tid[§]
Children[†]	Ciprofloxacin (Cipro) 10-15 mg/kg PO tid[§]	Doxycycline (Vibramycin): >8y and >45 kg: adult dose; >8y and ≤45 kg: 2.2 mg/kg PO tid; ≤8y: 2.2 mg/kg PO bid

*Use of trade names and commercial sources is for identification only and does not imply endorsement by the U.S. Department of Defense.
[†]Duration of therapy is 60 days in all cases. DHHS also offers options of extending the duration of prophylaxis to 100 days, with or without postexposure vaccination under and investigational new drug protocol.
[‡]Includes immunocompromised persons.
[§]According to CDC recommendations, amoxicillin is suitable for postexposure prophylaxis only after 10 to 14 days of fluoroquinolone or doxycycline (Vibramycin) treatment and then only if there are contraindications to these two classes of medications (e.g., pregnancy, lactating mother, or intolerance of other antimicrobials)
[†]Ciprofloxacin (Cipro) dose not to exceed one g/d.
Abbreviations: bid = twice daily; CDC = Centers for Disease Control and Prevention; IV = intravenously; PO = orally; tid = three times daily; DHHS = U.S. Department of Health and Human Services.
From Investigation of anthrax associated with intentional exposure and interim public health guidelines. Morb Mortal Wkly Rep 2001;50:889-893.

remains, particularly during autopsies. Guidelines for handling remains have been developed by the DHHS.

Future Prospects

Potential modalities for future investigation include immune modulators (immune serum globulin, tumor necrosis factor inhibitors), and agents to inhibit toxin synthesis or activity (protease inhibitors, soluble toxin receptor, calcium channel blockers, angiotensin converting enzyme inhibitors). Internet-based resources on diagnosis and management are provided by the CDC at http://www.bt.cdc.gov/, and the Infectious Diseases Society of America (IDSA) at http://www.idsociety.org/.

REFERENCES

Bell DM, Kozarsky PE, Stephens DS: Clinical issues in the prophylaxis, diagnosis, and treatment of anthrax. Emerg Infect Dis 2002;8:222-225.
Centers for Disease Control and Prevention: Update: Investigation of anthrax associated with intentional exposure and interim public health guidelines, October 2001. MMWR Morb Mortal Wkly Rep 2001;50:889-893.
Centers for Disease Control and Prevention: Update: Investigation of bioterrorism-related anthrax and interim guidelines for exposure management and antimicrobial therapy, October 2001. MMWR Morb Mortal Wkly Rep 2001;50:909-919.
Centers for Disease Control and Prevention: Considerations for distinguishing influenza-like illness from inhalational anthrax, November 2001. MMWR Morb Mortal Wkly Rep 2001;50:984-986.
Centers for Disease Control and Prevention: Update: Investigation of bioterrorism-related anthrax—Connecticut, 2001. MMWR Morb Mortal Wkly Rep 2001;50:1049-1051.
Centers for Disease Control and Prevention: Notice to readers: Additional options for preventive treatment for persons exposed to inhalational anthrax, December 21, 2001. MMWR Morb Mortal Wkly Rep 2001;50:1142.
Centers for Disease Control and Prevention: Medical examiners, coroners, and biologic terrorism. A guidebook for surveillance and case management. MMWR Recomm Rep 2004;53:RR-08;1-27.
Friedlander, AM: Anthrax. In Sidell FR, Takafuji ET, Franz DR (eds): Textbook of Military Medicine. Part I: Warfare, Weaponry, and the Casualty: Medical Aspects of Chemical and Biological Warfare. Washington, DC: TMM Publications, Borden Institute, 1997, pp 467-478.
Inglesby TV, O'Toole T, Henderson DA, et al: Anthrax as a biological weapon, 2002: Updated recommendations for management. JAMA 2002;287:2236-2252.
Jernigan JA, Stephens DS, Ashford DA, et al: Bioterrorism-related inhalational anthrax: The first 10 cases reported in the United States. Emerg Infect Dis 2001;7:933-944.
Kanafani ZA, Ghossain A, Sharara AI, et al: Endemic gastrointestinal anthrax in 1960s Lebanon: Clinical manifestations and surgical findings. Emer Infect Dis 2003;9:520-525.
Lucey D: Bacillus anthracis (anthrax). In Mandell GL, Bennett JE, Dolin R (eds): Philadelphia: Elsevier Churchill Livingstone, 2005, pp 2485-2491.

Psittacosis (Ornithosis)

Method of
Burke A. Cunha, MD

General Concepts

Psittacosis is caused by *Chlamydia psittaci,* an obligate intracellular parasite of birds and animals. Psittacosis is a zoonotic infection in man, and is acquired by inhalation of aerosolized organisms from the respiratory secretions or feces of birds. In birds, psittacosis is a disease primarily involving the liver and spleen without lung involvement. In contrast, in humans, *C. psittaci* infection begins in the liver and spleen initially, and hematogenously is spread to the lungs, which are responsible for its primary manifestation, namely, pneumonia. The incubation period of psittacosis is 1 to 2 weeks and is most common in individuals in close contact with birds (pet owners, veterinarians, workers in pet shops, and workers in poultry processing plants).

Clinical Features

In humans, psittacosis presents as atypical community-acquired pneumonia (CAP). The onset of psittacosis often resembles an influenza-like illness with fever, chills, malaise, nonproductive cough, and severe headache. Although severe headache is the most common central nervous system (CNS) manifestation of psittacosis, patients may rarely present with meningitis, meningoencephalitis, or encephalitis. The dry and unproductive cough is occasionally blood tinged. While patients have a pneumonia, they are not usually short of breath, and chest pain is an infrequent part of the clinical presentation. On physical examination, the patient may have pink macular lesions on the face, which resemble the rose spots of typhoid fever in size and color. These are known as Horder's spots and are pathognomonic for psittacosis. Epistaxis may also be present, which in the presence of CAP and the absence of an alternative explanation should suggest psittacosis as the diagnosis. On physical examination, chest findings are usually unremarkable, even if lobar consolidation is present.

Cardiac involvement with psittacosis is common and is manifested as a pulse temperature deficit, that is, relative bradycardia. Less commonly seen is myocarditis, and, rarely, pericarditis. Culture negative endocarditis may complicate psittacosis. Examination of the abdomen may reveal liver enlargement. The liver may be slightly tender to palpation. Splenomegaly is uncommon and occurs in less than 10% of patients. However, the presence of hepatosplenomegaly in a patient with CAP should suggest psittacosis.

Nonspecific Laboratory Findings

Routine laboratory findings include a normal white blood cell (WBC) count and platelet count. Leukocytosis or leukopenia argue against the diagnosis of psittacosis. Mild anemia is not uncommon, but erythrophagocytosis has rarely been present in patients with psittacosis. Patients with meningitis, meningoencephalitis, or encephalitis may have a mild lymphocytic pleocytosis. Examination of the sputum, if present, reveals few mononuclear organisms with no bacteria or normal flora being present. Serum transaminases are mildly and transiently elevated, and less frequently the alkaline phosphatase or total bilirubin may be slightly increased. Chest radiograph in psittacosis typically is that of a single, lobar-consolidating CAP. Multilobar involvement may occur. Lobar consolidation resembles that seen with the typical pathogens that cause CAP. The lobar consolidation on the chest radiograph is less dense than consolidation from a bacterial lobar pneumonia, such as from *Streptococcus pneumoniae* or *Haemophilus influenzae*.

Pleural effusions are not part of the presentation of psittacosis.

Diagnostic Considerations

Psittacosis should be considered a diagnostic possibility in a patient presenting with CAP with extrapulmonary findings, who has had a recent contact with birds or bird products. During the first week of the illness, the patient may feel unwell with low-grade fevers, but respiratory manifestations are not usually present until the second week of the illness. Patients presenting with a CAP accompanied by extrapulmonary findings have an atypical CAP. A positive zoonotic contact history virtually excludes legionnaires' disease and *Mycoplasma pneumoniae* or *Chlamydia pneumoniae* pneumonia from diagnostic consideration in a patient with an atypical CAP. Among the zoonotic atypical pneumonias, psittacosis must be differentiated from Q fever and tularemia. Atypical pneumonia presenting with a severe headache should suggest psittacosis, *Legionella* infection, or Q fever. The presence of Horder's spots on the face would clinch the diagnosis of psittacosis in a patient with an atypical pneumonia and recent contact with birds. The presence of relative bradycardia in a patient with an atypical CAP immediately limits diagnostic possibilities to legionnaires' disease, Q fever, or psittacosis. Mild/transient increases

 CURRENT DIAGNOSIS

- Suspect an atypical community-acquired pneumonia (CAP) when a patient has extrapulmonary features in addition to lung findings.
- Suspect psittacosis in a patient with an atypical CAP and with a history of recent contact with psittacine birds.
- Each atypical CAP has a characteristic pattern of extrapulmonary organ involvement, which provides an accurate working diagnosis.
- In addition to CAP, psittacosis is characterized by one or more findings indicating central nervous system, liver, splenic, cardiac, skin, or vascular involvement.
- A cardiac finding with psittacosis CAP is a pulse-temperature deficit (relative bradycardia).
- Doxycycline (Vibramycin) therapy is ordinarily continued for 2 weeks in the treatment of psittacosis CAP.
- If doxycycline cannot be used, a quinolone may be used instead for the treatment of psittacosis, but therapeutic experience is limited at the present time.
- With effective therapy, headache, relative bradycardia, and serum transaminases improve or resolve in 5 to 7 days. Horder's spots, if present, resolve in 1 to 2 weeks.

in the serum transaminases in a patient with an atypical CAP also limits possibilities to legionnaires' disease, psittacosis, or Q fever. The presence of liver enlargement in a patient with an atypical CAP should suggest the diagnosis of psittacosis. Although legionnaires' disease, Q fever, and psittacosis all may have slight increases in transaminase levels early in the illness, only psittacosis is frequently accompanied by mild hepatic enlargement/tenderness. In a patient with an atypical pneumonia and splenomegaly, Q fever is the most probable diagnosis, but psittacosis should also be considered. The presence of hepatosplenomegaly in a patient with atypical CAP limits diagnostic possibilities to psittacosis. The patient with psittacosis may complain of mild nonspecific abdominal pain, but diarrhea is not a feature of psittacosis.

The typical causes of CAP are not accompanied by extrapulmonary features. The zoonotic and nonzoonotic atypical pneumonias are accompanied by a variety of extrapulmonary features. The extrapulmonary pattern of organ involvement is characteristic for each of the atypical causes of CAP. There is a characteristic pattern of organ involvement in psittacosis. CNS involvement is common (e.g., severe headache, meningitis, meningoencephalitis, or encephalitis). Epistaxis may be present in the early phases of psittacosis. There may be skin involvement (e.g., Horder's spots on the face), lung involvement (e.g., lobar consolidation without cavitation or pleural effusions), cardiac involvement (e.g., relative bradycardia, myocarditis, pericarditis, or culture-negative endocarditis), reticuloendothelial system involvement (e.g., hepatic enlargement, mildly elevated serum transaminases, splenomegaly).

During convalescence, psittacosis may be accompanied by otherwise unexplained lower extremity phlebitis. There may be mild abdominal pain, but the presence of diarrhea or renal involvement argues against the diagnosis of psittacosis.

Laboratory Diagnosis

C. psittaci requires cell culture and does not grow on conventional laboratory media. *C. psittaci* is readily transmitted via aerosolization and is easily transmitted to laboratory personnel. For these reasons, psittacosis is not cultured in routine clinical laboratories. The diagnosis of psittacosis is usually based on serologic tests. The most common test employed is the complement fixation (CF) test. Psittacosis CF titers of 1:4 to 1:16 are common in the general population and are nondiagnostic. Psittacosis CF titers of 1:16 to 1:32 are commonly seen in workers of poultry processing plants, veterinarians, or pet shop owners, and are not, *per se*, diagnostic of psittacosis. If a patient presents with an atypical pneumonia and with a history of recent bird contact, an acute titer equal to 1:64 is diagnostic. Alternatively, a fourfold or greater rise between acute and convalescent *C. psittaci* CF titers, is also diagnostic of psittacosis. In a patient with bird contact with a clinical illness compatible with psittacosis, and without chronic exposure to birds (discussed previously), the probable

diagnosis of psittacosis is suggested by an acute CF titer to *C. psittaci* of 1:32, whereas a definitive diagnosis of psittacosis is provided by a fourfold rise in titer or an acute titer equal to 1:64.

Therapy

Chlamydiae are obligate cellular parasites like rickettsiae. Chlamydiae are surrounded by cell membranes rather than cell walls as in the bacteria, and for this reason cell wall active antibiotics are not effective against chlamydiae. *C. psittaci* is one of four chlamydial species and the only one that is a zoonosis. Both *C. psittaci* and *C. pneumoniae* are causes of atypical CAPs, that is, zoonotic and nonzoonotic atypical CAPs, respectively. Susceptibility to antimicrobial therapy varies among the species of *Chlamydia*. Sulfonamides are useful in *Chlamydia trachomatis* infection. *C. trachomatis* pneumonia is limited to infants, but in adults, two main chlamydial species responsible for atypical pneumonias are *C. pneumoniae* and *C. psittaci*.

 CURRENT THERAPY

- Atypical community-acquired pneumonias (CAPs) are not responsive to β-lactam antimicrobial therapy.
- Atypical CAPs have been treated with macrolides, tetracyclines, and quinolones.
- *Chlamydia psittaci,* the organism causing psittacosis, is relatively insensitive to macrolide (erythromycin) therapy.
- Hepatic involvement with psittacosis is manifested by a mild or transient increase in serum transaminases (not alkaline phosphatase).
- Headache is the usual CNS feature of psittacosis.
- Splenomegaly in a patient with an atypical CAP suggests Q fever and, less commonly, psittacosis. Splenomegaly is not a feature of other atypical or typical causes of CAP.
- Horder possessive spots are the characteristic skin finding of psittacosis. Horder possessive spots are found on face and are faint, discrete, maculopapular lesions resembling the rose spots of typhoid fever.
- Epistaxis and phlebitis are the vascular manifestations that may accompany psittacosis.
- Phlebitis is obscure (without another explanation) and usually occurs during convalescence in patients recovering from psittacosis.
- *C. psittaci* is not readily culturable in most microbiology laboratories.
- Psittacosis is definitively diagnosed serologically. An initial high titer (>1:64) or a fourfold rise between acute and convalescent titers to *C. psittaci* is diagnostic.
- Doxycycline is the preferred tetracycline to use for any typical or atypical CAP, particularly psittacosis.

Doxycycline (Vibramycin) is the preferred anti-microbial agent for both *C. psittaci* and *C. pneumoniae*. Although clinical experience is limited with quinolones, they are effective in vitro and in animal studies. As with sulfonamides, erythromycin is effective in *C. trachomatis* infections but is less effective in *C. psittaci* infections. Therefore, unless contraindicated, doxycycline (Vibramycin) is the preferred antimicrobial to treat *C. psittaci* CAP. Erythromycin[1] should be used only if it is not possible to use doxycycline. If erythromycin is used, erythromycin glucceptate (Ilotycin) or lactobionate (Erythracin) may be given as a 1-g intravenous (IV) dose every 6 hours. If given orally, any erythromycin preparation given as a 500-mg dose by mouth (PO) every 6 hours is an acceptable alternative or transition from parenteral erythromycin. In patients with severe psittacosis, doxycycline (Vibramycin) should be administered beginning with a loading regimen, that is, doxycycline (Vibramycin), 200 mg (IV or PO) every 12 hours for 72 hours, and then 100 mg (IV or PO) every 12 hours for the remainder of therapy—usually 2 weeks. Psittacosis may be severe but is usually nonfatal with effective therapy (<1% of cases are fatal). Without antimicrobial therapy, the mortality rate for psittacosis is from 20% to 40%.

Obscure phlebitis may complicate psittacosis and usually occurs during the convalescent period. Patient symptoms promptly respond to effective treatment. The temperature decreases over 3 days, and the headache decreases in intensity over the first week. Chest radiograph findings lag behind clinical improvement and may persist for weeks.

REFERENCES

Bacon AE III, Holloway WJ: *Chlamydia psittaci* (psittacosis). In Schlossberg D (ed): Current Therapy of Infectious Diseases. St. Louis: Mosby-Yearbook, 1996, pp 399-400.
Crosse BA: Psittacosis—a clinical review. J Infect 1990;21:251.
Cunha BA: Diagnostic and therapeutic approach to the atypical pneumonias. J Postgrad Med 1991;90:89-101.
Cunha BA: The chlamydial pneumonias. In Chmel H (ed): Pulmonary Infections and Immunity. New York: Plenum Press, 1994, pp 183-196.
Cunha BA: Atypical pneumonias. In Conn RB, Borer WZ, Snyder JW (eds): Current Diagnosis 9. Philadelphia: WB Saunders, 1996, pp 311-313.
Cunha BA: Psittacosis. In Cunha BA (ed): Infectious Disease Pearls. Philadelphia: Hanley & Belfus, 1999.
Cunha BA, Klein NC: Psittacosis. In Marrie TJ (ed): Community-Acquired Pneumonia. New York: Kluwer Academic/Plenum Publishers, 2001, pp 849-853.
Garo B, Garre M, Boles JM, et al: Severe pneumopathy and acute renal insufficiency disclosing *Chlamydia psittaci* infection: Resistance to the treatment with erythromycin. Ann Med Interne (Paris) 1987;138:296.
Gregory DW, Schaffner W: Psittacosis. Semin Respir Infect 1997; 12:7-11.
Grayston JT, Thom DH: The chlamydial pneumonias. Curr Clin Top Infect Dis 1999;11:1.
Hammers-Berggren S, Granath F, Julander I, Kalin M: Erythromycin for treatment of ornithosis. Scand J Infect Dis 1991;23:159.
Yung AP, Grayson ML: Psittacosis: A review of 135 cases. Med J Aust 1988;148:228-233.

---

[1]Not FDA approved for this indication.

Q Fever

Method of
Pere Domingo, MD, PhD

Epidemiology

Q fever is a zoonosis with a worldwide distribution that may present in humans with acute or chronic manifestations. It is caused by *Coxiella burnetii*, a gram-negative bacterium previously classified in the Rickettsiales order, but now considered as belonging to the gamma subdivision of Proteobacteria. The Q fever reservoir includes many wild and domestic mammals, birds, and arthropods such as ticks, although domestic ruminants represent the most common source of human infection. The aerosol route (inhalation of infected fomites) is the primary mode of human contamination with *C. burnetii*, whereas ingestion (mainly drinking raw milk) and person-to-person transmission (transplacental, during autopsies, via intradermal inoculation, or via blood transfusion) are extremely rare. The primary mode of transmission of Q fever has recently raised concern about the potential use of *C. burnetii* as an agent of bioterrorism. The true incidence of Q fever is unknown, because *C. burnetii* infection in humans is usually asymptomatic or manifests as a mild disease with spontaneous recovery, and it is rarely a notifiable disease. However, current epidemiologic studies indicate that Q fever should be considered a public health problem in France, the United Kingdom, Italy, Spain, Germany, Israel, Greece, and Canada (Nova Scotia).

Clinical Features

C. burnetii infection may present with acute or chronic clinical manifestations. The incubation period may last from 2 to 3 weeks. The most frequent clinical manifestation of acute Q fever is a self-limited febrile illness associated with severe headache. Other major clinical presentations include atypical pneumonia and hepatitis, and, more rarely, myocarditis, pericarditis, maculopapular or purpuric rashes, and meningoencephalitis. Less common manifestations of acute Q fever include hemolytic anemia, mediastinal lymphadenopathy, erythema nodosum, thyroiditis, pancreatitis, mesenteric panniculitis, epididymitis, orchitis, priapism, inappropriate secretion of antidiuretic hormone, optic neuritis, Guillain-Barré syndrome, extrapyramidal neurologic disease, and splenic rupture. During pregnancy, *C. burnetii* infection may result in miscarriage, neonatal death, premature birth, or death in utero. Chronic Q fever represents 0.2% of all the cases of *C. burnetii* infection and most commonly presents as culture-negative endocarditis. It supervenes almost exclusively in patients with previous cardiac valve defects. Its diagnosis is often delayed because of the negativity of conventional blood cultures and because cardiac vegetations are small and visible on echocardiography in only 12%

of patients. Other, less common manifestations of chronic Q fever include vascular infections (aneurysms and vascular grafts), osteoarticular infections (osteomyelitis and osteoarthritis), chronic hepatitis, chronic pulmonary infections, amyloidosis, mixed cryoglobulinemia, malignancy-like presentations (such as pseudotumor of the lung), and central nervous system manifestations. These presentations occur months or years after the acute disease, and they represent long-term sequelae of untreated (and possibly undiagnosed) acute Q fever infection.

Diagnosis

Q fever diagnosis is based on serologic methods because culture and molecular biology techniques are available only in reference laboratories. Serologic diagnosis is easy to establish, although antibodies are mostly detected only after 2 to 3 weeks from the onset of the disease. Thus, serologic tests should be performed on both acute- and convalescent-phase sera, and serology allows the differentiation[1] of acute and chronic *C. burnetii* infections. Seroconversion or a fourfold rise in antibody titers can be diagnostic of Q fever. The immunofluorescent assay (IFA) is the reference technique for Q fever diagnosis. During acute Q fever, seroconversion is usually detected from 7 to 15 days after the onset of clinical symptoms and antibodies are detected by the third week in approximately 90% of cases. An IgG anti–phase II antibody titer of 1:200 and an IgM anti–phase II antibody titer of 1:50 are diagnostic of acute infection. However, such results are observed only in 10% of patients during the second week following the onset of symptoms, with 50% observed during the third week, and 70% during the fourth week. Antibody titers reach their highest levels approximately 4 to 8 weeks after the onset of acute Q fever, with gradually decreasing levels over the subsequent 12 months. A persistence of high levels of anti–phase I antibodies despite therapy, or the reappearance of antibodies in a high titer after previously being undetectable or only present in low titers, may herald the development of chronic Q fever infection. If acute Q fever has been diagnosed, recommendations are for repeat serologic testing, monthly, for at least

---

[1]Not FDA approved for this indication.

   CURRENT DIAGNOSIS

- *Acute Q fever*: A flu-like illness together with atypical pneumonia, hepatitis, or both, accompanied by disproportionate headache and seroconversion or a fourfold rise in IgG anti–phase II antibody titers against *Coxiella burnetii*.
- *Chronic Q fever*: Intermittent fever, cardiac failure, hepatomegaly, and splenomegaly, together with an IgG anti–phase I antibody titer against *C. burnetii* of 1:800.

6 months. An IgG anti–phase I antibody titer of 1:800 is highly predictive (98%) of chronic infection. Phase I IgA, which was first considered useful for the diagnosis of chronic Q fever, is now used only for serologic follow-up. Cross-reactions are the biggest source of confusion when interpreting serologic results, and have been described between *C. burnetii* and *Legionella pneumophila*, *Legionella micdadei*, and *Bartonella quintana* or *Bartonella henselae*. PCR-based methods are commonly applicable only to tissue samples, especially cardiac valve specimens, and are not usually necessary for routine diagnosis. Nonspecific laboratory findings of Q fever include leukocytosis, elevated erythrocyte sedimentation rate, elevated creatine kinase, thrombocytopenia, moderate hepatic transaminase elevations (2 to 10 times normal values), and autoantibodies (antiphospholipid antibodies, anti–smooth muscle antibodies, antimitochondrial antibodies).

Treatment

Acute Q fever is most often a mild disease that resolves spontaneously within 2 weeks. Thus, clinical assessment of pharmacologic treatment is difficult. Doxycycline (Vibramycin) at 100 mg every 12 hours for 14 days is the current recommended regimen for acute Q fever. Fluoroquinolones are considered to be a reliable alternative and have been advocated for patients with Q fever meningoencephalitis, because they penetrate the cerebrospinal fluid. Although a macrolide compound or cotrimoxazole (Bactrim)[1] may be effective alternatives, no reliable antibiotic regimen can be currently recommended for children and pregnant women. Anecdotal reports indicate that lincomycin (Lincocin)[1], co-trimoxazole (Bactrim)[1], and chloramphenicol (Chloromycetin)[1] may be effective in the treatment of Q fever pneumonia. Erythromycin is ineffective in vitro against *C. burnetii*, but in vivo clinical efficacy has been suggested. The slow regression of symptoms in patients with Q fever hepatitis has led to anecdotal reports of the benefit of a short, tapering, 1-week course of prednisone therapy together with antibiotic therapy. Adjunctive prednisone therapy may be considered in patients with Q fever hepatitis who have persistent fevers, persistent high elevations of erythrocyte sedimentation rate, and high titers of autoantibodies, especially when these occur despite adequate antibiotic therapy.

Combination antibiotic therapies are the most effective therapy for Q fever endocarditis. Combination regimens include lincomycin (Lincocin)[1], rifampin (Rifadin)[1], pefloxacin (Pefocin),[2] or ofloxacin (Floxin)[1] plus doxycycline. The combination of doxycycline with an alkalinizing agent of phagolysosomes, such as hydroxychloroquine (Plaquenil),[1] is bactericidal in vitro. In a comparison with doxycycline-ofloxacin, the doxycycline-hydroxychloroquine combination significantly diminished the relapse rate; patients improved more rapidly, and

---

[1]Not FDA approved for this indication.
[2]Not available in the United States.

CURRENT THERAPY

Disorder	Recommended treatment	Alternative treatment*	Comments
Acute Q fever	Doxycycline (Vibramycin) 100 mg PO or IV every 12h for 14d	■ Ofloxacin (Floxin)[1] 200 mg PO every 8h for 14d ■ Pefloxacin (Pefocin)[2] 400 mg PO or IV every 12h for 14d ■ Erythromycin[1] 500 mg PO every 6h for 14d	Erythromycin is not recommended for severe cases. Corticosteroids may be used in Q fever hepatitis unresponsive to antibiotics alone.
Chronic Q fever	Doxycycline 100 mg PO every 12h *plus* hydroxychloroquine (Plaquenil)[1] 200 mg PO every 8h for 18m	Doxycycline 100 mg PO every 12h *plus* ofloxacin 200 mg PO every 8h for approximately 4y	Valvular replacement frequently required.
Q fever in pregnancy	Co-trimoxazole (Bactrim)[1] 160/800mg PO every 12h until term	Rifampicin (Rifampin)[1] 600 mg PO four times per day (length not known)	Doxycycline and fluoroquinolones are contraindicated in pregnancy.
Q fever in children	Co-trimoxazole (Bactrim)[1] based on 2.2-4 mg/kg of trimethoprim IV or PO every 12h for 14d	Chloramphenicol (Chloromycetin)[1] 25 mg/kg PO every 12h	Recommendations for treatment of chronic Q fever in children have not been established.

*In cases where more than one treatment is listed, choose only one.
[1]Not FDA approved for this indication.
[2]Not available in the United States.
Abbreviations: d = days; IV = intravenously; h = hours; m = months; PO = by mouth; y = years.`

2

treatment duration could be shortened to 18 months (compared to 3 years with doxycycline-ofloxacin) to prevent most relapses. The optimum duration of antibiotic therapy cannot be accurately determined because no definite criteria for a Q fever cure are currently available. Suggestions have ranged from 1 year to indefinite administration of antibiotics. The surveillance of chronically infected patients should include titration of phase I IgG and IgA antibodies, and its decrease to a titer to 1:200 or less is the main predictive criterion of a clinical cure. Clinical and laboratory evaluation, including Q fever serology, should be performed monthly for the first 6 months of therapy, then every 3 months to assess the duration of treatment. An echocardiogram should be performed every 3 months. For patients on chloroquine therapy, regular ophthalmologic examination are warranted, and chloroquine serum levels should be regularly monitored. Valve replacement has been proposed in Q fever endocarditis as a result of hemodynamic failure.

Chemoprophylaxis

Postexposure prophylaxis after a biological attack might be considered for individuals or groups who have essential roles, and for those classified as being at high risk of acute disease in epidemiologic analyses, but is not recommended for the general public. Chemoprophylaxis is effective if begun 8 to 12 days after exposure and should be performed with tetracycline (Sumycin), 500 mg every 6 hours, or doxycycline (Vibramycin), 100 mg every 12 hours, for 5 to 7 days. Chemoprophylaxis is not effective and may prolong the onset of disease if given earlier than 7 days after exposure.

REFERENCES

Domingo P, Muñoz C, Franquet T, et al: Acute Q fever in adult patients. Report on 63 sporadic cases from an urban area. Clin Infect Dis 1999;29:874-879.
Madariaga MG, Rezai K, Trenholme GM, Wienstein RA: Q fever: A biological weapon in your backyard. Lancet Infect Dis 2003; 3:709-721.
Maurin M, Raoult D: Q fever. Clin Microbiol Rev 1999;12:518-553.
Raoult D, Houpikian P, Dupont HT, et al: Treatment of Q fever endocarditis. Comparison of 2 regimens containing doxycycline and ofloxacin or hydroxychloroquine. Arch Intern Med 1999; 159:167-173.
Raoult D, Tissot-Dupont H, Foucault C, et al: Q fever 1985-1998. Clinical and epidemiologic features of 1,383 infections. Medicine (Baltimore) 2000;79:109-123.

Rabies

Method of
*Millicent Eidson, MA, DVM, DACVPM(Epid),
and Charles V. Trimarchi, MS*

With all mammalian species susceptible and close to a 100% fatality rate, rabies is one of the world's most feared diseases. It is one of the World Health Organization's priority diseases for control, with an estimated annual human death toll of 35,000 to 50,000. If a disability-adjusted life year standardization is used to compare its relative impact, rabies scores higher than onchocerciasis, Chagas, dengue, and leprosy.

Etiology

The disease is caused by infection with rabies virus, which is the prototype species (genotype 1) RNA virus of the genus *Lyssavirus* in the family Rhabdoviridae. Six other rabies-related *Lyssavirus* genotypes are recognized outside the Western Hemisphere that also cause encephalomyelitis in mammals indistinguishable from rabies: Lagos bat virus, Mokola virus, and Duvenhage virus in Africa; and the European bat lyssavirus types 1 and 2 and Australian bat lyssavirus. Recently, four genetically distinct additional lyssaviruses have been isolated from bats in Eurasia.

Routes of Transmission

With such a high case-fatality rate, it is fortunate that rabies transmission usually requires the bite of a rabid mammal. Virus present in the saliva or nervous tissue of an infected animal gains entry via a bite wound or contact with a break in the skin or mucous membrane. Other than in the laboratory (2 cases), there is no definitive evidence for aerosol transmission. Human transmission has occurred through the transplantation of corneas (10 cases), liver (1 case), kidney (2 cases), and a segment of iliac artery (1 case).

Pathogenesis

The virus is introduced at the bite wound, infecting nerve cells directly, or after initial amplification in myocytes. The viral RNA progresses by retrograde axoplasmal transport to the central nervous system (CNS). Only after reaching the brain does it spread in an anterograde fashion to peripheral nerves and other tissues, including, most importantly, the salivary glands. The impact on behavior of infected animals induces biting behavior synchronized with infectious virus in saliva, facilitating bite transmission. The incubation period, from exposure to onset of clinical manifestations, is highly variable, ranging between 1 week and many years but typically from 2 to 12 weeks.

Clinical Features

The clinical features of rabies may be indistinguishable from those of other CNS diseases, metabolic conditions, psychological disorders, or injuries. Nonspecific flulike signs are common during the clinical prodrome, including fever and gastrointestinal symptoms. Within several days of onset, paresthesia at the site of exposure has been reported in up to half of human cases. Cases may be classified as the *dumb* form, characterized primarily by weakness, paralysis, and nonresponsiveness, or the *furious* form, characterized by agitation and aggression. The classic sign of hydrophobia may develop because of nerve dysfunction in the face and throat. Periods of lucidity may alternate with periods of altered mental status and hallucinations. The mean duration between symptom onset and death is 12 days with a range of 5 to 19 days. Because of the nonspecific signs plus a lack of an animal bite history, more than half of the recent U.S. human cases have been diagnosed only after death.

Epizootiology of Animal Rabies

Rabies exists in nature compartmentalized in specific animal host populations, in discrete geographically and temporally defined cycles. Each of the cycles is maintained by host-to-host transmission in the characteristic primary vector species for which the cycle and the rabies virus variant is named. These variants can be antigenically and genetically distinguished in the laboratory. Other mammals, including humans, can be infected with each of these variants, but adaptive attributes of the virus related to transmission within the primary host species rarely permit a sustained *species jump*. Rabies in animals can be discussed in three general categories: domestic canine rabies, terrestrial wildlife rabies epizootics, and rabies in bats.

Rabies in domesticated dogs was nearly pandemic until Western Europe and North America controlled rabies in dog populations by widespread vaccination programs during the 1950s and 1960s. The disease persists in dog populations in developing nations in Africa, Asia, Eastern Europe, and South America. Rabies is also present in a wide range of terrestrial (nonbat) wildlife species almost globally. In North America, rabies cycles exist regionally in raccoons, foxes, and skunks. Wherever rabies exists in terrestrial animal populations, spillover occurs to wildlife and unvaccinated domestic species, mainly in cats and dogs but also livestock. Rabies cycles in bats exist throughout the world, either as genotype 1 in Western Hemisphere insectivorous and hematophagous species, or as one of the rabies-related lyssaviruses in insectivorous or fruit-eating bats of

Eurasia, Australia, and Africa. Spillover of bat rabies to terrestrial species is infrequently recognized.

Epidemiology of Human Rabies

Worldwide, most human rabies deaths result from rabid dog bites. The areas that have controlled dog and fox variants are experiencing human rabies primarily from unreported or unrecognized bat bites. Of the 1990 to 2004 U.S. human rabies deaths, 28 of 31 were because of bat variants (2 were from the dog/coyote variant, and 1 was from the raccoon variant). Although a bat bite was not established for 19 of the bat-variant cases, inapparent or unreported bat bites appear the most likely source of exposure. These human deaths have been disproportionately caused by variants associated with two relatively rare small bats, the silver-haired (*Lasionycteris noctivagans*) and the eastern pipistrelle (*Pipistrellus subflavus*). Experimental evidence indicates that these variants may have evolved increased infectivity for transmission through more superficial contact, with viral replication in surface skin tissues and at lower skin-surface temperatures.

Diagnostic Evaluation

Rabies diagnosis is most commonly performed for the postmortem evaluation of animals that have bitten or otherwise possibly exposed humans or domestic animals. The primary procedure is a direct fluorescent antibody (DFA) of fresh brain tissue. The rabies DFA is fast, sensitive, and specific. Attributes of the pathogenesis of rabies infection and the high sensitivity of the test (achievable with strict adherence to a standard protocol)

 CURRENT DIAGNOSIS

- Nonspecific prodrome may include pain or paresthesia at the site of exposure.
- Rabies is an acute, progressive encephalitic disease, involving fever, autonomic dysfunction, periods of altered mental status, and cranial nerve signs including impaired swallowing and hydrophobia, leading to paralysis and death.
- A history of bite or other animal exposure may be absent.
- Antemortem laboratory diagnosis of human rabies may be performed on saliva, nuchal skin biopsy, serum, and CSF.
- For management of human exposures, there is no reliable antemortem rabies diagnostic test of the exposing animal.
- Immunofluorescence microscopic examination of fresh brain tissue is used for postmortem diagnosis in animals and humans.

Abbreviation: CSF = cerebrospinal fluid.

allow health care providers to withhold rabies treatment based on negative results from the public health laboratory. Most laboratories confirm DFA results by virus isolation in cell culture or by inoculation of laboratory rodents. Similar methods are employed for postmortem testing in suspected human rabies cases.

Antemortem rabies testing for human encephalopathy relies on a battery of tests: demonstration of rabies-specific antibody in serum and cerebrospinal fluid (CSF); demonstration of rabies antigen by DFA on nuchal skin biopsy and sometimes corneal impressions; isolation of virus from saliva; and demonstration of rabies virus RNA by reverse transcription polymerase chain reaction and product analysis performed on saliva. However, many of these procedures may remain negative well into the clinical period.

The most important use of rabies antibody assays is in the estimation of vaccination efficacy, although they are also employed in the antemortem diagnosis of human rabies and in surveillance for disease prevalence in animal populations. Because vaccination efficacy is largely dependent on the production of virus neutralizing humoral antibody, the 1999 Advisory Committee on Immunizations Practices (ACIP) *Human rabies prevention* guidelines recommend the virus neutralization test, generally performed in cell culture. Results are reported as reciprocal titers, or preferably, they are converted to International Units (IUs) through comparison with an international standard immune globulin.

Assessing Rabies Exposures

Efforts should be made to determine the rabies status of the exposing animal to avoid unnecessary rabies treatments following contact with nonrabid animals. Pets and domestic animals were not actively transmitting rabies at the time of exposure if they do not develop rabies signs during a subsequent 10-day confinement and observation period. Animals with rabies signs at the time of exposure or during the observation period must be promptly tested. For wildlife species, even if captive, problems with the recognition of early rabies signs and uncertainty about their viral shedding period necessitate euthanasia and prompt testing, if rabies is to be definitively ruled out at the time of exposure.

When the rabies status of encountered animals cannot be definitively established, the exposure probability must be determined based on evidence such as the species of the exposing animal, the epidemiology of rabies in that geographic area, the exposure history for the exposing animal itself, and the degree of contact witnessed or suspected based on wounds. Because of the small, sometimes undetectable wounds left by bat bites, incidents in which there is a *reasonable probability* of exposure must also be evaluated. Reasonable probability bat exposures include skin contact in which contact by the bat's mouth cannot be ruled out, and bats in close proximity to anyone who may be unaware of or unable to report contact. The latter include a bat in a room with someone sleeping, or close to an unattended child, or a mentally impaired or intoxicated person.

Rabies Postexposure Management

The ACIP guidelines and any relevant state guidelines should be followed when providing human rabies treatment after a suspect rabies exposure (Table 1). Immediate wound management is important, to reduce infectious virus at the wound site. However, for specific rabies treatment, exposures are rarely medical emergencies, except for head wounds from a likely rabid animal.

Rabies treatments are costly, and adverse reactions include localized pain and swelling in 75% of vaccine recipients, and flulike signs in almost half. Immune complex reactions are reported, particularly in those revaccinated, or on the fourth or fifth doses of postexposure treatment. A small number of severe neurologic illnesses, including Guillain-Barré syndrome, have been reported.

Immunosuppressive disease or drugs (including corticosteroids) and antimalarial drugs may reduce the immunologic response to the rabies vaccine, leading to treatment failure and death. In these cases, a rabies titer may be obtained 2 to 4 weeks after treatment has been completed to verify immunologic response; however, a detectable titer does not provide a guarantee of treatment efficacy. Avoid use of immunosuppressive or antimalarial drugs during rabies treatment.

The National Association of State Public Health Veterinarians' *Compendium of Animal Rabies Prevention and Control*, updated annually, should be consulted for the specific details of animal rabies management. Typically, pets and domestic animals possibly exposed to a rabid animal are either euthanized or quarantined for 6 months, unless they are currently on rabies vaccinations and can be given a booster shot within 5 days of exposure. The effectiveness of animal postexposure treatment has not been definitively established.

Rabies Preexposure Immunization

Consult the ACIP guidelines for details of rabies preexposure immunization (see Table 1 for summary). Immunization should be considered for anyone who has frequent live or dead animal contact and may have inadvertent exposures to rabies; this includes rabies laboratory workers. The ACIP schedule for obtaining titers should be followed, and booster vaccinations should be provided if antibody levels become undetectable. Because of their frequent exposure to rabies vaccine, persons receiving preexposure immunization boosters are the group at highest risk for rabies vaccine adverse reactions.

Infection Control

All activities that may result in exposure to potentially infectious fluids, tissues, or aerosols, including clinical management of patients, collection and submission of human or animal specimens, and performance of autopsies and necropsies, should be performed according to standard guidelines and practices. Particular care should be taken to avoid percutaneous injury, contact of mucous membranes, and creation of aerosols with infectious material. Rabies virus is characterized as a biosafety level II pathogen in diagnostic settings, but it is considered a biosafety level III agent for certain high-risk research and vaccine-production activities. Fortunately, the virus is fragile outside a mammalian host, and areas potentially contaminated with virus-containing saliva or nervous tissue can be cleaned with the use of gloves and 10% bleach. Instruments should be autoclaved. Infected animal carcasses may be buried away from a water supply, landfilled, or incinerated.

Prevention and Control

Primary rabies prevention requires avoidance of contact with potentially rabid mammals. Educational programs, particularly directed at children, are critical to inform the general public that they should avoid handling wildlife. Education must also focus on recognizing and reporting all potential rabies exposures, including the reasonable probability exposures to bats. If an exposure has occurred, verification of the rabies status of the exposing animal is key to avoiding unnecessary medical treatment for the exposed person.

Immunization programs are required to reduce the frequency of occurrence of rabid mammals. Most U.S.

TABLE 1   Use of Rabies Biologics in the United States

Biologics*	Postexposure†	Pre-exposure	Administration‡
HDCV, PCEC RIG	5 doses: days 0, 3, 7, 14, 28 1 dose: day 0	3 doses: days 0, 7, 21, or 28 None	1 mL IM in deltoid 20 IU/kg body weight infiltrated in wound area

*See ACIP guidelines (1999) for details.
†For those with prior immunization (see ACIP), only two vaccine doses are provided, on days 0 and 3 (no RIG).
‡For RIG, if exposure site is unknown (e.g., reasonable probability bat exposures) or located in a mucous membrane, or if it is impossible to fully infiltrate the wound, the remaining RIG should be provided IM at a site distant from the vaccination site (e.g., deltoid of opposite arm).
Abbreviations: ACIP = Advisory Committee on Immunizations Practices; HDCV = human diploid cell vaccine (Imovax); IM = intramuscular administration; IU = International Unit; PCEC = purified chick embryo cell vaccine (RabAvert); RIG = rabies immune globulin.

CURRENT THERAPY

- Consult the ACIP's *Human Rabies Prevention* guidelines (1999).
- Immediately clean wounds with soap and water to reduce the risk of infection.
- Administer rabies immune globulin *at the wound site* as well as five vaccine doses intramuscularly over the period of a month. (This is the usual rabies treatment.)
- Give animal bites the highest priority for rabies treatment, including *reasonable probability* of an undetected bat bite, such as when a person was asleep or is incapable of reporting bat contact, because of youth, mental problems, or intoxication.
- Determine exposing animal's rabies status to avoid unnecessary rabies treatments for the patient.
- Avoid administration of immunosuppressive or antimalarial drugs during rabies treatment.

Abbreviation: ACIP = Advisory Committee on Immunizations Practices.

jurisdictions require rabies vaccinations for dogs, with fewer requiring cat vaccinations. Vaccination may be considered for other species, and may even be provided off-label by a veterinarian for those species without a licensed vaccine product, if the mammals will be in contact with the public at fairs, petting zoos, educational exhibits, and the like. Considerable research is occurring worldwide on the use of wildlife vaccination programs to reduce rabies. In the United States and Canada, several oral bait formulations have been used to successfully reduce rabies in coyotes, foxes, and raccoons.

REFERENCES

Centers for Disease Control and Prevention: Human rabies prevention: Recommendations of the Advisory Committee on Immunizations Practices (ACIP). MMWR Morb Mortal Wkly Rep 1999;48(RR-1).
Centers for Disease Control and Prevention: Update: Investigation of rabies infections in organ donor and transplant recipients—Alabama, Arkansas, Oklahoma, and Texas, 2004. MMWR Morb Mortal Wkly Rep 2004;53:615-616.
Coleman PG, Fevre EM, Cleaveland S: Estimating the public health impact of rabies. Emerg Infect Dis 2004;10:140-142.
Gibbons RV: Cryptogenic rabies, bats, and the question of aerosol transmission. Ann Emerg Med 2002;39:528-536.
Jackson, AC: Pathogenesis. In Jackson AC, Wunner WH (eds): Rabies. New York, Academic Press, 2002.
Kaplan, MM: Safety precautions in handling rabies virus. In Meslin FX, Kaplan MM, Koprowski H (eds): Laboratory Techniques in Rabies, 4th ed. Geneva, Switzerland, World Health Organization, 1996.
Krebs JW, Wheeling JT, Childs JE: Rabies surveillance in the United States during 2002. J Am Vet Med Assoc. 2003;223:1736-1748.
Linhart SB, Wlodkowski JC, Kavanaugh DM, et al: A new flavor-coated sachet bait for delivering oral rabies vaccine to raccoons and coyotes. J Wildl Dis. 2002;38:363-377.
Messenger SL, Smith JS, Orciari LA, et al: Emerging pattern of rabies deaths and increased viral infectivity. Emerg Infect Dis 2003;9:151-154.
National Association of State Public Health Veterinarians. Compendium of animal rabies prevention and control, 2004. MMWR Morb Mortal Wkly Rep 2004;53(RR-9).
Trimarchi CV, Smith JS: Diagnostic evaluation. In Jackson AC, Wunner WH (eds): Rabies. New York, Academic Press, 2002.
World Health Organization: World Survey of Rabies No. 34 for the year 1998 (WHO/CDS/APH/99.6). Geneva, Switzerland, World Health Organization, 2000.

Rat-Bite Fever

Method of
Terrance P. McHugh, MD

Because rats live in or near human habitations, they transmit many diseases to people. One such disease is rat-bite fever (RBF). This term refers to two similar, yet distinct, disease syndromes: an acute form caused by *Streptobacillus moniliformis* and a subacute form caused by *Spirillum minus*. Their untreated mortality rates are 12% and 6.5%, respectively. Recognition and early treatment is vital in preventing a fatal outcome. Unfortunately, arriving at the correct diagnosis is hampered by the nonspecific clinical presentation, a broad differential diagnosis, and the difficulty in identifying the responsible organisms. Therefore, physicians must keep a high index of suspicion and actively seek a history of occupational, recreational, or incidental exposure to a rodent scratch or bite.

Epidemiology and Bacteriology

The rat is the major vector and the natural reservoir of RBF. As many as 50% to 100% of wild and laboratory rats carry *S. moniliformis* as a commensal organism in their nasopharynx and excrete it in their urine; 25% of tested rats harbor *S. minus* in their conjunctival secretions or blood. RBF may be transmitted following a bite or scratch, handling a dead rat, handling materials from a cage, or even a scratch from the cage itself. RBF has also been reported following the bites of mice, squirrels, hamsters, weasels, and rat-eating carnivores, such as dogs, cats, and pigs.

RBF occurs worldwide. Because it is not a reportable disease, it is hard to determine its true incidence. One to three million animal bites occur annually in the United States; approximately 2% to 3% of these are thought to be rodent bites. The people most at risk of contracting RBF include those who handle rats as part of their occupation (laboratory workers, vets, pet shop employees); confined individuals (infants in cribs and some elderly patients); and people of lower socioeconomic status (because of homelessness, overcrowding, and poor sanitation). In the United States, nearly half of all reported cases have involved laboratory personnel who handle rats and the other half have involved children. Rats seem particularly attracted to residual food particles found on the hands and faces of infants. Because the child is often sleeping, there may be neither history nor evidence of a bite.

S. moniliformis, the organism responsible for most North American and European cases of RBF, is a gram-negative rod. It is nonencapsulated, nonmotile, and capable of spontaneously forming stable cell wall–deficient L-forms. It is responsible for epizootics of respiratory, arthritic, and septicemic illnesses among wild and laboratory rodents. *S. minus*, the major cause of RBF in Asia and Africa, is a gram-negative, spiral-shaped bacterium with flagella at each pole.

Diagnosis

Streptobacillary RBF has a normal incubation period of 2 to 5 days, but it may range up to 3 weeks. It is characterized by rapid healing of the bite site and minimal regional signs of inflammation, such as cellulitis or lymphadenopathy. Clinically, it is associated with irregularly relapsing fevers, shaking chills, headache, sore throat, and vomiting. Severe diarrhea and weight loss are common in infants and young children. Within the first week of illness, nearly 50% of patients develop arthralgias or arthritis. Joint involvement tends to be asymmetric, migratory, and typically involves the large joints. Up to 75% of patients develop a rash within 1 to 8 days of the onset of fever. This can be maculopapular, pustular, petechial, or purpuric, and commonly involves the extremities, especially the palms and soles. Approximately 20% of these rashes desquamate. Hemorrhagic pustules can also involve the pharynx. Complications of streptobacillary RBF include anemia, tenosynovitis, bronchitis, bronchopneumonia, endocarditis, myocarditis, pericarditis, splenic or renal infarcts, and localized abscesses involving the soft tissues or brain.

Haverhill fever, a related syndrome, is also caused by *S. moniliformis*. In this instance, the organism is transmitted by the ingestion of milk or ice cream that has been contaminated by rodent excrement. Because Haverhill fever frequently occurs in epidemics and causes rashes and arthritis, it is also known as *erythema arthriticum epidemicum*. Symptoms of upper respiratory tract infection and an increased incidence of vomiting are prominent in this food-borne variant.

Spirillary RBF, also known as Sodoku in Japan, has an incubation period of 1 to 4 weeks, but averages 2 weeks. Although the initial bite frequently heals, the hallmark of infection is the later development of a chancre-like lesion at the bite site, which is typically associated with regional lymphadenopathy and lymphangitis. Patients develop alternating cycles of 2 to 4 days of fever followed by 2 to 4 days of defervescence. These cycles generally repeat 6 to 8 times before the illness ends. During this period, chills, vomiting, photophobia, and other systemic signs are common. A macular rash, usually involving the extremities, develops in approximately 50% of patients. Complications of spirillary RBF include meningitis, myocarditis, hepatitis, nephritis, epididymitis,

and splenomegaly. Arthritis and endocarditis are unusual. Spontaneous cures usually occur in 4 to 8 weeks; however, some cases have smoldered for years.

The differential diagnosis of RBF includes the following broad categories:

- Bacterial diseases (disseminated gonococcal disease, meningococcemia, streptococcal toxic shock syndrome [STSS or Strep TSS], brucellosis)
- Rickettsial diseases (Rocky Mountain spotted fever [RMSF], ehrlichiosis)
- Viral diseases (mononucleosis, coxsackie and enteroviral infections)
- Diseases secondary to spirochetal agents (secondary syphilis, Lyme disease, leptospirosis)
- Diseases associated with relapsing fevers (malaria, typhoid fever, *Borrelia recurrentis* infection)
- Miscellaneous disease states (acute rheumatic fever, collagen vascular diseases, and drug reactions)

Key Diagnostic Points

Routine laboratory tests are of little diagnostic help. Gram staining does not detect *S. minus* and may easily overlook the highly pleomorphic *S. moniliformis*. False-positive serologic tests for syphilis occur in 25% of patients with streptobacillary RBF and 50% of patients with spirillary RBF. Enzyme-linked immunosorbent assays, polymerase chain reaction amplification and gene sequencing have been used at certain centers but are of no help in a typical clinical situation. *S. moniliformis* can be isolated from blood, pus, and joint or ascitic fluid, but it is highly fastidious and difficult to recover. To optimize the chance of growth, normal culture medium must be supplemented with blood, serum, or ascitic or joint fluid, and needs to incubate in an atmosphere of 5% to 10% carbon dioxide. The presence of sodium polyanethol sulfonate, a substance found in most aerobic blood culture bottles, inhibits growth. No serologic or molecular tests exist to identify *S. minus*, nor can it be cultured. This organism can occasionally be seen in a Wright or Giemsa–stained specimen but is best demonstrated using darkfield microscopy. Animal inoculation tests may also be helpful.

 CURRENT DIAGNOSIS

- Obtain a history of environmental or occupational exposure to rodents.
- Consider the diagnosis even in the absence of a history or evidence of a bite.
- Screen for relapsing fever, joint involvement, rash, or any nonhealing ulcer.
- Use enhanced growth media if cultures are obtained.

Key Treatment Points

Treatment of any rat bite begins with meticulous local care. The wound should be cleaned, thoroughly irrigated, and tetanus toxoid administered as indicated by the patient's immunization history. A rodent bite almost never calls for antirabies prophylaxis. The efficacy and benefit of prophylactic antibiotic administration remains controversial, however, many authors recommend oral penicillin V (Pen-Vee K)[1].

Treatment of established cases of RBF requires parenteral penicillin. The Centers for Disease Control and Prevention (CDC) recommends aqueous penicillin G administered intravenously for 7 days; once a clinical response is noted, the patient may be switched to oral medication. If an intravenous (IV) line cannot be established, procaine penicillin (Wycillin) can be administered intramuscularly every 12 hours for 10 to 14 days. Serious clinical complications usually require 15 to 20 million units per day of intravenous aqueous penicillin G administered over a 4- to 6-week period, with exact dosages calculated using serum bactericidal levels. Including an additional antibiotic, such as streptomycin[1] or tetracycline,[1] is often recommended because of its added bactericidal effects and activity against L-forms. Other antibiotics reported to be potentially useful include erythromycin (E-Mycin),[1] chloramphenicol (Chloromycetin),[1] cephalosporins, ciprofloxacin (Cipro),[1] ofloxacin (Floxin),[1] and clindamycin (Cleocin),[1] although none of these have been subjected to any clinical trial.

Prevention

As long as people and rats coexist, the complete prevention of RBF is impossible. Protective gloves and proper handling techniques might decrease the incidence of bites among high-risk laboratory workers and pet shop employees. Although rodent eradication programs are potentially beneficial in urban areas, they are neither effective nor economical in rural areas.

---

[1]Not FDA approved for this indication.

CURRENT THERAPY

- Clean the wound and administer tetanus toxoid as indicated.
- Consider prophylactic administration of oral penicillin V following a recent bite.
- Administer parenteral antibiotics (aqueous penicillin G) in established cases.
- Consider using a second antibiotic for additional bactericidal activity, as well as activity against L-forms.

REFERENCES

Berger C, Altwegg BC, Nadal D: Broad range polymerase chain reaction for diagnosis of rat-bite fever caused by *Streptobacillus moniliformis*. Pediatr Infect Dis J 2001;20:1181-1182.

Boot R, Oosterhuis A, Thuis HC: PCR for the detection of *Streptobacillus moniliformis*. Lab Anim 2002;36:200-208.

CDC Report: Rat-bite fever—New Mexico, 1996. MMWR 47: 89-91, 1998.

Freels LK, Elliott SP: Rat-bite fever: Three case reports and a literature review. Clin Pediatr (Phila) 2004;43:291-295.

Hockman DE, Pence CD, Whittler RR, et al: Septic arthritis of the hip secondary to rat-bite fever. Clin Ortho 2000;380:173-176.

Hudsmith L, Weston V, Szram J, et al: Clinical picture: Rat-bite fever. *Lancet Infect Dis* 2001;1(2):91.

Stehle P, Dubuis O, Dedler J: Rat-bite fever without fever. Ann Rheum Dis 2003;62:894-896.

Thong BY, Barkham TM: Suppurative polyarthritis following a rat-bite. Ann Rheum Dis 2003;62:805-806.

Relapsing Fever

Method of
David T. Dennis, MD, MPH

2

Etiology

Relapsing fever refers to disease caused by blood-borne infection with a subgroup of spirochetes of the genus *Borrelia*. It comprises two distinct entities: epidemic louse-borne relapsing fever (LBRF) and endemic tick-borne relapsing fever (TBRF). Both are characterized by recurring acute episodes of spirochetemia and fever alternating with short periods of immune suppression of spirochetes and apyrexia. This cyclical pattern is caused by the spontaneous emergence of new spirochetal serotypes resulting from DNA rearrangement within genes on linear plasmids, which encode for variable major proteins (VMPs) on the spirochete's outer-membrane surface. The diverse antigenic variability permits borreliae to intermittently escape immune sequestration in reticuloendothelial tissue, leading to a return of spirochetemia and febrile illness.

Epidemiology

LBRF, caused by infection with *Borrelia recurrentis*, was once widely distributed around the world, especially among persons living under conditions with crowding and poor hygiene. Historically, it has been associated with epidemics of fever among lice-infested refugees, defeated armies, the homeless and destitute. Today it is found only in the northeastern horn of Africa, especially among stressed populations in Ethiopia, Eritrea, and occasionally neighboring Somalia and Sudan. The body louse acquires infection by feeding on spirochetemic persons, passing on the infection when it moves to another person and is crushed, typically by scratching of pruritic louse bite sites, allowing its infectious fluids to pass through minor breaks in the skin. Relapsing fevers are acute and incapacitating; LBRF is generally more severe than TBRF with a mortality rate of 20% or higher among untreated patients and approximately 5% among patients in treatment series. Casual visitors to endemic areas such as tourists are at almost no risk of LBRF, but persons who have close contact with infected populations, such as relief workers and care providers, can acquire the illness from lice, accidental needle sticks, or other direct contact with a patient's blood.

TBRF is caused by various closely related species of *Borrelia* and is found in scattered endemic foci throughout most regions of the world, excluding Australia and other areas of the South Pacific. It is transmitted by the bite of soft ticks (ticks with a leathery cutis and lacking a hard scutum) of the genus *Ornithodoros*. TBRF borreliae are usually named for the specific *Ornithodoros* tick that transmits them. With one exception, TBRF spirochetes are zoonotic, with small rodents typically serving as sources of blood meals for vector ticks and as reservoirs for the infecting borreliae. The exception is *Borrelia duttoni*, the principal cause of TBRF in sub-Saharan Africa, which infects only humans. In the United States, TBRF is endemic in far western states, especially in mountainous and forested areas above 5000 feet, where the agent *Borrelia hermsii* is transmitted by *Ornithodoros hermsi*. In the United States human infection occurs most often in spring and summer months from staying in rustic cabins infested by rodents, such as chipmunks, mice, and wood rats. In this circumstance *Ornithodoros* ticks acquire infection by feeding on rodents nesting in foundations, walls, or attics of dwellings and typically pass on the infection to persons while they are sleeping in nearby rooms. Camping near rodent nests in hollow logs, woodpiles, or other outdoor nesting sites can also result in exposure. Ticks can remain infectious through many generations and can survive for years without taking a blood meal. They are generally nocturnal and feed quickly and surreptitiously in the manner of bedbugs, so that patients are often not aware of having been bitten. In the southwestern United States, TBRF caused by *Borrelia turicatae* occurs rarely among persons exposed to rodent and tick infested caves. Although the TBRF is endemic and sporadic in nature, clusters of cases are common among persons sharing infested dwellings, and larger outbreaks can occur when groups of dwellings are affected. Fewer than 100 cases a year are reported in North America, and most cases are reported from Washington, California, Colorado, Idaho, Oregon, and British Columbia. TBRF is generally not as severe as LBRF, and treated patients almost always recover without serious complication. Relapsing fever may be severe in pregnant women, and TBRF is a significant cause of abortion, fetal death, and neonatal infection in some endemic areas of Africa.

Clinical Manifestations

The clinical manifestations of LBRF and TBRF are similar. Table 1 lists the common signs of TBRF in the United States. The mean incubation period is 7 days (2 to 18 days), and the onset of illness is sudden, manifest as fever above 38°C (100.4°F), headache, chills and rigors, sweats, lethargy, and aches and pains in muscles and joints. Headache and arthralgia can be severe. Inappetence, nausea and vomiting are common. The temperature remains high, generally in the range of 38°C (100.4°F) to 39.5°C (103.1°F), and the patient becomes withdrawn, dehydrated, weak, and listless, leading to prostration, as the untreated illness progresses. Orthostatic hypotension is typical. Tachycardia and mild tachypnea are common. Meningism may be present, and the patient is often photophobic. Scattered petechiae develop on the trunk, extremities, and mucous membranes in one third or more of patients with LBRF and in a lower proportion of patients with TBRF. Epistaxis and blood-tinged sputum are common complications in LBRF, whereas gastrointestinal or intracranial bleeding rarely occurs. Thrombocytopenia (<75,000 platelets/mm^3 peripheral blood) is usual. A nonproductive cough is common, as are pleuritic pain and an accompanying pleural rub on auscultation. Cardiac findings are those associated with a high output state, tachycardia, and summation gallop. Spirochetes are sequestered in reticuloendothelial tissues as well as in the blood; patients may have tender enlargement of the liver and spleen and be mildly jaundiced. Other complications of lesser incidence are iridocyclitis, optic neuritis, aseptic meningitis, coma, facial nerve palsy, pneumonitis, myocarditis, and rupture of the spleen. Infection during pregnancy is life-threatening to the fetus.

In untreated patients symptoms intensify over 2 to 7 days (mean of 5 days in LBRF and 3 days in TBRF), ending in a spontaneous crisis during which spirochetes rapidly disappear from the circulation and the fever breaks. Following the crisis, spirochetemia and symptoms may return after a period of several days or weeks (mean interval to first relapse is 9 days in LBRF and

TABLE 1 Signs and Symptoms of Tick-Borne Relapsing Fever Reported in Northwestern United States and Southwestern British Columbia

Sign or Symptom	%	Sign or Symptom	%
Headache	94	Photophobia	25
Myalgia	92	Neck pain	24
Chills	88	Rash	18
Nausea	76	Dysuria	13
Arthralgia	73	Jaundice	10
Vomiting	71	Hepatomegaly	10
Abdominal pain	44	Splenomegaly	6
Confusion	38	Conjunctival injection	5
Dry cough	27	Eschar	2
Eye pain	26	Meningitis	2
Diarrhea	25	Nuchal rigidity	2
Dizziness	25		

From Dworkin MS, Schwan TG, Anderson DE Jr: Tick-borne relapsing fever in North America. Med Clin North Am 2002;86:417.

7 days in TBRF). Characteristically, 1 or 2 relapses occur in untreated LBRF and as many as 10 (mean of 3) occur in untreated TBRF patients.

Diagnosis

Suspicion of diagnosis is most often triggered by the pattern of relapsing illness and a history of recent possible exposure to ticks or lice in endemic areas. Confirmation is most commonly made by observing the typical long, wavy, helical-shaped spirochetes in stained films of peripheral blood, sometimes in enormous numbers. The organisms are most numerous in the blood during periods of high fever; they can also be recovered from bone marrow, cerebrospinal fluid, and urine. Relapsing fever spirochetes can be cultured on modified BSK media, the media commonly used to isolate spirochetes causing Lyme borreliosis. A recently developed Western immunoblot test using a species-specific recombinant glycerophosphodiester phosphodiesterase (GlpQ) as antigen is the immunodiagnostic test of choice. Differential diagnostic possibilities, depending on circumstances of exposure, include malaria, typhus, dengue, salmonellosis, leptospirosis, viral hemorrhagic fevers, and Colorado tick fever.

Treatment

Patients with relapsing fever are acutely ill and should be managed in hospital during the early treatment period. An intravenous line should be established and vital signs monitored closely until spirochetes have been

cleared from the blood and the patient has recovered from a possible post-treatment reaction. Relapsing fever spirochetes are highly sensitive to a wide range of antimicrobial agents. Treatment with a tetracycline (such as doxycycline [Vibramycin]), erythromycin (E-Mycin),[1] chloramphenicol (Chloromycetin),[1] ceftriaxone (Rocephin),[1] or a short-acting penicillin produces a rapid clearance of spirochetes and remission of symptoms (Table 2). Erythromycin or penicillin is recommended for treating pregnant women and children younger than 8 years of age. Although single-dose treatment is highly effective against LBRF, less is known about single-dose treatment of TBRF, and an empirical course of 7 days is recommended to prevent post-treatment relapse of TBRF. Treatment may be given orally unless the patient is vomiting or unable to swallow. Spirochete clearance from the circulation typically begins within 1–3 hours of administration of the first treatment dose, often associated with a violent Jarisch-Herxheimer reaction (JHR) of several hours' duration. This reaction occurs in a higher proportion of LBRF than TBRF patients, and it is likely to be most severe in LBRF patients. Children are less likely to experience a reaction than adults, and if it occurs at all it is usually mild. The severity of the reaction is positively correlated with spirochete density in the peripheral circulation. The reaction comprises a chill (pressor) phase of 1 to 2 hours with body temperature often rising to 40.5°C (104.9°F) or higher, and marked by

---

 CURRENT DIAGNOSIS

- There may be recurring brief episodes, lasting as long as days, of high fever, headache, shaking chills, sweats, and weakness ending in lysis of fever by crisis. They may be complicated by bleeding, mild jaundice, meningitis, and facial nerve palsy. Intrafebrile periods generally last from 1 to 2 weeks.
- For TBRF there may be a history of possible exposure to soft ticks in rodent-infested dwellings, especially in rustic cabins in forested mountainous areas of the far western United States. For LBRF there may be a history of work with homeless, destitute populations in Ethiopia, or neighboring countries of northeastern Africa.
- Characteristic spirochetal forms on stained peripheral blood smears may be present.
- A JHR may occur within hours of first dose of antimicrobial treatment.

 CURRENT THERAPY

- Relapsing fever borreliae are highly sensitive to a range of broad-spectrum antimicrobials, including tetracyclines, erythromycin (E-Mycin),[1] chloramphenicol (Chloromycetin),[1] penicillins, and ceftriaxone (Rocephin).[1] Erythromycin (E-Mycin)[1] or penicillins are drugs of choice for children younger than 8 years of age as well as pregnant women.
- Treatment may be administered orally. Parenteral treatment is used in persons unable to reliably ingest or absorb medication; oral administration can be substituted as condition indicates.
- Single-dose treatment is adequate for treating LBRF; a 7-day course is recommended for treatment of TBRF.
- Patients should be monitored carefully during a JHR, a sometimes violent reaction that typically develops within a few hours of first antimicrobial dose. Signs of myocardial overload are of special concern. JHR management problems may include hyperpyrexia, bleeding, ineffective circulating blood volume, and pulmonary edema.

---

[1]Not FDA approved for this indication.

Abbreviations: JHR = Jarisch-Herxheimer reaction; LBRF = louse-borne relapsing fever; TBRF = tick-borne relapsing fever.

Abbreviations: JHR = Jarisch-Herxheimer reaction; LBRF = louse-borne relapsing fever; TBRF = tick-borne relapsing fever.

TABLE 2 Antibiotic Treatment of Louse-Borne and Tick-Borne Relapsing Fever in Adults

Medication	Louse-Borne Relapsing Fever (Single Dose)	Tick-Borne Relapsing Fever (7-day Schedule)
PO		
Erythromycin (E-Mycin)[1]	500 mg	500 mg q6h
Tetracycline	500 mg	500 mg q6h
Doxycycline (Vibramycin)	100 mg	100 mg q12h
Chloramphenicol (Chloromycetin)[1]	500 mg	500 mg q6h
Parenteral*		
Erythromycin (E-Mycin)[1]	500 mg	500 mg q6h
Tetracycline	250 mg	250 mg q6h
Doxycycline (Vibramycin)	100 mg	100 mg q12h
Chloramphenicol (Chloromycetin)[1]	500 mg	500 mg q6h
Penicillin (procaine)	600,000 IU	600,000 IU daily
Penicillin G	4 million IU	4 million IU q4h
Ceftriaxone (Rocephin)[1]	2 g	2 g daily

*For tick-borne relapsing fever, oral therapy may replace parenteral therapy as soon as it can be tolerated.
[1]Not FDA approved for this indication.
Abbreviation: PO = by mouth.

rigors, agitation, confusion, and sometimes delirium. The chill phase is followed over the next few hours by a flush phase of drenching sweats, rapidly falling temperature, a decrease in effective circulating blood volume, and a fall in arterial pressure. Patients need to be monitored carefully during this period, especially for signs of myocarditis and cardiac overload, evidenced by a prolonged QT corrected for heart rate (QT_C) interval on the electrocardiogram, a third heart sound, elevated central venous pressure, arterial hypotension, and pulmonary edema. The management of patients with myocardial dysfunction requires careful attention to fluid balance and rarely, a need for rapid digitalization. The JHR reaction is completed within 6 to 8 hours, leaving the patient exhausted but recovering. Delayed-release intramuscular penicillin (Bicillin L-A)[1] has been used in attempts to avoid or ameliorate the JHR in LBRF; but the treatment response may be delayed, and relapses have occurred following its use. Anti-inflammatory agents such as glucocorticoids[1] and aspirin[1] have not been shown to be effective in controlling the post-treatment reaction, which is associated with release of cytokines and other pro-inflammatory proteins, including interleukins, C-reactive protein, and large amounts of tumor necrosis factor-α (TNF-α). Experimental pretreatment of LBRF patients with antibody to TNF-α has been shown to suppress the JHR but is impractical for general use. Heparin[1] has no positive effect against bleeding, which is caused by transient thrombocytopenia rather than a disseminated intravascular coagulopathy. Hyperpyrexia can be ameliorated by using a cooling blanket, ice packs in the axillae, and sponging the patient with tepid water and alcohol.

Prevention

LBRF is controlled and prevented by improved sanitation and hygiene, delousing, and administration of antimicrobial agents to patients and close contacts. TBRF is controlled by removing rodent nests and rodent proofing dwellings, and by applying acaricides to affected premises. In hyperendemic areas of Africa, persons have been known to seed new dwellings with ticks from previous homes to ensure continuing protective immunity.

REFERENCES

Barbour AG: Relapsing Fever. In Goodman JL, Dennis DT, Sonenshine DE (eds): Tick-Borne Diseases of Humans. Washington, D.C., ASM Press, 2005.
Barbour AG, Restrepo BI: Antigenic variation in vector-borne pathogens. Emerg Infect Dis 2000;6:449.
Cadavid, D, Barbour AG: Neuroborreliosis during relapsing fever: Review of clinical manifestations, pathology, and treatment of infections in humans and experimental animals. Clin Infect Dis 1998;26:151.
Dworkin MS, Schwan TG, Anderson DE Jr: Tick-borne relapsing fever in North America. Med Clin North Am 2002;86:417.
Fekade D, Knox K, Hussein A, et al: Prevention of Jarisch-Herxheimer reactions by treatment with antibodies against tumor necrosis factor α. N Engl J Med 1996;335:311.
Perine PL, Teklu B: Antibiotic treatment of louse-borne relapsing fever in Ethiopia: A report of 377 cases. Am J Trop Med Hyg 1983; 32:1096.
Paul WS, Maupin G, Scott-Wright AO, et al: Outbreak of tick-borne relapsing fever at the north rim of the Grand Canyon: Evidence for effectiveness of preventive measures. Am J Trop Med Hyg 2002;66:71.
Porcella SF, Raffell SJ, Schrumpf ME, et al: Serodiagnosis of louse-borne relapsing fever with glycerophosphodiester phosphodiesterase (GlpQ) from *Borrelia recurrentis*. J Clin Microbiol 2000;38:3561.

---

[1]Not FDA approved for this indication.

Lyme Disease

Method of
Robert T. Schoen, MD

First recognized in 1975, Lyme disease is now the most common vector-borne illness in the United States. Since 1982, when surveillance was initiated by the Centers for Disease Control and Prevention (CDC), there has been a 19-fold increase in reported cases. Most cases in North America occur in the coastal northeastern states (Massachusetts to Virginia), the Midwest (Minnesota and Wisconsin), and the western states (California, Oregon, and parts of Nevada). Lyme disease is a spirochetal infection caused by a newly recognized organism, *Borrelia burgdorferi,* and transmitted primarily by ticks of the *Ixodes ricinus* complex, including *Ixodes scapularis.* In association with increased disease incidence and geographic expansion, there has also been widespread media interest, often sensationalizing Lyme disease. Although Lyme disease is underreported, perhaps by a factor of as much as 10, the disease and its complications are often overdiagnosed and overtreated.

Diagnosis

Lyme disease has characteristic clinical features with confirmatory diagnostic tests, yet many treatment-related difficulties in Lyme disease arise from errors in diagnosis. As a generalization, the most common reason for treatment failure in Lyme disease, particularly late Lyme disease, is misdiagnosis. Thus, a well-grounded understanding of the clinical manifestations of Lyme disease will solve many treatment problems.

The most important diagnostic principle in understanding the clinical features of Lyme disease is the recognition that the disease is divided into early-stage and late-stage disease. Early disease may be localized or disseminated.

 CURRENT DIAGNOSIS

- Assess risk of Lyme disease based on geographic location, time of year, and potential for deer tick exposure.
- Differentiate early-stage from late-stage Lyme disease.
- Avoid indiscriminate serologic testing, which will increase false positives.
- Consider the differential diagnosis for both early disease (flu-like illnesses in the summertime) and late disease (inflammatory arthritis, central nervous system disease).

Early Disease

EARLY LOCALIZED INFECTION

In early infection, most patients (perhaps 85%) develop an erythema migrans (EM) rash. If early disease is localized, other significant manifestations will be lacking. These patients may have mild fever and constitutional symptoms. Presumably in such individuals, spirochetal infection does not spread beyond the skin.

EM is an expanding erythematous rash, often with a well-demarcated outer border. The primary lesion occurs at the site of the deer tick bite with centrifugally expanding erythema. The lesion is often raised, sometimes indurated, warm, and itchy. It is usually not painful. EM develops within several days to up to 30 days after a deer tick bite but rarely occurs beyond this time. It is large (greater than 5 cm) and may expand within days or sometimes within hours. In untreated patients, the rash disappears without scarring several days to several weeks after onset.

EARLY DISSEMINATED DISEASE

In some patients, EM is associated with hematogenous dissemination of the organism to more widely metastatic sites, such as:

- Skin (secondary skin lesions)
- Liver and spleen (hepatitis)
- Peripheral nervous system and the brain (cranial and peripheral neuropathies, meningitis, and encephalitis)
- Heart (myocarditis)
- Joints (arthritis)

In early, localized disease, patients have only minor constitutional symptoms such as a low-grade fever or myalgias in addition to EM. In contrast, patients with early disseminated disease can be quite ill with high fever, headache, stiff neck, significant arthralgias, and malaise. Secondary skin lesions can cover the entire body, numbering up to 100. These tend to be smaller than the primary lesion, wax and wane over time, and resolve independently from the primary lesion. Lyme disease causes mild hepatitis in 15% of patients with early disseminated infection. Typically, there is a mild to moderate transaminitis (aspartate transaminase [AST] approximately 400 units) that resolves over several weeks.

LYME CARDITIS

In the United States, Lyme carditis occurs in 10% to 15% of patients with untreated early disseminated Lyme disease. Lyme carditis is a well-characterized clinical syndrome. Patients have mild myocarditis and variable degrees of atrioventricular nodal conduction disease, approximately 50% developing complete heart block, which is always reversible. Lyme carditis does not affect the heart valves and does not cause other arrhythmias such as atrial fibrillation or distal conduction system disease (for example, left bundle branch block pattern). Lyme carditis has been suggested as a cause of chronic cardiomyopathy in Europe, but there have been no such cases of Lyme disease causing chronic cardiomyopathy in the United States. Strain heterogeneity of *B. burgdorferi* may account for the different clinical manifestations in Europe and North America.

NEUROLOGIC DISEASE

The neurologic manifestations of Lyme disease present the most difficult diagnostic problems, but the neurologic features of early disseminated Lyme disease are often characteristic:

- Patients may have disease of the peripheral nervous system.
- Cranial neuropathies, particularly facial palsy, are common.
- Facial palsy may be unilateral or bilateral.
- Patients may have external ophthalmoplegia and present with diplopia.

These manifestations can wax and wane, occur with other manifestations of early disseminated Lyme disease, and may be associated with Lyme meningitis or encephalitis. Many patients with early disseminated Lyme disease have headache, fever, and stiff neck. A significant percentage will be found to have Lyme meningitis with a mild to moderate lymphocytic pleocytosis, cerebrospinal fluid (CSF) protein elevation, and increased CSF index (ratio of CSF to serum *B. burgdorferi* antibody titers of greater than 1). Some patients have a pattern consistent with meningoencephalitis and have acute cognitive difficulties, emotional lability, or other alterations in higher cortical function. These manifestations will usually resolve promptly with antibiotic treatment, whereas in the preantibiotic-era patients with Lyme meningoencephalitis often took months to recover.

Lyme arthritis is a late manifestation of Lyme disease, but many patients have arthralgias early in the illness, and some patients develop frank arthritis within days after disease onset, overlapping with other early features of the disease.

Late Disease

LYME ARTHRITIS

Lyme disease was recognized in the United States in patients with Lyme arthritis, a late manifestation of the disease. Sixty percent of individuals with early disease that is not treated will develop Lyme arthritis. Approximately half of these patients have characteristic frank arthritis of one or several joints, usually including the knee. Lyme arthritis is an asymmetric, oligoarticular arthritis usually affecting less than five joints, typically the large joints. The arthritis tends to occur in intermittent attacks lasting from several days to several weeks, although in roughly 10% of patients the arthritis is continuous (lasting more than 1 year). Large joint effusions are common in the knees. Baker's cysts occur and rupture early. The arthritis is often not painful and usually resolves with surprisingly little joint dysfunction.

A minority of patients have chronic unremitting arthritis and permanent joint destruction. Lyme arthritis can also present as arthralgias or migratory musculoskeletal pain. Antibiotic therapy clearly improves the natural history of Lyme arthritis, but not all patients respond immediately to treatment. It may require several months for arthritis to resolve after successful antibiotic treatment.

LATE NEUROLOGIC DISEASE

Late Lyme disease can occasionally affect the central nervous system (CNS). Patients may have cognitive dysfunction such as memory loss, fatigue syndromes, and in some cases upper motor neuron disease. These patients usually have earlier manifestations of the disease such as EM, cranial nerve palsies, or oligoarticular arthritis. They have confirmatory Lyme disease–specific antibodies measured by enzyme-linked immunosorbent assay (ELISA) in peripheral blood serologic studies. As with the early disease, the CSF often shows a mild lymphocytic pleocytosis, increased protein, and CSF index (ratio of CSF to serum *B. burgdorferi* antibodies by ELISA) greater than 1.

SEROLOGIC TESTING

Serologic testing is useful in Lyme disease, but because it relies on the patient's immune response, it has inherent limitations. Many, if not the majority of patients with early localized disease are seronegative for *B. burgdorferi* antibodies by ELISA when they present with EM. Because the goal of treatment at this stage is to shorten the duration of EM and prevent late manifestations of the disease, it is appropriate to treat such individuals with antibiotics based on clinical suspicion, even in the absence of serologic confirmation. It is easy to treat EM with oral antibiotic therapy, and it should resolve in less than 2 weeks. These patients will not only have complete recovery, but they may never make a detectable serologic response against *B. burgdorferi*. However, such individuals are not immune and may be reinfected. Most patients with early disseminated Lyme disease have *B. burgdorferi*–specific antibodies by ELISA. It may take up to 2 months for a detectable immune response to develop after disease exposure. In these individuals, treatment decisions are based on recognition of characteristic clinical syndromes. For example, Lyme disease can be diagnosed in a patient with complete heart block associated with EM in the spring or summer, even if serologic testing is initially negative. Atypical syndromes can also occur. Lyme hepatitis might occur in the absence of EM in an individual who is seronegative early in the course of their illness.

Patients with late Lyme disease almost always (greater than 95% of patients) develop anti–*B. burgdorferi* antibodies by ELISA. In individuals who present with questions about late Lyme disease, it is important to determine whether signs and symptoms fit the clinical syndrome. Serologic testing can be used to establish or exclude the diagnosis in such patients.

Testing should not be indiscriminate, however. Both false-negative results and, even more commonly, false-positive results occur. The predictive value of the test will be greatly influenced by the prevalence of the disease in the population being studied. At the present time, hundreds of thousands of Lyme disease serologic studies are being done to find hundreds of cases. As a result, the predictive value of Lyme disease serologic testing has been diminished and false-positive tests are a common clinical problem.

Treatment and Prevention

KEY TREATMENT POINTS

Early Lyme disease is routinely cured with oral antibiotics, typically doxycycline (Vibramycin)[1] and amoxicillin (Amoxil)[1]. Late manifestations of Lyme disease, arthritis, and neurologic manifestations require more intensive therapy, but there is no validity to long-term antibiotic therapy for chronic Lyme disease. Table 1 lists recommendations for the prevention and treatment of Lyme disease.

PREVENTION

Currently available preventive measures include the use of repellents, protective clothing (light-colored clothing makes ticks easier to identify), and skin inspection for ticks because ticks removed within 24 hours after attachment are relatively unlikely to transmit disease. A Lyme disease vaccine consisting of a recombinant outer surface protein A (OspA) with adjuvant is no longer available.

Whether asymptomatic persons should be given prophylactic antibiotic treatment after deer tick bites is still controversial. Although infection rates among ixodid ticks from endemic areas are high (typically 10% to 35%), the likelihood of acquiring Lyme disease after a deer tick bite in an endemic area is much lower, presumably because experimental studies suggest that ticks must remain attached for more than 48 hours for effective transmission of infection to occur. Prophylactic antibiotic treatment has a small risk of adverse effects, and in controlled clinical trials, such treatment has not been shown to confer a major benefit. In one study, the administration of single-dose doxycycline (Vibramycin)[1] (200 mg) after a deer tick bite reduced the incidence of

---

[1]Not FDA approved for this indication.

CURRENT THERAPY

- Most early-stage disease is treated with oral antibiotics (amoxicillin and doxycycline).
- Lyme arthritis is treated both orally and parenterally, depending on its chronicity.
- Most neurologic disease is treated with parenteral antibiotic therapy.

EM from 3.2% in the control population to 0.4% in the treated group.

EARLY DISEASE

For early-stage disease (local and disseminated), the goal of antibiotic therapy is to shorten the duration of EM and associated symptoms as well as to prevent the development of later stages of the illness. During early-stage disease, Lyme disease can be cured in more than 90% of individuals with a simple course of oral antibiotic therapy. Parenteral antibiotic therapy is usually unnecessary in the absence of neurologic or cardiac disease. Evidence-based treatment recommendations for Lyme disease have been developed by the Infectious Diseases Society of America and the American College of Physicians (see Table 1).

For EM the drug of choice for adults (except pregnant women) and children with permanent dentition is doxycycline[1] (100 mg orally [PO] twice daily for 14 to 21 days). The range of treatment duration suggested reflects the variability of severity of associated symptoms at disease onset. Severe disease at onset correlates with a greater risk for late complications such as arthritis. In general, because antibiotic therapy is most effective early in the illness, it is appropriate to treat most patients with more-than-mild illness at onset for a full 3-week course of antibiotic therapy. An advantage of doxycycline is its efficacy against the agent of human granulocytic ehrlichiosis, because some patients may be co-infected with this tick-transmitted infection. As an alternative, Amoxicillin (Amoxil)[1] may be just as effective as doxycycline for early Lyme disease and should be used in children who do not have permanent teeth and pregnant women. In patients who are allergic to either of these drugs, cefuroxime axetil (Ceftin)[1] is a third choice. Erythromycin (E-Mycin)[1] or its congeners, which are fourth-choice alternatives, are recommended only for patients who are unable to take doxycycline, amoxicillin, or cefuroxime axetil. Maternal-fetal transmission of *B. burgdorferi* seems to occur rarely, if at all. Therefore, it is recommended that pregnant women receive standard therapy, but they should avoid doxycycline. First-generation cephalosporins such as cephalexin (Keflex)[1] are an ineffective treatment for Lyme disease.

NEUROLOGIC MANIFESTATIONS

In patients with mild disease (for example, facial palsy alone), oral doxycycline (Vibramycin)[1] may be adequate therapy for acute neuroborreliosis. For most patients with objective evidence of neurologic abnormalities, however, intravenous ceftriaxone (Rocephin)[1] given for 2 to 4 weeks is recommended. Parental therapy with cefotaxime (Claforan)[1] or penicillin G[1] may be satisfactory alternatives. The signs and symptoms of acute neuroborreliosis usually resolve within weeks and objective evidence of relapse is rare after a 4-week course of therapy.

---

[1]Not FDA approved for this indication.

TABLE 1 Prevention and Treatment of Lyme Disease

Prevention

Asymptomatic deer tick bites	Prompt tick removal
	Doxycycline (Vibramycin)[1] 200 mg PO (single dose)

Treatment*

Early infection (local or disseminated)

Adults	Doxycycline (Vibramycin),[1] 100 mg PO bid for 14–21d
	Amoxicillin (Amoxil),[1] 500 mg PO tid for 14–21d
In case of doxycycline or amoxicillin allergy	Cefuroxime axetil (Ceftin),[1] 500 mg PO bid for 14–21d
	Erythromycin (E-Mycin),[1] 250 mg PO qid for 14–21d
Children	Amoxicillin (Amoxil),[1] 250 mg PO 3 times a day or 50 mg/kg/d in 3 divided doses for 14–21d
In case of penicillin allergy	Cefuroxime axetil (Ceftin),[1] 125 mg PO twice daily or 30 mg/kg/d in 2 divided doses for 14–21d
	Erythromycin,[1] 250 mg PO tid or 30 mg/kg/d in 3 divided doses for 14–21d

Neurologic abnormalities (early or late)

Adults	Ceftriaxone (Rocephin),[1] 2 g IV qd for 14–28d
	Cefotaxime (Claforan),[1] 2 g IV every 8h for 14–28d
	Penicillin G,[1] 3.3 million U IV every 4h (20 million U per day) for 14–28d
In case of ceftriaxone or penicillin allergy	Doxycycline (Vibramycin),[1] 100 mg PO bid for 30d[†]
Facial palsy alone	Oral regimens may be adequate
Children	Ceftriaxone (Rocephin),[1] 75–100 mg/kg (maximum, 2 g) IV qd for 14–28d
	Cefotaxime (Claforan),[1] 150 mg/kg/d in 3 or 4 divided doses (maximum, 6 g) for 14–28d
	Penicillin G[1] sodium, 200,000–400,000 U/kg/d in 6 divided doses for 14–28d

Arthritis (intermittent or chronic)	Oral regimens listed above for 30–60d or IV regimens listed above for 14–28d
Cardiac abnormalities	
First-degree atrioventricular block	Oral regimens listed above for 14–21d
High-degree atrioventricular block	IV regimens listed above and cardiac monitoring (PR interval >0.3 sec)
Pregnant women	Standard therapy for manifestation of the illness; except doxycycline

*The recommendations for antibiotic treatment are based on the guidelines of the Infectious Diseases Society of America.
[†]This regimen may be ineffective for late neuroborreliosis.
[1]Not FDA approved for this indication.
Abbreviations: bid = twice daily; d = days; h = hours; IV = intravenous; PO = by mouth; qd = daily; qid = four times daily; tid = three times daily; U = units.

CARDIAC DISEASE

Patients with first-degree heart block and PR interval of less than 0.3 second may be treated orally like other individuals with EM. In patients with atrioventricular nodal block and a PR interval of greater than 0.3 second, parenteral antibiotic therapy with one of the regimens listed in Table 1 and cardiac monitoring are recommended. Because Lyme carditis resolves without conduction system damage, a permanent pacemaker, even in patients with transient complete heart block, can almost always be avoided.

ARTHRITIS

Several oral regimens are successful treatments for Lyme arthritis in approximately 50% to 75% of patients and avoid the morbidity and expense of intravenous antibiotic therapy. In adults, these include doxycycline (Vibramycin)[1] 100 mg orally twice daily for 30 to 60 days and amoxicillin (Amoxil)[1] 500 mg 3 times day for 30 to 60 days. In patients who do not respond to oral therapy, the intravenous regimens described in

Table 1 (ceftriaxone [Rocephin][1] or penicillin G[1]) are an alternative. Despite either oral or intravenous antibiotic therapy, approximately 10% of patients in the United States have persistent joint inflammation for months or even several years after antibiotic therapy. These patients may benefit from anti-inflammatory agents or arthroscopic synovectomy.

CHRONIC LYME DISEASE

One of the most significant challenges in the management of Lyme disease is the treatment of patients with a well-documented antecedent history of Lyme disease treated according to standard regimens who continue to have subjective symptoms such as musculoskeletal pain, neurocognitive difficulties or fatigue syndrome (similar to chronic fatigue syndrome or fibromyalgia). Whatever the mechanism of this *post-Lyme disease syndrome*, there is no evidence that long-term antibiotic therapy,

---

[1]Not FDA approved for this indication.

intravenous or oral, benefits these patients. Supportive care, reassurance, and in many instances, treatment of underlying depression should be considered.

REFERENCES

Dattwyler RJ, Halperin JJ, Volkman DJ, Luft BJ: Treatment of late Lyme borreliosis—randomized comparison of ceftriaxone and penicillin. Lancet 1988;1:1191-1194.

Klempner MS, Hu LT, Evans J, et al: Two controlled trials of antibiotic treatment in patients with persistent symptoms and a history of Lyme disease. N Engl J Med 2001;345:85-92.

Logigian EL, Kaplan RF, Steere AC: Successful treatment of Lyme encephalopathy with intravenous ceftriaxone. J Infect Dis 1999; 180:377-383.

Massarotti EM, Luger SW, Rahn DW, et al: Treatment of early Lyme disease. AM J Med 1992; 92:396-403.

Nadelman RB, Nowakowski J, Fish D, et al: Prophylaxis with single-dose doxycycline for the prevention of Lyme disease after an *Ixodes scapularis* tick bite. N Engl J Med 2001;345:79-84.

Reid MC, Schoen RT, Evans J, et al: The consequences of overdiagnosis and overtreatment of Lyme disease: An observational study. Ann Intern Med 1998; 128:354-362.

Sood SK, Salzman MB, Johnson BJ, et al: Duration of tick attachment as a predictor of the risk of Lyme disease in an area in which Lyme disease is endemic. J Infect Dis 1997;175:996-999.

Steere AC: Lyme disease. N Engl J Med 2001;345:115-125.

Steere AC, Levin RE, Molloy PJ, et al: Treatment of Lyme arthritis. Arthritis Rheum 1994;37:878-888.

Wormser GP, Nadelman RB, Dattwyler RJ, et al: Practice guidelines for the treatment of Lyme disease. The Infectious Diseases Society of America. Clin Infect Dis 2000;31(Suppl 1):1-14.

Wormser GP, Ramanathan R, Nowakowski J, et al: Duration of antibiotic therapy for early Lyme disease. A randomized, double-blind, placebo-controlled trial. Ann Intern Med 2003;138:697-704.

Rubella and Congenital Rubella Syndrome

Method of
*Dennis Cunningham, MD, and
Jennifer Meddings, MD*

Rubella is Latin for "little red." It was considered a less severe variant of measles. The rash typically lasts 3 days, hence the name "three-day measles." Physicians in 18th century Germany recognized rubella as a distinct clinical entity and extensively studied the disease, also known as German measles.

Background and Epidemiology

Rubella virus consists of single-stranded RNA surrounded by a lipid-rich envelope. Classified in the family Togaviridae, rubella virus is the sole member of the genus *Rubivirus*. Infection is limited to humans. Incubation lasts 14 to 23 days. Rubella infections peak in the late winter and early spring with an increased number of cases occurring every 6 to 9 years. The last major epidemic in

the United States occurred in 1965. Vaccination, started in 1969, has dramatically reduced the incidence of rubella.

Between 10% and 20% of people in the United States are susceptible to rubella. Those at highest risk of disease include nonvaccinated immigrants, particularly those born in Mexico and Central America. Religious groups opposed to vaccinations are also at higher risk. The estimated attack rate in susceptible populations ranges from 50% to 80%. Transmission is via large respiratory droplets. An infected person is contagious from 7 days prior to 14 days after appearance of the exanthem.

Clinical Features

Children rarely have symptoms other than tender lymphadenopathy and a rash. Coryza and conjunctival hyperemia may accompany the rash. Adolescents and adults often have symptoms prior to appearance of the rash. Pain on movement of the eyes (myalgia) is a common feature of rubella. Systemic symptoms include headache, fatigue, mild fever, arthralgias, and cough. Jaundice is uncommon. Fevers resolve soon after appearance of a rash. Skin may desquamate as the rash fades. Classically, patients have tender lymphadenopathy involving the cervical, postauricular, and suboccipital chains. The rash starts on the face and spreads to the torso. The rash consists of discrete erythematous macular-papular eruptions. In adolescents and adults, the rash, which resolves over 3 to 5 days, may be accompanied by severe pruritus. Most patients will have an enanthem consisting of erythematous macules on the soft palate (Forchheimer spots). Forchheimer spots are not pathognomonic for rubella. A complete blood count may demonstrate transient lymphopenia. Approximately one third to one half of all primary infections are asymptomatic. Reinfection is possible, but it is usually asymptomatic and without clinical significance.

Diagnosis

Serology is the preferred method to diagnose disease. IgM does suggest recent infection, but false-positive results may occur with Epstein-Barr virus (EBV), cytomegalovirus (CMV), parvovirus, *Toxoplasma*, or rheumatoid factor. A fourfold increase in IgG titers suggests infection if acute and convalescent sera are tested concurrently. Polymerase chain reaction (PCR) assay is available but has limited clinical utility. Viral culture can detect rubella in blood, saliva, tears, breast milk, and urine. Diagnosis of congenital rubella infection requires isolation of virus from culture.

Complications

In healthy people, rubella is of little consequence. Arthralgias or arthritis of the fingers, wrists, and knees may develop within a week of the rash's appearance. This is much more common in adults but may occur in adolescents. Arthritis typically occurs in adult females,

CURRENT DIAGNOSIS

- Diagnosis is based on detailed history and physical
- Rubella unlikely if patient vaccinated
- Two doses of vaccine recommended
- Vaccine available as single vaccine (Meruvax II) or combination vaccine (MMR)
- Congenital rubella is rare
- Most cases in United States occur in immigrants from Central and South America
- Acute and convalescent serology confirms the diagnosis
- PCR used for research, but limited clinical utility at this time

and symptoms last 2 to 4 weeks. Rubella does not cause chronic arthritis. Thrombocytopenia and purpura may develop in children, probably because of an autoimmune reaction triggered by infection. The incidence of thrombocytopenia is approximately 1 in 3000 infected children. Encephalitis is a rare complication in 1 in 6000 infected individuals. The mortality rate of encephalitis is not clear, as evidenced by estimates of 0% to 50% in various reports. If patients survive encephalitis, recovery is usually complete. Rare reports of myocarditis and hepatitis have been described. The most significant complication of infection is congenital rubella syndrome (CRS).

Congenital Rubella

Primary infection of pregnant women in early gestation is devastating to the fetus. Reinfection of a gravid female usually does not cause CRS although a few cases have been reported. Rubella virus is a known teratogen and is thought to result in a vasculitis, which disrupts organogenesis. Rubella virus may also produce a protein-inhibiting mitosis. Infection during the first trimester can result in spontaneous abortion, stillbirth, or CRS. Risk is much lower when infection occurs in the second trimester and is negligible in the third trimester. Symptoms and signs of CRS may include growth retardation, pneumonitis, cataracts, retinopathy, glaucoma, persistent ductus arteriosus, peripheral pulmonary artery stenosis, mental retardation, organomegaly, thrombocytopenia, behavioral issues, and jaundice. The skin of CRS infants may have a "blueberry muffin" appearance secondary to extramedullary erythropoiesis in the skin. Radiographs of long bones typically show radiolucent metaphyses. The mortality rate for severe disease (CRS with organomegaly and thrombocytopenia) is 20% during the first year of life. Diagnosis of CRS requires isolation of the virus from culture and evaluation by many pediatric subspecialists. CRS is a reportable disease, and five to six cases of CRS occur in the United States each year. Typically the parents of infected infants were not born in the United States and never vaccinated. Some children with CRS have low serum levels of IgG. The clinical significance of this low

IgG is unknown, but regular intravenous immunoglobulin (IVIG) (Gamimune N)[1] infusions are probably reasonable. Infants with CRS may shed virus for up to 1 year. These patients are at increased risk for developing diabetes and thyroid disease.

Management of Exposure during Pregnancy

Prevention of CRS by vaccination is the best strategy. Pregnant women should avoid children with rashes whenever possible. If a confirmed exposure has occurred, the woman's serum should be tested. If IgG is present, the woman is considered immune, and the fetus is not at risk. If the test result is negative, it is prudent to repeat rubella titers at 3 and 6 weeks postexposure. Development of IgM or IgG indicates primary infection. If titers are negative, no infection occurred. There is no proven therapy for an infection during early pregnancy. Families should receive counseling and education on the risk of CRS and expected outcomes. Risk is highest during the first 4 weeks of gestation (85%) and is 20% to 30% during the second month. Many experts would recommend therapeutic abortion for primary infection in the first trimester. Treatment with IVIG (Gamimune N)[1] within 72 hours of exposure may be offered (0.55 mL/kg) only if abortion is not an option. The efficacy of IVIG in this setting is controversial. It may mask symptoms of illness but probably does not stop viremia.

Treatment

There is no proven therapy for rubella, which emphasizes the importance of prevention. Disease is limited to humans, and eradication is theoretically possible with widespread vaccination. Treatment is targeted toward specific symptoms. Nonsteroidal anti-inflammatory drugs are recommended for arthritis following infection. Antihistamines may benefit those with pruritic rashes. IVIG is helpful for thrombocytopenia following rubella. There is no role for glucocorticoids. Supportive care is indicated for rubella encephalitis.

---

[1]Not FDA approved for this indication.

CURRENT THERAPY

- There is no effective therapy
- Vaccination provides excellent protection
- Many experts recommend therapeutic abortion for primary infection in first trimester
- *Unclear if IVIG[1] is beneficial in this setting

[1]Not FDA approved for this indication.

Rubella Vaccine

Currently the United States has one licensed rubella vaccine, which uses a live attenuated virus. It may be administered singly (Meruvax II) or combined with measles and mumps vaccine (MMR). The immunization schedule recommends a dose of MMR between 12 and 15 months of age and again between 4 and 6 years of age. After one dose of vaccine, 95% of individuals will be seropositive, indicating protection from disease. Protection is usually life-long. Reinfection after wild type disease or immunization does occur, but is usually asymptomatic. Because it contains a live virus, rubella vaccine should not be administered to immunocompromised patients, except for those with well-controlled HIV infection. Vaccination of pregnant women is not recommended. The Centers for Disease Control and Prevention (CDC) has a registry of pregnant women inadvertently vaccinated against rubella. None of the children born to these mothers had findings of symptomatic infection. Pregnancy termination is not indicated if a pregnant woman is inadvertently immunized with MMR.

REFERENCES

American Academy of Pediatrics: Rubella. In Pickering LK (ed): Red Book: 2003 Report of the Committee on Infectious Diseases, 26th ed. Elk Grove Village, Ill, American Academy of Pediatrics, 2003, pp 536-541.
Centers for Disease Control and Prevention: Epidemiology & Prevention of Vaccine-Preventable Diseases (The Pink Book), 8th ed., 2nd printing. Atlanta, Author. Available online at http://www.cdc.gov/nip/publications/pink/def_pink_full.htm
Ezike E, Ang J: Rubella. Boston Med E Med J 2004;2(7).
Feigin RD, Cherry JD, Demmler GJ, Kaplin S: Textbook of Pediatric Infectious Diseases, Vol 2, 5th ed. Philadelphia, WB Saunders, 2004, pp 2134-2162.
Ray P, Black S, Shinefield H, et al: Risk of chronic arthropathy among women after rubella vaccination. JAMA 1997;278(7):551-556.

Measles (Rubeola)

Method of
John R. Stephenson, PhD

Measles (rubeola) has probably been responsible for the deaths of more children than any other single cause. Its normal presentation is as an acute childhood exanthematous illness, but severe complications including encephalitis, deafness, and pneumonia are frequently reported. Since the introduction of a live, attenuated vaccine (Attenuvax), it is rarely seen in North America and Europe, but it is still a major cause of childhood mortality in developing countries, especially in sub-Saharan Africa.

Etiology

Measles is caused by a negative-stranded RNA virus belonging to the Paramyxoviridae family and the *Morbillivirus* genus. It consists of a single strand of RNA incorporated into a morphologically distinct *herringbone* nucleocapsid. The nucleocapsid also contains the N, P, and L proteins. The outer layer of the virion contains two envelope glycoproteins embedded in a lipid bilayer that is bordered internally by the M protein. The H glycoprotein contains the virus receptor and hemagglutinin, and the F protein is responsible for fusion between the virion and cell membranes, and between the plasma membranes of infected cells. Infected cells also contain the C and V proteins.

Epidemiology

Measles virus is probably the most infectious transmissible agent causing human disease. Transmission occurs mainly in the early clinical phase through aerosols generated by the characteristic *brassy* cough. Before the introduction of measles vaccine, nearly every child had become infected before the age of 10 years, resulting in around 130 million cases and more than 8 million deaths per year. The introduction of live attenuated vaccines has dramatically reduced the global occurrence of disease and in countries where vaccine uptake is high, indigenous disease has been virtually eliminated. Although current vaccines are efficient, they do have limitations. Children are most at risk during the first year of life; while maternal antibody protects from infection during the perinatal period, declining antibody levels in the second half of the first year of life are not protective but can prevent effective immunization. In vaccinated populations this effect is more marked because most women of childbearing age have never been in contact with *wild* measles. In these populations, maternal antibody wanes faster than in populations whose immunity has been derived from or boosted by wild measles virus.

In recent years vaccination rates in some industrial countries have been adversely affected by inadequate vaccination protocols, complacency, and fears of adverse reactions. In the United States during the early 1980s, there were fewer than 4000 cases per year, but within a few years the annual incidence had risen to nearly 27,000. It became apparent that the current single-dose vaccination strategy was inadequately protecting significant numbers of children from urban ethnic and racial minority groups who had depended on vaccination rather than natural disease for their immunity. Lower levels of maternal antibody, coupled with continued low vaccine uptake in inner cities probably conspired to produce the dramatic rise in measles cases. Significant numbers of cases were also seen in vaccinated populations of school age children and in college students. Consequently in 1989 the U.S. Public Health Service Advisory Committee on Immunization Practices (ACIP) recommended that a two-dose schedule be adopted, preferably using the combined measles-mumps-rubella (MMR) vaccine (MMR II). More recently vaccination rates have been adversely affected, especially in the United Kingdom, through fears that measles vaccines are linked to inflammatory bowel disease and autism. Although there is no conclusive evidence to support these fears, they remain and probably contribute to poor vaccine uptake in some regions and some sections of society.

The Pan American Health Organization set a target date to eliminate measles in the western hemisphere by 2000. Although this target was not met, there were less than 5000 cases in 2004 and no indigenous measles transmission has been reported in this area since 2002. Progress in other areas has been less promising, and recent WHO estimates indicate that total global vaccine coverage is close to 80%, but 32 countries still have coverage rates below 60%.

Clinical Manifestations

ACUTE INFECTION

Measles infection can normally be divided into three phases: incubation or catarrhal, prodromal enanthem, and exanthem. Infection starts in the nasal mucosa, resulting in fever, coryza, cough, conjunctivitis, photophobia, and an erythematous maculopapular rash followed by a characteristic enanthem. The incubation period lasts 10 to 15 days with a prodromal period of 1 to 3 days during which respiratory and ocular symptoms (chiefly photophobia and conjunctivitis) appear. Viral transmission is thought to occur at this time. Toward the end of this time, Koplik's spots, the pathognomonic sign of measles, appear. These are small, greyish-white dots, approximately the size of a grain of sand appearing opposite the lower molars and irregularly over the remainder of the buccal mucosa. The typical measles exanthem appears around day 14 when respiratory symptoms are at their peak and the patient's temperature frequently exceeds 39°C (102.2°F). The exanthem usually appears behind the ears and at the hairline and spreads down throughout the body, reaching the lower extremities approximately 3 days later. It frequently reaches confluence on the face and upper trunk and begins to clear after approximately 3 days, following the same course as its appearance. Disease severity is correlated with the extent and confluence of rash, and in severe cases the skin can be completely covered and the face disfigured. Splenomegaly and cervical lymphadenopathy may occur. Mesenteric lymphadenopathy may cause abdominal pain, and virus-induced pathology in the mucosa of the appendix may result in appendicitis. Gastrointestinal (GI) symptoms, otitis media, and bronchopneumonia are more common in infants and young children, especially if undernourished.

MODIFIED MEASLES

This presentation usually occurs in the presence of maternally acquired antibodies, after the administration of immune globulin to a susceptible child or occasionally as the result of vaccine failure. This illness is normally mild, but it follows the same course as typical measles. The prodromal phase is shortened, Koplik's spots are rare, and the rash is seldom confluent.

ATYPICAL MEASLES

Following the success of the formalin-fixed Salk polio vaccines, two similar measles vaccines were produced in the United States and licensed for use in 1961. After several reports of untoward effects, this vaccine was withdrawn from use in the United States in 1966, but its use was continued for several years in Canada and Germany. In those individuals who had received killed vaccine and were then given live attenuated vaccine, local reactions consisting of mild to severe swelling and maculopapular or vesicular rash were common. In patients who had contracted natural measles after receiving killed vaccine, a variety of clinical forms were seen, but pulmonary complications, abdominal pain, headache, and unusual purpuric or vesicular rashes were more common in atypical measles than in natural measles. The appearance of rash was unlike classical measles, starting on the palms, wrists, soles, and ankles and spreading in a centripetal direction. However Koplik's spots, conjunctivitis, and coryza were not present and antibody responses were usually tenfold higher than in natural measles. The exact nature of this effect is still unknown, but the most plausible hypothesis suggests that both virus and antibody circulate in the blood and form large immune complexes, which could be trapped in the pulmonary vessels. Immunologic tissue damage would result, manifesting itself as pneumonia.

COMPLICATIONS

Measles infection is frequently associated with several severe complications, which can give rise to high levels of morbidity and mortality in immunocompromised or malnourished individuals. Measles infection has been known to be associated with a transient immune suppression for many years, which is probably the cause of the most frequent complications, pneumonia and otitis media. These usually arise from secondary bacterial infections, of which *Staphylococcus aureus, Haemophilus influenzae,* pneumococci, and the group A streptococci (GAS) are the most common. Measles infection may also exacerbate tuberculosis and AIDS, with measles pneumonia being frequently fatal in the latter patient group. Pulmonary involvement resulting from measles virus infection is also common and in its most severe form, giant cell pneumonia, frequently fatal. Neurologic complications occur more frequently during measles than in any other exanthem, but there is no observable correlation between the severity of the initial infection, neurologic involvement, the severity of the encephalitis, and prognosis. Encephalitis usually occurs 2 to 3 weeks after the onset of the exanthem, sometimes ending in permanent neurologic impairment, coma, or death. Early onset of encephalitis is usually associated with viral invasion of the CNS, but late-onset disease is thought to be an immunologic event. Other neurologic complications such as Guillain-Barré syndrome, hemiplegia, retrobulbar neuritis, and cerebral thrombophlebitis are less common. A rare and invariably fatal neurologic complication of measles is subacute sclerosing panencephalitis (SSPE). Curiously, this complication occurs on average 3 to 4 years after the initial infection, with a significantly higher prevalence in males. Onset is frequently associated with an insidious change in personality and deterioration in intellectual performance. Myoclonic jerks of the head, trunk, and limbs occur after a few months, and the patient slowly and progressively deteriorates over a period of approximately 2 years into a decorticate state, coma, and death. GI complications occur often in acute measles, and in recent outbreaks in the United States around 8% of patients reported with diarrhoea. Less frequently, myocarditis, pericarditis, hemorrhage, glomerulonephritis, hepatitis, appendicitis, ileocolitis, and mesenteric lymphadenitis have been reported as complications associated with measles.

Diagnosis

Clinical diagnosis has been traditionally based on presentation with coryza, a distinctive brassy cough, and conjunctivitis, in association with high fever and a typical rash. However, measles is now rarely seen by physicians in North America and Europe, and differential diagnosis based on clinical presentation alone can be difficult. Therefore, laboratory confirmation of a raised measles-specific IgM is usually required to confirm diagnosis. IgM levels can be low during the first few days following the appearance of rash and testing may need to be repeated. Traditionally, hemagglutination inhibition (HI) and complement fixation (CF) tests, and virus neutralization have been used for laboratory diagnosis, but these were slow and insensitive and have been replaced by IgM enzyme-linked immunosorbent assays (ELISAs). The virus can be isolated from blood, urine, and nasopharyngeal secretions during the early stages of infection, but it is time-consuming and slow.

CURRENT DIAGNOSIS

- Coryza, a distinctive *brassy* cough, and conjunctivitis in association with high fever and a typical rash
- Koplik's spots in the buccal cavity in the early stages of infection
- Raised measles-specific IgM, usually determined by ELISA
- Virus isolation from blood, urine, and nasopharyngeal secretions during the early stages of infection; when possible RT-PCR can determine the genetic clade of the virus in outbreaks
- Low WBC counts, with evidence of lymphocytosis
- Patients with encephalitis, but normal glucose levels in their CSF
- Rash differentiated from that associated with infections caused by other viruses

Abbreviations: CSF = cerebrospinal fluid; ELISA = enzyme-linked immunoabsorbent assay; RT-PCR = reverse transcriptase polymerase chain reaction; WBC = white blood cell.

Recently reverse transcriptase–polymerase chain reaction (RT-PCR) methods have greatly improved the reliability and sensitivity of virus detection in bodily fluids. White blood cell (WBC) counts are usually low, with evidence of lymphocytosis. Patients with encephalitis have raised protein but normal glucose levels in their cerebrospinal fluid (CSF).

KEY DIAGNOSTIC POINTS

Laboratory confirmation of raised serum IgM levels is now required in most developed countries. All suspected cases must be reported immediately to local and national centers, such as the Centers for Disease Control and Prevention (CDC) in the United States and the Health Protection Agency in the United Kingdom.

DIFFERENTIAL DIAGNOSIS

Measles-associated rash must be differentiated from that associated with infections caused by adenovirus, coxsackievirus, echovirus, Epstein-Barr virus, human herpesviruses 6 and 8, meningococci, *Rickettsia,* rubella virus, and streptococci, as well as rashes associated with adverse reactions to drugs, vaccines, and passive immunization.

Treatment

Because no measles-specific antiviral therapy is available, treatment is usually limited to supportive therapy. Antipyretics, maintenance of fluid intake and bed rest are indicated, with reduced lighting for patients with photophobia. Complications caused by secondary bacterial infections (e.g., otitis media and pneumonia) can normally be successfully treated with antibiotics.

Oral or intrathecal ribavirin (Virazole)[1] has been used as an experimental treatment on occasion, especially with cases of SSPE, but the toxicity of this drug prevents its widespread use. In developing countries, oral vitamin A supplementation[1] can significantly reduce

[1]Not FDA approved for this indication.

CURRENT THERAPY

There is no measles-specific antiviral therapy or treatment available. Patient care is usually limited to supportive therapy and antipyretics maintenance of fluid intake and bed rest are indicated. Reduced lighting is recommended for patients with photophobia. Complications caused by secondary bacterial infections (e.g., otitis media and pneumonia) can normally be successfully treated with antibiotics. In cases where malnutrition is apparent, oral vitamin A[1] can frequently improve recovery.

the morbidity and mortality of severe measles. In these countries vitamin A supplementation is recommended for children in the first 3 years of life who are hospitalized with measles or its complications, and for all children with measles and evidence of vitamin A deficiency or immunodeficiency. (Vitamin A has not been approved by either the U.S. FDA or the EU MCA for this indication.)

Prognosis

Improved socioeconomic conditions and the successful treatment of secondary bacterial infections have dramatically reduced the case-fatality rates for all age groups in industrialized countries. Despite this improvement, case-fatality rates can still reach 1:1000, mainly from pneumonia or bacterial infection. In developing countries the situation is much worse, especially in infants, in whom case-fatality rates can reach 1:4. Malnutrition almost certainly plays a role, but cannot completely account for these high death rates. Most of the 800,000 deaths per year occur in sub-Saharan Africa where other local factors such as parasite burden may also contribute.

Prevention

Measles is very easily transmitted in enclosed environments and therefore institutional isolation should occur from the seventh day after exposure to at least the fifth day following the appearance of rash.

VACCINATION

A combined vaccine containing live attenuated MMR II was introduced in the United States in 1975 and many other countries quickly followed. In most developed countries, the first dose is given from 12 to 15 months of age and a second dose to children from 3 to 6 years old. In the United States all children should have received two doses by 11 to 12 years of age, as should all entrants into college or full-time employment. During outbreaks vaccination can be given to infants as young as 6 months of age. MMR is not recommended for children with primary immunodeficiency, pregnant women, patients with untreated tuberculosis, cancer, or those receiving immunosuppressive therapy or undergoing organ transplantation. Individuals with asymptomatic or mild HIV infection can be vaccinated, but not those with severe disease.

Immunoglobulin interferes with vaccination, and anergy to tuberculin antigen frequently develops and persists for several weeks after vaccination. Consequently children with active tuberculosis should start on a course of treatment before the vaccine is administered.

POSTEXPOSURE PROPHYLAXIS

Passive immunization is effective if given within 6 days after exposure and immunocompromised individuals should receive intramuscular immunoglobulin, regardless of their levels of immunity.

REFERENCES

Atkinson WL, Orenstein WA: The resurgence of measles in the United States, 1989-1990. Annu Rev Med 1992;43:451-463.

Centers for Disease Control: Measles prevention: Recommendations of the Immunization Practices Advisory Committee (ACIP). MMWR Morbid Mortal Wkly Rep 1990;38:1-18.

Children's Vaccine Initiative Ad Hoc Committee on an Investment Strategy for Measles control: A Bellagio consensus. J Infect Dis 1994;170:S63-S64.

Clements CJ, Cutts FT: The epidemiology of measles: Thirty years of vaccination. In ter Meulen V, Billiter MA (eds): Measles Virus. Berlin, Springer-Verlag, 1995, pp 13-34.

De Quadros CA, Olive JM, Hersh BS, et al: Measles elimination in the Americas, evolving strategies. JAMA 1996;275:224-229.

Johnson RT, Griffin DE, Hirsch RL: Measles encephalomyelitis: Clinical and immunologic studies. N Engl J Med 1984;310:137-141.

Julkunen I, Davidkin I, Oker-Blom C: Methods for detecting anti-measles, mumps and rubella virus antibodies. In Stephenson JP, Warnes A (eds): Diagnostic Virology Protocols. Totowa, New Jersey, Humana Press, 1998, pp 142-158.

Katz M: Clinical spectrum of measles. In ter Meulen V, Billiter MA (eds): Measles Virus. Berlin, Springer-Verlag, 1995, pp 1-12.

Metcalf J: Is measles infection associated with Crohn's disease? The current evidence does not support a causal link. BMJ 1998; 316:166.

O'Donovan C, Barua KN: Measles pneumonia. Am J Trop Med Hyg 1973;22:73-77.

Rall GF: Measles virus 1998-2002: Progress and controversy. Annu Rev Med 2003;57,343-367.

ter Meulen V, Stephenson JR, Kreth HW: Subacute sclerosing panencephalitis. In Fraenkel-Conrat H, Wager RR, (eds): Comprehensive Virology, vol 18. New York, Plenum Press, 1983, pp 105-160.

Tetanus

Method of
Ramesh K. Khurana, MD, FAAN, and
James P. Richardson, MD, MPH

Tetanus, one of the oldest and most preventable afflictions of humankind, results from infection by the anaerobic gram-positive organism *Clostridium tetani.* Tetanospasmin, the neurotoxin produced by the organism, blocks spinal and brainstem inhibitory pathways, leading to localized or generalized muscle spasms. It often presents itself as the increased tone of the masseter muscles, or trismus—hence the former name *lockjaw.*

Etiology

The causative organism of tetanus, *C. tetani,* exists as spores that are resistant to boiling for 20 minutes and to disinfectants, and, hence, it is nearly ubiquitous. Spores have been found in animal and human feces, as well as soil, dust, human dwellings, and hospitals.

Vegetative cells, however, are susceptible to heat, antiseptics, and several antibiotics.

Epidemiology

Tetanus is a rare disease in the United States, with an annual incidence of approximately 0.02 per 100,000 people. Less than 50 cases are reported to the Centers for Disease Control and Prevention (CDC) each year. However, many cases of tetanus probably go unreported. In recent cases reported to the CDC, 55% of the patients were 20 to 59 years old; 36% were 60 years old and older. There is a slightly higher incidence of tetanus in men, older adults, recent immigrants, and parenteral drug users. Serologic surveys document lower levels of protective antibody levels in older adults, women, Hispanic Americans, and those with lower incomes and educational levels. Untreated, tetanus is usually fatal. Even with treatment, the overall case-fatality rate is greater than 10%, increasing with age to 40% in those older than 60 years in the most recent report from the CDC. It is well worth noting, however, that in the United States since 1989, no deaths have occurred in individuals with current tetanus immunization.

The disease is much more common worldwide because of lower levels of immunization. The World Health Organization (WHO) estimates that in the year 2000, 309,000 people died of tetanus, including 200,000 neonates.

Pathogenesis

Tetanus spores gain entrance to the body through skin injuries. These injuries are often so minor that they do not result in any medical attention (e.g., a prick from a thorn bush or a minor puncture wound). Because *C. tetani* is an obligate anaerobe, the spores will grow only in areas of low oxygen tension, such as occurs with pressure sores, puncture wounds, or gangrene. Reports of tetanus following abortion, animal bites and stings, splinters, and body piercing are documented. The portal of entry in the newborn is usually through the contaminated umbilical stump. Growing or vegetative *C. tetani* organisms produce tetanospasmin, one of the most potent neurotoxins known, which reaches the nervous system via two routes: blood-borne delivery to peripheral nerves and retrograde intraneuronal transport. The toxin exerts its effects on the peripheral nerves, neuromuscular junction, muscle, spinal cord, brainstem, and possibly the hypothalamus.

Tetanospasmin is recognized by high-affinity receptors located on the surface of the peripheral nerve endings, is internalized and retrogradely transported to the neurons in the spinal cord and brainstem. The toxin then migrates transsynaptically to presynaptic terminals and blocks the release of the inhibitory neurotransmitters gamma-aminobutyric acid (GABA) and glycine. Loss of inhibition affects the alpha motor neurons and preganglionic sympathetic neurons, producing muscle spasms and autonomic hyperactivity, respectively.

Recovery involves synthesis of new presynaptic components and their transport to the distal axons.

Clinical Presentation

The incubation period of tetanus is usually from 3 days to 3 weeks, but tetanus can occur several months after an injury. Cases with shorter incubation periods and rapid generalization of spasms tend to be the most severe. There are three clinical forms of tetanus based on the site of toxin action and the age of the patient: generalized, localized, and neonatal.

Generalized disease is the most common of the forms (Box 1). Typical presenting complaints include trismus, neck rigidity, stiffness, dysphagia, restlessness, and reflex spasms. Tetanus patients may display risus sardonicus (a characteristic grimace manifested as raised eyebrows and a wrinkled forehead with the corners of the mouth pulled up). Muscle rigidity usually starts with the jaw and facial muscles and then spreads to the trunk (opisthotonos) and extensor muscles of the limbs. Hands and feet are relatively spared. Spasms may occur spontaneously or may be provoked by external stimuli such as noise, touch, lights, and parenteral injections. Tetanic spasms differ from grand mal seizures in that patients with tetanic spasms remain conscious. These spasms affect agonist and antagonist muscle groups together and are extremely painful. Violent paroxysms of generalized spasms may result in fractures, muscle rupture and rhabdomyolysis, and laryngospasm and apnea, both of which preclude ventilation and feeding.

Autonomic dysfunction usually complicates severe cases, occurring some days after spasms. This dysfunction may be one of overactivity or underactivity of the sympathetic and parasympathetic nervous systems. Sympathetic disturbances may manifest as labile or sustained hypertension, tachycardia, dysrhythmia, peripheral vasoconstriction, profuse sweating, glycosuria, and elevated plasma and urinary catecholamines. Parasympathetic manifestations include profuse salivation, increased bronchial secretions, gastric stasis,

---

BOX 1 Presentation of Tetanus

Generalized Disease
Trismus
Risus sardonicus
Dysphagia
Opisthotonos
Isolated cranial nerve palsies
Rigidity or stiffness in an extremity
Neck stiffness
Restlessness
Tetanic seizures
Poor sucking (newborns)
Localized Disease
Rigidity or stiffness in an extremity
Cephalic Disease
Single or multiple cranial nerve palsies

---

and ileus. Hypotension, bradycardia, and cardiac arrest may occur.

Two less common types of tetanus are localized tetanus and cephalic tetanus. Localized tetanus is characterized by painful spasms of muscles near the site of injury. This disorder is usually self-limiting and lasts less than 2 weeks, but progression to generalized disease can occur if untreated. Cephalic tetanus is a frequently severe form of localized tetanus. The bacillus enters through minor head trauma or chronic otitis media. Cephalic tetanus may present as single or multiple, often unilateral, cranial nerve palsies before the development of trismus, dysphagia, dysarthria, head tilt, and possible generalization.

Neonatal tetanus presents as an inability to suck and irritability 3 to 10 days after birth. It is usually a generalized form characterized by muscle rigidity, opisthotonos, apnea, and cyanosis.

Diagnosis

Tetanus is a clinical diagnosis; there is no specific confirmatory laboratory test. A history of a predisposing injury in an inadequately immunized host is helpful. As noted earlier, however, a history of injury is not always present. A well-documented history of primary immunization and a booster immunization within the last 10 years makes the diagnosis of tetanus less likely. The diagnosis is based on the observation of characteristic clinical features. Apte and colleagues, in administering a spatula test to diagnose tetanus, observed that 94% of 359 patients with tetanus involuntarily bit the spatula because of the reflex spasm of masseter muscles, instead of gagging and expelling it. Absence of sensory deficits and a clear sensorium supports the diagnosis of tetanus. Laboratory tests such as complete blood counts and routine blood chemistry tests are not helpful. Creatine kinase may be elevated. Cultures are positive in only 32% to 50% of patients, and, in any event, treatment cannot wait for their completion. Tetanus antitoxin antibody levels are not usually available quickly and are not reliable after the administration of human tetanus immune globulin (HTIG). Electromyography of the involved muscles, or the masseter muscle, shows continuous motor unit discharge. Laboratory tests can,

however, be useful in excluding other conditions. For example, a urine screen may be positive in cases of strychnine poisoning.

Established generalized tetanus is easily recognized, whereas the diagnosis of cephalic tetanus can pose some difficulty. Cranial nerve involvement is common and may confuse the physician. Trismus may result from intraoral disease or an acute dystonic reaction to phenothiazines or metoclopramide (Reglan). Muscular stiffness can also be a manifestation of strychnine poisoning, meningitis, hepatic encephalopathy, rabies, hypocalcemic tetani, stiff-man syndrome, and conversion reaction. A delay in the diagnosis of tetanus has occurred in patients presenting with dysphagia. Rigid abdominal muscles may simulate an acute abdomen.

Treatment

Whenever possible, patients with suspected tetanus should be transferred to a facility that has experience with this disease. Patients should be kept in a quiet and dark environment to minimize sensory stimulation. Treatment has the following goals:

- Neutralization of the circulating toxin that has not yet entered the nervous system
- Elimination of the source of the toxin by careful surgical débridement and by antibiotic administration to inhibit growth of the bacilli
- Prevention of respiratory and metabolic complications
- Prevention of muscle spasms
- Management of cardiovascular complications caused by autonomic instability

Tetanus antitoxin should be given to prevent further fixation of the toxin to the central nervous system,

---

 CURRENT THERAPY

- Tetanus antitoxin[2] and/or human tetanus immune globulin (BayTet) should be given immediately, followed by débridement and appropriate antibiotic therapy (e.g., metronidazole [Flagyl]).
- Tetanus immunization with tetanus and diphtheria toxoid (Td) should also be given.
- Tetanic spasms should be controlled with benzodiazepines.
- Fentanyl (Sublimaze)[1] may help control autonomic cardiovascular instability (manifested as hypertension and tachycardia) by attenuating the sympathetic efferent discharge.
- Supportive care includes protection of the airway, management of fluids and electrolyte balance, nutrition, bowel and bladder functions, skin care, deep venous thrombosis prophylaxis, and physiotherapy.

[1]Not FDA approved for this indication.
[2]Not available in the United States.

 CURRENT DIAGNOSIS

- The diagnosis is clinical; laboratory tests are not helpful, except in eliminating other diagnoses.
- A history of adequate tetanus immunization makes the diagnosis much less likely.
- Involuntary biting of a spatula because of masseter muscle spasm is highly suggestive.
- Generalized disease is the most common form of tetanus and may present as trismus, neck rigidity, stiffness, dysphagia, restlessness, reflex spasms, and risus sardonicus.

although it will not reduce manifestations already present. Between 3000 and 6000 units of HTIG (or Hyper-Tet) should be given intramuscularly as soon as possible and definitely before manipulating the wound. Some authorities recommend giving some of the HTIG near the site of the wound. Tetanus does not confer immunity. Therefore, active immunization with tetanus and diphtheria toxoid (Td) or diphtheria toxoid–pertussis vaccine–tetanus toxoid (DPT) or DTaP, as appropriate, also should be given, at a site contralateral from that for tetanus immune globulin (TIG) (Table 1).

Débridement is important for several reasons. It removes live organisms, creates an aerobic environment unfavorable for further growth, and secures specimens for culture. Débridement should be delayed until several hours after the administration of antitoxin because tetanospasmin may be released into the bloodstream. Antibiotic therapy is essential to sterilize the wound and eradicate the bacilli in their vegetative form. The antibiotic of choice is metronidazole (Flagyl), given at a dose of 7.5 mg per kg every 6 hours up to a maximum of 500 mg. Acceptable alternatives are doxycycline (Vibramycin) and imipenem cilastatin (Primaxin).[1] Penicillin, once the drug of choice, should not be used because it acts as a competitive antagonist to GABA and promotes hyperexcitability and convulsions.

Oxygenation is ensured by protecting the airway. In all but the mildest of cases, prophylactic intubation should be initiated early. Intubation will usually require sedation with a benzodiazepine (e.g., lorazepam [Ativan],[1] 2 mg intravenously) and neuromuscular blockade (e.g., vecuronium [Norcuron], 0.08 to 0.1 mg per kg). Patients in whom orotracheal intubation precipitates laryngeal spasms, require more than 10 days of intubation, or have generalized seizures should undergo elective tracheostomy. An oropharyngeal airway will allow removal of secretions and prevent biting in mild cases that do not require intubation.

Control of tetanic spasms and rigidity is best achieved with the benzodiazepines. Additional benefits are that

[1]Not FDA approved for this indication.

TABLE 1 Routine Diphtheria and Tetanus Immunization Schedule for Persons 7 Years of Age and Older

Dose	Age/Interval	Product
Primary 1	First dose	Td
Primary 2	4–8 weeks after the first dose*	Td
Primary 3	6–12 months after second dose*	Td
Boosters	Every 10 years after last dose	Td

*Prolonging the interval does not require restarting series.
Abbreviation: Td = tetanus and diphtheria toxoid.
From Immunization Practices Advisory Committee: Diphtheria, tetanus, and pertussis: Recommendations for vaccine use and other preventive measures-recommendations of the Immunization Practices Advisory Committee (ACIP). MMWR 1991;40(No. RR-10).

Rakel and Bope: *Conn's Current Therapy 2006*

these drugs produce sedation and amnesia. Diazepam (Valium)[1] can be given at a large dose of 0.5 mg per kg to 15 mg per kg per day[3] intravenously. Alternatively, continuous infusions of lorazepam (Ativan) at a dose of 0.1 to 2.0 mg per kg per hour,[3] midazolam (Versed)[1] at a dose of 0.01 to 0.10 mg per kg per hour, or propofol (Diprivan)[1] at a dose of 3.5 to 4.5 mg/kg per hour can be given. The intrathecal administration of baclofen (Lioresal)[1] has been found useful, but it is both costly and invasive.

In patients whose muscle spasms do not respond to sedation, neuromuscular blocking agents, such as vecuronium (Norcuron),[1] are often necessary. The patients will require assisted ventilation, often for several days or weeks. Because neuromuscular agents prevent skeletal muscle movements only and do not reduce pain or provide sedation, it is essential that patients be monitored very closely for adequate pain relief.

Later in the course of the disease, autonomic cardiovascular instability may develop. Both morphine[1] and fentanyl (Sublimaze)[1] may control hypertension and tachycardia by attenuating the sympathetic efferent discharge. Fentanyl (Sublimaze)[1] is considered superior because it does not depress myocardium. Previously used agents phentolamine (Regitine) and metoprolol (Lopressor) for treatment of hypertension and tachycardia are no longer recommended. Hypotension induced by phentolamine may be difficult to reverse, and β-adrenergic blockers may contribute to cardiac failure and high mortality. Hypotension may require monitoring of cardiac output and intravenous fluids or pressor agents. Bradycardia may develop, requiring placement of a pacemaker.

Complications

Supportive care is critical to the prevention of complications. It includes management of fluids and electrolyte balance, nutrition, bowel and bladder functions, skin care, and physiotherapy. Most of the complications are those that are common to immobile patients. Frequent turning of the patient will prevent pressure sores. Low-dose heparin or enoxaparin (Lovenox) should be administered to prevent deep venous thrombosis and formation of pulmonary emboli. Physical therapy should be given as soon as possible to prevent contractures. Orthopedic management may be required for fractures and dislocations resulting from tetanic seizures.

Prognosis

The severity of illness, age of the patient, and the facilities available are the most important factors determining prognosis. In the developing world where mechanical ventilation is unavailable, asphyxia is the most common

[1]Not FDA approved for this indication.
[3]Exceeds dosage recommended by the manufacturer.

cause of death. Those who survive the acute phase may succumb to autonomic dysfunction. With expanding facilities for intensive care, most patients eventually make a full recovery over 4 to 6 weeks, but some patients remain hypertonic; some patients remain amnestic for the event, whereas others have unpleasant memories of painful tetanic spasms, physiotherapy to the chest, and tracheal suction. Tracheal stenosis as a sequel to prolonged intubation and tracheostomy is common. It is important that recovering patients complete a primary series of immunizations because having had the disease does not confer immunity (Table 2).

Prevention

Prevention of tetanus through immunization is the key to the elimination of tetanus. It is useful to distinguish between primary and booster immunization. A patient 7 years old or older who has never been immunized requires two additional doses of Td beyond that given when the wound is treated (see Table 2). Wounded patients who have never been immunized may require HTIG (see Table 1). The elderly are particularly susceptible if they have never been immunized or if their immunity has lapsed.

Physicians should use a case-finding approach to increase tetanus immunization rates. System changes (such as clinical pathways that allow immunization without a physician's order) are the most effective means of increasing immunization rates. Reminders placed at physicians' desks or computer-generated reminders attached to charts or patients' bills have also increased immunization rates. Td should be given whenever

tetanus immunization is necessary to ensure immunity to diphtheria as well as to tetanus.

Td is a safe vaccine. Adverse reactions consist primarily of local edema, tenderness, and fever. Anaphylactoid reactions are rare. Most adverse reactions occur in persons with evidence of hyperimmunization. The only contraindications of Td are a history of a neurologic sequela or a severe hypersensitivity reaction following a previous dose.

To reduce neonatal tetanus and protect the mother, pregnant women who are due for a booster should receive Td, preferably during the last two trimesters. HTIG should be given to pregnant women only when clearly indicated. The WHO recommends that women attending prenatal clinics in developing countries be given two doses:

- During the first pregnancy
- In the third trimester at least 4 weeks before delivery

These should be followed by one dose in each subsequent pregnancy, up to a total of five doses. Needless to say, promoting clean delivery and hygienic cord care practices constitutes a key element in the prevention of neonatal tetanus.

REFERENCES

Apte NM, Karnad DR: Short report: The spatula test: A simple bedside test to diagnose tetanus. Am J Trop Med Hyg 1995;53(4):386-387.

Borgeat A, Popovic V, Schwander D: Efficiency of a continuous infusion of propofol in a patient with tetanus. Critical Care Medicine 1991; 19(2):295-297.

Cook TM, Protheroe RT, Handel JM. Tetanus: A review of the literature. Br J Anaesth 2001;87(3):477-487.

Farrar JJ, Yen LM, Cook T, et al: Tetanus. J Neurol Neurosurg Psychiatry 2000;69:292-301.

Hsu SS, Groleau G. Tetanus in the emergency department: A current review. J Emerg Med 2001;20(4):357-365.

Moughabghab AV, Prevost G, Socolovsky C: Fentanyl therapy controls autonomic hyperactivity in tetanus. Br J Clin Practice 1996; 50(8):477-478.

Pascual FB, McGinley EL, Zanardi LR, et al: Tetanus surveillance—United States, 1998-2000. MMWR 2003;52(No. SS-3):1-8.

Richardson, JP, Knight AL: The management and prevention of tetanus. J Emerg Med 1993;11:737-742.

Schon F, O'Dowd L, White J, Begg N: Tetanus: Delay in diagnosis in England and Wales. J Neurol Neurosurg Psychiat 1994;57: 1006-1007.

Vandelaer J. Birmingham M, Gasse F, et al: Tetanus in developing countries: An update on the maternal and neonatal tetanus elimination initiative. Vaccine 2003;21:3442-3445.

TABLE 2   Guide to Tetanus Prophylaxis in Routine Wound Management

History of Adsorbed Tetanus Toxoid (doses)	Clean, Minor Wounds		All Other Wounds*	
	Td†	TIG†	Td†	TIG†
Unknown or <Three	Yes	No	Yes	Yes
≥Three‡	No§	No	No‖	No

*Such as, but not limited to, wounds contaminated from dirt, feces, soil, saliva; puncture wounds; avulsions; and wounds resulting from missiles, crushing, burns, or frostbite.

†For children under 7 years old, DTaP, DTP, or DT if pertussis vaccine is contraindicated is preferred to TT alone. For persons 7 years of age and older, Td is preferred to TT alone.

‡If only three doses of fluid toxoid have been received, a fourth dose of toxoid, preferably an adsorbed dose, should be given.

§Yes, if more than 10 years since last dose.

‖Yes, if more than 5 years since last dose. (More frequent boosters are not needed and can accentuate side effects.)

Abbreviations: DT = pediatric diphtheria and tetanus toxoid; DTaP = diphtheria and tetanus toxoid and acellular pertussis vaccine; DTP = diphtheria and tetanus toxoid and whole-cell pertussis vaccine; Td = tetanus and diphtheria toxoid; TIG = tetanus immune globulin; TT = tetanus toxoid.

From Immunization Practices Advisory Committee: Diphtheria, tetanus, and pertussis: Recommendations for vaccine use and other preventive measures—recommendations of the Immunization Practices Advisory Committee (ACIP). MMWR 1991;40(No. RR-10).

The Infectious Diseases

Whooping Cough (Pertussis)

Method of
A. Larry Simmons, MD, and J. Gary Wheeler, MD

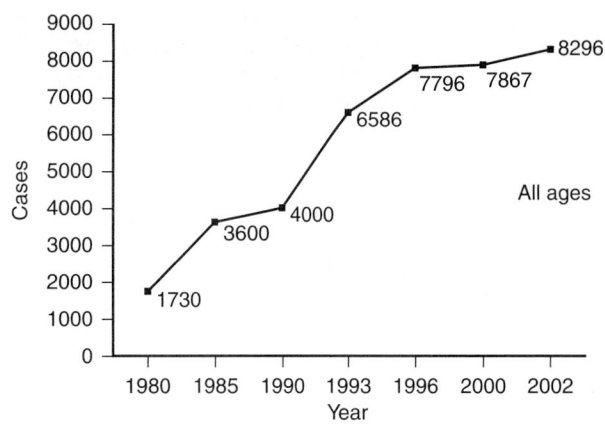

FIGURE 1. Incidence of pertussis disease in the United States from 1980 to 2002. (From Centers for Disease Control and Prevention, Pertussis Technical Information, February 2004.)

Pertussis is a highly communicable disease caused by *Bordetella pertussis.* It typically produces prolonged paroxysmal spasms of severe coughing followed by a forceful inspiratory whoop and post-tussive emesis. However, the characteristic inspiratory whoop may not be present in infants and young children. Complications and mortality are greatest in infants younger than 4 months old. In older children, adolescents, and adults, persistent cough, without the whoop, is a more common manifestation of the disease. Even though complications are fewer, infected individuals in these populations frequently transmit infection to incompletely and unimmunized infants and children. Pertussis is caused by *Bordetella pertussis,* a gram-negative coccobacillus. Treatment halts spread of disease but has limited impact on symptoms. Vaccination is the main tool that limits spread of disease and morbidity. Other infectious agents may produce a similar prolonged cough syndrome.

Epidemiology

Pertussis outbreaks were first described in the 16th century, and the organism was first isolated in 1906. Prior to introduction of pertussis vaccine in the 1940s, more than 200,000 cases were reported annually in the United States. Thereafter, the incidence fell dramatically to a historic low of 1010 cases in 1976. Since 1980, however, the incidence has increased significantly to between 5000 and 8000 cases each year. In 2002, 8296 cases of pertussis were reported in the United States, an incidence of 3.01 per 100,000 people. There were 13 deaths from pertussis in the United States in 2003. Pertussis epidemics have occurred every 3 to 5 years in the United States since 1980. The incidence has increased since 1980 in incompletely immunized children and in infants too young to have received the first three doses of the vaccine. The mean annual incidence reported in infants during the 1990s increased by 49% compared to the previous decade.

There has been a disproportionate increase in cases in adolescents and adults since 1990. A 62% increase in adolescents and a 60% increase in adults have been reported. During this same period (1990 to 1996), the rate increased by 11% in infants and 8% in children between 1 and 4 years of age (Figure 1).

These increases may be caused by true increases in disease incidence, improved diagnostic technology (polymerase chain reaction [PCR]), or changes in reporting. A combination of these and other factors may be related to the reported increases in incidence since 1990.

Rakel and Bope: *Conn's Current Therapy 2006*

Pathogens and Pathogenesis

Humans are the only known hosts of *B. pertussis.* Pathogenesis is dependent on local and systemic effects (Box 1). Transmission occurs by close contact from aerosolized droplets from infected patients. As many as 80% of nonimmune household contacts may acquire the disease after exposure. Patients are most contagious prior to coughing, the catarrhal stage, and during the first 2 weeks after the onset of cough (Boxes 2 and 3). Older children, adolescents, and adults often manifest mild or atypical disease (rhinorrhea or persistent cough with absence of inspiratory whoop), but these individuals represent an important source of transmission to infants and unimmunized children. Young unimmunized and untreated infants may be contagious for 6 weeks or more after the onset of cough. Treatment with appropriate therapy reduces infectivity within 5 days in most cases. Although *B. pertussis* is the primary pathogen, *Bordetella parapertussis, Mycoplasma pneumoniae, Chlamydia trachomatis, Chlamydia pneumoniae, Bordetella bronchiseptica,* and some adenoviruses may cause similar cough illnesses.

BOX 1   CDC Pertussis Technical Information, February, 2004
Pertussis Pathogenesis

- There may be attachment to ciliated epithelial cells in the respiratory tract.
- Pertussis antigens allow evasion of host defenses (induce lymphocytosis and impair chemotaxis).
- There may be local tissue damage in respiratory tract.
- Systemic disease may be toxin mediated.

From the Centers for Disease Control and Prevention, Division of Bacterial and Mycotic Diseases, Pertussis Technical Information, February 2004.

2

Clinical Features

The clinical course of the disease is divided into three stages. The disease typically begins with mild, upper respiratory tract symptoms (catarrhal stage) followed by cough and then paroxysms of cough, the *paroxysmal stage*. In children the cough episodes may be followed by the characteristic inspiratory whoop, commonly followed by emesis. In infants less than 6 months of age, apnea is common, and the inspiratory whoop is often absent. In older children, adolescents, and adults, prolonged cough, with or without paroxysms and no whoop, is more common; otherwise healthy adults who cough to the point of emesis are believed to have pertussis until proven otherwise (see Boxes 2 and 3).

The disease is often suspected during the *paroxysmal stage* during which the characteristic symptoms of cough paroxysms, with or without the inspiratory whoop and post-tussive emesis, occur (age dependent). Cyanosis at the end of the paroxysms may occur, and there may be an average 15 *attacks* per 24 hours, occurring more frequently at night. Young children and infants often appear distressed during these episodes and may be exhausted after attacks subside. Between paroxysms, patients may appear normal. The paroxysmal stage usually lasts from 1 to 6 weeks, occasionally lasting up to 10 weeks.

During the *convalescent stage*, recovery is gradual. Subsequent respiratory infections may trigger recurrent

paroxysms for many months after the initial onset of pertussis.

Complications

Young infants are at highest risk for complications. Between 1997 and 2000 63% of infants younger than 6 months of age required hospitalization, and 62 deaths were reported, 90% occurring in infants younger than 6 months of age. Most pertussis-associated deaths are caused by secondary bacterial pneumonia. Pressure-related complications following severe paroxysms include pneumothorax, epistaxis, subdural hematomas, hernias, head and neck petechiae, and rectal prolapse. Less serious complications include otitis media and dehydration (Table 1).

Diagnosis

The diagnosis of pertussis is often made on the basis of the clinical characteristics. An elevated absolute lymphocyte count often exceeding 20,000 may be seen. In mild cases, cases modified by partial immunity, and cases in infants and young children, there may be no lymphocytosis. The Centers for Disease Control and Prevention (CDC) definition of a *clinical case* is a cough illness lasting 2 weeks or longer with at least one of the following: paroxysms of cough, inspiratory whoop,

 CURRENT DIAGNOSIS

Clinical Case

Cough illness for 2 weeks or more in duration with at least one of the following (for which there is no other obvious cause):

- Paroxysms of cough
- Inspiratory whoop
- Post-tussive vomiting

Confirmed Case

- Clinical case confirmed by PCR assay
- Culture-positive cough illness of any duration

or post-tussive vomiting, without other obvious cause. A *confirmed case* is a clinical case confirmed by PCR, or a culture-positive acute cough illness of any duration. Because of inadequate specificity and sensitivity, the direct fluorescent antigen (DFA) test for pertussis has fallen out of favor and is not used by the CDC for case confirmation. The availability of PCR and the ability to isolate and culture *B. pertussis and B. parapertussis* vary by facility or community.

Medical Management

The medical management of pertussis is primarily supportive. Infants and patients with severe disease commonly require hospitalization, and intensive care facilities may be required to address and treat serious complications. Appropriate antimicrobial agents given during the catarrhal stage may ameliorate the disease. After the cough develops, however, antimicrobials may not affect the course of the disease, but they may be helpful in limiting infectivity and for chemoprophylaxis. Erythromycin estolate (Ilosone), given for 14 days, is the traditional drug of choice. Infantile hypertrophic pyloric stenosis (IHPS) has been reported in association with orally administered erythromycin in neonates younger than 2 weeks of age, but because pertussis can be life-threatening at this age, the American Academy of Pediatrics (AAP) recommends the use of erythromycin for treatment and prophylaxis of pertussis in neonates. Parents should be advised, however, of the potential risk and signs of IHPS. Azithromycin dihydrate (Zithromax)[1] and clarithromycin (Biaxin)[1] may be as effective, with fewer side effects and improved compliance. Penicillins and first- and second-generation cephalosporins are not effective against *B. pertussis* (Table 2).

Control Measures

Immunization and chemoprophylaxis may be helpful in controlling the spread of the disease following diagnosis and treatment of an index case. For hospitalized patients,

 CURRENT THERAPY

Erythromycin estolate (Ilosone)
- 40 to 50 mg/kg per day, in four divided oral doses for 14 days
- Maximum dose: 2 g per day

Azithromycin dihydrate (Zithromax)
- 10 to 12 mg/kg per day, in one oral dose per day, for 5 days
  Do not step down doses on days 2 to 5
- Maximum dose: 600 mg per day

Clarithromycin (Biaxin)
- 15 to 20 mg/kg per day, in two divided oral doses, for 7 days
- Maximum dose: 1 g per day

Trimethoprim-sulfamethoxazole (Bactrim)
- Trimethoprim-sulfamethoxazole (Bactrim) in patients intolerant of erythromycin or infected with erythromycin-resistant strains
- Pediatric dose: 8 mg/kg per day trimethoprim and 40 mg/kg per day sulfamethoxazole, in two divided oral doses

droplet precautions are recommended until 5 days after treatment is begun (Table 3).

IMMUNIZATION

Universal immunization with diphtheria, tetanus toxoids, and acellular pertussis vaccine (DTaP) is recommended for children younger than 7 years of age. Doses are recommended at 2, 4, 6, and 15 to 18 months of age, with a booster dose between 4 and 6 years of age. However, pertussis vaccines are among the least effective. In a U.S. elementary school outbreak in 1997, the effectiveness in preventing infection was 80% in children who had received the complete series. Because of waning immunity, older children and adolescents may

[1]Not FDA approved for this indication.

TABLE 2 Antimicrobial Treatment/Chemoprophylaxis Recommendations	
Antibiotic	**Recommended Dose**
Erythromycin estolate (Ilosone)	40-50 mg/kg/d, 4 divided doses PO for 14 days; maximum dose: 2 g/d
Azithromycin dihydrate (Zithromax)[1]	10-12 mg/kg/d, one dose/d PO for 5 days (do not step down on days 2-5); maximum dose 600 mg/d
Clarithromycin (Biaxin)[1]	15-20 mg/kg/d, 2 divided doses PO for 7 days; maximum dose: 1 g/d
Trimethoprim-sulfamethoxazole (Bactrim)[1]	alternative for patients intolerant of erythromycin or infected with erythromycin-resistant strains Pediatric dose: 8 mg/kg/d trimethoprim and 40 mg/kg/d sulfamethoxazole in 2 divided doses PO

Modified from 2003 Report of the Committee on Infectious Diseases, ed 26. 2003, American Academy of Pediatrics, Elk Grove, IL.
Abbreviations: d = day; PO = by mouth.
[1]Not FDA approved for this indication.

TABLE 3 Control Measures for Exposed Household and Close Contacts*

Immunization

- Unimmunized close contacts younger than 7 years of age or children who have received fewer than 4 doses of DTaP should have pertussis immunization initiated or continued according to the recommended schedule.
- Children who have received their third dose 6 months or more prior to exposure should receive a fourth dose.
- Children who have had 4 doses of DTaP should receive a booster dose unless a dose has been given within 3 years or the child is older than 7 years of age.

Chemoprophylaxis

- Antimicrobial chemoprophylaxis is recommended for all household and close contacts regardless of age and immunization status to limit secondary transmission (see Table 2). Persons who have had household or close contact with an infected patient should be monitored closely for 21 days.

Return to Child Care/School

- Children and staff should be excluded from attending child care or school facilities until completion of 5 days of recommended antimicrobial treatment (see Table 2).

---

*According to the CDC, close contacts include all household members, child care or school direct face-to-face contacts with a symptomatic index patient, or those who have shared a confined space for a prolonged time with a symptomatic index patient.
Modified from 2003 Report of the Committee on Infectious Diseases, ed 26. 2003, American Academy of Pediatrics, Elk Grove, IL.
Abbreviation: DTaP = diptheria, tetanus, and acellular pertussis.

be susceptible to infection 5 to 15 years after the last DTaP dose. Clinical trials are in progress to evaluate the effectiveness of adding acellular pertussis vaccine to tetanus/diphtheria vaccines in adolescents, thereby reducing contact between these usually atypical cases and at-risk infants and children.

REFERENCES

Centers for Disease Control and Prevention, Division of Bacterial Mycotic Diseases, Pertussis Technical Information, February, 2004.
Centers for Disease Control and Prevention: School Associated Pertussis Outbreak. MMWR 2004;53:216-219.
Centers for Disease Control and Prevention: Pertussis. MMWR 2002;51(4):73-76.
Centers for Disease Control and Prevention: Case definitions for infectious conditions. MMWR Recomm Rep 1997;46(RR10:1-55).
Khetsuriani N, Bisgard K, Prevots D, et al: Pertussis outbreak in an elementary school with high vaccine coverage. Pediatr Infect Dis J 2001;20(12):1108-1112.
Red Book, 2003 Report of the Committee on Infectious Diseases, American Academy of Pediatrics, 26th ed, pp 473-486, Elk Grove, IL.
Tanaka M, Charles R, Pascual F, et al: Trends in pertussis among infants in the US, 1980-1999. JAMA 2003;290(22):2968-2975.

Office-Based Immunization Practices

Method of
Barbara P. Yawn, MD

Administering immunizations to children is one of the most successful activities performed in primary care offices. The rates of most vaccine-preventable diseases have fallen to record lows in the United States, with several of those diseases, such as paralyzing polio and diphtheria, now close to extinction. Childhood chickenpox and its related complications have declined 77.6% since the introduction of the vaccine. However, two vaccine-preventable diseases continue to increase in the United States: Pertussis in both children and adults has doubled in prevalence since 1992, and influenza rates wax and wane, depending on the predominant strain and vaccine availability. New adolescent and adult vaccines have become available recently, including an adolescent and adult pertussis vaccine that may solve the problem of pertussis resurgence.

The estimated rates of vaccine coverage for children ages 19 to 35 months was greater in 2003 than in 2002 but continues to vary widely among the states. The basic immunization coverage (four diphtheria, tetanus toxoid, acellular pertussis vaccine [DTaP], three inactivated polio vaccine [IPV], and one measles-containing vaccine [MMR]) increased from 78.5% in 2002 to 82.2% in 2003. The rates of complete vaccine coverage (four DTaP, three IPV, one MMR, three hepatitis B [HepB], three pneumococcal conjugate vaccine [PCV], and one varicella) increased from 65.5% in 2002 to 72.5% in 2003. Many factors contribute to incomplete immunization of children, including barriers to access, missed opportunities, parents' fears, and financial and transportation limitations. Immunization registries, electronic health records, and recall and reminder systems have all increased immunization rates among those with a usual source of health care. Preservative-free vaccines have reduced parents' fears, as has the publication of several studies that have found no link between vaccinations and neurologic problems. However, other innovations are required if the Healthy People 2010 childhood immunization goals are to be met.

Immunizations are also important for adolescents and adults (Figure 1). Immunization rates in adults lag significantly behind those in infants and children. Boosters for tetanus and diphtheria (Td) are seldom up to date, influenza vaccinations are administered to less than 50% of those considered at high risk and less than 70% of health care workers, and the 23-valent pneumococcal vaccine (Pneumovax 23) is administered to less than 50% of adults older than age 65 years. Strategies for linking influenza immunization to adolescent and adult immunizations such as Td and DTaP may increase immunization coverage.

Diphtheria, Tetanus, and Pertussis Vaccines

Diphtheria and tetanus continue to be sporadic and rare diseases in the United States, occurring primarily in older children and adults who have not been fully immunized with the recommended booster doses. Pertussis prevalence has doubled since 1992 and continues to increase (Table 1). Diphtheria is toxin-mediated and is caused by *Corynebacterium diphtheriae*. When attacked by the appropriate bacteriophages, *C. diphtheriae* that is colonizing the nose releases toxin that causes local tissue inflammation, destruction, and membrane formation, blocking the airway with resultant respiratory collapse. The toxin also can spread systemically, causing myocarditis, neuritis, and otitis media. Case-fatality rates range up to 10% in preschool children and adults older than age 40 years.

Like diphtheria, tetanus is a toxin-mediated disease. *Clostridium tetani* is a common gram-negative organism in the environment that is killed easily by oxygen and heat. However, *C. tetani* spores can exist for extended periods, and in a deep puncture wound or a surgically closed contaminated wound, the spores germinate and toxin is produced. The toxin interferes with the release of brain neurotransmitters, increasing muscle tone and resulting in lockjaw, neck stiffness, difficulty swallowing, laryngospasm, and muscle spasms severe enough to fracture vertebrae and long bones. The case-fatality rate is 11% overall and almost 100% in patients older than age 60 years.

Pertussis, or whooping cough, is caused by several toxins produced by *Bordetella pertussis*, an aerobic gram-negative bacterium. The disease-producing agents include toxins, hemagglutinin, and agglutinogens. Pertussis begins with 10 to 14 days of upper respiratory infection (URI)-like symptoms, progressing to the whooping phase with episodes of continuous hacking cough and then a prolonged inspiratory phase with a high-pitched whoop. The coughing attacks can be severe, with marked respiratory effort, cyanosis, vomiting, and exhaustion. The case-fatality rate is 0.2% in patients of all ages but more than 10 times higher in young children.

All three conditions are prevented effectively by the DTaP vaccine (Infanrix). The pertussis vaccine was changed from a whole-cell vaccine to an acellular vaccine to reduce the side effects. The primary series for children consists of an initial series of four DTaPs beginning at 6 to 8 weeks of age and then three more at 4- to 8-week intervals (Figure 2). A fourth dose is given at 12 to 18 months. The fifth dose is given at 4 to 6 years of age and usually is required for school entry. Td vaccine previously was recommended only for children older than 7 years of age and younger children with severe adverse reactions. The availability of the newer adult pertussis vaccine combinations should solve this problem. Boosters are recommended every 10 years after completion of the initial series and at the time of major trauma. A pertussis vaccine for adolescents and adults has been approved by the FDA to be used as a booster dose.

Polio Vaccine

Paralytic polio has a rare and sporadic occurrence in the United States, but cases have been brought into the country and spread to unimmunized, incompletely immunized, or immunosuppressed children and adults. The use of inactivated polio vaccine (IPV, IPOL) has reduced the small risk of transmission of polio from the oral polio vaccine (vaccine-associated paralytic polio [VAPP]). The virus is spread by fecal–oral contamination and airborne droplets from coughing and sneezing. The virus multiples in the oral and gastrointestinal (GI) tract, spreading systemically. Most polio cases are asymptomatic, with fewer than 1% of patients developing paralysis related to the central nervous system after destruction of neurons in the brainstem and anterior horn cells. The overall case-fatality rate is approximately 2% to 5% in those with paralytic polio but is higher in adults and those with bulbar involvement.

The primary series of IPV begins at 6 weeks and consists of three doses given at 8-week intervals. A fourth dose is recommended for preschool children ages 4 to 6 years and usually is required for school entry. Reactions to IPV are mild, with local redness or inflammation at the injection site. Contraindications include allergies to streptomycin, polymyxin B, and neomycin. IPV and DTaP can be given simultaneously.

Haemophilus influenzae Type B Vaccines

Haemophilus influenzae type B (Hib) can be associated with meningitis, epiglottitis, septic arthritis, pneumonia, cellulitis, osteomyelitis, purulent pericarditis, endocarditis, and neonatal sepsis. Hib disease is most common around 6 to 8 months of age and uncommon after age 5 years. The Hib organism is a gram-negative coccobacillus with six capsular subtypes that all must be included in the vaccine. Infection is spread primarily from the respiratory tract and colonizes the oral pharynx, where it can spread to the bloodstream to produce invasive disease at several sites.

Conjugate vaccines (HibTITER, ActHIB, PedVaxHIB) have been available since 1990, and the Hib series should begin no earlier than age 6 weeks. Earlier use of Hib may produce immunologic tolerance to later doses. The total number of doses depends on the vaccine used and the age at initiation. Children who receive the first dose after 7 months of age may not require the full series, and if the series is begun after age 15 months, only one dose is required. However, delaying the first dose to 7 months or later misses the prime period of infection and is not recommended. Adverse reactions are unusual other than minor local inflammation at the injection site. Hib can be administered with DTaP and IPV.

RECOMMENDED CHILDHOOD AND ADOLESCENT IMMUNIZATION SCHEDULE • UNITED STATES • 2005

Vaccine ↓ Age →	Birth	1 month	2 months	4 months	6 months	12 months	15 months	18 months	24 months	4–6 years	11–12 years	13–18 years
Hepatitis B[1]	HepB #1	HepB #2			HepB #3						Hep3 series	
Diphtheria, tetanus, pertussis[2]			DTaP	DTaP	DTaP		DTaP	DTaP		DTaP	Td	Td
Haemophilus influenzae type b[3]			Hib	Hib	Hib	Hib						
Inactivated poliovirus			IPV	IPV		IPV				IPV		
Measles, mumps, rubella[4]						MMR #1				MMR #2	MMR #2	MMR #2
Varicella[5]						Varicella	Varicella			Varicella		
Pneumococcal[6]			PCV	PCV	PCV	PCV	PCV		PCV	PPV	PPV	
Influenza[7]					Influenza (yearly)	Influenza (yearly)				Influenza (yearly)		
Hepatitis A[8]										Hepatitis A series		

Vaccines below this line are for selected populations

Legend:
- Range of recommended ages
- Preadolescent assessment
- Only if mother HBsAg(–)
- Catch-up immunization

This schedule indicates the recommended ages for routine administration of currently licensed childhood vaccines, as of December 1, 2004, for children through age 18 years. Any dose not given at the recommended age should be given at any subsequent visit when indicated and feasible.

■ Indicates age groups that warrant special effort to administer those vaccines not previously given. Additional vaccines may be licensed and recommended during the year. Licensed combination vaccines may be used whenever any components of the combination are indicated and the vaccine's other components are not contraindicated.

Providers should consult the manufacturers' package inserts for detailed recommendations. Clinically significant adverse events that follow immunization should be reported to the Vaccine Adverse Event Reporting System (VAERS). Guidance about how to obtain and complete a VAERS form can be found on the internet: www.vaers.org or by calling 800-822-7967.

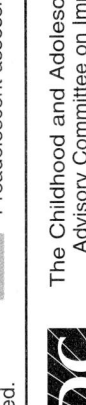

The Childhood and Adolescent Immunization Schedule is approved by:
Advisory Committee on Immunization Practices www.cdc.gov/nip/acip
American Academy of Pediatrics www.aap.org
American Academy of Family Physicians www.aatp.org

Department of Health and Human Services
Centers for Disease Control and Prevention

CDC
SAFER • HEALTHIER • PEOPLE™

Footnotes
Recommended Childhood and Adolescent Immunization Schedule
United States • 2005

1. **Hepatitis B (HepB) vaccine.** All infants should receive the first dose of hepatitis B vaccine soon after birth and before hospital discharge; the first dose may also be given by age 2 months if the infant's mother is hepatitis B surface antigen (HBsAg) negative. Only monovalent HepB can be used for the birth dose. Monovalent or combination vaccine containing HepB may be used to complete the series. Four doses of vaccine may be administered when a birth dose is given. The second dose should be given at least 4 weeks after the first dose, except for combination vaccines which cannot be administered before age 6 weeks. The third dose should be given at least 16 weeks after the first dose and at least 8 weeks after the second dose. The last dose in the vaccination series (third or fourth dose) should not be administered before age 24 weeks.

Infants born to HBsAg-positive mothers should receive HepB and 0.5 mL of Hepatitis B Immune Globulin (HBIG) within 12 hours of birth at separate sites. The second dose is recommended at age 1–2 months. The last dose in the immunization series should not be administered before age 24 weeks. These infants should be tested for HBsAg and antibody to HBsAg (anti-HBs) at age 9–15 months.

Infants born to mothers whose HBsAg status is unknown should receive the first dose of the HepB series within 12 hours of birth. Maternal blood should be drawn as soon as possible to determine the mother's HBsAg status; if the HBsAg test is positive, the infant should receive HBIG as soon as possible (no later than age 1 week). The second dose is recommended at age 1–2 months. The last dose in the immunization series should not be administered before age 24 weeks.

2. **Diphtheria and tetanus toxoids and acellular pertussis (DTaP) vaccine.** The fourth dose of DTaP may be administered as early as age 12 months, provided 6 months have elapsed since the third dose and the child is unlikely to return at age 15–18 months. The final dose in the series should be given at age ≥4 years. **Tetanus and diphtheria toxoids (Td)** is recommended at age 11–12 years if at least 5 years have elapsed since the last dose of tetanus and diphtheria toxoid–containing vaccine. Subsequent routine Td boosters are recommended every 10 years.

3. *Haemophilus influenzae* **type b (Hib) conjugate vaccine.** Three Hib conjugate vaccines are licensed for infant use. If PRP-OMP (PedvaxHIB or ComVax [Merck]) is administered at ages 2 and 4 months, a dose at age 6 months is not required. DTaP/Hib combination products should not be used for primary immunization in infants at ages 2, 4 or 6 months but can be used as boosters following any Hib vaccine. The final dose in the series should be given at age ≥12 months.

4. **Measles, mumps, and rubella vaccine (MMR).** The second dose of MMR is recommended routinely at age 4–6 years but may be administered during any visit, provided at least 4 weeks have elapsed since the first dose and both doses are administered beginning at or after age 12 months. Those who have not previously received the second dose should complete the schedule by the visit at age 11–12 years.

5. **Varicella vaccine.** Varicella vaccine is recommended at any visit at or after age 12 months for susceptible children (i.e., those who lack a reliable history of chickenpox). Susceptible persons aged ≥13 years should receive 2 doses, given at least 4 weeks apart.

6. **Pneumococcal vaccine.** The heptavalent **pneumococcal conjugate vaccine (PCV)** is recommended for all children aged 2–23 months. It is also recommended for certain children aged 24–59 months. The final dose in the series should be given at age ≥12 months. **Pneumococcal polysaccharide vaccine (PPV)** is recommended in addition to PCV for certain high-risk groups. See *MMWR* 2000;49(RR-9):1–35.

7. **Influenza vaccine.** Influenza vaccine is recommended annually for children aged ≥6 months with certain risk factors (including but not limited to asthma, cardiac disease, sickle cell disease, HIV, and diabetes), health care workers, and other persons (including household members) in close contact with persons in groups at high risk (see *MMWR* 2004;53[RR-6]: 1–40) and can be administered to all others wishing to obtain immunity. In addition, healthy children aged 6–23 months and close contacts of healthy children aged 0–23 months are recommended to receive influenza vaccine, because children in this age group are at substantially increased risk for influenza-related hospitalizations. For healthy persons aged 5–49 years, the intranasally administered live, attenuated influenza vaccine (LAIV) is an acceptable alternative to the intramuscular trivalent inactivated influenza vaccine (TIV). See *MMWR* 2004;53(RR-6):1–40. Children receiving TIV should be administered a dosage appropriate for their age (0.25 mL if 6–35 months or 0.5 mL if ≥3 years). Children aged ≤8 years who are receiving influenza vaccine for the first time should receive 2 doses (separated by at least 4 weeks for TIV and at least 6 weeks for LAIV).

8. **Hepatitis A vaccine.** Hepatitis A vaccine is recommended for children and adolescents in selected states and regions and for certain high-risk groups; consult your local public health authority. Children and adolescents in these states, regions, and high-risk groups who have not been immunized against hepatitis A can begin the hepatitis A immunization series during any visit. The 2 doses in the series should be administered at least 6 months apart. See *MMWR* 1999;48(RR-12):1–37.

FIGURE 1. Recommended Childhood and Adolescent Immunization Schedule. (Source: Advisory Committee on Immunization Practices, American Academy of Pediatrics, American Academy of Family Physicians.)

Continued

Rakel and Bope: *Conn's Current Therapy 2006*

RECOMMENDED IMMUNIZATION SCHEDULE FOR CHILDREN AND ADOLESCENTS WHO START LATE OR WHO ARE MORE THAN ONE MONTH BEHIND
UNITED STATES • 2005

The tables below give catch-up schedules and minimum intervals between doses for children who have delayed immunizations. There is no need to restart a vaccine series regardless of the time that has elapsed between doses. Use the chart appropriate for the child's age.

CATCH-UP SCHEDULE FOR CHILDREN AGED FOUR MONTHS THROUGH SIX YEARS

Vaccine	Minimum age for dose 1	Minimum interval between doses			
		Dose 1 to dose 2	Dose 2 to dose 3	Dose 3 to dose 4	Dose 4 to dose 5
Diphtheria, tetanus, pertussis	6 weeks	4 weeks	4 weeks	6 months	6 months[1]
Inactivated poliovirus	6 weeks	4 weeks	4 weeks	4 weeks[2]	
Hepatitis B[3]	Birth	4 weeks	8 weeks (and 16 weeks after first dose)		
Measles, mumps, rubella	12 months	4 weeks[4]			
Varicella	12 months				
Haemophilus influenzae type b[5]	6 weeks	4 weeks if first dose given at age <12 months 8 weeks (as final dose) if first dose given at age 12–14 months No further doses need if first dose given at age ≥15 months	4 weeks[6] if current age <12 months 8 weeks (as final dose)[6] if current age ≥12 months and second dose given at age <15 months No further doses need if first dose given at age ≥15 months	8 weeks (as final dose) This dose only necessary for children aged 12 months–5 years who received 3 doses before age 12 months	
Pneumococcal[7]	6 weeks	4 weeks if first dose given at age <12 months and current age < 24 months 8 weeks (as final dose) if first dose given at age ≥12 months or current age 24–59 months No further doses need for healthy children if first dose given at age ≥24 months	4 weeks if current age <12 months 8 weeks (as final dose) if current age ≥12 months No further doses needed for healthy children if previous dose given at age ≥24 months	8 weeks (as final dose) This dose only necessary for children aged 12 months–5 years who received 3 doses before age 12 months	

CATCH-UP SCHEDULE FOR CHILDREN AGED 7 YEARS THROUGH 18 YEARS

Vaccine	Minimum interval between doses		
	Dose 1 to dose 2	Dose 2 to dose 3	Dose 3 to booster dose
Tetanus, diphtheria	4 weeks	6 months	6 months[8] if first dose given at age <12 months and current age <11 years 5 years[8] if first dose given at age ≥12 months and third dose given at age <7 years and current age ≥11 years 10 years[8] if third dose given at age ≥7 years
Inactivated poliovirus[9]	4 weeks	4 weeks	IPV[2,9]
Hepatitis B	4 weeks	8 weeks (and 16 weeks after first dose)	
Measles, mumps, rubella	4 weeks		
Varicella[10]	4 weeks		

Footnotes

Children and Adolescents Catch-up Schedules • United States • 2005

1. **DTaP.** The fifth dose is not necessary if the fourth dose was given after the fourth birthday.

2. **IPV.** For children who received an all-IPV or all-oral poliovirus (OPV) series, a fourth dose is not necessary if third dose was given at age ≥4 years. If both OPV and IPV were given as part of a series, a total of 4 doses should be given, regardless of the child's current age.

3. **HepB.** All children and adolescents who have not been immunized against hepatitis B should begin the HepB immunization series during any visit. Providers should make special efforts to immunize children who were born in, or whose parents were born in, areas of the world where hepatitis B virus infection is moderately or highly endemic.

4. **MMR.** The second dose of MMR is recommended routinely at age 4–6 years but may be given earlier if desired.

5. **Hib.** Vaccine not generally recommended for children aged ≥5 years.

6. **Hib.** If current age <12 months and the first 2 doses were PRP-OMP (PedvaxHIB or ComVax [Merck]), the third (and final) dose should be given at age 12–15 months and at least 8 weeks after the second dose.

7. **PCV.** Vaccine is not generally recommended for children aged ≥5 years.

8. **Td.** For children aged 7–10 years, the interval between the third and booster doses is determined by the age when the first dose was given. For adolescents aged 11–18 years, the interval is determined by the age when the third dose was given.

9. **IPV.** Vaccine is not generally recommended for persons aged ≥18 years.

10. **Varicella.** Give 2-dose series to all susceptible adolescents aged ≥13 years.

Report adverse reactions to vaccines through the federal Vaccine Adverse Event Reporting System. For information on reporting reactions following immunization, please visit www.vaers.org or call the 24-hour national toll-free information line at 800-822-7967. Report suspected cases of vaccine-preventable diseases to your state or local health department.

For additional information about vaccines, including precautions and contraindications for immunization and vaccine shortages, please visit the National Immunization Program Web site at www.cdc.gov/nip or call the National Immunization Information Hotline at
800-232-2522 (English) or 800-232-0233 (Spanish).

FIGURE 1. cont'd

TABLE 1 Vaccine-Preventable Disease Prevalence Over the Last 15 Years

Disease	1992 Rate per 100,000 People	2002 Rate per 100,000 People
Pertussis	1.60	3.47
Hepatitis B	6.32	2.84
Measles	0.88	0.02
Mumps	1.03	0.10
Polio	0.00	0.01
Tetanus	0.02	0.01

Measles, Mumps, and Rubella Vaccine

No recent measles epidemics have occurred in the United States, and the immunization rate for measles appears to be at an all-time high. Measles is a paramyxovirus that spreads primarily through the respiratory tract. A prodromal phase of cough, runny nose, conjunctivitis, and whitish Koplik spots inside the cheeks proceeds to a rash that begins around the hairline and spreads distally. Death related to measles, encephalitis, or pneumonia is more likely to occur in children younger than 1 year of age and older adults. The prognosis is also poor in people with AIDS and other immunocompromising conditions.

Rubella is very uncommon in the United States, and congenital rubella is almost nonexistent. Rubella is caused by a togavirus that is spread mainly by the respiratory route and sustained personal contact. The symptoms include a 3-day rash (3 day measles) with little or no prodrome and generalized lymphadenopathy. A person with rubella is contagious for up to 10 days before and after the rash appears and clears. Infants with congenital rubella may excrete the virus in their urine for up to 6 months. Fatalities are rare and usually are caused by encephalitis or cardiac abnormalities of congenital rubella. Congenital rubella also is associated with eye defects, including cataracts, retinitis, and glaucoma.

Cases of mumps have declined 10-fold since 1992, with fewer than 300 cases in the United States in 2002. Mumps virus is a paramyxovirus, and humans are the natural host. Mumps infections primarily consist of nonsuppurative parotitis; they are highly contagious and spread by droplets from the respiratory tract. Complications include aseptic meningitis, encephalitis, and orchitis. Although orchitis is rare in boys, it occurs in 15% to 35% of postpubertal males, accompanied by testicular atrophy but rarely sterility.

The MMR vaccine (M-M-RI) is given at age 12 to 15 months with a booster in the preschool period and usually is required for school entry. Adverse reactions include a low-grade fever and a noncontagious rash 7 to 10 days after the immunization. The MMR vaccine should not be given to pregnant women, people with allergies to gelatin or neomycin, or immunosuppressed people such as those with AIDS and those taking more than 20 mg of steroids per day. Postvaccination febrile seizures may occur but are not related to an increase in epilepsy. MMR may be administered with IPV, DTaP, and Hib.

Hepatitis B Vaccine

Hepatitis B causes both acute and chronic liver inflammation. Long-term complications of chronic active hepatitis B include hepatoma and cirrhosis. Hepatitis B is caused by a hepadnavirus (family Hepadnaviridae) that is transmitted by blood and body fluids, including during oral, vaginal, or anal intercourse, and by vertical transmission from mother to fetus. Acute hepatitis has an incubation period of 6 weeks to 6 months with a short prodromal period of fatigue, anorexia, nausea, and abdominal pain followed by a period of 1 to 3 weeks of jaundice and continuation of the prodromal symptoms. Resolution requires weeks to months. Young children may be asymptomatic but still contagious and are at increased risk for late complications. Chronic hepatitis occurs in approximately 2% to 7% of adults who are infected, and fulminating hepatitis is rare but appears in clusters associated with the e antigen–negative virus.

Hepatitis B vaccine (Recombivax HB, Engerix-B) is recommended for all infants. All pregnant women are candidates for hepatitis B (HBV) screening. In children of mothers who are HBV-negative, the hepatitis B immunization series can begin at 6 to 8 weeks of age with three doses at least 4 weeks apart and the third dose at 6 months or later. For adolescents who were not vaccinated at birth, a series of three vaccinations is recommended before age 10 years. Nonimmune adults who engage in high-risk behaviors or work in the health care profession should receive the series of three immunizations over a period of not less than 4 months. High-risk individuals include men who have sex with men, people with multiple (>6) sexual partners, sex industry workers, intravenous (IV) drug users, prison inmates, people on hemodialysis, people who live in the households of HBV carriers, and those from endemic areas (including Pacific Islanders and Alaskan natives).

For infants of HBV-positive mothers, HBV immunizations should begin before discharge from the hospitalization for delivery and should be accompanied by an immediate dose of hepatitis B immunoglobulin (HBIG, BayHep B). Contraindications to hepatitis B vaccine are few and consist primarily of a severe adverse reaction to previous doses. No studies have proved the hypothesized link between this vaccine and demyelinating, autoimmune, or rheumatologic diseases.

Varicella Vaccine

Chickenpox (varicella) and shingles are caused by a herpesvirus. Transmitted by the respiratory tract and conjunctival fluids, chickenpox is a disease primarily of childhood, with a secondary reactivation in adulthood that is known as shingles. The primary infection begins with a low-grade fever, fatigue, and a rash characterized by papules, vesicles, and crusted lesions that are

RECOMMENDED ADULT IMMUNIZATION SCHEDULE
UNITED STATES • OCTOBER 2004–SEPTEMBER 2005

Summary of Recommendations Published by

The Advisory Committee on
Immunization Practices

Department of Health and Human Services
Centers for Disease Control and Prevention

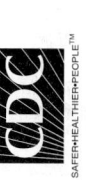

SAFER•HEALTHIER•PEOPLE™

RECOMMENDED ADULT IMMUNIZATION SCHEDULE BY VACCINE AND AGE GROUP
UNITED STATES • OCTOBER 2004–SEPTEMBER 2005

Vaccine	Age groups (years) 19–49	50–64	65
Tetanus, diphtheria (Td)*	1 dose booster every 10 years[1]		
Influenza	1 dose annually[2]		1 dose annually
Pneumococcal (polysaccharide)	1 dose annually[3,4]		1 dose[3,4]
Hepatitis B*	3 doses (0, 1–2, 4–6 months)[5]		
Hepatitis A*	2 doses (0, 6–12 months)[6]		
Measles, mumps, rubella (MMR)*	1 or 2 doses[7]		
Varicella*	2 doses (0, 4–8 weeks)[8]		
Meningococcal (polysaccharide)	1 dose[9]		

*Covered by the Vaccine Injury Compensation Program.
See Footnotes for Recommended Adult Immunization Schedule on back cover.

For all persons in this group

For persons lacking documentation of vaccination or evidence of disease

For persons at risk (i.e., with medical/exposure indications)

The Recommended Adult Immunization Schedule is approved by the Advisory Committee on Immunization Practices (ACIP), the American College of Obstetricians and Gynecologists (ACOG), and the American Academy of Family Physicians (AAFP)

This schedule indicates the recommended age groups for routine administration of currently licensed vaccines for persons aged 19 years. Licensed combination vaccines may be used whenever any components of the combination are indicated and when the vaccine's other components are not contraindicated. Providers should consult manufacturers' package inserts for detailed recommendations.

Report all clinically significant postvaccination reactions to the Vaccine Adverse Event Reporting System (VAERS). Reporting forms and instructions on filing a VAERS report are available by telephone, 800-822-7967, or from the VAERS Web site at http://www.vaers.org.

Information on how to file a Vaccine Injury Compensation Program claim is available at http://www.hrsa.gov/osp/vicp or by telephone, 800-338-2382. To file a claim for vaccine injury, contact the U.S. Court of Federal Claims, 717 Madison Place, N.W., Washington DC, 20005, telephone 202-219-9657.

Additional information about the vaccines listed above and contraindications for immunization is available at http://www.cdc.gov/nip or from the National Immunization Hotline, 800-232-2522 (English) or 800-232-0233 (Spanish).

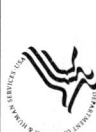

FIGURE 2. Recommended Immunization Schedule for Adolescents Who Start Late or are More than One Month Behind. (Source: Advisory Committee on Immunization Practices, American Academy of Pediatrics, American Academy of Family Physicians.)

RECOMMENDED ADULT IMMUNIZATION SCHEDULE BY VACCINE AND MEDICAL AND OTHER INDICATIONS
UNITED STATES • OCTOBER 2004–SEPTEMBER 2005

Vaccine / Indication	Pregnancy	Diabetes, heart disease, chronic pulmonary disease, chronic liver disease (including chronic alcoholism)	Congenital immunodeficiency, cochlear implants, leukemia, lymphoma, generalized malignancy, therapy with alkylating agents or antimetabolites, CSF** leaks, radiation or large amounts of corticosteroids	Renal failure/end stage renal disease, recipients of hemodialysis or clotting factor concentrates	Asplenia (including elective splenectomy and terminal complement component deficiencies)	HIV*** infection	Health-care workers
Tetanus, diphtheria (Td)*,1							
Influenza2		A, B			C		
Pneumococcal (polysaccharide)3,4		B	D		D, E, F	D, G	
Hepatitis B*,5				H			
Hepatitis A*,6		I					
Measles, mumps, rubella (MMR)*,7							
Varicella*,8			K			J	

Legend:
- For all persons in this group
- For persons lacking documentation of vaccination or evidence of disease
- For persons at risk (i.e., with medical/exposure indications)
- Contraindicated

*Covered by the Vaccine Injury Compensation Program.
**Cerebrospinal fluid.
***Human immunodeficiency virus.
See Special Notes for Medical and Other Indications below. Also see Footnotes for Recommended Adult Immunization Schedule on next page.

Special Notes for Medical and Other Indications

A. Although chronic liver disease and alcoholism are not indications for influenza vaccination, administer 1 dose annually if the patient is aged ≥50 years, has other indications for influenza vaccine, or requests vaccination.
B. Asthma is an indication for influenza vaccination but not for pneumococcal vaccination.
C. No data exist specifically on the risk for severe or complicated influenza infections among persons with asplenia. However, influenza is a risk factor for secondary bacterial infections that can cause severe disease among persons with asplenia.
D. For persons aged <65 years, revaccinate once after ≥5 years have elapsed since initial vaccination.
E. Administer meningococcal vaccine and consider Haemophilus influenzae type b vaccine.
F. For persons undergoing elective splenectomy, vaccinate ≥2 weeks before surgery.
G. Vaccinate as soon after diagnosis as possible.
H. For hemodialysis patients, use special formulation of vaccine (40 g/mL) or 20 g/mL doses administered at one body site. Vaccinate early in the course of renal disease. Assess antibody titers to hepatitis B surface antigen (anti-HB) levels annually. Administer additional doses if anti-HB levels decline to <10 mIU/mL.
I. For all persons with chronic liver disease.
J. Withhold MMR or other measles-containing vaccines from HIV-infected persons with evidence of severe immunosuppression (see MMWR 1998;47 [No. RR-8]:21–2 and MMWR 2002;51 [No. RR-2]:22–4).
K. Persons with impaired humoral immunity but intact cellular immunity may be vaccinated (see MMWR 1999;48 [No. RR-6]).

Rakel and Bope: *Conn's Current Therapy 2006*

Footnotes

Recommended Adult Immunization Schedule • United States • October 2004–September 2005

1. **Tetanus and diphtheria (Td).** Adults, including pregnant women with uncertain history of a complete primary vaccination series, should receive a primary series for adults is 3 doses; administer the first 2 doses at least 4 weeks apart and the 3rd dose 6–12 months after the second. Administer 1 dose if the person received the primary series and if the last vaccination was received 10 years previously. Consult recommendations for administering Td as prophylaxis in wound management (see *MMWR* 1991;40 [No. RR-10]). The American College of Physicians Task Force on Adult Immunization supports a second option for Td use in adults: a single Td booster at age 50 years for persons who have completed the full pediatric series, including the teenage/young adult booster.

2. **Influenza vaccination.** The Advisory Committee on Immunization Practices (ACIP) recommends inactivated influenza vaccination for the following indications, when vaccine is available. *Medical indications:* chronic disorders of the cardiovascular or pulmonary systems, including asthma; chronic metabolic diseases, including diabetes mellitus, renal dysfunction, hemoglobinopathies, or immunosuppression (including immunosuppression caused by medications or by human immunodeficiency virus [HIV]); and pregnancy during the influenza season. *Occupational indications:* health-care workers and employees of long-term–care and assisted living facilities. *Other indications:* residents of nursing homes and other long-term–care facilities; persons likely to transmit influenza to persons at high risk (i.e., in-home caregivers to persons with medical indications, household/close contacts and out-of-home caregivers of children aged 0–23 months, household members and caregivers of elderly persons and adults with high-risk conditions); and anyone who wishes to be vaccinated. For healthy persons aged 5–49 years without high-risk conditions who are not contacts of severely immunocompromised persons in special care units, either the inactivated vaccine or the intranasally administered influenza vaccine FluMist®) may be administered (see *MMWR* 2004;53 [No. RR-6]).

Note: Because of the vaccine shortage for the 2004–05 influenza season, CDC has recommended that vaccination be restricted to the following priority groups, which are considered to be of equal importance: all children aged 6–23 months; adults aged >65 years; persons aged 2–64 years with underlying chronic medical conditions; all women who will be pregnant during the influenza season; residents of nursing homes and long-term–care facilities; children aged <6 months–18 years on chronic aspirin therapy; health-care workers involved in direct patient care; and out-of-home caregivers and household contacts of children aged <6 months. For the 2004–05 season, intranasally administered, live, attenuated influenza vaccine, if available, should be encouraged for healthy persons who are aged 5–49 years and are not pregnant, including health-care workers (except those who care for severely immunocompromised patients in special care units) and persons caring for children aged <6 months (see *MMWR* 2004;53:923–4).

3. **Pneumococcal polysaccharide vaccination.** *Medical indications:* chronic disorders of the pulmonary system (excluding asthma); cardiovascular diseases; diabetes mellitus; chronic liver diseases, including liver disease as a result of alcohol abuse (e.g., cirrhosis); chronic renal failure or nephrotic syndrome; functional or anatomic asplenia (e.g., sickle cell disease or splenectomy); immunosuppressive conditions (e.g., congenital immunodeficiency, HIV infection, leukemia, lymphoma, multiple myeloma, Hodgkin's disease, generalized malignancy, or organ or bone marrow transplantation); chemotherapy with alkylating agents, antimetabolites, or long-term systemic corticosteroids; or cochlear implants. *Geographic/other indications:* Alaska Natives and certain American Indian populations. *Other indications:* residents of nursing homes and other long-term–care facilities (see *MMWR* 1997;46[No. RR-8] and *MMWR* 2003;52:739–40).

4. **Revaccination with pneumococcal polysaccharide vaccine.** One-time revaccination after 5 years for persons with chronic renal failure or nephrotic syndrome; functional or anatomic asplenia (e.g., sickle cell disease or splenectomy); immunosuppressive conditions (e.g., congenital immunodeficiency, HIV infection, leukemia, lymphoma, multiple myeloma, Hodgkin's disease, generalized malignancy, or organ or bone marrow transplantation); or chemotherapy with alkylating agents, antimetabolites, or long-term systemic corticosteroids. For persons aged 65 years, one-time revaccination if they were vaccinated 5 years previously and were aged <65 years at the time of primary vaccination (see *MMWR* 1997;46 [No. RR-8]).

5. **Hepatitis B vaccination.** *Medical indications:* hemodialysis patients or patients who receive clotting factor concentrates. *Occupational indications:* health-care workers and public-safety workers who have exposure to blood in the workplace; and persons in training in schools of medicine, dentistry, nursing, laboratory technology, and other allied health professions. *Behavioral indications:* injection-drug users; persons with more than one sex partner during the previous 6 months; persons with a recently acquired sexually transmitted disease (STD); all clients in STD clinics; and men who have sex with men. *Other indications:* household contacts and sex partners of persons with chronic hepatitis B virus (HBV) infection; clients and staff members of institutions for the developmentally disabled; inmates of correctional facilities; or international travelers who will be in countries with high or intermediate prevalence of chronic HBV infection for >6 months (http://www.cdc.gov/travel/diseases/hbv.htm) (see *MMWR* 1991;40 [No. RR-13]).

6. **Hepatitis A vaccination.** *Medical indications:* persons with clotting factor disorders or chronic liver disease. *Behavioral indications:* men who have sex with men or users of illegal drugs. *Occupational indications:* persons working with hepatitis A virus (HAV)-infected primates or with HAV in a research laboratory setting. *Other indications:* persons traveling to or working in countries that have high or intermediate endemicity of hepatitis A. If the combined Hepatitis A and Hepatitis B vaccine is used, administer 3 doses at 0, 1, and 6 months (http://www.cdc.gov/travel/diseases/hav.htm) (see *MMWR* 1999;48 [No. RR-12]).

7. **Measles, mumps, rubella (MMR) vaccination.** *Measles component:* adults born before 1957 can be considered immune to measles. Adults born during or after 1957 should receive 1 dose of MMR unless they have a medical contraindication, documentation of 1 dose, or other acceptable evidence of immunity. A second dose of MMR is recommended for adults who 1) were recently exposed to measles or in an outbreak setting, 2) were previously vaccinated with killed measles vaccine, 3) were vaccinated with an unknown vaccine during 1963–1967, 4) are students in postsecondary educational institutions, 5) work in health-care facilities, or 6) plan to travel internationally. *Mumps component:* 1 dose of MMR vaccine should be adequate for protection. *Rubella component:* Administer 1 dose of MMR vaccine to women whose rubella vaccination history is unreliable and counsel women to avoid becoming pregnant for 4 weeks after vaccination. For women of childbearing age, regardless of birth year, routinely determine rubella immunity and counsel women regarding congenital rubella syndrome. Do not vaccinate pregnant women or those planning to become pregnant during the next 4 weeks. For women who are pregnant and susceptible, vaccinate as early in the postpartum period as possible (see *MMWR* 1998;47 [No. RR-8] and *MMWR* 2001;50:1117).

8. **Varicella vaccination.** Recommended for all persons lacking a reliable clinical history of varicella infection or serologic evidence of varicella zoster virus (VZV) infection who might be at high risk for exposure or transmission. This includes health-care workers and family contacts of immunocompromised persons; persons who live or work in environments where transmission is likely (e.g., teachers of young children, child care employees, and residents and staff members in institutional settings); persons who live or work in environments where VZV transmission can occur (e.g., college students, inmates, and staff members of correctional institutions, and military personnel); adolescents aged 11–18 years and adults living in households with children; women who are not pregnant but who might become pregnant; and international travelers who are not immune to infection. **Note:** Approximately 95% of U.S.-born adults are immune to VZV. Do not vaccinate pregnant women or those planning to become pregnant during the next 4 weeks. For women who are pregnant and susceptible, vaccinate as early in the postpartum period as possible (see *MMWR* 1999;48 [No. RR-6]).

9. **Meningococcal vaccine (quadrivalent polysaccharide for serogroups A, C, Y, and W 135).** *Medical indications:* adults with terminal complement component deficiencies or those with anatomic or functional asplenia. *Other indications:* travelers to countries in which meningococcal disease is hyperendemic or epidemic (e.g., the "meningitis belt" of sub-Saharan Africa and Mecca, Saudi Arabia). Revaccination after 3–5 years might be indicated for persons at high risk for infection (e.g., persons residing in areas where disease is epidemic). Counsel college freshmen, especially those who live in dormitories, regarding meningococcal disease and availability of the vaccine to enable them to make an educated decision about receiving the vaccination (see *MMWR* 2000;49 [No. RR-7]). The American Academy of Family Physicians recommends that colleges should take the lead on providing education on meningococcal infection and availability of vaccination and offer it to students who are interested. Physicians need not initiate discussion of meningococcal quadrivalent polysaccharide vaccine as part of routine medical care.

FIGURE 2. cont'd

present simultaneously. Minor superinfections and scarring are common complications. Severe complications, including encephalitis, severe bacterial skin infections, arthritis, hepatitis, pneumonia, and thrombocytopenia, occur in immunocompromised person. All these complications have decreased significantly since the introduction of the varicella vaccine.

Varicella vaccine (Varivax) is a live, attenuated vaccine that is given to infants in a single dose between 12 and 18 months of age. Nonimmune children and adolescents can receive the vaccine at any time, and those older than age 13 should receive two doses at least 4 weeks apart. Contraindications to varicella vaccine are similar to those for the other live, attenuated vaccines and include pregnancy, immunosuppression, and severe allergy to a first dose.

Influenza Vaccine

Influenza is an acute febrile respiratory illness caused by a member of the Orthomyxoviridae family and is divided into types A, B, and C. Influenza is usually abrupt in onset, with fever, chills, headache, myalgia, malaise, arthralgias, cough, and nasal discharge. Because many other conditions may mimic influenza, sentinel-case identification requires antigen-specific testing. The combination of A, B, and C types used in the influenza vaccine varies from year to year and requires new formulation and testing each year. The complex processing has resulted in vaccine shortages, including one during the 2004–2005 season. In infants and older adults, influenza often is complicated by lower respiratory infections such as pneumonia with high rates of hospitalization and increased mortality, especially among those with co-morbid conditions such as chronic obstructive pulmonary disease (COPD), frailty, cardiac disease, and diabetes.

Beginning in 2005, influenza immunization was recommended for all infants ages 6 to 24 months as well as high-risk adolescents and adults, including all those older than age 65 years. Chronic diseases, including diabetes, cardiac disease, asthma, and COPD, and conditions associated with immunosuppression are considered risk factors. Immunization for health care workers, day-care personnel, and others in close contact with high-risk individuals is also recommended. Universal influenza immunization recommendations are anticipated.

The dose of influenza vaccine (Fluzone) is 0.25 mL in infants 6 to 35 months of age and 0.5 mL for all others. Children up to age 9 years who are receiving their first influenza immunization should get two doses at least 2 weeks and preferably 4 weeks apart. Yearly immunizations are required. The injectable vaccine is recommended for use in children younger than age 6 years and adults older than age 49 years as well as high-risk individuals, including pregnant women in the third trimester during the influenza season. A cold-adapted live, attenuated influenza vaccine (FluMist) administered by nasal spray is available for low-risk schoolchildren and adults but is less effective after age 65 years. The nasal vaccine should not be given to pregnant women and people with immunosuppression, including those with AIDS and those using more than 20 mg of steroids daily.

Pneumococcal Vaccines

The pneumococcal vaccines are used to prevent diseases from *Streptococcus pneumoniae*, a gram-negative bacterium that causes pneumonia, bacteremia, and meningitis. Because many serotypes exist, the available vaccines are polyvalent. The 7-valent vaccine (Prevnar) is given to infants, and the 23-valent vaccine (Pneumovax 23) is used in children older than age 2 years and adults. Pneumococcal disease is most devastating to very young infants and immunosuppressed or asplenic individuals of any age. Pneumococcal pneumonia also has a high mortality rate in the elderly.

The 7-valent vaccine (Prevnar) is begun in children at 6 to 8 weeks of age and includes three doses 6 to 8 weeks apart and a booster dose at 12 to 15 months of age. If it is begun at 6 to 12 months of age, only two doses and a booster are required. From 12 to 23 months the initial series consists of only two doses, and after age 2 years only one dose is required. The catch-up schedule has been historically important because of the chronic shortage of the infant vaccine from the time of its approval by the U.S. Food and Drug Agency until November 2004.

The 23-valent vaccine (Pneumovax 23) should be given to anyone older than age 2 years who is immunosuppressed or asplenic or has chronic cardiac, renal, or liver disease as well as all adults older than age 65 years and residents of chronic care facilities. The initial dose consists of a single injection, and this is considered sufficient for most people. However, those older than age 65 years who received the vaccine before age 65 years and more than 5 years earlier should be given a second dose. The recommendations for reimmunization of other groups remain vague. Reactions to the vaccine are uncommon, and the only contraindication is a severe allergic reaction to a previous dose.

Hepatitis A Vaccine

Hepatitis A is a picornavirus that is spread by the fecal–oral route and after an incubation period of 15 to 50 days causes the abrupt onset of fever, malaise, anorexia, nausea, and jaundice. More than 30% of infected children (<6 years of age) are asymptomatic but contagious. Hepatitis A immunization is recommended only for children and adults in regions with high prevalence rates, primarily the western United States (Washington, Oregon, California, Arizona, and New Mexico).

Hepatitis A vaccine (Havrix, Vaqta) is an inactivated whole-virus vaccine licensed for children older than 23 months. The series consists of an initial dose followed by a booster in 6 to 12 months. Adverse reactions are mild and include local redness or pain at the injection site and, rarely, low-grade fever and malaise.

Contraindications include a severe allergic reaction to a previous dose and allergy to alum or to 2-phenoxyethanol.

Smallpox Vaccine*

Smallpox is currently a concern only in regard to potential bioterrorism events. Recent smallpox immunization programs for first responders have been delayed because of small but increased rates of postvaccine myocarditis and pericarditis.

Vaccine Administration

For a few vaccines, such as the varicella vaccine, storage is critical. Thawing of the varicella vaccine during transport may result in decreased efficacy. All vaccine-containing refrigerators and freezers should be monitored to maintain temperatures at the recommended levels. Vaccine effectiveness has been shown to improve with longer needles (25-mm, 25-gauge needles), and intradermal administration may improve the immunogenicity of some vaccines, such as influenza vaccine.

The Future of Vaccines

Vaccination describes the induction of a protective immune response against infectious diseases and antigen-specific immunotherapy for allergy, cancer, and autoimmunity. The hope for future vaccines is broad, including vaccines for the prevention of more infectious diseases, such as tuberculosis, HIV/AIDS, dental caries, human papillomavirus infection, and chlamydial infection, as well as other common chronic diseases, such as arteriosclerosis, malignancies, autoimmune disease, allergy, glaucoma, and perhaps even the common cold.

REFERENCES

Centers for Disease Control and Prevention National Immunization Program online. Available at http://www.cdc.gov/nip. Last modified 11/29/04 (accessed December 1, 2004).
National Immunization Information Hotline. Available at 800-232-2522 (English) or 800-232-0233 (Spanish).
Centers for Disease Control and Prevention, Vaccine Adverse Event Reporting System online. Available at http://www.vaers.org (accessed December 1, 2004).
Centers for Disease Control and Prevention Difference in Estimated Vaccination Coverage table online. Available at http://www.cdc.gov/nip/coverage/nis/03/tab34_diff.xls (accessed December 1, 2004).

*Not available in the United States for the general public.

Travel Medicine

Method of
Kenneth R. Dardick, MD

All our patients travel. It is estimated that 40 million Americans will travel abroad each year; 8 to 10 million Americans and more than 1 million Canadians will visit underdeveloped or tropical areas. Many more will stay within the United States or visit nearby destinations such as Mexico, Canada, or Europe. Physicians must be prepared to identify travel-related issues when they arise. Some patients will ask, "What shots do I need?" which is not the best starting point. Other patients are simply in the office for a cold or sprained ankle. Only by taking a complete history will the physician discover that the patient is about to take a long trip. Maybe the patient with diarrhea has just returned from a stay in the tropics. The practice of travel medicine comprises pretravel counseling, risk assessment for travelers with unique needs, and the care of travelers who return home with symptoms of illness or injury.

Physicians with expertise in travel medicine may be found among members of the American Society of Tropical Medicine and Hygiene's (ASTMH) clinical interest group, the American Committee on Clinical Tropical Medicine and Traveler's Health (ACCTMTH), or the International Society of Travel Medicine (ISTM). The ACCTMTH offers an examination leading to a Certificate in Clinical Tropical Medicine and Traveler's Health under the auspices of the American Society of Tropical Medicine and Hygiene. The ISTM offers a Certificate of Knowledge Examination leading to a Certificate in Travel Health.

Sources of Information

There are more than 200 countries and international entities worldwide. Each has its own unique set of factors including geography, climate, regulations, illnesses, and social customs, which may impact the traveler. The physician providing medical care to the traveler cannot possibly keep all this in memory. Outbreaks occur and are reported on an almost daily basis. Books and guides, even those published monthly or yearly, cannot keep track of all this. It is essential to have access to an online source or sources of reliable information. Some are free; others require a paid subscription (Box 1).

Pretravel Counseling

Health issues while traveling are common. Overall, 20% of travelers may become ill, but as many as 39% in one recent study had at least one medical or health problem, and 9% consulted a health professional while abroad. More than 50% of travelers to the tropics become ill, but only 0.2% to 0.5% require hospitalization. Frequency of illness is not related to the duration of the trip.

Depending on the trip and the individual's itinerary and medical history, it may require as much as 6 months to 1 year or as little as 1 to 2 days to prepare the traveler. A formal consultation is an excellent way to begin. Plan to spend about 30 to 45 minutes with the traveler. Many patients do not object to this, but one study found that 60% to 80% of patients in Great Britain would pay nothing for travel health advice. Health insurance may not cover expenses for medical consultations, immunizations, or prescriptions related to travel.

Avoid the temptation to give advice over the telephone. You will probably not have enough time to get into all the issues in the depth required. Remember, it is not good enough to simply state whether "shots are needed"; that is only a small part of the process. Avoid the temptation to schedule patients just for a shot; invariably there will be questions about other travel health concerns, and either your nurse, your assistant, or you will then be in the delicate position of telling the patient there isn't time to discuss these other important issues right then and there. It is much better to schedule the visit as a formal *travel consult* right up front.

Even so, much of the advice physicians give to prospective travelers will be ignored. We must pay special attention to giving health advice in ways it will be understood and acted upon. A recent study of Dutch travelers to malarious areas found that only 16% followed advice to avoid mosquito bites during the trip. Those who failed to follow doctors' advice tended to

be younger, more experienced, and going on adventure trips.

Pretravel advice includes:

- General issues for any traveler
- Environmental health, vector-borne illnesses
- Immunizations, both recommended and required
- Personal issues for individual circumstances

General Issues

ACCIDENTS

Accidents are common both at home and on the road. In a 1987 study of 90 deaths among Swiss travelers, most were related to accidents, drowning, or the act of travel. Accidents are the most common cause of death for Peace Corps workers. Morbidity and mortality rates from accidents are worse than those in the United States for comparable accidents (roughly twice the accident mortality—80% of deaths occur out of hospital). Prevention can be difficult for many reasons:

- Seat belts are not always available.
- Others may do the driving.
- Alcohol use is common.
- A sense of adventure and invulnerability often prevails.
- Driving on the "other side" of the road creates confusion.

INSURANCE AND MEDICAL ASSISTANCE

Insurance is not the same as medical assistance. Insurance pays for medical bills and hospital expenses after the fact, while medical assistance helps obtain care and coordinates services such as finding a doctor, paying up-front fees, communicating with the traveler's own physician at home, and arranging the return home. Many insurance companies provide medical assistance coverage (see the United States Department of State Web site for a comprehensive listing of these companies at www.travel.state.gov/medical.html). These policies are often coupled with other coverages sold by travel agents.

Note that Medicare is not valid outside the United States. Supplemental travel policies are essential for medical coverage of Medicare beneficiaries while traveling. Commercial health insurance coverage outside the United States may have other limitations such as the need for prior authorization for diagnosis and treatment as well as issues of out-of-network coverage. In any case the traveler will have to pay for any services first and then attempt to be reimbursed by his or her medical policy. Supplemental health insurance policies can cover these and other gaps.

TRAVEL KIT

Prepare a list of generic drug names, doses, and indications for your patient in case a replacement prescription is needed. Medications should be carried with the traveler, not checked through with luggage. All medications should be carried in original pharmacy bottles (not loose in a zip-lock plastic bag, very suspicious). Those traveling with needles and syringes should have a letter on the medical practice letterhead indicating the need for the injectable drugs (e.g., diabetes). Travelers should take an extra pair of glasses, contact lenses, and a copy of their vision prescription. Those with a cardiac condition should carry a copy of a recent electrocardiogram (ECG) and, if relevant, pacemaker information. Other items are related to the duration of travel and availability of common supplies at the destination (e.g., bandages, antibacterial ointment, antidiarrheal medication, antibiotics for presumptive treatment of skin or respiratory infections).

JET LAG

Jet lag is caused by an imbalance between the traveler's diurnal rhythm and the real time at the destination. It is not a problem with north-south travel, only east-west travel across more than 5 time zones. The biological clock prefers a longer day, so westward travel is usually handled better. Common symptoms of jet lag are fatigue, malaise, headache, anorexia, and difficulty concentrating. Jet lag is compounded by the fatigue that all travelers experience and by dehydration. There is no easy way to avoid jet lag; most travelers do not have the luxury of breaking up their trip with intermediate stops to allow the biological clock to adjust. The use of short-acting hypnotic drugs is controversial; amnesia has been reported with triazolam (Halcion), especially when mixed with alcohol. Melatonin[1],* may be effective in reducing symptoms of jet lag, but may take 2 to 3 days of daily administration to reach full effect. Typical doses for eastward travel are 3 to 5 mg daily at destination bedtime on the day of travel, and then nightly for 3 to 5 nights. When traveling westward omit the dose on the day of travel, but continue melatonin 3 to 5 mg nightly for 3 to 5 nights after arrival.

DEEP VENOUS THROMBOSIS

There is good evidence that jet travelers on long-haul flights (>8 hours' duration) are at increased risk of developing deep venous thrombosis (DVT), which may be symptomless. This can be prevented by wearing moderate compression (20-30 mm Hg) elastic stockings. High-risk travelers (prior history of DVT, pregnant women, hypercoagulable states) should be advised to wear elastic stockings, drink ample fluids, and walk up and down the aisles every 30 to 60 minutes, if possible.

MOTION SICKNESS

All forms of travel may induce the familiar symptoms of motion sickness (nausea, diaphoresis, anorexia, lethargy, vomiting). These symptoms are triggered by an imbalance among visual, rotatory, and kinesthetic cues in the inner ear (labyrinth) and brain. All travelers are

susceptible to motion sickness in certain circumstances, but some are clearly more susceptible than others. Those at greatest risk are children 5 to 12 years of age and women. Travel in small aircraft, small boats, and cars may pose the greatest risks. Motion sickness is often aggravated by up and down movements of the head and neck. A number of strategies are known to help reduce the symptoms of motion sickness (Box 2).

There are many effective medications but no one solution is best for all travelers. Children do best with common antihistamines such as dimenhydrinate (Dramamine), diphenhydramine (Benadryl), or promethazine (Phenergan). Drowsiness is the most common side effect for all of these drugs. A little-known fact is that dimenhydrinate is actually the theophylline salt of diphenhydramine, a pharmacological attempt to make it less sedating. The antihistamines are highly effective if taken before the onset of symptoms.

Adults can use the same antihistamines as children, as well as meclizine (Bonine or Antivert, ages 12 and older). The most effective single medication for prevention of motion sickness is scopolamine. The transdermal patch (Transderm Scop), introduced in 1981, was the first transdermal medication. A single patch provides 72 hours of prevention and is applied at least 6 to 8 hours before travel. For longer trips, additional patches should be applied every 72 hours. Scopolamine cannot be used by those younger than 12 years of age or by those with glaucoma, urinary retention, or pyloric obstruction. Elderly patients may develop hallucinations. More than 60% of patients using scopolamine develop dry mouth. Other side effects may include blurred vision and bradycardia. Sedation is seen much less commonly with scopolamine than with antihistamines.

Nonpharmacologic measures to prevent motion sickness, such as ginger[1],* and acupuncture (at the

---

[1]Not FDA approved for this indication.
*Available as a dietary supplement.

> **BOX 2 Strategies for Minimizing Motion Sickness Symptoms**
>
> - Sit in the front seat of a car (note that this is not acceptable for children, who must sit in car seats in the back for safety reasons).
> - Avoid strong odors, perfumes, colognes, or smoke; maintain adequate ventilation.
> - Sit over the wings in a plane or amidships in a boat (the most stable areas).
> - Eat and drink lightly, if at all.
> - Do not read or play video games; look at the distant horizon.
> - On a boat stay on deck, watch the horizon, do not lie down; the ideal position is in a deck chair with a pillow around the neck for stability.
> - Children may benefit from a cushion to raise them up to look out the window.

---

[1]Not FDA approved for this indication.
*Available as a dietary supplement.

Rakel and Bope: *Conn's Current Therapy 2006*

P6/Neiguan acupuncture point), may reduce symptoms but have not been shown to prevent motion sickness. Wristband acupressure has not been shown to be effective.

HIGH ALTITUDE (ALSO SEE HIGH ALTITUDE SICKNESS ARTICLE)

High altitude is not just a problem for mountain climbers. Many who travel to hike or sightsee are susceptible to the clinical syndromes of altitude illness. There are no reliable screening tests for altitude illness, but those who have had problems in the past are more likely to have problems in the future. Anyone traveling to destinations above 1219 m (4000 ft) may be at risk for acute mountain sickness (AMS), but the risk is greatest with abrupt ascent above 2743 m (9000 ft).

Symptoms are variable and include headache, fatigue, anorexia, nausea, and vomiting. AMS can be prevented with acetazolamide (adult dose 125 mg twice a day, starting 2 days before ascent and continuing for 2 to 3 days after reaching maximal altitude). Ginkgo biloba[4,*] (various preparations; 100 mg twice a day, starting 5 days prior to ascent and continuing for 2 to 3 days after reaching maximal altitude) may also be effective for prevention.

High-altitude cerebral edema (HACE) is more severe than AMS, comprising symptoms of severe lethargy, confusion, and ataxia. AMS may progress to HACE.

High-altitude pulmonary edema (HAPE) is manifested by dyspnea on exertion, progressing to dyspnea at rest. HAPE and HACE may occur alone or in tandem. Rapid descent is critical in managing both HAPE and HACE. Medications including dexamethasone (Decadron) and nifedipine (Adalat)[1] are effective treatments for HAPE and HACE. A pressurization (Gamov) bag can simulate a descent of 1500 to 1800 m (5000-6000 ft), which can be lifesaving if actual emergency descent cannot be achieved.

SEXUALLY TRANSMITTED DISEASES

The relationship between sexually transmitted diseases (STDs) and travel is not a new one. Columbus was said to have brought syphilis home to the Old World from the New World. U.S. military personnel brought home penicillin-resistant gonorrhea (PPNG) from Southeast Asia. Travelers on jet aircraft from Africa to Europe and the Americas spread HIV rapidly. Condoms and abstinence (not necessarily in that order) are the most effective means of prevention. In a study of Dutch expatriates in HIV-endemic areas, 41% of the men and 31% of the women had sex with casual or steady local partners, and 23% had unprotected sex with local partners. It is important to remind travelers of their responsibility to practice "safe sex" to protect themselves from acquiring or spreading venereal diseases worldwide.

Environmental Health (Enteric, Vector-Borne)

Travel exposes the individual to a variety of infectious diseases. Some are related to poor sanitation or hygiene; others are acquired by exposure to vectors. Many of these diseases are not vaccine preventable. The traveler must be educated about other preventive measures to avoid disease; these include behavioral measures as well as preventive or presumptive treatment medication in some cases.

TRAVELER'S DIARRHEA

Traveler's diarrhea (TD) is one of the major illnesses causing significant morbidity in travelers. Most illness is caused by enterotoxigenic *Escherichia coli*; some is caused by other enteric bacteria. There is no generally agreed-upon definition of TD, but most people "know it when it happens," an abrupt onset of an increase in watery stools with or without fever, and cramps, and usually lasting 3 to 5 days. More than 90% of cases last less than 1 week, but nearly 1% may last 3 months or longer. TD is rarely life threatening, but in an area where cholera is present, a TD syndrome may be the early clinical presentation of cholera. Fluid replacement is an important part of the early management of all cases of TD. Prevention of TD and other enteric infections is based on a number of well-established principles (Box 3).

Self-treatment of mild traveler's diarrhea can promptly relieve symptoms of most cases. Up to 80% of patients will be cured with as little as a single dose of antibiotics. If there is no fever, the person can take both an antibiotic and loperamide (Imodium AD) (see list that follows this paragraph). If there is fever, the person should take only the antibiotic. In most parts of the world a fluoroquinolone is an excellent choice, but in Southeast Asia, because of an increasing prevalence of quinolone-resistant *Campylobacter* infection, azithromycin (Zithromax)[1] is a better choice.

The dosages for self-treatment of TD are:

1. Antibiotic
   - Ciprofloxacin (Cipro) 500 mg, two tablets initially, then one tablet twice a day.
   - Doxycycline monohydrate (Monodox)[1] 100 mg, one tablet twice a day.
   - Azithromycin (Zithromax) 250 mg, one tablet daily.
   - Take the antibiotic until symptoms are gone (as little as a single dose of antibiotics may be curative). Do not exceed 3 days of treatment. There is no clear preference among these antibiotics except that azithromycin may be favored in areas of Southeast Asia where there is increasing resistance to fluoroquinolones and an increase in prevalence of *Campylobacter* infection. Azithromycin may also

---

[4]Not yet approved for use in the United States.
*Available as a dietary supplement.

---

[1]Not FDA approved for this indication.

be preferred for children and women who might be pregnant.

2. Loperamide
   - Take 4 mg (two capsules or 4 teaspoons) initially, followed by 2 mg (one capsule or 2 teaspoons) after each loose stool, up to a maximum of 16 mg (eight capsules or 16 teaspoons) per day.
   - Do not take loperamide in the presence of fever or bloody dysentery syndrome.

MALARIA

Malaria is one of the most significant health risks to travelers, not because of the large number of cases or morbidity, but because it can be fatal and should be largely preventable. From 1985 to 2001, the Centers for Disease Control and Prevention (CDC) reported an average of approximately 600 cases of malaria per year in the United States civilians, with four fatalities per year. Approximately 94% of the U.S. malaria cases were caused by *Plasmodium falciparum*, and 71% were contracted in sub-Saharan Africa. Transmission is predominantly by the bite of an infected anopheline mosquito (usually in the dusk-to-dawn hours), but malaria can also be transmitted by blood transfusion. It is estimated that worldwide there are 300 to 500 million cases annually with up to 1 million deaths. The risk of acquiring malaria while traveling is specific to location and itinerary. For example, two visitors to the same location will have very different risks if one hikes and sleeps outdoors at night while the other remains predominantly in an air-conditioned environment, uses adequate repellents, and wears long sleeves and trousers.

Education of the traveler is paramount. The use of personal protective measures—applying insect repellents on the skin (diethyltoluamide [DEET] or picaridin [Cutter Advanced]) and clothing (permethrin), sleeping under bed nets (even more effective if treated with permethrin), remaining in screened areas, and wearing long sleeves and pants—greatly reduces the likelihood of being bitten by mosquitoes. Recent publications have emphasized the safety and effectiveness of DEET repellents.

Malaria, dengue, leishmaniasis, filariasis, and other vector-borne infections are best prevented by avoiding insect bites. Protective measures to avoid mosquito exposure are advised by the CDC in addition to taking prophylactic antimalarial medication (Box 4).

MEDICATION

Travelers to areas at high risk for malaria transmission must be counseled about proper preventive medication.

BOX 3   "Boil It, Peel It, Cook It, or Forget It!"—Advice for the Prevention of Traveler's Diarrhea

- Cooked food that has been held at room temperature for several hours constitutes one of the greatest risks of food-borne illness. Make sure your food has been thoroughly cooked and is still hot when served.
- Avoid any uncooked food, apart from fruits and vegetables that can be peeled or shelled. Avoid fruits with damaged skin.
- Ice cream from unreliable sources is frequently contaminated and can cause illness. If in doubt, avoid it.
- In some countries, certain species of fish and shellfish may contain poisonous biotoxins even when they are well cooked. Local people can advise you about this.
- Unpasteurized milk should be boiled before consumption.
- When the safety of drinking water is doubtful, have it boiled or disinfect it with reliable, slow-release, disinfectant tablets. These are generally available in pharmacies. Iodine tablets may be effective for purification, but efficacy is affected by the temperature and clarity of the water and the iodine may impart an objectionable taste. Or, drink bottled water.
- Filters may be used to purify water in some settings (hiking), but be aware that small filter pore size (0.1-0.3 micron) can remove bacteria and protozoa, but not viruses. Filters with a small pore size are readily clogged and less effective for large volumes of water; they are not effective in water with heavy sediment. Neither the FDA nor the CDC certifies filters, but the following are useful sources of information:
  - http://www.cdc.gov/ncidod/dpd/parasites/cryptosporidiosis/factsht_crypto_prevent_water.htm
  - http://www.NSF.org/certified/dwtu (click on "cyst reduction")
- Avoid ice unless you are sure that it is made from safe water.
- Beverages such as hot tea or coffee, wine, beer, and carbonated soft drinks or fruit juices that are either bottled or otherwise packaged are usually safe to drink.

Adapted from WHO and CDC publications.

BOX 4   Personal Protective Measures to Avoid Insect Bites

- Sleep inside screened areas.
- Wear clothing that covers arms and legs.
- Avoid outdoor activities in the evening when mosquitoes are most active. (Note that day-biting mosquitoes may transmit dengue, yellow fever, filariasis, and Japanese encephalitis. Sandflies, which transmit leishmaniasis; deerflies, which transmit onchocerciasis; and tsetse flies, which transmit African trypanosomiasis, may also bite during the day.)
- Apply repellent as follows:
  DEET (diethyltoluamide) is now available in low-concentration slow-release formulations that keep the DEET on the skin surface and prevent absorption. Ultrathon, Sawyer controlled release, and Sawyer Family are products that contain DEET in nonabsorbable formulations.
  Picardin (Cutter Advanced) is as effective for 3–4 hours as low concentration DEET but has no odor and is not a plasticizer.
  Permethrin (Permanone) is a synthetic derivative of chrysanthemum. It is applied to clothing; one soaking application may last up to 4-8 wks or longer, even with laundering.
  Use a pyrethrum-containing insect spray in living and sleeping areas at night.

The decision about which medication is best for each individual traveler depends on factors such as the local pattern of malaria transmission, season of the year, activities of the traveler, presence of drug resistance (Table 1), availability of competent local medical care, and contraindications to a particular drug. A 2002 CDC summary of malaria in travelers documented that less than 20% of those infected with malaria had taken proper medication. Travelers returning home to visit friends or relatives have a high risk of developing malaria.

Various medications are available for the prevention of malaria among travelers. An understanding of the factors listed above is critical in being able to properly prescribe the optimal medication for each traveler (Table 2).

DENGUE

Dengue is a flavivirus infection found in most tropical countries and many tropical urban centers; more than 2.5 billion people live in areas at risk for dengue infection. Dengue is transmitted by the bite of an infected day-biting *Aedes aegypti* mosquito, the same mosquito vector as for yellow fever. There are four serotypes of dengue (DEN1-4) and no cross-immunity among them. In fact, it is the subsequent infection with different serotypes that may increase the risk of developing dengue hemorrhagic fever (DHF). There are an estimated 50 to 100 million cases per year with 200 to 500,000 cases of DHF, which has a case-fatality rate (CFR) of 5%. Repellents are an effective preventive measure (see Box 4). Dengue infection produces an acute febrile illness with a typical incubation period of 4 to 7 days (range: 3-14 days). High fever is accompanied by headache, myalgias, and arthralgias ("breakbone fever"); a rash may appear 3 to 5 days after the onset of fever.

LEISHMANIASIS

Leishmaniasis is a protozoal infection transmitted by the bite of an infected phlebotomine sandfly. These flies

TABLE 1 Malaria-Preventive Medication According to Travel Destination

Region of Travel	Preferred Medication for Malaria Prevention
Areas of the world with chloroquine-sensitive malaria (Central America west of the Panama Canal, the Middle East, and Egypt)	Chloroquine
Mefloquine-resistance areas of Southeast Asia (Thailand-Myanmar and Thailand-Cambodia borders, eastern Myanmar)	Atovaquone/proguanil (Malarone) or doxycycline
All other areas	Atovaquone/proguanil, mefloquine (Lariam), or doxycycline

From World Health Organization (WHO)/Department of Immunization, Vaccines and Biologicals.

are quite small and easily pass through typical mosquito netting. They cannot bite through most clothing. Preventive measures include using repellents and wearing trousers and long-sleeved shirts. All nonhealing papular-ulcerative lesions in travelers who have visited endemic countries should be considered suspicious for diagnosis of leishmaniasis. Leishmaniasis can also manifest as a systemic syndrome of splenomegaly, anemia, fever, and weight loss. Contact the CDC Division of Parasitic Diseases (770-488-7775) for assistance in the diagnosis and treatment of suspected cases of leishmaniasis.

SCHISTOSOMIASIS

Schistosomiasis is a potentially serious systemic infection. It is acquired by swimming in fresh water inhabited by certain species of snails carrying the infective cercariae. These cercariae penetrate the skin and subsequently invade various body organs including the lungs, spinal cord, portal veins, and the urinary bladder. Although there is some evidence that application of DEET repellent on the skin may prevent infection, the most important advice for travelers is to be aware of the presence of this infection in certain freshwater areas (not saltwater) and to avoid swimming or wading in these locations.

Immunizations

Although the first question asked is often "I'm taking a trip—what shots do I need?" it must be understood that advice for travelers may or may not include immunizations. There are only limited situations in which vaccination is required for entry to a country. Yellow fever vaccine (YF-VAX) may be a legal requirement for some travelers; some visitors to Saudi Arabia on Haj (pilgrimage) may be required to have proof of meningococcal vaccination.

All other vaccine advice should be based on factors such as these:

- Prevalence of a vaccine-preventable disease
- Itinerary and risk behaviors that increase the traveler's risk of acquiring a particular disease
- Effectiveness and side effects of the vaccine
- Personal medical history of the traveler, which may increase susceptibility to a particular disease or increase risk from the vaccine (immune status, pregnancy, age). It is important to obtain accurate, up-to-date information for the traveler. Because books become quickly out of date, the Internet and a subscription service (see Box 1) remain the most reliable sources of such information for proper health advice, including immunizations, for the traveler.

Routine immunizations such as tetanus-diphtheria-pertussis (in children), *Haemophilus influenzae*, measles-mumps-rubella (MMR), polio, varicella, hepatitis B, and influenza should all be maintained according to the usual schedules. The risk of acquiring these diseases is generally no greater while traveling than while at home,

TABLE 2 Drugs Used in Malaria Prophylaxis

Drug	Usage Contraindications	Adult Dose	Pediatric Dose	Adverse Reactions	Contraindications
Chloroquine phosphate (Aralen)	In areas with chloroquine-sensitive *P. falciparum*	300 mg base (500 mg salt) orally 1/wk	5 mg/kg base (8.3 mg/kg salt), orally 1/wk, up to max adult dose of 300 mg base	Mild nausea, blurred vision, headache, psoriasis flare-ups; itching in dark-skinned persons; very rarely agranulocytosis, photosensitivity, neuropsychiatric effects	Patients hypersensitive to 4-aminoquinolone derivatives; patients with retinal or field changes attributable to drug therapy; patients with psoriasis; use with caution in patients with liver disease, and/or alcoholism.
Atovaquone/ proguanil (Malarone)	In areas with chloroquine-resistant *P. falciparum*	Each tablet contains atovaquone 250 mg/ proguanil 100 mg; adults, adolescents, and children ≥3 years of age weighing >40 kg: 1 tablet orally1/d	Each pediatric tablet contains atovaquone 62.5 mg/ proguanil 25 mg; children ≥3 y . and 31-40 kg: 3 oral tablets 1/d; <3 y and 21-30 kg: 2 oral tablets 1/d; ≥3 y and 11-20 kg: 1 tablet orally 1/d; children ≥3 y or <11 kg: safety and efficacy not established	Abdominal pain, nausea/vomiting, headache, diarrhea, asthenia, anorexia, dizziness, pruritus	Any known hypersensitivity to proguanil or atovaquone.
Mefloquine HCl (Lariam)	In areas with chloroquine-resistant *P. falciparum*	228 mg base (250 mg salt) orally, 1/wk	<15 kg, 4.6 mg/kg base (5 mg/kg salt), orally 1/wk; 15-19 kg: 1/4 tab/wk; 20-30 kg: 1/2 tab/wk; 31-45 kg: 3/4 tab/wk; >45 kg: 1 tab/wk	Adverse reactions include nausea/vomiting, diarrhea, dizziness, difficulty sleeping, and bad dreams	Patients who are hypersensitive to related compounds, such as quinine; patients with active depression or with history of seizures or severe psychiatric disorders; use with caution in patients with cardiac conduction abnormalities. Do not combine with halofantrine (Halfan).

Continued

TABLE 2 Drugs Used in Malaria Prophylaxis—cont'd

Drug	Usage Contraindications	Adult Dose	Pediatric Dose	Adverse Reactions	Contraindications
Doxycycline monohydrate (Adoxa) or hyclate (Vibramycin) (monohydrate may be better tolerated)	In areas with chloroquine-resistant *P. falciparum*	100 mg orally 1/d	>8 years of age: 2 mg/kg orally 1/d, up to adult dose of 100 mg	Photosensitivity reactions to doxycycline after sunlight (ultraviolet). Discontinue at first sign of erythema; skin reactions can increase when used with sulfonamide, sulfonylureas, or thiazide diuretics; gastrointestinal upset.	Patients hypersensitive to any of the tetracyclines; some commercially available preparations contain sulfites that can result in increased asthmatic attacks in such persons, as well as anaphylaxis.
Hydroxychloroquine sulfate (Plaquenil)	Alternative to chloroquine	310 mg base (400 mg salt) orally 1/wk	5 mg/kg base (6.5 mg/kg salt), orally 1/wk, up to max adult dose of 310 mg base	Same as for chloroquine.	Same as for chloroquine.

Adapted with permission from Dardick K: Educating travelers about malaria: Dealing with resistance and patient noncompliance. Cleve Clin J Med 2002;69(6):469.

but infants who are not protected against measles may be exposed to a greater risk of measles in many parts of the world where infant vaccination is less complete than in the United States. Travelers have been known to import measles back to the United States. There have been outbreaks of diphtheria (Eastern Europe) and influenza (late summer on cruises), and the prevalence of hepatitis B in East Asia is far greater than in North America or Europe.

Other immunization considerations more directly associated with travel (Table 3) are:

- Conditions of poor hygiene and sanitation increase the risk of hepatitis A and typhoid.
- Hepatitis A is perhaps the most common vaccine-preventable disease among travelers, with considerable morbidity and some mortality in those older than 40 years of age.
- Typhoid fever is most commonly acquired on the Indian subcontinent, often by those returning to their native land to visit family.
- Japanese encephalitis is a risk for travelers who will be spending extended time in certain rural areas of Asia where exposure to mosquitoes is considerable, especially in areas devoted to rice farming and pig farming.
- Meningococcal disease is found in the sub-Saharan belt of Africa; vaccination may be appropriate for those spending extended periods in crowded cities during epidemic periods.

- Rabies vaccine should be strongly advised for those who will spend extended periods of time in developing countries or rural areas other than North America, Europe, Australia, Japan, and other islands designated as "rabies-free." Pre-exposure vaccination precludes the need for postexposure human rabies immunoglobulin (BayRab), which may be difficult to obtain or of questionable safety. It also reduces the number of postexposure shots from 5 to 2.
- Vaccines against diseases such as cholera, anthrax, and plague are of limited effectiveness and rarely advised for travelers except for unique circumstances such as field biologists or laboratory workers.
- Tick-borne encephalitis vaccine is not available in the United States. It may be obtained in Canada or in Europe for a traveler who will be exposed in areas of Eastern or Central Europe while hiking or camping.

The CDC offers the following vaccine information:

- Except for oral typhoid vaccine (Vivotif Berna), it is unnecessary to restart an interrupted series of vaccine or toxoid, or to add extra doses. Simply pick up with the next dose in the series.
- It is okay to give any combination of vaccines on the same day including all live virus vaccines and yellow fever vaccine (YF-VAX).
- Live virus vaccines not given concurrently should be given more than 28 days apart. If live virus vaccines are given less than 28 days apart, the second vaccine should be readministered after 4 to 6 weeks.

Rakel and Bope: *Conn's Current Therapy 2006*

TABLE 3 Travel Immunization Doses

Vaccine Name	Dosage	Comments
Inactivated or Recombinant Antigens		
Hepatitis A vaccine—Havrix	Age 2-18 y, 720 EL.U., 0.5 mL, 2 doses at 0, 6-12mo; age ≥19 y, 1440 EL.U., 1.0 mL, 2 doses at 0, 6-12 mo	2 doses provide lifelong immunity; Havrix or Vaqta may be substituted for the 2nd dose of the other. Giving the 2nd dose at a longer interval does not interfere with immune response; it may give an even better result.
Hepatitis A vaccine—Vaqta	Age 2-18 y, 25 U, 0.5 mL, 2 doses at 0, 6-18 mo; age ≥19 y, 50 U, 1.0 mL, 2 doses at 0, 6-12 mo	
Hepatitis B vaccine—Engerix-B	Age 0-19 y, 10 μg, 3 doses at 0, 1, 6 mo, or 4 doses at 0, 1, 2, 12 mo; age ≥20 y, 20 μg, 3 doses at 0, 1, 6 mo, or 4 doses at 0, 1, 2, 12 mo	May also be given in a non–FDA-approved schedule of 0, 7, 14 d with a booster 6 mo later. No need to restart a series that has been interrupted. Engerix-B and Recombivax-HB may be used interchangeably in the 3-dose schedule only.
Hepatitis B vaccine—Recombivax-HB	Age 0-19 y, 5 μg, 3 doses at 0, 1, 6 mo; age 11-15 y 10 μg; 2 doses at 0, 4-6 mo; age ≥20 y, 10 μg; 3 doses at 0, 1, 6 mo	
Hepatitis A/hepatitis B—Twinrix (combined vaccine)	Age ≥18 y, 720 EL.U./20 μg, 1.0 mL, 3 doses at 0, 1, 6 mo	
Meningococcal polysaccharide vaccine—Menomune (quadrivalent A,C,Y,W-135)	Age ≥2 y, but may be given for short-term protection against group A to infants >3 mo, 1 dose, 0.5 mL	Revaccination of a single 0.5 mL dose administered subcutaneously may be indicated for individuals at high risk of infection, particularly children who were first vaccinated when they were less than 4 y of age; such children should be considered for revaccination after 2 or 3 y if they remain at high risk. Although the need for revaccination in older children and adults has not been determined, antibody levels decline rapidly over 2-3 y, and if indications still exist for immunization, revaccination may be considered within 3-5 y.
Meningococcal polysaccharide diptheria toxoid conjugate vaccine (Menactra, Quadrivalent A,C,Y,W-135)	Age 11-55 y, 0.5 mL IM	The need for or timing of a booster dose has not been determined.
Typhoid vaccine, injectable—Typhim Vi	Age ≥2 y, 0.5 mL	Booster dose every 2 y.
Japanese encephalitis virus vaccine—JE Vax	Age 1-2 y, 0.5 mL; ≥3 y 1.0 mL, 3 doses on d 0, 7, 30	Adverse reactions to JE vaccine manifesting as generalized urticaria or angioedema may occur within minutes following vaccination. Most reactions occur in 48 h, but can be as late as 17 d after vaccination. Vaccinated persons should be observed for 30 min after vaccination and warned about the possibility of delayed generalized urticaria, often in a generalized distribution or angioedema of the extremities, face, and oropharynx, especially of the lips. They should be advised to remain in areas where they have ready access to medical care and should not embark on international travel within 10 d after receiving a dose of JE vaccine. Booster dose: 1 dose at 24 mo, but the full duration of protection is not known.
Rabies vaccine—Imovax (human diploid cell vaccine); HDCV; RVA (rabies vaccine adsorbed); RabAvert (purified chick embryo cell vaccine [PCEC])	All ages, 1.0 mL, 3 doses at 0, 7, and 21 or 28 d	The full course should be given with the same product. Travelers who are immunosuppressed should avoid travel to areas at risk for rabies and postpone vaccination. If this cannot be avoided, antibody titers should be checked after vaccination. Booster doses are not advised for travelers other than those with frequent exposure to rabies (spelunkers, veterinarians, rabies diagnostic laboratory workers, animal control workers in rabies-epizootic areas).

Continued

TABLE 3 Travel Immunization Doses—cont'd

Vaccine Name	Dosage	Comments
Live-Attenuated Vaccines		
Typhoid vaccine, oral (attenuated bacteria)	Age ≥6 y, 1 capsule, 4 doses on d 0, 2, 4, 6	Booster dose, same as the initial 4-capsule dose after 5 years. Do not take with antibiotics, which kill the attenuated Vivotif bacterium. Booster dose every 10 years.
Yellow fever (attenuated virus vaccine)—YF-VAX	Age ≥9 mo, 0.5 mL	Yellow fever vaccination may be required for international travel. Some countries in Africa require evidence of vaccination from all entering travelers and some countries may waive the requirements for travelers staying less than 2 wks who are coming from areas where there is no current evidence of significant risk for contracting yellow fever. Some countries require an individual, even if only in transit, to have a valid International Certificate of Vaccination if the individual has been in countries either known or thought to harbor yellow fever virus. The certificate becomes valid 10 d after vaccination with YF-VAX.

From CDC and package inserts.

- Immunoglobulin is now given infrequently. If it is administered it may interfere with the immune response to certain vaccines. Refer to Table 1-1 in *CDC Health Information for International Travel 2005-2006* for detailed information on the use of immunoglobulin.
- Immunosuppressed travelers should not receive live virus vaccines (yellow fever, measles, mumps, rubella, varicella), including patients with AIDS, leukemia, lymphoma, or generalized malignancy or those taking systemic steroids, alkylating drugs, antimetabolites and radiation therapy.
- The following patients are *not* considered immunosuppressed and may receive live virus vaccines:
  Patients taking low-dose steroids (<20 mg prednisone per day)
  Patients on short-term (<2 weeks) steroid therapy
  Patients receiving steroid injections in joints, tendons, or bursae
  Patients who have asymptomatic HIV infection with established laboratory verification of adequate immune system function (CD4$^+$ >200)

Yellow fever is a flavivirus transmitted by the bite of the *A. aegypti* mosquito. It exists in both South America (approximately 10% of the cases) and sub-Saharan Africa (approximately 90% of the cases). The World Health Organization (WHO) reports that in 2003 there were 200,000 cases with 30,000 deaths. Lately there may be an increased risk of yellow fever infection to the 3 million who visit endemic areas annually because the infection is spreading and is under-reported. It has been estimated that an unvaccinated traveler spending 2 weeks in a yellow fever zone in Africa has a 1 in 267 chance of contracting the illness and 1 in 1333 risk of death. Rates in South America are one-tenth the rates in Africa.

The yellow fever vaccine (YF-VAX) is an attenuated strain (17D), which has been in widespread use for more than 60 years. More than 400 million doses have been given with an excellent safety record. A single dose yields protective antibodies in more than 99% of recipients in 1 month; the immunity may last for decades, but repeat vaccination is required every 10 years. Mild adverse effects may be seen in up to 25% of recipients (fever, myalgias), with 1% of recipients curtailing daily activities. Immediate hypersensitivity reactions are seen in less than 1 per 100,000; these are mostly because of egg protein allergies. Disseminated systemic reactions (viscerotropic) have been seen lately with seven cases (six deaths) reported from 1996 to 2000. It is estimated that there is a viscerotropic or neurotropic reaction risk of 1/400,000 to 1/500,000 vaccine recipients older than 60 years of age. The vaccine is contraindicated during pregnancy and in infants younger than 6 months of age, but there is limited data on its use during lactation. It is not recommended for infants 6 to 8 months of age except during outbreaks. Those who are immunosuppressed should not receive yellow fever vaccine.

Simultaneous administration of yellow fever vaccine with all others is acceptable, but data are not available on interactions of the yellow fever vaccine with the rabies vaccine and the Japanese encephalitis vaccine. If other live virus vaccines cannot be given at the same time as the yellow fever vaccine, they should be given more than 4 weeks later.

HEPATITIS A (SEE "ACUTE AND CHRONIC VIRAL HEPATITIS" ARTICLE)

Hepatitis A is an enteric viral infection that is a risk to travelers visiting tropical or poorly developed areas. Infections are usually asymptomatic (>70%) in those younger than 6 years of age, and the CFR is low (<0.3%). Those older than 50 years of age have both greater morbidity and mortality (CFR 1.8%). Completion of the two-dose series of hepatitis A immunization appears to provide life-long protection. The vaccine (Havrix, Vaqta) is a recombinant DNA vaccine and should be offered to all travelers to tropical or underdeveloped areas outside of the United States, Canada, Western Europe, Australia, New Zealand, and Japan.

HEPATITIS B (SEE ACUTE AND CHRONIC VIRAL HEPATITIS ARTICLE)

Hepatitis B is a blood-borne viral infection that poses a risk to travelers who have blood and body-fluid exposure in areas of the world with rates of hepatitis B infection in excess of 2%. These areas comprise much of the world except North America, northern and western Europe, Australia, New Zealand, and southeast South America. The usual dosing schedule is three doses given in a 6- to 12-month period, but there is a non–FDA-approved accelerated schedule. Adolescents, 11 to 15 years old, may receive a two-dose schedule. A combination hepatitis A–hepatitis B vaccine (Twinrix) is also available. This vaccine is contraindicated for those allergic to yeast, but may be given during pregnancy or lactation.

INFLUENZA (SEE INFLUENZA ARTICLE)

Influenza is a common viral respiratory infection worldwide. Outbreaks may occur among travelers out of the usual seasonal pattern. There have been well-documented outbreaks among passengers on cruise ships during the summer months. North American travelers may be at risk of influenza infection while traveling to the southern hemisphere from April to September. Influenza vaccine is recommended for all travelers during the influenza season (including the North American summer for travel to the southern hemisphere).

MENINGOCOCCAL DISEASE

Neisseria meningitidis is an encapsulated gram-negative bacterium that can produce both meningitis and disseminated sepsis (meningococcemia). Travelers to Saudi Arabia on Haj (pilgrimage) may be required to show proof of this vaccination. Areas of sub-Saharan Africa in the so-called meningitis belt have both endemic and epidemic meningococcal disease. Travelers to these countries with extended itineraries may be at increased risk and should consider vaccination with the polysaccharide capsular meningococcal vaccine (Menomune-A/C/Y/W-135) or polysaccharide conjugate meningococcal vaccine (Menactra-A/C/Y/W-135.

RABIES (SEE RABIES ARTICLE)

Perhaps the most important things to remember about rabies are these:

- Rabies infection is invariably fatal.
- There is no treatment for rabies infection, only prevention; there is a limited time window of opportunity for vaccination after suspected exposure.

- Pre-exposure immunization and postexposure immunization (and rabies immunoglobulin, if needed), when followed properly, protect against rabies infection.
- After suspected rabies exposure, those who have been properly prepared with pre-exposure immunization do not require rabies immunoglobulin (RIG) (BayRab) and require only two doses of rabies vaccine instead of the usual five doses.

TYPHOID (SEE TYPHOID FEVER ARTICLE)

Typhoid is a member of the *Salmonella* family that produces both intestinal and enteric fever syndromes. There are an estimated 2.6 cases per 1 million U.S. citizens or residents traveling abroad. Two vaccines are available, oral (Vivotif Berna) and injectable (Typhim Vi). Both have equivalent efficacy, about 70% protection; and the side effects of the two vaccines are comparable. The advantage of the injectable vaccine is that it is given in the office with no concerns about compliance or interference from antibiotics. These are both possible problems with the oral vaccine, which must be taken as four doses during a 7-day period—noncompliance is common. Also, the injectable vaccine can be given to children who cannot swallow the oral capsule; it cannot be crushed or broken because that would destroy the enteric coating, which is important for its dissolution. The oral vaccine provides protection for 5 years as opposed to only 2 years for the injectable vaccine. Pregnant women should not receive the oral vaccine; it is a live, attenuated bacterial vaccine.

Individual Health Considerations

HEALTH CARE WORKERS

Health care workers at risk of blood and body-fluid exposure should receive hepatitis B vaccinations and consider carrying a 1- to 2-week course of highly active retroviral therapy (HAART) with them in case they cannot receive prompt care after exposure.

HIV-INFECTED AND IMMUNOSUPPRESSED TRAVELERS

Travel to tropical and developing destinations may pose an increased risk of infectious diseases especially to those with $CD4^+$ counts less than $200/mm^3$. The CDC advises these travelers to pay particular attention to:

- Knowledge of the diseases present in the destination country
- Sources of medical care and need for supplemental insurance
- Adequate supply of medications which may not be available in the travel destination
- Chemoprophylaxis for traveler's diarrhea, a fluoroquinolone for nonpregnant persons, azithromycin for pregnant women and children
- Safe sex practices
- Risk from live virus vaccines (measles, varicella, yellow fever) balanced against the risk of the disease

PREGNANCY

According to the American College of Obstetrics and Gynecology, the safest time to travel during pregnancy is during weeks 18 to 24. Travel no more than 300 miles from home during the third trimester. Be sure that health insurance covers pregnancy-related health problems while traveling as well as delivery, complications, and newborn care. The CDC advises that the greatest risks for the pregnant traveler are motor vehicle accidents (be sure to wear seat belts), hepatitis E (follow food and water precautions), and scuba diving (risk of decompression). It is safe for pregnant women to travel up to 36 weeks of gestation. International travel may be allowed until week 32 of gestation, depending on each airline's individual policy. Those with placental abnormalities, severe anemia, sickle disease or trait, or a history of DVT probably should not fly. Getting up to walk frequently and wearing 20- to 30-mm compression stockings will help to prevent thrombosis.

Malaria is a more severe infection in pregnancy. Travel to a malarial zone should be deferred until after pregnancy if possible. If travel cannot be avoided, then the usual principles of mosquito avoidance and chemoprophylaxis should be followed. There is no evidence of any risk to the pregnant woman or developing fetus from recommended use of DEET or permethrin. Antimalarial chemoprevention with standard doses of chloroquine and mefloquine (Lariam) is not believed to be a significant risk to the mother or developing fetus or child. It is malaria that kills, not the preventive measures.

BREAST-FEEDING

Breast-feeding should be encouraged for infants who are traveling. Breast milk is a safe and convenient source of food. Women who are breast-feeding should obtain any necessary immunization, as there is no evidence of any risk from immunization in this setting. Although some immunity may be passed to the unimmunized infant, it cannot be relied upon for protection of the child. The infant should receive any necessary immunizations, but some (meningococcal, yellow fever, typhoid) cannot be administered; therefore, risk of infection in the young infant must be considered. Traveler's diarrhea can pose a particular risk if the mother becomes dehydrated. Breast-feeding should be continued, oral rehydration solution administered, and antibiotics considered for treatment. Bismuth must be avoided. The use of iodine for water treatment is acceptable but must be limited in time to avoid thyroid toxicity.

POST-TRAVEL

All who travel must be educated about which signs or symptoms following travel require evaluation. This is particularly important for those who have visited malarial zones. The majority of life-threatening malaria cases manifest themselves within 1 month of the traveler's return home, but some cases of *P. falciparum* malaria may take longer to develop.

Other parasitic diseases, including tapeworms and helminths, may not be apparent for months or years after the return home. Cutaneous leishmaniasis typically develops 2 to 6 months after the return home. Some infections, such as tuberculosis or strongyloidiasis, may only be apparent years later when the patient's immune system is impaired by malignancy, immunosuppressant drugs, or age. Symptoms of cough and fever, which would ordinarily be considered a routine respiratory infection, may take on new significance if the traveler has visited an area of the world experiencing an outbreak of a "new" infection such as severe acute respiratory syndrome (SARS). Physicians must always include a travel history in the evaluation of unusual symptoms.

There is no indication for routine laboratory testing for returned travelers. Those who have lived abroad for an extended period of time (missionaries, Peace Corps and other humanitarian volunteers, expatriates) may benefit from tuberculin testing, a complete blood count (CBC) (to check for eosinophilia, a sign of intestinal helminth infection), and stool testing for parasites (three samples taken during a few days). Those who have lived in areas endemic for relapsing (vivax or ovale) malaria should be considered for terminal prophylaxis with primaquine.

Toxoplasmosis

Method of
Thomas T. Ward, MD

Toxoplasmosis is the disease caused by infection with the obligate intracellular protozoan *Toxoplasma gondii*. Toxoplasmosis is a worldwide zoonosis and causes infection in both birds and mammals. Cats, the definitive hosts for *T. gondii*, are the animals in which the parasite maintains an enteroepithelial sexual cycle. Human beings and domestic animals are secondary hosts and are important in maintaining an extraintestinal asexual cycle of transmission. Although most human infection is asymptomatic, self-limited clinical disease can infrequently occur after primary infection in immunocompetent persons. Because of the persistence of dormant cyst forms, all infection becomes chronic and latent. Primary infection during pregnancy can result in transplacental transmission of infection to the fetus; resultant congenital toxoplasmosis has varied clinical manifestations. Reactivation of dormant cysts is an important cause of infection in immunocompromised patients with defective T-cell–mediated immunity, including those patients with advanced HIV infection, hematologic malignancies, and bone marrow and solid-organ transplants.

T. gondii exists in three forms: the oocyst, the tissue cyst, and the tachyzoite. Oocysts are formed only in infected felines; these cats excrete large numbers of cysts for approximately 2 weeks after infection. Oocysts may remain viable in the soil for months and are an important environmental reservoir for infection of incidental hosts. Tachyzoites occur with acute infection in incidental hosts; their presence is required for the histologic confirmation of active disease. Tissue cysts occur after replication of tachyzoites and likely persist for the life of the incidental host. Dormant cysts are most commonly located in skeletal and smooth muscle, heart, brain, and eye. The presence of tissue cysts in histologic sections is indicative of past infection, but by itself it does not signify active infection.

The human incidence of seropositivity for *T. gondii* antibody varies greatly throughout the world. Within the United States, seropositivity increases with age, and the overall seroprevalence is approximately 15%. Within Western Europe, seroprevalence ranges between 50% and 70%. Human transmission occurs by oral exposure to oocysts that have contaminated water sources, vegetables, or other food products or, even more commonly, by ingesting poorly cooked or raw meat that contains tissue cysts. As many as 25% of lamb or pork samples contain tissue cysts.

After human ingestion of either oocysts or tissue cysts, specialized forms of *T. gondii* emerge that penetrate the intestinal mucosa, establish intracellular infection within white blood cells, and enter the blood and lymphatic circulations to result in widespread dissemination throughout the body. Intact cell-mediated immunity leads to clearance of intracellular tachyzoites and the formation of dormant tissue cysts. Impaired cell-mediated immunity leads to either uncontrolled, primary infection (as in the fetus) or reactivation of infection later in life (as in AIDS and other immunosuppressed conditions).

Diagnosis

The diagnosis of *T. gondii* infection can be established by serologic tests, amplification of specific nucleic acid sequences, or histologic demonstration of the parasite or its antigens. Rarely employed reference or research methods for diagnosis include isolation of the organism, specific IgG avidity tests, various antigen detection tests, and lymphocyte transformation tests.

IgG antibodies appear in immunocompetent individuals within 2 to 3 weeks after infection. A negative IgG test essentially excludes previous or past infection with *T. gondii*. IgG antibody may persist in high titers for years after infection; therefore, a single positive IgG titer does not differentiate whether infection is recently acquired, chronic and latent, or chronic and reactivated. Sequential IgG antibody tests that increase by more than two tube dilutions are consistent with recent infection. Specific IgM and IgA antibody tests are usually positive during the first 6 months after acquisition of infection, and negative tests have a high predictive value for excluding recent infection. A positive IgM test

can indicate recent onset of infection; however, both false-positive results and persistently positive IgM antibody test results in chronically infected individuals can occur. When therapeutic decisions will be based on the interpretation of a positive IgM antibody test, confirmatory testing by a reference laboratory should be performed if feasible. Serologic tests can be more difficult to interpret in immunocompromised patients.

Polymerase chain reaction (PCR) for detection of specific *T. gondii* nucleic acid sequences has been successfully employed using vitreous and aqueous humor, bronchoalveolar lavage fluid, peripheral blood buffy coat preparations, cerebrospinal fluid, and amniotic fluid after 18 weeks of gestation. False-positive results on brain tissue PCR tests may occur in patients with HIV infection and suspected toxoplasmic encephalitis.

Specific histopathologic findings on resected lymph nodes can be strongly suggestive of the diagnosis of toxoplasmosis in immunocompetent patients. Demonstration of tachyzoites in tissue is invariably diagnostic of active infection. Although the presence of a single cyst does not differentiate between active and chronic or latent infection, multiple cysts present on cytopathologic examination suggest the presence of active disease. Staining for specific antigens (e.g., immunoperoxidase techniques) is highly specific for active infection when positive, and it is much more sensitive than hematoxylin and eosin or Wright-Giemsa staining alone. Tests employing direct fluorescent antibody tests can be nonspecific and are best avoided.

Clinical Manifestations

Most patients with acute *T. gondii* infection do not have symptomatic disease. Clinical manifestations of acute infection occasionally occur in immunocompetent adults, as does reactivation of infection within the retina of the eye. Infection during pregnancy results in congenital toxoplasmosis at an incidence of approximately 1 in 8000 live births in the United States; the frequency in which *T. gondii* causes spontaneous abortion is unknown. Reactivation infection from dormant cysts is the cause of toxoplasmic infections in patients with AIDS, patients with bone marrow or solid-organ transplants, and other immunosuppressed hosts. The clinical syndromes in each of the foregoing settings are sufficiently distinct to warrant separate comment.

ACUTE INFECTION IN IMMUNOCOMPETENT PATIENTS

Approximately 15% of immunocompetent patients who become infected have either regional lymphadenopathy or a mononucleosis-like syndrome characterized by generalized adenopathy and constitutional symptoms. Toxoplasmic lymphadenopathy is largely a self-limited disease in immunocompetent patients, and it rarely requires therapy. Epstein-Barr virus and cytomegalovirus infections are much more common causes of the mononucleosis syndrome. Other causes of lymphadenopathy that need to be considered include cat-scratch disease, lymphoma or metastatic malignancy, sarcoidosis, tuberculosis, and the deep mycoses. Serologic testing and lymph node biopsy are most beneficial in establishing a diagnosis. Infections acquired by blood transfusion or through a laboratory accident may be severe and should be treated.

OCULAR TOXOPLASMOSIS IN IMMUNOCOMPETENT PATIENTS

Approximately 33% of all cases of chorioretinitis within the Unites States are caused by *T. gondii*. Most cases are believed to result from unrecognized congenital infection that reactivates, most commonly during the second and third decades of life. Retinal clinical findings are highly suggestive of *T. gondii* infection when evaluated by ophthalmologists experienced in managing this infection. Serologic testing is usually positive for prior exposure to toxoplasmosis, but in difficult cases, PCR testing may be performed on samples of aqueous or vitreous humor to confirm the diagnosis. Control of the host inflammatory response by the concomitant use of corticosteroids may be required in some patients receiving therapy for toxoplasmosis. Relapse of infection requiring repeated treatment is not uncommon.

CONGENITAL TOXOPLASMOSIS

Congenital toxoplasmosis results from transplacental spread of *T. gondii* infection that is asymptomatically acquired either during pregnancy or shortly before the onset of gestation. The risk of fetal infection varies with the stage of trimester; it is highest during the second and third trimesters. Approximately 60% of maternal infections acquired during the third trimester will result in fetal infection. Fetal infection occurring during the first trimester is believed to result frequently in spontaneous abortion. Clinical manifestations of congenital toxoplasmosis are varied. There may be no sequelae, or clinical disease may become manifest at birth or at various times after birth. Children may be born with the nonspecific manifestations of the TORCH (toxoplasmosis, other infections, rubella, cytomegalovirus, and herpes simplex) syndrome, including chorioretinitis, hydrocephalus, intracranial calcifications, hepatosplenomegaly, rash, anemia, and/or jaundice. Other infectious causes such as herpes simplex, cytomegalovirus infection, rubella, and syphilis should be considered and excluded. In those infants born with subclinical congenital infection, studies suggest that most will eventually demonstrate evidence of clinical disease even though they appear normal at birth. Years or decades later, previously subclinically infected children may develop chorioretinitis, seizure disorders, or psychomotor and mental retardation. Early recognition and treatment of congenital infection reduce the likelihood of subsequent sequelae; therefore, congenital *T. gondii* infection should always be treated regardless of whether there are symptoms at birth. Treatment of acute maternal infection diagnosed during pregnancy reduces the risk of fetal infection by approximately 60%.

Because congenital toxoplasmosis occurs almost exclusively in women infected during pregnancy, it is important that such infection be recognized and treated aggressively. In some countries where there is a higher seroprevalence of *T. gondii* infection (e.g., France), routine screening for acquisition of infection during pregnancy is performed. Routine pregnancy screening is not currently advocated in the United States. Women who have IgG antibody but who lack specific IgM antibody are believed to have evidence of past, chronic infection and are not at risk of transmitting congenital infection. A positive IgM test requires further confirmatory testing through a reference laboratory to determine whether infection has been recently acquired. Confirmation of acutely acquired maternal infection during pregnancy mandates testing during and after pregnancy to determine whether fetal or congenital infection has occurred. PCR testing of amniotic fluid at 18 weeks of gestation and beyond is approximately 60% sensitive and 100% specific in diagnosing fetal infection. Diagnosis of congenital toxoplasmosis at birth is usually confirmed by the presence of specific IgA (or IgM) in fetal serum, with careful attention to exclusion of maternal contamination of fetal blood. In children with suspected congenital toxoplasmosis, it is important to perform ophthalmologic evaluation and neuroimaging studies and to examine the cerebrospinal fluid for pleocytosis or elevated protein concentrations.

TOXOPLASMOSIS IN AIDS AND IMMUNOCOMPROMISED PATIENTS

In immunocompromised patients, toxoplasmosis almost always occurs as reactivation infection. One exception is infection after heart transplantation, in which primary infection can occur when a seronegative host receives a donor heart from a seropositive donor. The central nervous system is the most commonly affected site, resulting in necrotizing focal or multifocal encephalitis and, less frequently, focal spinal cord involvement. Other forms of infection include chorioretinitis, myocarditis, and pneumonia. Active toxoplasmosis in immunodeficient patients can cause significant morbidity and mortality and always requires therapy. The duration of therapy is largely dependent on the degree of chronic immunosuppression, and, on occasion, lifelong maintenance therapy is indicated.

In natural history studies of HIV infection performed before effective antiretroviral therapy, it was observed that approximately one third of toxoplasmosis-seropositive patients with AIDS developed toxoplasmic encephalitis before death. Daily receipt of one tablet of double-strength trimethoprim (160 mg)-sulfamethoxazole (800 mg) (Bactrim DS) largely eliminates the risk of disease. Most episodes of toxoplasmic encephalitis complicating AIDS occur in patients with CD4$^+$ counts of less than 100 cells/mm^3, and infection is uncommon if the CD4$^+$ count exceeds 200 cells/mm^3. Patients with toxoplasmic encephalitis most commonly present with focal neurologic abnormalities of subacute (weeks) onset, often with fevers, headache, or subtle mental status or memory changes. Motor palsies are the most common focal abnormalities, although cranial nerve abnormalities, visual field defects, and seizure disorders can be the major presenting symptoms. Neuroradiologic imaging is best performed using magnetic resonance imaging, with the most common finding being multiple, ring-enhancing cerebral lesions. Involvement of the basal ganglion area is common. Computed tomography is, in general, less sensitive in defining disease and its extent. Single lesions on magnetic resonance imaging are unusual in toxoplasmic encephalitis and suggest possible central nervous system lymphoma. Multifocal leukoencephalopathy resulting from JC virus can also cause neuroradiologic findings that resemble toxoplasmosis. PCR can be performed on cerebrospinal fluid for Epstein-Barr virus, JC virus, and toxoplasmosis.

A definitive diagnosis of toxoplasmic encephalitis is made by brain biopsy and by the histologic demonstration of tachyzoites. However, to avoid the morbidity associated with brain biopsy, in patients with HIV infection who are toxoplasmosis seropositive and who have consistent neuroradiologic findings, it is now standard practice to treat these patients for toxoplasmosis empirically and to observe the clinical response. Although neuroradiologic resolution is delayed, most patients with toxoplasmic encephalitis demonstrate clinical improvement within 7 days of initiating therapy. Failure to respond clinically to empirical therapy, seronegativity to *T. gondii* antibody, and the presence of a single lesion on magnetic resonance imaging all are findings that suggest the possibility of an alternative diagnosis and warrant consideration of performing a brain biopsy.

Tissue biopsies with histologic examination are usually necessary for diagnosing toxoplasmosis at other sites in immunocompromised patients. PCR testing on bronchoalveolar lavage fluid can be positive in cases of pneumonitis. Endomyocardial biopsy should be performed if toxoplasmosis is a consideration in the seronegative heart recipient of a seropositive donor.

Therapy

Treatment of toxoplasmosis is summarized in Table 1. Most infections in immunologically normal adults are self-limited and do not require therapy. In ocular, central nervous system, and congenital toxoplasmosis, first-line therapy is the combination of pyrimethamine (Daraprim), and sulfadiazine, with folinic acid (leucovorin, not folic acid). Treatment duration is based on time of clinical resolution, but it is usually approximately 6 weeks in ocular and central nervous system infections and 12 months in congenital infection. In patients with AIDS who have persistently low CD4+ counts (less than 200 cells/mm³), and in other patients with continued profound immunosuppression, long-term maintenance therapy with pyrimethamine–sulfadiazine–folinic acid should be continued at the same doses used for primary therapy. Spiramycin[1],* (3 g per day) is the drug of choice for pregnant women with acquired primary *T. gondii* infection. Spiramycin should be continued until term if there is no evidence of fetal infection. Spiramycin does not cross the placenta and will not treat infection in the fetus. If fetal infection is demonstrated to be present by amniotic fluid PCR, pyrimethamine–sulfadiazine–folinic acid should be administered during the second and third trimesters. Pyrimethamine is potentially teratogenic and should not be administered during the first 16 weeks of pregnancy.

Allergic reactions to sulfonamides are common in patients with HIV infection. Alternative drugs to sulfadiazine that may be employed in combination therapy

---

[1]Not FDA approved for this indication.
*Not available in the United States except from the FDA (call 301-827-2335).

TABLE 1 Therapy of Toxoplasmic Infection

	Adult Doses	Pediatric Doses
Immunologically Normal		
Acute lymphadenopathy	No treatment	No treatment
Acute chorioretinitis	Pyrimethamine (Daraprim) 100 mg PO bid on day 1, then 25 mg PO qd + sulfadiazine 1 g PO qid + folinic acid (leucovorin) 5 mg PO qd	
Pregnancy	Spiramycin* 1.0 g PO q8h (see text)	
Congenital toxoplasmosis		Pyrimethamine 2 mg/kg for 2 d, then 1 mg/kg PO qd + sulfadiazine 50 mg/kg PO bid + folinic acid 10 mg 3 × wk PO
AIDS and Immunologically Impaired		
Encephalitis and other tissue sites of infection	Pyrimethamine 200 mg PO × one dose, then 75 mg PO qd + sulfadiazine 1 g PO qid ?+ folinic acid 5-10 mg PO qd	

*Not available in the United States except from the FDA (call 301-827-2335).
Abbreviations: bid = twice daily; PO = orally; q = every; qd = every day; qid = four times daily.

Rakel and Bope: *Conn's Current Therapy 2006*

include clindamycin (Cleocin),[1] 600 to 1200 mg every 6 hours intravenously or orally; clarithromycin (Biaxin),[1] 1 g every 12 hours orally; atovaquone (Mepron),[1] 750 mg every 6 hours orally; azithromycin (Zithromax),[1] 1200 to 1500 mg per day orally; and dapsone,[1] 100 mg per day orally. Alternatively, increasing experience suggests that trimethoprim-sulfamethoxazole (Bactrim, Septra),[1] 5 mg/kg trimethoprim component every 6 hours orally or intravenously (20 mg/kg per day total), is as effective as the pyrimethamine-containing combination regimens in patients who are not allergic to sulfa agents.

Corticosteroids can be administered to patients with ocular toxoplasmosis in whom a brisk inflammatory response is believed to be contributing to ocular pathology. Similarly, in toxoplasmic encephalitis with cerebral edema or significant mass effect, short-duration corticosteroids may be concomitantly employed with antitoxoplasmic antimicrobial therapy.

Prevention

Prevention of *T. gondii* infection is of major importance in pregnant women and immunodeficient patients who have not been previously exposed. Risk of primary infection can be reduced by not eating undercooked meat and by taking proper precautions when disposing of or cleaning cat litter material. Cysts in meat are killed at 60°C (140°F) or higher. Hands should be thoroughly washed after soil contamination, and all fruits and vegetables should be washed before they are eaten.

Primary prophylaxis should be administered in patients with AIDS who have CD4[+] counts of less than 100 cells/mm³ and who are seropositive for toxoplasmosis antibody. Trimethoprim (160 mg)-sulfamethoxazole (800 mg),[1] one double-strength tablet daily, is highly effective for prevention of toxoplasmosis infection. Alternative prophylactic regimens include either (a) pyrimethamine, 50 to 75 mg orally per week, plus dapsone,[1] 50 mg per day or 200 mg per week; or (b) pyrimethamine-sulfadoxine (Fansidar),[1] three tablets every 2 weeks. Dapsone alone is not effective at preventing toxoplasmosis.

---

[1]Not FDA approved for this indication.

Cat-Scratch Disease

Method of
*Andrew P. Steenhoff, MBBCh, and
Samir S. Shah, MD*

Bartonella henselae (formerly *Rochalimaea henselae*), a fastidious gram-negative bacterium, is the principal causative organism of cat-scratch disease (CSD). CSD is a common cause of chronic lymphadenopathy; atypical manifestations such as neuroretinitis, osteomyelitis, endocarditis, and fever of unknown origin occur in 5% to 10% of reported cases.

Epidemiology

There are an estimated 24,000 cases of CSD annually in the United States with a majority of patients being diagnosed in the fall and winter. CSD affects individuals of any age, although 80% of patients are 18 years of age or younger. Approximately 60% of cases occur in males. *B. henselae* is transmitted from cat to cat by the flea, *Ctenocephalides felis*. The bacterium is transmitted to humans via a cat scratch or, less commonly, a bite or lick. Contact with a domestic cat, or more typically a kitten, is seen in 90% of patients. Kittens scratch more frequently and are more likely to be bacteremic with *Bartonella* species than older cats. Cats that transmit CSD are not ill and have no distinctive features.

Clinical Manifestations

LYMPHADENITIS

CSD lymphadenitis starts with papules at the inoculation site 7 to 12 days after the scratch (Figure 1). The nontender, red-brown papules last 1 to 4 weeks and then spontaneously resolve. A papule identifies the site of inoculation in more than half of cases—often an overlooked feature. Lymphadenitis appears in the regional nodes as the papules begin to resolve. In as many as 20% of cases, additional lymph node groups are enlarged. The upper extremity (46%) is the site most commonly involved, followed by the neck and jaw (26%), groin (18%), and supraclavicular (2%) areas. More than half of the patients report mild constitutional symptoms including low-grade fever, malaise, anorexia, fatigue, and headache. In 90% of patients, CSD lymphadenitis is indolent and self-limiting with full resolution by 2 to 6 months. In approximately 10% of patients, however, the affected nodes develop overlying erythema and fluctuance requiring surgical drainage.

ATYPICAL MANIFESTATIONS

Atypical manifestations of cat-scratch disease occur in 5% to 10% of cases. Parinaud's oculoglandular syndrome,

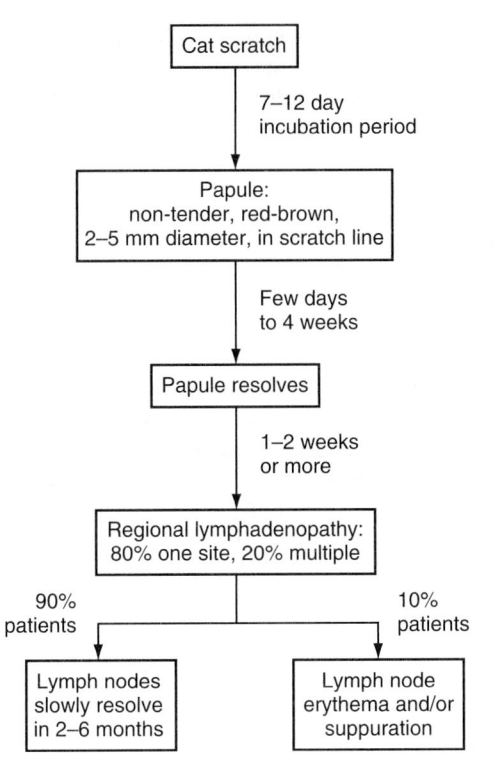

FIGURE 1. Typical clinical course of cat-scratch lymphadenitis.

reported in up to 6% of patients, occurs when the site of inoculation is the eyelid. It presents as a unilateral, nonexudative, granulomatous conjunctivitis with ipsilateral preauricular lymphadenopathy. Most patients recover spontaneously from Parinaud's syndrome in 2 to 4 months without residual damage.

Hepatosplenic CSD is an important cause of prolonged fever in children. CSD accounted for 5% of cases of fever of unknown origin in a series by Jacobs and colleagues. Prolonged or relapsing fever also occurs in immunocompromised patients. Weight loss and abdominal pain are common; and patients may also complain of joint pain and headache. Clinically, half of the patients have either hepatomegaly or splenomegaly. Ultrasound or computed tomography usually demonstrates multiple hepatic or splenic microabscesses.

Neurologic manifestations are reported in 1% to 7% of patients with CSD. In one series of 76 patients with neurologic symptoms, encephalopathy occurred 1 to 6 weeks after the onset of adenopathy and most commonly began with a headache that rapidly progressed to altered mentation and unresponsiveness. Seizures occurred in 46% of these patients and transient behavior change occurred in 39%; however, recovery is usually rapid without neurologic sequelae. Less common neurologic manifestations of CSD include aseptic meningitis, stellate macula retinitis, endophthalmitis, ataxia, transient hemiplegia, hearing loss, and bilateral sixth nerve palsy.

Skeletal involvement in CSD includes osteomyelitis of vertebrae, pelvic bones, skull, and long bones; osteolytic lesions; and paravertebral masses. Skin involvement is reported in 3% of patients with CSD; cutaneous

manifestations include erythema nodosum, maculopapular rash, and thrombocytopenic purpura. Other rare systemic manifestations of CSD include laryngitis, hemolytic anemia, atypical pneumonia, pulmonary nodules, endocarditis, mononucleosis syndrome, and disseminated bartonellosis.

BACILLARY ANGIOMATOSIS AND PELIOSIS

In the immunocompromised patient, *B. henselae* may cause bacillary angiomatosis or bacillary peliosis. Bacillary angiomatosis is a vasoproliferative disorder characterized by verrucous, papular, or pedunculated skin lesions on an erythematous base. The lesions may exist singly or cover the entire body and usually enlarge if untreated. Less commonly, bacillary angiomatosis presents as deep soft tissue masses or as tender and erythematous subcutaneous nodules. In AIDS patients, these lesions may be mistaken for Kaposi's sarcoma. Bacillary angiomatosis may also be caused by *Bartonella quintana*, the agent of trench fever.

Bacillary peliosis is an extracutaneous presentation of bacillary angiomatosis; the two may coexist. It affects organs of the reticuloendothelial system, particularly the liver (peliosis hepatis), but the spleen, bone marrow, and abdominal lymph nodes may also be involved. Findings include fever, nausea, vomiting, diarrhea, abdominal distention, and hepatosplenomegaly.

Diagnosis

In the past, the diagnosis of CSD required three of the following four classic criteria:

1. History of animal contact (usually a cat) and an abrasion, scratch, or ocular lesion
2. A positive CSD skin antigen test result
3. Regional lymphadenopathy for which other causes have been excluded
4. Characteristic histopathologic changes consistent with CSD in a lymph node biopsy

With the advent of newer diagnostic tools as well as safety and standardization concerns, however, the cat-scratch antigen test is no longer recommended.

LABORATORY DIAGNOSIS

Specific serologic diagnostic tests can support the diagnosis of CSD. One of these, the indirect fluorescent

 CURRENT DIAGNOSIS

- Antecedent cat exposure in most but not all cases
- Serologic testing for antibodies to *Bartonella henselae* to confirm diagnosis in most cases
- PCR detection of *B. henselae* in blood or involved tissue to confirm atypical manifestations of CSD

Abbreviations: CSD = cat-scratch disease; PCR = polymerase chain reaction.

antibody (IFA) test, was shown to be 98% sensitive and 98% specific in a population of patients who met the classic case definition of CSD. Enzyme immunoassay (EIA) testing for IgM and IgG antibodies to *B. henselae* is also commercially available. A high antibody titer (more than 1:64) suggests recent infection. An elevation in titer between acute and convalescent sera may be confirmatory. Paired sera are particularly useful in cat owners who may have a background rate of *Bartonella* antibody seropositivity greater than the general population (2% to 6%).

The most sensitive technique currently available to diagnose *B. henselae* infection is polymerase chain reaction (PCR) assay. This species-specific test detects *B. henselae* DNA in blood or tissue specimens (e.g. lymph nodes, bone). The Centers for Disease Control and Prevention (CDC) and some commercial laboratories perform *B. henselae* PCR testing. This test should be considered when an atypical manifestation is suspected. It is also useful to diagnose CSD in immunocompromised patients who may be unable to mount a significant antibody response.

MICROSCOPIC DIAGNOSIS

The Warthin-Starry silver stain occasionally detects bacilli in tissue specimens but is not specific for *B. henselae*. Histologic findings vary depending on the stage of the disease. Early histologic changes in lymph nodes consist of lymphocytic infiltration with epithelioid granuloma formation. Later changes consist of polymorphonuclear leukocyte infiltration with necrotic granulomas, followed by large, pus-filled sinuses that eventually rupture through the node capsule into surrounding tissue. Biopsy of bacillary angiomatosis lesions shows proliferating small vessels with prominent endothelial cells and varying numbers of neutrophils. Unlike their spindle-shaped counterparts in Kaposi's sarcoma, the epithelial cells of bacillary angiomatosis are protuberant without slit-like spaces. *B. henselae* can be isolated from bacillary angiomatosis lesions using a variety of techniques including Warthin-Starry staining and PCR.

RADIOLOGIC DIAGNOSIS

In hepatosplenic CSD, ultrasonography or computed tomography scan often reveals multiple round, oval, or irregular lesions of 3 to 30 mm in diameter. Although other diseases can cause similar lesions, the presence of these lesions in the appropriate context strongly suggest CSD.

Treatment

LYMPHADENITIS

Because CSD lymphadenitis is typically self-limited, no specific treatment is recommended for the majority of patients with mild or moderate disease. Only one randomized placebo-controlled trial has been performed. In this study by Bass and colleagues, patients received 5 days of azithromycin (Zithromax)[1] or placebo. At 1 month, the primary outcome measure (an 80% decrease in lymph node volume by ultrasound) was achieved in 7 of 15 patients in the azithromycin group and 1 in 14 patients in the placebo group. However, no difference was seen in the treated and untreated groups in the ultimate length of time to resolution. Affected lymph nodes infrequently require surgical drainage or fine-needle aspiration.

ATYPICAL MANIFESTATIONS

Treatment of atypical manifestations of CSD in immunocompetent persons has not been adequately evaluated. The benefit of therapy in these patients remains uncertain. Retrospective reviews describe treatment in some atypical presentations of CSD. Margileth retrospectively reviewed the therapeutic outcome in 268 patients diagnosed with CSD. Patients with typical and atypical manifestations were included. Improvements in fever, constitutional symptoms (malaise, anorexia), and erythrocyte sedimentation rate were noted with rifampin (Rifadin),[1] ciprofloxacin (Cipro),[1] trimethoprim-sulfamethoxazole (Bactrim),[1] and gentamicin (Garamycin).[1] Beta-lactam agents (e.g., ampicillin, cephalosporins), despite in vitro susceptibility of *B. henselae*, were not clinically effective. In other series treatment with doxycycline (Vibramycin, Doryx, or Monodox) reduced intraocular inflammation associated with CSD neuroretinitis, and treatment with rifampin (Rifadin)[1] relieved fever and constitutional symptoms in hepatosplenic CSD. With this limited evidence, the decision to commence antimicrobial therapy is made on a case-by-case basis. The long-term outcome for the immunocompetent host is usually favorable. Immunocompromised patients can experience severe and disseminated disease and, therefore, warrant treatment for either typical or atypical manifestations of CSD. Table 1 lists potential therapeutic agents and dosing information.

BACILLARY ANGIOMATOSIS AND PELIOSIS

Antibiotic therapy is recommended uniformly for immunocompromised patients (see Table 1). Erythromycin (E-Mycin) is the antibiotic of choice. Tetracycline,[1] minocycline (Minocin),[1] and azithromycin (Zithromax)[1] also appear to be effective. If a second drug is needed,

---

[1]Not FDA approved for this indication.

CURRENT THERAPY

- CSD lymphadenitis usually does not require treatment in the immunocompetent patient.
- Treat all immunocompromised patients with CSD.
- Consider therapy in atypical CSD.

Abbreviation: CSD = cat-scratch disease.

The Infectious Diseases

TABLE 1 Potential Antibiotic Therapy for *Bartonella henselae* Infection

Antibiotic	Dose/Route	Notes
Cat-Scratch Disease		
Azithromycin (Zithromax)[1]	Children (<45 kg): 10 mg/kg PO on day 1 and 5 mg/kg on days 2-5 Adults: 500 mg PO on day 1 and 250 mg PO on days 2-5	-
Ciprofloxacin (Cipro)[1]	20-30 mg/kg/d PO divided into 2 doses 7-14 d Adults: 500-750 mg PO bid 7-14 d	For children ≥12 y
Rifampin (Rifandin,[1] Rimactane, Rifocin)	10-20 mg/kg/d PO divided into 2 or 3 doses 7-14 d	Maximum dose, 600 mg
Trimethoprim-sulfamethoxazole (Bactrim)[1]	10 mg/kg of the trimethoprim dose PO bid for 7 d	-
Gentamicin (Garamycin)[1]	5 mg/kg/d IV or IM in divided doses q8h	For severely ill patients Monitor serum gentamicin levels
Bacillary Angiomatosis and Peliosis[2]		
Erythromycin (E-Mycin)	500 mg PO qid 6-8 wk	Duration of therapy depends on clinical response; some immunocompromised patients require long-term therapy
Doxycycline (Vibramycin, Doryx, Monodox)	100 mg PO bid 6-8 wk	
Clarithromycin (Biaxin)	500 mg PO bid 6-8 wk	
Azithromycin (Zithromax)[1]	250 mg PO qd 6-8 wk	
Ciprofloxacin (Cipro)[1]	500-750 mg PO bid 6-8 wk	

[1]Not FDA approved for this indication.
[2]Adult dosages.
Abbreviations: bid = twice a day; d = day; IV = intravenous; PO = by mouth; q = every; qd = every day; wk = week; y = year.

rifampin (Rifadin)[1] or intravenous gentamicin (Garamycin)[1] is used in combination with either erythromycin (E-Mycin) or doxycycline (Vibramycin). Patients with only cutaneous lesions should be treated for at least 2 months, and those with visceral lesions should receive at least 4 months of treatment. However, with suboptimal clinical response in an immunocompromised person, longer therapy may be required.

REFERENCES

Arisoy ES, Correa AG, Wagner ML, Kaplan SL: Hepatosplenic cat-scratch disease in children: Selected clinical features and treatment. Clin Infect Dis 1999;28:778-784.
Bass JW, Freitas BC, Freitas A, et al: Prospective randomized double blind placebo-controlled evaluation of azithromycin for treatment of cat-scratch disease. Pediatr Infect Dis J 1998;17:447-52.
Bass JW, Vincent JM, Person DA: The expanding spectrum of *Bartonella* infections: II. Cat-scratch disease. Pediatr Infect Dis J 1997;16:163-179.
Carithers HA: Cat-scratch disease: An overview based on 1200 patients. Am J Dis Child 1985;139:1124-1133.
Goldstein DA, Mouritsen L, Friedlander S, et al: Acute endogenous endophthalmitis caused by *Bartonella henselae*. Clin Infect Dis 2001;33:718-721.
Jacobs RF, Schutze GE: *Bartonella henselae* as a cause of prolonged fever of unknown origin in children. Clin Infect Dis 1998;26:80-84.
Koehler JE: *Bartonella*-associated infections in HIV-infected patients. AIDS Clin Care 1995;7:97-102.
Margileth AM: Antibiotic therapy for cat-scratch disease: Clinical study of therapeutic outcome in 268 patients and a review of the literature. Pediatr Infect Dis J 1992;11:474-478.
Mirakhur B, Shah SS, Ratner AJ, et al: Cat-scratch disease presenting as orbital abscess and osteomyelitis. J Clin Microbiol 2003;41:3991-3993.
Ridder GJ, Boedeker CC, Technau-Ihling K, et al: Role of cat-scratch disease in lymphadenopathy in the head and neck. Clin Infect Dis 2002;35:643-649.
Robson JMB, Harte GJ, Osborne DRS, McCormack JG: Cat-scratch disease with paravertebral mass and osteomyelitis. Clin Infect Dis 1999;28:274-8.

Salmonellosis

Method of
Clifford L. S. Leen, MBChB, MD

Until recently all *Salmonella* species were given names based on the Kaufmann-White typing system, with the species defined by the O antigens (the polysaccharide component of their lipopolysaccharide [LPS]) and the H antigens (flagella). The genus has now been reorganized into two species, *Salmonella bongori* and *Salmonella enterica*. *S. enterica* is divided into additional subgroups. All salmonellae that are isolated from humans and other warm-blooded animals, including *Salmonella typhi*, are included in the *S. enterica* subgroup 1. The other subgroups are made up of *Salmonella* serotypes that are usually isolated from cold-blooded hosts or the environment. However, because no general agreement has been reached on a new naming convention, and because most clinicians are familiar with the old serologically defined names,

[1]Not FDA approved for this indication.

the old nomenclature will be used in this article. *Salmonella typhimurium* and *Salmonella enteritidis* are the most common species causing human disease.

Epidemiology

The number of cases of nontyphoid *Salmonella* infections has increased during the past few years, with a threefold increase in the United States. This may be an underestimate because most cases of gastroenteritis are managed without diagnostic stool cultures, and there is under-reporting of diagnosed cases.

Almost all *Salmonella* infections are acquired orally, although infection transmitted via contaminated blood products has been reported.

Host Factors

The infective dose of nontyphi salmonellae is very low, approximately 10^5 organisms. Conditions that lead to low gastric acid, such as pernicious anemia, or the use of antacids, H_2 blockers, or proton pump inhibitors predispose individuals to salmonellosis. Other risk factors include extremes of age, recent use of antibiotics, increased gastric transit (as in gastroenterostomy), diabetes, malignancy, rheumatologic disorders, sickle cell disease, HIV, and iatrogenic immunodeficiency.

Clinical Features

The four clinical syndromes arising from infection with nontyphoid salmonellae are gastroenteritis, bacteremia, enteric fever, and asymptomatic fecal excretion. Enteric fever is not discussed in this chapter.

Gastroenteritis

This is the most common manifestation of *Salmonella* infection and occurs after an incubation period of 12 to 96 hours. Gastroenteritis caused by *Salmonella*

BOX 1 Risk Factors for Salmonellosis
• Low gastric acid, for example, pernicious anemia, use of antacids, H_2 blockers, or proton pump inhibitors • Extreme age • Recent use of antibiotics • Increased gastric transit as in gastroenterostomy • Diabetes • Malignancy • Rheumatologic disorders • Sickle cell disease • HIV • Iatrogenic immunosuppression

---

cannot be reliably distinguished from that caused by other pathogens. The illness is usually self-limiting and consists of nausea, vomiting, crampy abdominal pain, and watery diarrhea.

Other symptoms include fever, urgency of defecation, and tenesmus. The stools may be frankly bloody, reflecting significant mucosal inflammation. The illness usually resolves within 4 to 6 days but may last up to 14 days. Fever may be present in 50% of patients and persist for 1 to 2 days. Approximately 5% of patients with gastroenteritis have positive blood cultures.

TREATMENT OF ACUTE NONTYPHOID SALMONELLA GASTROENTERITIS

Salmonellae are facultative, intracellular pathogens, and although they are susceptible to most antibiotics that are active against gram-negative organisms, only the antibiotics that are highly active intracellularly, such as the quinolones, tend to be useful in the treatment of salmonellosis. There is an increasing prevalence of antibiotic-resistant *Salmonella* strains throughout the world; these include resistance to ampicillin and trimethoprim-sulfamethoxazole. Furthermore, 6% of all *Salmonella* cases in England proved to be quinolone resistant in 1995. A study of stored *Salmonella* isolates shows that resistance to nalidixic acid is a predictor for poor clinical response to other quinolones. An outbreak of salmonellosis caused by multidrug- and quinolone-resistant *Salmonella* linked to a swine herd lends supporting evidence of a link between antimicrobial resistance in human isolates with agricultural use of antibiotics. The emergence of *Salmonella* resistant to third-generation cephalosporins and other extended-spectrum beta-lactamases (ESBLs) is of major concern. In a case report, all but one of the resistances to 13 antibiotics were carried on a conjugative plasmid, and the clinical isolate from the child was indistinguishable from one that was isolated from the family's cattle. Resistance to third-generation cephalosporins is a growing concern for children, for whom the cephalosporin antibiotics are the current drugs of choice for the treatment of invasive salmonellosis.

The quinolone group of antimicrobial agents are active against salmonellae because they have the following:

- High bactericidal activity against *Salmonella*, including multiresistant strains.
- Rapid oral absorption resulting in wide tissue distribution with high concentrations in bile, the gallbladder wall, and feces.
- Excellent intracellular penetration and concentration in neutrophils and macrophages.

Cephalosporins have high serum levels and long serum half-lives but have poor intracellular penetration. However, they are particularly helpful for treating systemic infections in children, in whom the therapeutic choices are very limited.

Because the illness is self-limiting, treatment is generally based on symptom relief and replacement of fluid and electrolyte losses. Antipyretics and antiemetics are usually effective, but antimotility agents are usually contraindicated, particularly when dysenteric symptoms are present. Antisecretory agents are not helpful because they have insignificant effects on stool water losses.

Studies indicate that oral treatment with ciprofloxacin (Cipro)[1] (500 mg twice daily for 5 days) or norfloxacin (Noroxin) (400 mg twice daily for 5 days) can shorten both the duration of fever and diarrhea and lessen the severity of the diarrhea; the benefit is greatest for those with severe illness. These studies were conducted within the first 3 days of onset of symptoms and may not be applicable if treatment with quinolone is started late, particularly when microbiological isolation is delayed. The effect of quinolones on fecal clearance of salmonellae is unclear, but they do not appear to prolong carriage. As a result, antibiotic therapy is not routinely recommended for the empirical treatment of mild-to-moderate, presumed or proven *Salmonella* gastroenteritis in healthy persons.

Empirical antibiotics are indicated for those who are severely ill and for high-risk patients who are prone to systemic invasive disease or severe local disease. However, management is complicated, as those with bloody diarrhea may have infection with other pathogens including shigellae or enterohemorrhagic *Escherichia coli* (EHEC), and antibiotic treatment of EHEC may increase the risk of hemolytic uremic syndrome. An algorithm for the possible use of empirical antibiotics is shown in Figure 1. Additional patients who could be considered at risk of severe complications include patients with underlying atherosclerotic lesions and infants younger than 3 months of age.

---

[1]Not FDA approved for this indication.

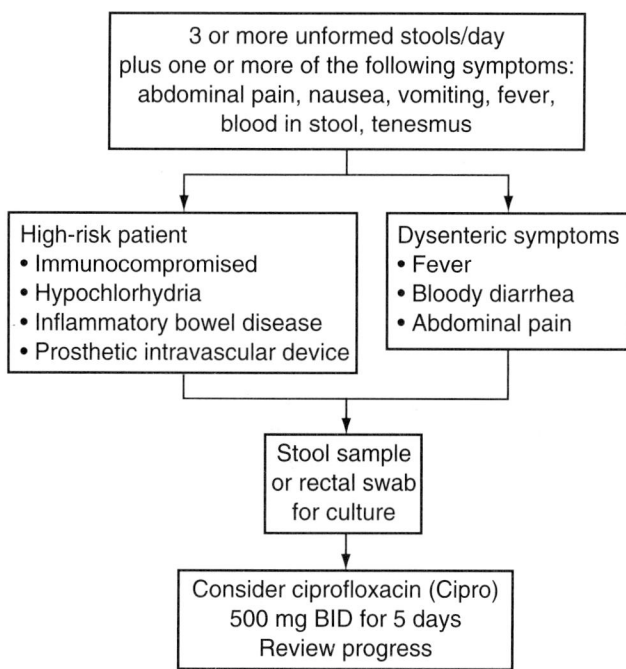

FIGURE 1. Algorithm for empirical therapy of gastroenteritis.

Rakel and Bope: *Conn's Current Therapy 2006*

Antibiotics are also useful when rapid interruption of fecal shedding is required to reduce transmission of *Salmonella* infection in institutions.

Follow-up fecal cultures are not routinely indicated, but meticulous personal hygiene is important to prevent spread of infection. Good hand hygiene and the firming up of stools are important criteria for return to work. Local health departments should be consulted about food handlers and health care workers with *Salmonella* as each department may have different criteria for return to work.

Bacteremia

Most nontyphoid *Salmonella* serotypes can cause a primary bacteremia and extraintestinal infections in the absence of diarrhea. Most invasive serotypes carry virulence plasmids. Extraintestinal infections are found in 10% to 20% of bacteremia cases. Although *Salmonella choleraesuis* can cause invasive infection in previously healthy persons, bacteremia can occur in persons with underlying immune defects. Host factors that are associated with invasive infections include defects in T-cell immunity. These include HIV infection, systemic lupus erythematosus (SLE), lymphomas, immunosuppression with steroids or for transplantation, conditions associated with iron overload, and congenital defects in interferon (IFN)-γ and interleukin (IL)-12 signaling. Metastatic infections include meningitis, osteomyelitis, septic arthritis, and, less frequently, aortitis, endocarditis, pyelonephritis, and pneumonia. Infection in other rare sites like the prostate and thyroid have also been reported.

A mycotic aneurysm results from *Salmonella* infection of an artery previously affected by arteriosclerosis. Diagnosis of endovascular infection is very difficult, but this disorder must be suspected in any person with bacteremia without an obvious source. Classic features such as fever, pain, and tender palpable mass are uncommon. If suspected, the diagnosis should be further explored using computed tomography (CT), magnetic resonance imaging (MRI), or white cell or gallium scanning.

Salmonella meningitis is a rare cause of bacterial meningitis, and usually occurs in children younger than 1 year of age. It carries a high mortality rate and high rates of complications including seizures and hydrocephalus. In young children with sickle cell disease, *Salmonella* osteomyelitis affects the long bones; but in

---

CURRENT DIAGNOSIS

- Nausea, vomiting.
- Crampy abdominal pain.
- Diarrhea, watery or bloody.
- Tenesmus.
- Endovascular infection must be suspected in patients with bacteremia without an obvious source.

adults with this condition, it tends to involve the vertebrae. Monoarticular infection caused by *Salmonella* tends to involve the knee or hip joints, which is usually a result of adjoining osteomyelitis. Approximately 5% of nontyphoid *Salmonella* cases involves the urinary tract, and this is more common in patients who have abnormal renal tracts, particularly those with obstructive uropathy.

Salmonellosis in AIDS can be an invasive disease presenting as bacteremia. The risk of nontyphoid bacteriemia increases as the $CD4^+$ cell count decreases, and AIDS patients have a 100-fold increased risk compared with HIV patients without AIDS. Metastatic complications occur at the same frequency as in other immunocompromised patients but may also involve very unusual sites such as muscles. Recurrent bacteremia is described, and before highly active antiretroviral therapy (HAART) it often required lifelong antibiotic therapy.

TREATMENT OF INVASIVE SALMONELLOSIS

Treatment of *Salmonella* bacteremia is usually with a single antibacterial agent, either a third-generation cephalosporin or a quinolone. In view of the changing resistance pattern in human *Salmonella* isolates, life-threatening infections should probably be treated with a combination of a quinolone and a third-generation cephalosporin until the susceptibility to antimicrobial agents is confirmed. If there is no suspicion of endovascular focus, *Salmonella* bacteremia can usually be successfully treated with a 14-day course of antibiotics.

Any suspicion of an endovascular infection warrants further investigation. If endocarditis or infectious arteritis is confirmed, surgery should be considered. However, for the hemodynamically stable patient, medical treatment alone may be considered for both native and prosthetic endocarditis in view of some case reports of successful prolonged medical treatment without surgery.

For endovascular infection, surgical intervention is recommended for patients who are able to have surgery. Antibiotic therapy should be continued for a minimum of 6 weeks after surgery, although many clinicians may elect to continue the antibiotics for a few months. In cases where the focus of infection cannot be removed surgically, lifelong suppressive treatment is recommended,

as there is a high risk of recurrence once the antibiotic is stopped. There is no consensus on whether the choice of antibiotics should be a third-generation cephalosporin or a quinolone. Some clinicians favor cephalosporins because high serum levels of cephalosporins relative to minimum bactericidal concentrations may lead to adequate antibiotic penetration and, therefore, kill the salmonellae in the vegetation or devitalized tissue. Other clinicians favor quinolones because of their intracellular activity against *Salmonella*. Unfortunately, it is unlikely that any clinical trial will be undertaken to resolve this issue. Certainly the long-term use of an oral quinolone after an initial period of treatment with an intravenous cephalosporin (ceftriaxone [Rocephin] 2 to 3 g twice daily) would be a good compromise.

Focal infections such as arthritis and abscesses should be drained or surgically treated whenever possible. Antibiotic treatment should be carried out for a minimum of 4 to 6 weeks.

The use of ceftriaxone or ciprofloxacin leads to adequate therapeutic concentration in the cerebrospinal fluid (CSF) even when the blood-brain barrier is intact. A minimum of 4 to 6 weeks of therapy with either agent is recommended for the treatment of *Salmonella* meningitis, brain abscess, or subdural empyema.

AIDS patients with invasive disease will benefit from long-term quinolone treatment until their immune systems can be reconstituted with the use of HAART. Because zidovudine (Retrovir) has been shown to have in vitro activity against gram-negative organisms, including *Salmonella*, it is possible that its inclusion in the HAART regimen may have additional benefits to its anti-HIV activity.

Asymptomatic Fecal Excretion

Following acute gastroenteritis, most patients will excrete salmonellae in their stools for a mean duration of 4 weeks for adults and 7 weeks for young children. However, up to 1% of patients may continue to excrete nontyphoid salmonellae for 1 year after acute infection. Patients older than 50 years of age with biliary tract disease are predisposed to long-term carriage. Management of chronic carriage of greater than a 1-year duration is extrapolated from experience with *S. typhi*. Quinolones are useful in eradicating chronic carriage, but the optimal duration and dose have not been established. Regimens that have been tried include ciprofloxacin (Cipro)[1] (500 mg twice a day for up to 28 days) and ofloxacin (Floxin)[1] (400 mg once daily for 7 days). Failure and relapse following treatment are not uncommon. Cholecystectomy may be considered, particularly when antibiotics have failed to eradicate carriage, and when gallbladder pathology is present.

During an outbreak of infection in an institution, antibiotics may be used to reduce fecal shedding to limit transmission and the need for prolonged isolation.

CURRENT THERAPY

- A single antibacterial agent, either a third-generation cephalosporin or a quinolone within 3 days of onset of diarrhea.
- Suspicion of an endovascular infection merits further investigation. If endocarditis or infectious arteritis is confirmed, then surgery should be considered.
- For endovascular infection, surgical intervention is recommended for patients who are able to have surgery.
- Focal infections such as arthritis and abscesses should be drained or surgically treated.

---

[1]Not FDA approved for this indication.

Special Consideration for Children and Pregnant Women

The finding of cartilage dysplasia in animal studies of quinolones has given rise to concerns regarding their use in children and pregnant women. However, there is now increasing evidence that they may be safely administered to children with severe, pathogen-resistant infections. For example, quinolones are now routinely given to children in areas of the world where multidrug-resistant *S. typhi* is common. Alternative agents include azithromycin (Zithromax)[1] and aztreonam (Azactam),[1] although experience with their use is limited. Where resistance is limited, third-generation cephalosporins are used rather than quinolone.

Antibiotic treatment is not usually indicated in young, healthy individuals with mild to moderate gastroenteritis caused by *Salmonella*. In the immunocompromised individual, *Salmonella* can cause severe, invasive disease in the form of bacteremia and focal disease. This needs careful clinical evaluation to identify the focus of infection. Management includes prolonged antibiotic use and surgical intervention for endovascular infections if possible. Resistance to current antimicrobial agents is increasing worldwide, and knowledge of antimicrobial susceptibility is essential for optimal management of invasive salmonellosis.

REFERENCES

Chui C, Ou JT: Risk factors for endovascular infection due to nontyphoidal salmonellae. Clin Infect Dis 2003;36:835-836.
Dunne E, Fey P, Kludt P, et al: Emergence of domestically acquired ceftriaxone-resistant *Salmonella* infections associated with AmpC[beta]-lactamase. JAMA 2000;284:3151-3156.
Fierer J, Swancutt M: Nontyphoid *Salmonella*: A review. Curr Clin Top Infect Dis 2000;20:134-157.
Hohmann EL: Nontyphoidal salmonellosis. Clin Infect Dis 2001; 32(2):263-269.
Parry CM: Antimicrobial drug resistance in *Salmonella enterica*. Curr Opin Infect Dis 2003;16(5):467-472.
Sirinavin S, Garner P: Antibiotics for treating salmonella gut infections. Cochrane Database Syst Rev 2000;(2):CD001167.
Trevejo RT, Courtney JG, Starr M, Vugia DJ: Epidemiology of salmonellosis in California, 1990-1999: Morbidity, mortality and hospitalization costs. Am J Epidemiol 2003;157:48-57.

[1]Not FDA approved for this indication.

Typhoid Fever

Method of
Zulfiqar A. Bhutta, MB, BS, PhD

Despite vast advances in public health and hygiene in much of the developed world, typhoid fever remains endemic in many developing countries. Probably because of the ease of modern travel, cases are also reported in most developed countries.

Etiology

Typhoid fever is caused by *Salmonella typhi*, a gram-negative bacterium. A very similar but often less severe disease is caused by *Salmonella* serotype *paratyphi* A. The ratio of disease caused by *S. typhi* to that caused by *S. paratyphi* is approximately 10:1, although the proportion of *S. paratyphi* infections is increasing in some parts of the world. Although *S. typhi* shares many genes with *Escherichia coli* and at least 90% with *Salmonella typhimurium,* several unique gene clusters known as pathogenicity islands and others were acquired during evolution. One of the specific genes is for the polysaccharide capsule Vi. This is present in approximately 90% of all freshly isolated *S. typhi* organisms and has a protective effect against the bactericidal action of the serum of infected patients.

Epidemiology

Although accurate community-based figures are unavailable, an estimated 16 million cases occur annually, with more than 0.6 million deaths. The vast majority of cases occur in Asia. Given the paucity of microbiologic facilities in developing countries, these figures may largely represent the clinical syndrome. Regional incidence rates vary from 100 to 1000 cases per 100,000 population, and there may be differences in the spectrum of the disorder. Recent population-based studies from south Asia also indicate that, contrary to previous views, the disease may largely affect children younger than 5 years of age. In contrast, data from sub-Saharan Africa and HIV-endemic areas indicate that nontyphoidal *Salmonella* bacteremia far outstrips typhoid fever as a cause of community-acquired bacteremia.

In recent years, typhoid fever is notable for the emergence of drug resistance. Following sporadic outbreaks of chloramphenicol-resistant typhoid, many strains of *S. typhi* developed plasmid-mediated multidrug-resistance to all of the three primary antimicrobials (ampicillin [Chloromycetin], chloramphenicol, and trimethoprim-sulfamethoxazole [Septra]). More troubling, chromosomally acquired quinolone resistance in *S. typhi* was recently described in various parts of Asia

2

and may be a consequence of widespread and indiscriminate use of these agents.

Pathogenesis

Typhoid fever occurs by the ingestion of the organism, and a variety of sources of fecal contamination are reported, including street vendor foods and contamination of water reservoirs. A larger infecting dose leads to a shorter incubation period and more severe infection. The organism crosses the intestinal mucosal barrier after attachment to the microvilli by an intricate mechanism involving membrane ruffling, actin rearrangement, and internalization in an intracellular vacuole. Once inside the intestinal cells, S. typhi find their way into the circulation and reside within the macrophages of the reticuloendothelial system. The clinical syndrome is produced by a release of proinflammatory cytokines (interleukin [IL]-6, IL-1β, and tumor necrosis factor [TNF]-α) from the infected cells. Some 1% to 5% of patients with acute typhoid infection may become chronic carriers of the infection in the gallbladder, depending on age, sex, and treatment regimen.

Clinical Features

Patients with typhoid fever usually present with high-grade fever and a wide variety of associated symptoms, such as abdominal pain, hepatosplenomegaly, diarrhea, and constipation. In the absence of localizing signs, the early stage of the disease may be difficult to differentiate from other endemic diseases including malaria and dengue fever. The classic stepladder rise of fever is relatively rare, but the presentation of typhoid fever may be tempered by coexisting morbidities and early administration of antibiotics. In malaria-endemic areas and in parts of the world where schistosomiasis is common, the presentation of typhoid may also be atypical.

Although data from South America and parts of Africa suggest typhoid may present as a mild illness in young children, this may vary in different parts of the world. Emerging evidence from south Asia indicates the presentation of typhoid may be more dramatic in children younger than 5 years of age, with comparatively higher rates of complications and hospitalization. Diarrhea, toxicity, and complications such as disseminated intravascular coagulopathy are also more common in infancy, with higher case fatality rates. Some of the other features of typhoid fever seen in adults, however, such as relative bradycardia, are rare, and rose spots may be visible only at an early stage of the illness in fair-skinned children.

It is also recognized that multidrug-resistant (MDR) typhoid is a more severe clinical illness with higher rates of toxicity, complications, and case fatality rates. This may be related to the increased virulence of MDR S. typhi as well as a higher number of circulating bacteria. These findings may have implications for treatment algorithms, especially in endemic areas with high rates of MDR typhoid.

CURRENT DIAGNOSIS

- In the absence of localizing signs, the early stage of the disease may be difficult to differentiate from other endemic diseases such as malaria or dengue fever.
- The presentation and diagnosis of typhoid fever may be tempered by coexisting morbidities and early administration of antibiotics.
- The presentation of typhoid may be more dramatic in children younger than 5 years of age, with comparatively higher rates of complications and hospitalization.
- The sensitivity of blood cultures in diagnosing typhoid fever may be limited in many developing countries because of antibiotic prescribing.
- Multidrug-resistant (MDR) typhoid is a more severe clinical illness with higher rates of toxicity and complications. In particular, recent cases of quinolone-resistant typhoid may be more severe.

Diagnosis

The mainstay of the diagnosis of typhoid fever is a positive culture from the blood or another anatomic site. But the sensitivity of blood cultures in diagnosing typhoid fever in many parts of the developing world is limited because widespread use of antibiotics may render bacteriologic confirmation difficult. Although bone marrow cultures may increase the likelihood of bacteriologic confirmation of typhoid, these are difficult to obtain and relatively invasive.

The serologic diagnosis of typhoid is also fraught with problems because results of a single Widal test may be positive in only 50% of cases in endemic areas, and serial tests may be required in cases presenting in the first week of illness. Newer serologic tests such as a dot enzyme-linked immunoabsorbent assay (ELISA) (TyphiDot) and the TUBEX tests are promising but require further evaluation in large-scale studies in community settings. In much of the developing world, the mainstay of diagnosis of typhoid remains clinical, and several diagnostic algorithms are being evaluated in endemic areas.

Therapy

An early diagnosis of typhoid fever and institution of appropriate treatment are essential. The vast majority of typhoid patients can be managed at home with oral antibiotics and close medical follow-up for complications or failure to respond to therapy. But patients with persistent vomiting, severe diarrhea, and abdominal distension may require hospitalization and parenteral antibiotic therapy. These are the general principles of typhoid management:

- Adequate rest, hydration, and attention to correction of fluid-electrolyte imbalance

CURRENT THERAPY

- The vast majority of typhoid patients can be managed at home with oral antibiotics and close medical follow-up for complications or failure to respond to therapy.
- Although newer quinolones are associated with better cure rates and clinical outcomes, there is insufficient evidence to recommend them as first-line agents in children.
- Recent emergence of quinolone resistance among *S. typhi* isolates requires treatment with alternatives such as third-generation cephalosporins and azithromycin.

- Antipyretic therapy (acetaminophen, 120 to 750 mg orally every 4 to 6 hours[3]) as required
- Soft, easily digestible diet unless the patient has abdominal distension or ileus
- Antibiotic therapy (the right choice, dosage, and duration)

[3]Exceeds dosage recommended by the manufacturer.

- Traditional therapy with either chloramphenicol (Chloromycetin) or amoxicillin,[1] associated with relapse rates of 5% to 15% and 4% to 8%, respectively; newer quinolones and third-generation cephalosporins associated with higher cure rates

Some authorities recommend treatment with second-line agents in all cases of typhoid. Others questioned this on the basis of adequate response to therapy among sensitive cases with first-line agents. Blanket administration of second-line agents such as fluoroquinolones and third-generation cephalosporins in all cases of suspected typhoid is expensive and may lead to the rapid development of further resistance. Table 1 gives the recommended therapy for typhoid fever based on a recent consensus document by the World Health Organization (2003).

Preventive Strategies for Typhoid

Of the major risk factors for outbreaks of typhoid, contamination of water supplies with sewage is the most important. During outbreaks, therefore, a combination

[1]Not FDA approved for this indication.

TABLE 1 Treatment of Typhoid Fever Based on Diagnosis, Treatment, and Prevention

	Optimal Therapy			Alternative Effective Drugs		
Susceptibility	Antibiotic	Daily Dose (mg/kg)	Days	Antibiotic	Daily Dose (mg/kg)	Days
Uncomplicated Typhoid Fever						
Fully sensitive	Fluoroquinolone (e.g., ofloxacin [Floxin][1] or ciprofloxacin [Cipro])	15	5-7*	Chloramphenicol (Chloromycetin) Amoxicillin[1] TMP-SMX (Bactrim)[1]	50-75[3] 75-100[1] 8/40	14-21 14 14
Multidrug resistance	Fluoroquinolone or Cefixime (Suprax)[1]	15 15-20[3]	5-7 7-14	Azithromycin (Zithromax)[1] Cefixime	8-10[3] 15-20[3]	7 7-14
Quinolone resistance[†]	Azithromycin (Rocephin)[1] or Ceftriaxone (Rocephin)[1]	8-10[3] 75[3]	7 10-14	Cefixime[1]	203	7-14
Severe Typhoid Fever						
Fully sensitive	Fluoroquinolone (e.g., ofloxacin)[1]	15	10-14	Chloramphenicol Ampicillin[1] TMP-SMX	100[3] 100[3] 8/40	14-21 14 14
Multidrug-resistant	Fluoroquinolone	15	10-14	Ceftriaxone[1] or Cefotaxime (Claforan)[1]	60[3] 80[3]	10-14
Quinolone-resistant	Ceftriaxone[1] or cefotaxime[1]	60[3] 80[3]	10-14	Fluoroquinolone	20[3]	14

[1]Not FDA approved for this indication.
[3]Exceeds dosage recommended by the manufacturer.
*Three-day courses are also effective and are particularly so in epidemic containment.
[†]The optimum treatment for quinolone-resistant typhoid fever is not determined. Azithromycin, the third-generation cephalosporins, or a 10- to 14-day course of high-dose fluoroquinolones is effective.
Abbreviation: TMX-SMZ = trimethoprim-sulfamethoxazole.
From World Health Organization (WHO)/Vaccines and Biologicals/03.07.

of central chlorination and domestic water purification is important. In endemic situations, consumption of street vendor foods, especially ice cream and cut-up fruit, is recognized as an important risk factor. The human-to-human spread by chronic carriers is also important, and attempts should be made to target food handlers and high-risk groups for *S. typhi* carriage screening.

The classic heat-inactivated whole cell vaccine is associated with an unacceptably high rate of side effects. Two newer vaccines that offer protection for school-age children and for adults are the Vi polysaccharide vaccine (Typhim Vi) and the orally administratable, attenuated Ty21a vaccine (Vivotif Berna). Both offer a protective efficacy of 70% to 80% for at least 3 to 5 years. In younger children, the experimental Vi-conjugate vaccine has a protective efficacy exceeding 90% and may offer protection in parts of the world where a large proportion of preschool children are at risk for the disease.

REFERENCES

Bhutta ZA: Impact of age and drug resistance on mortality in typhoid fever. Arch Dis Child 1996;75:214-217.
Chinh NT, Parry CM, Ly NT, et al: A randomized controlled comparison of azithromycin and ofloxacin for treatment of multidrug-resistant or nalidixic acid-resistant enteric fever. Antimicrob Agents Chemother 2000;44:1855-1859.
Communicable Disease Surveillance and Response Vaccines and Biologicals, World Health Organization: Treatment of Typhoid Fever. Background Document: The Diagnosis, Prevention and Treatment of Typhoid Fever, 2003, pp. 19-23. Available online at http://www.who.int/entity/vaccine_research/documents/en/typhoid_diagnosis.pdf)
Crump JA, Luby SP, Mintz ED: The global burden of typhoid fever. Bull World Health Organ 2004;82:346-353.
Gasem MH, Keuter M, Dolmans WM, et al: Persistence of salmonellae in blood and bone marrow: Randomized controlled trial comparing ciprofloxacin and chloramphenicol treatments against enteric fever. Antimicrob Agents Chemother 2003;47:1727-1731.
Luby SP, Faizan MK, Fisher-Hoch SP, et al: Risk factors for typhoid fever in an endemic setting, Karachi, Pakistan. Epidemiol Infect 1998;120:129-138.
Parry CM, Hien TT, Dougan G, et al: Typhoid fever. N Engl J Med 2002;347:1770-1782.
Sinha A, Sazawal S, Kumar R, et al: Typhoid fever in children aged less than 5 years. Lancet 1999;354:734-737.
Thaver D, Zaidi AK, Critchley J, et al: Fluoroquinolones for treating typhoid and paratyphoid fever (enteric fever) (CD004530.pub2). Cochrane Database Syst Rev 2005;2.

Rickettsial and Ehrlichial Infections

Method of
David H. Walker, MD

Vector-borne transmission of obligately intracellular bacteria occurs in persons exposed to infected ticks, mites, fleas, and lice in endemic areas of the United States, as well as in returning international travelers (Table 1).

Rocky Mountain Spotted Fever and Other Rickettsioses

Rocky Mountain spotted fever (RMSF) is the most severe rickettsiosis, with a case-fatality rate of 23% unless treated with an appropriate antimicrobial agent sufficiently early in the course. Infection is highly seasonal (May through September) according to the activity of the American dog tick in the eastern and Pacific coastal United States and the wood tick in the Rocky Mountain states. Because the tick bite is painless, a history of tick attachment is often not available.

After inoculation of *Rickettsia rickettsii* in tick saliva into the skin during feeding, the organisms spread hematogenously and enter endothelial cells throughout the body where they grow and spread contiguously from cell to cell. Rickettsial infection injures endothelial cells, particularly in the microcirculation, leading to increased vascular permeability, edema, hypovolemia, acute renal failure, noncardiogenic pulmonary edema, and meningoencephalitis. Host factors including age, glucose-6-phosphate dehydrogenase (G6PD) deficiency, alcohol use, and underlying diseases such as diabetes mellitus are associated with enhanced severity of rickettsial disease. Delay in treatment with a tetracycline or chloramphenicol (Chloromycetin) greater than 5 days worsens the outcome dramatically.

After an incubation period of 2 to 14 days days, the onset is characterized by fever, headache, myalgia, nausea, vomiting, and often abdominal pain. Rash usually does not appear until the third to fifth day of illness, and in 10% of cases there is no rash. Cough, confusion, ataxia, focal neurologic signs, stupor, coma, and seizures reflect life-threatening pulmonary edema and encephalitis.

Clinical laboratory data usually include a normal white blood cell count, progressive thrombocytopenia, hyponatremia, and elevated serum transaminases and urea. True disseminated intravascular coagulation is rare.

The differential diagnosis of RMSF and other rickettsioses and ehrlichiosis in the absence of a rash includes influenza, enteroviral infection, infectious mononucleosis, viral hepatitis, leptospirosis, typhoid fever, bacterial sepsis, toxic shock syndrome, and malaria. Bacterial and viral enterocolitis, acute surgical abdomen, bronchitis,

TABLE 1 Diseases, Etiologic Agents, Geographic Distribution, Ecology, and Transmission of Rickettsioses and Ehrlichioses Presenting for Medical Care in the United States

Disease	Agent	Geographic Distribution	Natural Cycle	Transmission to Humans
Rocky Mountain spotted fever	*Rickettsia rickettsii**	47 states, especially southeastern, south central, and mid-Atlantic states; Mexico; Central and South America	Transovarian maintenance in *Dermacentor variabilis* and *Dermacentor andersoni* ticks and horizontal from rickettsemic rodents	Tick bite
Murine typhus	*Rickettsia typhi**	Tropical and subtropical coastal regions; in U.S., particularly Texas and California	*Ctenocephalides felis* (cat flea)–opossum and *Xenopsylla cheopis* (rat flea)–rat cycles	Flea feces
Typhus	*Rickettsia prowazekii**	Eastern U.S.; Andes and other poverty-burdened highlands	Flying squirrel species-specific flea and louse cycle; human–body louse cycle	Flea feces; louse feces
Rickettsialpox	*Rickettsia akari*	New York City and other urban and rural foci	*Liponyssoides sanguineus* (mite)–domestic mouse	Feeding mite
American tick-bite fever	*Rickettsia parkeri*	Southern U.S. to Uruguay	Transovarian maintenance in *Amblyomma* ticks	Tick bite
African tick-bite fever[†]	*Rickettsia africae*	Sub-Saharan Africa; French West Indies	Transovarian maintenance in *Amblyomma* ticks	Tick bite
Flea-borne spotted fever	*Rickettsia felis*	Worldwide	Transovarian maintenance in *C. felis* fleas	Unknown
Scrub typhus[†]	*Orientia tsutsugamushi*[†]	Eastern Asia, Northern Australia	Transovarian in trombiculid mites	Feeding mite
Human monocytotropic ehrlichiosis	*Ehrlichia chaffeensis*	47 states, predominantly south central and southeastern U.S.	Tick (mainly *Amblyomma americanum*)–vertebrate host (mainly white-tailed deer) cycles	Tick bite
Ehrlichiosis ewingii	*Ehrlichia ewingii*	South central and southeastern U.S.	Tick (mainly *Amblyomma americanum*)–vertebrate host (mainly white-tailed deer) cycles	Tick bite
Human granulocytotropic anaplasmosis	*Anaplasma phagocytophilum*	Northeastern, upper Midwest, Pacific coast of U.S.; Eurasia	Tick (*Ixodes scapularis, Ixodes pacificus, Ixodes ricinus*), rodent and ruminant cycles	Tick bite

*Agents potentially dispersed as low-dose stable aerosol by bioterrorists.
[†]Diseases occurring in international travelers after return.

pneumonia, meningitis, or encephalitis may be suspected with prominent gastrointestinal, respiratory, or neurologic manifestations. When a rash is observed, the differential diagnosis often includes drug eruption, measles, rubella, meningococcemia, disseminated gonococcal infection, secondary syphilis, idiopathic or thrombotic thrombocytopenic purpura, Kawasaki syndrome, immune complex disease, dengue, and arenaviral or filovirus hemorrhagic fever.

In most cases, patients are treated empirically for RMSF if the clinical manifestations and likelihood of tick exposure suggest the possibility of the disease. Laboratory testing that is effective in the acute stage when therapeutic decisions are made (e.g., immunohistochemical detection of rickettsiae in biopsy of a rash lesion) is often inconvenient and unavailable. Immunohistochemical diagnosis has 70% sensitivity and 100% specificity. Polymerase chain reaction detection of rickettsial DNA has been applied as an investigative

diagnostic method, and rickettsial isolation is performed only in research centers. Antibodies are detected by indirect immunofluorescence or enzyme immunoassay in the second week of illness or later and are unreliable for diagnosis at the time of presentation.

The drug of choice for RMSF in nonpregnant adults and children of all ages, who do not have hypersensitivity to tetracyclines, is doxycycline (Vibramycin). Doxycycline (Vibramycin), 100 mg, is given orally every 12 hours, for adults and children weighing more than 45 kg. If the patient is vomiting or in a coma, the same dosage is administered intravenously. Children weighing less than 45 kg are given 2.2 mg/kg body weight of doxycycline (Vibramycin) twice daily. Although no studies of the optimal duration of study have been published, doxycycline (Vibramycin) treatment is usually continued for 5 to 10 days or until the patient has been clinically improved and afebrile for at least 48 hours. The risk of dental staining with short courses of doxycycline

CURRENT DIAGNOSIS

- Because diagnostic antibodies are not present during the first week of illness in rickettsioses, ehrlichioses, and anaplasmosis, a presumptive diagnosis must be made and empirical treatment given on a clinical and epidemiologic basis.
- For RMSF, HME, and HGA, the possibility of tick exposure and presence of thrombocytopenia are useful clues. Patients frequently do not recall a tick attachment but are more often aware of exposure to ticks.
- A rash will seldom be present early in RMSF and is usually absent in HGE and HGA. Never wait for rash involvement of the palms and soles or the appearance of petechiae to consider RMSF.
- Always collect acute and convalescent sera, test for antibodies against *Rickettsia rickettsii, Rickettsia typhi, Ehrlichia chaffeensis,* and *Anaplasma phagocytophilum,* and report the case to the state health department.

Abbreviations: HGA = human granulocytotropic anaplasmosis; HGE = human granulocytic ehrlichiosis; HME = human monocytotropic ehrlichiosis; RMSF = Rocky Mountain spotted fever.

(Vibramycin) in children younger than 8 years of age[1] is minimal and does not justify use of the less effective antibiotic chloramphenicol (Chloromycetin). However, pregnant women should be treated with chloramphenicol (Chloromycetin), 500 mg intravenously every 6 hours.

RMSF is prevented by avoidance of tick bites by tucking pants into boots; permethrin treatment of clothing; and daily bodily tick search. Ticks are removed with tweezers or fingers protected by a cloth, tissue paper, or paper towel using firm traction to avoid leaving tick mouth parts in the skin.

---

[1]Not FDA approved for this indication.

CURRENT THERAPY

- Treat RMSF, HGE, HGA, and *Ehrlichia ewingii* infections in nonpregnant persons of all ages with doxycycline (Vibramycin), 100 mg orally every 12 hours for adults. Children less than 45 kg body weight are given 2.2 mg/kg body weight of doxycycline (Vibramycin) twice daily.
- Treat pregnant women with RMSF with chloramphenicol (Chloromycetin), 500 mg every 6 hours.
- In pregnant women with HGA or HME, consider treatment with rifampin unless the severity is life-threatening, in which case doxycycline (Vibramycin) should be used.

Abbreviations: HGA = human granulocytotropic anaplasmosis; HGE = human granulocytic ehrlichiosis; HME = human monocytotropic ehrlichiosis; RMSF = Rocky Mountain spotted fever.

Murine typhus, flying squirrel–associated typhus, rickettsialpox, American and African tick-bite fevers and scrub typhus are distinguished by the epidemiology of exposure including travel history and, for the latter three diseases, the potential presence of an eschar. Antigenic cross-reactivity between *Rickettsia typhi* and *Rickettsia prowazekii* and among *Rickettsia akari, Rickettsia africae, Rickettsia parkeri,* and *R. rickettsii* impedes a specific serologic diagnosis. The treatment for all is the same with the reservation that scrub typhus resistant to doxycycline (Vibramycin) and chloramphenicol (Chloromycetin) has been observed in northern Thailand.

Ehrlichiosis

Ehrlichia are obligately intracellular bacteria that grow within a cytoplasmic vacuole in monocytes or macrophages (*Ehrlichia chaffeensis*) or neutrophils (*Ehrlichia ewingii* and *Anaplasma phagocytophilum*). They have evolved to manipulate their phagocytic host cells to their advantage. Transmitted by ticks, these organisms are not maintained transovarially from one generation to the next in ticks, but their survival requires horizontal transmission by ticks and persistent infection in a wild vertebrate host to survive (see Table 1).

Infection by *E. chaffeensis,* human monocytotropic ehrlichiosis (HME), has an incidence as high as 100 cases per 100,000 people in areas where white-tailed deer and Lone Star ticks are abundant. Infection is highly seasonal with 68% of cases occurring from May through July. Patients usually manifest headache, myalgia, and malaise. Less than 40% have rash, gastrointestinal, respiratory, or central nervous system (CNS) abnormalities. Leukopenia, thrombocytopenia and mildly to moderately elevated hepatic transaminases are frequently observed. Half of the patients are hospitalized. Severely ill patients may develop meningoencephalitis, toxic shock–like syndrome, respiratory insufficiency, and acute renal failure. The case-fatality rate is 3%. Immunocompromised patients are prone to develop overwhelming fatal infection. It is unclear whether in the rural southeastern and south central states this highly prevalent life-threatening infection is being treated empirically with doxycycline (Vibramycin), possibly as suspected RMSF, and thus aborting severe disease, or not.

Infection with *E. ewingii* is milder than HME and has been diagnosed mainly in immunocompromised patients.

Infection by *A. phagocytophilum,* human granulocytotropic anaplasmosis (HGA), has an incidence greater than 50 cases per 100,000 population in the upper Midwest and southern New England. Most cases occur between May and July when nymphal *Ixodes scapularis* ticks are active. HGA is usually an undifferentiated febrile illness with headache, myalgias, rigors, and malaise. Rash is rare. Leukopenia, thrombocytopenia, and elevated serum hepatic transaminases occur frequently. Severely ill patients may develop shock, confusion, pneumonitis, acute renal failure, hemorrhages, and opportunistic infections, which are the major cause of death. CNS infection is rare, and the case-fatality rate is less than 1%.

Diagnosis generally relies on indirect fluorescent antibody serology, which should test with both antigens in regions where both *E. chaffeensis* and *A. phagocytophilum* are circulating. Cross-reactive antibodies occur in some patients with the higher titer directed against the causative organism. Seroconversion or a fourfold rise in titer in a patient with a consistent illness is supportive of the diagnosis. Authorities' opinions of the value for a diagnostic single titer vary between 1 in 64 and 1 in 256. In most cases, the acute serum does not contain antibodies. *E. chaffeensis* serves as a surrogate antigen for *E. ewingii*, which has never been cultivated. Polymerase chain reaction assay is a relatively sensitive diagnostic test in the acute stage, is highly specific, and can distinguish *E. chaffeensis*, *E. ewingii*, and *A. phagocytophilum*. Microcolonies of organisms are seldom observed in peripheral blood monocytes (*E. chaffeensis*) and neutrophils (*E. ewingii*) except in some immunocompromised patients, but vacuoles containing *A. phagocytophilum* are observed in many patients with HGA.

The drug of choice for HME, HGA, and *E. ewingii* infections in adults and children weighing more than 45 kg is doxycycline (Vibramycin) given orally or intravenously in doses of 100 mg twice daily. Children weighing less than 45 kg are given doxycycline (Vibramycin) orally or intravenously at a dose of 2.2 mg/kg body weight twice daily. Defervescence usually occurs within 24 to 48 hours after starting this treatment. Treatment is continued for at least three days after defervescence. The organisms have been demonstrated to be resistant to chloramphenicol (Chloromycetin) in vitro. Pregnant women with life-threatening HME or HGA should be treated with doxycycline (Vibramycin).[1] Although there are no clinical trials to support the use of rifampin (Rifadin)[1], it has been used to treat HGA in pregnancy with a favorable outcome and could be used if the patient was only mildly ill and had an absolute contraindication against doxycycline (Vibramycin).[1] In vitro testing has shown that *E. chaffeensis* is also sensitive to rifampin.

Prevention relies on protection from transmission by ticks as for RMSF.

REFERENCES

Bakken JS, Dumler JS: Human granulocytic ehrlichiosis. Clin Infect Dis 2000;31:554.
Buller RS, Arens M, Hmiel SP, et al:, a newly recognized agent of human *Ehrlichia ewingii*. N Engl J Med 1999;341:148.
Dumler JS, Taylor JP, Walker DH: Clinical and laboratory features of murine typhus in South Texas, 1980 through 1987. JAMA 1991;266:365.
Elghetany MT, Walker DH: Hemostatic changes in Rocky Mountain spotted fever and Mediterranean spotted fever. Am J Clin Pathol 1999;112:159-168.
Fishbein DB, Dawson JE, Robinson LE: Human ehrlichiosis in the United States, 1985 to 1990. Ann Intern Med 1994;120:736.
Helmick CG, Bernard KW, D'Angelo LJ: Rocky Mountain spotted fever: Clinical, laboratory, and epidemiological features of 262 cases. J Infect Dis 1984;150:480.
Holman RC, Paddock CD, Curns AT, et al: Analysis of risk factors for fatal Rocky Mountain spotted fever: Evidence for superiority of tetracyclines for therapy. J Infect Dis 2001;184:1437.
Kaplowitz LG, Fischer JJ, Sparling PF: Rocky Mountain spotted fever: A clinical dilemma. Curr Clin Top Infect Dis 1981;2:89.
Olano JP, Masters E, Hogrefe W, et al: Human monocytotropic ehrlichiosis, Missouri. Emerg Infect Dis 2003;9:1579.
Paddock CD, Childs JE: *Ehrlichia chaffeensis*: A prototypical emerging pathogen. Clin Microbiol Rev 2003;16:37.
Raoult D, Ndihokubwayo JB, Tissot-Dupont H, et al: Outbreak of epidemic typhus associated with trench fever in Burundi. Lancet 1998;352:353.
Walker DH: Principles of the malicious use of infectious agents to create terror: Reasons for concern for organisms of the genus *Rickettsia*. Ann N Y Acad Sci 2003;990:1.
Watt G, Walker DH: Scrub typhus. In Guerrant RL, Walker DH, Weller PF (eds): Tropical Infectious Diseases: Principles, Pathogens, & Practice, 2nd ed. Philadelphia, Elsevier.

Smallpox: A Twenty-First Century View

Method of
Richard J. Whitley, MD

2

The events of September 11, 2001, along with the subsequent identification of anthrax in the United States Postal System, have generated a new sense of awareness for the potential of biological terrorism, if not warfare. Among the agents identified as "Class A Bioterrorist Threats" by the U.S. Centers for Disease Control and Prevention (CDC), smallpox is one of the most dangerous. The ease of transmission of smallpox, the lack of immunity in the population at large to this agent, and the rapidity of its spread, if released, all have generated significant concern for its deployment. A vaccine directed against smallpox* is available, but it is also associated with significant adverse events, some of which are life-threatening. No antiviral drug has proved efficacious for therapy of human disease, although one licensed drug, cidofovir (Vistide),[1] does have in vitro activity. Heightened awareness should lead to the development of a vaccine without significant adverse events as well as safe and efficacious antiviral drugs. The availability of a vaccine and antiviral drugs that are safe would significantly remove any major threat of smallpox deployment by terrorists.

History

Smallpox is one of the oldest recorded infections of mankind. Likely, this agent, also known as variola, evolved by adaptation to humans from a rodent cowpox-like virus through an intermediate host, such as cattle.

---

[1]Not FDA approved for this indication.

Rakel and Bope: *Conn's Current Therapy 2006*

*Licensed for restricted use and available only from the CDC.
[1]Not FDA approved for this indication.

The earliest descriptions of smallpox date back to 10,000 BC in Asia and India. The infection's subsequent spread can be traced eastward to Pacific Rim countries and westward to Europe and North Africa. By the 17th century, smallpox was introduced into North America from Europe. At its peak, namely when the World Health Organization (WHO) decided to initiate an eradication program, 10 to 15 million cases occurred annually, with an attendant fatality rate estimated to be 20% to 40%.

The WHO program against smallpox became one of the first effective preventive measures for an infectious disease, namely immunization. Interestingly, as early as 1000 AD, dried smallpox scab material was used in China for intranasal inhalation in order to develop protective immunity. In India, the same material was used to generate pustules to cause variolation, resulting in disease protection. Importantly, and surprisingly, the mortality following vaccination by such procedures, even if the material contained live virus, was approximately 2% rather than the customary 30%. Prevention by vaccination, however, was not introduced as a standard procedure until the late 18th century when Edward Jenner recognized that milkmaids who acquired cowpox were resistant to smallpox. By the middle to late 19th century, the use of vaccinia for the prevention of smallpox was routine. By the 1950s most industrialized countries had eliminated endemic smallpox by the use of vaccine prepared on the skin of either cattle or sheep and suspended in bactericidal concentrations of glycerol.

As early as 1958, the possibility of global eradication was suggested. Eradication was accomplished in a few developing countries by 1965, and in 1967 WHO launched its *Intensified Eradication Program*. Using the unique epidemiologic intervention principle of Foege and colleagues known as ring vaccination, cases gradually decreased in West Africa. The success of ring vaccination can be attributed to several factors, including:

- An intense societal desire to be rid of this scourge
- A very long incubation period (12 days) during which a vaccine can induce immune responses
- The lack of an animal reservoir
- Henderson and colleagues facilitated the WHO program leading to global eradication, with the last case occurring in Somalia in October of 1977. Routine smallpox vaccination of civilians was discontinued in the United States in 1972.

With the worldwide eradication of smallpox, the WHO launched an effort to destroy the remaining stocks of virus known to exist at the CDC in the United States and in Koltsovo, Russia, at the State Center of Virology and Biotechnology (VECTOR). As the issues concerning smallpox destruction were publicly debated, societies of the western world developed an increasing concern that stocks of smallpox existed in the hands of individuals for its clandestine use in an offensive biowarfare program, particularly in countries such as Iraq, Korea, Iran, and Libya. Polar positions existed in the United States regarding the destruction of the smallpox samples. Ultimately, following an Institute of Medicine Advisory Committee, a recommendation to maintain the stocks for purposes of antiviral and vaccine development was put forward by then President Clinton and supported by the Department of Defense and the United States Congress. This recommendation receives continued support from the Department of Health and Human Services and the Department of Defense.

Initially, scientists believed that the possibility of the reappearance of smallpox was miniscule; however, the safety of the population at large changed dramatically after the events of September 11, 2001, with the complete destruction of the World Trade Centers in New York City and the other tragic events of that day. Further, the subsequent deaths related to anthrax in postal workers and community members heightened awareness of the possibility that disease-causing microbes for bioterrorism could be deployed, particularly in developed societies. Because of waning immunity to smallpox, it is one of the most likely for consideration as a microbe of bioterrorism.

Bioterrorist Use

Likely, smallpox was first deployed as a biological weapon during the French and Indian Wars (1754-1767) by British forces in North America. Apparently, blankets contaminated with smallpox virus (obtained from infected patients) were distributed to American Indians. The resulting epidemics led to a mortality of greater than 50% in the affected tribes.

More recently, the potential spread of smallpox, if used as a biological weapon, was illustrated by two European smallpox outbreaks in the 1970s. These outbreaks were not thought to be intentional. The first occurred in Meschede, Germany, in 1970 when aerosol deployment led to a widespread outbreak, even when low doses of smallpox were released.

The second outbreak occurred in Yugoslavia in 1972. In spite of routine immunization, a single case led to a logarithmic increase in the number of person-to-person transmissions. From these two European events, it is anticipated that exposure of a limited number of individuals would result in an expansion factor of 10- to 20-fold. Inactivation of aerosol virus takes place during a period of approximately 48 hours.

Epidemiology

At the beginning of the 20th century, smallpox existed worldwide; however, its distribution was not uniform-areas of endemicity existed. Two principal forms of the disease exist, variola major and, the much milder form, variola minor (or alastrim). In 1970, 1300 new cases of variola major occurred in 1000 villages in Southwest India and in 1973, an additional 10,000 new cases occurred in India.

Smallpox is a viral disease that is unique to humans; no known animal reservoirs exist. To sustain itself, the virus must be transmitted from person to person.

It is caused by variola virus, a large DNA virus that belongs to the *Orthopoxvirus* family. The mechanism of spread is by droplet, aerosol, or direct person-to-person contact. Typically, an infected individual will cough or sneeze, which transmits the virus to the oral mucosa of a susceptible host. Direct contact is also a route of transmission, including contact with contaminated clothing or bed linens. The incubation period is, on average, 12 to 14 days with a range of 7 to 17 days. The disease is characterized by seasonal distribution with spread occurring during the late winter and early spring, a time when chickenpox is prevalent in most communities. However, it can be transmitted in any climate and in any part of the world. As would be expected, transmission within families is increased by overcrowding during rainy periods. On the other hand, transmission between communities increases during dry periods because of the greater mobility of individuals. The transmission of smallpox among populations is slower than that of chickenpox or measles. As noted, spread is primarily to family members and friends who are in close contact, but not among classroom contacts. The reason for this latter observation is that transmission did not occur until the onset of rash. Because disease onset was abrupt with fever and malaise, confinement occurred early in the course of illness.

After the early descriptions of smallpox, the distinction between variola major and variola minor was defined on epidemiologic grounds. In Asia, for example, variola major was associated with a mortality rate of 30% or higher. In contrast, in South America and sub-Saharan Africa, a similar clinical entity resulted in a mortality rate of 1% or lower, and was designated variola minor. Importantly, through the end of the 19th century, variola major predominated throughout the world. However, at the turn of the century, variola minor was detected at the very southern extremes of Africa and, subsequently, Florida. The distinction between these two strains relates to genetic and growth characteristics of the causative viruses in vitro.

Smallpox was typically a disease of children; nearly 33% of cases occurred in children younger than 5 years of age, and nearly 75% in individuals younger than 14 years of age. However, in rural communities where vaccination and natural infection were less common, disease incidence paralleled the age distribution. Both sexes are equally affected. The incidence of smallpox was higher in lower socioeconomic groups, presumably secondary to overcrowding.

Patients suffering from smallpox are most infectious during the early stages of illness, namely the first 7 to 10 days after the onset of lesions but not before. Transmission occurs most frequently 4 to 6 days after the onset of cutaneous lesions. At that time, the skin lesions are in a papulovesicular stage. However, as scabs form, infectivity wanes rapidly. Patients are considered infectious until all the crusts have separated.

Clinical Manifestations

Table 1 summarizes the issues relevant to clinical variola. Infection is initiated by viral replication on the respiratory mucosa. Primary viremia leads to seeding of the reticuloendothelial system. Secondary viremia results in clinical disease associated with fever, malaise, and myalgia. Virus localizes in small blood vessels of the dermis. The incubation period for smallpox is

TABLE 1 Smallpox

Clinical signs	Flulike symptoms with 2- to 4-day prodrome of fever and myalgia. Rash prominent on face and extremities including palms and soles. Pustular lesions become scabs over 1 to 2 weeks. Rash onset is synchronous.
Mode of transmission	Person-to-person.
Incubation period	1 day to 8 weeks (average 5 days).
Communicability	Contagious at onset of rash and remains infectious until scabs separate (approximately 3 weeks).
Infection control practices	Contact and airborne precautions. N95 respirator. Private room or cohort. Discharge when noninfectious.
Prevention	Live-virus intradermal vaccine that does not confer lifelong immunity. Contact CDC. Previously vaccinated person should be considered susceptible.
Supply assessment	Number of airborne precautions rooms available. Number of N95 respirators available. Vaccine availability.
Postexposure prophylaxis	Smallpox vaccine within 3 days of exposure. If greater than 3 days, vaccine and vaccinia immune globulin (VIG). Instruct exposed individuals to monitor self for flulike symptoms or rash for 7 to 17 days.
Treatment	There is no licensed antiviral for smallpox (cidofovir [Vistide][1] is experimental). Supportive care.

[1]Not FDA approved for this indication.
From Whitley RJ: Smallpox: A potential agent of bioterrorism, Antiviral Res 2003;57:7-12.

characteristically 12 days. The first clinical sign of infection is a prodromal illness that lasts 2 to 4 days, characterized by malaise, headache, high fever, vomiting, and delirium. Likely, prodrome coincides with the phase of secondary viremia. As prodrome progresses to the third or fourth day, buccal and pharyngeal lesions begin to appear. Rash begins on the face, spreads to the forearms and hands, and then to the lower limbs and trunk. Lesions are always more numerous on the face than other areas of the body. Lesions begin as macules and quickly evolve to papules and, subsequently, to vesicles by about the fifth day of illness. Pustules appear about the eighth day of illness. The pustules are usually round and tense and deeply embedded in the dermis. Pustules are followed by scabs and, ultimately, scars.

Hemorrhagic smallpox does occur; it is the most serious form of disease and is usually fatal. As would be anticipated, hemorrhages into the skin or mucous membranes characterize this clinical presentation. Secondary bacterial infection is not common. Death usually occurs during the second week and is attributed to immune complex mediated shock.

The illness associated with variola minor is less severe with few constitutional symptoms and a less pronounced rash.

The disease most commonly confused with smallpox is chickenpox. During the first 2 to 3 days of rash, it may be difficult to distinguish these two entities. Chickenpox is characterized by the development of a rash that involves lesions in all stages of development—maculopapules, vesicles, pustules, and scabs. Nevertheless, smallpox lesions do not demonstrate all stages of evolution simultaneously. The lesions of chickenpox tend to involve the extremities to a greater extent than the trunk.

Diagnosis

The identification of a single suspected case of smallpox should be treated as an international health emergency and brought immediately to the attention of national officials through local and state health departments. As discussed above, the clinical findings resemble those encountered with chickenpox. Laboratory confirmation of the diagnosis in a smallpox outbreak is important. Specimens should only be collected by someone who has been recently vaccinated. Vesicular/pustular fluid should be harvested and transmitted immediately to state or local health department laboratories for confirmation. Laboratory examination requires high containment (BL-4) facilities and should be undertaken only by experienced personnel. Typical approaches to the identification of the agent include electronmicroscopy, polymerase chain reaction assay, and isolation in cell culture. Differentiation from chickenpox can be accomplished by staining of scraped skin lesions with monoclonal antibodies directed against varicella zoster virus. A potentially confusing diagnosis, and one that occurs with global travel, is that of monkeypox, which would be identified in typical diagnostic assays. From 1970 to 1986, there were 400 cases of monkeypox worldwide with recent outbreaks in sub-Saharan Africa. This disease

closely resembles chickenpox but has a 5% to 10% mortality rate. Monkeypox is indistinguishable from smallpox with the exception of the enlargement of cervical and inguinal lymph nodes. Also, monkeypox resolves more promptly.

Vaccination

In the United States, vaccination against smallpox was discontinued in 1972. Thus, a significant portion of the American population is susceptible to smallpox. Persistence of detectable antibodies as detected by enzyme-linked immunoabsorbent assay (ELISA), particularly for older individuals, is approximately 5 to 10 years. However, persistence of neutralizing antibody has been documented in a few individuals for longer than 10 years after vaccination. Regardless, the following can be concluded. First, immunity is not lifelong. Second, some persistence of immunity has been documented in a limited number of individuals. In studies performed in Scandinavia, individuals exposed to smallpox but immunized as children had a lower mortality upon exposure to variola major than those not vaccinated. The implications of these findings are unclear.

Vaccination consists of the administration of vaccinia virus grown on scarified scabs of calves. Vaccine production for smallpox is, likely, the crudest for all vaccines available. After purification, virus is freeze-dried in rubber-stopped vials that contain enough vaccine for at least 50 doses. Vaccine is administered with a bifurcated needle. Vaccine should be stored at $-20°C$ ($-4°F$). Currently, there are approximately 90 to 100 million doses of vaccine* available for administration in the United States.

Vaccination is not without complications. First, and most importantly, no immunocompromised host should be vaccinated, as illustrated by an immunocompromised military recruit who was inadvertently vaccinated. Second, the rate of postvaccine encephalitis is approximately 2.3 to 2.9 cases per 1 million vaccinations with an associated 25% mortality. In addition, vaccinia gangrenosum occurs in approximately 2.6 cases per 1 million vaccinations and is associated with a high mortality. Generalized vaccinia is usually not fatal but occurs in as many as 290 individuals per 1 million vaccinations. Table 2 summarizes vaccine complications.

Postexposure Prophylaxis and Treament

Postexposure vaccine prophylaxis is the ideal method for disease prevention. However, given the vaccines currently available, it is not without both contraindications (immunocompromised hosts) and complications (encephalitis, etc.). However, adequate protective immune responses appear to be induced in the normal host within 4 days. For individuals in whom the vaccine

---

*Available only from the CDC.

TABLE 2 Complications of Smallpox Vaccination in the United States for 1968

Vaccination Status	Estimated No. of Vaccinations	Postvaccinial Encephalitis*	Progressive Vaccinia *	Eczema Vaccinia*	Generalized Vaccinia	Accidental Infection	Other	Total
Primary vaccination[†]	5,594,000	16 (4)	5 (2)	58	131	142	66	418
Revaccination	8,574,000	0	6 (2)	8	10	7	9	40
Contacts	. . .[‡]	0	0	60 (1)	2	44	8	114
Total	14,168,000	16 (4)	11 (4)	126 (1)	143	193	83	572

*Data in parentheses indicate number of deaths attributable to vaccination.
[†]Data include 31 patients with unknown vaccination status.
[‡]Ellipses indicate contacts were not vaccinated.
From Henderson DA, Inglesby TV, Gartlett JG, et al. and the Working Group on Civilian Biodefense: Smallpox as a biological weapon. JAMA 1999;281:2127-2137.

is contraindicated, there is a limited supply of vaccinia immune globulin (VIG)* that is available through the CDC.

At the present time, no antiviral drug has been shown to be effective in the prevention or treatment of smallpox. However, cidofovir (Vistide),[1] a licensed phosphonate analog, has in vitro activity against monkeypox, vaccinia, and variola, and is active against other poxviruses as well. While this drug is active in vitro, cidofovir does have significant nephrotoxicity. In addition, lipid products of cidofovir that are orally bioavailable are being investigated. Cidofovir administration should be by physicians experienced with its use. In the opinion of this author, cidofovir is a logical current choice of treatment. With the availability of vaccinia immune globulin, smallpox would at least be ameliorated if an outbreak occurred.

Development of New Vaccines

The original smallpox eradication campaigns used vaccines that were derived from many vaccinia virus strains, including the New York calf lymph virus, a New York City chorioallantoic membrane strain; EM-63 (USSR); and Temple of Heaven (China). By the late 1960s, more than 70 manufacturers used 15 principal strains of vaccinia virus for the development of vaccines. The Lister, or Elestree, strain, derived from sheep in the United Kingdom, became the most prevalently used throughout the world. Historically, most of these vaccines were produced in live animals. More recently, the use of primary cell substrates, particularly embryonated chicken egg–produced smallpox vaccine, avoids some of the potential problems associated with vaccine production in animals. These problems include harvesting, contamination, adventitious agents, allogenicity, and accompanying animal proteins. In addition, the Food and Drug Administration (FDA) has licensed live-virus vaccines that are produced in diploid cell substrates (e.g., MRC-5, WI-38). The MRC-5 cell line was used for the

preparation of a vaccine evaluated in a phase I clinical trial. Likely, the FDA will consider acceptable the production of live smallpox vaccines produced in these diploid cell substrates.

Alternatively, the continuous Vero cell line has been used to prepare inactivated virus vaccines, particularly the inactivated polio vaccine. While the FDA has not yet licensed this substrate for live-virus production, international experience suggests that it may be a suitable substrate for a smallpox vaccine. The selection of cell substrates of vaccine production in Vero cells has recently been addressed in an FDA letter (http://www.fda.gov/cber/letters.htm).

Strains selected for vaccine production warrant note. The LC16m8, an attenuated vaccinia virus strain, was developed in Japan for primary vaccination in 1975. It was derived by passing the Lister strain 36 times through primary rabbit kidney cells at low temperature. Initial studies indicated lower reactive genicity with acceptable immunogenicity. Of note, there was lower neurovirulence in a monkey assay. The most highly attenuated vaccinia strain is the Ankara. It has been passaged more than 570 times in chicken embryo fibroblasts. This virus is host restricted, being unable to replicate in human and other mammalian cells. Thus, for all intents and purposes it behaves like an inactivated virus, making it acceptable in high-risk individuals. It has been safely used in more than 100,000 persons in Turkey and Germany; however, its effectiveness in the prevention of smallpox is unknown.

Each of these constructs, as well as genetically engineered viruses, is being considered for use in humans. Of note, the recent availability of vaccinia pools at the Adventis Laboratory in Swiftwater, Pennsylvania, removes some of the intense pressure for the immediate development of new constructs.

Management of a Smallpox Outbreak

As soon as a diagnosis of smallpox is entertained, suspected infected individuals should be isolated and all household contacts vaccinated, if vaccine is available. Because of the potential of aerosol transmission, if

*Investigative drug in the United States.
[1]Not FDA approved for this indication.

feasible, patients should be managed in the home environment to prevent person-to-person spread. Vaccination administered within the first few days after exposure (up to 4 days) may prevent or significantly ameliorate subsequent illness. Currently, the more effective method of vaccine deployment to prevent the appearance of new cases, namely ring vaccination versus universal, is under discussion.

Because of aerosol transmission, smallpox transmission within the hospital environment has been recognized as a problem for some time. As a consequence, many health care providers have established two facilities for the delivery of health-related services during epidemics of smallpox with standby hospitals that deal only with patients having smallpox.

The potential use of smallpox has ominous implications, particularly given its rapidity of spread among susceptible individuals. As we have learned from the deployment of anthrax in North America during the fall of 2001 and early 2002, aerosol release of a potentially life-threatening agent is both feasible and devastating. Because improved vaccines take time to develop and there currently is no antiviral therapy for smallpox, research efforts to develop treatments and improve vaccines should be and are a high priority to the United States research establishment. As reported in *Emerging Infectious Diseases* in July 2002, all of the vaccines and treatments discussed in this article are actively being investigated by a team of researchers from the CDC.

Diseases of the Head and Neck

Vision Correction Procedures

Method of
Douglas D. Koch, MD, and
Thomas M. Harvey, MD

Most ophthalmic procedures share the goal of improving vision and visual functioning (Table 1). A select few, however, are used solely to correct refractive disorders such as nearsightedness and astigmatism. The goal of minimizing dependence on glasses and contact lenses is not a new one, and an ever-expanding array of surgeries is making this a reality for many people.

In the last decade, more than 8 million refractive laser eye procedures have been performed in the United States. Laser-assisted in situ keratomileusis (LASIK) has been an available procedure for years, but there are also many new refractive surgeries. Cutting-edge laser and nonlaser technologies are available to treat a multitude of refractive disorders safely. A summary of current refractive surgical options is given in this article.

Cornea Procedures

LASER MODALITIES

The U.S. Food and Drug Administration (FDA) approved the excimer laser for the treatment of myopia in 1995. This introduced to the United States a modality of laser vision correction that has become the mainstay for the treatment of low to moderate levels of myopia and hyperopia with or without astigmatism. The procedure uses a 193-nm wavelength and has demonstrated excellent safety, accuracy, reproducibility, and stability. The rise in popularity of this type of laser has led to the declining use of several procedures, including radial keratotomy.

A recent advance in excimer laser surgery has been the introduction of wavefront technology. The eye's wavefront (optical "fingerprint") provides objective measurements of refractive error on which LASIK and photorefractive keratectomy (PRK) treatments can be based. Custom or wavefront-guided surgery has improved the accuracy and safety of excimer procedures. FDA approval data for wavefront-guided LASIK for three different laser platforms showed that depending on the magnitude of myopia and astigmatism, more than 90% of operated eyes had 20/20 or better uncorrected vision 6 months after surgery.

Lamellar Treatment

LASIK uses a mechanical microkeratome or infrared laser to create a hinged lamellar flap of anterior corneal tissue. Ideally, this is done without damaging the adjacent epithelium. The flap is lifted, excimer energy is applied to the corneal stroma, and the flap is repositioned. The high level of satisfaction with this procedure in part is due to (1) rapid visual recovery, with most patients fully functional by 1 day postoperatively, and (2) little or no discomfort.

As with many refractive procedures, success with LASIK depends on a thorough screening process. Relative contraindications to LASIK include significant dry eye, abnormalities of corneal curvature, certain ocular and systemic diseases, and excessive refractive errors. Most surgeons try to preserve at least 250 µm of residual cornea under the flap, and so corneal thickness is one of many important preoperative measurements.

Surface Treatment

Excimer laser treatment of the corneal surface requires the removal of the corneal epithelium, which is approximately 50 µm thick. This can be done manually, mechanically, or with the laser. Ideally, it will leave a dry, uniform Bowman's membrane for ablation. PRK and related surface ablation procedures conclude with the placement of a temporary soft contact lens to aid

TABLE 1 Terms and Definitions

Term	Definition
Optics	
Accommodation	Process in which the refractive power of the eye increases with near stimulus by lens and ciliary body movement
Astigmatism	Steeper meridians in a cornea or lens that bend light more strongly, preventing a single point of focus
Hyperopia	Farsightedness; a condition in which parallel light rays focus posterior to the retina, making near objects blurry
Monovision	Therapeutic technique in presbyopia for contact lenses or refractive surgery, allowing one eye to be focused for distance and the other for near
Multifocal	Having more than one focal area in a cornea or lens, allowing objects to be seen clearly at varying distances
Myopia	Nearsightedness; a condition in which parallel light rays focus anterior to the retina, making distant objects blurry
Presbyopia	Age-related decrease in accommodation; often makes near objects blurry
Wavefront	Shape of light reflected off retina; used to describe elements of aberration or blur
Procedures	
Conductive keratoplasty (CK)	Radiofrequency energy applied to paracentral cornea to steepen centrally; used to treat hyperopia or induce myopia for reading vision
Corneal relaxing incision	Incision in peripheral cornea using a sharp blade with preset depth; used to reduce astigmatism
Epi-LASIK	Surface ablation technique similar to PRK; preserves a mechanically made epithelial flap for placement over the cornea at the end of the procedure; used to treat myopia, hyperopia, astigmatism, and higher levels of aberration
Intracorneal ring segments	Lamellar polymethylmethacrylate inserts; used to improve myopia or progressive corneal protrusion
Laser epithelial keratomileusis (LASEK)	Surface ablation technique similar to PRK; preserves an alcohol-mediated epithelial flap for placement over the cornea at the end of the procedure; used to treat myopia, hyperopia, astigmatism, and higher levels of aberration
Laser in situ keratomileusis (LASIK)	Excimer laser energy applied to anterior cornea under a preserved flap of epithelium and stroma; used to treat myopia, hyperopia, astigmatism, and higher levels of aberration
Phakic intraocular lens	Implantation of an intraocular lens without removal of the crystalline lens to treat high myopia or hyperopia
Photorefractive keratectomy (PRK)	Excimer laser energy applied to anterior cornea after epithelial removal; used to treat myopia, hyperopia, astigmatism, and higher levels of aberration
Radial keratotomy	Rarely used technique with deep spokelike corneal incisions; used to treat myopia
Refractive lens exchange	Crystalline lens removal before cataract formation for intraocular lens placement; used to treat hyperopia, presbyopia, and myopia

comfort and epithelial healing. Surface treatments have the primary advantage of avoiding the risks of the lamellar flap used in LASIK surgery. Their disadvantages include an increased likelihood of immediate postoperative discomfort as well as subepithelial haze.

PRK, the most common and time-tested form of surface ablation, has shown efficacy and longevity on a par with LASIK. A meta-analysis of PRK versus LASIK procedures performed before 2002 showed that approximately 50% of patients in each group saw 20/20 or better (uncorrected) for myopia up to 15.0 diopters (D). PRK patients have demonstrated refractive stability for 12 years and beyond.

Recently, some surgeons have attempted to preserve epithelium for repositioning after surface excimer treatment with the hope of limiting postoperative discomfort and the risk for subepithelial haze. Laser epithelial keratomileusis (LASEK) creates an alcohol-assisted epithelial flap, whereas epi-LASIK creates a mechanically separated epithelial flap. The theoretic advantages of each technique will require further clinical verification.

NONLASER MODALITIES

Radiofrequency Keratoplasty

Low degrees of hyperopia as well as presbyopia are being treated by radiofrequency energy (conductive keratoplasty [CK]). This technology creates a central steepening of the cornea by means of the application of circumferential spots at 450 μm depth in the corneal stroma, using a small probe. Patients seeking help for presbyopia typically are treated in one eye as a form of monovision. Some surgeons have found that the treated eye maintains good distance acuity, probably because of induced multifocality of the cornea.

Intracorneal Inserts

Intracorneal polymethylmethacrylate inserts (Intacs) have been used to correct low degrees of myopia and excessive corneal steepening, as is seen in keratoconus. Two 150-degree arc length inserts are placed in the midperipheral corneal stroma at greater than 50%

Rakel and Bope: *Conn's Current Therapy 2006*.

thickness to produce central flattening. They have the advantages of tissue preservation and reversibility, both of which can be useful in thinner or ectatic corneas.

Corneal Relaxing Incisions

For patients with higher levels of astigmatism and those with astigmatism and concomitant cataract, an excimer laser procedure may not result in satisfactory vision. Such patients may benefit from corneal relaxing incisions that are made with a guarded blade of preset depth. Incisions are aligned along the steep corneal meridian outside the optical zone to encourage a more spherical shape. Relaxing incisions have been used successfully in conjunction with multiple forms of keratorefractive procedures and intraocular surgeries or as the sole refractive treatment. The introduction of toric intraocular lenses has created another option to complement relaxing incisions for the reduction of corneal astigmatism.

RISKS OF CORNEA PROCEDURES

Overcorrection, undercorrection, irregular astigmatism, dry eye, and infection are all possible after corneal refractive surgery. Risks specific to LASIK are related to the creation and repositioning of the lamellar flap. Wrinkles, inflammation, and epithelial growth beneath the flap can degrade vision. Although the flap adheres firmly within hours to days after LASIK surgery, late dislocation as a result of trauma has been reported. Mild glare is relatively common and often short-lived after an excimer procedure.

Management of the most severe complications may require cornea transplantation in an attempt to regain best corrected vision. Fortunately, catastrophic outcomes are rare with both laser and nonlaser modalities.

Intraocular Procedures

Most candidates for intraocular refractive surgery have extreme myopia, high hyperopia, and/or significant presbyopia. For such patients, laser ablation of corneal tissue may not be the best option. The risk of corneal instability, dry eye, and bothersome visual side effects makes excimer therapy suboptimal for high refractive errors. Although cornea-based procedures have dominated the refractive surgery market, newer intraocular techniques are presenting options for select patients seeking independence from glasses and contact lenses.

All intraocular procedures use implantation of an artificial lens to focus light. The practice of lens implantation originally was developed for cataract surgery. Lens implantation has multiple potential advantages over corneal refractive procedures, including (1) accuracy for extreme refractive errors, (2) fewer visual side effects, and (3) preservation of normal corneal architecture. Intraocular lenses are used in conjunction with the patient's own natural lens (phakic intraocular lens) or as a replacement for it.

PHAKIC INTRAOCULAR LENS

Anterior Chamber

The first intraocular lens (Verisyse) for use without removal of the crystalline lens gained FDA approval in September 2004. The implant corrects 5 to 20 D of myopia by affixing the rigid lens to the anterior iris. Results have been excellent, with 85% of participants seeing 20/40 or better (uncorrected) 6 months after the procedure. Patients retain the ability to accommodate naturally, and some have demonstrated better corrected vision than was possible preoperatively.

Posterior Chamber

Another phakic intraocular lens, the Visian ICL (Implantable Collamer Lens), is designed for placement behind the iris. It is inserted with a folding technique that minimizes incision size and potential astigmatism. FDA approval data for myopia between 3 and 20 D showed that at 3 years after surgery, 59% of patients had 20/20 or better and 95% had 20/40 (uncorrected) acuity. Fewer than 1% of patients lost greater than or equal to two lines of best corrected visual acuity.

Although phakic intraocular lens technologies have brought surgical vision correction to patients with extreme refractive errors, some important considerations merit mention. The Verisyse requires a peripheral corneal incision of at least 5 mm, which is closed with sutures. The incision for the Visian ICL is approximately 3 mm and typically does not require sutures. Both phakic intraocular lenses necessitate deep anterior chambers and peripheral iridectomies to equalize pressure on both sides of the iris. The complications that can occur with phakic intraocular lenses are similar to those seen with other intraocular procedures.

REFRACTIVE LENS EXCHANGE

With the recent success of smaller incisions, high-frequency ultrasound, and superior lens implants, cataract surgery has become a refractive procedure. Some surgeons are using the same skills to offer refractive correction through lens removal with implant placement before cataract formation. Refractive lens exchange has been especially useful for patients with higher levels of hyperopia. Multiple options exist for the intraocular lens implant, which is selected after careful patient interview, examination, and lens removal.

Monofocal Implant

The vast majority of implants today are monofocal, allowing a clear image to be formed on the retina from a specific distance. Most patients choose to have an implant that will correct for distance but necessitate the use of reading glasses for closer work. Occasionally, monovision or planned myopia is used so that near and intermediate distances are clear without glasses. Monovision may be an option in motivated patients who are likely not to be bothered by a mild decrease in depth perception.

Multifocal Implant

Certain implants contain concentric rings of varying powers along the visual axis, thus providing excellent near and distance acuities. Newer designs may create less halo side effect and loss of contrast sensitivity, which limited the use of multifocal lenses in the past.

Accommodating Implant

The Crystalens is a silicone monofocal implant with a flexible structure that is believed to allow a forward accommodative motion. FDA approval data at 1 year postoperatively demonstrated that 92% of eyes were 20/25 or better for uncorrected distance and 89% could read at 20/40 at near and intermediate distances without magnifying spectacles. The implant has shown superb stability for all ranges of vision in patients implanted at least 4 years earlier. Studies are ongoing to verify its intraocular movement with near effort.

RISKS OF INTRAOCULAR PROCEDURES

The complications of intraocular refractive procedures may be uncommon, but their consequences can be devastating. Hemorrhage, infection, retinal detachment, and persistent edema of the cornea or retina are all possible with lens implantation procedures. Phakic intraocular lens procedures carry the additional risk of cataract formation, although this occurred in fewer than 5% of patients in the FDA trials.

Although refractive procedures have benefited millions of people, it should be evident that no single procedure is correct for every patient. Those interested in pursuing refractive surgery should have a thorough eye examination with pertinent screening by a qualified surgeon. Only after a complete discussion of risks, benefits, and alternatives to surgery should a procedure be performed.

REFERENCES

Findl O, Kiss B, Petternel V, et al. Intraocular lens movement caused by ciliary muscle contraction. J Cataract Refract Surg 2003;29(4): 669-676.

Güell JL, Velasco F, Sánchez SI, et al. Intracorneal ring segments after laser in situ keratomileusis. J Cataract Refract Surg 2004;20:349-355.

Heickell AG, Vesaluoma MH, Tervo TM, et al. Late traumatic dislocation of laser in situ keratomileusis flaps. J Cataract Refract Surg 2004;30(1):253-256.

Johnson SB, Coakes RL, Brubaker RF. A simple photogrammetric method of measuring anterior chamber volume. Am J Ophthalmol 1978;85(4):469-474.

Kershner RM. Refractive keratotomy for cataract surgery and correction of astigmatism. In Kershner RM (ed): Refractive Keratotomy for Cataract Surgery and Astigmatism, Thorofare, NJ, Slack, 3-5,1994.

Maloney RK, Nguyen LH, John ME. Artisan phakic intraocular lens for myopia: Short-term results of a prospective, multicenter study. Ophthalmology 2002;109(9):1631-1641.

McDonald MB, Durrie D, Asbell P, et al. Treatment of presbyopia with conductive keratoplasty: Six-month results of the 1-year United States FDA clinical trial. Cornea 2004;23(7):661-668.

Rajan MS, Jaycock P, O'Brart D, et al. A long-term study of photorefractive keratectomy, 12 year follow-up. Ophthalmology 2004;111: 1832-1839.

Solomon KD, Fernandez de Castro LE, Sandoval HP, et al. Refractive surgery survey 2003. J Cataract Refract Surg 2004;30(7): 1556-1569.

Wang L, Misra M, Koch DD. Peripheral corneal relaxing incisions combined with cataract surgery. J Cataract Refract Surg 2003;29: 712-722.

Wang L, Swami A, Koch DD. Peripheral corneal relaxing incisions after excimer laser refractive surgery. J Cataract Refract Surg 2004;30:1038-1044.

Werner L, Izak AM, Pandey SK, et al. Correlation between different measurements within the eye relative to phakic intraocular lens implantation. J Cataract Refract Surg 2004;30(9)1982-1988.

Yang XJ, Yan HT, Nakahori Y. Evaluation of the effectiveness of laser in situ keratomileusis and photorefractive keratectomy for myopia: A meta-analysis. J Med Invest 2003;50(3-4):180-186.

Conjunctivitis

Method of
Steven E. Katz, MD, and Amy M. Kopp, MD

The conjunctiva is a mucous membrane layer that covers the anterior surface of the eye from the corneal edge to the superior and inferior cul-de-sacs then reflects to line the inner surface of the eyelid margin. Beneath the transparent conjunctiva, connective tissue layers known as the episclera and sclera constitute the rigid white wall of the eye. The conjunctival layer is highly vascular with vessels readily visible with penlight examination; this layer functions to lubricate the eye due to its many mucin-secreting cells and to protect the eye against bacteria and foreign particles.

Primary care physicians regularly encounter "red eye" complaints, and this article provides a logical pattern to diagnosing and treating common forms of conjunctivitis and differentiating them from other forms of red eye. Conjunctivitis is infectious (i.e., bacterial, viral, chlamydial) or noninfectious (i.e., allergy, chemical exposure).

A three-step approach to the red eye is helpful in determining the most likely cause of conjunctivitis.

1. Symptoms—Symptoms range from increased redness, irritation, tearing, discharge, or photophobia. Itching is more specific for allergic conditions. Decreased vision and pain are not typical complaints of conjunctivitis and indicate a more serious process. The presence of pain is indicative of corneal epithelial involvement.

2. Signs—Conjunctival injection (redness) and edema (chemosis) are common. Watery discharge is often found in viral conjunctivitis while white, ropey discharge is more common in allergic types. Purulent discharge suggests a bacterial infection; copious amounts of purulent discharge usually indicates a more serious infection such as gonococcus.

3. Physical examination—Vision normal or near normal and pupils react bilaterally. The cornea is transparent allowing a clear view of the anterior chamber and iris. Severe conjunctival injection of one or both eyes can

Rakel and Bope: *Conn's Current Therapy 2006.*

Diseases of the Head and Neck

be encountered in combination with chemosis and/or subconjunctival hemorrhages. When exposing the palpebral surface of the conjunctiva by everting the upper lid or gently pulling down on the lower eyelid, follicles or papillae may be seen. Follicles are small, round, slightly elevated lesions that appear blister-like with blood vessels circumferentially around the base of the lesion; follicles are typical of allergic, viral or chlamydial involvement of the conjunctiva. Papillae are elevated red lesions typically found on the inner surface of the upper lid with a vessel found centrally in the lesion; papillae can identify such causes as allergic, bacterial, or contact-lens–related conjunctivitis. Preauricular and submandibular lymph nodes are enlarged or tender, especially in viral conjunctivitis; however, gonococcal and chlamydial infections should also be considered.

Infectious Conjunctivitis

VIRAL CONJUNCTIVITIS

Often referred to as the highly infectious "pink eye," viral conjunctivitis is transmissible through ocular and respiratory secretions as well as fomites (towels or medical equipment) and community swimming pools. Adenovirus is the most likely cause with an 8-day incubation period and a 10 to 12 day viral shedding period; it is even associated with systemic symptoms such as pharyngitis and fever. Patients typically develop bilateral sequential involvement due to self-inoculation of the opposite eye.

Presentation of viral conjunctivitis includes acute redness and watering of the involved eye. The patient complains of foreign body irritation or photophobia. Conjunctival injection, follicular changes, watery discharge, and eyelid edema are common. A tender, enlarged preauricular lymph node is typical. If corneal infiltrates are seen on exam (notably small white dots on the cornea surface), referral to an ophthalmologist should be made within 24 hours.

Treatment of viral conjunctivitis is mainly supportive in nature. Remind patients of the infectious potential of this disease; they should keep hands clean, keep towels or sheets clean, and avoid work 3 to 4 days if in a health care setting. Cool compresses help with lid edema (making sure the patient uses clean compresses); acetaminophen (Tylenol) is helpful if fever or malaise is present. Symptoms typically resolve spontaneously over a 2-week period.

BACTERIAL CONJUNCTIVITIS

Streptococcus and *Staphylococcus* are the two most common causative organisms. *Haemophilus influenzae* is more common in the pediatric population. Transmission for this type of bacterial conjunctivitis is through direct contact. The presentation is acute/subacute and consists of redness, irritation, and thick mucous discharge associated with mattering of the eyelid margin.

Treatment includes a broad-spectrum antibiotic solution or ointment. Ointments may relieve foreign body sensation; however, they also blur vision, which limits use during daytime hours. Recommended agents include the fluoroquinolone class such as ciprofloxacin (Ciloxan), ofloxacin (Ocuflox), or levofloxacin (Quixin), which are used four times daily. Ciprofloxacin is available in ointment form as well and can be used at bedtime to alleviate irritation. If the patient is allergic to fluoroquinolones, consider use of polymyxin-trimethoprim (Polytrim) at the same frequency. Gentamicin (Gentak) and tobramycin (Tobrex)[1] should not be a first-line therapy because it is highly likely to cause further conjunctival injection and irritation, but it can be considered if gram-negative organisms are strongly suspected (i.e., contact lens related).

We make a special note here regarding gonococcal conjunctivitis caused by a genitourinary infection with *Neisseria gonorrhoeae.* This hyperacute conjunctivitis is considered an ophthalmologic emergency because of this organism's virulence and propensity to cause corneal perforation. The patient presents with red, irritated eye and copious amounts of purulent, white-yellow discharge. After cleaning the patient's eye, the discharge is redeposited almost immediately. The patient may have concurrent urethritis symptoms. The exam reveals the excessive, purulent discharge with lid edema, chemosis, and a tender, preauricular lymph node. The cornea is often involved early in the course of the disease and can appear white or hazy. Treatment is emergent requiring immediate ophthalmologic consultation. Conjunctival cultures (cotton swab over conjunctival surface) are recommended using chocolate agar to confirm this diagnosis. Initial therapy should be ceftriaxone (Rocephin)[1] 1 g intravenously every 12 to 24 hours and topical ciprofloxacin or tobramycin every 2 hours (every 1 hour if the cornea is involved). Because bacterial toxins reside in the discharge, frequent eye irrigation is necessary. Also consider treatment for a likely concurrent chlamydial infection.

CHLAMYDIAL CONJUNCTIVITIS

Adult chlamydial conjunctivitis is caused by *Chlamydia trachomatis* serotypes D-K. This infection is found most often in young adults with concurrent genital infections. Transmission occurs from hand-to-eye contact, and the incubation period is approximately 1 week in duration.

Patients present with intermittent conjunctival injection and mucopurulent discharge. This condition can present during the previous 3 to 12 months. Direct monoclonal fluorescent antibody microscopy can be performed on conjunctival smears to confirm diagnosis.

Treatment involves systemic therapy for both the eye and genital infections. Azithromycin (Zithromax), 1 g as a single dose, is most commonly used, but doxycycline (vibramycin) 100 mg twice daily for 1 to 2 weeks can be used if macrolide allergy is present. Tetracycline ophthalmic ointment[2] can be used for treatment of the

---

[1]Not FDA approved for this indication.
[2]Not available in the United States.

Rakel and Bope: *Conn's Current Therapy 2006.*

conjunctivitis but requires four times daily dosage for 6 weeks and does not address any genital involvement.

NEONATAL CONJUNCTIVITIS

Etiology of neonatal conjunctivitis is dependent upon timeline and birth history. It can be caused by chemical irritation, bacterial infection, viral infection, or chlamydia. Chemical conjunctivitis is rapid onset (within 24 hours) redness because of irritation from silver nitrate ointment (no longer commonly used in the United States). *N. gonorrhoeae* conjunctivitis develops 24 to 48 hours after birth with lid edema, conjunctival swelling, and copious amounts of purulent discharge. Treatment is required immediately if suspected and includes penicillin eye drops 10,000 to 20,000 U every hour and intravenous penicillin G 100,000 U/kg daily in four divided doses for 7 days. Bacterial conjunctivitis caused by *Staphylococcus, Streptococcus*, and *Haemophilus* species has onset approximately 2 to 5 days postpartum. Conjunctival scraping and Gram stain may be needed to determine a causative organism. Treatment includes erythromycin ointment four times daily for 7 days if gram-positive infection is suspected; if gram-negative organism is suspected then use tobramycin (Tobrex) or fluoroquinolone drops four times daily for 7 days. Onset of conjunctivitis because of herpes simplex viruses type 1 and 2 is typically 3 to 15 days postpartum and can be associated with erythematous vesicles on the skin near the eye. Viral cultures should be performed to confirm the etiology. Treatment includes trifluorothymidine 1% (Viroptic) ophthalmic solution every 2 hours for 7 days or acyclovir ointment (Zovirax)[1] five times daily for 7 to 10 days. Ophthalmologic consultation is recommended if herpes is suspected because of early involvement of the corneal surface as well as intraocular inflammation or optic neuritis. Chlamydial infection occurs 5 to 14 days postpartum and is caused by *C. trachomatis*. The neonate may present with watery discharge that becomes mucopurulent with time. If diagnosed postpartum, therapy is oral erythromycin[1] 50 mg/kg daily in four divided doses for 14 days. However, with the use of erythromycin[1] ointment bilaterally immediately after birth, the incidence of chlamydial infection in the postpartum period has been dramatically reduced.

---

[1]Not FDA approved for this indication.

Non-Infectious Conjunctivitis

ALLERGIC CONJUNCTIVITIS

Allergic conjunctivitis is a hypersensitivity reaction to airborn agent causing IgE release and mast-cell destabilization releasing histamine. Most commonly associated with seasonal allergies and high pollen counts in spring and summer seasons, patients may already be on oral antihistamines or steroid nasal sprays. However, the systemic therapies do not always aid in the intense eye reaction that includes watery discharge, itching, and redness. Treatment should simply focus on controlling symptoms until after pollen counts have decreased, although treatment can be required year round if the patient suffers from indoor allergies such as dust mites or pet dander. A topical mast cell stabilizer is recommended first-line therapy; olopatadine (Patanol) or ketotifen (Zaditor) given one drop to both eyes twice daily will provide relief in 2 to 3 weeks after initiating therapy. Oral antihistamines may be used as a temporary measure while waiting for topical therapy to take effect.

CHEMICAL CONJUNCTIVITIS

Toxin Conjunctivitis

Chronic or overuse of over-the-counter ocular decongestants containing local vasoconstrictive agents (phenylephrine or naphazoline) may cause irritation, redness, and burning when discontinuation is attempted. Diagnosis must be that of exclusion of the other causes of conjunctivitis and must be based on the patient's history that includes use of such products. Patients present with diffuse redness, conjunctival follicles, and occasionally lid edema. Treatment is aimed at discontinuation of over-the-counter products and education of the patient. Cool compresses may be used to minimize symptoms; however, irritation and follicles may persist for 2 to 4 weeks after discontinuation especially if the product was used chronically. A low-dose steroid drop such as loteprednol 0.2% (Alrex) given three to four times daily for up to 2 weeks may provide symptomatic relief.

Acid/Base Exposure Conjunctivitis

When the patient arrives, begin irrigation of the eyes immediately even if the patient has started irrigation at home. Use of pH paper can be helpful to guiding how long irrigation is required (goal is pH of 7). Acid injury leaves the eye extremely injected as conjunctival vessels aim to

---

 CURRENT DIAGNOSIS

	Likely Organism	Type of Discharge
Viral conjunctivitis	*Adenovirus*	Watery discharge
Bacterial conjunctivitis	*Staphylococcus, Streptococcus*	Mucopurulent discharge
Chlamydial conjunctivitis	*Chlamydia trachomatis*	Mucopurulent discharge
Allergic conjunctivitis	Pollen, household irritants (e.g., dust)	Ropey, white discharge
Contact-lens–related conjunctivitis	Numerous organisms	Usually mucopurulent discharge

CURRENT THERAPY

	First-Line Therapy	Other Keys to Diagnosis/Treatment
Viral conjunctivitis	Supportive; proper hygiene	May have associated upper respiratory symptoms
Bacterial conjunctivitis	Fluoroquinolone four times daily	
Chlamydial conjunctivitis	Azithromycin 1 g orally	Usually in young adults with concurrent genital infection
Allergic conjunctivitis	Olopatadine (Patanol) twice daily; oral antihistamines	Patient may already be on nasal spray or oral allergy agent from primary care clinician
Contact-lens–related conjunctivitis	Fluoroquinolone four times daily; requires referral to ophthalmologist for continued care	Ask patient about lens care and routine

bring extra blood to the injured tissues. Alkali exposure may have a worse prognosis because of ongoing damage and deeper penetration into ocular tissues; blanched conjunctival vessels and corneal opacification may develop soon after the insult. These patients should be evaluated by an ophthalmologist as soon as possible after irrigation is completed.

Differential Diagnosis of the Red Eye

If the patient has decreased vision, cloudy cornea, or intense pain, diagnoses other than conjunctivitis should be considered:

- Episcleritis is unilateral sectoral redness with mild irritation usually seen in young adults. Treatment is not necessary (topical and oral nonsteroidal anti-inflammatory drugs [NSAIDs] are helpful in controlling inflammation).
- Scleritis is unilateral diffuse injection of deeper scleral vessels (do not blanch with phenylephrine 2.5% drops). It includes decreased vision, deep, boring eye pain with surrounding headache, and usually it is associated with systemic autoimmune diseases such as rheumatoid arthritis or Wegener's granulomatosis.
- Subconjunctival hemorrhage is bright red, usually sectoral hemorrhage obstructing view of the white sclera. It is painless and can be caused by valsalva maneuvers like vomiting or constipation. Question the patient on bleeding risk factors. If there are no risk factors, follow conservatively. It will spontaneously resolve in 1 to 2 weeks (patient may use artificial tears for any irritation).
- Corneal abrasion plus history of traumatic insult presents with decreased vision and increased tearing; painful, red eye with fluorescein dye uptake seen with blue light and Wood's lamp. Symptoms improve with anesthetic drops (do not dispense anesthetic drops to patient for home use as corneal melting may result).
- Herpes simplex keratitis presents with red, irritated eye with finger-like staining defects on the cornea with the use of fluorescein and Wood's lamp. Patients may have a history of current cutaneous skin eruptions.

- Acute glaucoma presents with diffuse, unilateral redness with mid-dilated pupil and likely corneal haziness; decreased vision, painful eye, and headache. Patients may have a history of taking antihistamines or cold remedies causing papillary dilation. Check the pressure of both eyes for comparison. Glaucoma is highly likely if the pressure of the red eye is greater than 35 mm Hg.
- Iritis presents with unilateral, diffuse red eye with a small pupil associated with decreased vision, photophobia, and headache. The patient may give history of recent trauma or autoimmune disorder.
- Bacterial keratitis is unilateral red eye with hazy, cloudy cornea causing a poor view of iris and pupil with penlight exam; discomfort and decreased vision are common symptoms. The patient may be a contact lens wearer.

For any of the previous symptoms or exam findings, referral to a local ophthalmologist is recommended especially if the patient wears contact lenses. Documentation of normal or near normal vision with a clear corneal surface often excludes any more serious ocular process.

REFERENCES

Arffa, C: Grayson's Disease of the Cornea, 4th ed. St. Louis, Mosby, 1997.
Kanski, J: Clinical Ophthalmology: A Systematic Approach, 5th ed. Edinburgh, Butterworth-Heinemann, 2003.
Pavan-Langston, D: Viral disease of the cornea and external eye. *In* Alber DM, Jakobiec FA (eds): Principles and Practice Ophthalmology, vol 2, 2nd ed. Philadelphia, Saunders, 2000, 846-892.
Vander J, Gault J: Ophthalmology Secrets, 2nd ed. Philadelphia, Hanley & Belfus, 2002.
Yanoff M, Duker J: Ophthalmology, 2nd ed. St. Louis, Mosby, 2004.

Optic Neuritis

Method of
Eric Eggenberger, DO

Optic neuritis refers to inflammation of the optic nerve; in the context of this article, optic neuritis refers to idiopathic or demyelinating origin and not to optic neuropathy related to infection or nondemyelinating origin such as sarcoidosis. Optic neuritis is a common condition with both visual and general neurologic implications, including a well-known association with multiple sclerosis.

Epidemiology

Optic neuritis is the most common optic neuropathy in younger patients. The annual incidence of optic neuritis is approximately 5 per 100,000 people, with a prevalence of 115 per 100,000 people in Olmstead County, Minnesota. The female-to-male ratio for optic neuritis is approximately 2 to 1 or 3 to 1. The average age at onset is the early 30s; however, cases occur in the pediatric age group as well as into the geriatric range.

Clinical Features and Diagnosis

Optic neuritis is just one of many processes that may affect the optic nerve. Several features of optic neuropathy are similar regardless of the etiology. The most common symptom of optic neuropathy is visual loss. Examination features of monocular optic neuropathy are similar regardless of etiology, and key portions include visual acuity, color vision, visual field, pupils, and the optic disc appearance. The archetypal monocular optic neuropathy produces decreased acuity and color, and a relative afferent papillary defect (RAPD); the configuration of the field defect does not assist the clinician in determining the cause of the optic neuropathy. Acutely, the disc appears either normal (retrobulbar or posterior optic neuropathy) or swollen (bulbar or anterior optic neuropathy). Focal swelling (or focal atrophy) is often associated with ischemic origin. Disc edema occurs in approximately 1 in 3 patients with optic neuritis and is typically nonfocal, mild, and without hemorrhage. Optic atrophy is the nonspecific end result of many optic nerve diseases.

Most of what is known about optic neuritis comes from the Optic Neuritis Treatment Trial (ONTT) and its follow-up study, the Longitudinal Optic Neuritis Study (LONS). The ONTT recruited 455 patients with acute optic neuritis between 1988 and 1991 at 15 centers in the United States. Eligibility for participation in the study included unilateral optic neuritis with visual symptoms for less than 8 days, age between 18 and 46 years, a relative afferent papillary defect, and visual field defect in the affected eye. Exclusion criteria included previous steroid-treated optic neuritis, history of optic

neuritis or pallor in the affected eye, the presence of macular exudate, or painless visual loss associated with disc edema and either hemorrhage or altitudinal defect. In the ONTT, the subjects were 77% female and 85% white, and had a mean age of 32 years.

Optic neuritis typically produces acute-subacute onset of monocular visual loss. The visual loss generally reaches a nadir within hours to days. Periorbital pain was reported in 92% of the ONTT subjects. Pain is typically mild and described as a soreness, ache, or discomfort. In most patients, the pain increases with eye movement and resolves within days. Most cases of optic neuritis are associated with central *blur* and a decline in visual acuity. Occasionally, cases present with peripheral field loss and preserved visual acuity. Color vision is often affected to a greater degree than visual acuity in optic neuritis. Demonstration of acquired dyschromatopsia through the use of pseudoisochromatic plates (and the presence of a RAPD) is an excellent method to confirm that a diminution of visual acuity is not related to refractive error or cataract change. RAPD is uniformly present in unilateral or asymmetric optic neuritis. Its magnitude is often larger in optic neuritis compared to other optic neuropathies with similar levels of visual acuity. Patients with monocular or asymmetric optic neuritis often report diminution of red saturation and the subjective brightness of light in the involved eye; this is an easy question to ask as the examiner performs the swinging flashlight test. Although classic teaching dictates that optic neuritis is associated with cecocentral scotomas, in the ONTT a wide range of field defects were noted. Altitudinal or other nerve fiber bundle-related defects occurred in 20% of ONTT participants, whereas cecocentral or central defects were noted in 8% and hemianopic defects were observed in 4%. Accordingly, the characteristics of the field defect alone cannot distinguish between inflammatory, demyelinating, ischemic, compressive, or other optic nerve pathophysiologies. In the ONTT, 35% of cases were bulbar (i.e., *papillitis* associated with disc edema acutely). Edema is typically mild, nonfocal, and generally unassociated with disc hemorrhage; severe edema, and hemorrhage should raise doubt about the diagnosis of optic neuritis and have prognostic importance. Most cases of optic neuritis (65%) are retrobulbar, and the disc acutely looks normal without edema, hemorrhage, or atrophy. Optic atrophy ensues as the visual function is improving, 4 to 6 weeks after optic neuritis onset in either the bulbar or retrobulbar forms. Photopsias commonly occur with optic neuritis, often taking the form of fleeting or flashing, colored or dark spots. A relatively high percentage of patients in the ONTT had asymptomatic fellow eye defects, including 14% visual acuity, 22% color vision, and 48% visual field defects. These abnormalities resolved over several months, suggesting subacute contralateral demyelination.

Prognosis and Evaluation

The ONTT found no value in routine lab tests including antinuclear antibody (ANA), fluorescent treponemal antibody (FTA), and chest radiograph in typical optic neuritis. Similarly, routine assessment of erythrocyte sedimentation rate (ESR), Lyme, Bartonella, ACE, or cerebral spinal fluid (CSF) is unwarranted in typical optic neuritis. Visual evoked potential (VEP), although sensitive for optic nerve dysfunction, rarely adds to the clinical diagnosis of optic neuritis, but it may be useful if diagnostic uncertainty or bilateral involvement is present.

The majority of patients with optic neuritis enjoy significant visual improvement. Improvement began within 3 weeks in 79% of ONTT patients; if no improvement occurs within 5 weeks, the clinician should rethink the diagnosis of optic neuritis. The majority of improvement occurs within 2 months, although further visual improvement often occurs over the first year following optic neuritis. Approximately 95% return to visual acuity, more than 20/40 at 12 months with or without steroid treatment. Final 12-month visual acuity of better than 20/20 occurred in 50% of patients, whereas less than 20/200 occurred in only 2% of all patients. Nonetheless, the majority of patients exhibit persistent examination evidence of the previous episode of optic neuritis, even if only the RAPD persists. Commonly, patients will notice difficulty with motion perception, a degree of decreased color, and diminished intensity of light in the affected eye. Following optic neuritis, some patients experience Uhthoff's phenomena, or transient visual decline following exposure to heat or exertion.

Optic neuritis is a common presenting event in multiple sclerosis (MS). The baseline magnetic resonance imaging (MRI) is the main prognosticator concerning the subsequent development of MS following a monosymptomatic episode of optic neuritis. A normal baseline MRI corresponds to a 16% MS risk at 5 years following optic neuritis, whereas a baseline MRI with more than 3 T2 lesions corresponds to a 5-year MS risk of 51%. At 10 years, a normal baseline MRI is associated with a 22% risk of MS, whereas an abnormal baseline MRI (>1 T2 lesion) corresponds to a 56% MS risk. Although intravenous (IV) methylprednisolone[1] as given in the ONTT transiently reduced the risk of clinically definite multiple sclerosis (CDMS) over 2 to 3 years, no effect was noted at 5 years.

Approximately 50% of patients with monosymptomatic optic neuritis will demonstrate abnormalities on a baseline MRI. MRI in typical optic neuritis is unlikely to reveal an alternative origin for visual dysfunction; only two patients with nonoptic neuritis origin for visual loss were detected in the ONTT (aneurysm and pituitary adenoma). The majority of patients with retrobulbar optic neuritis demonstrate abnormal optic nerve enhancement on MRI if fat suppressed gadolinium-enhanced images are obtained in the first several weeks after onset.

In the face of an abnormal MRI, CSF analysis adds very little to the MS prognosis. CSF analysis can help define a very low risk population for MS if both CSF and MRI are normal. Only 1 of 29 patients in the ONTT with a negative MRI and normal CSF analysis developed MS at 5 years (negative predictive value = 96%).

A subgroup of 388 patients in the ONTT/LONS did not have a clinical diagnosis of MS at study entry. Among this cohort, several clinical features in the context of a normal baseline MRI constituted a low MS risk factor group. Among 18 patients with normal MRI and painless optic neuritis, none developed MS at 10-year follow-up. None of the 21 patients with severe disc edema and a normal baseline MRI developed MS at 10 years. None of the 16 patients with disc hemorrhage, nor the 8 patients with a macular star developed MS at 10 years. These clinical characteristics in concert with a normal MRI are important because of the very low risk of MS in this group.

Therapy

Concerning visual function, acute treatment options for optic neuritis include intravenous methylprednisolone (IVMP)[1] or observation alone. IVMP enhances the *rate* of visual recovery but not the final visual function. In addition, an ONTT course of IVMP appears to decrease the chances of MS over the first 2 to 3 years following monosymptomatic optic neuritis if the baseline MRI is abnormal. The ONTT IVMP protocol is:

- 250 mg methylprednisolone[1] IV every 6 hours for 3 days, then
- 1 mg/kg prednisone orally (PO) each day for 11 days, followed by 20 mg prednisone PO every day for 1 day, then
- 10 mg prednisone PO every day for 1 day, then
- 0 mg prednisone PO each day for 1 day, then 10 mg prednisone PO every day for 1 day.

Most clinics have modified the initial intravenous (IV) portion to 1000 mg intravenously each day for 3 days to allow for single daily dosing on an outpatient basis. There is no role for long-term steroid therapy in optic neuritis.

IVMP as used in the ONTT is generally well tolerated, but mild steroid-related side effects are common including insomnia, weight gain, mild mood alteration, and gastrointestinal (GI) distress. More serious side effects such as psychosis, hyperglycemia, pancreatitis, depression, or avascular necrosis of the femoral head may also occur. The ONTT and LONS reported an increased incidence of recurrent optic neuritis (approximately twofold) in patients treated with the prednisone[1] orally at a 1 mg/kg per day regimen. Because of this finding, and that PO prednisone was no better than placebo in improving visual function, our practice (in accord with the American Academy of Neurology [AAN] practice parameter statement) advocates avoidance of this PO prednisone[1] regimen in optic neuritis.

Several studies have demonstrated the higher MS risk with a clinically isolated syndrome associated with T2 lesions on MRI. The CHAMPS trial (Controlled High Avonex MS Prevention Study) randomized patients with clinically isolated syndromes and a high risk MRI to interferon beta-1a (Avonex)[1] 30 µg IM every

[1]Not FDA approved for this indication.

Rakel and Bope: *Conn's Current Therapy 2006.*

[1]Not FDA approved for this indication.

CURRENT DIAGNOSIS

- Monocular decrease in visual acuity, field, and color
- Periorbital pain 92%, often increased with eye movements
- RAPD
- Normal optic disk acutely in 65%

Abbreviations: RAPD = relative afferent pupillary defect.

week or placebo, with clinically definite MS (CDMS) as the primary outcome. The CHAMPS criteria included monosymptomatic optic neuritis with at least two T2 hyperintensities greater than 3 mm on MRI. In this population, institution of interferon beta-1a (Avonex)[1] 30 mcg IM each week was associated with a 44% reduction in the occurrence of CDMS. In addition, all MRI parameters (T2 number, T2 volume and gadolinium enhancing lesions) favored interferon therapy at all imaging time points in the study (6, 12, and 18 months). Interferon beta-1a (Avonex)[1] was well tolerated in this population with a very low rate of neutralizing antibody formation (1%–2%). Using a combined outcome of CDMS or T2 change on follow up MRI, no low-risk subgroup of the CHAMPS cohort was identified (all had >65% risk of the combined outcome regardless of clinical and MRI features). Because of these data, and the lack of a precise

[1]Not FDA approved for this indication.

CURRENT THERAPY

- Secure the diagnosis. The diagnosis of optic neuritis can be made clinically in the majority of patients. In patients with typical optic neuritis, no ancillary lab testing is required.
- Consider high-dose steroid treatment acutely. The decision to treat with ONTT-style IV methylprednisolone (Solu-Medrol)[1] is individualized based on visual function, medical history, steroid risk, quality of pain, and MRI results, combined with patient input, realizing therapy will not change the ultimate visual acuity.
- Obtain an MRI, which is essential to stratify the risk for CDMS and serves a minor purpose of eliminating alternative diagnoses. We offer an MRI to all patients with optic neuritis unless a scanning contraindication exists, or the patient refuses imaging or declines possible therapy irrespective of MRI results.
- Consider interferon beta-1a (Avonex).[1] If a patient with typical optic neuritis exhibits an MRI consistent with CHAMPS entrance criteria, we discuss the results of this study and offer IFN beta-1a therapy unless a contraindication exists.

[1]Not FDA approved for this indication.
Abbreviations: CDMS = clinically definite multiple sclerosis; CHAMPS = Controlled High MS-Risk Avonex MS Prevention Study; MRI = magnetic resonance imaging; ONTT = Optic Neuritis Treatment Trial.

and accurate diagnostic test for MS, we discuss interferon[1] therapy with all monosymptomatic patients exhibiting a high risk MRI. A trial to assess the effect of glatiramer acetate in similar monosymptomatic patients has been initiated.

Subclinical optic neuritis is relatively common in the MS population; it is not unusual to find subtle evidence of an optic neuropathy (presence of a RAPD, slight decline in acuity and color) in this patient population in the absence of an identifiable episode of clinical visual decline. Chronic optic neuritis is rare and should be considered only after a thorough search for compressive causes of optic neuropathy.

Optic neuritis is a common cause of visual decline in younger patients, typically presenting with monocular visual loss and periorbital pain. Visual function generally improves over weeks (95% of patients return to better than 20/40 in 12 months with or without high-dose steroid treatment). Optic neuritis has an important relationship with MS, and the initial MRI helps stratify this risk in monosymptomatic optic neuritis patients. The 5-year MS risk in this group with more than 3 T2 MRI lesions is 51%, whereas a normal MRI in this setting equates to a 16% 5-year MS risk; the 10-year risk with more than 1 T2 MRI lesion is 56%, whereas the 10-year MS risk with a normal baseline MRI is 22%. A normal MRI in concert with painless optic neuritis, severe disc edema, peripapillary hemorrhage, or a macular star defines a very low MS risk subgroup. High-dose steroids such as methylprednisolone[1] IV hasten the rate (but not the final extent) of visual recovery in optic neuritis. Interferon beta-1a (Avonex)[1] therapy should be considered in patients with a high risk for MS.

REFERENCES

CHAMPS Study Group: Interferon β-1a for Optic Neuritis patients at high risk for multiple sclerosis. Am J Ophthalmol 2001; 132(4):463-471.

Jacobs LD, Beck RW, Simon JH, et al: Intramuscular interferon beta-1a therapy initiated during a first demyelinating event in multiple sclerosis. N Engl J Med 2000;343:898-904.

Kaufman DI, Trobe JD, Eggenberger ER, Whitaker JN: Practice parameters: The role of corticosteroids in the management of acute monosymptomatic optic neuritis. Neurology 2000;54:2039-2044.

Optic Neuritis Study Group: The 5-year risk of MS after optic neuritis: Experience of the optic neuritis treatment trial. Neurology 1997; 49:1404-1413.

Optic Neuritis Study Group: The clinical profile of acute optic neuritis: Experience of the optic neuritis treatment trial. Arch Ophthalmol 1991;109:1673-1678.

Rodriguez M, Siva A, Cross SA, et al: Optic Neuritis: A population-based study in Olmstead County, Minnesota. Neurology 1995;45:244-250.

[1]Not FDA approved for this indication.

Glaucoma

Method of
Robert N. Weinreb, MD

The glaucomas are a group of progressive optic neuropathies (disorders of the optic nerve) that have in common a slow progressive degeneration of retinal ganglion cells (RGCs) and their axons, resulting in a distinct appearance of the optic disk and a concomitant pattern of visual loss. The biologic basis of the disease is not fully understood, and the factors that contribute to its progression are not fully characterized. However, intraocular pressure is the only risk factor that has proved to be treatable. Without adequate treatment, glaucoma can progress to visual disability and eventual blindness.

It is estimated that glaucoma affects more than 66 million individuals worldwide, with at least 6.8 million of those patients being bilaterally blind. Vision loss caused by glaucoma is irreversible, and glaucoma is the second leading cause of blindness in the world. Among the many types of glaucoma, primary open-angle glaucoma (POAG), the main subject of this article, is perhaps the most common, particularly in populations of European and African ancestry. It is the leading cause of blindness in African Americans. It is expected that the magnitude of the problem will increase as the population ages. A significant proportion of individuals with glaucoma are undiagnosed or inadequately treated. Further, the number of individuals suspected of having glaucoma, usually those with either elevated intraocular pressure (ocular hypertension) or asymmetric optic disk appearance, far exceeds the number of people who have been diagnosed with glaucoma.

Anatomy and Physiology

Intraocular pressure (IOP) is regulated by a balance between the secretion and drainage of aqueous humor. The aqueous humor is secreted posterior to the iris by the ciliary body and then flows anteriorly to the anterior chamber. Aqueous humor provides nutrients to the iris, lens, and cornea. It exits the eye into the venous circulation through the trabecular meshwork and independently through the uveoscleral outflow pathway.

Axons of RGCs constitute the retinal nerve fiber layer (RNFL), the innermost layer of the retina. The human optic nerve contains approximately 1 million nerve fibers. These axons converge upon the optic disk (also known as the optic nerve head) and form the optic nerve. The convergence of the axons forms a central depression in the disk that is known as the cup. Most, but not all, optic nerves have a visible physiologic cup. The neuroretinal rim of the optic nerve head is pink and surrounds the cup. After exiting the eye, the fibers synapse in the lateral geniculate nucleus (LGN) of the brain.

Pathophysiology

Glaucoma is a neurodegenerative disease that is characterized by the slow, progressive degeneration of RGCs. With glaucoma, the size of the neuroretinal rim decreases, with concomitant enlargement of the cup. Other optic neuropathies usually result in pallor of the optic nerve head but for unknown reasons rarely cause enlargement of the optic disk cup. Neurons in the LGN and the visual cortex also are lost in glaucoma. Although the level of IOP unquestionably is related to RGC and optic nerve fiber death in some, if not all, patients with glaucoma, the pathophysiology of glaucomatous neurodegeneration is not fully understood.

Key Diagnostic Points

POAG is a chronic, generally bilateral but often asymmetric disease that is characterized by progressive optic nerve damage such as optic disk, RNFL, and/or visual field changes. The disease has an adult onset with open, normal-appearing anterior chamber angles and the absence of other known explanations for the optic nerve change. If the disease is detected early, progression frequently can be arrested or slowed with medical and surgical treatment.

OPTIC DISK EVALUATION

Optic disk examination is the single most valuable method of diagnosing early glaucoma, because the appearance of the optic nerve often changes before visual field loss is detectable. As many as half of RGCs and their axons can be lost before the visual field test shows evidence of glaucoma. Therefore, vision loss usually is not perceived until the disease is quite advanced. Optic disk changes consist of diffuse or focal narrowing or notching of the disk rim, especially at the inferior or superior poles, progressive cupping, asymmetric cupping, hemorrhage, acquired pit, and parapapillary RNFL loss.

VISUAL FIELD ASSESSMENT

Central visual acuity is relatively resistant to glaucomatous damage and therefore is decreased late in the course of glaucoma. Because peripheral vision is more susceptible to glaucomatous damage, there are marked changes in the peripheral field of vision before any changes in central visual acuity are noted. Standard automated perimetry, which employs a white stimulus on a white background, is the clinical test that is used routinely to quantify a patient's visual field. Although useful both for diagnosing glaucoma and for determining whether glaucoma is progressing, it is insensitive to loss of RGCs, particularly early in the course of the disease.

RECOGNIZED RISK FACTORS FOR GLAUCOMA

The overall risk of developing glaucoma increases with the number and strength of risk factors. It increases substantially with an increasing level of IOP elevation and with increasing age. African Americans are at greater risk than are white Americans: The onset of optic nerve damage comes at an earlier age, the damage is more severe at the time of detection, and surgery may be less successful. Other strong risk factors include certain visual field abnormalities, high myopia, and a family history of glaucoma. First-degree relatives of individuals affected with POAG have up to an eightfold increase in the risk of developing POAG compared with the general public. A thin cornea (central corneal thickness < 540 ∝m) and a vertical or horizontal cup-to-disk ratio greater than 0.4 also are strong risk factors. Weaker risk factors include systemic hypertension, cardiovascular disease, myopia, migraine headache, and peripheral vasospasm.

DETECTION AND SCREENING

In most cases, the loss of vision caused by glaucoma can be limited or prevented by the use of currently available therapies if the disease is identified in the early stages. However, most cases of glaucoma are not discovered until vision has been lost permanently. This may be related to the fact that the measurement of IOP alone is not an effective method for screening populations for glaucoma and because clinical signs of early glaucoma are subtle even to an eye specialist. Determining IOP, evaluating the optic disk, and assessing visual function provide complementary information; they can be used effectively to diagnose most individuals with glaucoma. Table 1 shows the recommended frequency of eye examinations for individuals in the general population on the basis of age and race.

Key Treatment

Glaucoma management is intended to enhance the patient's health and quality of life by preserving visual function without causing untoward effects from therapy. Specific goals consist of:

- Documenting the status of the optic disk and visual field upon presentation
- Estimating and maintaining through appropriate therapeutic intervention an IOP below which further optic nerve damage is unlikely to occur (the target IOP)

- Resetting the target IOP to a lower level if the glaucoma worsens
- Minimizing the side effects of management and their impact on the patient's vision, general health, and quality of life (including the cost of treatment)
- Educating the patient in the management of the disease

At present, treatment of POAG is directed at lowering IOP, which continues to be the only proven and treatable risk factor for the disease. There are three treatment modalities for lowering IOP—drugs, laser surgery, and incisional surgery—and they generally are applied in a stepped regimen.

Current management of glaucoma is directed at establishing and maintaining a target IOP: the level of IOP that prevents further glaucomatous damage. It is difficult to assess accurately and in advance the IOP level at which further damage may occur in each individual patient and individual eye. Further, there is no single IOP level that is safe for every patient. In general, the initial target is to achieve a 20% to 50% reduction from the initial pressure at which damage occurred. The least amount of medication and the fewest side effects in achieving the therapeutic response is a desirable goal. The greater the preexisting glaucoma damage is, the lower the target IOP should be. Progressive damage is more likely with higher IOP, more severe preexisting damage, and more risk factors. The target IOP of an individual should be re-evaluated periodically to assess its appropriateness by comparing optic nerve status with that in previous (including baseline) examinations.

With ocular hypertension, the decision to treat depends on the risk of the individual patient progressing as well as patient preference for treatment. Patients with established glaucoma generally are treated, and they certainly should be treated if they have demonstrated worsening or if their IOP exceeds the target.

MEDICAL TREATMENT

Glaucoma medications generally lower IOP by one of two mechanisms: a reduction in aqueous secretion or an increase in aqueous outflow through one or both of the drainage outflow pathways—the trabecular meshwork and the uveoscleral pathway. For most patients, topical administration of an eyedrop, generally a prostaglandin-like drug, is the first line of treatment. These drugs (latanoprost [Xalatan], travoprost [Travatan], and bimatoprost [Lumigan]) lower IOP by increasing aqueous humor outflow primarily through the uveoscleral pathway. These drugs generally have become the first line of therapy because of their once-daily application, minimal systemic side effects, and effectiveness in lowering IOP. Each can have unusual side effects, including a gradual irreversible darkening of the iris that is most commonly visible in patients with hazel irides and increased growth and darkness of eyelashes. Their use should be avoided if possible in patients with current or prior intraocular inflammation.

Several other classes of medications are employed to lower IOP in patients with glaucoma and usually are

TABLE 1 Frequency of Examinations to Identify Patients at Risk

Age (years)	Asymptomatic African Americans	Other asymptomatic patients
20–29	Every 3–5 y	At least once
30–39	Every 2–4 y	At least twice
40–64	Every 2–4 y	Every 2–4 y
>65	Every 1–2 y	Every 1–2 y

Rakel and Bope: *Conn's Current Therapy 2006.*

administered topically to the eye as second-line treatments. The α_2-adrenergic agonists appear to reduce the secretion of aqueous humor initially and then primarily increase aqueous outflow. They are not as effective at lowering IOP as are the prostaglandin analogues. Brimonidine (Alphagan P) is associated with allergic conjunctivitis and can cause sedation. It should be used with caution in children because of the potential for respiratory arrest. Carbonic anhydrase inhibitors reduce aqueous secretion. Topical forms of this medication (dorzolamide [Trusopt] and brinzolamide [Azopt]) have few systemic side effects compared with oral acetazolamide (Diamox). However, the IOP-lowering effect of the topical forms is not as effective as is that of the oral medication, and these forms should not be used in individuals with known sulfa allergy. β-Blockers, which still are widely used, also reduce aqueous secretion. They can have significant cardiovascular and respiratory side effects, particularly in the elderly. The use of a combination drop (two drugs in one bottle) such as the dorzolamide-timolol (Cosopt) fixed combination can reduce the total number of drops administered. Cholinergic agonists (e.g., pilocarpine [Isopto Carpine]) increase aqueous outflow but have significant ocular side effects, particularly blurring of vision because of the small pupil and induced myopia, which limit their use. The systemic side effects of these drugs can be reduced considerably with the use of punctual occlusion or gentle lid closure for 2 minutes to minimize drug absorption into the systemic circulation.

LASER TRABECULOPLASTY

In eyes judged to have an inadequate IOP-lowering response to medications and for patients in whom medications are poorly tolerated or are thought to be unsafe because of potential side effects, laser trabeculoplasty often is a second step in treatment. Because it is a minimally invasive office procedure with few complications, it also can be used early for patients who cannot use drops because of physical or mental handicaps or noncompliance with medical therapy as well as for individuals who prefer not to use drops. With this technique, small spots of laser light are directed at the trabecular meshwork to reduce the resistance to aqueous humor outflow and increase aqueous outflow. Although a high percentage of patients respond well in the first few months after laser treatment, 50% gradually lose this effect after 5 years. Although various wavelengths have been used to carry out laser trabeculoplasty, there is no convincing evidence that any specific wavelength is superior in lowering IOP.

CURRENT DIAGNOSIS

- Glaucoma is a chronic disease.
- It is generally bilateral.
- Often it is asymmetric.
- It is characterized by progressive optic nerve damage.

CURRENT THERAPY

- Document the status of the optic disk and visual field.
- Estimate and maintain the target intraocular pressure (IOP).
- Reset the target IOP if there is progression.
- Minimize side effects of treatment to maintain quality of life.
- Educate the patient and family about glaucoma.

SURGICAL TREATMENT

For individuals in whom the target IOP cannot be achieved despite the use of eyedrops and after laser trabeculoplasty, surgery with trabeculectomy is generally the next step. Trabeculectomy, a surgical procedure that consists of the excision of a minute portion of the trabecular meshwork and/or surrounding tissue, is the type of incisional surgery that is performed most widely to enhance aqueous humor drainage. With this procedure, a new outflow pathway is created surgically that bypasses the inadequately functioning in situ one.

The most common cause for failure of trabeculectomy is episcleral fibroproliferation that blocks the egress of aqueous humor. Anticancer agents such as 5-fluorouracil (Adrucil)[1] and mitomycin C (Mutamycin)[1] have been applied intraoperatively as single applications on a cellulose sponge for a few minutes or with postoperative subconjunctival injection to reduce the proliferative response. These agents inhibit scarring and increase the likelihood of long-term filtration and IOP lowering. They also increase the complication rate for the surgery.

Glaucoma drainage devices that direct aqueous humor to a subconjunctival reservoir that is sutured to the sclera also can be employed. Typically, they have been reserved for use in patients who have failed trabeculectomy or in whom trabeculectomy cannot be performed because of conjunctival scarring.

REFERENCES

American Academy of Ophthalmology, Preferred Practice Patterns Committee, Glaucoma Panel. Preferred Practice Pattern: Primary Open-Angle Glaucoma. San Francisco: American Academy of Ophthalmology, 2000.

European Glaucoma Society: Terminology and Guidelines for Glaucoma, 2nd ed. Svona, Italy: Editrice DOGMA, 2003.

Fremont AM, Lee PP, Mangione CM, et al: Patterns of care for open-angle glaucoma in managed care. Arch Ophthalmol 2003;121: 777-783.

Weinreb RN, Khaw PT: Primary open angle glaucoma. Lancet 2004; 363:1711-1720.

Weinreb RN, Toris CB, Gabelt BT, et al: Effects of prostaglandins on the aqueous humor outflow pathways. Surv Ophthalmol 2002; 47(Suppl 1):S53-S64.

[1]Not FDA approved for this indication.

Otitis Externa

Method of
David S. Haynes, MD

Otitis externa affects 4 of every 1000 Americans with approximately 10% of the population developing otitis externa in their lifetime. Known also as external otitis or *swimmer's ear,* it is an infectious or inflammatory process that involves the external auditory canal (EAC). Otitis externa may be divided into acute and chronic processes. Acute otitis externa generally results from an infectious process, primarily of bacterial origin. Chronic otitis externa is not fully understood and may have several contributing factors including infectious, inflammatory, idiopathic, and underlying dermatopathologic conditions.

The lateral one-third of the external canal is cartilaginous; the medial two-thirds of the canal are osseous. The entire EAC is lined with skin; the tympanic membrane is also lined on the external surface with squamous epithelium. The skin of the lateral aspect of the EAC contains sebaceous glands and modified sweat glands, the products of which mix with desquamated epithelial cells to form cerumen. A large proportion of cerumen consists of these desquamated epithelial cells from the skin of the EAC. The acidic pH of the cerumen in the external canal produces an acidic environment with a pH around 6.1. Cerumen also produces immunoglobulins, lysozyme, and polyunsaturated acids, which together with the acidic pH, are bacteriostatic. Cerumen is also beneficial to the external canal from its water repellent properties, preventing intrusion of water into the internal auditory canal (IAC) and maceration of the ear canal.

The EAC is colonized with multiple organisms, primarily skin organisms, such as diphtheroids, alpha-hemolytic streptococci, micrococci, and staphylococci. A variety of fungal organisms also exists as normal flora in the EAC, but *Pseudomonas aeruginosa,* the primary pathogen in otitis externa, is conspicuously absent.

Acute Otitis Externa

Acute otitis externa is thought to develop as a result from a break in the integrity of the integumental barrier with resultant infection. Water exposure, higher humidity, trauma, and high temperature all are commonly recognized as predisposing factors to developing otitis externa by violating the integumental barrier. Existing dermatologic conditions such as seborrheic dermatitis also contribute to the development of otitis externa.

In a recent study, 2049 ears with external otitis were cultured. By far, the most common causative organism recovered from patients with acute otitis externa was *P. aeruginosa* (38%). Other organisms recovered were *Staphylococcus epidermidis* (9.1%), *Staphylococcus aureus* (7.8%), *Microbacterium otitidis* (6.6%), and *Microbacterium alconae* (2.9%). Gram-negative organisms such

as *Pseudomonas* species, are not recovered from the normal external auditory canal. Most of the organisms that are considered causative organisms in otitis externa prefer a pH of 7.2 to 7.6, much higher than the normal pH of 6.1. The elimination of the acidic environment in the EAC creates an opportune environment for causative organisms to thrive.

Like most medical disorders, the diagnosis of otitis externa is made by careful history and physical examination. Pain (otalgia), otorrhea, and a prior history of swimming are all suggestive of a diagnosis of otitis externa. Pain is a significant and common feature of otitis externa and most often brings the patient to seek medical attention. The physical examination will commonly reveal edema of the EAC, otorrhea, and erythema of the skin. The otorrhea is generally not profuse and may be relatively thin and milky rather than profuse and purulent. Tenderness to the examination and manipulation of the auricle is marked and almost universally present, as are small micro-abscesses and skin changes such as a *cobblestone* appearance. An increase in EAC skin exfoliation is common during the active disease process. The tympanic membrane (TM), which is difficult to fully visualize in most cases, is intact.

The differential diagnosis of otitis externa includes chronic suppurative otitis media, acute otitis media with perforation and otorrhea, acute mastoiditis, dermatologic disorders of the EAC skin including dermatitis, keratosis obturans, malignant external otitis, and malignancy of the external ear canal. The most common diagnosis confused with external otitis is chronic suppurative otitis media (CSOM). Patients with CSOM will have otorrhea in the presence of a tympanic membrane perforation secondary to a chronic middle ear and mastoid infection. Pain, tenderness, and edema are infrequent in this condition. A history of prior ear surgery, cholesteatoma, and otorrhea of greater than 6 weeks or longstanding otorrhea are common in patients with CSOM and can help to differentiate from patients with otitis externa. The tympanic membrane is difficult to examine in either of the conditions secondary to the otorrhea; however, patients with CSOM tend to lack tenderness and edema of the EAC. The presence of a tympanic membrane perforation excludes, for the most part, the diagnosis of otitis externa. Acute mastoiditis will present with EAC edema and pain but will have postauricular swelling and fluctuance, a physical finding not encountered in otitis externa.

The treatment of otitis externa consists of cleaning the EAC, also called *aural toilet,* and the application of antimicrobial ototopical preparations. Acidification (or reacidification) is also a commonly employed treatment regimen. Aural toilet is an essential component to the treatment regimen, as removal of discharge and debris facilitates drop delivery. Aural toilet can be achieved via several mechanisms including a technique termed *dry mopping,* which involves gentle removal of debris at the external meatus with a cotton-tipped applicator. Gentle irrigation (only when the TM is intact) to remove purulent debris in the EAC is considered a more effective method of aural toilet. Hydrogen peroxide, acetic acid, and alcohol—alone or in combination—have all been used to irrigate the EAC. Cleaning the ear canal in the office under the microscope with microsuction is the most reliable, safe, and effective technique for aural toilet. The frequency of office cleaning varies among practitioners, but daily cleaning is not uncommon, especially in refractory cases.

A variety of ototopical agents have historically and successfully been used in the treatment of otitis externa. Ototopical agents that do not contain antibiotics (often referred to as *antiseptic agents*) depend on the mechanical properties of irrigation, as well as acidification for bacteriostatic or bacteriocidal activity. One advantage of most antiseptic agents is the relatively broad spectrum of activity against potential pathogens. Most ototopical preparations in use today contain antibiotics effective against both gram-positive and gram-negative organisms. Consequently, most ototopical preparations contain an aminoglycoside or fluoroquinolone, alone or in combination with other antibiotics or steroids (dexamethasone, hydrocortisone).

The most common ototopical agent used for external otitis has been a combination product that contains neomycin, polymyxin B, and hydrocortisone (Cortisporin Otic Suspension). Neomycin, as well as other aminoglycosides, gentamicin (Garamycin ophthalmic)[1], and tobramycin (Tobrex, TobraDex ophthalmic preparations)[1] have been used for years as ototopical agents despite potential ototoxicity. These agents were necessary for their spectrum of activity notably against gram-negative organisms. There is a trend toward using the more recently introduced fluoroquinolone drops, ciprofloxacin/dexamethasone (Ciprodex), and ofloxacin (Floxin Otic) in treating otitis externa. The fluoroquinolone drops have an excellent spectrum of activity against ear pathogens, including *P. aeruginosa,* and have demonstrated no evidence of ototoxicity. Technically, ototoxicity should not be an issue if the tympanic membrane is intact; however, an intact tympanic membrane is not always easy to determine secondary to edema and otorrhea. Hypersensitivity to neomycin is an adverse effect that is being encountered more regularly. The reaction to topical neomycin may range from mild skin erythema to severe excoriation and skin blistering.

Failure of drop delivery is the most common reason for persistent infection as opposed to resistant organisms. The high concentration of antibiotics delivered to the ear with commercially prepared drops prevents the development of resistant organisms. Drop delivery remains problematic despite good aural toilet if significant edema, or profuse otorrhea (less common), is present. Placement of a wick can be useful when significant edema is present. A wick is a small, commercially available sponge that can be placed in the EAC to maintain the patency of the canal and improve drop delivery. The wick also has the added advantage of keeping the antibiotics in contact with the skin for prolonged periods between dosing. A wick is not necessary in all cases of otitis externa. The standard Otowick is not absorbable and must be removed, most being retained from 2 to 7 days.

[1]Not FDA approved for this indication.

Rakel and Bope: *Conn's Current Therapy 2006.*

Cultures are rarely needed to direct therapy and are obtained only for refractory cases. If cultures are obtained, caution should be used regarding the interpretation of *resistance* and *sensitivity*. The resistance of an organism is determined based on the concentrations of antibiotics that can be reasonably achieved in tissues following *systemic* administration. Standard resistance and sensitivity determinations do not apply when antibiotics are delivered *topically* secondary to the high concentration that can be achieved with this method of delivery. A 3% solution of antibiotics such as seen with ciprofloxacin/dexamethasone (Ciprodex) or ofloxacin (Floxin Otic) contains an antibiotic concentration of 3000 µg/mL. This concentration is 1000 times the concentration that can be achieved with systemic administration of ciprofloxacin and ofloxacin, respectively, far exceeding the minimal inhibitory concentration (MIC) of any known ear pathogen. Therefore those organisms labeled as *resistant* by sensitivity testing to an antibiotic will actually be susceptible at the high concentrations delivered to the ear.

Ototopical agents alone are indicated for uncomplicated cases of otitis externa. Systemic antibiotics are still prescribed inappropriately for external otitis, especially in children; they are rarely required except in special circumstances such as treatment failures, diabetics, and immunocompromised patients. Systemic antibiotics are also indicated in patients with cellulitis, adenopathy, or signs of systemic infection (fever). As previously mentioned, pain is common and severe, often necessitating oral narcotics for pain relief.

Treatment failures or prolonged morbidity may arise from several causes:

- Poor compliance. Failure to use prescribed therapy and reexposure to causative agents (swimming) are potential causes for failure. Although compliance with drops is generally good, occasionally patients do not appreciate the significance and strength of topical therapy, which leads to poor compliance.
- Failure of drop delivery secondary to edema or otorrhea.
- Identification of *fungal* pathogens, as opposed to bacterial.
- Development of topical sensitization. Sensitivity to neomycin is relatively common. The skin reaction ranges from florid erythema and skin excoriation to mild erythema and edema. The latter reaction may be perceived as a persistent or refractory infection as opposed to a true skin reaction. Discontinuation of the offending drops, with application of topical steroids with or without systemic antihistamines and/or systemic steroids, is the treatment of choice; many *refractory* cases of external otitis are treated this way.
- Diagnosis of malignant otitis externa, or skull base osteomyelitis, osteoradionecrosis, or malignancy.
- Development of resistant organisms during the course of therapy. This, as mentioned previously, is unlikely given the high concentration of antibiotic existing in ototopical preparations.
- Presence of a primary dermatologic disorder.

Otomycosis (Fungal External Otitis)

Otitis externa is rarely the result of fungal pathogens in the nonimmunocompromised host. Fungi are normal saprophytes encountered in the EAC. Fungal elements may be seen on examination of the infected ear without necessarily being the true primary pathogen. Fungi may play a role as secondary pathogens after changes in pH and bacterial flora occur during the course of the infection and therapy.

If fungi are considered a true pathogen or significant copathogen, aural toilet, irrigation, and reacidification remain effective methods of therapy. If these methods fail, antifungal agents may be used. Currently the Food and Drug Administration (FDA) has not approved any antifungal ototopicals. Current antifungals nystatin (Mycostatin),[1] clotrimazole (Lotrimin),[1] ketoconazole (Nizoral),[1] amphotericin B (Fungizone),[1] and tolnaftate (Tinactin)[1] have been used in the EAC for otomycosis. Antifungal lotions are preferred because they may be administered as drops. Ointments or creams may be instilled into the aural canal with a blunt-tipped catheter or angiocatheter. These agents, although not FDA approved for this use, have been shown to be nonototoxic.

Chronic External Otitis

Chronic external otitis remains a frustrating and complex disorder for otologists to treat. The disorder is more than an acute otitis media that develops into a chronic process. The etiology of this process remains unclear. Several features distinguish chronic external otitis from acute otitis externa other than the chronicity which occurs over months to years. Chronic external otitis is generally painless, and pruritus is a prominent feature. The disease is bilateral in 50% of cases. The disease is unrelenting despite therapy, usually leading to stenosis and blunting of the ear canal with associated conductive hearing loss. Once the disease progresses to this stage, surgical repair of the external canal is indicated.

---

[1]Not FDA approved for this indication

CURRENT DIAGNOSIS

- Obtain medical, social, and family history, especially diabetes and prior history of malignancy.
- Obtain otologic history including ear pain, ear drainage, vertigo, and swimming history.
- Obtain history of prior ear surgery.
- Obtain history of prior treatment for ear drainage and length of symptoms.

Malignant External Otitis

Otitis externa may spread from the skin of the external canal to involve the bone of the external canal and the base of the skull. This disorder is also known as necrotizing external otitis and skull base osteomyelitis. It is rarely encountered in nonimmunocompromised individuals and is most likely to develop in elderly diabetics. As in acute otitis externa, *P. aeruginosa* is the causative agent.

The diagnosis of malignant external otitis is clinical, with a high index of suspicion necessary to make a prompt, correct diagnosis. Elderly diabetics who do not respond to initial therapy should be considered to have this diagnosis until proved otherwise. The erythrocyte sedimentation rate (ESR) is elevated (80 mm/hour or greater). A high resolution tomography (CT) scan of the temporal bone is helpful in establishing the diagnosis and for ruling out other disorders. A technetium-99m bone scan may be obtained to confirm the diagnosis of skull base osteomyelitis and determine the extent of disease. A gallium-67 (67Ga) study usually is obtained to determine the response to therapy and guide cessation of antibiotics. The technetium (Tc)-99m study will remain positive for many years and is not useful to follow for resolution of disease, therefore the 67Ga study is used for this purpose. MRI also is used for establishing the initial diagnosis and for long-term follow-up given the superior ability of MRI to image soft tissue. Currently, there is a trend for using anatomic imaging (CT, MRI) for diagnosis and monitoring of malignant external otitis over radionuclide studies (Tc-99m, 67Ga).

There has been an evolution in the standard therapy prescribed for these patients over the past two decades, which has decreased morbidity and improved overall survival. Where once treatment with a 6- to 8-week course of dual intravenous (IV) antipseudomonal antibiotics was standard, current therapy suggests that 6 weeks of oral antipseudomonal medications (fluoroquinolones) can achieve a cure in 90% of cases. Given the deep extension of the disease along the skull base, surgical débridement has no role and may further devascularize tissue-decreasing antibiotic delivery. Biopsies, however, may be indicated to rule out other diagnoses, notably

CURRENT THERAPY

- Examine the external ear canal for edema, otorrhea, erythema, and granulation tissue.
- Examine the tympanic membrane for perforation or cholesteatoma.
- Topical therapy alone is sufficient therapy in the absence of periauricular cellulitis.
- Culture otorrhea only when refractory to therapy. No need to culture initially.
- Consider biopsy to rule out malignancy when clinically appropriate (refractory erythema or edema, prolonged pain and persistent granulation tissue, or ulcerative areas).

squamous cell carcinoma of the temporal bone. Therapy is continued until a clinical response is achieved, pain is alleviated, and the ESR has reverted to normal. Intravenous antipseudomonal agents are indicated for treatment failures, especially given the critical patient population in which this disorder develops.

REFERENCES

Beers SL, Abramo TJ: Pediatr Emerg Care 2004;20(4):250-256.
Dohar JE: Evolution of management approaches for otitis externa. Pediatr Infect Dis J 2003;22(4):299-305.
Grandis R, Branstetter BF, Yu VL: The changing face of malignant (necrotizing) external otitis: Clinical, radiological, and anatomic correlations. Lancet Infect Dis 2004;4(1):34-39.
McCoy SI, Zell ER, Besser RE: Antimicrobial prescribing for otitis externa in children. Pediatr Infect Dis J 2004;23(2):181-183.
Roland PS: Chronic external otitis. ENT J 2001;80(6):12-16.
Roland PS, Stewart MG, Hannley M, et al: Consensus panel on role of potentially ototoxic antibiotics for topical middle ear use: Introduction, methodology, and recommendations. Otolaryngol Head Neck Surg 2004;130(3 Suppl):S51-S56.
Roland PS, Stroman DW: Microbiology of acute otitis externa. Laryngoscope 2002;112(7 Pt 1):1166-1177.
Slattery WH III, Saadat P: Postinflammatory medial canal fibrosis. Am J Otol 1997;18:294-297.
Tom LWC: Ototoxicity of common antimycotic preparations. Laryngoscope 2000;110:509-516.
Weber PC, Roland PS, Hannley M, et al: The development of antibiotic resistant organisms with the use of ototopical medications. Otolaryngol Head Neck Surg 2004;130(3 Suppl):S89-S94.

Otitis Media

Method of
Richard Propp, MD, and
Richard M. Rosenfeld, MD, MPH

One of the most important and common childhood illnesses, otitis media, requires special efforts to achieve diagnostic accuracy, manage uncertainty, and avoid unnecessary antibiotic prescriptions. A new management paradigm, the Dutch observation option, was explored in an Albany, New York, project in 1998 and incorporated into the 2000 Practitioner's Guideline. The New York Region Otitis Project (NYROP) developed an Observation Option Toolkit published in 2002. Both are on the New York Web site (http://www.health.state.ny.us/nysdoh/antibiotic/antibiotic.htm).

The NYROP toolkit was adopted into an American Academy of Pediatrics/American Academy of Family Physicians (AAP/AAFP) Clinical Practice Guideline in 2004 to help reduce the side effects of unnecessary antibiotics, including drug resistance. The new guideline also speaks to necessary initial pain management as distinct from infection. Moreover, clinicians have the option to observe children for up to 72 hours without antibiotics, because more than 80% will cure their infection naturally without any increase in complications

Rakel and Bope: Conn's Current Therapy 2006.

if appropriate follow-up is provided. The guideline is on the AAP Website (http://pediatrics.aappublications.org/cgi/content/full/113/5/1451). This new option requires increased attention to education of the parents (Figure 1).

Diagnosis

Ear examination requires a clear view of the tympanic membrane. Cerumen removal may require time and effort. The best methods are to clean gently with a blunt curette or wire loop under direct vision (through an open otoscope or binocular microscope) or to irrigate the ear canal with body-temperature water (assuming a perforation is not present). Deeply impacted or very hard cerumen can be removed safely by an otolaryngologist.

Without a clear view of the anatomy and function of the tympanic membrane, the diagnosis must be dealt with as uncertain, or the patient can be referred to an otolaryngologist for consultation where available. Most uncertainty arises from inability to clearly visualize middle ear effusion or to reliably assess tympanic membrane mobility with the pneumatic otoscope.

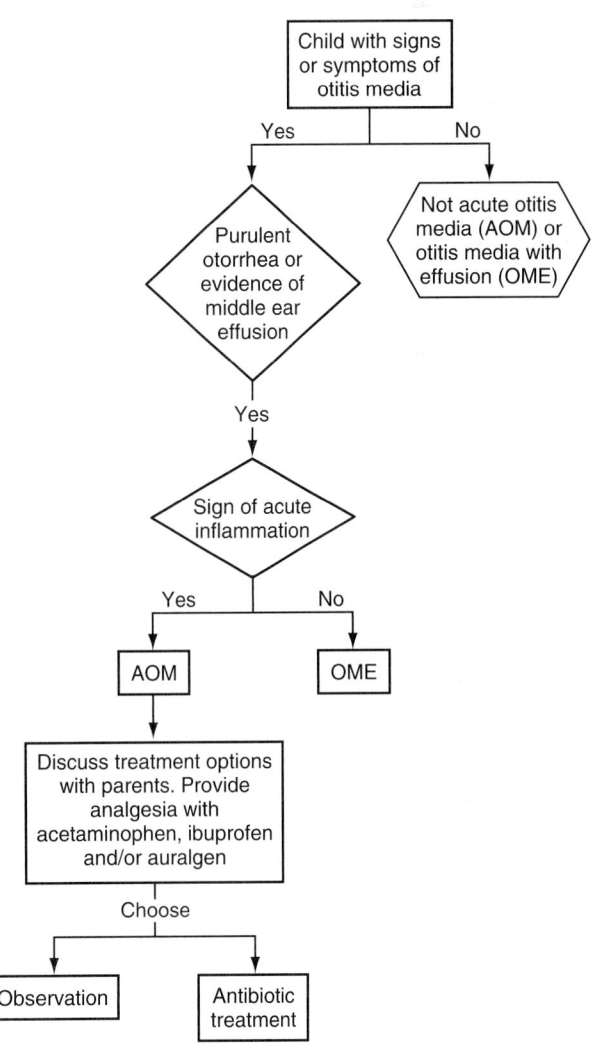

FIGURE 1. Clinical decision flowchart.

Diagnostic uncertainty is acceptable and should be shared with the parent. It requires closer follow-up and re-examination. Parents will accept an honest explanation.

Middle ear effusion (MEE) may be indicated by otorrhea, an obvious air-fluid level behind the tympanic membrane, or a bulging tympanic membrane with distinctly reduced mobility. Conversely, redness is a nonspecific finding that may or may not indicate effusion or infection. Pneumatic otoscopy is strongly recommended for diagnosing MEE, with tympanometry or acoustic reflectometry as confirmatory tests when necessary.

Treatment

Although antimicrobials have proven efficacy for acute otitis media (AOM), initial observation of selected children can also achieve excellent outcomes (as described in the following paragraph). Similarly, delaying interventions for recurrent AOM by 6 months will often provide relief. Otitis media with effusion (OME) is initially managed with watchful waiting for 3 months, but extending this to 6 months increases resolution by 30% to 50%. Recent widespread use of pneumococcal vaccination has provided an extra measure of security for the observation option.

The *observation option* for AOM allows selected children to fight the infection on their own for 48 to 72 hours before starting antibiotics. Children are best suited for observation if age 2 years or older with nonsevere AOM or an uncertain diagnosis. In contrast, observation is not advised for children younger than age 6 months, AOM treatment failures, or AOM relapses (within 30 days), or if children have immune deficiency, craniofacial anomalies, or coexisting streptococcal pharyngitis or bacterial sinusitis.

PAIN MANAGEMENT

All children should receive adequate analgesics (acetaminophen or ibuprofen), especially for the first 24 hours after the diagnosis of AOM. Analgesics, not antibiotics, are the cornerstone of initial pain relief, because the incremental benefit of antibiotics over placebo on natural history is not apparent until day 2 or later. Children who are initially observed should receive prompt antibiotics if symptoms worsen or fail to improve at 48 to 72 hours, which occurs in approximately 25% to 35% of cases. A safety net antibiotic prescription can be given to the family at the initial encounter with instructions to wait 48 to 72 hours before obtaining medication, and to call the physician's office if the prescription is filled.

ANTIBIOTICS

The primary role of antibiotic therapy for AOM is to reduce the risk of suppurative complications in at-risk children. Suppurative complications have an incidence of approximately 1:600 and include mastoiditis, meningitis, facial paralysis, and brain abscess. The guidelines for antibiotic therapy in Table 1 are intended to ensure that

TABLE 1 Criteria for Initial Antibiotics Versus Observation with Acute Otitis Media

Child age	Certain diagnosis or definite acute otitis media*	Uncertain diagnosis or suspected acute otitis media*
Younger than 6 mo	Antibiotics	Antibiotics
6 mo to 2 y	Antibiotics	Antibiotics if severe‡ illness Observe§ if nonsevere‡ illness
2 y or older	Antibiotics if severe‡ illness Observe§ if nonsevere‡ illness	Observe§

*Certain diagnosis implies definitive middle ear effusion plus recent onset of signs and symptoms of middle ear inflammation; uncertain diagnosis implies nondefinitive effusion or signs and symptoms.
†Nonsevere illness is mild otalgia and fever less than 39°C orally (approximately 102°F) or less than 39.5°C (103.1°F) (rectally in the past 24 hours; severe illness is higher fever, moderate to severe otalgia, or both.
‡Observation option is appropriate *only when* follow-up can be assured (by telephone or office visit) and antibiotics started if symptoms worsen or persist by 48 to 72 hours.
Adapted from Lieberthal AS, Ganiats TG, Cox EO, et al: Clinical practice guideline: Diagnosis and management of acute otitis media. Pediatrics 2004;113:1451-1465. *Official AAP/AAFP guideline.*

children at greatest risk for suppurative complications from AOM receive initial antibiotic therapy.

When a decision is reached to treat AOM with antibiotics, a drug should be used that is most likely to eradicate common pathogens. Approximately 25% to 50% of AOM is caused by *Streptococcus pneumoniae*, 15% to 30% by nontypeable *Haemophilus influenzae*, and 3% to 20% by *Moraxella catarrhalis*, of which approximately 0%, 50%, and 100% produce β lactamase. The prevalence of pneumococcal resistance to penicillin is approximately 30% (range 15% to 50%), of which 50% are highly resistant strains. Risk factors for resistant pneumococcus are antibiotic use, young age, day-care attendance, and prior hospitalization.

The optimum duration of AOM therapy is controversial. Short-course therapy (5 days of the amoxicillin and other antibiotics) is an option for children ages 2 years or older, and full-course treatment (7 to 10 days of amoxicillin and other antibiotics) is better for younger children (especially when attending group child care). Better outcomes with full-course therapy have also been demonstrated for children with AOM in the preceding month. Table 2 shows first-line antibiotic choice and dose.

INTRAMUSCULAR ANTIBIOTICS

A single intramuscular dose of ceftriaxone has comparable efficacy to a 7- to 10-day course of oral antibiotics for AOM, but use of ceftriaxone as *initial* therapy should be discouraged.

Rakel and Bope: *Conn's Current Therapy 2006.*

TABLE 2 Recommended Antibiotics for Children with Acute Otitis Media

Clinical situation	Nonsevere illness*	Severe illness*
Initial antibiotic therapy of AOM or clinical failure of observation option at 48–72h	• Amoxicillin 80–90 mg/kg/d • PCN allergy nontype I: cefdinir (Omnicef), Cefuroxime (Ceftin), cefpodoxime† (Vantin) • PCN allergy type I: azithromycin (Zithromax), clarithromycin† (Biaxin) • Amoxicillin-clavulanate (Augmentin), 90 mg/kg/d of amoxicillin with 6.4 mg/kg/d of clavulanate • PCN allergy nontype I: ceftriaxone 3 days† • PCN allergy type I: clindamycin†¹ (Cleocin)	• Amoxicillin-clavulanate (Augmentin), 90 mg/kg/d of amoxicillin with 6.4 mg/kg/d of clavulanate • PCN allergy nontype I: ceftriaxone (Rocephin) 1 or 3 days† • Ceftriaxone (Rocephin) 3 days • PCN allergy type I: tympanocentesis, clindamycin†¹ (Cleocin)

*Nonsevere illness is mild otalgia and fever <39°C orally (approximately 102°F) or <39.5°C (103.1°F) rectally in the past 24 hours; severe illness is higher fever, severe otalgia, or both.
†Type I PCN allergy, or hypersensitivity, is urticaria or anaphylaxis.
Abbreviation: PCN = penicillin.
Adapted from Lieberthal AS, Ganiats TG, Cox EO, et al: Clinical practice guideline: Diagnosis and management of acute otitis media. Pediatrics 2004;113: 1451-1465. *Official AAP/AAFP guideline.*

SURGERY

Children with recurrent AOM who receive tympanostomy tubes avoid 2.0 AOM/child-year, have 67% less AOM than controls, and can generally be managed with antibiotic eardrops. Children with chronic OME who receive tympanostomy tubes have 161 fewer days with effusion during the first year of intubation, a relative decrease of 72% versus no surgery or myringotomy alone. Tubes also improve hearing while patent. Ventilation tubes have no or only marginal beneficial effects on language developmental outcomes in otherwise healthy children who are not at risk for developmental delay.

Surgical candidacy for otitis media depends largely on the following:

• Associated symptoms (e.g., otalgia, hearing loss)
• Frequency and severity of AOM
• Child's risk of developmental delays
• Chance of timely spontaneous resolution of OME

Duration of OME *should not* be the sole operative criteria. A healthy child with chronic bilateral OME but normal development could be safely observed for months (or even years) until spontaneous resolution occurs, but a child with developmental delays could be a surgical candidate after weeks or months depending on individual circumstances.

Initial surgery consists of myringotomy and tympanostomy tube placement; adenoidectomy is withheld unless nasal obstruction is present. *Repeat surgery* consists of adenoidectomy and myringotomy with or without tube placement. Adenoidectomy will reduce the need for future surgery by approximately 50%. Tonsillectomy alone (without adenoidectomy) and myringotomy alone (without tube insertion) are ineffective.

ANTIBIOTIC EARDROPS

Acute tympanostomy tube otorrhea (TTO) in children ages 2 years or younger is most frequently caused by typical AOM pathogens. *Pseudomonas aeruginosa* and *Staphylococcus aureus* are more prevalent in older children, when TTO is related to water exposure or when ear odor is present. Most acute TTO is painless; initial management should consist of daily cleaning of the ear canal by the parents with a cotton wick or a nasal aspirator to remove secretions.

Topical antibiotic eardrops are indicated for persistent or symptomatic TTO, unless there is another bacterial infection that would warrant oral antibiotics (streptococcal pharyngitis, bacterial rhinosinusitis). Antibiotic drops have similar clinical efficacy to oral antibiotics, yet offer higher pathogen eradication and fewer adverse effects. Topical antibiotics achieve middle ear drug levels that are 1000 times higher than those achieved by oral drug. This maximizes efficacy and minimizes selective pressure for bacterial resistance.

Eardrops containing ofloxacin or ciprofloxacin are the only FDA-approved products for topical therapy of TTO. Neomycin and polymyxin are not recommended because they are ototoxic and are poorly effective against common pathogens. Ear drops with a steroid (ciprofloxacin plus dexamethasone) are preferred for TTO with significant otalgia, severe inflammation, or granulation tissue. Antibiotic eardrops overuse can result in fungal overgrowth in the ear canal.

 CURRENT DIAGNOSIS

■ Acute otitis media (AOM) is the presence of middle ear effusion (MEE) with the rapid, usually abrupt, onset of one or more symptoms or signs of inflammation of the middle ear (e.g., otalgia, fever, irritability, distinct bulging or retraction of the tympanic membrane, otorrhea).
■ Otitis media with effusion (OME) is MEE without symptoms or signs of acute middle ear inflammation.
■ Diagnostic accuracy is enhanced by evaluating tympanic membrane movement using pneumatic otoscopy or tympanometry.

CURRENT THERAPY

- More judicious antibiotic use is essential to limit bacterial resistance.
- Strategies for judicious use of antibiotics include: watchful waiting in otitis media with effusion (OME), selective use of the observation option with pain management in acute otitis media (AOM), amoxicillin for severe AOM or in children less than 2 years, surgical prevention (e.g., tubes) in selected cases of children with very frequent AOM, and antibiotic eardrops for AOM with tympanostomy tubes.
- Children with OME who are at risk for delays in speech, language, learning, or development should have prompt evaluation of hearing and may need surgical intervention.
- Pain management must be dealt with as an initial need separate from infection resolution.

Communication and Counseling

Parents should appreciate that otitis media is an almost universal component of early childhood, but one whose incidence disappears slowly between ages 3 and 8 years. Otitis media is best approached by striving for diagnostic accuracy and explaining, acknowledging, and transparent management of uncertainty. Early attention must be paid to discomfort as the natural healing is allowed to occur. Appropriate use of antibiotics and surgery improve quality of life for children with frequent or persistent illness. Educational materials for parents include high-quality brochures from the American Academy of Pediatrics, Centers for Disease Control and Prevention, and the New York State Department of Health. Studies of complementary and alternative medicine currently do not show benefits beyond the already favorable natural history.

REFERENCES

Goldblatt EL, Dohar J, Nozza RJ, et al: Topical ofloxacin versus systemic amoxicillin/clavulanate in purulent otorrhea in children with tympanostomy tubes. Int J Pediatr Otorhinolaryngol 1998;46:91-101. *Study showing comparable clinical efficacy, but better bacteriologic efficacy, for eardrops.*

Gurnaney H, Spor D, Johnson DG, Propp R: Diagnostic accuracy and the observation option in otitis media: The Capital Region Otitis Project: Int J Pediatr Otorhinolaryngol 2004;68:1315-1325. *Results of a multifaceted educational intervention on AOM management attitudes in clinicians.*

Lieberthal AS, Ganiats TG, Cox EO, et al: Clinical practice guideline: Diagnosis and management of acute otitis media. Pediatrics 2004; 113:1451-1465. *Official AAP/AAFP guideline.*

New York Region Otitis Project: Observation Option Toolkit for Acute Otitis Media (State of New York, Department of Health Publication No. 4894). Albany: State of New York, Department of Health, March 2002. *Contains a laminated decision chart and parent education materials.*

Roberts JE, Rosenfeld RM, Ziesel SA: Otitis media and speech and language: A meta-analysis of prospective studies. Pediatrics 2004;113:e238-e248. *Meta-analysis of prospective studies and randomized trials.*

Roland PS, Kreisler LS, Reese B, et al: Topical ciprofloxacin/dexamethasone otic suspension is superior to ofloxacin otic solution in the treatment of children with acute otitis media with otorrhea through tympanostomy tubes. Pediatrics 2004;113:e40-e46. *Comparative efficacy study of two FDA-approved eardrops for treating tympanostomy tube otorrhea.*

Rosenfeld RM: A Parent's Guide to Ear Tubes. Hamilton, Ontario: BC Decker, 2005. *Educational guide for parents that emphasizes shared decision making and appropriate antibiotic use.*

Rosenfeld RM, Bluestone CD (eds.): Evidence-Based Otitis Media, 2nd ed. Hamilton, Ontario: BC Decker, 2003. *Comprehensive overview including extensive evidence-tables.*

Rosenfeld RM, Culpepper L, Doyle KJ, et al. Clinical practice guideline: Otitis media with effusion. Otolaryngol Head Neck Surg 2004; 130:S95-S118. *Official AAP/AAFP/AAO-HNS guideline.*

Rosenfeld RM, Kay DJ: Natural history of untreated otitis media. Laryngoscope 2003;113:1645-1657. *Meta-analysis of cohort studies and placebo groups from randomized trials.*

Siegal RM, Kiely M, Bien JP, et al: Treatment of otitis media with observation and a safety-net antibiotic prescription. Pediatrics 2003;112:527-531.

Episodic Vertigo

Method of
Lorne S. Parnes, MD

For many, if not most, clinicians, assessing a patient with episodic vertigo, which is defined as episodic misperception of the self moving relative to the environment or vice versa, can be daunting. Much of the angst stems from the difficulties and inconsistencies patients have in describing their symptoms, leaving the clinician without a path to follow in corroborating a diagnosis. Thus, obtaining an accurate history is by far the most important but also the most challenging aspect of assessing these patients; however, it gets easier with practice. For many patients, vertigo often is described as a frightening experience. Thus, for those who have recurrent, episodic vertigo, the first bout is often the most memorable because many think they have experienced a graver event, such as a stroke. The term *vertigo* is merely a descriptor, with its physiologic or pathologic source in any part of the nervous system that contributes to spatial orientation. The major contributors to these neurologic signals are the vestibular, visual, and proprioceptive systems, all of which integrate at several levels throughout the brainstem, cerebellum, and cortex.

Everyone experiences normal physiologic bouts of vertigo. One example is the optokinetic-induced vertigo induced by the IMAX theater experience. The visual-vestibular mismatch creates the false perception of the self moving, and the nervous system treats the conflicting signals as a noxious stimulus, resulting in heightened vagal tone with nausea and even vomiting. Another example of vertigo occurs with the common childhood game of spinning around and around and then stopping suddenly. The resulting vestibular-induced vertigo is the sensation of the environment turning around, when of course neither it nor the self is moving at all.

Pathophysiology

There are many physiologic and pathologic causes of vertigo. For a better understanding of the pathophysiology of vestibular-induced vertigo, it is best to think of vertigo as resulting from a steady-state malfunction. The normal physiologic vestibular receptors in the bony labyrinth monitor the motion and position of the head in space by detecting angular and linear acceleration forces. Inside the bony labyrinth is the perilymphatic space, within which there is the membranous labyrinth and its contained endolymphatic space. The two otolith organs, one in the utricle and one in the saccule, in each inner ear monitor linear acceleration forces, including gravity, whereas the three semicircular canals in each inner ear detect angular acceleration. The canals are positioned at near right angles to each other so that they sense movements in any and all planes in space, with the left and right sides complementing each other. Thus, there is redundancy built into this system, which, as will be discussed later in this article, is an important concept in the outcome and treatment of the disease state. Each canal is filled with endolymph and has a swelling at the base that is called the ampulla. The ampulla contains the cupula, a gelatinous mass with the same density as endolymph, which is attached to polarized hair cells.

With the head at rest, the hair cells from both labyrinths emit a steady baseline rate of discharges that induces a steady rate of vestibular nerve impulses. As long as the nerve input at the level of the vestibular nuclei is equal from both labyrinths, the perception will be one of no (head) movement. It is the function of the vestibular end organs to modulate these steady-state signals and interact with the ocular motor system, the locomotive system, and the cognitive region of the brain to stabilize vision with head movements, maintain a stable upright posture against gravity and movement, and produce a conscious three-dimensional awareness of where the head and body are in space. As always, there are feedback loops from each of these systems, and the signals are modulated further by the cerebellum.

Displacement of the neutrally positioned cupula by head turning (an angular acceleration or deceleration) causes either a stimulatory or an inhibitory response of any or all semicircular canals bilaterally, depending on the direction and plane of the motion (Figure 1). It should be noted that the cupula forms an impermeable barrier across the lumen of the ampulla. The term *utriculofugal* refers to cupular movement away from the utricle, whereas *utriculopetal* refers to cupular movement toward the utricle. In the superior and posterior semicircular canals, utriculofugal deflection of the cupula is stimulatory and utriculopetal deflection is inhibitory. The opposite is true for the lateral semicircular canal.

Nystagmus is defined as the repeated and rhythmic oscillation of the eyes. Stimulation (or inhibition) of the semicircular canals most commonly causes jerk nystagmus, which is characterized by a slow phase (slow movement in one direction) followed by a fast phase (rapid movement in the other direction). Although it is the modulated vestibular signal that induces the slow phase, the nystagmus is named according to the direction of the fast phase. The fast phase is in fact a saccade generated by the reticular activating system; this is why nystagmus is more evident during states of heightened consciousness. Nystagmus can be horizontal, vertical, oblique, torsional (rotatory), or any combination and may be induced by vestibular signal asymmetries or disturbances that arise more centrally. The Current Diagnosis section summarizes the important key

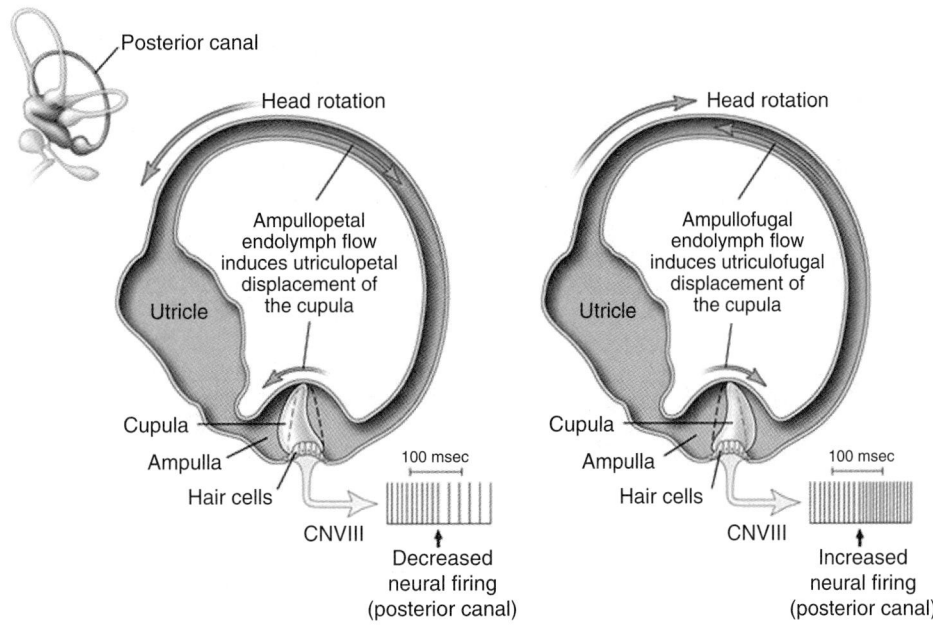

FIGURE 1. Semicircular canal physiology (posterior canal example). (From Parnes LS, Agrawal SK, Atlas J: Diagnosis and management of benign paroxysmal positional vertigo (BPPV). CMAJ 2003;169(7):681-693. Used with permission.)

clinical features that help differentiate peripheral (inner ear) from central causes of vertigo.

Disorders

There are a host of peripheral, central, and other disorders that can cause vertigo (Table 1). Although there is some controversy about whether clinicians should make this differentiation, it is a useful exercise to help make the differential diagnosis. This will help direct the workup, guide the treatment, and, if indicated, direct the patient to the proper specialist. Peripheral disorders induce vertigo through their evoked, nonphysiologic asymmetric central input. Therefore, not surprisingly, the peripheral disorders listed in Table 1 are all typically unilateral.

Ultimately, these disorders resolve with time, returning the system to the normal steady state; alternatively, if the vestibular end organ remains dysfunctional, the system (brain) adjusts to a new norm (vis-á-vis the new steady state). This process is mediated by the cerebellum and brainstem and occurs automatically in most individuals as long as the contralateral vestibular organ remains normal (the redundancy described earlier in this article). The process is facilitated greatly by head, visual, and body motion/stimulation and can be inhibited by vestibular suppressant medication and immobility. Thus, even though patients favor sedentary activity because it tends to minimize the vestibular "asymmetry," anyone with an acute vestibular disorder should be encouraged to ambulate as much and as soon as possible and avoid taking vestibular suppressants such as the benzodiazepines. For many individuals, a formal course of vestibular rehabilitation physiotherapy greatly facilitates the process.

As a result of impaired central compensation, virtually all these acute or episodic inner-ear disorders can become chronic. It therefore is important for the clinician to differentiate between cases of "true" episodic vertigo brought on by head movement (as in benign paroxysmal positional vertigo [BPPV]) and the dysequilibrium arising from the asymmetry of an uncompensated loss that is aggravated by motion.

In addition to an uncompensated unilateral vestibular loss, chronic (vestibular) dysequilibrium may result from bilateral vestibular hypofunction (Box 1). Bilateral disorders provide no backup, without any future possibilities for vestibular compensation. When both sides are affected simultaneously, as is often the case, there is no resultant vestibular asymmetry and thus no initial period of vertigo. The hallmark features, all of which are derived from the absent vestibular input, are gait ataxia, oscillopsia (visual blurring with head movement), and the absence of symptoms with the head at rest. The hallmark vestibular-ocular test findings include reduced caloric responses and abnormal lateral head thrusts bilaterally. Unfortunately, there are few treatments to offer these patients; however, their long-term safety should be considered when they are advised about the operation of heavy machinery and automobiles and counseled on assistive living devices (canes, walkers, and railings). They also must learn to rely more on their visual and proprioceptive systems.

TABLE 1 Causes of Vertigo

	Peripheral	Central	Mixed/other

Single vertigo attack > 24h	• Vestibular neuronitis
	• Viral labyrinthitis
	• Bacterial labyrinthitis
	• Trauma
	• Surgically destructive procedure
		• Vertebrobasilar infarct
		  PICA
		  AICA
		• Cerebellar/brainstem hemorrhage
		• Multiple sclerosis
		• Trauma	

Recurrent (episodic) vertigo	• BPPV
	• Ménière's disease
	• Recurrent vestibulopathy
	
	• Perilymphatic fistula
	  Oval/round window
	  Semicircular canal erosion from cholesteatoma
	  Dehiscent superior semicircular canal syndrome
	• Autoimmune inner-ear disease
	• Large vestibular aqueduct syndrome and other inner-ear malformations
		• Migraine (may have peripheral component)
		  Benign paroxysmal vertigo of childhood
		• Vertrobasilar TIAs
		• Multiple sclerosis
		• Seizures
		• Familial periodic ataxia
		• Arnold-Chiari malformation
			• Psychogenic
			• Cardiac
			• Cervicogenic
			• Microvascular eighth nerve compression

Abbreviations: AICA = anterior inferior cerebellar artery; BPPV = benign paroxysmal positional vertigo; PICA = posterior inferior cerebellar artery; TIAs = transient ischemic attacks.

Rakel and Bope: *Conn's Current Therapy 2006.*

BOX 1 Causes of Chronic Vestibular Dysequilibrium

- Uncompensated unilateral loss
- Vestibulotoxicity (aminoglycosides)
- Congenital/hereditary
- Bilateral Ménière's disease
- Autoimmune disorders
- After meningitic labyrinthitis
- Trauma
- Presbyastasis (aging)
- Chronic radiation effects
- Bilateral acoustic neuromas (neurofibromatosis type 2)
- Idiopathic

BOX 2 Key Considerations in Treatment of Vertigo

- Psychologic (common)
  Stress
  Anxiety
- Lifestyle (common)
  Sleep
  Diet
  Exercise
- Other coexisting illnesses
- Physical therapy (very common)
  Vestibular rehabilitation
  Repositioning maneuvers
- Medication (common)
  Oral
  Intratympanic
  Intravenous (rarely)
- Devices (see Ménière's disease article)
- Surgery
  Nondestructive
  Destructive

Assessment and Management

The article by Eggers and Zee provides a review of bedside and laboratory assessment of patients with vestibular disorders. Box 2 and the Current Therapy box list the important overall and specific medical treatment considerations.

Among all the disorders listed in Table 1 that can cause episodic dizziness and/or vertigo, BPPV is by far the most common, accounting for approximately 20% of patients seen in specialized dizziness clinics. The two other most common disorders that cause episodic vertigo, Ménière's disease and migraine, both have articles in this edition and will not be discussed here. Most of the other listed disorders are uncommon, and in those cases, imaging can be helpful in making a diagnosis. For example, high-resolution temporal bone computed tomography (CT) is useful in the diagnosis of perilymph fistula or large vestibular aqueduct syndrome, whereas magnetic resonance imaging (MRI) is more helpful with central disorders such as multiple sclerosis and vertebrobasilar artery disease.

Recurrent vestibulopathy is relatively common and is essentially a diagnosis of exclusion. These patients have recurrent bouts of vertigo that each last less than 24 hours, similar to Ménière's disease vertigo attacks but without any associated hearing loss, tinnitus, aural fullness, or any other symptoms aside from the vegetative response. This is usually a self-limited disorder, and there is no treatment except symptomatic relief of the acute attacks.

Benign Paroxysmal Positional Vertigo

BPPV is a condition that usually is easy to diagnose and, more important, is readily treated with a simple office-based procedure. BPPV can be caused by either canalithiasis (free-floating endolymph debris) or cupulolithiasis (debris stuck to the cupula) and can affect each of the three semicircular canals, though the vast majority of cases are of the posterior canal variant. Most posterior canal BPPV cases result from canalithiasis because free-floating endolymph debris tends to

gravitate to the posterior canal, which is the most gravity-dependent part of the vestibular labyrinth in both the upright and supine positions. Once debris enters the posterior canal, the cupular barrier at the shorter, more dependent end of the canal blocks the exit of the debris. Therefore, the debris becomes "trapped" and can exit only at the nonampullated end. Once in the canal, the canalith mass moves to a more dependent position when the orientation of the semicircular canal is modified in the gravitational plane. The drag that is created must overcome the resistance of the endolymph in the semicircular canal and the elasticity of the cupular barrier to deflect the cupula. The time needed for this to occur, plus the original inertia of the particles, explains the latency seen during the Dix-Hallpike maneuver.

In the head-hanging position, the canalith mass will move away from the cupula to induce ampullofugal cupular deflection. In the vertical canals, ampullofugal deflection produces an excitatory response. This causes an abrupt onset of vertigo and the typical torsional nystagmus in the plane of the posterior canal. In the left head-hanging position (left posterior canal stimulation), the fast component of the nystagmus beats clockwise as viewed by the examiner. Conversely, the right head-hanging position (right posterior canal stimulation) results in counterclockwise nystagmus. These nystagmus profiles correlate with the known neuromuscular pathways that arise from stimulation of the posterior canal ampullary nerves in an animal model.

This nystagmus is of limited duration because the endolymph drag ceases when the canalith mass reaches the limit of descent, and the cupula then returns to its neutral position. Reversal nystagmus occurs when the patient returns to the upright position; the mass moves in the opposite direction, thus creating a nystagmus in the same plane but in the opposite direction. The response is fatigable because the particles are dispersed along the canal and become less effective in creating endolymph drag and cupular deflection.

LATERAL CANAL BPPV

There is no doubt that by far BPPV most commonly affects the posterior semicircular canal. However, reports on the frequency of the horizontal canal variant vary. The posterior canal hangs inferiorly and has its cupular barrier at its shorter, more dependent end. Any debris that enters the canal essentially becomes trapped within it. Conversely, the lateral canal slopes upward and has its cupular barrier at the upper end. Therefore, free-floating debris in the lateral canal tends to float back out into the utricle with natural head movements, and this probably accounts for the quicker resolution of lateral canal BPPV. By the same token, its incidence probably is underestimated because usually it has resolved by the time the patient is examined.

Although cupulolithiasis is thought to play a greater role in lateral canal BPPV, canalithiasis is still more common. The vertigo is more intense, leading to more nausea, and the induced nystagmus is purely horizontal. Testing for lateral canal BPPV is done with the patient supine, turning the head to one side for a minute or two and then to the other. Depending on the underlying mechanism (cupulolithiasis or canalithiasis), the induced nystagmus can be apogeotropic (fast phase away from the ground) or geotropic (toward the ground), with one side producing a stronger response. Lateral canal testing, diagnosis, and treatment should be carried out in a specialized vestibular clinic.

ETIOLOGY

In most cases, BPPV is found in isolation and is termed primary or idiopathic BPPV, accounting for approximately 50% to 70% of cases. Secondary BPPV can result from head trauma, vestibular neuronitis, Ménière's disease, and migraine and as a complication of inner-ear surgery.

SYMPTOMS

Patients describe sudden, severe attacks of either horizontal or vertical vertigo or a combination of both that is precipitated by certain head positions and movements. The most common movements include rolling in bed, extending the neck to look up, and bending forward. Patients often can identify the affected ear by stating the direction of movement that precipitates the majority of the attacks (e.g., when rolling in bed to the right but not the left precipitates the dizziness, that indicates right ear involvement). The attacks of vertigo typically last less than 30 seconds, but some patients overestimate the duration by several minutes. The reasons for this discrepancy may include the fear associated with the intense vertigo and the nausea and disequilibrium that may follow the attack. Most patients experience several attacks per day.

In addition to vertigo, many patients complain of light-headedness, nausea, imbalance, and, in severe cases, sensitivity to all directions of head movement. Many patients also become extremely anxious for two main reasons: Some fear that the symptoms may represent a sinister underlying disorder such as a brain tumor; for others, the symptoms can be so unsettling that they go to great lengths to avoid the movements that bring on the vertigo. Some may not realize when the condition has resolved, as it often does over time without any treatment. BPPV can be described as self-limited, recurrent, or chronic.

As the name implies, BPPV is most often a benign condition. However, in certain situations it can be dangerous. For example, a painter looking up from the top of a ladder may suddenly become vertiginous and lose his or her balance, risking a bad fall. The same is true for underwater divers, who may get very disoriented

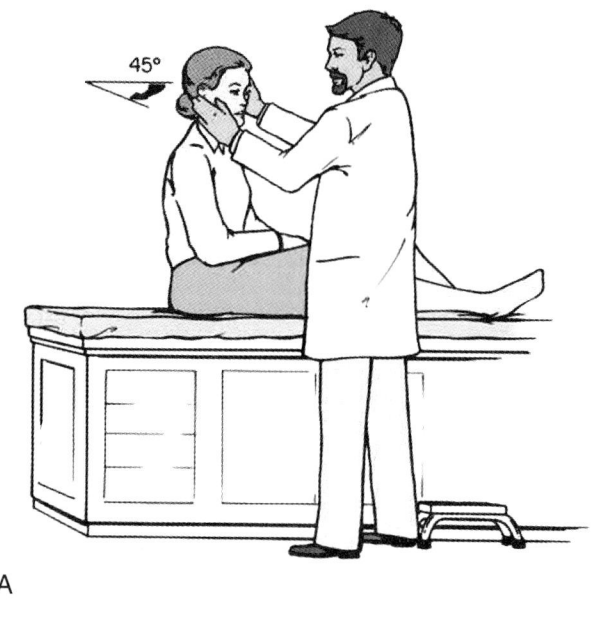

A

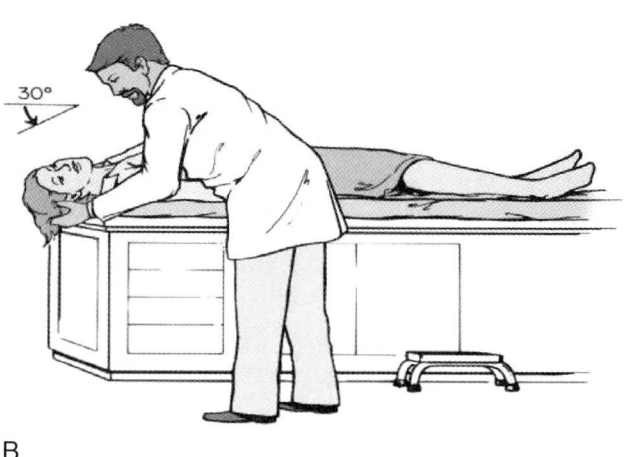

B

FIGURE 2. Dix-Hallpike maneuver (right ear). In this case, with the right side being tested, in position B the examiner should expect to see a fast-phase counterclockwise nystagmus. To complete the maneuver, the patient is returned to the seated position (position A) and the eyes are observed for reversal nystagmus, in this case a fast-phase clockwise nystagmus. (From Parnes LS, Agrawal SK, Atlas J: Diagnosis and management of benign paroxysmal positional vertigo (BPPV). CMAJ 2003;169(7):681-693. Used with permission.)

from acute vertigo. Heavy machinery operators should use great caution, especially if the job involves significant head movement. Most people can drive a car safely as long as they are careful not to tip the head back when checking the blind spot.

The diagnostic maneuver for posterior canal BPPV was described by Dix and Hallpike in 1952 (Figure 2). The patient is seated and positioned so that the head will extend over the edge of the table in the supine position. The head is turned 45 degrees toward the ear that is being tested, and the patient quickly is lowered into the supine position with the head extending below the level of the table. The patient's head is held in this position, and the examiner observes the eyes for nystagmus. After lowering of the head, the typical nystagmus onset has a brief latency (1 to 5 seconds) and a limited duration (typically less than 30 seconds). With the eyes in the midposition (neutral), the nystagmus has a slight vertical component, the fast phase of which is upbeating. There is a stronger torsional component, in the fast phase of which the superior pole of the eye beats toward the affected (dependent) ear. The direction of the nystagmus reverses when the patient is brought into the upright position, and the nystagmus will fatigue with repeat testing. Along with the nystagmus, the patient will describe feeling vertiginous; the intensity of that symptom parallels the nystagmus response. It should be emphasized that the two posterior canals are tested independently, the right with the head turned right and

the left with the head turned left. Overall, the history and eye findings during positional testing are the gold standards for diagnosing BPPV and additional testing is not normally necessary.

MANAGEMENT

The management of BPPV has changed dramatically in the last 20 years as understanding of the condition has progressed. Because medications were found to be largely ineffective, traditionally patients were instructed to avoid positions that induced the vertigo. Although BPPV is usually self-limited, with most cases resolving within 6 months, as the theories of cupulolithiasis and canalithiasis emerged, several noninvasive techniques were developed to correct the pathology directly. Figure 3 demonstrates a maneuver that is called the particle repositioning maneuver (PRM), a variant of the so-called Epley maneuver. With proper understanding of inner-ear anatomy and the pathophysiology of BPPV, appropriately trained health professionals, including family doctors and physiotherapists, should be able to carry out the PRM in most straightforward cases. Atypical cases, nonresponders, and patients with presumed lateral or anterior canal variants should be referred to a tertiary care "dizzy" clinic.

Overall, the PRM should take less than 5 minutes to complete. Studies using the repositioning maneuvers are difficult to compare because they vary considerably

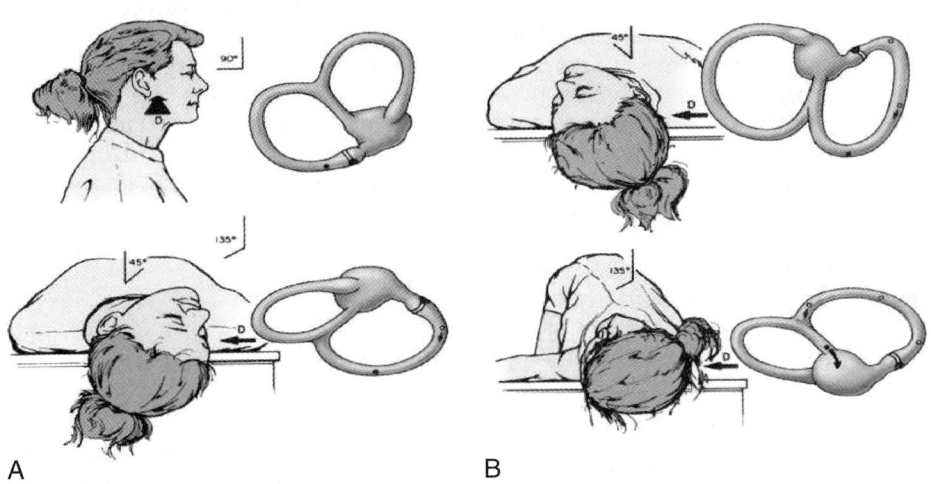

A   B

FIGURE 3. Particle repositioning maneuver (right ear). Schema of patient and concurrent movement of posterior and superior semicircular canals and utricle. The patient is seated on a table as viewed from the right side (**A**). The remaining parts show the sequential head and body positions of a patient lying down as viewed from the top. Before moving the patient into position B, turn the head 45° to the side being treated (in this case the right side). The patient in the normal Dix-Hallpike head-hanging position (**B**). Particles gravitate in an ampullofugal direction and induce utriculofugal cupular displacement and subsequent counterclockwise rotatory nystagmus. This position is maintained for 1 to 2 minutes. The patient's head then is rotated toward the opposite side with the neck in full extension through position C and into position D in a steady motion by rolling the patient onto the opposite lateral side. The change from position B to position D should take no longer than 3 to 5 seconds. Particles continue to gravitate in an ampullofugal direction through the common crus into the utricle. The patient's eyes are observed immediately for nystagmus. If the particles continue to move in the same ampullofugal direction, that is, through the common crus into the utricle, this secondary-stage nystagmus should beat in the same direction as the primary-stage nystagmus. Position D is maintained for another 1 to 2 minutes, and then the patient sits back up to position A. With a successful maneuver there should be no nystagmus or vertigo when the patient returns to the sitting position because the particles already will have been repositioned into the utricle. D = direction of view of labyrinth; *dark circle* = position of particle conglomerate; *open circle* = previous position. (From Parnes LS, Agrawal SK, Atlas J: Diagnosis and management of benign paroxysmal positional vertigo (BPPV). CMAJ 2003; 169(7):681-693. Used with permission.)

CURRENT DIAGNOSIS

	Peripheral	Central
Onset of vertigo	Usually sudden	Sudden or gradual
Severity of vertigo	Often intense and disabling	Less distinct and disabling
Pattern of vertigo	Single self-limited or episodic	Episodic or constant
Vertigo aggravated by head movement	Yes	Not usually
Associated nausea, vomiting, diaphoresis	Frequent and prominent	Infrequent and less severe
Nystagmus type	Horizontal or torsional (or mixed); never vertical	Horizontal, torsional, or vertical
Nystagmus direction	Unidirectional with fast phase usually away from the affected ear (irrespective of direction of gaze)	May be bidirectional; may change direction with changes in direction of gaze
Nystagmus intensity affected by fixation	Intensity decreased or totally suppressed by visual fixation (except torsional variant)	Intensity unaffected or, rarely, enhanced by visual fixation
Nystagmus intensity affected by direction of gaze	Nystagmus intensity may be increased when patient looks in direction of fast phase	Nystagmus intensity usually not affected by direction of gaze
Hearing loss and facial weakness	May be present	Very uncommon
Central nervous system symptoms/signs	Absent	Often present
Gait	Mild to moderate ataxia with tendency to fall toward side of lesion	Moderate to severe ataxia with tendency to fall to either side

in terms of the technique, length of follow-up, number of treatment sessions, number of maneuvers per session, use of sedation, and use of mastoid vibration, but the overall response rate is on the order of 90% to 95%. In the author's clinic, physicians normally do not use sedation and typically perform only one maneuver per session as long as the nystagmus response is favorable (see Figure 3). Contrary to the original recommendations, recent studies suggest that the use of mastoid (skull) oscillation or postmaneuver head movement limitation is unnecessary. Recent evidence suggests that as many as 50% of patients will have at least one long-term recurrence.

For those with troublesome symptoms who have frequent recurrences or do not respond initially to the

PRM, surgical occlusion of the posterior semicircular canal is a safe, reliable alternative. Before the institution of the PRM, free-floating endolymph debris often was seen during these operations, and in one instance it was removed and subjected to electron microscopy and found to be consistent with degenerating otoconia. Presumably, then, otoconia becomes detached from the otolithic membrane in the utricle and migrates downward into the posterior canal, resulting in a case of canalithiasis. This mechanism can result from trauma, inflammation, Ménière's disease, and even migraine but usually occurs spontaneously and probably accounts for the vast majority of BPPV cases.

REFERENCES

Dieterich M: Dizziness. Neurologist 2004;10(3):154-164.

Eggers SD, Zee DS: Evaluating the dizzy patient: Bedside examination and laboratory assessment of the vestibular system. Semin Neurol 2003;23(1):47-58.

Minor LB. Labyrinthine fistulae: Pathobiology and management. Curr Opin Otolaryngol Head Neck Surg 2003;11(5):340-346.

Neuhauser H, Lempert T: Vertigo and dizziness related to migraine: A diagnostic challenge. Cephalalgia 2004;24(2):81-82.

Parnes LS, Agrawal SK, Atlas J: Diagnosis and management of benign paroxysmal positional vertigo (BPPV). CMAJ 2003;169(7):681-693.

Ruckenstein MJ: Autoimmune inner ear disease. Curr Opin Otolaryngol Head Neck Surg 2004;12(5):426-430.

Strupp M, Zingler VC, Arbusow V, et al: Methylprednisolone, valacyclovir, or the combination for vestibular neuritis. N Engl J Med 2004;351(4):354-361.

Welling DB, Parnes LS, O'Brien B, et al: Particulate matter in the posterior semicircular canal. Laryngoscope 1997;107(1):90-94.

CURRENT THERAPY

Target symptom	Medication type
Motion sickness prevention	• Motion sickness medications
Vertigo prevention	• Diuretics • Vasodilators • Vestibular suppressants
Nausea and vomiting	• Antiemetics • Vestibular suppressants
Co-morbid conditions, symptoms	• Anxiolytics • Antidepressants • Sedatives
Autoimmune, inflammatory	• Corticosteroids—oral and intratympanic
Destructive	• Aminoglycosides—intratympanic (rarely intravenous)

Ménière's Disease

Method of
Ronald K. de Venecia, MD, PhD, and
Joseph B. Nadol Jr., MD

Ménière's "disease" is more accurately termed Ménière's "syndrome" because a single causative agent is unknown, and in fact, is unlikely. It is characterized by episodic vertigo; fluctuating, sensorineural hearing loss; aural fullness; and tinnitus. In 1861, Prosper Ménière first attributed the symptoms to a disorder of the semicircular canals rather than the central nervous system. In 1938, Yamakawa, and then Hallpike and Cairns independently reported the histopathologic finding of endolymphatic hydrops in the inner ears of patients with Ménière's syndrome (Figure 1). With this associated "lesion," the term Ménière's disease came to be applied when the syndrome could not be specifically attributed to another disorder. Although the pathophysiologic mechanism underlying Ménière's disease likely involves a disruption of homeostasis of inner ear fluid, the mechanism and the pathophysiology of the symptoms remain uncertain. The description of endolymphatic hydrops in patients *without* Ménière's syndrome and animal studies that demonstrate typical cytochemical abnormalities in the cochlea before hydrops develops suggest that endolymphatic hydrops may be an epiphenomenon rather than directly responsible for the symptoms. Ménière's syndrome can be caused by otosyphilis, involvement of the inner ear in collagen vascular diseases, as a delayed posttraumatic syndrome, obstruction of the endolymphatic duct, or may be idiopathic.

The natural history of Ménière's syndrome is highly variable. The classic triad of spontaneous episodic rotational vertigo, fluctuating hearing loss, and tinnitus are often accompanied by aural fullness and pressure. Although vertiginous attacks are the most debilitating

symptom, they can vary in frequency with intervals of hours to months. Clusters of attacks may be separated by periods of long remission. Balance function between attacks can be normal, although a sense of disequilibrium often persists later in the clinical course. An estimated 2% to 6% of patients with Ménière's syndrome of long duration can experience "drop attacks" (otolithic crisis of Tumarkin), characterized by being abruptly thrown to the ground without loss of consciousness and with little or no vertigo. Increases in aural pressure, tinnitus, and hearing loss classically precede or accompany attacks of vertigo. A previously described variant termed "vestibular Ménière's disease" (episodic vertigo without cochlear symptoms) is best recognized as recurrent vestibulopathy or recurrent vestibular neuritis. Spontaneous remission of vertigo has been reported in up to 70% of patients within 8 years.

The hearing loss in Ménière's syndrome is a fluctuating, low-frequency sensorineural loss early in the clinical course. Eventually, the loss becomes irreversible, often progressing in severity with involvement of higher frequencies and loss of speech discrimination. In contrast, in Lermoyez syndrome, occurring in 1% of Ménière patients, attacks of vertigo are accompanied by transient improvement in hearing. The tinnitus in Ménière's syndrome is commonly described as a low-pitched roaring or similar to a seashell noise. So-called cochlear Ménière's disease (fluctuating hearing loss and tinnitus without vertigo) may represent a different disease process if the symptoms do not evolve into a classic Ménière pattern.

The prevalence rate of Ménière's syndrome in the United States is 15 per 100,000 persons. However, reported rates per 100,000 persons in other countries vary widely from 4 in Japan, to 46 in Sweden, to 157 in Great Britain. The peak incidence is in the 40- to 60-year-old age group, with a nearly equal female to male ratio (1.3:1). Estimates of symptoms arising in the opposite ear vary from 2% to 50%. Whether the variability in prevalence rates is caused by differences in environment, genetics, or diagnostic criteria is unclear.

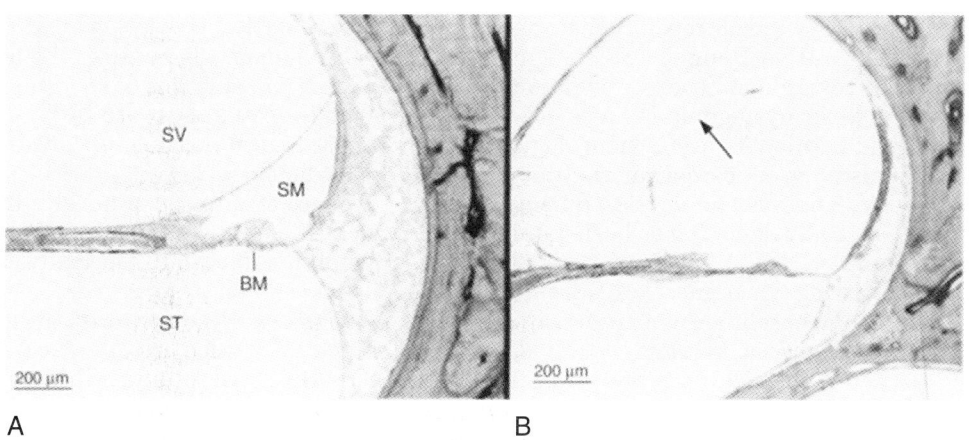

FIGURE 1 Photomicrographs of sections through the cochlea of (**A**) a 43-year-old man showing the normal appearance of the membranous labyrinth, and (**B**) a 79-year-old man with Ménière's syndrome during life showing pathologic distension of Reissner membrane *(arrow)* into the scala vestibuli *(SV)* characteristic of endolymphatic hydrops. *Abbreviations*: BM = basilar membrane below the organ of Corti; SM = scala media; ST = scala tympani.

Diagnosis

The diagnosis of Ménière's syndrome is primarily based on the medical history. According to established guidelines, a definite diagnosis requires the following:

- Two or more definitive episodes of spontaneous rotational vertigo lasting at least 20 minutes
- Low frequency sensorineural hearing loss documented by audiometry
- Tinnitus or aural fullness in the affected ear
- Exclusion of other causes for the symptoms

Importantly, the constellation of vertigo, hearing loss, and tinnitus does not automatically confirm a diagnosis of Ménière's disease. The definitive vertiginous attack is sudden in onset, lasts 20 minutes but abates by 24 hours, and is often prostrating with nausea and vomiting. Typically, any movement during an attack aggravates the vertigo. The presence of neurologic signs or symptoms such as syncope, visual aura, and motor weakness suggest another diagnosis. Perceived hearing loss can be difficult to verify without audiometry, especially during an exacerbation of tinnitus or aural pressure. Asking patients to log their symptoms and perceived triggers helps to confirm a characteristic Ménière pattern. Disorders that can present with similar symptoms include migraine, acoustic neuroma, perilymphatic fistula, dehiscence of the superior semicircular canal, labyrinthitis, otosyphilis, autoimmune inner ear disorder, Cogan's syndrome, and multiple sclerosis.

The findings on physical examination are remarkably normal in most patients with Ménière's syndrome. A detailed head and neck exam should be performed to exclude other disorders. Otoscopic evaluation typically reveals a normal external and middle ear. Testing with a tuning fork (Rinne and Weber tests) confirms a sensorineural hearing loss. The Hallpike maneuver helps to exclude positional vertigo. Useful signs of inner ear pathology, although not specific for Ménière's syndrome, include diplacusis and Hennebert's sign. Diplacusis is present if the frequency of a tone differs between ears or is perceived as two tones in one ear. Testing for Hennebert's sign involves application of positive and negative pressure to an intact tympanic membrane using a pneumatic otoscope. A positive Hennebert's sign in Ménière's syndrome is induction of ocular deviation although induction of a rapid nystagmus is more suspicious for perilymphatic fistula. A careful neurologic evaluation usually reveals no gross cerebellar dysfunction or other focal deficit. The nystagmus seen during an attack of vertigo is classically described as horizontal or horizontal/rotary.

Extensive laboratory testing for Ménière's syndrome is usually not warranted. A baseline audiogram with pure-tone average and speech discrimination is required. Because hearing fluctuates early during the clinical course, the audiogram may be normal. If so, a second audiogram should be obtained when the patient is experiencing a decrease in hearing. Additional diagnostic studies are obtained only if clinical suspicion of an alternative diagnosis exists. Serology for syphilis should be obtained if bilateral symptoms are present or if

suspected by history. Magnetic resonance imaging with gadolinium contrast is the most useful initial imaging study to rule out retrocochlear pathology, such as acoustic neuroma, in atypical cases. Auditory brainstem response testing also can detect retrocochlear disease. Vestibular testing (electronystagmography, caloric and rotational testing, and dynamic posturography) is used judiciously to differentiate peripheral vestibular hypofunction from a central disorder, but may be completely normal, particularly early in the course of the disorder. Elevation of the ratio of summating potential and action potential (SP/AP) on electrocochleography may provide objective evidence of the presence of endolymphatic hydrops. However, the diagnostic utility of the test is limited by the variability of the ratio both in Ménière patients and in normal individuals.

Treatment

There is no cure for Ménière's syndrome. The principal therapeutic objective is control of vertigo. Current medical treatments to reduce the symptoms are empirical in nature, based on the objective of maintaining homeostasis of inner ear fluid. Dietary salt restriction and diuretics are the mainstays of therapy. Sodium restriction to less than 1.5 g per day is the primary therapy. A food guide helps patients to monitor salt intake and adjust dietary habits. Caffeine and alcohol consumption are also discouraged. If salt restriction fails to control symptoms, then a combination thiazide and triamterene diuretic such as Dyazide[1] (one tablet daily) is added until symptoms abate. For acute control of severe attacks of vertigo that may be accompanied by nausea and vomiting, we prescribe lorazepam (Ativan),[1] 0.5 to 1 mg, taken

---

[1]Not FDA approved for this indication.

 CURRENT DIAGNOSIS

- Diagnosis primarily based on detailed history and physical
- Definite diagnosis requires the following:
  At least two episodes of spontaneous vertigo lasting 20 minutes to 24 hours
  Sensorineural hearing loss documented by audiometry
  Presence of tinnitus or aural fullness
  Exclusion of other causes for the symptoms
- Symptoms fluctuate, especially early in the clinical course.
- Attacks of vertigo are prostrating in intensity.
- Attacks of vertigo are often accompanied by increased aural fullness, tinnitus, or hearing loss.
- Early hearing loss is typically low frequency sensorineural.
- General physical and otoscopic exam is usually normal, other than hearing loss and the presence of nystagmus during an attack.

Rakel and Bope: *Conn's Current Therapy 2006.*

CURRENT THERAPY

- Primary goal of treatment is to control vertiginous attacks.
- Mainstay of medical treatment is dietary salt restriction to less than 1.5 grams daily.
- Diuretics (typically a thiazide) are used as necessary to control frequency of vertiginous attacks.
- Sublingual lorazepam (Ativan)[1] can be used acutely to alleviate vertigo during an attack.
- Long-term daily use of vestibular suppressants (e.g., meclizine [Antivert],[1] benzodiazepines) are not recommended.
- Surgical treatments are reserved for failure of medical treatment and start with the least invasive procedures (e.g., intratympanic gentamicin[1] injection).

[1]Not FDA approved for this indication.

Carey J: Intratympanic gentamicin for the treatment of Ménière's disease and other forms of peripheral vertigo. Otolaryngol Clin North Am 2004;37:1075-1090.

Claes J, Van de Heyning PH: A review of medical treatment for Ménière's disease. Acta Otolaryngol Suppl 2000;544:34-39.

Committee on Hearing and Equilibrium, American Academy of Otolaryngology–Head and Neck Surgery: Ménière's disease: Criteria for diagnosis and evaluation of therapy for reporting. Otolaryngol Head Neck Surg 1995;113:181-185.

Gianoli GJ, Larouere MJ, Kartush JM, Wayman J: Sac-vein decompression for intractable Ménière's disease: Two-year treatment result. Otolaryngol Head Neck Surg 1998;118:22-29.

Glasscock ME III, Gulya AJ, Pensak ML, Black JN: Medical and surgical management of Ménière's disease. Am J Otolaryngol 1984; 5:536-542.

Jackson CG, Glasscock ME III, Hughes GB, et al: Medical management of Ménière's disease. Ann Otol Rhinol Laryngol 1981;90: 142-147.

Merchant SN, Adams JC, Nadol J Jr: Pathophysiology of Ménière's syndrome: Are symptoms caused by endolymphatic hydrops? Otol Neurotol 2005;115:74-78.

Van Deelen GW, Huizing EH: Use of a diuretic (Dyazide) in the treatment of Ménière's disease: A double-blind cross-over placebo-controlled study. ORL Head Neck Nurs 1986;48:287-292.

sublingually to assure rapid systemic drug delivery. Long-term use of vestibular suppressants such as diazepam (Valium)[1] and meclizine (Antivert)[1] is not recommended because they retard central vestibular compensation. Although high-dose oral steroids and intratympanic steroid injection have been anecdotally reported as helpful in controlling frequent vertigo attacks with severe drops in hearing, the efficacy of these treatments was not proved and not routinely recommended. Patients with persistent baseline disequilibrium may benefit from vestibular physical therapy.

For patients who fail medical management of vertigo, a chemical or surgical ablative therapy is recommended. Low dose intratympanic injection of gentamicin[1] partially ablates the vestibular labyrinth with a low risk of hearing loss and a 60% to 90% rate of controlling vertigo. In selected bilateral cases, intramuscular aminoglycoside injections may control attacks of vertigo but bear the risk of creating chronic imbalance and oscillopsia. Decompression of the endolymphatic sac is said to control vertigo in 60% of cases with minimal risk to hearing and balance. However, some clinical trials suggest that this procedure has only a placebo effect. Labyrinthectomy and vestibular neurectomy have 95% control rates but sacrifice vestibular function. Labyrinthectomy additionally results in total hearing loss. Bilateral disease is a relative contraindication for these ablative procedures. The 1% to 2% of Ménière patients who develop bilateral severe-profound sensorineural hearing loss may benefit from cochlear implantation.

REFERENCES

Bretlau P, Thomsen J, Tos M, Johnsen NJ: Placebo effect in surgery for Ménière's disease: A nine year follow-up. Am J Otolaryngol 1989;10:259-261.

[1]Not FDA approved for this indication.

Rakel and Bope: *Conn's Current Therapy 2006.*

3

Sinusitis

Method of
Scott C. Manning, MD

Background and Diagnosis

Rhinosinusitis is the most commonly reported chronic condition of adults on health surveys, affecting up to 14% of the U.S. population. On validated general health outcome measures, a history of sinusitis is associated with significant increases in scores for body pain, impaired social functioning, and general health problems. As with respiratory tract disease in general, health statistics show an increasing prevalence of sinusitis as an ambulatory clinic primary diagnosis over the past 2 decades. Rhinosinusitis accounts for approximately 12% of all antibiotic prescriptions in the United States, and it represents the fifth most common diagnosis for which antibiotics are prescribed.

Despite its prevalence, no specific symptom or sign defines sinusitis. For adults, the most common symptoms include congestion, facial pressure, nasal discharge, dental pain, cough, loss of smell, and headache. Headache as the principal symptom actually correlates with a greater likelihood of normal sinus imaging findings. For children, the most common symptoms include congestion, nighttime cough, fatigue, and irritability. Persistence of symptoms beyond the usual 7- to 10-day course of a viral upper respiratory infection most commonly defines clinical rhinosinusitis.

Imaging studies are helpful to confirm (or rule out) sinusitis, but they must be interpreted in light of clinical signs and symptoms. Air-fluid levels, frontal or sphenoid disease, and complete sinus opacification correlate more strongly with clinical symptoms. The finding of clear sinuses on imaging correlates with the absence of symptoms (except headache). Computed tomography (CT) demonstrates sinus anatomy in more detail than plain radiographs, but findings of mucosal thickening on CT in general do not correlate well with clinical signs and symptoms, especially in children. In fact, up to 70% of young children undergoing CT for non–sinus-related diagnoses in the winter have findings of sinus mucosal thickening.

Children and adults are estimated to average eight and four viral upper respiratory tract infections, respectively, per year, and approximately 2% of these episodes are believed to progress to bacterial infections of the sinus cavities. The second most common predisposing condition is allergic rhinitis, present in at least 60% of patients with chronic or recurrent rhinosinusitis. Gastroesophageal reflux, cigarette smoking, other environmental pollutants, and immunodeficiency also are potential predisposing conditions. Healthy sinuses are a consequence of adequate local and systemic immune defenses, mucociliary function, and sinus drainage and ventilation.

Acute Sinusitis

Acute sinusitis is usually defined as upper respiratory signs and symptoms persisting beyond the usual course of a viral illness, but for less than 3 weeks. In placebo-controlled studies, the rate of spontaneous resolution of symptoms is at least 40%. The most commonly cultured organisms in radiographically documented acute sinusitis cases are *Streptococcus pneumoniae* and nontypeable *Haemophilus influenzae*. While unusual in adults, *Moraxella catarrhalis* is cultured from approximately 20% of pediatric cases. *Staphylococcus aureus* can be cultured from approximately 30% of healthy noses, but it is unusual in specimens obtained from maxillary sinus taps in acute sinusitis. The usual recommendation for initial antibiotic therapy for uncomplicated pediatric acute sinusitis is still amoxicillin (Amoxil), although at higher doses (80 mg/kg/day for pediatric patients), in order to overcome the intermediate penicillin resistance of *S. pneumoniae*. The fact that studies usually fail to show improved outcomes for acute pediatric sinusitis with other drugs despite a growing incidence of β-lactamase resistance with *M. catarrhalis* and *H. influenzae* may in part be because of the lower virulence and higher spontaneous resolution rates of those organisms versus *S. pneumoniae*. Backup drugs for amoxicillin failure for acute sinusitis include amoxicillin/clavulanate, cefuroxime, cefdinir, and macrolides. The usual recommended treatment time course is 10 days.

Chronic Sinusitis

Chronic sinusitis is classically defined as persistence of symptoms beyond 3 months, but a far more common history is that of symptoms that improve with therapy and then recur. In contrast to acute sinusitis, nontypeable *H. influenzae* is more commonly cultured in maxillary tap studies along with *S. aureus,* gram-negative bacteria, and anaerobes. Chronic infections are also much more likely to be polymicrobial. Although maxillary sinus puncture and culture remain the gold standard for antimicrobial selection, it is not commonly performed in routine clinical settings. However, culture of purulent secretions from the middle meatus or nasal vestibule under direct visualization with an endoscope or otoscope correlates well with maxillary tap results and should be performed routinely to identify the organism(s) and sensitivity profile(s). For empirical therapy of adult chronic sinusitis, after considering prevailing resistance patterns, drug concentrations in sinus fluid and other pharmacodynamic and pharmacokinetic properties, a recent practice management consortium has recommended fluoroquinolones, amoxicillin/clavulanate, high-dose amoxicillin, or cefdinir as initial therapy. Patients with chronic sinusitis are commonly treated for 2 to 3 weeks (poor concentration levels in sinus fluid) to achieve bacterial eradication and recovery of mucosal defense.

Although study data are limited, topical antibiotic therapy holds promise as a way to potentially overcome microbial resistance with high antibiotic concentration. One empirical regimen is mupirocin[1] ointment or cream (Bactroban) (5 g in 45 mL nasal saline), at a dose of two squirts in each nostril twice a day. Some clinicians recommend gentamicin (Garamycin)[1] (1 g in 1 L of saline) nasal irrigation if the patient is demonstrated to have a gram-negative infection. A few commercial enterprises have begun supplying compounded antibiotic powder or solution (based upon culture and sensitivity results) delivered nasally via a nebulizer.

Care must be used in targeting appropriate antimicrobial therapy to identified organisms for limited defined periods. Antibiotic overuse and shotgunning multiple antibiotics without culture guidance have been shown to alter normal flora competitive inhibition and to increase the potential for resistant polymicrobial infection.

Perhaps the most significant new insights into chronic sinusitis involve the concept of the upper and lower airways as a unified system with eosinophilic inflammation in the background of a large percentage of cases of respiratory tract illness. Chronic or recurrent sinusitis is strongly associated with allergic rhinitis and bronchial hyperreactivity. Strategies designed to help reduce nasal inflammation can improve mucociliary function and improve sinus ventilation and are often necessary to break a cycle of recurrent disease. Daily nasal saline lavages can help to remove allergens and bacteria. Topical cromolyn sodium (Intal)[1] can help by stabilizing mast cells but works best when started before a known allergy season. Topical nasal steroids are the most potent treatment for nasal congestion and have been shown to potentiate the treatment benefit of antibiotics in placebo-controlled trials of adult

---

[1]Not FDA approved for this indication.

chronic sinusitis. Azelastine hydrochloride (Astelin)[1] is approved by the Food and Drug Administration (FDA) for age 12 years and older as an antihistamine nasal spray; it is particularly beneficial for symptoms of eustachian tube dysfunction. Leukotriene inhibitors (montelukast [Singulair]) recently received FDA approval for seasonal rhinitis, and study data show particular benefit when these medications are combined with oral antihistamines. Immunotherapy is generally considered for documented allergens when patients desire greater symptom relief after trying pharmacologic therapy.

Fungal disease has received significant attention recently as a possible cause of chronic sinusitis in immunocompetent patients. This conclusion is based upon the culture of fungal organisms from nasal secretions of affected patients. All normal control patients also grew fungi from nasal secretions using careful culturing techniques, which is not surprising given the ubiquitous nature of fungal spores. True allergic fungal sinusitis is characterized by nasal polyps, atopic history, and allergic mucin within sinus cavities (eosinophils, scattered fungal elements, and Charcot-Leyden crystals). Treatment usually consists of surgery, topical and systemic steroids, and immunotherapy.

---

[1]Not FDA approved for this indication.

BOX 1   Treatment Options for Chronic Rhinosinusitis

Reduce Viral Exposure
- Handwashing, alcohol hand lotions
- Smaller daycare

Environmental Irritants
- Daily use of nasal saline lavages
- Cessation (or avoidance) of smoking (cigarette smoke)
- Avoidance of paint, perfume, chlorine (patients with chemical sensitivities)

Allergy Management
- Environmental measures for dustmites and mold
- Oral antihistamines
- Nasal antihistamines
- Leukotriene receptor antagonists (montelukast [Singulair])
- Nasal steroids
- Systemic steroid burst
- Allergy immunotherapy

Gastroesophageal Reflux Management
- H$_2$ blockers
- Proton pump inhibitors

Antibiotic Therapy
- Topical antibiotic sprays
- High-dose amoxicillin (Amoxil)
- Fluoroquinolones
- Amoxicillin/clavulanate (Augmentin)
- Cefdinir (Omnicef)

Surgery
- Adenoidectomy (usually young children)
- Inferior turbinate reduction (chronic congestion)
- Endoscopic ethmoidectomy, middle meatus antrostomies

Rakel and Bope: *Conn's Current Therapy 2006.*

CURRENT DIAGNOSIS

- Allergic rhinitis is present in at least 60% of patients with chronic or recurrent sinusitis.
- The most common cause of sinusitis is viral upper respiratory infections that progress to bacterial sinus infections.
- No specific symptom or sign is diagnostic of sinusitis. The most common symptoms are nasal congestion and discharge, facial pressure, dental pain, cough, loss of smell, and headache.
- Computed tomography is better than plain radiographs for showing mucosal thickening, but this thickening does not correlate well with clinical signs and symptoms, especially in children.

Adjunctive Therapy

Common oral decongestants include phenylpropanolamine[2] and pseudoephedrine. They have not been shown to change the course of clinical respiratory tract disease, and they must be used with caution in patients younger than 3 years and older than 65 years of age, and those with a history of thyroid disease, hypertension, or depression (interaction with monoamine oxidase inhibitors). Similarly, the topical alpha agonists, such as oxymetazoline (Afrin), have not been shown to shorten the course of sinusitis, and they can lead to symptomatic rebound congestion within 1 week of use.

Guaifenesin (Robitussin) is the most commonly used mucolytic, and it is often found in combination with decongestants. High doses (up to 2400 mg per day in adults) are required for a mucous thinning effect, but side effects such as abdominal pain and nausea are common at those doses.

Daily use of nasal saline has been shown to be better than no therapy in prospective controlled studies for relief of nasal symptoms. Among nutritional therapies,

---

[2]Not available in the United States.

CURRENT THERAPY

- Spontaneous resolution occurs in at least 40% of patients with acute sinusitis
- If amoxicillin, the first choice antibiotic in acute sinusitis, fails go next to amoxicillin/clavulanate (Augmentin), cefuroxime (Ceftin), cefdinir (Omnicef), or a macrolide.
- Management of chronic sinusitis should be guided by culture. Recommended antibiotics include a fluoroquinolone, amoxicillin/clavulanate, high dose amoxicillin, or cefdinir for 2 or 3 weeks.
- Topical antibiotics into each nostril twice daily may be useful in chronic sinusitis.

vitamin C[1] and echinacea[1] have mild antihistamine effects at high doses, but, along with zinc[1] and goldenseal,[1] they have not been shown to prevent or to speed resolution of sinusitis.

Sinusitis is a potential endpoint of many etiologic pathways. The problem of chronic sinusitis is rarely solved simply by trying to match an antibiotic to the suspected bacterial culprit. Strategies to reduce underlying mucosal inflammation to help restore sinus ventilation and local mucociliary defense are necessary to break a cycle of recurrent infection. Referral to an otolaryngologist should be considered for refractory symptoms, persistent polyposis, disease in an immunocompromised patient, or concern for developing orbital or intracranial infection. In general, surgery is reserved for the small percentage of patients with image-documented, persistent symptomatic disease after completing an appropriate hierarchy of medical options (Box 1).

---

[1]Not FDA approved for this indication.

Nonallergic Rhinitis

Method of
Laura Waikart, MD, and Phillip Lieberman, MD

Epidemiology

Rhinitis is defined as inflammation of the membranes lining the nose. The symptoms include sneezing, nasal congestion, postnasal drainage, and anterior rhinorrhea. Chronic rhinitis may be either allergic or nonallergic in origin. Nonallergic rhinitis is distinguished from its allergic counterpart by the absence of a clinically relevant IgE antibody response to aeroallergens. Thus, the diagnosis of chronic nonallergic rhinitis is one of exclusion. Nonallergic rhinitis is not a single disorder; it consists of a variety of syndromes that manifest the above-mentioned symptoms and share a single characteristic: the absence of allergy.

The frequency of nonallergic rhinitis and of the various syndromes that make up this broad class of disease is estimated to be 17% to 57% of all rhinitis patients worldwide (Table 1). Based on the findings of one of the studies conducted by the National Rhinitis Classification Task Force, a nationwide epidemiologic survey of patients in the outpatient setting is currently underway. This survey, which uses a patient-screening tool for rhinitis, is being conducted in 25,000 office-based nonallergy practices nationwide. The goal of this study is to develop better epidemiologic data on the incidence of allergic, nonallergic, and mixed (allergic and nonallergic) disease

and to assess the diagnostic usefulness of the rhinitis screening tool. Interim data in 3500 patients show that 32% of patients have allergic rhinitis, 22% have nonallergic rhinitis, and 46% have mixed rhinitis.

Nonallergic rhinitis is more prevalent in adults older than the age of 20 years (approximately 70%), whereas allergic disease is more common in patients younger than 20 years of age. Female gender may also be a risk factor for nonallergic rhinitis.

Pathophysiology and Classification

VASOMOTOR RHINITIS

Nonallergic rhinitis is classified into distinct syndromes based on etiologic and cytologic features (Table 2). Vasomotor rhinitis (VMR), or idiopathic perennial nonallergic rhinitis, is the most common of these syndromes (61%). The term *vasomotor* implies a vascular or neurologic dysfunction but is perhaps a misnomer because no mechanism of production has been established. The syndrome is unrelated to allergy, infection, structural lesions, systemic disease, or drug use. VMR probably results from multiple causes. The symptoms are similar to those of allergic rhinitis without the pruritus. VMR is characterized by nonspecific nasal hyperreactivity on exposure to nonimmunologic stimuli. Mucosal biopsy may reveal an increase in mast cells similar to allergic rhinitis but without an increase in goblet cells. Stimuli include changes in temperature or relative humidity, ingestion of alcohol, strong odors (perfumes, hair spray, paint products), and airborne irritants (chemical cleaning products, tobacco smoke, and automobile exhaust fumes). Hyperreactivity of the nasal mucosa to capsaicin (Zostrix), histamine, and methacholine in vivo has been demonstrated.

NONALLERGIC RHINITIS EOSINOPHILIA SYNDROME

Nonallergic rhinitis with eosinophilia syndrome (NARES), first described in 1981, is characterized by increased nasal eosinophilia and makes up 15% to 20% of nonallergic rhinitis cases. The pathophysiology is unknown. Patients present with profuse watery rhinorrhea and nasal pruritus. Patients may also report hyposmia or anosmia. Eosinophilia, the hallmark of this syndrome, may contribute to nasal mucosal dysfunction owing to the release of major basic protein and eosinophil cationic protein. These toxins damage nasal ciliated epithelium and prolong mucociliary clearance. Nasal polyps are often associated with nasal eosinophils; consequently, concerns have been raised that nasal eosinophilia may be a precursor to the aspirin-induced tetrad syndrome (NARES, asthma, sinusitis, and nasal polyps). Blood eosinophilia nonallergic rhinitis syndrome (BENARS), a related disorder that accounts for approximately 4% of all nonallergic rhinitis cases, is associated with an increase in blood eosinophils.

TABLE 1 Frequency of Occurrence of Rhinitis

Investigator (year)	N	Allergic rhinitis	Nonallergic rhinitis	Mixed rhinitis
Mullarkey (1980)	142	48%	52%	Not studied
Enberg (1989)	152 (128)	54%	30%	16%
Togias (1990)	362	83%	17%	Not studied
ECRHS (1999)	1412	75%	25%	Not studied
NRCTF (1999)	975	43%	23%	34%

Abbreviations: N = Number of patients.

BASOPHILIC/METACHROMATIC NASAL DISEASE

A subcategory of nonallergic rhinitis is basophilic/metachromatic cell nasal disease, or nasal mastocytosis. Mast cell infiltration (>2000/mm^3) requires, like NARES, a histologic diagnosis. Likely symptoms include profuse rhinorrhea and congestion without significant sneezing or pruritus. The cause of this syndrome is unknown.

DRUG-INDUCED RHINITIS

Multiple drugs can cause nonallergic rhinitis symptoms (Box 1). Rhinitis medicamentosa commonly describes the rebound nasal congestion that occurs with overuse of decongestant nasal sprays as well as cocaine abuse. Underlying rhinitis can lead to this type of overuse. The rebound swelling of this disorder can be the result of interstitial edema without vasodilation. A number of oral agents, such as antihypertensives, hormones, and other drugs, also can cause rhinitis. In addition, eyedrops, via transit through the nasal-lacrimal duct, also can produce this syndrome.

ENDOCRINE-INDUCED OR HORMONALLY INDUCED RHINITIS

Oral contraceptives, estrogen replacement therapy, pregnancy, hypothyroidism, and acromegaly can cause rhinitis. Pregnancy can produce rhinitis characterized mainly by congestion because of increased blood volume in combination with hormonally induced vasodilation. Rhinitis has been estimated to affect up to 30% of pregnant women. It most commonly develops at approximately the second month of pregnancy and frequently persists until after delivery or the cessation of breastfeeding. Hypothyroidism and acromegaly both can cause turbinate hypertrophy.

TABLE 2 Classification of Nonallergic Rhinitis Based on Etiologic and Cytologic Features

Nonallergic rhinitis, inflammatory	Nonallergic rhinitis, noninflammatory	Nonallergic rhinitis, structurally related
Eosinophilic nasal disease (NARES, BENARS)	Rhinitis medicamentosa	Septal deviation
Basophilic/metachromatic nasal disease	Topical decongestants	Septal perforation
Infections (viral, bacterial)	Systemic medications	Foreign body
Nasal polyps	Vasomotor rhinitis	Obstructive adenoid hyperplasia
Aspirin intolerance	Physical rhinitis	Nasal valve dysfunction
Chronic sinusitis	(Cold air or bright-light induced)	Trauma
Churg-Strauss syndrome		Malformation
Young's syndrome (sinopulmonary disease,	Gustatory rhinitis	Tumors/neoplasms
azoospermia)	Irritant rhinitis	CSF leak
Cystic fibrosis	Rhinitis sicca	
Kartagener's syndrome (bronchiectasis, chronic	Endocrine/metabolic	
sinusitis, nasal polyps)	Pregnancy or estrogen-related	
Atrophic rhinitis	rhinitis	
Immunologic nasal disease (non-IgE mediated or	Hypothyroidism	
secondary to systemic immunologic disorders)	Acromegaly	
Sjögren's syndrome		
Systemic lupus erythematosus		
Relapsing polychondritis		
Churg-Strauss syndrome		
Sarcoidosis		
Wegener's granulomatosis		

Abbreviations: BENARS = blood eosinophilia nonallergic rhinitis syndrome; CSF = cerebral spinal fluid; NARES = nonallergic rhinitis with eosinophilia syndrome.

GUSTATORY RHINITIS OR PHYSICAL RHINITIS

Rhinitis can be caused by exposure to certain triggers including eating (gustatory rhinitis), cold air (skier's or jogger's nose), or sunlight. This form of rhinitis is characterized by profuse, watery rhinorrhea because of an overly sensitive cholinergic reflex. It begins within minutes of eating or exposure to cold air; spicy foods and alcoholic beverages are frequent culprits.

ATROPHIC RHINITIS

Atrophic rhinitis is more common in elderly patients, but it can occur at any age. Symptoms may include dryness of the nasal mucosa, a sensation of nasal congestion, and a bad smell (ozena) in the nose. In industrialized countries this condition is rare and mostly associated with complications of an overly aggressive removal of nasal tissue during surgery. In other areas of the world, atrophic rhinitis is frequently associated with *Klebsiella* colonization, and the symptoms of epistaxis, crusting, stuffiness, and a foul odor are more prominent.

RHINITIS ASSOCIATED WITH AUTOIMMUNE OR GRANULOMATOUS DISEASES

Rhinitis can occur with systemic autoimmune diseases such as Churg-Strauss vasculitis, Sjögren's syndrome, systemic lupus erythematosus, and relapsing polychondritis. Wegener's granulomatosis and sarcoidosis also can cause upper airway symptoms including rhinitis.

GASTROESOPHAGEAL REFLUX DISEASE ASSOCIATED RHINITIS

Upper airway symptoms, including rhinitis, have recently been associated with gastroesophageal reflux disease (GERD). This association was confirmed in a study by Theodoropoulos and colleagues. Interestingly, rhinitis and other upper airway symptoms occurred even when the GERD was limited to the distal esophagus. This finding implies direct contact with the upper airway or occult aspiration is not required. The pathogenesis is not currently understood but may involve a neurogenic mechanism.

Diagnosis

The differential diagnosis of rhinitis can be difficult given the often indistinguishable symptoms of nonallergic and allergic rhinitis, the number of patients presenting with mixed rhinitis, and the multiple syndromes that make up nonallergic rhinitis (see Box 1).

Although historically classic physical examination findings are described with several forms of rhinitis, these are nonspecific findings. For example, allergic rhinitis is frequently characterized by pale, boggy turbinates; infectious rhinitis is suspected by the presence of purulent nasal discharge; and rhinitis medicamentosa may have erythematous or hemorrhagic mucosa. However, NARES, nasal polyposis, and nasal mastocytosis frequently appear indistinguishable from allergic rhinitis. The appearance of vasomotor rhinitis can vary and often overlaps with several other types of rhinitis. As a result, physical examination is generally unhelpful in distinguishing between allergic and nonallergic disease, but it is essential in the evaluation of structural problems such as septal deviations, septal perforations, polyps, and tumors.

Anatomic abnormalities represent approximately 5% to 10% of chronic nasal disorders. Nasal septal deviation is common and often aggravated by other coexisting forms of rhinitis. Nasal polyps may be associated with other disorders including the aspirin tetrad syndrome (nasal polyposis, aspirin intolerance, sinusitis, and asthma), cystic fibrosis, Kartagener's syndrome, Churg-Strauss syndrome, or chronic sinusitis. Very rare structural causes of rhinitis include tumors and neoplasms such as chordoma, neurofibroma, angiofibroma, squamous cell carcinoma, sarcoma, lymphoma, teratoma, encephaloceles, meningoceles, and inverting papilloma. Another rare but serious cause of rhinorrhea is a cerebral spinal fluid (CSF) leak, which can occur as a result of trauma, surgical complications, or even spontaneously. CSF leaks occur after approximately 5% of all basilar skull fractures. The diagnosis requires a high index of suspicion and can be confirmed by the detection of β_2-transferrin in the fluid.

The features that distinguish nonallergic from allergic disease in terms of the history are seen in Table 3. The definitive diagnosis rests on the presence or the absence of clinically important IgE-mediated reactions to aeroallergens. The test of choice in this regard is the allergy skin test; however, a positive test does not rule out the presence of nonallergic disease and must be evaluated for significance in light of the history. However, negative tests establish the presence of nonallergic rhinitis by exclusion.

Management

Management of chronic nonallergic rhinitis can be difficult because some cases are relatively resistant to therapy. The mainstay of treatment is pharmacologic,

TABLE 3 Differential Diagnosis of Rhinitis

Manifestation	Allergic rhinitis	Chronic nonallergic rhinitis
Age of onset	<20 years of age	>20 years of age
Seasonality	Seasonal variations: spring and fall	Usually perennial, but can be worse with weather changes
		Irritant exposure, weather changes
Exacerbating factors	Allergen exposure	Rare
Nature of symptoms		
Pruritus	Common	Common
Congestion	Common	Usually not prominent, but dominant in some cases
Sneezing	Prominent	
Postnasal drainage	Not prominent	Prominent
Other related manifestations (e.g., allergy, conjunctivitis, atopic dermatitis)	Often present	Absent
Family history	Usually present	Usually absent
Physical appearance	Variable, classically described as pale, boggy, swollen mucosa but may appear normal	Variable, erythematous
Allergy testing	Allergy testing always positive	Allergy testing negative or not clinically significant
Nasal eosinophilia	Usually present	Present 15%-20% of the time (NARES)

Abbreviations: NARES = nonallergic rhinitis with eosinophilia syndrome.

3

but of course avoidance of triggers is helpful. Two pharmacologic approaches can be taken to treat vasomotor rhinitis: nonspecific, broad-based therapy aimed at multiple symptoms or therapy tailored to specific symptoms (Table 4). Owing to the variability of vasomotor symptoms, nonspecific treatment may be preferable.

NONSPECIFIC, BROAD-BASED TREATMENT

Broad-based treatment includes the topical antihistamine azelastine (Astelin) or topical corticosteroids, the only two forms of therapy demonstrated to be of use for the management of nonallergic rhinitis. Azelastine is the only antihistamine approved for use in both allergic and nonallergic rhinitis. The antihistamine and anti-inflammatory activities of azelastine produce a high response rate (82% to 85%) in vasomotor rhinitis, improve all associated rhinitis symptoms (congestion, rhinorrhea, postnasal drainage, and sneezing), and have a rapid onset of action. In addition, three topical corticosteroids have been approved for use in the treatment of nonallergic rhinitis: budesonide (Rhinocort Aqua),[1] fluticasone (Flonase), and beclomethasone (Beconase AQ). Budesonide has only been approved for this condition in its aerosol form, which is no longer available. However, it is not unreasonable to assume that the aqueous form would also be effective. There are no comparative studies that assess the relative efficacy of any of these drugs, and the choice of therapy remains speculative. Possible side effects are generally mild and include local irritation, mucosal bleeding, and, rarely, septal perforation. Long-term treatment with beclomethasone dipropionate was shown to be safe and did not produce nasal atrophy after 5 years of

continuous treatment. Using the proper technique for administration of nasal steroids can minimize the risk of any significant side effects.

SYMPTOM-SPECIFIC THERAPY

For treatment tailored to specific symptoms, decongestants are first-line therapy for patients whose symptoms are obstructive. Decongestants, however, have no effect on other manifestations such as rhinorrhea or sneezing. Commonly used oral decongestants include pseudoephedrine[1] and phenylephrine.[1] Potential side effects include insomnia, nervousness, urinary hesitancy, palpitations, and elevated blood pressure. They are generally considered safe to use in patients with stable, controlled hypertension. However, they are contraindicated in patients taking MAO-inhibitors. Relative contraindications include thyroid disease, glaucoma, and coronary artery disease. They are not recommended for use during pregnancy. Topical decongestants such as oxymetazoline (Afrin)[1] and phenylephrine (Neo-Synephrine)[1] can be used effectively in certain situations as a temporary measure. However, their use should be strictly limited to less than 3 to 5 days to avoid the rebound symptoms of rhinitis medicamentosa.

The topical anticholinergic agent ipratropium bromide (Atrovent) is first-line treatment for vasomotor rhinitis with a predominant symptom of rhinorrhea. Anticholinergics primarily affect rhinorrhea with only modest effects on congestion. The only intranasal anticholinergic agent available in the United States is ipratropium bromide in a 0.03% solution for use in chronic nonallergic rhinitis. An anticholinergic agent is a particularly effective choice of therapy for physical

[1]Not FDA approved for this indication.

[1]Not FDA approved for this indication.

TABLE 4 Examples of Some Typical Medications Used to Treat Nonallergic Rhinitis

Generic name	Trade name(s)	Dosage
Broad-based treatments		
Azelastine*	Astelin	2 sprays each nostril qd-bid
Fluticasone*	Flonase	2 sprays each nostril qd or 1 spray each nostril bid
Budesonide*	Rhinocort AQ	1 spray each nostril bid to 4 sprays each nostril qd
Beclomethasone*	Beconase AQ	1-2 sprays each nostril bid
	Vancenase AQ	1-2 sprays each nostril qd
Symptom-specific treatments		
Ipratropium bromide*	Atrovent	0.03%, 2 sprays each nostril bid-qid
Decongestants†		
Pseudoephedrine	Multiple formulations	varies
Phenylephrine	Multiple formulations	varies
Saline nasal spray	SeaMist, Ocean, Pretz	1-3 sprays each nostril prn

*Examples provided are typical adult dosages.
†There are multiple formulations and dosage schedules for the decongestants.
Abbreviations: bid = twice daily; prn = as needed; qd = every day.

rhinitis symptoms (gustatory or cold induced rhinitis) requiring treatment. It can be used approximately 1 hour prior to exposure to cold air or eating. Ipratropium bromide can be used alone or in combination with topical nasal corticosteroids. The benefits of this particular therapeutic combination appear to be additive compared with the use of either drug alone. Ipratropium has minimal side effects (infrequent episodes of nasal dryness and minor epistaxis).

Topical saline solution alone or in combination with other therapies may provide additional relief from the symptoms of postnasal drainage, sneezing, and congestion in vasomotor rhinitis. In patients who do not respond to pharmacotherapy, several surgical approaches have been tried successfully.

OTHER THERAPEUTIC APPROACHES AND CONSIDERATIONS

Surgical approaches that divide the parasympathetic supply to the nasal mucosa, thereby reducing nasal secretion, are endoscopic vidian nerve section and electrocoagulation of the anterior ethmoidal nerve. In cases in which the predominant symptom is congestion, turbinectomy is a treatment option. However, there may be a recurrence of symptoms after surgery.

CURRENT DIAGNOSIS

- The diagnosis of nonallergic rhinitis encompasses a variety of syndromes that share common symptoms, such as sneezing, nasal congestion, postnasal drainage, and anterior rhinorrhea.
- Nonallergic rhinitis is distinguished from allergic rhinitis by the lack of a clinically relevant IgE response to aeroallergens.
- Nonallergic rhinitis is a diagnosis of exclusion. To distinguish this condition from allergic rhinitis the diagnostic test of choice is allergy skin testing. However, results must be properly interpreted and clinically correlated with the patient's history.
- Physical examination findings are nonspecific in nonallergic rhinitis and cannot be used exclusively to distinguish between allergic and nonallergic rhinitis.
- Mixed rhinitis (allergic and nonallergic) occurs in a significant number of patients.
- Vasomotor rhinitis or idiopathic perennial nonallergic rhinitis is the most common subtype of nonallergic rhinitis, approximately 61% of nonallergic rhinitis syndromes.
- Vasomotor rhinitis is characterized by nasal hyperreactivity on exposure to nonimmunologic stimuli including temperature or humidity changes, strong odors, and airborne irritants.
- Nonallergic rhinitis with eosinophilia syndrome (NARES) represents approximately 15% to 20% of nonallergic rhinitis and is characterized by increased nasal eosinophilia. The pathophysiology of this disorder is poorly understood.
- Multiple drugs can cause rhinitis, especially antihypertensive medications, hormones, and cocaine.
- The overuse of topical nasal decongestants is a common cause of rebound nasal congestion, rhinitis medicamentosa.
- Endocrine disorders can lead to rhinitis, including hypothyroidism and acromegaly.
- Rhinitis of pregnancy is a common condition affecting up to a third of pregnant women.
- Many autoimmune or granulomatous diseases can be associated with rhinitis.
- Rhinitis symptoms can be related to multiple structural problems. A deviated septum, turbinate deformation, nasal valve dysfunction, or obstructive adenoid hypertrophy may be identified as the cause of rhinitis symptoms.
- Other rare, but serious, conditions can cause rhinitis symptoms including tumors, neoplasms, and trauma.

CURRENT THERAPY

- Treatment for nonallergic rhinitis can be generally divided into nonspecific broad-based treatment or symptom-specific treatment options.
- Nonspecific broad-based options include topical corticosteroids and azelastine (Astelin).
- Topical corticosteroids shown to be effective in nonallergic rhinitis include budesonide (Rhinocort),[1] fluticasone (Flonase), and beclomethasone (Beconase AQ).
- Obstructive symptoms can be treated symptomatically with decongestants. These agents do not affect rhinorrhea or sneezing.
- The topical anticholinergic, ipratropium bromide (Atrovent) can be used to treat rhinorrhea, with minimal effect on congestion.
- Topical saline solution can provide some benefit in the treatment of postnasal drainage, sneezing, and congestion because of vasomotor rhinitis.
- Rhinitis of pregnancy can be resistant to therapy. Treatment options are often limited by safety concerns.
- Surgical options exist for nonallergic rhinitis but are mainly reserved for those patients who do not respond to pharmacotherapy.

[1]Not FDA approved for this indication.

Rhinitis of pregnancy is a particularly challenging therapeutic problem. The major principle that guides therapy for this disorder is caution in medication use. First-line treatment should include the safest therapies, such as steam inhalation, saline solution nasal sprays, and avoidance of irritants. Unfortunately, rhinitis of pregnancy can often be recalcitrant, responding only to topical corticosteroids. At present there are two class B antihistamines, cetirizine (Zyrtec) and loratadine (Claritin); one class B topical nasal steroid, budesonide (Rhinocort AQ); and one class B leukotriene modifier, montelukast (Singulair) approved for use in allergic rhinitis. Only one of these, budesonide (Rhinocort AQ),[1] has shown efficacy in nonallergic rhinitis.

Treatment of rhinitis medicamentosa requires withdrawal from the topical decongestant, the oral agent, or the eyedrops as well as treatment of the underlying rhinitis. This is often best accomplished with a 1-week tapering course of an oral glucocorticoid, with gradual discontinuation of the decongestant spray beginning on the second or third day of treatment. Administration of a topical corticosteroid spray also can begin on the third day of treatment and should be maintained subsequently. Oral decongestants can be used as needed.

The presence of nasal eosinophilia in patients with chronic nonallergic rhinitis is generally regarded as a good prognostic indicator for response to treatment with topical corticosteroids. Patients with NARES and massive

eosinophilic infiltration also may require intermittent use of oral glucocorticoids to control symptoms.

TREATING MIXED RHINITIS

Once a differential diagnosis of mixed rhinitis has been confirmed, empirical treatment with a topical broad-based agent effective in both allergic and nonallergic rhinitis (e.g., azelastine or an intranasal corticosteroid) is a reasonable choice for first-line therapy. Other agents such as oral decongestants or ipratropium (Atrovent) can be used adjunctively as indicated.

REFERENCES

Banov C, Laforce C, Lieberman P: Double-blind trial of Astelin nasal spray in the treatment of vasomotor rhinitis. Ann Allergy Asthma Immunol 2000;84:138.

Dockhorn R, Aaronson D, Bronsky E, et al: Ipratropium bromide nasal spray 0.03% and beclomethasone nasal spray alone and in combination for the treatment of rhinorrhea in perennial rhinitis. Ann Allergy Asthma Immunol 1999;82:349-359.

Dykewicz MS, Fineman S, Skoner DP, et al: Diagnosis and management of rhinitis: Complete guidelines of the Joint Task Force on Practice Parameters in Allergy, Asthma, and Immunology. American Academy of Allergy, Asthma and Immunology. Ann Allergy Asthma Immunol 1998;81:478-518.

Graf P, Hallen H, Juto JE: The pathophysiology and treatment of rhinitis medicamentosa. Clin Otolaryngol 1995;20:224-229.

Incaudo GA, Schatz M: Rhinosinusitis associated with endocrine conditions: Hypothyroidism and pregnancy. In Schatz M, Zeigler RS, Settipane GA (eds.): Nasal Manifestations of Systemic Diseases. Providence, RI, OceanSide Publications, 1991, p 54.

Moneret-Vautrin DA, Hsieh V, Wayoff M, et al: Nonallergic rhinitis with eosinophilia syndrome a precursor of the triad: Nasal polyposis, intrinsic asthma, and intolerance to aspirin. Ann Allergy 1990;64:513-518.

Settipane RA, Lieberman PL: Update on nonallergic rhinitis. Ann Allergy Asthma Immunol 2001;86(5):494-507.

Theodoropoulos DS, Ledford DK, Lockey RF, et al: Prevalence of upper respiratory symptoms in patients with symptomatic gastroesophageal reflux disease. Am J Respir Crit Care Med 2001;164(1):72-76.

Togias A: Age relationships and clinical features of nonallergic rhinitis. J Allergy Clin Immunol 1990;85:182.

Turkeltaub PC, Gergen PJ: The prevalence of allergic and nonallergic respiratory symptoms in the U.S. population: Data from the second national health and nutrition examination survey 1976-1980 (NHANES II). J Allergy Clin Immunol 1988;81:305.

Zeiger RS: Differential diagnosis and classification of rhinosinusitis. In Schatz M, Zeiger RS, Settipane GA (eds.): Nasal Manifestations of Systemic Diseases. Providence, RI, OceanSide Publications, 1991.

Zlab MK, Moore GF, Daly DT, Yonkers AJ: Cerebrospinal fluid rhinorrhea: A review of the literature. Ear Nose Throat J 1992;71:314-317.

3

[1]Not FDA approved for this indication.

Rakel and Bope: *Conn's Current Therapy 2006.*

Hoarseness and Laryngitis

Method of
Paul C. Bryson, MD, and Robert Buckmire, MD

Hoarseness is a nonspecific complaint that connotes a subjective change in voice quality. As a presenting complaint, it often means something different to patients than it does to a clinician. Further questioning is required to determine the patient's specific voice-related complaint. Common specific complaints include:

- Complete intermittent voice loss (aphonia)
- Decreased vocal range
- Vocal fatigue
- Voice breaks (cracking)
- Generalized voice quality change (dysphonia)

If the patient is a singer, a more complete delineation of voice symptoms and complaints is warranted. The voice complaints of singers often involve loss of singing endurance, pitch control, and vocal range. These discrete deficits may not be as readily apparent in the speaking voice.

Laryngitis is another nonspecific complaint that connotes a generalized, persistent change in voice quality. When used in a medical context, laryngitis suggests an inflammatory process of the vocal folds commonly caused by infection or phonotrauma (behaviors damaging to the vocal mechanism; i.e., coughing, screaming).

There are many benign causes of a voice change, which are discussed in this article. In a larger medical context, however, hoarseness and laryngitis are the most common early symptoms of laryngeal cancer. Therefore, any persistent voice change lasting longer than 2 weeks in duration requires a detailed otolaryngologic evaluation to ascertain the etiology. This article focuses on the most common causes of persistent hoarseness and their treatments.

Acute Laryngitis

DIAGNOSIS

Laryngitis refers to a nonspecific inflammatory condition affecting the larynx and resulting in dysphonia. The causes of this condition are myriad and include all forms of infection, inflammation, or injury affecting the respiratory tract. These causes include viral and bacterial pathogens, intubation trauma, neck trauma, and phonotrauma, as well as the upper respiratory tract effects of allergy and laryngopharyngeal reflux disease. By far the most common transient cause of this condition is inflammation associated with a viral upper respiratory infection (URI). In this setting the duration of dysphonia should be appropriate for the presumed cause. Therefore, hoarseness associated with a URI would be expected to resolve along with the other symptoms. In general, an acute voice change persisting

for longer than 2 weeks is an indication for a laryngeal examination.

TREATMENT

The recommended therapeutic modality is entirely dependent on the suspected cause of the laryngitis. Treatment for viral URI symptoms should be expectant with attention to good hydration and reduced voice use (not voice rest). Bacterial and fungal laryngotracheitis are diagnosed by findings during laryngeal visualization in association with appropriate symptoms. Bacterial infection should be suspected with prolonged symptoms of dysphonia in temporal association with a productive cough and fever. It is generally well treated by a full course of therapy with a broad-spectrum oral antibiotic that covers oropharyngeal flora. Treatment of fungal laryngitis typically requires a systemic antifungal such as fluconazole (Diflucan, 200 mg orally every day for the first day followed by 100 mg daily for the rest of the prescribed course). These infections are uncommon and generally arise in the setting of antibiotic or steroid use, or when some form of immunosuppression/immunocompromise is present.

Laryngopharyngeal Reflux Disease

DIAGNOSIS

Laryngopharyngeal reflux disease (LPRD) is caused by the effect of gastric secretions on the mucosal lining of the larynx. The described laryngeal changes include interarytenoid edema and erythema, vocal fold erythema, as well as infraglottic edema affecting the lower lip of the vocal folds. In severe cases, posterior glottic ulceration and granulation tissue are visible. These changes may be associated with symptoms of heartburn or dyspepsia, but absence of symptoms in no way excludes the clinical diagnosis. Commonly associated pharyngeal symptoms include excessive thick pharyngeal mucus, cough, throat clearing, globus sensation, and mild dysphonia. Dysphonia results from altered glottic closure and inflammatory changes of the posterior glottis. Objective confirmation of pathologic reflux disease may be established by means of multiple channel, ambulatory pH probe testing.

TREATMENT

Ideal treatment of reflux laryngitis is multifactorial. Lifestyle changes such as elevating the head of the bed, avoiding meals several hours before recumbency, and weight reduction programs are important in the management of this condition. These changes in conjunction with dietary control, including avoidance of acidic foods and those promoting reflux (tomato-based foods, caffeine, alcohol, etc.) forms the core of treatment. Adjuvant medical therapy involves lowering the amount of gastric acid production. Antacids, H_2 blockers, and proton pump inhibitors (PPIs) are effective medications, but cases of medication resistance are

Rakel and Bope: *Conn's Current Therapy 2006.*

occasionally seen. Aggressive medical therapy might begin with a twice daily oral dose of a PPI (i.e., omeprazole 20 mg to 40 mg) in conjunction with lifestyle and dietary modifications. Surgical intervention addressing the lower esophageal sphincter is also available, but it is generally reserved for cases refractory to medical management.

Muscle Tension Dysphonia

DIAGNOSIS

Muscle tension dysphonia (MTD) is a common voice disorder characterized by inappropriate or excessive use of the intralaryngeal and extralaryngeal musculature during speech. Patients with this disorder typically present with hoarseness and vocal fatigue as primary complaints. Other associated symptoms may include loss of vocal range and frequent sore throats exacerbated by voice use. The cause of this disorder is unknown, but it is often associated with periods of vocal overuse, abuse, or periods immediately following viral upper respiratory infections with associated laryngitis. It may present in associated conditions that create a *weak* voice such as muscular atrophy or vocal fold paresis.

TREATMENT

Muscle tension dysphonia is most often successfully treated with behavioral voice therapy administered by a speech language pathologist (voice therapist). The therapeutic regimen is designed to produce a more efficient and appropriate technique for voice production. The prognosis for improvement of dysphonia from MTD with voice therapy is excellent. A typical course of therapy requires only 8 to 12 sessions.

Neurologic Voice Disorders

DIAGNOSIS

There are a variety of neurologic disorders that affect voice quality and voice production. Parkinson's disease, essential tremor, and spasmodic dysphonia are all fairly common neurogenic causes of dysphonia. Parkinson's disease causes a classic constellation of communication difficulties consisting of soft voice and rapid and slurred speech. One of the major communication disorder components of Parkinson's disease is an inability of the patient to monitor one's own vocal loudness.

TREATMENT

The Lee Silverman Voice Training Program (LSVT) was specifically developed to address improving the communication disorder associated with Parkinson's disease and is efficacious. LSVT is administered by a speech pathologist and requires a specialized form of speech therapy four times per week for 1 month (approximately 16 to 20 sessions). The improvement

gained from the LSVT program is best maintained when the patient continues the home exercises on a long-term basis.

Essential Tremor

DIAGNOSIS

Essential tremor (ET) is the most common movement disorder. It can involve the larynx, upper aerodigestive tract, and the head and neck region. This causes a periodic alteration (tremor) to the voice production that is often erroneously attributed to the normal aging process. When this tremor is severe, it can significantly disrupt normal communication fluency and intelligibility.

TREATMENT

ET is primarily treated with systemic pharmacologic agents in coordination with a neurologist. Adjunctive treatment with voice therapy techniques and intralaryngeal botulinum toxin injections are helpful in some patients with this disorder.

Spasmodic Dysphonia

DIAGNOSIS

Spasmodic dysphonia (SD) is a focal dystonia of the laryngeal musculature, with an unknown etiology. The voice symptoms of this disorder are characterized by severe disruption of the normal fluency of voice production. Patients typically feel as if they cannot "get their voice out" and have a "strained/strangled" voice quality and sensation.

TREATMENT

This disorder is most often treated successfully with repeated intralaryngeal botulinum toxin injections. The specific laryngeal muscular site of injection is determined by the specific variety of SD diagnosed (adductor versus abductor type). Typical intramuscular doses range from 1.25 to 10 units in a unilateral or bilateral injection. Adjunctive voice therapy helps produce an optimal voice outcome and therapeutic longevity following injections.

Voice Disorders Associated With Aging

DIAGNOSIS

Voice disorders related to the aging process have recently gained greater visibility. These voice problems are typically related to *atrophy,* a loss of muscle bulk, of the vocal fold musculature, resulting in a weak voice, decreased vocal range, and vocal fatigue.

Rakel and Bope: *Conn's Current Therapy 2006.*

3

TREATMENT

After exclusion of focal neurologic or specific anatomic voice pathology, the initial treatment for this condition is voice therapy. In general, 8 to 10 sessions of voice therapy are highly successful (>85%) for improving specific symptoms of vocal fold atrophy. Patients with severe symptoms and/or significant vocal demands may require surgical intervention in addition to voice therapy for symptom relief. When necessary, vocal fold augmentation by means such as medialization thyroplasty or injection laryngoplasty is usually successful.

Vocal Fold Lesions

Vocal fold nodules, polyps, and cysts are common benign lesions of the true vocal folds causing dysphonia. They can reliably be distinguished from one another only by a thorough laryngoscopic examination including videostrobolaryngoscopy.

VOCAL NODULES

Diagnosis

Vocal nodules (often referred to by singers as *nodes*) are localized, benign, superficial growths on the medial surface of the true vocal cords that are commonly believed to be the result of a pattern of vocal misuse and abuse (phonotrauma). Nodules are bilateral in nature and are classically located at the junction of the anterior third and the middle third of the vocal fold. They are most often seen in women ages 20 to 50 years but are also common in children, particularly boys, who are prone to excessive loud talking or screaming.

Treatment

Treatment for nodules always involves a course of behavioral voice therapy. Patient compliance is paramount because the therapy is designed to correct the etiologic vocal behaviors. Surgical intervention is an inappropriate first-line therapy for most vocal fold nodules. It may be considered, however, for cases in which the patient strictly complies with the prescribed course of therapy but is still left with an unacceptable vocal impairment. (If performed, surgery should be limited to the most superficial layers of the vocal fold, preserving the uninvolved surrounding lamina propria.)

VOCAL FOLD POLYPS

Diagnosis

Vocal fold polyps are generally unilateral and have a broad spectrum of appearances from pedunculated to sessile. They, too, are believed to result from phonotrauma; however, they can arise from a single episode of abusive behavior or hemorrhage. Polyps arise in the superficial lamina propria layer and typically involve the free (medial) edge of the vocal fold mucosa.

Their mass causes altered vocal fold vibration and interferes with glottic closure. Both deficits contribute to the symptom of dysphonia.

Treatment

Treatment for vocal fold polyps is aimed at correcting the underlying causative factors, largely through voice therapy and vocal education. Following voice therapy, if significant dysphonia persists, surgery is indicated. The recommended technique is a minimally invasive, microlaryngoscopic procedure, preserving the uninvolved epithelial cover and surrounding submucosal tissue. When voice therapy and surgery are used appropriately and combined with a compliant patient, the voice outcome is usually excellent.

VOCAL FOLD CYSTS

Diagnosis

Vocal fold cysts are a focal abnormality of the superficial lamina propria and are predominantly unilateral. Intracordal mucus retention cysts are believed to arise after blockage of a glandular duct. Another type of cyst found in the vocal folds, an epidermoid cyst, is similar to those found in the skin and tends to be smaller. Both varieties appear as a well-circumscribed, spherical mass beneath intact, normal appearing epithelial lining.

Treatment

Treatment of these lesions consists of a surgical microlaryngoscopic approach with creation of a flap of the overlying epithelium that will be preserved and returned after removal of the lesion. This approach allows for the expedient return of proper glottic closure and vocal fold vibration previously interrupted by this intracordal mass lesion. Preoperative and postoperative voice therapies are key components to successful treatment.

Recurrent Respiratory Papilloma

DIAGNOSIS

Recurrent respiratory papilloma (RRP) is a histologically benign neoplastic lesion with a broad range of symptoms and unpredictable natural history. Most commonly affecting the glottis, this papillomatous alteration of the squamous epithelium affects both children and adults and is caused by the human papilloma virus (HPV). Subtypes 6 and 11 are the most common among respiratory tract lesions. Lesions may be self-limited or progressive, and, depending on the site of involvement as well as the size of the patient's airway, symptoms may range from mild dysphonia to frank stridor and airway obstruction. Malignant transformation to squamous cell carcinoma is exceedingly rare but has been documented. The course of disease typically involves recurrence and unpredictable remissions. Death from this disease is usually associated with complications of repeated surgical therapy or respiratory failure caused by pulmonary spread of extralaryngeal disease. Aggressive cases in children may require extremely frequent surgical treatment (1 to 2 per month) and/or tracheotomy to preserve the airway.

TREATMENT

Surgical excision of RRP lesions is the mainstay of therapy with either CO_2 laser, cold steel excision, or the microdebrider. These therapies have been effective but are not without soft tissue morbidity such as thermal damage to nonpapillomatous tissue, vocal fold scarring, and anterior commissure web formation. The 585-nm pulsed-dye laser is an evolving technology and may facilitate papilloma removal with less soft tissue complications. The energy from this laser penetrates normal epithelium (roughly 2 mm) and is selectively absorbed by the subepithelial microvasculature, causing angiolysis and ischemia of the overlying papilloma. Long-term safety and effectiveness data are not yet available.

Both topical and systemic adjuvant medical therapies are also available. The most common of these medications has become cidofovir, a nucleoside analogue, antiviral agent. Administered by injection, cidofovir has shown some significant success in topical treatment of recurrent papillomatous lesions. Several different concentrations of the medication have been used clinically in both adults and children.

Alpha-interferon is another adjuvant therapy for RRP. Typical doses include 5 million units per meter squared of body surface in a daily subcutaneous injection to initiate therapy, and then 3 million units per meter squared 3 days per week over 6 months. This treatment regimen effectively slows RRP growth, but it is not curative. Other treatments that have been attempted with varying success include indole-3-carbinol (substance found in cruciferous vegetables such as broccoli, cauliflower, and cabbage), topical chemotherapy, and vaccines.

Laryngeal Carcinoma

DIAGNOSIS

Laryngeal carcinoma accounts for approximately 1% of new cancers each year and can involve the structures above and below the true vocal cords as well as the true vocal cords themselves. The most common variant is squamous cell carcinoma. The carcinogenic properties of tobacco smoke and alcohol are the typical etiologic agents and risk factors. The most common early symptom is hoarseness. Dyspnea and airway obstruction may present at later stages of the disease.

TREATMENT

Laryngeal cancer staging is based on tumor size, lymph node involvement, and the presence of metastasis. Early-stage lesions are typically treated with a single modality such as transoral endoscopic resection; external beam radiation; or open, partial laryngeal resection. In later stages of the disease, combinations of radiation,

Rakel and Bope: *Conn's Current Therapy 2006.*

CURRENT DIAGNOSIS

- History of hoarseness (dysphonia) should include the details of onset, duration, recent illnesses, recent injuries including any recent intubations, presence of acid reflux symptoms, and recent or chronic neurologic or vascular events.
- If hoarseness persists more than 2 weeks, laryngeal examination is recommended.
- Laryngeal EMG may be warranted if neurogenic causes of dysphonia are suspected.

Abbreviations: EMG = electromyelogram.

extirpative surgery, and chemotherapy are routinely employed. There is a current trend toward multimodality therapy with organ sparing protocols.

Vocal Fold Paralysis (Vocal Fold Immobility)

DIAGNOSIS

Normal vocal fold motion involves wide abduction (away from the midline) during inspiration as well as coordinated glottic closure during phonation and swallowing. When a unilateral vocal fold is found to be immobile, the glottis is generally incompetent in adduction resulting in some level of dysphonia. Associated vocal fatigue and potential aspiration during swallowing may also be present. When this condition is diagnosed, a search for the cause should be undertaken. Imaging of the course of neural supply to the larynx including chest radiograph and computed tomography (CT) or magnetic resonance imaging (MRI) from the skull base through the mediastinum is necessary to rule out occult neoplastic lesions. Common etiologies of vocal fold immobility include paralysis secondary to vagal or recurrent laryngeal nerve injury from thyroid, carotid, or chest surgery. Vocal folds may also be immobile secondary to cricoarytenoid joint dysfunction despite an intact nerve supply. Laryngeal electromyelogram (EMG) prior to 6 months after the onset of immobility is helpful in establishing the status of the neural innervation as well as providing important prognostic information regarding spontaneous recovery.

TREATMENT

Swallowing and voice deficits are treated with a combination of nonsurgical and surgical techniques. Aspiration refractory to nonsurgical swallowing techniques is an indication for surgical intervention whether temporary or permanent in scope. In these patients procedures to improve closure are employed early in the course of the disease to avoid the potentially devastating complications of aspiration pneumonia.

Dysphonia in the absence of aspiration may be amenable to either voice therapy or surgical intervention. The therapeutic decision-making is generally based on the patient's desire for an improved voice and the glottic

CURRENT THERAPY

- A suspected viral cause may be managed expectantly with hydration and reduced voice use.
- Antibiotics are not indicated for hoarseness without infectious symptoms (but may be used when fever, productive cough, purulent rhinorrhea, etc. are present).
- Reflux may call for lifestyle modifications with H_2 antagonist/proton pump inhibitor as adjuvant therapy is effective in most instances.
- Muscle tension dysphonia and vocal nodules may necessitate behavioral therapy.
- Vocal cord polyps and cysts require behavioral voice therapy with or without surgical excision.
- For respiratory papillomatosis, surgical excision is effective with or without topical cidofovir injections.
- Neurologic abnormality—including spasmodic dysphonia, tremor, and Parkinsonism—may require a referral to a speech pathologist, neurologist, or ENT (possible role for intralaryngeal Botox injection depending on specific disease process).
- Vocal cord paralysis/paresis voice therapy may call for a neurologic evaluation with laryngeal electromyography or surgical augmentation/medialization.
- Laryngeal carcinoma may necessitate a referral to an ENT for some combination of surgical excision, chemotherapy, and/or radiation therapy.

Abbreviations: ENT = ear, nose, and throat.

configuration on laryngoscopic exam. Small glottic gap associated with an immobile vocal fold in a favorable paramedian position may often be treated successfully with voice therapy alone. Significant dysphonia secondary to a larger glottic gap may be treated by injection laryngoplasty (fat, Gelfoam, or collagen) or medialization laryngoplasty. Larger levels of glottic incompetence are more likely to require medialization thyroplasty (laryngeal framework surgery) designed to statically position the immobile vocal fold in a phonatory posture.

REFERENCES

Baumgartner CA, Sapir S, Ramig TO: Voice quality changes following phonatory-respiratory effort treatment (LSVT) versus respiratory effort treatment for individuals with Parkinson disease. J Voice 2001;15(1):105-114.
Co J, Woo P: Serial office-based intralesional injection of cidofovir in adult-onset recurrent respiratory papillomatosis. Ann Otol Rhinol Laryngol 2004;113(11):859-862.
Franco RA Jr, Zeitels SM, Farinelli WA, Anderson RR: 585-nm pulsed dye laser treatment of glottal papillomatosis. Ann Otol Rhinol Laryngol 2002;111(6):486-492.
Gibbs SR, Blitzer A: Botulinum toxin for the treatment of spasmodic dysphonia. Otolaryngol Clin North Am 2000;33(4):879-894.
Maronian NC, Waugh PF, Robinson L, Hillel AD: Tremor laryngeal dystonia: treatment of the lateral cricoarytenoid muscle. Ann Otol Rhinol Laryngol 2004;113(5):349-355.
Silverman DA, Pitman MJ: Current diagnostic and management trends for recurrent respiratory papillomatosis. Curr Opin Otolaryngol Head Neck Surg 2004;12(6):532-537.

Streptococcal Pharyngitis

Method of
Burke A. Cunha, MD

Group A streptococcal pharyngitis depends an accurate diagnosis. The demonstration/recovery of group A streptococci (GAS) from the pharynx does not differentiate colonization from infection. Ordinarily, colonization is not treated while GAS infection may be treated. To further compound the diagnostic dilemma, group A streptococcal colonization frequently accompanies viral pharyngitis. For this reason, the recovery of GAS from a patient with clinical pharyngitis does not indicate a causal relationship. If the patient does have group A streptococcal pharyngitis, the object of treatment is to decrease the possibility of suppurative and nonsuppurative complications. The most important of these is acute rheumatic fever, which is the rarest manifestation of untreated group A streptococcal pharyngitis.

The clinical approach is further compounded by the fact that most patients who go on to develop acute rheumatic fever following group A streptococcal pharyngitis have a mild pharyngitis and are not seen by their physicians. The aphorism that the more severe the throat's appearance in group A streptococcal pharyngitis, the less likely the patient will develop acute rheumatic fever remains correct. GAS pharyngitis is primarily a disease of children and young adults and is rare after age 30.

Diagnostic Considerations

The correct therapeutic approach is based on an accurate presumptive diagnosis. The appropriateness of therapy for any infectious disease cannot be properly assessed unless based on an accurate diagnosis. The clinical features of patients presenting with pharyngitis are somewhat helpful in differentiating viral from bacterial pharyngitis. In general, an erythematous pharynx without the presence of exudates suggests a viral pharyngitis. The presence of an exudative pharyngitis favors a group A streptococcal etiology. Exudative pharyngitis also presents with other bacterial infections (e.g., *Corynebacterium diphtheriae,* gonorrhea or *Arcanobacterium haemolyticum)* as well as some viral infections (Epstein-Barr virus [EBV], infectious mononucleosis). The presence of palatal petechiae suggests the presence of group A streptococcal infection or EBV pharyngitis.

Uveal edema favors the diagnosis of group A streptococcal pharyngitis. Patients with viral or bacterial pharyngitis may have fever, chills, myalgias, or pain on swallowing. Bilateral anterior cervical adenopathy is common with pharyngitis of any etiology and does not discern between viral and bacterial pharyngitis. In contrast, bilateral posterior cervical adenopathy immediately points to a systemic infectious process, which in the presence of pharyngitis, should suggest EBV, cytomegalovirus (CMV), or toxoplasmosis. If the patient with pharyngitis has a scarlatiniform rash, then diagnostic possibilities are limited to *A. haemolyticum* or GAS (scarlet fever). The presence of membranes with pharyngitis should suggest the possibility of *C. diphtheriae*. Other clinical associations with pharyngitis may suggest a particular diagnosis (Table 1).

Group A Streptococcal Colonization Versus Infection

Bacterial pharyngitis is most commonly caused by GAS. Streptococcal pharyngitis may also be attributable to groups C or G streptococci, whereas groups B and D streptococci are rarely, if ever, associated with acute bacterial pharyngitis. Group A streptococcal pharyngitis is best diagnosed by combining characteristic clinical findings and demonstrating the presence of GAS in a patient with acute pharyngitis. The mere demonstration/ recovery or growth of GAS in a throat culture does not differentiate streptococcal colonization from infection in

a patient with pharyngitis. Several ways have been used to differentiate colonization from infection, but each is associated with particular problems. The rapid antigen tests (RATs) do not differentiate colonization from infection. Furthermore, there is a problem with false-positive results using RATs. Approximately 15% of patients with culture-negative group A streptococcal pharyngitis have positive group A streptococcal rapid antigen tests, because of antigenic reactions to *Streptococcus milleri* antigens. Culture of the pharynx for GAS remains the gold standard but does not differentiate colonization from infection. The Gram stain of the pharynx has been used to differentiate colonization from infection but requires someone to perform or interpret the Gram stain smear. The Gram stain smear of the pharynx is not done to identify GAS or other bacteria but rather to demonstrate the presence or absence of intense polymorphonuclear response to infection.

In a patient with pharyngitis, positive throat cultures and/or positive rapid antigen testing for GAS with a Gram stain of pharyngeal secretions demonstrating an intense polymorphonuclear (PMN) predominance, indicates infection. Patients with pharyngitis who have a group A streptococcal positive throat culture and positive RAT, but have no or few white blood cells (WBCs) present in the Gram stain of pharyngeal secretions, have streptococcal colonization, not infection.

THERAPEUTIC APPROACH

If the patient has a lower respiratory tract infection in conjunction with pharyngitis, then diagnostic possibilities are limited to *Chlamydia pneumoniae* or *Mycoplasma pneumoniae*. Doxycycline (Vibramycin)[1] is the preferred therapy for both *C. pneumoniae* pharyngitis and community-acquired pneumonia (CAP), as well as *M. pneumoniae* CAP/pharyngitis. The duration of therapy for these systemic infections with a pharyngitis component in normal hosts is usually 2 weeks. Pharyngitis caused by *Neisseria gonorrhoeae*, *C. diphtheriae*, or *A. haemolyticum* may be treated with β-lactams or respiratory quinolones for a duration of 2 weeks (Table 2).

Because most cases of acute pharyngitis are viral, no specific therapy is available for such patients. If GAS can be demonstrated to be present by culture or RAT testing in the pharyngeal secretions, then the clinician must still decide whether this represents colonization or infection. Clinicians should remember that approximately 30% of patients with acute EBV pharyngitis are colonized with GAS. Streptococcal colonization is also common with pharyngitis caused by respiratory viruses. Patients who have viral pharyngitis and are colonized with GAS should not be treated; these patients are analogous to the chronic carrier state with streptococci. It is difficult to eradicate GAS from pharyngeal secretions with antibiotics such as penicillin commonly used to

TABLE 1 Diagnostic Considerations in Pharyngitis

Clinical syndrome	Diagnostic considerations
Pharyngitis + laryngitis	Respiratory viruses *Chlamydia pneumoniae*
Pharyngitis without exudates	Respiratory viruses *Mycoplasma pneumoniae* Nonexudative EBV CMV *Neisseria gonorrhoeae* *Arcanobacterium haemolyticum* *Corynebacterium diphtheriae*
Pharyngitis + exudates	Streptococcal pharyngitis EBV CMV *N. gonorrhoeae* *A. haemolyticum* *C. diphtheriae*
Pharyngitis + bilateral anterior cervical adenopathy only	Streptococcal pharyngitis HSV-1 Coxsackie A virus
Pharyngitis + bilateral posterior cervical adenopathy ± anterior cervical adenopathy	EBV CMV Toxoplasmosis
Pharyngitis + maculopapular rash	GAS *A. haemolyticum* EBV
Pharyngitis + ulcerations	HSV-1 Coxsackie A virus
Pharyngitis + conjunctivitis	Adenovirus
Pharyngitis + pneumonia	*M. pneumoniae* *C. pneumoniae* Influenza

Abbreviations: CMV = Cytomegalovirus; EBV = Epstein-Barr virus; GAS = group A streptococci; HSV-1 = herpes simplex virus 1.

[1]Not FDA approved for this indication.

Rakel and Bope: *Conn's Current Therapy 2006.*

TABLE 2 Treatment for Pharyngitis

Cause	Treatment
GAS	Amoxicillin (Amoxil) 1 g (PO) q24h × 5d or Cefadroxil (Duricef) 1 g (PO) q24h × 5d or Clindamycin (Cleocin) 150 mg (PO) q6h × 10d
Mycoplasma pneumoniae or *Chlamydia pneumoniae*	Doxycycline (Vibramycin) 100 mg (PO) q12h × 10d
EBV/CMV infectious mononucleosis	No treatment

Abbreviations: CMV = cytomegalovirus; d = day; EBV = Epstein-Barr virus GAS = group A streptococci; h = hour; PO = by mouth; q = every.

treat pharyngitis. There is no need to eliminate GAS carriage from patients with EBV pharyngitis or viral pharyngitis. Patients with EBV mononucleosis treated with penicillin or ampicillin for presumed streptococcal infection (actually group A streptococcal colonization) may develop a maculopapular skin rash that may be confused with scarlet fever.

Patients with group A streptococcal pharyngitis will have a normal or slightly elevated peripheral WBC count without a lymphocytosis or atypical lymphocytes. The erythrocyte sedimentation rate (ESR) in group A streptococcal pharyngitis is within normal limits. With EBV infectious mononucleosis, the WBC count is normal or decreased and followed by lymphocytosis. Atypical lymphocytes in EBV infectious mononucleosis increase over time and may not be present initially. Thrombocytopenia may accompany EBV infectious mononucleosis but is not a feature of streptococcal pharyngitis. The serum transaminases are mildly elevated early in the course of EBV infectious mononucleosis but are not a clinical feature of group A streptococcal pharyngitis.

If the patient has group A streptococcal pharyngitis, it still presents a treatment dilemma. If the streptococcal pharyngitis is exudative and the patient has a severe sore throat, treatment may not be necessary to prevent rheumatic fever. The likelihood of rheumatic fever is inversely proportionate to severity of the sore throat with group A streptococcal pharyngitis. Treatment may be initiated to prevent suppurative complications, which is not unreasonable. Many available antibiotics have good activity against GAS; however, the antibiotics selected must not only be active against GAS but also must be able to effectively penetrate the respiratory secretions to eliminate the organism in the pharynx.

 CURRENT DIAGNOSIS

- The most common causes of acute pharyngitis are viral due to the common upper respiratory tract viruses.
- Uncomplicated viral pharyngitis may be accompanied with fever, chills, myalgias, pain on swallowing, and bilateral anterior cervical adenopathy, but no other systemic manifestations.
- Viral pharyngitis with fatigue, abdominal findings, hematologic abnormalities, an elevated ESR or slightly increased serum transaminases, and postbilateral posterior cervical adenopathy should suggest a systemic viral infection with pharyngitis, such as EBV or CMV.
- Acute pharyngitis with pneumonia should suggest *Mycoplasma pneumoniae* or *Chlamydia pneumoniae* as a cause of the pharyngitis.
- Pharyngitis with laryngitis should suggest a respiratory viral etiology or less commonly C. pneumoniae.
- Pharyngitis plus a scarlatiniform should suggest scarlet fever or *Arcanobacterium haemolyticum* pharyngitis.
- Exudative pharyngitis should suggest group A streptococcal pharyngitis or EBV.
- Nonexudative pharyngitis should suggest a viral etiology.

- Pharyngitis with palatal petechiae suggests group A streptococcal infection or EBV.
- Group A streptococcal colonization is common in viral pharyngitis. The streptococcal carriage rate in EBV pharyngitis is approximately 30%. There is no easy way to tell group A streptococcal colonization from infection. Gram stain of oropharyngeal secretions for PMNs and positive throat culture is diagnostic of group A streptococcal pharyngitis.
- The demonstration or recovery of GAS from the oropharynx by culture or RAT antigen testing indicates that GAS are present but does not differentiate colonization and infection.
- RATs have a high false-positive rate (up to 15%) and are highly sensitive, but they are not highly specific.
- GAS commonly persist in the oropharynx after treatment of group A streptococcal pharyngitis, particularly following treatment with β-lactam antibiotics. Group A streptococcal carriage in the oropharynx is suggested by an underlying viral pharyngitis. GAS culture/RAT positivity and the lack of an exudate PMNs in a gram stain of the oropharynx.

Abbreviations: CMV = cytomegalovirus; EBV = Epstein-Barr virus; ESR = erythrocyte sedimentation rate; GAS = group A streptococci; PMN = polymorphonuclear; RAT = rapid antigen test.

BOX 1 **Cases of Penicillin Treatment Failures in Group A Streptococcal Pharyngitis**

- Poor compliance because of frequency of dosing or length of regimen
- Poor penetration into oropharyngeal secretions
- Misdiagnosis (viral cause)
- Treatment of colonization rather than infection
- Inactivation by β-lactamases produced by mouth flora

PENICILLIN FAILURES IN GROUP A STREPTOCOCCAL PHARYNGITIS

It is well known that penicillin treatment in approximately 15% of patients with group A streptococcal pharyngitis fails. The reasons for this include the presence of β-lactamase-producing organisms in the oral flora and/or lack of penetration into oropharyngeal secretions (Box 1). Therefore, if a β-lactam is selected to treat group A streptococcal pharyngitis, amoxicillin (Amoxil) is preferred to penicillin because of its superior ability to penetrate into respiratory secretions and eradicate the organism. Among oral cephalosporins, cefadroxil (Duricef) is preferred to other cephalosporins on the basis of excellent penetration into respiratory secretions. Macrolides should be avoided because they do not penetrate secretions well and may induce resistance in strains of *S. pneumoniae* in the oral flora. Doxycycline (Vibramycin) penetrates well into oropharyngeal secretions and is effective against 85% of GAS. It may be used as alternative therapy in group A streptococcal pharyngitis. Patients who are allergic to penicillin and have nonanaphylactoid reactions, such as maculopapular rash or fever, may be safely treated with cefadroxil (Duricef). Patients with group A streptococcal pharyngitis, who have had anaphylactic reactions to penicillin (laryngospasm, bronchospasm, hypotension, or hives/urticaria) may be treated with a respiratory quinolone, such as levofloxacin (Levaquin),[1] gatifloxacin (Tequin),[1] moxifloxacin (Avelox),[1] gemifloxacin (Factive),[1] or with clindamycin (Cleocin).[1] The duration of antibiotic therapy to treat streptococcal pharyngitis is 1 to 2 weeks.

GROUP A STREPTOCOCCAL CARRIER STATE

Group A streptococcal carriage in the pharynx is common following the treatment of group A streptococcal

---

[1]Not FDA approved for this indication.

 CURRENT THERAPY

- Because most cases of pharyngitis are viral, no treatment is necessary.
- Patients with EBV mononucleosis and streptococcal colonization should not be treated for group A streptococcal pharyngitis.
- A patient with nonexudative pharyngitis and a positive culture for GAS or positive RAT need not be treated.
- Patients with pharyngitis and laryngitis have a viral infection and need not be treated even if GAS colonization is present by culture or RAT.
- Patients with pharyngitis, laryngitis, and respiratory symptoms may be treated with doxycycline (Vibramycin)[1] based on the presumptive diagnosis of *Chlamydia pneumoniae* as the causative organism.
- Nonexudative pharyngitis plus respiratory symptoms may either be caused by a virus or *Mycoplasma pneumoniae*. Empiric treatment with doxycycline (Vibramycin) is not unreasonable because there is no rapid test to readily differentiate viral from *Mycoplasma* pharyngitis, and *Mycoplasma* pharyngitis is treatable with doxycycline (Vibramycin).
- Patients with an exudative pharyngitis should be presumed to have diphtheria until proved otherwise and treated accordingly.

- Patients with scarlet fever should be treated with a β-lactam. Penicillin-allergic patients may be treated with clindamycin (Cleocin).[1]
- The preferred treatment for patients with group A streptococcal pharyngitis (exudative) with bilateral anterior cervical adenopathy, pain on swallowing, and fever/chills is amoxicillin (Amoxil), 1 g PO every 8 hours for 1 to 2 weeks. Children may be given amoxicillin (Amoxil), 20 mg/kg per day oral suspension given in three divided doses every 8 hours for 1 to 2 weeks.
- Macrolides and TMP-SMX (Bactrim) should be avoided if possible.
- Patients who have nonanaphylactic reactions to penicillin may be treated with an oral cephalosporin, preferably cefadroxil (Duricef). Patients with group A streptococcal pharyngitis unable to take β-lactam antibiotics or who have anaphylactic reactions to penicillin may be treated with a respiratory quinolone[1] or oral clindamycin (Cleocin).[1]
- The persistence of streptococci in respiratory secretions following group A streptococcal pharyngitis is common and need not be treated.
- If elimination of group A streptococcal carriage is desired, then respiratory quinolones[1] or clindamycin (Cleocin)[1] have the greatest likelihood of eradicating the carrier state.

---

[1]Not FDA approved for this indication.
Abbreviations: EBV = Epstein-Barr virus; GAS = group A streptococci; RAT = rapid antigen test; TMP-SMX = trimethoprim-sulfamethoxazole.

Rakel and Bope: *Conn's Current Therapy 2006.*

pharyngitis, particularly with agents that do not penetrate respiratory secretions well, such as penicillin. There is no need clinically to eliminate the persistence of streptococci in respiratory secretions following the resolution of acute group A streptococcal pharyngitis with antimicrobial therapy. If eradication of streptococci from the oropharynx is desired, then it is most likely to be achieved with antimicrobials that are both highly effective against the organism and penetrate respiratory secretions effectively. The best antibiotics to use to eliminate group A streptococcal carriage from oropharyngeal secretions are an oral respiratory quinolone[1] or oral clindamycin (Cleocin).[1]

REFERENCES

Adam D, Scholz H, Helmerking M: Short course antibiotic treatment of 4,782 culture-proven cases of group A streptococcal tonsillopharyngitis and incidence of poststreptococcal sequelae. J Infect Dis 2000;182:509.

Bisno AL: Diagnosing strep throat in the adult patient: Do clinical criteria really suffice? Ann Intern Med 2003;139:150-151.

Block SL: Short-course antimicrobial therapy of streptococcal pharyngitis. Clin Pediatr (Phila) 2003;42:663-671.

Brook I: β-lactamase-producing bacteria recovered after clinical failures with various penicillin therapy. Arch Otolaryngol 1984;110:228-231.

Cohen S, Centor R: Diagnosis and management of adults with pharyngitis. Ann Intern Med 2004;140:763.

Cooper RJ, Hoffman JR, Bartlett JG, et al: Principles of appropriate antibiotic use for acute pharyngitis in adults: Background. Ann Intern Med 2001;134:509.

Cunha BA: Group A streptococcal pharyngitis versus colonization. Intern Med 1994;15:18-19.

Cunha BA: Acute pharyngitis. *In* Conn RB, Borer WZ, Snyder JW (eds): Current Diagnosis 9. Philadelphia, WB Saunders, 1996, pp 291-293.

Cunha BA: Antibiotic selection for the treatment of sinusitis, otitis media, and pharyngitis. Inf Dis Clin Practice 1998;7:S324-S326.

Feder HM, Gerber MA, Randolph MF, et al: Once-daily therapy for streptococcal pharyngitis with amoxicillin. Pediatrics 1999;103:47.

Gastanaduy AS, Kaplan EL, Huwe BB, et al: Failure of penicillin to eradicate group A streptococci during an outbreak of pharyngitis. Lancet 1980;2:498-502.

Glezen WP, Clyde WA Jr, Senior RJ, et al: Group A streptococci, mycoplasmas, and viruses associated with acute pharyngitis. JAMA 1967;202:455.

Gonzales R, Cooper RJ, Hoffman JR. Strategies to diagnose and treat group A streptococcal pharyngitis. JAMA 2004;292:167-168.

Johnson DR, Kaplan EL: False-positive rapid antigen detection test results: Reduced specificity in the absence of group A streptococci in the upper respiratory tract. J Infect Dis 2001;183:1135-1137.

Kafetzis DA, Liapi G, Tolia M, et al: Failure to eradicate group A β-haemolytic streptococci (GABHS) from the upper respiratory tract after antibiotic treatment. Int J Antimicrob Agents 2004;23:67-71.

Kaplan EL, Gastanaduy AS, Huwe BB: The role of the carrier in treatment failures after antibiotic therapy for group A streptococci in the upper respiratory tract. J Lab Clin Med 1981;98:326.

Kaplan EL, Johnson DR: Eradication of group A streptococci from the upper respiratory tract by amoxicillin with clavulanate after oral penicillin V treatment failure. J Pediatr 1988;113:400.

Kaplan EL, Johnson DR: Unexplained reduced microbiological efficacy of intramuscular benzathine penicillin G and of oral penicillin V in eradication of group A streptococci from children with acute pharyngitis. Pediatrics 2001;108:1180-1186.

Neuner JM, Hamel MB, Phillips RS, et al: Diagnosis and management of adults with pharyngitis. A cost-effectiveness analysis. Ann Intern Med 2003;139:113-122.

Pichichero ME: The rising incidence of penicillin treatment failures in group A streptococcal tonsillopharyngitis: An emerging role for the cephalosporins? Pediatr Infect Dis J 1991;10(Suppl 10):550-555.

Pichichero ME, Casey JR, Mayes T, et al: Penicillin failure in streptococcal tonsillopharyngitis: Causes and remedies. Pediatr Infect Dis J 2000;19:917-923.

Pichichero ME, Cohen R: Shortened course of antibiotic therapy for acute otitis media, sinusitis and tonsillopharyngitis. Pediatr Infect Dis J 1997;16:680-695.

Shulman ST, Gerber MA: So what's wrong with penicillin for strep throat? Pediatrics 2004;113:1816-1819.

Snow V, Mottur-Pilson C, Cooper RJ, Hoffman JR: Principles of appropriate antibiotic use for acute pharyngitis in adults. Ann Intern Med 2001;134:506.

Standaert BB, Finney K, Taylor MT, et al: Comparison between cefprozil and penicillin to eradicate pharyngeal colonization of group A beta-hemolytic streptococci. Pediatr Infect Dis 1998;17:39-43.

Tanz RR, Poncher JR, Corydon KE, et al: Clindamycin treatment of chronic pharyngeal carriage of group A streptococci. J Pediatr 1991;119:123.

---

[1]Not FDA approved for this indication.

The Respiratory System

Acute Respiratory Failure

Method of
Max M. Weder, MD, and James F. Donohue, MD

Myriad underlying conditions can cause respiratory failure. Depending on whether the predominating problem is oxygenation or ventilation, respiratory failure is divided into *hypoxic* respiratory failure and *hypercapnic* respiratory failure, or a combination of the two. As a practical approach, we will first summarize basic principles in the evaluation of respiratory failure and briefly outline the pathophysiology. Then we will focus on the most common disorders that result in hypoxic and hypercapnic respiratory failure, namely acute respiratory distress syndrome (ARDS), cardiogenic pulmonary edema (CPE), chronic obstructive pulmonary disease (COPD), and asthma. This article does not provide insight into the principles of mechanical ventilation, which would exceed the limits of this article.

Clinical Evaluation of Respiratory Failure

PHYSICAL EXAMINATION AND HISTORY

Respiratory failure may develop acutely, subacutely, or chronically, depending on the underlying process. The symptomatic hallmark of respiratory failure is dyspnea. Usually the sensation of dyspnea is more pronounced when respiratory failure develops acutely, although a decreased level of consciousness, either caused by the underlying disease process or drugs, may blunt the perception of respiratory distress. Furthermore, dyspnea is difficult to quantify, and the level of dyspnea correlates poorly with the severity of respiratory failure. Other symptoms such as cough, sputum production, fever, and chest pain may provide clues to the etiology of respiratory failure, but they are not very specific.

A patient's general appearance provides important guidance to the initial approach of respiratory failure. Cyanosis, especially when central, may indicate hypoxia. The patient's respiratory rate, use of accessory muscles,

diaphoresis, and ability to speak in full sentences may help assess the severity of respiratory failure, but those parameters are influenced by numerous other factors. These clinical features also may be helpful to assess response to treatment. Pulsus paradoxus, i.e., decreased blood pressure with inspiration, correlates with the degree of airway obstruction and dynamic hyperinflation, especially in patients with asthma. The lung exam can also provide important clues to the etiology of respiratory failure. Expiratory wheezing may occur with airway obstruction but correlates poorly with the degree of obstruction. In fact, severely impaired airflow may be insufficient to produce wheezing.

LABORATORY TESTING

Arterial blood gas analysis is the most useful test in the evaluation of respiratory failure. It is an important tool in the triage of patients, aids in the assessment of the acid-base status, and helps distinguish between hypoxic and hypercapnic respiratory failure. Calculating the alveolar-arterial oxygen gradient ($[A-a]O_2$) reflects the degree of hypoxia more accurately than just looking at the arterial partial pressure of oxygen (P_{O_2}):

$$(A-a)O_2 = FiO_2 \text{ (atmospheric pressure} - 47) - (pCO_2 \times 0.8) - P_{O_2}$$

FiO_2, fraction of inspired oxygen; pCO_2, pressure of carbon dioxide

A normal A-a gradient (A-a) is less than 10 torr but has to be adjusted for age:

$$\text{Normal A-a gradient} = (\text{age in years} + 10)/4$$

Pathophysiology

PATHOPHYSIOLOGY OF OXYGEN DELIVERY

Critically ill patients are susceptible to anaerobic metabolism, either related to insufficient oxygen delivery or impaired oxygen extraction. Oxygen delivery depends on the arterial oxygen content and cardiac output. In a normal patient, a normal resting cardiac output of 5 L per minute delivers approximately 1000 mL per minute of oxygen to the tissues. The tissues then extract approximately 25% of the delivered oxygen, which corresponds to a mixed venous oxygen saturation of 75% or a mixed venous P_{O_2} of 40 mm Hg.

Respiratory failure is often associated with conditions that result in increased oxygen demand. On the other hand, oxygen delivery may be impaired because of decreased cardiac contractility, an abnormal hemoglobin concentration, or a fall in arterial oxygen saturation. An oxygen uptake sufficient to maintain aerobic metabolism may still be accomplished through a physiologic increase in cardiac output and/or increase in peripheral oxygen extraction, but those compensatory mechanisms have limitations. Measuring *mixed venous saturations* through the pulmonary artery or the central venous catheter in critically ill patients provides important information about the status of oxygen delivery. A decrease in mixed venous saturation reflects increased peripheral oxygen extraction and occurs when oxygen demand exceeds delivery, such as in cardiogenic shock or hypovolemia. Critical illness may increase oxygen demand in peripheral tissue to such a degree that it cannot be met even when cardiac output and volume status are appropriate (high cardiac output state in a septic patient with adequate volume resuscitation). An abnormally high mixed-venous saturation may be seen in early sepsis, where abnormal distribution of blood flow may prevent oxygen extraction by the tissue. The mixed-venous P_{O_2} approximates the P_{O_2} surrounding capillary blood vessels and can be regarded as the driving pressure for oxygen diffusion from the capillaries into metabolizing cells. Low pV_{O_2} therefore may result in anaerobic metabolism and lactic acidosis.

Hypoxic Versus Hypercapnic Respiratory Failure

The underlying pathophysiology leading to hypoxic and hypercapnic respiratory failure is distinctly different. In hypoxic respiratory failure, blood flow is directed toward nonventilated alveoli (shunt perfusion), leading to hypoxia that is relatively refractory to supplemental oxygen. In hypercapnic respiratory failure, alveolar ventilation is insufficient for CO_2 elimination. The alveolar gas equation shows that with pure hypoventilation the alveolar oxygen level drops proportionally as CO_2 levels rise:

$$Pa_{O_2} = (FiO_2 \times [patm - pH_2O] - (pCO_2/0.8)]$$

patm, atmospheric pressure; pH_2O, partial pressure of water vapor

This may occur even with normal or increased minute ventilation, as a result of airflow to alveoli with poor circulation (dead space ventilation). Hypercapnia may also be the result of increased CO_2 production. In hypercapnic respiratory failure, hypoxia can easily be corrected with supplemental oxygen.

Hypoxic Respiratory Failure

In hypoxic respiratory failure, gas exchange is usually impaired by the alveoli filling with water, pus, or blood. Accordingly, blood passes nonventilated alveoli without

effective oxygen exchange, resulting in right-to-left intrapulmonary shunting. Alveolar collapse (microatelectasis) may also contribute to hypoxia. Commonly, hypoxic respiratory failure is caused by cardiogenic or noncardiogenic pulmonary edema.

Differentiating Cardiogenic Versus Noncardiogenic Pulmonary Edema

Pulmonary edema can occur as the result of increased hydrostatic pressure. This is commonly seen in left ventricular failure, where increased end-diastolic, left-ventricular pressures are transduced to the pulmonary vasculature and lead to alveolar filling. This may also occur with valvular disease, particularly mitral stenosis. Alternatively, pulmonary edema may occur when lung injury results in increased capillary permeability, which is seen in ARDS.

Distinguishing cardiogenic from noncardiogenic pulmonary edema is not always straightforward. Physical findings suggestive of heart failure or valvular disease may be helpful but fairly nonspecific. *Electrocardiogram (ECG) changes* and cardiac enzymes should be obtained to evaluate for possible cardiac ischemia. Reviewing the patient's fluid balance may provide further clues to the volume status. ARDS often occurs in the context of certain clinical scenarios, most commonly sepsis, lung injury secondary to aspiration or inhalation of toxic fumes, and massive resuscitation with blood products in trauma patients (Table 1).

Although quick and easy to obtain, unfortunately the *chest radiograph* is inaccurate in the diagnosis of cardiogenic versus noncardiogenic pulmonary edema. Findings suggestive of cardiogenic pulmonary edema include increased heart size; increased diameter of the vascular trunk; cephalization of blood flow; septal lines; and perihilar, symmetric distribution of infiltrates. In ARDS infiltrates tend to be patchy, extending to the lateral lung margins.

Echocardiography provides helpful information regarding ventricular function. The findings of left-ventricular dilatation with associated mitral regurgitation and wall-motion abnormalities are supportive of cardiogenic pulmonary edema. However, depressed

TABLE 1 Causes of Acute Respiratory Distress Syndrome

Direct Lung Injury	Indirect Lung Injury
Pneumonia	Sepsis
Toxic inhalation	Shock
Aspiration	Multiple blood transfusions
	Drug overdose
	Trauma
	Pancreatitis
	Massive fat embolus
	Brain injury

Rakel and Bope: *Conn's Current Therapy 2006.*

myocardial function commonly also may be seen in conditions leading to noncardiogenic pulmonary edema, most importantly in sepsis.

It is a matter of ongoing controversy whether *invasive hemodynamic monitoring* is helpful in the differential diagnosis of pulmonary edema and the management of patients with respiratory failure. Although it has been assumed that a pulmonary capillary wedge pressure greater than 18 to 20 mm Hg promotes fluid shift across the capillary membrane and causes hydrostatic pulmonary edema, studies have suggested that the central venous pressure and pulmonary artery occlusion pressure correlate poorly with volume and cardiac performance status, even in healthy subjects. Furthermore, alveolar flooding can occur at much lower pulmonary capillary pressure levels when capillary or alveolar damage is present, as seen in ARDS. In addition, there is considerable inter- and intraobserver variability when it comes to interpretation of data obtained through right heart catheterization. This is not to say that such data are useless, but they have to be interpreted with great caution in the proper clinical context. Following mixed venous hemoglobin saturations may provide important information regarding the patient's tissue oxygenation, and hemodynamic parameters may aid in adequate volume resuscitation and guide treatment with inotropes. Recently, a blood test for measuring the level of *pro-brain natriuretic peptide* (pro-BNP) has become readily available. Its level correlates with left-ventricular dysfunction and can help in the evaluation of hypoxic respiratory failure. It is less helpful in the evaluation of shock in the intensive care unit and does not supplement data obtained with right heart catheterization, because pro-BNP levels are commonly elevated in sepsis.

Management of Hypoxic Respiratory Failure

ACUTE RESPIRATORY DISTRESS SYNDROME

ARDS has been defined by an international consensus statement, outlining three diagnostic criteria:

1. A P_{O_2} to FiO_2 ratio of less than 200 (a ratio of less than 300 is defined as acute lung injury)
2. Bilateral pulmonary infiltrates
3. Pulmonary capillary wedge pressure (PCWP) of less than 18 mm Hg, or absence of elevated right atrial pressure if no right heart catheterization is performed

The definition of ARDS is intentionally broad, and it is important to recognize that not every patient who has ARDS is critically ill: A stable patient without heart failure with a P_{O_2} of 100 mm Hg on 50% oxygen with bilateral infiltrates meets ARDS criteria.

The course of ARDS is characterized by different stages (Fig. 1). Microscopically, the pulmonary lesions have been defined as diffuse alveolar damage (DAD). During the early *exudative stage* of DAD, pulmonary

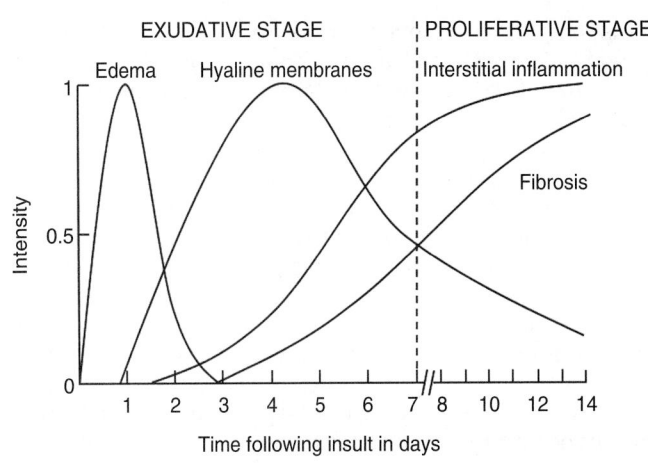

FIGURE 1. Representation of the time course of ARDS. The early stage is primarily characterized by alveolar filling. Alveolar exudates eventually organize and form hyaline membranes, triggering interstitial inflammation and fibrosis. (Redrawn from Katzenstein AA, Askin FB: Surgical Pathology of Non-Neoplastic Lung Diseases. Philadelphia, WB Saunders, 1982.)

capillary leakage predominates. The alveoli are flooded with proteinaceous fluid and cellular injury is minimal. The exudative stage of ARDS lasts for approximately 3 to 5 days. Later, protein material in the alveoli aggregates to form hyaline membranes, and inflammatory cells in the interstitium become more prominent. During the later or *proliferative stage* of ARDS, intense necrosis of type I alveolar cells occurs. The disorganized healing process with proliferation of type II alveolar epithelial cells and predominance of myofibroblasts and fibroblasts may lead to extensive pulmonary fibrosis (*fibrotic stage*). This process may begin as early as within 7 to 10 days.

Clinically, the exudative stage of ARDS is characterized by profound hypoxia and shunt perfusion. Over time, the shunt perfusion may improve as alveolar filling diminishes, and patients tend to be less responsive to extrinsic positive end-expiratory pressure (PEEP). The increase in dead space ventilation that occurs in the later stages of ARDS may result in substantial minute ventilation requirements.

ARDS itself is not a diagnosis but a descriptive term that may be related to numerous underlying conditions. Thus, the search for and treatment of the underlying cause of ARDS is the mainstay of therapy.

Most patients with ARDS require *mechanical ventilation*. Substantial research has been performed to develop strategies to improve the outcome of patients with ARDS. High-resolution computed tomography (HRCT) studies in ARDS patients have revealed that the alveolar filling process is heterogeneous; certain areas of the lung may show extensive alveolar filling, whereas others are relatively spared. Accordingly, the compliance of these areas will depend on the extent of the alveolar filling, and the summative volume of ventilated alveoli can be substantially smaller than total alveolar volume. The air delivered with mechanical ventilation will follow the path of least resistance and primarily ventilate areas of the lung with higher compliance.

This may lead to overdistension and barotrauma of "good" alveoli that still participate in oxygen exchange and cause further alveolar damage, a concept that has led to the use of lower tidal volumes and avoidance of high-plateau pressures in ARDS patients. A substantial body of evidence is available to support that such *lung-protective ventilation* actually improves outcome in ARDS patients. Based on these data, a tidal volume around 6 mL per kg of body weight should be used, and plateau pressures should remain less than 30 cmH$_2$O. Ideal or predicted rather than actual body weight should be used when calculating the tidal volume. This may become important in patients with obesity or massive edema secondary to third-space fluid, which commonly occurs in patients with sepsis.

It may be challenging to match a patient's ventilation requirements with such ventilator settings, particularly in the later stages of ARDS, when dead space ventilation (and minute ventilation requirements) may be substantial. The resulting respiratory acidosis is considered acceptable (*permissive hypercapnia*), as long as the pH is above critical levels (generally greater than 7.20). It has even been suggested that hypercapnia may be lung protective, but there are insufficient data to support induction of hypercapnia that is independent of lung-protective ventilation strategies.

The application of positive end-expiratory pressure (PEEP) may be of particular benefit during the early exudative phase of ARDS. In patients with ARDS, the qualitative and quantitative surfactant defect leads to considerable end-expiratory alveolar collapse. Repetitive cycles of alveolar collapse and redistension result in considerable shear stress, which can lead to further lung injury. PEEP can prevent alveolar collapse, help alveolar recruitment, and improve oxygenation in ARDS patients. Whether the addition of high PEEP levels to lung-protective ventilator strategies in ARDS prevents alveolar derecruitment and further improves outcome has recently been addressed in a large multicenter trial. No significant mortality differences were found between high (14 cmH$_2$O) versus low (8 cmH$_2$O) PEEP levels, but these results cannot be regarded as the final answer.

Cardiogenic Pulmonary Edema

This article does not cover the management of heart failure; however, we would like to comment on some specific aspects regarding the management of hypoxic respiratory failure associated with cardiogenic pulmonary edema. The application of continuous positive airway pressure (CPAP) can help with alveolar recruitment, improve oxygenation, reduce left-ventricular preload and afterload, improve left-ventricular function, and reduce the work of breathing. Similar effects are achieved with mechanical ventilation and PEEP. Discontinuation of mechanical ventilation in patients with congestive heart failure may be particularly difficult, because it results in increased preload and afterload. These effects may be aggravated by stress and anxiety that occur during this process. Therefore, it is important to optimize cardiac therapy prior to discontinuing mechanical

ventilation. A transition from invasive to noninvasive positive pressure ventilation may facilitate the weaning process.

Hypercapnic Respiratory Failure

Hypercapnic respiratory failure is seen in conditions that cause alveolar hypoventilation, either related to decrease in respiratory drive (for example, narcotic overdose), neuromuscular disease (Guillain-Barré syndrome, myasthenia gravis, etc.) or obstructive airways disease (decompensated asthma, COPD).

In a drug overdose, the indication for mechanical ventilation is usually based on airway protection and respiratory acidosis related to a suppressed respiratory drive. Direct pulmonary complications are usually absent unless the consumed drug has pulmonary toxicity. Cocaine inhalation, for example, may cause noncardiogenic pulmonary edema by mechanisms that are incompletely understood. Lung injury in drug overdose may also occur as the result of aspiration. The care for patients with drug overdose is largely supportive and may include measures to decrease absorption of ingested substances, such as gastric lavage and activated charcoal. Patients with neuromuscular disease may benefit from noninvasive positive-pressure ventilation (NPPV).

Obstructive Airways Disease: Asthma and Chronic Obstructive Pulmonary Disease

CHRONIC OBSTRUCTIVE PULMONARY DISEASE

Patients with exacerbated COPD often present with a mixture of hypoxia, which is worse than at baseline, and hypercapnia. Hypoxia is the result of nonuniform airway obstruction and may result in ventilation/perfusion mismatch. In addition, there may be areas of pulmonary consolidation with alveolar filling, which can result in hypoxia. Hypercarbia is the result of alveolar hypoventilation from airway obstruction. In addition, respiratory muscle fatigue may result in decreased minute ventilation, and the increased work of breathing can increase CO$_2$ production.

COPD exacerbations are most commonly caused by infections (bacterial or viral), followed by environmental factors (air pollution, etc.), and reflux disease (including aspiration). In up to one-third of all patients, an underlying cause cannot be identified. Bacterial organisms frequently associated with COPD exacerbations include *Haemophilus influenzae*, *Streptococcus pneumoniae*, *Moraxella catarrhalis*, and *Chlamydia pneumoniae*; with more advanced disease, patients are also at risk of developing infections with *Pseudomonas*.

The mortality risk for COPD exacerbations requiring hospital admission is high and continues to rise after hospital discharge. Mortality for patients requiring admission to the intensive care unit can be as high as 20%.

Rakel and Bope: Conn's Current Therapy 2006.

Factors that have been associated with increased mortality in patients with COPD exacerbations include older age, severity of illness, lower-body mass index, coexisting congestive heart failure and cor pulmonale, prior functional status, serum albumin level, lower P_{O_2}/FiO_2 ratio, and prior use of corticosteroids.

The administration of *supplemental oxygen* is a major supportive intervention in the management of COPD exacerbations. Hypoxia may be easily correctable with low-flow oxygen via nasal canula because $\dot{V}/\dot{Q}$ mismatch is usually the main underlying mechanism in COPD exacerbations. The risk of worsening hypercapnia in this setting is usually low and has to be balanced against the benefit of maintaining adequate oxygen delivery. Patients with severe respiratory acidosis and those who require high-flow oxygen (suggesting a process other than, or in addition to $\dot{V}/\dot{Q}$ mismatch, as causing hypoxia) are at higher risk for worsening hypercapnia and should be monitored closely with arterial blood gases. The P_{O_2} should be targeted around 60 mm Hg, which corresponds to a hemoglobin saturation of approximately 90%.

Bronchodilators are crucial in the management of COPD exacerbations. Combination therapy with β agonists and anticholinergics is feasible and safe and can be administered via nebulizer or metered dose inhaler. The routine use of theophylline (e.g., Theo-Dur, Uniphyl), once considered standard therapy, should be discouraged because of its limited efficacy in the acute setting, narrow therapeutic window, and side effects. The addition of *corticosteroids* may decrease airway inflammation and is recommended in COPD exacerbations requiring hospital admission. The best dose regimen is unknown, but giving 30 to 40 mg of oral prednisone per day for 10 to 14 days is a reasonable compromise between efficacy and safety. *Antibiotics* should be used when increased sputum volume and purulence indicate an underlying infection and should reflect local sensitivity profiles of likely organisms.

NONINVASIVE MECHANICAL VENTILATION IN CHRONIC OBSTRUCTIVE PULMONARY DISEASE

To avoid respiratory muscle fatigue and improve alveolar ventilation, NPPV is well established in patients with COPD exacerbations (further information follows). If NPPV is contemplated, one should consider its use early in the course of respiratory failure and before severe acidosis develops, to avoid the need for endotracheal intubation. Dyspneic patients may experience a certain degree of claustrophobia when the mask is put on. This can be mediated by good communication and a slow titration to target pressure levels.

ASTHMA

Patients with asthma exacerbations typically present with a combination of mild hypoxia (average P_{O_2} around 69 mm Hg), hypocapnia, and respiratory alkalosis. The hypoxia is the result of $\dot{V}/\dot{Q}$ mismatching. Respiratory alkalosis develops because most patients with asthma exacerbations are dyspneic and hyperventilate.

Therefore, normocapnia is usually indicative of severe airflow limitation and should be viewed as impending respiratory failure. Hypercapnia and respiratory acidosis may develop as a consequence of severe airways obstruction, decreased cardiac output with lactic acidosis (as a consequence of dynamic hyperinflation), and increased CO_2 production by respiratory muscles.

Short-acting β agonists like albuterol (Proventil, Ventolin, Volmax) and terbutaline (Brethine) are rapid in onset, provide superior bronchodilatation compared to anticholinergics and methylxanthines, and can be considered first line in the treatment of asthma exacerbations. Although long-acting β agonists such as salmeterol (Serevent) and formoterol (Foradil) are effective and safe in the treatment of stable asthma, they are generally not recommended in the emergency treatment of asthma exacerbations. There is some data to suggest that long-acting β agonists have a role in the postemergency department treatment of acute asthma. The therapeutic effect of albuterol depends on the administered dose, not on the mode of delivery. Usually, three 2.5 mg treatments of albuterol are given by nebulizer every 20 minutes. A total dose of 10 mg restores peak expiratory flow rates to 60% of predicted in approximately 60% of patients presenting with asthma exacerbations. The response to albuterol is not influenced by the chronic use of long-acting β agonists. Levalbuterol (Xopenex) may offer some advantages over albuterol in the emergency room treatment of asthma exacerbations. Reserve therapy with subcutaneous terbutaline (Brethine) or epinephrine can be considered in patients where inhalation therapy cannot be administered because of altered mental status or in patients with refractory bronchospasm.

Anticholinergics like ipratropium (Atrovent) are less potent, have a slower onset of action, and are considered second line. They can be used in combination with β agonists. Theophylline (Uniphyl, Theo-Dur) has limited efficacy in acute asthma and probably should not be used.

Because asthma exacerbations are commonly associated with intense airway inflammation, the use of *corticosteroids* in the management of acute asthma is the established standard of care. Because corticosteroids have a delayed onset of action of at least 6 hours, they should be instituted early in the treatment course. A dose-response relationship for corticosteroids could not be established, and higher quantities do not offer additional advantage over more conventional dosing schedules. The U.S. guidelines recommend 120 to 180 mg of intravenous methylprednisolone (Solu-Medrol), divided into 3 to 4 doses per day for the first 2 days in asthma exacerbations requiring hospitalization, followed by 60 to 80 mg per day until peak expiratory flow reaches 70% of predicted. Oral preparations are similarly efficacious, and 30 to 60 mg of prednisone per day can be given instead of intravenous corticosteroids.

Asthma exacerbations are often triggered by noninfectious etiologies; thus the routine use of *antibiotics* is much less established than in exacerbations of COPD.

Issues regarding invasive and noninvasive mechanical ventilation in patients with asthma are discussed further on in the article.

Invasive Mechanical Ventilation in Obstructive Airways Disease

When patients with obstructive airways disease fail to respond to conservative therapy and/or noninvasive positive-pressure ventilation, intubation may be life-saving. There are no set criteria to guide in the decision when to intubate a patient with obstructive airways disease. However, progressive hypercapnia despite therapy, worsening mental status with obtundation, refractory hypoxemia, and impending cardiopulmonary collapse are generally accepted indications. Managing patients with obstructive airways disease on invasive mechanical ventilation can be challenging. Airway inflammation, obstruction, and hyper-responsiveness can be extreme, particularly in status asthmaticus. Airflow limitation slows lung emptying, and exhalation is incomplete when the next breath is already initiated. The accumulating air that remains in the lung creates a pressure gradient between the alveoli and the airways, which is termed *dynamic hyperinflation* or *auto-PEEP*. In an intubated patient, dynamic hyperinflation can be identified by simply observing flow curves on the ventilator. If the flow fails to reach zero at the end of expiration, dynamic hyperinflation is usually present (Fig. 2). The level of auto-PEEP is measured by performing an occlusion at end expiration.

Dynamic hyperinflation may worsen with the application of positive pressure ventilation. This poses a risk for hemodynamic collapse (once the intrathoracic pressure raises enough to impede venous return) and barotrauma. Ventilator management therefore has to be aimed at limiting dynamic hyperinflation. The amount of hyperinflation is determined by the minute ventilation, tidal volume and expiratory time. Therefore, dynamic hyperinflation can be limited by choosing relatively small tidal volumes (6 to 10 mL/kg), lower respiratory rates (8 to 12 breaths/min), and higher inspiratory flow rates (80 to 100 L/min) with the goal to keep static inspiratory pressures (plateau pressures)

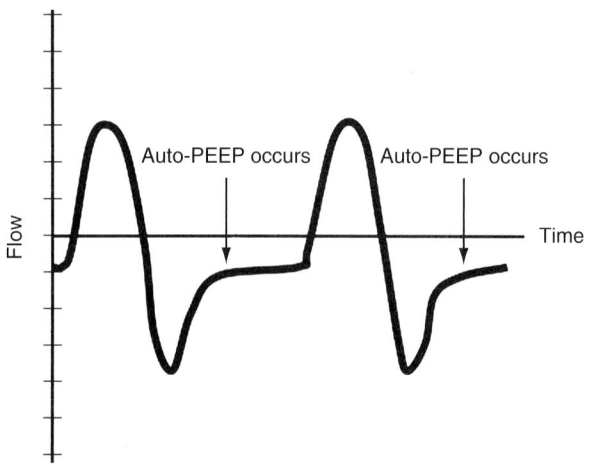

FIGURE 2. Flow-curve demonstrating auto-PEEP on a mechanically ventilated patient. The flow fails to reach zero at the end of expiration.

below 30 cmH$_2$O. This may result in high peak inspiratory pressures that can usually be tolerated.

Because the patient has to counterbalance auto-PEEP to initiate patient-triggered breaths, dynamic hyperinflation may also increase the work of breathing. In this situation the increased effort can be alleviated by applying *extrinsic PEEP*, which decreases the pressure gradient between airways and alveoli that is created by dynamic hyperinflation. The level of extrinsic PEEP should be around 80% of the measured auto-PEEP.

Approaches to reduce dynamic hyperinflation reduce minute ventilation and may cause or worsen respiratory acidosis. Respiratory acidosis is usually tolerated as long as it develops gradually and the pH stays above 7.20. However, this mode of ventilation may be extremely uncomfortable for the patient and usually requires deep sedation. Sometimes airway obstruction can be so severe that the use of *paralytics* cannot be avoided. It is important to realize that the combination of paralytics and systemic corticosteroids is associated with a high risk of neuropathy and myopathy. Therefore, the use of paralytics should be limited as much as possible.

Decision to Extubate

The timing of discontinuing mechanical ventilation is of considerable consequence, because both delayed and failed extubation can add to a patient's morbidity and mortality risk. Factors associated with a higher risk for extubation failure include co-morbidities, older age, length of mechanical ventilation, continuous use of sedatives, and severity of illness at the time of extubation. Patients receiving mechanical ventilation should undergo daily *spontaneous breathing trials* to assess extubation potential, if the following criteria are met:

1. Evidence of some improvement of the underlying cause of respiratory failure
2. Adequate oxygenation and acid-base status (i.e., P$_{O_2}$ to FiO$_2$ ratio >150 to 200 or FiO$_2$ requirement of less than 50%, PEEP between 5 and 8 cm H$_2$O, pH greater than 7.25)
3. Hemodynamic stability (i.e., not dependent on vasopressors and absence of hypotension, no evidence of myocardial ischemia)
4. Ability to initiate spontaneous breaths

The decision to extubate is usually preceded by a successful spontaneous breathing trial, which should be performed on a T-piece or with low levels of pressure support ventilation. No clear guidelines exist as to how long the patient needs to sustain a spontaneous breathing trial to predict successful extubation, but time frames between 30 and 120 minutes are reasonable. A successful, spontaneous breathing trial indicates a probability of extubation success in excess of 75%. Of the specific parameters to assess a patient's performance and the likelihood of successful extubation, a respiratory rate to tidal volume ratio (*rapid shallow breathing index*) of less than 105 is perhaps the most reliable. Other *weaning parameters* include negative inspiratory force (NIF), minute ventilation, and tidal volume (Table 2).

Rakel and Bope: Conn's Current Therapy 2006.

TABLE 2 Weaning Parameters Associated With a Higher Chance of Successful Extubation

	Threshold Value	Normal (Not Mechanically Ventilated)
FiO$_2$	<0.60	Roomair (0.21)
P$_{O_2}$/FiO$_2$ ratio	>240	>450
Vital capacity	>10 mL/kg	60 to 80 mL/kg
Tidal volume	>300 mL	450 mL
Respiratory rate	<30	<20
Minute ventilation	<10 L/min	6 L/min
NIF	≥20 cmH$_2$O	≥100 cmH$_2$O
Rapid shallow breathing index (respiratory rate/tidal volume in liters)	<105	<30

Abbreviations: FiO$_2$ = fraction of inspired oxygen; NIF = negative inspiratory force; P$_{O_2}$ = pressure of oxygen.

BOX 1 Selection Criteria for NPPV in the Acute Setting

Appropriate diagnosis with potential reversibility
Establish need for ventilator assistance
- Moderate to severe respiratory distress
- Tachypnea
- Accessory muscle use or abdominal paradox
- Blood gas derangement pH <7.35, pCO$_2$ >45 mm Hg or P$_{O_2}$/FiO$_2$ <200

Exclude patients with contraindications to NPPV:
- Respiratory arrest
- Medically unstable
- Unable to protect airway
- Excessive secretions
- Uncooperative or agitated
- Unable to fit mask
- Recent upper airway or gastrointestinal surgery

From Liesching T, Kwok H, Hill NS: Acute Applications of Noninvasive Positive Pressure Ventilation. Chest 2003;124:699-713.
Abbreviations: FiO$_2$ = fraction of inspired oxygen; NPPV = noninvasive positive pressure ventilation; P$_{O_2}$ = pressure of oxygen.

Patients failing spontaneous breathing trials should be kept on a mode of ventilation that provides sufficient support to rest the respiratory muscles for 24 hours before undergoing the next spontaneous breathing trial.

Noninvasive Positive Pressure Ventilation

PATIENT SELECTION

In appropriately selected patients (Box 1), NPPV can obviate the need for intubation, decrease the risk of infections, shorten hospital stay, and allow earlier extubation of mechanically ventilated patients. NPPV should not be used in patients that are medically unstable; had respiratory arrest; or are unable to protect their airway, either from altered level of consciousness or excessive secretions. The use of NPPV requires a certain amount of understanding and cooperation from the patient. NPPV should not be used if the patient's facial anatomy does not allow appropriate fitting of the NPPV interface.

The strongest evidence for the use of NPPV is available for exacerbation of chronic obstructive pulmonary disease, for which it is a standard of care. Patients with severe COPD exacerbations and respiratory acidosis (pH <7.30) seem to benefit the most. In contrast to COPD, there is insufficient evidence to support the routine use of NPPV in patients with asthma. Whether NPPV should be used in patients with hypoxic respiratory failure without hypercapnia remains controversial, and the data from available studies are conflicting, likely because hypoxic respiratory failure represents such a heterogeneous group of diagnoses. High failure rates have been reported in patients with pneumonia and ARDS, except for patients with COPD and pneumonia. Immunocompromised patients can benefit from NPPV because they are at particularly high risk to develop nosocomial infections.

Use of NPPV in acute cardiogenic pulmonary edema is also controversial. Although continuous positive airway pressure (CPAP) is beneficial for hypoxic patients with acute cardiogenic pulmonary edema, evidence that NPPV raises the incidence of myocardial infarction in this population is of concern, but these findings were unconfirmed in a subsequent trial. NPPV can benefit patients with cardiogenic pulmonary edema that are also hypercapnic. In normocapnic patients, CPAP seems to be as effective as NPPV and should be the preferred mode of therapy until more conclusive data become available.

Limited data are available about whether NPPV allows earlier extubation, and the role of NPPV in the peri-extubation period remains to be determined. It seems reasonable, however, to consider NPPV in patients with acute or chronic respiratory failure that do not meet extubation criteria but would otherwise be good candidates. There is only a limited role for the use of NPPV in patients who fail planned extubation; two trials conducted in this setting produced negative results.

FACTORS PREDICTING SUCCESS OF NONINVASIVE POSITIVE PRESSURE VENTILATION

Not every patient responds favorably to NPPV, and approximately 25% of patients that receive NPPV will eventually require intubation. Factors associated with NPPV failure include greater severity of illness and acidosis, the presence of pneumonia, excessive secretions, pursed-lip breathing, and inadequate sealing of the NPPV interface. Patients are also more likely to fail NPPV treatment if blood gases and/or level of consciousness fail to improve after one hour, which underlines the importance of close clinical monitoring.

4

CURRENT DIAGNOSIS

Physical exam findings may provide important clues to etiology and severity of acute respiratory failure, but they may be nonspecific and generally unreliable. An arterial blood gas is the single most important test in the evaluation of acute respiratory failure to differentiate between hypoxia and hypercapnia. Following arterial blood gases also helps to assess response to therapeutic interventions. Chest radiograph, electrocardiogram (ECG), echocardiogram, and pro-brain natriuretic peptide (pro-BNP) levels provide additional information and may help differentiate between cardiogenic and noncardiogenic pulmonary edema.

NONINVASIVE POSITIVE PRESSURE VENTILATION INTERFACE SELECTION

Different devices are available to apply NPPV. Often nasal or oronasal interfaces are used. Although nasal devices offer the potential advantage of greater patient comfort, decreased risk of aspiration and less interference with speech, they also have a higher tendency to leak, because the mouth needs to remain closed in order for the positive pressure to be delivered effectively. In the acute setting, it may therefore be preferable to use oronasal devices. Helmet devices that fit entirely over the patient's head and snugly around the neck have recently been introduced, but there is limited experience in acute respiratory failure. The large air volume within the circuit raises concerns of effective triggering and cycling of the ventilator and increases the risk of rebreathing. Thus, helmet devices cannot be recommended in acute respiratory failure until these issues have been adequately addressed.

VENTILATOR SELECTION

Any ventilator that is used for invasive mechanical ventilation can also deliver NPPV. Most commonly, portable pressure ventilators are used. Typically, these machines deliver inspiratory positive airway pressure (IPAP) and expiratory positive airway pressure (EPAP). The level of EPAP is equivalent to PEEP on conventional ventilator devices, whereas the difference between IPAP and EPAP equals pressure support (i.e., an IPAP of 10 cmH$_2$O and an EPAP of 5 cmH$_2$O equals 5 cmH$_2$O of PEEP and 5 cmH$_2$O of pressure support on a conventional ventilator).

In general, oxygenation mostly will be affected by the level of EPAP, whereas ventilation is affected by the level of pressure support, i.e., the difference between IPAP and EPAP. Most portable pressure ventilators do not have an oxygen control, and oxygen is added into the circuit. The actual fraction of inspired oxygen cannot be determined under those circumstances, because room air is mixed with supplemental oxygen, and the concentration of delivered oxygen also depends on the flow,

 CURRENT THERAPY

Therapeutic interventions largely depend on the underlying etiology of acute respiratory failure. In acute respiratory distress syndrome (ARDS), identification and treatment of the underlying cause must be attempted. Ventilator management should follow lung-protective strategies. Optimizing heart failure therapy is crucial to ensure successful extubation in patients requiring mechanical ventilation for cardiogenic pulmonary edema. Supplemental oxygen, bronchodilator therapy with beta-agonists and anticholinergics, corticosteroids, and appropriate use of antibiotics are the key therapeutic elements in the management of acute respiratory failure in patients with chronic obstructive pulmonary disease (COPD). The use of noninvasive positive pressure ventilation in these patients is well established. In comparison, the role of anticholinergics, antibiotics and noninvasive positive pressure ventilation in patients with asthma is much less established. If mechanical ventilation has to be used in patients with obstructive airway disease, the management should focus on prevention of dynamic hyperinflation. Daily spontaneous breathing trials are proven to shorten the duration of mechanical ventilation. Being able to sustain a spontaneous breathing trial for 30 to 120 minutes has a high positive predictive value for successful extubation.

that is, lower concentrations can be expected with higher pressure levels. Some newer generation devices have an oxygen blender and combine the convenience of portability with the ability to control the FiO$_2$.

It is important to realize that patients with acute respiratory failure often present with anxiety and agitation, and it is crucial to carefully explain the NPPV procedure to the patient, ensure comfortable and appropriate mask fitting, and gently adjust the pressure settings to the desired target levels. This may be very time consuming, particularly when NPPV is first initiated.

REFERENCES

Bach PB, Brown C, Gelfand SE, et al: Management of acute exacerbations of chronic obstructive pulmonary disease: A summary and appraisal of published evidence. Ann Intern Med 2001;134:600-620.

Blanch L, Bernabe F, Lucangelo U: Measurement of air trapping, intrinsic positive end-expiratory pressure, and dynamic hyperinflation in mechanically ventilated patients. Respir Care 2005;50:110-124.

Brower RG, Lanken PN, MacIntyre N, et al: Higher versus lower positive end-expiratory pressures in patients with the acute respiratory distress syndrome. N Engl J Med 2004;351:327-336.

Fabbri LM, Hurd SS: Global strategy for the diagnosis, management and prevention of COPD: 2003 update. Eur Respir J 2003;22:1-2.

Hall JS, Schmidt GA, Wood L: Principles of Critical Care, 2nd ed. New York: McGraw-Hill, 1998.

Hess DR: The evidence for noninvasive positive-pressure ventilation in the care of patients in acute respiratory failure: A systematic review of the literature. Respir Care 2004;49:810-829.

Hospenthal MA, Peters JI: Long-acting beta(2)-agonists in the management of asthma exacerbations. Curr Opin Pulm Med 2005;11:69-73.

Kumar A, Anel R, Bunnell E, et al: Pulmonary artery occlusion pressure and central venous pressure fail to predict ventricular filling volume, cardiac performance, or the response to volume infusion in normal subjects. Crit Care Med 2004;32:691-699.

Laffey JG, O'Croinin D, McLoughlin P, et al: Permissive hypercapnia—Role in protective lung ventilatory strategies. Intensive Care Med 2004;30:347-356.

Liesching T, Kwok H, Hill NS: Acute applications of noninvasive positive pressure ventilation. Chest 2003;124:699-713.

MacIntyre NR, Cook DJ, Ely EW Jr, et al: Evidence-based guidelines for weaning and discontinuing ventilatory support: A collective task force facilitated by the American College of Chest Physicians; the American Association for Respiratory Care; and the American College of Critical Care Medicine. Chest 2001;120:S375-S395.

McFadden ER Jr: Acute severe asthma. Am J Respir Crit Care Med 2003;168:740-759.

Ram FS, Picot J, Lightowler J, et al: Non-invasive positive pressure ventilation for treatment of respiratory failure caused by exacerbations of chronic obstructive pulmonary disease. Cochrane Database Syst Rev 2004;CD004104.

Schumaker GL, Epstein SK: Managing acute respiratory failure during exacerbation of chronic obstructive pulmonary disease. Respir Care 2004;49:766-782.

The Acute Respiratory Distress Syndrome Network. Ventilation with lower tidal volumes as compared with traditional tidal volumes for acute lung injury and the acute respiratory distress syndrome. N Engl J Med 2000;342:1301-1308.

Tung RH, Garcia C, Morss AM, et al: Utility of B-type natriuretic peptide for the evaluation of intensive care unit shock. Crit Care Med 2004;32:1643-1647.

Atelectasis

Method of
David R. Jones, MD and Brian K. Rundall, DO

Background

The diagnosis of atelectasis refers to collapse of alveoli leading to hypoventilation of a segment, lobe, or the entire lung. The condition can be acute or chronic and may or may not result in symptoms. Lobar atelectasis occurs in 8.5% of adult surgical intensive care unit (SICU) patients. The incidence of atelectasis in the postoperative patient is well studied and varies from 15% to 98%. It is as high as 64% to 65% in the postoperative cardiac patient and only 20% to 30% following abdominal surgery. Atelectasis is the most common complication following thoracic surgery, and the more severe form, lobar atelectasis, is reported in 5% to 8% postoperatively. Rounded atelectasis is most often asymptomatic, and in one report the yearly incidence was 5 to 15 cases in a 100,000 population (Table 1).

Rakel and Bope: *Conn's Current Therapy 2006.*

TABLE 1 Atelectasis: Incidence by Patient Population

Type of atelectasis	Incidence
All Types	
Surgical patients	15%-98%
Cardiac surgery	64%-65%
Abdominal surgery	20%-30%
Lobar	
Intensive care unit patients	8.5%
Thoracic surgery	5%-7.8%
Rounded	
Men older than 40 y	5-15/100,000

Types of Atelectasis

The several types of atelectasis can be easily classified by mechanism or by radiographic patterns. Resorptive or obstructive atelectasis is caused by mucus, foreign bodies, endobronchial tumors, lymph nodes, or extrapulmonary masses causing compression of major or multiple small bronchi. Passive atelectasis occurs secondary to a space-occupying process in the chest, particularly pneumothorax or hydrothorax. Adhesive atelectasis denotes collapse occurring secondary to loss of surfactant, as seen in association with pneumonia, hyaline membrane disease, or acute respiratory distress syndrome (ARDS). Compression atelectasis is a localized compression of parenchyma, as seen in lung adjacent to a chest wall, pleural, or intraparenchymal mass, loculated fluid collection, or bulla. Cicatrization atelectasis results from idiopathic pulmonary fibrosis, chronic tuberculosis, fungal infections, or radiation fibrosis. Rounded or folded atelectasis, seen in lung adjacent to the pleura, is associated with asbestosis, tuberculosis, or parapneumonic effusions. The following are types organized by radiographic patterns. They are subsegmental or platelike, segmental, lobar, whole lung, or generalized.

Causes

Common causes for atelectasis are retained secretions, hypoventilation, oversedation, decreased patient mobilization, and ineffective cough from pain as occurs in the elderly with rib fractures, chest trauma, or following upper abdominal or chest surgery.

Presentation

Common signs and symptoms of atelectasis are tachypnea, tachycardia, hypoxia, fever, diminished breath sounds, and dullness to percussion over the affected area. If developed over a longer period, symptoms may not be present, as in the case of rounded atelectasis. The radiographic changes on chest roentgenogram are categorized as direct or indirect. Direct signs are displaced pulmonary vessels, air bronchograms, and displacement of the fissures. Indirect signs are pulmonary opacification, diaphragmatic elevation, hyperexpansion of unaffected lung, tracheal, heart, and mediastinal shift toward the atelectatic side, shift of the hilum toward the collapsed lobe or segment, and ipsilateral rib approximation. The most reliable sign of collapse is the displacement of interlobar fissures. Radiographic patterns of lower lobe collapse are similar on the right and left sides, and one study reports a twofold higher incidence of left lower lobe collapse than right. The less common upper lobe collapse demonstrates radiographic differences between right and left lobes. The radiographic diagnosis of rounded atelectasis demonstrates a peripheral location that has the following site predilections: right upper lobe, 2%; right middle lobe, 11%; right lower lobe, 47%; left upper lobe, 3%; lingula, 10%; left lower lobe, 27%.

Diagnosis

Early diagnosis of a patient with acute lobar collapse requires radiographic evaluation of a hypoxemic and tachypneic patient, then identification of pulmonary opacification, diaphragmatic elevation, displacement of interlobar fissures, and mediastinal shift.

Treatment

The treatment for atelectasis is aimed at clearing secretions, as in chest percussion, vibration, nasotracheal and bronchoscopic suctioning, and reexpansion of the lung with incentive spirometry, hyperinflation, continuous positive airway pressure (CPAP), intermittent positive pressure breathing, and ambulation. Adequate pain control in the patient with thoracic trauma can be difficult to manage, but significant reductions in the incidence of lobar collapse are achieved with epidural analgesia. These treatment modalities are generally accepted, but the most effective combination lacks a consensus. In one study, lobar atelectasis treated with hyperinflation and suction only was better resolved when vibration and positioning were added. In a prospective study, the addition of bronchoscopy to a respiratory therapy regimen added no benefit in resolving lobar atelectasis. A meta-analysis of postoperative analgesia and prevention of atelectasis showed that administration of opiate and/or local anesthetic via epidural catheter and local infiltration of the wound is superior to systemic opioids. The management of rounded atelectasis usually involves careful radiographic follow-up to rule out a

CURRENT DIAGNOSIS

- Tachypnea
- Hypoxia
- Fever
- Diminished breath sounds
- Dullness to percussion or affected area
- Radiographic changes

CURRENT THERAPY

Prevention and Treatment of Atelectasis
- Encourage deep breathing and coughing
- Incentive spirometry
- Early ambulation
- Adequate pain control
- Chest percussion therapy
- Positive pressure breathing
- Nasotracheal suctioning
- Bronchoscopic suctioning

bronchogenic carcinoma. A biopsy of the lesion occasionally is required if the diagnosis is in question. Prevention remains the most effective treatment modality to improve outcomes.

Key Treatment Points

Treatment is aimed at clearing secretions and reexpansion. The most common modalities are chest percussion, nasotracheal suctioning to clear secretions, incentive spirometry, positive pressure breathing, adequate pain control in thoracic trauma and postoperative patients, and early ambulation to aid reexpansion. Prevention remains the cornerstone treatment and, as such, includes deep breathing, coughing, incentive spirometry, early ambulation, and adequate pain control.

REFERENCES

Ballantyne J, Carr DB, deFerranti S, et al: The comparative effects of postoperative analgesic therapies on pulmonary outcome: Cumulative meta-analyses of randomized, controlled trial. Anesth Analg 1998;86:598-612.

Goodman LR: Postoperative chest radiograph: I. Alterations after abdominal surgery. AJR Am J Roentgenol 1980;134:533-541.

Hillerdal G: Rounded atelectasis: Clinical experience with 74 patients. Chest 1989;95(4):836-841.

Magnusson L, Zemgulis V, Wicky S, et al: Atelectasis is a major cause of hypoxia and shunt after cardiopulmonary bypass. Anesthesiology 1996;87:1153-1163.

Marini JJ, Pierson DJ, Hudson LD: Acute lobar atelectasis: A prospective comparison of fiberoptic bronchoscopy and respiratory therapy. Am Rev Respir Dis 1979;119:971-978.

Miller WT: Radiographic evaluation of the lungs and chest. In Shields TW (ed): General Thoracic Surgery, vol 1, 4th ed. Philadelphia, Williams and Wilkins, 1994, pp 145-148.

Pasquina P, Tramer MR, Walder B: Prophylactic respiratory physiotherapy after cardiac surgery: Systematic review. BMJ 2003;327: 1-6.

Stiller K, Geake T, Taylor J, et al: Acute lobar atelectasis: A comparison of two chest physiotherapy regimens. Chest 1990;98:1336-1340.

Uzieblo M, Welsh R, Pursel SE, Chmielewski GW: Incidence and significance of lobar atelectasis in thoracic surgical patients. Am Surg 2000;66(5):476-480.

Wisner D: A stepwise logistic regression analysis of factors affecting morbidity after thoracic trauma: Effect of epidural analgesia. J Trauma 1990;30(7):799-804.

Management of Chronic Obstructive Pulmonary Disease

Method of
Juan Armando Garcia, MD, and
Stephen G. Jenkinson, MD

Chronic obstructive pulmonary disease (COPD) is characterized by airflow limitation that is not fully reversible. The airflow limitation is usually both progressive and associated with an abnormal inflammatory response of the lungs to noxious particles of gases. Under the direction of the National Heart, Lung, and Blood Institute (NHLBI) and the World Health Organization (WHO), collaborative guidelines on the diagnosis and management of chronic obstructive pulmonary disease (COPD) have been assembled by an expert panel: the Global Initiative for Chronic Obstructive Lung Disease (GOLD). These guidelines define the classifications of COPD on the basis of both severity and type of symptoms and explore all new information on the diagnosis and treatment of COPD. The GOLD initiative aims to improve prevention and management of COPD through a concerted worldwide effort of people involved in all facets of health care policy and to encourage a renewed research interest in this extremely prevalent disease.

To assure that recommendations for management of COPD are based on current scientific literature, the GOLD program established a science committee to update the sections of the report on recommendations for management of COPD each year. Although the update of these sections will occur each year and will be posted on the Web site (http://www.goldcopd.com), the full report will be updated and printed every 5 years. The latest update, including new modifications of management, was published in late 2003.

Pathophysiology

The pathophysiology of COPD is somewhat different in various patients, and the terms *emphysema* or *chronic bronchitis* were used in the past. Both of these disorders cause airway obstruction. Emphysema is defined pathologically as abnormal permanent enlargement of airspaces distal to the terminal bronchioles, accompanied by destruction of their walls and without obvious fibrosis. This tissue destruction results in enlargement of proximal and distal airspaces and can ultimately form bullae in the lung parenchyma. These bullae result in loss of surface area for gas exchange in the involved lungs. There is also a genetically inherited form of emphysema which is caused by the α_1-antitrypsin (AAT) deficiency. This disorder accounts for less than 1% of COPD cases in the United States. AAT is a protease inhibitor produced by the liver that circulates into tissues. Active proteases are released into the lung by lung macrophages, which can contribute to the development

of emphysema. When patients smoke cigarettes, they also recruit a neutrophil population into their lungs. These neutrophils release neutrophil elastase (another type of protease) and other toxic molecules, which can destroy alveolar walls and may also contribute to the production of emphysema. AAT offers protection from these effects, but the protection found in normal people is inadequate in patients with AAT deficiency. Patients who develop emphysema despite normal levels of AAT usually develop emphysema in the fifth or sixth decades of life, whereas patients with AAT deficiency can develop emphysema as early as the third or fourth decades of life, depending on the extent of their deficiency and smoking history.

All patients developing emphysema who form bullae before the age of 45 years should be evaluated for AAT deficiency. A normal serum level of AAT is greater than 11 mmol/L (>80 mg/dL). Patients with low levels of AAT should be evaluated by a pulmonologist and may be candidates for AAT replacement therapy.

Chronic bronchitis is defined clinically as the presence of chronic, productive cough for 3 months during each of 2 consecutive years, and for which other causes of chronic cough are excluded. The other most common causes of chronic cough include asthma, gastric reflux, or postnasal drip secondary to sinus disease. The pathologic findings of chronic bronchitis are enlargement of tracheobronchial mucus glands, variable amounts of airway smooth-muscle hyperplasia, inflammation, and bronchial wall thickening. Abnormalities of small airways may be present as well and are accompanied by fibrosis and the presence of a mononuclear inflammatory process. The forced expiratory volume at 1 second (FEV_1) of a COPD patient is inversely proportional to the number of inflammatory cells in the airways. Patients with chronic bronchitis also have increased mucus hypersecretion, goblet cell metaplasia, increased submucosal gland formation, and abnormal matrix deposition.

The use of the terms *emphysema* or *chronic bronchitis* is no longer specified in the GOLD definition of COPD. The inflammation seen in COPD is different from that seen in asthma, but some obstructive lung disease patients do have pathologic changes that can be seen in both diseases, so some overlap does occur.

Epidemiology and Risk Factors

In the United States COPD is presently the fourth leading cause of death and affects more than 21 million people. Death rates have risen more than 22% in the last decade and the disease is responsible for approximately 700,000 hospital stays each year. The disease is now almost equal in men and women because of increasing amounts of tobacco in the female population. The primary risk factor associated with the development of COPD, cigarette smoking increases the death rate and disability caused by COPD and causes lung function to deteriorate over time much more rapidly than in a nonsmoker. Cigar and pipe smokers have greater COPD incidence than nonsmokers. Approximately 20% of smokers will develop COPD. The risk of development of COPD is increased in first-degree relatives of patients with COPD, which suggests the importance of genetic factors, but AAT deficiency is the only proved genetic risk factor in COPD. Exposures other than smoking that have been associated with COPD development include passive smoking, ambient air pollution, occupational dust and chemical exposure, and severe respiratory childhood infections.

Diagnosis

The diagnosis of COPD is suggested on the basis of symptoms, which may include those caused by the airway irritation (cough and sputum production) and those reflecting altered lung mechanics (dyspnea, wheezing, and occasionally chest pain). Individuals usually experience cough and sputum production years before the development of airflow limitation, while not all individuals with cough and sputum production go on to develop COPD.

Physical examination of individuals with COPD can reveal hyperinflation, wheezing, diminished breath sounds, hyperresonance, or prolonged expiration. Visual inspection during an examination can reveal signs of increased respiratory rate, increased anteroposterior (AP) chest diameter, hyperresonance to chest percussion, and impaired respiratory muscle function. Patients with COPD commonly have a respiration rate greater than 16 breaths per minute, and often this is proportional to disease severity; patients with COPD severe enough to exhibit hypercapnia (partial pressure of arterial carbon dioxide [$PaCO_2$] greater than 45 mm Hg) may have breathing rates of greater than 25 breaths per minute. Absence of wheezing does not exclude COPD. Patients with end-stage COPD may adopt body positions that help relieve dyspnea, such as leaning forward or expiring through pursed lips. Use of accessory muscles for respiration, such as the use of the abdominal rectus muscle on expiration, is a sign of advanced disease. Other signs of hyperinflation may include decreased diaphragm movement, tracheal tug, or pulsus paradoxus greater than 20 mm Hg.

Patients with advanced COPD may also have central cyanosis, peripheral edema, and signs of cor pulmonale associated with right heart failure. Other objective findings often include arterial blood gas changes demonstrating hypercapnia, severe hypoxemia, compensated respiratory acidosis with elevated carbon dioxide (CO_2), tension and a normal pH, and elevated serum bicarbonate level. Morning headaches in COPD patients may be indicative of hypercapnia.

The diagnosis of COPD is confirmed by spirometry. The standard pulmonary function test used to measure airway obstruction is the forced expiratory spirogram. This test assesses the rate of change in volume that occurs as a function of time. Pulmonary functions useful in the evaluation of patients presenting with symptoms of COPD include FEV_1, the forced vital capacity (FVC), and the ratio of FEV_1/FVC, which is also called the *timed vital capacity*. The FVC provides a measure of lung volume and the FEV_1 and FEV_1/FVC

both provide a measure of obstruction. In most of these patients, other abnormal lung volumes that may exist include increases in both the total lung capacity (TLC) and the residual volume (RV). These increases in lung volumes are caused by hyperinflation of the lungs.

An FEV_1/FVC less than 70% of predicted confirms the presence of airflow obstruction. The FEV_1 serves as a marker of severity of the airflow obstruction. Other pulmonary function tests such as the flow volume loop or diffusing capacity for carbon monoxide (DL_{CO}) can help rule out other types of airway obstruction or help quantitate a patient's risk for surgery. Chest radiographs are only helpful for diagnosis in COPD if there are signs of bullous disease or severe hyperinflation or loss of vascular markings. Computed tomography (CT) scanning can show the location of bullous disease which can be helpful in narrowing the differential diagnosis of a patient with airway obstruction and also may be used to help determine if a patient is a candidate for lung reduction surgery.

COPD Classification

The GOLD committee presented a new classification of COPD. The management of COPD is largely symptom driven, and there is only an imperfect relationship between the degree of airflow limitation and the presence of symptoms. The staging therefore is aimed at practical implementation and should be only regarded as an educational tool, and a general indication of the approach to management. All FEV_1 values refer to postbronchodilator FEV_1.

This classification includes stages 0 to IV (Figure 1).

Stage 0: At Risk—Characterized by chronic cough and sputum production. Lung function, as measured by spirometry, is still normal.

Stage I: Mild COPD—Characterized by mild airflow limitation (FEV_1/FVC <70% but FEV_1 >80% predicted) and usually, but not always, chronic cough and sputum production. At this stage, the individual may be unaware of abnormal lung function.

Stage II: Moderate COPD—Characterized by worsening airflow limitation (<50% FEV_1 <80% predicted) and usually the progression of symptoms, with shortness of breath typically developing on exertion. This is the stage at which most patients typically first seek medical attention because of dyspnea or an exacerbation of their disease.

Stage III: Severe COPD—Characterized by further worsening of airflow limitation (<30% FEV_1 <50% predicted), increased shortness of breath, and repeated exacerbations which have an impact on the patient's quality of life.

Stage IV: Very Severe COPD—Characterized by severe air-flow limitation (FEV_1 <30% predicted) or the presence of chronic respiratory failure. Patients may have very severe (Stage IV) COPD even if the FEV_1 is greater than 30% predicted, if respiratory failure is present. At this stage, quality of life is appreciably impaired and exacerbations may be life-threatening.

THERAPY AT EACH STAGE OF COPD

	0: At risk	I: Mild	II: Moderate	III: Severe	IV: Very severe
Characteristics	• Chronic symptoms • Exposure to risk factors • Normal spirometry	• $FEV_1/FVC < 70\%$ • $FEV_1 \geq 80\%$ • With or without symptoms	• $FEV_1/FVC < 70\%$ • $50\% \leq FEV_1 < 80\%$ • With or without symptoms	• $FEV_1/FVC < 70\%$ • $30\% \leq FEV_1 < 50\%$ • With or without symptoms	• $FEV_1/FVC < 70\%$ • $FEV_1 < 30\%$ or $FEV_1 < 50\%$ predicted plus chronic respiratory failure
	Avoidance of risk factor(s); influenza vaccination				
		Add short-acting bronchodilator when needed			
			Add regular treatment with one or more long-acting bronchodilators *Add* rehabilitation		
				Add inhaled glucocorticosteroid if repeated exacerbations	
					Add long-term oxygen if chronic respiratory failure. Consider surgical treatments

FIGURE 1. Therapy for different stages of COPD.

Management of Stable COPD

The general guidelines to management of COPD include the avoidance of risk factors to prevent disease progression and pharmacotherapy as needed to control symptoms. In addition, patient education including counseling about smoking cessation, instruction in physical exercise, and nutritional advice are necessary components of a comprehensive COPD management plan. The goals of management are to relieve symptoms, increase exercise tolerance, improve quality of life, prevent and treat complications, and decrease disease progression.

Smoking cessation is the single most effective (and cost-effective) intervention to reduce the risk of developing COPD and stop its progression. Comprehensive tobacco elimination policies and programs with clear and repeated nonsmoking messages should be delivered through every feasible system possible. Legislation to establish smoke-free schools, public facilities, and work environments should be encouraged by working with government officials, public health workers, and the public. Guidelines for smoking cessation were published by the U.S. Agency for Health Care Policy and Research (AHCPR) in 2000.

There are numerous effective pharmacotherapies for smoking cessation. Except in the presence of special circumstances, pharmacotherapy is recommended when counseling is insufficient. Nicotine replacement therapy in any form (nicotine gum, inhaler, nasal spray [Nicotrol NS], transdermal patch [Nicoderm], sublingual tablet [Nicorette Microtab],[2] or lozenge [Commit]) reliably increases long-term smoking abstinence rates. The antidepressants bupropion (Zyban) and nortriptyline (Pamelor)[1] have also been shown to increase

long-term quit rates. The antihypertensive drug clonidine (Catapres)[1] can also be used to help a patient quit smoking, but side effects should be carefully reviewed with each patient. Special consideration should be given before using pharmacotherapy in selected populations including patients smoking fewer than 10 cigarettes per day, pregnant patients, and adolescent smokers.

The overall approach to managing stable COPD should be characterized by a stepwise increase in treatment, depending on the severity of the disease. The management strategy is based on an individualized assessment of disease severity and response to various therapies. Disease severity is determined by the severity of symptoms and airflow limitation (using pulmonary function measurements) and other factors such as the frequency and severity of exacerbations, complications, respiratory failure, co-morbidities (cardiovascular disease and sleep-related disorders), and the general health status of the patient. Different types of pharmacologic agents treat patients with COPD (Box 1). Pharmacologic therapy is used to prevent and control symptoms, reduce the frequency and severity of exacerbations, improve health status, and improve exercise tolerance. Initial use should decrease airway obstruction and decrease dyspnea. None of the existing medications for COPD had been shown to alter the inevitable long-term decline in lung function that occurs with COPD; however, they can decrease morbidity and may also delay disability and mortality in some patients. Medications may also decrease the number of exacerbations of COPD occurring per year.

Bronchodilators are primary medications for symptomatic management of COPD. Bronchodilator drugs commonly used include anticholinergics (short and long acting), β_2 agonists (short and long acting), and

[1]Not FDA approved for this indication.
[2]Not available in the United States.

[1]Not FDA approved for this indication.

<table>
<tr><td>

BOX 1   Current Drugs Used to Manage Chronic Obstructive Pulmonary Disease

- SABAs
- Albuterol (salbutamol) (Proventil)
- LABAs
- Formoterol (Foradil)
- Salmeterol (Serevent)
- Short-acting anticholinergics
- Ipratropium (Atrovent)
- Long-acting anticholinergics
- Tiotropium (Spiriva)
- Combination SABA + anticholinergic in 1 inhaler
- Albuterol/ipratropium (Combivent)
- Methylxanthines
- Theophylline (Theo-Dur)
- Inhaled corticosteroids
- Beclomethasone (QVAR)
- Budesonide (Pulmicort)
- Fluticasone (Flovent)
- Triamcinolone (Azmacort)
- Combination LABA + ICS in 1 inhaler
- Formoterol/budesonide (Symbicort)
- Salmeterol/fluticasone (Advair)
- Systemic corticosteroids
- Prednisone
- Methylprednisolone (Medrol)

Abbreviations: LABAs = Long-acting β$_2$ agonists; SABAs = short-acting β$_2$ agonists.

</td></tr>
</table>

long-acting methylxanthines. All of these medications have been shown to improve exercise capacity in COPD patients even if the FEV$_1$ is insignificantly changed. Inhaled drugs tend to have fewer side effects than oral drugs. Short-acting bronchodilators on an as-needed basis are recommended for mild (Stage I) COPD. The GOLD guidelines recommend the use of regular daily treatment with bronchodilators for moderate (Stage II) or severe (Stages III and IV) COPD and long-acting bronchodilators are preferred to short-acting drugs because of better compliance because of longer duration of action (Box 1). Regular use of a long-acting anticholinergic (tiotropium [Spiriva]) or a long acting β$_2$-agonist (salmeterol [Serevent] or formoterol [Foradil]) improves health status. Theophylline (Theo-Dur) is effective in COPD, but because of its potential toxicity, inhaled bronchodilators are preferred when available. All studies that have shown efficacy of theophylline (Theo-Dur) in COPD were done with slow-release preparations (theophylline [Theo-Dur]). Each of the inhaled bronchodilators requires a delivery device which must be used correctly. Each type of device requires patient education and monitoring, and the GOLD guidelines recommend consideration of the delivery device as part of the selection process for drug treatment in a single patient. As symptoms of COPD worsen, several different types of COPD therapy are given simultaneously, and deletion of drug therapy is usually not possible. In general nebulized therapy for a stable patient is unnecessary unless it has been demonstrated to be more effective than conventional metered dose or dry powder inhaler dose therapy in that patient.

Combinations of bronchodilators with different mechanisms and durations of action tend to increase the degree of bronchodilation in COPD patients with increases in FEV$_1$, FEV$_1$/FVC, and peak expiratory flow (PEF). Changes in pulmonary function are indirectly additive with increasing the number of bronchodilators being administered, but combinations usually increase pulmonary function more than each agent alone. Short-acting β$_2$ agonists (SABAs) are quick-relief medications for use only when necessary rather than on a daily, regular schedule. The regular use of a SABA results in twice as much β$_2$ agonist use without any noted clinical benefits. Increasing use or daily use of a SABA for rescue indicates the need for additional therapy to achieve long-term control. Inhaled SABAs include albuterol (Proventil, Ventolin), bitolterol (Tornalate), pirbuterol (Maxair), and terbutaline (Brethaire). These medications are effective for 4 to 6 hours after use. Adverse effects of SABAs include palpitations, chest pain, tachycardia, tremor, unstable coronary artery disease or nervousness. Patients with coronary artery disease or cardiac dysrhythmias should also be monitored closely. Use caution in giving these medications to patients receiving monoamine oxidase inhibitors or tricyclic antidepressants. The short-acting anticholinergic agent, ipratropium bromide (Atrovent), causes bronchodilation by competitive inhibition of muscarinic receptors. This agent reverses cholinergically mediated bronchospasm and may decrease mucus-gland secretions. It is effective for 4 to 6 hours after use.

The most recent addition to the long-acting bronchodilators is tiotropium (Spiriva), a long-acting anticholinergic agent that lasts 24 hours, allowing for once-daily administration. Tiotropium (Spiriva) has shown in several recent studies with COPD patients to result in significant improvement in lung function compared with ipratropium (a short-acting anticholinergic) or salmeterol (Serevent, a long-acting β$_2$ agonist [LABA]). Inhaled LABAs are highly preferred than the extended-release oral formulation because of longer action and fewer side effects. Salmeterol (Serevent) and formoterol (Foradil) are both long-acting, inhaled β$_2$ agonists, and extended-release albuterol (Proventil Repetabs) are long-acting, β$_2$ agonists available as oral agents. The long-acting inhaled agents have a slower onset of action and longer duration of action, remaining active for more than 12 hours. The onset of action of formoterol (Foradil) is more rapid than salmeterol (Serevent), but it should not be used for rescue during episodes of acute shortness of breath. It remains a chronic bronchodilator therapy. Like the short-acting inhaled β$_2$ agonists, the long-acting agents produce bronchodilation by smooth muscle relaxation as a result of adenylate cyclase activation and increasing cyclic AMP in smooth muscle cells. Combining β$_2$ agonists and anticholinergics may increase the effects of these agents. Several studies have shown superior efficacy for either a SABA or LABA in combination with an anticholinergic.

Theophylline (Theo-Dur) inhibits phosphodiesterase action, which causes smooth muscle relaxation and leads to bronchodilation. It also increases central respiratory drive, diaphragm strength, promotes venous pooling in

Rakel and Bope: *Conn's Current Therapy 2006.*

the legs, and may have some mild anti-inflammatory activity. Therapy with theophylline (Theo-Dur) should be individualized, taking into account such factors as drug interactions, current smoking, the patient's age, and the presence of congestive heart failure or liver disease. Serum theophylline (Theo-Dur) concentrations should be maintained at levels between 5 and 15 µg/mL. Dosage adjustment is based on the patient's clinical response, tolerance to the agent, and serum theophylline (Theo-Dur) levels. Some patients metabolize theophylline (Theo-Dur) very rapidly. Although theophylline (Theo-Dur) is not a preferred first line agent in the management of COPD, it may be a second-line agent in patients with severe COPD.

Inhaled corticosteroids (ICSs) are not recommended as single agents for chronic use in COPD management, which is quite different from the recommendations in asthma. They are recommended in combination therapy with other bronchodilators in severe COPD, and the only Food and Drug Administration (FDA)-approved combinations of ICS and a LABA are fluticasone plus salmeterol (Advair) or formoterol (Foradil) plus budesonide (Symbicort)[4] (see Box 1). Systemic steroids are clinically beneficial to patients hospitalized with COPD exacerbations and maximum effects of oral steroids after 3 days of intravenous (IV) steroids are achieved by 2 weeks of therapy. Longer use of oral steroids increases side effects without increasing pulmonary functions. Long-term treatment with oral glucocorticosteroids is not recommended in COPD. There is no evidence of a long-term benefit from this treatment. Moreover, a side effect of long-term treatment with systemic glucocorticosteroid is steroid myopathy, which contributes to muscle weakness, decreased functionality, and respiratory failure in patients with advanced COPD. Oral glucocorticosteroid use for long periods of time can also complicate control of diabetes and hypertension as well as causing bone demineralization.

Other pharmacologic treatments have been evaluated by the GOLD committee with some being beneficial. Use of influenza vaccines can reduce serious illness and death in COPD patients by approximately 50%. Use of the influenza vaccine has also been shown to reduce outpatient visits for influenza and reduces both hospital costs and death. Vaccines containing killed (Fluzone) or live, inactive viruses (FluMist)[1] are recommended and should be given once (in autumn) or twice[3] (in autumn and winter) each year. A pneumococcal vaccine containing 23 virulent serotypes (Pneumovax-23) has been used in an effort to decrease the number of cases of pneumococcal pneumonia in COPD patients but evidence supporting its effectiveness in COPD patients is lacking. An oral vaccine* using a strain of nontypeable *Haemophilus influenzae* has been shown to produce short-lived reduction in the number of exacerbations in some groups of COPD patients. The use of antibiotics, other than in treating infectious exacerbations of COPD or other bacterial infections such as pneumonia, is not recommended. Although a few patients with viscous sputum may benefit from mucolytics, the overall benefit is small. Therefore, the widespread use of these agents cannot be recommended.

Cough, although sometimes a troublesome symptom in COPD, has a significant protective role and the regular use of antitussives is contraindicated in stable COPD. The use of doxapram (Dopram), a nonspecific respiratory stimulant available as an intravenous formulation, is not recommended in stable COPD. Almitrine bismesylate (Duxil) also is not recommended for regular use in stable COPD patients. Narcotics are contraindicated in COPD because of their respiratory depressant effects and potential to worsen hypercapnia. Clinical studies suggest that morphine use to control dyspnea may have serious adverse effects, but it may provide benefits to a few select limited patients. Codeine and other narcotic analgesics should be avoided. Nonsteroidal anti-inflammatory agents (Nedocromil [Tilade]) and leukotriene modifiers have not been adequately tested in COPD patients and are not recommended for use. Alternative healing methods including herbal medicine, acupuncture, and homeopathy are not recommended for treatment in COPD.

Nonpharmacologic management of COPD patients includes pulmonary rehabilitation and long-term oxygen therapy. The principal goals of pulmonary rehabilitation are to improve quality of life, decrease symptoms, and increase physical participation in everyday activities. To accomplish these goals, pulmonary rehabilitation addresses a range of nonpulmonary problems, including exercise deconditioning, relative social isolation, altered mood states (especially depression), muscle wasting, and weight loss. COPD patients at all stages of disease benefit from exercise training programs and improve with respect to both exercise tolerance and symptoms of dyspnea and fatigue. These benefits can be sustained even after a single pulmonary rehabilitation program. Benefits have been reported from rehabilitation programs conducted in inpatient, outpatient, and home settings. Ideally, a comprehensive pulmonary rehabilitation program includes exercise training, nutrition counseling, and education. Baseline and outcome assessments of each participant in a pulmonary rehabilitation program should be made to quantify individual gains and target areas for improvement and include a detailed medical history and physical exam; measurement of spirometry before and after a bronchodilator drug; assessment of exercise capacity; measurement of the impact of breathlessness and/or health status; and assessment of inspiratory and expiratory muscle strength and lower limb strength (e.g., quadriceps) in patients who suffer from muscle wasting.

The long-term administration of oxygen (more than 15 hours per day) to COPD patients with chronic respiratory failure has been shown to increase survival. In studies done in Britain by the Medical Research Council Trial and in the United States in the Nocturnal Oxygen Therapy Trial, patients receiving continuous oxygen therapy had increased survival as compared with patients that did not receive oxygen or received

---

*Investigational drug in the United States.
[1]Not FDA approved for this indication.
[3]Exceeds dosage recommended by the manufacturer.
[4]Not yet approved for use in the United States.

oxygen only at night. Oxygen also has a beneficial impact on hemodynamics, hematologic characteristics, exercise capacity, lung mechanics, and mental state. Oxygen therapy also should be used if the patient has evidence of pulmonary hypertension, peripheral edema suggesting either right- or left-sided heart failure or evidence of polycythemia (hematocrit greater than 55%). Therapy can be given continuously, acutely to combat acute dyspnea, or intermittently during exercise. It is recommended to perform arterial blood gas measurement in patients with FEV_1 less than 40% predicted or with clinical findings suggestive of respiratory failure or cor pulmonale.

Management of Exacerbations

Patients with COPD will have usually two to three exacerbations of symptoms of their disease each year with some requiring hospitalization. The economic and social burden of COPD exacerbations is extremely high. The most common causes of an exacerbation are pulmonary infections (acute bacterial bronchitis) and air pollution. The exact cause of approximately one-third of severe exacerbations cannot be identified and may be related to reactive airway disease. Other conditions that may produce the symptoms of an acute exacerbation of COPD include pneumonia, myocardial ischemia, congestive heart failure, pneumothorax, formation of a pleural effusion, pulmonary embolism, cardiac arrhythmias, esophageal reflux, or noncompliance with medications. The clinical diagnosis of a COPD exacerbation is an increase in amount of sputum production, change in color of sputum, or increase in dyspnea. Exacerbations may also be accompanied by a number of nonspecific complaints such as malaise, insomnia, sleepiness, fatigue, anxiety, depression, confusion, or panic attacks. Patients with exacerbations of COPD may require hospital admission, and some patients will require ICU admission. There is a high incidence of *H. influenzae* infections in patients with a COPD exacerbation caused by infection. Other important bacterial causes include *Streptococcus pneumoniae, Moraxella catarrhalis,* and *Pseudomonas aeruginosum.* Hospital admission must be considered in COPD with an exacerbation if they have marked increase in symptoms, failure to respond to outpatient treatment, confusion, lethargy and coma, worsening oxygenation, or development of respiratory acidosis. Oxygen therapy is usually required in a hospitalized patient with an acute exacerbation of COPD; but this may lead to CO_2 retention and acidosis, which in turn could lead to either noninvasive mechanical ventilation, or mechanical ventilation depending on the cause of the exacerbation and the patient's wishes. Hospital mortality for patients with COPD admitted for an acute exacerbation is approximately 10%. Ventilator associated pneumonia is also an important risk in a COPD patient treated with invasive mechanical ventilation.

The primary objectives of mechanical ventilatory support in patients with acute exacerbations of severe COPD are to decrease mortality and morbidity and relieve symptoms. Ventilatory support can be given through an orotracheal or nasotracheal tube or tracheostomy connection, which is referred to as invasive (conventional) mechanical ventilation and is particularly suitable in severe acute exacerbations occurring in patients with end-stage disease. Ventilatory support can also be given through a noninvasive means using either negative or positive pressure devices. Fewer complications occur with noninvasive ventilation, but many patients presenting with severe exacerbations of COPD, including respiratory acidosis, may not be candidates for noninvasive ventilation. Noninvasive positive-pressure ventilation (NPPV) involves using a mechanical ventilator connected by tubing to an interface that allows airflow into the nose or the nose and mouth by using a mask or a mouthpiece. Head straps are used to secure the mask tightly to the patient. NPPV allows ventilation without the use of an endotracheal tube. Use of NPPV in acute respiratory failure has been studied in both uncontrolled and randomized controlled trials. The studies show consistently positive results with success rates of 80% to 85%. Taken together they provide evidence that NPPV increases pH, reduces $PaCO_2$, reduces the severity of breathlessness in the first 4 hours of treatment, and decreases the length of hospital stay. More importantly, mortality and intubation rates are reduced by this intervention. However, NPPV is not appropriate for all patients and invasive mechanical ventilation may still be needed to maximize arterial blood gases values. NPPV can be delivered by different types of ventilators: volume-controlled, pressure-controlled, bilevel positive airway pressure, or continuous positive airway pressure. The use of NPPV together with long-term oxygen therapy has been shown to result in a significant improvement in daytime arterial blood gases, total sleep time, sleep efficiency, quality of life, and overnight $PaCO_2$.

Other treatments that can be useful in COPD patients who must be hospitalized include fluid administration as needed to keep the patient normovolemic; nutrition supplementation as needed with careful attention to the amount of carbohydrates given because excessive amounts can increase CO_2 production; and the use of low molecular weight heparin in immobilized patients with or without a history of thromboembolic disease. Manual or mechanical chest percussion and postural drainage may also be beneficial in patients producing greater than 25 mL sputum per day or those with lobar atelectasis.

Surgical Options

Surgical treatments of COPD include bullectomy, lung volume reduction surgery, and lung transplantation. In carefully selected patients, bullectomy can be effective in reducing dyspnea and improving lung function. A thoracic CT scan, arterial blood gases measurement and comprehensive respiratory function tests are essential before making a decision regarding a patient's suitability for resection of a bulla. Specific large bullae may be removed if they are compressing significant amounts of normal lung tissue.

Lung volume reduction surgery (LVRS) is another option for COPD patients and involves removing 20% to

30% of the upper lobes to improve airway mechanics and increase FEV_1. The National Emphysema Treatment Trial (NETT) study was a randomized controlled trial in 1218 patients with severe emphysema who received either LVRS or medical therapy. The results showed no overall survival benefit with LVRS compared with medical therapy, but improved exercise capacity and quality of life. The best outcome of this surgery was in patients with predominately upper lobe emphysema and initial low exercise capacity. The surgery was prohibitive in patients with an FEV_1 of up to 20% and either a homogeneous distribution of emphysema or a concomitant diffusing capacity of lung for carbon monoxide (DL_{CO}) of up to 20%.

In appropriately selected patients with very advanced COPD, lung transplantation has been shown to improve quality of life and functional capacity. The average 3-year survival rate is approximately 60% when performed by highly skilled medical or surgical teams that specialize in lung transplantation. Appropriate criteria for lung transplantation recipients include FEV_1 of up to 35% of predicted, $PaCO_2$ greater than 55 mm Hg, PaO_2 less than 60 mm Hg on room air, or the presence of secondary pulmonary hypertension.

Cystic Fibrosis

Method of
Robert L. Zanni, MD

Cystic fibrosis (CF) is a complex, multisystem clinical syndrome involving exocrine glands, including sweat glands, the pancreas, and mucous glands of the respiratory, gastrointestinal, and reproductive tracts. It is characterized by elevated sweat electrolyte content, chronic obstructive pulmonary disease, and exocrine pancreatic insufficiency. CF is the most common lethal genetic disease among the white population. The disorder is autosomal recessive, and the incidence is 1 in 3200 in the white population. CF is less common in African Americans with an incidence of 1 in 15,000 and in Asian Americans with an incidence of 1 in 31,000. Initially CF was thought to be a rare and invariably fatal disease. As a result of refined diagnostic techniques and improved therapeutic approaches, however, there has been an increase in life expectancy. Emphasis on early diagnosis, prevention of lung disease, and improving nutrition are the current areas of concentration on diagnosis and therapy. The median predicted survival is currently 32.9 years.

Pathophysiology

The isolation and cloning of the gene mutation causing CF occurred in 1989. The CF gene is located on the long arm of human chromosome 7. The CF gene codes for the production of a membrane transport protein termed cystic fibrosis transmembrane regulator (CFTR). This protein is expressed in all the epithelial cells affected in CF. This includes the lung, pancreas, sweat glands, liver, large intestine, and testes. CFTR acts as an apical chloride conductance channel resulting in reduced activation of chloride ion transport. CFTR is important in controlling other ions as well. It has been shown that CFTR secondarily regulates sodium absorption in the CF airways. The combined function of CFTR as a chloride channel and regulator of sodium channels suggests that CFTR is the trigger that balances the rates of chloride secretion and sodium absorption to properly hydrate airway secretions in normal airway epithelial cells.

To date, more than 1000 mutations have been identified to cause CF. Progress has been made in understanding the molecular mechanisms by which CF-associated mutations cause dysfunction of the CFTR protein. Depending on the type of mutation, one of five mechanisms may come into play. Five different class mutations result in different degrees of chloride channel defects causing different degrees of disease severity. Class I mutations are associated with defective CFTR production resulting in a lack of production of full length or functional protein. In class II mutations, the protein is not correctly processed and unable to progress through the biosynthetic pathway to the cell membrane. Class III mutations cause defects in chloride channel regulation. Class IV mutations result in reduced flow of chloride through the channel. Class V mutations result in decreased amounts of functional CFTR. In general, individuals with class I and II mutations are pancreatic insufficient, whereas classes III, IV, and V are pancreatic sufficient.

PULMONARY MANIFESTATIONS

As a result of the dysfunctional CFTR, the secretions of the airway become abnormally thick and tenacious. This situation leads to chronic obstruction of the bronchial airways. The inspissation of secretions causes chronic infection and inflammation to progress. This cyclic process progresses to bronchiectasis, fibrosis, and eventual respiratory failure (Figure 1). Infection is initially caused by *Staphylococcus aureus* and *Haemophilus influenzae*. As patients age, infection with *Pseudomonas aeruginosa* becomes most prominent. The rate of progression of lung disease is variable among patients. Factors associated with acceleration in decline of lung function are poor nutritional status, infection with *P. aeruginosa*, tobacco exposure, pancreatic insufficiency, and lack of consistent medical care. The key clinical manifestation of the upper respiratory tract is pansinusitis. Approximately 25% of patients with CF will develop nasal polyps.

GASTROINTESTINAL/NUTRITIONAL MANIFESTATIONS

As many as 90% of patients with CF are pancreatic insufficient. Inspissation of thick secretions within the pancreatic ducts causes insufficient or total absence of

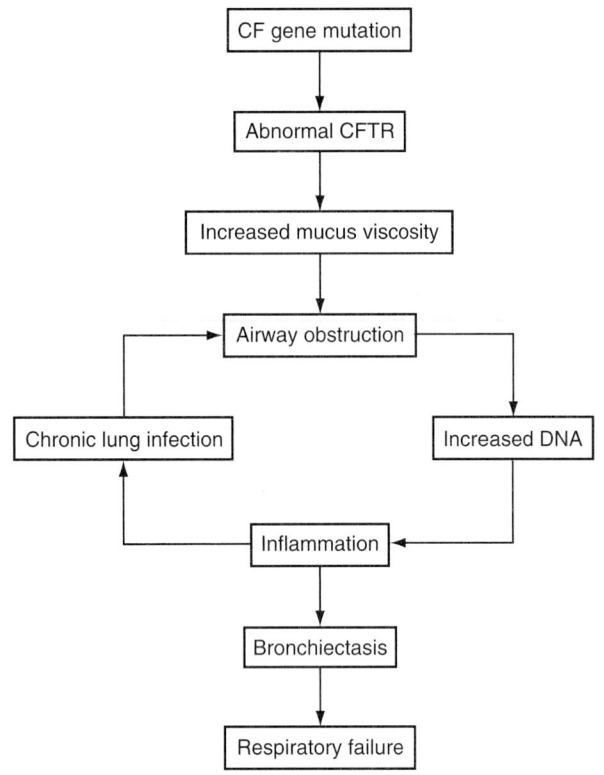

FIGURE 1. A vicious cycle of chronic airway obstruction, infection, and inflammation leads to progressive pulmonary damage. *Abbreviations:* CF = cystic fibrosis; CFTR = cystic fibrosis trans-membrane regulator.

CURRENT DIAGNOSIS

Diagnosis is based on:

- Presence of one or more characteristic phenotypic features or
- A history of CF in a sibling or
- Positive newborn screening test

  Plus

- Elevated sweat chloride concentrations (chloride > 60 mmol/L) or
- Identification of two CF mutations or
- Characteristic abnormalities in ion transport across the nasal epithelium

Characteristic Phenotypic Features:

1. Chronic sinopulmonary disease
   - Chronic cough and sputum production
   - Clinical findings consistent with airway obstruction (wheezing, air trapping)
   - Pansinusitis, nasal polyps
   - Persistent pulmonary infection with typical CF pathogens (*Staphylococcus aureus, Haemophilus influenzae, Pseudomonas aeruginosa*)
   - Persistent chest radiograph abnormalities (bronchiectasis, atelectasis, infiltrates, hyperinflation)
   - Digital clubbing
2. Gastrointestinal and nutritional abnormalities
   - Intestinal: Meconium ileus, DIOS, rectal prolapse
   - Pancreatic: Pancreatic insufficiency, recurrent pancreatitis
   - Hepatic: Focal biliary cirrhosis
   - Nutritional: Protein-calorie malnutrition; hypoproteinemia and edema; complications secondary to fat-soluble vitamin deficiency
3. Salt loss syndrome
   - Acute salt depletion
   - Chronic metabolism alkalosis
4. Male urogenital abnormalities resulting in obstructive azoospermia

Abbreviations: CF = cystic fibrosis; DIOS = distal intestinal obstructive syndrome.

secretion of pancreatic enzymes, which leads to maldigestion and malabsorption of fats and protein. This is clinically manifested by steatorrhea and failure to thrive.

There are other manifestations of CF related to the gastrointestinal (GI) tract. CF-related diabetes mellitus occurs in approximately 17% of patients. Approximately 20% of infants with CF present at birth with meconium ileus. This is an obstruction of the distal small bowel with viscous, thick meconium. Children, adolescents, and adults with CF may suffer from distal small bowel obstruction (distal intestinal obstruction syndrome [DIOS]). Approximately 5% of CF patients develop liver disease characterized by focal biliary cirrhosis.

Diagnosis

Approximately 50% of patients are diagnosed by 6 months of age and 68% by the age of 1 year. The key to diagnosing patients with CF is to have a high index of suspicion based on presenting symptoms. Classic clinical features include chronic sinopulmonary disease and GI symptoms. A small percentage of patients present with less-than-classic symptoms. These patients tend to be pancreatic sufficient.

Confirmation of the diagnosis can be obtained through a sweat test. To avoid false-positive or false-negative results, the sweat test should be performed by experienced laboratory personnel using the iontophoresis pilocarpine technique (Gibson-Cooke method). Positive sweat tests yield sweat chlorides of more than 60 mmol/L. Diagnosis also can be confirmed through DNA analysis by finding two known CF mutations. Difficult diagnostic cases may require testing by nasal transepithelial potential difference.

Prenatal and carrier testing may be offered where there is a family history. More states have mandated newborn screening for CF by measuring immunoreactive trypsinogen (IRT) in a dried blood sample. An elevated IRT is then followed by CF mutation analysis. When the newborn screen is positive, confirmation of the diagnosis is recommended by sweat testing.

Rakel and Bope: *Conn's Current Therapy 2006.*

Management

GENERAL

A comprehensive, multidisciplinary approach to the care of CF patients improves their health and life expectancy. The Cystic Fibrosis Foundation accredits CF care centers around the United States. Accredited CF care centers employ physicians, nurses, nutritionists, social workers, and respiratory and physical therapists trained in the care of CF patients. Patients who enter comprehensive treatment programs before the onset of symptomatic lung disease do better than patients who begin treatment after lung disease has manifested itself clinically.

PULMONARY DISEASE

The prognosis of patients with CF depends on the progression of pulmonary disease. The main goals of therapy focus on efforts to reduce the frequency of pulmonary exacerbations, prevent the decline in pulmonary function, and delay irreversible lung damage. Clinically these goals can be achieved by controlling pulmonary infection, relieving airway obstruction through various modalities, and minimizing inflammation of the airway epithelium. The progression of pulmonary disease can be monitored by serial pulmonary function testing, yearly chest radiographs, and routine clinical follow-up of the patient.

CURRENT THERAPY

Drug	Dosage
Antibiotics: Oral	
Amoxicillin/clavulanate (Augmentin)	45 mg/kg/d divided q 12h
Azithromycin (Zithromax)	10 mg/kg/d on day 1
	5 mg/kg/d on days 2–5
Cephalexin (Keflex)	25–100 mg/kg/d divided q 6h
Cefuroxime (Ceftin)	30 mg/kg/d divided q 6h
Ciprofloxacin (Cipro)	30–40 mg/kg/d divided q12h
Levofloxacin (Levaquin)	500 mg/d
Tetracycline (Sumycin)	25–50 mg/kg/d divided q 12h
Trimethoprim/sulfamethoxazole (Bactrim)	8–10 mg/kg/d of trimethoprim divided q 12h
Antibiotics: Aerosolized*	
Tobramycin for inhalation (TOBI)	300 mg bid
Colistin (Coly-Mycin M)[1]	150 mg bid
Antibiotics: Parenteral	
β-lactam penicillins	
Nafcillin (Nafcil)	50–100 mg/kg/d divided q 6h
Piperacillin (Pipracil)	400–500 mg/kg/d divided q 6h
Piperacillin/tazobactam (Zosyn)	400–500 mg/kg/d divided q 6h
Ticarcillin (Ticar)	200–400 mg/kg/d divided q 6–8h
Other β-lactams	
Ceftazidime (Fortaz)	150–200 mg/kg/d divided q 6–8h
Meropenem (Merrem)	120 mg/kg/d divided q 8h
Aztreonam (Azactam)	150-200 mg/kg/d divided q 6–8h
Aminoglycosides†	
Amikacin (Amikin)	15 mg/kg/d divided q 8–12h
Gentamicin (Garamycin)	7.5–15 mg/kg/d divided q 8–12h
Tobramycin (Nebcin)	7.5–10 mg/kg/d divided q 8–12h
Mucolytics	
Dornase alfa (Pulmozyme)	Inhalation of 2.5 mg per dose once daily
Anti-inflammatory	
Azithromycin (Zithromax)[1]	Ages 6 years and older
	<40 kg, 250 mg tiw
	>40 kg, 500 mg tiw
Pancreatic Enzymes	
Pancrelipase (Creon, Pancrease, Ultrase)	1000–2000 lipase U/kg/meal
Nutritional	
Multivitamins (A, D, E, K [ADEK]; Vitamax; A, B, D, E, K [ABDEK])	Dose varies according to age

[1]Not FDA approved for this indication.
*Aerosolized antibiotics may be used for 2 to 3 weeks for acute exacerbation or for 28 days on, 28 days off as chronic therapy.
†Monitor serum peak and trough levels and for renal toxicity and ototoxicity.
Abbreviations: d = daily; h = hour; q = every; tid = three times a day; tiw = three times a week; U = unit.

Rakel and Bope: *Conn's Current Therapy 2006.*

ANTIBIOTICS

Antibiotics are used to treat pulmonary exacerbations. A pulmonary exacerbation for CF is defined as a change in respiratory signs and symptoms from one's baseline. Commonly these can be an increase in chest congestion, a decrease in exercise tolerance, and the onset of new or an increase in crackles on chest examination. Patients may experience an increase in frequency or duration in cough, an increase in sputum production, and a change in sputum color. Dyspnea, decreased appetite, and hemoptysis may also herald a pulmonary exacerbation.

Most patients require antibiotics intermittently for treatment of exacerbations; few require continuous antibiotic therapy. The choice of antibiotics is based on sputum or oropharyngeal culture and sensitivities. The most common organisms are *S. aureus,* generally found in younger patients, and *P. aeruginosa,* which predominates in older patients.

The treatment of a mild exacerbation can be achieved with the use of an oral antibiotic, an inhaled antibiotic, or both. Generally patients will return to their baseline within 14 days. If patients fail to improve or if the exacerbation is more complex, intravenous antibiotic therapy is advised. Intravenous therapy and frequent airway clearance should be continued until the patient reaches his or her best pulmonary function. This is generally achieved within 14 days. When intravenous antibiotics are used, a combination of an aminoglycoside with an antipseudomonal penicillin, cephalosporin, or antistaphylococcal agent is recommended. The choice of intravenous antibiotics also is based on culture and sensitivity results. Combination therapy helps to avoid the development of bacterial resistance.

Recent evidence supports the use of inhaled tobramycin (TOBI) in patients who are chronically infected with *P. aeruginosa.* TOBI is used on a cycle of 28 days on, 28 days off. Its use can minimize pulmonary exacerbations and improve lung function.

BETA 2 AGONISTS

Although not all patients with CF have airway hyperreactivity, it has become accepted practice to use aerosolized bronchodilators prior to the initiation of airway clearance techniques. Albuterol (Proventil) or levalbuterol (Xopenex) are commonly used.

MUCOLYTICS

The airway secretions of CF patients are extremely thick, tenacious, and viscous. This is because of the increased amount of DNA present from neutrophils. Inhaled dornase alfa (Pulmozyme) is a purified solution of recombinant human deoxyribonuclease I (DNAse I). This enzyme cleaves extracellular neutrophil-derived DNA resulting in the thinning of airway secretions allowing them to be expectorated more easily. Studies support that the once-daily use of dornase alfa (Pulmozyme) preserves lung function and decreases pulmonary exacerbations.

ANTI-INFLAMMATORY THERAPY

Chronic infection is associated with chronic inflammation. Inhaled anti-inflammatory agents such as cromolyn (Intal), nedocromil (Tilade), and inhaled corticosteroids have been used but not studied adequately. Use of alternate day oral corticosteroids and ibuprofen (Motrin) has been studied sufficiently and shows improvement in lung function. Serious side effects have limited their widespread use in CF patients. A recent trial of azithromycin (Zithromax)[1] given three times per week has shown pulmonary benefits. Although the use of azithromycin (Zithromax)[1] for this purpose is off-label, it is a recommended therapy for CF patients 6 years of age and older who have chronic infection with *P. aeruginosa.*

AIRWAY CLEARANCE

Daily airway clearance is recommended for all CF patients. There are various techniques that can be offered to patients. Chest physical therapy using percussion and postural drainage is effective for infants and young children. Older children, adolescents, and adults mostly prefer the various mechanical devices that are available. These devices offer levels of independence for the patients. Examples of such devices are positive expiratory pressure devices (Flutter, Therapep), vibratory positive expiratory pressure devices (Acapella), and high-frequency, chest wall oscillation devices (Vest).

NUTRITIONAL MANAGEMENT

The basis for malnutrition in CF patients is multifactorial. The majority of patients with CF are pancreatic insufficient and unable to digest fats and proteins. CF patients also have increased caloric needs because of an increase in metabolism. The increased metabolic state results from chronic pulmonary infection and increased work of breathing.

Pancreatic enzyme replacement, along with high-calorie, high-fat diets and fat-soluble vitamins, provides adequate nutrition for many patients with CF. If the patient fails to gain weight, high-calorie oral supplements or enteral feeds at nighttime are helpful.

COMPLICATIONS

Respiratory, gastrointestinal, and other organ system complications can occur in patients with CF. Box 1 lists the more common complications encountered in the care of patients with CF.

Research

As the understanding of the genetic and molecular basis for the disease increases, new therapeutic approaches will become available. Current therapeutic approaches

---

[1]Not FDA approved for this indication.

The Respiratory System

BOX 1   Clinical Complications

Pulmonary
- Hemoptysis
- Pneumothorax
- Allergic bronchopulmonary aspergillosis

Gastrointestinal/Nutritional
- Distal intestinal obstructive syndrome
- Protein-caloric malnutrition
- Pancreatitis
- Focal biliary cirrhosis

Endocrine
- Cystic fibrosis-related diabetes mellitus (CFRDM)
- Osteopenia/osteoporosis

Rheumatologic
- Arthropathy
- Arthritis

Urogenital
- Congenital bilateral absence of vas deferens
- Male infertility

Abbreviations: CF = cystic fibrosis; DM = diabetes mellitus.

Obstructive Sleep Apnea

Method of
Brian A. Boehlecke, MD, MSPH

Obstructive sleep apnea syndrome (OSAS) comprises a constellation of symptoms and physiologic changes associated with recurrent episodes of apnea and/or hypopnea during sleep. Bed partners are often more aware of a sleep disturbance than the patient and report loud snoring; gasping, choking, or pauses in breathing followed by *snorting*; and/or body jerking. The patient usually has excessive daytime somnolence (EDS) and may complain of nonrefreshing sleep, morning headaches, decreased ability to concentrate, poor memory, irritability or frank mood disturbance, and/or impotence. Evidence is accumulating that OSAS is associated with increased risk for hypertension, cardiovascular disease, stroke, and insulin resistance. Patients with OSAS report reduced quality of life on standardized questionnaires and have an increased risk of motor-vehicle crashes. These consequences are related to the sleep disturbance (recurrent microarousals as well as reduced deep and rapid eye movement [REM] sleep) and the oxyhemoglobin (HbO_2) desaturation associated with the apneas and hypopneas. The most commonly used measure of severity is the number of apneas plus hypopneas per hour of sleep, the apnea-hypopnea index (AHI), during an overnight sleep study (polysomnogram [PSG]). Also clinically important is the severity of HbO_2 desaturations indicated by the lowest arterial oxyhemoglobin saturation (SpO_2) and percentage of time below 90% saturation. The objective of treatment is to ameliorate current symptoms and physiologic abnormalities with the goal of reducing the risk of future morbidity and mortality.

involve correcting the genetic defect (gene therapy); regulation of ion transport, which will affect abnormal mucus production; and novel anti-infective and anti-inflammatory therapies. An unprecedented number of therapies for CF are being tested in well-designed clinical trials.

REFERENCES

Boat T, Cantin A, Cutting G, et al: The diagnosis of cystic fibrosis: Consensus statement. Consensus Conferences, Concepts in Care, Cystic Fibrosis Foundation, Bethesda, MD, March 25, 1996; Volume VII, Section 1, 1-15.

Borowitz D, Baker R, Stallings V: Consensus report on nutrition for pediatric patients with cystic fibrosis. J Pediatr Gastroenterol Nutr 2002;35:246-259.

Cystic Fibrosis Foundation: Cystic Fibrosis Foundation Patient Registry, annual data report to the center directors for 2003. Cystic Fibrosis Foundation, Bethesda, MD, 2004.

Farrell P, Korosok M, Rock M, et al: Early diagnosis of cystic fibrosis through neonatal screening prevents severe malnutrition and improves long term growth. Pediatrics 2001;107:1-13.

Farrell P, Zanhai L, Korosok M, et al: Bronchopulmonary disease in children with cystic fibrosis after early and delayed diagnosis. Am J Respir Crit Care Med 2003;168:1100-1108.

Gibson R, Burns J, Ramsey B: Pathophysiology and management of pulmonary infections in cystic fibrosis. Am J Respir Crit Care Med 2003;168:918-951.

Gross S, Boyle C, Batkin J, et al: Newborn screening for cystic fibrosis. MMWR 2004;53:1-36.

Basis for Treatment

Recurrent, sleep-related, upper-airway narrowing or complete closure causes the hypopneas and apneas characteristic of OSAS. Both anatomic abnormalities (e.g., large tongue and/or tonsils, *redundant* pharyngeal tissue and/or submucosal fat deposition, or retrognathia) and inadequate upper-airway muscle tone during inspiration (increased *collapsibility*) can compromise upper-airway patency. Maintaining adequate airway patency ameliorates obstructive apneas and hypopneas and reduces or eliminates the associated arousals and HbO_2 desaturations. Reduction of the AHI to near-normal levels and maintaining HbO_2 saturation at 90% or greater for most of the night has been shown to reduce daytime somnolence and improve self-rated quality of life in patients with OSAS. Although less consistently demonstrated, there also have been improvements in cognition and mood. Likewise reduction in nocturnal and daytime blood pressure, especially in those classified as

4

hypertensive, often occurs within a relatively short time of starting effective treatment. From these findings it is postulated, but not yet proved, that risk for cardiovascular disorders also will be decreased.

Whom to Treat

The severity of sleep-disordered breathing (SDB) has been graded using the AHI as mild (>5 to 15), moderate (>15 to 30) or severe (>30). Although patients with higher grades of SDB tend to have more severe symptoms, each patient's symptoms are often inconsistent with the grade of SDB demonstrated on PSG. This may be because of perceptual differences, individual variability in susceptibility to the effects of sleep disturbance and hypoxemia and/or contributions by factors other than the events tallied in the AHI. The latter might include arousals associated with increased respiratory effort without airflow reduction (upper airway resistance syndrome [UARS]) or poor quality sleep from pain or psychological distress. Likewise, although it is logical to assume that those with the most severe SDB are at greatest risk for long-term adverse consequences and mortality, this has yet to be definitively demonstrated. Therefore decisions on whom to treat and the optimal modality must still rely on clinical judgment applied to each patient's overall circumstances. Guidelines for determining initial management based on the AHI and the presence or absence of symptoms and/or co-morbid conditions potentially caused or aggravated by SDB are given below. Because nasal continuous positive airway pressure (CPAP) is the most efficacious therapy for OSAS, has few serious side effects, and is easily discontinued if the patient cannot tolerate it or does not improve, it is the initial specific therapy of choice for OSAS. General measures to reduce sleep disturbance and SDB are always indicated and may suffice in some instances. Alternate therapies discussed below may be indicated if CPAP is not tolerated or is not fully effective.

Treatment Guidelines

- *AHI less than 5:* No specific treatment for OSAS. (SDB is unlikely to account for symptoms or significantly increase risk for cardiovascular disease or insulin resistance.) Recommend general measures (good sleep hygiene, avoid sleeping supine, weight loss if indicated, avoidance of respiratory depressants and alcohol, oxygen if clinically significant hypoxia not because of OSAS is present). Evaluate for UARS if symptoms and risk factors consistent with this diagnosis are present.
- *AHI greater than 5 to 15:* If there are symptoms (e.g., EDS, morning headaches) or co-morbid conditions (e.g., hypertension, heart failure, insulin resistance, impotence, depression) possibly because of or aggravated by SDB present, start nasal CPAP after adequate titration. If there is no improvement in symptoms or objective improvement in co-morbid conditions demonstrated in 2 months, evaluate for

causes of treatment failure (described later in the article) and consider reverting to basic measures. If no symptoms or co-morbid conditions present at baseline, recommend general measures.
- *AHI greater than 15 to 30:* Start nasal CPAP after adequate titration. If there is no subjective improvement (e.g., improved alertness or mood even if not recognized as a problem before treatment) or objective improvement in co-morbid conditions (e.g., reduction in need for antihypertensive medication or improved insulin sensitivity) in 2 months, evaluate for causes of treatment failure (described later in this article). Consider reverting to general measures.
- *AHI greater than 30:* Start nasal CPAP after adequate titration. If there is no subjective or objective improvement in 2 months, evaluate for causes of treatment failure (described later in this article). Consider reverting to general measures if no symptoms are present. However, if co-morbid conditions are present and/or there is a strong family history of early cardiovascular disease and the patient is tolerating therapy, consider continuing CPAP for 6 months and re-evaluate.

Optimal CPAP pressure for a patient is best identified by an in-laboratory titration attended by a qualified sleep technologist. Because a patient's initial experience with CPAP is a major determinant of long-term use, the technician should be attentive to correcting any difficulty the patient experiences during titration and should provide encouragement and support to facilitate adaptation. Ideally one would like to identify a pressure that abolishes all sleep-related disordered breathing events and prevents significant HbO_2 desaturations. However, the pressure needed to achieve this endpoint may not be tolerable for the patient. If prescribed at this pressure, CPAP may be rejected outright, underused, or discontinued later. Therefore, the optimal pressure for effective treatment is often a compromise lying between the lowest level producing a clinically significant but incomplete reduction in the frequency of SDB events and the highest one likely to be accepted and adhered to by the patient. Selection of this level requires clinical judgment and readjustment based on patient response during the first few weeks of treatment. Identify a pressure that reduces the AHI to below 15 and abolishes HbO_2 desaturations below 88%. In some cases supplemental oxygen will be needed to maintain adequate saturation at a tolerable CPAP pressure.

Problems that could compromise patient acceptance or adherence to treatment should be addressed promptly. Discomfort from the interface or air leaks because of poor mask fit are common initial problems amenable to adjustments or changes in equipment. If use of a chin strap cannot prevent mouth opening, a full face mask is indicated. If the patient has a sense of claustrophobia or cannot tolerate a nasal mask for other reasons, substitute nasal pillows or a nasal cannula type interface. Humidification reduces nasal drying and congestion; some patients, especially those with pre-existing nasal problems, may require a heated humidifier. Persistent rhinitis may respond to nasal steroids. Oral nonsedating antihistamine therapy may be added if allergic rhinitis is present. Significant rhinorrhea may respond to ipratropium (Atrovent) nasal spray. If anatomic nasal obstruction is present (e.g., deviated nasal septum or marked turbinate enlargement) referral for evaluation for surgery or radiofrequency ablation by an otorhinolaryngologist is indicated. There is no evidence that external or internal nasal dilators or nasal lubricants are effective for ameliorating obstructive sleep apnea (OSA).

If the patient cannot tolerate the pressure required to achieve an acceptable AHI, tolerance may improve with use of machines that reduce the pressure during part of the exhalation (*flexible* CPAP) or have separately adjustable pressures during inhalation and exhalation (*bilevel* positive airway pressure). Autotitrating CPAP machines that continuously adjust the pressure based on automated detection of apneas and flow limitation may be efficacious when significant changes in optimal pressure occur with position changes or varying nasal obstruction throughout the night. Some patients find these machines more tolerable than conventional CPAP if the average pressure is significantly lower than that required for adequate therapy for the most severe airway compromise during sleep. Improvement in compliance or overall therapeutic outcomes has not been clearly demonstrated, however, and some patients have their sleep disturbed when changes in pressure are initiated by the machine.

It is important to see the patient for a follow-up visit early in the course of CPAP treatment to address any problems. In some cases temporary use of a benzodiazepine medication or short-acting hypnotic may ease acclimatization to CPAP.

General measures, including weight loss if indicated, should be recommended for all patients with OSAS. In some cases relatively modest weight loss will significantly improve sleep quality and reduce the CPAP pressure required. Bariatric surgery may be indicated and effective when morbid obesity precludes adequate treatment with other measures. Sedatives and alcohol should be avoided. Good sleep hygiene with relatively constant bedtime and rise times as well as adequate time in bed is important. If airway obstruction is significantly worse in the supine position, efforts to maintain sleep in the lateral position are useful. A foam wedge or body pillow behind the back is most effective. Elevating the head of the bed also is helpful and can ameliorate symptoms of gastroesophageal reflux commonly present in patients with OSAS.

Other Therapies

Oral devices to hold the tongue forward or reposition the mandible to increase airway size have been used with variable success. They are more easily tolerated than CPAP by some patients. However, they are less efficacious than CPAP for reducing the AHI and maintaining HbO_2 saturation. They should generally be considered only for patients with mild to moderate OSAS who are intolerant of CPAP. Patients must have adequate dentition to use mandibular repositioning devices.

Several surgical procedures to reduce upper airway narrowing have been developed. Uvulopalatopharyngoplasty (UPPP) removes the uvula and *redundant* pharyngeal tissue. It appears to be most effective in milder cases of OSAS and results in a *cure* in up to 50% of cases. Use of CPAP after UPPP may be complicated by increased mouth leaks because of lack of a seal of the soft palate against the back of the tongue.

Genioglossus/hyoid advancement has produced significant reduction in the AHI but complete success rate has been similar to that of UPPP. Maxillomandibular advancement can increase upper airway dimensions and improve OSAS especially in patients with significant retrognathia. However this is extensive surgery and may require adjustment of dental occlusion. Laser-assisted uvulopalatoplasty is not recommended. In general, surgical procedures should be considered second line therapy for those who do not respond to basic measures and cannot tolerate CPAP.

Residual Sleepiness on Continuous Positive Airway Pressure

Significant improvement in subjective sleepiness and objective measures of alertness (e.g., performance on a driving simulator) have been demonstrated after 3 to 7 days of effective CPAP therapy. Excessive daytime sleepiness despite patient report of compliance with CPAP requires careful evaluation to determine appropriate management. Attempt documentation of CPAP use with a recording CPAP device, or at least a patient log. Equipment should be checked for function and correct pressure setting. The patient should be carefully questioned regarding possible mask leaks or mouth opening (often suggested by morning dry mouth and nose) causing inadequate pressure maintenance. Adequate sleep hygiene with sufficient time in bed

 CURRENT DIAGNOSIS

Symptoms/Signs

- Frequent loud snoring
- Witnessed apneas, gasping or choking during sleep
- Excessive daytime sleepiness and/or nonrefreshing sleep

Risk Factors

- Male sex or postmenopausal female
- 40 to 70 years of age
- Obesity, especially central (large neck circumference and/or high waist/hip ratio)
- Nasal obstruction (structural or functional)
- Anatomic upper airway compromise (e.g., large tongue or tonsils, retrognathia)
- Genetic predisposition (family history of snoring/OSAS, African American)

Abbreviations: OSAS = obstructive sleep apnea syndrome.

CURRENT THERAPY

- Patients often are poorly cognizant of sleep disordered breathing; their bed partners are more aware.
- CPAP is the most effective therapy.
- Adequate titration of CPAP is important to determine effective pressure and tolerance.
- CPAP pressure below that completely abolishing sleep disordered breathing events may be clinically the most effective if higher pressures are poorly tolerated.
- Initiate prompt intervention to ameliorate any problems with CPAP that might be critical for long-term adherence (e.g., heated humidifier and/or nasal steroid for nasal congestion, chin strap or full face mask for mouth opening, or proper mask fit to reduce leaks).
- Bilevel continuous positive airway pressure or auto-titrating CPAP may improve tolerance, but adherence is not definitely improved.
- Oral appliances that are less effective than CPAP may be better tolerated by some patients.
- Upper airway surgical procedures may be indicated if CPAP is not tolerated or fully effective but often do not produce complete resolution of sleep disordered breathing.
- General measures are always indicated (good sleep hygiene, avoid supine sleep and respiratory depressants, treatment for nasal congestion if present, weight loss if overweight or obese).

Abbreviations: CPAP = continuous positive airway pressure.

REFERENCES

Ayes NT, Patel SR, Malhotra A, et al: Auto-titrating versus standard continuous positive airway pressure for the treatment of obstructive sleep apnea: Results of a meta-analysis. Sleep 2004;27:249-253.

Barnes M, McEvoy RD, Banks S, et al: Efficacy of positive airway pressure and oral appliance in mild to moderate obstructive sleep apnea. Am J Respir Crit Care Med 2004;170:656-664.

Breugelmans JG, Ford DE, Smith PL, Punjabi NM: Differences in patient and bed partner-assessed quality of life in sleep-disordered breathing. Am J Respir Crit Care Med 2004;170:547-552.

Buchwald H, Avidor L, Braunwald E, et al: Bariatric surgery: A systematic review and meta-analysis. JAMA 2004;292:1724-1737.

Dinges DF, Weaver TE: Effects of modafinil on sustained attention and quality of life in OSA patients with residual sleepiness while being treated with NCPAP. Sleep Med 2003;4:393-402.

Ferguson KA, Heighway K, Ruby RRF: A randomized trial of laser-assisted uvulopalatoplasty in the treatment of mild obstructive sleep apnea. Am J Respir Crit Care Med 2003;167:15-19.

Kaneko Y, Floras JS, Usui K, et al: Cardiovascular effects of continuous positive airway pressure in patients with heart failure and obstructive sleep apnea. N Engl J Med 2003;348:1233-1241.

Lim J, Lasserson TJ, Fleetham J, Wright J: Oral appliances for obstructive sleep apnea. Cochrane Database Syst Rev 2003;(4): CD004435.

Mansfield DR, Gollogly NC, Kaye DM, et al: Controlled trial of continuous positive airway pressure in obstructive sleep apnea and heart failure. Am J Respir Crit Care Med 2004;169:361-366.

Meoli AL, Rosen CL, Kristo D, et al: Non-prescription treatments of snoring or obstructive sleep apnea: An evaluation of products with limited scientific evidence. Report of the AASM Clinical Practice Review Committee. Sleep 2003;26:619-624.

Meston N, Davis RJ, Mullins R, et al: Endocrine effects of nasal continuous positive airway pressure in male patients with obstructive sleep apnea. J Intern Med 2003;254:447-454.

Turlington PM, Sircar M, Saralaya D, Elliott MW: Time course of changes in driving simulator performance with and without treatment in patients with sleep apnea hypopnea syndrome. Thorax 2004;59:56-59.

should be evaluated by a patient log maintained for 2 weeks. Other factors that may contribute to inadequate or nonrefreshing sleep should be considered, such as chronic pain, psychologic conditions (e.g., anxiety or mood disorders), medications, need for frequent nocturnal urination, or periodic limb movements during sleep (PLMS). If no clear cause is identified, a repeat PSG on CPAP will evaluate prescribed pressure adequacy and identify other causes of sleep disturbance such as PLMS. Persistent *spontaneous* arousals on CPAP at the prescribed pressure may be indicative of UARS, and attempts to eliminate them with increased pressure may be warranted. The PSG may be followed by a multiple sleep latency test (MSLT) to evaluate daytime sleepiness and look for multiple episodes of sleep-onset REM suggestive of narcolepsy. Lack of short sleep latency may indicate misperception of fatigue as sleepiness by the patient.

Lengthening of the sleep period by 30 minutes to 1 hour may be helpful. If excessive sleepiness is documented despite adequate sleep with no recognized disruptions, treatment with a stimulant may be indicated. Modafinil (Provigil) 100 to 400 mg in the morning may increase daytime alertness without causing overstimulation or sleep disturbance. Scheduled naps up to 30 minutes often improve alertness without residual grogginess interfering with rapid resumption of activities or interfering with sleep onset at the usual bedtime.

Current Therapy for Lung Cancer

Method of
Corey J. Langer MD

Epidemiology

Lung cancer remains a health-care debacle of growing, global proportions. Although the incidence in the United States has reached a plateau, its incidence worldwide continues to grow steadily. Because of improved antibiotic therapy for common infectious illnesses, better nutrition in many countries, and improved public health, denizens of the second and third world are now living longer and, consequently, are experiencing a sharp rise in cancer incidence and deaths. This pattern parallels the experience of the first world during the past 50 to 60 years.

In 2005, nearly 170,000 individuals in the United States (roughly 90,000 men and 80,000 women) were diagnosed with lung cancer. Although the survival rates have improved from 6% in the 1960s to 15% currently, lung cancer remains the leading cause of cancer death in the United States, ahead of both breast cancer and prostate cancer, even though the latter two malignancies are diagnosed more often.

In men, the incidence has begun to decrease slightly; however, in women, both the incidence of lung cancer and the mortality rate continue to climb, largely because of increased women's smoking rates that first manifested during World War II and have continued to rise during the postwar period. This in turn has translated into a devastating statistic: 50% more women die of lung cancer than of breast cancer, even though far more attention is paid to the latter by grassroots coalitions.

Approximately 80% to 85% of lung cancers are directly attributable to cigarette smoking. A third of the remainder, roughly 5%, are caused by secondhand smoke. The other 10% are likely attributable to environmental toxins or genetic factors. Environmental exposure to arsenic, asbestos, bischloromethyl ether, chromium, nickel, radon, and vinyl chloride have been implicated in the causation of lung cancer. In addition, increased risk has been noted in patients who have received external beam radiation for Hodgkin's disease, breast cancer, or childhood malignancies. Research has just begun to focus on the genetic factors that may contribute to increased risk, including genotypes that induce the synthesis of high levels of 4-debrisoquin hydroxylase and the relative deficiency of the mu phenotype of glutathione transferase, which has been shown to protect epithelial cells from external toxins. In those who continue to smoke after initial treatment for either lung cancer or head and neck cancer, the risk of subsequent thoracic malignancies increases 10- to 15-fold. Polycyclic hydrocarbons and N-nitrosamines in cigarette smoke are believed to induce DNA damage by methylation; in turn, DNA methylation leads to altered gene expression, and ultimately contributes to the neoplastic process.

Symptoms and Signs

Lung cancer patients who present with symptoms of their primary malignancy have a reduced chance of surviving their illness. Hence, recent efforts have focused on low dose spiral computed tomography (CT) screening, which may potentially detect pulmonary malignancy long before symptoms occur, or lesions are visible on chest film. An ongoing, prospective, randomized, nationwide phase III trial is comparing CT screening to conventional chest radiograph (CXR); the study has completed accrual with more than 50,000 individuals enrolled. Results should be available in the next 3 to 5 years.

The most common symptoms of lung cancer include new or altered cough, dyspnea, hemoptysis, chest pain, pleurisy, and shoulder pain with or without tingling or numbness in the arm (often associated with apical lesions). In addition, a number of physical examination findings often are present. Those with superior sulcus tumors often manifest Horner syndrome, including meiosis, anhidrosis, and ptosis. Patients with mediastinal

nodal disease often will demonstrate supraclavicular or cervical adenopathy.

More advanced tumors are frequently associated with persistent pneumonitis and chest wall pain and, in the case of liver metastases, abdominal pain. Central nervous system (CNS) metastases are often manifested by headache, paresis, confusion, ataxia, and seizures. Systemic symptoms, regardless of stage, may include fatigue, weight loss, and cachexia.

A number of paraneoplastic syndromes have been associated with pulmonary malignancy, including hyperparathyroidism (squamous malignancy), dermatomyositis, acanthosis nigricans, and in small cell malignancy, syndrome of inappropriate antidiuretic hormone (SIADH) secretion, ectopic adrenocorticotropic hormone (ACTH) production, and Eaton-Lambert syndrome.

Histologic Classification

It is hypothesized that virtually all lung cancers arise from a common, pluripotential stem cell, and that the phenotypic (histologic) appearance is a function of all genetic expression. Lung cancer is grouped into two basic pathologies: small cell carcinoma and non-small cell carcinoma. Small cell carcinoma accounts for a declining percentage of lung cancer in the United States. In the past, 20% to 25% of those diagnosed with pulmonary malignancy had small cell histology, whereas currently it accounts for no more than 15%. Histologically these cells are small and dense, with high N:C ratio, nuclear and cellular molding, and the presence of neurosecretory granules on electromicroscopy. Overexpression of neural cell adhesion molecules, including neuron-specific enolase (NSE), chromogranin, and synaptophysin is characteristic of small cell carcinoma of the lung (SCLC). Clinically, SCLC generally is characterized by subacute onset, progressive dyspnea, hoarseness, and cough, and, less frequently, hemoptysis. Tumors generally present centrally with hilar or mediastinal adenopathy. More than two thirds manifest metastatic disease at presentation.

The vast majority of patients in the United States have NSCLC, and adenocarcinoma accounts for more than 50% of all lung cancer now diagnosed in the United States. Its incidence is growing, and it is particularly frequent in women. It usually is associated with cigarette smoking and secondary pulmonary injury, although of all non-small cell carcinoma of the lung (NSCLC) histologies, adenocarcinoma is the most likely to be found in nonsmokers. Adenocarcinomas can arise both centrally and peripherally. Adenocarcinoma of the lung is more prone to metastasize compared with squamous cell carcinoma, and other NSCLC histologies.

Bronchoalveolar carcinoma (BAC) is a unique subtype of adenocarcinoma, often characterized by multifocal and multilobar, lapidal spread. The neoplastic cells in BAC are type II pneumocytes; hence, the propensity of alveolar infiltrates and lobar consolidation. These tumors may often grow quite slowly, though, and are generally less likely to metastasize outside the chest. Bronchorrhea and dyspnea are frequent symptoms.

The percentage of all lung cancers attributed to squamous cell carcinoma is currently declining. In the past, 30% to 40% had squamous histology; now only 25% have it. This decline has been attributed in part to a decrease in popularity of unfiltered cigarettes. Histologically, these tumors stain positively for keratin, and generally manifest centrally, with frequent cavitation. Symptoms often suggest pneumonitis or abscess.

Large cell carcinomas account for 5% to 7% of all lung cancers, and frequently have an anaplastic appearance. They may resemble neuroendocrine tumors, but morphologically they look distinct from carcinoid or small cell. Unlike the latter two entities, these tumors are grouped with NSCLC and tend to behave very aggressively.

Finally carcinoid tends to be the least aggressive of all lung cancers, often manifesting endobronchially. Carcinoid tumors, even without treatment, tend to be fairly indolent. Although histologically these cells exhibit many of the same staining characteristics as SCLC, the cells tend to be bland and monomorphic.

Over the past 5 to 10 years, increasing use of immunohistochemical stains, including carcinoembryonic antigen, cytokeratin, and thyroid transcription factor-1 (TTF1), have enabled us to accurately differentiate epithelial malignancies, particularly adenocarcinoma of the lung, from malignancies that originate outside the thorax.

Biology of Primary Lung Cancer

Mutations in the bronchial epithelium over the course of a person's life are responsible for the development of thoracic malignancies. It is speculated that 10 to 20 mutational events on average ultimately precipitate lung cancer. Allelic loss in the short arm of chromosome 3 (3p) is one of the earliest events leading to epithelial hyperplasia. Tumor suppressor genes are found at this locus. Dysplasia is associated with allelic loss of 3p as well as allelic loss in the short arm of chromosome 9 (9p). Mutations of the gene for P53 (chromosome 17) and mutational activation of the K-*ras* oncogene (chromosome 12) can convert epithelial dysplasia into carcinoma in situ or frank malignancy. Additional mutational events will generally determine the ultimate phenotypic appearance (histologic type) of the malignancy. For instance, deletion of 3p coupled with the *myc* oncogene (N-c-L *myc*, chromosome 8 q24) activation, mutation of the gene encoding retinoblastoma (chromosome 13), and the loss of K-*ras* activation are generally associated with SCLC phenotype. Conversely, persistence of K-*ras* activation, allelic loss of chromosome 1, and overexpression of the *c-erb*B-2 and/or bcl2 oncogenes can lead to the NSCLC phenotype.

In turn, multiple growth factors can stimulate tumor growth. Gastrin releasing peptide and cholecystokinin are paracrine promoters of cellular growth of SCLC, whereas epidermal growth factor, IGFr type 1 (insulin growth factor) and transforming growth factor beta are associated with NSCLC. These growth factors are now proving to be targets for anticancer agents.

Screening for Lung Cancer

Unlike prostate cancer, for which prostate-specific antigen (PSA) has a role, or breast cancer, for which mammograms are clearly established, there is no definitive screening procedure for lung cancer. Currently, however, intensive research focuses on low-dose, spiral CT scans as a means of detecting early, asymptomatic cancers. The Early Lung Cancer Action Project (ELCAP) demonstrated efficacy in detecting early stage malignancy in high-risk patients in which 1000 at-risk patients (60 years old; 10 pack-years) underwent both CXR and low-dose chest CT. On CT, 23% had non-calcified pulmonary nodules versus only 7% on CXR. Those with small, equivocal nodules had 3-month, followup examinations. The CT scan proved four times as likely to find malignancy than the CXR (2.7% vs. 0.7%), and these cancers were six times as likely to be early stage (85% stage I). Consequently, case fatality rates appear to have dropped. However, the impact on cancer mortality is unclear. A major prospective, nationwide phase III study comparing conventional CXR to low-dose, spiral CT has completed accrual with more than 50,000 accrued; participants are in the follow-up stage.

Diagnostic Methods and Staging of Lung Cancer

Patients with lung cancer, almost by definition, will have abnormal chest films and CT scans. Carcinoma in situ is extraordinarily rare and, generally, presents as an incidental finding in a patient undergoing bronchoscopy for other indications. In rare instances, patients with negative chest films or CT scans may present with hemoptysis and have endobronchial disease, with minimal or no overt invasion.

If CXR discloses a suspicious lesion, obtaining old chest films for comparison is essential. If a lesion has been stable on CXR for 2 years or more, further workup is *likely* not necessary, although relatively indolent tumors, such as low-grade adenocarcinomas and early stage BACs, may often manifest this way. New lesions demand evaluation. A diligent history is key to assessment, as is physical exam. It is imperative that the supraclavicular region be examined carefully; small nodes are often present, and a positive fine needle aspirate or biopsy often will yield both diagnosis and stage. Pulmonary exam may reveal evidence of bronchial obstruction (wheezing), or pleural effusion (dullness to percussion with or without adventitious sounds). The presence of a Horner syndrome will frequently indicate the presence of an invasive Pancoast tumor. Enlargement of the liver and/or neurologic abnormalities are generally signs of distant spread. The presence of lymph node enlargement or organomegaly yields critical staging information, and helps locate potential areas for biopsy, if histologic diagnosis is not yet established.

If physical exam findings are entirely normal, the next step includes a CT of the chest with inclusion of the liver and adrenals. CT scan will confirm the presence and extent of the pulmonary mass, evaluate the mediastinum for the presence or absence of lymphadenopathy, rule out pleural effusions, and detect otherwise asymptomatic hepatic or adrenal metastases. It will also confirm or exclude the presence of other pulmonary nodules.

In the last 10 years, positron emission tomography (PET) with 2-fluorodeoxyglucose (2-FDG) has become an almost standard component of the work-up, necessary for assessment of solitary pulmonary nodules (SPNs) and for the evaluation of any patient with stage I-IIIa disease. PET scanning, particularly in the chest, is generally more sensitive and specific than routine CT imaging, and the standard uptake values (SUVs) may have prognostic implications. The sensitivity and specificity of PET scans in the hilum and mediastinum are 85% and 90%, respectively. In addition, PET scans often can detect extrathoracic disease that is not appreciated on CT. Unlike CT scans, PET scans will often divulge asymptomatic osseous metastases that would otherwise require bone scan, and many investigators substitute PET scan for bone scan in the assessment of the skeletal architecture. The absence of any uptake of FDG on PET scan excludes a malignant neoplastic process with nearly a 99% level of confidence.

Headaches or other neurologic complaints should prompt CT imaging of the brain or magnetic resonance imaging (MRI) of the brain. Most clinicians will advocate CNS imaging for stage II or III lesions, and many will even include routine CNS imaging in the presence of clinical or pathologic stage IB disease. In the absence of abnormalities on PET scan, complaints of bony discomfort or back pain, call for a technetium-99m bone scan. Additional evaluation may include plain films or MRIs of specific bones, or CT scans of particular regions, generally based on symptoms and physical findings. At the completion of clinical staging, patients are segregated by TNM status into stages I, II, IIIA or B, and IV. The presence of distant spread beyond the thorax, whether the patient is diagnosed with NSCLC or SCLC, warrants the institution of upfront systemic treatment.

Pathologic Staging

In the absence of disease outside the chest, fiberoptic bronchoscopy or CT-guided fine needle aspirates are generally standard. Fiberoptic bronchoscopy is an accurate and generally safe technique to render the diagnosis of lung cancer, particularly for central and perihilar lesions. Bronchoscopy can directly visualize the proximal tracheobronchial tree; hilar masses can be sampled by direct biopsy or brushings. In addition, enlarged mediastinal nodes are often accessible by Wang needle biopsy. The location of the mass relative to the carina is determined, and the carina and otherwise normal-appearing bronchial epithelium can be inspected and, if necessary, biopsied.

Initial clinical staging of the mediastinum is provided by chest CT scan. Nodes 2 cm or larger are usually pathologic. Those smaller than 1 cm, particularly if

they are isolated, are generally negative, in which case mediastinoscopy has relatively low yield. However, nodes between 1 and 2 cm are considered intermediate in size, and predicting involvement often is difficult, if not impossible. These nodes may be reactive or may contain metastases. For nodes of indeterminate size, PET scanning of the mediastinum often will confirm the presence or absence of metastases. If PET scan shows uptake, then pathologic confirmation by mediastinoscopy or Wang needle biopsy is desirable, if not mandatory, particularly if the presence or absence of mediastinal nodal involvement alters the therapeutic decision. Likewise, a negative PET scan does not necessarily rule out microscopic involvement.

If a patient presents with clinical stage IA disease, and otherwise has a negative CT scan and PET scan, further pathologic work-up prior to surgery is probably unnecessary. These patients can undergo thoracotomy and resection as long as adequate mediastinal sampling or dissection is performed. If a patient has clinical stage IB, or stage II disease, then pathologic assessment in mediastinal nodes is warranted. Most mediastinal nodes are accessible by mediastinoscopy. Those in the aortopulmonary (AP) window or in the left periaortic region often will require mediastinotomy (Chamberlain procedure) for pathologic confirmation. Mediastinoscopy is a surgical procedure performed under general anesthesia in which a hollow, rigid instrument is introduced through a small incision in the suprasternal notch, and advanced along the pretracheal plane to the level of the carina. Enlarged nodes can be visualized and sampled for biopsy. On the right side, the upper margin of the hilum is accessible, whereas the aortic arch on the left precludes access to the left hilum. Contraindications to mediastinoscopy include superior vena cava (SVC) obstruction, prior mediastinal surgery, and to a great extent, prior radiation.

Once pathologic staging has been accomplished and patients have been segregated into clinical/pathologic stages I through IV, then the treating physician is capable of making rational, therapeutic recommendations. Without proper staging, any therapeutic decision becomes suspect. Patients who have not been adequately staged often will receive inappropriate treatment.

Preoperative Assessment

Before considering surgical intervention, or aggressive combined modality therapy in the case of locally advanced disease, it is imperative to assess the overall health of the patient, the patient's physiologic age, and presence or absence of co-morbidities. This may entail additional cardiac evaluation. At a minimum, preoperative assessment mandates a careful evaluation of pulmonary function, and best estimation of postoperative pulmonary function. Ideally, patients should have a minimum preoperative forced expiratory volume in 1 second (FEV_1) of greater than 1.2 L and a DL_{CO} (diffusing capacity for carbon monoxide) of 80% or greater. There should be no evidence of hypercapnia or cor pulmonale. Baseline assessment of FEV_1 is necessary to establish a comfort zone in anticipation of pulmonary resection, and even higher baseline FEV_1s are desirable in anticipation of pneumonectomy. Patients with a baseline FEV_1 of 0.5 L or less are medically inoperable. Those with a baseline FEV_1 of 0.8 to 1.2 L or DL_{CO} less than 60% are considered borderline. In these individuals, thoracotomy and resection raises the risk or perioperative and postoperative morbidity and mortality; and there are clear limits to the feasible extent of resection. These individuals generally undergo quantitative ventilation and profusion lung scans to more precisely gauge postoperative pulmonary function. Those with an estimated postoperative FEV_1 of less than 0.6 to 0.8 L generally will prove medically inoperable.

In addition, lung cancer patients, most of whom are current or former smokers, will generally require some sort of cardiac screening, and in certain circumstances, a full cardiac evaluation including stress perfusion scans or angiography if there is evidence of active coronary disease or questionable ejection fraction. Finally, it is imperative that all operative candidates quit smoking or cut down as much as possible prior to thoracotomy. Those who continue to smoke have disturbances of mucociliary clearance and often have increased risk of postoperative complications like pneumonitis.

Non-Small Cell Lung Cancer Treatment of Stages IA, IB, IIA, and IIB Disease

Pathologically proven stage I lesions (T1 or T2 N0M0) are clearly in the province of surgery. However, stage I disease accounts for less than 20% of all newly diagnosed NSCLC. T1 lesions by definition include the prototypical solitary pulmonary nodule (<3 cm) confined to a single lobe with no evidence of pleural invasion. T2 lesions include 1 or more of the following characteristics: greater than 3 cm in size, invasion of the mainstem bronchus (but more than 2 cm from the carina), or involvement of the visceral pleura.

Stage II NSCLC, by definition, generally stipulates N1 disease, which includes either peribronchial nodal involvement or involvement in adjacent hilar nodes ipsilateral to the primary tumor. Stage II is further segregated into IIA (T1N1) and IIB (T2N1) based on primary tumor size.

Finally, selected patients with T1-3N2 disease may prove resectable. N2 NSCLC denotes ipsilateral mediastinal or subcarinal nodal involvement; and T3 lesions include those arising in the mainstem bronchus within 2 cm of the carina or invasion of the parietal pleura or chest wall.

The preferred treatment for stage I-IIIA patients who are medically fit remains surgical resection, and the preferred surgical resection is lobectomy, if possible, with sampling or dissection of mediastinal lymph nodes. Segmental pulmonary resection is a reasonable alternative in patients who do not have adequate pulmonary reserve to tolerate lobectomy, although it should be

noted that several randomized series have demonstrated higher local recurrence rates after segmental resection compared with standard lobectomy. Pneumonectomy confers absolutely no advantage over lobectomy, and it is indicated only if lobectomy would result in incomplete resection. The operative mortality rates (including the 30-day postoperative period) associated with pneumonectomy, lobectomy, and segmental resection are 6.2%, 2.9%, and 1%, respectively. Death in this period is generally caused by pneumonia, respiratory failure, myocardial infarction, intractable arrhythmias, pulmonary emboli, broncho-pleural fistula, or empyema. Video assisted thoracoscopic resection or lobectomy continues to undergo prospective evaluation, but it is generally reserved for patients in whom full anatomic resections are not feasible.

The 5-year survival rate for patients with pathologically proven stage I NSCLC is generally 60% to 80%; and for those with stage II NSCLC, it is generally 35% to 50%. Patients with stage I or II squamous cell carcinoma have generally improved disease-free survival rates compared with those with adenocarcinoma and equivalent stage; the latter are more likely to manifest distant metastases at some point during follow-up. Additional prognostic factors predicting increased risk of recurrence or compromised survival have variously included K-*ras* mutations at codon 12 (a factor indicating poor prognosis in adenocarcinoma) and the absence of *Bcl*-2 expression.

Patients with stage I or II NSCLC who are medically unfit or who for other co-morbid reasons are deemed poor surgical candidates should be treated with radiation: 60 Gy or more in 2 Gy fractions × 30. In this regard, stereotactic and three-dimensional approaches are undergoing investigation. The disease-free survival rate for patients with stage I or II NSCLC treated with radiation alone is 15% to 30% at 5 years; this compromised percentage reflects both a higher propensity for relapse, as well as the adverse prognostic effects of co-morbidities.

Emergence of Adjuvant Therapy

Until recently, adjuvant therapy or postoperative radiation had absolutely no role in patients with stage I, II, or IIIA NSCLC. However, in 1995, a meta-analysis of nearly 1400 patients enrolled on adjuvant cytotoxic, platinum-based trials, demonstrated in aggregate, a 5% improvement in 5 year survival rates ($p = 0.08$) compared with standard observation postresection. To confirm this putative 5% survival advantage in a prospective trial large enough to show statistically significant therapeutic benefit, investigators led by T. LeChevalier spearheaded the International Adjuvant Lung Trial (IALT) over a 5-year period ending in 2000. Nearly 1900 patients worldwide were randomized after surgical resection to platinum-based combinations with either etoposide or vinca alkaloids or to standard observation. Radiation was given electively to selected patients with stage II or III NSCLC. The vast majority of patients on this study (80%) were male. The mean age was 59 (all were ≤75 years); squamous cell histology was noted in nearly half of those enrolled (47%), whereas adenocarcinoma was diagnosed in 40%. Of those enrolled, 36% had stage I disease, 25% stage II NSCLC, and 39% stage III NSCLC.

The 5-year survival rate in the adjuvant arm was 44.5%, compared with 40.4% in the control group ($p = <0.03$). Treatment-related mortality occurred in fewer than 1% of enrollees, and grade greater than or equal to 4 toxicity occurred in only 23%. A therapeutic benefit was observed regardless of gender, performance status, age, type of surgery, stage, choice of chemotherapy, or the institution or omission of radiation. The greatest benefit was observed in stage III patients, who had a 5-year survival rate of 37.4% versus 29.9% in the control group. Benefits were less pronounced in those with T1 disease, those older than 65 years of age, and those with compromised performance status. The IALT effort represented one of the first large-scale adjuvant trials to show a survival benefit. However, a number of criticisms have been leveled at this study: Staging was heterogeneous and not precisely prescribed. The nature of cytotoxic therapy and the application of radiation were not standardized. Although the study was the largest adjuvant trial to date in NSCLC, it actually closed earlier than planned and did not meet its accrual goal of 3300 patients. In addition, those older than age 75 years were explicitly excluded from this trial. Finally, there were a number of contemporaneous trials, including the Adjuvant Lung Project Italy (ALPI), Big Lung Trial (BLT), and the joint Eastern Cooperative Oncology Group/Radiation Therapy Oncology Group (ECOG/RTOG) effort, each of which failed to show a survival advantage for adjuvant chemotherapy compared with standard observation.

Hence, until 2004, most practitioners did not routinely administer adjuvant treatment to resected patients. But as of the American Society of Clinical Oncology (ASCO) meeting in 2004, two additional adjuvant efforts have demonstrated even more striking therapeutic benefits. The National Cancer Institute-Canada (NCI-C), in collaboration with the Eastern Cooperative Oncology Group and the Southwest Oncology Group (SWOG), mounted a phase III trial comparing combination cisplatin and vinorelbine during a 4-month period to standard observation in patients with resected stage IB and II NSCLC. During a 7-year period 482 patients were accrued; those receiving systemic chemotherapy enjoyed a statistically significant improvement in 5-year survival: 69% versus 54% ($p = 0.01$). There were only two treatment related deaths in the adjuvant arm. However, delivery of the adjuvant regimen was difficult. Of those enrolled, 13% were taken off treatment because of toxicity; an additional 29% declined to complete treatment, primarily because of side effects. Toxicity withdrawals were more common in those who had undergone pneumonectomy: 27% versus 8%, ($p = >0.001$).

A similar trial by Strauss and colleagues from the Cancer and Leukemia Group B (CALGB) focused specifically on resected stage IB NSCLC in which patients were randomized to either standard observation or to combination paclitaxel and carboplatin every 3 weeks for four cycles. In this effort, compliance was superior

to that observed in the NCI-C trial, with more than 80% of patients completing all scheduled treatment; 65% of these completed treatment at full dose without modification. Patients were stratified based on tumor histology (squamous versus other), differentiation (poorly versus moderately/well differentiated), and the use or omission of preoperative mediastinoscopy versus lymph node sampling. During a 7-year period, 344 patients were accrued: 64% were male; median age was 61 years. Nearly 90% underwent lobectomy. At 4 years, a statistically significant improvement in survival emerged favoring the adjuvant group: 71% versus 59% ($p = 0.028$). This improvement was directly attributable to a decrease in lung cancer deaths: 19 in the adjuvant group versus 34 in the control group ($p = 0.018$).

These two trials, in the context of the previous IALT effort, which demonstrated a similarly significant, albeit numerically more modest, improvement in survival, have recalibrated the therapeutic thermostat for most clinicians treating resected NSCLC. At this point, adjuvant, platinum-based combination treatment has emerged as a standard approach in fit patients who have undergone R0 surgical resections. Therapeutic benefit, at this point, appears unequivocal.

Alternative Adjuvant Concepts

In Japan, nonplatinum approaches, including oral fluorinated pyrimidines, have demonstrated therapeutic benefit compared with observation in patients with resected stage I-IIIA NSCLC. In addition, a number of clinical trials have demonstrated the feasibility and potential benefit for induction chemotherapy, which has a number of theoretic advantages:

- Improved drug delivery through intact vasculature
- Enhanced treatment compliance and tolerance compared with adjuvant therapy
- Early application of systemic treatment in an illness in which the majority of patients succumb to disseminated disease
- Potential early eradication of occult regional and distant micrometastases
- Potential facilitation of local treatment, including the implementation of less radical surgical procedures

Objective responses to induction therapy range from 40% to 70%, with pathologic complete remission rates of 5% to 20%; the pathologic complete remission (pCR) rate is generally higher in patients receiving induction chemoradiation. Compliance with induction cytotoxics is generally better than conventional adjuvant therapy, although concerns exist regarding the potential exacerbation of perioperative morbidity and mortality. Two small randomized phase III trials in patients with stage III NSCLC suggested a survival benefit, but a much larger phase III effort comparing induction therapy with mitomycin, ifosfamide, and cisplatin followed by surgery to surgery alone failed to show a statistically significant survival advantage, even though a relative survival benefit was seen at 3 years: 49% versus 41% ($p = 0.09$). Although patients with stage IIIA disease derived no benefit, those with N0 or N1 disease enjoyed a statistically significant survival benefit ($p = 0.27$).

Because of the therapeutic benefit demonstrated by recent adjuvant trials, a phase III intergroup trial (SWOG 9900) comparing surgery alone to surgery preceded by induction chemotherapy was closed to accrual; however, in Europe, similar trials continue to accrue patients, and a critical trial from Spain directly compares surgery alone with surgery combined with either neoadjuvant (induction) or conventional adjuvant chemotherapy.

Second Primary Tumors

Patients who have undergone successful treatment for stage I or II NSCLC have a 2% to 3% risk per year of developing other smoking-related tumors, usually in the lung or head and neck region. At 10 years, the cumulative risk can be as high as 20% to 30%. Hence, sedulous follow-up is mandatory. Phase III trials assessing the capacity of *cis*-retinoic acid for up to 5 years have failed to demonstrate a significant capacity to reduce the risk of second primary tumors (SPTs) in this population. An ongoing, placebo-controlled, randomized, prospective, phase III intergroup trial is assessing the role of selenium in resected stage I NSCLC patients. Most clinicians advocate monitoring every 3 to 4 months for the first 24 months and then every 6 months thereafter for this high-risk group. At a minimum, periodic CXR is mandatory; ongoing studies are evaluating the role of low-dose spiral CT imaging at regular intervals.

Treatment of IIIA and IIIB NSCLC

Patients with IIIA disease are a highly heterogeneous group and can be divided into three general categories.

1. Incidental N2 involvement appreciated only during mediastinal node dissection or sampling after a negative or equivocal preoperative assessment by PET and/or mediastinoscopy.
2. Nonbulky, potentially resectable N2 (mediastinal) involvement with nodes appreciated on CT scan or at mediastinoscopy, but not on CXR or bronchoscopy.
3. Bulky N2 disease with paratracheal nodes clearly visible on chest radiograph or splaying of the carina at bronchoscopy, indicating bulky subcarinal adenopathy.

Under these circumstances a uniform treatment approach to patients with stage IIIA NSCLC cannot be recommended. For patients with NSCLC and incidental nodal involvement at the time of resection, R0 surgical resection is still key, and adjuvant therapy is now indicated. The 5-year survival rates in such patients approach 40% to 50%. There is no proven role for adjuvant radiation (RT), although studies from the Lung Cancer Study Group (LCSG) have demonstrated a reduction in local recurrence rates in patients with N2 or hilar N1 squamous carcinoma. Nor is there an established role for preoperative RT with

one exception: patients with T3, N0-1, M0 Pancoast (superior sulcus) tumors who receive preoperative radiation to 45 Gy or concurrent chemoradiation with etoposide and cisplatin in the preoperative setting followed by lung resection can expect 5-year survival rates of 40% to 50%. There are no randomized trials in the Pancoast setting to support the routine use of radiation and chemotherapy, but outcome compared with historic controls appears substantially better. In the broader group of patients with resectable stage IIIA disease, an upcoming phase III intergroup trial will compare induction chemoradiation to induction chemotherapy alone, thereby isolating the role, if any, of RT in this setting.

Bulky IIIA (T1-3, N2M0) Stage IIIB NSCLC

For those with bulky IIIA disease, radical thoracic radiation (≥ 60 Gy in 30 Fx) has been the historic "standard"; unfortunately long-term survival rates were only 3% to 7%. More recently, combined modality therapy has shown a survival advantage, particularly in fit individuals. Neoadjuvant or induction chemotherapy followed by radiation has demonstrated a clear-cut advantage compared with radiation alone in four separate, mature, prospective, randomized phase III trials, generally confined to patients with good performance status and less than or equal to 5% weight loss. In the Dillman (CALGB) effort, induction therapy with cisplatin and vinblastine during a 5-week period followed by conventional RT yielded a 6-year survival rate of 16%, compared with only 6% in the radiation control group. The RTOG confirmed the benefit of induction cisplatin and vinblastine prior to radiation and demonstrated a statistically significant improvement in median, 2-year, and 5-year survival rates, although the 5-year survival rate of 8% observed in the combined modality arm was less impressive than that observed in the CALGB study. A French effort comparing high-dose radiation alone to platinum-based chemotherapy both preceding and following high-dose RT demonstrated a doubling of long-term survival: 6% versus 3% in a mixed group of good and poor prognosis patients. Finally, a randomized phase III trial from the UK demonstrated an increase in 5-year survival from 4% to 10% in patients receiving platinum-based chemotherapy followed by radiation versus radiation alone, with a significant improvement in quality of life.

Concurrent chemoradiation with cisplatin administered on a daily basis has proved beneficial in a critical European Organization for Research and Therapy of Cancer (EORTC) effort, although other cisplatin-based studies have not shown a benefit. Two other clinical trials comparing hyperfractionated radiation alone to combined hyperfractionated radiation and either weekly or daily etoposide and carboplatin demonstrated a statistically significant survival benefit for combined modality, with 4- and 5-year survival rates approaching 20%.

More recently, three separate phase III trials have shown a benefit for concurrent chemoradiation compared with sequential or asynchronous chemotherapy followed by radiation. A Japanese effort in which the majority of patients had stage IIIB disease demonstrated superiority for concurrent chemoradiation using mitomycin, vindesine, and cisplatin, compared with induction chemotherapy followed by RT: 5-year survival rates were 16% and 8% respectively. RTOG 9410, the largest phase III trial to date in locally advanced unresectable NSCLC, demonstrated a similar survival advantage for concurrent, uninterrupted chemoradiation with vinblastine and cisplatin versus sequential chemotherapy and radiation using identical cytotoxic agents. A smaller trial from Eastern Europe demonstrated a similar, marked improvement in median survival (21 vs. 13 months) for patients receiving concurrent chemoradiation with more modern agents (vinorelbine and cisplatin) versus sequential therapy with identical chemotherapy for four cycles followed by RT.

Although virtually all patients with stage IIIB disease are considered categorically unresectable, those who present with pathologically documented IIIA disease, even many with relatively bulky disease, may be rendered resectable. Based on a phase II study mounted by the SWOG showing feasibility for this approach and a long-term survival rate exceeding 20%, a large, prospective randomized phase III intergroup trial comparing chemoradiation alone to chemoradiation followed by surgical resection in stage IIIA NSCLC was completed. This effort demonstrated a significant improvement in progression-free survival (14 vs. 11.7 months) and 3-year, progression-free survival (29% versus 19%) for the trimodality approach, but no significant improvement in overall survival at 3 years (38% versus 33%). The incidence of perioperative morbidity and mortality was also higher in the trimodality arm. A followup trial will compare chemotherapy followed by surgery to concurrent chemoradiation followed by surgery and will hopefully isolate the role of RT in the induction setting. Treatment mortality rates for the trimodality approach as high as 7% to 15% have been cited.

Treatment of Stage IV NSCLC

Unfortunately, nearly half the patients with newly diagnosed NSCLC in 2005 will have stage IV disease. For such patients, with rare exception (isolated CNS metastases or adrenal metastases), there is no curative therapy. The goal under these circumstances is palliation, improvement in quality of life, and extension of survival. During the past 10 to 15 years, several meta-analyses of randomized efforts comparing chemotherapy to best supportive care have shown in aggregate.

- Nondebilitated patients with NSCLC and good performance status can sustain a 27% to 35% reduction in mortality at 3 to 6 months, although the benefits diminish with time.
- Median survival increases from less than 4 months to nearly 7 months, with improvement in 1-year survival rates from 15% to 30%.
- With cytotoxic therapy, 50% to 75% will sustain symptomatic improvement.

Rakel and Bope: *Conn's Current Therapy 2006.*

Multiple analyses have consistently demonstrated that prognosis is worse in those with impaired performance status, declining appetite or weight, male gender, as well as metastatic involvement of the brain, bone, or subcutaneous tissue. Older, second-generation regimens including etoposide and platinum, mitomycin and vinblastine have generally yielded median survival times of 6 to 8 months and 1-year survival rates of roughly 25%. Unfortunately, improvements in response rate do not necessarily translate into improved survival. More recently, platinum combinations with third-generation cytotoxics including paclitaxel, docetaxel, gemcitabine, vinorelbine, irinotecan, and topotecan have yielded response rates and survival rates as good as, if not better than, older combinations. At this point, established agents to treat NSCLC include the following older agents:

- Cisplatin
- Carboplatin
- Etoposide
- Vinblastine
- Mitomycin
- Ifosfamide
and newer agents:L
- Paclitaxel
- Docetaxel
- Vinorelbine
- Gemcitabine
- Irinotecan
- Topotecan
- Pemetrexed
- Gefitinib
- Erlotinib

In performance status (PS 0-2) patients with advanced or recurrent NSCLC, chemotherapy has a clear-cut, well established role. Standard of practice dictates a platinum combination. Cisplatin or carboplatin have proved almost equally effective in combination with any of the following newer agents: taxanes, gemcitabine, vinorelbine. Third generation chemotherapy regimens in combination with cisplatin have generally proved superior to cisplatin alone, and there are multiple examples of superiority for third-generation regimens compared to older second-generation regimens. New agent/nonplatinum combinations are reasonable alternatives in selected patients who are unable to tolerate cisplatin. Single-agent therapy is a reasonable alternative in PS 0-2 patients, and at least one nested analysis in the context of a phase III trial has shown a potential advantage for combination carboplatin/paclitaxel versus paclitaxel alone. There is no indication for systemic chemotherapy in PS 3 or 4 patients.

Two agents have generally shown superiority to one agent, whereas three agents in combination have generally yielded increased toxicity, without survival benefit. There is no evidence to suggest that extending treatment beyond 4 to 6 cycles (12 to 18 weeks) enhances survival. Nor is there any evidence that a planned switch to a non-cross-resistant regimen can improve outcome. With extended treatment, we generally witness a plateau in therapeutic benefit at the expense of cumulative toxicity.

SECOND-LINE THERAPY

In patients who have experienced disease progression either during or after their first-line treatment, either single agent docetaxel or pemetrexed has emerged as a reasonable standard of comparison. Docetaxel has yielded therapeutic superiority compared to best supportive care in a critical NCI-C sponsored trial; a separate trial showed an advantage for docetaxel compared to either vinorelbine or ifosfamide. Pemetrexed has shown de facto equivalency to docetaxel, with less toxicity, particularly myelosuppression.

In addition, the Epidermal Growth Factor receptor (EGFr) tyrosine-kinase inhibitor (TKI) erlotinib, has recently been approved for second-line treatment based on a phase III trial showing superiority versus best supportive care with median survival of 6.7 versus 4.8 months and 1-year survival rates of 31% versus 22%. In the third-line setting both erlotinib (Tarceva) and gefitinib (Iressa) are approved.

There is no evidence that combining targeted agents such as gefitinib or erlotinib with conventional cytotoxic regimens in the first-line setting can enhance survival compared to cytotoxic therapy alone. However, nested analyses suggest a potential up-front benefit in nonsmokers with advanced disease who receive cytotoxics and EGFr inhibitors, and in those who harbor the activation or gain of function mutation in the catalytic domain of the EGFr chromosome. There is also emerging evidence to suggest that these agents may work best as consolidation or maintenance after cytotoxic therapy has been completed. Follow-up phase II and III studies are investigating these leads.

Small Cell Carcinoma of the Lung

The incidence of small cell carcinoma of the lung (SCLC) has declined during the past 20 to 25 years. This histology previously constituted 20% to 25% of all cases in the United States, but now represents roughly 13% to 15%. Currently, an estimated 25,000 men and women are diagnosed with SCLC yearly. SCLC is a distinct clinical pathologic entity. It almost always is associated with cigarette smoking. Of all lung cancer histologies, it has the tightest link to cigarette exposure. It also has a characteristic histologic appearance. Cells are generally smaller than observed in other epithelial cancers, with fairly pronounced apposition to other cells, nuclear molding, and relatively high N:C ratios. SCLC is distinguished by the presence of electron-dense neuroendocrines granules on electron microscopy, and fairly distinct cytogenetic alterations, including the deletion of the short arm of chromosome 3 (3p14-21). SCLC also is associated with peptide secretion, including gastrin releasing peptide; unlike most NSCLC, it stains positively for neuron specific enolase, synaptophysin, and chromogranin.

SCLC is characterized by relatively rapid tumor growth and progression. SCLC also is marked by paraneoplastic syndromes, including SIADH and corticotropins (ACTH). It is considered relatively more cytoresponsive than NSCLC, at least initially, with response rates as high as 70% to 80%. In addition, unlike NSCLC, complete responses are observed in 10% to 30% of individuals.

As with NSCLC, standard evaluation includes a thorough history and physical exam, chest films, CT of the chest including the liver and adrenals, and either CT or MRI of the brain, as well as bone scan. PET scans as in NSCLC, are extraordinarily sensitive in detecting occult metastases, and may potentially substitute for bone scan. Previously, bone marrow aspirate biopsy was considered part of standard staging, but, in the presence of other sites of extrathoracic disease, it is unnecessary, and even in those with otherwise limited disease, it discloses metastatic involvement less than 5% of the time. Unless an otherwise limited-disease patient has an elevated alkaline phosphatase, or symptoms that point to possible occult marrow involvement (e.g., anemia, or bone achiness) bone marrow biopsy is unnecessary.

Treatment of SCLC is determined by stage. Patients with extensive disease constitute more than two thirds of those diagnosed with SCLC, and chemotherapy is the mainstay of treatment. Standard combinations include etoposide and platinum, either carboplatin or cisplatin. More recently, a phase III trial from Japan showed therapeutic superiority for irinotecan and cisplatin compared to etoposide and cisplatin with a fourfold improvement in 2-year survival rate: 19.5% versus 5.2%. Confirmatory studies in the United States and elsewhere in the world are underway. Median survival with standard cytotoxic combinations ranges from 7 to 11 months, with 1-year survival rates of 30% to 40%. Patients with extensive SCLC and reasonable performance status should receive a platinum based combination. In extensive disease, carboplatin and cisplatin appear equivalent with respect to response rates and survival. Ongoing studies are assessing the role of consolidative therapy with non-cross-resistant approaches, including targeted agents. More recently, phase III trials in chemosensitive relapse (previous response, with greater than 60 to 90 day hiatus from prior chemotherapy) showed therapeutic superiority for topotecan compared to cyclophasphamide, doxirubicin (Adriamycin), and vincristine (CAV): identical response rates and survival rates, but improved symptomatic control.

Future Directions

Patients diagnosed with limited disease are best served by combined modality therapy, preferably concurrent chemoradiation. In the past 10 to 15 years, a number of critical trials have established the beneficial role of radiation and chemotherapy in combination. The Pignon meta-analysis showed a clear-cut survival advantage for radiation in combination with chemotherapy versus chemotherapy alone. A Japanese trial demonstrated a twofold improvement in survival (30% versus 15%) for patients receiving concurrent chemoradiation upfront compared to sequential chemotherapy followed by radiation. An NCI-C study similarly showed a benefit for early concurrent versus delayed concurrent chemoradiation using alternating regimen of CAV and etoposide and cisplatin (EP), with similar, statistically significant, twofold improvement in long term survival: 20% versus 10%. Finally, a domestic trial jointly managed by the ECOG and RTOG demonstrated therapeutic superiority for hyperfractionated radiation (45 Gy), in combination with etoposide and cisplatin versus more conventional once-daily RT, with a 10% absolute improvement in long-term survival: 26% versus 16%. The bulk of data at this point underscore the importance of concurrent upfront chemoradiation in eligible individuals, although those with bulky disease may be better served by chemotherapy for two to three cycles followed by concurrent chemoradiation.

To date, single, daily fractionation to higher doses (e.g., 60 Gy) has not been compared to standard twice-daily RT (45 Gy). Continuation of chemotherapy beyond 4 to 6 cycles has not enhanced survival benefit. However, prophylactic cranial irradiation (PCI) in another critical meta-analysis has in aggregate demonstrated an improvement in long-term survival rates that roughly equals the improvement seen with radiation added to chemotherapy, by decreasing the frequency and delaying the onset of CNS relapse. Concurrent radiation and EP leads to a 60% to 90% complete remission rate. Median survival for patients with limited SCLC historically has been 16 to 20 months, but has now improved to 22 to 24 months, with 2-year survival rates of 40% to 50%, and 5-year survival rates of 15% to 25%. But the improvement in survival comes with some cost, including enhanced myelosuppression, esophagitis, and pulmonary toxicity. Ongoing studies are evaluating the role of concomitant boost RT toward the end of the chemoradiation course, as well as the integration of irinotecan with cisplatin and RT in the limited SCLC setting.

Late relapse beyond 3 years is highly unusual. Those with limited SCLC who do relapse generally do so within the first 24 to 36 months. Survival after relapse is poor, generally no more than 4 to 6 months.

Fewer than 3% of patients with SCLC are candidates for surgery. To date, no randomized study has demonstrated a therapeutic benefit for surgery in addition to standard chemoradiation. However, surgery may benefit the rare patient who presents with a solitary pulmonary nodule, or those who have undergone definitive treatment, and who develop a limited pulmonary relapse.

Conclusions

We have made significant headway during the past 15 to 20 years in the therapy of lung cancer. In SCLC, concurrent chemoradiation has improved outcome in patients with limited SCLC, and irinotecan may portend therapeutic advantage in extensive disease.

In the adjuvant setting in NSCLC, platinum-based chemotherapy has increased survival rates by 5% to 15%. In locally advanced disease in patients who are reasonably fit, concurrent chemoradiation can yield long-term survival rates of 15% to 20%. Finally, in advanced disease, third-generation platinum-based chemotherapy combinations reliably produce median survival rates of 8 to 10 months, 1-year survival rates of 30% to 35%, and

Rakel and Bope: *Conn's Current Therapy 2006*.

2-year survival rates of 10% to 15%. For the first time, there is evidence of benefit for second- and, even, third-line therapy that was virtually unthinkable before 1990. And in the last year, we have witnessed the emergence of evidence-based data supporting the use of EGFr TKIs in the salvage setting compared to BSC.

It is imperative that eligible patients be placed on therapeutic trials. Unfortunately, fewer than 2% of Americans enroll in clinical trials. Without clinical trials, there will be absolutely no headway in improving survival. Progress in the treatment of lung cancer cannot occur without clinical research.

Coccidioidomycosis

Method of
Robert Libke, MD

4

Coccidioidomycosis is an illness caused by the fungus *Coccidioides immitis*. This fungus grows in soil in conditions found in the arid and semiarid regions of the southwestern United States and in a few places in Central and South America. Under proper conditions the fungus produces an abundance of arthroconidia, which are very light and easily carried in the air. Infection occurs when arthroconidia are inhaled and converted in the host to spherules, which reproduce by endosporulation. The primary infection is, therefore, almost always in the lung. In the great majority of cases the infection is quickly contained by host defenses and remains confined to a limited area of the lung. In a few cases, the organism is more aggressive and rapidly produces a diffuse pneumonia with an adult respiratory distress syndrome (ARDS)-like picture that may be fatal. In other cases the pulmonary legions heal but the organism is spread to other organs in the body through the blood or lymphatic channels. When this happens, the disease is considered to be disseminated and takes on a different character.

The pathology of infection with *C. immitis* is dimorphic. The initial reaction of the body to the arthroconidia and to the endospores is an acute inflammatory reaction similar to that seen in acute bacterial infections. Reaction to the mature coccidioidal spherules is a granulomatous one similar to that seen in tuberculosis. Clinically, coccidioidomycosis reflects both of those processes; it can have features of both acute and chronic infection.

Clinical Manifestations

The primary infection in the lung is asymptomatic in the majority of instances. When symptomatic, it resembles many other acute lower respiratory tract infections. In some cases, however, clues are present that raise the suspicion of coccidioidomycosis. These include a radiologic finding of hilar adenopathy on the side of the airspace consolidation, significant eosinophilia in the differential leukocyte count, certain dermatoses (erythema nodosum, erythema multiform, or a morbilliform maculopapular eruption), and a failure to show a clinical response to conventional antibiotic therapy. Recovery from the primary pulmonary infection may be complete or may leave chronic residuals of either a cavity or a granuloma. Some cavities heal spontaneously within 2 years of the primary infection. Others are complicated by secondary infection, recurrent hemoptysis, or, rarely, rupture into the pleural space. Occasionally these complications are severe enough to warrant lobectomy, but this is the exception rather than the rule (except in cavity rupture). Unlike tuberculosis, the chronic cavitary residuals of primary pulmonary coccidioidomycosis rarely progress. When they do, the progressive fibrocavitary disease may be indistinguishable from tuberculosis in radiographs.

The residual granuloma is significant because of the difficulty of distinguishing it from a carcinoma of the lung when it is first discovered on a routine chest radiograph. If the patient is younger than 40 years of age or the lesion is calcified (coccidioidal granuloma calcify in less than 20% of cases), the lesion can be considered benign and possibly followed with serial chest radiographs. Occasionally organisms recovered from the lesion by computed tomography (CT)-guided fine-needle aspiration allow the pathologist to make the diagnosis without tissue biopsy. Otherwise, enough tissue must be obtained by transbronchial, thoracoscopic, or open biopsy to allow the pathologist to make a diagnosis.

Dissemination is considered to occur when clinically apparent lesions are found outside the thoracic cavity. The most common sites of dissemination are the skin, lymph nodes, skeleton, synovia, and central nervous system (CNS). Almost any organ, however, can be involved. Dissemination may be focal, multifocal, or diffuse. The two most serious forms are diffuse dissemination and focal dissemination to the CNS. Before the advent of effective therapy, those two forms were almost always fatal. Even now, with effective antifungal agents, these two conditions carry a significant mortality. Dissemination usually occurs with the primary infection and only rarely as a late complication of a chronic pulmonary lesion. Cumulative clinical experience since the first description of coccidioidomycosis now allows the clinician to predict with some accuracy the likelihood of dissemination. Coccidioidomycosis is unique among infectious illnesses in that humans have a genetically determined resistance to dissemination of the organism. This resistance is found most commonly in whites and least frequently in Filipinos. In between, in descending order of frequency of inherited resistance, are Asians, Native Americans, Hispanics, and African Americans. Infection in infancy and infection in the second or third trimester of pregnancy carry a high risk of dissemination, as does infection in persons with immunocompromised status. Clinical clues to the development of dissemination are (one or more of) a rapid rise in complement-fixing antibodies to a titer of 1:32 or greater, a prolonged febrile primary illness (greater than 4 weeks), and the development of mediastinal adenopathy on the chest radiograph. The risk of dissemination is so high in the latter two circumstances that treatment is advisable before clinically overt evidence of dissemination occurs. The same can be said for infection in infants and in immunocompromised patients. Otherwise, the risk of dissemination is a matter of clinical judgment in weighing the number of unfavorable factors such as race, pregnancy, co-morbid illnesses, and complement-fixation titers.

Diagnosis

The diagnosis of coccidioidomycosis is established by finding the distinctive organism microscopically, by culture of tissue or body fluids, or by serology. Skin test results were used in the past but reagents are no longer available. Serologic reactions are the tests most frequently used for the diagnosis of coccidioidal infection. The best are both specific and sensitive. Some of the serologic tests are designed to detect IgM antibodies (the earliest and most evanescent); others detect IgG antibodies (which persist much longer and are quantitatively related to the severity of the infection), and others detect both. The most reliable techniques for detecting IgM antibodies are the tube precipitin test, the immunodiffusion technique, and an enzyme immunoassay. The most reliable tests for IgG antibodies are the complement fixation test and an immunodiffusion test. The magnitude of the complement fixation titer or IgG quantitative immunodiffusion has the great advantage of being related to the severity of infection and, therefore, is useful in following the progression or resolution of the disease. In patients with extra pulmonary spread, biopsy of lesions or aspiration of fluid from abscesses or joints not only establishes the diagnosis of coccidioidomycosis but also confirms the presence of dissemination in some cases. Cerebrospinal fluid (CSF) examinations are needed to evaluate for coccidioidal meningitis. Differential and total cell counts and glucose and protein measurements, along with CSF complement fixation titers, should be done. Fungal cultures of CSF are rarely positive in patients with proven meningitis and should not be relied upon for diagnosis.

Treatment

PRIMARY PULMONARY DISEASE

Treatment is not usually necessary for patients with uncomplicated primary infection. However, patients who:

- Have prolonged signs and symptoms
- Have diabetes
- Are in the third trimester of pregnancy
- Are of Filipino ancestry
- Are immunocompromised

should receive treatment for primary coccidioidomycosis with an azole. If the infection appears to be unusually severe and is progressing to an ARDS-like picture, however, it is prudent to undertake immediate diagnostic tests and initiate treatment with intravenous amphotericin B (Fungizone) or, if pre-existing renal disease is present, a lipid complex form of amphotericin (Abelcet). After control of toxicity and disease progression is arrested, change to an oral form of therapy if possible (Table 1).

DISSEMINATED DISEASE

Disseminated disease is always an indication for treatment. There are several classes of antifungal agents available, including amphotericin B, lipid complex forms of amphotericin, azoles, and echinocandins. The azoles have the advantage of being sufficiently absorbed from the gastrointestinal tract to achieve serum concentrations that are effective. Fluconazole (Diflucan)[1] is not dependent on gastric acidity for absorption and has the additional theoretic advantage of readily passing the blood-brain barrier to achieve good concentration in the CSF. Itraconazole (Sporanox)[1] and fluconazole appear to be equally effective for nonmeningeal disseminated disease.

Treatment with fluconazole (Diflucan) should start with 400 mg per day and be gradually increased to a tolerable dose up to a maximum of 800 mg per day.[3] Patients with meningitis may be treated with doses up to 2000 mg per day.[3] Itraconazole (Sporanox) is usually given at 400 mg per day but may be increased to 800 mg per day.[3] Because the half-lives of both of those drugs are very long, they can be administered in one dose or divided into a twice daily dosage schedule. The length of treatment is entirely dependent on the clinical course and probably should be continued for several months following complete clinical resolution. Relapse following cessation of therapy is common, and some patients may require lifelong treatment. When given for threatened rather than clinically evident dissemination, the course of treatment often can be shortened. Fluconazole[1] is preferred in the treatment of coccidioidal meningitis in

---

[1]Not FDA approved for this indication.
[3]Exceeds dosage recommended by the manufacturer.

TABLE 1 Antifungal Agents

Drug	Dose (mg/d)	Route
Ketoconazole (Nizoral)	200-400	PO
Fluconazole (Diflucan)[1]	200-2000[2]	PO/IV
Itraconazole (Sporanox)[1]	200-800[2]	PO/IV
Amphotericin B (Fungizone)	0.3-1.5 mg/kg	IV
Lipid complex Amphotericins (AmBisome, Abelcet, Amphotec)	3-6 mg/kg	IV

[1]Not FDA approved for this indication.
[2]Exceeds dosage recommended by the manufacturer.
Abbreviations: IV = intravenously; PO = orally.

doses of 600 to 2000 mg per day.[3] Control of disease with improvement in CSF parameters has occurred in the majority of patients, but relapse has been frequent when therapy has been stopped. When treating patients who have coccidioidal meningitis with fluconazole, it is prudent to continue the treatment indefinitely, possibly lifelong.

When dissemination is diffuse and rapid or an ARDS-like pulmonary picture develops, mortality is high regardless of the type of therapy used. Initial control of severe dissemination with intravenous amphotericin B is recommended because it may have more rapid onset of action than agents. Amphotericin B is given intravenously in a concentration of 0.1 mg/mL during a period of 1 to 2 hours daily. It is customary to start with a small dose of 10 mg and increase it by 20 mg increments up to a daily dose of 50 mg. The dosage can be escalated more rapidly when the patient is desperately ill or when the clinical course is deteriorating rapidly. Toxic side effects are almost universal and should be anticipated by giving premeditation of acetaminophen, 650 mg, and diphenhydramine (Benadryl), 50 mg, to lessen the rigors that frequently accompany the intravenous infusion. When this combination fails to control rigors, 25 mg of meperidine (Demerol)[1] given as a slow intravenous bolus is often successful. Nausea and vomiting frequently can be ameliorated with antiemetics such as prochlorperazine (Compazine) or trimethobenzamide (Tigan). Renal tubular acidosis with hypokalemia, hypomagnesemia, mild metabolic acidosis, and azotemia are also predictable results of continued amphotericin treatment. The metabolic acidosis is rarely significant enough to require attention, but the serum potassium, magnesium, and creatinine levels must be monitored frequently until the response to treatment appears to be stable. Potassium can be replaced orally but sometimes requires very large doses. Magnesium replacement may also be required and usually can be done orally. Daily amphotericin should be discontinued when the serum creatinine exceeds 3.0 and can be restarted and given less frequently when the creatinine drops below 2.5. After an accumulated dose of 0.5 gram of amphotericin has been given and disease control is apparent, administration often can be reduced to three times a week instead of daily. This makes outpatient administration quite practical for most patients. The clinical course and response to treatment should determine the total dosage of amphotericin. For disseminated disease, anywhere from 1 to 4 or more grams may be required.

Newer lipid complex forms of amphotericin (Abelcet, Amphotec, and AmBisome) have reduced side effects compared with the older colloidal dispersion form of amphotericin B (Fungizone). These forms of amphotericin may be considered if patients have severe immediate reactions such as hypotension, bronchospasm, and persistent uncontrollable rigors to the standard form of amphotericin. In addition, patients with pre-existing renal dysfunction may be candidates for treatment with these newer agents since they are less nephrotoxic.

---

[3]Exceeds dosage recommended by the manufacturer.
[1]Not FDA approved for this indication.

Doses of 3 to 6 mg/kg of the liposomal formulations are given IV for 1 to 2 hours daily. The possibility of reduced side effects must be balanced with the dramatic increase in cost of the lipid forms.

When patients fail to respond to azole therapy for meningitis, intrathecal (cisternal or intraventricular)* amphotericin B[1] may be necessary. Cisternal injection is the preferred route of administration whenever possible. The starting dose is 0.05 mg, and this is increased daily by 0.1 mg to a maximum of 0.5 mg per day for an indefinite period of time as determined by the lumbar fluid parameters as well as the clinical response. It is desirable to continue intrathecal therapy until the lumbar fluid returns to normal and then for an additional 3 to 6 months. After achieving a stable dose, the frequency of administration can be reduced to three times a week and after lumbar fluid parameters have returned to normal, to once or twice a week.

The newer azoles (voriconazole [Vfend][1] and posaconazole[†]) and the echinocandins (caspofungin [Cancidas][1]) have promising in vitro and animal data regarding *C. immitis*, but experience in treatment of human infections is limited.

---

*Not FDA approved for this route of administration.
[1]Not FDA approved for this indication.
[†]Investigational drug in the United States.

Histoplasmosis

Method of
Jose Martagon-Villamil, MD and
Sherif B. Mossad, MD

Samuel Taylor Darling, a young American pathologist working at the Panama Canal Zone in 1906, is credited with the first description of histoplasmosis, in a young black man emigrating from Martinique. It remains a fascinating disease and a paradigm of the complex interactions between the host immune system and the organism inherent abilities.

Key Clinical Points

Figure 1 summarizes the spectrum of clinical manifestations produced by *Histoplasma capsulatum*. Although a detailed review of the finer clinical points regarding histoplasmosis is beyond the scope of this article, the following provides basic information:

• From epidemiologic observations in endemic areas, anywhere between 50% and 90% of infections with *H. capsulatum* are asymptomatic or clinically so mild that they go undiagnosed.

• The degree of symptoms of acute pulmonary histoplasmosis will depend on the inoculum size. After a heavy respiratory inoculum, diffuse, patchy infiltrates with mediastinal adenopathy can occur. A lighter exposure may produce a more subacute flulike illness with or without a localized infiltrate.

• Some patients with acute disease may have secondary, immune-mediated manifestations: A polyarticular, symmetric arthritis is evident in up to 5% to 10% of patients, and a subset of these may also have erythema nodosum. Acute pericarditis occurs in an additional 10% of acute cases.

• Another clinically distinct subset of patients may experience what could be termed *sequelae* of prominent acute histoplasmosis: large mediastinal granulomatous adenopathy causing obstruction or compression of vessels or esophagus, evolving over months to years; erosion of calcified lymph nodes into bronchi (broncholithiasis).

• A rare complication (affecting less than 1% of symptomatic patients), termed *fibrosing mediastinitis*, represents an aberrant, excessive fibrosing response to the presence of *Histoplasma* antigens in mediastinal lymph nodes.

• Chronic pulmonary histoplasmosis tends to occur only in patients with a preexisting chronic lung disease. It resembles reactivation tuberculin tuberculosis (TB) both clinically and radiologically.

• Disseminated histoplasmosis, which can involve essentially any organ system in the body and have a

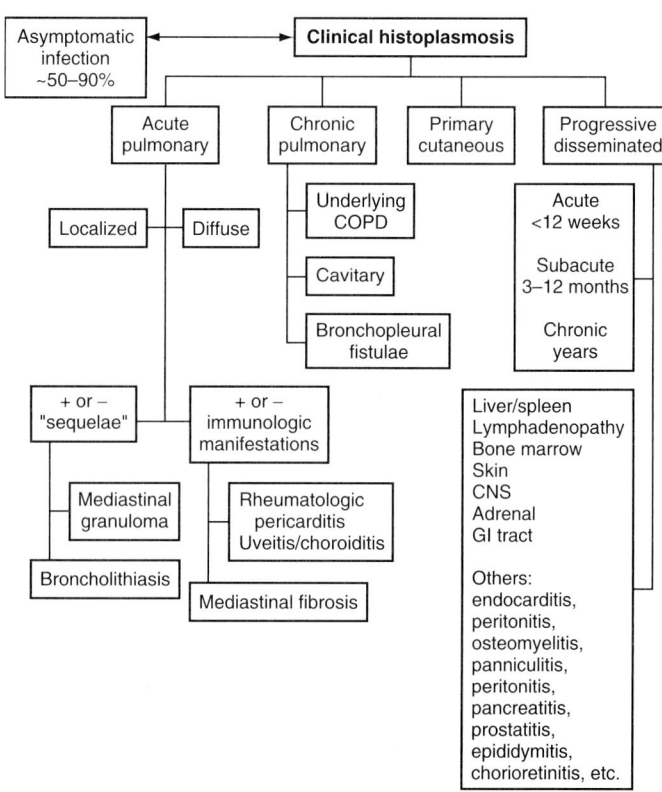

FIGURE 1. The clinical spectrum of histoplasmosis. COPD = chronic obstructive pulmonary disease.

Rakel and Bope: *Conn's Current Therapy 2006.*

substantial mortality, represents the most severe end of the disease spectrum, and usually affects people with underlying immune suppression or in the extremes of age.

Treatment

A substantial majority of patients with *H. capsulatum* infection will recover without treatment. Therefore, it remains essential to appropriately define which patients benefit from therapy.

Let's first consider the antifungal options available.

AMPHOTERICIN B AND LIPID PREPARATIONS

Amphotericin B (Fungizone) remains the agent of first choice for severe forms of the disease. It is fungicidal against *H. capsulatum* and has MIC90s (minimum inhibitory concentrations against 90% of isolates; the lower the number, the more active the agent) in the range of 0.5 to 1.0 µg/mL. Needless to say, the use of amphotericin B (Fungizone) implies intravenous (IV) administration with all its potential complications and side effects, including infusion-related toxicity, nephrotoxicity, and potassium wasting. Amphotericin B (Fungizone) should be used at a dose of 0.7 mg/kg per day and the lipid preparations (liposomal amphotericin B, [AmBisome]) at 3 mg/kg per day.

AZOLES

Itraconazole (Sporanox) is the agent in this family with the most clinical experience against *H. capsulatum*. It demonstrates in vitro MIC90s of around 0.02 to 0.06 µg/mL and remains the most active azole against this fungus. It can be used orally or intravenously, but the oral formulations have some important points to consider: The capsule needs to be given with food or acid beverage and the suspension on an empty stomach. The recommended dose is 200 mg once or twice daily, depending on levels (described later in this article). Itraconazole (Sporanox) is a potent cytochrome P-450 inhibitor and therefore has multiple drug interactions. These, and the potentially unpredictable absorption, make it advisable to check serum concentration at some early point during therapy, such as during the second week, when a steady state is reached. The guidelines from the Infectious Disease Society of America (IDSA) suggest that a level obtained 2 to 4 hours after administration that is equal to or above 1 µg/mL should be therapeutic. Alternatively, levels can be measured as a trough, just before the next dose. In this case, levels of 0.5 µg/mL are probably therapeutic. If levels are ≥ 3 µg/mL, twice per day dosing can be reduced to once per day.

Voriconazole (Vfend)[1] is active against *H. capsulatum*, with MIC90 of 0.25 µg/mL and may emerge as a good alternative therapy. Fluconazole (Diflucan)[1] is only recommended when itraconazole (Sporanox) cannot be

taken or tolerated because there are reports of resistance developing during therapy, with MICs going from 0.625 to 20 µg/mL. Posaconazole[*] and ravuconazole[*] both have been shown to have low MICs and clinical efficacy in murine models for the treatment of histoplasmosis, but clinical experience in humans is lacking.

ECHINOCANDINS

In vitro, *H. capsulatum* exhibits higher MICs with caspofungin (Cancidas)[1] than with other antifungal agents. Experience with murine models shows decreased survival in comparison to amphotericin B.

CHITIN SYNTHASE INHIBITORS

These are agents in the antifungal pipeline, not yet in clinical use. Nikkomycin Z[*] has shown some promising data in murine models. The use of high doses results in reduction of organism burden and better survival, but lower doses are inferior to other agents. One study showed synergism with fluconazole (Diflucan).[1] There is no clinical experience in humans.

COMBINATION ANTIFUNGAL THERAPY

At this point data to support combination therapy for histoplasmosis come only from animal models, in vitro data, and very little clinical experience and cannot be considered standard by any means. In a murine model, fluconazole (Diflucan)[1] and amphotericin B (Fungizone) actually appeared antagonistic.

Specific Treatment Recommendations

ACUTE PULMONARY HISTOPLASMOSIS

Patients with localized disease usually improve without therapy. Treatment is recommended when there is lack of improvement after 4 weeks, when there is radiographically diffuse disease, or when fever persists for more than 3 weeks. For patients ill enough to require hospitalization or who are hypoxemic, amphotericin B (AmBisome) is preferred. Patients with diffuse disease probably benefit from adjunctive corticosteroid therapy (equivalent to 60 mg of prednisone for 7 to 14 days). On the other hand, in patients that are mildly to moderately ill but have an indication for therapy, itraconazole (Sporanox) can be used from the beginning. The target course is 6 to 12 weeks of therapy. When amphotericin B (AmBisome) is used, it can be switched to oral itraconazole (Sporanox) once the patient is clinically stable.

RHEUMATOLOGIC SYNDROMES

Antifungal therapy is not indicated for rheumatologic syndromes. Symptoms resolve with nonsteroidal

---

[1]Not FDA approved for this indication.

[*]Investigational drug in the United States.
[1]Not FDA approved for this indication.

anti-inflammatory drugs (NSAIDs), usually over a few weeks. Occasionally, when there is a recurrence, anti-inflammatory therapy may be required for 3 to 6 months.

PERICARDITIS

Mild to moderate cases of pericarditis usually respond to NSAIDs alone, for 2 to 12 weeks. The presence of hemodynamic abnormalities probably warrants the use of corticosteroids. In this case, the use of concurrent oral itraconazole (Sporanox) is suggested, to prevent disseminated disease. For cases refractory to corticosteroids or in tamponade picture, surgical or percutaneous drainage is recommended.

FIBROSING MEDIASTINITIS

There is considerable controversy in the literature about the benefit of antifungal therapy for fibrosing mediastinitis—a rare, late, immune-mediated complication—and it is very difficult to make general recommendations. On a case-by-case basis, treatment probably should be considered for patients with evidence of active progression, elevated serology titers, or erythrocyte sedimentation rate (ESR). Similarly, the length of therapy is controversial. A 12-week course of itraconazole (Sporanox) is suggested, possibly extending further if there is evidence of response. There is no evidence for any benefit from corticosteroid therapy. Advanced cases may need surgical or endovascular palliative measures, but only physicians experienced in this disease should attempt such measures.

MEDIASTINAL GRANULOMA

Treating mediastinal granuloma seems to be beneficial in reducing inflammation and its resultant obstructive symptoms. The choice of agent depends on the severity of illness. Patients with severe obstructive manifestations probably need initially IV amphotericin B (AmBisome), which may later be switched to oral itraconazole (Sporanox). Patients with milder illness may respond well to oral itraconazole (Sporanox) from the start. There are data supporting the use of corticosteroids for severe airway obstruction, for the initial 1 to 2 weeks of therapy.

CHRONIC PULMONARY HISTOPLASMOSIS

Treatment is always recommended for chronic pulmonary histoplasmosis, to prevent progression, loss of function, and, ultimately, death. Itraconazole (Sporanox), for a target period of 12 to 24 months, would be the primary choice. However, in patients who are severely ill, needing ventilatory support, or unable to take by mouth, an initial induction course with amphotericin B (AmBisome) would be appropriate.

DISSEMINATED HISTOPLASMOSIS

In a multicenter study of 81 patients with AIDS and disseminated histoplasmosis, liposomal amphotericin B

(AmBisome) had better survival and tolerability than conventional amphotericin B (Fungizone). Although there is no similar comparative study in HIV-negative patients, in cases with moderate to severe disseminated disease, regardless of the HIV status, liposomal amphotericin B (AmBisome) probably is preferred. Once an initial induction course of 2 to 4 weeks has resulted in clinical improvement, it is reasonable to switch to oral itraconazole (Sporanox) to complete a course of 12 to 18 months, or until the *Histoplasma* antigen assay reverts to negative or to less than 2 units. IDSA guidelines suggest that if amphotericin B (AmBisome) is to be used for the entire course, the target is a total dose of 35 mg/kg over 2 to 4 months.

In a patient whose clinical presentation is stable enough to consider oral therapy from the start, IV induction is not mandatory.

It is unclear whether a patient recovering from disseminated histoplasmosis needs maintenance or lifelong therapy. Some data in HIV-positive patients with clinical and immunologic response to highly active antiretroviral therapy (HAART), suggest that a CD4+ cell count equal to 150 cells/mL makes it safe to discontinue prophylactic therapy. Conversely, a decrease to less than 100 CD4+ probably requires reinstitution of maintenance itraconazole.

CENTRAL NERVOUS SYSTEM HISTOPLASMOSIS

Within the spectrum of disseminated disease, central nervous system (CNS) involvement deserves special mention because of its high mortality, relapse rate, and poor penetration of antifungal drugs to CSF. Liposomal amphotericin B (AmBisome) seems to achieve higher neural tissue concentrations than regular amphotericin B (Fungizone) and therefore, an initial course of liposomal amphotericin B (AmBisome) at a dose of 3 to 5 mg/kg per day, for 12 to 16 weeks is recommended. This should be followed by maintenance therapy for at least a year, and differently from other forms of the disease, high-dose fluconazole (Diflucan)[1] (800 mg/day)[3] probably is preferred to itraconazole (Sporanox), because although intrinsically less active against *H. capsulatum*, it penetrates to cerebrospinal fluid (CSF) much better. Patients with relapse or failure to therapy may become candidates to salvage with voriconazole (Vfend),[1] which penetrates CSF well. The use of intrathecal amphotericin B is discouraged, because it has marginal benefit, if any, and may be associated with complications.

INCIDENTAL SURGICAL FINDING OF *HISTOPLASMA*

Occasionally, a resected lung nodule is found to be an old *Histoplasma* granuloma. There are no prospective data in the follow-up of these patients, but no treatment is recommended because it probably represents remote, burnt-out infection.

---

[3]Exceeds dosage recommended by the manufacturer.
[1]Not FDA approved for this indication.

CURRENT DIAGNOSIS

Diagnosing histoplasmosis requires a honed clinical suspicion and the selection of the appropriate test(s) for a particular clinical scenario. Recommended tests are:

- *Histoplasma* Antigen: The sensitivity of the assay is superior in urine than in blood or BAL fluid. Sensitivity also is dependent on the clinical presentation, because it correlates with fungal burden: as high as 95% for disseminated disease in HIV/AIDS, around 80% for acute pulmonary disease or disseminated disease in HIV-negative patients, but as low as 14% in chronic pulmonary disease. There is a degree of cross-reactivity with *Blastomyces, Paracoccidioides,* and *Penicillium.*
- Serology: Antibodies against *Histoplasma* can be measured by CF or ID assays. CF is more sensitive than ID but less specific. There are several caveats to serologic testing: Mounting an appropriate antibody response requires 2 to 6 weeks; patients with immune suppression may not respond reliably; there may be a background rate of positivity in endemic areas; there is some cross-reactivity with other fungi as well. Serology is most sensitive for chronic pulmonary disease (>95%), disseminated disease (around 70%), and fibrosing mediastinitis (67%).
- Culture of the organism from a tissue or body fluid may take up to 4 to 6 weeks to grow, with a median of 20 days. Sensitivity, again, will depend on the clinical presentation: less than 10% in the immunologically mediated manifestations, around 15% in acute, self-limited illness, around 85% in disseminated disease. If a blood culture is requested, it needs to be done by lysis-centrifugation technique.
- Histopathologic examination of tissue, with fungal stains, while occasionally the defining diagnostic test, requires an experienced pathologist because other fungi and parasites may be misidentified as *Histoplasma* and granulomas can be caused by many different etiologies.
- Most molecular methods, including traditional and real-time PCR assays, are considered investigational at this time and require validation in clinical series. A DNA probe is commercially available and has been used for diagnosis directly in tissue (e.g., a heart valve).

Abbreviation: BAL = bronchoalveolar lavage; CF = complement fixation; ID = immunodiffusion; PCR = polymerase chain reaction.

MONITORING THE RESPONSE TO THERAPY

Ideally, clinicians treating histoplasmosis would like to have a test that accurately and promptly follows disease activity. The urine antigen assay may be helpful for this purpose because it should decrease progressively with therapy, but it lags behind clinical response, and may remain positive for weeks to months. A decline in titers,

CURRENT THERAPY

In the big picture, a majority of patients with *Histoplasma capsulatum* infection recover without the need for treatment. If treatment is required:

- Choose the route of therapy depending on the severity of illness.
- Use Amphotericin B (Fungizone) at 0.7 mg/kg per day or lipid formulations (liposomal AmphoB, [Ambisome]) at 3 mg/kg per day.
- Use itraconazole (Sporanox) at 200 mg once or twice daily, depending on serum therapeutic levels. Be aware of drug interactions, side effects and administration requirements.

followed by a new elevation, does suggest the possibility of relapse.

Angiotensin-converting enzyme (ACE) levels, which may be elevated in histoplasmosis, do correlate with response to therapy.

REFERENCES

Goldman M, Zackin R, Fichtenbaum CJ, et al: Safety of discontinuation of maintenance therapy for disseminated histoplasmosis after immunologic response to antiretroviral therapy. Clin Infect Dis 2004;38:1485-1489.
Johnson PC, Wheat J, Cloud GA, et al: Safety and efficacy of liposomal amphotericin B compared with conventional amphotericin B for induction therapy of histoplasmosis in patients with AIDS. Ann Intern Med 2002;137:105-109.
Wheat J, Garringer T, Brizendine E, Connolly P: Diagnosis of histoplasmosis by antigen detection based upon experience at the histoplasmosis reference laboratory. Diagn Microbiol Infect Dis 2002;43:29-37.
Wheat J, Sarosi G, McKinsey D, et al: Practice guidelines for the management of patients with histoplasmosis. Clin Infect Dis 2000;30:688-695.
Wheat LJ, Batteiger BE, Sathapatayavongs B: *Histoplasma capsulatum* infections of the central nervous system: A clinical review. Medicine (Baltimore) 1990;69:244-260.
Wheat LJ, Connolly-Stringfield PA, Baker RL, et al: Disseminated histoplasmosis in the acquired immune deficiency syndrome: clinical findings, diagnosis and treatment. Medicine (Baltimore) 1990;69:361-374.
Wheat LJ, Kauffman CA: Histoplasmosis. Infect Dis Clin N Am 2003;17:1-19.

Blastomycosis

Method of
Candace L. Mitchell, MD

Originally called Gilchrist's disease, blastomycosis is an environmentally acquired infection caused by the fungus *Blastomyces dermatitidis.* The fungus is dimorphic and naturally occurs as a mold, but it converts to a yeast at body temperature. Although the disease is somewhat uncommon, infections can vary in severity from acute, self-limited illness to severe disseminated infection.

Epidemiology

Our knowledge of the epidemiology of blastomycosis is based primarily on analysis of cases of human and canine disease and limited environmental investigations. *B. dermatitidis* is responsible for point-source outbreaks as well as sporadic infection in endemic areas. Individuals entering woodsy areas with a plethora of warm, moist, decaying vegetation are at highest risk. In most areas, males are infected twice as often as females, perhaps because males are more likely to encounter the appropriate habitat through hunting, fishing, or logging. North American endemic areas include states bordering the Mississippi and Ohio River basins and areas bordering the Great Lakes; the bulk of cases originate from Mississippi, Arkansas, Kentucky, Tennessee, and Wisconsin. Sporadic case reports, however, continue to challenge the defined areas of endemicity with observations of disease in drier climates such as Nebraska and South Dakota.

Pathogenesis and Immunity

The mold consists of mycelia with branching hyphae and terminal fruiting structures called *conidia*. The conidia, which are easily inhaled when mycelia are disturbed during environmental foraging, undergo mycelial-to-yeast phase conversion within the airways and cause a primary pulmonary infection. Neutrophils, monocytes, and alveolar macrophages are the first line of defense against inhaled conidia. Antibodies against fungal antigens are synthesized but are not protective and do not accelerate recovery. Protective acquired immunity is exclusively cell mediated, and infections are more severe in patients who have undergone transplants, are prescribed chronic steroids, or suffer from AIDS or sarcoidosis.

Clinical Manifestations

After sufficient inhalation of conidia, pulmonary infection ensues. Acute self-limited pulmonary infection does occur but is uncommonly encountered and difficult to diagnose. The yeast may then spread hematogeneously from the lung to the skin, bone, male genitourinary (GU) tract, and, rarely, other sites including the central nervous system (CNS). Discovery of blastomycosis at any site should prompt a thorough evaluation to identify other infected systems. Treatment ultimately depends on clinical status and whether CNS disease is present. Table 1 lists the radiographic presentations associated with pulmonary blastomycosis.

The skin is the most common site of dissemination, and three forms of infection have been described: verrucous, subcutaneous, and ulcerative. Verrucous lesions begin as raised papules that develop an irregular border

TABLE 1 Chest Radiograph Observations

Pattern	Comment
Alveolar infiltrate	48% of cases
Mass-like infiltrate	32% of cases
Miliary, reticulonodular, or cavitary disease	Rarely observed
Pleural effusion	Rarely observed
ARDS	Usually secondary to inhalation of high inoculum or bronchogenic or miliary spread;high mortality

Abbreviations: ARDS = Acute respiratory distress syndrome.

with subsequent crusting and drainage confusing their diagnosis with skin carcinomas or pyoderma gangrenosum. Ulcerative lesions have sharp, heaped-up borders and a central exudate. Often verrucous and ulcerative lesions will connect with a subcutaneous cold abscess through a sinus tract; however, subcutaneous nodular infection without overlying skin changes can occur and resemble panniculitis. Histology is consistent among the forms: papillomatosis with intraepidermal pyogranulomatous abscess formation and a dermal inflammatory infiltrate. Although appropriately stained biopsy specimens frequently demonstrate the yeast cells, extensive necrosis or granulomatous changes can make visualization of organisms challenging.

Osseous involvement is observed next in frequency with vertebral bodies, and long bones are the most common sites of dissemination. Overlying skin changes or a septic arthritis bring involved sites to the practitioner attention, whereas radiographic appearance suggests nonspecific osteomyelitis. Histology of affected bone may reveal suppurative granulomas or only necrosis, making culture a necessity for diagnosis. In most cases, chest radiographs will reveal pulmonary involvement even if the patient has no respiratory symptoms. However, case reports describe patients without endemic exposures or pulmonary involvement who presented with culture-positive skin and bone infection after soil-contaminated injuries raising the question of direct inoculation as a means of infection. Hematogeneous dissemination from a primary focus is observed most commonly, but local inoculation of fungus should be considered in soil-contaminated traumatic injuries. Débridement of any sequestrum is standard in addition to medical therapy, but controlled trials have not been performed to determine the necessity.

GU infection is observed in 10% to 30% of men with disseminated blastomycosis and manifests as prostatitis, epididymitis, or orchitis, while asymptomatic disease also occurs. A digital exam may reveal a nodular prostate, and direct examination of prostatic secretions may demonstrate yeast forms. Postprostatic massage urine cultures are sometimes positive even in asymptomatic patients. Positive results from the GU tract may exclude a need for other diagnostic procedures and should be pursued in male patients in whom disseminated blastomycosis is suspected. Medical therapy alone should be sufficient to treat GU blastomycosis unless an abscess requiring drainage is present.

The CNS is involved in 5% to 10% of disseminated blastomycosis. Epidural or intracranial abscess is more common than is meningitis. Abscesses present as focal neurologic deficits with obvious lesions on contrasted neuroimaging studies. Direct microscopy of purulence often reveals yeast cells, and growth of the mold in culture is rapid, on average within 2 weeks from inoculation. Meningitis is typically a result of fulminate dissemination, and patients are very ill with widespread disease at presentation. Cerebrospinal fluid is rarely diagnostic, and investigations conclude that direct ventricular fluid specimens are of higher yield and are suggested if a diagnosis cannot be made from other clinical specimens.

Blastomycosis rarely involves other organs, but it can present with associated hormonal perturbations (Table 2). Dissemination to the larynx, although infrequent, histologically mimics skin disease, and it is sometimes misdiagnosed as squamous cell cancer because of its gross appearance.

Immune-suppressed, pregnant, and pediatric patient populations are at risk for aggressive blastomycosis with a higher mortality or rate of relapse. However, the incidence of infection in these groups is intriguingly less than that observed with *Candida* and other endemic fungi. Immunosuppressed patients often are strikingly ill at presentation and have a high rate of acute respiratory distress syndrome (ARDS) with primary pulmonary disease. Moreover, up to 40% of AIDS patients (CD4 count < 200 cells/mm^3) with blastomycosis demonstrate CNS involvement.

Key Treatment Points

The Infectious Diseases Society of America (IDSA) practice guidelines exist for initiating medical treatment. All cases of identified blastomycosis should receive therapy except for resolving cases of acute, apparently self-limited

pulmonary infection. Withholding treatment is controversial, and if these cases are not treated, patients should receive intensive follow-up for a minimum of 3 years to observe for dissemination. Pharmacologic treatment options include amphotericin B (AmB) deoxycholate (Fungizone), various lipid preparations of AmB, ketoconazole (Nizoral), itraconazole (Sporanox), and fluconazole (Diflucan)[1]. Itraconazole (Sporanox) has proved to be the drug of choice for non-CNS, non-life-threatening infection, whereas AmB should be used primarily in patients with life-threatening disease, CNS infection, immunodeficiency states, and in pediatric patients. In some cases, switching to an oral azole formulation after initial stabilization with AmB has proved efficacious. Low-dose itraconazole (Sporanox) cures most patients, so initial dosing should start at 200 mg per day; the dose may be increased in 100-mg daily increments to a maximum of 400 mg per day in cases of disease progression. Itraconazole (Sporanox) requires gastric acid for absorption and should not be coadministered with any medications that reduce gastric acid production or increase gastric pH. Fluconazole (Diflucan) is less effective than the other azoles; however, its penetration into the CNS is superior to any of the other agents, and its use may be appropriate for difficult-to-treat CNS disease. Drug interactions are common with the azole drug class, and a careful review of concomitantly administered drugs should be performed to avoid toxicity. Although liposomal preparations of AmB are expected to provide comparable results to AmB

---

[1]Not FDA approved for this indication.

CURRENT DIAGNOSIS

- In suggestive clinical syndromes, consider the diagnosis, even without endemic exposures.
- Completely evaluate all potentially involved sites.
- Perform neuroimaging if evaluation suggests CNS involvement.
- Clinical specimens for direct visualization of yeasts are often positive and permit a rapid diagnosis. KOH smears of respiratory specimens, skin exudates, joint fluid, brain tissue, prostatic secretions.
  GMS and PAS stains, in addition to routine H&E stain of biopsy material.
- Culture requires mycelial-to-yeast conversion for definite identification unless genetic probe is employed.
- Submit clinical specimens for both culture and histology for greatest diagnostic success.
- Colonization does not exist; identified organisms are conisdered pathogens.
- Serologies and skin testing are not useful in diagnostics due to a lack of specificity.
- Canine infection may serve as a sentinel event and suggests a common environmental source.

TABLE 2 Sites of Blastomycosis

Site	Frequency (%)
Lungs	70–100
Skin	40–80
Bones	25
Genitourinary, male	10–30
CNS	
Overall	5
AIDS	40
Larynx, myocardium, pericardium, orbit, sinuses, reticuloendothelial system organs, uterus	Very rare
Adrenals (adrenal insufficiency), thyroid (hypothyroidism), pituitary (diabetes insipidus), granulomatous hypercalcemia	Very rare

Abbreviations: AIDS = Acquired immunodeficiency syndrome; CNS = central nervous system.

Abbreviations: CNS = central nervous system; KOH = potassium hydroxide; GMS = Gomori methenamine silver; PAS = periodic acid Schiff; H&E = hematoxylin and eosin.

CURRENT THERAPY

Disease	Primary Regimen	Alternative Regimen
Pulmonary		
Acute self-limited	Close observation, minimum 3 years	
Mild to moderate	ITR 200–400 mg/d*	KTC 400–800 mg/d[†]
		FLU[1] 400–800 mg/d[†]
		AmB initially and ITR after stabilization
Life-threatening	AmB 0.7–1 mg/kg/d, cumulative dose 1.5–2.5 g[†]	
Disseminated		
Non-CNS		
Mild to moderate	ITR 200–400 mg/d*	KTC 400–800 mg/d[†]
		FLU[1] 400–800 mg/d[†]
Life-threatening	AmB 0.7–1 mg/kg/d, cumulative dose 1.5–2.5 g[†]	AmB initially and ITR after stabilization
CNS	AmB, cumulative dose minimum 2 g[†]	For patients unable to tolerate full course AmB, FLU[1] 800 mg/d[†]
Special populations		
Pregnancy	AmB, cumulative dose 1.5–2.5 g[†]	Azole drugs teratogenic
Pediatrics	AmB, cumulative dose ≥30 mg/kg/d[†]	ITR 5-7 mg/kg/d*
Immunocompromised	AmB, cumulative dose 1.5–2.5 g[†] followed by chronic suppression ITR 200–400 mg/d (non-CNS) or FLU[1] 800 mg/d (CNS or ITR-intolerant)	

Modified from Chapman, Bradsher, Campbell, et al: Practice guidelines for the management of patients with blastomycosis. Clin Infect Dis 2000;30:679-683.
*Optimal treatment duration for azoles is minimum of 6 months.
[†]Extended duration of AmB administration can be given 0.6-0.8 mg/kg or tiw every other day after initial stabilization.
Abbreviations: Amb = Amphotericin B deoxycholate (Fungizone); CNS = central nervous system; d = day; FLU = Fluconazole (Diflucan); ITR = Itraconazole (Sporanox); KTC = Ketoconazole (Nizoral); tiw = three times a week.

deoxycholate, comparative studies have not been performed, and their use should be relegated only to populations intolerant of conventional AmB. Two newer antifungals, caspofungin (Cancidas)[1] and voriconazole (Vfend)[1] have demonstrated in vitro activity against *B. dermatitidis*, but clinical experience is nonexistent at the time of this writing. Treatment should be managed in accordance with the IDSA guidelines.

REFERENCES

Bradsher RW, Chapman SW, Pappas PG: Blastomycosis. Infect Dis Clin North Am 2003;17:21-40.
Chapman SW: Blastomyces dermatitidis. In Mandell GL, Bennett JE, Dolin R (eds.): Principles and Practice of Infectious Diseases, Philadelphia, Churchill Livingstone 2000, pp 2733-2744.
Chapman SW, Bradsher RW, Campbell GD, et al: Practice guidelines for the management of patients with blastomycosis. Clin Infect Dis 2000;30:679-683.
Lemos LB, Soofi M, Amir E: Blastomycosis and pregnancy. Ann Diagn Pathol 2002;6(4):211-215.
Veligandla SR, Hinrichs SH, Rupp ME, et al: Delayed diagnosis of osseous blastomycosis in two patients following environmental exposure in nonendemic areas. Am J Clin Pathol 2002;118:536-541.
Ward BA, Parent AD, Raila F: Indications for the surgical management of central nervous system blastomycosis. Surg Neurol 1995;43:379-388.

[1]Not FDA approved for this indication.

Pleural Effusion and Empyema Thoracis

Method of
Jeffrey Rentz, MD, and Robert L. Thurer, MD

The pleural space normally contains 0.1 to 0.3 mL/kg of serous fluid. Each day, the parietal pleura produces 0.25 mL/kg of fluid, essentially all of which is absorbed by the pleural lymphatics. Because the normal pleura and lungs have a large absorptive capacity (approximately 5-10 mL/kg/day), any fluid collection in the pleural space is abnormal. When effusions do occur, patients may have symptoms such as dyspnea, chest pain, fatigue, and cough. Fever and weight loss are symptoms of pleural space infection.

Pleural effusions are categorized as transudates or exudates. Altered osmotic or hydrostatic forces cause transudative effusions. Notably, transudates contain low protein. Treatment of transudative effusions is initially directed toward correction of the causative disorder. Exudative effusions develop from alterations in lymphatic drainage or abnormalities of the capillary permeability of the pleura itself. These effusions contain higher levels of protein. Treatments of exudative effusions also may deal with the underlying disorder, but pleural interventions are necessary more often. Common causes of both transudates and exudates are shown in Box 1.

Various imaging studies are appropriate for evaluating a patient with suspected or known pleural effusion. Upright posterior-anterior and lateral chest radiographs should be always obtained but do not reliably identify pleural fluid collections of less than 500 mL. Lesser amounts of fluid may be detected as blunting of the costophrenic angle on the lateral film. Decubitus films are more sensitive for identifying minimal effusions and can help determine whether the fluid is loculated. Thoracic ultrasound is useful to define loculated collections and is associated with a reduction in complications during thoracentesis. Chest computed tomography (CT) scans are relied on to define and characterize fluid collections and assess the underlying lung. They are very helpful in following the course of treatment of patients with pleural effusions or empyema. Magnetic resonance imaging (MRI) offers little more information than chest CT.

Thoracentesis is typically performed for initial evaluation of patients with pleural effusion. As much fluid as possible should be drained because adequate drainage may be therapeutic as well as diagnostic. CT scanning provides better visualization of the lung parenchyma and pleural process when done after rather than before initial drainage. Thoracentesis is the simplest method of pleural drainage and can be performed at the bedside with or without image guidance. Proper fluid analysis begins with gross observation (for clarity, cloudiness, blood, or foul smell), Gram stain, culture with sensitivity, pH, cell count and differential, cytology, protein, lactate dehydrogenase (LDH), and glucose. Bilirubin levels are appropriate when hepatic diseases are suspected. Elevated amylase is present in patients with effusions related to pancreatic disorders.

If targeted treatments fail or if symptoms require management before those treatments are effective, therapeutic drainage of the pleural space is required. For most patients, bedside or ultrasound-guided thoracentesis will suffice. Video-assisted thoracentesis allows a thorough examination of the lung and pleural space with biopsies if necessary as well as enhanced drainage of loculated effusions. Patients usually require general anesthesia and single lung ventilation, whereas diagnostic thoracoscopy can be done with conscious sedation and local anesthesia in good-risk patients. Chemical pleurodesis is appropriate for patients with recurrent effusions (especially malignant effusions) as long as the lung expands well following drainage. We typically use talc (Sclerosal) introduced as an aerosol (5 g) during thoracoscopy or as a *slurry* (5 g suspended in 100 mL normal saline) placed through chest drains for patients with malignant effusions. Diluted doxycycline (Vibramycin)[1] (10 mg/kg diluted in 100 mL normal saline) is appropriate for patients with benign disorders because the incidence of late fibrothorax may be less with doxycycline (Vibramycin)[1] than with talc. For patients with lung entrapment because of malignancy, an indwelling silastic catheter that can be intermittently drained as an outpatient (Pleurx) may help control dyspnea. Hepatic hydrothorax is difficult to treat with pleurodesis unless the underlying disease has been treated. Reexpansion pulmonary edema occurs if more than 1.5 L are drained at one time, however, this is uncommon.

Empyema

Empyema refers to infected pleural fluid or frank pus in the pleural space. It is related usually to bacterial pneumonia, but other causes include chest trauma, esophageal perforation, seeding from systemic infection, and complications of thoracic procedures. Parapneumonic effusions frequently are present in patients hospitalized for pneumonia. Most are uninfected *sympathetic* effusions, but up to 20% progress to empyema. Light has described criteria that define empyema based on pleural fluid analysis (Box 2).

Although generally divided into three phases, the pathophysiology of empyema should be thought of as a continuum. The first or acute exudative phase is characterized by thin, purulent fluid and expandable underlying lung. During the second transitional or fibrinopurulent phase, fibrin organizes on the lung. The fluid is more turbid and the cellularity increases. A thick, organized fibrous peel that envelops the visceral

---

[1]Not FDA approved for this indication.

BOX 1	**Common Etiologies of Transudative and Exudative Effusions**

Transudates
Congestive heart failure
Renal disease
Nephrotic Syndrome
Uremia
Peritoneal dialysis
Cirrhosis
Myxedema
Exudates
Malignancy
Infection
Pancreatitis
Subphrenic abscess
Collagen vascular diseases
Methotrexate exposure
Asbestos exposure
Postcardiotomy and post infarction syndromes
Hemothorax
Chylothorax

BOX 2	**Light's Criteria for Exudative Effusions**

Pleural fluid protein to serum protein ratio greater than 0.5
Pleural LDH greater than 200 or pleural LDH/ serum LDH greater than 0.6

Abbreviations: LDH= lactate dehydrogenase.

CURRENT DIAGNOSIS

- Transudates are characterized by low protein and low LDH.
- Exudates are characterized by high protein and high LDH.
- Chest CT scans should be obtained after therapeutic thoracentesis.
- Direct observation of the pleural fluid is important for diagnosis.

Abbreviations: CT = computed tomography; LDH= lactate dehydrogenase.

pleura and effectively *traps* the lung typifies the third or chronic organizational phase.

The principles of management for patients with empyema are drainage of the infected fluid, reexpansion of the underlying lung with obliteration of free spaces in the pleura (no space—no problem) as well as systemic administration of appropriate antibiotics. Percutaneous drains (small *pigtail* catheters or larger chest tubes) adequately treat most early stage patients. No further instrumentation is needed if the fluid is removed, the lung expands, and there is no additional fluid accumulation. Tube thoracostomy with a 28-F to 32-F chest tube is preferable to a small catheter when the fluid is thick or turbid.

During the transitional phase, the fluid becomes loculated and more complicated to drain. Tubes may be placed using image guidance and fibrinolytics can be instilled to promote drainage. The majority of patients in this stage are best treated by video-assisted decortication and drainage. With this method, loculations can be lysed, the fluid drained completely and lung expansion improved by debridement of the visceral pleura. Video-assisted drainage has a higher rate of success, and results in fewer intensive care unit days and fewer hospital days of care than treatment with fibrinolytics. Mortality increases with delays in drainage.

When an empyema progresses to the organized stage with *trapped* lung, thoracoscopic surgery is difficult, and open thoracotomy is needed for adequate decortication. If the lung expands well and there is only a small residual effusion, the chest tubes may be removed in 3 to 4 days. If the lung fails to expand, the residual space can be managed by removing the tubes slowly over several weeks or by daily irrigation with antibiotic solution followed by primary closure (Clagett procedure). For patients unable to tolerate thoracotomy, open drainage by rib resection and marsupialization (Eloesser flap) is preferable to prolonged closed drainage.

Special consideration is needed for patients with empyema and bronchopleural fistula. Initial therapy requires drainage of the infected fluid to prevent aspiration of purulent material through the fistula. Definitive treatment ranges from open repair with vascularized flap coverage (chest wall muscle or omentum), if the fistula is discovered promptly, to open drainage with an Eloesser flap. This may be followed by a Clagett procedure if the fistula heals.

CURRENT THERAPY

- Thoracentesis always should remove as much fluid as possible.
- Early drainage is indicated for patients with parapneumonic effusions.
- Video assisted procedures are more effective than drainage with small or large bore tubes.
- Prompt decortication is more effective than lesser operations.

The authors wish to thank Dr. David Feller-Kopman for his helpful review of the manuscript.

REFERENCES

Clagett OT, Geraci JC: A procedure for the management of postpneumonectomy empyema. J Thorac Cardiovasc Surg 1963;45:141.
Erickson KV, Yost M, Bynoe R, et al: Primary treatment of malignant pleural effusions: video-assisted thoracoscopic surgery poudrage versus tube thoracostomy. Am Surg 2002;68(11):955-959.
Hasley PB, Albaum MN, Li YH, et al: Do pulmonary radiographic findings at presentation predict mortality in patients with community-acquired pneumonia? Arch Intern Med 1996;156(19):2206-2212.
Kennedy L, Rusch VW, Strange C, et al: Pleurodesis using talc slurry. Chest 1994;106(2):342-346.
Light RW, MacGregor MI, Luchsinger PC, et al: Pleural effusions: The diagnostic separation of transudates and exudates. Ann Int Med 1972;77:507.
Yim AP, Chan AT, Lee TW, et al: Thoracoscopic talc insufflation versus talc slurry for symptomatic malignant pleural effusions. Ann Thorac Surg 1996;62:1655.

Primary Lung Abscess

Method of
Matthew E. Levison, MD

Definition

Lung abscess is a necrotizing infection that results in one or more discrete cavities, each 2 cm or larger in diameter. If there are multiple, small cavities, each smaller than 2 cm in diameter, the process is usually referred to as necrotizing pneumonia, although the pathogenesis and microbiology of both lung abscess and necrotizing pneumonia are thought to be the same.

Pathogenesis

Respiratory pathogens can reach the lung by one of several routes: airways, blood stream, spread from contiguous infection, or traumatic entry (e.g., knife wound). The most common routes are the airways and the blood stream. Lung abscess developing as a consequence of bronchogenic spread to the lung is usually referred to as primary, and hematogeneous lung abscess is referred to as secondary, because in the latter instance the primary infection (bacteremia, endocarditis, or suppurative thrombophlebitis) is usually clinically evident.

The most common risk factor for primary lung abscess is aspiration of secretions from various surfaces of the oropharynx, such as the periodontal pocket, tonsillar crypts, and buccal and lingula mucosa. The periodontal pocket-fluid microflora is normally predominantly anaerobic and gram-positive; the predominant anaerobic species is *Actinomyces*. However, most patients with primary lung abscess usually also have periodontitis, in which case the periodontal pocket deepens as the epidermal dentine junction recedes toward the tooth apex, and the bacterial flora in the abnormal periodontal pocket becomes predominantly anaerobic and gram-negative; the predominant gram-negative species in the abnormal periodontal pocket include the anaerobic gram-negative bacilli *Porphyromonas, Prevotella, Bacteroides,* and *Fusobacterium*. More than 200 microbial species are found in the crevicular fluid in enormous numbers (e.g., 10^{12} colony-forming unit [CFU]/g). Aspirated oropharyngeal secretions contain these periodontal organisms as well as other organisms that colonize the nasopharynx, such as known facultative pulmonary pathogens (e.g., *Streptococcus pneumoniae* and *Haemophilus influenzae*).

Aspiration occurs among normal people, especially during deep sleep, but in certain patients aspiration may be of sufficient magnitude or frequency, or the aspirated material may contain adjuvants, such as necrotic tissue, food or foreign bodies, or particularly virulent pathogens or synergistic combinations of microorganisms to overcome lung defenses. Patients with lung abscess usually have underlying conditions that predispose to aspiration, such as loss of consciousness from any cause or neurologic or esophageal defects in swallowing. Concurrent presence of periodontal disease would favor aspiration of necrotic periodontal tissue along with large numbers of periodontal pathogens in aspirated oropharyngeal secretions. The development of primary lung abscess in patients who are edentulous should prompt a search for a neoplastic process in the oropharynx or lower respiratory tract that would result in obstruction of the airways and provides a focus of anaerobic microbial proliferation in necrotic neoplastic tissue.

Initially the pathologic process that follows aspiration is infiltrative (aspiration pneumonia), but cavitation develops 1 to 2 weeks following rupture of the abscess into a bronchus, if there is no resolution at the infiltrative stage.

Microbiology

Multiple bacteriologic studies establish that a polymicrobial anaerobic flora present in the oral cavity, particularly the abnormal periodontal pocket, causes primary lung abscess. When aspirated into the lower respiratory tract there is a marked simplification of the microflora, so that only the most virulent anaerobic species, such as *Prevotella melaninogenica, Fusobacterium* *nucleatum,* and *Peptostreptococcus* species, predominante. Microaerophilic and facultative streptococci also are frequently present.

In some patients, the anaerobes are mixed with facultative respiratory pathogens, such as *S. pneumoniae, Staphylococcus aureus, H. influenzae,* or *Klebsiella pneumoniae*. The anaerobic bacterial etiology of primary lung abscess is frequently putative, based on the clinical presentation, especially the pungent, putrid odor of the breath or infected material, such as sputum or pleural fluid, that is characteristically produced by anaerobes.

Some facultative pulmonary pathogens alone can cause primary lung abscess, and should be suspected in certain clinical settings. For example, *S. aureus,* usually following influenza, can cause a necrotizing pulmonary infection; facultative gram-negative bacilli, such as *K. pneumoniae* or *Pseudomonas aeruginosa*, nocardia, or fungi, such as aspergillus, can cause cavitary pneumonia, usually in immunocompromised patients or in a nosocomial setting; *Histoplasma* or *Coccidioides* can cause cavitary pneumonia in patients living in certain geographic areas of the United States, and *Mycobacterium tuberculosis* or *Mycobacterium kansasii* can produce cavities that usually are located in the upper lobes or in any pulmonary location in the immunocompromised as patient.

Clinical Presentation

Approximately 75% of patients with primary lung abscess have an indolent febrile, wasting illness with respiratory symptoms (cough, sputum production, pleuritic chest pain, blood-streaked sputum) of several weeks' duration, similar to that of tuberculosis or lung cancer. More than 50% of patients have putrid sputum. Pleuritic chest pain may indicate penetration into the pleural space, at times producing a pyopneumothorax as a result of a bronchopleural fistula. A more acute illness similar to that of pneumococcal pneumonia presents in 25% of patients.

Diagnosis

Patients who present with typical features of primary lung abscess that include a predisposition for aspiration, periodontal disease, a sputum with pungent, foul odor, one or more thick-walled cavities in dependent bronchopulmonary segments with air-fluid levels, need little further initial diagnostic workup and can be treated presumptively for a polymicrobial anaerobic infection. In these patients, expectorated sputum is of no value for detecting anaerobes because of contamination with oral flora, but it is useful to exclude the presence of other organisms capable of causing necrotizing pulmonary infection.

Febrile patients should have blood cultures and pleural fluid, if present, should be obtained for stains and cultures. Hematogenous *S. aureus* dissemination from infected intravenous catheters or right-sided

4

endocarditis, usually causes bilateral multifocal non-contiguous lung abscesses and blood cultures positive for *S. aureus*. Similarly, anaerobic bacterial suppurative thrombophlebitis can cause multifocal lung abscesses because of septic pulmonary emboli in Lemierre syndrome (*Fusobacterium* bacteremia, suppurative jugular thrombophlebitis, and lung abscesses) or pelvic anaerobic infection.

Upper lobe cavities without air-fluid levels suggest tuberculosis and require exclusion of *M. tuberculosis* with three morning sputum collections for mycobacterial stains and cultures. In patients who fail to respond to empiric therapy for putative anaerobic lung abscess, are suspected of having a pulmonary neoplasm, or are immunocompromised, more rigorous diagnostic testing is usually indicated, including:

- Bronchoscopy
- Protected brushing and collection of bronchoalveolar lavage fluid for stain and cultures for routine bacteria
- *Rhodococcus equi* (in patients with AIDS)
- *Legionella*, nocardia and fungi, if expectorated sputum studies fail to disclose the presence of these organisms

Computed tomography (CT) of the chest may be important to define pathologic anatomy in patients with a pyopneumothorax. CT and bronchoscopy also are important for exclusion of noninfectious conditions, such as cystic bronchiectasis, cavitating neoplasms, and Wegener's granulomatosis, all of which may be confused with lung abscess in some patients. Percutaneous CT-guided aspiration for culture and histology with special stains for fungi and other organisms should be performed, especially for peripheral, easily accessible lesions in problematic clinical situations (i.e., no clinical or radiologic response or relapse to empiric antimicrobial therapy).

Treatment

Penicillin or tetracycline were the standard antimicrobial agents used in empiric regimens to treat putative anaerobic lung abscess. However, many anaerobic gram-negative respiratory pathogens are now found to be penicillin resistant as a consequence of β lactamase production and are also tetracycline resistant. Two prospective trials of clindamycin versus penicillin in the treatment of putrid lung abscess have demonstrated the superiority of clindamycin. Clindamycin (Cleocin) can be used intravenously in doses of 600 mg every 8 hours initially in hospitalized patients unable to tolerate oral therapy, or otherwise orally in doses of 300 mg every 6 hours. Other agents active against both the oral anaerobes and microaerophilic streptococci include the carbapenems, imipenem (Primaxin) or meropenem (Merrem), cefoxitin (Mefoxin), β lactamase/β lactam antibiotic combinations (e.g., amoxicillin/clavulanate [Augmentin], ampicillin/sulbactam [Unasyn], ticarcillin/clavulanate [Timentin] or piperacillin/tazobactam [Zosyn], or a penicillin plus metronidazole (Flagyl) combination. However, most of these have not been evaluated in clinical trials. Metronidazole (Flagyl) alone is

CURRENT DIAGNOSIS

- Chronic, febrile wasting illness with respiratory symptoms
- Aspiration-prone patient
- Presence of periodontal disease
- Pungent, putrid sputum
- One or more lung cavities, with or without air-fluid levels, in dependent portions of the lungs

inadequate therapy, apparently because it is inactive against microaerophilic streptococci, although it is reliably active against anaerobes. Antibiotic therapy should be modified to cover facultative respiratory pathogens, such as *S. aureus, H. influenzae*, or *K. pneumoniae*, when isolated.

In addition to these older drugs, several newer antimicrobial agents (e.g., ertapenem [Invanz], gatifloxacin [Tequin], moxifloxacin [Avelox], gemifloxacin [Factive],

CURRENT THERAPY*

- Antimicrobial agents with activity against β lactamase producing anaerobic gram-negative bacilli and anaerobic gram-positive cocci. Modify therapy to cover facultative pulmonary pathogens, such as pneumococci and *Haemophilus influenzae*, if isolated from sputum.
  - Clindamycin (Cleocin) 600 mg IV every 8 hours or 300 mg orally every 6 hours
  - Ampicillin/sulbactam (Unasyn) 3 g IV every 6 hours or amoxicillin/clavulanate (Augmentin XR) 2 g orally every 12 hours
  - Penicillin 3 million U IV every 6 hours plus metronidazole (Flagyl) 500 mg IV every 6 hours or
  - Amoxicillin (Amoxil) 875 mg orally every 6 hours plus metronidazole (Flagyl) 500 mg orally every 6 hours
- Defervescence and clinical improvement should occur within approximately 1 week.
- Antimicrobial therapy is continued until pulmonary lesions resolve or there is a small, stable residual scar. Most patients require 6 to 8 weeks of therapy.
- Percutaneous aspiration under CT-guidance for drainage and culture should be attempted in patients unresponsive to medical therapy.
- Bronchoscopy is reserved for patients in whom an underlying malignancy is suspected or to remove an aspirated foreign body.
- Surgery is reserved for massive hemoptysis, empyema, bronchopleural fistula, and in those patients in whom an underlying malignancy is suspected.

*Antibiotic dosing for adults with normal renal function.
Abbreviations: CT = Computed tomography; IV = intravenous.

Rakel and Bope: *Conn's Current Therapy 2006*.

telithromycin [Ketek], and linezolid [Zyvox] have received Food and Drug Administration (FDA) approval for treatment of community-acquired pneumonia. However, none of these drugs has been studied in series of patients with putative or confirmed anaerobic pleuropulmonary infections. Although these drugs show in vitro activity against oral anaerobes isolated from bite wound infections, when the source of the pathogen is other than pleuropulmonary, the published in vitro data are not predictive of efficacy for infection caused by anaerobic pleuropulmonary pathogens.

Patients on effective therapy will defervesce within 1 week. Chest radiographic findings will take weeks to resolve. The duration of therapy is controversial. The recommended duration of therapy for anaerobic lung abscess is usually at least 4 to 6 weeks to prevent relapse, or until the abscess completely resolves, or there is a small, stable residual scar. Failure to adequately respond should prompt more intensive investigation to exclude the presence of resistant pathogens or a noninfectious etiology.

Surgery is rarely indicated for putrid lung abscess, except for the rare complication of massive hemoptysis or concurrent lung cancer. Postural and bronchoscopic drainage and chest physiotherapy traditionally were recommended to enhance antimicrobial therapy. However, caution should be exercised to avoid potentially fatal, sudden massive emptying of pus-filled cavities into the airways and previously uninvolved bronchopulmonary segments. Percutaneous drainage may be necessary for unresponsive large cavities, as well as for empyema.

REFERENCES

Bartlett JG: Anaerobic bacterial infections of the lung and pleural space. Clin Infect Dis 1993;16 (Suppl 4): S248-S255.
Bartlett JG, Gorbach SL: Treatment of aspiration pneumonia and primary lung abscess: Penicillin G vs clindamycin. JAMA 1975; 234:935-937.
Gonzalez CL, Calia FM: Bacteriologic flora of aspiration-induced pulmonary infections. Arch Intern Med 1975;135:711-714.
Gudiol F, Manresa F, Pallares R, et al: Clindamycin vs. penicillin for anaerobic lung infections. High rate of penicillin failures associated with penicillin-resistant *Bacteroides melaninogenicus*. Arch Intern Med 1990;150:2525-2529.
Ha HK, Kang MW, Park JM, et al: Lung abscess: percutaneous catheter therapy. Acta Radiologica 1993;34:362-365.
Levison ME, Bran JL, Ries K: Treatment of anaerobic bacterial infections with clindamycin 2 phosphate. Antimicrob Agents Chemother 1974;5:276-280.
Levison ME, Mangura CT, Lorber B, et al: Clindamycin compared with penicillin for the treatment of anaerobic lung abscess. Ann Intern Med 1983;98:466-471.
Lorber B, Swenson RM: Bacteriology of aspiration pneumonia, a prospective study of community and hospital acquired cases. Ann Intern Med 1974;81:329.
Marina M, Strong CA, Civen R, et al: Bacteriology of anaerobic pleuropulmonary infection. Preliminary Report. Clin Infect Dis 1993;16 (Suppl 4):S256-S262.
Perlino CA: Metronidazole vs clindamycin treatment of anaerobic pulmonary infection: failure of metronidazole therapy. Arch Intern Med 1981;141:1424-1427.
Slots J: Subgingival microflora and periodontitis. J Clin Periodontol 1979;6:351-382.
Sosenko A, Glassroth J: Fiberoptic bronchoscopy in the evaluation of lung abscesses. Chest 1985;87:489-494.

Acute Bronchitis

Method of
Jeffrey A. Linder, MD, MPH

Acute bronchitis is an acute respiratory infection of fewer than 3 weeks' duration in a patient without underlying cardiopulmonary disease in which cough, with or without phlegm production, is the predominant feature.

Traditionally, antibiotics were prescribed for acute bronchitis, but given evidence that antibiotics are not effective and carry a real risk of adverse drug events for individual patients, acute bronchitis is a major target of efforts to reduce inappropriate antibiotic prescribing. Acute bronchitis accounted for approximately 10% of all antibiotic prescriptions in the United States in 1996. From 1991 to 1999, physicians decreased antibiotic prescribing from 76% to 59% of acute bronchitis visits. Studies detect no disease in pneumonia in populations in which the antibiotic prescribing rate is markedly reduced.

Epidemiology and Microbiology

Acute bronchitis is one of the most common reasons for seeking ambulatory care, accounting for approximately 3 million ambulatory visits annually. A pathogen can be identified in a minority of cases of acute bronchitis even when using highly sensitive techniques. Acute bronchitis has a nonbacterial cause in more than 90% of cases. The most common viruses associated with acute bronchitis are influenza A, influenza B, parainfluenza, respiratory syncitial virus, coronavirus, adenovirus, and rhinovirus. Bacteria are associated with acute bronchitis in only 5% of cases. Bacteria isolated from patients with acute bronchitis include *Mycoplasma pneumoniae*, *Bordetella pertussis*, and *Chlamydia pneumoniae*.

Pathophysiology

Bacterial and viral infection causes hyperemia of the airways, followed by increased mucus production, and desquamation of the lung epithelium. Purulence is caused by peroxidase from leukocytes and is not an indication of bacterial infection. Coughing helps clear debris from the irritated, damaged airways. Pulmonary function testing shows obstructive findings that can last 6 to 8 weeks. Obstruction is caused by enlargement of airway walls from hyperemia, debris in the airways, failure of ciliary clearance of debris, and bronchial muscle spasm.

Evaluation

HISTORY

Adults with acute bronchitis generally present with a cough that can be accompanied by mild dyspnea, low-grade fever, and malaise. The primary goal in the evaluation of adults with acute bronchitis is to rule out pneumonia. Indications of pneumonia include high fever, severe dyspnea, and pleuritic chest pain.

Pertussis should be considered in the presence of documented outbreaks. Unfortunately, there are no clinical features that allow clinicians to distinguish patients with persistent cough who have pertussis. Purulent or colored sputum is not helpful in differentiating acute bronchitis from pneumonia and does not change the approach to treatment.

Acute bronchitis also is one of the most common causes of hemoptysis. Hemoptysis associated with acute bronchitis usually is minimal in amount, and hemoptysis associated with acute bronchitis should resolve promptly. Persistent hemoptysis should prompt a search for alternative diagnoses.

PHYSICAL EXAMINATION

As with the history, the principal goal of the physical examination in adults with acute bronchitis is to rule out pneumonia. Studies show that if a patient has a temperature of less than 38°C, (100.4°F), heart rate less than 100 beats per minute, respiratory rate less than 24, and a normal lung examination, pneumonia is sufficiently unlikely that a chest radiograph is not warranted. Patients with acute bronchitis may have abnormal lung findings such as rhonchi and crackles.

TESTING

Routine testing is not necessary in the vast majority of cases for the diagnosis and management of adults with acute bronchitis. Clinicians should only order a chest radiograph if pneumonia is suspected or if it will change management. For example, if physicians are going to diagnose pneumonia and prescribe antibiotics to a relatively well-appearing patient with normal vitals signs and minimal lung abnormalities on physical examination, a chest radiograph is probably not warranted.

During influenza season and when influenza is known to be circulating, rapid influenza testing may aid in diagnosis and guide treatment. Several different kits are available to identify influenza. Testing for pertussis should be only performed in the setting of known or suspected outbreak as it rarely affects the management of individual patients.

Differential Diagnosis

The differential diagnosis of acute bronchitis includes nonspecific upper respiratory tract infections, pneumonia, asthma, and other causes of cough. Nonspecific upper respiratory tract infection is characterized by the acute onset of respiratory symptoms, including fever, congestion, sinus pain or pressure, rhinorrhea, sore throat, and myalgias without one particular symptom predominating. Bacterial pneumonia is characterized by the acute onset of cough, chest pain, and high fever. As noted earlier, patients with bacterial pneumonia generally have vital sign abnormalities or abnormalities on lung examination.

Asthma is difficult to differentiate acutely from acute bronchitis as the pathophysiology and findings on pulmonary function testing are similar. Pulmonary function testing is not helpful for acute bronchitis, but clinicians can consider pulmonary function testing in patients who have coughs for longer than 3 months. Other causes of acute and chronic cough include gastroesophageal reflux, sinusitis with postnasal drip, and medications, especially angiotensin-converting enzyme inhibitors.

Treatment

Antibiotics are not appropriate for adults with acute bronchitis. A guideline from the Centers for Disease Control and Prevention, American Academy of Family Physicians, the American College of Physicians, and the Infectious Diseases Society of America states, "Routine antibiotic treatment of uncomplicated acute bronchitis is not recommended, regardless of the duration of cough." Antibiotics are not indicated for patients with purulent sputum or for smokers without underlying cardiopulmonary disease. Antibiotics for suspected pertussis do not hasten resolution of symptoms, but do decrease shedding of pertussis to others.

β-Agonists such as albuterol (Proventil)[1] show promise in the treatment of acute bronchitis. Some studies show trends toward reduced cough, night cough, productive cough, and early return to work. Results appear to be better for adults with airflow obstruction as evidenced by wheezing. Common adverse effects of β-agonists are tremor, shakiness, or nervousness.

There is a general lack of evidence for or against the use of over-the-counter medications. There are no data to support the use of analgesics and antipyretics like acetaminophen (Tylenol) and ibuprofen (Motrin and others), but they may help patients feel better. Antihistamines are no better than placebo. Results have been at best mixed for expectorants, mucolytics, and decongestant-antihistamine combinations. Although evidence is mixed, antitussives such as guaifenesin with codeine (Robitussin AC) help coughing patients sleep at night. Patients should be encouraged to rest and drink plenty of fluids. Vaporizers and humidifiers may help patients feel better.

For patients with influenza, four antiviral medications are available. All must be started within 48 hours of symptom onset to be effective. Amantadine (Symmetrel) and rimantadine (Flumadine) are effective against influenza A. Oseltamivir (Tamiflu) and zanamivir (Relenza) are effective against both influenza A and B.

Patient Education

Patient education plays an important role in the management of adults with acute bronchitis. Proper education has the potential to improve health, set

---

[1]Not FDA approved for this indications.

CURRENT DIAGNOSIS

- Clinical diagnosis
- Rule out pneumonia: Chest radiograph probably not necessary if:
  - Temperature less than 38°C (100.4°F)
  - Heart rate less than 100 beats per minute
  - Respiratory rate less than 24
  - Normal lung examination
- Consider rapid influenza test if influenza season and influenza is circulating.
- Consider pertussis test if there is a known or suspected pertussis outbreak.

expectations, and improve patients' use of the health system. Studies show that patients who previously received antibiotics are much more likely to want them in the future. Other studies show that patient satisfaction is dependent on patients' perception that the physician spent enough time with them and that the illness and treatment was adequately explained, regardless if antibiotics were prescribed.

Patients should be informed that the cough from acute bronchitis generally lasts 10 to 14 days but can last 3 to 4 weeks. Any patient with acute bronchitis who is a smoker should be urged to quit. For smokers, the duration of cough from acute bronchitis is much longer, smokers appear to be more susceptible to acute

CURRENT THERAPY

- Albuterol MDI[1], (Proventil)[1] two puffs three times daily for 7 days for patients with evidence of airflow obstruction
- Analgesics/antipyretics:
  - Acetaminophen, 1 gm orally three times daily for 5 to 7 days, or
  - Ibuprofen 400 to 600 mg orally three times daily for 5 to 7 days
- Guaifenesin with codeine (Rubitussin AC) 10 ml orally every 4 hours as needed at night
- Antiviral treatment for patients with influenza:
  - Amantadine (Symmetrel) 100 mg orally twice daily for 5 days
  - Rimantadine (Flumadine) 100 mg orally twice daily for 5 days
  - Oseltamivir (Tamiflu) 75 mg orally twice daily for 5 days
  - Zanamivir (Relenza) 10 mg inhaled twice daily for 5 days
- Patient education
  - Antibiotics are not beneficial and pose risks to the individual patient.
  - Cough usually lasts 10 to 14 days, but occasionally longer.
  - Smoking cessation is important.

[1]Not FDA approved for this indication.

Rakel and Bope: *Conn's Current Therapy 2006.*

bronchitis, and smokers are at risk of developing chronic pulmonary disease.

Patients should be educated about the inefficacy of antibiotics for acute bronchitis and the individual risk of inappropriate antibiotic use, such as adverse reactions and development of antibiotic-resistant bacteria. Although studies show that referring to acute bronchitis as a "chest cold" reduces patients' expectation for antibiotics, it makes more long-term sense to educate patients about the inefficacy of antibiotics for acute bronchitis.

REFERENCES

Gonzales R, Bartlett JG, Besser RE, et al: Principles of appropriate antibiotic use for treatment of uncomplicated acute bronchitis: Background. Ann Intern Med 2001;134(6):521-529.
Schroeder K, Fahey T: Over-the-counter medications for acute cough in children and adults in ambulatory settings. Cochrane Data Base Syst Rev 2004; 4:CD 001831.
Snow V, Mottur-Pilson C, Gonzales R: Principles of appropriate antibiotic use for treatment of acute bronchitis in adults. Ann Intern Med 2001;134(6):518-520.
Steinman MA, Gonzales R, Linder JA, et al: Changing use of antibiotics in community-based outpatient practice, 1991-1999. Ann Intern Med 2003;138:525-533.

4

Bacterial Pneumonia

Method of
*William Kevin Green, MD, and
John A. Vande Waa, PhD, DO*

Pneumonia is a serious infection with significant morbidity and mortality. It is the sixth leading cause of death in the United States and the leading cause of infection-related mortality. It is a common infection, one of the leading reasons for hospital admission, more than 1.1 million patients are admitted each year for community-acquired pneumonia (CAP) alone, and treatment costs exceed $8 billion annually. It affects the young and the old; one third of patients are elderly, with the most serious infections occurring at the extremes of age and those with co-morbidities including immunosuppression.

Despite all the advances in modern medicine, the diagnosis of most bacterial pneumonias is made clinically, management has changed little since the introduction of antibiotics, and therapy is usually empiric. The bacterial pathogens responsible for the vast majority of cases have changed little and often are determined by host and environmental factors. However, the emergence of antibiotic resistance of these bacterial pathogens has become a major problem. *Streptococcus pneumoniae* remains the major cause of community-acquired pneumonia in nearly all populations, young, old, or infirm.

Community-acquired bacterial pneumonia may be categorized by clinical presentation, typical versus atypical. Other categories of patients and clinical scenarios also are useful in determining the most likely pathogens and, subsequently, which empiric antimicrobial therapy should be initiated: CAP in the elderly, CAP in patients with co-morbidities, pneumonia in nursing-home patients, hospital-associated pneumonia (HAP), and ventilator-associated pneumonia (VAP).

Despite our best efforts and appropriate therapy, the mortality from CAP in most series ranges from 10% to 15%, and ventilator-associated pneumonia ranges from 15% to 50% (in most series). Many patients without co-morbidities or extremes of age usually can be treated on an outpatient basis, others may require hospitalization, or, if severe, intensive care often requiring intubation and mechanical ventilation for respiratory failure. Treatment and management strategies of bacterial pneumonia remain a serious challenge due in great part to the rapid change in resistance to multiple antibiotics, changing demographics, and economic pressures. Unfortunately, the emergence of antibiotic resistance among most pathogens including drug-resistant *S. pneumoniae* (DRSP), community-acquired, methicillin-resistant *Staphylococcus aureus* (MRSA), and multidrug resistant, gram-negative bacilli appears to be outpacing our development of new therapies and further complicating our treatment strategies.

Diagnosis, Clinical Manifestations, and Etiology

The diagnosis of pneumonia remains problematic and often depends upon bacterial and host factors (Box 1). In general, the diagnosis of pneumonia is made on clinical presentation and laboratory and radiologic evidence. It is important but often difficult to differentiate it from less invasive upper respiratory tract infections. The clinical presentation of pneumonia is unfortunately variable and dependent upon both pathogen and host factors. Because therapy for pneumonia is usually empiric and critical to initiate promptly, it is important to make the diagnosis and identify the suspected pathogens responsible for the infection. The possible pathogens responsible for the pneumonia can be suspected based upon patient's history and clinical and associated risk factors (Table 1).

CAP can be categorized as being either typical or atypical in presentation, and, although these distinctions are frequently blurred, it still may be useful. Typical pneumonia is characterized by an abrupt onset of fever and chills, with a productive cough, classically rust-tinged, that evolves over several days, usually less than 1 week. As with nearly all pneumonias, it may be associated with headache, malaise, nausea, vomiting, abdominal pain, and diarrhea. Altered mental status, dyspnea, and pleuritic chest pain are concerning for more serious disease. Laboratory evaluation often reveals a leukocytosis usually greater than 15×10^9 per liter, often with left shift. Leukopenia also may be seen and

often is associated with severe symptoms and poorer outcome. Sputum specimens were traditionally used for diagnosis and advocated by many, but problems with sensitivity and specificity of the test have limited its usefulness. However, a good expectorated specimen that is mucopurulent can be an early guide to the etiology particularly when the Gram stain is consistent with a suspected pathogen. Blood cultures are helpful and specific when positive, which may further guide therapeutic choices, but only grow out organisms in less than 16% of the cases. There are no specific signs that identify the offending organism, but most patients are febrile and tachycardic, usually there are localized crackles and, less frequently, signs of lobar consolidation. The chest radiograph is essential for the diagnosis of CAP and, most frequently, shows lobar or segmental opacification in typical pneumonia. Risk factors for typical CAP include: common co-morbidities of chronic obstructive pulmonary disease (COPD), alcohol abuse, cardiovascular disorders, neurologic or cerebrovascular disorders, diabetes mellitus, renal failure, liver disease, malnutrition, residence in chronic-care facilities, immunosuppression, and HIV-1 infection. The common bacterial etiologies of typical CAP include *S. pneumoniae*, *Haemophilus influenzae*, enteric gram-negative bacilli including *Klebsiella pneumoniae*, gram-negatives such as *Pseudomonas aeruginosa*, *S. aureus*, and anaerobes (if aspiration is suspected). DRSP also has emerged, and risk factors are listed in Table 1. Community-acquired methicillin-resistant *S. aureus* also appears to be emerging as an etiology of CAP, particularly when associated with viral influenza. It is also important to note that some of the atypical pneumonia pathogens, particularly *Legionella* species may also present in a typical pneumonia presentation with an acute onset and often severe infection, and consequently, therapy for *Legionella* species is given for any severe pneumonia regardless of presentation.

In contrast, atypical pneumonia begins more insidiously with fever and a nonproductive cough. Symptoms may be present for 2 to 3 weeks before the patient seeks medical treatment. Dyspnea on exertion often occurs before shortness of breath at rest is experienced. Headache, confusion, and impaired consciousness are also seen and suspect for *Legionella* species. Sore throat is common with *Mycoplasma* and *Chlamydia*. Laboratory findings may reveal a mild leukocytosis; no other laboratory evaluations are specific, although *Legionella* species are associated with hyponatremia (50% of cases) and elevated liver enzymes. Sputum specimens and blood cultures are negative for the atypical pneumonia pathogens. Serology for the atypical bacterial pathogens and *Legionella* urinary antigen may be useful, but the results are not routinely available until well after therapy has begun or patient is ready for discharge from the hospital. Examination often reveals fever, tachypnea, and lung findings most commonly with bilateral inspiratory crackles, but they may be absent. The chest radiograph is typically bilateral ground glass or diffuse nodular opacification but also may be negative. Risk factors and the associated pathogen of atypical pneumonia include those of typical pneumonia but are associated with

TABLE 1 Risk Factors and Agents of Bacterial Pneumonia

Risk factors	Bacterial pneumonia and common associated pathogens
Age (> 60-65)	CAP,* HAP,[†] DRSP,[¶] gram-negatives
Alcohol	CAP,* gram-negatives including *Klebsiella*, DRSP[¶]
Antibiotic use (prior)	HAP,[†] DRSP,[¶] *Pseudomonas*
Aspiration	CAP,* anaerobes
Coronary artery disease (CAD)	CAP,* *S. pneumoniae*
Congestive heart failure (CHF)	CAP,* *S. pneumoniae*
Chronic liver disease	CAP*
COPD, chronic lung disease	CAP,* HAP,[†] *S. pneumoniae, H. influenzae, M. catarrhalis, M. pneumoniae, C. pneumoniae*
Cystic fibrosis	*Pseudomonas, S. aureus*
Dementia	CAP,* *S. pneumoniae*
Diabetes mellitus	CAP,* HAP,[†] *S. aureus*
Exposure to birds	*C. psittaci*
Exposure to contaminated water systems, aerosols	*L. pneumophila*
Exposure to cats, cattle, sheep, goats	*C. burnetti*
Exposure to daycare	DRSP[¶]
HIV-1, AIDS	CAP,* *S. pneumoniae, Legionella, M. tuberculosis, Mycobacterium* species, *Pseudomonas, Nocardia, R. equi*
Hospital admission (>48 hours)	HAP[†]
Intensive care unit	HAP[†]
Impaired swallowing	Anaerobes, gram-negatives
Institutionalized (e.g., nursing home)	CAP,* HAP,[†] *S. pneumoniae, M. catarrhalis*, gram-negatives including *Pseudomonas*, anaerobes (if aspiration risks present)
Immunosuppression, including steroid use, or malnutrition	HAP,[†] VAP,[§] DRSP,[¶] *Pseudomonas, Legionella*
Influenza infection	*S. aureus* (including MRSA[‡])
Intubation	VAP,[§] *Pseudomonas*
Malignancy	CAP,* HAP,[†] *Legionella*
Neutropenia	HAP,[†] *Pseudomonas*
Neurologic disease, CVA, reduced consciousness	HAP,[†] *S. pneumoniae*, gram-negatives, anaerobes
Surgery: prolonged	HAP,[†] VAP[§]
Surgery: Recent thoracoabdominal	HAP,[†] anaerobes
Tobacco use	HAP,[†] *H. influenzae*

*CAP core pathogens: *Streptococcus pneumoniae, Haemophilus influenzae, Mycoplasma pneumoniae, Moraxella catarrhalis, Staphylococcus aureus, Legionella pneumophila.*
[†]HAP core pathogens: *Streptococcus pneumoniae, Haemophilus influenzae, Staphylococcus aureus.*
[‡]MRSA, enteric gram-negative bacilli, *Enterobacter* species, *Pseudomonas aeruginosa, Acinetobacter* species, *Legionella.*
[§]VAP core pathogens: *Staphylococcus aureus*, mixed infections, *Pseudomonas aeruginosa, Acinetobacter* species, enteric gram-negative bacilli.
[¶]DRSP: Drug-resistant *Streptococcus pneumoniae.*
Abbreviations: *C. burnetti* = Coxiella burnetti, *C. pneumoniae* = Chlamydia pneumoniae, *C. psittaci* = Chlamydia psittaci, *H. influenzae* = Haemophilus influenzae, *L. pneumophila* = Legionella pneumophila, *M. catarrhalis* = Moraxella catarrhalis, *M. pneumoniae* = Mycoplasma pneumoniae, *M. tuberculosis* = Mycobacterium tuberculosis, *P. aeruginosa* = Pseudomonas aeruginosa, *R. equi* = Rhodococcus equi, *S. aureus* = Staphylococcus aureus, *S. pneumoniae* = Streptococcus pneumoniae pneumophila, COPD = chronic obstructive pulmonary disease, CAP = community-acquired pneumonia, CVA = cerebrovascular accident, HAP = hospital acquired pneumonia.

Rakel and Bope: *Conn's Current Therapy 2006.*

epidemics (*Mycoplasma, Legionella*); COPD (*Chlamydia, Mycoplasma*); bird exposure (*Chlamydia*); cat, cattle, sheep, goats exposure (*Coxiella burnetii*); exposure to contaminated water system (*Legionella*); and immunosuppression (*Legionella, Mycobacteria*).

The elderly are at increased risk for pneumonia and impose unique problems for diagnosis of pneumonia due in part to the highly variable clinical presentation. Fifty to sixty percent of elderly patients do not have the classic fever, cough, and dyspnea. Chills or rigors are rarely seen, and these patients are more likely to present with confusion, falling, depression, anorexia, and worsening of co-morbid conditions. The signs of pneumonia are also altered in the elderly; apyrexia, delirium, hypotension, tachypnea, or tachycardia may

be the only findings. Laboratory findings include a low, normal, or elevated leukocyte count, an isolated left-shift, hyper- or hyponatremia, although blood cultures are more likely to be positive (30% to 60% of cases in most series). The chest radiographs are commonly normal at onset, but show progression of infiltrates with sequential films, and when present are associated with an increase in severity of the pneumonia.

The diagnosis and clinical manifestation of pneumonia among nursing-home residents merits specific mention because of numerous risk factors for developing pneumonia and with hospital-associated pathogens. This population has higher rates of colonization with *S. aureus, K. pneumoniae,* and *Escherichia coli.* The clinical manifestations are similar to the elderly but often complicated by poorer health and debilitating co-morbidities. Risk factors for pneumonia in addition to the co-morbidities include: swallowing disorders and suspicion for aspiration, malnutrition, prior antibiotic use, and poor quality of life. The pathogens responsible for the pneumonia are similar to those in the elderly: Nearly 50% are caused by *S. pneumoniae*, but include a higher risk for anaerobes from aspiration, susceptible and antibiotic-resistant, gram-positives including DRSP, MRSA, and gram-negatives including *P. aeruginosa.*

HAP, any pneumonia developing more than 48 hours after admission to a hospital is another presentation that has unique diagnostic features, clinical presentations, and risks for nosocomial pathogens. Co-morbid conditions and prior antibiotic use may alter the clinical presentation of pneumonia and increase the exposure to nosocomial pathogen colonization and subsequent infection. The diagnosis based on fever, cough, dyspnea, and an abnormal chest radiograph is confounded by altered signs and symptoms caused by the use of antipyretics, antibiotics, or underlying medical or surgical problems and may be present to some degree prior to the onset of the pneumonia. The chest films are frequently abnormal; underlying lung, heart, or chest surgery may mask an infiltrate or often affects the ability of the patient to have a good quality chest radiograph. Chest computed tomography (CT) scans have been useful and proven sensitive under these circumstances. Diagnosis is further aided with expectorated sputum, which has a high sensitivity but low specificity, particularly if the patient is not on antibiotics; or positive blood cultures (but positive in only 25% to 50% of cases); induced sputum; or bronchoscopy. Bronchoscopy with a protected brush has a 30% to 100% sensitivity and specificity, and bronchoalveolar lavage (BAL) has a 40% to 100% sensitivity and 69% to 100% specificity in most series. The criteria for diagnosis of HAP includes rales or dullness to percussion on physical examination plus any (1) new onset purulent sputum or a change in sputum character; (2) organism isolated from blood; (3) isolation of pathogen from transbronchial aspirate bronchial brush, BAL, or biopsy *or* chest radiograph with new or progressing infiltrate, consolidation, cavitation, or pleural effusion plus any 1, 2, or 3, *or* (4) isolation of virus or viral antigen in respiratory secretions; (5) diagnostic IgM or fourfold increase in IgG for a pathogen; (6) histopathologic evidence of pneumonia. Risk factors for nosocomial pneumonia include: admission to ICU, prior antibiotics use (which changes colonization), prior prolonged surgery (especially requiring postoperative intubation), chronic lung disease, renal failure, advanced age (>60 years old), and any immunosuppression. The common etiologies of nosocomial pneumonia include *E. coli, Klebsiella* species, *Proteus* species, *Serratia marcescens, Enterobacter* species (the enteric gram-negative bacilli), *H. influenzae* and *S. pneumoniae* (usually within the first 5 days of hospitalization), *S. aureus* including MRSA, anaerobes (when impaired swallowing or aspiration is suspected), *Pseudomonas, Acinetobacter,* and *Legionella* species (associated with immunosuppression and endemic in many hospital environments).

The diagnosis and clinical manifestations of VAP also are often difficult, and clinical manifestations are variable because of the severity of underlying illness or surgery that resulted in the ventilator-dependent condition. Patients frequently have baseline fever, cough/sputum production, limited oxygenation and ventilation, leukocytosis, abnormal lung examination, and abnormal chest radiographs prior to the development of pneumonia. The criteria for diagnosis are the same as for nosocomial pneumonia described previously. Diagnosis may be aided by an endotracheal suction specimen, which has a good correlation of what may be causing the pneumonia, but unfortunately, it is more likely to be false positive than negative because of bacterial colonization. Bronchoscopy with protected brush or BAL can improve the yield and, for heavy secretions, also may be therapeutic. The most common bacterial pathogens for VAP are the same as mentioned earlier for HAP, but because patients are confined to intensive care units (ICUs), they are more likely to be colonized and then infected with more antibiotic-resistant gram-positives such as MRSA and gram-negatives such as multidrug resistant *Pseudomonas, Acinetobacter,* or resistant *Enterobacteriaceae* (with extended-spectrum, beta-lactamase production) that may be endemic in that specific ICU. Antibiotic selection is directed against these resistant pathogens, and, in the cases of MDR gram-negatives, the choices can be frustratingly limited.

Risk Stratification for Community-Acquired Pneumonia

After the diagnosis of CAP has been made, the next critical step is to determine whether or not the patient should be hospitalized. Physicians often rely on their clinical impression of severity of illness in making this decision, but this approach has been shown to overestimate the risk of death, thus hospitalizing many patients who are at low risk for complications or death. Also, hospitalization rates vary widely region to region, suggesting that inconsistent criteria are used to determine the need for admission. Many investigators have attempted to devise models that stratify patients with pneumonia into risk categories, thus improving the decision-making process regarding hospitalization. Most of these are limited by retrospective design, the need for complex calculations, focus on mortality as a measure of outcome, or lack of validation in independent patient populations.

However, Fine and colleagues devised the prediction tool to accurately identify patients with CAP at low risk for death within 30 days of presentation that was derived and prospectively validated in large numbers of patients. Their Pneumonia Severity Index (PSI) is a two-step scoring system combining demographic information, co-morbid conditions, and physical and laboratory findings. Patients without defined demographic factors, co-morbid conditions, or specific physical findings were assigned to Risk Category 1 and had the lowest 30-day mortality. Patients with these defined factors were

TABLE 2 CAP 30-Day Mortality by Class and PSI score

Class	PSI Score	30-Day Mortality (%)
I	No factors	0.1
II	≤70	0.6
III	71-90	0.9
IV	91-130	9.3
V	>130	27

stratified into four additional categories (II-V) based on a cumulative score and had increasing 30-day mortality rates (Table 2). Although not the primary goal of the study, these data suggest that patients in classes I-III could be managed as outpatients, whereas patients in classes IV and V should be managed in the hospital. Few studies have adequately addressed whether such predictive rules alter management and outcome, but most suggest benefits in using predictive rules to reduce both hospital admissions for low-risk patients and length of hospital stays.

Treatment

Initial therapy in most cases of pneumonia is empiric and is directed toward the most likely causative organisms. In the United States, CAP treatment guidelines have been published by the Infectious Disease Society of America (IDSA) and the American Thoracic Society (ATS). These guidelines are summarized in the Current Therapy box (Box 1). The guidelines differ in their approach to patient risk stratification and recommended therapies. The IDSA guidelines stratify patients by location of treatment. Combination therapy with β-lactams and macrolides or fluoroquinolones is included to provide adequate therapy for *S. pneumonia* and *Legionella*, the leading causes of fatal cases of pneumonia. The ATS guidelines stratify patients by location of treatment and by cardiopulmonary co-morbid conditions (COPD and congestive heart failure [CHF]) and risk factors for drug-resistant *S. pneumonia* and *Pseudomonas*. The risk factors for *Pseudomonas* and drug-resistant *S. pneumonia* are outlined in Table 1. The IDSA and ATS are currently working on a unified guideline to resolve these differences. In patients presenting with severe, necrotizing pneumonia, or who developed pneumonia concurrently with influenza infection, therapy (e.g., vancomycin [Vancocin]) or linezolid (Zyvox) for community-acquired MRSA must be considered.

CAP in elderly patients, particularly those who reside in nursing homes, may be the result of aspiration of oral secretions. Empiric therapy should include coverage for oral *Streptococci*, anaerobes, and gram-negative rods. Therapy including Clindamycin (Cleocin) or a β-lactam/β-lactamase combination—ampicillin/sulbactam (Unasyn) or piperacillin/tazobactam (Zosyn) is an excellent choice.

Rakel and Bope: *Conn's Current Therapy 2006.*

Empiric therapy for HAP should be directed toward multidrug-resistant organisms and anaerobes, including MRSA, *Pseudomonas,* and oral flora. Antibiotic sensitivity patterns vary widely, therefore, local antibiograms should be consulted. Typical agents that are chosen for empiric therapy in HAP include vancomycin or linezolid combined with an antipseudomonal β-lactam (piperacillin [Pipracil]) or β-lactam/β-lactamase inhibitor combination (piperacillin/tazobactam [Zosyn])), an extended spectrum carbapenem (imipenem/cilastatin [Primaxin] or meropenem [Merrem]) or a late generation cephalosporin (ceftazidime [Fortaz] or cefepime [Maxipime]) combined with clindamycin. Guidelines for the treatment of HAP were released in early 2005. In patients with both CAP and HAP, if a causative organism is recovered, the patient should receive therapy specifically directed at that organism. When the patient becomes stable and is eating and drinking, an automatic switch to oral agents with good bioavailability should occur.

Length of therapy for both CAP and HAP has traditionally been 7 to 14 days, however, there are few data to support this practice. Recently, several well-designed studies have investigated abbreviated treatment courses with good results.

Complications

The most common complication of bacterial pneumonia is pleural effusion, and the incidence varies with the etiologic agent. Pleural effusions occur in approximately 10% of pneumonococcal pneumonias, 50% to 70% with gram-negative rod pneumonias and up to 90% with group A streptococcal pneumonias. Effusions begin as transudates composed of serum, and contain low numbers of neutrophils, and normal values of pH, lactate dehydrogenase (LDH), and glucose. Cultures are usually negative at this stage. An empyema forms as the process continues and more neutrophils accumulate, LDH and protein increase, and pH and glucose fall. Over time, the fluid usually becomes loculated, and there is deposition of fibrin over the pleura. In the final stage, a thick, fibrous rind forms that encases the lung. Pleural effusions account for 40% to 60% of empyemas.

Pleural effusion or empyema should be considered when a patient with pneumonia has persistent symptoms of fever, shortness of breath, cough, and chest pain despite adequate antibiotic therapy. On examination, the patient may have decreased breath sounds over the affected area, with dullness to percussion and crackles present. Plain chest radiography, including posterior-anterior, lateral and lateral decubitus views, is the best initial approach to detecting and evaluating a pleural effusion. Blunting of the costophrenic angle may be visible on posterior-anterior views but occurs only after significant fluid accumulation. Lateral decubitus radiographs, however, can detect smaller collections. Ultrasound is more sensitive for estimating fluid volumes and can localize fluid collections for guided thoracentesis. Ultrasound also has been shown to have a lower rate of pneumothorax than traditional thoracentesis methods. Computed tomography is the imaging modality of choice for complex, loculated effusions as it allows for differentiation between pleural effusion and lung abscess.

Pleural effusions should be sampled if adequate fluid is present or if the effusion is loculated. Cultures of pleural fluid may result in recovery of the causative bacterium, and laboratory testing will help distinguish between simple effusion and empyema. Fluid should be examined for total and differential cell count, glucose, total protein, LDH, and pH and be sent for gram strain and culture. The application of Light's criteria aids in distinguishing transudates from exudates (Table 3).

The primary indications for drainage include an effusion pH less than 2, or persistent symptoms despite adequate therapy. Studies have shown that a pH less than 2 is most accurate in detecting complicated effusions and need for drainage. Drainage using tube thoracostomy is successful in many patients and the success of this method may be improved with use of fibrinolytic agents. Video-assisted thoracoscopy (VATS) or open thoracotomy with decortication remains the definitive surgical therapy for complicated pleural effusions.

TABLE 3　Light's Criteria for Interpreting Pleural Effusions

Characteristic	Transudate	Exudate
Appearance	Translucent	Opaque
pH	>7.2	<7.2
WBC count	<10,000/mm³	>50,000/mm³
Glucose	≥60 mg/dL	<60 mg/dL
Total protein	<3 g/dL	>3 g/dL
Fluid/serum ratio	<0.5	>0.5
LDH	<200 IU/L	>200 IU/L
Fluid:serum ratio	<0.6	>0.6

Abbreviations: LDH = lactase dehydrogenase; WBC = white blood cell count.

 CURRENT THERAPY

The following provides a summary of IDSA and ATS CAP treatment guidelines.

IDSA Group	IDSA Therapy	ATS Group	ATS Therapy
Outpatients	Macrolide,[1] or doxycycline (Vibramycin) or FQ[2] *or* alternative[1]	I (no CPD[3] or DRSP[4] risk)	Macrolide *or* doxycycline (Vibramycin)
		II (CPD, DRSP risk or enteric GNR)	β-lactam[5] + macrolide *or* FQ
Inpatient non-ICU[6]	β-lactam + macrolide *or* FQ	IIIa (CPD or DRSP risk or enteric GNR)	IV β-lactam + macrolide *or* FQ
		IIIb (no CPD, DRSP risk or enteric GNR)	IV azithromycin (β-lactam + doxycycline (Vibramycin) for azithromycin allergy) *or* IV FQ
Inpatient ICU	β-lactam + macrolide *or* β-lactam + FQ (Clindamycin-Cleocin for β-lactam in case of allergy	Iva (no *Pseudomonas* risk)	IV β-lactam + IV azithromycin *or* FQ
		Ivb (*Pseudomonas* risk)	Antipseudomonal β-lactam[7], cephalosporin[8], or Carbapenem[9] + FQ *or* antipseudomonal β-lactam + AG[10] + IV macrolide *or* IV FQ (Aztreonam [Azactam] for β-lactam allergy)
Alternatives: amoxicillin/ clavulanate (Augmentin), cefuroxime (Ceftin), cefpodoxime (Vantin), cefprozil (Cefzil)			

[1]Macrolide = azithromycin (Zithromax) or clarithromycin (Biaixin)
[2]FQ = Fluoroquinolone-levafloxacin (Levaquin), moxifloxacin (Avelox), gatifloxacin (Tequin), gemifloxacin (Factive)
[3]CPD = cardiopulmonary disease—COPD or CHF (chronic obstructive pulmonary disease, congestive heart failure.)
[4]DRSP = risk factors for drug-resistant *S. pneumonia*
[5]Recommended β-lactam: ceftriaxone (Rocephin), cefotaxime (Claforan), ampicillin/sulbactam (Unasyn), piperacillin/tazobactam (Zosyn)
[6]ICU = intensive care unit
[7]Antipseudomonal β-lactam: piperacillin (Pipracil), piperacillin/tazobactam (Zosyn)
[8]Antipseudomonal cephalosporin: cefepime (Maxipime), ceftazidime (Fortaz)
[9]Carbapenem: Imipenem (Primaxin), meropenem (Merem)
[10]AG = aminoglycoside: gentamicin (Garamicin), tobramycin (Tobrex), amikacin (Amikin)

Rakel and Bope: *Conn's Current Therapy 2006.*

Prevention

Only one pneumococcal vaccine (Pneumovax 23) is approved for use in adults in the United States and is composed of capsular polysaccharides from 23 common disease-causing serotypes of *S. pneumoniae*. Currently, vaccination is recommended for persons older than 65 years or those who have underlying medical conditions including chronic pulmonary disease, cardiovascular disease, chronic liver disease, chronic kidney disease or hemodialysis, diabetes mellitus, functional or anatomic asplenia, immunosuppressive conditions, and residents of nursing homes or other long-term care facilities. Revaccination after 5 years is recommended for those with chronic renal disease, functional or anatomic asplenia, immunosuppressive conditions, and those older than 65 years who received the vaccine more than 5 years earlier and were older than 65 years at the time. Retrospective studies have shown a reduction in pneumonia and invasive disease, but few prospective studies have confirmed this effect. However, vaccination remains an important intervention in the prevention of pneumonia.

REFERENCES

Alfageme I, Munoz F, Pena N, et al: Empyema of the thorax in adults: Etiology, microbiologic findings, and management. Chest 1993; 103:839-843.

Clave-Sanchez AJ, Giron-Gonzalez JA, Lopez-Prieto D, et al: Multivariate analysis of risk factors for infection caused by penicillin resistant and multidrug resistant *Streptococcus pneumoniae*: A multicenter study. Clin Infect Dis 1997;24:1052-1059.

Colice GL, Curtis A, Deslauriers J, et al: Medical and surgical treatment of para-pneumonic effusions: an evidence-based guideline. Chest 2000;118:1158-1171.

Dennesen PJW, van der Ven AJAM, Kessels AGH, et al: Resolution of infectious parameters after antimicrobial therapy in patients with ventilator-associated pneumonia. Am J Respir Crit Care Med 2001;163:1371-1375.

Dunbar LM, Wunderink RG, Habib MP, et al: High-dose, short-course levofloxacin for community-acquired pneumonia: A new treatment paradigm. Clin Infect Dis 2003;37(6):752-760.

Eibenberger KL, Dock WI, Ammann ME, et al: Quantification of pleural effusions: sonography versus radiography. Radiology 1994; 191:681-684.

Fine MJ, Auble TE, Yealy, DM, et al: A prediction rule to identify low-risk patients with community-acquired pneumonia. N Engl J Med 1997;336(4):243-250.

Light RW: Pleural effusions. N Engl J Med 2002;346:1971-1977.

Mandell LA, Bartlett JB, Dowell SF, et al: Update of practice guidelines for the management of community-acquired pneumonia in immunocompetent adults. Clin Infect Dis 2003;37(11):1405-1433.

Niederman MS, Craven DE, et al: Guidelines for the management of adults with hospital acquired, ventilator associated, and health-care associated pneumonia. Am J Respir Crit Care Med 2005; 171:388-416.

Niederman MS, Mandell LA, Anzueto A, et al: Guidelines for the management of adults with community-acquired pneumonia. Am J Respir Crit Care Med 2001;163:1730-1754.

Raptopoulos V, David LM, Lee G, et al: Factors affecting the development of pneumothorax associated with thoracentesis. AJR Am J Radiol 1991;156:917-920.

Woodhead DM: Community-acquired pneumonia: severity of illness evaluation. Infect Dis Clin North Am 2004;18:791-807.

Viral Respiratory Infections

Method of
Ronald B. Turner, MD

Viral infections of the respiratory tract are among the most common infections of humans. Rhinovirus, coronavirus, parainfluenza virus, influenza virus, adenovirus, metapneumovirus, and respiratory syncytial virus (RSV) are all important pathogens that cause viral respiratory syndromes. Although some of these pathogens are traditionally associated with distinctive clinical syndromes, there is considerable overlap in the illnesses caused by these viruses. The treatment of viral respiratory infections is, with only a few exceptions, limited to symptomatic therapies.

The seasonal increase in viral respiratory infection begins with an increase in rhinovirus infections from September through October. Outbreaks of parainfluenza virus infection (types 1 and 2) tend to occur in the late fall and are then followed by RSV, metapneumovirus, and influenza in the winter and early spring months. A less predictable increase in rhinovirus infections may occur in the late spring. Coronavirus and adenovirus have a less distinctive seasonal pattern.

Common Cold

The clinical syndrome most frequently associated with viral respiratory infection is the common cold. The rhinoviruses are responsible for the majority of these illnesses, but the other viral respiratory pathogens can cause an indistinguishable syndrome. The characteristic common cold associated with rhinovirus infection usually begins with a sore or *scratchy* throat. This symptom is quickly followed by development of nasal obstruction and rhinorrhea. These symptoms increase in severity over the next 24 to 48 hours before gradually resolving. The nasal symptoms of obstruction and rhinorrhea are most often identified as the most bothersome symptoms of the cold. Cough, reported by 30% to 40% of patients, tends to occur later in the course of the illness and may persist as other symptoms resolve. Systemic symptoms of fever or myalgia are usually not associated with rhinovirus colds, but they may be more frequent during common cold illnesses caused by other viral respiratory pathogens.

The common cold is a benign and self-limited illness but may be associated with medically important complications. The sinuses are abnormal in a majority of patients with a common cold. These abnormalities resolve without antibiotic treatment and occur with sufficient frequency that they should be considered a part of the common cold syndrome rather than a complication. The middle ear is also frequently affected by the common cold. As many as 60% of children with common cold symptoms have abnormal middle ear pressure and up to 30% of children with colds are diagnosed with otitis media.

Many of these patients appear to have viral otitis media, which presumably would resolve without antibiotics, whereas others have bacterial otitis media as a complication of their underlying viral illness. Other complications associated with viral upper respiratory illnesses in specific patient populations include exacerbations of asthma, cystic fibrosis, and chronic bronchitis.

The treatment of the common cold is limited to symptomatic therapy. Studies in adults have demonstrated the beneficial effects of the adrenergic decongestants, antihistamines, and analgesics. Studies in children have not found similar benefits, and it is unclear whether this is because of the difficulty of assessing symptom severity in children or to real age-related differences in therapeutic response. The use of the symptomatic therapies should be directed at specific symptoms and must take into account the expected benefits and known side effects of these medications. None of the symptomatic treatments has been shown to prevent otitis media, sinusitis, or exacerbations of underlying pulmonary disease.

TREATMENT OF NASAL OBSTRUCTION

Oral adrenergic agents such as pseudoephedrine (Sudafed) and topical adrenergic agents such as oxymetazoline (Afrin) have demonstrated effects on nasal obstruction. The oral agents reduce obstruction by approximately 20% compared with placebo. These agents also have systemic effects and can cause side effects such as increased blood pressure, nervousness, and insomnia. The topical adrenergic agents reduce obstruction by approximately 80% compared with placebo. The side effects of these agents include nasal irritation and rebound congestion with prolonged use.

TREATMENT OF RHINORRHEA

The runny nose associated with the common cold can be treated with either oral first-generation antihistamines or topical anticholinergic agents. The first-generation antihistamines such as clemastine (Tavist) reduce rhinorrhea by approximately 25% compared with placebo. The mechanism of the treatment effect appears to involve anticholinergic rather than antihistaminic activity because second-generation antihistamines such as loratadine (Claritin) have no effect. The side effects of the first-generation antihistamines also are associated with their anticholinergic activity and include sedation and drying of the nose and mouth. Administration of ipratropium bromide (Atrovent 0.06%) as a nasal spray has an effect comparable to that of the antihistamines for treatment of rhinorrhea. Nasal irritation is the primary side effect.

TREATMENT OF SORE THROAT, HEADACHE, AND MYALGIA

Pain symptoms associated with the common cold can be treated with cyclooxygenase inhibitors such as ibuprofen (Advil) or acetaminophen (Tylenol).

CURRENT DIAGNOSIS

- Knowledge of which pathogen is circulating in the community together with a distinctive clinical syndrome can provide insight into the likely viral pathogen, which is sufficiently accurate for most clinical situations.
- Rapid diagnostic testing is available for influenza and RSV, but this testing is generally unnecessary for the management of patients.

Abbreviation: RSV = respiratory syncytial virus.

TREATMENT OF COUGH

Although commonly used, cough suppression with either codeine or dextromethorphan (Benylin) has not been shown to be effective for treatment of cough caused by the common cold. Very limited data suggest that treatment with first-generation antihistamines or antihistamine-decongestant combinations may have a modest effect on cough. This potential effect must be balanced against the known side effects of these agents.

There has been significant interest in zinc[1] and echinacea[1] as potential treatments for the common cold. Although the results of different studies have been somewhat inconsistent, it appears that these treatments have little effect on common cold symptoms.

Influenza

Influenza is another important clinical syndrome caused by viral respiratory infection. This syndrome is caused only by the influenza viruses, but other viral pathogens may be associated with an influenza-like illness. Influenza refers to an illness characterized by the abrupt onset of fever, chills, headache, and myalgia. Respiratory symptoms may be present, but the most bothersome symptoms are usually headache and myalgia. The fever generally lasts 3 to 4 days and resolves along with the other symptoms. Complete recovery may require 1 to 2 weeks.

Treatment of influenza is generally symptomatic, but effective, specific antiviral therapy is available. Four different antiviral drugs are available. The neuraminidase inhibitors such as oseltamivir (Tamiflu) are most frequently used, but M2 inhibitors such as rimantadine (Flumadine) also are effective against the influenza A viruses. The recommended dose of oseltamivir (Tamiflu)

[1]Not FDA approved for this indication.

CURRENT THERAPY

Treatment of viral respiratory infections is primarily symptomatic. Specific antiviral treatment is available only for influenza.

for treatment of adults is 75 mg twice each day for 5 days. Specific antiviral treatment modestly reduces the duration of illness and may reduce associated otitis media in children.

Croup

Croup is most commonly caused by the parainfluenza viruses and is primarily an illness of young children. This illness begins with common cold symptoms that progress to development of a barky cough and inspiratory stridor. Treatment is focused on appropriate management of the airway obstruction with hospitalization if necessary. Treatment with dexamethasone (Decadron)[1] as a single dose of 0.6 mg/kg given either orally or intramuscularly shortens the duration of the illness.

REFERENCES

Akerlund A, Klint T, Olen L, Rundcrantz H: Nasal decongestant effect of oxymetazoline in the common cold: An objective dose-response study in 106 patients. J Laryngol Otol 1989;103:743-746.

Ausejo M, Saenz A, Pham B, et al: Glucocorticoids for croup. Cochrane Database Syst Rev 2004;(1):CD001955; PMID:14973975.

Curley FJ, Irwin RS, Pratter MR, et al: Cough and the common cold. Am J Respir Crit Care Med 1988;138:305-311.

Diamond L, Dockhorn RJ, Grossman J, et al: A dose-response study of the efficacy and safety of ipratropium bromide nasal spray in the treatment of the common cold. J Allergy Clin Immunol 1995; 95:1139-1146.

Gwaltney JM Jr, Druce HM: Efficacy of brompheniramine maleate for the treatment of rhinovirus colds. Clin Infect Dis 1997; 25:1188-1194.

Muether PS, Gwaltney JM Jr: Variant effect of first- and second-generation antihistamines as clues to their mechanism of action on the sneeze reflex in the common cold. Clin Infect Dis 2001; 33:1483-1488.

Taverner D, Danz C, Economos D: The effects of oral pseudoephedrine on nasal patency in the common cold: A double-blind single-dose placebo-controlled trial. Clin Otolaryngol 1999;24:47-51.

Treanor JJ, Hayden FG, Vrooman PS, et al: Efficacy and safety of the oral neuraminidase inhibitor oseltamivir in treating acute influenza: A randomized controlled trial. US Oral Neuraminidase Study Group. JAMA 2000;283:1016-1024.

Turner RB, Sperber SJ, Sorrentino JV, et al: Effectiveness of clemastine fumarate for treatment of rhinorrhea and sneezing associated with the common cold. Clin Infect Dis 1997;25:824-830.

Van Voris LP, Betts RF, Hayden FG, et al: Successful treatment of naturally occurring influenza A/USSR/77 H1N1. JAMA 1981;245:1128-1131.

---

[1]Not FDA approved for this indication.

Rakel and Bope: *Conn's Current Therapy 2006.*

Viral and Mycoplasmal Pneumonia

Method of
Stephen B. Greenberg, MD

Viral and mycoplasmal pneumonias are reported in otherwise healthy patients and in immunocompromised hosts. The most common viral causes of pneumonia in adults are influenzavirus types A and B. Proven viral pneumonias in immunocompromised hosts are most likely caused by cytomegalovirus, herpes simplex viruses, varicella-zoster virus, adenovirus, and measles virus. Specific populations such as the military may have more prevalent viral pneumonias secondary to adenovirus. *Mycoplasma pneumoniae* can cause either tracheobronchitis or pneumonia in children and young adults.

Mycoplasma Pneumoniae

M. pneumoniae is associated with up to 30% of community-acquired pneumonia (CAP) cases in adults. It is most common in young adults and in those more than 65 years of age. Less than 10% of hospitalized cases are caused by proven *M. pneumoniae*, however, *M. pneumoniae* is transmitted by the aerosol route—person to person. The most common clinical presentation of *M. pneumoniae* infections is pharyngitis or tracheobronchitis. Only 5% to 10% of cases progress to pneumonia. Cough can be a major chronic symptom. Fever, malaise, and headache are other common symptoms and signs. Extrapulmonary manifestations include erythema multiforme, meningoencephalitis, hemolytic anemia, IgA nephropathy, as well as nonspecific ear symptoms.

M. pneumoniae can elicit an interstitial mononuclear inflammation in the lungs. Radiographically, diffuse, reticular infiltrates in the perihilar regions or lower lobes are common. Although unilateral infiltrates are most common, 20% of cases have bilateral involvement. Lobar consolidation with bilateral alveolar involvement is reported. The degree of consolidation may be worse than the severity of clinical manifestations suggest. Pleural effusions may occur but are usually small.

Histopathologic findings in *M. pneumoniae* pneumonia include lesions of the epithelial lining of the mucosal surfaces with ulceration and destruction of ciliated epithelium of bronchi and bronchioles. Macrophage infiltration, bronchial wall edema, and bronchiolitis obliterans are described. Immunosuppressed patients may lack pulmonary infiltrates.

In *M. pneumoniae* infection, laboratory findings are rarely diagnostic. Although cold agglutinin titers were used in the past as a diagnostic test, the availability of specific antibody tests make these titers less useful and reserved for cases in which mycoplasmal pneumonia is a likely possibility. Culture of *M. pneumoniae* is expensive, takes a long time, and therefore is not routinely recommended. Rapid assays for direct antigen detection have limited use because of low sensitivity. Polymerase chain reaction (PCR) assays may prove sensitive and specific, but currently they are not standardized, unavailable for routine use, and expensive.

M. pneumoniae is inhibited by tetracyclines, macrolides, ketolides, and fluoroquinolones. All mycoplasmas are resistant to all β-lactam and glycopeptide antibiotics. Macrolides and tetracyclines are bacteriostatic against *M. pneumoniae*. Fluoroquinolones are bacteriocidal. However, macrolides are considered the treatment of choice in both adults and children. Clarithromycin (Biaxin) and azithromycin (Zithromax) are equally effective, with cure rates exceeding 90%. Newer fluoroquinolones, such as levofloxacin (Levaquin) and moxifloxacin (Avelox), are effective clinically.

Viral Pneumonia

Influenzavirus types A and, more rarely, B are the most common causes of viral pneumonia. During outbreaks, influenza virus may be the cause of 10% of CAP requiring hospitalization. Influenzavirus infection can present as a primary pneumonia with diffuse interstitial infiltrates, hypoxia, and high mortality rates. This complication is rare. More commonly, acute influenza illness leads to superimposed or subsequent bacterial pneumonia secondary to *S. pneumoniae* or *Staphylococcus aureus*.

The most prominent histologic changes in viral pneumonia are observed in the epithelium and interstitial tissue. Parenchymal involvement involves the lung adjacent to the terminal and respiratory bronchioles. Rapidly progressive pneumonia can have diffuse alveolar damage with interstitial lymphocyte infiltration, air-space hemorrhage, edema, and fibrin type 2 cell hyperplasia and hyaline pneumonia formation.

Radiographically, viral pneumonia demonstrates small nodules and patchy areas of peribronchial ground-glass opacities and air-space consolidation. Hyperinflation is also common. With progression of the pneumonia, there is confluence of consolidation leading to diffuse alveolar damage.

Diagnosis can be made presumptively during known community-wide outbreaks based on clinical presentation. Specific diagnosis of influenzavirus infection can be confirmed by viral culture, rapid antigen assay, and PCR. Several antigen detection assays are commercially available and useful if positive. These rapid antigen assays for influenzavirus are more sensitive in children than adults because of the increased quantity of influenzavirus shedding in nasopharyngeal secretions.

Specific anti-influenza agents include the M2 ion channel inhibitors, amantadine (Symmetrel) and rimantadine (Flumadine), and the neuraminidase inhibitors, zanamivir (Relenza) and oseltamivir (Tamiflu). Amantadine and rimantadine are effective only against influenzavirus A. The neuraminidase inhibitors are effective against both influenzaviruses A and B. The best clinical results with either of these antiviral agents are found when they are initiated within the first

48 hours of symptom onset. None of these agents is approved for the treatment of influenza pneumonia, although anecdotal evidence supports their use and possible benefits. Prevention of influenza is best provided with yearly administration of the influenza vaccine.

Respiratory syncytial virus (RSV) has a similar epidemiology to influenza with outbreaks occurring during the winter months. RSV is a major cause of morbidity in children younger than 5 years of age and in persons older than 65 years of age. Bronchiolitis is the most common presentation in young children clinically, but it can cause pneumonia as well. RSV pneumonia occurs in premature infants, in children with bronchopulmonary dysplasia and cystic fibrosis, and in adults with chronic obstructive pulmonary disease (COPD) or post-transplantation. Diagnosis can be made by antigen detection or viral culture. A rapid enzyme immunoassay with good sensitivity and specificity is commercially available.

Treatments with ribavirin (Virazole), corticosteroids, and bronchodilators do not demonstrate significant improvement in outcomes for RSV pneumonia. Prophylaxis with RSV immunoglobulin (RespiGam) or monoclonal antibody to IgE (Xolair)[1] reduces the incidence of RSV hospitalizations, but treatment of RSV pneumonia with these agents is not effective.

Parainfluenza virus types 1, 2, and 3 do cause lower respiratory tract infections in young children. Serotype 3 is associated more with bronchiolitis and pneumonia, and serotypes 1 and 2 are associated more with croup. In elderly and immunosuppressed adults, parainfluenza viruses rarely cause pneumonia. Diagnostic tests include viral cultures, antigen detections assays, PCR, or serology. No specific approved antivirals are available for parainfluenza virus infections.

Adenovirus pneumonia is reported in young children and military recruits, but rarely in immunosuppressed patients post-transplantation. Diagnostic tests include viral culture, antigen detection, PCR, and serology. No specific antiviral agents are approved for use. An approved adenovirus type 4 and type 7 vaccine is currently not being manufactured.

Immunosuppressed patients are most likely to develop pneumonia secondary to the herpesvirus family, which includes cytomegalovirus (CMV), varicella-zoster virus (VZV), and herpes simplex virus (HSV). Diagnosis of CMV requires bronchial samples and detection of viral DNA, intranuclear inclusions, or culture. Patients with these pneumonias are usually on immunosuppressive drugs or receiving cytotoxic chemotherapy. Antiviral treatments are available and depend on the specific herpesvirus detected. These viral pneumonias are best cared for after consultation with an infectious disease specialist.

---

[1]Not FDA approved for this indication.

Legionellosis (Legionnaires' Disease and Pontiac Fever)

Method of
Miguel Sabria, MD, PhD

Legionnaires' disease is a pneumonic illness caused by *Legionella* bacteria. *Legionella* include more than 49 species, such as *Legionella pneumophila,* which is responsible for up to 80% of the cases of pneumonia. Other species causing legionnaires' disease are *Legionella micdadei, Legionella bozemanii, Legionella dumoffii,* and *Legionella longbeachae.* Pontiac fever is a nonpneumonic, self-limited infection caused by *Legionella* species not requiring antimicrobial treatment.

Clinical Presentation

High fever, shivering, headache, and myalgia appear after 2 to 10 days of incubation. Respiratory symptoms such as productive cough or thoracic pain are not prevalent. Dyspnea is infrequent except in severe cases of legionnaires' disease. Physical examination shows involvement of the general status of the patient, prostration, obnubilation, and high fever. Radiologic findings are nonspecific. Despite appropriate antibiotic therapy, however, progression of pulmonary infiltrates is suggestive of legionnaires' disease. A common cause of severe pneumonia requiring admission to the intensive care unit (ICU), legionnaires' disease ranks among the three most common causes of severe pneumonia in the community setting.

Diagnosis

From a clinical point of view, it is very difficult to distinguish pneumonia by *Legionella* from other community- or hospital-acquired pneumonias. Suspicion of legionnaires' disease should be raised by an adequate epidemiologic context, the presence of headache, confusion, hyponatremia, elevated creatine kinase (CK), and/or severe pneumonia. A history of smoking, unresponsiveness to β-lactamic drugs, and sputum full of neutrophils with scarce microorganisms are indicative data. A chest radiograph almost always shows a pulmonary infiltrate at the time of clinical presentation.

Definitive diagnosis of legionnaires' disease is established by recovery of the microorganism from respiratory secretions on selective media (buffered charcoal yeast extract [BCYE]-alpha supplemented with polymyxin B, ansamycin, and cefamandole). The detection of the *Legionella* urinary antigen is a useful technique for the diagnosis of legionnaires' disease. The urinary antigen appears very early during the course of the disease and usually disappears within 2 months, but its excretion may be longer in patients receiving immunosuppressive

treatment or corticoids. The main limitation of the urinary antigen is that it detects only the soluble antigen of *L. pneumophila* serogroup 1. Other specific laboratory tests are direct fluorescent antibody stain and seroconversion of antibodies to *L. pneumophila.*

Pontiac fever is diagnosed by seroconversion in a patient with the typical clinical manifestations of headache, fever, and myalgias.

Therapy

Because *Legionella* is an intracellular pathogen, the optimal antibiotic therapy for legionnaires' disease are those antibiotics that penetrate white blood cells (WBCs) and alveolar macrophages. β-Lactam antibiotics such as penicillins and cephalosporins are ineffective because of their poor intracellular penetration. Macrolides, fluoroquinolones, rifampin (Rifadin),[1] trimethoprim-sulfamethoxazole (Bactrim),[1] and tetracyclines have excellent intracellular penetration.

The newer macrolides (azithromycin [Zithromax],[1] clarithromycin [Biaxin][1]), and quinolones (levofloxacin [Levaquin],[1] moxifloxacin [Avelox][1], or gemifloxacin [Factive][1]) are the antibiotics of choice for legionnaires' disease.

Azithromycin (Zithromax)[1] has been found to be the most active macrolide against *Legionella.* It has an excellent macrophage penetration, good distribution on lung tissue, and potent intracellular activity. Azithromycin (Zithromax)[1] produces prolonged inhibition of *Legionella* growing in the intracellular model. This prolonged inhibition may be of importance in immunosuppressed patients in whom the intracellular clearance of *Legionella* is presumably slower.

Quinolones are the most active drugs against *Legionella* in intracellular and animal models. Like azithromycin (Zithromax),[1] fluoroquinolones produce prolonged inhibition of *Legionella* growing in the intracellular model. Time to apyrexia and hospital discharge used to be shorter in patients receiving fluoroquinolones compared to those receiving macrolides. Moreover, unlike the macrolides, they do not interact with cyclosporine (Neoral) or tacrolimus (Prograf), which are administered to transplant recipients.

Other antibiotics that may be effective include tetracycline,[1] doxycycline (Vibramycin),[1] and trimethoprim-sulfamethoxazole (Bactrim).[1] Rifampin (Rifadin)[1] combined with another antibiotic has been used in patients with severe legionnaires' disease who are not responding to monotherapy. However, the combination of a quinolone (levofloxacin [Levaquin][1] or ciprofloxacin [Cipro][1]) with a macrolide (azithromycin) may be especially considered in this context.

The initial administration should be intravenous (IV) because the oral route may be unreliable in patients with gastrointestinal symptoms. Once an objective response has occurred, oral therapy can be given. Duration of therapy can be 7 to 10 days in immunocompetent

---

[1]Not FDA approved for this indication.

CURRENT THERAPY

Antimicrobial agent	Dosage*
Macrolides	
Azithromycin (Zithromax)[1‡]	500 mg PO or IV q24h
Clarithromycin (Biaxin)[1]	500 mg PO or IV[†] q12h
Quinolones	
Levofloxacin (Levaquin)	750 mg[†] IV q24h
	500 mg*[‡] IV q24h
	500 mg[‡] PO q24h
Ciprofloxacin (Cipro)[1]	400 mg IV q8h
	750 mg PO q12h
Ofloxacin (Floxin)[1]	400 mg PO or IV q12h
Moxifloxacin (Avelox)[1]	400[‡] PO q24h
Tetracyclines	
Doxycycline (Vibramycin)[1‡]	100 mg PO or IV q12h
Minocycline (Minocin)[1]	100 mg PO or IV q12h
Tetracycline	500 mg PO or IV q6h
Others	
Trimethoprim/	160 and 800 mg IV q8h
Sulfamethoxazole (Bactrim)[1]	160 and 800 mg PO q12h
Rifampin (Rifadin)[1§]	300-600 mg PO or IV q12h

*Dosages are based on clinical experience and not on controlled trials.
[†]750 mg dose form unavailable in some countries.
[‡]We recommend doubling the first dose.
[§]Rifampin should be only used as part of combination therapy with a quinolone or a macrolide.
[1]Not FDA approved for this indication.
Abbreviations: IV = intravenously; PO = orally.

patients. In immunosuppressed patients treatment with a quinolone or azithromycin and longer therapy (21 days) are recommended.

The newer macrolides and respiratory tract quinolones are also ideal antibiotics for empiric therapy of community-acquired pneumonia in the immunocompetent patient; they cover both the *typical* microorganisms such as *Streptococcus pneumoniae* and *Haemophilus influenzae* as well as the *atypical* microorganisms such as *L. pneumophila, Chlamydia pneumoniae,* and *Mycoplasma pneumoniae.* Antibiotic therapy is not necessary for Pontiac fever.

Pulmonary Embolism

Method of
Victor F. Tapson, MD

Venous thromboembolism (VTE) represents the spectrum of deep venous thrombosis (DVT) and the potentially fatal entity of pulmonary embolism (PE) with the latter responsible for as many as 60,000 to 200,000 deaths in the United States every year. Most commonly, PE results from DVT that develops in the legs, but

upper extremity thrombosis is common, particularly in patients with central venous catheters, and these clots may embolize also. The risk of PE is higher in patients with proximal DVT than in patients with only calf-vein thrombosis. The diagnosis should be suspected in patients presenting with dyspnea, chest pain (particularly, but not only, pleuritic), hemoptysis, and syncope; other nonspecific symptoms and signs may be present as well, and the diagnosis may be particularly elusive in patients with underlying cardiopulmonary disease. Leg pain, tenderness, swelling, and Homans' sign may suggest the diagnosis of DVT (with or without PE) but these findings are neither sensitive nor specific. The presence of risk factors for DVT, and thus PE, such as prior VTE, cancer, older age, obesity, surgery, trauma, and acute medical illness should raise the suspicion for DVT and PE if a consistent clinical scenario is present. Such risk factors also should prompt the use of prophylactic measures. Hospitalized patients are frequently at risk because such individuals have underlying disease that may increase the risk for VTE, and because they are immobilized to varying degrees, rendering them susceptible.

The Diagnostic Approach to Acute Pulmonary Embolism

The chest radiograph and electrocardiogram (ECG) may offer clues to alternative diagnoses, but they are nonspecific for PE. For suspected PE, ventilation-perfusion scanning followed by pulmonary arteriography has been the gold-standard approach for decades. Spiral (helical) computed tomography (CT) scanning is used increasingly, and in many hospitals is the procedure of choice for suspected PE. When PE is suspected, leg studies may be useful if a scan cannot be easily obtained or interpreted. There should be a low threshold for proceeding with a diagnostic evaluation when PE is suspected. In severely ill patients who may be candidates for aggressive treatment, such as thrombolytic therapy or open embolectomy, bedside echocardiographic evaluation for massive central emboli and evaluation of right ventricular function may hasten therapeutic interventions. For the diagnosis of suspected DVT, ultrasound is the appropriate initial test with magnetic resonance imaging (MRI), or a venography is sometimes necessary. D-dimer testing is most useful when there is a relatively low suspicion for DVT or PE. The enzyme-linked immunoabsorbent assay (ELISA)-based tests are the most sensitive. A negative test in the latter setting may eliminate the need for further evaluation. If clinical suspicion is higher, objective radiographic imaging is crucial.

Initial Therapy for Acute Pulmonary Embolism

When there is a high clinical suspicion for acute DVT or PE, initiation of therapy should be considered even before confirmation of the diagnosis, as long as the risk of anticoagulation appears to be minimal. Confirmatory diagnostic testing should be arranged as soon as possible if anticoagulation is to be continued. The issue of bedrest is frequently raised in patients with acute DVT and/or PE. At present, there is no convincing data suggesting that bedrest is necessary, although in patients with extensive, symptomatic DVT, bedrest is advisable until the initial inflammation and swelling begin to subside.

Options for initial treatment include anticoagulation with heparin or low-molecular-weight heparin (LMWH), thrombolytic therapy, and inferior vena cava filter (IVCF) placement. The approaches to anticoagulation for DVT and for PE are essentially the same. Massive PE may occasionally be treated with surgical embolectomy. Each therapeutic approach has specific indications as well as advantages and disadvantages.

UNFRACTIONATED HEPARIN

By accelerating the action of antithrombin III, heparin and LMWH exert a prompt antithrombotic effect that prevents thrombus extension. They do not directly dissolve the thrombus, but allow the fibrinolytic system to proceed unopposed and more readily reduce the size of the thromboembolic burden. While thrombus growth can be prevented, early recurrence sometimes may develop even when anticoagulation is therapeutic. Specific settings may require alternative therapies as when direct thrombin inhibitors are used for heparin-induced thrombocytopenia with or without proven thrombosis.

When continuous intravenous unfractionated heparin (UFH) is initiated, the activated partial thromboplastin time (aPTT) must be followed at 6-hour intervals until it is consistently in the therapeutic range of 1.5 to 2.0 times the control value. This range corresponds to a heparin level of 0.2 to 0.4 µ/mL as measured by protamine sulfate titration. Because achieving a therapeutic aPTT within 24 hours after PE reduces the recurrence rate, it is clear that the traditional heparin regimen, consisting of a 5000 unit bolus at 1000 units/hour, is often inadequate. Heparin should be administered in one of several ways. An intravenous bolus of 5000 units followed by a maintenance dose of 30,000 to 40,000 units per 24 hours by continuous infusion is one approach. The lower dose is administered if the patient is considered at high risk for bleeding. This aggressive approach decreases the risk of subtherapeutic anticoagulation. An alternative regimen, consisting of a bolus of 80 U/kg followed by 18 U/kg per hour is recommended by the American College of Chest Physicians in their 2001 Consensus Conference on Antithrombotic Therapy. Subsequent adjusting of heparin also should be weight-based.

Warfarin (Coumadin) generally is initiated the same day as parenteral anticoagulation unless the risk of bleeding suggests that the longer acting oral anticoagulant should be temporarily withheld. It is possible that early initiation of warfarin, *without* heparin or LMWH may intensify hypercoagulability and increase the clot burden caused by the short half-life of anticoagulation factors that are inhibited by warfarin. Factor VII is the primary clotting factor affecting the prothrombin time; it has a half-life of approximately 6 hours. Definitive anticoagulation requires the depletion of factor II (thrombin), which takes approximately 5 days. Thus, at least 5 days of intravenous heparin or subcutaneous LMWH is recommended. Heparin is maintained at a therapeutic level until two consecutive therapeutic international normalized ratio (INR) values of 2.0 to 3.0 have been documented at least 24 hours apart. The first several doses of warfarin should be 5 or 10 mg, depending on the size of the patient, and generally it is administered in the evening. Subsequent dosing is based upon the INR value.

LOW-MOLECULAR-WEIGHT HEPARIN

The LMWH preparations have tremendous advantages compared with unfractionated heparin and have had a substantial impact upon the treatment of thromboembolic disease. Among the differences between these two substances is the greater bioavailability of the LMWHs and more predictable dosing. They can be subcutaneously administered once or twice per day even at therapeutic doses and do not require monitoring in most settings. Intravenous LMWH is never required for therapy of DVT or PE. Subcutaneous LMWH is replacing standard heparin in many settings. Numerous clinical trials strongly suggest the efficacy and safety of LMWH for treatment of established acute DVT and PE. These trials, which used recurrent symptomatic VTE and bleeding as outcome measures, indicate that LMWH preparations are at least as effective and as safe as unfractionated heparin. At least one meta-analysis suggests that LMWH preparations result in less bleeding and lower mortality than unfractionated heparin for the treatment of acute VTE. The lower mortality is not entirely explained by a reduction in fatal PE. Presently, the two LMWH preparations that are FDA-approved for treatment of DVT with or without PE are enoxaparin (Lovenox) and tinzaparin (Innohep). A comparison of LMWH with standard, unfractionated heparin is provided in Table 1.

Unlike unfractionated heparin, LMWHs do not require monitoring in most settings. This is supported by extensive experience from large clinical trials. However, monitoring appears appropriate in a few clinical settings such as in morbidly obese patients (>150 kg [331 lb]), very small patients (<40 kg [88 lb]), pregnant patients, and those with renal insufficiency. Because these drugs are renally metabolized, monitoring is particularly important when the creatinine clearance is less than 30 mL/minute. A patient might be expected to require a dose of two thirds of the usual dose when the creatinine clearance is less than 30 mL/minute. With more severe renal insufficiency, standard heparin should be considered. The LMWHs have a more profound effect with regard to inhibiting clotting factor Xa relative to thrombin, and when patients on these drugs are monitored, it is the anti-Xa level (sometimes referred to as an LMWH level) that should be checked and not the aPTT. The steps for anticoagulating with LMWH are outlined in Box 1.

TABLE 1 Comparison of LMWH with Unfractionated Heparin

Characteristic	UFH*	LMWH
Mean molecular	12,000-15,000	4,000-6,000 weight
Protein binding	Substantial	Minimal
Bioavailability	Substantial	Much lower/less predictable
Heparin-induced	Incidence 3%-4%	Much less common[†] thrombocytopenia
Anti-Xa activity	Substantial	Substantial
Anti-IIa activity	Substantial	Minimal
Monitoring	aPTT every 6h	None in most settings[†]
Outpatient therapy	Difficult	Simplified

*LMWH should not be used for treatment of established heparin-induced thrombocytopenia (HIT).
[†]In certain circumstances, the anti-Xa level is appropriate to monitor. This should be considered when weight ≥150 kg or ≤40 kg, creatinine clearance <30 mL/min, and in pregnant patients.
Abbreviations: aPTT = activated partial thromboplastin time; LMWH = low-molecular-weight heparin; UFH = unfractionated heparin.

OTHER AGENTS FOR INITIAL THERAPY

A very-low-molecular-weight (pentasaccharide) heparin (fondaparinux [Arixtra][1]) has proved effective for the treatment of both DVT and PE in two separate large, randomized trials. Like the LMWHs, fondaparinux is administered subcutaneously. It is a pure factor Xa inhibitor. However, at present this agent does not have the FDA-approved indication for treatment of acute DVT or PE. Another agent, an oral direct thrombin inhibitor called ximelagatran (Exanta),* has proved effective for the treatment of acute DVT and PE, both for long-term management instead of warfarin, and as initial therapy. It has not yet been evaluated for FDA approval in the United States.

---

[1]Not FDA approved for this indication.
*Investigational drug in the United States.

BOX 1   Initiation of LMWH for Therapy of Acute Deep Venous Thrombosis (DVT) and Pulmonary Embolism (PE)

- Begin LMWH by subcutaneous administration.*
- Determine whether monitoring is needed (extremes of weight, renal insufficiency, pregnancy).
- Administer warfarin from day 1; initial dose 5-10 mg, adjusted according to INR.
- Check platelet count between days 3 and 5.
- Stop LMWH after ≥5 days of combined therapy and when INR is ≥2.0 for 2 consecutive days.
- Anticoagulate with warfarin for ≥3 months (goal, INR = 2.0-3.0).

*Enoxaparin (Lovenox) and tinzaparin (Innohep) are the two LMWHs that are FDA-approved for treatment of VTE. While LMWH preparations sometimes are used for patients presenting with PE in the United States, and while clinical trials support this use, the FDA approval reads "established DVT with or without PE."
Abbreviations: INR = international normalized ratio; LMWH = low-molecular-weight heparin. DVT = deep venous thrombosis. PE = pulmonary embolism.

OUTPATIENT THERAPY OF ACUTE DEEP VENOUS THROMBOSIS AND PULMONARY EMBOLISM

Patients with acute DVT can be treated as outpatients if they meet certain criteria. While outpatient treatment of PE has been studied and is feasible, it is not commonly practiced in the United States. A Canadian clinical trial evaluated patients with proved PE for possible outpatient treatment. Criteria for admission included hemodynamic instability, hypoxemia requiring oxygen therapy, admission for another medical reason, severe pain requiring parenteral analgesia, or high risk of major bleeding. Certainly, in the setting of either DVT or PE when inpatient therapy is initiated, therapy may be completed in the outpatient setting in appropriate, stable individuals. It is clear that at least 30% to 40% of patients with acute, proximal DVT have *silent* PE. Many patients treated for DVT also have asymptomatic PE, unknown to the treating clinician. The criteria for outpatient therapy for acute DVT are given in Box 2.

BOX 2   Criteria for Outpatient Therapy of Acute Deep Venous Thrombosis and Pulmonary Embolism*

- DVT/PE that is stable and not massive/extensive
- Low risk of bleeding
- Education complete/compliance with injections
- Follow-up assured
- Other medical problems stable
- Reimbursement available

*Patients with symptomatic PE are generally treated as inpatients. However, the use of low-molecular-weight heparin (LMWH) as a bridge can facilitate earlier hospital discharge. The two LMWH preparations approved for treatment of acute venous thromboembolism (VTE) are approved for acute DVT with or without PE. Thus, although data support the use of LMWH preparations for acute PE, treatment of acute PE may be considered off-label in the United States.
Abbreviations: DVT = deep venous thrombosis; PE = pulmonary embolism.

PREGNANCY AND ACUTE VENOUS THROMBOEMBOLISM: LOW-MOLECULAR-WEIGHT HEPARIN

Increasing experience suggests that LMWHs are safe and effective for VTE in pregnancy. The advantages of these preparations compared with UFH include the same advantages evident in the nonpregnant population. These include a longer plasma half-life coupled with substantially increased bioavailability and, thus, a more predictable dose response. Once- or twice-daily subcutaneous administration facilitates treatment. While anti-factor Xa monitoring is not generally required with LMWH use, it is appropriate in pregnancy, particularly in view of the usual progressive weight gain. Evidence indicates that LMWHs do not cross the placenta.

Long-Term Therapy for Pulmonary Embolism

The duration of therapy is the same for acute DVT and for PE. Anticoagulant therapy should be stopped when the benefit no longer clearly outweighs the risk. This assessment needs to be individualized. Patients with VTE provoked by a transient risk factor have a lower (approximately 33%) risk of recurrence than those with an unprovoked VTE or a persistent risk factor. Three months of anticoagulation is adequate treatment for VTE provoked by a transient risk factor; the subsequent risk of recurrence is approximately 3% per patient-year. Three months of anticoagulation is inadequate for an unprovoked (idiopathic) episode of VTE; the subsequent early risk of recurrence varies from 5% to 25% per patient-year. Idiopathic VTE can be somewhat difficult to define in some settings. Clearly, VTE in the complete absence of any temporary or permanent risk factor would be classified as idiopathic. Prolonged travel appears to be a risk factor for acute VTE. However, it would be unusual for an otherwise healthy young patient without VTE risk factors to develop PE, for example, after a 6-hour car ride. Such a patient might be considered for more prolonged treatment. Idiopathic VTE should be treated for at least 6 months to 1 year, with the shorter duration reserved for patients considered at higher risk of bleeding. If patients are not candidates for long-term anticoagulant therapy, it is reasonable to stop therapy for an unprovoked VTE after 6 months and to use aggressive prophylaxis at times of superimposed high risk.

INTENSITY OF WARFARIN THERAPY

While lower INR values (range of 1.5 to 2.0) have proved superior to placebo for long-term therapy, normal-intensity warfarin with a target INR of 2.5 (range of 2.0 to 3.0) is shown to result in less recurrences than low-intensity warfarin. Thus, current evidence suggests that normal-intensity warfarin is appropriate for long-term anticoagulation. It is reasonable to stop therapy for an unprovoked VTE after 6 months and to use aggressive prophylaxis at times of superimposed high risk.

Rakel and Bope: *Conn's Current Therapy 2006.*

Other Forms of Therapy

INFERIOR VENA CAVA FILTER PLACEMENT

Placement of an IVCF is the standard of care when a patient fails therapeutic anticoagulation or develops significant bleeding while being anticoagulated for acute VTE. If a patient is felt to have suffered a recurrent event, it is important to be certain that the anticoagulation was truly in the therapeutic range before proceeding with a filter. Temporary filters are now available that can be removed within two weeks if a bleeding complication has resolved and a patient can be safely anticoagulated. Lifetime anticoagulation, when deemed safe, is appropriate when a filter must remain in place.

THROMBOLYTIC THERAPY

Based upon the potential for serious bleeding complications, thrombolytic therapy must be used cautiously. These agents activate plasminogen to form plasmin, which then results in fibrinolysis as well as fibrinogenolysis. Because anticoagulants do not actively lyse emboli, thrombolytic agents are considered in certain settings to hasten the reduction in thromboembolic burden. Clinical studies have culminated in the approval of streptokinase (Streptase), urokinase (Abbokinase), and recombinant tissue-type plasminogen activator (tPA) (Activase) for the treatment of massive PE. The specific regimens are shown in Box 3.

For several decades, the clearly accepted scenario in which thrombolytic therapy was recommended was for patients with hemodynamic instability (hypotension). Those with severely compromised oxygenation also have been considered. Although thrombolytic therapy may result in rapid improvement of right ventricular function in patients with acute PE, it remains controversial as to whether or not patients with echocardiographic right ventricular dysfunction but without hypotension should receive this form of treatment. Several large studies suggest that such patients should be considered. There are no clear data proving that one thrombolytic agent is superior to the others, but in massive PE more rapidly infused regimens may be favored.

Coagulation assays are unnecessary during thrombolysis because the approved regimens are administered

---

> **BOX 3** **Thrombolytic Therapy for Acute Pulmonary Embolism: Approved Regimens**
>
> - Streptokinase (Streptase): 250,000 U IV (loading dose over 30 minutes); then 100,000 U per hour for 24 hours*
> - Urokinase (Abbokinase): 2000 U/lb IV (loading dose over 10 minutes); then 2,000 U/lb per hour for 12 to 24 hours
> - Tissue-type plasminogen activator (Activase): 100 mg IV for 2 hours
>
> ---
> *Streptokinase administered over 24 to 72 hours at this loading dose and rate has been also approved for use in patients with extensive DVT.
> *Abbreviations:* DVT = deep venous thrombosis; IV = intravenously.

as fixed doses. Heparin is generally withheld until the thrombolytic infusion is completed. The aPTT is then determined and heparin is initiated without a loading dose if this value is less than twice the upper limit of normal. If the aPTT exceeds this value, the test is repeated every 4 hours until it is safe to proceed with heparin. While a number of investigators have employed standard or low-dose intrapulmonary arterial thrombolytic infusions in order to deliver a high concentration of drug in close proximity to the clot, intravenous therapy appears adequate in most cases. Thrombolytic therapy for DVT is more controversial. Local thrombolytic therapy can be considered in patients with proximal occlusive DVT associated with significant swelling and symptoms when there are no contraindications. Many vascular radiology or vascular medicine departments have established protocols for this form of therapy.

Hemorrhage is the primary adverse effect associated with thrombolytic therapy. If possible, invasive procedures should be minimized. The most devastating complication associated with thrombolytics is the development of intracranial hemorrhage, which occurs in less than 1% of patients. Retroperitoneal hemorrhage may result from a vascular puncture above the inguinal ligament and may be life-threatening. Thrombolytic therapy is contraindicated in the presence of any previous intracranial surgery or pathology, in patients having surgery in the previous 10 to 14 days, and in patients with active bleeding or recent significant bleeding.

HEMODYNAMIC MANAGEMENT OF MASSIVE PULMONARY EMBOLISM

Massive PE always should be suspected in the setting of the sudden onset of hypotension or extreme hypoxemia. The presence of electromechanical dissociation or sudden cardiac arrest always should make massive embolism a consideration. Once PE associated with hypotension and/or severe hypoxemia is suspected, supportive treatment is immediately initiated. Intravenous saline should be infused rapidly but cautiously because right ventricular function often is markedly compromised. Dopamine (Intropin) and norepinephrine (Levophed) (one or the other) are the favored choices of vasoactive therapy in massive PE and should be administered if the blood pressure is not rapidly restored. Dobutamine (Dobutrex) may offer inotropy, but hypotension is one of the potential risks. Oxygen therapy is administered, and thrombolytic therapy is considered as described above. Intubation and mechanical ventilation are instituted as needed to support respiratory failure.

PULMONARY EMBOLECTOMY

A candidate for acute embolectomy should meet the following criteria:

- Massive PE (detected by ventilation-perfusion scan, angiography, or CT scan)
- Hemodynamic instability (shock) despite anticoagulation/resuscitative efforts

- Failure of thrombolytic therapy or a contraindication to its use

Operative mortality in the era of rapidly available cardiopulmonary bypass ranged from 10% to 75% in an uncontrolled, retrospective case series. Embolectomy should be only undertaken when a patient meets all three criteria and an experienced surgical team is immediately available. Catheter-directed embolectomy (fragmentation, suction, low-dose thrombolytic therapy) is sometimes performed at experienced centers.

The treatment of acute venous thromboembolism should be aggressive, with caution regarding the potential for bleeding. Therapy for PE unequivocally reduces mortality.

Sarcoidosis

Method of
Marc A. Judson, MD

Sarcoidosis is a multisystem, granulomatous disease of unknown cause. The lung is most commonly affected, but any organ may be involved. The clinical presentation of sarcoidosis is variable for two main reasons. First, the manifestations of pulmonary sarcoidosis are variable and may range from an asymptomatic state to significant pulmonary dysfunction. Second, extrapulmonary indications of sarcoidosis are common and may cause the prominent presenting symptoms of the disease. This variability in disease presentation often makes the diagnosis of sarcoidosis problematic.

Epidemiology

Sarcoidosis occurs worldwide and affects all races and ages. Although the disease shows a predilection for the third decade of life, a smaller second peak in diagnosis occurs in people older than 50. There is a slightly higher disease rate in women. The highest prevalence of sarcoidosis is found in whites in Scandinavia and in persons of African descent in the United States. In the United States, the lifetime risk of sarcoidosis is 0.85% in whites and 2.4% in African Americans, with an age-adjusted incidence rate of 10.9 per 100,000 people for the white population and 35.5 per 100,000 people for African Americans. The relative risk for having sarcoidosis increases significantly if a family member has it as well. In the United States, nearly 20% of African Americans with sarcoidosis have an affected first-degree relative compared with 5% in whites.

The clinical presentation and severity of sarcoidosis varies among racial and ethnic groups. The disease tends to be more severe in African Americans, whereas whites are more likely to be asymptomatic at presentation.

Extrathoracic manifestations are more common in certain populations, such as ocular and cardiac sarcoidosis in Japanese populations, chronic uveitis in African Americans, and erythema nodosum in Europeans. There is increasing evidence that genetic polymorphisms affect the risk and manifestations of the disease. This is consistent with the current theory that sarcoidosis does not have a single cause but is the result of an abnormal host (granulomatous) response to one of many potential antigens in a genetically susceptible individual.

Immunopathogenesis

The exact immunopathogenesis of sarcoidosis is unknown, but it is thought to be similar to other granulomatous diseases. That is, antigen-presenting cells (APCs), usually either macrophages or dendritic cells, process and present an antigen via a human leukocyte antibody (HLA) class II molecule to T lymphocytes and their receptors. These T lymphocytes are usually of the CD4 T-helper 1 (Th1) class. The antigen involved in this reaction is unknown; and as previously mentioned, there may be many putative antigens that are each associated with a specific HLA class II molecule and T cell receptor. This may explain the inability to determine one specific cause of sarcoidosis and the varied phenotypic expression of the disease. The interaction of APCs and T lymphocytes activates the APCs to produce tumor necrosis factor-α (TNF-α), and other cytokines. A proliferation of CD4 Th1 lymphocytes also ensues that results in the secretion of interferon gamma (INF-γ), interleukin (IL)-2, IL-12, and other cytokines. These cytokines activate and recruit monocytes and macrophages and transform them into giant cells, which are important building blocks of the granuloma.

The typical sarcoidosis lesion is a noncaseating (nonnecrotic) granuloma. The sarcoid granuloma consists of a compact core of macrophage-derived epithelioid and multinucleated giant cells surrounded by a perimeter of monocytes, lymphocytes, and fibroblasts. Granulomas may resolve spontaneously or with therapy; however, they may also persist and lead to peripheral hyalinization and fibrosis. The development of such fibrosis may cause permanent organ damage and in large part determines the prognosis.

Clinical Features/Clinical Course

PULMONARY SARCOIDOSIS

Between 30% and 60% of patients with pulmonary sarcoidosis are asymptomatic, such that sarcoidosis is detected as an incidental chest radiographic finding. Patients may also present with nonspecific pulmonary symptoms, such as dyspnea, cough, wheezing, and chest pain. Respiratory failure from sarcoidosis is extremely rare at presentation. Unlike many other interstitial lung diseases, crackles are rarely heard on chest auscultation.

Abnormalities on the chest radiograph occur in more than 90% of patients with pulmonary sarcoidosis.

Rakel and Bope: *Conn's Current Therapy 2006.*

TABLE 1 Chest Radiograph Stages of Sarcoidosis

Stage	Lymph node enlargement	Parenchymal disease
0	No	No
1	Yes	No
2	Yes	Nonfibrotic
3	No	Nonfibrotic
4	No or yes	Fibrotic

Adapted from Judson MA, Baughman RP: Sarcoidosis. *In* Diffuse Lung Disease: A Practical Approach. London: Arnold, 2004, pp 109-129.

Bilateral hilar adenopathy occurs in 50% to 85% at disease presentation, and 25% to 50% have parenchymal infiltrates. Sarcoid granulomas have a predilection for the bronchovascular bundles, subpleural locations, intralobular septa, and the airways. A radiographic staging system was developed several decades ago (Table 1). Groups of patients with higher radiographic stages have more severe pulmonary dysfunction, lower remission rates, and greater mortality. However, there is significant overlap between these groups such that predictions concerning individual patients based on stage are highly inaccurate.

Advanced pulmonary stage IV sarcoidosis displays destruction of the lung architecture with upward traction of the hila, lung distortion, upper lobe volume loss, fibrocystic disease, honeycombed cysts, and decreased lung volumes. Aspergillomas may develop in these large cystic lesions and may be associated with life-threatening hemoptysis. Bronchiectasis from airway distortion also may occur and is an additional potential cause of hemoptysis.

The majority of patients with pulmonary sarcoidosis have a vital capacity of greater than 70% of predicted at diagnosis. There is frequently discordance between pulmonary function and the chest radiographic findings. In pulmonary sarcoidosis patients with a normal lung parenchyma (stage 1), the vital capacity, diffusing capacity, partial pressure of oxygen, arterial (PaO_2) at rest, PaO_2 with exercise, and lung compliance are abnormal in 20% to 40% of cases. Patients with abnormal lung parenchyma have abnormal pulmonary function tests 50% to 70% of the time. Patients with stage IV fibrocystic sarcoidosis tend to have the most severe pulmonary dysfunction.

Sarcoidosis is an interstitial lung disease with a restrictive ventilatory defect often found on spirometry. It is underappreciated, however, that endobronchial involvement is common in sarcoidosis; and therefore airflow obstruction may be the major abnormality found on pulmonary function testing. Wheezing may be the prominent presenting symptom of sarcoidosis, and many sarcoidosis patients are misdiagnosed as having asthma. Airflow obstruction is also common in chronic pulmonary sarcoidosis, where it is caused by airway distortion from fibrosis.

The cause of dyspnea in pulmonary sarcoidosis is multifactorial. It may be the result of abnormalities of gas exchange or lung mechanics, weakness of the respiratory muscles, obesity from corticosteroid therapy, or sarcoidosis involvement of the heart.

Only 3% to 5% of patients die of sarcoidosis. In the United States, 75% of these deaths are the result of pulmonary involvement. Death from pulmonary involvement is rarely acute but an insidious process that develops over 5 to 25 years with the development of progressive pulmonary fibrosis. Several studies have suggested that pulmonary hypertension is a major risk factor for death from pulmonary sarcoidosis. Patients with aspergillomas and stage IV fibrocystic sarcoidosis are also at risk of death from episodes of life-threatening hemoptysis. Other organs that result in fatalities from sarcoidosis include the heart and the central nervous system (CNS). In Japan death from sarcoidosis is more commonly caused by cardiac rather than pulmonary involvement.

EXTRAPULMONARY SARCOIDOSIS

Sarcoidosis is a multisystem disease that may affect any organ in the body. The extrapulmonary manifestations of sarcoidosis may predominate in many patients. The presence of extrapulmonary disease may affect the prognosis and treatment options for sarcoidosis. The eye and skin are the most common extrapulmonary organs involved with sarcoidosis. Ocular manifestations occur in 25% to 50% of patients; anterior uveitis is the most common manifestation. Symptoms of anterior uveitis include red eyes, painful eyes, and photophobia. However, in one-third of patients with anterior uveitis from sarcoidosis, the eye is *quiet,* and without symptoms. In addition, an intermediate or posterior uveitis may cause vision problems or be asymptomatic. For this reason, all patients diagnosed with sarcoidosis should undergo an eye examination by an ophthalmologist. Other ocular manifestations of sarcoidosis include conjunctivitis, keratoconjunctivitis sicca (dry eyes), scleritis, and optic neuritis.

Skin lesions in sarcoidosis can be classified into two categories: specific lesions that demonstrate noncaseating granulomas on biopsy and nonspecific lesions that do not. The specific skin lesions are often papular and have a predilection for areas of previous scars and tattoos. Lupus pernio is a type of specific skin lesion causing disfiguring lesions on the face, often with erythema and significant induration. These lesions have a predilection for the nose, cheeks, medial and lateral sides of the eyes, and lateral sides of the mouth. Lupus pernio lesions are relatively recalcitrant to therapy and often respond only partially to corticosteroids. The most common nonspecific skin lesion is erythema nodosum that is often seen with an acute sarcoidosis presentation of fever, arthritis (especially in the ankles), pulmonary symptoms, and bilateral hilar adenopathy on chest radiograph. This syndrome is known as *Löfgren's syndrome* and tends to have a good long-term prognosis.

Cardiac and neurologic sarcoidosis can be life-threatening and is therefore important to recognize. Cardiac involvement is detected clinically in 5% of sarcoidosis patients premortem but in 25% at autopsy. Cardiac sarcoidosis may cause left ventricular dysfunction and cardiac arrhythmias possibly resulting in sudden death. All patients with sarcoidosis are recommended to have a 12-lead electrocardiogram; and if this test is abnormal it should prompt further evaluation. The diagnosis of cardiac sarcoidosis is problematic because the disease is patchy and diagnosed less than 25% of the time by endomyocardial biopsy because of sampling error. Often the diagnosis is made noninvasively, if a typical clinical presentation is coupled with detection of abnormalities on echocardiography, gallium scanning, thallium scanning, or cardiac magnetic resonance imaging (MRI) with gadolinium enhancement.

Clinically apparent neurosarcoidosis occurs in less than 10% of sarcoidosis patients. Palsy of the seventh cranial nerve is the most common manifestation of neurosarcoidosis, and it often predates the diagnosis of the disease. Sarcoidosis can affect any part of the peripheral nervous system (PNS) and CNS and may cause a cranial nerve palsy, mononeuropathy or polyneuropathy, aseptic meningitis, seizures, mass lesions in the brain and spinal cord, and encephalopathy.

Sarcoidosis causes clinically apparent peripheral lymphadenopathy in more than 10% of patients. Splenic involvement may be present in up to 50% of patients, but it is usually asymptomatic and rarely causes hypersplenism. Bone involvement is occasional, usually presenting as small cysts or cortical defects found in the small bones of the hands and feet. An acute sarcoid arthritis often is present at disease onset and has a good prognosis. This is commonly found in the ankles of patients who present with Löfgren's syndrome. Chronic sarcoid arthritis is rare. It is usually a nondestructive arthropathy of the shoulders, wrists, knees, ankles, and small joints of the hands and feet. Sarcoidosis of the sinuses is underappreciated. It may occur in the nasopharynx, hypopharynx, larynx, or any of the sinuses and is known as *sarcoidosis of the upper respiratory tract* (SURT). SURT is often relatively recalcitrant to therapy. Histologic evidence of hepatic sarcoidosis is present in 50% to 80% of sarcoidosis patients, although most are asymptomatic and have normal liver function blood tests. Hepatomegaly, abdominal pain, and pruritus are the most common symptoms associated with hepatic sarcoidosis but are present only in 15% to 25% of patients with hepatic involvement. Elevation of the serum alkaline phosphatase is the most common liver function test abnormality. Hypercalcemia or hypercalciuria leading to nephrolithiasis and renal dysfunction may occur with sarcoidosis. These phenomena are the result of the enzyme, 1-α hydroxylase in activated macrophages that convert 25-hydroxyvitamin D to 1,25-dihydroxyvitamin D, the active form of the vitamin. This results in increased gut absorption and increased renal excretion of calcium that can cause nephrolithiasis. Sarcoidosis rarely involves the thyroid, renal parenchyma, and GI tract.

Constitutional symptoms such as fever, night sweats, weight loss, malaise, and fatigue may occur at presentation. These symptoms occasionally are associated with hepatic sarcoid involvement but together may be a sign of the systemic nature of the disease, presumably from cytokine release, rather than specific organ involvement.

Patients who present with Löfgren's syndrome or with asymptomatic bilateral hilar adenopathy on chest radiograph have a good prognosis. African Americans tend to have a worse prognosis than whites with lower forced vital capacity and more new organ involvement within 2 years of diagnosis. Box 1 lists risk factors associated with a poor prognosis.

Diagnosis/Initial Workup

The diagnosis of sarcoidosis requires a compatible clinical picture, histologic demonstration of noncaseating granulomas, and exclusion of other diseases capable of producing a similar histologic and clinical picture. Mycobacterial and fungal diseases always must be considered as alternative diagnoses. Therefore, stains and cultures of tissue specimens for mycobacteria and fungi always should be obtained when the diagnosis of sarcoidosis is considered.

Because sarcoidosis is a diagnosis of exclusion (granulomatous inflammation of unknown cause), bear a healthy degree of skepticism in the diagnosis and follow the patient closely for additional clues supporting an alternate diagnosis. Sarcoidosis is a systemic disease, so the signs or symptoms of extrathoracic disease such as uveitis, skin lesions, or an elevated serum alkaline phosphatase should be sought. The diagnosis in a patient with granulomas on lung biopsy who has interstitial infiltrates without adenopathy on radiographic studies is suspect. In this situation, granulomatous infections and bioaerosol exposure causing hypersensitivity pneumonitis should be strongly considered.

Because of the varied clinical presentation of sarcoidosis, there is no single diagnostic algorithm. It is prudent to select a biopsy site associated with less morbidity, such as the skin if a lesion is present. Transbronchial lung biopsy has a diagnostic yield of 40% to more than 90% in pulmonary sarcoidosis. It is recommended that at least four lung biopsy specimens be collected to maximize the diagnostic yield. Endobronchial biopsy has 40% to 60% sensitivity and adds to the yield of

CURRENT DIAGNOSIS

- The diagnosis of sarcoidosis is one of exclusion.
- Tissue biopsy, confirming noncaseating granulomatous inflammation is required in most cases.
- Efforts should be made to search for the least invasive biopsy site.

transbronchial biopsy. Bronchoalveolar lavage (BAL) with examination of lymphocyte populations has been used in the evaluation of possible pulmonary sarcoidosis. In sarcoidosis, there is an increased number of BAL lymphocytes, and these are predominantly CD4 positive. It has been proposed that an increase in BAL lymphocytes and a BAL CD4/CD8 ratio of greater than 3.5 make the diagnosis of sarcoidosis highly likely. Although serum angiotensin-converting enzyme (SACE) often is elevated in active sarcoidosis, the specificity and sensitivity of this test is inadequate for it to be used diagnostically. SACE may be used as supportive evidence for the diagnosis, and it also may be used in some instances to follow disease activity. Gallium-67 (67Ga) scanning is cumbersome because it takes several days to complete and is infrequently used as a diagnostic test. However, bilateral hilar uptake and right paratracheal uptake (lambda sign) coupled with lacrimal and parotid uptake (panda sign) with 67Ga strongly suggest a diagnosis of sarcoidosis.

Ideally, the diagnosis of sarcoidosis requires demonstration of noncaseating granulomas in at least one organ. However, certain clinical presentations are so specific for the diagnosis of sarcoidosis that the diagnosis may be accepted without tissue biopsy. Extreme caution must be taken in these situations to ensure that there is no clinical information that would suggest an alternative diagnosis that should prompt a tissue biopsy. Clinical or laboratory findings that would strongly support the diagnosis of sarcoidosis without a tissue biopsy are listed in Box 2.

Treatment

Therapy is not mandated for sarcoidosis because the disease may remit spontaneously. Therapy is indicated

---

BOX 1   Factors Associated With a Poor Prognosis of Sarcoidosis

African American race
Extrathoracic disease
Stage II-III versus stage I CXR
Age older than 40
Splenic involvement
Lupus pernio
Disease duration >2 years
FVC <1.5 L
Stage IV CXR/aspergilloma

Abbreviations: CXR = chest radiograph; FVC = forced vital capacity.
From Judson MA, Baughman RP: Sarcoidosis. *In* Diffuse Lung Disease: A Practical Approach. London: Arnold, 2004, pp 109-129. (Used with permission.)

BOX 2   Clinical or Laboratory Findings That Strongly Support a Sarcoidosis Diagnosis Without a Tissue Biopsy

Löfgren's syndrome
Heerfordt's syndrome (uveoparotid fever)
Asymptomatic bilateral hilar adenopathy on chest radiograph
BAL lymphocytosis with a CD4/CD8 ratio >3.5
67Ga scan showing a lambda sign and panda sign

Abbreviation: BAL = bronchoalveolar lavage; 67Ga = Gallium-67.

---

for potentially dangerous disease that includes neurosarcoidosis, cardiac sarcoidosis, hypercalcemia that does not respond to dietary measures, ocular sarcoidosis that does not respond to topical (eyedrop) therapy, and other life- or organ-threatening disease. Therapy also should be considered when the disease is progressive. Relative indications for therapy include arthritis that fails to respond to nonsteroidal, anti-inflammatory agents; a systemic inflammatory response syndrome of fever, night sweats, fatigue, and arthralgias; and symptomatic hepatic disease.

In general, treatment is discouraged for asymptomatic elevations of serum liver function tests, specific levels of angiotensin converting enzyme, or asymptomatic uptake on 67Ga scan (except if found in the heart or brain).

The decision to treat sarcoidosis can be problematic, because the disease has a variable prognosis that must be weighed against the potential side effects of therapy. It is often most prudent to monitor patients without therapy if they are asymptomatic or have only mild organ dysfunction.

For pulmonary sarcoidosis, asymptomatic patients and those with mild disease that may spontaneously remit usually are not treated. For patients with clinical findings that predict spontaneous remission (e.g. erythema nodosum), the benefits of treatment often are exceeded by the toxicity of therapy. Often these patients can be managed with palliative therapy such as nonsteroidal anti-inflammatory agents for arthralgias and fever, and bronchodilators and inhaled corticosteroids for wheezing and cough. It is recommended that patients with mild to moderate pulmonary sarcoidosis be observed for 2 to 6 months, if possible. Patients who improve will have avoided the toxicity of corticosteroids, whereas patients who deteriorate over this period should be considered for treatment. Patients with pulmonary dysfunction who neither improve nor deteriorate during the observation period often are given a corticosteroid trial, or they may be observed further. Patients with severe pulmonary dysfunction or pulmonary symptoms causing significant impairment should be treated.

Corticosteroids often are used to treat sarcoidosis, but the dose, duration of therapy, and method by which one can assess effectiveness have not been standardized. Topical corticosteroid therapy should be used whenever possible in an attempt to minimize systemic complications. This would include corticosteroid eyedrops for anterior sarcoid uveitis and corticosteroid creams and injections for localized skin lesions.

 CURRENT THERAPY

- Many cases of sarcoidosis do not require treatment.
- All patients should be evaluated for possible pulmonary, eye, and cardiac disease.
- When therapy is indicated, corticosteroids are most commonly used.
- Topical corticosteroids should be given whenever possible.

Pulmonary sarcoidosis usually is treated initially with 20 to 40 mg per day of prednisone or its equivalent. Higher doses may be required for neurosarcoidosis and cardiac sarcoidosis. The patient usually is evaluated within 2 to 12 weeks for a response. Patients failing to respond to therapy within 3 months are unlikely to respond to a more protracted course of therapy or a higher dose. Among the responders, the corticosteroid dose is tapered to 5 to 10 mg/day of prednisone equivalent or an every-other-day regimen. Treatment is usually continued for 12 months. The relapse rate after corticosteroid therapy is withdrawn may be as high as 70%, and therefore patients need to be followed closely as the corticosteroid dose is tapered and discontinued. In some patients, there may be recurrent relapses requiring long-term, low-dose therapy. On occasion the chronic prednisone dose needed to prevent relapse may be less than 5 mg per day.

Patients who relapse after corticosteroids have been withdrawn should be retreated with corticosteroids. In addition, alternative agents should be considered *corticosteroid-sparing agents* to control the patient on a chronic low dose of prednisone. On occasion, alternative agents may completely replace corticosteroid therapy. In general, corticosteroid-sparing agents should not be considered unless the patient requires more than 7.5 mg per day of daily prednisone to control the disease.

Methotrexate (Rheumatrex)[1] and hydroxychloroquine (Plaquenil)[1] are the most studied alternative sarcoidosis medications. They are usually used as corticosteroid-sparing agents but at times can be used as replacement therapy. Methotrexate is most useful for pulmonary, skin, joint, and eye sarcoidosis. Hydroxychloroquine is used often for skin, joint, neurosarcoidosis, and hypercalcemia from sarcoidosis. Azathioprine (Imuran)[1] may be useful for sarcoid uveitis, but usually it is added to corticosteroid plus methotrexate in this instance. Monocycline (Minocin)[1] and doxycycline (Vibramycin)[1] may be useful for skin sarcoidosis. Cyclophosphamide (Cytoxan)[1] is used occasionally and seems to have a potential role for neurosarcoidosis. Recently anti–TNF-α therapies have shown promise in the treatment of sarcoidosis. Such agents include pentoxifylline (Trental),[1] thalidomide (Thalomid),[1] and monoclonal antibodies against TNF-α, such as infliximab (Remicade).[1]

REFERENCES

Baughman RP, Teirstein AS, Judson MA, et al: Clinical characteristics of patients in a case control study of sarcoidosis. Am J Respir Crit Care Med 2001;164:1885-1889.
Gibson GJ, Prescott RJ, Muers MF, et al: British Thoracic Society Sarcoidosis study: Effects of long term corticosteroid treatment. Thorax 1996;51:238-247.
Hunninghake GW, Costabel U, Ando M, et al: ATS/ERS/WASOG statement on sarcoidosis. Am J Respir Crit Care Med 1999;160:736-755.
Hunninghake GW, Gilbert S, Pueringer R, et al: Outcome of treatment for sarcoidosis. Am J Respir Crit Care Med 1994; 149:893-898.

---

[1]Not FDA approved for this indication.

Rakel and Bope: *Conn's Current Therapy 2006.*

Judson MA: An approach to the treatment of pulmonary sarcoidosis with corticosteroids. Chest 1999;111:623-631.

Judson MA, Baughman RP: Sarcoidosis. *In* Diffuse Lung Disease: A Practical Approach. London: Arnold, 2004, pp 109-129.

Judson MA, Baughman RP, Teirstein AS, et al: Defining organ involvement in sarcoidosis: The ACCESS proposed instrument. Sarcoidosis Vasc Diffuse Lung Dis 1999;16:75-86.

Lower EE, Baughman RP: Prolonged use of methotrexate in refractory sarcoidosis. Arch Intern Med 1995;155:846-851.

Lynch JP, Kazerooni EA, Gay SE: Pulmonary sarcoidosis. Clin Chest Med 1997;755-785.

Newman LS, Rose CS, Maier LA: Sarcoidosis. N Engl J Med 1997;1224-1234.

Sharma OP: Pulmonary sarcoidosis and corticosteroids. Am Rev Respir Dis 1993;147:1598-1600.

Silicosis and Asbestosis

Method of
Germania Pinheiro, MD, MSc, PhD,
and John E. Parker, MD

Pneumoconioses are diseases caused by inhalation and deposition of mineral dust in the lungs. Silica, coal mine dust, and asbestos can lead to pulmonary fibrosis and other types of respiratory diseases.

Silicosis

Silicosis is the oldest pneumoconiosis known in the world. Only respirable dust (0.5 to 5 μm) containing crystalline silica is able to reach the lungs and cause fibrosis. The three most important crystalline forms of silica are quartz, tridymite, and cristobalite. Quartz is the most common and commercially available form of this mineral, but tridymite and cristobalite are more fibrogenic. Exposure to silica dust occurs in many occupations such as mining, quarrying, drilling, and tunneling operations. It is also a hazard to stonecutters and refractory brick, pottery, foundry, and sandblasting workers. Silica flour added to porcelain, cosmetics, and soap also represents a risk.

Precise information on the incidence and prevalence of silicosis worldwide is unknown, but it seems to be decreasing in industrialized countries because of improvements in working conditions and dust-control measures. Nevertheless, silicosis persists as a serious public health problem, especially in developing countries, where occupational diseases are frequently misclassified and underdiagnosed. In the United States, there are more than two million workers exposed to silica at a potential risk of developing the disease.

In terms of pathology, the fundamental lesion is a concentric silicotic nodule. The pathogenesis is complex,

Rakel and Bope: *Conn's Current Therapy 2006.*

with four basic mechanisms involved:

1. Direct cytotoxicity that can release enzymes
2. Activation of oxidant production by pulmonary phagocytes
3. Activation of mediator release from alveolar macrophages and epithelial cells, causing recruitment of polymorphonuclear leukocytes and macrophages and also resulting in production of proinflammatory cytokines and reactive species
4. Secretion of growth factors from alveolar macrophages and epithelial cells, stimulating fibroblast proliferation

These different mechanisms can lead to eventual cell injury and lung scarring. Many studies have demonstrated that freshly fractured silica is more toxic to the lungs, which can be explained by the presence of free radicals.

Three important criteria are generally sufficient for a diagnosis of silicosis:

1. A careful occupational history documenting silica exposure with an appropriate latency period
2. A chest radiograph interpreted as 1/0 or greater in accordance with International Labour Organization (ILO) classification of radiographs of pneumoconioses
3. The absence of diseases that can mimic silicosis such as tuberculosis, sarcoidosis, or pulmonary fungal infections

Pulmonary biopsy typically is not necessary. High-resolution computed tomography (CT) can be useful in achieving more accurate categorization of the parenchymal changes in each type of pneumoconiosis, but these findings are not standardized and the procedure is expensive for medical screening purposes.

CLINICAL FEATURES

All four forms of this pneumoconiosis—chronic, complicated, accelerated, and acute—are related to the degree or intensity of silica exposure.

Patients with chronic silicosis are often asymptomatic. The chest radiograph presents with small (less than 10 mm), rounded opacities mainly in the upper zones that appear more than 15 years after onset exposure. These parenchymal abnormalities may occur without significant changes in pulmonary function or may lead to mild restriction. Because of smoking habits or the presence of dust, an obstructive pattern may be observed in the spirometry. Carbon monoxide diffusing capacity (DLCO) measures the transfer of a diffusion-limited gas (carbon monoxide [CO]) across the alveolo-capillary membrane. The carbon monoxide diffusing capacity also may be decreased because of silicotic changes.

Progressive massive fibrosis also is known as complicated silicosis. The most common symptom is exertional dyspnea. Cough can occur as a result of superimposed infections or chronic obstructive pulmonary disease (COPD). The radiograph is characterized by the presence of large opacities greater than 1 cm in diameter. The spirometry usually presents a restrictive pattern caused by fibrosis or mixed pattern with associated obstruction, because of emphysema causing hyperinflation of the lungs. Carbon monoxide diffusing capacity is reduced. These patients are at risk for tuberculosis, nontuberculous mycobacterioses, and bacterial infections, and may present with bronchiectasis. Because of extensive areas of fibrosis and gas exchange abnormalities, with hypoxemia, cor pulmonale and respiratory failure may be present in the final stage of the disease.

Accelerated silicosis occurs with high levels of exposure of shorter duration (usually 5 to 10 years). The radiographic patterns are similar to chronic silicosis, but the progression of disease is more rapid. Patients present symptoms early, and the lung function deteriorates very quickly with a rapid decline in forced expiratory volume in 1 second (FEV_1).

Acute silicosis may develop within 6 months to 2 years after massive silica exposure. The symptoms are severe dyspnea, weight loss, and weakness. The chest radiograph shows a completely different pattern from other types of silicosis with alveolar spaces flooded with exudates. This pattern is very similar to alveolar proteinosis. Pulmonary fibrosis is not a prominent finding in acute silicosis. The prognosis is guarded, and the disease usually progresses resulting in severe hypoxemia, respiratory failure, and death. Superimposed bacterial infections, tuberculosis, and nocardia infections may be present.

MANAGEMENT

All forms of the disease are irreversible, often progressive (even after the exposure has ceased), and potentially fatal, although completely preventable. Many experimental studies have been conducted to establish a treatment for this disease, but, because of their toxicity, they are not available for humans. Tetrandrine, an extract of the root of *Stephania tetranda,* used in traditional Chinese medicine, was approved by State Drugs Administration of China as a drug for the treatment of silicosis. It exhibits anti-inflammatory, antifibrogenetic, and antioxidant effects. Tetrandrine is not available in the United States and additional research must be conducted before it is considered safe and effective. Because there is no specific drug to reverse the fibrosis, the treatment of silicosis should be focused on alleviating symptoms and remediating the complications of the disease. A common complication is the association between silicosis and pulmonary tuberculosis. Tuberculosis can be present in up to 15% of the cases in some countries. Clinical symptoms compatible with tuberculosis should prompt bacteriologic confirmation of the diagnosis. The current recommended treatment is a course of pyrazinamide, rifampin (Rifadin), ethambutol (Myambutol), and isoniazid (INH) for 2 months, followed by 6 to 7 months of isoniazid and rifampin. Some authors suggest that the treatment with at least two drugs should be prolonged for 12 months. Long-term-follow-up with bacteriologic culture and radiographs is mandatory. Nontuberculous mycobacteria account for an increased proportion of the mycobacterial diseases in those with silicosis in the industrialized countries. *Mycobacterium kansasii* or

Mycobacterium avium-intracellulare can occur, and cultures should be performed. The treatment will need to be modified according to the type of mycobacterium grown. *M. kansasii* usually responds well to therapy. Rifampin and ethambutol should be given for a period of 9 months. Silicosis also is associated with connective tissue disorders, mainly scleroderma and rheumatoid arthritis. Treatment of sclerodermatous involvement of the skin and internal organs is a challenge. Immunosuppressive drugs such as prednisone, azathioprine (Imuran),[1] chlorambucil (Leukeran),[1] cyclosporine (Neoral),[1] and many others have been used as an attempt to treat this disease. Calcium channel blockers, mainly nifedipine (Procardia),[1] are indicated for treating Raynaud's phenomenon. Some physicians recommend α-adrenergic receptor blockers. Many drugs are available to control and manage rheumatoid disease, such as steroids, methotrexate (Rheumatrex), or other disease-modifying agents. Lupus erythematosus has been described in sandblasters with silicosis; pleuritic pain and effusions can occur, and usually there is a significant response to steroids and resolution of effusion within 2 weeks. Spontaneous resolution does not occur. The use of immunosuppressives can trigger infections, and purified protein derivative must be checked before treatment, although a negative skin test will not rule out infection.

COPD occurs more frequently in workers exposed to silica than in the general population. Classification of severity of this obstructive disease is the basis for treatment. Use of an inhaled short-acting bronchodilator on demand is useful in all stages. Long-acting bronchodilators such as formoterol (Foradil) or salmeterol (Serevent), given twice daily, may be used from stage II as continuous medication. Tiotropium bromide (Spiriva) is a long-acting anticholinergic bronchodilator that maintains bronchodilation for at least 24 hours, allowing once-daily administration. Inhaled steroids (budesonide [Pulmicort], fluticasone [Flovent]) are indicated in severe stages. Systemic steroids should be used during exacerbations as short-course therapy. Theophylline (Slo-Phyllin) achieves small changes in FEV_1 with long-term use. Pulmonary hypertension is the underlying cause of cor pulmonale. Supplemental oxygen is necessary to prevent pulmonary hypertension and cor pulmonale if hypoxemia is present. Oxygen therapy should be prescribed when the arterial partial pressure of oxygen (PaO_2) is less than 55 mm Hg or arterial oxygen saturation (SaO_2) is less than 88% and partial pressure of oxygen 56 to 59 mm Hg with electrocardiogram (ECG) evidence of P pulmonale, pedal edema, and/or secondary erythrocytosis. Patients using oxygen for at least 15 hours per day had an important decrease in their pulmonary artery pressures and enhanced cardiac output. Noninvasive positive pressure ventilation has a significant role in the treatment of severe COPD exacerbations. Mechanical ventilatory support for respiratory failure is indicated when it is caused by a treatable complication. A pulmonary rehabilitation program has a role to improve dyspnea and enhance quality-of-life scores.

---

[1]Not FDA approved for this indication.

Rakel and Bope: *Conn's Current Therapy 2006.*

Episodes of acute bronchitis can occur and are usually caused by *Haemophilus influenzae, Streptococcus pneumoniae, Pseudomonas aeruginosa,* and *Moraxella catarrhalis.* Antibiotics should be prescribed for purulent exacerbations. Viral infections and *Mycoplasma pneumoniae* also can be investigated. After dust exposure is controlled, smoking cessation remains the most effective intervention to reduce the risk of COPD and to slow its progression.

The International Agency for Research on Cancer (IARC) has classified crystalline silica as a potential human lung carcinogen; however, the issue remains controversial in the medical literature. Other conditions such as chronic renal disease also have been linked with silica exposure in some populations, although the overall levels of morbidity and mortality are too low to justify medical screening for this health outcome. Pneumothorax may occur spontaneously or may be ventilator related, and a chest tube generally is required urgently.

Acute silicosis has been treated with whole-lung lavage to remove the inflammatory exudates and reduce the lung dust burden. The benefits are uncertain, and serious bacterial infections can occur after this procedure. Some reports suggest using prednisone[1] as an attempt to treat acute silicosis. The initial doses can vary from 40 to 60 mg per day for 1 month, and if benefits can be documented, the treatment can be maintained with lower doses (15 to 20 mg per day) for 6 months. Steroids are potentially dangerous if coexistent tuberculosis (TB) or other infectious agents are not recognized.

After an initial evaluation, based on guidelines for recipient selection, single or bilateral lung or lung-heart transplantation should be considered for selected patients with end-stage silicosis. Once a patient is selected as a potential candidate for lung transplantation, further studies, including pulmonary function tests, high-resolution CT scan, complete cardiac evaluation, serologic tests for hepatitis and HIV, and renal and liver function, are often required to be performed at the referring center.

PREVENTION

In the absence of specific treatment for silicosis, primary prevention is the key to avoid the disease. Dust control and use of efficient respirators for brief periods when exposure might occur are essential in preventing this disease, combined with specific programs to educate workers regarding the risks of silica dust exposure. Engineering controls such as dust suppression, local exhaust and appropriate general ventilation, and wet techniques are effective when vigorously implemented in workplaces.

Although silicosis reporting is required in many states to assure investigation of continuing workplace hazards, a national surveillance is essential to obtaining knowledge of the extent and distribution of the disease,

thereby facilitating elimination of this disease in the United States.

Asbestosis

Asbestosis is an interstitial pneumonitis and fibrosis caused by the inhalation of asbestos fibers. In the United States, the number of asbestosis deaths increased from 77 (annual age-adjusted death rate: 0.54 per million population) in 1968 to 1493 deaths (6.88 per million) in 2000 as an historical legacy of asbestos exposure; during the same period, deaths for all other pneumoconioses decreased. The geographic distribution of mortality indicates that asbestosis increased particularly in the coastal states, where asbestos was frequently used in shipbuilding. Other occupations with potential risk for asbestosis are mining, insulation application and removal, and use of asbestos-containing material in construction, and manufacturing of cement products.

Other nonmalignant outcomes associated with asbestos are pleural plaques, acute pleural effusion, pleural thickening, rounded atelectasis, and chronic airway obstruction. Lung cancer and mesothelioma (a type of pleural cancer) are malignant diseases related to asbestos exposure. The type of fiber (length and dimension) and its biopersistence are very important variables in determining the development of disease, as well as the dose-response and latency period. The most common type of asbestos is chrysotile, although amphiboles (crocidolite, amosite, and anthophyllite) are more fibrogenic and carcinogenic.

The latency period for the development of asbestosis is usually around 15 to 20 years after initial exposure to this mineral. It is essentially an occupational disease related to the intensity of exposure; nevertheless, environmental and nonoccupational exposures to this fiber may cause other types of asbestos-related diseases such as mesothelioma.

The criteria recommended for the clinical diagnosis of asbestosis are a history of asbestos exposure, dyspnea, bibasilar crackles, and pulmonary function showing a restrictive or mixed pattern or reduced lung volumes, and radiographic abnormalities consistent with irregular opacities 1/1 predominant in lower fields. In advanced phases of this disease, middle and upper lobes can be affected, and the presence of honeycombing can be noted. If there are doubts about the diagnosis, a high-resolution CT should be performed. An open lung biopsy is required only in special cases to establish the differential

---

 CURRENT DIAGNOSIS

- Obtain a detailed medical and working history, including all past exposures.
- Obtain a chest radiograph.
- Exclude other diseases that may mimic radiographic appearance of pneumoconiosis.
- Perform lung function tests to assess severity of disease.

---

[1]Not FDA approved for this indication.

Rakel and Bope: *Conn's Current Therapy 2006.*

CURRENT THERAPY

- There is no specific treatment for pneumoconiosis.
- Primary prevention is the key to avoid disease.
- Complications such as infections, chronic bronchitis, and cor pulmonale should be treated.
- A pulmonary rehabilitation program may help the patient.
- Lung transplantation is appropriate in selected cases.

diagnosis with other interstitial diseases if the history does not clearly document sufficient occupational exposure or the latency period is not compatible with the disease. The presence of asbestos bodies in sputum or bronchoalveolar lavage (BAL) would be helpful in this differentiation. The disease often remains or progresses after cessation of exposure.

MANAGEMENT

There is no effective treatment for this disease. Some patients can develop pulmonary hypertension or cor pulmonale, and oxygen should be provided. Respiratory infections may occur and antibiotics should be given. Mechanical ventilatory support for respiratory failure should be evaluated with careful consideration for the presence of reversible complications or co-morbidities.

PREVENTION

Asbestosis is a preventable disease, and efforts to eliminate it should be constant. According to the Environmental Protection Agency, there is no safe level for asbestos exposure to avoid cancer. Engineering controls to eliminate dust in the workplace, material replacement, and selection of an appropriate respirator for different levels of exposure are important measures. Smoking cessation is also an important approach to reduce the risk for asbestos-related lung cancer.

REFERENCES

Akira M: High-resolution CT in the evaluation of occupational and environmental disease. Radiol Clin North Am 2002;40:43-59.

American Thoracic Society: Adverse effects of crystalline silica exposure. American Thoracic Society Committee of the Scientific Assembly on Environmental and Occupational Health. Am J Respir Crit Care Med 1997;155:761-768.

American Thoracic Society: Diagnosis and initial management of nonmalignant diseases related to asbestos. Am J Respir Crit Care Med 2004;170:691-715.

Becklake MR: Occupational exposures: Evidence for a causal association with chronic obstructive pulmonary disease. Am Rev Respir Dis 1989;140:S85-S91.

Castranova V, Vallyathan V: Silicosis and coal workers' pneumoconiosis. Environ Health Perspect 2000;108(Suppl 4):675-684.

Centers for Disease Control and Prevention: Changing patterns of pneumoconiosis mortality—United States, 1968-2000. MMWR Morb Mortal Wkly Rep 2004;53:627-632.

Centers for Disease Control and Prevention: Silicosis screening in surface coal miners—Pennsylvania, 1996-1997. MMWR Morb Mortal Wkly Rep 2000;49:612-615.

Centers for Disease Control and Prevention: Treatment of tuberculosis. MMWR Morb Mortal Wkly Rep 2003;52:1-74.

Harkin TJ, McGuinness G, Goldring R, et al: Differentiation of the ILO boundary chest roentgenograph (0/1 to 1/0) in asbestosis by high-resolution computed tomography scan, alveolitis, and respiratory impairment. J Occup Environ Med 1996;38:46-52.

Huuskonen O, Kivisaari L, Zitting A, et al: Emphysema findings associated with heavy asbestos-exposure in high resolution computed tomography of Finnish construction workers. J Occup Health 2004;46:266-271.

International Agency for Research on Cancer: Silica and some silicates. IARC Monographs on the Evaluation of Carcinogenic Risks to Humans, vol 42. Lyon, France, International Agency for Research on Cancer, 1987.

National Institute for Occupational Safety and Health (NIOSH): Work-Related Lung Disease Surveillance Report 2002 (DHHS [NIOSH] Publication No. 2003-111), U.S. Department of Health and Human Services, Cincinatti, OH, 2003.

Wagner GR: Screening and surveillance of workers exposed to mineral dusts. Geneva, Switzerland, World Health Organization, 1996.

Wilt JL, Parker JE, Banks DE: The diagnosis of pneumoconiosis and novel therapies. In Banks DE, Parker JE (eds): Occupational Lung Disease. New York, Chapman & Hall, 1998, pp 119-138.

Xie QM, Tang HF, Chen JQ, Bian RL: Pharmacological actions of tetrandrine in inflammatory pulmonary diseases. Acta Pharmacol Sin 2002;23:1107-1113.

Hypersensitivity Pneumonitis

Method of
Yvon Cormier, MD

Hypersensitivity pneumonitis (HP) is a respiratory disease caused by a hyperimmune response to a variety of inhaled antigens. These antigens include animal proteins, bacterial or fungal particles, and nonorganic compounds that act as haptens with human albumin. The clinical manifestations vary from an acute form characterized by fever, shortness of breath, and chest tightness, which start 3 to 8 hours after exposure, to a more insidious presentation in which the patient will develop progressive shortness of breath with cough and weight loss. Physical examination is unremarkable with inspiratory crackles, sometimes a fever, and, in some chronic cases, digital clubbing. Early in the disease, the physiologic abnormalities are restrictive and a marked reduction in lung diffusion capacity with a decrease in lung volumes. In acute cases or after a lengthy subacute presentation, hypoxemia is usually present. Lung functions can revert to normal when the disease is diagnosed early and prevented from progressing. If, however, the disease is allowed to continue for repeated bouts of acute reactions or for a prolonged period of time, irreversible lung damage can occur. The long-term outcome can be either in the form of lung fibrosis with restrictive lung functions or present as emphysema with associated irreversible airflow obstruction and hyperinflation.

Diagnostic Points

There are no robust diagnostic criteria for HP. Previously published criteria were based on expert opinions and on the characteristics of the disease. These criteria were not validated. In 2003 Lacasse and colleagues published a simple predictive rule for the diagnosis or exclusion of HP. This predictive rule can be sufficient to rule in or out HP in typical settings, but additional investigative procedures often will be required. Additional procedures include a bronchoalveolar lavage in which the absence of a typical high-intensity lymphocytic alveolitis will rule out active HP. Chest radiographs, especially high-resolution computed tomography (CT), can be very useful. Typically, one sees patchy alveolitis and ground-glass infiltrations on the high-resolution CT. Chest radiographs can be normal in up to 20% of cases. Lung biopsy sometimes is required in difficult cases to confirm the diagnosis of HP or rule out other diseases. According to Coleman and Colby, a "diagnostic triad" of HP includes:

1. Cellular infiltrates of lymphocytes and plasma cells of varying density along airways
2. Interstitial infiltrates of lymphocytes and plasma cells varying from mild to very dense
3. Single, non-necrotizing, randomly scattered granulomata in the parenchyma with some in bronchiolar and alveolar walls, but without mural vascular involvement

Eosinophils are scant or absent.

Treatment

The treatment of HP is based on contact avoidance when possible. Complete elimination of antigenic exposure often is difficult. This is especially obvious when the antigen is in the workplace (e.g., dairy farm) or when a patient lives in an area where pigeons are part of the living environment. Even when the responsible source can be eliminated and cleaning measures applied, a significant amount of antigen can persist for months. Wearing a protective respirator can be effective but respirators are uncomfortable and cumbersome and always must be worn when the patient is in contact with the offending environment. It is likely that if all

CURRENT DIAGNOSIS

Clinical findings that can predict the presence or, in their absence, exclude the likelihood of hypersensitivity pneumonitis:

- Exposure to a known antigen
- Serum antibodies to that antigen
- Weight loss
- Inspiratory crackles
- Recurrent symptoms
- Symptoms occurring 4 to 8 hours after exposure

CURRENT THERAPY

- Prevention
  Primary: Decreaseing the risks of developing Hypersensitivity pneumonitis
  Secondary: Avoidance of contact with subjects with the disease
- Pharmaceutical
- Oral corticosteroids
- Short course, high dose (50 mg prednisolone per day)
- Maintenance low dose (20 mg prednisolone per day)

contact is eliminated, the disease will stop progressing and some or total recovery will occur. The amount of recovery will depend on the extent of irreversible damage present (destruction or fibrosis) when the contact is eliminated.

Corticosteroids are the only drugs currently recognized for the treatment of HP. There is no evidence that inhaled steroids are beneficial unless some reversible airflow obstruction is present. Oral steroids are often used. These compounds will attenuate the clinical symptoms and are as effective as contact avoidance in the early outcome of HP. The long-term outcome is probably not altered by corticosteroid use. An empirical recommendation is to give high-dose prednisolone (Prednisone 50 mg/day) in acute severe cases, for example, a patient with a class IV or V shortness of breath and hypoxemia. In this setting, the steroids usually can be withdrawn within a few days, as soon as the acute manifestations have waned. One could also consider giving oral prednisolone at lower doses (20 mg per day) over a longer period of time as a maintenance treatment (a month or two) when contact cannot be avoided (e.g., a dairy farmer). Appropriate treatment of potential side effects of long-term corticosteroids also must be considered when this approach is used.

REFERENCES

Coleman A, Colby TV: Histologic diagnosis of extrinsic allergic alveolitis. Am J Surg Pathol 1988;12:514-518.
Cormier Y, Israel-Assayag E, Desmeules M, Lesur O: Effect of contact avoidance or treatment with oral prednisolone on bronchoalveolar lavage. Can Respir J 1994;1:223-228.
Hodgson MJ, Parkinson DK, Karpf M: Chest X-rays in hypersensitivity pneumonitis: A meta-analysis of secular trends. Am J Ind Med 1989;16:45-53.
Lacasse Y, Selman M, Costabel U, et al: Clinical diagnosis of active hypersensitivity pneumonitis. Am J Respir Crit Care Med 2003;158:952-958.
Lalancette M, Carrier G, Laviolette M, et al: Farmer's lung. Long-term outcome and lack of predictive value of bronchoalveolar lavage fibrosing factors. Am Rev Respir Dis 1993;148:216-221.
Monkare S, Haahtela T: Farmer's lung—A 5-year follow-up of eighty-six patients. Clin Allergy 1987;17:143-151.
Pérez-Padilla R, Salas J, Chapela R, et al: Mortality in Mexican patients with chronic pigeon breeder's lung compared to those with usual interstitial pneumonitis. Am Rev Respir Dis 1993;148:49-53.
Richerson HB, Bernstein IL, Fink JN, et al: Guidelines for the clinical evaluation of hypersensitivity pneumonitis. Report of the Subcommittee on Hypersensitivity Pneumonitis. J Allergy Clin Immunol 1989;84:839-844.

Schuyler M, Cormier Y: The diagnosis of hypersensitivity pneumonitis. Chest 1997;111:534-536.

Silver SF, Muller NL, Miller RR, et al: Computed tomography in hypersensitivity pneumonitis. Radiology 1989;173:441-445.

Terho E: Diagnostic criteria for farmer's lung disease. Am J Ind Med 1986;10:329.

Tuberculosis and Other Mycobacterial Diseases

Method of
Christopher J. Lahart, MD

Tuberculosis (TB) is a curable and preventable disease, but it is the cause of more deaths each year worldwide than any other infectious disease. Although apparently contradictory, both of these statements about TB are accurate and, unfortunately, will remain accurate for years to come. The World Health Organization (WHO) estimates that during 2001 there were 8.5 million new cases of TB with 1.9 million deaths. The vast majority of these cases and deaths occur in the developing world. In the United States, the Centers for Disease Control and Prevention (CDC) reported a total of 14,874 cases in 2003 and 802 deaths in 2002. Within the United States TB cases are unevenly distributed, with a concentration in urban and medically underserved areas. The top five states in numbers of TB cases (California, Texas, New York, Florida, and Illinois) account for more than 53% of the national cases, whereas the five states with the lowest occurrence have less than 1%. There are fewer than 50 cases in each of 15 states. In 2002, for the first time since nation-of-birth data were collected, persons born outside of the country accounted for more than 50% of the TB cases in the United States. This highlights the worldwide issues of resource distribution and the ability of infectious diseases to transcend national borders and natural boundaries. In recognition of this, CDC has increased efforts of collaboration with international organizations to improve TB control in countries heavily impacted by the disease.

Case identification and treatment are essential elements of TB control efforts. Another is identification of individuals with latent TB infection who are at high risk of progressing to active disease. With an estimated 25% of the human population infected by *Mycobacterium tuberculosis,* this is an enormous task. It is even more important in areas with a low prevalence of active TB, such as the United States, where a high percentage of the annual cases arise from these latently infected people. Approximately 10% of the U.S. population has latent TB infection, providing a reservoir of more than 25 million individuals from which active cases may arise. Primary care physicians are on the front line of this challenge and must learn to assess a patient's risk and then test for latent TB infection when warranted.

An additional challenge to TB control in the United States is presented by the increasing infrequency of the disease itself. Fewer cases mean fewer physicians familiar with the disease's presentation, complications, and treatment. Despite a decreasing chance of encountering TB, practitioners must remind themselves to *think TB* when confronted with patients who have symptoms and signs suggestive of TB.

Pathogenesis of Tuberculosis

The human disease termed *tuberculosis* is caused by the organism *M. tuberculosis.* Archeologic findings have determined the presence of this disease since before recorded history, and it is more prevalent now than ever before. Transmission of *M. tuberculosis* is from person to person with no intermediate host or environmental reservoir. A person with respiratory tract TB expels airborne particles that contain *M. tuberculosis* during coughing and sneezing but also during normal speech and respiration. The particles of greatest importance are generally only 1 to 5 μm in size and can remain suspended in air for a considerable period of time. Another individual inhales them along with ambient air. After inhalation, organism-containing particles of appropriate size come to rest in pulmonary alveoli where the organisms are promptly ingested by alveolar macrophages. *M. tuberculosis* can survive and multiply within macrophages, is released with cell death, and spreads to regional lymph nodes and hematogeneously to other well-perfused organ systems. The resulting immune response from this initial infection induces cell-mediated immunity as well as granuloma formation. Delayed-type hypersensitivity reaction is developed to certain tuberculin antigens and forms the basis of tuberculin skin testing. Latent TB infection (LTBI) is thus established. This is the condition present in 25 million persons in the United States and 1.5 billion persons worldwide.

The immune response generated by this initial infection is able to perpetuate this latency as a lifelong condition in 90% of those infected. Only 10% will progress from latent infection to active disease. Half of this progression (5% of the infected total) will occur within the first 2 years following initial infection. The other half will occur during the remaining lifetime, often associated with the development of other medical complications such as diabetes, malignancy, renal failure, or immunosuppressive diseases or therapy. The proportions progressing to active disease and the time course of progression are dramatically altered by HIV infection. This interaction between TB and HIV is a critical driving force of the TB epidemic in the developing world, but also of major importance in the United States. This is elaborated on in a separate section of this article, highlighting the recommendations for HIV testing and special considerations for both TB and HIV therapy.

Rakel and Bope: *Conn's Current Therapy 2006.*

Diagnosis of Latent Tuberculosis Infection

TUBERCULIN SKIN TESTING

Although 25 million persons in the United States have LTBI, mass screening is not recommended. Rather, practitioners must assess the risk an individual has to progress to active disease if latently infected and then test for latent infection in those at high risk. The diagnosis of LTBI is based on purified protein derivative (PPD) tuberculin skin testing to elicit the delayed-type hypersensitivity reaction. This reaction is usually present within 2 to 12 weeks following infection. Tuberculin is injected intradermally on the volar aspect of either forearm, and the intensity of the reaction is assessed within 48 to 72 hours by measuring the amount of induration around the injection site. Prior vaccination with bacilli Calmette-Guérin (BCG) is not a contraindication to tuberculin skin testing, and a significant reaction should not be ascribed to such vaccination. Persons receive this vaccination because they reside in a country with a high burden of TB, and the significant tuberculin reaction is more likely a reaction to LTBI than to BCG.

Because of the sensitivity and specificity of the tuberculin skin test, as well as the prevalence of LTBI in different groups, the interpretation of the skin test reaction incorporates three different cutpoints for significance of reaction (Table 1). For those at highest risk of developing active TB and those with immunosuppressive conditions that may impair their response, 5 mm of induration indicates a significant reaction. Persons with an increased likelihood of recent infection or other social or clinical conditions associated with higher risk of progression exhibit a significant reaction at the 10 mm level. For those with no perceived risk factors or who are entering into a longitudinal screening program such as for employment, 15 mm is a significant reaction size. Results of tuberculin skin testing should be recorded in millimeters of induration and not as positive or negative. Depending on certain life events, what was once considered to be an insignificant reaction could be significant with the development of a new clinical diagnosis (e.g., HIV infection).

If sequential tuberculin skin testing is anticipated, such as annual screening in the health care industry, special consideration must be given to the boosting phenomenon. In some individuals the cellular immune response to tuberculin may be lost over a period of years. The initial application of tuberculin may not elicit a significant response but the second application may. If this second tuberculin exposure is part of the annual re-examination, it may be misinterpreted to signify recent TB infection during the past year of employment. Repercussions of such a misinterpretation include investigations of lapses in TB control within the facility and placement of the individual in a high-risk category for progression because of recent infection. However, the infection may have been remote, the risk of progression low, and there may have been no TB transmission in the facility. To prevent this mishap,

a two-stage approach to the initial tuberculin screening needs to be used. A second tuberculin test should be done shortly following the initial one to assess the presence or absence of boosting.

CHEST RADIOGRAPHS

Once the diagnosis of LTBI has been considered, care must be taken to not miss a diagnosis of active disease. A missed diagnosis can have serious consequences; the treatment regimens for LTBI are inadequate for active

TABLE 1 Targeted Skin Testing to Identify Persons With Latent Tuberculosis Infection Who Would Benefit From Treatment: Criteria for Purified Protein Derivative Positivity for Specific Disease Risk Factors

Positive result	Risk for disease after infection*
5 mm	HIV infection
5 mm	Fibrotic changes on chest radiograph consistent with old healed TB
5 mm	Recent contact with infectious TB case
5 mm	Organ transplantation or other immunosuppression[†]
10 mm	Medical conditions Diabetes mellitus End-stage renal disease Silicosis Immunosuppressive therapy Hematologic or reticuloendothelial diseases Cancers of the head, neck, and lung Intestinal bypass or gastrectomy Chronic malabsorption Body weight 10% or more below ideal
10 mm	History of inadequately treated TB in the past
10 mm	TB infection within 2 y (skin test increase by ≥10 mm)
10 mm	Illicit injection of drugs or cocaine use
10 mm	Children age <4 y, children and adolescents exposed to high-risk adults
10 mm	Foreign individuals from high-prevalence countries who have resided in the United States <5 y
10 mm	Prolonged travel/residence in a high-prevalence region
10 mm	Residents or employees of high-risk group settings[‡]
10 mm	Health care workers serving high-risk persons
10 mm	Mycobacteriology laboratory personnel
15 mm	No risk factors[§]

*Includes individuals with a high likelihood of recent infection and thus more at risk for disease.
[†]Prednisone doses of ≥15 mg/d for ≥1 mo.
[‡]Prisons, jails, shelters, health care facilities, nursing homes; low-risk individuals being tested for the first time for longitudinal screening programs are not included.
[§]Includes those being tested for the first time as part of a longitudinal screening program.
Abbreviations: TB = tuberculosis.

Rakel and Bope: *Conn's Current Therapy 2006.*

disease and would foster drug resistance. All persons diagnosed with LTBI in whom treatment is being considered should have a chest radiograph performed. A single posterior-anterior exposure is appropriate for children older than 5 years of age. For those younger than 5 years the only manifestation of active TB may be small pleural effusions or adenopathy, so a lateral projection of the chest also should be obtained. Pregnant women with LTBI or with recent contact with active TB cases are at risk for progression to active disease and congenital TB in the infant. Chest radiography should be performed with the use of proper shielding in the radiology suite.

SPUTUM EXAMINATION

In a person with LTBI and a chest radiograph that is clear of changes for TB, no sputum examination for mycobacterial smear or culture is necessary. However, a special consideration is the HIV-infected person with or without respiratory symptoms. If symptoms are present, sputum specimens from 3 consecutive days should be submitted unless the respiratory symptoms are explained by an alternate diagnosis and resolve with treatment. If no symptoms are present but the HIV infection is advanced, as indicated by an AIDS diagnosis, sputum should be examined if recent contact with a TB case is suspected.

Persons with chest radiographs that are suggestive of prior or healed TB infection, but with no history of prior TB treatment, should have sputum samples sent for examination on 3 consecutive days. Initiation of treatment for LTBI can await the results of these examinations, or treatment for active TB disease can be initiated and subsequently tapered to treatment of LTBI once results are final and negative.

Treatment of Latent Tuberculosis Infection

Because the decision to test for LTBI should be based on the identification of those at high risk of progression to active disease, the decision to test is also a decision to treat those in whom LTBI is diagnosed. The primary contraindication to the treatment of LTBI with a recommended single-drug regimen is the inability to rule out active TB disease. If active TB remains a clinical consideration, multidrug therapy should be initiated and maintained until active disease is no longer a consideration. Other contraindications to treatment are the presence of active hepatitis or end-stage liver disease.

PRETREATMENT EVALUATION

The major pretreatment evaluation is to eliminate active disease from consideration. The evaluation in preparation of LTBI treatment is an assessment of the risk of hepatic disease. Persons with a history or physical examination indicative of liver disease or regular excessive use of alcohol should have baseline liver function tests (LFTs). The presence of risk factors for hepatitis B or C infection or diagnosed HIV infection also should prompt baseline LFTs. Pregnant women and those in the immediate postpartum period also should undergo such testing. Routine baseline testing is not indicated. If rifampin (Rifadin) is to be used, a baseline complete blood count (CBC) should be obtained.

TREATMENT REGIMENS

A common misunderstanding is that isoniazid (INH) therapy for LTBI is not recommended for persons older than 35 years of age. Current recommendations do not include consideration of age. Individuals at high risk of progression, regardless of age, should receive treatment of LTBI because the risk of active TB is higher than the risk of treatment-related complications. Practitioners must assess individual patients for their risk of a treatment-related complication.

There are four recommended regimens for treatment of LTBI. Medications used to treat LTBI are the same as those used to treat active TB. The preferred regimen consists of INH given daily for 9 months (which can be self-administered by the patient), or alternately, the drug may be taken on a twice-weekly dosing schedule given as part of a directly observed protocol. It should be emphasized that because of the concern for the development of drug resistance, any intermittent therapy, whether for latent or active TB, should be only prescribed as part of a directly observed therapy. A second but less preferred regimen is INH given for 6 months. This also can be given daily or twice weekly but should be reserved for those unable to complete a full 9-month course. It also is not preferred for those with HIV infection or fibrotic lesions on chest radiograph. The 6-month regimen results in slightly higher rates of active disease despite treatment of LTBI.

A third regimen, better studied in the HIV-infected population, consists of rifampin (Rifadin) plus pyrazinamide administered for 2 months. This also can be prescribed as daily therapy or twice weekly. Caution must be taken with this regimen because of its higher rate of hepatotoxicity, especially in the non–HIV-infected patient. This regimen can be considered for patients who are close contacts with a person who has INH-resistant TB. Patients should be evaluated every 2 weeks while on this regimen to minimize the chance of continued treatment administration during development of hepatitis. Although well studied in the HIV infected, the use of rifampin (Rifadin) can complicate treatment of HIV infection because of the significant drug–drug interactions between rifampin (Rifadin) and many HIV medications. The fourth regimen consists of rifampin (Rifadin) alone, administered for 4 months as daily therapy.

MONITORING DURING TREATMENT OF LATENT TUBERCULOSIS INFECTION

After the initial clinical evaluation and the initiation of treatment for LTBI, patients should receive monthly follow-up evaluations if they are receiving INH or rifampin (Rifadin) alone. If they are receiving rifampin

(Rifadin) and pyrazinamide, they should be evaluated at weeks 2, 4, 6, and 8. The evaluation should include examination for symptoms and signs of hepatitis. Routine laboratory monitoring is not recommended. Only patients with abnormal baseline LFTs or those at risk for hepatic disease should be retested routinely during therapy. Follow-up chest radiographs are not indicated.

Diagnosis of Active Tuberculosis Disease

Control of TB depends on the prompt recognition of active TB disease and the initiation of effective therapy. Because TB is generally a slowly progressive disease of an indolent nature, it is uncommon for the individual suspected of TB to require hospitalization. Patients suspected of infectious TB should preferably be evaluated as outpatients, remaining in the environment in which they have resided instead of bringing them into a new environment with potential new contacts, many of whom may be immunosuppressed. Should a patient suspected of having TB need hospitalization because of the severity of illness, co-morbidities, or to facilitate evaluation, he or she should be placed in strict respiratory isolation until three sputum specimens are smear negative for acid-fast bacilli. Unfortunately, studies show significant delays in the diagnosis of active TB in hospitalized patients with up to 50% of the cases unsuspected at admission. Consideration of TB must remain prominent in clinicians' minds.

CLINICAL FEATURES

Active TB typically presents as a chronic illness with progression of symptoms occurring over a period of weeks to months. Symptoms often include chronic cough, fever, night sweats, and weight loss. Some patients may minimize these symptoms, but will present themselves within days of the development of hemoptysis. Roughly 80% of TB cases have pulmonary involvement; 72% have pulmonary alone and 8% have both pulmonary and extrapulmonary. Approximately 20% have only extrapulmonary disease, which is characterized by constitutional symptoms plus symptoms referable to the organ system involved. Many of the so-called extrapulmonary cases actually involve intrathoracic sites that are separate from the pulmonary parenchyma, such as mediastinal lymph nodes and pleural disease. Other sites include bones and joints, the genitourinary system, the central nervous system (CNS), the meninges, and peritoneal TB. Granulomas may be seen in the liver or spleen.

RADIOGRAPHS

The typical chest radiograph of active TB shows unilateral or bilateral upper lobe involvement with fibronodular disease and/or cavitation. Such findings should always raise suspicion of TB. Although this is the typical appearance of adult reactivation disease from the latent state, TB disease caused by progression of initial infection may be seen in children or the immunosuppressed,

especially advanced HIV infection. This picture includes middle and lower lobe infiltrates, pleural effusions, and hilar adenopathy.

SPUTUM EXAMINATION

In pulmonary TB, sputum specimens have positive acid-fast bacilli (AFB) smears in 45% of the cases and cultures positive for *M. tuberculosis* in 70% of the cases. When pulmonary TB is considered, sputum should be submitted for examination. Because of specimen quality issues and test sensitivity, a sputum specimen from each of 3 consecutive days is recommended. The initial culture-positive specimen should have drug susceptibility testing performed as a routine procedure. Most mycobacteriology laboratories will do this without a specific request, but the practitioner must confirm this. Up to 17% of TB cases in the United States are based on clinical and radiographic suspicions when sputum specimens remain smear and culture negative. In these instances, appropriate diagnostic studies should be performed to evaluate other possible diagnoses; however, if TB remains the leading diagnostic concern, therapy should be initiated. Clinical and radiographic responses to TB treatment at 2 months should be assessed to provide further support for the TB diagnosis.

Treatment of Active Tuberculosis

Current regimens for treatment of active TB have a 97% success rate in the initial treatment and less than a 5% relapse rate. The success of these regimens depends on the use of appropriate multidrug therapy to eliminate the emergence of drug-resistant organisms, the extended duration of therapy to reach the slowly replicating mycobacteria and to prevent later relapse, and maximum adherence to the regimen dosing and duration. Adherence is best addressed through the use of directly observed therapy. Directly observed therapy uses the resources of the local public health authority to deliver therapy to the patient with the public health worker observing the patient taking the medication. In addition to verifying treatment administration, the worker also inquires about potential side effects and serves as a resource for the patient, further enhancing adherence.

PRETREATMENT EVALUATION

Much like treatment of LTBI, active TB patients must be assessed for the presence or potential for hepatic disease. Baseline LFTs should be obtained along with a CBC and platelet count. Most patients also receive ethambutol (Myambutol) as part of their initial regimen, so testing of visual acuity and color vision should be performed and recorded.

TREATMENT REGIMENS

There are four recommended regimens for treating active TB. Three of the regimens use typical four-drug therapy, including INH, rifampin (Rifadin), pyrazinamide, and ethambutol (Myambutol). The fourth regimen is for patients who are unable to take pyrazinamide (severe liver disease, gout, and pregnancy) and includes the remaining three drugs. Each regimen has a 2-month initial phase followed by a 4- or 7-month continuation phase. The minimal acceptable duration of treatment for any case of culture-positive TB is 6 months. The differences between the regimens are how intermittent some of the dosing frequencies are and how soon in the course of treatment the intermittent administration begins. For all treatment, directly observed therapy is recommended, but for any intermittent therapy it is absolutely necessary.

Regimen 1 is the daily administration of all four drugs for the initial 2 months of treatment. In regimen 2 the same medications are administered daily for the first 2 weeks, followed by twice-weekly dosing for 6 weeks. Regimen 3 consists of the same four drugs administered three times weekly for 8 weeks. Regimen 4 is INH, rifampin (Rifadin), and ethambutol (Myambutol) administered daily for 8 weeks. Patients with advanced HIV infection are an exception. These patients should never receive medications less than three times per week because of the higher rate of relapse seen in that setting. The usual prescription for these patients is daily therapy for 2 weeks followed by thrice-weekly dosing to completion.

After the initial 2-month phase there is a second decision point. By this time drug susceptibility results should be known and if the organism is pansensitive, both pyrazinamide and ethambutol (Myambutol) should be discontinued. Pyrazinamide is used to hasten early sterilization, and the early phase is completed. Ethambutol (Myambutol) is used to protect the other medications in the setting of possible drug resistance and actually can be discontinued as soon as susceptibility results demonstrate no resistance. Most patients will continue therapy for 4 additional months (regimens 1, 2, and 3). Those who should continue for 7 months include persons with cavitary disease whose sputum culture obtained at the 2-month interval remains positive and those who did not receive pyrazinamide (regimen 4). For all four regimens, the continuation phase can consist of INH and rifampin (Rifadin) given daily, twice weekly, or thrice weekly; the exceptions are regimen 3, which continues on the thrice-weekly schedule, and the patient with advanced HIV infection who should never receive twice-weekly dosing.

Rifapentine (Priftin) is a recently approved anti-TB medication that allows for once-weekly dosing in the continuation phase of therapy. Rifapentine (10 mg/kg, 600 mg maximum) can be given with INH (900 mg) once per week for the final 4 months in persons known to be HIV-negative, AND with noncavitary pulmonary disease, AND with negative sputum cultures after the initial 2 months. This can be only done via directly observed therapy.

MONITORING THERAPY

Therapy is often initiated before culture results are finalized. Drug susceptibility results will further lag the culture results. A sputum specimen for AFB smear and culture should be submitted at monthly intervals until two consecutive cultures are negative. If a culture obtained after 3 months of treatment is reported as positive, drug susceptibility testing should be repeated on that isolate to assess acquired drug resistance. If AFB cultures have been negative throughout the evaluation, a repeat chest radiograph at 2 months should be done to check for response to therapy. No other chest radiographs are needed during the course of therapy. A chest radiograph at the time of completion of therapy should be done to serve as the new baseline study with which future radiographs will be compared.

PARADOXICAL REACTIONS

Although more typically seen in the current era with HIV co-infection, paradoxical reactions had been described with anti-TB therapy before the HIV epidemic. A paradoxical reaction appears to indicate a worsening of the disease or failure of treatment when in actuality it is occurring during adequate therapy. Symptoms occur weeks into therapy and may include a return of cough or fever, enlarging lymph nodes, a chest radiograph with worsening of prior infiltrates or development of new infiltrates, effusions, or adenopathy. In the HIV-infected TB case, paradoxical reactions are related to the initiation of effective anti-HIV therapy. They may occur in the early, middle, or late stages of TB treatment but are more common when HIV therapy initiation is closer to the initiation of TB therapy. In the more advanced HIV infected, care must be taken not to assume these symptoms are related to TB. They also may signify an immune reconstitution reaction to other disseminated infections such as histoplasmosis, *Cryptococcus,* or *Mycobacterium avium* complex (MAC). These events should prompt a review of all data, including laboratory results of cultures and sensitivities, and assessment of adherence to therapy. In patients with no prior HIV testing, it should be recommended again at this time. Records of adherence from public health administered directly observed therapy are invaluable to evaluate the possibility of treatment failure. If all other etiologies are ruled out, consideration may be given to administration of steroids to moderate the reaction.

Tuberculosis and HIV Co-Infection

HIV infection alters the natural history and presentation of TB. In the non–HIV-infected person there is a 10% lifetime risk of developing TB after infection. If a person with LTBI becomes infected with HIV, the risk for active TB approaches 7% per year. A person without HIV who is newly infected by TB has a 5% risk of developing TB in the next 1 to 2 years. Depending on the degree of immunosuppression, an HIV-infected person has up to a 40% risk of developing active TB within the first year after infection. Additionally, HIV-related TB is more likely to present as primary infection with noncavitating pulmonary infiltrates in the middle and lower lobes, pleural effusions, and hilar adenopathy. Because of this dramatic alteration of ability to control TB infection, many active cases of TB are in persons with HIV infection. Thus, all patients with active TB should be tested for HIV infection. In many U.S. urban areas, the HIV rate in TB cases may be 20%. Also, to properly interpret a tuberculin skin test, a person's risk for HIV needs to be assessed. As noted in Table 1, a 5-mm reaction is significant if HIV infection is known but is insignificant for the majority of those tested.

Performing HIV testing in TB cases can help make an earlier diagnosis of HIV infection, preventing an opportunistic infection in the future. Should a person with TB be diagnosed with HIV, a question about the timing of therapy for HIV arises. The therapies for HIV and TB have multiple drug–drug interactions. If a person with HIV/TB does not have an imminent need for HIV therapy, it likely is best to complete treatment of TB prior to starting HIV therapy. If it is determined that HIV therapy is necessary before the completion of TB therapy, treatment should be done in consultation with a health care provider experienced in such dual therapy. The primary concern in dual therapy is the interaction of rifampin (Rifadin) with HIV medications in the protease inhibitor and non-nucleoside reverse transcriptase inhibitor classes. Rifampin (Rifadin) induces the hepatic cytochrome P450 metabolic pathway, which results in accelerated metabolism and reduced drug levels of these HIV medications. Such lowered drug levels can result in treatment failure because of HIV drug resistance. In general, rifabutin (Mycobutin)[1] can be substituted for rifampin (Rifadin) without altering the anti-TB efficacy, but it greatly reduces the degree of enzyme induction. There is still much to be learned about these drug interactions; the practitioner supervising the treatment of either TB or HIV, or both, needs to consult the most recent guidelines available through the CDC or the AIDS Treatment Information Service of the National Institutes of Health (NIH) at www.AIDSinfo.nih.gov/.

Disease Caused by Nontuberculous Mycobacteria

Once considered the realm of pulmonary consultants, nontuberculous mycobacteria (NTM) are becoming more important causes of pulmonary disease, especially as TB becomes less common, the general population ages, and the prevalence of chronic obstructive pulmonary disease (COPD) increases. Many of the NTM are ubiquitous in the environment and can colonize airways, may cause transient infection, or even contaminate clinical specimens. A decision to make a diagnosis of disease caused by NTM involves an analysis of symptoms, radiographic findings, and culture data.

CLINICAL AND RADIOGRAPHIC FEATURES

Much like TB, disease caused by NTM is characterized by a slow progression over time and is symptomatic with chronic cough, fever, night sweats, and weight loss. Hemoptysis also may occur. Radiographic findings also are similar to TB with the most common finding being upper lobe pulmonary disease that is fibrotic and/or cavitary. There is often evidence of underlying pulmonary disease such as COPD, healed TB, silicosis, or even malignancy. Tuberculin skin tests may exhibit some cross-reactivity to NTM, but the recommended cutpoints (see Table 1) take this into consideration. A significant reaction to tuberculin skin testing should be interpreted to indicate LTBI, even in the setting of confirmed NTM. On presentation NTM and TB usually are indistinguishable. In the interest of the patient and public health, anti-TB therapy often is initiated before receiving the laboratory report of the final culture results. Respiratory isolation should be maintained in institutional settings until TB is ruled out.

TREATMENT REGIMENS

Like the treatment of active TB, treatment of NTM requires prolonged multidrug therapy. Because of the lack of person-to-person transmission and thus any public health concerns, there is no option for directly observed therapy via local public health authorities. Often, TB is initially suspected and such therapy will be initiated; this can be done through directly observed therapy. Once NTM is the final diagnosis, directly observed therapy will no longer be available. The two most common disease-causing NTM are MAC and *Mycobacterium kansasii*. Both can be successfully controlled by any of the four-drug anti-TB regimens, but therapy can be tailored to the causative organism once it is identified. MAC therapy uses a macrolide antibiotic, either clarithromycin (Biaxin) (500 mg twice daily) or azithromycin (Zithromax) (250 mg once daily), plus ethambutol (Myambutol) (25 mg/kg once daily) plus either rifampin (Rifadin) (600 mg once daily) or rifabutin (Mycobutin)[1] (300 mg once daily). In HIV-infected patients with disseminated MAC, effective therapy has been only a macrolide plus ethambutol (Myambutol), which allows for the more important anti-HIV therapy to continue without the drug interactions of the rifamycins. *M. kansasii* is treated with antituberculous doses of INH[1] plus rifampin (Rifadin)[1] plus ethambutol (Myambutol).[1]

Duration of therapy is generally recommended to be for 12 months after culture conversion, which often occurs around month 6. Thus, 18 months of therapy is usually taken as a full course. With the amount of underlying lung disease present in many patients, therapy is often extended because of persistent positive cultures. In patients with advanced HIV infection, lifelong therapy formerly was considered likely. The increasing

[1]Not FDA approved for this indication.

[1]Not FDA approved for this indication.

Rakel and Bope: *Conn's Current Therapy 2006*.

CURRENT THERAPY
(First-Line Antituberculosis Drugs)

Drug	Form	Dose: mg/kg (Maximum)*					
		Daily		2×/wk†		3×/wk†	
		Adults	*Children*	*Adults*	*Children*	*Adults*	*Children*
Isoniazid	100,300-mg tablets Intramuscular syrup, 50 mg/5 mL	5 (300 mg)	10-20**	15 (900 mg)	20-40	15 (900 mg)	20-40
Rifampin (Rifadin)	150,300-mg capsules Intravenous syrup, 50 mg/5 mL	10 (600 mg)‡§	10-20‡	10 (600 mg)‡§	10-20‡	10 (600 mg)‡	10-20‡
Rifabutin (Mycobutin)[1]	150-mg capsules Intravenous[2]	5 (300 mg)‡	10-20‡	5 (300 mg)‡	10-20‡	5 (300 mg)‡	Unknown
Pyrazinamide	500-mg tablets	15-30 (2 g)	15-20	50-70 (4 g)	50-70	50-70** (4 g)	50-70
Rifamate	Fixed-combination capsules containing 150 mg Isoniazid, 300 mg rifampin (Rifadin) 2 capsules						
Rifater	Fixed-combination capsules containing 50 mg Isoniazid capsules containing 120-mg Rifampin (Rifadin) capsules containing 150 mg isoniazid, 50 mg isoniazid, 300 mg pyrazinamide, 300 mg rifampin <45 kg: 4 tablets 45-54 kg: 5 tablets >54 kg: 6 tablets						
Ethambutol (Myambutol)	100,400-mg tablets 300 mg pyrazinamide	15-25	15-25** (1 g)	50	50 (4 g**)	25-30	25-30
Streptomycin	Intramuscular 100-400-mg tablets Intravenous	15 (1 g) Age >60 y	20-40 (1 g) 10 (750 mg)	25-30 (1.5 g)	25-30	25-30 (1.5 g) (1.5 g)	25-30

Maximal doses for children are the same as those for adults.
**Exceeds manufacturer recommended dose.
†Directly observed therapy should be used with intermittent dosing.
‡Complex drug interactions occur with many medications, including those used for HIV infection; refer to the text.
§Not FDA approved for this indication.
[1]Not available in the United States.
[2]Not available in the United States.
Abbreviations: IM = intramuscular; INH = Isoniazid; IV = intravenous.

Rakel and Bope: *Conn's Current Therapy 2006.*

CURRENT DIAGNOSIS

Mycobacteria* in HIV-Positive and HIV-Negative Individuals

Symptoms

- Cough, fatigue, sputum, weight loss, hemoptysis not solely explained by an underlying condition.

Radiographic Abnormalities

- Cavities, infiltrates, nodules.
- High-resolution computed tomography, and multifocal bronchiectasis and/or multiple tiny nodules.
- Radiographic findings not explained by another condition.

Sputum

- 3 sputum/bronchial washing specimens from previous 12 months *and*
- 3 washings grow positive cultures, but AFB smears are NTM negative *or*
- 2 cultures are positive and 1 AFB smear is positive *or*
- 1 bronchial washing is available *and* culture is positive with a 2+, 3+, or 4+ AFB smear *or* 2+, 3+, or 4+ growth on solid media.

Lung biopsy

- Culture positive for NTM *or*
- Lung biopsy shows granulomas *and/or*
- Positive AFB and one or more sputum/bronchial washing is culture-positive for NTM.

*These criteria best apply to disease caused by MAC, *Mycobacterium kansasii,* and *Mycobacterium abscessus.*

Abbreviations: AFB = acid-fast bacillus; MAC = *Mycobacterium avium* complex; NTM = nontuberculous mycobacteria.

efficacy of anti-HIV therapy has allowed recovery of some immune function and these relatively low-grade pathogens are often contained by the reconstituted immunity. Still, therapy is continued as long as cultures are positive; discontinuation is considered after at least 12 months of therapy, with negative cultures, and on recovery of the CD4+ lymphocyte count.

REFERENCES

Blumberg HM, Burman WJ, Chaisson RE, et al: American Thoracic Society/Centers for Disease Control and Prevention/Infectious Diseases Society of America: Treatment of tuberculosis. Am J Respir Crit Care Med 2003;167:603-662.

Centers for Disease Control and Prevention: Targeted tuberculin testing and treatment of latent tuberculosis infection. MMWR Recomm Rep 2000;49(No. RR-6):1-51.

Centers for Disease Control and Prevention: Updated guidelines for the use of rifabutin or rifampin for the treatment and prevention of tuberculosis among HIV-infected patients taking protease inhibitors or nonnucleoside reverse transcriptase inhibitors. MMWR Morb Mortal Wkly Rep 2000;49:185-189.

National Center for HIV, STD, and TB Prevention at the Centers for Disease Control and Prevention. Available online at http://www.cdc.gov/nchstp/tb/. This Web site posts information as soon as it is released.

4

The Cardiovascular System

Acquired Diseases of the Aorta

Method of
Imran T. Mohiuddin, MD, and
Ruth L. Bush, MD

The first aortic operations occurred in the early 1800s and were performed on middle-aged men with aneurysmal disease secondary to syphilis. In 1817, Sir Astley Cooper did the first aortic ligation for a patient with a ruptured iliac artery aneurysm. Unfortunately, the patient soon died after the operation. The first successful ligation of the abdominal aorta for aneurysmal disease with long-term survival of the patient was performed by Dr. Rudolph Matas in 1923. Matas is also credited for improving and refining the technique of endoaneurysmorrhaphy.

The difficulties with early aortic surgery and complete aortic interruption led to the development of the aortic prosthesis. The early aortic prostheses were homografts. Jaretzki, Voorhees, and Blakemore were the first to report the use of Vinyon-N cloth tubes to replace the aorta in 17 patients with aortic aneurysms in 1952. In 1953, widespread application of this concept was brought about by the introduction of the Dacron velour graft by Dr. DeBakey, which is still in use. The development of the synthetic, arterial bypass graft heralded what is regarded as contemporary vascular surgery. However, vascular disease management is currently in the midst of an evolution with the advent of catheter-based technologies. The development of percutaneous angioplasty by the Swiss radiologist, Dr. Andreas Gruntiz, eventually led to the development of the first intravascular stent by Dr. Julio Palmaz in 1985. Arguably, the greatest advance in endovascular aortic surgery came by Dr. James Parodi who reported his results with 11 patients of endovascular repair of abdominal aortic aneurysms in 1991.

Acquired diseases of the aorta can be divided into three broad subtypes: aortoiliac occlusive disease, aneurysmal disease, and aortic dissection. Degeneration due to atherosclerosis has been implicated as a likely common etiology. The disease initially progresses silently in the aorta but will eventually lead to clinical manifestations after significant vessel-wall damage has occurred. Atherosclerosis is a disease of the intima in medium and large arteries. It is characterized by the accumulation of smooth muscle cells and lipid within the vessel wall. This accumulation leads to the development of a fatty streak and eventually a fibrous plaque. On a macroscopic level, this is manifested by luminal narrowing, thrombosis, and eventual occlusion. There are several risk factors that are associated with atherosclerosis including smoking, hypertension, hyperlipidemia, and family history.

Early detection using improved screening modalities such as ultrasound and computed tomography (CT) has led to improved surgical outcomes. In addition, advances in perioperative monitoring and anesthetic management have dramatically reduced the morbidity and mortality of complex aortic operations. The modern vascular surgeon has not only open surgical techniques but now also has a wide array of endoluminal procedures available as minimally invasive treatment modalities.

Epidemiology

The incidence of acquired diseases of the aorta is related to age. In the United States, the aging of the baby-boomer generation along with improved diagnostic imaging will likely result in an increased prevalence of aortic diseases. Conservative estimates indicate an incidence of at least 30% in patients older than age 70 years. In general, risk factors for aortic disease are similar to those of all vascular disease and include: age, smoking, hypertension, and family history. The increase of cigarette smoking in women has led to a rise in the incidence of aortic disease in women. The prevalence of abdominal aortic aneurysms is currently estimated to be about 5% to 7% of the population who are age 65 years or older. It is now the 10th leading cause of death with 15,000 deaths annually. This disease has a 4:1 male predominance. Although the exact incidence of aortoiliac occlusive disease is unknown, its incidence is common among patients with peripheral arterial disease and is second only to superficial femoral artery (SFA) disease. Aortic dissection occurs less frequently with approximately 2 of every 10,000 people affected. It can be seen in all age groups, but is most often seen in men 40- to 70-years old. Over the past 20 years, the mortality rates

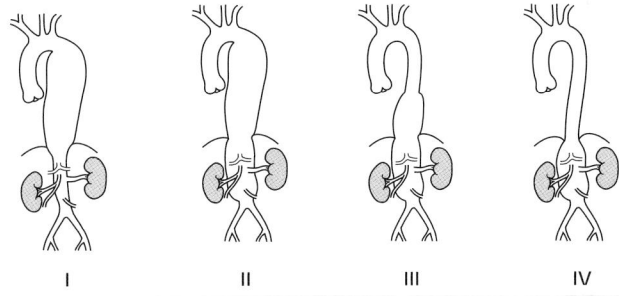

FIGURE 1. Crawford's classification system of aortic aneurysms.

I   II   III   IV

TABLE 1 Rupture Risk (%/y) Correlated With Size (cm)	
AAA Size (cm)	**Rupture risk (%/y)**
<4	0
4-5	0.5-5
5-6	3-15
6-7	10-20
7-8	20-40
>8	30-50

Adapted from Brewster DC, Cronenwett JL, Hallett JW, et al: Guidelines for the treatment of abdominal aortic aneurysms. Report of a subcommittee of the Joint Council of the American Association for Vascular Surgery and Society for Vascular Surgery. J Vasc Surg 2003;37(5): 1106-1117.

of aortic dissection have improved presumably as a result of improved management. In 1990, the average mortality rate per 100,000 was 1.2 in men and 0.6 in women.

Natural History

ANEURYSMAL DISEASE

The natural history of an aortic aneurysm is to expand and rupture. A classification system based on extent has been used often to describe aortic aneurysms (Figure 1). Symptoms are infrequent and a "staccato" pattern of growth is seen, where periods of relative quiescence may alternate with expansion. Therefore, although an individual pattern of growth cannot be predicted, average aggregate growth is approximately 3 to 4 mm per year. There is some evidence to suggest that larger aneurysms may expand faster than smaller aneurysms. Rupture risk appears to be directly related to aneurysm size as predicted by Laplace's law. Although more sophisticated methods of assessing rupture risk based on finite element analysis of wall stress is under active investigation, maximum transverse diameter remains the standard method of risk assessment for aneurysm rupture. Gender studies have shown that aneurysms in women have a higher rate of rupture when size-matched with men. The rupture risk is quite low below 5.0 cm and begins to rise exponentially thereafter. Based on risk-of-rupture studies, current guidelines from the United States dictate that once an aneurysm reaches 5.5 cm in size, it should be fixed in an "average" patient. Table 1 delineates the rupture risk with regard to size. Although data is less compelling, a pattern of rapid expansion of greater than 0.5 cm within 6 months can be considered a relative indication for elective repair. Other factors, which increase the risk of rupture are chronic obstructive pulmonary disease (COPD) and diastolic hypertension. Aneurysms that fall below these diameter indications may be safely followed with CT or ultrasound at 6-month intervals, with long-term outcomes equivalent to earlier surgical repair. Crawford reported a decline in the mortality rate from 19.2% to 1.9% over a 25-year period despite increasingly complex repairs in higher-risk patients.

AORTOILIAC OCCLUSIVE DISEASE

In aortoiliac occlusive disease, atherosclerotic narrowing often is centered on the aortic bifurcation. The symptoms and natural history of aortoiliac occlusive disease is influenced by the anatomic distribution and extent. In general, there are three frequently seen patterns (Figure 2). Type I disease is localized to the distal aorta and common iliac arteries. Type II is seen in patients with disease confined to the abdomen. Type III is the most common with a more widespread pattern. Approximately 65% of patients will have type III disease, whereas 25% of patients have disease that is confined to the abdomen. The majority of type III patients have multisegment disease, which is much more common in males. These patients generally have a higher incidence of co-morbidities including diabetes and hypertension. Progression to complete occlusion is more common with a higher percentage of patients requiring revascularization for limb-salvage rather than claudication. Symptoms can be equal in both extremities, but generally

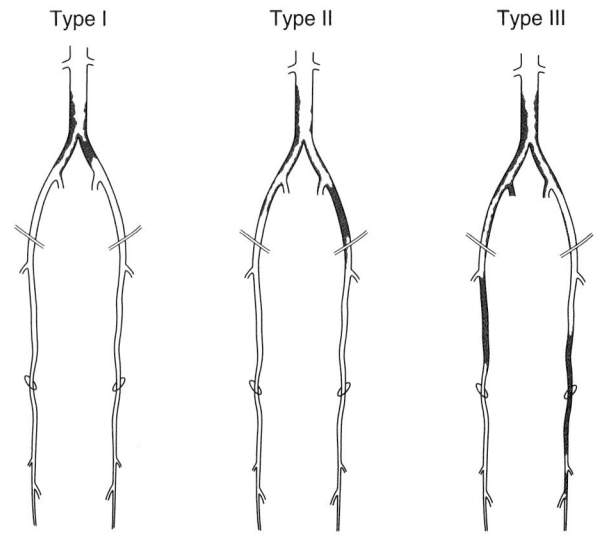

Type I   Type II   Type III

FIGURE 2. Types of aortoiliac disease. Type I: Disease is limited to aortic bifurcation. Type II: Disease is limited to intra-abdominal. Type III: Disease is extra-abdominal involving femoral arteries. Adapted from Brewster, DC: Direct reconstruction for aortoiliac occlusive disease. In Rutherford R (ed): Vascular surgery. Philadelphia, WB Saunders, 1995, pp 766-789.

one side is more affected than the other. In addition to calf and thigh claudication, presenting symptoms often include rest pain and ischemic tissue loss. However, type I or localized aortoiliac disease is seen infrequently in about 5% to 10% of patients. These patients are typically younger with a relatively low incidence of hypertension and diabetes but an increased likelihood of inherited lipid abnormalities. Patients typically present with claudication of the thigh, buttock, or hip with one extremity often being affected more than the other. Tissue loss is rare. In men, impotence is a frequent complaint and is seen in varying degrees from 30% to 50% of patients. In addition, about 50% of localized aortoiliac disease is seen with female patients where it has been implicated in early menopause and sexual dysfunction.

Aortic Dissection

Aortic dissection is characterized by the separation of the aortic wall layers by extraluminal blood that enters the wall through a tear in the intima. The most simple classification system is the Stanford types described by Daily in the 1970s in which all dissections that involve the ascending aorta are type A, whereas those that do not involve the ascending aorta are type B. It is generally acknowledged that the risk of early death is much greater with type A, whereas type B dissections have a more chronic course. If left untreated, type A dissections are often lethal. The early complications of intrapericardial rupture, acute aortic insufficiency, and occlusion of the coronary arteries rapidly leads to death and is well described in the literature. Type B aortic dissections are generally more chronic in nature; however, complications of rupture and ischemia can be seen and account for a mortality rate of up to 30% in the acute phase. Most ruptures occur in the left pleural cavity, and a massive hemothorax is seen. Although infrequent, ruptures also can be seen into the mediastinum and right hemithorax. Ischemic complications occur as a result of involvement of any of the branches of the descending thoracic and abdominal aorta. This is generally due to narrowing caused by compression of the true lumen by the false lumen. When compression is severe or circumferential, complete obstruction may occur leading to a coarctation-like picture with absence of distal pulses. There is an increased risk of rupture, and emergency surgery becomes imperative for survival. Chronic complications of aortic dissection are primarily due to aneurysm formation and account for the risk of late rupture after dissection. The risk of progressive dilation of the false lumen leading to aneurysm formation is estimated to be about 35%. These generally occur in the thorax opposite the site of the intimal flap or in the infrarenal aorta.

Key Diagnostic Points

The management of aortic disease is aided by adequate imaging. There are several imaging techniques that are currently used to image the aorta: ultrasound (US), CT scan, arteriogram, magnetic resonance angiography (MRA), transesophageal echocardiography (TEE), and intravascular ultrasound (IVUS). Ultrasound is the diagnostic screening modality of choice and is especially useful for aneurysms. It is cost-effective, noninvasive, and accurate. It also can be used to follow patients anually after repair. Ultrasound has the distinct advantage of providing physiologic information about the lesion. Anatomic limitations and experience of the ultrasonographer, however, can limit its use and quality. Because cross-sectional imaging is required for definitive evaluation of aortic disease, CT scan has become the most commonly used imaging modality. Thin cut (3-mm) CT scanning with contrast has become the principal technique for evaluating patients preoperatively for endograft placement. CT permits measurement of the neck diameter, detection of neck thrombus, measurement of neck length, aneurysm diameter, iliac diameter, and measurement of aneurysm length. It is particularly useful when combined with some of the newer techniques for CT reconstruction. Although more invasive, angiography is still used by most vascular surgeons who plan endovascular interventions. When performed with safe techniques, angiography provides the surgeon with the ultimate roadmap to successfully treat aortic disease. With the use of digital subtraction and timed bolus chases, the amount of contrast and radiation exposure can be minimized. Although adherence to strict technique minimizes the risks associated with angiography, this diagnostic modality is still not risk free. The desire for less invasive imaging has led to the emergence of MRA in the evaluation of the aorta. MRA is a safe but expensive alternative to angiography. MRA is the primary choice in patients with contrast allergies. However, there is some controversy regarding its accuracy when compared to angiography. When evaluating aortic dissection, transesophageal echo is also very useful. It can be used to document the presence and location of an intimal flap. In addition, the presence of pericardial fluid with TEE usually indicates rupture. A new imaging modality that has become useful in endovascular aortic procedures is IVUS, which provides real time information about aortic branch anatomy and the intima. It is used often in the operating room for precise positioning and placement of aortic endografts.

Key Treatment

There are several options in the management of aortic disease. Medical management is used to help prevent progression of disease. It also can be used in high-risk patients who are otherwise not candidates for surgery. Surgical management is divided into either operative or endovascular treatment.

MEDICAL MANAGEMENT

The medical management of aortoiliac occlusive disease is similar to that for atherosclerotic arterial disease elsewhere in the body. The cornerstone of medical management is reduction of vascular risk factors such as smoking cessation, control of blood pressure, reduction of blood lipid levels including statin therapy, correction of elevated homocysteine levels, and tight control of blood sugar in diabetics. Smoking cessation is by far the most important factor in determining the outcome of patients with aortoiliac occlusive disease. Control of blood pressure improves outcome in vascular disease. Interestingly, in patients with type III aortoiliac occlusive disease, control of blood pressure often incites claudication. It is not uncommon for hypertensive patients with aortic disease to develop claudication when high blood pressure is first detected and treated. Control of blood pressure is vital in patients with aortic dissection who are being prepared for the operating room. A short course of intravenous beta-blockade helps to delay rupture. Exercise therapy is also an important component of the treatment for aortoiliac occlusive disease. Other medical therapies directed specifically at peripheral disease rather than its risk factors include pentoxifylline (Trental)[1] and cilostazol (Pletal).[1] Clopidogrel (Plavix) and aspirin are effective antiplatelet agents that also have been successfully used to treat atherosclerotic disease. Their efficacy in coronary artery disease has been proved by multiple clinical trials.

Operative Management

The choice of operation is determined by the type of aortic disease. Regardless of etiology, the initial surgical approaches to the aorta are similar. Either a midline transperitoneal abdominal incision or a retroperitoneal approach can be used. The latter is particularly valuable in patients anticipated to have intra-abdominal adhesions and/or have abdominal stoma and may have value in patients with severe COPD. For some surgeons, this is the preferred approach for most infrarenal aortic surgery. However, there are two limitations: inability to reach the right renal artery and possible difficulty in exposing the right distal common iliac artery. Most surgeons still prefer the conventional midline incision. The ligament of Treitz is divided in order to mobilize the duodenum laterally. We prefer using a self-retaining retractor to maintain a clear field. The peritoneum anterior to the aorta is then incised to further dissect the infrarenal portion of the aorta. Once the aorta is exposed, the patient is anticoagulated using 100 U/kg of heparin. Clamps are carefully placed to achieve proximal and distal control.

With aneurysmal disease, the aneurysm is opened along its length, and a tube or bifurcated graft is sewn end-to-end inside the aneurysm using 3-0 Prolene suture for the aortic anastomosis. After hemostasis is achieved, anticoagulation is reversed using protamine sulfate. Prior to leaving the operating room, the surgical team must ensure that there is adequate perfusion to the feet by checking Doppler signals or presence of palpable pulses in the mesocolon. Patients are observed in the intensive care unit (ICU) overnight with most patients being hospitalized for 4 to 5 days post procedure.

[1]Not FDA approved for this indication.

Follow up is at 1 month, 6 months, then yearly. A CT scan is performed 3 years after the procedure, to look for evidence of pseudoaneurysm formation. Thoracic and thoracoabdominal aneurysms are better approached by using a thoracoabdominal incision with complete exposure of the aorta both above and below the diaphragm. Morbidity in these complex cases is best minimized by using a multidisciplinary team consisting of the surgeon, anesthesiologist, critical care specialist, perfusionist, and nursing staff. Descending aneurysms are repaired with standard techniques in which the aorta is replaced by a Dacron graft. Aneurysms that involve the visceral branches should be done in conjunction with afterload reduction usually using atrial-femoral bypass circuit. The renal arteries can be perfused in order to minimize ischemia. Care must be given to the critical zone of T9-L1 in which the vast majority of anterior spinal arteries arise from the aorta. Vessels in this area should be considered for reimplantation to a patch of the Dacron graft as described by Crawford. Careful postoperative care in the ICU by a critical-care team is essential for a good outcome.

With aortoiliac occlusive disease, the choice of operation is dependent on the distribution of disease. Disease limited to the aortic bifurcation may be treated with a simple endarterectomy. In most modern practices, endarterectomy is reserved only for carefully selected younger patients who have soft, ulcerated plaque and in the occasional septic patient in whom use of prosthetic material is contraindicated. Endarterectomy involves removal of the plaque in its entirety. Using a similar approach to the aorta as described previously in this section, proximal and distal clamps are applied, an arteriotomy is made, and the plaque is carefully dissected from the arterial wall leaving an intact adventitia. The arteriotomy is then reapproximated usually with a patch of either bovine pericardium or Dacron. More commonly, bypass grafting of the aortoiliac occlusive disease is performed using either aortobiiliac or bifemoral bypass. There are advantages to both as outlined in Table 2. Despite a single incision with avoidance of a groin incision, we prefer the aortobifemoral approach. This technique usually can be performed within the same time as the single-incision approach. It also prevents the impotence that is often seen with complete dissection of the aortic bifurcation when using the aortobiiliac approach. Aortoiliac disease progresses to eventually involve the femoral artery. By using an aortobifemoral approach, there are far fewer reoperations for outflow

TABLE 2 Comparison of Location of Distal Anastomosis: Iliac Versus Femoral

Bi-iliac	Bifemoral
Avoids groin incision	Allows for profundaplasty
Earlier ambulation	Lower rate of distal obstruction
Less pelvic ischemia	

Rakel and Bope: *Conn's Current Therapy 2006.*

obstruction (16% vs. 4%), which has established this approach as the gold standard. The choice between whether to perform an end-to-side versus end-to-end anastomosis remains unclear. There are some inherent advantages and disadvantages to each as outlined in Table 3. However, there are no comparative studies in the literature that have found any significant differences in patency rates between the two types of anastomoses. We believe that neither type of anastomosis should be used exclusively. For example, if an aneurysmal infrarenal aorta is encountered then the end-to-end anastomosis should be used. Conversely, if diseased external iliac arteries are encountered where proximal perfusion needs to be maintained, an end-to-side anastomosis would be more appropriate.

Most type B dissections are treated medically with operative repair reserved for emergent cases where there is rupture or the presence of neurologic symptoms. In addition, aneurysmal degeneration of chronic dissections must be repaired when discovered. In both of these cases, the approach is similar to standard aneurysms in this area. Because of the high risk of rupture in type A dissection, they must all be repaired early during hospitalization using cardiopulmonary bypass by an experienced cardiac surgeon. The aorta is replaced with Dacron with resuspension or replacement of the aortic valve.

Endovascular Management

Endovascular repair for aortic disease primarily consists of treatment for aortoiliac disease, aneurysm, and dissection. With the advent of the intravascular stent by Palmaz, more and more aortoiliac disease is being treated with iliac stents. Access is obtained with a 6- to 8-French sheath, the device is then deployed over a guidewire. When treating a distal or long-segment lesion, we use self-expanding stents. When the iliac lesion is close to the bifurcation, it is useful to place kissing stents in both common iliac arteries. This prevents compression of the uninvolved iliac artery by the stent. This technique involves obtaining bilateral access and simultaneous placement of stents. In this situation, we recommend using balloon expandable stents because of the need for precise placement. Arguably one of the most important advances in aortic surgery, the stent graft has revolutionized the practices of modern vascular surgeons. It is primarily used for the treatment of aortic aneurysms, but it also can be used to treat dissections although their use for this purpose has not been approved by the FDA. The stent graft is a covered stent device that is fixed proximally and distally to the nonaneurysmal aortic or iliac segment and thereby endoluminally excludes the aneurysm from the true aortic circulation. Unlike open surgical repair, neither the aneurysm sac nor its branches are resected or ligated. Currently three devices are available for elective repair of intact infrarenal abdominal aortic aneurysm (AAA):

1. Medtronic AneuRx (Santa Rosa, CA)
2. W.L. Gore Excluder (Flagstaff, AZ)
3. Cook Zenith (Bloomington, IN)

Despite some differences in physical appearance, mechanical properties, and materials, they will be discussed collectively for this chapter. They are all bimodular devices consisting of a primary device or main body and one or two iliac limbs that insert into the main body to complete the repair. Depending on the device, there are varying degrees of flexibility in the choice of iliac limbs that can be matched to the main body, which can impact the customizability for a particular anatomy. For thoracic aneurysms, several devices are currently being tested in clinical trials. One such device is the Talent stent graft. This thoracic device is unimodular and consists of a single stent graft that is deployed similarly to the currently available infrarenal devices.

Anatomic eligibility for endovascular aortic repair is mainly based on three areas: the proximal aortic neck, common iliac arteries, and the external, which relate to the proximal and distal landing zones or fixation sites respectively. It should be emphasized that prior to any endovascular aortic procedure, careful measurement of the aorta using both CT scan and a marker pigtail is imperative. When strict anatomic criteria are adhered to, 60% of AAA can be treated using an endovascular approach. The requirements for the proximal aortic neck are a diameter of 18 to 28 mm and a minimum length of 15 mm. The usual distal landing zone is the common iliac artery. The external iliac artery may serve as an alternate site when the ipsilateral common iliac artery is aneurysmal or ectatic. Once all the measurements have been made, the next step in the preoperative planning is device selection. Typically, the proximal diameter of the main device is oversized by 10% to 20% of the nominal diameter of the aortic neck. Distally, the iliac limbs are oversized by 1 to 4 mm depending on the individual device's instructions for use.

Although endovascular AAA repair may be performed in any venue with appropriate digital fluoroscopic imaging capability, due to the need for absolute sterility and aseptic technique, it is most safely performed in a surgical suite. Although a fixed floor or ceiling mounted fluoroscopic equipment, as in a dedicated endovascular surgical suite, may provide some benefit in terms of image quality and duration of fluoroscopy without radiograph tube burnout, most endovascular AAA repairs can be safely performed with portable C-arm fluoroscopic equipment.

TABLE 3 End-to-End Versus End-to-Side Proximal Aortic Anastomosis

End to end	End to side
Better hemodynamics	Less dissection/faster
Less embolization with distal aortic occlusion	Bigger anastomosis
Less likely to become kinked	Preserves flow to pelvis
Easier thrombectomy in juxtarenal occlusion	No worse off with occlusion of graft
Avoids competition between graft limb and native artery	

Rakel and Bope: *Conn's Current Therapy 2006.*

The patient is prepped and draped just as with an open AAA repair. Bilateral transverse oblique incisions are made just below the inguinal ligament to expose approximately 2 to 3 cm of common femoral arteries and obtain proximal control. Special attention is paid to avoid the groin crease to decrease the risk of wound complications.

Transfemoral access is obtained, and the Bentsen wire is placed into the aorta. This soft-tipped guidewire is then exchanged for stiffer guidewires (Amplatz), which are advanced to the thoracic arch. Intravenous heparin at 80 IU/kg is administered, and the ACT (activated clotting time) is maintained at 200 to 250 seconds. These guidewires provide the necessary support for the subsequent introduction of the large diameter delivery catheters and devices. In the absence of special anatomic considerations, the primary device is inserted through the right side, and the contralateral iliac limb is inserted through the left side. After administration of heparin, the delivery catheter or the introducer sheath is advanced to the L1-L2 vertebral space, which typically marks the location of the renal arteries. An angiographic catheter is advanced from the contralateral femoral artery to the same level. A road-mapping aortogram is obtained to localize the renal arteries. The primary device is rotated to the desired orientation and deployed immediately below the lowest renal artery. The contralateral limb on the main device is then cannulated, and a stiff guidewire is placed. The contralateral iliac limb is inserted into the docking opening of the primary device and deployed. For the Zenith device, there is a separate ipsilateral iliac limb that must be deployed to complete the repair. Depending on the accuracy of preoperative measurements, device selection, native anatomy, and technique, additional extenders may be required to achieve complete aneurysm exclusion and adequate fixation proximally and distally. Retrograde iliac angiograms are performed through the sheaths to locate the hypogastric arteries to prevent their inadvertent coverage. A completion angiogram is performed looking for patency of the renal and hypogastric arteries, the device limbs, proximal and distal fixation, and endoleak. Endoleaks are sealed using balloon angioplasty or extension cuffs. The procedure is concluded with routine repairs of the femoral arteries and closure of the groin incisions. The patients are recovered in the recovery room for 2 to 4 hours and admitted to the general care floor. Most patients can be started on a regular diet that evening and discharged the next morning.

Complications

Although in the past, aortic surgery was associated with significant risks, modern techniques have led to a significant decrease in the postoperative morbidity and mortality seen with aortic surgery. Currently, with perioperative mortality rates of 1% to 5%, and as low as 1:25 in high-volume institutions, intervention is recommended for all aneurysms greater than 5.5 cm. Crawford reported a decline in the mortality rate from 19.2% to 1.9% over a 25-year period despite increasingly complex

repairs in higher-risk patients. Complications encountered when treating aortic disease can be further divided into two groups: open surgery complications and endovascular complications.

OPEN SURGERY COMPLICATIONS

These complications include renal failure, lower extremity ischemia, colonic ischemia, graft complications, aortoenteric fistula, and spinal cord ischemia.

Renal failure can occur for several reasons, the most common being inadequate volume replacement. However, an aortic clamp close to the renal arteries can result in an embolic shower to the kidneys. Occasionally accessory renal arteries arise from the aneurysm. Although accessory renal arteries often can be sacrificed, they should be reimplanted in patients with compromised renal function. Preoperative impairment of renal function is the greatest predictor of postoperative renal insufficiency.

The absence of a femoral pulse suggests acute occlusion of the limb of the graft. This usually is due to a technical error such as a poor anastomosis, graft kinking, or compression, or it can be due to a clamp injury to the iliac artery beyond the anastomosis. This usually requires immediate surgical correction. If the femoral pulse is present, the limb is most likely ischemic either due to a distal embolus or acute thrombosis of the infrainguinal vessels because of pre-existing plaque or inadequate anticoagulation. Once again surgical exploration, thrombectomy, or bypass may be necessary.

Prosthetic grafting of the abdominal aorta for aneurysmal or occlusive disease is a common vascular procedure. It has a high patency rate at 5 years and a low complication rate. Complications include anastomotic aneurysms, graft infection, graft thrombosis, and aortoenteric fistulae (AEF). Anastomotic aneurysms involving the femoral or iliac arteries at the distal anastomosis are common. Para-anastomotic aneurysms involving the abdominal aorta (PAAA) also occur, but their incidence may be underestimated since routine screening after open aortic grafting is presently not the standard of care.

Colonic ischemia is reported as occurring with an incidence of 1% to 9%. However, with routine checking of the sigmoid perfusion at the completion of the case, the incidence has been significantly reduced. Diagnosis of colon ischemia is often delayed because of sedation, analgesia, or misdiagnosis as an ileus. Bloody diarrhea, elevated white cell count (WCC), or distension should prompt an aggressive search. The definitive diagnosis is established by colonoscopy. Early laparotomy and resection with colostomy is the only hope of survival in these critically ill patients.

An aortoenteric fistula is an uncommon (0.5%-2.3%) occurrence where the proximal aortic graft erodes into the overlying duodenum. The patient presents with gastrointestinal (GI) bleeding, which can be massive. Any patient with an upper GI bleed and a history of aortic surgery is presumed to have an aortoenteric fistula until proven otherwise. Positive diagnosis can be difficult, but upper GI endoscopy has the greatest yield.

CT scanning and angiography also may be helpful. Treatment is by graft excision and closure of the duodenum. Vascular reconstruction can be performed using either extra-anatomic bypass (bilateral axillopopliteal grafts, axillobifemoral graft) or by in situ replacement with antibiotic-impregnated Dacron grafts, or autogenous composite vein graft utilizing the superficial femoral vein.

Paraplegia is a rare (1:10,000) but devastating complication of abdominal aortic surgery. It is multifactorial in etiology and occasionally is due to contributions from a sacrificed lumbar artery to the spinal cord. However, more commonly, it is a manifestation of pelvic ischemia because of hypoperfusion (sacrifice of pelvic circulation) or embolization. Reimplantation of the inferior mesenteric artery or ensuring perfusion of an internal iliac artery will minimize the risk of this dreaded complication. The highest risk of spinal cord ischemia is with thoracoabdominal aneurysms (5.8%). Crawford reported that type II aneurysms were associated with the highest risk where the entire thoracic aorta needs to be replaced. This dire complication can be avoided by paying careful attention in the operating room to the location of the spinal artery. Although there are conflicting reports in the literature of its benefit, most surgeons reimplant patent intercostal vessels in the T8-L1 area to avoid this problem. In addition, cerebrospinal fluid (CSF) drainage and various pharmacologic techniques have been used with varying degrees of success.

ENDOVASCULAR COMPLICATIONS

The most common endovascular complications are access-related complications that are similar to those seen with all endovascular procedures. In decreasing order of frequency, these complications include groin hematoma, retroperitoneal hematoma, pseudoaneurysm, and arteriovenous fistula. Other general complications include dissection, perforation, distal embolization, occlusion, infection, and restenosis. The prevention of all of these can be best accomplished by adhering to meticulous techniques and is beyond the scope of this chapter.

Endovascular complications that are specific to aortic surgery are generally related to aortic-stent graft placement. These include endoleaks, hypogastric artery occlusion, and endotension.

An endoleak is an extravasation of contrast outside the stent graft and within the aneurysm sac. It can be present in up to 20% to 30% of all endovascular AAA repairs in the early postoperative period. In general, over half of these endoleaks will resolve spontaneously during the first 6 months resulting in a 10% incidence of chronic endoleaks in all cases beyond the first year of follow-up. Endoleaks can be detected using conventional angiography, contrast CT, MRA (magnetic resonance angiography), and color-flow duplex ultrasound. Although there is no recognized gold standard, in practice, angiography is considered the least sensitive but most specific for characterizing the source of the endoleak, whereas the CT scan is the most sensitive but least specific. Widespread availability and reliability that is relatively independent of technique have made the CT scan

the de facto standard imaging modality for postoperative surveillance. In this era of cost-sensitive medicine, duplex ultrasound has also emerged as an excellent imaging modality used to follow patients after an endograft. In the hands of a trained operator, ultrasound can provide valuable physiologic information. New techniques of ultrasound utilizing contrast agents are currently being evaluated.

Four types of endoleaks have been described. Type I endoleak refers to fixation-related leaks that occur at the proximal or distal attachment sites. These represent less than 5% of all endoleaks and are seen as an early blush of contrast into the aneurysm sac from the proximal or distal ends of the device during completion angiography. Although seen as markers of poor patient selection or inadequate repair, more than 80% of these leaks spontaneously seal in the first 6 months. Persistent type I endoleaks, on the other hand, require prompt treatment. Type II endoleak refers to retrograde flow originating from a lumbar, inferior mesenteric, accessory renal, or hypogastric artery. They are the most common type of endoleak accounting for 20% to 30% of all cases, and about half resolve spontaneously. On angiography, they are seen as a late filling of the aneurysm sac from a branch vessel(s). Type II endoleaks carry a relatively benign natural history and do not merit intervention unless associated with aneurysm growth. Type III endoleaks refer to failure of device integrity or component separation from modular systems. If detected intraoperatively or in the early perioperative period, it is usually from inadequate overlap between two stent grafts, whereas in the late period, it may be from a fabric tear or junctional separation from conformational changes of the aneurysm. Regardless of the etiology or timing, these should be promptly repaired. And last, type IV endoleak refers to the diffuse, early blush seen during completion angiography due to graft porosity and/or suture holes of some Dacron-based devices. It does not have any clinical significance and usually cannot be seen after 48 hours and heparin reversal. Endoleaks that have initially been considered type IV but persist become type III endoleaks by definition, as it indicates a more significant material defect than simple porosity or a suture-hole.

Incorrect measurement of the location of the hypogastric artery can lead to inadvertent coverage of the hypogastric artery by a long iliac limb. When one limb is affected, one incurs a 40% risk of ipsilateral hip and

 CURRENT DIAGNOSIS

- Obtain medical, cardiac, family, and social history
- Ultrasound evaluation for diameter evaluation
- Computed tomography scan for diameter, angulation, iliac involvement, and neck evaluation
- Aortogram prior to endovascular intervention
- Magnetic resonance arteriography for patients with contrast allergies
- Intravascular ultrasound during endovascular interventions with contrast restrictions

CURRENT THERAPY

- Control of hypertension, smoking cessation, tight blood sugar control, exercise therapy, and antiplatelet agents
- Selection of therapeutic approach
- Operative repair
- Endovascular repair
- Early and late complications
- Postoperative surveillance

buttock claudication. Often, patients with severe concomitant aortoiliac disease may have only one patent hypogastric artery. Although there is usually a good collateral blood supply, occasionally, occlusion of the remaining hypogastric artery in these patients can lead to severe pelvic ischemia. Pelvic ischemia also can result when the hypogastric artery is embolized in order to prevent or treat a type II endoleak.

In approximately 5% of cases, after an apparently successful endovascular repair, the aneurysm continues to grow without any demonstrable endoleak. This phenomenon has been described as endotension. Although it was initially thought that an endoleak was really present but simply not detected, cases have been reported where the aneurysm has been surgically opened, and the contents were completely devoid of any blood and no extravasation could be found. The mechanism of continued pressurization of the aneurysm sac following successful exclusion from the arterial circulation remains unsolved at this time. One putative mechanism has been linked to a transudative process related to certain expanded polytetrafluoroethylene (e-PTFE) graft materials. More importantly, however, the natural history of these enlarging aneurysms without endoleaks is unknown, but, to date, there has been no evidence to suggest that they carry an increased risk of rupture. Conservatively speaking, until further long-term data become available, if the patient is a suitable surgical risk, elective open conversion should be considered.

REFERENCES

Brewster DC: Direct reconstruction for aortoiliac occlusive disease. In Rutherford R (ed): Vascular surgery. Philadelphia, WB Saunders, 1995, pp. 766-789.

Brewster DC, Cronenwett JL, Hallett JL, et al: Guidelines for the treatment of abdominal aortic aneurysms. Report of a subcommittee of the Joint Council of the American Association for Vascular Surgery and Society for Vascular Surgery. J Vasc Surg 2003;37(5):1106-1117.

Brewster DC, Franklin DP, Cambria RP, et al: Intestinal ischemia complicating abdominal aortic surgery. Surgery 1991;109(4): 447-454.

Brock RC: The life and work of Sir Astley Cooper. Guys Hosp Rep 1968;117(3):147-168.

Brown LC, Powell JT: Risk factors for aneurysm rupture in patients kept under ultrasound surveillance. UK small aneurysm trial participants. Ann Surg 1999;230(3):289-296; discussion 296-297.

Cannon CP: Effectiveness of clopidogrel versus aspirin in preventing acute myocardial infarction in patients with symptomatic atherothrombosis (CAPRIE trial). Am J Cardiol 2002;90(7): 760-762.

Crawford E: Thoraco-abdominal and abdominal aortic aneurysms involving renal, superior mesenteric, celiac arteries. Ann Surg 1974;179(5):763-772.

Crawford ES, Crawford JL, Safi HJ, et al: Thoracoabdominal aortic aneurysms: preoperative and intraoperative factors determining immediate and long-term results of operations in 605 patients. J Vasc Surg 1986;3(3):389-404.

Cronenwett JL, Davis JL Jr, Gooch JB, et al: Aortoiliac occlusive disease in women. Surgery 1980;88(6):775-784.

Curci JA, Sanchez LA: Medical treatment of peripheral arterial disease. Curr Opin Cardiol 2003;18(6):425-430.

Daily PO, Trueblood HW, Stinson EB, et al: Management of acute aortic dissections. Ann Thorac Surg 1970;10(3):237-247.

Darling RC, Brewster DC, Hallett JW, et al: Aorto-iliac reconstruction. Surg Clin North Am 1979;59(4):565-579.

DeBakey ME: Clinical application of a new flexible knitted Dacron arterial substitute. Arch Surg 1958;77(713):15-20.

Gilling-Smith G, Brennan J, Harris P, et al: Endotension after endovascular aneurysm repair: Definition, classification, and strategies for surveillance and intervention. J Endovasc Surg 1999;6(4):305-307.

Gillum RF: Epidemiology of aortic aneurysm in the United States. J Clin Epidemiol 1995;48(11):1289-1298.

Gruntzig A, Hopff H: Percutaneous recanalization after chronic arterial occlusion with a new dilator-catheter (modification of the Dotter technique) [in German]. Dtsch Med Wochenschr 1974;99(49):2502-2510, 2511.

Hallin A, Bergqvist D, Holmberg L: Literature review of surgical management of abdominal aortic aneurysm. Eur J Vasc Endovasc Surg 2001;22(3):197-204.

Kato M, Bai H, Sato K, et al: Determining surgical indications for acute type B dissection based on enlargement of aortic diameter during the chronic phase. Circulation 1995;92(9 Suppl):II107-112.

Lemos DW, Raffetto JD, Moore TC, et al: Primary aortoduodenal fistula: a case report and review of the literature. J Vasc Surg 2003;37(3):686-689.

Lindsay J Jr, Hurst JW: Clinical features and prognosis in dissecting aneurysm of the aorta. A re-appraisal. Circulation 1967;35(5): 880-888.

Matas R: Personal experiences in vascular surgery: A statistical synopsis. Ann Surg 1940;112:802.

McIntyre K: Aortoiliac occlusive disease. In Kaufman J, Talavera FT, Phifer TJ, et al. (eds): Emedicine, pp 1-11, Las Vegas, 2003.

Palmaz J: Expandible intraluminal graft: A preliminary study. Radiology 1985;156:72-77.

Parodi J, Palmaz J, Barone H: Transfemoral intraluminal graft implantation for abdominal aortic aneurysm. Ann Vasc Surg 1991;5:491-499.

Roberts WC: Aortic dissection: Anatomy, consequences, and causes. Am Heart J 1981;101(2):195-214.

Rutherford RB: Options in the surgical management of aorto-iliac occlusive disease: A changing perspective. Cardiovasc Surg 1999;7(1):5-12.

Svensjo S, Bengtsson H, Bergqvist D: Thoracic and thoracoabdominal aortic aneurysm and dissection: an investigation based on autopsy. Br J Surg 1996;83(1):68-71.

Tran H, Anand SS: Oral antiplatelet therapy in cerebrovascular disease, coronary artery disease, and peripheral arterial disease. JAMA 2004;292(15):1867-1874.

Veith FJ, Braum FJ, Ohki T, et al: Nature and significance of endoleaks and endotension: Summary of opinions expressed at an international conference. J Vasc Surg 2002;35(5):1029-1035.

von Kodolitsch Y, Csosz SK, Koschyk OH, et al: Intramural hematoma of the aorta: predictors of progression to dissection and rupture. Circulation 2003;107(8):1158-1163.

Vorhees J: Use of tubes constructed from Vinyon-N cloth in bridging arterial defects: experimental and clinical. Ann Surg 1952;140: 324-334.

Webb TH, Williams GM: Thoracoabdominal aneurysm repair. Cardiovasc Surg 1999;7(6):573-585.

The Cardiovascular System

Angina Pectoris

Method of
Charles R. Lambert, MD, PhD

Evaluation of the Patient With Chest Pain

Evaluation of the patient with chest pain is a common task for the practicing physician, whether generalist or specialist. Differentiation of cardiac from noncardiac pain is of primary importance in such situations. Angina pectoris is usually described as a heavy chest pressure with a squeezing or burning characteristic that can be associated with difficulty breathing. It can be associated with radiation to the neck, left shoulder, arm, or jaw. Typical stable angina builds over several minutes and is usually associated with physical activity or psychologic stress. This type of angina is usually caused by a mismatch between myocardial oxygen supply and demand and is most commonly secondary to significant obstructive atherosclerotic coronary artery disease. The principal clinically measurable determinants of myocardial oxygen demand are heart rate and blood pressure. The importance of these simple physiologic parameters in treatment of patients with myocardial ischemia cannot be overestimated. Myocardial oxygen supply is determined primarily by coronary blood flow and the oxygen-carrying capacity of blood.

Characteristics of chest pain not usually related to myocardial ischemia include a pleuritic nature, primary localization to the abdomen with radiation to the chest, and radiation to the lower extremities. Pain that can be localized with a single finger over the left ventricular apex or that is present and persists for many hours or lasts for seconds is usually not caused by myocardial ischemia. It should be noted, however, that many episodes of ischemia in patients with documented coronary artery disease occur without symptoms and that even myocardial infarction can occur without symptoms. Indeed, the most significant litigation issue in emergency room evaluation of patients with myocardial ischemia is missed myocardial infarction.

Several grading systems have been developed to characterize angina pectoris; the most commonly used was developed by the New York Heart Association and the Canadian Cardiovascular Society (Table 1). These are very useful in describing the clinical status of a patient and documenting any changes that occur with natural history of the disease or with therapy. The differential diagnoses of chest pain include esophageal motility disorders, biliary colic, costosternal syndromes, severe pulmonary hypertension, pulmonary embolism, aortic dissection, myocardial infarction, and pericarditis.

Evaluation of the patient with chest pain of unknown cause or established angina pectoris begins with a complete and thorough physical examination as well as electrocardiogram (ECG) and chest radiograph. A resting ECG during an episode of chest pain can be particularly useful in establishing a diagnosis. Biochemical testing is done to define risk factors for development of coronary artery disease including hypercholesterolemia, other dyslipidemias, carbohydrate intolerance, and insulin resistance. Other markers such as C-reactive protein are also useful in clinical management of patients with coronary artery disease.

Echocardiography is performed in patients with stable angina who have a systolic murmur suggestive of aortic stenosis, mitral regurgitation, or hypertrophic cardiomyopathy. Echocardiography or radionuclide angiography is used to assess left ventricular function in patients with a history of prior myocardial infarction, pathologic Q waves, symptoms or signs of heart failure, or complex ventricular arrhythmias. Exercise ECG testing, with or without an imaging modality, is used for diagnostic purposes in patients with an intermediate pretest probability of coronary artery disease based on age, gender, and symptoms. It is also used for risk assessment and prognosis in patients undergoing initial evaluation. Stress testing is less useful in patients with either a high– or low–pretest probability of coronary artery disease. Dipyridamole (Persantine) or adenosine (Adenocard) myocardial perfusion imaging or exercise echocardiography is used in patients with left-bundle-branch block, a paced rhythm, and inability to exercise or with other baseline electrocardiographic abnormalities.

Direct referral for coronary angiography is appropriate when noninvasive imaging is contraindicated or unlikely to be adequate, when patients' occupations could pose a risk to themselves or others, or when the pretest probability of coronary artery disease is high. Patients who are in Canadian Cardiovascular Society classes III and IV, despite medical therapy, should undergo coronary angiography, as should patients who have survived sudden cardiac death or who have angina with associated congestive heart failure. Coronary angiography is also considered for patients with an uncertain diagnosis after noninvasive testing in whom the possible benefits of a certain diagnosis outweigh the risks of catheterization. Coronary angiography is also considered in patients with inadequate prognostic information after diagnostic testing or who cannot undergo such testing because of disability, illness, or body habitus. The extent and severity of coronary artery disease and left ventricular dysfunction identified during cardiac catheterization remain the most powerful predictors of long-term outcome for patients with coronary atherosclerosis and angina pectoris.

Medical Management

Once clinical evaluation of the patient with angina is complete, a treatment strategy is individualized for each patient that includes reduction of risk factors, treatment of exacerbating diseases, pharmacologic therapy, revascularization, and alterations related to general psychosocial and lifestyle issues. Associated diseases or conditions that can exacerbate angina pectoris include anemia, thyroid disease, fever, infections, tachycardia, and weight gain. These generally alter the myocardial

5

TABLE 1 Grading Systems for Angina Pectoris

Class	New York Heart Association functional classification	Canadian Cardiovascular Society functional classification	Specific activity scale
I	Patients with cardiac disease but without resulting limitations of physical activity. Ordinary physical activity does not cause undue fatigue, palpitation, dyspnea, or anginal pain.	Ordinary physical activity, such as walking and climbing stairs, does not cause angina. Angina with strenuous or rapid or prolonged exertion at work or recreation.	Patients can perform to completion any activity requiring ≤7 metabolic equivalents (e.g., can carry 24 lb up eight steps; carry objects that weigh 80 lb; do outdoor work [shovel snow, spade soil]; do recreational activities [skiing, basketball, squash, handball, jog/walk at 5 mph])
II	Patients with cardiac disease resulting in slight limitation of physical activity. They are comfortable at rest. Ordinary physical activity results in fatigue, palpitation, dyspnea, or anginal pain.	Slight limitation of ordinary activity. Walking or climbing stairs rapidly, walking uphill, walking or stair climbing after meals, in cold, in wind, or when under emotional stress, or only during the few hours after awakening. Walking more than two blocks on the level and climbing more than one flight of ordinary stairs at a normal pace and in normal conditions.	Patients can perform to completion any activity requiring ≤5 metabolic equivalents (e.g., have sexual intercourse without stopping, garden, rake, weed, roller skate, dance fox trot, walk at 4 mph on level ground) but cannot and do not perform to completion activities requiring ≥7 metabolic equivalents.
III	Patients with cardiac disease resulting in marked limitation of physical activity. They are comfortable at rest. More than ordinary physical activity causes fatigue, palpitation, dyspnea, or anginal pain.	Marked limitation of ordinary physical activity. Walking one to two blocks on level ground and climbing more than one flight of stairs in normal conditions.	Patients can perform to completion any activity requiring ≤2 metabolic equivalents (e.g., shower without stopping, strip and make bed, clean windows, walk 2.5 mph, bowl, play golf, dress without stopping) but cannot and do not perform to completion any activities requiring ≥5 metabolic equivalents
IV	Patient with cardiac disease resulting in inability to carry on any physical activity without discomfort. Symptoms of cardiac insufficiency or of the anginal syndrome may be present even at rest. If any physical activity is undertaken, discomfort is increased.	Inability to carry on any physical activity without discomfort; anginal syndrome *may be* present at rest.	Patients cannot or do not perform to completion activities requiring ≥2 metabolic equivalents. *Cannot* carry out activities listed above (Specific Activity Scale, class III).

From Goldman L, Hashimoto B, Cook EF, Loscalzo A: Comparative reproducibility and validity of systems for assessing cardiovascular functional class: Advantages of a new specific activity scale. Circulation 1981;64:1227. Copyright 1981, American Heart Association.

oxygen supply–demand ratio, as do sympathomimetic drugs. Any condition that increases left ventricular wall stress such as worsening heart failure, valvular dysfunction, or tachyarrhythmias can also worsen anginal symptoms through increasing myocardial oxygen demand in the face of limited supply.

Risk factor reduction and associated education should be stressed to all angina patients. Hypertension is a well-established effector linked to coronary heart disease mortality and severity. Left ventricular hypertrophy is an even stronger predictor of adverse outcome in

hypertensive patients. Rigorous blood pressure control is essential in management of patients with coronary artery disease and angina pectoris. Tight diabetes control is also essential in managing the patient with coronary artery disease. Weight reduction should be stressed and pursued in obese patients. Cigarette smoking is one of the most powerful predictors for the development of coronary artery disease in all age groups. In patients with coronary artery disease, smoking is associated with a higher 5-year risk of sudden death, myocardial infarction, and all-cause mortality than patients who have quit smoking. Smoking appears to increase myocardial oxygen demand, decrease coronary blood flow, stimulate progression of atherosclerosis, and reduce the efficacy of drug therapy. Clearly, discontinuation of smoking should be a primary target of antianginal therapy.

The National Cholesterol Education program guidelines suggest use of cholesterol-lowering therapy in all patients with coronary artery disease to 100 mg/dL or less. Most cardiologists target levels less than 80 mg/dL supported by other clinical studies. Lipid-lowering therapy with statins reduces the level of circulating C-reactive protein, improves endothelial responses, and favorably influences the composition of atheroma. Lipid-reduction therapy is associated with a reduction in coronary events and improvement in survival for patients with coronary artery disease and is a mainstay of therapy in patients with angina pectoris. Low HDL cholesterol represents an additional risk factor for coronary events. Therapy includes diet and exercise with LDL-cholesterol reduction in patients with concomitant elevation. The Veterans Affairs High Density Lipoprotein Cholesterol Intervention Trial demonstrated a 24% reduction in death, nonfatal myocardial infarction, and stroke with gemfibrozil therapy in patients with low HDL but no elevation in LDL cholesterol. Lipid-lowering therapy also improves outcome after coronary artery bypass surgery where LDL cholesterol is a risk factor for development of graft-occlusive disease.

Although past studies are conflicting, current evidence does not suggest using hormone replacement therapy in women for cardiovascular prevention. However, it is generally suggested that exercise is beneficial in patients with angina pectoris if begun under supervision and increased gradually. Exercise improves cardiopulmonary conditioning, aids in weight loss and cigarette discontinuation, and supplies other pathophysiologic benefits in patients with coronary artery disease and angina pectoris.

Aspirin therapy is associated with reductions in acute myocardial infarction and sudden death in patients with coronary artery disease. In the absence of contraindications, 75 to 325 mg of aspirin should be given every day to patients with stable angina pectoris and/or coronary artery disease. Clopidogrel (Plavix) can be substituted for aspirin in patients with aspirin hypersensitivity or intolerance. This agent offers additional long-term benefit in patients with non–sinus tachycardia (ST) elevation coronary syndromes or who underwent percutaneous coronary intervention.

In the absence of contraindication, β-adrenergic blockers are generally considered first-line therapy for treatment of patients with coronary artery disease. They are effective in prevention or delay of exercise-induced angina pectoris and reduce death and recurrent myocardial infarction in patients who sustained a previous myocardial infarction. β-Blockers also have beneficial effects on certain arrhythmias and in patients with left ventricular dysfunction. They are also very effective agents in management of hypertension. β-Blockers exert their favorable effects in angina pectoris primarily by reducing heart rate, blood pressure, myocardial contractile

state, myocardial wall stress, and subsequently myocardial oxygen demand. Patients with obstructive coronary artery disease can exercise longer and at a higher level before reaching the double product of heart rate and blood pressure that precipitates angina without therapy.

Calcium antagonists are used in combination with β-blockers when the efficacy of the former is incomplete or as a substitute for β-blockers when they are not tolerated because of adverse effects. Although verapamil (Calan) has the most negative chronotropic and inotropic effects of the class, the dihydropyridines such as nifedipine (Procardia) and nicardipine (Cardene) have the most vascular selective and least chronotropic and inotropic effects. Diltiazem (Cardizem) lies between these classes. When combined with β-blocker therapy, the least adverse effects are usually seen when using the dihydropyridines. A reflex tachycardia is seen when the latter are used alone without β-blockade.

Sublingual nitroglycerin should be given to all patients with angina pectoris with appropriate education on how and when to use it for treatment of acute angina episodes. Long–acting nitrates—oral, sublingual, or topical—can be used either in addition to β-blockers and calcium antagonists, or as monotherapy in patients with coronary artery disease and angina pectoris.

Angiotensin-converting enzyme (ACE) inhibitors are not indicated specifically for the treatment of angina pectoris; however, they appear to have very beneficial effects in reducing the incidence of future ischemic events in coronary artery disease patients. They are currently indicated in patients with left ventricular systolic dysfunction and/or diabetes. Data clarified after development of these guidelines, we feel, support treating most coronary artery disease patients with ACE inhibitors even in the absence of left ventricular dysfunction if no contraindications exist.

Although conflicting evidence was presented in the past, current recommendations do not include therapy with supplemental vitamin E, vitamin C, chelation therapy, or beta carotene for treating coronary artery disease. However, treatment of depression, including pharmacotherapy, should be considered integral to management of patients with coronary artery disease and angina pectoris. Changes in lifestyle with respect to both work and recreation in association with education, weight loss, stress reduction therapy, and structured exercise can all benefit the angina patient. Often, the best place to start such an effort is not in a busy physician's office but in a good cardiac rehabilitation program. It is not rare to see a patient who underwent hundreds of thousands of dollars' worth of interventional procedures without ever having any exposure to the basic educational programs and support available in cardiac rehabilitation.

Percutaneous Coronary Intervention

Percutaneous coronary intervention (PCI) therapy for coronary artery disease has changed dramatically since the initial introduction of balloon angioplasty. Advances in technology, pharmacotherapy, and stent development along with formal training programs, augmented– quality management, and adjunctive therapies have fueled dramatic expansion in the number of procedures performed. Conversely, a reduction in the number and increase in the complexity of cardiac surgical revascularization has emerged, especially with the advent of drug eluting stents with their associated lower restenosis rate. Interventional cardiology is a recognized subspecialty of cardiology, and it is beyond the scope of this article to explore the many criteria for selection of patients and lesions, as well as performance of interventions and probable outcomes. In general, however, it can be stated that patients with chronic stable angina who are ideal for PCI have symptoms or objective evidence for ischemia despite intensive medical therapy, are at low risk of complications, and have anatomy associated with high technical success.

Current guidelines recommend PCI for patients with stable angina pectoris with double- or triple-vessel disease including proximal left anterior descending (LAD) involvement with suitable anatomy, normal left ventricular function, and no diabetes. PCI is also suitable for single- or double-vessel disease without LAD involvement but with a large area of myocardium at risk and high-risk criteria on noninvasive testing. PCI is indicated for recurrent stenosis with a significant area of myocardium at risk and for patients who have failed medical therapy and can undergo intervention with acceptable risk. PCI is also used for patients with focal-vein-graft stenosis where the area of myocardium at risk is significant, and medical therapy is ineffective. PCI is not indicated in borderline lesions (50% to 60%) without evidence of ischemia. PCI is not yet established as primary therapy for left main coronary artery disease in patients who are candidates for coronary artery bypass surgery.

Coronary Artery Bypass Graft Surgery

Coronary artery bypass graft (CABG) surgery is a mainstay of therapy for patients with chronic stable angina as well as other coronary syndromes. Currently, CABG is considered to be primary therapy for patients with left main coronary artery disease although increasing evidence suggests that PCI with drug-eluting stents offers comparable efficacy and durability. CABG is indicated for patients with triple-vessel disease and offers an additional survival benefit in such patients with impaired left ventricular function. In other patient subsets, as listed earlier for PCI, CABG offers an alternative revascularization therapy and must be individualized with respect to risk of the respective procedure, the probability of achieving complete revascularization, the expected durability of the result, and informed patient preference. Revascularization therapy is not considered in patients with hemodynamically insignificant lesions (<50%) and where there is a small area of viable myocardium supplied by the target artery.

Patient Follow-Up

Coronary artery disease is a chronic condition, and patient follow-up with careful attention to the measures reviewed under medical management earlier are very important. In general, patients with chronic stable angina should have follow-up evaluations every 4 to 6 months during the first year and at least annually thereafter. Patients need to understand that more frequent evaluation must occur should symptoms change. The guidelines for use of testing during follow-up are generally conservative. We individualize stress testing and echocardiographic or radionuclide testing based on clinical status, the severity of underlying disease, the presence of stents and whether they are drug eluting, also considering risk factors and general patient compliance. For patients who had PCI, we generally do yearly functional assessments with stress testing for a period after initial treatment. For CABG patients, the initial interval is generally 1 year as well. If patients have other confounding conditions, such as valvular dysfunction, hypertrophic cardiomyopathy, severe hypertension, or arrhythmias, more frequent follow-up and testing are needed.

Unstable Angina

In contrast with stable angina pectoris, unstable angina pectoris is characterized by one or more of the following clinical characteristics:

- Symptoms occurring at rest or with minimal exertion
- New onset
- A crescendo pattern

Symptoms in unstable angina are often more severe than for stable angina and often persist until nitroglycerin is administered. Patients with unstable angina comprise a very heterogeneous population, and classification schemes are useful in considering pathophysiology and treatment. The progression or transition of stable angina to unstable angina and myocardial infarction occurs because of a number of processes. The most common of these is probably plaque erosion or rupture with superimposed nonocclusive thrombus. This can be associated with dynamic coronary vasoconstriction such as that seen in Prinzmetal's angina. Unstable angina develops with a simple progression of obstructive coronary artery disease, inflammation, or with factors affecting the demand side of myocardial energetics such as anemia, tachycardia, hypertension, or hyperthyroidism. The line between unstable angina and non–ST elevation myocardial infarction is thin and defined by the presence of infarction. It is not surprising that these patients share many clinical characteristics.

Unstable angina patients frequently have ST-T changes on the electrocardiogram. Continuous monitoring shows labile ST segments even in the absence of symptoms indicating ongoing ischemia and is in general an indicator of poor outcome. In general, patients with unstable angina have severe coronary artery disease, although nonobstructive disease can be seen and can implicate dynamic coronary constriction or microvascular dysfunction.

Treatment goals for patients with unstable angina are to stabilize the unstable nature of the clinical syndrome, presumably by "passivating" the unstable coronary lesion and exacerbating conditions. Ischemia should be alleviated followed by appropriate invasive or noninvasive testing and then institution of revascularization, if indicated, and secondary presentation measures. A mainstay of initial therapy in unstable angina is antithrombotic and includes aspirin, clopidogrel (Plavix), unfractionated or fractionated heparin, and platelet glycoprotein IIb/IIIa receptor antagonists.

Anti-ischemic therapy not only serves to review ongoing ischemia but also to stabilize the unstable atherosclerotic plaque. With active pain, nitrates are initially given by sublingual administration followed by intravenous infusion. Care is taken to avoid hypotension that can compromise coronary perfusion pressure. Early intravenous administration of β-blockers is used to optimize heart rate and blood pressure while reducing contractile state. Care should be taken in patients with significant reduction in left ventricular function and bradycardia or conduction disturbances. β-Blockers such as pindolol (Visken), with intrinsic sympathomimetic activity, should be avoided.

After nitrates, β-blocker, and anticoagulation therapy is instituted, calcium antagonists can be used for adjunctive antithetic therapy or for rhythm control if indicated. These agents are also useful in patients who do not tolerate β-blockers. Short-term acute use of ACE inhibitors does not seem to add significant benefit in unstable angina therapy, although later chronic therapy as discussed in the stable angina section earlier is indicated. Lipid-lowering therapy should be started as initial therapy in unstable angina and can be associated with improved outcome most probably because of stabilization of the evolving atherosclerotic lesion.

Two strategies have evolved involving evaluation of patients with unstable angina. These include an aggressive or invasive strategy with early angiography and revascularization with PCI or CABG and a conservative strategy with medical management followed by noninvasive risk stratification. These strategies have been tested in multiple clinical trials with current recommendations for an early invasive strategy when feasible in high-risk patients. These include individuals with ST changes, positive troponin, recurrent ischemia, or congestive heart failure. An invasive strategy is also advised in patients who have a history of PCI or CABG or an earlier episode of unstable angina or myocardial infarction within 6 months. Noninvasive testing is generally used to stratify patients who are at low risk, to guide conservative strategy, to assess prognosis and residual ischemia and left ventricular function, and to direct chronic management and cardiac rehabilitation.

In general, the same considerations apply to selection of revascularization strategies in unstable angina as in stable angina. Technical and procedural factors in these cases differ because of the high prevalence of thrombus in these lesions and frequent active ongoing ischemia. Adjunctive pharmacotherapy, device therapy such

as aspiration thrombectomy or distal protection, and intraaortic balloon counterpulsation are more commonly used in the catheterization laboratory treatment of patients with unstable ischemic syndromes when compared to more stable patients.

Therapy of the patient with angina pectoris requires coordination of noninvasive and invasive diagnostic strategies, medical therapy, lifestyle, risk factor modification, revascularization, support, and education. The goals are to minimize myocardial ischemia and maximize long-term clinical outcomes and quality of life. Although tremendous advances have been made in all of these areas, our efforts remain lifelong and palliative.

REFERENCES

Gibbons RJ, Abrams J, Chatterjee K, et al: ACC/AHA 2002 guideline update for the management of patients with chronic stable angina—summary article: A report of the American College of Cardiology/American Heart Association Task Force on Practice Guidelines (Committee on the Management of Patients with Chronic Stable Angina). J Am Coll Cardiol 2003;41:159-168.

Hamm CW, Braunwald E: A classification of unstable angina—revisited. Circulation 2000;102:118.

Sudden Cardiac Death

Method of
Brian J. O'Neil, MD, and James E. Skinner, PhD

Sudden cardiac death (SCD) is defined as the sudden, unexpected loss of detectable signs of life, usually occurring within 1 hour of symptom onset. Sudden death is generally defined as death within 24 hours from symptom onset. These later deaths are primarily caused by sepsis or postarrest complications. Other causes of sudden death are intracranial catastrophes, asphyxia, and trauma. Up to 60% of all cardiac deaths are sudden, with deaths defined from all diseases of the heart, including congenital malformations. In the West, coronary heart disease (CHD) is the primary cause of sudden cardiac death. Healed myocardial infarction was found in 40% to 72% of autopsy studies, with up to 77% revealing at least one 90% occluded coronary artery. The risk for sudden death is four to six times higher in patients with prior acute myocardial infarction (AMI) compared to the general population. Sudden death also occurs from cardiac nonatherosclerotic disease, such as spastic coronary artery spasm, congenital coronary artery lesions, vasculitis, and coronary artery emboli (Box 1).

The Centers for Disease Control and Prevention (CDC) estimates that 340,000 people die in the United States annually of CHD either before or very shortly after arrival at the emergency department. Moreover, for people under the age of 65 years, approximately 80% of CHD mortality occurs without previous warnings. In total, 50% of men and 64% of women who die suddenly from CHD had not reported any previous symptoms. Sudden cardiac death accounts for 19% of sudden deaths in children ages 1 to 13 years and 30% of sudden deaths in young people ages 14 to 21 years. Recent data show a 30% increase in the death rate for young women, with death rates remaining higher in African Americans compared to whites.

Ventricular tachycardia and fibrillation accounts for 75% of SCDs, with other causes including bradyarrhythmias. Disorders of impulse formation or impulse conduction, or a combination of the two, may cause arrhythmias. The three main mechanisms of arrhythmogenic sudden death are triggered activity, reentry, and ischemia-induced arrhythmias.

Triggered activity occurs when the membrane attempts to repolarize before depolarization is complete, the so-called *R on T phenomenon*. These early afterdepolarizations can result from class 1A antiarrhythmics, acidosis, hypokalemia, and excess catecholamines. The electrocardiogram (ECG) in these patients may reveal a long QT syndrome, which is associated with torsades de pointes. Alpha$_1$-adrenergic stimulation, which occurs in states like ischemia, results in increased intracellular calcium that results in afterdepolarizations. Delayed afterdepolarizations are associated with digitalis toxicity and post-AMI. Magnesium sulfate[1] is a natural calcium antagonist that decreases afterdepolarizations and is effective in the treatment of torsades de pointes.

Reentry occurs as a result of a unidirectional block, which is the etiology of many ventricular tachyarrhythmias. There are three types of reentry: anatomic, such as Wolff-Parkinson-White syndrome (WPW); anisotropic reentry, which is caused by variable cell-to-cell coupling; and functional or leading circle reentry. Arrhythmias during postischemic reperfusion are often caused by acute changes imposed on a previously damaged heart. In particular, cardiac hypertrophy appears to predispose the heart to reperfusion arrhythmias. Ischemia causes abnormalities in calcium and potassium currents, which predispose the heart to ventricular ectopy with the potential to induce ventricular fibrillation (VF) or tachycardia.

The Heart-Brain Interaction

Ebert and colleagues in 1970 showed that if *all* of the nerves projecting to the heart are severed, including the intrinsic ones, the complete occlusion of the left anterior descending (LAD) coronary artery simply does *not* result in VF. In contrast, if the nerves are left intact, ligation of the LAD coronary artery resulted in VF 100% of the time. Soon after, coronary occlusion sensory neurons in the heart are activated and send impulses to the brain, triggering reactive autonomic outflow that results in descending neural activity, which is both necessary and sufficient to cause the lethal arrhythmogenesis.

The consideration of cardiovascular disorders should include the concept that regulation occurs at higher brain centers and not just by the more reflexive peripheral autonomic nervous system. Elevations in blood pressure are maintained by the same cerebral system that regulates vulnerability to arrhythmogenesis during myocardial ischemia. Skinner and colleagues revealed the underlying process is noradrenergic mediated through the second-messenger cyclic adenosine monophosphate (cAMP) and an altered slow outward potassium channel. It is known that the β-blockade, which competitively inhibits the postsynaptic effects of norepinephrine, has a salutary effect on SCD. Moreover, the more lipophilic β-blockers, which therefore enter the brain at higher concentrations, have shown the greatest antimortality benefit.

---

[1] Not FDA approved for this indication.

The neurocardiac interactions are complex but central to the pathophysiology of sudden death. Ample compelling evidence suggests that the autonomic nervous system regulates the electrostability of the myocardium. Sympathetic and parasympathetic imbalance may predispose to arrhythmias, particularly in the face of other factors such as electrolyte abnormalities. It is well known that central nervous system disease, such as subarachnoid hemorrhage or cerebral infarcts, may be associated with nearly every electrocardiographic change, reflecting abnormal depolarization and repolarization as a result of altered autonomic conditions. Sudden cardiac death in these states is infrequent, however. Excessive sympathetic simulation is known to induce dispersed subendocardial necrosis after stimulation of the stellate ganglion or prolonged infusions of catecholamines.

Psychosocial Stress

Psychosocial stress is associated with SCD. Rahe and colleagues studied the impact of defined psychosocial stressors on SCD and found that job insecurity, marital strife, a recent move, and death of a spouse are all psychosocial stressors significantly correlated with the incidence of SCD. Skinner and colleagues showed the importance of stress leading to an increase in VF in pigs after the coronary artery was occluded. More recently, the INTERHEART trial (a standardized case-control study of acute myocardial infarction in 52 countries representing every inhabited continent) showed the adjusted risk for acute myocardial infarction is highest for the ratio of apolipoprotein B to apolipoprotein A-1 at a risk of 49.2, next was current smoking at 35.7, and contrary to Western-dominated literature, psychosocial factors had a risk of 32.5, using a population-attributable risk model.

Blood Pressure Elevation

Blood pressure elevations are harbingers of arrhythmic death in humans. Skinner and colleagues showed that cryoblockade of fibers arising from the frontal cortex quickly normalize the blood pressure in hypertensive animals. This result explains why reducing blood pressure elevations with β-blockers also has an antimortality efficacy, whereas reducing the blood pressure with other hypertensives has little effect on mortality. Further, the sedative effects of β-blockers, likely caused by its effects on the frontal lobe, are also well known.

Sudden Cardiac Death in Conditions Other Than Coronary Heart Disease

In ventricular hypertrophy-related deaths, 50% to 70% are caused by ventricular tachycardia or fibrillation. Further, hypertrophic cardiomyopathy, which includes

conditions such as idiopathic hypertrophic subaortic stenosis, is a leading cause of SCDs in patients younger than 30 years of age. In some studies, hypertrophic cardiomyopathy accounted for 22% of the sudden deaths in patients younger than 20 years old and in 13% of patients ages 20 to 29 years. These patients are difficult to identify prospectively because relatively few have historical identifiers such as unprovoked syncope or sudden death in close relatives. Most sudden cardiac death victims younger than 35 years old have some form of hypotropic cardiomyopathy or other myopathy as their underlying disease.

Sudden death in heart failure patients is usually caused by interactions involving myocardial structural abnormalities, neurohumoral influences, and electrolyte disturbances. In acute decompensated heart failure, the stretch on the myocardium can result in conduction abnormalities and also arrhythmias via triggering activity.

Myocarditis is the origin of sudden death in many children, adolescents, and young adults. Sudden death associated with myocarditis is often exertional; therefore increased catecholamines in combination with inflammatory myocardial irritability and conduction abnormalities certainly play a role in this phenomenon. This observation led to the recommendation to decrease physical activity after periods of upper respiratory tract infections. In addition to viral myocarditis, other cardiac infectious diseases may also lead to SCD including endocarditis, Chagas' disease, and syphilitic compromise of the coronary ostia.

Dilated cardiomyopathies are responsible for approximately 10% of SCD. Causes include both idiopathic and dilated cardiomyopathies with a defined etiology. Autopsies demonstrate interstitial and perivascular fibrosis and myocardial hypertrophy in these patients, all of which are substrates for ventricular arrhythmias.

VALVULAR HEART DISEASE

Valvular heart disease such as aortic stenosis is a well-known cause of SCD. In cases of severe stenosis, the incidence of SCD is relatively high in symptomatic and relatively low in asymptomatic patients. Marked mitral valve prolapse or prolapse associated with significant mitral regurgitation is reported as an etiology of SCD in a very small percentage of patients. Seven-year follow-up of patients with prosthetic valve replacement reveals an incidence of SCD between 2% and 4%.

CONGENITAL HEART DISEASE

Congenital heart disease as an etiology of SCD is reported primarily in four congenital heart conditions: transposition of great arteries, tetralogy of Fallot, aortic stenosis, and pulmonary vascular obstruction. SCD also has been reported with anomalous left main coronary artery. It should be noted that a QRS interval greater than 170 milliseconds is predictive of ventricular tachycardia (VT) in patients with tetralogy of Fallot after surgical repair.

WOLFF-PARKINSON-WHITE SYNDROME

In patients with Wolff-Parkinson-White syndrome (WPW), 0.1%, or 1 per 1000, experience sudden death. The main mechanism is believed to be atrial fibrillation with very rapid conduction down the accessory pathway, which degenerates into ventricular fibrillation. Patients with WPW should be evaluated for ablation by an electrophysiologist because those with conduction rates of more than 230 beats per minute (bpm) down the accessory pathway are at greater risk for SCD. Other syndromes, such as arrhythmogenic right ventricular dysplasia, as the name suggests, have a risk for sudden death of approximately 2%. The pathology is caused by fatty and fibrofatty infiltration into the right ventricle with concomitant infiltration in the left ventricle occurring one half to two thirds of the time. Expected ECG findings include right bundle branch block, T-wave inversions in leads V1 to V3, and an epsilon wave, which is a terminal notch in leads V1 and V2.

BRUGADA SYNDROME

The Brugada syndrome, as described in 1992, is a syndrome associated with right bundle branch block and ST elevation in leads V1 to V3 and SCD. The pathology lies in a genetic defect within the cardiac sodium channel. One of the dilemmas of this syndrome in these ECG changes can be transient and may be worsened by drugs that block the sodium channel. This disease is suspected in the sudden death of young Thai men, particularly during sleep. The precipitating arrhythmia is thought to be a polymorphic VT, which can result in syncope or sudden cardiac death.

The QT interval is measured from the beginning of the QRS complex to the end of the T wave, which represents the duration of the activation and recovery of the ventricle. Increased recovery duration contributes to the increased likelihood of dispersion of refractoriness when some part of the myocardium may be refractory to subsequent depolarization. Subsequently, the excitation wave may follow a path around the refractory focus within the myocardium (circus reentrant rhythm), leading to ventricular tachycardia and potentially sudden death. Heart rate–corrected QT_c values above 0.44 seconds generally are considered abnormal, although these change slightly with age and sex. Hereditary or acquired long QT syndromes are known risks for lethal arrhythmias. Patients with congenital forms of long QT syndromes consist of the Jervell and Lange-Nielsen syndrome, which has an effect primarily on potassium channels, and the Romano-Ward syndrome, which has an effect primarily on potassium and sodium channels. The acquired QT syndrome may be caused by electrolyte and metabolic abnormalities including states of hypokalemia, hypocalcemia, or hypomagnesia, in addition to medications including tricyclic antidepressants, antihistamines such as terfenadine (Seldane) (removed from the market in 1998); anticholinergic drugs such as cisapride (Propulsid) (removed from the U.S. market in 2000); macrolide antibiotics such as erythromycin, antifungals, and fluoroquinolone antibiotics that are metabolized in the liver; and type IA antiarrhythmics such as quinidine and disopyramide (Norpace).

Multiple other etiologies may contribute to a terminal arrhythmic event, including any states that cause excess catecholamines or electrolyte or metabolic abnormalities including hypothermia. Metabolic and endocrine disorders also can lead to arrhythmias such as adrenal insufficiencies, hypokalemia from Cushing's syndrome, and cardiomyopathy caused by hemochromatosis. Lethal arrhythmias in these patients are rare. Many toxins render the heart vulnerable to lethal arrhythmias, including cocaine and anabolic steroids, toluene inhalations, nicotine, alcohol (such as in holiday heart syndrome), and drugs that have potential for proarrhythmic effects.

Iatrogenic causes of SCD include electrolyte imbalances such as hypokalemia caused by diuretic therapy and QT prolongation caused by the medications described earlier, with women, those over 65 years of age, and patients with ventricular hypertrophy, in particular, predisposed to QT prolongation.

Sudden cardiac arrest can occur in concert with or secondary to respiratory complications such as bronchoconstriction because of severe asthma, anaphylaxis, or obstruction. The heart in these states is exposed to an arrhythmogenic milieu of hypoxia and excess catecholamines. Sudden death in asthma is linked to vasovagally mediated bradycardia and hypotension. Asphyxia asthma is seen more often in men than women and carries an extremely poor neurologic prognosis, probably because of the continued flow of glucose-laden hypoxic blood that results in anaerobic glycolysis and increased brain lactic acid.

Sudden cardiac death associated with seizures has been ascribed to sympathetic overactivity, causing cardiac arrhythmias. Sudden death caused by epilepsy accounts for 15% of the cases of sudden death from ages 1 to 22 years when accidental and traumatic causes are excluded. Hypoxia and increased catecholamine levels may play a major role in the cardiac abnormalities that occur during seizures, however. Noncoronary vascular disease precipitates of sudden death include cerebral vascular catastrophes, aortic dissection, and pulmonary emboli.

Sudden Cardiac Death Prevention

Effective prevention requires a two-pronged approach. The first is to identify and evaluate those at highest risk and then to provide systems to treat SCD effectively when it occurs, for example emergency medical services (EMS) and cardiopulmonary resuscitation (CPR) training. Preventive therapy needs to concentrate on structural and acute substrate changes that make the heart more susceptible to arrhythmogenic triggers. The main factors that lead to these abnormalities include ischemia with reperfusion, systemic factors, neural input, and toxins. The Cardiac Arrhythmia Suppression Trial (CAST) revealed the proarrhythmic potential of many antiarrhythmic drugs.

RISK STRATIFICATION AND MANAGEMENT

Post-AMI patients are at the highest risk for SCD, although not all AMIs set the stage for lethal arrhythmogenesis, and differentiating patients who are at risk for arrhythmogenic SCD is the challenge. Figure 1 illustrates some major risk factors for sudden death and the inverse relationship between progressively higher risk groups and the decreasing occurrence rate for events.

All cardiac arrest survivors should be thoroughly evaluated with a complete history, physical exam, and ancillary testing, including laboratory and provocative testing. The history should focus on possible drug abuse or misuse, drug interactions, family history of arrest, preceding symptoms of chest pain or syncope, and shortness of breath or palpitations. The preceding symptoms can be difficult to obtain because antegrade or retrograde amnesia is common after arrest. The area responsible for forming new memories, the hippocampus, is one of the most vulnerable brain regions.

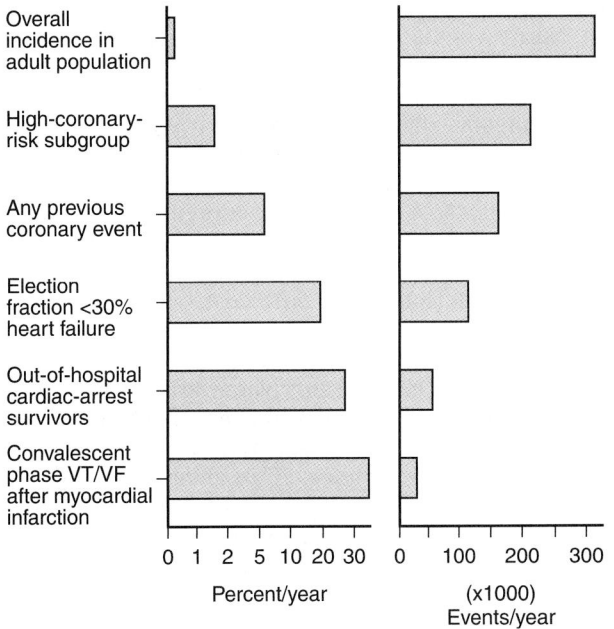

FIGURE 1. Sudden cardiac death among population subgroups. Estimates of incidence (percentage per year) and total number of sudden cardiac death per year are shown for the overall adult population in the United States and for higher-risk subgroups. The overall estimated incidence is 0.1% to 0.2% per year, totaling more than 300,000 deaths per year. Within subgroups, identified by increasingly powerful risk factors, the increasing incidence is accompanied by progressively decreasing total numbers. Practical interventions for the larger subgroups require identification of higher-risk clusters within the groups. The horizontal axis for the incidence figures is nonlinear. EF = ejection fraction; MI = myocardial infarction; VT/VF = ventricular tachycardia/ventricular fibrillation. (From Myerburg RJ, Kessler KM, Castellanos A: Sudden cardiac death: Epidemiology, transient risk and interventional assessment. Ann Intern Med 1993;119:1187-1197. Reproduced with permission from the American Heart Association.)

Rakel and Bope: *Conn's Current Therapy 2006.*

Physical examination should focus primarily on the cardiovascular and central nervous systems. ECGs should be evaluated for conditions like prolonged QTs, Brugada syndrome, and WPW. Electrophysiologic assessment, Holter monitoring, and tilt-table testing may occasionally provide additional information in these patients.

Reduced heart rate variability following myocardial infarction indicates sympathetic predominance and is the single best predictor of ventricular fibrillation and sudden death. The prognostic ability of tests of autonomic function was demonstrated in the Azimilide Post Infarct Survival Study, which associated impaired beat-to-beat variability with increased mortality. These results fueled the recent interest in the analysis of heartbeat dynamics to predict arrhythmogenic SCD. The choice of an appropriate analytic algorithm for the study of heartbeat dynamics should consider what is being measured physiologically. The older heart rate variability algorithms were based on linear stochastic models that measure sympathetic-parasympathetic balance (as in power spectral ratios or T wave alternans). The newer algorithms based on nonlinear deterministic models measure the dynamics imposed on the heartbeats by all levels of the nervous system. The nonlinear PD2i algorithm used on heartbeat data (15-minute ECGs) can accurately predict the lack of vulnerability (no false-negative predictions with 1-year follow-up). In a study of high-risk ER patients presenting with chest pain, a positive PD2i test predicted all cases of arrhythmic death within the next 180 days. Again, when comparing the nonlinear analysis of the heartbeat intervals of the patients who later died of arrhythmic death (i.e., VF) with their nearest controls who did not die, the results were 100% for sensitivity and 100% for specificity.

DEVICES

Current recommendations for placement of implantable cardiac defibrillators (ICDs) include:

- American College of Cardiology (ACC) class I recommendations for cardiac arrest caused by VF or VT not because of a transient or reversible cause (level A)
- Spontaneous sustained VT (level B)
- Syncope of undetermined origin with clinically relevant sustained VT or VF induced by an electrophysiologic study when drug therapy is ineffective (level B)
- Nonsustained VT with coronary disease, prior MI, and left ventricle (LV) dysfunction

The many class II indications include:

- Nonsustained VT with coronary artery disease
- Prior MI and LV dysfunction
- Inducible sustained VT or VF by an electrophysiologic study (level B) and class III patients with coronary artery disease with LV dysfunction and prolonged QRS duration in the absence of spontaneous or inducible sustained or nonsustained VT who are undergoing coronary bypass surgery (level of evidence: B)

The recent Multicenter Autonomic Defibrillator Implantation Trial 2 (MADIT-2) shows that placement of implantable defibrillators in high-risk patients sustains improvement in overall survival with a relative risk ratio of 0.69 for death. In the Comparison of Medical Therapy, Pacing, and Defibrillation in Chronic Heart Failure (COMPANION) Trial, the combination of implantable defibrillator and cardiac resynchronization improved survival and reduced hospitalization in patients with both ischemic and nonischemic cardiomyopathies and in patients with New York heart failure classes III and IV. The Defibrillator in Acute Myocardial Infarction Trial (DINAMIT) investigators performed a randomized open label comparing ICD versus no ICD in patients who were 6 to 40 days post-AMI, with LVEF equal to 35% and depressed heart rate variability or elevated average heart rate over 24 hours. The results showed no decrease in overall mortality; it did demonstrate a significant decrease in arrhythmogenic death in the ICD group with a hazard ratio of 0.42 and P value of 0.009.

PHARMACOLOGIC AGENTS

None of the antiarrhythmic drugs show efficacy in reducing mortality when compared to implantable cardiac defibrillators. Nonetheless, antiarrhythmic drugs such as amiodarone (Cordarone) still have a role in patients with a history of sustained VT. The evidence to date supports their use in combination with an ICD. Evidence also supports discharge therapy with β-blockers, angiotensin-converting enzyme (ACE) inhibitors, and aspirin in eligible patients.

Regarding prevention from sudden cardiac death, particularly in Western society, risk factors should be targeted, in particular smoking, cholesterol, and weight reduction. As noted in recent publications such as the INTERHEART study, reduction in psychological stressors should be attempted.

Management of Cardiac Arrest

Survival after cardiac arrest is still woefully inadequate, particularly in large cities with reported hospital discharge rates from 1% to 2% in out-of-hospital cardiac arrest victims. Recent trials demonstrate encouraging discharge-from-hospital rates in both the treatment and placebo groups. In a study of amiodarone (Cordarone) versus placebo in out-of-hospital VF arrest, 13% of patients were discharged from hospitals alive, with an impressive 50% to 55% able to resume an independent lifestyle or return to their former employment. In the study of amiodarone (Cordarone) versus lidocaine for shock-resistant VF, 28% of the patients survived to hospital admission in the amiodarone (Cordarone) group with approximately 15.3% surviving in the lidocaine group. Current trials of hypothermia after cardiac arrest are even more optimistic, with 49% good neurologic outcome in hypothermic and 26% good neurologic outcome in the normothermic in patients discharged from the hospital. Data from the hypothermia-after-cardiac-arrest study group corroborate a reported 55% of hypothermic and 39% normothermic cardiac arrest

survivors were discharged from the hospital with favorable outcomes.

Survival after cardiac arrest is increased when the initial rhythm is VF or VT. In contrast, resuscitation rates with pulseless electrical activity (PEA) and asystole are much worse. There appears to be a current trend toward increased incidence of PEA and asystolic presenting rhythms in recent studies of out-of-hospital cardiac arrest. The decreased rate of resuscitation is understandable, given that VF and VT require intact high-energy phosphate stores and asystole is a depolarized myocardium with depleted energy stores. Reentry is considered the mechanism for episodes of both ventricular tachycardia and ventricular defibrillation. Typically this occurs in myocardial abnormalities of the heart, both at the macroscopic level, such as a scar from previous infarction, and at the microscopic level, for example with a long QT syndrome.

The use of automatic external defibrillation in cardiac arrest patients increases resuscitation rates. In arrest durations of more than 5 minutes, however, it is still controversial whether the correct sequence is initially three defibrillations or 3 to 5 minutes of CPR followed by defibrillation. Efficacy of amiodarone (Cordarone) in patients with and without VF is provided against placebo and lidocaine in the Arrest and Alive trials, respectively. The use of vasopressin (Pitressin)[1] versus epinephrine remains controversial with conflicting studies regarding efficacy currently reported. The survival links for cardiac arrest particularly emphasize early recognition, early activation, and basic cardiopulmonary resuscitation, with a decrease in emphasis on the breathing portion of airway, breathing, circulation (ABC) and an increase in emphasis on early defibrillation, then management of airway circulation, with finally administration of medications. The recent trial that tested outcomes with public access defibrillation (PAD), shows a small but statistically significant difference in hospital discharge (30/128 versus 15/107; $P = 0.03$). Only two survivors were reported in residential areas, with a low likelihood of bystander recognition, whereas bystanders showed improved outcomes for placement of automated external defibrillators (AEDs) in casinos and in airports because both areas have a high likelihood of recognition. Figure 2 displays the odds ratio for survival comparing various variables and likelihood of survival.

POSTRESUSCITATION CARE

The most successful therapy in postresuscitation care to date is hypothermia postarrest to a temperature of 33°C (91.4°F). However, multiple other factors can improve survival. It has been known since the Trial of ORG 10172 in Acute Stroke Treatment (TOAST) study that hyperglycemia at stroke presentation is a predictor of poor outcomes. The study by Parsons and colleagues of magnetic resonance (MR) imaging and MR spectroscopy proved a mechanistic link between hyperglycemia and

---

[1]Not FDA approved for this indication.

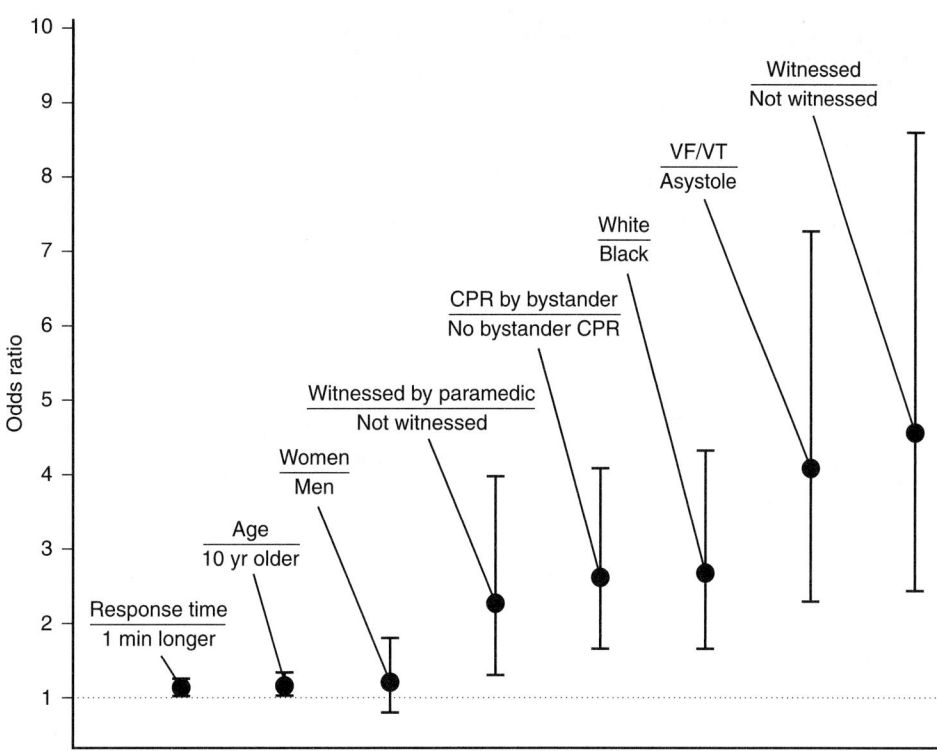

FIGURE 2. Association between eight variables and the likelihood of survival. Odds ratios and 95% confidence intervals *(vertical bars)* were calculated for eight paired risk factors. The likelihood of a patient's survival given the more favorable risk factor in each category (shown as the numerator) is divided by the likelihood of the patient's survival given the less favorable category (shown as the denominator). For example, the patient's actual response time (more favorable) is compared to an interval that is 1 minute longer (less favorable). The age factor compares the patient's current age with an age of 10 additional years. Similarly, women were compared with men, patients whose arrests were witnessed by paramedics with patients whose arrests were not so witnessed, patients receiving cardiopulmonary resuscitation (CPR) from a bystander with patients not receiving CPR from a bystander, white patients with black patients, patients with ventricular fibrillation (VF) or ventricular tachycardia (VT) with patients with asystole, and patients with witnessed arrests with patients with arrests that were not witnessed. Odds ratios for each variable are shown after adjustment for the other variables included in the model. (From Becker LB, Han BH, Meyer PM, et al: CPR Chicago: Racial difference in the incidence of cardiac arrest and subsequent survival. N Engl J Med 1993;329[9]:600-606.) Copyright © 1993 Massachusetts Medical Society. All rights reserved.

increased infarct volume and lactate production in stroke. Additional studies have shown that tight glucose control in the range of 120 m/dL improves outcomes after stroke and also reduces the mortality by 50% of intensive care unit (ICU) patients. The reason for this exact effect is unknown postevent; decreased lactic acidosis and the fact that insulin is a growth factor are

two potential mechanisms. As a corollary to hypothermia, postresuscitation care should avoid it because the cerebral metabolic rates increase 4% with each increase in degree centigrade. As with most critical patients, tight electrolyte control should be practiced. During postarrest states the adrenals are nonfunctional, and therefore most experts recommend stress doses of steroids

---

CURRENT DIAGNOSIS

- Thorough electrocardiogram analysis should be performed to look for potential proarrhythmic conditions such as prolonged QT and Brugada syndrome.
- Analysis of heart rate variability with devices like the nonlinear PD2i algorithm should be performed on patients at high risk for sudden cardiac death.
- Post–acute myocardial infarction patients and cardiac arrest survivors should be thoroughly evaluated with a complete history, physical exam, and ancillary testing, including laboratory and provocative testing.

CURRENT THERAPY

- Implantable cardiac defibrillators are the most effective therapies to date for sudden cardiac death in the high-risk patients noted in the article. These devices should be placed alone or in combination with antiarrhythmic drugs such as amiodarone (Cordarone).
- Therapy with β-blockers, angiotensin converting enzyme inhibitors, and aspirin should be included in high-risk patients.
- In post–cardiac arrest patients, hypothermia, tight glucose control, stress dose steroids, and monitoring for seizures are recommended.

(hydrocortisone,[1] 100 mg, IV push). Many experts also recommend monitoring for seizures and/or seizure prophylaxis because postresuscitation seizures portend a poor outcome. During postresuscitation care, cerebral autoregulation is usually lost, and therefore cerebral profusion pressure depends directly on mean arterial pressure. Maintaining a good arterial pressure is recommended. Simple care, such as elevating the head of the bed to 30 degrees and other standard ICU therapies are also recommended.

REFERENCES

Bernard SA, Gray TW, Buist MD, et al: Treatment of comatose survivors of out of hospital cardiac arrest with induced hypothermia. N Engl J Med 2002;346;557-563.

Camm AJ, Pratt CM, Schwartz PJ, et al: Mortality in patients after a recent myocardial infarction: A randomized, placebo-controlled trial of azimilide using heart rate variability for risk stratification. Circulation 2004;109:990-996.

Dorian P, Cass D, Schwartz B, et al: Amiodarone as compared with lidocaine for shock-resistant ventricular fibrillation. N Engl J Med 2002;346(12):884-890.

Ebert PA, Vanderbeck RB, Allgood RJ, Sabiston DC Jr: Effect of chronic cardiac denervation on arrhythmias after coronary artery ligation. Cardiovasc Res 1970;4:141-147.

Echt D, Liebson P, Mitchell L, et al: Mortality and morbidity in patients receiving flecainide or placebo: The Cardiac Arrhythmia Suppression Trial. N Engl J Med 1991;324:7881-7888.

Kleiger RE, Bigger JT, Bosner MS, et al: Stability over time of variables measuring heart rate variability in normal subjects. Am J Cardiol 1919;68:626-630.

Kudenchuk PJ, Cobb LA, Copass MK, et al: Amiodarone for resuscitation after out-of-hospital cardiac arrest because of ventricular fibrillation. N Engl J Med 1999;341(12):871-878.

Kuller I, Coper M, Perper J: Epidemiology of sudden cardiac death. Arch Int Med 1972:129;714-719.

Myerburg RJ, Kessler KM, Bassett AL, et al: A biographical approach to sudden cardiac death; structure, function, and cause. Am J Cardiol 1989;63;1512-1516.

Newman WB, Strong JP, Johnson WD, et al: Community pathology of atherosclerosis and coronary artery disease in New Orleans: Morphologic findings in young black and white men. Lab Invest 1981;41:496-501.

Parish DC, Dinesh Chandra KM, Dane FC: Success changes the problem: Why ventricular fibrillation is declining, why pulseless electrical activity is emerging, and what to do about it. Resuscitation 2003;58:31-35.

Rahe RH, Hervig L, Romo M, et al: Coronary behavior in three regions of Finland. J Psychosom Res 1978;22(5):455-460.

Schaffer W, Cobb L: Recurrent ventricular fibrillation and modes of cardiac death in survivors of out-of-hospital ventricular fibrillation. N Engl J Med 1975;293:259-262.

Skinner JE, Lie JT, Entman ML: Modification of ventricular fibrillation latency following coronary artery occlusion in the conscious pig: The effects of psychological stress and beta- adrenergic blockade. Circulation 1975;51:656-667.

Skinner JE, Pratt CM, Vybiral T: A reduction in the correlation dimension of heartbeat intervals precedes imminent ventricular fibrillation in human subjects. Am Heart J 1993;125:731-743.

Skinner JE, Welch KMA, Reed JC, Nell JH: Psychological stress reduces cyclic 3′, 5′-adenosine monophosphate level in the parietal cortex of the conscious rat. J Neurochem 1978;30:691-698.

Sudden cardiac arrest in U.S. young adults, 1989-96. CDC, 2001.

Szilagyi JE, Taylor AA, Skinner JE: Cryoblockade of ventromedial frontal cortex reverses hypertension in the rat. Hypertension 1987;9:576-581.

Wik L, Hansen TB, Fyling F: Delaying defibrillation to give basic cardiopulmonary resuscitation to patients with out-of-hospital

ventricular fibrillation. A randomized trial. JAMA 2003;289: 1389-1395.

Yusuf S, Hawken S, Ounpuu S, et al: Effect of potentially modifiable risk factors associated with myocardial infarction in 52 countries (the INTERHEART study). Lancet 2004. Available at http://image.thelancet.com/extras/04art8001web.pdf

Zheng ZJ, Croft JB, Giles WH, et al: State-specific mortality from sudden cardiac death—United States 1999. MMWR 2002; 51(6): 123-126.

Zipes DP, Levy MN, Cobb LA, et al: Task force 2: Sudden cardiac death. Neural-Cardiac interactions. Circulation 1987;76(Suppl): I 202-I 207.

Atrial Fibrillation

Method of
Mathias L. Stoenescu, MD, and
Peter R. Kowey, MD

Definition

Atrial fibrillation (AF) is a disorganized atrial rhythm that usually originates in the left atrium. Because the atrial rate can be as high as 600, the atrioventricular (AV) node does not transmit all the stimuli from the atria to the ventricles, and this variable protects the ventricles from very rapid rates.

Mechanisms

Moe's multiple wavelet theory is widely accepted as the mechanism sustaining AF. The theory postulates that a number of wavelets swirl around in the atria, sometimes colliding with each other and the anatomic boundaries of the chambers, thus extinguishing themselves, and sometimes dividing and perpetuating the rhythm. More recently discovered triggers, which represent foci of automaticity and triggered activity, commonly but not exclusively originating in the pulmonary veins, can act as initiators of the wavelets. A process of structural and electrical remodeling of the atria takes place with time and becomes more advanced the longer the tachycardia persists. It induces changes that favor the perpetuation of fibrillation.

Classification

Camm's proposed 3P classification describes the three stages of clinical manifestation:

1. Paroxysmal: self-terminating episodes
2. Persistent: requires termination by electrical or chemical cardioversion
3. Permanent: arrhythmia is refractory to cardioversion

---

[1]Investigational drug in the United States.

The remodeling process explains how longer paroxysms are gradually replaced by persistent and eventually permanent atrial fibrillation. Aging, associated with fibrosis of the atrial myocardium, plays a prominent role in this remodeling process. From an electrophysiologic standpoint, shortening of the atrial refractoriness and its lack of rate adaptation, together with an increase in automaticity and triggered activity of some cells, underlie the favorable substrate of the arrhythmia.

Epidemiology

The prevalence of AF increases with age from approximately 1% at age 20 years to more than 5% at age 70 years and older, according to epidemiologic investigations such as the Framingham Heart Study and the Cardiovascular Health Study. In 1995 an estimated 2 million individuals were affected, and an increasing trend is projected that will raise this number to 3 million by the year 2020. The aging of the population, combined with an increase in the prevalence of coronary artery disease (CAD), congestive heart failure (CHF), diabetes, and hypertension, is responsible.

The probability of developing AF after age 40 years is 25%. The number of hospitalizations from the diagnosis of AF has risen sharply in the past 2 decades.

AF is not a benign condition as previously thought. The most common arrhythmia, it accounts for large numbers of cardioembolic strokes and is a major contributing factor in exacerbating heart failure. The Framingham data suggest an increased mortality for patients with AF, after adjusting for other cardiovascular co-morbidities and age, which remain increased even in those without manifest heart disease.

Clinical Manifestation

Patients with AF often are asymptomatic. AF frequently is associated with embolic stroke, commonly the first symptom. When patients are symptomatic, the arrhythmia can cause palpitations, tiredness, lightheadedness, dyspnea, chest discomfort, and syncope.

Hemodynamically, the atrial contraction in sinus rhythm (SR) makes up 30% of the stroke volume, and in certain conditions associated with diastolic dysfunction, it makes up an even higher proportion. The loss of mechanical atrial systole can markedly decrease cardiac output, especially in the setting of a rapid ventricular rate, and heart failure may ensue or worsen if already present. Sustained rapid ventricular rates often result in tachycardia-induced cardiomyopathies, underlining the importance of ventricular rate control in AF.

Electrocardiographically, there is an absence of P waves, which are replaced by fibrillation waves. These low-amplitude irregular waves often have the appearance of an unruly baseline. The ventricular rhythm is irregular, and QRS electrical alternans may be observed as a rate-related phenomenon when the ventricular rate is rapid.

The pulse is irregular with a detectable pulse deficit between the actual heart rate measured by the apical impulses and the peripheral pulse rate caused by contractions of the left ventricle, which because of a shortened diastolic phase has not had adequate time to fill and hence does not generate a high enough stroke volume in the ejection phase. The heart sounds vary in intensity because of the beat-to-beat variability in the filling and contractility of the heart chambers.

Management

The management of AF is complex and depends on many variables. AF can exist in the absence of any structural heart disease (called "lone AF"), or it can be associated with a number of other cardiac and systemic conditions. Because patients with AF can be completely asymptomatic or severely symptomatic and can have different co-morbidities, a highly individualized treatment plan is usually necessary.

STROKE PREVENTION

Of foremost concern in treating AF is stroke prevention; the American College of Cardiology (ACC), American Heart Association (AHA), and European Society of Cardiology (ESC) have published elaborate consensus guidelines addressing this issue. They are under constant revision. The current guidelines (March 2001) recognize several risk factors for thromboembolism in AF: age over 60 years, heart failure, decreased systolic function (ejection fraction is ≤35%), hypotension, prior history of thromboembolism, rheumatic heart disease, atrial thrombus seen on transesophageal echocardiogram (TEE), prosthetic heart valves, thyrotoxicosis, and diabetes. For all those who have any of these conditions, oral anticoagulation with warfarin (Coumadin) is advocated. For those younger than age 60 years, with no heart disease or with heart disease that does not include the risk factors just listed, and for those between ages 60 and 75 years who have no risk factors, aspirin, 325 mg daily, is recommended. Patients age 75 years or older, especially women, should receive warfarin (Coumadin).

Recently an entirely new class of drugs—direct thrombin inhibitors-have stirred interest, but they remain somewhat controversial at this stage. Ximelagatran[1] is one of the better known representatives in this class. Potential advantages of thrombin inhibitors are fixed daily dosages, eliminating the need for blood tests for dose adjustments and more rapid onset of action. One potential drawback may be liver toxicity. Clinical trials studying their comparative efficacy to warfarin (Coumadin) and their side-effect profile are under way.

RATE-CONTROL STRATEGY

For patients with AF who are asymptomatic and for those who do not have significant symptoms of heart

---

[1]Not yet approved for use in the United States.

failure, controlling the ventricular rate by influencing AV node conduction pharmacologically or by AV node ablation may be a good option. Stroke prevention is essential. This strategy has been demonstrated in several studies, the largest of which was the Atrial Fibrillation Follow-up Investigation of Rhythm Management (AFFIRM), to be equivalent to a more aggressive rhythm-control strategy with regard to mortality and symptom relief. Rhythm control was slightly superior in controlling symptoms of heart failure, but overall freedom from AF was successful only in 62% of patients with drug therapy in this arm. No good data exist on what the optimal ventricular rate should be when rate control is attempted.

The drugs used for rate control slow conduction in the AV node and belong to several classes (Box 1). The calcium channel blockers (CCBs) diltiazem (Cardizem) and verapamil (Calan, Isoptin) in intravenous and oral formulations are effective in slowing ventricular rates acutely and chronically. β-Blockers (BBs) such as metoprolol (Lopressor, Toprol)[1] have the same effect. They can exacerbate bronchospasm but may be the preferred choice when used for chronic rate control in patients with coronary artery disease (CAD) and/or heart failure. Digoxin (Lanoxin) via its vagotonic effects on the AV node may be useful for rate control, especially in those over 65 years of age and inactive patients. Its drawback is poor rate control with exercise when compared to rest, which may require the addition of a CCB or BB. It should be used with caution in renal impairment where accumulation can lead to toxicity. It is beneficial when systolic left ventricular (LV) dysfunction is present and when hypotension makes the use of CCBs and BBs problematic. When rate control is more difficult to achieve and/or some of the previously mentioned drugs are contraindicated, amiodarone (Cordarone)[1] may prove useful as a stand-alone agent or in conjunction with a BB or CCB.

Radiofrequency catheter ablation of the AV node in conjunction with a pacemaker is a viable alternative, particularly in those over 65 years of age whose

---

[1] Not FDA approved for this indication.

BOX 1	**Drug Options for Rate Control**

- β-Blockers:
    Metoprolol (Lopressor) 25-100 mg bid PO; (Toprol XL)
      25-200 mg qd PO
    Atenolol (Tenormin) 25-100 mg bid PO
    Propranolol (Inderal) 10-30 mg tid/qid PO
    Nadolol (Corgard) 60-160 mg qd PO
- Calcium channel blockers
    Diltiazem SR (Cardizem CD) 120-480 mg qd
    Verapamil SR (Calan SR) 120-480 mg qd
    Digoxin (Lanoxin) 0.0625-0.5 mg qd
    Amiodarone (Cordarone)[1] 200-400 mg qd

[1]Not FDA approved for this indication.
Abbreviations: bid = twice daily; tid = three times per day; PO = by
  mouth; qd = every day; qid = four times per day.

---

ventricular rates are difficult to control with several agents or who manifest side effects of these drugs. This "ablate and pace" strategy does not eliminate the need for stroke prevention therapy, however.

RHYTHM-CONTROL STRATEGY

In selected groups of patients, maintaining sinus rhythm (SR) is desirable. These include patients who are symptomatic in AF despite appropriate rate control, patients less than 65 years of age who are active and have lone atrial fibrillation, patients whose ventricular rate is difficult to control in AF, and more controversially those who are not candidates for anticoagulation. In these patients the first step is cardioversion, which can be electrical or pharmacologic.

Direct current (DC) cardioversion is very effective and safe in restoring SR when certain precautions are taken. The risk of embolism after cardioversion is increased if AF has been present for longer than 48 hours because the resumption of the mechanical atrial systole lags behind the electrical restoration of SR. This phenomenon is called "atrial stunning." It seems to be a consequence of the atrial fibrillation and its termination and not of the modality of termination itself (DC shock versus pharmacologic intervention). Anytime the onset of AF is uncertain or more than 48 hours prior, full systemic anticoagulation with warfarin (Coumadin) for 4 weeks with weekly confirmation of therapeutic international normalized ratio (INR) should be undertaken before any type of cardioversion (chemical or electrical) is attempted. This should be followed by another 4 weeks of warfarin (Coumadin). An alternative is to perform TEE prior to cardioversion to rule out left atrial appendage thrombus and follow with 4 weeks of anticoagulation.

Anticoagulation can be safely discontinued only if good evidence indicates that no recurrence has occurred, which is often difficult to document because recurrences are fairly frequent and often without symptoms. In patients with other risk factors for stroke, medication for anticoagulation should probably be continued with warfarin (Coumadin).

Pharmacologic cardioversion represents another option to restore SR (Box 2). In the case of structurally normal hearts, single oral doses of class IC drugs (flecainide [Tambocor] and propafenone [Rythmol]) have been proved successful and safe—the so-called "pill-in-the-pocket" approach—even on an outpatient basis. Intravenous ibutilide (Corvert) is an effective alternative in a hospital setting. For patients with structural heart disease, ibutilide (Corvert) may effect conversion to SR. Intravenous amiodarone (Cordarone)[1] and oral dofetilide (Tikosyn) offer safe alternatives.

Because recurrences of AF are common, antiarrhythmic drugs (AAD) are often necessary to maintain SR (Box 3). AFFIRM demonstrated that the success rate of any currently available drug is no higher than 62%, challenging the wisdom of discontinuing

---

[1]Not FDA approved for this indication.

BOX 2 Drugs Used for Chemical Cardioversion

- Normal Heart
    Flecainide (Tambocor) 300 mg PO (single dose)
    Propafenone (Rythmol) 600 mg PO (single dose)
    Ibutilide (Corvert) 1 mg IV (can repeat once)
    Procainamide (Pronestyl) 15-17 mg/kg IV loading dose
        over 30-60 min
- Abnormal Heart (↓LVEF, CAD, severe LVH)
    Ibutilide (Corvert)[1] 1 mg IV (may repeat once)
    Amiodarone (Cordarone), 150 mg IV bolus, then
        1 mg/min for 6 h, followed by 0.5 mg/min for 18 h
    Dofetilide (Tikosyn) 0.125-0.5 mg bid PO

[1]Not FDA approved for this indication.
Abbreviations: bid = twice daily; CAD = coronary artery disease;
    IV = intravenous; LVEF = left ventricular ejection fraction; LVH = left
    ventricular hypertrophy; PO = by mouth.

---

warfarin (Coumadin) after successful conversion to SR. Because long-term drug treatment is required with this strategy, the choice of drug has to focus not only on efficacy but also on potential organ toxicities and the side-effect profile. Some of the sodium channel blocking drugs, especially those in the IC group (flecainide [Tambocor] and propafenone [Rythmol]), are very effective and generally well tolerated long term, but they can be pro-arrhythmic in the setting of structural heart disease (moderately to severely decreased LV [left ventricle] function, CAD, marked LVH [left ventricular hypertrophy]). They should be avoided in these cases. In structurally normal hearts, they play a role in chemically terminating AF, as well as in the maintenance of SR. The class III drugs sotalol (Betapace) and dofetilide (Tikosyn) are potassium channel blockers, which prolong the action potential. By increasing the QT interval, they may predispose to torsades de pointes. If prescribed and monitored correctly, they can be valuable in prevention of AF recurrences. Ibutilide (Corvert), another class III agent, is effective in terminating AF and atrial flutter, when given intravenously, with the same caveats of potential QT prolongation and torsades. Amiodarone (Cordarone) combines class I, II, III, and IV effects and

---

BOX 3 Drug Options for Maintenance of Sinus Rhythm

- Normal Heart
    Flecainide 50-200 mg bid PO
    Propafenone* 150-300 mg tid PO
    Sotalol 80-160 mg bid PO
    Dofetilide 0.125-0.5 mg bid PO
- Abnormal Heart
    Amiodarone† 200 mg qd (after loading dose of
        usually 600 mg daily for 1 wk)
    Dofetilide 0.125-0.5 mg bid PO
    Sotalol 80-160 mg bid PO (avoid if LVEF ↓)

*Propafenone SR (Rythmol SR) is available in doses of 225-425 mg bid.
†Amiodarone is not approved by the FDA for use in AF.
Abbreviations: bid = twice daily; LVEF = left ventricular ejection fraction;
    PO = by mouth; tid = three times per day; qd = every day

 CURRENT DIAGNOSIS

The differential diagnosis of atrial fibrillation (AF) based on the electrocardiogram includes:

- Atrial fibrillation: The ventricular rhythm is usually irregular unless complete heart block with a regular escape rhythm is present. The isoelectric line is unruly, with fibrillation waves that are unequal in amplitude and width.
- Sinus rhythm with frequent premature atrial contractions (PACs): This rhythm can be irregular like AF, but usually a clear isoelectric line is distinguished and several P waves with identical morphology are detectable.
- Multifocal atrial tachycardia: This is also irregular but a clear isoelectric line exists, and P waves of at least three different morphologies are present.
- Atrial flutter: The ventricular rhythm can be regular or irregular. Flutter ("f") waves equal in amplitude and width are distinguishable in all or most leads. No clear isoelectric baseline can be found between them, with the exception of lead V1.

---

is effective in maintaining SR. It can have potentially severe organ toxicities when used chronically, especially in higher doses. Corneal deposits, liver toxicity, lung fibrosis, and thyroid abnormalities are some of the possible side effects, and this drug should be used judiciously with close monitoring of the patient. It is not FDA approved for treatment of AF, but it is used off license mainly when impaired LV systolic function precludes the use of other AAD. Dronaderone,[1] a related compound, has not been released yet but holds the promise of an improved side-effect profile while maintaining a similar efficacy to amiodarone.

In the last decade, a new invasive catheter-based procedure has been developed that currently is undergoing a

---

[1]Not yet approved for use in the United States.

 CURRENT THERAPY

- Stroke prevention (relevant to both rate and rhythm-control strategies)
- Rate-control strategy
    Drugs (see Box 1)
    Ablate and pace
- Rhythm-control strategy
    Cardioversion
    Direct current shock
    Drugs (see Box 2)
- Maintenance of sinus rhythm
    Drugs (see Box 3)
    Ablation

---

rapid and promising evolution. AF ablation started as an intervention targeted at using radiofrequency (RF) to cauterize foci of automaticity inside the pulmonary veins. This approach has been abandoned because of the high incidence of pulmonary vein stenosis. Newer techniques are designed to encircle the pulmonary vein ostia with RF point lesions, thus isolating the veins from conducting impulses into the left atrium, or to draw anatomic lines of RF in the left atrium following different patterns. Both techniques claim equivalent success rates, which can be as high as 80% in patients with paroxysmal AF and somewhat lower in persistent AF. Long-term data and comparisons to drug therapy are not yet available. Epicardial pulmonary vein isolation techniques are also being developed. They are generally performed thoracoscopically. Surgical endocardial ablations performed at the time of other open heart procedures are also under evaluation replacing "the maze" procedure in which the left atrium is cut and reanastomosed following a particular pattern of lines, thus making the wide propagation of AF wavelets difficult. Ablative techniques are constantly and rapidly being modified and refined. In conjunction with newer and more efficacious drugs with improved side-effect profiles, they offer promise in the quest for a cure of this common arrhythmia.

REFERENCES

ACC/AHA/ESC guidelines for the management of patients with atrial fibrillation. J Am Coll Cardiol 2001;38:1231-1265.

Carlsson L, Miketic S, Windeler J, et al: Randomized trial of rate control versus rhythm-control in resistant atrial fibrillation (STAF) study. J Am Coll Cardiol 2003;41:1690-1696.

Hohnloser SH, Kuck KH, Lilienthal J, et al: Rhythm or rate control in atrial fibrillation—pharmacological intervention in atrial fibrillation (PIAF): A randomized trial. Lancet 2000;3356:1789-1794.

Kowey PR, Naccarelli GV: Atrial fibrillation. New York, Marcel Dekker, 2005.

Roy D, Talajic M, Dorian P, et al: Amiodarone to prevent recurrence of atrial fibrillation. The Canadian Trial of Atrial Fibrillation (CTAF). N Engl J Med 2000;342(13):913-920.

Singh H, Zoble R, Yellen L, et al: Efficacy and safety of oral dofetilide in converting to and maintaining sinus rhythm in patients with chronic atrial fibrillation or atrial flutter: The symptomatic atrial fibrillation investigative research on dofetilide (SAFIRE-D) study. Circulation 2000;1029(19);2000:2385-2390.

Stoenescu M, Kowey PR: Selection of drugs in pursuit of a rhythm control strategy. Prog Cardiovasc Dis 2005 (in press).

The atrial fibrillation follow-up investigation of rhythm management (AFFIRM) investigators. A comparison of rate control and rhythm control in patients with atrial fibrillation. N Engl J Med 2002;347:1825-1833.

Wiffles M, Crijns H: Recent advances in drug therapy for atrial fibrillation. J Cardiovasc Electrophysiol 2003;14(Suppl):540-547.

Premature Beats

Method of
*John A. Yeung-Lai-Wah, MB, ChB, and
Bandar Al Ghandi, MD*

Premature beats are beats that occur early in the cardiac cycle and originate from a site other than the sinus node. They are termed "supraventricular" if they arise from anywhere from the atria (premature atrial contractions [PACs]), or atrioventricular (AV) junction (i.e., AV node or bundle of histidine [His]). Premature beats that originate from below the His bundle are termed "premature ventricular contractions (PVCs). By definition, an ectopic beat must arise earlier than the next normally timed beat would be expected. Thus the interval between the ectopic beat and the proceding beat is shorter than the cycle length of the dominant rhythm. This is important to differentiate premature beats from other abnormal beats such as escape beats or intermittent bundle branch block.

Premature Supraventricular Complexes or Contractions

DEFINITION

An atrial premature beat (atrial ectopic beat, PAV) is an extra heartbeat caused by electrical activation of the atria from an abnormal site before a normal heart beat occurs.

DESCRIPTION

The P wave morphology of PACs differs from sinus beats. Depending on the prematurity of the atrial impulse and refractoriness of the AV node, the P wave may conduct with normal or prolonged PR interval. The electrocardiographic wave (QRS) complex becomes wide as in bundle branch block, when one of the bundle branches is still refractory when the impulse conducts down the Purkinje system. If the impulse blocks, the P wave is not followed by a QRS complex. Runs of three or more premature beats are considered tachycardia.

CLINICAL FEATURES

PACs occur in many healthy people and rarely cause symptoms. They have been recorded in up to 60% of young adults without heart disease, but only 2% had more than 100 PACs per 24 hours. The prevalence increases with age. More than 80% of patients older than 90 years of age had more than 100 PACs per 24 hours. PACs are common among people who have lung disorders. They may be worsened by emotional upset, coffee, tea, or alcohol and by using sympathomimetic drugs.

In symptomatic patients, PACs are usually perceived by patients as "palpitations," and sometimes are of concern

CURRENT DIAGNOSIS

The following summarizes the ECG criteria for premature beats. Premature supraventricular complexes or contractions:

- Premature and abnormal P wave morphology as compared to the sinus P wave activity. (The premature P wave is obvious, or it is buried in the T wave.)
- Premature P wave is or is not conducted, and when conducted is followed by a narrow or wide QRS complex.

Premature ventricular complexes or contractions:

- QRS is abnormal looking and usually broadened to more than 0.12 second.
- P waves: the sinus P wave is usually obscured by the QRS, or it may be recognized as a notching on the ST segment or T wave. While the P wave is often dissociated from the QRS complex, retrograde P waves may occur consistently after QRS.

Abbreviations: ECG = electrocardiogram; QRS = electrocardiagraphic wave.

to patients who notice "skipped" beats or "fluttering" that is frightening. Rarely, frequent PACs can give rise to dizziness, which might be aggravated by anxiety and hyperventilation.

KEY TREATMENT

PACs do not usually require treatment. Rarely, when these beats occur frequently and cause intolerable symptoms, treatment is necessary. Aggravating factors should be eliminated. We start with a β-blocker such as atenolol (Tenormin)[1], 25 to 50 mg once daily, or verapamil SR (Isoptin SR)[1], 120 to 240 mg once daily. An anxiolytic agent such as clonazepam (Klonopin)[1], 0.5 to 1 mg twice daily orally, may be required.

Propafenone (Rythmol), 150 mg to 300 mg three times daily, or sotalol (Betapace), with a dose ranging from 80 mg to 160 mg three times daily orally, may be used. These drugs must be avoided in patients with heart failure or with left ventricular ejection fractions (LVEF) less than 40%. Blocked PACs may cause bradycardia and are sometimes misdiagnosed as sinus node dysfunction. Pacing therapy should be considered only if the patient is very symptomatic. Radiofrequency (RF) ablation of PACs may be used.

Premature Ventricular Complexes or Contractions

DEFINITION

Premature ventricular complexes or contractions (PVC) is an extra beat originating in the ventricle before the next expected sinus beat. This beat is also called a

[1]Not FDA approved for this indication.

Rakel and Bope: *Conn's Current Therapy 2006.*

ventricular ectopic beat (VEB) or ventricular premature depolarization (VPD).

DESCRIPTION AND TERMINOLOGY

PVCs can result from the firing of an automatic focus, reentry, or triggered activity. Because they originate in the ventricle, the sequence of ventricular depolarization is altered, compared to sinus rhythm. Impulse conduction occurs more slowly through the myocardium than through specialized conduction pathways. This results in a wide and bizarre-appearing QRS. PVCs arise from different areas within the ventricles (polymorphic) or from a single focus (monomorphic).

PVCs occur as isolated complexes, or they occur in pairs (two PVCs in a row), which are called couplets. When three or more PVCs occur in a row ventricular tachycardia (VT) is present. When VT lasts for more than 30 seconds or causes hemodynamic instability such as presyncope or syncope it is arbitrarily defined as sustained VT. If every other beat is a PVC, ventricular bigeminy is present. If every third or fourth beat is a PVC, the term ventricular trigeminy or quadrigeminy is used respectively.

CLINICAL FEATURES

PVCs are common and occur in patients with or without structural heart disease. They are more frequent in men than women, in African Americans compared to whites, and in those with organic heart disease. The prevalence of PVCs increases with duration of observation, age, and the presence of other factors, such as hypokalemia, hypomagnesemia, and hypertension.

A single PVC has little effect on the pumping ability of the heart and usually does not cause any symptoms. It may be felt as a strong or skipped beat, often described as a thump or flip-flop. Sometimes, the sensation is referred to as "fullness in the neck" because of cannon waves. If PVCs are frequent as in bigeminy or VT, they may cause more severe symptoms such as lightheadedness and syncope. PVCs may be worsened by medications such as aminophylline, sympathomimetic drugs, electrolyte abnormalities (e.g., hypokalemia), heart failure or other cardiac disease, emotional upset, stress, and excess of caffeine and alcohol.

Premature Ventricular Contractions without Heart Disease

In a resting 12-lead electrocardiogram (ECG), PVCs are infrequent in patients with no known heart disease. When 24-hour ambulatory monitoring is used, up to 80% of healthy men or women have PVCs.

SPECIFIC TYPES OF PVCS

PVCs that have right ventricular outflow tract with tachycardia (RVOT-VT) are common arrhythmias in young patients, mostly women. While the vast majority of cases are benign and occur without structural heart disease, they can rarely be associated with sudden death in the presence of arrhythmogenic right ventricular dysplasia (ARVD). The arrhythmia has left bundle-branch block (LBBB) and right axis QRS morphology. IT is usually sensitive to catecholamines and occurs during stress, exercise, or cool-down postexercise. In women, the arrhythmia may worsen with hormonal flux such as onset of menses or during pregnancy. Other PVCs have right bundle-branch block (RBBB) with left axis morphology and can lead to development of VT. This is called verapamil-sensitive idiopathic left fascicular VT. Of persons developing this 60% to 80% are males, usually 15 to 40 years of age.

MANAGEMENT

In the absence of heart disease, the risk-benefit ratio of antiarrhythmic therapy does not support routine treatment. For the patient who complains of disturbing palpitations, the clinician can attempt to relieve the symptom. Reassurance and avoidance of potentially aggravating factors (e.g., tobacco and caffeine-containing drinks) should be tried before specific pharmacologic therapy. Beta blockers, such as atenolol (Tenormin)[1] 25 to 50 mg orally once daily, are the safest initial pharmacologic choice. Mexitil (Mexiletine) is the next drug of choice. The next agents to be tried would be flecainide (Tambocor), sotalol (Betapace) and amiodarone (Cordarone). Quinidine is avoided because of risk of torsades de pointes.

For RVOT PVCs, treatment is started with beta blockers followed by calcium channel blockers. Type I drugs such as procainamide or flecainide can be useful. Sotalol and amiodarone are also effective. Radiofrequency (RF) ablation is the treatment of choice of RVOT-VT and fascicular VT.

---

[1]Not FDA approved for this indication.

Premature Ventricular Contractions with Heart Disease

CORONARY ARTERY DISEASE

In patients with acute myocardial infarction (MI), PVCs in general are not predictors of ventricular fibrillation (VF). R-on-T PVCs trigger VF in only a small minority. Thus, *no* treatment is recommended for peri-infarction PVCs unless the are occurring so frequently that they cause hemodynamic compromise. In any event, a beta blocker should be given (IV) to all patients with acute MI unless a contraindication is present. Use of antiarrhythmic agents should be restricted to only a few days because long-term benefit has not been shown. In the (CCU), lidocaine is loaded at a dose of 1 to 2 mg/kg at a rate of 25 to 50 mg per minute, followed by a maintenance infusion of 2 to 4 mg per minute. If the initial bolus is ineffective, up to two more boluses, of 25 mg can be given at 5 to 10 minute intervals. The maintenance dose can be reduced by approximately half in patients with low-cardiac output, with hepatic disease, or receiving drugs that decrease metabolism of lidocaine such as cimetidine (Tagamet) and propranolol.

If lidocaine fails to suppress PVCs or if the patient has VT, a loading dose of procainamide of 15 mg/kg is administered as a slow infusion over 25 to 30 minutes or 100 to 200 mg/dose repeated every 5 minutes as needed to a total dose of 1 g, followed by a maintenance dose of 1 to 4 mg per minute by continuous infusion. Up to two more boluses of 25 mg can be given at 5 to 10-minute intervals. The maintenance dose can be reduced by approximately half in patients with low cardiac output, hepatic disease, or receiving drugs that decrease metabolism of lidocaine such as cimetidine and propranolol.

Amiodarone (Cordarone) is given as an initial intravenous loading dose of 150 mg over 10 minutes, followed by a continuous infusion of 0.5 to 1 mg per minute. The total cumulative dose must not exceed 1.2 g over 48 hours. The use of a higher dose of amiodarone was

TABLE 1 Vaughan Williams Classification of Antiarrhythmic Drugs

Class	Action	Drugs	Side Effects
I	Sodium-channel blockade		
IA	Prolong repolarization	Quinidine, procainamide, disopyramide	Torsades de pointes, proarrhythmia
IB	Shorten repolarization	Lidocaine, mexiletine, tocainide, phenytoin	Proarrhythmia
IC	Little effect on repolarization	Encainide, felcainide, propafenone	Proarrhythmia, bradycardia, AV block Negative inotropic effect
II	β-adrenergic blockade	Propranolol, atenolol, acebutolol, sotalol	Bradycardia, worsen asthma and AV block
III	Prolong repolarization (potassium-channel blockade; other)	Ibutilide, dofetilide, sotalol (d,l), amiodarone, bretylium	Torsades de pointes, bradycardia
IV	Calcium-channel blockade	Verapamil, diltiazem, bepridil	Negative inotropic effect, AV block, sinus bradycardia
Misc.	Miscellaneous actions	Adenosine, digitalis, magnesium	

Abbreviation: AV = atrioventricular.

associated with increased mortality. Blood pressure must be carefully monitored because intravenous amiodarone can cause hypotension.

Post-MI, in the presence of a left ventricular ejection fraction (LVEF) less than or equal to 40%, treatment with encainide,[1] flecainide (Tambocor), and moricizine (Ethmozine) increases mortality. These drugs are contraindicated. Class IC antiarrhythmic drugs are best avoided even if LVEF is normal.

The role of amiodarone (Cordarone) in treatment of PVCs after MI was evaluated in European Myocardial Infarct Amiodarone Trial (EMIAT) and Canadian Amiodarone Myocardial Infarction Trial (CAMIAT) studies. Amiodarone reduced arrthythmic death but did not reduce overall mortality. A positive interaction with beta blockers was demonstrated in both studies.

Post-MI β-blockers clearly improve survival. In addition, they are effective in suppressing repetitive forms of PVCs in many patients and significantly reduce total PVC frequency in some. They should be used indefinitely.

PVCs with Noncoronary Artery Disease

ACUTE AND SUBACUTE MYOCARDITIS

Myocarditis is commonly accompanied by PVCs and sustained VT, and VF can occur infrequently, even in the absence of heart failure. Frequent PVCs, or nonsustained VT, are usually treated until the carditis has resolved. In those patients who have not had sustained VT or VF, conventional antiarrhythmic agents are given orally and titrated to suppression of PVCs if possible or at least to suppression of salvos.

Antiarrhythmic therapy is continued 2 months and then the patient is monitored off arrhythmic drugs. In case of recurrence, the patient should be considered for an implantable cardioverter-defibrillator (ICD) (Table 1).

IDIOPATHIC DILATED CARDIOMYOPATHY AND HYPERTROPHIC CARDIOMYOPATHY

Chronic PVCs are very common in patients with advanced idiopathic dilated cardiomyopathy and in patients with hypertrophic cardiomyopathy. Both groups have a high risk of arrhythmic sudden death. In some reports, 90%

[1]Not available in the United States.

 CURRENT THERAPY

- It is initially important to determine frequency and severity of symptoms.
- Obtain family history of sudden cardiac death.
- Establish the presence or absence of structural heart disease (e.g., echocardiogram).

ANot for approved for this indication.

Rakel and Bope: *Conn's Current Therapy 2006.*

of patients with dilated cardiomyopathy have frequent PVCs, and more than 50% have ventricular couplets or nonsustained VT. Antiarrhythmic therapy is ineffective for prevention of VF. In the absence of contraindications, patients with dilated cardiomyopathy should receive a beta blocker such as carvedilol (Coreg)[1] 3.125-50 mg twice daily, metoprolol (Lopressor)[1] 12.5 to 25 mg twice daily or bisoprolol (Zebeta)[1] 1.25 to 10 mg per day.

ARRHYTHMOGENIC RIGHT VENTRICULAR DYSPLASIA/CARDIOMYOPATHY

Arrhythmogenic right ventricular dysplasia (ARVD) is a heart muscle disease that is characterized by structural and functional abnormalities caused by replacement of myocardial tissue by fat and fibrosis. This disease affects mostly the right ventricle (RV) and, to a lesser extent, the left ventricle (LV). The left ventricular involvement is usually late and carries poor prognosis. Initial manifestations of the disease include various arrhythmias generally of right ventricular origin including isolated extrasystoles, nonsustained or sustained VT, and VF. PVCs from the RV have LBBB morphology. Investigation requests should emphasize examination of RV (e.g., magnetic resonance imaging [MRI] scan, measurement of RV ejection fraction by radionuclear scan, and RV size and wall motion by echocardiography).

There are no well-established guidelines for the management of patients. Patients with non–life-threatening ventricular arrhythmias are usually treated empirically with antiarrhythmic drugs including sotalol (Betapace)[1], blockers, propafenone (Rhythmol)[1], and amiodarone (Cordarone)[1] alone or in combination therapy. Radiofrequency ablation is reserved for those patients with more frequent symptomatic PVCs. An implantable cardioverter-defibrillator (ICD) which represents the only effective safeguard against sudden death from VF or rapid VT, should be strongly considered in patients who have a strong family history of premature sudden death and who have structural abnormalities or VT.

PVCS AND EXERCISE STRESS TEST

A recent study shows that PVCs more frequent than 7 per minute or of higher grades during recovery post-exercise are independent predictors of higher all-cause mortality than similar arrhythmias that occur during exercise. These patients need further investigation.

REFERENCES

Boutitie F, Boissel, J-P, Connolly, SJ, et al., and the EMIAT and CAMIAT Investigators: Amiodarone interaction with B-blockers: Analysis of the merged EMIAT (European Myocardial Infarct Amiodarone Trial) and CAMIAT (Canadian Amiodarone Myocardial Infarction Trial) databases. *Circulation* 1999:2268.

Bordsky M, Wu D, Denes P, et al: Arrhythmias documented by 24 hour continuous electrocardiographic monitoring in 50 male medical students without apparent heart disease. Am J Cardiol 1977; 39:390-395.

Cairns J, Connolly SJ, Roberts R, et al: Randomised trial of outcome after myocardial infarction in patients with frequent or repetitive

[1]Not FDA approved for this indication.

ventricular premature depolarisations. CAMIAT. Lancet 1997; 349:675.

CAMIAT Investigators. Randomised trial of outcome after myocardial infarction in patients with frequent or repetitive ventricular premature depolarizations (Canadian Amiodarone MI Arrhythmia Trial). Lancet 1997:675-682.

Daoud E MF: Catheter ablation of ventricular tachycardia. Curr Opin Cardiol 1995: 21-25.

Domenico Corrado CB, Gaetano T: Arrhythmogenic right ventricular cardiomyopathy: diagnosis, prognosis, and treatment. *Heart* 2000:588-595.

Frolkis JPP, Claire E, Blackstone EH, et al: Frequent ventricular ectopy after exercise as a predictor of death. N Engl J Med 2003; 348(9):781-790.

Hiss RL: LE. Electrocardiographic findings in 122,043 individuals. Circulation 1962; 947-961.

Janse M, Malik M, Camm AJ, et al., on behalf of the EMIAT Investigators: Identification of post acute myocardial infarction patients with potential benefit from prophylactic treatment with amiodarone: A substudy of EMIAT (the European Myocardial Infarct Amiodarone Trial). Eur Heart J 1998:85.

Marchlinski FE DM, Zado ES: Sex-specific triggers for right ventricular outflow tract tachycardia. Am Heart J 2000: 1009-1013.

Sobotka PA, Mayer JH, Bauernfeind RA, Kanakis C, Jr, Rosen KM: Arrhythmias documented by 24-hour continuous ambulatory electrocardiographic monitoring in young women without apparent heart disease. Am Heart J 1981;101:753-759.

Heart Block

Method of
Anne Hamilton Dougherty, MD

The term *heart block* describes a group of bradyarrhythmias resulting from delay or block in atrioventricular (AV) propagation of excitatory impulses. Conduction abnormalities may occur either at the level of the AV node or more distally in the His-Purkinje system. The consequences of resultant arrhythmias range from benign to severe, even life threatening, depending on the level and severity of block and the adequacy of escape rhythms emerging distal to the block.

Anatomy and Electrophysiology of Atrioventricular Conduction

STRUCTURE AND FUNCTION OF THE AV CONDUCTION SYSTEM

A complex sequence of structures, beginning with the AV node and extending through the penetrating bundle of His, the bundle branches, and the Purkinje fiber network, forms an electrical bridge between atrial and ventricular myocardium. Conduction velocity is slowest in the AV node, providing a functional interval for active ventricular filling during atrial systole. AV node conduction velocity is the primary determinant of the PR interval, normally 120 to 200 milliseconds. More rapid propagation through the His-Purkinje system results in a relatively uniform wave front of biventricular activation

and a narrow (60 to 100 milliseconds) electrocardiographic wave (QRS) complex.

The compact AV node lies in the interatrial septum at the apex of the triangle of Koch, an anatomic area bounded by the tendon of Todaro, the tricuspid valve annulus, and the eustachian valve. The AV node potential is characteristic of slow-response calcium-dependent tissue. Spontaneous diastolic depolarization during phase 4 of the action potential provides latent pacemaker capability that may become manifest during sinus bradycardia or proximal AV nodal block, providing a junctional escape rhythm. The low density of gap junctions between nodal cells contributes to its decremental conduction; increasing heart rates and premature impulses produce progressive delay. With incremental atrial pacing, second-degree AV block (Wenckebach) can be demonstrated in normal individuals; the rates at which this block occurs vary widely, however. Rich sympathetic and parasympathetic innervation modulates nodal function from moment to moment.

The posterior descending branch of the right coronary artery supplies the AV node in 90% of the population; in others, the AV nodal artery arises from the left circumflex. Thus the AV node is vulnerable to ischemia in the event of inferior or posterior myocardial infarction (MI). Transient complete heart block may occur in 10% to 15%; collateral supply from other penetrating branches of the posterior descending artery and septal perforators usually restores function within a few days after inferior infarction.

The common bundle of His lies within the connective tissue of the central fibrous body at the apex of the membranous interventricular septum and measures approximately 1 cm in length. Within the septum it bifurcates into the right and left bundle branches. The right bundle branch is a discrete structure coursing toward the right ventricular apex and crossing over to the right free wall within the moderator band. In contrast, the left bundle branch forms a broad fan over the subendocardial surface of the left ventricle, usually in two or three major fascicles subject to individual variation. Perhaps because of significant anatomic variability, surface electrocardiographic (ECG) patterns of left anterior and left posterior fascicular blocks correlate poorly with actual anatomic lesions. His-Purkinje cells are sodium-channel dependent with linear orientation promoting rapid conduction velocity. A dual blood supply is provided by the left and right coronary arteries. Innervation of the bundle of His, less dense than that of the AV node, is predominantly sympathetic.

NORMAL ELECTROPHYSIOLOGY OF THE ATRIOVENTRICULAR CONDUCTION SYSTEM

Invasive intracardiac His bundle recordings can be helpful in analyzing AV conduction (Figure 1). During sinus rhythm, the AH interval represents AV nodal conduction time, 50 to 130 milliseconds in normal individuals. The HV interval reflects conduction time from the proximal bundle of His to ventricular myocardium, normally 35 to 55 milliseconds. Intracardiac recordings

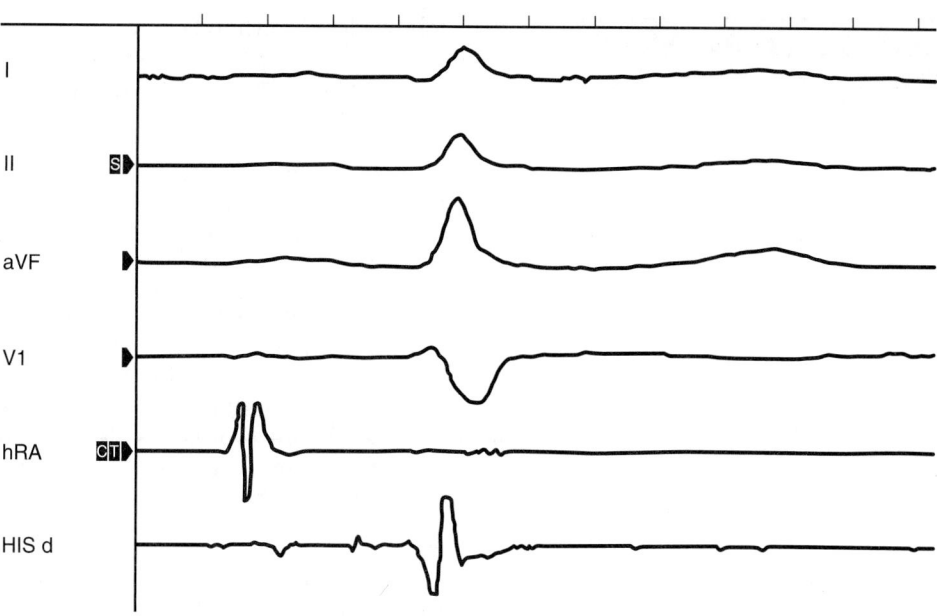

FIGURE 1. Normal intracardiac His bundle recording during sinus rhythm. Surface electrocardiogram (ECG) leads I, II, and aVF are shown, as well as a high right atrial recording (hRA). A catheter straddling the tricuspid valve at the level of the distal bundle of His is labeled as His d. A (low right atrial), H (His), and V (right ventricular) complexes are shown on the latter electrogram.

during sinus rhythm and atrial pacing can be helpful in identifying the anatomic substrate for AV block. When performed during spontaneous AV block, they can demonstrate the level of block.

PATHOLOGY OF THE ATRIOVENTRICULAR CONDUCTION SYSTEM

It is important in the management of AV block to determine whether or not reversible or remediable causes exist. In adults, the most common causes of AV block are pharmacologic, autonomic, ischemic, and degenerative processes of the conduction system (Box 1). Drugs that slow or block conduction in the AV node include digitalis, beta-blockers, and nondihydropyridine calcium channel antagonists. Class I and III antiarrhythmic agents and other membrane-active drugs can produce infranodal block. Neurally mediated block in the AV node may occur in vagotonic states and can usually be recognized both by the clinical setting and by concomitant sinus bradycardia. Complete AV block in the setting of acute inferior MI is usually self-limited, caused by collateral blood supply and the transience of the heightened parasympathetic state. In contrast, heart block is less common in acute anterior MI but more likely to be permanent. It confers a poor prognosis, implying a large volume of infarcted tissue.

AV block in children is frequently congenital and associated with structural heart defects in approximately one half of cases. Maternal lupus is a common etiologic factor in others, particularly when antiribonucleoprotein antibodies are present. There is a higher incidence of ostium primum atrial septal defect and transposition of the great vessels in individuals with congenital heart block.

Electrocardiographic Diagnosis of Heart Block

FIRST-DEGREE ATRIOVENTRICULAR BLOCK

First-degree AV block, defined as a PR interval exceeding 200 milliseconds in an adult (180 milliseconds in adolescents), is more accurately described as first-degree AV conduction delay. A 1:1 AV relationship is maintained. In most instances the conduction delay occurs at the level of the AV node (prolonged AH interval). Intra-atrial and His-Purkinje conduction delay may rarely result in the same ECG pattern. In patients with a widened QRS or bundle branch block, the likelihood of distal intra-His (HH') and infra-His (increased HV) is higher and implies a poorer prognosis.

SECOND-DEGREE ATRIOVENTRICULAR BLOCK

Intermittent AV conduction failure defines second-degree AV block. ECG patterns show regular sinus P waves, some of which are not followed by a QRS complex, resulting in an A to V ratio of more than 1:1. Second-degree AV block is classified further into Mobitz I (Wenckebach) and Mobitz II types, terms useful in predicting the anatomic level of block and potential risk.

AV Wenckebach results from decremental conduction in the AV node, producing cycles of progressive AV

Rakel and Bope: *Conn's Current Therapy 2006.*

Pharmacologic
- Cardiac glycosides
- β-Blockers
- Calcium channel antagonists
- Membrane-active antiarrhythmics
- Edrophonium

Autonomic
- Vagotonia
- Carotid sinus hypersensitivity

Degenerative
- Lev's disease (calcific or fibrotic)
- Lenègre's disease (sclerodegenerative)
- Calcific aortic stenosis

Ischemia
- Acute myocardial infarction
- Chronic coronary disease

Infiltrative
- Amyloidosis
- Sarcoidosis
- Hemochromatosis
- Tumors

Congenital
- Maternal lupus
- Ostium primum atrial septal defect
- Transposition of the great vessels

Infectious and Inflammatory
- Endocarditis
- Parasitic (Chagas' disease)
- Bacterial (Lyme disease, diphtheria, rheumatic fever, tuberculosis, syphilis)
- Viral (measles, mumps)
- Collagen/vascular (scleroderma, Reiter's syndrome, ankylosing spondylitis, systemic lupus erythematosus, rheumatoid arthritis, dermatomyositis)

Traumatic
- Catheter ablation
- Alcohol septal ablation
- Catheter trauma
- Valvular surgery
- Radiation

Metabolic
- Hyperkalemia
- Hypermagnesemia
- Hypothyroidism
- Hypothermia
- Addison's disease

Neuromyopathic
- Myotonic dystrophy
- Erb's dystrophy
- Kearns-Sayre syndrome
- Peroneal muscular atrophy

conduction delay punctuated by intermittent block. The surface ECG features regular PP intervals with progressive PR interval prolongation, culminating in a dropped QRS complex with each Wenckebach cycle. The overall pattern of group beating (clusters of beats with decreasing RR intervals, separated by pauses) is distinctive. The QRS complex is usually normal. Intracardiac ECG recordings during typical Mobitz I show progressive prolongation in the AH interval with fixed HV intervals; the nonconducted A wave is followed by neither H nor V. As with first-degree AV block, Wenckebach is usually a benign finding in healthy individuals, especially under conditions of enhanced vagal tone.

Mobitz II AV block is characterized on the surface ECG by sudden absence of a QRS following a P wave without heralding PR prolongation. Type II block usually occurs in patients with other evidence of His-Purkinje disease, usually bundle branch block, and confers a worse prognosis than type I. Sudden 2:1 AV block may not be classifiable by Mobitz type on the surface ECG; the presence of a widened QRS increases the likelihood of the infra-His block, however. The infra-His or intra-His level of conduction block can be documented on intracardiac recordings by demonstrating an AH without subsequent V in the nonconducted beat. The HV interval is typically prolonged during sinus rhythm.

Some refer to a more severe form of second-degree AV block as high-degree AV block. In this state, two or more consecutive P waves are not conducted, whereas the atrial and ventricular rhythms are still otherwise associated.

THIRD-DEGREE ATRIOVENTRICULAR BLOCK

Third-degree, or complete, AV block results from the total failure of propagation of atrial impulses to the ventricles. Atrial and ventricular rhythms are fully dissociated with the atrial rate exceeding an independent junctional or ventricular escape rate. The ECG appearance depends on the anatomic site of the block (Figure 2). Most congenital heart block is intranodal. Like acquired AV blocks that arise from drugs or ischemia affecting the AV node, it is associated with a narrow QRS complex escape rhythm at 40 to 60 beats per minute (bpm). The escape rhythm originating from the AV junction increases with exercise, isoproterenol (Isuprel), or atropine. An intracardiac His bundle recording shows regular A complexes dissociated from the slower HV complexes.

In contrast, most acquired complete heart block occurs within the His-Purkinje network (infra-His or rarely intra-His). The escape rhythm is ventricular in origin, resulting in a wide QRS rhythm between 20 and 40 bpm. Thus intracardiac recordings show AH complexes dissociated from V complexes. Long ventricular pauses may occur if the escape rhythm is unreliable.

BUNDLE BRANCH BLOCKS

Relative conduction delay or complete block in one of the bundle branches or its fascicles produces the ECG criteria for bundle branch or fascicular block. The widened QRS complex (120 milliseconds) results from inhomogeneous ventricular activation, the ventricle ipsilateral to the block receiving late activation. Right bundle branch block is the most common and most benign; it is recognized by the characteristic RSR' pattern in V_1; HV interval prolongation is usually minimal. Left bundle branch block is characterized by a broad, sometimes notched, R wave in V_6 with a wide, deep S wave in V_1. It is frequently associated with structural heart disease

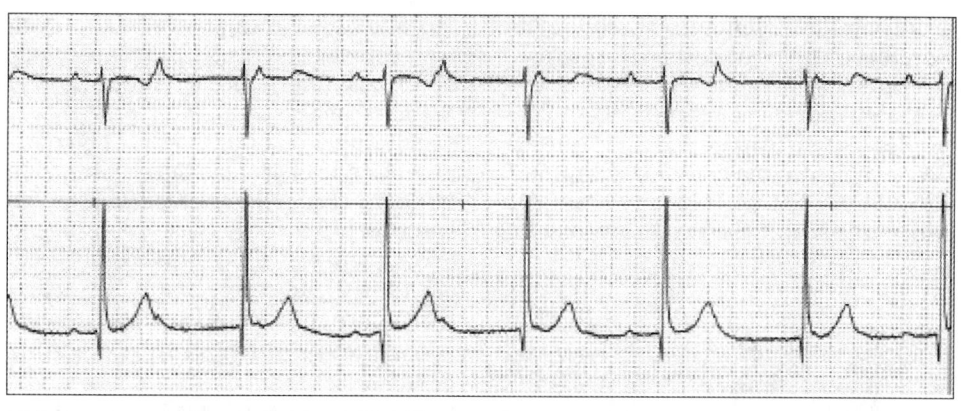

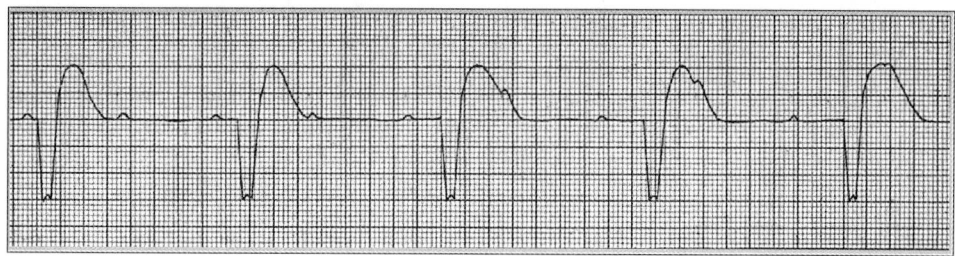

FIGURE 2. Two types of complete AV (atrioventricular) block. A, Congenital AV block in an asymptomatic 9-year-old girl. The junctional escape rhythm at rest was 50 beats per minute (bpm) but rose to 110 bpm with exercise. B, Acquired complete AV block in an adult patient with a slow ventricular escape rate of 35 bpm, resulting in syncope.

and significant HV prolongation. Because of the variability in the distribution of the left bundle and its fascicles, left anterior and posterior fascicular blocks correlate poorly with actual anatomic lesions. The combination of right bundle branch block with either left anterior or left posterior fascicular block is termed *bifascicular block,* and *trifascicular block* refers to the additional finding of first- or second-degree AV block.

Clinical Manifestations

SIGNS AND SYMPTOMS OF ATRIOVENTRICULAR BLOCK

Symptoms related to first-degree AV block are rare and only observed in cases where PR prolongation is extreme (>300 milliseconds). Fatigue or dyspnea may result from the equivalent of a pacemaker syndrome in which the hemodynamic benefit of AV synchrony is lost because of the excessive delay. Patients with significant systolic or diastolic dysfunction are most prone to this condition. Convincing proof of the causal relationship between the symptoms and the ECG abnormality should be sought. Relief of symptoms with temporary dual-chamber pacing and establishment of physiologic intervals suggest causality.

Bundle branch block may complicate congestive heart failure (CHF) by producing or aggravating ventricular dyssynchrony and producing functional mitral regurgitation; it serves as a marker of adverse outcomes. Resynchronization with atriobiventricular pacing has

been demonstrated to improve symptoms, functional status, and quality of life in affected patients. On the average, an improvement in left ventricular ejection fraction of 5% results from cardiac resynchronization.

Dizziness, fatigue, presyncope, and syncope may result from second- or third-degree AV block. The severity of symptoms depends largely on the degree of bradycardia produced as well as on underlying cardiac or cerebrovascular disease. Sudden and significant bradycardia because of complete heart block can result in an Adams-Stokes attack, a sudden and catastrophic loss of consciousness that may be fatal.

Objective findings of conduction block can be found on the physical exam. Paradoxical splitting of the second heart sound (S2) occurs with left bundle branch block. AV dissociation because of complete heart block produces variation in the intensity of the first heart sound as a result of the variable position of the mitral valve at the onset of ventricular systole. Careful examination of the jugular veins also reveals intermittent cannon A waves because of the occasional atrial contraction against a closed tricuspid valve.

NATURAL HISTORY OF ATRIOVENTRICULAR BLOCK

First-degree and Mobitz I blocks are typically benign. Mobitz II AV block is more commonly associated with underlying cardiac disease; the incidence of symptoms and the probability of progression to complete AV block are high. Acquired complete block may be fatal if not treated swiftly and effectively. Heart block may be complicated by bradycardia-dependent torsades de pointes. Unless reversible causes can be discovered, permanent pacing is required.

In contrast to acquired forms, congenital complete heart block is better tolerated and carries a more favorable prognosis. Some affected children may develop symptoms in infancy or even in utero, but many remain asymptomatic until adolescence because of the responsiveness of the junctional escape rhythm to sympathetic influence with activity and stress. Permanent pacemaker implantation at the first notice of effort intolerance and/or slowing of the escape rhythm helps prevent syncope and myocardial dysfunction and improves outcomes.

Mobitz II block, left bundle branch block, and left posterior fascicular block occurring in the setting of acute anterior MI each increase the probability of progression to complete heart block and serve as markers of increased mortality. But even complete heart block associated with acute inferior MI is usually self-limited.

Management of Heart Block

DIAGNOSIS

ECG documentation of the arrhythmia and correlation with symptoms and underlying cardiac status are necessary to guide management. The intermittency of second- and third-degree AV blocks may make ECG documentation challenging. In patients with suspected conduction disease, ambulatory ECG monitoring and loop-format transient symptomatic event recording can be useful in documenting the culprit arrhythmia. Implantable loop recorders are particularly useful in patients with rare clinical events. This process may be too tedious, however, for patients with severe, asymptomatic, or infrequent events. In those cases, invasive electrophysiologic study is useful in identifying abnormalities in AV node and His-Purkinje function. It is also helpful in determining the site of block when risk cannot be determined with certainty from the surface ECG. Some cardiologists advocate the diagnostic use of intravenous procainamide[1] as a provocative test for infra-His conduction disease. Patients with syncope of undetermined etiology associated with structural heart disease can also benefit from formal electrophysiologic testing, not only to assess the integrity of the conduction system but also to determine whether ventricular arrhythmias may account for symptoms.

INDICATIONS FOR PACEMAKER THERAPY

Although symptomatic AV block can frequently be palliated with emergency use of intravenous atropine, its use in infranodal block may aggravate the level of block by accelerating the sinus rate. The use of isoproterenol (Isuprel) to accelerate the junctional or ventricular escape rhythm or reverse block is more predictable. Temporary pacing may be accomplished with transcutaneous or intravenous electrodes. Permanent pacemaker therapy is the standard of care for symptomatic and high-risk patients when there is no reversible cause. Guidelines for implantation of permanent pacemakers have recently been updated by a joint task force of the American College of Cardiology, American Heart Association, and North American Society of Pacing and Electrophysiology (now known as the Heart

---

BOX 2   Indications for Permanent Pacemaker Implantation in Adult Patients With AV Block and Fascicular Blocks

Class I: Conditions for which there is general agreement that pacing is beneficial and effective.
- Third-degree and advanced second-degree AV block at any level, associated with symptomatic bradycardia, required drug therapy, asystole >3.0 seconds or escape rates <40 bpm while awake, AV junction ablation, postoperative AV block not expected to resolve, high-risk neuromuscular diseases (Kearns-Sayre syndrome, Erb's dystrophy, and peroneal muscular atrophy)
- Second-degree AV block with symptomatic bradycardia
- Type II second-degree AV block or alternating bundle branch block in patients with chronic bifascicular or trifascicular block
- Persistent infranodal second- or third-degree AV block after acute MI
- Transient second-or third-degree infranodal AV block and bundle branch block after acute MI
- Persistent and symptomatic second- and third-degree AV block

Class II: Conditions for which there is conflicting evidence and/or divergence of opinion about pacing benefit.

Class IIa: Evidence and/or opinion favors benefit.
- Asymptomatic third-degree AV block with awake heart rates ≥40 bpm
- Asymptomatic type II second-degree AV block with a narrow QRS
- Asymptomatic type I second-degree AV block at intra- or infra-His levels documented at invasive electrophysiologic study
- First- or second-degree AV block with symptoms of pacemaker syndrome
- Syncope in patients with chronic bifascicular and trifascicular block after exclusion of other causes, especially ventricular tachycardia
- Medically refractory, symptomatic NYHA class III and IV patients with LVEF ≤35% and QRS interval ≥130 milliseconds (atriobiventricular pacing).

Class IIb: Benefit is less-well established.
- First-degree AV block (>0.30 seconds) in patients with CHF after demonstration of hemodynamic improvement with shortening of the AV interval
- Neuromuscular diseases (Kearns-Sayre syndrome, Erb's dystrophy, peroneal muscular atrophy) with first-, second-, or third-degree AV block
- Persistent infranodal second- and third-degree AV block

Class III: Other conditions for which there is evidence and/or general agreement that pacing is ineffective.

Abbreviations: AV = atrioventricular; CHF = congestive heart failure; LVEF = left ventricle ejection fraction; MI = myocardial infarction; NYHA = New York Heart Association; QRS = electrocardiographic wave.

---

[1]Not FDA approved for this indication.

Rakel and Bope: *Conn's Current Therapy 2006.*

Rhythm Society). Box 2 summarizes the indications related to heart block.

PACEMAKER PRESCRIPTION

Although the most basic ventricular demand pacemaker can prevent bradycardia, modern pacemakers provide more physiologic pacing to optimize functional capacity. AV universal (DDD) pacing requires leads in both atrium and ventricle and provides AV synchrony, a feature that contributes approximately 10% to cardiac output in a structurally normal heart. The atrial contribution to ventricular filling is even more significant in patients with ventricular hypertrophy or CHF; thus dual-chamber pacing provides even more hemodynamic benefit in affected individuals. Dual-chamber pacing reduces the frequency of paroxysmal atrial fibrillation but is inappropriate in patients with chronic atrial fibrillation. Automatic mode switching to ventricular pacing may be a very useful feature in individuals with uncontrolled paroxysmal atrial fibrillation, preventing rapid atrial tracking and inappropriately rapid pacing rates.

Right ventricular pacing is not ideal for all pacemaker recipients and can exacerbate CHF. The addition of a third lead, usually placed in a posterolateral or lateral branch of the coronary sinus for left ventricular pacing, provides synchronous biventricular pacing that can improve CHF symptoms in two thirds of patients with QRS duration exceeding 130 milliseconds. The MIRACLE trial established its usefulness as an adjunctive treatment for patients with CHF and bundle branch block, even in the absence of bradycardia-related indications for pacing.

Sensor-driven rate-responsive pacing is particularly effective in patients with chronotropic incompetence. Physical activity, acceleration, minute ventilation, core blood temperature, and evoked responses each are used in commercial biosensors as indexes of metabolic activity to determine the appropriate pacing rate on a minute-by-minute basis.

Pacemaker devices can be programmed to tailor function and address the needs of the individual, but the function is limited by the choice of implanted hardware and by thoughtful programming to suit the needs of the individual patient. Careful consideration of the arrhythmia history and hemodynamic profile of the individual recipient should be rendered at the time of initial implant in choosing a device that optimizes comfort and performance.

CURRENT DIAGNOSIS

- Electrocardiogram documentation of the symptomatic arrhythmia is essential.
- Identification of the anatomic level of block is useful in assessing the risk of the arrhythmia.
- Invasive electrophysiologic studies can be useful in identifying the arrhythmia substrate and assessing the level of risk.

CURRENT THERAPY

- Identification and management of all potentially reversible causative factors is advised.
- Emergency treatment of symptomatic heart block may include intravenous isoproterenol (Isuprel) or temporary transcutaneous or transvenous pacing.
- Permanent pacemakers are indicated for patients with irreversible symptomatic and/or high-risk atrioventricular block.
- Proper prescription of permanent pacemaker hardware and software can maximize patient benefit.

REFERENCES

Abraham WT, Fisher WG, Smith AL, et al: Cardiac resynchronization in chronic heart failure. N Engl J Med 2002;346:1845-1853.

Barold SS: Indications for permanent cardiac pacing in first-degree AV block: Class I, II, or III? Pacing Clin Electrophysiol 1996;19:261-264.

Gregoratos G, Abrams J, Epstein AE, et al: ACC/AHA/NASPE 2002 guideline update for implantation of cardiac pacemakers and antiarrhythmia devices—summary article: A report of the American College of Cardiology/American Heart Association Task Force on Practice Guidelines (ACC/AHA/NASPE Committee to Update the 1998 Pacemaker Guidelines). J Am Coll Cardiol 2002;40:1703-1719.

Gregoratos G, Cheitlin MD, Conill A, et al: ACC/AHA Guidelines for implantation of cardiac pacemakers and antiarrhythmia devices: Executive summary: A report of the American College of Cardiology/American Heart Association Task Force on Practice Guidelines (Committee on Pacemaker Implantation). Circulation 1998;97:1325-1335.

Kim YH, O'Nunain S, Trouto T et al: Pseudo-pacemaker syndrome following inadvertent fast pathway ablation for atrioventricular nodal reentrant tachycardia. J Cardiovasc Electrophysiol 1993;4:178-182.

Lamas GA, Lee KL, Sweeney MO, et al: Ventricular pacing or dual-chamber pacing for sinus node dysfunction. N Engl J Med 2002;346:1854-1862.

Michaelsson M, Jonzon A, Riesenfeld T: Isolated congenital complete atrioventricular block in adult life. A prospective study. Circulation 1995;92:442-449.

Shamim W, Francis DP, Yousufuddin M, et al: Interventricular conduction delay: A prognostic marker in chronic heart failure. Int J Cardiol 1999;70:171-178.

Tachycardias

Method of
Richard H. Hongo, MD, and
Nora Goldschlager, MD

Tachycardia in the adult is defined as a heart rate of more than 100 beats per minute (bpm) and can be characterized as either supraventricular or ventricular. *Supraventricular* tachycardias (SVTs) are abnormal rhythms that originate from structures above the ventricles, including the atria, the sinoatrial nodal tissue, and the atrioventricular (AV) node. SVTs also involve accessory pathways that are abnormal electrical connections between supraventricular and ventricular tissue separate from the AV node left behind during embryonic development. *Ventricular* tachycardias (VTs) originate in, and involve, either the His-Purkinje conduction system or the ventricular myocardium.

There are three electrophysiologic mechanisms of tachycardia:

1. Abnormal Automaticity: An abnormal increase in depolarization rate of pacemaker cells, or spontaneous depolarization of non-pacemaker cells.
2. Reentry: A repetitive loop of electrical activation around a circuit formed by barriers to rapid conduction (such as scar tissue).
3. Triggered Activity: An abnormal cell depolarization triggered by oscillations in membrane potential during, or immediately following, normal depolarization (early or delayed "after depolarizations").

A tachycardia is generally described as *focal* when the mechanism is either abnormal automaticity or triggered activity; however, reentry can also appear focal if the activation circuit is small.

Tachycardias present clinically as palpitations, dizziness, presyncope, or frank syncope. Sudden cardiac death (SCD) can be the presenting manifestation of ventricular tachyarrhythmias, and much more rarely, of supraventricular tachycardia. Patients can also be asymptomatic, and the tachycardia is discovered incidentally.

The analysis of a 12-lead electrocardiogram (ECG) obtained during tachycardia, when available, is the first step in defining the tachycardia mechanism (Figure 1). The tachycardia is first assessed as regular or irregular. An irregular rhythm to the QRS complexes without a pattern to the irregularity (called an *irregularly irregular rhythm*) is the hallmark of atrial fibrillation (AF). If the tachycardia is regular, the next step is assessing the QRS complex duration as narrow or wide. A narrow (<120 milliseconds) QRS complex tachycardia is invariably supraventricular in origin. A wide (≥120-millisecond) QRS complex tachycardia can be either ventricular or supraventricular with preexisting bundle branch block, aberrant conduction, or preexcitation.

Approximately 80% of wide QRS complex tachycardias are VT. A history of heart disease in a patient with

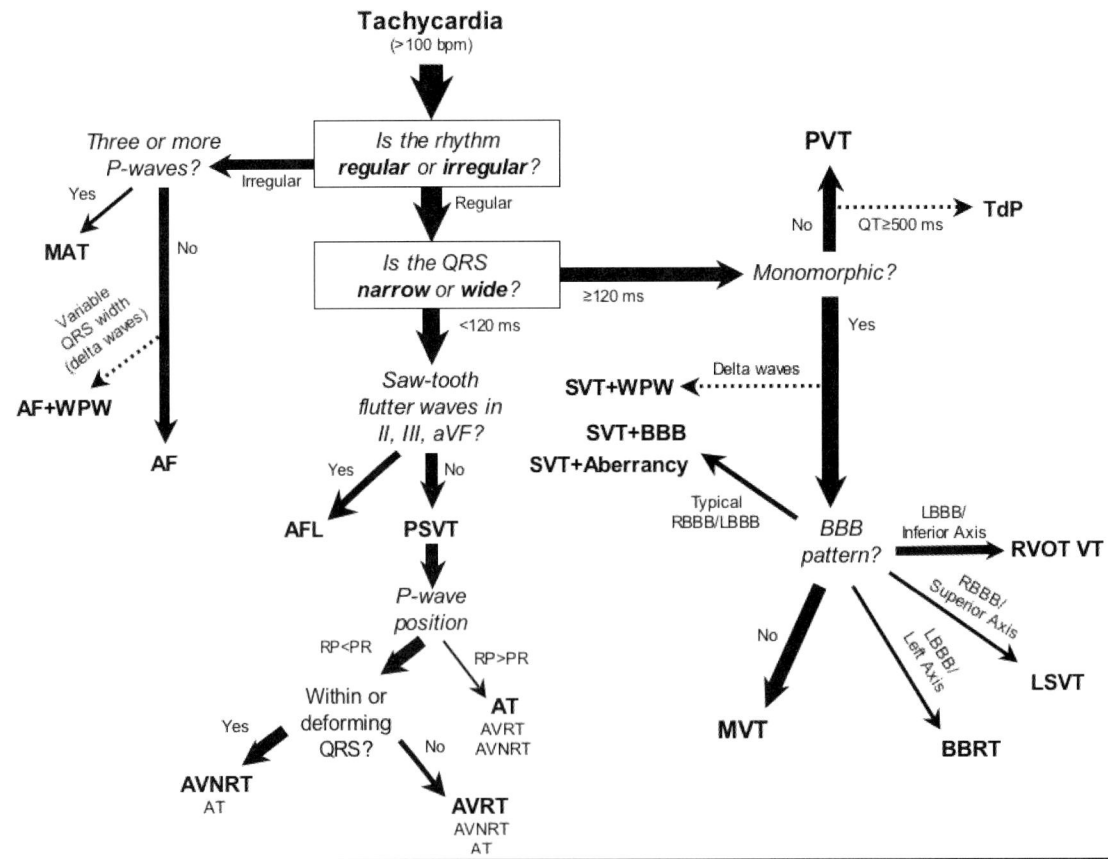

FIGURE 1. General algorithm for diagnosing tachycardias by electrocardiographic criteria. The relative weight of the arrows approximates the frequency of arrhythmias. AF = atrial fibrillation; AFL = atrial flutter; AT = atrial tachycardia; AVNRT = atrioventricular nodal reentrant tachycardia; AVRT = atrioventricular reciprocating tachycardia; BBB = bundle branch block; BBRT = bundle branch reentry tachycardia; LBBB = left bundle-branch block; LSVT = left septal ventricular tachycardia; MAT = multifocal atrial tachycardia; MVT = monomorphic ventricular tachycardia; PSVT = paroxysmal supraventricular tachycardia; PVT = polymorphic ventricular tachycardia; RBBB = right bundle-branch block; RVOT = right ventricular outflow tract; SVT = supraventricular tachycardia; TdP = torsades de pointes; VT = ventricular tachycardia; WPW = Wolff-Parkinson-White syndrome.

wide QRS complex tachycardia has a positive predictive value of 95% for VT. Typical bundle branch block patterns are observed in patients with SVT when there is a fixed or aberrant (rate-related) conduction block within the Purkinje system. Although a QRS morphology atypical for bundle branch block, or a QRS duration of more than 160 milliseconds makes VT more likely, these findings can be seen in patients with SVT who have hyperkalemia or severe dilated cardiomyopathy. AV dissociation, established by identifying either P waves dissociated from QRS complexes, capture beats, or fusion beats, is diagnostic of VT. A *capture beat* is a sinus beat that conducts down the AV node and captures (depolarizes) the entire ventricle before its depolarization from the VT source. It appears as a narrow QRS complex in the midst of wide complexes. A *fusion beat* is a sinus beat that conducts down the AV node and fuses with depolarization from the VT source, resulting in a beat intermediate in width and morphology between normal and wide complexes. A preexcited SVT is suspected when a slurred upstroke of QRS complexes resulting in shortened PR interval (delta waves) is present during sinus rhythm.

Hemodynamic stability must be established in patients with sustained tachycardia. Any tachyarrhythmia should be immediately treated with electrical cardioversion if the blood pressure is excessively low or consequences of hypoperfusion (cognitive impairment, chest pain, heart failure) are present. VT tends to lead to hemodynamic instability because it generally occurs in patients with structural heart disease. Because a delay in treating VT can be life threatening, a wide QRS complex tachycardia of unclear origin should be considered VT until proved otherwise. Antiarrhythmic drugs can be administered as initial therapy to stable patients (Table 1).

TABLE 1 General Guide to Antiarrhythmic Therapy

Vaughn Williams class	Specific Agent	Preparation/dosage	Typical use	Comments
Class IA Na⁺ channel blockade (prolongs RP, QT)			Prevention of SVT in patients without SHD	Rarely used to prevent VT; increased mortality in patients with SHD
	Procainamide (Pronestyl)	IV: load = 1 g IV: infusion = 1-4 mg/min PO: 250-500 mg q6h	Termination of VT or AF; prevention of SVT	Especially appropriate for stable preexcited AF
	Quinidine (Quinaglute)	PO: 324-648 mg q8-12h	Prevention of SVT	
	Disopyramide (Norpace)	PO: 200-400 mg bid	Prevention of SVT	
Class IB Na⁺ channel Blockade	Lidocaine (Xylocaine)	IV: load = 1 mg/kg IV: infusion = 1-4 mg/min	Termination of VT; prevention of VT	Probably less effective than amiodarone or procainamide except during active ischemia
	Mexiletine (Mexitil)	PO: 200-300 mg q8h	Prevention of VT	Contraindicated in heart block
Class IC Na⁺ channel Blockade			Prevention of SVT in patients without SHD	Increased mortality in patients with SHD or ischemia
	Flecainide (Tambocor)	PO: 50-150 mg q12h	Prevention of SVT	Contraindicated in heart block
	Propafenone (Rythmol)	PO: 150-300 mg q8h	Prevention of SVT	May be used prn to terminate AF or AFL
Class II β-Blockade	Metoprolol (Lopressor)	PO: 25-100 mg bid	Decreases VR in SVT; prevention of SVT	Multiple oral β-blockers available. Metoprolol is shown as an example
	Esmolol (Brevibloc)	IV: load = 500 µg/kg IV: infusion = 50-200 µg/kg/min	Decreases VR in SVT	Preferred IV preparation because of short half-life

Continued

TABLE 1 General Guide to Antiarrhythmic Therapy—cont'd

Vaughn Williams class	Specific Agent	Preparation/dosage	Typical use	Comments
Class III K⁺ channel blockade (prolongs RP, QT)	Sotalol (Betapace)	PO: 80-160 mg bid	Prevention of SVT or VT	Dosage interval decreased with renal failure
	Amiodarone (Cordarone)	IV: load = 150 mg, then 1 mg/min × 6 h, then 0.5 mg/min × 18 h PO: 200-400 mg qd	Termination of VT; prevention of SVT or VT	Often started with an oral load (800-1200 mg qd)
	Dofetilide (Tikosyn)	PO: 125-500 μg bid	Prevention of AF	Dosage decreased with renal failure
	Ibutilide (Corvert)	IV: 0.01 mg/kg up to 1 mg over 10 min	Cardioversion of AF, AFL	
Class IV Ca⁺⁺ channel blockade				Dihydropyridines have no significant AV nodal blocking effect
	Verapamil (Calan)	PO: 120-240 mg bid	Decreases VR in SVT; prevention of SVT	Should be avoided in patients with WPW
	Diltiazem (Cardizem)	IV: infusion = 5-15 mg/h PO: 120-360 mg qd	Decreases VR in SVT; prevention of SVT	Should avoid if tachycardia is possibly VT
Miscellaneous	Digoxin (Lanoxin)	IV: load = 0.5 mg, then 0.25 mg q6h × 2 doses PO: 0.25-0.625 mg qd	Decreases VR in SVT	Should be avoided in patients with WPW
	Adenosine (Adenocard)	IV: 6-12 mg rapid bolus	Termination of SVT	Diagnostically useful

Abbreviations: AF = atrial fibrillation; AFL = atrial flutter; AV = atrioventricular; RP = refractory period; SHD = structural heart disease; SVT = supraventricular tachycardia; VR = ventricular rate; VT = ventricular tachycardia; WPW = Wolff-Parkinson-White syndrome.
Reproduced and modified with permission from Rakel RE, Bope ET (eds): Conn's Current Therapy 2004. Philadelphia, Elsevier, 2004, p 330.

Adenosine (Adenocard) is an especially useful drug in managing narrow QRS complex tachycardia because of its selective blocking effect on the AV node and its elimination by cellular uptake within seconds. AV nodal reentrant tachycardia (AVNRT) and AV reciprocating tachycardia (AVRT) (see later) are reliably terminated by adenosine (Adenocard) because the AV node is critical to the circuit of these tachycardias (Table 2). Some types of VT, especially right ventricular outflow tract (RVOT) VT, are also adenosine (Adenocard) sensitive (Table 3). Termination of a tachycardia with adenosine (Adenocard) is not always diagnostic of the type of arrhythmia because of the wide range of adenosine-sensitive rhythms. Transient AV nodal block with continuation of an atrial arrhythmia, such as atrial flutter or atrial tachycardia, however, is diagnostic (Figure 2).

Ongoing advances in catheter ablation of tachyarrhythmias and establishment of the efficacy of implantable cardioverter defibrillators (ICDs) has changed the chronic management of tachycardias. Whereas the mainstay of tachycardia management has been suppression with antiarrhythmic drugs, most tachycardias are now amenable to cure with catheter ablation. Patients with severe dilated cardiomyopathy are at increased risk for SCD and can be protected with ICD implantation. Recurrent VT, requiring frequent ICD shocks, is treated with antiarrhythmic drug suppression. Catheter ablation, aimed at disrupting reentry circuits within a ventricular scar, also can be performed to decrease VT episodes and thus the frequency of ICD shocks.

Supraventricular Tachyarrhythmias

SINUS TACHYCARDIAS

Enhanced automaticity of the sinus node appropriate to physiologic demand results in physiologic sinus tachycardia. The P-wave morphology and frontal plane axis is that of sinus rhythm, and gradual (rather than abrupt) changes in heart rate are characteristic of normal sinus node function. Sinus tachycardia is not an arrhythmia, and therapy is thus directed toward the underlying

TABLE 2 Electrocardiographic Features of Supraventricular Tachycardia

Tachycardia	P Morphology	AV Relationship	RP interval*	AV node dependence†	Response to adenosine (Adenocard)‡
Sinus tachycardia	Same as sinus	1:1	Long RP	No	Transient suppression of sinus and/or AV block
Atrial tachycardia	Different from sinus	Usually 1:1 or 2:1	Long RP, can be short RP	No	Transient suppression, termination, or AV block
MAT	≥3 different P waves	Usually 1:1	Long RP, variable	No	Transient AV block
Atrial fibrillation	No discrete P waves	Variable	Not applicable	No	Increased AV block
Atrial flutter	Flutter, sawtooth	Usually 2:1, variable	Not applicable	No	Flutter waves with AV block
AVNRT	Retrograde§, within, or distorting QRS	Usually 1:1, may be 2:1 AV or VA block	Very short RP	Yes	Usually terminates with AV block
AVRT	Retrograde§	1:1	Short RP	Yes	Usually terminates with AV block

*The RP interval is termed long RP if RP > PR, and short RP if RP > PR.
†AV node dependence indicates that the AV node is an obligate component of the tachycardia mechanism.
‡Adenosine (Adenocard) is not FDA approved for diagnosing supraventricular tachycardia.
§A retrograde P wave, caused by retrograde conduction from either the AV node or an accessory pathway, is negative in leads II, III, aVF.
Abbreviations: AV = atrioventricular; AVNRT = atrioventricular nodal reentrant tachycardia; AVRT = atrioventricular reciprocating tachycardia; MAT = multifocal atrial tachycardia; VA = ventriculoatrial.
Reproduced and modified with permission from Rakel RE, Bope ET (eds): Conn's Current Therapy 2004. Philadelphia, Elsevier, 2004, p 328.

5

cause, such as fever, anemia, hypotension, hypoxemia, thyrotoxicosis, myocardial ischemia, and pain.

In contrast, increase in sinus node automaticity disproportionate to the level of exertion can be caused by inappropriate sinus tachycardia, of which the mechanism is not fully understood. Treatment can be attempted with beta- or calcium channel blockers but is often inadequate despite large doses. Modification of the sinus node region with catheter ablation is occasionally effective (<25% of cases), but the recurrence of symptoms is high and thus the procedure has been virtually abandoned. The diagnosis of inappropriate sinus tachycardia

TABLE 3 Electrocardiographic Features of Ventricular Tachycardia

Tachycardia	QRS morphology	RS interval	QT Interval	Response to adenosine (Adenocard)	Response to verapamil (Calan)
Scar-related VT	Variable, not typical BBB pattern, multiple morphologies common	>100 msec	Normal	–	–
BBRT	LBBB/LAD		Normal	–	–
LS VT	RBBB/superior axis	60-80 msec	Normal	–	+
RVOT VT	LBBB/inferior axis		Normal	+	+
ARVC VT	Usually LBBB pattern, multiple morphologies common		Normal	–	–
Polymorphic VT	Variable amplitude		Normal	–	–
Torsades de pointes	Variable amplitude, "turning on point"		Prolonged	–	–

Abbreviations: + = sensitive; – = no response; ARVC = arrhythmogenic right ventricular cardiomyopathy; BBB = bundle branch block; BBRT = bundle branch reentry tachycardia; LAD = left axis deviation; LBBB = left bundle-branch block; LS = left septal; RBBB = right bundle-branch block; RVOT = right ventricular outflow tract; VT = ventricular tachycardia.

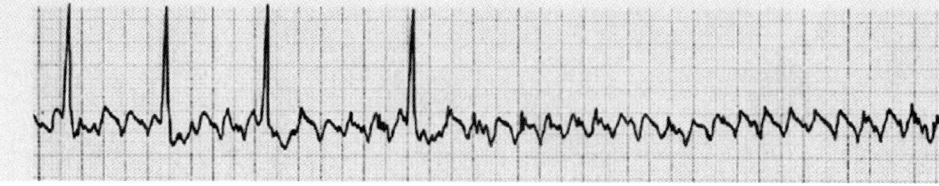

FIGURE 2. Adenosine (Adenocard)-induced atrioventricular block revealing an underlying atrial flutter.

should be made only after other causes of tachycardias that originate in and around the sinus node, such as sinus node reentry tachycardia, are excluded. Sinus node reentry tachycardia is diagnosed by its abrupt onset and reproducibility with pacing during electrophysiology (EP) study, and it can be cured with catheter ablation in the majority of cases. Calcium channel blockers and digoxin (Lanoxin) may prevent sinus node reentry tachycardia; beta-blockers have been reported to be less effective.

ATRIAL TACHYCARDIAS

In focal atrial tachycardia, the impulse originates from a location within the atria separate from the sinus node (called "ectopic"). The underlying mechanism can be abnormal automaticity, reentry using a discrete but small circuit, or triggered activity. The P wave morphology differs from that of sinus rhythm and depends on the location of the focus. The PR interval is normal (unless there is associated AV block), and thus a long RP interval, relative to the PR interval, is present during tachycardia. The demonstration of atrial tachycardia during induced AV block (e.g., by carotid sinus massage, Valsalva maneuver, adenosine [Adenocard]) is diagnostic. Digoxin toxicity can cause a unique combination of AT and AV block, which is rarely seen today because of the decreasing use of digoxin (Lanoxin).

The management of atrial tachycardias can be challenging. Class IC[1] and III[1] antiarrhythmic drugs can be tried, but suppression of atrial tachycardia is often difficult. Even without complete suppression of the atrial arrhythmia, AV nodal blocking agents can be used to try and control ventricular rate and symptoms. The success of catheter ablation of a focal atrial tachycardia ranges between 70% and 90% and depends on the ability to reproduce the tachycardia and localize the atrial focus during EP study.

The presence of multiple active atrial foci results in multifocal atrial tachycardia (MAT). This arrhythmia is an irregularly irregular rhythm with three or more discrete P wave morphologies and PR intervals; nonconducted P waves are common. MAT frequently occurs in the setting of severe pulmonary disease, and therapy is directed toward the underlying disease because the arrhythmia itself is generally not destabilizing hemodynamically. AV nodal blocking agents can be used to slow an excessively rapid heart rate; reactive airway disease often limits the use of beta-blockers.

---

[1]Not all are FDA approved for this indication.

ATRIAL FIBRILLATION

Atrial fibrillation (AF) is an atrial arrhythmia that lacks organized atrial activity or organized input into the AV node His-Purkinje system, resulting in an irregularly irregular QRS rhythm without discrete P waves. The clinical presentation of AF varies and depends on an interplay between focal atrial triggers and diseased atrial myocardium. In younger (e.g., age <75), more symptomatic patients, the suppression of AF with antiarrhythmic drugs is initially pursued. Catheter ablation techniques that can isolate electrically the regions within the atria that are important to the initiation and maintenance of AF are available, and they have demonstrated success rates of up to 90% in selected patients. In older (e.g., age >60), less symptomatic patients, ventricular heart rate control with AV nodal blocking agents is the preferred approach. If adequate rate control cannot be achieved, catheter ablation of the AV node with implantation of a permanent ventricular pacemaker can be performed. Warfarin (Coumadin) is recommended for all patients with risk factors for thromboembolic stroke: congestive heart failure, hypertension, age 75 years or older, diabetes, and history of transient ischemic attack or stroke.

ATRIAL FLUTTER

Atrial flutter is an intra-atrial reentry tachycardia with a circuit that involves a large portion of one of the atria. Typical (right atrial) flutter is the most common type of atrial flutter and uses a circuit around the tricuspid annulus. Continuous activation of a portion of the atria via this reentry circuit results in a characteristic undulating baseline likened to a sawtooth pattern (see Figure 2) in ECG leads II, III, and aVF. In other forms of atrial flutter (atypical atrial flutters), the undulations are less distinct.

The atrial rate in flutter is 250 to 300 bpm; the ventricular rate depends on the degree of AV conduction block (e.g., 2:1, 3:1, etc.). Ventricular rate control can be achieved with AV nodal blocking agents, but unlike AF, good control is often difficult. As with AF, the risk of a thromboembolic stroke is a concern if the arrhythmia persists beyond 48 hours. Unless cardioversion is urgently indicated because of hemodynamic instability, the patient should be anticoagulated for more than 3 weeks (international normalized ratio [INR] of 2 to 3) or have intracardiac thrombus excluded by transesophageal echocardiogram before cardioversion. Cardioversion can be performed either by external shock or with medications such as ibutilide (Corvert) infusion. The risk of postconversion stroke is considered the same with either modality.

In typical flutter, the reentry circuit passes through an isthmus of atrial tissue bordered by the inferior vena cava and tricuspid annulus. This isthmus is readily accessible during EP study, and catheter ablation of the isthmus has become the mainstay of therapy for typical flutter with success rates exceeding 90%. Atypical atrial flutters involve less well-defined reentry circuits, and thus catheter ablation is less successful.

PAROXYSMAL SUPRAVENTRICULAR TACHYCARDIAS

Episodes of paroxysmal supraventricular tachycardia (PSVT) have abrupt onset and termination. The sudden onset of palpitations, difficulty breathing, and anxiety in PSVT not infrequently leads to an erroneous diagnosis of panic attacks. Because the episodes can be transient and PSVT typically occurs in patients without structural heart disease or an abnormal ECG, the arrhythmia may remain undiagnosed for years. PSVT typically is a regular, narrow QRS complex tachycardia with a rate between 150 and 250 bpm.

Atrioventricular nodal reentrant tachycardia (AVNRT) is the most common PSVT (approximately 60%), and the number of women affected is twice that of men. AVNRT is a reentry tachycardia that involves a slow and fast conducting pathway connecting the AV node to the atrium. The central location of the AV node results in simultaneous, or near-simultaneous, excitation of the atria and ventricles. Although the P waves are most commonly obscured and buried within the QRS complexes, at times the P waves can deform the QRS morphology, manifesting as pseudo R' waves in lead V_1 or as pseudo S waves in leads II, III, and aVF. The complaint of neck pounding is a sensitive (93%) and specific (100%) symptom of AVNRT and is caused by right atrial contraction occurring against a closed tricuspid valve during ventricular systole.

Atrioventricular reentry tachycardia (AVRT) accounts for approximately 30% of PSVTs the number of men affected is twice that of women. AVRT is a reentry tachycardia that uses an accessory pathway between atrium and ventricle. Approximately 90% of AVRT conducts antegradely through the AV node His-Purkinje system (orthodromically) and retrogradely through the accessory pathway to the atrium; this results in a narrow QRS complex tachycardia with P waves distinct from the QRS complexes. Conduction over the accessory pathways is typically rapid, and therefore the RP interval is short relative to the PR interval. Reverse activation of the reentry circuit, or antidromic (retrograde conduction through AV node) AVRT, results in a wide QRS complex tachycardia with maximal delta waves because of exclusive excitation of the ventricules through the accessory pathway. Because both the atrium and ventricle are part of the reentry circuit, loss of 1:1 AV relationship during tachycardia excludes AVRT as the diagnosis. Most of the remaining 10% of patients with PSVT have atrial tachycardias.

When medical management is preferred for the treatment of PSVTs, AV nodal blocking agents can be used. Digoxin[1] and verapamil (Calan)[1] should be avoided in the chronic management of patients with AVRT and preexcitation because these drugs are associated with serious hemodynamic decompensation during preexcited AF, should this occur. Both class I and III antiarrhythmic drugs can be used to treat AVNRT and AVRT. Infrequent episodes of AVNRT that are well tolerated and responsive to vagal maneuvers can be observed without chronic therapy.

Currently, fewer patients with PSVT are managed with chronic drug therapy. Catheter ablation of SVT is a safe and curative procedure that can be offered as first-line therapy. The slow pathway in AVNRT and the accessory pathway in AVRT are targeted for ablation with a success rate between 95% and 98%. Major complications are rare and include complete AV block (1%), pericardial tamponade (0.6%), and stroke (0.2%).

WOLFF-PARKINSON-WHITE SYNDROME

In Wolff-Parkinson-White (WPW) conduction, ventricular preexcitation (early activation of the ventricle) occurs over an accessory pathway that electrically connects the atrium directly to the ventricle. This results in a loss of the isoelectric PR segment and in a slurring of the initial portion of the QRS complex that is termed the delta wave (Figure 3). Ventricular preexcitation appears to be a benign condition in asymptomatic patients. But patient with symptoms of palpitations, dizziness, or syncope have an approximate 1 in 1000 annual risk of SCD. The diagnosis of WPW syndrome is ventricular preexcitation accompanied by symptoms, thus implying a SCD risk.

In addition to orthodromic and antidromic AVRT, other SVTs can occur in WPW syndrome. The most concerning, and a cause of SCD, is preexcited AF, an arrhythmia recognized by an irregularly irregular rhythm with varying QRS width (Figure 4). The width of the QRS complex reflects the degree of ventricular preexcitation relative to normal AV nodal His-Purkinje conduction. Antegrade conduction over the accessory pathway can result in AF-inducing ventricular fibrillation (VF). The risk of VF is higher with more rapid antegrade accessory pathway conduction; an accessory pathway is characterized as malignant if the shortest RR interval during preexcited AF is less than 250 milliseconds. In contrast, the loss of delta waves during sinus rhythm, either spontaneously or with treadmill testing, is evidence of a poorly conducting accessory pathway that is benign.

Hemodynamic instability during preexcited AF should prompt immediate external cardioversion. The use of AV nodal blocking agents can be deleterious because they do not slow conduction over the accessory pathway. Verapamil and digoxin have been associated with precipitation of hemodynamic collapse and death, and should be avoided. Intravenous procainamide (Pronestyl)[1] is the pharmacologic treatment of choice because of its ability to block conduction in the accessory pathway.

Rakel and Bope: *Conn's Current Therapy 2006.*

[1]Not FDA approved for this indication.

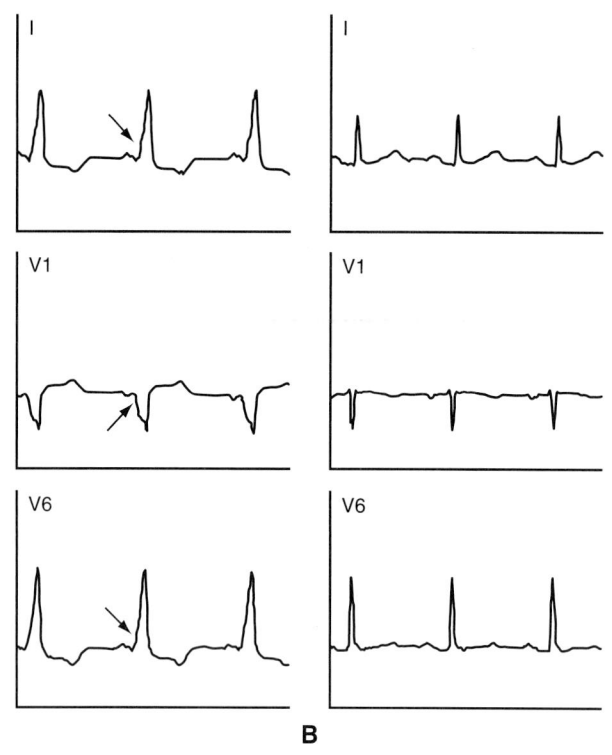

FIGURE 3. Electrocardiogram leads I, V_1, and V_6, before and after catheter ablation of an atrioventricular accessory pathway. *A,* Arrows indicate delta waves. *B,* Delta waves no longer present.

EP study with catheter ablation of the accessory pathway is recommended for patients with WPW and AF. Catheter ablation of the accessory pathway eliminates the risk of SCD, and can cure the AF, in some (<5%) patients. EP study and prophylactic ablation of the accessory pathway should also be considered in patients with WPW syndrome, especially if their occupations pose a hazard, such as pilots, bus drivers, and professional athletes.

Ventricular Tachyarrhythmias

VENTRICULAR ARRHYTHMIAS AND STRUCTURAL HEART DISEASE

In both ischemic and nonischemic dilated cardiomyopathy, ventricular scar-related reentry tachyarrhythmias are a major cause of death. Ventricular tachycardia, defined as three or more ventricular beats at a tachycardia rate, is considered sustained when persistent for longer than 30 seconds. The QRS complex morphology can be unchanging (monomorphic) or variable (polymorphic). VF is chaotic ventricular activity recognized by variable ventricular undulations. Spontaneous termination of either VT or VF results in dizziness or syncope; sustained tachyarrhythmias can result in SCD. Antiarrhythmic drugs are ineffective in improving survival in patients at risk for SCD, but multiple studies have established the efficacy of ICDs in preventing death in cardiac arrest survivors. Recent trials also demonstrate the effectiveness of ICDs in primary prevention of SCD in patients with depressed left ventricular ejection fraction (35%) due to either ischemic or nonischemic heart disease.

When patients with structural heart disease present with ventricular tachyarrhythmia, the general approach is to recommend ICD implantation to prevent SCD. Antiarrhythmic drugs, such as amiodarone (Cordarone), are used in patients who experience frequent ICD shocks. Although amiodarone (Cordarone) does not impact overall survival, it can decrease the number of arrhythmic events and has not been associated with excess mortality. Catheter ablation can target and disrupt VT reentry circuits in and around a scar. Although the elimination of all reentry circuits is not usually a realistic goal because of the complex nature of cardiomyopathic scars, catheter ablation can be effective in decreasing the number of VT episodes in selected cases.

Sustained monomorphic VT in nonischemic dilated cardiomyopathy frequently turns out to be *bundle branch reentry tachycardia.* This form of reentry tachycardia

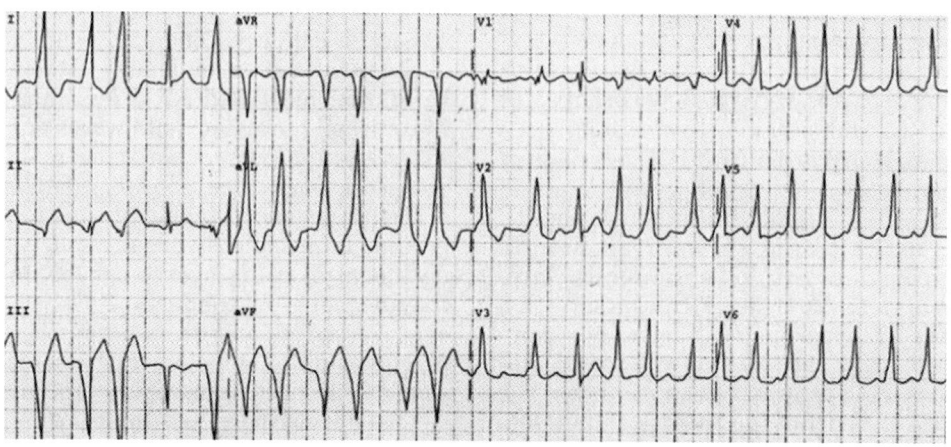

FIGURE 4. Twelve-lead electrocardiogram, preexcited atrial fibrillation. The arrhythmia is characterized by an irregularly irregular rhythm with variable QRS width.

involves diseased bundle branches and most commonly manifests as a left bundle-branch block pattern with left axis deviation. Catheter ablation targeting one of the involved bundle branches can be performed with relative ease, curing a tachycardia that is typically rapid and recurrent. ICDs should still be considered in these patients since they are still at risk for SCD because of underlying cardiomyopathy.

IDIOPATHIC VENTRICULAR TACHYCARDIA

VT occurring in the absence of structural heart disease is termed idiopathic. In general, the risk of SCD is low. More than 80% of idiopathic VT originates from the RVOT and characteristically has a left bundle branch block pattern with an inferior mean frontal plane QRS axis. RVOT VT presents either as repetitive bursts of nonsustained VT or episodes of sustained VT brought about by physical or emotional stress. In most patients, the mechanism is catecholamine-induced cyclic adenosine monophosphate (cAMP)-mediated intracellular calcium increase, resulting in triggered activity. Because adenosine (Adenocard) decreases cAMP levels in ventricular cells and is effective in terminating RVOT VT, response to adenosine is useful in distinguishing RVOT VT from other forms of idiopathic VT.

RVOT VT is responsive to a wide range of antiarrhythmic drugs. Beta-blockers are usually tried first, and effectiveness of therapy can be assessed with treadmill testing. Diltiazem (Cardizem)[1] and verapamil[1] appear equally effective. The accessibility of the RVOT makes RVOT VT amenable to catheter ablation as well. The focus is usually found just below the pulmonary valve on the septal aspect of the RVOT, but variant foci can be found in the left ventricular outflow tract or epicardium. The success rate of catheter ablation exceeds 90%. Sotalol (Betapace) or flecainide (Tambocor) can also be considered in patients unresponsive to beta-blockers or calcium channel blockers who are not amenable to catheter ablation.

An important condition to exclude in patients presenting with a right ventricular (RV) VT is arrhythmogenic right ventricular cardiomyopathy (ARVC). In ARVC there is gradual fibrofatty displacement of the RV myocardium, resulting in scar-facilitated reentrant VT that is potentially life threatening. A gold standard diagnostic test currently is lacking; the diagnosis is made from multiple clinical criteria and results from various tests, which include echocardiography looking for RV dilation, and gated cardiac magnetic resonance imaging looking for intramyocardial fat. ICDs are considered in patients with ARVC who are inadequately treated with antiarrhythmic drugs.

The most common idiopathic left VT originates from the left ventricular septum and presents with a right bundle branch block pattern with superior axis. The tachycardia mimics a focal tachycardia with an origin in the region of the left posterior fascicle, but the mechanism has been revealed to be reentry involving a circuit that includes the left posterior fascicle and

abnormal verapamil-sensitive tissue (presumably Purkinje fibers) that runs adjacent to the fascicle. Catheter ablation of the diseased Purkinje fibers is curative. Although this VT is sensitive to intravenous verapamil,[1] less data are available on chronic oral verapamil for long-term arrhythmia suppression.

---

[1]Not FDA approved for this indication.

 CURRENT DIAGNOSIS

- A narrow (≥120 milliseconds) QRS complex tachycardia is supraventricular; a wide (120 milliseconds) QRS complex tachycardia is either ventricular or supraventricular with bundle branch block, aberrant intraventricular conduction, or ventricular preexcitation.
- Typical right atrial flutter is recognized by a unique undulating baseline likened to a sawtooth pattern in ECG leads II, III, and aVF.
- Transient block of the AV node (vagal maneuvers, adenosine [Adenocard]) with continuation of an atrial arrhythmia, such as atrial flutter or atrial tachycardia, is diagnostic.
- Multifocal atrial tachycardia is defined as an irregularly irregular rhythm, more than 100 beats per minute, with three or more discrete P wave morphologies and PR intervals. These features distinguish it from atrial fibrillation.
- The sensation of neck pounding is a sensitive (93%) and specific (100%) symptom of atrioventricular nodal reentrant tachycardia.
- Distortion of the terminal portion of the QRS complex during supraventricular tachycardia, by negative P waves in ECG leads II, III, aVF (pseudo S waves) or upright P waves in V$_1$ (pseudo R' waves), is highly suggestive of atrioventricular nodal reentry tachycardia.
- Preexcited atrial fibrillation is associated with induction of ventricular fibrillation and recognized by an irregularly irregular rhythm with varying QRS width because of delta waves of varying duration. An accessory pathway is malignant when it conducts rapidly (shortest RR interval during atrial fibrillation less than 250 milliseconds). Catheter ablation of the accessory pathway eliminates the risk of sudden death.
- A history of heart disease in a patient with wide QRS complex tachycardia has a positive predictive value of 95% for ventricular tachycardia.
- Ventricular-atrial dissociation, established by dissociated P waves, capture beats, or fusion beats, is diagnostic of ventricular tachycardia.
- Right ventricular outflow tract ventricular tachycardia characteristically has a left bundle branch block pattern with inferior frontal plane QRS axis and is distinguishable from other idiopathic ventricular tachycardias by its sensitivity to adenosine (Adenocard).

---

[1]Not FDA approved for this indication.

CURRENT THERAPY

- For any tachyarrhythmia, if the blood pressure is excessively low or consequences of hypoperfusion (cognitive impairment, chest pain, heart failure) are evident, immediate electrical cardioversion should be performed.
- Because a delay in therapy of ventricular tachycardia can be life threatening, a wide QRS complex tachycardia should be considered ventricular tachycardia until proved otherwise.
- Persistence of atrial fibrillation or atrial flutter for more than 48 hours is associated with an increased risk for thromboembolic stroke, and exclusion of intracardiac thrombus should precede cardioversion unless hemodynamic instability dictates urgent therapy.
- Adenosine (Adenocard) reliably terminates atrioventricular nodal reentry tachycardia and atrioventricular reciprocating tachycardia.
- Infrequent episodes of atrioventricular nodal reentry tachycardia that are well tolerated and responsive to vagal maneuvers can be managed with observation. Episodes that are frequent and/or poorly tolerated are best treated with catheter ablation.
- Verapamil and digoxin have been associated with precipitating hemodynamic collapse and death when administered during preexcited atrial fibrillation. Intravenous procainamide is the treatment of choice because of its ability to block the accessory pathway.
- Fewer patients with supraventricular tachycardias are chronically managed with drugs. Catheter ablation is effective in curing atrial flutter, atrioventricular nodal reentry tachycardia, atrioventricular reciprocating tachycardia, some forms of atrial tachycardia, Wolff-Parkinson-White syndrome, and selected patients with atrial fibrillation.
- Implantable cardioverter defibrillators are effective in preventing sudden cardiac death in patients with depressed left ventricular function.
- Frequent implantable cardioverter defibrillator shocks resulting from recurrent ventricular tachycardia can be treated with antiarrhythmic drugs, which reduce the number of tachycardia episodes. Catheter ablation can target and disrupt ventricular tachycardia reentry circuits in and around scar tissue, and can decrease ventricular tachycardia episodes in selected patients.
- Intravenous magnesium[1] is the initial treatment of choice for nonsustained torsades de pointes.

[1]Not FDA approved for this indication.

LONG QT SYNDROMES AND TORSADES DE POINTES

Prolongation of the QT interval denotes an abnormality in ventricular repolarization that can lead to triggered activity. This can result in torsades de pointes, a polymorphic VT with continuously changing QRS amplitude and polarity that has the appearance of "twisting around a point" along the isoelectric baseline. Long QT syndrome (LQTS) encompasses congenital and acquired forms. An extensive list of drugs is recognized to cause QT prolongation and includes class IA and III antiarrhythmic drugs, various antipsychotic agents, and some antibiotics. Continually updated lists of QT prolonging drugs are available for reference (e.g., http://www.torsades.org).

Intravenous magnesium[1] is the initial treatment for nonsustained torsades de pointes. Lidocaine (Xylocaine)[1] infusion can also be effective. To suppress further episodes of tachycardia, the heart rate can be increased with temporary atrial or ventricular pacing; the increase in heart rate is accompanied by shortening of the QT interval. Isoproterenol (Isuprel)[1] can also be used for this purpose, but exacerbation of ventricular arrhythmia can occur, especially in patients with ischemic heart disease. Any potential causes for QT prolongation must be identified and eliminated. Certain types of congenital LQTS can be treated chronically with beta-blockers. ICDs are employed in patients at high risk for SCD (e.g., syncope, aborted SCD).

A growing number of other genetic tachyarrhythmia syndromes are recognized. These syndromes are rare, but their unique presentations aid in diagnosis and management. Genetic testing is increasingly available for definitive diagnosis, as well as for risk assessment of family members.

REFERENCES

Akhtar M, Shenasa M, Jazayeri M, et al: Wide QRS complex tachycardia: Reappraisal of a common clinical problem. Ann Intern Med 1988;109:905-912.
Baerman JM, Morady F, DiCarlo LA, et al: Differentiation of ventricular tachycardia from supraventricular tachycardia with aberration: Value of the clinical history. Ann Emerg Med 1987;16:40-43.
Bardy GH, Lee KL, Mark DB, et al: Amiodarone or an implantable cardioverter-defibrillator for congestive heart failure. N Engl J Med 2005;352:225-237.
Calkins H, Yong P, Miller JM, Olshansky B, et al: Catheter ablation of accessory pathways, atrioventricular nodal reentrant tachycardia, and the atrioventricular junction: Final results of a prospective, multicenter clinical trial. The Atakr Multicenter Investigators Group. Circulation 1999;99:262-270.
Echt DS, Leibson PR, Mitchell LB, Peters RW, et al: Mortality and morbidity in patients receiving encainide, flecainide, or placebo. The Cardiac Arrhythmia Suppression Trial. N Engl J Med 1991;324:781-788.
Ferguson JD, DiMarco JP: Contemporary management of paroxysmal supraventricular tachycardia. Circulation 2003;107:1096-1099.
Gürsoy S, Steurer G, Brugada J, Andries E, et al: The hemodynamic mechanism of pounding in the neck in atrioventricular nodal reentrant tachycardia. N Engl J Med 1992;327:772-774.
The Antiarrhythmics versus Implantable Defibrillators (AVID) Investigators: A comparison of antiarrhythmic-drug therapy with implantable defibrillators in patients resuscitated from near-fatal ventricular arrhythmias. N Engl J Med 1997;337:1576-1583.

[1]Not FDA approved for this indication.

The Cardiovascular System

Wellens HJ: Contemporary management of atrial flutter. Circulation 2002;106:649-652.
Wellens HJ: Cardiac arrhythmias: The quest for a cure: A historical perspective [Review]. J Am Coll Cardiol 2004;44:1155-1163.
Wellens HJ: Catheter ablation for cardiac arrhythmias. Circulation 2004;351:1172-1174.

Congenital Heart Disease

Method of
John P. Cheatham, MD,
and Stephen C. Cook, MD

CURRENT DIAGNOSIS

- Thorough history and physical examination
- Cardiac examination, including palpation of the pulses, blood pressure measurements in all four extremities, and pulse oximetry
- Electrocardiogram
- Chest radiograph
- Pediatric cardiology consultation
    - Children with Down syndrome, chromosomal abnormalities, multiple anomalies
    - Pathologic findings on exam (diastolic, holosystolic, or harsh murmurs more than grade III to VI in intensity)
    - Exam findings of heart failure/tachypnea/cyanosis

The incidence of congenital heart disease (CHD) in the general population is approximately 8 per 1000 live births. Several factors can lead to an underestimation of reported CHD, however, including the inability to diagnose congenital heart defects accurately and to identify defects that produce relatively few symptoms and might otherwise go undetected, plus the lack of information on infants who die shortly after birth whose cause of demise may have been secondary to CHD. Regardless of these limitations, advances in fetal ultrasound to diagnose CHD prenatally, as well as rapid referral to a pediatric cardiologist to evaluate the newborn with a murmur, cyanosis, or symptoms consistent with CHD, aid in rapid detection.

Cardiac Examination

In addition to a thorough history, a systematic physical examination in conjunction with chest radiography and electrocardiogram aid in the detection of CHD. Inspection begins with general appearance of the child and recognition of dysmorphic facial features as well as cyanosis and clubbing. Palpation of the pulses and blood pressure measurements in all four extremities are essential. Palpation also includes assessment of the cardiac impulse.

Auscultation of the first heart sound in children is usually single. The second heart sound, which varies with respiration, is best appreciated at the left upper sternal border. Abnormalities of the second heart sound are frequently associated with CHD. Murmurs are best described by intensity, timing, location, and radiation. The intensity of the murmur is graded I (barely audible) to VI (audible with stethoscope off the chest). Innocent murmurs are relatively soft in intensity, vary in position of the patient, and are described frequently as vibratory. Murmurs that are either harsh, holosystolic, or diastolic are rarely innocent and warrant further investigation.

Examination of the back and abdomen is equally important in assessing a child with suspected CHD. Finding rales at the bases of the lung fields and hepatomegaly may suggest congestive heart failure (CHF) encountered in certain types of CHD. Transthoracic echocardiography

in experienced hands has greatly facilitated the accurate and rapid diagnosis of CHD, regardless of complexity.

Once the diagnosis of CHD has been made in conjunction with echocardiography, the broad spectrum of the disease can be categorized further based on the presence or absence of cyanosis and the degree of pulmonary circulation. Cyanosis is seen with right-to-left shunts. Right-to-left shunts also occur in combination with obstructive-type right-sided cardiac lesions. Pulmonary overcirculation is seen in patients with left-to-right shunts and obstructive left-sided cardiac lesions. Restriction to pulmonary flow is seen in obstructive-type defects. Thus a thorough understanding of cardiac physiology is crucial to the successful management of each unique defect.

Acyanotic Lesions

PATENT DUCTUS ARTERIOSUS

The patent ductus arteriosus (PDA), a naturally occurring vascular structure, connects the aorta and the pulmonary artery and is vital in fetal life. After birth, the response to increased blood oxygen levels leads to constriction of the smooth muscle within the walls of the ductus. Ongoing constriction and ischemia leads to full structural closure within the first few days of life.

In the premature infant, however, the PDA may not undergo complete closure. The presence of a PDA enables left-to-right shunting to occur that results in increased pulmonary blood flow. The volume overload placed on the pulmonary vascular bed and the left ventricle is manifested by signs of CHF, tachypnea, and tachycardia. Physical exam findings include a hyperdynamic precordium, bounding peripheral pulses, and widened pulse pressure. The classic continuous machinery murmur is not frequently encountered in the newborn with a PDA. The diastolic component of the murmur may be absent because of the relatively elevated pulmonary vascular resistance (PVR) still present at birth. As the PVR begins to fall, the diastolic component of the murmur is heard.

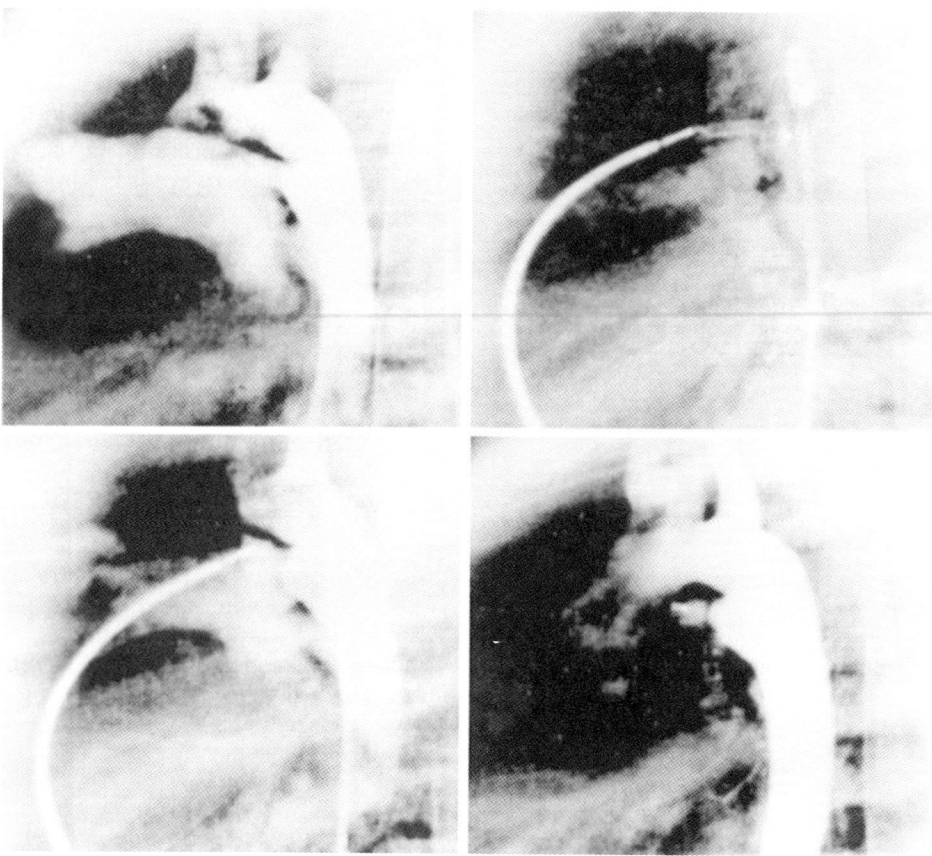

FIGURE 1. An aortic angiogram in this 18-month-old demonstrates a large type A patent ductus arteriosus (PDA). An 8- to 6-mm AMPLATZER Duct Occluder is delivered percutaneously with complete closure demonstrated within 10 minutes of implantation.

Management in the preterm infant with PDA remains controversial. Strategies used to approach the PDA include pharmacologic management with prostaglandin inhibitors that promote ductal closure or surgical ligation. Advances in interventional catheterization techniques provide additional methods of ductal closure in infants, children, and adults using Gianturco coils, including detachable coils (small PDA) and the Amplatzer Duct Occluder, the only FDA-approved device for this purpose (Figure 1). The Nit-Occlud Spiral Coil is also available in selected centers under an FDA-sponsored clinical trial. Clinical decisions surrounding treatment of the ductus should be individualized and based on the gestational age of the infant, the respiratory status, and the degree of the ductal shunt. The older child (beyond one year of age) is frequently asymptomatic. The classic continuous murmur is present on examination. PDA closure in these patients is recommended. Options available include surgical ligation as well as transcatheter closure. The current recommended treatment of choice in centers with experienced personnel is transcatheter closure using the devices just described.

ATRIAL SEPTAL DEFECT

Abnormalities in the development of the atrial septum lead to communications between the left and right atria known as atrial septal defect (ASD). Embryologic abnormalities may occur anywhere along the length of the septum and account for the different subtypes. Centrally located defects, secundum ASD, are the most common and account for 75% of these defects. Studies have shown that secundum ASD smaller than 3 mm in diameter in the first 3 months of life nearly always close, and those greater than 8 mm in diameter are unlikely to close. Defects in the atrial septum that occur at the level of the atrioventricular valves are the second most common at 15% and known as primum defects. A cleft in the anterior leaflet of the mitral valve is associated with this defect and may lead to mitral regurgitation. These defects rarely close spontaneously. Another 10% of defects, which occur at the junction of the superior vena cava and the atrial septum, are known as sinus venosus defects. This type of defect is seen in combination with anomalous drainage of the right upper pulmonary vein. Defects rarely occur near the orifice of the coronary sinus, suitably named the coronary sinus ASD.

Children with small ASD are rarely, if ever, symptomatic. The larger ASD eventually leads to right atrial and right ventricular enlargement and pulmonary overcirculation. This increased volume load generates a systolic ejection murmur best heard at the left upper sternal border, accompanied by a widely fixed-split second heart sound. The chronic volume overload on the right heart eventually produces symptoms of fatigue, dyspnea on exertion, and palpitations. In addition, the unrepaired

ASD is associated with an increased risk of developing atrial arrhythmias and pulmonary hypertension (<10%) in the fifth and sixth decades of life.

Most ASD are electively closed during childhood to reduce these risks. Defects may be surgically closed with sutures (primary repair) or with a patch, depending on the size and location of the defect. However, most patients with secundum ASD are suitable candidates for nonsurgical closure. Percutaneous transcatheter implantation of the Amplatzer Septal Occluder, now FDA approved, revolutionized the approach to these defects, having evolved into a well-tolerated, efficient, and cost-effective method of treatment with minimal discomfort for the patient and is considered the treatment of choice (Figure 2). In experienced centers, surgery is seldom necessary to close secundum ASD. Other devices are currently being evaluated under FDA-sponsored clinical trials (e.g., HELEX Septal Occluder and STARFlex Septal Occluder). Currently surgery is the only therapeutic option available for primum and sinus venosus defects.

VENTRICULAR SEPTAL DEFECT

The development of the ventricular septum is rather intricate, and ventricular septal defect (VSD) results from failure of complete formation of the primary septum, failure of fusion of the atrioventricular cushions, malalignment of the outlet septum, or failure of the septum that contributes to the membranous septum to form completely. These errors in development account for the different subtypes of VSD. Defects may occur alone or in combination with ASD, PDA, or aortic arch obstruction (coarctation, aortic arch interruption).

Most commonly (70%), VSD is perimembranous, located in the upper fibrous region of the septum beneath the septal leaflet of the tricuspid valve and aortic valve. Muscular defects (20%) are located along the muscular septum between the left and right ventricles. Inlet defects (5%) are situated posteriorly along the ventricular septum beneath the tricuspid valve. Outlet defects (5%), also referred to as subpulmonary or supracristal defects, are located between the left and right ventricular outflow tracts just below the pulmonary valve.

The clinical presentation of the child with a VSD is determined by the size, location, and the ratio of pulmonary to systemic arterial resistance. Smaller defects present with relatively few symptoms and a grade II to III high-pitched holosystolic murmur on examination. Moderate to large size defects may not become apparent until 4 to 6 weeks of life. As PVR continues to fall postnatally, the degree of left-to-right shunting increases, which leads to the development of symptoms. These infants often present with signs of CHF and poor feeding. The examination may demonstrate a grade III to IV harsh holosystolic murmur, prominent second heart sound, gallop rhythm, and diastolic flow rumble over the mitral valve.

Management also depends on the size, location, and physiology that accompany each type of defect. Asymptomatic patients with small muscular or perimembranous VSD must be followed regularly because

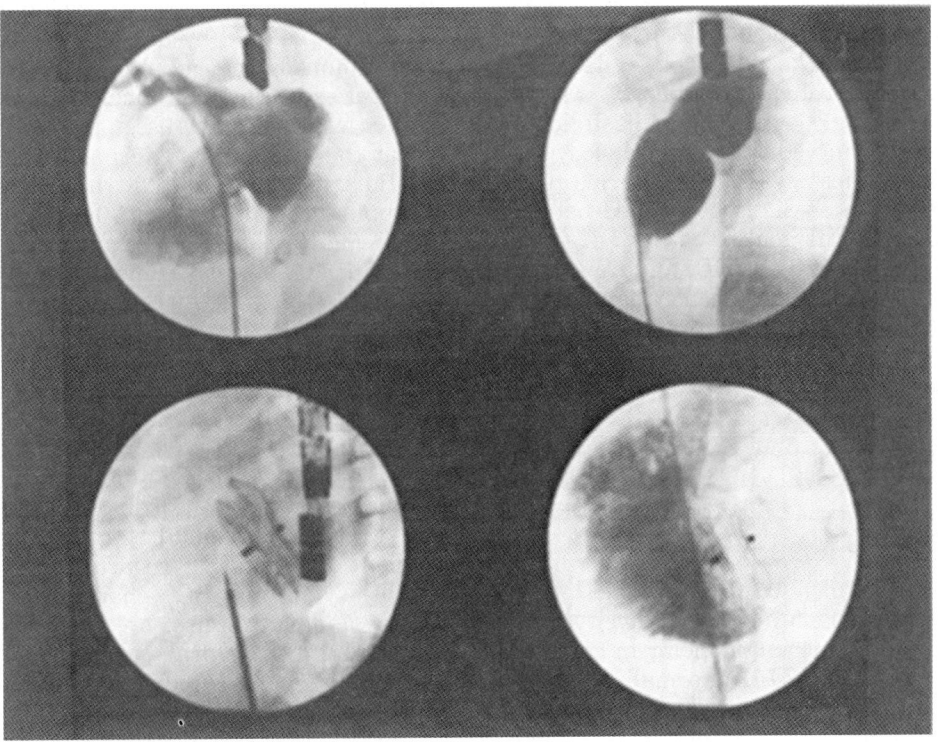

FIGURE 2. A right upper pulmonary vein angiogram nicely defines a large secundum atrial septal defect (ASD) measuring 18 mm in diameter in this 2-year-old with Down syndrome weighing 10 kg. After balloon sizing the defect, a 20-mm AMPLATZER Septal Occluder is implanted with complete closure.

many of these defects close spontaneously. Symptomatic patients with larger defects initially require medical management that includes digitalis, diuretic therapy, and afterload reduction. These defects are unlikely to close spontaneously and warrant closure. Historically, these defects were treated by age 2 years to avoid pulmonary vascular obstructive disease (PVOD). More contemporary treatment closes the defect surgically in early infancy. Inlet and outlet defects are unlikely to close spontaneously and should be repaired surgically. Defects adjacent to the aortic valve (outlet, perimembranous) may be associated with valve prolapse. The right coronary cusp herniates into the VSD, and aortic insufficiency ensues. These defects should be repaired early to prevent this known complication.

Transcatheter closure techniques are also applied to perimembranous and muscular VSD. FDA-sponsored clinical trials evaluating the Amplatzer Membranous and Muscular VSD Occluders (AGA Medical Corp.) show excellent closure rates and low mortality. These devices are currently only available in FDA-approved centers, however.

ATRIOVENTRICULAR SEPTAL DEFECT

Atrioventricular septal defect (AVSD) results from abnormalities in the development of the endocardial cushions. This malformation creates abnormalities in the atrial septum, ventricular septum, and the atrioventricular (AV) valves. A strong genetic component is associated with these defects, and they are commonly seen in patients with Down syndrome. The clinical presentation depends on the degree of anatomic anomalies, but most children with complete AVSD present with symptoms of CHF at or near 4 weeks of life as PVR decreases. On exam, the precordium is hyperdynamic, S_1 is single, S_2 is narrowly split or single, and an S_3 or diastolic flow rumble may be present in addition to the holosystolic murmur of mitral insufficiency. Early operative repair of symptomatic complete AVSD is performed between 3 and 6 months of age. The goal of earlier surgery in these patients is to prevent PVOD and to restore normal growth and development. Reoperation is sometimes required to address residual mitral valve stenosis or insufficiency.

Obstructive Lesions

PULMONARY STENOSIS AND AORTIC STENOSIS

Pulmonary stenosis (PS) may occur below the level of the valve (subvalvar), at the level of the valve (valvar), or above the valve (supravalvar), alone or in combination with other forms of CHD. Abnormalities of the distal bulbus cordis during fetal development result in the dysplastic appearance of the pulmonary valve, which becomes dome shaped and dysplastic. The prevalence of this disease in families and its association with syndromes (e.g., Noonan's syndrome) suggest an underlying genetic component. Most pulmonary valve stenosis is nondysplastic, however, and not related to an underlying systemic disorder.

Mild valvar PS rarely produces symptoms. The exam is significant for an early systolic ejection click that is accentuated during expiration, accompanied by a systolic ejection murmur at the left upper sternal border. As the severity increases, symptoms of dyspnea and fatigue may appear. A palpable heave and late peaking murmur indicate severe obstruction.

The degree of valvar stenosis is determined by the peak transvalvar gradient estimated by echocardiography or measure during cardiac catheterization or the systolic pressure ratio of right ventricle (RV) compared to systemic arterial pressure. Mild PS is defined as a gradient smaller than 40 mm Hg or RV pressure less than one-half systemic pressure. Moderate PS is defined as a gradient equal to 40 mm Hg or RV pressure of one half, but less than systemic pressure. Severe PS is defined as a transvalvar gradient of 80 mm Hg or RV pressure more than systemic pressure. Since 1982, the treatment of valvar PS has resided in the cardiac catheterization lab using balloon valvuloplasty techniques. The indications for balloon therapy include gradient higher than 40 mm Hg pressure estimated by echocardiography and RV pressure equal to half systemic arterial pressure. Balloon valvuloplasty provides excellent medium-term relief for patients with nondysplastic valvar stenosis. Surgery is usually required for significant sub- and supravalvar stenosis.

Abnormalities in the development of the aortic valve lead to aortic valve stenosis (AS). Bicuspid aortic valve is the most frequently encountered abnormality. Patients with mild AS may be relatively asymptomatic. Mild AS is defined by a Doppler gradient of less than 30 to 40 mm Hg and catheter gradient of 25 to 30 mm Hg. Physical exam findings include an ejection click and a systolic crescendo-decrescendo ejection murmur present at the right upper sternal border radiating to the carotid arteries. Patients with moderate AS, defined as a Doppler gradient of 40 to 70 mm Hg and catheter gradient equal to 50 mm Hg, may become symptomatic. The murmur may become louder, but more importantly, the splitting of the second heart sound becomes less audible. Critical AS, particularly in the newborn period, presents with heart failure, tachycardia, and poor peripheral pulses, and it requires urgent therapy to relieve the obstruction.

Therapeutic options include balloon aortic valvuloplasty or surgical valvotomy. Transcatheter balloon valvuloplasty, the initial procedure of choice over the last two decades, should be considered with a catheter gradient of 70 mm Hg, regardless of symptoms, 50 mm Hg with symptoms, ECG changes indicative of ischemia at rest and/or exercise, or significant left ventricular hypertrophy. Surgical valvotomy is reserved for patients in whom balloon valvuloplasty is unsuccessful. Although balloon valvuloplasty remains the preferred technique, occasionally progressive valvar insufficiency requires valve replacement. Surgical options include use of a prosthetic aortic valve that requires lifelong anticoagulation. Alternatively, a pulmonary autograft in the aortic position, known as the Ross procedure, does not require anticoagulation and is preferred in the growing child.

Infants presenting with critical AS remain the most problematic. Acceptable outcomes with current therapies may be difficult with a small aortic valve annulus. The presence of a small left ventricle and mitral valve, endocardial fibroelastosis, and mitral insufficiency from infarcted papillary muscles strongly influence outcomes. The presence of one or more of these findings may ultimately guide transcatheter versus surgical therapy.

COARCTATION OF THE AORTA

The embryologic abnormality associated with coarctation of the aorta (CoA) is not completely defined. Suggested hypotheses include aberration in the media of the aortic arch and/or anomalous ductal tissue present in the arch. Associated defects include VSD and aortic and mitral valve abnormalities. Shone syndrome is the finding of CoA in combination with subaortic stenosis and mitral stenosis.

The clinical presentation depends on the age of the patient, severity of coarctation, and associated anomalies. Newborns with severe coarctation frequently present within the first few weeks of life with tachypnea, poor feedings, and CHF symptoms. Discrepant blood pressure measurements between upper and lower extremities and diminished femoral pulses are classic findings. Older patients are frequently asymptomatic but present with severe systolic arterial hypertension in the upper

extremities. Cardiac examination reveals a systolic ejection murmur along the left sternal border with radiation to the interscapular region posteriorly. A continuous murmur may also be present in the older child as a result of well-developed collaterals that bypass the coarctation segment. A systolic ejection click is encountered in the presence of a bicuspid aortic valve because these lesions frequently coexist with one another.

Surgical repair is recommended for newborns who present with severe CoA. Surgical techniques, such as resection with an end-to-end anastomosis, patch aortoplasty, and subclavian flap aortoplasty, have been used to address the coarctation segment. Late outcomes of the patch aortoplasty technique have demonstrated aneurysm formation at the site of repair. In the left subclavian flap technique, the surgeon must sacrifice the major vascular supply to the left upper extremity. Thus the end-to-end approach is the preferred technique.

When CoA presents outside of the neonatal age group, balloon aortic angioplasty is widely accepted as a suitable alternative therapy. A recurrence rate of residual obstruction makes it a less favorable alternative in the neonate. Primary intravascular stent implantation in older children (weight greater than 20 kg), adolescents, and adults with CoA is gaining popularity and provides a suitable alternative to surgery (Figure 3).

Long-term follow-up of patients after treatment of CoA is mandatory. Late complications such as aortic aneurysms, hypertension, aortic valve stenosis, and recoarctation are well described. Balloon angioplasty

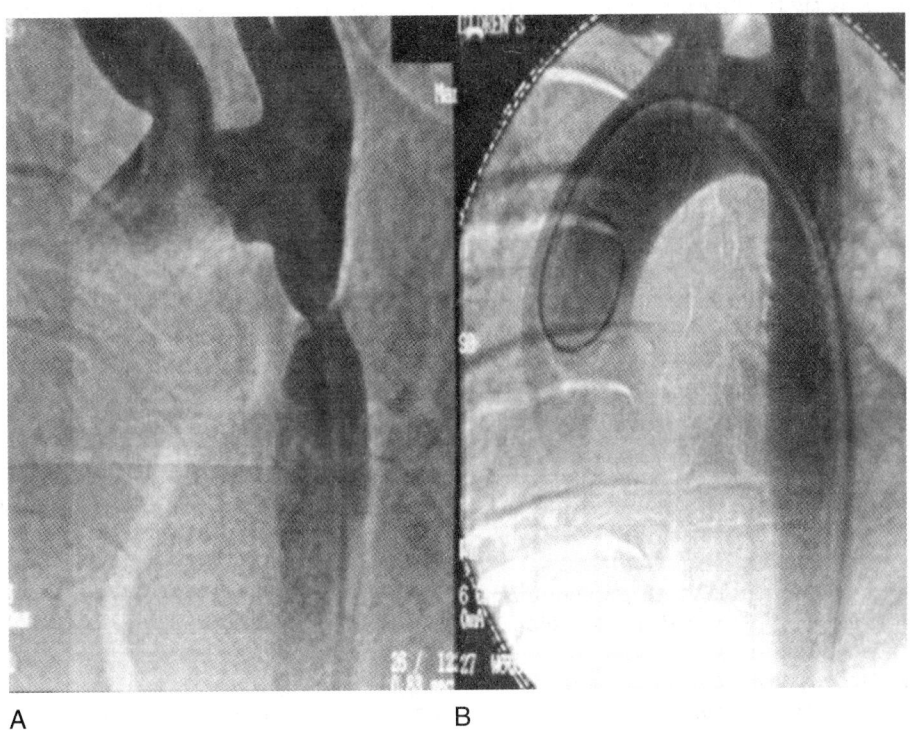

A   B

FIGURE 3. A 12-year-old presents with hypertension, and aortic angiography confirms coarctation of the aorta. After stent implantation, there is complete relief of obstruction with normalization of blood pressure. Long-term follow-up is required.

Rakel and Bope: *Conn's Current Therapy 2006.*

and/or stent implantation is the treatment of choice in recoarctation. Indications for therapy include resting hypertension proximal to the CoA and/or a resting systolic blood pressure gradient of 20 mm Hg across the narrowed segment.

HYPOPLASTIC LEFT HEART SYNDROME

The term *hypoplastic left heart syndrome* (HLHS) describes a series of left-sided lesions involving hypoplasia/atresia of the mitral and aortic valves and hypoplasia of the left ventricle, representing the most severe form of obstructive CHD. Systemic blood flow depends on the presence of a PDA. Constriction of the PDA in the first few days of life leads to systemic hypoperfusion. Newborns rapidly deteriorate and present with a clinical picture of shock. Initial medical therapy requires establishing ductal patency with a prostaglandin E_1 (PGE_1) infusion. The several treatment options include a staged surgical reconstruction, cardiac transplantation, and palliative care.

The goal of the staged reconstruction is to separate pulmonary and systemic circulations supported by a single ventricle, provide stable systemic cardiac output, regulate pulmonary blood flow, and provide unrestricted flow from the left atrium. Patients initially undergo a systemic to pulmonary artery shunt procedure to provide a stable form of pulmonary blood flow, aortic arch reconstruction, and atrial septectomy, commonly known as the stage I Norwood procedure. A cavopulmonary anastomosis in which venous flow from the upper extremities is directed to the pulmonary arteries and the shunt is ligated follows (stage II procedure). The final stage, or Fontan completion, directs all venous blood flow directly to the pulmonary arteries by connecting the inferior vena cava (IVC) flow to the pulmonary arteries. Since its original description, several modifications over the last two decades have led to improved surgical outcomes. During the highest risk stage I repair, the aortopulmonary shunt is replaced by a right ventricle to pulmonary artery nonvalved conduit, the so-called Sano modification. For Fontan completion with or without fenestration, the lateral tunnel procedure, in which IVC flow is directed to the pulmonary arteries via an intracardiac baffle along the free wall of the right atrium, is commonly performed. The extracardiac Fontan conduit uses a Gore-Tex tube to redirect IVC flow outside the heart to the right pulmonary artery.

Cardiac transplantation, which restores normal cardiac physiology, is performed in several centers for HLHS, although the shortage of neonatal heart donors remains a major obstacle. Post-transplant care requires lifelong immunosuppression, potential for rejection, infections, graft vasculopathy, and lymphoproliferative diseases.

A new hybrid palliative approach is gaining in popularity in which the high-risk stage I procedure is replaced by surgical right and left pulmonary artery bands without cardiopulmonary bypass, transcatheter PDA stent, and balloon atrial septostomy. A comprehensive stage II procedure is performed at 4 to 6 months of age, and the Fontan completion accomplished at 2 years of age.

A prospective randomized clinical trial is under way to evaluate these management strategies.

Cyanotic Lesions

Cyanosis is the physical sign of blue discoloration of the mucous membranes, nail beds, and skin. It occurs when the level of deoxygenated hemoglobin reaches 3 to 5 g/dL. Cyanosis is less likely to occur in an anemic neonate in whom the hemoglobin levels may be too low to produce a cyanotic appearance.

TRANSPOSITION OF THE GREAT ARTERIES (TGA)

In transposition of the great arteries (TGA), the aorta arises from the right ventricle and the pulmonary artery arises from the left ventricle. Because the two circulations are in parallel, oxygenated blood returns to the lungs and desaturated blood returns to the body. Thus these infants depend on intracardiac mixing to survive. The physical exam may be unremarkable except for a single S_2. Initiation of PGE_1 infusion to maintain ductal patency and balloon atrial septostomy are strategies available to improve mixing in the severely cyanotic newborn.

In the past, the atrial switch procedure, known as the Mustard or Senning, was performed. An intracardiac baffle was created to redirect desaturated blood toward the left ventricle where it is pumped to the pulmonary arteries. Oxygenated blood is directed toward the right ventricle where it is pumped to the aorta. Long-term complications such as tricuspid insufficiency, right ventricular failure, arrhythmias, and sudden death are described.

As a result of these late outcomes, the arterial switch procedure is now performed. In this procedure, the great arteries are transected and the pulmonary artery is anastomosed to the aortic root anteriorly and the aorta is brought posteriorly and anastomosed to the pulmonary root. The coronary arteries are then transferred to the aorta, resulting in an anatomic correction. Results from long-term follow-up have been favorable, but patients should be evaluated lifelong for coronary artery stenosis and any obstruction at the great artery anastomoses.

TETRALOGY OF FALLOT

Unequal conotruncal septation during cardiac development leads to the common findings of ventricular septal defect, pulmonary stenosis, overriding aorta, and right ventricular hypertrophy found in tetralogy of Fallot (TOF). Approximately 25% of patients also have a right-sided aortic arch. Cyanosis occurs with right-to-left shunting through the VSD. The degree of hypoxemia depends on the severity of right ventricular outflow tract (RVOT) obstruction. Patients with mild obstruction appear relatively pink (so-called pink TOF). The murmur generated by the right ventricular outflow tract obstruction is a high-pitched systolic crescendo-decrescendo at the left upper sternal border that radiates to the back.

Timing for complete repair depends on the size and distribution of the pulmonary arteries and presence/absence of associated anomalies. Newborns with severe cyanosis, acidosis, and hypoxemia may require a palliative shunt. A modified Blalock-Taussig shunt (Gore-Tex tube that communicates between the subclavian and pulmonary arteries) augments pulmonary blood flow until complete repair can be performed. Balloon pulmonary valvuloplasty and/or stents of the PDA are performed as a nonsurgical palliation to provide additional pulmonary blood flow. Otherwise, definitive repair of TOF usually occurs around 3 to 6 months of age and includes VSD closure and relief of RVOT obstruction. Lifelong evaluation is required because severe pulmonary insufficiency, right ventricular enlargement, residual RVOT and PA obstruction, ventricular arrhythmias, and sudden death have been reported.

PULMONARY ATRESIA WITH INTACT VENTRICULAR SEPTUM AND CRITICAL PULMONARY VALVE STENOSIS OF THE NEWBORN

Pulmonary atresia with intact ventricular septum (PA/IVS) may occur early or late in fetal development, resulting in varying degrees of RV hypoplasia. The same can be said of critical pulmonary valve stenosis of the newborn. These patients present with cyanosis, a loud holosystolic murmur of tricuspid valve regurgitation, and cardiomegaly on chest radiograph (CXR). PGE_1 infusion is necessary to maintain patency of the ductus arteriosus to provide pulmonary blood flow. Modern-day treatment includes cardiac catheterization to determine the presence or absence of RV-dependent coronary circulation and to perform catheter-based perforation of the atretic pulmonary valve or guidewire manipulation through the critical valve narrowing, followed by balloon valvuloplasty. In approximately 50% of these neonates, additional pulmonary blood flow is required, which can be accomplished by a surgical aorticopulmonary shunt or stenting of the PDA (Figure 4). Ultimately, either a single or biventricular repair is performed, depending on the adequacy of the right-sided cardiac structures.

TRUNCUS ARTERIOSUS

This conotruncal abnormality consists of a VSD and one great artery arising from the heart and is classified into several subtypes based on the origin of the pulmonary arteries. Abnormalities of the truncal valve result in either severe stenosis or insufficiency. This defect is frequently associated with DiGeorge syndrome (22q11 deletion), and chromosomal analysis should be performed. Newborns present with cyanosis, and symptoms of CHF develop as PVR decreases. Medical management should include anticongestive medications. Surgical repair should be considered early to prevent the development of pulmonary vascular disease. Surgical correction involves patch closure of the VSD and placement of a valved homograft from the right ventricle to the pulmonary arteries. Follow-up is mandatory to evaluate the homograft integrity and truncal valve stenosis/insufficiency.

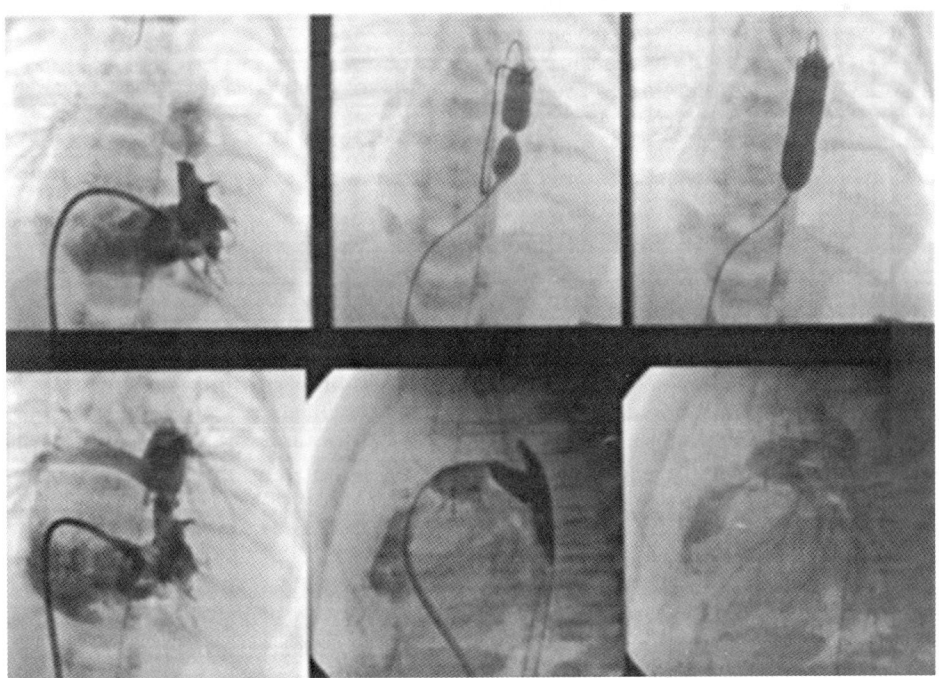

FIGURE 4. A right ventricle angiogram in a 1-day-old weighing 2.2 kg demonstrates critical pulmonary valve stenosis of the newborn. Successful balloon valvuloplasty was performed resulting in excellent antegrade flow through the valve. Failing to be weaned from prostaglandin E_1 infusion after 2 weeks, however, the neonate required stenting of the patent ductus arteriosus to provide additional pulmonary blood flow.

BOX 1 Improved Survival and Long-term Outcomes are the Result of Several Key Points

- Advances in fetal ultrasound provide earlier detection of congenital heart disease (CHD).
- A systematic approach and comprehensive knowledge of cardiac physiology facilitates the management of various forms of CHD.
- Earlier surgical repair and improvements in transcatheter interventions for infants and children with CHD.

TRICUSPID ATRESIA

Tricuspid atresia is defined as complete agenesis of the tricuspid valve without communication between the right atrium and right ventricle that is further categorized based on the relationship of the great arteries and presence of a VSD. Obligatory right-to-left shunting is required at the atrial level for survival. Infants typically present with cyanosis, but the clinical presentation, physiologic manifestations, and treatment depend on the relationship of the great arteries and the presence or absence of pulmonary atresia. Separation of systemic and pulmonary circulations is accomplished through staged surgical palliation, resulting in single-ventricle physiology.

TOTAL ANOMALOUS PULMONARY VENOUS RETURN

Total anomalous pulmonary venous return (TAPVR) is a rare form of CHD. Incomplete incorporation of the pulmonary veins into the left atrium results in abnormal communications between the pulmonary and systemic venous systems. The four types of TAPVR describe the location of the pulmonary venous connection to the systemic veins: supracardiac, cardiac, infracardiac, and mixed. It is further classified based on the presence or absence of obstruction. Newborns with obstruction present with severe cyanosis, respiratory distress, and rapid deterioration. This situation represents a surgical emergency, and immediate repair is required.

Single Ventricle

The single ventricle embodies an anatomically complex group of congenital heart diseases with one identifiable ventricle and another chamber, when present, representing the outlet chamber. This group includes the

CURRENT THERAPY

- Advances in surgical and transcatheter techniques to address complex forms of congenital heart disease (CHD) have led to improved survival.
- Long-term follow-up is mandatory in all forms of CHD to evaluate late complications.

single left ventricle, single right ventricle, and the so-called common ventricle with deficient ventricular septum. These defects present early in the newborn period with cyanosis or CHF. Separation of systemic and pulmonary circulations is accomplished through staged surgical palliation and eventual Fontan completion (Box 1).

REFERENCES

Cheatham JP: Pulmonary stenosis. *In* Garson A, Bricker JT, Fisher DJ, Neish SR (eds): The Science and Practice of Pediatric Cardiology. Baltimore, Williams & Wilkins, 1998, pp 1207-1256.

Hijazi ZM, Hakim F, Haweleh AA, et al: Catheter closure of perimembranous ventricular septal defects using the new Amplatzer membranous VSD occluder: Initial clinical experience. Catheter Cardiovasc Interv 2002;56(4):508-515.

Hoffman JIE: Congenital heart disease: Incidence and inheritance. Pediatr Clin North Am 1990;37(1):25-43.

Holzer R, Balzer D, Cao QL, Lock K, et al: Amplatzer muscular ventricular septal defect investigators. Device closure of muscular ventricular septal defects using the Amplatzer muscular ventricular septal defect occluder: Immediate and mid-term results of a U.S. registry. J Am Coll Cardiol 2004;43(7):1257-1263.

Knight DB: The treatment of patent ductus arteriosus in preterm infants. A review and overview of randomized trials. Semin Neonatol 2001;6(1):63-73.

Radzik D, Davignon A, van Doesburg N, Fournier A, et al: Predictive factors for spontaneous closure of atrial septal defects diagnosed in the first 3 months of life. J Am Coll Cardiol 1993;22(3):851-853.

Rao PS: Indications for balloon pulmonary valvuloplasty. Am Heart J 1988;116(6 Part 1):1661-1662.

Rao PS: Interventional pediatric cardiology: State of the art and future directions. Pediatr Cardiol 1998;19(1):107-124.

Wilkinson JL: Interventional pediatric cardiology: Device closures. Indian J Pediatr 2000;67(3 Suppl):S30-S36.

Hypertrophic Cardiomyopathy

Method of
Michael P. Frenneaux, MB, BS, MD, and Lynne K. Williams, MB, BCh

Hypertrophic cardiomyopathy (HCM) is diagnosed on the basis of left ventricular hypertrophy (LVH) for which there is no or insufficient explanation (e.g., mild hypertension or mild aortic stenosis with marked hypertrophy). This phenotypic definition encompasses a range of pathologic processes. In adolescents and adults, the disorder frequently exhibits autosomal dominant inheritance and is attributed to a mutation in a gene coding for sarcomere proteins. However, sporadic causes account for 50%. Occasionally, adults with unexplained LVH have other causes. In healthy young competitive athletes with mild LVH, the distinction from athlete's heart may be difficult. In infants and small children, the phenotype is usually attributed to inherited metabolic disorders and neuromuscular disorders.

Epidemiology

In the past, HCM was considered a rare disorder associated with a poor prognosis. Recent population screening studies suggest that it is actually very common (1:500 individuals).

Pathology

The hallmark of HCM is unexplained LVH, which may be marked. However, in some affected individuals, hypertrophy may be mild; indeed, wall thickness may be within normal limits. The hypertrophy is usually asymmetric (usually affecting the upper anterior interventricular septum). Occasionally the hypertrophy may be concentric, localized to the apex, or may involve the right ventricle. The histologic hallmark of the disease is the presence of marked and extensive myocyte disarray. Ultrastructurally there is disarray of the myofibrils. Small areas of myocyte disarray may be present in normal hearts and the disarray is patchy in HCM, making endomyocardial biopsy unhelpful in diagnosis. Thickening of the intramural microvessels and interstitial fibrosis are also seen.

Pathophysiology

The clinical features of HCM are generally attributed to the following:

- *Diastolic dysfunction*—This is the result of impairment of active relaxation and an increase in passive left ventricular stiffness (caused by hypertrophy and fibrosis). Abnormalities of diastolic filling impair the ability to increase stroke volume during exercise and cause an increase in left ventricular end-diastolic pressure (LVEDP) especially during exercise.
- *Obstruction*—Approximately 25% to 30% of patients demonstrate left ventricular outflow tract "obstruction." Anterior motion of the anterior (and occasionally posterior) mitral leaflet and chordae occurs, making contact with the septum and obstructing the narrowed outflow tract in mid-to-late systole. This is usually associated with mitral regurgitation. The magnitude of the pressure gradient may be highly variable and is influenced by inotropic status and central blood volume (a sudden increase in LV volume increases the degree of obstruction). Systolic anterior motion of the mitral valve is caused by "drag forces" associated with anterior displacement of the mitral valve apparatus, and/or to a Venturi effect. In a minority of patients, there is obstruction at midcavity level.
- *Myocardial ischemia*—This is the result of increased myocardial muscle mass, reduced trans-coronary perfusion gradient (a result of the increased LVEDP), and thickening of the coronary microvessels. Unfortunately, "standard" clinical measures of ischemia (electrocardiogram [ECG] changes during exercise and perfusion defects on nuclear scintigraphy) seem to correlate poorly with ischemia as documented by

changes in coronary sinus pH during rapid atrial pacing, suggesting that they may not be particularly helpful. The majority of patients with "typical" angina probably have underlying ischemia.
- *Vascular instability*—Approximately 33% patients demonstrate abnormal blood pressure responses during maximal upright exercise. In such patients, systolic blood pressure fails to increase or may even decrease with exercise. Although this may be attributed to a marked impairment in the cardiac output response to exercise, in the majority it is attributed to an exaggerated decrease in systemic vascular resistance believed to be the result of inappropriate firing of stretch-sensitive receptors in the left ventricle (LV mechanoreceptors). These patients often also exhibit impaired vasoconstriction or paradoxical vasodilator responses to orthostatic stress (e.g., application of lower-body negative pressure). Abnormal vascular control mechanisms also have a role in the genesis of presyncope and syncope in some patients.
- *Arrhythmias*—Supraventricular arrhythmias are frequent in HCM (approximately 30% of patients). Atrial enlargement is a predictor of the development of atrial fibrillation (AF), and is caused by obstruction, diastolic dysfunction, or mitral regurgitation. Nonsustained ventricular tachycardia is also common, occurring in 15% to 20% of adults. Although rarely asymptomatic, it is associated with an increased risk of sudden cardiac death and reflects "electrical instability" of the myocardium caused by myocyte disarray and fibrosis. Sustained monomorphic ventricular tachycardia is rare, and may be associated with apical left ventricular aneurysms.
- *Systolic dysfunction*—Classically, patients have a small ventricular cavity and often systolic cavity obliteration. Recent data derived from tagged MRI and tissue Doppler echocardiography has suggested that despite "supranormal" LVEF, myocardial contractile function may actually be impaired, and it has been suggested that the hypertrophy may be a compensatory phenomenon. Although LVEF is usually normal or supranormal, in a small subset (10% to 15%), progressive wall thinning and impairment of LVEF occurs ("end stage"/"burnt-out" HCM).

Genetics

SARCOMERE DISEASE

Approximately 50% to 60% of adults have been shown to have mutations in genes encoding for one of eight sarcomere proteins (Box 1). Mutations in a further three genes have also been suggested but not proved. It is believed that sarcomere gene mutations will ultimately be shown to be responsible for the vast majority of HCM. There is considerable interest in genotype-phenotype correlation. In some families with troponin T mutations, individuals have minimal hypertrophy but a high risk of sudden cardiac death. In many families with cardiac myosin binding protein C gene mutations, the development of LVH is delayed until middle age and beyond. However, genotype-phenotype correlations are not as clear-cut as initially suggested.

NON–SARCOMERE DISEASE

In infants and young children, LVH is often not associated with mutations of genes encoding sarcomere proteins. Some adults presenting with HCM also have alternate causes (Box 2). Recent reports suggest that a number of males presenting with HCM who are older than 40 years of age have Anderson-Fabry's disease. This X-linked disorder can be diagnosed in males by demonstrating reduced plasma activity of the enzyme α-galactosidase. In females, enzyme activity may be within the normal range and DNA analysis is necessary. Enzyme replacement therapy is available (although expensive). Pheochromocytoma may produce marked LVH. Amyloidosis may cause marked thickening of the left ventricular wall, and in the early stages ventricular function may be preserved. Highly competitive athletes may have LVH. This is rarely more than 15 mm in whites, but may be greater in Afro-Caribbean people.

Clinical Features

SYMPTOMS

Many patients are asymptomatic or minimally symptomatic. Major symptomatic limitation refractory to medical therapy occurs in a small proportion. Chest pains may be typical of exertional angina (often worse postprandially), atypical, or a combination of the two. Although many patients do not complain of breathlessness, almost all patients have reduced peak oxygen consumption, and some may experience marked limitation. Worsening breathlessness may be associated with the development of AF or a progressive impairment of left ventricular systolic function, which may be insidious. Presyncope and syncope may occur during exertion or at rest (Box 3).

CLINICAL EXAMINATION

The classical findings are described in Box 4. However, in many patients without obstruction, clinical examination may be normal.

INVESTIGATIONS (Box 5)

- ECG—In the majority of patients the ECG is abnormal, but the pattern is highly heterogeneous.
- *Echocardiogram*—Apical HCM may be difficult to visualize, and the use of contrast agents may aid diagnosis. Approximately 25% of patients have outflow tract pressure gradients that may be highly labile. The majority of these patients have associated mitral regurgitation. Diastolic dysfunction is demonstrated on the transmitral filling pattern and tissue Doppler long axis velocities. As in other diseases, the ratio of transmitral E wave to the long axis early diastolic tissue Doppler filling velocity (E′) has been shown to correlate well with LVEDP in patients with HCM. Recently it has become apparent that HCM can occur with normal left ventricular wall thickness, which can be problematic when undertaking clinical family screening. In this context, the presence of impaired long axis tissue Doppler systolic velocities, particularly if there are ECG abnormalities, makes the diagnosis probable.

Rakel and Bope: *Conn's Current Therapy 2006*.

BOX 4   Findings on Clinical Examination

Obstructive HCM

Arterial pulse	Jerky (rapid upstroke and downstroke)
Jugular venous pressure	Prominent α waves
	Increased pressure in patients with heart failure
Apical impulse	Sustained
	Double impulse (palpable atrial impulse)
	Triple impulse (late systolic impulse)
Ejection systolic murmur	Left sternal edge
	Radiates to axilla and up the sternum (not into the neck)
	Increase in intensity with standing, amyl nitrate, Valsalva maneuver (caused by reduction in LV cavity size)
Pansystolic murmur	Associated mitral regurgitation
	Radiates to axilla

Nonobstructive HCM

Normal examination

Abbreviations: HCM = hypertrophic cardiomyopathy.

BOX 5   Abnormalities on Investigation

Electrocardiogram

Atrial fibrillation
Left atrial enlargement
Repolarization abnormalities
Increased left ventricular voltages
Pathologic Q waves
Giant negative T waves
Preexcitation (short PR interval and delta wave)

Echocardiogram

Maximum wall thickness more than 15 mm
Normal (<13 mm) wall thickness (troponin T and cardiac myosin binding protein C mutations)
Small left ventricular size with normal left ventricular ejection fraction
Outflow tract pressure gradient (in 20% to 30% of patients)
Systolic anterior motion of the mitral valve
Mitral regurgitation (usually posteriorly directed)
Thickened mitral valve leaflets and chordae
Abnormal diastolic function (reversal of E/A ratio on transmitral filling, prolonged deceleration time)
Pseudonormal or restrictive transmitral filling pattern (if LVEDP is increased)

Ambulatory ECG monitoring

Supraventricular arrhythmias (atrial fibrillation/flutter)
Nonsustained ventricular tachycardia

Exercise testing

Abnormal BP response (less than 25 mm Hg increase in systolic BP, or an initial increase followed by a decrease)
Reduced peak oxygen consumption

Abbreviations: LVEDP = left ventricular end-diastolic pressure.

- *Cardiac MRI*—This may provide better delineation of the pattern and magnitude of hypertrophy in patients with poor echocardiographic windows.
- *Ambulatory ECG monitoring*—Forty-eight-hour ambulatory ECG monitoring forms part of routine risk factor stratification as short runs of nonsustained ventricular tachycardia confer an increased risk for sudden cardiac death.
- *Exercise testing*—Assessment of the blood pressure response during maximal upright exercise forms part of the routine risk factor stratification process, as an abnormal response (failure of systolic blood pressure to increase by at least 25 mmHg) predicts an increased risk of sudden cardiac death. ST segment changes developing during exercise seem to be poorly predictive of the presence of reversible myocardial ischemia. Metabolic exercise testing with measurement of respiratory gas exchange may be useful in documenting the extent of, and mechanism of, exercise limitation. Profound impairment of peak oxygen consumption combined with a severe and early lactic acidemia increase the possibility of an underlying mitochondrial myopathy.
- *Coronary angiography*—In patients with typical angina ages older than 40 years (or younger if a smoker), the presence of atheromatous coronary artery disease should be excluded.
- *Etiologic testing*—A thorough search for non–sarcomere disorders should be undertaken (see Box 2). Renal function should also be routinely assessed.

Rakel and Bope: *Conn's Current Therapy 2006*.

Natural History

- *Sudden cardiac death*—This event may be the first manifestation of the disease, and is less common than previously believed (annual incidence of less than 1% in large unselected series). Nevertheless, HCM is the most common etiologic cause in most series of sudden cardiac deaths occurring in young adults (including athletes). The challenge is to identify the minority at high risk and to reassure the majority at low risk. Several risk factors have been described which are associated with an increased risk of sudden cardiac death (Box 6). The positive predictive accuracy of each of these risk factors is low, but evidence suggests that they are additive in terms of risk. In one series, the annual incidence of sudden cardiac death was less than 1% in patients with one risk factor and 3.5% in those with two risk factors.
- *Progressive impairment of systolic function*—This occurs with an incidence of 1% per year.
- *Stroke*—Patients with AF (paroxysmal or established) have an increased risk of stroke.
- *Infective endocarditis*—The risk is low (approximately 4 cases per 1000 person years) and almost always in patients with "obstruction."

Clinical Management

The aims of clinical management are outlined in Box 7.

TREATMENT OF SYMPTOMS AND PREVENTION OF STROKE IN PATIENTS WITH ATRIAL FIBRILLATION

Patients With Obstruction

β-Blocker monotherapy should be initiated, and if unsuccessful disopyramide (Norpace)[1] may be added, initially at low dose and then up-titrated (contraindicated in patients taking amiodarone [Cordarone]). In refractory patients or in those with a contraindication to β-blockade, verapamil (Calan) may relieve symptoms. It should be initiated and up-titrated cautiously (symptoms can worsen in association with an increase in the magnitude of the obstruction in some cases). In drug-refractory highly symptomatic patients, septal myectomy produces excellent long-term symptomatic results in most patients. Recently, alcohol septal ablation has been shown to be an alternative. The technique reduces the degree of obstruction and improves symptoms, but should only be undertaken at this stage by expert centers. The procedural mortality and periprocedural complication rate (principally heart block) in expert centers is similar to that of surgery (less than 1%), but recovery is generally more rapid. There has been no randomized comparison of the longer-term benefits of the two therapies. Concerns have been raised that the infarct produced by the alcohol ablation technique may increase the risk of arrhythmias in the longer term and that progressive remodeling may increase the risk of systolic heart failure. Long-term

---
[1]Not FDA approved for this indication.

follow-up data are required to exclude these possibilities. Short atrioventricular delay dual-chamber pacing reduces gradients and may improve symptoms in some patients. Two large trials suggested that much of the symptomatic benefit was a placebo effect.

Patients Without Obstruction

Verapamil[1] or diltiazem (Cardizem) should be used first line and may be titrated up to high doses (480 mg of verapamil). In patients refractory to these therapies, β-blockers are sometimes helpful.

Patients With Systolic Impairment

Conventional heart failure therapy should be administered. Systolic impairment is progressive and some patients require cardiac transplantation.

Management of Atrial Fibrillation

Amiodarone (Cordarone)[1] is the most effective agent for reducing the occurrence of paroxysmal AF and for maintaining sinus rhythm after cardioversion in patients with new-onset AF. In patients with established AF, rate control can usually be achieved with verapamil or β-blockers. Occasionally, AV nodal ablation with permanent pacemaker implantation is required. Unless contraindicated, patients with established or paroxysmal AF should receive anticoagulation.

Pregnancy and Hypertrophic Cardiomyopathy

Serious complications (including death) are relatively rare during pregnancy/delivery. Symptoms may worsen, especially in those with marked symptoms before pregnancy. Epidural analgesia can theoretically increase

---
[1]Not FDA approved for this indication.

 CURRENT DIAGNOSIS

- Clinical features
- Family history
    Electrocardiogram—
        Rule out atrial fibrillation.
        LV voltage and repolarization abnormalities
    Echocardiogram—
        Maximum LV wall thickness greater than 15 mm
        Systolic anterior motion of the mitral valve
        Mitral regurgitation
        Diastolic dysfunction
- Forty-eight-hour ambulatory ECG monitoring
- Metabolic exercise testing and assessment of blood pressure response
- Etiologic testing
- Cardiac catheterization—if history of angina

CURRENT THERAPY

- Medical therapy
    - Nonobstructive HCM—
        - Verapamil
    - Obstructive HCM—
        - β-Blockers ± disopyramide
        - Verapamil if β-blockers contraindicated
        - Alcohol septal ablation/septal myectomy
        - (drug-refractory cases)
- Risk factor stratification
- Infective endocarditis prophylaxis
- Family screening/genetic counseling

obstruction via a reduction in systemic vascular resistance. Antibiotic prophylaxis should be administered to obstructive HCM patients undergoing instrumental delivery.

ASSESSMENT AND REDUCTION OF RISK OF SUDDEN CARDIAC DEATH

In high-risk patients (usually those with two risk factors, but in some cases only one risk factor), an automated implantable cardioverter defibrillator (AICD) should be considered. In those who have had a previous resuscitation from averted sudden cardiac death, AICD should be strongly considered. Nevertheless, the annual discharge rate in HCM patients with AICDs is low (11% in those with previously documented ventricular tachycardia/ventricular fibrillation and much lower in those implanted because of an adverse risk factor profile). The balance of risks of sudden cardiac death versus risks of lifelong AICD therapy (including serious infection) should be carefully considered and discussed with the patient. Some uncontrolled data suggest that amiodarone may reduce the risk of sudden cardiac death in high-risk patients, but this remains controversial.

PREVENTION OF INFECTIVE ENDOCARDITIS

Antibiotic prophylaxis should be administered for dental and surgical procedures in patients with obstructive HCM.

FAMILY/GENETIC COUNSELING

Although this area is controversial, given the emerging evidence that subjects at high versus low risk of sudden cardiac death can be differentiated and effective therapy (AICD) is available, screening should be offered after counseling about the potential insurance and employment implications of a positive diagnosis. Clinical ECG and echocardiographic screening of families can sometimes identify individuals with borderline LVH with or without ECG abnormalities. Unfortunately, genetic testing is not yet widely available, in large part because of the marked genetic heterogeneity of the disorder. In the past, clinical screening was discontinued in early adult life, but in pedigrees with a history of late presentation, it should be

continued until middle age. Counseling on the genetic implications of the disease and supportive counseling are important aspects of disease management.

REFERENCES

Elliott P, McKenna WJ: Hypertrophic cardiomyopathy. Lancet 2004; 363:1881-1891.
Frenneaux MP: Assessing the risk of sudden cardiac death in a patient with hypertrophic cardiomyopathy. Heart 2004;90: 570-575.
Hess OM, Sigwart U: New treatment strategies for hypertrophic obstructive cardiomyopathy alcohol ablation of the septum: The new gold standard? J Am Coll Cardiol 2004;44:2054-2055.
Maron BJ (ed): Diagnosis and Management of Hypertrophic Cardiomyopathy. Malden, MA, Blackwell Futura, 2004.
Maron BJ: Hypertrophic cardiomyopathy: A systematic review. JAMA 2002;287:1308-1320.
Maron BJ, McKenna WJ, Danielson GK, et al: American College of Cardiology/European Society of Cardiology clinical expert consensus document on hypertrophic cardiomyopathy. A report of the American College of Cardiology Foundation Task Force on Clinical Expert Consensus Documents and the European Society of Cardiology Committee for Practice Guidelines. J Am Coll Cardiol 2003;42:1687-1713.
Prasad K, Atherton J, Smith GC, et al: Echocardiographic pitfalls in the diagnosis of hypertrophic cardiomyopathy. Heart 1999; 82(Suppl 3): III8-III15.

5

Heart Failure

Method of
Marc A. Silver, MD

Heart failure is an epidemic in the United States. Every day, clinicians face the task of caring for more patients with heart failure in all its forms. Heart failure is the primary reason for hospitalization of Americans older than 65 years, and although 6 million Americans are estimated to have symptomatic heart failure, that number is expected to double over the next 7 years. Many millions more have asymptomatic left ventricular dysfunction or existing medical conditions that make it quite likely heart failure will develop and they will die.

It is truly in the hands of primary care physicians, who care for most heart failure patients, as well as those with common precursors of heart failure, to understand heart failure and its natural history better and thereby make an impact on this challenging epidemic. With this concept in mind, heart failure is discussed here from the perspective of understanding its natural history or stages, as well as a chronic disease process amenable to strategic planning.

Definitions

All clinicians define heart failure differently. Some choose to think about heart failure only when the patient has advanced disease characterized by significant volume overload and exercise limitation. Others consider heart failure to be present only when the left ventricle is dilated. Although broad by intent, *heart failure* is usually defined as a complex clinical syndrome that affects cardiac function (its ability to fill and/or eject blood) and is often preceded by and certainly accompanied by systemic neurohormonal abnormalities that participate in and perpetuate the dysfunction of the heart as well as other target organs, including the vasculature and muscles.

Although a wide range of signs and symptoms may accompany the heart failure syndrome of whatever cause, once symptomatic, patients usually have evidence of dyspnea, fatigue, and sodium and water retention manifested as congestion in the lungs, legs, and gut. It is useful, however, to think about heart failure not only as a symptomatic disease but also as a disease whose development begins decades before the patient crosses the threshold of clinical symptoms.

Classification and Stages of Heart Failure

Although many clinicians bristle at the concept of prescribed sets of recommendations or guidelines applied to a diverse disease process such as heart failure, these guidelines are frequently a place where available evidence is evaluated in a critical way and balanced with consensus to provide a distillation of what might work when caring for a patient with a disease process.

One of the well-accepted standard guidelines for heart failure recently was revised. Within the 2001 Revision of the American College of Cardiology/American Heart Association Guidelines for the Evaluation and Management of Chronic Heart Failure for the Adult (executive summary and full text available online at http://www.acc.org/clinical/guidelines/failure/hf_index.htm), aside from detailed information on the testing and therapies currently supported by evidence, appears a new classification for heart failure (Table 1).

The classification most clinicians are familiar with is that of the New York Heart Association (NYHA) (Box 1). The NYHA classification is generally applied to patients who at some point become symptomatic. Although they may revert to a symptom-free status (NYHA functional class I), it is still implied the patient has overt heart failure. Even though the NYHA classification is of great value and carries prognostic value, it also tends to allow us to think of a patient with mild or moderate symptoms (i.e., NYHA functional class II to III) as having a mild or moderate disease, but indeed, patients in this category have a markedly shortened life span and by definition less than optimal functional status.

The new classification (Box 2), in contrast, identifies four stages of heart failure based on the spectrum of common clinical syndromes from which they have evolved. By so doing, it is hoped the clinician recognizes the patient's increased risk for the clinical syndrome and then acts aggressively to reduce the risk and/or intervene earlier just as one would with a patient at risk for cancer.

The classification addresses four stages. Unlike the NYHA classification, in which a patient may easily pass back and forth through several functional classes over a period of days to weeks, as the patient passes through each stage of the new classification, there is no longer any hope of reverting to an earlier stage, which should act as an impetus to capture the patient at the earliest stage and prevent progression to the next stage by using the proper diagnostics and therapeutics.

Stage A refers to patients who by virtue of having other common clinical conditions are at increased risk of heart failure ultimately developing. These conditions include hypertension, diabetes mellitus, and coronary artery disease. Similarly, patients with a family history of heart failure have an increased risk. The heart failure syndrome clearly does not develop in all these patients, but acknowledging their at-risk status gives the clinician and the patient fair warning of the potential risk of development of heart failure and may serve as an early warning detection system for the insidious progression to more advanced heart failure.

TABLE 1 Common Heart Failure Drugs and Their Therapeutic Targets

Drug	Dose	Comment
Loop diuretics (expressed as furosemide [Lasix] equivalent units)	40-100 mg once or twice daily	Many factors affect the doses required, such as patient compliance with dietary restrictions, fluid intake, and associated titration of other medication, including ACE inhibitors and β-blockers.
ACE inhibitors (expressed as enalapril [Vasotec] equivalent units)	10-20 mg twice daily	Higher doses seem to have an impact on hospitalization rates. Be aware of adverse events that will limit use, including hyperkalemia. To allow adequate titration of β-blockers, reduced doses may be used.
β-Blockers (expressed as carvedilol [Coreg] equivalent units)	25-50 mg twice daily	Dependent on body size. Although data suggest clinical improvement and decreased mortality with smaller doses, the target remains full dose.
Digoxin	0.125-0.25 mg daily	Adjustment needed for renal function. Routine measurement of serum levels is not required unless done to confirm toxicity.

Abbreviation: ACE = angiotensin-converting enzyme.

Progression to the next stage is preventable, and disease progression is usually measured in years or decades.

Stage B refers to patients in whom structural and even functional abnormalities in heart function are already developed, but because of enormous cardiac reserve, the signs or symptoms that usually bring these patients to medical attention are not yet developed. This stage has also been referred to as "asymptomatic left ventricular dysfunction." Progression to the next stage may be slowed and again may be measured in years.

BOX 2 **Stages of Heart Failure**

Stage A
• Patients who are at increased risk for heart failure because of associated medical conditions (e.g., hypertension, coronary artery disease, or diabetes mellitus).
• Heart structure and function: Not yet affected.
• Potential therapies: Treatment of hypertension, smoking cessation, and weight loss; ACE inhibitors in appropriate patients.

Stage B
• Patients who have abnormal heart structure and/or function but who have not manifested signs or symptoms.
• Heart structure and function: Abnormal.
• Potential therapies: Same as for stage A, plus ACE inhibitors and β-blockers in all appropriate patients.

Stage C
• Patients with symptomatic heart failure. These patients indeed have advanced heart failure. Note that signs and symptoms develop as late phenomena after significant perturbation of many homeostatic mechanisms and the consumption of large cardiac reserves.
• Heart structure and function: Abnormal.
• Potential therapies: Same as for stages A and B, plus ACE inhibitors, β-blockers, and digoxin and diuretics in most patients; also, coronary revascularization and repair of mitral regurgitation in select patients.

Stage D
• Patients with extremely advanced heart failure.
• Heart structure and function: Extremely abnormal.
• Potential therapies: Same as for stages A, B, and C, plus consideration of advanced therapies including investigational therapies, consideration for left ventricular assist devices, heart transplantation for appropriate patients, as well as end-of-life counseling and hospice.

Abbreviation: ACE = angiotensin-converting enzyme.

Stage C represents most of what is called heart failure today: specifically, a patient who has structural and functional disease but who has now progressed and used up enough cardiac reserve actually to have signs and symptoms of the disease. By looking at heart failure in this perspective, it becomes clear that any symptomatic heart failure indeed represents a serious condition that the clinician must diagnose and treat accordingly. In this stage of the disease, clinicians can intervene to improve symptoms and quality of life, as well as improve, but not completely abolish, the increased mortality. Progression to the next stage is quite variable but is usually measured in months to years.

Stage D represents very advanced disease in which even standard measures cannot overcome its severity and advanced measures need to be undertaken. During this stage, despite best efforts, patients usually have increased use of resources, decreased quality of life, and progressive limitation. Although many advanced resources are applied during this stage, including heart transplantation and ventricular restraint and assist devices, generally these patients ultimately die of either progressive heart failure or sudden cardiac death.

Steps for Appropriate Heart Failure Management

Physicians often take a reflex approach to initiating drug therapy in a patient with symptomatic heart failure. For example, a patient who is volume overloaded might be treated with diuretics as monotherapy while overlooking the need not only to treat the current symptoms but also plan a strategy to limit progression of disease. Thus a useful approach in planning patient care involves two broad steps. The first is assessing the information needed to create a management plan, and the second is understanding the therapeutic targets in heart failure treatment.

An assessment of what is known or yet needed to be known to best make the diagnosis and treat a patient with heart failure is a very useful step. This assessment generally involves an understanding of the etiology of the heart failure, the current stage or functional class, and so forth. Even after a detailed history and physical examination and collection of some diagnostic data, however, a gap can remain in the information needed to complete the therapeutic plan. Generally, the clinician can group the areas that need to be completed into three main categories: diagnostics, therapeutics, and prognostics. In fact, these three areas are useful to consider each time a patient is seen in the office or hospital. Even though treatment is often initiated without complete information in each of these areas, not asking what other information is needed often leads to an incomplete understanding of the disease syndrome, as well as suboptimal therapy.

Diagnostics refers to any additional information that allows a better understanding of the etiology, status, degree of limitation, and signs and symptoms of a patient. For example, an echocardiogram allows assessment of the nature and degree of left ventricular function and may lead to consideration of myocardial ischemia (wall motion abnormalities) or valvular disease (valvular regurgitation or stenosis) as a therapeutic target. Often in this category are tests that might reveal an easily addressable cause of the heart failure and even a form of heart failure that is potentially reversible (such as hyperthyroidism).

Therapeutics refers to the design of the treatment strategy based on what is currently known about the patient and that patient's disease. It is also useful to write down a therapeutic plan, including the one or two next steps that might be taken should the patient's signs or symptoms not abate with the current regimen. For example, the clinician might begin with using angiotensin-converting enzyme (ACE) inhibitors but indicate that if the patient is found to have underlying coronary artery disease, the addition of long-acting nitrates should be considered.

Prognostics refers to focusing in on what is known about the patient's heart failure in terms of predicting what might be the path of progression in the near future. Although imperfect, many pieces of information are closely linked to survival and disease progression, including functional status, exercise tolerance, and left ventricular ejection fraction. In considering any additional prognostics, the clinician should always ask what might be done differently given the result. Over the years we have become more willing to intervene earlier with therapeutics, which can alter progression of the disease, and therefore we depend less on a bad set of prognostic markers to make these decisions. Nevertheless, awareness of a low peak oxygen consumption, a low right ventricular ejection fraction, or a markedly elevated neurohormonal marker often serves to alert the physician and the patient and family to review the current therapeutic plan and broaden considerations to include the next level of care and treatment, which might consist of investigational therapies and evaluation for heart transplantation. The role of measurement of B-type natriuretic peptide in this regard is of some interest and may prove to be a prognostic marker against which to target our therapies.

TREATMENT TARGETS

In designing the drug treatment plan, the following treatment targets for patients with heart failure should be considered: improved survival, improved symptoms, slowing and/or reversal of disease progression, improved functional status and quality of life, avoidance of troublesome adverse events, and decreased use of resources, including hospitalization. With the recognition that not all these targets are concordant or attainable, the drug regimen reflects these targets and our understanding of the ability of drugs to address them.

In general, patients with symptomatic heart failure are managed with a core group of four drug classes, including diuretics, an ACE inhibitor, a β-blocker, and, usually, digoxin. The former and the latter are generally applied to relieve symptoms or to improve functional status or exercise tolerance, whereas the middle

two are also administered with the specific intention of altering disease progression, reversing the structural and/or functional abnormalities of the heart and other target organs, and improving medium- and long-term survival.

Increasing evidence supports the initiation of ACE inhibitors and β-blocker jointly when caring for a symptomatic patient. Diuretics often need to be adjusted up or down, depending on a patient's level of compensation, as well as where they are in terms of other (β-blocker) titration. Target doses for most of the commonly used drugs come from clinical trials suggesting their benefit (ACE inhibitors) or from tradition, as well as from attempts to balance drug efficacy with drug safety (digoxin and diuretics). Target doses are listed in Table 1. Excellent details and practical considerations of implementing and titrating heart failure drugs can be found in recent guidelines (http://www.acc.org/clinical/guidelines/failure/ hf_index.htm).

NONPHARMACOLOGIC MEASURES

An enormous armamentarium outside routine drug therapy is available to clinicians caring for patients with heart failure. In general, most nonpharmacologic measures should be used in a simultaneous fashion with the initiation and titration of drug therapy. Although most of these therapies either have not or will not undergo rigorous clinical investigation, they nonetheless remain therapeutic cornerstones of complete heart failure care. Dramatic functional improvement can often be observed with more careful attention to nonpharmacologic therapies. Of particular interest is an understanding that sleep-disordered breathing (including obstructive and central forms of sleep apnea) may be present in nearly 40% of heart failure patients. Increasing evidence suggests therapy that includes continuous positive airway pressure may alter symptoms, disease progression, and even survival (Box 3). As far as dietary advice, generally admonitions for avoidance of excessive sodium intake and fluid are given along with specific information on lowering dietary saturated fat. Emerging information is that the patient with heart failure

---

BOX 3   Nonpharmacologic Therapies for Patients with Heart Failure

Definitely Helps Reduce Symptoms or Improve Functional Status
- Salt restriction (target: 2.3 g of salt per day)
- Exercise
- Stress reduction
- Screening for depression
- Smoking cessation
- Weight loss
- Treatment of documented sleep-disordered breathing

May Be of Use in Selected Patients
- Fluid restriction
- Avoidance of alcohol

---

suffers a significant energy imbalance, however, and may well benefit from nutritional assessment, including measurement of nitrogen balance.

Use of Disease Management and Other Resources

Perhaps one of the greatest tools at hand for clinicians caring for patients with heart failure, as well as for their families, is providing a thorough understanding of the heart failure syndrome and how self-empowered actions may have a significant impact on how they feel, what they can do, and how long they might live. Studies have repeatedly demonstrated the benefits of a structured disease management program in reducing symptoms, improving functional status, and, in particular, reducing heart failure hospitalizations. The clinician frequently can best serve the patient by fostering and supporting a heart failure disease management program. Although not present in all communities yet, the resources required (a physician and/or a nurse champion) are often accessible. Abundant educational patient-oriented books and materials are available to support these programs.

Disease management programs are often part of a larger specialized heart failure center. Within these structures are advanced strategies, including investigational therapies. It is incumbent on clinicians to be aware of these local and regional resources and refer patients when appropriate. Even with advanced disease, these centers can often offer improved outcomes and strategies not available to all clinicians.

Another area within the disease management spectrum is the home care programs that exist in most communities. These services frequently provide a link between intensive hospital-based care and infrequent, less intensive office-based care. In addition, for many patients with advanced disease, home care meets the constraints of patients and families.

For patients with advanced disease, physicians often begin discussions surrounding end-of-life issues too late. Patients who have advanced disease requiring frequent hospitalization and treatment generally are aware of their likelihood of death and, in fact, they value regaining some control of their lives through discussion of end-of-life planning and preferences. For some, hospice care is the choice made, whereas for others, referral to specialized centers and participation in emerging therapies through clinical trials might be the correct choice. Understanding comes only with an open and frank discussion with each patient and family.

Emerging and Emerged New Therapeutic Areas

Because of the intense interest in heart failure, a variety of important additional therapies are undergoing clinical investigation. These therapies include new application of biventricular pacemakers, aggressive mitral valve

CURRENT DIAGNOSIS

- Determine the etiology. It is critical to determine the underlying cause of a patient's heart failure; common clinical conditions including hypertension, diabetes mellitus, and coronary artery disease increase the risk of developing heart failure.
- Assess a patient's stage and functional class (see text). These are good guides to help recognize disease severity and guide treatment. Symptoms include evidence of dyspnea, fatigue, and sodium and water retention as congestion in the lungs, legs, and gut; these are usually late symptoms.
- Assess the volume status on every patient at every visit. Inability to assess volume carefully often leads to errors in therapeutics.
- Use additional tests and biomarkers such as peak oxygen consumption, ventricular ejection fraction, and elevated neurohormonal markers (B-type natriuretic peptide), which may provide early clues to disease severity.

repair for patients with ongoing mitral valve regurgitation, and the use of left ventricular assist devices as bridges to heart recovery, as well as destination or permanent therapies. Moreover, several new cardiac restraint devices are being applied with some success. Within years, genomic therapies will broaden, as will areas of vascular and myogenic regeneration. Again, although most clinicians are not aware of all these

CURRENT THERAPY

Targets
- Improved survival
- Improved symptoms
- Slowing and/or reversal of disease progression
- Improved functional status, quality of life
- Avoidance of adverse events
- Decreased use of resources including hospitalization

Care for Patients With Heart Failure
- Treatment of hypertension
- Smoking cessation
- Dietary counseling
- Exercise
- Weight loss
- Treatment of sleep-disordered breathing
- Angiotensin-converting enzyme (ACE) inhibitors (at target doses)
- β-Blockers (at target doses)
- Digoxin and diuretics
- Coronary revascularization
- Repair of mitral regurgitation
- Investigational therapies
- End-of life counseling and hospice

5

newly emerging therapies, they can offer their patients referrals to specialized centers where suitable therapies can be sought.

REFERENCES

Gattis WA, O'Connor CM, Gallup DS, et al: Predischarge initiation of carvedilol in patients hospitalized for decompensated heart failure: Results of the Initiation Management Predischarge: Process for Assessment of Carvedilol Therapy in Heart Failure (IMPACT_HF) trial. J Am Coll Cardiol 2004;43:1534-1541.

Hunt SA, Baker DW, Chin MH, et al: ACC/AHA guidelines for the evaluation and management of heart failure in the adult: A report of the American College of Cardiology/American Heart Association Task Force on Practice Guidelines (Committee to Revise the 1995 Guidelines for the Evaluation and Management of Heart Failure), 2001. American College of Cardiology Web site. Available online at http://www.acc.org/clinical/guidelines/failure/hf_index.htm

Konstam MA: Systolic and diastolic dysfunction in heart failure? Time for a new paradigm. J Card Fail 2003;9:1-3.

Pitt B, Remme W, Zannad F, et al: Eplerenone, a selective Aldosterone blocker in patients with left ventricular dysfunction after myocardial infarction. N Engl J Med 2003;348:1309-1321.

Poole-Wilson PA, Swedberg K, Cleland JG, et al: Comparison of carvedilol and metoprolol on clinical outcomes in patients with chronic heart failure in the Carvedilol or Metoprolol European Trial (COMET): Randomized controlled trial. Lancet 2003;362:7-13.

Redfield MM: Heart failure—an epidemic of uncertain proportions. N Engl J Med 2002;347:1442-1444.

Mitral Valve Prolapse

Method of
Richard B. Devereux, MD

The term mitral valve prolapse (MVP) describes displacement of the mitral leaflets in superior and posterior directions from their normal location during systole, in keeping with the dictionary definition of prolapse as "the slipping of a body part from its normal position in relation to other body parts." Mitral valvular function in MVP may range from mild leaflet displacement without regurgitation to marked leaflet "billowing" and severe regurgitation.

Pathogenesis and Etiology of Mitral Valve Prolapse

The mitral valve motion abnormalities that characterize MVP result from enlargement of the valve's connective tissue elements (leaflets, annulus, and chordae tendineae) relative to the supporting papillary muscles and left ventricular myocardium. Generalized enlargement, localized distortion, and abnormal distensibility of the valve are all documented in patients with MVP. Although MVP may be a secondary component of many conditions, these are uncommon. The best documented of these, the Marfan syndrome, accounts for

only approximately 1 of every 500 cases of MVP. In most instances, therefore, MVP is a primary condition. Its frequency (2% to 3% of the general population) makes it the most common heart-valve abnormality in the United States.

Although the precise cause of primary MVP remains undefined, most instances of MVP are inherited in an autosomal dominant mode, with linkage to several chromosomal regions without identification yet of the responsible genes. The MVP genes appear to be fully expressed in adult women younger than 50 years of age, with less consistent gene expression in adult men, older women, and children of both sexes. The genetic defects causing MVP are likely to involve as-yet-undefined components of connective tissue.

The pattern of abnormal mitral leaflet motion in patients with MVP causing significant valvular regurgitation is characterized by systolic billowing of mitral leaflets into the left atrium, whereas dynamic systolic expansion of the mitral annulus may cause posterior displacement of the leaflets in systole as well as systolic clicks and murmurs. Strong familial patterns of these forms of MVP suggest that they reflect separate genetic entities. Mitral valve enlargement and leaflet thickening, markers of increased risk of complications, occur in a subset of MVP patients with leaflet billowing. The disproportionate occurrence of complications or severe pathologic abnormalities in older subjects with MVP suggests an additional role of "wear and tear" superimposed on the underlying gene defects.

Diagnosis of Mitral Valve Prolapse

Because of the potential to induce anxiety about nonexistent heart disease or about the presence of a more serious condition if MVP is over- or underdiagnosed, respectively, the most important step in patient management is determining whether MVP is present.

The most useful auscultatory features of MVP are (a) midsystolic clicks that move earlier in systole with sitting, standing, or other interventions that reduce ventricular size or later with those that increase chamber size, such as squatting; and (b) late systolic murmurs in individuals too young to be at risk for mitral annular calcification or papillary muscle dysfunction. The clicks and murmurs caused by prolapsing mitral valves may be made louder by isometric handgrip exercise (clenching both fists), which raises arterial blood pressure and thus increases the intensity of left-sided heart auscultatory events. One must be attentive to the timing of auscultatory abnormalities because we have found widely split first-heart sounds and midsystolic, rather than late-systolic, murmurs to be present in a high proportion of patients with false-positive diagnoses of MVP. It is also noteworthy that auscultatory manifestations are highly variable in subjects with echocardiographic MVP, with both fluctuation among audible clicks, murmurs, and combinations thereof, as well as shifts back and forth between typical auscultatory findings and "silent" mitral prolapse. As a result, several examinations are needed to determine whether an individual intermittently has a murmur of mitral regurgitation, an important consideration in determining whether to recommend antibiotic prophylaxis.

Role of Echocardiography

Because of its ability to visualize the anatomy and function of the mitral valve, echocardiography is a nearly ideal method to detect and characterize MVP. MVP was initially diagnosed echocardiographically by M-mode recordings that showed late systolic posterior motion, by at least 2 mm, of continuous mitral leaflet interfaces behind the line connecting the valve's closure and opening points. Diagnosis of mitral prolapse by this criterion is reproducible, provided that tracings are of high technical quality, and is more sensitive for detection of MVP in patients with typical systolic clicks and murmurs than currently accepted two-dimensional (2D) echocardiographic criteria.

Two-dimensional echocardiography now plays a central role in recognition of MVP. MVP should be diagnosed by 2D echocardiography only when systolic billowing of mitral leaflets is demonstrated in parasternal or apical long-axis views. This is because the mitral annulus is not flat, but rather has a saddle shape. The mitral annulus is farthest from the left ventricular apex in its anterior and posterior portions, where the hinging points of the anterior and posterior mitral leaflets are seen in long-axis views, and is closest to the apex in its medial and lateral portions, where it is seen in the apical four-chamber view. Because of this, mitral leaflets that lie clearly on the left ventricular side of the mitral annulus during systole in long-axis views may appear to protrude artifactually into the left atrium in the apical four-chamber view. This artifact has been found in up to one third of normal adolescents.

Diagnosis of MVP in 2D long-axis views is highly specific but is somewhat insensitive, because it detects billowing into the left atrium of enlarged central scallops of the posterior and/or anterior mitral leaflet but yields negative results in individuals with auscultatory evidence of MVP in whom there is isolated anatomic deformity of the medial or lateral portion of the mitral leaflets. Correct recognition of such localized MVP requires expert echocardiographic interpretation.

Clinical Features of Mitral Valve Prolapse

Although MVP was first recognized by its auscultatory features and by abnormal mitral-valve motion revealed by angiography and echocardiography, reports soon appeared of a high prevalence of nonanginal chest pain, dyspnea, and anxiety-related symptoms in patients with MVP. The concept of an inclusive "MVP syndrome" has proved clinically useful because it provides an explanation for common, troublesome, and otherwise confusing cardiovascular and psychologic symptoms that is acceptable to patients and clinicians alike. However, controlled studies have documented similar prevalences of chest pain, dyspnea, and psychologic symptoms, as well as prolongation of the electrocardiographic Q-T interval among prolapse patients and cardiovascularly normal individuals evaluated in the same clinical or epidemiologic setting. MVP also appears to be no more common among patients with panic and anxiety disorders than control subjects when similar precautions are taken. Our own studies compared affected relatives (relatively unselected individuals with MVP) to unaffected relatives and spouses in more than 100 families of patients with MVP (who constitute genetically related and unrelated control groups). Affected relatives were more likely than control subjects to have thoracic bony abnormalities (pectus excavatum, scoliosis, and straight back syndrome), low body weight and systolic blood pressure, and palpitations. In contrast, we found no difference between MVP and control relatives in the prevalence of nonanginal chest pain, dyspnea, panic attacks, high levels of anxiety, or electrocardiographic repolarization abnormalities. We showed that MVP and panic attacks were associated with contrasting patterns of autonomic dysfunction. More MVP subjects than control subjects exhibited orthostatic hypotension and syncope, possibly related to reduced blood volume, whereas the group with panic attacks exhibited hyperreactive heart rate and blood pressure increases in response to orthostatic stress. Thus, MVP and panic disorders are biologically distinct as well as statistically unassociated.

Thus, controlled studies show a relatively narrow spectrum of clinical features associated with MVP. Even features truly associated with MVP, such as thoracic bony abnormalities, low body weight, or palpitations, are not sufficiently specific to be useful diagnostic features. Furthermore, we found that patients in whom nonspecific symptoms led to consideration of MVP are particularly likely to have false-positive diagnoses because of misattribution to MVP of panic attacks and midsystolic murmurs.

Complications of Mitral Valve Prolapse

Patients with MVP are at risk for infective endocarditis, mitral regurgitation, serious arrhythmias, and sudden death; a possible association with stroke has been suggested. MVP has been found more commonly among patients with these complications than expected from its prevalence of 2% to 3% in unselected populations. Among patients with severe mitral regurgitation in industrialized countries, from 38% to 64% have MVP as the underlying cause, whereas the proportion ranged from 11% to 29% among patients with infective endocarditis. The data for neurologic ischemic episodes have been quite variable, with MVP found in 2% to 35% of patients, leaving it uncertain whether this is a true association. Sudden death occurs with discernible frequency only among MVP patients with severe mitral regurgitation, although MVP also occurs in a

Rakel and Bope: *Conn's Current Therapy 2006.*

disproportionate number of the small minority of sudden-death patients who are free of obstructive coronary artery disease.

Identifying Mitral Valve Prolapse Patients At Risk of Complications

By comparing the characteristics of MVP patients with infective endocarditis and a control group of adults found to have MVP in our family studies, we were able to show that male gender, age (45 years of age or older), and a history of preexisting heart murmur were independently associated with infective endocarditis. Compared with an average incidence of 1 per 20,000 people per year in the general population, we estimated that infective endocarditis would occur each year in 1 of every 1920 MVP patients with a late or holosystolic murmur of mitral regurgitation versus 1 of every 21,950 without a mitral systolic murmur. Similar calculations would suggest annual incidences of infective endocarditis of 1 of every 3640 among affected men and 1 of every 2930 among individuals 45 years of age or older with MVP. The facts that major morbidity (death or need for valve replacement) occurred in one third of our MVP patients with endocarditis during short-term follow-up and that endocarditis appeared to be of dental origin in one third suggests that infective endocarditis as a complication of MVP is both dangerous and partially preventable.

In long-term follow-up studies, we found the risk of complications of MVP, principally mitral valve repair or replacement but also including infective endocarditis, heart failure, and sudden death, to be increased by male gender, by age (45 years of age or older), and most markedly by a holosystolic or nearly holosystolic murmur and left ventricular or left atrial dilatation. These findings result in overall rates of complications that ranged from well below 0.5% annually in MVP subjects with a midsystolic click and normal heart size to nearly 7% per year among MVP patients (principally men) with clinical and echocardiographic evidence of moderate or severe mitral regurgitation. Among all patients with MVP, it has been calculated that the lifetime risk of needing mitral valve replacement is approximately 4% to 5% among men and 1.5% among women. For sudden, presumably arrhythmic death, the estimated annual risk may be as high as 1 in 100 among MVP patients with important mitral regurgitation, but only 1 in 5000 or less in subjects with little or no mitral regurgitation.

Treatment

Appropriate care of an individual with MVP depends on accurate diagnosis of the valvular abnormality and on matching the intensiveness of evaluation and treatment to the level of risk.

INITIAL DIAGNOSIS AND SCREENING

Auscultation remains the most common method by which MVP is recognized. When both a midsystolic click and late systolic murmur are present and vary appropriately in timing and intensity with maneuvers, or a loud midsystolic click exhibits appropriate mobility, the diagnosis is definitive. If there are less specific auscultatory features, such as a soft or immobile midsystolic click or a late systolic murmur in a middle-aged (>45 years) or older individual, echocardiographic confirmation of MVP is desirable. Diagnosis of MVP by echocardiography is based on either unequivocal systolic billowing of one or both mitral leaflets across the mitral annulus in 2D long-axis views or on 2 mm or more late systolic posterior displacement of continuous mitral leaflet interfaces in high-quality 2D targeted M-mode recordings (which can have the advantage of visualizing the medial and lateral portions of the posterior mitral leaflet). Echocardiographic screening for MVP in unselected populations or symptomatic patients without typical auscultatory features is not cost effective because of its low yield and disproportionate identification of subjects at low risk. Echocardiography may, however, be useful as an objective means to expunge a dubious diagnosis of MVP and free a patient from unfounded concerns about heart disease and unwarranted treatment. Echocardiographic screening of adolescent and adult first-degree relatives of patients with unequivocal MVP is likely to be cost effective, because approximately 30% of such individuals also have MVP. MVP is too rare among children younger than 10 years of age to warrant screening.

MANAGEMENT OF UNCOMPLICATED MITRAL VALVE PROLAPSE

Management of the patient with MVP should be matched to the risks of infective endocarditis and progressive mitral regurgitation. Because these risks are related to the presence of at least mild mitral regurgitation, no specific treatment may be needed for subjects with MVP, particularly women younger than 45 years of age, who do not have a mitral systolic murmur on any of several examinations that include auscultation in multiple positions and with isometric handgrip exercise or evidence of more than trivial mitral regurgitation by Doppler echocardiography. We reassure such individuals that the outlook is benign and may even be enhanced if they have low body weight and blood pressure; antibiotic prophylaxis is not routinely recommended unless the individual wishes maximum protection against even the remotest risk. Re-evaluation by auscultation and echocardiogram is recommended at moderate intervals (perhaps every 5 years) to be certain the patient has not passed into a higher risk group.

On the basis of current evidence, patients with echocardiographic MVP who even intermittently or with simple maneuvers such as sitting or handgrip exercise have soft late systolic murmurs of mitral regurgitation appear to be at modestly increased risk of endocarditis or progressive mitral regurgitation. We recommend antibiotic prophylaxis to such patients, following the 1997 American Heart Association's recommendations of amoxicillin (Amoxil and other brands), 2 g orally 1 hour before dental procedures (Table 1). Clindamycin, 600 mg 1 hour before dental procedures, is recommended for patients allergic to penicillin. In view of suggestive evidence that elevated blood pressure may predispose to chordal rupture and progressive mitral regurgitation in patients with MVP, we recommend antihypertensive treatment for all MVP patients with mild mitral regurgitation with even very mild established systemic hypertension. Doppler echocardiography is an important adjunct to imaging techniques in defining precisely the extent of mitral regurgitation, and this evaluation as well as auscultatory examination is warranted at more frequent intervals (every 2 to 3 years) to assess possible progression of mitral regurgitation.

MITRAL VALVE PROLAPSE WITH HEMODYNAMICALLY IMPORTANT MITRAL REGURGITATION

MVP patients who have hemodynamically important mitral regurgitation are at greatest risk of endocarditis, sudden death, and need for mitral valve surgery. This group constitutes 2% to 4% of adults with MVP. Severe regurgitation is suggested on physical examination by a holosystolic or nearly holosystolic mitral regurgitant murmur, commonly accompanied by a left ventricular third heart sound and leftward displacement of a dynamic left ventricular impulse, and is confirmed by the demonstration of significant mitral regurgitation by Doppler color flow mapping and calculation of regurgitant volume in conjunction with imaging echocardiographic evidence of MVP and left heart chamber enlargement. Infective endocarditis prophylaxis is mandatory, with amoxicillin in the absence of a specific allergy, and it is theoretically attractive although not of proven value to treat even borderline systemic hypertension with antihypertensive drugs in such patients. Angiotensin-converting enzyme (ACE) inhibitors (e.g., ramipril [Altace] starting at 2.5 to 5.0 mg daily) or other agents that reduce peripheral resistance and enhance arterial compliance may be especially valuable in reducing stress in prolapsed mitral valve. Regular follow-up is required with annual imaging and Doppler echocardiograms and selected use of other methods such as nuclear angiograms and treadmill exercise tests being recommended. Corrective valvular surgery, by valve repair rather than by valve replacement in an increasing proportion of cases is recommended when patients either develop dyspnea of class II or greater New York Heart Association severity or when left ventricular systolic performance falls into the lower part of the normal range in the absence of symptoms. A simple partition value for recognition of the latter is an M-mode echocardiographic left ventricular fractional shortening of less than 31%, reported to predict a suboptimal outcome after mitral-valve surgery for severe mitral regurgitation. Frankly, subnormal ventricular performance should not preclude corrective valvular surgery, which may improve the poor survival associated with medical management of patients with severe mitral regurgitation and ventricular dysfunction.

TREATMENT OF ARRHYTHMIAS

Arrhythmias in MVP may require treatment to relieve symptoms or to reduce risk of sudden death. Palpitations and salvos of atrial premature complexes and brief bursts of atrial tachycardia are found slightly more commonly in subjects with MVP than in normal individuals. Suggested mechanisms of arrhythmogenesis include (a) stimulation of atrial pacemakers by the impact of prolapsing leaflets or mitral regurgitant jets and (b) origin of impulses from electrically active cells, shown to have β-adrenoceptors, in the mitral leaflets. However, many episodes of palpitation reflect forceful heart beating during sinus rhythm, and many episodes of atrial arrhythmia are asymptomatic. Awareness of palpitation in other prolapse subjects may coincide with simple ventricular premature complexes, but the prevalence of ventricular arrhythmias in controlled studies of MVP is not strikingly higher than in normal subjects.

In our experience, many cases of atrial arrhythmia and some instances of ventricular premature contractions will respond to treatment with β-blocking drugs (e.g., nadolol [Corgard] beginning at a dose of 40 mg daily).

TABLE 1 Endocarditis Prophylaxis: American Heart Association Recommendations for Dental, Oral, Respiratory Tract, or Esophageal Procedures*

Drug	Dose
Oral: Amoxicillin (Amoxil and other brands)	2.0 g (children 50 mg/kg) PO 1 h before procedure
Parenteral: ampicillin	2.0 g (children 50 mg/kg) IV or IM within 30 min of procedure
Penicillin-allergic patients:	
Oral: clindamycin (Cleocin)*	600 mg (children 20 mg/kg) PO 1 h before procedure
Parenteral: clindamycin (Cleocin)*	600 mg (children 20 mg/kg) IV within 30 min of procedure

*Further information concerning endocarditis prophylaxis for other procedures and additional alternative medications can be obtained at: http://www.americanheart.org
Abbreviations: IM = intramuscular injection; IV = intravenous; PO = orally.

Rakel and Bope: *Conn's Current Therapy 2006.*

However, periods of remission and of exacerbation of symptoms may continue to occur in these subjects, as often occurs in untreated subjects. Some patients with atrial arrhythmias may respond favorably to digitalization (digoxin [Lanoxin], 0.25 mg daily, or reduced doses in the presence of renal dysfunction) or to administration of verapamil (240 to 480 mg daily of long-acting Calan, Isoptin, or Verelan). Episodes of supraventricular tachycardia in MVP patients are usually because of reentry in the atrioventricular node. If episodes are recurrent and disruptive to the patient, we offer electrophysiologic study and potentially corrective ablation of the extra electrical pathway as a treatment option. Because of their frequent side effects and occasional proarrhythmic activity, we use type I agents (e.g., quinidine, procainamide [Pronestyl], flecainide [Tambocor], and amiodarone [Cordarone]) only when simpler regimens have failed in highly symptomatic subjects.

Whether and when to use antiarrhythmic drugs to prevent sudden death in patients with MVP remains controversial. Sudden death appears strongly concentrated in the 2% to 4% of patients with hemodynamically severe mitral regurgitation, but even in this high-risk group there is no evidence that antiarrhythmic drug treatment is beneficial. Individuals with MVP who experience sustained ventricular tachycardia or are resuscitated from near sudden death are best evaluated with electrophysiologic testing followed by use of medications shown to be protective or, more frequently, an implantable antitachycardia device. The occurrence of arrhythmic death among the large population of subjects with otherwise uncomplicated MVP is too rare for either potentially toxic antiarrhythmic agents or expensive antitachycardia devices to represent cost-effective management strategies.

TREATMENT OF NONSPECIFIC CARDIOVASCULAR SYMPTOMS

Management of the patient with MVP and symptoms other than palpitations or dyspnea related to mitral regurgitation may require varied approaches. Chest pain, palpitations, and dyspnea may occur concurrently with severe anxiety and other symptoms, including tremor, dizziness, and diaphoresis in repeated episodes termed panic attacks. If panic attacks occur spontaneously or in response to emotionally stressful situations such as elevators or crowded places, treatment directed toward either pharmacologic or behavioral therapy for panic disorder under the guidance of an experienced psychiatrist is often effective. Patients with these complaints generally do not respond well to standard cardiac medications. Meticulous attention to details of the clinical history is important, for in some anxiety-prone individuals the sudden onset of rapid palpitations because of paroxysmal atrial tachycardia or fibrillation may lead to other cardiovascular symptoms and secondary panic; this situation often responds well to appropriate medications (e.g., digoxin, β-blockers) and reassurance. Both panic disorders and repeated paroxysms of atrial arrhythmia may remit spontaneously or recur after a period of quiescence. Other chest pain syndromes with

 CURRENT DIAGNOSIS

Auscultation
Definitive
   Midsystolic click(s) alone or with late systolic murmur that move(s) earlier with sitting/standing and become(s) louder with handgrip.
Suggestive
   Midsystolic click that does not vary with maneuvers.
   Late systolic murmur alone.
Echocardiography
Definitive
   Leaflet billowing in long-axis (parasternal or apical views).
   Greater than 2 mm late systolic prolapse by two-dimensionally guided M-mode echocardiography.
Suggestive
   Marked late systolic billowing in other apical two-dimensional views.

features suggestive of angina, esophageal disorders, or a musculoskeletal origin should not be attributed to MVP but rather should lead to appropriate further evaluation and specific treatment if clinically indicated.

MANAGEMENT OF AUTONOMIC DYSFUNCTION

A variety of autonomic dysfunction syndromes may occur in patients diagnosed or considered to have MVP. The most common of these in our experience consists of recurring episodes ranging from dizziness through presyncope, requiring the individual to sit or lie down, to even frank syncope that occurs most commonly with variably prolonged standing or with exercise on a hot day. These episodic symptoms may be associated with physical fatigue and a sense of being emotionally drained but occur in the absence of evidence of generalized autonomic failure or specific metabolic defects. In such patients, orthostatic hypotension (>10 mm Hg fall in diastolic blood pressure) or tachycardia (>10 beats per minute increase in heart rate) are usually provoked by 5 minutes of quiet standing. Nausea, mild chest constriction, and bradycardia may precede actual syncope. Detailed investigation commonly reveals a deficit in blood volume, and most such patients respond favorably to dietary supplementation or addition of NaCl tablets (1 g, 1 to 4 tablets daily). Fludrocortisone acetate (Florinef), 0.05 to 0.1 mg daily, or clonidine hydrochloride (Catapres), 0.1 to 0.2 mg daily, may be added if necessary, with careful monitoring of blood pressure responses; individuals with features of neurocardiogenic syncope may benefit from treatment with atenolol (Tenormin), beginning at a dose of 25 mg daily. Orthostatic hypotension in women with MVP may also remit during the natural volume expansion that occurs during pregnancy.

Rakel and Bope: *Conn's Current Therapy 2006.*

CURRENT THERAPY

The following are guidelines for matching risk and management in mitral valve prolapse:

Lowest Risk

Subjects without mitral regurgitant murmurs or Doppler regurgitation, especially women younger than 45 years of age.

Management includes reassurance, no clear need for antibiotics, re-evaluation, and echocardiogram at moderate intervals (5 years).

Modest Risk

Subjects with intermittent or persistent mitral murmurs, mild Doppler regurgitation, and enlarged or thickened valves.

Management includes antibiotic prophylaxis (see doses in Table 1) with clindamycin or alternatives; treatment of even mild established hypertension; re-evaluation and echocardiography done more frequently (2 to 3 years).

High Risk

Patients with moderate or severe mitral regurgitation.

Management includes antibiotic prophylaxis with clindamycin or alternatives; optimization of afterload (arterial pressure); re-evaluation with Doppler echocardiogram and other tests if needed annually. Consider valve repair or replacement for exertional dyspnea, decline of left ventricular function into low-normal range, or detection of a flail mitral leaflet segment or a large regurgitant orifice (>40 mm^2) by Doppler echocardiogram.

A variety of other syndromes of autonomic dysfunction, characterized by evidence of sympathetic or parasympathetic overactivity, appear to occur with nearly equal frequency in individuals with and without MVP. Their evaluation commonly requires specialized testing, the results of which should guide therapy.

REFERENCES

Dajani AS, Taubert KA, Wilson W, et al: Prevention of bacterial endocarditis: Recommendations by the American Heart Association. JAMA 1997;277:1794-1801.

Devereux RB, Brown WT, Kramer-Fox R, et al: Inheritance of mitral valve prolapse. Effect of age and sex on gene expression. Ann Intern Med 1982;97:826-832.

Devereux RB, Jones EC, Roman MJ, et al: Prevalence and correlates of mitral valve prolapse in a population-based sample: The Strong Heart Study. Am J Med 2001;111:679-685.

Devereux RB, Kramer-Fox R, Brown WT, et al: Relation between clinical features of the "mitral prolapse syndrome" and echocardiographically documented mitral valve prolapse. J Am Coll Cardiol 1986;8:763-767.

Devereux RB, Kramer-Fox R, Shear MK, et al: Diagnosis and classification of severity of mitral valve prolapse: Methodologic, biologic, and prognostic considerations. Am Heart J 1987;113:1265-1280.

Disse S, Abergel E, Berrebi A, et al: Mapping of a first locus for autosomal dominant myxomatous mitral-valve prolapse to chromosome 16p11.2-p12.1. Am J Hum Genet 1999;65:1242-1251.

Enriquez-Sarano M, Avierinos JF, Messika-Zeitoun D, et al: Quantitative determinants of the outcome of asymptomatic mitral regurgitation. N Engl J Med 2005;352:928-929.

Frary CJ, Devereux RB, Kramer-Fox R, et al: Clinical and health-care cost consequences of infective endocarditis in mitral valve prolapse. Am J Cardiol 1994;73:263-267.

Gilon D, Duonanno FS, Joffe MM, et al: Lack of evidence of an association between mitral-valve prolapse and stroke in young patients. N Engl J Med 1999;341:8-13.

Grayburn PA, Berk MR, Spain MG, et al: Relation of echocardiographic morphology of the mitral apparatus to mitral regurgitation in mitral valve prolapse: Assessment by Doppler color flow imaging. Am Heart J 1990;119:1095-1102.

Levine RA, Stathogiannis E, Newell JB, et al: Reconsideration of echocardiographic standards for mitral valve prolapse: Lack of association between leaflet displacement isolated to the apical four chamber view and independent echocardiographic evidence of abnormality. J Am Coll Cardiol 1988;11:1010-1019.

Levine RA, Triulzi MO, Harrigan P, et al: The relationship of mitral anular shape to the diagnosis of mitral valve prolapse. Circulation 1987;75:756-767.

Weissman NJ, Pini R, Roman MJ, et al: In vivo mitral valve morphology and function in mitral valve prolapse. Am J Cardiol 1994;73:1080-1088.

Zuppiroli A, Mori F, Favilli S, et al: "Natural" histories of mitral valve prolapse: Influence of patient selection on event rates. Ital Heart J 2001;2:107-114.

Zuppiroli A, Rinaldi M, Kramer-Fox R, et al: Natural history of mitral valve prolapse. Am J Cardiol 1995;75:1028-1032.

Infective Endocarditis

Method of
Navin M. Amin, MD

Epidemiologic Changes

Infective endocarditis denotes microbial infection of the cardiac valves and, less frequently, infection of the mural endocardium or of septal defects. At present, infective endocarditis accounts for 1 case per 1000 hospital admissions. The age of patients with endocarditis has increased. In the preantibiotic era, the average age of patients with endocarditis was 32 to 39 years old; currently more than half the cases occur in patients older than 60 years of age. Men are affected twice as often as women; the ratio increases to 5:1 in men older than 60 years of age.

Three major epidemiologic changes are observed in endocarditis:

1. The pattern of infective organisms has changed. Early in the antibiotic era, group A *Streptococci* (β hemolyticus), *Pneumococci, Gonococci,* and *Meningococci* were the predominant pathogens. *Streptococcus viridans, Staphylococcus aureus* (methicillinsensitive [MSSA] or methicillin resistant [MRSA]), coagulase—negative *Staphylococcus epidermidis* or *lugdunensis*—and gram-negative organisms are more common today.

2. Certain signs and symptoms, once characteristic of endocarditis, are seen in less than 5% of cases today: peripheral lesions involving skin, nails, and eyes—petechiae, subungual hemorrhage, Janeway lesions, Osler nodes, or Roth's spots.

3. Surgical procedures can be both a cause and a cure of endocarditis. Prosthetic valves inserted to improve mechanically malfunctioning valves can predispose recipients to endocarditis. But surgery can be lifesaving in patients with refractory congestive heart failure (CHF) or resistant infections.

Forms of Endocarditis

Endocarditis is classified as acute or subacute on the basis of its clinical course. The acute form, which evolves over days to weeks, is diagnosed within 2 weeks. Invasive organisms such as *Staphylococcus aureus*, *Streptococcus pneumoniae*, group A streptococci, *Neisseria gonorrhoeae*, *Haemophilus influenzae*, *Salmonella,* other Enterobacteriaceae, and *Pseudomonas aeruginosa* are usually the cause. Clinically acute endocarditis is associated with high fever, systemic toxicity, and leukocytosis with rapid destruction of the valves. It carries high morbidity and mortality.

Subacute endocarditis has a duration of more than 6 weeks and an indolent course. The most common agents are streptococcal species, with *Streptococcus viridans* the most predominant: *Enterococcus,* HACEK *(Haemophilus, Actinobacillus, Cardiobacterium, Eikenella, Kingella)* organisms, fungi, and *Coxiella burnetii*. Clinically subacute endocarditis is associated with prolonged low-grade fever (fever of unknown origin [FUO]), night sweats, weight loss, and vague symptoms such as generalized weakness, lethargy, and myalgia.

Infective endocarditis can also be grouped into three categories:

1. *Native valve endocarditis* usually develops when there is structural damage to the heart valve. Rheumatic/syphilitic valvular disease is responsible in 20% to 40% of the cases. The mitral valve is involved in 85%, and the aortic valve is affected in 50% of the cases. In patients older than age 60 years, 30% of cases occur with degenerative cardiac lesions such as calcified mitral valve annulus and calcified nodular lesions secondary to atherosclerosis or post-myocardial infarction thrombus. Twenty percent of cases with mitral valve prolapse (with thickened leaflets or significant mitral regurgitation) and obstructive cardiomyopathy can predispose to endocarditis. In 6% to 25% of cases, congenital heart disease is a risk factor as is evident in ventricular septal defect (VSD), patent ductus arteriosus (PDA), tetralogy of Fallot, or coarctation of the aorta. It can also occur with a stenotic or regurgitant valve such as bicuspid aortic valve and pulmonary stenosis. Endocarditis is rare in patients with atrial septal defect (secundum type) because of the low-pressure gradient between the atria. Finally is a group of patients without any structural defect who are susceptible to endocarditis. Tricuspid valve endocarditis can develop in intravenous drug abusers and immunocompromised patients (with chronic renal failure, severe burns, chronic active hepatitis, collagen vascular disease, or neoplasm involving the pancreas, lung, or stomach).

2. *Prosthetic valve endocarditis* (PVE) at present constitutes 20% of all cases of endocarditis. It occurs in 2% to 4% of patients with a prosthetic valve. It can be early or late. Early PVE occurs within 60 days of the valve replacement, and predominant organisms are *Staphylococcus epidermidis* and *S. aureus* (MSSA or MRSA). In the case of late-onset endocarditis, which occurs after 2 months, *Streptococcus viridans* are the main offending pathogens.

3. *Nosocomial endocarditis* commonly affects patients older than age 60 years and serious ill hospitalized patients. These individuals are subjected to invasive procedures such as insertion of central venous pressure, monitoring lines, hyperalimentation catheters, or intracardiac pacemaker wires that represent nidus of infection. Box 1 summarizes the factors predisposing to endocarditis.

BOX 1   Factors Predisposing to Endocarditis

Native Valve Endocarditis
- Structural Damage
    Rheumatic valvular disease
    Syphilitic valvular disease
    Degenerative
        Calcified mitral/aortic valve
        Calcified post-MI thrombus
    Mitral valve prolapse
    IHSS
    Congenital heart disease
        Regurgitant or stenotic valve, bicuspid aortic valve, PS, Ebstein's anomaly, Marfan's syndrome
        High-pressure shunt, VSD, PDA, coarctation of the aorta, tetralogy of Fallot
- No Structural Damage
    IVDA
    Immunocompromised

Prosthetic Valve Endocarditis
- Early (<2 mo)
    Staphylococcus epidermidis
    Staphylococcus aureus
- Late (>2 mo)
    Staphylococcus viridans

Nosocomial Endocarditis
- Invasive procedures

Abbreviations: IHSS = idiopathic hypertrophic subaortic stenosis; IVDA = intravenous drug abuse; MI = myocardial infarction; PDA = patent ductus arteriosus; PS = pulmonary stenosis; VSD = ventricular septal defect. Adapted with permission from Amin NM: Infective endocarditis. Consultant 1994;34(3):319-343.

Microbiology

Any microorganism can cause endocarditis (Table 1). Certain pathogens have increased ability to adhere to valvular leaflets, thereby establishing infection. Approximately 70% of the cases are caused by streptococci and staphylococci.

Staphylococci (MSSA or MRSA) are encountered predominantly in intravenous drug abuse (IVDA), in early PVE, in an immunocompromised host, and in nosocomial endocarditis. *S. viridans* is more commonly seen in native valve endocarditis and in late PVE. Gram-negative bacilli commonly cause right-sided endocarditis as in IVDA and in patients with intravascular catheters.

Approximately 10% of patients with endocarditis have a negative blood culture after 48 to 72 hours of incubation. Factors that produce culture-negative endocarditis are (1) antibiotic therapy before cultures are obtained; (2) a low level of bacteremia (common with right-sided and mural endocarditis); (3) infection with fastidious or nutritionally deficient bacteria that require prolonged cultures (2 to 3 weeks) or additional supplements (e.g., pyridoxine) for growth; this group includes HACEK organisms, *Brucella*, and nutritionally deficient streptococci; (4) nonbacterial infectious agents such as fungi, viruses, spirochetes, *Rickettsia*, *Chlamydia*, or parasites; and (5) noninfectious causes: left atrial myxoma, Libman-Sacks endocarditis, systemic lupus erythematosus, Löffler's hypereosinophilic endocarditis, carcinoid syndromes, and marantic endocarditis associated with malignancies of the pancreas, stomach, or lung.

TABLE 1 Microbiology of Infective Endocarditis

Type of Infection	Specific Associated Risk Factors
Bacterial	
Gram Positive	
Streptococci (40%-60%)	
S. viridans, S. pneumoniae, S. bovis, S. pyogenes, S. sanguis	NVE, late-onset PVE
Enterococci (Group D) (5%-20%)	
S. faecalis, S. faecium, S. durans	Gastrointestinal malignancies
Staphylococci (17%-40%)	IVDA, early PVE
S. aureus, S. epidermidis, S. lugdunensis	
Diphtheroids	
Listeria	IVDA, early PVE
Gram Negative	
Cultured easily	
Pseudomonas aeruginosa, Serratia marcescens, Salmonella, Proteus mirabilis, Shigella, Providencia, Enterobacter, Neisseria gonorrhoeae, Escherichia coli	IVDA, immunocompromised, nosocomial endocarditis
Difficult to culture	
(HACEK) (1%-10%)	
Haemophilus, Actinobacillus, Cardiobacterium, Eikenella, Kingella	
(not HACEK)	
Brucella, Legionella	
Nonbacterial	
Fungi (2%-4%)	
Candida, Aspergillus, Histoplasma, Coccidioides, Blastomyces	IVDA, PVE, cardiac surgery, IV catheters, immunosuppressed
Viruses	
Coxsackie B, adenovirus	
Spirochetes	
Borrelia burgdorferi	Tick bite
Spirillum minus	Rat bite
Rickettsiae	
Coxiella burnetii	Infected livestock or unpasteurized milk
Chlamydia	
C. psittaci	Infected birds
Parasites	
Trypanosoma cruzi (Chagas' disease)	Kissing bug bite

Abbreviations: IVDA, intravenous drug abuse; NVE, native valve endocarditis; PVE, prosthetic valve endocarditis.
Modified from Amin NM: Infective endocarditis. Consultant 1994;34(3):319-343.

Clinical Manifestations

The clinical manifestations of infective endocarditis are extremely diverse and can mimic pulmonary, neurologic, renal, or bone and joint disease. The classic manifestations of fever, heart murmur, splenomegaly, and petechiae of the skin and the mucous membranes help establish the diagnosis.

The onset may be abrupt or insidious. The early manifestations may be vague flulike symptoms that occur within 3 weeks after an invasive procedure. The patient may complain of malaise, fatigue, weakness, myalgia, arthralgia, low-grade fever, night sweats, or weight loss. Anorexia is almost universal. When the onset is acute, as in intravenous (IV) drug abuse, PVE, or nosocomial endocarditis, there may be evidence of severe infection heralded by high fever (90% to 95%), shaking chills and rigors, or, more ominous, symptoms of frank heart failure or embolic phenomena.

In patients older than age 60 years, diagnosis is often delayed because 5% may not have fever or are admitted with diagnosis of cerebral vascular accident (CVA), pneumonia, occult neoplasm, degenerative joint disease, or osteomyelitis. Infective endocarditis should always be considered in patients older than age 60 years who have fever and associated unexplained CHF, CVA, renal failure, weight loss, anemia, new-onset murmur, or confusional state.

In 85% of the cases, cardiac manifestations include a heart murmur. In right-sided endocarditis and mural infection, murmur is absent. A new or changing murmur (usually of aortic regurgitation) occurs in 5% to 10% of patients and is a very helpful diagnostic sign. Persistent or progressive CHF is indicative of a serious complication that carries a high mortality rate.

Peripheral cutaneous manifestations take a variety of forms: skin pallor caused by secondary anemia; petechiae found in 20% to 40% of cases concentrated on the conjunctiva, palate, buccal mucosa, and distal extremities; clubbing of nails in 10% to 20% if infection is long-standing; splinter hemorrhages as linear red-to-brown streaks in the middle of the nail bed of fingers and toes; Osler nodes (5% to 20% cases), which are small painful, tender, purplish subcutaneous nodules in the pads of fingers and toes; and Janeway lesions, which are small macular, painless, erythematous or hemorrhagic plaques on the palms or soles.

Ocular manifestations include Roth's spots, which occur in 5% of the patients and appear as oval or boat-shaped white or pale retinal lesions surrounded by hemorrhage and located near the optic disk. In a few cases there may be presence of cotton-wool exudates, petechiae, or flame-shaped hemorrhages.

Embolization can occur in 15% to 35% of cases. A cerebral emboli may produce hemiplegia, monoplegia, aphasia, or unilateral blindness. Mesenteric emboli can result in acute abdominal pain, ileus, or melena. Splenic emboli may cause left upper quadrant pain that radiates to the left shoulder of the chest with a small pleural effusion or splenic frictional rub. Flank pain with hematuria indicates a renal infarction. Peripheral arterial emboli may produce pain or gangrene. Large arterial occlusions are frequently seen with fungal endocarditis. Very rarely, emboli to coronary arteries cause acute myocardial infarction, myocardial abscess, or mycotic aneurysm.

Neurologic complications (30% to 40%) include CVA from embolization, mycotic aneurysm causing cerebral of subdural hemorrhage and seizure, and brain abscess or toxic encephalopathy with confusion and nonspecific obtundation.

Renal manifestations are accompanied by microscopic or frank hematuria secondary to renal infarct, diffuse membranoproliferative glomerulonephritis, focal embolic glomerulonephritis, or renal abscess.

Splenomegaly occurs in 25% to 45% of the patients and is more common in subacute than in acute endocarditis.

Diagnosis

Infective endocarditis may mimic any systemic disorder. For this reason and because of its high morbidity and mortality, the diagnosis should be kept in mind whenever a high-risk patient has an unexplained fever, constitutional symptoms, or multiple systemic involvement with a changing or new heart murmur. A high index of suspicion for endocarditis in certain clinical situations is very helpful:

- Intravenous drug abusers with high fever
- Patients older than age 60 years with nonspecific vague symptoms with a calcified mitral valve annulus
- Unknown source of embolization
- Certain virulent infections caused by organisms such as *Staphylococcus* or *Enterococcus*

A thorough history, complete examination, and laboratory tests should establish the correct diagnosis. Box 2 outlines the various laboratory abnormalities in infective endocarditis.

A baseline electrocardiogram (ECG) is helpful to detect chamber enlargement or possible conduction defect that may indicate underlying valvular or congenital anomalies. Later development of first-degree atrioventricular (AV) block, new bundle branch block, or new ectopic beats may indicate a myocardial abscess, especially in aortic valve endocarditis.

Echocardiography (transesophageal [TEE], M mode, two-dimensional, or Doppler) can confirm the diagnosis, detect complications, and help assess the prognosis. The echocardiogram can detect vegetations larger than 2 to 3 mm on mitral or aortic valves. Sensitivity in detecting vegetations is approximately 87% to 90% with TEE, 30% to 75% with M-mode, 40% to 50% with two-dimensional, and 50% with Doppler echocardiography. False-positive results are seen with old healed vegetations, myxomatous valvular degeneration, arterial myxoma, or a thrombus.

Echocardiogram can detect complications such as torn or perforated valves, ruptured chordae tendineae, myocardial abscess, or pericardiac effusion that may require surgical intervention. Large-sized vegetations

BOX 2 Laboratory Abnormalities in Endocarditis

- Hematologic
  - Leukocytosis
  - Anemia of chronic disorder
  - Thrombocytopenia (10% SBE)
  - Elevated ESR
- Urinalysis
  - Hematuria, microscopic
  - Proteinuria
- Cardiac abnormality
  - ECG: chamber enlargement, conduction defect
- Chest radiograph
  - Cardiomegaly
  - Evidence of congestive heart failure
  - Nodular infiltrate (staphylococcal endocarditis)
- Diagnostic gold standards
  - Echocardiography (transesophageal [TEE] preferred)
  - Three sets of blood (embolus) cultures
- Immunologic abnormalities
  - Rheumatoid factor (disappears after treatment)
  - Hypergammaglobulinemia
  - Cryoglobulinemia
  - Circulating immune complexes
  - Low complement levels

Abbreviations: ECG = electrocardiogram; ESR = erythrocyte sedimentation rate; SBE = subacute bacterial endocarditis.

in the left side of the heart or in the aortic valve, or myocardial abscess, suggest a relatively poor prognosis, and surgery may be indicated.

Serial blood cultures are required to establish the diagnosis by isolating the offending bacterium or fungus. A minimum of three blood samples should be drawn 30 to 60 minutes apart before initiating empiric antibiotic therapy. If the patient has taken antibiotics in the preceding 2 weeks, two or three additional sets of blood cultures should be taken. Cultures of arterial blood offer no additional advantage over venous blood. Ninety percent of the blood cultures become positive within 7 days of incubation. Negative blood cultures are likely seen in patients who have received prior antibiotics or who have endocarditis caused by fastidious gram-negative (HACEK) bacilli, fungi, or nutritionally deficient streptococci. The microbiology laboratory should be alerted to the suspected endocarditis, and a report for prolonged incubation for 2 weeks included.

In fungal endocarditis, in which there is embolization of large arteries, a culture of the removed embolus can establish the diagnosis. Serologic studies can be helpful in fungal infection (histoplasmosis or coccidioidomycosis) or when rickettsial (Q fever) *Legionella* or *Chlamydia* infections are suspected.

Treatment of Infective Endocarditis

The main goal is eradicating the infecting pathogens as quickly as possible to reduce the risks of morbidity and mortality. This can be achieved with antibiotic therapy, surgical intervention, or both.

Rakel and Bope: *Conn's Current Therapy 2006.*

ANTIBIOTIC THERAPY

In using antibiotics to treat infective endocarditis, the following guidelines are helpful:

- Parental antibiotics are used to sustain bactericidal activity.
- Bactericidal antimicrobials are used for complete eradication of the pathogens. Synergistic bactericidal activity is achieved with combination therapy such as ampicillin and aminoglycosides in treatment of enterococcal endocarditis.
- The drug regimen and appropriate duration of course, 2 to 6 weeks, must be tailored to prevent relapse.
- The bactericidal activity of the antibiotic is monitored by determining the minimum inhibitory concentration (MIC) and the minimum bactericidal concentration (MBC) against the infecting organisms.
- Antibiotic therapy is initiated as quickly as possible. When endocarditis is severe and/or complicated, empiric treatment should be instituted immediately with antibiotics effective against *S. aureus* and enterococci. A combination of vancomycin (Vancocin) and gentamicin (Garamycin) is recommended. Once a specific organism is identified, appropriate bactericidal antibiotics should be used.

Most streptococci other than enterococci are exquisitely sensitive to penicillin. If MIC is less than 0.2 μg per mL, high-dose penicillin alone or in combination with either gentamicin (Garamycin) or streptomycin or ceftriaxone (Rocephin) can be used for 4 weeks. If the MIC is below 0.1 μg per mL, treatment should be for 2 weeks. If MIC is greater than 0.2 μg per mL or the MBC to MIC ratio exceeds 10:1, as it occurs in 15% to 20% of cases with *S. viridans* infection, higher dose of penicillin with aminoglycoside should be used. In penicillin-allergic patients, vancomycin is the best alternative with or without aminoglycoside (Table 2).

In enterococcal endocarditis, ampicillin is recommended in combination with an aminoglycoside. Gentamicin is preferred because 40% of the isolates are resistant to streptomycin. In penicillin-allergic patients, vancomycin with an aminoglycoside is the best choice.

In *S. aureus* infection, semisynthetic penicillin or first-generation cephalosporins are the agents of first choice. Addition of gentamicin or rifampin (Rifadin)[1] during the first few days rapidly reduces bacteremia. Vancomycin is recommended for patients allergic to penicillin or if the organism is methicillin resistant (MRSA). Addition of rifampin, although controversial, is recommended in patients demonstrating poor bactericidal activity during therapy with beta-lactams or vancomycin and for patients with suppurative complication, such as a valve ring abscess.

Endocarditis with *S. epidermidis*, which commonly develops on prosthetic valves, is ideally treated with vancomycin and rifampin.[1] An aminoglycoside may be added for 2 weeks.

[1]Not FDA approved for this indication.

5

TABLE 2 Antibiotic Regimens for Bacterial Endocarditis

Infecting Organism	Antibiotic	Dosage, Route, and Frequency	Duration in Weeks
Penicillin susceptible *Streptococcus viridans, and S. bovis* (MIC <0.2 µg/dL	*Preferred Regimen* Penicillin G	12-16 million U/d IV in 6 divided doses	4
	or Penicillin G	12-16 million U/d IV in 6 divided doses	4
	PLUS Gentamicin	1 mg/kg IM or IV q8h	2
	or Penicillin G	Dosages same as above regimen	2
	PLUS Gentamicin		
	or Ceftriaxone	2g IV or IM q24h	4
	Alternative Regimen Vancomycin	0.5 g IV q6h	4
Relative penicillin-resistant streptococci (MIC >0.2 µg/dL)	*Preferred Regimen* Penicillin G	20-30 million U/d IV in 6 divided doses	4
	PLUS Gentamicin	1 mg/kg IV or IM q8h	4
	Alternative Regimen Vancomycin	0.5 g IV q6h	4
Staphylococcus epidermidis	*Native Valve* Vancomycin	0.5 g IV q6h	4
	Prosthetic Valve Vancomycin	0.5 g IV q6h	4-6
	PLUS Gentamicin	1 mg/kg IV or IM q8h	2
	or Rifampin	300 mg PO/IV q12h	2
Enterococcus (S. faecalis, S. faecium, S. durans)	*Preferred Regimen* Penicillin G	20-30 million U/d IV in 6 divided doses	4-6
	PLUS Gentamicin	1 mg/kg IM or IV q8h	4-6
	or Ampicillin	2g IV q4h	4-6
	PLUS Gentamicin	1mg/kg IM or IV q8h	4-6
	Alternative Regimen Vancomycin	0.5 g IV q6h	4-6
	PLUS Gentamicin	1 mg/kg IM or IV q8h	4-6
Staphylococcus aureus (methicillin sensitive)	*Preferred Regimen* Nafcillin or Oxacillin	2 g IV q4h	4-6
	or Oxacillin	2 g IV q4h	4-6
	PLUS Gentamicin	1 mg/kg IM or IV q8h	2
	or plus Rifampin	300 mg PO/IV q12h	2
	Alternative Regimen Cefazolin	2 g IV q6h	4-6
	or Vancomycin	0.5 g IV q6h	
S. aureus (methicillin resistant [MRSA])	Vancomycin	0.5 g IV q6h	4-6
	PLUS Gentamicin	1 mg/kg IM or IV q8h	2
	OR/PLUS		

Continued

Rakel and Bope: *Conn's Current Therapy 2006.*

TABLE 2 Antibiotic Regimens for Bacterial Endocarditis—cont'd

Infecting Organism	Antibiotic	Dosage, Route, and Frequency	Duration in Weeks
HACEK group *(Haemophilus, Actinobacillus, Cardiobacterium, Eikenella, Kingella)*	Rifampin[1]	300 mg PO/IV q12h	2
	Ampicillin or	2 g IV q6h	4
	Ampicillin PLUS	2 g IV q6h	4
	Gentamicin or	1 mg/kg IM or IV q8h	4
	Ceftriaxone	2 g IV q24h	4
Culture negative	Vancomycin PLUS	0.5 g IV q8h	6
	Gentamicin	1 mg/kg IM or IV q8h	6

Abbreviations: MIC = minimum inhibitory concentration
Modified from Amin NM: Infective Endocarditis. Consultant 1994;34(3):319-343.
[1]Not FDA approved for this indication

TABLE 3 Preprocedural Antibiotic Prophylaxis for At-Risk Patients

Type of Procedure and Situation	Antibiotic	Dosage, Route, and Frequency
Dental, oral respiratory tract, and esophageal procedures		
Standard prophylaxis	Amoxicillin	2 g PO 1 h before procedure
Patient unable to take oral medication	Ampicillin	2 g IM/IV within 30 min before procedure
Patient allergic to penicillin	Clindamycin (Cleocin*) or	600 mg PO 1 h before procedure
	cefadroxil (Duricef*) or	2 g PO 1 h before procedure
	cephalexin (Keflex*) or	2 g PO 1 h before procedure
	azithromycin (Zithromax*) or	500 mg PO 1 h before procedure
	clarithromycin (Biaxin*)	500 mg PO 1 h before procedure
Patient allergic to penicillin and unable to take oral medication	Clindamycin (Cleocin*) or	600 g IV within 30 min of starting procedure
	cefazolin (Ancef) or	1 g IV within 30 min of starting procedure
	vancomycin (Vancocin)	1 g IV over 1-2 h within 60 min of starting procedure
Genitourinary/gastrointestinal procedures		
Moderate-risk patient	Amoxicillin or	2 g PO 1 h before procedure
	ampicillin	2 g IM/IV within 30 min of starting procedure
Moderate-risk penicillin-allergic patient	Vancomycin	1 g IV over 1-2 h infusion completed within 30-60 min of starting procedure
High-risk patient	Ampicillin PLUS	2 g IM/IV given within 30 min of starting procedure
	gentamicin *6 h later*	1.5 mg/kg IV given within 30 min of starting procedure
	Ampicillin or	1 g IM or IV
	amoxicillin	1 g PO
High-risk penicillin-allergic patients	Vancomycin PLUS	1 g IV over 1-2 h
	gentamicin	1.5 mg/kg IV given within 30 min of starting procedure

Modified from Dajani AS, Taubert KA, Wilson W, et al: Prevention of bacterial endocarditis: Recommendation by the American Heart Association. JAMA 1997;277(22):1794-1801.
*Not FDA approved for this indication

TABLE 4 Indications for Endocardial Prophylaxis

Cardiac Conditions	Procedures
High-risk category Prosthetic valve Previous endocarditis Complex cyanotic disease Tetralogy of Fallot, single ventricle Surgically conducted systemic-pulmonary shunt	**Dental** Dental extraction Periodontal procedures: surgery, scaling, root planing Dental implant replacement Subgingival placement of antibiotic fibers Intraligamentary local anesthetic injection Cleaning of teeth or implants
	Respiratory Tonsillectomy/adenoidectomy Rigid bronchoscopy
Moderate-risk category Congenital heart disease: VSD, PDA, AS, PS Acquired valvular dysfunction Rheumatic/syphilitic Hypertrophic cardiomyopathy MVP with MR or thickened leaflets	
	Gastrointestinal Sclerotherapy Esophageal stricture dilation ERCP with biliary obstruction Biliary tract surgery Surgery involving intestinal mucosa
	Genitourinary Prostatic surgery Cystoscopy Urethral dilation Septic abortion

Abbreviations: AS = aortic stenosis; ERCP = endoscopic retrograde cholangiopancreatography; MVP = mitral valve prolapse; MR = mitral regurgitation; PDA = patent ductus arteriosus; PS = pulmonary stenosis; VSD = ventricular septal defect.
Modified from Dajani AS, Taubert KA, Wilson W, et al: Prevention of bacterial endocarditis: Recommendations by the American Heart Association. JAMA 1997;277(22):1794-1801.

TABLE 5 Endocardial Prophylaxis Not Recommended

Cardiac Conditions	Procedures
Isolated secundum ASD Surgical repair of ASD, VSD, PDA (without residue > 6 mo) Previous CABG surgery MVP without valvular dysfunction Functional murmur Kawasaki disease without valvular dysfunction Previous rheumatic fever without valve dysfunction Cardiac pacemaker and implanted defibrillators Cardiac catheterization, balloon angioplasty Coronary stent placement	**Dental** Restorative dentistry Local anesthetic injections Intracanal treatment Postoperative suture removal Oral impression/radiograph Fluoride treatment Shedding of primary teeth
	Respiratory Endotracheal intubation Fiberoptic bronchoscopy Tympanostomy tube insertion
	Gastrointestinal TEE* Endoscopy with/without biopsy*
	Genitourinary Vaginal delivery/hysterectomy* Cesarean section Urethral catheterization Uterine dilation and curettage Insertion/removal of IUD Circumcision

*Prophylaxis optional for high-risk category.
Abbreviations: ASD = atrial septal defect; CABG = coronary artery bypass graft; IUD = intrauterine device; MVP = mitral valve prolapse; PDA = patent ductus arteriosus; TEE = transesophageal echocardiogram; VSD = ventricular septal defect.
Modified from Dajani AS, Taubert KA, Wilson W, et al: Prevention of bacterial endocarditis: Recommendations by the American Heart Association. JAMA 1997;277(22):1794-1801.

Gram-negative infections causing high mortality are best treated with broad-spectrum penicillin or, preferably, a third-generation cephalosporin with an aminoglycoside. In most of these patients, valve replacement is necessary.

SURGICAL INTERVENTIONS

Approximately 25% of patients with severe or complicated endocarditis undergo surgery. The chief indications for surgery are refractory moderate or severe CHF; perivalvular invasion or myocardial abscess as evident by persistent fever despite antibiotics or electrocardiographic changes of conduction defects; systemic or arterial embolization; fungal endocarditis; PVE of early onset; large bulky vegetations that increase risk of CHF; persistent infection (particularly with gram-negative bacilli) that does not respond to 7 to 10 days of antibiotic therapy; and staphylococcal endocarditis in IV drug abusers that does not respond to antimicrobials.

PREVENTION OF BACTERIAL ENDOCARDITIS

Transient bacteremia that develops after a variety of manipulations or surgical procedures in patients with structural heart defects causes endocarditis. Prophylactic antibiotics in this situation can be highly effective when given before the procedure. Administration of these agents only once is required 30 minutes to 2 hours before the procedure (Table 3).

In choosing prophylactic therapy, the following questions (Table 4) are useful:

- Is the patient at increased risk for endocarditis with underlying structural defect?
- Is there a high risk the procedure will produce bacteremia with organisms that cause endocarditis, such as *S. viridans* infection with oral cavity procedures or enterococcal with gastrointestinal or genitourinary procedures?

Antibiotic prophylaxis is recommended for patients with VSD, PDA, pulmonary or aortic stenosis, tetralogy of Fallot, or coarctation of the aorta. Such therapy is needed for patients with rheumatic or syphilitic valvular defects, prosthetic valves, calcified valves, obstructive cardiomyopathy, or mitral valve prolapse with either regurgitant murmur or with thickened mitral valve leaflets.

Endocarditis prophylaxis is not advised for patients with isolated secundum atrial septal defect or those who have undergone surgical repair for VSD or PDA and have no residual defect beyond 6 months. The same is true for those who have coronary artery bypass graft, previous rheumatic fever, or Kawasaki disease without any valve dysfunction. Prophylaxis is not recommended for those who have mitral valve prolapse (MVP) without mitral regurgitation (MR) and for persons with a cardiac pacemaker or implanted defibrillator (Table 5).

Procedures for which antibiotic prophylaxis is needed are those in which transient bacteremia develops when mucosal surfaces colonized with microorganisms are traumatized. For example, bacteremia may occur following dental manipulation in 80% of cases or in 20%

Rakel and Bope: *Conn's Current Therapy 2006*.

 CURRENT DIAGNOSIS

- High index of suspicion
- Febrile patient (temperature >38°C [100.4°F]) with
   Valvular or congenital heart defects
   Intravenous drug abuse
   Prosthetic or vascular access
   New onset or changing cardiac murmur
   Unknown source of embolization
- Positive blood cultures on at least two different specimens.
- Presence of vegetation detected on echocardiography (transesophageal [TEE] preferred)

of patients after urethral instrumentation. Prophylactic antimicrobials are recommended for high-risk patients who are scheduled to have certain dental, oropharyngeal, gastrointestinal, or genitourinary manipulations.

Standard antibiotic prophylaxis for patients undergoing oral, dental, or upper respiratory tract manipulations include oral amoxicillin. Clindamycin (Cleocin),[1] cefadroxil (Duricef),[1] cephalexin (Keflex),[1] or azithromycin (Zithromax)[1] or clarithromycin (Biaxin)[1] should be given to those who cannot tolerate or are allergic to penicillin.

Parenteral ampicillin is recommended for patients who cannot take oral antibiotics and for those at high risk for infective endocarditis, such as patients with a prosthetic valve, previous endocarditis, or surgical systemic pulmonary shunts. Clindamycin[1] or cefazolin (Ancef) can be used as an alternative. Patients undergoing gastrointestinal or genitourinary instrumentation should be given vancomycin.

---

[1]Not FDA approved for this indication.

 CURRENT THERAPY

- Empiric antibiotics should be started immediately with vancomycin and gentamicin.
- Specific therapy should be started once the pathogen is identified:
   Use combination therapy for synergetic activity.
   Monitor MIC/MBC level whenever possible.
   Administer therapy for 2 to 6 weeks.
- Surgical interventions should be undertaken for severe, refractory, and complicated endocarditis.
- Prophylactic antibiotics are recommended in patients with structural heart defects undergoing surgical procedures or manipulations that can cause transient bacteremia, as recommended by the American Heart Association.
- Administration of antibiotic is usually once and 30 minutes to 1 to 2 hours before the procedure.

Abbreviations: MBC = minimum bactericidal concentration; MIC = minimum inhibitory concentration.

As recommended by the American Heart Association, all prophylactic antibiotics should be used only once before the procedure. There is no need for additional antibiotic administration except in high-risk patients who are undergoing gastrointestinal or genitourinary manipulation and who are given an ampicillin and gentamicin combination.

REFERENCES

Amin NM: Infective endocarditis. Consultant 1994;34(3):319-343.

Bansal RC: Infective endocarditis. Med Clin North Am 1995;79: 1205-1220.

Bayer AS, Bolger AF, Taubert KA, et al: Diagnosis and management of infective endocarditis and its complications. Circulation 1998;98:2936-2948.

Bayer AS, Ward JI, Ginzton LE, Shapiro SM: Evaluation of new clinical criteria for diagnosis of infective endocarditis. Am J Med 1994;96:211-219.

Cunha BA, Gill MV, Lazar JM: Acute infective endocarditis. Infect Dis Clin North Am 1996;10(4):811-834.

Dajanai AS, Taubert KA, Wilson W, et al: Prevention of bacterial endocarditis. Recommendations by American Heart Association. JAMA 1997;277:1794-1801.

Giessel BE, Koenig CJ, Blake RL: Management of bacterial endocarditis. Am Fam Physician 2000;61:1725-1732.

Karchner AW: Infections on prosthetic valves and intravascular infections. In Mandell GL, Bennett JE, Dolin R (eds): Mandell, Douglas and Bennett's Principles and Practice of Infectious Diseases, 5th ed. Philadelphia, Churchill Livingstone, 2000, pp 903-917.

Li JS, Sexton DJ, Mick N, et al: Proposed modification to Duke criteria for diagnosis of infective endocarditis. Clin Infect Dis 2000; 30:633-638.

Mylonakis E, Calderwood SB: Infective endocarditis in adults. N Engl J Med 2001;345(18):1318-1330.

Hypertension

Method of
Patrick J. Mulrow, MD

Hypertension, or elevated blood pressure, is a worldwide epidemic. In Western Europe and North America, the prevalence for this condition is more than 20% of the adult population, and it increases with age. In the United States, more than 50% of the population 65 years of age or older has hypertension, and this approaches 90% for those older than 80 years of age. Thus, approximately 50 million people in the United States and approximately 1 billion people worldwide have hypertension. Hypertension is the most common diagnosis for patient office visits in the United States.

The relationship between blood pressure and cardiovascular disease is continuous and independent of other risk factors. The higher the blood pressure, the greater the risk of stroke, heart attacks, heart failure, and kidney failure. An increase of 20 mm Hg systolic blood pressure or 10 mm Hg diastolic blood pressure doubles the risk of cardiovascular disease from the blood pressure range of 115/75 to 185/115 mm Hg.

The health benefits of lowering blood pressure have been demonstrated time and time again. In clinical trials, antihypertensive treatment has reduced stroke incidence by approximately 40%, heart attacks by approximately 25%, and heart failure by more than 50%. Despite the demonstration of health benefits, in study after study the control of hypertension to goal levels of less than 140/90 mm Hg is only approximately 30% in the United States and much less in many countries around the world. This failure to adequately treat hypertension persists despite the availability of multiple drugs and lifestyle modifications known to be effective in preventing and treating hypertension.

This failure to apply the fruits of clinical science to clinical practice is because of many factors, but it is clear that physicians are part of the problem. Physicians frequently do not follow up and aggressively treat hypertension. In clinical trials—notably the Antihypertensive and Lipid Lowering Treatment to Prevent Heart Attack Trial (ALLHAT study)—approximately 66% of hypertension patients can be treated to reach goal blood pressure levels. The success of clinical trials in achieving a higher patient success rate is because of the health care team approach to the management and follow-up of the hypertensive patient.

Classifications of Blood Pressures

The definition of hypertension has changed over the years. A blood pressure of greater than 160/95 mm Hg was often used as the cutoff point, but it is clear from numerous epidemiologic studies that there is a continuous cardiovascular disease risk in blood pressure from 120 mm Hg systolic on up. The consensus is that 140/90 mm Hg in the general population is a cutoff point and a treatment goal. However, in certain conditions, such as diabetes mellitus or underlying renal disease, 130/80 mm Hg or lower is the goal.

Table 1 summarizes the recommendations from the Seventh Report of the Joint National Committee on Prevention, Detection, Evaluation, and Treatment of High Blood Pressure (JNC 7). A new category, called prehypertensive, has been added because patients with prehypertension are at twice the risk of developing hypertension compared with those with lower levels. For this extremely large population of potential hypertensive patients, prevention of hypertension by lifestyle modification is strongly recommended. It should be remembered that even a controlled hypertensive patient has more cardiovascular events than someone who has never had hypertension. Therefore, it is best to prevent the development of hypertension.

Measurement of Blood Pressure

Blood pressure is an extremely variable hemodynamic measurement. Its measurement is the basis for diagnosing and classifying hypertensive patients. We can measure many blood elements very accurately, but frequently

TABLE 1 Classification and Management of Blood Pressure for Adults

BP classification	Systolic BP (mm Hg)	Diastolic BP (mm Hg)	Lifestyle modification	Initial Drug Therapy	
				Without compelling indications	With compelling indications*
Normal	<120	<80	Encourage		
Prehypertension	120-139	80-89	Yes	No antihypertensive drug indicated	Drug(s) for compelling indications
Stage 1 hypertension	140-159	90-99	Yes	Thiazide-type diuretics for most May consider ACEI, ARB, BB, CCB, or combination	Drug(s) for the compelling indications Other antihypertensive-drugs (diuretics, ACEI, ARB, BB, CCB) as needed
Stage 2 hypertension	>160	>100	Yes	Two-drug combination for most (usually thiazide-type diuretic and ACEI, ARB, BB, or CCB)	

*Compelling indications are diabetes mellitus, heart failure, coronary artery disease, and chronic kidney disease.
Abbreviations: ACEI = angiotensin-converting enzyme inhibitor; ARB = angiotensin-receptor blocker; BB = beta-blocker; BP = blood pressure; CCB = calcium channel blocker.
Modified from: U.S. Department of Health and Human Services, National Heart Institutes of Health, National Heart, Lung, and Blood Institute: JNC 7 Express, The Seventh Report of the Joint National Committee on Prevention, Detection, Evaluation, and Treatment of High Blood Pressure (Publication No. 03-5233), May 2003, p 3. JAMA 2003;289:2560-2572.

the results are of no consequence or are unimportant. Blood pressure measurement is often poorly measured in the doctor's office or clinic. There are two important components to measuring blood pressure, the preparation of the patient and the actual measurement. Here are some suggestions:

- Patients should be seated quietly for 5 minutes with feet on the floor and the arm supported at the level of the heart. The blood pressure in both arms should be measured at the first visit. Standing blood pressure is indicated sometimes, especially in those patients older than 65 years of age and those prone to postural hypotension, such as diabetics.
- Patients should refrain from smoking or ingesting caffeine for at least 30 minutes before the measurement.
- An appropriate size arm cuff should be used. The cuff bladder should encircle at least 80% of the arm.
- A properly calibrated instrument should be used, and the instrument should be validated at regular intervals.
- An average of two or more readings should be taken at each sitting.
- If the auscultatory method is used, systolic blood pressure is the point at which the first of two or more successive sounds are heard. Diastolic pressure is the point before the disappearance of sounds.

- The physician should inform the patient of the blood pressure level.

AMBULATORY AND SELF-MEASUREMENT OF BLOOD PRESSURE

A number of publications have reported the usefulness of ambulatory blood pressure monitoring (ABPM) in certain conditions. The measurement is somewhat complex and should be done in the office of the specialist. ABPM is warranted for patients who need evaluation for white-coat hypertension and resistant hypertension, and in patients with unusual reactions to blood pressure medications. The ambulatory blood pressure values are lower than clinical readings. A blood pressure measured by ABPM that is more than 135/85 mm Hg is defined as hypertension. There should be a nocturnal dip in blood pressure.

Self-measurement of blood pressure is more practical and useful in monitoring the response to antihypertensive medication and in evaluating white-coat hypertension. I have many of my patients measure their blood pressure at least weekly at home, record the results, and bring the record to the office for evaluation. Oscillometric blood pressure measurement instruments are becoming more reliable and easy to use. The patient needs to be instructed in the office on how to measure the blood pressure at home.

Rakel and Bope: *Conn's Current Therapy 2006.*

Types of Blood Pressure: Systolic or Diastolic

Traditionally, hypertension has been classified based on the diastolic blood pressure. Numerous reports, especially from the Framingham study, have emphasized that *systolic* hypertension is a greater risk for causing cardiovascular disease than *diastolic* hypertension. A combination of a high systolic and low diastolic blood pressure (widened pulse pressure) is a major predictor of cardiovascular disease. The widened pulse pressure reflects atheromatous thickening and stiffening of the major capacitance vessels. With aging, systolic blood pressure tends to increase even in the normotensive patient, while diastolic tends to fall. Most elderly (65 years of age or older) hypertensive patients have primarily systolic hypertension with only minor elevations of diastolic blood pressure. It is imperative, therefore, to control systolic hypertension to below goal levels of 140. A blood pressure of 150/80 mm Hg is too high in a 65-year-old patient.

Evaluation of the Hypertensive Patient

To make the diagnosis of hypertension, an accurate blood pressure measurement should be made on at least two separate occasions, one or more weeks apart. Obviously, if the blood pressure is very high under non-stress conditions, a diagnosis can be made on one visit and treatment started.

DIAGNOSTIC EVALUATION

There are two components to the diagnostic workup:

1. Evaluation of the patient for the presence of cardiovascular risk factors (Box 1) and organ damage
2. Evaluation for secondary causes of hypertension

A thorough medical history, physical examination, and routine laboratory studies should be performed. Before starting treatment, I usually include a urinalysis, serum electrolytes including calcium, creatinine, blood glucose, hematocrit, a fasting lipid profile, and an electrocardiogram.

Secondary causes of hypertension also should be evaluated. How extensive the evaluation should be is a subject of debate. Unless there is some obvious reason to suspect a secondary cause or the patient has resistant hypertension, or there is sudden onset of type 2 hypertension in the young (younger than 30 years) or in the patient older than 55 years of age, I do not routinely do special diagnostic tests. Recently, the evidence is becoming compelling that approximately 7% to 8% of the hypertensive population has primary aldosteronism. Blood tests for measuring the serum aldosterone to renin ratio are being recommended by many experts. A ratio greater than 25 should be pursued with more extensive testing. I have been doing these ratios recently, but my practice is more a tertiary rather than a primary practice, where many patients have stage 1 hypertension. Secondary causes of hypertension should be pursued when the above criteria are noted (Box 2).

Treatment of the Hypertensive Patient

The goal of therapy is to reduce cardiovascular complications. In the usual hypertensive patient, the blood pressure goal is less than 140/90 mm Hg. However, in patients with diabetes or renal disease and hypertension, the blood pressure goal is less than 130/80 mm Hg.

LIFESTYLE MODIFICATION

Lifestyle modification such as weight reduction, low-sodium diet, reduced alcohol intake, cessation of smoking, and increased physical activity should be an adjunct to all drug therapy. In the hypertensive patient, lifestyle modifications can reduce blood pressure, enhance the blood pressure lowering effects of antihypertensive drugs, and decrease cardiovascular risk. As little as 10 to 20 pounds weight loss can significantly reduce blood pressure. A low-sodium diet of less than 100 mEq per day can be quite effective. Reduction in excess alcohol intake can also lower the blood pressure. Physical activity, such as brisk walking for 30 minutes daily, can reduce blood pressure. Certain diets (Dietary Approaches to Stop Hypertension [DASH]) that are high in fruits, vegetables, and low-fat dairy products may be as effective as monotherapy in lowering the blood pressure. Smoking cessation may not lower the blood pressure, but it does decrease the cardiovascular complications.

BOX 1   Major Cardiovascular Risk Factors

Obesity (body mass index >30 kg/m^2)
Dyslipidemia
Cigarette smoking
Diabetes mellitus
Family history of premature cardiovascular disease (CVD)
Age (men >55 years, women >65 years)
Microalbuminuria
Decreased renal function
Left ventricular hypertrophy (LVH)

BOX 2   Causes of Secondary Hypertension

Coarctation of the aorta
Cushing's syndrome
Drug induced (e.g., nonsteroidal anti-inflammatory drugs, estrogen, sympathomimetics, certain herbal medications)
Hyperparathyroidism
Hyperthyroidism
Pheochromocytoma
Primary aldosteronism
Renal disease
Renovascular disease
Sleep apnea

Although lifestyle modifications can be extremely effective, every physicians knows how difficult it is for some patients to adhere to these lifestyle changes. I give patients in stage 1 hypertension (140-159/90-99 mm Hg), without diabetes or other cardiovascular risk factors or end-organ damage, a 4-month trial of lifestyle changes. If goal blood pressure is not achieved, I start pharmacologic therapy.

WHITE-COAT HYPERTENSION

Some patients have a blood pressure that is high in the office, but normal when measured at home or at work. However, to be certain of the diagnosis of this benign condition, the blood pressure should be monitored frequently over several months. Patients with true white-coat hypertension show little if any evidence of end-organ damage from the blood pressure. If the diagnosis is not certain, drugs that diminish sympathetic activity such as β-blockers or α-adrenergic drugs may be effective. Ambulatory blood pressure measurement can be helpful in making the diagnosis, because these patients on 24-hour monitoring show normal blood pressures. In my opinion, one should err on the side of treating the patient if there is doubt about the diagnosis.

DRUG TREATMENT OF HYPERTENSION

The efficacy of various antihypertensive agents in lowering blood pressure is about the same when the proper dose is used. A single drug usually reduces blood pressure 8 to 12 mm Hg compared with placebo.

Clinical outcome trials demonstrate the ability of angiotensin-converting enzyme (ACE) inhibitors, angiotensin receptor blockers (ARB), β-blockers, calcium channel blockers, and thiazide diuretics to reduce the complications of hypertension.

Classes of Antihypertensive Drugs (Box 3)

Thiazide Diuretics

Thiazide diuretics have been shown in many studies to be useful in lowering blood pressure and preventing cardiovascular complications. In low doses they have few complications, hypokalemia being the most serious. In my opinion, it is the first-line drug in most hypertensive patients; if two or more drugs are needed, a thiazide

---

BOX 3   Classes of Antihypertensive Drugs

Diuretics
β-Blockers
Calcium channel blockers (CCBs)
Angiotensin-converting enzyme (ACE) inhibitors
Angiotensin receptor blocker (ARB)
α-Adrenergic blocking drugs
Central α-adrenergic agonists
Direct vasodilators
Combination products

Rakel and Bope: *Conn's Current Therapy 2006.*

diuretic is usually one of the drugs. Loop diuretics are good diuretics, but poor antihypertensive agents unless renal failure is present. In patients with chronic renal disease, loop diuretics can be used instead of thiazide diuretics, because thiazides are ineffective in producing a diuresis. Volume retention plays an important role in the development of hypertension in the patient with chronic renal failure. All thiazide diuretics appear to be equally effective. Potassium-sparing compounds such as triamterene (Dyrenium), amiloride (Midamor), and spironolactone (Aldactone) are sometimes added alone or in a combination pill to lessen the potassium-losing effect of diuretics, especially when large doses are used. I usually start with 12.5 mg of hydrochlorothiazide. To avoid cutting the 25 mg pill in half, 15 mg of chlorthalidone can be used.

ADVERSE EFFECTS. Hypokalemia is a common problem when large doses of thiazide diuretics are used. The mechanism is diuresis $\rightarrow$ volume depletion $\rightarrow$ increased renin $\rightarrow$ increased aldosterone $\rightarrow$ increased kidney loss of potassium. With low doses, especially in the elderly and diabetics with low renin levels, hypokalemia is not as common. When needed, I usually recommend a combination pill, triamterene plus hydrochlorothiazide (Dyazide) or amiloride plus hydrochlorothiazide (Moduretic) to prevent the hypokalemia. If several drugs are needed, ACE inhibitors or angiotensin-receptor blockers (ARBs) can block the renin-angiotensin system and lessen K loss. K supplements, 10 to 20 mEq per day, may be useful in some patients, but serum levels of K should be monitored to prevent serious hyperkalemia when multiple K-sparing drugs are used.

Hyponatremia is seen in the elderly, especially women. Some patients are exquisitely sensitive to very low doses of thiazides, and the hyponatremia can cause serious neurologic problems. Mild hyponatremia with a serum concentration of sodium of more than 130 mEq/L usually is of no consequence. Hyperuricemia can occur and lead to gout, especially in males. This complication may cause the discontinuation of diuretics; but if a diuretic is needed, allopurinol (Zyloprim) can be added to the regimen to reduce uric acid production.

β-*Blockers*

β-Blockers are not usually a first-line drug except in people younger than 30 years of age with a hyperdynamic circulation or in hyperthyroidism. β-blockers are included in the treatment of patients with ischemic heart disease, postmyocardial infarction, and patients with certain arrhythmias. I do not use them unless there is some cardiovascular reason for adding it to the blood pressure regimen. Labetalol (Trandate), a combination of α and β drugs, may be used. Labetalol combines an α-adrenergic receptor blockade and a β-blocker. It lowers blood pressure faster than other β-blockers. Carvedilol (Coreg) is another α-blocker and nonselective β-blocker that lowers blood pressure by a peripheral vasodilatation while maintaining cardiac output. It is promoted as especially effective in treating patients with hypertension and congestive heart failure.

These patients are usually on multiple drugs, including a diuretic and an ACE inhibitor.

ADVERSE EVENTS. The major adverse events are bronchospasm, fatigue, and Raynaud's phenomenon. There is some concern that long-term treatment of patients with β-blockers may cause a higher incidence of type 2 diabetes.

Calcium Channel Antagonist

Calcium channel blockers (CCBs) are very effective in treating hypertension in patients, especially in patients older than 65 years of age and African Americans. They cause vasodilatation, which decreases peripheral resistance. Short-acting CCBs such as nifedipine (Procardia) should not be used to treat hypertensive patients. There is concern that the reflex tachycardia may lead to cardiovascular events. However, the long-acting dihydropyridines, such as amlodipine (Norvasc), and nondihydropyridines, such as verapamil (Calan), and diltiazem (Cardizem), are effective. There is debate over the use of CCBs in diabetic patients with proteinuria, because the CCBs may increase protein excretion. I do not use them except as a third add on in patients with proteinuria. Usually I give an ACE inhibitor or an ARB plus a thiazide diuretic, and if the blood pressure is not controlled, I add a CCB or a β-blocker.

Verapamil, diltiazem, and amlodipine cause little or no reflex increase in heart rate. However, verapamil and diltiazem can actually slow the heart rate and have an adverse effect on atrioventricular (AV) conduction. They should be used with caution in patients taking a β-blocker. Amlodipine causes significant peripheral edema, especially in high doses, but combining it with an ACE inhibitor reduces the edema.

I prefer CCBs such as amlodipine as a second drug, usually added to a diuretic in elderly patients and in African Americans. However, if significant proteinuria is present, an ACE inhibitor or ARB should be used instead.

Angiotensin-Converting Inhibitors

ACE inhibitors were originally introduced as antihypertensive drugs, but are now considered to have significant effects in preventing cardiovascular events in patients with underlying cardiovascular disease. They are now recommended as an adjunct therapy for patients with left ventricular dysfunction, recent myocardial infarction, or stroke; and to preserve renal function in diabetic patients. They also appear to increase sensitivity to insulin and reduce the development of diabetes mellitus. The ACE inhibitors are less effective in lowering blood pressure in African American patients. However, there is a broad range of response with many African Americans showing good hypotensive effects. Furthermore, ACE inhibitors confer renal protection in African Americans.

ADVERSE EVENTS. A common adverse effect of an ACE inhibitor is a dry cough. Approximately 10% of the patients note a dry cough, and in a few patients it is especially annoying at night, requiring the drug to be discontinued. Cough is a side effect for all ACE inhibitors and is not related to dose.

Angioedema is an uncommon but serious side effect. Patients with bilateral renal vascular disease may develop acute renal failure from ACE inhibitors. Also, hyperkalemia may occur, especially in the patient taking K supplements or K-sparing diuretics, or who has poor renal function. I measure serum K and creatinine levels about 1 week after starting an ACE inhibitor. I measure creatinine and electrolytes periodically thereafter. ACE inhibitors are contraindicated in pregnancy.

There are numerous ACE inhibitor preparations on the market. I believe they are all equally effective when given in the proper dose. I prefer the ones that are long acting and need only once-a-day medication. This applies to most of the ACE inhibitors. In patients with diabetes, renal disease, and proteinuria, I recommend increasing the dose to the maximum dose to reduce proteinuria and protect the kidneys.

Angiotensin Receptor Blocker

By blocking the binding of angiotensin II to its receptor (AT_1), ARBs can lower blood pressure. They have few side effects. In contrast to ACE inhibitors, ARBs do not cause a cough. The ARBs have been shown to have renal protection in patients with diabetes mellitus type 2. Compared with the β-blocker atenolol (Tenormin), the ARB losartan (Cozaar) is more effective in reducing left ventricular hypertrophy (LVH) and the incidence of stroke in patients with hypertension and LVH. However, this protective effect is not seen in African Americans. Like ACE inhibitors, the beneficial cardiovascular effects of ARBs appear to be beyond just lowering blood pressure. Usually ARBs are given with a diuretic.

As with ACE inhibitors, all ARBs seem to be equally effective when the proper dose is used. Perhaps the only unique feature of one of the ARBs is the mild uricosuric effect of losartan.

α-Adrenergic Blocking Drugs

α-Adrenergic blocking drugs were once considered to be heart friendly because of their favorable effects on blood lipids and glucose metabolism. However, in the ALLHAT study, the doxazosin (Cardura) arm was discontinued because of the twofold increase in the risk of heart failure when compared with diuretics. Therefore, α-adrenergic drugs are not recommended as first-line drugs. In patients who do not have the risk for heart failure, they may be beneficial as an add-on drug or be useful for symptomatic relief of prostatism in men. However, they may cause significant hypotension. I rarely use these drugs.

Central α-Adrenergic Agonists

Central α-adrenergic agonist drugs are not recommended as first-line drugs. They are not used as much today because of their side effects of sedation, dry mouth, and depression. Clonidine (Catapres) is used more frequently because it can be applied to the skin as a patch, but there is some concern about reflex tachycardia and rebound hypertension when it is discontinued. Occasionally I will use guanfacine (Tenex) at bedtime because it is a longer acting drug. It would be a fourth-line add-on in patients with resistant hypertension. In other words, I do not recommend these drugs as routine medications, but do add them as a third- or fourth-line add-on in certain patients.

Peripheral Adrenergic Neuron Antagonists

Reserpine in low doses is the only drug in this category that is still in use. Low doses are effective as antihypertensive drugs with few significant side effects. The reported side effects of depression and sedation were overemphasized by physicians because too large a dose was used. Reserpine is cheap and often combined with a diuretic. However, no outcome studies have been performed with reserpine. Nevertheless, this is a commonly prescribed drug in many developing countries because it is inexpensive.

Direct Vasodilators

Direct vasodilators such as hydralazine (Apresoline) cause reflex tachycardia, and when used should be given with a β-blocker to prevent the tachycardia. Hydralazine has to be given 3 or 4 times each day and is rarely used today. Minoxidil (Loniten), a potent drug, is reserved for severe resistant hypertension. It can cause significant fluid retention and its chronic use can cause disfiguring hirsutism.

Combination Products (Box 4)

More than 50% of hypertensive patients need two or more antihypertensive drugs to attain goal blood pressures. In diabetics with a lower goal, three or more drugs may be needed. Also, patients with stage 2 hypertension (blood pressure greater than 160/ 100 mm Hg) usually require two drugs as initial therapy. Combination products may improve compliance. Also, combining antihypertensive drugs with different mechanisms of action may allow smaller doses of each drug to be used and thus lessen dose-dependent side effects.

BOX 4 Combination Drugs

Diuretics and potassium-sparing drugs such as hydrochlorothiazide plus triamterene (Maxzide) or amiloride (Moduretic) or spironolactone (Aldactazide)

Various ACE inhibitors plus thiazide

Various ARBs plus thiazide

Various β-blockers plus thiazide

Centrally acting drugs such as clonidine or methyldopa plus thiazide diuretics

Reserpine plus thiazide

Calcium channel blockers plus ACE inhibitors in various combinations

Abbreviations: ACE = angiotensin-converting enzyme; ARB = angiotensin-receptor blocker.

Although there are no prospective drug studies comparing the efficacy of combination therapy with monotherapy, in most monotherapy trials the majority of the subjects are taking one or more drugs in addition to the study drug. Diuretics plus ACE inhibitors or ARBs are frequent combinations. The combination of an ACE with a CCB lessens the edema seen with the large doses of dihydropyridine CCBs. Of course, for many years potassium-sparing drugs have been combined with thiazide diuretics.

Compliance

Good blood pressure control requires patient and physician compliance. The physicians must educate the patients, prescribe appropriate medication, and follow the patient carefully. Hypertensive patients usually have several cardiovascular risk factors that need to be assessed and treated. All members of the health care team physician, nurse, and other health professionals— must work together to improve lifestyle and detect and control blood pressure. We have the knowledge and the modalities to control hypertension if we apply what we know to our clinical practice.

First Choice of Drug

The recent JNC7 guidelines in hypertension recommend low-dose diuretics as the first step in treatment for most hypertensive patients, including those at risk such as elderly hypertensives and hypertensives with cardiovascular risk factors. Diuretics are also recommended as the second drug choice when the initial drug does not lower the blood pressure to goal levels. Because most patients require two or more drugs, a diuretic is usually a component of the regimen. These recommendations are based on a number of long-term clinical studies that demonstrate the beneficial effects of diuretics in preventing cardiovascular complications in hypertensive patients. However, despite the evidence the use of diuretics declined in the United States until the recent ALLHAT study gave a major boost to diuretics. In this study, thiazide was compared with a CCB, an ACE inhibitor, and an α-adrenergic blocker. The latter drug was discontinued early in the study because of poor outcome compared with a diuretic. The major finding of this study is that the diuretic is as good as, if not better than, other drugs in lowering blood pressure and preventing cardiovascular complications. Thiazide diuretics are cheap and, in low doses, relatively free of side effects. A thiazide diuretic is my first-line drug for treating hypertension. I usually start with 12.5 mg of hydrochlorothiazide and occasionally the longer acting one, chlorthalidone. I emphasize thiazide diuretics because nonthiazide diuretics have not been shown to be effective antihypertensive agents.

HYPERTENSION AND CO-MORBID CONDITIONS

Patients with hypertension tend to have multiple metabolic abnormalities such as diabetes mellitus, obesity, dyslipidemia and insulin resistance, as well as underlying vascular disease. Therefore, in addition to antihypertensive medication, these patients receive several other medications and diets to decrease the cardiovascular complications.

Diabetes

Two or more drugs are usually needed to meet the target goal of less than 130/80 mm Hg in diabetic patients. ACE inhibitors and ARBs, in addition to lowering blood pressure, also slow the progression of diabetic nephropathy. Diuretics are usually required as a second-line drug to reduce the blood pressure to goal levels. There is some concern that CCBs may increase proteinuria. Nevertheless, all these drugs—thiazide diuretics, ARBs, ACE inhibitors, and CCBs—have been shown in clinical trials to reduce cardiovascular disease and stroke in diabetic subjects. Although ACE inhibitors and ARBs may have beneficial vascular effects, it is important to control the blood pressure to goal levels. This may mean the use of two or more medications. I usually recommend starting with an ACE inhibitor and then adding a small dose of a thiazide diuretic, if necessary. If a third drug is needed, I usually add either the CCB amlodipine (Norvasc) or the β-blocker atenolol (Tenormin), depending upon the cardiovascular situation.

Ischemic Heart Disease

In patients with hypertension and ischemic heart disease, the first-line drug therapy is usually a β-blocker. CCBs are a reasonable alternative drug. For patients with a myocardial infarction and hypertension, a β-blocker and an ACE inhibitor should be started and other drugs then added to control the blood pressure to goal levels.

Heart Failure

In patients with hypertension and heart failure, loop diuretics along with ACE inhibitors and β-blockers are recommended. ARBs may be substituted for ACE inhibitors, and small doses of the aldosterone antagonist spironolactone (Aldactone) should be added. Close monitoring of the serum K levels is required.

BOX 5   Causes of Resistant Hypertension

Volume overload
Failure to take drugs
Inadequate drug doses
Drug-induced hypertension (nonsteroidal anti-inflammatory
   drugs, sympathomimetics, estrogens, oral contraceptives,
   adrenal glucocorticoids, amphetamines, cyclosporine,
   erythropoietin, over-the-counter drugs such as ephedra)
Excess adrenal glucocorticoid production
Excess adrenal glucocorticoid administration
Excess alcohol intake
Poor blood pressure measurement, especially in obese
   subjects
Secondary causes of hypertension

Chronic Renal Disease

Hypertensive male patients with creatinine greater than 1.5 mg/dL and hypertensive female patients with creatinine greater than 1.3 mg/dL will progress to chronic renal failure unless treated aggressively. Treatment with ARBs and ACE inhibitors show favorable responses in both diabetic and nondiabetic kidney disease. The blood pressure goal is less than 130/80. When renal failure is more advanced (creatinine 2.5 to 3), loop diuretics such as furosemide (Lasix) may be needed for diuresis. The renin angiotensin system inhibitors may cause a limited rise in serum creatinine, but blood pressure drugs should be maintained unless there is a doubling of the creatinine or significant hyperkalemia.

RESISTANT HYPERTENSION

Resistant hypertension is defined as the failure to reach goal blood pressure on three blood pressure medications. Adding an adequate diuretic dose to the drug regimen usually controls resistant hypertension. In addition, the physician should obtain a history for the possibility of certain drugs and over-the-counter medications that may contribute to hypertension, as well as excessive alcohol intake. Box 5 indicates some of the causes of resistant hypertension.

Acute Myocardial Infarction

Method of
Kevin A. Bybee, MD,
and Stephen L. Kopecky, MD

During the 20th century, acute myocardial infarction (AMI) became the leading cause of death in the United States and in other developed regions of the world including Europe. Individual mortality rates from AMI have recently decreased in both men and women because of modern therapeutic advances and increasing public awareness of AMI symptoms and the need for emergent evaluation. Despite advances in the diagnosis and treatment of AMI, however, it will likely remain the leading cause of death well into the future, given the aging of the population and the increasing prevalence of type II diabetes mellitus. Information obtained from clinical trials has revolutionized the modern approach to patients with AMI, emphasizing early and accurate diagnosis, early risk stratification, and prompt reperfusion therapy in those with ST-segment-elevation myocardial infarction (STEMI).

Rakel and Bope: *Conn's Current Therapy 2006.*

Diagnosis

In 2000 the American College of Cardiology (ACC) and the European Society of Cardiology (ESC) issued a joint recommendation that redefines the diagnosis of AMI, thus replacing the World Health Organization definition. The ACC/ESC definition requires the typical rise and fall of troponin or more rapid rise and fall of creatinine kinase myocardial band (CK-MB) in addition to one of the following:

- Symptoms consistent with myocardial ischemia
- Electrocardiogram (ECG) changes indicating myocardial ischemia (ST-segment depression or elevation)
- New pathologic Q waves
- Percutaneous coronary intervention (PCI)

Pathologic findings of AMI at autopsy are also considered diagnostic. Additionally, any patient presenting with a clinical history consistent with AMI and new left bundle branch block should be triaged as STEMI. Based on the ACC/ESC guidelines, as well as recommendations issued by the ACC and American Heart Association (AHA) in 2002, differentiating between unstable angina (UA) and non-ST-segment-elevation myocardial infarction (NSTEMI) is based on whether biomarkers of myocardial injury are elevated, denoting myocardial necrosis. Detectable elevations of troponin and CK-MB may not be apparent in those who present within the first 4 to 6 hours following symptom onset. Thus distinguishing between UA and NSTEMI may not be possible at the time of initial evaluation and may require serial measurements of cardiac biomarkers.

PATHOPHYSIOLOGY

AMI occurs when myocardial necrosis results from prolonged myocardial ischemia. Acute coronary syndromes (ACS) represent a spectrum of clinical presentations including UA, NSTEMI, and STEMI. Despite this spectrum of presentations, the underlying pathophysiologic mechanisms are similar in most cases. The most common initiating mechanism responsible for AMI is acute plaque rupture, with subsequent exposure of thrombogenic substances with the lipid-laden plaque core to circulating blood and consequent coronary thrombus formation. STEMI is almost always a result of complete thrombotic coronary occlusion. Subtotal coronary occlusion often results in UA or NSTEMI. Myocardial necrosis in the setting of NSTEMI may result from transient complete coronary occlusion with spontaneous partial recanalization, persistent near-complete coronary occlusion, and distal embolization of plaque debris and platelet-rich thrombi with associated vascular spasm. Most plaque ruptures involve relatively small, vulnerable nonobstructive coronary plaques. Studies using intravascular ultrasound document the presence of multiple ruptured plaques in many patients presenting with AMI. AMI can also result from endothelial erosion and in situations of prolonged increases in myocardial oxygen demand in the setting of a stable, yet high-grade coronary lesion. Other rare mechanisms of AMI include coronary artery spasm, coronary artery embolism, coronary artery dissection, and coronary injury from trauma.

HISTORY

Initial assessment of patients with suspected ACS should begin with a focused history, physical examination, and 12-lead ECG (Figure 1). Patients with AMI can present with a variety of symptoms—from crushing substernal chest pain to no pain at all. This variability in symptoms can make initial diagnosis challenging in some patients and reinforces the importance of physicians remaining astute. The discomfort classically associated with AMI is described as a crushing, squeezing, or tightness in the anterior left chest. These symptoms can radiate to the jaw, teeth, shoulders, arms, and back and usually last for at least 20 minutes. Older (age >75 years) patients, diabetics, and female patients are more likely to present with dyspnea as their primary symptom. Patients with AMI usually do not have pleuritic chest pain, which suggests an alternative diagnosis such as pericarditis, pulmonary embolism, pneumothorax, or pneumonia. Patients with tearing pain may have aortic dissection.

PHYSICAL EXAMINATION

The physical examination usually does not help significantly in the diagnosis of AMI, but it does it aid in the risk stratification of patients with suspected AMI and in an evaluation for non-AMI etiologies responsible for patient symptoms. Hemodynamic stability should be assessed. Evaluation of jugular venous pressure and wave form can give clues to right ventricular infarction and right atrial pressure as well as indirect information about left heart function and intravascular volume status. Lung evaluation should note the presence of rales, indicating left heart failure. Cardiac palpation can give clues to underlying cardiomyopathy. A soft S_1 suggests reduced left ventricle (LV) systolic function or first-degree atrioventricular (AV) block. A holosystolic murmur could indicate mitral regurgitation resulting from ischemic papillary muscle dysfunction or ventricular septal defect. An S_4 gallop is often present, indicating abnormal left ventricular relaxation, whereas an S_3 gallop suggests elevated left ventricular end-diastolic pressure. Hypotension at the time of presentation is usually caused by large areas of ischemic myocardium. Hypotension and rales greater than one third of the lung field are indicators of increased morbidity and mortality during hospitalization. Unstable patients should also be assessed for mechanical complications of AMI such as papillary muscle rupture, ventricular septal defect, and left ventricular free-wall rupture.

Alternative etiologies responsible for the patient's presentation should also be sought during the physical examination. Symmetry of pulses in all extremities and symmetry of blood pressure in both arms should be assessed in evaluating for aortic dissection. A pericardial rub suggests pericarditis, whereas a pleural rub suggests pulmonary embolism or pneumonia. Palpation of the chest wall may be helpful in identifying

5

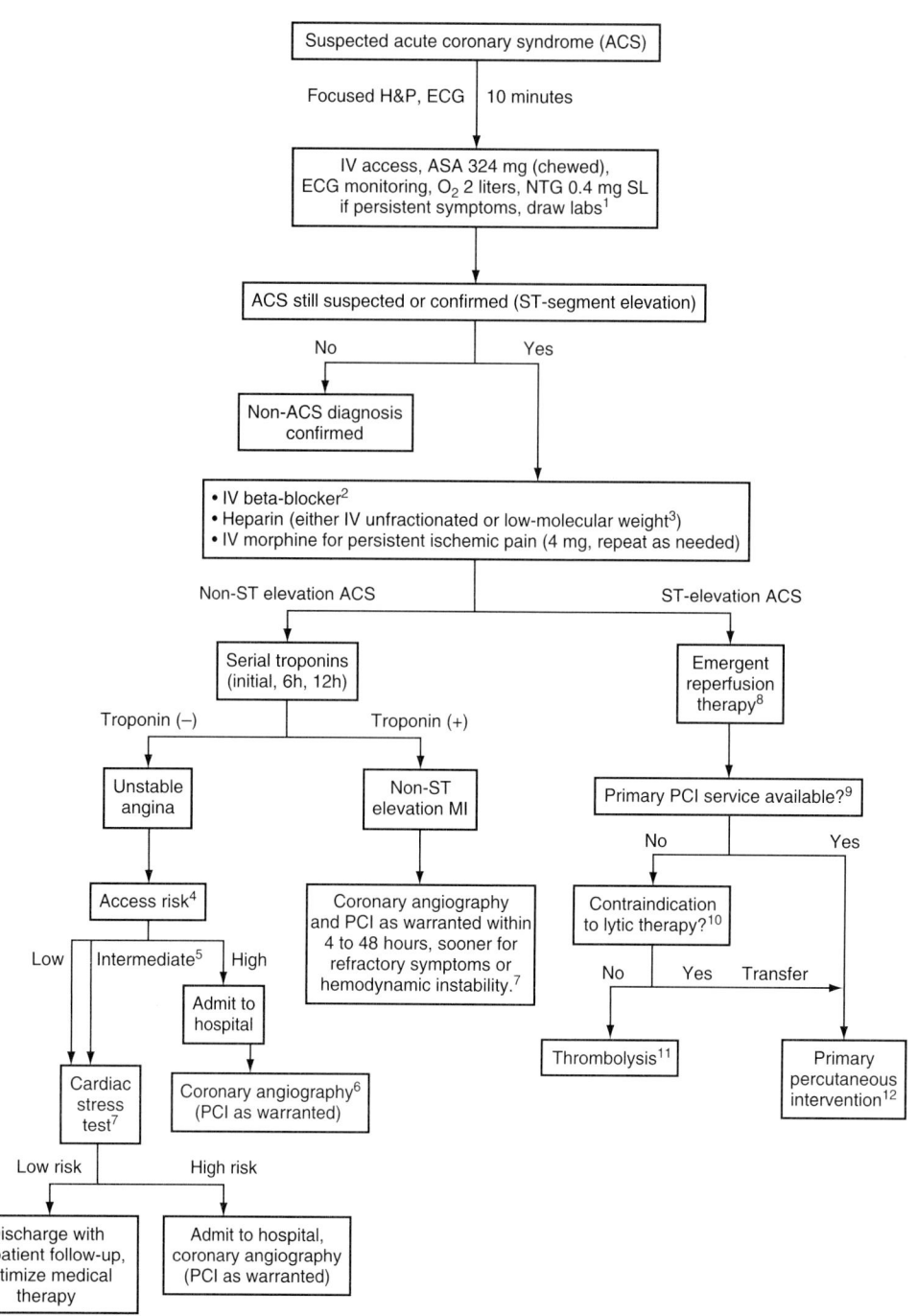

FIGURE 1. Algorithm for evaluation and treatment of patients with suspected acute coronary syndromes. ACS = acute coronary syndrome; ALT = alanine amino transferase; ASA = aspirin; CBC = complete blood count; CXR = chest radiograph; ECG = electrocardiogram; H&P = history and physical; IV = intravenous; MI = myocardial infarction; NSTEMI = non-ST-segment-elevation myocardial infarction; NTG = nitroglycerin; PCI = percutaneous coronary intervention; SL = sublingual.
[1]Troponin, CBC , electrolytes, creatinine, ALT, CXR.
[2]Metoprolol, 5 mg IV × 3 every 5 minutes, until heart rate 55 to 65 bpm; hold for hypotension or pulmonary edema.
[3]Low-molecular-weight heparin appears superior to IV unfractionated heparin in patients with unstable angina with high risk features and those with NSTEMI. Some interventionists prefer IV unfractionated heparin in patients undergoing coronary angiography/PCI.
[4]See Table 1 for risk assessment.
[5]For intermediate-risk patients, consider risk stratification if the chest pain unit is available.
[6]Consider addition of glycoprotein (GP) IIb/IIIa inhibitor. GP IIa/IIIb inhibitor can be initiated upon admission or just prior to PCI in the cardiac catheterization laboratory.
[7]Exercise electrocardiogram preferred; exercise imaging study if baseline ST changes present or if patient is on digoxin; pharmacologic imaging study if unable to walk on treadmill to acceptable workload.
[8]Administer reperfusion therapy if symptom onset within 12 hours. Refer for coronary angiography if symptom onset more than 12 hours and persistent chest symptoms or hemodynamic instability.
[9]Can consider transport to primary PCI facility if door-to-balloon time still less than 90 minutes.
[10]See Table 2 for absolute and relative contraindications to thrombolytic therapy.
[11]Door-to-needle time should be less than 30 minutes.
[12]Door-to-balloon time should be less than 90 minutes; goal is less than 60 minutes.

musculoskeletal etiologies. However, for unclear reasons, patients with documented AMI may have increased pain with chest wall palpation.

ELECTROCARDIOGRAM

The initial ECG plays an important role in the diagnosis, risk stratification, and management of patients with AMI and should be performed on all patients with chest pain and/or dyspnea immediately upon presentation. Patients presenting with AMI should be classified as non-ST-elevation ACS or ST-segment-elevation ACS. This nomenclature is preferred because ST-segment elevation at the time of presentation indicates ongoing myocardial injury and identifies patients who can benefit from prompt reperfusion therapy. The ECG is normal at the time of presentation in 10% of patients with AMI and therefore should be used as a supportive tool in addition to the clinical history, physical examination, and laboratory evaluation.

ST-Segment-Elevation Myocardial Infarction

STEMI is characterized by at least 1 mm of ST-segment elevation in two or more contiguous ECG leads. Reciprocal ST-segment depression may be present in leads remote from those with ST elevation and is associated with higher risk. The distribution of ST-segment elevation on the ECG can give clues to the coronary artery responsible for the ischemia (Table 1). A right-sided ECG should be obtained in all patients with inferior STEMI to evaluate for evidence of right ventricular infarction manifest by ST-segment elevation in lead V_3R and/or V_4R. Marked ST depression in leads V_1 to V_3 is the hallmark of acute posterior infarction, which can be confirmed by ST-segment elevation in posteriorly placed leads (V_7R to V_9R), and should be treated as an STEMI. Patients presenting with symptoms consistent with AMI and a new left bundle branch block should be triaged and managed as an STEMI.

Other disease entities with associated ST-segment elevation should be kept in mind when assessing a patient with suspected STEMI. These include pericarditis, myocarditis, left ventricular aneurysm, early repolarization, coronary artery spasm, intracranial bleeding, head trauma, and transient left ventricular apical ballooning syndrome.

Non-ST-Segment-Elevation Myocardial Infarction

Patients with NSTEMI can present with marked or minimal ST-segment depression, isolated T wave changes, or with no ST-segment or T wave changes at all. ST-segment depression identifies patients at higher risk who subsequently benefit most from an aggressive management strategy.

BIOMARKERS OF CARDIAC INJURY

Because of their high sensitivity and specificity for myocardial necrosis, cardiac troponin T and troponin I assays are preferred in the initial evaluation of patients with suspected AMI. Detectable troponin elevations usually occur 3 to 6 hours following onset of myocardial necrosis and thus may not be abnormal at the time of initial presentation. As a result, troponin may not be useful in the early diagnosis of STEMI and is most helpful in discerning UA and NSTEMI. Troponin remains elevated for 7 to 14 days following AMI.

Creatine kinase (CK) and CK-MB are less sensitive and less specific for myocardial necrosis. Elevated CK levels are detectable 4 to 6 hours following AMI and peak around 24 hours following the onset of necrosis. CK concentrations return to normal by 72 hours and thus may be useful in the diagnosis of reinfarction. CK-MB is not entirely specific for myocardial muscle and can be elevated in situations of skeletal muscle, bowel, and prostate injury.

Risk Stratification

Several characteristics are associated with a worse prognosis in patients with unstable angina (Table 2), NSTEMI, and STEMI, including advanced age, female gender, hemodynamic alterations (hypotension, tachycardia), left heart failure (pulmonary rales, S3 gallop, elevated BNP [brain natriuretic peptide]), cumulative extent of

TABLE 1 Infarct-related Artery and Associated Distribution of Electrocardiographic ST-Segment Elevation

Location of coronary occlusion	Distribution of ST-segment elevation	30-Day Mortality with Successful Reperfusion*
Proximal LAD (proximal to first septal perforator)	V_1-V_6, aVL, I, new LBBB common	19.6%
Mid-LAD (distal to first septal perforator and proximal to first large diagonal branch)	V_1-V_6, aVL, I,	9.2%
Distal LAD (distal to first large diagonal branch) or diagonal branch	V_1-V_4, or aVL, I, V_{5-6}	6.8%
Right coronary artery	II, III, aVF, V_{5-6} (V_3R, V_4R with RV infarction)	6.4%
Left circumflex	V_{5-6}, III, II, aVF (can have minimal ECG changes)	4.5%

*Derived from Global Utilization of Streptokinase and t-PA for Occluded Coronary Arteries-I (GUSTO-I) cohort population of patients receiving successful reperfusion therapy.
Abbreviations: ECG = electrocardiogram; LAD = left anterior descending; LBBB = left bundle branch block; RV = right ventricle.

Rakel and Bope: *Conn's Current Therapy 2006.*

TABLE 2 Risk Stratification in Patients With Unstable Angina

High risk (20% event rate*)	Intermediate risk (~6% event rate*)	Low risk (~<1% event rate*)
Presence of at least one of the following:	No *high-risk* features but at least one of the following:	No *high intermediate risk* features but may present with one of the following:
- Acceleration of ischemic symptoms in last 48 h - Ongoing rest pain > 20 min - Age >75 y - New or worsening MR murmur - Pulmonary edema or evidence of worsening heart failure. - Hemodynamic instability - Rest angina associated with dynamic ST-segment deviation >0.05 mV - New bundle branch block - Ventricular tachycardia	- Known atherosclerotic vascular disease (prior MI/PCI/CABG, peripheral, cerebrovascular) - Rest pain (>20 min) now resolved with moderate or high likelihood of CAD - Rest angina <20 min relieved with NTG - Age >70 y - Prior aspirin usage - T wave inversions > 0.2 mV - Q waves	- New-onset angina within 2 wk to 2 mo - Increasing frequency of exertional angina without rest pain. - Normal or unchanged ECG

*Risk for death, unfatal MI at 6 months.
Abbreviations: CABG = coronary artery bypass graft; CAD = coronary arterial disease; ECG = electrocardiogram; MI = myocardial infarction; MR = mitral regurgitation; MV = millivolt; NTG = nitroglycerin; PCI = percutaneous coronary intervention.

ST-segment deviation, new bundle branch block, proximal or mid-LAD (left anterior descending coronary artery) occlusion, aspirin use at the time of AMI, elevated C-reactive protein, diabetes mellitus, prior myocardial infarction or prior coronary artery bypass grafting, concomitant peripheral vascular disease, and underlying renal insufficiency. The thrombolysis in myocardial infarction (TIMI) risk scores for STEMI and NSTEMI are prognostically useful (Tables 3 and 4). Intermediate-risk UA patients may be risk stratified over 6 to 9 hours with serial biomarkers and an exercise ECG. If biomarkers become positive or the stress test is positive, the patient should be admitted. If negative, the patient should be dismissed with follow-up in 72 hours for re-evaluation and coronary artery disease (CAD) risk factor modification.

Treatment

The goals of initial treatment of patients presenting with AMI are:

- Obtain intravenous (IV) access and stabilize hemodynamics if unstable.

- Relieve ischemic discomfort using IV morphine and sublingual or IV nitroglycerin.
- Minimize myocardial oxygen supply-and-demand mismatch with IV β-blockers (goal: heart rate less than 70 beats per minute as blood pressure tolerates) and supplemental oxygen.
- Maintain or restore myocardial perfusion using aspirin and heparin (either IV unfractionated or subcutaneous low molecular weight).

Patients with STEMI should receive prompt reperfusion therapy (thrombolysis or primary percutaneous intervention). Table 5 outlines the recommended dosing regimens of medications commonly used in ACS.

Aspirin

All patients presenting with a proved or suspected AMI should receive 324 mg of aspirin (four 81 mg tablets chewed and swallowed or as a rectal suppository if unable to take orally) and continue at 81 mg daily thereafter. Aspirin significantly reduces mortality in AMI. In patients with STEMI, aspirin reduces mortality to a similar extent as thrombolytic therapy, with additive

TABLE 3 TIMI Risk Score for Unstable Angina/Non-ST-Segment-Elevation Myocardial Infarction

One point for each of the following:	Score	Risk of Adverse Event*
Age ≥65 y	0/1	4.7%
Presence of ≥3 CV risk factors[†]	2	8.3%
Recent (<24 h) severe angina	3	13.2%
Known coronary stenosis ≥50%	4	19.9%
ST-segment deviation on admission ECG ≥0.5 mm	5	26.2%
Use of aspirin within past 7 d	6/7	40.9%
Elevated biomarkers of cardiac injury (troponin, CK-MB)		

*Death, MI, or urgent revascularization within 14 days.
[†]Family history of premature coronary artery disease, hypertension, hyperlipidemia, diabetes mellitus, active smoker.
Abbreviations: CV = cardiovascular; ECG = electrocardiogram.

Rakel and Bope: *Conn's Current Therapy 2006.*

TABLE 4 TIMI Risk Score for ST-Segment-Elevation Myocardial Infarction

Risk factor	Points	Score	30-Day Mortality (%)
Age ≥75 y	3	0	0.8
Age 65-74 y	2	1	1.6
Systolic BP <100 mm Hg	3	2	2.2
Heart rate >100 beats/min	2	3	4.4
Killip class >1	2	4	7.3
Anterior MI or LBBB	1	5	12.4
Diabetes mellitus, HTN, or angina	1	6	16.1
Weight <67 kg	1	7	23.4
Symptom onset to treatment >4 h	1	8	26.8
		>8	35.9

Abbreviations: BP = blood pressure; HTN = hypertension; LBBB = left bundle branch block; MI = myocardial infarction.

benefits of both. Aspirin-allergic patients should receive 300 mg of clopidogrel (Plavix).

Clopidogrel

Clopidogrel (Plavix) blocks the platelet ADP receptor and can be given in place of aspirin in aspirin-allergic patients. A 300-mg loading dose is administered with 75 mg daily administered thereafter. Clopidogrel is as efficacious as aspirin in AMI. Clopidogrel is beneficial in those undergoing primary percutaneous intervention for STEMI. Clopidogrel in addition to aspirin, compared with aspirin alone, reduces the risk of cardiovascular death, myocardial infarction, or stroke in patients with NSTEMI who do not undergo percutaneous revascularization (CURE [Clopidogrel in Unstable Angina to Prevent Recurrent Events] trial) and in those who do undergo percutaneous revascularization (PCI-CURE [Percutaneous Coronary Intervention-Clopidogrel in Unstable Angina to Prevent Recurrent Ischemic Events] and CREDO [Clopidogrel for the Reduction of Events During Observation] trials). The decision to give clopidogrel prior to coronary angiography in patients with AMI should take into account the ultimate requirement of coronary artery bypass graft (CABG) in some patients, which would delay CABG for 5 to 7 days following the administration of clopidogrel. Clopidogrel, 75 mg daily, should be continued for at least 6 and preferably 12 months following percutaneous coronary revascularization in the setting of AMI. If coronary angiography is not anticipated, clopidogrel should be initiated and also continued for 9 to 12 months. A recent study suggests

TABLE 5 Dosage of Medications Commonly Used in the Treatment of Myocardial Infarction

Medication	Dosing and administration
Aspirin	• 324 mg chewed and swallowed (81 mg × 4) upon presentation, then 81 to 325 mg daily. • If unable to take PO, crush and administer via NG tube or as 325-mg rectal suppository.
Clopidogrel (Plavix)	• 300-mg oral loading dose, then 75 mg PO daily for 9 to 12 mo or indefinitely in high-risk patients.
Heparin	
• IV unfractionated	• 60 U/kg IV bolus (max: 5000 U), then 12 U/kg/h (max: 1000 U/h) for 48 h or PCI (goal aPTT 1.5 = 2.5 × control).
• Low-molecular-weight Enoxaparin (Lovenox)	• 1 mg/kg SC Q12 h for 48 to 72 h or until PCI. Initial 30-mg IV bolus can be given.
(Dalteparin (Fragmin)	• 120 IU/kg SC (max 10,000 IU) Q12 h.
β-Blockers	
• Metoprolol (Lopressor)	• 5 mg IV Q5 min × 3 to goal heart rate 60-65/min or hypotension, then 50 mg PO Q12 h.
• Atenolol (Tenormin)	• 5 mg IV Q5 min × 3 to goal heart rate 60-65/min or hypotension, then 50-100 mg PO daily.
• Esmolol (Brevibloc)	• 500 µg/kg IV bolus, then 50 µg/kg/min titrating to HR.
Nitroglycerin	0.4 mg sublingual Q5 min × 3 for persistent ischemic pain or IV infusion starting at 5-10 µg/min with up titration for persistent ischemic pain.
Morphine sulfate	4 to 6 mg IV; repeat as needed.
GP IIb/IIIa inhibitors	
• Eptifibatide (Integrelin)	• 180 µg/kg IV bolus, then infuse at 2.0 µg/kg/min × 72 h to 96 h
• Tirofiban (Aggrastat)	• 0.4 µg/kg/min IV for 30 min, then 0.1 µg/kg/min × 48 to 96 h
• Abciximab (ReoPro)	• Use ony if PCI planned or likely; 0.25 mg/kg bolus followed by infusion at 0.125 µg/kg/min (max 10 µg/min) for 12 to 24 h.

Abbreviations: IV = intravenous; HR = heart rate; NG = nasogastric; PCI = percutaneous coronary intervention; PO = by mouth; SC = subcutaneous.

Rakel and Bope: *Conn's Current Therapy 2006.*

that clopidogrel imparts incremental benefit when given in combination with thrombolytic therapy in the setting of STEMI.

Heparin

Patients presenting with AMI should be treated with either IV unfractionated heparin (IVUFH) (60 IU/kg bolus, then 12 IU/kg per hour infusion) or subcutaneous low-molecular-weight heparin (LMWH), except for STEMI patients receiving streptokinase. In STEMI, IVUFH is required to maintain vessel patency in those receiving a fibrin-specific thrombolytic agent (alteplase, reteplase, and tenecteplase). The use of LMWH in combination with thrombolytic therapy is still being evaluated in clinical trials and is not currently recommended. Administration of LMWH reduces the risk of death and ischemic events compared with IVUFH in patients with NSTEMI and in unstable angina when high-risk features are present (see Table 2). LMWH appears safe when continued up until the time of coronary angiography and percutaneous intervention; however, individual PCI operator preference should be taken into account. LMWH should not be given to patients with significant renal insufficiency (creatinine clearance less than 30 mL per minute) or morbid obesity.

β-Blockers

β-Blockers should be given to all patients presenting with AMI unless hypotension, bradycardia, or other contraindications exist. Metoprolol (Lopressor) or atenolol (Tenormin), 5 mg IV, should be given every 3 to 5 minutes to achieve a resting heart rate of less than 70 beats per minute (bpm). Oral metoprolol (Lopressor) or atenolol (Tenormin) should then be administered 30 minutes following the last IV dose and continued indefinitely. β-Blockers reduce oxygen supply-and-demand mismatch in the setting of AMI by lowering heart rate, reducing myocardial contractility, and reducing afterload through systemic blood pressure reduction. In addition to reducing mortality in AMI, β-blockers also reduce the risk of atrial and ventricular arrhythmias and free wall rupture. If a patient's tolerance of β-blockers is uncertain, short-acting IV esmolol (Brevibloc) may be used initially.

Nitroglycerin

Nitroglycerin can be administered as a sublingual formulation or as an IV infusion and is given if symptoms of ongoing myocardial ischemia persist. Nitroglycerin does not improve prognosis in AMI and should be used with caution in patients with right ventricular infarction that could result in hypotension. Nitroglycerin should not be administered to patients who have taken Viagra or other phosphodiesterase inhibitor within 24 hours.

Glycoprotein IIb/IIIa inhibitors

Glycoprotein (GP) IIb/IIIa inhibitors block the GP IIb/IIIa platelet receptor, which functions as the receptor

for fibrinogen adherence. GP IIb/IIIa inhibitors reduce ischemic complications associated with PCI and should be administered in patients for whom an early invasive strategy is planned. It is not clear if upstream GP IIb/IIIa administration upon admission is superior to initiation in the catheterization laboratory just prior to PCI. Benefit is shown with eptifibatide (Integrilin) and tirofiban (Aggrastat) in patients with non-ST-elevation ACS who do not undergo early PCI. This benefit appears isolated to high-risk patients including those with troponin elevation, ST-segment depression more than 0.5 mV, diabetes mellitus, and LV ejection fraction less than 40%. Post hoc analyses suggest a potential differential benefit of GP IIb/IIIa therapy in men versus women, and it is an area of continued investigation.

REPERFUSION THERAPY IN ST-SEGMENT-ELEVATION MYOCARDIAL INFARCTION

Patients presenting with STEMI represent a true medical emergency and require accurate, yet expeditious evaluation and treatment directed at reperfusion of ischemic myocardium. Regardless of the modality of reperfusion used, the time from symptom onset to establishment of myocardial reperfusion is the strongest predictor of myocardial salvage, recovery of myocardial function, and reperfusion-mediated improvements in mortality. Patients receiving successful reperfusion within 2 hours of symptom onset derive the greatest benefit from reperfusion therapy.

Thrombolysis

Thrombolytic therapy is the most commonly utilized method of reperfusion worldwide. The fibrin-specific t-PA derived thrombolytic agents (alteplase [Activase], reteplase [Retavase], and tenecteplase [TNKase]) have proven superior but significantly more expensive than the fibrin-nonspecific agents such as streptokinase. The fibrin-specific agents reduce 30-day mortality rates by 15% compared with streptokinase and appear to provide similar rates of successful reperfusion and mortality reduction. They differ primarily in the manner in which they are given and subsequently the ease of administration (Table 6). Clinically, successful thrombolysis is associated with resolution of chest symptoms and reduction of ST-segment elevation by at least 50%. Patients with persistent symptoms, persistence of ST-segment elevation, and/or hemodynamic instability following thrombolysis should be referred for emergent coronary angiography. The absence of contraindications to thrombolytic therapy should be assured prior to administration (Box 1).

The benefit of routine predischarge coronary angiography in all patients with apparent successful thrombolysis is not substantiated in clinical trials. Many PCI-capable centers, however, do routinely perform coronary angiography following successful thrombolysis to better delineate coronary anatomy and evaluate for multivessel obstructive coronary disease. Patients who successfully reperfuse following thrombolysis and do not undergo in-hospital coronary angiography should undergo a submaximal exercise stress test or pharmacologic stress

TABLE 6 Thrombolytic Agents

Thrombolytic	Dosing/administration	Fibrin specific
Alteplase (t-PA) (Activase)	15 mg IV bolus, then 0.75 mg/kg over 30 min (max 50 mg), then 0.5 mg/kg over 60 min (max 35 mg)	Yes
Reteplase (rPA) (Retevase)	10 U IV bolus over 2 min then second 10-U IV bolus 30 min later	Yes
Tenecteplase (TNK) (TNKase)	0.5 mg/kg single IV bolus (max 50 mg), or weight <60 kg, 30 mg; 60-69 kg, 35 mg; 70-79 kg, 40 mg; 80-89 kg, 45 mg; ≥90 kg, 50 mg	Yes
Streptokinase (Streptase)	1.5 million U IV over 60 min	Yes

Abbreviation: IV = intravenous.

test prior to hospital discharge. Patients with an abnormal predischarge stress test, recurrent symptoms, or ECG changes, and those with an LV ejection fraction less than 40%, should undergo coronary angiography with PCI as warranted prior to discharge.

Early Invasive Versus Conservative Therapy in Unstable Angina/Non-ST-Segment-Elevation Myocardial Infarction

Patients with NSTEMI usually do not have complete occlusion of the culprit coronary artery. Thus emergent revascularization is generally not indicated except in patients with hemodynamic instability or persistent symptoms despite initial medical therapy. Whether or not patients with UA/NSTEMI benefit from an early invasive approach (i.e., routine coronary angiography and PCI as indicated during hospitalization) was evaluated in three studies using modern antithrombotic/

BOX 1 Contraindications for Thrombolytic Administration

Absolute
- Prior intracranial hemorrhage
- Ischemic stroke within prior 3 mo
- Ongoing active bleeding (not including menses)
- Significant head injury or facial trauma within 3 mo
- Possible or suspected aortic dissection
- Intracranial neoplasm
- Intracranial vascular structural abnormality

Relative
- Recent internal bleeding (within 4 wk)
- Major surgery within 3 wk
- History of ischemic stroke
- Traumatic or prolonged (>10 min) CPR
- Pregnancy
- Current use of warfarin (Coumadin) with INR >2.0
- Noncompressible vascular puncture
- Significant hypertension on presentation (SBP >180 mm Hg or DBP >110 mm Hg)
- History of chronic, severe, poorly controlled hypertension
- Active peptic ulcer disease
- Prior streptokinase exposure (for repeat streptokinase administration)

Abbreviations: CPR = cardiopulmonary resuscitation; DBP = diastolic blood pressure; INR = international normalized ratio; SBP = systolic blood pressure.

antiplatelet therapy and current PCI technology. The FRISC II (Fragmin and Fast Revascularization During Instability in Coronary Artery Disease), TAC-TICS-TIMI 18 (Treat Angina With Aggrastat and Determine Cost of Therapy With Invasive or Conservative Strategy-Thrombolysis in Myocardial Infarction), and RITA 3 (Randomized Intervention Trial of Unstable Angina 3) trials demonstrate improved outcomes with an early invasive strategy in intermediate- and high-risk patients with unstable angina and in patients with NSTEMI. In response to the accumulating data demonstrating a benefit from an early invasive approach using contemporary medical management and modern interventional techniques, the ACC/AHA guidelines now recommend an early invasive approach in patients with NSTEMI.

ELECTRICAL COMPLICATIONS ASSOCIATED WITH ACUTE MYOCARDIAL INFARCTION

Conduction abnormalities are common in patients with AMI and should be assessed in all patients. Ischemia-mediated alterations in cardiac conduction can manifest as AV block (first, second, and third degree), bundle branch block, and fascicular block. Conduction abnormalities at the AV node level in the setting of inferior AMI are usually transient and usually do not require transvenous pacing, even in the setting of high-grade AV block. AV block as well as new bundle branch block in patients with anterior STEMI portends a worse prognosis and is associated with a high risk of progression to complete heart block. Temporary transvenous pacing should be considered in those with anterior myocardial infarction (MI) and Mobitz 2 AV block, third-degree AV block, or new left bundle-branch block (LBBB).

Ventricular fibrillation can complicate myocardial infarction and should be treated promptly with unsynchronized electrical shock as per current ACLS guidelines. Table 7 lists recommendations for the approach and treatment of ventricular tachycardia in the setting of AMI.

ADJUNCTIVE THERAPY/HOSPITAL DISCHARGE MEDICATIONS

Aspirin, 81 mg to 325 mg, should be continued indefinitely in all ACS patients. An angiotensin-converting enzyme inhibitor (ACEI) should be started within

TABLE 7 Treatment of Ventricular Arrhythmias Associated With Acute Myocardial Infarction

Arrhythmia	Electrical shock*	Other therapeutic measures
Sustained polymorphic VT	Yes, 200 J, 300 J, 360 J	As per current ACLS recommendations Normalize electrolyte abnormalities
Sustained monomorphic VT: with symptoms or hemodynamic compromise	Yes, 100, 200, 300, 360	As per current ACLS recommendations
Sustained monomorphic VT: without symptoms or hemodynamic compromise	No	Amiodarone (Cordarone), 150 mg IV infused over 10 min, then 360 mg over 6 h (1 mg/min) then 540 mg over 18 h (0.5 mg/min) (max 2.2 g over 24 h)
Nonsustained VT (within 48 h of MI)	No	No treatment recommended unless symptomatic or associated with hemodynamic compromise
Nonsustained VT (>48 h following MI)	No	Electrophysiology study with programmed stimulation. If sustained VT inducible, then insertion of AICD.
Accelerated idioventricular rhythm	No	None

Abbreviations: ACLS = Advanced Cardiac Life Support; AICD = Automatic Implantable Cardioverter Defribrillator; MI = myocardial infarction; VT = ventricular tachycardia.
*Energy is for monophasic defibrillators.

24 hours in all hemodynamically stable patients with large anterior infarctions and in patients with LV ejection fraction less than 40%. We prefer starting with a short-acting ACEI such as captopril (Capoten), 3.125 mg by mouth every 8 hours, with titration upward as tolerated. Upon discharge, a longer acting ACEI can be substituted. Statin therapy in the setting of ACS improves short- and long-term outcomes and should be initiated before discharge in all ACS patients regardless of cholesterol levels. The recent PROVE-IT (Pravastatin or Atorvastatin Evaluation and Infection Therapy) trial showed that intensive statin therapy (mean LDL [low-density lipoprotein]: 62 mg/dL) following ACS reduces adverse cardiac events compared with less intensive statin therapy (mean LDL: 95 mg/dL). All patients with ACS should be discharged on a β-blocker unless a contraindication exists. One randomized trial (COMET [Carvedilol Or Metoprolol European Trial]) suggests that carvedilol (Coreg) at optimal doses is superior to short-acting metoprolol tartrate (Lopressor) in patients with symptomatic chronic heart failure and LV ejection fraction of less than 35%.

CURRENT DIAGNOSIS

Acute myocardial infarction is defined as the typical rise and fall of cardiac troponin or creatine kinase myocardial band in addition to one of the following:
- Symptoms consistent with myocardial ischemia
- Electrocardiogram changes indicating myocardial ischemia (ST-segment depression or elevation)
- New pathologic Q waves
- Percutaneous coronary intervention

CARDIAC REHABILITATION/SECONDARY PREVENTION/RISK FACTOR MODIFICATION

All patients should undergo cardiovascular risk factor assessment and modification during and following hospitalization. Blood pressure readings should ideally be lower than 120/80 mm Hg. Smoking cessation should be addressed and glycemic control optimized in diabetic patients. Patients should be instructed on an AHA step II low-fat diet, and statin therapy should be initiated and/or modified to achieve an LDL lower than 70 mg/dL. The goal of cardiac rehabilitation is to help the patient safely return to and maintain normal daily activities and promote secondary prevention measures. This generally includes a staged approach with patients attending monitored exercise sessions for the first 6 to 8 weeks following MI during which levels of exercise are gradually increased. Following an uncomplicated MI, patients are instructed to return to work in 14 to 28 days, with driving allowed within 7 to 14 days. Patients with complicated MI, including those with significant ventricular arrhythmias, require a more gradual return to normal daily activities.

HOSPITAL FOLLOW-UP VISIT

Patients should generally be seen in follow-up between 3 and 6 weeks following hospital discharge. They should be evaluated for recurrence of symptoms, evidence of heart failure, and medication intolerance or noncompliance. Medications should be reviewed individually and the rationale for each discussed. Modification of cardiovascular risk factors should continue. A transthoracic echocardiogram should be obtained to assess LV function 4 to 6 weeks following discharge. Patients with an LVEF of less than 30% should be considered for prophylactic internal defibrillator insertion. Patients with an LVEF between 31% and 40% should undergo 48-hour

The Cardiovascular System

5

 CURRRENT THERAPY

- All patients with suspected AMI should immediately receive aspirin, 324 mg chewed and swallowed, with subsequent administration of β-blockers, heparin, and nitrates as indicated.
- Administration of adjuvant antithrombotic therapy using low molecular weight heparin, clopidogrel, and GP IIb/IIIa inhibitors should be used in high-risk patients including those with NSTEMI.
- Those with STEMI should receive either thrombolysis (if within 12 hours of symptom onset) or undergo emergent primary percutaneous intervention (if within 24 hours of symptom onset).
- Patients with NSTEMI and those with unstable angina with high-risk features benefit from an early invasive treatment strategy that includes coronary angiography and percutaneous coronary intervention as warranted.
- Patients younger than age 75 years presenting with AMI and cardiogenic shock should preferentially undergo emergent coronary angiography with percutaneous coronary intervention.

Abbreviations: AMI = acute myocardial infarction; GP = glycoprotein; MI = myocardial infarction; NSTEMI = non-ST-segment-elevation myocardial infarction; STEMI = ST-segment-elevation myocardial infarction.

Holter monitoring with subsequent referral to an electrophysiologist if nonsustained ventricular tachycardia (VT) is present.

REFERENCES

Antman EM, Anbe DT, Armstrong PW, Bates ER, et al: ACC/AHA guidelines for the management of patients with ST-elevation myocardial infarction: A report of the American College of Cardiology/American Heart Association Task Force on Practice Guidelines, 2004. Available at www.acc.org/clinical/guidelines/stemi/index.pdf

Boersma E, Harrington RA, Moliterno DJ, et al: Platelet glycoprotein IIb/IIIa inhibitors in acute coronary syndromes: A meta-analysis of all major randomized clinical trials. Lancet 2002;359:189-198.

Braunwald E, Antman EM, Beasley JW, Califf RM, et al: ACC/AHA 2002 guideline update for the management of patients with unstable angina and non-ST-segment elevation myocardial infarction: Summary article: A report of the American College of Cardiology/American Heart Association Task Force on Practice Guidelines (Committee on the Management of Patients with Unstable Angina). J Am Coll Cardiol 2002;40:1366-1374.

Cannon CP, Weintraub WS, Demopoulos LA, et al: Comparison of early invasive and conservative strategies in patients with unstable coronary syndromes treated with the glycoprotein IIb/IIIa inhibitor tirofiban. N Engl J Med 2001;344:1879-1887.

Cohen M, Demers C, Gurfinkel EP, et al: A comparison of low-molecular-weight heparin with unfractionated heparin for unstable coronary artery disease. Efficacy and Safety of Subcutaneous Enoxaparin in Non-Q-Wave Coronary Events Study Group. N Engl J Med 1997; 337:447-452.

Fox KA, Poole-Wilson PA, Henderson RA, et al: Interventional versus conservative treatment for patients with unstable angina or non-ST-elevation myocardial infarction: The British Heart Foundation RITA 3 randomised trial. Randomized intervention trial of unstable angina. Lancet 2002;360:743-751.

Hochman JS, Sleeper LA, Webb JG, et al: Early revascularization in acute myocardial infarction complicated by cardiogenic shock. N Engl J Med 1999;341:625-634.

Schwartz GG, Olsson AG, Ezekowitz MD, et al: Effects of atorvastatin on early recurrent ischemic events in acute coronary syndromes: The MIRACL study: A randomized controlled trial. JAMA 2001; 285:1711-1718.

Yusuf S, Zhao F, Mehta SR, et al: Effects of clopidogrel in addition to aspirin in patients with acute coronary syndromes without ST-segment elevation. N Engl J Med 2001;345:494-502.

Acute Pericarditis

Method of
Ralph Shabetai, MD

A common cause of acute pericarditis is viral infection. In many cases, even exhaustive investigation fails to disclose the cause, and clinicians generally do not include viral studies in their evaluation. Thus, for practical purposes, viral and idiopathic forms of pericarditis are considered the same, so treatment is also the same. Acute pericarditis may conveniently be divided into simple and complicated (Box 1). Antiviral therapy has yet to find a place in the treatment of acute pericarditis; therefore treatment of simple pericarditis comprises anti-inflammatory and analgesic agents. Treatment of complicated pericarditis requires, in addition, recognition and management of the etiology and treatment of complications such as persistent pericardial effusion, cardiac tamponade, tuberculosis, or purulent infection, discussed later.

Simple Pericarditis

Simple pericarditis frequently is a benign condition that often affects the relatively young and responds quickly to simple treatment. Hospital admission is unnecessary, provided the patient can be observed closely as an outpatient for the ensuing several days and at decreasing intervals thereafter. Furthermore, detailed evaluation to determine etiology or to exclude other conditions,

---

BOX 1 Features Suggesting Acute Pericarditis Require Hospital Admission

- Persisting large pericardial effusion
- Cardiac tamponade, elevated jugular pressure
- Suspected purulent pericardial effusion
- Tuberculous pericarditis, known or suspected
- Failure to respond promptly to anti-inflammatory treatment
- Large pericardial effusion in end-stage renal disease or dialyzed patients
- Traumatic pericardial effusion

---

such as ischemic heart disease, is not justified. Nonsteroidal agents should be employed. Steroid treatment is not only unnecessary but invites complications. The choice of agent can be left to the practitioner and often is influenced by the patient's prior experience with this class of drug. Although newer nonsteroidal agents are often recommended by so-called experts, evidence that they are more effective than aspirin is lacking. Very few patients should be treated with expensive COX-2 (isoform of cyclooxygenase) drugs in view of recent evidence that they increase the risk of cardiovascular death, especially in subjects at high risk for coronary arterial heart disease.

Aspirin should be started at a high dose (e.g., 1 g three or four times daily for a week or 10 days). Ibuprofen (Motrin), starting with 800 to 1200 mg three times daily, or indomethacin (Indocin), starting with 50 mg three times daily, is an acceptable alternative. Whichever drug is selected, resolution of chest pain, ST elevation and PR depression, and fever should be anticipated within 48 hours or less. After 2 weeks, the dose can be halved, tapered over the ensuing 2 to 4 weeks, and then stopped. If the patient relates gastric intolerance to these drugs or a history of gastrointestinal problems, prophylaxis with a mucosal protective agent such as omeprazole (Prilosec), 20 mg, or misoprostol (Cytotec), 100 to 200 μg four times daily, with food, is prescribed.

Complex and High-Risk Acute Pericarditis

Most patients who are diagnosed with complex and high-risk acute pericarditis (see Box 1) should be admitted to the hospital for close observation, including, where indicated, hemodynamic monitoring. Many, perhaps the majority, do not have idiopathic or viral pericarditis; therefore, a thorough search for the etiology is required. Patients who fail to respond to anti-inflammatory immunosuppressive treatment after 24 hours should be treated as cases of complicated acute pericarditis.

RECURRENT PERICARDITIS

In 20% to 30% of cases, acute pericarditis recurs. The recurrences may be single or multiple and occur soon after the initial episode or after months or years. It is considered an autoimmune phenomenon. Pain is often severe and tries the patience of patient and practitioner alike. The patient should be informed the illness is not another infection, long-term sequelae are rare, and recurrences eventually cease. As with the initial episode, every effort should be made to avoid treatment with prednisone, but resort to steroidal treatment cannot always be avoided. When prednisone must be given, the starting dose, 1 to 2 mg/kg/day, is maintained for approximately 3 weeks, after which it is tapered by 5 mg every 3 days. If another recurrence is diagnosed, the patient is returned to the lowest dose that suppressed pericardial pain and maintained there for 3 weeks, after which tapering is attempted again. Patients who

require long or repeated courses of high-dose prednisone should have bone density monitored. A nonsteroidal anti-inflammatory drug (NSAID) should be given as well. Some reports claim that colchicine, 1 mg daily, facilitates avoidance of and weaning from prednisone. After multiple recurrences over a period of years, some patients report recurrence of pain, but all objective evidence of pericarditis is absent. Although the explanation is not clear, these patients should be treated for pain, often with help from a pain clinic.

PURULENT PERICARDITIS

Patients with purulent pericarditis are very sick, often with multisystem disease, and they frequently are already in an intensive care unit before the diagnosis is suspected. The correct diagnosis is often missed or made too late. A high index of suspicion is the key to improving this situation. Mortality is alarmingly high, even in the antibiotic era. Any reasonable suspicion of purulent pericarditis mandates exploration of the pericardium via pericardiocentesis or surgery. When the diagnosis is confirmed, an infectious disease specialist and a cardiac surgeon must immediately be added to the treating team. When thick pus is found, and especially if adhesions and organization of the effusion are present, surgical drainage is usually optimal. Cardiologists should defer to the infectious disease specialist for both identification and classification of the infecting organism and direction of the antibiotic regimen, whether it is supplementary to surgical treatment or the primary modality. The sooner in the course that treatment is begun and the more thorough its supervision, the less likely the infection is to proceed to constrictive pericarditis.

TUBERCULOUS PERICARDITIS

Clues to the correct diagnosis of tuberculous pericarditis include immunosuppressed patients, especially those with AIDS, immigrants from countries where the prevalence of tuberculosis is high, failure to respond to NSAID therapy, patient contact with known cases, and a recent conversion to a positive tuberculin test. Pericardial effusion is present in the majority. The effusion may be large and can cause cardiac tamponade. Treatment of large or persistent pericardial effusion and cardiac tamponade is reviewed later. Samples should be taken for microscopic examination, culture, and, where suspicion is high, polymerase chain reaction (PCR). In view of the emergence of resistant strains of *Mycobacterium tuberculosis*, and the possibility of infection by mimics such as the bacillus of avian tuberculosis, a cardiologist and an infectious disease specialist ideally should also participate in management.

A recommended regimen for adults comprises isoniazid (Rifamate) (300 mg daily), rifampin (Rifadin) (600 mg daily), pyrazinamide (15 to 30 mg/kg daily to a total of 2 g/day), and either ethambutol (Myambutol) (15 to 25 mg/kg/day), or streptomycin (20 to 40 mg/kg up to 1 gram/day). After 8 weeks treatment is only with isoniazid and rifampin daily or twice weekly. If the twice-weekly regimen is selected, drug administration should be monitored. Empirical treatment for suspected tubercular pericarditis is seldom warranted but may be appropriate in immunosuppressed patients. The acute phase frequently leads to effusive-constrictive pericarditis and subsequent constrictive pericarditis. Prednisone is thought to lessen the chance of this complication.

Pericardial Effusion

Any pericarditis can cause pericardial effusion, and any effusion may cause cardiac tamponade. The volume of effusion varies from small to massive. Not all effusions need specific treatment. Examples are small effusion during acute viral pericarditis and small effusion during acute myocardial infarction.

Management of a large chronic pericardial effusion, *not compromising hemodynamics* and for which the cause cannot be elucidated, is tailored to the patient's circumstances and the physician's preferences. Treatment can be expectant, but it is critically important that the primary care physician following the case be skilled in detecting the early signs of tamponade. In practice, this generally means the patient is referred to a cardiologist. The patient must be highly reliable, keep medical appointments faithfully, and not travel frequently or for long periods to places where state-of-the-art cardiology is not readily accessible; otherwise, pericardiectomy is the safest option. The patient is followed for increase in jugular pressure and other signs of tamponade, which, when found and if at least of moderate severity, calls for removal of pericardial fluid. Should the effusion recur after one or two extensive draining procedures, pericardiectomy is a reasonable option.

Cardiac Tamponade

Normal pericardial pressure is zero or a few mm Hg lower. Cardiac tamponade is the result of pericardial effusion that creates a significant increase in pericardial pressure, thereby impairing diastolic filling. The increase in pericardial pressure ranges from 3 to 10 to as much as 40 or more mm Hg. Diastolic function is impaired in direct proportion to the severity of this abnormal constraint on chamber filling and compliance. Pericardial pressure of approximately 7 mm Hg denotes mild tamponade. Often pericardiocentesis is not indicated for mild tamponade, but the patient should be observed and, in cases of borderline severity, monitored until it is clear the situation is stable. Many such cases respond to NSAIDs.

Severe tamponade, pericardial pressure of 15 to 40 mm Hg, may be acute, in which case the effusion is *small* because the normal pericardium is extremely stiff and quickly limits the volume of effusion and fiercely resists distension in the face of a rapid effusion of fluid or blood. For the same reason, aspiration of a small amount of fluid dramatically improves the patient

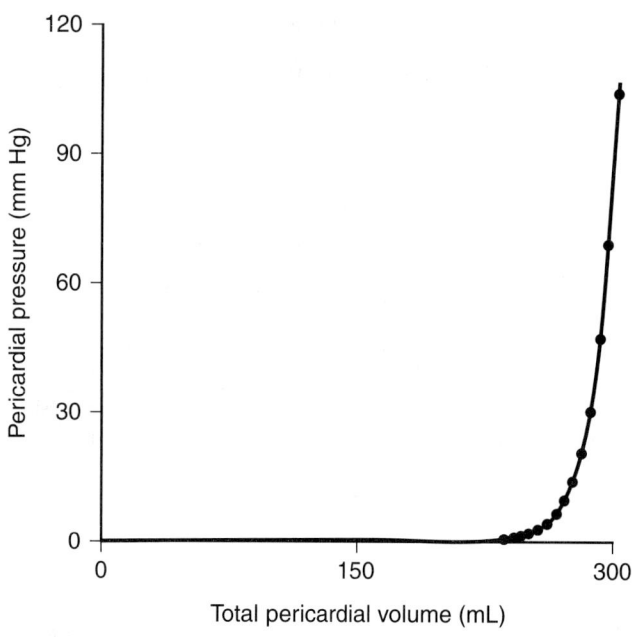

FIGURE 1. Pericardial pressure-volume curve of normal canine pericardium. The volume does not begin at zero because the volume of the heart has been added. The curve was constructed by infusing fluid into the pericardium. Its J shape shows the pericardium is compliant when slightly stretched but rapidly loses compliance and resists with increasing pressure any attempt to increase its volume. Removing a small volume of fluid produces dramatic relief.

(Figure 1). When tamponade is not acute, the elevation of pericardial pressure can be just as high as it is in acute tamponade. The effusion varies enormously in size, depending on the rate at which the effusion has accumulated, because over weeks or months, the pericardium remodels and becomes more compliant (Figure 2). As with acute tamponade, it is the earlier aliquots of pericardial fluid aspirated that cause pericardial pressure to drop substantially, but the volume removed is much more than in acute tamponade.

Circulation cannot be maintained when pericardial pressure significantly exceeds cardiac diastolic pressures. The patient with severe tamponade (pericardial pressure 18 or more mm Hg) has severe diastolic dysfunction with dyspnea, anxiety, hypotension, and tachycardia and a profound drop of blood pressure with each inspiration (severe pulsus paradoxus). Inspection of the neck veins shows the central venous pressure identical to pericardial pressure and thus provides direct evidence of the severity of tamponade. When pericardial pressure is lowered to a nearly normal value, the symptoms and signs disappear quickly and dramatically. Pericardiocentesis for severe acute tamponade is urgent and lifesaving but hazardous, and therefore only a physician experienced in treating this syndrome should undertake it. The alternative is surgical drainage. Less severe and acute tamponade, in which the findings are often less dramatic, is treated by

Rakel and Bope: *Conn's Current Therapy 2006.*

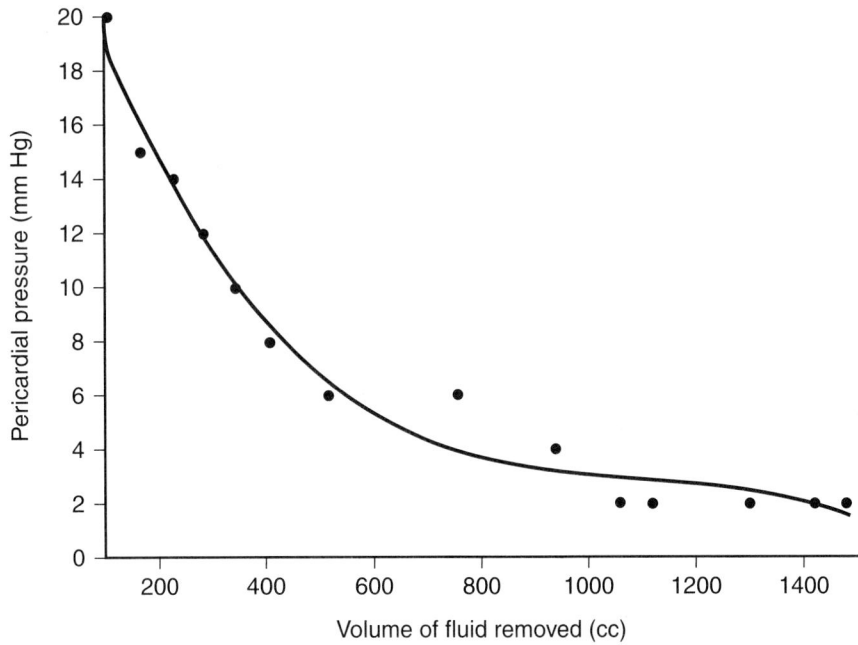

FIGURE 2. Pericardial pressure curve constructed from data obtained during pericardiocentesis of subacute cardiac tamponade. The direction of the curve is opposite from that of the normal curve, as shown in Figure 1, because fluid is being infused in the former but aspirated in the latter. Note that the pericardial pressure is severely elevated, but the volume of the effusion is much greater than could be infused into a normal pericardium. Removal of several hundred milliliters lowered pericardial pressure to 6 mm Hg. The residual effusion did not impair diastolic function.

elective pericardiocentesis. Again, only those skilled and experienced with the technique should perform the procedure unsupervised.

UREMIC- AND DIALYSIS-RELATED PERICARDIAL EFFUSION AND TAMPONADE

Preexisting heart disease and hypertension and the volume status greatly modify the findings in uremic- and dialysis-related pericardial effusion and tamponade (Table 1). Uncomplicated effusion often responds well to increased dialysis intensity. Large nonresponsive effusion may require pericardiocentesis or subxiphoid pericardiotomy.

Patients receiving dialysis may be either hypovolemic or hypervolemic. Hypovolemia is responsible for the paradox of low-pressure tamponade in which central venous pressure is normal or only modestly elevated because central pressure was very low before tamponade supervened, and thus pericardial pressure need not be very high before it compresses the heart. These patients respond to fluid infusion and subsequent pericardiocentesis. Unlike patients with classic tamponade, increased dialysis intensity *worsens* the tamponade. The correct therapeutic choice depends on accurate evaluation of the clinical and echocardiographic findings and often is beyond the scope of even highly competent primary care physicians.

TABLE 1 Tamponade in Renal Disease Compared With Typical Tamponade

Variable	Classic tamponade	Tamponade in renal disease
Jugular pressure	Elevated	May be low (low pressure tamponade)
Pulsus paradoxus	Usually present	Often absent
Diastolic pressures equalized	RA = pericardial = wedge	RA = pericardial; wedge considerably higher
Reason for atypical findings	Usually absent except in localized tamponade after cardiac surgery	BP+, LVH, CAD, dialysis shunt

Abbreviations: BP+ = hypertension; CAD = coronary artery disease; LVH = left ventricular hypertrophy; RA = right atrial pressure; wedge = pulmonary wedge pressure.

Constrictive Pericarditis

In constrictive pericarditis, cardiac volume is restrained and diastolic function impeded by a rigid, often abnormally thick, and sometimes calcified pericardium (Figure 3). As with tamponade, central venous pressure is elevated in proportion to the severity of compression. Euvolemic patients with a venous pressure less than 10 mm Hg do not need specific treatment, but they should be followed for increasing pericardial constriction. Those with venous pressure in the vicinity of 10 cm H_2O who develop edema require salt restriction and occasionally a low-dose diuretic. Those with higher venous pressure and more impressive edema are best treated by pericardiectomy. Venous pressure of 15 or more cm H_2O is often associated with anasarca and demands radical pericardiectomy. It is a mistake to treat patients with escalating doses of a diuretic. The need for a high-dose diuretic is an indication for pericardiectomy. The operative mortality in good hands has dropped to 5%.

It is critically important to distinguish anasarca caused by cirrhosis or other noncardiovascular cause from constrictive pericarditis, but all too often this distinction is not made. The clue lies in the jugular pressure. In anasarca secondary to constrictive pericarditis, pulsation of the internal jugular veins is visible to the earlobes when the patient is sitting straight up. In patients in whom it is difficult to determine the jugular pressure at the bedside, an echocardiogram quickly shows a dilated inferior vena cava when the jugular pressure is greatly elevated. In patients with anasarca not caused by cardiac or pericardial disease, jugular pressure is normal, or

CURRENT THERAPY

- Simple cases of acute and recurrent pericarditis
  Nonsteroidal anti-inflammatory drug (NSAID) treatment is used
  Steroids are used only as a last resort
  Hospital admission is not required
- Complicated cases (with tamponade and purulent infection)
  Hospital admission is required
  Etiology should be investigated
- Uremic- and dialysis-related pericardial effusion and tamponade
  Confirmation is done with echo-Doppler cardiography
  Pericardial and ventricular diastolic pressures are equally elevated
  When mild and associated with acute pericarditis (<10 cm), responds to NSAID
  In other cases: fluid should be drained, usually by pericardiocentesis
  Acute traumatic cases constitute an emergency
- Neoplastic pericardial disease
  Presentation may be tamponade
  Pericardial effusion is present, sometimes without malignant cells in fluid or pericardium
  Etiology is constrictive pericarditis
  Treatment should be individualized, with the patient, primary caregiver, and oncologist participating

nearly normal, and the size of the inferior vena cava is normal.

Patients with late-stage constrictive pericarditis with anasarca, cachexia, and atrial fibrillation are at high operative risk, and even when the operation is successfully accomplished, the outcome often is disappointing. Consideration should be given to managing them with salt restriction, larger diuretic doses, and control of the heart rate. Aspiration of pleural effusion or ascites may be a useful adjunct. The primary care physician is often ideally suited for managing these patients.

Ionizing radiation is a cause of severe constrictive pericarditis but also injures the myocardium. Thus the outcome of pericardiectomy also generally becomes less satisfactory. Physicians referring these patients for treatment should be aware of this unfortunate fact and conduct frank discussions with the cardiac surgeon and the patient's family. The characteristics of severe constrictive pericarditis are as follows:

- Heart constrained by a fibrotic or calcific rigid pericardium
- Equalized pressures, as in tamponade
- Dip and plateau ventricular diastolic pressure contour

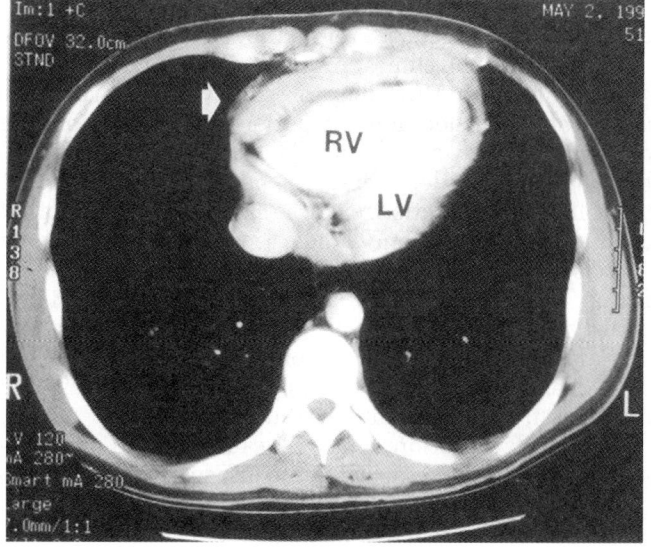

FIGURE 3. Severe constrictive pericarditis. Computed tomography (CT) shows an extremely thick pericardium caused by mesothelioma. The jugular pressure was 25 mm Hg. As in tamponade, the abnormal external restraint greatly impairs diastolic function. There is no fluid to aspirate; therefore, pericardiectomy is the only effective remedy.

Rakel and Bope: *Conn's Current Therapy 2006.*

The differential diagnosis is restrictive cardiomyopathy (e.g., cardiac amyloidosis), with these features:

- Prominent descent of venous pressure
- Pericardiectomy indicated except in mild and end stage (increased risk, poorer outcome in postradiation cases)

Neoplastic Pericardial Disease

Malignancy may cause either pericardial effusion with or without tamponade, constrictive pericarditis, or even both (effusive-constrictive pericarditis). Technical details are not relevant here. Pericardiocentesis may be required for patient comfort. The drainage catheter should be left in place until its yield is 50 mL per day to prevent recurrence. This step may also obviate the need to inject a sclerosing agent into the pericardium. In patients expected to survive several months or longer, surgical or balloon pericardiotomy is often performed when pericardial effusion recurs.

The topic of how to manage neoplastic pericardial disease is of paramount importance to family physicians. For far advanced cases with poor prognosis, it is sometimes legitimate to withhold all procedures. Left to the cardiologist, emergency room physician, or the cardiac surgeon, inappropriately radical treatment may be advised, even carried out, before the primary care physician is consulted. In patients with advanced neoplastic pericardial disease, the oncologist, but more especially the physician who best knows the patient and the family, should retain firm control to the end.

REFERENCES

Adler Y, Finkelstein Y, Guindo J, et al: Colchicine treatment for recurrent pericarditis. A decade of experience. Circulation 1998;97:218-223.

Imazio M, Demichelis B, Parrini I, et al: Day-hospital treatment of acute pericarditis: A management program for outpatient therapy. J Am Coll Cardiol 2004;43:1042.

Ling LH, Oh JK, Schaff HV, et al: Constrictive pericarditis in the modern era: Evolving clinical spectrum and impact on outcome after pericardiectomy. Circulation 1999;100:1380.

Liu G, Crump M, Goss PE, et al: Prospective comparison of the sclerosing agents doxycycline and bleomycin for the primary management of malignant pericardial effusion and cardiac tamponade. J Clin Oncol 1996;14:3141.

Maisch B, Seferovic PM, Ristic AD, et al: Guidelines on the diagnosis and management of pericardial diseases executive summary: The task force on the diagnosis and management of pericardial diseases of the European society of cardiology. Eur Heart J 2004;25:587.

Permanyer-Miralda G, Sagrista-Sauleda J, Soler-Soler J: Primary acute pericardial disease: A prospective series of 231 consecutive patients. Am J Cardiol 1985;56:623.

Rajagopalan N, Garcia MJ, Rodriguez L, et al: Comparison of new Doppler echocardiographic methods to differentiate constrictive pericardial heart disease and restrictive cardiomyopathy. Am J Cardiol 2001;87:86.

Reddy PS, Curtiss EI, Uretsky BF, et al: Spectrum of hemodynamic changes in cardiac tamponade. Am J Cardiol 1990;66:1487.

Sagrista-Sauleda J, Ange J, Permanyer-Miralda G, Soler-Soler J: Long-term follow-up of idiopathic chronic pericardial effusion. N Engl J Med 1999;341:2054.

Shabetai R: Pericardial effusion: Haemodynamic spectrum. Heart 2004;90:255.

Tsang TS, Seward JB, Barnes ME, et al: Outcomes of primary and secondary treatment of pericardial effusion in patients with malignancy. Mayo Clin Proc 2000;75:248.

Peripheral Arterial Disease

Method of
Peter C. Spittell, MD

Peripheral arterial disease (PAD), because it is most commonly caused by atherosclerosis, is a relatively common disorder in current medical practice. Occlusive and aneurysmal diseases are the most frequently encountered disorders, but less common types of arterial disease can present an interesting diagnostic challenge. Although the clinical findings of PAD are often characteristic, readily available noninvasive tests provide objective quantification of both the location and severity of the disease. Effective medical and surgical therapies for most types of PAD are widely available, further emphasizing the importance of familiarity with these diseases.

Chronic Occlusive Peripheral Arterial Disease

Because occlusive PAD is usually caused by atherosclerosis, persons with recognized cardiovascular risk factors (age greater than 70 years, male gender, tobacco use, hyperlipidemia, hypertension, and/or diabetes mellitus) are more commonly affected. An estimated 10% to 15% of persons older than age 70 years have intermittent claudication, although a significant number are not diagnosed. The lower extremities are affected more frequently than the upper extremities, and given the diffuse nature of atherosclerosis, coronary artery disease and carotid occlusive disease are also commonly present. Less common causes of intermittent claudication (post-traumatic, prior radiation therapy, vasculitis, ergotamine use) are usually apparent from the clinical history.

Patients with PAD may present with intermittent claudication, although many patients are asymptomatic or have atypical symptoms. The degree of functional limitation varies depending on the amount of stenosis, the collateral circulation, exercise capacity, and co-morbid conditions. Intermittent claudication, always induced by exercise, is a discomfort (aching, cramping, or tightness). It may involve one or both legs, and symptoms occur at a fairly constant walking distance. Relief is obtained by standing still (minutes). When more severe ischemia develops, pain at rest (ischemic rest pain) and ischemic ulceration, even with minor trauma, can occur.

Pseudoclaudication, caused by lumbar spinal stenosis, is the condition most often confused with intermittent claudication, although several clinical features help differentiate the two disorders (Table 1).

Physical examination in patients with PAD is important because a significant number of patients are asymptomatic or have atypical leg symptoms. Reduced or absent pulsation of one or more peripheral pulses is the classic physical finding in PAD, although the physical examination may be normal. Proximal arterial narrowing may

TABLE 1 Differential Diagnosis of Intermittent Claudication

	Intermittent claudication	Pseudoclaudication
Onset	Walking	Standing, walking, other
Character	Discomfort (muscular)	Paresthetic
Bilateral	±	+
Walking distance	Fairly constant	Variable
Relief	Standing still	Sit down, lean forward
Cause	Atherosclerosis	Lumbar spinal stenosis
Diagnosis	ABI pre- and postexercise	CT, MRI of lumbar spine
		Electromyography

Abbreviations: ABI = ankle-brachial index; CT = computed tomography; MRI = magnetic resonance imaging.

cause audible systolic bruits over large arteries (carotid, subclavian, aorta, and femoral arteries), and when the lumen becomes severely narrowed (more than 80% stenosis), the bruit may extend into diastole. A useful clinical estimate of the degree of lower extremity ischemia can be obtained by observing the development of pallor on elevation of the extremity and the time required for the return of color to the skin and the superficial veins to fill on dependency of the extremities after elevation (Tables 2 and 3). In the upper extremities, brachial blood pressures should be determined bilaterally to detect subclavian artery stenosis or occlusion. In the presence of a significant subclavian artery stenosis, simultaneous radial artery palpation reveals a delay in the radial pulse ipsilateral to the subclavian stenosis. The Allen test, which evaluates the circulation in the hand, and the thoracic outlet maneuvers, which uncover dynamic subclavian artery compression, are additional useful tests in patients with symptoms of upper extremity or digital arterial disease.

Noninvasive diagnosis of PAD, using supine ankle-to-brachial systolic pressure indexes (ABI [ankle-brachial index]), taken with a standard blood pressure cuff and a hand-held Doppler, ABI provides an objective measure of the severity of PAD (resting ABI: normal, more than 1.0; mild disease, 0.8 to 0.9; moderate disease, 0.5 to 0.8; severe disease, less than 0.5). ABI testing before and following exercise is the screening test of choice for patients with intermittent claudication, providing both a functional as well as semiquantitative assessment of the severity of occlusive arterial disease (Table 4).

Limitations of the ABI include noncompressible arteries (resulting in erroneously high ABI values), bilateral subclavian artery stenosis, and inability to localize arterial lesions precisely. Duplex ultrasonography can provide both anatomic and functional information regarding the location and severity of PAD and is useful if the ABI is nondiagnostic. Magnetic resonance angiography is an accurate alternative to standard angiography and useful in patients with contraindications to invasive angiography (i.e., renal insufficiency and/or severe allergy to contrast media). Angiography is indicated when surgical or endovascular intervention is warranted or when an unusual type of occlusive arterial disease is suspected. Angiography is not required to establish a diagnosis of PAD.

The overall 5-year mortality rate in patients with intermittent claudication is 29%, largely caused by complications of associated coronary artery disease and carotid artery disease. The rate for major lower extremity amputation at more than 5 years is 4%, with 55% of patients having stable or improved symptoms. Concurrent use of tobacco results in a 10-fold increase in the risk for major amputation and a greater than 2-fold increase in mortality. The effect of diabetes on patients with intermittent claudication is also significant, resulting in a 12-fold increased risk of below-knee amputation and a cumulative risk of major amputation exceeding 11%. Additional clinical features that predict an increased risk of limb loss in patients with peripheral arterial occlusive disease include ischemic rest pain, ischemic ulceration, and/or gangrene.

TABLE 2 Elevation Pallor Testing in Peripheral Arterial Disease

Grade of pallor	Duration of elevation*
0	No pallor in 60 sec
1	Pallor in 60 sec
2	Pallor in 30-60 sec
3	Pallor in less than 30 sec
4	Pallor on the level

*Elevation of the lower extremities to 60 degrees for 1 minute.

TABLE 3 Color Return and Venous Filling Time in Peripheral Arterial Disease

	Time for color return (sec)	Venous filling time (sec)
Normal	10	15
Moderate ischemia	15-20	20-30
Severe ischemia	>40	>40

Rakel and Bope: *Conn's Current Therapy 2006.*

TABLE 4 Ankle-Brachial Systolic Pressure Index (ABI) Interpretation

Disease severity	ABI (rest)	ABI (after exercise)*
Minimal	>0.9	>0.8
Mild	>0.8	>0.5
Moderate	<0.8	<0.5
Severe	<0.5	<0.2

*Treadmill exercise (2 mph, 10-degree incline, 5 min, symptom limited) or active pedal plantarflexion (50 repetitions or symptom limited).

Initial medical management of intermittent claudication involves three modalities:

1. Risk factor reduction (discontinuation of tobacco, treatment of hypertension, diabetes, and hyperlipidemia)
2. Exercise training
3. Pharmacologic therapy

In addition, weight reduction (if obese), foot care and protection, and avoidance of vasoconstrictive drugs are beneficial.

Exercise training is of significant benefit to patients with intermittent claudication. A regular walking program for patients with intermittent claudication (level ground, walking the distance to claudication, stopping to rest for relief, repeatedly for 45 to 60 minutes per session, 4 or more days a week, continued for 6 months), can result in a significant (often greater than 180%) improvement in initial claudication distance in many patients. Aspirin,[1] 81 to 325 mg per day, is effective in PAD, resulting in a decreased risk of limb loss and reduced need for vascular surgery, as well as a decreased incidence of major coronary and cerebrovascular events. Clopidogrel (Plavix),[1] 75 mg per day, is more effective than aspirin in preventing major atherosclerotic vascular events. For persons with disabling intermittent claudication who do not respond adequately to a walking program, two pharmacologic agents, pentoxifylline (Trental) and cilostazol (Pletal), may be useful. Pentoxifylline, a methylxanthine derivative, has vasoactive properties that result in the relaxation of vascular smooth muscle, a weak antithrombotic effect, and rheologic activity. Unfortunately, the beneficial effect of pentoxifylline on maximal walking distance is only modest (a 12% increase). Cilostazol, a phosphodiesterase III inhibitor, results in a more significant improvement in walking ability (an approximate doubling of initial and absolute claudication distance), compared to placebo and pentoxifylline. Cilostazol is contraindicated in patients with heart failure. Statins[1] should be considered in patients with PAD; they improve the symptoms of intermittent claudication as well as reduce the incidence of adverse cardiovascular and cerebrovascular events. Angiotensin-converting[1] enzyme inhibitors may also reduce the risk of ischemic events in patients with PAD.

[1]Not FDA approved for this indication.

Patients with PAD who have disabling symptoms, diabetes mellitus with progressive symptoms, ischemic rest pain, ischemic ulceration, and/or gangrene should be considered for revascularization (surgical or endovascular) if their general medical condition permits.

Endovascular treatment of PAD is most effective in patients with proximal arterial occlusive disease, short partial occlusions, and good distal runoff. For example, iliac artery percutaneous transluminal angioplasty (PTA) with selective stent placement has initial and long-term outcomes comparable to open surgical procedures (if distal runoff is good). PTA of femoropopliteal stenoses has an initial overall success rate of 88%, but the 2-year patency rate is only 50%. PTA of the infrapopliteal arteries may be considered in selected patients with critical limb ischemia who are not surgical candidates or to avoid amputation. Advantages of PTA over surgery include lower morbidity and mortality, shorter convalescence, lower cost, and preservation of the saphenous vein for the future. PTA in aortic or iliac disease may also allow for an infrainguinal surgical procedure to be performed at reduced perioperative risk (as compared to procedures requiring aortic cross-clamp application). Surgical therapy remains the treatment of choice for most patients with diffuse symptomatic atherosclerotic disease of the lower extremities.

Acute Arterial Occlusion

Acute arterial occlusion remains a clinical challenge. Cardiopulmonary complications cause significant morbidity and mortality, and limb loss rates are significant, underscoring the importance of early diagnosis and prompt treatment. The symptoms of acute arterial occlusion (pain, numbness, and/or coldness of the involved extremity or extremities) are usually sudden in onset (less than 5 hours). Physical findings include pallor, absent pulses, and neurologic deficits (decreased fine touch and/or motor deficits).

An embolic cause of acute arterial occlusion is suggested by the presence of cardiac disease (arrhythmia, valvular heart disease, cardiomyopathy), proximal aneurysm, and proximal atherosclerosis. Features suggesting a thrombotic cause of acute arterial occlusion include prior occlusive disease in the involved limb, occlusive disease involving other extremities, acute aortic dissection, hematologic disease, arteritis, inflammatory bowel disease, neoplasm, and drugs (ergotism, cocaine, amphetamines).

Based on the clinical examination, acute arterial disease is classified into one of three categories:

1. Viable limb without imminent threat of tissue loss
2. Threatened limb with reversible ischemia
3. Nonviable limb with irreversible ischemia

Initial treatment includes intravenous heparin and protection of the ischemic limb. Subsequent treatment varies depending on the viability of the limb and the patient's overall medical condition. If thrombolytic therapy is used initially, PTA or surgical therapy is often indicated to treat underlying stenosis, if present, to improve patency. Patients with nonviable extremities should undergo prompt amputation.

Peripheral Artery Aneurysms

Similar to PAD, arterial aneurysms are most commonly caused by atherosclerosis. Therefore, peripheral arterial aneurysms are more frequent in men and are more common in the lower extremities. Additional predisposing factors for aneurysmal disease include systemic hypertension, inherited disorders, connective tissue disease, trauma, infection, chronic obstructive pulmonary disease, and inflammatory diseases.

Most aneurysms are asymptomatic, frequently discovered incidentally during a test performed for another reason (e.g., abdominal ultrasound, computed tomography). The sensitivity of the physical examination in detecting an aneurysm depends on the location of the aneurysm. Abdominal aortic aneurysms (AAAs) are often occult on examination unless they have achieved a diameter larger than 4 cm and the patient is not obese. For this reason, a onetime screening ultrasound for AAA by ultrasonography is indicated in men age 65 to 75 years who have ever smoked. Aneurysms of the subclavian, iliac, femoral, and popliteal arteries are frequently palpable as a pulsating mass.

Complications of aneurysms include peripheral embolization, pressure on surrounding structures, infection, and rupture. Aneurysms of certain arteries develop one complication more often than others (e.g., the most common complication of aortic aneurysms is rupture, whereas embolism is a more common complication of femoral and popliteal artery aneurysms). (The article, "Acquired Diseases of the Aorta," provides additional information on AAA.)

An iliac artery aneurysm usually occurs in association with abdominal aortic aneurysm but may occur as an isolated finding. Iliac artery aneurysm may cause obstructive urologic symptoms, unexplained groin or perineal pain, iliac vein obstruction, or embolization. Computed tomography with intravenous contrast is the preferred diagnostic procedure. Surgical resection is indicated when an iliac aneurysm is causing symptoms or it exceeds 3.0 cm in diameter.

Popliteal artery aneurysms are bilateral in 50% of patients with 40% of patients having one or more aneurysms at other sites, most often the abdominal aorta. Although thromboembolism is the most common complication of popliteal artery aneurysm, venous obstruction, venous thrombosis, neuropathy, infection, and rupture (rarely) can also occur. The diagnosis is readily made with ultrasonography, but angiography is necessary prior to surgical treatment to evaluate the proximal and distal arterial circulation. Prophylactic surgery for popliteal aneurysms in asymptomatic limbs has significantly better results than surgery on limbs with ischemic symptoms, but the aneurysm size at which to recommend surgery is still not settled.

Atheroembolism, which is secondary to peripheral arterial aneurysms, is characterized by livedo reticularis, blue toes, palpable pulses, hypertension, renal insufficiency,

elevated sedimentation rate, and eosinophilia (transient). Atheroembolism may occur spontaneously or secondary to medication (warfarin or thrombolytic therapy) or angiographic or surgical procedures. Lower extremity atheroembolism is most commonly caused by an abdominal aortic aneurysm or diffuse atherosclerotic disease. In such patients, livedo reticularis and blue toes are bilateral. Unilateral blue toes suggest the embolic source is distal to the aortic bifurcation. Treatment of choice for atheroembolism is identification of the source of embolism and surgical resection, if feasible.

Uncommon Types of Peripheral Arterial Disease

The less common types of occlusive PAD include thromboangiitis obliterans (Buerger's disease), arteritides (giant cell arteritis and connective tissue disorders), extrinsic arterial compression (popliteal artery entrapment and thoracic outlet compression of the subclavian artery), and traumatic (repetitive blunt type) arterial occlusive disease in the hand. An uncommon type of occlusive PAD is suggested by occurrence in young persons; by acute, often digital, ischemia; and/or associated systemic symptoms. In connective tissue disorders, the occlusive disease is usually digital; giant cell (temporal, cranial) arteritis affects persons older than 60 years of age whose dominant symptoms are headache and those of a systemic illness; whereas Takayasu's arteritis typically affects the branches of the aortic arch of young women. In occlusive arterial disease caused by arteritis, the

 CURRENT DIAGNOSIS

- Patients with PAD are often asymptomatic or have atypical symptoms.
- Ankle-brachial index measurement detects occult PAD.
- The overall 5-year mortality rate in patients with PAD is high, largely because of complications of associated coronary artery disease and carotid artery disease.
- Angiography is not required to establish a diagnosis of PAD.
- Disabling symptoms, diabetes mellitus with symptoms, ischemic rest pain, and ischemic ulceration are indications for angiography and revascularization.
- Peripheral artery aneurysms are frequently palpable as a pulsating mass (excluding abdominal aortic aneurysm).
- Popliteal artery aneurysms are bilateral in 50% of patients, with 40% having aneurysms at other sites, most often the abdominal aorta.
- An uncommon type of occlusive arterial disease is suggested by occurrence in young persons, acute (often digital) ischemia, and/or associated systemic symptoms.

Abbreviations: PAD = peripheral arterial disease.

CURRENT THERAPY

- Medical treatment is effective in most patients with PAD.
- An antiplatelet agent should be used in all patients.
- Cardiovascular risk factor reduction is of paramount importance in PAD patients.
- Associated coronary and carotid artery diseases must be checked for and treated, if present, in PAD patients.
- Endovascular treatment is effective in proximal, focal peripheral arterial stenoses.
- Initial treatment for acute arterial occlusion includes intravenous heparin and protection of the ischemic limb.
- Intra-arterial thrombolysis or surgical treatment for acute arterial occlusion depends on the degree of ischemia and viability of the involved limb.
- Surgery for asymptomatic popliteal aneurysms has significantly better results compared to surgery in symptomatic patients.

Abbreviations: PAD = peripheral arterial disease.

frequency of limb loss depends on the severity of ischemia at the time of diagnosis and the control of the arteritis achieved. Management should include therapy of the systemic process and general measures to protect the ischemic limb. In thromboangiitis obliterans, the risk of limb loss is greater than atherosclerosis and depends mainly on the severity of the ischemia at the time of diagnosis and whether the patient stops using tobacco permanently. In chronic occlusive arterial disease caused by repetitive blunt trauma to the hand, loss of digits can occur if the cause is not recognized and corrected. Measures to protect the hand (regular use of gloves and avoiding blunt trauma) are important to prevent progression. If ischemic ulceration has already occurred, an alpha blocking agent (i.e., doxazosin (Cardura)[1] 1 mg at bedtime) or sympathectomy can be used to hasten healing and provide longer term protection of the ischemic digit. Limb or digital loss can occur with arterial compression syndromes as a result of embolization from mural thrombus that develops in the poststenotic aneurysm that chronic arterial compression can cause. The appropriate management of arterial compression syndromes is surgical relief.

REFERENCES

Peripheral Arterial Occlusive Disease
Aquino R, Johnnides C, Makaroun M, et al: Natural history of claudication: Long-term serial follow-up study of 1244 claudicants. J Vasc Surg 2001;34:962-970.
CAPRIE Steering Committee: A randomized, blinded trial of clopidogrel versus aspirin in patients at risk of ischemic events (CAPRIE). Lancet 1996;348:1329-1339.
Hiatt WR: Medical treatment of peripheral arterial disease and claudication. N Engl J Med 2001;344:1608-1621.

---

[1]Not FDA approved for this indication.

Hirsch AT, Criqui MH, Treat-Jacobson D, et al: Peripheral arterial disease detection, awareness, and treatment in primary care. JAMA 2001;286:1317-1324.
McDaniel MD, Cronenwett JL: Basic data related to the natural history of intermittent claudication. Ann Vasc Surg 1989;3:273.
McPhail IR, Spittell PC, Weston SA, Bailey KR: Intermittent claudication: An objective office-based assessment. J Am Coll Cardiol 2001;37:1381-1385.
Selvin E, Erlinger TP: Prevalence of and risk factors for peripheral arterial disease in the United States: Results from the National Health and Nutrition Examination Survey, 1999-2000. Circulation 2004;110:738.
Acute Arterial Occlusion
Ouriel K, Veth FJ, Sasahara AA, for the Thrombolysis or Peripheral Artery Surgery (TOPAS) Investigators: A comparison of recombinant urokinase with vascular surgery as initial treatment for acute arterial occlusion of the legs. N Engl J Med 1998;338:1105.
Peripheral Artery Aneurysms
U.S. Preventive Services Task Force. Screening for abdominal aortic aneurysm: Recommendation statement. Ann Int Med 2005;142:198-202.
Uncommon Types of Peripheral Arterial Disease
Olin JW: Thromboangiitis obliterans (Buerger's disease). N Engl J Med 2000;343:864-869.
Spittell PC, Spittell JA: Occlusive arterial disease of the hand due to repetitive blunt trauma: A review with illustrative cases. Int J Cardiol 1993;281-292.

Venous Thrombosis

Method of
Ali F. AbuRahma, MD, and Patrick A. Stone, MD

In 1846 Rudolph Virchow recognized that deep venous thrombosis (DVT) is associated with embolic sequelae in the lungs. Prior to the 20th century, venous ligation was the predominant therapy for DVT. Heparin was introduced in 1937, and the diagnosis and treatment of DVT continued to progress. Despite the increased awareness of this disease and improvement in prophylaxis, approximately 80 cases per 100,000 people are diagnosed annually in the United States. Approximately 600,000 patients are hospitalized yearly with a diagnosis of DVT and/or pulmonary emboli (PE). Thrombosis of the deep venous system results in fatal PE in 200,000 patients each year, and it is the leading cause of preventable in-hospital mortality. Of those patients who do not succumb to PE, continued morbidity from chronic venous insufficiency occurs in up to 66%, with at least a 5% ulceration rate during an 8-year follow-up. Health care costs are more than $2 billion each year in acute treatment alone.

Pathophysiology and Risk Factors

Virchow formulated the triad of venous stasis, endothelial injury, and hypercoagulable state. Usually two of the three inciting events are needed for venous thrombosis to occur. Evidence is accumulating that an inflammatory response is related to thrombosis by initiation or amplification. Once thrombosis occurs within a deep vein, the vein either recanalizes or scars, or the thrombus dislodges and embolizes. The most common site of DVT is in the soleal veins within the calf or behind the valve pockets. Determining those at highest risk is important in the decision to use DVT prophylaxis.

Epidemiologic findings thoroughly evaluate the recognized risk factors for developing thrombus in the deep venous system. As previously published in the *Handbook of Venous Disorders* by Gloviczki and colleagues, and modified by the American Venous Forum, the highest risk factors are age, surgery, malignancy, trauma, immobilization, previous DVT, primary hypercoagulable states, oral contraceptives, hormone therapy, and pregnancy. Multiple risk factors have an exponential rather than additive risk of developing thrombosis.

AGE

DVT occurs in both the young and the elderly. The risk with age appears to increase nearly two times for each 10 years of increasing age. The influence of age on the incidence of venous thrombosis is likely multifactorial. The number of risk factors increases with age; three or more risk factors are generally present in the small percentage of hospitalized patients who are younger than 40 years but in more than 30% of patients ages 40 years and older. Venous thrombosis is generally rare in children younger than 10 years of age and almost always is associated with recognized thrombotic risk factors. Multiple risk factors are often required to precipitate DVT in children, including spinal cord injuries, prolonged orthopedic immobilization, and hypercoagulable states.

SURGERY

The increased risk of DVT with surgery depends on the length and type of surgery (i.e., general surgery, neurosurgery, orthopedic surgery, gynecologic surgery, etc.) and the duration of postoperative immobilization. The overall incidence of DVT is approximately 20% in patients undergoing general surgical procedures, 25% for elective neurosurgical procedures, and 50% to 60% among those undergoing orthopedic procedures, such as hip fractures and hip and knee replacements. Accordingly, patients can be classified as at low, moderate, or high risk for thromboembolic complications (Table 1). Approximately 50% of postoperative lower extremity DVT cases develop at the time of surgery, with the remaining one half occurring primarily in the next several days. The risk of thromboembolic events does not end at hospital discharge, however, and may be delayed up to 6 weeks after surgery. Surgery is generally accompanied by a transient hypercoagulable state secondary to the release of tissue factor and increased plasminogen activator inhibitor levels, which are also associated with a decrease in fibrinolytic activity on the first postoperative day.

Rakel and Bope: *Conn's Current Therapy 2006.*

TABLE 1 Risk of Postoperative Deep Venous Thrombosis

Category	Characteristics
Low	Age <40 years, no other risk factors; uncomplicated abdominal/thoracic surgery; age >40 years, no other risk factors, minor elective abdominal/thoracic surgery <30 min
Moderate	Age >40 years; abdominal/thoracic surgery >30 min
High	History of recent thromboembolism; abdominal or pelvic procedure for malignancy; major lower extremity orthopedic procedure

From Hull RD, Raskob GE, Hirsh J: Prophylaxis of venous thromboembolism. Chest 1986;89(5)(Suppl):374S-383S.

MALIGNANCY

DVT may be a herald for undetected malignancy and found in up to 25% of those with idiopathic DVT. Approximately 15% of malignancies are complicated by venous thromboembolism. Carcinoma of the lung is more prevalent and considered the most common malignancy associated with venous thromboembolism, accounting for 25% of cases. An association between mucin-secreting gastrointestinal malignancy and thrombosis also is recognized. Another wide variety of malignancies is associated with DVT, including genitourinary malignancies. Thrombotic events during malignancy are likely to involve multiple factors, including the release of substances that activate coagulation. Tissue factor and cancer procoagulant, cysteine protease activator of factor X, are the primary tumor cell procoagulants; associated macrophages may also produce procoagulants as well as inflammatory cytokines. Approximately 90% of patients with malignancies have abnormal coagulation studies, including elevation of coagulation factors (e.g., fibrinogen or fibrin degradation products and thrombocytosis). In addition, the level of coagulation prohibitors (antithrombin, protein C, and protein S) may also be reduced in malignancy. Chemotherapeutic agents used for treatment of some malignancies are also associated with an increasing incidence of DVT.

TRAUMA

Trauma patients have a significantly increased risk for DVT, especially those with increased age, blood transfusions, fracture of the femur or tibia, and spinal cord injury. The prevalence of DVT among autopsied trauma patients is a reported 60% to 65%, compared with a 58% incidence in injured patients in a modern series using venography. Lower DVT rates of 4% to 20% are noted in studies using duplex ultrasonography, although many of these patients were receiving prophylaxis. Several risk factors may be responsible for a high incidence of DVT in trauma patients, including immobilization by skeletal fixation, paralysis, venous stasis in critically ill patients, mechanical injury, and central venous cannulation. Trauma patients may also be associated with hypercoagulable states following depletion of coagulation inhibitors and components of the fibrinolytic system.

IMMOBILIZATION

The longer the immobilization, the higher the risk of thrombosis. Advancing age and inactivity of the calf muscle pump exacerbates stasis in the soleal veins and behind the valve cusps. Both preoperative and postoperative immobilization are associated with an increasing incidence of DVT. The disease among stroke patients is significantly more common in paralyzed limbs than in nonparalyzed limbs. The definition of immobilization is extended to include prolonged travel, the so-called economy-class syndrome, which arises after sitting in a cramped position during extended aircraft flights. Further evidence includes PE as the second leading cause of death in those traveling.

HISTORY OF VENOUS THROMBOEMBOLISM

Approximately 25% of patients presenting with an acute DVT have a previous history of venous thrombosis. Several population-based studies demonstrate that recurrent thromboembolic events occur once in every 10 to 50 patients with a previous episode of thromboembolism, depending on age and sex. Primary hypercoagulable states appear to have a significant role in many recurrences.

PRIMARY HYPERCOAGULABLE STATES

Deficiencies of antithrombin III, protein C, and protein S can cause hypocoagulable states. Also, resistance to activated protein C (factor V Leiden) is considered the most common cause of hypercoagulable states. Overall, 40% to 50% of patients with lower extremity DVT can be characterized as thrombophilic on this basis, and a family history is associated with a relative risk of 2.9 for venous thromboembolism. Primary deficiencies of protein C, protein S, and antithrombin are present in approximately 0.5% of healthy subjects. Approximately 25% of individuals with factor V Leiden mutation sustain a thrombosis by the age of 50 years, and the prevalence of activated protein C resistance among DVT patients varies from 10% to 65%.

ORAL CONTRACEPTIVES AND HORMONE THERAPY

The use of oral contraceptives is established as an independent risk factor for DVT. Most reports indicate an odds ratio of 3:11.0 for idiopathic thrombosis with an unweighted summary relative risk among 18 controlled studies of 2.9. The increased risk of thromboembolic events appears to decrease soon after these contraceptives are discontinued. The use of third-generation oral contraceptives may act synergistically with factor V Leiden mutation, increasing the thromboembolic risk 30- to 50-fold. Hormonal therapy also increases the risk of venous thromboembolic events when used for lactation suppression, treatment for carcinoma of the prostate, or postmenopausal replacement therapy.

CENTRAL VENOUS CATHETERS

The increasing use of central venous catheters for hemodynamic monitoring, infusion catheters, and pacemakers is associated with increasing incidences of thromboembolic events. This is particularly noticeable in upper extremity venous thrombosis, in which as many as 60% of thrombi are related to central venous cannulation.

Diagnosis

Clinical evaluation is notoriously inaccurate in the diagnosis of DVT. Pain with plantar extension is traditionally taught as a classic finding of DVT, as described by Homan, but also has minimal usefulness. Approximately 50% of patients with DVT are asymptomatic. Findings suggestive of thrombus in the deep veins include more than 3 cm calf or thigh swelling, tenderness along the distribution of the deep veins, unilateral pitting edema, erythema, and dilated nonvaricose veins in the symptomatic extremity only. Massive thrombosis of the deep and superficial system can result in phlegmasia alba dolens (pale or white leg) and phlegmasia cerulean dolens (blue leg), with the latter presenting a high risk of limb loss if not addressed promptly.

Wells and colleagues demonstrate that categorizing the patient's pretest probability of DVT into low, moderate, or high probability improves diagnostic accuracy. They show that combining the use of a model of clinical probability of DVT with venous duplex ultrasound examination decreases the number of false-positive and false-negative diagnoses, and they use ascending venography as the definitive diagnostic test. Box 1 indicates that patients with a high clinical suspicion of DVT have an 85% chance of venography-proven DVT. Wells and colleagues also suggest that patients with low pretest probability and a negative noninvasive test result do not require treatment or additional testing and those with high pretest probability and positive noninvasive test results should be treated.

Overall, the ultimate test to diagnose DVT should be accurate, inexpensive, and noninvasive. Blood tests were performed for the past two decades to try and find a reliable marker to identify those with DVT. D-dimer was extensively evaluated and found to have an extremely high negative predictive value. Most recently, Wells and colleagues report that d-dimer has a negative predictive value of nearly 100% of those with low risk as determined by clinical predictors. Except in this small group of patients, an objective test is needed to assess these patients.

Venous duplex imaging is the study of choice for evaluation of DVT. Duplex findings suggestive of acute DVT include enlargement of the vein, noncompressible vein, absence of spontaneous phasic signal, and the presence of echogenic thrombus in the lumen. The sensitivity

5

BOX 1 Clinical Signs, Symptoms, and Risk Factors of Deep Vein Thrombosis (DVT)*

Major
- Acute cancer
- Paralysis/paresis
- Recent cast immobilization of lower extremities
- Bedridden for 3 days
- Major operation within 4 weeks
- Tenderness in distribution of the deep venous system
- Swelling of thigh or calf (>3 cm)
- Family history of DVT (≥first-degree relatives)

Minor
- History of recent trauma to symptomatic leg
- Unilateral pitting edema (symptomatic leg)
- Dilated (nonvaricose) superficial veins, symptomatic leg only
- Hospitalization within the prior 6 months
- Erythema

Clinical Probability
High
- ≥3 major points and no alternative diagnosis
- ≥2 major points and ≥2 minor points and no alternative diagnosis

Low
- 1 major point and ≥2 minor points and an alternative diagnosis
- 1 major point and ≥1 minor point and no alternative diagnosis
- 0 major points and ≥3 minor points and an alternative diagnosis
- 0 major points and ≥2 minor points and no alternative diagnosis

Moderate
- All other combinations

*Used to develop a clinical model for predicting the pretest probability of DVT.

---

and specificity are near 100% in detecting thrombus from the groin to the popliteal vein; however, the veins above the inguinal ligament and calf veins are more difficult to visualize. Despite the mentioned drawbacks, duplex is extremely safe, painless, and easy to repeat. Magnetic resonance venography (MRV) is used increasingly in the evaluation of suspected DVT. Some authors recommend MRV as the study of choice for suspected iliac vein or inferior vena caval thrombosis. Gadolinium, as a contrast agent, extravasates into the area of inflammation with acute thrombi. The limitations of its use are the cost and contraindications in patients with metallic implants and those with claustrophobia.

Venography is used as the gold standard for evaluation of extremity DVT, but it has many disadvantages, including contrast-induced phlebitis and high cost, so its use has become extremely selective. In recent years, duplex technology is increasingly considered the gold standard for the diagnosis of DVT.

DIAGNOSTIC STRATEGIES

Patients with clinical suspicion of DVT should initially be examined using venous duplex imaging. If the test is

positive, the patient should be treated for DVT. If the test is negative, the patient should then be classified according to the level of clinical suspicion for DVT (see Table 1). A low clinical suspicion of DVT accompanied by a negative duplex image can effectively exclude DVT, and no further evaluation is necessary. For patients with moderate clinical suspicion, a negative duplex test should be followed by another test in a few days or a d-dimer test. A negative d-dimer test most probably excludes the presence of DVT. A positive d-dimer test following a normal venous duplex image, however, requires further evaluation with ascending venography or MRV. Patients with a high clinical suspicion of DVT, despite a negative venous duplex image, should undergo an additional investigation using ascending venography, MRV, or a second venous duplex image. For those patients with inconclusive venous duplex imaging, which is infrequent, the following can be pursued:

- For patients with a low clinical suspicion, a second duplex image in a few days is appropriate.
- For those with a moderate or high clinical suspicion, the d-dimer test, MRV, or ascending venography can be used.
- If the d-dimer test is negative and the patient's clinical status remains stable or improved, the patient can be observed.
- If the clinical suspicion of DVT increases with time or if the d-dimer test is positive, ascending venography or MRV is indicated.

Treatment

Once the diagnosis of DVT is made, the treatment and treatment duration are determined based on the site of thrombosis. Isolated calf vein thrombosis has been an area of controversy for some time. But increasing evidence supports the use of anticoagulation therapy secondary to the risk of propagation up to 30% and an increase in recurrence as well as post-thrombotic syndrome in those without anticoagulation. Femoral-popliteal DVT carries a more complicated natural history, with up to 40% of patients having asymptomatic PE by routine ventilation/perfusion scans. These patients are generally treated with routine anticoagulation. Anticoagulation does not lyse the thrombus but allows for physiologic fibrinolysis of the affected vein. Iliofemoral DVT, which has the most serious manifestation of this DVT, is also associated with severe post-thrombotic sequelae. Eliminating the thrombus by either thrombectomy or thrombolysis improves both the short- and long-term venous function and overall morbidity. Vena cava filters may be placed in those patients with a free-floating thrombus or nonocclusive thrombus in their vena cava before thrombolysis. Anticoagulation is the mainstay of treatment in the United States unless contraindications are present. Heparin, low-molecular-weight heparin (LMWH), and warfarin (Coumadin) compounds are used in the treatment of DVT.

Heparin is an unfractionated product that binds to antithrombin III and augments the inhibition of Xa and thrombin. The anticoagulation effect varies widely in those treated and thus requires measurement of response to treatment by a partial thromboplastin time (PTT) level, with titration based on laboratory results. An elevation in the PTT to a level of 1.5 to 2 times that of the control value is needed for treatment. There is a proved decrease in recurrent thrombosis, if a therapeutic level is achieved within the first 24 hours of diagnosis, by as high as six times that of patients taking longer to achieve therapeutic levels.

More recently, LMWH has become very popular for prophylaxis and treatment, with a longer half-life, 90% bioavailability, and a more predictable anticoagulation response than unfractionated heparin. This class of anticoagulation can be administered once or twice daily, without the need for routine laboratory monitoring. In a meta-analysis comparison between LMWH and unfractionated heparin, patients with LMWH had a decrease in major bleeding. With these findings, the use of this class of drugs allows for safe outpatient treatment of DVT and for use as a bridge to therapeutic oral anticoagulation in those patients who are in the hospital for no other reason. Heparin is generally given for 5 days while oral anticoagulation is initiated.

Warfarin (Coumadin) therapy is inexpensive and used for long-term treatment after the patient is discharged. The drug is started after therapeutic effect with heparin or LMWH, secondary to the paradoxical effect on the coagulation cascade, until therapeutic levels are obtained, which are verified with a prothrombin time (PT) and international normalization ratio (INR). The mechanism of action of warfarin is inhibition of the vitamin K–dependent carboxylation of the clotting factors II, VII, IX, and X. The time to peak effect is up to 72 hours after administration, and close evaluation of the PT is needed. A troublesome consequence of this drug is its high level of interaction with other medications; therefore, close evaluations must be made of all new and old medications. The recommended goal of therapy is to achieve an INR of 2.0 to 3.0. Warfarin compounds cross the placenta and are contraindicated during pregnancy, secondary to teratogenic effects. Both unfractionated heparin and LMWH can be used in this population.

The recommended length of treatment depends on the etiology and presence of recurrence. The length of treatment for a first episode of DVT is 3 to 6 months, and those with recurrence require lifelong anticoagulation, particularly those with cancer or hypercoagulable states. Ultrasound follow-up in patients with DVT revealed a statistically significant increase in recurrence in those with residual thrombus. The ongoing incidence of recurrent DVT is 5% to 6% per year. A recent multicenter study, the Prevention of Recurrent Venous Thromboembolism (PREVENT) trial, shows a reduction of recurrent DVT or PE by 64% in those with low-dose warfarin therapy, compared with those taking placebo. An INR goal of 1.5 to 2.0 was achieved in the studied patients, with an average follow-up of 2 years.

The major adverse effect of all anticoagulation therapy is bleeding. Other complications of heparin therapy include osteoporosis and thrombocytopenia. Patients with bleeding while on heparin require cessation of

anticoagulation, use of fresh-frozen plasma, and the use of protamine. A dreaded possible complication of heparin-induced thrombocytopenia (HIT) is venous as well as arterial thrombosis, resulting in limb loss or death. This complication is secondary to IgG antibodies binding to the platelet membrane, with a stimulating effect on platelets. HIT occurs in up to approximately 2% of patients receiving heparin and typically develops 2 to 10 days after therapy is initiated. A drop of more than 50% of the platelet count should raise a high level of suspicion for this complication. In these patients, direct thrombin inhibitors (lepirudin [Refludan]) are used, and warfarin therapy is instituted after several days of treatment. With warfarin therapy, skin necrosis can develop, usually within 10 days of therapy and most often in women in areas of abundant subcutaneous tissue. Patients with congenital deficiencies of protein C and malignancies are especially prone to warfarin-induced skin necrosis. Prompt cessation of warfarin therapy and initiation of alternative anticoagulants are required.

Prevention

Prophylaxis in high-risk patients is used to decrease the incidence of DVT. The importance of prevention is paramount; as seen in orthopedic patients in the National Confidential E[I]nquiry into Perioperative Deaths (NCEPOD) study, which indicates PE as the cause of death in 35% of patients at autopsy following hip replacement. Graduated compression stockings and intermittent leg compression devices decrease the incidence of DVT in moderate-risk surgical patients. Their use is routine in surgical and trauma patients, with good reason, because approximately 50% of DVT occurs intraoperatively. With the ease of administration of LMWH products, and with no need for frequent laboratory work to assess the level of anticoagulation, anticoagulation therapy has become increasingly popular as a means of prophylaxis. Randomized control trials show LMWH to have an equal or greater effectiveness and similar or less bleeding complications than traditional unfractionated heparin. Even subtherapeutic doses of oral anticoagulation show a decreased incidence of thrombosis in patients with indwelling catheters.

SPECIFIC DEEP VENOUS THROMBOSIS PROPHYLAXIS RECOMMENDATION
Low-Risk Patients

Patients who are at low risk for DVT do not usually need specific prophylactic measures, except for ambulation.

Moderate-Risk Patients
General Surgical, Thoracic, or Gynecologic Procedures

The use of subcutaneous low-dose unfractionated heparin (5000 U every 8 to 12 hours) or subcutaneous LMWH is recommended in patients who have undergone general surgical, thoracic, or gynecologic procedures. Intermittent pneumatic compression (IPC) devices can also be effective. Neurosurgical patients should receive IPC, but a low-dose heparin is also an acceptable alternative.

High-Risk Patients

High-risk patients with elective hip replacement can be treated with LMWH or warfarin adjusted to maintain an INR of 2 to 3. Other effective approaches include adjusted-dose subcutaneous unfractionated heparin and IPC. For patients with elective knee replacement, the prophylaxis of choice is LMWH once or twice daily postoperatively. For patients with hip fractures, either warfarin with an INR of 2 to 3 or a fixed dose of subcutaneous LMWH started preoperatively is effective. The combined use of IPC with LMWH or warfarin may prove of additional benefit in certain patients with hip fractures.

Multiple Trauma

LMWH is the prophylaxis of choice in multiple trauma. IPC is recommended, when feasible, because it eliminates any risk for bleeding. Other alternatives include low-dose unfractionated heparin or warfarin. Insertion of an inferior vena cava (IVC) filter is recommended for very high-risk patients when anticoagulation may be contraindicated.

Acute Spinal Cord Injury Associated With Paralysis

LMWH is the most effective prophylaxis in these patients with spinal cord injury.

Other Medical Conditions

Medical patients should be classified as low, moderate, or high risk for venous thromboembolic events, and depending on their medical condition and risk, they can be treated based on the previous outlines as suggested.

Pregnancy

Subcutaneous low-dose heparin is the prophylaxis of choice for pregnant patients who are at high risk for DVT and PE. For those undergoing an emergency caesarean section, prophylaxis with low-dose unfractionated heparin is recommended.

Superficial Thrombophlebitis

Some consider thrombosis of the superficial veins a benign process. The most common etiologies include direct injury, stasis within varicose veins, and an association with malignancy. The incidence of DVT is reported to be 11% in these patients. This diagnosis is easier to make in the superficial system than in the deep system. A painful cord is often palpated with erythema along the course of the underlying vein. Duplex is accurate

and critical in assessing the extension of the thrombus. Anti-inflammatory agents are the mainstay of treatment and compression, and bed rest and warm compresses are also part of first-line therapy. If extension occurs to the saphenofemoral junction, ligation or anticoagulation with warfarin can be performed with the known concomitant presence of DVT in 40% of patients. The prognosis depends on etiology, deep venous involvement, and thrombus load. Follow-up duplex is recommended, and if the process persists, a hypercoagulable state workup and malignancy search should be sought.

Axillary-Subclavian Vein Thrombosis

Axillary-subclavian vein thrombosis (ASVT), which accounts for 1% to 2% of all DVT, can be either primary (effort vein thrombosis) or secondary. Primary ASVT is more commonly reported in men 40 years of age or younger, but it may occur at any age or in any sex. Secondary ASVT may be related to these situations:

- Iatrogenic (secondary to insertion of Hickman catheters, pacemakers, central venous pressure lines, or other vascular catheterizations)
- Malignancy (both from direct obstruction by tumor or metastatic nodes or secondary to hypercoagulability states associated with certain tumors)
- Direct trauma
- Heart disease (stasis) and nephrotic syndrome
- Infections

In a review of reported phlebograms in patients with permanent pacemaker electrodes, evidence of venous thrombosis was observed in 31%. Total occlusion was present in 15%, but arm or facial edema was reported in only 5%.

EFFORT SUBCLAVIAN VEIN THROMBOSIS

The most frequently reported examples of subclavian venous thrombosis are those related to effort, or positioning of the arm and external compression of the vein in the costoclavicular space.

Paget, in 1875, and von Schroetter, in 1884, described cases of upper arm swelling attributable to thrombosis of the main veins of the upper extremity. Hughes, in his excellent collective review of 320 reported cases, coined the term *Paget-Schroetter syndrome*. The thrombosis may occur in the axillary or subclavian vein and be related to injury or effort, but it can also be spontaneous. This syndrome is therefore best described as a primary ASVT.

The pathophysiology of effort vein thrombosis is postulated to be multifactorial. First, external compression of the axillary-subclavian vein contributes to stasis of blood flow. Factors causing external compression include anomalous subclavius or anterior scalene muscle, congenital fibromuscular bands, or narrowing of the costoclavicular space from depression of the shoulder. Second, the stress of exercise may temporarily cause hypercoagulability. Third, repetitive shoulder-arm motion may cause microscopic intimal tears in the vessel wall. These three factors satisfy Virchow's classic triad for thrombosis: stasis, hypercoagulability, and intimal damage. The most important factor in explaining the high thrombosis rate in the axillary-subclavian vein, compared with other major veins, seems to be its relatively fixed position in the thoracic outlet, exposing it to repeated trauma during arm movement.

The commonly observed activities are those associated with hyperabduction and external rotation of the arm or with activities in which the shoulders are held in the backward and downward positions. Hyperabduction actions described include throwing a baseball or football, playing tennis, painting ceilings, chopping wood, rowing a boat, and washing walls. Depression of the shoulder, which occurs with carrying heavy objects or in a figure-eight splint, has preceded thrombosis. It has also been observed following positioning of the arms during sleep or under anesthesia in which the arm is positioned in hyperabduction or the shoulders are depressed. Direct compression of the axillary vein by hanging on a ladder rung or falling asleep with an arm over the back of a chair is described. But some cases are described in which no inciting effort or position is remembered. Roos emphasizes the central role of the first rib as the major limiting structure in the thoracic outlet.

Effort vein thrombosis presents clinically, predominantly in middle-age men, with abrupt swelling of the involved upper extremity. The involved extremity is most often the person's dominant arm. Recent trauma or unusual exertion can be documented in the majority of cases. Venous hypertension of the upper extremity after the onset of subclavian vein thrombosis causes long-term disability consisting of arm pain and swelling exacerbated by exercise. These symptoms persist for a long time in a large percentage of patients and appear uninfluenced by standard anticoagulant therapy. Venous duplex imaging is used in the diagnosis of this entity with excellent accuracy. Venography can be used to confirm the diagnosis.

Several investigators employ oral anticoagulation as the sole therapy for patients with subclavian vein thrombosis, with a reported clinical success rate of 4% to 100% (mean 49%). With early conservative therapy of effort vein thrombosis, complete resolution of symptoms occurs in 15% to 30% of patients. Adams and DeWeese report residual symptoms in up to 70% of conservatively treated patients, including swelling, pain, disability, and even a rare case of venous gangrene. PE is also observed in 12% to 36% of patients with ASVT.

The use of lytic therapy may ultimately improve the efficacy of oral anticoagulation therapy and may partially explain the improved results of more current oral anticoagulation series compared with historical studies. Although thrombolytic therapy is costly, its use is justified considering the potential loss of productivity in relatively young men with effort ASVT who are treated with anticoagulation therapy.

Symptoms associated with effort subclavian vein thrombosis are sufficiently dramatic that most patients present promptly for treatment. Lytic therapy can reduce the size or completely lyse the clots, and it is most effective for fresh clots (5 to 7 days old). The results of lytic therapy in clot resolution of ASVT is somewhat mixed, however. Some authorities report good results, with clot resolution ranging from 57% to 100%, whereas others have limited success. In our series, initial thrombolysis was achieved in the majority (93%) of patients. When using adjunctive therapy, 13 (87%) patients who had initial lytic therapy experienced complete resolution of their symptoms and patent veins. More objective data regarding subclavian vein lumen patency following lytic therapy and anticoagulation are needed, however, including a comprehensive follow-up with duplex scanning of the subclavian vein, before any recommendation regarding surgery versus lytic therapy can be made.

Although initial lytic therapy is gaining wider acceptance, proponents of early surgical thrombectomy and initial surgical repair remain. At the other end of the spectrum, some authorities suggest treating the thrombotic process alone, without addressing the underlying anatomical abnormality. Machleder refutes this approach, however, arguing that if the underlying anatomical abnormality is not corrected, the recurrence rate and/or residual symptoms will be rather high.

First rib resection may seem the logical treatment for effort vein thrombosis because the major cause of this disorder seems to be a fixed position of the axillary-subclavian vein in the thoracic outlet. But no anatomical abnormality is apparent in some cases. For this reason, first rib resection should be reserved for patients in whom an anatomic abnormality can be identified or if reocclusion of the vein occurs after treatment. In our series, 7 of 23 patients had supplementary first rib or cervical rib resection in the present series, and all symptoms were resolved.

The timing of first rib resection following initial successful lytic therapy is controversial. Some authorities advocate first rib resection shortly after the vein is opened and a few days after heparin therapy. The rationale for this sequence is to decompress the vein before it reoccludes. The second option, chosen in our series, is to maintain warfarin therapy for 2 to 3 months and then perform a first rib resection for persistent and significant symptoms. At this time, there is insufficient data for favoring one option over the other.

The clinical outcome is very good following effort subclavian vein thrombosis treatment that includes at least catheter-directed lytic and oral anticoagulation therapy. Balloon angioplasty appears ineffective regardless of etiology. Stent placement may enhance the results of angioplasty in selected patients without effort vein thrombosis, and surgery may improve symptom resolution in effort vein thrombosis patients with external compression or intrinsic venous abnormalities.

Deep Venous Thrombosis in Pregnancy

The incidence of antepartum DVT is estimated to occur in 0.5% or less of deliveries. Postpartum DVT is three to five times more common than antepartum. One out

CURRENT DIAGNOSIS

Approximately 50% of patients with DVT are asymptomatic. Findings suggestive of DVT include:
- \>3 cm calf or thigh swelling
- Tenderness along the distribution of the deep veins
- Unilateral pitting edema
- Erythema
- Dilated nonvaricose veins in the symptomatic extremity only

Other diagnostic considerations include:
- Categorizing pretest probability of DVT into low, moderate, or high probability improves diagnostic accuracy.
- Combining the use of a model of clinical probability of DVT with venous duplex ultrasound exam decreases the number of false-positive and false-negative diagnoses.
- Patients with a high clinical suspicion of DVT have an 85% chance of having venography-proven DVT.
- D-dimer has a negative predictive value of nearly 100% of those with low risk as determined by clinical predictors.
- Venous duplex imaging is the study of choice for initial evaluation of DVT.

Abbreviation: DVT = deep venous thrombosis.

CURRENT THERAPY

- Treatment and duration are determined by the site of thrombosis.
- Increasing evidence supports the use of anticoagulation therapy for isolated calf vein thrombosis.
- Femoral-popliteal DVT is generally treated with routine anticoagulation.
- Eliminating the thrombus by either thrombectomy or thrombolysis improves both the short- and long-term venous function and overall morbidity for patients with iliofemoral DVT.
- Vena cava filters may be placed in patients with a free-floating thrombus or nonocclusive thrombus in their vena cava before thrombolysis.
- Heparin, low-molecular-weight heparin, and warfarin compounds are used in treatment of DVT.
- Recommended length of treatment depends on the etiology and presence of recurrence.
- Length of treatment for first episode of DVT is 3 to 6 months.
- Patients with recurrence require lifelong anticoagulation, particularly those with cancer or hypercoagulable states.

Abbreviation: DVT = deep venous thrombosis.

of 2000 pregnancies is complicated by a PE. Twenty percent of untreated DVT may be complicated by a PE, which carries a 15% mortality rate. In contrast, if treated, the incidence of PE is less than 5% with less than a 1% mortality rate.

Pregnancy is considered an acquired hypercoagulable state or a low grade of chronic disseminated intravascular coagulation (DIC) within the placenta. Increases of several clotting factors (factors I, V, VII, VIII, IX, X, and XII) are associated with decreased fibrinolytic activities and increased fibrinolytic inhibitors. Decreases in antithrombin III and proteins C and S are observed.

A clinical diagnosis is generally invalid in 50% of cases, and the diagnosis is primarily made using a color duplex ultrasound.

TREATMENT

The choice of therapy is widely debated. Warfarin passes through the placenta to the fetus and may cause fetal complications and/or death. Heparin, in contrast, does not cross the placenta, but its long-term use may be impractical and increase the risk of complications.

Conventional Therapy (for Proximal Iliofemoral Popliteal Deep Vein Thrombosis)

Full-dose intravenous (IV) heparin is administered for several days followed by subcutaneous heparin

every 12 hours until delivery. Then subcutaneous heparin or warfarin is used for 6 weeks postpartum. Distal below-knee isolated DVT can be treated using compression stockings and heat with follow-up duplex ultrasounds.

Peripartum Management

Several options can be considered for peripartum management:

- Continue heparin treatment as antepartum for high-risk patients.
- Decrease heparin dose to 5000 U subcutaneous every 12 hours (PTT of 1.5) for recent thromboembolic disease.
- Discontinue IV heparin 4 to 6 hours before delivery and insertion of IVC filter.
- Resume heparin 6 hours after delivery and continue for 6 to 8 weeks.
- Administer warfarin therapy in nonlactating mothers as needed.

Alternative Therapies in Pregnancy

Alternative therapies of DVT during pregnancy include low-dose heparin and IVC filter, iliofemoral venous thrombectomy, and LMWH. A recent Medline review of LMWH concludes they are generally safe and effective, but the benefits remain inconclusive.

REFERENCES

AbuRahma AF, Mullins DA: Endovascular caval interruption in pregnant patients with deep vein thrombosis of the lower extremity. J Vasc Surg 2001;33:375-378.

Hull RD, Raskob GE, Pineo GF, et al: Subcutaneous low-molecular weight heparin compared with continuous intravenous heparin in the treatment of proximal vein thrombosis. N Engl J Med 1992; 326:975-982.

Hyers TM, Agnelli G, Hull RD, et al: Antithrombotic therapy for venous thromboembolic disease. Chest 2001;119:176S-193S.

Koch A, Bouges S, Ziegler S, et al: Low-molecular weight heparin and unfractionated heparin in thrombosis prophylaxis after major surgical intervention: Update of previous meta-analysis. Br J Surg 1997;84:750-759.

Nicolaides AN, Bergquist D, Hull RD, et al: Prevention of venous thromboembolism: International consensus statement. Int Angiol 1997;16:3-38.

Weitz JI, Hirsh J: New anticoagulant drugs. Chest 2001;119: 95S-107S.

The Blood and Spleen

Aplastic Anemia

Method of
Deborah Chirnomas, MD, and Eva Guinan, MD

Definition and Epidemiology

Aplastic anemia (AA) is defined as peripheral pancytopenia with a hypocellular bone marrow but without increased reticulin or abnormal marrow infiltration. It is classified into three categories: nonsevere (or moderate), severe, and very severe. Severe aplastic anemia (SAA) is defined as having bone marrow cellularity less than 25% or 25% to 50% with less than 30% residual hematopoietic cells and two of the following: an absolute neutrophil count (ANC) less than 500/mm^3, a platelet count less than 20,000/mm^3, and/or a reticulocyte count less than 60,000/mm^3. Very severe AA is defined as having the previous findings with an ANC less than 200/mm^3. Patients who do not meet the above criteria fall into the category of nonsevere AA. AA can be further distinguished as either being idiosyncratic and acquired, which comprises the majority of cases, or congenital, which is rare. The incidence of acquired AA is 2 per 1 million general population each year in North America and Europe with a two- to threefold higher incidence in East Asia. There is a biphasic age distribution, the first peak being between 10 and 25 years of age and the later peak being in people greater than 60 years of age. The most common type of congenital AA is Fanconi anemia, which is inherited in an autosomal recessive or X-linked manner. It has an incidence of 1 in 300,000 with a carrier frequency as high as 1 in 300 in certain communities. Other rare congenital AA syndromes include dyskeratosis congenita and Shwachman-Diamond syndrome.

Pathogenesis

Most cases of acquired AA are idiopathic, but there are several drugs and toxins that have been associated with AA (Table 1). These associations, however, are rarely established for individuals and have mostly been

documented by case reports rather than controlled studies. There are also viruses that have been associated with AA such as Epstein-Barr virus (EBV), cytomegalovirus (CMV), and the hepatitis viruses. Autoimmune diseases have also been implicated, including autoimmune hepatitis. Pregnancy has been associated with the onset of AA and may predispose women to have recurrence of previously diagnosed AA.

The pathophysiology of AA remains unknown. There is little evidence for acquired stromal defects. Based in part on response to immunosuppressive therapy, abnormal immune regulation is a major factor. Dissection of potential immune defects has been hampered by the confounding effects of transfusion and transfusional sensitization. In vitro, interferon-γ (IFN-γ), and tumor necrosis factor-α (TNF-α), cytokines produced in part by circulating activated suppressor T cells, have been shown to inhibit production of hematopoietic stem cells. Some human studies have shown increased levels of these cytokines in AA patients, suggesting that they may be a contributing factor to the pathogenesis of the disease. Increased apoptosis of hematopoietic stem cell precursors also may have a role in the etiology of AA. It has been observed that people with AA have increased expression of Fas antigen, which is associated with apoptosis, on their CD34+ bone marrow cells (a phenotype felt to reflect a progenitor cell population). IFN-γ and TNF-α may upregulate Fas expression on normal CD34+ cells, leading to increased apoptosis of these cells.

Intrinsic stem cell abnormalities (acquired or germline) have also been postulated to contribute to this clinical phenotype. Molecular abnormalities consistent with paroxysmal nocturnal hemoglobinuria (PNH) can be found in many AA patients. PNH is a monoclonal process characterized by hematopoietic stem cells that are deficient in glycosylphosphatidylinositol (GPI)-linked proteins in the cell membrane. This deficiency is caused by an acquired defect in the phosphatidylinositol glycan-class A (PIG-A) gene. The resulting loss of GPI proteins on the membrane targets the cells for complement-mediated hemolysis. Patients with PNH may have isolated hemolytic anemia, or they may have concurrent marrow failure. Recently, shortened telomeres and mutations in telomerase-related genes (similar to those found in the congenital marrow-failure syndrome, dyskeratosis congenita) have been reported in patients with AA. The molecular lesions underlying many of the congenital

TABLE 1 Etiologic Agents in Acquired Aplastic Anemia*

Pharmacologic agents

Cancer chemotherapeutic agents
  Alkylating agents (e.g., busulfan), anthracyclines (e.g., daunorubicin), antimetabolites (e.g., methotrexate), antimitotic agents (e.g., colchicine), levamisole[†]
Antibiotics
  Chloramphenicol, penicillins, cephalosporins, sulfonamides[†]
Anti-inflammatory drugs
  Phenylbutazone,[§] indomethacin, ibuprofen, sulindac, diclofenac, gold compounds, penicillamine
Antiepileptic agents
  Felbamate, phenytoin, carbamazepine, ethosuximide, and others
Antithyroid agents
  Methimazole, prophylthiouracil
Hypoglycemic agents
  Chlorpropamide, tolbutamide
Antimalarial agents
  Quinacrine,[§] chloroquine
Neuroleptic agents
  Chlorpromazine,[†] clozapine[†]
Cardiac medications
  Captopril,[†] procainamide[†]

Chemicals and toxins

Pesticides, benzene, other aromatic hydrocarbons

Infections

Viral hepatitis, Epstein-Barr virus (infectious mononucleosis), cytomegalovirus, brucellosis, miliary tuberculosis, parvovirus B19[††]

Rheumatologic and autoimmune diseases

Systemic lupus erythematosus (SLE), rheumatoid arthritis, cryoglobulinemia, graft-versus-host disease

Paroxysmal nocturnal hemoglobinuria

Ionizing radiation

Thymoma

Pregnancy

Idiopathic

---

*Listed are agents more commonly associated with aplastic anemia. This list is not intended to be exhaustive.
[†]More commonly associated with agranulocytosis than with aplastic anemia.
[††]More commonly associated with aplastic crises in patients with underlying hemolytic disorders.
[§]Not available in the United States.
From Nimer SD, Araten DJ: The blood and spleen. In Rakel RE, Bope ET: *Conn's Current Therapy 2004*, ed 56. Philadelphia, 2004, Saunders.

TABLE 2 Diagnostic Studies for the Evaluation of a Patient With Pancytopenia

CBC with a manual differential, smear, and reticulocyte count
Bone marrow aspirate and biopsy with cytogenetics
Viral studies: hepatitis A, B, C; EBV; CMV
Liver function tests
Fanconi anemia test for chromosome breakage in patients younger than 30 years
Flow cytometry for PIG-AP or acidified serum (Ham's) test for PNH clone
HIV
ANA and anti-dsDNA
As indicated: HBF in children, vitamin B_{12} and folate, other marrow failure syndrome, genetic testing

---

Abbreviations: ANA = anti-nuclear antibody; anti-dsDNA = anti–double-stranded deoxyribonucleic acid; CBC = complete blood count; CMV = cytomegalovirus; EBV = Epstein-Barr virus; HBF = fetal hemoglobin; PIG-AP = phosphatidylinositol glycan-anchored proteins.

myelodysplastic syndrome (MDS), acute leukemias, and occasionally other hematologic malignancies. Other rare causes of severe marrow suppression include mycobacterial infections, HIV, and anorexia nervosa (AN). The most common presenting symptoms of AA patients are mild mucosal bleeding and fatigue from anemia. The physical exam may demonstrate pallor, petechiae, and purpura and is notable for the absence of splenomegaly and lymphadenopathy, but findings of congestive heart failure (CHF), including hepatomegaly, are occasionally present. A thorough history of infectious symptoms may suggest hepatitis or infectious mononucleosis. If there is a history of suspicious medication or toxic exposure, immediate cessation of the agent is recommended. AA caused by drugs such as chemotherapeutics may be fully reversible. Initial screening with a complete blood cell count (CBC), reticulocyte count, and peripheral blood smear will rapidly confirm the presence or absence of pancytopenia. If there is evidence of one or more affected cell lines, promptly refer to a hematologist. Further recommended laboratory studies for the evaluation of AA include bone marrow aspirate and biopsy with cytogenetics, liver function tests (LFTs), viral studies (hepatitis A, B, C; EBV; CMV; HIV), and Fanconi anemia and PNH testing. Additional genetic testing for marrow failure syndromes in children and evaluation for autoimmune diseases and malignant states should be considered individually.

Treatment

BONE MARROW TRANSPLANT

A human leukocyte antibody (HLA)-matched, sibling-donor stem-cell transplant is the generally accepted first-line therapy for children and adults younger than age 30 years with AA. Between 30 and 40 years of age, a clinical decision must be made based on the severity

syndromes are being increasingly better defined, yet the relationship of these mutations to marrow failure remains incompletely understood.

Diagnosis

Because there is no definitive diagnostic test, it is important to exclude other processes that can present with pancytopenia and hypocellularity (Table 2). Those include

of the disease, the general health of the patient, and the availability and quality of the donor. Alternative donor transplants are used in the case of severe AA with poor response to immunosuppressive therapy. The most common current ablative regimen with a sibling donor is cyclophosphamide (Cytoxan),[1] antithymocyte globulin (ATG) (Atgam), and methylprednisolone (Depo-Medrol),[1] whereas regimens for alternative donor transplant range widely.

The major cause of transplant failure is graft rejection/failure. Graft rejection may be related to the underlying immune etiology of some AA, transfusional sensitization, or the relatively low intensity of the conditioning regimen. The major long-term toxicities are those of transplant in general, including toxicities related to chronic graft-versus-host disease (GVHD) and the regimen used. Recent prophylactic modifications have reduced the risk of GVHD, but it is still a major cause of death in adults and accounts for the disparity between pediatric and adult survival for this disease. Recent studies report between 75% and 94% disease-free survival in all patients.

IMMUNOSUPPRESSIVE THERAPY

The major components of immunosuppressive therapy for AA are ATG (Atgam), corticosteroids, and cyclosporine (Sandimmune).[1] This treatment regimen is associated with a 60% to 80% response rate and 5-year overall survival of 75%. Combination therapy is significantly more beneficial than any agent alone. The risk of relapse has been reduced with the longer use and slower tapering of cyclosporine (Sandimmune)[1] over many months. The use of hematopoietic stem cell stimulants has not proven to be of significant benefit to overall survival, but they may have a role in decreasing the number of infections and duration of neutropenia. However, there have also been studies showing that prolonged use of granulocyte colony-stimulating factor (G-CSF) was associated with more clonal disease and malignancy. Not all studies support these findings. Autologous recovery after conditioning with high-dose cyclophosphamide (CY) was first observed years ago and is currently being evaluated as an alternative immunosuppressive regimen. Initial regulated studies suggested efficacy and a lower relapse rate with less clonal evolution than other immunosuppressive approaches. A randomized 2002 study did not support these observations, in part because the study was closed early, secondary to excess morbidity and mortality in the CY-treated group. This area is still being actively investigated.

SUPPORTIVE CARE

Patients with AA must be supported with blood products as needed. Generally, platelets should be transfused for a platelet count less than $10 \times 10^9/L$ to limit the risk of spontaneous intracranial hemorrhage. However, thresholds for bleeding have not been rigorously studied in this setting and should be individualized to tolerance

[1]Not FDA approved for this indication.

Rakel and Bope: *Conn's Current Therapy 2006.*

and situation. Transfusions will affect the likelihood of graft failure after transplant and contribute to iron- and infection-related co-morbidity. In particular, transfusions from family members prior to stem cell transplantation may increase the risk of graft rejection. It is also recommended that the transfusions be leuko-reduced, irradiated (or washed), and CMV negative.

INFECTION

Fever should be aggressively addressed in patients with SAA. Broad-spectrum intravenous (IV) antibiotics should be administered until infection is ruled out, and empiric fungal coverage should be added for persistent fever. Prophylactic antibiotics in afebrile, neutropenic patients are not recommended, but use of *Pneumocystis carinii* pneumonia (PCP) prophylaxis in patients undergoing aggressive immunosuppressive therapy is warranted. Diagnostic studies should be performed as needed to identify infectious sources.

Long-Term Outcome

CLONAL EVOLUTION

The evolution of a detectable clonal process has long been recognized in AA. A small percentage of patients have chromosomal aberrations at the time of their initial diagnosis, raising the question of whether they should be considered to have MDS or AA. Some studies have indicated these abnormalities do not necessarily predict for malignant transformation and may not predict response to treatment, but this is very controversial. Such findings are currently difficult to interpret in a therapeutic sense, and practice is highly divergent.

Long-term outcomes data have confirmed a risk for late development of clonal hematopoiesis in AA. Since the initiation of ATG therapy, the survival of patients with SAA has markedly improved. Along with improved survival has come the recognition that the risk of developing hematopoietic clonal diseases such as leukemia, MDS, and/or PNH approaches 20% or more at 10 years from diagnosis. These data are collected from studies looking at patients treated with immunosuppressive therapy alone and not transplantation. The most common clonal aberrations are monosomy 7 and trisomy 8, but small series have reported several cases of trisomy 6. According to a recent National Institutes of Health study, the implications of specific abnormalities may vary depending on the underlying disease (MDS versus SAA). The monosomy 7 clone continues to be a poor prognostic indicator with mortality approaching 50% at almost 4 years after development of the clone. Annual patient screening seems prudent. Relapse is rarely observed after transplant but does occur after immunosuppressive therapy. The frequency ranges from 10% to 50%.

QUALITY OF LIFE

Patients who respond to immunosuppressive therapy generally have a good quality of life, particularly if

CURRENT DIAGNOSIS

- Decrease in two or more cell lines with low reticulocyte count
- Referral to hematologist/oncologist
- Requires a bone marrow biopsy and cytogenetics for diagnosis and to exclude malignancy
- Exclude infectious causes: HIV, cytomegalovirus, Epstein-Barr virus
- Evaluate for congenital bone marrow failure syndromes and paroxysmal nocturnal hemoglobinuria

they are no longer transfusion dependent. Prolonged cyclosporine (Sandimmune)[1] use can have multiple side effects including hypertension, hypomagnesemia, and hirsutism, all of which are reversible with cessation of cyclosporine (Sandimmune).[1] Exposure to steroids may result in complications including cataracts, osteopenia, and avascular necrosis. Risk of MDS and leukemia is reviewed previously in the article, and there is an increased lifetime risk of certain other malignancies, including skin cancers. Transplant is associated with similar effects from immunosuppressive medication. The differential morbidity of transplant relates to the occurrence of acute and/or chronic GVHD with their protean and debilitating effects on skin, GI tract, and liver. Time-limited or long-lived effects can range in severity from imperceptible to fatal. Other late complications of transplant include the development of solid tumors related to the conditioning regimen chosen.

Summary

AA is a syndrome of bone marrow failure that is frequently immune-mediated and is incurable without

---

[1]Not FDA approved for this indication.

CURRENT THERAPY

- Refer patient to AA-experienced AA transplant center.
- Implement bone marrow transplants for patients younger than 30 to 40 years of age with HLA-matched sibling.
- If there is no matched sibling and/or the patient is younger than 30 to 40 years of age, consider cyclosporine, steroids, and ATG (IST) first, with transplant or other modalities if IST fails.
- Support with CMV, leukoreduced transfusions as needed, but if the patient is a candidate for early transplant, discuss transfusion parameters with the transplant team.
- Implement aggressive therapy for fever and infection but avoid use of prophylactic antibiotics.

Abbreviations: AA = aplastic anemia; ATG = antithymocyte globulin; CMV = cytomegalovirus; HLA = human leukocyte antibody; IST = immunosuppressive therapy.

treatment. With prompt referral to a medical center experienced in treating SAA with immunosuppressive therapy (IST) and/or transplant, children and adults now have markedly improved outcomes.

REFERENCES

Kojima S: Use of granulocyte colony-stimulating factor for treatment of aplastic anemia. Nagoya J Med Sci 1999;62(3-4):77-82.
Kurre P, Johnson FL, Deeg HJ: Diagnosis and treatment of children with aplastic anemia. Pediatr Blood Cancer 2005;44:1-11.
Marsh JC, Ball SE, Darbyshire P, et al: Guidelines for the diagnosis and management of acquired aplastic anemia. Br J Haematol 2003;123(5):782-801.
Maciejewski JP, Anderson S, Katevas P, Young NS: Phenotypic and functional analysis of bone marrow progenitor cell compartment in bone marrow failure. Br J Haematol 1994;87:227-234.
Nash RA: Allogeneic HSCT for autoimmune diseases: Conventional conditioning regimens. Bone Marrow Transplant 2003;32 Suppl 1: S77-S80.
Polychronopoulou S, Koutroumba P: Telomere length variation and telomerase activity expression in patients with congenital and acquired aplastic anemia. Acta Haematol 2004;111(3):125-131.
Tisdale J, Maciejewski JP, Nunez O, et al: Late complications following treatment for severe aplastic anemia with high dose cyclophosphamide: Follow-up of a randomized trial. Blood 2002;100(13): 4668-4670.
Young NS: The problem of clonality in aplastic anemia: Dr. Dameshek's riddle, restated. Blood 1992;79(6):1385-1392.

Iron Deficiency

Method of
Jay Umbreit, MTS, MD, PhD

Iron deficiency is the most common nutritional deficiency. In children 1 to 2 years of age the prevalence is 7%; in females 16 to 19 years of age it can be as high as 19%. Iron deficiency increases in minority populations and can reach 22% of Hispanic women. Iron deficiency in its most severe form results in iron deficiency anemia. In infants and preschool children iron deficiency anemia results in decreased motor activity, social inattention, and decreased social interaction. Among pregnant women in their first two trimesters, iron deficiency anemia results in increased incidence of preterm labor and low-weight births. The prevalence of anemia in low-income pregnant females in the first, second, and third trimesters is 9%, 14%, and 37%, respectively. There is strong evidence that iron deficiency anemia results in decreased work productivity, increased child mortality, increased maternal mortality, and slowed child development. The effects of mild to moderate anemia are not well established, nor are the effects on susceptibility to infectious disease.

There are data that indicate neuropsychologic effects of iron deficiency occur without overt anemia and may respond to iron therapy. Nonanemia iron deficiency likely reduces work capacity. This suggests that iron deficiency anemia is only part of the overall syndrome of iron deficiency.

Diet predicts iron status into infancy and early childhood. Between 20% and 40% of infants fed unfortified formula or cow's milk, and 15% to 20% of breast-fed infants are at risk. After 24 months of age, the risk of iron deficiency decreases with the decreased dependence on milk. In older children the risk for deficiency is related to limited access to food because of family income, low-iron diets, or medical conditions such as bleeding or inflammatory disease. During adolescence (12 to 18 years of age), iron requirements increase because of growth. Among females menstrual blood loss becomes an issue, and heavy loss (greater than 80 mL per month) is a significant risk factor. Other risk factors for this population include use of an intrauterine device, high parity, and low iron intake. Data from the Health and Nutrition Examination Survey (HANES) III indicated that 11% of nonpregnant women aged 16 to 49 years have iron deficiency and 3% to 5% have iron-deficiency anemia. Among pregnant women the expansion of the blood volume, growth of the fetus, and other maternal tissues increase the demand for iron threefold. In the absence of iron supplements many pregnant women are unable to maintain iron stores, but prevalence data across the entire population are not available. Although some iron is returned by contraction of the blood volume after delivery, the iron in the fetal and supportive tissues is lost.

The worldwide problem of anemia is magnified. In children younger than 5 years of age, it may reach 49% and is likely to reach 25% of adult females.

Dietary iron is present as inorganic iron and heme iron. Fifty percent of the iron in meat is heme, of which 15% to 35% is bioavailable. Although most iron in the diet is inorganic iron, its absorption ranges from 2% to 20% so that most dietary iron is from heme. In developed countries perhaps 66% of the iron intake is derived from heme. Men absorb and excrete approximately 1 mg daily. During their childbearing years, women need to absorb approximately 2 mg each day because of menstrual bleeding and childbirth losses. Nonheme (inorganic) iron absorption is facilitated by meat and ascorbic acid but inhibited by phytates, some dietary fibers and lignins, phenolic polymers, and calcium. Gastric acid is required to maintain the common ferric form of inorganic iron soluble, and achlorhydria may be a significant cause of iron deficiency in the elderly. Perhaps 30% of the elderly have achlorhydria. Gastric atrophy and *Helicobacter pylori* gastric infestation may result in altered pH and iron deficiency. Pharmacologic iron is ferrous iron that is soluble at a neutral pH, and its absorption is unaffected by low gastric acidity. Unusual dietary habits resulting in ingestion of chelators such as starch or clay are still found in clinical practice.

The most common etiology of iron deficiency is bleeding, and a bleeding source should be investigated in all cases of iron deficiency. There are 0.5 mg of iron contained in 1 mL of blood. Occult bleeding may be because of gastrointestinal (GI) loss, but the usual stool test requires loss of 20 mL per day for detection. Bleeding into the hip joint space or intra-abdominally may be initially undetected. Menstrual loss may not be reported as bleeding. Rarely hemosiderinuria may cause iron deficiency. Pregnancy by itself can result in iron deficiency. During a full-term pregnancy, the fetus takes up approximately 400 mg of iron, and placenta and uterus take up approximately 150 mg. Additionally, 300 to 400 mg is needed to increase the red cell mass. Iron lost in milk during lactation is approximately 30 mg per month. During the first 6 months of life, approximately 50 g of new hemoglobin are made. A growing child maintains this by absorbing approximately 0.5 mg of iron in excess of body losses to ultimately achieving 4000 mg in adulthood (70-kg man). The majority (66%) is hemoglobin and approximately 1000 mg is ferritin or hemosiderin. A woman has a smaller body store of iron (approximately 300 mg) because of menstrual losses and childbirth.

Failure to absorb iron can occur in gastric disease with extremely high transient time such as celiac disease. A recent cause of iron deficiency is the use of erythropoietin (Epogen) to treat chemotherapy-induced and renal failure–related anemia.

Iron is transported in the plasma bound to transferrin. This protein binds a specific receptor on the cell surface, the transferrin receptor (TfR), with high affinity, and the complex is internalized via a clathrin-coated pit. A small amount of TfR is found in a soluble form in the plasma (serum transferrin receptor [sTfR]). The body is able to detect iron deficiency and compensate to a limited extent by increased intestinal absorption. Hepcidin may be the communicator between iron stores and the intestinal absorption mechanism.

The pathophysiology of iron deficiency is largely unknown. In iron deficiency there is an increase in red-cell-free porphyrin. Ribonucleotide reductase (RR) is a nonheme-iron protein commonly stated to be the most sensitive enzyme to iron deficiency, and lack of iron is reported to stop DNA synthesis. Other essential heme proteins might be involved, in particular those of the respiratory chain in the genesis of loss of energy and central nervous system (CNS) function. Severely anemic rats with a 50% decrease in hemoglobin have an almost 50% reduction in myoglobin and cytochrome c, and decreased iron-sulfur content, pyruvate dehydrogenase, and other tricarboxylic acid (TCA) cycle enzymes. Perinatal iron deficiency in rats decreases cytochrome c oxidase activity in the neonatal brain. In contrast, in milder anemias, which would be more physiologic with hemoglobins in the 6 to 12 g/dL range, there was increased platelet count and increased serum transaminase consistent with cell damage but no decrease in the activities of TCA enzymes or cytochrome oxidase activity, suggesting this is not an important mechanism. On the other hand, abnormalities in lipid composition were observed, consistent with effects on the lipid desaturase activities.

A variety of genes are increased in iron deficiency based on limited DNA microarray data, including Rb, p21, cdk2, cyclins A, D3, E1, myc, iNOS, FasL, none of which is intuitively related to iron metabolism, but may help account for the symptoms and signs. Many of the proteins involved in iron homeostasis may be regulated at the translational (rather than transcriptional) level.

The messenger RNAs (mRNAs) of ferritin, transferrin receptor, aminolevulinic acid synthetase, ferroprotein, m-aconitase, and divalent metal transporter-1 (DMT-1) are regulated by an iron responsive element (IRE) on the mRNA.

Individuals with iron deficiency may experience no symptoms. Findings common to all anemias may be present, or those rather specific to iron's effects on rapidly turning over epithelial cells; glossitis gastric atrophy, stomatitis, ice eating (pagophagia), and leg cramping. The esophageal web syndrome (Plummer-Vinson syndrome) is still reported, and at least some cases appear to respond to iron therapy. Koilonychia or spoon nails may be more commonly caused by fungal infection or hereditary variation.

Definitive diagnosis requires laboratory tests (Table 1). A bone marrow smear with no stainable iron is definitive. A low serum iron level, elevated total iron-binding capacity (TIBC), and a low serum ferritin concentration are considered diagnostic for iron deficiency. Serum iron-binding capacity should be less than 10%. In advanced iron deficiency, the ferritin levels are 0.6 to 12 ng/mL, serum iron is 7 to 60 μg/dL, and TIBC is increased to 450 to 500 μg/dL with absent stores in the marrow. However, serum iron is subject to diurnal variations, with higher concentrations late in the day, and may be increased after meat ingestion. Oral contraceptives increase serum transferrin and result in low transferrin saturation. The serum ferritin reflects body stores and is unaffected by recent iron ingestion. When present as a microcytic anemia, the anemia of chronic disease may be mistaken for iron deficiency. This anemia classically has low serum iron, low iron-binding capacity, elevated ferritin, and saturation of the iron-binding capacity more than 10%.

Perhaps a better estimate of body stores is obtained by the ratio of sTfR-to-serum ferritin (R/F ratio). Studies of the R/F ratio show age dependence, and in males there is a gaussian distribution but in females a bimodal distribution. Ferritin is an *acute phase reactant* and in the presence of infection or inflammation the ferritin may be high and the serum iron and transferrin low. The R/F ration would also be affected by inflammation. In the elderly the R/F ratio may be more sensitive than the classic blood tests and may be more sensitive in distinguishing iron deficiency anemia from anemia of chronic disease. A major problem is the lack of standardization of the sTfR assay.

In individuals treated with recombinant erythropoietin (Epogen) the increased production of red blood cells (RBCs) exhausted iron stores rapidly, resulting in a reduction of serum iron and desaturated transferrin. A functional deficiency resulting from decreased body stores without anemia is suggested by rapid development of the phenotype of iron deficiency on erythropoietin (Epogen) therapy. In healthy individuals iron stores determine the response to erythropoietin (Epogen), and baseline ferritin values less than 1000 μg/L have been associated with a *functional* iron deficiency. But ferritin concentrations are not correlated to body stores in the setting of hyperthyroidism, malignancy, inflammation, hepatocellular disease, alcohol, and oral contraception use. The percentage of hypochromic RBC and reticulocyte hypochromic cells may be useful in identification of functional iron deficiency and in predicting response to erythropoietin (Epogen) and intravenous iron treatments. The percentage is not useful in the settings of thalassemia or chemotherapy patients.

Oral iron is the preferred treatment for nutritional iron deficiency (Table 2). Ferrous iron salts are preferred because of their increased solubility and availability at the pH of the duodenum and jejunum. Standard therapy for iron deficiency anemia in adults is oral administration of a 300-mg tablet of ferrous sulfate (60 mg of elemental iron) three or four times daily. Absorption is enhanced by administration of the iron on an empty stomach. The major side effects of oral iron therapy are epigastric distress, heartburn, nausea, vomiting, and diarrhea. Administering the tablets with meals, decreasing the dose, or gradual dose escalation can reduce these symptoms. Other preparations containing less iron, such as ferrous gluconate tablets (320 mg with 36 mg of elemental iron) or the oral administration of carbonyl iron (Ircon) may reduce the intolerance. Pediatric liquid preparations of iron (Fer-In-Sol) can be used with the dose modified to avoid side effects. The response of the anemia to iron deficiency should be determined (Figure 1). Reticulocytosis may be observed as early as 4 days after treatment and will reach a maximum in 7 to 10 days. Ferritin responds within a few days. An increase in the hematocrit and hemoglobin is delayed. Therapy needs to continue for 2 to 3 months after correction of the anemia to restore the body's store of iron.

Noncompliance is the usual cause of failure to respond. Inability to absorb enteric-coated iron tablets or malabsorption of iron caused by high transit times may occasionally cause treatment failure. True malabsorption of ferrous sulfate is extremely rare. It may be

---

TABLE 1 Differential Diagnoses for Iron Deficiency

Anemia of chronic inflammatory or neoplastic disease
Unresponsive to iron, but may be associated with
    diseases causing blood loss and iron deficiency
Requires >1-2 months of infection
Usually serum iron decreased, TIBC reduced, saturation
    decreased (in iron deficiency, TIBC increased)
Not found in uncomplicated diabetes
Disorders of globin synthesis
α-Thalassemia hemoglobin A2 may normalize if iron
    deficiency coexists
α-Thalassemia low MCV even with normal hemoglobin
    level
Microcytic hemoglobinopathies
Sideroblastic anemia
Hypochromic blood picture, but marrow shows ringed
    sideroblasts (requires marrow biopsy)
Usually normocytic
Folate or vitamin B$_{12}$ Usually have macrocytic anemia, but
    if coexisting with iron deficiency may be normalized

Abbreviations: MCV = mean corpuscular volume; TIBC = total iron-binding capacity.

TABLE 2 Common Oral Replacement Therapies

Type	Dose	Iron content	Dose recommended
Iron Tablets			
Ferrous sulfate	330 mg Capsule (extended release) 250 mg Enteric coated 324, 325 mg Elixir 200 mg/5mL Tabs 195, 300, 324, 325 mg	60 mg	3 per d
Ferrous gluconate	325 mg Enteric coated 325 mg Tabs 200, 300, 325, 350 mg	37 mg	5 per d
Ferrous fumarate	200 mg Chewable tabs 100 mg Suspension 100 mg/5 mL Tabs 200, 300, 325, 350 mg	66 mg	3 per d
Liquid			
Ferrous gluconate (300 mg/tsp)	35 mg/tsp	2 tsp tid	(adult); 1 mg/kg (pediatric)
Ferrous sulfate Elixir (220 mg/tsp) (Adult), 1 mg/kg iron (pediatric)	44 mg/tsp	2 tsp bid-tid	

Abbreviations: bid = twice daily; PO = orally; tid = three times daily.

6

diagnosed by administering an oral dose of liquid ferrous sulfate (50 to 60 mg of iron) in a fasted state and obtaining a serum iron level before administration and 1 and 2 hours later. An increase in the serum iron concentration of 100 μg/100 mL should be observed. Iron for intramuscular or intravenous administration was available in the form of iron dextran (Watson Pharmaceuticals), but it had a high toxicity rate and is now rarely indicated. In contrast, iron sucrose appears safer. The iron is delivered to endogenous iron-binding proteins with a half-life of 90 minutes and it becomes rapidly available for erythropoiesis. Some formulations can cause anaphylactic reactions. Some parenteral preparations such as ferric gluconate and ferric citrate deliver iron to many proteins rather than specifically iron-binding proteins and are deposited in the parenchyma of the liver resulting in necrosis. Oral iron products have been largely abandoned in patients with end-stage renal disease, most of whom are treated with erythropoietin (Epogen). Parenteral iron can be administered by slow intravenous injection, intravenous drip infusion or injection into dialyzer. The most frequently adverse effects reported during treatment in hemodialysis patients are hypotension, cramps, and nausea. Some dialysis centers have tried oral heme iron. Some authorities are recommending the combination

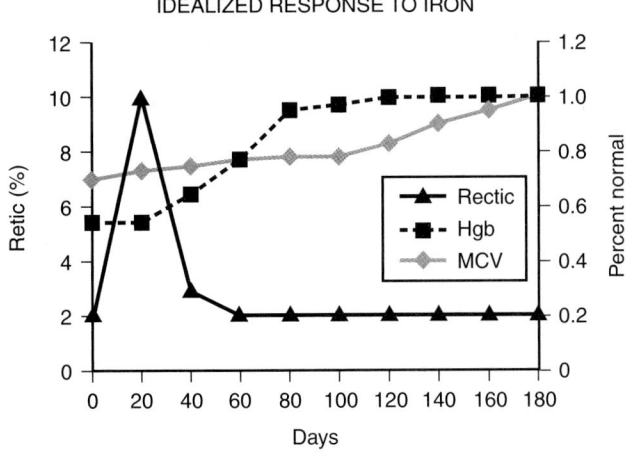

FIGURE 1. Response to iron replacement therapy in iron deficient anemia. The response to iron depends on the degree of deficiency, but reticulocyte count increases almost immediately and peaks at 7 to 10 days, the hemoglobin and hematocrit improve over 2 to 3 months but the MCV lags the correction in hemoglobin. MCV = mean corpuscular volume. (Data from Wintrobe, et al:)

CURRENT DIAGNOSIS

- Microcytic anemia (low mean corpuscular volume), low reticulocyte count
  Absent thalassemia
  Absent lead intoxication
- Low serum iron, low iron saturation (reflects current situation)
  Also low in anemia of chronic disease
- Low ferritin (reflects body stores)
  Ferritin: acute phase reactant, elevated in inflammation
- Elevated total iron-binding capacity (or transferrin)
  Low in anemia chronic disease
- Soluble transferring receptor
  In cases with inflammation

Rakel and Bope: *Conn's Current Therapy 2006.*

CURRENT THERAPY

- Determine source of blood loss or inability to absorb iron. Usual causes are:
  Heavy menstrual loss
  Gastrointestinal bleeding (polyps, ulcers, cancer)
  Achlorhydria
  Gastrointestinal malabsorption
- Prescribe oral iron, 325 mg orally, three times daily. Start with low dose (once a day) and increase over 2 to 3 weeks to improve compliance.
- Monitor for response. The usual cause of lack of response is noncompliance.
- Administer intravenous iron in special cases, including:
  Renal failure
  Severe depletion of iron store and inability to tolerate oral iron
  Need for rapid reversal
  Some cases of erythropoietin administration

---

of erythropoietin (Epogen) and intravenous iron (iron sucrose, 200 mg intravenously, and recombinant erythropoietin [rh-EPO], 300 U/kg twice a week) for rapid reversal of anemia in pregnant patients.

REFERENCES

Annibale B, Capurso G, Lahner E, et al: Concomitant alterations in intragastric pH and ascorbic acid concentration in patients with *Helicobacter pyloris* gastritis and associated iron deficiency anemia. Gut 2003;52:496-501.

Beryman C. Iron deficiency and anemia in pregnancy: Modern aspects of diagnosis and therapy. Blood Cells Mol Dis 2002;29:506-516.

Brugnara C: Iron deficiency and erythropoiesis: New diagnostic approaches. Clin Chem 2003;49:1573-1578.

Carpenter CE, Mahoney AW: Contribution of heme and non-heme iron to human nutrition. Crit Rev Food Sci Nutr 1992;31:333-337.

Cook JD, Flowers CH, Skikne BS: The quantitative assessment of body iron. Blood 2003;101:3359-3364.

Pollitt E: Iron deficiency and cognitive function. Annu Rev Nutr 1993;13:521-537.

Autoimmune Hemolytic Anemia

Method of
Katharine A. Downes, MD,
and Ira A. Shulman, MD

Autoimmune hemolytic anemia (AIHA) is characterized by a decrease in circulating erythrocytes resulting from autoimmune-mediated hemolysis. AIHA occurs when autoantibodies bind to the erythrocyte membrane and cause premature clearance of red blood cells (RBCs)

BOX 1 Possible Mechanisms for Loss of Immunologic Tolerance of Red Blood Cell Self-Antigen in Autoimmune Hemolytic Anemia

- Ignorance of erythrocyte self-antigen
- Molecular mimicry between self-and non–self-antigens
- Activation of polyclonal B and/or T cell
- Immunoregulatory disturbances altering the cytokine network

From: Fagiolo E: Immunological tolerance loss vs. erythrocyte self-antigens and cytokine network disregulation in autoimmune hemolytic anaemia. Autoimmun Rev 2004;3(2):53-59.

---

from the circulation, which results in decreased circulating RBCs when the bone marrow fails to compensate for shortened RBC survival. Several mechanisms have been postulated to account for the loss of immunologic tolerance for erythrocyte self-antigens and autoantibody formation (Box 1).

Clinical data and laboratory findings define six different types of AIHA: warm (WAIHA), cold (CAIHA), paroxysmal cold hemoglobinuria (PCH), combined/mixed, drug-induced, and Evans syndrome (ES) (Box 2, Table 1). WAIHA and CAIHA are further subdivided based on the absence (primary or idiopathic) or presence (secondary) of concomitant disease (Table 2).

Laboratory Diagnosis

The diagnosis of AIHA requires the diagnostic triad of anemia, hemolysis, and an immune etiology (Table 3 and Figure 1). Hemoglobin or RBC count that falls below the reference range establishes the diagnosis of anemia. Reticulocytosis, increased unconjugated bilirubin and

---

BOX 2 Types of Autoimmune Hemolytic Anemia

WAIHA
Typical autoantibody characteristics: IgG, which reacts at body temperature

CAIHA
Typical autoantibody characteristics: IgM, which reacts at 4°C (39.2°F) but has some reactivity at 30°C (86°F)
Mixed/combined WAIHA and CAIHA
Typical autoantibody characteristics: IgG and IgM
Paroxysmal cold hemoglobinuria
Bithermal hemolysis with anti-P specificity
Evans syndrome (if thrombocytopenic)
Typical autoantibody characteristics: IgG, which reacts at body temperature
Drug induced
Autoantibody mechanism
Typical autoantibody characteristics: IgG, which reacts at body temperature

Abbreviations: AIHA = autoimmune hemolytic anemia; CAIHA = cold autoimmune hemolytic anemia; WAIHA = warm autoimmune hemolytic anemia.

TABLE 1 Essential Features of Autoimmune Hemolytic Anemias*

Subtype	Percentage of AIHA cases	Incidence	Autoantibody	Clinical features	Laboratory findings	Pediatric considerations	Other
WAIHA	60%–70%	1:50,000–80,000; Females > males.	Panagglutinin Usually IgG	Severe anemia (see Box 5). Chronic pattern. Acute pattern.	Positive DAT: Anti-IgG+ and anti-C3+ 67%. IgG+ only: 20%. C3+ only: 13% Negative ~1%* *because of inadequate sensitivity of test to detect low levels of bound autoantibodies.	Typically sudden onset. Associated with complications. Exertional dyspnea, progressive weakness, and dark urine occur in rapidly progressing cases. Usually preceded by acute infection or immunization; often history of recent vaccination. Not associated with an underlying systemic illness. Patients usually successfully managed with corticosteroids and/or immunoglobulin infusions and recover within 6 months. Relapse associated with acute infections.	70% secondary; 30% idiopathic.
CAIHA	20%–30%	1:100,000–200,000; Older adults, Peak incidence 70 years of age; Females > males.	Usually IgM Specificity for I blood group antigen Titers (measured at 4°C[39.2°F]) >1:8000	Positive DAT: Anti-C3+ only 91%–98%. Anti-IgG and anti-C3: rare. Anti-IgG only:** rare. ** Lack of detectable C3 may be caused by: 1) Poor sensitivity of anti-C3 reagent 2) Failure to read the anti-C3 DAT result after incubation step. Peripheral blood smear: Rouleaux and RBC agglutination.	Rarely affects children.	Synonyms are cold hemagglutinin disease and cold agglutinin syndrome.	

Continued

6

TABLE 1 Essential Features of Autoimmune Hemolytic Anemias*—cont'd

Subtype	Percentage of AIHA cases	Incidence	Autoantibody	Clinical features	Laboratory findings	Pediatric considerations	Other
PCH	1%	1:600,000–800,000.	Biphasic IgG DL	Acute attacks. High fever, chills, abdominal cramping. Constitutional symptoms may subside in hours. Hemolysis may be severe and life-threatening.	DAT positive for C3. DL test is pathognomonic for PCH.	Predominantly affects children. Leading cause of hemolytic anemia in children. Often antecedent respiratory infection.	
Combined/mixed	7%–8%	Rare.	Both IgG and IgM	Severe acute anemia.	DAT positive for IgG and C3. RBC eluate positive for panreactive IgG.	Corticosteroids demonstrate success.	
Drug-induced			IgG	See Table 5.	RBC eluate positive for IgG.		
ES				Lymphadenopathy. Hepatomegaly. Splenomegaly.	Extremely common.	Diagnosis of exclusion. Rule out confounding disorders before establishing diagnosis.	

*Except where indicated, features listed pertain to the adult patient population.
Abbreviations: AIHA = autoimmune hemolytic anemia; CAIHA = cold autoimmune hemolytic anemia; DAT = direct antiglobulin test; DL = Donath-Landsteiner; ES = Evans syndrome; PCH = paroxysmal cold autoimmune hemolytic anemia; RBC = red blood cell; WAIHA = warm autoimmune hemolytic anemia.

Rakel and Bope: *Conn's Current Therapy 2006.*

TABLE 2 Autoimmune Hemolytic Anemia Secondary to Other Diseases

Type of AIHA	Coexisting conditions	Type of AIHA	Coexisting conditions
WAIHA	Immune disorders	CAIHA	Infectious agents
	AIDS		Viral
	Antiphospholipid syndrome		CMV
	Agammaglobulinemia		EBV
	Ulcerative colitis		Mumps
	Wiskott-Aldrich syndrome		Infectious mononucleosis
	Hematologic		Bacterial agents
	Lymphoma (Hodgkin's & non-Hodgkin's)		*Mycoplasma pneumoniae*
	Leukemia (chronic lymphocytic leukemia)		Hematologic disorders
	Lymphoproliferative syndromes		Leukemia
	Connective tissue disease		Lymphoma
	Dermatomyositis		Monoclonal IgM gammopathies
	Periarteritis nodosa		Collagen vascular disorders
	Rheumatoid arthritis		Malignancy
	Scleroderma	PCH	Recent vaccination
	Systemic lupus erythematosus		Secondary to infectious disease
	Infectious agents		Syphilis
	Viral		Measles
	Atypical pneumonia		Chickenpox
	CMV		Influenza
	Coxsackie B		Infectious mononucleosis
	EBV (mono)		*Mycoplasma pneumoniae*
	Hepatitis		Smallpox vaccination
	Herpes simplex virus		Mumps
	Influenza A		CMV
	Measles		*E. coli, Haemophilus influenzae, Klebsiella pneumoniae*
	Varicella		
	Bacterial	Combined/ mixed	Systemic lupus erythematosus Lymphoproliferative disorders
	Escherichia coli sepsis	Drug-induced	See in Table 5
	Streptococcal	Evans syndrome	Autoimmune lymphoproliferative syndrome
	Typhoid		

Abbreviations: AIHA= autoimmune hemolytic anemia; CAIHA = cold autoimmune hemolytic anemia; CMV = cytomegalovirus; EBV = Epstein-Barr virus; ES = Evans syndrome; PCH = paroxysmal cold autoimmune hemolytic anemia; WAIHA = warm autoimmune hemolytic anemia.

TABLE 3 Key Laboratory Findings in Diagnostic Triad of Autoimmune Hemolytic Anemia

Key feature	Laboratory findings
Anemia	RBC count↓
	Hemoglobin↓
	Hematocrit↓
Hemolysis	
General	Hyperbilirubinemia
	Serum LDH↑
Intravascular	Free hemoglobinemia
	Serum haptoglobin↓
	Hemosiderinuria
	Hemoglobinuria
Extravascular	Spherocytes on peripheral blood smear
	Urine urobilinogen↑
Bone marrow response	Reticulocytosis
	Polychromasia
	Erythroid hyperplasia
Immune etiology	DAT (positive)

Abbreviations: DAT = direct antiglobulin test; LDH = lactate dehydrogenase; RBC = red blood cell.

lactate dehydrogenase, and decreased haptoglobin are consistent with the presence of hemolysis. The direct antiglobulin test (DAT) (Coombs test), which detects autoantibodies bound to the RBC membrane in the patient's circulation, establishes an immune etiology for the hemolysis. When the diagnosis of AIHA is suspected, specialized immunohematologic tests (described in this article) are often needed to select the most appropriate donor RBC units, in the event the patient requires a transfusion.

Step 1: Determination of immune etiology for hemolysis

A positive DAT is critical to establishing the diagnosis of AIHA in a patient with hemolytic anemia. Both a positive DAT and clinical evidence of hemolysis are required to support an immune-mediated hemolytic process and shift the diagnosis away from nonimmune etiologies of hemolytic anemia (see Figure 1;). Because a positive DAT without hemolysis is *not* diagnostic of AIHA, the clinical significance and interpretation of a positive DAT must be assessed in the context of the patient's medical history and clinical presentation (Table 4).

Rakel and Bope: *Conn's Current Therapy 2006.*

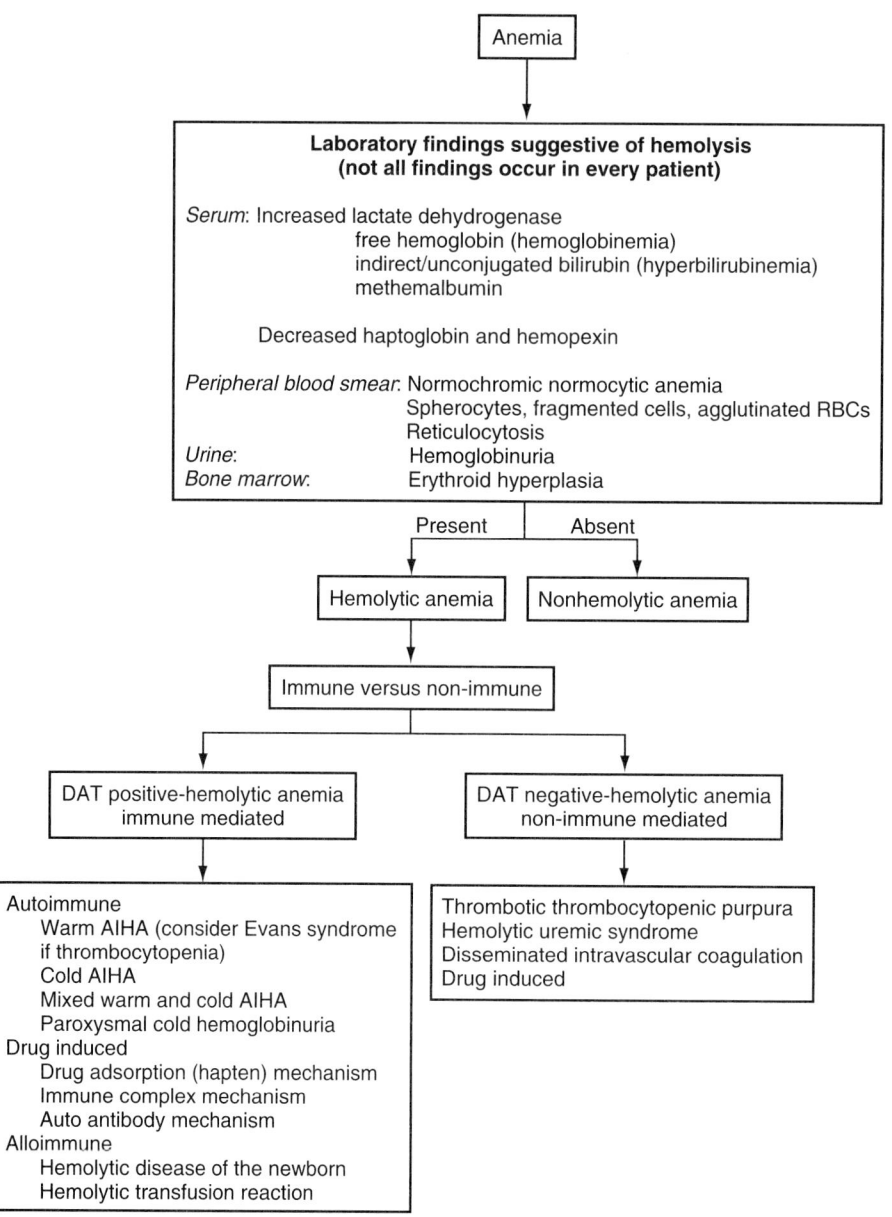

FIGURE 1. Diagnostic algorithm to determine cause of anemia.

TABLE 4 Clinical Situations That May Result in a Positive Direct Antiglobulin Test

Clinical situation	Antibody type	Antibody source	Antigen source	Why is DAT positive?
Autoimmune hemolytic anemia	Autoantibody IgG and/or IgM	Patient	Patient's RBCs	Autoantibody bound to patient's RBC
Transfusion reaction	Alloantibody IgG and/or IgM	Patient	Transfused RBC	Transfusion recipient antibody bound to transfused donor RBCs
Hemolytic disease of the newborn	Alloantibody IgG	Maternal	Fetus/neonate RBC	Maternal antibody bound to fetal/neonatal RBCs
Drug-related mechanism	Autoantibody	Patient	Patient RBC/drug	See Table 5

Abbreviations: DAT = direct antiglobulin test; RBC = red blood cell.

Rakel and Bope: *Conn's Current Therapy 2006.*

DAT Methodology

The sample for a DAT should be collected in an ethylenediaminetetraacetic acid (EDTA) purple-top or pink-top test tube, because EDTA negates in vitro complement pathway activation, which may occur during storage of clotted blood in a red-top plain tube and result in false-positive DATs. Three types of reagents are used in the DAT:

1. Polyspecific antihuman globulin (AHG)-containing antibodies directed against IgG and complement 3 (C3),
2. Monospecific AHG containing anti-IgG
3. Monospecific–AHG-containing antibodies directed against complement (C3)

A positive DAT indicates that the patient's RBCs are coated in vivo with antibodies. The initial DAT may be performed by testing the patient's RBCs with polyspecific AHG reagent. Because a positive polyspecific DAT indicates nonspecifically that RBCs are antibody coated in vivo, a positive polyspecific AHG DAT is followed by testing with monospecific reagents (anti-IgG and anti-C3) to determine whether complement and/or IgG is coating the patient's RBCs. Some laboratories use monospecific anti-IgG and anti-C3 reagents for initial DAT testing. A DAT result may be positive for polyspecific AHG, for anti-IgG or anti-C3 only, or for both anti-IgG and anti-C3 (Figure 2).

Differential Diagnosis of Positive DAT

An elution, which removes antibody bound to RBC, is used to determine the cause of a positive DAT when a delayed hemolytic transfusion reaction (DHTR), drug dependent antibody, or a combination of autoantibodies and alloantibodies is suspected. DHTRs mimic AIHA, but they are caused by an anamnestic antibody response that occurs hours to days after RBC transfusion. In such cases, the DAT is positive, and the eluate shows an alloantibody with a particular specificity (i.e., anti-Jk[a]) rather than a panagglutinating autoantibody. When autoantibodies coat a patient's RBC, an eluate prepared from those cells often reacts with all RBC tested (panagglutinating) without specificity for a particular antigen; thus, other eluates are not performed routinely to establish a diagnosis of AIHA except in the clinical situations described above.

Step 2: Determination of the presence of autoantibodies

ANTIBODY SCREENING TEST

The patient's sample should be tested for autoantibodies in the same manner as screening for alloantibodies prior to blood transfusion.

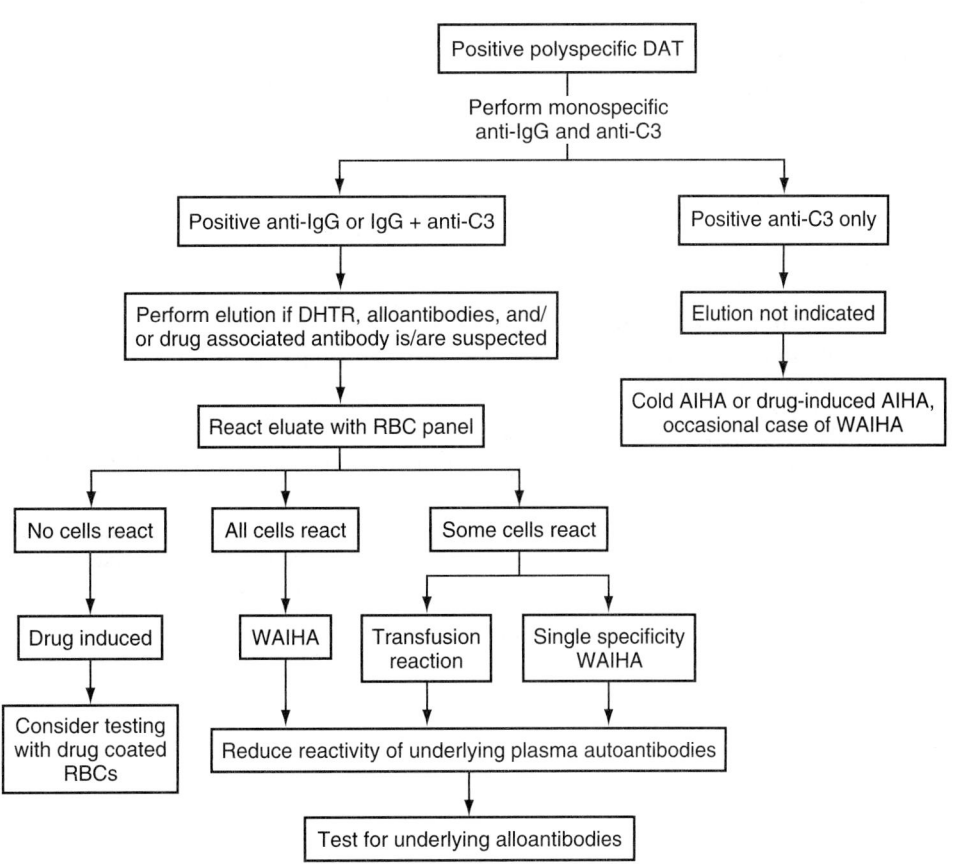

FIGURE 2. Testing algorithm for positive direct antiglobulin test [DAT].

Rakel and Bope: *Conn's Current Therapy 2006.*

Step 3: Determination of the presence of alloantibodies

Before transfusing a patient with AIHA it is crucial to determine if coexisting RBC alloantibodies are present in a patient's serum or plasma. Alloantibodies develop as a result of previous exposure to RBC antigens, such as in transfusion or pregnancy, are directed against RBCs antigens from non-ABO blood group systems, and may cause hemolytic transfusion reactions (HTR). Alloantibodies have been detected in up to 32% of patients with AIHA. Alloantibody detection is performed to prevent alloantibody-induced HTR. Undetected alloantibodies may cause hemolysis following transfusion, which might be attributed incorrectly to an increase in the severity of AIHA. Because autoantibodies interfere with the detection of alloantibodies, steps must be taken to reduce or eliminate the strength of reactivity of the autoantibodies in the test system before proceeding with testing for alloantibodies. Methods for diminishing the reactivity of autoantibodies include adsorption of autoantibody by patient or reagent RBC and dilution of autoantibody strength, a less sensitive method.

ALLOANTIBODY DETECTION

After the autoantibody reactivity has been reduced, alloantibodies can be detected and identified. The patient's sample is tested against a RBC panel of known antigenic phenotypes.

Step 4: Selection of RBC for transfusion

Transfusion of RBCs requires performing a series of pretransfusion compatibility tests (Box 3). If a patient has an alloantibody that is capable of causing a hemolytic reaction, RBC units lacking the antigen to which the antibody is directed are selected. A crossmatch assesses the in vitro compatibility between the patient's serum or plasma and the donor RBC unit selected for transfusion. Because autoantibodies react with common antigens intrinsic to the RBC membrane, incompatible crossmatches are common when testing RBC units selected for transfusion. For cold-reacting autoantibodies the crossmatch procedure can be modified by warming the patient sample and RBC, which reduces the reactivity of the autoantibody (*prewarm technique*) and may result in a *compatible crossmatch*. Warm-reacting autoantibodies generally result in incompatible crossmatches with donor RBC unless the autoantibody

---

BOX 3 Pretransfusion Compatibility Testing

- ABO group
- RhD type
- Antibody detection
- Antibody identification
- Phenotyping of RBC unit for antigens (if alloantibody is present)
- Crossmatch (patient serum/plasma and donor RBCs)

Abbreviations: RBC = red blood cell; RhD = rhesus D antigen.

BOX 4 Controversy Surrounding Nomenclature of Red Blood Cell Units Incompatible for Transfusion Caused by Autoantibodies*

- The term *least incompatible* is used in medical parlance but is undefined in medical literature.
- It is used to suggest the selection of an RBC unit for transfusion that gives weaker reactions in vitro than other incompatible units.
- *Least incompatible* is a historical term from a time when testing was less advanced.
- The term should be avoided because:
  It is undefined in the medical literature.
  Interpretation varies between transfusion services.
  It does not convey meaningful information.
  It implies that it is an acceptable alternative to standard serologic evaluations.

*For a discussion of controversy surrounding *least incompatible* terminology, see http://www.cbbsweb.org/enf/incompat_term.html/; last accessed August 30, 2005.
Abbreviations: RBC = red blood cell.

---

reactivity has been diminished by an adsorption method or dilution. Controversy surrounds the terminology used to describe RBC units that show in vitro incompatible crossmatches caused by autoantibodies (Box 4).

Types of Autoimmune Hemolytic Anemia

This section describes the pathogenesis, clinical features, and management of the primary AIHA subtypes; for secondary AIHA the treatment of the underlying disease is the preferred approach.

WARM AUTOIMMUNE HEMOLYTIC ANEMIA

Pathogenesis

Autoantibodies are directed against intrinsic RBC surface antigens. A risk factor stimulates an autoimmune phenomenon, which results in reticuloendothelial tissue destruction of autoantibody coated RBCs.

Clinical Features

Patients present with severe anemia and its complications (Box 5). Disease acuity parallels initial presentation.

BOX 5 Complications Associated With Severe Anemia

- Weakness
- Dizziness
- Pallor
- Jaundice
- Splenomegaly
- Hepatomegaly and lymphadenopathy
- Hemodynamic compromise leading to shock
- Congestive heart failure
- Acute renal failure
- Dehydration

When symptoms develop over a few months (chronic pattern), the patient may have adjusted to low-grade hemolysis, but patients with acute onset and rapid hemolysis (acute pattern) usually present with more severe symptoms. The chronic pattern has an insidious onset of signs and symptoms with hemolysis lasting months to years and is associated with an underlying systemic illness.

Management

Acute Pattern

Management involves medications and supportive measures (RBC transfusions and fluid resuscitation) to treat hemodynamic compromise caused by precipitous, severe anemia. If necessary, patients should be transfused with appropriate RBC (further discussed later in this article). Prednisone (1 to 2 mg/kg per day) has been demonstrated to have an excellent response with the acute transient pattern but a variable response with the chronic pattern. Prednisone has been shown to downregulate fragment, crystallizable (of immunoglobulin) gamma (Fcγ) receptor expression potentially decreasing the phagocytosis of IgG-coated RBCs by the reticuloendothelial system, which has Fcγ receptors. Patients should be monitored closely for complications of corticosteroids (Box 6) and tapered slowly from prednisone after hemolysis ceases but restarted on a full dose if relapse occurs.

Chronic Pattern

Management of chronic WAIHA may involve splenectomy, immunosuppressive agents (azathioprine, danazol, intravenous immune [serum] globulin [IVIG]), and in some cases plasmapheresis. Splenectomy is a second line of therapy for patients who are unresponsive to corticosteroid therapy but useful only for patients with IgG autoantibody; those who initially respond to splenectomy may relapse and require further immunosuppressive therapy. Patients should receive folate supplementation to compensate for increased erythropoiesis.

COLD AUTOIMMUNE HEMOLYTIC ANEMIA

Pathogenesis

The autoantibody is typically IgM, reacts with the I or RBC antigen, and binds optimally at near-freezing temperatures. Attachment of IgM on the RBC membrane activates complement; complement-coated RBCs are phagocytosed by C3b receptor-bearing macrophages.

Clinical Features

Patients have severe anemia and with exposure to cold may have hemoglobinuria and hemoglobinemia.

Management

Fluid resuscitation is used to treat hemodynamic compromise. Although advisable it is not required to warm intravenous (IV) solutions and blood prior to administration, because many CAIHA patients undergo surgical procedures while hypothermic. However, if a patient has intravascular hemolysis following exposure to the cold, such a patient should receive warmed solutions and blood products. Patients should avoid the cold, which may precipitate attacks. Corticosteroid therapy is less effective. Splenectomy has no role because the liver clears complement-coated red cells.

PAROXYSMAL COLD HEMOGLOBINURIA

Pathogenesis

PCH is a form of CAIHA mediated by the Donath-Landsteiner (DL) autoantibody, which is an IgG auto–anti-P biphasic hemolysin. In vitro DL initially binds to RBCs at cold temperatures, but when the temperature is raised to 37°C (98.6°F), it causes complement-mediated hemolysis. In vivo DL attaches to RBCs in the colder extremities, but when RBCs circulate centrally, complement is activated lysing RBC.

Clinical Features

History of exposure to the cold or a prodromal flulike illness is often reported. Patients may present with acute attacks of shaking chills, fever, and abdominal, back, and leg pain with hemoglobinuria detected afterwards.

Laboratory Investigation

PCH is diagnosed identifying the DL in patient's plasma using a bithermal antibody test. Patient serum is incubated with RBCs at 4°C (39.2°F) and the cold-reacting antibody binds to RBCs; when heated to 37°C (98.6°F), RBCs hemolyze from complement activation initiated by the DL antibody. Approximately 2% of cold agglutinins give false positive DL tests.

Management

Patient should be kept warm. Most require only supportive care.

MIXED OR COMBINED AUTOIMMUNE HEMOLYTIC ANEMIA

Patients have cold agglutinins with low titers at 4°C (39.2°F) but with high thermal amplitude (up to 30°C

BOX 6	**Complications of Corticosteroid Therapy**

- Osteoporosis
- Avascular necrosis
- Susceptibility to infections
- Posterior subcapsular cataracts
- Increased intraocular pressure
- Abnormalities of glucose and lipid metabolism

Rakel and Bope: *Conn's Current Therapy 2006.*

[86°F] or higher). Both warm-reacting IgG autoantibodies and cold-reacting IgM autoantibodies may be present in the serum. Patients often present with acute severe anemia. Like WAIHA, use of corticosteroids demonstrates success.

DRUG-ASSOCIATED AUTOIMMUNE HEMOLYTIC ANEMIA

Pathogenesis

Drugs may induce an IgG warm autoantibody, which presents like WAIHA (Table 5). Other drug-related mechanisms for autoantibody production include drug adsorption and immune complexes, which are beyond the scope of this article.

Clinical Pattern

The presenting symptoms range from asymptomatic to rapidly progressive hemolysis. Patients may report a recent change in medication though some medications after prolonged administration cause AIHA (i.e., methyldopa).

Management

Treatment is cessation of the medication.

EVANS SYNDROME

Pathogenesis

ES is characterized by autoimmune-mediated destruction of at least two hematologic cell types. In AIHA, related subtype RBCs and platelets are destroyed. The underlying pathogenesis remains unknown, but immune dysregulation is thought to play a role.

Clinical Pattern

ES is a chronic relapsing disease associated with significant morbidity and mortality.

Management

Overall treatment results are unsatisfactory. Corticosteroid therapy controls acute episodes and results in a transient remission in most patients; subsequent

TABLE 5 Drug-Associated Autoimmune Hemolytic Anemia

Drug mechanism	Mechanism and hemolysis	Laboratory investigation and findings	Implicated medications
Autoantibody mechanism (drug independent; autoantibody induction)	*Mechanism:* Drug stimulates production of IgG autoantibodies that react with all RBCs (in the absence of any drug bound neoantigen). *Hemolysis:* Mild to moderate extravascular hemolysis.	Drug stimulates production of IgG autoantibodies that react with all RBCs. DAT is positive for IgG alone. Drug is not required for in-vitro demonstration of antibody.	Methyldopa Mefenamic acid Interferon-α Moxalactam Apazone[2] Nomifensine[2] Catergen[2] Phenacetin[2] Cephalosporins (second and third generation) Chaparral Procainamide Chlorpromazine Streptomycin Cyanidanol[2] Sulindac Cyclofenil[2] Suprofen Cyclosporine Teniposide Diclofenac Tolmetin Fenoprofen Zomepirac[2] Glafenine[2] Tacrolimus (Prograf) Ibuprofen Fludarabine* Levodopa Cladribine (Leustatin)*

*Chronic lymphocytic leukemia (CLL) patients.
[2]Not available in the United States.

splenectomy seldom results in complete remission. Persistent cytopenia requires prolonged corticosteroid treatment with alternate-day dosing if possible. IVIG, plasmapheresis, and immunosuppressive agents have shown limited success. Recent data suggest a high prevalence of autoimmune lymphoproliferative syndrome (ALPS) in patients with ES. Elevated levels of double-negative T cells (CD4–/CD8–), and defective Fas-mediated apoptosis of mitogen-stimulated T cells characterize ALPS. Because management of ALPS differs from ES, patients with ES should be tested for ALPS.

Transfusion Therapy for Patients with Autoimmune Hemolytic Anemia

RBC transfusion should never be withheld from a patient because of in vitro serologic RBC incompatibility resulting from autoantibodies. Transfusion-medicine physicians provide guidance for how to balance the risks of morbidity and mortality from not transfusing a patient with severe anemia against the potential risks of acute and/or delayed HTR from transfusing in vitro incompatible blood (Box 7). If coexisting alloantibodies have been excluded or have been identified and RBC units have been selected that are negative for the antigen to which the alloantibody is directed, transfusion of RBCs that show incompatibility in vitro because of an autoantibody is relatively safe. Overall, morbidity/mortality of severe hemorrhage or anemia outweighs the risks of HTR. For practical aspects of transfusing *incompatible* blood see Box 8.

> **BOX 7   Clinical Assessment for Red Blood Cell Transfusion in Autoimmune Hemolytic Anemia**
>
> - Clinical assessment should consider:
>   Expectation of continued blood loss
>   Patient's age
>   Co-morbid conditions
> - Hemoglobin at which RBC transfusion is clinically indicated depends on clinical factors unique for each patient:
>   Cardiovascular, cerebrovascular, and pulmonary status
> - Clinical indications for transfusing a patient with AIHA:
>   Rapid, ongoing blood loss or RBC destruction
>   Symptomatic anemia with hemoglobin of <5g/dL
>   Hemoglobin of <7g/dL for patients with a history of cardiac, pulmonary, or cerebrovascular disease
>   For patients older than 65 years of age with acute MI, hemoglobin should not be allowed to fall below 10 g/dL
>
> *Abbreviations:* AIHA = autoimmune hemolytic anemia; MI = myocardial infarction; RBC = red blood cell.

> **BOX 8   Key Steps in Administration of Incompatible Red Blood Cells in Autoimmune Hemolytic Anemia**
>
> - Transfuse incompatible RBCs slowly.
> - Hydrate the patient and monitor closely for signs of hemolysis throughout the transfusion.
> - If coexisting alloantibodies have not been excluded, one method is:
>   Transfuse 50 mL of RBCs slowly
>   Stop the transfusion
>   Draw a sample from the patient and send it to the laboratory for examination for hemolysis
>   Restart the transfusion if hemolysis is absent
> - Document the transfusion of crossmatch incompatible blood in the patient's medical record

New Frontiers in Treatment of Autoimmune Hemolytic Anemia

Preliminary studies suggest that off-label usage of monoclonal antibodies (MoAbs) directed against the CD20 antigen (rituximab [Rituxan],[1] MabThera) and CD52 antigen (alemtuzumab [Camoath-1H][1]) may be a possible new treatment for AIHA. Rituximab (Rituxan)[1] causes in vivo destruction of B lymphocytes with consequent cessation of antibody production. Rituximab (Rituxan)[1] may be an effective treatment for WAIHA, CAIHA, and ES. However, case series are limited by small size and off-label usage for the drug, and the drug should be used with caution without FDA approval. The drug's manufacturers (Biogen Idec and Genentech) notified health care professionals of revisions to the *warnings* section of the prescribing information because of reports of hepatitis B virus (HBV) reactivation with fulminant hepatitis, hepatic failure, and

---

[1]Not FDA approved for this indication.

 CURRENT DIAGNOSIS

- Establish presence of immune-mediated hemolysis
- Notify transfusion service of suspected case of AIHA
- Determine if hemolysis is immune mediated; perform DAT
- Establish reason for positive DAT
- Confirm presence of autoantibodies
- Determine if alloantibodies are present
- Select RBCs for transfusion that lack the antigen against which the antibody is directed if alloantibodies are present
- Transfuse appropriately tested RBCs

Abbreviations: AIAH = autoimmune hemolytic anemia; DAT = direct antiglobulin test; RBC = red blood cell.

6

CURRENT THERAPY

Treatment of autoimmune hemolytic anemia varies depending on the subtype.

Idiopathic or Primary AIHA

- WAIHA.

    Initial management should consist of corticosteroids such as prednisone at 1 to 2 mg/kg per day orally.

    Second-line therapies to consider after failure to respond to corticosteroids are IV immunoglobulin, danazol, and plasma exchange (all with variable benefits).

    Splenectomy should be considered for patients who do not respond to second-line treatments.

Cold Agglutinin Syndrome

- Patients should avoid exposure to cold.
- Corticosteroid therapy is less effective than in AIHA.
- Plasma exchange yields primarily temporary benefit.
- Splenectomy is considered ineffective.
- Cytotoxic drugs cause improvement in minority of patients.

    Fludarabine has limited effectiveness and significant adverse effects.

    Chlorambucil usually used with daily doses of 2 to 4 mg per day.

    Biweekly blood counts including a reticulocyte count should be performed.

    Patient should be monitored for adverse effects of bone marrow suppression, anorexia, and nausea.

Paroxysmal Cold Hemoglobinuria

- Aggressive supportive therapy should be implemented.

Mixed/combined AIHA

- Corticosteroid therapy is effective.

Evans Syndrome

- Corticosteroid therapy controls acute episodes and often results in a transient remission.
- IVIG, plasmapheresis, and immunosuppressive agents have shown limited success.

Secondary AIHA

- Therapy for the underlying disorder may result in remission of hemolysis.

Abbreviations: AIHA = autoimmune hemolytic anemia; IV = intravenous; IVIg = intravenous immunoglobulin; WAIHA = warm autoimmune hemolytic anemia.

death in some patients with hematologic malignancies. Patients at high risk for HBV infection should be screened before initiation of rituximab (Rituxan),[1] and HBV carriers should be monitored closely for signs of active HBV infection during and for several months after therapy. Clinical experience with alemtuzumab is

---

[1]Not FDA approved for this indication.

even more limited. Further studies with these MoAb and longer follow-up of patients for efficacy and side effect profiles are warranted.

REFERENCES

Engelfriet CP, Reesink HW, Garratty G, et al: The detection of alloantibodies against red cells in patients with warm-type autoimmune haemolytic anaemia. Vox Sang 2000;78(3):200-207.

Fagiolo E: Immunological tolerance loss vs. erythrocyte self antigens and cytokine network disregulation in autoimmune hemolytic anaemia. Autoimmun Rev 2004;3(2):53-59.

Mantadakis E, Danilatou V, Stiakaki E, Kalmanti M: Rituximab for refractory Evans syndrome and other immune-mediated hematologic diseases. Am J Hematol 2004;77(3):303-310.

Petz LD: A physician's guide to transfusion in autoimmune haemolytic anemia. Br J Haematol 2004;124(6):712-716.

Robak T: Monoclonal antibodies in the treatment of autoimmune cytopenias. Eur J Haematol 2004;72(2):79-88.

Rosse WF, Hillmen P, Schreiber AD: Immune-mediated hemolytic anemia. Hematology (Am Soc Hematol Educ Program) 2004;48-62.

Shanafelt TD, Madueme HL, Wolf RC, Tefferi A: Rituximab for immune cytopenia in adults: Idiopathic thrombocytopenic purpura, autoimmune hemolytic anemia, and Evans syndrome. Mayo Clin Proc 2003;78(11):1340-1346.

Teachey DT, Manno CS, Axsom KM, Andrews T, et al: Unmasking Evans Syndrome: T cell phenotype and apoptotic response reveal autoimmune lymphoproliferative syndrome (ALPS). Blood 2004; 105(6):2443–2448.

Wright MS, Smith LA: Laboratory investigation of autoimmune hemolytic anemias. Clin Lab Sci 1999;12(2):119-122.

Zecca M, Nobili B, Ramenghi U, et al: Rituximab for the treatment of refractory autoimmune hemolytic anemia in children. Blood 2003; 15;101(10):3857-3861.

For information on Rituxan see July 12, 2004—Letter—Genentech/Biogen at http://www.fda.gov/medwatch/SAFETY/2004/Rituxan_dearhcp.pdf/; last accessed August 30, 2005; See June 2004 Label—Genentech/Biogen at http://www.fda.gov/medwatch/SAFETY/2004/rituxan-prescribing.pdf/; last accessed August 30, 2005.

For a discussion concerning *least incompatible terminology* see http://www.cbbsweb.org/enf/incompat_term.html/; last accessed August 30, 2005.

Nonimmune Hemolytic Anemia

Method of
Ted Wun, MD

There are several congenital and acquired diseases that result in the premature destruction of red blood cells by non-antibody–mediated mechanisms. The method of categorization varies by clinician. I have found it most useful to separate these diseases into abnormalities internal to the red blood cell, those affecting the erythrocyte membrane, and those causes of hemolysis that are external to the red cell.

Rakel and Bope: *Conn's Current Therapy 2006.*

Internal Red Cell Defects

The two major disorders in this category are red cell enzyme deficiencies (enzymopathies) and unstable hemoglobins.

RED CELL ENZYME DEFECTS

Although defects in all of the enzymes of the glycolytic pathway and the pentose monophosphate shunt have been described, pyruvate kinase (PK) and glucose-6-phosphate dehydrogenase (G6PD) deficiencies are the most common. Of these, G6PD is the most common by far.

The red blood cell is dependent on the glycolytic pathway for the production of ATP, important in maintaining membrane integrity via energy-dependent membrane pumps. PK catalyzes an essential step in ATP synthesis: the ATP deficiency results in a loss of membrane integrity with resultant hemolysis. Increases in glycolytic pathway intermediates proximal to the defect lead to a marked increase in red blood cell 2,3-diphosphoglycerate (or bisphosphoglycerate) that increases oxygen release from hemoglobin.

Protection of the red cell from oxidant-mediated damage that might result in hemolysis is dependent on an adequate pool of reduced intermediates such as nicotinamide adenine dinucleotide phosphate (NADPH). NADPH is essential for the regeneration of reduced glutathione (GSH) from oxidized glutathione and the activity of catalase, which degrades hydrogen peroxide, and is produced by the pentose monophosphate shunt. G6PD catalyzes the first step in this pathway.

GLUCOSE-6-PHOSPHATE DEHYDROGENASE DEFICIENCY

Prevalence and Pathophysiology

G6PD deficiency occurs with high incidence in parts of Africa (and in African Americans), the Mediterranean basin, the Middle East, and Southeast Asia. It has been estimated that more than 200 million people have these mutations. Persistence of the genotype is thought related to partial protection from falciparum malaria. More than 500 mutations in this X-linked gene have been described that result in qualitative or quantitative abnormalities of enzyme function; therefore, the phenotype may vary and some authors have divided the disease into five major types. Although this X-linked disease affects mainly males, because of the high prevalence of the gene, symptomatic females are not rare. Red blood cells deficient in G6PD are unable to regenerate sufficient quantities of GSH to compensate for oxidized glutathione that results from oxidant damage. When GSH is depleted, sulfhydryl groups of hemoglobin are oxidized and denatured hemoglobin precipitates on the inner side of the erythrocyte membrane. The red blood cell becomes less deformable, is unable to traverse the microcirculation and reticuloendothelial system, and is therefore cleared from the circulation (e.g., hemolyzed).

Rakel and Bope: *Conn's Current Therapy 2006.*

Clinical Manifestations

In the absence of illness (usually febrile) or exposure to oxidant drugs, the vast majority of patients with G6PD deficiency have no evidence of hemolysis. The typical presentation is that of rapid onset of fatigue accompanied by jaundice, dark urine, and anemia that typically follow the offending agent by a day or two. The provocation can be a febrile illness or drugs such as antimalarials, sulfonamides and sulfones, nitrofurans, antihelminthics, and ribavirin. Favism is a hemolytic episode that follows the ingestion of fava beans and is classically characterized by severe symptomatic anemia, fever, abdominal pain, and nausea. Sensitivity to fava beans typically occurs in the Mediterranean types of G6PD deficiency. The hemolytic episodes usually resolve within a few days with full recovery of hemoglobin levels within a few weeks. Neonatal jaundice can also occur as the result of G6PD deficiency. Chronic hemolysis, unrelated to identifiable provocation, is rare.

Laboratory Features

During hemolytic episodes, the patient will have biochemical evidence for red cell destruction (elevated serum lactate dehydrogenase, total and indirect bilirubin, low serum haptoglobin, and hemoglobinuria) along with a moderate to severe anemia. Heinz bodies, which are precipitates of denatured hemoglobin, can be seen with methyl violet stain of a peripheral blood smear. Reticulocytosis is usually found in patients without bone marrow suppression attributed to another process.

Semiquantitative screening tests and quantitative tests are available for the diagnosis of G6PD deficiency. A caveat to these tests is that the activity of G6PD may be normal or nearly normal in reticulocytes and young red blood cells. This is especially true in the type most prevalent in African Americans. Whereas a low level can be considered diagnostic, a normal test result shortly after a hemolytic episode may be a false negative. Thus, it is prudent to wait 3 to 4 weeks after a hemolytic episode to order the enzyme level. Alternatively, some laboratories synchronously determine the activity of another age-dependent enzyme, such as hexokinase, and calculate an activity ratio relative to G6PD.

Treatment

Treatment consists of supportive measures for the acute hemolytic episode that includes maintaining adequate urine flow and transfusion for severe anemia. Drugs and/or other provoking agents should be avoided. There is no role for splenectomy.

PYRUVATE KINASE DEFICIENCY

Despite being the second most common red cell enzymopathy, fewer than 1000 patients with PK deficiency have been reported. It affects people mostly of Northern European and Mediterranean ancestry. The transmission is autosomal, and only homozygotes have hemolysis severe enough to result in anemia. The hemolysis is chronic, with exacerbations seen with infections and pregnancy. Besides biochemical evidence for hemolysis, one can also find burr cells on examination of a Wright-stained peripheral blood smear. Severe anemia may develop with transient bone marrow suppression as a result of infection with parvovirus B19. The degree of anemia varies, and some patients may be transfusion dependent. Splenomegaly may be present, and splenectomy may ameliorate the anemia in some patients.

UNSTABLE HEMOGLOBINS

Many structural abnormalities of globin have now been described that enhance the tendency of the hemoglobin to denature, form precipitates within the erythrocyte (Heinz bodies), decrease deformability, and lead to hemolysis in response to, or exacerbated by, oxidant stress. Thus, the hemolysis may be clinically episodic as in patients with G6PD deficiency, and this is included in the differential diagnosis. However, some variants result in a chronic hemolytic anemia. The screening test for unstable hemoglobin is incubation in 17% isopropanol, which will cause unstable hemoglobin to precipitate. Variant hemoglobins may also migrate abnormally on hemoglobin electrophoresis. An example of unstable hemoglobin is hemoglobin Hammersmith.

Membrane Defects

Although there are several congenital membrane defects, hereditary spherocytosis (HS) is by far the most common. Hereditary elliptocytosis (HE) can result from abnormalities of some of the same membrane proteins that lead to the HS phenotype. Paroxysmal nocturnal hemoglobinuria (PNH) and spur cell hemolytic anemia are acquired membrane defects.

The structural and functional integrity of the red blood cell depends on several integral membrane proteins and their interaction with the underlying cytoskeleton. Inherited mutations in genes encoding these proteins can result in abnormal membrane integrity, reduced red cell survival with hemolytic anemia, and characteristic red cell morphology.

HEREDITARY SPHEROCYTOSIS AND ELLIPTOCYTOSIS

The basic structure of the red cell cytoskeleton is a hexagonal lattice of the protein spectrin. In turn, spectrin consists of α and β chains. Interactions between spectrin chains with one another and with the lipid bilayer are mediated by proteins such as ankyrin, band 3, glycophorin, protein 4.1, and actin. Mutations in the genes coding for these proteins can lead to HS or HE; the most common abnormalities that result in HS are in spectrin. Quantitative or qualitative defects in these proteins result in a cytoskeleton that may be nondeformable and/or lack structural integrity. Membrane vesiculation and hemolysis result.

The incidence of HS in North America and Europe is estimated to be between 1 in 2000 to 5000. It is less common in persons of African descent. The mode of inheritance is autosomal dominant in 75% of the cases and autosomal recessive in most of the others (de novo mutations have been described).

Clinical Manifestations

HS and HE are marked by a chronic hemolytic anemia that varies as to degree in the presence of spherocytes or elliptocytes, respectively. Mild disease, denoted by a hemoglobin level more than 11 g/dL and bilirubin levels of 1 to 2 mg/dL, comprises approximately 30% of the cases. Neonates often have jaundice, and hemoglobin levels may decrease precipitously in the first 3 weeks of life. As with other chronic hemolytic anemias, splenomegaly and bilirubin gallstones are frequent. In severe forms, red cell morphology can be extreme with extensive poikilocytosis and bizarre-shaped red cells.

Laboratory Features

Biochemical evidence for chronic hemolysis will be present. In HS, the mean corpuscular hemoglobin concentration (MCHC) may be increased, denoting the presence of spherocytes (low surface-to-volume ratio). If there is an abundance of microspherocytes, the mean corpuscular volume may be low. The peripheral blood smear may reveal spherocytes and microspherocytes, and elliptocytes in the case of HE. However, these red cell abnormalities may be difficult to locate even in patients with well-documented HS. The osmotic fragility test, which determines the susceptibility of erythrocytes to lysis in progressively more hypotonic solutions, reveals increased fragility compared with normal red blood cells. The sensitivity of the test can be increased by a 24-hour incubation step. Red cells in some cases of HE (the extreme form of which is called hereditary pyropoikilocytosis) will exhibit increased thermal sensitivity with fragmentation at temperatures of 44°C to 46°C (111.2°F to 114.8°F).

Treatment

The spleen is the major site of sequestration and hemolysis in the vast majority of patients with HS/HE and anemia. Thus, in patients with moderate to severe anemia, splenectomy will effectively cure the anemia. Because of concerns surrounding the risk for postsplenectomy sepsis and thrombotic complications, especially in older individuals, the necessity of splenectomy in patients with mild disease has been questioned. Patients should be preoperatively vaccinated with pneumococcal, meningococcal, and *Haemophilus influenzae* vaccines. Prophylactic penicillin should be given for at least 1 year postsplenectomy, and perhaps longer in young children. Concern regarding postsplenectomy sepsis has prompted the use of subtotal splenectomy in young children. This procedure removes sufficient spleen to ameliorate the anemia, whereas leaving enough splenic tissue for adequate phagocytic function.

PAROXYSMAL NOCTURNAL HEMOGLOBINURIA

Paroxysmal nocturnal hemoglobinuria (PNH) is an acquired, clonal hematopoietic stem cell disorder that results in a red cell membrane defect that classically presents as periodic episodes (paroxysms) of hemolytic anemia signified by jaundice and dark urine (hemoglobinuria from intravascular hemolysis). Despite the name, most hemolytic episodes do not occur at night. Venous thrombosis, particularly at unusual sites such as mesenteric and portal vein, can also complicate the course of illness. Varying degrees of bone marrow failure can also be present, from mild cytopenias to frank aplastic anemia. Indeed, it is being increasingly recognized that patients with otherwise classic aplastic anemia oftentimes have "PNH-like" cells and develop a PNH clinical picture after successful therapy with immunosuppressive drugs.

Pathogenesis

Glycosyl phosphatidylinositol (GPI) anchors are vital for the proper attachment of many proteins to the cell membrane. The phosphatidylinositol glycan complementation group A, coded by the *PIG-A* gene, is critical in the biosynthesis of GPI anchors. Somatic mutations in the *PIG-A* gene have been demonstrated in most patients with PNH. This gene is present on the X chromosome: a single defective gene can result in the PNH phenotype. Complement-inactivating proteins on red blood cells (such as CD55, CD59, and C-8 binding protein) are GPI anchored and thus lacking or deficient in the red blood cells on patients with PNH. These erythrocytes are more susceptible to complement-mediated damage, resulting in a chronic hemolytic anemia with intermittent clinical exacerbations.

The pathogenesis of the thrombosis and aplasia in PNH are less clear. Although it has been speculated that the abnormal red cell membrane leads to thrombin generation, platelet hyperreactivity may also have a role. The aplasia seems to result from autoreactive T cells because it often responds to immunosuppressive therapy as in classic aplastic anemia.

Clinical Manifestations

Although the hemolysis in PNH is chronic, clinical paroxysms marked by jaundice and hemoglobinuria occur with variable frequency. The onset is often heralded by crampy abdominal and back pain. This has been variously attributed to esophageal spasm or mesenteric ischemia. These episodes typically persist for a few days. Thrombosis is generally venous and, as noted, can involve unusual sites. Some authorities have advocated routine anticoagulation in patients with PNH; others would reserve this only for patients with objectively proven

thrombosis. Patients can also present with signs and symptoms associated with pancytopenia.

Laboratory Findings

There is often biochemical evidence for ongoing hemolysis in between clinical episodes. The serum haptoglobin is often undetectable because the predominant site of hemolysis with PNH is intravascular. Urine hemosiderin is typically positive. After an acute exacerbation, the peripheral blood smear may reveal polychromasia (indicating reticulocytosis); there are typically no detectable morphologic abnormalities of leukocytes and platelets. Historically, the sugar water test was used as the screening test for PNH with confirmation with the acidified serum acid lysis (or Ham's) test. A low leukocyte alkaline phosphatase (LAP) score provided corroborating evidence. These have now been supplanted by determination of the surface expression of CD55 and CD59 using fluorescent-labeled monoclonal antibodies and flow cytometry, which are both more sensitive and specific for PNH. This assay is now widely available via large referral clinical laboratories.

Treatment

In the past, therapy was supportive. During acute exacerbations, adequate urine flow to protect the kidneys from hemoglobin-mediated damage, analgesia, and transfusion of red blood cells were the mainstays of therapy. For patients with thrombosis, anticoagulation is given, although the efficacy of this in preventing recurrence has been questioned. In patients with an aplastic presentation, immunosuppressive therapy as for classic aplastic anemia is associated with a relatively high response rate. Allogeneic stem cell transplants have also been done for aplasia; much less often for recurrent thrombosis. Recently, an anti-C5 monoclonal antibody has been shown to be effective in preventing hemolytic episodes.

 CURRENT DIAGNOSIS

- Biochemical evidence for hemolysis includes an increased indirect hemoglobin, increased serum lactate dehydrogenase, and reduced serum haptoglobin.
- The Coombs test is negative, denoting the lack of immune etiology.
- Review of the peripheral blood smear may reveal diagnostic clues such as the presence of spherocytes, elliptocytes, or schistocytes.
- The MCHC may be increased in the presence of spherocytes.
- Once an immune-mediated process has been excluded, specialized tests for the presence of spherocytes, intraerythrocytic enzyme deficiencies, unstable hemoglobin, or PNH cells can be obtained.

CURRENT THERAPY

- The decision to transfuse is based on the severity of the anemia and the degree to which the patient is symptomatic.
- Patients with an inadequate compensatory response, as denoted by severe anemia and reticulocytopenia, are in the most danger for anemia-related adverse events.
- Avoidance of oxidant drugs is the mainstay of "therapy" for most patients with enzymopathies and unstable hemoglobins.
- Patients with hereditary spherocytosis and anemia typically respond to splenectomy.
- Recently, an anti-C5 monoclonal antibody has been shown to decrease hemolysis in patients with paroxysmal nocturnal hemoglobinuria (PNH).
- Moderate to severe intravascular hemolysis from faulty prosthetic heart valves generally responds to valvuloplasty and/or replacement.

However, it is too early to know whether long-term use of this antibody will be feasible.

SPUR CELL HEMOLYTIC ANEMIA

Acanthocytes, or spur cells, are often seen in patients with severe liver disease. The presence of these cells is thought to reflect an altered phospholipid/sphingomyelin ratio in the red cell membrane. Rarely, this acanthocytosis can lead to a severe hemolytic anemia, and usually denotes end-stage liver disease and a grave prognosis. There is no known effective therapy for this disorder other than liver transplantation.

Extraerythrocytic (Extrinsic) Causes of Hemolysis

Occasionally, hemolytic anemia can occur as a result of mechanical damage to red blood cells: this process is referred to as microangiopathic hemolytic anemia (MAHA). The predominant clinical concern in disseminated intravascular coagulation (DIC) and thrombotic thrombocytopenic purpura (TTP) is generally not hemolysis, although the degree of MAHA can become quite profound in these disorders (discussed in other articles). Patients with malignant hypertension can also have MAHA.

A dysfunctional prosthetic mechanical cardiac valve may result in MAHA. This is unusual in patients who have received xenograft replacements and native, stenotic valves. The turbulent flow that causes hemolysis is typically the result of leakage around the valve ring, rather than around the actual valve surface. Rarely, significant hemolysis may be present in those with patent ductus arteriosus and ventricular septal defects. Biochemical evidence of chronic hemolysis will be present, iron deficiency may be present because of chronic hemoglobinuria (denoted by a positive urine hemosiderin), and

schistocytes will be present on the peripheral blood smear. Iron replacement may partially ameliorate the anemia, but many patients with persistent moderate-to-severe anemia will require valve repair or replacement.

REFERENCES

Bolton-Maggs PH, Stevens RF, Dodd NJ, et al: Guidelines for the diagnosis and management of hereditary spherocytosis. Br J Haematol 2004;126:455-474.

Bolton-Maggs PH: The diagnosis and management of hereditary spherocytosis. Baillieres Best Pract Res Clin Haematol. 2000; 13:327-342.

Gallagher PG, Tse WT, Forget BG: Clinical and molecular aspects of disorders of the erythrocyte membrane skeleton. Semin Perinatol. 1990;14:351-367.

Hillmen P, Hall C, Marsh JC, et al: Effect of eculizumab on hemolysis and transfusion requirements in patients with paroxysmal nocturnal hemoglobinuria. N Engl J Med. 2004;350:552-559.

Lam BK, Cosgrove DM, Bhudia SK, Gillinov AM: Hemolysis after mitral valve repair: Mechanisms and treatment. Ann Thorac Surg 2004;77:191-195.

Mecozzi G, Milano AD, De Carlo M, et al: Intravascular hemolysis in patients with new-generation prosthetic heart valves: A prospective study. J Thorac Cardiovasc Surg 2002;123:550-556.

Mehta A, Mason PJ, Vulliamy TJ: Glucose-6-phosphate dehydrogenase deficiency. Baillieres Best Pract Res Clin Haematol 2000; 13:21-38.

Nurse GT, Coetzer TL, Palek J: The elliptocytoses, ovalocytosis and related disorders. Baillieres Clin Haematol 1992;5:187-207.

Smith LJ: Paroxysmal nocturnal hemoglobinuria. Clin Lab Sci 2004;17:172-177.

Tchernia G, Bader-Meunier B, Berterottiere P, et al: Effectiveness of partial splenectomy in hereditary spherocytosis. Curr Opin Hematol 1997;4:136-141.

Pernicious Anemia and Other Megaloblastic Anemias

Method of
Dan L. Longo, MD

Megaloblastic anemia is the name used to describe anemias in which the red blood cells (RBCs) are larger than normal, usually greater than 100 fL (10^{-15} L) in mean corpuscular volume (MCV). The term *megaloblastic* is from the Greek words *megas* meaning large and *blastos* meaning germ or bud. Megaloblastic anemias are caused by impaired DNA synthesis. Historically, 95% of cases of megaloblastic anemia were caused by folate and/or vitamin B_{12} deficiency. Since the advent of folate food supplementation in January 1998, however, the incidence of folate deficiency has declined (current incidence is estimated at 4 per 100,000 population). Precise incidence figures for pernicious anemia, the most common form of vitamin B_{12} deficiency, are lacking; however, the condition increases in incidence with age, and estimates are as high as 2% of people older than age 60 years. When asymptomatic patients older than age 65 years are screened, 10% to 15% or more may have biochemical evidence for vitamin B_{12} deficiency in the absence of anemia. Box 1 lists the causes of megaloblastic anemia.

Clinical Presentation

Anemia is associated with weakness, fatigue, shortness of breath, headache, exercise intolerance, or palpitations. On physical examination, the patient may have pallor or even a lemon-yellow cast from the combination of anemic pallor and low-grade icterus from the destruction of megaloblastic erythroid precursors in the marrow. The pulse is rapid and increases with even mild exertion. The effects of the nutritional deficiency may be manifest in the gastrointestinal (GI) tract in approximately 25% of patients; such symptoms may include a smooth or sore tongue (glossitis) and diarrhea.

The pattern of clinical presentation from vitamin B_{12} deficiency seems to have changed in the last 30 years.

Classically, vitamin B_{12} deficiency was caused by pernicious anemia and patients presented with anemia. However, 75% to 89% of patients also had neurologic signs and symptoms including paresthesias, peripheral neuropathy, unsteady gait, and balance problems because of posterior column dysfunction called *combined systems disease*. Patients often had loss of vibration sense on physical examination. In addition, vitamin B_{12} deficiency was found to be associated with memory impairment or even frank dementia, irritability, personality change, depression, and psychosis. In series beginning in the late 1960s, however, neurologic signs and symptoms have accompanied the anemia in only approximately 44% of patients. In part this may be because of earlier diagnosis of anemia. Other evidence supporting a change in pattern is the occurrence of vitamin B_{12}-deficiency neurologic symptoms in the absence of anemia. Up to 25% of patients with B_{12} neuropathy are not anemic. Because a mechanism for the neurologic damage has not been defined, the reasons for the differential manifestations of vitamin B_{12} deficiency are unknown.

BOX 1 Causes of Megaloblastic Anemia*

Cobalamin Deficiency
1. Inadequate ingestion: Strict vegetarian
2. Malabsorption
   - Gastric disorders
     Pernicious anemia: Atrophic gastritis type A, antibodies to parietal cells or intrinsic factor
     Achlorhydria: Defective release of cobalamin from food
     Partial or total gastrectomy
   - Terminal ileum disorders
     Tropical and nontropical sprue
     Regional enteritis
     Bowel resection
     Tumors or granulomatous disorders (rare)
   - Pancreatic disease
     Trypsin and bicarbonate essential for absorption
     ZES: pH too acidic for absorption
   - Competition for cobalamin
     Blind loop/bacterial overgrowth syndromes
     Fish tapeworm (*Diphyllobothrium latum*)
   - Drug-induced malabsorption (see following text)
   - Inherited defects in absorption (see following text)
3. Congenital defects (rare)
   - Imerslund-Graesbeck syndrome (inherited selective B_{12} malabsorption)
   - Transcobalamin II deficiency
   - Intrinsic factor defects
4. Drug effects
   - **Block acid secretion:** Proton pump inhibitors such as omeprazole and H_2 blockers to a lesser degree
   - Block absorption at terminal ileum: Metformin, calcium channel blockers, para-aminosalicylate, colchicine
   - Destroy cobalamin: Nitrous oxide, large doses of ascorbic acid
5. Increased requirements: Hyperthyroidism

Folic Acid Deficiency
1. **Inadequate ingestion:** Malnutrition, alcoholism, imbalanced diet (no vegetables)
2. Increased requirements
   - Pregnancy
   - Increased hematopoiesis in chronic RBC disorders like sickle cell anemia, hemolytic anemia
   - Hemodialysis
   - Malignancy
   - Growing children
3. Malabsorption
   - Tropical and nontropical sprue
   - Drug effects (see text following)
4. Drug effects
   - Antifols: Methotrexate, trimethoprim pentamidine, sulfasalazine, triamterene
   - Block absorption in proximal small intestine: Phenytoin, barbiturates, ethanol, oral contraceptives, metformin
5. Congenital defects (rare)

Other Causes
1. Drug effects
   - Inhibitors of DNA synthesis
     Purine inhibitors: Thioguanine, azathioprine, 6-mercaptopurine
     Pyrimidine inhibitors: Azidothymidine, 5-fluorouracil, capecitabine
     Ribonucleotide reductase inhibitors: Cytosine arabinoside, hydroxyurea
     Other mechanisms: Procarbazine,
   - Other mechanisms: L-asparaginase, protein synthesis inhibitor; benzene, unknown mechanism
2. Congenital defects (rare)
   - Orotic aciduria/Lesch-Nyhan syndrome
3. Megaloblastic anemia of unknown etiology
   - Refractory megaloblastic anemia
   - Congenital dyserythropoietic anemia

*The more common causes are in **bold type.**
Abbreviations: RBC = red blood cell; ZES = Zollinger-Ellison syndrome.

Vitamin B_{12} and folate deficiency differ in several respects. Because the body stores sufficient folate reserves to last approximately 3 to 4 months, if intake ceases completely anemia usually develops over a period of 10 to 15 weeks. By contrast, the body stores sufficient vitamin B_{12} that depletion does not occur for 4 or more years. If enterohepatic circulation is normal, the manifestations of vitamin B_{12} anemia may not occur for 20 years. Because the anemia may develop slowly, low levels of hemoglobin may be tolerated. Another important clinical difference between folate and vitamin B_{12} deficiency is that neurologic symptoms are an uncommon feature of folate deficiency. However, folate deficiency may occur in the setting of alcoholism, which can cause neurologic symptoms from thiamine deficiency that can mimic vitamin B_{12} deficiency. In addition, diabetic patients who develop folate deficiency may have neurologic manifestations of their diabetes that confuse the diagnosis. Thus, the differential diagnosis of megaloblastic anemia rests with laboratory testing or a therapeutic trial rather than clinical signs and symptoms. The important distinguishing features are based on understanding folate and B_{12} biochemistry and the physiology of their absorption.

Biochemistry and Physiology of Folate and Vitamin B_{12}

Folate and vitamin B_{12} biochemistry overlap in the de novo thymidylate synthesis pathway (Figure 1). Deoxyuridylate (deoxyuridine [dU] monophosphate) is converted to deoxythymidylate by the action of thymidylate synthase. A reduced folate, 5,10-methylene tetrahydrofolate (5,10-methylTHF), is the methyl donor, and dihydrofolate is a product of the reaction. The supply of reduced folate is replenished by the action of dihydrofolate reductase to form tetrahydrofolate (THF), and the methyl donor form of folate (5,10-methylene THF) is regenerated by the action of serine hydroxymethyl transferase, an enzymatic reaction that requires pyridoxal phosphate (vitamin B_6). The predominant form of folate in food is methylTHF polyglutamate. Conjugases in the gut remove the extra glutamates and the methylTHF is absorbed. After absorption methylTHF requires vitamin B_{12} to enter cells; methylTHF is demethylated to THF by methionine synthase in a reaction that converts homocysteine to methionine and depends on the action of methylcobalamin (vitamin B_{12}). In reactions not shown in Figure 1, 5,10-methenylTHF participates in chemical reactions that contribute the 2 and 8 carbons to the purine rings of guanine and adenine.

Nearly all the manifestations of folate deficiency and the hematologic manifestations of vitamin B_{12} deficiency are because of an inadequate supply of reduced folate for thymidylate synthesis. In the absence of thymidylate, DNA synthesis slows and deoxyuridylate may be incorporated in its place. This can lead to abnormal base pairing (uridylate binding to cytosine residues instead of adenine residues) and mutations.

Figure 1 also illustrates where 5-fluorouracil and methotrexate act on this pathway and how folinic acid and pteroylglutamic acid can overcome blocks in the pathway. The dependence of the methylTHF demethylation step on vitamin B_{12} also illustrates how homocysteine levels can increase in vitamin B_{12} deficiency. In the absence of vitamin B_{12}, methylTHF levels in the serum usually increase (so-called methyl folate trap).

The second biochemical pathway involving vitamin B_{12} is the synthesis of succinyl CoA (coenzyme A) from methylmalonyl CoA in a reaction that requires adenosylcobalamin. Because neurologic dysfunction is more commonly associated with vitamin B_{12} than with folate deficiency, it has been hypothesized that a deficiency in adenosylcobalamin underlies the neurologic symptoms in vitamin B_{12} deficiency, which are characterized by demyelination and axon loss. However, evidence for a role for a defect in fatty acid synthesis because of inadequate levels of succinyl CoA or excess levels of methylmalonyl CoA in the pathogenesis of vitamin B_{12}–deficiency-associated neuropathy has been inconsistent. The pathogenesis of the neurologic disease is undefined.

Nearly all folate deficiency is caused by inadequate dietary intake of vegetables and fruit. In patients with malabsorption syndromes because of small intestinal disease, other symptoms (diarrhea, weight loss) are more prominent before folate deficiency appears. After ingestion, food folate polyglutamates are deconjugated down to one glutamate group by intestinal enzymes and absorbed in the proximal third of the small intestine. Phenytoin (Dilantin) blocks folate absorption in the gut. After absorption, the monoglutamate form is taken up by cells in a vitamin B_{12}-dependent process and glutamates are added again; they aid in keeping the folate in the cell.

DE NOVO THYMIDYLATE SYNTHESIS

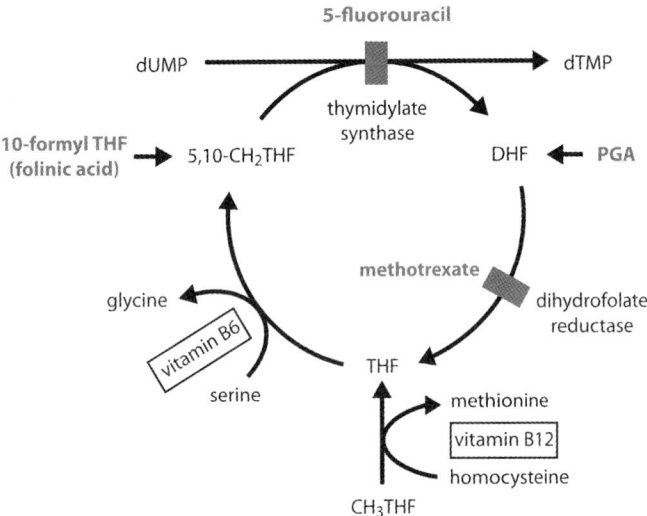

FIGURE 1. Vitamin B_{12} deficiency and folate deficiency both produce anemia by causing a cellular deficiency of thymidylate that inhibits DNA synthesis. The major food form of folate, methyl folate (CH_3 THF), requires demethylation in order to enter cells and this step requires vitamin B_{12}. Thus, large amounts of folate can overcome the hematologic effects of vitamin B_{12} deficiency. Folate cannot correct the neurologic effects of vitamin B_{12} deficiency.

Rakel and Bope: *Conn's Current Therapy 2006.*

By contrast, most vitamin B_{12} deficiency is caused by inadequate absorption. Because vitamin B_{12} is in meats, milk, and eggs, dietary deficiency is rare. Food vitamin B_{12} is generally protein bound. Gastric acid releases it from food, and it is bound by R proteins (cobalophilins) in saliva and gastric juice. In the duodenum, the cobalamin-R binder complex is digested by pancreatic enzymes, and cobalamin is bound to intrinsic factor, a 60 kD protein made by gastric parietal cells. This cobalamin-intrinsic factor complex travels to the terminal ileum where it is absorbed by cells bearing specific receptors for the complex. Inside the intestinal mucosa, the intrinsic factor is degraded and cobalamin is bound to transcobalamin II, which transports the cobalamin through the blood to the liver for storage and marrow for use.

The most common causes of vitamin B_{12} deficiency are related to gastric disorders. Pernicious anemia is a familial autoimmune disease that attacks the parietal cells of the gastric fundus and body. H^+/K^+ ATPase is the most common target. Approximately 20% of the relatives of people with pernicious anemia have pernicious anemia. The gastric mucosa is infiltrated with inflammatory cells and the consequence of the chronic inflammation is atrophic gastritis. Atrophic gastritis is of two types, the antral-sparing type A associated with antibodies to parietal cells and intrinsic factor that cause achlorhydria and elevated gastrin levels, and the pangastritis (antrum involved) type B that occurs as a consequence of *Helicobacter pylori* infection associated with hypogastrinemia. Vitamin B_{12} deficiency is infrequent in type B gastritis, occurring only after many years of achlorhydria. Pernicious anemia may be associated with other autoimmune disorders including Hashimoto's thyroiditis, diabetes, Addison's disease, primary ovarian failure, Graves' disease, vitiligo, myasthenia gravis, Eaton-Lambert syndrome, and primary hypoparathyroidism. Patients are also at risk for gastric cancer and gastric carcinoid tumors. Chronic use of proton pump inhibitors (omeprazole [Prilosec]) and H_2 blockers to control gastroesophageal (GE) reflux is an increasingly common cause of achlorhydria and the inability to release vitamin B_{12} from food.

The recommended daily allowance for food folate is 400 µg (600 µg in pregnancy, 500 µg during lactation) and for vitamin B_{12} is 2.4 µg. Total body stores of folate are normally around 5 mg; vitamin B_{12} stores amount to approximately 4 mg.

Laboratory Testing in the Differential Diagnosis of Megaloblastic Anemia

The laboratory feature that most often identifies a patient with megaloblastic anemia is an elevated MCV on the automated complete blood count (CBC) in the setting of anemia. It is important to examine a peripheral blood smear in this setting. Macrocytosis is said to occur in two morphologic varieties: Megaloblastic erythropoiesis produces macro-ovalocytes (oval-shaped, large RBCs), but the presence of large RBCs of normal round shape is associated with alcoholism, renal or liver disease, or hypothyroidism in the absence of megaloblastic erythropoiesis. In megaloblastic anemia, anisocytosis and poikilocytosis are common. Another important reason for routinely examining the peripheral blood smear of an anemic patient is that 25% or greater of patients with vitamin B_{12} or folate deficiency may have concurrent iron deficiency. In this setting, the RBCs may be normal in size (the inhibition of hemoglobin synthesis compensates for the slow DNA synthesis), but a clue to the correct diagnosis will be apparent in the presence of hypersegmented neutrophils. Neutrophil hypersegmentation can be discerned in several ways: counting the lobes of 100 cells and dividing by 100 (level >3.5 is abnormal), finding 5% of the cells with five lobes (*rule of fives*), or finding a single cell with six or more lobes. Because folate deficiency and vitamin B_{12} deficiency are generally systemic problems affecting all dividing cells, patients with vitamin B_{12}- or folate-deficiency anemia have coincident pancytopenia in approximately 40% of cases. Furthermore, megaloblastic changes are apparent in the intestinal mucosa, oral mucosa, and cervical epithelium.

The first set of tests in the setting of a megaloblastic anemia is a serum vitamin B_{12} level, a red cell folate level, and a reticulocyte count. Folate and vitamin B_{12} deficiency states develop over time with tests becoming abnormal before the actual onset of anemia (Tables 1 and 2). Serum folate is a poor measure of tissue folate stores; RBC folate is a more reliable measure of folate availability for DNA synthesis. Folate deficiency is ruled out by an RBC folate level higher than 160 ng/mL, and folate deficiency is confirmed by levels less than 120 ng/mL. Vitamin B_{12} deficiency is ruled out by a serum level greater than 300 pg/mL and confirmed by

TABLE 1 Laboratory Features of Folate Deficiency

	Normal	Folate depletion	Folate deficient hematopoiesis	Folate deficient anemia
RBC folate (ng/ml)	>200	<160	<120	<100
PMN lobe average	<3.5	<3.5	>3.5	>3.5
RBC morphology	Normal	Normal	Normal	Macroovalocytes
MCV	Normal	Normal	Normal	>100 fL
Hemoglobin	Normal	Normal	Normal	<12 g/dL

Rakel and Bope: *Conn's Current Therapy 2006.*

TABLE 2 Laboratory Features of Vitamin B$_{12}$ Deficiency

	Normal	Vitamin B$_{12}$ depletion	Vitamin B$_{12}$ deficient hematopoiesis	Vitamin B$_{12}$ deficiency anemia
Holotranscobalamin II (pg/ml)	>50	<40	<40	<40
Serum B$_{12}$ level (pg/ml)	>300	<300	<300	<150
Serum homocysteine	Normal	Normal or elevated	Elevated	Elevated
PMN lobe average	<3.5	<3.5	>3.5	>3.5
RBC morphology	Normal	Normal	Normal	Macroovalocytes
MCV	Normal	Normal	Normal	>100 Fl
Hemoglobin	Normal	Normal	Normal	<12 g/dL
Serum methylmalonate (µmol/L)	<0.4	<0.4	>0.4	>0.4

levels less than 200 pg/mL. Reticulocyte counts are low. Marrow examination is generally not indicated unless folate and vitamin B$_{12}$ levels are normal; in such a setting, a myelodysplastic syndrome must be ruled out by morphologic examination. In usual megaloblastic anemia, the marrow will be normocellular or hypercellular and erythroid precursors will be large with nuclear-cytoplasmic dissociation; that is, mature hemoglobinized cytoplasm with nuclei containing open rather than condensed chromatin. The effect on the granulocyte lineage is manifested by the presence of giant metamyelocytes. In maturation disorders (leukemias, myelodysplasias) that also affect cytoplasmic maturation, one can get delayed nuclear condensation together with slower than normal hemoglobinization. This morphologic change has been called *megaloblastoid*. This does not mean slightly megaloblastic; it refers to a particular picture of delayed nuclear and cytoplasmic maturation.

Other tests that support the diagnosis of megaloblastic anemia are elevated lactate dehydrogenase (LDH) and indirect bilirubin levels reflecting the intramedullary hemolysis of ineffective erythropoiesis.

Much has been written about the value of measuring homocysteine and methylmalonic acid levels in settings where the results of the vitamin measurements are equivocal. It is said that both of these metabolites are elevated in cobalamin deficiency whereas folate deficiency is more likely if homocysteine levels are elevated (>14 µM) and methylmalonic acid levels are normal (<270 nM or 0.4 µmol/L). However, in one study, 63% of cobalamin responsive patients did not have low cobalamin and high homocysteine and methylmalonic acid levels. Thus, as in many areas of medicine, clinical judgment is an important component of interpreting the laboratory tests.

Patients with cobalamin deficiency require additional testing to discern the cause. Antibodies to intrinsic factor that block binding to cobalamin are specific for pernicious anemia but are insensitive (positive in 70% of patients); antibodies to parietal cells are sensitive (positive in 90%) but not specific.

Unfortunately, the three most useful tests for diagnosing cobalamin deficiency and determining its cause are not routinely performed or available. The most sensitive indicator of cobalamin deficiency is serum levels of holotranscobalamin II (transcobalamin II bound to vitamin B$_{12}$). Levels below 40 pg/mL are the first

indication of vitamin B$_{12}$ deficiency (see Table 2). Another extremely useful diagnostic test is the dU suppression test performed on bone marrow in vitro. As in Figure 1, for exogenously added dU to be able to suppress the incorporation of radiolabeled thymidine into DNA, the folate and vitamin B$_{12}$ pathways need to be intact. In the setting of megaloblastic anemia, dU fails to optimally block thymidine incorporation. The particular nutrient that is lacking can be directly assessed in vitro by adding back either vitamin B$_{12}$ or folate. The nutrient that restores the capacity of dU to inhibit thymidine incorporation is the deficient nutrient.

The third valuable and therapeutic diagnostic test is the Schilling test. This test and its variations can determine the mechanism of cobalamin malabsorption. The test involves injecting the cobalamin-deficient patient with a large dose of cobalamin intravenously or intramuscularly. The patient is then fed a radiolabeled dose of cobalamin (usually Co[57] labeled). If less than 8% of the oral dose of radioactivity appears in the urine within 24 hours, the patient has a defect in absorption. If the feeding of intrinsic factor together with the labeled cobalamin results in an increased urinary excretion of labeled cobalamin (>8% in 24 hours), the patient has pernicious anemia. If not, the patient can be treated with antibiotics for 10 days to treat bacterial overgrowth.

CURRENT DIAGNOSIS

- RBC morphology: macro-ovalocytes and hypersegmented neutrophils
- Vitamin levels assessment: Serum B$_{12}$, RBC folate
- Measurement of homocysteine and methylmalonic acid levels if vitamin levels are equivocal:
  If both are elevated, probably cobalamin deficiency
  If only homocysteine is elevated, probably folate deficiency
- Diagnosis of PA: In cobalamin deficiency, serumblocking antibodies to intrinsic factor
- Empiric clinical trial may be indicated

Abbreviations: PA = pernicious anemia; RBC = red blood cell.

Rakel and Bope: *Conn's Current Therapy 2006.*

If this does not correct the malabsorption, ileal causes must be ruled out. Patients with the inability to release cobalamin from food may have normal excretion of oral labeled vitamin B_{12}. A variation on this test has been devised—but not yet clinically validated—in which one looks for a defect in releasing cobalamin from food by adding labeled vitamin B_{12} to a scrambled egg and assessing urinary excretion. People with achlorhydria excrete less than 8% in 24 hours.

Because of the unavailability of labeled vitamin B_{12} and the difficulty of 24-hour urine collections, the Schilling test is rarely performed. As a consequence of the general inadequacy of diagnostic tests, many clinicians favor an empiric therapeutic trial to confirm the diagnosis.

Treatment of Megaloblastic Anemia

An empiric therapeutic trial involves administering replacement doses of vitamin B_{12}[1] for 10 days while following the reticulocyte count. If daily intramuscular (IM) injections of 100 μg of cyanocobalamin[1] fail to produce a reticulocytosis, the process is repeated with oral folic acid in daily doses of 1 to 5 mg. If reticulocytosis is undocumented after the second 10 days, a bone marrow is performed looking for an alternative diagnosis such as myelodysplasia. Rare patients may have deficits in both nutrients (but it would be very unusual for none of the lab tests to suggest this possibility). Another cause of failure to respond might be inadequate levels of iron or erythropoietin to support vigorous red blood cell production.

---

[1]Not FDA approved for this indication.

 CURRENT THERAPY

Cobalamin Deficiency
- Replenishment of stores: Cyanocobalamin 1 mg IM daily × 7, weekly × 3
- Chronic therapy: Cyanocobalamin 1 mg IM monthly or 2 mg PO daily

Folate Deficiency
- Oral folate 1-5 mg per day until full recovery
- Prophylaxis in:
  Women contemplating pregnancy or lactating
  Women who have had a child with neural tube defects in the past
  People with hemolytic anemia or hemoglobinopathy
  People on renal dialysis
  Patients on methotrexate for a chronic inflammatory or autoimmune condition
- General Consideration
- Adequate iron stores and erythropoietin to support erythropoiesis
- Monitoring for hypokalemia and thrombocytosis

Abbreviations: IM = intramuscular injection; PO = orally.

Rakel and Bope: *Conn's Current Therapy 2006.*

For chronic replacement therapy in cobalamin deficiency, use either monthly IM injections of 1 mg[3] of cyanocobalamin (after initial daily therapy for 1 week and weekly therapy for 3 weeks) or daily oral administration of 2 mg. Oral therapy works because even without the normal mechanism of absorption, a small amount of a large dose will be absorbed by diffusion. Each approach has advantages and disadvantages; intramuscular injection is painful but reliable, oral medication is easier to take but adherence may be more erratic. Either approach should be monitored with serum B_{12} levels to assure compliance. Lifelong treatment is essential unless a reversible cause is detected. Neurologic symptoms usually resolve over several months. Those that have not improved after one year are unlikely to be reversed.

Oral folate supplementation (1- to 5-mg tablet daily) should be provided until complete hematologic recovery is confirmed. Women who may become pregnant should take at least 400 μg of folate daily to prevent neural tube defects in the first trimester; usually pregnancy is not detected until after the risk period for these defects. Lactating women and people with hemolytic anemias, hyperproliferative hematologic states, or on dialysis and those on methotrexate for chronic inflammatory diseases like rheumatoid arthritis and psoriasis may need supplementation.

Replenishment of the deficient nutrient will produce a reticulocytosis in 3 to 7 days. During recovery of hematopoiesis, the rapid synthesis of new cells can produce hypokalemia. Therefore, serum K^+ should be followed and potassium supplements provided as needed. A more unusual response to therapy is thrombocytosis, which can lead to thrombotic complications in patients with other predisposing factors if the platelet count exceeds 1 million/μL.

Patients with pernicious anemia should be monitored for the development of other autoimmune diseases and should have stool guaiac tests at least annually to screen for gastric cancer.

REFERENCES

Baik HW, Russell RM: Vitamin B_{12} deficiency in the elderly. Annu Rev Nutr 1999;19:357-377.

Carmel R (ed.): Beyond megaloblastic anemia. Semin Hematol 1999;36:1-100.

Klee GG: Cobalamin and folate evaluation: Measurement of methylmalonic acid and homocysteine vs vitamin B_{12} and folate. Clin Chem 2000;46:1277-1283.

Solomon LR: Cobalamin-responsive disorders in the ambulatory care setting: Unreliability of cobalamin, methylmalonic acid, and homocysteine testing. Blood 2005;105:978-985.

Toh B-H, van Driehl IR, Gleeson PA: Pernicious anemia. N Engl J Med 1997;337:1441-1448.

---

[3]Exceeds dosage recommended by the manufacturer.

Thalassemia

Method of
Susan P. Perrine, MD, and Valia Boosalis, MD

Pathophysiology: Basic Mechanisms of Hemoglobin Synthesis

The sequential expression of the globin genes results in production of specific types of hemoglobins at different stages of development. At 12 weeks of gestation, a transition from embryonic to fetal hemoglobin ($\alpha_2\gamma_2$) occurs; and at 28 weeks of gestation, increasing amounts of β-globin and of adult hemoglobin (Hb A, $\alpha_2\beta_2$) are produced. For intact hemoglobin tetramers to form, α-like globin proteins must equal β-like globin proteins. Thalassemia syndromes result from deficiencies in either α-globin (α-thalassemia) or β-like globin (β-thalassemia) chains. The diseases become apparent when the affected globin is required during development. During gestation, α-thalassemia is symptomatic, because α-globin is required for fetal hemoglobin (Hb F, $\alpha_2\gamma_2$). Because β-globin is not required in large amounts before birth, β-thalassemia is asymptomatic until 6 months after birth. Mutations that cause prolonged production of fetal γ-globin chains may manifest later, at 2 to 4 years of age.

The major pathologic process of thalassemia is caused by the imbalance of α and non–α chain accumulation. The unaffected chains, produced in normal amounts, precipitate during erythropoiesis. In β-thalassemia, the precipitated α-globin chains are particularly toxic, damaging cell membranes and causing rapid cell death (apoptosis). Red blood cell life span is further shortened by removal of abnormal cells in the reticuloendothelial system. In response to the hypoxia, erythropoietin levels increase, causing erythroid hyperplasia. Hypersplenism causes more severe anemia. An increase in plasma volume, from marrow and splenic expansion, also lowers hemoglobin levels.

In α-thalassemic fetuses, the unbalanced fetal (γ)-globin chains form tetramers (γ_4, hemoglobin Bart's); excess β-globin (β_4, hemoglobin H) accumulates after birth. Hemoglobin Bart's and hemoglobin H result in milder ineffective erythropoiesis but have abnormal oxygen binding. If all four α-globin genes are deleted, only hemoglobin Bart's is formed, with a massively left-shifted oxygen dissociation curve that provides almost no oxygen delivery to tissues and results in a lethal intrauterine condition, hydrops fetalis. Decreased production of α-globin from three or four abnormal α-globin genes results in a moderate hemolytic anemia, hemoglobin H disease. Deletion of only one (α-thalassemia-2) or two (α-thalassemia-1) loci is asymptomatic.

Thalassemia syndromes are graded according to severity of the anemia. *Thalassemia major*, in which severe anemia manifests during infancy, is caused by inheritance of two severely impaired β-globin alleles. This homozygous or doubly heterozygous state may have a milder manifestation when there is a higher-than-usual increase in fetal chain production or when the co-inheritance of β-thalassemia decreases the net imbalance of the synthesis of α-globin to β-globin. *Thalassemia trait* (thalassemia minor), which is caused by the inheritance of a single defective allele, is characterized by mild hypochromic, microcytic anemia. *Thalassemia intermedia* manifests as moderate anemia with total hemoglobin levels of 6.0 to 10.0 g/dL. These patients require occasional transfusions with concomitant infections, but do not require chronic transfusions.

Diagnosis

The diagnosis of severe thalassemia is usually straightforward in ethnic groups at risk (Mediterranean, African, Asian, Middle Eastern, East Indian). Thalassemia major and thalassemia intermedia are marked by severe microcytic anemia; hyperbilirubinemia, elevated lactate dehydrogenase levels, and splenomegaly appear in the first few years of life (β-thalassemia). Hydrops fetalis (α-thalassemia with classic four-gene deletion) manifests as polyhydramnios and fetal distress during the second trimester. Thalassemia trait is characterized by mild anemia (hematocrit >30), low mean corpuscular volume (<75 fL), and erythrocytosis (red blood cell [RBC] count $>5 \times 10^6$ per mm^3). Quantitative hemoglobin electrophoresis demonstrates elevated hemoglobins A_2 and F. Hemoglobin A is absent in β°-thalassemia and decreased in $\beta+$-thalassemia. α-Thalassemia is best diagnosed by the presence of hemoglobin Bart's in cord blood. Hemoglobin H is unstable, and electrophoresis of fresh specimens is required for its detection. In most, but not all, β-thalassemia heterozygotes, hemoglobin A_2 levels are elevated. Basophilic stippling, target cells, fragmented cells (schistocytes), and nucleated RBCs are typical of the severe thalassemias. The reticulocyte count may be relatively low because of ineffective erythropoiesis, and MCV may become high from rapid emergence of erythroid precursors. Prenatal diagnosis of thalassemia is performed by direct polymerase chain reaction (PCR) analysis of fetal DNA obtained by amniocentesis or chorionic villus sampling. This procedure is being explored for use in preimplantation diagnosis and in vitro fertilization procedures.

Transfusion Therapy

In β-thalassemia major, RBC transfusion is the mainstay of supportive therapy. Transfusions should maintain a hemoglobin level ideally above 10.5 to 11 g/dL (range: 10.5 to 13 g/dL) to suppress endogenous erythropoiesis, with the least amount of transfused blood required. Regular transfusions are begun for a persistent decline in hemoglobin below 7 g/dL in children with two β-thalassemic mutations. A complete genotype of the patient's RBCs should be performed before transfusions are begun to facilitate identification of involved antigens in the event of isoimmunization. Ideally, transfusions of 15 mL/kg of packed RBCs (in children) should be given at 3- to 4-week intervals using fresh compatible blood from a limited donor pool, and filtered to remove white blood cells and viruses inhabiting these cells. Cytomegalovirus (CMV)-negative preparations should be used for transplantation candidates. Administering acetaminophen (Tylenol) and diphenhydramine (Benadryl) before transfusions prevents febrile reactions. Transfusion records should be meticulously maintained to assess mean pre- and post-transfusion hemoglobin levels and annual blood consumption. An increase in transfusion requirements suggests hypersplenism, isoimmunization, or an accessory spleen.

Transfusions can transmit blood-borne infections, including hepatitis viruses, HIV, and CMV. In regions where hepatitis C is endemic, 90% of patients on chronic transfusions may develop hepatitis C within 5 years; chronic infection eventually advances to cirrhosis in 85%. Patients should be vaccinated against hepatitis A and B and monitored for elevated transaminase levels and for hepatitis C antibodies, with referral to consultants for management if found. Combined therapy with interferon alfa-2a (Roferon-A) and ribavirin (Rebetol) can produce sustained responses in hepatitis C; transfusion requirements often increase during treatment. HIV testing should be performed annually.

Partial exchange transfusion by erythrocytapheresis (PET-E), in which older red blood cells are exchanged for fresh-packed red cells by pheresis, reduces iron accumulation significantly compared to simple transfusion with deferoxamine chelation. PET-E exposes patients to more units of packed RBCs and minor side effects related to citrate, but reduces transfusional iron burden, which is the long-term cause of early mortality.

Splenectomy

Massive splenomegaly is avoidable by transfusion, but splenic sequestration of donor cells can cause excessive transfusion requirements. Splenectomy should be performed if a 40% or greater increase in the transfusion requirement occurs during a 1-year period, or if a transfusion of more than 200 mL/kg per year of packed RBCs is required without isoimmunization, or if the patient develops thrombocytopenia. Splenectomy increases the risk of overwhelming sepsis with encapsulated organisms and *Yersinia,* especially in young children, so ideally should be deferred until 4 to 5 years of age. Polyvalent pneumococcal vaccine should be given at least 1 month before splenectomy. Prophylactic oral penicillin VK should be used in children younger than 10 years and for invasive (dental) procedures. Immediate medical attention should be sought and broad-spectrum antibiotics given emergently for significant fever (greater than 38.3°C [101°F]), as asplenic patients are at risk for a fulminant course and death within hours.

Complications of Transfusion Therapy

Approximately 1 mg of iron per mL of packed RBCs is administered in packed RBC transfusions, with no mechanism for elimination. Iron deposition from transfusional hemosiderosis causes dysfunction in the heart, liver, and endocrine organs. Glucose intolerance with insulin-dependent diabetes mellitus, primary hypothyroidism, hypoparathyroidism, delayed puberty, amenorrhea, and other endocrinopathies are not uncommon; digoxin refractoriness and arrhythmias result from cardiac iron deposition and hypocalcemia secondary to hypoparathyroidism. Growth retardation may respond to growth hormone before 13 years of age. Hepatic hemosiderosis and hepatitis C lead to fibrosis and cirrhosis. Cardiac dysfunction (detectable first by magnetic resonance T2* measurement of less than 20 milliseconds and reduced ejection fractions) typically presents with fatigue, arrhythmias, or pericarditis, advancing to congestive heart failure. Cardiac disease remains the major cause of death in transfused patients (60%), with infections (13%) and liver disease, including cancer (6%), following. Osteopenia may be severe and cause fractures, especially in thalassemia intermedia. Patients should be maintained on elemental calcium (1500 mg per day) and vitamin D (400 IU per day) in adults. Osteoporosis may require bisphosphonates, such as pamidronate (Aredia)[1] or alendronate (Fosamax), and monitoring with calcium, phosphate, 1,25-hydroxyvitamin D levels, 24-hour urinary calcium and hydroxyproline, and bone mineral density (dual-energy x-ray absorptiometry scan [DEXA]) measurements annually.

Monitoring and Treatment of Iron Overload (Box 1)

The parenteral iron chelator deferoxamine mesylate (Desferal) is the only first-line chelator approved in the United States and Europe for more than 30 years. Deferoxamine can maintain negative iron balance relative to the transfusion burden, when administered five to seven times per week as a continuous subcutaneous or intravenous infusion or as twice-daily bolus subcutaneous (not intramuscular) injections of the same total dose. Urinary iron excretion is used to adjust the dosage to maintain negative iron balance. When begun within 2 years of beginning transfusions and faithfully administered, deferoxamine prolongs survival. If a significant iron burden is present before chelation therapy is begun, progressive cardiac dysfunction may not be completely prevented or reversed.

Iron overload should be documented by a challenge test or begun after 12 to 18 months of regular transfusions, as children require iron for growth, and chelation

[1]Not FDA approved for this indication.
*Investigational drug in the United States.

is detrimental for patients who are not overloaded with iron. To begin chelation, iron in a 24-hour urine after injection of 500 mg of deferoxamine should exceed 1 mg, or the serum ferritin level should exceed 1000 ng/mL. Small infusion pumps are used to administer doses of 25 to 40 mg/kg per day over 12 hours subcutaneously. Irritation from hypertonicity and local reactions can be prevented by increasing the diluent to produce a 10% solution, adding hydrocortisone (2 mg/mL), or with topical diphenhydramine. A topical anesthetic cream should be applied 30 to 60 minutes before insertion of the needle. Intravenous administration through an indwelling port device is often more tolerable, because such devices can be accessed once weekly without repeated needle sticks. Intravenous chelation is more effective than subcutaneous chelation, so fewer treatment days may suffice. Arrhythmias and congestive heart failure have been temporarily reversed with high-dose deferoxamine (15 mg/kg per hour maximum for 24 hours per day, 7 days per week). Anaphylactic reactions can be treated with desensitization; idiosyncratic acute respiratory distress syndromes are rare but life-threatening, necessitating rapid recognition and intensive care. Excessive doses can cause optic and acoustic neuritis, so ophthalmologic and hearing evaluations should be performed annually. Iron overload causes depletion of vitamin C, which inhibits iron release from reticuloendothelial cells. Sudden availability of vitamin C can cause a massive release of iron and serious cardiotoxicity. Vitamin C (50 mg per day in children and 100 mg per day in adults) should be given only after the first cycle of deferoxamine. Despite available deferoxamine therapy, 50% to 60% of transfused thalassemia patients die of cardiac disease before age 35 years.

New oral and long-acting iron chelators (still in clinical trials in the United States) offer major advantages and less onerous therapy. The oral chelator deferiprone[1] (L1) crosses cell membranes more readily than does deferoxamine, and, in a recent British study, prevented the onset or progression of myocardial dysfunction more effectively. Combined use of deferoxamine (2 days per week) with daily deferiprone (75 mg/kg) produces higher iron excretion than deferoxamine alone. An international trial demonstrated that deferiprone does not promote hepatic fibrosis, which had been raised previously in a trial that was confounded by hepatitis C. A new oral chelator, ICL670,* requires administration once daily and has shown efficacy similar to deferoxamine in ongoing clinical studies. The experimental chelator 40SD02,* containing deferoxamine chemically attached to a modified starch polymer, has favorable pharmacokinetics with once-weekly intravenous administration.

Serial ferritin levels should be followed every 3 months, but *do not correlate directly with cardiac iron*. Liver biopsy is used to assess hepatic iron content and fibrosis, but also does not correlate with *cardiac* iron burden. Noninvasive technology is available in a few medical centers, including a superconducting quantum interference device (SQUID) and T2*, a magnetic resonance method that assesses myocardial iron and ventricular function in the same study and can detect myocardial iron before ventricular dysfunction occurs, which facilitates earlier treatment. T2* can detect hepatic iron burden, albeit with more variability when fibrosis is present.

---

[1]Not FDA approved for this indication.
*Investigational drug in the United States.

Rakel and Bope: *Conn's Current Therapy 2006.*

Thalassemia Intermedia

Patients with β-thalassemia who do not develop debilitating anemia should not be committed to a lifelong transfusion regimen. When the hemoglobin levels remain above 8 g/dL, patients generally can lead a normal life. Most specialists avoid regular transfusions at hemoglobin levels higher than 7 g/dL, particularly in regions where the blood supply predictably results in hepatitis C transmission, although intermittent transfusions are often necessary for more severe anemia with infections. Patients should be monitored closely for signs of marrow expansion, facial deformity, splenomegaly, or growth retardation. Facial deformity can be severe, and is an indication for regular transfusions. Hypertransfusion can often be avoided by splenectomy. Anemia in thalassemia intermedia patients, particularly those with high baseline Hb F levels, often responds to experimental therapies that stimulate fetal globin production.

The hyperplastic marrow in thalassemia intermedia stimulates intestinal iron absorption and iron overload, which eventually results in the same endocrine deficiencies that occur in thalassemia major, and requires chelation therapy. The same clinical manifestations, including splenomegaly, gallstones, osteopenia, and iron overload develop more slowly in thalassemia intermedia, but cardiomyopathy does not typically develop in untransfused patients. Avoidance of iron-rich meats and regular consumption of tea can reduce iron absorption. Folic acid and antioxidant supplements should be given. Spinal cord compression syndromes from thoracic or vertebral paraspinal bone marrow masses should be suspected with acute or increasing weakness, numbness, and diminished reflexes in the lower extremities—this is a medical emergency. Diagnosis is made by magnetic resonance imaging (MRI) or computed tomography (CT); radiation therapy and steroids should be instituted emergently.

α-Thalassemia

The homozygous form of α-thalassemia is usually lethal in utero. However, prenatal diagnosis and milder variants have enabled affected fetuses to be supported to term with intrauterine transfusions, followed by postnatal transfusions. For milder hemoglobin H disease, only folic acid, antioxidants, and monitoring for severe anemia during infections or with increasing splenomegaly are necessary. Because hemoglobin H is sensitive to oxidant stress, drugs such as sulfonamides should be avoided, particularly with coexistent glucose-6-phosphate dehydrogenase (G6PD) deficiency. Iron status should be monitored.

Transplantation

Allogeneic bone marrow or stem cell transplantation is curative by replacing the patient's hematopoietic stem cells with normal stem cells that contain two normal genes or one normal and one thalassemic globin gene.

Transplantation from a human leukocyte antigen (HLA)-identical related donor in patients younger than 8 years of age, without hepatic fibrosis, and with a good iron chelation history (risk class 1), has an excellent prognosis. Still, the overall mortality rate of transplantation in experienced centers is 15%. Significant morbidity may result from graft-versus-host disease (GVHD). Unrelated donors and cord blood as sources of donor cells have increased risks of GVHD and graft rejection, but provide broader availability. Relapses (graft rejection) occur in 8% of patients receiving related donor transplants. Many patients do well clinically even with mixed chimeric states. The serious risks of this curative treatment modality must be weighed against the lifelong burden of hypertransfusion and chelation. This balance may be shifted with the new oral iron chelators.

Stimulation of Fetal Globin Gene Synthesis and Erythropoiesis

A large body of evidence shows that expression of endogenous fetal globin to approximately 70% of α-globin chain synthesis ameliorates anemia in β-thalassemia enough to eliminate transfusion requirements. Chemotherapeutic agents (5-azacytidine[1] or decitabine,[1] hydroxyurea[1]), short chain fatty acid derivatives (SCFADs), and human recombinant (rhu) erythropoietin (EPO) are being evaluated in phase II trials, with best responses observed in patients with baseline endogenous (untransfused) Hb F levels of greater than 50%. Combinations of these agents will likely be required to completely eliminate transfusion requirements in severe β-thalassemia patients. SCFADs, which are not mutagenic or cytotoxic, are preferable over chemotherapy for lifelong treatment. Sodium phenylbutyrate (Buphenyl)[1] and arginine butyrate,[1] which require large numbers of tablets or IV infusion, respectively, have increased total hemoglobin by 1 to 4 g/dL above baseline in untransfused patients with active erythropoiesis. Patients with β+-thalassemia with baseline erythropoietin levels less than 40 mU/mL have responded best to combined therapy with butyrate and EPO. The long-acting EPO preparation, darbepoetin (Aranesp),[1] may also increase hemoglobin in some. These therapies require supplementation with oral iron to be effective, even in the presence of elevated ferritin levels, as stored iron may not be available for erythropoiesis, and several months of treatment are often required for responses to EPO. New oral short chain fatty acid derivatives, which are currently being evaluated, appear more tolerable and promising.

Gene Transfer

Gene therapy for β-thalassemia requires both a transfer of the fetal (γ) or a normal β-globin gene into repopulating hematopoietic stem cells and a high-level expression

---

[1]Not FDA approved for this indication.

of transferred genes solely in erythrocytes throughout life, a formidable challenge. Major DNA regulatory elements must also be introduced, and transferred genes must be integrated at sites that allow high-level expression. Problems that must be surmounted include:

- Need and production of safe, effective vectors for long-term treatment
- Prevention of silencing of transduced genes
- Difficulty in transducing rare pluripotent repopulating stem cells
- Selective expansion of transduced stem cells
- Selection of ablative chemotherapy prior to infusion of transfected cells (to create space in the marrow for expansion of transduced stem cells)

Clinical trials of gene therapy with limited endpoints are projected to begin in years 2006 to 2007.

Management Issues in Sickle Cell Disease

Method of
Kenneth R. Bridges, MD

Nature of the Problem

Sickle cell disease (SCD) reflects substitution of a valine residue for glutamic acid at position 6 in the beta subunit of hemoglobin. With a few minor exceptions, people with one gene for hemoglobin S (Hb S) are phenotypically normal (sickle trait). Two Hb S genes produce sickle cell disease. Two important compound heterozygous states, sickle–β-thalassemia and sickle/hemoglobin C, also produce sickle disease pathology.

The mechanism by which these changes in the physical properties of the hemoglobin molecule produce the clinical manifestations of the disease is not unequivocally proven. The most widely accepted hypothesis is that erythrocytes deform as they release their oxygen in the capillaries and are trapped in the microcirculation. The blockade of blood flow produces areas of tissue ischemia, leading to the myriad of clinical problems seen with sickle cell disease.

Other cells in the circulation probably moderate the severity of sickle cell disease manifestations. High neutrophil counts correlate with a worse prognosis in sickle cell disease. Platelets and abnormally circulating endothelial cells might also adversely affect severity. Chronic damage to endothelial cells lining vessel walls could increase the risk of injury because of erythrocyte adhesion. Inflammatory cytokines also seem to mediate some problems in sickle cell disease.

Sickle cell disease is extremely varied in its manifestations. A study of the natural history of the disorder indicated that approximately 5% of patients account for nearly 33% of hospital admissions. Although the disease

---

> **BOX 1   Factors That Correlate With a Severe Clinical Course in Sickle Cell Disease**
>
> - An episode of dactylitis before 1 year of age
> - A hemoglobin level of less than 7 g/dL before age 2 years
> - Persistent leukocytosis in the absence of infection

can be incapacitating, many people have few admissions and live productive and relatively healthy lives. The average life expectancy with sickle cell disease is below normal for the population, however, reflecting increased mortality attributed to the complications of the disease. Fortunately, improved care is lengthening life span.

Clinically, sickle cell disease is best thought of as two disorders, one involving children and one involving adults. With the exception of acute crisis pain, the manifestations of the two are largely different. Pediatric sickle cell disease is more of a purely hematologic disorder in which the pathophysiology derives directly from erythrocyte sickling. Because sickling is reversible, many of the associated problems are reversible, including vaso-occlusive pain episodes, splenic sequestration, and aplastic crisis. Chronic, fixed-organ damage comes to dominate the adult clinical picture. Renal dysfunction, avascular necrosis of bone, and chronic lung disease are gargantuan issues reflecting chronic injury. Therapeutic approaches must factor in these differences.

The advent of therapies that can significantly ameliorate the clinical course of sickle cell disease opens the possibility of early intervention. Multivariate clinical analysis of nearly 400 children followed at comprehensive sickle cell centers between infancy and 10 years of age uncovered several factors that augured a severe clinical course (Box 1). Children who manifest these characteristics should be considered for aggressive early treatment of their sickle cell disease. The special relationship of stroke risk to high blood velocity in the intracranial arteries is discussed later.

The Hydroxyurea Era of Sickle Cell Disease Management

Hydroxyurea (Hydrea) is the most important advancement in the care of people with sickle cell disease since the 1986 introduction of prophylactic penicillin. No message is more important than the need to assess *all* patients for possible treatment with hydroxyurea. The drug is neither investigational nor an esoteric intervention that is the province of sickle cell disease specialists. Hydroxyurea therapy is not appropriate for all people with sickle cell disease nor is it effective in everyone for whom it is tried. The medication can dramatically alter the clinical course of many patients, however. No vaticinator can augur which patients will respond to hydroxyurea. Consequently, the clinician is obliged to affirm that no patient who might benefit from hydroxyurea is neglected.

Rakel and Bope: *Conn's Current Therapy 2006.*

Every physician who cares for people with sickle cell disease must freshly visit the broad clinical picture of their patients with an eye toward a possible trial of hydroxyurea. Only when every patient has been considered for hydroxyurea, whether the drug is eventually used or not, will management attain standard-of-care status. The facts are that in a cohort of patients:

- Hydroxyurea reduces painful crises by half.
- Hydroxyurea reduces hospital stays for painful crises by half.
- Hydroxyurea reduces acute chest syndrome (ACS) by half.
- Hydroxyurea reduces transfusion requirements.

Hydroxyurea seems to lower mortality in sickle cell disease. Table 1 is a broad template against which each patient should be compared. For patients not needing hydroxyurea, the issue should be reviewed yearly. Pediatric studies confirm hydroxyurea safety in children 5 years of age and older. The drug seems more efficacious in children than in adults, and hydroxyurea should be a major focus in the management of pediatric sickle cell disease.

Although thrombocytopenia and/or neutropenia are relative contraindications, close monitoring allows nearly all patients to tolerate the medication. Bimonthly blood counts are required when patients are started on hydroxyurea. Occasionally, the hematocrit increases to the high 30s or even low 40s in response to hydroxyurea therapy necessitating dose reduction. No conclusive evidence exists to support hydroxyurea as prophylaxis against stroke, chronic leg ulcers, priapism, or other complications of sickle cell disease.

The dose of hydroxyurea needed to prevent painful crises is unknown. In the Multicenter Study of Hydroxyurea in Sickle Cell Anemia (MSH), patients received the maximum tolerated dose (MTD). The dose administered was increased stepwise until signs of toxicity, such as mild neutropenia, developed. The dose of hydroxyurea was then reduced slightly. Whether such intense treatment is required is unknown. Some specialists use lower doses of hydroxyurea (e.g., 25 mg/kg/day) with good success. Most patients treated with hydroxyurea develop macrocytosis (e.g., mean corpuscular volume = 110). Fleetingly few patients have thrombocytopenia or neutropenia at this medication dose. The therapeutic window is excellent for hydroxyurea in sickle cell disease.

Management of Acute Problems

PAIN

Vaso-occlusive pain episodes experienced by patients with sickle cell disease vary tremendously in frequency and severity. The cooperative study of the natural history of sickle cell disease showed that approximately 5% of patients accounted for 33% of hospital days devoted to pain control. To complicate matters further, the pattern of pain varies over time, so that a patient who has particularly severe problems one year might later have a prolonged period characterized by only minor pain.

The onset of sickle cell pain crises likewise varies in pattern. Patients can develop agonizingly severe pain in as little as 15 minutes without prevenient problems. In other cases, the pain gradually evolves over hours or even days. Patients manage most episodes of pain at home. Oral analgesics along with rest and fluids often allow people to "ride out" the pain episode. Some patients report that warm baths or warm compresses applied to aching joints ameliorate the severity of the pain.

The sites affected in acute painful crises vary. Pain usually occurs in the extremities, thorax, abdomen, and back. Pain tends to recur at the same site for a particular person. For each person, the quality of the crisis pain is usually similar from one crisis to another. During the evaluation, the provider should inquire whether the pain feels like "typical" sickle cell pain. Most patients can distinguish back pain caused by pyelonephritis or abdominal pain caused by cholecystitis, for instance, from their typical sickle cell pain. If the quality of the pain is not typical of their sickle cell disease, other causes should be investigated before ascribing it to vaso-occlusion.

No reliable objective index of pain exists. The provider depends solely on the patient's report. One of the most difficult problems that patients with sickle cell disease face is seeking treatment for pain in a setting in which they are unknown. Some providers mistakenly believe that the number of deformed sickle cells on the peripheral blood smear reflects the degree of patient pain. Other providers look to parameters such as blood pressure and heart rate. Although the latter measures provide more information than the peripheral smear, they do not reliably reflect pain severity. Trust in the patient report is key to the management of sickle cell pain crises.

Opioids

Vaso-occlusive sickle pain typically is severe in character. Most patients describe a major crisis as the most intense pain that they have ever experienced relative even to childbirth, the general touchstone of pain intensity. Pain control often requires large quantities of opioid analgesics. The exact amount varies, and depends in part on the frequency with which the person

TABLE 1 Hydroxyurea Therapy in Sickle Cell Disease

Eligibility for hydroxyurea	Clinical indications for hydroxyurea
Five years of age or older	Recurrent vaso-occlusive pain crises. Patients with three or more pain crises per year should be considered for hydroxyurea management.
Not pregnant	Recurrent acute chest syndrome Frequent or chronic transfusion requirement

requires opioids. For many patients, 4 to 8 mg[3] of hydromorphone (Dilaudid) can be given as an intravenous bolus over 15 to 20 minutes followed by another 4 mg in 30 minutes if pain control is inadequate. More restrained dosing of opioids is indicated for patients naive to this class of drug. Two to four milligrams of hydromorphone every 30 to 45 minutes often suffices.

Pain relief occurs more slowly with intramuscular injections, and the injections themselves can produce substantial discomfort. Consequently, intravenous administration of analgesics is usually preferable. As pain control improves, the analgesia should be maintained to prevent symptom rebound. "PRN"(as needed) analgesic administration should be avoided. After stabilization of the emergency situation with intravenous boluses of opioids, the patient should be transferred to the floor and prescribed a maintenance regimen. Patient-controlled analgesia (PCA) often works well for pain relief. Patients can become drowsy as their pain is controlled. Often, this reflects the fatigue that comes with one or more sleepless nights with pain at home. The analgesics should not be discontinued automatically for somnolence as long as the patient is easily aroused. In addition to analgesia, patients with painful crises should also receive supplemental oxygen and intravenous fluids. Once the pain is under control, oral hydration can replace the intravenous fluids.

Meperidine (Demerol) can present problems for pain control with sickle cell disease. The half-life of the drug in the circulation is approximately 4 hours. The liver converts meperidine to normeperidine, a derivative that has analgesic activity but which also is toxic. Grand mal seizure is a particularly serious complication that occurs with the administration of large amounts of meperidine. Normeperidine likely is the primary culprit. Other opioid analgesics, therefore, are preferable to meperidine. The American Pain Society recommends that meperidine no longer be used to control pain requiring long-term or recurrent opioid analgesic treatment.

Eventually the patient should be switched to oral opioid analgesics, which might be necessary for a week or more after discharge. The parenteral analgesics should be tapered after the oral medication starts. Abrupt termination of parenteral analgesics when oral medications are begun can cause resurgence in sickle cell crisis pain. Patients should have a supply of analgesics at home (that might include opioids) to control less severe episodes of pain.

Epidural analgesia clearly controls acute sickle cell crisis pain. This approach is most effective when the major discomfort is below chest level. Although some patients receive good relief with epidural analgesia alone, others continue to require systemic analgesics, albeit at lower doses. Some patients have a psychological aversion to having infusion hardware introduced into their backs and balk at epidural analgesia, despite its superior pain relief relative to systemic analgesics.

Undermedication in emergency care settings is the most prevalent problem with respect to sickle cell disease pain management. Further antagonizing matters, patients often wait hours for attention before receiving inadequate doses of analgesics. Health care providers must guard against this fault and provide timely and adequate analgesic care to these vulnerable patients.

Nonsteroidal Anti-Inflammatory Drugs (NSAIDs)

Recently, NSAIDs have been added to the management algorithm of acute sickle cell pain with ketorolac tromethamine[1] (Toradol) occupying a prominent place. Existing clinical reports are largely anecdotal. Although some are positive, others show no effect of ketorolac in the treatment of acute vaso-occlusive pain crises. Ketorolac can produce gastritis and bleeding. The drug should be used cautiously in patients with peptic ulcer disease or a history of gastrointestinal bleeding. NSAIDs can impair kidney function and accelerate the renal injury intrinsic sickle cell disease. Consequently, an increasing number of specialists eschew NSAIDs in sickle cell disease management.

Transfusion

The complex pathophysiology of sickle cell disease confounds this intuitively rational approach to a problem deriving from deformed erythrocytes. Vaso-occlusive sickle cell crises are probably fueled, at least in part, by sluggish blood flow through the microcirculation. Slow blood flow promotes deoxygenation of hemoglobin and exacerbates red cell deformation. Although the oxygen-carrying capacity of blood increases with hematocrit, so does viscosity. As the hematocrit increases beyond the range of the low 30s, increased viscosity might outweigh enhanced oxygen delivery conferred by allogeneic blood transfusion and swing the dynamics toward sickling.

Sporadic transfusion is not an effective intervention for the management of acute painful episodes in patients with sickle cell disease. Exchange transfusion has been used in attempts to alleviate bouts of severe, intractable pain with better effect, overall. Chronic transfusion for pain is more effective in children, for whom erythrocyte sickling is the dominant issue, than among adults, for whom fixed-organ damage is often a primary cause of pain.

Corticosteroids[1]

Reports exist of significant improvement in pain profile among children receiving large doses of intravenous steroids on each of the first 2 days of their painful sickle crises. Opioid analgesic requirements halved. The rate of pain relapse was significantly higher among patients who received steroid treatment, however. This intriguing observation awaits confirmation, particularly in adults with sickle cell disease. The observation is consistent with the idea that inflammatory cytokines are important in the pathophysiology of sickle cell disease.

---

[3]Exceeds dosage recommended by the manufacturer.

[1]Not FDA approved for this indication.

> **BOX 2** **Red Cell Antigens* That Alloimmunize Chronically Transfused Sickle Cell Disease Patients**
>
> Kell
> C
> E
>
> ---
>
> *Phenotype matching for these antigens significantly reduces the incidence of alloimmunization in patients with sickle cell disease who receive chronic red cell transfusions. (Adapted from Vichinsky E, Luban N, Wright E, et al: Prospective RBC phenotype matching in a stroke-prevention trial in sickle cell anemia: A multicenter transfusion trial. Transfusion 2001;41:1086-1092.)

Chest Syndrome"). Kell, E, and C are the most problematic minor antigens. The rate of alloimmunization approaches 40% in some reports of chronic transfusion in sickle cell disease. Occasionally, patients develop such severe problems with alloantibodies that transfusion becomes nearly impossible. Phenotype matching for these antigens markedly reduces the incidence of alloimmunization (Box 2). Routine use of blood from black donors for black patients with sickle cell disease is not warranted, however. The likelihood of finding matched units for patients with sickle cell disease is greater when black people are in the donor pool. Matching is necessary, nonetheless, because antigen variation among black people, as with all other humans, is great. An expanded donor pool substantially improves the chance of a match with antigen testing.

Age and Severity of Anemia

The severity of the anemia in sickle cell disease sometimes increases gradually with age. The basis of this marrow exhaustion phenomenon is unknown. Many patients have end-organ damage, such as a dilated cardiomyopathy, that can limit tolerance of severe anemia. Recombinant human erythropoietin[1] (rHuEPO; Procrit, Epogen) and hydroxyurea can improve the hemoglobin picture for some patients. Dosing can be adjusted from starting levels of 1000 mg daily of hydroxyurea and 40,000 U weekly of rHuEPO depending on patient response.

INFECTION PROPHYLAXIS

Antibiotics

The penicillin[1] prophylaxis trial completed in 1986 prompted the recommendation that all children be given prophylactic penicillin[1] (or equivalent) at a dose of 250 mg twice a day. A second study involving older children showed no difference in the incidence of severe infection among 5- to 12-year-olds. The role of prophylactic penicillin[1] in adults with sickle cell disease is undocumented, but the intervention is probably superfluous.

Immunization

Immunization with pneumococcal vaccine (Pneumovax 23) is standard practice both in adults and children with sickle cell disease. Several studies suggest that immunization provides some protection, although incomplete, against pneumococcal infection. The vaccine seems to be effective even in adults whose splenic function is lost. The more recently available 7-valent vaccine provides improved coverage of specifically problematic bacterial subtypes relative to the earlier 23-valent vaccine. Although the duration of protection is unknown, most specialists reinoculate patients once every 5 to 7 years.

More recently, a vaccine against *H. influenzae* Type b (HibTITER) entered the clinical arena. The efficacy of this vaccine in sickle cell disease is unknown. Given the serious nature of *H. influenzae* infections in these patients, many specialists, particularly pediatricians, now routinely immunize patients against this organism.

Viral influenza is potentially deadly for older people and those with several chronic illnesses including sickle cell disease. Because bacterial infection and other problems often complicate influenza, prevention of the disease by immunization is a practical intervention (FLUMIST).

The need for hepatitis B immunization (Engerix-B vaccine) for patients with sickle cell disease reflects the high likelihood of transfusion at some point.

AVASCULAR NECROSIS OF BONE

Avascular necrosis of bone is a common and debilitating problem in sickle cell disease. This process differs totally from the acute bone marrow necrosis discussed earlier. With acute bone marrow necrosis, the pathology involves damage to hematopoietic elements within the bone marrow cavity. Bone is living tissue that can die as a result of poor blood circulation within the wall of the bone itself. The areas of bone most frequently affected are the acetabulum and the head of the humerus. The etiology of avascular necrosis of bone is unknown. One hypothesis posits that marrow hyperplasia in the femoral head crowds tissue and secondarily reduces blood flow through bony trabeculae.

The quality of the pain associated with avascular bone necrosis differs substantially from sickle cell pain. The articular cartilage thins and often disappears as the process progresses. The joints can deteriorate producing a bone-on-bone interface. Movement then becomes wrenchingly painful. Early on, nonsteroidal anti-inflammatory agents can be useful. With more severe situations, particularly those that involve the shoulder, corticosteroid injection into the joint articular space can relieve symptoms. Finally, decompression of the marrow tissue in the head of the humerus or the head of the femur is used by some orthopedic surgeons. This invasive procedure should be reserved for patients with more advanced avascular necrosis. No definitive data address the efficacy of the procedure.

These interventions slow osteonecrosis without halting the process, leading sometimes to joint replacement. Some patients with sickle syndromes tolerate

---

[1]Not FDA approved for this indication.

artificial joints poorly. As many as 33% of patients require a second surgery within 4 years of joint replacement. Also, these patients, for unclear reasons, are vulnerable to infections of their orthopedic hardware. The unfortunate result can be a destroyed articular interface and a flail joint that, in the case of the femur, produces wheelchair confinement.

MR imaging is a promising addition to the diagnostic armamentarium that exceeds by far the sensitivity of plain bone films. The technique detects very early evidence of damage and holds the hope of earlier detection and improved management of this most debilitating of sickle cell disease complications.

OSTEOMYELITIS

Nearly three quarters of cases of osteomyelitis with sickle cell disease are attributed to *Salmonella* species. Local pain and fever are the most common indicators of chronic osteomyelitis. In the early stages of the disorder, bone roentgenograms and even bone scans frequently are unrevealing. Gallium scans can provide early evidence of the condition. The addition of MRI to the diagnostic arsenal is a promising development. Bone biopsy gives the definitive diagnosis. This procedure sometimes is not an option, depending on the location of the infection, however. Once the diagnosis is made, 4 to 6 weeks of intravenous antibiotic therapy are needed.

SKIN ULCERS

The 1% incidence of skin ulcers in the United States is low relative to the 30% reported incidence in Jamaica. The basic of the strikingly different figures is unknown. The most common site of skin ulceration is over the lateral malleoli. The ulceration often lacks clear-cut antecedent trauma and progresses over a period of weeks to the point that the lesions penetrate into the dermis and often into the underlying subcutaneous tissue. Breakdown in protection provided by the integument leaves patients susceptible to infections and other complications.

Treatment of ankle ulcers should be conservative. Rest, elevation, and dry dressings with antimicrobial ointments by far are the best approaches to this problem. Attempts at skin grafting are frequently frustrated by poor blood flow to the affected region. Healing usually requires weeks to months. The area should be protected against trauma when the patient is up and about. Socks or other clothing that cover the area should be avoided, to reduce friction injury. A simple dry dressing provides additional protection. Reports of enhanced healing of ulcers associated with chronic transfusion therapy are anecdotal.

RENAL DYSFUNCTION

The most common renal defect in sickle cell disease is impaired urine-concentrating ability (hyposthenuria) that often appears by 2 or 3 years of age. The condition can produce bedwetting in children or embarrassing wetting in public places such as classrooms. Hyposthenuria

also occurs with compound heterozygous states (e.g., sickle-β-thalassemia). The extremely high osmolality in the distal tubule produces renal medullary sickling even in people with sickle trait. Consequently, hyposthenuria is the most common abnormality associated with sickle cell trait.

Medullary ischemia and papillary necrosis occur frequently. Sometimes, the necrotic papillae slough into the collecting system, obstructing the outflow tract. No effective specific intervention exists for this problem. Increasing BUN and creatinine values herald sickle glomerulonephropathy. The most important intervention is limiting protein consumption, as is recommended for many types of renal dysfunction including that associated with diabetic nephropathy. One report suggested that angiotensin-converting enzyme inhibitors[1] (e.g., enalapril [Vasotec]) might retard nephropathy progression in sickle cell disease. Unfortunately, confirmatory studies were never conducted.

Patients with sickle cell disease usually have *low* serum creatinine and BUN levels. This reflects the high glomerular filtration rate along with a high rate of creatinine secretion in the distal tubule. BUN values of 7 mg/dL and creatinine values of 0.5 mg/dL are typical for patients with sickle cell disease. Creatinine clearance often exceeds 150 mL/minute/1.73 m^2 surface area. A formal evaluation of glomerular filtration should be considered for patients in whom the serum creatinine increases above the level of approximately 1.0 mg/dL.

Limited experience exists on the efficacy of dialysis with sickle cell disease. Reports that hemodialysis is problematic in patients with sickle cell disease are anecdotal. Every effort should be undertaken to prevent renal deterioration. Microscopic hematuria is common with sickle cell disease (as well as some patients with sickle cell trait). Hematuria per se requires no intervention unless blood loss is massive. Some patients with sickle cell disease and renal failure have successfully received renal allografts.

Massive hematuria occasionally develops in people with sickle cell trait. Interestingly, the bleeding often comes from the left kidney. Hydration and alkalization of the urine are frequently used interventions. Anecdotal reports of the use of desmopressin[1] (DDAVP) in this situation are encouraging. Epsilon aminocaproic acid[1] (Amicar) has been used in some patients with refractory bleeding from the kidney. Bleeding can continue for weeks. Iron replacement may be necessary as treatment interventions continue. Nephrectomy has been performed, but this frightful intervention should be a last-ditch approach to a life-threatening situation.

RETINOPATHY

Retinopathy is a significant problem for 10% to 20% of people with sickle cell disease. The peak age of onset is in the 20s. For unknown reasons, the condition develops more frequently with hemoglobin sickle cell disease than with homozygous sickle cell disease. The problem

---

[1]Not FDA approved for this indication.

CURRENT DIAGNOSIS

Problem	Manifestation	Treatment
Acute chest syndrome	Decreasing oxygen saturation with partial pressure of oxygen less than 80 mm Hg on room air Chest radiograph infiltrates Fever Leukocytosis	Simple transfusion Exchange transfusion Antibiotics Ventilation support Bronchodilators
Splenic sequestration crisis	Enlarging spleen on examination Left upper quadrant pain Decreasing hemoglobin	Simple transfusion
Stroke	Acute hemiplegia/hemiparesis Severe headache Nausea, vomiting	Exchange transfusion
Aplastic crisis	Reticulocyte count low or zero Decreasing hemoglobin Fever, vaso-occlusive pain	Simple transfusion
Septicemia	Fever Leukocytosis Peripheral blood bands Lethargy Confusion	Cultures Broad-spectrum antibiotics

resembles diabetic retinopathy both clinically and pathologically with retinal thinning and neovascularization. The areas affected, at least initially, are in the periphery of the retina with indirect ophthalmoscopy required for detection. Laser photocoagulation has been used in an effort to prevent retinal hemorrhage. A retina specialist is the preferred provider, particularly if diabetic retinopathy is a practice focus. Annual evaluation is key to early detection of lesions and prevention of complications. Retinopathy has no correlation with sickle cell disease pain profile. All patients must have retinal examination irrespective of clinical status.

HEART

Cardiomegaly is often caused by a sustained high cardiac output state. Whereas high output failure occurs in

CURRENT THERAPY

- Hydroxyurea—Daily oral administration in children older than 5 years of age and adults who fit the appropriate treatment profile
- Penicillin prophylaxis—Daily penicillin or equivalent in children from ages 6 months to 7 years
- Pneumococcal immunization—Children and adults. Repeat every 5 to 7 years
- Hepatitis B immunization—Children and adults
- Viral influenza immunization—Adults every year
- Limited phenotype matched red cell transfusion—Children and adults when transfusion is needed
- Severe acute pain crisis—Parenterally administered, short-acting opioids
  - Patient-controlled analgesia (PCA)
  - Avoid meperidine

some patients with sickle cell disease, the heart usually is hyperdynamic. Pulmonary congestion caused by fluid overload during hydration for painful crisis is uncommon in young patients, but can be an issue in older adults. Careful monitoring of cardiovascular status can prevent serious problems with pulmonary congestion.

PREGNANCY

Women with sickle cell disease can carry pregnancies to term, but the process sometimes is complicated. The frequency of painful crises usually increases during pregnancy. Women who have painful crises during pregnancy should receive analgesics as necessary, including narcotics. The newborns with intrauterine opioid exposure must undergo opioid withdrawal. Warned of this issue, neonatologists can easily manage the problem. Routine transfusion is not indicated during pregnancy.

BONE MARROW TRANSPLANTATION

Bone marrow transplantation can cure SCD. This promising but complex intervention remains in the domain of highly specialized care groups who manage many such patients. The intervention is far more effective in children than in adults.

Without major breakthroughs in gene therapy or bone marrow transplantation that make these treatments applicable to many patients, drug intervention will remain the major therapeutic option for sickle cell disease. Currently, all patients must be assessed for possible treatment with hydroxyurea.

REFERENCES

Adamkiewicz T, Sarnaik S, Buchanan G, et al: Invasive pneumococcal infections in children with sickle cell disease in the era of penicillin prophylaxis, antibiotic resistance, and 23-valent pneumococcal polysaccharide vaccination. J Pediatr 2003;143:438-444. Pneumococcal sepsis remains a problem despite penicillin prophylaxis and vaccination with the 23-valent vaccine. Early aggressive treatment of suspected sepsis is vital.

Charache S, Terrin M, Moore R, et al: Effect of hydroxyurea on the frequency of painful crises in sickle cell anemia. Investigators of the Multicenter Study of Hydroxyurea in Sickle Cell Anemia. N Engl J Med 1995;332:1317-1322. The article presents the data on hydroxyurea for prophylactic treatment of sickle cell disease. This remains the only intervention proven to prevent problems, specifically acute vaso-occlusive pain crisis, crisis-related hospitalization, and acute chest syndrome. The drug also lowers transfusion requirements.

Falletta J, Woods G, Verter J, et al: Discontinuing penicillin prophylaxis in children with sickle cell anemia. Prophylactic Penicillin Study II. J Pediatr 1995;127:685-690. Penicillin prophylaxis can be safely stopped at 5 years of age.

Kinney T, Helms R, O'Branski E, et al: Safety of hydroxyurea in children with sickle cell anemia: Results of the HUG-KIDS study, a phase I/II trial. Pediatric Hydroxyurea Group. Blood 1999; 94:1550-1554. This Phase I/II trial shows that hydroxyurea therapy is safe for children with sickle cell disease when treatment is directed by a pediatric hematologist.

Quinn C, Rogers Z, Buchanan G: Survival of children with sickle cell disease. Blood 2004;103:4023-4027. Childhood mortality from SCD is decreasing, the mean age at death is increasing, and a smaller proportion of deaths is from infection.

Scothorn D, Price C, Schwartz D, et al: Risk of recurrent stroke in children with sickle cell disease receiving blood transfusion therapy for at least five years after initial stroke. J Pediatr 2002; 140:348-354. The absence of an antecedent or concurrent medical event associated with an initial stroke is a major risk factor for subsequent stroke while receiving regular transfusions.

Tahhan H, Holbrook C, Braddy L, et al: Antigen-matched donor blood in the transfusion management of patients with sickle cell disease. Transfusion 1994;34:562-569. Approximately 33% of patients who received chronic transfusion with blood that was not matched for extended phenotype developed alloantibodies. None of the matched patients developed alloantibodies. A cost saving also existed with the extended phenotype-matched blood because of lower subsequent laboratory testing expenses.

Vichinsky E, Neumayr L, Earles A, et al: Causes and outcomes of the acute chest syndrome in sickle cell disease. N Engl J Med 2000;342:1855-1865. The article provides the most extensive information available on the causes and treatment of acute chest syndrome. In particular, the study shows that although infection and fat emboli are the leading proven causes of acute chest syndrome, the etiology is mysterious in more than 33% of patients. Transfusions and bronchodilators are keys to treatment.

Zimmerman R: Pneumococcal conjugate vaccine for young children. Am Fam Physician 2001;63:1991-1998. The American Academy of Family Physicians recommends routine vaccination of infants, catch-up vaccination of children younger than 24 months, and catch-up vaccination of children 24 to 59 months of age with high-risk medical conditions such as sickle cell disease and congenital heart disease.

Neutropenia

Method of
Peter E. Newburger, MD

Neutropenia is defined as a below-normal number of peripheral blood neutrophils, as determined by calculation of the absolute neutrophil count (ANC). The ANC equals the total white blood cell count multiplied by the proportion of neutrophils (including both segmented and band forms) on the differential count. The clinical significance of neutropenia depends on the level of depression of the ANC (Table 1). Severe neutropenia, with ANC less than 200, is also termed "agranulocytosis," even though eosinophils and basophils (which are also granulocytes) may remain normal in number, and monocytes may be normal or increased. The normal range for the ANC extends to 1000/mm^3 in persons of African ethnic origin.

Fever in the setting of ANC less than 500 is a medical emergency that compels immediate evaluation and antibiotic treatment.

Clinical Presentation

Neutropenia causes no clinical symptoms or signs per se, so that the clinical presentation derives only from secondary infections. Patients may be asymptomatic but usually present with fever with or without localizing signs of infection. Gingivitis or ulcerative stomatitis, often with thrush, occurs commonly; periodic stomatitis occurring every 21 days is a hallmark of cyclic neutropenia. Predictable but often asymptomatic neutropenia follows 7 to 14 days after administration of myelosuppressive cancer chemotherapy.

Neutropenic patients can develop infection in virtually any organ system. The most common forms are cellulitis; pneumonia and lung abscess; enteritis, which can progress rapidly to peritonitis; perirectal abscess; lymphadenitis; and sepsis, which is particularly likely in patients with indwelling central venous catheters, mucositis, or additional defects in host defense (such as chemotherapy-induced immunosuppression). With agranulocytosis, clinical signs can be limited to fever, which occurs even in the complete absence of granulocytes; local inflammation is attenuated or absent. Common pathogens include *Staphylococcus aureus* and enteric gram-negative bacilli. Fungi and opportunistic or multiple antibiotic-resistant bacteria generally cause infection only after prolonged neutropenia and broad-spectrum antibiotic therapy, but need to be considered even at initial presentation. Isolated neutropenia does not impair host defense against viral infection.

Evaluation

Box 1 presents a differential diagnosis of neutropenia, which can serve as a guide for diagnostic evaluation. In an acutely ill patient, the initial evaluation for infection needs to be completed rapidly (within hours at the most) and should include assessment of potential sites and causes of infection but with minimal or no manipulation of the anus and rectum, where minor trauma could induce a perirectal abscess. The diagnostic approach requires a step-by-step evaluation of a differential diagnosis based on the history, severity, and duration of neutropenia, leukocyte and bone marrow morphology, associated hematologic or congenital abnormalities, and tests for specific disorders.

Rakel and Bope: *Conn's Current Therapy 2006.*

TABLE 1 Clinical Significance of Absolute Neutrophil Counts

ANC (neutrophils/mm³)	Clinical significance	Treatment
>1500	Normal	None
1000-1500	Not clinically significant	None
500-1000	Very slight predisposition to infection	Outpatient antibiotic treatment for febrile illness
200-500	Significant predisposition to infection	G-CSF if symptomatic; inpatient IV antibiotics for febrile illness
<200 (agranulocytosis)	Very high risk of infection, decreased local signs of inflammation	G-CSF if responsive; aggressive IV antibiotics for febrile illness

Abbreviations: G-CSF = granulocyte colony-stimulating factor; IV = intravenous.

Acquired neutropenia often accompanies viral infection and requires only monitoring of blood counts until recovery. However, depletion of bone marrow reserves can also reduce the ANC in bacterial sepsis in the newborn or in overwhelming bacteremia, as with meningococcus. Drug-induced neutropenia can be associated with a large number of agents including, but by no means limited to, antibiotics, anticonvulsants, anti-inflammatories, antithyroid drugs, diuretics, and phenothiazines. Antineutrophil antibodies are detected by flow cytometry or agglutination assays, but false-negative and borderline-positive results obscure the diagnosis of immune neutropenia. Careful review of the peripheral blood smear reveals blasts or nucleated erythrocytes indicative of bone marrow involvement by malignancy, large granular lymphocytosis, or specific neutrophil morphology associated with a congenital disorder, such as the giant granules of Chédiak-Higashi syndrome.

Bone marrow examination, including cytogenetics, is indicated in cases of severe neutropenia or when other bone marrow lineages are abnormal. In some of the less severe forms of congenital neutropenia, such as familial benign neutropenia, adequate bone marrow reserves of mature granulocytes can be demonstrated by steroid stimulation of neutrophil release into the peripheral blood, evaluated by white blood cell and differential counts before and 6 hours after prednisone,[1] 1 to 2 mg/kg orally (or methylprednisolone[1] intravenously). Serial blood counts, twice weekly over 6 to 9 weeks, are necessary to make the diagnosis of cyclic neutropenia and to document the period of the cycles and the depths of the nadirs. Several of the syndromes listed in the table include unique phenotypic features that aid in the diagnosis; most pediatric hematology texts and the Online Mendelian Inheritance in Man Web site (http://www.ncbi.nlm.nih.gov/Omim/) provide detailed descriptions. Evaluation of cellular immunity and quantitative measurements of IgG, IgA, and IgM not only contribute to the diagnosis of neutropenia associated with immunologic abnormalities but also indicate a need for more aggressive management if other arms of host defense are impaired. In newborns or infants with hypoglycemia or neurologic abnormalities, blood and urine testing reveals a metabolic disorder such as glycogen storage disease type 1b, Barth's syndrome, hyperglycinemia, tyrosinemia, or an organic acidemia. Excessive neutrophil margination in benign "pseudoneutropenia" can be demonstrated by epinephrine administration.

BOX 1 Differential Diagnosis of Neutropenia

Acquired
- Viral bone marrow suppression
- Bacterial or fungal sepsis with exhaustion of bone marrow storage pool
- Drug-induced
    Impaired production (chemotherapy, phenothiazines, other drugs)
    Antibody-mediated (aminopyrine, other drugs)
- Immune-mediated (alloimmune and autoimmune)
- Bone marrow aplasia, dysplasia, or replacement
- Hypersplenism
- Nutritional (folate, vitamin B₁₂)

Congenital
- Congenital neutropenia
    Severe congenital neutropenia (Kostmann's neutropenia)
    Cyclic neutropenia
    Myelokathexis
    Familial benign neutropenia
    Syndromes including neutropenia
    Cartilage-hair hypoplasia
    Chédiak-Higashi syndrome
    Dyskeratosis congenita
    Fanconi anemia
    Reticular dysgenesis
    Shwachman-Diamond syndrome
- Neutropenia associated with immunologic abnormalities (e.g., X-linked hyper-IgM)
- Neutropenia associated with metabolic disorders (e.g., glycogen storage disease type 1b, organic acidurias)
- Pseudoneutropenia

Treatment

SUPPORTIVE CARE

Fever or other signs of infection require immediate, aggressive antibiotic therapy in the neutropenic patient

---

[1]Not FDA approved for this indication.

with ANC less than 500. Antibiotics tailored to the susceptibility of identified organisms provide ideal treatment for infections with positive cultures. However, the initial treatment of most febrile illnesses and the entire therapy of many with negative cultures will rely on an empiric choice of antibiotics. Empirical therapy consists of a single broad spectrum antibiotic (such as a third generation cephalosporin) or a combination of broad spectrum antibiotics such as an aminoglycoside (e.g., gentamicin [Garamycin],[1] tobramycin [Nebcin][1]) and either a third generation cephalosporin (e.g., ceftazidime [Fortaz][1]) or a semisynthetic penicillin with anti-*Pseudomonas* activity (e.g., piperacillin [Pipracil][1], ticarcillin [Ticar][1]). Patients with indwelling central venous catheters require substitution of an agent with better gram-positive coverage (e.g., nafcillin [Unipen][1] or vancomycin [Vancocin][1]) for the aminoglycoside. Each institution needs to base its empirical antibiotic selection on the identity and antibiotic susceptibilities of micro-organisms in the community or hospital (depending on the likely site of acquisition of infection), with the final choices made in consultation with the local microbiology or infectious disease division. Fever persisting for more than 5 days generally indicates the need for modification of antibiotic coverage, generally including addition of empirical antifungal therapy such as amphotericin B (Fungizone),[1] caspofungin (Cancidas),[1] or a triazole agent.

For hospitalized patients, hand washing needs to be strictly enforced. More aggressive reverse precautions do little to prevent the majority of infections, which derive from the patient's own skin, mucosa, and gastrointestinal flora. Careful oral, perianal, and skin hygiene help reduce the prevalence of infection in patients with acute or chronic neutropenia.

Prophylactic antibiotics can be useful in uncorrected chronic neutropenia, particularly for the prevention of *S. aureus* colonization and infection. Cephalosporins or trimethoprim-sulfamethoxazole (Bactrim)[1] are appropriate for this indication. The latter, widely used combination provides broad spectrum coverage with very little toxicity but can cause neutropenia.

SPECIFIC THERAPY

Granulocyte colony-stimulating factor (G-CSF), marketed as filgrastim (Neupogen), is the most important, highly specific drug for the treatment of neutropenia. FDA-approved indications for G-CSF include neutropenia associated with cancer chemotherapy and severe congenital neutropenia. The pegylated, long-acting form of the drug (pegfilgrastim [Neulasta]) provides a single-dose formulation that can be administered once in each chemotherapy cycle.

Treatment with G-CSF can correct the ANC to the normal range in most patients with severe congenital neutropenia or cyclic neutropenia. Successful correction of the peripheral blood count also prevents stomatitis and other infection-related symptoms and risks.

---

[1]Not FDA approved for this indication.

 CURRENT DIAGNOSIS

- The clinical significance of neutropenia depends on the level of depression of the ANC.
- Fever in the setting of ANC less than 500 is a medical emergency that compels immediate evaluation and antibiotic treatment.
- Patients may be asymptomatic, but usually present with fever, with or without localizing signs of infection, which may be attenuated or absent.
- Common complications include gingivitis, ulcerative stomatitis, cellulitis, pneumonia, lung abscess, enteritis, peritonitis, perirectal abscess, lymphadenitis, and sepsis.
- Common pathogens include *Staphylococcus aureus* and enteric gram-negative bacilli. Infections with fungi and other opportunistic organisms may appear in the setting of prolonged neutropenia and antibiotic therapy.
- The diagnostic approach requires a step-by-step evaluation of a differential diagnosis based on the history, severity, and duration of neutropenia; leukocyte and bone marrow morphology; associated hematologic or congenital abnormalities; and tests for specific disorders.
- Bone marrow examination, including cytogenetics, is indicated in cases of severe neutropenia or when other bone marrow lineages are abnormal.
- Evaluation of cellular immunity and Ig abnormalities, but may also indicate a need for more aggressive management.

Abbreviation: ANC = absolute neutrophil count.

At the initiation of therapy, or if the ANC rises far above normal, expansion of myelopoiesis may cause bone pain or splenomegaly. The major long-term risk in these patients is a conversion to myelodysplasia or leukemia. Most reported cases of myelodysplasia or secondary myeloid leukemia in severe congenital neutropenia patients, both treated and untreated, have been associated with an acquired deletion or abnormality of chromosome 7. Therefore, bone marrow cytogenetics need to be examined prior to initiation of G-CSF and yearly during its chronic administration. Sensitivity to G-CSF varies considerably in severe congenital neutropenia; dosage needs to be titrated for each patient, usually within a range of 1 to 20 μg/kg daily, but occasionally much higher. Patients with cyclic neutropenia generally respond to lower doses of G-CSF and do not appear to have an increased risk of myelodysplasia or leukemia.

The use of G-CSF for acquired neutropenia is more controversial. Although it hastens recovery in drug-induced neutropenia, discontinuation of the offending drug is usually sufficient. An empiric trial of G-CSF in other acquired forms of chronic neutropenia may be

CURRENT THERAPY

- Fever or other signs of infection require immediate, aggressive antibiotic therapy in the neutropenic patient with ANC less than 500.
- Antibiotics tailored to the susceptibility of identified organisms provide ideal therapy, but empirical antibiotics are usually necessary for the initial treatment of febrile neutropenia.
- Prophylactic antibiotics can be useful in uncorrected chronic neutropenia.
- Granulocyte colony-stimulating factor (filgrastim [Neupogen]) is the most important, highly specific drug for the treatment of congenital and some forms of acquired neutropenia. A pegylated formulation (pegfilgrastim [Neulasta]) permits single-dose administration once in each cycle to alleviate chemotherapy-induced neutropenia.
- Granulocyte transfusion may be indicated for patients with agranulocytosis complicated by persistent, life-threatening bacterial or fungal infections.

Abbreviation: ANC = absolute neutrophil count.

warranted for symptomatic patients. Patients with autoimmune neutropenia often respond to low doses of G-CSF and may experience considerable bone pain at the standard dosage used for postchemotherapy myelosuppression.

Granulocyte transfusions, although rarely indicated, provide additional therapeutic support for newborns with sepsis and bone marrow neutrophil depletion as well as for older children or adults with agranulocytosis complicated by life-threatening bacterial or fungal infections that persist after adequate trials of appropriate antibiotic therapy.

Patients with systemic rheumatologic disorders, including Felty's syndrome, may benefit from therapy with glucocorticosteroids (e.g., prednisone),[1] but there is rarely any indication for their use in other forms of neutropenia. Administration of steroids to a patient with neutropenia may do more harm than good, particularly if there is little or no response. Steroids add immunosuppression to an already compromised host defense system and predispose patients to fungal infection. However, a single dose is safe as a diagnostic test for mobilization of bone marrow neutrophils.

REFERENCES

Bhatt V, Saleem A: Drug-induced neutropenia—pathophysiology, clinical features, and management. Ann Clin Lab Sci 2004;34(2):131-137.
Boxer L, Dale DC: Neutropenia: Causes and consequences. Semin Hematol 2002;39(2):75-81.
Dale D: Current management of chemotherapy-induced neutropenia: The role of colony-stimulating factors. Semin Oncol 2003;30(4 Suppl 13):3-9.

[1]Not FDA approved for this indication.

Dale DC, Cottle TE, Fier CJ: Severe chronic neutropenia: Treatment and follow-up of patients in the Severe Chronic Neutropenia International Registry. Am J Hematol 2003;72(2):82-93.
Petitti DB, Contreras R, Glowalla M, et al: Most severe neutropenia in individuals with no chronic condition did not result in a specific diagnosis. J Clin Epidemiol 2004;57(11):1182-1187.
Walsh TJ, Teppler H, Donowitz GR, et al: Caspofungin versus liposomal amphotericin B for empirical antifungal therapy in patients with persistent fever and neutropenia. N Engl J Med 2004;351(14):1391-1402.

Hemolytic Disease of the Newborn

Method of
James W. Kendig, MD

Hemolytic disease of the fetus and newborn refers to a spectrum of problems that were formerly classified as four separate entities: erythroblastosis fetalis, congenital anemia, icterus gravis neonatorum, and hydrops fetalis. Further studies demonstrated that these entities are all manifestations of a single disease caused by red blood cell isoimmunization (alloimmunization).

The major red blood cell surface antigen responsible for this process is the $Rh_o(D)$ antigen. Because there is no corresponding "d" antigen, the term "d" refers only to the absence of the $Rh_o(D)$ antigen. $Rh_o(D)$-negative individuals (dd) have no $Rh_o(D)$ antigens on their red blood cells. $Rh_o(D)$-positive individuals may be homozygous (DD) or heterozygous (Dd) for the $Rh_o(D)$ gene, which is located on the short arm of chromosome 1. In addition to the $Rh_o(D)$ gene, the Rh blood group system includes the related Cc Ee structural gene, which encodes four specific antigens (C, c, E, and e) on the red blood cell surface. Zygosity for $Rh_o(D)$ may be predicted on the basis of classic serologic tests for the antigens C, c, D, E, e, and the known incidence of various phenotypes in different racial and ethnic groups.

$Rh_o(D)$ alloimmunization occurs when fetal $Rh_o(D)$-positive red blood cells (inherited from the father) cross the placenta and enter the circulation of an $Rh_o(D)$-negative (dd) mother. The maternal immune system is stimulated to produce $Rh_o(D)$ antibodies (IgG). ABO incompatibility (mother 0 and fetus A or B) helps to protect against the $Rh_o(D)$ sensitization of the $Rh_o(D)$-negative mother.

The maternal $Rh_o(D)$ antibodies cross the placenta of the current or a subsequent pregnancy and cause the destruction of the $Rh_o(D)$-positive fetal red blood cells. The fetus responds to this hemolytic anemia with extramedullary hematopoiesis involving the liver and spleen. The hepatic production of fetal albumin is compromised, leading to hydrops with edema, ascites, and pericardial and pleural effusions. Bilirubin, produced by the hemolysis of fetal red blood cells, readily crosses the placenta and is excreted by the maternal liver. After delivery, however, neonatal hyperbilirubinemia develops,

6

which may lead to an acute encephalopathy (kernicterus). Other red blood cell antigen–antibody systems (Kidd, Kell, Duffy, the C/c and E/e alleles of the Rh system, and, rarely, the ABO system) may occasionally result in hemolytic disease of the fetus and newborn. In the case of anti-Kell isoimmunization, fetal anemia is caused by a suppression of erythropoiesis in addition to hemolysis.

Prevention of Rh$_o$(D) Alloimmunization

The development, commercial production, and widespread use of commercially prepared Rh$_o$(D) immunoglobulin (RhoGAM) for the prevention of Rh$_o$(D) alloimmunization are among the greatest scientific and medical achievements of the 20th century. This is an example of passive immunization preventing active immunization, but the precise mechanism by which the administration of the Rh$_o$(D) antibody blocks the mother's production of the same antibody is still not fully understood. RhoGAM is not beneficial to the Rh$_o$(D)-negative woman after alloimmunization has taken place, and it does not prevent sensitization because of the C/c and E/e antigens of the Rh blood group system. Box 1 gives a list of events and procedures that may lead to the Rh$_o$(D) alloimmunization of the Rh$_o$(D)-negative woman. An intramuscular dose of RhoGAM (300 µg) should be administered after these events and procedures. In the event of a severe fetal-to-maternal hemorrhage at delivery, more than 300 µg of RhoGAM may be required.

Blood type (ABO and Rh$_o$(D)) and an antibody screen (the indirect Coombs test) should be obtained on the first prenatal visit. The antibody screen detects Rh$_o$(D) antibodies as well as antibodies directed against the other red blood cell antigens, such as Kell, Duffy, C/c, and E/e. If the antibody screen is positive, alloimmunization has already occurred, and serial titers should

be obtained. If the antibody titer is 1:16 or greater by 20 weeks' gestation, further testing is necessary.

ANTEPARTUM PREVENTION

At 28 weeks' gestation, all Rh$_o$(D)-negative mothers should have an antibody screen (indirect Coombs test). If the test is negative, a prophylactic intramuscular dose of RhoGAM (300 µg) should be administered, unless the father of the infant is definitely known to be Rh$_o$(D)-negative (dd). The purpose of this prophylactic antepartum dose is to prevent alloimmunization during the pregnancy. The half-life of this dose is 12 weeks. This antepartum dose may lead to a weakly positive indirect Coombs test in the mother at the time of delivery and a weekly positive direct Coombs test in the infant.

POSTPARTUM PREVENTION

Every Rh$_o$(D)-negative mother who has not undergone Rh$_o$(D) alloimmunization should receive an intramuscular dose of *at least* 300 µg of RhoGAM after the delivery of an Rh$_o$(D)-positive newborn. This critical step in the prevention of Rh$_o$(D) disease requires careful communication among the labor and delivery area, the hospital blood bank, and the postpartum floor. These communication issues are particularly important when early discharge from the hospital is being considered and when the birth has occurred outside the hospital.

A single dose of RhoGAM (300 µg) neutralizes approximately 30 mL of Rh$_o$(D)-positive fetal whole blood or 15 mL of packed fetal red blood cells. If a large fetal-to-maternal transfusion should occur at the time of delivery, a single dose of RhoGAM may be inadequate to prevent alloimmunization. Because of this possibility, the hospital blood bank should check the mother's blood after delivery to determine the presence and the magnitude of a fetal-to-maternal bleed. The rosette test is used to screen maternal blood for the presence of fetal red blood cells, and the Kleihauer-Betke stain is used to evaluate the magnitude of a fetal-to-maternal bleed. This information is used to determine the need for a larger (more than 300 µg) dose of intramuscular RhoGAM. RhoGAM should be administered within 72 hours of delivery. If administration has been inadvertently omitted, it may still be given up to 4 weeks after delivery. The Rh$_o$(D)-negative mother who is already Rh$_o$(D) alloimmunized at the time of delivery will not benefit from the administration of RhoGAM.

Obstetric Management of the Mother With a Positive Initial Antibody Screen

All pregnant women should have an antibody screen (indirect Coombs test) at the first prenatal visit. If the result is positive, the blood bank identifies the antibody and determines its titer. The blood bank examines the father's red blood cells for the corresponding antigen. If the father's result is negative for the antigen, and if the

---

BOX 1   Reproductive Events and Procedures That Can Lead to Alloimmunization of the Rh$_o$(D)-Negative Woman

Events
- Threatened abortion and antepartum hemorrhage
- Spontaneous abortion
- Delivery at any gestational age
- Ectopic pregnancy
- Hydatidiform molar pregnancy
- Abdominal trauma and motor vehicle accidents during pregnancy
- Inadvertent transfusion with Rh-positive blood

Procedures
- Cordocentesis
- Chorionic villous sampling
- Induced abortion
- Amniocentesis any time during pregnancy
- External cephalic version
- Delivery at any time

Rakel and Bope: *Conn's Current Therapy 2006.*

mother has absolutely no doubts regarding paternity, no further studies are required. If the father's result is positive for the involved antigen, the mother should have serial antibody titers at 1-month intervals. Early ultrasonography should also be done for gestational age assessment. If a critical antibody titer of 1:16 is reached, there is a risk of the development of erythroblastosis fetalis and hydrops, and further investigation and interventions are required (Figure 1).

The $Rh_o(D)$-alloimmunized mother with a history of a previous pregnancy requiring an intrauterine transfusion or a neonatal exchange transfusion is at a high risk for hydrops. With this history, serial ΔOD_{450} evaluations of amniotic fluid are recommended, starting at 20 to 22 weeks' gestation, even if the antibody titer has not reached the critical level of 1:16.

PATERNAL ZYGOSITY

If the maternal antibody is $Rh_o(D)$, and the father has the corresponding $Rh_o(D)$ antigen, the blood bank determines whether he is homozygous (DD) or heterozygous (Dd). This prediction is based on the classic serologic tests for the C, c, E, and e antigens and the known incidence of various phenotypes in different racial and ethnic groups. If the father is heterozygous, there is a 50% chance that the fetal red blood cells are $Rh_o(D)$-negative (dd) and that the fetus is not at risk for the development of erythroblastosis fetalis. If the father is heterozygous, it is useful to determine the fetal blood type.

DETERMINATION OF FETAL BLOOD TYPE

Techniques for obtaining samples of fetal blood from the umbilical vessels, using ultrasound guidance, have been perfected and are available at large regional perinatal centers. This procedure, known as cordocentesis, involves obvious risks and should be performed only by specialists experienced in fetal and maternal medicine. Several centers have used the polymerase chain reaction (PCR) to identify the fetal $Rh_o(D)$ genotype. This new technique is based on the amplification of the DNA from a few fetal red blood cells found in a centrifuged sample of amniotic fluid. If the mother has $Rh_o(D)$ antibodies and the fetus is $Rh_o(D)$-negative (by cordocentesis of a fetal blood sample or by PCR of fetal red blood cells from amniotic fluid), no further studies are indicated.

AMNIOTIC FLUID ΔOD_{450} MEASUREMENTS

If the maternal antibody titer reaches a critical titer of 1:16 and if there is a possibility that the fetal red blood cells are positive for the corresponding antigen, serial measurements of amniotic fluid ΔOD_{450} (optical density at 450 nm) should be done every 10 to 14 days to evaluate the level of bilirubin in the amniotic fluid. These values are plotted on the modified Liley curve (Figure 2).

INTRAUTERINE FETAL TRANSFUSION

When ΔOD_{450} values climb to the upper indeterminate zone or anywhere in the $Rh_o(D)$-positive (affected) zone on the modified Liley curve, cordocentesis should be done to measure the fetal hematocrit. If this value is less than 30%, an intravascular fetal transfusion (via cordocentesis) of packed red blood cells should be carried out at a regional perinatal center by specialists experienced in maternal and fetal medicine. For severe hydrops, more than one intrauterine transfusion may be required. The timing of delivery should be based on gestational age estimates and the determination of fetal lung maturity.

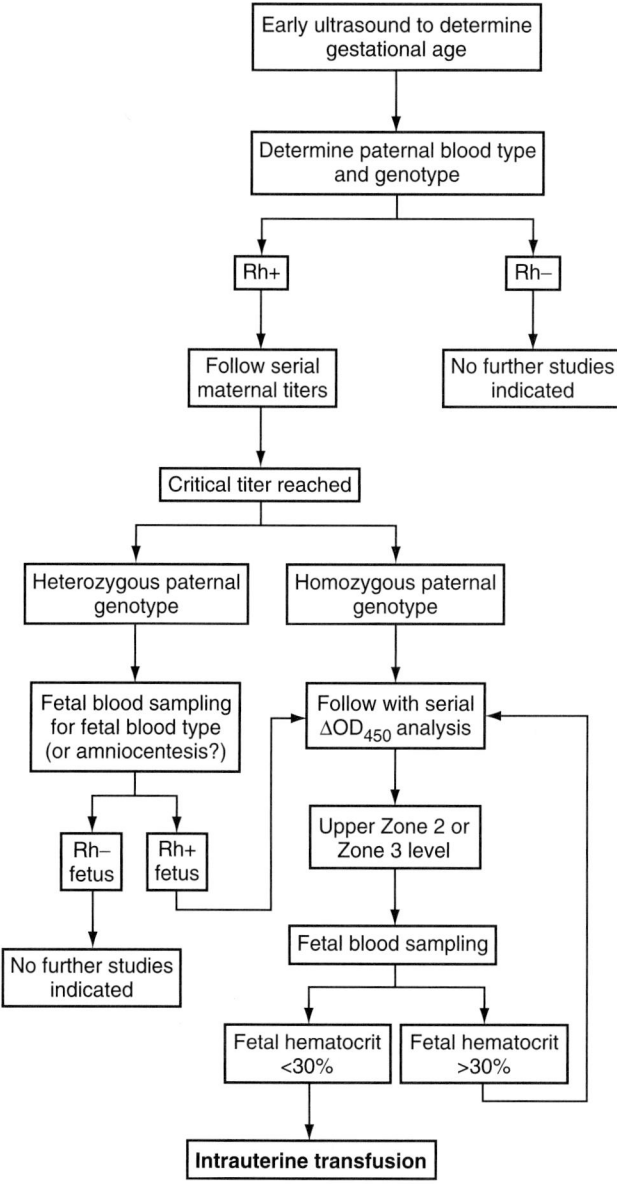

FIGURE 1. Algorithm used at Baylor College of Medicine, Houston, for the management of newly diagnosed, red blood cell $Rh_o(D)$ alloimmunization in pregnancy. (From Moise KJ: Changing trends in the management of red blood cell alloimmunization in pregnancy. Arch Pathol Lab Med 1994;118:421-428. Copyright 1994, American Medical Association. Used with permission.)

Rakel and Bope: *Conn's Current Therapy 2006.*

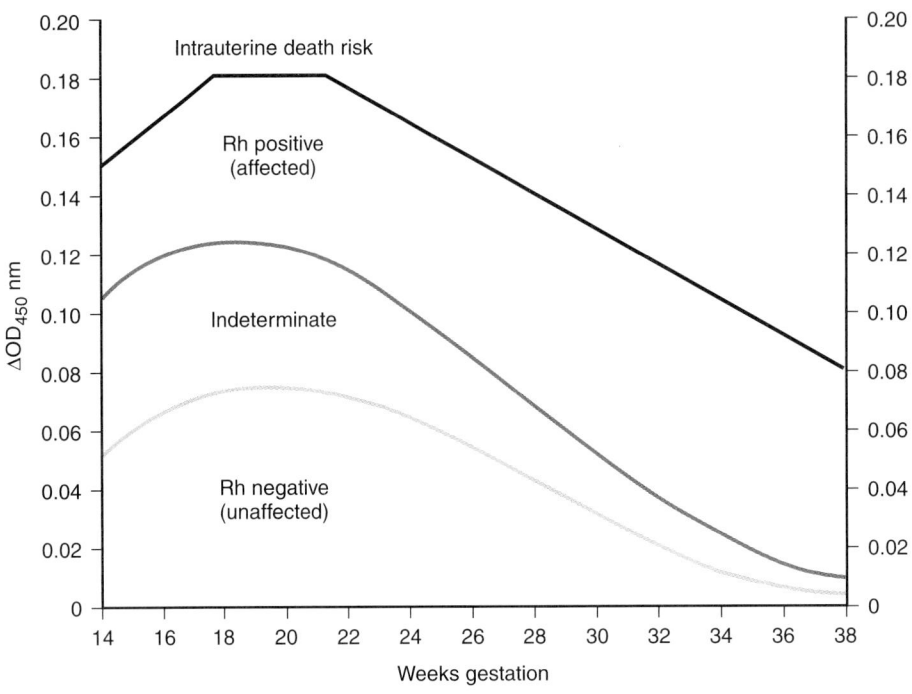

FIGURE 2. Amniotic fluid optical density (ΔOD_{450}) zones for management of pregnancy complicated by $Rh_o(D)$ alloimmunization. (From Queenan JT, Tomai TP, Ural SH, King JC: Deviation in amniotic fluid optical density at a wavelength of 450 nm in Rh-immunized pregnancies from 14 to 40 weeks' gestation: A proposal for clinical management. Am J Obstet Gynecol 1993;168:1370-1376. Used with permission.)

Management of the Newborn With Erythroblastosis Fetalis

DELIVERY ROOM MANAGEMENT

With advances in the field of maternal–fetal medicine and the use of intravascular fetal transfusions, it is unusual for an infant to be delivered with severe erythroblastosis and hydrops secondary to $Rh_o(D)$. When this does occur, however, three teams of neonatologists, pediatricians, and nurse practitioners must be immediately available to initiate multiple interventions.

One team is responsible for airway management, including intubation, and the initiation of positive-pressure ventilation. This team also monitors the heart rate and initiates chest compressions, if needed. A second team is responsible for securing immediate intravascular access, usually via the umbilical vein. A hematocrit value is obtained immediately, and if it is less than 30%, a partial exchange transfusion using 25 to 80 mL per kg of packed red blood cells is carried out within 30 minutes of birth to raise the hematocrit to 40% or higher. A third team should be available to perform paracentesis and thoracentesis, if needed. With severe hydrops, effective pulmonary ventilation frequently cannot be achieved until large collections of pleural and ascitic fluid have been removed.

Immediately after umbilical cord clamping, the obstetric team should obtain a sample of cord blood, which is sent to the laboratory for a direct Coombs test and determination of hematocrit, reticulocyte count, total and direct bilirubin levels, cord pH, and blood gas tension values.

INTENSIVE PHOTOTHERAPY

Upon admission to the neonatal intensive care nursery, the infant with erythroblastosis fetalis should be placed immediately under intensive phototherapy. This can be achieved by using multiple banks of special blue fluorescent tubes (e.g., F20T12/BB manufactured by General Electric, Westinghouse, and Sylvania).

Place the full-term infant in a bassinet rather than an incubator, and line the sides of the bassinet with white linens or aluminum foil to maximize surface area exposure.

Obtain serial serum bilirubin values (total and direct) at 2- to 3-hour intervals to establish the rate of rise under intensive phototherapy, and plot the levels, as shown in Figure 3.

INTRAVENOUS GAMMA GLOBULIN

The administration of intravenous immune globulin (IVIG) (0.5 g/kg over 2 hours) is recommended if the total serum bilirubin is rising in spite of intensive phototherapy or if the total serum bilirubin is within 2 to 3 mg/dL of the exchange level shown in Figure 3.

NEONATAL DOUBLE-VOLUME EXCHANGE TRANSFUSION

With the widespread use of RhoGAM to prevent the alloimmunization of $Rh_o(D)$-negative women, coupled with advances in fetal intravascular transfusion therapy, neonatal double-volume exchange transfusions are becoming rare procedures. When neonatal exchange

Rakel and Bope: *Conn's Current Therapy 2006.*

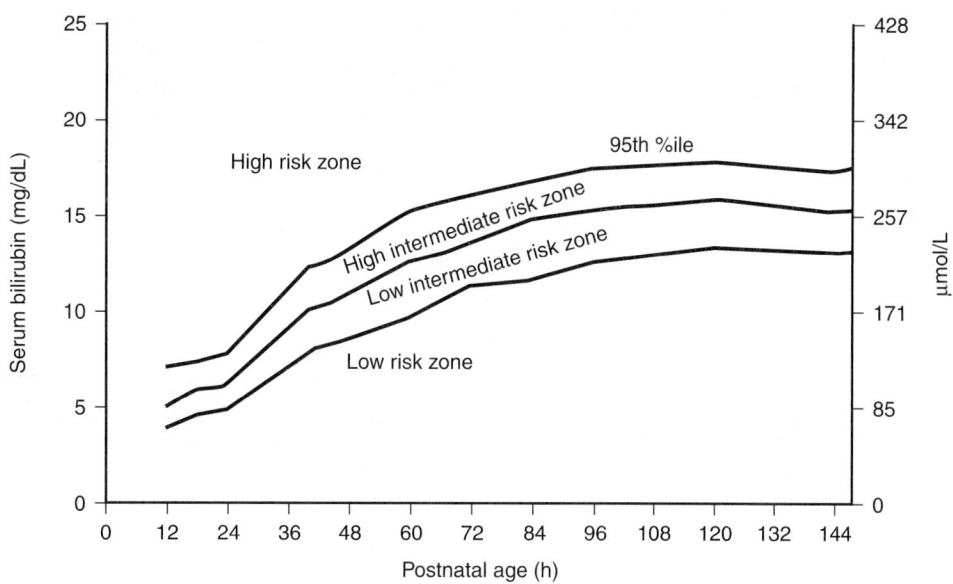

FIGURE 3. Nomogram for designation of risk in 2840 well newborns at 36 or more weeks' gestational age with birth weight of 2000 g or more, or 35 or more weeks' gestational age and birth weight of 2500 g or more based on the hour-specific serum bilirubin values. The serum bilirubin level was obtained before discharge, and the zone in which the value fell predicted the likelihood of a subsequent bilirubin level exceeding the 95th percentile (high-risk zone). (From Pediatrics 2004;14(1):301, American Academy of Pediatrics. Used with permission.)

6

transfusions are required, they should be done by experienced neonatologists and pediatricians working in neonatal centers that are prepared to deal with the various complications of the procedure, which include hypoglycemia, thrombocytopenia, necrotizing enterocolitis, and infection.

After the delivery of an infant with erythroblastosis fetalis, serial serum bilirubin values (total and direct) should be obtained at 2- to 3-hour intervals to establish the rate of rise. A serum indirect bilirubin level that is climbing by more than 0.5 mg per dL per hour indicates that there is a relatively brisk hemolytic process that may require a double-volume exchange transfusion within the first 12 hours after birth. Recently published guidelines for exchange transfusions are shown in Figure 3. In addition to lowering the serum bilirubin level, an early double-volume exchange transfusion helps to correct the fetal anemia and removes a significant portion of the antibody-coated red blood cells before they hemolyze. The blood sample for routine metabolic screens for hypothyroidism, inborn errors of metabolism, and hemoglobinopathies should be drawn before the exchange transfusion is performed.

Serial serum bilirubin levels should be continued even if an early double-volume exchange transfusion is not mandated by the rate of rise. It is impossible to determine exactly what level of indirect bilirubin constitutes a risk for encephalopathy (kernicterus on neuropathology) in any given infant at any given time. Prematurity, hypoxia, asphyxia, acidosis, sepsis, and hypoalbuminemia may increase the risk of bilirubin encephalopathy. Various drugs, such as the sulfa preparations and ceftriaxone, displace bilirubin from albumin-binding sites and increase the risk for encephalopathy.

 CURRENT DIAGNOSIS

- Blood type—ABO and $Rh_o(D)$—and an antibody screen (the indirect Coombs test) should be obtained on the first prenatal visit. If the antibody screen is positive, alloimmunization has already occurred, and serial titers should be obtained. If the titer reaches a critical level of 1:16 or greater, additional testing such as determination of paternal zygosity, amniocentesis, and cordocentesis will need to be done by a specialist in maternal–fetal medicine.
- All $Rh_o(D)$-negative mothers who deliver an $Rh_o(D)$-positive infant should be screened with a rosette test or a Kleihauer-Betke test to detect an excessive fetal–maternal hemorrhage. Those mothers with evidence of an excessive fetal–maternal hemorrhage may need more than the standard 1 vial of $Rh_o(D)$-immunoglobulin (RhoGAM).
- There is no single simple test to tell what level of bilirubin is dangerous to any given infant at any given time.
- Following intensive phototherapy and/or exchange transfusion for moderate to severe erythroblastosis fetalis, serial hematocrit values must be followed carefully for 4 to 8 weeks to determine the need for a top-up transfusion of packed red blood cells.

CURRENT THERAPY

- The unsensitized, $Rh_o(D)$-negative patient should receive prophylactic anti-D immunoglobulin (RhoGAM) at 28 weeks' gestation and again post-delivery at any gestational age if newborn infant is $Rh_o(D)$ positive.
- The unsensitized, $Rh_o(D)$-negative patient should receive prophylactic RhoGAM after any of the following events and procedures: Ectopic gestation, abruption of placenta, abortion, abdominal trauma, amniocentesis, cordocentesis, chorionic villous sampling, and external cephalic version.
- The combined use of intensive phototherapy and intravenous immunoglobulin may reduce the need for an exchange transfusion.

In the otherwise healthy, full-term newborn with hemolytic disease, the indirect bilirubin level should not be permitted to climb above 20 mg per dL. With prematurity and hemolytic disease, lower threshold levels for exchange transfusion, based on gestational age, birth weight, chronologic age in days, and the presence or absence of other risk factors for bilirubin encephalopathy are recommended. Premature newborns with hemolytic disease should be managed by experienced neonatologists working in regional perinatal centers. Phototherapy is used as an adjunct to exchange transfusion, and in the case of mild hemolytic disease, phototherapy alone may be sufficient to control the bilirubin level.

DELAYED NEONATAL RED BLOOD CELL TRANSFUSIONS

A slow hemolysis frequently continues for up to 6 to 8 weeks after delivery in those infants who received a fetal intravascular transfusion or an exchange transfusion after delivery and in those infants with a mild hemolysis requiring only phototherapy. These infants should be followed up with serial hematocrit determinations at 1- to 2-week intervals during the first 6 to 8 weeks after birth. A transfusion of packed red blood cells (10 to 15 mL per kg) may be necessary to correct severe anemia. With severe hemolytic anemia, particularly in infants who received intrauterine transfusions, fetal and neonatal iron stores are elevated. Neonatal iron therapy should be withheld until the serum ferritin level returns to normal.

REFERENCES

American Academy of Pediatrics: Clinical practice guidelines for management of hyperbilirubinemia in the newborn infant 35 or more weeks of gestation. Pediatrics 2004;114(1):297-316.
American College of Obstetricians and Gynecologists: Prevention of RhD Alloimmunization. ACOG Practice Bulletin 4. Washington, DC, ACOG, 1999.

Gottstein R, Cooke RWI: Systematic review of intravenous immunoglobulin in haemolytic disease of the newborn. Arch Dis Child Fetal Neonatal Ed 2003;88:F6-F10.
Harkness UF, Spinnato JA: Prevention and management of RhD isoimmunization. Clin Perinatol 2004;31(4):721-742.
Maisels MJ: Why use homeopathic doses of phototherapy? Pediatrics 1996;98:283-287.
McKenna DS, Nagaraja HN, O'Shaughnessy: Management of pregnancies complicated by anti-Kell isoimmunization. Obstet Gynecol 1999;93:667-673.

Hemophilia and Related Conditions

Method of
Roshni Kulkarni, MD and Jeanne Lusher, MD

Hemophilia A (Factor VIII Deficiency) and Hemophilia B (Factor IX Deficiency)

The hemophilias A and B are X-linked bleeding disorders caused by a deficiency of clotting factors (Fs) VIII and IX, respectively. The manifestations are almost exclusively in males, whereas females are often asymptomatic carriers. Hemophilia affects 18,000 persons (primarily males) in the United States and, in conjunction with von Willebrand's disease (VWD), represents approximately 80% to 85% of the inherited bleeding disorders. Deficiencies of fibrinogen, prothrombin, FV, FVII, FX, FXI, FXIII, and combined FV and FVIII account for 15% of congenital bleeding disorders. Hemophilia A occurs in 1:5000 and hemophilia B in 1:30,000 males, respectively. The prevalence of hemophilia A is 20.6 cases per 100,000 males, with 60% having severe disease. The prevalence of hemophilia B is 5.3 cases per 100,000 males, with 44% having severe disease.

PATHOPHYSIOLOGY

The FVIII and FIX genes are located at the tip of the long arm of the X chromosome. The gene for FVIII is one of the largest known genes and spans more than 180 kb. Inversion mutations account for 40% of cases of severe hemophilia A; and deletions, point mutations, and insertions account for the remaining 50% to 60% of cases of hemophilia A.

The site of synthesis of FVIII is unclear and thought to be the endothelial cells (in the liver and other sites). FVIII, a cofactor for FIX, is a complex glycoprotein containing 2351 amino acids organized into distinct domains. The heavy chain, composed of A1-a1-A2-a2-B domains, and the light chain, composed of a3-A3-C1-C2, are covalently linked. The function of the B domain is unclear, and it is not required for coagulant activity. vWf binds to the C2 domain, and FIX interactive sites are in the A2 and A3 domains. Thrombin cleaves to sites in both the heavy and light chains. FVIII has a half-life of approximately 12 hours (shorter in infants and children), and VWf protects it from proteolytic degradation in the plasma and concentrates it at the site of injury.

The gene for FIX is 34 kb long, and the mature protein is a vitamin K–dependent serine protease composed of 415 amino acids. Gene deletions and point mutations are seen in hemophilia B. FIX is synthesized in the liver and requires vitamin K for gamma carboxylation. Plasma concentration is approximately 50 times that of FVIII, and it has a half-life of 24 hours.

ROLE OF FACTORS VIII AND IX IN COAGULATION

After an injury, encrypted tissue factor (TF) is exposed and forms a complex with FVIIa. The TF-FVIIa complex activates FIX to FIXa (that moves to the platelet surface) and FX to FXa. The latter generates small amounts of thrombin that activates platelets, platelet FV to FVa, converts FXI to FIXa, releases FVIII from vWf and activates it. The FXIa activates plasma FIX to FIXa on the platelet surface. FVIII is a cofactor for FIXa and forms a tenase complex (FVIIIa/FIXa) that converts large amounts of FX to FXa on the platelet surface. The FXa forms a "prothrombinase" complex with FVa that converts large amounts of prothrombin to thrombin, the so-called thrombin burst. This results in the conversion of sufficient fibrinogen to fibrin to form a firm and stable hemostatic clot. (An interactive animation on "cell-based coagulation" is available for online viewing at http://www.hemostasiscme.org.) In hemophilia, deficiency of FVIII or FIX results in insufficient thrombin generation because of the lack of formation of "tenase" complex; primary platelet plug formation and initiation phases of coagulation are normal. Any clot that is formed (because of small amounts of thrombin in the initiation phase) is friable and porous.

CLINICAL FEATURES

The diagnosis of hemophilia is often made after a bleeding episode or because of a known family history. In approximately 33% of the cases, there is no known family history. Based on the plasma levels of FVIII or FIX (normal levels are 50% to 150%) that correlate with severity and predict bleeding risk, hemophilia is classified as mild (>5%), moderate (1% to 5%), and severe (<1%) (Table 1). Approximately 66% of persons with hemophilia have severe disease, 15% have moderate disease, and 20% have mild disease. Although most severe hemophiliacs manifest by 4 years of age, those with moderate and mild disease are often diagnosed later in life, often after bleeding secondary to trauma or surgery.

The hallmark of hemophilia is hemarthrosis (joint bleeds) that may occur with or without obvious trauma. Joint and muscle bleeds account for 60% and 30%, respectively, of all bleeding episodes in severe hemophiliacs. Besides being excruciatingly painful and tender, if not promptly treated, these bleeds lead to chronic and debilitating arthropathy. Debilitating arthropathy is characterized by synovial thickening, chronic inflammation, and repeated hemorrhages resulting in a "target joint." The most common joints affected are the knees, elbows, ankles, hips, and shoulders. Accompanying disuse atrophy of surrounding muscles leads to further joint instability. Limitation of joint range of motion caused by hemarthrosis often correlates positively with older age, people of color, and increased body mass index; and it severely impacts quality of life.

Muscle hematomas, another characteristic site of bleeding in hemophiliacs, may lead to compartment syndrome with eventual fibrosis and peripheral nerve damage. Iliopsoas bleeds often present with pain and flexion deformity. Central nervous system (CNS) hemorrhage, although rare, is the most serious complication, with a 10% recurrence rate, and is the leading cause of mortality in hemophiliacs.

Gastrointestinal bleeding and hematuria are less frequent manifestations. Although most newborns with severe hemophilia experience an uneventful course after vaginal delivery, vacuum extraction has been reported to be associated with an increased CNS bleeding risk. The incidence of intracranial hemorrhage in newborns with hemophilia is 1% to 4%.

The life expectancy of hemophiliacs has steadily increased over the years, except during the 1980s when transfusion-transmitted HIV accounted for 55% of hemophilia deaths. Older individuals with hemophilia may manifest end-stage liver disease caused by transfusion-transmitted hepatitis C virus (HCV) or may have HIV/HCV co-infection.

TABLE 1 Hemophilia Severity and Clinical Manifestations

Characteristics	Severe (50%-70%)	Moderate (10%)	Mild (30%-40%)
Factor VIII or IX activity (normal 50%-150%)	<1%	1%-5%	>5%
Age of diagnosis	Birth to 2 years of life	Childhood or adolescence	Adolescence or adulthood
Bleeding patterns	2-4 per month	4-6 per year	Rare
Clinical manifestations	Hemarthroses, muscle, central nervous system, gastrointestinal bleeding, hematuria	Bleeding into joints or muscle after minor trauma, surgical procedure, dental bleeding; rarely spontaneous	Surgical procedures (including dental) and major trauma

Rakel and Bope: *Conn's Current Therapy 2006.*

Hemophilia A and B are clinically indistinguishable, and specific factor assays are the only way to differentiate between them and confirm the diagnosis. Both should be differentiated from vWD. The prothrombin time (PT), platelet function analyzer (PFA-100, a platelet function screening test that is replacing bleeding time, because the latter has low sensitivity and specificity and is operator dependent), and fibrinogen are normal. The activated partial thromboplastin time (APTT) is often prolonged (especially when the factor levels are <30%). Table 2 gives the details about the characteristics and differences between the hemophilias and vWD. Female carriers in general are asymptomatic except those in whom extreme lyonization results in low levels of FVIII or FIX. Levels of FVIII increase throughout pregnancy and drop to prepregnancy levels after delivery; FIX levels, however, remain constant throughout pregnancy. Prenatal diagnosis by various methods (preimplantation genetic diagnosis, chorionic villus sampling) to determine fetal sex and mutation may aid in the management of pregnancy and delivery.

MANAGEMENT

Replacement therapy to achieve hemostatic levels for treatment of bleeding episodes is accomplished using recombinant factor concentrates produced in mammalian cell lines or concentrates derived from normal pooled plasma. Both products seem to have equivalent clinical efficacy and are virally inactivated.

TABLE 2 Hemophilias and von Willebrand's Disease: Key Characteristics and Differences

	Hemophilia A	Hemophilia B	von Willebrand's disease
Incidence	1:5000	1:30,000	1%-3% of U.S. population
Abnormality	FVIII deficiency.	FIX deficiency.	von Willebrand's factor (VWF) (qualitative and quantitative defect).
Inheritance	X-linked, affects males. Gene at the tip of X chromosome.	X-linked, affects males. Gene at the tip of X chromosome.	Autosomal dominant (gene: chromosome 12). Some are recessive or compound heterozygotes.
Production site	Unknown; liver endothelium (?).	Liver (vitamin K-dependent).	Megakaryocytes and endothelial cells.
Function	Cofactor; forms complex with FIX and activates FX leading to "thrombin burst" that results in conversion of large amounts of fibrinogen to fibrin.	Serine protease (inactive form: zymogen) activated by FXI or FVIIa; forms a tannase complex with FVIII and activates FX.	Platelet adhesion to site of injury or damaged endothelium. Protects FVIII from proteolysis.
Classification (normal levels 50%-150%)	Mild (>5%). Moderate (1%-5%). Severe (<1%).	Mild (>5%). Moderate (1%-5%). Severe (<1%).	Types 1. Type 2 (2A, 2B, 2M, 2N). Type 3.
Clinical presentation	Positive family history (30% new mutation). Hemarthroses, hematomas, hematuria, intracranial hemorrhage, gastrointestinal hemorrhage, etc.	Positive family history (30% new mutation). Milder disease, although has identical hemorrhage sites as hemophilia A.	Positive family history. Mucocutaneous bleeding (epistaxis, menorrhagia, postdental bleeding). Type 3 may present as hemophilia A.
PFA/bleeding time	Normal.	Normal.	May be prolonged.
PT	Normal.	Normal.	Normal.
APTT	Prolonged.	Prolonged.	Prolonged or normal.
FVIII assay	Decreased or absent.	Normal.	Decreased or normal (absent type 3).
FIX assay	Normal.	Decreased or absent.	Normal.
VWF: antigen	Normal.	Normal.	Decreased or absent (type 3).
VWF R: Co	Normal.	Normal.	Decreased or abnormal.
VWF multimers	Normal.	Normal.	Abnormal (types 1, 2A, 2B, absent type 3).
Specific treatment	rFVIII (preferred). Pathogen-safe plasma-derived concentrates. DDAVP for mild cases.	rFIX, pathogen-safe plasma-derived concentrates. DDAVP ineffective.	DDAVP (intranasal or intravenous) VWF concentrates (pathogen-safe plasma-derived).
Inhibitor patients	Immune tolerance, rFVIIa, APCC.	Immune tolerance, rFVIIa.	Inhibitors are rare.
Adjunct therapy	Antifibrinolytics.	Antifibrinolytics.	Oral contraceptives, antifibrinolytics.

Abbreviations: APCC = activated prothrombin complex concentrates; APTT = activated partial thromboplastin time; DDAVP = 1-deamino (8-D-arginine) vasopressin; F = factor; PFA = platelet function analyzer; PT = prothrombin time; rFIX = recombinant activated factor IX; rFVIII = recombinant activated factor VIII; rFVIIa = recombinant activated factor VIIa.

Recombinant factor concentrates are recommended but, if unavailable, pathogen-safe plasma-derived concentrates can be used. Cryoprecipitate is no longer recommended because of concerns regarding pathogen safety.

The goal of treatment of hemophilia is to raise factor levels to approximately 30% or more for minor bleeds (such as hematomas or joint bleeds) and 100% for major bleeds (such as CNS or surgery). This is accomplished by administration of appropriate FVIII or FIX concentrates; 1 IU/kg increases plasma FVIII levels by 2% and FIX levels by 1.5%, respectively (except with the only available recombinant FIX product, the recovery is approximately 0.8%). The half-life of FVIII is approximately 8 to 12 hours and FIX is up to 24 hours. Factor concentrates can be administered either as a bolus dose or continuous infusion (3 to 4 IU/kg/hour). The bolus dose varies from 25 to 50 IU/kg depending on the severity, site, and type of bleeding, and is dosed to the closest vial because of the cost of the products. Table 3 lists the dosing schedule for various types of bleeds.

For short-term therapy, such as before dental procedures and for minor bleeding episodes in individuals with mild hemophilia A and vWD, the synthetic vasopressin analogue desmopressin acetate (1-deamino [8-D-arginine] vasopressin, DDAVP or Stimate) is useful. It increases plasma concentrations of coagulation FVIII and vWf threefold to fivefold. A "DDAVP trial" to determine response is helpful in selecting individuals who may benefit from such therapy. For hemostatic purposes, intravenous (IV) (0.3 μg/kg in 50 mL of normal saline infused over 15 to 30 minutes) or intranasal dose can be used. The intranasal dose is 15 times larger than that recommended for diabetes insipidus. A multidose intranasal spray formulation (Stimate nasal spray, manufactured for ZLB Behring by Ferring Pharmaceuticals,

Malmo, Sweden) includes a metered-dose spray pump that delivers 150 μg per activation (spray) of the pump. The recommended dosage is one spray for patients weighing less than 50 kg and two sprays (one in each nostril) for those weighing more than 50 kg. Desmopressin[1] is ineffective in hemophilia B. Aspirin and aspirin-containing compounds should be avoided in individuals with bleeding disorders because they interfere with platelet function and may further exacerbate bleeding.

Antifibrinolytics such as epsilon-aminocaproic acid (Amicar)[1] (ε-aminocaproic acid or EACA) and tranexamic acid (Cyklokapron)[1] are used as adjunct therapies, and in mild hemophilia obviates the need for factor. The recommended dosage for EACA is 75 to 100 mg/kg/dose IV or orally every 4 to 6 hours (maximum 30 g/24 hours), and for tranexamic acid,[1] 10 mg/kg/dose IV or 25 mg/kg body weight orally, three times daily.

Prophylactic administration of concentrates (FVIII 25 to 40 IU/kg every other day; FIX 25 to 40 IU/kg twice weekly because of the longer half-life of FIX) is aimed at preventing debilitating effects of joint disease and often begun at 1 to 2 years of age and continued throughout life. Self-infusion before any planned strenuous activity should be encouraged. Because of the complications of central venous catheters (infections, thrombosis, and mechanical), use of a peripheral vein is encouraged.

COMPLICATIONS OF HEMOPHILIA TREATMENT

Approximately 5% to 10% of individuals with hemophilia A and as many as 30% with severe disease develop neutralizing IgG inhibitory antibodies. The incidence of

---

[1]Not FDA approved for this indication.

TABLE 3 Treatment of Bleeding Episodes and Desired Plasma Levels in Hemophilia A and B

Type of bleeding	Desired factor level (%)	Factor VIII dose (IU/kg)	Factor IX dose (IU/kg)	Duration of treatment (days)	Comments (dose factor to the closest vial)
Persistent or profuse epistaxis. Oral mucosal bleeding (including tongue and mouth lacerations)	20-30	10-15	20-30	1-2	Local pressure, antifibrinolytics, fibrin glue for local control, Nosebleed QR for epistaxis. Sedation in small children with tongue laceration
Dental procedures	30-50	15-25	30-50	1h before procedure	Antifibrinolytics for 7-10d
Acute hemarthrosis, intramuscular hematomas. Physical therapy (PT)	30-60 30-50	15-50 15-25	30-60 30-50	1-3 Treat before PT	Use lower doses if treated early. Non-weight bearing on affected joint. Consider synovectomy (surgical, radioisotope, or chemical) for target joints.
Life-threatening bleeding such as intracranial hemorrhage, major surgery, and trauma	80-100	40-50	80-100	10-14	Bolus dose followed by continuous infusion (3-4 IU/kg/h); may switch to bolus before discharge
Gastrointestinal bleeding	30-50	15-25	30-50	2-3	May use oral antifibrinolytics
Persistent painless gross hematuria	30-50	15-25	30-50	1-2	Increased PO or intravenous fluids (low-dose antifibrinolytics)

Rakel and Bope: *Conn's Current Therapy 2006.*

inhibitors in hemophilia B is lower (1% to 3%). Inhibitors arise, on an average, after 10 exposure days to FVIII or FIX concentrates and can be transient or permanent and should be suspected if a patient does not respond to an appropriate dose of clotting factor concentrate. Inhibitors can further exacerbate bleeding episodes and hemophilic arthropathy. Inhibitor levels measured using Bethesda units (BU) are classified as high titer (>5 BU) or low titer (<5 BU). Current modalities for treatment of bleeding episodes in inhibitor patients include the use of higher than normal doses of FVIII or FIX, use of agents that bypass the need for FVIII or FIX, such as recombinant activated FVII (rFVIIa), and, in the case of hemophilia A, activated prothrombin complex concentrates[2] (APCC) and recombinant porcine FVIII[2] (currently in prelicensure clinical trials). Immune tolerance induction (ITI), a long-term approach designed to eradicate inhibitors, is effective in 70% to 85% of selected patients with severe hemophilia A; the most important predictor of success of ITI is an inhibitor titer of less than 10 BU at the start of ITI.

Although inhibitors are rare in hemophilia B eradication, using ITI is more difficult to achieve and is effective in only 40% of the cases. Furthermore, several hemophilia B patients with inhibitors have developed severe anaphylaxis to infusions of FIX concentrates and some have developed nephrotic syndrome approximately 8 to 9 months after starting ITI.

Another complication of treatment is transmission of blood-borne pathogens. In the 1980s, approximately 95% of hemophiliacs exposed to pooled plasma concentrates became infected with HIV and or HCV. Two thirds of these patients have died and some survivors continue to be on antiretroviral therapy for HIV and/or pegylated interferon and ribavirin (Rebetol) therapy for HCV. Although the currently available products are safe with regard to enveloped viruses (such as HIV, hepatitis B and C), the potential for transmission of blood-borne pathogens such as parvovirus, hepatitis A virus, and prions remains with products that contain human or animal proteins. By eliminating the use of human- or animal-derived proteins in the cell culture, stabilization, and final formulation of the new generation recombinant factor concentrates, the risk of pathogen transmission is virtually eliminated. Routine vaccination against hepatitis A and B is encouraged because many of these patients are at risk for exposure to blood and blood products.

Individuals with bleeding disorders should be encouraged to attend the regional hemophilia treatment centers (HTCs) where, besides education, patients are trained to self-infuse, calculate dosage, maintain treatment logs, and call the center for serious bleeding episodes. The mortality rate among patients who receive care at HTCs is lower than those who do not: 28.1% versus 38.3%, respectively. Gene therapy offers promise of cure with sustained factor release. However, as of January 2005, there are no ongoing clinical trials of gene therapy in persons with hemophilia.

---

[2]Not available in the United States.

von Willebrand's Disease

von Willebrand's disease (VWD) is a hereditary disorder of von Willebrand's factor (VWf), a large multimeric glycoprotein that is produced in endothelial cells and megakaryocytes. The defect in VWf may be quantitative or qualitative. VWD is the most common of the hereditary coagulation disorders, affecting 1% or more of the population. It is usually inherited as an autosomal dominant trait. It is worldwide in distribution, and affects all racial groups. There are several different variants of VWD (type I, types 2A, 2B, 2N, 2M, and type 3), with type I being the most common.

CLINICAL PRESENTATION

Persons with VWD characteristically have mucous membrane-type bleeding (e.g., menorrhagia, epistaxis) and excessive bruising. Because the degree of bleeding manifestations varies considerably, with some having no recognizable increase in bleeding, the diagnosis may never be suspected until excessive bleeding occurs with a surgical procedure or invasive dentistry. In some young women, excessive menstrual bleeding may be the first manifestation. Unfortunately, the possibility of VWD is often not thought of, and thus the diagnosis is not made.

In the rare occurrence of infants or small children with type 3 (severe) VWD, excessive bruising and even joint bleeding (caused by very low levels of FVIII) may mimic hemophilia A.

DIAGNOSIS

Once suspected, laboratory evaluation for VWD often requires several assays to quantitate VWD and to characterize its structure and function. Screening tests (such as APTT and bleeding time) are often normal in those with mild or moderate VWD; thus, more specific tests must be done. These include the ristocetin cofactor assay, which measures the activity of VWf, an FVIII assay, and an assay for VWf antigen (VWf:Ag). Because VWf circulates with FVIII, and protects it from rapid proteolytic degradation in the circulation, low levels of VWD (as well as some qualitative defects of VWf) will result in low levels of FVIII.

Many variables may affect VWf assay results. These include the patient's ABO blood type. Persons of blood group AB have a 60% to 70% higher level of VWf than do those of blood group O. Thus, some laboratories interpret VWf levels referenced to specific normal ranges for blood types. Clinical conditions and disorders can also affect VWf levels. For example, in the third trimester of pregnancy, levels of VWf (and FVIII) increase. Because VWf acts as an acute-phase reactant protein, levels also increase in collagen-vascular disorders, postoperatively, in liver disease, and in disseminated intravascular coagulation. Levels decrease in hypothyroidism.

If a diagnosis of VWD seems probable on the basis of the above tests, it is important to determine the type of VWD the individual has, because treatment varies depending on the type. Most affected persons have type I VWD, in which VWf is subnormal in amount, but normal in structure (as determined by multimeric analysis or agarose gel and staining of the multimers with radiolabeled antibody to VWf). Those with types 2A and 2B VWD lack the higher-molecular-weight multimers, which are the most important hemostatically.

In type 2B, the VWf produced has a heightened affinity for platelets, often resulting in some degree of thrombocytopenia from platelet aggregation. A useful laboratory test for type 2B is the low-dose ristocetin-induced platelet aggregation assay.

In type 3 (severe) VWD, the affected individual has inherited a gene for type I VWD from each parent, resulting in very low levels (3%) of VWf (and FVIII, because there is practically no VWf to protect FVIII from rapid proteolytic degradation). Less often, a person with type 3 is doubly heterozygous.

MANAGEMENT

Proper management of VWD requires a specific diagnostic laboratory workup and proper classification of the type of VWD that the individual has.

In type I VWD (characterized by subnormal levels of normally functioning VWf), the treatment of choice for most situations is 1-deamino (8-D-arginine) vasopressin (desmopressin; DDAVP). This synthetic agent causes a rapid release of VWf from its storage sites. It can be given parenterally (usually IV) or by the intranasal route. The recommended dose for IV use is 0.3 µg/kg, given in saline over 10 minutes. Most persons with type I VWD have a twofold-to-fourfold increase in plasma

levels of VWf within 15 to 30 minutes after infusion. The IV route is often used for surgical coverage, or for a severe bleeding episode requiring hospitalization. When necessary, repeat doses can be given at 12- to 24-hour intervals. Tachyphylaxis is seen less often in VWD than it is when desmopressin is used in hemophilia.

A concentrated form of desmopressin for intranasal use (Stimate nasal spray) is also effective for many bleeding episodes. The recommended dosage is the same as that used in hemophilia described earlier. Once the patient has been properly instructed in its use, Stimate nasal spray is particularly useful for home use. Some young women with menorrhagia have benefited from its use at the onset of menses, with a second dose being used the following day. Others have used it approximately 45 minutes before invasive dentistry, with good results.

In the type 2 variants (in which the VWf produced is abnormal), desmopressin may result in an increase in VWf levels, but it will be the abnormal VWf. Although some persons with type 2A may respond, desmopressin is seldom useful on type 2 and may even be contraindicated (as in type 2B). In type 3 VWD, there is no VWf to be released from storage sites; thus, desmopressin is ineffective. For these types, an intermediate purity plasma-derived concentrate rich in the hemostatically effective high-molecular-weight multimers of VWf (such as Humate P, ZLB Behring) should be used for treatment of moderately severe or severe bleeding episodes, and for surgical coverage. Humate P contains nearly normal VWf multimers, and is licensed for use in VWD. In persons with type I VWD who do

 CURRENT DIAGNOSIS

- The hemophilias together with von Willebrand disease (VWD) account for 80% to 85% of inherited bleeding disorders. Hemophilia A and B are X-linked, whereas VWD and rare bleeding disorders (RBDs) are autosomal disorders.
- The diagnosis of hemophilia and other inherited bleeding disorders should be confirmed by specific assays, because screening tests such as prothrombin time (PT), and activated partial thromboplastin time (APTT) may be normal. Plasma levels of deficient factor determine clinical severity and management.
- Hemarthrosis is the most common and debilitating complication and central nervous system (CNS) bleeding is the most common cause of mortality in hemophilia. Mucosal bleeding and menorrhagia are the most common manifestation of VWD. Bleeding manifestations of RBDs are mild although homozygotes can present with severe disease.
- Newborns have normal levels of FVIII; therefore, the diagnosis of hemophilia A can be established at birth. Vacuum delivery should be avoided to prevent head bleeds.

 CURRENT THERAPY

- Early and effective treatment and prophylaxis may prevent repeated hemarthrosis and joint destruction in individuals with hemophilia. Patients should be tested annually for the presence of inhibitors.
- Wherever available and indicated, recombinant factor concentrates are preferred over plasma-derived products because of potential risk of pathogen transmission. Cryoprecipitate is not recommended. For mild and moderate hemophilia A and VWD, the use of desmopressin coupled with antifibrinolytics may obviate the use of concentrates. Continued vigilance should be implemented for new and emerging blood-borne pathogens.
- All patients with inherited bleeding disorders should be immunized against hepatitis A and B and followed in close collaboration with the local Hemophilia Treatment Center (http://www2a.cdc.gov/ncbddd/htcweb/index.asp). The National Hemophilia Foundation's (http://www.hemophilia.org) Medical and Scientific Advisory Committee (MASAC) guidelines for updated recommendations and product choice should be followed.

not respond adequately to desmopressin, Humate P can be used.

As in hemophilia (see earlier discussion), an effective adjunctive treatment for invasive dental procedures or other bleeding in the oropharyngeal cavity is the use of antifibrinolytic agents, such as ε-aminocaproic acid (EACA) or tranexamic acid. These synthetic agents are useful when used alone in some VWD women with menorrhagia. For epistaxis, oral contraceptives or hormone releasing intrauterine device (Mirena) may also be helpful for the treatment of menorrhagia. Topical agents such as Nosebleed QR (Biolife, LLC Florida), a hydrophilic powder, may help.

An interactive VWD animation that includes types of VWD, laboratory diagnosis, clinical features, and treatment is available on the National Hemophilia Foundations Web site for Project Red Flag at http://www.hemophilia.org/projectredflag for online viewing.

PREGNANCY

As noted earlier, VWf (and FVIII) levels increased during the third trimester of pregnancy, and women with type I VWD often note a decrease in bruising or other bleeding symptoms. However, those with type 2 VWD will have an increase in the abnormal form of VWD, and thus no lessening of bleeding tendency. Similarly, in type 3 VWD, there will be no improvement, because there will be no increase in VWf.

Even in type I VWD, VWf levels will decrease after delivery, so treatment (with IV desmopressin, or Humate P) may be needed.

ACQUIRED VON WILLEBRAND DISEASE

Acquired VWD may occur in an individual who does not have a lifelong bleeding disorder. Such persons may

TABLE 4 Rare Bleeding Disorders: Inheritance, Clinical Features, and Treatment

Type of disorder, prevalence (homozygous), and inheritance	Manifestation and diagnosis	Treatment	Hemostatic levels	Half-life
FI: 1:1,000,000 Afibrinogenemia AR Dys/hypofibrinogenemia AD	Mild bleeding, CNS bleeding, umbilical, joint, recurrent miscarriage, PT/APTT, TT prolonged. Low fibrinogen (FI) levels. Paradoxical thrombosis.	Fresh-frozen plasma (FFP), 15-20 mL/kg. cryoprecipitate (cryo), 1 bag/5-10 kg. Plasma-derived concentrate not available in the U.S. Treat every 3-5 days.	50 mg-1 g/dL	2-5d
FII (hypo or dysprothrombinemia): 1:2,000,000, AR Type I: hypo, type II: dys	Hematomas, hemarthroses menorrhagia, CNS, umbilical, PPH. PT abnormal.	FFP, prothrombin complex concentrates (PCCs), 20-30 IU/kg; used for prophylaxis or treatment.	20%-30%	3-4d
FV (parahemophilia, labile factor, proaccelerin Owren's disease): 1:1,000,000, AR	Mucosal bleeding, PPH, CNS. Platelet FV deficiency more reflective of bleeding potential. Prolonged PT, APTT; normal TT.	FFP (as above), platelet transfusions (Plt Tx). Antiplatelet antibodies may develop with repeated platelet transfusions.	15%-20%	36h
FVII (proconvertin or stable factor): 1:500,000, AR	Mucosal, menorrhagia, muscle, intracranial bleeds (15%-60%), hemarthrosis. Prolonged PT; normal APTT, TT, FI, and liver functions.	Recombinant FVIIa, 15-30 µg/kg q 2h for major bleeds. FFP, PCC (as above). Plasma-derived FVII concentrates available in Europe.	15%-20%	4-6h
FX: 1:1,000,000, AR	Umbilical, joint, mucosal, muscle, menorrhagia, intracranial bleeding. Prolonged PT/APTT.	FFP, PCCs (20-30 IU/kg).	15%-20%	24-48h
FXI: 1:1,000,000, AR Common in Ashkenazi Jews	Post-traumatic bleeding, menorrhagia. Prolonged APTT, normal PT.	Hemoleven (available in Europe), FFP 15-20 mL/kg. Inhibitors may occur.	15%-20%	
Factor XIII: 1:2,000,000, AR	Intracranial, joint, umbilical, delayed wound healing, recurrent miscarriages. PT, APTT normal; ↓FXIII assay.	Fibrogammin P (compassionate use in the U.S.), 10-20 IU/kg, FFP 15-20 mL/kg or Cryo1bag/5-10 kg q 3-4wk.	2%-5%	11-14d
Combined factors V and VIII: 1:2,000,000	Mucosal bleeding. Prolonged PT, APTT (disproportionately).	FVIII concentrates and FFP.	15%-20%	
Vitamin K-dependent multiple deficiencies: 1:2,000,000	Umbilical stump; intracranial, postsurgical bleeding; skeletal abnormalities, hearing loss.	Oral vitamin K, FFP, PCC.	15%-20%	

Abbreviations: AD = autosomal dominant, APTT = activated partial thromboplastin time; AR = autosomal recessive; CNS = central nervous system; d = days; F = factor; h = hours; PPH = postpartum hemorrhage; PT = prothrombin time; q = every; TT = thrombin time; U.S. = United States; wk = weeks.

Rakel and Bope: *Conn's Current Therapy 2006.*

have an underlying autoimmune disease such as hypothyroidism, lymphoproliferative disorders, and in association with certain drug reactions. Removal of the underlying condition will often correct the individual's VWf; if treatment of bleeding is necessary, one can try desmopressin, Humate P, rFVIIa,[1] or plasma exchange.

Rare Bleeding Disorders

The rare bleeding disorders (RBDs) comprise 3% to 5% of inherited coagulation deficiencies, other than FVIII, FIX, or VWf deficiencies, are autosomal recessive, and affect both sexes. The prevalence of RBDs ranges from 1:500,000 to 1:2 million. Bleeding manifestations are restricted to individuals who are homozygous or compound heterozygotes. RBDs are common in countries such as Iran where consanguineous marriages are frequent. Ashkenazi Jews are particularly affected by FXI deficiency. Deficiency of FXII is not associated with bleeding manifestations; instead, it is a risk factor for thrombosis. Most cases of RBDs are identified by abnormal screening tests coupled with specific factor assays. Concentrates (recombinant or plasma-derived) are available for some of the deficiencies (mostly in Europe, but not in the United States). Fibrogammin P,* a plasma-derived virally purified FXIII concentrate, is not yet licensed in the United States but is available under an Investigational New Drug (IND) protocol of the Food and Drug Administration through Dr. Diane Nugent, Children's Hospital of Orange County, 500 So. Main St., Orange, CA 92868. The advantages of concentrates are pathogen safety and small volume. The use of antifibrinolytics and fibrin glue as adjunct therapy for bleeding manifestations is encouraged. Table 4 lists the inheritance, frequency, manifestations, and treatment of the RBDs.

REFERENCES

Arnold WD, Hilgartner MW: Hemophilic arthropathy: Current concepts of pathogenesis and management. J Bone Joint Surg Am 1977;59:287-305.
Bolton-Maggs P, Pasi KJ: Haemophilias A and B. Lancet 2003;36:1801-1809.
Kulkarni R, Lusher J: Treatment of congenital coagulopathies. In Mintz PD (ed): Transfusion Therapy: Clinical Principles and Practice, 2nd ed. Bethesda, Md, AABB Press, 2005, pp 121-157.
Kulkarni R, Reddy UM: Cell based coagulation. Interactive animation. Available at http://www.hemostasiscme.org and http://www.msu.edu/user/phd/under Dr. Kulkarni's research (accessed December 2004).
Kulkarni R, Reddy UM, Evatt BL, Miller CM: An overview of von Willebrand's disease. An interactive animation. Available at http://www.hemophilia.org/projectredflag or http://www.projectredflag.com (accessed December 2004).
Mannucci PM, Duga S, Peyvandi F: Recessively inherited coagulation disorders. Blood 2004;104(5):1243-1252.
Montgomery RR, Cox Gill J, Scott JP: Hemophilia and von Willebrand disease. In Magee DJ, Nathan DG, Orkin SH, Ginsburg D, Look AT (eds): Hematology of Infancy and Childhood, 6th ed. New York, Elsevier Science, 2003, pp 1547-1576.
National Hemophilia Foundation's Medical and Scientific Advisory Committee (MASAC): MASAC recommendations concerning the treatment of hemophilia and other bleeding disorders (MASAC Document No. 151). New York, National Hemophilia Foundation. Available at http://www.hemophilia.org (accessed November 2003).
Soucie JM, Cianfrini C, Robert L, et al: Joint range-of-motion limitations among young males with hemophilia: Prevalence and risk factors. Blood 2004;103:2467-2473.
Soucie JM, Nuss R, Evatt B, et al: Mortality among males with hemophilia: Relations with source of medical care. The Hemophilia Surveillance System Project Investigators. Blood 2000;96:437-442.
Veldman A, Hoffman M, Ehrenforth S: New insights into the coagulation system and implications for new therapeutic options with recombinant factor VIIa. Curr Med Chem 2003;10(10):797-811.

Platelet-Mediated Bleeding Disorders

Method of
Joel S. Bennett, MD

An insufficient number of platelets (thrombocytopenia) or disorders of platelet function can produce bleeding. Both situations are encountered frequently in clinical practice, engendering substantial and appropriate concern about the risk and prevention of bleeding.

Elements of Platelet Function

When the vascular endothelium that separates circulating platelets from adhesive substrates in the subendothelial connective tissue is breached, platelets tether to and translocate upon exposed collagen, fibronectin, and laminin. However, at the higher shear rates of blood in arteries and in the microcirculation, efficient platelet adhesion requires the presence of vWF. The hemostatic plugs that form on the layer of adherent platelets are composed of aggregated platelets. Platelet aggregation occurs when signaling pathways initiated by agonists such as thrombin, ADP, thromboxane A_2, and collagen enable the platelet integrin GPIIb/IIIa complex ($\alpha IIb\beta3$) to bind soluble fibrinogen or von Willebrand's factor (vWF). Fibrinogen and vWF bound to GPIIb/IIIa crosslinks platelets into a hemostatic plug.

Platelets contain four types of granules that are secreted coincident with platelet aggregation. Dense (δ) granules contain adenosine 5′-diphosphate (ADP), adenosine 5′-triphosphate (ATP), calcium, serotonin, and pyrophosphate; α granules contain a variety of proteins including fibrinogen, vWF, factor V, platelet-derived growth factor (PDGF), and IgG; lysosomes contain acid hydrolases; and microperoxisomes contain peroxidase activity. Secreted ADP propagates primary platelet responses, PGDF participates in wound repair, and platelet factor V contributes to thrombin generation. The function of many of the other granule

[1]Not FDA approved for this indication.
*Investigational drug in the United States.

Rakel and Bope: *Conn's Current Therapy 2006.*

substances is unclear. Nonetheless, platelet secretion disorders produce mild to moderate bleeding, indicating that secretion is essential role for normal hemostasis.

Membranes of activated platelets provide a surface for the assembly of the "tenase" and "prothrombinase" complexes that generate active coagulation factor X and thrombin, respectively. Expression of platelet procoagulant activity requires an agonist-stimulated rise in intraplatelet Ca^{2+} and the translocation of acidic phospholipids to the platelet surface.

Quantitative Platelet Disorders

A sufficient number of platelets are required for primary hemostasis. Thrombocytopenia can result from decreased platelet production by bone marrow megakaryocytes, accelerated platelet removal, or platelet sequestration in an enlarged spleen, but there is no readily available test to differentiate between these possibilities. Thus, the clinical context of thrombocytopenia is crucial to decide which mechanism pertains. Nonetheless, in the absence of splenomegaly, the presence of megakaryocytes in an otherwise normal bone marrow implies that thrombocytopenia occurs because of accelerated platelet removal.

The cutaneous bleeding time, a measure of in vivo platelet function, prolongs when the platelet count decreases to less than 100,000/μL. Nonetheless, hemorrhage following trauma or surgery generally does not occur if the platelets count is greater than 50,000/μL. Moreover, in an otherwise hemostatically normal patient, significant spontaneous bleeding generally does not occur until the platelet count declines to less than 5000 to 10,000. However, there is no absolute threshold for spontaneous bleeding because of thrombocytopenia, and it can occur at higher platelet counts when fever, sepsis, severe anemia, and other hemostatic defects are present or when platelet function is impaired by medication.

THROMBOCYTOPENIA CAUSED BY DECREASED PLATELET PRODUCTION

Decreased platelet production occurs in diseases such as acute leukemia and aplastic anemia; myelophthisic processes in which bone marrow is replaced by metastatic carcinoma, fibrosis, or multiple myeloma; following chemotherapy and/or radiation therapy; because of ethanol toxicity; and during infections with viruses such as HIV, measles, cytomegalovirus (CMV), and varicella. Thrombocytopenia also occurs when megakaryocyte proliferation is impaired by myelodysplasia and paroxysmal nocturnal hemoglobinuria. Overt bleeding in these disorders, occurring clearly because of thrombocytopenia, is treated by platelet transfusion. Prophylactic platelet transfusion, however, is an area of controversy and is complicated by the short life span of platelets (10 days), the 5-day shelf-life of untransfused platelets, and by platelet immunogenicity. Thus, when the cause of decreased platelet production cannot be readily reversed, long-term prophylaxis requires frequent transfusions and the risk of developing platelet alloantibodies.

In patients undergoing treatment for acute leukemia, outcome is unchanged when platelet counts of 5000 to 10,000/μL are used as the threshold for prophylactic transfusion. Because most chronic conditions rarely result in this degree of thrombocytopenia, prophylactic platelet transfusions are not usually necessary. When they are, using single donor apheresis platelets and/or platelet donors who are HLA-identical to the recipient should be considered to prevent alloimmunization.

THROMBOCYTOPENIA CAUSED BY INCREASED PLATELET DESTRUCTION

Nonimmune and immune processes can lead to a shortened platelet life span. Nonimmune causes include sepsis, disseminated intravascular coagulation, thrombotic thrombocytopenic purpura–hemolytic uremic syndrome (TTP-HUS), preeclampsia/eclampsia, cardiopulmonary bypass, and giant cavernous hemangiomas (Kasabach-Merritt syndrome). Thrombocytopenia in these disorders resolves as the disorders resolve and platelet transfusion is rarely necessary. In TTP-HUS, thrombocytopenia is associated with thrombosis rather than bleeding, and there are reports of clinical deterioration, even death, following platelet transfusion.

Immune-mediated platelet destruction can occur because of medication, alloimmune sensitization following transfusion or pregnancy, and autoimmunity. The list of medications reported to cause antibody–mediated platelet destruction is long, but drugs that clearly cause antibody–meditated thrombocytopenia include quinine and quinidine, sulfonamides, and gold salts. Nonetheless, medications should always be considered as a possible etiology for thrombocytopenia. Besides stopping the offending medication, emergent treatment for severe thrombocytopenia with bleeding in this situation includes platelet transfusion, as well as corticosteroids and intravenous immunoglobulin[1] G (IV IgG [Gamimune N]), similar to emergent treatment for autoimmune thrombocytopenia (see following paragraphs).

Heparin-induced thrombocytopenia (HIT) is a special case of drug-induced thrombocytopenia. HIT can occur in 2% to 5% of patients given unfractionated heparin for 5 to 10 days by any route. It is caused by antibodies to a complex of heparin and the platelet α granule protein platelet factor 4. Patients with HIT rarely bleed, but rather the HIT immune complex activates platelets, causing thrombosis in both the arterial and venous circulations. HIT must always be considered when thrombocytopenia is detected in a hospitalized patient. If HIT is a possibility, all heparin administration must be stopped, and alternative anticoagulation instituted, at least until the platelet count returns to normal. Alternative anticoagulants approved for HIT include the direct thrombin inhibitors recombinant hirudin and argatroban. Warfarin (Coumadin)[1] should not be used for acute HIT because several days are required for its anticoagulant effect, and it can be associated with a syndrome of venous limb gangrene leading to amputation.

---

[1]Not FDA approved for this indication.

Alloimmune thrombocytopenia, because of sensitization to alloantigens such as Pl[A1], results from transfusion (post-transfusion purpura [PTP]) or maternal sensitization during pregnancy (neonatal alloimmune thrombocytopenia, NATP). PTP causes profound thrombocytopenia 7 to 10 days after transfusion and can be treated with IVIG[1] or plasma exchange. NATP can cause severe thrombocytopenia and bleeding in neonates and is treated with platelet transfusion, corticosteroids, and IVIG.[1]

Autoimmune thrombocytopenia, also known as idiopathic thrombocytopenic purpura (ITP), occurs because of circulating antiplatelet autoantibodies. An ITP-like picture can also occur in autoimmune diseases such as systemic lupus erythematosus, in patients with low-grade lymphoproliferative disorders such as chronic lymphocytic leukemia and well-differentiated lymphocytic lymphoma, and in patients with HIV infections. ITP can occur at any age in either sex and presents with either spontaneous mucocutaneous bleeding or unexplained asymptomatic thrombocytopenia. Red cell and white cell counts are normal, splenomegaly is absent, and peripheral blood smears are only remarkable for a decreased number of platelets, some of which may be larger than normal. Megakaryocytes are present in ITP bone marrow, but a bone marrow examination is rarely necessary in the absence of other findings suggesting myelodysplasia. Assays are available to detect antiplatelet antibodies, but they lack sensitivity and specificity and are rarely helpful diagnostically.

Treatment of ITP is guided by symptoms and platelet count. Bleeding is usually minimal to absent until platelet counts decline to less than 30,000/μL. Thus, asymptomatic patients with platelet counts more than 30,000 can be followed without treatment. When bleeding is present, and/or the platelet count is less than 30,000/μL, treatment is initiated with prednisone at a dose of 1mg/kg body weight. Most patients respond, and platelet counts increase toward normal over days to weeks. When the platelet count increases to more than 100,000, the dose of prednisone is tapered slowly with three possible outcomes. First, the platelet count may remain normal after prednisone is discontinued. Second, the platelet count may decrease, but it remains greater than 30,000 at prednisone doses of 10 mg or less. Third, the disease either relapses or prednisone doses greater than 10 mg daily are required to maintain an acceptable platelet count. The latter group of patients, as well as patients who initially fail to respond, are candidates for splenectomy because 60% to 75% enter remission following this procedure. The small number of patients continuing to experience symptomatic thrombocytopenia after splenectomy are candidates for various immunosuppressive agents including azathioprine,[1] cyclophosphamide,[1] rituximab,[1] and cyclosporine.[1]

When patients with ITP present emergently with severe thrombocytopenia (<5.000/μL) and/or internal bleeding, the patients should be treated with high doses of corticosteroids (methylprednisolone [30 mg/kg per day] and/or IV IgG [1 g/kg per day times 2]). Platelet transfusion can be given concurrently with IV IgG for critical bleeding. Anti-D immunoglobulin (WinRhoSDF) may be substituted for IVIG in Rh-positive patients who have not undergone splenectomy.

THROMBOCYTOPENIA CAUSED BY PLATELET SEQUESTRATION IN AN ENLARGED SPLEEN

Approximately 30% of the circulating platelet mass is normally present in the spleen. Additional platelets can be sequestered when the spleen enlarges because of portal hypertension or infiltrative diseases. Platelet counts in patients with hypersplenism are generally in the range of 40,000 to 50,000/μL, but bleeding because of thrombocytopenia alone is unusual.

Qualitative Platelet Disorders

A prolonged bleeding time in a patient with a normal platelet count suggests a diagnosis of von Willebrand's disease or a qualitative platelet disorder.

6

ACQUIRED QUALITATIVE PLATELET DISORDERS

Acquired disorders of platelet function are relatively common, but are usually asymptomatic or mild. Nonetheless, they can be of substantial clinical importance when they are engrafted on another hemostatic abnormality. They can be subclassified into disorders attributed to medications, to systemic illnesses, and to hematologic disorders. Although a wide variety of medications impair platelet function in vitro, only a small number produce clinically significant bleeding. These include aspirin, the thienopyridines ticlopidine (Ticlid) and clopidogrel (Plavix), and the GPIIb/IIIa antagonists abciximab (ReoPro), tirofiban (Aggrastat), and eptifibatide (Integrilin). Aspirin, by preventing platelet synthesis of thromboxane A_2, is an important cause of platelet dysfunction. Although aspirin has a minimal effect on hemostasis in normal individuals, it causes a substantial prolongation of the bleeding time, and can precipitate hemorrhage, in individuals with other hemostatic defects such as von Willebrand's disease and hemophilia.

Nonhematologic disorders in which platelet dysfunction can be a prominent feature include uremia and cardiopulmonary bypass. Platelet dysfunction in uremia is usually corrected by dialysis. When it persists, the vasopressin analog desmopressin acetate[1] (DDAVP) is the treatment of choice, but conjugated estrogens[1] and cryoprecipitate can also improve hemostasis. DDAVP causes the release of vWF from tissue stores and at a dose of 0.3 μg/kg IV over 15 to 30 minutes (maximum dose 20 μg) shortens the bleeding time in 50% to 75% of patients with uremia for approximately 4 hours.

---

[1]Not FDA approved for this indication.

---

[1]Not FDA approved for this indication.

Dosing can be repeated at 12- to 24-hour intervals, but tachyphylaxis can occur. The prolonged bleeding time in uremia can also be shortened, and hemostasis can be improved by the correction of anemia using red cell transfusion or erythropoietin (Procrit).[1] Platelet dysfunction following cardiopulmonary bypass results from the interaction of platelets with the bypass circuit and from hypothermia induced during bypass. It generally resolves spontaneously in 2 to 24 hours, but persistent bleeding may require platelet transfusion.

Platelet dysfunction occurs in chronic myeloproliferative disorders such as polycythemia vera and essential thrombocythemia, in dysproteinemias such as multiple myeloma and macroglobulinemia, in myelodysplasia and leukemia, and in acquired forms of von Willebrand's disease. Platelet dysfunction in the myeloproliferative disorders occurs because of intrinsic platelet defects, as well as substantial increases in platelet count. Reducing the platelet count to near the normal range with hydroxyurea (Droxia)[1] or anagrelide (Agrylin) reduces the risk of bleeding or thrombosis in patients older than 60 years

---

[1]Not FDA approved for this indication.

 CURRENT DIAGNOSIS

- Thrombocytopenia can result from decreased platelet production, accelerated platelet removal, or platelet sequestration in an enlarged spleen.
- The cutaneous bleeding time can be prolonged when the platelet count is less than 100,000/µL, but a prolonged bleeding time does not predict clinical bleeding.
- In an otherwise hemostatically normal patient, significant spontaneous bleeding generally does not occur until the platelet count declines to less than 5000 to 10,000/µL.
- Heparin-induced thrombocytopenia must always be considered when thrombocytopenia is detected in a hospitalized patient.
- Idiopathic thrombocytopenic purpura presents as otherwise unexplained spontaneous mucocutaneous bleeding or asymptomatic thrombocytopenia and is a diagnosis of exclusion.
- A prolonged bleeding time in a patient with a normal platelet count suggests a diagnosis of von Willebrand's disease or a qualitative platelet function disorder.
- Although many medications impair platelet function in vitro, only a few, including aspirin, the thienopyridines, and the GPIIb/IIIa antagonists induce clinically significant bleeding.
- Although hereditary disorders of platelet adhesion and aggregation are very rare, hereditary disorders of platelet secretion are not uncommon causes of easy bruising, menorrhagia, and excessive postoperative and postpartum blood loss.

of age and in patients with symptomatic platelet dysfunction regardless of age. Aspirin is helpful in patients with thrombosis, but its routine use in asymptomatic patients can increase the risk of bleeding. Platelet dysfunction in the dysproteinemia is because of the associated paraprotein and improves when the paraprotein concentration is decreased by plasmapheresis or chemotherapy. Acquired von Willebrand's disease is a rare complication of myeloproliferative disorders, autoimmune diseases, and dysproteinemias. DDAVP,[1] vWF concentrates, and IV IgG reportedly improve hemostasis in these patients.

HEREDITARY QUALITATIVE PLATELET DISORDERS

The Bernard-Soulier syndrome (BSS) and Glanzmann thrombasthenia (GT) are rare autosomal recessive disorders of the platelet membrane glycoproteins GPIb-IX and GPIIb/IIIa, respectively. These disorders present with mucocutaneous bleeding in infancy or childhood. Patients with BSS are also thrombocytopenic and have very large platelets that do not agglutinate when exposed to ristocetin. Platelet counts and platelet morphology are normal in GT, but the platelets cannot aggregate in response to ADP or thrombin. Reliable treatment of bleeding in both conditions requires platelet transfusion.

---

[1]Not FDA approved for this indication.

 CURRENT THERAPY

- In the absence of bleeding, platelet counts of 5000 to 10,000/µL are used as the threshold for prophylactic transfusion.
- Because bleeding in patients with idiopathic thrombocytopenic purpura (ITP) is usually minimal to absent until platelet counts decline to less than 30,000/µL, asymptomatic patients with platelet counts greater than 30,000 usually can be followed without treatment.
- Treatment for ITP is initiated with prednisone; patients who fail to enter clinical remission are candidates for splenectomy or treatment with immunosuppressive agents.
- High doses of corticosteroids and/or intravenous IgG are indicated for the emergent treatment of ITP. Platelet transfusion given concurrently with intravenous IgG can be effective for critical bleeding.
- When heparin-induced thrombocytopenia is a possibility, stop all heparin administration and institute alternative anticoagulation, at least until the platelet count returns to normal.
- Although the treatment of hereditary disorders of platelet adhesion and aggregation usually requires platelet transfusion, hereditary disorders of platelet secretion may respond to desmopressin acetate (DDAVP)[1] infusion.

---

[1]Not FDA approved for this indication.

Hereditary disorders of platelet secretion are not uncommon causes of easy bruising, menorrhagia, and excessive postoperative and postpartum blood loss and can occur because of granule deficiency, for example, gray platelet syndrome ([α granule deficiency] or δ storage pool disease [δSPD; dense granule deficiency]) or biochemical abnormalities of the platelet secretory mechanism. δSPD is the most common platelet secretion disorder and can be subclassified into δSPD associated with albinism (the Hermansky-Pudlak and Chédiak-Higashi syndromes) and δSPD in otherwise normal individuals. Patients with δSPD have normal platelet counts and usually prolonged bleeding times and abnormal platelet aggregation studies. An increased ratio of platelet ATP to ADP, because of the absence of platelet dense granule ADP, is diagnostic. Although bleeding in patients with secretion disorders can be controlled by platelet transfusion, this is seldom necessary because DDAVP[1] can shorten the bleeding times and improve hemostasis.

REFERENCES

Bennett JS: Novel platelet inhibitors. Annu Rev Med 2001;52:161-184.
Beutler E: Platelet transfusion: the 20,000/μL trigger. Blood 1993;81:1411-1413.
Cines DB, Blanchette VS: Immune thrombocytopenic purpura. N Engl J Med 2002;346:995-1008.
George JN, Caen JP, Nurden AT: Glanzmann thrombasthenia: The spectrum of clinical disease. Blood 1990;75:1383-1395.
Huizing M, Boissy RE, Gahl WA: Hermansky-Pudlak syndrome: Vesicle formation from yeast to man. Pigment Cell Res 2002;15:405-419.
Lind SE: The bleeding time does not predict surgical bleeding. Blood 1991;77:2547-2552.
Lopez JA, Andrews RK, Afshar-Kharghan V, et al: Bernard-Soulier syndrome. Blood 1998;91:4397-4418.
Mannucci PM: Desmopressin (DDAVP) in the treatment of bleeding disorders: The first 20 years. Blood 1997;90:2515-2521.
Patrono C: Aspirin as an antiplatelet drug. N Engl J Med 1994;330:1287-1294.
Pearson TC: The risk of thrombosis in essential thrombocythemia and polycythemia vera. Semin Oncol 2002;29:16-21.
Tefferi A, Nichols WL: Acquired von Willebrand disease: Concise review of occurrence, diagnosis, pathogenesis, and treatment. Am J Med 1997;103:536-540.
Warkentin TE: Heparin-induced thrombocytopenia: pathogenesis and management. Br J Haematol 2003;121:535-555.

Disseminated Intravascular Coagulation

Method of
Deborah Brown, MD, and William K. Hoots, MD

Disseminated intravascular coagulation (DIC) is an acquired syndrome characterized by the systemic intravascular activation of coagulation. A variety of conditions may cause DIC, including sepsis, trauma, malignancy, obstetrical calamities, vascular malformations, severe hepatic failure, and severe toxic or immunologic reactions. The hallmark of DIC is diffuse microvascular fibrin deposition that leads to thrombotic occlusion of small and midsize vessels, contributing to organ failure and depletion of platelets and coagulation proteins, increasing the risk of bleeding. DIC that accompanies sepsis is a poor prognostic risk factor, with a mortality rate as high as 70%.

Pathophysiology of Disseminated Intravascular Coagulation

In the systemic inflammatory response syndrome (sepsis), increased thrombin generation occurs primarily through the tissue factor (TF)-FVIIa pathway. The source of TF is presumed to be endothelial cells and monocyte-derived microparticles that transfer TF to activated platelets. Depletion of the thrombin inhibitor antithrombin III is caused by consumption, degradation by elastase, and impaired synthesis. Low levels of antithrombin III are associated with increased mortality in DIC. Inflammatory cytokines down-regulate thrombomodulin expression on endothelial cells, reducing activation of the endogenous anticoagulant protein C, thus enhancing the procoagulant state. The factor V Leiden mutation, which causes activated protein C (APC) resistance, and inherited protein C deficiency, both contribute to the morbidity and mortality from sepsis-induced DIC. During this heightened activation of coagulation, fibrinolysis is impaired by increased amounts of circulating plasminogen activating inhibitor-1 (PAI-1). Mutations in the PAI-1 gene contribute to worsened clinical outcome in meningococcal septicemia.

Activated coagulation proteins may also mediate inflammatory responses in a two-way interaction between coagulation and inflammation. The coagulation proteases FXa and thrombin can induce signaling pathways on endothelial cells, eliciting the synthesis of proinflammatory cytokines and growth factors. The family of protease-activated receptors (PARs) are G-protein–coupled transmembrane receptors that are thrombin receptors (PARS 1, 3, and 4) or are activated by the TF-FVIIa complex and FXa (PARs 1 and 2). In addition, APC inhibits endotoxin-induced production of cytokines mediated by the endothelial protein C receptor (EPCR) on monocytes and macrophages.

[1]Not FDA approved for this indication.

Diagnosis

The diagnosis of DIC is based on a combination of laboratory test results in a patient with an underlying disease known to be associated with DIC. No single laboratory test is sufficiently sensitive or specific to establish the diagnosis. In clinical practice, the diagnosis can be made with reasonable accuracy if the patient has a clinical condition known to be associated with DIC, a platelet count of less than 100,000 per μL or a rapid decline in platelet count, prolongation of the prothrombin time, and fibrin degradation products in plasma. Other causes of thrombocytopenia and coagulopathy should be excluded. Review of the peripheral blood smear usually reveals schistocytes (red cell fragments) and spherocytes. Fibrinogen is an acute-phase reactant, and plasma levels may remain in the normal range despite disseminated consumption. Assay systems measuring fibrin degradation products (FDPs or d-dimer) are highly variable in sensitivity and specificity for the diagnosis of DIC and cannot be relied on to establish or exclude the diagnosis.

The Scientific Subcommittee on DIC of the International Society of Thrombosis and Hemostasis (ISTH) has developed an algorithm for the diagnosis of overt DIC in which the presence of an underlying disorder known to be associated with DIC is a precondition. The clinical assessment of organ failure and bleeding is not included in the scoring system because the DIC score itself may form part of scores for organ failure. Commonly available coagulation assays (platelet count, prothrombin time, fibrinogen, and a marker for soluble fibrin or FDPs) are scored daily. A score of 5 or greater is compatible with overt DIC. A score less than 5 may be suggestive of nonovert DIC and should be repeated daily. Nonovert DIC represents hemostatic dysfunction before it is at the stage of frank decompensation. In the ISTH scoring system for nonovert DIC, the trend over time of the coagulation assays is also evaluated as a component of the scoring. Additional laboratory tests, which may not be available in local laboratories, are optional.

Treatment

Management of DIC depends primarily on treatment of the underlying disorder and general supportive care. Inhibition of disseminated coagulation with anticoagulation therapy is theoretically beneficial, and positive results are reported in small noncontrolled case series, but no benefit on outcomes is seen in the few well-controlled clinical trials that are published. Low-dose heparin[1] may be helpful to reduce the risk of venous thromboembolism and to treat thromboembolic complications such as purpura fulminans.

Patients with severe thrombocytopenia or coagulopathy who have active bleeding symptoms or require invasive procedures should be treated with platelet concentrates and fresh-frozen plasma. Prophylactic

transfusions in patients only with laboratory abnormalities do not improve outcomes. Likewise, the mythology that plasma and platelet infusions "fuel the fire" of patients with DIC who are bleeding is largely discredited. Transfused platelets are likely to have reduced survival because of consumption and sequestration. Large volumes of plasma may be required to overcome coagulation factor deficiencies and ongoing consumption. Because the half-life of the shortest acting coagulation factor, factor VII, is less than 6 hours, dosing frequency of plasma should be every 6 hours or less. Cryoprecipitate infusions may correct severe fibrinogen deficiency. Specific coagulation factor concentrates are rarely indicated, given the pervasive deficiencies of both procoagulant and anticoagulant proteins, and they may be specifically contraindicated because of increased thrombogenic potential. For example, activated prothrombin complex concentrates have small amounts of activated procoagulant factors and are associated with thrombotic complications when administered to patients with hemophilia. Recombinant factor VIIa[1] (Novo Seven) has not been formally tested in patients with DIC and should be avoided in this context until further studies are completed.

Antifibrinolytic treatment is contraindicated in most patients with DIC because deficient fibrinolysis is believed to be an important contributor to the development of microvascular occlusion and organ failure. The coagulopathy associated with acute promyelocytic leukemia, however, is associated with hyperfibrinolysis, and bleeding symptoms may respond to treatment with antifibrinolytic therapy.

---

[1]Not FDA approved for this indication.

 CURRENT DIAGNOSIS

The following presents the International Society of Thrombosis and Hemostasis (ISTH) diagnostic algorithm for the diagnosis of overt disseminated intravascular coagulation (DIC). Before using this algorithm, however, determine if the patient has an underlying disorder known to be associated with overt DIC.
If yes, proceed; if no, do not use this algorithm.
- Order global coagulation tests (platelet count, prothrombin time [PT], fibrinogen, soluble fibrin monomers, or fibrin degradation products).
- Score global coagulation test results:
  Platelet count (>100 = 0; <100 = 1; <50 = 2)
  Elevated fibrin-related marker (no increase = 1, moderate increase = 2, strong increase = 3)
  Prolonged prothrombin time (<3 seconds = 0; >3 seconds but <6 seconds = 1; >6 seconds = 2)
  Fibrinogen level (>1.0 g/L = 0; <1.0 g/L = 1)
- Calculate score:
  If >5, compatible with overt DIC; repeat score daily.
  If <5, suggestive (not affirmative) for nonovert DIC; repeat next 1 to 2 days.

---

[1]Not FDA approved for this indication.

CURRENT THERAPY

Treatment	Indication	Dose	Frequency	Monitor
Fresh-frozen plasma	Bleeding or high risk of bleeding and PT >18 s.	10 mL/kg BW	6 h	PT q6h
Random donor platelets	Bleeding or high risk of bleeding and platelets <100 × 10³/μL.	1 U/10 kg BW	prn platelets <100	Platelet count bid
Red blood cells	Anemia (Hgb <8 g/dL).	10 mL/kg BW	prn Hgb <8 g/dL	Hgb/Hct bid
Cryoprecipitate	Fibrinogen <100 mg/dL.	1 U/10 kg BW	prn fibrinogen <100 mg/dL	Fibrinogen bid
Activated protein C	Severe sepsis.	24 μg/kg BW/h	Continuous infusion for 96 h	Protein C level (optional)
Antithrombin III	No proven indication: Consider if AT level <50%.	50 μg/kg	Daily	Antithrombin III level
Heparin	Thromboembolism, purpura fulminans, acral cyanosis. Consider for VTE prophylaxis.	10 U/kg BW/h	Continuous infusion	PTT q6h

Abbreviations: AT = antithrombin; bid = twice daily; BW = body weight; Hgb = hemoglobin; Hct = hematocrit; prn = as needed; PT = prothrombin time; q = every; VTE = venous thromboembolism.

6

In situations associated with DIC, such as sepsis, the majority of patients have reduced levels of protein C, which is related to an increased risk of death. In a large randomized controlled trial in patients with severe sepsis (the PROWESS [Recombinant Human Activated Protein C Worldwide Evaluation in Severe Sepsis] trial), treatment with APC reduces mortality with an absolute risk reduction of 6.1%. Plasma d-dimer and interleukin (IL)-6 levels are significantly lower in days 2 through 7 after initiating treatment with APC. There is an increased incidence of serious bleeding in the APC-treated patients (3.5% versus 2.0%), whereas risk of thrombotic events is similar (2.0% versus 3.0%). The use of APC for patients with DIC with causes other than sepsis awaits further study.

Plasma levels of antithrombin (AT) are also decreased in DIC associated with sepsis, but the benefit of AT replacement[1] in sepsis is less clear. A meta-analysis of controlled clinical trials using AT for sepsis suggests a decreased mortality in treated patients; however, in a large randomized controlled trial, a clear benefit was not seen. Subgroup analysis suggests that patients not also treated with heparin[1] may show benefit with AT replacement. Although AT appears safe and well tolerated, because of lack of proven benefit in the treatment of DIC associated with sepsis, AT replacement should be considered optional for patients with severely decreased levels.

Future Directions

Pharmacologic agents that are currently in phases I and II of clinical trials for the treatment of DIC include inhibitors of the TF pathway such as tissue factor pathway inhibitor and the recombinant nematode[1] anticoagulant protein c2. Direct thrombin inhibition with hirudin[1] shows promising results in animal studies and phase I clinical trials. The synthetic serine protease inhibitors gabexate[1] mesilate and nafamostat[1] mesilate are used in Japan for the treatment of patients with DIC. Replacement therapy with the endogenous anticoagulants recombinant thrombomodulin[1] and protein S concentrates is a promising area of research not yet subject to clinical trials. Improvements in survival of patients with DIC will undoubtedly originate from advances in critical care management combined with strategies for regulating excessive inflammation and thrombin generation.

REFERENCES

Bernard GR, Vincent JL, Laterre PF, et al: Efficacy and safety of recombinant human activated protein C for severe sepsis. N Engl J Med 2001;344:699-709.

Davidson BL, Geerts WH, Lensing AWA: Low-dose heparin for severe sepsis. N Engl J Med 2002;347:1036-1037.

Levi M: Current understanding of disseminated intravascular coagulation. Br J Haematol 2004;124:567-576.

Lorente JA, Garcia-Frade, Landin L, et al: Time course of hemostatic abnormalities in sepsis and its relation to outcome. Chest 1993;103:1536-1542.

Spero JA, Lewis JH, Hasiba U: Disseminated intravascular coagulation: Findings in 346 patients. Thromb Haemost 1980;43(1):28-33.

Taylor FB, Toh CH, Hoots WK, et al: Towards definition, clinical and laboratory criteria, and a scoring system for disseminated intravascular coagulation. Thromb Haemost 2001;86:1327-1330.

---

[1]Not FDA approved for this indication.

[1]Not FDA approved for this indication.

Thrombotic Thrombocytopenia Purpura

Method of
Laura Cooling MD, MS

Thrombotic thrombocytopenia purpura (TTP) is a pro-thrombotic, microvascular occlusive disorder characterized by thrombocytopenia, microangiopathic hemolytic anemia (MAHA), neurologic findings, fever, and renal failure. TTP should be considered in any patient presenting with thrombocytopenia and MAHA. Untreated, TTP has a mortality of 80% to 90%.

Etiology and Pathogenesis

Idiopathic TTP is a relatively rare disorder, with approximately 1000 new cases diagnosed per year. TTP can occur at any age but is more common in younger (<35 years of age) adults and women. Many patients have a history of recent infection, such as a cold or gastrointestinal illness. Active infections with HIV, shiga toxin–producing *Escherichia coli,* and tick-borne illnesses (Rocky Mountain spotted fever, granulocytic ehrlichiosis) can also precipitate TTP. In addition to infection, TTP can be triggered by metastatic cancer, autoimmune disease, pregnancy, drugs, and bone marrow and organ transplantation. Drugs specifically linked to TTP include quinine, clopidogrel (Plavix), ticlopidine (Ticlid), mitomycin C, cyclosporin (Sandimmune), and tacrolimus (Prograf). There is also a rare inherited form of the disease.

Histologically, TTP is characterized by bland microvascular thrombi, composed of platelets and von Willebrand's factor (vWf), occluding small arterioles and capillaries. The latter results in MAHA, a consumptive thrombocytopenia; ischemia; and organ dysfunction. Recent studies have uncovered a central role for vWf, and particularly ultralarge von Willebrand's factor (ULvWf) multimers, in the pathogenesis of TTP. Synthesized by vascular endothelium, ULvWf multimers are released after endothelial injury and activation, facilitating both platelet adherence and aggregation at the site of injury. Because of its proclivity to adhere and induce platelet aggregation, circulating ULvWf is normally broken down into smaller, lower molecular weight forms by the metalloprotease ADAMTS-13 (a disintegrin and metalloproteinase with thrombospondin motif-13). In idiopathic (and familial) TTP, there is a deficiency in ADAMTS-13 activity (less than 5% to 10% normal), accompanied by increased circulating ULvWf, because of autoantibodies against ADAMTS-13. The latter are also implicated in autoimmune and drug-associated TTP. In contrast, hemolytic uremic syndrome and TTP secondary to cancer, chemotherapy, and transplantation typically have normal ADAMTS-13 activity and vWf multimers.

Diagnosis

The classic pentad for TTP is thrombocytopenia, MAHA, fever, acute renal failure, and neurologic signs. In reality, few patients present with all five symptoms. Thrombocytopenia and MAHA are nearly always present. Neurologic findings are present in 70% of patients and may present as confusion, lethargy, delirium, or seizures. Many patients report an antecedent viral illness.

The diagnosis of TTP must be distinguished from other microangiopathic disorders. Useful laboratory studies are a complete blood count (CBC) with white blood count (WBC) differential, peripheral blood smear, direct antiglobulin test (DAT), coagulation studies (PT [prothrombin time], PTT [partial thromboplastin time], fibrinogen, d-dimers), haptoglobin, lactate dehydrogenase (LDH), electrolytes, and urinalysis. Based on the patient's history, laboratory studies to exclude autoimmune disease, infection, and illicit drugs may also be required.

Sentinel findings in TTP are the presence of anemia, thrombocytopenia, and fragmented red blood cells (RBCs), (schistocytes) on CBC and peripheral blood smear. In general, the WBC should be normal or only slightly elevated (less than 20,000/μL). Intravascular hemolysis is confirmed by a low haptoglobin, hemoglobinemia, elevated LDH, and increased indirect bilirubin. Unlike autoimmune hemolytic anemia and disseminated intravascular coagulation (DIC), the DAT and coagulation studies are normal in TTP. Differentiating TTP from vasculitis, systemic viral infections, and acute graft-versus-host disease (GVHD) can be difficult. Commercial assays for ADAMTS-13 activity and/or anti-ADAMTS-13 autoantibodies could be extremely helpful in this group of patients and may be available in the near future. A vWf multimer assay is available at many institutions and commercial laboratories.

Note that all diagnostic serologic tests, including vWf multimers, rheumatology tests, and viral serologies, must be drawn before initiating therapeutic plasma exchange (TPEX). TPEX removes the patient's plasma by automated continuous centrifugation, replacing the patient's plasma with homologous plasma from the blood bank. As a result, serologic studies drawn after initiating TPEX may be falsely negative.

Treatment

The mainstay of treatment is plasma exchange (TPEX), which has reduced the morbidity of TTP from more than 80% to 10% to 20%. In idiopathic TTP, TPEX presumably removes anti-ADAMTS-13 autoantibodies while replenishing ADAMTS-13 activity. Not surprisingly, TPEX is less effective in TTP because of other causes such as bone marrow transplantation, cancer, and vasculitis. TPEX is effective in HIV-associated TTP. In the future, recombinant ADAMTS-13 may be available for treatment.

TPEX should be initiated as soon as possible. If a lengthy delay is unavoidable (more than 24 hours), the patient can receive fresh-frozen plasma (FFP) infusions

Rakel and Bope: Conn's Current Therapy 2006.

(25 to 30 mL/kg/day) until TPEX is available. A standard treatment course is a series of daily 1–blood volume TPEX using FFP as the replacement fluid. To minimize donor exposures, many institutions give a mixture of albumin and FFP, with equivalent clinical results. With few exceptions, most patients require placement of a double-lumen dialysis catheter for venous access. Despite the presence of profound thrombocytopenia, platelet transfusion is *contraindicated* in these patients, unless there is active bleeding. In addition to TPEX, steroids and folate[1] may be given to suppress autoantibody formation and support endogenous hematopoiesis, respectively. Response to treatment is based on clinical improvement and daily LDH and platelet counts. Disease remission is defined as either a normal LDH and platelet count or when the platelet count exceeds the LDH.

On average, most patients respond to TPEX within 2 weeks, with a total course lasting from 1 to 4 weeks. Patients who fail to respond can be given a trial of cryopoor FFP, which is depleted of vWf. Corticosteroids and pulse immunosuppression[1] may also be required (Figure 1 and Table 1). Because refractoriness is often the result of underlying infection, all refractory patients should be carefully assessed for sources of infection

___

[1] Not FDA approved for this indication.

CURRENT DIAGNOSIS

Differential diagnosis of thrombotic thrombocytopenia purpura is as follows:

- Hemolytic uremic syndrome (HUS)
- Pregnancy
  Preeclampsia/eclampsia
  Hemolysis-elevated liver enzymes-low platelet
      syndrome (HELLP syndrome)
- Malignant hypertension
- Disseminated intravascular coagulation
- Infection
- Sepsis (viral, fungal)
  HIV
  Rocky Mountain spotted fever and other
      rickettsial-like infections
  Granulocytic ehrlichiosis
  Shiga toxin–producing Enterobacteriaceae
      (hemolytic uremic syndrome [HUS])
- Autoimmune disease
  Vasculitis
  Evans syndrome
  Antiphospholipid syndrome
  Scleroderma
  Systemic lupus erythematosus (SLE)
- Disseminated malignancy
- Transplant rejection/acute graft-versus-host
  disease
- Cocaine intoxication
- Severe folate/vitamin B_{12} deficiency (e.g., HIV
  antiviral medications)

Rakel and Bope: *Conn's Current Therapy 2006.*

including dental infections and colonized indwelling catheters. On occasion, refractory thrombocytopenia is secondary to TPEX itself, which removes 20% to 30% of circulating platelets and can outpace endogenous platelet production. Refractoriness can also be mimicked or exacerbated by severe hypertension, erythropoietin, and nutritional deficiencies. TTP secondary to metastatic cancer and bone marrow transplantation is often resistant to TPEX.

Despite an initial good response to TPEX, approximately 30% of patients suffer an exacerbation (less than 2 weeks after discontinuing TPEX) or relapse (more than 2 to 4 weeks). As before, patients are treated by daily 1–blood volume TPEX using either FFP or cryopoor FFP (see Table 1). Unlike the initial course of TPEX, most centers taper the frequency of TPEX once clinical remission is achieved. A typical taper course is 2 to 3 TPEX per week for another 1 to 2 weeks. Patients with repeated exacerbations and/or relapses may require a course of IVIgG (intravenous immunoglobulin G) (Gammagard), rituximab (Rituxan),[1] or splenectomy to sustain remission (see Table 1).

___

[1] Not FDA approved for this indication.

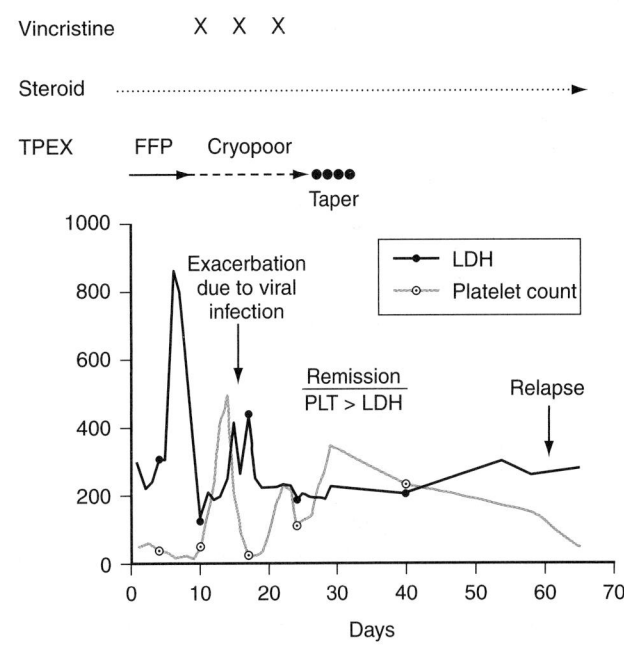

FIGURE 1. A course of TTP in a 13-year-old boy with autoimmune disease. Note the inverse relationship of the platelet count and LDH in TTP. As shown, the patient was initially refractory to treatment, with no significant increase in platelet count. A response was observed after switching to cryopoor plasma and pulse vincristine. Following an upper respiratory tract infection, the patient suffered an exacerbation of his TTP, requiring a total of 30 days of daily TPEX to achieve clinical remission (platelet count higher than LDH). Because of his long course, TPEX was tapered in this patient. The patient's platelet count slowly dropped over the next month, and he eventually suffered a relapse 65 days after his initial diagnosis. The patient responded quickly to a second course of TPEX using FFP replacement. *Abbreviations:* FFP = fresh-frozen plasma; LDH = lactate dehydrogenase; TPEX = therapeutic plasma exchange; TTP = thrombotic thrombocytopenia purpura.

TABLE 1 Evaluation and Management of TTP by Therapeutic Plasma Exchange (TPEX)

Pre-TPEX evaluation	Standard therapy (at first diagnosis)	Salvage therapy (refractory/exacerbation or relapse)
Laboratory Studies: (draw before first TPEX)	**Treatment***	**Treatment***
CBC with WBS differential	Plasma Exchange (TPEX)	TPEX +/– taper
Peripheral blood smear	Daily (TPEX)	Daily TPEX
DAT	1 blood volume	1 blood volume
Haptoglobin	Replacement Fluid:	Replacement Fluid:
LDH, LFTs	FP (100%) or	trial cryo-poor FFP or
Coagulation studies	Albumin + FFP	FFP +/– albumin
Electrolytes	Premedication†	Premedication
Type and screen		
Other diagnostic laboratories e.g., ANA. vWF multimers, etc.	Laboratories	Laboratories
	Daily CBC	Daily CBC
	Daily LDH	Daily LDH
Medications:	**Ancillary Treatment**	**Ancillary Treatment**
ACE inhibitors‡	Folate	Folate
Protein-bound drugs	Immunosuppression steroids	Immunosuppression:
Anti-arrythmics		Steroids
Anti-seizure		Vincristine (Oncovin)
Antibiotics		Cyclophosphamide (Cytoxan)
Vascular Access:		Medical Evaluation:
Double lumen, dialysis catheter		Exclude infection or other
Medical History:		precipitating etiology
Vitals: Ht, Wt, BP, HR, RR		
Allergies		
Cardiac disease		**Alternate Therapy**
Pulmonary disease		IVIgG (Gammagard)
Renal function		Rituximab (Rituxin)
Hx transfusion reactions¶		Splenectomy
		Protein A column

*Remission: Clinical improvement and platelet count >150,00/µL or platelet count >LDH.
†Because of the increasing risk of allergic reactions to FFP replacement, patients are typically premedicated with diphenhydramine (25-50 mg) prior to procedure.
‡ACE inhibitors are contraindicated in patients undergoing TPEX and must be discontinued.
¶Highly protein-bound drugs willl be removed during TPEX.

Overall, the incidence of adverse events associated with TPEX is estimated to be between 30% and 60% in TTP patients. Allergic transfusion reactions are common because of massive exposure to homologous FFP over the course of treatment. Volume overload, hypotensive reactions, and transfusion-related acute lung injury (TRALI) are also reported. Because of their potential to precipitate severe hypotensive reactions, angiotensin-converting enzyme (ACE) inhibitors are contraindicated for all patients undergoing TPEX and must be discontinued immediately. Although rare, transfusion-transmitted infections remain a risk in these patients because of the large amount of blood product support during their treatment.

Other adverse reactions include hypocalcemia, hypotension, metabolic alkalosis, and citrate toxicity, which are exacerbated in TTP patients because of hepatic dysfunction, renal failure, and use of plasma replacement. In patients with TTP and preexisting lung injury, TPEX can further aggravate pulmonary dysfunction with increased Fi_{O2} requirements. Finally, TPEX can effectively decrease therapeutic concentrations of protein-bound drugs and globulin-based therapies. Because of the complexity of medical issues in these patients, there should be a discussion and review of the patient's medical history, current medications, and laboratory values with the apheresis physician.

 CURRENT THERAPY

- Initiate daily plasma exchange with FFP or FFP/albumin replacement. If significant delay, start FFP infusion (25-30 mL/kg/day) until apheresis available.
- Restrict platelet transfusions.
- Consider steroids and folate supplementation.
- If refractory, consider the addition of vincristine and/or plasma exchange with cryopoor FFP.
- Follow efficacy with daily LDH and platelet counts.

Abbreviations: FFP = fresh-frozen plasma; LDH = lactate dehydrogenase.

REFERENCES

Bandarenko N, Brecher ME, US TTP Apheresis Study Group: United States thrombotic thrombocytopenia purpura apheresis study group (US TTP ASG): Multicenter survey and retrospective analysis of current efficacy of therapeutic plasma exchange. J Clin Apheresis 1998;13:133-141.
Fontana S, Kremer Hovinga JA, Studt J-D, et al: Plasma therapy in thrombotic thrombocytopenia purpura: Review of the literature

The Blood and Spleen

and the Bern experience in a subgroup of patients with severe acquired ADAMTS-13 deficiency. Sem Hematol 2004;41:48-59.

George JN, Li X, McMinn JR, et al: Thrombotic thrombocytopenia purpura-hemolytic uremic syndrome following allogeneic HPC transplantation: A diagnostic dilemma. Transfusion 2004;44: 294-304.

Kiprov DD, Golden P, Rohe R, et al: Adverse reactions associated with mobile therapeutic apheresis: Analysis of 17,940 procedures. J Clin Apheresis 2001;16:130-133.

Kremer Hovinga JA, Studt J-D, Alberio L, Lammle B: Von Willebrand factor-cleaving protease (ADAMTS-13) activity in the diagnosis of thrombotic microangiopathies: The Swiss experience. Sem Hematol 2004;41:75-82.

McLeod BC, Price TH, Weinstein R (eds): Apheresis: Principles and Practice, 2nd ed. Bethesda, Md, AABB Press, 2003.

Moake JL: Thrombotic microangiopathies. New Engl J Med 2002; 247:589-600.

Hemochromatosis

Method of
Paul C. Adams, MD

Hemochromatosis is the most common genetic disease in populations of European ancestry. The diagnosis can be elusive because of the nonspecific nature of the symptoms. With the discovery of the hemochromatosis gene (*HFE*) in 1996, comes new insights into the pathogenesis of the disease and new diagnostic strategies.

A fundamental issue that arose since the discovery of the *HFE* gene is whether the disease "hemochromatosis" should be defined strictly on phenotypic criteria such as the degree of iron overload (i.e., transferrin saturation, ferritin, liver biopsy, hepatic iron concentration, iron removed by venesection therapy), or whether the condition should be defined as a familial disease in Europeans most commonly associated with the C282Y mutation of the *HFE* gene and varying degrees of iron overload. Because the genetic test was increasingly used as a diagnostic tool, most studies now use a combination of phenotypic and genotypic criteria for the diagnosis of hemochromatosis.

Clinical Features of Hemochromatosis: Liver Disease

Although hemochromatosis is often classified as a liver disease, it should be emphasized that it is a systemic genetic disease with multisystem involvement. The liver is central both in the diagnosis and prognosis in hemochromatosis. Hepatomegaly remains one of the more common physical signs in hemochromatosis but is always present in the young asymptomatic homozygote. In a study of 717 homozygotes from Australia, 8% of men and 1.7% of women had cirrhosis of the liver at the time of diagnosis. The prevalence of cirrhosis in asymptomatic or screened patients is much lower. It is likely

that there are factors other than iron overload that contribute to cirrhosis in hemochromatosis. This can include the effects of alcohol and/or comodifying genes. The effect of iron depletion therapy is usually stabilization of the liver disease, and fibrosis improves with repeat liver biopsy after iron depletion. This accounts for the relatively small number of C282Y homozygotes that require liver transplantation. The other common clinical manifestations are arthralgias, pigmentation, diabetes, congestive heart failure, impotence, and fatigue.

Diagnosis of Hemochromatosis

A paradox of genetic hemochromatosis is that the disease is underdiagnosed in the general population and overdiagnosed in patients with secondary iron overload.

UNDERDIAGNOSIS OF HEMOCHROMATOSIS

Preliminary population studies using genetic testing demonstrate a prevalence of homozygotes of approximately 1 in 227 in whites. The fact that many physicians consider hemochromatosis to be rare implies either a lack of penetrance of the gene (nonexpressing homozygote) or a large number of patients that remain undiagnosed in the community.

DIAGNOSTIC TESTS FOR HEMOCHROMATOSIS

Transferrin Saturation

An elevated transferrin saturation has a sensitivity of greater than 90% for hemochromatosis in family studies. The sensitivity of transferrin saturation is lower in population-screening studies designed to detect C282Y homozygotes (genotypic case definition) and can be in the normal range in young female homozygotes.

Unsaturated Iron Binding Capacity

The unsaturated iron binding capacity (UIBC) is a one-step colorimetric assay that is used in many reference laboratories to calculate the transferrin saturation. It is an inexpensive test compared to transferrin saturation and performs as well as transferrin saturation at the lower cost.

Serum Ferritin

The relationship between serum ferritin and total body iron stores was clearly established by strong correlations with hepatic iron concentration and the amount of iron removed by venesection. However, ferritin can be elevated secondary to chronic inflammation and histiocytic neoplasms. A major diagnostic dilemma in the past was whether the serum ferritin was related to hemochromatosis or another underlying liver disease such as alcoholic liver disease, chronic viral hepatitis, or nonalcoholic steatohepatitis. It is likely that most of these difficult cases can now be resolved by genetic testing.

Liver Biopsy

Liver biopsy was previously the gold standard diagnostic test for hemochromatosis; however, it has shifted from a major diagnostic tool to a method of estimating prognosis and concomitant disease. The need for liver biopsy seems less clear now in the young asymptomatic C282Y homozygote where there is a low clinical suspicion of cirrhosis based on history, physical examination, and liver biochemistry. A large study conducted in France and Canada suggested that C282Y homozygotes with a serum ferritin of less than 1000 µg/L, a normal aspartate transaminase (AST), and without hepatomegaly have a very low risk of cirrhosis. C282Y homozygotes with a ferritin greater than 1000 µg/L, an elevated AST, and a platelet count less than 200,000 have a 80% chance of having cirrhosis. Patients with cirrhosis have a 5.5-fold relative risk of death compared to the noncirrhotic hemochromatosis patients. Cirrhotic patients are also at increased risk of hepatocellular carcinoma. Although early detection is clearly demonstrated by serial ultrasound and α-fetoprotein determination, curative treatment options remain limited. Liver biopsy is considered in typical C282Y homozygotes with liver dysfunction and in potentially iron-overloaded patients without the typical C282Y mutation. Simple C282Y heterozygotes, compound heterozygotes (C282Y/H63D), H63D homozygotes, and patients with other risk factors (e.g., alcohol abuse, chronic viral hepatitis) with moderate to severe iron overload (ferritin > 1000 µg/L) may be considered for liver biopsy. Prior to genetic testing, hepatic iron concentration was useful in the diagnosis of hemochromatosis. The hepatic iron concentration (µmol/g) divided by age (years) is the hepatic iron index. The hepatic iron index becomes less useful with the advent of genetic testing. It remains a tool to aid clinicians with their clinical judgment about an individual case. It is most useful in the unusual hemochromatosis patient who is negative by conventional genetic testing but clinically seems to have genetic hemochromatosis.

Genetic Testing for Hemochromatosis

A major advance stemming from the discovery of the hemochromatosis gene is the use of a diagnostic genetic test. Most studies report that more than 90% of typical hemochromatosis patients were homozygotes for the C282Y mutation. A second minor mutation, H63D, was also described in the original report. Compound heterozygotes (C282Y/H63D) and, less commonly, H63D homozygotes resemble C282Y homozygotes with mild to moderate iron overload. Genetic mutations involving ferroportin, hemojuvelin, transferrin repector-2, ceruloplasmin, and hepcidin are associated with iron overload. It is likely that as more mutations are found, they will only be relevant to a minority of patients. There are patients with clinical pictures indistinguishable from genetic hemochromatosis that are negative for the C282Y mutation. Most of these patients are isolated cases, although a few cases of familial iron overload were reported with negative C282Y testing. A negative C282Y test should alert the physician to question the diagnosis of genetic hemochromatosis and reconsider secondary iron overload related to cirrhosis, alcohol, viral hepatitis, or iron-loading anemias. If no other risk factors are found, the patient should begin venesection treatment similar to any other hemochromatosis patient. The interpretation of the genetic test in several settings is shown in Box 1. Genetic discrimination is a concern with the widespread use of genetic testing. In the case of hemochromatosis, the advantages of early diagnosis of a treatable disease outweigh the disadvantages of genetic discrimination.

FAMILY STUDIES IN HEMOCHROMATOSIS

Once the proband case is identified and confirmed with the genetic test for the C282Y mutation, family testing is imperative. Siblings have a 1 in 4 chance of carrying the gene and should be screened with the genetic test (C282Y and H63D mutation), transferrin saturation, and serum ferritin. A cost-effective strategy now possible with the genetic test is to test the spouse for the C282Y mutation to assess the risk in the children. If the spouse is not a C282Y heterozygote or homozygote, the children will be obligate heterozygotes. This assumes paternity and excludes another gene or mutation causing hemochromatosis. This strategy is particularly advantageous where the children are geographically separated or in different health care systems.

TREATMENT OF HEMOCHROMATOSIS

The therapy of hemochromatosis continues to use the medieval therapy of periodic bleeding. At our center, patients attend an ambulatory care facility, and the venesections are performed by a nurse using a kit containing a 16-gauge straight needle and collection bag.* Blood is removed with the patient in the reclining position over 15 to 30 minutes. A hemoglobin is done at the time of each venesection. If the hemoglobin decreased to less than 10 g/dL the venesection schedule is modified

---

*Blood Pack MR6102, Baxter, Deerfield, IL

 CURRENT THERAPY

- Iron overload from hemochromatosis is treated by the weekly removal of 500 mL of blood until the serum ferritin is in the low normal range of approximately 50 µg/L.
- Some patients will require maintenance therapy of three to four phlebotomies per year. In some countries this can be a voluntary blood donation.
- Excess alcohol, high doses of vitamin C, and iron supplementation should be avoided, but strict dietary restrictions are not recommended.
- Siblings and children of patients should be tested for hemochromatosis with transferrin saturation, ferritin, and genetic testing.

Abbreviation: UIBC = Unsaturated iron binding capacity.

Rakel and Bope: *Conn's Current Therapy 2006.*

BOX 1 Interpretation of Genetic Testing for Hemochromatosis

C282Y Homozygote

This is the classic genetic pattern seen in more than 90% of typical cases. Expression of disease ranges from no evidence of iron overload to massive iron overload with organ dysfunction. Siblings have a 1 in 4 chance of being affected and should have genetic testing. For children to be affected, the other parent must be at least a heterozygote. If iron studies are normal, false-positive genetic testing or a nonexpressing homozygote should be considered.

C282Y/H63D – Compound Heterozygote

This patient carries one copy of the major mutation and one copy of the minor mutation. Most patients with this genetic pattern have normal iron studies. A small percentage of compound heterozygotes are found to have mild to moderate iron overload. Severe iron overload is usually seen in the setting of another concomitant risk factor (e.g., alcoholism, viral hepatitis).

C282Y Heterozygote

This patient carries one copy of the major mutation. This pattern in seen in approximately 10% of the white population and is usually associated with normal iron studies. In rare cases, the iron studies are high in the range expected in a homozygote rather than a heterozygote. These cases may carry an unknown hemochromatosis mutation, and liver biopsy is helpful to determine the need for venesection therapy.

H63D Homozyote

This patient carries two copies of the minor mutation. Most patients with this genetic pattern have normal iron studies. A small percentage of these cases have mild to moderate iron overload. Severe iron overload is usually seen in the setting of another concomitant risk factor (e.g., alcoholism, viral hepatitis).

H63D Heterozygote

This patient carries one copy of the minor mutation. This pattern is seen in approximately 20% of the white population and is usually associated with normal iron studies. This pattern is so common in the general population that the presence of iron overload can be related to another risk factor. Liver biopsy is required to determine the cause of the iron overload and the need for treatment in these cases.

No *HFE* Mutations

If iron overload is present without any *HFE* mutations, a careful history for other risk factors must be reviewed, and liver biopsy can be useful to determine the cause of the iron overload and the need for treatment. Most of these cases are isolated, nonfamilial cases. There are cases described with genetic mutations in ferroportin, hemojuvelin, transferrin receptor-2, ceruloplasmin, and hepcidin genes. These genetic tests are not widely available.

Abbreviations: HFE = hemochromatosis gene.

6

to 500 mL every other week. Venesections are continued until the serum ferritin is approximately 50 µg/L. The concomitant administration of a salt-containing sport beverage (e.g., Gatorade) is a simple method of maintaining plasma volume during the venesection. Maintenance venesections after iron depletion of three to four venesections per year are done in most patients, although the rate of iron reaccumulation is highly variable. The transferrin saturation will remain elevated in many treated patients and will not normalize unless the patient becomes iron deficient. In some countries, patients with mild iron abnormalities are encouraged to become voluntary blood donors.

Chelation therapy with desferrioxamine[1] is not recommended for hemochromatosis. Patients are advised to avoid oral iron therapy and alcohol abuse, but there are no dietary restrictions. Patient support groups are

---

[1]Not FDA approved for this indication.

 CURRENT DIAGNOSIS

- Consider the diagnosis.
- Initial testing is transferrin saturation or UIBC and serum ferritin.
- Secondary testing is the C282Y genetic test.
- If the genetic test is not typical, reassess the diagnosis.
- Not all patients need a liver biopsy.
- Siblings are at highest risk in a family study.

discouraged by the practice of iron fortification of foods, but much of this iron is in an inexpensive form with poor bioavailability.

POPULATION SCREENING FOR HEMOCHROMATOSIS

Early diagnosis and treatment of hemochromatosis leads to a long-term survival rate similar to the general population. Many prospective and retrospective studies demonstrate that genetic mutations are much more common than clinical illness, and many C282Y homozygotes do not develop progressive iron overload. The natural history of untreated disease remains the most difficult component in an assessment of the cost effectiveness of screening, and it is unlikely to be resolved because of ethical concerns about withholding therapy. Targeted screening in high risk groups, improved physician and patient education initiatives, and extended family studies are more likely to be considered than mass population screening.

Hemochromatosis is a common and often underdiagnosed disease. Early diagnosis and treatment results in an excellent long-term prognosis. The development of a diagnostic genetic test improved the feasibility of the goal of prevention of morbidity and mortality from hemochromatosis.

REFERENCES

Adams PC, Reboussin DM, Barton JC, et al: Hemochromatosis and iron overload screening (HEIRS) study: screening in a racially diverse of primary care population. N Engl J Med 2005. 352: 1769-1778.

Adams P, Zaccaro D, Moses G, et al: A comparison of the unsaturated iron binding capacity of transferrin saturation as a screening test to detect C282Y homozygotes for hemochromatosis in 101,168 participants in the HEIRS study. Hepatology 2004;40:232A.

Andersen R, Tybjaerg-Hansen A, Appleyard M, et al: Hemochromatosis mutations in the general population: Iron overload progression rate. Blood 2004;103:2914-2919.

Beaton M, Guyader D, Deugnier Y, et al: Non-invasive prediction of cirrhosis in C282Y-linked hemochromatosis. Hepatology 2002;36: 673-678.

Beutler E, Felitti V, Koziol J, et al: Penetrance of the 845G to A (C282Y) HFE hereditary haemochromatosis mutation in the USA. Lancet 2002;359:211-218.

Guyader D, Jacquelinet C, Moirand R, et al: Non-invasive prediction of fibrosis in C282Y homozygous hemochromatosis. Gastroenterology 1998;115:929-936.

Pietrangelo A: Hereditary hemochromatosis: A new look at an old disease. N Engl J Med 2004;350:2383-2397.

Powell L, Dixon J, Ramm G, et al: The penetrance of HFE-associated hemochromatosis as assessed by clinical evaluation and liver biopsy in subjects identified by health checks, family screening and population screening. Hepatology 2004;40:574A.

Wojcik J, Speechley M, Kertesz A, et al: Natural history of C282Y homozygotes for haemochromatosis. Can J Gastroenterol 2002;16:297-302.

Hodgkin's Disease: Chemotherapy

Method of
David J. Straus, MD

The use of radiotherapy and chemotherapy for Hodgkin's disease is one of the major success stories in medical oncology. An understanding of the clinical features and course of the disease aided this success. Extended field radiation therapy (EF RT), introduced nearly 40 years ago by Kaplan, was a major advance in the treatment of patients with early-stage Hodgkin's disease. DeVita and colleagues introduced combination chemotherapy to the treatment of advanced stages of Hodgkin's disease in the mid 1960s, and this was the second major advance in treatment. Combinations of chemotherapy with radiation therapy were widely used during the past 20 years, and further improvements in outcome were seen with this approach, particularly in patients with early stages of Hodgkin's disease. More recently, chemotherapy alone was employed for many patients with excellent results. Less late toxicity may be seen in patients cured of their Hodgkin's disease with reduction in the amount of radiation therapy in combination with chemotherapy, or its complete elimination when it is not required.

Histopathology

Currently, the Rye modification of the Lukes and Butler classification is in use throughout the world. The *lymphocyte predominant* subtype is characterized by an abundance of small lymphocytes with occasional, often atypical, Reed-Sternberg (R-S) cells of lymphocytic-histiocytic variety (L and H or popcorn cells) with vesicular, polylobulated nuclei and small nucleoli. Unlike the other forms Hodgkin's disease, the atypical cells usually have B-cell antigens (CD19,20,22,79a). The growth pattern is usually nodular, although less commonly, a diffuse pattern may be seen. The classic presentation is in a high cervical node in a young asymptomatic male. It is associated with a favorable prognosis, although late recurrences have been reported in some series.

Nodular sclerosis is the most common subtype in North America and Western Europe. There is often abundant fibrosis in the node dividing tumor nodules containing inflammatory cells and the "lacunar cell" variant of R-S cells with a clear area surrounding the cells. The typical presentation is in a young female with mediastinal involvement with or without symptoms. Although it has classically been felt to carry a relatively favorable prognosis, this seems to be dependent on the stage of the disease, the bulkiness of the tumor masses, and the presence or absence of systemic symptoms. The new World Health Organization (WHO) classification of neoplastic diseases of the hematopoietic and lymphoid tissues adds two histologic grades of nodular sclerosis Hodgkin's disease according to the British National Lymphoma Investigation criteria (grade 1, few R-S cells; grade 2, many R-S cells). Some studies demonstrated a worse outcome associated with grade 2 cases, and others showed no difference in outcome. For now, the grading is not required for clinical purposes but should be the subject of future investigations.

Mixed cellularity is characterized by a pleomorphic cellular infiltrate of plasma cells, eosinophils, lymphocytes, histiocytes, and R-S cells. Subdiaphragmatic and extranodal presentations and the presence of B systems may be somewhat more frequent than with the nodular sclerosis subtype. It is the second most common histologic subtype in North America and Western Europe and is more common in the poorer parts of the world and among indigent populations in this country. It is also somewhat more common among older patients. It has been associated with a worse prognosis than nodular sclerosis, but this may be because of the association of this subtype with the unfavorable clinical prognostic features.

The lymphocyte depletion subtype has a paucity of cellular elements and an increased reticular network. It is associated with advanced age, systemic symptoms, retroperitoneal lymphadenopathy, and extranodal involvement. It is a diagnosis that is now made infrequently because modern immunophenotyping and molecular genetic studies have demonstrated that many cases formerly thought to be lymphocyte depletion Hodgkin's disease are actually T-cell non-Hodgkin's lymphomas. Lymphocyte depletion Hodgkin's disease has the worst prognosis of the four histologic subtypes.

The R-S cells, in the cases of nodular sclerosis, mixed cellularity, and lymphocyte depletion Hodgkin's disease, carry the CD30 surface antigen, an antigen that is expressed on activated and proliferating lymphocytes.

They also stain with antibodies to CD15, more commonly a myeloid marker. Recent cloning of this molecule has enabled its identification as a new member of the tumor necrosis factor (TNF) receptor superfamily. Single cell polymerase chain reaction (PCR) of classic R-S cells literally scraped from slides shows a follicular center B-cell origin for these cells with clonally rearranged but crippled V heavy chain genes presumably leading to a block in apoptosis.

The R-S–like cells in the nodular variant of lymphocyte predominant Hodgkin's disease are weakly reactive or nonreactive with antibodies to CD30, and, unlike those in the other Hodgkin's disease subtypes, demonstrate a mature B-cell marker phenotype with CD20 and also pan-lymphocyte antigen (CD45, leukocyte common antigen) expression. Molecular genetic studies also have demonstrated the clonal B-cell origin of the nodular variant of lymphocyte predominant Hodgkin's disease. The R-S cells of the diffuse variant of lymphocyte predominant Hodgkin's disease have the phenotypic features of classic R-S cells.

Staging

The current staging classification was established by the Ann Arbor Workshop in 1971. There are both clinical staging (CS), which consists of all staging procedures short of staging laparotomy, and pathologic staging (PS), which refers to the findings at staging laparotomy during which liver biopsies, splenectomy, and excisional biopsies of retroperitoneal nodes are performed. Staging laparotomies are performed infrequently at the present time because fewer patients are treated with radiation therapy alone and more patients with systemic treatment with chemotherapy alone or in combination with radiation therapy.

The Ann Arbor classification divides Hodgkin's disease into four stages: Stage I refers to disease limited to a single lymph node or lymph node group. Stage II refers to disease in two or more noncontiguous lymph node groups and/or spleen on the same side of the diaphragm. Stage III refers to disease in two or more lymph node groups and/or spleen on both sides of the diaphragm. Stage IV refers to disease in extranodal sites, usually lung, liver, bone or bone marrow, and more rarely other sites. Extranodal involvement by extension from lymph node disease to such sites as the lung, bone, pleura, or skin may occur in stages IE and is not considered to increase the stage to IV. Such disease is designated by a subscript E (IE, IIE, IIIE). For each stage, the absence of systemic symptoms is designated by the suffix A, whereas the presence of unexplained fevers to 38°C (100.4°F) or higher, night sweats, and/or weight loss greater than 10% over 6 months is designated by a B suffix. In general, the prognosis worsens with higher stage, and, within each stage, the presence of symptoms (B) carries a worse prognosis than absence of such symptoms (A). A mediastinal tumor greater than one third of the thoracic diameter or lymph node disease greater than 10 cm is defined as bulky; a subscript X is added to the numerical stage if such disease is present

(e.g., I_xB, II_xA, II_xB, III_xA, III_xB). Stage IIIA1 refers to subdiaphragmatic disease in spleen and/or high abdominal node, whereas IIIA2 indicates disease in lower retroperitoneal nodes.

Staging procedures include chest radiograph, computerized tomography (CT) of the chest, abdomen, and pelvis with oral and intravenous contrast, complete blood counts with platelet and differential counts, bone marrow aspiration and biopsy, serum liver biochemistries including alkaline phosphatase, and erythrocyte sedimentation rate. The latter test has been shown to carry prognostic significance. A CT of the abdomen and pelvis will show enlarged retroperitoneal, mesenteric, and pelvic lymph nodes that are involved by disease.

If there are masses in the liver on CT scan, positron emission tomography (PET) scan, or liver-spleen scintigram or if there are gross abnormalities of serum liver biochemical studies, a liver biopsy should be performed under CT-guided or laparoscopic visualization if the masses are accessible. Slight elevations of serum alkaline phosphatase may be seen without liver involvement.

Gallium 67 scanning is a useful imaging procedure for following mediastinal disease, but it can be associated with false negatives and false positives. It is of value in the decision of whether to biopsy a residual mass following treatment to determine the presence or absence of residual disease. A PET scan provides similar and even more detailed information. $[^{18}F]$fluoro-2-deoxy-D-glucose (FDG) PET scanning is useful in predicting recurrences in residual masses following treatment for Hodgkin's disease. False-negative studies are less common (the negative predictive value is 95%) than false-positive studies (the positive predictive value is 60%).

A CT of the chest may show disease, particularly retrosternal disease, missed by a plain chest radiograph. Also, some patients with bulky mediastinal and hilar nodal disease will have peripheral lung nodules that can only be detected by chest CT. Although traditional radiotherapy treatment seems rarely affected by these findings, CT does allow for refinements in radiotherapy treatment planning.

Treatment

STAGES IA/B AND IIA/B, NONBULKY

The work of Gilbert, Peters, and, later, Kaplan demonstrated that recurrences rarely occur within the treated lymph node areas with doses of radiation therapy (RT) to 3500 to 4500 cGy. The use of the linear accelerator made it possible to deliver these doses to large fields. The *mantle* port (cervical, supraclavicular, mediastinal, and axillary regions—an area like the mantle on a suit of armor) and the *inverted Y* port (para-aortic nodes, spleen [if not removed], splenic pedicle, and iliac, inguinal, and femoral nodes) and combinations of the two were developed in the 1960s. Total lymphoid irradiation (TLI) refers to combinations of the two that have also at times included low dose irradiation of liver and lung. Subtotal lymphoid irradiation (STLI) includes the mantle port with irradiation of para-aortic nodes, splenic pedicle, and spleen if it was not removed.

Local irradiation is probably adequate for high-cervical-stage IA disease and lymphocyte-predominant or nodular sclerosis histology in a young patient. Lymphocyte-predominant Hodgkin's disease is often clinically localized, is usually effectively treated with irradiation alone, and may relapse late (a clinical feature reminiscent of low-grade lymphoma). The 15-year disease-specific survival is excellent (>90%).

There is also general agreement that bulky mediastinal disease with a mediastinal mass diameter more than one third of the chest diameter should be treated with combined modality treatment with chemotherapy and RT. Recently some groups have treated selected patients with bulky mediastinal masses whose disease is well defined on CT scan with RT only using ports designed with the aid of the CT scan.

The prognostic importance of contiguous extension of disease from hilar nodes into the lung parenchyma is controversial. Some centers employing radiotherapy only report good results using low dose irradiation also administered to the entire affected lung aided by thin lung blocks. However, these patients are usually treated with combined chemotherapy and less complex involved field RT (IF RT).

The European Organization for Research and Treatment of Cancer (EORTC) found elevations of erythrocyte sedimentation rate (ESR) (>50 mm/hour for stages IA and IIA, >30 mm/hour for stages IB and IIB) to be a powerful adverse prognostic factor among patients treated with RT only. However, this is not an adverse prognostic factor for patients treated with chemotherapy or combined modality treatment.

There are several treatment options for the majority of patients with stages IA and IIA Hodgkin's disease.

Subtotal lymphoid irradiation, which can include the spleen, to doses of at least 3500 cGy in $3^1/_2$ weeks has resulted in complete remission (CR) percentage in excess of 90% with a 20% to 40% relapse rate in pathologically staged patients, probably depending upon radiotherapy technique and/or patient selection. The likelihood of salvage of these patients into a second durable CR may be in excess of 50%. This approach is rarely employed because of the long-term potential toxicities of extensive RT, and the lower relapse rates seen after treatment with combined modality treatment or chemotherapy alone.

Combination chemotherapy alone and when combined with radiotherapy has resulted in a CR percentage of greater than 90% with a relapse rate of approximately 10% or less. This was achieved in the past with six cycles of chemotherapy with MOPP (mechlorethamine [nitrogen mustard], vincristine [Oncovin], procarbazine, and prednisone) or similar regimens.

When radiotherapy is also used, fewer cycles of chemotherapy may give similar results. A protocol at Memorial Hospital randomized patients to four cycles of either MOPP or thiotepa, bleomycin, and vinblastine (TBV) combined with modified extended field RT. The results with a median follow-up time of 65 months (7 to 96 months) were similar in both arms of this trial and also similar to the results achieved with six cycles of MOPP and similar radiotherapy.

Two French studies suggest that three cycles of MOPP may be sufficient in combination with radiotherapy. The H8-F trial of the EORTC demonstrated the superiority of three cycles of a MOPP/Adriamycin (doxorubicin), bleomycin, and vincristine/vinblastine (ABV) hybrid plus IF RT (36-40 Gy) (4-year, treatment failure-free survival [TTFS] rate 99%) to EF RT at the same dose (TTFS rate 77%, $P < 0.001$) in favorable early stage Hodgkin's disease.

The Southwest Oncology Group (SWOG) demonstrated a superior failure-free survival for three cycles of doxorubicin and vinblastine plus STLI (94%) as compared to STLI alone (81%, $P < .001$). The German Hodgkin's Lymphoma Study Group HD-7 study compared two cycles of doxorubicin, bleomycin, vinblastine, and dacarbazine (ABVD) plus EF RT (30 Gy)/IF RT boost (10 Gy) to EF RT (30 Gy)/IF RT (10 Gy) in favorable stage I and II patients. The freedom from treatment failure was 96% for combined modality treatment compared to 84% for EF RT alone.

From February 1990 to July 1996, in a randomized trial of patients with clinically staged early Hodgkin's disease (I bulky and/or B; IIA, IIA bulky, and IIEA), a comparison was made of four cycles of ABVD followed by STLI, versus the same regimen followed by IF RT. There were 136 patients assessable, with the main characteristics fairly well balanced between the two arms. After a median follow-up of 87 months (range 8 to 123), treatment outcome was as follows: complete remission 100% after ABVD plus STLI versus 97% after ABVD plus IF RT; FFP 97% versus 94%, and total survival 93% versus 94%, respectively. These results indicate that four cycles of ABVD followed by IF RT can achieve results comparable to the same regimen followed by extensive RT. This effective and safe regimen can be considered to be a standard option for most patients with early-stage Hodgkin's disease.

The results of a randomized trial from Memorial Hospital of chemotherapy with ABVD alone or combined with RT in clinical stages I, II, and IIIA disease without bulky mediastinal or peripheral nodal involvement has been recently reported. Although this trial was not statistically powered to show equivalence of the two treatment approaches, no differences in CR percentage, freedom from progression, or overall survival were seen. The results of a randomized phase III trial of standard treatment (STLI, favorable; two cycles of ABVD plus STLI, unfavorable) versus experimental treatment (four to six cycles of ABVD alone) in stage IA and IIA patients without high risk factors was recently reported from the National Cancer Institute of Canada Clinical Trial Group (NCIC-CTG) and the Eastern Cooperative Oncology Group (ECOG). The estimated progression-free survival (PFS) was 93% for the patients on the standard treatment arm and 87% for those in the experimental treatment arm, a result that was statistically significant. There was no difference in overall survival. Somewhat less than 30% of patients on the experimental arm received four cycles of ABVD alone, although it is not clear that an excess of relapses were seen in this group. In view of the high rate of salvage-ability of patients who might relapse after this type of chemotherapy, and the late morbidity of treatment that is mostly attributable to RT, the clinical meaning of a 6% difference in PFS is unclear. On the basis of these results, chemotherapy alone with six cycles of ABVD alone, which is more standard than four cycles, for non-bulky early stage Hodgkin's disease, is also a treatment option, although, as mentioned earlier, there may be a slightly higher risk of relapse.

STAGES II$_X$, III, AND IV

The major advance for patients with advanced Hodgkin's disease came from the use of MOPP by DeVita and colleagues. Eighty-four percent of 188 patients achieved a CR, and 66% of these were free of disease for more than 10 years. Ninety percent of these patients had stage IIIB or IVB disease. There are many modifications of the MOPP regimen that achieved similar results.

The groups at Memorial Hospital and at the National Tumor Institute in Milan pioneered the use of alternating potentially non–cross-resistant drug combinations and low-dose RT. Santoro, Bonadonna, and their colleagues developed the ABVD combination and demonstrated similar CR percentages as seen with MOPP. Also, it was demonstrated that at least some patients relapsing after MOPP could be put into second remissions, although the duration of these remissions is not as long as with primary treatment. They suggested that the ABVD combination might be potentially non–cross-resistant with MOPP in that tumors resistant to MOPP might be sensitive to ABVD.

Following this suggestion, a program of alternating monthly MOPP and ABVD combined with reduced-dose RT was developed at Memorial Hospital. Adjuvant reduced-dose RT to the initially involved bulky lymph node regions was employed to prevent relapses in these areas. A protocol was designed in 1975 in which MOPP and ABVD were alternated monthly for eight cycles in combination with reduced-dose RT to bulky sites In 1979, a new trial was started in which MOPP/ABVD/RT (8-drug regimen) was randomized against three alternating potentially non–cross-resistant combinations (10-drug regimen) and RT. The third combination was lomustine (CCNU), melphalan (Alkeran), and vindesine (DVA), following the demonstration of activity of vindesine alone and in this combination for relapsed patients. The same reduced dose RT was administered as in the initial trial.

The results for the initial 8 drug/RT protocol and the subsequent 8 drug/RT versus 10 drug/RT protocol were the same. Between 1975 and 1988, 270 patients were treated with either two or three alternating drug combinations and low-dose RT. Two hundred twenty-two patients (82%) achieved a CR, 38 (14%) a PR, and 10 (4%) progressed. At 10 years, the relapse-free survival for the patients achieving a CR was 80%, overall survival was 74%, and progression-free survival was 70%. The relapse-free survival for CS IIB patients was 89% and at 10 years was 73% each for CS IIIB and IV patients.

Similar results have been achieved in a number of trials with alternating monthly chemotherapy with or without RT. The cancer and acute leukemia group B (CALGB) conducted a randomized trial in patients with stages IIIA2, IIIB, and IV disease with assignment to MOPP, ABVD, or alternating MOPP/ABVD. Response and failure-free survival rates were superior for both MOPP/ABVD and ABVD as compared with MOPP alone. Similar results have also been achieved using a compressed schedule hybrid approach in which the nitrogen mustard and vincristine are given on day 1 along with oral procarbazine, prednisone, doxorubicin, bleomycin and vinblastine on day 8 (MOPP/ABV hybrid). Recently, the results of an intergroup (CALGB, Southwest Oncology Group [SWOG], ECOG, NCIC-CTG) randomized trial established ABVD as equivalent in treatment outcome to MOPP/ABV hybrid with less acute toxicity, myelodysplastic syndrome, and leukemia.

A number of short-course, dose-intense chemotherapy regimens combined with RT were introduced over the past decade. The Stanford V is a 12-week chemotherapy program consisting of doxorubicin, vinblastine, bleomycin, nitrogen mustard, vincristine, etoposide,[1] and prednisone followed by RT to bulky sites (adenopathy = 5 cm, macroscopic splenic nodules). In a phase 2 trial conducted by ECOG in 47 patients with bulky mediastinal stage I/II or stages III/IV disease, the FFP was 85% and overall survival 96% at 5 years. Grade 3 or 4 neutropenia was seen in 59% of patients, and there was one acute monocytic leukemia. This regimen is strongly dependent on the RT to achieve maximal results.

The German Hodgkin's Lymphoma Study Group conducted a three-arm randomized trial, using a combination of bleomycin, etoposide, Adriamycin (doxorubicin), cyclophosphamide, vincristine, and prednisone (BEACOPP) versus dose-escalated BEACOPP with aid of granulocyte colony-stimulating factor (G-CSF) versus cyclophosphamide, Oncovin (vincristine), procarbazine, and prednisone (COPP)/ABVD (× 8). After chemotherapy, RT was administered to initially bulky nodal sites or sites of residual disease. The freedom from treatment failure rates at 5 years were 69% for COPP/ABVD, 76% for standard BEACOPP, and 87% for dose-escalated BEACOPP ($P < 0.001$ for COPP/ABVD vs. dose-escalated BEACOPP). The 5-year survival rates were 83% for COPP/ABVD, 88% for standard BEACOPP, and 91% for dose-escalated BEACOPP ($P = 0.002$ for COPP/ABVD vs. dose-escalated BEACOPP). There was a considerable amount of acute toxicity including grade 4 neutropenia in 90% of patients and grade 4 thrombocytopenia in 47% with dose-escalated BEACOPP. The rate of secondary acute leukemias at 5 years was 2.5%, significantly higher than in the other two arms of the trial. The toxicity of this regimen and the possibility of successful salvage of resistant or relapsed patients after ABVD have somewhat tempered the enthusiasm for its use in this country.

However, another randomized trial showed a benefit for a conventional hybrid regimen over a shortened

---

[1]Not FDA approved for this indication.

dose-intensified regimen using doxorubicin, cyclophosphamide, etoposide, vincristine, bleomycin, and prednisone (VAPEC-B) versus chlorambucil, vinblastine, procarbazine, prednisone/etoposide, vinblastine, and doxorubicin (ChlVPP/EVA) hybrid: A British and Italian cooperative trial of 225 patients with bulky or stage B I and II or stages III and IV were randomized to either 11 weekly cycles of VAPEC-B or ChlVPP/EVA hybrid. This trial also included RT to initial bulky nodal sites or sites of residual disease after chemotherapy. At a median follow-up time of 25 months, there was almost a three times increased progression rate in VAPEC-B arm as compared with the ChlVPP/EVA hybrid arm.

Until recently, our policy was to administer adjuvant RT to all initially involved lymph node sites, whether or not they are bulky, in combination with alternating chemotherapy regimens for patients with advanced stages of Hodgkin's disease. The results of a large definitive randomized trial conducted by the EORTC showed no benefit to IF RT in patients achieving a CR after six to eight cycles of MOPP/ABV hybrid in patients with stages III and IV Hodgkin's disease, although a benefit for RT was seen in patients who only achieved a PR. At a median follow-up time of more than 6 years, there was an excess of deaths because of other causes including secondary malignancies approaching statistical significance in the group of patients in CR who received IF RT.

The issue of combined modality treatment as opposed to chemotherapy alone in most patients is being further addressed in a phase III randomized trial of short-course, intensive chemotherapy combined with involved field RT with the Stanford V regimen versus ABVD with RT only to bulky mediastinal sites in patients with locally extensive or stages III/IV Hodgkin's disease that is being conducted by ECOG and CALGB.

Based on the results with alternating chemotherapy with CS IIB, IIIB, and IV patients, a prognostic model was constructed in which five pretreatment characteristics emerged as having adverse prognostic importance in a multivariable analysis:

1. Low hematocrit
2. High-serum lactic acid dehydrogenase (LDH)
3. Older than age 45 years
4. Inguinal node involvement (a reflection of extensive subdiaphragmatic disease)
5. Bulky mediastinal disease greater than 0.45 of the thoracic diameter

Approximately 60% of the patients had none or only one of these adverse factors, and their survival was greater than 95%. Patients with two or more of these factors had a dramatically inferior survival rate. The utility of this model has been confirmed by others.

Hasenclever and Diehl for the International Prognostic Factors Project on advanced Hodgkin's disease published a prognostic model based on a retrospective analysis of 1618 patients from 25 centers. In the final model, seven factors were used:

1. Albumin less than 4 g/dL
2. Hemoglobin (Hgb) less than 10.5 g/dL
3. Male sex
4. Stage IV
5. Age ≥45 years
6. White blood cell (WBC) count ≥15,000 mm^3
7. Lymphocyte count less than 600 mm^3 or less than 8% of WBC

The worst prognostic group (7% = five, six, or seven factors) had a 5-year overall survival (OS) of 56% and a FFP of 42%. This model does not separate out a group with a very poor prognosis. A recently made comparison of seven prognostic models for Hodgkin's disease was retrospectively applied to 516 patients with advanced Hodgkin's disease. Three models were found to be the most predictive of outcome: the International Prognostic Factors Project Index (employing albumin, hemoglobin, gender, stage, age, WBC, and lymphocyte count), the Memorial Sloan-Kettering Cancer Center model (employing age, L-lactate dehydrogenase [LDH], hematocrit, inguinal nodal involvement, and mediastinal mass bulk), and the International Database on Hodgkin's disease (employing stage, age, B symptoms, albumin, and gender). Integration of the three models in a linear model improved their predictive power: Between 19% and 25% of patients fell into groups with either a 10% or a 50% risk of failure.

Salvage Treatment

Because of the high relapse rates seen following conventional salvage chemotherapy after primary chemotherapy, most groups are using high-dose chemotherapy with or without RT depending on the prior treatment with autologous bone marrow or peripheral stem cell rescue. The results are promising in selected patients with more than half the patients achieving remission of varying durations transplanted in second or subsequent remission. Results of high dose chemoradiotherapy with autologous stem cell transplantation in 65 patients with relapsed or refractory Hodgkin's disease treated between 1994 and 1998 at Memorial Sloan-Kettering Cancer Center have been recently reported. At a median follow-up time of 43 months, estimates of the proportion of patients alive are 73% and event-free are 58% by intent-to-treat analysis. In a multivariable logistic regression model, there were three adverse prognostic factors: extranodal sites of relapse or refractory disease, complete remission duration of less than 1 year, or refractory disease and B symptoms. Patients with zero or one adverse factor had an OS of 90% and an event-free survival (EFS) of 83%. Patients with two adverse factors had an OS of 57% and an EFS of 27%, and those with three adverse factors had an OS of 25% and an EFS of 10%.

Toxicity

Most long-term toxicity of chemotherapy seems to be related to alkylating agent and procarbazine-containing regimens of the MOPP type. There is approximately a 3% lifetime risk of acute leukemia following MOPP-type chemotherapy. Among solid tumors, only alkylating agent–based regimens are associated with an increased risk of lung cancer. Azoospermia occurs in approximately 80% of men treated with six cycles of MOPP, and another 10% are rendered oligospermic. Sperm banking with cryopreservation is encouraged for male patients who may wish to have children in the future. Female patients younger than 30 years of age are less likely to become permanently infertile than those older than 30 years of age. The risks of infertility and secondary myelodysplastic syndromes or acute leukemias are less with ABVD than with MOPP-type regimens.

Vascular damage to coronary and peripheral arteries is a concern with RT. Carotid stenosis risk is increased after cervical RT. Patients who receive mantle field RT have a threefold increased risk of fatal myocardial infarction. Heart-valve fibrosis requiring surgical replacement, and more subtle abnormalities such as restrictive cardiomyopathy and conduction abnormalities have also been reported following mediastinal RT. The actuarial risk of second malignancies is 22% to 27% at 25 to 30 years following treatment for Hodgkin's disease. Most of this risk seems to be related to RT.

Neuromuscular problems are another late complication related to RT. Neck muscle atrophy resulting in neck pain and difficulty in neck extension occurs in some patients. Symptomatic radiation pulmonary and pericardial fibrosis and brachial plexopathies occur, but less frequently than in the past with current RT techniques. Secondary hypothyroidism is usually manageable with thyroid replacement therapy.

Pulmonary toxicity from bleomycin treatment is a problem with the ABVD regimen. The major nonhematologic toxicity is pulmonary and related to bleomycin.

CURRENT THERAPY

- Clinical stages I and II without bulky disease— Four cycles of ABVD with IF RT or six cycles of ABVD alone would both be acceptable. Although the equivalence of the outcome of chemotherapy alone to chemotherapy plus RT has not yet been definitively proven, chemotherapy alone would probably reduce the late toxicities of treatment, most of which are related to RT.
- Clinical stages II_xA/II_xB—Six cycles of ABVD plus IF RT or Stanford V
- Clinical stage IIIA—Six cycles of ABVD
- Clinical stages IIIB and IV—Six cycles of ABVD, Stanford V, or BEACOPP regimens
- Relapsed/refractory disease—Salvage chemotherapy followed by high-dose chemotherapy with peripheral blood stem cell support for most cases.

Abbreviations: ABVD = doxorubicin, bleomycin, vinblastine, and dacarbazine; BEACOPP = bleomycin, etoposide, doxorubicin, cyclophosphamide, vincristine, and prednisone; RT = radiation therapy; IF RT = involved field radiation therapy; Stanford V = 12-week chemotherapy program consisting of doxorubicin, vinblastine, bleomycin, nitrogen mustard, vincristine, etoposide,[1] and prednisone followed by RT to bulky sites (adenopathy = 5 cm, macroscopic splenic nodules).
[1]Not FDA approved for this indication.

Rakel and Bope: *Conn's Current Therapy 2006*.

In the trial conducted at Memorial Hospital, 33 patients (22%) discontinued bleomycin because of a decrease in DLCO. Ten of the symptomatic patients received brief courses of corticosteroids, and there was one death because of bleomycin during treatment.

REFERENCES

Adams MJ, Lipsitz SR, Colan SD et al: Cardiovascular status in long-term survivors of Hodgkin's disease treated with chest radiotherapy. J Clin Oncol 22(15);2004:3139-3148.

Aleman BM, Raemaekers JM, Tirelli V, et al: Involved-field radiotherapy for advanced Hodgkin's lymphoma. N Engl J Med 348(24); 2003:2396-2406.

Bhatia S, Yasui Y, Robison LL, et al: High risk of subsequent neoplasms continues with extended follow-up of childhood Hodgkin's disease: report from the Late Effects Study Group. J Clin Oncol 21(23);2003:4386-4394.

Bonadonna G, Bonfante V, Viviani S, et al: ABVD plus subtotal nodal versus involved-field radiotherapy in early-stage Hodgkin's disease: long-term results. J Clin Oncol 22(14);2004:2835-2841.

Diehl V, Franklin J, Pfreundschuh M, et al: Standard and increased-dose BEACOPP chemotherapy compared with COPP-ABVD for advanced Hodgkin's disease. N Engl J Med 348(24);2003: 2386-2395.

Hasenclever D, Diehl V: A prognostic score for advanced Hodgkin's disease. International Prognostic Factors Project on Advanced Hodgkin's Disease. N Engl J Med 339(21);1998:1506-1514.

Horning SJ, Hoppe RT, Breslin S, et al: Stanford V and radiotherapy for locally extensive and advanced Hodgkin's disease: mature results of a prospective clinical trial. J Clin Oncol 20(3);2002: 630-637.

Hull MC, Morris CG, Pipine CJ, et al: Valvular dysfunction and carotid, subclavian, and coronary artery disease in survivors of Hodgkin lymphoma treated with radiation therapy. JAMA 290(21);2003:2831-2837.

Radford JA, Rohatiner AZ, Ryder WD, et al: ChlVPP/EVA hybrid versus the weekly VAPEC-B regimen for previously untreated Hodgkin's disease. J Clin Oncol 20(13);2002:2988-2994.

Straus DJ, Gaynor JJ, Myers J, et al: Prognostic factors among 185 adults with newly diagnosed advanced Hodgkin's disease treated with alternating potentially noncross-resistant chemotherapy and intermediate-dose radiation therapy. J Clin Oncol 8(7);1990:1173-1186.

Straus DJ, Portlock CS, Qin J, et al: Results of a prospective randomized clinical trial of doxorubicin, bleomycin, vinblastine, and dacarbazine (ABVD) followed by radiation therapy (RT) versus ABVD alone for stages I, II, and IIIA nonbulky Hodgkin disease. Blood 104(12);2004:3483-3489.

Hodgkin's Lymphoma: Role of Radiation Therapy

Method of
Joachim Yahalom, MD

Radiation is considered by many oncologists to be the most effective single agent for the treatment of Hodgkin's lymphoma (HL). Indeed, for several decades, radiation therapy (RT) alone cured most patients with HL who presented in stages I, II, and III. Over the last 25 years, with the advent of effective and safe chemotherapy (CT) for HL, the standard of care has changed, and in recent

6

years most patients with HL are treated with combined modality programs, namely CT followed by radiation to a limited volume of the original and/or residual disease.

Radiation alone remains the treatment of choice for patients with lymphocyte-predominant HL, a less common subtype of HL with a typical early-stage presentation and rare involvement of the mediastinal lymph nodes. Obviously, patients with classical HL (all other subtypes) who are at high risk for complications of CT may still be cured with RT alone, using the traditional principles of RT for HL (extended-field RT).

It is important to emphasize several points that are sometimes ignored in an era when CT is the primary treatment of classical HL:

- RT as a part of a combined modality program is radically different from the extended-field RT that was used in the past as a single modality. The volume that requires RT after CT is significantly smaller, and the RT dose is markedly reduced. Further, the planning and delivery of RT has considerably improved over the last two decades.
- Adding RT not only improves disease control but also allows the administration of shorter and less toxic CT in all stages of HL, including salvage therapy.
- The new *mini-radiotherapy* for HL is well tolerated and unlikely to result in the same extent of long-term morbidities that were associated with wide-field RT, often used as a single therapy for HL in the 1960s through the 1980s.

Lymphocyte-Predominant Hodgkin's Lymphoma

It is important to distinguish between the two well-defined entities of HL: classical HL and the less common nodular lymphocyte-predominant Hodgkin's lymphoma (LPHL). The radiation approach to each entity is different. Most patients with LPHL are potentially curable with radiation alone, whereas combined modality therapy is the standard approach for the majority of patients with classic HL.

Most patients with LPHL (>75%) present at an early stage; the disease is commonly limited to one peripheral site (neck, axilla, or groin), and involvement of the mediastinum is extremely rare. The treatment recommendations for LPHL differ markedly from those for classic HL. The American National Comprehensive Cancer Network (NCCN) guidelines, the German Hodgkin's Lymphoma Study Group (GHSG), and the European Organization for Research and Treatment of Cancer (EORTC) currently recommend involved-field (IF) radiation alone as the treatment of choice for early-stage LPHL. It should be emphasized that even if regional radiation fields are selected, the uninvolved mediastinum should not be irradiated, thus avoiding the site most prone for radiation-related short- and long-term side effects. Although there has not been a study that compared extended-field RT (commonly used in the past) with involved-field RT (IFRT), retrospective data suggest that IF is adequate. The radiation dose

recommended is between 30 to 36 Gy with an optional additional boost of 4 Gy to a (rare) bulky site.

Classical Hodgkin's Lymphoma

EARLY STAGE (FAVORABLE AND UNFAVORABLE)

The New Role of Radiation Therapy

As discussed previously, the treatment of early-stage classical HL has drastically changed. Combined modality therapy consisting of short-course CT (most often doxorubicin [Adriamycin], bleomycin, vinblastine, and dacarbazine [ABVD]) consolidated by reduced-dose radiation carefully directed only to the involved-lymph node(s) site successfully replaced radiation alone as treatment of choice. Although no longer the primary treatment, radiotherapy (RT) limited to smaller volumes, administered to a reduced dose with improved targeting that is achieved with new imaging technology, and supported by modern delivery systems remains an important component of effective treatment programs for HL.

The *old* (1950s to 1980s) treatment strategy for HL maximized the use of radical RT, because it was considered the optimal curative modality in early-stage HL. Even in later years radiation fields remained extensive to reduce the need for the less effective (as compared to ABVD) and relatively toxic CT combination of that time: mechlorethamine, vincristine (Oncovin), procarbazine, and prednisone (MOPP).

Over the last 5 decades, RT alone cured most early stage patients. For example, long-term follow-up of 392 pathologically staged patients without large mediastinal adenopathy treated by the Harvard group demonstrated 10- and 20-year freedom-from-treatment failure (FFTF) rates of 84% and 82%, respectively. The 10- and 20-year overall survival rates were 92% and 82%, respectively. The Harvard group documented, like many others, the late increase in the incidence of second solid tumors as the main cause for decrease in survival rate after 10 years.

The lesson from the RT period in HL should not be limited to the increasing awareness of long-term risks associated with the use of large-field RT. We should appreciate that RT alone as a single agent was (and still is) a highly effective tool in curing HL. Yet, RT should be adapted to its new role as consolidating treatment using a low dose and a smaller field to maximize cure while reducing the toxicity of either prolonged or potentially toxic regimens of CT. The development of this concept is described below.

The improved efficacy of combining doxorubicin (Adriamycin)-based CT with traditional large-field RT compared to the same RT alone was shown in the GHSG HD7 study and Southwest Oncology Group (SWOG) #9133 of favorable patients. Patients on the combined modality arm had a significantly better FFTF. Overall survival remained the same, probably reflecting good salvage or still too short a follow-up period.

The EORTC/Groupe d'Etude des Lymphomes de l'Adulte (GELA) H7F and H8F trials significantly reduced the irradiated volume in the combined-modality arm to include only the site of the originally involved-nodes (involved field) as opposed to treatment of all lymph node sites (and the spleen) on the radiation alone arm. Still, the combined modality arm yielded significantly better relapse-free survival rate than radiation alone.

Several recent studies showed that when combined with CT, IFRT is as effective as a combination of the same CT followed by extended-field radiation.

Randomized studies performed by several groups have clearly indicated that reducing the radiation field has not detracted from the excellent disease FFTF or RFS rates (84% to 95%) or overall survival (92% to 94%) in patients with favorable or unfavorable (GHSG, EORTC/GELA, and Milan) early stage HL. The detailed analysis of the GHSG H8 study demonstrated that a smaller radiation field was associated with a reduction in acute side effects and a trend for a lower risk of second malignancies (2.8% versus 4.5%) that may possibly strengthen with more time of follow-up.

Combined modality therapy allows not only for a drastic restriction of the irradiated volume, it also permits a meaningful reduction (by up to 50%) in the effective prescribed radiation dose. The GHSG studies of combined modality therapy in unfavorable early stage patients indicated that disease control with 20 Gy was as effective as with 40 Gy, provided that bulky disease sites were irradiated to 40 Gy. The recently completed GHSG study HD10 for favorable patients randomized patients to either 20 Gy IFRT or 30 Gy IFRT following a short course (two or four cycles) of ABVD. At a median follow-up of 24 months, the overall results are excellent (FFTF of 97%), with no difference between the four arms. The GHSG study of unfavorable patients (HD11) with similar RT dose design and 24-month FFTF of 90%, also suggests that radiation dose reduction is safe. More mature and detailed results are expected soon. The EORTC/GELA current trial for favorable patients (H9F) is evaluating six cycles of epirubicin, bleomycin, vinblastine, and prednisone (EBVP) to complete remission (CR) followed by either IFRT of 36 Gy or IFRT of 20 Gy. The third arm of patients with CR after six cycles of EBVP and no radiation was closed early because of an excessive number of relapses. The combined modality arms have remained open until the study completed accrual.

The conversion from large multisite radiation fields to a smaller and better-defined radiation field allowed also for accurate conformal RT. The large fields of the past limited the radiation technique to simply two opposed anterior and posterior fields. The conversion to smaller and better-defined radiation volumes allowed the use of more conformal RT, based on better imaging, computerized planning programs, and when indicated, advanced tools such as intensity-modulated radiation therapy (IMRT). Modern breakthroughs in RT technology can now be implemented in HL to increase accuracy even further, avoid normal organ irradiation, and thus improve the therapeutic ratio.

Rakel and Bope: *Conn's Current Therapy 2006.*

Chemotherapy Alone for Early-Stage Hodgkin's Lymphoma?

The standard treatment for early-stage favorable and unfavorable classical HL recommended by the large European HL groups and by the NCCN is CT followed by IFRT. Yet, the idea of eliminating RT from the treatment program in all stages of HL has been advocated by some. This article review some of the recent studies addressing the issue.

Two decades ago, two prospective randomized studies evaluated MOPP CT in early stage HL alone as an alternative to the standard of that time: subtotal lymphoid irradiation (STLI). The Netherlands Cancer Institute (NCI) study showed that in nonbulky patients, MOPP CT was at least as effective as STLI. The Italian study, however, demonstrated that although freedom from progression was similar in both treatment groups, the overall survival of the irradiated patients was significantly ($P < .001$) better (93% versus 56%) compared to the MOPP-treated group. The inferior survival was the result of the poor response to salvage of the MOPP-treated group. The toxicity profile of MOPP and the previously mentioned conflicting results hindered its consideration for primary treatment of early-stage HL.

When the aforementioned MOPP studies were reported, Adriamycin (doxorubicin)-containing regimens such as ABVD had already demonstrated a lower toxicity profile and superior efficacy compared to MOPP in both advanced-stage and early-stage HL. The EORTC conducted a randomized trial in unfavorable early-stage HL comparing a combination of MOPP and mantle field irradiation to ABVD with the same radiation. At 10 years, failure-free survival was better in the ABVD/RT treated patients compared to the MOPP/RT group (88% versus 77%, $P < .0001$). There was no difference in overall survival.

The next step was to evaluate the efficacy of ABVD (or similar combinations) alone, omitting radiation if a CR has been obtained at the end of the CT program. A study group for cancer in children tested the role of RT in young patients (younger than 21 years) who attained a CR with risk-adapted CT (mostly cyclophosphamide, vincristine [Oncovin], procarbazine, and prednisone [COPP]/Adriamycin [doxorubicin], bleomycin, and vinblastine [ABV], four to six cycles). They enrolled 829 patients into the study (68% were early stage); 501 patients who achieved a CR were then randomized to receive either low-dose (21 Gy) IFRT or no further treatment. The accrual was stopped earlier than planned because of a significantly higher number of relapses on the no-RT arm.

The 3-year event-free survival (EFS) with an intent-to-treat analysis was 92% for patients randomized to receive RT and 87% for those randomized to no further treatment ($P = .057$). Because 30 patients switched their treatment after randomization, an analysis *as treated* was performed and showed a 3-year EFS of 93% for those who received radiation and only 85% for those who were only observed ($P = .0024$). At this early analysis, no survival difference was detected.

A large prospectively randomized study from the main cancer center in Mumbai, India, included 251 patients with HL (55% early stage) who received six cycles of ABVD CT. Of those, only 179 patients (71%) who achieved a CR were randomized to either IFRT of 30 Gy (+10 Gy boost to bulky sites) or to no further therapy.

At a median follow-up of 63 months, the 8-year EFS and overall survival were significantly better for the patients who received consolidation with IFRT compared to those who received ABVD alone (EFS 88% versus 76%, $P = .01$; OS 100% versus 89%, $P = .002$). Most relapses in the ABVD-alone arm were early and systemic, whereas in the ABVD+RT arm, the relapses were late and localized.

A North American intergroup (National Cancer Institute of Canada [NCIC]/Eastern Cooperative Oncology Group [ECOG]) study included 405 patients with nonbulky stage I and II patients. They were randomized to either receive *standard therapy,* namely, subtotal nodal irradiation (STNI) for favorable patients, and ABVD (two cycles) followed by STNI for unfavorable (B, elevated erythrocyte sedimentation rate [ESR] = 3 sites, age = 40 years, mixed cellular (MC) histology) patients, or to the experimental arm that consisted of six cycles or four cycles (if CR was attained after two cycles) of ABVD and no RT.

At a median follow-up of 4.2 years, progression-free survival (PFS) with ABVD alone was significantly inferior ($P = .006$; HR = 2.6; 5-year PFS estimates 87% versus 93%). At this early point no survival difference has been detected. Although the *standard* arm that included RT alone for favorable patients is no longer considered the standard of care, the inferior performance of ABVD alone compared to standard therapy in nonbulky early-stage patients cannot be ignored.

The EORTC/GELA groups conducted a large randomized trial in favorable early-stage patients with classic HL. All patients receive six cycles of epirubicin, bleomycin, vinblastine, and prednisone (EBVP). Only patients who achieve a CR are randomized to either IFRT of 36 Gy, IFRT of 20 Gy, or to no radiation. In 2003, the EORTC/GELA groups closed the no-RT arm because of an excessive number of relapses in this group. The study remained open for randomization on the two combined modality arms and is awaiting analysis.

The Memorial Sloan-Kettering (MSK) trial started in 1990 and included 152 patients with nonbulky early-stage HL. Patients were randomized upfront to either receive six cycles of ABDV alone or six cycles of ABVD followed by RT. At 60 months CR duration, freedom from progression (FFP), for ABVD+RT versus ABVD alone was 91% versus 87% ($P = 0.61$), and 86% versus 81% ($P = 0.61$), respectively. Overall survival was 97% with ABVD+RT versus 90% with ABVD alone ($P = 0.08$). Although the differences between the outcomes of the two treatment groups were statistically insignificant, it is important to emphasize that it was not powered to detect differences between the treatment strategies that were smaller than 20% because of the small number of patients and events. The superior overall survival ($P = 0.08$) of the ABVD+RT group is also difficult to explain and is possibly a result of the small size of this trial.

Advanced-Stage Hodgkin's Lymphoma

Although the role of consolidation RT after induction CT remains controversial, irradiation is often added in patients with advanced-stage HL who present with bulky disease or remain in uncertain complete remission after CT. Retrospective studies have demonstrated that adding low-dose RT to all initial disease sites after CT-induced complete response decreases the relapse rate by approximately 25% and significantly improves overall survival. Interpretation of the impact of radiation in prospective studies has been controversial. However, a SWOG randomized study of 278 patients with stage III or IV Hodgkin's disease suggested that the addition of low-dose irradiation to all sites of initial disease after a complete response to mechlorethamine, vincristine (Oncovin), prednisone, bleomycin, doxorubicin (Adriamycin), and procarbazine (MOP-BAP) CT improves remission duration in patients with advanced-stage disease. An intention-to-treat analysis showed that the advantage of combined-modality therapy was limited to patients with nodular sclerosis. No survival differences were observed. A meta-analysis of several randomized studies demonstrated that the addition of RT to CT reduces the rate of relapse but did not show survival benefit for combined-modality compared to CT alone.

Recently, EORTC reported the results of a randomized study that evaluated the role of IFRT in patients with stage III/IV Hodgkin's disease who obtained a CR after MOPP/ABV. Patients received six or eight cycles of MOPP/ABV CT (number of cycles depended on the response). Patients who did not receive a CR (only 40% of patients) were not randomized to receive CT and received IFRT. Of the 418 patients who reached a CR, 85 patients were not randomized to receive treatment for various reasons. A total of 161 patients were randomized to receive no RT and 172 patients were randomized to receive IFRT. The authors concluded that IFRT does not improve the treatment results in patients with stage III/IV Hodgkin's disease who reached a CR after six to eight courses of MOPP/ABV CT. The 5-year overall survival rates were 91% and 85%, respectively ($P = 0.07$). The data indicated that in comparison with CT alone, there were more cases of leukemia second tumors on the CR combined modality but surprisingly not on the PR combined modality arm. In partial responders after six cycles of MOPP/ABV, the addition of IFRT yielded overall survival and EFS rates that were similar to those obtained in CR to CT patients. Among the 250 patients in partial remission after CT, the 5-year event-free and overall survival rates were 79% and 87%, respectively. The EORTC study has several limitations that detract from its applicability to many advanced-stage patients. First, a relatively small fraction of patients were determined to be in CR and thus eligible for randomization on the study. The regimen of six to eight cycles of MOPP/ABV is quite toxic, and this regimen is no longer used in North America. Second, few patients with bulky disease were randomized on the EORTC study. Lastly, the claim that added RT caused more secondary malignancies on the combined modality has not been evident in patients with PR receiving even higher doses of RT to multiple areas after MOPP/ABV.

The only randomized study questioning the role of consolidation RT after CR to six cycles of ABVD (the most common regimen currently used for advance-stage HL) was performed at Tata medical center in India. The study included patients of all stages, but almost half were stages III and IV. A subgroup analysis of the advanced-stage patients showed a statistically significant improvement of both 8-year EFS and 8-year overall survival with added RT compared to ABVD alone (EFS 78% versus 59%; P <0.03 and OS 100% versus 80%; P <0.006).

When advanced-stage HL is treated with the new highly effective and less-toxic treatment program of Stanford V, it is imperative to follow the brief CT program with IFRT to sites originally larger than 5 cm or to a clinically involved spleen. When RT was fully or partially omitted on this program the results were inferior.

In summary, patients in CR after a full-dose CT program like MOPP/ABV may not need RT consolidation. Yet, patients with bulky disease, incomplete or uncertain CR, or patients treated on brief CT programs will benefit from IFRT to originally bulky or residual disease.

Salvage Programs for Refractory and Relapsed Hodgkin's Lymphoma

High-dose therapy supported by autologous stem cell transplantation (ASCT) has become a standard salvage treatment for patients who relapsed or remained refractory to CT or to combined-modality therapy. Many of the patients who enter these programs have not received prior RT or relapsed at sites outside the original radiation field. These patients could benefit from integrating RT into the salvage regimen.

The team at Stanford analyzed the efficacy and toxicity of adding cytoreductive (pretransplant; n = 18) or consolidative (post-transplant; n = 6) RT to 24 of 100 patients receiving high-dose therapy. This study showed that most (69%) relapses after ASCT occurred in sites known to be involved immediately before transplantation. When these sites were irradiated prior to transplantation, no in-field failures occurred. Although only a trend in favor of IFRT could be shown for the entire group of transplanted patients, for patients with stages I through III freedom from relapse was significantly improved. Limiting the analysis to patients who received no prior RT also resulted in a significant advantage to IFRT. Fatal toxicity in this series was not influenced significantly by IFRT.

At Memorial Sloan-Kettering Cancer Center (MSKCC), we have developed a program that integrated RT into the high-dose regimen for salvage of HD almost 20 years ago, and modified it every several years. We schedule accelerated hyperfractionated irradiation (twice daily fractions of 1.8 Gy each) to start after the completion of reinduction CT and stem cell collection and prior to the high-dose CT and stem cell transplantation. Patients who have not been previously irradiated

received IFRT (18 Gy in 5 days) to sites of initially bulky (>5 cm) disease and/or residual clinical abnormalities followed by total lymphoid irradiation (TLI) of 18 Gy (1.8 Gy per fraction, twice daily) within an additional 5 days. Patients who had prior RT received only IFRT (when feasible) to a maximal dose of 36 Gy. This treatment strategy has been in place since 1985 with over 350 patients treated thus far. The first-generation program demonstrated the feasibility and efficacy of the high-dose combined modality regimen, resulting in an EFS of 47% for the patients receiving TLI followed by cyclophosphamide-etoposide CT. The recent report of the second-generation, two-step, high-dose chemoradiotherapy program indicated that after a median follow-up of 34 months the intent-to-treat EFS and overall survival were 58% and 88%, respectively. For patients who underwent transplantation, the EFS was 68%. Treatment-related mortality was 3% with no treatment-related mortality over the last 8 years. The results of this treatment program in refractory patients were similar to those that we had in relapsed patients. Both groups showed favorable EFS and overall survival compared to most recently reported series. Most failures in this salvage program occurred in either unirradiated extranodal sites or in nodal sites that could not be further irradiated. Although the pattern of failure may suggest that the extensive use of nodal irradiation in our program contributed to its overall success, randomized cooperative group studies would be needed to determine whether integrating RT, such as TLI and/or IFRT, contributes to the success of a salvage program of HL.

Radiation Fields: Principles and Design

In the past, radiation-field design attempted to include multiple involved and uninvolved lymph node sites. The large fields known as *mantle, inverted Y,* and *TLI* were synonymous with the radiation treatment of HL and non-Hodgkin's lymphoma (NHL). These fields should rarely be used nowadays. The IF—or its slightly larger version, the regional field—encompasses a significantly smaller, but adequate volume when RT is used as consolidation after CT in HL. Even when radiation is used as the only treatment in lymphocyte predominant HL, the field should be limited to the involved site or to the involved sites and immediately adjacent lymph node groups. Further, even more limited radiation fields restricted to the originally involved lymph node are currently under study by several European groups.

The many terminologies given to radiation field variations in HL caused significant confusion and difficulties in comparing treatment programs. Although the final determination of the field may vary from patient to patient and depends on many clinical, anatomic, and normal tissue tolerance considerations, general definitions and guidelines are available and should be followed.

The following sections provide definitions of types of radiation fields used in HL.

INVOLVED FIELD

The involved field is limited to the site of the clinically involved lymph node group. For extranodal sites—the field includes the organ alone (if no evidence for lymph node involvement). The grouping of lymph nodes is not clearly defined, and involved-field borders for common presentation of HL are discussed later in this article.

REGIONAL FIELD

The regional field includes the involved lymph node group field plus at least one adjacent clinically uninvolved group. For extra nodal disease it includes the involved organ plus the clinically uninvolved lymph node region.

EXTENDED FIELD

The extended field includes *multiple* involved and uninvolved lymph node groups. If the multiple sites are limited to one side of the diaphragm, the upper field is called the *mantle* field. The extended field that includes all lymph node sites below the diaphragm (with or without the spleen) is called after its shape—*inverted Y*.

When radiation treatment includes all lymph nodes on both sides of the diaphragm, these are combined, the resulting field is *TLI* or *total nodal irradiation (TNI)*, if the pelvic lymph nodes are excluded the field is *STLI*.

INVOLVED LYMPH NODE(S) FIELD

The involved lymph node field is the most limited radiation field, and has just recently been introduced. The clinical treated volume (CTV) includes only the originally involved lymph node(s) volume (prechemotherapy) with the addition of 1 cm margin to create planned treatment volume (PTV).

Considerations in Designing Involved-Field Radiotherapy

Although it is understood that the IF should address an area smaller than the classical extended fields of mantle or inverted Y, it is not entirely clear how small the field should remain. Should only the area of the enlarged lymph node (with margins) be irradiated? Should a region of lymph nodes be addressed? And if yes, what are the borders of this region? Many use the lymph node region diagram that was adopted for staging purposes at the 1966 Rye symposium to define a region of lymph nodes. However, this diagram was not developed for individual radiation field design and strangely enough the chart distinguishes between a mediastinal and a hilar region, has a separate infraclavicular lymph region, and does not provide borders of the individual sites. Other questions relate to the change in size (or complete resolution) of the lymph node after CT. Should the prechemotherapy volume be irradiated? Or should the tissues (such as lung) that are no longer involved by the disease be spared by irradiating the postchemotherapy residual abnormality alone?

There are no definitive answers to these questions, and it is often the individual clinical situation that affects the field design. At the same time, uniform general guidelines are important for assuring high standards of treatment and are essential for collaborative group studies.

SUGGESTED GUIDELINES FOR DELINEATING THE INVOLVED FIELD TO NODAL SITES

- IFRT is treatment of a region, not of an individual lymph node.
- The main IF nodal regions are neck (unilateral), mediastinum (including the hilar regions bilaterally), axilla (including the supraclavicular [SCL] and infraclavicular lymph nodes), spleen, para-aortic lymph nodes, and inguinal (including the femoral and iliac) nodes.
- In general, the fields include the involved prechemotherapy sites and volume, with an important exception that involves the transverse diameter of the mediastinal and para-aortic lymph nodes. For the field width of these sites, it is recommended to use the reduced postchemotherapy diameter. In these areas the regression of the lymph nodes is easily depicted by computed tomography imaging, and the critical normal tissue is saved by reducing the irradiated volume.
- The SCL lymph nodes are considered part of the cervical region, and if involved alone or with other cervical nodes, the whole neck is unilaterally treated. The upper neck (above the larynx) is spared only if the SCL involvement is an extension of mediastinal disease and the other neck areas are not involved (based on computed tomography imaging with contrast and gallium/positron emission tomography [PET] imaging when appropriate). This is to save on irradiating the salivary glands when the risk for the area is low.
- All borders should be easy to outline (most are bony landmarks) and plan on with a 2D standard simulation unit. Computed tomography data are required for outlining the mediastinal and para-aortic region and will also help in designing the axillary field.
- Prechemotherapy and postchemotherapy information (both computed tomography and PET) regarding lymph node localization and size is critical and should be available at the time of planning the field.

INVOLVED-FIELD GUIDELINES FOR COMMON NODAL SITES

Unilateral Cervical/Supraclavicular Region

For involvement at any cervical level with or without involvement of the SCL nodes:

Arm Position: Akimbo or at sides.
Upper Border: 1 to 2 cm above the lower tip of the mastoid process and midpoint through the chin.
Lower Border: 2 cm below the bottom of the clavicle.

Lateral Border: To include the medial two thirds of the clavicle.

Medial Border: (a) If the SCL nodes are uninvolved, the border is placed at the ipsilateral transverse processes, except when medial nodes close to the vertebral bodies are seen on the initial staging neck CT scan. For medial nodes the entire vertebral body is included. (b) When the SCL nodes are involved, the border should be placed at the contralateral transverse processes. For stage I patients the larynx and vertebral bodies above the larynx can be blocked (assuming no medial cervical nodes).

Blocks: A posterior cervical cord block is required only if cord dose exceeds 40 Gy. Midneck calculations should be performed to determine the maximum cord dose, especially when the central axis is in the mediastinum. A laryngeal block should be used unless lymph nodes were present in that location. In that case the block should be added at 20 Gy.

Bilateral Cervical/Supraclavicular Region

Both cervical and SCL regions should be treated as described previously regardless of the extent of disease on each side. Posterior cervical cord and larynx blocks should be used as described above. Use a posterior mouth block if treating the patient supine (preferably with an extended travel couch at greater than 100 cm face straight down [FSD]) to block the upper-field divergence through the mouth.

Mediastinum

For involvement of the mediastinum and/or the hilar nodes (In HL this field includes also the medial SCL nodes even if not clinically involved. In NHL, the volume is limited to the mediastinum.):

Arm Position: Akimbo or at sides. The arms-up position is optional if the axillary nodes are involved.

Upper Border: C5-C6 interspace. If SCL nodes were also involved, the upper border should be placed at the top of the larynx, and the lateral border should be adjusted as described in the section on treating neck nodes.

Lower Border: The lower of (a) 5 cm below the carina or (b) 2 cm below the *prechemotherapy* inferior border.

Lateral Border: The *postchemotherapy* volume with 1.5 cm margin.

Hilar Area: To be included with 1 cm margin unless initially involved where the margin should be 1.5 cm.

Mediastinum With Involvement of the Cervical Nodes

When both cervical regions are involved, the field is a mantle without the axilla using the guidelines described previously. If only one cervical chain is involved, the vertebral bodies, contralateral upper neck, and larynx can be blocked as previously described. Because of the increased dose to the neck (the isocenter is in the upper mediastinum), the neck above the lower border of the

larynx should be shielded at 30.6 Gy. If paracardiac nodes are involved, the whole heart should be treated to 14.4 Gy and the initially involved nodes should be treated to 30.6 Gy.

Axillary Region

The ipsilateral axillary, infraclavicular, and SCL areas are treated when the axilla is involved. Whenever possible use CT-based planning for this region:

Arm Position: Akimbo or up

Upper Border: C5-C6 interspace

Lower Border: The lower of the two of: (a) the tip of the scapula or (b) 2 cm below the lowest axillary node

Medial Border: Ipsilateral cervical transverse process. Include the vertebral bodies only if the SCL are involved

Lateral Border: Flash axilla

Spleen

The spleen is treated only if abnormal imaging was suggestive of involvement. The *postchemotherapy* volume is treated with 1.5 cm margins.

Abdomen (Para-aortic Nodes)

Upper Border: Top of T11 and at least 2 cm above prechemotherapy volume

Lower Border: Bottom of L4 and at least 2 cm below prechemotherapy volume

Lateral Border: Edge of the transverse processes and at least 2 cm from the postchemotherapy volume

Inguinal/Femoral/External Iliac Region

These ipsilaterally lymph node groups are treated together if any of the nodes are involved:

Upper Border: Middle of the sacroiliac joint.

Lower Border: 5 cm below the lesser trochanter.

Lateral Border: The greater trochanter and 2 cm lateral to initially involved nodes.

Medial Border: Medial border of the obturator foramen with at least 2 cm medial to involved nodes. If common iliac nodes are involved, the field should extend to the L4-L5 interspace and at least 2 cm above the initially involved nodal border.

Involved-Field Radiotherapy of Extranodal Sites

In most cases, the whole involved organ is the target and draining lymph nodes are not included unless involved. The optimal plan is 3D-conformal and CT-simulation based. The margins for the planned treatment volume depend on quality of imaging and reliability of immobilization, and most importantly, should account for organ motion during respiration. Typically, organs in the head and neck require margins of 1 cm, and organs in the mediastinum, abdomen, and pelvis require margins of 2 cm.

Rakel and Bope: *Conn's Current Therapy 2006.*

New Aspects of Radiation Field Design and Delivery

As the notion of treating large areas of involved and uninvolved areas has changed in favor of treating only the involved lymph node group or extra nodal organ, new options of more conformal RT have opened up. The old extensive radiation fields like mantle or inverted Y included multiple sites at various depths (from the body surface), and each site had different limitations of access and tolerance of normal tissue. The only way to include these sites in one radiation field (and avoid overlaps and gaps when radiation fields were matched) was to treat the whole field from only two opposed directions: anterior and posterior. This technique assured the inclusion of most lymph nodes in one field, yet it also resulted in exposure of large volumes of normal organs (e.g., heart, lungs, breasts, and spinal cord) to the full prescribed radiation dose.

The RT of the IF alone as is practiced today avoids this shortcoming in most cases by allowing the use of 3-dimensional conformal radiotherapy (3-D CRT). For example, 3-D CRT of an anterior mediastinal mass could avoid radiation of the spine and much of the heart and lung tissue located behind the mass.

The change in the lymphoma RT paradigm coincided with substantial improvement in imaging and treatment planning technology, which have revolutionized the field of RT over the last 15 years. The integration of fast high-resolution computerized tomography into the simulation and planning systems of radiation oncology has changed how treatment volumes and relationship to normal critical structures are determined and planned. In the recent past, tumor volume determinations were made with fluoroscopy-based simulators that produced less than optimal chest radiograph films that obviously resulted in a need to include wide safety margins that detracted from accuracy and sparing of critical organs. The most modern simulators arc in fact high resolution CT scanners with capabilities and software that allow accurate conformal treatment planning with detailed information on the dose-volume delivered to normal structures in each individual optional plan and the homogeneity of dose delivered to the target. More recently, these simulators are integrated also with a PET scanner that provides additional tumor volume information for consideration during radiation planning.

IMRT is the most advanced planning and radiation delivery mode and is mainly used for small volume cancers that require high radiation doses (e.g., prostate and head neck cancers) or are adjacent to critical organs. IMRT allows for accurately enveloping the tumor with either a homogenous radiation dose (*sculpting*) or delivering higher doses to predetermined areas in the tumor volume (*painting*). The end result of this new modality is highly accurate treatment with maximal sparing of normal tissues. In the RT of lymphoma, there are several clinical situations where IMRT provides a benefit: treatment of large or complicated tumor volumes in the mediastinum and abdomen, head, and neck lymphomas. IMRT also allows reirradiation of sites prior to high-dose salvage programs that otherwise will be prohibited by normal tissue tolerance, particularly of the spinal cord.

Side Effects and Complications of Radiotherapy

Side effects of RT depend on the irradiated volume, dose administered, and technique employed. They are also influenced by the extent and type of prior CT, if any, and by the patient's age. Most of the information that we use today to estimate risk of RT is derived from strategies that used radiation alone. The field's size and configuration, doses, and technology have all drastically changed over the last decade. So it is probably misleading to judge current RT for lymphomas and inform patients solely on this basis of different past practice of using RT in treating lymphomas.

It is of interest that most of the data of long-term complications associated with RT and particularly second solid tumors and coronary heart disease were reported from databases of HL patients treated more than 25 years ago. We have scant information on NHL patients treated with combined modality or with radiation alone and their potential long-term complications. The difference between the two diseases with regard to increased risk reported may be a result of differences in age group treated, length of follow-up, and smaller volumes of RT fields used in NHL. It is also important to note that we have very limited long-term follow-up data on patients with HL or on NHL patients who were treated with CT alone. Yet, increased incidence of lung cancer following treatment with CT alone was reported for both HL and NHL.

ACUTE EFFECTS

Radiation, in general, may cause fatigue, and areas of the irradiated skin may develop mild sun exposure–like dermatitis. The acute side effects of irradiating the full neck include mouth, dryness, change in taste, and pharyngitis. These side effects are usually mild and transient. The main potential side effects of subdiaphragmatic irradiation are loss of appetite, nausea, and increased bowel movements. These reactions are usually mild and can be minimized with standard antiemetic medications.

Irradiation of more than one field, particularly after CT, can cause myelosuppression, which may necessitate short treatment interruption and rarely administration of granulocyte colony–stimulating factor (G-CSF).

EARLY SIDE EFFECTS

Lhermitte's Sign

Fewer than 5% of patients may note an electric shock sensation radiating down the backs of both legs when the head is flexed, known as Lhermitte's sign, 6 weeks to 3 months after mantle-field RT. Possibly secondary to transient demyelinization of the spinal cord, Lhermitte's sign resolves spontaneously after a few months and is

Rakel and Bope: *Conn's Current Therapy 2006.*

not associated with late or permanent spinal cord damage.

Pneumonitis and Pericarditis

During the same period, radiation pneumonitis and/or acute pericarditis may occur in fewer than 5% of patients; these side effects occur more often in those who have extensive mediastinal disease. Both inflammatory processes have become rare with modern radiation techniques.

LATE SIDE EFFECTS

Subclinical Hypothyroidism

Irradiation of the neck and/or upper mediastinal can induce subclinical hypothyroidism in approximately one third of patients. This condition is detected by elevation of thyroid-stimulating hormone (TSH). Thyroid replacement with levothyroxine (T4) is recommended, even in asymptomatic patients, to prevent overt hypothyroidism and decrease the risk of benign thyroid nodules.

Infertility

Only irradiation of the pelvic field may have deleterious effects on fertility. In most patients this problem can be avoided by appropriate gonadal shielding. In females, the ovaries can be moved into a shielded area laterally or inferomedially near the uterine cervix. Irradiation outside of the pelvis does not increase the risk of sterility.

Secondary Malignancies

Hodgkin's disease patients who were cured with RT and/or CT have an increased risk of secondary solid tumors (most commonly, lung, breast, and stomach cancers, as well as melanoma) and NHL 10 or more years after treatment. Unlike MOPP and similar CT combinations or etoposide, RT for Hodgkin's disease is not leukemogenic.

Lung Cancer

Patients who are smokers should be strongly encouraged to quit the habit because the increase in lung cancer that occurs after irradiation or CT has been detected mostly in smokers.

Breast Cancer

For women whose HD was successfully treated at young age, the main long-term concern is the increased risk of breast cancer. During the last decade, multiple studies have documented and characterized the risk of breast cancer after HD, and have established that the increase in breast cancer risk is undoubtedly associated with the use of radiation. The magnitude of the risk is unclear, and different methods of risk reporting and data are found in the literature with relative risk ratios (RRs) ranging from 2 to 450. Unfortunately, RR, absolute risk,

and actuarial risks are often cited without detailing specifics that could have influenced the findings (i.e., length of follow-up for the group and for the individuals; age group, age-incidence and actuarial risk of the malignancy in an untreated population; and quality of follow-up, which may result in event overestimation). In the largest long-term follow-up study of second neoplasms in survivors of HD, which included data from 16 cancer registries of more than 35,000 patients, the RR for breast cancer in women was 2 and the absolute excess risk (AER) was 10.5.

The increase in breast cancer risk is inversely related to the patient's age at Hodgkin's disease treatment; no increased risk has been found in women irradiated after 30 years of age. It is also inversely related to the radiation dose to the breast and the volume of breast tissue exposed. In a recent study, Travis and colleagues from 13 centers in 7 countries reported a large case-control study that included 105 women who developed breast cancer within a cohort of more than 3800 1-year female survivors of HD diagnosed at age 30 years or younger. Unique to this study is the use of patients who received a very low radiation dose (<4 Gy) or no radiation to the breast area where breast cancer developed. This approach allowed isolating treatment factors and analyzing the radiation dose– and CT dose–risk relationships. For all patients who received RT alone (<4 Gy) the relative risk (RR) of breast cancer is 3.2 and increases to 8 in the highest radiation dose group. The results reported by Travis and colleagues clearly demonstrate the influence of radiation dose on the risk of breast cancer. Within the range of doses to which the breast was exposed in past years, more radiation translates into a higher risk of developing breast cancer. This information, as well as data from earlier publications showing a significantly lower risk of second tumors when radiation was reduced from 40 Gy to 20 Gy, support the notion that *lower is better* as long as the radiation dose used augments HD cure rate.

RT alone had been the standard treatment and primary curative modality for HD through the 1970s and early 1980s. Irradiating all lymph node regions, regardless of clinical involvement with HD, has been standard practice, and relatively high doses (more than 40 Gy) have been used. Consequently, a substantial amount of breast tissue has been exposed to either the full prescribed dose or to an attenuated dose (at field margins or under the lung shields) in almost all women irradiated for HD. Most breast exposure in the *mantle* era, resulted from the radiation of the axillae (65% of tumors in this study developed in the outer part of the breast), and to a lesser extent from wide mediastinal and hilar irradiation. Approximately two thirds of women with early-stage HD do not require radiation of the axillae, and additional protection to the upper and medial aspects of the breast could be provided by further reducing field size using careful CT-based planning which usually allows for smaller mediastinal volumes, especially post-CT exposed to radiation on the risk of breast cancer. During the last decade, reduction in field size has been the most important change in RT of HD. Reduction in the volume of exposed breast tissue together with dose

6

reduction (from more than 40 Gy to a dose in the range of 20 to 30 Gy) is likely to dramatically change the long-term risk profile of young male and female patients cured of HD. Emerging data from trials using smaller fields and lower doses support the expectation that the modern application of mini-RT will be associated with a significantly lower risk of breast cancer as well as other solid tumors and cardiac sequelae. Yet, longer follow-up of studies that employ smaller fields and lower doses is necessary.

Breast cancer is curable in its early stages, and early detection has a significant impact on survival. Breast examination should be part of the routine follow-up for women cured of Hodgkin's disease, and routine mammography should begin approximately 8 years after treatment.

Coronary Artery Disease

An increased risk of coronary artery disease has recently been reported among patients who have received mediastinal irradiation. To reduce this hazard, patients should be monitored and advised about other established coronary disease risk factors, such as smoking, hyperlipidemia, hypertension, and poor dietary and exercise habits. There are data supporting the notion that reduced fields and lower doses to the mediastinum have reduced the risk of heart disease in irradiated patients.

Effects on Bone and Muscle Growth

In children, high-dose irradiation will affect bone and muscle growth and may result in deformities. Current treatment programs for pediatric Hodgkin's disease are CT based; radiotherapy is limited to low doses.

RT is an invaluable tool for the curative treatment of HL. RT can also provide important palliation for many patients who failed CT. Like most cancer treatments, radiation may have long-term side effects, particularly second solid tumors. These risks are related to the volume of normal tissue irradiated and to the radiation dose delivered. The use of RT has drastically changed over the last two decades, the radiation fields are

markedly smaller, the doses are lower, and improved technology of planning and delivery improved the identification of the appropriate target and the precision of delivery, resulting in reduced short- and long-term risks to normal structures. Radiation when used smartly can reduce the amount of CT and length of treatment and its optimal integration in treatment programs for HL should continue to be pursued.

REFERENCES

Aleman BM, Raemaekers JM, Tirelli U, et al: Involved-field radiotherapy for advanced Hodgkin's lymphoma. N Engl J Med 2003;348:2396-2406.
Bonadonna G, Bonfante V, Viviani S, et al: ABVD plus subtotal nodal versus involved-field radiotherapy in early-stage Hodgkin's disease: Long-term results. J Clin Oncol 2004;22:2835-2841.
Diehl V, Stein H, Hummel M, et al: Hodgkin's lymphoma: Biology and treatment strategies for primary, refractory, and relapsed disease. Hematology (Am Soc Hematol Educ Program) 2003;225-247.
Diehl V, Thomas RK, Re D: Part II: Hodgkin's lymphoma—Diagnosis and treatment. Lancet Oncol 2004;5:19-26.
Engert A, Schiller P, Josting A, et al: Involved-field radiotherapy is equally effective and less toxic compared with extended-field radiotherapy after four cycles of chemotherapy in patients with early-stage unfavorable Hodgkin's lymphoma: Results of the HD8 trial of the German Hodgkin's Lymphoma Study Group. J Clin Oncol 2003;21:3601-3608.
Hoppe RT, al. e: NCCN physician guidelines: Hodgkin Disease 2004 vol 1. Available online at http://www.nccn.org/
Laskar S, Gupta T, Vimal S, et al: Consolidation radiation after complete remission in Hodgkin's disease following six cycles of doxorubicin, bleomycin, vinblastine, and dacarbazine chemotherapy: Is there a need? J Clin Oncol 2004;22:62-68.
Moskowitz CH, Nimer SD, Zelenetz AD, et al: A 2-step comprehensive high-dose chemoradiotherapy second-line program for relapsed and refractory Hodgkin disease: Analysis by intent to treat and development of a prognostic model. Blood 2001;97:616-623.
Nachman JB, Sposto R, Herzog P, et al: Randomized comparison of low-dose involved-field radiotherapy and no radiotherapy for children with Hodgkin's disease who achieve a complete response to chemotherapy. J Clin Oncol 2002;20:3765-3771.
Yahalom J, Mauch P: The involved field is back: Issues in delineating the radiation field in Hodgkin's disease. Ann Oncol 2002;13 (Suppl 1):79-83.

 CURRENT THERAPY

- Use RT alone for lymphocyte-predominance HL subtype.
- In early-stage (favorable and unfavorable) classical HL, RT consolidation (low-dose, involved field) is the preferred standard-of-care following CT.
- In advanced-stage following chemotherapy, use IFRT for incomplete responders.
- After CR to brief CT like Stanford V
- For an original bulky disease site.
- For refractory/relapse patients, RT should be an integral component of a salvage program.

Abbreviations: CR = complete remission; CT = chemotherapy; HL = Hodgkin's lymphoma; IFRT = involved-field radiotherapy; RT = radiation therapy.

Acute Leukemia in Adults

Method of
Hans W. Grünwald, MD

Key Diagnostic Points

The prognosis of acute leukemia in adults is not yet as good as that achieved by newer treatments in children. However, enormous strides have been made in adults in the last few years with intensive induction and postremission combination chemotherapy (CT) and the use of stem cell transplantation in selected patients. With currently available therapeutic measures, the projected cure rate of acute leukemia (predicted from the freedom from relapse rate in the first 3 years) is expected to be

30% to 40% of all adults, and in selected subsets of patients with good prognostic features the cure rate may be as high as 50% to 60%. In addition to more intensive regimens of treatment, the reason for improved results can be ascribed to better supportive care and the increasing use of newer methods for the identification of characteristics of the disease, which better guide therapeutic decisions. Currently it is essential to obtain cytochemical markers of the leukemic cells as well as their biochemical, immunologic, and especially cytogenetic characteristics. These may frequently be complemented by the investigation of molecular alterations at the DNA level using well-defined probes.

The use of growth factors (colony-stimulating factors [CSFs]) in the management of patients with acute leukemia is beneficial in shortening hospital stays by enhancing recovery from severe cytopenias induced by cytotoxic CT. They have been shown not to stimulate the regrowth of the leukemic cells that carry receptors for such growth factors, which is a concern in the acute myeloid leukemias. Other major scientific advances that may yield a higher proportion of cures of acute leukemia in the future include the identification of minimal residual disease after completion of intensive postremission therapy using immunologic and/or molecular markers, and the potential for eradication of the residual disease by the use of biologic response modifiers (monoclonal antibodies, interleukins, and other cytokines) singly, in combination, or even combined with cytotoxic chemotherapeutic agents, or by the use of monoclonal antibodies either alone or attached to either toxins or radioisotopes. These investigational advances require that as many patients as possible participate in clinical trials. All new patients with acute leukemia should first be evaluated for entry eligibility on investigational protocols. They can be treated off-protocol if proved not to be eligible or if the patient refuses to participate. The intensive therapy needed both during remission induction and during postremission consolidation is associated with a high rate of complications and even a significant mortality. Therefore, all such patients should be treated in a major medical center capable of providing the needed supportive measures for such critically ill patients.

Acute Myeloid Leukemia

PRESENTATION

The clinical manifestations of acute myeloid leukemia (AML) are related mostly to bone marrow failure. The lack of erythropoietic activity manifested by anemia of varying severity causes fatigue, palpitations, lightheadedness, and dyspnea on exertion. The lack of megakaryocytic activity, manifested by thrombocytopenia, leads to purpura and mucosal bleeding. The lack of normal myeloid maturation, manifested by granulocytopenia, frequently leads to infections, which are often life-threatening. Common infections at presentation include pneumonia, perirectal abscesses, sinusitis, and otitis; however, fever and bacteremia without a localizing site of infection are common.

Rakel and Bope: *Conn's Current Therapy 2006.*

Some patients with hyperleukocytosis (>80,000 $M_1/\mu L$) can have mental symptoms characterized by confusion and even loss of consciousness (cerebral leukostasis) or pulmonary symptoms characterized by dyspnea and inadequate gas exchange (pulmonary leukostasis). Caution must be used in the interpretation of the results of an arterial blood gas specimen obtained in a patient with high leukocyte counts: The laboratory report may suggest extreme hypoxia in the patient; this pseudo-hypoxia is because of in vitro oxygen consumption by the white cells (*leukocyte oxygen larceny*). This laboratory abnormality can be avoided by adding fluoride to the heparin in the syringe loaded with arterial blood, thus arresting glycolysis. Many patients with high leukocyte counts have been inappropriately intubated and placed on respirators for this reason.

Some patients with the myelomonocytic or monocytic variety of AML may present with severe gingival hyperplasia, marked tendency to gum bleeding, and skin and/or subcutaneous (SC) infiltrates.

Patients with the promyelocytic variant of AML frequently present with serious hemorrhagic manifestations and are found to have consumption coagulopathy (disseminated intravascular coagulation [DIC]) because of release of proteolytic (thrombin-like) enzymes into the circulation. These patients require close monitoring including all their coagulation parameters. Such patients may benefit from the administration of heparin in addition to fresh-frozen plasma (FFP) and/or cryoprecipitate until the coagulopathy is arrested by the treatment of the leukemia.

PROGNOSTIC FACTORS

Patients with a history of cytopenias caused by marrow dysplasia (myelodysplastic syndrome), exposure to aromatic hydrocarbons such as benzene, or treatment with alkylating and/or topoisomerase inhibitory chemotherapeutic agents (secondary myeloid leukemias) have a low remission induction rate (approximately half the complete remission [CR] rate of comparable patients with de novo AML). These remissions, when achieved, are rarely durable. Thus in patients younger than 40 years of age with *secondary AML* and an HLA-matched sibling donor, early bone marrow transplantation should be considered.

Age is the second important prognostic feature in AML. The CR and the cure rates are higher in patients younger than 40. In spite of the poorer prognosis of AML in the elderly, CR can be achieved even in the 8th and 9th decades of life, and treatment with curative intent should always be offered to the elderly provided they understand the risk involved. The risk-to-benefit ratio must be clearly presented to the patient to allow an informed decision to be made concerning treatment.

Certain subsets of patients with AML using the French-American-British (FAB) classification of leukemias (based on morphology and cytochemical features of the leukemic cells) are associated with a better prognosis (M4 with marrow eosinophilia, M3 hypergranular promyelocytic, etc.). These rare patients can often be better identified by their characteristic cytogenetic abnormality. Therefore, it is better to rely on the karyotype for therapeutic decisions after CR has been achieved (postremission therapy). The chromosome analysis (karyotype) is one of the best methods to identify subsets of AML that have a higher probability of prolonged remissions and cures. Such subsets include chromosomal inversions (inv) and translocations (t) such as inv(16), t(15;17), t(8;21). Chromosome analysis is also the best method to identify subsets of AML with a poor prognosis such as trisomy 8, abnormalities or loss of chromosome 5 or 7, abnormalities of chromosome 11q, or multiple translocations or trisomies. These abnormalities not only predict a short remission duration but also refractoriness to standard remission induction CT. More intensive regimens incorporating high-dose cytarabine (Cytosar-U) may be warranted for such patients, and allogeneic stem cell transplantation may be considered once a remission is attained.

Finally, immunophenotypic markers can identify patients with poorer prognosis. Patients whose blasts have the CD34 antigen on their surface (an antigen of early hematopoietic progenitors) have a high probability of being refractory to conventional induction CT, and warrant trials with a more intensive regimen.

Acute Lymphoblastic Leukemia

PRESENTATION

Most patients with acute lymphoblastic leukemia (ALL) present with manifestations of bone marrow failure: anemia, thrombocytopenia (with the characteristic purpura and mucosal bleeding), and granulocytopenia (with infections of all kinds). In addition, such patients often have bone pain and tenderness, generalized lymphadenopathy and/or splenomegaly. Fever at presentation can be because of the high leukemic cell turnover, but should always be considered to be of infectious origin until exhaustive investigations prove negative.

PROGNOSTIC FACTORS

Age is a very important prognostic factor in ALL. Young adults have a cure rate of approximately 70%, whereas in the elderly the prognosis of ALL is not much better than for AML (i.e., 20%).

The initial white blood cell (WBC) count is a major prognostic factor in ALL. Patients with leukocytosis above 50,000/μL readily achieve a CR, but usually have an early relapse. Such patients warrant more intensive postremission therapy or stem cell transplantation.

The morphology of the leukemic blasts in peripheral blood and bone marrow smears can identify the Burkitt's type (FAB L3) of ALL. Such blasts are characteristically large with deep blue cytoplasm and with cytoplasmic vacuoles. This type of leukemia has a much lower CR rate than the L1 and L2 varieties of ALL and warrants the use of different, more intensive, therapeutic regimens. The Burkitt's type of leukemia can also be identified by the surface immunoglobulin of the blast

cells, a characteristic of B cells, and by the characteristic chromosomal translocations [t(8;14) or t(8;22)] involving the *c-myc* oncogene on chromosome 8.

Chromosome analysis in ALL also can yield important prognostic clues. One or more translocations, especially t(4;11) and t(9;22), predicts for a high probability of early relapse after a remission has been attained. This justifies more intensive postremission CT or allogeneic stem cell transplantation if a suitable donor is available.

Initial Evaluation in the Patient with Acute Leukemia

Initial evaluation of the patient begins with a complete history and physical examination. Next is a careful and accurate evaluation of the peripheral blood and bone marrow smears for the morphology and classification of the leukemia. The bone marrow aspirate and biopsy stained with Wright or Giemsa yield the exact cytologic type and subtype (AML or ALL and its FAB class) in 80% to 90% of patients. It is also essential to perform a full cytochemical panel on the blood and marrow smears, assay for terminal deoxynucleotidyl transferase (TDT), immunophenotyping, and cytogenetic analysis on the bone marrow cells. This not only serves to confirm the morphologic classification but also to identify the prognostic subtypes mentioned previously.

Also part of the initial evaluation of the patient is a careful analysis of the coagulation system, including prothrombin time (PT), activated partial thromboplastin time (APTT), plasma fibrinogen level and serum fibrin degradation product (FDP), or d-dimer assay. These tests can identify the DIC present in most patients with acute promyelocytic leukemia (AML FAB M3) and in some patients with myelomonocytic and monocytic leukemia (FAB M4 and M5).

Renal, hepatic, pulmonary, and especially cardiac function should also be assessed. Most antileukemic drugs are excreted by the kidneys and/or detoxified by the liver and are potentially toxic to these organs. Cardiac dysfunction diagnosed before treatment is begun can obviate the use of anthracyclines, which may lead to potentially fatal cardiac insufficiency in patients with poor cardiac function.

Multiple cultures should be obtained from blood and excreta and also from various mucosae prone to colonization by bacteria, fungi, and viruses (pharynx, nose, and rhinopharynx). Such cultures should be obtained not only in patients with suspected infection and fever but also in asymptomatic and afebrile patients to predict the possible microorganism responsible for an infection occurring later in the patient's course (*surveillance cultures*).

Finally, histocompatibility leukocyte antigen (HLA) typing should be performed in every new patient to identify potential stem cell donors among the patient's siblings (or even from the unrelated donor data banks) as well as to provide HLA-matched platelet transfusions if and when the patient becomes refractory to unmatched platelet transfusions because of alloimmunization. It is usually impossible to HLA-type the patient at the time alloimmunization is detected because there usually are few or no leukocytes in the peripheral blood to type as a result of the cytotoxic CT.

Treatment

Chemotherapeutic drugs should be started as soon as possible after the diagnosis of AML or ALL is made. There is rarely a need to initiate such treatment as an emergency, and there is usually sufficient time to perform all the aforementioned pretreatment evaluations. Biochemical, hemostatic, or other abnormalities should be corrected before initiation of cytotoxic CT. Hyperleukocytosis (>80,000 blast cells per µL), however, constitutes a medical emergency requiring immediate leukapheresis (removal of leukocytes by blood centrifugation at the bedside) and the rapid initiation of the cytotoxic CT to avoid pulmonary and/or cerebral leukostasis, which may be fatal.

Before CT, patients with acute leukemia should be hydrated and given allopurinol (Zyloprim) oral doses of 300 mg per day to avoid the development of hyperuricemia and urate nephropathy. Optimally, the allopurinol (Zyloprim) should be started 36 hours before the initiation of cytotoxic CT and continued for a total of 10 days. Thereafter, the risk of urate nephropathy is minimal, and the frequency of cutaneous hypersensitivity to the drug increases.

Venous access for the duration of treatment and the period of severe cytopenias that follows should be assured prior to initiation of the treatment. Many patients have adequate peripheral veins to permit administration of all required drugs and blood products. However, many patients eventually develop venous access problems during induction CT. Therefore, it is common to centrally implant a Silastic catheter (Hickman or Broviac) that is exposed to the outside. Alternatively, a port may be attached to the catheter and remain permanently under the skin (requiring a noncoring needle to access). Another method of achieving venous access is by means of a peripherally inserted central catheter (PICC) line, which does not require use of operating room facilities for insertion but can only remain in place for 3 to 6 weeks.

Another important issue before the initiation of cytotoxic CT is the control of infections. Appropriate bactericidal antibacterial, antiviral, and/or antifungal agents are used because needed. The use of bacteriostatic antibiotics (macrolides, etc.) *must* be avoided because they are ineffective in a granulocytopenic patient and may antagonize bactericidal antibiotics.

Finally, severe anemia and thrombocytopenia are corrected by packed red blood cell (RBC) and platelet transfusions, and FFP and heparin are given to correct the hemostatic abnormalities of the consumption coagulopathy. All blood cell transfusions (RBC and platelets) should incorporate a WBC retaining filter to minimize the exposure to allogeneic HLA antigens and reduce the

risks of eventual platelet refractoriness and presensitization for an eventual allogeneic stem cell transplant. For the same reason, family members of a patient deemed suitable for allogeneic stem cell transplantation should *not* be used as donors for RBC or platelet transfusions.

If evidence of a consumption coagulopathy is detected (prolonged PT and PTT; increased fibrin degradation products or d-dimers; prolonged thrombin time; decreased factors I, II, V, and VIII), prompt initiation of differentiation agent therapy (all-trans-retinoic acid [ATRA]), and/or heparinization in addition to administration of FFP and/or cryoprecipitate; this reduces the incidence of fatal hemorrhage. Heparin can be started with a bolus of 8 to 10,000 intravenous (IV) units, followed by a continuous IV infusion of 1000 units per hour during the first 48 hours, thereafter reduced to 700 units per hour until correction of the coagulopathy (rise in fibrinogen is the best marker for this).

ACUTE MYELOID LEUKEMIA

The majority of patients with AML of all types (FAB M1 through M7) respond to the standard induction combination CT of cytarabine (Cytosar-U) and an anthracycline given in the 7+3 regimen. Cytarabine (Cytosar-U) is given as a continuous IV infusion of 100 to 200 mg per m^2 per day for 7 days, and daunorubicin (Cerubidine) is administered in doses of 45 mg/m^2 per day as a slow IV bolus for the first 3 days. An alternative anthracycline, with similar therapeutic spectrum to daunorubicin (Cerubidine), is idarubicin (Idamycin) given at a dose of 12 mg/m^2 per day as a slow IV bolus for 3 days. These doses are given irrespective of the initial blood count, because the goal is to achieve temporary marrow aplasia to be followed by normal marrow regeneration (achievement of a CR). However, if initial liver function tests demonstrate major impairment (bilirubin >3 mg per dL, ALT >3 times normal), the doses of both drugs should be reduced to half and the cytarabine (Cytosar-U) infusion stopped after 5 days if the liver function tests have not improved. Antiemetics such as ondansetron (Zofran), metoclopramide (Reglan), or prochlorperazine (Compazine) may be used liberally.

Patients older than 70 years of age should have the anthracycline dose decreased by 33% (30 mg/m^2 per day for 3 of daunorubicin [Cerubidine] or 8 mg/m^2 per day for 3 of idarubicin [Idamycin]). Patients with a history of coronary artery disease, heart failure, or who have a decreased cardiac ejection fraction on multigated angiogram (MUGA) scan can be given mitoxantrone (Novantrone) instead of daunorubicin (Cerubidine) (lower risk of heart failure) at a dose of 12 mg/m^2 per day, given as a 1-hour IV infusion for the first 3 days, together with the 7-day cytarabine (Cytosar-U) infusion. An alternative for such high-risk patients is the use of continuous IV cytarabine (Cytosar-U) (100 mg/m^2 per day) plus daily oral thioguanine (Tabloid) (2 mg/kg per day) until marrow aplasia is achieved. A bone marrow examination is performed on the day immediately following the conclusion of the cytarabine (Cytosar-U) infusion to assess the extent of cytoreduction. If the marrow cellularity on biopsy has not decreased to 20% or less and the proportion of leukemic blasts has not decreased by 80% or more, it is improbable that a CR will result. Additional CT consisting of 3 days of mitoxantrone (Novantrone), etoposide (VePesid), or high-dose cytarabine (Cytosar-U) (at dosages to be discussed in this article for refractory or recurrent AML) may then be considered, but at the cost of increased toxicity (mucositis, pancytopenia of greater duration, etc.). An exception to the discussed recommendations is acute promyelocytic leukemia (FAB M3) with the t(15;17), where the ability of the leukemic blast cells to differentiate when exposed to retinoids has led to the use of ATRA as the mainstay of remission induction therapy. This has yielded not only an increase in the rate of CRs but also a dramatic prolongation of survival and a significant increase in the number of long-term, disease-free surviving patients (projected to be more than 75%). The treatment with tretinoin (Vesanoid) (ATRA) is given orally, 45 mg/m^2 per day (in 2 doses) in addition to the standard 7+3 induction treatment with cytarabine (Cytosar-U) and daunorubicin (Cerubidine) (or idarubicin [Idamycin]) as described previously for myeloblastic leukemia. A not uncommon complication of ATRA administration is the development of the *retinoic acid syndrome,* consisting of dyspnea, fluid retention, pleural and/or pericardial effusions, and occasionally even pulmonary edema. The retinoic acid syndrome usually improves with the administration of corticosteroids. Dexamethasone (10 mg orally twice daily for 3 to 5 days) should be initiated as soon as the first symptoms of the syndrome appear.

Daily blood count monitoring during and after induction CT is essential as a measure of the cytoreduction induced. Close platelet count monitoring guides the administration of platelet transfusions. Hemoglobin levels guide the administration of packed RBC transfusions. Frequent monitoring of serum electrolyte levels is needed to detect the occurrence (fortunately rare) of a tumor lysis syndrome.

A second postinduction bone marrow aspiration and biopsy should be performed 1 week after completion of the course of CT to help make the decision regarding need for a second course of induction CT. If the proportion of leukemic blasts in the aspirate remains above 5% and the cellularity on biopsy is more than 10%, a second course of the same drugs used initially should be given. However, the duration of the second CT course should be shorter, with a 5-day infusion of cytarabine (Cytosar-U) and two daily doses of the anthracycline at the same daily doses given for the first course (5+2). If the bone marrow shows a cellularity of less than 10%, but the majority of cells are blasts, it is advisable to wait 3 to 5 days and repeat the bone marrow aspiration and biopsy, since it is virtually impossible to differentiate between residual leukemia and very early marrow regeneration. A subsequent marrow can reveal further lineage differentiation (appearance of promyelocytes, myelocytes and even metamyelocytes) if it is early regeneration. A persistently leukemic marrow shows a further increase in blasts. If, after a second course of cytarabine (Cytosar-U) plus anthracycline (5+2) the marrow remains leukemic, one has to characterize the patient as *refractory* to the induction CT.

REFRACTORY OR RELAPSED ACUTE MYELOID LEUKEMIA

Patients who are refractory to induction CT or who relapse after having attained a CR require more intensive induction CT, usually the high-dose cytarabine (HiDAC) (Cytosar-U) regimen consisting of 1 to 3 g/m^2 of cytarabine (Cytosar-U) every 12 hours for 6 days (a total of 12 doses) given as a 75-minute infusion each. Because HiDAC (Cytosar-U) concentrates in tears and can cause keratitis, it is important to wash the eyes with saline or artificial tears at least six times each day. Patients must also be closely monitored for cerebellar toxicity involving coordination and speech. The drug must be discontinued at the first sign of ataxia or slurred speech. Less common toxicities of HiDAC (Cytosar-U) include hemorrhagic enterocolitis and noncardiac pulmonary edema (acute respiratory distress syndrome [ARDS]).

After the 6 days of cytarabine (Cytosar-U) infusions have been completed, bone marrow aspiration and biopsy are performed. If the marrow still shows more than 20% leukemic blasts, it is advisable to give 3 days of mitoxantrone (Novantrone), 12 mg/m^2 per day as a 1-hour infusion.

An alternative regimen for refractory or relapsed AML is the use of mitoxantrone (Novantrone) and etoposide (VePesid);[1] etoposide (VePesid)[1] is given as a 5-day infusion of 150 mg/m^2 per day, mitoxantrone (Novantrone) is given as a 1-hour intravenous infusion of 12 mg/m^2 per day for the first 3 days. If, after completing this 5-day regimen, the marrow shows reduction but not disappearance of the leukemic blasts, a second 5-day course of these two drugs can be administered. These drugs require hepatic function for detoxification and should thus not be used if the patient has abnormal liver function tests (ALT >3 times normal, bilirubin >3 mg/dL).

For elderly or poor-performance status patients with refractory or relapsed AML, an alternative regimen consists of the administration of gemtuzumab ozogamicin (Mylotarg) 9 mg/m^2 per dose for two IV doses 14 days apart as a single agent. This drug, a monoclonal anti-CD33 antibody linked to the cytotoxic antibiotic calicheamicin, can induce remissions in refractory AML but usually of only short duration, so this therapy must be followed by some other antileukemic regimen, usually a nonmyeloablative allogeneic stem cell transplant.

Patients with relapsed or refractory acute promyelocytic leukemia (APL) (no longer responding to ATRA) can be treated with arsenic trioxide (Trisenox) at a daily IV dose of 0.15 mg/kg per day (most often given 5 days per week to allow ambulatory administration in units open only Monday through Friday) until a remission is achieved.

---

[1]Not FDA approved for this indication.

Rakel and Bope: *Conn's Current Therapy 2006.*

POSTREMISSION CONSOLIDATION

Once CR has been achieved (normal bone marrow, reticulocyte, platelet, and granulocyte counts) and the patient is deemed free of infections and aftereffects of the induction CT (attainment of a near-normal performance status), postremission therapy is planned. A significant advance in recent years is the attainment in a significant proportion of patients of long relapse-free survival (and thus possible cure of the leukemia), by the institution of very intensive postremission consolidation CT. The intensity of treatment is similar or greater than that used for remission induction. Such treatment, however, may produce life-threatening toxicities. Most patients can be treated on an ambulatory basis (provided they live at a reasonable distance from the hospital). The regular need for platelet transfusions requires an ambulatory transfusion center. Furthermore, because most patients remain markedly neutropenic for periods ranging from 10 to 30 days following each consolidation course, they are advised to avoid external sources of infection (crowds, animals, vases with stagnant water, etc.) and to come to the hospital for prompt initiation of antibiotic therapy at the first evidence of chills, fever, or infection. Complete blood counts (CBCs) to monitor hemoglobin, leukocyte, and platelet counts are performed every other day (until recovery of adequate granulocyte and platelet counts), and blood biochemical monitoring is done weekly.

Drugs used for consolidation are the same as those used in induction and at doses similar to or higher than those used for induction. Patients with the better prognostic karyotypes (core binding factor defects such as t;8:21 or inv;16) should receive at least 3 courses of HiDAC (Cytosar-U) 1 to 3 g/m^2 every 12 hours for a total of 6 to 10 doses per course. Patients with the less favorable karyotypes who are not scheduled to receive a stem cell transplant are usually given consolidation courses, which may consist of cytarabine (Cytosar-U) and an anthracycline used in the 7+3 induction regimen followed by at least one course of the HiDAC (Cytosar-U) regimen, and a third consolidation course, which might consist of the combination of etoposide (VePesid)[1] and mitoxantrone (Novantrone)[1] (as described previously for refractory or relapsed AML). The total number of consolidation courses ranges between 3 and 6, depending on the patient's tolerance to the drugs, the rate of recovery from each course of consolidation (if the hematologic depression from a course is greater than 3 weeks, the probability for prolonged or even irreversible cytopenias after an ensuing course increases) and the initial prognostic category (patients with high relapse risk should receive the highest possible number of consolidation courses).

Patients at high risk for early relapse (high initial WBC count or other sign of high leukemic burden such as very high LDH, trisomy 8, abnormalities of chromosome 5 or 7, etc.) should be considered for a stem cell transplant if they attain a CR. Patients younger than 45 years of age with an HLA-matched sibling should receive an allogeneic stem cell transplant from that sibling. If an HLA-matched sibling is unavailable, a search for a voluntary unrelated donor (VUD) should be initiated through the National Marrow Donor Registry. For patients between 45 and 60 years of age, a nonmyeloablative allogeneic stem cell transplant should be considered.

Patients with less-than-optimal performance status or who are older than the age of 70 years should be considered for an autologous stem cell transplant; this procedure involves harvesting bone marrow or peripheral blood stem cells shortly before a planned intensive consolidation CT course. The marrow or peripheral blood stem cells may be subjected to in vitro purging (either using drugs or antibodies with complement) and frozen. Thereafter, the patient is given the preparative regimen of high-dose cyclophosphamide (Cytoxan)[1] plus total body irradiation (or busulfan) followed by infusion of the thawed marrow or peripheral blood cells.

Patients with APL who attained a remission with ATRA, cytarabine (Cytosar-U), and daunorubicin (Cerubidine) are given consolidation with cytarabine (Cytosar-U) and daunorubicin (Cerubidine) as for patients with AML without the t;15:17. However, the HiDAC, etoposide (VePesid),[1] and mitoxantrone (Novantrone) consolidations are omitted, and the patients are given maintenance oral ATRA on alternating weeks for at least 1 year at a dose of 45 mg/m^2 daily (the addition of methotrexate and mercaptopurine [Purinethol] to this maintenance is currently being evaluated).

Patients with relapsed or refractory APL who responded to arsenic trioxide (Trisenox) as second-line therapy are given a second consolidation course of IV arsenic trioxide (Trisenox) 0.15 mg/kg per day for 25 doses more than 5 weeks (5 days per week). Thereafter, they should be considered for a possible allogeneic stem cell transplant.

ACUTE LYMPHOBLASTIC LEUKEMIA

The majority of patients with ALL achieve a remission following vincristine (Oncovin) and prednisone induction therapy. Significant increases in both remission rates and their duration can be attained by the addition of anthracyclines, L-asparaginase (Elspar), and alkylating agents. The presently recommended remission induction regimen for adults with ALL consists of the following drugs:

- One dose of cyclophosphamide (Cytoxan) 1 g/m^2 by slow IV injection
- Vincristine (Oncovin) 2 mg by slow IV injection weekly for 4 doses
- Prednisone 100 mg per day orally for 21 days (no need to taper)
- Daunorubicin (Cerubidine) 45 mg/m^2 per day by slow IV injection for 3 days

---

[1]Not FDA approved for this indication.

---

[1]Not FDA approved for this indication.

- L-asparaginase (Elspar) 6000 U/m^2 intramuscularly (IM) (SC if the platelet count is below 50,000/µL) every 4 days for six doses

For patients older than the age of 65 years, the cyclophosphamide (Cytoxan) dose is reduced to 700 mg/m^2, the daunorubicin (Cerubidine) to 30 mg/m^2, and the duration of prednisone administration is reduced to 10 days. The administration of filgrastim (Neupogen), a granulopoiesis stimulant, at the dose of 5 µg/kg body weight should be initiated on day 5 and continued until a granulocyte count of 10,000/µL is attained. Blood counts are performed daily to monitor cytoreduction and to evaluate the need for RBC and platelet transfusions. Bone marrow aspiration and biopsy are performed 4 weeks after the start of CT. If the leukemic blasts have not disappeared, an alternative induction regimen with teniposide, cytarabine (Cytosar-U), and prednisone should be initiated. If the marrow on day 28 shows disappearance of the leukemic blasts, but is not yet normal, an additional 7 to 10 days off CT may lead to the signs of remission (normalization of marrow, reticulocyte, granulocyte, and platelet counts).

Once remission has been documented, central nervous system (CNS) prophylaxis is given with 15 mg of intrathecal methotrexate (be careful to use preservative-free drug) every week for 4 weeks combined with cranial radiation (24 Gy). During this 4-week period, the patient is also given 6-mercaptopurine (6-MP) (Purinethol) 60 mg/m^2 daily by mouth and methotrexate 20 mg/m^2 weekly by mouth. Blood counts are done at least twice weekly, and the dosage of 6-MP (Purinethol) and methotrexate is reduced if cytopenias occur. Liver function tests should also be closely monitored and the dosage of both drugs reduced if abnormalities occur.

After completion of the CNS prophylaxis, and only if and when the blood counts and blood chemistries are normal, an intensive 2-month consolidation CT is initiated as follows:

- Cyclophosphamide (Cytoxan) 1 g/m^2 IV on weeks 1 and 5
- Cytarabine (Cytosar-U) 75 mg/m^2 per day SC for 4 days on weeks 1, 2, 5 and 6
- 6-MP (Purinethol) 60 mg/m^2 per day orally during weeks 1, 2, 5, and 6
- Vincristine (Oncovin) 2 mg IV per week on weeks 3, 4, 7 and 8
- L-asparaginase (Elspar) 6000 units IM (SC if platelet count is below 50,000/µL) twice weekly on weeks 3, 4, 7, and 8

Patients usually require frequent platelet and occasional RBC transfusions during this period of consolidation, but the treatment can be accomplished on an ambulatory basis if an ambulatory transfusion and CT unit is available. If at the start of week 5 there is persistent thrombocytopenia and/or neutropenia (below 50,000 and 1000/µL), the scheduled CT should be postponed for 1 week. For patients with Ph$^+$ ALL (t;9:22), the addition of imatinib (Gleevec)[1] is currently being evaluated as an additional agent during consolidation to eliminate minimal residual disease.

After completion of this intensive consolidation CT, repeat bone marrow aspiration and biopsy are performed to confirm continued remission. Then the 2-year maintenance phase is initiated, consisting of 6-MP (Purinethol) 60 mg/m^2 by mouth daily, methotrexate 20 mg/m^2 by mouth weekly, vincristine (Oncovin) 2 mg IV monthly and prednisone 80 mg per day for 5 days every month (starting on the day of vincristine [Oncovin] administration). Blood counts are performed weekly and blood chemistries biweekly. If significant cytopenias and/or liver dysfunction occur, the maintenance CT is dose reduced or temporarily withheld until acceptable values are achieved.

Patients with prognostic indicators for early relapse (initial WBC count of 50,000/µL or higher, t(9;22) or t(4;11) translocations, etc.) may be considered for allogeneic bone marrow transplantation after achieving a remission if an HLA compatible sibling is available.

Patients with B-cell ALL (Burkitt cell leukemia, FAB = L3) may be treated with a more intensive, shorter, aggressive lymphoma-like induction CT followed by CNS prophylaxis, without a prolonged maintenance phase. The regimen includes the use of high doses of cyclophosphamide (Cytoxan) and methotrexate (with leucovorin reversal) plus vincristine (Oncovin), dexamethasone,[1] cytarabine (Cytosar-U), etoposide (VePesid),[1] and doxorubicin.

SUPPORTIVE CARE

In addition to the proper chemotherapeutic agents, all other aspects of the patient's care must be optimal. The major reason for failure to achieve CR is the death of the patient because of complications of the disease and/or the CT. Primary resistance to CT is infrequent.

A most important clinical consideration is the assurance of adequate hemostasis; thrombocytopenia associated with acute leukemia and that resulting from the use of cytotoxic drugs is the most common cause of hemorrhage. Platelet transfusions have markedly reduced morbidity and mortality from bleeding. Platelets should be given whenever the platelet count is 10,000/µL or fewer, although hemorrhage can occur even with higher levels. Some patients may have very low platelet counts (below 10,000/µL) without bleeding. Patients who require an invasive intervention (insertion of a Hickman catheter, performance of a spinal tap, etc.) should have their platelet count increased to 50,000/µL with platelet transfusions. The presence of signs of DIC as manifested by prolonged PT, PTT, elevated FDP, and/or decreased fibrinogen in addition to thrombocytopenia mandates the administration not only of platelet transfusions (to bring the platelet count above 30,000/µL) but also of FFP and/or cryoprecipitate to restore the hemostatic function to normal. In addition, heparin given to such patients (as described previously) has sometimes proven helpful in this situation. Finally,

---

[1]Not FDA approved for this indication.

Rakel and Bope: *Conn's Current Therapy 2006.*

prolongation of PT and/or PTT well into the course of treatment may occur in some patients as a consequence of vitamin K deficiency. The latter may be because of poor oral food intake and prolonged antibiotic therapy that alters the intestinal flora. Hemostatic function must thus be monitored and supplementary vitamin K given as needed.

After a few weeks of treatment, some patients may become totally refractory to platelet transfusions as shown by a lack of increase in platelet count 1 hour after completion of the transfusion. This situation is usually because of HLA alloimmunization, and can be overcome if one obtains HLA-matched platelets for transfusion. The use of filters, which remove WBCs from all transfused blood products (red cells and platelets) from the start, reduces (but does not eliminate) the incidence of HLA alloimmunization. This benefit not only decreases the incidence of platelet refractoriness, but also reduces the risk of an eventual graft rejection after bone marrow transplantation.

The main cause of morbidity and mortality in patients with acute leukemia is infection, both during induction CT and later during the intensive consolidation phases of treatment. Prophylactic antibacterial therapies with a quinolone such as ciprofloxacin (Cipro) or with trimethoprim-sulfamethoxazole (Bactrim),[1] and/or antifungal prophylaxis with fluconazole (Diflucan)[1] have not yet been proven to decrease the risk of such infections. However, it is advisable to initiate antibiotic and/or antifungal therapy as soon as fever occurs, especially if the granulocyte count is less than 500/μL. Fever in the neutropenic patient requires prompt and intensive attention: cultures for bacteria, fungi, and viruses should be obtained from all potential sites of infections. Immediately thereafter, treatment with broad-spectrum bactericidal antibiotics such as a semisynthetic penicillin like piperacillin (Pipracil)[1] and an aminoglycoside such as gentamicin (Garamycin)[1] should be initiated. For the possible cutaneous entry of hospital bacteria such as methicillin-resistant *Staphylococcus aureus,* or for catheter colonization by *Corynebacterium* of the JK subtype, the addition of vancomycin (Vancocin)[1] is recommended. If the patient remains febrile after 72 hours of such triple antibiotic therapy, antifungal therapy with amphotericin B (Fungizone)[1] should be started on an empiric basis. Therapy of infections is guided and modified according to results of cultures obtained prior to the initiation of the antibiotic therapy.

Although uncommon, viral infections must also be addressed. Serology for herpes simplex virus (HSV) and cytomegalovirus (CMV) should be obtained prior to the start of induction CT. Changes are then monitored during febrile episodes if mucosal lesions suggesting herpes simplex appear. Treatment with IV acyclovir (Zovirax)[1] may be highly effective. CMV can cause interstitial pneumonia as well as esophagitis, enterocolitis, and hepatitis, all of which can be treated with ganciclovir (Cytovene).

PSYCHOSOCIAL ASPECTS

Caution must be used in addressing the patients with acute leukemia and their families. They may not be prepared for the major lifestyle alterations that the disease and its treatment will require. In addition to calm counseling and explanation of all planned phases of treatment, it is important to reinforce these concepts repeatedly. An excellent source of information for both patient and family is a patient with a similar diagnosis who has already undergone a treatment similar to the one planned and can provide the information in terms easily understood by laypersons.

Once the induction CT has led to a CR and the patient has returned home, the availability of a group of patients with successfully treated hematologic neoplasms (such as *Candlelighters*) has proven helpful to make the adjustments required by the disease and its therapy more tolerable. These groups are led by a trained professional, and provide the wherewithal for physical and psychologic adjustment. The availability of a social worker and a psychiatrist with oncologic orientation as team members helps greatly in patient management.

REFERENCES

Byrd JC, Ruppert AS; Mrózek K, et al: Repetitive cycles of high-dose cytarabine benefit patients with acute myeloid leukemia and inv(16)(p13q22) or t(16;16)(p13;q22): Results from CALGB 8461. J Clin Oncol 2004;22(6):1087-1094.
Carey RW, Ribas-Mundo M, Ellison RR, et al: Comparative study of cytosine arabinoside therapy alone and combined with thioguanine, mercaptopurine, or daunorubicin in acute myelocytic leukemia. Cancer 1975;36(5):1560-6.
Daenen S, Löwenberg B, Sonneveld P, et al: Efficacy of etoposide and mitoxantrone in patients with acute myelogenous leukemia refractory to standard induction therapy and intermediate-dose cytarabine with Amsidine. Dutch Hematology-Oncology Working Group for Adults (HOVON). Leukemia 1994;8(1):6-10.
Herzig RH, Wolff SN, Lazarus, HM, et al: High-dose cytosine arabinoside therapy for refractory leukemia. Blood 1983;62(2):361-369.
Larson RA, Dodge RK, Linker CA, et al: A randomized controlled trial of filgrastim during remission induction and consolidation chemotherapy for adults with acute lymphoblastic leukemia: CALGB study 9111. Blood 1998;92(5):1556-1564.
Larson RA, Boogaerts M, Estey E, et al: Antibody-targeted chemotherapy of older patients with acute myeloid leukemia in first relapse using Mylotarg (gemtuzumab ozogamicin). Leukemia 2002;16(9):1627-1636.
Preisler H, Davis RB, Kirshner J, et al: Comparison of three remission induction regimens and two postinduction strategies for the treatment of acute nonlymphocytic leukemia: A cancer and leukemia group B study. Blood 1987;69(5):1441-1449.
Shen ZX, Chen GQ, Ni JH, et al: Use of arsenic trioxide (As2O3) in the treatment of acute promyelocytic leukemia (APL): II. Clinical efficacy and pharmacokinetics in relapsed patients. Blood 1997;89(9):3354-3360.
Tallman MS, Andersen JW, Schiffer CA, et al: All-trans retinoic acid in acute promyelocytic leukemia: long-term outcome and prognostic factor analysis from the North American Intergroup protocol. Blood 2002;100(13):4298-302.
Yates J, Glidewell O, Wiernik P, et al: Cytosine arabinoside with daunorubicin or Adriamycin for therapy of acute myelocytic leukemia: A CALGB study. Blood 1982;60(2):454-462.

[1]Not FDA approved for this indication.

Rakel and Bope: *Conn's Current Therapy 2006.*

Acute Leukemia In Childhood

Method of
Raymond J. Hutchinson, MS, MD

The acute leukemias comprise approximately 30% to 35% of all malignant diseases diagnosed in children younger than 15 years of age. Approximately 2400 new cases of acute lymphoblastic leukemia (ALL) are diagnosed annually in the United States among children and adolescents younger than 20 years of age. An additional 800 to 900 cases of acute myelogenous leukemia (AML) are diagnosed annually in U.S. children and adolescents. Of the acute leukemias of childhood, ALL accounts for 75% to 80% of the total and AML for 20% to 25% of the total. Both disease processes continue to be the subject of intense biologic and epidemiologic study and the focus of comprehensive clinical investigation searching for optimal therapy.

The cellular proliferation characteristic of acute leukemias often occurs in association with key molecular events resulting from chromosomal translocations, inversions, and/or additions/deletions with corresponding genetic mutations. Mutations may be germinal arising in utero or acquired occurring in individual somatic cells; individual mutations may be both necessary and sufficient to promote leukemic proliferation or they may be necessary but not sufficient, implying that at least one more genetic event must occur to promote expansion of a preleukemic clone. Certain chromosomal translocations (t) are consistently associated with specific subtypes of acute leukemia and have significant impact upon prognosis and hence upon choice of treatment; for example:

- In ALL, t(9;22), t(4;11), t(12;21), and t(1;19)
- In AML, chromosomal additions, deletions, rearrangements, and translocations such as trisomy 8, monosomies 5 and 7, inversion 16, and translocations t(8;21) and t(15;17)

With further refinements in molecular techniques, the genetic events contributing to or actually responsible for leukemic cell proliferation will be more fully defined. The future holds promise that novel understanding of these events will lead to new treatment approaches that will be much more specific for the leukemia cells than has conventional chemotherapy.

Diagnosis

Patients with acute leukemia are generally well until they or their parents notice the onset of acute symptomatology, including otherwise unexplained fever, bruising, bone pain, and/or lethargy. With persistence of any of these symptoms, medical care is sought. Often the physician notes physical findings, including fever, signs of cutaneous bleeding (petechiae, ecchymoses), splenomegaly, and lymphadenopathy. The astute physician will obtain a complete blood count with a white blood cell (WBC) differential count and a chest radiograph. If two or more blood cell cytopenias are observed (e.g., anemia with leukopenia, leukopenia with thrombocytopenia, etc.), a bone marrow aspirate and biopsy are called for. The bone marrow aspirate typically reveals displacement of normal hematopoietic precursors by leukemic blast cells, which generally have a high nuclear/cytoplasmic ratio, often exhibit nucleoli, and sometimes demonstrate vacuoles in the cytoplasm and occasionally in the nucleus. This test is the definitive test needed to establish the diagnosis of acute leukemia, even in the presence of what appear to be circulating leukemic blasts. When the diagnosis of acute leukemia is apparent, necessary additional studies include examination of the cerebrospinal fluid (CSF) for leukemic blasts; a chest radiograph looking for a mediastinal mass; serum chemistries including blood urea nitrogen (BUN), creatinine, electrolytes, calcium, and phosphorus to assess for tumor lysis syndrome; and coagulation studies (prothrombin time [PT], partial thromboplastin time [PTT]) to rule out a leukemia-associated coagulopathy.

Classification

The acute leukemias of childhood are initially separated into two broad categories, ALL and AML. Historically, this classification was done by light microscopic histologic review, employing special stains such as periodic acid-Schiff (PAS), myeloperoxidase, and the esterase stains. This classification had significant ramifications as treatment varies widely for these two primary categories of acute leukemia; in addition, treatment outcomes were significantly better for children with ALL than was true for those with AML. In the 1980s, immunophenotyping of leukemic blasts became a mainstay of classification, using monoclonal antibodies, which marked cells expressing their cognate antigen. The antigens were given cluster designation (CD) nomenclature to allow for consistency in analysis and in reporting results (Table 1). Thus, certain CD antigens were characteristic of ALL and others were characteristic of AML:

- ALL—CD2, CD5, and CD7 for ALL of T-cell origin and CD10, CD19, CD20, and CD22 for ALL of pre-B-cell and B-cell origin
- AML—CD11, CD13, and CD33

Establishing the immune phenotype of acute leukemias added greatly to more definitive classification, especially when separating ALL from AML and T-cell ALL from pre-B-cell ALL. Immunophenotypic characterization of acute leukemias enhanced the classification established by the French-American-British (FAB) systems for classifying ALL and AML. The combined approach of using blast cell morphology and blast cell immunophenotype has facilitated the delivery of specific treatment to children with each of the major subtypes of acute leukemia; it has also augmented the application of risk-directed therapies to patients with subclasses of ALL and AML, particularly the former.

TABLE 1 Immunophenotypes of Major
Categories of Acute Leukemia

Phenotype	Antigens expressed	Frequency
Acute Lymphoblastic Leukemia		
B precursor	CD19, CD20, CD22, CD24, CD10	65%
Pre-B cell	As above plus cytoplasmic Ig	20%
Mature B cell	CD19, CD20, CD21, surface Ig	2%
T cell	CD2, CD5, CD7, CD1, CD4, CD8, CD3	13%
Acute Myelogenous Leukemia		
Myeloid	CD11, CD13, CD15, CD33, CD34, CD65	

Further advances in classification have been achieved with refinements in cytogenetic and molecular classification of acute leukemias. Several well-known cytogenetic changes in blast cells are associated with important prognostic differences in outcome; the translocations t(9;22) and t(4;11) impart poor outcomes to those individuals whose leukemia cells contain them, while the t(12;21) translocation imparts a very good prognosis to children with blasts containing that translocation. The same is true in AML, wherein t(8;21), inversion of chromosome 16, and t(15;17) impart favorable outcomes; while monosomy 7, absence of the long arm of chromosome 5, and 11q23 abnormalities signal a poor prognosis. In summary, the classification of childhood acute leukemias, much the same as in adult leukemias, is accomplished using morphology under the light microscope, immunophenotypic features, and blast cell cytogenetic and molecular features; the result of this sophisticated classification impacts both choice of treatment and outcome.

Supportive Care

Improvements in supportive care continue to enhance outcomes for all patients with acute leukemia. Many of these advances have come in the area of infectious disease. Anti-infective drugs developed for bacteria resistant to conventional antibiotics have made significant inroads in the treatment of both gram-positive and gram-negative infections. New antifungal drugs, in particular, offer promise for some of the most deadly infections that patients with leukemia face. Modified hematopoietic growth factors now allow for fewer painful administrations, while maintaining longer-lasting effects. A new drug designed to reduce uric acid levels has found a place in the management of fulminant tumor lysis syndrome. High-quality transfusional support facilitates oxygen delivery and reduces bleeding in leukemia patients, while minimizing the transmission of infectious agents.

Rakel and Bope: *Conn's Current Therapy 2006.*

HYPERLEUKOCYTOSIS

At presentation, children with acute leukemia often have WBC counts in excess of 100,000/μL. When they do, consideration is given to leukapheresis or to administration of single-agent corticosteroid therapy to rapidly reduce the blood count and, specifically, the number of circulating leukemic blasts. Hyperleukocytosis may be associated with decreased cerebral and/or pulmonary blood flow, with consequent stroke-like symptoms or respiratory distress and hypoxia. Patients with AML appear to be at higher risk of such adverse physiology than patients with ALL. In general, leukapheresis is recommended when the WBC reaches or exceeds 200,000/μL. The use of single-agent corticosteroids in patients with ALL is discouraged unless part of an established treatment protocol. In fact, indiscriminant use of corticosteroids at the time of diagnosis often precludes patient entry onto one of the current national frontline investigational treatment protocols for ALL.

TRANSFUSION THERAPY

Support of the plasma hemoglobin level and of the platelet count are essential ingredients in the successful management of patients with acute leukemia. Without adequate oxygen delivery, organ dysfunction may occur, impacting negatively upon the patient's ability to tolerate aggressive chemotherapy. Red blood cell (RBC) transfusion, employing irradiated cells, is implemented when the patient's hemoglobin value falls below a value of approximately 8.0 g/dL; in very young children, the threshold for RBC transfusion may be 7.0 g/dL or even somewhat lower. Patient symptoms may also influence the decision of when to transfuse RBCs; dizziness, headache, fatigue, and shortness of breath, when present, should result in a lower threshold for transfusion.

To prevent the bleeding to which thrombocytopenic patients are predisposed, irradiated platelet transfusions are administered to nonbleeding patients for platelet counts below 5000/μL. For patients who are thrombocytopenic and actively bleeding, there is no specific platelet transfusion threshold; the degree of bleeding drives decisions about the timing of platelet transfusions. For all leukemic patients, transfusions should be done only with irradiated, leukocyte-depleted products, thereby to reduce risks of transfusion-associated graft-versus-host disease (GVHD) and of exposure to transfused cytomegalovirus.

TUMOR LYSIS SYNDROME

When leukemic cell cytoreduction begins with the onset of administration of chemotherapy, byproducts of cell death, including uric acid, potassium, and phosphorus, are released into the bloodstream. If the uric acid level exceeds its solubility in the blood, it will precipitate in the form of crystals in the kidneys, resulting in uric acid nephropathy. Thereafter, clearance of potassium and phosphorus in the kidneys can be impaired with threatening consequences for the patient. Allopurinol at 10 mg/kg (maximum dose 600 mg/day) is given orally in two or three divided doses for the first several days of antineoplastic therapy. For most patients, this is sufficient to prevent uric acid nephropathy and tumor lysis syndrome.

For patients with:

- Peripheral blood WBC counts in excess of 100,000/mL,
- Significant organomegaly,
- Elevated levels of serum potassium and/or phosphorus, and
- Preexistent kidney dysfunction,

the uric acid oxidase, rasburicase, may offer the advantage of very rapid reduction of serum uric acid levels, thereby reducing the risk of developing hyperkalemia and subsequently of cardiac arrhythmia. It should be kept in mind, however, that uric acid oxidase is currently very expensive, and for most patients allopurinol is more than sufficient.

INFECTION

Infection remains the primary cause of death in patients with acute leukemia undergoing chemotherapy. When patients are neutropenic with fever, as often occurs during induction, intensification, or reinduction/reintensification therapy, they require rapid evaluation. They should have blood samples and other target fluids/tissues collected for culture, and they should be started promptly on broad-spectrum antibiotic coverage. Most data indicate that chest radiographs are not necessary for febrile patients presenting with no pulmonary symptomatology. Antibiotic coverage typically consists of dual-agent coverage, such as gentamicin and Zosyn, to provide good gram-negative coverage along with reasonable gram-positive coverage. In some centers, single-agent coverage with a drug demonstrating broad-ranging efficacy, such as Cefepime or ciprofloxacin, is initiated, adding additional agents or changing coverage as dictated by culture results and clinical course. Other physicians prefer to add vancomycin initially to achieve excellent gram-positive coverage, important in an era when gram-positive organisms account for a majority of the infections occurring in patients receiving chemotherapy. Usually, the febrile patient is managed as an inpatient for the first 2 days of the illness; however, strategies are being developed and tested, either for total outpatient management of these patients or for rapid discharge from the inpatient unit once initial cultures are negative and fevers disappear. When specific organisms are identified, the therapy should be refined to provide the most active antibiotics for the identified organism. In the face of continuing fevers and neutropenia without positive culture results, antifungal agents, usually amphotericin-B or one of the related lipid formulations, are started. The new agent, voriconazole, offers relatively broad antifungal coverage, while reducing the risk of nephrotoxicity. However, voriconazole interacts with many drugs, altering blood levels of those drugs; it also can cause retinal and liver toxicity. Another new choice among antifungal agents is caspofungin; this agent is well tolerated and has excellent activity

against *Candida* and *Aspergillus* infections. Fever occurring during non-neutropenic periods also requires careful management, since many patients have poor cell mediated immunity and often have indwelling plastic central venous catheters. When the latter is the case and also when patients appear ill, it is wise to obtain blood cultures and to initiate antibiotic therapy.

Most patients undergoing therapy for acute leukemia are maintained on prophylactic antibiotics. All patients who are not allergic to trimethoprim-sulfamethoxazole should be placed on this drug at 5 to 6 mg/kg per day (of the trimethoprim component) in two divided doses for 2 to 3 successive days each week in order to prevent *Pneumocystis carinii* pneumonia. For intense induction regimens, the use of oral nystatin (Mycostatin) or of fluconazole reduces the incidence of candidal infections.

GROWTH FACTORS

The hematopoietic growth factor, granulocyte colony-stimulating factor (G-CSF), has been used greatly in patients with solid tumors to facilitate recovery from chemotherapy. However, in patients with acute leukemia, the use of G-CSF and other growth factors has been limited. In part, concerns over expanding leukemic blast cell populations have limited use of G-CSF, particularly for patients with AML. In general, use of G-CSF has largely been limited to treatment of patients when febrile and neutropenic. The development of pegylated growth factors (pegfilgrastim, darbepoetin alfa) offers the prospect of using these agents in children with less discomfort because of the increased interval between injections.

VENOUS ACCESS

The use of indwelling venous access devices has become prevalent in the management of pediatric oncology patients. These catheters offer easy access for blood draws, for administration of chemotherapy and other medications, for transfusions, and for administration of parenteral nutrition, while minimizing pain for the children. Therefore, most leukemia patients have them placed early in the course of their evaluation and before the initiation of therapy. Their use, however, is associated with risks of infection, thrombosis in the used vein, and failure to work properly, most troublesome when patients have low blood counts making line replacement difficult. After the intensive part of therapy has been completed, consideration should be given to removing the catheter, weighing the disadvantages of not having easy venous access against the risk of infection if the catheter remains in place.

Treatment

ACUTE LYMPHOBLASTIC LEUKEMIA

The treatment of ALL has historically been divided into three phases—induction of remission, consolidation or intensification of that remission, and maintenance of the remission. With the advent of reintensifying therapy, additional phases of treatment have come into play (Table 2). One typical scheme of therapy, which is used in the Children's Cancer Group/ Children's Oncology Group and is modified from the Berlin-Frankfurt-Munster (BFM) Leukemia Study Group, includes induction, intensification, interim maintenance, delayed intensification, and maintenance phases of therapy. Contemporary therapy of ALL produces 70% to 80% 5-year disease-free survival, with outcomes varying according to risk group (Table 3).

Induction

During induction therapy, a combination of vincristine, corticosteroid (prednisone or dexamethasone), and asparaginase (L-asparaginase or PEG-asparaginase) with or without an anthracycline (usually daunorubicin) is employed to achieve several logs of cytoreduction, thereby inducing remission. The induction phase lasts 4 to 6 weeks. Remission is defined by the results of marrow aspiration; individuals with fewer than 5% blasts are considered in complete remission (CR) (M_1 status), those with 5% to 24% blasts in partial remission (M_2 status), and those with greater than 25% blasts in relapse (M_3 status). Typically, remission status also implies that the peripheral blood counts have returned to normal, as has the physical exam.

Approximately 98% of pediatric patients with ALL achieve remission. Early marrow response at day 7 is an important indicator of long-term disease-free survival (DFS). For patients with M_3 marrow status at day 7, intensification of induction therapy with the addition of an anthracycline will often enhance the probability of achieving remission and long-term disease-free survival. If a patient continues to demonstrate M_3 marrow status at day 28 of induction therapy or later, the prognosis with conventional therapy is very poor. These individuals should be considered for alternative induction therapy and for allogeneic hematopoietic stem cell transplantation (HSCT). The use of HSCT for patients with ALL in first CR is limited to individuals with the t(9;22) and

6

TABLE 2 Treatment Approach for Acute Lymphoblastic Leukemia*

Risk group	Induction	Consolidation	Interim maintenance
Standard risk	VCR, PRED or DEXA, ASPARA, IT ARA-C/MTX	CYCLO, ARA-C, TG or IDMTX, MP, VCR, PRED/DEXA, IT MTX	VCR, PRED/DEXA, MP, MTX, IT MTX
High risk	VCR, PRED or DEXA, ASPARA, ± DAUNO, IT ARA-C/MTX	CYCLO, ARA-C, TG or IDMTX, MP, VCR, PRED/DEXA IT MTX	VCR, PRED/DEXA, MP, MTX, IT MTX
Very high risk	VCR, PRED or DEXA, ASPARA, ± DAUNO, IT ARA-C/MTX	IFOS, ETOP, IT MTX, ± STI571, HDARA-C, HDMTX	(Proceed to HSCT or to reinduction)
T cell	VCR, PRED, DAUNO, ASPARA, MP, ARA-C, CYCLO, ± 506U78, IT MTX	MP, HDMTX, IT MTX	(Proceed to reinduction)

Risk group	Reinduction/reintensification	Maintenance	
Standard risk	VCR, DEXA, ASPARA, DOXO, IT MTX, CYCLO, ARA-C, TG	VCR, PRED/DEXA, MP, MTX, IT MTX	
High risk	VCR, DEXA, ASPARA, DOXO, IT MTX, CYCLO, ARA-C, TG	VCR, PRED/DEXA, MP, MTX, IT MTX	
Very high risk	VCR, DEXA, DAUNO, PEG-ASPARA, CYCLO, IT MTX, ± STI571, HDMTX, ETOP, CYCLO, HDARA-C, ASPARA	HDMTX, VCR, DEXA, MP, IT MTX, MTX, ETOP, CYCLO, ± STI571, ± CR XRT	
T cell	VCR, DEXA, DOXO, ASPARA, TG, CYCLO, ARA-C, ± 506U78, IT MTX, CR XRT	VCR, PRED, MP, MTX, ± 506U78	

Risk group	Induction/intensification	Reinduction/reintensification	
Infants		VCR, DEXA, DAUNO, CYCLO, ASPARA, ITT, HDMTX, ETOP	VCR, DEXA, DAUNO, CYCLO, ASPARA, ITT, IT ARA-C, VHDMTX, ETOP

	Consolidation	Intensification/maintenance	Maintenance
	ARA-C, ASPARA, VHDMTX, VCR, IT ARA-C,	VCR, DEXA, MTX, MP, IT ARA-C, ETOP, CYCLO	VCR, PRED, MTX, MP

*Recommendations are based upon the following protocols: B-precursor standard risk—Children's Cancer Group (CCG) 1991; B-precursor high risk—CCG 1961; B-precursor very high risk—Children's Oncology Group (COG) AALL0031; infants—CCG 1953; and T cell—COG AALL00P2.

Abbreviations: ARA-C = cytosine arabinoside (Cytosar-U); ASPARA = L-asparaginase (Elspar); CR XRT = cranial radiation therapy; CYCLO = cyclophosphamide (Cytoxan); DAUNO = daunorubicin (Cerubidine); DEXA = dexamethasone; DOXO = doxorubicin (Adriamycin); ETOP = etoposide (VePesid)[1]; HDARA-C = high-dose cytosine arabinoside; HDMTX = high-dose methotrexate; HSCT = hematopoietic stem cell therapy; IDMTX = intermediate dose methotrexate; IFOS = ifosfamide (Ifex)[1]; IT = intrathecal; ITT = triple drug intrathecal (methotrexate, hydrocortisone, cytosine arabinoside); MP = 6-mercaptopurine (Purinethol); MTX = methotrexate, PEG-ASPARA = peg-asparaginase (Oncaspar); PRED = prednisone; STI571 = imatinib (Gleevec)[1]; TG = 6-thioguanine (Tabloid); VCR = vincristine (Oncovin); VHDMTX = very-high-dose methotrexate.

[1]Not FDA approved for this indication.

TABLE 3 Risk Classification of B-Cell and T-Cell Acute Lymphoblastic Leukemia

NIH Consensus Risk Definitions

Standard	WBC <50,000 cells/mm³ and age 1 to <10 years
High	WBC ≥50,000 cells/mm³ or age ≥10 years

Other Factors Modifying Risk

Factor	Better risk	Worse risk
Gender	Female	Male
DNA index	>1.16	≤1.16
Cytogenetics	Hyperdiploid	Hypodiploid
	Trisomies 4, 10, 17	t(9;22)
	t(12;21)	MLL gene (11q23) disruption
CSF status	No blasts	Blasts present
Treatment response*	Rapid	Slow

*Determined by bone marrow status at day 7 or 14 or by peripheral blood status at day 7.
Abbreviations: CSF = cerebrospinal fluid; MLL = mixed lineage leukemia; WBC = white blood cell count.

t(4;11) translocations, to infants less than 1 year of age, and to patients with high WBC counts (>200,000/mm³) at diagnosis.

Intensification

Intensification therapy is designed to solidify the remission achieved during induction, with a goal of reducing further the remaining logs of leukemic cells. Various strategies are used in centers around the world. Intravenous cyclophosphamide, pulses of cytosine arabinoside with or without 6-thioguanine, and intravenous methotrexate and/or 6-mercaptopurine have been used. An additional goal of this phase of therapy is the initiation of therapy directed at sanctuary sites of disease, either to prevent central nervous system (CNS) relapse or to treat existent disease in the CNS, in the testes, or in other extramedullary sites. The intensification phase of therapy lasts 4 to 8 weeks.

Interim Maintenance

This phase of therapy is designed to allow a respite from intensive therapy, after induction/intensification but before reintensification, while at the same time providing maintenance therapy that will prevent relapse. This phase of therapy often begins with a dose of vincristine and a pulse of corticosteroid. Oral maintenance agents used include 6-mercaptopurine (or 6-thioguanine) and methotrexate. This phase of therapy lasts for 8 weeks.

Reintensification

During reintensification, induction therapy and intensification therapy are recapitulated, with the goal being eradication of any residual leukemia that has escaped the first three phases of therapy. The initial portion of this therapy includes three weekly doses of intravenous vincristine and doxorubicin, a 3-week course of oral dexamethasone or two 7-day courses of oral dexamethasone (days 1-7 and 15-21), and intramuscular asparaginase. The second segment of therapy consists of a single

dose of intravenous cyclophosphamide, eight doses of subcutaneous or intravenous cytosine arabinoside given over 2 weeks, and two 4-day courses of oral 6-thioguanine. This phase of therapy is one in which the risks of low blood counts and infection must be considered; patients often require transfusions and sometimes admission because of fever with neutropenia. The duration of this phase is 7 to 8 weeks.

Maintenance

Maintenance therapy is given over an extended period to bring the total duration of therapy to 2 to 3 years. Monthly pulses of vincristine and prednisone or dexamethasone are complemented with daily oral doses of 6-mercaptopurine and weekly oral doses of methotrexate. Some maintenance regimens employ pulses of chemotherapy agents rather than continuous oral maintenance agents.

Prophylaxis of Central Nervous System Leukemia

Because of a high propensity for extramedullary recurrence of ALL in the CNS, it is necessary to provide preventive treatment. Historically, this treatment has consisted of a combination of cranial radiation therapy and intrathecal chemotherapy. However, standard-risk patients with ALL do not need to receive cranial radiation therapy, provided the intrathecal therapy is given throughout maintenance therapy. The standard intrathecal medication used is methotrexate; the dose is age-adjusted and ranges from 6 to 15 mg. For patients with high-risk ALL, cranial radiation therapy to a dose of 1260 to 1800 cGy is given along with intrathecal methotrexate.

Treatment of Extramedullary Leukemia

When present at diagnosis, CNS leukemia is managed with cranial radiation of 1800 cGy plus weekly intrathecal methotrexate for at least six doses; intrathecal methotrexate is also continued during maintenance therapy, being given once every 8 to 12 weeks. If the CNS leukemia fails to respond to the single-drug intrathecal methotrexate, triple drug therapy employing cytosine arabinoside, hydrocortisone sodium succinate, and methotrexate should be initiated. With CNS leukemia poorly responsive to intrathecal methotrexate, the radiation field should be expanded to a craniospinal field, using 2400 cGy. Treatment of CNS relapse occurring while on therapy should consist of triple drug intrathecal therapy followed by 2400 cGy craniospinal radiation therapy.

Management of extramedullary leukemia outside of the CNS varies depending upon the location of the relapse, time of occurrence of the relapse, and response to systemic induction therapy. When present at diagnosis, soft tissue leukemia (such as can be seen in the testes, kidneys, ovaries, and skin) often responds well to standard induction therapy; lack of response to induction is managed with radiation therapy of 2400 to 3000 cGy. Extramedullary relapse on therapy should be managed with radiation therapy of 2400 to 3000 cGy plus institution of systemic reinduction therapy. The required total duration of therapy after such an isolated extramedullary relapse is controversial, with most patients receiving therapy for 2 years after relapse.

Treatment of Marrow Relapse

The timing of a marrow relapse of ALL is critical in treatment planning. Early marrow relapses occurring within 18 months of diagnosis carry a poor prognosis, with a high risk of treatment failure following salvage therapy. For patients with early marrow relapse, histocompatibility testing should be done on the patient, the patient's parents, and on any siblings. If a related donor who is compatible at human leukocyte antigens (HLA)-A, -B, -C, and -DR loci can be identified, then plans to undergo HSCT following reinduction therapy should be made. Some oncologists recommend pursuing unrelated donor stem cell transplantation after an early marrow relapse when a matched related donor is unavailable. This entails undertaking an unrelated donor search through the National Marrow Donor Program and other hematopoietic stem cell registries.

For marrow relapses that are either intermediate (18 to 35 months) or late (36 months or more) postdiagnosis, application of reinduction, intensification, and maintenance chemotherapies constitute the standard approach. Whether hematopoietic stem cell transplantation should be recommended for such patients remains a topic of discussion; clinical trials are needed to define the role of HSCT in the care of intermediate-to-late marrow relapses.

Treatment of Central Nervous System Relapse

Initial, isolated CNS relapses require both regional and systemic therapy. Because most patients experiencing such a relapse currently will not have received cranial radiation therapy as part of their prophylactic regimen,

craniospinal radiation therapy to a dose of 2400 cGy is a mainstay of therapy. Typically, patients receive either intrathecal methotrexate or triple intrathecal therapy (methotrexate, hydrocortisone sodium succinate, cytosine arabinoside) for four to six doses to clear the CSF of leukemic blasts. This will then be followed by radiation therapy delivered over 2 to 3 weeks. In addition, systemic chemotherapy is usually given for 2 years as experimental studies following isolated CNS relapse indicate the presence of subliminal disease in the marrow and elsewhere.

Treatment of Testicular Relapse

With testicular relapse, radiation to the testes has been delivered to a dose of 2400 cGy; historically, both testes have been irradiated, even when the relapse appears confined to one testis. However, recent data from Holland have challenged the necessity of administering testicular irradiation for late isolated testicular relapses (>8 months after completion of chemotherapy). For some patients with large testicular masses or with slow response to the radiation therapy, the treatment dose has been increased to 3000 cGy. As in isolated CNS relapse, patients with isolated testicular relapse receive systemic chemotherapy for 2 years.

ACUTE MYELOID LEUKEMIA

The management of acute myelogenous leukemia has evolved during the last 20 years to a point where more than 50% of newly diagnosed patients are expected to be alive and disease-free 5 years after diagnosis. The improvement from less than 30% to 50% has occurred because of intensification of therapy, particularly during the consolidation phase of therapy (Table 4). To some degree, the improvement relates to improved algorithms for defining risk groups (Table 5) and predicting outcomes following chemotherapy, with the decision on whether to include hematopoietic stem cell transplantation in therapy being based on the presence or absence of certain high-risk features.

Induction

Once the diagnosis of AML is established, chemotherapy is initiated employing an anthracycline (daunorubicin, doxorubicin, or idarubicin) and cytosine arabinoside with or without other agents, such as etoposide and/or thioguanine. A typical induction course consists of anthracycline daily for 3 days, cytosine arabinoside for 5 to 7 days, and, when used, etoposide or thioguanine for 3 to 4 days. Remissions are successfully induced 80% to 90% of the time.

Consolidation

Once remission is induced, the therapeutic emphasis becomes one of solidifying and maintaining the remission. Most consolidation/intensification strategies center on the use of high-dose cytosine arabinoside with amsacrine, etoposide, mitoxantrone, or L-asparaginase.

TABLE 4 Treatment Approach for Acute Myelogenous Leukemia*

Subtypes[†]	Induction	Consolidation	Intensification
M1, M2, M4-M7	IDAR or DAUNO, ARA-C, ± ETOP, ± TG, ± DEXA, IT ARA-C ± HSS ± MTX	IDAR or DAUNO, ARA-C, ± ETOP, ± TG, ± DEXA, IT ARA-C ± HSS ± MTX, and/or FLUD, ARA-C, IDAR	HDARA-C, ASPARA or MITOX, IT ARA-C ± HSS ± MTX or HSCT
M3	ATRA, DAUNO, ARA-C	DAUNO, ARA-C	ATRA maintenance

*Recommendations are based upon the following protocols: Children's Cancer Group (CCG) 2891, CCG 2961.
[†]From the French-American-British (FAB) classification system.
Abbreviations: ARA-C = cytosine arabinoside (Cytosar-U); ATRA = all-transretinoic acid (Vesanoid)[1]; DAUNO = daunorubicin (Cerubidine)[1]; DEXA = dexamethasone; ETOP = etoposide (VePesid)[1]; FLUD = fludarabine (Fludara)[1]; HDARA-C = high-dose cytosine arabinoside; HSCT = hematopoietic stem cell transplantation; HSS = hydrocortisone sodium succinate; IDAR = idarubicin (Idamycin)[1]; MITOX = mitoxantrone (Novantrone)[1]; MTX = methotrexate[1]; TG = 6-thioguanine (Tabloid).
[1]Not FDA approved for this indication.

Often two or three consolidation courses are administered in sequence. Hematopoietic stem cell transplantation is often used as one of these consolidation courses for children who have HLA-matched related donors.

Maintenance

The use of maintenance therapy in AML remains controversial. Randomized studies have failed to demonstrate benefit from maintenance therapy, provided the induction therapy and consolidation therapy are very intense.

Hematopoietic Stem Cell Transplantation

The use of matched related-donor hematopoietic stem cell transplantation in the treatment of newly diagnosed

TABLE 5 Risk Classification of Acute Myelogenous Leukemia (AML)

Morphologic Classification (FAB)

M0	Undifferentiated leukaemia
M1	Myeloblastic, no maturation
M2	Myeloblastic, with maturation
M3	Promyelocytic, hypergranular type
M3v	Promyelocytic, microgranular variant
M4	Myelomonocytic
M4Eo	Myelomonocytic, with eosinophilia
M5a	Monocytic
M5b	Monocytic, with differentiation
M6	Erythroleukemia
M7	Megakaryoblastic

Other Factors Modifying Risk

Factor	Better risk	Worse risk
White blood count	<100,000 cells/mm³	≥100,000 cells/mm³
Chromosomes	t(8;21) t(15;17) Inversion 16	Deletion of 5 or 7
Other	Down syndrome	Secondary AML* Previous myelodysplasia

*Secondary leukemia occurs following chemotherapy for a prior malignancy.
Abbreviation: FAB = French-American-British.

patients with AML, while having found a central role in the United States, is not universally accepted elsewhere for all risk groups. In the United Kingdom, for children with favorable blast cytogenetics (t[8;21], t[15;17], and inv16 with eosinophilia) who also have a rapid early response to chemotherapy, matched related-donor stem cell transplantation is not recommended. The growing trend appears to center on an effort to define high-risk criteria, which, when present, would dictate proceeding with matched related-donor stem cell transplantation in first CR. The use of unrelated donors for HSCT in first CR is limited only to patients with extremely high-risk AML, that is, those with monosomy 7 or 7q–, and those with poor response to induction therapy.

After relapse, stem cell transplantation has a major role in therapy. Both related donors when available and unrelated donors otherwise are used to provide the necessary stem cells. As the prognosis following relapse is so dismal with conventional chemotherapy, little debate surrounds the application of hematopoietic stem cell transplantation to these patients. Typical preparative regimens employed include:

- BuCy4—busulfan for 4 days followed by cyclophosphamide for 4 days
- BuCy2—busulfan for 4 days followed by cyclophosphamide for 2 days
- BAC—busulfan for 4 days followed by cytosine arabinoside for 2 days and then cyclophosphamide for 2 days
- CyTBI—cyclophosphamide for 4 days either before or after total body irradiation (1200 to 1440 cGy in divided doses over 3 to 4 days)

Chloroma

Occasionally patients with AML present with or later develop soft tissue collections of leukemic cells; these collections are called chloromas. At diagnosis, isolated chloromas are managed with systemic chemotherapy, with or without radiation therapy; recent data suggest a similar outcome for those receiving radiation therapy as for those not receiving it. Additional data suggest that the prognosis of patients with isolated chloromas as their presenting feature of AML have better prognoses than do patients presenting with marrow involvement. If a chloroma is present at relapse, local radiation therapy may be appropriate, especially if the relapse occurs while the patient is still receiving chemotherapy.

Relapse

Marrow is the typical site of relapse. Reinduction therapy following marrow relapse typically consists of a combination of high-dose cytosine arabinoside and etoposide, mitoxantrone, and/or L-asparaginase. Amsacrine and idarubicin have been used in place of mitoxantrone. The combination of topotecan and 2-chloro-deoxyadenosine (2-CDA) has activity in relapsed AML. Newer experimental approaches now being evaluated include the use of an anti-CD33 monoclonal antibody conjugated to an antitumor antibiotic (gemtuzumab ozogamicin) and the use of agents that block the activity of mutated FLT3, found in 10% to 15% of childhood AML cases. The use of the latter two biologic therapies requires the expression of CD33 on leukemic blasts for the gemtuzumab and FLT3-ITD (internal tandem duplications) in leukemic cells for the FLT3 mutation blockers. Furthermore, the clinical use of gemtuzumab is limited by an associated risk of veno-occlusive disease of the liver; this is particularly relevant for individuals eligible for HSCT following reinduction therapy, which includes gemtuzumab. Once remission is achieved, stem cell transplantation is an important consideration, using either a matched related donor if available, a mismatched related donor (5/6), or a well-matched unrelated donor (6/6 or 5/6). The availability of cord blood stem cells allows for a greater degree of HLA disparity in the matching process, with less risk of GVHD, but also less benefit from graft-versus-leukemia effect (GVL). The use of cord blood as a stem cell source is limited by the size of the cord blood units available and the weight of the patient, as the cell number per kilogram of weight infused is critical to successful engraftment.

Relapse in Sites Other Than Marrow

CNS relapses require the administration of intrathecal chemotherapy (cytosine arabinoside ± hydrocortisone sodium succinate and methotrexate) and 2400 cGy craniospinal radiation therapy, plus the administration of reinduction and consolidation chemotherapy. Allogeneic stem cell transplantation should be considered for consolidation of remission following a CNS relapse. Similarly, relapse in a soft-tissue site requires radiation at a comparable dose to the affected soft tissues, provided that the field of treatment does not encompass too much normal tissue. Once again, reinduction and reconsolidation chemotherapy are essential, and stem cell transplantation should be considered.

LATE EFFECTS OF THERAPY

The successful management of acute leukemia must take into consideration the side effects of the therapy delivered, as these will significantly impact the quality

of life not only during therapy but also after therapy. Oftentimes, the negative impact of therapy is seen years after completion of therapy, and occasionally death results from these late effects of therapy. During treatment, patients experience nausea, vomiting, hair loss, mouth sores, low blood counts with risks of infection and bleeding, liver injury, and renal dysfunction; fortunately, most of these pass quickly and completely once the patient has completed taking the offending drug or receiving radiation therapy. However, deleterious effects on the CNS, such as leukoencephalopathy and radiation injury to the brain, may have lasting ramifications for the patient's well-being. Similarly, growth impairment from radiation therapy; cardiomyopathy from anthracyclines; osteonecrosis from corticosteroids; pituitary, thyroid, and gonadal hormonal insufficiency from radiation therapy; pulmonary injury from chemotherapy or radiation therapy; and the late sequelae of infertility and second malignancy will have lasting impacts on quality of life. As pediatric oncologists achieve improved control of acute leukemia, with higher rates of remission induction and longer disease-free intervals, and, particularly as the long-term cure rate rises, one compelling goal of investigative efforts must be to lessen the long-lasting and late sequelae of treatment. This mission is indeed already being implemented in the management of the lower risk groups of patients with ALL, following trends established in the successful treatment of Wilms tumor and Hodgkin disease. Finally, the establishment of *late effects* clinics in cancer centers around the country allows practitioners to focus on assessing the total impact of the therapy they previously delivered to leukemia patients. With 70% to 80% of children with ALL and 40% to 50% of children with AML surviving for more than 5 years, pediatric oncologists must now deal with treatment-related issues

---

 CURRENT DIAGNOSIS

- History (including a family history of blood disorders) and physical examination
- Complete blood count with a manual white blood cell differential count and review of the peripheral smear
- Chest radiograph (PA and lateral views)
- Serum electrolytes, BUN, creatinine, uric acid, calcium, phosphorus, LDH, ALT, bilirubin
- Coagulation studies—prothrombin time, partial thromboplastin time
- Varicella titer (IgG)
- Bone marrow aspirate and biopsy for morphology, cytochemistry, blast cell immunophenotype, blast cell cytogenetics
- Lumbar puncture with CSF cell count, morphology on a spun preparation, protein, and glucose

Abbreviations: ALT = alanine aminotransferase; BUN = blood urea nitrogen; CSF = cerebrospinal fluid; LDH = lactate dehydrogenase; PA = posteroanterior.

arising in schools and in workplaces, as well as in the homes, of these surviving children. Many of these survivors need guidance and assistance in the educational arena, in job placement, in social adjustment, and in obtaining health insurance coverage. The good news of longer durable remissions and of cures for many patients with acute leukemia must be balanced against the need for achieving greater success in treating high-risk patients with ALL and a majority of patients with AML, as well as against the imperative of evaluating late sequelae of therapy and developing strategies to prevent and assist in managing these problems.

Chronic Leukemias

Method of
Helen Enright, MD, and
Jonathan Bond, MB, BCh

Chronic Lymphocytic Leukemia

Chronic lymphocytic leukemia (CLL) is the most common leukemia in the Western world with an incidence of thirty per million per year. Two thirds of patients are male. The median age at presentation is 65 to 70 years of age.

Nearly 50% of patients are asymptomatic at presentation with the diagnosis made incidentally following a routine blood count. Symptomatic presentation relates to consequences of bone marrow failure, lymphadenopathy and/or hepatosplenomegaly, constitutional symptoms, or autoimmune complications such as hemolytic anemia.

DIAGNOSIS

The presence of peripheral blood lymphocytosis of greater than 5×10^9/L is required for the diagnosis of CLL. The blood film typically shows small mature lymphocytes in addition to fragile cells damaged in the film-spreading process called smudge cells. Immunophenotyping shows a clonal population of mature B lymphocytes that aberrantly express CD5.

Diagnostic evaluation should include direct Coombs test (DCT) (positive in 35%) and serum immunoglobulin estimation.

Bone marrow aspiration and biopsy is important in delineating the extent and pattern of marrow involvement (nodular, diffuse, or interstitial) and to evaluate response to treatment. Cytogenetic analysis may reveal important prognostic information.

Two main staging systems exist (Box 1). These are based on the extent of disease and degree of bone marrow failure.

BOX 1 The Rai and Binet Staging Systems for Chronic Lymphocytic Leukemia (CLL)

Rai System
- 0: No anemia, thrombocytopenia, or physical signs
- I: Lymphadenopathy only
- II: Splenomegaly and/or hepatomegaly but no anemia or thrombocytopenia
- III: Anemia (Hb < 11.0 g/dL)
- IV: Thrombocytopenia (platelet count <100 × 10⁹/L)

Binet System
- A: 0 to 2 areas* involved—can be further subdivided into A(0), A(I), and A(II)
- B: 3 to 5 areas involved
- C: Anemia (Hb <10.0 g/dL) or thrombocytopenia (<100 × 10⁹/L)

*Each general lymph node region, the liver, and the spleen constitutes an area.
Abbreviation: Hb = hemoglobin

PROGNOSIS

CLL has an extremely variable clinical course. Ideally, prediction of the likely rate of progression of disease would direct therapeutic intervention.

The staging systems of Rai and Binet are the longest-standing means of assessing the prognosis of individual patients with CLL. These have inherent limitations, notably to predict if patients presenting with early stage disease would still have rapid clinical progression. Recent studies on prognostic indicators have focused on biological and molecular characteristics of leukemic cells.

Adverse cytogenetic features at diagnosis include trisomy 12 and anomalies affecting the tumor suppressor gene p53 on chromosome 17p, the latter predicting a poor response to chemotherapy.

Gene expression profiling has identified two distinct subgroups of disease based on the presence or absence of somatic mutation in the specific immunoglobulin heavy-chain variable region (IgV_H) genes in leukemic cells. Although technically difficult to analyze, this information has important prognostic significance, with a median survival of 25 years in *mutated* cases versus 8 years in *unmutated* cases.

Levels of expression of ZAP-70 (which normally functions as a T cell signaling molecule) by CLL cells have been shown to correlate inversely with IgV_H gene mutation status. This is evaluated by flow cytometry and thus could theoretically be available as a prognostic marker in most routine hematology laboratories.

The prognostic significance of levels of CD38 expression, beta₂-microglobulin, lactate dehydrogenase (LDH), thymidine kinase, and soluble CD23 remains under investigation.

INDICATIONS FOR TREATMENT

CLL is a heterogeneous disease with a variable and often indolent course; a proportion of patients never require treatment for their disease. CLL is not curable

BOX 2   Indications for Treatment of Chronic Lymphocytic Leukemia (CLL) Suggested by the National Cancer Institute Working Group (1996)

- Progressive bone marrow failure
- Massive (>10 cm) or progressive lymphadenopathy
- Massive (>6 cm) or progressive splenomegaly
- Progressive lymphocytosis (doubling time <6 months or > 50% rise in lymphocyte count within 2 months)
- Systemic symptoms, e.g., debilitating night sweats, fevers, fatigue, weight loss
- Autoimmune cytopenias

by conventional treatment approaches, although reports of long-term disease-free survival (DFS) with newer treatment regimens including transplantation have led to some reconsideration of this tenet. The objective of treatment in the majority of cases, however, is disease control and palliation of symptoms.

Indications for treatment were published by the National Cancer Institute (NCI) Working Group in 1996 (Box 2). These include all Binet stages B and C and some stage A patients. Isolated lymphocytosis or hypogammaglobulinemia are not indications for treatment.

Supportive Treatment

Regular intravenous immunoglobulin (400 mg/kg every 3 to 4 weeks) should be considered in hypogammaglobulinemic patients with recurrent infections. The incidence of viral and fungal infections in CLL patients increases with the use of more intensive therapy, especially with purine analogues and alemtuzumab (Campath). Prophylaxis against *Pneumocystis carinii* is indicated in these patients. Autoimmune complications are treated in the same manner as in non-CLL associated cases, that is, usually with steroids—most patients will also require treatment of CLL in this setting. Erythropoietin may be useful in anemic patients.

Initial Treatment

The traditional first-line option for patients requiring treatment was the alkylating agent chlorambucil (Leukeran), which induces partial responses (PR) in 60% to 70% of patients. Treatment of early-stage disease does not confer a survival benefit, and there appears no difference in effect of continuous compared with intermittent dosing in patients needing treatment. There is no demonstrable therapeutic advantage to the addition of prednisone to chlorambucil, whereas combination regimens such as cyclophosphamide, hydroxydaunomycin (doxorubicin), Oncovin (vincristine), and prednisone (CHOP), despite higher overall response rates (ORR), show no relative survival benefit.

More recently, treatment with the purine analogue fludarabine (Fludara) has been shown to result in ORR of 70% to 80% in untreated disease with complete response (CR) rates of 20%, and these results have led

to its increased use as a first-line agent. Intravenous treatment is given at a dose of 25 mg/m^2 for 5 days, usually for six courses at four weekly intervals. Treatment with the oral formulation of the drug (40 mg/m^2) yields comparable response rates.

Comparative studies of fludarabine and alkylator-based regimens have consistently shown increased ORR, CR, and duration of response in fludarabine-treated groups. This has, however, not translated to an increase in overall survival, possibly because of crossover in study designs and high response rates to second-line treatment.

Fludarabine has potent immunosuppressive effects, causing increased susceptibility to serious infections. Defects in lymphocyte function may persist for months and even years after discontinuation of treatment. Transfusion should be with cytomegalovirus (CMV) seronegative and gamma-irradiated blood products. Purine analogues may also trigger autoimmune complications including refractory hemolysis and so are contraindicated in patients with a positive DCT.

Combination treatment with fludarabine with cyclophosphamide (Cytoxan) results in higher CR rates than with fludarabine alone with responses in 40% of cases previously resistant to fludarabine. The combination regimen fludarabine (25 mg/m^2) and cyclophosphamide (250 mg/m^2) (FCR) for 3 days with the anti-CD20 monoclonal antibody rituximab (Rituxan)[1] (375 mg/m^2, day 1 only) has resulted in ORR of more than 90% and CR rates of 70% in previously untreated patients.

Second-Line Treatment

Most patients who initially respond to first-line therapy have subsequent further progression of CLL requiring retreatment. Alkylating agents may be reintroduced, but responses are usually short-lived. Patients relapsing after initial fludarabine treatment are unlikely to respond to single agent alkylator therapy.

Fludarabine produces impressive results in patients previously treated with chlorambucil with ORR of 60% to 70% in patients responsive to alkylators and 20% to 50% in those previously resistant. Retreatment with fludarabine results in approximately 85% ORR in previously sensitive patients.

Combination treatment with cyclophosphamide, vincristine, and prednisone (CVP)[1] gives ORR in 31% of previously treated patients and is commonly used in patients with bulky disease. There is little evidence that anthracycline-based regimens confer therapeutic advantage over fludarabine in patients with relapsed disease. Responses have been seen, however, in fludarabine-resistant cases, and these may be considered in this setting.

The use of alemtuzumab (Campath), a monoclonal anti-CD52 antibody that specifically targets lymphocytes, has given ORR of 33% to 40% when studied in heavily pretreated patients. The achievement of CR in

---

[1]Not FDA approved for this indication.

this setting may be associated with long-term DFS in selected patients. Bulky lymphadenopathy is poorly responsive to this treatment. Alemtuzumab is potently immunosuppressive with a high risk of infective complications, notably CMV reactivation (seen in 10%).

Rituximab (Rituxan)[1] as a single agent has yielded disappointing results. Its use in the combination FCR, however, has shown impressive ORR of greater than 70%, with CR rates as high as 25% reported.

Patients with p53 mutations who are resistant to treatment have a particularly poor prognosis. Responses to both alemtuzumab and high-dose methylprednisolone[1] have, however, been demonstrated in this setting.

Stem Cell Transplantation

Peripheral blood stem cell (PBSC) and marrow transplant remain experimental in CLL. PBSC mobilization followed by high-dose therapy and stem cell rescue is feasible, although extensive pretreatment with fludarabine may compromise stem cell mobilization and harvesting.

Allogeneic transplant offers the only current potential for cure of CLL, and long-term DFS is possible, even in poor risk patients, with three-year survival rates of 46% reported, although treatment-related mortality (TRM) of 46% is also seen. The encouraging response rates seen with fludarabine-based regimens with much lower attendant morbidity means myeloablative allogeneic transplant is usually reserved for young patients with poor prognostic features.

Attempts have been made to decrease transplant toxicity while harnessing beneficial graft-versus-leukemia (GVL) effects by using nonmyeloablative conditioning regimens. These regimens have resulted in CR rates of approximately 40% with chronic graft-versus-host disease (GVHD) occurring in 75% of patients and TRM of 15% to 20%.

Richter's Syndrome

Transformation to a high-grade, usually diffuse, large-cell lymphoma, occurs in 5% to 10% of CLL. Prognosis is poor with low response rates to therapy and very short survival rates (2 to 8 months).

T cell prolymphocytic leukemia (T-PLL) typically follows an aggressive clinical course with survival usually less than 1 year. It is slightly more common in males with a median age at presentation of 65 years of age. Patients usually have hepatosplenomegaly and lymphadenopathy with skin involvement in 20% of cases. There is typically a marked lymphocytosis (>100 × 10^9/L).

Treatment responses are usually disappointing. Chlorambucil, pentostatin (Nipent), or combination regimens such as CHOP are usually ineffective or give a transient short-lived PR. Recent encouraging responses have been seen with alemtuzumab with ORR of 51% to 76%, although infusion-related adverse events and infective complications are common.

T cell large granular lymphocytic (LGL) *leukemia* is characterized by a persistent increase in clonal large granular lymphocytes in the peripheral blood that may infiltrate the bone marrow, liver, and spleen.

The median age at presentation is 50 to 60 years of age with males and females equally affected. The commonest clinical presentations relate to neutropenia and splenomegaly (seen in 50% of cases).

The abnormal lymphocytes usually have a mature T cell immunophenotype—expression of natural killer cell markers (e.g., CD56) is associated with a more aggressive clinical course.

Complications of neutropenia and (more rarely) red cell aplasia are believed to be cytokine-mediated. Immunologic abnormalities are common, including clinical and/or serologic evidence of rheumatoid arthritis in 30% of cases.

T-LGL leukemia usually follows an indolent clinical course, and treatment is not indicated in asymptomatic cases. Recurrent infection because of neutropenia is the commonest indication for intervention. Neutropenia may respond to corticosteroids whereas granulocyte colony-stimulating factor (G-CSF) (Neupogen)[1] may be effective in some cases.

Cyclosporine A (Neoral)[1] (5 to 10 mg/kg/day) and low-dose oral methotrexate (Rheumatrex)[1] (usually 7.5 mg/week) are used. Cyclophosphamide (Cytoxan)[1] (100 mg/day) has shown efficacy in pure red (blood) cell aplasia (PRCA).

Treatment responses in the more aggressive forms of the disease (including combination chemotherapy) have been almost universally disappointing.

Hairy cell leukemia is characterized by malignant proliferation of mature B lymphocytes with cytoplasmic projections, giving it a characteristic morphologic appearance. Patients usually present with splenomegaly and/or pancytopenia (with monocytopenia characteristic).

Bone marrow aspiration is typically difficult because of increased fibrosis. Tartrate-resistant acid phosphatase (TRAP) stain is usually positive. The bone marrow biopsy shows an interstitial infiltrate of widely spaced lymphoid cells.

Variant cases have distinct morphology and tend to have a poorer response to treatment.

Cladribine (Leustatin) is the treatment of choice, usually given as a continuous infusion over 7 days at 0.1 mg/kg/day. CR rates of 50% to 91% with progression-free survival (PFS) and DFS at 4 years of up to 84% and 96%, respectively, are reported. Alternative dosing schedules have also been used successfully.

Pentostatin (Nipent) produces ORR of 84% with CR of 64% when given at doses of 5 mg/m^2 for 2 days every 2 weeks until maximum response.

---

[1]Not FDA approved for this indication.

[1]Not FDA approved for this indication.

Interferon alfa-2a (Roferon-A) (3 µ/day by subcutaneous injection for 16 to 24 weeks initially) may be considered in cases refractory to purine analogues. Splenectomy may be considered where splenomegaly is the dominant clinical feature and other treatments have failed.

Chronic Myeloid Leukemia

Chronic myeloid leukemia (CML) is characterized by a specific chromosomal translocation resulting in the generation of an aberrant tyrosine kinase, which fuels proliferation of a malignant clone of myeloid cells.

Most patients present in chronic phase with proliferation of well-differentiated myeloid cells. Some present with more advanced disease or in blast crisis, similar to acute leukemia.

CML has an annual incidence of 1 to 2 cases per 100,000 population (accounting for 15% to 20% of all leukemia) with a slight male preponderance. Typical age of presentation is 40 to 60 years of age.

CLINICAL FEATURES

Up to 20% to 50% of cases are diagnosed incidentally following blood tests performed for other reasons. Symptomatic presentation includes:

- Systemic symptoms such as sweats, fatigue and malaise
- Symptoms referable to splenomegaly, that is, abdominal discomfort or early satiety
- Rarely, may present with acute gout, priapism, or with symptoms of hyperviscosity because of very high leukocyte counts

LABORATORY FEATURES

CML usually presents with neutrophil leukocytosis. There is a "left shift" with increased myelocytes and metamyelocytes in the peripheral blood and bone marrow. The differential diagnosis includes a leukemoid reaction to infection, inflammation, or malignancy. There is typically basophilia and often eosinophilia. The platelet count is normal or elevated and mild anemia is common. Biochemical markers of increased cell turnover, such as LDH and urate, are typically elevated.

Bone marrow aspiration and biopsy show myeloid hyperplasia, but dysplastic features are not prominent.

In chronic phase, the blast count is typically less than 5%. The transition to accelerated and blast phases is defined by increasing blast percentages and other hematologic abnormalities (Box 3).

PROGNOSIS

The median survival of patients in chronic phase is 4 to 6 years. Patients with more advanced disease have much shorter life expectancy with median survival of

BOX 3 World Health Organization Definitions of Accelerated and Blast Phases of Chronic Myeloid Leukemia (CML)

Accelerated Phase (One or more features is required for diagnosis)
- Blasts 10% to 19% (PB/BM)
- PB basophils > 20%
- Platelet count <100 × 10⁹/L (Unrelated to therapy)
- Platelet count > 1000 × 10⁹/L
- Increasing splenic size
- Increasing WCC (All unresponsive to therapy)
- Cytogenetic evidence of clonal evolution

Blast Phase (One or more features is required for diagnosis)
- Blasts > 20% (PB/BM)
- Extramedullary blast proliferation (i.e., chloromata)
- Large foci or clusters of blasts in bone marrow biopsy

Abbreviations: BM = bone marrow; CML = chronic myeloid leukemia; PB = peripheral blood; WCC = white cell count.

less than 1 year in accelerated phase and 3 to 6 months in blast phase.

The classic prognostic scoring system for CML is that of Sokal, devised in 1984, which includes patient age, splenic size, peripheral blood blast percentage, and platelet count at diagnosis. Other scoring systems have also been used that consider parameters such as basophil and eosinophil counts. More recently, there is increasing interest in risk assessment based on the achievement of cytogenetic and molecular responses with treatment.

MOLECULAR BIOLOGY

CML is characterized by a chromosomal translocation involving chromosomes 9 and 22, which results in the fusion of the *ABL* oncogene on chromosome 9 with the breakpoint cluster region (BCR) of chromosome 22.

In 90% to 95% of cases, this results from a t(9;22)(q34;q11) translocation resulting in the formation of the Philadelphia chromosome (Figure 1). In rare cases, variant translocations involving other chromosomes or cryptic translocations may occur. These anomalies may be detected by conventional karyotyping of metaphase cells, fluorescence in situ hybridization (FISH), or by polymerase chain reaction (PCR) techniques. Rarely, no translocation is detectable and these patients tend to have more rapid disease progression.

The abnormal *BCR/ABL* fusion gene in CML encodes an abnormal tyrosine kinase that is constitutively activated and phosphorylates proteins in signaling pathways involved in cellular proliferation and apoptosis. The resultant inhibition of apoptosis and abnormal proliferation results in the accumulation of excessive myeloid cells in the bone marrow.

Rakel and Bope: *Conn's Current Therapy 2006.*

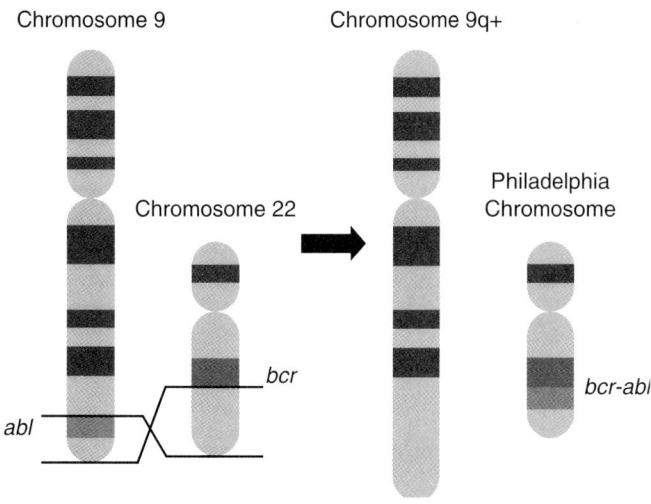

FIGURE 1. The Philadelphia chromosome. (From Mughal TI, Goldman JM: Chronic leukemias. In Rakel RE, Bope ET: Conn's Current Therapy 2004, 56th ed. Philadelphia, WB Saunders, 2004.)

TREATMENT

Nontransplant treatment options in the pre-imatinib era included hydroxyurea, busulphan, and interferon (IFN) with or without cytarabine.

Both hydroxyurea (Hydrea) and busulphan (Busulfex) suppress myeloid hyperplasia with reduction of the leukocyte count, although cytogenetic responses are rare, with no evidence of prolongation of overall survival.

Interferon alfa-2a (Roferon-A) (5 million U/m^2/day by subcutaneous injection) when used as a single agent produces hematologic responses in a majority of patients with complete cytogenetic remission (CCR) in 13% to 27%. IFN has well-recognized flulike adverse effects at time of injection that frequently limit dose escalation.

The combination of interferon plus cytarabine (Cytosar-U) results in increased rates of cytogenetic response compared with single agent IFN (41% versus 24% major cytogenetic response [MCR] at 12 months in one study), with improved overall survival. This combination was considered the standard of care for initial treatment of CML prior to the introduction of imatinib.

Imatinib (Gleevec) selectively inhibits the tyrosine kinase activity of *BCR/ABL* by binding its ATP-binding site, thereby inhibiting protein phosphorylation by the enzyme and blocking downstream signaling.

Following impressive preclinical and early clinical data, the International Research Information Service (IRIS) study was the first to compare the use of imatinib (400 mg/day) with conventional treatment (IFN and cytosine arabinoside [ara-C] in combination) in previously untreated patients in a randomized controlled setting. Imatinib treatment was superior in newly diagnosed chronic phase patients in several areas, notably achievement of cytogenetic responses (with MCR and CCR of 87% and 76% respectively with imatinib versus

35% and 14% in the combination group), whereas achievement of major molecular response (defined as at least a 3-log reduction in *BCR/ABL* by PCR) was seen in 39% of the imatinib group with only 2% in the combination arm achieving this response.

Significant quality of life benefits were also seen, attributable to the relative ease of administration (oral) and reduced incidence of side effects in the imatinib group. A survival benefit was not demonstrated; perhaps because of the crossover design of the study, a majority of patients in the combination group switched to imatinib treatment.

The latest data after 30 months of treatment show a still impressive MCR rate of 90% with a CCR rate of 82%.

Studies of the use of imatinib in accelerated phase disease have shown CCR in 24% of patients whereas activity has also been demonstrated in blast crisis with ORR of 55% to 70% seen. The incidence and severity of side effects seems consistent across treatment groups. These include nausea, ankle edema, skin rash, and cytopenias, all of which are usually mild to moderate in severity.

Fifteen percent to twenty percent of CML patients exhibit primary resistance to imatinib. Secondary resistance following initially successful treatment is seen in approximately 8% to 15% of chronic phase patients after 18 to 24 months.

Resistance is thought to occur by a number of mechanisms, including enhanced tyrosine kinase activity via chromosome or gene amplification, mutations within the ATP-binding site, or the development of new clonal cytogenetic abnormalities.

Ongoing studies include investigation of optimal dosage (400 mg vs. 800 mg) and the role of imatinib in combination with IFN[1] or ara-C.[1]

TREATMENT MONITORING

Response to treatment in CML has traditionally been monitored by full blood count and cytogenetic analysis. Latest data from the IRIS study suggest that CCR is associated with a decreased risk of disease progression. In addition, there is good evidence that achievement of a good molecular response as measured by quantitative PCR may result in improved PFS. Monitoring for ABL kinase domain mutations may be useful in determining likelihood of or emergence of resistance.

A broad consensus currently supports three-monthly monitoring of *BCR/ABL* mRNA levels by quantitative PCR with six-monthly assessment of cytogenetic status. A rising *BCR/ABL* level should trigger search for kinase domain mutations.

Stem cell transplantation currently provides the only proven means of achieving long-term DFS in CML. A suitable donor may not, however, be available, whereas medical co-morbidity or advanced patient age may provide unacceptable mortality risks.

---

[1]Not FDA approved for this indication.

CURRENT DIAGNOSIS

Chronic Myeloid Leukemia
- Neutrophil leukocytosis
- Splenomegaly
- Demonstration of t(9;22) translocation/BCR/ABL by PCR

Chronic Lymphocytic Leukemia
- Lymphocytosis (lymphocytes coexpress CD5 and CD19)
- Lymphadenopathy
- Splenomegaly
- Anemia/thrombocytopenia

Abbreviation: PCR = polymerase chain reaction

 CURRENT THERAPY

- Imatinib is the initial treatment of choice for most patients.
- Other nontransplant approaches include hydroxyurea, busulphan, and interferon (+/− ara-C).
- Allogeneic transplant should be considered in young patients presenting in chronic phase.
- Autologous and nonmyeloablative transplant remain experimental.

Success of allogeneic transplantation is determined by several factors, notably patient age and stage of disease at time of transplant. Chronic phase patients transplanted within a year of diagnosis have significantly improved survival (70% versus 40%) than those transplanted later in the course of disease. Overall, mortality posttransplant approaches 20% in the first 100 days, mainly because of infection and GVHD.

Donor lymphocyte infusion (DLI), by inducing a GVL effect, can reestablish remission in patients relapsing following transplant, often with molecular remission and prolonged survival in responders. This maneuver may be associated with exacerbation or triggering of GVHD, and optimum dosing and scheduling remains under investigation.

Nonmyeloablative transplantation using less intensive pretransplant preparative regimens aims to harness more beneficial GVL effects with reduced transplant-related morbidity, and, to date, mortality has been studied in relatively small series and is currently regarded as suboptimal treatment in fit patients where a suitable donor is available. It may be used in patients medically unfit for a myeloablative procedure but remains experimental.

Transplantation using matched unrelated donor (MUD) grafts may be considered for young patients who lack a sibling donor. Improvements in transplant outcome are attributable to improved molecular typing of donors, supportive care, and GVHD prophylaxis. Data from the National Marrow Donor Program show DFS for patients younger than 35 years of age comparable to that seen with sibling donors, although rates of GVHD are higher.

The use of autologous transplant remains largely experimental. Data from UK centers show low morbidity and mortality with a suggestion of increased duration of chronic phase and prolonged survival.

TREATMENT OPTIONS IN THE IMATINIB ERA

The advent of imatinib has heralded a major change in treatment approaches to CML. This has been accompanied by increased complexity of therapeutic decisions with several ongoing areas of investigation. It is unknown if prolonged prior treatment with imatinib and consequent delayed transplant will compromise transplant outcome. Although CCR is common with imatinib, most patients do not achieve a molecular remission as measured by current techniques. It is as yet unclear if this has meaningful clinical consequences or if prolonged DFS with molecularly positive disease may prove a valid therapeutic target for many patients.

Most centers institute imatinib in all patients older than 50 years of age and most patients older than 40 years of age. Failure of or resistance to treatment may be considered an impetus to transplant in medically fit patients. The use of nonmyeloablative transplant regimens may expand the eligible patient population. The proven efficacy of transplant in younger patients (especially those younger than 30 years of age) with a suitable donor makes this still the preferred treatment option in these patients. MUD transplantation is also a valid option in this group.

Evaluation of patient wishes and expectations with regard to potential morbidity, mortality, and survival benefits is an integral part of the decision-making process. It is hoped that the evolving data on the use of imatinib and ongoing experience with transplant may aid therapeutic decisions and facilitate consistent management approaches in the years to come.

REFERENCES

Crespo M, Bosch F, Villamar N, et al: ZAP-70 expression as a surrogate for immunoglobulin-variable-region mutations in chronic lymphocytic leukemia. N Engl J Med 2003;348:1764.

Gabor EP, Mishalani S, Lee S: Rapid response to cyclosporine therapy and sustained remission in large granular lymphocyte leukemia. Blood 1996;87:1199.

Gratwohl A, Hermans J, Goldman JM et al: Risk assessment for patients with chronic myeloid leukaemia before allogeneic blood or marrow transplantation. Chronic Leukaemia Working Party of the European Group for Blood and Marrow Transplantation. Lancet 1998;352:1087.

Jaffe ES, Harris NL, Stein H, et al (eds): World Health Organization Classification of Tumours. Pathology and Genetics of Tumours of Haemopoietic and Lymphoid Tissues. Lyon, IARC Press, 2001.

Jehn U, Bortl R, Dietzfelbinger H, et al: An update: 12-year follow-up of patients with hairy cell leukemia following treatment with 2-chlorodeoxyadenosine. Leukemia 2004;18(9):1476.

Keating MJ, O'Brien S, Lerner S, et al: Long-term follow-up of patients with chronic lymphocytic leukemia (CLL) receiving fludarabine regimens as initial therapy. Blood 1998;92:1165.

Kurzrock R, Kantarjian HM, Druker BJ, et al: Philadelphia chromosome-positive leukemias: From basic mechanisms to molecular therapeutics. Ann Intern Med 2003;138:319.

O'Brien SG, Guilhot F, Larson RA, et al: Imatinib compared with interferon and low-dose cytarabine for newly-diagnosed chronic-phase chronic myeloid leukemia. N Engl J Med 2003;348:994.

Paneesha S, Milligan DW: Stem cell transplantation for chronic lymphocytic leukemia. Br J Haematol 2005;128(2):145.

Non-Hodgkin's Lymphomas

Method of
Garrett Lynch, MD, and Tasha Stevens, BS

The non-Hodgkin's lymphomas are a relatively common malignancy. They consist of a heterogeneous group of disorders that may be B cell, T cell, and natural-killer (NK) cell in origin. B-cell lymphomas (BCLs) are overwhelmingly the most common. The follicular small–cleaved-cell lymphoma is the most common of all the non-Hodgkin's lymphomas, accounting for up to 25% of cases. Although the non-Hodgkin's lymphomas may affect persons of all ages, they are most common in patients older than age 50 years. They are especially common in the elderly. Certain lymphomas have a predilection for teenagers and young adults, especially Burkitt's lymphomas and acute lymphoblastic lymphoma.

A number of possible etiologies for non-Hodgkin's lymphomas have been postulated. The overall theme of the etiology of the BCLs is immune dysregulation. Immunodeficiency is the most well-established risk. Patients with hereditary immune deficiency diseases, those undergoing organ transplantation, and those with HIV all have an increased incidence of non-Hodgkin's lymphomas. In the case of HIV and organ-transplant recipients, the incidence of high-grade B-cell lymphomas is increased 20-fold; the lymphomas in these patients often involve extranodal sites, such as the gastrointestinal (GI) tract and the central nervous system (CNS). Immune stimulation has also been implicated in the development of lymphomas. Patients with rheumatological disorders are at increased risk for BCLs, especially patients with Sjögren's syndrome, with which the incidence of non-Hodgkin's lymphomas approaches 10% of patients over time. Occupational and industrial exposure may also play a role in the development of lymphomas; an increased incidence of follicular small–cleaved-cell lymphomas has been observed in farmers.

Infections, especially viruses, have been implicated in the development of non-Hodgkin's lymphomas. In addition to HIV, the Epstein-Barr virus (EBV) has been associated with Burkitt's lymphoma, especially in African children. EBV has also been implicated in NK-cell lymphoma, an aggressive lymphoma involving the nasal sinuses and nasal cavity. Herpesvirus 8 has been associated with a primary serous cavity lymphoma in patients with HIV. Human T lymphotropic virus 1 (HTLV-1) has been associated with an aggressive T-cell lymphoma characterized by organomegaly, skin infiltration, hypercalcemia, and lytic bone disease. HTLV-2 has been implicated in the etiology of mycosis fungoides, a primary T-cell lymphoma involving the skin. Some studies suggest an increased incidence of non-Hodgkin's lymphomas in patients with hepatitis C infection. Finally, *Helicobacter pylori* has been associated with mucosa-associated lymphoid tissue (MALToma), a low-grade lymphoma of the stomach that can often be eradicated with *H. pylori* therapy.

Specific chromosomal translocations have been identified through molecular biology techniques that have helped elucidate the pathogenesis of these disorders; these may someday serve as targets for therapy. The overall theme of the translocations identified in the B-cell non-Hodgkin's lymphomas is a translocation to chromosome 14 at the locus of the heavy immunoglobulin gene. In the most common follicular small–cleaved-cell lymphoma, the BCL oncogene on chromosome 18 is translocated to chromosome 14 t(14;18). BCL is involved in the regulation of apoptosis. The translocation results in an interruption of apoptosis and an accumulation of the malignant B cells. In the case of Burkitt's lymphoma, the c-myc oncogene on chromosome 8 is translocated next to the heavy immunoglobulin gene on chromosome 14 t(8;14), leading to uncontrolled cell proliferation. Mantle cell lymphoma is relatively chemotherapy-refractory lymphoma that is associated with the translocation of the gene for cyclin D1 on chromosome 11 to the heavy immunoglobulin gene on chromosome 14 t(11;14). Cyclin D1 is a cell cycle-checkpoint gene regulating progression of the cells through the cell cycle.

The classification schemes to categorize the non-Hodgkin's lymphomas has undergone multiple revisions though the years as our understanding of the biology, natural history, and cell of origin of these lymphomas has evolved. The common classification schemes today include the REAL (Revised European American Classification of Lymphoid Neoplasms) and the World Health Organization (WHO) classification (Box 1).

BOX 1   Working Formulation of Non-Hodgkin's Lymphomas

Low Grade
- Small lymphocytic
- Follicular small-cleaved cell
- Follicular, mixed small-cleaved and large cell
- Intermediate grade
- Follicular large cell
- Diffuse small-cleaved cell
- Diffuse small-cleaved, and large cell
- Diffuse large cell

High Grade
- Large cell, immunoblastic
- Lymphoblastic
- Small, noncleaved cell

Rakel and Bope: *Conn's Current Therapy 2006.*

> **BOX 2   Ann Arbor Staging Classification**
>
> Stage 1: Involvement or a single lymph node region or a single extranodal organ site (Ie)
> Stage 2: Involvement of 2 or more lymph node regions on the same side of the diaphragm or localized involvement of an extranodal site or organ (IIe) and one or more lymph node regions on the same side of the diaphragm
> Stage 3: Involvement of lymph node regions on both sides of the diaphragm, which may be accompanied by localized involvement of an extranodal organ or site (IIIe) or spleen (IIIs) or both (IIIse)
> Stage 4: Diffuse or disseminated involvement of two or more extranodal organs with or without associated lymph node involvement

On the other hand, the staging system for the non-Hodgkin's lymphomas has remained stable for more than 30 years. The Ann Arbor staging system remains in effect (Box 2).

Clinical Findings

SIGNS AND SYMPTOMS

Patients with non-Hodgkin's lymphomas may present with painless lymphadenopathy. The lymphomas may be localized to a given lymph node region, such as the neck, axilla, or groin, or they may be widespread. Paradoxically, the low-grade, indolent lymphomas often involve multiple nodal regions at diagnosis. The lymph nodes in patients with low-grade or indolent lymphomas are often small to moderate in size and may progress slowly. These nodes may actually wax and wane in size and number. On occasion, a spontaneous remission of the lymphoma may occur in the low-grade lymphomas, in particular the follicular small–cleaved-cell variant. The intermediate- and high-grade lymphomas are frequently associated with a sudden appearance of a lymph node with a relatively rapid increase in size of the node. The lymph node involvement in patients with high-grade lymphomas is often localized to one or two nodal regions. Unlike Hodgkin's disease, the lymph node involvement in the non-Hodgkin's lymphoma is often noncontiguous; frequently, peripheral lymph nodes are involved, including the epitrochlear nodes. Although peripheral lymphadenopathy often brings the patient with non-Hodgkin's lymphoma to attention, lymph node involvement of the mediastinal, hilar, celiac, peripancreatic, retroperitoneal, and pelvic lymph nodes is not uncommon. These patients often present with abdominal or back pain or with B symptoms.

B symptoms, defined as a weight loss of greater than 10% body weight, fever, and night sweats, are common and may be the presenting symptom of lymphoma. B symptoms are present in 40% of non-Hodgkin's lymphoma patients. They tend to be more common in the higher stage higher-grade patients but not exclusively. Pruritus, while not a B symptom per se, is a common associated symptom.

In approximately 30% of cases of low-grade lymphomas, the lymphoma may suddenly undergo a change in the natural history of the disease. Sudden rapid growth of new or preexisting lymph nodes or the sudden appearance of B symptoms may herald a Richter's transformation, which is the transformation of a low- to a high-grade lymphoma. Any time such a change occurs, a new lymph node biopsy is in order. Overall, the transformed lymphomas do poorly with therapy and have a limited survival.

Extranodal involvement is common in the non-Hodgkin's lymphomas, occurring in 25% of cases at presentation and up to 50% of cases during the course of the illness. Common extranodal sites of involvement include the GI tract, liver, bone, skin, and CNS. Virtually any extranodal site may be involved. Extranodal involvement is commonly noted in the high-grade BCLs complicating HIV.

Laboratory Findings

A tissue diagnosis is essential in establishing the diagnosis of a non-Hodgkin's lymphoma. Because their architectural pattern and the size of the malignant lymphocytes characterize the non-Hodgkin's lymphomas, an excisional biopsy is preferable to fine-needle aspiration or core-needle biopsy. The biopsy specimen should be sent for morphology, immunotyping/flow cytometry, and molecular genetic analysis. Flow cytometry may help subclassify the non-Hodgkin's lymphomas. The tissue should be examined for CD20 expression, a B-cell surface marker that may determine if rituximab (Rituxan), a monoclonal antibody to CD20, is used in lymphoma therapy.

Workup of a non-Hodgkin's lymphoma should include a complete history and physical, a complete blood count, BUN, creatinine, electrolytes, liver function tests, an LDH, a β_2-microglobulin, and a uric acid level. A chest radiograph and a computerized axial tomogram of the neck, chest, abdomen, and pelvis are in order. A bone marrow aspirate and biopsy are an essential part of staging.

Patients are often noted to be anemic at diagnosis. Pancytopenia is not uncommon, especially with bone marrow involvement. Bone marrow involvement is very common in the indolent or low-grade lymphomas; 80% to 90% of patients with follicular small–cleaved-cell lymphoma will have bone marrow involvement at diagnosis. In the case of diffuse large-cell lymphoma, only 15% of patients have bone marrow involvement at diagnoses; these patients have a worse prognosis and are at high risk for CNS relapse.

The LDH level is often increased in these patients and is associated with tumor bulk. The LDH level correlates with prognosis. The β_2-microglobulin is another prognostic marker in BCLs. It is the light chain of the MHC complex and is present on the majority of B cells. With a high burden of clonal B cells, it is shed into the peripheral blood and correlates with tumor bulk. An elevated uric acid level relates to increased cell turnover and may be a clue to high risk of tumor lysis.

Rakel and Bope: *Conn's Current Therapy 2006.*

CT scanning may detect disease in the chest and abdomen. It may detect nodal involvement as well as involvement of the visceral organs. The low-grade lymphomas tend to have widespread nodal disease, including visceral organ involvement. CT scanning is often used in the diagnosis of occult lymphomas.

With treatment, especially in the case of bulky lymphomas, there may be residual disease after therapy that may or may not represent active lymphoma. PET CT scanning may be useful in these situations, where a negative PET in the presence of residual lymph nodes may mean that the nodes are likely not clinically active.

Treatment

The low-grade or indolent lymphomas can be treated on a watch and wait basis. Waiting to treat until the patient is symptomatic does not adversely affect survival. Although combination chemotherapy has a higher response rate, acceptable treatment includes radiation, single-agent chemotherapy such as cyclophosphamide or combination chemotherapy with regimens such as COP (cyclophosphamide [Cytoxan], vincristine, prednisone), CHOP (cyclophosphamide, doxorubicin [Adriamycin],[1] vincristine, and prednisone), or FND (fludarabine [Fludara],[1] mitoxantrone [Novantrone][1] and dexamethasone [Decadron]).[1] Rituximab (Rituxan),[1] a monoclonal antibody to CD20, induces remissions in patients who relapse or are refractory to chemotherapy. A 40% response rate with this agent has been reported. Significant complete remission rates approaching 70% to 80% have been reported combining CHOP and rituximab (Rituxan)[1] or FND and rituximab (Rituxan)[1] in patients with follicular small–cleaved-cell lymphomas. Although prolonged remissions, including molecular remissions, have been reported, follow-up is not long enough to know if this will translate into long-term, disease-free survival. Targeted radioimmunotherapy combining a radioisotope with an antibody to CD20 (tositumomab [Bexxar] or ibritumomab [Zevalin]) may induce remission in patients refractory to the combination therapy; some of these remissions have been prolonged.

Although a number of regimens have been studied in diffuse large-cell lymphoma, the most common of the intermediate and high grade tumors, no regimen is superior to CHOP, with a 60% complete response rate and a 40% to 50% long-term survival rate. Studies adding rituximab (Rituxan)[1] to CHOP, especially in the elderly, resulted in an improvement of the response rate to 80%. Patients failing CHOP/rituximab (Rituxan)[1] can be considered for bone marrow transplantation if candidates otherwise a variety of second-line chemotherapy regimens may produce short-term remissions.

Although chemotherapy is the mainstay of therapy, radiation therapy may increase the remission rate when added to chemotherapy for early-stage (I and II) lymphomas and may provide palliation of symptoms in advanced stages.

---

[1]Not FDA approved for this indication.

Prognosis

Prognosis of the non-Hodgkin's lymphomas is highly variable. Patients with indolent lymphomas have a median survival of 7 to 10 years; survival beyond 10 years is not infrequent. In these lymphomas, treatment may reduce nodal size and may relieve symptoms, but does not affect overall outcome. Delaying therapy until symptoms occur does not affect outcome, as this disease is considered incurable with current treatment modalities.

In the case of high-grade lymphomas, the prognosis is 50/50. Approximately 50% of patients may be cured with current therapy and become long-term survivors. Patients not cured have a median survival of 1 to 2 years. Untreated, the survival of intermediate-grade lymphomas is a matter of only months, and in high-grade lymphomas it may be a matter of only weeks. Additional patients with high-grade lymphomas who do not obtain a complete remission or who relapse on therapy may obtain remission with bone marrow transplantation. Patients who have an especially poor prognosis with large-cell lymphoma include patients older than age 60 years, those with stage III or IV disease, B symptoms, liver and bone marrow involvement, a tumor mass of 10 cm or greater, and elevations of the LDH and/or β_2-microglobulin.

REFERENCES

Ceiffier B, Lepage E, Briere J, et al: CHOP chemotherapy plus rituximab compared with CHOP alone in elderly patients with diffuse large B-cell lymphoma. N Engl J Med 2002;346:235-242.

Chiu BC, Weisenburger DD: An update of the epidemiology of non-Hodgkin's lymphoma. Clin Lymphoma 2003;4:161.

Jaffe ES, Harris NL, Stein H, Vardiman JW: World Health Organization classification of tumours. Pathology and genetics of tumours of haematopoietic and lymphoid tissues. Lyon, France, IARC Press, 2001.

Staudt LM: Molecular diagnosis of the hematologic cancers: N Engl J Med 2003;348:1777.

Multiple Myeloma

Method of
Robert A. Kyle, MD, and
S. Vincent Rajkumar, MD

Multiple myeloma is characterized by the neoplastic proliferation of a single clone of plasma cells producing a monoclonal (M) protein in the serum or urine. In the United States, multiple myeloma constitutes 1% of all malignant diseases and slightly more than 10% of hematologic malignancies. The annual incidence is 4 per 100,000; the incidence in African Americans is twice that in whites. The apparent increase in rates is probably caused by increased availability and use of medical facilities and improved diagnostic techniques, particularly in the older population. The median age at diagnosis is

65 to 70 years, and only 2% of patients are younger than 40 years.

Weakness, fatigue, bone pain, recurrent infections, and symptoms of hypercalcemia or renal insufficiency should alert the physician to the possibility of multiple myeloma. Anemia is present in 70% of patients at the time of diagnosis. An M protein is found in the serum or urine in 97% of patients with multiple myeloma. Lytic lesions, osteoporosis, or fractures are present at diagnosis in 80%. Technetium bone scanning is inferior to conventional radiography and should *not* be used. Magnetic resonance imaging (MRI) or computed tomography (CT) is helpful in patients who have skeletal pain but no abnormality on radiographs or when spinal cord compression is suspected. Hypercalcemia is present in 25% of patients, and the serum creatinine value is 2 mg/dL or greater in almost 20% of patients at diagnosis.

Diagnosis

If multiple myeloma is suspected, the patient should have, in addition to a complete history and physical examination:

- Determination of values for hemoglobin, leukocytes with differential count, platelets, serum creatinine, calcium, and uric acid
- A radiographic survey of bones, including humeri and femurs
- Serum protein electrophoresis with immunofixation
- Quantitation of immunoglobulins
- Bone marrow aspirate and biopsy
- Routine urinalysis
- Electrophoresis and immunofixation of an adequately concentrated aliquot from a 24-hour urine specimen

Measurement of β_2-microglobulin, C-reactive protein, and lactate dehydrogenase values is helpful for prognosis. Cytogenetics and measurement of the plasma cell labeling index are also important from a prognostic standpoint.

Minimal criteria for the diagnosis of multiple myeloma consist of more than 10% plasma cells in the bone marrow or a plasmacytoma and one of the following: (a) M protein in the serum (usually more than 3 g/dL), (b) M protein in the urine, or (c) lytic bone lesions. In addition, the usual clinical features of multiple myeloma must be present. Metastatic carcinoma, lymphoma, leukemia, and connective tissue disorders may resemble multiple myeloma and must be considered in the differential diagnosis. Patients with multiple myeloma must be differentiated from those with monoclonal gammopathy of undetermined significance (benign monoclonal gammopathy) and smoldering (asymptomatic) multiple myeloma because they may remain stable for long periods (Box 1). The plasma cell labeling index is helpful in differentiating monoclonal gammopathy of undetermined significance or smoldering multiple myeloma from multiple myeloma. The patient's symptoms, physical findings, and all laboratory and radiographic data must be considered in the decision to begin therapy. If there are doubts about

whether to begin treatment, therapy should be withheld and the patient reevaluated in 2 to 3 months. There is no evidence that early treatment of multiple myeloma is advantageous.

BOX 1	Mayo Clinic Criteria for the Diagnosis of MGUS, SMM, and MM
MGUS	Serum M protein <3 g/dL and bone marrow plasma cells <10% and absence of anemia, renal failure, hypercalcemia, and lytic bone lesions
SMM	Serum M protein ≥3 g/dL and/or bone marrow plasma cells ≥10% and absence of anemia, renal failure, hypercalcemia, and lytic bone lesions
MM	Presence of a serum or urine M protein, bone marrow plasmacytosis and anemia, renal failure, hypercalcemia, or lytic bone lesions; patients with primary systemic amyloidosis and ≥30% bone marrow plasma cells are considered to have both multiple myeloma and amyloidosis

Abbreviations: M = monoclonal; MGUS = monoclonal gammopathy of undetermined significance; MM = multiple myeloma; SMM = smoldering multiple myeloma.
From Rajkumar SV, Dispenzieri A, Fonseca R, et al: Thalidomide for previously untreated indolent or smoldering multiple myeloma. Leukemia 2001;15:1274-1276. (Used with permission from Nature Publishing Group.)

Treatment

If the patient is eligible for an autologous peripheral blood stem cell transplant, the hematopoietic stem cells should be collected before the patient is exposed to alkylating agents. Patients who are ineligible for stem cell transplantation should be treated with standard alkylating agent therapy (discussed later in this article).

AUTOLOGOUS PERIPHERAL BLOOD STEM CELL TRANSPLANTATION

If a patient is eligible, the physician should seriously consider autologous peripheral blood stem cell transplantation. Some patients older than age 70 years are physiologically younger, whereas some patients younger than age 70 years may have medical problems such as heart disease, pulmonary insufficiency, or renal failure and are not suitable candidates for an autologous stem cell transplant. The patient should first be treated with an induction chemotherapy regimen that is nontoxic to the hematopoietic stem cells. Some physicians initially treat with VAD therapy:

- Vincristine[1] (Oncovin) 0.4 mg/m^2 and doxorubicin (Adriamycin),[1] 9 mg/m^2 intravenously (IV) each day for 4 days
- Plus dexamethasone (Decadron),[1] 40 mg orally on days 1 to 4, 9 to 12, and 17 to 20 each month for 3 to 4 months

---

[1]Not FDA approved for this indication.

However VAD therapy is less commonly used now because of its toxicity and the need for intravenous administration. Most physicians usually treat with the oral regimen of:

- Thalidomide (Thalomid),[1] 200 mg/day
- Plus dexamethasone (Decadron),[1] 40 mg/day on days 1 to 4, 9 to 12, and 17 to 20 in odd cycles
- And dexamethasone (Decadron),[1] 40 mg/day on days 1 to 4 in the even cycles

This treatment produces response rates similar to those of VAD. Venous thrombosis, sedation, constipation, and rash constitute the most frequent side effects of thalidomide (Thalomid).[1] Patients should be anticoagulated with low-molecular-weight heparin or warfarin in therapeutic doses. Aspirin may reduce the risk of thromboembolic complications, but that has not yet been proved. Another option is the use of oral dexamethasone (Decadron)[1] as a single agent. A randomized trial comparing dexamethasone (Decadron)[1] alone to thalidomide (Thalomid)[1] plus dexamethasone (Decadron)[1] revealed a superior response rate for thalidomide (Thalomid)[1] plus dexamethasone (Decadron)[1] (58% versus 42%) but a higher incidence of deep venous thrombosis. Although induction chemotherapy is important, we proceed with stem cell transplantation even if the patient has not responded to such treatment.

Most physicians use granulocyte colony-stimulating factor (GCSF)[1] for stem cell collection. After stem cell collection, autologous stem cell transplantation can proceed as soon as the patient has recovered or the transplantation can be delayed and the patient treated with standard alkylating agent therapy, the transplantation being reserved for relapsed disease. There is no difference in overall survival among patients who receive an autologous stem cell transplant immediately after collection and those who receive it at first relapse. We recommend autologous stem cell transplantation as soon as the patient has recovered from the stem cell collection because the patient is saved the inconvenience of prolonged chemotherapy and the potential risk of myelodysplasia from treatment with alkylating agents. Currently, approximately 50% of patients receiving an autologous stem cell transplant are treated as outpatients.

Melphalan (Alkeran), 200 mg/m^2, is the most widely used preparative regimen for autologous stem cell transplantation. Melphalan (Alkeran) plus total body irradiation is rarely used because it produces more side effects, particularly mucositis, and is not more effective.

In two studies from France and the United Kingdom, peripheral stem cell transplantation was superior to combination chemotherapy. Progression-free survival was longer, and median overall survival was increased by approximately 1 year in the transplant group.

It is not known whether maintenance therapy after transplantation is advantageous. Most physicians do not give therapy after transplantation and simply follow the patient for evidence of relapse. Maintenance options

are interferon alfa-2b (Intron A),[1] prednisone every 48 hours, or low-dose thalidomide (Thalomid),[1] but prospective studies are needed to demonstrate benefit. The role of double or tandem autologous stem cell transplantation is controversial. In a randomized study from France, there was no difference in event-free or overall survival between the single and double autologous stem cell transplant groups when evaluated at 2 years, but at 7 years both event-free and overall survival were superior in the double transplant group. The investigators recommended a tandem transplant for patients who did not have a complete response or at least an excellent partial response with the first transplant. However, results of additional randomized trials are pending, and an alternative approach is to collect enough stem cells so the patient may have a second transplant at relapse.

Fortunately, the mortality rate with autologous stem cell transplantation is approximately 1% to 2%. However, the two major shortcomings are that multiple myeloma is not eradicated even with large doses of chemotherapy, and in addition, the autologous peripheral stem cells are contaminated by myeloma cells or their precursors. In an effort to improve the preparative regimen, the addition of bone-seeking radioisotopes that provide increased radiation to the bone marrow (such as holmium-166 DOTMP[2] and samarium Sm 153 EDTMP[1]) is being investigated. In an effort to reduce the contamination of hematopoietic stem cells, CD34 selection was studied. Although contaminating tumor cells were reduced by three logs, there was no prolongation of event-free or overall survival with this approach.

SYNGENEIC OR ALLOGENEIC BONE MARROW TRANSPLANTATION

Bone marrow transplantation from an identical twin donor (syngeneic) is the treatment of choice if a donor is available. Results are superior to allogeneic transplantation.

Allogeneic bone marrow transplantation is advantageous in that the graft contains no tumor cells, and there is a graft-versus-tumor effect. However, subsequent graft-versus-host disease is troublesome. Furthermore, only 5% to 10% of patients with multiple myeloma are eligible for allogeneic transplantation because an HLA-compatible donor is available in only one third of patients and 90% are 50 years of age or older. Currently, allogeneic transplantation is associated with too high a mortality and cannot be recommended. However, efforts are under way to reduce allogeneic transplant-related mortality using T-cell depletion or nonmyeloablative regimens.

Nonmyeloablative (*mini-allo*) allogeneic protocols following autologous stem cell transplantation are being pursued. It is hoped that the benefits of an allograft may be realized while the toxicity associated with the procedure is decreased. The mortality is 10% to 15%, and graft-versus-host disease remains troublesome.

---

[1]Not FDA approved for this indication.

[1]Not FDA approved for this indication.
[2]Available for study but not FDA approved.

Efforts are being made to reduce the toxicity of this approach. Currently, we believe that nonmyeloablative approaches should be limited to protocol studies.

STANDARD ALKYLATING AGENT THERAPY

Alkylating agent-based chemotherapy with oral administration of melphalan (Alkeran) and prednisone produces an objective response in 50% to 60% of patients and a median survival of 2 to 3 years. We prefer to give melphalan (Alkeran) orally in a dosage of 8 to 10 mg daily for 7 days and prednisone in a dosage of 20 mg three times a day orally for the same 7 days. If the serum creatinine value is more than 2 mg/dL (177 mmol/L), the initial dose of melphalan (Alkeran) should be reduced by 25%. Melphalan (Alkeran) should be given when the patient is fasting because absorption is reduced after food is eaten. Leukocyte and platelet counts must be determined at 3-week intervals after the start of therapy and the melphalan (Alkeran) dosage altered until midcycle cytopenia occurs. The melphalan (Alkeran) and prednisone regimen should be repeated every 6 weeks. If the neutrophil count is less than 1500/mm^3 or the platelet count is less than 100,000/mm^3 at 6 weeks, chemotherapy should be delayed and the counts determined at weekly intervals until the pretreatment level is reached. If the neutrophil or platelet counts remain low or if the counts are unduly low at 3 weeks, the melphalan (Alkeran) dose in the next 7-day course must be reduced. Unless the disease progresses rapidly, at least three courses of melphalan (Alkeran) and prednisone should be given before this therapy is abandoned. An objective response may not be achieved for 6 to 12 months or longer in some patients. The natural course of multiple myeloma is one of progression, and if the patient's pain is alleviated and there is no evidence of progressive disease, the therapeutic regimen is beneficial despite the failure to reach an objective response.

Chemotherapy should be continued for at least 1 year or until the patient is in a plateau state. This is defined as stable serum and urine M-protein levels and no evidence of progression. Continued chemotherapy is not recommended because it may lead to the development of a myelodysplastic syndrome or acute leukemia. Patients should be followed closely during the plateau state, and the same chemotherapy should be reinstituted if relapse occurs more than 6 months later.

Because of the obvious shortcomings of melphalan (Alkeran) and prednisone, various combinations of therapeutic agents have been tried. A large meta-analysis, based on data from 6633 patients in 30 trials comparing melphalan (Alkeran) and prednisone with various combinations of chemotherapy, was performed by the Myeloma Trialists Collaborative Group. Although the response rate was higher with combination chemotherapy, there was no survival benefit over melphalan (Alkeran). This meta-analysis also failed to find any category of patients in which combination chemotherapy had a significantly different mortality rate from that with melphalan (Alkeran) and prednisone. There was no evidence that poor-risk patients did better with combination chemotherapy than with melphalan (Alkeran)

and prednisone. Consequently melphalan (Alkeran) and prednisone remains standard treatment outside of clinical trials for patients who are not candidates for autologous stem cell transplantation.

TREATMENT FOR REFRACTORY MULTIPLE MYELOMA, INCLUDING THE USE OF NOVEL AGENTS

Almost all patients with multiple myeloma who survive eventually have relapse. If relapse occurs more than 6 months after the plateau state has been reached, the initial chemotherapy regimen should be reinstituted. Most patients will respond again, but the duration and quality of response are usually inferior to the initial response. Patients who are initially refractory or who become refractory to alkylating agent therapy generally have a low response rate to subsequent chemotherapy and a short survival. The highest response rates in such patients have been with VAD[1] given via IV or bolus injection. Many physicians choose single-agent dexamethasone (Decadron)[1] instead because it accounts for approximately 80% of the effect of VAD. Methylprednisolone, 2 g IV three times weekly for a minimum of 4 weeks, is helpful for patients with pancytopenia, and we find fewer side effects than from dexamethasone (Decadron).[1] Other regimens, including VBMCP (vincristine,[1] BiCNU, melphalan [Alkeran], cyclophosphamide, and prednisone[1]) or VBAP (vincristine[1], BiCNU, Adriamycin[1] IV, and prednisone[1] orally) are useful in relapsed disease. Interferon alfa-2b (Intron A)[1] as a single agent for refractory disease has been disappointing, with objective responses of 10% to 20%.

Novel agents for the treatment of multiple myeloma include thalidomide (Thalomid)[1] and its analog lenalidomide CC-5013 (Revimid),[1] and the proteasome inhibitor bortezomib (Velcade, PS-341). Thalidomide (Thalomid)[1] is usually given in a dosage of 200 mg daily with an increase to 400 mg daily as tolerated. Objective responses occur in approximately one third of patients and last for a median duration of approximately 12 months. The addition of dexamethasone (Decadron)[1] to thalidomide (Thalomid)[1] increases the response rate. Side effects from thalidomide (Thalomid)[1] include weakness, fatigue, constipation, and somnolence. Rashes, thrombotic events, and sensorimotor peripheral neuropathy are more troublesome side effects. Thalidomide (Thalomid)[1] alone or in combination with dexamethasone (Decadron)[1] is now a standard therapy for relapsed or refractory multiple myeloma.

The immunomodulatory thalidomide (Thalomid)[1] derivative lenalidomide (Revimid)[2] CC-5013 has shown activity in previously treated patients but is not yet commercially available. Phase II studies produce response in 30% of patients, and constipation, somnolence, and neuropathy have not been troublesome.

Bortezomib produced objective response in 35% of patients with relapsed, refractory myeloma who had received at least two prior therapeutic regimens. It is

---

[1]Not FDA approved for this indication.
[2]Not available in the United States.

administered as an intravenous bolus dose of 1.3 mg/m^2 twice weekly for 2 weeks, followed by a 10-day rest period for a maximum of eight 21-day cycles. The median duration of response is approximately 12 months. Adverse events include fatigue, anorexia, nausea, and vomiting, fever, diarrhea, constipation, anemia, asthenia, peripheral neuropathy, neutropenia, and thrombocytopenia. The agent has been given accelerated approval by the Food and Drug Administration (FDA) for the treatment of relapsed, refractory myeloma in patients in whom two or more prior regimens have failed.

SUPPORTIVE THERAPY

Radiotherapy

Palliative radiation in a dose of 20 to 30 Gy should be limited to patients with disabling pain who have a well-defined, focal process that has not responded to chemotherapy. Analgesics in combination with chemotherapy usually can control the pain. This approach is preferred to local radiation because pain frequently occurs at another site, and local radiation does not benefit the patient with systemic disease. In addition, the myelosuppressive effects of radiotherapy and chemotherapy are cumulative and may restrict future therapy.

Hypercalcemia

Hypercalcemia must be suspected if the patient has anorexia, nausea, vomiting, polyuria, increased constipation, weakness, confusion, stupor, or coma. If it is untreated, renal insufficiency usually develops. Hydration, preferably with isotonic saline and prednisone (25 mg orally 4 times daily) is effective in most patients. The dosage of prednisone must be reduced and discontinued as soon as possible. After hydration has been achieved, furosemide (Lasix) may be helpful. If these measures fail, a bisphosphonate such as zoledronic acid (Zometa) or pamidronate (Aredia) should be tried.

Renal Insufficiency

Approximately 20% of patients with multiple myeloma have a serum creatinine level of 2.0 mg/dL or more at diagnosis. *Myeloma kidney* and hypercalcemia are the two major causes. Myeloma kidney is characterized by the presence of large, waxy, laminated casts in the distal and collecting tubules. Some light chains are very nephrotoxic, but no specific amino acid sequence of the light chain has been identified.

Dehydration, infection, nonsteroidal anti-inflammatory agents, and radiographic contrast media may contribute to acute renal failure. Hyperuricemia or amyloid deposition may produce renal insufficiency. Nephrotic syndrome rarely occurs in multiple myeloma unless amyloidosis is present.

Maintenance of a high fluid intake producing 3 L of urine per 24 hours is important for preventing renal failure in patients with Bence Jones proteinuria.

Intravenous pyelography or preparation for barium enema can be performed with little risk if dehydration is avoided. If hyperuricemia occurs, allopurinol (Zyloprim) in doses of 300 mg daily provides effective therapy.

Acute renal failure should be treated promptly with appropriate fluid and electrolyte replacement. Patients with acute or subacute renal failure should be treated with dexamethasone (Decadron),[1] or thalidomide (Thalomid)[1] plus dexamethasone (Decadron),[1] or VAD[1] to reduce the tumor mass as quickly as possible. A trial of plasmapheresis is recommended in an attempt to prevent chronic dialysis. Hemodialysis and peritoneal dialysis are equally effective and are necessary for patients with symptomatic azotemia. Renal transplantation for myeloma kidney has been followed by prolonged survival.

Anemia

Almost every patient with multiple myeloma eventually becomes anemic. Increase of plasma volume from the osmotic effect of the M protein may produce hypervolemia and spuriously lower the hemoglobin and hematocrit values. Erythropoietin (Epogen, Procrit) reduces the transfusion requirement and increases hemoglobin concentration in more than half of patients. Those with low serum erythropoietin (Epogen, Procrit) values are more likely to respond. Most physicians proceed with a trial of erythropoietin (Epogen, Procrit) 150 U/kg three times weekly or 40,000 units once a week. Darbepoetin, a long-lasting erythropoietin (Aranesp), may be given weekly or biweekly.

Skeletal Lesions

Bone lesions manifested by pain and fractures are a major problem. A skeletal radiographic survey should be repeated at 6-month intervals or sooner if pain develops. Patients should be encouraged to be as active as possible because confinement to bed increases demineralization of the skeleton. Trauma must be avoided because even mild stress may result in a fracture. Fixation of long bone fractures or impending fractures with an intramedullary rod and methyl methacrylate has given excellent results. All patients with multiple myeloma who have lytic lesions, pathologic fractures, or severe osteopenia should receive intravenous bisphosphonates. Zoledronic acid (Zometa) 4 mg IV over 15 minutes every 4 weeks or pamidronate (Aredia) 90 mg IV over 2 hours every 4 weeks are equally efficacious. The dosage of bisphosphonates should be reduced with renal insufficiency. Because renal insufficiency or nephrotic-range proteinuria may occur, serum creatinine and 24-hour urine protein monitoring is necessary. Osteonecrosis of the jaw has been reported in patients receiving bisphosphonates. Although the relationship is unclear, it is prudent to avoid dental surgery while taking bisphosphonates. Vertebroplasty or kyphoplasty may be helpful for patients with compression fracture of the spine.

---

[1]Not FDA approved for this indication.

Rakel and Bope: *Conn's Current Therapy 2006.*

CURRENT DIAGNOSIS

- Complete history and physical examination
  Determination of values for hemoglobin, leukocytes with differential count, platelets, serum creatinine, calcium, and uric acid
  Radiographic survey of bones including humeri and femurs
  Serum protein electrophoresis with immunofixation
  Quantitation of immunoglobulins
  Bone marrow aspirate and biopsy
  Routine urinalysis
  Electrophoresis and immunofixation of an adequately concentrated aliquot from a 24-hour urine specimen
- Measurement of β_2-microglobulin, C-reactive protein, lactate dehydrogenase values
- If available, cytogenetics—FISH and plasma cell labeling index

Abbreviation: FISH = fluorescence in situ hybridization.

Infections

Bacterial infections are more common in patients with myeloma than in the general population. Pneumococcal and influenza immunization should be given to all patients despite their suboptimal antibody response. Substantial fever is an indication for appropriate cultures, chest radiography, and consideration of antibiotic therapy. The greatest risk for infection is during the first 2 months after initiation of chemotherapy. Prophylactic trimethoprim-sulfamethoxazole (Bactrim, Septra)[1] may be useful during the first 2 months of chemotherapy. Prophylactic daily oral penicillin[1] may benefit patients with recurrent pneumococcal infections.

CURRENT THERAPY

Newly Diagnosed Symptomatic Myeloma
- Eligible for stem cell transplant
  Thalidomide[1] plus dexamethasone[1]
  VAD[1]
  Dexamethasone[1]
  Novel agents
- Ineligible for stem cell transplant
  Melphalan (Alkeran) and prednisone[1]
  Combinations of alkylating agents
  Novel agents
Refractory or Relapsed Myeloma
- Thalidomide[1] plus dexamethasone[1]
- Dexamethasone[1]
- VAD[1]
- Bortezomib (Velcade)
- Combinations of alkylating agents
- Novel agents

Abbreviations: VAD = Vincristine[1] plus doxorubicin[1] (Adriamycin)[1] plus dexamethasone.
[1]Not FDA approved for this indication.

Rakel and Bope: *Conn's Current Therapy 2006.*

IV-administered Ig[1] may be helpful for patients with recurrent infections, but it is too expensive for long-term therapy.

Hyperviscosity Syndrome

The symptoms of hyperviscosity may include oronasal bleeding, gastrointestinal bleeding, blurred vision, neurologic symptoms, or congestive heart failure. Most patients have symptoms when the serum viscosity measurement is more than 4 cp but the relationship between serum viscosity and clinical manifestations is imprecise. The decision to perform plasmapheresis, which promptly relieves the symptoms of hyperviscosity, should be made on clinical grounds rather than serum viscosity levels. Hyperviscosity is more common in IgA myeloma than in IgG myeloma.

Extradural Myeloma (Cord Compression)

The possibility of cord compression must be excluded if weakness of the legs or difficulty in voiding or defecating occurs. The sudden onset of severe radicular pain or severe back pain is suggestive of compression of the spinal cord. MRI or CT is most helpful for diagnosis. Radiation therapy in a dose of approximately 30 Gy is beneficial. Dexamethasone (Decadron) should be administered during radiation therapy to reduce edema.

Emotional Support

All patients with multiple myeloma need substantial and continuing emotional support. The physician's approach must be positive in emphasizing the potential benefits of therapy. It is reassuring for patients to know that some survive for 10 years or more. It is vital that the physician caring for patients with multiple myeloma has the interest and capacity for dealing with incurable disease over the span of years with assurance, sympathy, and resourcefulness.

REFERENCES

Attal M, Harousseau JL, Facon T, et al: Single versus double autologous stem-cell transplantation for multiple myeloma. N Engl J Med 2003;349:2495-2502. (Erratum appears in N Engl J Med. 2004 Jun17;350[25]:2628.)

Child JA, Morgan GJ, Davies FE, et al: High-dose chemotherapy with hematopoietic stem-cell rescue for multiple myeloma. N Engl J Med 2003;348:1875-1883.

Myeloma Trialists' Collaborative Group: Combination chemotherapy versus melphalan plus prednisone as treatment for multiple myeloma: An overview of 6,633 patients from 27 randomized trials. J Clin Oncol 1998;16:3832-3842.

Kyle RA, Rajkumar SV: Multiple myeloma: Drug therapy (review article). N Engl J Med 2004;351:1860-1873.

Rajkumar SV, Blood E, Vesole DH, et al: Thalidomide plus dexamethasone versus dexamethasone alone in newly diagnosed multiple myeloma (E1A00): Results of a phase III trial coordinated by the Eastern Cooperative Oncology Group. Blood 2004;63a (abst #205).

Rajkumar SV, Gertz MA, Kyle RA, Greipp PR: Current therapy for multiple myeloma. Mayo Clin Proc 2002;77:813-822.

[1]Not FDA approved for this indication.

6

Rajkumar SV, Hayman S, Gertz MA, et al: Combination therapy with thalidomide plus dexamethasone for newly diagnosed myeloma. J Clin Oncol 2002;20:4319-4323.

Richardson PG, Barlogie B, Berenson J, et al: A phase 2 study of bortezomib in relapsed, refractory myeloma. N Engl J Med 2003; 348:2609-2617.

Singhal S, Mehta J, Desikan R, et al: Antitumor activity of thalidomide in refractory multiple myeloma. N Engl J Med 1999;341: 1565-1571. (Erratum appears in N Engl J Med 2000 Feb 3; 342[5]:364.)

Polycythemia Vera

Method of
Magda Elkabani, MD, Kenneth S. Zuckerman, MD, and Harold H. Davis, MD

Polycythemia vera (PV) is a chronic myeloproliferative disorder in which the most prominent abnormality is a marked increase in number of red blood cells. This proliferation of red blood cells is not driven by the normal physiologic regulator of number of red blood cells, erythropoietin, which in turn is regulated by tissue oxygenation. Platelet and granulocyte numbers also are increased frequently. The cause of PV is presumed to be an undiscovered mutation or mutations in a multipotent hemopoietic progenitor cell that results in impaired programmed cell death and subsequent clonal accumulation of hemopoietic cells in the bone marrow and blood, which have acquired this selective advantage over normal bone marrow cells.

Epidemiology

PV is a disease that occurs primarily in patients older than 50 years of age, with the median age at diagnosis 60 years of age. The incidence is 1.9 per 100,000, males being slightly more commonly afflicted than females. The median survival appears to be at least 15 to 20 years, which is slightly less than that of the age-matched general population. Arterial and venous thromboses, particularly pulmonary embolism, ischemic stroke, and coronary artery thrombosis, are the most common causes of serious morbidity and mortality in PV. Progression to severe myelofibrosis occurs in approximately 15% of patients, and transformation to acute myeloid leukemia has been reported in 1.4% to 6.3% of patients with PV, but may be 10% to 15% in patients treated with alkylating agents or radioactive phosphorus. The overall death rate of patients with PV was reported to be 2.9 per 100 patient years in Polycythemia Vera Study Group

(PVSG) studies, but probably has decreased with more recent therapeutic approaches.

Clinical Manifestations

Many patients are diagnosed incidentally because of plethora or elevated hematocrit and/or hemoglobin on routine blood count. Other patients present with arterial or venous thrombosis, pruritus (especially after a warm shower or bath), palpable splenomegaly, gouty arthritis, erythromelalgia (acral dysesthesia with erythema, pallor, or cyanosis of hands and feet), headaches, dizziness, or gastrointestinal symptoms (gastric erosions, increased incidence of *Helicobacter pylori*, and peptic ulcer disease).

Diagnosis

The hallmark of PV is persistently elevated red cell mass and a low erythropoietin level. The vast majority of patients with a hematocrit greater than 60 have an elevated red cell mass. A red cell mass greater than 36 mL/kg in men or greater than 32 mL/kg in females is considered elevated. However, currently there is a great deal of controversy over the necessity and value of red cell mass measurements. These studies have become very difficult to obtain in most centers, and even when available, there are many extraneous factors affecting the proper calculation and interpretation of the results. Serum erythropoietin level can be extremely helpful in making or excluding the diagnosis of PV. A low serum erythropoietin level in an untransfused polycythemic patient with a prior history of normal hemoglobin and hematocrit levels makes the diagnosis of PV highly likely. An elevated erythropoietin level makes the diagnosis of PV very unlikely. A normal serum erythropoietin level does not help to distinguish between PV and other causes of erythrocytosis. Abnormally increased leukocyte (granulocytes) and platelet counts are frequently seen and support the diagnosis of PV but are not required for diagnosis. Other commonly encountered laboratory abnormalities include microcytosis from iron deficiency, elevated vitamin B_{12} levels, and elevated leukocyte alkaline phosphatase score. These are neither sensitive nor specific enough to be of great diagnostic value.

The bone marrow of patients with PV shows hyperplasia with decreased or absent iron stores, varying degrees of reticulin fibrosis, increased erythroid lineage cells, and usually increased numbers of granulocyte lineage cells and megakaryocytes. Clustering of abnormal-appearing megakaryocytes is almost diagnostic of a myeloproliferative disorder, but it does not distinguish PV from other myeloproliferative disorders. Bone marrow examination is not essential to making the diagnosis of PV. However, it may be very useful in patients with borderline criteria for diagnosis and to establish baseline levels of marrow hyperplasia and fibrosis in all patients.

Endogenous erythroid colony (EEC) formation in vitro is determined by the generation of colonies of maturing erythroid cells derived from single erythroid precursor cells in the bone marrow, called colony-forming units-erythroid (CFUs-E), in the absence of exogenous erythropoietin. Normal erythroid precursors do not form erythroid cell colonies in the absence of erythropoietin. Increased spontaneous EEC formation has a sensitivity and specificity approaching 100% for PV when there are any other findings of a myeloproliferative disorder. However, it is a research procedure and is not widely available clinically for diagnostic testing.

Cytogenetic abnormalities associated with PV include deletion of the long arm of chromosome 20, trisomy 8, trisomy 9, and loss of heterozygosity of chromosome 9. Elevated expression of the polycythemia rubra vera-1 gene (PRV-1) in granulocytes has been described recently as a potentially useful test for distinguishing PV from secondary polycythemias, although increased PRV-1 expression also is found in patients with other myeloproliferative disorders. A majority (69% to 91%) of PV patients overexpress the PRV-1 gene. One recent report indicates that level of PRV-1 expression may be highly correlated with the leukocyte alkaline phosphatase (LAP) score, which is a simple, widely available test. Other investigational techniques that may aid in establishing the diagnosis of PV include overexpression of Bcl-xL, reduced numbers of thrombopoietin receptor on platelets, and hypersensitivity of erythroid precursors to insulin-like growth factor-1. Finally, there has been a recent breakthrough finding of a somatic mutation, V617F in the Janus Kinase 2 (JAK2) gene on chromosome 9, which results in a gain of function of this tyrosine kinase. This mutation apparently is present in at least 65% of patients with PV, and less frequently in other myeloproliferative disorders. PV patients with this mutation were found to have a longer duration of disease and a higher rate of complications. While still mainly a research tool, analysis of this mutation in patients with suspected PV may be an important diagnostic finding in the future.

PSVG was created in 1967 to develop a set of guidelines for the optimal approach to diagnosis and treatment of PV. The diagnostic criteria have evolved over the last 35 years as certain criteria were found to be insufficiently specific and sensitive, and new tests, especially measurement of serum erythropoietin level, became available. For patients with a hemoglobin/hematocrit consistently above the reference range of normal on at least two independent measurements (Hb [hemoglobin] > 18.5 in men, Hb > 16.5 in women), the diagnostic criteria listed in the Current Diagnosis box may be used. Any patient with a history of chronic volume depletion, hypoxic pulmonary disease, sleep apnea, massive obesity (pickwickian syndrome), smoking, living at high altitude, erythropoietin-producing neoplasms, methemoglobinemia, or familial polycythemia without other signs of a myeloproliferative disorder should be evaluated for secondary or relative polycythemia. The presence of hypoxemia, elevated carboxyhemoglobin, elevated erythropoietin, or normal red cell mass indicates that secondary or relative erythrocytosis is a more likely diagnosis. One reasonable algorithm that may be used for patients with suspected PV is shown in Figure 1.

CURRENT DIAGNOSIS

- Polycythemia is defined as Hb greater than 18.5 g/dL in men and greater than 16.5 g/dL in women on at least two measurements, and/or red blood cell mass greater than 36 mL/kg for men and greater than 32 mL/kg for women.
- Secondary polycythemia should be excluded by documenting: arterial oxygen saturation more than 92%, Pao_2 greater than 60, carboxyhemoglobin level less than 5%, no history of living at high altitude recently, no use of exogenous erythropoietin injections, no erythrocyte hypertransfusion, and no high oxygen affinity hemoglobin mutation.
- Serum erythropoietin level is low or normal.
- Increased formation of endogenous erythroid colonies (EECs) has high sensitivity and specificity.
- Bone marrow examination shows erythroid and usually granulocyte and megakaryocyte hyperplasia, iron deficiency, variable fibrosis, and clustering of abnormal megakaryocytes; cytogenetics may show abnormalities in chromosome 8, 9, and 20.
- Thrombocytosis (platelet > 400,000) and leukocytosis (white blood cells > 10,000) are variably present.
- Splenomegaly, elevated B_{12} levels, and elevated leukocyte alkaline phosphatase score may be present and are supportive of a diagnosis of PV, but are not specific for PV.
- Increased expression of PRV-1 gene may be useful in distinguishing polycythemia vera from secondary polycythemias.

Abbreviations: EECs = endogenous erythroid colonies; Hb = hemoglobin; PV = polycythemia vera; PRV-1 = polycythemia rubra vera-1 gene.

Treatment

More than 1600 PV patients were evaluated in the European collaboration on low-dose aspirin (ECLAP) study, and 38% of those enrolled had a history of thrombosis. Therapy has been aimed at reducing thrombotic risk in these patients through the use of phlebotomy, cytoreductive therapy, and aspirin[1] at a dose of 81 to 100 mg per day. It is widely assumed that reduction of an elevated platelet count with cytoreductive therapy to the normal range or to a level less than 600,000 reduces the incidence of thromboses, although there are no firm experimental data that support that assumption. The Current Therapy box provides a summary of treatment considerations.

PHLEBOTOMY

The most commonly used therapy to treat erythrocytosis in PV patients is phlebotomy. This is not an effective treatment for thrombocytosis, which is unaffected or may even increase transiently after phlebotomy. The risk of

---

[1]Not FDA approved for this indication.

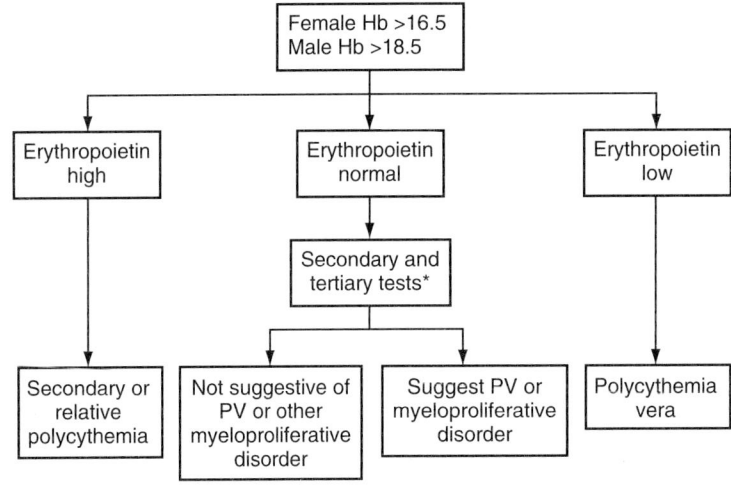

FIGURE 1. Simplified general algorithm for diagnosis of polycythemia vera.

thrombosis dramatically and progressively increases for all hematocrit levels more than 44%. Thus, the PVSG has recommended that a threshold hematocrit of 45% be used for phlebotomy therapy. A threshold hematocrit of 42% has been suggested for females, but without clear supporting data. One unit of blood (450 to 500 mL) is generally removed at a time. Elderly patients or

 CURRENT THERAPY

- All patients should receive phlebotomy to keep Hct at less than 45% for men and less than 42% for women.
- All patients should receive low dose aspirin[1] therapy (81 to 100 mg) unless there is a contraindication to treatment.
- Cytoreductive therapy should be considered for patients at high risk of thrombosis, including patients older than 60 years of age, with a history of previous thrombosis, or with presence of cardiovascular risk factors.
- Hydroxyurea (Hydrea)[1] almost always is the cytoreductive therapy of choice, resulting in decreased morbidity and mortality associated with thrombosis, although it may be associated with a minimally increased risk of leukemic transformation.
- Anagrelide (Agrylin)[1] is an alternative cytoreductive therapy that does not alter erythropoiesis, but it lowers platelet counts and results in decreased incidence of thrombosis without risk of leukemia transformation.
- Bone marrow transplantation, imatinib,[1] and other experimental therapies are reserved for specific patient populations at this time

[1]Not FDA approved for this indication.
Abbreviation: Hct = hemocrit

patients with compromised cardiovascular function may have half a unit of blood removed on a more frequent basis. Weekly phlebotomies may be required initially until the iron stores have been depleted, and hemoglobin and hematocrit fail to rebound, but, subsequently, the frequency of phlebotomies is reduced.

CYTOREDUCTIVE THERAPY

Patients with progressive erythrocytosis requiring frequent phlebotomy, progressive or painful splenomegaly, significant thrombocytosis, or those at high risk of thrombosis usually benefit from the addition of cytoreductive therapy to phlebotomy. Those considered to be at high risk for thrombosis are patients older than 60 years of age, previous history of thrombosis, or known cardiovascular risk factors. Cytoreductive therapies that have shown effectiveness in PV include ^{32}P,[2] busulfan (Myleran),[1] chlorambucil (Leukeran),[1] pipobroman (Vercyte),[1] hydroxyurea (Hydrea),[1] interferon alfa-2a (Roferon-A),[1] interferon alfa-2b (Intron A),[1] and anagrelide (Agrylin).[1]

PSVG and European trials in the 1970s and 1980s showed that chlorambucil,[1] ^{32}P,[2] pipobroman,[1] and busulfan[1] were effective at reducing the incidence of thrombosis as compared to patients treated with phlebotomy alone. However, an excess mortality occurred with ^{32}P[2] or alkylating agents, because of the substantially increased risk of acute leukemia, gastrointestinal tumors, and skin cancers, leading to reduced survival. Because of the late increased risk of developing treatment-associated acute myeloid leukemia, these agents are generally now recommended only for patients at increased thrombotic risk, who are intolerant of or unresponsive to other treatments, and whose life expectancy is limited to less than 5 to 10 years.

[1]Not FDA approved for this indication.
[2]Not available in the United States.

Rakel and Bope: *Conn's Current Therapy 2006.*

Interferon-alpha (IFN-α) (Intron A, Roferon-A)[1] has been used in the treatment of PV because of its myelosuppressive effect and lack of leukemogenic potential. In a review of several small trials using IFN-α, overall response rates were 50% for hematocrit reduction and 77% for reduction in spleen size. However, IFN-α requires parenteral administration, and most patients suffer from variable severity of fatigue, sleep problems, myalgias, fever, flulike symptoms, depression, weight loss, hair loss, gastrointestinal symptoms, and cardiovascular symptoms, which results in discontinuation of interferon therapy in 25% to 35% of patients. Because it is nonteratogenic, IFN-α is a possible treatment modality for women who are pregnant. The starting dose is 3 million U subcutaneously three times per week.

Hydroxyurea (Hydrea)[1] is an antimetabolite inhibitor of DNA synthesis, which was developed in the 1970s as a noncarcinogenic drug and is the most commonly used cytoreductive drug in PV. It is usually very well tolerated, with the most common side effects being fatigue, cytopenias, and macrocytosis. Skin lesions, leg ulcers, oral ulcers, hepatotoxicity, and fever occur infrequently. The PVSG reported 51 patients with PV who were treated with hydroxyurea[1] and were compared to patients treated with phlebotomy alone (control group). The hydroxyurea group had fewer deaths and less myelofibrosis compared to historical controls, but there was a slight tendency (not statistically significant) to more acute leukemias (6% versus 1.5%). Subsequent studies also have shown no or minimal (less than 3%) absolute increase in risk of developing acute myeloid leukemia, compared with PV patients who do not receive hydroxyurea or alkylating agent therapy. The starting dose ranges from 500 to 3000 mg/kg orally, depending on the urgency of reducing erythrocyte and platelet counts. The dose can be titrated, with an optimal goal of normalization of the platelet count and marked decrease or elimination of the need for therapeutic phlebotomy. Most patients require a long-term dose of 500 to 1000 mg per day for optimal therapeutic benefit without significant side effects.

A newer treatment for thrombocytosis associated with myeloproliferative disorders, including PV, is anagrelide (Agrylin).[1] The mechanism by which it reduces platelet counts is not completely understood, but it inhibits megakaryocyte maturation and platelet production. Approximately 85% to 90% of patients with thrombocytosis in myeloproliferative disorders achieve a platelet count less than 600,000 or 50% reduction in initial platelet count. The most common side effects include headache, fluid retention, atrial tachyarrhythmias, and diarrhea, resulting in 15% to 20% of patients discontinuing therapy. Experience with essential thrombocythemia suggests decreased risk of thrombosis and resolution of erythromelalgia with reduction of platelet counts to normal. The starting dose is 0.5 mg orally four times per day, but the dose is titrated to achieve a goal platelet count of less than 600,000, or in the normal range, if possible.

ASPIRIN

The use of aspirin[1] had been limited until recently because of the concern for gastrointestinal bleeding. A PVSG trial published in 1986 reported an increased incidence of significant gastrointestinal hemorrhage and no reduction in incidence of thrombosis with 975 mg of aspirin daily. The ECLAP trial reported in 2004 on 518 patients with PV, who had no previous history of thrombosis and were randomized to receive low dose aspirin or placebo. All patients were treated with either phlebotomy, cytoreductive therapy, or both. In patients receiving 100 mg of aspirin daily, there was a statistically significant reduction in frequency of nonfatal myocardial infarction, nonfatal stroke, pulmonary embolism, deep vein thrombosis, and death from any cardiovascular cause, and there was no increased risk of clinically significant bleeding. Unless there is a contraindication to aspirin[1] treatment, all patients with PV should receive 81 to 100 mg of aspirin[1] per day.

EXPERIMENTAL THERAPIES

Imatinib mesylate (Gleevec)[1] has been reported to treat successfully two patients with PV who were unable to tolerate hydroxyurea[1] or interferon.[1] The mechanism is unknown, although it has been proposed that inhibition of c-Kit may play a role. Allogeneic bone marrow transplantation has been used in select patients, with some reports of cure. Given the risks associated with transplantation, this modality is generally reserved for patients who develop PV at a young age and progress rapidly.

REFERENCES

Berk P, Goldberg J, Donovan P, et al: Therapeutic recommendations in polycythemia vera based on Polycythemia Vera Study Group protocols. Semin Hematol 1986;23:132-143.

Cotes P, Dore C, Yin J, et al: Determination of serum immunoreactive erythropoietin in the investigation of erythrocytosis. N Engl J Med 1986;315:283-287.

Fruchtman S, Mack K, Kaplan M, et al: From efficacy to safety: a polycythemia vera study group report on hydroxyurea in patients with polycythemia vera. Semin Hematol 1997;34:17-23.

Jones C, Michael M, Dickinson T: Polycythemia vera responds to imatinib mesylate. Am J M Sci 2003;325(3):149-152.

Klippel S, Strunck E, Temerinac S, et al: Quantification of PRV-1 mRNA distinguishes polycythemia vera from secondary erythrocytosis. Blood 2004;102(10):3569-3574.

Kravolics R, Passamonti F, Buser A, et al: A gain of function mutation of Jak2 in myeloproliferative disorders. N Engl J Med 2005;352[17]:1779-1790.

Landolfi R, Marchioli R, Kutti J, et al: Efficacy and safety of low dose aspirin in polycythemia vera. N Engl J Med 2004;350(2):114-124.

Spivak J: Polycythemia vera: myths, mechanisms, and management. Blood 2002;100:4272-4290.

Streiff M, Smith B, Spivak J: The diagnosis and management of polycythemia vera in the era since the Polycythemia Vera Study Group: A survey of American Society of Hematology member's practice patterns. Blood 2002;99(4):1144-1149.

Tartagilia A, Goldberg J, Berk P, et al: Adverse effect of antiaggregating platelet therapy in the treatment of polycythemia vera. Semin Hematol 1988;23:172-176.

Tefferi A: Polycythemia vera: A comprehensive review and clinical recommendations. Mayo Clin Proc 2003;78(2):174-194.

6

---

[1]Not FDA approved for this indication.

Rakel and Bope: *Conn's Current Therapy 2006.*

---

[1]Not FDA approved for this indication.

The Porphyrias

Method of
Claus A. Pierach, MD

The *porphyrias* present a group of mostly inherited diseases where disturbances along the heme biosynthetic pathway to heme lead to accumulations of metabolic intermediaries. Porphyria cutanea tarda can present without discernible inheritance; it can also be induced by chemicals (see the following). All steps of heme synthesis are enzymatically regulated and all porphyrias are a result of specific impasses along these transitions. Not all enzymatic defects result in clinically relevant or recognizable disease manifestations in every patient. On the one hand, the severity of the enzymatic defect plays a role. On the other, some poorly understood revealing or unveiling cofactors are operational. The prevalence of the porphyrias is not known and fluctuates in different parts of the world.

The porphyrias can be divided between neurovisceral (acute) and cutaneous manifestations. Two types, the very rare delta-aminolevulinic acid-dehydratase deficiency porphyria and acute intermittent porphyria (AIP) have only neurological symptoms (acute attacks). Hereditary coproporphyria (HCP) and variegate porphyria (VP) may have both neurologic and dermatologic signs and symptoms. Congenital erythropoietic porphyria, porphyria cutanea tarda (PCT), and erythropoietic protoporphyria (EPP) exhibit only skin lesions but can be complicated by other problems (anemia, hepatic insufficiency).

Heme Synthesis

Succinyl coenzyme-A and glycine are the initial building blocks, subsequently transformed through eight enzymatic steps to the end product, heme, in itself essential not only for hemoglobin but also for other hemoproteins such as cytochromes, myoglobin, and other enzymes (catalase, nitric oxide synthase, and tryptophan pyrrolase). Heme synthesis happens in all cells but mostly in the liver and in the bone marrow. It is controlled by heme through feedback inhibition of the first step, delta-aminolevulinic acid synthase. Figure 1 shows the various steps, intermediaries, and resulting porphyrias. Porphyrins and their precursors, delta-aminolevulinic acid (ALA) and porphobilinogen (PBG), are only generated during heme synthesis and not during heme catabolism toward bilirubin. Specific enzymatic defects result in specific patterns of heme precursors and are of high diagnostic value when determining the type of porphyria. Although enzyme and DNA measurements are of great interest, at present their availability is limited. The excretory pattern of heme precursors is influenced by their water solubility, which decreases toward heme; ALA and PBG are highly water soluble and measured

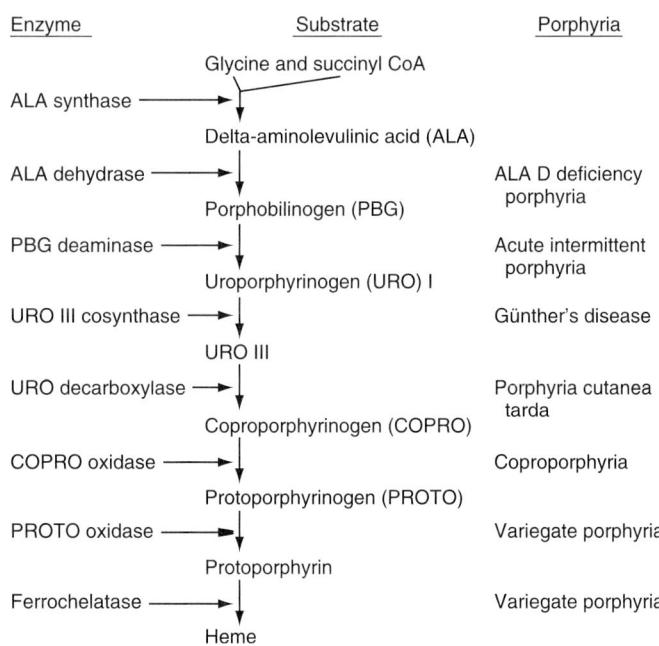

FIGURE 1. Heme biosynthetic pathway. Enzymes that have defects or deficiencies that cause the various porphyries are listed on the left side, heme and precursors are in the middle, and the resulting porphyrias are on the right side.

in urine, whereas protoporphyrin is so hydrophobic that it is only excreted in stool and not in urine.

There is not just one porphyria and not just one single test revealing all porphyrias. Furthermore, the porphyric symptomatology can differ from type to type and can have considerable overlap between the various porphyrias (see previous paragraphs). Thus, highly specific and sensitive laboratory tests are necessary. All porphyrias with acute manifestations present with similar attacks, responding to similar treatment but exhibit different biochemical patterns according to their specific enzyme defect. A clinically useful grouping splits the porphyrias between acute and cutaneous.

The Acute Porphyrias

There are four types of acute porphyrias to consider:

1. The very rare ALA-dehydratase deficiency porphyria is inherited in an autosomal recessive fashion.
2. AIP, an autosomal dominant disorder, is the most common of the acute porphyrias (except for South Africa where variegate porphyria is more common).
3. HCP, again an autosomal dominant disease, is frequently misdiagnosed because coproporphyrin is often moderately and nonspecifically increased in many disorders.
4. VP is autosomal dominant and probably the mildest of the acute porphyrias.

All acute porphyrias are sensitive to a multitude of drugs and circumstances (Box 1). HCP and VP can also present with skin lesions resembling PCT. Skin lesions

> **BOX 1   Short List of Safe and Unsafe Drugs in the Acute Porphyrias**
>
> | Unsafe | Safe |
> |---|---|
> | Alcohol | Acetaminophen |
> | Barbiturates | Aspirin |
> | Carbamazepine | Atropine |
> | Carisoprodol | Bromides |
> | Clonazepam | Cimetidine |
> | Danazol | Erythropoietin |
> | Diclofenac | Gabapentin |
> | Ergotamines | Glucocorticoids |
> | Estrogens, progesterones | Insulin |
> | Ethchlorvynol | Narcotic analgesics |
> | Glutethimide | Penicillins |
> | Griseofulvin | Phenothiazine |
> | Mephenytoin, phenytoin | Ranitidine |
> | Meprobamate | Streptomycin |
> | Methyprylon | Digoxin |
> | Metoclopramide | Labetalol, propranolol |
> | Primidone | Paraldehyde |
> | Pyrazinamide | Bupivacaine |
> | Pyrazolone | Chloral hydrate |
> | Rifampin | Tetracycline |
> | Sulfonamides | Vitamins |
> | Valproic acid | |
>
> *Drugs not listed cannot be considered safe or unsafe.

and acute attacks may happen at the same time or one after the other, or only one manifestation may ever be present in a given patient.

The Porphyric Attack

DIAGNOSIS

Diagnosis of the porphyric attack hinges mainly on a keen sense of suspicion. Any inexplicable symptom complex involving abdominal pain, tachycardia, and psychological findings should be suspect for porphyria. However, no clinical presentation can be called *porphyric* unless biochemically supported. Small deviations from the narrow normal range for heme precursors are fairly common and nonspecific. PBG and/or ALA must be markedly elevated, at least fivefold above the normal range, and, if not, porphyria is an unlikely explanation for the patient's symptoms.

Older screening mechanisms such as the Watson-Schwartz test and the Hoesch test have been replaced by easier, more specific tests such as the Trace PBG kit, still relying on the color reaction with Ehrlich's aldehyde. A *random* urine sample is highly sufficient for the initial diagnostic evaluation and if positive must be later followed up by more detailed tests such as quantitative measurements of porphyrins and precursors in a 24 hour urine collection. Fecal porphyrin measurements may also be called for, but enzyme tests are only indicated if family studies can employ that test. Because the porphyrias are almost always hereditary, family studies are highly appropriate. The proper interpretation of

Rakel and Bope: Conn's Current Therapy 2006.

any test result is best done with consideration for the clinical information.

CLINICAL PRESENTATION

Clinical presentations of porphyric attacks vary so much, that the term *the little imitator* has been used. No signs or symptoms are always present, but severe and poorly localized abdominal pain and unexplained tachycardia are so prevalent that their absence further complicates the diagnosis of an acute porphyric attack. The genesis of the attack is not well understood, but acutely increased demand for heme seems to be the foundation. This increased demand can be because of a wide variety of circumstances, from drugs through hormones (premenstrual phase) to stress, infection, fasting, and starvation. However, most carriers of the genetic defect for an acute porphyria remain asymptomatic for all their lives. Some have only one or two attacks, and very few suffer from many attacks.

The clinical picture with pain, fast heart rate, and neurovisceral symptoms can be complicated by, at times, severe hyponatremia, heralding seizures with therapeutic dilemmas (see Box 1) and respiratory paralysis necessitating ventilatory support. Death is rare nowadays, especially when the diagnosis is made early. The recovery is usually complete but at times prolonged, up to 1 year after a severe attack.

Superb nursing care, initially preferable in an intensive care unit, is necessary, and meticulous attention has to be paid to *all* problems. Dehydration from vomiting is common; ileus and urinary retention are not infrequent; hyponatremia occurs in approximately half of the porphyric attacks. Muscle strength must be tested frequently. Twice daily measurement of vital capacity helps to assess the necessity for tracheal intubation. High blood pressure and tachycardia deserve careful attention and, if appropriate, cautious treatment with a β-blocker. A negative caloric balance must be avoided, initially best treated with carbohydrates (if necessary intravenously with glucose), later with a balanced diet.

THERAPY

Therapy must always start with a careful look at the drugs recently taken by the patient. It is best to discontinue as many drugs as possible, especially those deemed unsafe (see Box 1). Appropriate lists of safe and unsafe drugs in porphyria are readily available via the Internet. An infection must be diligently searched for and at once be treated. Seizure precautions are especially indicated if hyponatremia is found. Analgesics should be adequately dispensed; opiates are frequently necessary in fairly large doses.

SPECIFIC THERAPY

Specific therapy was introduced a generation ago in the form of hematin* (Panhematin). This has largely replaced

*Hematin can be obtained as Panhematin from Ovation Pharmaceuticals, Inc. by calling (888) 514-5204.

glucose (300 g/day), which had the main advantages of ready availability, relatively low cost, and the possibility of curbing an early or mild attack. But one must not wait for quick changes in a patient's condition and should at once take steps to obtain the definitive medication, hematin (Panhematin). This represents the equivalent to the end product, heme, and exerts its beneficial effect through repression of the deranged, and in the porphyric attack, markedly activated pathway to heme. It is still unclear whether the quick suppression of potentially toxic heme precursors (in 1 to 2 days) or a postulated replenishment of an assumed heme deficiency is the effective principle. *Early* administration of hematin (Panhematin) is strongly advocated because the course of a porphyric attack is unpredictable, and a point of no return can unfortunately be reached quickly. The infusion of hematin (Panhematin) must start as soon as possible. A daily dose of 3 to 4 mg/kg body weight is recommended for up to 4 days. Longer treatment periods are of questionable value but may be tried in severe cases for up to 2 weeks. The infusion must be strictly intravenous and with ample flushing because hematin (Panhematin) can cause thrombosis and phlebitis as it is a pro- and anticoagulant. This also makes frequent measurements of coagulation parameters advisable. Anticoagulants like coumarin should if possible be avoided. Admixture of 5% human serum albumin has been advocated to stabilize the final hematin solution and to lessen side effects. Hematin is available in many countries as heme arginate (Normosang). Its effectiveness is similar to Panhematin.

A beneficial clinical effect can be expected in 1 to 2 days, accompanied by a decrease in all heme precursors, most notably ALA and PBG. Many patients have received many treatment courses with hematin without apparent loss of effectiveness. Prophylactic use of hematin (Panhematin) can be helpful in the treatment of women with regular premenstrual exacerbations of their porphyria. Hematin should never be given as a diagnostic test to see if unexplained symptoms lessen. The diagnosis of a porphyric attack must be as precise and as certain as possible, especially in new cases. Partial liver transplantation has been successfully undertaken and found to be curative in a patient with unrelenting porphyric attacks.

Prophylaxis of porphyric attacks is of great importance and can be accomplished to a large extent by avoidance of unsafe drugs, by stable caloric intake, and by prompt attention to intercurrent illnesses. It is a difficult decision if unsafe drugs have to be administered for a vital indication such as seizures. Here, consultation with an expert in porphyria is strongly advised.

The Cutaneous Porphyrias

The symptomatology of cutaneous porphyrias is mainly photosensitivity, often combined with skin fragility and blisters. All these findings occur because of porphyrin toxicity, resulting in cutaneous light absorption at the wavelength of 400 to 410 nm and subsequent formation of damaging reactive oxygen species. Thus, two therapeutic approaches are plausible: decrease of porphyrins and protection of the skin from light. The usual sunscreens are, however, ineffective, and reflective agents containing zinc or titanium, although better, are less popular because of their appearance.

In three porphyrias—PCT, HCP, and VP—the skin lesions are rather similar, but EPP and congenital erythropoietic porphyria can lead to very painful skin lesions, and, in the latter, even to mutilations.

PORPHYRIA CUTANEA TARDA

PCT is the most common porphyria and occurs because of uroporphyrinogen-decarboxylase deficiency and accumulation of mostly uroporphyrin. It can be inherited autosomal dominantly or may occur sporadically. It can also occur because of toxins such as halogenated aromatic hydrocarbons.

The most prominent skin manifestations are seen on the dorsa of the hands and on the face, consisting of blisters filled with mostly clear fluid, shallow, slow healing ulcers, whitish plaques, and tiny inclusion bodies, *milia*. Hypertrichosis and hyperpigmentation are frequently seen.

Unveiling factors promote the manifestation of the disease and consist mainly of liver disease, commonly because of alcohol. Hepatitis, frequently type C, and HIV infections are also common revealers. The drug list (see Box 1) is not applicable to the cutaneous porphyrias. The diagnosis is easily suspected at inspection and confirmed by measurement of urinary uroporphyrin excretion, typically manifold increased more than the normal range.

There are two treatment options with different principles but rather similar effectiveness. Repeat phlebotomies of 350 to 450 mL at 1 to 2 weeks intervals are performed and followed by hemoglobin and ferritin measurements. Overt anemia should be avoided. Ferritin usually reaches the lower end of the normal range after approximately 8 to 10 phlebotomies, and clinical remission can be expected after approximately half a year. Remission can be long lasting, especially when unveiling factors are avoided; total abstinence from alcohol is advocated. Patients should not take iron enriched vitamins because iron plays a critical role in PCT.

If phlebotomies are contraindicated (anemia, pulmonary or cardiac disease) or very inconvenient, low-dose chloroquine[1] (125 mg twice weekly) can be given orally. This flushes porphyrins from the liver and can be continued until remission is reached. In such low doses, the drug is virtually free from side effects.

Patients on chronic dialysis can develop PCT and also *pseudoporphyria*. Plasma porphyrin measurements establish the correct diagnosis. Patients with PCT and end stage renal disease respond well to erythropoietin, probably via iron (Fe) depletion through incorporation of Fe into hemoglobin. Pseudoporphyria is also seen as a side effect of many drugs, mostly nonsteroidal

---

[1]Not FDA approved for this indication.

Rakel and Bope: *Conn's Current Therapy 2006.*

CURRENT DIAGNOSIS

- There is not just one porphyria, but there are at least six (and a few very rare ones because of homozygosity and dual porphyrias).
- There is not one test covering *all* porphyrias. For suspected acute porphyria, screening for excessive porphobilinogen is the test of choice.
- If cutaneous porphyria is in the differential diagnosis, quantitative measurements of porphyrins in urine and stool are recommended.
- Family studies are always indicated in these hereditary diseases.

anti-inflammatory drugs and diuretics, but although phenotypically identical to PCT, does not respond to phlebotomies or chloroquine. Patients with PCT have a higher incidence of hepatocellular carcinoma and should be checked twice annually with hepatic imaging and measurement of alpha-fetoprotein.

CONGENITAL ERYTHROPOIETIC PORPHYRIA (GÜNTHER DISEASE)

Congenital erythropoietic porphyria (Günther disease), a rare autosomal recessive disorder, is usually apparent shortly after birth when brick-colored urine in diapers is observed because of excessive amounts of uroporphyrin (even more impressive under UV light). This porphyria and the rare homozygous PCT, hepatoerythropoietic porphyria, can be progressive and severely mutilating. Therapy is limited to sun protection and blood transfusion if hemolytic anemia is present.

ERYTHROPOIETIC PROTOPORPHYRIA

Erythropoietic protoporphyria is an autosomal dominant disorder that occurs because of deficiency of ferrochelatase, the last enzyme in heme biosynthesis. Urinary porphyrins are normal, but protoporphyrin is markedly elevated in red cells and in stool. These patients suffer from painful sun sensitivity, followed by edema and wrinkles in the thickened, light-exposed

CURRENT THERAPY

- Prophylaxis is mandatory and depends on the type of porphyria.
- Abstinence from alcohol is always indicated.
- The drug list should be respected in the acute porphyrias.
- Glucose therapy for the acute attack has mostly been superseded by the more effective, definitive treatment with hematin (Panhematin), to be instituted as soon as possible once the diagnosis has been made.

Rakel and Bope: *Conn's Current Therapy 2006.*

skin. Approximately one fifth of these patients develop progressive liver disease secondary to hepatic accumulation of protoporphyrin. Liver transplantation can become necessary.

Therapy is often beneficial with oral β-carotene (up to 400 mg/day for adults). This leads to a harmless slight orange-yellow discoloration of the skin and often effective sun protection. Ideally, the β-carotene dose should be adjusted to a plasma level between 11 and 15 mmol/L.

REFERENCES

American Porphyria Foundation online available at: www.porphyriafoundation.com
Anderson KE, Bloomer JR, Bonkovsky HL, et al: Recommendations for the diagnosis and treatment of the acute porphyrias. Ann Intern Med 2005;142:439-450.
Anderson KE, Sassa S, Bishop DF, et al: Disorders of heme biosynthesis: X-linked sideroblastic anemia and the porphyrias. In Scriver CR, AL Beaudet, WS Sly, et al. (eds): The Molecular and Metabolic Bases of Inherited Disease, vol 1, 8th ed. New York, McGraw-Hill, 2001, pp 2961-3062.
Badminton MN, Elder GH: Management of acute and cutaneous porphyrias. Int J Clin Pract 2002;56:272-278.
Chemmanur AT, Bonkovsky HL: Hepatic porphyrias: diagnosis and management. Clin Liver Dis 2004;8:807-838.
European Porphyria Initiative online. Available at: http://www.porphyria-europe.com
Kauppinen R: Porphyrias. Lancet 2005;365:241-252.

6

Therapeutic Use of Blood Components

Method of
Sally A. Campbell-Lee, MD, and
Paul M. Ness, MD

With the discovery of the blood groups A, AB, B, and O, development of anticoagulant preservative solutions, and the ability to manufacture various components, transfusion therapy evolved rapidly during the 20th century. During this period of growth, new risks associated with transfusion were also identified. The decision to use blood components should be evidence based and include an evaluation of risks versus benefits for each patient. Presented here are our practice parameters for using red blood cells (RBCs), platelets, plasma, cryoprecipitate, and granulocytes.

Red Blood Cells

Whole blood is rarely used because component therapy has become quite advantageous, supplying recipients with only the blood components required and maximizing the availability of a limited resource. Whole blood is collected into a plastic bag containing a preservative solution.

Although available in several formulations, common to all is the provision of glucose for metabolic energy, adenine for adenosine triphosphate production, to enhance survival, and citrate as an anticoagulant. The more commonly used preservatives in the United States are citrate phosphate dextrose adenine (CPDA-1), which provides 35 days of storage, and citrate phosphate dextrose (CPD), which allows storage for 21 days. As an adjunct, additive solutions such as Adsol (AS-1) containing additional adenine, dextrose, sodium chloride, and mannitol are widely used to extend the storage life up to 42 days.

Biochemical changes still occur even with the proper use of preservative or additive solutions during storage of red blood cells. This *storage lesion* includes an increase in plasma potassium, hemoglobin, and a decrease in 2,3 diphosphoglycerate (DPG). For most patients, even in massive transfusion, these changes have little, if any, effect.

A unit of RBCs, also referred to as *packed red blood cells,* is prepared by removal of most of the plasma from a 500-mL unit of whole blood. RBC may also be collected using automated erythrocytapheresis, which is capable of collecting two units of red cells from a single donor, relieving the donor of less than 15% of his red cell mass. A unit of RBCs contains red blood cells and smaller amounts of white blood cells, platelets, and plasma in its unmodified state. It has an average volume of 300 mL, with a hematocrit (Hct) ranging between 65% and 80%. These contents may be modified into the following components to fit the needs of various patients: leukocyte reduced RBCs, washed RBCs, irradiated RBCs, and frozen deglycerolized RBCs.

LEUKOCYTE REDUCED RBCs

Leukocyte reduced RBCs are prepared by filtration though a device made from fibers that trap the white blood cells (WBCs), resulting in fewer than 5×10^6 residual leukocytes. This component is indicated for transfusion when the recipient has had more than one febrile nonhemolytic transfusion reaction (FNHTR) and for the prevention of alloimmunization to HLA antigens. FNHTRs are characterized by a greater than 1°C (2.0°F) rise in temperature up to 6 hours post-transfusion, often accompanied by chills and/or rigors. FNHTRs result from contaminating leukocytes. In some cases it is the interaction between recipient cytotoxic anti-HLA antibodies and the component leukocytes, or the release of biologically active cytokines by leukocytes, which can lead to the reaction. Leukoreduction, particularly prestorage, is effective in decreasing FNHTRs associated with the transfusion of allogeneic RBCs. Leukoreduction of RBCs has also been thought to reduce the incidence of HLA alloimmunization. Because HLA alloimmunization leads to decreased efficacy of platelet transfusions, its prevention is important for patients who may require substantial platelet transfusion support. Prevention of HLA alloimmunization is also important for patients who may require bone marrow or solid organ transplantation such as kidney transplantation.

Transfusion-transmitted cytomegalovirus (CMV) is a concern for immunocompromised patients. CMV-seronegative RBCs are often requested for CMV-negative bone marrow transplant candidates or recipients, in utero transfusions, low-birthweight, premature infants of CMV-negative mothers, CMV-negative pregnant women, and the rare HIV-positive, CMV-negative patient. CMV is known to be carried by leukocytes. A study comparing CMV transmission rates in patients with acute leukemia who received either bedside leukoreduced transfusions or CMV seronegative transfusions, published by Bowden and colleagues in 1995, concluded the two methods were equivalent. Leukoreduced components, largely because of the difficulty in obtaining sufficient quantities from CMV seronegative donors, have also become commonly used in the prevention of CMV transmission by blood transfusion.

WASHED RBCs

Washed RBCs are prepared by centrifugation of RBCs with a sterile isotonic saline wash fluid, which is then removed, while the remaining RBCs are resuspended in saline. This process removes 99% of the plasma proteins and electrolytes contained within the RBC component. Unfortunately up to 20% of the RBCs are also lost in the procedure, depending on whether manual or automated techniques are employed. If RBCs are prepared in an open system, the washed RBCs must be used within 24 hours. These RBCs are indicated for patients who have suffered recurrent severe allergic transfusion reactions that are not prevented by antihistamines. Recipient IgE antibodies to donor plasma proteins mediate these reactions. Washed RBCs are also indicated for IgA-deficient patients who have formed anti-IgA antibodies. In these patients, transfusion of blood products containing plasma with IgA can result in anaphylaxis.

IRRADIATED RBCs

The purpose of irradiation of cellular blood components is to inactivate immunocompetent lymphocytes. RBCs are commonly irradiated using a cesium-137 source. A dose of 2500 centigray (cGy) must be delivered to each unit. After irradiation, storage time is decreased to a maximum of 28 days because of shortened RBC survival and increased potassium leakage.

Irradiated RBCs are indicated for the prevention of transfusion-associated graft-versus-host (GVH) disease in immunocompromised patients, a frequently fatal complication. Neonates, patients with hematologic malignancies, aplastic anemia, bone marrow transplants, or congenital immune deficiency are susceptible to transfusion-associated GVH disease; irradiated cellular blood components are indicated for these patients. Irradiated RBCs are also required for patients receiving directed donations from first degree relatives because of the increased risk of transfusion associated GVH disease.

FROZEN RED BLOOD CELLS

RBCs can be frozen for long-term storage, up to 10 years, and probably longer for certain indications. After RBCs are prepared from whole blood, they are treated with glycerol as a cryoprotective agent. The most common method in the United States is the high-glycerol method (40% to 50% glycerol). After adding the glycerol solution, the cells are frozen and stored at −65°C (−85°F) or below. To be transfused, the cells must be thawed and deglycerolized by washing with saline. The remaining product contains few white blood cells or platelets, and 99.9% of the plasma has been removed.

The major advantage of frozen RBCs is that rare blood types can be stored. Patients with rare phenotypes may make autologous donations that can be frozen for later use. For patients who become alloimmunized to multiple clinically significant RBC antigens, frozen RBCs from donors with compatible, rare phenotypes are useful. Because 99.9% of plasma is removed in processing frozen RBCs, patients who may have adverse events related to plasma components may also benefit from the use of frozen RBCs. Because of the high cost and cumbersome nature of freeze-thaw procedures, however, other more routine uses of frozen RBCs are difficult to justify.

INDICATIONS FOR TRANSFUSION OF RBCs

One unit of RBCs should raise the hemoglobin of an average adult by 1 g/dL and the hematocrit by 3%. For pediatric patients the usual dose is 3 mL/kg to raise the hemoglobin by 1 g/dL and the hematocrit by 3%. Transfusion of RBCs is indicated in the treatment of anemia with symptomatic deficits of oxygen-carrying capacity and hemorrhagic shock when administered with volume expanders. That said, much discussion continues regarding the suitability of RBC transfusion thresholds for patients in certain settings, particularly nonsurgical, critical care. Many studies have shown that there is no universal level of hemoglobin at which one must transfuse a patient, but that the decision to transfuse should be based on evaluation of each patient's circumstances. Nonetheless, most published guidelines agree that transfusion is rarely beneficial when the hemoglobin is more than 10 g/dL; and transfusion is generally indicated, even in stable patients without cardiovascular deficits, when the hemoglobin approaches 6 g/dL. In surgical patients the decision to transfuse is often mitigated by the presence of microvascular hemorrhage or coexistent coagulopathy, which may require a lower threshold for transfusion of RBCs.

TRANSFUSION METHOD

Transfusion safety is dependent on collaboration between the medical director of the transfusion service, clinical service directors, and nursing staff. Procedures should be in place and periodically reviewed with all staff involved in transfusion. This process is necessary to ensure that the highest levels of patient safety, including appropriate identification of the patient and blood specimen as well as the correct component, have taken place, in addition to monitoring during the transfusion. Informed consent should be obtained before initiating transfusion therapy; every patient or family should

have a discussion with their practitioner regarding all aspects of transfusion risk.

Premedication with antihistamines occasionally helps patients with a history of allergic transfusion reactions; ideally an oral antihistamine should not be given more than 30 minutes prior to the start of the transfusion. The use of antipyretics prior to transfusion is usually restricted to patients with a history of nonhemolytic febrile transfusion reactions because the use of antipyretics can mask a fever, which is the main symptom of a hemolytic transfusion reaction. The increasing use of leukoreduced RBCs for all patients has reduced the reasons for administering antipyretics on a prophylactic basis.

Proper identification of the patient and validation of information included on the transfusion form or requisition are critical. In the United States, patient and blood component identification is performed by two people in an effort to discover any errors. Once identification is confirmed, the transfusionist should take and record vital signs.

Intravenous access should be in place before the components are released from the blood bank. There are no strict rules for the size of needles used in intravenous access for transfusion. Patients with good venous access should have the largest-size needle placed that can be tolerated for the best flow rates. For peripheral access, an 18-gauge needle can usually be used unless the patient's veins are too small, such as in children. It should be noted that high-pressure flow through much smaller needles can result in hemolysis. Therefore, slower flow rates may be necessary when using smaller needles. Central venous catheters are also suitable for transfusion.

Blood infusion sets with in-line filters should be used for all transfusions. The filter should be designed to remove blood clots and other particles such as cellular aggregates and debris that may form during storage. Standard blood transfusion filters have pore sizes of 170 to 260 μ.

To avoid hemolysis, only compatible solutions can come into contact with red blood cells in an infusion set. Solutions such as dextrose, hypotonic saline, or lactated Ringer's should not be added to blood or infused by the same line.

The transfusionist should observe the patient closely during the first 15 minutes of the transfusion. The transfusion should be started slowly during this period, and the rate may be increased to that specified in the order. The infusion rate should take into account the patient's cardiac status and hemodynamic condition. Although reactions because of acute hemolysis or anaphylaxis tend to occur at the onset of the transfusion, the patient should continue to be monitored even up to an hour after completion of the transfusion so that any signs or symptoms of an adverse reaction can be reported and investigated.

Platelets

Platelet concentrates for transfusion may be prepared by one of two methods. They may be produced from whole blood that is not allowed to cool after collection with separation by centrifugation. These components are commonly referred to as *random donor* or whole blood-derived platelets. The second method is to collect the platelets by processing of donor blood using apheresis technology (*single-donor* or apheresis platelets).

A platelet concentrate made from whole blood contains at least 5.5×10^{10} platelets in 45 to 65 mL of donor plasma, which also contains stable coagulation factors. Pheresis platelets contain at least 3×10^{11} platelets in approximately 300 to 500 mL of donor plasma. Unmodified, platelet components also contain leukocytes. Platelet components may also be modified in the same manner as RBCs for various patient requirements: leukoreduced, washed, and irradiated platelets.

LEUKOREDUCED PLATELETS

As stated earlier, leukoreduced blood components have proven beneficial for three indications:

1. Prevention of febrile nonhemolytic transfusion reactions
2. Reduction of infectious risks from cell-associated viruses such as CMV
3. Reduction of alloimmunization in transfusion recipients

There has been considerable debate regarding the additional immunomodulatory effects of transfusion, such as a potential increase in postoperative infections and cancer recurrence. The effect of leukoreduced blood components on these complications is highly controversial.

Regardless of whether leukoreduction is applied universally or on a case-by-case basis, most patients will require leukodepleted platelet components. Current apheresis equipment can provide leukoreduced products at the time of collection. The advantage of this *process leukodepletion* is a decrease in the amount of cytokines, which cause FNHTR, released during storage.

WASHED PLATELETS

Platelets are washed with sterile normal saline using manual or automated equipment as for RBCs to remove 99% of plasma. After washing the platelets are resuspended in saline. Up to 30% of the platelets contained in the component can be lost during washing, and the post-transfusion survival of the remaining platelets is mildly affected. This processing occurs in an open system, so washed platelets must be used within 4 hours of preparation. Patients who require washed platelets are those who have had severe allergic or anaphylactic reactions during transfusion, or who are IgA deficient with IgA antibody.

IRRADIATED PLATELETS

Platelets may also be irradiated, like RBCs. However, the effects on platelet function after irradiation are the limiting factor in irradiation dosage. The current dose of 2500 cGy is used because it inactivates leukocytes but does not affect platelet function.

Irradiated platelets should be used for the prevention of transfusion-associated GVH disease in the same patients who require irradiated RBCs, who are neonates and patients with hematologic malignancies, aplastic anemia, bone marrow transplants, or congenital immune deficiency.

Indications for Platelet Transfusion

Platelet transfusion is indicated when a patient develops bleeding with thrombocytopenia or a deficiency in platelet function. If the platelet count is more than $50,000/\mu L$, bleeding is unlikely because of thrombocytopenia. Many patients are transfused platelets prophylactically. At platelet counts between $10,000/\mu L$ and $50,000/\mu L$, bleeding generally does not occur unless there is a hemostatic challenge such as surgery or an invasive procedure. There is a greater risk of spontaneous bleeding at platelet counts between $5,000/\mu L$ and $10,000/\mu L$; it is at these platelet counts that prophylactic transfusion of platelets is commonly used. When bleeding is because of platelet dysfunction, however, the platelet count is not germane. For patients who have received antiplatelet drugs that block the platelet IIb/IIIa receptor—such as abciximab, tirofiban, and eptifibatide—and are bleeding or need to have emergent surgery, stopping the drug along with transfusion of platelets can decrease blood loss.

PLATELET TRANSFUSION METHOD

The same patient and component identification steps should be taken prior to platelet transfusion as were described in the section on RBC transfusion methods. An infusion set with a filter intended for use in platelet transfusion should be used. Platelets can be infused from 30 to 60 minutes; the patient should be monitored during this time period for signs of adverse events.

PLATELET REFRACTORINESS

One unit of platelets can be expected to increase the platelet count by approximately $5000/\mu L$. When a patient repeatedly responds poorly to allogeneic platelets, platelet refractoriness should be considered. However, the post-transfusion platelet count can also be negatively affected by the presence of splenomegaly, fever, neutropenia, disseminated intravascular coagulation, or sepsis; these reasons for refractoriness should be considered prior to further evaluation. Post-transfusion platelet counts can be drawn between 10 minutes and 1 hour after completion of the transfusion; these counts are the most helpful in evaluating a patient for refractoriness. A post-transfusion corrected count increment (CCI) can be calculated to aid in defining the cause of refractoriness:

$$CCI = \frac{Platelet\ increment \times BSA\ (m2)}{Number\ of\ platelets\ transfused}$$

Rakel and Bope: *Conn's Current Therapy 2006.*

(BSA= body surface area; number of platelets transfused is using minimum number of platelets per unit as 3×10^{11} for apheresis platelets and 5.5×10^{10} for random donor platelets)

A CCI of less than 4500 using a post-transfusion platelet count collected 18 to 24 hours after transfusion, particularly following a normal CCI at 1 hour post-transfusion often represents a nonimmune cause, such as splenomegaly, for refractoriness. A CCI of less than 7500 using 10-minute to 1-hour post-transfusion platelet counts correlates with only 20% to 30% recovery of transfused platelets and points to an immune cause for refractoriness. The most likely reasons for immune mediated platelet refractoriness are HLA alloimmunization or, less commonly, platelet specific antigen alloimmunization. Because platelets express HLA A and B antigens, prior exposure by pregnancy, transfusion with nonleukoreduced cellular components, or transplantation are usually the immunizing events. Platelets alone are poor immunogens, and antigen recognition requires HLA class I and II antigens, which are expressed on leukocytes. If the patient's serum demonstrates HLA antibodies, then a trial of HLA matched platelets may be appropriate. However, only 80% of HLA-alloimmunized patients who are refractory to allogeneic platelet transfusions are responsive to HLA matched platelets. For patients who do not respond, or lack HLA antibodies but show clear signs of immune mediated refractoriness, alloimmunization to platelet specific antigens should be investigated by screening patient serum for antibodies. There are 13 human platelet antigen (HPA) systems identified; the most commonly involved antibodies are to the antigen HPA-1a (also known as Pl^{A1}). Platelets lacking the offending antigen may be obtained in some cases, but there is frequently no correlation between platelet specific antigen alloimmunization and transfusion refractoriness.

Fresh Frozen Plasma

Fresh-frozen plasma (FFP) is manufactured from whole blood by centrifugation and separation or collected via apheresis. FFP is then stored at –18°C (–0.4°F) or less for up to 12 months. It must be thawed in a 37°C (98.6°F) water bath prior to transfusion. One unit of FFP has a volume of approximately 220 to 250 mL. FFP contains all labile and nonlabile coagulation factors, as well as other plasma proteins. Factors V and VIII decay most rapidly, leaving fractions of prestorage levels after a few days storage. Levels of all other factors are more stable.

INDICATIONS FOR FFP TRANSFUSION

FFP is the only available component for treatment of specific deficiencies of factors II, V, X, and XI. FFP is used as replacement for plasma removed during plasmapheresis in the treatment of thrombotic thrombocytopenic purpura. FFP is most commonly indicated for patients with multiple factor deficiencies—usually

because of liver disease, dilution or consumption—who either are bleeding or at increased risk of bleeding. The patients at greatest risk of bleeding usually have a prothrombin time at least 1.5 times the midpoint of the normal range. FFP is also indicated for reversal of warfarin effect in patients who require invasive procedures or develop bleeding. If warfarin reversal is not emergent, vitamin-K therapy offers a better alternative that does not carry a risk of infectious disease. There is little evidence to support prophylactic use of FFP in patients with mild prolongation of the prothrombin time, defined as less than 1.5 times the midpoint of the normal range. FFP is also not indicated as a volume expander; crystalloid or fractionated albumin solutions that do not carry any infectious risks are better choices.

FFP is given at a dose of 10 to 15 mL/kg and can be infused as rapidly as the patient's volume status will allow. ABO-compatible FFP should be administered, but compatibility testing is unnecessary.

CRYOPRECIPITATE

Cryoprecipitate is prepared by thawing frozen plasma at 4°C (39.2°F), removing the supernatant and then refreezing the remaining cold precipitant. It is stored at –18°C (–0.4°F) for 1 year. Cryoprecipitate contains von Willebrand's factor (vWf), factor VIII, fibrinogen, fibronectin, and factor XIII. Each unit contains a minimum of 80 IU of factor VIII and 150 mg of fibrinogen with a volume of approximately 10 mL. Several units are usually pooled for an adult dose, and once pooled it must be transfused within 4 hours.

Cryoprecipitate is indicated for transfusion when congenital or acquired hypofibrinogenemia or dysfibrinogenemia result in bleeding. In congenital hypofibrinogenemia or afibrinogenemia, cryoprecipitate is used during bleeding episodes to increase the fibrinogen level to between 50 and 100 mg/dL. However, the most common use of cryoprecipitate is for acquired hypofibrinogenemia, which can be seen in liver disease, massive transfusion, and disseminated intravascular coagulopathy. In these cases transfusion of cryoprecipitate should be considered when fibrinogen levels fall to below 100 mg/dL.

Cryoprecipitate has also been used to make fibrin sealant, which is used to enhance local surgical hemostasis. This usage has largely been replaced by a commercial product. This product consists of fibrinogen and thrombin, which when mixed together form a fibrin clot over the wound surface. Cryoprecipitate is no longer indicated in the therapy of hemophilia A. Most patients with von Willebrand disease use factor concentrates that provide replacement of the diminished factors, or DDAVP [1-deamino (8-D-arginine) vasopressin] to stimulate production; neither therapy carries any infectious disease risk.

Cryoprecipitate requires approximately 30 minutes to thaw and pool before release from the blood bank. It contains very little anti-A or anti-B isohemagglutinins and is usually given without regard to ABO or Rhesus (Rh) group in adults. Cryoprecipitate can be transfused as rapidly as the patient can tolerate the volume, usually

10 to 15 minutes. Dosage can be estimated using an empiric dose of 1 U/5 kg, or calculated by the formula:

$$\text{Fibrinogen increase (g/L)} = \frac{(0.2 \times \text{number of units})}{\text{Plasma volume}}$$

Granulocytes

Granulocyte concentrates are collected by apheresis techniques that yield a mean of 20 to 30×10^9 granulocytes per collection. The product also contains 200 to 400 mL of donor plasma and 10 to 30 mL of donor RBC as well as platelets. Granulocytes are stored at room temperature without agitation. There is rapid decline in cell function and survival; therefore granulocytes must be transfused within 24 hours of collection.

Granulocyte concentrate usage requires coordination and communication with blood bank staff and with the donor center as well. A granulocyte donor must be recruited from the community for each product desired, usually from among previous frequent donors or plateletpheresis donors. Donors must be ABO compatible with the recipient because of the large contamination of the product with RBC. To get the best yield of granulocytes at donation, the donor must take either the granulocyte colony-stimulating factor (G-CSF) filgrastim (Neupogen) or corticosteroids to increase the circulating granulocyte count. G-CSF can induce side effects such as bone pain and headache, but in most donors it is well tolerated. Collection time usually takes approximately 3 hours. Consideration must also be given to recruiting CMV-negative donors if the recipient is CMV negative, because these products obviously cannot be leukoreduced.

Granulocytes are indicated for neutropenic patients with an otherwise good prognosis and who have documented infections or a clinical course highly suspicious for infection, which are unresponsive to antibiotic or antifungal therapy. Granulocytes should be transfused daily until the infection clears or the patient is no longer neutropenic. Recipients with HLA alloimmunization or previously documented severe febrile or allergic transfusion reactions are ineligible for granulocyte transfusions. Patients with HLA alloimmunization will rapidly clear the granulocytes before the cells would have an opportunity to fight the infection. There is also a high risk of pulmonary complications in this patient population.

Prior to administration, premedication with antipyretics and/or corticosteroids may be beneficial for patients who have previously had fever or chills during granulocyte transfusion. Amphotericin B (Abelcet) should be administered either several hours before or after granulocyte transfusion. There have been some published reports of severe pulmonary reactions when the drug is given in close proximity to granulocytes. To prevent GVH disease, the granulocytes should be irradiated directly before release from the blood bank. The concentrate should be transfused through a standard blood administration set over 1 to 2 hours.

Transfusion Alternatives

In recent years, progress in the development of artificial oxygen carriers has accelerated. Currently, the most promising RBC substitutes consist of extracted hemoglobin from lysed RBCs, referred to as hemoglobin-based oxygen carriers (HBOCs). These products have undergone major evolution since Sellards and Minot first infused lysed RBCs into humans in 1916. Although no products have been approved in the United States for any indication, several are currently undergoing phase II and III testing. In addition, several case reports have been published regarding the use of these products in patients with anemia unresponsive to standard RBCs (sickle cell anemia, autoimmune hemolytic anemia), or in patients with other contraindications to transfusion (for example, Jehovah's Witnesses).

Although much progress has been gained with HBOCs, issues regarding safety and efficacy of these products have delayed Food and Drug Administration (FDA) approval. Safety concerns have been addressed with clinical and preclinical investigations throughout the past 10 years. However, efficacy endpoints have remained ill defined. Although doubtless that current HBOCs under study carry oxygen effectively, comparisons with RBCs on morbidity and mortality have been difficult to pursue; RBCs are considered to be both effective and safe. The only endpoint the FDA has publicly suggested has been transfusion avoidance. Therefore, this is the endpoint

 CURRENT DIAGNOSIS

Platelet Refractoriness
- Post-transfusion platelet count is affected by factors such as splenomegaly, fever, DIC, and sepsis.
- Post-transfusion platelet count at 10 minutes to 1 hour after transfusion is helpful in diagnosing refractoriness.
- CCI is useful in determining an immune versus a nonimmune cause of refractoriness.
- CCI less than 4500 at 18 to 24 hours post-transfusion indicates a nonimmune cause for refractoriness.
- CCI less than 7500 at 10 minutes to 1 hour post-transfusion indicates an immune cause for refractoriness.
- The most common immune cause of refractoriness is HLA alloimmunization.
- If the HLA antibody screen is positive in a patient who demonstrates platelet refractoriness, HLA antigen matched platelets should be used for platelet transfusion.
- Patients unresponsive to HLA-matched platelets or lacking HLA antibodies but who have signs of immune refractoriness should be evaluated for platelet specific antibodies.

Abbreviations: CCI = corrected count increment; DIC = disseminated intravascular coagulation.

CURRENT THERAPY

Red Blood Cells
- One unit of RBCs will increase the hemoglobin of an adult by 1 g/dL and the hematocrit by 3%.
- The pediatric dosage of RBCs is 3 mL/kg.
- RBC transfusion is only indicated for the treatment of symptomatic anemia.
- The decision to transfuse must be based on each individual patient's circumstances.

Platelet Concentrates
- Bleeding secondary to thrombocytopenia (platelet count <50,000/µL) or platelet function deficiency indicated.
- Prophylactic platelet transfusion indicated at platelet counts between 5 and 10,000/µL.
- Leukoreduced platelets decrease the incidence of febrile nonhemolytic reactions, alloimmunization, and can reduce the risk of transfusion-transmitted cytomegalovirus infection.

Fresh-Frozen Plasma
- FFP is the only available component for factors II, V, X, and XI replacement.
- FFP is indicated in patients with bleeding because of multiple factor deficiencies usually because of liver disease, dilution or consumption.
- FFP is indicated when the protime (PT) is at least 1.5 times the midpoint of the normal range.
- FFP is also indicated for emergent reversal of warfarin effect.
- FFP is not indicated as a volume expander.
- FFP dosage is 10 to 15 mL/kg.

Cryoprecipitate
- Contains factors VIII and XIII, fibrinogen, fibronectin, and vWf.
- Contains a minimum of 80 IU of factor VIII and 150 mg fibrinogen per unit.
- Most commonly indicated for acquired hypofibrinogenemia (fibrinogen <100 mg/dL).

Granulocytes
- Indicated for neutropenic patients with otherwise good prognosis, with a documented infection or clinical course highly suspicious for infection that has not responded to antibiotics or antifungals.
- Must be transfused daily until the infection clears or the patient is not neutropenic.
- Must not transfuse HLA-alloimmunized patients under most circumstances.
- Must be irradiated to prevent GVH disease.

Abbreviations: FFP = fresh-frozen plasma; GVH = graft-versus-host; RBC = red blood cell; vWf = von Willebrand's factor.

6

to which most manufacturers have gravitated. The use of large doses of HBOC in trauma has been reported and a randomized trial in trauma is currently in progress.

Finally, some experts argue that not one of these current products has so far satisfied market demands for a product that can compete in price with donated blood. This issue has been complicated also by the increased safety of the blood supply over the past 15 to 20 years.

Although regulatory approval for HBOCs has been slow in coming, it is anticipated that these products will have an important role in transfusion practice in the future. For some patients, such as patients with no compatible blood immediately available, HBOCs would have obvious clinical advantages over RBCs. In the coming years, clinicians will eventually have a menu of HBOCs from which to tailor individual therapy.

REFERENCES

Corwin H, Gettinger A, Pearl R, et al: The CRIT study: Anemia and blood transfusion in the critically ill—current clinical practice in the United States. Crit Care Med 2004;32(1):39-52.

DeLoughery T, Liebler J, Simonds V, Goodnight S: Invasive line placement in critically ill patients: do hemostatic defects matter? Transfusion 1996;36:827-831.

Development Task Force of the College of American Pathologists: Practice parameters for the use of fresh frozen plasma, cryoprecipitate and platelets. JAMA 1994;271:777.

McVay P, Toy P: Lack of increased bleeding after paracentesis and thoracocentesis in patients with mild coagulation abnormalities. Transfusion 1991;21:164.

Simon T, Alverson D, auBuchon J, et al: Practice parameter for the use of red blood cell transfusions: Developed by the Red Blood Cell Administration Practice Guideline Development Task Force of the College of American Pathologists. Arch Pathol Lab Med 1998;122:130-138.

Slichter S: Relationship between platelet count and bleeding risk in thrombocytopenic patients. Transfus Med Rev 2004;18(3):153-167.

Strauss R: Neutrophil (granulocyte) transfusions in the new millennium. Transfusion 1998;38:710-712.

Wandt H, Frank M, Ehninger G, et al: Safety and cost effectiveness of a 10×10^9/L trigger for prophylactic platelet transfusions compared with the traditional 20×10^9/L trigger: A prospective comparative trial in 105 patients with acute myeloid leukemia. Blood 1998;91(10):3601-3606.

Adverse Effects of Blood Transfusion

Method of
Phillip J. DeChristopher, MD, PhD

In the United States, an estimated 5 million recipients are transfused annually with approximately 22 million blood components, derived from approximately 5 million blood donations. These statistics position the transfusion of blood components as the most prevalent allogeneic tissue transplants practiced in medicine. Because blood components are both derived from human donors and manufactured, they are defined by the U.S. Food and Drug Administration (FDA) as both biologics and drugs. Thus it is expected that blood components have inherent, nonreducible risks of living tissues from other individuals, such as alloimmunization risks or infectious disease transmission, as well as certain limitations of drugs, such as variations in purity, potency, storage lesions, and limited shelf lives.

The safety of blood transfusion is upheld and maintained by several interlacing pillars, which include standardized blood banking operations and processes controlling transfusion administration. All U.S. blood donors are volunteers; they are currently screened by a nationally uniform Donor History Questionnaire that identifies relevant donor eligibility information, such as medical illnesses, and other disqualifying conditions, such as lifestyle and travel risks and medications. All collected blood is tested for the presence of markers for numerous transmissible infectious agents (Box 1); the application of quality management systems for the preparation, testing, storage, transportation, ordering, compatibility testing (including serologic testing, crossmatching, and serologic history checks), and administration of blood; and the use by clinicians of practice guidelines for blood transfusion. Current Good Manufacturing Practices (cGMPs) are implemented to track and indemnify blood components from the vein of the donor to the vein of the recipient.

Overall, adverse effects of transfusion are reported in approximately 0.2% of all transfusions (albeit recognizing that clinically silent adverse effects occur much more commonly). But much higher rates for specific adverse effects are observed in chronically or heavily transfused patient cohorts. Although the risks of infectious complications of transfusion were markedly reduced in the United States over the last 25 years, a zero-risk blood supply is still not available. The constellations of

clinical signs and symptoms, as well as the times to onset of symptoms (or disease), are commonly used to categorize most adverse effects of blood transfusion. The classification schemas of adverse effects are typically divided into either immune mediated or nonimmune mediated. Both categories have acute or delayed varieties, and both can have noninfectious or infectious adverse complications. The most frequent immune-mediated noninfectious transfusion hazards clearly are predicated on the fact that donor-recipient pairs in transfusion are allogeneic to one another. Such inherent genotypic/phenotypic discrepancies as well as residual or emerging infectious disease transmission risks label the practice of blood transfusion unavoidably unsafe.

The most dramatic progress over the last quarter century to improve the safety of donated blood was made in controlling viral disease transmission and other nonimmune mediated risks. These incremental improvements in the provision of a safer blood resource were made chiefly via key control steps prior to making blood available for transfusion in the clinical setting. Advances in blood preservation, storage, shipment, computerized inventory and tracking systems, regularly updated blood donor qualification schema, as well as discovery and implementation of new disease testing methods for known and emerging diseases, have all added to safeguarding donated blood. Box 1 notes the current compilation of tests applied to all blood components collected for transfusion in the United States. Table 1 gives estimates of the residual infectious disease risks of blood transfusion. (Treatment considerations for transfusion-transmitted diseases are omitted because they are the same as if the diseases were contracted outside the blood transfusion setting.) Transmission of infectious diseases—some of which can be chronic, acute, or even fatal—is not further discussed, except as noted:

- Nucleic acid test (NAT) methods for hepatitis C virus (HCV) and HIV were FDA licensed and implemented nationwide in early 2003. Application of this methodology is expected to include other analytes such as hepatitis B virus (HBV) and to continue to improve the already low levels of viral disease transmission.
- By comparison, the bacterial contamination of platelet concentrates has reemerged as a much more significant transfusion risk, with detection rates in the 1 case in the 1000 to 2000 population range. In early 2004, the American Association of Blood Banks (AABB) implemented new standards to limit and detect bacteria in platelet concentrates, which are stored at room temperature. The impact of these new standards is expected to improve the safety of platelet transfusions.
- In the summer of 2002, the United States experienced the largest arbovirus epidemic ever recorded in the Western Hemisphere because of the imported and emerging West Nile Virus (WNV). That year documented the first ever transmission of WNV by both blood transfusion and solid-organ transplantation. By mid-2003, NAT testing of the nation's blood supply for WNV began as an FDA investigational new

---

BOX 1   Required Testing of All Blood Components Collected for Transfusion in the United States

- ABO blood group and Rh type
- Antibody screening for clinically significant RBC alloantibodies
- Serologic test for syphilis
- Serologic tests, typically using an EIA technique:
- HBsAg
- Anti-HB$_c$
- Anti-HCV
- Anti-HIV-1/2
- Anti-HTLV-I/II
- Nucleic acid testing (NAT) using genomic amplification methods:
- HIV-1
- HCV
- WNV (in pilot testing under FDA IND since 2003)

Abbreviations: EIA = enzyme immunosorbent assay; FDA = Food and Drug Administration; HB$_c$ = hepatitis B$_c$ (virus); HCV = hepatitis C virus; HTLV = human T-cell lymphotrophic virus; IND = investigational new drug/device; RBC = red blood cell; WNV = West Nile Virus.

TABLE 1 Residual Infectious Disease Risks of Blood Transfusion in the United States

Infectious agent	Estimated frequency/unit transfused or comment
Viruses	
Hepatitis B	1:220,000 to 1:488,000.
Hepatitis C	1:1,935,000.
HTLV–I/II	1:2,993,000.
HIV-1	1:2,135,000.
HIV-2	Transfusion-related cases never reported.
Hepatitis A	<1:1,000,000.
Hepatitis E	Transfusion-related cases never reported.
B19 parvovirus	1:3300 to 1:40,000 donors are viremic.
CMV	<1% of seropositive components transmit CMV; protect selected seronegative recipient populations.
EBV	Rare.
HHV-6	Seroprevalence in adults ~100%; blood transmissible, but no disease associations after transfusion.
HHV-8 (also known as KSHV)	~10% of donors are seropositive; transfusion transmission not yet documented.
GBV-C, TTV, SEN-V (putative hepatitis viruses)	Transfusion-transmissible viruses with high seroprevalence rates in asymptomatic donors; *actual clinical disease transmissions are nil*; screening not currently recommended.
Bacteria	
Gram-positive organisms (RD platelets)	1:1000 (detected by culture); 1:2500 results in clinical sepsis.
Gram-negative organisms (RD platelets)	1:2000 (detected by culture).
Platelets pheresis	1:2000 (detected by culture); 1:13,400 results in clinical sepsis.
GP or GN in RBC	1:1000 (detected by culture); 1:10,000,000 fatal sepsis.
Treponema pallidum	No transfusion transmissions reported in the last 35 years.
Borrelia burgdorferi	No transfusion-related Lyme disease case yet reported.
Parasites	
Plasmodium (all species)	0.25 per 1,000,000; 1 to 5 cases reported per year; transfusion transmission fatal in ~10% of recipients.
Babesia microti	*Rare*; ~50 cases reported, only in the United States; high seroprevalence in northeastern United States.
Trypanosoma cruzi	Transfusion-transmitted Chagas' disease *rare*; however, *T. cruzi* seroprevalence 1:9000 in Southern California.
Leishmania species	Transfusion-related cases never reported.

Abbreviations: CMV = cytomegalovirus; GBV-C = GB virus C (formerly hepatitis G virus [HGV]); GN = gram-negative; GP = gram-positive; HHV = human herpesvirus; HTLV = human T-lymphotrophic virus; KSHV = Kaposi's sarcoma–associated herpesvirus; RBC = red blood cell (unit); RD = random donor, derived from whole-blood donation; TTV and SEN-V = acronyms for patient propositi.

drug (INV). In 2004 nearly 1000 units of donor blood contaminated with WNV were intercepted.

- Provision of cytomegalovirus (CMV)–reduced-risk cellular blood components remains a challenge because most adult donors are CMV-seropositive. In most clinical settings, reduction in CMV risk is accomplished by using either CMV-seronegative or leukoreduced components interchangeably. Both are equally safe and effective in preventing CMV transmission.
- Emerging infectious agents will certainly continue to pose threats to the blood supply. Such pressures will continue until methods are developed to sterilize donor blood. Although pathogen inactivation technologies using chemical and photochemical methods are actively being pursued in the research setting, no such methodology is licensed or available for transfusable cellular components at this time.
- Specialized blood components (such as CMV–reduced-risk, leukoreduced, and gamma irradiated) are usually reserved for specific patient populations who require reduction or removal of risk (Box 2).

Acute Adverse Effects

Table 2 shows a classification scheme for acute adverse effects of blood transfusion.

IMMUNOLOGIC

Acute (Intravascular) Hemolysis

Most acute hemolytic transfusion reactions (AHTR) are caused by the transfusion of ABO-incompatible red blood cells (RBCs). The cardinal signs and symptoms include fever and chills, burning along the vein, restlessness/anxiety, and pain anywhere, as well as, ironically, being clinically silent. They can occur after the

---

Rakel and Bope: *Conn's Current Therapy 2006.*

BOX 2   Typical Major Indications for the Selective Use of Specialized Blood Components to Protect Patients at Risk

CMV-Reduced-Risk Component Support
- All intrauterine transfusions (IUT)
- Very-low-BW infants (<1200 g) born to SN mothers
- SN allograft recipients of SN solid organs or SN hematopoietic stem cells
- All SN patients with oncologic diagnoses receiving chemotherapy
- All SN candidates for any transplantation procedure
- SN pregnant women
- SN HIV-infected patients

Gamma Irradiation of Cellular Blood Components
- IUTs and exchange after IUT
- Congenital cell-mediated immunodeficiency syndromes
- Childhood solid tumors
- All BMT or PBPC recipients
- Hodgkin's lymphoma
- ALL
- Patients with leukemias, lymphomas, other malignancies requiring immunosuppressive chemoradiotherapy
- All directed blood donations
- All HLA- or crossmatch-compatible platelet components (for recipients who share a haplotype with related or unrelated HLA-homozygous donors)

Leukoreduced Cellular Blood Components
- Decreases incidence of platelet refractoriness because of HLA alloimmunization
- Prevents FNHTRs in patients
- Provides alternative supply of blood components with reduced risks for CMV transmission
- Decreases incidence of HLA alloimmunization in solid-organ transplant candidates

Abbreviations: ALL = acute lymphocytic leukemia; BMT = bone marrow transplant; BW = birth weight; CMV = cytomegalovirus; FNHTR = febrile nonhemolytic transfusion reaction; HLA = human leukocyte antigen(s); IUT = intrauterine transfusion; PBPC = peripheral blood progenitor cells; SN = (CMV–) seronegative.

transfusion of only a small volume of blood or manifest after 1 or more units of RBCs are given. In the anesthetized patient, the only signs may be hypotension, so-called red urine, and unexpected oozing. The transfusion must be stopped immediately and the institutional policy and procedures followed for a transfusion reaction (TR) workup (see Table 2).

Although ABO-incompatible TRs occur very infrequently, improper specimen and/or patient identification all too commonly cause them. Completely enforced and documented procedures from specimen collection and labeling through to blood administration are the key preventive strategies.

The severity of an AHTR is directly proportional to the volume of incompatible blood transfused. The first essential steps in treatment include early recognition, stopping the transfusion, and preventing the transfusion of additional incompatible RBCs. Prompt and vigorous treatments for hypotension and cardiovascular support as well as maintenance of renal blood flow are the mainstays of therapy. Pressor agents may be necessary for maintenance of blood pressure, and component therapy

may be necessary if the TR is complicated by disseminated intravascular coagulation (DIC).

Anaphylactic Reactions

The immediate and systemic anaphylactic reactions are mediated by an acute hypersensitivity response to proteinaceous plasmatic constituents, which trigger mast cell degranulation in multiple organ systems, including the skin, the gastrointestinal (GI) tract, the respiratory tract, and the cardiovascular system. Respiratory distress, shock, angioedema, and GI symptoms characterize this abrupt life-threatening response. The TR can occur in any clinical setting and after the administration of even vanishing small amounts of blood. Early recognition is mandatory because a combination of upper airway obstruction (laryngeal edema and bronchospasm) and severe cardiovascular collapse can occur within minutes of the first symptoms. The transfusion must be stopped immediately. Prompt administration of epinephrine (0.3 mL to 0.5 mL subcutaneously of a 1:1000 solution; injections can be repeated), volume expansion with normal saline, airway and cardiovascular support, and supplemental oxygen for patients in respiratory distress are absolutely essential. Intravenous (IV) epinephrine may be necessary for intractable hypotension. (Etiologically, the solitary identifiable protein implicated in this TR is class-specific anti-IgA in recipients who are IgA deficient; most anaphylaxis is not associated with anti-IgA in an IgA-deficient recipient.)

Fever Without Hemolysis

Febrile nonhemolytic transfusion reaction (FNHTR) is a diagnosis of exclusion that must be distinguished from AHTR and bacterial contamination. FNHTRs are characterized by fever (defined by an increase in temperature of more than 1°C above pretransfusion baseline), sometimes accompanied by chills or rigors, usually within 1 or 2 hours of transfusion. Because the differential diagnosis includes AHTR and bacterial sepsis, the transfusion is commonly suspended and discontinued. FNHTRs occur very frequently in multiply and heavily transfused recipients. Most FNHTRs are likely attributed to either cytokine showers (a storage lesion in RBC and platelets, in which proinflammatory cytokines such as IL-1, IL-6, IL-8, and tissue necrosis factor are released into the supernatant) or to preformed white blood cell (WBC) antibodies to residual WBC in the component. Treatment with antipyretic agents, either prophylactically or therapeutically, provides symptomatic relief; more severe FNHTRs can be treated more intensively with agents such as hydrocortisone (Solu-Medrol) or meperidine (Demerol). FNHTRs can be minimized in patients who experience repeated documented TRs or who are chronically or heavily transfused by using leukoreduced components (Table 3).

Transfusion-Related Acute Lung Injury

Transfusion-related acute lung injury (TRALI) is a clinical diagnosis of exclusion characterized by worsening

TABLE 2 Acute Adverse Effects of Transfusion: Classification and Frequency of Occurrence

Adverse effect	Estimated frequency/unit or comments
Immune Mediated	
Fever without hemolysis (FNHTR)	1:100 to 1:200 in adults; 6% and 12% in adult and pediatric hematologic malignancies, respectively.
Cutaneous hypersensitivity ("*allergic*")	1% to 3% of plasma transfusions.
Transfusion-related acute lung injury (TRALI) (Noncardiogenic pulmonary edema)	1:5000 to 1:7500.
Acute hemolysis, *nonfatal* (ABO incompatibility)	1:6000 to 1:33,000.
Hypotension	Incidence remains unknown; small numbers reported.
Anaphylaxis	1:20,000 to 1:47,000.
Acute hemolysis, *fatal* (ABO)	1:587,000 to 1:630,000.
Nonimmune Mediated	
Transfusional hypervolemia	Uncertain, but common, ~1:700 to 1:3000.
Bacterial contamination	1:150 to 1:2500.*
Transfusion-associated bacterial sepsis (platelets)	1:435 to 1:13,500.
Transfusion-associated bacterial sepsis (RBC)	1:1,000,000.
Fatal: transfusion-associated bacterial sepsis (RBC)	1:10,000,000.
Nonimmune hemolysis	Infrequent.
Citrate toxicity	Uncommon.†
Metabolic derangements (low Ca^{++}, Mg^{++}, K^+, etc.)	Uncommon.†
Coagulopathy, hypothermia	Uncommon

*Laboratory evidence, usually by Gram stain or culture.
†Typically associated with massive transfusion or therapeutic hemapheresis.
Abbreviations: FNHTR = febrile, nonhemolytic transfusion reaction; TRALI = transfusion-related acute lung injury; RBC = red blood cell unit.

6

TABLE 3 Delayed Adverse Effects of Blood Transfusion: Classification and Frequency of Occurrence

Adverse effect	Estimated frequency/unit or comments
Immune Mediated	
Alloimmunization to class I HLA on WBC and platelets	1:100 to 1:1000†; common in multiparous women.
Platelet refractoriness, clinical (can be associated with FNHTRs)	1:3,300 to 1:10,000; very high in heavily transfused patients.
To RBC antigens, serologic only, with delayed hemolysis	1:1500
To RBC antigens, clinical symptoms, with delayed hemolysis	1:4000; significant in heavily transfused patients.
Graft-versus-host disease	~1:400,000.‡
Post-transfusion purpura	Rare; fewer than 400 cases reported worldwide; more common in multiparous women.
Immune modulation/suppression	Unknown.
Nonimmune Mediated	
Transfusional iron overload (RBCs only)	Variable, dose related; very common in chronically transfused patients with congenital hemolytic anemias.
Infectious disease transmission	Variable; see Table 2.

Abbreviations: FNHTR = febrile nonhemolytic transfusion reactions; HLA = human leukocyte antigen(s); RBC = red blood cell; WBC = white blood cell.
*Additional "relative" indications of each kind of component are matters of clinical judgment and should be individualized and clinically correlated.
†Incidence among selected, heavily transfused patient populations is very high (50%-100%).
‡Only selected patient populations are at high risk for this complication; they require prophylactic protection using gamma irradiation for cellular blood components (see Table 3).

Rakel and Bope: *Conn's Current Therapy 2006*.

respiratory distress, dyspnea, and bilaterally symmetric pulmonary edema with hypoxemia usually developing within 2 to 8 hours after transfusion. The diagnosis of TRALI requires an interval change in the chest radiograph (demonstrating "white-out" by alveolar or interstitial infiltrates) in which cardiogenic or other causes of pulmonary edema are ruled out. Other frequent manifestations include fever and mild hypotension. Differential diagnostic considerations include anaphylactic TR, bacterial contamination, and circulatory overload. TRALI is associated with passive transfer of donor human leukocyte antibody (HLA) (class I and class II) and/or granulocyte-specific antibodies. Its pathophysiology probably involves complement-mediated neutrophil lysis and pulmonary capillary leakage. Other patient-specific risk factors and component constituents also appear involved in its presentation, but its complete etiology is still under study. TRALI is associated with any blood component containing plasma. TRALI is a relatively mild form of acute respiratory distress syndrome (ARDS), and although fatal outcomes occur (usually in patients who are already sick or have co-morbidities), recovery within 48 hours is the rule. The mainstay of treatment is reversal of the progressive hypoxemia using supplemental oxygen. Aggressive treatment for respiratory failure in a critical care setting may be required. No clear preventive strategies are available.

Simple Allergic Reactions

Acute cutaneous hypersensitivity, characterized by urticaria (hives) and pruritus (itching), occur commonly after IV exposure to plasmatic components; patients requiring frequent transfusions or large amounts of plasma can experience allergic TRs in 1% to 3% of transfusion episodes. Transfused allergens in plasma cause tissue mast cell degranulation. If this TR is limited to the skin without other signs and symptoms, antihistamine administration is usually sufficient to provide symptomatic relief. The transfusion can be interrupted and if the TR does not progress, the transfusion can be restarted. These mild allergic reactions are TRs that do not need to be reported or evaluated as possible hemolytic transfusion reactions (HTRs). Transfusions can usually be safely resumed.

NONIMMUNOLOGIC

Bacterial Sepsis

Bacterial sepsis in transfusion is most commonly associated with platelet concentrates. Patients are symptomatic with very high fevers early in the transfusion episode, associated with rigors and profound hypotension, and they often experience nausea and/or diarrhea. The transfusion must be stopped and not restarted, and a TR investigation started at once (Box 3). Importantly, blood cultures must be drawn on the recipient (and later compared to blood cultures of the component). Broad-spectrum antibiotics should be administered immediately upon suspicion of bacterial sepsis because of the high likelihood of fatality. Definitive preventive measures are the current standard of practice to reduce incidence of such contaminations of platelet concentrates.

Transfusional Hypervolemia

Transfusional hypervolemia (circulatory fluid overload) is characterized by dyspnea, tachycardia, distended neck veins, hypertension, occasional cyanosis, and headache, associated with cardiogenic pulmonary edema. It is seen most frequently in patients at the age extremes and in patients who were massively transfused. Volume overload is best prevented by transfusing smaller aliquots of blood at slower rates and by close monitoring of patient's inputs/outputs and volume status. Mainstays of management include stopping the transfusion, vigorous diuresis, use of

---

BOX 3   Immediate Responses to Acute Adverse Effects of Blood Transfusion

STOP (Interrupt) the Transfusion
The transfusionist performs assessment and evaluative functions
Related to patient
1. Repeat documented clerical RECHECK of ID.
2. Keep IV line open with 0.9% saline; if an HTR or other life-threatening reaction is suspected, *discontinue and disconnect* component from patient.
3. Contact treating physician for directions on patient care.
4. Administer supportive/definitive care.

Related to blood component
1. Repeat documented clerical RECHECK of label(s) on blood container(s).
2. Send administration set, blood bag, and IV fluid bag to TS.
3. Contact TS for directions for investigation.
4. Obtain blood/urine specimens from patient; send to TS with appropriate request forms and labels.

Laboratory Functions to Rule Out Acute Hemolysis
CLERICAL CHECK: Examine label on blood containers, all other records, and patient's specimen.
Check visually for hemolysis of pre- and post-transfusion serum or plasma (reliable when [Hgb] ≥50 mg/dL is present).
Perform DAT on post-transfusion sample.
Report findings to TS supervisor and medical director.
Report interpretation of transfusion reaction workup evaluation in the patient's medical record.
Perform additional studies per TS policies and procedures, clinically correlated to event.

Abbreviations: DAT = direct antiglobulin test; HTR = hemolytic transfusion reaction; Hgb = hemoglobin concentration; ID = identification; IV = intravenous; TS = transfusion service.

supplemental oxygen, and, less commonly, phlebotomy (in 250-mL increments).

Chemical Effects

Citrate Toxicity

Citrate is the anticoagulant used both in all blood components for transfusion and for extracorporeal manipulations involving most forms of hemapheresis. Massive transfusion or large-volume hemaphereses place patients at risk for hypocalcemia, characterized by numbness, tingling, muscular spasm, seizures, and even cardiac arrhythmias. Iatrogenic hypocalcemia is best managed by serially following ionized serum calcium and by calcium repletion using either solutions of calcium carbonate or calcium gluconate.

Hyperkalemia or Hypokalemia

Hyperkalemia is of concern usually with very small infants (occasionally in patients with renal failure) who are exchange transfused using RBCs that are near outdating. A common strategy is to use fresher units of RBCs, which have lower absolute amounts of supernatant potassium. In patients who undergo either massive transfusion or prolonged hemapheresis procedures using citrate anticoagulant, hypokalemia is common. Citrate metabolism causes a metabolic alkalosis that causes potassium to be transported intracellularly. Electrolyte monitoring and appropriate repletion, as indicated, are recommended.

Nonimmune Hemolysis Without Symptoms

Patients may develop so-called red urine because of hemoglobinuria or because transfused RBCs were lysed by thermal extremes, mechanical means, or by chemical means (e.g., by admixture with hypo- or hypertonic drugs or parenteral solutions). All reports of red urine or findings of hemoglobinuria need to be distinguished carefully from immune hemolysis and bacterial contamination. A TR workup should aggressively seek an etiology, which usually can be traced to a remediable incident, error, or accident. Strict adherence to all standards of practice regarding the storage, transportation, and administration of blood components is the best preventive strategy.

Delayed Adverse Effects

Table 3 notes a classification list and frequency estimates of delayed adverse effects of blood transfusion.

IMMUNOLOGIC

Alloimmunization

RBC alloimmunization is possible whenever recipients are exposed to RBC antigens they lack. Because routine compatibility testing detects only the A, B, and D

Rakel and Bope: *Conn's Current Therapy 2006.*

antigens on RBCs, transfusion recipients are at risk for alloimmunization. Risks for alloimmunization to any blood group antigen on all formed elements of blood increase in proportion to transfusion frequency. Patients can also become alloimmunized through pregnancy and transplantation. Up to 30% of heavily transfused populations, such as patients with congenital hemolytic anemias, can become alloimmunized to one or more clinically significant RBC antigens, which mandates provision of antigen-negative RBC. For patients with a history of multiple alloantibodies, the provision of appropriately antigen-negative RBCs becomes more and more problematic, ultimately requiring the finding of rare or very rare donor units to realize therapeutic benefits. An additional consideration is the disappearance of alloantibodies, which commonly happens. When this occurs, a patient transfused with an apparently compatible antigen-positive unit mounts an anamnestic humoral response and experiences a DHTR. HLA and/or other WBC alloimmunization are also frequently seen in patients who are alloimmunized to RBC antigens.

Delayed Hemolytic Transfusion Reaction

When a recently transfused patient experiences an unexplained anemia, possibly associated with hyperbilirubinemia and mild fever, within approximately 14 days of transfusion, delayed hemolysis should be suspected. DHTRs are associated with clinically significant IgG antibodies to all of the antigens of the Rh, Kell, MNSs, Duffy, and Kidd Blood Group Systems. Such hemolysis is usually antibody mediated, slow in onset, with the RBCs removed extravascularly (liver or spleen). Uncommonly, IgG-mediated hemolysis may present as an AHTR because some antibodies bind complement. RBC alloantibodies are usually demonstrable either in the patient's serum/plasma or from eluates prepared from the antigen-positive RBCs still in circulation. Except for having to transfuse again for symptomatic anemia, DHTRs generally require no specific treatment. However, an important consequence of such TRs is that all future RBC transfusions must use RBCs that lack the implicated antigen(s). When alloimmunization to multiple RBC alloantigens occurs, provision of compatible RBC becomes more difficult and can delay indicated therapy.

Platelet Refractoriness

Platelet refractoriness is suspected clinically whenever a patient's platelet count does not increase appropriately after receiving an adequate platelet transfusion dose. The refractoriness may be on an immune or nonimmune basis; nonimmune causes are the most common. If sources of platelet loss, destruction, or consumption (such as active bleeding, fever, infection, sepsis, DIC, splenomegaly, numerous drugs) can be eliminated, immune destruction may be occurring. Serial post-transfusion platelet counts, 30 to 60 minutes after transfusion, showing no platelet increment, supports immune destruction; so does a positive screen for HLA antibodies. Patients requiring chronic or heavy platelet transfusion

CURRENT DIAGNOSIS

The table below gives the signs and symptoms of *acute transfusion reactions* occurring within 24 hours or less of transfusion.

Reaction type	Component risk	Usual etiology or clinical correlate	Common signs/symptoms
Acute hemolysis, *with symptoms*	RBC; platelets; granulocyte concentrates	*ABO incompatibility,* caused by management or clerical error (specimen or patient *misidentification*); immune-mediated intravascular hemolysis because of anti-A and anti-B, from out-of-group plasma	Fever*; chills/rigors; hypotension; *pain* anywhere (chest, flank, limbs); *burning along* the vein; hemoglobinuria (*red* urine); hemolyzed serum in lab specimens; oliguria; bleeding, oozing (skin punctures)
Acute hemolysis, *usually without symptoms*	RBC	Physical disruption of RBCs because of mechanical physical forces or exposure to *nonisotonic* fluids or other parenteral drugs	Hemoglobinuria (*red* urine); might be asymptomatic
Anaphylaxis	All[†]	Antibody to unspecified plasma protein; anti-IgA in IgA-deficient patients; *systemic* mast cell degranulation	Hypotension; respiratory stridor/wheezing/arrest; shock and cardiovascular collapse; abdominal pain, nausea, vomiting, diarrhea; skin flushing, urticaria, pruritus
Hypotension	Plasma-containing components	Mediated by bradykinin; prekallikrein-activating factors in patients on ACE inhibitor drugs Hypovolemia	Volume resuscitation or pressor support as necessary Avoid or discontinue ACE inhibitors in patients requiring therapeutic hemapheresis procedures
Bacterial sepsis	Platelets; RBC	Bacterially contaminated components; components containing bacterial toxins	Rapidly rising, high fever; rigors; profound hypotension; nausea and/or diarrhea
Simple "allergic" reaction	All[†]	Antibody to unspecified plasma protein; type I hypersensitivity response	Virtually always limited to the skin; skin flushing; urticaria (hives); pruritus (itching);
Fever *without* hemolysis (*febrile, nonhemolytic*)	RBC; platelets; granulocytes	*Storage lesion* proinflammatory *cytokines;* preformed WBC antibodies in recipient	Fever* and/or chills/rigors
Transfusion-related acute lung injury	All except cryoprecipitate	*Donor* antibody to patient's WBC; acute, noncardiogenic pulmonary edema because of capillary leakage	Acute respiratory distress; shortness of breath; progressive hypoxemia; interval chest radiograph changes with symmetrical bilateral infiltrates
Transfusional hypervolemia; volume overload	All except cryoprecipitate	Circulatory overload; nonrecognition of patients at risk (age extremes)	Shortness of breath; dyspnea/cyanosis; distended neck veins; peripheral edema
Acute hypothermia	All except cryoprecipitate	Associated with massive transfusion; nonwarmed IV fluids	Chills/rigors
Citrate toxicity	All[†]	Often associated with massive transfusion or therapeutic apheresis procedures	Numbness, tingling (perioral, extremities); tetanic muscle cramping; seizures; cardiac arrhythmias

*Fever defined as >1°C above baseline.
[†]*All* includes any kind of RBC, fresh-frozen or other plasma, any platelet or granulocyte concentrates, and cryoprecipitate.
Abbreviations: ACE = angiotensin-converting enzyme; IV = intravenous; RBC = red blood cell; WBC = white blood cell.

support are at high risk for immune-mediated platelet refractoriness or may already be immunized (50% to 100% develop HLA antibodies for some period of time) because of multiparity or previous treatment. Optimally, platelet (HLA class I) alloimmunization is best prevented. In nonalloimmunized patients, immune-mediated platelet refractoriness can effectively be minimized or avoided by using leukoreduced blood components (see Table 2). In HLA alloimmunized myelosuppressed patients requiring daily platelet transfusion, obtaining suitable components could be difficult to impossible. They are at very high risk for significant bleeding complications, including death. Options to consider in the support of HLA-alloimmunized patients include use of crossmatch-compatible platelets or HLA-matched platelets if they are available.

Rakel and Bope: *Conn's Current Therapy 2006.*

CURRENT THERAPY

Reaction type	Usual etiology	Treatment considerations
Acute hemolysis *with symptoms*	RBC incompatibility; intravascular hemolysis, immune- or complement-mediated; circulating immune complexes	To treat renal failure: hydration, 1 L, 0.9% saline over 1-2 h; to maintain urine flow >1 mL/kg/h; administer diuretic, such as furosemide (Lasix) mg, IV; consider low-dose dopamine or other pressor support. If DIC is present: consider heparinization, 5000-U loading dose and 1500 U/h continuous infusion, to be continued for 6 to 24 h; consider component therapy, as indicated. *Under no circumstances should the transfusion be restarted.*
Anaphylaxis	Antibody to *unspecified* plasma protein(s); anti-IgA in IgA-deficient patients (less commonly)	Epinephrine (1:1000), 0.3 mL, SC; supportive measures for BP, respiratory and cardiac functions. *Under no circumstances should the transfusion be restarted.*
Hypotension	Extracorporeal volume depletion, such as in therapeutic hemapheresis; ACE inhibitor drugs	
Bacterial sepsis	Bacterially contaminated components; *sterile* components containing bacterial endo- or exotoxins	*The transfusion must be stopped and not restarted;* initiate transfusion reaction workup to include culture of component bag and IV fluids; obtain blood cultures on patient; supportive care to include antimicrobial therapy.
Fever *without* hemolysis	*Storage lesion* proinflammatory cytokines; recipient antibody to donor WBC	Acetaminophen, 650 mg, PO; rule out hemolysis and sepsis; for repeated episodes, consider prophylactic antipyretic therapy; for heavily transfused recipients, consider leukocyte reduction; for fevers with *rigors*, consider adding hydrocortisone (Hydrocortone Phosphate), injected, 50-100 mg, IVP and/or meperidine (Demerol), injected, 50 mg, IVP.
TRALI (noncardiogenic pulmonary edema)	Donor antibody (HLA or granulocyte-specific) to recipient WBC causing ARDS; possible role of patient risk factors and storage-lesion lipids in components	Reverse progressive hypoxemia, using supplemental O_2; if respiratory failure develops, intubation and mechanical ventilation, critical care support; without cardiac failure, roles for use of digoxin and diuretics unclear.
Simple allergic reactions (cutaneous hypersensitivity), urticaria and pruritus, *without* other signs and symptoms	*Type I hypersensitivity* response to plasma proteins, other allergens	Diphenhydramine (Benadryl), 25-100 mg, PO, IM, or IV; if recurrent, consider prophylactic antihistamine prior to next indicated transfusion; if urticaria is nonprogressive, may restart blood 15-30 min after antihistamine administration.
Transfusional hypervolemia (circulatory fluid overload)	Volume overload	Best prevented by transfusing smaller volumes or at slower rates (e.g., 1 mL/kg/h); consider rapid diuresis and supplemental O_2; uncommonly, therapeutic phlebotomy may be necessary.
(Nonimmune) hemolysis without symptoms	Transfusion of hemolyzed, but compatible RBC; hemolysis because of physical, chemical, drug *adulteration* of components	Cautiously rule out immune hemolysis or sepsis; perform transfusion reaction investigation to elicit etiology; watchful inaction; monitor for urine output, renal function, and evidence of DIC.
Chemical effects and derangements	Citrate toxicity; serum potassium abnormalities; hypomagnesemia; dilutional coagulopathy	Monitor for evidence of hypokalemic metabolic alkalosis; replete serum (ionized) calcium, total serum magnesium, and potassium with oral or IV preparations, as indicated; replace coagulation factors using appropriate component therapy.

Abbreviations: ARDS = acute respiratory distress syndrome; BP = blood pressure; DIC = disseminated intravascular coagulation; HLA = human leukocyte antigen; IM = intramuscular; IV = intravenous; IVP = intravenous push; O_2 = oxygen; PO = by mouth; RBC = red blood cell; SC = subcutaneous; TRALI = transfusion-related acute lung injury; WBC = white blood cell.

Immunomodulation and Suppression

A growing body of literature supports transfusion-associated immunomodulation as a real biologic phenomenon associated with clinically significant deleterious effects in recipients of allogeneic blood. For example, in selected surgical patients, blood transfusions are associated with earlier recurrences of malignancy after resection and/or increased rates of postoperative infections. The evaluation of such information and how to control this apparent biologic phenomenon are a matter of controversy in transfusion medicine. Although the use of leukoreduced blood components is suggested as a possible fix, currently no established preventive strategies exist.

Transfusion-Associated Graft-Versus-Host Disease

Transfusion-associated graft-versus-host disease (TA-GVHD) is an ominous and near universally fatal complication of blood transfusion. It is caused by engraftment of viable donor T lymphocytes into recipients who either cannot or do not mount a cytotoxic cellular immune response against foreign cells. Patients develop an acute syndrome within 4 to 30 days of transfusion characterized by high fever, whole body erythematous skin rash, severe GI and hepatic toxicities, and ultimately death because of bone marrow failure (bleeding and infection). Because no effective therapy is known, TA-GVHD must be prevented in susceptible populations (see Table 2). This is accomplished by gamma irradiation of cellular blood components, using at least 25 Gy (2500 rads) dose of delivered radiation, to inhibit mitotic potential of donor lymphocytes that contaminate all cellular blood components.

Post-Transfusion Purpura

The typical patient with post-transfusion purpura (PTP) is a previously transfused or multiparous middle-age woman (the female-to-male ratio is 26:1) who develops profound thrombocytopenia within 5 to 10 days of transfusion. Because of the rarity of this syndrome, the pathophysiology of PTP is only partly understood. The platelet destruction is immune mediated, caused initially by platelet-specific alloantibodies; anti-HPA-1a is a common, but not exclusive, specificity associated with this syndrome and clearance of allogeneic platelets or circulating platelet antigens. However, platelet autoantibodies also develop that destroy autologous platelets as well; the cause of thrombocytopenia in PTP remains unexplained. The duration of thrombocytopenia is typically approximately 2 weeks. Urgent treatment is necessary because the severe thrombocytopenia can last for days to weeks and has led to hemorrhagic deaths. No randomized controlled studies to optimize the treatment of PTP are available, but the optimal first-line therapy appears to be infusions of high-dose IV immunoglobulins. Plasma exchange using fresh-frozen plasma as replacement fluid is also effective. Because of its partial autoimmune nature, high-dose steroids are also used, but there is little convincing evidence for efficacy. After recovery, prognosis of PTP is good, and it usually does not recur following subsequent transfusion.

NONIMMUNOLOGIC

Transfusional Iron Overload

Individuals who require chronic or prolonged RBC transfusion therapy, such as those with thalassemias and sickle hemoglobinopathies, inexorably accumulate excessive parenchymal iron, a complication that is ultimately life-threatening. Each unit of transfused RBC contains approximately 250 mg of iron, which saturates the monocyte-macrophage system and then deposits in the heart, liver, and endocrine system. The cardiac sequelae are the most dreadful, accounting for the majority of deaths from iron overload because of cardiac failure and conduction defects with lethal arrhythmias. Treatment with the only FDA-licensed iron chelator, deferoxamine, is currently the most effective therapy for transfusional iron overload. Its effectiveness owes to preventing cardiac toxicity, thus helping prolong survival. Compliance with chelation therapy is a real and chronic problem because deferoxamine must be administered parenterally. Oral iron chelating agents are eagerly anticipated.

REFERENCES

Brecher ME (ed): Technical Manual, 14th ed. Bethesda, Md, American Association of Blood Banks Press, 2002. (See especially Chapter 18, "Pretransfusion Testing"; Chapter 21, "Blood Transfusion Practice"; Chapter 27, "Noninfectious Complications of Blood Transfusion"; Chapter 28, "Transfusion-Transmitted Diseases.")
Brecher ME (ed): Bacterial and Parasitic Contamination of Blood Components. Bethesda, Md, American Association of Blood Banks Press, 2003.
Busch MP, Kleinman SH, Nemo GJ: Current and emerging infectious risks of blood transfusions. JAMA 2003;289(8):959-962.
DeChristopher PJ, Anderson RR: Practice parameters for transfusion medicine. Lab Med 2001;32(4):193,200-204.
Dodd RY, Notari EP, Stramer SL: Current prevalence and incidence of infectious disease markers and estimated window-period risk in American Red Cross donor population. Transfusion 2002;42(8):975-979.
Klein HG: Pathogen inactivation technology: Cleansing the blood supply. J Intern Med 2005;257(3):224-237.
Popovsky MA (ed): Transfusion Reactions, 2nd ed. Bethesda, Md, American Association of Blood Banks Press, 2001.
Prezepiorka D, LeParc GF, Stovall MA, et al: Use of irradiated blood components. Practice parameter. Am J Clin Pathol 1996;106:6-11.
Prezepiorka D, LeParc GF, Werch J, Lichtiger B: Prevention of transfusion-associated cytomegalovirus infection. Practice parameter. Am J Clin Pathol 1996;106:163-169.
Ratko TA, Cummings J, Oberman HA, et al: Evidence-based recommendations for the use of WBC-reduced cellular blood components (Conference Report). Transfusion 2001;41:1310-1319.
Silva MA (ed): Standards for Blood Banks and Transfusion Services, 23rd ed. Bethesda, Md, American Association of Blood Banks Press, 2004, pp 37-41.

The Digestive System

Cholelithiasis and Cholecystitis

Method of
Oscar Ruiz, MD

Gallstone disease is one of the most common diseases in the world. It is estimated that in the United States, more than 20 million people have gallstones. The incidence is higher in patients that are obese, diabetic, older, that have a family history of gallstones, and in certain ethnic groups (e.g., Native Americans).

Gallstone disease has always plagued humans. Gallstones were found in Chilean mummies that date back to 300 AD. The Greeks described biliary stones in the 5th century AD. Clinical jaundice related to gallstones was first described by Vesalius in the 16th century. Bile composition, physiology, and circulation were studied in the 1800s. The first cholecystectomy was performed in Berlin by Langenbach in 1882.

Most gallstones remain asymptomatic, but the gallstones that become symptomatic may cause very serious problems. Patients may develop acute cholecystitis, choledocholithiasis (with or without jaundice), gallstone ileus, gallstone pancreatitis, and/or ascending cholangitis. In these situations, prompt recognition of the problem is essential, as this leads to earlier treatment and better outcomes. For good surgical candidates, cholecystectomy remains the treatment of choice. It is estimated that more than 300,000 laparoscopic cholecystectomies are performed annually in the United States. The laparoscopic approach has become the surgical treatment of choice for gallbladder disease, leaving the open technique, cholecystostomy tubes, or endoscopic decompression, for more complicated cases.

Anatomy

The gallbladder is located between the divisions of right and left liver lobes. It is formed by the fundus (composed of smooth muscle), body (elastic tissue), infundibulum, and neck, which are connected with the cystic duct. The blood supply comes from the cystic artery that originates from the right hepatic artery. The blood return is through small vessels into the liver, and the cystic vein will drain into the portal vein. The cystic duct joins the common bile duct, where there are variations that are important to recognize for surgical approach. The lymphatic drainage goes directly into the liver and also drains into periportal lymph nodes.

Physiology

The gallbladder has a 20- to 50-mL capacity. Nearly half of the bile produced by the liver enters the duodenum directly. When the common bile duct pressure increases, the rest of the bile enters the gallbladder where water is passively absorbed over approximately 4 hours. The gallbladder then delivers the concentrated bile into the duodenum in response to cholecystokinin (CCK), secretin, and vagal stimulation from ingested food. The gallbladder relaxation is mediated by vasoactive intestinal polypeptide (VIP), pancreatic polypeptide, and somatostatin.

Gallstone Composition

The formation of gallstones is multifactorial (obstruction, inflammation, decreased solubility of bile, cholesterol crystals, etc.). The most common gallstones in the Western hemisphere are cholesterol gallstones, followed by bile pigment, the majority of which is bilirubin. The third most common are calcium, which occur predominantly as bilirubinate. There are other substances that can be found in gallstones, like carbonate, sodium, potassium, phosphate, copper, and iron, and so on.

Symptomatic and Asymptomatic Cholelithiasis

Based on numerous studies, it is generally believed that patients with asymptomatic gallstones do not require treatment. Physicians must be careful to recognize clear symptoms of gallbladder disease. The risk of observation in asymptomatic patients compared to surgical approach is definitely less. However, there are select groups of asymptomatic patients that may benefit from cholecystectomy, including patients with large gallstones (>2.5 cm), hemolytic anemia, children, and morbidly obese patients with rapid weight loss. Incidental cholecystectomies are mainly left as a decision of the surgeon, depending on the individual circumstances. Identifying the different clinical presentations of symptomatic cholelithiasis, such as biliary colic, chronic cholecystitis, or acute cholecystitis, is critical for deciding the best timing of treatment.

Biliary colic, which is caused by temporary cystic duct obstruction of bile flow, is the most common manifestation of cholelithiasis. This process begins soon after meals and manifests as constant, right-upper-quadrant pain that can last for several hours. The pain often radiates to the shoulder or back. These attacks are self-limiting, and timing of recurrence is unpredictable. In addition to the previously mentioned symptoms, patients with chronic cholecystitis have more frequent attacks than in biliary colic, and are at greater risk for complications of gallstone disease. Patients with acute acalculous or calculous cholecystitis require admission to the hospital. These patients present with fever, elevated white blood count, elevated liver function tests, nausea, vomiting, and positive Murphy's sign. There is a special group of patients with the presumptive diagnosis of biliary dyskinesia that present with typical symptoms of biliary colic, but no gallstones. These individuals require a more extensive workup to rule out other etiologies for their symptoms. A paraisopropyliminodiacetic acid (PIPIDA) scan with ejection fraction (EF) will help considerably in making a diagnosis. Approximately 80% of patients with biliary dyskinesia will benefit from cholecystectomy.

Chronic Cholecystitis

Chronic attacks and inflammation of the gallbladder are most often associated with gallstones and the typical history of biliary colic. Usually, there is an obstruction in the neck of the gallbladder by a gallstone. This can produce a hydrops (mucocele), which may become secondarily infected with *Salmonella typhi*, *Streptococci*, and *Klebsiella*. The patient usually presents with postprandial, right-upper-quadrant pain with radiation to the right shoulder, chest, or epigastrium. Significant back pain is a concern for possible choledocholithiasis. The image modality of choice is undoubtedly an ultrasound, which shows gallstones in 90% of patients. In addition, the ultrasound may reveal thickening of the gallbladder wall, evidence of pericholecystic fluid, as well as an excellent visualization of the biliary tree, liver, pancreas, and kidney (Figure 1). Other modalities can be used to rule out additional sources of gastrointestinal pain, including computerized tomography (CT) scan of the abdomen, upper endoscopy, upper or lower gastrointestinal (GI) studies, and hepatobiliary iminodiacetic acid (HIDA) scan. If the diagnosis is made with no complications, and there is resolution of the pain, the patient will be prepared for elective cholecystectomy.

TREATMENT

Cholecystectomy is one of the most common abdominal surgeries in the United States, and it is the treatment

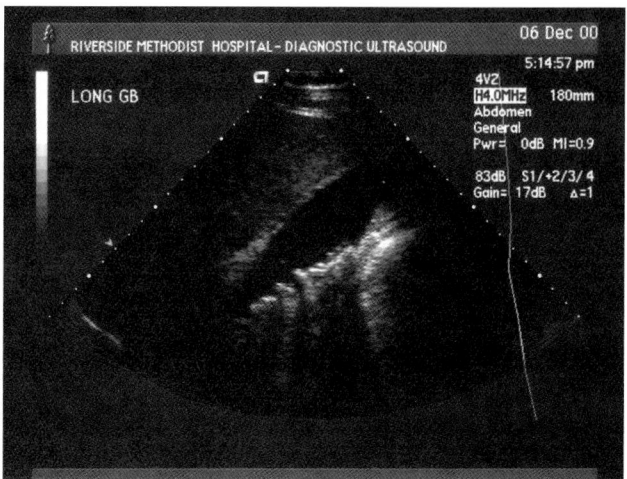

FIGURE 1. Gallbladder ultrasound demonstrates thickening of the wall, cholelithiasis.

of choice for patients with symptomatic cholelithiasis. At the present time, the laparoscopic technique is the standard of care, with very low morbidity, mortality, and an incidence of clinically significant bile leaks between 1% and 3%. The decision of using the laparoscopic approach or converting to an open technique will depend on the circumstances that the surgeon encounters. The conversion rate to open cholecystectomy in elective cases of chronic cholecystitis is very low (<2%). The most common reasons for conversion are previous upper abdominal procedures, congenital ductal anomalies (5% to 7% of the general population), unexpected inflammatory processes, and Mirizzi's syndrome.

Acalculous Cholecystitis

Acute or chronic cholecystitis can occur without cholelithiasis. The incidence of chronic acalculous cholecystitis in this country is less than 5% of all cases, and occurs mainly in children. The causes are various, including anatomic anomalies, tumors that can cause obstruction, thrombosis of blood vessels, diabetes mellitus, collagen diseases, or infections (mycotic, typhoid fever, parasites). However, acute acalculous cholecystitis usually is a complication of sepsis, diabetes, multiple organ dysfunction, burns, or post–major surgical procedures. The treatment of choice is cholecystectomy, but in some cases, because of the associated disease processes, cholecystostomy tube placement (open or percutaneous) may be effective.

Acute Cholecystitis

Acute cholecystitis is usually associated with an obstruction in the infundibulum or neck of the gallbladder by stones. After direct pressure from the stones on the mucosa, the local area develops ischemia, edema, necrosis, and ulceration, which may result in a wall perforation. The etiology of acute cholecystitis may be bacterial (*Klebsiella, E. coli, Streptococci, Salmonella, Clostridia*), sepsis from mechanical impaction of a stone, trauma, or after surgery. Less than 1% of the cases are secondary to tumors. Emphysematous cholecystitis is very rare, and is a secondary infection with gas-forming bacilli. Because of the rapid progression of this process with early perforation, the treatment of choice is early operation. Acute cholecystitis presents clinically and, by history, similarly to chronic cholecystitis and cholelithiasis. It may happen at any age, but it is most common between the 4th and 8th decades of life. The patients present with fever, elevated white blood count, positive Murphy's sign, and the gallbladder may be palpable. Mild jaundice is suggestive of extrinsic compression from the inflammatory process or choledocholithiasis. Usually leukocytosis with a shift to the left is noted. The preoperative workup includes a chest radiograph to rule out pneumonic processes, as well as a right-upper-quadrant ultrasound and HIDA scan, if needed (Figures 2 and 3).

TREATMENT

Acute cholecystitis is the indication for laparoscopic cholecystectomy in approximately 20% of cases. There are different opinions about the optimal time for surgical intervention. Most surgeons favor early surgery (24 to 48 hours). The acute inflammation, edematous and thick gallbladder wall and sometimes gangrene of the gallbladder wall pose technical difficulties with dissection. As a result, the conversion rate to open cholecystectomy may be higher than in elective cases. The incidence of bile leak using cholescintigraphy following

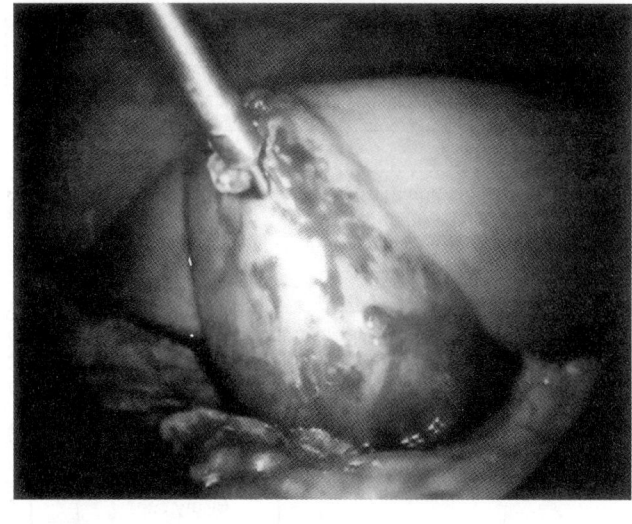

FIGURE 3. Intra-operative laparoscopic picture of acute gangrenous cholecystitis.

laparoscopic cholecystectomy for acute cholecystitis reveals a subclinical bile leak rate of 4%, similar to those for elective cases.

Choledocholithiasis

Stones in the common bile duct, single or multiple, are one of the most common and serious complications of gallstones. The incidence is difficult to determine but definitely increases with age. Common bile duct stones may be present in as many as 7% to 15% of patients that require cholecystectomy, and less than 5% may not be diagnosed before surgery. Common bile duct stones can cause acute or chronic obstruction, which may dictate the resulting clinical presentation and symptoms. The patient will typically present with right-upper-abdominal pain, jaundice, pale stools, and dark urine. The attack usually is sudden, and often precipitated by ingestion of a fatty meal. If the patient has associated ascending cholangitis, the clinical presentation is more severe. In addition to the pain and jaundice, there is also a high fever (Charcot intermittent fever). This group of patients often requires emergency removal of the common bile obstruction by endoscopic retrograde cholangiopancreatography (ERCP) and sphincterotomy, in combination with full support in the intensive care unit. If the endoscopic procedure is unsuccessful, open common bile duct exploration is necessary.

The differential diagnoses of choledocholithiasis include carcinoma of the common bile duct, viral hepatitis, drug-induced jaundice, peptic ulcer disease, myocardial infarction, pancreatitis, and pancreatic carcinoma. The main noninvasive diagnostic studies include hematology studies and evaluation of alkaline phosphatase, serum glutamic-oxaloacetic transaminase (SGOT), serum glutamic-pyruvic transaminase (SGPT), and bilirubin. The imaging studies include ultrasound, CT scan of the abdomen, magnetic resonance cholangiopancreatography

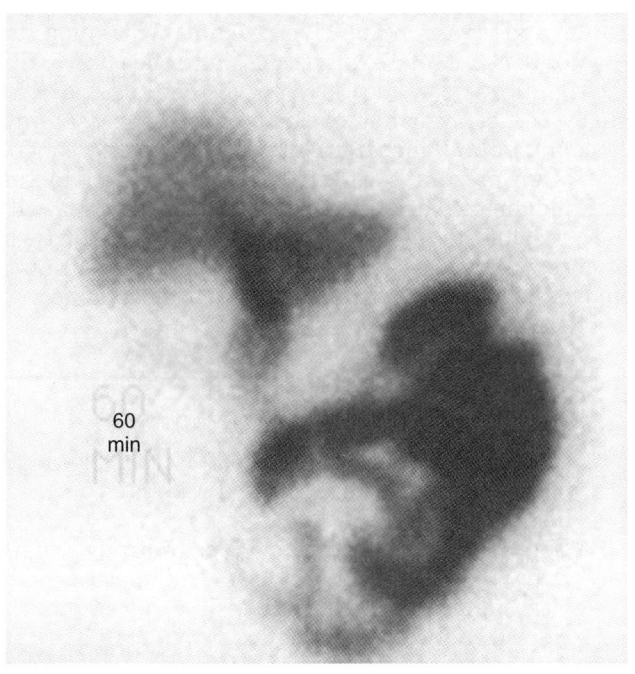

FIGURE 2. Positive HIDA scan, non visualization of gallbladder in 60 min.

Rakel and Bope: *Conn's Current Therapy 2006.*

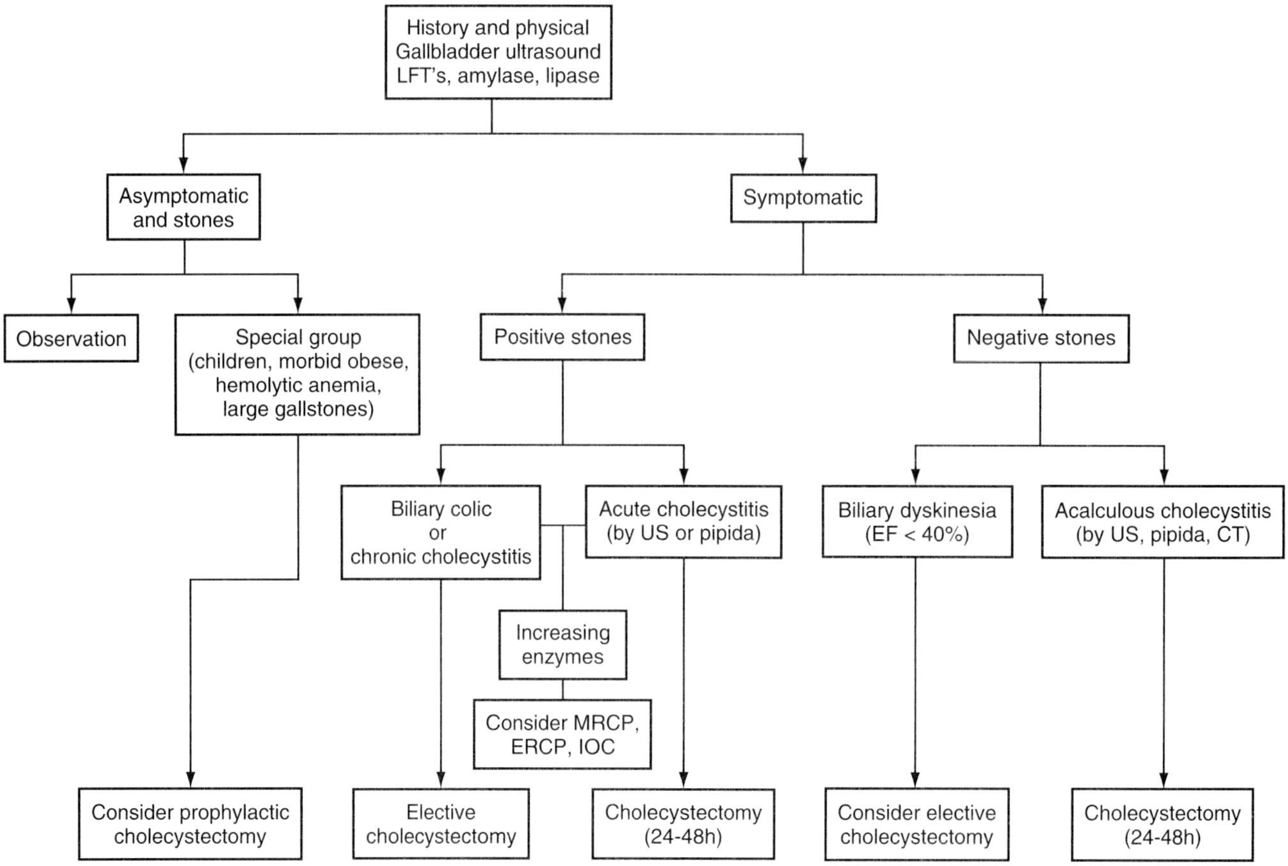

```
                          ┌──────────────────────┐
                          │ History and physical  │
                          │ Gallbladder ultrasound│
                          │ LFT's, amylase, lipase│
                          └──────────────────────┘
```

FIGURE 4. Protocol of management of gallbladder disease.

(MRCP), ERCP, intraoperative cholangiogram, or transhepatic cholangiogram. For the group of surgeons that advocate routine use of intraoperative cholangiogram in cholecystectomies, the incidence of common bile duct injuries and retained bile duct stones is significantly lower. The previously mentioned radiologic studies may demonstrate a stone in the common bile duct, or dilated intra- and extrahepatic bile ducts and, importantly, exclude any tumor mass in the duct, head of the pancreas, or liver. Recently the increased use of MRCP has been a very useful noninvasive tool in the diagnosis of common bile duct stones. After the diagnosis is made, the decision is to select the best approach for each case to relieve the obstruction. This can be accomplished endoscopically with a transhepatic technique, or with a surgical approach, open or laparoscopically (Figure 4).

Other Complications of Cholelithiasis

The early diagnosis of symptomatic gallstones is essential to prevent the many complications that can occur. Delay in diagnosis can lead to emphysematous cholecystitis, gallbladder perforation, gangrene, or empyema; sepsis that ensues may be difficult to counteract.

Associated illnesses in this group of patients can make diagnosis difficult. Patients often need aggressive resuscitation and invasive intensive care unit (ICU) monitoring prior to abdominal exploration. Gallstone pancreatitis is a significant complication of gallstone disease. This usually occurs after one of the stones has passed into the common bile duct. Patients with gallstone pancreatitis often present with peritonitis and an acute surgical abdomen. These attacks may be transient with quick resolution of symptoms; however, 20% of these patients will need some type of surgical intervention to remove the stones. Gallstone ileus is a rare complication

CURRENT DIAGNOSIS

- Obtain a complete medical history (i.e., previous biliary colic attacks associated with fatty meals, history of jaundice).
- Determine pain location and type (Murphy's sign).
- Evaluate WBC, LFT, amylase, and lipase.
- Use radiologic diagnostic tools (i.e., ultrasound, HIDA scan with or without EF, CT scan).

Abbreviations: CT = computerized tomography; EF = ejection fraction; HIDA = hepatobiliary iminodiacetic acid; LFT = liver function test; WBC = white blood cell count.

CURRENT THERAPY

Surgical Candidate

- Consider surgical therapy (laparoscopic cholecystectomy) for patients with diagnosis of chronic cholecystitis, acute calculous or acalculous cholecystitis, biliary dyskinesia, or gallstone pancreatitis.
- Place on low-fat diet until date of elective cholecystectomy.

Poor Surgical Candidate

- With acute cholecystitis, consider percutaneous cholecystostomy.
- With chronic cholecystitis, use conservative management.
- Prophylactic cholecystectomy should be considered in patients with gallstones, who are morbidly obese, have large gallstones, or are children with hemolytic anemia.
- If patient is pregnant, conservative management is preferred.

of cholelithiasis. This can occur when a large gallstone penetrates the wall of the gallbladder and enters the duodenum or colon forming a fistula. The stone can migrate to the terminal ileum where it becomes lodged causing a small bowel obstruction. If the patient is severely ill, the fistula between the bowel and the gallbladder may be treated in a second operation.

Another rare complication of cholelithiasis is a condition known as Mirizzi's syndrome. Mirizzi's syndrome is described as external compression of the common hepatic duct by a stone impacted in the neck of the gallbladder or in the cystic duct. This stone can erode directly through the ducts and become lodged in common bile duct causing an obstruction. In the unlikely scenario that the diagnosis is made preoperatively, the ideal management is to treat the patient conservatively. If the patient presents with an acute inflammatory process, following diagnosis with ERCP, the treatment is to proceed with cholecystectomy. This usually requires the open technique because of the challenging anatomy and the difficult dissection.

REFERENCES

Dominguez E, Ruiz O, Giammar D, et al: A prospective study of bile leaks after laparoscopic cholecystectomy in acute cholecystitis. Submitted for Publication, Riverside Methodist Hospital Department of Surgery.

Flum DR, Koepsell T, Heagerty P, et al: Common bile duct injury during laparoscopic cholecystectomy and use of intraoperative cholangiography. Arch Surg 2001;136:1287-1292.

Flum DR, Flowers C, Veenstra DL: A cost effectiveness analysis of intraoperative cholangiography in the prevention of bile duct injury during laparoscopic cholecystectomy. J Am Coll Surg 2003; 196:385-393.

Friedman GD: Natural history of asymptomatic and symptomatic gallstones. Am J Surg 1993;165(4):399.

Hasl DM, Ruiz OR, Baumert J, et al: A prospective study of bile leaks after laparoscopic cholecystectomy. Surg Endosc 2001;15:1299-1300.

Rakel and Bope: *Conn's Current Therapy 2006.*

Phillips EH: Routine versus selective intraoperative cholangiography. Am J Surg 1993;165:505-507.

Young-Fadok TM, Smith CD, Sarr MG: Laparoscopic minimal-access surgery: Where are we now? Where are we going? Gastroenterology 2000;118:148-65.

Yu P, De Petris G, Biancani P, et al: Cholecystokinin-coupled intracellular signaling in gallbladder muscle. Gastroenterology 1994; 106(3):763.

Cirrhosis

Method of
*David S. Kotlyar, BS, and
K. Rajender Reddy, MD*

Cirrhosis is the 10th most common cause of death in the United States, and one of the leading causes of death in the world. The condition is characterized by nodular regeneration and fibrosis. Neither nodular regeneration nor fibrosis alone is synonymous with cirrhosis. The most common causes of cirrhosis include:

- Alcohol abuse
- Infection with hepatitis C virus (HCV)
- Infection with hepatitis B virus (HBV)
- Nonalcoholic steatohepatitis
- Cholestatic disorders such as primary biliary cirrhosis and primary sclerosing cholangitis
- Inborn errors of metabolism such as Wilson's disease and hemochromatosis
- Vascular disorders such as hepatic vein thrombosis
- Autoimmune chronic hepatitis

Symptoms and Diagnosis

There are several nonspecific symptoms of cirrhosis including fatigue, malaise, weight loss, skin fragility, easy bruising, and abdominal discomfort. A physical exam may reveal jaundice and parotid gland swelling, and the spleen (left upper quadrant) may be enlarged. The right upper quadrant may be tender, and an enlarged liver may be palpable. Also, the patient may have gynecomastia and palmar erythema. There may be spider angiomas on the face, neck, and torso.

Dullness on tapping of the abdomen or distension of the abdomen is an indication that there may be ascites, which suggests the possibility of severe liver disease. Patients may also have slight confusion, which may be a feature of encephalopathy. Generalized pruritus can also be indicative of chronic liver disease, and this is more common in patients with cholestatic liver disease.

Laboratory investigations can further help to narrow down a diagnosis of cirrhosis of the liver. The most common initial investigations are the alanine aminotransferase (ALT) test, aspartate aminotransferase (AST) test, serum bilirubin test, and alkaline phosphatase test. Elevated ALT or AST levels may indicate generalized liver disease without pinpointing a cause. Cirrhosis may be indicated by the presence of a higher AST over ALT. Additional tests include serum albumin and the measurement of the prothrombin time. In the context of elevated aminotransferase levels, low levels of serum albumin and a prolonged prothrombin time suggest significant liver injury. Blood counts should also be performed; the presence of cytopenia supports portal hypertension secondary to chronic liver disease, which is often cirrhosis. High alkaline phosphatase levels relative to aminotransferase levels strongly suggest a cholestatic process as opposed to hepatocellular injury. Table 1 lists common causes of cirrhosis and basic diagnostic testing.

Complications

Many patients with cirrhosis have no serious outward complications from the disease. These patients are described as having compensated cirrhosis. For the remaining patients several classic complications arise, which are described as decompensated cirrhosis. The major complications include ascites, bleeding from esophageal varices, and hepatic encephalopathy. Other common and serious complications include spontaneous bacterial peritonitis, which may progress to hepatorenal syndrome, and hepatocellular carcinoma.

ASCITES

Manifestations

Ascites is the most common complication to evolve from cirrhosis. In 33% to 50% of patients with compensated cirrhosis, ascites will develop within 10 years. Portal hypertension is a prerequisite for the formation of ascites. In response to portal hypertension there is vasodilation of the arterioles of the splanchnic circulation; and to compensate, there is activation of the renin-angiotensin system. This causes massive sodium retention and, when coupled with an increase in hydrostatic pressure in the portal system and a decrease in oncotic pressure caused by hypoalbuminemia, leads to ascites. The formation of ascites secondary to cirrhosis is one of the indications for consideration of liver transplant.

Clinical examination is unreliable in the detection of small to moderate amounts of ascites, particularly if patients are obese. Therefore ultrasonography is the ideal test to detect small to moderate amounts of ascites. Further ultrasonography can be used to rule out thromboses of the hepatic vasculature and hepatocellular carcinoma. On detection of ascites, a paracentesis should be performed and the fluid examined for total protein, polymorphonuclear leukocyte (PMN) count, and albumin. A same-day serum albumin should also be obtained. The serum ascites-albumin gradient (SAAG [serum albumin]-[ascitic albumin]) is an excellent diagnostic tool for confirming portal hypertension as the cause of the ascites (>97% accuracy). A SAAG value greater than

or equal to 1.1 g/dL is confirmatory for portal hypertension as the cause of ascites. Paracentesis carries a very small risk of bowel perforation or abdominal wall hematoma (<1:1000).

Treatment

Ascites can be graded in severity, and treatment can be tailored based on the grade of ascites. If ascites is solely seen on ultrasound (US), it is categorized as grade 1. Sodium restriction may be sufficient without the need for diuretics. However, additional diuretics may hasten resolution. If the abdomen becomes distended, then this ascites is categorized as grade 2. Most cases of grade 1 ascites progress to grade 2. Tense ascites is considered grade 3 ascites. Figure 1 is a guide to treatment of ascites.

For ascites of grade 2 or higher, sodium restriction to 2 g (88 mEq) per day is recommended, as well as the initiation of diuretics. The recommended diuretics are oral spironolactone (Aldactone) and furosemide (Lasix)[1] with initial doses of 100 mg and 40 mg, respectively, taken once in the morning. Painful gynecomastia may result from taking spironolactone (Aldactone) and if this occurs, amiloride (Midamor)[1] can be substituted (5 to 20 mg per day). However, amiloride (Midamor)[1] is less effective in reducing ascites. If initial doses of spironolactone (Aldactone) and furosemide (Lasix)[1] do not

[1]Not FDA approved for this indication.

TABLE 1 Common Causes of Cirrhosis

Condition	Diagnostic testing*
Hepatitis C	Anti-HCV (EIA), HCV RNA, genotype, quantitative HCV RNA
Hepatitis B	HBsAg, HBeAg, HBeAb, HBV DNA
Autoimmune chronic	ANA, ASMA, Anti-LKM, quantitative hepatitis IgG
Hemochromatosis	Serum iron and total iron binding capacity, serum ferritin, HFE gene analysis
Primary biliary cirrhosis	AMA, quantitative IgM
Primary sclerosing	p-ANCA, combination of chemical, cholangitis biochemical, and radiological features
Alcohol abuse	AST/ALT ratio >2:1, ALT and AST usually <500 IU/dL, liver biopsy
Wilson's disease	Serum ceruloplasmin, serum copper, hepatic copper content, Kayser-Fleischer rings

*These are some of the basic tests; further testing may be required based on the clinical situation.
Abbreviations: ALT = alanine aminotransferase; AMA = antimitochondrial antibody; ANA = antinuclear antibody; ASMA = anti–smooth-muscle antibody; AST = aspartate aminotransferase; EIA = enzyme immunoassays; HBeAb = hepatitis B e antibody; HBeAg = hepatitis B e antigen; HBsAg = hepatitis B surface antigen; HBV DNA = hepatitis B DNA detection; HCV = hepatitis C virus; LKM = liver-kidney microsome; p-ANCA = pericytoplasmic antineutrophil nuclear antibodies.

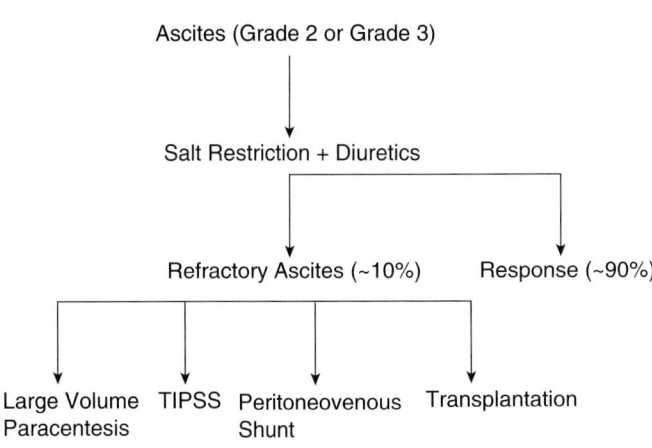

FIGURE 1 A guide to the treatment of ascites.

resolve the ascites, the dosage can be increased every 3 to 5 days up to a maximum of 400 mg per day for spironolactone (Aldactone) and 160 mg per day[3] for furosemide (Lasix).[1] Grade 3 ascites should be treated first with therapeutic paracentesis, followed by administration of diuretics and salt restriction.

A key indicator of response to diuretics is a random spot urine test to see if the ratio of the sodium-to-potassium concentration has reversed and is greater than 1. If so, then it is approximately 90% certain that the patient is satisfactorily excreting enough sodium (minimum of 78 mmol per day). Ideal target weight loss because of a decrease in ascites should be approximately 0.5 kg per day in patients without edema, and approximately 1 kg per day in patients with leg edema. If it is observed that there is no weight loss, but patients have good sodium clearance, then noncompliance with sodium restriction should be considered and discussed with the patient. Patients who are sensitive to diuretics can be treated with sodium restriction and oral diuretics without the need for therapeutic paracentesis.

Inpatient treatment should be initiated on the evolution of encephalopathy, bacterial infection, or gastrointestinal hemorrhage. However, if patients do not have these complications and are steadily losing weight they can be followed in the outpatient setting. Also, fluid restriction is unnecessary unless the patient's serum sodium level falls below 120 mmol/L.

If ascites proves resistant to diuretics, two other treatments are available:

1. Serial paracenteses
2. Transjugular intrahepatic portosystemic stent shunt (TIPSS)

Paracentesis is highly effective. Two possible complications are postparacentesis circulatory disturbance (PPCD) and renal impairment. PPCD usually occurs in paracentesis greater than 5 L, and therefore in such procedures it is recommended that albumin be given at 8 to 10 g/L of ascites removed.

[1]Not FDA approved for this indication.
[3]Exceeds dosage recommended by the manufacturer.

Rakel and Bope: *Conn's Current Therapy 2006.*

TIPSS is a radiologically placed shunt that relieves portal hypertension by shunting blood between the portal and the hepatic veins. Ascites resolves in 66% of patients with this procedure. There is no difference in survival between patients who undergo large-volume paracentesis as opposed to TIPSS. Thus, TIPSS is recommended more than large volume paracentesis when it becomes necessary more than two times a month, or if paracentesis is impractical. The major complication to TIPSS is hepatic encephalopathy (20% incidence), particularly in patients with advanced liver disease; it is, therefore, recommended with caution in Child class C patients. Some of the requirements for successful placement of TIPSS include a cardiac ejection fraction of at least 55%, patency of the portal vein, and absence of severe hepatic encephalopathy. Liver transplantation is the only definitive therapy for refractory ascites and should be considered for all appropriate candidates. Another possible treatment for patients ineligible for transplant, TIPSS, or paracentesis is the placement of a peritoneovenous shunt.

ESOPHAGEAL VARICES

Please see the esophageal varices article in this volume for more information.

HEPATORENAL SYNDROME

Approximately 40% of all patients with ascites will develop hepatorenal syndrome (HRS) within 5 years. It occurs when there is continued sodium retention, activation of the renin-angiotensin system, and arterial filling remains too low. The kidneys have an inherent vasodilation system. When this is overcome because of massive systemic vasoconstriction, which commonly occurs with long-term presence of ascites, the renal blood flow and glomerular filtration rates (GFR) plummet, and renal failure evolves. One precipitator of HRS is nonsteroidal anti-inflammatory drugs, such as ibuprofen. These should be scrupulously avoided by a patient with ascites. In the diagnosis of HRS several key criteria are almost always present (Table 2).

There are two types of HRS, type I and type II. In type I HRS, there is a rapid increase in serum creatinine (>2.5 mg/dL within 2 weeks). The prognosis for type I HRS is dismal, with 80% mortality within 2 weeks. Type II HRS is a more slowly progressive form and can evolve to type I. Type II also has a poor prognosis, with only 50% survival after 6 months. Type II presents with moderate levels of renal deterioration with serum creatinine between 1.5 and 2.5 mg/dL that has evolved in more than 2 weeks.

The most successful treatment for HRS is liver transplantation, with survival rates greater than 80% over 1 year. The next most effective treatment for type I HRS is albumin infusion (20 to 40 g per day for 20 days) with arterial vasoconstrictors. Albumin, rather than synthetic volume expanders, should be used in this treatment. Octreotide (Sandostatin)[1] at a dose of 200 µg

[1]Not FDA approved for this indication.

TABLE 2 Criteria of the International Ascites Club for Diagnosing the Hepatorenal Syndrome

Major criteria (all criteria must be met)	Additional criteria (usually present)
Chronic or acute liver disease with advanced hepatic failure and portal hypertension	Urine volume <500 mL/d
Low glomerular filtration rate, as indicated by a serum creatinine of >1.5 mg/dL or 24-h creatinine clearance <40 mL/min	Urine sodium <10 mEq/L
Absence of shock, ongoing bacterial infection, and current or recent treatment with nephrotoxic drugs; absence of gastrointestinal fluid losses (e.g., vomiting or diarrhea) or renal fluid losses (e.g., overaggressive diuresis)	Urine osmolality greater than plasma osmolality
No sustained improvement of renal function (i.e., a decrease of serum creatinine <1.5 mg/dL or increase in creatinine clearance to >40 mL/min) following removal of diuretic therapy and volume expansion with 1.5 L of normal saline intravenously	Urine red blood cells <50 per high-power field
Proteinuria <500 mg/dL and no ultrasound evidence of either obstructive uropathy or parenchymal renal disease	Serum sodium concentration <130 mEq/L

Adapted from Arroyo V, Gines P, Gerbes AL, et al: Definition and diagnostic criteria of refractory ascites and hepatorenal syndrome in cirrhosis. International Ascites Club. Hepatology 1996;23(1):164-76.

should be given subcutaneously three times per day along with midodrine (ProAmatine)[1] titrated up to 12.5 mg three times per day to achieve an increase in mean blood pressure (BP) of 15 mm Hg. TIPSS treatment is experimental for HRS.

HEPATOCELLULAR CARCINOMA

Patients with cirrhosis have a marked increased risk for the development of hepatocellular carcinoma (HCC)—10% to 15% of cirrhosis patients develop HCC over a 10-year period. Patients who successfully undergo orthotopic liver transplant (OLT) for HCC that have ideal criteria for transplantation have a 50% to 70% 5-year survival rate.

Screening is best accomplished through both α-fetoprotein (AFP) tests and US examination of the abdomen every 6 months in the cirrhotic patient. The α-fetoprotein test is less specific, being only definitive for HCC when levels exceed 1000 ng/mL. However, levels of AFP between 300 and 500 ng/mL can be considered suspicious for HCC development. AFP levels are usually elevated in pregnant women and can be elevated in patients with chronic hepatitis. Thus, the specificity of an AFP at low levels is minimal; therefore, there is a dependence on imaging studies and the sequential course of AFP. Other investigational tumor markers are des-γ-carboxy prothrombin (DCP) and lectin-reactive AFP (AFP-L3).

Treatment for HCC includes both surgical and nonsurgical modalities; surgical treatments are the most successful. Surgery includes resection of the tumor and liver transplantation. Few candidates meet the criteria for successful and safe resection because often they have decompensated cirrhosis, which contraindicates surgical resection. Nonsurgical methods include embolization and ablation of the tumor. Either embolization or ablative therapies might be appropriate in HCC patients with nonresectable tumors. The role of chemotherapy (CT) is unclear.

The earlier HCC is detected, the greater the likelihood of successful outcomes with transplantation. To be a candidate for liver transplantation, the patient must not have vascular invasion, metastatic disease, or more than three suspected lesions in the liver. If there are multiple lesions, all must be less than 3 cm in diameter; if only one lesion is present, it must be less than 5 cm in diameter.

ENCEPHALOPATHY

Hepatic encephalopathy (HE) is characterized by neurologic and neuromuscular abnormalities, which are primarily caused by accumulation of nitrogenous compounds, endogenous ligands for benzodiazepine receptors, and other unknown neurotoxins released by bacteria from the colon that are not well metabolized by the cirrhotic liver.

HE has five stages, with stage 0 representing no abnormal psychiatric effects of cirrhosis. Patients in stage 0 may have moderate insomnia, with an inversion of the normal night/day sleep cycle. Loss of fine coordination and moodiness indicate a progression to stage 1. Stage 2 patients suffer from ataxia and serious memory problems with possible ankle clonus, whereas stage 3 patients suffer confusion, incoherence, paranoia, and seizures. Stage 4 patients represent the most severe encephalopathy, with complete coma. Asterixis can be a part of any of these stages.

Precipitating causes of HE include infection, gastrointestinal (GI) bleeding, hypokalemia, progression of cirrhosis, and recent TIPSS placement. Other causes include dehydration or diuretic-induced prerenal azotemia. Use of benzodiazepines, particularly for treatment of stage 0 insomnia, will significantly worsen HE and must be avoided. Other tranquilizers and sedatives can have a similar effect and must not be used.

Most cases of HE are avoidable, and a good awareness of the precipitating causes will help prevent it. Reduction and modification of ingested protein (e.g., no red meat) is suggested for patients who manifest

---

[1]Not FDA approved for this indication.

features of encephalopathy. An effective treatment for HE is lactulose (Cephulac) with a goal of achieving three to four soft bowel movements a day. Avoid excessive use leading to diarrhea, because it can cause prerenal azotemia and other electrolyte imbalances. In patients who have profound encephalopathy and are unable to take medication orally, lactulose (Cephulac) can be administered as a retention enema at a dose of 300 mL in 700 mL of tap water, to be administered two to three times per day. Opiate analgesics, calcium, and iron supplements can all exacerbate HE; all should be avoided if possible. Also, antibiotics such as neomycin[1] (1 to 2 g per day) and metronidazole (Flagyl)[1] (250 mg two or three times per day) can help alleviate HE and can be used in conjunction with lactulose (Cephulac), particularly in cases where dietary modification and lactulose (Cephulac) alone do not adequately treat HE.

SPONTANEOUS BACTERIAL PERITONITIS

Spontaneous bacterial peritonitis (SBP) is a proliferation of bacteria in the ascitic fluid. Hospitalized patients with decompensated cirrhosis have a 10% to 30% chance of SBP. Once it occurs, SBP has approximately 20% mortality per episode. Also, SBP recurs in approximately 70% of patients in 1 year.

Patients with cirrhosis and ascites as well as sudden onset of fever, encephalopathy of unknown origin, abdominal pain, renal failure, acidosis, or peripheral leukocytosis should receive immediate antibiotic therapy before the data from paracentesis and ascitic fluid cultures are available. A polymorphonuclear leukocyte (PMN) count of 250 cells/mm^3 suggests SBP. If secondary bacterial infection is suspected, lactate dehydrogenase, total protein, and glucose should be evaluated. Blood and urine cultures should be done, and ascites cultures should always be in blood culture bottles.

Treatment involves primarily the antibiotic cefotaxime (Claforan). It is recommended that 2 g of cefotaxime (Claforan) be given intravenously (IV) every 8 hours. A paracentesis should be repeated after 48 hours and a PMN count performed again. In SBP the PMN count should be 50% of its previous level, whereas in other sources of peritonitis the PMN count may be higher or unchanged. Treatment with cefotaxime (Claforan) for 5 days is sufficient to clear SBP. Alternatively, the patient can take oral ofloxacin (Floxin)[1] if the patient has no vomiting, shock, or hemorrhage; has a serum creatinine of less than 3 mg/dL; and has stage 1 or stage 0 encephalopathy. An optimal dose is 400 mg every 12 hours. Albumin[1] administration decreases mortality following an episode of SBP; the suggested dose is 1.5 g albumin/kg of body weight within 6 hours after starting antibiotic therapy and readministered at 1 g/kg on the third day of treatment.

SBP can be prevented by administration of prophylactic treatment. Norfloxacin (Noroxin)[1] (400 mg per day) is useful and is indicated for patients who have already had an episode of SBP or who have low ascitic protein levels (<1 g/dL). Norfloxacin (Noroxin)[1] prophylaxis has reduced SBP occurrence by 60% and is highly cost effective. For patients admitted to the hospital for cirrhosis and GI hemorrhage, Norfloxacin (Noroxin)[1] can be given for prevention of SBP twice per day (total of 800 mg per day) for 7 days, or ofloxacin (Floxin)[1] can be given instead (400 mg per day).

SECONDARY BACTERIAL INFECTIONS

Peritonitis can also be caused by other infections from perforations in the gut or from nonperforated infections elsewhere in the peritoneum. If the ascitic fluid protein is more than 1 g/dL, the lactate dehydrogenase higher than normal, and glucose less than 50 mg/dL, there is a strong (50%) probability of secondary, rather than spontaneous infection. If the carcinoembryonic antigen (CEA) is more than 5 ng/mL and the ascitic fluid alkaline phosphatase (AP) is more than 240 U/L, there is an 88% chance the infection is caused by a perforation of the gut. For nonperforation, secondary peritonitis, a second PMN count 48 hours later confirms nonperforated secondary peritonitis if:

- PMN is the same or higher even after antibiotic treatment.
- Tests for perforated peritonitis (ascites CEA and AP) are negative.

Surgery and antibiotics have a good chance of clearing the infection if it is found in time.

HEPATOPULMONARY SYNDROME AND PORTOPULMONARY HYPERTENSION

Patients with chronic liver disease may have pulmonary manifestations of either hepatopulmonary syndrome (HPS) or pulmonary hypertension (PPH). HPS is characterized by hypoxemia commonly with levels of PO$_2$ below 70 mm Hg and can affect as many as 33% of all patients with liver disease. This is a consequence of inappropriate vasodilation in the lungs. These patients essentially have an intrapulmonary shunt physiology. No effective treatment exists for HPS except for liver transplantation.

PPH is another lung disorder associated with chronic liver disease. Depending on the severity of this manifestation, an overall 30% survival rate over 5 years has been observed. Liver transplantation alone may reverse minor or moderate degrees of pulmonary hypertension. Transplantation is contraindicated in patients with severe pulmonary hypertension because of high postoperative mortality related to cardiac failure. Experimental approaches include vasodilators and combined lung-liver transplant.

Causes and Treatments

HEPATITIS VIRUSES

More information on these viruses and their etiologic outcomes are available in the hepatitis article in this volume.

---

[1]Not FDA approved for this indication.

---

[1]Not FDA approved for this indication.

ALCOHOL

Laboratory features can be specific for alcoholic hepatitis. An AST value more than two times the level of ALT is a good indication of liver damage caused by alcohol. Aminotransferases usually do not exceed 500 IU/L. An AST/ALT ratio of less than 2 indicates that alcohol is unlikely to be the cause of liver injury. One key marker for severity of alcoholic hepatitis is the discriminant function $(4.6 \times [PT_{patient} - PT_{control}] + bilirubin)$. A value greater than 32 predicts 50% mortality in 1 month.

The best treatment for alcoholic liver disease is total abstinence from alcohol. In severe, life-threatening hepatitis caused by alcohol (a discriminant function >32; HE; and the absence of renal failure, infection, or pancreatitis) administration of prednisone[1] (40 mg per day for 28 days) is the main treatment. Pentoxifylline (Trental)[1] may also be used (400 mg every 8 hours for 4 weeks) and has significant survival benefit. Liver transplantation is controversial in alcoholic hepatitis.

AUTOIMMUNE HEPATITIS

Autoimmune hepatitis (AIH) is usually progressive with liver parenchyma destruction and eventual cirrhosis. AIH can be subdivided into three main types. In type I AIH, antibodies to nuclei (ANA or antinuclear antibodies) or to smooth muscle (SMA) are present. In type II AIH, anti–liver/kidney microsome-1 (ALKM-1) antibodies are most common, and in this form the disease predominantly strikes children or young women. A third type associated with anti-SLA (soluble liver antigen) may be a subset of type I.

Other autoimmune diseases such as childhood-onset diabetes and thyroiditis should trigger suspicion for AIH. Many patients present asymptomatically. AST, ALT, and bilirubin are commonly elevated in AIH. A particularly indicative diagnostic sign is a high level of globulins, especially IgG. Liver biopsy characteristically shows an increase in plasma cells with other features of chronic hepatitis. In most cases, lifelong therapy with low levels of prednisone[1] or azathioprine (Imuran)[1] are needed to prevent relapses.

For initial induction of remission, adults should be on 20 to 30 mg of prednisone per day, whereas in children it should be 2 mg/kg per day up to 60 mg per day. Azathioprine (Imuran)[1] can also be given at a dose of 50 mg per day. Once transaminases fall 50%, prednisone[1] can be reduced to 15 mg per day in 5 mg decrements every 2 weeks. Once normalized, both azathioprine (Imuran)[1] and prednisone[1] can be continued at 50 to 75 mg per day and 15 mg per day, respectively, for 2 months. Then prednisone[1] can be held at 12.5 mg per day for 3 months, and then 10 mg per day for the next 3 months. Most patients require a combination of prednisone[1] and azathioprine (Imuran)[1] for a year, at which time attempts can be made to attain remission with azathioprine (Imuran)[1] (2 mg/kg body weight) alone. A full blood count should be performed every 2 weeks to ensure no myelosuppression occurs for the first 2 months.

There is controversy regarding long-term therapy versus an attempt to discontinue therapy in the hope of sustained remission. Treatment can be stopped, but recurrence rates approach 90% and may need to be aggressively treated.

PRIMARY BILIARY CIRRHOSIS

Primary biliary cirrhosis (PBC) is an autoimmune disease characteristically found in women older than 40 years of age. PBC results in progressive granulomatous destruction of bile ducts. Complications of the disease include severe generalized pruritus, osteoporosis, skin xanthomata, sicca disease, vitamin deficiencies, and recurrent urinary tract infection. PBC may progress to cirrhosis, and in some cases liver failure. There are four histologic stages to PBC. First, there is granulomatous destruction of the bile ducts, followed by periportal hepatitis and proliferation of bile ducts. The third stage has fibrous septae and bridging necrosis, and the fourth stage features cirrhosis.

Most patients who are discovered to have PBC have no symptoms. PBC can first be suspected in cases where alkaline phosphatase (AP) is elevated. By cross-checking the γ-glutamyl transpeptidase (γGT), the origin of the rise of AP can be traced to being either of liver or non-liver origin. A positive antimitochondrial antibody (AMA) is seen in 95% of patients with PBC. Markers for AIH such as anti–smooth-muscle antibodies (SMA) are found 25% of the time in PBC patients.

The first-line treatment for PBC is typically ursodiol (Actigall). It is a safe drug that lowers toxic bile acid levels and has a protective effect on the membranes of liver cells. The typical administration of ursodiol (Actigall) is 13 to 15 mg/kg per day. AP, bilirubin, and γGT all typically fall to normal or near-normal levels while a patient takes ursodiol (Actigall). Immunosuppressive therapy is not recommended.

Pruritus is one of the most disabling and difficult to manage complications of PBC. For this complication the first-line therapy is cholestyramine (Questran), a bile salt-binding resin. Patients should take cholestyramine (Questran) 4 hours before taking other medication. The dose is 4 g to be taken before breakfast and dinner with extra doses at bedtime or before lunch. Second-line therapies include naltrexone (ReVia)[1] (50 mg per day) and rifampicin (Rifadin)[1] (150 mg bid). In extreme cases, plasmapheresis can be performed. Liver transplantation is the only definitive therapy for pruritus and can be considered in the rare case of debilitating pruritus.

Bone disease and deficiency of fat-soluble vitamins (A, D, E, and K) may occur in PBC. As a consequence of bone disease, fractures of the spine and ribs can occur readily in PBC. Osteopenia can be detected with a bone density scan; between 30% and 50% of patients with PBC have low mineral density in their ribs and vertebrae. To treat this vitamin D and calcium (1 to 1.5 g per day) are recommended, but only liver transplantation can treat this complication fully. If levels of 25-hydroxy vitamin D are low, supplementation at a dose of 20 µg

---

[1]Not FDA approved for this indication.

---

[1]Not FDA approved for this indication.

per day is ideal. Calcitonin (Miacalcin)[1] or alendronate (Fosamax)[1] can also be considered in these patients. Also, malabsorption of the fat-soluble vitamins may occur. It is therefore reasonable to place these patients on 400 IU per day of vitamin E. Vitamin A levels can be monitored and if low, up to 15,000 IU per day can be used; otherwise, it is recommended that a maintenance regimen of 5000 IU per day be used. Vitamin K supplementation is generally not given unless the patient is deeply icteric or has a tendency to bleed from the gums, skin, and so forth.

PRIMARY SCLEROSING CHOLANGITIS

Primary sclerosing cholangitis (PSC) is an uncommon disease (incidence of 10 to 50 cases per million population) affecting both the intra- and extrahepatic bile ducts. In PSC, the bile ducts are intermittently strictured and dilated. In approximately 70% of cases PSC is accompanied by chronic ulcerative colitis; it is less commonly accompanied by Crohn's colitis. PSC is progressive and eventually leads to portal hypertension, cirrhosis, and liver failure. Patients with PSC have a 15% cumulative risk of eventually developing cholangiocarcinoma.

Patients are predominantly males older than 20 years of age. However, women are seen with this condition approximately 33% of the time. Many patients present with significant fatigue, intermittent right upper quadrant abdominal pain, generalized pruritus (itching), and jaundice. Approximately 25% of patients have no symptoms. The most common abnormal laboratory finding is often an elevated alkaline phosphatase (AP) in relation to the transaminases. ALT and AST are also usually elevated in this disease to about two to five times normal. The presence of pericytoplasmic anti-neutrophil nuclear antibodies (p-ANNA, also known as p-ANCA) is associated (70% to 80%) with both PSC and inflammatory bowel disease. Imaging via endoscopic retrograde cholangiopancreatography (ERCP) can confirm PSC by showing multiple strictures in both the extra- and intrahepatic bile ducts.

The progression of PSC is variable, but in general four main stages arise. In the first stage the portal triad becomes inflamed. In the second stage inflammation spreads to the periportal area, and progresses to septa formation, which is characteristic of the third stage. The fourth stage features regenerative nodules and cirrhosis. These features can be ascertained through biopsy and histology.

Treatment is limited. Currently ursodiol (Actigall)[1] is commonly given for the condition. Doses of 20 to 30 mg/kg per day have shown modest improvement in hepatic biochemical tests. However, unlike in PBC, ursodiol (Actigall)[1] has not been shown to have a benefit on survival when used for patients with PSC. Also, liver transplantation has been successfully accomplished in patients with PSC, but if patients have a cholangiocarcinoma, their outcomes are poor. The overall survival rate after transplant is approximately 70% to 80% after 5 years.

---

[1]Not FDA approved for this indication.

Rakel and Bope: *Conn's Current Therapy 2006.*

HEMOCHROMATOSIS

Hemochromatosis is defined as excessive iron deposition in major organs such as the kidney and liver. The main cause is hereditary hemochromatosis (HHC), the most common genetic mutation found in people of European descent. Approximately 10% of all northern European men are carriers of the HHC allele. For HHC, there are two main genetic recessive mutations, both on the short arm of chromosome 6. One gene is termed *HFE.*

Iron absorption is usually regulated in normal people where there is little absorption of iron in the gut if serum iron is satisfactory. In HHC iron absorption is constitutively active, driving serum iron levels too high. In this case, excess iron is stored by the hepatocytes in the liver. Excess iron storage causes eventual activation of hepatic stellate cells initiating the fibrosis-cirrhosis chain of events. Most patients present with liver disease in their forties to fifties. Typical symptoms include severe fatigue, impotence (in men), pain in the abdomen, and arthralgia. Patients usually have an enlarged liver and spleen and skin pigmentation. Cirrhosis occurs in more than 60% of patients with HHC. From a biopsy, it is possible to determine the hepatic iron concentration (HIC).

An effective treatment for HHC is serial phlebotomy. By doing phlebotomies, the serum iron decreases, and even severe liver damage can reverse. HHC patients must be rigorously screened for hepatocellular carcinoma. Vitamin C supplements should be avoided because they increase absorption of iron. Liver transplantation can be considered for patients with end-stage liver disease; however, a careful evaluation is needed for cardiac involvement before determining their candidacy.

NONALCOHOLIC STEATOHEPATITIS

Nonalcoholic steatohepatitis (NASH) presents almost identically as alcohol-induced hepatitis, with the exception that the patient drinks less than 40 g of ethanol

---

 CURRENT DIAGNOSIS

- Bilirubin
- Alanine aminotransferase and aspartate aminotransferase (ALT and AST) alkaline phosphatase
- Lactate dehydrogenase
- Anti-hepatitis C antibody (enzyme immunoassay [EIA])
- Hepatitis B surface antigen (HBsAg), hepatitis B e antigen (HBeAg), hepatitis B e antibody (HBeAb), hepatitis B viral DNA
- Anti-nuclear antibody (ANA), anti–smooth-muscle antibody (ASMA)
- Serum iron, total iron binding capacity, serum ferritin
- Serum ceruloplasmin, serum copper

per week. NASH is correlated with obesity, hyper-triglyceridemia, and type II diabetes. It can be diagnosed when histology confirms steatosis and inflammation in the absence of the well-recognized causes of liver dysfunction and alcohol abuse. It progresses to cirrhosis between 15% and 40% of the time.

Usually ALT and AST levels are elevated. Interestingly, the ALT level is usually the same or greater than the AST level. This finding is important because it generally rules out alcohol-induced hepatitis. Imaging can also be helpful. First, on US examination, the parenchyma of a fatty liver is significantly more echogenic than a normal liver. The first-line treatment for NASH should be weight reduction within 10% of ideal body weight in those with obesity as an underlying cause for this

condition. Weight loss should not exceed 1.6 kg per week. Rapid weight loss, including bariatric surgery in patients with significant fibrosis/cirrhosis, is ill advised because it may precipitate liver failure. On the other hand, bariatric surgery in carefully selected patients in early stage liver disease is effective. Pilot trials with thiazolidinediones and metformin (Glucophage)[1] (drugs that increase insulin sensitivity), vitamin E (antioxidant), and ursodiol (Actigall),[1] taken 13 to 15 mg/kg per day, have demonstrated limited success in small trials. These, however, should not be considered the standard of care.

---

[1]Not FDA approved for this indication.

TABLE 3 Commonly Used Medications and Procedures for Cirrhosis

Medications and procedures	Indications	Special considerations
Diuretics, such as spironolactone (Aldactone) (100-400 mg/d) and furosemide (Lasix)A (40-160 mg/d)	Ascites	Avoid prerenal azotemia. Emphasize salt restriction (2 g/d.) Avoid NSAIDs.
Lactulose (Cephulac) (30 mL qd-qid)	Hepatic encephalopathy	Avoid red meat. Titrate to 2-3 soft bowel movements/d.
Norfloxacin (Noroxin)[1] (400 mg/d)	Spontaneous bacterial peritonitis; prevention of recurrence	Consider in patients with low ascites protein to prevent a first episode of SBP.
Prednisone[1] and azathioprine (Imuran)[*,1]	Autoimmune hepatitis	Be cautious for bone marrow suppression. Watch for steroid side effects.
Cholestyramine (Questran) (4-12 g bid, before breakfast and dinner)	Pruritus	GI disturbances possible. Use no other drugs within 4 h.
Rifampicin (Rifadin)[1] (150 mg bid)		GI disturbances possible.
Ursodiol (Actigall)[*,1]	NASH, cholestatic liver disease	
Phlebotomy	Hemochromatosis	
D-Penicillamine (Cuprimine)	Wilson's disease	Neuropathy; Cytopenia.
Trientine HCl (Syprine), Zinc[1], BAL	Wilson's disease	Rash.
Liver transplant	Indicated for decompensated cirrhosis, HCC, fulminant liver failure	Referral needed. Careful selection of candidates by multidisciplinary team at tertiary transplant center.
HRS cocktail: Octreotide (Sandostatin)[1] (200 g tid subcutaneous), Midodrine (ProAmatine)[1] (12.5 mg tid, orally), Albumin (20-40 g/d for 20 d)	Hepatorenal syndrome	Avoid NSAIDs. Consider referral for liver transplant.
TIPSS	Refractory ascites, esophageal varices[†]	Encephalopathy common. Use caution in advanced liver disease.
β blockers[†]	Esophageal varices[†]	
Esophageal banding		
Pegylated interferon (2a or 2b)[‡] or interferon-α (2a or 2b)	Hepatitis C infection[‡]	
Ribavirin (Virazole)		
Interferon-α (2a or 2b)[‡]	Hepatitis B infection[‡]	
Lamivudine (Epivir)		
Adefovir (Hepsera)		

[1]Not FDA approved for this indication.
[*]See text for dosing.
[†]See "Esophageal Varices" article in this volume.
[‡]See "Viral Hepatitis" article in this volume.
Abbreviations: BAL = British anti-Lewisite therapy; GI = gastrointestinal; HCC = hepatocellular carcinoma; HRS = hepatorenal syndrome; NASH = nonalcoholic steatohepatitis; NSAIDs = nonsteroidal anti-inflammatory drugs; qd = once per day; qid = four times per day; SBP = spontaneous bacterial peritonitis; tid = three times per day; TIPSS = transjugular intrahepatic portosystemic stent shunt.

CURRENT THERAPY

- Diuretics (such as spironolactone and furosemide for ascites)
- Lactulose (for encephalopathy)
- Norfloxacin (for prevention of spontaneous bacterial peritonitis [SBP])
- Immunosuppressants (such as prednisone and azathioprine, used in autoimmune hepatitis)
- Ursodeoxycholic acid (for cholestatic liver diseases)
- Penicillamine (for Wilson's disease)
- Transjugular intrahepatic portosystemic stent shunt (TIPSS) (for ascites and other complications of bleeding esophagogastric varices)
- Antiviral medication (for hepatitis B, hepatitis C viral infections)

OTHER DISEASES

Wilson's Disease (Copper Overload)

Wilson's disease is the inability to properly excrete copper, and thus results in inappropriate copper storage in both liver and central nervous system (CNS). Once treatment is initiated the prognosis is excellent. Wilson's disease is quite possible if ceruloplasmin (CP) levels are below 20 mg/dL. Another key diagnostic exam is a slit-lamp examination for Kayser-Fleischer rings. If rings are present with low CP levels, then Wilson's disease is present. If rings are not present, a liver biopsy should be done. Intrahepatic levels of copper greater than 250 µg/g are indicative of Wilson's disease. The drug of choice is D-penicillamine (Cuprimine). Other drugs used are trientine (Syprine) and zinc,[1] but the latter is used more as a maintenance therapy. British anti-Lewisite (BAL) therapy is seldom used today.

α₁-Antitrypsin Deficiency

This deficiency is found in patients with the PiZZ (protease inhibitor phenotype ZZ homozygous) genotype. In this disease, the α_1-antitrypsin deficiency (AT) causes production of a mutant protease inhibitor. This causes liver damage in 10% to 15% of individuals afflicted with this mutation. Most patients with AT-induced liver disease are children. An effective treatment is liver transplantation, and the 5-year survival rate approaches 80%. Hepatocyte transplantation is a theoretical treatment that holds much promise in this disease. Table 3 summarizes the commonly used treatments for cirrhosis and their indications.

REFERENCES

Arroyo V, Gines P, Gerbes AL, et al: Definition and diagnostic criteria of refractory ascites and hepatorenal syndrome in cirrhosis. International Ascites Club. Hepatology 1996;23(1):164-176.

Blei AT, Cordoba J, Practice Parameters Committee of the American College of Gastroenterology: Hepatic encephalopathy. Am J Gastroenterol 2001;96(7):1968-1976.
Czaja AJ: Chronic nonviral hepatitis. In Friedman SL, McQuaid KR, Grendell JH (eds): Current Diagnosis & Treatment in Gastroenterology, 2nd ed. New York, Lange Medical Books, 2003.
Fitz JG: Approach to the patient with suspected liver disease. In Friedman SL, McQuaid KR, Grendell JH (eds): Current Diagnosis & Treatment in Gastroenterology, 2nd ed. New York, Lange Medical Books, 2003.
Hunt CM, Carson KL: Management of pruritus. In Krawitt EL (ed): Medical Management of Liver Disease. New York, Marcel Dekker, 1999.
Moore KP, Wong F, Gines P, et al: The management of ascites in cirrhosis: Report on the consensus conference of the International Ascites Club. Hepatology 2003;38(1):258-266.
Runyon BA: Practice Guidelines Committee, American Association for the Study of Liver Disease (AASLD). Management of adult patients with ascites due to cirrhosis. Hepatology 2004;39(3):841-856.
Schiano TD, Bodenheimer HC: Complications of chronic liver disease. In Friedman SL, McQuaid KR, Grendell JH (eds): Current Diagnosis and Treatment in Gastroenterology, 2nd ed. New York, Lange Medical Books, 2003.

Bleeding Esophageal Varices

Method of
Greg V. Stiegmann, MD

Esophageal varices are present in 30% to 60% of patients with hepatic cirrhosis. The outlook for these patients can be stratified using the Child-Pugh scoring system (Table 1). Child-Pugh classes A and B patients have relatively well-compensated liver disease, and approximately 30% have esophageal varices. Their risk of bleeding from esophageal varices is approximately 30% over a 2-year period. Child-Pugh class C patients have poorly compensated liver disease, and approximately 60% have esophageal varices. The risk of bleeding for any patient with esophageal varices is directly proportional to the size of the varices. The risk of bleeding is further increased when so-called red color signs are observed at endoscopy. These are small dilated blood vessels on the surface of the varix. Child-Pugh class C patients with large varices and red color signs have approximately 60% risk of bleeding from esophageal varices over a 2-year period.

Pressure within the portal venous system is also related to the risk of bleeding from esophageal varices.

TABLE 1 Child-Pugh Classification*

Parameter	1 Point	2 Points	3 Points
Serum bilirubin (mg/dL)	<2	2-3	<3
Albumin (g/dL)	>3.5	2.8-3.5	<2.8
Prothrombin time (↑,s)	1-3	4-6	>6
Ascites	None	Slight	Moderate
Encephalopathy	None	1-2	3-4

*Grades: A, 5 to 6 points; B, 7 to 9 points; C, 10 to 15 points.

---

[1]Not FDA approved for this indication.

Rakel and Bope: *Conn's Current Therapy 2006.*

Normal portal vein pressures are less than 10 mm Hg. Portal pressure is seldom measured directly. A surrogate for direct portal venous pressure measurement is the hepatic venous pressure gradient (HVPG). This is determined by passing a balloon-tipped catheter (usually via a transjugular route) into one of the hepatic veins and measuring the pressure within the vein. The balloon is then inflated to occlude the vein, and the pressure that results (similar to obtaining a wedged pulmonary artery pressure) is the hepatic venous wedged pressure. This value is subtracted from the free hepatic venous pressure to result in the HVPG. Normal HVPG is 2 to 6 mm Hg. Pressures greater than 12 mm Hg are considered portal hypertension. Patients with HVPG less than 12 mm Hg seldom bleed from esophageal varices. The HVPG is usually an accurate reflection of pressure in the portal venous system in patients with cirrhosis. Patients who have other causes for esophageal varices (e.g., portal or splenic vein thrombosis), however, may have normal HVPG pressure determinations.

Bleeding from esophageal varices is currently associated with mortality in 20% to 30% of patients in the year following the index bleed. The risk of dying is directly proportional to the severity of the underlying liver disease (Child-Pugh class). These results are greatly improved from only a few decades ago (Figure 1) and reflect advances in resuscitation, intensive care, and new pharmacologic, endoscopic, and radiologic treatments. Patients who have one episode of bleeding from esophageal varices have a 70% chance of a second episode of variceal bleeding within 1 year if untreated. It is generally agreed that these patients, as well as those with large esophageal varices that have never bled, should be actively treated to prevent an initial or recurrent bleeding episode.

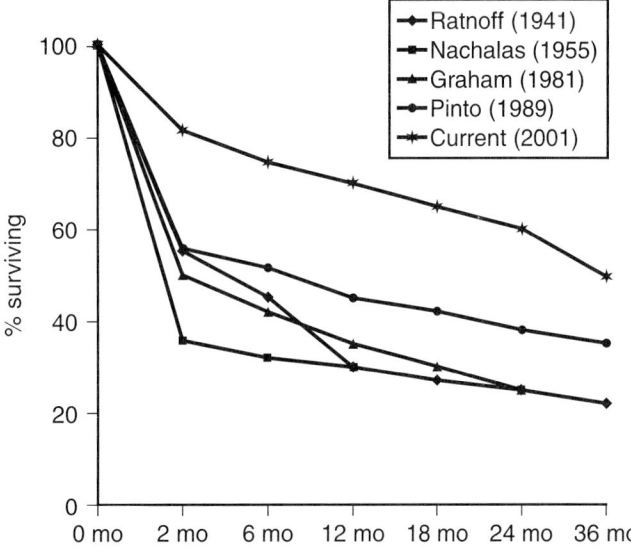

FIGURE 1. Comparison of survival curves of acute variceal bleeding reported over 6 decades. (Reprinted from Chalasani, Kahi C, Francois F, et al: Improved patient survival after vesiceal bleeding: A multicenter cohort study. Am J Gastroenterol 2003;98:656. With permission from the American College of Gastroenterology.)

Acute Bleeding From Esophageal Varices

Hematemesis and melena are the usual clinical presentation of upper gastrointestinal hemorrhage including bleeding from esophageal varices. In many cases a history of liver disease or findings of stigmata of cirrhosis/portal hypertension on initial physical examination suggest the possibility of bleeding from esophageal varices. Resuscitation should proceed rapidly with two large-bore intravenous lines, bladder catheterization for monitoring urine output, and transfusion of red blood cells, fresh-frozen plasma, and platelets as needed to achieve hemodynamic stability. Uncooperative patients, such as those with hepatic encephalopathy, may benefit from early endotracheal intubation both to assure adequate ventilation and to protect against tracheal aspiration. Patients suspected of bleeding from portal hypertensive causes benefit from early administration of drugs that reduce portal venous pressure. Octreotide (Sandostatin) is given intravenously in an initial 50-μg bolus followed by continuous intravenous infusion at 25 to 50 μg per hour. Vasopressin (Pitressin) is an alternative agent that should be given intravenously starting at 0.2 U per minute. The dose may be increased up to 0.4 to 0.6 U per minute. Electrocardiographic monitoring is essential because this drug produces systemic vasoconstriction that can result in myocardial ischemia. Intravenous nitroglycerine is frequently administered in conjunction with vasopressin to lessen these effects. Drugs given to lower portal pressure should be continued for 3 to 5 days after variceal bleeding is controlled. They may be stopped immediately if endoscopic examination finds a nonvariceal (e.g., peptic ulcer, Mallory-Weiss tear) cause of hemorrhage. Patients with cirrhosis and acute bleeding from esophageal varices have a high incidence of infection-related complications (e.g., subacute bacterial peritonitis, pneumonia, urinary tract infection) and have better outcomes, including a lower incidence of early recurrent bleeding, when treated with prophylactic antibiotics. Fluoroquinolone drugs (e.g., norfloxacin [Noroxin] or levofloxacin [Levaquin]) should be administered intravenously at first and converted to oral administration when feasible. Antibiotic treatment should continue for 5 to 7 days.

Upper gastrointestinal endoscopy should be performed as soon as possible after the patient with suspected variceal bleeding is hemodynamically stable. Gastric lavage, using a large-bore tube to remove blood and clots from the stomach, may enhance visualization. Uncooperative or combative patients require endotracheal intubation to assure adequate ventilation during endoscopy and to protect their airway. Bleeding from esophageal varices is confirmed if bleeding from a varix is observed directly, if a platelet plug is observed on the surface of a varix, or if large varices are present and no other potential source of bleeding is identified after conducting a complete examination of the stomach and duodenum. A thorough diagnostic endoscopic examination is important because approximately 25% of patients with known esophageal varices and upper gastrointestinal bleeding have a nonvariceal source of hemorrhage. If bleeding varices are discovered in a patient with no history of liver disease, diagnostic evaluations should be done when bleeding is controlled and the patient is stabilized. These investigations should include an imaging study, such as contrast-enhanced computed tomography (CT), to rule out thrombosis of the portal or splenic vein as the cause of portal hypertension.

Endoscopic therapy to control variceal bleeding should be started, if possible, at the time of diagnostic endoscopy. Endoscopic band ligation is the preferred treatment (Figure 2) and results in control of bleeding in approximately 90% of cases. Endoscopic sclerotherapy (Figure 3) is also acceptable treatment for acutely bleeding varices. Sclerotherapy has efficacy similar to band ligation, although it is associated with a higher risk of complications such as esophageal stricture and deep esophageal ulceration.

Patients whose bleeding varices are not controlled by endoscopic/pharmacologic treatment should be considered for transjugular intrahepatic portal systemic shunt (TIPS) (Figure 4). If active bleeding is ongoing, a Sengstaken-Blakemore balloon tamponade tube may be inserted to control bleeding and stabilize the patient (Figure 5). After passage of the tube into the stomach, 50 mL of air is used to inflate the gastric balloon. Then an abdominal radiograph is taken to assure correct position in the stomach. When correct positioning is confirmed, the gastric balloon is inflated to 250 mL and drawn up against the gastroesophageal junction and then secured in place. This maneuver controls bleeding in most situations. If inflation of the esophageal balloon is needed to control bleeding, pressure in the esophageal balloon should not exceed 40 mm Hg as measured by a blood pressure manometer. A nasogastric tube should be passed into the proximal esophagus

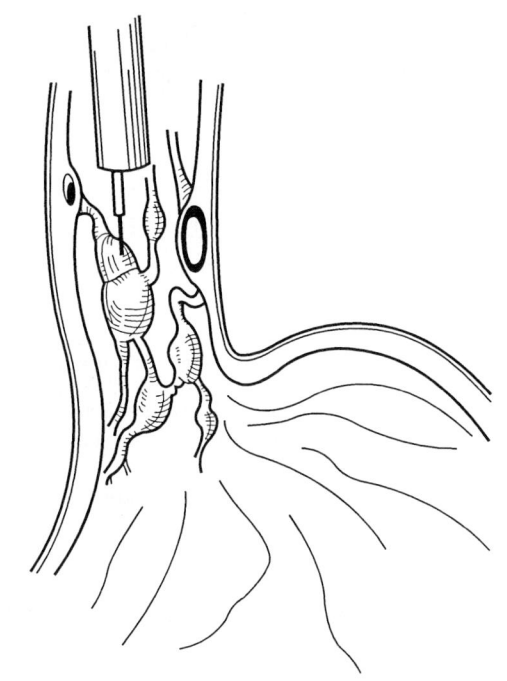

FIGURE 3. Endoscopic sclerotherapy performed with a flexible endoscope. A flexible injection needle is used to inject sclerosant into the varix. (From Schaefer J. In GI/Liver Secrets, Philadelphia, Hanley and Belfus, 1996, p 355. Reprinted with permission.)

to aspirate secretions that pool above the inflated balloons of the tamponade tube to prevent tracheal aspiration. Patients treated with balloon tamponade should have definitive portal venous decompression (TIPS) as soon as they are hemodynamically stable.

Prevention of Recurrent Bleeding

The most accurate predictor of future bleeding from esophageal varices is a history of a past episode of variceal bleeding. Treatments to prevent recurrent bleeding include pharmacologic, endoscopic, surgical, and radiologic shunt insertion and hepatic transplantation. Drug therapy is based on administration of nonselective β-blocking drugs (e.g., Nadolol), usually titrated to reduce the resting heart rate by 25% or to a heart rate of 60. More sophisticated regimens that titrate drug dosage based on measurements of HVPG appear to be more effective than relying on reduction in resting pulse rate alone. Agents such as isosorbide mononitrate (Monoket) may be added to the β-blocker regimen to produce further reduction in portal pressure. Problems with pharmacologic therapy include intolerance to side effects of the medication in 10% to 20% of patients and inability of some patients to maintain compliance with the medication schedule. Patients need to continue β-blocker therapy indefinitely because rapid cessation results in a rebound effect with increased risk of variceal bleeding. Compliance with β-blocker therapy reduces the risk of recurrent hemorrhage from esophageal varices from 70% to approximately 40% over a 1-year period following an index bleeding episode. Patients treated exclusively

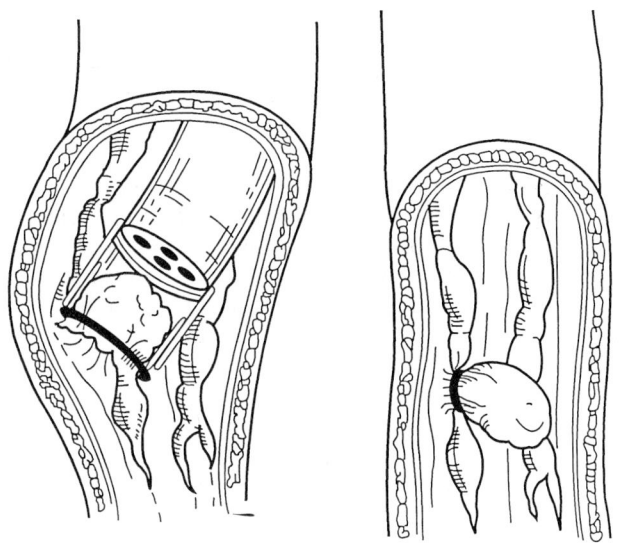

FIGURE 2. Endoscopic band ligation performed with a flexible endoscope. A varix is aspirated into the device using endoscopic suction and ensnared with an elastic band. (From Schaefer J. In GI/Liver Secrets, Philadelphia, Hanley and Belfus, 1996, p 355. Reprinted with permission.)

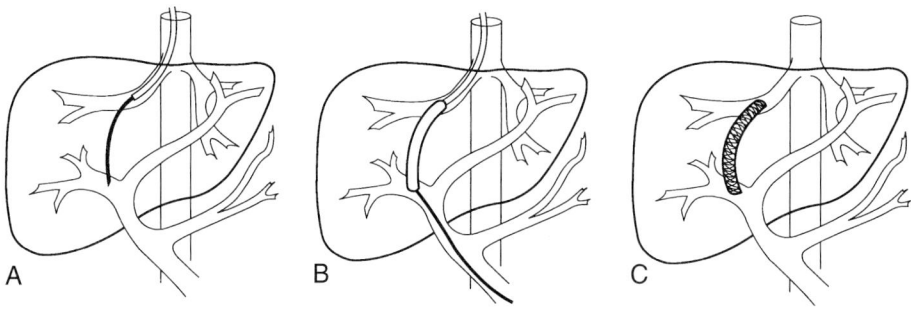

FIGURE 4. Transjugular intrahepatic portal systemic shunt (TIPS). **A**, A needle is used to puncture from an hepatic vein into the portal vein. **B**, The liver parenchyma is dilated with a balloon catheter. **C**, A metal stent is inserted to complete the shunt. (From Schaefer J. In GI/Liver Secrets, Philadelphia, Hanley and Belfus, 1996, p 355. Reprinted with permission.)

with pharmacologic therapy who experience recurrent bleeding from varices should receive endoscopic treatment.

Endoscopic band ligation is the treatment used at most centers to prevent recurrence of bleeding from esophageal varices. Serial endoscopic treatments are done on an outpatient basis at 10- to 14-day intervals until varices in the distal esophagus are obliterated, which requires an average of three to four sessions. After varices are obliterated, follow-up endoscopy is done every 3 to 6 months to detect and treat any varices that recur. Complications associated with band ligation therapy are few when compared with those resulting from endoscopic sclerotherapy, and the number of endoscopic sessions needed to eradicate varices is less. Patients treated with endoscopic band ligation alone have approximately a 30% risk of experiencing recurrent bleeding from esophageal varices. Patients treated simultaneously with both β-blockade and endoscopic band ligation have approximately a 15% risk of recurrent bleeding from esophageal varices. Patients in whom endoscopic therapy fails to control bleeding (e.g., one, or at most two, major episodes of recurrent bleeding from varices after initiation of treatment) should have decompression of their portal hypertension.

Surgical portosystemic shunts are effective at decompressing portal hypertension and preventing recurrent

bleeding from esophageal varices. Recurrent variceal bleeding occurs in approximately 10% of patients so treated. Selective shunt operations decompress only the esophageal varices (maintaining high pressure in the portal vein to perfuse the liver). Central shunts decompress the entire portal system. The selective shunt is associated with a somewhat lower incidence of hepatic encephalopathy and a slightly greater risk of recurrent variceal bleeding than central shunts. Partial shunt operations (using small-diameter vascular grafts) aim to lower portal vein pressure enough to prevent variceal bleeding while still maintaining some portal vein flow to the liver. Failures of endoscopic therapy, good-risk patients (Child-Pugh A and B) who live in remote areas, or patients who are not compliant with endoscopic or pharmacologic treatments are the best candidates for elective shunt operations. Central shunt operations should be used sparingly in patients who are candidates for liver transplantation because the subsequent transplant operation is made more difficult as a result of previous dissection in the area of the porta hepatis.

TIPS eliminates the morbidity associated with the laparotomy necessary for surgical shunt construction. The trade-off is the need to monitor flow regularly through the intrahepatic stent and revise (usually dilate) the stent in a high percentage of patients. TIPS results in decompression of the entire portal venous system. The interventional radiologist can control the magnitude of decompression of the portal system, however, by altering the diameter of the shunt. TIPS is effective in preventing recurrent bleeding from esophageal varices, but the risk of hepatic encephalopathy is similar to that of a surgical shunt. TIPS is best suited for patients who do not want to have pharmacologic/endoscopic therapy or those awaiting liver transplantation who are willing to return for regular follow-up studies.

Patients who experience bleeding from esophageal varices should all be considered potential candidates for liver transplantation. Most Child-Pugh A and B patients can be managed effectively by the measures just outlined, but progression of liver disease is unpredictable. Patients who remain in Child-Pugh class C after recovery from an episode of bleeding varices are usually candidates for liver replacement, provided they meet criteria such as abstinence from alcohol consumption.

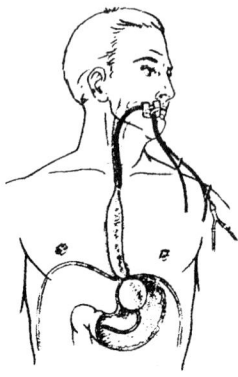

FIGURE 5. Sengstaken-Blakemore balloon tamponade. (From Sun JH and Steigmann GV. In Abernathy's Surgical Secrets, Philadelphia, Hanley and Belfus, 2004, p 155. Reprinted with permission.)

Rakel and Bope: *Conn's Current Therapy 2006.*

CURRENT DIAGNOSIS

- Diagnosis of esophageal varices (patients who have not bled) should be considered in any patient with known liver disease.
- Diagnosis is established using upper gastrointestinal endoscopy.
- Patients with liver disease who experience upper gastrointestinal bleeding have a 25% chance of the bleeding arising from a nonvariceal source.

Prevention of a First Variceal Bleed

Patients diagnosed with cirrhosis of the liver who have not experienced upper gastrointestinal bleeding should undergo diagnostic upper gastrointestinal endoscopy to determine presence or absence of esophageal varices. Patients with cirrhosis have approximately a 6% chance per year for developing varices. Treatment to prevent a first episode of variceal bleeding for patients who have small esophageal varices is controversial. These patients may be best served by serial endoscopic examinations with institution of treatment if varices enlarge. Treatment should be recommended for patients found to have large esophageal varices and certainly for those that have red color signs or who are in Child-Pugh class C (i.e., patients at greater risk for a first variceal bleed). Pharmacologic therapy with β-blocking drugs titrated to reduce the resting pulse rate by 25% or to a heart rate of 60 reduces the risk for a first variceal bleed from approximately 30% to approximately 10%. Side effects of the medication and compliance with the medication schedule are the main deterrents to this therapy. Endoscopic band ligation is as effective as β-blocker therapy in lowering the risk of a first variceal bleed. Treatment is done as an outpatient with the goal of obliterating varices in the distal esophagus. When distal esophageal varices are eradicated, surveillance endoscopy should be done at 6- to 12-month intervals to detect and treat recurrent varices. No studies have addressed the efficacy of combining β-blocker therapy with band ligation to prevent a first variceal bleed. Results in patients treated with combined drug and endoscopic therapy to

prevent recurrent bleeding from varices suggest the combined treatment may be advantageous.

REFERENCES

Garcia-Tsao G: Portal hypertension. Curr Opin Gastroenterol 2004; 20(3):254-263.
Gotzsche P, Hrobjartsson A: Somatostatin analogues for acute bleeding oesophageal varices. Cochrane Database Syst Rev 2005;1:CD000193.
Hou MC, Lin HC, Liw TT, et al: Antibiotic prophylaxis after endoscopic therapy prevents rebleeding in acute variceal hemorrhage: A randomized trial. Hepatology 2004;39(3):746-753.
Lubel JS, Angus PW: Modern management of portal hypertension. Intern Med J 2005;35(1):45-49.
Rosemurgy AS, Bloomston M, Clark WC, et al: H-graft portacaval shunts versus TIPS: Ten-year follow-up of a randomized trial with comparison to predicted survivals. Ann Surg 2005;241(2):238-246.
Sarin SK, Agarwal SR: Extrahepatic portal vein obstruction. Semin Liver Dis 2002;22(1):43-58.
Schepke M, Kleber G, Nurnberg D, et al: Ligation versus propranolol for the primary prophylaxis of variceal bleeding in cirrhosis. Hepatology 2004;40(1):65-72.
Stiegmann G: Update of endoscopic band ligation therapy for treatment of esophageal varices. Endoscopy 2003;35(8):S5-S8.

Dysphagia and Esophageal Obstruction

Method of
Kenneth R. DeVault, MD

Dysphagia, from the Greek *phagia* ("to eat") and *dys* ("difficulty," "disordered"), refers to the sensation of food being hindered in its passage from the mouth to the stomach. Most patients say that food "sticks," "hangs up," or "stops" or they feel that the food "just won't go down right." Occasionally they complain of associated pain. Dysphagia always indicates a malfunction of some type in the esophagus, although associated psychiatric disorders can amplify this symptom. It is a symptom to be respected and should always trigger a focused search for its etiology. Dysphagia is a common symptom, present in 12% of patients admitted to an acute care hospital and in more than 50% of those in chronic care facility. Dysphagia becomes more common with aging and affects aging and up to 15% of individuals aged 65 or older.

Pathophysiology

The inability to swallow in usually caused either by a problem with the strength or coordination of the muscles required to move material from the mouth to the stomach or by an obstruction somewhere between the mouth and the stomach. Some patients may experience a combination of the two processes. The oropharyngeal swallowing mechanism and the primary and secondary peristaltic contractions of the esophageal body that

CURRENT THERAPY

- Patients with bleeding esophageal varices should be adequately resuscitated prior to having diagnostic upper gastrointestinal endoscopy.
- Vasoactive drugs (Octreotide) may be started prior to endoscopy.
- Patients with bleeding and cirrhosis benefit from prophylactic antibiotic administration.
- Prompt endoscopic treatment is desirable.
- Endoscopic treatment should be repeated until esophageal varices are eradicated.

follow usually transport solid and liquid boluses from the mouth to the stomach within 10 seconds. If these orderly contractions fail to develop or progress, the accumulated bolus of food distends the lumen and causes the discomfort that is dysphagia. Some patients, particularly the elderly, generate low-amplitude primary or secondary peristaltic activity that is insufficient for clearing the esophagus. Another group has primary or secondary motility disorders that grossly disturb the orderly contractions of the esophageal body. Because these motor abnormalities may not be present with every swallow, dysphagia may wax and wane.

Mechanical narrowing of the esophageal lumen may interrupt the orderly passage of a food bolus despite adequate peristaltic contractions. Symptoms vary with the degree of luminal obstruction, associated esophagitis, and type of food ingested. Although minimally obstructing lesions cause dysphagia only with large, poorly chewed boluses of such foods as meat and dry bread, lesions that totally obstruct the esophageal lumen are symptomatic for both solids and liquids. Gastroesophageal reflux disease (GERD) may produce dysphagia related to an esophageal stricture, but it has become increasingly clear that some patients with GERD have dysphagia in the absence of a demonstrable stricture and perhaps even without esophagitis. Finally, abnormal sensory perception within the esophagus may lead to dysphagia. Because some normal subjects experience the sensation of dysphagia when the distal esophagus is distended by a balloon, as well as by other intraluminal stimuli, an aberration in visceral perception could explain dysphagia in patients who have no definable cause. This mechanism also may apply to the amplification of symptoms in patients with spastic motility disorders, among whom the prevalence of psychiatric disorders has increased.

Approach to Diagnosis and Treatment

When faced with a patient complaining of dysphagia, it is helpful to approach the problem in a systematic way. Most patients can localize their dysphagia to either the upper or the lower portion of the esophagus (although occasional patients with esophageal dysphagia present with symptoms referred only to the suprasternal notch or higher). For the purpose of this review, we have divided the approaches into oropharyngeal and esophageal dysphagia, with the knowledge that there may be considerable overlap in certain groups of patients. In addition, it is important to try to determine whether the patient has trouble only with solid boluses or with both liquids and solids.

OROPHARYNGEAL DYSPHAGIA

Processes that affect the mouth, hypopharynx, and upper esophagus produce a distinctive type of dysphagia. The patient is often unable to initiate swallowing and repeatedly has to attempt to swallow. Patients frequently describe coughing or "choking" when they attempt to eat. When a food bolus cannot be propelled successfully from the hypopharyngeal area through the upper esophageal sphincter into the esophageal body, the resulting symptom is oropharyngeal, or transfer, dysphagia. The patient is aware that the bolus has not left the oropharynx and specifically locates the site of symptoms to the region of the cervical esophagus. Dysphagia occurring immediately or within 1 second of swallowing is suggestive of an oropharyngeal abnormality. At times, a liquid bolus may enter the trachea or the nose rather than the esophagus. Some patients describe recurrent bolus impactions that require manual dislodgment. In severe cases, saliva cannot be swallowed, and the patient drools. Speech abnormalities such as dysarthria or nasal speech may be associated with oropharyngeal dysphagia.

There are many potential causes for oropharyngeal dysphagia (Box 1). After an adequate history is obtained, the best initial test for patients with these symptoms is a carefully performed barium examination. Often this is performed with a swallowing therapist (modified barium swallow). If the results of liquid portion of the examination are normal, the patient should be fed a bolus to attempt to bring out their symptoms and localize the pathologic condition. If the oropharyngeal portion of the study is normal, it is often helpful to visualize the remainder of the esophagus. This simple test usually allows localization of the problem and development of a plan for initial therapy.

BOX 1   Common Causes of Oropharyngeal Dysphagia

Neuromuscular Causes*
Stroke
Parkinson's disease
Multiple sclerosis
Myasthenia gravis
Amyotrophic lateral sclerosis (ALS or Lou Gehrig's disease)
Idiopathic upper esophageal sphincter (UES) dysfunction
Central nervous system tumors (benign or malignant)
Postpolio syndrome
Muscular dystrophy
Poly- or dermatomyositis
Thyroid dysfunction
Manometric dysfunction of the UES or pharynx[†]
Structural
Carcinomas
Osteophytes and other spinal disorders
Zenker's diverticula
Proximal esophageal webs
Prior surgery or radiation therapy
Infection of pharynx or neck
Thyromegaly
Cervical osteophytes

---

*Any disease that affects striated muscle or innervation may result in dysphagia.
[†]Many manometric disorders (hypertensive and hypotensive UES, coordination issues, and incomplete UES relaxation) have been described, although their true relationship to the symptom is often unclear.

Symptoms and the results of a barium examination may then be used to direct the approach to these patients. For example, swallowing associated with a gurgling noise may suggest the presence of *Zenker diverticulum*. These diverticula are occasionally asymptomatic when discovered, and treatment should be reserved for those who are experiencing symptoms. A limited number of patients who are not surgical candidates have been treated by the injection of botulinum toxin[1] (Botox) (80–100 units) in the muscle just distal to the diverticulum, but this approach is certainly unproven. Most patients are treated surgically. In the past this usually consisted of an open myotomy of the muscle just distal to the diverticulum with or without an actual resection of the pouch. More recently, endoscopic myotomy with an opening of the septum between the diverticulum and the esophagus has become the operation of choice. The barium examination may also reveal a proximal esophageal stenosis that may be due to either an inflammatory or a muscular cause. Patients with such stenoses often respond to dilation of their esophagus using orally passed dilators or balloons, which are best employed in combination with upper gastrointestinal endoscopy. Endoscopy also allows any suspicious areas to be biopsied. Recurrent bouts of *pulmonary infection* may reflect spillover of food into the trachea from inadequate laryngeal protection. *Hoarseness* may result from recurrent laryngeal nerve dysfunction or intrinsic muscular disease, both of which cause ineffective vocal cord movement. Weakness of the soft palate or pharyngeal constrictors causes *dysarthria* and *nasal speech* as well as *pharyngonasal regurgitation*. If there is no mechanical cause (such as a Zenker diverticulum or other obstruction), patients are best managed with swallowing therapy that is coordinated by a speech therapist with special training in swallowing disorders. These specialists can often teach patients, even those with profound swallowing problems including aspiration, to swallow safely. Finally, *unexplained weight loss* may be the only clue to a swallowing disorder; patients avoid eating because of the difficulties encountered. If patients cannot maintain their weight or swallow without aspiration, long-term nutritional therapy via a gastrostomy tube may be needed.

ESOPHAGEAL DYSPHAGIA

Most patients with esophageal dysphagia localize their symptoms to the lower sternum or even the epigastric region at times. A smaller number of patients describe a sensation in the suprasternal notch or even higher, despite the actual bolus stopping in the lower esophagus. When esophageal dysphagia develops, it frequently can be relieved by various maneuvers, including repeated swallowing, raising the arms over the head, throwing the shoulders back, and using the Valsalva maneuver. Motility disorders or mechanical obstructing lesions can cause esophageal dysphagia. To better clarify the origin of symptoms of esophageal dysphagia, the answers to three questions are crucial: (1) What type of food or liquid causes symptoms?, (2) Is the dysphagia intermittent or progressive?, and (3) Does the patient have heartburn? On the basis of these answers, it often is possible to distinguish the causes of esophageal dysphagia (Box 2) as either a mechanical or a neuromuscular defect and to postulate the cause accurately.

After obtaining a focused history of the patient's symptoms, an initial barium examination, including a solid bolus challenge, is often advocated as the initial first test. This should include a solid bolus challenge. Many experts have advocated endoscopy as an alternative first test, especially in patients with intermittent solid food dysphagia suggestive of a lower esophageal ring or in patients with significant reflux symptoms. The choice of which test to offer first should be based on local expertise and the preference of individual health care providers. If the barium examination demonstrates an obstructive lesion, endoscopy is usually required to visualize and potentially biopsy the area of concern. Endoscopy also allows for dilation of strictures, rings, and other obstructing lesions. If the barium examination result is normal, then an esophageal manometry test is often used to screen for significant motility disorders. Finally, some patients with reflux and dysphagia respond to a trial of acid suppression, even if the results of their barium study, endoscopy, or both are normal.

Patients who report dysphagia with both solids and liquids are more likely to have an esophageal motility disorder. *Achalasia* is the prototypical esophageal motility disorder in which, in addition to dysphagia, many patients complain of bland regurgitation of undigested food, especially at night, and of weight loss.

> **BOX 2 Common Causes of Esophageal Dysphagia**
>
> **Motility (Neuromuscular) Disorders**
> Primary Disorders
>   Achalasia
>   Diffuse esophageal spasm (DES)
>   Nutcracker (high-pressure) esophagus
>   Hypertensive lower esophageal sphincter
>   Ineffective esophageal motility (IEM)
> Secondary Disorders
>   Scleroderma and other rheumatologic associations
>   Reflux-related dysmotility
>   Chagas' disease
> **Structural (Mechanical) Disorders**
> Intrinsic
>   Peptic stricture
>   Lower esophageal (Schatzki's) ring
>   Other esophageal rings and webs
>   Diverticula
>   Carcinoma and benign tumors
>   Medication-induced strictures
>   Foreign bodies
> Extrinsic
>   Vascular compression
>   Mediastinal masses
>   Spinal osteophytes

---

[1]Not FDA approved for this indication.

Rakel and Bope: *Conn's Current Therapy 2006.*

The treatment of achalasia can be divided into four possibilities. The first is pharmacologic therapy designed to relax the lower esophageal sphincter and allow the bolus to pass. Possible agents include nifedipine[1] (Procardia), 10–20 mg, or nitroglycerin[1] (either by spray or tablet) sublingually before meals. Neither of these choices has been shown to provide long-term control in most patients. A second "medical therapy" is the use of botulinum[1] toxin (Botox) (80–100 units) injected into the lower esophageal sphincter via an endoscope. Forceful pneumatic dilation to the esophagus has long been considered the best, albeit somewhat risky (perforation rates of up to 5%), treatment for this disorder. Recently, laparoscopic myotomy of the lower esophageal sphincter has become the treatment of choice in many centers.

Patients with other spastic motility disorders such as diffuse esophageal spasm (DES) may also complain of chest pain and sensitivity to either hot or cold liquids. The treatment of the other spastic disorders is similar to that for achalasia, beginning with the sublingual use of nitrates and calcium channel blockers and the endoscopic application of botulinum toxin. Surgical myotomy of the esophageal muscle is almost never performed in patients with esophageal motility disorders except for those with achalasia. Patients with *scleroderma* of the esophagus usually have Raynaud's phenomenon and severe heartburn. In these patients, mild complaints of dysphagia can be caused by either a motility disturbance or an esophageal inflammation, but severe dysphagia may signal the presence of a peptic stricture. If a stricture is present, it should be dilated endoscopically. Patients with strictures usually have severe acid reflux and should be treated with a standard dose of proton pump inhibitor (omeprazole [Prilosec], 20 mg, lansoprazole [Prevacid], 30 mg, rabeprazole [Aciphex], 20 mg, pantoprazole [Protonix], 40 mg, or esomeprazole [Nexium], 40 mg[3] twice daily, taken before the morning and evening meals.

In patients who report dysphagia only after swallowing solid foods and never with liquids alone, a mechanical obstruction is suspected. When a luminal obstruction is of sufficiently high grade, however, it may be associated with dysphagia for both solids and liquids. If food impaction develops, the patient frequently must regurgitate for relief. Patients who continue to drink liquid after the bolus impaction may regurgitate large amounts of that liquid. In addition, hypersalivation is common during an episode of dysphagia, providing even more liquid to regurgitate. Episodic and nonprogressive dysphagia without weight loss is characteristic of an *esophageal web* or a *distal esophageal ring* (i.e., Schatzki ring). The first episode typically occurs during a hurried meal, often with alcohol. The patient notes that the bolus of food sticks in the lower esophagus; it often can be passed by drinking large quantities of liquids. Many patients finish the meal without difficulty after relieving the obstruction. The offending food frequently is a piece of bread or steak, hence the description

"steakhouse syndrome." Initially, the episode may not be repeated for weeks or months, but then episodes recur more frequently. Daily dysphagia, however, is likely not caused by a lower esophageal ring. Patients with daily dysphagia are best treated with endoscopically directed dilation of the ring (either with a balloon or an oral dilator). The goal should be to have the ring dilated to at least 16–20 mm. It has been suggested, but not proven, that acid suppression may delay the recurrence of dysphagia from esophageal rings. In patients with symptoms out of proportion to the degree of narrowing noted by barium examination or endoscopy, esophageal manometry may reveal a coexisting motility disturbance.

If solid food dysphagia is clearly progressive, the major differential diagnosis should include *peptic esophageal stricture* and *carcinoma*. Benign peptic esophageal strictures develop in up to 10% of patients with GERD. Most of these patients have a long history of associated heartburn. Weight loss seldom is noticed with benign lesions because these patients have a good appetite and convert their diet to high-calorie soft and liquid foods to maintain weight. Esophageal strictures should be dilated to a diameter of 16–20 mm and should be routinely biopsied because up to 50% of these strictures have coexisting Barrett's esophagus (a premalignant risk factor for esophageal carcinoma). It is clear that acid suppression with standard doses of proton pump inhibitors (see above for doses) given once daily decreases the need for repeated dilations in patients with reflux-related esophageal strictures.

> **BOX 3   Common Ingestions and Infections Causing Dysphagia**
>
> Caustic ingestion
>   Acid
>   Alkali (lye)
> Pill-induced injury
>   Alendronate and other bisphosphonates
>   Empronium bromide
>   Tetracycline and derivatives
>   Potassium chloride (especially slow release)
>   Quinidine
>   Nonsteroidal anti-inflammatory drugs and aspirin
>   Zidovudine
>   Iron preparations
> Infectious esophagitis
>   Viral
>   Herpes simplex
>   Cytomegalovirus
>   Human immunodeficiency virus
>   Epstein-Barr virus
>   Bacterial
>   *Mycobacterium tuberculosis* or *Mycobacterium avium-intracellulare*
>   Fungal
>   *Candida albicans*
>   *Histoplasma*
>   Protozoan
>   *Cryptosporidium*
>   *Pneumocystis*

---

[1]Not FDA approved for this indication.
[3]Exceeds dosage recommended by the manufacturer.

Patients with carcinoma differ from those with peptic stricture in several ways. As a group, the cancer patients are older and present with a history of rapidly progressive dysphagia. They may or may not have a history of heartburn, and it may be a symptom of the past but not the present. Most cancer patients have anorexia and weight loss. Treatment depends on the stage of the cancer and may include surgery, radiation therapy, chemotherapy, endoscopic dilation, application of laser or other types of heat energy, placement of intralumenal stents, or (often) a combination of several of these. A new treatment for esophageal malignancy is photodynamic therapy, which is a "drug and device" treatment that combines a photosensitizer drug and laser light energy to induce a photochemical reaction triggering mucosal ablation. True dysphagia may be seen in patients with *pill esophagitis;* however, the predominant complaint of patients with these acute esophageal injuries is usually odynophagia (painful swallowing). Treatment involves

avoidance of the offending agent (Box 3) and dilation of any persistent strictures. There are many infectious causes of dysphagia (see Box 3), the majority of which are diagnosed by endoscopic biopsy. Specific therapy directed against the organism involved usually results in resolution of dysphagia.

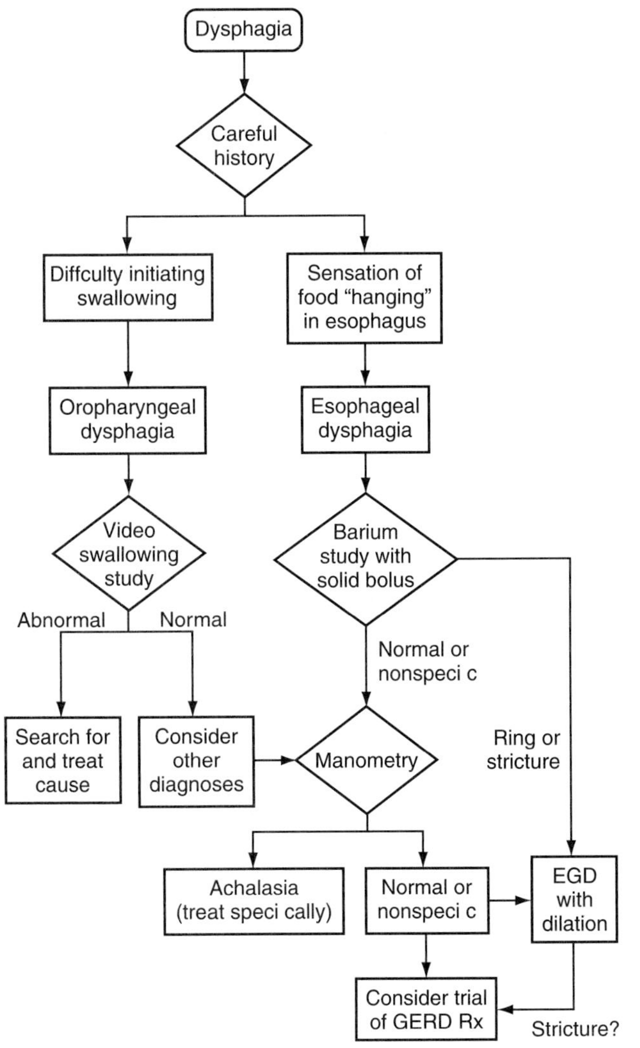

Summary

A carefully obtained history followed by the application of selective tests allows for a specific diagnosis in the majority of patients with dysphagia. Fortunately, many of these diagnoses are readily treatable with medication, endoscopy, and/or surgery. Malignancy is a rare cause of dysphagia but must be respected and checked in appropriate patients. A suggested approach to these patients is outlined in Figure 1.

REFERENCES

Bloem BR, Lagaay AM, van Beek W, et al: Prevalence of subjective dysphagia in community residents aged over 87. BMJ 1990; 300:721-722.
Clouse RE, Lustman PJ: Psychiatric illness and contraction abnormalities of the esophagus. N Engl J Med 1983; 309:1337.
Clouse RE, McCord GS, Lustman PJ, Edmundowicz SA: Clinical correlates of abnormal sensitivity to intraesophageal balloon distension. Dig Dis Sci 1991;36:1040.
Edwards DA: Discriminative information in the diagnosis of dysphagia. JR Coll Physicians Lond 1975;9:257.
Kahrilas PJ, Dodds WJ, Hogan WJ: Effects of peristaltic dysfunction on esophageal volume clearance. Gastroenterology 1986;91:987.
Marks RD, Richter JE, Rizzo J, et al: Omeprazole versus H2-receptor antagonists in treating patients with peptic stricture and esophagitis. Gastroenterology 1994;106:907-915.
Pross RL, Wolfsen HC, Gahlen J: Photodynamic therapy for esophageal diseases: A clinical update. Endoscopy 2003;35:1059–1068.
Schatzki R, Gary JE: Dysphagia due to a diaphragm-like localized narrowing in the lower esophagus. AJR 1953;70:911.
Triadifilopoulos G: Nonobstructive dysphagia in reflux esophagitis. Am J Gastroenterol 1989;84:614.

FIGURE 1. Diagnostic algorithm for patients with dysphagia. For details of the approach to each type of dysphagia, see the text and tables. (Less specific motility disorders include nutcracker esophagus, diffuse esophageal spasm, and other disorders of ineffective esophageal motility.)

Rakel and Bope: *Conn's Current Therapy 2006.*

Diverticula of the Alimentary Tract

Method of
R. Craig Nodurft, MD, and John G. Kuldau, MD

A diverticulum is an outpouching of a tubular structure. A *true diverticulum,* which contains all layers of the intestinal wall, is typically considered congenital, whereas a *false diverticulum,* or *pseudodiverticulum,* is the result of herniation of mucosa and submucosa through the muscular wall and is considered an acquired lesion.

Diverticula are most common in the colon but can be found in all intestinal segments. Although generally asymptomatic, they can cause significant complications, as described in this article.

Zenker's Diverticulum

Zenker's diverticula occur in the distal posterior hypopharynx just above the upper esophageal sphincter (UES). A Zenker's diverticulum is the result of herniation of hypopharyngeal mucosa through Killian's triangle, which is formed by the cricopharyngeus muscle and the oblique fibers of the inferior constrictor muscle. A Zenker's diverticulum is caused by incomplete relaxation of the UES during deglutition, which generates elevated pressure above the UES and thus predisposes to mucosal outpouching.

Zenker's diverticula are present in an estimated 0.01% to 0.1% of the population. They usually develop in the 7th or 8th decades of life and are twice as common in men as in women.

Symptoms include dysphagia, halitosis, regurgitation of undigested food, cough, and recurrent episodes of aspiration pneumonia. The pathogenesis of dysphagia is multifactorial. The anatomy of the hypopharynx is often distorted by the presence of the diverticulum, which can push the opening of the esophagus off to one side. In addition, large diverticula can become filled with food, which can impress on the esophagus and result in obstructive dysphagia.

Air-fluid levels are sometimes seen in the neck on plain radiographs. But the diagnostic test of choice is an esophagram, during which the diverticulum may fill with contrast material.

TREATMENT

Therapy is primarily surgical with resection of the diverticulum, combined with a myotomy of the cricopharyngeus muscle to prevent elevated pressures above the UES and recurrent diverticular formation. Surgery should be offered only to symptomatic patients or to the asymptomatic patient with a very large diverticulum. A diverticulopexy is another treatment option that involves suspending the free end of the diverticulum in a cranial position so food (and medical instruments) cannot become lodged within. This procedure is associated with less surgical morbidity and can also be effective. Surgical treatment results in complete resolution of symptoms in more than 90% of patients.

Esophageal Diverticula

Diverticula of the esophagus are uncommon. When present, they usually occur in the middle esophagus at the level of the carina or just above the diaphragm (epiphrenic diverticulum). Pulsion diverticula of the esophagus are caused by increased intraluminal pressure and usually associated with underlying motility disorders such as diffuse esophageal spasm or achalasia. Traction diverticula of the esophagus are typically associated with

an inflammatory process in the mediastinum (e.g., tuberculosis) that adheres to the esophagus and pulls outward. Esophageal diverticula are usually asymptomatic but can present with dysphagia and regurgitation, both of which could be secondary to an underlying motility disturbance.

TREATMENT

Treatment is surgical excision, but surgery should only be considered in patients whose symptoms are clearly linked with the presence of diverticula. Symptomatic patients should undergo upper endoscopy and esophageal manometry prior to any surgery.

Gastric Diverticula

Gastric diverticula are rare, occurring in only 0.02% of autopsy specimens. The most common type is the juxtacardiac diverticula, accounting for 75% of cases. They are usually small, ranging from 1 to 3 cm.

Most patients with gastric diverticula have no symptoms. Patients occasionally report mild upper abdominal pain. Bleeding and perforation are very rare. Diagnosis is easily made on upper endoscopy, although barium radiographs, if carefully performed, are useful.

TREATMENT

Diverticulectomy is the treatment of choice but almost never indicated because of the rarity of symptoms, bleeding, or perforation. If the diverticulum is near the pylorus, partial gastric resection may be necessary.

Duodenal Diverticula

Found in approximately 25% of the population, duodenal diverticula arise where a vessel penetrates the duodenal wall or in the region where the dorsal and ventral pancreas fuse during embryologic development. Approximately 75% of duodenal diverticula are found within 2 cm of the major duodenal papilla (juxtapapillary diverticula). It is common to find the major duodenal papilla contained within a diverticulum. Most are asymptomatic and picked up incidentally during an upper gastrointestinal (GI) series or endoscopic retrograde cholangiopancreatogram (ERCP). Symptoms can include duodenal diverticulitis, hemorrhage, obstruction, perforation, and small bowel bacterial overgrowth syndrome. Periampullary diverticula are associated with recurrent pancreatitis, sphincter of Oddi dysfunction, and common bile duct stones.

TREATMENT

Surgical treatment is indicated only if complications, such as perforation, occur. Surgical should be carefully performed to avoid damaging the bile and pancreatic ducts.

Rakel and Bope: *Conn's Current Therapy 2006.*

Jejunoileal Diverticula

Diverticula of the jejunum and ileum have a prevalence anywhere from 0.2%, if based on small bowel series, to 4.5%, if based on autopsy series. They can be located anywhere in the small intestine but are most common in the proximal jejunum. Wide, or fished-mouthed, diverticula are seen in patients with scleroderma. Small bowel follow-through and enteroclysis are the most accurate imaging studies for diagnosis. Computed tomography (CT) scan often reveals a mass with an air-fluid level within it.

Patients with small bowel diverticula are typically asymptomatic, but they can present in a variety of ways, including vague and nonspecific abdominal pain, intestinal hemorrhage, diverticulitis, and perforation. Small bowel bacterial overgrowth can occur in many of the cases of jejunoileal diverticula. Patients can have symptoms such as early satiety, bloating, and abdominal pain or more serious conditions such as malabsorption, weight loss, and steatorrhea. Jejunoileal diverticula can also lead to intestinal obstruction secondary to volvulus, intussusception, and adhesions from prior episodes of diverticulitis or extrinsic compression by a large fluid-filled saccular diverticulum.

TREATMENT

Surgery is indicated for cases of bowel perforation, obstruction, uncontrolled bleeding, or diverticulitis that does not respond to antibiotic therapy. Small bowel bacterial overgrowth is treated with long-term oral antibiotics. A typical first choice for treatment is tetracycline,[1] 250 mg by mouth four times daily, but many other antibiotics are effective.

Meckel's Diverticulum

Representing the most common congenital abnormality of the GI tract (present in approximately 2% of the population), a Meckel's diverticulum is the result of a failure to obliterate properly the omphalomesenteric duct, or vitelline duct, during embryologic development. During early fetal development, the fetal midgut is attached to the yolk sac by the omphalomesenteric duct. This duct is usually obliterated by the 8th week of gestation. Failure to do so properly can result in a Meckel's diverticulum. Meckel's diverticula are found in the distal ileum, typically within 60 to 100 cm of the ileocecal valve. They can be lined by normal ileal mucosa, although roughly 50% harbor heterotopic tissue. Gastric mucosa is the most common type of heterotopic mucosa contained within a Meckel's diverticulum. Heterotopic gastric mucosa produces acid, which can lead to diverticular or small intestinal ulceration and gastrointestinal bleeding. A variety of others mucosal types can also be found, such as colonic, hepatobiliary, and pancreatic acinar tissue.

---

[1]Not FDA approved for this indication.

Meckel's diverticula are usually asymptomatic. A common presentation, especially in children, is painless large-volume intestinal hemorrhage. A Meckel's diverticulum can cause intestinal obstruction by way of volvulus, intussusception, or herniation (Littre's hernia). Diverticulitis is a rare presentation. There are rare reports of neoplastic tissue arising within Meckel's diverticula.

TREATMENT

A Meckel's diverticulum is often incidentally diagnosed at the time of laparotomy. In patients with occult gastrointestinal bleeding, a noninvasive diagnostic modality is the technetium-99m pertechnetate scintigraphic study, or "Meckel's scan." The labeled tracer is picked up by the heterotopic gastric mucosa in the diverticulum.

Surgical excision is the treatment of choice for all symptomatic Meckel's diverticula. Debate surrounds the issue of whether to resect an incidentally found Meckel's diverticulum, especially in an adult.

Colonic Diverticula

Colonic diverticulosis is a very common acquired condition, present in more than 50% of individuals older than 80 years of age. Diverticula tend to form in areas of weakness such as along the edges of the taenia coli and also where a penetrating artery enters the bowel. It is believed that elevated intraluminal pressure predisposes to the formation of these pseudodiverticula. A commonly observed motor pattern in the colon is that of segmental contractions. These serve to compartmentalize the colon, which slows transit and allows for greater water absorption. These segmental contractions also dramatically increase the pressure within each compartment and transmit the forces radially to the bowel wall rather than producing propulsive forces, and this predisposes to the formation of diverticula.

The overall prevalence of colonic diverticulosis in the United States is 10%, which increases dramatically with age. The prevalence is less than 10% in those younger than age 40 years, and between 50% and 66% in those older than age 80 years. In the United States, most colonic diverticulosis is left sided. Only 15% of cases of colonic diverticulosis in the United States involves the right colon, but 70% of Asians with diverticulosis have right-sided involvement.

Colonic diverticulosis is usually asymptomatic but can be associated with nonspecific abdominal complaints such as pain, bloating, excessive flatulence, and irregular defecation. Complications primarily revolve around diverticulitis and diverticular hemorrhage, as discussed later.

Colonic diverticulosis is readily diagnosed by barium enema, which shows the characteristic outpouchings. They can also be seen on CT scanning with the use of oral contrast and are easily observed during colonoscopy, where it can often be difficult to readily discriminate true lumen from diverticular opening in severe cases.

No specific therapy exists for uncomplicated and asymptomatic diverticulosis. A diet high in fiber is promoted to decrease colonic transit time and intraluminal pressure in an attempt to decrease the incidence of diverticular complications and formation of new diverticula.

Diverticulitis

Diverticulitis represents inflammation and infection, usually of just one diverticulum. Diverticulitis arises as a complication in 10% to 25% of patients with colonic diverticulosis. The pathogenesis involves abrasion and impaction of a fecalith within the opening of the diverticulum. Inflammation and focal necrosis can occur, leading to a contained microperforation. A subsequent inflammatory reaction or phlegmon follows. Diverticulitis is associated with a number of complications, including the development of an abscess or fistulizing disease. Free perforation can occur with pneumoperitoneum, peritonitis, and sepsis. In addition, the inflammation and edema associated with diverticulitis can be severe enough to cause intestinal obstruction.

Because the sigmoid colon is the most common site of diverticulitis, symptoms usually consist of left lower quadrant pain. Fever is seen in the majority of patients but may be absent with a contained microperforation. Because the site is usually low in the pelvis, in close proximity to the bladder and ureters, urinary complaints are possible, including increased urinary frequency and dysuria. Pneumaturia and fecaluria are signs that a colovesical fistula has developed. Examination typically reveals left lower quadrant tenderness. There may be a palpable inflammatory mass in this region. Leukocytosis is seen in roughly 75% of cases of diverticulitis.

Evaluation of a patient with suspected diverticulitis should include a complete blood count (CBC) and urinalysis, and it may include acute abdominal radiographs to rule out perforation and obstruction. The diagnostic test of choice is a CT of the abdomen and pelvis with both oral and intravenous contrast, which often demonstrates inflammatory thickening of a segment of the colon with pericolonic graying of the fat secondary to edema. Areas of the colon adjacent to the inflammation may reveal diverticulosis. A CT scan can also evaluate for abscess formation.

Abscesses complicate diverticulitis in approximately 15% of cases. Those of suitable size require drainage. Substantial improvements in CT-guided percutaneous aspiration and drainage are evident in the last 10 years. This is usually the best initial option for patients with a diverticulitis-associated abscess that is focal and walled off. A small catheter, usually left in place to bulb suction, can be used periodically to inject water-soluble contrast and investigate for a fistula to the bowel or for a persistent abscess cavity that may require repositioning of the catheter. Surgery is required for patients not amenable to CT-guided drainage. Approximately 15% to 30% of patients require surgery for their current episode of diverticulitis if it does not resolve with medical therapy or if there is fistula or abscess formation.

After a first episode of diverticulitis, approximately one third of patients have a recurrence of the disease. After a second episode, the chance of a third episode is well more than 50%. Thus, for two or more episodes of documented uncomplicated diverticulitis, it becomes reasonable to consider elective surgical resection of the involved area.

TREATMENT

Treatment depends on the severity of the underlying disease. In uncomplicated diverticulitis, patients are advised to go on a clear liquid diet and should be given a 10-day course of oral antibiotics to treat the most common pathogens, including gram-negative rods and anaerobes. The combination of ciprofloxacin (Cipro),[1] 500 mg by mouth twice daily, and metronidazole (Flagyl),[1] 500 mg by mouth three times daily, is adequate first-line therapy for uncomplicated diverticulitis. Patients with high fever, significant leukocytosis, nausea and vomiting, or with significant tenderness on examination should be considered for inpatient management with bowel rest, intravenous hydration, and broad-spectrum intravenous antibiotics with good coverage against *Escherichia coli* and *Bacteroides*. Piperacillin/tazobactam (Zosyn),[1] 3.375 g intravenously every 6 hours, is a reasonable choice. Patients who have ongoing tenderness or recrudescence of fevers after an initial period of improvement should be evaluated for the development of an abscess.

Diverticular Hemorrhage

Another significant complication of colonic diverticulosis is diverticular hemorrhage, which classically presents as a sudden onset of painless lower GI bleeding. Diverticulosis is the most common cause of lower gastrointestinal bleeding, accounting for 30% to 50% of cases of massive rectal bleeding. Bleeding is often large volume, brisk, and hemodynamically significant, especially in

---

[1]Not FDA approved for this indication.

    CURRENT DIAGNOSIS

- Zenker's and esophageal diverticula are best diagnosed with barium radiographs.
- Gastric and duodenal diverticula are often found incidentally during endoscopy but rarely warrant treatment.
- Small bowel diverticula are found most easily with small bowel follow-through or enteroclysis.
- Colonic diverticulosis are easily seen on barium enema or colonoscopy.
- Computed tomography (CT) scan is the best modality for diagnosing diverticulitis of the gastrointestinal (GI) tract, especially colonic diverticulitis.

CURRENT THERAPY

- In general, most intestinal diverticula are asymptomatic and do not require treatment.
- When symptoms such as bleeding, perforation, or recurrent diverticulitis do occur, surgical resection is usually indicated.
- For dysphagia associated with Zenker's diverticulum, therapy is primarily surgical with resection of the diverticulum, combined with a myotomy of the cricopharyngeus muscle.
- If small bowel bacterial overgrowth is associated with small bowel diverticula, treatment with antibiotics such as tetracycline,[1] 250 mg PO qid, is indicated.
- For bleeding colonic diverticulosis, urgent colonoscopy can find a bleeding source in a minority of cases. If a bleeding source is found, endoscopic therapy is generally successful.
- For uncomplicated diverticulitis, a conservative approach with a combination of ciprofloxacin (Cipro),[1] 500 mg PO bid, and metronidazole (Flagyl),[1] 500 mg PO tid, is adequate first-line therapy.
- For cases of diverticulitis associated with abscess, fistula, peritonitis, or sepsis, surgical intervention is usually required.

[1]Not FDA approved for this indication.
Abbreviations: bid = two times per day; PO = by mouth; qid = four times per day; tid = three times per day.

the older population with medical co-morbidities, in which diverticulosis is so common.

Severe diverticular bleeding occurs in 5% to 15% of patients with diverticulosis. Although diverticulosis is more common in the sigmoid colon, diverticular hemorrhage can originate from any segment of the colon, including the right side. Diverticular bleeding is possibly associated with aspirin and nonsteroidal anti-inflammatory drug (NSAID) use. Many believe it can be triggered by ingestion of nuts, berries, seeds, popcorn, or other relatively indigestible material, although this theory has never been adequately studied. Bleeding usually originates from the neck of the diverticulum where the penetrating artery is covered by the thinnest layer of mucosa.

Diverticular bleeding stops spontaneously approximately 80% of the time. Recurrence of bleeding after spontaneous cessation occurs in 22% to 38% of cases.

Definitive diagnosis requires endoscopic visualization of blood emanating from a diverticulum. Unfortunately, this is rarely seen. More often, colonoscopy shows blood in the colon along with diverticulosis, and no other causative lesions are identified.

TREATMENT

Therapy is primarily supportive because most cases stop spontaneously. However, colonoscopy is usually performed in attempt to visualize a bleeding diverticulum,

Rakel and Bope: *Conn's Current Therapy 2006.*

evaluate the most proximal extent of diverticula, and rule out other lesions such as colitis, arteriovenous malformations, and tumors. Unfortunately, colonoscopy only finds the bleeding source in a minority of patients. Endoscopic therapy via electrocoagulation or placement of a hemoclip is useful if a bleeding diverticulum can be found.

If colonoscopy fails to localize the source of active bleeding, angiography and nuclear medicine tagged red blood cell scan are often employed. Embolization can be performed if the site is identified on angiography. Ultimately, if bleeding does not stop or is recalcitrant to therapy, surgical resection becomes necessary. The general site of bleeding ideally should be identified preoperatively with angiography or tagged red blood cell scan because it guides a segmental resection. If a specific site cannot be localized, a subtotal colectomy is necessary to ensure the bleeding site is removed.

REFERENCES

Afridi SA, Fichtenbaum CJ, Taubin H: Review of duodenal diverticula. Am J Gastroenterol 1991;86(8):935-938.
Casarella WJ, Kanter IE, Seaman WB: Right-sided colonic diverticula as a cause of acute rectal hemorrhage. N Engl J Med 1972;286(9):450-453.
Feldman M, Friedman LS, Sleisenger MH (eds): Gastrointestinal and Liver Disease, 7th ed. Philadelphia, WB Saunders, 2002.
Longo WE, Vernava AM: Clinical implications of jejunoileal diverticular disease. Dis Colon Rectum 1992;35:381-388.
Martin JP, Connor PD, Charles K: Meckel's diverticulum. Am Fam Physician 2000;61(4):1037-1042.
McGuire HH: Bleeding colonic diverticula: A reappraisal of natural history and management. Ann Surg 1994;220(5):653-656.
Simpson J, Scholefield JH, Spiller RC: Pathogenesis of colonic diverticula. Br J Surg 2002;89(5):546-554.
Stollman NH, Raskin JB: Diverticular disease of the colon. J Clin Gastroenterol 1999;29(3):241-252.
Tobin RW: Esophageal rings, webs and diverticula. J Clin Gastroenterol 1998;27(4):285-295.

Inflammatory Bowel Disease

Method of
Rahul K. Chhablani, MD, and
Gary R. Lichtenstein, MD

Inflammatory bowel disease (IBD) constitutes multisystem diseases of idiopathic origin. Since Drs. Wilks and Moxon's original description of ulcerative colitis in 1875, and Drs. Crohn, Ginzburg, and Oppenheimer's initial description of Crohn's disease in 1932, much has been learned about these two disorders. Both are found worldwide and spare no socioeconomic group. Recent scientific and technologic advances have not only led to greater understanding of the pathogenesis underlying these disorders, but have also led to the discovery and use of new medications in the treatment of inflammatory bowel disease.

Medical therapies for IBD aim to induce and maintain disease remission; decrease disease-associated complications, including malnutrition, osteoporosis, and colon cancer; and, ultimately, improve the patient's quality of life. This article discusses drug therapies, including indications and adverse effects, nutritional therapy, and management strategies for the various site-specific presentations of ulcerative colitis (UC) and Crohn's disease (CD).

Drug Therapy

AMINOSALICYLATES

Sulfasalazine

Sulfasalazine (Azulfidine) is composed of mesalamine (5-aminosalicylate [5-ASA]) joined by an azo-bond to a sulfapyridine moiety. This bond is cleaved by colonic bacterial azo-reductase, separating mesalamine from the sulfapyridine carrier. These molecules inhibit arachidonic acid production; interleukin (IL)-1, IL-2, and nuclear factor-κ B (NF-κB) activity; tumor necrosis factor-α (TNF-α); and reactive oxygen metabolites.

Initially used to treat rheumatoid arthritis by Dr. Nana Svartz of the Karolinska Institute in the 1930s, sulfasalazine[1] was found to reduce diarrhea in patients with coexisting UC. It is now used to treat mildly to moderately active UC and to maintain remission (Table 1). Sulfasalazine is known to benefit patients with mild to moderate CD, especially ileocolonic and colonic CD, but not patients with isolated small bowel disease. It is not effective for maintenance therapy of CD, as results from the National Cooperative Crohn's Disease Study (United States) and the European Cooperative Crohn's Disease Studies in the late 1970s and early 1980s failed to show maintenance benefit from reduced doses of sulfasalazine.

The sulfapyridine moiety of sulfasalazine contributes to most of this drug's adverse effects (see Table 1), including headache, nausea, vomiting, pancreatitis, and impaired folate metabolism. Patients on sulfasalazine should receive concurrent folic acid supplementation (1 mg/day).

Sperm abnormalities (dysmorphic sperm and sperm motility abnormalities) are another common, reversible side effect that has been reported with sulfasalazine. Male patients should be informed of the potential adverse effect of reduced fertility prior to using sulfasalazine.

Mesalamine Derivatives

Given the toxicity and the frequent intolerance that many patients experience with sulfasalazine (15% of individuals taking sulfasalazine are unable to tolerate the use of this medication), mesalamine derivatives without the sulfapyridine moiety have been created.

Asacol is made of a special coating that ensures a pH-dependent release in the ileocecal region and allows for approximately 15% to 30% of the mesalamine to be released in the small bowel. Pentasa is composed of sustained-release, ethylcellulose-coated microgranules that allow for equal release of mesalamine in the small bowel (50%) and the colon (50%). Olsalazine (Dipentum) is a mesalamine dimer linked by a diazo bond, formulated as gelatin capsules that is released primarily in the colon. Balsalazide (Colazal), a newer mesalamine derivative, is bound to an inert carrier molecule. Once cleaved from its carrier by colonic bacterial azo-reductase, approximately 99% of the mesalamine is delivered to the colon.

Topical mesalamine can be delivered in the form of enema or suppository. The use of enemas allows mesalamine to be delivered up to the splenic flexure. The suppository is effective in treating disease up to 15 to 20 cm from the anal verge. Topical mesalamine has been proven to be effective in treating distal UC and proctitis. It may be used in patients with colonic CD. However, there have been no randomized, controlled trials to evaluate its efficacy in the setting of colonic CD.

Table 1 lists the indication, dose, route, and adverse effects of these mesalamine derivatives. Neutropenia, agranulocytosis, hypersensitivity reactions (serum sickness, skin rash, pneumonitis, hepatitis, pancreatitis) are rarely seen with mesalamine derivatives. Up to 10% of patients treated with olsalazine experience drug-related diarrhea. This effect is significantly reduced when the drug is taken with meals. Topical mesalamine use has been associated with anal irritation and pruritus, occasionally precluding patients from continuing topical therapy.

CORTICOSTEROIDS

Corticosteroids have multiple effects on the immunomodulatory pathway, including:

- Inhibiting the release of proinflammatory cytokines such as IL-1, IL-2, IL-6, IL-8, γ-interferon, TNF-α
- Down-regulating NF-κB activity
- Reducing plasma exudation from postcapillary venules at inflammatory sites
- Interfering with phagocytic activity
- Decreasing chemotaxis of monocytes, eosinophils, and neutrophils

Corticosteroids continue to serve as a frequently used therapy for active IBD, regardless of disease distribution. Corticosteroids are not effective for maintenance of remission. Prednisone, in doses equivalent to 40 to 60 mg per day, has been proven effective in treating moderately to severely active UC and CD. Intravenous methylprednisolone, at a dose of 32 to 60 mg daily, is indicated in hospitalized patients with severe UC or CD, or for patients who have failed oral therapy. Hydrocortisone enemas are effective therapy for induction of remission in patients with active UC distal to the splenic flexure, and CD involving the distal colon.

Budesonide (Entocort EC) is a newer corticosteroid that is associated with fewer systemic side effects and less adrenal insufficiency. This is because of its low systemic bioavailability and extensive first-pass metabolism in the liver and erythrocytes. At a dose of 9 mg per day,

---

[1]Not FDA approved for this indication.

TABLE 1 Indication, Dose, Route, and Adverse Effects of Drugs Used in Inflammatory Bowel Disease

Agent	Indication	Dose	Route	Adverse Effects
Azo-bonded mesalamine derivatives Sulfasalazine (Azulfidine) Balsalazide (Colazal) Olsalazine (Dipentum)	**CD:** *Sulfasalazine:* Induction of remission for mildly to moderately active disease (especially Ileocolonic and colonic disease) *Balsalazide and Olsalazine:* No current approved use **UC:** *Sulfasalazine:* Induction of remission for mildly to moderately active disease *Balsalazide:* Induction of remission for active UC Maintenance of remission *Olsalazine:* Induction of remission for active UC Maintenance of remission for active UC	*Sulfasalazine:* 4 to 6 g/d* 2 to 4 g/d† *Balsalazide:* 2 to 6.75 g/d *Olsalazine:* 1.5 to 3 g/d	PO	*Sulfasalazine:* Nausea, vomiting, anorexia, headache, fever, rash, agranulocytosis, pancreatitis, hepatitis, folate malabsorption, sperm abnormalities *Balsalazide:* Headache, abdominal pain, nausea, vomiting, diarrhea, arthralgias, respiratory depression *Olsalazine:* Diarrhea, abdominal pain, cramps
Mesalamine derivatives (Asacol, Pentasa)	**CD:** Induction of remission for mildly to moderately active disease Induction of remission for active disease treated with corticosteroids (reducing steroid dependency) Maintenance of remission (especially surgically induced remission) **UC:** Induction of remission for mildly to moderately active disease Maintenance of remission	4 to 4.8 g/d* 2 to 4.8 g/d†	PO, topical	Nausea, dyspepsia, headache, rare hypersensitivity reactions (fever, rash, agranulocytosis); anal irritation and pruritus possible with topical use
Topical aminosalicylates	**UC:** Induction of remission for acute distal colitis (enema) and proctitis (suppository) Maintenance of remission for acute distal colitis (enema) and proctitis (suppository)	1 to 1.5 g/d	Topical	Anal irritation and pruritus
Corticosteroids	**CD:** *Oral* Induction of remission for moderately to severely active disease *Topical*: Induction of remission of distal Crohn's colitis/proctitis	PO: 40 to 60 mg/d‡ IV: 32 to 60 mg/d Topical: 100 mg§	PO, IV, topical	Fat redistribution, acne, weight gain, mood changes, hyperglycemia, myopathy, osteoporosis; with prolonged use, osteonecrosis, cataracts

Continued

Rakel and Bope: *Conn's Current Therapy 2006.*

TABLE 1 Indication, Dose, Route, and Adverse Effects of Drugs Used in Inflammatory Bowel Disease—cont'd

Agent	Indication	Dose	Route	Adverse Effects
Metronidazole (Flagyl)[1]	**UC**: *Oral:* Induction of remission for moderately to severely active disease: *Topical*[1]: Induction of remission of distal ulcerative colitis/proctitis **CD**: Induction of remission for active colitis Induction of remission for active perianal disease (closure of fistula) Maintenance of remission for surgically induced remission **UC**: No current approved indication	10 to 20 mg/kg/d	PO	Nausea, abdominal pain, metallic taste; disulfiram-like reaction with concurrent alcohol use; peripheral neuropathy (seen in prolonged use)
Ciprofloxacin (Cipro)[1]	**CD**: Induction of remission for active colitis Induction of remission for active perianal disease (closure of fistula) **UC**: No current approved indication **CD**: Induction of remission for active disease Induction of remission for steroid-dependent disease (allowing for steroid withdrawal) Fistulous disease	1 g/d	PO	Dyspepsia, diarrhea, headaches, abdominal pain; rarely, hepatotoxicity, seizures, rash, interstitial nephritis, Achilles tendon rupture (unilateral or bilateral)
Azathioprine (Imuran)[1] 6-Mercapto-purine (6-MP Purinethol)[1]	Maintenance of remission for medically and surgically induced remission **UC**: Induction of remission for active disease Induction of remission for steroid-dependent disease (allowing for steroid withdrawal) Maintenance of remission for medically induced remission	AZA: 2.0 to 2.5 mg/kg/d 6-MP: 1.0 to 1.5 mg/kg/d	PO	Nausea, vomiting, allergic reactions, pancreatitis, abnormal liver function tests, bone marrow toxicity
Cyclosporine[1] (Sandimmune, Neoral, Gengraf)	**CD**: Fistulous disease refractory to other medical therapies (antibiotics, AZA/6-MP, infliximab) **UC**: Severe UC refractory to or intolerant of other medical therapies (corticosteroids, AZA/6-MP)	4 mg/kg/d	IV, PO	Hypertension, headache, paresthesias, electrolyte and liver function abnormalities, nephrotoxicity, gingival hyperplasia; rarely, seizures, opportunistic infections

Rakel and Bope: *Conn's Current Therapy 2006.*

TABLE 1 Indication, Dose, Route, and Adverse Effects of Drugs Used in Inflammatory Bowel Disease—cont'd

Agent	Indication	Dose	Route	Adverse Effects
Methotrexate[1] (Rheumatrex, Trexall)	**CD:** Induction of remission for active disease Induction of remission for steroid-dependent disease (allowing for steroid withdrawal) Disease nonresponsive to other medical therapies (infliximab, AZA/6-MP) Maintenance of remission **UC:** No current approved use	25 mg/wk* 15 mg/wk[†]	PO, IM, SC	Stomatitis, esophagitis, oral ulcerations, nausea, vomiting, diarrhea; bone marrow suppression (anemia, leukopenia, thrombocytopenia); elevated liver function tests, portal fibrosis, and cirrhosis (can be seen in patients who have received cumulative dose of 1.5 g)
Infliximab (Remicade)	**CD:** Induction of remission for moderately to severely active disease Induction of remission for active fistulous disease Maintenance of remission for infliximab-induced remission **UC:** No current approved use	5 mg/kg or 10 mg/kg	IV	Upper respiratory tract infections, headache, nausea, myalgias, vomiting, diarrhea; infusion reaction, possibly delayed hypersentivity response; CHF exacerbation; tuberculosis, histoplasmosis, listeriosis, aspergillosis

[1]Not FDA approved for this indication.
*Dose for induction of remission.
[†]Dose for maintenance of remission.
[‡]For ileocecal Crohn's disease; includes budesonide at 9 mg/day.
[§]Hydrocortisone enema.
[¶]High relapse rate upon transition to oral cyclosporine.
Abbreviations: 6-MP = 6-mercaptopurine; AZA = azathioprine; CD = Crohn's disease; CHF = congestive heart failure; IM = intramuscular; IV = intravenous; PO = by mouth; SC = subcutaneous; UC = ulcerative colitis.

budesonide is comparable to traditional corticosteroids for the induction of remission for moderately active CD. Studies have not shown oral budesonide[1] to be effective for treating active UC.

There are multiple, potentially serious side effects associated with corticosteroid use (see Table 1), often correlating with dose and duration of therapy. These include the potential of promoting or masking intestinal microperforations. It is critical to evaluate for and exclude the presence of an abscess or other potential sources of infections before using corticosteroids (in the correct clinical setting).

Patients receiving steroids should receive supplemental oral daily calcium (1200 to 1500 mg/day) and vitamin D (400 to 800 IU/day). In addition, patients on chronic steroid therapy should undergo baseline and periodic bone densitometry studies (DEXA scans); in appropriate patients, the use of bisphosphonates may aide in preventing and potentially treating bone loss.

ANTIMICROBIALS

Experimental and clinical evidence indicates that bacterial flora may play a role in the pathogenesis of inflammatory bowel disease. The intestinal mucosal wall, as a result of the inflammatory response, becomes increasingly permeable and vulnerable to bacterial cell wall antigens, like lipopolysaccharides. These antigens are thought to either initiate or sustain an inflammatory response in host tissue. Abnormal intestinal flora has been found in the bowel wall and mesenteric lymph nodes of patients with CD. In addition, diversion of the fecal stream has been shown to delay postoperative recurrence of CD and minimize the severity of inflammation seen in recurrent disease.

Antimicrobials are primarily used in the treatment of active CD and perianal CD, and for maintenance of surgically induced remission. Although clinical trials fail to demonstrate benefit in treating UC, intravenous, broad-spectrum antibiotics are empirically used in patients with severe UC and in those with signs of systemic toxicity or fulminant colitis with or without megacolon.

The two most commonly used antibiotics for treatment of active CD are metronidazole (Flagyl)[1] and ciprofloxacin (Cipro) (see Table 1). Peripheral neuropathy, commonly seen with prolonged use of metronidazole, is typically reversible if recognized early and the dose is decreased

[1]Not FDA approved for this indication.

[1]Not FDA approved for this indication.

or discontinued. Ciprofloxacin is generally better tolerated; however, Achilles tendon rupture and secondary fungal infections have been reported with ciprofloxacin therapy. A recent study has assessed the efficacy of ornidazole (Avrazor)[2] in the maintenance of postoperative remission. The intention was to use an antibiotic with fewer related adverse events. This antibiotic was effective for the maintenance of postoperative recurrence clinically and endoscopically as long as the medication was taken. There was a significant side-effect profile similar to that of metronidazole. Hence the search for other agents continues.

IMMUNOMODULATORS

Azathioprine and 6-Mercaptopurine

Azathioprine (Imuran)[1] and 6-mercaptopurine (6-MP) (Purinethol)[1] are purine analogues that alter the immune system by inhibiting nucleic acid biosynthesis and the cytotoxicity of natural killer and T cells. Azathioprine is nonenzymatically converted to 6-MP within erythrocytes; 6-MP is then enzymatically cleaved to a group of active end products, called 6-thoiguanine nucleotides. A competing enzyme, thiopurine methyltransferase (TPMT), also converts 6-MP to another metabolite, 6-methylmercaptopurine (6-MMP).

Azathioprine and 6-MP are indicated for induction of remission for active CD and UC, facilitating steroid withdrawal in steroid-dependent UC and CD, and facilitating maintenance of remission in CD and UC. Preliminary data suggest that 6-MP may be effective in preventing postoperative relapse of CD.

In retrospective cohort series, the elevation of this metabolite has been found in association with abnormal alanine aminotransferase (ALT) and aspartate aminotransferase (AST), as well as asymptomatic elevation of serum amylase and lipase. The incidence of lymphoma and leukemia does not seem to be increased in patients with IBD treated with azathioprine and 6-MP.

Bone marrow suppression is a common, dose-dependent toxicity that occurs in 2% to 5% of patients using azathioprine and 6-MP. This potentially significant toxicity should be monitored by obtaining complete blood counts biweekly for the first 8 weeks and then every 1 to 3 months for the remainder of therapy.

Methotrexate

Methotrexate[1] (Rheumatrex, Trexall) inhibits the enzymes dihydrofolate reductase and thymidine synthetase, as well as other enzymes critical to DNA synthesis; it interferes with the production of proinflammatory cytokines IL-1, IL-2, TNF-α, and γ-interferon; and it impairs histamine release from basophils and decreases neutrophil chemotaxis.

Methotrexate is primarily indicated for maintenance of remission and induction of remission for active CD or steroid-dependent CD (allowing for steroid withdrawal).

It can also be considered in patients with CD that have not adequately responded to azathioprine, 6-MP, or infliximab (Remicade). The route of administration that has been effective for patients with CD is either subcutaneously or intramuscularly. The efficacy of orally ingested methotrexate has not been demonstrated. Randomized clinical trials have yet to demonstrate the efficacy of methotrexate in the treatment or maintenance of UC.

Potential toxicities of methotrexate are listed in Table 1. Many of these can be minimized with folic acid supplementation. Bone marrow suppression can be minimized by the concurrent use of leucovorin (Wellcovorin). Hepatic fibrosis is one of the most serious potential sequela of long-term methotrexate therapy. While the utility of liver biopsy in the management of patients on methotrexate remains controversial, a pretreatment liver biopsy should be considered in patients at increased risk for hepatic toxicity (i.e., obese patients or those who consume alcohol).

During the induction period of treatment, patients should receive frequent evaluations of their complete blood counts and liver function tests, initially perhaps every 2 to 4 weeks. This frequency can be reduced during the maintenance period. While some clinicians recommend follow-up liver biopsy in patients who have received a cumulative dose of 1.5 g, it is currently not recommended universally or widely accepted as the standard of care.

Cyclosporine

Cyclosporine[1] (Sandimmune, Neoral, Gengraf) is a cyclic undecapeptide (polypeptide) that inhibits IL-2 production and T-helper-cell function. It also decreases recruitment of cytotoxic T helper cells and blocks the activity of IL-3, IL-4, γ-interferon, and TNF-α.

Randomized controlled trials do not show cyclosporine to be beneficial in patients with CD; however, data from uncontrolled studies suggest that intravenous cyclosporine may be beneficial in the treatment of fistulous CD unresponsive to corticosteroids, antibiotics, or other immunomodulators such as azathioprine or 6-mercaptopurine. In patients with UC, cyclosporine has been used to treat severe disease that is refractory to corticosteroids; in addition, cyclosporine may be used as a bridge for control of disease until azathioprine or 6-MP reaches therapeutic levels or until elective surgery is performed.

Cyclosporine can be administered orally or parenterally. Its absorption is dependent on several factors, including the small bowel transit time, length of small bowel, and integrity of the intestinal mucosa. The microemulsion formulation of cyclosporine (Neoral, Gengraf, Sandimmune) has similar bioavailability and efficacy to that of intravenous cyclosporine.

Monitoring cyclosporine blood levels is suggested as a means of reducing drug toxicity. Patients receiving oral cyclosporine should have weekly trough cyclosporine levels checked and maintained between

---

[2]Not available in the United States.
[1]Not FDA approved for this indication.

[1]Not FDA approved for this indication.

200 and 300 ng/mL, as measured by high-pressure liquid chromatography.

Adverse effects (see Table 1) that may occur with cyclosporine include nephrotoxicity, hypertension, electrolyte abnormalities, seizures, paresthesias, and tremor. Patients receiving cyclosporine may be susceptible to opportunistic infections, therefore *Pneumocystis carinii* pneumonia prophylaxis is recommended with one double-strength dose of trimethoprim-sulfamethoxazole (Bactrim OS) three times a week.

Antitumor Necrosis Factor Therapy

Cytokines, or glycosylated proteins synthesized by various cell types in response to inflammation, can be categorized either as proinflammatory (IL-1, IL-2, IL-6, IL-8, IL-12, TNF-α) or anti-inflammatory (IL-4, IL-10, IL-11, IL-13). An imbalance between the proinflammatory and anti-inflammatory cytokines may play an integral part in the severity of inflammatory bowel disease. Efforts to correct this imbalance have led to the formulation of newer therapy directed at blocking the proinflammatory actions of specific cytokines.

INFLIXIMAB

Infliximab (Remicade) is a chimeric immunoglobulin (Ig) G-1 subclass monoclonal antibody directed against TNF-α. It also inhibits IL-1, IL-6 production, endothelial cell and leukocyte expression of adhesion molecules, fibroblast proliferation, and prostaglandin synthesis. In IBD patients, infliximab reduces TNF-α production and inflammatory cell proliferation in inflamed areas of the intestine. Infliximab is also known to induce apoptosis in lymphocytes and monocytes.

In 1998, the Food and Drug Administration (FDA) approved infliximab for the treatment of patients with moderately to severely active CD refractory to conventional therapy and with draining enterocutaneous fistulae. Based on recent data, infliximab is indicated for induction of remission for moderately to severely active CD, induction of remission for active fistulous CD, and maintenance of remission in patients with quiescent CD induced by infliximab. Concurrent use of infliximab with azathioprine or 6-MP may be associated with prolonged remission of CD. While infliximab is not FDA approved for the treatment of active UC, preliminary uncontrolled studies show modest benefit in the treatment of severe steroid-refractory UC. Two large randomized, controlled trials are currently being conducted to confirm these preliminary findings.

Infliximab is administered as an infusion and has a rapid onset of action (2 to 4 weeks). The most common adverse effect is headache, seen in approximately 23% of patients. Other effects seen include nausea, vomiting, and abdominal pain (see Table 1). Some patients may develop antibodies against infliximab (formerly known as human antichimeric antibodies [HACA]). Individuals who receive infliximab as an episodic therapy (as opposed to a maintenance therapy given in a specified periodicity) are more prone to develop antibodies against infliximab. The presence of these antibodies at a high level has been correlated with a shorter duration of action and a higher rate of infusion reactions. Individuals who receive infliximab at a specified periodicity after receiving three induction doses (typically at weeks 0, 2, 6) are less likely to develop antibodies than the aforementioned population. Serious infections such as tuberculosis, histoplasmosis, listeriosis, and aspergillosis can occur in patients treated with infliximab. A screening purified protein derivative (PPD) test (and we advocate a chest radiograph as well) is recommended before infliximab therapy is initiated. The long-term risk of developing lymphoma or other malignancies following infliximab therapy is currently being followed. At present, it is believed that the risk of developing lymphoma is not higher in those receiving infliximab than the risk in the general population.

Investigational Therapies

ETANERCEPT AND THALIDOMIDE

Two additional anti-TNF agents that are currently being investigated in the treatment of CD are etanercept (Enbrel) and thalidomide (Thalomid). While etanercept has yet to show benefit in treating CD (when used at a dose of 25 mg twice weekly in a subcutaneous fashion), studies using thalidomide show its benefit in the treatment of intestinal and fistulizing CD that are unresponsive to standard therapies. Neither of these agents can be recommended for the routine care of patients with CD until controlled clinical trials can be completed. Their use should be reserved for clinical trials. The use of thalidomide is complicated by the development of peripheral neuropathy and sedation in a large percentage of treated patients. There currently are second generation thalidomide congeners under investigation that hopefully will not possess the adverse effects seen in the first generation of compounds.

NICOTINE

The observation that smoking appears to have a protective effect in patients with UC has led to therapeutic trials of nicotine in these patients. Based on the results of randomized, placebo-controlled trials, nicotine may be beneficial in patients with active and steroid-dependent UC who recently stopped smoking. Patients who never smoked are frequently unable to tolerate this therapy, given its side effects of nausea and headache. A maintenance trial for patients with ulcerative colitis has failed to demonstrate efficacy over placebo.

HEPARIN

Prothrombic abnormalities within the circulatory system and the presence of inflammatory vasculitis and microthrombi with the bowel mucosa suggest that a hypercoagulable state may contribute to the pathogenesis of IBD. Based on results of several uncontrolled trials, unfractionated heparin (Hepalean) reduces symptoms and improves healing in patients with steroid-resistant UC, but not in treating moderate-to-severe UC. Results from several multicenter, randomized, controlled trials using heparin have failed to demonstrate efficacy for patients with active ulcerative colitis.

PROBIOTICS

Probiotics are living organisms in foods and dietary supplements that help reestablish normal intestinal flora. They create an environment that is unfavorable for the growth of potentially pathogenic bacteria and maintain the integrity of the gut mucosal barrier. In vitro studies suggest that probiotics stimulate the intestinal mucosal immune system by enhancing macrophage and natural killer cell activities, and by augmenting the proliferation of lymphocytes.

Uncontrolled clinical trial results show that probiotics may have a modest benefit in the treatment of CD and in the maintenance of quiescent UC. Placebo-controlled trials are needed before probiotics can be recommended in the management of IBD patients.

Two trials show efficacy of a probiotic called VSL-3 (from VSL Pharmaceuticals, Inc.), which is a conglomerate of three different bacteria. This agent has been shown to lessen the development of pouchitis (inflammation of a surgically created ileoanal pouch after patients have undergone total proctocolectomy) when taken either as postoperative prophylaxis or when taken after an antibiotic-induced remission in patients who have had a chronic course of recurrent pouchitis.

Nutritional Therapy

Total parenteral nutrition (TPN) should be reserved for patients with obstructive CD or CD with a high-output fistula. Even though this treatment has not been proven effective in UC, hospitalized patients with severe colitis receiving parenteral therapy who cannot tolerate oral intake or patients who are severely malnourished may benefit from TPN.

Short-chain fatty acids (SCFA) serve as primary energy substrate for colonic mucosal cells, and disrupted delivery of this substrate can result in mucosal inflammation. The primary component of SCFAs is butyrate. Butyrate accounts for approximately 70% of the energy source for the colonocyte. UC patients may have decreased levels of this substrate, and delivery of SCFA in the form of enemas may aid in the treatment of active distal colitis, a finding that has yet to be warranted by large, randomized, controlled clinical trials.

Despite the fact that food may serve as a major source of intraluminal antigens, food elimination diets or highly restrictive diets have not proved effective in the treatment of IBD. Lactose restriction may be helpful in eliminating symptoms that can be confused with those of CD in some patients, but is not mandatory in all patients. Patients with symptomatic fibrostenotic disease may benefit from a low-residue diet and avoidance of particular foods that may cause obstruction, such as nuts, seeds, and corn.

Periodic monitoring of electrolytes and appropriate supplementation of potassium, magnesium, zinc, and vitamin B_{12} may be required in patients with chronic diarrhea or extensive ileal disease, ileal resection, or bacterial overgrowth. Calcium, fat-soluble vitamin, and iron supplementation may be necessary in patients with fat malabsorption and iron deficiency anemia.

Medical Management of Inflammatory Bowel Disease

Appropriate management of ulcerative colitis and Crohn's disease requires defining the extent and severity of disease. While endoscopic evidence is valuable in defining the extent of disease, severity of disease is based on a variety of findings including the patient's symptoms, the impact of disease on daily function, pertinent physical examination findings (e.g., fever, abdominal tenderness), and abnormal laboratory values (e.g., anemia, hypoalbuminemia).

The Truelove and Witts' Activity Index (Box 1) continues to be one of the standard systems used for assessing systemic severity in patients with UC. Patients with toxic megacolon, a life-threatening form of UC, present with signs of toxicity (fever >101°F [38.3°C], tachycardia, abdominal distension, and signs of localized or generalized peritonitis) with leukocytosis (i.e., white blood cell count greater than 11,000 THO/mL) and dilated loops of bowel on plain abdominal radiograph. Standardized instruments (including the Crohn's Disease Activity Index [CDAI]) have been developed to assess disease severity in patients with CD, but most of these are inconvenient for daily practice and are best reserved for clinical trials. From a practical perspective, patients are considered to have mildly to moderately active CD when they are ambulatory; able to tolerate an oral diet; and exhibit no signs of dehydration, toxicity, abdominal tenderness, mass, or obstruction. Patients who have failed treatment for mildly to moderately active disease or patients presenting with fever, weight loss, anemia, nausea, vomiting, abdominal pain, and tenderness (without obstruction)

BOX 1   Truelove and Witts' Activity Index for Ulcerative Colitis

Severe
- More than six bowel movements a day with blood
- Temperature greater than 37°C (98.6°F)
- Heart rate greater than 90 beats per minute
- Anemia with hemoglobin less than 75%
- Erythrocyte sedimentation rate (ESR) greater than 30 mm per hour

Mild
- Less than four bowel movements a day without blood
- No fever
- Heart rate less than 90 beats per minute
- Mild anemia
- ESR less than 30 mm per hour

Moderate
- Features between those of mild and severe

Rakel and Bope: *Conn's Current Therapy 2006.*

are considered to have moderately to severely active CD. Severe or fulminant CD defines patients with persistent symptoms despite corticosteroid therapy or patients exhibiting high fevers, persistent vomiting, evidence of intestinal obstruction or an abscess, rebound tenderness, cachexia, and profound anemia. Patients are considered to be in remission when they are asymptomatic, either spontaneously or after medical or surgical intervention.

The clinical management of patients with UC and CD classified by extent and severity is discussed below.

ULCERATIVE COLITIS

Proctitis and Proctosigmoiditis

Patients with proctitis have inflammation limited to the rectum (approximately the distal 15 cm of the colon), while patients with proctosigmoiditis have disease involving the distal 30 to 40 cm of the colon. Symptoms of proctitis include rectal bleeding, tenesmus, and multiple frequent small bowel movements, often associated with mucus. Patients with proctosigmoiditis often have a similar presentation, but may also have minimal systemic symptoms such as fever, weight loss, and anorexia.

Topical aminosalicylates, in the form of twice daily 500 mg mesalamine suppositories (Canasa) or nightly 4 g mesalamine enemas, are among the first-line agents to be considered for treating patients with active proctitis and proctosigmoiditis, respectively (Figure 1). A combination of oral and topical aminosalicylates is usually required for patients who present with severe proctitis or proctosigmoiditis. Treatment is continued for at least 2 to 3 weeks to evaluate for efficacy. For patients who have an inadequate response at this time, another topical aminosalicylate, or hydrocortisone enema (Cortenema)[1] (100 mg) can be added to the regimen.

Corticosteroids (oral prednisone at 40 to 60 mg/day) are often ineffective for treating ulcerative proctitis, but can be used for patients with severe proctosigmoiditis who are symptomatic or have an inadequate response to the aforementioned therapy. A response to corticosteroid treatment is usually seen within 10 to 14 days.

When remission is achieved, corticosteroids should be tapered, as they play no role in the maintenance of disease remission. Patients initially treated with topical corticosteroid preparations should be transitioned to topical mesalamine and gradually tapered off the topical corticosteroid. Maintenance therapy is not required for patients who experienced their first disease exacerbation that responded promptly to treatment. Other patients achieving remission may benefit from maintenance therapy, consisting of continuing the specific combination of mesalamine therapy that was successful in inducing remission. Fewer relapses may occur with twice-daily mesalamine suppositories than compared to once daily doses. Over time, most patients are able to reduce topical mesalamine therapy to once at night and eventually to every third night.

[1]Not FDA approved for this indication.

Rakel and Bope: *Conn's Current Therapy 2006.*

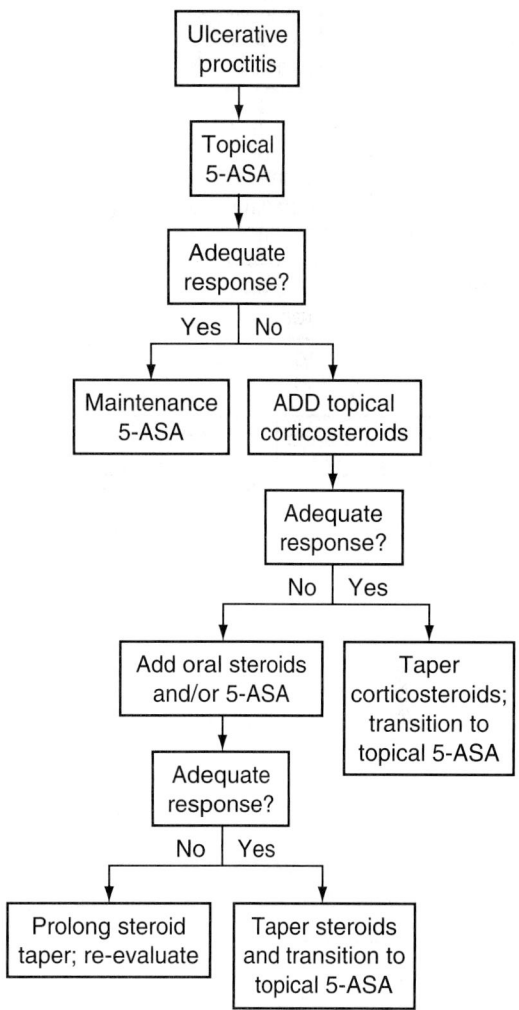

FIGURE 1. Management of ulcerative proctitis and proctosigmoiditis. (Modified from: Srinivasan R, Su CG, and Lichtenstein GR: Medical Therapy for Ulcerative Colitis. In Lichtenstein GR: The Clinician's Guide to Inflammatory Bowel Disease. Thorofare, NJ, SLACK Incorporated, 2003, pp 255-289. Used with permission.)

Left-Sided Colitis

Ulcerative colitis extending up to but not beyond the splenic flexure (up to 60 cm from the anal verge) is defined as left-sided colitis. These patients often present with bloody diarrhea, tenesmus, and rectal urgency. Initial therapy is determined by the severity of disease symptoms.

Topical therapy with mesalamine enemas, 4 g every hour, can be used as initial therapy for mildly to moderately active disease (Figure 2). Patients with moderately to severely active left-sided colitis may benefit from twice-daily mesalamine enemas with alternating corticosteroid enema, especially in patients who are unable to tolerate aminosalicylate enemas. Combining oral and topical aminosalicylates is usually required for inducing remission in patients with severe left-sided colitis. This combination may be more effective in producing a quicker and more complete relief of symptoms. Therapeutic response should be evident within 4 weeks of therapy and may be seen at maximal doses of aminosalicylates

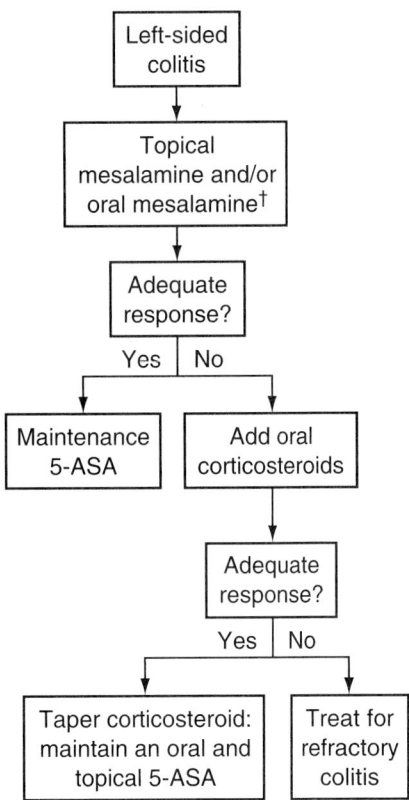

†Oral and topical 5-ASA are usually required for treating patients with severe left-sided colitis

FIGURE 2. Management of left-sided colitis. (Modified from: Srinivasan R, Su CG, and Lichtenstein GR: Medical Therapy for Ulcerative Colitis. In Lichtenstein GR: The Clinician's Guide to Inflammatory Bowel Disease. Thorofare, NJ, SLACK Incorporated, 2003, pp 255-289. Used with permission.)

(sulfasalazine [Azulfidine], 6 g/day; oral mesalamine [Asacol], 4 to 4.8 g/day; olsalazine [Dipentum], 3 g/day[3]).

Corticosteroids (e.g., oral prednisone, 40 to 60 mg/day) should be reserved for patients who have an inadequate response to aminosalicylate therapy or patients with severe disease that may benefit from a more rapid response as compared to that of amino salicylate therapy. When in remission, prednisone should be tapered to reduce steroid-related adverse effects. It is important to ensure that patients have inactive disease before initiating this corticosteroid taper. Even though there are no studies to formally evaluate the rate of corticosteroid taper, a potential regimen may include reducing prednisone by 5 mg per week and then 2.5 mg per week after 20 mg, if deemed appropriate. It is imperative to maintain oral aminosalicylates at their maximal doses while corticosteroids are being tapered.

Once remission is achieved, an oral 5-ASA maintenance therapy with the same drug is recommended. Often, doses similar to what was used to induce remission may be required, as the efficacy of these agents in maintaining remission is dose dependent. A combination

---

of oral and topical mesalamine may be more effective than just oral mesalamine in the maintenance of remission in patients with left-sided colitis.

Extensive Colitis or Pancolitis

Ulcerative colitis that has extended beyond the splenic flexure is termed extensive colitis; when the inflammation reaches the cecum, it is then referred to as pancolitis. For mildly to moderately active disease, oral sulfasalazine (3 to 4 g/day) or mesalamine (2.4 to 4.8 g/day) are the first-line therapy (Figure 3), as the inflammation extends beyond the reach of topical preparations. However, topical aminosalicylates can be added to treat left-sided symptoms such as tenesmus or fecal urgency.

Systemic corticosteroids (oral prednisone, 40 to 60 mg/day) should be used to treat patients who have not achieved remission with maximal doses of oral and topical aminosalicylates. Steroids do not have a role in maintaining remission, but should not be tapered until the symptoms are controlled completely. Long-term maintenance therapy with oral sulfasalazine and the newer mesalamine derivatives at standard maintenance doses should be used once a patient has achieved remission. The addition of maintenance topical 5-ASA may further decrease the risk of disease exacerbation.

Some patients may continue to be symptomatic, despite maximal 5-ASA and oral prednisone therapy.

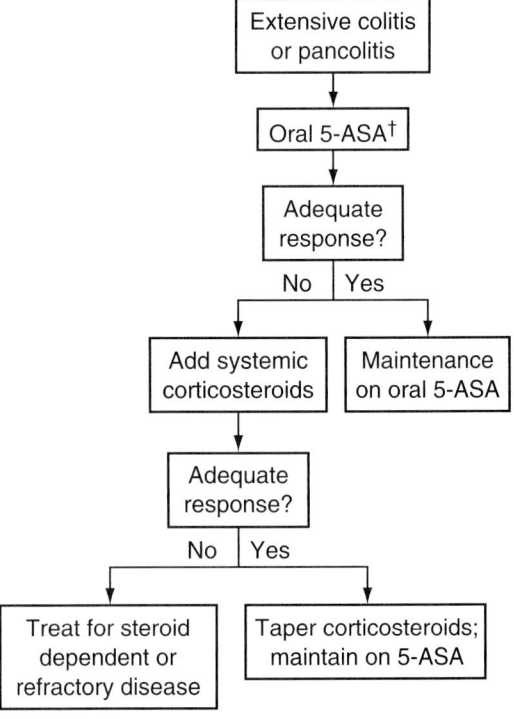

†Topical 5-ASA or corticosteroids can be added for symptomatic treatment of tenesmus or urgency

FIGURE 3. Management of extensive colitis or pancolitis. (Modified from: Srinivasan R, Su CG, and Lichtenstein GR: Medical Therapy for Ulcerative Colitis. In Lichtenstein GR: The Clinician's Guide to Inflammatory Bowel Disease. Thorofare, NJ, SLACK Incorporated, 2003, pp 255-289. Used with permission.)

---

[3]Exceeds dosage recommended by the manufacturer.

These patients, considered to have refractory disease, may need to be hospitalized and treated with intravenous corticosteroids. The treatment of patients with refractory disease is discussed in the subsequent section on refractory colitis.

Severe Colitis

Patients with severe colitis present with more than six bloody bowel movements per day, fever, hypotension, dehydration, tachycardia, anemia, abdominal pain/tenderness, and an elevated erythrocyte sedimentation rate.

Initial treatment requires hospitalization and initiation of intravenous corticosteroids (prednisolone 40 to 60 mg/day, methylprednisolone 32 to 48 mg/day, or hydrocortisone 300 to 400 mg/day) either as continuous infusion or in divided doses every 8 hours (Figure 4). Topical therapy (hydrocortisone enema [Cortenema], 100 mg every hour) can be offered to patients with significant rectal symptoms such as tenesmus or fecal urgency.

Supportive care with fluid resuscitation, electrolyte repletion, and transfusion to correct anemia should be initiated early in the hospital course. Patients should be placed on bowel rest; anticholinergics, antidiarrheals, and narcotics should be held to decrease the potential for initiation of toxic megacolon. Total parenteral nutrition (TPN) should be used in malnourished patients who do not improve quickly or are unable to tolerate

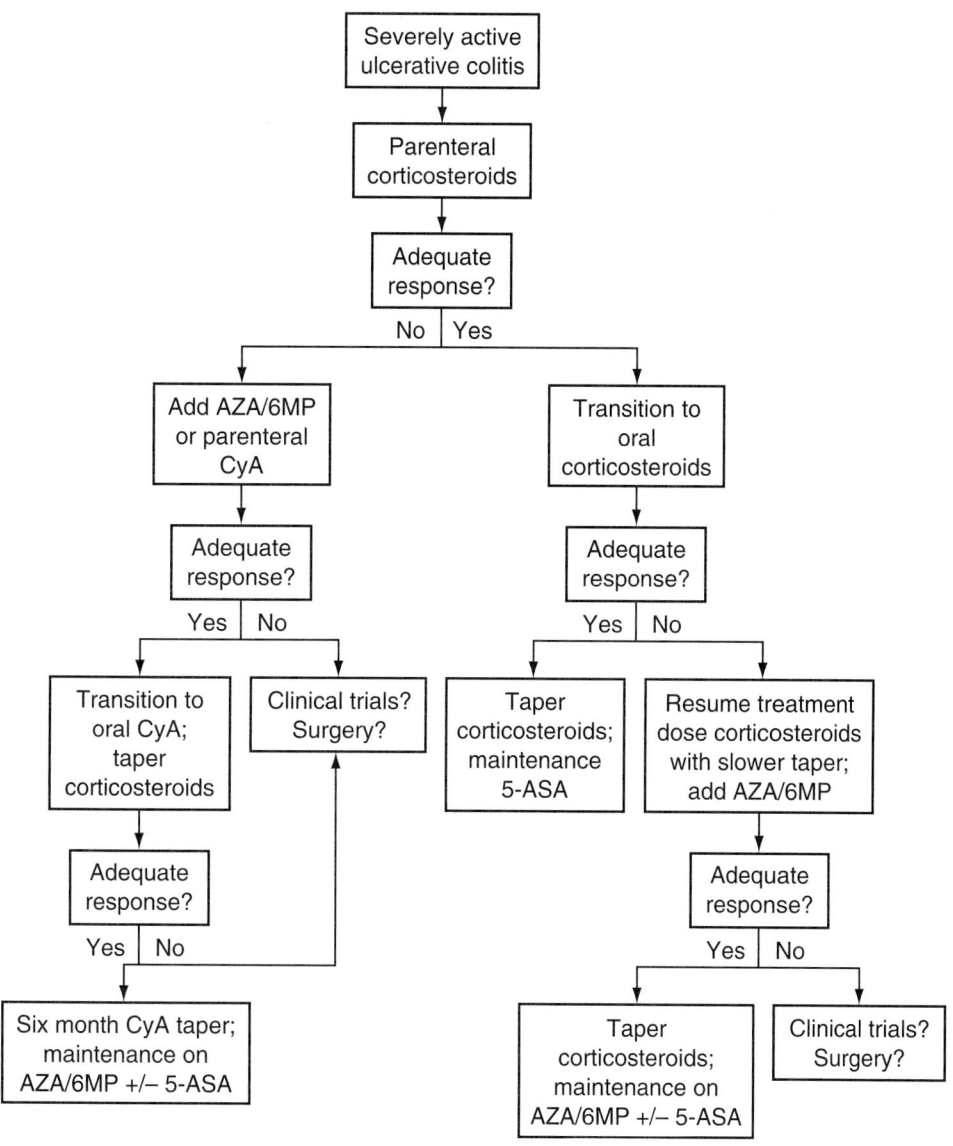

AZA = Azathioprine; 6MP = 6-Mercaptopurine; CyA = Cyclosporine

FIGURE 4. Management of severely active ulcerative colitis. (Modified from: Srinivasan R, Su CG, and Lichtenstein GR: Medical Therapy for Ulcerative Colitis. In Lichtenstein GR: The Clinician's Guide to Inflammatory Bowel Disease. Thorofare, NJ, SLACK Incorporated, 2003, pp 255-289. Used with permission.)

Rakel and Bope: *Conn's Current Therapy 2006.*

oral intake; as symptoms improve, patients can be transitioned from TPN to a low-residue diet.

Patients should generally improve within 7 days of intravenous corticosteroid therapy. When patients begin to have more formed bowel movements without blood, pain, or urgency and can tolerate oral intake, oral corticosteroids can be substituted (prednisone, 40 mg/day) and aminosalicylate therapy initiated. A slower taper should be initiated if patients remain in remission after the transition to oral steroids. Recurrence of disease at any time during the taper should be treated promptly with increase of steroids to previous dose and a slower taper once symptoms are controlled.

Patients who do not improve during the first week of intravenous corticosteroids generally have a low probability of future improvement; surgical intervention or cyclosporine therapy should be considered to treat these patients. Cyclosporine (Neoral)[1] has several potentially serious adverse effects and its use should be limited to medical centers with access to same-day or next-day cyclosporine levels, and appropriate surgical backup.

Intravenous cyclosporine at a dose of 4 mg/kg per day is given in conjunction with intravenous corticosteroids. Frequent cyclosporine levels should be checked in the treatment phase, and the dose adjusted to maintain a high-pressure liquid chromatography blood level between 250 to 350 ng/mL. Patients receiving cyclosporine should respond within the first 5 days. Surgical intervention should be considered if this response is not seen or if the patient's condition worsens. Patients who respond to and achieve remission on IV cyclosporine should be transitioned to oral cyclosporine twice daily at a total dose twice that of the final IV dose (5 to 7 mg/kg).

Cyclosporine is intended only for short-term use, with long-term maintenance therapy on azathioprine (AZA) (Imuran),[1] 2.0 to 2.5 mg/kg per day, or 6-MP (Purinethol),[1] 1.0 to 1.5 mg/kg per day. The addition of AZA or 6-MP allows for tapering of corticosteroids, improves the potential of long-term maintenance of remission, and reduces the likelihood of future surgery. *Pneumocystis carinii* prophylaxis should be administered to all patients on cyclosporine. Prednisone should first be tapered, followed by cyclosporine over the next 3 to 6 months. AZA or 6-MP should be continued to maintain disease remission.

Fulminant Colitis/Toxic Megacolon

Patients with fulminant colitis present with a toxic appearance and evidence of fever, abdominal tenderness and distention, leukocytosis, and anemia. Rapid extension of inflammation through the bowel wall into the serosa may result in toxic megacolon, manifested by colonic dilatation greater than 6 cm and evidence of systemic toxicity.

Patients should be kept on nothing by mouth (NPO), aggressively fluid resuscitated, and transfused to correct anemia. They should receive perioperative intravenous corticosteroids (methylprednisolone, 40 to 60 mg/day), and broad-spectrum antibiotics. Serial abdominal films should be followed in cases of fulminant colitis to evaluate for colonic dilatation or perforation.

[1]Not FDA approved for this indication.

Frequently repositioning the patient from supine to decubitus to prone position may aid in passing trapped gas and decompressing the dilated colon. Surgery is indicated in patients with either fulminant colitis or toxic megacolon who do not respond to the aforementioned medical therapy within 72 hours.

Pouchitis

Approximately 25% of patients with medically uncontrolled UC require surgery. In such cases, a total abdominal colectomy with ileal pouch anal anastomosis (IPAA) is performed. Chronic inflammation of this pouch, or pouchitis, is the most common long-term complication of this procedure. Symptoms of pouchitis include increased stool frequency, hematochezia, fever, abdominal pain, and tenesmus. Up to 50% of patients will develop at least one episode of pouchitis and 15% of these patients will need maintenance therapy and are thought to have chronic pouchitis.

The first-line therapy for the treatment of pouchitis is metronidazole (Flagyl),[1] 10 to 20 mg/kg per day, or ciprofloxacin (Cipro),[1] 1000 mg per day, for a 14-day course (Figure 5). Symptomatic response is usually seen after 1 to 2 days of therapy. Amoxicillin/ clavulanic acid (Augmentin)[1] is an alternative antibiotic choice,

[1]Not FDA approved for this indication.

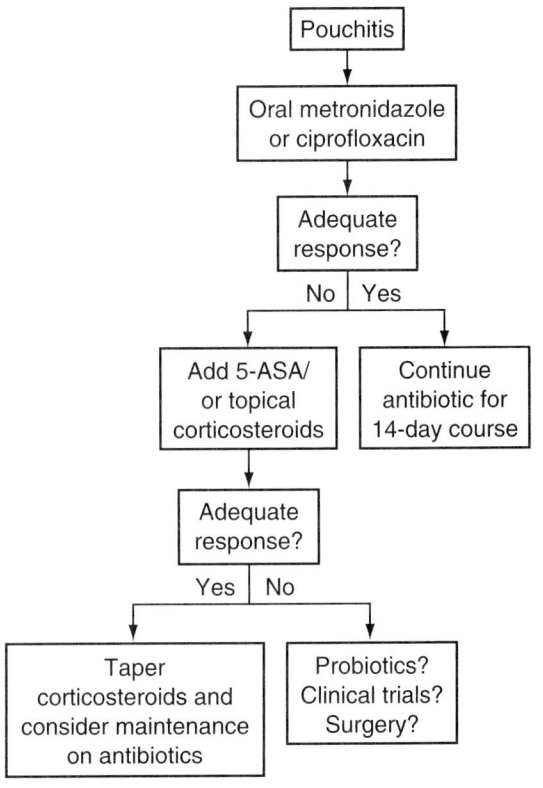

FIGURE 5. Management of pouchitis. (Modified from: Lee T, Buchman AL: Medical Therapy for Ulcerative Colitis. In Lichtenstein GR: The Clinician's Guide to Inflammatory Bowel Disease. Thorofare, NJ, SLACK Incorporated, 2003, pp 125-140. Used with permission.)

although there have been no controlled trials using this antimicrobial agent.

Patients with pouchitis unresponsive to the 14-day course of metronidazole may benefit from repeating the course of antibiotics. If symptoms still persist, oral or topical mesalamine therapy may be used. Data from uncontrolled studies show that bacterial concentrations in the pouch are sufficient to break down the azo bond of sulfasalazine. Other potential investigational agents include topical corticosteroids, probiotics, short-chained fatty acid enemas, and bismuth carbomer enemas. Further research is needed to determine if these agents may be beneficial for select patients.

Some patients may require long-term maintenance therapy on metronidazole. These patients should be closely monitored for adverse effects. Cycling of multiple antibiotics at weekly intervals may help prevent bacterial resistance.

Usually pouchitis is mild and effective to medical therapy, but some patients do not respond to therapy or have frequent recurrences. Occasional complications in these cases include pouch failure requiring removal of the pouch. The risk of dysplasia and malignancy is unclear at this point and warrants further investigation.

CROHN'S DISEASE

Oral Lesions

Aphthous ulcers, deep linear ulcers with associated edema and ulceration are the most common oral manifestations of Crohn's disease. Topical applications of triamcinolone dental paste, hydrocortisone in a pectin or gelatin carrier, or lidocaine lozenges may benefit in reducing the pain and oral discomfort. Refractory disease may require corticosteroids (oral prednisone, 20 mg/day for 1 week), but systemic therapy aimed at treating the underlying Crohn's disease may be required.

Esophagogastroduodenal Crohn's Disease

Fewer than 5% of patients with Crohn's disease present with disease involving the stomach, distal antrum, or duodenum. These patients often present with epigastric pain, postprandial nausea, and vomiting. Because of their distal site of release, aminosalicylates may not be effective, but some patients have been known to occasionally ingest mesalamine in the form of Rowasa enemas. Proton pump inhibitors (omeprazole [Prilosec][1]), 40 mg per day, have been reported to be helpful in inducing and maintaining remission. Moderate-to-severe disease may require treatment with corticosteroids, immunomodulatory agents (azathioprine/6-MP, methotrexate), or infliximab.

Ileocolitis/Colitis

Based on the site of bowel involvement, aminosalicylates are the first-line therapy in mildly to moderately

active disease (Figure 6). While Pentasa has historically been used to treat active disease proximal to the terminal ileum, either Pentasa or Asacol can treat distal ileitis and ileocolitis. Once maximal doses are reached, clinical improvement should be seen within 2 to 4 weeks. If not, either ciprofloxacin[1] (1 g/day) or metronidazole[1] (10 to 20 mg/kg/day) should be considered. If patients improve, usually within 3 to 4 weeks, the antibiotic dose can be tapered over the next few weeks to months. Some patients may require long-term antibiotics to maintain disease remission, although no controlled trials have been performed to ascertain the efficacy of antibiotics for maintenance of remission in Crohn's disease.

Corticosteroids should be reserved for patients whose disease remains unresponsive to aminosalicylate and antibiotic therapy, or who present with moderate-to-severe disease. Oral prednisone (40 to 60 mg/day) or budesonide (9 mg/day) can be administered and tapered slowly once the symptoms are controlled. AZA or 6-MP, when used concomitantly with corticosteroids, may induce remission more rapidly and with lower prednisone doses. Patients who do not respond to the aforementioned therapies should be treated for refractory disease, as described later. Once remission is achieved, corticosteroids should be tapered and patients should be maintained on AZA/6-MP either with or without aminosalicylates.

Severe Crohn's Disease

Patients with severe Crohn's disease often present with fever, abdominal pain and tenderness, bloody diarrhea, hypotension, and leukocytosis. Because of transmural inflammation with serosal involvement, these patients may be prone to microperforation with resulting localized peritonitis.

Patients with severe Crohn's disease should be hospitalized and resuscitated with intravenous fluids. CT of the abdomen should be performed to evaluate for abscess or phlegmon, which requires broad-spectrum antibiotics and, potentially, surgical drainage. Corticosteroids are withheld in this setting.

Once infection is excluded, intravenous corticosteroids (methylprednisolone, 40 to 60 mg/day) should be administered. The addition of AZA or 6-MP to corticosteroid therapy may accelerate remission with lower doses of corticosteroids. Patients who do not respond adequately to this combination therapy should be treated for refractory disease, as discussed later.

Fistulous/Perianal Crohn's Disease

As a result of transmural inflammation, patients with Crohn's disease are prone to developing internal and external fistulas. Internal fistulas often require surgical intervention, as there are little data on the pharmacologic therapy for internal fistulas.

First-line therapies for perianal fistulas include metronidazole[1] (10 to 20 mg/kg/day) or ciprofloxacin[1] (1 g/day). Combining the two antibiotics may also be

---

[1]Not FDA approved for this indication.

[1]Not FDA approved for this indication.

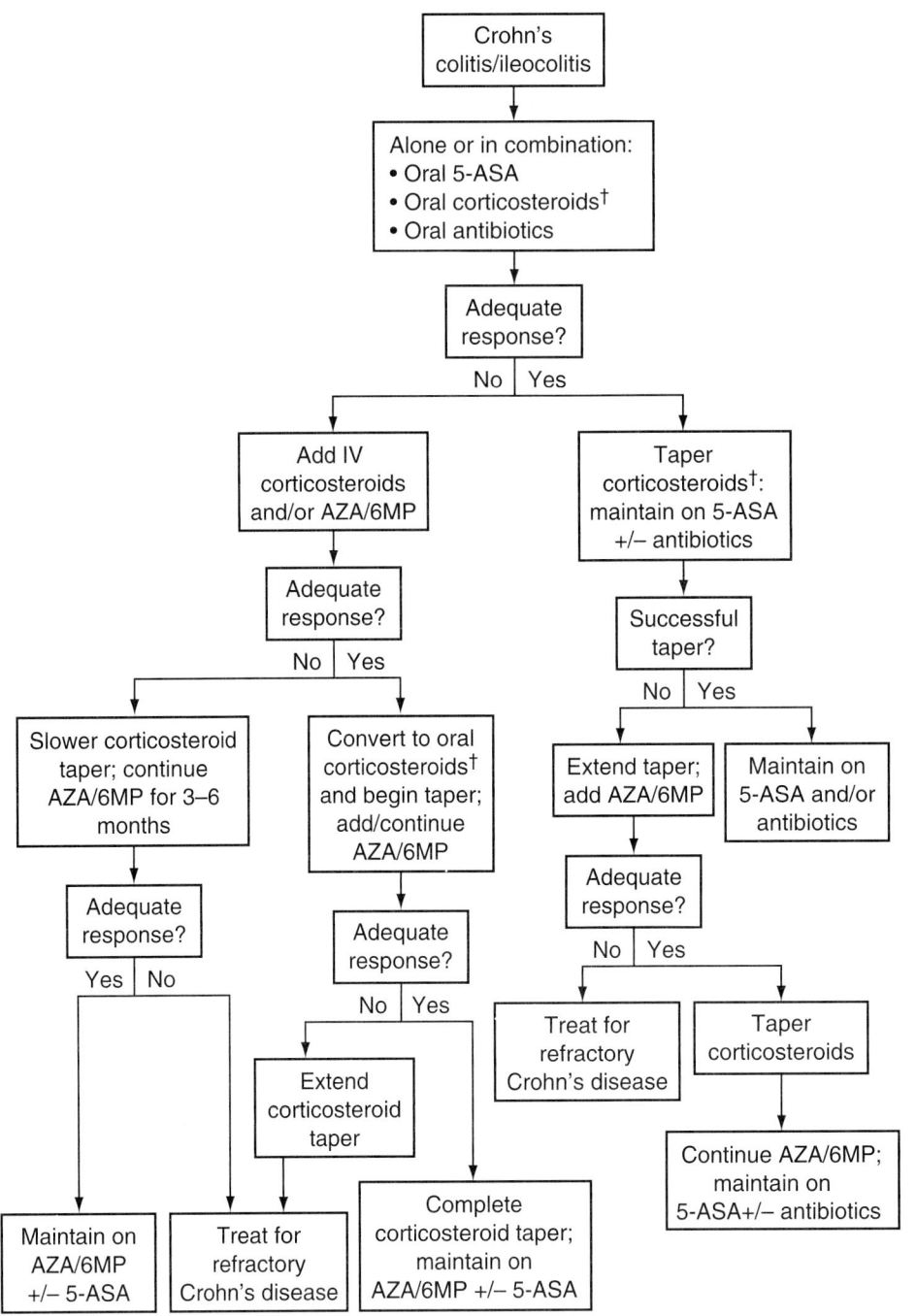

†May include oral budesonide

FIGURE 6. Management of Crohn's colitis or ileocolitis. (Modified from: Han P, Cohen RD: Medical Therapy for Ulcerative Colitis. In Lichtenstein GR: The Clinician's Guide to Inflammatory Bowel Disease. Thorofare, NJ, SLACK Incorporated, 2003, pp 343-370. Used with permission.)

effective if monotherapy fails. Antibiotics can be tapered once these fistulas close, although some patients may require chronic antibiotic therapy. AZA[1] or 6-MP[1] can be used to treat fistulous CD that does not respond to antibiotics. Infliximab, infused at a dose of 5 mg/kg at 0, 2, and 6 weeks with subsequent maintenance therapy (usually at 5 mg/kg every 8 weeks thereafter) can be used as an alternative to AZA or 6-MP, or in conjunction with these medications. Because of the significant toxicity of cyclosporine, intravenous cyclosporine[1] (4 mg/kg) should be reserved for patients whose disease remains unresponsive to the aforementioned therapies.

[1]Not FDA approved for this indication.

Rakel and Bope: *Conn's Current Therapy 2006*.

Refractory Disease

Despite the numerous efficacious medical therapies currently available, some IBD patients may remain symptomatic while on maximal 5-ASA, antibiotic, and corticosteroid therapy.

Patients who respond to corticosteroids but who are unable to discontinue them are considered to have steroid-dependent disease. Others may have steroid refractory disease, defined as disease that remains active despite high-dose corticosteroids.

The management of refractory UC and CD is outlined in Figures 7 and 8, respectively. While on maximal dose corticosteroids, AZA or 6-MP are initiated at 50 to 100 mg and slowly increased by 25 mg over the next 2 weeks if tolerated to the maximum of 2.5 mg/kg per day for AZA and 1.5 mg/kg per day for 6-MP. Alternatively, AZA or 6-MP can be initiated at maximum doses with careful subsequent monitoring for toxicity. Treatment for at least 3 to 6 months is required to evaluate for an adequate response. Corticosteroids should be tapered if an adequate response is noted on AZA or 6-MP. These agents have several potentially toxic adverse effects, including leukopenia and aminotransferase elevation, which should be closely monitored by following patients' complete blood counts and liver-associated laboratory chemistries. There is conflicting evidence as to the duration of treatment with AZA/6-MP. While some suggest discontinuing AZA/6-MP after 4 years, others recommend continuing AZA/6-MP beyond 5 years—even indefinitely.

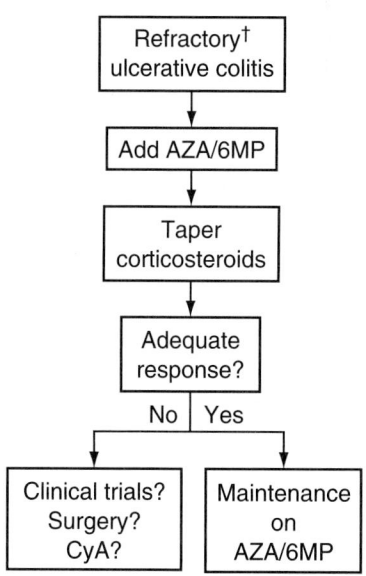

AZA = Azathioprine; 6MP = 6-Mercaptopurine;
CyA = Cyclosporine
†Refractory = No response to equivalent
glucocorticoid dose (prednisone, 40 to 60 mg/d)

FIGURE 7. Management of refractory ulcerative colitis. (Modified from: Han P, Cohen RD: Medical Therapy for Ulcerative Colitis. In Lichtenstein GR: The Clinician's Guide to Inflammatory Bowel Disease. Thorofare, NJ, SLACK Incorporated, 2003, pp 343-370. Used with permission.)

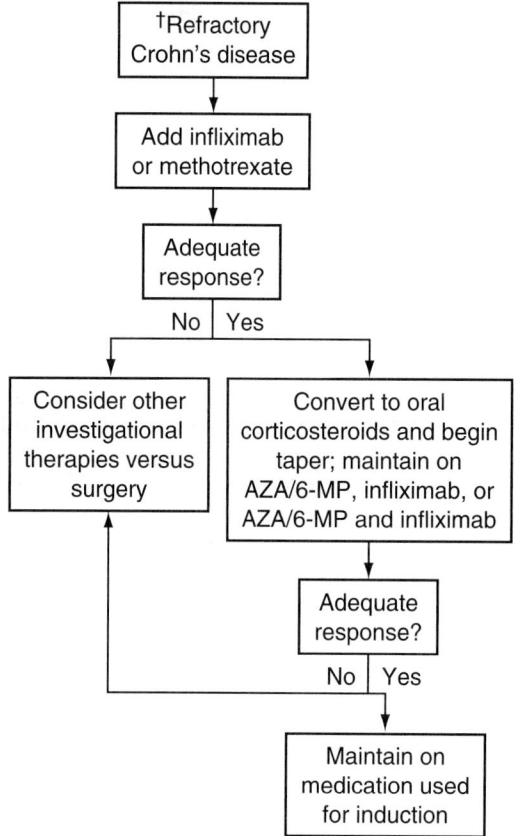

†Symptomatic despite maximal doses of
corticosteroids and azathioprine/6-mercaptopurine

FIGURE 8. Management of refractory Crohn's disease. (Modified from: Han P, Cohen RD: Medical Therapy for Ulcerative Colitis. In Lichtenstein GR: The Clinician's Guide to Inflammatory Bowel Disease. Thorofare, NJ, SLACK Incorporated, 2003, pp 343-370. Used with permission.)

Lifelong therapy, however, should be reserved for patients with aggressive disease or those who are at high risk for relapse (e.g., patients whose disease began at an earlier age, or who required more than 6 months of immunomodulator therapy to achieve disease remission).

Results from a recent study suggest that intravenous cyclosporine may be beneficial in treating steroid-refractory UC. In addition, cyclosporine may serve as a bridge until AZA or 6-MP have reached therapeutic levels or until elective surgery is performed. Cyclosporine has not proven beneficial in the treatment of refractory CD.

Methotrexate, at a dose of 25 mg per week intramuscularly, can be used to treat patients with refractory CD who are intolerant, allergic, or unresponsive to AZA/6-MP. Frequent monitoring of complete blood counts and liver function tests are required to monitor for potential toxicity associated with methotrexate. Methotrexate should be continued for at least 1 to 3 months to assess for an adequate response. If remission and steroid withdrawal are successful, methotrexate can be continued as maintenance therapy at an intramuscular dose of 15 mg per week. Frequent, subcutaneous dosing is administered because of the untested belief that subcutaneous administration is equally as efficacious as intramuscular administration. Randomized clinical trials demonstrated methotrexate to have no benefit in the treatment of UC.

Infliximab can be used to treat patients with refractory CD unresponsive to maximal doses of immunomodulator therapy. Given as 5 mg/kg infusion at 0, 2, and 6 weeks with repeat infusions every 8 weeks thereafter, infliximab has been shown to allow for steroid withdrawal in refractory CD. It also has been shown to prolong disease remission when used concurrently with AZA/6-MP. Patients on infliximab therapy should be monitored for development of infectious complications.

Patients who continue to have active disease despite immunomodulator and infliximab therapy should be evaluated for surgery. However, some patients may choose to participate in ongoing clinical trials of experimental therapies prior to surgery.

As our knowledge expands on the pathophysiology underlying inflammatory bowel disease, better and more efficacious therapies can be expected. The medical therapies and management of site-specific presentations of ulcerative colitis and Crohn's disease aim at inducing and maintaining disease remission, while helping patients maintain an excellent quality of life. Living with inflammatory bowel disease is often challenging, and the Crohn's and Colitis Foundation of America (*http://www.ccfa.org*) offers social support and educational resources that may help patients cope with these potentially debilitating disorders.

Irritable Bowel Syndrome

Method of
James Christensen, MS, MD

Inexplicable gastrointestinal symptoms are generally blamed on the irritable bowel syndrome (IBS; also called spastic colon, mucous colitis, and functional bowel syndrome). This common diagnosis remains scientifically undefined after more than a century of study. A recent clinical redefinition mainly provides a basis for investigation.

The Clinical Definition

People often blame various unexplained chronic gastrointestinal complaints (abdominal pain, diarrhea, constipation, nausea, vomiting, gas, and bloating) on IBS. Authorities also used to accept various genitourinary, cardiovascular, and emotional symptoms as those of IBS. The list shortened over time to the current

definition, the Rome II criteria (Box 1), proposed by a panel of authorities convened in Rome to revise previous definitions.

This latest definition requires *abdominal discomfort or pain* that is related to defecation. To support the diagnosis, it also accepts *bloating* and certain *abnormal features of the defecation.*

Centuries of clinical-pathologic correlation taught physicians and surgeons how to interpret abdominal pain by considering certain characteristics: Its *character, location, chronology, aggravating and relieving factors,* and *associated symptoms* (see http://www.vh.org/adult/provider/internalmedicine/BedsideLogic/index.html). The Rome II definition of IBS fails to consider such features.

Clinical-pathologic correlation also taught doctors how to use the characteristics of the stool (*consistency, color, presence of overt or occult blood, odor,* and *daily volume*) and of disordered defecation (*frequency of defecation, changes over time, aggravating and relieving factors,* and *associated symptoms*) to guide the diagnostic process. The Rome II definition of IBS neglects these matters as well.

The Physiologic Definition

Most physicians and patients accept that IBS reflects dysfunction of the nerves of the gut. Even the newest information and technologies fail to confirm the various theories that are offered to explain IBS: spasm and dysrhythmia in the colon, irritability (hypersensitivity) of the gastrointestinal tract, primary autonomic nerve dysfunction, and food allergy.

The absence of a uniformly accepted clinical definition of the syndrome still limits the selection of patient groups for study. The complexity of gastrointestinal neurophysiology (neurogastroenterology) hampers the search for a pathogenesis. For both reasons, no physiologic definition of IBS is established.

BOX 1   Rome II Symptom Criteria for a Diagnosis of the Irritable Bowel Syndrome

- At least 12 weeks (not necessarily consecutive) in the preceding 12 months of abdominal pain or discomfort that has two of the following three features:
    Relief with defecation
    Onset associated with a change in stool frequency
    Onset associated with a change in the form (appearance) of the stool
- Other symptoms not required but supportive include:
    Abnormal stool frequency (more than three stools per day or less than three stools per week)
    Abnormal stool form (lumpy/hard or loose/watery)
    Abnormal stool passage (straining, urgency, feeling of incomplete evacuation)
    Passage of mucus
    Bloating or a feeling of abdominal distension

The Differential Diagnosis

IBS constitutes a set of *symptoms*—which are individual and personal—without *signs*, the objective evidence of defined diseases. Thus the diagnosis is subjective, depending on the communication skills of both patient and physician.

The diagnosis remains a diagnosis of exclusion. That is, the physician must exclude all other reasonable explanations for the symptoms that come to mind. The finding of a rational explanation yields an established and defined pathophysiologic diagnosis based on current knowledge and understanding; the failure to find such a defined disease entity or process leads to the diagnosis of IBS.

The vast array of defined diseases that can produce abdominal pain demands a systematic method for the efficient exploration of the complaint. A thoughtful and thorough analysis of the character, location, chronology, aggravating and relieving factors, and associated symptoms in respect to abdominal pain is the necessary first step in the orderly diagnostic process. A similar analytic method is necessary for all the other gastrointestinal complaints that might be interpreted as a part of IBS, including diarrhea, constipation, nausea, vomiting, gas, and bloating.

Making a diagnosis of exclusion, such as IBS, demands the consideration of such matters as the family history (e.g., looking for gastrointestinal cancer or celiac disease), the past medical history (e.g., looking for a history of abdominal operations), and the dietary history. The diagnosis also calls for an expert physical examination seeking evidence for all the possibilities suggested by the account of the symptoms. It demands, in sum, the most skillful use of the established clinical methods and the proven methods of history taking and physical examination to guide the further investigation.

Some authorities suggest certain minor features of the symptom complex that seem to characterize IBS, especially the persistence of the symptoms without change for more than 2 years, the onset of symptoms in young adulthood, and the presence of a family history of the diagnosis of IBS. More usefully, one should take the *absence* of such so-called *soft* features as warning against the diagnosis.

Beyond the history and physical examination, the modern investigation of gastrointestinal complaints commonly employs a battery of blood tests, endoscopic procedures, and radiographic examinations. The routine use of simple lists of those tests required for a diagnosis of IBS does not substitute for a thoughtful analysis of symptoms and a careful physical examination. Blind routine testing may fail to show the rarer or subtler organic pathology that would explain symptoms otherwise attributed to IBS. With a set of specific organic diagnoses (the differential diagnosis) firmly in mind, doctors must direct such investigations more specifically to find disordered function.

Warning signs, such as unexplained weight loss and gastrointestinal bleeding, signal many serious or life-threatening gastrointestinal disorders, but such diseases in their early stages can mimic IBS without such red flags. That is, they can produce only abdominal pain or discomfort coupled with bloating or a disturbed pattern of defecation.

When the most thorough analysis fails to explain a set of gastrointestinal symptoms, a diagnosis of IBS seems in order. However, even then the physician must not consider IBS a single homogeneous entity. It could represent many kinds of neural or neuromuscular dysfunction in the gut, considering how much remains unknown about gastrointestinal physiology. The gut is a mechanical device in which a complex and obscure nervous system drives the musculature. Much remains to be learned about this system before ways can be found to test adequately its manifold operations.

Some Conditions With a High Risk for Misdiagnosis

The risk of an erroneous diagnosis of IBS seems especially likely in some particular conditions (Box 2). The proliferation of organisms in the small intestine causes gas, bloating, and abdominal cramps. Giardiasis produces

---

BOX 2   Some Conditions Presenting a High Risk of Misdiagnosis as Irritable Bowel Syndrome

Conditions in which diarrhea, constipation, gas, and bloating may be readily misinterpreted as irritable bowel syndrome (IBS)
- Organisms growing in the gut that should not be there
  Giardiasis
  Bacterial overgrowth in the small intestine
- Abnormalities in the lining of the intestine
  Intolerance to lactose
  Celiac disease (sprue)
  Inflammatory bowel disease (especially lymphocytic colitis)
- Dietary practices
  Intolerance to fructose
  Intake of laxative substances (sorbitol, mannitol, xylitol)
  Food intolerances
- Unconscious swallowing of air from
  Poor dentition
  Nervous habit
- Systemic diseases
  Diffuse systemic sclerosis
  Thyroid disease

Conditions in which abdominal pain may be misinterpreted as IBS
- Abdominal wall pain
  Neuropathies
  Trigger points
  Incisional neuromas and hernias

Conditions in which nausea and vomiting may be misinterpreted as IBS
- Disordered emptying of the stomach
  The neuropathy of diabetes
  Viral neuropathy
- Partial small intestinal obstruction

Rakel and Bope: *Conn's Current Therapy 2006.*

such symptoms. The propagation of coliform bacteria in the small intestine, *small bowel bacterial overgrowth* (which has several causes, including diabetes), does as well.

Abnormalities in the intestinal epithelium may not be apparent in the usual examinations. Intolerance to dietary lactose from mucosal *lactase deficiency* produces symptoms like those of IBS. Mild *celiac disease* (or *sprue*) may produce mainly abdominal discomfort with little other symptomatology. *Inflammatory bowel disease* can be very subtle, especially lymphocytic colitis and the related disorder, collagenous colitis.

IBS symptoms may arise from unorthodox dietary practices or unrecognized food intolerances that lead to osmotic diarrhea. The most common such cause is *intolerance to fructose*. This natural and poorly absorbed monosaccharide, often called "corn sweetener," now finds such widespread use in the sweetening of commercially prepared beverages and foods that daily intake can be enormous. Normal persons may also chronically ingest other sorts of laxative substances, such as the noncaloric sugar alcohol sweeteners (sorbitol, mannitol, and xylitol) and similar artificial sweeteners. Other specific *food intolerances* may be unrecognized by patients. Some common foods such as beans, beer, cabbage, onions, and nuts variably produce gas and bloating in many people, for unknown reasons. Other foods may produce diarrhea.

Excessive air swallowing sometimes occurs with poor dentition as well as part of a nervous habit. Many *systemic diseases*, such as diffuse systemic sclerosis and thyroid disease, can produce IBS symptoms and remain undiagnosed for a long time.

Many people forget that abdominal pain can arise from the abdominal wall as well as from the abdominal cavity. *Sensory somatic neuropathies* (as in complicated diabetes) and *trigger points* in the abdominal wall are common and easily proved with the appropriate techniques of physical examination. Pain from *neuromas* and tiny *hernias* in incisional scars and from rare abdominal wall hernias such as *Richter's hernia* can easily be misconstrued as IBS pain.

Disordered emptying of the stomach is now recognized as common. The abnormality arises from defective operation of the gastric innervation, an *autonomic neuropathy* that is a complication of diabetes or the result of a *viral neuropathy*. Too rapid gastric emptying ("dumping") and delayed emptying ("gastroparesis") can produce similar symptoms. *Incomplete obstruction of the distal small bowel*, also a mimic of IBS, can be very difficult to diagnose.

Major Psychological Issues

No specific psychopathology correlates with the diagnosis of IBS. The specific psychological determinants that dictate the health-seeking behavior of patients with all sorts of chronic illnesses also determine the health-seeking behavior in IBS.

In the normal mind–body relationship, depression and anxiety can elicit gastrointestinal symptoms that resemble IBS. This normal cause-and-effect relationship makes

use of normal physiologic mechanisms. It does not signify gastrointestinal disease and responds best to treatment of the cause.

Many drugs used in modern psychiatry act on neurotransmitter mechanisms in the brain that also operate in the enteric nervous system. Thus unexplained gastrointestinal symptoms could possibly represent the effects of drugs used to treat emotional and mental disorders.

Management

THE DOCTOR–PATIENT RELATIONSHIP

How does the physician, ethically compelled to explain the pathophysiology of disease to patients, explain IBS? Obviously, when an understood cause of the IBS symptoms is discovered, in the form of a trigger point in the abdominal wall for example, the diagnosis is no longer IBS, and a pathogenesis can be readily explained. In the case of IBS, however, the best that can be done is a general attribution of the symptoms to nerve trouble. Some patients, not accepting uncertainty or confessions of ignorance in their physicians, may seek others who may seem more certain they know the truth. This makes for a problematical clinical relationship for which there is no easy solution.

DIETARY ADVICE

Dietary changes should form the mainstay of therapy because they are effective and harmless. This constitutes essentially symptomatic therapy. The commonsense advice to avoid specific foods that worsen symptoms and to eat three balanced meals daily may be necessary for those who have unorthodox patterns of eating. When diarrhea is dominant, advice to curtail or eliminate high-fructose beverages and foods (essentially all soft drinks and many so-called *diet* foods) seems reasonable because the intake of large amounts of fructose produces symptoms in normal people. The same can be said of foods prepared as low-calorie sweets for diabetic patients and persons trying to lose weight.

Bulking agents help those with unexplained constipation; they make for normal patterns of defecation

CURRENT DIAGNOSIS

- Exclusion of all disorders capable of producing the symptoms, especially
    Gastrointestinal disorders
    Neurologic disorders
    Psychological disorders
- Such exclusion requires
    A complete and thoughtful history
    A complete and thoughtful physical examination
    Normal results of the tests justified by the
        history and physical examination

Rakel and Bope: *Conn's Current Therapy 2006.*

CURRENT THERAPY

- Admission of ignorance as to pathophysiology
- Reassurance as to the absence of serious disease
- Dietary therapy: avoidance of foods recognized to exacerbate symptoms
- Bulking agents to regularize defecation

in general. Ordinary dietary food fiber may not be enough, and bran supplementation is difficult to make wholly palatable. The many preparations of psyllium seed offer good therapy in the treatment of IBS in which defecatory disturbances, both diarrhea and constipation, are troublesome. The dosage can be increased gradually until the desired effect is achieved. The addition of a small daily dosage of milk of magnesia can soften hard stools with fiber supplementation when that remains a problem.

ANTIDIARRHEAL AGENTS AND ANTICHOLINERGICS

The synthetic nonabsorbed opioid loperamide (Imodium) can control diarrhea temporarily, but its long-term use requires a particularly thorough search for organic disease first. The addition of bulking agents also can facilitate the treatment of chronic diarrhea.

Preparations of anticholinergic agents have been used in IBS for more than a century for the temporary suppression of abdominal cramps or colicky pain. The side effects of such agents make their chronic administration in IBS unwise.

NEW DRUGS

Some advocates currently promote new agents directed to the neural 5-HT3 and 5-HT4 receptors for serotonin to treat IBS. Their utility remains untested in practice, and because the pathogenesis of IBS remains unknown, there is no logic in their use. Experience to date indicates that alosetron, a 5-HT3 antagonist, carries some risk of potentially fatal side effects.

REFERENCES*

Azpiroz F: Gastrointestinal perception: Pathophysiological implications. Neurogastroenterol Motil 2002;14:229-239.
Azpiroz F: Hypersensitivity in functional gastrointestinal disorders. Gut 2002;51(Suppl I):i25-i28.
Christensen J: Defining the irritable bowel syndrome. Perspect Biol Med 1994;38:21-35.
Gregersen H, Kassab GS: Biomechanics of the gastrointestinal tract. Neurogastroenterol Motil 1996;8:277-297.
Thompson WG, Longstreth GF, Drossman DA, Heaton KW: Functional bowel disorders and functional abdominal pain. Gut 1999;45(Suppl II):II43-II47.

*The sheer number of publications on the subject every year attests to the absence of agreement on the subject. The references listed here only begin to indicate the many trends in thought in the past, including the troubled history of the most recent, that of gastrointestinal hypersensitivity. This latter concept is related to the biomechanics of the gut, a subject treated in one article cited here from 1996 but still widely ignored.

Hemorrhoids, Anal Fissure, Anorectal Abscess, and Fistula

Method of
Matthew D. Vrees, MD, and Eric G. Weiss, MD

The anal canal is a site of diverse pathology. Benign diseases arising from the anal canal are typically easy to diagnose, but the reluctance by many physicians to thoroughly examine the area and the embarrassment on the part of the patient often lead to late diagnosis and considerable, unnecessary discomfort. The anal canal begins at the level of the puborectalis muscle and ends distally at the anal ectoderm or skin. The length of the anal canal is 3 to 4 cm in length. It consists of a sphincter muscle complex, multiple types of mucosa rich in sensory fibers, and anal glands; vascular cushions known as *hemorrhoids* can all be sites of benign anorectal conditions.

History

Patients routinely blame any problem in the anorectal area as hemorrhoids. A focused history with directed questions in regard to the duration of symptoms, the presence or absence of pain, bleeding, or discharge can indicate the exact pathology prior to any examination in the vast majority of patients. Always keep in mind that any complaints in the anorectal area may be secondary to a more proximal gastrointestinal problem, and it is imperative to inquire about changes in bowel habits and whether the patient has had a recent sigmoidoscopic or colonoscopic examination.

PHYSICAL EXAMINATION

Examination of the perianal area, the anus, and the distal rectum requires good lighting, appropriate equipment, and a cooperative patient. The best position to examine the patient is in the prone-jackknife or the left lateral–decubitus position. The first part of this examination is a complete inspection of the perianal region. This part of the examination is often overlooked, but it is crucial to making the appropriate diagnosis. The examiner should be looking for skin tags, erythema, fluctuant masses, tenderness, scars, and tears of the tissue. The next part of the examination is the digital rectal examination. Because many patients present with pain in the anal area, reassurance is imperative. The digital examination allows for estimation of sphincter tone, the detection of a low rectal or anal carcinoma, diagnosis of an abscess, and assessment of pain. After the digital exam is complete, anoscopy should be performed, which is the best maneuver for visualization of internal hemorrhoids. Although second- and third-degree hemorrhoids are easily observed, first-degree hemorrhoids may require a Valsalva maneuver to reproduce. Other tests such as rigid or flexible sigmoidoscopy, colonoscopy, barium enema, or defecography should be performed on a patient-to-patient basis.

Hemorrhoids

Hemorrhoids are submucosal cushions of tissue made up of arterial and venous plexuses, a rich supply of nerves, smooth muscle, and connective tissue that lie above and below the dentate line of the anal canal. Hemorrhoids are a normal component of the anal canal and are typically located in the right-anterolateral, right-posterolateral, and left lateral position. Although many variations exist, the hemorrhoids most commonly receive their blood supply from both a systemic (internal iliac) and mesenteric (inferior mesenteric) arterial supply, allowing for a potential portosystemic shunt.

CLASSIFICATIONS

Hemorrhoids are divided into two categories: internal and external. Internal hemorrhoids arise above the dentate line, are covered by transitional or columnar epithelium, and are classified based on the degree of prolapse. External hemorrhoids arise distal to the dentate line and are covered by anoderm, opposed to skin tags, which are covered by true squamous cell epithelium.

SYMPTOMS

Bleeding is the most common symptom associated with internal hemorrhoids. The bleeding is episodic and described as bright red blood seen either on the toilet tissue or in the toilet bowel after an otherwise normal bowel movement. The blood may or may not be mixed with stool, found just on the toilet paper, or of a larger quantity. If these symptoms are ignored long enough, the patient may present with severe anemia. Prolapse or protrusion of the hemorrhoidal tissue produces a feeling of pressure or a mass in the anal canal. Patients may also complain of moisture or irritation from the mucus produced by the hemorrhoidal mucosa residing outside the anal canal. Internal hemorrhoids are not painful unless they are unable to be reduced and thrombosis sets in.

Complaints from external hemorrhoids range from acute to chronic symptoms. The most typical presentation is during the acute phase of thrombosis, which is associated with severe pain and a hard nodule. If patients do not seek medical attention quickly, the symptoms may resolve on their own when the overlying anoderm sloughs and the clot is evacuated. At this time some bleeding may be observed. Healing following resolution of a thrombosed hemorrhoid may lead to the development of anal skin tags. Except in rare cases of dermatitis, the significance of these skin appendages are limited to cosmesis and hygiene.

TREATMENT

The initial treatment for all patients with nonthrombosed hemorrhoids should be an increase in noncaffeinated beverages and the addition of a bulking agent (fiber) to help reach a goal of 25 to 30 grams of fiber a day. If patients complain of mild discomfort, soaking the perineal region in warm water known as sitz baths may bring relief. Some patients find treatment with hydrocortisone suppositories efficacious for symptomatic relief, but long use of any product containing steroids may contribute to the risk of fungal infections.

If conservative treatment fails, one of the office-based therapies is employed. Regardless of which therapy is chosen, they all shrink the hemorrhoids and fix them back into the anal canal by scarring. Rubber band ligation is one of the most frequently used methods in the United States. This procedure is indicated for first-, second-, and selected third-degree internal hemorrhoids that are a continued source of bleeding. This method of treatment is only indicated for internal hemorrhoids and care must be taken to place the band well above the dentate line to minimize discomfort. Complications of the procedure are uncommon but include pain, bleeding, and urinary retention. Bleeding may occur 5 to 7 days after the procedure when the banded hemorrhoid sloughs; to minimize this risk patients should avoid any anticoagulation or antiplatelet medication for 1 week. Pelvic sepsis, although very rare, has been reported and must be considered when pain and urinary retention are associated with fever. In this setting patients should undergo an examination under anesthesia.

Infrared photocoagulation and sclerotherapy are two other methods of obliterating hemorrhoidal tissue. Both of these methods are much more costly than rubber band ligation and have not been shown to be superior. One advantage of sclerotherapy is its potential use in patients who require antiplatelet and anticoagulation medicine. Unfortunately it is associated with a higher incidence of oleomas and abscesses.

The procedure for prolapsing hemorrhoids (PPHs), otherwise referred to as a stapled hemorrhoidectomy, was first described by Longo in 1998 and is a revolutionary approach to the treatment of third-degree hemorrhoids as well as second-degree hemorrhoids that have failed rubber band ligation. The PPH procedure, unlike standard hemorrhoidectomy, does not remove the hemorrhoidal tissue. Instead, a circular stapling device divides the hemorrhoidal blood supply and in the process restores the hemorrhoidal bundles to their normal physiologic position. This procedure was criticized by some for its expense and early complications but has since been shown to be as safe and associated with much less pain than a surgical hemorrhoidectomy. Because the PPH does not remove the hemorrhoidal bundles, it does not remove the external hemorrhoids.

Surgical hemorrhoidectomy should be reserved for patients who present with acutely thrombosed external hemorrhoids, thrombosed prolapsed internal hemorrhoids, and third- and fourth-degree internal hemorrhoids with a significant external hemorrhoidal component. If patients present with an acutely thrombosed–external hemorrhoid, excision in the office with local anesthesia is the preferred treatment. Excision with alleviate the associated pain immediately and eliminate the risk of recurrence. We do not recommend

The Digestive System

treatment by incision and drainage because of the risk of recurrence, infection of the retained clot, and almost certain development of an unsightly skin tag.

The treatment of acutely prolapsed and thrombosed internal hemorrhoids or second-degree hemorrhoids with large external components are best approached in the operating room with systemic anesthesia. In the closed technique described by Ferguson, the hemorrhoid tissue is excised taking great care to visualize and preserve the internal and external sphincter fibers as well as to maintain sufficient intact anoderm between each hemorrhoidal bundle to avoid anal stenosis. Although excisional hemorrhoidectomy achieves a better success rate than any other form of treatment, it is associated with severe pain that usually leaves the patient severely uncomfortable for 2 to 3 weeks.

Anal Fissure

An acute anal fissure is a split in the anoderm of the anal canal. The vast majority of anal fissures are in the posterior and anterior midline, 83% and 16% respectively. Chronic anal fissures are the result of nonhealing. There is a full thickness defect in the anoderm with exposed muscle fibers, a hypertrophied internal papilla at its base, and an associated perianal skin tag.

Anal fissures typically occur after passage of a hard bowel movement that is thought to be because of a traumatic tear of the anal skin. Among theories behind the anterior/posterior location of most fissures, there is inherent weakness in the sphincter muscles resulting in increased distribution of force in these locations. Others postulate that because the anterior and posterior skin is tethered to the sphincters, it is unable to evert with bowel movements, creating tension and potential tearing. Lastly, elevated anal canal pressure along with the lateral course of the blood supply to the anal canal may result in decreased blood flow and possible ischemia to the anoderm. Physiologic tests in patients with anal fissures have demonstrated higher-than-normal internal anal sphincter muscle pressures with postrelaxation pressures exceeding resting tone and known as an overshoot phenomena. When fissures are found in atypical positions, pathologic fissures from tumors, Crohn's disease, infectious etiologies, or states of immunodeficiency can be suspected.

Patients presenting with a fissure classically report excruciating pain on defecation with blood found on the toilet paper. Following defecation the patient complains of a dull ache or spasm in the anal canal of significant intensity that usually resolves within a few hours. Rarely do patients complain of any significant bleeding.

The diagnosis of a fissure is made by spreading the patient's buttocks and examining the distal anal canal. If the fissures appear as small tears in the anoderm, no further examination should be performed at this time. If any additional examination is necessary, it should be done in the operating room with sedation or general anesthesia.

Most patients with anal fissures will respond to medical therapy. Medical management consists of sitz bath,

bulking agents, and medications to relax the internal anal sphincter. *Pharmacologic* sphincterotomy can be accomplished with nitroglycerin,[1] diltiazem,[1] or botulism toxin A (Botox).[1] Nitroglycerin ointment (0.2%) and diltiazem ointment (2%) have been shown in nonrandomized and randomized trials to be efficacious in healing anal fissures. Although each medication works through a different mechanism, they accomplish relaxation of the internal anal sphincter, which aids in healing. Nitroglycerin,[1] unlike diltiazem,[1] has been criticized because of the systemic side effects of severe headaches in some patients, which affects compliance. Diltiazem[1] has also been shown to be efficacious in patients who failed treatment with nitroglycerin.[1] Thus, the first line therapy uses the calcium channel blocker diltiazem[1] 2% ointment. The medicine is applied by placing a pea-sized amount of the ointment around the anoderm three times a day for 3 to 6 weeks. Botulinum toxin A (Botox)[1] injection of the sphincter muscle has improved healing rates when compared to the aforementioned agents. However, it is associated with a higher rate of temporary incontinence, pain and expense than topical ointments. We reserve botulinum A (Botox)[1] toxin for patients who have failed treatment with topical ointments and are at high risk of incontinence with surgical intervention.

With the advent of these topical ointments along with dietary modifications, surgical management is usually unnecessary. Surgical management or sphincterotomy is reserved for patients who fail to respond to medical management. Lateral, internal sphincterotomy is the standard surgical technique used. The procedure can be performed on either the right or left side of the sphincter, but the right side avoids the left lateral hemorrhoidal bundle. Before performing a sphincterotomy, the patient should be aware of the possibility of incontinence observed in the early postoperative period (typically to gas) and a long-term incontinence rate, which has been reported in the literature as being between 0% and 13%. Special considerations must be addressed when treating women who have had external sphincter injuries from childbirth trauma and patients with Crohn's disease.

Abscesses and Fistula-in-Ano

Perianal or perirectal abscesses are the result of obstruction of the glands in the anal canal. The glands can extend into the submucosa, internal sphincter, and the intersphincteric plane, hence abscesses can form in multiple anatomic locations. If the tract from which the abscess originates does not close, a fistula-in-ano will exist.

Abscesses are classified by their location. The most common location is the perianal region followed by the ischiorectal, intersphincteric space and least commonly the supralevator region. The horseshoe abscess is rare but important to recognize when it occurs. It is thought to originate as a posterior intersphincteric abscess, which then spreads to the ischiorectal and supralevator spaces.

[1]Not FDA approved for this indication.

CURRENT DIAGNOSIS

- Obtain detailed history of present illness including presence of incontinence
- Obtain obstetrical history in women and inquire about traumatic births and episiotomies
- Obtain family history of inflammatory bowel disease
- Use good lighting, which is imperative to differentiate pathology
- Refrain from digital rectal exam or anoscopy without anesthesia if severe pain is associated with the problem
- Remember that unless hemorrhoids are acutely thrombosed, they are not associated with pain
- Observe whether prolapsing tissue from anal canal is a polyp or a tumor
- Utilize colonoscopy prior to any surgical intervention, and do not be fooled by a more proximal bleeding source

 CURRENT THERAPY

- Increase fiber in the diet with supplements to approach 25g/day
- Drain all abscesses
- Attempt conservative, dietary therapy of hemorrhoids prior to surgical therapy
- Individualize surgical therapy of hemorrhoids on the patient's complaints and degree of prolapse
- Attempt medical (topical) treatment of fissures prior to considering surgery
- Avoid internal and external sphincter injury to maintain continence regardless of the anal disease
- Consider the presence of inflammatory bowel disease or a malignancy when healing is slower than expected

The patient presents with pain in the area of the abscess associated in some cases with fevers. Examination of the area will reveal an erythematous, swollen, tender mass with perianal and ischiorectal abscesses. Intersphincteric abscesses have no changes to the skin of the perineum but are associated with exquisite tenderness on digital rectal exam. When suspected, endorectal ultrasound or computed tomography (CT) can be used to diagnose these complex abscesses, but one should have a low threshold to examine the patient under anesthesia to diagnose and treat the problem.

The treatment of any abscess requires drainage regardless of the location. Drainage should be performed rapidly to minimize the risk of sepsis and necrotizing soft tissue infections. Adequate drainage requires that the cavity must not close prematurely. Prevention of early skin closure can be accomplished by packing the cavity with gauze or placing an appropriately sized mushroom catheter and securing it to the skin with a simple suture, eliminating the need for postoperative dressing care. Postdrainage use of antibiotics should be reserved for patients with cellulitis of the surrounding skin, signs of systemic infection, the presence of a prosthesis, diabetes, or the immunosuppressed.

If the patient has continued or recurrent drainage a fistula may exist. A fistula is an abnormal tract with the internal opening in the anal canal or distal rectum and the external opening in the skin. Fistulas are classified by the path they take in regard to the anal sphincter muscles. Maintaining the integrity of the sphincter muscles and preserving fecal continence is essential when dealing with a fistula that traverses the sphincter. Even the smallest division of the internal or external sphincter muscle in certain patients (typically women who have had vaginal deliveries) may result in incontinence. Physical examination cannot always assess the level of the fistula, and ancillary tests such as endorectal ultrasound with the use of hydrogen peroxide or magnetic resonance imaging (MRI) can be helpful. If a fistulotomy is unsafe, the treatment options include a cutting seton or a noncutting seton followed by injection of fibrin glue or an endorectal advancement flap. Although these procedures preserve sphincter function, the success rate ranges from 50% to 80%, and the patient must be educated that resolution may require multiple operations. If a patient with Crohn's disease presents with a fistula or perianal Crohn's disease, medical management, including the use of infliximab (Remicade), is instrumental. If perianal sepsis is uncontrollable in a patient with Crohn's disease, fecal diversion or a proctectomy may be required.

REFERENCES

Ambrose NS, Hares MM, Alexander-Williams J: Prospective randomized comparison of photocoagulation and rubber band ligation in treatment of hemorrhoids. BMJ 1983;286:1389-1391.

Buls JG, Goldberg SM: Modern management of hemorrhoids. Surg Clin North Am 1978;58:469.

Gamalainen KP, Sainio AP: Incidence of fistulas after drainage of acute anorectal abscesses. Dis Colon Rectum 1998;41:1357-1361.

Gorfine S: Treatment of benign anal diseases with topical nitroglycerin. Dis Colon Rectum 1995;48:453-456.

Ho YH, Tan M, Chui CH: Randomized controlled trial of primary fistulotomy with drainage alone for perianal abscesses. Dis Colon Rectum 1997;40:1435-1438.

Jost WH, Schimrigk K: Use of botulinum toxin in anal fissure. Dis Colon Rectum 1993;36:974.

Lund JN, Scholefield JH: A randomized prospective, double-blind, placebo controlled trial of glycerol trinitrate ointment in the treatment of anal fissure. Lancet 1997;349:11-14.

Nelson R: Meta-analysis of operative techniques for fissure in ano. Dis Colon Rectum 1999;42:1424-1428.

Saheer S, Reilly WT, Pemberton Jh, Ilstrup D: Urinary retention after operations for benign anorectal diseases. Dis Colon Rectum 1998;41:696-704.

Senagore AJ: A prospective, randomized, controlled multicenter trial comparing stapled hemorrhoidectomy and Ferguson hemorrhoidectomy: Perioperative and one year results. Dis Colon Rectum 2004;47:1824-1836.

Topical diltiazem ointment in the treatment of chronic anal fissures. Br J Surg 2001;88:553-556.

Rakel and Bope: *Conn's Current Therapy 2006.*

Gastritis and Peptic Ulcer Disease

Method of
Barry J. Marshall, MD

Gastritis

Gastritis literally means inflammation of the stomach. Gastritis is a nonspecific term because it can be used to describe:

- Symptoms related to the stomach
- An endoscopic appearance of the gastric mucosa
- Histologic change characterized by infiltration of the epithelium with inflammatory cells such as polymorphonuclear leukocytes (PMNs)

The last description is the most correct.

CLINICAL GASTRITIS

In lay terms, nausea and vomiting with epigastric pain might be called "an attack of gastritis," even though the exact pathology affecting the stomach is unknown. Use of the term gastritis in this situation is to be discouraged as symptoms correlate rather poorly with actual pathology present in the stomach.

ENDOSCOPIC GASTRITIS

Mucosal Redness (Erythema)

The appearance of the mucosa at endoscopy does not correlate well with the histologic diagnosis determined from a biopsy. Confusion can arise because almost every abnormality of the gastric mucosa is called gastritis by endoscopists.

The normal color of the gastric mucosa is pink, similar to the palm of your hand. An appearance of redness probably represents increased capillary blood flow in the mucosa, but does not necessarily mean that inflammatory cells are present. When bile is present, the redness often appears to be diffusely present throughout the stomach.

Redness (erythema) in the gastric mucosa may be localized to the antrum or the corpus. It may be homogeneous or mottled, or present in spots from petechia size to a few millimeters. Sometimes redness is present on the top of the gastric folds of the corpus. Often, red streaks radiate upward from the pylorus. In all cases it is appropriate for the endoscopist to refer to the appearance as *endoscopic gastritis*, accompanied by a description of gastric mucosa. General treatment of endoscopic gastritis is to treat the patient's symptoms, usually with acid reduction therapy and avoidance of foods or medications that might aggravate the problem. Specific treatment of endoscopic gastritis depends on a histologic

diagnosis. Therefore, biopsies of the gastric mucosa are necessary.

Surface Irregularity (Chicken Skin, Gooseflesh, Cobblestones)

The cause of small lumps on the antral mucosa, which are referred to as *chicken skin*, *gooseflesh*, and *cobblestones*, is usually *Helicobacter pylori* gastritis.

Erosive Gastritis

Erosions are breaks in the mucosa that do not extend beyond the muscularis mucosa. All lesions less than 1 mm deep are erosions. The distinction between ulcers and erosions might not have much effect on patient management, because both can bleed and both are usually healed with acid blocking therapy.

Umbilicated lumps may be a variant of erosive gastritis. As with all erosive mucosal lesions of the gastrointestinal (GI) tract, viral causes should be considered in immunosuppressed patients.

Atrophic Gastritis and Gastric Atrophy

After many years of chronic gastritis, the gastric mucosa can become atrophic (i.e., thin and translucent), with the submucosal veins easily visible. In severe cases, the folds normally present in the upper half of the stomach (the corpus) are diminished or absent (gastric atrophy). Acid secretion diminishes and the condition predisposes to adenocarcinoma of the stomach. *H. pylori* and pernicious anemia are the two main causes.

Hypertrophic Gastritis (Ménétrier's Disease)

Rarely, gastric folds are massively increased in size because of hyperplasia and hypertrophy of the specialized acid-secreting mucosa. Excessive mucus secretion leads to a syndrome of hypoalbuminemia with diarrhea, edema, or a hypercoagulable state. *H. pylori* infection is one cause, other causes are idiopathic (so far).

Portal Gastropathy and Angiodysplasia

The red lesions caused by portal gastropathy and angiodysplasia give a pattern of *snake skin* and *watermelon stomach*, respectively, when severe. They may cause GI blood loss, but are usually asymptomatic. The former is associated with portal hypertension. The latter is idiopathic and is treated, when necessary, with argon plasma coagulation.

HISTOLOGIC GASTRITIS

Histologic gastritis is present when inflammatory cells infiltrate the mucosa. Diagnostic biopsies for detection of gastritis should be taken from intact mucosa, away from any focal lesion. At least one antrum and one corpus biopsy should be examined by histology because diseases can selectively affect only the mucus-secreting mucosa of the antrum, or only the parietal cell mucosa of the corpus.

Rakel and Bope: *Conn's Current Therapy 2006*.

If mononuclear cells are increased, chronic gastritis is present. If the PMNs are also increased, the gastritis is termed as active. In typical *H. pylori* infection, PMNs infiltrate the necks of the mucus-secreting glands of the gastric antrum causing active chronic gastritis.

Helicobacter pylori Gastritis

In the first week after infection, many PMNs and a few eosinophils infiltrate the mucosa. These are gradually replaced with the mononuclear cells. The presence of lymphoid follicles is called mucosa-associated lymphoid tissue (MALT). Rarely, MALT may become autonomous to form a low-grade, B-cell lymphoma called MALT lymphoma. When gastric tissue exists in the duodenal bulb (normally present in approximately 60% of persons), *H. pylori* may also colonize that location leading to active duodenitis.

When *H. pylori* is eradicated with antibiotics, PMNs disappear in a week or so, but reduction in the mononuclear cells is slow, often leaving mild chronic gastritis several years after *H. pylori* has disappeared.

In most countries with a high prevalence of *H. pylori*, gastric cancer is common, although diet probably also modulates the risk so that the association is not universal. Because *H. pylori* causes peptic ulcer and gastric cancer, nearly everyone with *H. pylori* chooses to be treated with antibiotics.

Non-*Helicobacter pylori* Gastritis

Because *H. pylori* is the most common cause of gastritis, and perhaps the most easily treated, non-*H. pylori* gastritis must be diagnosed with caution. Usually the *H. pylori* has been missed because of low numbers of organisms. This occurs when patients have recently taken antibiotics, or are taking proton pump inhibitors (PPIs), or have a patchy infection caused by intestinal metaplasia in the stomach (to which *H. pylori* cannot adhere). Therefore, as well as taking biopsies for urease test, histology, and culture, the physician should check serology before claiming a patient has *H. pylori*-negative histologic gastritis. Laboratory-based serologic tests are quite sensitive so can be used to confirm that *H. pylori* is not present and that the negative biopsy diagnosis is correct.

Rare causes of *H. pylori*-negative histologic gastritis are Crohn's disease, eosinophilic gastritis, gastric MALT lymphoma, as well as (very rarely) other viral and bacterial infections.

NONSTEROIDAL-INDUCED EROSIVE GASTRITIS AND ULCERS

Aspirin and nonsteroidal anti-inflammatory drugs (NSAIDs) are corrosive. Aspirin and NSAIDs inhibit prostaglandin synthesis, which is essential for maintenance of the mucus and bicarbonate barrier in the stomach. The resulting gastric erosions are often asymptomatic but sometimes lead to gastric ulcer or duodenal ulcer.

The harmful effects of NSAIDs and *H. pylori* are not synergistic because *H. pylori* boosts the prostaglandin levels, thus partially negating the deleterious effect of the NSAID.

Eradication of *H. pylori* before or at the beginning of NSAID therapy is worthwhile. Once NSAID patients have developed an ulcer, provided that treatment of the ulcer with a PPI is continued, eradication of *H. pylori* is neither urgent nor essential.

DYSPEPSIA VERSUS GASTRITIS

Dyspepsia is defined here as discomfort in the upper half of the abdomen and lower chest that is somehow related to food. Symptoms and descriptions vary widely so the patient's ethnicity needs to be taken into account when taking a history.

Regurgitation refers to reflux of gastric contents into the mouth without discomfort. Gnawing is a feeling halfway between hunger and nausea, in which case the patient tends to have small snacks to ease the symptom without vomiting. Fullness and bloating are feelings of distension that contribute to early satiety in some patients so that they are unable to finish a normal-sized meal. Burning epigastric and lower thoracic pain that is quickly relieved by antacid is likely to be caused by gastroesophageal reflux disease (GERD), although it is wise to exclude a cardiac cause.

In general, dyspepsia correlates poorly with endoscopic findings. When endoscopy is freely available at no cost to the patient, endoscopy quickly defines a management plan and gives greater patient satisfaction, according to questionnaires given to patients 12 months later. However, endoscopy-first strategies are about 20% more expensive.

The alternative strategy is called test and treat, where patients are selected for initial endoscopy only if they have alarm signs, are older than 50 years of age, or are in a high-risk category for gastric cancer. Alarm signs are dysphagia, vomiting, weight loss, blood in the stool, a family history of gastric cancer, an abdominal mass, or virtually any abnormal laboratory test.

When dyspepsia is diagnosed but there is no peptic ulcer, the condition is called nonulcer dyspepsia (NUD) or functional dyspepsia. Many NUD patients actually have GERD. If GERD is suspected, a 7-day trial of double-dose PPI therapy is worthwhile.

For patients not obviously suffering from GERD, the possibility of peptic ulcer should be considered. Because most peptic ulcers are related to *H. pylori* infection, noninvasive tests for *H. pylori* can be used to determine ulcer risk. Patients who are *H. pylori*-negative on serology are unlikely to have peptic ulcer. This means that they can be managed by trial and error until symptoms respond to therapy. On the other hand, patients who are *H. pylori*-positive on serology should be regarded as possible ulcer candidates and should have the bacterium eradicated as the first step in management.

For patients who actually do have an ulcer, antibiotic therapy for *H. pylori* leads to clinical cure in approximately 70% of cases. Of the 30% who do not respond clinically, 50% have persistent *H. pylori* and the remainder have *H. pylori*-negative dyspepsia (GERD, etc.). To differentiate these groups it is necessary to confirm cure of *H. pylori* in all patients who do not completely respond to *H. pylori* eradication. Cure is confirmed with a urea breath test. Follow-up breath test is also necessary in all patients with known peptic ulcer because these patients are at risk of ulcer relapse, with all its possible complications, if *H. pylori* persists. Because a nonendoscopic strategy does not separate ulcer from nonulcer patients at the beginning, there is a case for confirmation of *H. pylori* eradication in all patients, so that ulcer relapse never occurs.

GASTROESOPHAGEAL REFLUX DISEASE

Gastroesophageal reflux disease and symptoms related to the esophagus may be treated initially with acid reduction therapy, as needed. Antacid is used for immediate relief, and histamine-$_2$ receptor antagonists (H$_2$RAs) or PPIs may be given at the same time to diminish acid secretion over the next few hours. Combinations of these two are available as over-the-counter (OTC) medications in the United States. If dysphagia is present (difficulty swallowing), immediate endoscopy is advised, as this could be an early symptom of esophageal cancer or an acid-induced stricture.

If GERD symptoms do not completely respond, or if the patient requires the above treatment on a daily basis, then endoscopy is required. Endoscopy will indicate whether the patient's symptoms correlate with the disease severity. It is important to control both clinical and endoscopic GERD, because continued heartburn raises the lifetime risk of esophageal adenocarcinoma.

GERD patients should be given the following commonsense advice. Eat smaller meals, control obesity, and avoid tight clothing around the abdomen. Avoid liquids with meals, especially tea, coffee, colas, and beer. Do not eat large meals during the working day. Avoid bending or heavy work after meals. Eat the evening meal at least 3 hours before bedtime. Raise the head of the bed and sleep on the left side. Tablets that might damage the esophagus (aspirin, doxycycline, alendronate) should be taken before meals to ensure that they do not linger in the esophagus.

In spite of the above management, many patients continue to have symptoms, and endoscopic assessment reveals acid-induced esophageal damage. In this case lifestyle measures are rarely curative and long-term acid reduction with PPI is required. Since PPIs have long half-lives, once-daily therapy is usually sufficient. For severe GERD, start at double the usual dose then decrease after 3 months to a single daily maintenance dose. The aim of medical therapy is complete control of acidic symptoms. Advise patients that long-term medical treatment is usually necessary.

OTHER DYSPEPSIA

Because chronic dyspeptic symptoms unrelated to GERD or ulcer do not have a specific cause or defined therapy, it is worthwhile initially to search for another, more treatable diagnosis. Be certain to exclude cardiac causes of chest pain. Intermittent pain could be esophageal spasm, which can be diagnosed with esophageal manometry. Treat with PPI to abolish any GERD component, smooth muscle relaxants for the acute episode, and calcium channel blockers (CCBs). Note that therapy for angina is quite similar, so cardiac disease needs to be ruled out before treating esophageal spasm. Some of the above medical therapy causes side effects that make treatment hardly worthwhile in patients with intermittent spasm.

EPIGASTRIC DYSPEPSIA AND GASTROPARESIS

Always try to find the definitive causes of epigastric dyspepsia and gastroparesis, as this allows better planning of therapy and more accurate prognosis. Endoscopy often rules out any macroscopic lesion such as an ulcer or a tumor, allowing trials of medical therapy to proceed.

If the patient has symptoms of GERD, but does not respond completely to therapy, he/she may be a rapid metabolizer of PPI. If starting with once-daily omeprazole (Prilosec), double the dose to twice daily, use a more powerful drug (esomeprazole [Nexium]), choose one with a longer half-life (pantoprazole [Protonix]), or use a drug that is less affected by metabolizer status (rabeprazole [AcipHex]). At endoscopy, avoid PPI on the day of the test and measure gastric-juice pH to see if the patient maintains a pH above 4 for the complete 24 hours after a dose. If pH is above 4.0, then the cause of the continued symptoms might not be acid reflux.

Symptoms of nausea and/or vomiting are unlikely to be caused by esophageal disease. Gastric mucosal problems or gastric outlet obstruction need to be considered. The two should be considered separately because disorders such as acute viral gastroenteritis and food poisoning cause nausea, but motility is normal. Similarly, patients with chronic gastroparesis are worse off if they also have a mucosal disease such as *H. pylori* causing the nausea.

If *H. pylori* is present it should be treated. If patients cannot take antibiotics because of nausea, try to settle them with high-dose PPI as this will suppress *H. pylori* in 50% of cases.

Delayed gastric emptying (gastroparesis) may be diagnosed with an isotope gastric emptying study. When present, gastroparesis is usually a chronic disorder with relapses and remissions. Eradication of *H. pylori* often decreases nausea and settles the condition somewhat, but relapses still occur in most patients. Promotility agents such as metoclopramide (Reglan) and cisapride (Propulsid)* should be used (cisapride is no longer available in the United States because it has caused fatal arrhythmias). Small doses of erythromycin[1] (25 mg per day before meals) may improve gastric peristalsis as this drug is a motilin agonist. As long as obstruction is not present, a soft or liquid diet will usually empty from

---

*Investigational drug in the United States.
[1]Not FDA approved for this indication.

the stomach, even when motility is poor. Posturing the patient to stay vertical after meals, with an inclination toward the right side, should help gastric contents drain through the pylorus. Avoid uncooked vegetables because skins and salad leaves take many hours to leave the stomach. A low-residue diet is preferred whenever motility is impaired.

Management of Dyspepsia

I usually include a *test and treat* strategy for *H. pylori* as part of any dyspepsia management plan. I also search for and treat GERD with PPI. Lesser symptoms of GERD or vague dyspepsia may respond (if needed) to H_2 blocker such as ranitidine (Zantac), 150 mg once or twice daily. In addition, patients can carry antacid tablets for immediate relief. Antacid-H_2RA combinations are available OTC in the United States, and these are very effective. The complete algorithm for management of dyspepsia is shown as Figure 1.

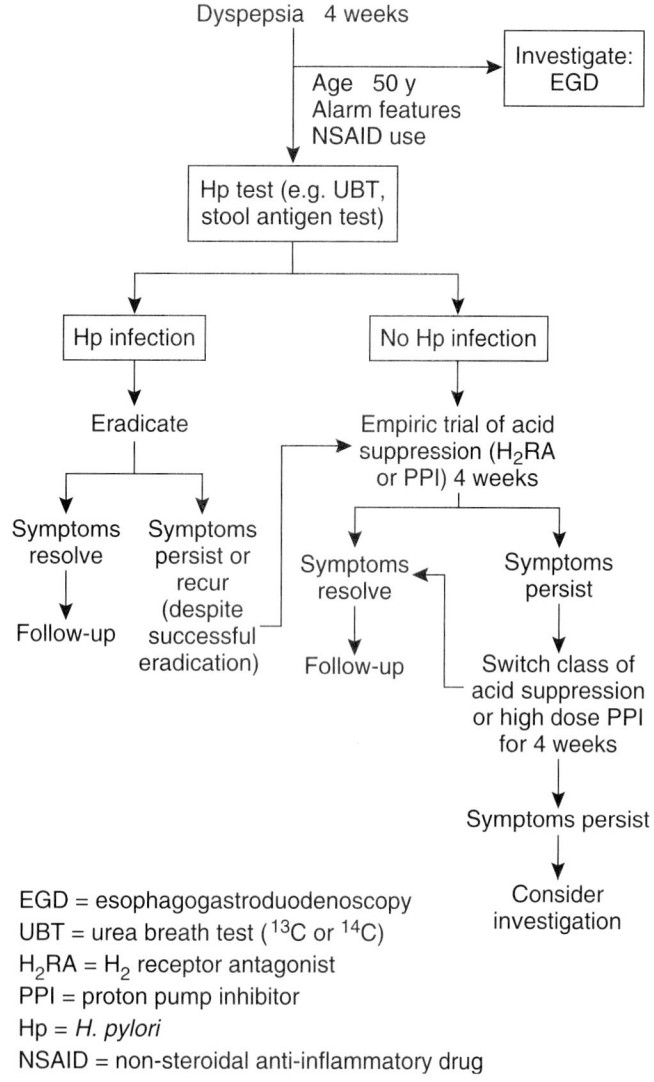

EGD = esophagogastroduodenoscopy
UBT = urea breath test (^{13}C or ^{14}C)
H_2RA = H_2 receptor antagonist
PPI = proton pump inhibitor
Hp = *H. pylori*
NSAID = non-steroidal anti-inflammatory drug

FIGURE 1. Management of uninvestigated dyspepsia.

Peptic Ulcer

Peptic ulcer is usually caused by *H. pylori*, NSAIDs, or a combination of the two. Rarely, hyperacidity is caused by a gastrinoma (Zollinger-Ellison syndrome) in which case a cause may not be found until serum gastrin is noted to be elevated. In any ulcer situation, resuscitate the patient and control acute bleeding endoscopically. At the first endoscopy, diagnostic biopsies should be taken for *H. pylori* (one urease test, one antrum, and one corpus for histology). If *H. pylori* is present, initiate treatment. *H. pylori* serology should be sent if the bacterium is not detected on biopsy because sometimes the acutely ill patient has taken medication, which suppresses *H. pylori* in the gastric mucosa, but has not eradicated the bacterium.

Ulcer patients without *H. pylori* usually have NSAIDs as the cause of the ulcer. In patients who have both *H. pylori* and NSAIDs, the sensible approach is to treat both. In most cases the NSAIDs will have been ceased and the patient given intravenous PPI, so antibiotic therapy is not the most important part of the acute therapy. Adding intravenous amoxicillin to an *H. pylori*-positive patient is an option to improve the healing rate of a dangerous ulcer. The normal oral *H. pylori* therapy can be completed a few days later when the patient tolerates a normal diet.

Peptic ulcers almost always heal once the initiating factor has been removed. However, it is usual to give H_2RA or PPI for 8 weeks to ensure a symptom-free healing period. During this time the *H. pylori* can be eradicated. At the end of 8 weeks, PPI can be changed to H_2RA, and a follow-up urea breath test can be done to confirm eradication of the bacterium. A stool antigen test is an alternative.

In patients who are unable to cease their NSAIDs, the drug should be changed to a cyclooxygenase (COX)-2 selective agent. In addition, full-dose PPI should be continued long term. Most ulcers will then heal and not relapse. Low-dose aspirin may remove the benefit of COX-2 selective NSAIDs so the relative benefits of aspirin should be reviewed in all patients. Prostaglandins are not a first choice ulcer therapy because of side effects, such as cramps (in women) and diarrhea; however, they do specifically protect against erosive gastritis and peptic ulcer caused solely by NSAIDs.

TREATMENT FOR *HELICOBACTER PYLORI*

In vitro testing does not correlate with in vivo success, so treatment combinations should be used that have been proven to work in each individual country. Treatment for less than 7 days has a low cure rate, but cure rates from day 7 to day 14 are similar, and more than 14 days of treatment is usually unnecessary. The first drug to use is a PPI in order to render the gastric pH neutral. This enhances the cure rate for the second drug, which is usually amoxicillin (Amoxil). Clarithromycin (Biaxin) is given as the third drug. Treatment and doses vary in each country; doses in Table 1 are typical for the United States and Australia.

TABLE 1 Treatment Options for *Helicobacter pylori*

Group		Duration
A*	**BISMUTH**	
	Ranitidine bismuth citrate[2] (RBC) 400 mg bid	14 days
	Bismuth subsalicylate (Pepto-Bismol)* 525 mg (2 tabs) qid	14 days
	Bismuth subcitrate[1,†] (De-Nol) 120 mg (1 tab) qid	14 days
B	**PENICILLIN**	
	Amoxicillin 1 g bid	7, 10 or 14 days
C	**MACROLIDE**	
	Clarithromycin (Biaxin) 500 mg bid	7, 10 or 14 days
	Josamycin[1,2,†] 1000 mg bid	7 days
D	**NITROIMIDAZOLE**	
	Metronidazole (Flagyl)[1] 500 mg bid or tid	7, 10 or 14 days
	Tinidazole[1,2] 1000 mg qd	7, 10 or 14 days
E	**TETRACYCLINE**	
	Tetracycline[1] 500 mg qid	14 days
F	**QUINOLONE**	
	Ofloxacin (Floxin)[1] 1000 mg[3] qd	7-14 days
	Levofloxacin (Levaquin) 500 mg qd	7-14 days
	Ciprofloxacin (Cipro)[1] 500 mg bid	14 days
G	**NITROFURAN**	
	Furazolidone (Furoxone)[1] 100 mg qid	7, 10 or 14 days
H	**ANSAMYCIN**	
	Rifabutin (Mycobutin)[1] 150 mg bid	14 days
I	Proton pump inhibitors (use double a normal dose)	
	Omeprazole (Prilosec) 20 mg bid	
	Esomeprazole (Nexium) 40 mg bid	
	Lansoprazole (Prevacid) 30 mg bid	
	Pantoprazole (Protonix) 40 mg bid	
	Rabeprazole (AcipHex) 20 mg bid	

[1]Not FDA approved for this indication.
[2]Not available in the United States.
[3]Exceeds dosage recommended by the manufacturer.
*When Pepto-Bismol is not available, substitute De-Nol, 1 tablet qid. RBC is not available in all countries.
Side effects are likely as doses of clarithromycin, metronidazole, and furazolidone increase.
Treatment combination priorities are normally: IBC → IBD → IBEG. For penicillin allergy choose ICD or IAED → IFH.
[†]Investigational drug in the United States.
Abbreviations: bid = twice daily; qd = once daily; qid = four times daily; tid = thrice daily.

One month after completing therapy, ensure that the patient is not taking PPI for 7 days, and then perform a urea breath test (UBT). Serology remains positive after treatment so it is not useful to prove eradication. If the UBT shows persistent infection, re-treat with a different regimen. As a second therapy, you may use PPI and amoxicillin again, since *H. pylori* does not develop resistance to amoxicillin. The third drug should change to metronidazole (Flagyl).[1] Always repeat the UBT after therapy.

If two therapies fail, the *H. pylori* is resistant to both clarithromycin[1] and metronidazole[1]; therefore, alternatives must be chosen. In addition, the motivation of the patient and physician need to be reassessed as compliance may be an issue. A third treatment changes the PPI to a much higher dose and/or a drug less affected by the metabolizer status of the patient.

Rabeprazole (AcipHex), 20 mg twice daily, might be a good choice. Amoxicillin is given as before. In addition, add ofloxacin (Floxin)[1] or levofloxacin (Levaquin)[1] plus rifabutin (Mycobutin),[1] with all four drugs being given for 14 days.

An alternative and inexpensive regimen is bismuth (Pepto-Bismol) with tetracycline,[1] metronidazole (Flagyl),[1] and a PPI. This is also called bismuth quad therapy. It is useful also when patients are allergic to penicillin. Allergic patients might also try PPI with clarithromycin (Biaxin)[1] and metronidazole[1] as the initial therapy. If patients are unable to take oral antibiotics because of nausea, start with a harmless drug such as PPI or bismuth, and then add tetracycline[1] or amoxicillin (Amoxil). After 1 week, by which time symptoms have improved, add the clarithromycin[1] or metronidazole.[1] If all else fails, high-dose PPI will suppress *H. pylori* in 30% to

[1]Not FDA approved for this indication.

[1]Not FDA approved for this indication.

Rakel and Bope: *Conn's Current Therapy 2006*.

50% of patients. Alternatively, because biopsy and culture with antibiotic sensitivity testing are necessary, refer patients to a gastroenterologist specializing in *H. pylori*.

After *H. pylori* eradication, symptoms are still present in most patients, but improve gradually over 3 to 6 months. GERD symptoms may temporarily worsen, so I treat these symptoms with H_2 blockers initially because this does not interfere with the follow-up UBT. If symptoms persist then the patient is managed as *H. pylori*-negative dyspepsia as per the algorithm in Figure 1.

Acute and Chronic Viral Hepatitis

Method of
Fritz-Henry Volmar, MD, and Dilip Moonka, MD

Outbreaks of acute hepatitis and the ever-increasing number of patients diagnosed with chronic liver disease, cirrhosis, and hepatocellular carcinoma continue to fuel interest in the field of viral hepatitis. Viral hepatitis is the leading cause of liver disease. The past decade has yielded significant advances in our understanding of the natural history and molecular biology of the hepatotrophic viruses. Expanding efforts to prevent and treat viral hepatitis have led to the development of effective vaccines and therapies. The current section will focus on these advances as well as identify areas where further progress is necessary.

Hepatitis can be caused by a number of viruses. The overwhelming majority of cases of viral hepatitis are caused by the human hepatotropic viruses designated by the letters A, B, C, D, and E (Table 1). Although each of these can cause acute hepatitis, the hepatitis A virus (HAV) and hepatitis E virus (HEV) infections do so exclusively. The hepatitis B virus (HBV) and the hepatitis C virus (HCV) primarily lead to morbidity in that they cause chronic infection and chronic liver disease.

Less common causes of viral hepatitis include herpes simplex, Epstein-Barr, cytomegalovirus, coxsackie, echovirus, adenovirus, rubella, and the mumps virus. Although these viruses will not be discussed in any detail, they should be included in the differential diagnosis of patients with acute hepatitis especially in those with compromised immune systems. It should also be noted the term hepatitis F was applied to a putative virus that was subsequently shown to be artifact. Hepatitis G virus (HGV) is present in 1% to 2% of the U.S. population but does not clearly cause disease in humans. Its primary distinction is that patients co-infected with HIV and HGV appear to have a more indolent form of the HIV infection.

Acute Hepatitis

All of the five lettered viruses listed previously can cause acute hepatitis, which is generally a self-limited illness. Although the majority of patients remain asymptomatic, those who develop symptoms will often attribute them to a nonspecific viral illness especially if jaundice is absent. The illness is clinically silent in most infected children and is more likely to be symptomatic in the elderly and immunocompromised. Symptomatic patients may complain of fever, malaise, fatigue, anorexia, nausea with or without vomiting, and abdominal discomfort localizing to the right-upper quadrant. Jaundice, if present, may be associated with darkening of the urine or pale stools. These symptoms will typically last several weeks. Rarely, acute hepatitis may lead to severe hepatic dysfunction manifesting as encephalopathy and coagulopathy. Mortality from fulminant hepatic failure is high, and the degree of liver injury may necessitate liver transplantation.

Chronic Hepatitis

Patients who have persistent symptoms or signs of liver disease 6 months after the acute infection are classified as having chronic hepatitis. As mentioned earlier, this is seen with HBV, HCV, as well as HDV. The clinical course of chronic viral hepatitis is highly variable and depends on viral and host factors. Persistent chronic inflammation can result in fibrosis, which can lead to cirrhosis and

TABLE 1 Common Hepatotropic Viruses

	HAV	HBV	HCV	HDV	HEV
Size	27-32 nm	42 nm	55 nm	35 nm	32 nm
Genome	ssRNA	dsDNA	ssRNA	ssRNA	ssRNA
Transmission	Fecal–oral	Percutaneous, sexual	Percutaneous, sexual	Percutaneous, sexual	Fecal–oral
Incubation	15-45 d	60-180 d	15-160 d	21-140 d	15-60 d
Acute infection	Yes	Yes	Yes	Yes	Yes
Chronic liver disease	No	<5% adults, >90% infants	70%-85%	Superinfection ~80%, coinfection <5%	No

Abbreviations: dsDNA = double-stranded DNA; HAV = hepatitis A virus; HBV = hepatitis B virus; HCV = hepatitis C virus; HDV = hepatitis D virus; HEV = hepatitis E virus; ssRNA = single-stranded RNA.

liver failure. Co-infection with HIV or other hepatotropic viruses and other causes of chronic liver disease such as alcohol will hasten the progression to cirrhosis. Cirrhotic patients, in particular, are at risk of developing hepatocellular carcinoma and require surveillance.

Hepatitis A

HAV is the most commonly reported hepatitis virus and does not lead to chronic infection. It is a positive-strand RNA virus. There is only one HAV serotype, which means immunity to all HAV is conferred with vaccination or infection with any HAV virus. HAV is transmitted via the fecal–oral route, and infection often results from contamination of food, water supplies, or seafood such as oysters. Rarely, transmission may occur percutaneously. Viral spread is favored by low standards of sanitation and close contact. Common sources of infection include household contacts of infected individuals and those connected to daycare centers.

The clinical course and severity varies with the age of the infected individual. Children, especially those younger than 2 years of age, are typically asymptomatic. However, a majority of adults have symptomatic infections often with jaundice that may persist for weeks. Affected individuals display symptoms of acute hepatitis after an incubation period of approximately 4 weeks (15 to 45 days). Fecal shedding of the virus, and thus infectivity of the individual, begins in the second week of incubation, increases until the prodromic phase, and declines once jaundice develops. Acute hepatitis can be more severe in patients with underlying liver disease, such as chronic HBV or HCV, and these individuals should be vaccinated against HAV. Complete recovery is the norm for the majority of patients. A minority of patients suffer relapses of HAV occurring weeks to months following the initial infection. Liver enzyme abnormalities are similar to the initial acute infection, and HAV may be recovered from the stools. These patients ultimately recover and have not been shown to be at risk for chronic liver disease. All patients with hepatitis A should be warned of this possibility of relapse. Less than 1% of patients may develop fulminant liver disease marked by coagulopathy and hepatic encephalopathy. Consultation with a liver transplant program should be initiated for any patient with a significant prolongation of the prothrombin time or with mental status changes. Skin rashes, renal dysfunction, and pancreatitis have all been reported in patients with acute HAV.

Investigations of symptomatic patients reveal abnormalities of liver aminotransferases (alanine transaminase [ALT], aspartate transaminase [AST]) that may peak in the thousands (IU/L). It is common to find elevations of the bilirubin as the appearance of jaundice was the factor that prompted the medical evaluation. By the time most patients present, virus is no longer detectable in the stool. Acute infection is diagnosed by the finding of the IgM antibody to HAV (IgM anti-HAV). The presence of this antibody will persist for 3 to 6 months and is eventually replaced by IgG anti-HAV,

which persists indefinitely and confers immunity. The IgM anti-HAV must be obtained to differentiate acute exposure from prior infection. The HAV total antibody combines both the IgG and IgM to HAV and is inadequate.

The mainstay of treatment for HAV is supportive care. Some patients remain cholestatic for extended periods of time but ultimately recover fully. A minority of patients in whom liver dysfunction (encephalopathy, coagulopathy) persists may require liver transplantation. Active and passive immunoprophylaxis have been employed in the prevention of HAV. Passive prophylaxis entails administration of pooled human Ig. It prevents or attenuates infection in 85% to 95% of individuals if given within 2 weeks of exposure. The standard dose is 0.02 mL/kg and provides protection for approximately 3 months. A 0.05-mL/kg dose may provide protection for up to 6 months. Passive immunization is advised in travelers to endemic areas and household contacts of patients with acute HAV, unless prior HAV infection has been documented for that person. Contacts outside the home are typically not required to receive immunoglobulin.

Active prophylaxis or vaccination is another method for conferring immunity. The HAV vaccine uses inactivated virus. Vaccines should be administered to travelers to endemic areas, men who have sex with men, illicit drug users, recipients of clotting factor concentrates, institutionalized individuals, and those with chronic liver disease. Immunity is conferred 4 weeks after administration of the first dose. Individuals traveling to endemic areas prior to 4 weeks should consider receiving Ig as well. Two vaccines licensed in the United States are Havrix and Vaqta. To attain seroconversion, two doses spaced 6 months apart are considered adequate.. Lower titers of anti-HAV may result when the vaccine is administered with immunoglobulin, and such patients may require booster doses. Twinrix, a combination vaccine for both HAV and HBV, is now available.

Hepatitis B

HBV is a member of the Hepadnaviridae family and is the only DNA virus of the five listed. HBV is classified into eight genotypes (A through H) based on DNA sequence differences. Genotypes A and G are more common in the United States. The relationship between genotype and the severity of liver disease and response to treatment is under investigation. HBV is a partially double-stranded virus that replicates via a reverse transcriptase in a manner similar to retroviruses. The virus encodes four major proteins (surface, polymerase, precore/core, and X protein, respectively). The hepatitis B surface antigen (HBsAg), or S protein is the major envelope protein of the virus. It is produced in large amounts and serves as the initial marker of infection. The core gene encodes two proteins, the hepatitis B core antigen (HBcAg) and the hepatitis B e antigen (HBeAg). The HBcAg helps compose the inner core of the virion. HBeAg has an unclear role but is commonly used as a marker of active viral replication. It should be noted that HBeAg

Rakel and Bope: *Conn's Current Therapy 2006.*

is not vital to viral replication, and a substantial percentage of patients have a mutant form of HBV that does not produce HBeAg but still causes significant liver disease. Mutations that prevent production of HBeAg occur in the "precore" region. Different treatment algorithms are used for patients with the precore mutant or HBeAg-negative disease.

Up to 400 million individuals are said to be infected with HBV worldwide, and approximately 1.25 million are in the United States. Approximately 15% to 40% of infected individuals will develop cirrhosis or hepatic decompensation. There is also a clearly increased risk of developing hepatocellular carcinoma (HCC), and HBV has been labeled as having oncogenic properties. HBV is found in body fluids including blood, saliva, sweat, breast milk, vaginal secretions, and semen. Transmission may be from mother to child (vertical or perinatal transmission) or from exposure to body fluids (horizontal transmission) most commonly through sex or injection drug use. In areas of lower prevalence of HBV, transmission is more commonly via horizontal transmission, whereas vertical transmission is the predominant mode of acquisition in high endemic areas. Because the virus is so infectious, proper infection control practices are of the utmost importance when caring for patients with HBV.

The age and immune status of the infected individual are important factors in determining the outcome of acute infection. The typical incubation period is from 60 to 180 days from acute exposure to clinical symptoms, which manifest more commonly in adult patients. When acquired early in life, 90% of cases of acute HBV are silent. Chronic infection is defined as persistence of the HBsAg for at least 6 months. Approximately 90% of those infected early in life or with compromised immune function will acquire chronic HBV as opposed to a minority of adults. Of individuals exposed to HBV as adults, more than 95% will have spontaneous resolution of their infection with resulting permanent immunity. It is important to appreciate the likelihood of a successful outcome when encountering jaundiced and anxious adults with acute HBV in the clinic setting. As with HAV, a small number of patients with acute HBV (<1%) can develop fulminant liver disease, and patients should be monitored for mental status changes and changes in the prothrombin time.

The diagnosis of the HBV infection involves the use of clinical, laboratory, and pathologic parameters. Identifying the correct stage of disease relies heavily on the correct interpretation of serologic markers. HBsAg is typically the first marker to appear after infection. It may appear prior to the onset of clinical symptoms in the acute infection and will typically disappear over a few weeks to months as patients recover from the illness. Patients are classified as having chronic HBV if HBsAg persists for more than 6 months. Its disappearance coincides with the appearance of the antibody to HBsAg (anti-HBs), which confers immunity to the virus. Anti-HBs is also seen when immunity is conferred through vaccination. HBcAg is a protein contained in the inner core of the virion and is not found in serum. The antibody to the core protein (anti-HBc) is found early during infection and persists indefinitely. The IgM to

the core protein (IgM anti-HBc) signifies acute HBV infection and may allow differentiation from chronic infection marked by anti-HBc of the IgG subtype. The presence of HBeAg typically correlates with active replication, although patients with the precore mutant can have active replication without detectable HBeAg. The HBV DNA is the most definitive test for viral replication, and patients positive for HBV DNA are said to have active infection. However, it should be noted that much of the work in this field relied on hybridization assays for HBV DNA that had a lower detection limit of 5 to 7 pg/mL. Current HBV DNA assays use the more sensitive polymerase chain reaction (PCR) assay, which is sensitive to 100 to 1000 copies/mL. One picogram is roughly equivalent to 150,000 copies. Currently, patients with HBV DNA levels greater than 100,000 copies/mL are considered to have active disease and are candidates for therapy.

Chronic infection with HBV can exist in several forms that allow sufficient room for confusion. Perhaps the most critical distinction to be made is between those patients with nonreplicating virus and those with replicating virus. Patients with nonreplicating virus were previously referred to as "inactive carriers." These individuals have HBsAg but are negative for the HBV DNA and HBeAg. These individuals are not considered to be at risk for progressive liver disease and are not currently candidates for therapy. They remain infectious, however, and are at risk for liver cancer. Patients with nonreplicating or inactive virus can spontaneously reactivate and should be monitored with blood work at least yearly. In addition, virus in these patients can become active if the patient is immunocompromised, which occurs most commonly through immunosuppressive medications including chemotherapy. Patients who are positive for the HBV DNA have active disease, are at risk for disease progression, and are potential candidates for therapy. Typically, these patients will have at least intermittent elevations of the AST/ALT and active inflammation on liver biopsy. Patients with an HBV DNA more than 100,000 copies/mL and a positive HBeAg are said to have HBeAg-positive chronic HBV; those with an HBV DNA more than 10,000 copies/mL and a negative HBeAg are said to have HBeAg-negative chronic HBV. The treatment algorithm is different for the two different forms of infection.

The treatment of HBV is by no means straightforward, and it is difficult to give definitive recommendations because no one agent is ideal or superior and because new agents are currently being evaluated. It should be noted that the goal of current therapy is not the loss of HBsAg per se because that is difficult to achieve. The goals of therapy are sustained viral suppression as measured by the sustained loss of HBV DNA and HBeAg and improvement in liver histology. Loss of HBeAg will be more durable if it is accompanied by the appearance of anti-HBe (seroconversion). Current agents approved for treatment of HBV include interferon alfa-2b (Intron A), lamivudine (Epivir), and adefovir dipivoxil (Hepsera); and each can be considered in initial therapy. Interferon alfa, an immunostimulatory protein, was the first drug approved for the treatment of HBV.

In the treatment of HBV, interferon is injected subcutaneously for a total of 16 weeks at a dose of 5 million U daily or 10 million U three times per week. The medication is typically safe but has significant side effects including fatigue, flulike symptoms, headaches, anorexia, and depression and anxiety. In addition, interferon can cause a decrease in both the neutrophil and platelet count. The principle advantages of interferon are that there is a finite duration of therapy, and up to a third of HBeAg-positive patients can have a sustained response (indefinite loss of HBeAg and HBV DNA). Interferon might be considered in individuals infected as adults with high ALTs and low levels of HBV DNA because it works best in these patients. It is significantly less effective in patients infected through vertical transmission. This group, which includes most Asian patients, often has a mildly elevated or normal ALT and high HBV DNA levels. It should be noted that pegylated (long-acting) interferon is being evaluated in patients with HBV and may be more effective with weekly dosing than standard interferon with daily dosing.

The alternatives to interferon are the orally available agents, lamivudine and adefovir dipivoxil. These agents effectively suppress viral suppression by interfering with viral replication and can significantly improve liver histology. Furthermore, they are very well tolerated with side effect profiles comparable to placebo. The primary limitation of these agents is that they usually do not result in sustained suppression of virus. Moreover, both agents can give rise to viral mutants that are resistant to the medication, although this occurs significantly more often with lamivudine (50% at 3 years) than with adefovir (6% at 3 years). Patients with HBeAg-positive chronic HBV should be treated with lamivudine at 100 mg a day or adefovir at 10 mg a day until there is loss of HBV DNA and HBeAg seroconversion and then for an additional 6 months. This occurs in less than 20% of patients with 48 weeks of treatment but can increase to up to 45% of patients after 144 weeks of therapy. For patients with HBeAg-negative disease, determining the duration of therapy is more problematic because HBeAg seroconversion cannot be used as an endpoint. For this reason, long-term therapy is frequently advocated.

There are several caveats about treatment with lamivudine and adefovir. Because of the potential long duration of therapy with these agents, it is often useful to document active disease with a liver biopsy prior to beginning treatment. Because of its lower rate of resistant mutants, adefovir is often preferred when long-term therapy is anticipated such as with HBeAg-negative patients. It should also be noted that these agents are particularly safe and potentially effective in patients with chronic HBV with decompensated liver disease (jaundice, ascites, encephalopathy), although these patients usually should be treated by staff at dedicated liver centers who can also anticipate the potential need for liver transplant. Finally, both lamivudine and adefovir appear, so far, to be active against mutations resistant to the other.

Patients with chronic HBV are at risk of developing HCC and should be screened with a blood test for α-fetoprotein (AFP) every 6 months and ultrasonography yearly. Patients with an elevated AFP should have more sensitive imaging either with an abdominal magnetic resonance imaging (MRI) scan or a dual phase computed tomography (CT) scan.

Significant progress has been made in the prevention of HBV with recombinant vaccines. Several vaccines are available for HBV (Engerix-B, Recombivax) including a combination vaccine for HAV and HBV (Twinrix). The universal vaccination of newborns prior to hospital discharge regardless of maternal status is expected to result in a significant decline in HBV infection. Individuals for whom vaccination is currently recommended include all infants and children, health care workers, injection drug users, those engaging in high-risk sexual behavior, inmates of correctional facilities, dialysis patients, recipients of blood products, household contacts of infected patients, those who live in or emigrated from high endemic areas, and patients with chronic liver disease. Approximately 95% of patients will respond to a single series of three injections, and a substantial number of the remainder will respond to a second series. Postvaccination testing for anti-HBs is unnecessary except in high-risk individuals such as health care workers. Booster injections are currently only recommended for dialysis patients. Unvaccinated patients who sustain an exposure to HBV and infants born to mothers who are HBsAg-positive should also receive HBV Ig as soon as possible in addition to starting vaccination.

Hepatitis C

Approximately 170 million individuals are infected with HCV worldwide, and up to 3 million people are infected in the United States. HCV accounts for close to half of the liver transplants performed in the United States. Although there is an increase in the number of patients presenting with HCV, the actual number of new cases has been decreasing since the early 1990s. The decline in new cases is because of effective screening of the blood supply and saturation of the injection drug–using population with prior HCV infection. The majority of patients diagnosed now were exposed to the virus in the 1960s through the 1980s through injection drug use and infected blood products.

HCV is a single-stranded RNA virus belonging to the Flaviviridae family. A single open reading frame encodes a large protein that is then cleaved into smaller ones. The study of this virus has allowed its categorization into six major genotypes, which have marked geographic variation. Although the genotypes do not clearly vary in the rate with which they cause hepatic fibrosis, they vary markedly in their response to therapy. Genotype 1, the more common form of HCV in the United States, tends to be more resistant to treatment than genotypes 2 and 3.

Unlike HBV, the HCV virus has not been found in body fluids other than blood, and the virus is transmitted primarily through exposure to blood and blood products. Individuals primarily at risk include those who have received blood products prior to 1992 and injection drug users. Other risk factors include the use of intranasal drugs, tattoos, and exposure to multiple sex partners. The virus is not spread efficiently in long-term monogamous relationships. The virus can be transmitted from mother to infant at birth, and this occurs in 1% to 2% of cases.

Acute infection with HCV is silent in the majority of individuals. It is often mistaken for a viral syndrome, and no further workup is pursued unless patients remain symptomatic for an extended period of time or develop jaundice. Approximately 70% to 85% of patients infected with HCV will develop the chronic form of the disease and are at risk of persistent liver inflammation and fibrosis that can progress over many years. The insidious nature of the infection helps explain why so many patients are being diagnosed now when they contracted the virus 20 to 30 years ago. Clinical features vary with the stage of disease. Many patients are diagnosed incidentally through blood donation or following the discovery of abnormal liver tests on routine laboratory examination. However, patients with advanced cirrhosis may present with fatigue, jaundice, ascites, variceal bleeding, or encephalopathy. The Centers for Disease Control and Prevention (CDC) notes no more than 20% of infected individuals will develop cirrhosis, and no more than 5% will die from chronic liver disease. Extrahepatic manifestations include cryoglobulinemia, membranoproliferative glomerulonephritis, lymphoproliferative disorders, arthritis, thyroid disease, lichen planus, and corneal ulcers. More serious extrahepatic manifestations are unusual.

Screening for HCV is achieved by checking for the antibody to the virus (anti-HCV). HCV is different from HAV and HBV in that the antibody to the virus is not protective and does not translate into immunity. It is in fact a marker of infection. The anti-HCV has excellent sensitivity, and false negative tests are unusual but may be seen in immunocompromised patients or those recently exposed. The diagnosis is confirmed by detecting HCV RNA in blood usually with the PCR assay. The actual HCV RNA level is valuable in monitoring and predicting the response to therapy, and we typically recommend that the quantitative HCV RNA be performed over qualitative assays. The HCV genotype should also be ordered routinely because it helps assess the likelihood of response to therapy and the duration of treatment. It is important to appreciate that patients consistently negative for HCV RNA are extremely unlikely to be infected.

The goal of current therapy for HCV is a sustained virologic response (SVR) as determined by the absence of detectable virus in blood 24 weeks after the completion of successful antiviral therapy. For almost all patients, a sustained response is synonymous with a cure. Thanks to rapid progress in the past decade, an SVR can now be achieved in more than 50% of patients (Table 2). The current best treatment for HCV is the combination of pegylated interferon and ribavirin (Rebetol). Interferon is an immune stimulating protein or cytokine, which also has direct antiviral activity. Pegylated interferon is a form of interferon with a polyethylene glycol (PEG) moiety attached. The pegylation of interferon decreases viral clearance and allows sustained serum levels of drug with once weekly dosing. There are two forms of pegylated interferon available. Pegylated interferon alfa-2a (Pegasys) is injected at a dose of 180 μg weekly and pegylated interferon alfa-2b (PEG-Intron) is injected at a dose of 1.5 μg/kg weekly. Ribavirin, a nucleoside analogue, is given as an oral pill twice a day with doses varying from 800 mg to 1200 mg per day. Patients are treated for 12 weeks and then assessed for an early virologic response (EVR), which is defined as a 2 log drop or more in the HCV RNA level. Patients who achieve this response then will receive a total of 48 weeks of therapy if they have genotype 1 or 4 and 24 weeks if they have genotype 2 or 3. Therapy is typically discontinued in patients who do not achieve the EVR.

Side effects of therapy are significant, and effective management of side effects is important in that treatment efficacy improves with compliance. Side effects of interferon include fatigue, flulike symptoms, nausea, weight loss, depression, and irritability. Neuropsychiatric side effects are an important cause of treatment discontinuation. Interferon can also cause neutropenia and thrombocytopenia and can cause or exacerbate autoimmune conditions. Ribavirin can cause hemolysis (with a drop in hemoglobin of 2 to 4 mg/dL) and skin rash and is teratogenic. Patient education is an important part of management. Antidepressant and analgesic medications help with many of the side effects. Erythropoietin (Procrit) and granulocyte colony-stimulating factor (G-CSF) (Neupogen) can help with anemia and neutropenia. Dose modifications are common, and it is important that practitioners know dose adjustment algorithms.

Therapy might be considered in all patients who do not have contraindications to interferon-based treatment. Relative contraindications include decompensated liver disease, preexisting cytopenias, active autoimmune conditions, and severe or unstable mental disease. Patients with renal insufficiency should not receive ribavirin. Given that treatment is difficult and that a minority of patients will develop cirrhosis, a liver biopsy may be helpful to some patients in determining the urgency or desire for therapy. Groups that are historically more challenging to treat include those with genotype 1 (the most common in the United States), African American patients, and those who have failed prior antiviral therapy.

TABLE 2   Sustained Virologic Response* for Different Hepatitis C Virus Patient Groups Treated With Pegylated Interferon and Ribavirin

All patients	54%-56%
Genotype 1	42%-46%
Genotype 2 or 3	76%-80%
Genotype 4	77%
Cirrhosis	43%-44%
African Americans	19%-26%
HCV and HIV co-infection	27%-40%

*The sustained virologic response (SVR) is defined as undetectable HCV RNA 24 weeks after stopping therapy.
Abbreviations: HCV = hepatitis C virus.

In addition to treating the virus in appropriately selected candidates, management of patients with HCV includes avoidance of hepatotoxins, especially alcohol. Patients with cirrhosis should undergo surveillance for hepatocellular carcinoma with monitoring of the AFP every 6 months and yearly liver imaging. Patients should be vaccinated against HAV and HBV, unless there is evidence of prior exposure. There is no vaccine against HCV. Prevention of HCV relies on counseling of infected individuals and those at risk. Patients should avoid sharing objects such as razors and toothbrushes and should cover open wounds. The risk of sexual transmission in long-term monogamous relationships is low and partners, in this setting, are not counseled to change their sex habits. As is the case with any other infection, universal precautions should be exercised when caring for HCV infected individuals.

Hepatitis D

The hepatitis D virus (HDV), or delta virus, is a defective virus that requires co-infection with HBV for long-term pathogenicity. Although HDV can potentially replicate autonomously, it uses the HBsAg to construct the outer envelope required for complete virion assembly and secretion. The HBsAg-containing envelope encloses a single-stranded RNA genome and a structural protein, the hepatitis delta antigen (HDAg). HDV is relatively unusual in the United States. It can be diagnosed in individuals from endemic areas, and outbreaks in communities of injection drug users have been described. HDV is endemic in parts of South America and the Mediterranean basin and, to a lesser degree, in East Asia and the Pacific Rim. Worldwide, approximately 5% of HBV infected individuals are co-infected with HDV, amounting to approximately 15 to 20 million cases.

HDV requires HBV for infection to occur, and the modes of transmission of HDV are similar to those of HBV. HDV may be acquired in individuals with previous HBV infection (superinfection) or may be acquired simultaneously with HBV (co-infection). Co-infected patients typically present with features of a self-limited acute HBV, and the majority recover fully with less than 5% developing chronic infection. Patients with superinfection may present with acute hepatitis in a previously unrecognized HBV carrier, or as an exacerbation of preexisting chronic HBV. Chronic HDV infection occurs in about 70% to 80% of superinfected patients. Traditionally, it is considered that patients infected with both HDV and HBV have more aggressive liver disease than those with HBV alone. However, more recent studies have shown HDV infection follows a highly variable course. Fulminant liver disease is more common with co-infection than superinfection.

The diagnosis of HDV is typically made through the detection of antibody to HDV (anti-HDV). The IgM anti-HDV is preferred. It is positive in acute infection, persists in chronic infection, and does a better job than anti-HDV IgG (or total anti-HDV) in distinguishing

---

CURRENT DIAGNOSIS

Diagnostic tests for the hepatitis viruses

Virus	Status	Tests						
Hepatitis A	Acute infection	IgM anti-HAV						
	Vaccination and previous infection	IgG anti-HAV						
Hepatitis B	Acute infection	HBsAg	HBeAg	IgM anti-HBc	IgG anti-HBc	Anti-HBs	Anti-HBe	HBV-DNA
	Early phase	+	+	+	−	−	−	+
	Window phase	−	−	+	−	−	+	+
	Recovery phase	−	−	−	+	+	+	−
	Chronic infection							
	Replicating	+	+	−	+	−	−	+
	Precore mutant	+	−	−	+	−	+	+
	Nonreplicating	+	−	−	+	−	+	−
	Previous exposure with immunity	−	−	−	+	+	+	−
	Vaccination	−	−	−	−	+	−	−
Hepatitis C	Acute infection	Anti-HCV (by EIA or RIBA), HCV RNA						
	Chronic infection	Anti-HCV, HCV RNA						
Hepatitis D	Acute infection	HDV antigen, IgM anti-HDV, HDV RNA						
	Coinfection with HBV	Above and HBsAg, IgM anti-HBc						
		Above and presence of chronic HBV						
	Superinfection with HBV	IgM anti-HDV, HDV RNA, HBsAg						
	Chronic infection							
Hepatitis E	Acute infection	IgM anti-HEV						
	Resolved infection	IgG anti-HEV						

Abbreviations: anti-HAV = antibody to hepatitis A virus; anti-HBc = antibody to hepatitis B core antigen; anti-HCV = antibody to hepatitis C virus; anti-HEV = antibody to hepatitis E virus; EIA = enzyme immunoassay; HBeAg = hepatitis B e antigen; HBsAg = hepatitis B surface antigen; HBV = hepatitis B virus; HCV = hepatitis C virus; HDV = hepatitis D virus; RIBA = recombinant immunoblot assay.

Rakel and Bope: *Conn's Current Therapy 2006.*

past from current infection. For the diagnosis of HDV to be accurate, HBsAg must also be detected. IgM anti-HBc is often a marker for acute HBV infection and can help distinguish HDV co-infection from superinfection. The most sensitive and accurate test for HDV is the HDV RNA measured by reverse transcriptase polymerase chain reaction (RT-PCR). The HDV RNA is also a reliable test for monitoring response to therapy.

The goals of therapy are suppression of HDV replication through undetectable HDV RNA, normalization of the ALT level, and improvement in liver histology. Seroconversion of HBsAg to anti-HBs is rarely attained. Patients who have cleared HDV but who remain HBsAg-positive remain at theoretical risk of reinfection with HDV. Therapy should be considered for patients with chronic HDV infection and active liver disease. Treatment is with interferon alfa-2a (Roferon-A)[1] administered at 9 million U 3 times a week for 48 weeks. Results from controlled trials have been variable. In the most encouraging study, 10 of 14 patients randomized to this regimen had normalization of the ALT, and the group overall had a significant decline in serum HDV RNA (compared to placebo). After 12 years, 7 patients had lost IgM anti-HDV. Lamivudine[1] is not effective against HDV.

Vaccination against HBV remains the most cost-effective means to prevent HDV infection. There is no successful vaccine against HDV. Infected patients are at risk of developing hepatocellular carcinoma and should be screened on a regular basis. Patients infected with HBV should be checked for HDV.

Hepatitis E

HEV is a small single-stranded RNA virus and is similar to HAV in its enteric mode of transmission. Like HAV, HEV causes acute but not chronic hepatitis.

---

[1]Not FDA approved for this indication.

HEV infection is rare in the United States and is almost always seen in patients who have recently returned from endemic areas. The virus is endemic in South and Central Asia, Africa, and Central America. In these areas, HEV is associated with hepatitis outbreaks and epidemics and is a leading cause of acute hepatitis. Outbreaks affecting more than 100,000 individuals were observed in China in the 1980s.

HEV is transmitted by the fecal–oral route commonly through consumption of contaminated water. Outbreaks often follow heavy rainfalls and flooding resulting in contamination of the water supply. Household contacts of patients with HEV become infected 1% to 2% of the time versus a 50% to 75% incidence for household contacts of HAV patients. The incubation period of HEV infection ranges from 15 to 60 days. Symptoms are similar to those seen in patients with other types of acute viral hepatitis and may include fatigue, malaise, anorexia, abdominal pain, nausea, and vomiting and generally resolve in 6 weeks. Jaundice may also be present and is accompanied by light-colored stools and dark urine. Less common complaints may include pruritus, urticarial rash, diarrhea, and arthralgias. Acute HEV typically causes a self-limited illness. The virus is most notorious for its impact on pregnant women in the third trimester of pregnancy in whom it has a mortality rate between 15% and 25%. The reason for this is not known. Patients with chronic liver disease infected with HEV are also at increased risk of fatal outcomes.

HEV is diagnosed through serologic testing. Acute infection is suggested by the finding of antibody to HEV (anti-HEV). As with HAV, the critical test is IgM anti-HEV which is detectable early in the infection and becomes undetectable by 6 months. IgG anti-HEV remains detectable for years and does not distinguish between recent and past infection. Abnormalities of liver function tests including elevations of the bilirubin, ALT, and AST are often seen. These return to normal as the illness subsides, typically in 1 to 4 weeks. A minority of

CURRENT THERAPY

Treatment regimens for chronic hepatitis

	Dosage	Duration	Drawbacks/side effects
Hepatitis B Virus			
Interferon alfa-2b (Intron-A)	5 million U daily of 10 million U SC 3 times per wk	16 wk.	SC administration: flulike symptoms, fatigue, depression, leukopenia, thrombocytopenia, anorexia, worsening of autoimmune disorders
Lamivudine (Epivir) Adefovir (Hepsera)	100 mg by mouth daily 10 mg by mouth daily	1 y.	Resistance
Hepatitis C Virus			
Pegylated alfa-2a (Pegasys)	180 µg SC once per week	Stop treatment at wk 12 if no EVR; continue until wk 24 (gen 2 and 3);	Similar to interferon
Pegylated alfa-2b (PEG-Intron)	1.5 µg/kg body weight SC once per week	continue until wk 48 (gen 1).	Similar to interferon
Ribavirin (Rebetol)	800-1200 mg daily by mouth in 2 divided doses		Teratogenicity; hemolytic anemia, rash

Abbreviations: EVR = early virologic response; gen = genotype; SC = subcutaneously.

Rakel and Bope: *Conn's Current Therapy 2006.*

patients may have prolonged cholestasis taking up to 6 months to resolve. Amplification techniques, which are limited to research purposes, have been employed to detect HEV RNA in the serum, the liver, and the stool.

The treatment of patients infected with HEV is largely supportive, and no specific intervention is required. The use of Ig[1] for postexposure prophylaxis is not effective in preventing infection. Prevention focuses on improved sanitation and avoiding the consumption of contaminated food and water. Investigations into the creation of a vaccine have yielded encouraging results. At least one vaccine for HEV is being field-tested in humans.

REFERENCES

Berk Paul (ed): Chronic hepatitis C. Semin Liver Dis 2004;24(Suppl 2):.
Berk P (ed): HBV viral kinetics and clinical management: Key issues and current perspectives. Semin Liver Dis 2004;24(Suppl 1):.
Emerson SU, Purcell RH: Hepatitis E virus. Rev Med Virol 2003; 13:145-154.
Farci P, Roskams T, Chessa L, et al: Long-term benefit of interferon therapy of chronic hepatitis D: Regression of advanced hepatic fibrosis. Gastroenterology 2004;126(7):1740-1749.
Farci P: Delta hepatitis: An update. J Hepatol 2003;39:S212-219.
Fried MW, Shiffman ML, Reddy KR, et al: Peginterferon alfa-2a plus ribavirin for chronic hepatitis C virus infection. N Engl J Med 2002;347(13):975-982.
Keefe EB, Dietrich DT, Han SHB, et al: A treatment algorithm for the management of chronic hepatitis B virus infection in the United States. Clin Gastroenterol Hepatol 2004;2:87-106.
Lok AS, McMahon BJ: Practice guidelines committee, American Association for the Study of Liver Diseases (AASLD). Chronic hepatitis B: Update of recommendations. Hepatology 2004;39(3): 857-861.
Manns MP, McHutchinson JG, Gordon SC, et al: Peginterferon alfa-2b plus ribavirin compared with interferon alfa-2b plus ribavirin for the treatment of chronic hepatitis C: A randomised trial. Lancet 2001;358:958-965.
Strader DB, Wright T, Thomas DL, et al: Diagnosis, management, and treatment of hepatitis C. AASLD practice guidelines. Hepatology 2004;39(4):1147-1171.

[1]Not FDA approved for this indication.

Malabsorption

Method of
Laura Harrell, MD, and Eugene Chang, MD

Intestinal malabsorption can arise from a number of clinical conditions and be protean in its presentation. Symptoms can be so minor that patients do not seek medical attention, but in other individuals, severe malnourishment and nutrient malabsorption may be blatant. In the former it is important to recognize the clinical condition before systemic complications occur, whereas in the latter the rapid identification and treatment of the malabsorption are indicated to prevent further decline of the patient's nutritional status. Therefore, in

approaching patients with malabsorption, it is essential to have a fundamental understanding of both physiologic and pathophysiologic mechanisms of intestinal digestion and absorption. These processes can be categorized by their sites of nutrient assimilation, which include: (a) intraluminal digestion; (b) mucosal absorption; (c) postabsorptive or delivery phase. Disruption of any of these phases can result in maldigestion and malabsorption.

Lipids

The average American diet consists of 120 to 150 g of dietary fat daily. Dietary lipids, a major source of energy, are mostly in the form of long-chain triglycerides but are also made up of cholesterol, phospholipids, and free fatty acids. Digestion begins with emulsification of dietary lipids through mastication and gastric contractions. Lipids are hydrophobic molecules and are insoluble in the aqueous environment of the intestinal lumen. Emulsification increases the surface area of the lipid droplets allowing greater contact between the lipid molecules and digestive enzymes (Figure 1). Lingual and gastric lipase, active in the presence of an acidic pH, begin hydrolyzing triglycerides to free fatty acids, monoglycerides, and glycerol. Fat then enters the small intestine resulting in the release of hormones, cholecystokinin, and secretin from mucosal cells in the duodenum and proximal jejunum. Cholecystokinin is a small peptide hormone that stimulates the gallbladder to contract and release bile into the duodenum and also stimulates the exocrine cells of the pancreas to release digestive enzymes. Secretin is released in response to the acidic pH of chyme entering the small intestines. Secretin stimulates the pancreas to secrete a solution rich in bicarbonate, raising the pH of the chyme, which in turn activates pancreatic enzymes. Pancreatic lipase, in the presence of colipase, is responsible for 70% of fat digestion.

Bile salts are necessary for the absorption of dietary lipids. Bile salts are amphipathic molecules capable of stabilizing hydrophobic molecules in an aqueous environment. Bile acids are synthesized from cholesterol in the liver to form chenodeoxycholic acid and cholic acid, primary bile acids. These primary bile acids are conjugated to form bile salts, which are secreted in the bile into the duodenum. Bile salts combine with the products of lipolysis forming mixed micelles. Cholesterol- and fat-soluble vitamins, the most water-insoluble lipids, are dependent on micellar formation and are therefore packaged in the core of the micelles. (NOTE: Short- and medium-chain fatty acids do not require micelle formation for their absorption across the brush-border membrane.)

Micelles are then delivered to the brush-border membrane of the villus epithelial cells where, through either passive diffusion or a carrier-mediated process, mucosal absorption occurs and lipids enter the epithelial cells. Bile salts remain in the intestinal lumen, and eventually are actively reabsorbed in the terminal ileum where they enter into the portal circulation and are resecreted

EVALUATION OF MALABSORPTION

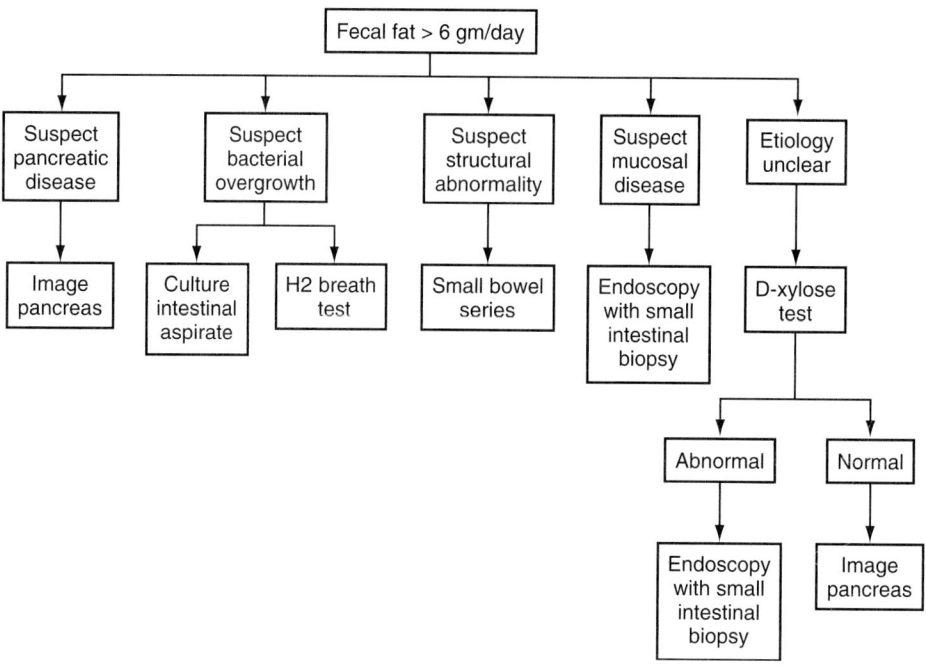

FIGURE 1. Algorithm for the evaluation of malabsorption.

into the bile. Approximately 15 to 30 g of bile salts are secreted in the bile daily. Only 0.5 g of bile is lost in the stool per day. Hepatic synthesis of bile acids maintains the bile acid pool, matching this loss of bile acids.

Inside the mucosal cells, fatty acids and monoglycerides are re-esterified and converted to triglycerides. The triglycerides, β-lipoproteins, cholesterol, and phospholipids form chylomicrons. The chylomicrons then exit the cell by exocytosis and are absorbed into the lymphatics where they eventually enter the blood via the thoracic duct.

Medium-chain triglycerides (MCT) can be absorbed intact and do not require micelle formation for absorption. If MCTs are hydrolyzed into medium-chain fatty acids (MCFA) in the intestinal lumen, MCFAs are readily absorbed. After absorption MCTs are hydrolyzed in the cell, forming MCFAs. These MCFAs are then released into the portal circulation and are delivered to the liver. Because MCTs are digested and absorbed through a different mechanism than long-chain triglycerides, MCTs are sometimes used as nutritional supplements in patients with severe malnutrition resulting from impaired lipid absorption secondary to impaired lipolysis, micelle formation, or uptake of lipids into the lymphatics.

Short-chain fatty acids (SCFAs) are not consumed in the diet but are synthesized in the colon. Carbohydrates, which are not absorbed in the small intestines, are delivered to the colon where they are fermented by colonic bacteria and form SCFAs and hydrogen gas. The most common SCFAs are acetate, propionate, and butyrate. Butyrate is an important nutrient for colonocytes, and if absent, colitis may result.

Carbohydrates

The average American consumes 300 g of carbohydrates every day. Carbohydrates in the diet include monosaccharides, disaccharides, polysaccharides, and fiber. Glucose, fructose, sucrose, and lactose are examples of monosaccharides and disaccharides found in the average diet. Starch is an example of a complex polysaccharide often found in plants, wheat, grains, beans, and vegetables. Dietary fiber, an undigestible form of carbohydrate, has many beneficial effects such as preventing diverticulosis, constipation, and colon cancer. Dietary fiber is found in bran, beans, whole grains, and some fruits and vegetables. There are soluble and insoluble fibers. Soluble fibers are believed to help reduce cholesterol levels and control blood sugar levels; insoluble fibers are responsible for increasing stool bulk. Dietary fiber remains undigested in the small bowel and is hydrolyzed in the colon to form SCFAs. Some dietary fibers such as pectin are better hydrolyzed to SCFAs than others. Cellulose and hemicellulose are hydrolyzed to a lesser extent in the colon.

Starch is hydrolyzed by salivary and pancreatic amylase to form oligosaccharides, maltose, maltotriose, and α-limit dextrins. Monosaccharides such as glucose are readily absorbed by enterocytes though oligo- and disaccharides are not. Brush-border enzymes break down oligo- and disaccharides into monosaccharides, which are absorbed via specific transport proteins and delivered into the portal circulation. Unabsorbed carbohydrates have an osmotic effect in the colon, causing intraluminal fluid accumulation resulting in diarrhea.

Rakel and Bope: *Conn's Current Therapy 2006*.

Colonic bacteria ferment unabsorbed carbohydrates forming SCFAs, hydrogen, and carbon dioxide gases. These gases are responsible for bloating and flatulence experienced with carbohydrate malabsorption.

Proteins

The average American diet consists of 70 to 100 grams of protein daily. Protein is initially digested by pepsin, which is secreted by gastric chief cells. However, proteins are mostly hydrolyzed and degraded by trypsin and other proteases in the small bowel. Enterokinase, a brush-border enzyme, cleaves pancreatic trypsinogen to trypsin, which in turn activates more trypsinogen and other precursor pancreatic proteases. The products of protein digestion yield oligopeptides, dipeptides, and amino acids. Oligopeptidases, present on the brush border, split these small peptides. Dipeptides are absorbed directly into the mucosal cell and are digested to amino acids in the cytoplasm by dipeptidases. Multiple specific transport systems are responsible for the uptake and absorption of amino acids.

Disorders of Malabsorption

The number and spectrum of diseases and disorders that can be associated with intestinal maldigestion and malabsorption are extensive. For this article, diseases and disorders will be classified by their predominant site in which malabsorption takes place. In some instances, however, it should be noted that multiple sites and mechanisms of actions are involved (Figure 2).

IMPAIRED INTRALUMINAL DIGESTION

Many diseases associated with malabsorption involve abnormalities of the intraluminal phase. The intraluminal phase of digestion is complex and involves many factors. Disruption of any of these factors, such as an impairment of lipolysis, a decrease in the concentration of conjugated bile salts, intestinal bacterial overgrowth, or ileal disease or resection can result in maldigestion or malabsorption.

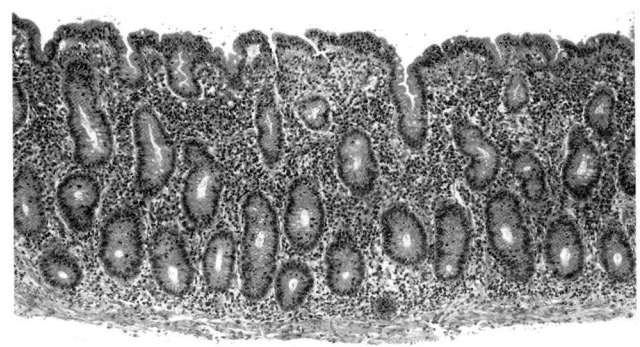

FIGURE 2. Duodenal biopsy in untreated celiac disease demonstrating severe blunting of villi, crypt hyperplasia and inflammatory infiltrate of the lamina propria.

Rakel and Bope: *Conn's Current Therapy 2006.*

Impaired Lipolysis

Defective lipolysis is often secondary to a decrease in pancreatic enzymes. Lipolysis is maintained as long as 5% of pancreatic lipase is secreted. Significant reduction of exocrine pancreatic function is required to affect lipolysis. Pancreatic insufficiency secondary to chronic pancreatitis is the most common cause of impaired lipolysis. Most cases of chronic pancreatitis in the United States are associated with excessive alcohol intake. These patients often present with steatorrhea, abdominal pain, and diabetes mellitus (DM). Their stools are often greasy and bulky with a tendency to float. These patients do not develop watery diarrhea because the malabsorbed triglycerides have very little secretory or osmotic effect in the colon. Gastric lipase allows for a small degree of lipolysis, maintaining fat-soluble vitamin levels. Brush-border disaccharidases and proteases typically preserve adequate carbohydrate and protein absorption.

The malabsorption associated with chronic pancreatitis can be treated with replacement of pancreatic enzymes, 30,000 units of lipase per meal. Patients may note an improvement of their chronic abdominal pain with pancreatic enzyme supplementation, likely because of a decrease in pancreatic secretions. Pancreatic supplements should have a pH-sensitive coating or be given with an acid-blocking agent to prevent inactivation of the enzymes in the acidic environment of the stomach.

Altered Intraluminal pH

Alteration in the intraluminal pH can also affect digestion and absorption of nutrients. An acidic pH in the duodenum and proximal jejunum irreversibly inactivates lipase. Zollinger-Ellison syndrome (ZES) is the classic example of a disorder causing an alteration of the intraluminal pH. Patients with chronic pancreatitis may also have an alteration of their intraluminal pH because of a decreased secretion of pancreatic bicarbonate into the duodenum. H_2-receptor antagonists or proton pump inhibitors (PPIs) may be useful for patients with increased secretion of gastric acid.

Mixing Abnormalities

Impaired mixing of emulsified lipids with pancreatic enzymes and bile salts prevents the absorption of fat and fat-soluble vitamins. Surgical resection of bowel, gastrojejunostomy, partial gastrectomy, and disorders causing alteration in transit time are examples of situations that can alter the normal pathway of nutrients and impair the mixing of nutrients with digestive enzymes and bile salts. If food is diverted away from the duodenum, stimulation of bile and pancreatic enzyme secretion is blunted. Stasis of intestinal contents in afferent limbs can also cause bacterial overgrowth leading to problems discussed later in this article.

Impaired Micelle Formation

Bile salts are necessary for the normal absorption of lipids. Bile salts are synthesized in the liver, excreted in bile into the small intestines and then reabsorbed in the ileum where they are carried through the portal vein back to the liver and the enterohepatic circulation of bile salts continues. Normal hepatic function is essential for the synthesis and conjugation of bile acids. A decrease in the formation of bile salts can occur in patients with cirrhosis of the liver. Impaired secretion of bile salts into bile can also be seen in patients with primary biliary cirrhosis and biliary duct obstruction. Patients who have undergone significant resection of the ileum or who have mucosal disease affecting the distal small bowel may have decreased reabsorption of bile salts leading to an overall decrease in their bile salt pool.

Intestinal Bacterial Overgrowth

Intestinal bacterial overgrowth can cause deconjugation of bile salts, leading to impaired micelle formation. Intestinal bacterial overgrowth occurs in patients with conditions such as diabetes, small bowel diverticulum, immunoglobulin deficiencies, AIDS, and other immunocompromised states. Intestinal bacterial overgrowth occurs when there is an increase of colonic bacteria in the small intestine, achieving concentrations greater than 10^3 organisms per milliliter. Intestinal stasis, loss of ileocecal valve competency, conditions altering the immune system and motility disorders can increase susceptibility to bacterial overgrowth. When bacterial overgrowth does occur, anaerobic bacteria release enzymes, which deconjugate bile salts. Deconjugated bile salts are passively absorbed in the jejunum, leading to a decrease in the concentration of the bile acid pool in the proximal small bowel, impairing micelle formation. Anaerobic bacteria also ingest vitamin B_{12} but synthesize folate, preventing folate deficiency while leading to a vitamin B_{12} deficiency in these patients, an important differentiating factor in the diagnosis of bacterial overgrowth. Colonic bacteria also release proteases, which destroy brush-border disaccharidases, most notably lactase, potentially causing carbohydrate malabsorption.

Patients with bacterial overgrowth often present with watery diarrhea, steatorrhea, abdominal pain, bloating, and weight loss. The watery diarrhea results from the osmotic effects of malabsorbed carbohydrates and the secretory effects of malabsorbed fatty acids. Fat-soluble vitamins and vitamin B_{12} may be deficient, but folate deficiency is rare. Patients are treated with antibiotics, ideally aimed to treat organisms isolated in cultured aspirates from the small intestines. Often a specific organism is not identified and broad-spectrum antibiotics with aerobic and anaerobic treatment is appropriate (i.e., fluoroquinolones and metronidazole [Flagyl]). Rotation of antibiotics is often useful. If vitamins A, D, E, K, and B_{12} are found to be deficient, supplementation is essential. If the bacterial overgrowth is secondary to a structural abnormality, surgical correction should be attempted if possible. Prokinetic agents, such as metoclopramide (Reglan),[1] erythromycin, and cisapride

(Propulsid)[*] are sometimes useful if bacterial overgrowth is secondary to a motility disorder. There has been some success with the use of octreotide (Sandostatin)[1] at low doses, (50 µg subcutaneously daily for 3 weeks) to improve intestinal motility in addition to antibiotics in patients with scleroderma.

Ileal Disease/Resection

Patients with extensive ileal disease or resection suffer from bile acid malabsorption. Crohn's disease is a common cause of ileal disease and resection. Upregulation of hepatic synthesis of bile acids can compensate for losses of bile acids up to 3 g/day. If the liver is unable to compensate for bile acid losses, the bile acid pool decreases and impaired micelle formation and steatorrhea result. Bile salts not absorbed in the ileum are delivered to the colon and excreted in the feces. If less than 100 cm of ileum is diseased or resected, bile acids that reach the colon stimulate water and electrolyte secretion causing watery diarrhea. Steatorrhea typically does not occur in these patients because the liver is able to compensate for bile acid losses. Cholestyramine (Questran)[1] is often effective in the treatment of bile acid diarrhea because it binds malabsorbed bile acids thereby reducing diarrhea. If more than 100 cm of ileum is diseased or resected, the liver is unable to maintain the bile salt pool and fatty-acid malabsorption and steatorrhea ensues. Cholestyramine (Questran)[1] is ineffective in these patients because it further depletes the bile acid pool leading to worsening fat malabsorption. These patients are best treated with a low-fat diet and antidiarrheal agents as needed. Vitamins A, D, E, K, and B_{12} levels and bone density should be monitored.

Short Bowel Syndrome

Short bowel syndrome describes a malabsorptive state following resection of a portion of the small bowel typically manifested by diarrhea and/or steatorrhea and nutrient and mineral deficiencies. The length and location of the resected bowel and the state of the residual bowel determines the manifested symptoms.

In the United States the most common reason for small bowel resection is the surgical treatment of Crohn's disease. Individuals with mesenteric vascular disease, trauma, or who have undergone obesity surgery may also develop short bowel syndrome. Structural and functional adaptations of the residual bowel occur after small bowel resection. Ingestion of nutrients leads to the stimulation of structural adaptations via direct nutrient contact with the mucosal surface, biliary and pancreatic secretions, and the release of intestinal hormones and growth factors. These factors stimulate hyperplasia, elongation, and upregulation of nutrient transporters of the mucosa, which allows for increased nutrient and fluid absorption.

Resection of the ileocecal valve can result in more severe diarrhea secondary to decreased transit time and

---

[1]Not FDA approved for this indication.

[*]Investigational drug in the United States.
[1]Not FDA approved for this indication.

reflux of colonic bacteria into the small intestines resulting in bacterial overgrowth. Patients with ileal resection may malabsorb bile acids resulting in bile acid diarrhea and possible fat malabsorption. These patients are also at risk for vitamin B_{12} deficiency. For reasons not entirely understood, hypersecretion of gastric acid also occurs in patients who have undergone large resections of the small intestines contributing to the diarrhea and malabsorption of nutrients through the deactivation of digestive enzymes in the acidic duodenal environment. The colon plays an important role in patients who have undergone small bowel resections. If the colon is diseased or has been resected, diarrhea may be more severe. The colon is important for fluid absorption and the conversion of malabsorbed carbohydrates into small chain fatty acids, salvaging energy provided by carbohydrates. Long-term complications of short bowel syndrome include mineral and nutrient deficiencies, bone loss, gallstones, oxalate kidney stones, and rarely D-lactic acidosis.

Management of short bowel syndrome depends on the severity of symptoms. In patients with sufficient adaptation of the remaining bowel, a diet high in complex carbohydrates and low in fat should be instituted. Supplementation with MCTs may be of benefit. Vitamin and mineral levels, including fat-soluble vitamins, folate, vitamin B_{12}, iron, calcium, magnesium, and zinc should be monitored and repleted. Antimotility agents can help reduce stool output. Treatment of gastric acid hypersecretion with H_2-receptor antagonists (H2RA) or PPIs and the treatment of bacterial overgrowth with antibiotics may be helpful when appropriate. When the above therapeutic approaches are insufficient, intravenous (IV) fluids and/or parenteral nutrition may be necessary. Small bowel transplant is considered in patients unable to tolerate parenteral nutrition.

IMPAIRED MUCOSAL ABSORPTION

The mucosal absorptive cells play an important role in the digestion and absorption of nutrients. A number of diseases or conditions affect these cells, impairing the absorption process. Diseases such as celiac disease, infection, tropical sprue, graft-versus-host (GVH) disease, radiation enteritis, ischemia, infiltrative diseases such as amyloidosis or collagenous sprue, and the effects of nonsteroidal, anti-inflammatory drugs are examples of disorders causing mucosal absorption impairment. Depending on the extent and location of disease involvement, patients may experience diarrhea, weight loss, and symptoms related to mineral or nutrient deficiencies. Although many nutrients are absorbed diffusely throughout the small bowel, some nutrients are absorbed in specific regions of the bowel. For example, diseases involving only the proximal bowel cause specific nutritional deficiencies of iron, calcium, and folate. Some diseases cause selective or specific impairment of mucosal cells. These diseases involve defects in specific transport or digestion of substances. Examples of such disorders include abetalipoproteinemia, enteropeptidase deficiency, and disaccharidase deficiencies.

Rakel and Bope: *Conn's Current Therapy 2006*.

Celiac Disease

Celiac disease is a chronic inflammatory disease of the small intestines induced by an immune mediated response to gluten, storage proteins found in wheat. Related proteins in barley and rye are also toxic to patients with celiac disease. Celiac disease usually involves the proximal intestines but can extend to the more distal bowel. Clinical manifestations of the disease are typically determined by the location and extent of inflammation. Inflammation leads to blunting of villi, decreasing the absorptive surface area of the small bowel. Patients with disease typically present with anemia secondary to nutrient deficiencies of iron and folate and bone loss secondary to vitamin D and calcium malabsorption. Diarrhea and severe nutrient malabsorption occurs in patients with more extensive disease involvement.

Extraintestinal manifestations may include neurologic symptoms such as peripheral neuropathy, ataxia, and epilepsy or psychiatric symptoms such as depression and schizophrenia. Rarely, clinical manifestations of celiac disease include arthritis, elevated liver transaminases, infertility, or dermatitis herpetiformis. Autoimmune diseases also occur more frequently in patients with celiac disease than in the general population.

The diagnosis of celiac disease is made based on characteristic histologic findings found on small intestinal biopsies. These characteristic findings include villous atrophy, crypt hyperplasia, and increased intraepithelial lymphocytes. Endoscopically, patients typically have scalloping of the mucosal folds and a reduction in the number of mucosal folds in the descending duodenum. Removal of gluten from the diet can result in reversal of these endoscopic and histologic abnormalities.

Serologic markers can also help diagnose celiac disease, but serologic markers alone are insufficient for the diagnosis. Markers are also useful for screening individuals at high risk for developing celiac disease, such as first-degree relatives of patients with celiac disease. Antibodies against gliadin, endomysial antibodies, and tissue transglutaminase antibodies are useful diagnostic markers for celiac disease.

Iron and folate levels should be monitored and supplemented in all patients with celiac disease. Bone density tests should be followed and calcium and vitamin D should be supplemented if bone loss is discovered. Patients should be referred for dietary counseling and given information regarding celiac support groups. Patients need to follow a strict gluten-free diet, avoiding wheat, barley, and rye. Oats are safe for celiac patients as long as there is no contamination of the oats with wheat. Continued ingestion of gluten should be considered in patients with refractory sprue. If patients with refractory symptoms are following a strict gluten-free diet but continue to have symptoms, other causes of malabsorption should be investigated. Immunosuppressive agents are occasionally helpful in the treatment of refractory sprue. There are reports of patients treated successfully with steroids, azathioprine[1] and infliximab (Remicade).[1]

---

[1]Not FDA approved for this indication.

Lymphoma and gastrointestinal (GI) carcinoma should be considered in patients who have recurrence or persistence of symptoms.

Tropical Sprue

Tropical sprue is a syndrome that affects visitors and natives of tropical areas. Patients affected with this syndrome often present with diarrhea, steatorrhea, weight loss, and megaloblastic anemia secondary to both folate and vitamin B_{12} deficiency. The etiology of tropical sprue is unknown. There is speculation that one or more infectious agents play a role in the etiology of this syndrome because most patients respond to antibiotic therapy. It is interesting that tropical sprue is not common in all tropical regions. Tropical sprue is most common in South India, the Philippines, and several Caribbean islands. For other unclear reasons, some patients may not develop symptoms until years after travel to an endemic area.

The diagnosis of tropical sprue is made based on the history of travel or residence in a tropical area, vitamin B_{12} and/or folate deficiency and an abnormal intestinal biopsy. The intestinal biopsy demonstrates mononuclear cells infiltrating the lamina propria and villus flattening involving the proximal as well as the more distal bowel. The villus atrophy seen in tropical sprue is often patchy and less severe than that seen with celiac sprue.

Treatment of tropical sprue consists of vitamin B_{12} and folate replacement and a 1 to 6 month course of broad-spectrum antibiotics. Folic acid alone induces some improvement in the histologic findings of tropical sprue.

Disaccharidase Deficiency

Lactose intolerance is a common problem resulting in clinical symptoms of diarrhea, abdominal pain, and flatulence after the ingestion of lactose-containing products. Lactose malabsorption can be because of an acquired lactase deficiency, congenital lactase deficiency, or a secondary lactase deficiency resulting from underlying intestinal disease.

Acquired lactase deficiency is the most common form of lactose intolerance and is more common among Native Americans, African Americans, Asians, and Hispanics. Preservation of intestinal lactase is most commonly seen in whites, particularly those of northern European descent. Individuals of all races maintain lactase activity until the age of 5 years. Lactase activity begins to decline during childhood although symptoms of lactose intolerance usually do not manifest until adulthood. Development of lactose malabsorption in early childhood should raise suspicions of congenital lactase deficiency. Congenital causes of disaccharidase deficiency are rare, and clinical symptoms manifest in infancy. These disorders include congenital lactase deficiency, congenital sucrase-isomaltase deficiency, and congenital glucose-galactose deficiency.

Diseases involving the mucosa of the bowel can result in a reduction of brush-border disaccharidases.

Lactase, the least abundant disaccharidase present in the intestinal brush border, is the most vulnerable disaccharidase to intestinal disease, explaining the development of secondary lactase deficiency in many diseases affecting the small intestine. Bacterial overgrowth can also cause lactose malabsorption. Lactose not digested in the small intestines is delivered to the colon where colonic bacteria convert lactose to short chain fatty acids and hydrogen gas. The small chain fatty acids are absorbed by the colonocytes, salvaging the energy provided by lactose. Lactose not converted to SCFAs exerts an osmotic effect in the colon resulting in watery diarrhea. Colonic bacteria can adapt to the presence of increased amounts of lactose in the colon, explaining the ability of some individuals with lactase deficiency to increase their tolerance to lactose containing products.

The association of symptoms with lactose ingestion leads to a suspected diagnosis of lactose intolerance. Because lactose intolerance can occur as a result of other malabsorptive small bowel disorders, it is sometimes difficult to differentiate between primary and secondary lactase deficiency.

Patients with lactose intolerance should follow a lactose-reduced or lactose-free diet. Bacterial-produced lactase is available commercially and may reduce symptoms when ingested with lactose-containing products. Predigested dairy products are also commercially available.

Congenital Enterokinase Deficiency

Enterokinase deficiency is a rare congenital disorder wherein there is an absence of the brush-border enzyme enteropeptidase, which converts the proenzyme trypsinogen to trypsin. Trypsin is necessary for the activation of more trypsinogen and other pancreatic proteases. Protein malabsorption results in hypoproteinemia and growth retardation.

Abetalipoproteinemia

After fatty acids and monoglycerides have been absorbed into the intestinal epithelial cells, they are re-esterified to form triglycerides. These re-esterified triglycerides, cholesterol, and apoprotein B then form chylomicrons, which cross the basolateral membrane of the intestinal epithelial cell into the lymphatics. A rare disorder, abetalipoproteinemia is an autosomal recessive disorder resulting in a mutation of the microsomal triglyceride transfer protein (MTP). This mutation leads to the failure of chylomicron formation and triglycerides accumulate in the enterocytes. These patients develop steatorrhea, diarrhea, and neurologic symptoms. Laboratory studies reveal abnormal erythrocytes, or acanthocytes, which develop because of cell membrane defects. These patients also have low levels of cholesterol, triglyceride, and apoprotein B. Intestinal biopsy reveals lipid-laden small intestinal epithelial cells, which become normal after a prolonged fast. These patients are treated with a low-fat diet and dietary supplementation of fat-soluble vitamins and medium-chain triglycerides.

Rakel and Bope: *Conn's Current Therapy 2006.*

ABNORMALITIES OF NUTRIENT TRANSPORTATION

Intestinal Lymphangiectasia

Intestinal lymphangiectasia can either be a congenital or an acquired disorder secondary to obstruction of the lymphatics. (Tuberculosis [TB], lymphoma, carcinoma, trauma, Whipple's disease, sarcoidosis, congestive heart failure, and retroperitoneal fibrosis are examples of causes of secondary intestinal lymphangiectasia.) Obstruction of the lymphatic channels results in increased intestinal lymphatic pressure and eventual rupture of the lymphatic vessels with loss of lymph containing fat, protein, and lymphocytes into the bowel lumen. Carbohydrates are absorbed through the portal circulation and are unaffected by the obstructed lymphatic channels. Patients typically present with fat malabsorption, fat-soluble vitamin deficiencies, hypoproteinemia, lymphopenia, and edema. Treatment of this condition includes treatment of the underlying cause of the disorder if appropriate and institution of a low-fat diet enriched with complex-carbohydrates with fat-soluble vitamin replacement. Supplementation with MCTs is often useful.

Whipple's Disease

Whipple's disease, first described in 1907 by G.H. Whipple, is an uncommon disease capable of affecting many organ systems of the body. Most often, the disease is characterized by weight loss, diarrhea, and generalized malabsorption. Clinical manifestations of the disease are not limited to the gastrointestinal system and can include a vast range of symptoms depending on the organ system involved. Examples of systemic symptoms include cardiac manifestations such as pleuritis, pericarditis, and valvular endocarditis; pulmonary involvement resulting in chronic cough and pleuritic pain; ocular symptoms; and neurologic symptoms including dementia, headache, myopathy, epilepsy, ataxia, sensory deficits, myoclonus, and cranial nerve impairment. Fever and arthritis are the most common extraintestinal symptoms. The arthritis, an intermittent migratory arthritis of the large and small joints, is often present years before development of gastrointestinal symptoms. Gastrointestinal symptoms, although common, need not be present in Whipple's disease.

Whipple's disease is caused by *Tropheryma whippelii*, a gram-positive actinomycete. The disease is more common in men and usually presents in the fourth through sixth decades of life. The epidemiologic pattern of this disease is unknown. Direct transmission of the infectious agent is unlikely, and host susceptibility factors are believed to play a role in patients who develop the disease. Diagnosis is made by the histologic findings of para-aminosalicylic acid–positive (PAS-positive) macrophages containing the organisms from biopsies of affected tissues. MAC can cause a similar histologic picture, but MAC organisms are acid-fast positive and *T. whippelii* organisms are not. Whipple's disease is treated with a prolonged course of antibiotics.

Diagnosis of Malabsorption

A detailed history is the most valuable diagnostic tool in determining the etiology of malabsorption. The causes of malabsorption vary greatly, and often a history can provide clues to its cause and help guide further diagnostic tests. Initial laboratory studies may provide additional diagnostic clues. Nutrients and minerals may be absorbed throughout the small bowel or absorbed at specific sites. For example, iron, calcium, and folic acid are absorbed in the proximal bowel, and vitamin B_{12} and bile acids are absorbed in the ileum. Deficiencies of these nutrients help identify areas of the bowel contributing to a patient's malabsorption. Other nutrients such as lipids, amino acids, and glucose are absorbed throughout the small bowel. Levels of many nutrients can be obtained through routine laboratory studies. Other abnormal laboratory studies may indirectly provide clues of nutrient deficiencies. An elevated prothrombin time may suggest a vitamin K deficiency in a patient who is not anticoagulated and has normal liver function. A macrocytic anemia may suggest vitamin B_{12} or folic acid deficiency. Iron-deficiency anemia in patients without evidence of gastrointestinal blood loss may suggest iron malabsorption as seen in celiac disease.

Examination of the stool for fat remains the best screening test available for malabsorption. Normally a person excretes less than 6% of ingested fat in the stool. If a patient ingests 100 g/day of fat, more than 6 g/day of fat is considered abnormal. Patients with steatorrhea often have more than 20 g/day of fat in their stool. A 72-hour quantitative stool fat determination in a patient consuming 100 to 120 g/day of dietary fat is the gold standard test for the detection of steatorrhea. A prolonged stool collection is impractical and often inaccurate; therefore, many practitioners will instead perform a 48-hour stool collection for fecal fat quantification. If this test suggests malabsorption, further studies are performed based on clues gained from history and initial laboratory studies. If pancreatic insufficiency is suspected, radiologic imaging of the pancreas is the next appropriate test. If bacterial overgrowth is suspected, a culture of intestinal aspirate should be obtained and a hydrogen breath test can be performed. Small bowel barium series is a valuable test when structural abnormalities are suspected as the cause of malabsorption. Small bowel series may also provide useful information in diagnosing Crohn's disease of the small bowel. When mucosal disease is suspected, endoscopy provides an opportunity to visualize small bowel mucosa and obtain biopsies providing histologic clues to the diagnosis. Small intestinal biopsies may be diagnostic in celiac disease, Crohn's disease, intestinal lymphoma, parasitic infections, amyloidosis, abetalipoproteinemia, Whipple's disease, and intestinal lymphangiectasia.

If the etiology of malabsorption is unclear, the urinary D-xylose absorption test can help differentiate whether malabsorption is secondary to mucosal disease or pancreatic insufficiency. The D-xylose absorption test is performed by giving 25 g of D-xylose, a pentose absorbed in the proximal small intestines. Urine is collected for

Rakel and Bope: *Conn's Current Therapy 2006.*

5 hours and the D-xylose excretion is measured. Serum levels are drawn after 1 hour and 3 hours. If the D-xylose absorption test is normal, evaluation of the pancreas should be performed. If the test is abnormal, evaluation for mucosal disease is indicated.

Treatment

Once the etiology of malabsorption is determined, the underlying disorder should be corrected or treated if possible. Caloric, protein, and volume needs should be assessed, and nutrient, vitamin, mineral, and electrolyte levels should be measured. The patient's quality of life should also be determined. The goals for treatment of malabsorptive disorders should include improvement and maintenance of the patient's quality of life, and the replacement of nutrients, minerals, vitamins, electrolytes, and fluids. Specific therapies are discussed previously in this article regarding specific malabsorptive disorders. The following section provides some general guidelines for the management of malabsorptive disorders.

Diarrhea in malabsorptive disorders may be the result of a number of factors including osmotic and secretory effects of malabsorbed nutrients and bile acids, alteration of intestinal transit time or increased gastric secretions as can be seen with intestinal resections. Treatment aimed to alter any of these factors may be successful in reducing stool or ostomy output.

Opiates are the most widely and successfully used antidiarrheal agents. These agents decrease intestinal motility. Loperamide (Imodium), in divided doses up to 16 mg/day, is an optimal treatment because of its low side-effect profile. Diphenoxylate combined with atropine (Lomotil) can also be given in doses up to 8 pills/day. Occasionally a more potent opiate is required to control diarrhea, such as deodorized tincture of opium, codeine,[1] or morphine.[1]

H_2-receptor antagonists or PPIs may be useful adjunctive medications through their ability to decrease acid secretion and reduce gastric secretions. Octreotide (Sandostatin)[1] is sometimes used because of its ability to decrease intestinal secretions. Octreotide (Sandostatin)[1] is not an optimal treatment because it is an expensive medication and must be given subcutaneously. Cholestyramine[1] is useful in treating bile acid diarrhea but can potentially worsen diarrhea in patients with fatty acid malabsorption. Patients with fatty acid malabsorption are best treated with a low-fat diet and bile-acid replacement. A lactose-free diet may also alleviate symptoms in many malabsorptive disorders. As discussed previously, secondary lactase deficiency is a common consequence of many intestinal disorders. MCTs are useful nutritional supplements for patients with fat malabsorption. MCTs are usually tolerated at doses of 1 tablespoon 3 to 4 times a day.

Patients should be instructed to eat frequent meals (at least 6/day) to increase contact time between food and the intestinal mucosa, improving overall absorption.

---

[1]Not FDA approved for this indication.

CURRENT DIAGNOSIS

Clinical Manifestation	Nutritional Deficiencies
General	
Weight loss, fatigue, amenorrhea, anorexia	Protein-calorie
Hair, Skin	
Pallor	Iron, folate, vitamin B_{12}
Alopecia	Protein, zinc
Ecchymoses	Vitamin K
Follicular hyperkeratosis	Vitamin A
Dermatitis	Zinc
Eyes	
Nightblindness	Vitamin A
Retinopathy	Vitamin E
Mouth	
Glossitis	Folate, niacin, riboflavin
Angular stomatitis or cheilosis	Iron, riboflavin, niacin
Bleeding gums	Vitamin K
Hypogeusia	Vitamin E
Neurologic	
Tetany	Calcium, magnesium
Paresthesias	Vitamin B_{12}, thiamine
Dementia	Vitamin B_{12}, niacin
Hyporeflexia, foot or wrist drop	Thiamine
Ataxia, loss of vibratory and position sense	Vitamin B_{12}, folate, vitamin E

Additional nutritional supplements can be given between meals or nocturnal tube feeds can be administered at night to increase caloric intake. Oral rehydration solutions can be beneficial to some patients with fluid and electrolyte losses. These solutions are typically given to patients with less than 100 cm of jejunum and an end jejunostomy or jejuno-colonic anastomosis. These solutions should contain 90 to 120 mmol of sodium, optimizing sodium and fluid absorption in the gut.

Nutrients, electrolytes and fluid status should be closely monitored and replaced. Fat-soluble vitamins and vitamin B_{12} are stored in the body and deficiencies develop with continuous losses. Vitamins A, D, and E are available in water-soluble forms and are more effective for replacement therapy. Vitamin B_{12}[1] should be given parenterally when more than 100 cm of the ileum is diseased or resected. Vitamin B_{12}[1] can be administered by intramuscular injection (IM), subcutaneously (SQ), or through a nasal gel. Repletion of magnesium is difficult because magnesium is poorly absorbed and can worsen diarrhea. Soluble magnesium salts, such as magnesium gluconate, are better tolerated. Magnesium can be added to oral rehydration solutions and sipped throughout the day minimizing its osmotic effect in the colon. Parenteral magnesium is also available. Calcium should be supplemented at doses of 1.5 to 2.0 g/day. Zinc is best given as zinc gluconate between meals. Most patients require up to 150 mg of elemental zinc/day, but the dose should be adjusted according to stool or ostomy output. Iron replacement is usually most successful

The Digestive System

CURRENT THERAPY

Condition	Treatment
Pancreatic insufficiency	Pancreatic enzyme supplements
Bacterial overgrowth	Surgical correction if appropriate
	Antibiotics
	Fat-soluble vitamins, vitamin B$_{12}$
	Prokinetics, octreotide (Sandostatin)[1]
Ileal disease/resection	<100 cm, cholestyramine[1]
	>100 cm, low-fat diet, antidiarrheal agents
	Fat-soluble vitamins, vitamin B$_{12}$
Short bowel syndrome	Antidiarrheal agents
	MCTs
	±H$_2$-receptor antagonist or PPI
	Low-fat diet
	Vitamin and mineral supplementation
	IVF or parenteral nutrition
Celiac disease	Gluten-free diet
	Iron, folate, calcium, and vitamin D
Tropical sprue	Long-course antibiotics
	Vitamin B$_{12}$, folate
Lactase deficiency	Lactose reduced/free diet
Lymphangiectasia	Low-fat diet
	MCTs
	Fat-soluble vitamins

[1]Not FDA approved for this indication.
Abbreviations: IVF = intravenous fluid; MCTs = medium-chain triglycerides; PPI = proton pump inhibitor.

when the dose is slowly titrated to a goal dose of 180 mg elemental iron/day in divided doses. Parenteral iron is useful for patients with severe depletion of iron or patients with chronic iron malabsorption not corrected with oral replacement.

Patients unable to maintain hydration with oral solutions or suffering from severe malnourishment despite oral supplementation may require intravenous fluids (IVFs) or parenteral nutrition. Institution of parenteral nutrition can sometimes drastically improve a patient's quality of life by decreasing diarrhea resulting from aggressive oral rehydration therapy and improving overall health.

REFERENCES

Drazen JM, Gill GN, Griggs RC, et al (Eds.): Cecil Textbook of Medicine. 21st ed. Philadelphia, WB Saunders, 2000.
Feldman M, Friedman LS, Sleisenger MH (Eds.): Sleisenger & Fordtran's Gastrointestinal and Liver Disease, vol. 2, 7th ed. Philadelphia, WB Saunders, 2002.
Fine KD, Schiller LR: AGA technical review on the evaluation and management of chronic diarrhea. Gastroenterology 1999;116(6): 1464-1486.
Sleisenger MH: Malabsorption syndrome. N Engl J Med 1969;281(20): 1111-1117.

Acute Pancreatitis

Method of
Vivek Gumaste, MD

Acute pancreatitis is an inflammatory disease of the pancreas characterized by severe epigastric pain and raised levels of amylase and lipase in the blood. Common causes of acute pancreatitis are gallstone disease and alcohol abuse. The incidence of acute pancreatitis in the United States ranges from 15 to 20 per 100,000 population. A mortality rate of 10% to 15% is often quoted in the literature, but this figure appears to be too high. A more realistic estimate is a rate of 3% to 5%. Although no definite gender predilection exists, alcoholic pancreatitis is more common in men, and gallstone pancreatitis is more frequent in women.

Definitions

In the past, pancreatitis was fraught with vague and conflicting nomenclature. These definitions, proposed at the Symposium on Acute Pancreatitis, held in Atlanta, Georgia, in 1992, are now widely accepted:

- *Mild acute pancreatitis:* Mild acute pancreatitis is defined as an episode with minimal or no organ dysfunction and an uneventful recovery.
- *Severe acute pancreatitis:* Severe acute pancreatitis is associated with organ failure (Box 1) and/or local complications such as necrosis, abscess, or pseudocyst.
- *Acute fluid collection:* Acute fluid collection is fluid bodies located in or near the pancreas that lack a definite fibrous wall and occur early in the course of the disease.
- *Acute pseudocyst:* Acute pseudocyst is a fluid collection encapsulated by a wall of fibrous tissue and usually occurs 4 to 6 weeks after the onset.
- *Pancreatic abscess:* Pancreatic abscess is a circumscribed intra-abdominal collection of pus close to the pancreas with little or no necrosis.
- *Pancreatic necrosis:* Pancreatic necrosis consists of diffuse or focal nonviable pancreatic parenchyma accompanied by peripancreatic fat necrosis

Etiology

Although there are myriad causes for acute pancreatitis, gallstones and alcohol account for more than 80%

BOX 1 Organ Failure

- Shock: systolic blood pressure <90 mm Hg
- Pulmonary insufficiency: Pao$_2$ <60 mm Hg
- Renal failure: serum creatinine >2 mg/dL
- Gastrointestinal bleeding: >500 mL/24 hr

Abbreviations: Pao$_2$ = partial pressure of alveolar oxygen

of all cases. In the United States, alcohol is the most likely etiology in large city or county hospitals, whereas gallstone pancreatitis is more common in community hospitals.

Alcoholic pancreatitis usually occurs in patients around 30 years of age who ingest a minimum of 150 grams of alcohol per day and who have been drinking heavily for at least 5 years. A bout of acute pancreatitis typically follows an alcoholic binge. In contrast, gallstone pancreatitis occurs in older patients.

Drugs form an important category. Although some drugs are clearly linked with acute pancreatitis, others have a more nebulous role (Box 2).

Post-endoscopic retrograde cholangiopancreatography (ERCP) pancreatitis accounts for 2% to 8% of all cases of pancreatitis. Female sex, age less than 55 years, and a previous history of acute pancreatitis are factors that predispose to post-ERCP pancreatitis. Other possible contributory factors include procedure-related factors such as sphincter of Oddi manometry, difficult cannulation, and precut sphincterotomy.

Certain infections can cause acute pancreatitis. These include viral infections such as mumps, mononucleosis, Coxsackie virus, enteric cytopathogenic human orphan (ECHO) viruses, varicella, and measles. Bacterial causes are *Mycoplasma pneumoniae*, salmonellosis, *Campylobacter* species, and tuberculosis. Parasitic worms such as *Ascaris lumbricoides* can induce acute pancreatitis by obstructing the papilla.

Serum triglyceride levels in excess of 1000 mg/dL are associated with acute pancreatitis and commonly seen in patients with type I, IV, and V hyperlipidemia.

Acute pancreatitis can be a presenting feature in tumors that obstruct the pancreatic duct such as

ampullary tumors and ductal adenocarcinomas. Pancreatic lymphoma can manifest as acute pancreatitis. Mucinous ductal ectasia is a premalignant condition that is increasingly recognized as a cause of recurrent acute pancreatitis. If detected early and treated, progression to cancer can be prevented.

Less than 1% of cases are hereditary in nature. Hereditary pancreatitis is an autosomal dominant disorder with 80% penetrance. Congenital anomalies such as pancreas divisum and annular pancreas may predispose to acute pancreatitis. Some experts are of the opinion that pancreas divisum is merely an incidental finding, however, and not a causative factor for acute pancreatitis.

In Trinidad, the sting of the scorpion *Tityus trinitatis* is the most common cause of acute pancreatitis. Other miscellaneous causes include hypercalcemia, trauma, and the postoperative state.

In approximately 10% to 20% of cases, the cause cannot be ascertained and the cases are labeled idiopathic.

Pathophysiology

Normally the pancreas is protected from auto-digestion by the following features:

- Synthesis of enzymes as inactive zymogens
- Presence of protease inhibitors
- Segregation of enzymes within membrane-bound compartments
- Activating enzyme (enterokinase) separated geographically from the pancreas

Inappropriate intracellular activation of trypsin is the key initiating factor. How this occurs is not clear. It is possible that reflux of duodenal contents into the pancreatic duct may play a role. Another possible mechanism implicates co-localization of lysosomal hydrolases, which are capable of activating trypsinogen.

Activation of trypsin in turn triggers the entire zymogen activation cascade, resulting in potent enzymes being extruded into the interstitium across the basolateral membrane. Neutrophils and macrophages are subsequently drawn into this process and further add to the damage by releasing other proteolytic enzymes and cytokines that mediate local and systemic inflammatory responses.

Clinical Presentation

Most patients with acute pancreatitis present with severe epigastric abdominal pain that radiates to the back and occasionally to the flanks. The pain is so severe that patients usually present to the emergency room; a patient with acute pancreatitis is unlikely to walk into the office or clinic. The pain is worsened by eating food and may be relieved by sitting up or assuming a fetal position. The majority of patients have associated nausea and vomiting. A fever in excess of 38.9°C (102°F) suggests the development of complications or cholangitis.

BOX 2   Drug-Induced Pancreatitis

Definite
- Asparaginase
- Azathioprine
- Didanosine
- Estrogens
- 6-Mercaptopurine
- Pentamidine

Probable
- Protease inhibitors
- Acetaminophen
- Sulfasalazine
- Furosemide
- Thiazide diuretics

Questionable
- Corticosteroids
- Erythromycin
- Octreotide
- Ketoprofen
- Ranitidine
- Cimetidine
- Valproate

Isoniazid
- Rifampicin

Dyspnea occurs in patients with acute respiratory distress syndrome (ARDS).

Physical examination is unrevealing except for mild epigastric tenderness. Dehydration, tachycardia, and jaundice may be present. Occasionally a pleural effusion or ascites may be detected. Ecchymotic patches in the body wall around the umbilicus (Cullen's sign) or in the flanks (Grey Turner's sign) are rarely seen in clinical practice. Erythematous skin nodules may result from focal subcutaneous fat necrosis. Purtscher's angiopathic retinopathy, a rare funduscopic finding in acute pancreatitis, results from ischemic injury to the retina caused by activation of complement and agglutination of blood cells within retinal vessels. Temporary or permanent blindness can be the consequence.

Diagnosis

SERUM AMYLASE

Despite several failings, serum amylase continues to be the key diagnostic test in cases of acute pancreatitis. A serum amylase level greater than three times normal is generally used as the cutoff threshold. But using serum amylase as a diagnostic test has the following limitations:

- Elevations of serum amylase are not specific to the pancreas. Amylase is found in a variety of organs, such as the salivary gland, fallopian tubes, and lungs. False elevations of amylase may be seen in perforated peptic ulcer, choledocholithiasis, mesenteric infarction, appendicitis, intestinal obstruction, and ruptured ectopic pregnancy. The degree of elevation of serum amylase in these patients with nonpancreatic abdominal pain, however, is usually less than three times normal.
- Serum amylase levels are extremely high (in the thousands) in gallstone pancreatitis and has a sensitivity of more than 90% in diagnosing this condition. With alcohol as the etiology, the elevations are much more modest; up to one third of patients have normal amylase levels. The sensitivity of serum amylase in detecting acute alcoholic pancreatitis, therefore, is significantly lower.
- Macroamylasemia is a condition characterized by falsely elevated serum amylase levels resulting from an abnormal amylase molecule. A normal serum lipase level and a normal urinary amylase level resolve the issue.
- High triglyceride levels interfere with the assay of serum amylase (probably because of the presence of an amylase inhibitor) and produce falsely normal amylase levels in 50% of patients with hypertriglyceridemia-induced acute pancreatitis.
- Asymptomatic elevations maybe seen in patients with AIDS. The precise cause remains unknown but could be the result of subclinical infection of the pancreas.
- Renal failure per se is known to produce serum amylase elevations up to but not greater than three times normal.

SERUM LIPASE

Difficulties in lipase assay techniques and standardization prevent the widespread use of serum lipase, although it is theoretically more specific than amylase. In the following situations, serum lipase is superior to serum amylase:

- Serum lipase levels tend to be extremely high in acute alcoholic pancreatitis (more than five times normal) and is a much more accurate test to diagnose acute alcoholic pancreatitis as long as appropriate cutoff levels are used.
- Serum lipase tends to remain elevated for longer periods of time than serum amylase and may be useful in patients who present late.
- Normoamylasemia pancreatitis can also be detected with the help of serum lipase.

SERUM TRYPSIN

Serum trypsin levels have a high sensitivity and a reasonable specificity in diagnosing acute pancreatitis, but problems with the assay technique limit its use in clinical practice. Attempts to use other enzymes (serum elastase-1, phospholipase A2, alpha 1-protease, antichymotrypsin, pancreas-specific protein) for diagnostic purposes are not fruitful.

STANDARD BLOOD TESTS

The white blood cell count may be elevated in cases of acute pancreatitis. Elevations in liver enzymes seen in gallstone pancreatitis caused by choledocholithiasis may also be seen in alcoholic pancreatitis when an edematous pancreas obstructs the bile duct. Hypocalcemia can occur.

ABDOMINAL PLAIN FILM

An abdominal radiograph is of little help in the diagnosis of acute pancreatitis. Very rarely one may see a sentinel loop, which is a localized ileus of a segment of small intestine, or the colon cutoff sign. More important, a plain radiograph may exclude other causes of abdominal pain. The presence of pancreatic calcification may provide a clue to the etiology of the acute pancreatitis.

ULTRASOUND

Despite being less sensitive than a computerized tomography (CT) scan, ultrasound exam is the initial imaging study of choice because it is noninvasive and inexpensive and should be routinely ordered in all suspected cases of acute pancreatitis. The presence of a swollen pancreas on an ultrasound confirms the diagnosis. Useful additional information, such as the presence of gallstones or a dilated common bile duct (CBD), can also be obtained from a sonogram. In approximately 25% to 30% of cases, however, the pancreas is obscured by gas and poorly visualized.

Rakel and Bope: *Conn's Current Therapy 2006.*

COMPUTERIZED TOMOGRAPHY SCAN

Although a CT scan is the best available method to visualize the pancreas, it is not cost effective to perform in all patients with acute pancreatitis. Neither is it necessary. As a diagnostic tool, a CT scan may be useful in rare instances when the diagnosis is in doubt. More central is its role in the stratification of severity and detection of complications. We recommend a CT scan only in those patients with severe pancreatitis or who have abdominal pain lasting greater than 5 days, persistently raised amylase levels, or a temperature higher than 38.9°C (102°F).

ENDOSCOPIC ULTRASONOGRAPHY AND MAGNETIC RESONANCE IMAGING

Endoscopic ultrasonography (EUS) and magnetic resonance imaging (MRI) have no definite role in the diagnosis of acute pancreatitis.

Severity Stratification

Assessment of the severity of the diseases at presentation is important for appropriate management and also for prognostication. In fact, failure to stratify patients accurately can result in potentially avoidable deaths. Several different grading systems exist. Some use purely clinical criteria or laboratory data; others use a combination of both. CT imaging is an important modality in severity stratification.

MULTIFACTORIAL SCORING SYSTEMS

Components of *Ranson's criteria* and the *Glasgow system*, two similar grading systems, are listed in Box 3. The presence of more than three criteria predicts a more severe course.

The *Acute Physiological And Chronic Health Evaluation II* (APACHE II) system is more complex than the Ranson's criteria, requires the aid of a computer, and is more suited to the intensive care setting. An advantage is that it can be used for daily assessment. The sensitivity and specificity depends on the cutoff threshold used. A score of 9 or more is indicative of severe disease, but the sensitivity is poor at this level. When 6 is used as a cutoff marker, the sensitivity reaches 95%; however, the positive predictive value dips to 50%.

SERUM MARKERS

C-reactive protein (CRP), a simple test that can gauge severity, is universally available. A level of more than 210 mg/L after 4 days or more than 120 mg/L after a week is as accurate in prognostication as the multifactorial systems. Its sensitivity in detecting necrotizing pancreatitis is 95%.

Other enzymes such as polymorphonuclear (PMN) elastase, serum RNase, α-macroglobulin, and interleukin-6 may in the future be used to predict severity of diseases, but at present their use is experimental.

BOX 3 Prognostic Criteria

Ranson's Criteria
- At admission
  Age older than 55 years
  WBC greater than 16,000/mm³
  Glucose greater than 200 mg/dL
  LDH greater than 350 IU/L
  AST greater than 250 U/L
- After 48 hours
  Hematocrit decrease of 10%
  BUN increase greater than 5 mg/dL
  Calcium less than 8 mg/dL
  Pao₂ less than 60 mm Hg
  Base deficit greater than 4 mEq/L
  Fluid sequestration greater than 6 L

Glasgow Scoring System
- Age older than 55 years
- WBC greater than 15,000/mm³
- Glucose greater than 180 mg/dL
- LDH greater than 600 U/L
- AST greater than 100 U/L
- BUN >45 mg/dL
- Pao₂ less than 60 mm Hg
- Calcium less than 8 mg/dL
- Albumin less than 3.2 g/dL

Abbreviations: AST = aspartate aminotransferase; BUN = blood urea nitrogen; LDH = lactate dehydrogenase; Pao₂ = partial pressure of alveolar oxygen; WBC = white blood count.

Similarly, attempts to use inflammatory markers such as interleukin-6, PMN elastase, trypsinogen activation peptide, and methemalbuminemia have limited success.

URINARY TESTS

Trypsinogen activation peptide (TAP) is cleaved from trypsinogen during activation and can be measured in the serum and urine. Urinary TAP, when measured within 48 hours, can discriminate between mild and severe cases of acute pancreatitis.

COMPUTED TOMOGRAPHY SCAN

All patients judged to have severe disease by any of the clinical or laboratory indexes need to undergo intravenous (IV) contrast-enhanced dynamic CT scanning. Although the other systems suggest severity, the CT scan actually confirms the presence of complications such as necrosis, fluid collections, or abscess formation. The grading system is outlined in Table 1. A CT severity index greater than 7 is associated with increased morbidity and mortality.

MAGNETIC RESONANCE IMAGING

MRI is as reliable as CT in the staging of acute pancreatitis. The advantages of MRI include the ability to detect necrosis without the use of contrast and to define pancreatic duct disruption without the use of secretin.

TABLE 1 Computed Tomography (CT) Severity Index

Computed Tomography Grading System

Grade	Computed Tomography Morphology
A	Normal
B	Focal or diffuse gland enlargement
C	Any of above plus peripancreatic inflammatory changes
D	Grade C plus associated single fluid collection
E	Grade C plus two or more peripancreatic fluid collections or gas in the pancreas or retroperitoneum

Computed Tomography Severity Index (CT Score + Necrosis Score)

CT Grade	Score	Necrosis	Score
A	0	None	0
B	1	<33%	2
C	2	33%-50%	4
D	3	>50%	6
E	4		

Adapted from Balthazar EJ, Robinson DL, Megibow AJ, Ranson JH: Acute pancreatitis: Value of CT in establishing prognosis. Radiology 1990;174:331-336.

Etiologic Assessment

HISTORY

Emphasis should be placed on a detailed history that records alcohol intake, previous history of gallstones, list of medications, prodromal illness, HIV disease, and recent surgery.

LABORATORY INDICATORS

Calcium levels and triglyceride estimation is routinely recommended. A serum alanine aminotransaminase (ALT) level greater than 150 IU/L has a sensitivity of more than 90% in diagnosing gallstone disease. In acute alcoholic pancreatitis, high lipase-to-amylase ratios (more than 2) are noted as opposed to gallstone pancreatitis.

ULTRASOUND

An ultrasound exam can confirm gallstones as the etiology. In a small percentage of patients, however, gallstones are not seen on the initial exam, and the exam has to be repeated after the acute episode subsides.

RECURRENT IDIOPATHIC PANCREATITIS

When adequate history, laboratory tests, and pancreaticobiliary imaging are not able to ascertain the etiology, the condition is termed *idiopathic pancreatitis*. Potential causes include missed biliary stones, microlithiasis, pancreas divisum, ampullary neoplasms, or sphincter of Oddi dysfunction. Further workup depends on the clinical situation. A mild episode may not warrant further

workup, but recurrent episodes or severe disease need added evaluation:

- *CT scan* may be necessary to exclude a tumor.
- Examination of the *duodenal aspirate* may reveal microlithiasis.
- Magnetic resonance cholangiopancreatography *(MRCP)* or *EUS* may detect CBD stones and microlithiasis.
- *ERCP without manometry* is useful only when pancreas divisum is suspected.
- *ERCP with manometry* may be considered when all other tests prove inconclusive.
- Other tests that may be necessary include *sweat electrolyte estimation* (cystic fibrosis), *genetic testing* (hereditary pancreatitis), and *immune markers* (autoimmune pancreatitis).

Treatment

The medical treatment of acute pancreatitis is mainly supportive in nature. Pain control, adequate fluid resuscitation, and careful monitoring are the mainstays of therapy. The ultimate goal is to decrease morbidity and mortality by the prevention, detection, and early treatment of complications such as infection, necrosis, and pseudocyst formation (Figure 1).

MILD PANCREATITIS

Most cases of acute pancreatitis fall into the mild category and have an excellent prognosis. These patients can be managed on regular hospital floors and have an uneventful recovery in 5 to 7 days. Nothing orally is the single most important intervention in all patients with acute pancreatitis. This approach must be clearly explained and emphasized to the patient. It can be an

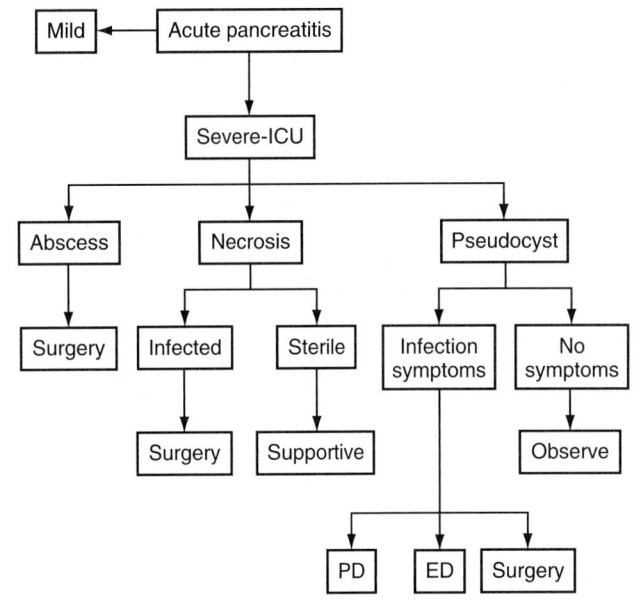

FIGURE 1. Management of acute pancreatitis. ED = endoscopic drainage; ICU = intensive care unit; PD = percutaneous drainage.

issue with alcoholic patients, who have a tendency to sneak in some foods.

Oral feeds are restarted when all symptoms, especially abdominal pain, are *completely resolved* (usually 3 to 5 days) and when serum amylase levels are down *to normal or near-normal levels*. Serum lipase, which can be an important diagnostic tool, tends to remain elevated for longer periods of time and is not important in deciding when to initiate oral feeding.

IV hydration and pain control are the other important measures. Pain can usually be controlled with meperidine (Demerol), 50 to 100 mg, given parenterally every 4 hours. Morphine or its derivatives are avoided because of the possibility of sphincter of Oddi spasm.

A nasogastric tube is not routinely inserted but can be useful in patients with an ileus or in those patients who have intractable vomiting. Proton pump inhibitors and H_2 blockers have shown no advantage, and antibiotic therapy does not provide any additional benefit in cases of mild pancreatitis.

SEVERE PANCREATITIS

Patients with severe pancreatitis are more likely to have complications such as organ failure, necrosis, and infection. These patients must be monitored in an intensive care setting.

Although studies do not show that fluid hydration prevents pancreatic necrosis, it is good clinical judgment to embark on a course of aggressive fluid resuscitation. Patients may require 5 to 10 liters of fluid per day. Albumin infusion may be given when the serum albumin level drops below 2 g/L. Hematocrit levels should be maintained at approximately 30%.

Adequate oxygenation is maintained, and in those who develop ARDS, endotracheal intubation and positive end-expiratory ventilation may be required.

Hypocalcemia is usually the result of low albumin levels and requires no treatment. Blood sugar levels fluctuate, and the patient is administered insulin or dextrose accordingly. Magnesium and potassium may need replacement.

Nutrition

Most patients with mild acute pancreatitis do not require any other form of nutritional support, apart from IV fluids. In patients with severe pancreatitis, prolonged nutritional supplementation, either through the enteral or parenteral route, is necessary. Total parenteral nutrition (TPN), the preferred mode of nutritional support for a long time, results in a high incidence of infection because it has a tendency to impair humoral and cell-mediated immunity. In enteral feeding, feeds are delivered to the jejunum using a nasojejunal tube with the aim of decreasing pancreatic stimulation. Enteral feeding, compared with TPN, decreases the incidence of infection, surgical intervention, and length of hospital stay and is the route of choice. In clinical practice, however, the physician is often tormented by an inability to maintain the location of the feeding tube.

Pancreatic Infection

Pancreatic infection is the single most important determinant of mortality in acute pancreatitis. Necrosis predisposes to infection, occurring in greater than 50% of patients with necrosis totaling more than 50%, and mortality rates reach 30% in this subset. Less than 5% of patients with interstitial pancreatitis develop infection, and mortality rates are negligible.

Infection is usually monomicrobial (70%) with *Escherichia coli* the most common organism. Other organisms isolated include *Pseudomonas, Klebsiella,* and *Enterococcus* species. Anaerobic infection and fungal infections can occur but are rare.

Prevention

Attempts to decrease pancreatic infection involve selective gut decontamination by nonabsorbable antibiotics, prophylactic systemic antibiotics, and enteral feeding. Selective decontamination, although promising in one study, is not routinely recommended.

Although earlier studies using less sophisticated systemic antibiotics failed to reveal any beneficial effect, recent studies using agents that penetrate the pancreas decrease infection, and a trend toward decreased mortality is noted. We recommend prophylactic antibiotic therapy for patients with severe pancreatitis, especially those with significant necrosis, presence of fluid collections, and/or organ dysfunction. Imipenem, 0.5 g IV every 8 hours, provides adequate coverage and should be administered for a minimum of 10 to 14 days.

Treatment

In patients with a high white cell count in excess of 20,000/mm³, a temperature of more than 38.9°C (102°F), or unresolved organ failure, a CT-guided needle aspiration of the pancreas is indicated. The aspirate is gram stained and cultured for aerobic as well as anaerobic bacteria and fungi. Patients with definite evidence of infection should undergo surgical debridement. The role of nonsurgical approaches such as endoscopic drainage or radiologic intervention requires further evaluation.

Pancreatic Abscess

A pancreatic abscess occurs approximately 4 weeks after the onset of acute pancreatitis and appears on a CT scan as a poorly marginated, low-density mass containing diffuse air bubbles. Surgical or percutaneous drainage is indicated.

Sterile Necrosis

Most patients with sterile necrosis respond to conservative nonsurgical medical management.

PANCREATIC PSEUDOCYST

Development of a pseudocyst should be suspected when an episode of acute pancreatitis fails to resolve or when a patient has persistently raised amylase levels or continued pain. Rarely can an epigastric mass be felt. The diagnosis is usually confirmed by sonography or a CT scan.

All pseudocysts do not require intervention. Up to 40% of all pseudocysts undergo spontaneous resolution. Pseudocysts smaller than 6 cm in size, as a rule, are more likely to resolve spontaneously, but in many instances cysts larger than 6 cm also regress without intervention. Thus it appears prudent to opt for a conservative approach, especially in the case of small asymptomatic pseudocysts or even larger asymptomatic ones that show signs of improvement. Serial ultrasound exams or CT scans done at intervals of 4 weeks are used to assess the progress of the pseudocyst.

Intervention is indicated in infected pseudocysts, those that are expanding rapidly, or if the patient's symptoms are worsening. Three options are available: surgery, percutaneous drainage, and endoscopic drainage. We favor radiologically guided percutaneous drainage as the initial approach because it is done under local anesthesia and has few contraindications and a low complication rate. After drainage, an indwelling catheter must be left in place because failure to do so results in a recurrence rate as high as 60%. Concomitant use of somatostatin[1] decreases the drainage period. Use of larger drains or multiple drains with frequent sterile saline lavage may be necessary to wash out thick necrotic material. Despite this, the chances of failure are high when large amounts of necrotic material are present. In pseudocysts associated with pancreatic duct disruption, placement of a pancreatic stent via ERCP may facilitate drainage by the percutaneous route.

Surgery should be reserved for those patients who fail percutaneous drainage, those for whom the method is contraindicated, those who have other associated conditions, such as gallstones, that favor a surgical option, or those for whom the diagnosis is uncertain. Surgical procedures for pancreatic pseudocyst include excision, external drainage, and internal drainage. Of these methods, internal drainage is the most frequent and can take the form of cystogastrostomy, cystoduodenostomy, or cystojejunostomy. Excision is the preferred method but is only feasible for cysts in the tail. External drainage is performed when the cyst wall is not thick enough to allow anastomosis to the gut wall.

Another approach uses a needle-knife inserted through an endoscope to create a fistula between the cavity and the lumen of the gut, thereby facilitating drainage. Prior EUS is strongly recommended to ensure a bloodless field for the site of intervention. A high degree of expertise on the part of the endoscopist, along with the lack of universal availability of EUS, makes this approach less practical. Evidence for this technique is too weak at the present time to advocate endoscopic drainage as a standard method of care.

A final decision about the right approach should be made depending on the overall condition of the patient, the characteristics of the pseudocyst, and the availability of local expertise.

 CURRENT DIAGNOSIS

- Presence of abdominal pain
- Serum amylase level more than three times normal
- Serum lipase: a better test for acute alcoholic pancreatitis
- Study of choice: ultrasound exam initial imaging
- CT (computed tomography) scan important to detect necrosis and grade severity
- CT-guided needle aspiration confirms infection in necrotic pancreas

SPECIFIC CONDITIONS

Gallstone Pancreatitis

ERCP has no role in mild biliary pancreatitis. Patients with severe disease, especially those with evidence of biliary obstruction or cholangitis, benefit from early ERCP (within 24 to 72 hours) with sphincterotomy and stone extraction.

Cholecystectomy must be performed in patients with gallstone pancreatitis after recovery from the acute episode but prior to discharge from the hospital. There is a 25% risk of developing another episode of acute pancreatitis within 6 weeks if cholecystectomy is not done.

Post–Endoscopic Retrograde Cholangiopancreatography Pancreatitis

Post-ERCP pancreatitis can be prevented by proper technique and appropriate patient selection. In high-risk patients, prophylactic pancreatic duct stenting is beneficial. The use of low or high osmolality contrast media has no bearing on the outcome. Gabexate,[2] a protease inhibitor, and somatostatin,[1] an antisecretory agent, show some promise in preventing post-ERCP pancreatitis but require further study. So is the case with agents such as diclofenac (Voltaren)[1] and nitroglycerine.[1]

Pancreas Divisum

Although no large randomized controlled trials exist, surgical sphincteroplasty and endoscopic therapy, like minor papilla sphincterotomy and stenting, may prove beneficial in patients with pancreas divisum (PD) who have acute recurrent pancreatitis (ARP). Results in patients with chronic pancreatitis as the predominant symptom are less promising.

Hyperlipidemic Pancreatitis

Treatment of hyperlipidemic pancreatitis includes dietary restriction of fat and lipid-lowering medications such as gemfibrozil (Lopid), mainly fibric acid derivatives. Anecdotal reports suggest that treatments such

---

[1]Not FDA approved for this indication.

[1]Not FDA approved for this indication.
[2]Not available in the United States.

CURRENT THERAPY

- Nothing orally, intravenous hydration, and pain control are the mainstay of therapy.
- Patients with severe disease must be monitored in an intensive care unit.
- Prophylactic antibiotics are recommended for severe acute pancreatitis.
- Early endoscopic retrograde cholangiopancreatography (ERCP) is beneficial in severe gallstone pancreatitis.
- Surgical debridement is the treatment for infected necrosis.
- Asymptomatic pseudocysts can be managed expectantly.
- Infected and symptomatic pseudocysts should undergo either percutaneous or surgical drainage.
- Evidence for endoscopic drainage of a pseudocyst is weak and requires expert hands.

as plasmapheresis, lipid pheresis, and extracorporeal lipid elimination may be successful. Further episodes can be prevented when triglyceride (TG) levels are maintained below 200 mg/dL.

REFERENCES

Baillie J: Pancreatic pseudocyst. II: Technological review. Gastrointest Endosc 2004;60:105-113.
Banks PA: Practice guidelines in acute pancreatitis. Am J Gastroenterol 1997;92:377-386.
Gumaste VV: Role of prophylactic antibiotic therapy in acute pancreatitis. J Clin Gastroenterol 2000;31:6-10.
Klein SD, Affronti JP: Pancreas divisum, an evidence-based review. Gastrointest Endosc 2004;60:585-589.
NIH State of the Science Conference statement: ERCP. Jan 14-16, 2002. (NIH Web site www.niddk.nih.gov).
United Kingdom guidelines for the management of acute pancreatitis. Gut 1998;42(Suppl 2):S1-S13.

Chronic Pancreatitis

Method of
Vivek Gumaste, MD

Chronic pancreatitis is an inflammatory disease in which progressive irreversible structural damage to the pancreas results in a permanent impairment of both the exocrine and endocrine functions. The annual incidence of chronic pancreatitis in the United States is approximately 4 per 100,000 population.

Clinical Features

ABDOMINAL PAIN

Abdominal pain is a prominent clinical feature in most patients. Usually the pain, described as dull, deep, and boring, is localized to the upper abdomen and may radiate to the back. Meals exacerbate the pain. Relief is obtained by sitting up or leaning forward. Although some patients complain of constant pain, others experience intermittent episodes of pain that are separated by pain-free intervals lasting from several days to months. In a minority of patients, chronic pancreatitis can be totally painless. The severity of the pain decreases or resolves over a period of 5 to 25 years.

STEATORRHEA

Steatorrhea is a manifestation of advanced disease and does not occur until the pancreatic secretion is reduced to less than 10% of normal. Patients notice their stools are bulky and malodorous. Leakage of oil per anus is pathognomonic of the condition. Weight loss may or may not occur, depending on the severity of the disease.

DIABETES

Secondary diabetes is a consequence of long-standing disease. The median time to develop diabetes ranges from 12 to 25 years.

COMPLICATIONS

Pseudocyst formation is a known complication of both acute and chronic pancreatitis and discussed in detail in "Acute Pancreatitis." Chronic pancreatitis is a definite risk factor for pancreatic cancer with a lifetime risk of 4%. With hereditary pancreatitis, the cumulative lifetime risk reaches 40%. Extensive fibrosis in the head of the pancreas may encase the bile duct, leading to obstruction and dilation of the common bile duct (CBD) with altered liver chemistry. In approximately 5% of patients with chronic pancreatitis, duodenal stenosis develops. Rupture of the pancreatic duct may lead to leakage of the pancreatic juice into the peritoneum or pleural space, resulting in ascites or pleural effusion, respectively.

Etiopathogenesis

Alcohol is responsible for 60% to 70% of all cases of chronic pancreatitis. Idiopathic chronic pancreatitis accounts for 20% and occurs in two forms: an early-onset variety that manifests in the late teens or 20s and a late-onset form that presents itself for the first time between 50 and 60 years of age.

Tropical pancreatitis is extremely common in certain areas of India and also reported in parts of Africa, Southeast Asia, and Brazil. The onset of the disease is in the teens or early adulthood. Patients present with abdominal pain, severe malnutrition, and secondary diabetes. Marked ductal dilation is a prominent feature, and pancreatic calculi are present in more than 90% of patients. Box 1 lists other causes of chronic pancreatitis.

The pathogenesis of chronic pancreatitis remains unclear. Several hypotheses are proposed based on studies in alcoholic patients. The *ductal obstruction* theory contends that stones formed as a result of rich proteinaceous material obstruct the ductular system and lead to parenchymal damage. In the *toxic-metabolic* concept, a direct injurious effect on the pancreatic ductal and acinar cells by alcohol is evoked. The *necrosis-fibrosis* hypothesis holds that repeated injury results in necrotic tissue being replaced by fibrosis.

Recent genetic research bolsters the necrosis-fibrosis theory of continuous injury. In hereditary pancreatitis, a mutation in the cationic trypsinogen gene (codons 29 and 122) is deciphered that produces a trypsin variant immune to autolysis. Serine protease inhibitor Kazal type 1 (SPINK1) mutations found in patients with idiopathic pancreatitis lead to ineffective inhibition of trypsin.

Diagnostic Tests

Strictly speaking, the diagnosis of chronic pancreatitis should be based on a combination of clinical, morphologic, functional, and histologic criteria. However, in actual practice, clinical and morphologic criteria alone suffice because function testing is cumbersome and not universally available. Only rarely is tissue required to make a diagnosis.

LABORATORY TESTS

Serum amylase and serum lipase levels are only modestly elevated in chronic pancreatitis. Fecal fat is increased. Low levels of serum trypsinogen, fecal chymotrypsin, and fecal elastase are found in cases of advanced disease.

PLAIN RADIOGRAPH

A plain radiograph may reveal pancreatic calcification in 30% of cases. When calcifications are noted, the diagnosis can be made with 90% certainty. Pancreatic calcification is a sign of advanced disease, however, and of little help in diagnosing early cases.

ULTRASOUND

Ultrasound has a sensitivity of 50% to 80% in diagnosing chronic pancreatitis. Findings indicative of chronic pancreatitis include ductal dilation, shadowing pancreatic stones, gland atrophy, and changes in the parenchymal echotexture.

COMPUTED TOMOGRAPHY SCAN

Increased sensitivity (vis-à-vis ultrasound), noninvasiveness (compared to ERCP [endoscopic retrograde cholangiopancreatography]), and reproducibility make a CT scan pivotal in the evaluation of patients with chronic pancreatitis. A helical CT scanner with a pancreas-optimized protocol provides the best images. Characteristic features of moderate to severe disease, such as calcification, a dilated main pancreatic duct, and cysts, are easily identified. The role of CT in identifying early changes is limited.

Endoscopic Retrograde Cholangiopancreatography

The most sensitive and specific test of pancreatic structure is ERCP; it is the gold standard for this purpose, but it is more invasive and expensive than a CT scan. Changes in the main pancreatic duct and its side branches are evaluated to make a diagnosis of chronic pancreatitis and grade its severity (Table 1). A massively dilated duct with alternating strictures (the chain of lakes) is pathognomonic of severe disease. ERCP has the advantage of identifying early changes seen in the small ducts.

Endoscopic Ultrasonography

Endoscopic ultrasonography (EUS) is noninvasive and has no radiation exposure. It has the added capability of obtaining pancreatic tissue and should be used prior to ERCP wherever it is available. The EUS criteria for

---

BOX 1	**Etiology of Chronic Pancreatitis: TIGAR-O* Classification**

Toxic/metabolic
- Alcohol
- Tobacco
- Hypercalcemia
- Hyperlipidemia
- Chronic renal failure
- Phenacetin

Idiopathic
- Early onset
- Late onset
- Tropical

Genetic
- Autosomal dominant
  Cationic trypsinogen
- Autosomal recessive
  CFTR mutation
  Serine protease inhibitor Kazal type 1 (SPINK1) mutation
  α_1-Antitrypsin deficiency

Autoimmune
- Recurrent and severe acute pancreatitis
  Postnecrotic
  Recurrent acute pancreatitis
  Postirradiation
- Obstructive
  Tumor
  Trauma
  Stricture
  Sphincter of Oddi dysfunction

*Toxic-metabolic, idiopathic, genetic, autoimmune, recurrent and severe acute pancreatitis, or obstructive.
Reprinted and adapted from Etemad B, Whitcomb DC: Chronic pancreatitis: Diagnosis, classification, and new genetic developments. Gastroenterology 2001;20:682-707, with permission from the American Gastroenterology Association.

TABLE 1 Grading of Chronic Pancreatitis by Endoscopic Retrograde Cholangiopancreatography

Grade	Main pancreatic duct	Side branches
Normal	Normal	Normal
Equivocal	Normal	<3 abnormal
Mild	Normal	≥3 abnormal
Moderate	Abnormal	>3 abnormal
Severe	Any one of the following: Large cavity (>10 mm) Duct obstruction Intraductal filling defect Severe dilation or irregularity	>3 abnormal

Adapted from Forsmark CE: Chronic pancreatitis. In Feldman M, Friedman L, Sleisenger MH, Scharschmidt BF (eds): Sleisenger and Fordtran's Gastrointestinal and Liver Disease. Philadelphia, WB Saunders, 2002, pp 943-967.

chronic pancreatitis are listed in Box 2. A minimum of three criteria are necessary to make a diagnosis; there is an 80% correlation with ERCP for moderate to severe disease. Early changes are not detected.

Magnetic Resonance Cholangiopancreatography

Although initial reports have been encouraging, more studies are necessary to define the role of magnetic resonance cholangiopancreatography (MRCP) in the diagnosis of chronic pancreatitis.

PANCREATIC FUNCTION TESTS

Direct

Direct testing of pancreatic function is cumbersome, not freely available, and it can be misleading when interpreted independent of other modalities. Low bicarbonate and enzyme levels in the pancreatic juice obtained after secretin stimulation is indicative of chronic pancreatitis. Pancreatic juice for this purpose traditionally was collected by means of a tube placed in the duodenum. Nowadays ERCP can be used.

BOX 2 Endoscopic Ultrasonography Criteria for Chronic Pancreatitis

- Echogenic foci within the gland
- Focal areas of reduced echogenicity within the gland
- Increased thickness and echogenicity of the main duct wall
- Accentuation of the gland's lobular pattern
- Cysts
- Irregular contour of the main pancreatic duct
- Dilation of the main pancreatic duct

Adapted from Bhutani MS: Endoscopic ultrasound in pancreatic disease. Gastroenterol Clin North Am 1999;28:747-770.

Indirect (Bentiromide Test)

The bentiromide test involves the administration of an oral substrate that is acted on by pancreatic enzymes to release a metabolite (N-benzoyl-L-tyrosyl-p-aminobenzoic acid) that can be measured in the urine.

Figure 1 provides an overview of the sequence of diagnostic testing in chronic pancreatitis.

Treatment

The two major treatment goals in chronic pancreatitis are control of the abdominal pain and amelioration of the exocrine pancreatic insufficiency.

ABDOMINAL PAIN

To treat the pain of chronic pancreatitis, the underlying mechanisms of pain in this disease must be understood. Increased intraductal and parenchymal pressure, neural inflammation, and continuous cholecystokinin (CCK) stimulation (because of a paucity of pancreatic enzymes in the small intestine) are some of the theories proposed. Complications like pseudocysts, duodenal obstruction, biliary obstruction, and pancreatic carcinoma may also contribute to the pain and need to be identified before embarking on other forms of therapy. Although several therapeutic modalities exist, the success of each therapy depends on appropriate patient selection.

General Measures

General measures indicated in all patients include abstinence from alcohol (which has been shown to reduce pancreatic pain and arrest the progression of the disease) and analgesics. Although some patients can be controlled with acetaminophen or aspirin, many patients require narcotic analgesics (propoxyphene equals acetaminophen

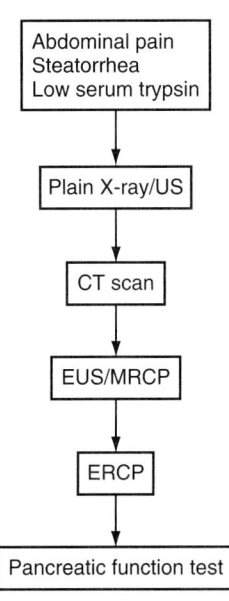

FIGURE 1. Sequence of diagnostic tests in chronic pancreatitis.

Rakel and Bope: *Conn's Current Therapy 2006.*

The Digestive System

[Darvocet-100], 1 tablet every 4 hours, or tramadol [Ultram], 50 to 100 mg every 4 to 6 hours).

Enzyme Therapy

Enzyme therapy is based on the assumption that delivery of pancreatic enzymes to the small intestine interrupts the CCK pathway, decreases CCK levels, and decreases pancreatic stimulation. Of the six randomized studies so far, beneficial results are noted in only two studies, both of which use non-enteric-coated preparations. The enzyme supplement should have a high protease content (>50,000 U). A typical prescription would involve four to eight tablets of Viokase, four times daily. This therapy is more likely to be effective in mild to moderate disease and the small duct variety.

Octreotide

Octreotide (Sandostatin)[1] targets the same mechanism by decreasing pancreatic secretion and CCK levels. Doses of 100 to 250 µg three times daily may decrease pain symptoms, but more studies are required to confirm this premise.

Endoscopic Therapy

Endoscopic therapy attempts to decrease the intraductal pressure by facilitating improved drainage of the duct. This can take the form of pancreatic duct sphincterotomy, stenting of strictures, and removal of pancreatic duct stones. Although a significant number of patients may experience symptom relief after the procedure, recurrence is common.

Surgery

Surgery is indicated in patients with intractable pain that is not amenable to medical or endoscopic therapy. Surgical procedures involve either duct drainage, resection, or a combination. The most commonly performed drainage procedure is the lateral pancreaticojejunostomy (modified Puestow). A duct diameter larger than 7 mm is a prerequisite and best suited for patients with big duct disease. Immediate pain relief is noted in 80% of patients, but only 60% remain pain free by 2 years.

Patients without ductal dilation are not candidates for drainage procedures but may benefit from pancreatic resection. Distal pancreatotomy alone has poor results, but a Whipple's resection in patients with a large inflammatory mass in the head is followed by pain relief in 85% of cases.

Celiac Plexus Block

Celiac plexus block is not routinely recommended because its effect lasts only 2 to 4 months, and there is a definite risk of paraplegia. When celiac block is performed under EUS guidance, its efficacy is slightly more prolonged.

---

[1]Not FDA approved for this indication.

Rakel and Bope: *Conn's Current Therapy 2006.*

TABLE 2 Commercially Available Enzyme Supplements	
Supplement	**Units of lipase/capsule or pill**
Enteric-coated	
Creon 5, 10, 20	5000, 10,000, 20,000, respectively
Pancrease MT 4, 10, 16, 20	4000, 10,000, 16,000, 20,000, respectively
Ultrase MT 12, 18, 20	12,000, 18,000, 20,000, respectively.
Non–enteric-coated	
Viokase 8, 16	8000, 16,000
Generic pancrelipase	8000

Adapted from Forsmark CE: Chronic pancreatitis. In Feldman M, Friedman L, Sleisenger MH, Scharschmidt BF (eds): Sleisenger and Fordtran's Gastrointestinal and Liver Disease. Philadelphia, WB Saunders, 2002, pp 943-967.

STEATORRHEA

The treatment of steatorrhea should include general measures such as a low-fat diet and specific pancreatic enzyme supplements. A minimum of 25,000 to 40,000 U of lipase must be supplied with each meal. This is achieved by 2 to 3 enteric-coated capsules (Creon and Pancrease) or 8 nonenteric tablets (Viokase). A list of commercially available enzymes is given in Table 2. When non–enteric-coated preparations are used, the efficacy can be increased by the concomitant use of proton pump inhibitors or H_2 blockers because gastric acid has the potential to destroy the enzyme.

COMPLICATIONS

Pancreatic Pseudocyst

Treatment is discussed in "Acute Pancreatitis."

Pancreatic Ascites and Pleural Effusion

Initial therapy should include nothing orally, parenteral nutrition, and octreotide.[1] If these measures fail, the rupture in the pancreatic duct can be bridged by means of an endoscopically placed pancreatic duct stent.

---

[1]Not FDA approved for this indication.

 CURRENT DIAGNOSIS

- Abdominal pain
- Increased fecal fat
- Pancreatic calcification
- Pancreatic duct dilation
- Pancreatic stones
- Low bicarbonate and enzymes in pancreatic juice
- Abnormal bentiromide test

CURRENT THERAPY

Abdominal Pain

- Pseudocyst, biliary, and duodenal obstruction, and gastroparesis excluded
- Abstinence
- Analgesics
- Non-enteric-coated enzymes
- Octreotide[1]
- Endoscopic therapy
    Sphincterotomy[*]
    Stenting[*]
    Stone extraction[*]
- Surgeryo
    Drainage procedures (Puestow)[*]
    Resection[*]

Steatorrhea[*]

- Enteric-coated enzymes

[*]Minimum of 25,000 to 40,000 U lipase per meal.
[1]Not FDA approved for this indication.

Surgical resection is an option in patients who fail or who are not candidates for endoscopic therapy.

Bile Duct Obstruction

Frequently, a dilated CBD may be encountered incidentally in an asymptomatic patient and no therapy is warranted. Surgical intervention is required for persistent symptoms, cholangitis, and worsening liver function tests.

Duodenal Stenosis

Duodenal stenosis requires surgical intervention.

REFERENCES

AGA Technical Review: Treatment of pain in chronic pancreatitis. Gastroenterology 1998;115:763-776.
Bhutani MS: Endoscopic ultrasound in pancreatic disease. Gastroenterol Clin North Am 1999;28:747-770.
Etemad B, Whitcomb DC: Chronic pancreatitis: Diagnosis, classification, and new genetic developments. Gastroenterology 2001;120:682-707.
Forsmark CE: Chronic pancreatitis. In Feldman M, Friedman L, Sleisenger MH, Scharschmidt BF (eds): Sleisenger and Fordtran's Gastrointestinal and Liver Disease. Philadelphia, WB Saunders, 2002, pp 943-967.
Greenberger NJ: Enzymatic therapy in patients with chronic pancreatitis. Gastroenterol Clin North Am 1999;28:687-693.

Gastroesophageal Reflux Disease

Method of
Jonathan F. Finks, MD, and John G. Hunter, MD

Epidemiology

Gastroesophageal reflux disease (GERD) is an increasingly important disease in the United States and other Western nations, with major impact on both quality of life and health care costs. In a 1988 Gallup Organization survey, 44% of U.S. adults reported monthly symptoms; 14% reported weekly symptoms and 7% reported daily symptoms. The annual cost of GERD treatment in the United States is an estimated $10 billion. Patients with GERD consistently score lower on quality-of-life surveys than patients with congestive heart failure and angina. GERD is also the most important risk factor for esophageal adenocarcinoma.

Nonerosive Reflux Disease Versus Gastroesophageal Reflux Disease

The term *GERD* applies to all individuals at risk for physical complications from gastroesophageal reflux or clinically significant impairment of health-related quality of life because of reflux-related symptoms. This definition applies equally to patients with erosive esophagitis and those with nonerosive reflux disease (NERD). This latter group accounts for approximately 70% of GERD patients. Despite the lack of endoscopic findings in patients with NERD, their symptoms are often as severe as and sometimes even more difficult to control than patients with esophagitis, and their quality of life is equally affected. Indeed, patients with NERD should be treated in a similar way to patients with erosive esophagitis.

Pathophysiology

The etiology of GERD is related to three primary mechanisms: lower esophageal sphincter (LES) incompetence, transient lower esophageal sphincter relaxation (TLESR), and hiatal hernia. Conditions such as esophageal dysmotility (achalasia, scleroderma) or impaired salivary secretion (Sjögren's syndrome) hinder esophageal clearance and can augment the injurious effect of acid reflux. Delayed gastric emptying may lead to gastric distension and distortion of the gastroesophageal (GE) junction, which may promote or intensify the symptoms of GERD.

Incompetence of the LES can result in GERD, although the LES resting pressure in most patients with reflux symptoms is normal. The most common cause of pathologic reflux disease is excessive frequency or duration of TLESRs. These events, associated with distension of the gastric fundus, are responsible for up to 70% of reflux episodes in patients with GERD.

The most important anatomic factor leading to GERD is hiatal hernia, which alters the three main components of the reflux barrier (LES, crural diaphragm, and angle of His). Hiatal hernia reduces LES pressure and leads to distension of the GE junction. Resultant stretching of the crural diaphragm impairs its ability to augment LES pressure. The herniated portion of the stomach acts as an acid reservoir, worsening the impact of reflux on the distal esophagus. Finally, upward distraction of the GE junction into the chest leads to loss of the acute cardioesophageal angle, which normally serves to prevent reflux.

Clinical Presentation

The presentation of GERD is often divided into esophageal (typical) and extraesophageal (atypical) symptoms. The most common symptoms of GERD are heartburn, a sensation of substernal burning pain, and regurgitation of swallowed food. Both symptoms typically occur in the postprandial period. Other esophageal complaints include excessive salivation (water brash) and a sensation of a foreign body in the posterior pharynx (globus hystericus).

Extraesophageal manifestations of GERD include symptoms arising from the oropharynx, airway, and respiratory tree: chronic cough, wheezing, hoarseness, choking, sinusitis, and dental caries. The presence of these atypical symptoms should prompt an evaluation for malignancy (including laryngoscopic exam) in a patient with suspected GERD. Aspiration pneumonia and asthma are also strongly associated with GERD.

So-called alarm symptoms (dysphagia, odynophagia, bleeding, anemia, and weight loss) suggest complicated disease (e.g., esophageal stricture, malignancy) and merit further evaluation.

Diagnosis

EMPIRICAL THERAPY

In patients presenting with typical reflux symptoms (heartburn or regurgitation), a trial of empirical therapy is appropriate provided the patient does not present with alarm symptoms or other indications for endoscopy (Box 1). A good response to empirical therapy is considered diagnostic of GERD, with accuracy comparable to that of 24-hour esophageal hydrogen ion concentration (pH) monitoring.

ENDOSCOPY

Box 1 lists the indications for upper gastrointestinal endoscopy upon initial presentation. Endoscopy is also indicated in patients with early or frequent relapses following an empirical trial of medical therapy. Endoscopy allows direct inspection of esophageal mucosa and is the only reliable means of diagnosing Barrett's esophagus (BE).

Rakel and Bope: *Conn's Current Therapy 2006.*

BOX 1	Indications for Endoscopy in Patients Presenting With Heartburn

- Presence of alarm symptoms: dysphagia, odynophagia, anemia, weight loss, gastrointestinal bleeding
- Duration of symptoms longer than 5 years
- Age more than 50 years
- Known infection with *Helicobacter pylori*
- Family history of gastroesophageal reflux disease
- Severe daily symptoms

BARIUM ESOPHAGRAM

Although the barium esophagram has low yield in the diagnosis of GERD, it is the first test to order in a patient presenting with dysphagia. The barium swallow is the best means of detecting esophageal strictures and diverticula and can help guide the endoscopist in patients with these complications. The esophagram also serves as a road map for the surgeon preparing for an antireflux procedure.

AMBULATORY ESOPHAGEAL HYDROGEN ION CONCENTRATION TESTING

Esophageal pH testing is not necessary to diagnose GERD in all patients. The combination of typical symptoms and endoscopic changes has a specificity of 97% for GERD. Ambulatory pH testing is a useful diagnostic tool for patients with NERD or those with entirely extraesophageal symptoms. The traditional catheter-based test is limited by patient discomfort as well as somewhat variable sensitivity and specificity. The newer capsule-based system is much better tolerated and gives up to 48 hours of data, significantly improving the accuracy of the test. Another recent advance is the combined acid and impedance monitor, which allows for detection of both acid and nonacid (volume) reflux. This test may prove useful in patients with persistent symptoms despite adequate medical therapy, particularly those with extraesophageal symptoms.

MANOMETRY

An esophageal motility study allows for a functional assessment of the LES and esophageal body. Its main utility in GERD is to rule out severe motility disorders, such as achalasia or scleroderma, prior to antireflux surgery.

Treatment

The goals of therapy for most GERD patients are relief of symptoms and long-term disease control. Mucosal healing is also an important endpoint in patients with significant esophagitis or complications (stricture, BE).

LIFESTYLE MODIFICATION

Data on the efficacy of lifestyle/dietary modifications are limited, but certain recommendations may prove useful.

These include smoking cessation, weight loss, avoidance of recumbency for 3 hours postprandially, and abstinence from foods known to lower LES pressure: chocolate, peppermint, coffee, and alcohol.

MEDICAL THERAPY

Over-the-counter (OTC) antacids and alginates are commonly used to treat milder forms of GERD. They offer instant relief but have a short duration of action. Prokinetic agents, such as metoclopramide (Reglan),[1] domperidone (Motilium),[1] and cisapride (Propulsid),[*] are used to enhance foregut motility, but to date little evidence suggests they are better than placebo in controlling GERD symptoms. Baclofen (Lioresal),[1] a γ-aminobutyric acid B receptor (GABA-B) agonist, works by reducing TLESRs and decreases both acid and nonacid postprandial reflux episodes and improves symptoms in patients with GERD. Baclofen[1] is limited, however, by its side-effect profile. H_2-receptor antagonists (H_2RAs) are proving effective in numerous placebo-controlled trials, offering symptomatic relief in 60% of GERD patients, with healing of esophagitis in 50%.

Proton pump inhibitors (PPIs) remain the most effective medical therapy for GERD, providing symptom relief and esophageal healing in 80% of patients. Several large controlled trials demonstrate the superiority of PPIs over H_2RAs in terms of symptom relief, esophageal healing, and cost effectiveness. In addition, PPIs normalize the impaired quality of life associated with GERD.

Upon initial presentation with typical GERD symptoms, patients not requiring endoscopy should undergo an empirical trial of standard-dose PPIs for 4 to 8 weeks. Patients who fail therapy or relapse soon after medication withdrawal should undergo further evaluation, including endoscopy. Patients whose symptoms are relieved following an initial trial of PPIs may benefit from on-demand therapy, in which PPIs are started at the onset of symptoms and discontinued after 24 hours of symptom relief. This treatment modality may also be appropriate for patients with NERD or mild erosive esophagitis because on-demand therapy is proven cost effective in this group of patients. Patients with frequent symptom relapse, however, should be started on continuous PPI therapy. Patients with moderate to severe esophagitis and those with extraesophageal symptoms should receive continuous maintenance therapy with standard or higher doses of PPIs.

ANTIREFLUX SURGERY

Although most patients with GERD can be managed effectively with PPIs, the therapy is lifelong, and up to 50% of patients experience symptom relapses and require dose escalation. Antireflux surgery is an attractive option for patients who do not wish to take medications chronically. Surgery is also effective for patients with persistent symptoms despite maximal therapy,

particularly those with volume reflux, or regurgitation. Antireflux surgery should also be considered in patients with complications of the disease such as strictures, BE, or laryngotracheal aspiration (Box 2).

Excellent results are achieved with traditional open procedures, including complete (Nissen) and partial (Toupet, Dor) fundoplications. In the last decade, however, the laparoscopic approach to antireflux surgery became the standard of care, with most surgeons favoring the so-called floppy Nissen fundoplication.

Patient selection is crucial to the success of antireflux surgery. Preoperative evaluation should include a detailed history to document reflux-associated symptoms. All patients considered for surgery should undergo endoscopy, both to confirm the presence of GERD and to assess for strictures, BE, or malignancy. Manometry must also be performed to rule out a severe motility disorder. An ambulatory pH study should be done on patients with NERD to confirm the diagnosis of reflux disease.

Relief of heartburn and regurgitation is seen in 90% to 95% of patients following antireflux surgery, and quality-of-life scores are normalized. The most consistent preoperative predictors of successful outcome are an abnormal ambulatory pH study and a good response to PPI therapy. The response of extraesophageal symptoms to surgery is more variable, with improvement rates ranging from 60% to 80%. The response of atypical symptoms to surgery is correlated with the response to medical therapy.

Laparoscopic antireflux surgery is generally well tolerated. Side effects such as gas bloat and dysphagia are common postoperatively but typically resolve within a few months. Infrequently, patients with dysphagia may require dilation or, rarely, reoperation. Long-term outcome from surgery is excellent, with symptom relief maintained in 85% to 90% of patients in most series with at least 5 years of follow-up. Reoperative rates range from 3% to 8%. Table 1 lists the most common reasons for failure.

BOX 2	**Indications for Antireflux Surgery in Patients With GERD**

- Failure of medical therapy
- Patient's desire for surgery despite successful medical management (because of lifestyle considerations, including age, time, or expense of medications)
- Patients with complications of GERD (e.g., BE, grade III or IV esophagitis, esophageal stricture)
- Medical complications attributable to a large hiatal hernia (e.g., bleeding, dysphagia)
- Atypical symptoms (asthma, hoarseness, cough, chest pain, aspiration) and reflux documented on 24-hour pH monitoring

---

Abbreviations: BE = Barrett's esophagus; GERD = gastroesophageal reflux disease; pH = hydrogen ion concentration.
Adapted from Society of American Gastrointestinal Endoscopic Surgeons (SAGES) Guidelines: Guidelines for surgical treatment of gastroesophageal reflux disease (GERD). Surg Endosc 1998;12(2): 186-188.

---

[1]Not FDA approved for this indication.
[*]Investigational drug in the United States.

TABLE 1 Causes of Fundoplication Failure in 1000 Laparoscopic Antireflux Procedures

Cause of failure	*n* = 39
Transdiaphragmatic herniation of fundoplication	29 (74%)
Twisted or slipped fundoplication	4 (10%)
Excessive tightness of fundoplication	3 (8%)
Esophageal motility disorder	2 (5%)
Disruption of fundoplication	1 (3%)

Adapted from Terry M: Outcomes of laparascopic fundoplication for gastroesophageal reflux disease and paraesophageal hernia. Surg Endosc 2001;15(7):691-699.

ENDOSCOPIC THERAPY

Several endoscopic therapies for treating GERD are available. Their use is limited to patients with esophageal symptoms, hiatal hernia smaller than 2 cm, esophagitis grade II or lower, and no evidence of BE. The Stretta procedure delivers radiofrequency energy to the distal esophagus and may act through reduction of TLESRs and alteration of neural pathways. A variety of devices work by internal plication of the stomach below the GE junction. Finally, a device approved by the Food and Drug Administration (FDA) acts to bulk up the GE junction by injection of a biocompatible polymer into the wall of the distal esophagus. Most of the data on these procedures comes from open-label trials with follow-up of a year or less. Although most series demonstrate improvement in GERD symptoms and quality-of-life scores, none of the devices normalize esophageal acid exposure. Long-term controlled trials are needed before the impact of these endoluminal therapies on GERD treatment can be assessed.

Esophageal Stricture

Excessive scar formation from erosive esophagitis can lead to stricture of the distal esophagus. The thin fibrous bands at the GE junction of a Schatzki's ring are usually amenable to endoscopic dilation, whereas longer fusiform strictures may prove refractory.

TABLE 2 American College of Gastroenterology Guidelines for Surveillance of Barrett's Esophagus

Dysplasia grade	Follow-up endoscopy
None	3 years
Low grade	1 year
High grade	
Focal	Every 3 months
Multifocal	Intervention (resection/ablation)
Mucosal irregularity	Endoscopic mucosal resection

Adapted from Sampliner RE: Updated guidelines for the diagnosis, surveillance and therapy of Barrett's esophagus. Am J Gastroenterol 2002;97(8):1888-1895.

CURRENT DIAGNOSIS

- Alarm symptoms suggest complications of GERD and include: dysphagia, odynophagia, anemia, weight loss, and gastrointestinal bleeding.
- Endoscopy at initial presentation is recommended for patients with alarm symptoms or other risk factors for Barrett's esophagus.
- Ambulatory esophageal pH testing is useful to confirm the diagnosis of GERD in patients with NERD or exclusively extraesophageal symptoms.
- Combined impedance and pH testing may be useful in patients with persistent symptoms despite adequate medical therapy, particularly those with extraesophageal symptoms.
- An empirical trial of PPI therapy has equivalent diagnostic accuracy to a 24-hour ambulatory esophageal pH study.
- Patients with Barrett's esophagus should be enrolled in a surveillance endoscopy program.

Patients should remain on continuous PPI therapy following dilation to promote mucosal healing. Antireflux surgery is usually indicated in the presence of a benign esophageal stricture.

Barrett's Esophagus

BE represents intestinal metaplasia of the distal esophagus and is a known precursor lesion of esophageal adenocarcinoma. The yearly incidence of adenocarcinoma in patients with BE is 0.5%, nearly 40 times higher than

CURRENT THERAPY

- Potentially effective lifestyle modifications include weight loss, smoking cessation, avoidance of postprandial recumbency and abstinence of foods known to lower LES pressure: chocolate, peppermint, alcohol, coffee.
- Proton pump inhibitors (PPIs) are the most effective and cost-effective medical therapy available for the treatment of GERD.
- On-demand therapy with PPIs is appropriate for patients with NERD or mild esophagitis who respond to an initial trial of PPIs.
- Patients with moderate to severe esophagitis or extraesophageal symptoms should be placed on continuous PPI therapy with standard or higher doses.
- The most consistent preoperative predictors of success following laparascopic antireflux surgery are an abnormal esophageal pH study and a good response to PPIs.
- The indications for antireflux surgery include patients whose symptoms are incompletely relieved with PPIs, as well as those who do not wish to remain on lifelong medical therapy.

that of patients without BE. Risk factors for BE are duration of reflux symptoms, presence of hiatal hernia, advanced age, and male gender. Patients with chronic GERD symptoms should undergo endoscopy to screen for BE, and those found to have BE should be entered into a surveillance program (Table 2). Continuous PPI therapy or antireflux surgery is recommended for patients with BE. Titration of PPIs to normalization of esophageal acid exposure may result in regression of BE, although to date no convincing evidence suggests medical or surgical therapy can prevent the development of cancer in patients with BE.

REFERENCES

Bytzer P, et al: Personal view: Rationale and proposed algorithms for symptom-based proton pump inhibitor therapy for gastro-oesophageal reflux disease. Aliment Pharmacol Ther 2004;20: 389-398.

DeVault K, et al: Updated guildelines for the diagnosis and treatment of gastroesophageal reflux disease. Am J Gastro 2005;100:190-200.

Galmiche JP, et al: Treatment of gastroesophageal reflux disease in adults: An individualized approach. Dig Dis 2004;22:148-160.

Gordon C, et al: Review article: The role of the hiatus hernia in gastroesophageal reflux disease. Aliment Pharmacol Ther 2004;20: 389-398.

Hunter JG, et al: A physiologic approach to laparoscopic fundoplication for gastroesophageal reflux disease. Ann Surg 1996;223(6): 673-687.

Kamolz T, et al: Laparoscopic Nissen fundoplication in patients with nonerosive reflux disease: Long-term quality of life assessment and surgical outcome. Surg Endosc 2005 February.

Lind T, et al: On demand therapy with omeprazole for the long-term management of patients with heartburn without esophagitis: A placebo-controlled randomized trial. Aliment Pharmacol Ther 1999;13:907-904.

Sampliner RE: Updated guidelines for the diagnosis, surveillance, and therapy of Barrett's esophagus. Am J Gastro 2002;97(8):1888-1895.

Sharma, P: Barrett Esophagus: Will effective treatment prevent the risk of progression to esophageal adenocarcinoma? Am J Med 2004; 117(5A):79S-85S.

Terry M, et al: Outcomes of laparascopic fundoplication for gastroesophageal reflux disease and paraesophageal hernia: Experience with 1,000 consecutive cases. Surg Endosc 2001;15:691-699.

Triadafilopoulos G, et al: GERD: The potential for endoscopic intervention. Dig Dis 2004;22:181-188.

Trus TL, et al: Improvement in quality of life measures after laparoscopic antireflux surgery. Ann Surg 1999;229(3):331-336.

Tumors of the Stomach

Method of
Steven Powell, MD, and Hester H. Choi, MD

Stomach tumors can be classified as benign or malignant according to their invasive potential. Adenocarcinoma comprises the vast majority of malignant stomach tumors, followed by primary gastric lymphoma, and less frequently, carcinoid and stromal tumors. The most common benign tumor is the hyperplastic polyp. This article focuses on our understanding of the pathogenesis, diagnosis, and treatment of the more common gastric tumors.

Gastric Adenocarcinoma

EPIDEMIOLOGY

Gastric adenocarcinoma, commonly referred to as gastric carcinoma or stomach cancer, accounts for 95% of all malignant tumors of the stomach. It is the second most common cause of cancer-related deaths worldwide despite declining incidences in many industrialized countries. The incidence is highest in Japan, China, South America, and Eastern Europe, reaching up to 100 per 100,000 persons each year in some regions. The annual incidence of gastric cancer in the United States, however, has markedly declined over the past 50 years, down to 3.8 per 100,000. This reduced temporal incidence in gastric cancer can be at least partially explained by a decline in the intestinal, distal type of tumors. On the other hand, the incidence of cancers in the proximal stomach and esophagogastric junction appears to be increasing over recent decades. Analysis on the influence of improvements in cancer site classification has found that the purported increase in cardia cancer incidence may be accounted for by improved specification of gastric cancer sites. The highest rates of gastric cancer continue to be observed in lower socioeconomic groups. The incidence and mortality rate also increases with age and peaks in the sixth to seventh decades.

PATHOLOGY

There are two distinct histolopathologic subtypes of gastric adenocarcinoma—intestinal (expansive or gland forming) and diffuse (infiltrative) types—as described by Lauren in 1965. The intestinal-type tumors predominate in highly endemic populations and elderly men. These often arise within an area of intestinal metaplasia or chronic atrophic gastritis, tend to occur more distally, and are characterized by distinct glandular structures. Diffuse-type gastric tumors are often observed in younger women without identifiable precursor lesions and are associated with a poor prognosis. These diffuse-type tumors tend to be infiltrating within the stomach without distinct margins and can harbor mucus-containing, signet-ring cells.

ETIOLOGY

Most cases of gastric cancer appear to occur sporadically, but a familial clustering is observed in approximately 10% of cases. First-degree relatives of patients with gastric cancer have a two- to threefold greater risk, but the contribution of genetics versus shared environmental factors is unclear. Gastric cancers have been associated with hereditary nonpolyposis colon cancer (HNPCC) syndrome. They have also been reported in extended Li-Fraumeni kindreds harboring an underlying germline p53 mutation. Several kindreds manifesting a highly penetrant diffuse-type gastric cancer have been shown to harbor cosegregating germline mutations in the gene for E-cadherin. Women in these families are also at risk of developing lobular breast cancer.

Cigarette smoking and low socioeconomic status are also associated with increased stomach cancer risk. Dietary factors that are associated with the development of gastric cancer include ingestion of highly salted and preserved foods containing nitrates as well as nitrites and a low intake of fruit and vitamins such as vitamin C and other antioxidants. Obesity and gastroesophageal reflux disease also appear to be risk factors for gastric cardia adenocarcinoma.

In 1994 the World Health Organization (WHO) classified *Helicobacter pylori* as a carcinogen. Case-control studies have suggested that the risk of gastric cancer is threefold to sixfold higher in persons seropositive for *H. pylori* infection. Uemura and colleagues have reported a prospective study of 1246 patients with *H. pylori* infection and 280 patients without *H. pylori* infection in Japan. After a mean follow-up period of 7.8 years, gastric cancer was diagnosed in 2.9% of the infected patients and in none of the uninfected patients. The mechanism that leads *H. pylori* infection to gastric cancer has not been fully delineated. However, current theories focus on chronic inflammation and atrophy of normal mucosa in association with hypochlorhydria and other sequential insults that result in chronic atrophic gastritis, intestinal metaplasia, and subsequently dysplasia in some cases. Previous partial gastrectomy for benign conditions, pernicious anemia, and hypertrophic gastropathy (Ménétrier disease) also contribute to an increased risk.

In recent years, our understanding of genetic alterations that occur in gastric tumorigenesis has improved with advances in molecular biology. There is no clear *gate-keeper* gene for gastric cancer identified. Loss of heterozygosity analyses has identified tumor suppressor genes such as p53 that are involved in the majority of gastric tumors. Microsatellite instability secondary to alterations in DNA mismatch repair genes have been implicated in HNPCC as well as significant portions (16%) of sporadic gastric cancers. Amplification and overexpression of growth promoting genes such as hyperglycemic-glycogenolytic factor (HGF), cMET, vascular endothelial growth factor (VEGF), and cyclooxygenase-2 (COX-2) have also been observed. Further characterizations of these alterations are anticipated to provide new opportunities for earlier diagnosis, better prognostication, and guide therapeutic strategies.

CLINICAL MANIFESTATIONS

The early symptoms of gastric cancer are generally nonspecific and vague. Patients may complain of dyspepsia, epigastric pain, anorexia with weight loss, and nausea. Dysphagia may occur in patients with cardia tumor extending through the esophagogastric junction. Early satiety may be because of diffusely infiltrative, tumor-causing loss of gastric wall distension. Overt or occult bleeding can occur and eventually result in iron-deficiency anemia. Persistent vomiting with signs of gastric outlet obstruction can occur with antral tumors obstructing the pylorus outlet. Gastric carcinoma

spreads by direct extension through the stomach wall to the peritoneum as well as by lymphatics or blood vessels. The liver is the most common site of hematogenous spread. Patients with disseminated disease may present with supraclavicular (Virchow), axillary, or periumbilical (Sister Mary Joseph's nodule) lymphadenopathy. They may also develop jaundice, hepatomegaly, or malignant ascites.

DIAGNOSIS

Advanced gastric adenocarcinoma is typically seen on upper endoscopy as an ulcerating lesion with irregular margins. Early gastric cancer may appear as a polypoid or flat lesion; it may also be raised, depressed or ulcerated. Double-contrast barium studies have been used for mass screening in Japan since 1957. However, fiberoptic endoscopy with biopsy remains the diagnostic procedure of choice and has an accuracy of greater than 95%. The accuracy increases with the number of specimens obtained. Once the diagnosis is established, the extent of disease may be assessed by computed tomography (CT) of the abdomen and chest. Stomach wall thickness of more than 2 cm typically indicates transmural extension of the tumor. Metastases to other organs such as liver and lung can be documented. The overall accuracy of preoperative CT staging ranges from 61% to 72%. However, CT scans are particularly unreliable in assessing regional lymph nodes and invasion of adjacent organs. Endoscopic ultrasound is able to increase the accuracy of preoperative staging by delineating the depth of wall involvement of the tumor and help further in determining the lymph node and adjacent structure status. Laparoscopy and peritoneal lavage have also been used for more accurate determination of resectabililty.

STAGING

The American Joint Committee on Cancer (AJCC) staging system is commonly used in the United States (Table 1). It is based on the depth of the primary tumor (T), regional lymph node involvement (N) and distant metastases (M). The most recent AJCC staging system in 2002 also reflects the importance of the number of lymph nodes retrieved in a specimen rather than just its location. The number of positive lymph nodes remains the most significant determinant of recurrence and survival. Staging was not found to be reliable if fewer than 10 nodes were examined and determined that at least 15 should be available for analysis. The 5-year survival rate for AJCC stage IA disease is 78% and declines to 7% for stage IV disease. Unfortunately, early gastric cancer represents only approximately 10% of diagnosed cases in the United States.

TREATMENT

The primary management of gastric cancer continues to be surgical resection and is potentially curative in localized lesions. Prophylactic gastrectomy has also been proposed for asymptomatic individuals at risk in families with highly penetrant hereditary diffuse gastric cancers.

TABLE 1 American Joint Committee on Cancer Sraging of Gastric Cancer, 2002

Definition of TNM

T

TX	Primary tumor cannot be assessed
T0	No evidence of primary tumor
Tis	Carcinoma *in situ*: intraepithelial tumor without invasion of the lamina propria
T1	Tumor invades lamina propria or submucosa
T2	Tumor invades muscularis propria or subserosa
T2a	Tumor invades muscularis propria
T2b	Tumor invades subserosa
T3	Tumor penetrates serosal (visceral peritoneum) without invasion of adjacent structures
T4	Tumor invades adjacent structures

N

NX	Regional lymph node(s) cannot be assessed
N0	No regional lymph node metastasis
N1	Metastasis in 1–6 regional lymph nodes
N2	Metastasis in 7–15 regional lymph nodes
N3	Metastasis in more than 15 regional lymph nodes

M

MX	Presence of distant metastasis cannot be assessed
M0	No distant metastasis
M1	Distant metastasis

Stage Grouping

0	Tis	N0	M0
IA	T1	N0	M0
IB	T1	N1	M0
	T2a/b	N0	M0
II	T1	N2	M0
	T2	N1	M0
	T3	N0	M0
IIIA	T2a/b	N2	M0
	T3	N1	M0
	T4	N0	M0
IIIB	T3	N2	M0
IV	T4	N1-3	M0
	T1-3	N3	M0
	Any T	Any N	M1

Abbreviations: M = distant metastasis; N = regional lymph nodes; T = primary tumor.
AJCC 6th Edition Staging Manual, 2002. Used with permission.

An algorithm for managing kindreds of familial gastric carcinoma has previously been proposed (Figure 1). Controversy remains on the optimal extent of gastric resection (total versus subtotal gastrectomy), the extent of lymphadenectomy (local versus extended) and the mode of deliverance of adjuvant chemoradiotherapy. Subtotal resection may offer similar survival benefits to that of total gastrectomy with less associated morbidity. For proximal tumors or diffusely infiltrative lesions, total gastrectomy is often required; occasionally with distal pancreatectomy and splenectomy if involved.

The Japanese have defined four levels of lymph node dissections (D1 to D4). A D2 dissection is more extensive than a D1 and may carry an increased mortality risk. However, less than a D2 resection may inadequately stage a significant population of patients especially with T3+ tumors. The clinical merits of extended D2 lymphadenectomy still remain to be proven. A Cochrane Review and a meta-analysis of randomized trials did not reveal any survival benefits of extended lymph node dissection.

The recent Intergroup 0116 study has shown that the combination of 5-fluorouracil (5-FU)/leucovorin chemotherapy with radiotherapy prolongs disease-free and overall survival when compared with no adjuvant treatment after gastric resection. The median overall survival in the surgery-only group was 27 months, compared with 36 months in the chemoradiotherapy group. Most of the patients enrolled in this study had T3 or T4 tumors and nodal metastases. Palliative radiation therapy has also been used to alleviate bleeding, pain or obstruction. Gastrojejunostomy may be performed to bypass distal stomach obstruction. Palliation of obstructing cancer at the distal esophagus and gastric outlet may even be performed endoscopically with wire mesh stents.

Endoscopic mucosal resection may now be considered for early staged gastric cancers in patients that are at a high risk for conventional operations. Local injection and electrocautery are generally employed; and multiple resections may be required. For raised lesions less than 2 cm, depressed lesions less than 1 cm without ulceration and lymphatic spread, this management approach has shown effectiveness in curing most patients.

Gastric Polyps

Gastric polyps are usually found incidentally during an endoscopic or radiologic examination. Most of these polyps are hyperplastic and typically asymptomatic. Adenomas are infrequent, but they carry distinct malignant potential. The incidence of adenocarcinoma in an adenoma greater than 2 cm in diameter may be up to 40%. Polypectomy and surveillance should be performed for adenomas because they also serve as a marker for increased risk for synchronous and metachronous carcinomas in the remaining gastric tissue. A wedge resection may be considered for sessile lesions and formal gastrectomy for more advanced lesions, multiple polyposis, or multiple recurrent adenomas.

Lymphoma

Gastric lymphoma is the second most common neoplasm in the stomach, yet only accounts for 3% to 5% of all gastric malignancies. The stomach is the most frequent extranodal site for lymphoma. It may occur as the primary site or as secondary involvement of the gastrointestinal tract in the setting of disseminated nodal disease. Hodgkin's disease rarely involves the gastrointestinal tract. Most of the gastric lymphoma is non-Hodgkin's lymphoma (NHL) of B-cell origin such as diffuse large B-cell NHL, gastric mantle cell lymphoma,

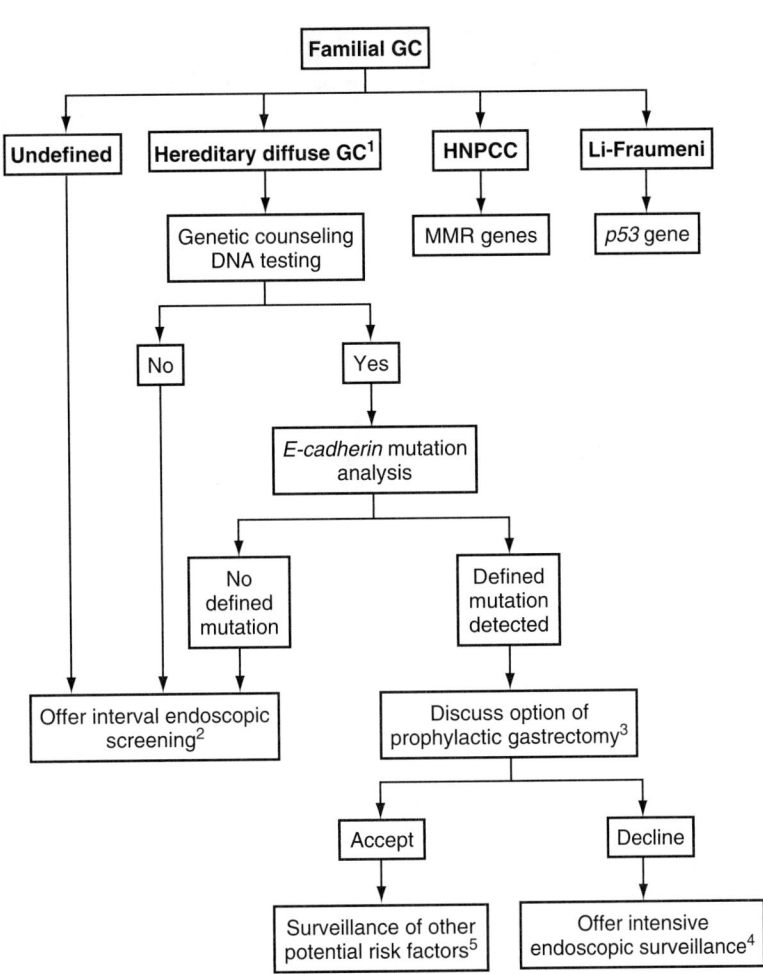

FIGURE 1. Algorithm for guidance in managing familial GC kindreds. Those identified to meet clinical criteria for HNPCC and the Li-Fraumeni syndrome are counseled for consideration of genetic testing. Microsatellite instability testing can aid in diagnosing HNPCC. This algorithm was initially formulated at the consensus of symposia with clinical criteria generated to define hereditary diffuse gastric cancer: two or more cases in first- and second-degree relatives, at least one diagnosed before the age of 50 years; or three or more cases of documented diffuse gastric cancer and first- and second-degree relatives. Consider individual age-dependent familial expression to determine the initiation, interval, and intensity of screening exams. Prophylactic gastrectomies have been performed in kindreds expressing highly penetrant phenotypes without prior knowledge of causative mutations. Consider age-dependent familial expressions in determining management. Endoscopic ultrasound and chromographic (methylene blue or indigo carmine staining) endoscopy can be applied in attempts to increase the sensitivity of detecting early lesions in the stomach. One should have a high index of suspicion for the potential development of other cancers such as that of the breast, colon, and endometrium. GC = gastric cancer; HNPCC = hereditary nonpolyposis colon cancer syndrome; MMR = mismatch repair. (From Powell SM, Smith MF Jr: Gastric cancer: Molecular biology. In Kelsen DP (ed): Gastrointestinal Oncology: Principles and Practice. Philadelphia, Lippincott Williams & Wilkins, 2002, pp 325–340. Used with permission.)

or the more common low-grade mucosa-associated lymphoid tissue (MALT) gastric lymphoma. *H. pylori* infection has been associated with a majority of MALT lymphoma. In response to *H. pylori* infection, an increase in gastric mucosal lymphoid cells accumulates and can form follicles that subsequently develop monoclonal B-cell populations and in some cases progress to more advanced high-grade malignant lymphomas.

The clinical manifestations of gastric lymphoma are nonspecific and difficult to distinguish from gastric adenocarcinoma. However, constitutional B-type symptoms such as fevers, weight loss, night sweats, massive splenomegaly, palpable peripheral adenopathy, and abdominal masses can be observed with advanced cases.

Other complications include bleeding, obstruction, perforation, and fistulization.

Primary gastric lymphoma may be seen on endoscopy as enlarged folds, ulcers, nodules, or a diffusely infiltrating lesion. Endoscopic diagnosis may also be difficult, and deep biopsies are often required to reveal submucosal involvement. Endoscopic ultrasonography can better define the depth of tumor infiltration and abnormal perigastric lymph nodes. CT of the abdomen and chest can determine the extent of nodal involvement and distant metastases.

The Ann Arbor staging system has been used for staging primary gastric lymphoma (Box 1). Because primary gastric lymphoma is uncommon, large, randomized,

Rakel and Bope: *Conn's Current Therapy 2006.*

BOX 1   Ann Arbor Staging System for Lymphoma

- *Stage I:* involvement of a single lymph node region (I) or a single localized extralymphatic site (IE)
- *Stage II:* involvement of two or more lymph node regions on the same side of the diaphragm (II) or with localized involvement of a single associated extralymphatic site (IIE)
- *Stage III:* involvement of lymph node regions on both sides of the diaphragm (III) or with localized involvement of an extralymphatic site (IIIE), the spleen (IIIS), or both (IIIES)
- *Stage IV:* disease that is diffusely spread throughout an extranodal site

The stages can be subclassified into A and B categories; the B designation is given to patients with constitutional symptoms of weight loss, fever, and night sweats.

 CURRENT DIAGNOSIS

- Gastric adenocarcinoma accounts for 95% of all malignant tumors of the stomach. It is typically diagnosed as an ulcerating mass on upper endoscopy. Early gastric cancer may appear as a polypoid, flat, raised, depressed, or ulcerated lesion.
- CT scans of the abdomen and chest in addition to endoscopic ultrasound may be helpful for preoperative staging and further characterizing the extent of gastric cancer.
- Most of the primary gastric lymphoma is NHL of B-cell origin such as diffuse large cell NHL and the more common low-grade MALT type.
- *Helicobacter pylori* infection has been associated with a majority of MALT lymphoma.
- Gastric carcinoid tumors are rare and may be associated with chronic atrophic gastritis (type I) or gastrinomas (type II) in the setting of Zollinger-Ellison syndrome or MEN type I. Sporadic gastric carcinoids (type III) tend to be aggressive in nature.
- GISTs are usually benign. Endoscopic ultrasound and fine needle aspiration may be helpful to make the diagnosis.

Abbreviations: CT = computed tomography; GIST = gastrointestinal stromal tumors; MALT = mucosa-associated lymphoid tissue; MEN = multiple endocrine neoplasia; NHL = non-Hodgkin's lymphoma.

---

controlled trials are unavailable to guide treatment plans. The diffuse large B-cell NHL is the most aggressive form of gastric lymphoma, accounting for more than 50% of these cases. Traditionally, surgery is the initial management of early stage diseases, followed by adjuvant radiation, chemotherapy, or both. Recent data have supported nonoperative management for early stage diseases. A 10-year survival rate can be greater than 80% after treatment in patients with early stage diseases.

Low-grade MALT lymphoma is slow growing and well differentiated. More than 70% of low-grade MALT lymphoma may regress after eradication of *H. pylori*. Serial follow-up endoscopic examinations at frequent intervals are required to document tumor regression and eradication. Specific chromosomal translocations have been observed in MALT lymphomas. The most frequent translocation observed is t(11;18)(q21;q21) with resultant API2-MALT1 chimeric gene formation and has been associated with resistance to cure with *H. pylori* treatment. The clinical significance of this finding is still unclear, and further studies may elucidate the proper management of these patients.

Carcinoid

Gastric carcinoid tumors are rare and account for only 2% of all gastrointestinal carcinoids and 0.3% of all gastric neoplasms. Gastric carcinoids are usually asymptomatic; however, they may cause abdominal pain or bleeding. Gastric carcinoid tumors are derived from histamine-secreting enterochromaffin-like (ECL) cells and the majority is associated with chronic atrophic gastritis and occasionally pernicious anemia (type I), which generate hypergastrinemic states. Lesions in these conditions can be multiple with low metastatic potential. Type II gastric carcinoids are associated with gastrinomas (i.e., Zollinger-Ellison syndrome [ZES] or multiple endocrine neoplasia [MEN] type I). Type III gastric carcinoids are sporadic in nature and are the most aggressive form, which may present with local or hepatic metastases. The malignant carcinoid syndrome

with symptoms characterized by flushing, diarrhea, bronchoconstriction, and cardiac valvular lesions is less often encountered.

Endoscopy and/or endoscopic ultrasound (EUS) with fine-needle aspiration (FNA) or polypectomy can provide the histologic diagnosis of gastric carcinoid tumors with sheets of argyrophilic ECL cells observed. CT of the abdomen may be obtained to evaluate tumor extension and metastases. For type 1 and type 2 gastric carcinoids tumors, local excision may be performed endoscopically and partial gastrectomy reserved for larger tumors or incomplete endoscopic resection. Partial gastrectomy or total gastrectomy with lymph node resection may be required for type III gastric carcinoid lesions.

Gastric Mesenchymal Tumors

Mesenchymal tumors of the stomach are slow-growing lesions that account for 1% of all gastric malignancies. Gastrointestinal stromal tumors (GISTs) are most common. Others include lipoma, leiomyoma/sarcoma, and schwannoma. Most of these tumors are small and benign. They are usually found incidentally on radiographic studies or endoscopy. However, they may present with abdominal pain or gastrointestinal bleeding. Routine endoscopic biopsy is usually insufficient to make the diagnosis as these are submucosal tumors. Endoscopic ultrasound may be helpful in determining the submucosal nature of the tumor and obtaining tissue through FNA for additional immunohistochemical analysis.

CURRENT THERAPY

- The primary management of gastric cancer remains surgical resection, and it is potentially curative with localized lesions.
- Adjuvant treatment with the combination of 5-fluorouracil/leucovorin[1] chemotherapy and radiotherapy has been shown to prolong disease-free and overall survival after gastric resection.
- Prophylactic gastrectomy has been proposed for consideration for at-risk asymptomatic individuals in families with highly penetrant hereditary diffuse gastric cancer and germline E-cadherin mutation carriers.
- Low-grade MALT lymphoma may regress after eradication of *Helicobacter pylori* infection. Follow-up endoscopic examinations are required to document tumor resolution.
- Surgical resection is the treatment of choice for GISTs, however, smaller lesions with benign features may be considered for endoscopic resection.
- Imatinib (Gleevec) is a selective tyrosine kinase inhibitor that has been shown to achieve a substantial response in treatment for patients with advanced/metastatic GIST with c-Kit mutations.

[1]Not FDA approved for this indication.
Abbreviations: GIST = Gastrointestinal stromal tumors;
MALT = mucosa-associated lymphoid tissue.

Tumor size greater than 3 cm, high mitotic index and tumor necrosis are factors that prognosticate malignant potential. Surgical resection is the treatment of choice, though smaller lesions with benign features may be monitored or be considered for endoscopic resection alone. Recurrence is quite common.

Recent advances in the understanding of GIST include its probable origin from the intestinal pacemaker cells (interstitial cells of Cajal). Activating mutations in the c-Kit gene, a tyrosine kinase has been observed in the majority of GISTs. Imatinib (Gleevec) a selective tyrosine kinase inhibitor, including c-Kit, has been shown to achieve a significant treatment response in patients with advanced/metastatic GIST, previously a fatal disease. Further advances in molecular and genetic biology should continue to facilitate research to develop novel agents and management strategies for this disease.

REFERENCES

Corley DA, Kubo A: Influence of site classification on cancer incidence rates: An analysis of gastric cardia carcinomas. J Natl Cancer Inst 2004;96(18):1383-1387.
Demetri GD, von Mehren M, Blanke CD, et al: Efficacy and safety of imatinib mesylate in advanced gastrointestinal stromal tumors. N Engl J Med 2002;347(7):472-480.
El-Rifai W, Powell SM: Molecular and biologic basis of upper gastrointestinal malignancy. Gastric carcinoma. Surg Oncol Clin N Am 2002;11(2):273-291, viii.

Fischbach W, Goebeler-Kolve ME, Dragosics B, et al: Long term outcome of patients with gastric marginal zone B cell lymphoma of mucosa associated lymphoid tissue (MALT) following exclusive *Helicobacter pylori* eradication therapy: experience from a large prospective series. Gut 2004;53(1):34-37.
McCulloch P, Nita M, Kazi H, Gama-Rodrigues J: Extended versus limited lymph nodes dissection technique for adenocarcinoma of the stomach. Cochrane Database Syst Rev 2004;18(4):CD001964.
Macdonald JS, Smalley SR, Benedetti J, et al: Chemoradiotherapy after surgery compared with surgery alone for adenocarcinoma of the stomach or gastroesophageal junction. N Engl J Med 2001; 345(10):725-730.
Pister PWT, Powell SM, Kelsen DP, Tepper JE: Cancer of the stomach. In DeVita VT, Hellman S, Rosenberg SA (eds): Cancer: Principles and Practice of Oncology, 7th ed. Philadelphia, Lippincott Williams and Wilkins, 2005.
Sobin LH, Wittekind CH: TNM Classification of Malignant Tumours, 6th ed. New York, Wiley, 2002.
Uemura N, Okamoto S, Yamamoto S, et al: *Helicobacter pylori* infection and the development of gastric cancer. N Engl J Med 2001; 345(11):784-789.

Tumors of the Colon and Rectum

Method of
Kirk A. Ludwig, MD

Colorectal cancer is a major public health issue, with approximately 140,000 new cases diagnosed every year in the United States. Approximately one third of these cases are rectal cancers. Cancer statistics consistently show that colorectal cancer is the number-two cancer killer in the United States for both men and women. Most cases (approximately 90%) are sporadic; that is, they occur in patients without any predisposing condition or genetic abnormality. Of these sporadic cases, however, approximately 30% of the patients have some family history of colorectal cancer. Approximately 5% to 10% of all cases are caused by the hereditary nonpolyposis colon cancer (HNPCC) syndrome, 1% are caused by familial adenomatous polyposis (FAP) or one of its variants, and a further 1% occur in patients with chronic inflammatory bowel disease: ulcerative colitis, or Crohn's disease.

Colorectal cancers, with few exceptions, start as the premalignant lesion known as a colorectal polyp or adenoma. This well-defined premalignant precursor lesion progresses to the malignant state over a prolonged period of time, generally many years. The existence of an adenoma-carcinoma sequence is based on both direct and indirect evidence:

- Patients who develop many polyps (FAP) inevitably develop colorectal cancer.
- Clearance of adenomas reduces the incidence of cancer.
- The risk of cancer within a polyp increases with the size of the polyp.

- Adenomas and cancers often coexist.
- Adenoma remnants are often found within resected cancers.
- Acquired genetic abnormalities common to adenomas are found in cancers.

Etiology of Colorectal Cancer

Although the exact etiology is not known, colorectal cancer seems to develop as a result of a combination of factors that are loosely categorized into genetic susceptibility and environmental factors. Colorectal cancer ultimately occurs as the result of a series of genetic abnormalities. The genes/mutations involved include the APC gene, the DCC gene, K-ras mutations, and p53 mutations or mismatch repair gene mutations. Much evidence now indicates that colorectal cancers develop along two distinct pathways depending on whether the initiating genetic event is an APC gene mutation (loss of heterozygosity [LOH] pathway) or a mutation of one of the mismatch repair genes (replication error [RER] pathway). There is increasing evidence that colorectal tumor behavior and response to therapy correlates to which pathway is involved. It is thought that approximately 70% to 80% of sporadic colorectal cancers develop through the LOH pathway and approximately 20% develop through the RER pathway.

A series of genetic events allow a polyp to develop and then progress to cancer. Although these events are often depicted as an orderly sequence, this is not the case. The cancer develops as a result of an accumulation of mutational events.

The environmental factors involved in colorectal cancer can be distilled down to a combination of Westernized diet and lifestyle. The most compelling evidence of the importance of these factors is taken from migrant studies showing that if large groups of people are moved from a low-incidence area (Africa, India, Mexico) to a high-incidence area (such as the United States), within a few generations the colorectal cancer incidence for this group of people is that of the indigenous population. So it would appear that lifestyle and dietary changes modify colorectal cancer risk. How these factors affect the development of colorectal cancer can be explained as an imbalance between neoplasia-promoting and protective constituents. The promoting factors would be high intake of fat, especially animal fat, high calorie intake, obesity, diets heavy in fried or charred foods, tobacco use, and excess intake of alcohol, especially beer. Protective factors would include adequate physical activity, high intake of dietary fiber, high fluid intake, high-calcium diet, and a high intake of fruit and vegetables and fish. In simplistic terms, the longer carcinogenic factors are in contact with the colonic mucosa, the more chance of them exerting their mutagenic influence on these cells. Factors such as fiber, adequate fluid intake, and exercise tend to speed transit through the colon, and micronutrients and bioactive substances protect the colonocytes from the carcinogens. In a general sense, then, patients can lower their risk of developing colon and rectal cancers by practicing the following behaviors:

- Eating a low fat diet
- Eating between 25 and 40 g of fiber each day from fruits, vegetables, whole grain breads, cereals, nuts, and beans
- Eating foods high in folate such as leafy green vegetables or supplementing the diet with a multivitamin with folate
- Drinking alcohol in moderation
- Refraining from smoking
- Exercising for 20 minutes, three to four times a week

Screening for Colorectal Cancer

Making dietary and lifestyle changes is difficult. Primary care physicians can make the biggest impact on colorectal cancer by encouraging their patients to undergo proper colorectal cancer screening. Clear and convincing evidence proves that screening is effective and the most important strategy in reducing the incidence of colon and rectal cancer.

Prevention of colorectal cancer is a matter of finding and removing polyps. This involves understanding and recommending screening for average-risk patients and taking a careful personal and family history from patients so high-risk individuals, by virtue of either a personal or family history of colorectal cancer or polyps, can be identified and screened appropriately. Colorectal cancer is a primarily a disease of older patients with the peak incidence in the seventh decade. More than 90% of cases occur in patients older than 50 years, with only 5% occurring in patients younger than 40 years.

Screening for average risk patients begins at age 50 years. Patients can be screened with one of five methods, each of which has its advantages and disadvantages that physicians and patients must weigh to make an appropriate choice. The five recommended screening techniques are:

1. Annual fecal occult blood testing (FOBT)
2. Flexible sigmoidoscopy every 5 years
3. Annual FOBT combined with flexible sigmoidoscopy every 5 years
4. Air-contrast barium enema (ACBE) every 5 to 10 years
5. Full colonoscopy every 10 years

The literature clearly indicates that combining a positive FOBT with colonoscopy reduces mortality from colorectal cancer. Although it is an inexpensive test shown effective in a number of large well-designed trials, compliance with testing is problematic (approximately 50%). The testing should be conducted on three consecutive stools, and for the 2 days before the testing and during the period of the testing, the patient must avoid red meats, aspirin, nonsteroidal anti-inflammatory drugs (NSAIDs), turnips, horseradish, and vitamin C. Any of these can cause a false-positive result. FOBT should be done at home. No evidence shows that random stool sampling in the physician's office is of any value. In fact, a recent study points out the very real deficiencies of FOBT done during random rectal exams in this setting. Although FOBT works on a large-scale population, its major problem is that, in reality, it fails to detect 50% of cancers and 90% of polyps.

Flexible sigmoidoscopy is designed to detect only those lesions found in the distal colon. One of the problems is that the amount of colon examined varies quite a bit from one examiner to the next. Although this type of exam may view the entire left colon up to the splenic flexure, at times patient discomfort and operator ability are such that the exam is terminated in the mid- to distal sigmoid. If an adenoma is found during this exam, colonoscopy should follow because almost one third harbor neoplastic lesions in the proximal colon. The effectiveness of the flexible sigmoidoscope in reducing mortality from colorectal cancer has never been demonstrated in a randomized controlled trial. The American Cancer Society recommends that if flexible sigmoidoscopy every 5 years is used for screening, it should be combined with annual FOBT. Unfortunately, even in patients with both a negative FOBT and flexible sigmoidoscopy, 15% to 25% have a proximal neoplasm detected at colonoscopy.

The ACBE is another screening option, although efficacy is inferred, not proven. The exam depends on a motivated and skilled radiologist. It fails to detect 50% to 80% of polyps smaller than 1 cm and 50% to 80% of stage I and stage II cancers. Single-column barium enemas are even less sensitive and not recommended for screening. If a barium enema is used as the screening tool, it should probably be combined with rigid proctoscopy so mid- and low rectal lesions are not missed.

The final screening technique is full colonoscopy. This study is the gold standard for evaluating the colonic mucosa. The ability of colonoscopy to reduce colorectal cancer mortality is demonstrated indirectly; that is, detecting and removing polyps reduces cancer risks and detecting cancers early lowers mortality. No trial as yet has looked at colonoscopy directly as a screening test. A normal colonoscopy at the age of 50 years, in the absence of intervening symptoms, does not need to be repeated until the age of 60 years, and there is no need for interval FOBT or flexible sigmoidoscopy during this period. In addition to its use as a screening tool, full colonoscopy is the common final pathway for any positive screen. A positive FOBT, a polyp found on flexible sigmoidoscopy, or a questionable lesion on an ACBE all require full colonoscopy for diagnostic and potentially therapeutic purposes.

The Office of Technology Assessment considers FOBT, flexible sigmoidoscopy, and colonoscopy equally cost effective as screening strategies. Screening for colorectal cancer makes sense from a public health standpoint, with an estimated cost of less than $20,000 per year of life saved (starting at age 50 years and ending at year 85). This cost compares favorably to many well-accepted screening programs, such as mammography for women older than 50 years of age. It is critically important for physicians to discuss colorectal cancer screening with their patients because the majority follow their primary care physician's recommendations if they are offered and plans put in place. Once screened, patients are three times more likely to get screened again. Although public awareness regarding colorectal cancer screening is improving, the majority of Americans do not name colorectal cancer as a serious disease that can be fatal, 20% cannot name one way to prevent colorectal cancer, and only 4% name screening as a way to protect themselves. Most patients believe it is the responsibility of their physicians to recommend screening. Currently, 63% of Americans older than age 50 years are not being screened for colorectal cancer.

The five screening strategies mentioned apply to the average-risk individual. There are others who require different strategies. Patients with chronic inflammatory bowel disease are at high risk for colorectal cancer. In patients with ulcerative colitis (or Crohn's colitis), beginning 7 to 8 years after the diagnosis of pancolitis or 12 to 15 years after the diagnosis of left-sided colitis (disease always confined to the colon distal to the splenic flexure), a full colonoscopy should be performed every 1 to 2 years with quadrant biopsies taken at multiple points throughout the colon and rectum to look for cancers, polyps, strictures, or dysplasia (an indication that the mucosa is becoming unstable and surgery may be indicated).

Then there are patients with a high risk based on a family history of colon cancer. Recommendations vary depending on whether the family history points to one of the two common syndromes, HNPCC or FAP. In general, however, for patients with a family history of colon cancer, screening should begin at the age of 40 years, or 10 years younger than the youngest affected family member. In these patients, screening should be conducted with colonoscopy. Interval studies are conducted at more frequent intervals than in average-risk patients.

Patients who have undergone resection for colorectal cancer should have a colonoscopy performed approximately 1 year after resection and then at regular intervals, 1 to 5 years, based on the findings and the given situation. Patients with a history of polyps should have follow-up surveillance scopes performed at intervals of 3 to 5 to 10 years, again based on findings (size, number, and type of polyp) and individual patient considerations.

Inherited Colorectal Cancer Syndromes

The two major inherited colorectal cancer syndromes are FAP and HNPCC. As stated earlier, colorectal cancer results from an accumulation of somatic mutations affecting cancer-related genes. These same genes and mutations are involved in these inherited syndromes, but the sequence of events is simply accelerated based on the fact that the initial mutation is germ line.

FAP is inherited in an autosomal dominant manner. The incidence is approximately 1 in 7000, with a prevalence of approximately 1 in 24,000 to 1 in 43,000. Essentially all who have the mutation manifest the syndrome; penetrance is 100%. FAP is caused by a germ line mutation of the APC gene located on 5q21. The APC gene is a tumor suppressor gene involved with apoptosis, or programmed cell death. Mutation of the APC gene results in a truncated protein product, and it is this truncated product that forms the basis of the commercially available serum test for diagnosing FAP.

A generalized disorder of cell growth, FAP has both colonic and extracolonic manifestations. The colonic manifestations, hundreds to thousands of colon and rectal polyps, are the hallmark of the syndrome. The absolute number of polyps varies, and the distribution varies based partly on where on the gene the mutation takes place. Mutations at various loci result in varying phenotypes. In general, polyp density tends to be greater in the left colon, although in attenuated FAP (marked by fewer polyps and later onset of polyps and cancer), polyp density is greater on the right. Recognizing this syndrome is vital because average patients with unrecognized FAP have colorectal cancer by the time they reach their mid- to late 30s. Screening for FAP should begin with a flexible sigmoidoscopic exam at approximately the age of 10 years. If polyps are found, a number should be biopsied to confirm the diagnosis, and a colonoscopic exam should follow to document the approximate number, size, and distribution of polyps and to rule out a cancer. Colorectal cancer before the age of 20 years in FAP patients is an unusual event. If no polyps are found and the patient declines genetic testing, screening exams should be repeated annually into the mid-20s and every 2 to 3 years thereafter. Surgery in young screen-detected patients is undertaken when convenient, whereas in older patients, who often present with a cancer, operation is usually conducted shortly after diagnosis.

The two most important extracolonic manifestations of FAP are duodenal polyps and desmoid tumors. Duodenal polyps arise in 80% to 90% of FAP patients. They tend to cluster around the ampulla of Vater. They are best viewed with a side-viewing endoscope, and patients should have an esophagogastroduodenoscopy (EGD) for screening starting in their early 20s and thereafter at 1- to 3-year intervals based on the polyp number, size, histology, and grade of dysplasia. Ultimately, it appears that from 5% to 12% of patients develop a malignancy as a result of these duodenal adenomas. Desmoid tumors are soft tissue tumors consisting of fibroaponeurotic tissue that can develop throughout the abdomen or the abdominal wall in 12% to 38% of patients with FAP. Desmoids that develop within the abdomen generally arise from the small bowel mesentery. They do not metastasize widely; rather they cause morbidity and mortality as a result of local growth characteristics resulting in small bowel obstruction, intestinal ischemia, and intestinal perforation. No standard cytotoxic chemotherapeutic regimen for treatment is available, and they do not respond well to attempts at surgical extirpation. NSAIDs[1] and antiestrogens[1] are generally used in an attempt to keep growth in check. In patients with FAP who have their colons and rectums managed properly,

[1]Not FDA approved for this indication.

duodenal cancer and desmoid tumors are the major causes of mortality today.

As mentioned, commercially available serum tests are available to detect an APC gene mutation so the diagnosis can be made without endoscopy. There are still issues regarding confidentiality, interpretation, psychology, and insurance that surround genetic testing, and as a general rule, this type of testing should be carried out in the context of a specialized registry or genetic disorder clinic so patients and their families have access to the personnel who can help resolve these sorts of issues.

HNPCC also has an autosomal dominant inheritance pattern, although the penetrance appears to be only 80% to 85%. This syndrome results from mutation in mismatch repair genes. At least six are implicated, but the two that result in the majority of cases are hMSH2 and hMLH1. Mismatch repair gene mutations result in replication error phenomena detected by testing for microsatellite instability.

The two types of HNPCC are referred to as Lynch syndrome I and Lynch syndrome II. Lynch syndrome I is a site-specific, early-age-of-onset (mean age 46 years) colorectal cancer syndrome. There is proximal colon predominance (70%), and these patients have an excess of synchronous (18%) and metachronous (40% within 10 years) cancers. Families with Lynch syndrome II also have colorectal cancer, but there is also familial clustering of other cancers, including endometrial and ovarian, small intestinal, stomach, pancreatic, and transitional cell cancers of the ureter and renal pelvis. The gynecologic tumors are the most common extracolonic cancers. Colorectal cancers in HNPCC, as compared to sporadic cancers, tend to be more mucinous, poorly differentiated, have a signet ring cell configuration, and they may incite an inflammatory response in the wall of the bowel. Despite what may appear to be an aggressive histology, these tumors less often invade through the bowel wall and spread to local lymph nodes, and they appear to have an overall better prognosis than similar sporadic colorectal cancers. Despite the term *nonpolyposis*, HNPCC patients develop polyps at a rate similar to the unaffected population, but their polyps tend to be larger, more villous, and more dysplastic. The cancer in HNPCC still arises from a polyp. The diagnosis of HNPCC is made by taking a careful family history or, in the index case, recognizing the features of the disease. Minimum criteria for making the diagnosis have been developed and revised. The most often used criteria for diagnosis are known as the Amsterdam criteria. By the criteria, the diagnosis should be considered if:

- Three relatives have confirmed colorectal cancer.
- Two successive generations are involved.
- One relative is a first-degree relative of the other two.
- One of the cancers was diagnosed before the age of 50 years.
- FAP is excluded.

Less strict guidelines, meant to be more clinically useful and taking into consideration extracolonic tumors, are known as the Bethesda guidelines. There are revisions of both guidelines as well. Screening of the colorectum in HNPCC starts at the age of 20 to 25 years, or 5 years younger than the youngest affected family member, and it is done with a full colonoscopy. The exam is repeated at 2-year intervals. In patients with family history of extracolonic cancers, screening of these systems is undertaken for the organs involved by history. Just as with FAP, genetic testing for HNPCC is available.

Surgical Treatment

Surgery is the basis of treatment in almost all cases of colon and rectal cancer, and curative treatment plans for colon and rectal cancer always have surgery as the primary mode of treatment. In fact, more than 50% of colon and rectal cancers are cured with surgery alone.

A number of staging systems are used for colorectal cancer. The TNM (tumor, node, metastasis) staging system is preferred. In this system, stage I tumors are confined to the bowel wall with no lymph node or distant spread, stage II tumors are outside the bowel wall but still with no lymph node or distant spread, stage III tumors are lymph node positive, and stage IV tumors have distant metastatic disease. In terms of the classic Dukes' classification system, stage I is Dukes' A, stage II is Dukes' B, and stage III is Dukes' C.

Most colorectal cancers grow silently, which is why screening is so important. When symptoms do arise, the most common are change in bowel habits and blood per rectum (usually caused by left-sided or rectal cancers), anemia (often seen in right-sided tumors), and abdominal pain (often an ominous sign of advanced disease). Approximately 50% of patients present with stage I or stage II disease, 25% present with stage III disease, and 25% present with stage IV cancers. Approximately 20% of patients present acutely with either obstruction or perforation. In either case, urgent or emergency resection is undertaken.

The diagnosis of colorectal cancer should be made, in the vast majority of cases, with a colonoscopic biopsy. After the diagnosis is made, clinical staging studies, including an abdominal and pelvic computed tomography (CT) scan and a posteroanterior (PA) and lateral chest radiograph, are obtained, as well as a complete set of laboratory tests, including a serum carcinoembryonic antigen (CEA) level, a complete blood count (CBC), and a chemistry and liver panel.

Most colon cancers are treated electively with an oncologic colon resection, which includes a proximal lymphovascular pedicle ligation and complete lymphadenectomy and a wide en bloc resection of the tumor-bearing bowel segment with adjacent soft tissue and mesentery. As a general rule, the extent of resection is guided by the major lymphatic drainage basin of the segment of bowel involved. This usually means that for any particular bowel segment, the major lymphovascular pedicle proximal and distal to the tumor is taken near its origin. Right colon tumors are treated with a right or extended right colectomy with an ileocolic anastomosis; descending colon tumors, with a formal left colectomy and colorectal anastomosis; and sigmoid tumors, with a sigmoid resection or anterior resection with a colorectal anastomosis. With the recent publication of two large

prospective randomized trials comparing conventional and laparoscopic colon surgery, it now appears that, at least in the hands of experienced laparoscopic surgeons, laparoscopic operation is comparable to the conventional approach and may offer short-term and possibly long-term advantages.

The surgical approach to the colon and rectum for patients with FAP takes into consideration the age of the patient, whether there is already a colon or rectal cancer, the distribution of polyps, whether there are many polyps (more than 20) or few (less than 20) in the rectum, and whether the patient is reliable for follow-up. In young patients with few polyps in the rectum who are willing to return yearly for surveillance of the rectum (to minimize the risk of developing rectal cancer) or in patients with attenuated FAP, a total abdominal colectomy with ileorectal anastomosis may be a good option. In patients with a high number of rectal polyps, in older patients, and in patients who are not reliable for rectal surveillance, a total proctocolectomy with ileal pouch anal anastomosis is the preferred operation. In unusual situations, FAP patients may be treated with a total proctocolectomy and an end ileostomy.

For patients with HNPCC who have colon cancer or a large polyp that cannot be removed colonoscopically, the preferred operation is a total abdominal colectomy with an ileorectal anastomosis. Yearly rectal surveillance is then undertaken with a flexible sigmoidoscope. In patients with HNPCC who have rectal pathology, a total proctocolectomy, with or without reconstruction, may be indicated. Prophylactic surgery for patients in HNPCC families is not generally undertaken. For female HNPCC patients with a family history of gynecologic pathology, strong consideration should be given to performing a prophylactic total abdominal hysterectomy and bilateral salpingo-oophorectomy at the time of any colon operation if the patient has completed her family or is postmenopausal.

Stage I cancers are typically treated with surgery alone, with a survival of 90% to 95% at 5 years. Stage II cancers are treated with surgery and, in specific instances, adjuvant chemotherapy with a 5-year survival of between 75% and 85%. Stage III cancers are treated with surgery followed by chemotherapy with a 5-year survival of 40% to 60%. Stage IV cancers are treated on an individual basis with either surgery, chemotherapy, palliative measures, or a combination, depending on symptoms, extent of disease, and functional status of the patient. In the setting of stage IV disease, the indications for resection of the primary tumor are generally bleeding or obstruction. In the case of isolated metastatic disease, in which potentially curative treatment is undertaken, resection of the primary tumor is also indicated. Survival for stage IV colon cancer is less than 10%. For a select group of stage IV patients with isolated and technically resectable metastatic disease, however, 5-year survival figures may be as high as 25% to 40%.

Tumors of the mid- and low rectum are treated differently than colon or upper rectal cancers. The difference in treatment is based on the fact that historically these tumors, unlike upper rectal cancers and colon

7

CURRENT DIAGNOSIS

- Average-risk patients start screening at age 50 years.
- High-risk patients (chronic inflammatory bowel disease, family or personal history of polyps or cancer, or documented or suspected nonpolyposis colon cancer [HNPCC] or familial adenomatous polyposis [FAP]) start screening earlier.
- Any positive finding on a noncolonoscopic screening test should lead to a full colonoscopy.
- For patients with a strong family history of colorectal cancer, the diagnosis of one of the inherited colorectal cancer syndromes and potential referral for genetic testing should be considered.

CURRENT THERAPY

- Diagnosis should be made with colonoscopic biopsy and tumor staged with chest radiograph, abdominal and pelvic CT scan, and for rectal cancer with endorectal ultrasound. A full set of labs and a CEA level should be drawn.
- Colon cancer is treated with an oncologic segmental or total colectomy using an open or laparoscopic technique.
- Stage III colon cancers and some high-risk stage II colon cancers are also treated with adjuvant chemotherapy.
- Locally advanced (stages II or III) mid- or low rectal cancers are treated with preoperative chemo/radiation therapy and then resection. Most patients can be treated with less than an abdominal perineal resection, without the need for a permanent colostomy.
- Follow-up of colorectal cancer patients includes evaluations every 3 to 6 months, with history and physical exam and CEA-level determination; chest radiograph every 6 to 12 months; and a colonoscopy 1 year after resection and thereafter, based on findings. Any abnormality is evaluated more fully with a CT scan or other appropriate imaging.

Abbreviations: CEA = carcinoembryonic antigen; CT = computed tomography.

cancers, have a stage-dependent high rate of local failure (recurrence within the pelvis). To manage this tendency for pelvic recurrence, stages II and III rectal cancers are treated with a combination of chemotherapy and radiation therapy, in addition to surgery. Rectal cancers are staged locally in the preoperative setting using endorectal ultrasound or pelvic magnetic resonance imaging (MRI). Although the chemotherapy and radiation therapy can be administered either preoperatively or in the postoperative setting, if the tumor can be accurately staged at diagnosis, there are many theoretic and practical advantages to using these treatments in the preoperative or neoadjuvant setting. This is generally the preferred approach. In patients with very low tumors that invade the pelvic floor muscles or the anal sphincters, an abdominal perineal resection with colostomy may be indicated. However, most rectal cancers can now be treated with a sphincter-preserving resection, avoiding a permanent colostomy and improving quality of life. For very select low-lying, superficially invasive rectal cancers, not associated with lymph node disease by endorectal ultrasound or MRI, transanal full-thickness local excision may be a treatment option. Specialized training and a high volume of rectal cancer experience strongly correlate with outcomes in the management of rectal cancer.

The follow-up for patients after resection of colorectal cancer varies, and data in the literature conflict about whether careful follow-up has any bearing on overall outcome. Therefore, follow-up schemes are individualized. In potentially curative situations, the follow-up plan might be:

- History and exam every 3 months for 2 years, then every 6 months for 3 years
- CEA level every 3 months for 2 years, then every 6 months for 3 years
- Colonoscopy 1 year after surgery and if normal repeated in 3 years
- Chest radiograph every 2 to 12 months

- CT scan for rising CEA or abnormal history or physical exam

Colorectal cancer is a common disease with approximately 50,000 deaths per year attributed to it in the United States alone. Because these cancers have polyps as precursor lesions and the lag time between polyp and cancer is so long, screening to detect and remove polyps should be the major emphasis for this disease. Screening programs reduce incidence and mortality. All patients 50 years of age and older should have regular screening. By taking a thorough personal and family history, high-risk individuals should be identified and proper surveillance programs should be put in place. Several screening options are available, so not screening is no longer an option. Once diagnosed and staged, treatment usually begins with surgical extirpation. Mid- and low rectal cancers require special attention in terms of appropriate preoperative staging and treatment to maximize oncologic outcome and quality of life.

REFERENCES

Beck DE (ed), Guillem JG (guest ed): Rectal Cancer. Clinics in Colon and Rectal Cancer, vol. 15. New York, Thieme, 2002.
Colon and Rectal Cancer Clinical Practice Guidelines in Oncology, wwww: J Natl Comp Cancer Network, www.nccn.org, 2003;1: 40-63.
Colorectal Cancer Screening Clinical Practice Guidelines in Oncology: J Natl Comp Cancer Network, www.nccn.org, 2003;1:72-93.
Ellis CN (ed): Inherited Cancer Syndromes: Current Clinical Management. New York, Springer-Verlag, 2004.

Jemal A, Thomas A, Murray T, et al: Cancer statistics, 2002. CA Cancer J Clin 2002;52:23-47.

Lacy AM, Garcia-Valdecasas JC, Delgado S, et al: Laparoscopy-assisted colectomy versus open colectomy for treatment of non-metastatic colon cancer: A randomized trial. Lancet 2002;359:2224-2229.

Nelson H, Sargent DJ, Weiand HS, et al: A comparison of laparoscopically assisted and open colectomy for colon cancer. N Engl J Med 2004;350:2050-2059.

Purves H, Pietroban R, Hervey S, et al: Relationship between surgeon caseload and sphincter preservation in patients with rectal cancer. Dis Colon Rectum 2005;48:195-204.

Winawer SJ, Fletcher RH, Miller L, et al: Colorectal cancer screening: Clinical guidelines and rationale. Gastroenterology 1997;112:594-642.

Intestinal Parasites

Method of
Linda Yancey, MD, and A. Clinton White, Jr., MD

Although many people in the United States mistakenly think that intestinal parasites are uncommon, current estimates suggest that 50% of all people worldwide harbor one or more intestinal parasite. Some parasitic diseases have been controlled in the developed world. For example, intestinal helminths such as *Ascaris* and hookworm are rarely acquired in the United States, whereas each infects more than 1 billion people worldwide. Even in industrialized areas some infections are more common than realized. For example, approximately one third of U.S. residents have serologic evidence of prior cryptosporidiosis by the time they reach adulthood; colonization with pinworms is common during childhood. Furthermore, global travel and immigration mean that even in nonendemic areas physicians will encounter patients harboring these organisms. The acquisition of most enteric parasites can be minimized by rigorous adherence to personal hygiene and safe eating and drinking habits. In developing countries where safe food and water are predominantly unavailable, precautions such as boiling or filtering contaminated water prior to usage, avoiding raw or undercooked food, using proper footwear, and not bathing in fresh water are effective preventive strategies. In suspected cases the mainstay of diagnosis has been examination of the stool specimens. However, many of the common protozoan parasites are only identified by special stains or immunologic assays. Unfortunately, these tests are only performed when specifically requested. The following is a brief overview of a few of the most common intestinal parasites worldwide. Concise and frequently updated guidelines on parasitic diseases are available from the Division of Parasitic Diseases, Centers for Disease Control and Prevention (CDC) at their Web site, http://www.dpd.cdc.gov/dpdx/.

Among the more common syndromes caused by intestinal parasites is diarrhea. Diarrheal syndromes can be separated into those associated with watery diarrhea and or dysentery. Frequent, small volume, bloody,

or mucoid stools are typically associated with colitis. Symptoms often include abdominal pain, tenesmus, hematochezia, and fever. Markers of inflammation such as fecal leukocytes, lactoferrin, or occult blood occur often in stool. Watery, large volume stools and malabsorption are typically associated with enteritis. Symptoms include watery stools, cramping, volume depletion, bloating, weight loss, and malodorous stools. Fever, hematochezia, and tenesmus are unusual, and fecal specimens show less pronounced inflammation. Parasites associated with each of these syndromes are listed in the Current Diagnosis box.

Protozoan Infections

Common protozoan enteric protozoan infections and associated diseases are listed in the Current Diagnosis box.

AMEBIASIS

The protozoan *Entamoeba histolytica* causes intestinal amebiasis. Amebiasis is a widespread condition; approximately 10% of the total world population is infected with an *Entamoeba* species. In addition to the pathogen *E. histolytica*, the genus also includes *Entamoeba dispar* and *Entamoeba moshkovskii*, which are indistinguishable from *E. histolytica* on microscopic examination but cause only asymptomatic colonization or mild illness. In Mexico, South and Central America, the Indian subcontinent, and southern and western Africa there is high prevalence of amebic disease. In developed countries, amebiasis is mainly a disease of immigrants and travelers. Clinical disease is sometimes noted in high-risk groups such as men who have sex with men (MSM), locations with poor sanitation, and institutionalized patients.

Infection is acquired by the fecal-oral route including consuming foods or water contaminated with amebic cysts. The cysts are surrounded by a chitinous cell wall, which allows them to remain viable in the environment for up to several weeks. Once in the small bowel, cysts release the trophozoites, which divide, mature, and travel down the gut to the colon, where they live on bacteria and colonic debris. Invasive disease is caused by invasion of the host tissues by the trophozoite forms, which can digest host tissues. They complete their life cycle when they encyst and are passed out of the host with the stool. The trophozoite forms can be excreted during episodes of brisk diarrhea, but they are delicate and do not survive long after leaving the host.

The spectrum of intestinal illness varies from asymptomatic infection to severe dysentery. Onset of infection is indolent with symptoms occurring 1 to 4 weeks after acquisition of the parasite. Patients often complain of diarrhea, abdominal pain, and tenesmus. The diarrhea commonly contains blood and mucus but is not usually voluminous. In mild cases the diarrhea may be described as watery. Weight loss is seen in approximately 50% of patients and fever is present in less than 33%. The more severe presentations including fulminant colitis, colonic perforation, and amebic peritonitis occur in less than 1% of cases but are associated with a high mortality rate.

Extraintestinal involvement primarily involves the liver. Hepatic amebiasis is caused by digestion of the liver tissue by the invasive trophozoites. The older term, *amebic liver abscess*, is incorrect in that the infection does not involve abscess formation, and the fluid typically contains few white blood cells (WBCs). Patients often present after an incubation period of weeks to months. The onset can be either indolent or acute. The clinical manifestations are very similar to those of biliary tract infection, with most patients presenting with abdominal pain, weight loss, and fever. Physical examination is characterized by fever and right upper quadrant tenderness. General laboratory tests reveal leucocytosis, often with a left shift and elevations of alkaline phosphatase and transaminases. Ultrasound (US) or computed tomography (CT) scans typically reveal hypodense lesions. Most patients have single lesions with a predominance of involvement of the right lobe.

Distinguishing between *E. histolytica* infections that require treatment even when not symptomatic and carriage of its nonpathogenic counterparts (*E. dispar* and *E. moshkovskii*), which require no treatment, has presented a challenge. Amebas containing red blood cells (RBCs), blood in the stool, or bowel ulcers with amoeba can be presumed to be *E. histolytica*. Serologic tests for antibody to *E. histolytica* can help in invasive infection. However, antibody (especially using older tests) can persist, such that serologic tests are not useful for distinguishing between acute and previous infection. However, the presence of antibody is associated with invasive disease, and in the correct context it can be diagnostic. Antigen kits have been developed to test specifically for *E. histolytica*. Antigen can be detected in stool in cases with intestinal infection. In liver disease, blood specimens obtained prior to treatment also usually contain amebic antigen. The clinical response to empiric therapy with metronidazole is rapid in liver disease and can be helpful in diagnosis.

All persons with *E. histolytica* infection, whether symptomatic or not, require treatment because the asymptomatic carriers can still transmit the disease. However, most patients passing cysts identified as *E. histolytica* may only have *E. dispar* or *E. moshkovskii*, which do not require treatment. Treatment of invasive amebiasis with the nitroimidazoles (metronidazole or tinidazole, which are currently available in the United States) results in a 90% cure rate. Side effects of metronidazole consist of a disulfiram-like reaction to alcohol, dizziness, and rarely paresthesias and a temporary neutropenia. Even after treatment with metronidazole or tinidazole, more than 50% of patients will have persistent carriage of *E. histolytica* and, like asymptomatic carries, will require treatment to eradicate the remaining cysts. The drugs of choice for both groups of patients are iodoquinol, paromomycin, and diloxanide furoate. Currently, diloxanide is not readily available in the United States. Nitazoxanide, a broad-spectrum antiparasitic agent, may also have activity against amebic cysts. In cases of fulminant amebic colitis there may be leakage of intracolonic bacteria, and broad-spectrum antibiotics can be added to the antiprotozoal regimen.

BALANTIDIUM COLI

Balantidium coli, a ciliated protozoan, is an infectious agent primarily in domesticated pigs but can rarely cause human colitis especially in those with concurrent disease or immunocompromise. The life cycle is similar to that of *E. histolytica* starting with the ingestion of infective cysts resulting in a spectrum of disease from asymptomatic carriage to acute bloody diarrhea and rarely a chronic infection with abdominal pain and diarrhea. Diagnosis, as is the case with most parasitic diseases, is via serial stool analysis for the large, 60 μ, motile-ciliated organisms or their cysts. Tetracycline is the drug of choice, but metronidazole or iodoquinol can also be used.

BLASTOCYSTIS HOMINIS

The protozoan *Blastocystis hominis* is commonly found in stool samples submitted for parasitic examination; its role as a human pathogen remains unclear. For many years it was considered an intestinal commensal and has only recently been studied as a possible cause of infectious diarrhea. Reports of disease related to *B. hominis* have been in the form of case reports and small series, though the literature is mixed with case series that failed to demonstrate pathogenicity in immunocompetent patients. Because the symptoms attributed to blastocystosis (including bloating, abdominal pain, diarrhea, fatigue, and nausea) occur in patients with irritable bowel syndrome (IBS), a link between the disorders has been theorized; however, most experts do not consider *Blastocystis* to be a human pathogen.

Blastocystosis is diagnosed on the basis of serial stool samples, and it is seen in 15% of samples submitted in the United States. Because the pathogenicity of the organism is still up for debate, there are no accepted standards for what samples, if any, constitute positive specimens. In most cases carriage of the organism is asymptomatic and does not require treatment. Patients with symptoms should be rigorously examined for an alternate diagnosis, because *B. hominis* is often found with other, more commonly accepted as pathogenic, intestinal parasites. Many agents have in vitro activity against *Blastocystis*, but none have proven clinical efficacy. Some authorities recommend treatment with metronidazole.

GIARDIA INTESTINALIS

The protozoan *Giardia intestinalis* is found in temperate and tropical regions worldwide. Much like other intestinal parasites, giardiasis is often acquired in areas of poor sanitation, but outbreaks can be seen in any environment that promotes crowding (such as daycare centers). Travelers to the former Soviet Union and many campgrounds in the western United States are at risk for the infection. *Giardia* infection and malnutrition in children have a close association.

Infection is acquired via the ingestion of infective cysts. The cysts can survive in cool, moist conditions for long periods of time and are infective to other vertebrates, which serve as reservoirs of infection. Once in the stomach and duodenum, excystation occurs and the motile organisms attach to the bowel wall within the small intestinal crypts. Here they divide and pass down the alimentary tract where encystation occurs.

Transmission is via person-to-person spread, waterborne, or food-borne routes. Person-to-person spread has been seen in settings such as daycare centers, where fecal contamination of fomites is common, and venereally in male homosexuals. Because the cysts are stable in water and resistant to chlorination, *Giardia* is associated with waterborne outbreaks of diarrhea. The temperatures used to cook food are sufficient to kill *Giardia* cysts, however, raw foods or foods that come into contact with an infective source after cooking can serve as sources of disease.

Giardiasis has a wide range of clinical manifestations ranging from asymptomatic infection seen in around 60% of those infected to a chronic illness with bloating, wasting and malabsorption. Patients with defective antibody responses (e.g., common variable immunodeficiency or IgA deficiency) are predisposed to chronic infection, but chronic infection is also reported in apparently normal hosts. Those who have been previously infected are less likely to develop the characteristic watery, foul-smelling, nonbloody diarrhea with abdominal cramping, flatulence, bloating, and nausea. Symptoms develop 1 to 2 weeks after exposure and can last from a week to months. Weight loss and dehydration are commonly seen and, especially in children, can necessitate hospital admission.

Diagnosis is made on the basis of a compatible clinical picture and cysts or trophozoites observed in the stool. Multiple specimens should be examined because the excretion of the parasite can be sporadic or difficult to detect. Stool antigen testing is available and more sensitive than traditional microscopic examinations. The immunoassays are incompatible with all stool preservatives, however, and ideally they should be performed on fresh or frozen specimens. For a small number of patients endoscopy may be needed to obtain duodenal samples; although this technique has a similar yield to stool studies, it can be used to evaluate for alternate diagnosis. Many cases require empiric therapy.

Because asymptomatic infection is common, not all patients with *Giardia* present in the stools require immediate treatment. Any patient with symptoms should be treated. Food handlers and children, especially those in daycare settings and requiring diaper changes, should be treated to prevent the spread of infection. Metronidazole has been the drug of choice for treatment; tinidazole has similar efficacy and may soon be available in the United States. Nitazoxanide has been recently approved for treatment. It shows efficacy at least as good as metronidazole with a shorter course of treatment (3 days versus 5 days). In comparative trials nitazoxanide was better tolerated. It is available as an oral suspension or tablets. Metronidazole-resistant cases have been described. They may respond to nitazoxanide or to the addition of quinacrine to metronidazole. Furazolidone and the oral unabsorbed aminoglycoside paromomycin are somewhat less effective alternative treatments. Furazolidone is available as a suspension. Paromomycin can be used in pregnancy. Although albendazole is indicated for giardiasis, its efficacy has been variable in clinical trials and is likely less effective.

Prevention of this, as with other intestinal parasites, hinges on breaking the fecal-oral contamination cycle. Although the organism is easily filtered from water, standard chlorination is relatively ineffective in prevention of infection and tap water can be contaminated. Hand washing and hygienic disposal of soiled diapers should be stressed in daycare settings. Travelers should follow standard precautions when in endemic areas. Because of the frequency at which *Giardia* is found in wilderness areas, hikers and campers should filter or boil water prior to use. Portable, light, and convenient filtration systems with a pore size of less than 2 μm are readily commercially available at camping supply stores. *Giardia* is sensitive to heat, thus even at high altitudes bringing water to a boil is an effective treatment as well.

THE COCCIDIANS: *CYCLOSPORA CAYETANENSIS* AND *ISOSPORA BELLI*

Cyclospora cayetanensis and *Isospora belli* have been recently recognized as important causes of diarrhea. Identified outbreaks have been associated with contaminated water or produce. In contrast to other intestinal parasites, the oocysts are not infectious when shed but need to sporulate before they become infectious. Approximately 1 week after ingestion of the oocysts, some patients experience a flulike illness with watery diarrhea, fatigue, and malaise. In those with symptoms illness can range from a brief course to a prolonged picture of chronic diarrhea and abdominal discomfort. Most patients experience a remittent illness lasting several weeks.

Diagnosis is made by stool examination. The oblong oocysts of *Isospora* are larger (typically 10×30 to 40 μ) and can often be identified on wet mounts. *Cyclospora* oocysts are smaller (approximately 8 to 10 μ) and round, and are more difficult to identify. Either may stain with modified acid-fast stains, but staining of *Cyclospora* is variable. The organisms autofluoresce with ultraviolet (UV) microscopy. Treatment in the form of double-strength trimethoprim-sulfamethoxazole (TMP-SMZ) twice daily for 1 week has shown benefit in immunocompetent patients. Those with symptomatic HIV infection have been treated at a higher dose of a double-strength TMP-SMZ four times daily followed by a maintenance dose of TMP-SMZ three times per week. Nitazoxanide has been used to treat both *Isospora* and *Cyclospora* and may work in patients allergic to sulfonamides. Ciprofloxacin was inferior to TMP-SMZ in AIDS patients with these organisms but may also have some efficacy.

There have been few outbreaks of *Cyclospora* or *Isospora*, so data on prevention are limited. Because outbreaks of *Cyclospora* have been associated with contaminated produce, carefully washing fresh fruits and vegetables could potentially have some benefit. Water purification is also likely important.

CRYPTOSPORIDIOSIS

Cryptosporidium species are intracellular parasites that inhabit the digestive tract of humans and various other vertebrates. Recent molecular studies have demonstrated that humans are infected by several different species, including organisms primarily infecting people *(Cryptosporidium hominis)*, ruminants including cattle and sheep *(Cryptosporidium parvum)*, dogs, cats, and even turkeys *(Cryptosporidium meleagridis)*. Spread is via the fecal-oral route from an infected person or animal, and few are needed to cause disease. Oocysts are very hardy, difficult to kill with common disinfectants, poorly removed by most filtration systems, and persist in the environment for months. Waterborne outbreaks have been associated with contaminated drinking water and recreational bodies of water such as swimming pools. Person-to-person transmission is likely the major route.

Cryptosporidium is a major agent in persistent diarrhea in children, causing approximately 33% of cases in developing countries and is associated with malnutrition. In the industrialized countries, epidemiologic studies suggest that childhood infection is common, especially in daycare centers. Cryptosporidiosis is mainly diagnosed in immunocompromised hosts and has been the major agent of diarrhea in HIV-positive patients.

Symptoms begin approximately 1 week after ingestion of oocysts and range from asymptomatic infection to severe enteritis. The classic presentation in immunocompetent people is mild to moderate watery diarrhea with associated malaise, crampy abdominal pain and, less frequently, fever. Illness usually resolves in 10 to 14 days without therapy, but a substantial portion of cases continue for 2 to 4 weeks. Oocysts are shed after resolution of symptoms and for long periods of time after recovery. In immunocompromised hosts, *Cryptosporidium* can cause a much more protracted syndrome of wasting and prolonged diarrhea. For patients with HIV, a CD4 count less than 100 is associated with this chronic infection whereas those with CD4 counts less than 50 are associated with a cholera-like illness with copious stools leading to volume depletion. Extraintestinal manifestations are mainly seen in severely compromised hosts and include biliary involvement.

Diagnosis is usually made by microscopic examination of the stool. *Cryptosporidium* oocysts are difficult to appreciate on routine stool examination. The oocysts can be identified by acid-fast staining, immunofluorescence testing, or antigen-detection methods. Unfortunately, most clinical laboratories only routinely perform these tests on request. Even if tested correctly, multiple stool samples may be needed. In severe disease more oocysts are shed so that the diagnosis may be made based on one sample.

Supportive care remains critically important and includes antimotility treatments (e.g., loperamide, diphenoxylate/atropine, and tincture of opium); rehydration, nutrition, and immune reconstitution where possible are the mainstays of treatment. Antiretroviral therapy is a key component of care in AIDS patients. Nitazoxanide is a broad-spectrum antiparasitic drug. Placebo-controlled trials demonstrated more rapid resolution of cryptosporidiosis in studies of children and adults in Egypt; HIV patients with CD4 counts greater than 50 in Mexico; and hospitalized, malnourished children in Zambia. In the latter study there was a significant improvement in mortality rate; however, the drug was insignificantly better than placebo in AIDS patients with low CD4 cell counts or in severely malnourished children infected with HIV. Nitazoxanide was approved by the FDA in 2002 for treatment of cryptosporidiosis and giardiasis in children and subsequently approved for giardiasis in adults. Paromomycin, a nonabsorbable aminoglycoside, has activity against *Cryptosporidium* in vitro and in animal models, but it is only partially effective in AIDS patients. The combination of paromomycin and azithromycin has some activity in AIDS patients.

Cryptosporidium species are stable in the environment if kept moist and completely resistant to potable concentrations of chlorine in water supplies. Those at risk for symptomatic infection should boil or filter all drinking water especially when traveling to areas with poor public sanitation. They should also avoid contact with farm animals, persons with diarrhea, and recreational water such as public swimming pools. Water filters should be capable of removing particles up to 1 μ in diameter. By contrast, iodine or other common decontaminants do not kill oocysts. In HIV-positive patients on prophylaxis for *Mycobacterium avium*, complex with rifabutin has been demonstrated to decrease the risk of developing cryptosporidiosis.

DIENTAMOEBA FRAGILIS

Dientamoeba fragilis is a small flagellated protozoan, related to *Trichomonas*. It lives in the human large intestine as a trophozoite form, and transmission is via the fecal-oral route. It has been implicated as a cause of diarrhea and other gastrointestinal (GI) complaints. Diagnosis depends on demonstration of the trophozoites in stool. Stools need to be examined or placed in preservatives promptly or the organisms may not be visible. The treatment of choice is metronidazole. Iodoquinol, paromomycin, and tetracycline may also be effective.

MICROSPORIDIOSIS (*ENTEROCYTOZOON BIENEUSI, ENCEPHALITOZOON INTESTINALIS,* AND OTHERS)

Microsporidia are small obligate intracellular organisms that are transmitted via specialized spores. The thick-walled spores contain a specialized polar tube that, when activated, injects parasite cytoplasm into the host cells, where they enlarge, divide, and form progeny spores. Two microsporidia species cause human enteric infection: *Enterocytozoon bieneusi* and *Encephalitozoon intestinalis* (formerly known as *Septata intestinalis*). Both *E. bieneusi* and *E. intestinalis* cause chronic diarrhea in HIV patients with low CD4 counts. Microsporidia have been reported as a rare cause of diarrhea in otherwise healthy adults. Recent studies have noted asymptomatic carriage is common in developing countries.

Spores can be identified in stool with Weber's modified trichrome or fluorochrome stains that have affinity for chitin (calcofluor, Uvitex 2B), but identification of the specific species requires electron microscopy or polymerase chain reaction (PCR). Infection of immunocompetent individuals is self-limited. AIDS patients with microsporidiosis may improve with effective antiretroviral therapy. Preliminary data suggest that albendazole may be used in the treatment of *E. intestinalis*. *E. bieneusi* responds poorly to albendazole, but in one study, AIDS and transplant patients with *E. bieneusi* and diarrhea improved with treatment with fumagillin, which is only available in the United States via expanded access.

Helminth Infections

For most of human history, intestinal helminth infections have been a normal part of life. Even today, most residents of developing countries are intermittently infected. Only during the last part of the 20th century have intestinal helminths become rare in developed countries. Now most cases in developed countries are seen in immigrants.

NEMATODES

Ascariasis

Ascaris lumbricoides infection affects an estimated 20% of the world's population. *Ascaris* is found commonly in the tropics where the warm, moist soil conditions are beneficial for year-round transmission. Cases were formerly common in the rural southern United States, but now the vast majority of cases in the country occur in immigrants from developing countries. Children are most commonly affected in endemic areas. Infection is acquired by ingestion of the parasite ova. The eggs are hardy and can survive in moist, shady soil for years. When eggs are ingested, the larvae hatch in the gut, penetrate though the wall of the stomach or small bowel, invade into the bloodstream, and migrate to the pulmonary capillaries. The larvae then exit the vessels and enter the alveoli. After crawling into the respiratory tree, the larvae are coughed up, swallowed, and then mature into adult worms mainly in the jejunum. The mature worms can survive in the intestines for years before being passed in the stool (Table 1).

Most carriers of disease are asymptomatic or may note mild abdominal symptoms or passing worms in their feces. Most symptomatic infections occur in the minority of patients with heavy infections. During passage of the larvae through the lungs, patients may present with bronchospasms and fleeting pulmonary infiltrates.

In patients with a high worm burden, there may be mechanical obstruction of the lumen of the gut with worm balls. The most widespread symptom of infection is the nutritional deficiency. The greater the worm burden, the more pronounced the deficiency and, conversely, the more difficult it is for the host to prevent further infestation. Recent studies have documented an adverse effect of worm burden on intellectual development in children in endemic areas.

Diagnosis is based on stool samples and the patient reports of adult worms passed in the stool. During the migratory phase, patients may present with eosinophilia and wheezing, but may have negative stool studies. In patients with mature worms, stool examinations are quite sensitive, particularly in patients with heavy worm burdens.

Mebendazole and albendazole are the most widely available treatments and are able to kill adult worms, eggs in the gut, and migratory stages in various tissues. Both have been shown to be highly effective and reasonably well tolerated. Ivermectin and nitazoxanide are also quite effective. Pregnant patients can be given pyrantel pamoate, which acts as a paralytic agent allowing the worm to be expelled. Because *Ascaris* worms are acquired from the environment, patients living in endemic areas are at a very high risk for reinfection and may require multiple courses of therapy.

Hookworm

More than 1 billion persons are infected with hookworms. The hookworm is found across several continents including the Americas, Africa, and Asia. The two genera that complete their life cycle in humans, *Ancylostoma* and *Necator*, thrive in areas of moist soil that support the development of larvae. The most common species are *A. duodenale,* which is found around the Mediterranean Sea and in China and northern India, and *N. americanus,* which is seen in the Western hemisphere. The dog hookworm *A. caninum* has also been reported to cause human disease. Hookworms were formerly common in the southern United States, but now most cases are imported.

Eggs hatch in moist soil, undergo several molting steps, and then the mature larvae enter the host through the skin, usually in the area of the foot. They may cause an inflammatory response at the site in entry. The larvae are carried by the circulatory system to the lungs where they become trapped in the pulmonary capillaries, move into the oropharynx, and are swallowed. The larvae mature into adult worms in the proximal small bowel where they feed on intestinal cells with the aid of proteases and anticoagulants. These actions result in minor blood loss (0.01 to 0.3 mL) for each actively feeding worm, which leads to iron deficiency anemia in those with high worm burden or low iron stores. Eggs are passed in the stool and contaminate soil. The larvae of *A. duodenale,* but not *N. americanus,* are infectious if consumed orally without the need to pass through the circulatory system and lungs. Although all stages of infection can cause symptoms, the major burden of disease is the chronic loss of blood with associated

TABLE 1 Drugs for the Treatment of Nematode Infections

Infection	Drug	Adult dosage	Pediatric dosage
Anisakiasis *(Anisakis):*			
Treatment of choice	Surgical or endoscopic removal		
Ascariasis *(Ascaris lumbricoides,* roundworm):			
Drugs of choice	Albendazole (Albenza) or Mebendazole (Vermox) or Ivermectin (Stromectol)	400 mg once 100 mg bid × 3 d or 500 mg once 150-200 µg/kg once	200-400 mg once 100 mg bid × 3 d or 500 mg once 150-200 µg/kg once
Enterobiasis *(Enterobius vermicularis,* pinworm):			
Drugs of choice	Albendazole (Albenza) or Mebendazole (Vermox) or Pyrantel pamoate (Antiminth)	400 mg once, repeat in 2 wk 100 mg once, repeat in 2 wk 11 mg/kg once (max, 1 g), repeat in 2 wk	200-400 mg once, repeat in 2 wk 100 mg once, repeat in 2 wk 11 mg/kg once (max, 1 g), repeat in 2 wk
Hookworm *(Ancylostoma duodenale, Necator americanus):*			
Drugs of choice	Albendazole (Albenza) or Mebendazole (Vermox) or Pyrantel pamoate (Antiminth)	400 mg once 100 mg bid × 3 d or 500 mg once 11 mg/kg once (max, 1 g) × 3 d	400 mg once 100 mg bid × 3 d or 500 mg once 11 mg/kg once (max, 1 g) × 3 d
Strongyloidiasis *(Strongyloides stercoralis):*			
Drug of choice	Ivermectin (Stromectol)	200 µg/kg/d × 2 d, repeat in 2 wk in hyperinfection	200 µg/kg/d × 2 d, repeat in 2 wk in hyperinfection
Alternative	Thiabendazole (Mintezol)	50 mg/kg/d in 2 doses × 2 d	50 mg/kg/d in 2 doses × 2 d
Trichuriasis *(Trichuris trichiura,* whipworm):			
Drug of choice	Mebendazole (Vermox)	100 mg bid × 3 d or 500 mg once	100 mg bid × 3 d or 500 mg once
Alternatives	Albendazole (Albenza) Nitazoxanide Ivermectin (Stromectol)	400 mg bid × 3 d 500 mg bid × 3 d 200 µg/kg qd × 3 d	400 mg bid × 3d 100-500 mg bid × 3 d 200 µg/kg qd × 3 d

Abbreviations: bid = twice daily; qd = daily.

nutritional deficiencies (e.g., iron deficiency anemia). In those at risk for anemia and poor nutrition, the impact of infection is related to total worm burden in the patient. Heavy infection also interferes with intellectual development in children. When people are infected with dog or cat hookworms, the larvae are unable to penetrate beyond the skin and form serpiginous areas of inflammation termed cutaneous larva migrans.

Diagnosis relies on the presence of hookworm eggs in serial stool samples. Because of the time required for the larvae to pass through the tissue, blood, and respiratory systems of the host prior to their arrival and sexual maturation in the gut, there is a lag of between 8 and 10 weeks before eggs can be detected in the stool. Eosinophilia is associated with infection and can persist for years in untreated cases, but the response will wane over time.

Treatment is with albendazole or mebendazole. Pyrantel pamoate may be used in pregnant patients. Nitazoxanide may also have activity. Cutaneous larva migrans can be treated with ivermectin or albendazole.

Strongyloidiasis

The helminth *Strongyloides stercoralis* is endemic to the tropical regions of the world. Filariform larvae in the soil pierce intact skin and enter the circulatory system where they travel to the lung and are caught in the pulmonary capillaries. From there they migrate into the alveoli and up the respiratory tree where they are coughed up and swallowed. In the gut they mature into adult worms that live within the mucosa of the small bowel. Infectious eggs are passed into the bowel wall where they hatch to release the noninfectious rhabditiform larvae that leave the host in the stool. Once in the soil, the rhabditiform larvae mature into filariform infectious larvae. Some of the larvae mature prior to passage of the stool. When that occurs, the filariform larvae can penetrate the wall of the gut or perianal skin and continue the life cycle leading to chronic infection of the host. In hyperinfection, large numbers of larvae mature and reinvade the host. Hyperinfection is associated with defects in host defenses, and is especially seen

Rakel and Bope: *Conn's Current Therapy 2006.*

with steroid therapy or human T cell lymphotropic virus type I (HTLV-I) coinfection.

On penetration of the skin the larvae may cause a local immune reaction visible as a serpiginous track that follows the migration of the filariform larvae through the dermis. This is termed *larva currens* (literally, larval *running*). The most common site for the reaction is the buttocks and if identified is diagnostic for strongyloidiasis. As the larvae pass though the pulmonary tree, they can elicit bronchospasms, fleeting pulmonary infiltrates, and even pulmonary hemorrhage in heavy infection. Once in the GI tract, the worms cause nonspecific symptoms of abdominal pain and bloating. Patients with a high worm burden may develop malabsorption and chronic enterocolitis. Hyperinfection syndrome occurs in patients with altered host responses who develop autoinfection with large numbers of filariform larvae. As the larvae migrate, they may drag intestinal bacteria with them, causing sepsis and meningitis, which can be polymicrobial. They can also cause localized symptoms including pulmonary and GI hemorrhage, bowel obstruction, and death.

Diagnosis of strongyloidiasis is difficult. Eosinophilia is usually present except in hyperinfection and can be a clue to infection in suspected cases. Most patients excrete relatively few larvae, however, which may not be seen with routine testing. Thus, many patients with strongyloidiasis will have negative stool studies. More than three specimens may be required to make the diagnosis. In some patients, duodenal aspirates may improve the diagnostic yield. Serologic tests can be used in suspected cases with negative stool studies. In the hyperinfection syndrome, larvae can be found in stool, sputum, and other organs.

Ivermectin is the drug of choice for treatment of strongyloidiasis and can be given in a single dose for limited infection. Patients with hyperinfection or patients with underlying HTLV-I or chronic steroid therapy should be retreated in 2 weeks. Thiabendazole was frequently used in the past, but ivermectin is as effective and better tolerated. Albendazole has been used to treat infection but is less effective than ivermectin. Although the most recent edition of *The Medical Letter* recommends albendazole as a treatment for strongyloidiasis, at least two randomized clinical trials have demonstrated its inferiority to ivermectin. In these studies cure rates with albendazole are approximately 50% that of ivermectin. Nitazoxanide may also have some activity.

Trichuriasis (Whipworm)

Trichuris trichiura (also called whipworm) is a common intestinal parasite worldwide with more than 1 billion people infected. The organisms are acquired by ingestion of embryonated eggs. The eggs hatch and the larvae mature in the small intestines. The mature worms live in the colon. Most cases are asymptomatic. However, heavy infection can be associated with bloody diarrhea, growth retardation, poor intellectual development, and rectal prolapse. Diagnosis is by demonstration of the characteristic eggs in stool. Mebendazole and albendazole are treatments of choice. Single-dose therapy, which can be used for *Ascaris* and hookworms, is ineffective for *Trichuris*. Nitazoxanide may also be effective.

Enterobiasis (Pinworm)

The pinworm, *Enterobius vermicularis*, is the most common helminthic infection in the United States with more than 20 million cases, mainly in children, reported per year. Infectious eggs are ingested and hatch in the lumen of the gut where they mature into adult worms over a period of weeks. The worms do not penetrate the wall of the gut and live in the large intestine in the area of the cecum. Mature female worms migrate through the anus to deposit their eggs in the perianal area, usually at night when the host is sleeping. The eggs cause perianal itching that transfers the eggs to the hands of the host where they can be ingested causing a cycle of autoinfection or spread to close contacts. The eggs are delicate and survive only a few days in the environment.

Symptoms of *E. vermicularis* infestation are usually mild with many asymptomatic cases. Perianal itching is the most common symptom. Occasionally worms can migrate to the female genital tract causing cases of vulvovaginitis and rarely salpingitis. Some patients may complain of seeing the adult worms. Case reports describe eosinophilic enterocolitis in patients with high worm burden, but this is a very rare manifestation of infection.

Diagnosis is made by recovering eggs or worms from the perianal area. Because neither worms nor eggs are passed in the feces stool studies will be negative. The cellophane tape test (consisting of swabbing the perianal skin with cellophane tape and then pressing the tape onto a glass slide) is commonly used for diagnosis. For best yield, the samples should be obtained at night or first thing in the morning; three swabs have approximately a 90% diagnostic yield.

The treatments of choice are the antihelminthics mebendazole or albendazole. A single dose of one of these agents has a greater than 95% cure rate, but a second dose in two weeks is useful to prevent reinfection. Ivermectin and nitazoxanide have also shown efficacy.

Because *Enterobius* infestations are common in close contacts, the entire household should be treated and all bed clothing and bedding material (including stuffed toys) should be laundered in hot water. Reinfection is common in children and recurrent infection likely represents a reacquisition of enterobiasis rather than relapse. The teaching of proper hand-washing techniques to children is beneficial; however, this infection remains very common in children younger than 10 years of age.

OTHER NEMATODES

Humans can occasionally be infected by a number of nematodes for which humans are not a normal host. *Angiostrongylus* species are strongylids normally found in rats. In humans, they can cause eosinophilic gastroenteritis and eosinophilic meningitis. Both can be treated with benzimidazoles such as albendazole or mebendazole, but there is limited evidence of clinical benefit. Steroids are the treatment of choice for eosinophilic meningitis. *Anisakis* is a fish ascarid.

Humans are infected by ingestion of infected raw fish. The parasites burrow into the stomach causing a painful syndrome termed *eosinophilic gastritis*. The infection is self-limited, but resolution is more rapid with endoscopic removal of the worms. Capillariasis is a rare intestinal infection acquired from ingestion of undercooked fish. The larvae invade the small intestines. The resultant adults can produce eggs and larvae, which can lead to an overwhelming infection associated with diarrhea, abdominal pain, and malabsorption. Treatment with mebendazole or albendazole is associated with improvement.

CESTODES

Taenia saginata (Beef Tapeworm)

The beef tapeworm *Taenia saginata* is seen primarily in sub-Saharan Africa and the Middle East, but it can occur in any area where raw or undercooked beef is eaten. The disease is acquired by the ingestion of the infective cysticercus in the skeletal muscle of cattle. Once in the human GI tract, the tapeworm attaches to the small bowel, usually in the region of the upper jejunum, and matures over a period of roughly 2 months. The point of attachment to the intestinal wall is the scolex with a chain of hermaphroditic proglottids, known as the strobila, extending behind the scolex to form the bulk of the tapeworm. Eggs are produced from the proglottids and are passed in the stool. Once in the environment, the eggs can last for several years until ingested by cattle. In the bovine intestine, the larvae penetrate the bowel wall and encyst in the muscle.

Mature proglottids break off the end of the tapeworm and can be noticed by the host at time of defecation. The proglottids are motile and cause irritation of the perianal area when they are passed but most beef tapeworm infections are asymptomatic or produce only vague abdominal discomfort, nausea, or weight loss.

Diagnosis can be made by examination of the stool for eggs or proglottids. Eggs can also be found in the perianal area and may be seen on a cellophane tape test as is used in pinworm infection. Because the eggs of *Taenia saginata* are indistinguishable from the eggs of *Taenia solium*, the pork tapeworm, speciation requires examination of the proglottids or the scolex.

A single dose of praziquantel is used for treatment after which the entire worm will be passed in the stool. Niclosamide is also effective, but it is no longer available in the United States. Nitazoxanide is an alternative that has proved effective in limited studies. The cysticerci are temperature sensitive, so cooking meat to 56°C (132.8°F) for 5 minutes or freezing to –10°C (14°F) for 9 days will prevent infection. The proper disposal of human waste, as in all parasitic infections, can break the cycle of infection.

Taenia solium (Pork Tapeworm)

The pork tapeworm, *Taenia solium*, is found in areas where pigs are raised with access to human fecal material. It is common in Mexico, Central and South America,

sub-Saharan Africa, and southern and southeast Asia. The life cycle is complicated by the fact that humans can serve as both the definitive and the intermediate host resulting in two distinct forms of the disease. *Taenia solium* encyst in the skeletal muscles of its intermediate host, the pig. When the cysticerci are ingested by humans, the tapeworm attaches to the jejunum and enlarges to form a segmented worm that can be up to 10 m long. As the worm matures, it will intermittently release the terminal proglottids, which can be passed in the stool. Eggs can be passed in the proglottid or released into the stool. The eggs are infections to both humans and animals. Infection of the intermediate host, pigs, results in the larvae penetrating the wall of the intestine and the completion of the life cycle with encystation in the muscle. If the eggs are consumed by a human, the larvae hatch in the bowel, penetrate the wall, and enter the bloodstream, where they migrate to the tissues. Although the larvae can migrate to a large range of tissues, they usually only mature in muscle, the central nervous system (CNS), skin, and eye. These cysticerci can survive for years, but they eventually die and calcify.

Symptoms of tapeworm infection, taeniasis, are mild and consist mainly of abdominal discomfort, some weight loss, and the passage of proglottids in the stool. Cysticercosis, the invasive infection from ingestion of eggs from a human carrier of the tapeworm, can take a variety of forms depending on the location of the cysticerci and the local immune response. Because the brain is a common site for neurologic manifestations such as new-onset seizures caused by inflammation around the cysticercus, hydrocephalus from mechanical obstruction of the flow of cerebrospinal fluid, and arachnoiditis can all be seen.

Diagnosis of taeniasis can be made by identification of the eggs or proglottids in the stool. The adult, intestinal pork tape worm can be effectively treated with a single dose of praziquantel. Niclosamide, although not readily available in the United States, is also effective. Prevention of infection centers on proper disposal of waste, both human and animal, careful attention to handwashing technique and the cooking of pork to kill cysticerci.

Hymenolepis nana (Dwarf Tapeworm)

The dwarf tapeworm is found worldwide in both temperate and tropical countries. Infection with this cestode is the most common of all the tapeworm infestations and is seen at an especially high frequency in institutional settings because it does not require an intermediate host outside the human. *Hymenolepis nana* eggs can be acquired from an infected human host or by the ingestion of insects such as larval fleas or mealworms. Once in the intestine, the oncosphere enters the wall of the villi where it develops into a cysticercoid larva; it later migrates back into the lumen of the gut as an adult tapeworm. The eggs are passed in the stool, but they can become infectious prior to exiting the host leading to a cycle of reinfection. Once in the environment, eggs can survive for approximately 10 days and are often passed from person to person.

Rakel and Bope: *Conn's Current Therapy 2006.*

The Digestive System

Infection with *H. nana* is usually asymptomatic and the life span of the tapeworm is from 4 to 10 weeks leading to a high spontaneous cure rate. Diagnosis is based on finding eggs in the stool, and the treatment of choice is one dose of praziquantel. Nitazoxanide is also effective. Prevention is aimed at breaking the chain of person-to-person transmission and a commitment to improved personal hygiene and environmental cleaning.

OTHER TAPEWORMS

Diphyllobothrium species are tapeworms acquired from ingesting undercooked fish infected with larval forms. After ingestion of the larva, the scolex attaches to the small intestines and forms segments or proglottids. The worms can reach a length of several meters. Most patients note no symptoms. They may experience minor intestinal symptoms such as bloating, mild abdominal pain, or loose stools. Because *Diphyllobothrium* can compete with the host for vitamin B_{12}, prolonged infection can cause pernicious anemia. Diagnosis is by demonstration of eggs or identification of proglottids in stool. Treatments include praziquantel or niclosamide.

Dipylidium caninum is a common intestinal parasite of domestic dogs. Infection is acquired from ingesting fleas, which contain the larval form of the parasite. Humans are accidental hosts, who are also infected by ingestion of fleas. Most human cases are in young children. The main clinical manifestation is passing segments of the parasite, which are similar in size and shape to grains of rice. Diagnosis is made by examination of the proglottids or demonstration of eggs in stool. Treatment is with praziquantel or niclosamide.

TREMATODES (FLUKES)

Schistosomiasis (*Schistosoma mansoni, Schistosoma japonicum, Schistosoma haematobium*)

Schistosomiasis results from infection with one of the blood flukes of the genus *Schistosoma*. Infection is

 CURRENT DIAGNOSIS

Diarrhea Syndromes Caused by Intestinal Parasites
Bloody diarrhea/dysentery
- *Entamoeba histolytica*
- *Balantidium coli*
- *Trichuris trichiura*
- *Schistosoma* spp.
- *Strongyloides*

Watery diarrhea/malabsorption
- *Cryptosporidium hominis, Cryptosporidium parvum,* and other species
- *Cyclospora cayetanensis*
- *Isospora belli*
- *Giardia intestinalis*
- Microsporidia (*Enterocytozoon bieneusi, Encephalitozoon intestinalis*)

Intestinal Protozoan Infections and Diarrhea

Infection	Parasite	Disease	Comments
Amebiasis	*Entamoeba histolytica*	Amebic dysentery, hepatic amebiasis	Infection may be asymptomatic.
Balantidiasis	*Balantidium coli*	Diarrhea, dysentery	Infections are usually asymptomatic.
Blastocystosis	*Blastocystis hominis*	Uncertain pathogenicity	Most experts do not believe *Blastocystis* is a pathogen.
Giardiasis	*Giardia intestinalis*		Acute or chronic enteritis
Cyclosporiasis	*Cyclospora cayetanensis*		Acute, remittent, or persistent enteritis
Dientamoebiasis	*Dientamoeba fragilis*	Diarrhea, abdominal cramps, flatulence	It is unclear whether it causes enteritis.
Cryptosporidiosis	*Cryptosporidium hominis* *Cryptosporidium parvum*	Acute or persistent enteritis or chronic in HIV	There are chronic and extraintestinal manifestations in immunodeficiencies.
Isosporiasis	*Isospora belli*	Acute, remittent or protracted enteritis	Chronic enteritis and malabsorption; in AIDS, associated with eosinophilia
Microsporidiosis	*Enterocytozoon bieneusi* and other species	Disease is rare in the immunocompetent	Chronic enteritis and extraintestinal manifestations in AIDS.

CURRENT THERAPY

Drugs for the Treatment of Protozoan Infections

Infection	Drug	Adult dosage	Pediatric dosage
Amebiasis (Entamoeba histolytica)			
Asymptomatic			
Drug of choice	Paromomycin (Humatin)	25-35 mg/kg/d in 3 doses × 7 d	25-35 mg/kg/d in 3 doses × 7 d
Alternatives	Diloxanide furoate (Furamide)	500 mg tid × 10 d	20 mg/kg/d in 3 doses × 10 d
	Iodoquinol (Yodoxin)	650 mg tid × 20 d	30-40 mg/kg/d (max, 2 g) in 3 doses × 20 d
Mild to moderate intestinal disease			
Drug of choice	Metronidazole (Flagyl)	500-750 mg tid 10 d	35-50 mg/kg/d in 3 doses × 10 d
	Tinidazole (plus paromomycin or diloxanide as luminal amebacide)	2 g/d × 3 d	50 mg/kg (max, 2 g) qd × 3 d
Severe intestinal disease, Hepatic abscess			
Drug of choice	Metronidazole (Flagyl)	750 mg tid or 500 mg IV q8h × 7-10 d	35-50 mg/kg/d in 3 doses × 7 d
	Tinidazole (plus paromomycin or diloxanide as luminal amebacide)	2 g/d × 5 d	50-60 mg/kg/d (max, 2 g) qd × 5 d
Cryptosporidiosis (Cryptosporidium hominis, Cryptosporidium parvum, other species)			
Not AIDS			
Drug of choice	Nitazoxanide	500 mg bid × 3 d	1-3 years: 100 mg bid × 3d; 4-11 years: 200 mg bid × 3 d
AIDS patients	Antiretroviral therapy plus nitazoxanide or paromomycin plus azithromycin	1 g bid × >14 d; 25-35 mg/kg in 2-3 qd doses; 600 mg qd	1 g bid × >14 d; 25-35 mg/kg in 2-3 qd doses; 10 mg/kg/d
Cyclosporiasis (Cyclospora cayetanensis)			
Drug of choice / Normal host	TMP-SMZ (Bactrim DS, Septra DS)	160 mg TMP, 800 mg SMZ bid × 7 d	5 mg/kg TMP, 25 mg/kg SMZ bid × 7 d
AIDS		160 mg TMP, 800 mg SMZ qid × 10 d, then bid × 3 wk, then qd	5 mg/kg TMP, 25 mg/kg SMZ × 10 d, then bid × 3 wk, then qd
Giardiasis (Giardia intestinalis)			
Drug of choice	Nitazoxanide	500 mg bid × 3 d	1-3 y: 100 mg bid × 3 d; 4-11 years: 200 mg bid × 3 d
	Metronidazole (Flagyl)	250 mg tid × 5 d	
Alternatives	Quinacrine	250 mg tid × 5 d	2 mg/kg PO tid × 5 d (max, 300 mg/d)
	Tinidazole	2 g once	50 mg/kg once (max, 2 g)
	Furazolidone (Furoxone)	100 mg qid × 7-10 d	6 mg/kg/d in 4 doses × 7-10 d
	Paromomycin	25-35 mg/kg/d in 3 doses × 7 d	25-35 mg/kg/d in 3 doses × 7 d
Isosporiasis (Isospora belli)			
Drug of choice / Normal host	TMP-SMZ (Bactrim DS, Septra DS)	160 mg TMP, 800 mg SMZ bid × 7 d 160 mg TMP, 800 mg SMZ qid × 10 d, then bid × 3 wk, then qd	5 mg/kg TMP, 25 mg/kg SMZ bid × 7 d
AIDS			5 mg/kg TMP, 25 mg/kg SMZ × 10 d, then bid × 3 wk, then qd
Microsporidiosis			
Drug of choice			
Encephalitozoon intestinalis	Combination antiretroviral therapy plus Albendazole (Albenza)	400 mg bid × 21 d	(no pediatric dose)
Enterocytozoon bieneusi	Combination antiretroviral therapy plus Fumagillin	60 mg qd × 21 d	(no pediatric dose)

Abbreviations: bid = twice daily; IV = intravenous; PO = orally; qd = daily; qid = four times daily; tid = three times daily; TMP-SMZ = trimethoprim-sulfamethoxazole.

TABLE 2 Drugs for the Treatment of Cestode and Trematode Infections

Infection	Drug	Adult dosage	Pediatric dosage
Tapeworms (*Taenia species, Diphyllobothrium, Dipylidium, Hymenolepis*):			
Drug of choice	Praziquantel (Biltricide)	5-25 mg/kg once	5-25 mg/kg once
	Nitazoxanide	500 mg bid × 3 d	1-3 yrs: 100 mg bid × 3 d
			4-11 yrs: 200 mg bid × 3 d
Alternative	Niclosamide	2 g once	50 mg/kg once
Schistosomiasis:			
Drug of choice	Praziquantel (Biltricide)	40 mg/kg/d in 2 doses × 1 d	40 mg/kg/d in 2 doses × 1 d
(*Schistosoma haematobium, Schistosoma mansoni*)			
(*Schistosoma japonicum, Schistosoma mekongi*)	Praziquantel (Biltricide)	60 mg/kg in 3 doses × 1 d	60 mg/kg in 3 doses × 1 d
Intestinal and biliary flukes (except for *Fasciola*):			
Drug of choice	Praziquantel (Biltricide)	75 mg/kg/d in 3 doses × 1 d	75 mg/kg/d in 3 doses × 1 d
Lung fluke (*Paragonimus*)	Praziquantel (Biltricide)	75 mg/kg/d in 3 doses × 2 d	75 mg/kg/d in 3 doses × 2 d
Fasciola hepatica	Triclabendazole	10 mg/kg once or bid × 1 d	10 mg/kg once or bid × 1 d

acquired when people enter water contaminated with the freshwater snails, which are intermediate hosts. The cercarial forms penetrate intact skin, migrate through the bloodstream, and migrate to the veins draining the intestines (*Schistosoma mansoni* and *Schistosoma japonicum*) or the urinary tract (*Schistosoma haematobium*). There the worms pair up and mate. Eggs shed by the female worm migrate to the intestine or urinary tract, where they induce formation of granulomas, which lead to shedding of the organisms into the stool or urine. Penetration of the skin can cause a localized rash (cercarial dermatitis). Acute schistosomiasis (also termed Katayama fever) develops at the time the parasites begin to lay eggs (2 to 8 weeks postinfection). Patients can present with fever, eosinophilia, diarrhea, and/or an urticarial rash. Other features may include spinal cord involvement or hematospermia. Most of the morbidity, however, results from chronic infections. *S. mansoni* and *S. japonicum* can cause hepatic fibrosis, which can lead to portal hypertension (esophageal varices, hemorrhoids, ascites). They also can cause GI disease with bloody diarrhea and a protein-losing enteropathy. *S. haematobium* can cause chronic urinary tract abnormalities (hematuria, hypotonic bladder, recurrent urinary tract infections, urinary obstruction, and carcinoma of the bladder). Diagnosis of chronic infection depends of demonstration of characteristic eggs in stool or urine. Multiple specimens may be required. Rectal biopsy may be required

for diagnosis in some cases. Acute infection may have negative studies for ova, but it is often diagnosed by demonstration of specific antibodies. The treatment of choice is praziquantel. Because immature parasites may respond poorly to treatment, patients with acute infection may require a second course of therapy (Table 2).

Other flukes

A number of trematodes can infect the human intestines, biliary tract, and even lung. All are associated with freshwater intermediate hosts and are acquired by ingestion. All can be treated with praziquantel with the exception of *Fasciola hepatica*, which responds poorly. Alternative treatments include triclabendazole (available via compassionate use programs). Nitazoxanide may work in chronic infection.

REFERENCES

Albonico M, Crompton DW, Savioli L: Control strategies for human intestinal nematode infection. Adv Parasitol 1999;42:277-341.
Haque R, Huston CD, Hughes M, et al: Amebiasis. N Engl J Med 2003;348(16):1565-1573.
Medical Letter on Drugs and Therapeutics: Drugs for Parasitic Infections. Med Lett Drugs Ther Aug 17, 2004;1189:1-12.
Petri WA: Treatment of giardiasis. Curr Treat Options Gasteroenterol 2005;8(1):13-17.
White AC: Nitazoxanide. A new broad spectrum antiparasitic agent. Expert Rev Anti Infect Ther 2004;2(1):43-49.

7

Metabolic Disease

Diabetes Mellitus in Adults

Method of
Shirwan A. Mirza, MD

Epidemiology

The prevalence of diabetes for all age groups worldwide was estimated to be 2.8% in 2000 and to increase to 4.4% in 2030. The total number of people with diabetes is projected to rise from 171 million in 2000 to 366 million in 2030. In the United States, the number of people with type 2 diabetes mellitus is growing to epidemic proportions. The number of people (20 years of age and older) in the United States who were diagnosed with diabetes in 1997 was estimated to be 10.2 million. The number of people who had undiagnosed diabetes was estimated to be 5.4 million. At diagnosis, 50% of patients have microvascular complications (diabetic neuropathy, nephropathy, or retinopathy). The risk of macrovascular complications is at least two times higher than that of the general population. Type 2 diabetes has become one of the most common chronic diseases in the United States. Recent data indicate that diabetes (diagnosed and undiagnosed combined) affects 8.7% of adults in the United States with rates reaching 18.8% at 60 years of age and older. This increase in prevalence portends that diabetes will continue to have a major impact on the health of the U.S. population. The risk of developing diabetes increases with age, obesity, and lack of physical activity. Type 2 diabetes is more common in individuals with a family history of the disease and in members of the minority groups in this country. It is more common in women with prior history of gestational diabetes and polycystic ovarian syndrome and in individuals with hypertension, dyslipidemia, impaired glucose tolerance, or impaired fasting glucose.

Diagnosis

One in five individuals in the United States has metabolic syndrome as defined by the Adult Treatment Panel III (ATP III) criteria. Insulin-resistance syndrome (IRS) is thought to be the underlying feature of the metabolic syndrome.

Prediabetes States

The American Diabetes Association (ADA) introduced the terminology of prediabetes to raise awareness to individuals who have increased risk of developing type 2 diabetes and cardiovascular disease. Prediabetes comprises both impaired fasting glucose (IFG) and impaired glucose tolerance (IGT), and it is associated with metabolic syndrome.

IMPAIRED FASTING GLUCOSE AND IMPAIRED GLUCOSE TOLERANCE

The Expert Committee on the Diagnosis and Classification of Diabetes Mellitus recognized an intermediate group of individuals whose glucose levels, although not meeting the criteria for diabetes, are nevertheless too high to be considered normal. This group is defined as having fasting plasma glucose (FPG) levels greater than or equal to 100 mg/dL but less than 126 mg/dL, or values in the oral glucose tolerance test (OGTT) of greater than or equal to 140 mg/dL but less than 200 mg/dL.

Thus:

- FPG levels less than 100 mg/dL are normal.
- FPG levels 100 to 125 mg/dL indicate impaired fasting glucose.
- FPG levels greater than or equal to 126 mg/dL indicate provisional diagnosis of diabetes (must be confirmed on an alternate day).
- Symptoms of diabetes (polyuria, polydipsia, and unexplained weight loss) plus casual plasma glucose concentration of greater than or equal to 200 mg/dL indicate diabetes.

When OGTT is used (FPG is less than 126 mg/dL, and there is high suspicion for diabetes):

- FPG values remain the same as previously listed.
- Two-hour postload glucose (75 g oral glucose) less than 140 mg/dL indicates normal glucose tolerance.
- Two-hour postload glucose 140 to 199 indicates IGT.
- Two-hour postload glucose greater than or equal to 200 mg/dL indicates provisional diagnosis of diabetes

that must be confirmed on an alternate day by measurement of FPG or 2-hour postload glucose.

The use of glycosylated hemoglobin (A1C) for the diagnosis of diabetes is not recommended at this time because of lack of standardization and its insensitivity for early diagnosis. Glucometers that use capillary blood are imprecise and must not be used for diagnostic purposes.

Insulin-Resistance Syndrome

IRS is a powerful and independent predictor of developing type 2 diabetes (Box 1). Insulin-resistant individuals maintain normal or near-normal glucose levels by secreting large amounts of insulin. IRS is considered a state of enhanced vascular inflammation and endothelial dysfunction accelerating atherosclerosis, and hence causing increased risk of cardiovascular disease. Insulin itself is not a risk factor for atherosclerosis. It is rather the elevated level of a dysfunctional insulin, an insulin unable to exert its physiologic vasodilatory and anti-inflammatory actions, which causes atherosclerosis. In insulin resistance, serum concentrations of triglycerides and free fatty acids, which are metabolic breakdown products of triglycerides, increase. These two substrates induce a state of lipotoxicity, reducing insulin production from the pancreatic β cells. Hypertriglyceridemia is also the underlying cause of nonalcoholic hepatic steatosis (fatty liver), which is now considered one of the diseases associated with IRS.

Pathophysiology

Type 2 diabetes is a multifactorial vascular disease with hyperglycemia and dyslipidemia as cardinal manifestations (Box 2). Diabetes has recently been recognized

---

BOX 1 Other Abnormalities Associated With Insulin-Resistance Syndrome

- Hypertriglyceridemia
- Low HDLC
- Increase in small dense atherogenic LDLC particles
- Increase in inflammatory markers (e.g., C-reactive protein)
- Increase in uric acid level
- Increase in procoagulant factors (fibrinogen and plasminogen activator inhibitor-1)
- Increase in androgens (polycystic ovary syndrome)
- Sleep-disordered breathing*
- Increase in sympathetic nervous system activity*
- Increase in renal sodium retention*
- Loss of vasodilatory effects of insulin.*

*The last four factors comprise the underlying mechanism for increased incidence of hypertension in IRS and type 2 diabetes.
Abbreviations: HDLC = high-density lipoprotein cholesterol; IRS = insulin-resistance syndrome; LDLC = low-density lipoprotein cholesterol

---

BOX 2 Pertinent Laboratory Data

Blood Count
TZDs can cause or exacerbate anemia. Biguanides might cause vitamin B_{12} deficiency and red-cell macrocytosis. Anemia might raise suspicion about cancers or malnutrition. Pancreatic cancer can cause secondary diabetes; sometimes such diabetes precedes pancreatic cancer by almost a year.

Metabolic Panel
- Renal insufficiency contraindicates metformin use, and it increases risk of hypoglycemia.
- Hepatic dysfunction contraindicates TZDs, statins, and fibrates.
- Elevated transaminase might indicate liver disease (e.g., fatty liver in hypertriglyceridemic patients).
- Severe hyperkalemia contraindicates ACEI and ARB use.
- Hypercalcemia might indicate hyperparathyroidism or malignancies.
- Hyponatremia might be because of sulphonylurea-induced syndrome of inappropriate antidiuretic hormone secretion.
- A low albumin level might indicate chronic illnesses or malnutrition.
- Thyroid panel assesses:
  Hyperthyroidism (exacerbates hyperglycemia).
  Hypothyroidism (exacerbates hypoglycemia).
- Lipid profile assesses cardiovascular risk.
- Microalbuminuria assesses renal manifestations. Microalbuminuria is an independent risk factor for CAD through loss of vasculoprotective proteins.
- Normaliron panel and ferritin can rule out hemochromatosis.
- C-peptide and anti-GAD assess insulin deficiency and LADA.
- A1C is the single most important test to assess glycemic control.

Glycemic Control Matters
The UKPDS concluded that intensive therapy with oral agents or insulin decreased risk of microvascular complications compared to diet therapy. A 1% reduction in A1C was associated with the following:
- Microvascular endpoints—35% reduction
- Myocardial infarction—18% reduction
- All-cause mortality—17% reduction

American College of Endocrinology Goals for Glycemic Control
- Target A1C is 6.5%.
- Preprandial plasma glucose target is less than 110 mg/dL.
- Two-hour postmeal plasma glucose target is less than 140 mg/dL.

Abbreviations: A1C = glycosylated hemoglobin; ACEI = angiotensin-converting enzyme inhibitor; ARB = angiotensin II receptor blocker; CAD = coronary artery disease; GAD = glutamic acid decarboxylase; LADA = Late-onset autoimmune diabetes of adults; TZD = thiazolidinediones; UKPDS = The United Kingdom Prospective Diabetes Study.

---

as a coronary artery disease (CAD) equivalent. Type 2 diabetes is characterized by a dual defect in insulin secretion and insulin action. Insulin is essential to enhance glucose uptake at the level of muscles and adipose tissue, and to reduce hepatic glucose production. Typically, insulin resistance precedes the diabetes by many years, during which insulin secretion from β cells is able to increase to counter insulin resistance. In genetically predisposed individuals, however, overt diabetes occurs when β cells are overworked and exhausted, and decreased insulin secretion can no longer overcome the individual's level of insulin resistance. The earliest change in insulin secretion occurs when β cells lose first-phase insulin secretion (first 5 to 6 minutes at a meal) designed to prevent postprandial hyperglycemia. At the onset of type 2 diabetes, on average 5 to 9 years have elapsed without diagnosis, chronic vascular complications are present, and 50% of β cell mass is already lost. Most people with type 2 diabetes show a phenotype of abdominal obesity, the majority have acanthosis nigricans and skin tags commonly around the neck and axillae. Insulin exerts its anabolic action on muscles, thus, individuals with type 2 diabetes have well-developed proximal muscle mass, especially the quadriceps. Individuals with diabetes who are slim and have wasted muscles, particularly the quadriceps, might have "type 1 diabetes," regardless of their age. Late-onset autoimmune diabetes of adults (LADA) is an insulin-deficient state of autoimmune nature occurring in 10% of adult populations with diabetes, including those of 60 years of age or older. The only difference from type 1 diabetes of childhood is that LADA has a slower onset and evolves over many years. Think of LADA in slim adults with diabetes, who do not respond to oral agents. Measurement of serum C-peptide (low or low normal) and/or glutamic acid decarboxylase (GAD) antibodies (usually elevated but not in all patients) would be useful diagnostic tools.

Malnutrition-Related Diabetes

This type of diabetes, once thought to be endemic in some poor developing countries in the tropical belt, is now seen sporadically in the United States, particularly in malnourished elderly patients residing in nursing homes. These patients usually respond only to insulin therapy because their β cells have been destroyed by prolonged protein-calorie deficiency.

The benefit of tight blood pressure control is not less important than that of glycemic control. The goal is to achieve a blood pressure less than 130/80 mm Hg with a regimen that includes either an angiotensin-converting enzyme inhibitor (ACEI) or an angiotensin II receptor blocker (ARB).

Microalbuminuria is an independent risk factor for CAD. It should be treated rigorously with either an ACEI or an ARB. In patients with type 2 diabetes, hypertension, renal insufficiency, and macroalbuminuria, an ARB is the drug of first choice. ACEI appears to have a class effect.

Lipid Management

The American College of Physicians recommends a statin for primary and secondary prevention of cardiovascular disease for all patients with type 2 diabetes. The serum low-density lipoprotein cholesterol (LDLC) goal is less than 100 mg/dL. Updated in 2004, ADA guidelines also include recommendation that a statin in adults with diabetes older than 40 years of age with a total cholesterol greater than or equal to 135 mg/dL, to achieve a 30% reduction in LDLC regardless of baseline level, may be appropriate. Triglycerides should be kept less than 150 mg/dL, and high-density lipoprotein (HDL) greater than 40 mg/dL (>50 mg/dL in women). The ADA recommends aspirin therapy (75 to 162 mg daily) for secondary prevention in the presence of macrovascular disease and for primary prevention in patients older than 40 years of age with family history of CAD, hypertension, smoking, dyslipidemia, and albuminuria.

Medical Nutrition Therapy

Both caloric restriction and weight loss benefit glucose metabolism. Weight loss of approximately 5% of initial body weight can significantly decrease fasting glucose and augment insulin sensitivity. There is no such thing as a "diabetes diet"; therefore, the terms "ADA diet," "no concentrated sweets," "no sugar added," and "low sugar" should no longer be used. The goal of medical nutrition therapy (MNT) is to achieve glucose, lipid, and blood pressure control. The total amount of carbohydrates is more important than the source or type. Expert consensus suggests a diet providing 60% to 70% of energy intake from both complex carbohydrates and monounsaturated fat. Sucrose and sucrose-containing foods should be eaten in the context of a healthy diet. There is not sufficient evidence of long-term benefit of low-glycemic index diets.

Low-Carbohydrate Diets

Negative energy balance produces weight loss regardless of macronutrient composition of the diet. Popular low-carbohydrate diets are in essence high-fat diets. Although safe in the short term, their long-term effects on metabolism and cardiovascular risk have not been established. A recent study compared the high-fat Atkins diet with a conventional low-fat diet. The high-fat diet produced a greater weight loss after 6 months, but at 1 year, weight loss was not significantly different between the two groups. An alternative approach to ad libitum high-fat diet is an ad libitum high-carbohydrate diet consisting of high-fiber foods with low caloric density. An example is the EatRight program employed at the University of Alabama at Birmingham. This program emphasizes the ingestion of high quantities of high-bulk, low-energy density foods (primarily vegetables, fruits, high-fiber grains, and cereals) and moderation in high-energy density foods (meats, cheeses, sugars, and fats). Participants lose on average 6.3 to 8.2 kg by the end of the 12-week program. Although nutritional counseling is usually delegated to the nutritionist, it is important for the physician to have a broad overview of the goals and problems. The dietary prescription should begin by obtaining full knowledge of the patient's dietary habits and preferences for which the patient should keep a detailed dietary log. The less flexible the dietary regimen, the less likely the patient is to comply. Choosing between a detailed exchange system, rigid meal planning, and a simpler regimen focusing on carbohydrate counting is made on an individual basis. Using dietary workshops for small groups of patients, where real food is used in educational settings, enhances patients' understanding. Giving pamphlets and theoretical information is not very effective.

Exercise

Promoting physical activity must be a core component of diabetes management. The benefit of physical activity in improving the metabolic parameters is greatest when it is used early in its progression from insulin resistance to IGT to overt diabetes. The benefits of exercise are substantial and include the following:

- Improves glycemia, lipid profile, blood pressure, and quality of life
- Prevents cardiovascular disease
- Affords modest weight loss
- Increases muscle strength and flexibility

Before starting an exercise program, one should rule out CAD, peripheral vascular disease, proliferative retinopathy, nephropathy, and neuropathy. A single bout of exercise increases insulin sensitivity for 2 days. Regular exercise results in lower average blood glucose and A1C without a significant effect on FPG. An exercise program should consist of moderately intense aerobic exercises for 30 minutes or longer at 60% to 70% maximum heart rate (subtract age from 220) three to four times per week. In the absence of hypertension or proliferative retinopathy, resistance exercise may also be well tolerated.

Pharmacologic Therapy

Pharmacologic treatments involve the following:

- Secretagogues to enhance insulin secretion (sulfonylureas and meglitinides)
- Drugs to enhance insulin sensitivity (thiazolidinedione [TZD] and biguanide)
- Drugs that delay carbohydrate absorption, e.g., glucosidase inhibitors (α-glucosidase inhibitors [AGIs])
- Insulin

SULFONYLUREAS

Sulfonylureas (SUs) act by stimulating insulin from pancreatic β cells (Table 1). They decrease fasting glucose by approximately 60 to 70 mg/dL and A1C by approximately 1.5% to 2%. Only 20% to 30% of newly diagnosed type 2 diabetes can be controlled on SU alone, and 75% of patients need a second agent to achieve A1C goal. Primary failures occur in 10% to 20% of individuals. Most of these patients have insulin deficiency and may have slowly evolving type 1 diabetes. Secondary failure occurs after an initial response at a rate of 5% to 7% per year. SUs are classified as either first- or second-generation. The latter are more commonly used because of their increased effectiveness and fewer side effects. With half to two thirds of the maximal dose (e.g., 10 mg glyburide or glipizide; 4 mg glimepiride), 80% to 90% of their effects are seen. When target A1C is not achieved with monotherapy, one can add either metformin, TZD, AGI, or insulin. Combination therapy may result in lower A1C and better preservation of endogenous insulin.

The typical starting dose is glyburide or glipizide (2.5 mg), or glimepiride (1 to 2 mg daily), taken 30 minutes before breakfast. The dose is to be titrated over 4 weeks to 5 to 10 mg daily (glyburide or glipizide), or 4 mg daily (glimepiride). Doses above this have little further effect. Hypoglycemia risk increases with increasing age, alcohol use, poor nutrition, and renal insufficiency. Glyburide has 19.9 episodes per person-years incidence of hypoglycemia, which could last for greater than 24 hours because this medication has active metabolites. A safer SU (such as glimepiride) should preferably be used in the elderly and in patients with renal insufficiency.

TABLE 1 Characteristics of Sulfonylureas

Sulfonylurea	Dose range (mg)	Peak level (h)	Duration of action (h)	Half-life (h)	Metabolites	Excretion
Tolbutamide (Orinase)	500-3000	3-4	6-10	5-7	Inactive	Renal
Chlorpropamide (Diabinese)	100-500	2-4	36-48	24-48	Active	Renal
Tolazamide (Tolinase)	100-1000	3-4	16-24	7	Weakly active	Renal
Glipizide (Glucotrol)	2.5-40	1-3	12-14	2-4	Inactive	Renal (80%) Hepatic (20%)
Glyburide (Micronase)	1.25-20	4	12-24	10	Weakly active	Renal (50%) Hepatic (50%)
Glimepiride (Amaryl)	1-8	2-3	16-24	9	Inactive	Renal (60%) Hepatic (40%)

Rakel and Bope: *Conn's Current Therapy 2006*.

8

> **BOX 3   Meglitinides**
>
> - Can be used in mild renal and hepatic insufficiency
> - Have low risk of severe hypoglycemia
> - Are useful in patients with erratic lifestyle
> - Should be skipped if the meal is missed

MEGLITINIDES

Meglitinides are short-acting insulin secretagogues, structurally different from SUs (Box 3 and Table 2). Both repaglinide and nateglinide restore the first phase of insulin secretion. Early insulin release inhibits hepatic glucose production, which attenuates postprandial hyperglycemia.

REPAGLINIDE

Repaglinide has a clinical efficacy similar to SUs. It can be given as monotherapy or in combination with metformin or TZDs. Risk of hypoglycemia is less than 50% of that seen with SUs.

NATEGLINIDE

Nateglinide is indicated as monotherapy in patients who have not been chronically treated with SUs or in combination with metformin or TZDs. Hypoglycemia occurs in 4.4% of nateglinide monotherapy and 2.9% of nateglinide plus metformin combination therapy.

BIGUANIDES

Metformin (Glucophage) is the only biguanide available in the United States. It enhances insulin sensitivity by inhibiting hepatic glucose output, which impacts FPG. It enhances muscle glucose uptake to a lesser degree. Metformin reduces FPG by 60 to 70 mg/dL and A1C by approximately 1.5%. An FPG of less than 140 mg/dL is achieved in 25% of patients with type 2 diabetes. A combination with sulfonylurea lowers glucose level more than either drug alone. It reverses secondary failure to sulfonylureas in more than 50% of patients. Metformin can also be combined with meglitinides, TZDs, or insulin. Other advantages include the following:

- Lower risk of hypoglycemia
- Lipid lowering effect
- Modest weight loss

Side effects include nausea, diarrhea, and abdominal discomfort but are usually transient. The maximum effective dose is usually 2000 mg daily. Doses up to 2500 mg are approved but with little additional advantage. Lactic acidosis is extremely rare, and the risk can be reduced by avoiding use when serum creatinine is greater than 1.4 mg/dL in women and 1.5 mg/dL in men and in hypoxic states such as congestive heart failure (CHF). The long-acting formulations have reduced gastrointestinal side effects. Metformin should not be used in patients older than 80 years of age, unless creatinine clearance is greater than or equal to 70 mL per minute. Withhold metformin before imaging with iodinated-contrast media. Creatinine should be measured before resuming metformin.

THIAZOLIDINEDIONES

TZDs are insulin-sensitizing drugs, which are selective ligands of the nuclear transcription factor peroxisomal proliferator-activated receptor (PPAR-γ) (Table 3). PPAR is abundant in adipose tissue, cells, and endothelium. It regulates the expression of several genes involved in metabolism. TZDs lower fasting and postprandial glucose concentration as well as free fatty acids. TZDs induce a "fatty acid steal" in the adipose tissue. The resulting decreased systemic availability of fatty acids, as an alternative source of fuel, will improve peripheral glucose uptake by skeletal muscles and thus ameliorate insulin resistance. That is, they force glucose use as a preferred fuel rather than free fatty acids. Considerable data have recently shown that TZDs have beneficial effects on the atherogenic process, lipid profile especially the high-density lipoprotein cholesterol (HDLC), hemostasis, endothelial function, microalbuminuria, and inflammatory markers. Long-term trials of the effect of TZDs on cardiovascular mortality are currently in progress. Rosiglitazone and pioglitazone are moderately effective in achieving glycemic control. At maximum doses, A1C is reduced on average 1% to 2%. TZDs can be used as monotherapy (equal in efficacy to SUs and biguanides) or added to other antidiabetic oral agents or insulin. Rosiglitazone and pioglitazone have been proven safe and effective for long-term therapy of type 2 diabetes. Low- and medium-dose pioglitazone and rosiglitazone (4 mg) also are indicated for use in combination with insulin but might increase the incidence of edema. These agents are contraindicated in patients with New York Heart Association (NYHA) class III or IV cardiac status. Pioglitazone should be initiated at the lowest approved dose if it is prescribed for patients with type 2 diabetes and NYHA class II CHF with an ejection fraction less than 40%.

TABLE 2   Meglitinide Therapy

Drug	Dose range	Maximum effective dose	Duration of action (h)	Clearance
Repaglinide (Prandin)	0.5-4 mg tid	4 mg tid	4-6	Liver
Nateglinide (Starlix)	60-120 mg tid	120 mg tid	2-4	Liver

Abbreviations: tid = three times daily.

Rakel and Bope: *Conn's Current Therapy 2006.*

TABLE 3 Thiazolidinedione Therapy

Drug	Daily dose range (mg)	Usage
Rosiglitazone (Avandia)	4-8 mg	Monotherapy combination with SUs, metformin, or insulin
Pioglitazone (Actos)	15-45 mg	Monotherapy or combination with SUs metformin or insulin

Abbreviations: SUs = sulfonylureas.

Full effects of TZDs may take weeks to be achieved. TZDs preserve β cell function, and they do not cause hypoglycemia when used as monotherapy or with metformin. Liver enzymes should be monitored at the start of therapy and periodically thereafter. The initial dose should be low (2 mg rosiglitazone or 15 mg pioglitazone daily). Escalate the dose slowly (over weeks), observe for signs of CHF, add diuretics judiciously as needed, reassess their usefulness, and adjust insulin doses on a regular basis.

α-GLUCOSIDASE INHIBITORS

Both acarbose (Precose) and miglitol (Glyset), two AGI agents, inhibit the upper gastrointestinal enzymes α-glucosidases that convert carbohydrates into monosaccharides. Although they delay digestion of carbohydrates, by shifting their absorption to distal parts of the bowel, they do not cause malabsorption. They improve postprandial blood glucose concentration. Both agents have comparable effects and are effective in monotherapy, in combination with SUs, metformin, or insulin. They decrease fasting glucose by 25 to 30 mg/dL, and the A1C by 0.7% to 1%. The postprandial glucose level is reduced by 50 to 60 mg/dL. They are most useful in patients with mild fasting hyperglycemia and predominant postprandial hyperglycemia. Such patients typically present with mild fasting hyperglycemia (110 to 140 mg/dL) but with a disproportionately high A1C (>8%). Side effects, which include abdominal discomfort and flatulence, tend to diminish with continued use. Hypoglycemia is typically not associated with monotherapy. Acarbose has been linked with elevated transaminases. AGIs are not recommended when serum creatinine exceeds 2 mg/dL. They are contraindicated in inflammatory bowel disease and in bowel obstruction. Therapy should be initiated with the lowest effective dose and titrated slowly over 2 to 4 weeks.

Combination Therapy

The availability of different classes of oral agents opened the opportunity to achieve glycemic targets in many patients, but at the same time added complexity to creating a therapeutic algorithm. Any of the oral agents discussed earlier could be used as initial therapy. No one agent is considered the best for all patients. Because type 2 diabetes is a progressive disease, even patients with initial good response to monotherapy eventually require a second agent with or without insulin. Substituting one agent for another is not a good strategy. However, combining oral agents from different classes has proven very beneficial. The current paradigm has recently shifted from a stepwise approach to combination therapy at the outset. Fixed combinations of metformin-SU and metformin-TZD are now available, and are very useful and cost effective. Addition of AGIs to a combined secretagogue-sensitizer has a modest supplementary effect and is costly. A combination of metformin-TZD is also effective if the patient still has a good endogenous insulin reserve. Triple oral therapy (secretagogue-metformin-TZD) has not been approved, although it might work in early stages of diabetes. However, when insulin secretion is deficient, such a combination becomes inferior to a regimen of adding insulin.

Insulin Therapy

Patients who remain hyperglycemic despite adequate oral antidiabetic agents, or individuals with severe hyperglycemia (glucotoxicity), may require insulin therapy. Based on the United Kingdom Prospective Diabetes Study (UKPDS), type 2 diabetes is associated with a progressive decline in β cell function; most patients eventually need insulin when endogenous insulin reserve is depleted. The natural history of type 2 diabetes is oral agent failure. The first step should be adding a bedtime long- or intermediate-acting insulin injection to the existing oral agents. Low doses of insulin at bedtime effectively suppress nocturnal hepatic glucose production, which will improve FPG. Adding insulin to a combination of metformin-TZD or metformin-SU is effective in reducing A1C level. If bedtime insulin plus daytime oral agent(s) are not sufficient, stop the secretagogues and start a full insulin regimen. Unless the patient has type 1 diabetes, continue metformin and/or TZDs with the insulin therapy. Keeping the insulin sensitizer(s) would lower insulin demand by more than 20% to 25%. The patient's attitude toward insulin reflects that of the physician's. Once insulin need is determined, we should be enthusiastic and not apologetic about insulin therapy. We should dispel the myths associated with insulin use, especially the notion that insulin is atherogenic. Many patients have had a relative who had to go on dialysis, or had had a limb amputation at or around the time insulin was started. We should emphasize that insulin does not cause any of these; in fact, poor glycemic control and delay in insulin therapy (when clearly needed) could lead to those complications. Once we determine that a patient needs insulin, we should start with a simple regimen using basal insulin glargine (Lantus). Neutral protamine Hagedorn (NPH), insulin zinc suspension (lente), or insulin zinc extended suspension (ultralente) could also be used once daily at bedtime. In the "Treat-to-Target" study, the initial glargine dose of 10 U at bedtime was adjusted on a weekly basis.

The author finds a weekly adjustment regimen (by 2- to 8-U increments) not very practical in a clinical setting. Research settings have the advantage of being closely controlled and monitored. Adding 8 U to a bedtime dose of glargine could cause hypoglycemia in some patients. We advise our patients to add 1 to 2 U of glargine every night to the 10 U at bedtime until the prebreakfast glucose reading approaches 120 mg/dL. For readings less than 70 mg/dL, we subtract 2 U. The goal is to achieve a fasting glucose of around 120 mg/dL. Nocturnal hypoglycemia is less frequent with glargine than with NPH.

Intensive insulin therapy is not appropriate for patients with:

- Symptomatic CAD
- Cardiac arrhythmias
- Debilitating diseases such as visual impairment and renal failure
- Advanced age

In severe diabetes (FPG > 220 mg/dL), a full-scale insulin regimen (basal + bolus) is usually indicated. Total daily insulin requirement is between 0.5 and 1.2 U/kg daily. Insulin analogs are superior to conventional insulin. Both insulin lispro (Humalog) and aspart (NovoLog) reduce postprandial hyperglycemia and cause lower incidence of hypoglycemia. Insulin glargine has virtually no peak in contrast to NPH, lente, and ultralente. In the basal plus bolus regimen, we usually discontinue the secretagogue and maintain the insulin sensitizer(s).

Calculate the total daily insulin at 0.5 to 1.2 U/kg. The total dose is divided by 2; half of this is to be given at bedtime as insulin glargine, the other half as insulin lispro or aspart (40% at breakfast, 30% at lunch, and 30% at supper). The patient checks blood glucose (sporadically) 2 hours after each meal. If 2-hour blood glucose is greater than 140 mg/dL, we will fine-tune

insulin lispro or aspart doses in increments of 2 U until target glucose readings are achieved. For example, a woman, 50 years of age, with an A1C of 9% on a combination of metformin-TZD plus glyburide 10 mg twice daily has a fasting glucose of more than 220 mg/dL. Her weight is 70 kg. Glyburide 10 mg daily is usually the maximum effective dose and should be given once a day. Splitting the dose is not necessary. Add 10 U of insulin glargine at bedtime. Adjust the dose by adding 2 U every night until next morning fasting glucose is around 120 mg/dL. If daytime glucose readings are still high, stop glyburide and add a full-scale insulin regimen. For example:

$$70 \text{ kg} \times 1 \text{ U} = 70 \text{ U total daily dose}$$
$$(50\% \text{ basal, } 50\% \text{ bolus})$$

$$= 35 \text{ U of glargine at bedtime}$$

$$= 35 \text{ U of lispro or aspart:}$$
$$35 \times 40\% = 14 \text{ U at breakfast}$$

$$35 \times 30\% = \text{approximately } 10 \text{ U at lunch}$$
$$\text{and } 10 \text{ U at supper}$$

If there is concern about hypoglycemia, reduce the initial doses and adjust them later on. In the previous example, give 25 U of glargine at bedtime and 6 U of aspart or lispro right before each meal and adjust aspart

---

CURRENT DIAGNOSIS

ATP III criteria for diagnosing metabolic syndrome*

- Abdominal obesity:
    Men: waist circumference greater than
        40 inches
    Women: waist circumference greater than
        35 inches
- Fasting plasma glucose greater than or equal to 110 mg/dL (recently changed to 100 mg/dL) and less than 126 mg/dL
- Blood pressure greater than or equal to 130/80 mm Hg
- Triglycerides greater than or equal to 150 mg/dL
- HDLC:
    Men: less than 40 mg/dL
    Women: less than 50 mg/dL

*The metabolic syndrome is present when three or more of these criteria are met.
Abbreviations: ATP III = Adult Treatment Panel III; HDLC = high-density lipoprotein cholesterol.

CURRENT THERAPY

- Any of the oral agents discussed in this article could be used as initial therapy.
- The current paradigm has recently shifted from stepwise approach to combination therapy at outset.
- Based on UKPDS, type 2 diabetes is associated with a progressive decline in β cell function; most patients eventually need insulin when the endogenous insulin reserve is depleted.
- The natural history of type 2 diabetes is oral agent failure. The first step should be adding a bedtime long- or intermediate-acting insulin injection to the existing oral agents. Adding insulin in combination with metformin-TZD or metformin-SU is very effective in reducing A1C level.
- When insulin deficiency prevails, a full-scale insulin regimen with or without insulin sensitizers (metformin-TZDs) should be started.
- Tight lipid and blood pressure control is of utmost importance. We should also treat microalbuminuria vigorously.
- At every visit we should remind our patients of the importance of adherence to balanced nutrition and physical activity and remind them of foot care and annual dilated eye exams.
- On September 7, 2004, the Food and Drug Administration approved duloxetine for the management of pain associated with diabetic neuropathy. The recommended dose is 60 mg at bedtime.

Abbreviations: A1C = glycosylated hemoglobin; SU = sulfonylurea; TZD = thiazolidinedione; UKPDS = United Kingdom Prospective Diabetes Study.

8

or lispro based on 2-hour blood glucose level. Adjust glargine as instructed earlier. An alternative regimen would be two injections of premixed insulin (analogs) twice daily.

REFERENCES

American Diabetes Association: Diagnosis and classification of diabetes mellitus. Diabetes Care 2004;27(Suppl 1):S5-S10.
Bell DS: Type 2 diabetes mellitus: What is the optimal treatment regimen? Am J Med 2004;8(116 Suppl 5A):23S-29S.
Calles-Escandon, Garcia-Rubi E, Mirza S, et al: Type 2 diabetes: One disease, multiple cardiovascular risk factors. Coron Artery Dis 1999;10:23-30.
DeFronzo RA: Pathogenesis of type 2 diabetes. Med Clin North Am 2004;88(4):787-835.
Leahy JL: What is the role for insulin therapy in type 2 diabetes? Current Opinion in Endocrinology and Diabetes 2003;10:99-103.
Lebovitz HE: Oral antidiabetic agents. Med Clin North Am 2004; 88(4):847-863.
Ritz E: Albuminuria and vascular damage: The vicious twins. N Engl J Med 2003;348:2349-2352.
Schoonjans K, Auwerx J: Thiazolidinediones: An update. Lancet 2000;355:1008-1010.
Steppel JH, Horton ES: Beta cell failure in the pathogenesis of type 2 diabetes mellitus. Curr Diab Rep 2004;4(3):169-175.
Weinstock RS: Treating type 2 diabetes mellitus: A growing epidemic. Mayo Clin Proc 2003;78:411-413.

Diabetes Mellitus in Children and Adolescents

Method of
Joseph I. Wolfsdorf, MB, BCh, and
Britta M. Svoren, MD

Diabetes mellitus (DM) is classified as type 1, type 2, and other specific types (Table 1). Type 1 is caused by progressive autoimmune destruction of β cells leading to absolute deficiency of insulin. Until recently, diabetes in children was virtually synonymous with type 1 DM, whereas type 2 diabetes was a disease of middle age and the elderly. Over the past 10 to 20 years, the prevalence of type 2 diabetes has increased in North America and elsewhere in the world. The worldwide epidemic of overweight and obese patients is responsible for the increase in prevalence of type 2 diabetes in children and adolescents. Patients with type 2 diabetes usually have normal or elevated serum insulin concentrations, but insulin secretion is impaired and insufficient to compensate for the degree of insulin resistance, resulting in reduced glucose disposal. Between 1% to 5% of white youth have a dominantly inherited genetic disorder of β-cell function that causes maturity-onset diabetes of the young (MODY). The life expectancy of patients with cystic fibrosis has increased dramatically, and cystic fibrosis related diabetes has become more common, especially in adolescents and young adults. Medications, such as tacrolimus (Prograf) and especially pharmacologic

TABLE 1 Classification of Diabetes Mellitus

Type 1 diabetes
Immune-mediated
Idiopathic

Type 2 diabetes
May range from predominantly insulin resistant to predominantly insulin deficient

Other specific types
Genetic defects of β-cell function
Genetic defects of insulin action
Diseases of endocrine pancreas
Endocrinopathies
Drug induced or chemical induced
Congenital rubella
Uncommon forms of immune-mediated diabetes
Other genetic syndromes sometimes associated with diabetes

Gestational diabetes

doses of glucocorticoids, are relatively common causes of DM in hospital practice. In addition, there are numerous miscellaneous, mostly rare, disorders that may be associated with diabetes in children. These children are treated like those with the more common types of diabetes depending on whether insulin deficiency or resistance is the predominant defect.

Diagnosis

DM is diagnosed in one of three ways. Symptoms of marked hyperglycemia typically include polyuria, polydipsia, and weight loss. Chronic hyperglycemia in girls and infants and toddlers of both genders commonly leads to perineal candidiasis. Severe insulin deficiency causes unrestrained lipolysis and ketoacid production leading to an anion gap acidosis characterized by nausea, vomiting, abdominal pain, and hyperpnea (Kussmaul's respiration). Hyperglycemia and ketonemia cause dehydration as a result of the osmotic diuresis induced by glucosuria and ketonuria. The diagnosis of type 1 diabetes is usually obvious because most children present with classic symptoms that have been present for a few days to weeks accompanied by marked hyperglycemia, or with diabetic ketoacidosis (DKA).

In contrast to adults with type 2 diabetes, in whom ketonuria is unusual, approximately 33% of adolescents with type 2 diabetes have ketosis at presentation and up to 25% present in DKA. With the current high prevalence of overweight and obese children and adolescents, distinguishing between type 1 and type 2 diabetes has become more difficult. The incidence of overweight, ketonuria, and DKA overlap considerably between the two major types of diabetes in children and adolescents. It may be necessary to rely on the measurement of pancreatic autoantibodies at diagnosis to make the distinction.

Treatment

INITIAL MANAGEMENT

The goals of initial management of the child with newly diagnosed DM depend on the clinical presentation; they are to restore fluid and electrolyte balance, stabilize the metabolic state with insulin, and provide basic diabetes education and self-care training for the child (when age and developmentally appropriate) and other caregivers (parents, older siblings, daycare providers, and babysitters).

At our center, most children are briefly hospitalized to initiate therapy. Even when the child is not gravely ill, the diagnosis of diabetes often causes great distress for the child and family. Therefore, we prefer to begin insulin replacement therapy, diabetes education, and self-care training in a safe and supportive environment. However, outpatient or home-based management is preferred at some centers with the appropriate resources. The most important factors to be taken into consideration when making the decision as to whether or not a child with newly diagnosed diabetes should be admitted to the hospital are the severity of the child's metabolic derangements, a psychosocial assessment of the family, and the resources available at the treatment center.

OUTPATIENT DIABETES CARE

The Diabetes Team

Optimal care of children with type 1 diabetes is complex and time consuming. Children should be managed by a multidisciplinary diabetes team consisting of a pediatric endocrinologist or pediatrician with training in diabetes, a pediatric diabetes nurse educator (DNE), a dietitian, and a mental health professional. A member of the team should always be available by telephone to respond to metabolic crises that require immediate intervention and to provide guidance and support to parents and patients.

Diabetes Education

The diabetes education curriculum should be adapted to the individual child and family. The education program for parents and children with newly diagnosed diabetes should be limited to essential *survival* skills (e.g., insulin administration, self-monitoring of blood glucose [SMBG], urine ketone measurement, basic meal planning, recognition and treatment of hypoglycemia) so the child can be safely cared for at home and return to daily routines as soon as possible. Frequent telephone contact, often daily, is initially needed to help parents interpret SMBG data and adjust insulin doses. Within a few weeks of diagnosis, many children enter a partial remission as evidenced by normal or near-normal blood glucose (BG) levels on a low dose (<0.25 units/kg/day) of insulin. At this stage patients and parents are often calmer and ready to begin to learn the details of intensive diabetes management.

In the first month, the patient is seen frequently by the diabetes team to review and consolidate the skills and principles learned in the first few days and to extend the scope of diabetes self-care training. Thereafter, follow-up visits with members of the diabetes team occur with a minimum frequency of every 3 months. Regular clinic visits are to ensure that the child's diabetes is being appropriately managed at home and therapy goals are being met. A focused history should obtain information about self-care behaviors, the child's daily routines, the frequency, severity and circumstances surrounding hypoglycemic events, and evidence of hyperglycemia (polyuria, polydipsia, nocturia, enuresis, weight loss, blurry vision, perineal candidiasis).

At each visit, height and weight are measured and plotted on a growth chart. The weight curve is especially helpful to assess adequacy of therapy because a significant weight loss usually indicates that the prescribed dose is insufficient or that the patient is omitting injections. A complete physical examination should be performed at least twice per year focusing on blood pressure, stage of puberty, evidence of thyroid disease, and examination of the injection sites for evidence of lipohypertrophy resulting from overuse.

Regular clinic visits also provide an opportunity to review, reinforce, and expand on the diabetes self-care training started at the time of diagnosis. At each visit the goal is to increase the patient's and family's understanding of diabetes management and to empower them, so that the child becomes more independent and can assume increasing responsibility for independent decision making and self-care.

Psychosocial Issues

A medical social worker should perform an initial psychosocial assessment of all newly diagnosed patients to identify families at high risk who need additional services. Thereafter, patients are referred to a mental health specialist when emotional, social, environmental, or financial concerns are suspected or identified as interfering with the ability to maintain satisfactory diabetes control.

GOALS OF THERAPY

The diabetes control and complications trial (DCCT) showed that treatment regimens reducing glycosylated hemoglobin (HbA_{1c}) to approximately 7% to 8% decrease the long-term risk of microvascular complications in adult and 13-year-old adolescent patients with diabetes. The American Diabetes Association (ADA) has recommended treatment goals for adolescents more than 13 years of age and for adults with DM: HbA_{1c} less than 7% (nondiabetic range 4% to 6%), preprandial plasma glucose 90 to 130 mg/dL, and peak postprandial plasma glucose less than 180 mg/dL. Because there are no clinical trial data to provide a basis for recommendations for children younger than 13 years of age, clinical judgment is required to determine appropriate goals for children of various ages.

Management of young children with diabetes, especially those younger than 5 years old, must balance opposing risks of hypoglycemia and future vascular complications. The risk for microalbuminuria increases steeply with HbA1c more than 8%. Based on these considerations, an HbA_{1c} = 7.5% to 8% is a reasonable general goal for children (younger than age 13 years) with diabetes. Because preschool-age children may be unable to recognize or interpret symptoms of hypoglycemia, we recommend stratifying the biochemical goals based on age (Table 2).

INSULIN THERAPY

The aim of insulin replacement therapy is to simulate, as closely as possible, the normal variations in plasma insulin levels that occur in nondiabetic individuals. No single insulin regimen can be used for all children with type 1 diabetes. The diabetes team has to design an insulin regimen that meets the needs of the individual patient and is acceptable to both the patient and family.

The initial route of insulin administration is determined by the severity of the child's condition at presentation. Insulin is preferably given intravenously for treatment of DKA. Children who are metabolically stable without vomiting or significant ketosis are treated with subcutaneous (SC) insulin administration. SC insulin treatment in the newly diagnosed child, who has recently recovered from DKA, usually begins with either a two- or three-injection-per-day regimen consisting of a mixture of human intermediate-acting and rapid- or short-acting insulin (Table 3). Some clinicians start intensive insulin management (i.e., basal-bolus insulin therapy) at the time of diagnosis (further discussion follows).

In addition to severity of biochemical disturbances, the child's age, weight, and pubertal status guide the selection of the initial insulin dose. When diabetes has been diagnosed early, before significant metabolic decompensation, 0.25 to 0.50 units/kg per day usually is an appropriate starting dose. When biochemical abnormalities are more severe (e.g., ketonuria without acidosis or dehydration) the initial dose typically is at least 0.5 units/kg per day. After recovery from DKA, prepubertal children usually require at least 0.75 units/kg per day, whereas adolescents require at least 1 unit/kg per day.

Insulin preparations are classified according to time course of action (Table 4). Several insulin regimens can be used; each has the same goal, namely to provide basal insulin throughout the day and more with meals (see Table 2). Clear superiority of any one regimen has not been demonstrated in children. When a two-dose

TABLE 2 Biochemical Goals of Treatment According to Age

Age (y)	Premeal blood glucose (mg/dL)	HbA$_{1c}$ (%)
<5	100-200	≤8.5-9.0
5-12	90-180	<7.-8.0
≥13	90-130	≤7.0

TABLE 3 Insulin Regimens Used to Treat Children and Adolescents

Doses	Breakfast	Lunch	Dinner	Bedtime
Two	S/R + N/L		S/R + N/L	
Three	S/R + N/L		S	S + N/L
	S/R + N/L		S	Glarg*
Four	S + N/L	S	S	S + N/L
	S + N/L	S + N/L	S	S + N/L
	S	S	S	Glarg
	S + Glarg	S	S	S
	S	S	S + Glarg	S
CSII†	S	S	S	S

*Insulin glargine is always given as a separate injection because it cannot be mixed with any other insulin.
†CSII (pump) boluses are given with meals and snacks together with basal insulin throughout the day and night.
Intensified insulin therapy is defined as use of at least three daily doses of insulin or CSII.
Abbreviations: CSII = continuous subcutaneous insulin infusion; Glarg = insulin glargine (Lantus); L = lente (insulin zinc suspension); N = neutral protamine Hagedorn (isophane); R = regular (soluble) insulin; S = short-acting insulin (insulin lispro [Humalog] or insulin aspart [NovoLog]).

regimen is used, the total daily dose is typically divided so that approximately 66% is given before breakfast and 33% is given in the evening. With a three-dose regimen, short- or rapid-acting insulin is administered before supper, and the second dose of intermediate-acting insulin is given at bedtime rather than before the evening meal. The initial ratio of rapid- to intermediate-acting insulin at both times varies from approximately 1:2 to 1:4 based on the patient's insulin sensitivity and the carbohydrate content of meals.

For toddlers and young children, we use 10 U (100 U insulin diluted to 1:10) rapid-acting insulin. Children of this age typically require a smaller fraction of rapid-acting insulin (10% to 20%) with proportionally more intermediate-acting insulin.

The optimal ratio of rapid- to intermediate-acting insulin for each patient is determined empirically guided by the results of frequent BG measurements. Five measurements daily: before each meal, before the bedtime snack, and at 2 to 4 AM, are initially required to determine the effects of each prescribed dose. Adjustments are made to each dose at 3- to 5-day intervals, usually in 5% to 10% increments or decrements, in response to patterns of consistently elevated or low blood–glucose levels, respectively.

Intensive insulin therapy, with at least three injections each day or with continuous subcutaneous insulin infusion (CSII) using a portable insulin pump, can more closely simulate normal diurnal insulin profiles and overcome some of the limitations inherent in a two- or three-dose regimen. A peakless long-acting insulin, insulin glargine (Lantus), can be used to provide basal insulin (typically 40% to 60% of the total daily dose). Insulin glargine (Lantus) has a duration of approximately 24 hours and is used with short- or rapid-acting insulin injected before each meal.

Rakel and Bope: *Conn's Current Therapy 2006.*

TABLE 4 Insulin Preparations Classified According to Their
Pharmacodynamic Profiles

	Onset of action (h)	Peak action (h)	Duration of action (h)
Rapid acting			
Insulin lispro (Humalog)*	0.25-0.5	0.5-2.5	≤5
Insulin aspart (NovoLog)*	<0.25	1-3	3-5
Short acting			
Regular (soluble) (Humulin R)	0.5-1	2-4	5-8
Intermediate acting			
NPH (isophane) (Humulin N)	1-2	2-8	14-24
Lente (insulin zinc suspension) (Humulin L)	1-2	3-10	20-24
Long acting			
Ultralente (Humulin U)	0.5-3	4-20	20-36
Insulin glargine (Lantus)*	2-4	peakless	20-24
Premixed combinations†			
50% NPH, 50% regular (Humulin 50/50)	0.5-1	dual	14-24
70% NPH, 30% regular (Humulin 70/30)	0.5-1	dual	14-24
70% NPA, 30% aspart (NovoLog Mix 70/30)	<0.25	dual	14-24
75% NPL, 25% lispro (Humalog Mix 75/25)	<0.25	dual	14-24

*Insulin analog developed by modifying the amino acid sequence of the human insulin molecule. Data are from the manufacturers. Pharmacodynamic effects
   appear to be equivalent. Both NPA and NPL are stable premixed combinations of intermediate- and short-acting insulins.
   Most of the human insulins and insulin analogs are available in insulin cartridges and/or disposable insulin pens.
†Premixed combinations, such as either 70% NPH and 30% regular or 70% NPA and 30% insulin aspart (NovoLog), or 75% NPL and 25% insulin lispro
   (Humalog), are usually used in twice-daily fixed dose insulin regimens.
These data are from human insulins and are approximations from studies in adult test subjects. Time action profiles are reasonable estimates only. The times
   of onset, peak, and duration of action vary within and between patients and are affected by numerous factors, including size of dose, site and depth of
   injection, dilution, exercise, and temperature.
Abbreviations: NPA = neutral protamine aspart; NPH = neutral protamine Hagedorn; NPL = insulin lispro protamine.

8

There has been a steady increase in the number of children and adolescents using pump therapy. An insulin pump is a sophisticated device that requires extensive training in its use; however, with appropriate education and training of parents and children (as appropriate), many children can manage the added responsibility of using an insulin pump and benefit from its advantages. Only rapid-acting insulin is used with CSII; therefore, any interruption in the delivery of insulin rapidly leads to metabolic decompensation. For this reason, meticulous care is necessary to ensure proper function of the infusion system and BG levels must be measured frequently (at least four times daily). Increased lifestyle flexibility, reduced BG variability, improved glycemic control, and reduced frequency of severe hypoglycemia are all documented advantages of CSII. To be successful, however, patients must understand that CSII therapy requires more time, effort, and active involvement in diabetes care.

Biochemical goals are impossible to achieve without strict attention to the other important factors that influence BG levels, namely, diet and physical activity.

MEDICAL NUTRITION THERAPY

Meal planning continues to be a cornerstone of the management of all types of DM. Starting with the initial hospitalization and continuing with intermittent visits in the outpatient setting, a registered dietitian is responsible for evaluating the patient's and family's knowledge of nutrition and formulating an individualized meal plan.

The nutritional needs of children with diabetes do not differ from those of otherwise healthy children. Therefore, nutrient recommendations are based on the requirements of healthy children and adolescents. The total intake of energy must be sufficient to balance the daily expenditure of energy and needs to be adjusted periodically to achieve an ideal body weight and to maintain a normal rate of physical growth and maturation. The main objective of dietary therapy in obese patients is to lose weight.

The ADA currently recommends that carbohydrates provide 50% to 60% of the total calories, with protein and fat making up 15% and 30%, respectively. Less than 10% of energy should come from saturated fat, and dietary cholesterol should be reduced to less than 300 mg per day. Fiber should be incorporated into the diet and may benefit the diabetic patient by blunting the rise in BG after meals. Unrefined or minimally processed foods (i.e., those with a low glycemic index) should replace highly refined carbohydrates as much as possible, and fruit juices should be reserved for treating episodes of hypoglycemia.

Formulation of the Meal Plan

The meal plan must take account of the child's usual eating habits and other lifestyle factors. Young children typically have three meals and two or three snacks daily, depending on the interval between meals, age of the child, and level of physical activity. The purpose of snacks is to prevent hunger and hypoglycemia between meals in children using intermediate-acting insulin preparations. Snacks are optional when a basal-bolus insulin regimen or insulin-pump therapy is used.

The meal plan must be simple, practical, easy to modify, and offer foods that are interesting, tasty, and inexpensive. Meal planning should be based on a combination of carbohydrate counting and the traditional exchange system, individualized to meet the particular circumstances of each family.

The exchange system is based on six food groups: milk, fruit, vegetable, bread/starch, meat/protein, and fat. The meal plan contains the number of exchanges from each food group to be included in each meal and snack. Parents are taught to calculate exchanges from the information on food labels.

Carbohydrate Counting

This refers to a meal planning method in which the amount of carbohydrate or number of carbohydrate servings eaten at each meal and snack are counted. Carbohydrate counting is the foundation of medical nutrition therapy (MNT) for patients who use basal-bolus insulin regimens or pumps. The patient's total daily dose and data from pre- and postprandial BG monitoring are used to formulate an individualized insulin-to-carbohydrate ratio. This ratio is then used to select insulin doses to match anticipated carbohydrate intake (e.g., 1 unit of rapid-acting insulin for each 10 g of carbohydrate consumed).

EXERCISE

Exercise acutely lowers the BG concentration by increasing use of glucose to a variable degree, depending on the intensity and duration of physical activity and the concurrent blood level of insulin. Children and teenagers with diabetes are encouraged to participate in sports and exercise throughout the year. In addition to normalizing the child's life and promoting self-esteem, exercise enhances insulin sensitivity, promotes good health, facilitates weight control, and may improve glycemic control.

Young children's activities tend to be spontaneous; therefore, bursts of activity are covered with a snack before, and if the exercise is prolonged, during the activity. A useful guide is to provide 5 to 15 g of carbohydrates, depending on the child's size, per 30 to 60 minutes of vigorous physical activity. Prolonged and strenuous exercise in the afternoon or evening should be followed by a 10% to 20% reduction in the presupper or bedtime dose of intermediate-acting insulin or an equivalent reduction in overnight basal delivery in patients using CSII. In addition, to reduce the risk of nocturnal or early-morning hypoglycemia caused by the lag effect of exercise, the bedtime snack should be larger than usual.

Older children who participate in organized sports are advised to reduce the dose of the insulin preparation most active during the period of sustained physical activity. The size of such reductions is determined by measuring BG levels before and after exercise and is generally on the order of 10% to 30% of the usual dose. Exercising the limb into which insulin has been injected accelerates the rate of insulin absorption. If possible, the insulin injection preceding exercise should be given in a site least likely to be affected by exercise.

Acute vigorous exercise in the child with poorly controlled diabetes can aggravate hyperglycemia and ketoacid production. Therefore, a child with ketonuria should not exercise until satisfactory biochemical control has been restored.

MONITORING DIABETES CONTROL

Self-monitoring of Blood Glucose

Most patients with type 1 diabetes should perform SMBG at least four times daily: before each meal and at bedtime. To minimize the risk of nocturnal hypoglycemia, BG should be measured between midnight and 4 AM once each week or every other week and whenever the evening dose of insulin is adjusted. Frequency of BG monitoring is an important predictor of glycemic control in children with type 1 diabetes. BG monitoring is also important for management of type 2 diabetes but need not be performed as frequently as in patients with type 1 diabetes. BG measurements before breakfast and intermittently before and after other meals usually provide sufficient data to guide adjustments in therapy. Periods of more frequent BG monitoring may be necessary when treatment is changed.

Ketone Testing

Urine ketones (acetoacetate and acetone) or blood ketone (β-hydroxybutyric acid) concentrations should routinely be measured during acute illness or stress, when BG levels are persistently elevated (e.g., two consecutive BG values >300 mg/dL), or when the patient feels unwell, especially with nausea, abdominal pain, or vomiting. Quantification of blood (beta-hydroxybutyrate [βOHB]), the predominant ketone body, on a drop of blood using a meter for home use is preferred over urine ketone testing for diagnosing and monitoring metabolic decompensation, as may occur with illness, and in ketoacidosis.

Glycated Hemoglobin or Hemoglobin A$_{1C}$

The level of glycated hemoglobin, formed when glucose is bound nonenzymatically to the hemoglobin molecule, is directly proportional to the time-integrated mean BG concentration during the preceding 2 to 3 months. Quarterly determinations of glycated hemoglobin are used to provide an objective measure of average glycemia in the intervals between office visits.

HYPOGLYCEMIA

Occasional episodes of hypoglycemia are an unavoidable consequence of insulin therapy aimed at maintaining BG levels near to normal. Patients and family members must be taught to recognize the early symptoms of hypoglycemia and to treat it promptly with a suitable form of concentrated carbohydrate. Because infants and toddlers are unable to recognize hypoglycemia and cannot verbalize their symptoms, parents are advised to measure the BG concentration whenever the child's behavior is unusual. Most episodes of hypoglycemia in children and adolescents are satisfactorily treated with 5 to 15 g of glucose; 5 grams is sufficient for infants or toddlers. Suitable forms of rapidly absorbed carbohydrate for treatment of hypoglycemia are glucose tablets, fruit juices, soft drinks, and candy. Family members are taught to use glucagon to treat an episode of severe hypoglycemia when the child is unconscious or unable to swallow or retain ingested carbohydrate. Glucagon (0.02 mg/kg, maximal dose 1.0 mg) is injected intramuscularly or subcutaneously and raises the BG level within 5 to 15 minutes. Nausea and vomiting may follow the administration of glucagon.

A medic alert bracelet or necklace should always be worn to identify the patient as having DM.

Screening for Other Autoimmune Diseases

Autoimmune thyroid disorders are common in patients with type 1 diabetes. Approximately 22% of patients have thyroid autoantibodies; however, the reported prevalence of thyroid dysfunction varies widely. Asymptomatic individuals should be screened annually for thyroid dysfunction with a sensitive thyroid-stimulating hormone (TSH) assay. Alternatively, some endocrinologists determine thyroid autoantibodies and measure TSH only in those with autoantibodies.

In Western Europe, North America, and Australia, the mean prevalence of celiac disease among children and adults with type 1 diabetes is approximately 5%. It has been suggested that all children with type 1 diabetes should be screened for celiac disease with either antiendomysial or tissue transglutaminase antibodies. The development of adrenocortical insufficiency in type 1 diabetes (approximately 1 in 200 patients) is characterized by recurrent unexplained hypoglycemia and decreasing insulin requirements and if suspected, serum adrenocorticotropic hormone (ACTH) level should be measured.

Type 2 Diabetes Mellitus in Children and Adolescents

Over the past 10 to 20 years, there has been an alarming increase in the prevalence of pediatric type 2 diabetes. Virtually all children with newly diagnosed type 2 diabetes are obese. Obesity in childhood is associated with insulin resistance, hyperinsulinism and decreased insulin-stimulated glucose metabolism compared to nonobese children. With the current high prevalence of overweight and obesity in children and adolescents, distinguishing between type 1 and type 2 diabetes has become more difficult. Measuring pancreatic autoantibodies, serum insulin and C-peptide levels at the time of

diagnosis is recommended to distinguish between these two forms of diabetes.

Goals of treatment of type 2 diabetes are the same as those outlined above for type 1 diabetes. Treatment aims to normalize fasting and postprandial BG concentrations and must address the common co-morbidities of type 2 diabetes, hypertension and dyslipidemia. Lifestyle changes that lead to weight loss, dietary modification, and exercise, should be the cornerstone of treatment for asymptomatic or mild symptomatic patients. Symptomatic patients who present with severe hyperglycemia, weight loss, and ketosis benefit from a period of intensive insulin therapy until fasting and postprandial normoglycemia have been restored. Because patients are insulin resistant, the dose of insulin initially required to achieve normal glucose levels may be up to 2 units/kg per day. The patient may later be weaned off insulin and switched to metformin (Glucophage).

PHARMACOLOGIC THERAPY

Approved pharmacologic treatment of diabetes in children is limited to insulin and metformin, a biguanide that decreases hepatic glucose production and increases insulin-mediated glucose uptake mainly in skeletal muscle. Metformin may aid weight loss because it has a mild anorectic effect in some patients and has the additional benefit of modestly lowering triglyceride and low-density lipoprotein (LDL) concentrations.

    CURRENT DIAGNOSIS

1. Symptoms of diabetes plus casual (any time of day without regard to time since last meal): plasma glucose ≥200 mg/dL (≥11.1 mmol/L). The classic symptoms of diabetes include polyuria, polydipsia, unexplained weight loss.
   or
2. Fasting (no calorie intake for at least 8 hours): plasma glucose ≥126 mg/dL (≥7.0 mmol/L)
   or
3. 2-hour plasma glucose ≥200 mg/dL (≥11.1 mmol/L) during an oral glucose tolerance test.
   The oral glucose tolerance test should be performed after at least 3 days of adequate (≥150 g/1.73 m) carbohydrate consumption and by using a glucose load containing the equivalent of 75 g anhydrous glucose dissolved in water for individuals who weigh >43 kg and 1.75 g/kg for individuals who weigh ≤43 kg. The OGTT is not recommended for routine clinical use; however, there are situations when it is indicated (e.g., in an asymptomatic child with incidentally discovered glucosuria or hyperglycemia).
   Criteria 2 and 3 should be confirmed by repeat testing on a separate day.

Modified from American Diabetes Association: Diagnosis and classification of diabetes mellitus. Diabetes Care 2004;27(Suppl 1):55-510.
Abbreviation: OGTT = oral glucose tolerance test.

8

Lactic acidosis is a rare, potentially fatal side effect of metformin. Provided that it is not administered to patients with renal insufficiency, poor tissue perfusion, or those undergoing procedures requiring contrast agents or anesthesia, the risk of lactic acidosis is not increased compared with that of other antihyperglycemic agents.

Metformin is available as 500, 850, and 1000 mg tablet strengths and as 500 and 750 mg extended-release tablets. For children 10 to 16 years of age, the recommended starting dose is 500 mg once daily. The dose may be increased to 500 mg twice daily, and further increases may be made weekly in 500 mg increments to a maximum daily dose of 2000 mg. The acute, reversible gastrointestinal adverse effects of metformin may be minimized by administration with or after food, and by using lower dosages, increased slowly, as necessary. The extended-release preparation should be initiated at a dose of 500 mg once daily, given with the evening meal. The maximum recommended dose of the extended-release product is 2000 mg per day. Clinical trials of thiazolidinediones and the rapid-acting insulin secretagogue, meglitinide, are currently in progress in pediatric patients with type 2 DM. An algorithm for the management of the asymptomatic or mildly symptomatic patient with type 2 diabetes (Figure 1).

Bedtime insulin glargine (Lantus) is an effective basal insulin in adults with type 2 diabetes, which, when combined with an oral agent, has less risk of nocturnal hypoglycemia than neutral protamine Hagedorn (NPH) insulin. If metformin alone dose not achieve BG goals, insulin glargine (Lantus) at bedtime should be the first choice insulin regimen in pediatric type 2 diabetes.

Because of the numerous cardiovascular risk factors associated with insulin resistance, it is reasonable to anticipate that inadequately treated patients will suffer considerable morbidity from both micro- and macrovascular complications at an earlier age than in childhood type 1 diabetes. Therefore, youth with type 2 diabetes must be treated aggressively, and concerted efforts should be made to maintain hemoglobin A_{1c} concentrations less than 7.0%.

Screening for Long-Term Complications

Development of diabetic complications is insidious; however, systematic screening can detect abnormality at an early stage, when intervention to arrest, reverse or retard the disease process will have the greatest impact. Diabetic retinopathy is rare before the onset of puberty or in patients who have had type 1 diabetes for less than

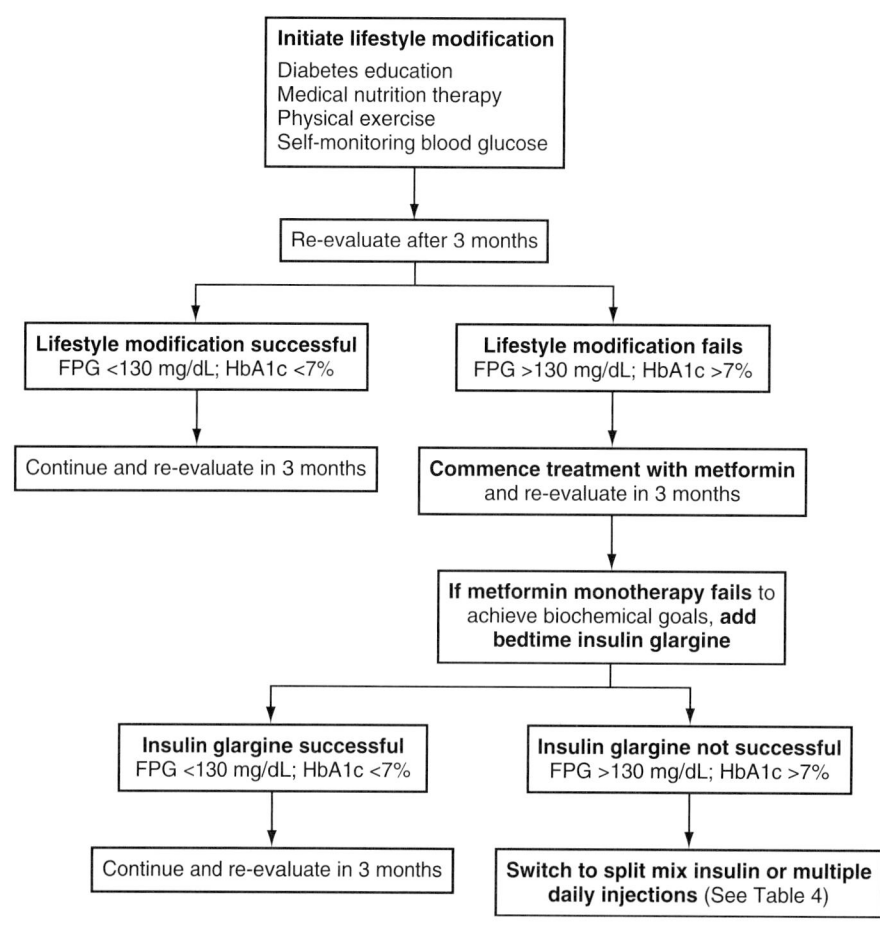

FIGURE 1. Management of asymptomatic or mildly symptomatic type 2 diabetes mellitus.

Rakel and Bope: *Conn's Current Therapy 2006.*

CURRENT THERAPY

- Restoration of fluid and electrolyte balance with metabolic stabilization at the time of diagnosis
- Provision of diabetes education and self-care training for child and caregivers
- Use of a multidisciplinary diabetes team
- Simulation of the normal variations in plasma insulin levels that occur in nondiabetic individuals by insulin therapy
- Formulation of an individualized meal plan
- Incorporation of exercise into daily care plan
- Performance of frequent blood glucose monitoring and ketone testing when indicated
- Recognition and prompt correction of hypoglycemic episodes

5 years. Therefore, annual dilated retinal examinations should begin 5 years after diagnosis or at the time of puberty. Renal disease is first detected by persistent albuminuria. After 5 years of diabetes, an annual screening measurement of urine albumin and creatinine concentrations should be performed to detect microalbuminuria. Circulatory and neurologic complications of diabetes are seldom clinically significant in the pediatric and adolescent population.

In contrast to the above recommendations for type 1 diabetes, monitoring lipids, urinary albumin excretion, and screening eye examinations should begin at the time of diagnosis in type 2 diabetes. Early onset type 2 diabetes is associated with a high incidence of diabetic nephropathy, and vascular disease may already be present at diagnosis.

In 1993 the Diabetes Control and Complications Trial (DCCT) recommended that most youth with diabetes should receive intensive therapy. Technologic innovations since then have made it possible to achieve tighter BG control with reduced risk of severe hypoglycemia in children and adolescents with diabetes. It is reasonable to expect that the benefits of sustained improvement in glycemic control will prevent or delay the appearance of the chronic complications of diabetes. The arduous task of controlling BG in a child is difficult and frustrating. Members of the diabetes team must set realistic and attainable goals for each patient while constantly providing encouragement and support. The resources of a multidisciplinary health care team are essential for the successful management of childhood diabetes. Unfortunately, in the past decade, type 2 diabetes has emerged as a major new challenge for those who provide care for children with diabetes.

REFERENCES

Alberti G, Zimmet P, Shaw J, et al: Type 2 diabetes in the young: The evolving epidemic. (Consensus statement). Diabetes Care 2004;27:1798-1811.
American Diabetes Association: Diagnosis and classification of diabetes mellitus. Diabetes Care 2004;27(Suppl 1):S5-S10.

Rakel and Bope: *Conn's Current Therapy 2006.*

American Diabetes Association: Standards of medical care in diabetes. Diabetes Care 2004;27:S15-S35.
Brand-Miller J, Hayne S, Petocz P, Colagiuri S: Low-glycemic index diets in the management of diabetes: A meta-analysis of randomized controlled trials. Diabetes Care 2003;26:2261-2267.
Clar C, Waugh N, Thomas S: Routine hospital admission versus outpatient or home care in children at diagnosis of type 1 diabetes mellitus. Cochrane Database Syst Rev 2003:CD004099.
Diabetes Control and Complications Trial Research Group: Effect of intensive diabetes treatment on the development and progression of long-term complications in adolescents with insulin-dependent diabetes mellitus: Diabetes Control and Complications Trial. J Pediatr 1994;125:177-188.
Diabetes Control and Complications Trial Research Group: The effect of intensive treatment of diabetes on the development and progression of long-term complications in insulin-dependent diabetes mellitus. N Engl J Med 1993;329:977-986.
Jones KL, Arslanian S, Peterokova VA, et al: Effect of metformin in pediatric patients with type 2 diabetes: a randomized controlled trial. Diabetes Care 2002;25:89-94.
Krolewski AS, Laffel LM, Krolewski M, et al: Glycosylated hemoglobin and the risk of microalbuminuria in patients with insulin-dependent diabetes mellitus. N Engl J Med 1995;332:1251-1255.
Libman IM, Pietropaolo M, Arslanian SA, et al: Changing prevalence of overweight children and adolescents at onset of insulin-treated diabetes. Diabetes Care 2003;26:2871-2875.
Liu E, Eisenbarth GS: Type 1A diabetes mellitus-associated autoimmunity. Endocrinol Metab Clin North Am 2002;31:391-410.
Weissberg-Benchell J, Antisdel-Lomaglio J, Seshadri R: Insulin pump therapy: A meta-analysis. Diabetes Care 2003;26:1079-1087.

Diabetic Ketoacidosis

Method of
Abbas E. Kitabchi, PhD, MD

Diabetic ketoacidosis (DKA) is an acute hyperglycemic emergency characterized by absolute or relative insulin deficiency, dehydration, elevated counterregulatory hormones, derangement of electrolytes and mineral metabolism, and severe alteration of carbohydrate, protein, and lipid metabolism. In general, DKA occurs in type 1 diabetes, but it is also associated with ketosis-prone type 2 diabetes, particularly in African Americans, as well as type 2 diabetic patients during certain catabolic conditions and acute illnesses.

The annual incidence of DKA is between 4 to 8 per 1000 patients with a primary diagnosis of diabetes and occurs in 4% to 9% of all hospital discharges of diabetic patients. There are approximately 100,000 annual hospital admissions for DKA at a cost of $13,000 per patient with associated costs in excess of $1 billion per year.

DKA consists of the triad of hyperglycemia, ketosis, and acidosis, each of which is also associated with other metabolic conditions in addition to DKA (Figure 1).

Based on the recent American Diabetes Association (ADA) Guidelines, DKA is now classified into mild, moderate, and severe (Table 1). Table 1 also presents various electrolyte and water deficits.

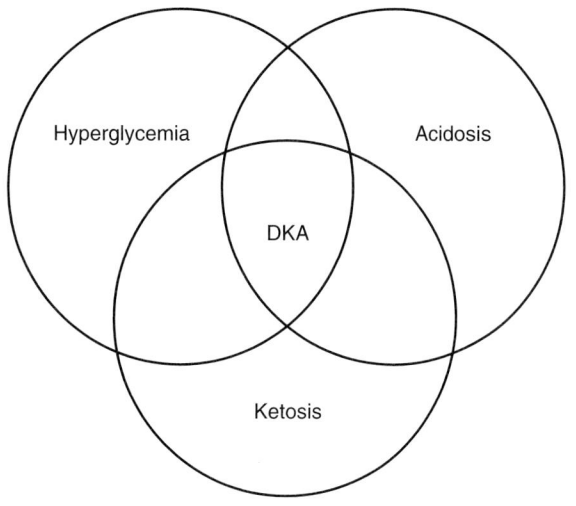

FIGURE 1. Other conditions associated with triad of DKA. **Other Hyperglycemic conditions**: Diabetes Mellitus, Hyperglycemic hyperosmolar state, Impaired glucose tolerance, Stress hyperglycemia. **Other Metabolic Acidotic States**: Lactic acidosis, Hyperchloremic acidosis, Drug-induced acidosis, Uremia. **Other Ketotic States**: Alcoholic ketoacidosis, Starvation ketosis, Ketotic hypoglycemia.

Factors most often associated with DKA vary from center to center depending on the clientele presenting to the emergency room. However, infection and omission or inadequate use of insulin are the two most common precipitating causes, each accounting for 30% to 35% of the cases. Previously unknown diabetes accounts for approximately 20% and miscellaneous illness and other causes account for the remaining 10% to 15% of the precipitating events.

Pathogenesis

The basic, underlying pathogenic mechanism in DKA is lack of adequate insulin (absolute or relative) in the presence of dehydration and elevated levels of stress hormones (cortisol, catecholamines, growth hormone, and glucagon). In the absence of adequate insulin, three pathways of glucose metabolism are affected that include increased glycogenolysis, decreased glucose use by peripheral tissues and increased gluconeogenesis. Of the three pathways gluconeogenesis plays the most prominent role because gluconeogenic pathways are stimulated in both the liver and kidneys, resulting in excess glucose production. When blood glucose is in excess of roughly 180 mg/dL, the glucose spills in the urine (glycosuria), which results in osmotic diuresis (polyuria) and increased thirst (polydipsia) and polyphagia.

Because insulin is an important anabolic and antilipolytic hormone, its lack in DKA along with excess availability of glucagon and catecholamines result in excess lipolysis and breakdown of triglycerides to free fatty acids (FFAs) and glycerol. The latter provides carbon skeleton, and the former provides reduced equivalents for gluconeogenesis. Gluconeogenesis is specifically stimulated as a result of increased glucagon/insulin ratio (a situation prevalent in DKA), stimulating multiple rate-limiting enzymes of gluconeogenesis. Ketogenesis is further enhanced by excess β-oxidation of FFA and

TABLE 1 Diagnostic Criteria and Typical Total Body Deficits of Water and Electrolytes in Diabetic Ketoacidosis

	DKA		
	Mild	**Moderate**	**Severe**
Diagnostic criteria and classification			
Plasma glucose (mg/dL)	>250	>250	>250
Arterial pH	7.25–7.30	7.00–<7.24	<7.00
Serum bicarbonate (mEq/L)	15–18	10–<15	<10
Urine ketone*	Positive	Positive	Positive
Serum ketone*	Positive	Positive	Positive
Effective serum osmolarity[†]	Variable	Variable	Variable
Anion gap[‡] (mEq/L)	>12	>12	>12
Mental status	Alert	Alert/Drowsy	Stupor/Coma
Typical deficits			
Total water (L)		6	
Water (mL/kg)		100	
Na+ (mEq/kg)		7–10	
Cl− (mEq/kg)		3–5	
K+ (mEq/kg)		3–5	
PO$_4$ (mmol/kg)		5–7	
Mg^{2+} (mEq/kg)		1–2	
Ca^{2+} (mEq/kg)		1–2	

*Nitroprusside reaction method.
[†]Calculation: Effective serum osmolality: 2 [measured Na+ (mEq/L)] + glucose (mg/dL)/18
[‡]Calculation: Anion Gap: [(Na+)+(K+) − (Cl− + HCO$^-_3$)]. Normal: <10 mEq/L
Abbreviations: DKA = diabetic ketoacidosis.
Adapted from Kitabchi AE, Umpierrez GE, Murphy MB, et al: Management of hyperglycemic crises in patients with diabetes. Diabetes Care 2001;24:241-269.

decreased concentration of malonyl-coenzyme A (CoA), which inhibits carnitine palmitoyltransferase (CPT) 1, the rate-limiting enzyme in the mitochondria for ketogenesis. Therefore, decreased malonyl-CoA stimulates CPT1 and leads to increased ketogenesis. The major ketone bodies (β-hydroxybutyrate and acetoacetate) will be neutralized by the body's buffer system, resulting in acidosis. Insulinopenia and cortisol in the presence of acidosis lead to increased proteolysis and, to a lesser degree, decreased protein synthesis. As a result of these two events, circulating levels of amino acids (particularly alanine) are increased (↑ blood urea nitrogen [BUN]) and serve as substrates for gluconeogenesis. Therefore, the metabolic hallmark of DKA consists of accelerated gluconeogenesis, lipolysis, glycogenolysis, ketogenesis, and proteolysis along with decreased protein synthesis, glycolysis, and glucose use by insulin-sensitive tissues (muscle, fat, and liver). Therefore, peripheral tissues such as muscle use FFA and ketone bodies as energy sources. FFA in the liver is converted to acyl-coenzyme A (acyl-CoA) in the muscle where it enters the Krebs cycle. β-Hydroxybutyrate in the muscle is converted to acetoacetate as it enters the Krebs cycle and is used as fuel.

Patient Evaluation

A prompt but complete history and physical examination should be performed as soon as the patient presents to the emergency room. Prior history of diabetes and possible events leading to DKA should be obtained from relatives or acquaintances if the patient is obtunded or comatose. DKA usually develops acutely (in less than 24 to 36 hours) and presents with abdominal pain, nausea, and vomiting, and then signs of dehydration (decreased skin turgor, tachycardia, dry mucous membranes, and hypotension) appear. Severe DKA is associated with deep, rapid respiration (Kussmaul's respiration). Despite volume depletion, patients have warm skin (because of acidosis-induced vasodilatation) and the breath often smells of acetone. Most patients are normothermic or hypothermic in spite of infection (owing to vasodilatation and diminishing of fuel-substrate). The laboratory tests should be obtained at once in the emergency room before treatment (Box 1).

Laboratory Evaluation and Pitfalls

Plasma sodium level is usually low because hyperglycemia draws water from intracellular space, diluting the plasma. In addition, severe hyperlipidemia leads to pseudohyponatremia and pseudonormoglycemia in DKA. On admission, plasma potassium may be high, low, or normal, despite total body potassium deficit. This is because of the shift of intracellular potassium to the extracellular compartment secondary to acidosis, hyperosmolarity, and lack of insulin. The majority of cases with hyperglycemic crises have leukocytosis even in the absence of infection, but a white blood cell (WBC) count greater than 25,000 signifies infection. Although the cause of leukocytosis is not established, recent study of patients

with hyperglycemic crises demonstrated increased levels of proinflammatory cytokines—interleukin-1β (IL-1β), interleukin-6 (IL-6), interleukin-8 (IL-8), tumor necrosis factor-α (TNF-α), and leukocytes—all of which returned to normal with insulin therapy and resolution of hyperglycemia. Creatinine levels in DKA may be falsely elevated because of interference of chemical reaction with ketone body determination. The amylase level may also be high because of its extrapancreatic sources (salivary glands). Triglyceride increase is because of decreased activity of lipoprotein lipase and elevation of very low density lipoprotein (VLDL) production. In follow-up of patients with DKA, venous pH instead of arterial pH may be used, but venous pH value is approximately 0.03 lower than arterial pH.

We do not recommend measurement of ketone bodies for assessment of treatment response because most clinical laboratories use the nitroprusside method for this measurement and nitroprusside only measures acetoacetate. Therefore, during the recovery phase as more β-hydroxybutyrate is converted to acetoacetate, the nitroprusside measurement indicates higher levels of *ketones*, which is misleading.

Treatment

The goals for treatment of DKA consist of improving the circulatory volume and tissue perfusion, reducing blood glucose and serum osmolality, clearing ketone bodies from the serum and urine, and correcting the electrolyte imbalances, while attempting to identify precipitating factors.

FLUID THERAPY

In general, in severe DKA there is a deficit of approximately 500 to 700 mEq of sodium and 700 mEq of potassium, which may not be obvious from the usual laboratory tests. Dehydration can be estimated by clinical examination and by calculating total serum osmolarity and corrected sodium concentration. The effective serum osmolarity is calculated as noted in Table 1 in which serum sodium is not corrected for hyperglycemia in DKA. For measurement of actual serum sodium concentration, however, correction is made in the presence of hyperglycemia. Therefore, for every 100 mg/dL of glucose above baseline (100 mg/dL), an additional 1.6 mEq/mL sodium has to be added to the measured sodium value. Approximately 30% of patients with DKA present in a hyperosmolar state, which is correlated to mental obtundation.

A priority in the treatment of DKA is restoration of the extracellular volume providing the first liter of solution as normal saline in the emergency room *after* withdrawal of blood for initial laboratory tests. Isotonic saline will restore intravascular volume, dilute the counterregulatory hormones, lower the blood glucose levels, and augment insulin sensitivity with little effect on restoration of intracellular volumes. After the first bottle of normal saline, the second bottle should consist of half normal saline. The hypotonic solution will expand contracted intracellular and interstitial volumes. Subsequent fluid infusion will be dictated by

---

BOX 1   Laboratory Evaluation

After a brief history and physical examination, initial laboratory evaluation should include determination of complete blood count, blood glucose, serum electrolytes, blood urea nitrogen, creatinine, serum ketones, osmolarity, arterial blood gases, and urinalysis. Admission ECG, chest radiograph, and cultures of blood, urine, and sputum may be ordered if clinically indicated. During therapy, capillary blood glucose should be determined every 1 to 2 hours at the bedside using a glucose oxidase reagent strip; and blood should be drawn every 4 hours for determination of serum electrolytes, glucose, blood urea nitrogen, creatinine, phosphorus, and venous pH.

Fluids

Give 1000 mL of normal saline (0.9% sodium chloride) in the first hour. Then normal or 0.45% saline at 500 to 1000 mL per hour next 2 hours, depending on serum sodium concentration and hydration, followed by 0.45% saline 250 to 500 mL/h. When plasma glucose is <200 mg/dL, change to D5% in {$\frac{1}{2}$} NSS at a rate of 250 mL/h to allow continued insulin administration (at 0.05 U/kg/h) until DKA is controlled, while avoiding hypoglycemia.

Insulin

Hold initial insulin until serum K value is known and is >3.3 mEq/L. Then give 0.1 U/kg of body weight insulin as intravenous bolus followed by 0.1 U/kg per hour as a continuous infusion. The goal is to achieve a rate of glucose decline between 50 and 70 mg per hour. When plasma glucose is <200 mg/dL, reduce insulin rate to 0.05 U/kg per hour. Thereafter, adjust insulin rate to maintain glucose levels between 150 to 200 mg/dL until ketoacidosis

is resolved. In patients with mild-to-moderate DKA, subcutaneous regular insulin or rapid-acting insulin analogs may be an alternative to intravenous insulin.

Potassium

- Serum K^+ = 5.0 mEq/L; no supplementation is required. Check serum K every 2 hours.
- Serum K^+ = 4 to 5.4 mEq/L; add 20 mEq/L to each liter of replacement fluid.
- Serum K^+ = 3.3 to 3.9 mEq/L; add 40 mEq/L to each liter of replacement fluid.
- Serum K^+ = <3.3 mEq/L; hold insulin and give 10 to 20 mEq/hour until K^+ >3.3, then add 40 mEq/L to each liter of replacement fluid.
- K may be given as one third KPO_4 and two thirds KCl.

Bicarbonate

Arterial pH <7.0 or bicarbonate <5 mEq; 50 mEq of bicarbonate in 200 mL of H_2O, infuse over 1 hour until pH is >7.0. Do not give bicarbonate if pH is >7.0.

Phosphate

If indicated (serum levels <1 mg/dL), 20 to 30 mmol potassium phosphate over 24 hours. Monitor serum calcium level.

Transition to subcutaneous insulin

Insulin infusion should be continued until resolution of ketoacidosis (glucose <200 mg/dL, bicarbonate >18 mEq/L, pH >7.30). When this occurs, begin subcutaneous insulin regimen.

To prevent recurrence of DKA during the transition period to subcutaneous insulin, intravenous insulin should be continued for 1 to 2 hours after subcutaneous insulin is given.

Abbreviations: DKA = diabetic ketoacidosis; ECG = electrocardiogram; IV = intravenous; KCl = potassium chloride; NSS = normal saline solution.

---

the state of hydration and serum sodium level, but in general half normal saline is the most common solution used along with supplemental potassium. It is also important to remember that replacement of urinary loss in DKA is a necessary aspect of fluid management.

INSULIN THERAPY

Evidence-based data have demonstrated that physiologic or low dose insulin therapy is as effective as higher dose with less incidence of hypokalemia or hypoglycemia. The current ADA guidelines recommend that insulin should be given intravenously at the rate of 0.1 U/kg per hour after the initial intravenous (IV) bolus dose 0.15 U/kg of insulin. Insulin should always be withheld until the serum potassium is either determined to be greater than 3.3 mEq/L or supplemented to that level when insulin can be started with supplemental potassium. Serum glucose should be determined hourly to ensure that glucose decremental rate is between 50 to 70 mg/dL per hour. If in the first hour of insulin therapy this change is not achieved, the insulin rate should be doubled until proper glucose decrement is obtained. Once blood glucose reaches 200 mg/dL, 5% glucose is to be added to the hydrating solution and insulin rate should be decreased to 0.05 U/kg per hour

to maintain blood glucose between 150 to 200 mg/dL until DKA is resolved (i.e., pH >7.3 and HCO_3 > 18 mEq/L). Two recent studies on the use of fast-acting insulin, (insulin lispro [Humalog] and insulin aspart [NovoLog]) demonstrated that in mild to moderate DKA subjects, subcutaneous insulin was as effective on the general wards as the use of IV insulin in the ICU. Therefore, such a protocol may be both cost effective and safe as long as there are resources available on the general wards to provide adequate nursing personnel and reliable glucometer measurement of glucose every 2 hours. The protocol for every 2-hour subcutaneous (SC) injection with aspart uses initial SC dose of 0.3 U/kg of insulin followed by SC injection of 0.2 U/kg every 2 hours.

Potassium Therapy

Potassium deficit in DKA is approximately 700 mEq, but most patients present with normal or high potassium because of insulinopenia, hyperosmolarity, or acidemia. As indicated in current therapy box however, this will correct with the infusion of insulin and hydrating solution, as potassium rapidly re-enters the intracellular compartment. The goal is to maintain the serum potassium in the range of 4 to 5 mEq/L.

BICARBONATE THERAPY

Evidence-based data suggest that bicarbonate therapy in DKA patients with pH more than 7.0 does not provide any advantage as compared to no bicarbonate. With pH less than 7.0, however, it is recommended that 50 mmol of bicarbonate be diluted with 200 mL of water to make the solution isotonic and be infused at the rate of 200 mL per hour with 10 mEq of potassium chloride.

PHOSPHATE THERAPY

In general, patients who present with DKA and severe dehydration have serum phosphate lower than normal. During insulin therapy, phosphate re-enters the intracellular compartment leading to further reduction in serum phosphate. Severe hypophosphatemia (serum phosphate concentration less than 1 mg/dL [0.32 mM]) is rare. One prospective randomized study demonstrated clinical benefit cannot be achieved with the use of phosphate replacement in the treatment of DKA. In fact, phosphate therapy may contribute to hypocalcemia and soft-tissue calcification. However, the recommendation has been made that to avoid chloride overload with KCl, one may use 33% of the solution as potassium phosphate and 66% as potassium chloride. This regimen might also prevent hyperchloremic acidosis and decrease the likelihood of development of hypophosphatemia during insulin therapy.

POSTHYPOGLYCEMIC CARE

DKA is initially treated with IV infusion of insulin, but the insulin may subsequently be given subcutaneously. However, because the half-life of regular insulin given intravenously is less than 10 minutes, to avoid relapse of DKA the first subcutaneous insulin should start 1 to 2 hours before IV insulin is discontinued with sliding scale regular insulin before each meal and at bedtime and long-acting insulin once a day. In patients who are unable to eat, 5% dextrose in hypotonic saline is continued at the rate of 100 to 200 mL per hour and blood glucose is monitored every 4 hours with the same sliding scale of regular insulin subcutaneously every 4 hour. A newly diagnosed diabetic patient may require insulin dose of 0.6 to 0.7 U/kg per day. A typical regimen would use approximately 30% to 40% of insulin as long-acting insulin such as glargine (Lantus) at bedtime and SC fast-acting insulin before each meal. Patients who are known diabetics can continue with their usual dose but need to be referred to their primary care physician for further adjustment of their insulin and education regarding further prevention of DKA recurrence.

COMPLICATIONS OF THERAPY

Hypokalemia and hypoglycemia are the two most common complications associated with insulin treatment of DKA. These problems may be avoided or decreased by use of physiologic doses of insulin in the therapy of DKA and addition of glucose to hydrating fluids after the patient's blood glucose reaches 200 mg/dL. DKA is

also associated with a hypercoagulable state and may result in thromboembolic complications. Therefore, prophylactic use of anticoagulant may be appropriate if there is no evidence of gastrointestinal bleeding.

Adult respiratory distress syndrome (ARDS) is reported during treatment of DKA because of adverse osmotic gradients resulting in interstitial edema of the lung. Patients with pulmonary rale in physical exam may be at increased risk of ARDS. Therefore, monitoring of PO_2 and $(A-a)O_2$ may be important in managing such patients.

Cerebral edema, a rarity in adult DKA patients, occurs in children, with a mortality rate of 40% to 70%, and may be related to rapid change in the extracellular and intracellular volume in the brain. The diagnosis of cerebral edema is made clinically by headache, decreased level of consciousness, papilledema, bradycardia, seizure, and respiratory arrest. Treatment includes intravenous mannitol (Osmitrol), reduction of fluid administration, and possible mechanical ventilation. A recent multicenter trial has suggested the possibility that brain ischemia and hypocapnia, as well as use of bicarbonate and initial bolus of IV insulin, in children may be associated with the risk of cerebral edema. It is prudent therefore to reduce the risk of cerebral edema by gradual replacement of sodium and water deficits and to avoid rapid lowering of blood glucose, keeping the blood glucose between 250-300 mg/dL, by addition of glucose to the hydrating solution.

Prevention

DKA admission may be reduced by as much as 50% with better educational programs for patients with type 1

 CURRENT DIAGNOSIS

- Obtain medical histories including history of antidiabetic medications, antibiotics, illicit drugs, symptoms, and time of appearance of uncontrolled diabetes as well as history of other systemic disorders. History of recent infections and recent discontinuations of any medications.
- Measure vital signs. Evaluate mental status, patency of airway, level of consciousness, dehydration, and status of cardiopulmonary, gastrointestinal, and genitourinary systems and possible presence of infection.
- Obtain immediate lab for complete blood counts with differential, urinalysis, blood glucose, BUN, electrolytes, chemistry profile, creatinine, amylase, lipase, arterial blood gases, serum osmolarity, and ketones. Obtain ECG, chest radiograph, and cultures, as needed.
- Classify as mild, moderate, or severe, based on blood bicarbonate, pH, and mental status.

Abbreviations: BUN = blood urea nitrogen; ECG = electrocardiogram.

CURRENT THERAPY

- After obtaining initial blood for laboratory tests, start IV fluid by giving 0.9% NaCl initially (15-20 mL/kg/h) followed by 0.9% or 0.45% NaCl at 250 to 500 mL per hour, depending on serum Na and hydration status.
- Add potassium to the second and subsequent IV bottles (if serum potassium is <5 mEq/L) to keep serum potassium between 4 to 5 mEq/L by giving potassium 66% as KCl and 33% as KPO_4 at a rate of 20 to 40 mEq of K per liter of fluid.
- Start IV insulin only when initial serum potassium is greater than 3.3 mEq/L, by giving 0.15 U of insulin/kg body weight as initial IV bolus, followed by 0.1 U/kg/h of IV insulin infusion.
- If blood pH is <7.0, give 50 mmol of bicarbonate in 200 mL of H_2O plus 10 mEq KCl to run for 1 hour.
- If blood pH is <6.9, give 100 mmol bicarbonate in 400 mL of H_2O plus 20 mEq KCl to run for 2 hours.
- Check blood glucose every hour and maintain blood glucose decrement between 50 to 70 mg/dL/h.
- When blood glucose reaches 200 mg/dL, switch to D5 {1/2} NSS and reduce insulin infusion rate to 0.05 U/kg/h to keep blood glucose between 150 to 200 mg/dL until resolution of DKA (defined as bicarbonate >18 mEq/L, anion gap is <12, pH is >7.3, and patient is alert).
- Check electrolytes, BUN and creatinine every 2 to 4 hours until stable. After resolution of DKA, continue IV infusion for 1 to 2 hours after subcutaneous insulin begins, to continue adequate insulin levels.
- Evaluate and address precipitating causes of DKA.

Abbreviations: DKA = diabetic ketoacidosis; IV = intravenous.

or ketosis-prone diabetes. The use of home blood β-hydroxybutyrate monitoring, which allows early detection of this ketone to help with proper use of insulin, may prevent additional hospitalization.

REFERENCES

American Diabetes Association: Hyperglycemic crisis in diabetes. Diabetes Care 2004;27:S94-S102. Position Paper.

Fisher JN, Kitabchi AE: A randomized study of phosphate therapy in the treatment of diabetic ketoacidosis. J Clin Endocrinol Metab 1983;57:177-180.

Glaser N, Barnett P, McCaslin I, et al: Risk factors for cerebral edema in children with diabetic ketoacidosis. N Engl J Med 2001;344:264-269.

Hillman K: Fluid resuscitation in diabetic emergencies: Our appraisal. Intensive Care Med 1987;13:4-8.

Kitabchi AE: Ketosis-prone diabetes—A new subgroup of patients with atypical type 1 and type 2 diabetes? J Clin Endocrinol Metab 2003;88:5087-5089.

Kitabchi AE, Ayyagari V, Guerra SM: Efficacy of low dose versus conventional therapy of insulin for treatment of diabetic ketoacidosis. Ann Intern Med 1976;84:633-638.

Kitabchi AE, Fisher JN: Insulin therapy of diabetic ketoacidosis: Physiologic versus pharmacologic doses of insulin and their routes of administration. In Brownlee M (ed): Handbook of Diabetes Mellitus. New York, Garland, 1981, pp 95-149.

Kitabchi AE, Umpierrez GE, Murphy MB, et al: Management of hyperglycemic crises in patients with diabetes. Diabetes Care 2001;24:241-269.

Morris LR, McGee JA, Kitabchi AE: Correlation between plasma and urine glucose in diabetes. Ann Intern Med 1981;4:469-471.

Stentz FB, Umpierrez GE, Cuervo R, Kitabchi AE: Proinflammatory cytokines, markers of cardiovascular risks, oxidative stress, and lipid peroxidation in patients with hyperglycemic crises. Diabetes 2004;53:2079-2086.

Umpierrez GE, Cuervo R, Karabell A, et al: Treatment of diabetic ketoacidosis with subcutaneous insulin aspart. Diabetes Care 2004;27:1873-1878.

Umpierrez GE, Latif K, Stoever J, et al: Efficacy of subcutaneous insulin lispro versus continuous intravenous regular insulin for treatment of diabetic ketoacidosis. Am J Med 2004;117:291-296.

Wagner A, Risse A, Brill HL, et al: Therapy of severe diabetic ketoacidosis. Diabetes Care 1999;22:674-677.

Umpierrez GE, Watts NB, Phillips LS: Clinical utility of beta-hydroxybutyrate determined by reflectance meter in the management of diabetic ketoacidosis. Diabetes Care 1995;18:137-138.

Tasker RC, Lutman D, Peter MJ: Hyperventilation in severe diabetic ketoacidosis. Ped. Crit. Care Med 2005;6:405-411.

Hyponatremia

Method of
Biff F. Palmer, MD

Hyponatremia is a common clinical disorder. Figure 1 outlines the approach to the patient with hyponatremia.

Is the Hyponatremia Representative of a Hypo-osmolar State?

There are two general causes of hyponatremia unassociated with a hypo-osmolar state. The first of these is pseudohyponatremia, which involves an abnormal measurement of the serum sodium. This occurs in patients with hyperglobulinemia or hypertriglyceridemia in whom plasma water relative to plasma solids is decreased in blood, leading to less sodium in a given volume of blood.

The other cause of hyponatremia in the absence of a hypo-osmolar state involves true hyponatremia but with elevations in the concentration of another osmole. Clinical examples include hyperglycemia as seen in

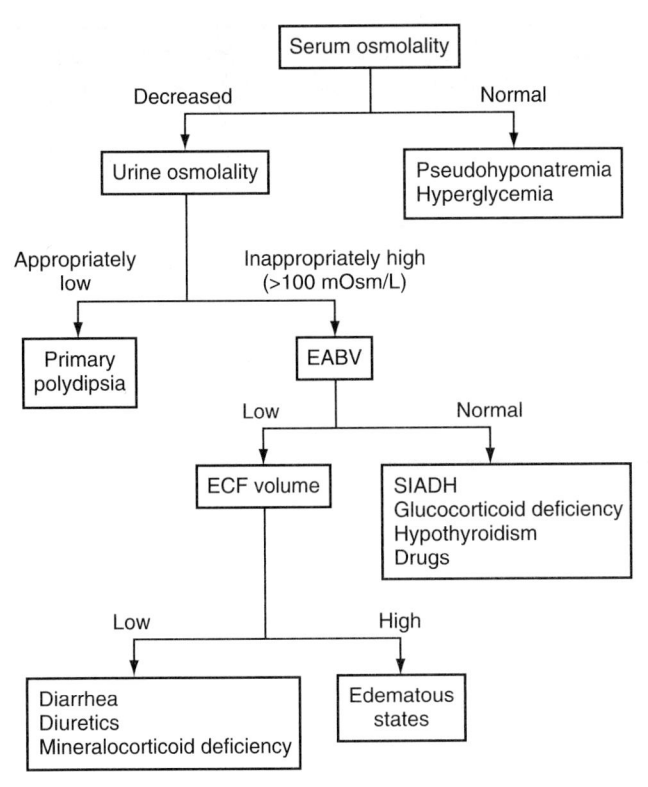

FIGURE 1. Approach to the patient with hyponatremia.

uncontrolled diabetes or, rarely, hypertonic infusion of mannitol used in the treatment of cerebral edema. The increases in plasma glucose raise serum osmolality, which pulls water out of cells and dilutes the serum sodium. For every 100 mg/dL rise in glucose or mannitol, the serum Na will quickly fall by 1.6 mEq/L. The increased tonicity will also stimulate thirst and arginine vasopressin (AVP) secretion, both of which contribute to further water retention. As the plasma osmolality returns toward normal, the decline in serum Na will be 2.8 mEq/L for every 100 mg/dL rise in glucose.

Is the Kidney's Ability to Dilute the Urine Intact?

The presence of hypotonic hyponatremia implies that water intake exceeds the ability of the kidney to excrete water. In unusual circumstances, this can occur when the kidney's ability to excrete free water is intact. However, because a normal kidney can excrete 20 to 30 L of water per day, the presence of hyponatremia with normal renal water excretion implies that the patient is drinking more than 20 to 30 L of water each day. This condition is referred to as *primary polydipsia*. These patients should have a urine osmolality less than 100 mOsm/L. Although primary polydipsia is a common condition that leads to polyuria and polydipsia, it is uncommon as a sole cause of hyponatremia.

In the absence of primary polydipsia, hyponatremia is associated with decreased renal water excretion and

urine that is inappropriately concentrated. It is important to note that in the presence of hyponatremia urine should be maximally dilute and a urine osmolality higher than this (>100 mOsm/L) reflects an impairment in renal water excretion. Inappropriately concentrated urine implies a defect in renal water excretion.

Excretion of water by the kidney is dependent on three factors. First, there must be adequate delivery of filtrate to the tip of Henle's loop. Second, solute absorption in the ascending limb and the distal nephron must be normal so that the tubular fluid will be diluted. Lastly, AVP levels must be low in the plasma. Of these three requirements for water excretion, the most important in the genesis of hyponatremia is the failure to maximally suppress AVP levels. In many conditions, decreased delivery of filtrate to the distal neuron also contributes.

What Is the Volume Status of the Patient?

In patients with hypotonic hyponatremia with inappropriately concentrated urine, it is necessary to define whether effective arterial volume is decreased. Most of the causes of hyponatremia result from a decrease in effective arterial volume, which causes baroreceptor stimulation of AVP secretion and leads to decreased distal delivery of filtrate to the distal neuron. If effective arterial volume is low, extracellular fluid volume can be low in the volume-depleted patient (hypovolemic hyponatremia) or high in the edematous patient (hypervolemic hyponatremia). If effective arterial volume is normal, one is dealing with the euvolemic causes of hyponatremia (isovolemic hyponatremia).

The clinical determination of effective arterial volume is usually straightforward. On physical examination the best index of effective arterial volume is the pulse and blood pressure. Urinary electrolytes are also extremely useful in the assessment of effective arterial volume. Patients with a low effective arterial volume will tend to have a low urinary sodium, urinary chloride, and fractional excretions of sodium and chloride in the urine. Patients with euvolemic hyponatremia, however, will be in balance and will excrete sodium and chloride at rates that reflect dietary intake of sodium and chloride. Thus, generally they have urinary sodium and chlorides more than 20 mEq/L and fractional excretions of these electrolytes more than 1%.

Plasma composition can also be used to assess effective arterial volume. The blood urea nitrogen (BUN) is particularly sensitive to effective arterial volume. In patients with normal serum creatinines, a high BUN suggests a low effective arterial volume, and a low BUN suggests a high effective arterial volume. The plasma uric acid can also be used as a sensitive index of effective arterial volume. In comparing patients with syndrome of inappropriate antidiuretic hormone secretion (SIADH) and other causes of hyponatremia, patients with low effective arterial volume tend to have an elevated serum uric acid. The serum urate is low in patients with SIADH. This is because of the fact that these patients

8

BOX 1   Disorders associated with SIADH

- Neoplasms
    Tumors
    Oat cell carcinoma
    Adenocarcinoma of the pancreas
    Hodgkin's disease
    Thymoma
- Pulmonary diseases
    Tuberculosis
    Lung abscess
    Viral and bacterial pneumonia
- CNS disorders
    Brain tumor
    Encephalitis
    Subarachnoid hemorrhage
    Acute intermittent porphyria

Abbreviations: CNS = central nervous system; SIADH = syndrome of
    inappropriate antidiuretic hormone secretion.

**BOX 2   Drugs Associated With Hyponatremia
According to Major Mechanism of Action**

- Stimulate ADH release
    Chlorpropamide
    Clofibrate
    Cyclophosphamide
    Vincristine
    Carbamazepine
    Amitriptyline
    Thiothixene, haloperidol, thioridazine
- Potentiation of ADH effect on kidney
    Chlorpropamide
    Carbamazepine
    Nonsteroidal anti-inflammatory drugs
    Cyclophosphamide
- ADH-like action
    Oxytocin
    DDAVP (1-deamino-D-arginine-vasopressin)

Abbreviations: ADH = antidiuretic hormone; DDAVP = desmopressin acetate.

---

are volume expanded, but it is clinically difficult to detect the degree of volume expansion.

Syndrome of Inappropriate Antidiuretic Hormone Secretion

SIADH is characterized by euvolemia, a concentrated urine, and increased levels of antidiuretic hormone (ADH). SIADH is generally associated with diseases of the central nervous system (CNS), usually those that affect the base of the brain, pulmonary diseases, and neoplasms (Box 1). These conditions lead to secretion of ADH, which is inappropriate both from the standpoint of plasma osmolality and effective arterial volume. A number of other etiologies cause a condition of hypo-osmolality associated with euvolemia and can mimic the syndrome of inappropriate ADH secretion, including isolated glucocorticoid deficiency (normal mineralo-corticoid activity), hypothyroidism, pain, nausea, acute psychosis, and a variety of drugs (Box 2). ADH levels are increased in these conditions.

Treatment of Hyponatremia

The principal danger of hyponatremia or hypernatremia relates to effects on CNS function because of changes in brain size. Hyponatremia initially leads to cell swelling driven by the higher intracellular osmolality. The net result is equilibration of intracellular and extracellular osmolality at the expense of increased brain volume. Cells, brain cells in particular, then respond by decreasing the number of intracellular osmoles; and as intracellular osmolality decreases, cell size returns toward normal despite the presence of hyponatremia. If the decrease in extracellular fluid (ECF) osmolality is slow, there will be no measurable cell swelling. This pathophysiologic sequence correlates well with clinical observations. If hyponatremia is slow in onset, neurologic symptoms and permanent brain damage are unusual, even if the decreases in Na concentration and ECF osmolality are large. Conversely, if hyponatremia is rapid in onset, cerebral edema and significant CNS symptoms and signs can occur with lesser changes in serum Na concentration.

TABLE 1   Treatment of Hyponatremia According to Volume Status and Rapidity of Development

Correction	Low ECF volume	Edematous state	Euvolemic
Acute Onset			
Slow	Normal saline	Fluid restriction	Fluid restriction
Rapid	Hypertonic saline	Hypertonic saline + furosemide	Hypertonic saline + furosemide (Lasix)[1]
Chronic	Remove cause	-Remove cause	-Remove cause
		-Demeclocycline[1] 600-1200 mg/day	-Discontinue drug
		-Vasopressin receptor antagonists when available	-Glucocorticoid or thyroid hormone replacement
			-Treat cause of SIADH

[1]Not FDA approved for this indication.
Abbreviations: ECF = extracellular fluid; SIADH = syndrome of inappropriate antidiuretic hormone secretion.

When treating a patient with hyponatremia, the Na concentration should be raised at the rate at which it fell (Table 1). In a patient whose serum Na concentration has fallen slowly, neurologic symptoms are generally minimal, brain size is normal, and the number of intracellular osmoles is decreased. Sudden return of extracellular fluid osmolality to normal values will lead to cell shrinkage, neurologic symptoms, and possible permanent brain damage. Specifically, rapid correction has been associated with central pontine myelinolysis. Thus, it is recommended that serum Na be corrected slowly in these patients. In a patient whose serum Na concentration has decreased rapidly, neurologic symptoms are frequently present and there is cerebral edema. In this setting there has been insufficient time to remove osmoles from the intracellular space in the brain, and rapid return to normal ECF osmolality merely returns brain size to normal. In general, the development of hyponatremia in the outpatient setting is more commonly chronic in duration and should be corrected slowly. By contrast, hyponatremia of short duration is more likely to be encountered in hospitalized patients receiving intravenous free water. In symptomatic patients, rapid correction may be necessary. The unusual patient with psychogenic polydipsia can also develop hyponatremia, which is of short duration and if symptomatic may similarly require rapid correction.

Rapid Correction of Hyponatremia

In patients with acute hyponatremia who are demonstrating CNS signs or symptoms, rapid correction is indicated. Rapid correction of hyponatremia involves intravenous administration of hypertonic saline (usually 3% NaCl). Generally, an infusion rate is used to raise serum Na concentration at a rate of 1 mEq/L per hour. Present evidence suggests that correction at a more rapid rate may be dangerous. To calculate the amount of Na required, one should use a volume of distribution of total body water. Although Na is confined to the ECF space, in disorders of osmolality one is replacing an osmolar deficit present throughout the total body water (TBW).

$$(\text{Desired Na} - \text{Actual Na}) \times \text{TBW}$$
$$= \text{amount of Na required}$$

Assume a patient presents with a serum Na of 110 mEq/L, has symptoms of stupor, and demonstrates

CURRENT DIAGNOSIS

- Determine if the hyponatremia represents a hypo-osmolar state.
- Determine if the kidney is responding appropriately to the excess free water by measuring the urine osmolality.
- Assess the volume status of the patient (check for orthostatic changes in blood pressure and pulse, presence or absence of edema, urine electrolytes, blood urea nitrogen/creatinine ratio).

Rakel and Bope: *Conn's Current Therapy 2006.*

CURRENT THERAPY

- Chronic hyponatremia should be corrected slowly and at a rate that does not exceed 1 mEq/L per hour.
- Normal saline is indicated in hyponatremic patients with decreased extracellular fluid volume.
- Fluid restriction is indicated in edematous patients with hyponatremia.

seizure activity. To raise the patient's serum Na to 130 mEq/L, one can calculate the amount of 3% saline needed.

$$\text{TBW} = 70 \text{ kg} \times 60\% = 42 \text{ L}$$

$$(130 \text{ mEq/L} - 110 \text{ mEq/L}) \times 42 \text{ L} = 840 \text{ mEq Na}$$

As each liter of 3% saline contains 513 mEq of Na, administer 1.6 L of 3% NaCl over 20 hours to raise the serum Na by 1 mEq/L per hour.

Use of hypertonic saline alone may be associated with volume expansion that would be dangerous in the elderly or patients with compromised cardiac function. Patients with impaired renal function are particularly prone to volume overload with such Na loads. In this instance a furosemide (Lasix)[1] diuresis can be used. Hypertonic saline is infused at a rate equal to the urinary loss of Na, chloride, and K that is induced by furosemide.

To calculate the total net negative fluid balance necessary to achieve the desired Na concentration one can use the following formulae:

$$\text{Body Weight} \times 60\% = \text{TBW}$$

$$\text{or } 70 \text{ kg} \times 60\% = 42 \text{ L}$$

$$\text{TBW} - (\text{actual Na/desired Na}) \times \text{TBW} = \text{amount of excess water}$$

$$\text{or } 42 - (110/130) \times 42 = 6.5 \text{ L}$$

When a serum Na concentration of 130 mEq/L is obtained, place the patient on fluid restriction. Thus, neurologic sequelae resulting from rapid correction of the serum Na can be avoided. It should be emphasized that these formulae are to be used as guidelines only, and frequent monitoring of the patient and serum Na need to be done during these rapid changes in fluid balance.

REFERENCES

Adrogue HJ, Madias NE: Hyponatremia. N Engl J Med 2000;342: 1581-1589.
Palmer BF: Hyponatremia in patients with central nervous system disease: SIADH or CSW. Trends Endocrinol Metab 2003;14:182-187.
Palmer BF, Gates JR, Lader M: Causes and management of hyponatremia. Ann Pharmacother 2003;37:1694-1702.
Spital A: Diuretic-induced hyponatremia. Am J Nephrol 1999;19: 447-452.

[1]Not FDA approved for this indication.

Gout and Hyperuricemia

Method of
Adel G. Fam, MD

Gout is characterized by chronic hyperuricemia, recurrent attacks of acute arthritis provoked by release of monosodium urate crystals into joint cavities, and development in some patients of gross urate deposit (tophi). It chiefly affects men older than 40 years of age, and the incidence in women increases after menopause. A familial occurrence is observed in approximately 40% (11% to 80%) of patients with gout. The overall prevalence of gout is estimated to be 6 per 1000 men and 1 per 1000 women. However, recent studies suggest a rising incidence of gout in New Zealand, the United States, and other countries. The reasons for this are unclear, but rising incidence of obesity and insulin resistance syndrome (IRS), increasing longevity, frequent use of both diuretics and prophylactic low-dose aspirin, more organ transplants and changing dietary trends (excess calories and purines), are implicated.

Gout occurs in three overlapping phases:

1. A long phase of asymptomatic hyperuricemia
2. A period of recurrent acute gouty attacks separated by symptom-free intervals (interval gout)
3. This is followed in approximately 10% to 20% of patients by the development of tophi and chronic tophaceous gouty arthritis.

Hyperuricemia, elevated serum urate more than 7.0 mg/dL (>450 µmol/L) in men and more than 6.0 mg/dL (>360 µmol/L) in women, is the biochemical hallmark of gout. In the majority of patients, gout is a primary disorder. Less commonly, hyperuricemia and gout are secondary to purine enzyme defects, myeloproliferative or lymphoproliferative disorders, renal failure, drugs, or other conditions (Box 1). Measurement of 24-hour urinary uric acid (UA) excretion in patients with primary gout, while on a low-purine diet for a week, can often indicate whether the hyperuricemia is the result of overproduction or underexcretion of UA. In most patients (>90%), hyperuricemia results from reduced renal tubular UA excretion (gouty underexcretors). These patients excrete either normal or reduced amounts of UA (<600 mg/day or <3.6 mmol/day on a purine-restricted diet for 1 week). Their urate clearance is reduced to less than 6 mL per minute (normal 6 to 11 mL per minute). They have a limited capacity to eliminate a urate (purine) load, and excretion of normal amounts of UA is accomplished only at inappropriately high serum urate levels. A genetic basis is suggested by the frequent presence of a similar proximal renal tubular abnormality in first-degree relatives. Whether this underexcretor status is related to structural heterogeneity of a specific proximal renal tubule urate anion exchanger/transporter, URAT1, is unclear.

In a minority of patients (<10%), hyperuricemia results from increased rate of de novo purine biosynthesis.

BOX 1   Classification of Hyperuricemia and Gout

Primary
    UA overproduction: <10%
    UA renal underexcretion: >90%
Secondary
UA Overproduction
Purine enzyme defects:
- HGPRT deficiency
- PRPP synthetase overactivity
- G6PD
- Fructose-1-phosphate aldolase deficiency
Increased nucleotide turnover:
- Myeloproliferative and lymphoproliferative disorders
- Hemolytic anemia
- Psoriasis
- Chemotherapy/radiotherapy: hematologic malignancies (tumor lysis syndrome)
Excessive dietary purines and ethanol abuse:
UA Renal Underexcretion
- Renal failure
- Acidosis: lactic, ethanol, diabetic ketoacidosis: dieting
- Drugs: low-dose aspirin, diuretics, cyclosporine A, pyrazinamide
- Chronic lead nephropathy (saturnine gout)
Uncertain Mechanisms
- Hypertension
- Hypothyroidism
- Pre-eclampsia and toxemia of pregnancy

Abbreviations: G6PD = glucose-6-phosphatase deficiency;
    HGPRT = hypoxanthine guanine phosphoribosyltransferase;
    PRPP = phosphoribosyl pyrophosphate; UA = uric acid.

These patients excrete excessive quantities of UA: more than 600 mg per day or more than 3.6 mmol per day on a low-purine diet for 1 week (gouty overproducer/overexcretors). Their UA clearance is either normal or increased with a UA/creatinine ratio of more than 6%. Studies using isotope-labeled UA invariably demonstrate an increased rate of de novo purine and UA biosynthesis.

Being a metabolic disorder, gout is significantly influenced by dietary, metabolic, and environmental factors. Included among these are overeating, obesity, dyslipidemia, diabetes mellitus, IRS (metabolic syndrome), and alcohol abuse. Hypertension is also common in patients with gout. Although hyperuricemia/gout is commonly associated with coronary artery disease (CAD), it is unlikely that hyperuricemia plays a causal role in the pathogenesis of CAD, and any apparent relationship is likely related to the frequent association of hyperuricemia with known risk factors for CAD: IRS, obesity, dyslipidemia, hypertension, and diabetes mellitus. Recent data suggest that hypertriglycidemia, obesity, and hypertension in patients with gout are often part of an underlying IRS or *metabolic syndrome*, estimated to occur in 76% to 95% of gout sufferers. Features of the syndrome include overall and abdominal obesity (waist circumference >102 cm in men, and >88 cm in women, waist:hip ratio >0.85), glucose intolerance with resistance to insulin and secondary compensatory hyperinsulinemia, and dyslipidemia characterized by hypertriglycidemia, increased levels of apolipoprotein B, low-density lipoprotein cholesterol (LDLC), and atherogenic small dense LDLC particles, and a decrease in high-density lipoprotein cholesterol (HDLC) levels. Both hypertension and hyperuricemia are frequently associated with IRS. Hyperinsulinemia has been shown to stimulate renal tubular sodium-hydrogen exchanger, thereby enhancing reabsorption of sodium, chloride, bicarbonate, and uric acid.

Acute Gouty Arthritis

Gouty attacks commonly affect the joints of the lower extremities, particularly the metatarsophalangeal (MTP) joint of the great toe (acute podagra). The intertarsal, ankle, knee, elbow, and wrist joints and olecranon bursae are next in order of frequency. The onset, which typically occurs at night, is rapid; and the acute arthritis often peaks within 24 hours, producing a painful, warm, red, tender, swollen joint, as well as diffuse erythema of the surrounding soft tissues, resembling cellulitis. In the early stages of gout, the attacks are few and far between with the affected joints returning to normal between attacks. Late in the course of the disease, the acute episodes become more frequent and longer lasting, with a tendency toward incomplete resolution and polyarticular involvement.

Chronic Tophaceous Gouty Arthritis

Before the introduction of effective urate-lowering drugs, approximately 20% to 40% of untreated patients developed chronic tophaceous gouty arthritis. Recent data suggest a much lower incidence (approximately 15% to 25%). However, every so often, one encounters patients in whom improper diagnosis or treatment has permitted full expression of the disease. The average time from the initial gouty attack to the development of tophi is 11 years. Tophi are typically located in the peripheral, cooler parts of the body: feet, fingers, and knees; in and around bursae (olecranon, prepatellar, and bunion); and in the subcutaneous tissues over the Achilles tendon and ear pinnae. Chronic gouty arthritis is characterized by persistent aching, stiffness, swelling, and often joint deformities. Superimposed episodes of acute gouty inflammation are common. Typical radiographic features include punched-out erosions with overhanging margins, and soft tissue swellings (tophi).

Diagnosis

Although hyperuricemia is a characteristic biochemical marker of gout, it is improper to equate the finding of hyperuricemia with gout. Many individuals who have life-long hyperuricemia do not develop gouty arthritis (asymptomatic hyperuricemia). Serum urate levels may be normal in some patients with gout, particularly during the early phases of gout, following alcoholic excesses or

withdrawal of diuretic therapy, and during initial therapy with allopurinol (Zyloprim) or uricosuric drugs.

A firm diagnosis of gout can be established by demonstration of intracellular or extracellular, needle-shaped, negatively birefringent, monosodium urate crystals in joint fluids, bursal effusions, or in aspirates from tophi using compensated polarized light microscopy. However, this may not be possible in all patients because of absence of a detectable joint effusion or visible tophi, an inaccessible joint, inexperience with either joint aspiration, or evaluation of synovial fluid for crystals, or presence of a few urate crystals or crystals too small (<1 μm) to be seen by light microscopy. Under these circumstances the diagnosis of gout can be made on the basis of a typical clinical history in association with documented hyperuricemia. In between gouty attacks, the diagnosis can sometimes be confirmed by demonstrating urate crystals in fluid aspirates from previously affected but asymptomatic knee or first MTP joint.

Treatment

Gouty arthritis nearly always occurs in the setting of chronic hyperuricemia. Consequently, management of a patient with gout requires that two objectives be considered independently: immediate control of the acute gouty episode and long-term treatment of chronic hyperuricemia to prevent both subsequent gout attacks and complications, including chronic tophaceous gouty arthritis, uric acid nephrolithiasis, and urate nephropathy.

ACUTE GOUTY ARTHRITIS

Treatment of acute gouty arthritis consists of rest, splinting of the joint, local ice application and drug therapy, including nonsalicylate nonsteroidal anti-inflammatory drugs (NSAIDs), colchicine, and corticosteroids (Box 2).

Nonsteroidal Anti-Inflammatory Drugs

Cyclooxygenase (COX-2) nonselective NSAIDs are preferred by most for the treatment of acute gout. They are generally better tolerated and more predictable in their therapeutic effects than oral colchicine. There is no clear advantage of any one preparation, but a large dose of indomethacin (Indocin), naproxen (Naprosyn), or diclofenac sodium (Voltaren) on the first 1 to 3 days, with a reduction thereafter is generally effective. Whatever drug is used, it should be started as early as possible after the onset of an acute episode. It is important, therefore, to supply the patient with the appropriate NSAID (preferably kept in a convenient pocket, for gout often strikes when the patient is far from home), and instructions on how to self-treat acute flares at the first *twinge* of an attack.

Although adverse reactions (e.g., nausea, dyspepsia, diarrhea, headache, confusion) can occur, the duration of NSAID therapy is usually short, and serious toxicity leading to drug withdrawal (e.g., gastrointestinal [GI] bleeding) is rare (<10% of patients).

<table>
<tr><td>

**BOX 2   Drugs in the Treatment of
Acute Gouty Arthritis**

- Nonsteroidal anti-inflammatory drugs
- Nonselective COX-2 inhibitors
  - Indomethacin (Indocin) 50 mg qid for 3-6 d
  - Naproxen (Naprosyn) 500 mg bid or tid for 3-6 d
  - Diclofenac sodium (Voltaren) 50 mg tid for 3-6 d
- Selective COX-2 inhibitors
  - Etoricoxib (Arcoxia) 120 mg/d for 3-6 d
  - Other selective COX-2 inhibitors: not evaluated
- Colchicine
  - 0.6 mg qh for 3 h (three tablets)
- Corticosteroids
  - Monoarticular or oligoarticular gouty attacks:
  - IA methylprednisolene acetate (Depo-Medrol)
    5-40 mg
- Polyarticular gouty attacks:
  - IM triamcinolone acetonide (Kenalog) 60 mg q1-4d
  - IM methylprednisolone acetate (Depo-Medrol)
    40 mg q1-4d *or* IM ACTH (corticotropin) 25-40 IU
    q12-24h
- Ambulatory treatment of gouty attacks: Oral prednisone
  20-40 mg first day, then taper in 4-8 d

Abbreviations: bid = twice daily; COX-2, cyclooxygenase-2; IA = intra-
articular; IM = intramuscular; qh = every hour; qid = four times daily;
tid = three times daily.

</td></tr>
</table>

A new selective COX-2 inhibitor, etoricoxib (Arcoxia) 120 mg per day, is as efficacious in the treatment of acute gouty arthritis as indomethacin (Indocin) 50 mg thrice daily, with etoricoxib (Arcoxia) demonstrating an improved safety profile. Whether the treatment of acute gout with etoricoxib (Arcoxia) and other selective COX-2 inhibitors [celecoxib (Celebrex), rofecoxib (Vioxx), valdecoxib (Bextra)], in place of the well-established, conventional NSAIDs, will prove to be more advantageous in terms of efficacy, GI safety, and cost-effectiveness remains to be established. However, recent concerns have been raised about the long-term safety and cardiovascular toxicity of this class of anti-inflammatory drugs, particularly in high-risk patients. NSAIDs, including selective COX-2 inhibitors, are potentially hazardous and should be used with caution for the treatment of acute gouty events in patients older than age 65 years and in those with co-morbid medical conditions, such as congestive heart failure, renal impairment, peptic ulcer disease, hepatic dysfunction, and treatment with anticoagulants.

Colchicine

Although colchicine has traditionally been rooted in the treatment of acute gouty arthritis, in recent years its use has steadily declined. Drawbacks include the following:

- Slow onset of action
- A narrow benefit-to-toxicity ratio, with approximately 80% of patients experiencing GI toxicity (nausea, diarrhea, and abdominal pain) after oral administration

- Reduced therapeutic efficacy when administered 24 hours or longer after the onset of acute gouty inflammation—not infrequent

It is administered orally in a dose of 0.6 mg every hour for up to 3 hours (maximum of three tablets). Given its toxicity, use of more extended regimens of oral colchicines, as primary treatment for acute gouty arthritis, is generally not recommended. Colchicine is efficacious in approximately two-thirds of patients. It is primarily useful for those without renal, hepatic, or bone marrow disease who are intolerant or hypersensitive to NSAIDs.

Recently, the role of intravenous (IV) colchicine in the treatment of acute gout has come under close scrutiny in light of growing concerns about its safety. A major drawback is the drug's potential for serious and sometimes lethal toxicity (bone marrow suppression, oliguric renal failure, hepatic necrosis, diarrhea, seizures, and death), particularly in patients older than age 65 years with renal and/or hepatic impairment. This controversy has led to the publication of a set of guidelines for the IV administration of colchicine. However, the guidelines are not widely recognized, inappropriate use of the drug occurs often, and many clinicians have advocated restriction or an outright ban on the use of IV colchicine.

Corticosteroids

Intra-articular (IA) corticosteroid therapy and both systemic corticosteroids and corticotrophin (ACTH) are indicated for the treatment of acute gouty episodes in patients with coexisting medical illnesses, contraindicating the use of NSAIDs and colchicine (Box 3). Such treatment is also efficacious in the management of acute gout occurring during the postoperative period, for those with NSAID hypersensitivity, and for severe gouty attacks refractory to both NSAIDs and colchicine. Intra-articular corticosteroid injections, such as methylprednisolone acetate (Depo-Medrol) 5 to 40 mg IA, are particularly useful for the treatment of acute monoarticular and oligoarticular gouty episodes in these patients. However, such therapy is impractical for those

<table>
<tr><td>

**BOX 3   Indications for Corticosteroid Drugs in
the Treatment of Acute Gouty Arthritis**

Co-morbid medical conditions:
- Cardiac failure, hypertension
- Renal insufficiency
- Peptic ulcer, gastrointestinal bleeding
- Hepatic insufficiency
- Chronic alcoholism
- Bleeding diathesis, anticoagulants
Advanced age
- Postoperative state
- NSAID hypersensitivity
- Severe attacks refractory to both NSAIDs and colchicine

Abbreviation: NSAID = nonsteroidal anti-inflammatory drug.

</td></tr>
</table>

Rakel and Bope: *Conn's Current Therapy 2006.*

with polyarticular gouty attacks. Concern about coexistent joint infection, concomitant anticoagulant therapy, and fear of needle injection may also preclude intra-articular corticosteroid administration. In these clinical situations, intramuscular (IM) triamcinolone acetonide (Kenalog) 60 mg, or IM methylprednisolone acetate 40 mg, repeated every 1 to 4 days as required, can be used to provide rapid control of acute attacks, thereby circumventing delayed absorption after oral administration. IV methylprednisolone sodium succinate (Solu-Medrol) 40 to 160 mg repeated every 1 to 4 days as required is indicated for those receiving anticoagulant therapy.

Oral prednisone, 20 to 40 mg on the first day, followed by gradual tapering over 4 to 8 days, is particularly useful for the ambulatory treatment of acute gouty flares in outpatients with co-morbid conditions contraindicating the use of NSAIDs.

The efficacy and safety of IM ACTH (Acthar), 25 to 40 IU repeated every 12 to 24 hours as required, in the treatment of acute gout has been demonstrated in a number of studies. ACTH produces a rapid relief of symptoms within hours. However, the drug is not universally available, and there is no convincing evidence that such therapy is superior to corticosteroids. Drawbacks of ACTH therapy include dependence of therapeutic effects on sensitivity of the adrenal cortex (it may be ineffective in subjects previously treated with corticosteroids); increased release of adrenal androgens and mineralocorticoids, which can lead to fluid overload; and a relatively short duration of action, with a greater potential for rebound attacks and treatment failures compared with IM corticosteroids.

CHRONIC GOUTY ARTHRITIS

Corrective measures constitute sufficient therapy for many patients with infrequent gouty attacks and mild hyperuricemia. These include weight reduction for obesity, elimination of drugs causing hyperuricemia (e.g., low-dose aspirin >325 mg per day, thiazide diuretics), restriction of alcohol intake and diet modification. The traditional, low-purine diet is rarely recommended because it is not palatable or practical for very long, it is high in both carbohydrates and dairy products rich in saturated fats, and it produces only 10% to 15% reduction of serum urate. Recent studies suggest a strong association between hyperuricemia/gout and IRS—abdominal obesity, glucose intolerance with compensatory hyperinsulinemia, hypertension, hyperuricemia, dyslipidemia, and increased risk of coronary heart disease. A pilot study of a weight-reducing diet, restricted in both carbohydrates (40% of energy), and saturated fats, with proportionate increase intake of protein (30% of energy) and unsaturated fats (30% of energy), resulted in a 37% reduction in serum urate, reduced frequency of gouty attacks, and improvement of IRS with decreased serum triglycerides, low-density lipoprotein C, glucose, and insulin levels. For patients with coexistent hypertension, losartan (Cozaar) may be used given its modest uricosuric effect, and for those with concomitant hyperlipidemia, fenofibrate (TriCor), also a mild uricosuric, may be prescribed.

The frequency of gouty attacks can be reduced by prophylactic administration of colchicine, 0.6 mg once or twice daily. However, such therapy does not correct the hyperuricemia, or prevent the silent progression of tophaceous lesions and cumulative joint damage. It can also lead to a number of toxic reactions, including neuromyopathy, myelotoxicity, alopecia, and malabsorption syndrome.

The ultimate treatment of established gout requires long-term control of hyperuricemia. Three types of urate-lowering drugs are available:

1. Uricostatic drugs (e.g., allopurinol [Zyloprim], a xanthine oxidase inhibitor that decreases uric acid synthesis)
2. Uricosuric agents, which act by competitive inhibition of postsecretory renal tubular reabsorption of urate, thus increasing urate excretion and lowering serum urate
3. Uricolytic drugs such as uricase (urate oxidase), which catalyzes the conversion of UA into the more soluble allantoin

Not every gout patient requires treatment with urate-lowering drugs (Box 4). The administration of a drug to normalize serum urate is usually a life-long commitment to regular daily therapy. Frequent measurement of serum urate concentrations is important in monitoring patients' compliance and the effectiveness of urate-lowering treatment. To prevent further gouty attacks and ongoing joint damage and to ensure resorption of the tophaceous deposits, serum urate should be reduced and sustained to less than 4 to 6 mg/dL or less than 250 to 350 μmol/L, well below the concentration at which urate saturates the extracellular fluid, approximately 6.8 mg/dL or 404 μmol/L at 37°C (98.6°F).

Initiation, dose reduction or interruption of urate-lowering therapy during an acute attack of gout is not recommended; a major change in serum urate levels, induced by starting or stopping allopurinol (Zyloprim) or a uricosuric drug, can in theory worsen an attack already in progress.

The sharp reduction in serum urate level that takes place early in the course of urate-lowering treatment may be associated with flares of gout. These flares may be mistaken for a poor response to treatment. Some physicians advocate prophylactic colchicine, 0.6 mg once or twice daily during the first 1 to 12 months of initiating antihyperuricemic therapy. However, this practice cannot be "routinely" recommended, given the potential toxicity of prolonged colchicine therapy (neuromyopathy, myelotoxicity, alopecia, malabsorption syndrome), and that only approximately one-third of patients develop flares of gouty arthritis after initiation of allopurinol (Zyloprim) or uricosuric treatment. Instead, many clinicians advocate the temporary use of a supplemental NSAID to control these attacks. Colchicine prophylaxis is of special value, however, in patients with continuing frequent gouty flares precipitated by urate-lowering therapy.

Allopurinol (Zyloprim)

Allopurinol (Zyloprim) is the urate-lowering drug of choice. As a xanthine oxidase inhibitor, it interferes

Rakel and Bope: *Conn's Current Therapy 2006.*

BOX 4   Urate-Lowering Drugs

- Indications for allopurinol therapy (Dose: allopurinol [Zyloprim] 100-600 mg/d, single dose):
  Frequent gouty attacks despite corrective measures (>2 attacks/y)
  Major overproduction of uric acid with hyperuricosuria including HGPRTase deficiency and PRPP synthetase overactivity
  Chronic tophaceous gouty arthritis
  Gout complicated by urate nephropathy, UA nephrolithiasis, or renal insufficiency
  Hyperuricemia secondary to lymphoma, leukemia, and other myeloproliferative disorders treated with cytotoxics or radiotherapy (to prevent tumor lysis syndrome)
  Failure of uricosuric drugs
  Recurrent calcium oxalate urinary calculi associated with hyperuricosuria
- Indications for uricosuric drugs (Dose: probenecid [Benemid], 1-3 g/d, divided doses):
  Sulfinpyrazone (Anturane): 100-800 mg/d (divided doses)
  Patients younger than 60 years of age with primary gout, underexcretion hyperuricemia, normal renal function, and no history of renal calculi or massive tophi
  Allergy or intolerance to allopurinol
  Combined allopurinol-uricosuric treatment for patients with massive tophaceous deposits.
- Indications for uricolytic (uricase) therapy (Dose: non–pegylated recombinant uricase, rasburicase [Elitek], 0.2 mg/kg/d IV infusion for 5-10 d):
  Short-term prevention and treatment of chemotherapy/radiotherapy-related malignant hyperuricemia and tumor lysis syndrome in patients with hematologic malignancies (lymphoma, leukemia, myeloma)

Abbreviations: HGPRTase = hypoxanthine guanine phosphoribosyltransferase; IV = intravenous; PRPP = phosphoribosyl pyrophosphate; UA = uric acid.

---

with the conversion of hypoxanthine to xanthine and of xanthine to UA, leading to a reduction of serum and urinary urate concentrations, and a concomitant increase in serum and urinary hypoxanthine and xanthine concentrations. Allopurinol (Zyloprim) is rapidly oxidized in the body to its principal metabolite, oxypurinol, which is also a potent xanthine oxidase inhibitor. The plasma half-life of allopurinol (Zyloprim) is 1 to 3 hours, whereas that of oxypurinol is 14 to 26 hours. Thus, allopurinol (Zyloprim) can be administered as a single daily dose. Because oxypurinol is excreted solely through the kidneys, reduction of allopurinol (Zyloprim) dose is indicated in patients older than 65 years and in those with renal impairment. The starting dose of allopurinol (Zyloprim) is 50 to 300 mg per day (100-mg, 200-mg, and 300-mg tablets), and the total daily dose ranges between 100 mg and 600 mg, with most patients requiring 300 mg per day. Reduction of serum urate concentration is noted within 2 days of starting therapy. The level usually falls to normal within 7 to 21 days, although it may take much longer in patients with extensive tophaceous deposits. Gouty attacks often cease within 3 to 6 months of continuous therapy, whereas dissolution of the tophi may take 6 to 24 months. Intermittent allopurinol (Zyloprim) therapy has been shown to be less efficacious. Discontinuation of allopurinol (Zyloprim) is followed by a rapid rise of serum urate concentration to pretreatment levels, although recurrence of acute gouty attacks may not occur for long periods. Box 4 outlines specific indications for the use of allopurinol (Zyloprim).

Allopurinol (Zyloprim) is well tolerated by the majority of patients, and adverse reactions are rare (approximately 3.5%). Precipitation of acute gouty arthritis and allergic dermatitis are the most frequent adverse reactions. Cautious reintroduction of allopurinol (Zyloprim) after cutaneous reactions may be possible using a schedule of gradually increasing doses. An initial oral dose of 50 μg, allopurinol (Zyloprim) daily is progressively increased every 3 to 7 days to 100 μg, 200 μg, 500 μg, 1 mg, 5 mg, 10 mg, 25 mg, and finally to a target dose of 50 to 100 mg daily. Further dose adjustments are based on the patient's serum urate and creatinine levels. This desensitization regimen is particularly useful in patients with renal insufficiency rendering uricosuric drugs ineffective.

Allopurinol (Zyloprim) hypersensitivity syndrome is a rare (0.1 to 0.4% of patients), life-threatening, toxic reaction characterized by fever, severe dermatitis (toxic epidermal necrolysis, erythema multiforme or exfoliative dermatitis), acute hepatitis, acute interstitial nephritis with renal failure, eosinophilia, and leukocytosis. It occurs most frequently in elderly patients with renal impairment in whom the dose of allopurinol (Zyloprim) has not been reduced appropriately, resulting in accumulation of oxypurinol. allopurinol (Zyloprim) desensitization is hazardous and is not recommended in these patients.

Uricosuric Drugs

Uricosuric drugs enhance renal excretion of urate, thereby reducing serum urate concentration. The intense initial uricosuria can result in the deposition of UA crystals in renal tubules and formation of urinary calculi, which in turn can cause renal colic or deterioration of renal function. To minimize this risk and to prevent the precipitation of acute gouty attacks associated with rapid decline in serum urate concentration, uricosuric drugs are started at low doses and gradually increased over 2 to 4 weeks. The risk of UA stones can be further reduced by maintenance of a high urine volume (>2 L per day) and/or alkalization of urine with sodium bicarbonate 1 g four times daily, particularly during the first 4 to 6 weeks of therapy when the uricosuria is greatest. As serum urate normalizes, the intense uricosuria subsides, and renal urate excretion approaches pretreatment levels.

Two uricosuric drugs are used to manage chronic gout. Probenecid (Benemid) is the most frequently used uricosuric. It is administered in a dose of 250 mg twice daily for 1 to 2 weeks, followed by 500 mg twice daily, increasing the dose thereafter to 1000 mg two or three times daily if required. Sulfinpyrazone (Anturane) 50 to 100 mg, is administered twice daily for 1 to 2 weeks, followed by 100 to 200 mg twice daily, increasing to

400 mg twice daily if needed. However, the drug is not universally available. Side effects of these drugs include nausea, abdominal pain, allergic rash, and fever.

In the absence of clear-cut indications for treatment with allopurinol (Zyloprim) (see Box 4), uricosuric drugs can be used in patients younger than 60 years old with primary gout, underexcretion hyperuricemia, normal renal function, and no gross tophi or a history of urinary calculi. Other indications for uricosurics include patients who are allergic or intolerant to allopurinol (Zyloprim), and those with massive tophaceous deposits who may require treatment with both allopurinol to block UA synthesis and a uricosuric to increase UA excretion (see Box 4).

Approximately 75% of patients respond to uricosuric drugs with normalization of serum urate, control of gouty attacks, and resorption of tophaceous deposits. Most failures in the remaining 25% of patients are because of declining renal function (uricosurics are ineffective at a creatinine clearance <50 to 60 mL per minute), intolerable side effects (particularly GI events and skin rash), concomitant intake of aspirin more than 325 mg per day (which antagonizes the uricosuric action), and poor compliance because of multiple daily doses.

Uricolytic Drugs

Uricase, or urate oxidase, is an enzyme that catalyzes the conversion of UA into allantoin, which is 5 to 10 times more soluble than UA and is more readily eliminated by the kidneys. Humans and certain higher primates lack uricase. Both native (nonrecombinant) and recombinant uricases have been used as short-term therapy for the prevention and treatment of malignancy-associated hyperuricemia and tumor lysis syndrome (TLS), resulting from chemotherapy and radiotherapy of hematologic malignancies, such as lymphoma, leukemia, and myeloma. Native uricases are no longer available, and recombinant uricases (such as rasburicase [fasturetic] and uricase-PEG 20), are preferred. These are faster and longer acting, more potent, and less immunogenic. Rasburicase has been approved in the United States only for the initial prevention and treatment of TLS in children with leukemia, lymphoma, and solid malignant tumors receiving anticancer therapy.

However, long-term uricase therapy for chronic gout is limited by the need for parenteral administration and side effects: pruritus, rash, nausea, headache, myalgia, edema, bronchospasm with respiratory distress and hemolysis, particularly in patients with glucose-6-phosphate dehydrogenase (G6PD) deficiency. Approximately 10% of patients develop antiuricase antibodies, which can potentially result in declining efficacy.

Patients with Massive Tophaceous Deposits

Patients with massive tophaceous deposits who do not respond to either allopurinol (Zyloprim) or a uricosuric drug alone may benefit from a combination of these drugs. Serum urate concentrations should be kept consistently less than 5 mg/dL or less than 300 µmol/L,

to ensure complete resolution of the tophaceous deposits. Surgical excision of bulky tophi may be required. Other helpful measures include restriction of alcoholic beverages and a weight-reducing diet, restricted in both carbohydrates (40% of energy) and saturated fats with proportionate increase intake of proteins (30% of energy) and of unsaturated fats (30% of energy).

Patients With Gout and Renal Impairment

Uricosuric drugs are generally ineffective in patients with renal insufficiency. Allopurinol (Zyloprim) therapy in these individuals is associated with an increased incidence of both cutaneous and severe hypersensitivity reactions. To minimize this risk, the drug is introduced in reduced doses, starting at 50 mg every 2 to 3 days and gradually increasing to a maximal daily dose based on the patient's creatinine clearance: 200 mg daily for clearance of 60 mL per minute, 100 mg daily for clearance of 20 mL per minute, and 50 to 100 mg on alternate days for clearance of 10 mL per minute or less.

GOUT IN THE ELDERLY

Co-morbid medical illnesses, including hypertension, cardiac failure, diabetes mellitus and renal impairment, are common in patients older than age 65 years with gout. NSAIDs are potentially hazardous and are not recommended for the treatment of acute gouty episodes in these patients. Oral colchicine is also poorly tolerated by the elderly and is best avoided. Oral, IM, IV, or intra-articular corticosteroids are increasingly being used for treating acute gouty flares in patients older than age 65 years with multiple medical conditions, contraindicating NSAID therapy.

Urate-lowering therapy should be approached with caution in the elderly. Because of the frequent presence of concomitant renal impairment, uricosuric drugs are unlikely to be efficacious and are best avoided. Allopurinol (Zyloprim) therapy is associated with an increased incidence of both cutaneous and severe hypersensitivity reactions. To minimize this risk, the doses of allopurinol (Zyloprim) must be kept low. A starting dose of 50 to 100 mg on alternate days to a maximum daily dose of 100 to 200 mg is recommended.

GOUT IN THE TRANSPLANT RECIPIENT

Both hyperuricemia and severe tophaceous gouty arthritis occur with increased frequency in cyclosporine-treated kidney, heart, or lung/heart allograft transplant recipients. Cyclosporine induces hyperuricemia by both inhibiting renal tubular urate secretion and enhancing postsecretory tubular urate reabsorption. Concurrent diuretic therapy and coexistent renal insufficiency are important contributing factors.

Both NSAIDs and colchicine are hazardous and are not recommended for the treatment of acute gouty arthritis in these patients. Corticosteroids, administered intra-articularly or systemically, are the preferred drugs. Resistance to ACTH from adrenal suppression by prior or current corticosteroid therapy is common.

Uricosuric drugs are generally ineffective in cyclosporine-treated transplant recipients with renal impairment. Allopurinol (Zyloprim) is the preferred urate-lowering drug. Its toxicity can be minimized by adjusting the initial dose according to the creatinine clearance.

Because azathioprine (Imuran) is inactivated by xanthine oxidase, inhibition of this enzyme by allopurinol (Zyloprim) markedly enhances allopurinol (Zyloprim) toxicity. Thus, in transplant patients receiving both azathioprine (Imuran) and allopurinol (Zyloprim), reduction of the initial doses of both drugs by approximately two thirds is recommended.

Asymptomatic Hyperuricemia

The exact implications of chronic asymptomatic hyperuricemia remain uncertain. Most individuals do not develop clinical gout, and there is no convincing evidence that hyperuricemia adversely affects renal function. For these reasons, and because of concerns about cost and potential hazards of unnecessary drug therapy, there seems to be no compelling rationale or clear benefit for treating these individuals with allopurinol (Zyloprim). Exceptions include acute urate overproduction because of tumor lysis syndrome, and patients with severe hyperuricemia (>12 mg/dL or >700 µmol/L) and hyperuricosuria who are at an increased risk of developing both gout and nephrolithiasis. For most other patients, corrective measures, including weight reduction; correction of an underlying IRS with a weight-reducing, carbohydrate-restricted diet with proportionate increase intake of proteins and unsaturated fats; restriction of alcoholic beverages; and elimination of drugs, such as low-dose aspirin more than 325 mg per day and thiazides, are important. The case for treating hyperuricemia is suggested by a recent study in rats showing that diet supplementation with oxonic acid (which inhibits uricase), can result in hyperuricemia, tubulointerstitial renal injury and renal hypertension, without intrarenal urate crystal deposition. Both hypertension and renal injury can be prevented by allopurinol (Zyloprim), which blocks the development of hyperuricemia.

Losartan (Cozaar), an angiotensin II converting enzyme (ACE) receptor antagonist antihypertensive drug,

CURRENT DIAGNOSIS

- Typical clinical history: Rapid-onset acute attacks of arthritis of first metatarsophalangeal and other lower extremity joints, tophi, punched-out joint erosions with *overhanging* margins
- Documented hyperuricemia: elevated serum urate more than 7.0 mg/dL (>450 µmol/L) in men and more than 6.0 mg/dL (>360 µmol/L) in women
- Confirmed by demonstration of monosodium urate crystals in joint or bursal effusions or in aspirates from tophi (by polarized light microscopy)

CURRENT THERAPY

- Control of acute gouty arthritis
  Colchicine
  NSAIDs
  Corticosteroids, corticotrophin (ACTH)
- Management of chronic hyperuricemia
  Urate-lowering drugs:
    Allopurinol (Zyloprim)
    Uricosurics
  Other nondrug therapies:
    Lifestyle modification: diet, control of IRS, decreased alcohol intake, weight reduction
    Restriction of diuretics, aspirin more than 325 mg per day, cyclosporin, niacin
    Dialysis: HD, PD, HF (TLS, CRF + refractory gout)
    Surgical excision, (debulking) of massive tophi

Abbreviations: CRF = chronic renal failure; HD = hemodialysis; HF = hemofiltration; IRS = insulin resistance syndrome; NSAIDs = nonsteroidal anti-inflammatory drugs; PD = peritoneal dialysis; TLS = tumor lysis syndrome.

is a mild uricosuric producing a modest lowering of serum urate. The drug may be particularly useful in treating patients with both hypertension and hyperuricemia, such as those with IRS.

Micronized fenofibrate (TriCor), a lipid-lowering fibric acid derivative, is also a mild uricosuric and a urate-lowering drug. It may be useful in individuals with both dyslipidemia and hyperuricemia, including those with IRS.

REFERENCES

Bomalaski JS, Clark MA: Serum uric acid-lowering therapies: Where are we heading in management of hyperuricemia and the potential role of uricase. Curr Rheumatol Rep 2004;6:240-247.

Choi HK, Atkinson K, Karlson EW, et al: Purine-rich foods, dairy and protein intake, and the risk of gout in men. N Engl J Med 2004; 350:1093-1103.

Emmerson BT: The management of gout. N Engl J Med 1996;334: 445-451.

Fam AG, Dunne SM, Iazzetta J, Paton TW: Efficacy and safety of desensitization to allopurinol following cutaneous reactions. Arthritis Rheum 2001;44:231-238.

Fam AG: Alternate urate-lowering drugs and the management of hyperuricemia in allopurinol-intolerant patients. Int J Adv Rheumatol 2003;1(4):122-130.

Fam AG: Gout in the elderly. Clinical presentation and treatment. Drugs Aging 1998;13:229-243.

Hande KR, Noone RM, Stone WJ: Severe allopurinol toxicity. Description and guidelines for prevention in patients with renal insufficiency. Am J Med 1984;76:47-56.

Mazzali M, Hughes J, Kim Y-G, et al: Elevated uric acid increased blood pressure in the rat by a novel crystal-independent mechanism. Hypertension 2001;38:1101-1106.

Rott KT, Ogudelo CA: Gout, JAMA 2003;289:2857-2860.

Terkeltaub RA: Gout. N Engl J Med 2003;349:1647-1655.

Dyslipoproteinemias

Method of
Peter P. Toth, MD, PhD

The complications of atherosclerotic disease remain the number one cause of death and disability for men and women in industrialized nations. Atherosclerosis is a complex, chronic disease with a multifactorial etiology. Considerable investigation demonstrates an unequivocal relationship between disturbances in cholesterol and lipoprotein metabolism and risk for atherogenesis within the coronary, peripheral, renal, and cerebral vasculature. Dyslipoproteinemias frequently develop in response to genetic and environmental factors and are modifiable through pharmacologic intervention and lifestyle charges. As demonstrated in the Framingham Study, Multiple Risk Factor Intervention Trial, and the Seven Countries Study, when serum levels of cholesterol increase, the lifetime risk for developing coronary artery disease (CAD) rises steadily. Consequently, cholesterol is one of the most important endogenous and exogenous toxins that humans are exposed to. The identification and aggressive management of dyslipidemias in both the primary and secondary prevention settings is pivotal to continued efforts to significantly reduce the prevalence of atherosclerotic disease and its clinical sequelae in populations throughout the world.

Lipoprotein Metabolism and Atherogenesis

Although it is pathogenic, cholesterol is also a critical modulator of cell membrane fluidity and is a precursor for steroid hormone biosynthesis. Consequently, a pool of cholesterol must be available for a variety of physiologic functions. Cholesterol, monoglycerides, free fatty acids, and phospholipids are absorbed from micelles in the intestinal lumen via a series of translocators located within the brush border of jejunal enterocytes. Absorbed cholesterol and lipid are assimilated with apolipoprotein (apo) B48 into chylomicrons. Chylomicrons are released into the lymph and ultimately transported to the central circulation via the thoracic duct. In serum, the triglycerides in chylomicrons are hydrolyzed by lipoprotein lipase. This lipolytic reaction produces chylomicron remnant particles that are taken up by the low-density lipoprotein (LDL) receptor-related protein and metabolized by the liver. The liver secretes very-low-density lipoprotein (VLDL), a lipoprotein enriched with triglycerides, cholesterol, and apoprotein B100. As the triglycerides in VLDL are hydrolyzed by lipoprotein lipase, the size of the lipoprotein particle decreases, eventually forming LDL. LDL particles are concentrated with cholesterol and cholesterol esters and relatively depleted of triglycerides. As the VLDL is progressively converted to LDL, it releases constituents from its surface coat (apoproteins AI, AII, and phospholipids) that are used to form high-density lipoprotein (HDL) in serum.

Patients with hypertriglyceridemia can have elevations in either serum chylomicron or VLDL levels, or both. Patients who consume very high fat diets or who are hyperabsorbers of dietary fat can be hyperchylomicronemic. In contrast, patients with excessive fat storage depots (most notably visceral adiposity) can develop elevated VLDL. Naturally occurring mutations in lipoprotein lipase and an insulin-resistant state can yield hypertriglyceridemia secondary to reduced lipolysis of chylomicrons and VLDL. Reduced lipolysis results in the formation of incompletely digested chylomicrons and VLDL, or "remnant particles" that are widely believed to be atherogenic. Patients with hypertriglyceridemia tend to have reduced serum levels of HDL because:

- There is a decreased release of surface coat constituents from chylomicrons and VLDL.
- As HDL becomes progressively more enriched with triglyceride, it becomes a better substrate for hepatic lipase, an enzyme that catabolizes HDL.

Serum VLDL remnant particles and LDL function as delivery vehicles of cholesterol to peripheral tissues, including blood vessel walls. These lipoproteins are atherogenic because they can traverse the endothelial cell barrier. Macrophages resident within the subendothelial space exposed to LDL oxidized by such enzymes as lipoxygenase or myeloperoxidase upregulate the expression of scavenger receptors (SR-A, CD-36) on their surface and actively take up excessive amounts of cholesterol. This process promotes foam cell and fatty streak development—events that precede atheromatous plaque formation. The activation of macrophages also promotes an inflammatory response with the elaboration of cytokines, interleukins, C-reactive protein, cell mitogens, matrix metalloproteinases, and reactive oxygen species that facilitate lesion progression and instability. LDL and VLDL remnants not taken up by peripheral tissues can be cleared from the circulation by hepatic LDL receptors. Therapies targeted at the upregulation of hepatic LDL receptors are antiatherogenic by virtue of their ability to reduce circulating levels of atherogenic lipoproteins.

HDL particles appear to protect the vasculature from progressive injury and atherogenesis. With few exceptions, in prospective epidemiologic and case-control studies conducted throughout the world, high HDL levels are protective against the development of CAD. For instance, patients with familial hypoalphalipoproteinemia (low HDL) have increased risk for premature CAD, whereas patients with familial hyperalphalipoproteinemia are relatively resistant to atherosclerotic disease. In contrast to LDL, which promotes cholesterol delivery to, and uptake by, vessel wall macrophages, HDL extracts excess cellular cholesterol and delivers it back to the liver for elimination through the gastrointestinal tract in a process referred to as "reverse cholesterol transport." HDL does the following:

- Reduces endothelial cell adhesion molecule (vascular cell adhesion molecule-1, intercellular adhesion molecule-1) expression

Rakel and Bope: *Conn's Current Therapy 2006.*

- Augments endothelial nitric oxide and prostacyclin production
- Reduces oxidized fatty acid components of LDL
- Decreases platelet aggregability
- Inhibits endothelial cell apoptosis

Recent studies suggest that among the elderly, low HDL is a better predictor of risk for cardiovascular disease than is high LDL. An HDL greater than 60 mg/dL is a negative risk factor. The higher the level of serum HDL, the lower the risk for CAD. Therapeutic maneuvers should not be undertaken to reduce circulating levels of HDL.

Identification of Lipoprotein Targets

Dyslipoproteinemias constitute a highly prevalent and heterogeneous class of disorders. Derangements in circulating levels of specific lipoprotein classes can be the result of abnormalities in gastrointestinal absorption, enzyme activities, and/or receptor expression. A complete fasting (12 to 14 hours) lipoprotein profile should be obtained from any patient being evaluated for dyslipidemia. Because of the relationship between specific lipoprotein fractions and risk for CAD, a total cholesterol level has little practical clinical utility.

The National Cholesterol Education Program Adult Treatment Panel III (NCEP ATPIII) has systematically defined risk-stratified target levels for atherogenic serum lipoproteins based on the best available evidence to date (Table 1). Risk stratification is performed by evaluating a patient's cardiovascular risk factor burden (number of risk factors) and, if two or more risk factors are present, calculation of the Framingham risk score. Among patients being treated for primary prevention, low risk is defined as a 0-1 risk factor. Moderate and moderately high risk are defined as 2 or more risk factors and a 10-year Framingham risk of less than 10% and 10% to 20%, respectively. In the high-risk category, patients either have CAD (defined as a history of myocardial infarction [MI], stable/unstable angina, revascularization with coronary artery bypass grafting, or percutaneous angioplasty) or a CAD risk equivalent (defined as diabetes mellitus, peripheral vascular disease, significant carotid artery disease [transient ischemic attack or stroke from carotid origin or greater than 50% obstructive atheromatous plaque in a carotid artery], abdominal aortic aneurysm, and a 10-year Framingham risk that exceeds 20%). Among patients with multiple risk factors and no history of CAD or a CAD risk equivalent, it is important to calculate the Framingham risk score so as to differentiate moderate, moderately high, and high risk. An electronic version of a Framingham risk calculator for men and women can be downloaded at www.nhlbi.nih.gov/guidelines/cholesterol. Risk factors recognized by NCEP are summarized in Box 1.

In ATPIII, the NCEP also instituted the following important changes:

- An optimal low-density lipoprotein cholesterol (LDLC) is defined as less than 100 mg/dL for all patients.
- An HDL less than 40 mg/dL is now defined as a categorical risk factor for CAD.
- It introduced target levels for non-high-density lipoprotein cholesterol (HDLC). Non-HDLC (total cholesterol – HDLC) is a measure of the burden of atherogenic lipoproteins in serum (LDL + VLDL).

The risk-stratified target for non-HDLC is the LDLC target plus 30. LDLC remains the primary target of antilipidemic therapy. However, in patients with baseline triglyceride levels greater than 200 mg/dL, non-HDL is the secondary priority for therapy.

Although it is well known by the majority of health care providers that a patient with CAD or a CAD risk

TABLE 1 Low-density Lipoprotein Cholesterol Goals and Thresholds for Initiating Lifestyle Change and Pharmacologic Intervention

Risk category*,†	LDLC goal	LDLC level at which to initiate TLC	LDLC level at which to consider drug therapy
CHD or CHD risk equivalents (10-year risk >20%)	<100 mg/dL (optional goal <70 mg/dL)‡	≥100 mg/d all patients regardless of LDL	≥130 mg/dL (100-129 mg/dL: drug optional) ≥100 mg/d§ (<100 mg/dL: drug optional)
2+ risk factors (10-year risk 10%–20%)	<130 mg/dL (optional goal <100)	≥130 mg/d all patients regardless of LDL	≥130 mg/dL (<100 mg/dL: drug optional§)
2+ risk factors (10-year risk <10%)	<130 mg/dL	≥130 mg/dL	≥160 mg/dL
0-1 risk factor	<160 mg/dL	≥160 mg/dL	≥190 mg/dL (160-189 mg/dL: LDL-lowering drug optional)

Modified from Grundy SM, Cleeman JI, Merz CN, et al: Implications of recent clinical trials for the National Cholesterol Education Program Adult Treatment Panel III guidelines. Circulation 2004;110(2):227-239.
*CHD risk equivalents include diabetes mellitus, peripheral vascular disease, carotid artery disease, abdominal aortic aneurysm and 10 yr Framingham risk >201.
†Risk factors included in Framingham risk evaluation are age, systolic blood pressure, total cholesterol, HDLC, and smoking status.
‡The optional goal of <70 mg/dL is particularly targeted at patients who are "very high" risk, i.e., patients with a recent acute coronary syndrome, poorly controlled diabetics with multiple risk factors, etc.
§When initiating statin therapy in these patients, the goal for LDLC reduction should be 30% to 40% from baseline.
Abbreviations: CHD = coronary heart disease; HDLC = high-density lipoprotein cholesterol; LDLC = low-density lipoprotein cholesterol; TLC = therapeutic lifestyle change.

BOX 1   National Cholesterol Education Program Risk Factors

Negative
HDLC > 60 mg/dL
Positive
Cigarette smoking
HDL < 40 mg/dL
Hypertension (blood pressure > 140/90 mm Hg or use of antihypertensive agents)
Family history of premature coronary artery disease (CAD in male first-degree relative < 55 yrs; CAD in female first-degree relative < 65 yrs)
Age (men ≥ 45 yrs; women ≥ 55 yrs)

Abbreviations: CAD = coronary artery disease; HDL = high-density lipoprotein; HDLC = high-density lipoprotein cholesterol.

TABLE 2   NCEP ATP III Criteria for Diagnosing the Metabolic Syndrome*

Risk factor	Defining level
Abdominal obesity	
Men	Waist > 40 inches
Women	Waist > 35 inches
Triglycerides	≥150 mg/dL
HDLC	
Men	<40 mg/dL
Women	<50 mg/dL
Blood pressure	≥130/≥85 mm Hg
Fasting glucose	≥100 mg/dL

*Patients having any three of the five risk factors meet criteria for the diagnosis of the metabolic syndrome.

equivalent should have an LDLC less than 100 mg/dL, a number of studies show that only 18% to 25% of these patients actually attain this target. An increasing amount of clinical trial evidence is demonstrating that, when it comes to LDLC reduction and CAD, "the lower, the better." In a recent addendum to ATPIII, the NCEP has suggested that physicians consider lowering LDLC to less than 70 mg/dL and non-HDLC to less than 100 mg/dL in very high risk patients (e.g., recent acute coronary syndrome or a diabetic with multiple poorly controlled cardiovascular risk factors). Other modifications of ATPIII include:

- Consider the initiation of pharmacologic intervention and therapeutic lifestyle change if baseline LDLC is greater than 100 mg/dL in patients with moderately high and high risk.
- Among patients at high risk with baseline LDLC less than 100 mg/dL, further reduction of LDLC by 30% to 40% with medication is a therapeutic option.

Such stringent criteria for LDLC and non-HDLC reduction require the institution of intensive lifestyle and pharmacologic interventions to ensure therapeutic success.

Therapeutic Lifestyle Change

Therapeutic lifestyle change (TLC) constitutes front-line therapy for all patients at risk for CAD. It is recommended that patients who smoke achieve smoking cessation. Smoking is associated with endothelial cell dysfunction as well as increased levels of oxidized LDLC and reduced serum HDLC. The amount of daily ingested cholesterol should not exceed 200 mg. The amount of saturated fat in the diet should be less than 7%, and the total fat intake should not exceed 25% to 35% of calories (Table 2). The distribution of calories from other nutrients should be as follows: 15% protein, 50% to 60% carbohydrates, 10% polyunsaturated fat, and 20% monounsaturated fat. Reductions in saturated fat and increased ingestion of mono- and polyunsaturated fats are associated with reductions in serum LDLC. The ingestion of plant stanols and viscous fiber

reduce cholesterol absorption. Patients should be encouraged to exercise for 20 to 30 minutes five times weekly. Exercise facilitates weight loss, which helps to relieve visceral adiposity and insulin resistance. These changes are associated with reduced serum triglycerides and elevations in HDLC.

Although many types of weight loss diets were introduced in recent years, the optimal long-term approach to weight reduction and maintenance is for patients to continue to exercise and restrict fat consumption to within recommended ranges (Table 3). Consultation with a dietitian increases the likelihood of success. For patients who are morbidly obese, bariatric surgery is emerging as an important therapeutic alternative when aggressive lifestyle and pharmacologic interventions fail. Bariatric surgery facilitates significant weight reduction and relieves insulin resistance, reduces blood pressure, and improves lipoprotein profiles. In the Swedish Obese Subjects Study, gastric bypass surgery was associated with a weight loss of 20 kg (44 lb) and decreased the incidence of new-onset type 2 diabetes mellitus by 81% compared to the usual standard of care over 8 years of follow-up. Once adequate weight loss is achieved, it can only be maintained if the patient remains in an isocaloric state through sustained lifestyle modification.

Therapeutic lifestyle change is a particularly important intervention in patients with the metabolic syndrome. Metabolic syndrome develops secondary to the effects of insulin resistance and obesity and is

TABLE 3   Dietary Recommendations for Therapeutic Lifestyle Change

Dietary component	Recommendation allowance
Polyunsaturated fat	Up to 10% of total calories
Monounsaturated fat	Up to 20% of total calories
Total fat	25%–35% of total calories
Carbohydrate	50%–60% of total calories
Dietary fiber	20–30 g/day
Protein	Approximately 15% of total calories
Dietary cholesterol	<200 mg/day

characterized by a set of five risk factors (Table 2). The diagnosis of metabolic syndrome is made when a patient has any three or more of these defining clinical features. Although the metabolic syndrome significantly increases risk for atherosclerotic disease and diabetes mellitus, it is not defined as a CAD risk equivalent. The Framingham risk score should be calculated on all of these patients. LDL and non-HDL goals should be defined by risk stratification. If triglycerides remain elevated (200 to 499 mg/dL) after the LDL goal is reached, then consideration is given to the addition of a triglyceride lowering drug. If triglycerides are greater than 500 mg/dL, patients should be treated aggressively with triglyceride-lowering medication and a very low fat diet with less than or equal to 15% of calories derived from fat to prevent the development of pancreatitis. Although the NCEP has not defined target levels for HDL, it is recommended that an effort be made to raise low HDL (<40 mg/dL in men, <50 mg/dL in women) through lifestyle modification and drug therapy. The Expert Group on HDL suggests that HDL be raised to greater than 40 mg/dL in patients at high risk or with metabolic syndrome. The American Diabetes Association recommends that HDL be raised to more than 40 mg/dL in diabetic men and to more than 50 mg/dL in diabetic women.

Pharmacologic Interventions

STATINS

The statins are reversible, competitive 3-hydroxy-3-methylglutaryl coenzyme A (HMG-CoA) reductase inhibitors. HMG-CoA reductase is the rate-limiting step for cholesterol biosynthesis. The statins provide the most potent means currently available by which to reduce serum levels of LDLC. In addition to reducing cholesterol biosynthesis, the statins augment the clearance of atherogenic apoB100-containing lipoproteins (VLDL, VLDL remnants, and LDL) by upregulating the expression of the LDL receptor on the surface of hepatocytes. These drugs stimulate apoA-I expression and hepatic HDL secretion secondary to weak peroxisomal proliferator-activated receptor-α (PPAR-α) agonism.

The statins exert benefit distinct from their ability to alter circulating levels of lipoproteins through their "pleiotropic effects." Statins inhibit the post-translational modification and activation of small G-proteins (Rho and Ras) by blocking the production of such isoprenoids as farnesyl-pyrophosphate and geranylgeranyl-pyrophosphate. This is associated with reductions in the production of a large number of atherogenic stimuli (C-reactive protein, reactive oxygen species, tissue factor, interleukins, adhesion molecules, monocyte chemoattract protein-1, angiotensin-II receptor, and endothelin-1), decreased platelet reactivity and smooth-cell proliferation, and a reversal of endothelial dysfunction, among other effects. Consequently, statins appear to modulate inflammation, oxidative status, vasodilation, thrombotic tendency, and the capacity of a variety of cell types in vessel walls to interact and drive atherogenesis.

The statins are highly efficacious medications. In a growing number of large-scale, placebo-controlled clinical trials, these agents significantly reduced rates of myocardial infarction, stroke, and coronary and all-cause mortality in both the primary and secondary prevention settings. Statins also decrease the frequency of stable and unstable angina and reduce the rate of atheromatous plaque progression and even stimulate some degree of plaque resorption. Statins reduce event rates in men and women, diabetics, smokers, hypertensives, as well as patients older than 70 years of age. Much of the risk reduction achieved with statin therapy is attributable to LDLC reduction. Studies now show that the greater the magnitude of LDLC reduction, the greater the reduction in risk for acute coronary events. The benefits of statin therapy are widely assumed to be a class effect.

Six different statins are currently available. These drugs differ by potency and a variety of pharmacokinetic properties. The specific choice of a statin is dictated by the magnitude of LDLC reduction required (baseline versus risk-stratified NCEP target). The LDLC reducing capacity of the statins is as follows:

1. Rosuvastatin (Crestor), 45% to 63% (5 to 40 mg daily)
2. Atorvastatin (Lipitor) 26% to 60% (10 to 80 mg daily)
3. Simvastatin (Zocor) 26% to 47% (10 to 80 mg daily)
4. Lovastatin (Mevacor) 21% to 42% (10 to 80 mg daily)
5. Fluvastatin (Lescol) 22% to 36% (10 to 80 mg daily)
6. Pravastatin (Pravachol) 22% to 34% (10 to 80 mg daily).

Each doubling of the statin dose yields an additional 6% reduction, on average, in serum LDLC (the rule of 6s). The statins provide dose-dependent reductions in serum triglyceride levels (typically 10% to 25%) and elevations in serum HDLC (2% to 14%). Atorvastatin has a tendency to be less and less effective at raising HDLC as the dose is titrated to higher levels. In patients with high baseline triglycerides (>300 mg/dL), the statins increase HDLC significantly more than in patients who are normotriglyceridemic. For instance, simvastatin and rosuvastatin can raise HDLC up to 18% and 22%, respectively, in these patients.

The statins have different pharmacokinetic profiles. Because of their relatively short half-lives (1 to 4 hours), lovastatin, pravastatin, fluvastatin, and simvastatin should be taken in the evening in order to intercept the peak activity of HMG-CoA-reductase that occurs around midnight. Atorvastatin and rosuvastatin can be taken at any time during the day because of their long half-lives (approximately 19 hours). The coadministration of cytochrome P450 3A4 inhibitors (azole type antifungals [ketoconazole, itraconazole], HIV protease inhibitors, macrolide antibiotics [erythromycin, clarithromycin], nefazodone [serzone], more than 1 quart of grapefruit juice daily, and cyclosporine) with simvastatin, lovastatin, and atorvastatin should be avoided as these statins are dependent on this P450 isozyme for metabolism. Concomitant dosing can lead to increased risk for toxicity. The dose of simvastatin should not exceed 20 mg daily in patients receiving verapamil or amiodarone.

Rakel and Bope: *Conn's Current Therapy 2006.*

The benefits of statin therapy significantly outweigh the risks. Hepatotoxicity is defined as an alanine aminotransferase elevation greater than or equal to 3 times the upper limits of normal (ULN), on two occasions at least one month apart. The average risk of this on statin therapy approximates 1%, but risk increases as a function of dose. Mild elevations in serum transaminases are relatively common, and they tend to spontaneously resolve. If transaminitis or hepatotoxicity develops, statin therapy should be discontinued until transaminase levels normalize and a different statin can be started at a lower dose. The most dreaded complication of statin therapy is rhabdomyolysis with skeletal muscle breakdown, myoglobinuria, and renal failure. The risk of this is less than 0.1%, but patients must be counseled about the possibility as well as warning signs for rhabdomyolysis (escalating muscle pain, proximal weakness, brownish-red discoloration of urine). Statins can induce myalgia. However, myalgias in general are common throughout the population. In the Heart Protection Study, among 20,536 patients randomized to either placebo or simvastatin, 40 mg daily, the incidence of myalgia was nearly identical in the two groups of patients. If a patient is experiencing significant myalgia or muscle weakness a serum creatine kinase level can be obtained. Myopathy is defined as a creatine kinase level that exceeds 10 times ULN. Statins are contraindicated in pregnant and nursing women.

EZETIMIBE

Dietary and biliary sources of cholesterol contribute substantially to circulating levels of this sterol. Although plant sterols and stanols can block cholesterol absorption, Ezetimibe (Zetia) is the first member of lipid-lowering drugs known as cholesterol absorption inhibitors. Ezetimibe inhibits a sterol transporter in the brush border of the jejunal enterocyte identified as Niemann-Pick C1 Like-1 protein that internalizes cholesterol and phytosterols from the intestinal lumen. After being glucuronidated, ezetimibe undergoes enterohepatic recirculation with negligible systemic exposure. The half-life of ezetimibe is approximately 22 hours and is dosed at 10 mg once daily. Ezetimibe reduces serum LDLC on average by 20%, but up to 24% of patients experience a reduction of greater than or equal to 25%. Ezetimibe also decreases triglycerides by up to 8% and raises HDLC by up to 4%. Ezetimibe does not decrease the absorption of bile acids, steroid hormones (ethinyl estradiol, progesterone), or such fat-soluble vitamins as vitamins A, D, E, or α- and β-carotenes.

The risk of hepatotoxicity with ezetimibe is nearly identical to placebo (0.5% vs. 0.3%), and there is no documented evidence of increased risk for myopathy. Fixed-dose ezetimibe is also available in combination with increasing doses of simvastatin (Vytorin; 10/10; 10/20; 10/40; 10/80 mg daily). Ezetimibe can also be safely used in combination with other statins and provides additive changes in lipoprotein levels to that observed with statin therapy. The addition of ezetimibe to a statin regimen substantially reduces the likelihood of having to titrate the statin.

BILE ACID BINDING RESINS

The bile acid sequestration agents (BASAs) are orally administered anion exchange resins that bind bile acids in the gastrointestinal tract and prevent them from being reabsorbed into the enterohepatic circulation. These drugs reduce serum LDLC by two mechanisms: (1) increased catabolism of cholesterol secondary to the upregulation of 7-α-hydroxylase, the rate-limiting enzyme for the conversion of cholesterol into bile acids; and (2) increased expression of LDL receptors on the hepatocyte surface that augments the clearance of apoB100-containing lipoproteins from plasma. At maximum doses, the BASAs can reduce serum LDLC by 15% to 30% and increase HDLC by 3% to 5%. It is recommended that these drugs be used in conjunction with a statin whenever possible because BASA therapy increases HMG-CoA reductase activity in the liver, which leads to increased hepatic biosynthesis of cholesterol, thereby offsetting the effects of the BASAs over time.

There are currently three different BASAs available. These include cholestyramine (Questran; 4 to 24 g daily in two to three divided doses daily), colestipol (Colestid; 5 to 30 g in two to four divided doses daily), and colesevelam (WelChol; 1250 mg two to three times daily). The development of constipation, flatulence, and bloating are relatively frequent, though colesevelam has the most favorable side-effect profile of the three available BASAs. Increasing water and soluble fiber ingestion ameliorates some of the difficulty with constipation. The BASAs bind negatively charged molecules in a nonspecific manner. Consequently, they can decrease the absorption of warfarin (Coumadin), phenobarbital, thiazide diuretics, digitalis, β-blockers, thyroxine, statins, fibrates, and ezetimibe. These medications should be taken 1 hour before or 4 hours after the ingestion of a BASA. The BASAs can reduce the absorption of fat-soluble vitamins.

FIBRATES

The fibrates are fibric acid derivatives that exert a number of effects on lipoprotein metabolism. These agents reduce serum triglycerides by 25% to 50% and raise HDLC by 10% to 20%. Fibrates activate lipoprotein lipase by reducing levels of apoprotein CIII (an inhibitor of this enzyme) and increasing levels of apoprotein CII (an activator of lipoprotein lipase). This stimulates the hydrolysis of triglycerides in chylomicrons and VLDL. Fibrates increase HDLC by two mechanisms. First, the fibrates are PPAR-α agonists and stimulate increased hepatic expression of apoproteins AI and AII. Second, by activating lipoprotein lipase, surface coat mass derived from VLDL is ultimately used to assimilate HDL in serum. In some patients, fibrate therapy may be associated with an increase in serum LDLC (the "β" effect) secondary to increased enzymatic conversion of VLDL to LDL. This effect may diminish over time as the patient increases the expression of hepatic LDL receptors.

The fibrates are particularly valuable for treating dyslipidemia in patients with a combination of hypertriglyceridemia and low HDLC. In this patient type, post-hoc evaluations of data from two studies (the Helsinki Heart Study and the Bezafibrate Infarction Prevention Study) have demonstrated substantial cardiovascular event rate reductions using fibrate therapy. In the Veterans Affairs High-Density Lipoprotein Intervention Trial (VA-HIT), men with CAD and low HDL (mean 31 mg/dL) were treated with either gemfibrozil (Lopid) 600 mg orally twice daily or placebo over a 5-year-follow-up period. With a 6% elevation in HDL, no change in LDL, and a 31% decrease in triglycerides, gemfibrozil therapy resulted in a 22% reduction in the composite endpoint of all-cause mortality and nonfatal MI compared to placebo. Gemfibrozil therapy also reduced the risk of stroke and transient ischemic attacks by 31% and 59%, respectively.

Among the diabetic patients in VA-HIT treated with gemfibrozil, there was a 32% reduction in the combined endpoint (41% in CHD death and 40% in stroke). Fibrates have been shown to exert many of the same pleiotropic effects as statins and reduce atheromatous plaque progression in native coronary vessels and in coronary venous bypass grafts.

Like the statins, fibrates are associated with a low incidence of myopathy and mild elevations in serum transaminases. Fibrate therapy can increase the risk for cholelithiasis and can raise prothrombin times by displacing warfarin from albumin binding sites. The periodic monitoring of serum transaminases (6 to 12 weeks after initiating therapy and twice annually thereafter) is recommended. The two most commonly used fibrates are gemfibrozil (Lopid; 600 mg twice daily) and fenofibrate (Tricor; 54 or 160 mg daily). Bezafibrate (Bezalip)[2] is available in Europe and is dosed at 400 mg daily. The use of therapies combining a statin and fibrate is becoming more commonplace in clinical practice, especially as the incidence of complex dyslipidemias increases. Gemfibrozil significantly reduces the glucuronidation of statins, which decreases their elimination. This increases the risk for myopathy/rhabdomyolysis and hepatotoxicity. When used in combination with gemfibrozil, the doses for simvastatin (Zocor), and rosuvastatin (Crestor), should not exceed 10 mg daily. In general, when embarking on combination therapy, fenofibrate is a safer choice, as it does not adversely impact the glucuronidation of the statins. There are no clinical trial data yet available to assess the effect of statin-fibrate combination therapy on cardiovascular morbidity and mortality.

Among patients in whom serum triglycerides do not normalize in response to a low-fat diet and fibrate therapy, consideration should be given to the addition of other agents. Patients with severe hypertriglyceridemia frequently possess mutations in lipoprotein lipase that reduce the lipolytic activity of this enzyme. In this scenario, the addition of orlistat (Xenical; 120 mg with meals) can reduce the absorption of dietary fat and hence the circulating levels of chylomicrons and triglycerides. Fish-oil capsules enriched with omega-3 (eicosapentaenoic acid) and omega-6 (docosahexaenoic acid) fatty acids can reduce serum triglyceride and VLDL levels and raise HDLC in a dose-dependent manner.

---

[2]Not available in the United States.

NIACIN

Niacin or nicotinic acid is a B vitamin that exerts multiple beneficial effects on lipoprotein metabolism. In contrast to statins and fibrates, niacin does not stimulate hepatic biosynthesis of HDL. Niacin appears to block HDL particle uptake and catabolism by hepatocytes without adversely impacting reverse cholesterol transport. This helps to increase circulating levels of HDL. Niacin reduces hepatic VLDL and triglyceride secretion according to two mechanisms: (1) decreasing the flux of fatty acids from adipose tissue to the liver by inhibiting lipase activity; (2) inhibiting triglyceride formation within hepatocytes by inhibiting diacylglycerol acyltransferase. Niacin also reduces serum LDLC concentrations by increasing the catabolism of apoB100. Consequently, niacin beneficially impacts all components of the lipoprotein profile.

When used as monotherapy at 3.0 g daily, crystalline niacin (Niaspan) significantly reduced the incidence of MI and stroke in patients with established CAD in the Coronary Drug Project. In the HDL-Atherosclerosis Treatment Study (HATS) combinations of high-dose niacin (2 to 4 g with simvastatin) reduced cardiovascular morbidity and mortality by up to 90% compared to placebo. This combination therapy also induced atheromatous plaque stabilization over a follow-up period of 3 years. Niaspan should be started at a low dose and gradually titrated upward based on the results of follow-up lipid panels. When evaluated as a function of dose (500 to 2000 mg daily), Niaspan induces the following changes

CURRENT DIAGNOSIS

- Dyslipidemia is a highly heterogeneous class of metabolic disorders with an etiology that can depend on abnormalities in the gastrointestinal absorption of cholesterol and lipids and mutations in cell surface receptors and enzymes in pathways regulating lipid metabolism.
- Dyslipidemia is a widely prevalent risk factor for CAD and is associated with elevations in serum LDLC and non-HDLC and low levels of HDLC.
- When making the diagnosis of dyslipidemia, it is important to rule out and treat secondary causes of dyslipidemia, such as thyroid dysfunction, alcoholism, diabetes mellitus, and nephrotic syndrome, among others.
- A complete fasting lipoprotein profile should be performed on anyone undergoing screening for dyslipidemia.
- The diagnosis of dyslipidemia requires comprehensive, global cardiovascular risk evaluation. Target levels for LDLC and non-HDLC are risk stratified. An HDLC of less than 40 mg/dL is a categorical risk factor for CAD.

Abbreviations: CAD = coronary artery disease; HDLC = high-density lipoprotein cholesterol; LDLC = low-density lipoprotein cholesterol.

in serum lipid levels: LDLC, 3% to 16% reduction; triglycerides, 5% to 32% reduction; HDLC, 10% to 24% elevation.

Niacin therapy is associated with a number of side effects. The most common side effect with niacin is cutaneous flushing. The incidence of this can be reduced by taking a 325-mg tablet of aspirin one hour before taking niacin. The flushing is prostaglandin mediated. Limiting fat intake for 2 to 3 hours before taking niacin also helps, as fat is a source of arachidonic acid, the substrate for cyclooxygenase. Niaspan is a sustained-release preparation of niacin associated with less flushing. Other side effects include bloating, pruritus, acanthosis nigricans, transient disturbances in glycemic control, and increased serum concentrations of uric acid. Niacin appears to increase rates of proximal tubular reuptake of urate from the glomerular ultrafiltrate. Niacin is available as a combination pill with lovastatin (Advicor; 500/20 mg, 750/20 mg, 1000/20 mg, and 2000/40 mg), and the two drugs give additive changes in the levels of serum lipoproteins.

Conclusion

Dyslipidemia is a widely prevalent risk factor for CAD. Specific target levels for atherogenic lipoprotein fractions are defined by the NCEP. The treatment of dyslipidemia with lifestyle modification and pharmacologic intervention is associated with significant reductions in cardiovascular morbidity and mortality.

CURRENT THERAPY

- Dyslipidemia is a modifiable risk factor.
- Lifestyle modification is first-line therapy for all patients with dyslipidemia.
- The intensity of pharmacologic intervention depends upon risk-stratified, NCEP targets for LDLC and non-HDLC. In patients with low HDLC, therapeutic effort should be made to raise the level of this lipoprotein as much as possible.
- Dyslipidemia can be treated with statins, fibrates, niacin, and combinations thereof. These drug classes have a substantial amount of end-point driven clinical trial data supporting their use.
- In patients unable to achieve their LDLC target with lifestyle modification and statin therapy, consider adding ezetimibe.
- Patients with severe hypertriglyceridemia unable to adequately reduce serum triglycerides with a low-fat diet and a fibrate likely have a lipoprotein lipase deficiency. These patients can benefit from the addition of orlistat to their pharmacologic regimen.
- The treatment of dyslipidemia in the context of both primary and secondary prevention must be coupled with the aggressive identification and management of all risk factors patients present with, including hypertension, diabetes mellitus, obesity, cigarette smoking, as well as nephropathy and chronic kidney disease.

Abbreviations: HDLC = high-density lipoprotein cholesterol; LDLC = low-density lipoprotein cholesterol. NCEP = National Cholesterol Education Program.

Rakel and Bope: *Conn's Current Therapy 2006.*

REFERENCES

American Diabetes Association: Dyslipidemia management in adults with diabetes. Diabetes Care 2004;27:S68-S71.

Brown G, Albers JJ, Fisher LD, et al: Regression of coronary artery disease as a result of intensive lipid-lowering therapy in men with high levels of apolipoprotein B. N Engl J Med 1990;323: 1289-1298.

Cannon CP, Braunwald E, McCabe CH, et al., for the Pravastatin or Atorvastatin Evaluation and Infection Therapy–Thrombolysis in Myocardial Infarction 22 Investigators: Comparison of intensive and moderate lipid lowering with statins after acute coronary syndromes. N Engl J Med 2004;350:1495-1504.

Expert Panel on Detection, Evaluation, and Treatment of High Blood Cholesterol in Adults: Executive summary of the third report of the National Cholesterol Education Program (NCEP) Expert Panel on Detection, Evaluation, and Treatment of High blood Cholesterol in Adults (Adult Treatment Panel III). JAMA 2001; 285:2486-2497.

Grundy SM, Cleeman JI, Merz CN, et al: Implications of recent clinical trials for the National Cholesterol Education Program Adult Treatment Panel III guidelines. Circulation 2004;110(2):227-239.

Heart Protection Study Collaborative Group: MRC/BHF Heart Protection Study of cholesterol lowering with simvastatin in 20,536 high-risk individuals: A randomised placebo-controlled trial. Lancet 2002;360:7-22.

Mosca L, Appel LJ, Benjamin EJ, et al: Evidence-based guidelines for cardiovascular disease prevention in women. Circulation 2004; 109:672-693.

Ridker PM, Bassuk SS, Toth PP: C-reactive protein and risk of cardiovascular disease: Evidence and clinical application. Curr Atheroscler Rep 2003;5:341-349.

Robins SJ, Collins D, Wittes JF, et al. VA-HIT Study Group. Veterans Affairs High-Density Lipoprotein Intervention Trial. Relation of gemfibrozil treatment and lipid levels with major coronary events. JAMA 2001;285:1586-1589.

Sacks FM and The Expert Group on HDL Cholesterol: The role of high-density lipoprotein (HDL) cholesterol in the prevention and treatment of coronary heart disease: Expert group recommendations. Am J Cardiol 2002;90:139-143.

Sever PS, Dahlöf B, Poulter NR, et al., for the ASCOT investigators: Prevention of coronary and stroke events with atorvastatin in hypertensive patients who have average or lower-than-average cholesterol concentrations, in the Anglo-Scandinavian Cardiac Outcomes Trial—Lipid Lowering Arm (ASCOT-LLA): A multicentre randomised controlled trial. Lancet 2003:361:1149-1158.

Sjostrum CD, Peltonen M, Wedel H, et al: Differentiated long-term effects of intentional weight loss on diabetes and hypertension. Hypertension 2000;36:20-25.

Toth PP: Clinician update: HDL and cardiovascular risk. Circulation 2004;109:1809-1812.

Toth PP: Low-density lipoprotein reduction in high risk patients: How low do you go? Curr Atheroscler Rep 2004;6:348-352.

8

Obesity

Method of
Robert F. Kushner, MD, and
Courtney A. Noble, MD

The epidemic of obesity continues to rise each year. According to the 1999 to 2000 National Health and Nutrition Examination Survey (NHANES) published by the Centers for Disease Control and Prevention (CDC), 65% of the U.S. adult population is overweight or obese (body mass index [BMI] >25 kg/m^2) and an estimated 30% are obese (BMI >30 kg/m^2). Although all demographic groups are affected by this epidemic, the prevalence of obesity among African American and Hispanic American women is particularly high at 38% and 35%, respectively.

Overweight and obesity have a negative impact on overall daily functioning (physical and psychological) and quality of life. Medical consequences are numerous and often life threatening. Obesity is a multiple organ disorder and a significant risk factor for type 2 diabetes, hypertension, dyslipidemia, obstructive sleep apnea, osteoarthritis, and some forms of cancer, among others (Box 1). The metabolic syndrome, a relatively recently described disorder, is also common in this patient population. It is defined by the National Cholesterol Education Program (NCEP) as the presence of three of the following five criteria: triglycerides more than 150 mg/dL; high-density lipoprotein (HDL) cholesterol less than 40 mg/dL (men) or less than 50 mg/dL (women); waist circumference more than 40 inches (men) or more than 35 inches (women); blood pressure (BP) more than 130/85 mm Hg; and fasting glucose more than 110 mg/dL. Patients with the metabolic syndrome have an increased risk of developing type 2 diabetes and coronary artery disease. As a result of the high prevalence of obesity and related co-morbidities, the U.S. Preventive Services Task Force now recommends that physicians "screen all adult patients for obesity and offer intensive counseling and behavioral interventions to promote sustained weight loss."

Assessment

A thorough history, physical examination, and laboratory evaluation based on the patient's risk factors needs to be performed prior to discussing and initiating treatment. The weight history should include an assessment of physiologic (medical illness, pharmacologic therapy) and environmental (social and psychological) factors that may contribute to weight gain. A family history is important to identify a potential genetic predisposition for obesity-associated co-morbid conditions. A history of weight loss attempts including patient's insight as to why attempts were or were not successful is particularly useful. Finally, nutritional knowledge, eating, activity, and coping patterns should be reviewed.

BOX 1   Symptoms and Diseases Associated With Obesity

Cardiovascular System
- Hypertension
- Congestive heart failure
- Cor pulmonale
- Varicose veins
- Pulmonary embolism
- Coronary artery disease

Endocrine System
- The metabolic syndrome
- Type 2 diabetes mellitus
- Dyslipidemia
- Polycystic ovary syndrome
- Infertility
- Amenorrhea

Musculoskeletal System
- Immobility
- Osteoarthritis
- Low back pain
- Gout
- Carpal tunnel syndrome

Respiratory System
- Dyspnea and fatigue
- Obstructive sleep apnea
- Hypoventilation (Pickwickian) syndrome
- Asthma

Gastrointestinal System
- Gastroesophageal reflux disease
- Nonalcoholic fatty liver disease
- Cholelithiasis
- Hernias
- Colon cancer

Psychosocial
- Work disability
- Social stigmatization
- Depression/low self-esteem
- Body image disturbance

Integument
- Venous stasis of legs
- Cellulitis
- Striae distensae (stretch marks)
- Intertrigo, carbuncles
- Lymphedema
- Acanthosis nigricans
- Hidradenitis suppurativa
- Acrochordon (skin tags)

Genitourinary Organs
- Urinary stress incontinence
- Hypogonadism (male)
- Breast and uterine cancer
- Obesity-related glomerulopathy
- Pregnancy complications

Neurologic
- Stroke
- Meralgia paresthetica
- Idiopathic intracranial hypertension

Physical assessment of the patient should include the evaluation of body mass index (BMI), waist circumference (for BMI <35 kg/m^2), and overall medical risk. BMI can be conveniently and routinely documented on all patients with use of a BMI height-weight table (Table 1). Alternatively, BMI can be calculated as

TABLE 1 Body Mass Index (BMI) Chart

Body Weight (pounds)

Height (inches) \ BMI	19	20	21	22	23	24	25	26	27	28	29	30	31	32	33	34	35
58	91	96	100	105	110	115	119	124	129	134	138	143	148	153	158	162	167
59	94	99	104	109	114	119	124	128	133	138	143	148	153	158	163	168	173
60	97	102	107	112	118	123	128	133	138	143	148	153	158	163	168	174	179
61	100	106	111	116	122	127	132	137	143	148	153	158	164	169	174	180	185
62	104	109	115	120	126	131	136	142	147	153	158	164	169	175	180	186	191
63	107	113	118	124	130	135	141	146	152	158	163	169	175	180	186	191	197
64	110	116	122	128	134	140	145	151	157	163	169	174	180	186	192	197	204
65	114	120	126	132	138	144	150	156	162	168	174	180	186	192	198	204	210
66	118	124	130	136	142	148	155	161	167	173	179	186	192	198	204	210	216
67	121	127	134	140	146	153	159	166	172	178	185	191	198	204	211	217	223
68	125	131	138	144	151	158	164	171	177	184	190	197	203	210	216	223	230
69	128	135	142	149	155	162	169	176	182	189	196	203	209	216	223	230	236
70	132	139	146	153	160	167	174	181	188	195	202	209	216	222	229	236	243
71	136	143	150	157	165	172	179	186	193	200	208	215	222	229	236	243	250
72	140	147	154	162	169	177	184	191	199	206	213	221	228	235	242	250	258
73	144	151	159	166	174	182	189	197	204	212	219	227	235	242	250	257	265
74	148	155	163	171	179	186	194	202	210	218	225	233	241	249	256	264	272
75	152	160	168	176	184	192	200	208	216	224	232	240	248	256	264	272	279
76	156	164	172	180	189	197	205	213	221	230	238	246	254	263	271	279	287

BMI \ Height (inches)	36	37	38	39	40	41	42	43	44	45	46	47	48	49	50	51	52	53	54
58	172	177	181	186	191	196	201	205	210	215	220	224	229	234	239	244	248	253	258
59	178	183	188	193	198	203	208	212	217	222	227	232	237	242	247	252	257	262	267
60	184	189	194	199	204	209	215	220	225	230	235	240	245	250	255	261	266	271	276
61	190	195	201	206	211	217	222	227	232	238	243	248	254	259	264	269	275	280	285
62	196	202	207	213	218	224	229	235	240	246	251	256	262	267	273	278	284	289	295
63	203	208	214	220	225	231	237	242	248	254	259	265	270	278	282	287	293	299	304
64	209	215	221	227	232	238	244	250	256	262	267	273	279	285	291	296	302	308	314
65	216	222	228	234	240	246	252	258	264	270	276	282	288	294	300	306	312	318	324
66	223	229	235	241	247	253	260	266	272	278	284	291	297	303	309	315	322	328	334
67	230	236	242	249	255	261	268	274	280	287	293	299	306	312	319	325	331	338	344
68	236	243	249	256	262	269	276	282	289	295	302	308	315	322	328	335	341	348	354
69	243	250	257	263	270	277	284	291	297	304	311	318	324	331	338	345	351	358	365
70	250	257	264	271	278	285	292	299	306	313	320	327	334	341	348	355	362	369	376
71	257	265	272	279	286	293	301	308	315	322	329	338	343	351	358	365	372	379	386
72	265	272	279	287	294	302	309	316	324	331	338	346	353	361	368	375	383	390	397
73	272	280	288	295	302	310	318	325	333	340	348	355	363	371	378	386	393	401	408
74	280	287	295	303	311	319	326	334	342	350	358	365	373	381	389	396	404	412	420
75	287	295	303	311	319	327	335	343	351	359	367	375	383	391	399	407	415	423	431
76	295	304	312	320	328	336	344	353	361	369	377	385	394	402	410	418	426	435	443

Abbreviations: BMI = body mass index.

Rakel and Bope: *Conn's Current Therapy 2006.*

([weight in kg]/[height in m]²). Waist circumference should be measured (at the end of normal expiration) around the abdomen at the level of the iliac crest. The importance of measuring and documenting waist circumference in patients with a BMI <35 kg/m² is because of the independent contribution of visceral fat to the development of co-morbid diseases (Table 2). BMI is used to define weight status with healthy weight BMI 18.5 to 24.9, overweight BMI 25.0 to 29.9, and obesity BMI more than 30 (Table 3). Obesity can be further classified as classes I, II, and III.

Therapies

The goals of obesity treatment are to:

- Stop the weight gain
- Reduce body weight
- Maintain a long-term lower body weight
- Improve obesity-related, co-morbid conditions and reduce the risk of future illness

The choice of treatment modalities is determined by the patient's risk status (defined previously), abilities and desires, and available resources. Table 3 provides a guide to selecting treatments based on the BMI category. The initial target goal of weight loss is to decrease body weight by approximately 10% of baseline weight over 6 months of therapy. Lifestyle management is used throughout the treatment continuum whereas pharmacotherapy and surgery are used as adjunctive modalities in accordance to increasing BMI levels. To provide guidance to the primary care practitioner and evidence for the effects of treatment, the National Heart, Lung, and Blood Institute (NHLBI) published the *Clinical Guidelines on the Identification, Evaluation, and Treatment of Overweight and Obesity in Adults* in 1998. *The Practical Guide to the Identification, Evaluation, and Treatment of Overweight and Obesity in Adults* was subsequently developed cooperatively by the NHLBI and North American Association for the Study of Obesity (NAASO) and published in 2001. In 2003, as part of their Roadmaps for Clinical Practice series, the American Medical Association (AMA) published *Assessment and Management of Adult Obesity: A Primer for Physicians*. These guidelines recommend proactive obesity care in the primary care setting, beginning with identification, classification, and categorization of risk.

LIFESTYLE MANAGEMENT

Because obesity is fundamentally a disease of energy imbalance, all patients must be counseled on the practical aspects of energy-in (dietary calories), energy-out (basal metabolic rate and physical activity), and how to incorporate this information into their daily life (behavior therapy). The NHLBI *Practical Guide* recommends that caloric intake should be reduced by 500 to 1000 kcal per day from the current level. This will result in a weight loss of approximately 1 to 2 lb per week. There is little value in calculating the patient's current dietary caloric intake because dietary records and the recall method are typically inaccurate. Rather the focus should be on where and how the patient will reduce daily calories. Similarly, a discussion of where and how the patient will increase physical activity to accumulate 30 minutes or more on most, if not all days of the week, should be the focus of counseling. In practice, it is more therapeutic to emphasize what patients should eat, drink, or do more often rather than admonishing them on what they should limit, avoid, or restrict. For example, simple targeted messages to drink more water, participate in moderate physical activity for 30 minutes per day, select leaner cuts of meat and skimmed dairy products, and use more healthful cooking methods are positive recommendations. Basic educational handouts reviewed with patients during the visit can be effective tools that reinforce these messages. Such materials are available in the NHLBI and North American Association for the Study of Obesity (NAASO) publications.

Diet

In 2005 the U.S. Department of Agriculture (USDA) revised its *Dietary Guidelines for Americans* based on

TABLE 2 Classification of Weight Status and Risk of Disease

| | | Risk of disease* | |
		Waist circumference†	Waist circumference†
		35″ or less (women)	More than 35″ (women)
		40″ or less (men)	More than 40″ (men)
Underweight	BMI <18.5		
Healthy weight	BMI 18.5-24.9		
Overweight	BMI 25.0-29.9	Increased	High
Class I obesity	BMI 30.0-34.9	High	Very high
Class II obesity	BMI 35.0-39.9	Very high	Very high
Class III (extreme) obesity	BMI 40 or more	Extremely high	Extremely high

*Relative to having a healthy weight and waist size.
†An increased waist circumference may indicate increased disease risk even at a normal weight.
Abbreviation: BMI = body mass index.
Modified from National Heart, Lung, and Blood Institute and National Institute for Diabetes and Digestive and Kidney Diseases: Clinical guidelines on the identification, evaluation, and treatment of overweight and obesity in adults. The Evidence Report. Obes Res 1998;6(Suppl 2):51S-210S.

TABLE 3 A Guide to Selecting Treatment

Treatment	Body mass index				
	25-26.9	*27-29.9*	*30-34.9*	*35-39.9*	*>40*
Diet, exercise, behavior therapy	With co-morbidities	With co-morbidities	+	+	+
Pharmacotherapy		With co-morbidities	+	+	+
Surgery				With co-morbidities	+

From National Heart, Lung, and Blood Institute and North American Association for the Study of Obesity: Practical guide on the identification, evaluation, and treatment of overweight and obesity in adults (NIH Publication No. 00-4084). Bethesda, Md, National Institutes of Health, 2000.

current evidence-based science. The guidelines, which focus on health promotion and risk reduction, can be applied to treatment of the overweight and obese patient as well keeping in mind the need for total caloric reduction. The dietary recommendations include maintaining a diet rich in whole grains, fruits, vegetables, and dietary fiber, consuming two servings (8 oz) of fish high in omega 3 fatty acids per week, decreasing sodium to less than 2300 mg per day, consuming 3 cups of milk (or equivalent low-fat or fat-free dairy products) per day, limiting cholesterol to less than 300 mg per day, and keeping total fat between 20% and 35% of daily calories and saturated fats to less than 10% of daily calories. The revised *Dietary Reference Intakes for Macronutrients* released by the Institute of Medicine recommends an adult diet where 45% to 65% of calories come from carbohydrates, 20% to 35% come from fat, and 10% to 35% come from protein. The guidelines also recommend daily fiber intake of 38 g (men) and 25 g (women) for persons older than 50 years and 30 g (men) and 21 g (women) for those younger than 50 years.

A current area of intense controversy is the use of low-carbohydrate diets for weight loss. Although the public and media tend to lump all of the low carbohydrate popular diets into one category, they actually represent a continuum of carbohydrate percentage levels and differ slightly in theory. As previously discussed, the Institute of Medicine recommends a diet in which 45% to 65% of calories come from carbohydrates. In contrast, most of the popular low-carbohydrate diets (South Beach, Zone, and Sugar Busters!) recommend a carbohydrate level of approximately 40% to 46%. The Atkins diet is 5% to 15% carbohydrate depending on the phase of the diet. Atkins believes that all carbohydrates are the primary cause of obesity and insulin resistance, whereas the other lower carbohydrate diets place a greater emphasis on choosing low glycemic index foods to reduce dietary insulin response.

Until recently the theories and arguments of popular lower-carbohydrate diet books have relied on poorly controlled, non–peer-reviewed studies and anecdotes. In recent years, several randomized, controlled trials have demonstrated greater weight loss at 6 months with improvement in coronary heart disease risk factors, including an increase in HDL cholesterol and a decrease in triglyceride levels. However, weight loss between groups did not remain statistically significant at 1 year.

A study that enrolled patients with diabetes and the metabolic syndrome showed relative improvements in glycemic control, insulin sensitivity, and dyslipidemia in those subjects randomized to the lower-carbohydrate diet. Because lower-carbohydrate diets are just now being scrutinized with greater scientific vigor, it is premature to make definitive conclusions regarding their role in the treatment of obesity and/or metabolic syndrome. However, conclusions from two comprehensive reviews are pertinent. The executive summary of a USDA conference on popular diets concluded that diets that reduce caloric intake result in weight loss *regardless* of macronutrient composition. A systemic review by Bravata and colleagues concluded that there is insufficient evidence to make recommendations for or against the use of low-carbohydrate diets and that participant weight loss was principally associated with decreased caloric intake and increased diet duration but not with reduced carbohydrate content.

Another dietary approach to consider is the concept of energy density. Dietary studies have demonstrated that people tend to ingest a constant volume of food, regardless of caloric or macronutrient content. The energy density approach to weight loss comes from this observation. Energy density refers to the number of calories (energy) a food contains per unit of weight. This value is affected by the water, macronutrient (fat, carbohydrate, and protein) and fiber content of the food. The theory holds that a smaller number of calories can be consumed for a given weight of food if the food is low in energy density. Adding water or fiber to a food decreases its energy density by increasing weight without affecting caloric content. Examples of foods with low-energy density include soups, fruits, vegetables, oatmeal, and lean meats. Dry and high fat foods such as pretzels, cheese, egg yolks, potato chips, and red meat have a high energy density. Studies on the topic suggest that diets containing low-energy dense foods control hunger and result in decreased caloric intake and weight loss.

Physical Activity

Increasing one's level of physical activity can be challenging. Overweight patients are often intimidated by or fearful of exercise. A simple walking regimen is a safe and usually well-tolerated way patients can begin to increase their activity. Progress can be monitored by using a pedometer to record number of steps walked per day. Depending on stride length, 10,000 steps is equivalent to approximately 3.5 to 5 miles. Using the pedometer, patients should assess their baseline activity level and then increase the distance walked by a small amount each week. Providing patients with distance goals or physical activity "prescriptions" are often effective motivational tools. It is also important to emphasize the value of both aerobic and resistance strength training, because the latter will maintain or enlarge muscle mass during weight loss and sustain a higher basal metabolic rate.

Many patients require more rigorous lifestyle education. Referral to a registered dietitian or exercise physiologist for further instruction can be an important key to success. Additional caveats of successful lifestyle counseling include the following:

- Aim for progress, not perfection. The patient's diet may need small changes, not a total makeover.
- It doesn't have to be all or nothing. All foods can be enjoyed in moderation and all physical activity counts.
- Have patients plan ahead. Thinking about what they are going to eat and do keeps them in control.
- Tailor your message to the patient. It should be straightforward, relevant, and action-oriented.

Cognitive behavior therapy (CBT) incorporates various strategies intended to help change and reinforce new dietary and physical activity behaviors. Strategies include self-monitoring techniques (e.g., journaling, weighing and measuring food, and activity), stress management, stimulus control (e.g., using smaller plates, not eating in front of the television or in the car), social support, problem solving, and cognitive restructuring such as helping patients develop more positive and realistic thoughts about themselves. These techniques can be learned and used by primary care physicians, but they do take time. Nonetheless, a few key behavioral principles should be used when possible. When recommending any behavioral lifestyle change, have the patient identify what, when, where and how the behavioral change will be performed, have the patient and yourself keep a record of the anticipated behavioral change, and follow-up progress at the next office visit.

Using Lifestyle Patterns as an Approach for Counseling

By allowing the patient an opportunity to describe personal eating, exercising, and coping habits; attitudes; and behaviors, recognizable patterns often emerge that can be used diagnostically and therapeutically. Although commonly used in other areas of medicine, it has not been previously applied to the management of obesity. Using this qualitative-lifestyle-personality-patterns approach, the initial emphasis of treatment is to identify and then provide targeted strategies to improve weight-gaining lifestyle patterns. Common eating patterns are hearty portioning, meal skipping, mindless munching,

and not eating enough fruits or vegetables. Common reasons for inadequate physical activity patterns are hate-to-move, lack of time, aches and pains, and self-consciousness. Common coping patterns are emotional eating, people pleasing, procrastinating, and over-reaching achievement. By tackling one pattern at a time, weight control is more manageable and remains patient-centered. For more information, see Dr. Kushner's *Personality Type Diet*, St. Martin's Griffin Press, 2004.

PHARMACOTHERAPY

Adjuvant pharmacologic treatments should be considered for patients with a BMI more than 30 kg/m^2 or with a BMI greater than 27 kg/m^2 who also have concomitant obesity-related risk factors or diseases and for whom dietary and physical activity therapy has not been successful. With the exception of the BMI cut points, these indications are identical to starting cholesterol-lowering agents, antihypertensives, or antidiabetic drugs. Similar to these otwher drugs, the patient must have realistic expectations regarding what the medication can accomplish and how to use it properly. What makes the use of antiobesity drugs different is the *absolute* need to use lifestyle modification as a foundation for drug action because of the importance of a drug-behavior interaction. Whether the antiobesity medication acts centrally to suppress appetite or peripherally to block the absorption of fat, patients must deliberately and consciously alter their behavior for weight loss to occur. In other words, for all antiobesity drugs, the pharmacologic action must be *translated* into behavior change. For anorexiants, a reduced sense of hunger and/or increased satiety must be translated into choosing smaller healthier meals and reduced snacking. Failure to sense and act on these inhibitory internal signals will result in modest or no weight loss. Similarly, if a patient takes an intestinal fat-blocking agent and does not limit the consumption of dietary fat to 30% or less, intolerable side effects will lead to discontinuation of the medicine. Moreover, failure to incorporate physical activity as part of the lifestyle change will seriously hinder maintenance of the initial weight loss. Thus, there is a bidirectional, mutually beneficial relationship between antiobesity drugs and lifestyle management, each therapy enhancing the efficacy of the other. In summary, when an antiobesity drug is prescribed, it must be accompanied by lifestyle counseling.

There are several potential targets of pharmacologic therapy for obesity, all based on the concept of producing a sustained negative energy (calorie) balance. The earliest and most thoroughly explored treatment has been suppression of appetite via centrally active medications that alter monoamine neurotransmitters. A second strategy is to reduce the absorption of selective macronutrients from the gastrointestinal tract, such as fat. These two mechanisms form the basis for all currently prescribed antiobesity agents. Box 2 summarizes the three agents approved for management of obesity, sibutramine (Meridia), orlistat (Xenical), and phentermine.

BOX 2 FDA-Approved Antiobesity Drugs

Sibutramine (Meridia)
- FDA approved 1997
- Acts centrally: anorexiant (SNRI)
- Induces feeling of satiety
- Daily with or without food
- Dosage: 5-, 10-, and 15-mg capsules
- Two years of clinical data

Orlistat (Xenical)
- FDA approved 1999
- Acts peripherally: lipase inhibitor
- Reduces absorption of 30% dietary fat
- Three times daily with meals and a vitamin supplement recommended
- Dosage: 120-mg capsules
- Four years of clinical data

Phentermine (multiple trade names, e.g., Adipex-P)
- FDA approved 1959
- Acts centrally: anorexiant (indirect sympathomimetic)
- Once daily (15 to 37.5 mg)
- Dosage: 15-, 30-, 37.5-mg capsules
- Six months of clinical data

Abbreviation: SNRI = serotonin-norepinephrine reuptake inhibitor.

Centrally Acting Anorexiant Medications

Appetite-suppressing drugs, or anorexiants, affect *satiation*—the processes involved in the termination of a meal, *satiety*—the absence of hunger after eating, and *hunger*—a biologic sensation that initiates eating. By increasing satiation and satiety and decreasing hunger, these agents help patients reduce caloric intake while providing a greater sense of control, more contentment with food intake, and with reduced feelings of deprivation. The target site for the actions of anorexiants is the ventromedial and lateral hypothalamic regions in the central nervous system. Their biologic effect on appetite regulation is produced by variably augmenting the neurotransmission of three monoamines: norepinephrine, serotonin (5-hydroxytryptamine,[5-HT]), and to a lesser degree, dopamine.

Sibutramine (Meridia) functions as a serotonin-norepinephrine reuptake inhibitor (SNRI). Unlike other previously Food and Drug Administration (FDA)-approved anorexiants, sibutramine (Meridia) is not pharmacologically related to amphetamine and has no addictive potential. Sibutramine (Meridia) produces a dose-dependent weight loss (available doses are 5, 10, and 15 mg capsules), with an average loss of approximately 8% of initial body weight at 6 months. The medication has also been demonstrated to be useful in maintenance of weight loss for up to 2 years. Start treatment at 10 mg per day and evaluate patients 4 weeks after therapy is initiated. At that time, dose can be titrated upward to a maximum of 15 mg per day or decreased to 5 mg per day. The most commonly reported adverse effects of sibutramine (Meridia) are headache, dry mouth, insomnia, and constipation. These are generally mild and well tolerated. The principal concern is a dose-related increase in BP and heart rate that may require discontinuation of the medication. A dose of 10 to 15 mg per day causes an average increase in systolic and diastolic blood pressure (DBP) of 2 to 4 mm Hg and an increase in heart rate of 4 to 6 beats per minute. For this reason, all patients should be monitored closely and seen back in the office within 1 month after initiating therapy. The risks of adverse effects on BP are no greater in patients with controlled hypertension than in those who do not have hypertension, and the drug does not appear to cause cardiac valve dysfunction. Absolute contraindications to sibutramine (Meridia) use include uncontrolled hypertension, congestive heart failure (CHF), coronary heart disease, cardiac arrhythmias, seizure disorder, renal impairment, liver disease, and history of stroke. Furthermore, patients on monoamine oxidase inhibitors (MAOIs) and women who are pregnant or breast-feeding should not take sibutramine (Meridia). Concomitant use of medications that increase serotonin effect put patients at risk of the serotonin syndrome. Similar to other antiobesity medications, weight reduction is enhanced when this drug is used along with behavioral therapy, and body weight increases once the medication is discontinued.

Phentermine (Adipex-P), an indirect sympathomimetic, increases release and inhibits reuptake of norepinephrine and dopamine. In use for the treatment of obesity since 1959, phentermine is currently FDA-approved for short-term use only (8 to 12 weeks). Current treatment strategy, however, dictates long-term administration of this medication. There are limited long-term data on the effectiveness of phentermine, and patients should be informed such use is not well studied. A 2002 review of six randomized, controlled trials using phentermine for weight control found that patients lost 0.6 to 6.0 kg of weight over 2 to 24 weeks of treatment. Treatment should start with 15 mg daily dose administered 30 minutes before or 1 to 2 hours after a meal. Medication effect can be evaluated 4 weeks after initiation and dose titrated up to maximum of 37.5 mg per day. Dose-related tolerance tends to occur after several weeks of therapy. When cessation of medication therapy is desired, dosage should be gradually tapered down. Abrupt discontinuation of the drug should be avoided because of potential physiologic dependence with prolonged use. The most common side effects of phentermine are restlessness, insomnia, dry mouth, and constipation. Phentermine can also increase BP and heart rate, so these parameters should be closely monitored. Absolute contraindications to phentermine use include coronary heart disease, history of cardiac arrhythmias, glaucoma, uncontrolled hypertension, hyperthyroidism, pulmonary hypertension, and valvular heart disease. Women should not use this medication while pregnant or breast-feeding, and patients should not take this medication if they are being treated with MAOIs. Phentermine is primarily excreted by the kidneys and should be used with caution in patients with abnormal renal function. Diabetic patients receiving phentermine should also be monitored closely as this drug can have hypoglycemic effects. Primary pulmonary hypertension (PPH) and

8

valvular heart disease have been reported in patients using a combination of phentermine with fenfluramine (Pondimin) or dexfenfluramine (Redux). The possible relationship of these disorders with use of phentermine alone cannot be ruled out. Patients should be closely monitored and medication discontinued if associated symptoms develop (dyspnea, syncope, decreased exercise tolerance, angina pectoris, or lower-extremity edema).

Peripherally Acting Medication

Orlistat (Xenical) is a synthetic hydrogenated derivative of a naturally occurring lipase inhibitor, lipostatin, produced by the mold *Streptomyces toxytricini*. Orlistat (Xenical) is a potent slowly reversible inhibitor of pancreatic, gastric, and carboxylesterase lipases and phospholipase A_2, which are required for the hydrolysis of dietary fat in the gastrointestinal tract into fatty acids and monoacylglycerols. The drug's activity takes place in the lumen of the stomach and small intestine by forming a covalent bond with the active serine residue site of these lipases. Taken at a therapeutic dose of 120 mg three times per day, orlistat (Xenical) blocks the digestion and absorption of approximately 30% of dietary fat. On discontinuation of the drug, fecal fat usually returns to normal concentrations within 48 to 72 hours.

Multiple randomized, 1- to 2-year double-blind, placebo-controlled studies have shown that after 1 year, orlistat (Xenical) produces a weight loss of approximately 9% to 10% compared with a 4% to 6% weight loss in the placebo-treated groups. When categorized by percent weight loss, more subjects randomized to orlistat (Xenical) compared to placebo lost more than 5% (average 55% versus 33%) and more than 10% (average 34% versus 16%) of body weight. Pooled data have also shown that early weight loss (>5% of initial weight after 3 months) predicts weight loss at 24 months. Another recent randomized placebo-controlled trial demonstrated that orlistat (Xenical) results in sustained weight loss at 4 years (5.8 kg versus 3.0 kg with placebo). Orlistat (Xenical) (120 mg) is administered three times per day with meals or up to 1 hour after a meal. Higher doses do not increase weight loss. Because orlistat (Xenical) is minimally (<1%) absorbed from the gastrointestinal tract, it has no systemic side effects. Tolerability to the drug is related to the malabsorption of dietary fat and subsequent passage of fat in the feces. Six gastrointestinal tract adverse effects have been reported to occur in at least 10% of orlistat (Xenical)-treated patients; oily spotting, flatus with discharge, fecal urgency, fatty/oily stool, oily evacuation, and increased defecation. The events are generally experienced early, diminish as patients moderate their dietary fat intake, and infrequently cause patients to withdraw from clinical trials. It has recently been shown that psyllium hydrophilic mucilloid is helpful in controlling the orlistat (Xenical)-induced gastrointestinal (GI) side effects when taken concomitantly with the medication.

Serum concentrations of the fat-soluble vitamins D and E and beta-carotene have been found to be significantly lower in some of the trials although generally remain within normal ranges. The manufacturer's package insert for orlistat (Xenical) recommends that patients take a vitamin supplement 2 hours before or after orlistat (Xenical) dose; to prevent potential deficiencies, orlistat (Xenical) is contraindicated in patients with cholestasis and malabsorptive syndromes and in women who are pregnant or breast-feeding. Orlistat (Xenical) can affect blood levels of cyclosporine and amiodarone, so patients on these medications should be closely monitored. International normalized ratio (INR) values should be followed closely in patients on warfarin during the first month of treatment with orlistat (Xenical) because it can decrease vitamin K levels. One additional caveat regarding orlistat (Xenical) is necessary. There are four sources of calories in the diet: fat, carbohydrate, protein, and alcohol. Orlistat (Xenical) partially blocks the absorption of only one of these sources. If patients increase the consumption of nonfat foods in place of the fatty foods they have to eliminate, they may actually increase total caloric intake and gain weight. Thus, attention to the whole diet, including reduction of total calories, must be carefully maintained for the medication to be effective.

SURGERY

Bariatric surgery can be considered for patients with severe obesity (BMI >40 kg/m^2) or those with moderate obesity (BMI >35 kg/m^2) associated with a serious medical condition. Two commonly performed operative approaches, the vertical banded gastroplasty (VBG) and Roux-en-Y gastric bypass (RYGB), limit the storage capacity of the stomach to 30 to 50 cm and reduce the pouch-emptying rate by creation of a 10-mm diameter anastomotic gastrointestinal stoma. These two gastric restrictive surgeries significantly reduce the total volume and rate at which food can be consumed. These procedures are generally effective in producing an average weight loss of approximately 30% to 35% of total body weight that is maintained in nearly 60% of patients at 5 years. In general, mean weight loss is greater after the RYGB operation than after the VBG. This is thought to be due, in part, to alteration of the gastrointestinal hormonal response to eating and development of the dumping syndrome. This syndrome represents a constellation of vasomotor and neuroendocrine events that collectively serve as negative reinforcers to the consumption of simple sugars. The syndrome, which is initiated by rapid emptying of food into the jejunum, results in a variety of unpleasant and distressing symptoms including nausea, abdominal cramping, diarrhea, lightheadedness, tachycardia, flushing, and syncope. Although the symptom-induced intolerance to sugar-containing foods is a powerful incentive after surgery, the dumping syndrome often disappears within 12 to 18 months in many patients. A third restrictive procedure was approved for use in the United States in 2001. In the laparoscopic adjustable silicone gastric banding (LASGB) procedure, a prosthetic band is placed around the upper portion of the stomach. A small gastric pouch is created, thus restricting storage capacity. Band diameter is adjusted by the subcutaneous injection or removal

CURRENT DIAGNOSIS

- Obtain medical, weight, and family/social histories.
- Measure BMI and waist circumference to ascertain risk.
- Screen for common obesity-related, co-morbid conditions (check BP, fasting glucose, lipid risk panel)
- Assess patient's readiness to make lifestyle changes

Abbreviations: BMI = body mass index; BP = blood pressure.

CURRENT THERAPY

- Recommend for diet: Well-balanced, calorie-restricted diet containing 45% to 65% carbohydrates, 10% to 35% protein, 20% to 35% fat, and daily fiber intake of at least 25 g/d.
- Accumulate at least 30 min/d of moderate physical activity.
- Consider pharmacotherapy for patients with BMI more than 30 or more than 27 and co-morbidities.
- Consider surgical therapy for patients with BMI more than 40 or more than 35 and co-morbidities.

Abbreviations: BMI = body mass index.

of saline solution in the band reservoir. Adjustment affects gastric outlet size and consequently volume and rate at which food can be consumed. Weight loss as a result of the LASGB is usually less than that with RYGB but the procedure is often preferred because it is less invasive, reversible, and associated with a more rapid recovery time than the RYGB or VBG surgeries.

If surgery is considered, the patient should be evaluated by a multidisciplinary team that incorporates medical, nutritional, and psychological care. Many surgeons are now performing these procedures using a laparoscopic approach, thus minimizing hospital stay and time of recovery. Significant and rapid improvement in diabetes control, sleep apnea, hypertension, gastroesophageal reflux disease, urinary incontinence, and osteoarthritis among others, are typically seen following surgery. The most common surgical complications include stomal stenosis or marginal ulcers (occurring in 5% to 15% of patients) that present as prolonged nausea and vomiting after eating or inability to advance the diet to solid foods. These complications are typically treated by endoscopic balloon dilatation and acid suppression therapy, respectively. Abdominal and incisional hernias (occurring in approximately 30% of patients) necessitate an operative repair, the timing of which is determined by symptoms and stabilization of body weight. For patients who undergo a VBG or LASGB, there are no intestinal absorptive abnormalities other than mechanical reduction in gastric size and outflow. Therefore, selective deficiencies uncommonly occur unless eating habits remain restrictive and unbalanced. In contrast the RYGB procedure produces a predictable increased risk for micronutrient deficiencies of vitamin B_{12}, iron, folate, and calcium based on surgical anatomical changes. The patients require lifelong supplementation with these micronutrients.

SPECIAL POPULATIONS: THE ELDERLY OBESE PATIENT

Age alone should not preclude evaluation and treatment for obesity. However, there are changing needs among the elderly that require special attention. In general, the BMI classification chart in Table 1 can be used to identify risk for the elderly patient with additional attention to muscle mass and muscle function. Aging is

associated with a small gradual loss in weight and height that is associated with reduction in BMI. Most importantly, skeletal muscle mass declines while fat accumulates in the abdominal (visceral) area. These changes respectively may lead to functional decline in daily and vigorous activities and risk of developing the metabolic syndrome. Although the relative risk (RR) between obesity and mortality declines with age, the absolute risk increases. Functional decline is particularly seen among the elderly obese when associated with a significant loss of muscle mass, called *sarcopenia*. The primary treatment for this age group is to promote an active lifestyle that includes both resistance strength training and aerobic activities. Studies have shown that approximately two decades worth of age-associated losses in strength and muscle mass can be regained within approximately 2 months of resistance strength training. Even small improvements in physical fitness are associated with a significant lowered risk of death.

LONG-TERM TREATMENT

Obesity is a chronic condition and is rarely cured. Therefore, the physician needs to help patients develop and use strategies that can be used for long-term control. Reinforcing behavioral changes in diet and physical activity and use of antiobesity medications when indicated has been shown to reduce weight regain. Referral to a registered dietitian, exercise specialist or commercial weight-loss program, and use of internet sites for additional guidance and support can also be considered. The physician can be effective in managing the patient with obesity by taking the initiative and providing targeted supportive strategies and skills.

REFERENCES

Arterburn DE, Crane PK, Veenstra DL: The efficacy and safety of sibutramine for weight loss: A systematic review. Arch Intern Med 2004;164:994-1003.

Kushner RF: Roadmaps for clinical practice: Case studies in disease prevention and health promotion-assessment and management of adult obesity: A primer for physicians. Chicago: American Medical Association; 2003. Available at http://www.ama-assn.org/ama/pub/category/10931.html

Kushner RF, Roth JL: Assessment of the obese patient. Endocrinol Metab Clin North Am 2003;32(4):915-934.

8

McTigue KM, Harris R, Hemphill B, et al: Screening and interventions for obesity in adults: Summary of the evidence for the U.S. Preventive Services Task Force. Ann Intern Med 2003;139: 933-949. *Appendix tables available at http://www.annals.org/*

National Heart, Lung, and Blood Institute and North American Association for the Study of Obesity: Practical guide on the identification, evaluation, and treatment of overweight and obesity in adults (NIH Publication No. 00-4084). Bethesda, Md, National Institutes of Health, 2000.

National Heart, Lung, and Blood Institute and National Institute for Diabetes and Digestive and Kidney Diseases: Clinical guidelines on the identification, evaluation, and treatment of overweight and obesity in adults. The Evidence Report. Obes Res 1998;6 (Suppl 2):51S-210S.

Padwal R, Li SK, Lau DCW: Long-term pharmacotherapy for overweight and obesity: A systematic review and meta-analysis of randomized controlled trials. Int J Obes Relat Metab Disord 2003; 27:1437-1446.

Torgerson JS, Hauptman J, Boldrin MN, Sjostrom L: XENical in the prevention of diabetes in obese subjects (XENDOS) study. Diabetes Care 2004;27(1):155-161.

Osteoporosis

Method of
Uriel S. Barzel, MD

Osteoporosis is a condition in which there is a propensity to fracture bones spontaneously or as a result of minimal trauma. In this condition that is present primarily among the aged, there is too little bone tissue to provide adequate skeletal support for the physical stresses of normal daily life and for commonly encountered minor accidents. Osteoporosis is not clinically apparent until the patient presents with a fracture. Its most common manifestation is wrist fracture, but much more disabling are hip fractures and vertebral collapses, all without a history of severe trauma. The destructive effect of this condition is made clear by the statistics of hip fractures, that is, 20% of patients with hip fractures, who number approximately 250,000 annually, die within 1 year of the event; 50% require nursing home care, 20% require help in the activities of daily living, and only 10% return to normal, self-sufficient life in their own homes.

There are some nonspecific radiologic findings associated with this condition, and some patients may be suspected of having osteoporosis as a result of incidental observations made in radiologic procedures. Measurement of bone-mineral density by dual-energy radiograph absorptiometry (DEXA) is the current gold standard for the early recognition of osteoporosis in clinical practice.

Achievement of Maximal Skeletal Growth

The achievement of maximal skeletal development requires the consumption of a normal diet with moderate amounts (4 oz per day) of animal proteins, copious amounts of fruits and vegetables, an adequate intake of vitamin D and calcium, and physical exercise. Vitamin D may be endogenously synthesized through the exposure of the skin to the ultraviolet rays of the sun for a few minutes a day. Vitamin D is available exogenously in cod liver oil, in deep-sea fish, and, in the United States, in nonskim milk that is fortified with vitamin D as well as some fortified fruit juices. It is also widely available singly or in therapeutic vitamin preparations. Recommended daily allowance (RDA) for vitamin D varies with age: It is 200 IU daily for children and adults through 50 years of age, 400 IU daily for adults between 50 and 70 years of age, and 600 IU daily for people older than 70 years of age. RDA for pregnant and for lactating women is 200 IU daily. RDA of calcium is also age dependent: Young children require 500 to 800 mg daily. The requirement increases at maturation, in the teens, to 1300 mg daily. For adults, 20 through 50 years of age, the recommended amount is 1000 mg daily. For adults older than 50 years of age, the recommended amount is 1200 mg daily. In pregnancy or lactation, it is 1000 to 1300 mg daily. Both vitamin D and calcium can be obtained in adequate amounts from the ingestion of nonskim milk—one quart of milk provides 1000 mg of calcium and 400 IU of vitamin D. Calcium is also easily available in multiple over-the-counter products, such as calcium carbonate, calcium citrate, and other calcium salts, and can be taken as a supplement. Maintenance of adequate muscle strength, by the performance of weight-bearing exercises such as walking or calisthenics for 30 to 60 minutes three times weekly, is also useful. Excessive exercise may induce amenorrhea and is, therefore, counterproductive because the cessation of estrogen production in this situation results in a negative calcium balance and decreased skeletal mass.

Maintenance of Skeletal Integrity and Prevention of Osteoporosis

Maintenance of the skeletal integrity, once maximal development has been achieved, requires continuation of the same regimen of normal diet, adequate intake of calcium and vitamin D, and maintenance of an exercise program. Furthermore, it is recommended that cigarette smoking and excessive alcohol consumption be avoided because these are associated with osteoporosis (as well as with other disabilities).

Epidemiologic studies, performed in postmenopausal white women, suggest that taking estrogen early in menopause reduces the risk of osteoporotic fractures by 50%. To eliminate the monthly bleeding associated with cyclic estrogen and progesterone therapy, a combined estrogen plus progesterone formulation, taken continuously, was widely accepted as an alternative hormonal treatment. *This fixed combination, however, was found in a recent large study, the Women's Health Initiative, to have risks that outweigh its benefits. Estrogen therapy alone, given in the same study to hysterectomized women, was also found to have risks that outweigh its benefit. Both studies were stopped prematurely because of these findings.* Soy phytoestrogens have not been shown to be of value in relieving menopausal symptoms or improving bone mineral density (BMD).

Pathogenesis of Osteoporosis

The origin of this condition is multifactorial: Increased bone resorption relative to bone formation is the basic underlying mechanism. In females, an important factor is the menopausal loss of estrogen that is universally associated with an increase in bone resorption without concomitant increase in bone formation (see previous section). Decreased physical activity may be a contributory factor, as well as a diet containing excessive or insufficient animal protein, little or no fruits and vegetables, and inadequate intake of calcium. Another factor is poor intestinal absorption of calcium that is frequently present in people over 60 years of age. In the physiologic process of bone turnover, newly laid bone matrix fails to calcify in the absence of vitamin D, leading to the development of osteomalacia in adults (and rickets in children). Bone densitometry cannot differentiate between osteomalacia and osteoporosis.

In some cases, osteoporosis is the result of an endocrinopathy or some other pathologic process. Hyperadrenocorticism, because of the administration of corticosteroids or abnormal adrenal function, is commonly associated with osteoporosis. Steroid hormones block recruitment of osteoblasts (bone-forming cells) and interfere with the absorption of calcium from the gut, thus interfering with the physiologic process of bone turnover. The failure to absorb calcium in the gut results in secondary hyperparathyroidism and accelerated bone resorption (insuring the maintenance of normal serum calcium). Hyperparathyroidism and excess growth hormone production may also result in osteoporosis. Testosterone-suppression therapy may also cause osteoporosis.

Other far less common causes of osteoporosis include exercise-induced amenorrhea, anorexia nervosa, chronic heparin administration, which stimulates resorption of bone by an unknown mechanism, chronic anemia, and immobilization as in poliomyelitis, paraplegia, or in space flight.

Osteoporosis is most commonly seen in the elderly, especially older women, in whom it is known as *postmenopausal osteoporosis*. In epidemiologic studies, it is more likely to occur in thin white women smokers of northern European extraction, but it is found in all segments of the U.S. population, including men. A large prospective follow-up study revealed that history of hyperthyroidism, history of a seizure disorder, poor general health, weakness of the lower extremities, and poor vision all contribute to the risk of osteoporotic fractures.

Rakel and Bope: *Conn's Current Therapy 2006.*

A specific vitamin D receptor allele may be causally related to the development of osteoporosis. A single recent report ties the blood level of RANKL (receptor activator of nuclear factor κ-B [NF κ-B] ligand) to the risk of osteoporotic fractures: Postmenopausal women, older than 60 years of age, in the low tertile of blood RANKL level had 10 times the risk of osteoporotic fracture, and those in the middle tertile had 4 times the risk of osteoporotic fractures than the women in the tertile with the highest blood level. RANKL blood level was equally, but less dramatically, associated with osteoporotic fractures in younger women and in older as well as younger men.

Differential Diagnosis

In the extreme, the diagnosis would be established when a patient presents with an osteoporotic fracture (Box 1). Wrist fracture (Colles fracture) is the most common presenting condition of osteoporosis, followed in frequency by collapse fractures of spinal vertebrae and hip fractures. In some cases, patients may sustain rib fractures as a result of leaning against a hard surface such as the side of a bathtub. Today, however, bone density (mg/cm^2) is easily measurable by DEXA, which allows us to stratify subjects in terms of likelihood of fractures. People whose bone density is lower than two standard deviations from that of 30-year-old persons of the same age, race, and sex controls (T score < −2.0) are classified as having osteopenia; those with a T score less than −2.5 are classified as having osteoporosis.

In osteopenia and osteoporosis, serum calcium, phosphorus, and alkaline phosphatase are normal, as are blood levels of parathyroid hormone and vitamin D metabolites. Urinary calcium excretion is in the normal range as well. Bones are histologically and biochemically normal. Fractures heal normally.

When patients have low bone density, with or without fractures, they have to be evaluated by history, physical examination, and appropriate laboratory tests for underlying conditions that may be responsible for the development of osteoporosis.

In a sample of 272 consecutive patients, mostly females, with low bone density consistent with osteoporosis,

---

BOX 1   Differential Diagnoses of Osteoporosis

- Osteomalacia
- Hypercalciuria
- Acromegaly
- Hyperparathyroidism
- Hyperthyroidism
- Hyperadrenocorticism
- Celiac disease
- Multiple myeloma
- Prolonged heparin therapy
- Lipid storage disease
- Liver disease
- Chronic anemia
- Testosterone suppression

we found that 17.9% had osteomalacia, 6.7% had hypercalciuria, and approximately 1% of the cases had primary hyperparathyroidism. (We had one case of osteoporosis secondary to heparin therapy.) Women with osteomalacia had low blood levels of 25-hydroxyvitamin D and elevated intact-parathyroid hormone. In some cases of hypercalciuria (24-hour urinary calcium greater than 250 mg), the latter was because of marked excess of salt intake, but in others it was because of renal leak of calcium. Other causes of osteoporosis were not found in our patient population. We concluded that, at the minimum, one must obtain determinations of blood calcium, 25-hydroxyvitamin D, parathyroid hormone (PTH), and a collection of 24-hour urine to determine total calcium and total sodium excretion. (Some physicians use the ratio of urinary calcium to creatinine as a differential diagnostic test. A ratio greater than 0.25 is associated with an increase in bone turnover, and a ratio less than 0.15 is indicative of malabsorption syndromes or disorders of vitamin D metabolism.) Thyroid-stimulating hormone (TSH) screening in the elderly patient may be appropriate.

Prevention and Treatment of Osteoporosis

The major thrust today is the prevention of clinical disease. For this reason, I believe that every woman who enters the menopause should have her bone density determined. If normal, it can be rechecked 5 to 7 years later, after the accelerated loss of bone, secondary to estrogen deficiency, has run its course. If still normal, it is probably reasonable not to be concerned about bone density until 65 years of age.

If bone density is found to be low at either of these two earlier time points, differential diagnostic studies are imperative. If those reveal no abnormality, preventive treatment is undertaken leisurely, because fractures rarely occur before 60 years of age. Thus, at this point, I stress the establishment of proper daily routines, including brisk walking for thirty minutes daily; adequate, but not excessive, animal protein intake; consumption of generous amounts of fruits and vegetables; and taking calcium and vitamin D at the proper RDA levels. In cases of vitamin D deficiency, repletion with vitamin D (Drisdol), 50,000 U weekly or biweekly for 12 weeks, is mandatory. In cases of hypercalciuria, low sodium intake and/or hydrochlorothiazide[1] therapy are in order. In these cases, the appropriate parameters are reexamined, and dosage adjustments made as indicated.

In special situations, medical intervention can prevent the development of osteoporosis. These include certain endocrine conditions, such as hyperadrenocorticism, acromegaly, and thyrotoxicosis, as well as ingestion of excess thyroid hormone, gastrectomy, and liver disease. To the extent possible, endocrine disease should be under optimal control. Patients receiving thyroxin replacement should be given this hormone in amounts that would maintain normal serum free thyroxin and serum TSH levels. Suppression of the serum TSH level

below the normal range should be avoided (except in cases of thyroid cancer in whom this is the therapeutic goal). If patients require pharmacologic doses of corticosteroids as a long-term therapy, bisphosphonate therapy (see the following paragraph) provides significant protection from osteoporosis. Some element of protection of the skeleton is achieved in these cases by the coadministration of pharmacologic doses (50,000 to 100,000 U per week) of vitamin D and an adequate calcium intake. In postgastrectomy states, osteomalacia may develop unless adequate vitamin D is given regularly to overcome a degree of malabsorption that is present in this condition.

In cases with a T score lower than –2.5, I resort to pharmacologic therapy. The available choices include nasal calcitonin (Miacalcin), oral antiresorptives (alendronate [Fosamax], risedronate [Actonel] and ibandronate [Boniva])), oral selective estrogen receptor modulator (SERM) (raloxifene [Evista]), and injection therapy with teriparatide (Fortéo). All but the latter function by limiting bone resorption, thus allowing bone formation to "catch up." Teriparatide, however, achieves its effect by stimulating bone formation.

In newly diagnosed patients with markedly low bone density (T score lower than –4.0), teriparatide is the treatment of choice. It stimulates bone formation and increases connectivity of bone trabeculae. When used in a medically naïve case, bone density can improve by as much as 12% per year. This costly medication is available in prefilled syringes and disposable needles and administered at a dose of 20 μg subcutaneously daily. Instruction has to be provided to patients who inject themselves daily. The Food and Drug Administration (FDA) approved the use of this drug for 18 months. It has a black box, disclosing the fact that there was an increase in osteosarcoma in rats given 3 to 60 times the exposure in humans. When given in conjunction with alendronate, the effectiveness of teriparatide is severely diminished, resulting in only 2% improvement in 1 year.

I use bisphosphonate therapy in cases with less severe osteoporosis (T score between –2.5 and –4.0). Alendronate was the first oral antiresorptive bisphosphonate to be approved by the FDA for treatment of osteoporosis (at a dose of 10 mg per day). Patients are instructed to take it with a large glass of water, remain upright, and take no food or medications for 30 minutes. Bone density improves in the first year by an average of 6% and by less in subsequent years. Some patients reach T scores of –2.0 or better when alendronate is added to the daily regimen of calcium and vitamin D supplementation and diet and exercise as described earlier, and they are able to discontinue the medication and maintain the new bone density on this regimen. The requirement to remain upright and avoid food or medication for 30 minutes daily was considered a hardship by some patients, and they welcomed the 70 mg alendronate formulation designed for once-a-week dosing. There is no evidence in the literature, however, that there is improved compliance with a once-a-week regimen. A major side effect is esophageal or gastrointestinal intolerance.

---

[1]Not FDA approved for this indication.

Rakel and Bope: *Conn's Current Therapy 2006.*

CURRENT DIAGNOSIS

- Serum calcium
- Serum 25-hydroxyvitamin D
- Serum PTH
- Serum TSH
- 24-hour urinary calcium, sodium, and creatinine
- N-telopeptide (second morning urine)*
- Serum osteocalcin*

*These are used as guides to therapy.
Abbreviations: PTH = parathyroid hormone; TSH = thyroid-stimulating hormone.

CURRENT THERAPY

- Adequate intake of animal proteins
- Generous amounts of fruits and vegetables
- Calcium supplements (as per RDA)
- Calcium carbonate
- Calcium citrate malate
- Calcium citrate*
- Adequate vitamin D intake (as per RDA)
- Exercise
- Teriparatide (Forteo)
- Alendronate (Fosamax)
- Risedronate (Actonel)
- Ibandronate (Boniva)
- Raloxifene (Evista)
- Calcitonin (Calcimar)
- Hydrochlorothiazide†
- Low sodium intake†

*Preferred preparation in hypochlorhydria.
†May be useful in controlling hypercalciuria.
Abbreviations: RDA = recommended daily allowance.

I believe that for treatment, adherence to the regimen of taking medication *daily*, physical activity, proper diet, and calcium and vitamin D supplements is mandatory. I do not want my patients to assume that just taking a pill once a week will miraculously cure them. With widespread advertising of once-a-week alendronate to the general public, I find it increasingly difficult to maintain the daily routine that I believe is necessary for therapeutic success. When 5 mg risedronate became available at the same time, I began using this medication daily with equal success. It also has to be taken with a large glass of water, and the patient has to remain upright and take no food or medications for 30 minutes. Its side-effect profile is similar to that of alendronate. There are differences in the rates of improvement of bone density and prevention of fractures between risedronate and alendronate, but I consider them to be essentially equal.

Recently, it was shown that the residence of risedronate in the body is measured in months, whereas that of alendronate is measured in years. This fact has potential importance in patients who fail the antiresorptive therapy and in whom teriparatide is the next best choice. It is theoretically likely that a drug holiday of only a few months would allow teriparatide to reach maximum effect in patients who have been on risedronate, but not on alendronate.

In patients with esophageal or gastrointestinal intolerance to the bisphosphonates, raloxifene (Evista) is the next choice. This SERM, given at a dose of 60 mg daily, has been shown to be effective in improving bone density without having breast- or uterine-stimulating effects. It achieves approximately half the rate of recovery of bone density as that of bisphosphonates, but has no gastrointestinal side effects. Its major side effects are hot flushes and thromboembolism. It is approved for treatment of reduced bone density, osteopenia, but not for established osteoporosis.

Calcitonin, a hormone with significant effect in Paget's disease, has been approved by the FDA for treatment of osteoporosis. Administered at a dose of 50 to 100 IU subcutaneously or intramuscularly daily or every other day, salmon calcitonin does have a salutary effect on bone density, but the studies are too short and contain too few subjects to prove that calcitonin treatment prevents fractures. I have little experience with nasal calcitonin, which replaced the injectable formulation. Its major side effect is nasal mucosal irritation.

Rakel and Bope: *Conn's Current Therapy 2006*.

A recent report identifies the rare earth mineral strontium, in the form of strontium ranelate, as another oral treatment that increases bone formation and reduces spinal fracture in osteoporotic women. It is not yet available commercially in the United States.

Fractures

When presented with a case of apparent osteoporosis and a fracture, we treat the actual fracture and at the same time review the differential diagnoses and initiate a treatment regimen for whatever underlying condition may be responsible for the development of osteoporosis. It must be remembered that patients who have experienced one osteoporotic fracture are at a very high risk for a second fracture. Colles, fracture is treated by casting. Spinal collapse is treated with injection of cement into the vertebra. This stabilizes the involved vertebra, but does not protect the adjacent vertebrae from potential future collapse. Previously, the only available treatment for collapse fracture of vertebrae was complete bed rest until the acute pain substantially diminished (72 hours to 2 weeks), followed by gradual mobilization, first to an inclined chair and later to full upright position and reambulation. Pain treatment in such cases should avoid narcotics, if possible, because of their tendency to produce constipation. A corset may be used for a few weeks to give the spine some support during the period of recovery, to be followed by physiotherapy. Hip fractures generally require surgical pinning or hip replacement, followed by aggressive physiotherapy. In addition to the regimen of diet, calcium plus vitamin D, and weight-bearing physical activity, hip-fracture patients, and those with gait disorders or neurologic diseases that predispose them to falls, may benefit from the wearing of a hip protector during waking hours.

REFERENCES

Barzel US, Aragaki A, Rittenbaugh C, et al: Increased risk of fractures is associated with acidogenic food intake among postmenopausal women enrolled in the observational study of the women's health initiative. (In preparation.)

Cranney A, Guyatt G, Griffith I, et al: Meta-analyses of therapies for postmenopausal osteoporosis. Endocr Rev 2002:23;570-578.

Freitag A, Barzel US: Differential diagnosis of osteoporosis. Gerontology 2002;48:98-102.

Miller PD, Bilezikian JP, Deal C, et al: Clinical use of teriparatide in the real world: Initial insights. Endocr Pract 2004;10:139-148.

Paget's Disease of Bone

Method of
Bart L. Clarke, MD

Paget's disease is a localized disorder of bone remodeling caused by an initial increase in osteoclast-mediated bone resorption, coupled to an increase in osteoblast-mediated bone formation. The increased resorption and formation process results in a disorganized mix of abnormal woven and normal lamellar bone with increased blood vessel flow at affected skeletal sites. Paget's disease is thought to be the second most common disorder affecting bone in the United States.

Epidemiologic surveys have demonstrated Paget's disease to be common in northern Europe, North America, Australia, and New Zealand but uncommon elsewhere. The highest prevalence rates are reported from Lancashire, England, where as many as 6% to 8% of the adult population older than 55 years may have radiographic evidence of the disease. Paget's disease probably affects approximately 3% of the U.S. population older than age 55 years, with most affected individuals having European ancestry.

Paget's disease affects slightly more men than women. The average age of diagnosis is in the fifth to sixth decade, but it may be diagnosed as early as the second decade. Most patients are asymptomatic and diagnosed incidentally on radiographic studies obtained for other purposes, but a small percentage have symptomatic disease.

The pathogenesis of Paget's disease remains unknown. Genetic predisposition to the disease, as reflected by positive family history, is found in as many as 15% to 30% of patients. Analysis of multiple affected families suggests an autosomal dominant pattern of inheritance. Individuals with an affected first-degree relative have been reported to have a sevenfold increased risk of developing the disease. Familial Paget's disease has been linked to a variety of chromosomal loci, including 18q, 6, and 5q. Previous studies showed linkage to HLA-DQW 1, even in patients without a family history of the disease. Linkage studies have shown linkage to chromosome 5q35-QTER in family studies from Quebec and elsewhere.

The gene on 5q35-QTER encodes a ubiquitin-binding protein called sequestasome-1. Sequestasome-1 serves as an anchor protein binding TRAF-6 in the IL-1 signaling pathway, or RIP-1 in the TNF signaling pathway to activate NFκB.

Current evidence suggests that genetically predisposed individuals develop Paget's disease after chronic paramyxoviral infections of their osteoclasts. Viral nucleocapsid antigens have been identified within pagetic osteoclasts from respiratory syncytial virus, measles virus, and canine distemper virus in some patients but not all. Virally infected osteoclasts form multinucleated giant cells rapidly, and cause increased bone resorption in affected skeletal sites. It remains unclear when chronic viral infection occurs, and the factors responsible for osteoclast susceptibility to chronic viral infection also remain unclear.

Clinical Features and Diagnosis

Paget's disease is usually diagnosed incidentally when radiographic studies are performed for other reasons. Few patients present with clinical symptoms and signs of active Paget's disease. Bone involvement may be monostotic or asymmetrically polyostotic. Paget's disease rarely spreads to bones other than those initially involved at diagnosis, but it may progress with bones over time. The most common sites of involvement are the pelvis, femur, spine, skull, and tibia. Bones of the upper extremities, clavicles, scapulae, ribs, and facial bones are less commonly involved.

The most common symptom of Paget's disease is bone pain, which may result from pagetic bone involvement or from degenerative arthritis in joints adjacent to pagetic bone. Pain may be because of microfractures or swelling of the cortices of bone because of advancing lytic lesions and is usually dull, aching, and fairly localized. Pain may occur at rest but is typically made worse with ambulation or activity. Pagetic bone is often swollen or warm because of hypervascularity; some patients perceive the increased warmth as uncomfortable. Weight-bearing bones, especially the femur, tibia or even both, may become deformed, resulting in gait abnormality. Degenerative arthritic changes may occur at joints adjacent to deformity or in joints in the contralateral lower limb.

Back pain may be because of pagetic involvement of vertebrae, vertebral collapse fractures because of coexisting osteoporosis, or spinal stenosis or neural compression. Skull pain may be associated with warmth, tenderness, bandlike headache, or increasing head size with or without frontal bossing or deformity. Hearing impairment may be because of isolated or combined conductive (because of otosclerosis) or neurosensory abnormalities. Nerve palsies may affect cranial nerves II, VI, VII, or others. Platybasia (flattening of the base of the skull) may occur with subsequent basilar invagination, resulting in brain stem compression or obstructive hydrocephalus. Facial bone involvement may result in deformity, dental problems, or rarely, narrowing of the airway.

Pagetic bone fractures more easily than normal bone. Fractures may be traumatic or pathologic, causing considerable blood loss. Long bones with advancing lytic lesions are most susceptible to fracture. Small, stable, asymptomatic partial cortical fractures along the convex surfaces of bowed, lower extremity bones may occasionally extend through the cortex and cause complete fractures. Pagetic fractures typically heal normally.

Late malignant transformation occurs rarely. Patients present with increased pain and swelling of pagetic bone. Sites most commonly affected are the pelvis, femur, and humerus, with lytic lesions superimposed on pagetic bone. Treatment is difficult, with the preferred course being wide local excision of tumor, followed by either chemotherapy or radiation therapy. Survival is usually limited to 1 to 3 years. Patients may also develop benign giant cell tumors in pagetic bone that usually respond well to glucocorticoid therapy.

Patients with newly diagnosed Paget's disease should have a total body bone scan, with roentgenograms of affected bones to document the extent of disease. This will eliminate confusion later regarding new pagetic activity if other bones become symptomatic. Follow-up bone scans or other roentgenograms are generally unnecessary unless the patient develops new or worsening symptoms.

Patients with active Paget's disease typically have increased serum alkaline phosphatase activity, which is a marker of osteoblast function. Because alkaline phosphatase activity may come from sources other than bone, it should always be fractionated during initial evaluation to make sure it is the bone fraction that is increased. Specific assays are now available to measure the bone isozyme. Evaluation of other biochemical markers of bone turnover, such as urinary pyridinoline, deoxypyridinoline, or NTx-telopeptide, is generally not useful unless these markers will be followed during treatment. Serum alkaline phosphatase correlates reasonably well with activity and extent of the disease. Patients having the highest levels of serum alkaline phosphatase often have polyostotic involvement, including the skull. Patients with mildly to moderately increased serum alkaline phosphatase levels may have monostotic involvement or relatively inactive, *burned-out,* Paget's disease. In some cases patients with long-standing, inactive disease or very mild disease may have completely normal serum alkaline phosphatase levels. During effective treatment markers of bone turnover typically decrease by 50% within the first few weeks or months of therapy. Urinary markers such as pyridinoline, deoxypyridinoline, or NTx-telopeptide decrease within days or weeks of therapy, whereas serum alkaline phosphatase decreases more slowly.

Serum calcium is typically normal in Paget's disease except when patients with relatively widespread disease are immobilized, or when Paget's disease and primary hyperparathyroidism coexist. Physiologic hyperparathyroidism may develop in 15% to 20% of Paget's disease patients with normal serum calcium and significantly increased serum alkaline phosphatase levels. Such individuals are advised to maintain an oral calcium intake of at least 1000 mg daily.

Treatment

All agents currently used to treat Paget's disease suppress osteoclast activity. Drugs approved for this indication by the U.S. Food and Drug Administration (FDA) include the very potent oral bisphosphonates alendronate (Fosamax), risedronate (Actonel), tiludronate (Skelid), and etidronate (Didronel). The potent intravenous (IV) bisphosphonate pamidronate (Aredia) is also approved for this indication. Salmon calcitonin (Miacalcin) is approved when given by subcutaneous injection, but not by nasal spray, although this is being used with much less frequency because the oral and IV bisphosphonates were approved.

Major indications for treatment of Paget's disease are relief of bone pain and prevention of fracture or deformity. Asymptomatic individuals generally do not require treatment. Bisphosphonates and subcutaneously injected salmon calcitonin (Miacalcin) are effective in decreasing bone pain and warmth, headache, and low back or hip pain because of pagetic activity. These agents may also improve compressive radiculopathies, slowly progressive brain stem or spinal cord compression, joint pain, and lytic lesions in long bones, thereby preventing pathologic fractures. Bone deformity or hearing loss will generally not improve with treatment, although hearing loss may be slowed. Other indications for treatment remain controversial.

The bisphosphonates are very potent, available both orally and intravenously, less expensive than subcutaneously injected salmon calcitonin (Miacalcin), and usually associated with tolerable side effects. Salmon calcitonin (Miacalcin) is used infrequently now, but it may occasionally relieve bone pain more quickly and decrease bone vascularity prior to surgery effectively. Initial therapy with either type of agent does not preclude use of the other agent at a later time.

BISPHOSPHONATES

Alendronate (Fosamax) is available in 40-mg tablets and is usually taken as one tablet each day for 6 months. Previous randomized, double-blind, placebo-controlled trials in patients with moderate-to-severe Paget's disease, defined as baseline serum alkaline phosphatase at least twice the upper limit of normal, showed alendronate (Fosamax) decreased serum alkaline phosphatase more effectively than etidronate (Didronel) 400 mg a day for 6 months. Approximately 85% of patients improved with alendronate (Fosamax), and the drug was effective regardless of age, gender, ethnicity, prior use of other bisphosphonates, or baseline serum alkaline phosphatase level. No osteomalacia was seen on bone histomorphometry in 33 patients treated with alendronate (Fosamax) for 6 months, and new bone formed had normal lamellar structure, suggesting that patients form new bone of normal quality and strength when treated with alendronate (Fosamax).

Risedronate (Actonel) is available in 30-mg tablets, and is usually taken as one tablet each day for 2 months. Tiludronate (Skelid) is available in 400-mg tablets and is usually taken as one tablet each day for 3 months. Randomized, double-blind, placebo-controlled clinical trials have shown these medications to be effective in treating Paget's disease, with shorter treatment courses than recommended for alendronate (Fosamax).

Etidronate (Didronel) is available in 200- and 400-mg tablets. Etidronate (Didronel) 5 mg/kg per day will usually reduce serum alkaline phosphatase by 50% and improve symptoms in as many as 70% of patients treated for 6 months. The major risk with etidronate (Didronel) is osteomalacia, which may develop if used in higher doses or for longer than 6 months. Osteomalacia presents with increased bone pain or stress fractures at sites of weakened bone.

Several courses of oral bisphosphonate therapy may be required to control symptoms and signs of Paget's disease effectively in many patients. Side effects, other than osteomalacia seen with etidronate (Didronel), include occasional upper gastrointestinal or esophageal distress or diarrhea, which usually resolves by withholding the drug for several days, and short-lived bone pain when first starting therapy, which usually resolves more than several days of continued therapy. Patients who develop a sudden or marked increase in pain while on therapy should temporarily stop the drug and be evaluated for progression of lytic lesions or impending fracture.

Pamidronate (Aredia) is approved in the United States for IV treatment of Paget's disease. A variety of regimens are used. One regimen involves giving 60 mg in 500 mL of normal saline over 2 hours, whereas the FDA-approved regimen gives three daily doses of 30 mg each day. Mild to moderate Paget's disease may respond to a single infusion of 60 or 90 mg, whereas moderate to severe Paget's disease may require several weekly or biweekly infusions over the course of weeks to months. Side effects include low-grade fever, myalgias, or bone pain that typically resolves spontaneously within 48 hours of the infusion. Some patients develop hypocalcemia, hypophosphatemia, hypomagnesemia, or lymphopenia within several days of the infusion. Venous irritation may occur if low fluid volumes are infused or the drug is infused too rapidly. Other IV bisphosphonates are being investigated for use in Paget's disease.

SALMON CALCITONIN (MIACALCIN)

Calcitonin (Miacalcin) is currently available as parenteral synthetic salmon calcitonin (Miacalcin) and synthetic salmon calcitonin intranasal spray (Miacalcin). Salmon calcitonin (Miacalcin) intranasal spray is approved in the United States for treatment of osteoporosis, but not for treatment of Paget's disease.

Parenteral salmon calcitonin (Miacalcin) is available in 2-mL vials containing 200 U/mL. The initial dose given for Paget's disease is usually 100 U (0.5 mL) injected subcutaneously each day, with reduction to 50 U (0.25 mL) each day as symptoms improve. Symptoms usually improve within a few weeks of beginning therapy, with biochemical parameters improving by 3 to 6 months of treatment. Once improvement has occurred, the maintenance dose may be reduced to 50 to 100 U

CURRENT DIAGNOSIS

- Increased serum total and bone alkaline phosphatase
- Characteristic radiographs showing lytic lesions, mixed lesions, or sclerotic lesions
- Bone scan showing monostotic or polyostotic Paget's disease
- Bone biopsy, if necessary, showing woven bone with marrow fibrosis

every other day or three times each week. The initial course of therapy is usually 6 months, although patients with severe involvement may benefit from more prolonged treatment. Despite salmon calcitonin (Miacalcin) being 20 times more potent than human calcitonin in humans, salmon calcitonin (Miacalcin) may lose effectiveness because of down-regulation of calcitonin (Miacalcin) receptors or development of neutralizing antibodies.

Side effects of parenteral salmon calcitonin (Miacalcin) include nausea and/or flushing about the face and neck lasting minutes to hours after the injections, and transient hypocalcemia during the first few months of therapy. Patients may minimize nausea or flushing by taking calcitonin (Miacalcin) at bedtime or with meals, decreasing the dose, or taking an aspirin 30 minutes before doses. The nausea or flushing is not harmful, and patients may develop tolerance to either.

OTHER TREATMENTS

Parenteral plicamycin (mithramycin [Mithracin][1]) has previously been used to treat patients with severe or refractory Paget's disease or individuals with neurologic syndromes requiring immediate relief, usually at 15 to 25 µg/kg over 6 to 8 hours. Doses are repeated every 2 to 3 days as required. Patients with spinal cord compression may have relief with a regimen combining plicamycin (mithramycin [Mithracin][1])and dexamethasone but should undergo surgical decompression if symptoms persist. Side effects include nausea, vomiting, hepatotoxicity, nephrotoxicity, thrombocytopenia, and mild transient hypocalcemia and hypophosphatemia.

Nonspecific treatments used to decrease pain associated with Paget's disease include nonsteroidal antiinflammatory drugs or narcotics. These may be used alone or in combination with specific antipagetic agents, especially to decrease arthritic symptoms. Shoe lifts, canes, or walkers may stabilize or improve gait disturbances. Patients should be advised against prolonged immobilization because of the risk of hypercalcemia.

Orthopedic surgery may stabilize or prevent impending fracture in long bones, and hips and knees affected by pagetic arthritis may be electively replaced. Deformed bone may be straightened with osteotomies. Neurosurgical decompression may relieve spinal cord compression,

---

[1]Not FDA approved for this indication.

CURRENT THERAPY

- Calcium and vitamin D supplementation as age appropriate
- Oral bisphosphonates
  Alendronate (Fosamax) 40 mg each day for 6 months
  Risedronate (Actonel) 30 mg each day for 2 months
  Tiludronate (Skelid) 400 mg each day for 3 months
  Etidronate (Didronel) 400 mg each day for 6 months
- Intravenous bisphosphonates
- Pamidronate (Aredia) 30 mg over 4 hours each day for 3 days
- Subcutaneous calcitonin (Miacalcin) 100 IU each day for 3 to 6 months, followed by 50 IU every other day as needed
- Plicamycin (mithramycin [Mithracin]), 15 to 25 µg/kg intravenously over 6 to 8 hours if needed
- Orthopedic or neurosurgical procedures if needed

neural foraminal syndromes, or basilar skull invagination with neural compromise. All cases of serious neurologic compromise should receive immediate neurologic and neurosurgical consultation.

The patient is often best served by a multidisciplinary approach to treatment. This includes the primary care practitioner and physical therapist, as well as the orthopedic surgeon and neurosurgeon when appropriate. Patients may also benefit from association with other patients with Paget's disease. The Paget Foundation (120 Wall Street, Suite 1602, New York, NY 10005-4001, http://www.paget.org) is an excellent resource of information about diagnosis and treatment of Paget's disease.

REFERENCES

Altman RD, Johnston CC, Khairi MRA, et al: Influence of disodium etidronate on clinical and laboratory manifestations of Paget's disease of bone (osteitis deformans). N Engl J Med 1973;289:1379-1384.
Brown JP, Hosking DJ, Ste-Marie L, et al: Risedronate, a highly effective, short-term oral treatment for Paget's disease: a dose-response study. Calcif Tissue Int 1999;64:93-99.
Cooper C, Dennison E, Schafheutle K, et al: Epidemiology of Paget's disease of bone. Bone 1999;24:3S-5S.
Eekhoff ME, van der Klift M, Kroon HM, et al: Paget's disease of bone in the Netherlands: A population-based radiological and biochemical survey—the Rotterdam Study. J Bone Miner Res 2004;19:566-570.
Good DA, Busfield F, Fletcher BH, et al: Identification of SQSTM1 mutations in familial Paget's disease in Australian pedigrees. Bone 2004;35:277-282.
Hocking LJ, Lucas GJ, Daroszewska A, et al: Novel UBA domain mutations of SQSTM1 in Paget's disease of bone: genotype phenotype correlation, functional analysis, and structural consequences. J Bone Miner Res 2004;19:1122-1127.

Langston AL, Ralston SH: Management of Paget's disease of bone. Rheumatology (Oxford) 2004;43:955-959.
Miller PD, Brown JP, Siris ES, et al: A randomized, double blind comparison of risedronate and etidronate in the treatment of Paget's disease of bone. Paget's Risedronate/Etidronate Study Group. Am J Med 1999;106:513-520.
Reid IR, Davidson JS, Wattie D, et al: Comparative responses of bone turnover markers to bisphosphonate therapy in Paget's disease of bone. Bone 2004;35:224-230.
Roux C, Gennari C, Farrerons J, et al: Comparative, prospective, double-blind, multicenter study of the efficacy of tiludronate and etidronate in the treatment of Paget's disease of bone. Arthritis Rheum 1995;38:851-858.
Siris E, Weinstein RS, Altman R, et al: Comparative study of alendronate vs. etidronate for the treatment of Paget's disease of bone. J Clin Endocrinol Metab 1996;81:961-967.
Walsh JP, Ward LC, Stewart GO, et al: A randomized clinical trial comparing oral alendronate and intravenous pamidronate for the treatment of Paget's disease of bone. Bone 2004;34:747-754.

Total Parenteral Nutrition in Adults

Method of
Gail Cresci, MS, RD, and
Robert Martindale, MD, PhD

The era of parenteral nutrition (PN) began in the 1960s when a technique to access the central venous circulation was demonstrated. Placement of a central venous catheter allows for the delivery of large volumes of hypertonic PN formulations, which are rapidly diluted in the high-flow central vein. Previously, the provision of PN was limited to isotonic or slightly hypertonic solutions infused through a peripheral vein. Limitations of peripheral PN are the need for large fluid volumes to meet the patient's nutritional needs leading to potential fluid overload and frequent loss of peripheral venous access. Extensive knowledge about the provision of total parenteral nutrition (TPN) has evolved over the past 45 years. There is now a multitude of commercial products available for inclusion in TPN formulations such as amino acids, carbohydrates, lipid emulsions, electrolytes, vitamins, minerals, and trace elements.

Indications

Like any invasive therapy, TPN has inherent risks (Table 1). TPN is indicated when nutrient provision via the enteral route is inadequate or not tolerated for periods greater than 7 days, the enteral route should be avoided, or when the enteral route may be detrimental to the disease process. A number of meta-analyses of the use of PN in different patient populations including intensive care, oncology, and surgery have not shown benefit and have generally reported increased complications. Therefore, careful patient selection for TPN is

8

TABLE 1   Indications for Total Parenteral Nutrition

Clinical condition	TPN indicated	Comments
Critical illness	EN preferred; TPN may be necessary during low flow states to supplement enteral feeding; prolonged ileus	PN glutamine shown benefit PN lipids containing n-3 FA, MCT, MUFA beneficial
Acute pancreatitis	EN preferred; TPN as alternative in those without jejunal enteral access, severe ileus; combined with EN when it's not fully tolerated, hemodynamic instability	PN lipids do not exacerbate disease; n-3 FAs, MCT lipids preferred
Hepatic failure	EN preferred; TPN if active GI bleeding, bowel obstruction, hemodynamic instability, supplement to enteral	High BCAA formulations for refractory HE
Renal failure	EN preferred; TPN if enteral contraindicated or needs supplementing	Use of standard amino acid solutions preferred more than those containing low amounts of nonessential amino acids
SBS	TPN initially until patient stable, fluid/electrolyte balance maintained; introduce enteral feeding slowly, monitor for tolerance, wean TPN accordingly	Additional vitamins and trace elements may be required for stool outputs >1 L/d
Enterocutaneous fistula	TPN initially until patient stable, fluid/electrolyte balance maintained; introduce enteral feeding slowly, monitor for tolerance, wean TPN accordingly	Additional vitamins, trace elements, protein, and fluid outputs >500 mL/d

Abbreviations: BCAA = branched-chain amino acid; EN = enteral nutrition; FA = fatty acid; GI = gastrointestinal; HE = hepatic encephalopathy; MCT = medium-chain triglyceride; MUFA = monounsaturated fatty acid; PN = parenteral nutrition; SBS = short bowel syndrome; TPN = total parenteral nutrition.

necessary and should only be considered when the enteral route is not an option.

TPN offers the obvious advantage that a functional gastrointestinal (GI) tract is not required. The parenteral route provides considerable ease in nutrient delivery, and as shown in several recent large series, the nutritional requirements are met more consistently. These *ease of delivery* advantages may be overshadowed by TPN's alleged disadvantages. The adverse effect of TPN on the mucosal barrier and gut-associated lymphoid tissue (GALT) has been extensively investigated. Other adverse effects often associated with TPN are hepatic impairment including steatosis, cholestasis and cholelithiasis, systemic immunosuppression, venous thrombosis, and local complications at the venous access site.

The proposed advantages of enteral nutrition (EN) over parenteral in surgical and critically ill patients are now well described. They include attenuation of the metabolic response to stress, improved nitrogen balance, better glycemic control, increased visceral protein synthesis, increased GI anastomotic strength, and increased collagen deposition. Other benefits of EN include decreased nosocomial infections, enhanced visceral blood flow, increased variety of nutrients available for delivery, and decreased risk of GI bleeding. Many of the proposed physiologic benefits of EN are based on animal studies with limited corroborating human data.

Recommendations for the use and specific indications for TPN are provided by several nutrition societies, including the American Society of Parenteral and Enteral Nutrition. When specialized nutrition support is indicated, TPN should only be used when the GI tract is not functional, cannot be safely accessed, or when adequate nutrients (approximately 60% nutritional needs) are not tolerated by oral diets and/or EN in which a combination of TPN and enteral feeding may

be provided. TPN should be initiated in the aforementioned patients in whom inadequate oral intake is expected over a 7- to 14-day period.

There are several disease states and clinical situations where TPN is preferred over EN because of hemodynamic instability and low visceral blood flow states, inadequate nutrient absorption, or enteral feeding intolerance.

Guidelines for Diseases

CRITICAL ILLNESS

Most critically ill patients exhibit one or more organ system dysfunctions necessitating active medical intervention. The systemic inflammatory response syndrome (SIRS) or sepsis is frequently present in critically ill patients. Metabolic alterations caused by cytokine, neuroendocrine, and hormone changes in response to the metabolic insult result in hypermetabolism, hyperglycemia and insulin resistance, and proteolysis with increased nitrogen losses. Nutrition intervention in these patients is supportive because it can slow the rate of net protein catabolism. Enteral feeding is the preferred route of nutrient delivery in critically ill patients. However, even with best efforts, adequate nutrient provision with enteral feeding is not always tolerated in the critically ill. Also, in early stages of critical care admissions, patients may often be hemodynamically unstable and require vasopressor support for stability, which results in decreased visceral blood flow. Therefore, TPN may be necessary to solely provide nutrient needs or supplement the patient's enteral intake if nutritional goals cannot be safely met after 7 to 10 days of attempts.

Supplementation with a variety of nutrients at pharmacologic doses has been investigated, primarily in trauma and surgical patients. Various TPN amino acid solutions have been reviewed in critically ill patients. Studies of branched-chain amino acid (BCAA)-enriched TPN solutions have not demonstrated a decreased catabolic rate or a reduction in morbidity or mortality. Although there are theoretical reasons for the use of BCAA-enriched solutions in the critical care population, they are not consistently superior to standard amino acid solution. Glutamine is a nonessential amino acid but may be essential in certain clinical settings (i.e., critical illness) because the body is unable to synthesize sufficient amounts. Glutamine[1] is not currently included in parenteral amino acid solutions because of limited solubility (3.5 g/dL) and stability (degradation with heat sterilization and prolonged storage). In the critically ill, decreased complications and hospital length of stay as well as improved survival have been associated with PN glutamine supplementation at doses from 0.26 to 0.57 g/kg per day. Intravenous (IV) lipids should be provided to critically ill patients to prevent essential fatty acid (FA) deficiency. However, because the solutions in the United States are very rich in n-6 FAs, provisions greater than 25% of total calories are associated with inflammation and immunosuppression. Outside the United States various parenteral lipid emulsions are available. Those containing omega-3 FAs, medium-chain triglycerides (MCT), and monounsaturated FAs (MUFAs) have shown beneficial effects such as decreased inflammatory responses and immune function.

ACUTE PANCREATITIS

Most patients with acute pancreatitis have a mild or self-limiting illness that resolves within 5 to 7 days. These patients can usually start with an oral diet within the first 3 days of onset if their pain is diminished, and the pancreatic enzymes have a tendency to return to normal. The patients who should be targeted for aggressive nutrition support are those at risk for developing severe necrotizing pancreatitis or infected pancreatic necrosis. Specific nutritional support depends on the severity of the disease. It is therefore essential to define the patients at risk and assess their nutritional needs throughout the course of the disease. Traditionally TPN was used to avoid stimulation of the exocrine pancreatic secretory response, or *pancreatic rest*. However, recent studies have shown that enteral feeding is superior to TPN in mild to severe necrotizing pancreatitis. EN when compared to TPN was found to attenuate the acute phase response in acute pancreatitis and attenuate disease severity and improve clinical outcome.

TPN is indicated in patients in whom a jejunal feeding tube near or distal to the ligament of Treitz cannot be placed, those with a severe ileus, as a supplement to enteral feeding, or in those who are hemodynamically labile. IV lipids have not been shown to exacerbate the disease and can be provided in the majority of patients with pancreatitis.

---

[1]Not FDA approved for this indication.

HEPATIC FAILURE

The liver plays a central role in metabolism, storage, and distribution of nutrients leading to protein calorie malnutrition and nutritional deficiencies in patients with hepatic failure. The pathophysiology of malnutrition is multifactorial and complex. Dietary restrictions and GI symptoms may limit nutrient intake, fat malabsorption may occur because of altered bile acid production, and total nutrient malabsorption may occur because of medication therapy (lactulose, neomycin). Therefore, the provision of nutritional support to patients with hepatic failure can be a life-saving treatment modality.

Altered amino acid metabolism is the hallmark of liver disease, characterized by low levels of circulating BCAA and elevated levels of aromatic amino acids (AAA). This altered amino acid profile is thought to be responsible for the production of *false neurotransmitters,* resulting in ineffective neurotransmission and the induction of hepatic encephalopathy (HE). Historically, the general recommendation for patients with HE has been to restrict protein intake to avoid excessive ammonia production. However, severe restriction of protein can worsen nutritional deficits and liver function. Trials have demonstrated that patients with hepatic failure can tolerate normal or increased protein intake of up to 70 g per day without exacerbating HE. Special amino acid formulations that are high in BCAA but low in AAA have been considered the alternative for protein intolerance in HE. They were initially administered to correct the abnormal serum amino acid profile and prevent the changes in blood brain barrier transport abnormalities and formation of *false neurotransmitters.* However, several randomized controlled trials of BCAA have not shown major beneficial effects on morbidity and mortality. A recent trial of 174 patients, comparing outcomes after 1 year of dietary supplements of BCAA versus lactalbumin or maltodextrin, showed significantly lower mortality, decreased hospital admission, and shorter hospital stay in the BCAA arm of the study.

PN is generally reserved for patients who cannot receive EN, as in cases of active GI hemorrhage or small bowel obstruction. The use of central PN is preferred over peripheral because less fluid volume is required to provide calories and protein because these patients are often fluid restricted. Parenteral BCAA solutions should be reserved for patients who have refractory HE.

RENAL FAILURE

Renal failure causes a variety of metabolic and clinical abnormalities that can affect a patient's nutritional status. The degree of actual nutritional impairment or risk of its development is dependent on the metabolic stress, the degree and duration of renal failure (acute versus chronic), and the medical intervention for its treatment. The type of medical intervention for treatment of renal failure greatly impacts nutrient delivery and its tolerance. Renal failure patients undergoing dialysis have elevated protein needs compared to those who do not. Often dialysis patients are malnourished because of nutrient restrictions and resultant inadequate consumption of allowed unpalatable foods.

Nutritional support is for those unable to consume adequate nutrients orally. Enteral feeding is preferred over parenteral. TPN is for patients unable to tolerate adequate enteral nutrients or where EN is contraindicated. There are several commercially available parenteral amino acid solutions designed for patients with renal compromise. These products contain predominantly essential amino acids as well as histidine. One product also contains arginine, which is important in the urea cycle, and another contains lower amounts of nonessential amino acids. The essential amino acid solutions for renal failure were based on the principles established for treating patients with chronic renal failure (CRF) with a low-protein diet and an essential amino acid supplement using the concept that the patient can endogenously produce the nonessential amino acids via transamination. Because of underlying differences in the metabolic response between chronic and acute renal failure, essential-only amino acid solutions may not meet protein needs. The benefits of modified amino acid solutions for renal failure over standard amino acids in acute renal failure remain controversial. For most patients with acute renal failure, a standard amino acid solution that contains both essential and nonessential amino acids should be used. In the event where dialysis is not used, protein should be restricted for a short period. Intradialytic TPN has been used as a supplement to protein and calorie intake for malnourished patients receiving maintenance hemodialysis. This therapy has several disadvantages and should be reserved for situations such as gut failure or when access problems exist inhibiting the ability to provide enteral feeding or TPN.

Intestinal Diseases

SHORT BOWEL SYNDROME

Short bowel syndrome (SBS) is secondary to either an anatomic or functional loss of mucosal absorptive surface resulting in malabsorption, and/or maldigestion, diarrhea, and steatorrhea. Although intestinal resection accounts for the majority of SBS cases, mucosal diseases such as Crohn's disease can result in functional SBS. With a normal small bowel length of 300 to 500 cm, symptoms of SBS typically begin when more than 50% of the small intestine is lost. Determinants of disease severity depend on the length of bowel resected or diseased, anatomic location of bowel affected (jejunum, ileum), and the presence or absence of the ileocecal valve.

Following resection, fluid, electrolyte, and nutrient absorption are compromised, and patients frequently become dehydrated. Most patients require TPN for a specific length of time; patients with less than 100 cm of small bowel distal to the ligament of Treitz and without a colon often require TPN indefinitely. Once the patient is stabilized and fluids and electrolytes are balanced, enteral feeding may be introduced. The goal is to maintain stool losses at less than 1 L per day. Often a combination of EN and TPN can be tolerated; early

attempts at enteral feeding are crucial because enteral feeding is trophic to gut mucosa. TPN is reduced gradually as enteral intake is tolerated, diarrhea decreases, and nutritional status is maintained. For patients with distal resections, fat-soluble vitamin supplementation and vitamin B_{12} injections may be required.

ENTEROCUTANEOUS FISTULA

Abdominal operations account for the majority of enterocutaneous fistulas (EF); other predisposing conditions include Crohn's disease, neoplasia, infection, and radiation. Fistulas are classified by their location in the GI tract and by their output (>500 mL per day is high output; <500 mL per day is low output). Early management of extracellular fluid (ECF) is similar to SBS with control of sepsis, drainage of abscesses, aggressive resuscitation by restoring intravascular volume and electrolyte abnormalities. Skin protection and aggressive nutrition support are the next main priorities because these patients are typically malnourished.

Although enteral feeding is the preferred method of nutrient provision, TPN is often provided in the early stages of ECF to promote bowel rest and control fistula output and potential spontaneous fistula closure. The spontaneous closure rate ranges from 30% to 70% depending on EC location, co-morbid factors, and nutritional state. Location of the fistula largely dictates the route of feeding. If at least 100 cm of bowel exists between the ligament of Treitz and the fistula, then enteral feeding should be attempted. Often a combination of TPN and enteral feeding is provided. Patients require additional vitamins, minerals, trace elements, fluids, protein, and electrolytes with high output fistulas.

Administration

ROUTE OF TOTAL PARENTERAL NUTRITION DELIVERY

Central venous access is the preferred route for infusion of TPN because it allows for maximizing nutrient delivery while minimizing volume. Peripherally inserted central catheters (PICCs) are inserted into a peripheral vein and advanced into a central vein. They also are useful for administering long-term home TPN or antibiotics. Peripheral lines are limited to parenteral solutions containing 900 mOsm/L or less, whereas central venous lines are for solutions greater than 900 mOsm/L. Incidence of phlebitis, pain, inflammation, and vessel thrombosis increases dramatically in peripheral veins once solution osmolality exceeds 900 mOsm/L. Other factors that can contribute to phlebitis besides osmolality include insertion site, vein size, duration of insertion, cannular size, material, and colonization. Peripheral lines should be rotated every 48 to 72 hours to prevent thrombosis and phlebitis.

ENERGY REQUIREMENTS

Provision of calories equal to energy expenditure is usually the goal, but under some circumstances hypocaloric

TABLE 2 Commonly Used Predictive Energy Equations

Name of equation	Equation	Explanation of abbreviations
Harris-Benedict equation BEE = kcal/d	BEE(male) = 13.7(W) + 5(H) − 6.8(A) + 66 BEE(female) = 9.6(W) + 1.7(H) − 4.7(A) + 655 Add injury/activity factor to BEE for total energy expenditure (10% to 40% above BEE)	W = weight in kg H = height in cm A = age in years
Penn State equation (for ventilated patients) RMR = kcal/d	RMR = RMR(healthy)(0.85) + V_E(33) + T_{max}(175) − 6433	RMR = BEE via Harris Benedict equation (actual body weight used), V_E = minute ventilation in L/min, T_{max} = maximum body temperature in the previous 24 hours (degrees centigrade)

Ireton-Jones equation EEE = kcal/d	Spontaneous breathing patients:
	  EEE(s) = 629 − 11(A) + 25(W) − 609(O)
	Ventilator-dependent patients:
	  EEE(v) = 1784 − 11(A) + 5(W) + 244(G) + 239(T) + 804(B)
		A = age in years
		W = weight (kg)
		O = presence of obesity; >30% above ideal body weight or BMI >27 (0 = absent, 1 = present)
		G = Gender (0 = female, 1 = male)
		T = Trauma diagnosis (0 = absent, 1 = present)
		B = Burn diagnosis (0 = absent, 1 = present)

General equation	20-35 kcal/kg	

Abbreviations: BEE = basal energy expenditure; EEE = estimated energy expenditure; RMR = resting metabolic rate.

feeding is acceptable or even desirable. Indirect calorimetry remains the *gold standard* method for determining a patients energy needs. However because of many factors (including expense), most facilities do not employ this technology and therefore rely on predictive equations. There are multiple predictive equations for determining energy requirements for patients, many of which have not been validated. Common practice for predicting resting metabolic rate in patients is to calculate healthy resting metabolic rate (often using the Harris-Benedict equations) and then to multiply this rate by a stress factor (Table 2). Total energy needs are then provided to the TPN patient with dextrose, protein, and lipids; the ratios of each depend on the medical situation.

PROTEIN REQUIREMENTS

Protein requirements will vary depending on the patient's metabolic state, wound-healing needs, and organ function (e.g., kidney, liver). In general most TPN patients will require more than the recommended daily allowance (RDA) (0.8 g/kg per day) for protein with limits up to 2.0 g/kg per day at which no further improvement in use occurs (Table 3). Providing amounts greater than this only increases the rate of ureagenesis or accumulates eventually producing additional clinical problems. However, this upper limit may not apply for those with protein-losing conditions such as open wounds, major thermal burns, or high-output EC fistulas. In those with organ dysfunction, the medical therapy dictates how much protein can be provided. Protein calories should be considered into the total energy provision.

NONPROTEIN CALORIES

The remaining energy needs, once protein calories are subtracted, are divided between dextrose and lipids. Box 1 shows a sample TPN calculation. Excessive amounts of

IV lipid are not only proinflammatory but also immunosuppressive as the solutions in the United States are rich in omega-6 FAs. Lipid infusion should comprise 10% to 30% of total calories and is better tolerated when infused over longer time periods (18 to 24 hours). Lipids should be withheld in those with serum triglyceride levels >400 mg/dL. Most patients can tolerate up to 10 days without lipids before concern for essential FA deficiency arises.

Carbohydrate, provided as dextrose, administered in excess can result in hyperglycemia, increased CO_2 production leading to increased ventilatory requirements, and hepatic steatosis. In addition to hyperglycemia, critically ill patients are commonly hyperinsulinemic and exhibit peripheral insulin resistance. Alterations in nutrient metabolism associated with critical illness often result in mobilization of FAs and therefore elevated triglyceride levels. The maximal total glucose oxidation rate in a human is 5 mg/kg per minute, or in a 70-kg human it is 500 g per day. Critical illness and resultant hypermetabolism can account for up to 3 mg/kg per minute endogenous glucose production; providing excessive exogenous glucose during hypermetabolism exacerbates hyperglycemia.

TABLE 3 Protein Requirements

Metabolic state	Recommended amounts
Normal condition, no stress	0.8 g/kg/d
Mild stress	1.0-1.2 g/kg/d
Moderate stress	1.2-1.5 g/kg/d
Severe stress	1.5-2.0 g/kg/d
Renal failure, predialysis	0.6-0.8 g/kg/d
Renal failure, dialysis	1.2-1.5 g/kg/d
Hepatic failure	0.8-1.2[*] g/kg/d

*If high branched-chain amino acid formulation used.

BOX 1   Sample Total Parenteral Nutrition Macronutrient Calculation

- Energy needs: 2000 kcal/d.
- Protein needs: 120 g/d.
- Fluid needs: 2400 mL/d.
- TPN:
    Protein contains 4 kcal/g, so 120 g protein = 480 kcal.
    2000 total kcal − 480 protein kcal = 1520 kcal
        (to provide as nonprotein kcal).
- Lipid: 1520 kcal × 0.25 = 380 kcal.
    Provided as 20% Intralipid: has 2 kcal/mL (380 kcal ÷ 2 kcal/mL) = 190 mL Intralipid.
- Dextrose: 1520 kcal × 0.75 = 1140 kcal.
    Dextrose has 3.4 kcal/g (1140 kcal ÷ 3.4 kcal/g) = 335 g dextrose.
    Volume (using 10% amino acid, and 70% dextrose solutions).
- Protein: 120 g ÷ 0.1 = 1200 mL.
- Dextrose: 335 g ÷ 0.7 = 478 mL.
- Lipid: 190 mL.
- Electrolytes and other additives: approximately 100 mL.
- Total volume = 1968 mL.
- Fluid needs: 430 mL sterile water.

Abbreviations: TPN = total parenteral nutrition.

INITIATION OF TOTAL PARENTERAL NUTRITION

Prior to initiating TPN patients should be adequately resuscitated and serum electrolytes should be normalized. Baseline laboratory values should be obtained (Table 4). Once the macronutrient composition goals have been determined (see Box 1), a formulation may either be provided via a nonstandard prescription, or many institutions may carry a standard TPN solution in which the dextrose and amino acid concentrations are preformulated, and the amount the patient will receive is dependent on the TPN volume provided; lipids can then be provided separately. A standard solution is often adequate for nonstressed patients and may be convenient and cost effective for community-based facilities where the number of TPN patients does not justify maintaining the necessary compounding equipment and staff.

The dextrose concentration in PN should be increased gradually to avoid hyperglycemia and electrolyte abnormalities with initial amounts of 100 to 150 g dextrose per day. It is imperative to take all dextrose-containing solutions into account when calculating daily carbohydrate intake. When serum glucose levels are controlled, preferably between 80 to 150 mg/dL, the dextrose concentration may be increased toward the goal. Calculated protein and lipid requirements can be provided at goal amounts initially. Electrolytes should be provided daily based on individual requirements (Table 5) and adjusted according to laboratory values. Vitamins and trace elements should be provided daily unless contraindicated based on medical condition.

METABOLIC COMPLICATIONS

Metabolic complications related to macronutrient and micronutrient composition of PN can be minimized by following published guidelines as well as fastidious monitoring.

HYPERVOLEMIA

Hypervolemia is more common in critically ill patients than hypovolemia because of fluid overload from increased vascular permeability associated with the SIRS. Hence, TPN volume restriction to as low as 1 L per day is sometimes necessary. Other patients at risk of hypervolemia include the elderly, and those with cardiac, renal, pulmonary, and hepatic failure. Using concentrated macronutrient substrates (15% amino acids, 70% dextrose, 30% lipid) with no additional sterile water allows for maximizing nutrient delivery while minimizing volume.

HYPERGLYCEMIA

Hyperglycemia is extremely common in the critical care setting. Causes include overly rapid advancement of dextrose delivery in the face of underlying metabolic stress, infection, sepsis, and diabetes mellitus. These high-risk patients should have capillary glucose measurements taken three to four times daily with a sliding

---

TABLE 4   Laboratory Values and Recommended Monitoring

	Baseline	Daily	Biweekly
CBC	X	X	
Basic metabolic panel (Na, K, Cl, CO$_2$, Ca, BUN, Cr)	X	X	
PO$_4$, Mg^{2+}	X	X	
Liver function tests (AST, ALT, ALK PHOS, T bili, D bili)			X
Visceral proteins (albumin, prealbumin)			X
Serum triglycerides			X

Abbreviations: ALK PHOS = alkaline phosphatase; ALT = alanine aminotransferase; AST = aspartate aminotransferase; BUN = blood urea nitrogen; Ca = calcium; CBC = complete blood count; Cl = chloride; CO$_2$ = carbon dioxide; Cr = chromium; D bili = direct bilirubin; K = potassium; Na = sodium; T bili = total bilirubin.

TABLE 5   Electrolyte Requirements for Adults

Substrate	Usual dose	Range
Sodium	2 mEq/kg/d	0.5-5 mEq/kg/d
Potassium	1 mEq/kg/d	0.5-2 mEq/kg/d
Chloride*	2 mEq/kg/d	0.5-4 mEq/kg/d
Acetate*	1 mEq/kg/d	0.5-2 mEq/kg/d
Calcium	10 mEq/d	5-15 mEq/d
Magnesium	16 mEq/d	8-32 mEq/d
Phosphorus	15 mmol/d	5-30 mmol/d

*Chloride and acetate to maintain acid-base balance.

scale insulin regimen provided with a goal of maintaining blood glucose at 80 to 150 mg/dL. Critically ill patients may require a continuous insulin infusion to maintain optimal blood glucose levels; for those on an insulin infusion, capillary glucose measurements should be hourly with adjustments made in the insulin delivery accordingly. In a large prospective intensive care unit (ICU) study, practising meticulous maintenance of blood glucose levels between 80 and 110 mg/dL resulted in significantly reduced mortality and morbidity. Dextrose concentrations should only be advanced to goal amounts when blood glucose levels are well maintained within desired ranges.

REFEEDING SYNDROME (HYPOKALEMIA, HYPOPHOSPHATEMIA, HYPERMAGNESEMIA)

Refeeding syndrome may result in malnourished patients with the initiation of aggressive specialized nutrition support as a result of the body's shifting from using stored body fat for energy to carbohydrates; it is a potentially lethal condition. As blood glucose levels rise, serum insulin levels also increase causing the intracellular movement of electrolytes from the systemic circulation. Circulating levels of potassium, phosphorus, and magnesium subsequently are reduced. Refeeding is associated with sodium retention and expansion of the extracellular space resulting in weight gain, thereby leading to an increase in cardiovascular demands. Fluid shifts can result in cardiac failure, dehydration or fluid overload, hypotension, prerenal failure, and sudden death. Patients at risk for developing refeeding syndrome include malnourished individuals, especially patients with an unexplained weight loss of more than 10% in <6 months, and critically ill patients who haven't been fed for 7 to 10 days. Overzealous feeding with specialized nutrition support should be avoided. Prior to initiating specialized nutrition support, electrolyte and mineral abnormalities should be corrected and fluid status adequately resuscitated. TPN dextrose should also be advanced slowly with patients monitored closely for signs of heart failure. Serum electrolytes, mineral, and glucose levels (e.g., potassium, magnesium, phosphorus) in addition to fluid status should be monitored closely for several days to allow for repletion of suboptimal

CURRENT DIAGNOSIS

- Obtain medical and surgical history.
- Obtain nutrition history, daily intake and output.
- Obtain pertinent laboratory parameters.
- Obtain current medications and fluids.
- Obtain height, actual body weight, and usual body weight.
- Obtain current interventions (e.g., mechanical ventilation, dialysis).
- Evaluate current access sites (e.g., central versus peripheral venous access).

levels, control of blood glucose should hyperglycemia occur, and restoration of fluid balance as needed.

LIVER DYSFUNCTION

Hepatic complications can occur if the patient is being overfed or receiving more carbohydrate than the liver can oxidize. Alterations in hepatic enzymes may not be seen for two to three weeks, but liver enzymes should be monitored on a weekly basis. Elevation of the serum transaminases and alkaline phosphatase can be seen within 1 week, whereas an increase in bilirubin usually occurs later. If elevations do occur, all etiologies of hepatic inflammation/dysfunction should be investigated before assuming PN is the culprit. PN administration has been associated with cholestasis, fatty changes, portal inflammation or triaditis, bile duct proliferation, and fibrosis. In the case of biliary sludge formation, providing some enteral feeding, particularly long-chain FAs, in combination with TPN may be beneficial to stimulate bile flow.

INFECTIOUS COMPLICATIONS

Many infections are related to the central venous catheter (CVC) with the incidence ranging from 3% to 20% in hospitalized patients. Rates are 2 to 5 times higher in the critically ill patient. Bacterial systemic infections related to the catheter occur in 3% to 7% of CVCs. Risk factors influencing sepsis include patient characteristics, therapy, catheter properties, and maintenance procedures. Because the glucose content in central PN is a good medium for bacterial growth, it is recommended that whenever possible, TPN be administered through a dedicated port of a central line that has not been used

CURRENT THERAPY

- Evaluate need for PN:
  Enteral feeding not indicated.
  Enteral nutrient provision inadequate (e.g., <60% nutritional needs tolerated for >7 days).
- Perform nutrition assessment:
  Calculate or measure energy requirements.
  Estimate protein requirements.
  Estimate fluid requirements.
- Calculate PN formulation:
  Protein: 1 to 2 g/kg per day (dependent on disease state and medical intervention).
  Dextrose: 40% to 60% kcal per day (2 to 5 mg/kg/min per day).
  Lipid: 10% to 30% kcal per day.
  Electrolytes per needs reflected in laboratory measurements and medical interventions.
  Vitamins, minerals based upon disease state.
  Extra fluid if need to meet fluid needs solely via parenteral feeding.
- Monitor daily clinical status, laboratory values, fluid status, and adjust parenteral formulation as needed.

Abbreviations: PN = parenteral nutrition.

for any other therapy. The maximum hang time for IV fat emulsions recommended by the Centers for Disease Control and Prevention (CDC) is 12 hours. This recommendation was subsequent to reports of increased microbial growth in contaminated IV fat emulsions hung for greater than 12 hours as well as reports of gram-negative sepsis associated with the administration of IV fat emulsion. TPN is associated with an increase in non–catheter-related infections that may be related to overfeeding, hyperglycemia, immunosuppression by n-6 fatty rich IV lipid, missing nutrients (e.g., taurine, choline, glutamine, vitamins, minerals), and nonluminal delivery of nutrients. Therefore to minimize these infections, changes in TPN therapy have been made over the years. Recommended calorie intake is less, more aggressive blood glucose control is becoming standard of therapy, EN is encouraged when possible, new lipid products are being evaluated, and a variety of missing nutrients are being studied for their usefulness in specialized nutrition support.

REFERENCES

ASPEN Board of Directors: Guidelines for the use of parenteral and EN in adult and pediatric patients. JPEN J Parenter Enteral Nutr 2002;26(Suppl):1SA-137SA.

Christensen M: Parenteral nutrition formulations. In Cresci G (ed): Nutrition Support for the Critically Ill: A guide to practice. Boca Raton, Fla, CRC Press, 2005.

Forbes A: Parenteral nutrition: New advances and observations. Curr Opin Gastroenterol 2004;20:114-118.

Pipkin W, Gadacz T: Nutritional considerations for dealing with intestinal disease in the intensive care unit. In Shikora S, Martindale R, Swaitzberg S (eds): Nutritional Considerations in the Intensive Care Unit. Dubuque, Iowa, Kendall/Hunt, 2002, pp 281-283.

Szeszeski E, Benjamin S: Complications of total parenteral nutrition. In Cresci G (ed): Nutrition Support for the Critically Ill: A Guide to Practice. Boca Raton, Fla, CRC Press, 2005.

Parenteral Fluid Therapy for Infants and Children

Method of
Thomas R. Welch, MD

The background behind our contemporary approach to parenteral fluid therapy in children is inextricably intertwined with the history of American pediatrics. The formulae and methods that have been used to calculate fluid requirements developed hand in hand with the evolution of our understanding of the physiology of dehydration.

The most common indication for parenteral fluid therapy originally was overwhelmingly diarrheal dehydration. Although this is still important, many children requiring such therapy today have complex disorders,

multiorgan system failure, parenteral nutrition requirements, and other complicating factors. Nonetheless, the principles underlying our approach today are largely unchanged. In fact, a solid grounding in these principles actually allows a more simplified approach than has classically been taught.

Normal Maintenance Fluid Requirements

The concept of *maintenance fluid therapy* quite simply implies that patients are to be maintained in a net fluid balance of zero: Fluid intake from all sources equals fluid output from all sources. The vast majority of healthy individuals manage to keep themselves in a net zero fluid balance every day, providing their own maintenance fluid therapy.

Parenteral maintenance fluid therapy is necessary when a child is unable to meet these needs orally. This could only occur today in limited situations such as children for whom oral feedings are being withheld awaiting a diagnostic or surgical procedure, children recuperating from surgery whose gastrointestinal tract is unable to tolerate oral feedings, or children unable to feed because of a recent change in neurologic status. Note that *by definition* maintenance fluid therapy does not apply to a child who is dehydrated or otherwise has a deficit, real or functional, in intravascular volume.

COMPONENTS OF NORMAL MAINTENANCE FLUID REQUIREMENTS

Understanding the usual requirements for maintenance fluid *input* requires knowledge of the usual sources of *output*, which generally are only *insensible* water loss from the skin and lung and urinary losses. Although a few additional sources of output exist (and at least one source of metabolic input), these are usually so trivial in magnitude that they may be ignored for purposes of calculating fluid therapy.

Insensible water loss and urine loss are calculated on caloric expenditure. Thus the first step in writing a prescription for maintenance fluid is estimating caloric expenditure. Other systems for calculating fluid therapy may be based on body surface area; surface area, which must be estimated from a nomogram, is only a surrogate for caloric expenditure.

Classic studies in hospitalized children have shown that caloric expenditure can be estimated closely by weight, using the calculation in Table 1. Thus, a 30-kg child is predicted to have a resting caloric expenditure of 1700 kcal per day.

Some factors operating in hospitalized children may raise the actual caloric expenditure above that estimated from body weight. The most obvious of these is the hypermetabolic state associated with fever; a 12% increase in basal caloric expenditure should be allowed for each degree centigrade above 37°C (98.6°F). Thus, if a 30-kg child has a temperature of 40°C (104°F), the estimated caloric expenditure will increase to approximately 2300 kcal per day.

TABLE 1 Estimation of Caloric Expenditure From Body Weight*

Body weight	Caloric expenditure
0 to 10 kg	100 kcal/kg/d
10 to 20 kg	1000 kcal plus 50 kcal/kg/d for weight >10 kg
>20 kg	1500 kcal plus 20 kcal/kg/d for weight >20 kg

*Note that for children with normal renal function who are euvolemic and who have no additional ongoing losses, the daily kcal expenditure translates into an approximation of mL fluid requirement.
Modified from Holiday MA, Segar WE: The maintenance need for water in parenteral fluid therapy. Pediatrics 1957;19:823-832.

Insensible Water Loss

The usual allowance for insensible water loss is 45 mL per 100 kcal, of which approximately one-third (15 mL/ 100 kcal) represents loss of water through expired air and two-thirds (30 mL/100 kcal) through the skin. It should be stressed that both of these represent *electrolyte-free* water; there is no appreciable sodium in insensible water loss. Insensible water loss from the skin is not to be confused with *sweat*. Insensible skin losses are constant evaporative losses of free water. Sweat is an adaptive process by which electrolyte-containing water is actively secreted by glands in the skin. Sweat losses are rarely encountered in hospitalized children today.

Urinary Water Loss

The allowance for urinary water losses is considerably less fixed than that provided for insensible water loss. Within a wide range of physiologic tolerance, the kidney is able to maintain a net zero fluid balance by excreting water taken in excess of daily need. To calculate a safe allowance for urine output, however, it is crucial to appreciate the role of the kidney in excreting solute. Two factors determine the required urine output: the *solute load* requiring excretion and the *urine concentration* at which these solutes are excreted.

Solute load consists of most of the daily intake of the electrolytes, sodium, potassium, and chloride, in addition to urea. The latter, as the ultimate breakdown product of protein metabolism, is more difficult to quantitate precisely, being determined by protein intake, the child's metabolic state, and the intake of nonprotein calories.

Using reasonably conservative assumptions regarding solute load and renal concentrating ability, 55 mL/100 kcal per day is suitable for the component of maintenance fluids related to obligatory urine output. Add to this amount 45 mL/100 kcal per day for insensible water loss, one derives a useful allowance for normal maintenance fluid of 100 mL/100 kcal per day. Because this formula fortuitously equates to 1 kcal/1 mL, the 100-50-20 rule (see Table 1) used to estimate caloric expenditure in kilocalorie per day can also be used to calculate the normal maintenance fluid requirement in milliliters per day.

Rakel and Bope: *Conn's Current Therapy 2006.*

MODIFICATIONS TO NORMAL MAINTENANCE FLUID REQUIREMENTS

By definition, maintenance fluids are provided for children who are euvolemic. The fluid therapy of dehydration, therefore, is *not* maintenance therapy and will be addressed separately in this article.

There are a variety of situations in which the *normal* requirements for maintenance fluid therapy may need to be adjusted. By understanding the physiologic principles on which the normal requirements are derived, it is relatively straightforward to make such adjustments. Note that this approach avoids such shorthand imprecisions as placing a child on *half maintenance* or *twice maintenance* fluid therapy.

Increased Metabolic Rate

Adjustments for the increased metabolic rate of fever were discussed previously. In this situation the estimated daily caloric expenditure is adjusted upward by 12% per degree centigrade. The usual allowance of 100 mL fluid per 100 kcal per day is still employed.

Altered Insensible Water Loss

Several factors may impact the allowance for insensible water loss. Children breathing humidified air, such as in a *croup tent* or on a ventilator, will have a lower volume of lung water loss than the 15 mL/100 kcal usually estimated. Reducing the normal maintenance allowance by this amount (i.e., from 100 to 85 mL/100 kcal/day) is rational in such settings, but the overall impact on fluid balance would be trivial.

Children with burns or other extensive denuding skin lesions have significant evaporative water losses from loss of the skin barrier, contributing to a substantial increase in cutaneous insensible water loss. The fluid therapy of severe burns, especially in the first few days, is complex and beyond the scope of this article. During recuperation, once intravascular volume has been returned and tissue edema reduced, an increase in the allowance for insensible loss beyond the 30 mL/kcal per day is required; the precise amount is directly related to the extent of the burns.

Altered Requirement for Urinary Loss

The allowance for urinary output may also require modification under specific circumstances. The major reason for such modification is a limitation on the kidney's ability to concentrate or dilute the urine. The 55 mL/kcal per day estimated urine allowance is based on the assumption of a normal dietary solute load and that urine concentration is in the range of 280 mOsm/L—easily achievable in virtually any child. Some intrinsic renal disorders (e.g., renal dysplasia, nephrogenic diabetes insipidus), however, may make even that degree of concentration impossible. A child with dysplastic kidneys and a maximal urine osmolality of 140 mOsm/L, for example, would probably become significantly dehydrated if provided normal maintenance fluids at 100 mL/kcal per day. Given that the child's urinary concentration is half that on which the 55 mL/kcal per day estimate is predicated, a more appropriate allowance would be 110 mL/100 kcal per day for urine loss. Adding in the (unchanged) 45 mL/100 kcal per day allowance for insensible water loss, the appropriate total maintenance fluid for this child would be 155 mL/100 kcal per day.

An opposite problem to a concentrating deficit occurs when a child is unable to dilute urine. Assuming that volume contraction has been excluded (in which case the fluid therapy would not be maintenance and isotonic volume resuscitation would be necessary), the most common cause of this would be the syndrome of inappropriate secretion of antidiuretic hormone (SIADH). This is a scenario that must be considered in children receiving parenteral fluids postoperatively and is likely consequent to pain, stress, and neurohormonal factors. Here again measurement of urine osmolality allows appropriate calculation of the allowance for urine output. A child with urine concentration of 540 mOsm/L, for example, would require *half* the usual allowance, which is based on a urine osmolality of approximately 270 mOsm/L. Thus the urine allowance for the child would be 27 mL/100 kcal per day, for a total daily maintenance fluid allowance of 72 mL/100 kcal per day.

Allowance for Other Continuing Losses

In most children requiring maintenance fluid therapy, only urinary and insensible losses need to be replaced. Occasionally, however, a child will have an additional, substantive loss, which needs to be replaced on an ongoing basis. Again, it must be stressed that ongoing replacement of continuing losses should not be confused with restoring accumulated loss; the latter is not maintenance therapy.

One of the most common sources of additional ongoing losses is gastric fluid loss from continuous nasogastric (NG) suction. Failure to replace NG losses can quickly result in metabolic alkalosis from chloride depletion. Ongoing losses such as this can be replaced milliliter for milliliter separate from the rest of the maintenance fluid. Typically, this is recalculated on a per shift basis, with total losses over the past shift replaced during the duration of the next. In very small infants with particularly voluminous losses, the interval for recalculation may need to be shorter than the usual 8- or 12-hour shift.

The content of these replacement fluids is driven by the measured electrolyte content of the fluid being lost. For gastric fluid this is usually approximately 50% isotonic saline. Some losses (chest tube drainage, for example) may contain substantial amounts of protein that, if the losses are substantial, may also need to be replaced.

Normal Maintenance Requirements for Electrolytes

SODIUM

The concept of a fixed daily maintenance requirement for sodium and its accompanying anions is frequently misunderstood. Although growing infants have a slightly positive sodium balance, reflecting net accretion, the fate of virtually all ingested sodium is to be excreted in the urine. Daily dietary intake of sodium virtually always matches urinary losses. Rather than being an essential nutrient, sodium is a ubiquitous accompaniment of most other nutrients, which must then be excreted. Thus, the concept of estimating a daily *requirement* for sodium by calculating the concentration of the element in foodstuffs such as milk is fundamentally flawed.

The frequently quoted daily sodium requirement of 2 to 4 mEq/kg per day actually derived from calculation of the average sodium intake of infants consuming equal caloric volumes of various milks. The relevance of such figures to the provision of brief courses of parenteral fluids to children of varying ages is questionable.

The danger of providing a fixed daily sodium allowance to a child receiving parenteral fluids is that the sodium intake may be considered in isolation from water intake. Consequently, a child whose total daily fluid intake has been restricted but who continues to receive a fixed sodium allowance could actually develop a free water deficit and be unable to excrete the solute load. Although this scenario would be unlikely in providing a brief course of normal maintenance fluid to a child with normal kidneys, it is a real concern in this provision of long-term total parenteral nutrition.

A more rational approach to the provision of sodium in maintenance fluid therapy is to index it to total fluid requirements rather than body weight. Providing parenteral fluid in the form of D_5 {1/4} isotonic saline (0.2% NaCl), ensures the provision of adequate sodium to address the trivial ongoing losses in a healthy child, while providing adequate free water to permit excretion of solute and replace insensible water losses.

POTASSIUM

As is the situation with sodium, there is no true fixed daily requirement for potassium. Children with no preexisting reason to have a potassium deficit (e.g., diarrheal dehydration, diuretic use) require no potassium during brief courses of parenteral maintenance fluid therapy. Children who have risk factors for potassium deficiency may have potassium chloride added to their parenteral fluids to achieve a concentration of 20 mEq/L.

CALCIUM, PHOSPHATE, AND OTHER ELECTROLYTES

Although provision of calcium and phosphate is essential for growing children and is a critical component of total parenteral nutrition, they are generally not provided during the course of normal maintenance fluid therapy. The same applies to trace minerals such as magnesium.

GLUCOSE

Although not an electrolyte, glucose is an important additive in intravenous fluids. It is impossible to provide sufficient calories to meet total daily needs solely by providing glucose in conventional maintenance fluids. Thus, children unable to take sufficient calories orally for more than a few days will require parenteral nutrition—a procedure outside the scope of this article.

Glucose serves two roles when used in normal maintenance fluid therapy. Solutions that are less than isotonic (e.g., {1/4} isotonic saline [0.2%] and {1/2} isotonic saline [0.45%]) can be provided in 5% glucose (D_5). In theory this will minimize the hypotonic lysis of erythrocytes in the immediate vicinity of the infusion if these dilute solutions did not contain glucose; the clinical importance of this is probably minimal. More importantly, the absorbed glucose from this fluid will provide some calorie intake (approximately 20 kcal for each 100 kcal expended, if the foregoing maintenance calculations are used) and may moderate ketosis.

Fluid Therapy for Children With Preexisting Deficits

The foregoing discussion applies to a child who is euvolemic at the time of beginning parenteral fluid therapy. In most hospitalized children requiring parenteral fluids, however, a deficit will be present. This may result from preexisting losses (e.g., diarrhea and vomiting from gastroenteritis), decreased intake (e.g., a febrile infant with an acute respiratory infection that has impaired feedings), or *third space* losses (e.g., movement of fluid out of the vasculature into the interstitial space following surgery). Using the maintenance scheme presented previously in such children would be inappropriate for two reasons. First of all, the rate of fluid administration would be inadequate to replace the deficit and restore circulation. Additionally, the free water provided in normal maintenance fluid is not excreted in states of volume contraction consequent to antidiuretic hormone (ADH) release and increased urinary concentration. This could result in the abrupt development of hyponatremia, which could have devastating neurologic consequences.

Some schemes for the parenteral fluid therapy of children with deficits are predicated on an estimation of the volume of the deficit, and provision of this volume over a fixed period of time; typically 8, 12, or more hours. There are two problems with this approach. First, none of the systems for estimating the volume of a deficit from physical findings has ever been validated

(but a uniform system for grading the *severity* of dehydration has been developed recently—Table 2). Second, if a fluid deficit compromising or potentially compromising circulation is present, there is no physiologic rationale for delaying its repair for several hours. It is for these reasons that the classical *deficit* approach to fluid therapy has recently been questioned.

The initial priority in managing a child with a fluid deficit is securing vascular access. If this cannot be accomplished expeditiously, the intraosseous route can be lifesaving. As this is being done, an objective assessment of the clinical signs of dehydration (see Table 2) should be obtained and recorded, to provide a baseline to assess response to therapy. A blood specimen for electrolyte determination should also be obtained, although initiation of therapy should never be delayed awaiting the results of this.

Once vascular access has been secured, restoration of the circulation with an isotonic solution is the next priority. Either isotonic (normal, 0.9%) saline or lactated Ringer's solution is appropriate. The latter has the advantage of providing some of its anion in the form of lactate. This may attenuate the transient worsening of acidosis that predictably accompanies volume expansion when chloride is the only anion. The usual dose of isotonic fluid is 20 mL/kg, given as rapidly as possible. Both of these solutions are also available with added dextrose, which may be important in small infants at risk for hypoglycemia.

After this initial dose of isotonic fluid, the child's response is assessed by such clinical measures as heart rate, capillary refill, urine output, state of consciousness, and the other measures of dehydration severity outlined in Table 2. Up to three additional such doses of isotonic fluid, to a total of 80 mL/kg, may be given. In most children with diarrheal dehydration, objective measures of circulatory restoration will be evident after this isotonic expansion. If not, careful assessment for confounding issues such as hypoglycemia, sepsis, or cardiac dysfunction may be required, and additional support such as pressors may be necessary.

If the child shows objective improvement after isotonic expansion, the next phase of therapy may be planned. Ideally this therapy can be provided orally. The likelihood of inducing dangerous osmotic shifts is much less when oral rehydration is employed. An oral electrolyte solution is one such option, formula or human milk is another.

TABLE 2 A Scale for the Quantitation of Dehydration Severity*

Characteristic	0	1	2
General appearance	Normal	Thirsty, restless, lethargic, but irritable when touched	Drowsy, limp, cold, sweaty, ± comatose
Eyes	Normal	Slightly sunken	Very sunken
Mucous membranes (tongue)	Moist	Sticky	Dry
Tears	Tears present	Tears decreased	Tears absent

*This scale results in total points ranging from 0 for no clinical evidence of dehydration to 8 for severe dehydration.
Modified from Friedman JN, Goldman RD, Srivastava R, Parkin PC: Development of a clinical dehydration scale for use in children between 1 and 36 months of age. J Pediatr 2004;145:201-207.

Rakel and Bope: *Conn's Current Therapy 2006.*

In the event that oral therapy is not an option, further parenteral fluids will be required, which will be designed to provide for normal maintenance requirements and to address any ongoing losses (e.g., persistent diarrhea). The volume of the maintenance component of therapy can be calculated as outlined above. Keep in mind that the allowance for urinary losses in these calculations was based on fairly dilute urine. In the event that urine is more concentrated than 280 mOsm/L, some of the 55 mL/100 kcal per day allowance for urinary losses will be retained. Thus, any remaining small deficit after the isotonic expansion will be restored with this maintenance fluid. In fact, occasional assessment of urine osmolality provides a measure of the adequacy of therapy. Once an intravascular fluid deficit has been repaired, the osmolality of urine in a child receiving normal maintenance fluids should be <300 mOsm/L. If timely urine osmolality measurements are not available, specific gravity is a useful surrogate, as long as glycosuria or proteinuria are not present (Table 3). Instead of providing maintenance therapy as D_5 {1/4} isotonic saline, it is prudent to provide D_5 {1/2} isotonic saline (0.45% NaCl) as long as urine concentration is >300 mOsm/L to avoid retention of free water and hyponatremia.

The only other modification to provide in this phase of therapy for dehydration is to provide potassium, typically by adding KCl to a final concentration of 20 mEq/L of fluid. This will begin replenishment of potassium lost during the acute phase of the illness.

Modification of Therapy in the Presence of Electrolyte Disturbances

ACID-BASE

Some degree of metabolic acidosis is very typical in diarrheal dehydration. Most often, this is a normal anion gap acidosis, resulting from stool bicarbonate losses. In severe dehydration, however, an elevated anion gap may reflect circulatory compromise and lactic acidosis.

Either type of acidosis will be corrected by the kidney once circulation has been restored. If the initial expansion is performed with isotonic saline, however, there may actually be a transient worsening of acidosis before

---

TABLE 3 Typical Correlations Between Urinary Specific Gravity and Urinary Osmolality*

Urine specific gravity	Urine osmolality
1.010	300 mOsm/L
1.020	600 mOsm/L
1.030	900 mOsm/L

*These approximations are appropriate in the absence of glycosuria and/or proteinuria.

CURRENT DIAGNOSIS

- Assess the child clinically for evidence of fluid deficit.
- Assess the child for coexisting metabolic abnormality: hypernatremia/hyponatremia, acidosis, and so on.
- Determine the extent and composition of any ongoing losses.
- Estimate the child's caloric expenditure.

---

correction occurs. This can usually be avoided if the initial expansion is with lactated Ringer's solution.

Persistence of serious acidosis after circulation and urine output have been restored for over 24 hours is unusual and should prompt further investigation for a complicating factor such as renal dysfunction or sepsis.

SODIUM DISORDERS

Most diarrheal dehydration today is *isotonic*, much as if the serum sodium is normal. Some children with diarrheal dehydration, however, may be *hyponatremic* at presentation. Typically, this results from consumption of low osmolality fluids in the face of the avid renal water retention, which characterizes dehydration. This situation should be viewed as a relative excess of free water rather than a relative deficit of sodium. Typically, once volume has been restored, the stimulus for urine concentration and renal water retention (ADH) is lost and the relative free water excess is excreted. With appropriate volume expansion, urine concentration should then fall and serum sodium rise. The correction of serum sodium is made by the coordinated activity of hypothalamic osmoreceptors, the pituitary, and the kidney. Thus, once the circulation has been restored, the process of correcting hyponatremia is not driven by the fluid therapy prescription but by the child's normal physiologic processes. The thought that the rate of correction of hyponatremia is under the control of the

---

CURRENT THERAPY

- Secure venous access. In urgent situations, if venous access is not easily obtained, immediately secure intraosseous access.
- Provide rapid volume expansion with an isotonic solution in 20 mL/kg increments if the child is assessed as volume depleted.
- Begin maintenance fluid therapy based on the child's estimated caloric needs, as well as any additional ongoing losses when volume depletion is repaired and if oral intake is not feasible.
- Monitor and adjust therapy based on objective changes in clinical status, urine output and concentration, and changes in measured serum chemistries.

Rakel and Bope: *Conn's Current Therapy 2006*.

prescriber of the fluid therapy reflects hubris rather than physiologic reality.

There have been reports of some individuals with severe hyponatremia developing demyelinating central nervous system (CNS) lesions during the course of repair. The bulk of these reports have been in adults, often in the perioperative setting, and usually with rapid movement of serum sodium concentrations to levels above normal. This should not be a concern in children with hyponatremic dehydration treated in the fashion described.

Some children with diarrheal dehydration may be *hypernatremic*. This is a much less common disorder and is unusual. It was more common in an era when the treatment of diarrhea included hyperosmolar liquids such as scalded skimmed milk. Today hypernatremic dehydration is most commonly seen in the context of breast-feeding insufficiency in infants.

The rapid correction of hypernatremia can result in significant osmotic shifts in the CNS and may precipitate cerebral edema. Treatment of hypernatremic dehydration with the protocol outlined above, in which rapid expansion of the circulation with an isotonic solution is the initial step, will avoid this complication. If the child is unable to tolerate oral feedings after isotonic volume expansion, the subsequent maintenance fluid should initially be more concentrated than usual, at least D_5 {1/2} isotonic saline (0.45% NaCl). More frequent reassessments of the serum sodium concentration may be needed to ensure that adequate free water is being provided to allow a correction of the hypernatremia.

REFERENCES

Finberg L: Hypernatremic (hypertonic) dehydration in infants. N Engl J Med 1973;289:196-198.

Friedman JN, Goldman RD, Srivastava R, Parkin PC: Development of a clinical dehydration scale for use in children between 1 and 36 months of age. J Pediatr 2004;145:201-207.

Holliday MA, Segar WE: The maintenance need for water in parenteral fluid therapy. Pediatrics 1957;19:823-832.

Holliday M: The evolution of therapy for dehydration: Should deficit therapy still be taught? Pediatrics 1996;98:171-177.

Winters RW: Maintenance fluid therapy. In Winters RW (ed): The Body Fluids in Pediatrics. Boston, Little, Brown, 1973, pp 113-133.

8

The Endocrine System

Acromegaly

Method of
Mark E. Molitch, MD

Pretreatment Evaluation

Acromegaly is an insidious disorder, usually present for years before the diagnosis is made. It is important to establish the activity of the disease prior to instituting therapy for two reasons:

1. A small percentage of growth hormone (GH)-secreting tumors spontaneously infarct. This causes the condition known as "burned-out" or "fugitive" acromegaly, in which GH levels are normal by the time the diagnosis is made and no therapy is indicated.
2. Tumor activity post-therapy can then be compared with the documented pretherapy to determine whether additional treatment is needed.

The definition of an abnormal basal serum GH level was difficult to ascertain in the past because of the poor sensitivity of GH assays and episodic secretion. Some patients with active acromegaly may have basal GH levels less than 2 µg/mL using conventional radioimmunoassays (RIAs). However, normal GH levels are even lower using immunoradiometric (IRMA) and enzyme-linked immunosorbent assays (ELISAs). Except for the episodic secretory surges, a level of 2 µg/mL may well be the upper limit of normal for basal GH levels. For establishing the diagnosis and clinical activity of acromegaly, it is necessary to document an elevated basal level of GH and the failure to suppress GH levels with an oral glucose load (75 to 100 g) to less than 1.0 µg/mL using an RIA and less than 0.4 µg/mL using the IRMA or ELISA assays. Elevation of levels of insulin-like growth factor-1 (IGF-1), using age-adjusted normal values, has also become accepted as a criterion for the diagnosis of active acromegaly. IGF-1 levels correlate with indexes of disease activity better than GH levels in most but not all studies. IGF-1 binding protein-3 (IGFBP-3) levels are also elevated in most patients with active disease, although there is some overlap with values in normal subjects and so this measurement is generally not used either for diagnosis or management. Rare patients with documented acromegaly may have GH levels less than 1.0 µg/mL and elevated IGF-I levels.

Approximately 35% to 40% of patients with acromegaly have elevated prolactin (PRL) levels. Uncommonly, patients present with symptoms caused by the hyper-prolactinemia, such as decreased libido, impotence, galactorrhea, or amenorrhea, rather than the normal presenting symptoms of acromegaly.

Almost all patients with acromegaly have GH-secreting pituitary adenomas. The size and degree of any extrasellar extension of the adenoma are best assessed by magnetic resonance imaging (MRI). Compression of the optic chiasm by the adenoma can be determined with Goldmann visual field testing when MRI shows that the tumor abuts the optic chiasm. Approximately 70% to 80% of patients have macroadenomas (more than 10 mm in diameter), and 15% to 20% have suprasellar extension of the adenoma. Large adenomas may cause hypopituitarism by directly compressing the normal pituitary or interfering with stalk function. A detailed evaluation of anterior and posterior pituitary function determines whether hormone replacement is necessary.

Acromegaly may cause hypertension, diabetes mellitus, hypertrophic cardiomyopathy, and sleep apnea. Colonic adenomatous polyps and colon cancer occur more frequently than expected, and colonoscopy is indicated. Should surgery be chosen as therapy, these complications may need treatment preoperatively.

Rarely, no evidence of pituitary adenoma is found, or, if surgery is performed, hyperplasia of the somatotropes may be found. Such patients may have a syndrome in which GH-releasing hormone (GHRH) is being secreted by a pancreatic, carcinoid, hypothalamic, or other tumor. If one of these GHRH-secreting tumors is suspected, GHRH blood levels can be measured.

Goals of therapy include:

- Elimination of effects caused by the mass of the tumor (hypopituitarism, visual field defects, etc.)
- Reduction of elevated GH levels and IGF-I levels to normal
- Amelioration of the end-organ effects of the elevated GH levels
- Avoidance of damage to remaining normal hypothalamic or pituitary function
- Minimizing other potential adverse effects of therapy

Treatment

TRANSSPHENOIDAL ADENOMECTOMY

Transsphenoidal surgery offers the patient a chance for cure. The newer technique of endoscopic endonasal transsphenoidal surgery is associated with fewer local symptoms postoperatively and a faster recovery time, but cure rates are no better than those using the standard approach. Even when so-called cure is not achieved, surgery may effect a significant reduction in GH levels and considerable amelioration of clinical symptoms. As would be expected, the smaller the tumor and the lower the basal GH levels, the better the surgical result. The actual cure rates depend on the criteria used. Using the criteria of postoperative glucose-suppressed GH levels less than 1 µg/mL, with a conventional RIA, or 0.4 µg/mL, with the newer two-site assays, and normal IGF-I levels (age adjusted), cure rates of 60% to 80% can be expected for intrasellar lesions and 25% to 50% for larger tumors when the operation is performed by experienced neurosurgeons. Studies show that the increased mortality of acromegaly can be reduced to normal and much of the morbidity reversed, however, where GH levels are maintained below 2 µg/mL (RIA). Relapses occur in approximately 5% of patients who initially achieve glucose-suppressed GH levels of less than 2 µg/mL but in less than 2% when 1 µg/mL is used. Approximately 25% of patients have discordant IGF-I and glucose-suppressed GH levels, and these patients appear to have a higher risk for relapse.

With microadenomas, the risks of surgery are very small. The mortality from surgery approaches that of anesthesia alone. Transient diabetes insipidus may occur in 10% to 20% of patients. Hypopituitarism occurs in less than 1%, and other complications such as meningitis and cerebrospinal fluid leak also occur in less than 1% of patients. The complication rate is higher for larger tumors, and loss of one or more anterior pituitary hormones occurs in 5% to 10% of patients.

Patients with very large tumors may sometimes need craniotomy and a subfrontal lobe approach. This may be necessary if the tumor has a large suprasellar extension with a dumbbell configuration. Risks are much higher with craniotomy, and mortality reaches 5% in some series.

Pituitary function tested 6 to 8 weeks postoperatively determines whether the patient is cured or whether there is persistent GH hypersecretion. Testing involves obtaining basal GH and IGF-I levels and showing suppression of GH with glucose. Those patients who appear cured need to be followed to detect potential relapse. Testing of other pituitary function detects other hormonal deficiencies that may need treatment. We routinely place patients with macroadenomas on maintenance glucocorticoids (5 to 7.5 mg daily of prednisone)[1] until the time of postoperative testing, in case loss of adrenocorticotropic hormone (ACTH) function has occurred. Because loss of ACTH is very unlikely

following surgery for microadenomas, we usually do not prescribe maintenance glucocorticoids unless the patient is symptomatic or is found deficient on the formal testing carried out at 6 to 8 weeks.

IRRADIATION

Irradiation is generally used in patients following surgery when a cure is not obtained. Many experienced clinicians also restrict this treatment modality to patients whose GH and IGF-I levels cannot be normalized with medical therapy. Irradiation is used as primary therapy generally only in those patients who are unable to tolerate surgery and who do not respond to medical therapy.

Conventional irradiation, given at a dose of 4500 cGy through two or three fields over 5 weeks, lowers GH levels substantially in more than 80% of patients. The destructive effects of the irradiation are cumulative over time, levels of GH continuing to decrease for up to 20 years of follow-up. GH levels decrease to less than 5 µg/mL in 15% to 20% of treated cases by 2 years, in approximately 40% by 5 years, and in approximately 70% by 10 years.

At the same time that irradiation affects tumor function, it also affects the normal pituitary. By 10 years after irradiation, approximately 20% of patients are hypothyroid, 35% to 40% are hypoadrenal, and approximately 50% are hypogonadal.

During irradiation therapy, some patients complain of fatigue. If a patient is deficient in ACTH and on glucocorticoid replacement therapy, a doubling of the glucocorticoid dose is sometimes needed during radiation therapy. In rare patients, irradiation may cause subtle but permanent cognitive and short-term memory deficits. Patients may complain of difficulty concentrating, a poor memory, and lack of initiative.

Tumor infarction may occur following irradiation and usually presents with the sudden onset of severe headache and often coma and vascular collapse, a syndrome referred to as *pituitary apoplexy*. Computed tomography (CT) or MRI usually shows evidence of hemorrhage. Such patients must be supported with glucocorticoids in stress doses, and consideration should be given to emergency transsphenoidal decompression. Lesser degrees of tumor infarction may also occur, and the patient may have either no symptoms or a mild headache—evidence of infarction found only later on scan or at surgery. With conventional radiotherapy, there is also an increased risk of stroke and brain tumors.

Stereotactic radiotherapy using the gamma-knife apparatus or linear accelerator (LINAC) is now the most common way to administer radiotherapy because it can be given over a single day and may have a somewhat better therapeutic benefit-to-risk ratio. The irradiation is given through multiple ports and shaped, at it were, to correspond with the tumor visible on MRI. With this treatment, GH levels less than 5 µg/mL are achieved in approximately 20% of patients by 1 year and in approximately 50% by 3 years. Complications of this type of radiotherapy appear to be much less than those with conventional radiotherapy, although the experience is much less and the follow-up periods are much shorter

[1]Not FDA approved for this indication.

thus far. Early results, however, indicate that hypopituitarism occurs in a similar proportion of patients as with conventional irradiation. The cranial nerves that pass through the cavernous sinus (i.e., III, IV, V_1, V_2, and VI) are relatively resistant to this form of irradiation, and thus this technique is particularly useful for residual tumor in the cavernous sinus. The optic nerves, tracts, and chiasm are more radiosensitive, and therefore this form of radiotherapy is less useful for tumors with considerable suprasellar extension.

MEDICAL THERAPY

Medical therapy is generally reserved for patients who maintain GH levels more than 2 μg/mL (RIA) and elevated IGF-I levels following surgery. In that population, it may be used alone or may be given following irradiation while awaiting the effects of the irradiation. A select group of patients may also be considered for primary medical therapy:

- Those who are medically unable to undergo surgery
- Those who have tumors that extend into the cavernous sinus and thus are not curable by surgery and who do not have a visual field deficit

In the latter group, somatostatin analogues often cause a 10% to 50% shrinkage of the tumor, and growth during such treatment occurs in less than 2% of patients.

Medical Therapy With Dopamine Agonists

Approximately one third of patients respond to cabergoline (Dostinex)[1] with a normalization of GH and IGF-I levels, although this drug is not approved by the U.S. Food and Drug Administration for this indication and published experience is limited. Patients with concomitant secretion of PRL may have a better chance of responding. Thus, although the chance of successful therapy is relatively low, a therapeutic trial with cabergoline is worth trying because it is generally well tolerated, given orally, and less expensive than other medical options. The starting dose is 0.5 mg twice weekly and increased by 1 mg per week at monthly intervals for 3 months. If there is a good response, the dose is increased further as needed until GH and IGF-I levels are normalized. If there is no response, another medical agent is tried. Side effects are uncommon but may include nausea and constipation.

Medical Therapy With Somatostatin Agonists

The somatostatin analogue octreotide (Sandostatin) results in substantial reductions of GH and IGF-I in 90% of patients; in approximately 60% of patients, IGF-I levels can be brought into the normal range. In most cases, a dosing frequency every 6 to 8 hours is usually necessary, beginning at 100 μg at each dose and increasing as necessary up to 1500 μg per day. Some patients

respond better to the combination of octreotide plus cabergoline than to either drug alone. MRI scans demonstrate 10% to 50% tumor size reduction as a result of therapy in approximately 20% to 30% of patients when used adjunctively following surgery and in up to 75% of patients when used primarily.

Side effects include mild abdominal bloating, nausea, moderate diarrhea, steatorrhea, and gastritis. Cholelithiasis and gallbladder sludge caused by poor gallbladder contractility occur in up to 25% of patients. Cholecystitis occurs in less than 1% of patients and is treated by laparoscopic cholecystectomy rather than stopping the drug if the patient is having a good GH/IGF-1 response. The glucose intolerance of acromegaly usually improves with treatment, but occasionally some patients worsen with octreotide use, and glucose levels should be monitored.

Two long-acting preparations of somatostatin agonists are available and the ones currently used in most patients. Octreotide-LAR (Sandostatin-LAR) is given monthly intramuscularly in 10-, 20-, or 30-mg doses, depending on the GH and IGF-1 responses. Higher doses are rarely necessary. Prior to starting the intramuscular preparations, octreotide should be given subcutaneously for 2 weeks to be sure no unacceptable side effects (mainly GI) occur. In patients who achieve normalization of GH and IGF-I with 10 mg per month, the interval between doses can sometimes be lengthened to 5 to 8 weeks. Lanreotide Autogel[1] is also given every 4 weeks subcutaneously. With both long-acting preparations, IGF-1 levels can be normalized in approximately 60% of patients and reduced considerably in most others. Tumor size reduction with octreotide-LAR is similar to that seen with the subcutaneous short-acting form, but size reduction with lanreotide appears to be less. Complications are similar to those seen with subcutaneous octreotide. Thus these long-acting preparations are greatly preferred to subcutaneous octreotide because of ease of use.

Medical Therapy With Pegvisomant

Pegvisomant (Somavert) is a biosynthetic GH analogue that is a GH-receptor blocker. It functions as a competitive inhibitor to GH, blocking its action in all tissues and decreasing the generation of IGF-I. It normalizes IGF-I levels in more than 95% of patients when given by daily subcutaneous injection. Because it does not directly work on the tumor, GH levels do not fall and actually rise because of loss of negative feedback by IGF-I. In a few patients treated with pegvisomant, tumor size increases, but it is uncertain whether this is caused by this lack of negative feedback or just to the natural history of tumor growth in those patients. Less than 5% of patients also have reversible liver function test abnormalities. Glucose intolerance usually improves with pegvisomant. Whether pegvisomant should be used as a first-line medical therapy or just in those patients who do not have adequate responses to octreotide

[1]Not FDA approved for this indication.

Rakel and Bope: *Conn's Current Therapy 2006.*

[1]FDA approval pending.

is controversial. At present, most clinicians reserve its use for patients who do not normalize GH and IGF-I levels with octreotide. There is very limited experience in using pegvisomant together with octreotide. Because of the risk of tumor size enlargement, MRI scans of the pituitary must be monitored, along with GH and IGF-I levels and liver function.

In patients with microadenomas and intrasellar macroadenomas, transsphenoidal surgery offers a 60% to 80% chance of cure, depending on the experience of the neurosurgeon. The recurrence rate after apparent cure is less than 5%. Thus this would appear to be the best choice as primary therapy for such patients. In patients with larger tumors, surgery can cause a considerable debulking of the tumor with a concomitant reduction in GH levels, but the cure rate decreases as tumor size increases.

Because radiotherapy may take several years to bring GH levels to normal, it should be regarded as third-line therapy to be used if an operation does not result in cure or is contraindicated and the response to medical therapy is poor.

Stereotactic radiotherapy appears to cause a considerably faster reduction of GH levels with less adverse effects, especially when the residual tumor is in the cavernous sinus, and it is now the preferred mode of irradiation. Hypopituitarism is the primary complication.

Medical therapy is generally reserved for patients not cured by surgery or in whom ablative therapy is contraindicated. When the parasellar extent of a tumor indicates it cannot be cured surgically and there is no visual field deficit, primary medical therapy with octreotide may be appropriate. Additionally, these drugs may be useful while awaiting the eventual destructive effects of irradiation.

Because of ease of use and lower cost, cabergoline (Dostinex)[1] can be tried first, realizing the success rates

---

[1]Not FDA approved for this indication.

CURRENT THERAPY

- Transsphenoidal surgery is generally the initial treatment for most patients.
    - Cure is defined as suppression of GH to less than 1 μg/mL (RIA) or less than 0.4 μg/mL (two-site assay) during a oral glucose tolerance test and normalization of IGF-I.
    - Adjunctive therapy is indicated for random GH levels more than 2 μg/mL and elevated IGF-I levels postoperatively.
- Gamma-knife stereotactic radiotherapy is reserved for patients not cured by surgery and often is used only when medical therapy also fails.
- Medical therapy is usually used in patients not cured by surgery.
    - Cabergoline (Dostinex)[1] results in normalization of GH/IGF-I levels in less than one third of patients but often is tried as initial therapy.
    - Octreotide-LAR (Sandostatin-LAR) is the mainstay of medical therapy and results in normalization of GH/IGF-I levels in approximately 60% of patients.
    - Tumor size reduction of 10% to 50% occurs in up to 75% of patients when octreotide is used primarily and approximately 25% when used adjunctively.
    - Pegvisomant (Somavert) results in normalization of IGF-I levels in more than 90% of patients but has no effect in decreasing tumor size.
- Octreotide-LAR may also be used primarily in patients whose tumors appear to be nonresectable.
- Patients must be carefully monitored with GH and IGF-I levels and MRI scans.

---

[1]Not FDA approved for this indication.
Abbreviations: GH = growth hormone; IGF-1 = insulin-like growth factor; RIA = radioimmunoassay.

CURRENT DIAGNOSIS

- Acromegaly diagnosed using the following criteria:
    - GH not suppressed below 1 μg/mL (conventional RIA) or 0.4 μg/mL (two-site assays) during a glucose tolerance test
    - IGF-I levels elevated (age corrected)
- Tumor size and extension assessed by MRI
- Visual fields performed if tumor found to be abutting optic chiasm on MRI
- Colonoscopy performed to rule out polyps/cancer
- Other pituitary functions assessed in patients with macroadenomas
- Prolactin measured to determine if the tumor co-secretes this hormone

Abbreviations: GH = growth hormone; IGF-1 = insulin-like growth factor; MRI = magnetic resonance imaging; RIA = radioimmunoassay.

for dopamine agonists are relative low. In those patients in whom dopamine agonists are ineffective, a long-acting somatostatin agonist such as octreotide-LAR (Sandostatin-LAR) can be given with good expectations of success at normalizing GH and IGF-1 levels. Pegvisomant has a very high rate of success in normalizing IGF-I levels and if tumor size is not an issue can be considered for early medical therapy or in patients who do not respond to octreotide.

In all cases, patients need to be followed carefully following surgery and/or radiotherapy and during medical treatment. GH and IGF-I levels need to be monitored as well as tumor size by MRI. Other pituitary functions may also need to be monitored and treated if there is hypopituitarism.

Rakel and Bope: *Conn's Current Therapy 2006.*

REFERENCES

Abs R, Verhelst J, Maiter D, et al: Cabergoline in the treatment of acromegaly: A study in 64 patients. J Clin Endocrinol Metab 1998; 83:374-378.

Beauregard C, Truong U, Hardy J, et al: Long-term outcome and mortality after transsphenoidal adenomectomy for acromegaly. Clin Endocrinol 2003;58:86-91.

Bevan JS, Atkin SL, Atkinson AB, et al: Primary medical therapy for acromegaly: An open, prospective, multicenter study of the effects of subcutaneous and intramuscular slow-release octreotide on growth hormone, insulin-like growth factor-I, and tumor size. J Clin Endocrinol Metab 2002;87:4554-4563.

Clemmons DR, Chihara K, Freda PU, et al: Optimizing control of acromegaly: Integrating a growth hormone receptor antagonist into the treatment algorithm. J Clin Endocrinol Metab 2003;88: 4759-4767.

Freda PU: Somatostatin analogs in acromegaly. J Clin Endocrinol Metab 2002;87:3013-3018.

Freda PU: How effective are current therapies for acromegaly? Growth Horm IGF Res 2003;13(Suppl A):S144-S151.

The Growth Hormone Research Society and The Pituitary Society Consensus Conference: Biochemical assessment and long-term monitoring in patients with acromegaly. J Clin Endocrinol Metab 2004;89:3099-3012.

Holdaway IM, Rajasoorya RC, Gamble GD: Factors influencing mortality in acromegaly. J Clin Endocrinol Metab 2004;89:667-674.

Melmed S, Vance ML, Barkan AL, et al: Current status and future opportunities for controlling acromegaly. Pituitary 2002;5:185-196.

Molitch ME: Clinical manifestations of acromegaly. Endocrinol Metab Clin N Am 1992;21:597-614.

Swearingen B, Barker FG II, Katznelson L, et al: Long-term mortality after transsphenoidal surgery and adjunctive therapy for acromegaly. J Clin Endocrinol Metab 1998;83:3419-3426.

Trainer PJ, Drake WM, Katznelson L, et al: Treatment of acromegaly with the growth hormone-receptor antagonist pegvisomant. N Engl J Med 2000;342:1171-1177.

Van der Lely AJ, Hutson RK, Trainer PJ, et al: Long-term treatment of acromegaly with pegvisomant, a growth hormone receptor antagonist. Lancet 2001;358:1754-1759.

Adrenal Insufficiency

Method of
David C. Aron, MD, MS

The clinical syndrome of adrenocortical insufficiency results from deficient levels of glucocorticoids and/or mineralocorticoids. Reduced adrenal production of these steroid hormones results from either the destruction/dysfunction of the cortex (primary adrenocortical insufficiency, or Addison's disease) or from deficient pituitary ACTH (adrenocorticotropin hormone) secretion (secondary glucocorticoid insufficiency). Primary adrenocortical insufficiency is uncommon but readily treatable. Survival now depends primarily on the underlying cause of the adrenal insufficiency. This section focuses on glucocorticoid deficiency.

Rakel and Bope: Conn's Current Therapy 2006.

Etiology

The etiology of primary adrenocortical insufficiency (Box 1) has changed over time; TB, once the major cause of adrenocortical insufficiency, has been superseded in frequency by autoimmune adrenalitis. Metastases from an extra-adrenal cancer to the adrenal glands are far more common than clinical adrenal insufficiency, but the latter is more common than previously believed. Primary adrenal insufficiency in AIDS is usually caused by opportunistic infections such as cytomegalovirus (CMV) and tuberculosis (TB), and adrenocortical insufficiency is usually a late manifestation of HIV infection. Because patients with malignant disease and HIV infection live longer, more cases of adrenal insufficiency will be seen. Adrenal hemorrhage typically occurs in the setting of anticoagulant therapy, the postoperative period, or the primary antiphospholipid antibody syndrome. Recent studies point to the possibility of adrenal insufficiency as a consequence of critical illness with severe inflammatory disorders (e.g., septic shock). Glucocorticoid therapy is the most common cause of secondary glucocorticoid insufficiency followed by pituitary tumors (see relevant articles).

Pathophysiology

Clinical manifestations of adrenocortical insufficiency usually occur only after the loss of more than 90% of both adrenal cortices. When adrenocortical destruction is gradual, a phase of decreased adrenal reserve (normal basal steroid secretion, but impaired response to stress) precedes frank adrenal insufficiency. Acute adrenal crisis can be precipitated during this initial phase by the stresses of surgery, trauma, or infection. As destruction of cortical tissue continues, even basal secretion of mineralocorticoids and glucocorticoids becomes deficient, leading to the manifestations of chronic adrenocortical insufficiency. If the destruction is rapid, a patient's first presentation may be crisis or impending crisis.

> **BOX 1 Causes of Primary Adrenocortical Insufficiency**
>
> - Autoimmune
> - Infectious—tuberculosis, cytomegalovirus, fungi (histoplasmosis, coccidioidomycosis), HIV, sepsis
> - Cancer—metastases, lymphoma
> - Adrenal hemorrhage
> - Infiltrative disorders—amyloidosis, hemochromatosis
> - Congenital adrenal hyperplasia
> - Miscellaneous—adrenoleukodystrophy, familial glucocorticoid deficiency and hypoplasia, drugs (ketoconazole, metyrapone, aminoglutethimide, trilostane,[2] mitotane, etomidate)
>
> [2]Not available in the United States.

Clinical Features

The clinical features (Table 1) depend on which steroids are deficient, the magnitude of the deficiency, the rate of development of the deficiency, and the presence or absence of intercurrent illness. Destruction of the adrenals results in deficiencies of both glucocorticoids and mineralocorticoids. In secondary glucocorticoid deficiency, ACTH deficiency is the primary event and leads to decreased cortisol and adrenal androgen secretion; aldosterone secretion is usually normal. Cortisol deficiency causes weakness, fatigue, anorexia, nausea and vomiting, hypotension, hyponatremia, and hypoglycemia. Mineralocorticoid deficiency produces renal sodium wasting and potassium retention and can lead to severe dehydration, hypotension, hyponatremia, hyperkalemia, and acidosis. The chief signs and symptoms of chronic primary adrenocortical insufficiency are weakness and fatigue, weight loss, anorexia, and gastrointestinal (GI) disturbances, especially nausea and vomiting and hyperpigmentation. Hyperpigmentation results from increased ACTH levels and may be generalized or localized to the buccal mucosa and gums, palmar creases, nail beds, or other areas. Hyperpigmentation is increased in sun-exposed areas and accentuated over pressure areas such as the knuckles, toes, elbows, and knees and may be accompanied by increased numbers of freckles. The GI symptoms may mimic a primary intra-abdominal process. Hypotension is most often accompanied by orthostatic symptoms. A minority of patients craves salt. Hypoglycemia is unusual in adults but may be provoked by fasting, fever, infection, or nausea and vomiting. Hypoglycemia occurs more commonly in secondary adrenal insufficiency. Decreased secretion of adrenal androgens can result in loss of axillary and pubic hair in women. Amenorrhea results from weight loss, chronic illness or associated primary ovarian failure. Autoimmune Addison's disease is frequently accompanied by other immune disorders (e.g., hypothyroidism, vitiligo). Hyponatremia and hyperkalemia are classic manifestations of the mineralocorticoid deficiency. Volume depletion results in azotemia. Laboratory findings of glucocorticoid deficiency include eosinophilia, relative lymphocytosis, and hypoglycemia. Acute adrenal (addisonian) crisis occurs in Addison's disease patients who are exposed to the stresses of infection, trauma, surgery, or dehydration caused by salt deprivation,

vomiting, or diarrhea. During this crisis, clinical features of adrenocortical insufficiency are exaggerated (e.g., volume depletion, hypotension); adrenal insufficiency should be considered in any patient with unexplained vascular collapse. Abdominal pain may mimic an acute intra-abdominal emergency. Weakness, apathy, and confusion are typical. Fever occurs because of infection or glucocorticoid deficiency per se. Shock and coma may rapidly lead to death in untreated patients. The diagnosis of acute adrenal hemorrhage should be considered in the deteriorating patient with unexplained abdominal or flank pain, vascular collapse, hyperpyrexia, or hypoglycemia. Secondary adrenal (glucocorticoid) insufficiency is usually chronic, and the manifestations may be nonspecific. However, acute crisis can occur in undiagnosed patients, in corticosteroid-treated patients who do not receive increased steroid dosage during periods of stress, or after surgical removal of a functional adrenal tumor. Features may include weakness, lethargy, easy fatigability, anorexia, nausea and occasionally vomiting, arthralgias, myalgias, and hypoglycemia. Because pituitary secretion of ACTH is deficient, hyperpigmentation is not present. In addition, mineralocorticoid secretion is usually normal so that volume depletion, dehydration, and hyperkalemia are frequently absent. Hypotension occurs only in acute presentations. Hyponatremia may occur as a result of water retention and an inability to excrete a water load; there is a lack of glucocorticoid negative feedback on antidiuretic hormone as well as the reduction in glomerular filtration associated with hypocortisolism. Acute decompensation with severe hypotension or shock unresponsive to vasopressors may occur. Patients with secondary adrenal insufficiency commonly have additional features that suggest the diagnosis (e.g., a history of glucocorticoid therapy or manifestations of deficiencies of other pituitary hormones).

Diagnosis

Therapy should not be delayed for the purpose of diagnostic testing. In the acutely ill patient, therapy should be instituted immediately and the diagnosis established when the patient is stable. The diagnosis of adrenal insufficiency requires the demonstration of inappropriately low cortisol production and involves assessment of

TABLE 1   Clinical Features of Adrenocortical Insufficiency

Chronic primary adrenocortical	Insufficiency	Acute adrenal crisis
Weakness, fatigue, anorexia	Hypotension, shock, weight loss	
Hyperpigmentation	Fever	
Hypotension	Dehydration, volume	Depletion
GI disturbances	Nausea, vomiting	Anorexia
Salt craving	Weakness, apathy	Depressed mentation
Postural symptoms	Electrolyte abnormalities	Hyperkalemia,
Electrolyte abnormalities	Hyponatremia, hyperkalemia	Hypoglycemia, hyponatremia
Hypercalcemia	Hypoglycemia, hypercalcemia	

Abbreviations: GI = gastrointestinal.

Rakel and Bope: *Conn's Current Therapy 2006.*

the pituitary-adrenal axis. Normally cortisol is secreted episodically from the adrenal cortex with a diurnal rhythm paralleling the secretion of ACTH. Consequently, normal levels of plasma cortisol constitute a broad range; the levels found in adrenal insufficiency may at any given time fall within the *normal* range. The hypothalamic-pituitary-adrenal (HPA) axis responds to *stress* with an increase in CRH (corticotropin-releasing hormone) secretion, followed by an increase in ACTH secretion, followed in turn by an increase in cortisol secretion. Such stress includes hypotension, hypoglycemia, and a variety of serious illnesses. The diagnostic usefulness of single plasma cortisol concentrations is limited by the episodic nature of cortisol secretion. However, an unstressed 8 AM plasma cortisol level of less than 3 µg/dL (80 nmol/L) is strongly suggestive of adrenal insufficiency, whereas a level greater than 20 µg/dL (550 nmol/L) at any time makes clinical adrenal insufficiency highly unlikely. Dynamic testing has been favored more than baseline measurements. In fact, severe acute illness constitutes a dynamic test, albeit unplanned. Elevated cortisol levels (>20 µg/dL [550 nmol/L]) would be the normal response. Similarly, ACTH levels should be elevated. Diagnostic tests used when the patient is stable include: ACTH administration that directly stimulates adrenal secretion; metyrapone that inhibits cortisol synthesis, thereby stimulating pituitary ACTH secretion; and insulin-induced hypoglycemia that stimulates ACTH release by increasing CRH secretion.

The rapid ACTH stimulation test measures the acute adrenal response to ACTH and is used to diagnose both primary and secondary adrenal insufficiencies. A synthetic human ACTH (cosyntropin [Cortrosyn]) is administered in a dose of 0.25 mg intramuscularly (IM) or intravenously (IV) after obtaining a baseline cortisol sample; additional samples are obtained 30 or 60 minutes following the injection. The peak cortisol response, 30 to 60 minutes later, should exceed 18 to 20 µg/dL (500 to 550 nm/L).

Use of a lower dose of ACTH, 1 µg, is believed to be a more sensitive indicator of adrenocortical insufficiency, but this is controversial. A normal response to the rapid ACTH stimulation test excludes both primary adrenal insufficiency (by directly assessing adrenal reserve) and overt secondary adrenal insufficiency with adrenal atrophy. However, a normal response does not rule out partial ACTH deficiency (decreased pituitary reserve). When the diagnosis remains uncertain, metyrapone testing can be used. Metyrapone blocks the pathway of cortisol synthesis, thus stimulating ACTH secretion, which increases the secretion and plasma levels of 11-deoxycortisol (a cortisol precursor). A normal response to adequate blockade (cortisol <5 µg/dL [135 nmol/L]) is a plasma 11-deoxycortisol level greater than 7 µg/dL (190 nmol/L) and a plasma ACTH level greater than 100 pg/mL (22 pmol/L). This test is not without risk, and it should not be performed in a patient who is already symptomatic from glucocorticoid deficiency. Insulin-induced hypoglycemia tests the entire HPA system. A normal cortisol response is a peak level greater than 18 to 20 µg/dL (485 to 540 nmol/L) and plasma ACTH greater than 100 pg/mL (22 pmol/L). This test is

associated with significant risk and is contraindicated in the presence of ischemic heart disease, cerebrovascular disease, seizure disorder, or in patients with low baseline cortisols (e.g., <3 to 5 µg/dL). When performed, the patient should be under constant medical supervision. It is rarely necessary in any patient in whom the likelihood of adrenal insufficiency is reasonably high.

If adrenal insufficiency is present, plasma ACTH levels are used to differentiate primary and secondary forms. The normal range for plasma ACTH, using a sensitive immunometric assay (IMA), is 9 to 52 pg/mL (2 to 11 pmol/L). In patients with primary adrenal insufficiency, plasma ACTH levels exceed the upper limit of the normal range (>52 pg/mL [11 pmol/L]) and usually exceed 200 pg/mL (44 pmol/L). Plasma ACTH concentration is usually less than 30 pg/mL (6.8 pmol/L) in patients with secondary adrenal insufficiency. Note that patients with secondary adrenal insufficiency exhibit inappropriately low plasma ACTH levels (i.e., levels are not elevated). A level in the *normal range* is inappropriate for someone with low cortisol levels. Patients with primary adrenal insufficiency should undergo imaging with an abdominal computed tomography (CT) scan. CT can detect adrenal calcification and adrenal enlargement. Adrenal calcification is found in approximately 50% of patients with tuberculous Addison's disease and in some patients with other invasive or hemorrhagic causes of adrenal insufficiency. Bilateral adrenal enlargement in association with adrenal insufficiency may be seen with TB, fungal infections, CMV, malignant and nonmalignant infiltrative diseases, and adrenal hemorrhage. Patients with secondary adrenal insufficiency should undergo anatomic evaluation of the hypothalamus and pituitary (e.g., visual field examination, magnetic resonance imaging [MRI]), and functional evaluations to assess for secondary hypothyroidism, gonadal deficiency, and growth hormone deficiency.

Suppression of the HPA axis may occur with doses of prednisone as low as 5 mg per day, but its development or degree is difficult to predict. In general, patients who develop clinical features of Cushing's syndrome or who have received glucocorticoids equivalent to 10 to 20 mg of prednisone per day for 3 weeks or more should be assumed to have clinically significant axis suppression. Evaluation of stress response is not performed until glucocorticoids have been tapered to physiologic replacement levels and morning cortisol exceeds 10 µg/mL. Even after the glucocorticoid dose has been reduced to physiologic levels, axis suppression (i.e., secondary adrenal insufficiency) can persist for months to years.

Treatment

The aim of treatment of adrenocortical insufficiency is to produce levels of glucocorticoids and mineralocorticoids equivalent to those achieved in an individual with normal HPA function under similar circumstances. Treatment for acute addisonian crisis should be instituted as soon as the diagnosis is suspected. Therapy includes administration of glucocorticoids; correction of dehydration, hypovolemia, hypoglycemia, and electrolyte

Rakel and Bope: *Conn's Current Therapy 2006.*

BOX 2   Management of Acute Adrenal Crisis

Glucocorticoid Replacement
- Administer hydrocortisone sodium phosphate or sodium succinate, 100 mg IV every 6 hours for 24 hours.
- When the patient is stable, reduce the dosage by 50% to 50 mg every 6 hours.
- Taper dosage to maintenance therapy by day 4 or 5 (assuming appropriate clinical response) and add mineralocorticoid therapy as required.
- Maintain or increase the dose to 200 to 400 mg per day if complications persist or occur.

General and Supportive Measures
- Correct volume depletion, dehydration, and hypoglycemia with intravenous saline and glucose.
- Evaluate and correct infection and other precipitating factors.

Abbreviations: IV = intravenously.

BOX 3   Regimen for Maintenance Therapy of Primary Adrenocortical Insufficiency

- Hydrocortisone, 10 to 15 mg in the morning, 5 mg in the afternoon, and 5 mg in the evening
- Fludrocortisone, 0.05 to 0.1 mg orally in the morning
- Clinical follow-up: maintenance of normal weight, blood pressure, and electrolytes with regression of clinical features
- Patient education plus identification card, medical alert bracelet or necklace (*dog tag*)*
- Increased hydrocortisone dosage during stress; doubling of the oral dose for mild illness[†]

---

*Useful patient education materials are available from the National Institutes of Health at http://www.cc.nih.gov/ccc/patient_education/pepubs/mngadrins.pdf/.
[†]Provide patient with injectable form of glucocorticoid for emergency use.

---

abnormalities; general supportive measures; and treatment of coexisting or precipitating disorders (Box 2). Cortisol (hydrocortisone hemisuccinate or phosphate) in IV doses of 100 mg is given every 6 hours for the first 24 hours. At these high doses hydrocortisone has sufficient sodium-retaining potency so that additional mineralocorticoid therapy is not required in patients with primary adrenocortical insufficiency. The response to therapy is usually rapid, with improvement occurring within 12 hours or fewer. If improvement occurs and the patient is stable, 50 mg every 6 hours is given on the second day, and in most patients the dosage may then be gradually reduced to approximately 10 mg three times daily by day 4 or 5. In severely ill patients, especially in those with additional major complications (e.g., sepsis), higher cortisol doses (100 mg IV every 6 to 8 hours) are maintained until the patient is stable. In primary adrenal insufficiency, mineralocorticoid replacement, in the form of fludrocortisone (Florincf) (discussed later), is added when the total cortisol dosage has been reduced to 50 to 60 mg per day. In secondary adrenocortical (glucocorticoid) insufficiency with acute crisis, only glucocorticoid replacement is needed. Cortisol can be used as above. However, if the salt-retaining properties of high doses of cortisol present a risk (e.g., in a patient with congestive heart failure prone to fluid overload), synthetic steroids with low mineralocorticoid activity, such as prednisolone or dexamethasone, can be used.

Intravenous glucose and saline are administered to correct volume depletion, hypotension, and hypoglycemia. Volume deficits may be severe in Addison's disease, and hypotension and shock may not respond to vasopressors unless glucocorticoids are administered. Hyperkalemia and acidosis are usually corrected with cortisol and volume replacement; however, an occasional patient may require specific therapy for these abnormalities. Therapy for the factors that precipitated the crisis (e.g., infection) is also necessary.

Patients with Addison's disease require lifelong glucocorticoid and mineralocorticoid therapy (Box 3).

Cortisol (hydrocortisone) is the glucocorticoid preparation of first choice. The basal production rate of cortisol is approximately 8 to 12 mg/m^2 per day. The maintenance dose of hydrocortisone is usually 15 to 25 mg daily in adults. The oral dose is usually divided to more closely mimic normal cortisol secretion. Thrice daily regimens (e.g., 10 mg in the morning, 5 mg in the afternoon, and 5 mg in the evening) are effective in maintaining well-being and normal energy levels. Twice-daily dosing regimens (e.g., 10 to 20 mg in the morning on arising and 5 to 10 mg later in the day) yield satisfactory responses in most patients. Insomnia is a side effect of glucocorticoid administration and can usually be prevented by administering the last dose at 4 PM to 5 PM. The daily dose of hydrocortisone should be doubled during periods of minor stress, and the dose needs to be increased to as much as 200 to 300 mg per day during periods of major stress, such as a surgical procedure.

Fludrocortisone (Florinef) is used for mineralocorticoid therapy; the usual doses are 0.05 to 0.2 mg per day orally in the morning. Because of its long half-life, a single morning dose is usually sufficient. Approximately 10% of addisonian patients can be managed with cortisol and adequate dietary sodium intake alone and do not require fludrocortisone (Florinef). Secondary adrenocortical insufficiency is treated with the cortisol dosages described for the primary form. Fludrocortisone (Florinef) is rarely required. The recovery of normal function of the HPA axis following suppression by exogenous glucocorticoids may take weeks to years, and its duration is unpredictable. Consequently, prolonged replacement therapy may be required. Recent studies have pointed to the potential benefits of dehydroepiandrosterone (DHEA) in doses of 50 mg per day, particularly in women, in terms of improvement in well-being.

Response to Therapy

Traditionally, assessment of the adequacy of glucocorticoid replacement in patients with adrenal insufficiency

CURRENT DIAGNOSIS

- Individuals with mass lesions involving both adrenals or involving the pituitary or hypothalamus should be evaluated for adrenal insufficiency.
- Adrenal insufficiency should be considered in the differential diagnosis of unexplained weight loss, in patients with hypotension and fever, and in patients withdrawn from high-dose glucocorticoids.
- Partial adrenal insufficiency may have subtle clinical manifestations.
- Biochemical diagnosis of adrenal insufficiency should be done using dynamic rather than static testing.
- Once the diagnosis of adrenal insufficiency is made, differentiation between primary and secondary causes and determination of specific etiology can be pursued.

has involved clinical, but not biochemical measures. These clinical signs include good appetite and sense of well-being. Adequate treatment results in the disappearance of weakness, malaise, and fatigue. Anorexia and other GI symptoms resolve and weight returns to normal. The hyperpigmentation invariably improves but may not entirely disappear. Inadequate cortisol administration leads to persistence of these symptoms of adrenal insufficiency, and excessive pigmentation will remain. Obviously, signs of Cushing's syndrome indicate overtreatment. Patients receiving excessive doses of glucocorticoids are also at risk for increased bone loss

CURRENT THERAPY

- Glucocorticoid therapy is required in both primary and secondary adrenal insufficiencies; mineralocorticoid is required only in primary.
- Glucocorticoid therapy should be administered so as to mimic normal secretory patterns, taking into account the normal diurnal rhythm and increased requirements during stress.
- Parental glucocorticoids are needed when oral intake is impaired (e.g., because of vomiting).
- Patient education and self-management (dose adjustment for stress) are critical. Patients should carry identification as having adrenal insufficiency so that glucocorticoids can be given even when their ability to give a history is impaired.
- Follow up of replacement therapy is primarily clinical. Mineralocorticoid can be adjusted based on PRA.

Abbreviations: PRA = plasma rennin activity.

and clinically significant osteoporosis. Therefore, the replacement dose of glucocorticoids should be maintained at the lowest amount needed to provide the patient with a proper sense of well-being. Potential risks, especially of overtreatment, have prompted more biochemical testing. Although the use of 24-hour urinary cortisol levels might seem an attractive method for following such patients, there are serious limitations. A high level of urinary cortisol would suggest over-replacement but by no means confirm it. Plasma cortisol day curves (i.e., multiple samples for plasma cortisol concentration) have been proposed, but they have not been widely adopted because of their inconvenience, expense, and variation among individuals in terms of the plasma levels of cortisol achieved with orally administered hydrocortisone or cortisol. The use of other glucocorticoids (e.g., prednisone) could not be assessed with these measures. Day curves are reserved for patients who appear to require higher than expected replacement doses. ACTH levels are not useful for monitoring even in treated primary adrenal insufficiency. Plasma ACTH levels fall toward the normal range, but because of the dose and timing of physiologic replacement, plasma ACTH levels usually remain in the high-normal to modest elevated range. Although undertreatment with mineralocorticoids may lead to fatigue and malaise, adequacy of mineralocorticoid replacement is usually assessed with measurements of blood pressure (BP) and electrolytes. Biochemical assessment of the renin-angiotensin system is not routinely performed. With adequate treatment, the BP is normal without orthostatic change, and serum sodium and potassium remain within the normal ranges. Hypertension and hypokalemia result if the fludrocortisone (Florinef) dose is excessive. Some endocrinologists monitor plasma renin activity (PRA) as an objective measure of fludrocortisone (Florinef) replacement.

Prevention of Adrenal Crisis

The development of acute adrenal insufficiency in previously diagnosed and treated patients is almost entirely preventable, with patient education, self-management, and increased glucocorticoid dosages during illness all playing roles. The patient should be informed about the necessity for lifelong therapy, the possible consequences of acute illness, and the necessity for increased therapy and medical assistance during acute illness. An identification card or bracelet should be carried or worn at all times. The cortisol dose should be doubled with the development of a minor illness; the usual maintenance dosage may be resumed in 24 to 48 hours if improvement occurs. Increased mineralocorticoid therapy is not required. If symptoms persist or become worse, the patient should continue increased cortisol doses and seek medical attention. Vomiting may result in an inability to ingest or absorb oral cortisol, and diarrhea in addisonian patients may precipitate a crisis because of rapid fluid and electrolyte losses. Patients must understand that if these symptoms occur, they should seek immediate medical assistance so that parenteral glucocorticoid therapy can be given. Patients can be given injectable forms of glucocorticoid (e.g., dexamethasone) as a temporizing measure until medical assistance can be obtained.

Steroid Coverage for Surgery

The normal physiologic response to surgical stress involves an increase in cortisol secretion. The increased glucocorticoid activity may serve primarily to modulate the immunologic response to stress. Thus, patients with primary or secondary adrenocortical insufficiency scheduled for elective surgery require increased glucocorticoid coverage. This problem is also encountered in patients with pituitary-adrenal suppression caused by exogenous glucocorticoid therapy. Box 4 outlines the principles of management. Recent clinical trials suggest a role for physiologic glucocorticoid replacement therapy in patients with sepsis syndrome.

Cushing's Syndrome

Method of
Kathryn G. Schuff, MD

The diagnosis of Cushing's syndrome is one of the most difficult but potentially most important that can be made in a patient. The consequences of pathologic hypercortisolism are significant, and excess mortality and morbidity improve with cure of the disease. Although the evaluation and management often involve specialty referral, the primary care provider plays a pivotal role in suspecting the diagnosis and initiating the workup.

Clinical Presentation

Although traditionally considered a rare disease with an incidence of 1 to 2 per 100,000, more recently Cushing's syndrome has been reported to occur in up to 3% to 4% of the obese, uncontrolled diabetic population. The classic presentation (moon facies, purple striae, central obesity) is uncommonly seen, and the presentation more commonly overlaps that of polycystic ovary syndrome, the metabolic syndrome, and depression. Given the nonspecific presentation, health care providers should have a low threshold for screening patients for the disease. More specific features (Table 1) that should prompt evaluation include difficult-to-control diabetes mellitus or hypertension, unexplained osteoporosis, and menstrual irregularities. In addition, physical signs that are disquieting include facial rounding, plethora, supraclavicular fat pad filling, central obesity, thin skin (including spontaneous ecchymoses), and proximal muscle weakness, particularly if a change in appearance can be demonstrated. Children exhibit poor linear growth, generalized obesity, and menstrual irregularities. The etiologies of hypercortisolism are varied (Box 1) and include both pathologic etiologies causing subclinical and overt Cushing's syndrome as well as pseudo-Cushing's syndrome, which is temporary, nonpathologic hypercortisolemia caused by concurrent medical or psychiatric illness.

SUBCLINICAL CUSHING'S SYNDROME

Subtle hypothalamic-pituitary-adrenal (HPA) axis abnormalities and autonomy have been demonstrated in 5% to 20% of patients with incidentally discovered adrenal masses. These patients do not exhibit frank signs, symptoms, or biochemical abnormalities of Cushing's syndrome, and thus this entity is termed subclinical Cushing's syndrome. However, there are higher rates of hypertension, impaired glucose tolerance, and diabetes in these patients, which often improve with removal of

TABLE 1 Clinical Features of Cushing's Syndrome (In Order of Decreasing Specificity)

Feature	Sensitivity (%)	Specificity (%)
Hypokalemia (K^+ <3.6)	25	96
Ecchymoses	53	94
Osteoporosis	26	94
Weakness	65	93
Diastolic blood pressure ≥105 mm Hg	39	83
Red or violaceous striae	46	78
Acne	52	76
Central obesity	90	71
Hirsutism	50	71
Plethora	82	69
Oligomenorrhea	72	49
Generalized obesity	60	38
Abnormal glucose tolerance	88	23

BOX 1 Etiologies of Hypercortisolism

- Pseudo-Cushing's syndrome (nonpathologic hypercortisolism)
    - Acute/chronic medical illness
    - Psychiatric illness
    - Alcoholism
- Subclinical Cushing's syndrome (subtle hypercortisolism without features of overt Cushing's syndrome)
    - Adrenal adenoma (incidentaloma)
    - Adrenal macronodular hyperplasia (rare)
    - Pituitary corticotroph adenoma (rare)
    - Aberrant receptor expression (rare)
- Cushing's syndrome (pathologic hypercortisolism)
    - Exogenous glucocorticoid use
        - Oral glucocorticoids (prednisone, dexamethasone [Decadron], hydrocortisone [Cortef])
        - Topical glucocorticoids (inhaled, intranasal, dermal)
        - Injected glucocorticoids (articular, periarticular, intramuscular)
        - Naturopathic preparations
    - Endogenous glucocorticoid production
        - ACTH-dependent
            - Pituitary corticotroph adenoma
                - MEN1 (rare, also includes hyperparathyroidism and pancreatic islet cell tumors)
            - Pituitary corticotroph hyperplasia (some because of ectopic CRH)
            - Ectopic ACTH syndrome
                - Oat-cell lung carcinoma
                - Foregut carcinoid tumors (bronchial, thymic, splenic)
                - Pheochromocytoma
                - Medullary thyroid carcinoma
                - Islet cell tumors
        - ACTH-independent
            - Adrenal adenoma
            - Adrenocortical carcinoma
            - Rare: micronodular hyperplasia
            - Macronodular hyperplasia
                - Aberrant receptor expression (gastric inhibitory peptide–food responsive, 5-hydroxytryptamine, angiotensin II, interleukin-1, luteinizing hormone and human chorionic gonadotropin, vasopressin, β-adrenergic)
            - Pigmented micronodular hyperplasia (Carney's triad)
            - Adrenal rests
            - McCune-Albright (activating mutations)

Abbreviations: ACTH = adrenocorticotropic hormone; CRH = corticotrophin-releasing hormone; MEN1 = multiple endocrine neoplasia, type 1.

the lesion, and a higher prevalence of cardiovascular dysfunction. Although this syndrome is considered a very mild form of Cushing's syndrome, there appears to be a low rate of progression to overt Cushing's syndrome, and therapeutic decisions must be individualized.

Diagnostic Evaluation

EXOGENOUS GLUCOCORTICOIDS

Cushing's syndrome caused by exogenous glucocorticoid use can be obvious, but careful investigation for

unsuspected or surreptitious use must be undertaken in all patients. Infrequently recognized culprits are intraarticular, epidural, topical (inhaled, intranasal, and dermal), and naturopathic preparations. Variations in the metabolic clearance of synthetic glucocorticoids can lead to markedly prolonged glucocorticoid exposure and development of Cushing's syndrome. Detection of the synthetic glucocorticoid may require tandem mass spectrometry evaluation.

ENDOGENOUS HYPERCORTISOLISM

Evaluation of suspected endogenous hypercortisolemia must follow a stepwise approach (Figure 1). The first step is to make the diagnosis of Cushing's syndrome. The second step is to determine if the abnormal cortisol secretion is adrenocorticotropic hormone (ACTH)-dependent (from either a pituitary adenoma (Cushing's disease) or the ectopic ACTH syndrome) or ACTH-independent (primary adrenal disease). Finally, in ACTH-dependent Cushing's syndrome, the health care provider must distinguish pituitary sources of ACTH from the ectopic ACTH syndrome. Proceeding in the evaluation in a stepwise approach is critical for correct interpretation of test results because the premise of many of the tests is that preliminary biochemical diagnoses have been confirmed. For example, Cushing's syndrome must be confirmed before the ACTH level can be interpreted. In addition, because of the high prevalence of incidental pituitary and adrenal lesions and the finding of nodular adrenal disease in some cases of Cushing's disease caused by pituitary adenomas, imaging should not be performed until the biochemical diagnoses have been established. Finally, as many as 15% of patients with Cushing's syndrome will have intermittent hypercortisolemia, and care must be taken that the evaluation is performed when the patient is symptomatic or has documented hypercortisolism.

STEP ONE: DIAGNOSE CUSHING'S SYNDROME

The first step in the evaluation is to establish the diagnosis of Cushing's syndrome by demonstrating pathologic hypercortisolism, either by measuring cortisol overproduction, abnormal HPA regulation, or absent diurnal variation. We recommend four tests for this purpose: the 1 mg overnight dexamethasone suppression (1 mg ON dex) test, measurement of 24-hour urine-free cortisol (24-hour UFC) excretion, assessment of diurnal variation with a midnight serum or salivary cortisol level, and the dexamethasone-suppressed corticotrophin-releasing hormone stimulation (dex-CRH) test.

One Milligram Overnight Dexamethasone Suppression Test

The 1 mg ON dex test has sensitivity sufficiently high to exclude the diagnosis of Cushing's syndrome; however, it lacks sufficient specificity to confirm the diagnosis, with false-positive rates from 5% to 30%. The test is simple to perform and involves administering 1 mg

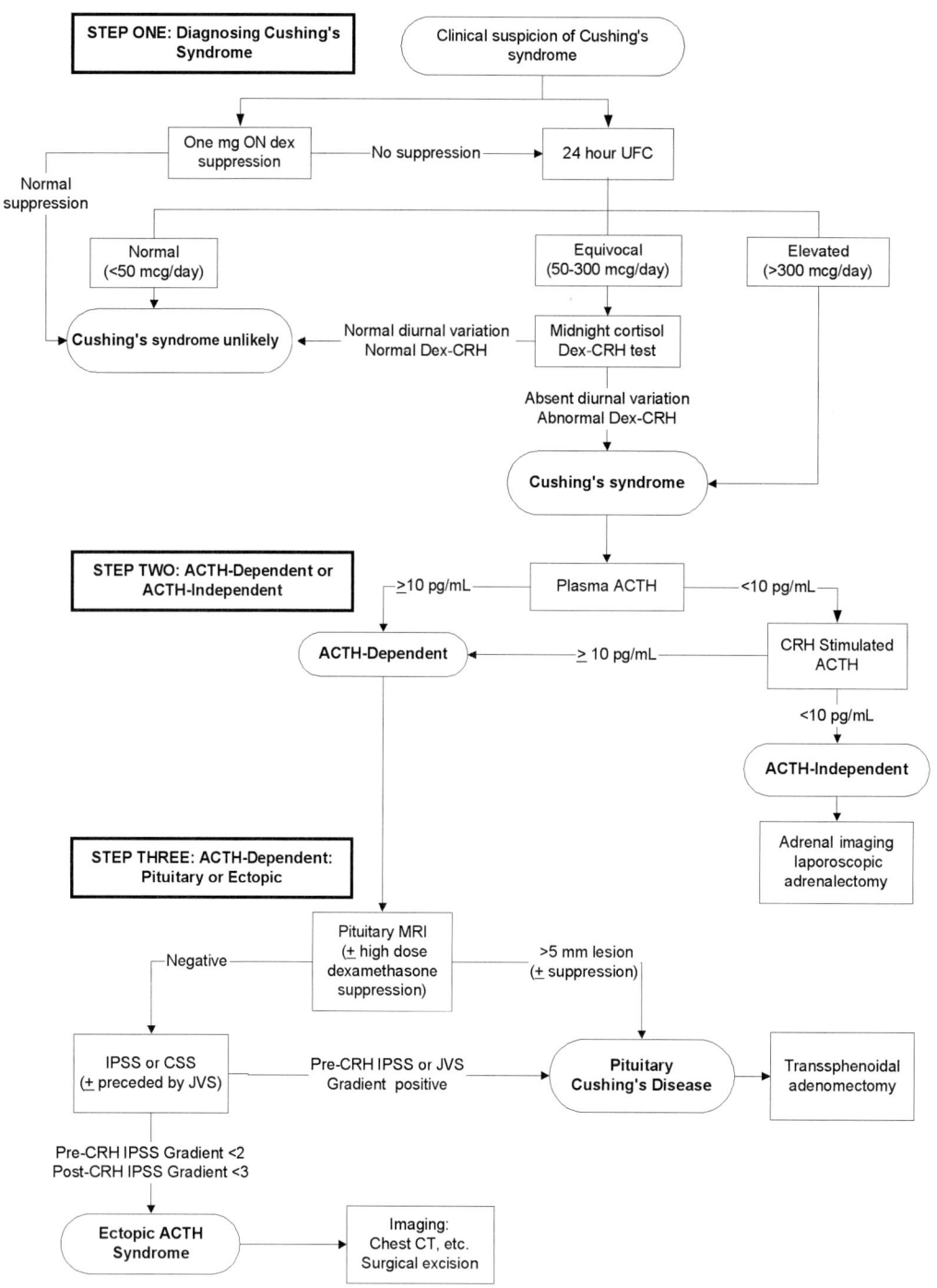

FIGURE 1. Stepwise approach to the diagnosis and differential diagnosis of Cushing's syndrome. ACTH = adrenocorticotropin; CRH = corticotrophin-releasing hormone; CSS = cavernous sinus sampling; CT = computed tomography; dex = dexamethasone; IPSS = inferior petrosal sinus sampling; JVS = jugular venous sampling; MRI = magnetic resonance imaging; ON = overnight; UFC = urine-free cortisol.

of dexamethasone (Decadron) by mouth at 11 PM. The serum cortisol at 8 AM the next morning should be less than 5 μg/dL; more strict criteria require suppression to less than 2.5 or 3 μg/dL. A simultaneous dexamethasone (Decadron) level can detect false positives that occur in patients taking medications that accelerate dexamethasone (Decadron) metabolism (phenytoin [Dilantin]), phenobarbital [Luminal], rifampin [Rifadin],

and primidone [Mysoline]). False positives may also be seen with estrogen therapy and tamoxifen (Nolvadex).

Measurement of 24-Hour Urine-Free Cortisol Excretion

Because of the high false-positive rate, an abnormal 1 mg ON dex test must be confirmed, usually by measurement

Rakel and Bope: *Conn's Current Therapy 2006.*

of 24-hour UFC excretion. Alternatively, a 24-hour UFC measurement may be the initial step in the evaluation. As shown in Figure 1, marked elevations in 24-hour UFC (>300 µg/day) confirm the diagnosis, but intermediate levels require additional evaluation. Because of potential problems with incomplete collections and intermittent hypercortisolemia, creatinine should be measured in the specimen, and normal 24-hour UFC excretion should be demonstrated on 2 or 3 occasions before the diagnosis of Cushing's syndrome is excluded. Acute medical illness can cause marked elevations in 24-hour UFC, false positives can occur with high urine volumes, and carbamazepine (Tegretol) can cross-react in the high-pressure liquid chromatography (HPLC) assay.

Midnight Serum or Salivary Cortisol Levels

Loss of the diurnal rhythm in cortisol secretion is a characteristic feature in Cushing's syndrome (Figure 2). Demonstration of a midnight serum cortisol greater than 7.5 µg/dL distinguishes patients with Cushing's syndrome from normal and pseudo-Cushing's patients with high sensitivity and specificity. More recent improvements in the salivary cortisol assay allow collection of a saliva sample at home, avoiding the logistic difficulties in arranging a blood draw at night. Cut-off values for salivary cortisol measurements vary by assay, but normal suppression is generally between less than 0.2 and 0.55 µg/dL.

Dexamethasone-Suppressed Corticotropin-Releasing Hormone Stimulation Test

The dex-CRH test detects the relative resistance to dexamethasone (Decadron) suppression and over-responsiveness to ovine corticotropin-releasing factor (oCRH [Acthrel]) in various tumors. It improves on the poor specificity of

the 1 mg ON dex test with a higher dose of dexamethasone (Decadron), 0.5 mg by mouth every 6 hours starting at 12 PM and ending at 6 AM on the second day. Because this dose of dexamethasone (Decadron) will suppress many pituitary adenomas, sensitivity of the test is retained by administration of oCRH (Acthrel)[1] 100 µg intravenously at 8 AM on the final day followed by cortisol and ACTH levels every 15 minutes for 1 hour. A plasma cortisol greater than 1.4 µg/dL distinguishes patients with Cushing's syndrome from those with pseudo-Cushing's with high accuracy.

STEP TWO: ACTH-DEPENDENT OR ACTH-INDEPENDENT DISEASE

Once the diagnosis of Cushing's syndrome has been established, the next step is to determine if the abnormal cortisol secretion is dependent on ACTH. A random ACTH level greater than 10 pg/mL confirms ACTH-dependent disease. However, because ACTH is secreted in a pulsatile, episodic fashion and is rapidly degraded, a low ACTH level must be confirmed by lack of stimulation to more than 10 pg/mL by oCRH (Acthrel),[1] 100 µg intravenously. When ACTH independent disease is confirmed, we then proceed with adrenal imaging, usually with high-resolution (3- to 5-mm sections), computed tomography (CT) to evaluate primary adrenal disease.

STEP THREE: DISTINGUISH PITUITARY FROM ECTOPIC SOURCES OF ACTH

Once ACTH-dependent disease has been confirmed, the health care provider must determine the source of excess ACTH secretion. Approximately 90% of patients have a

_____

[1]Not FDA approved for this indication.

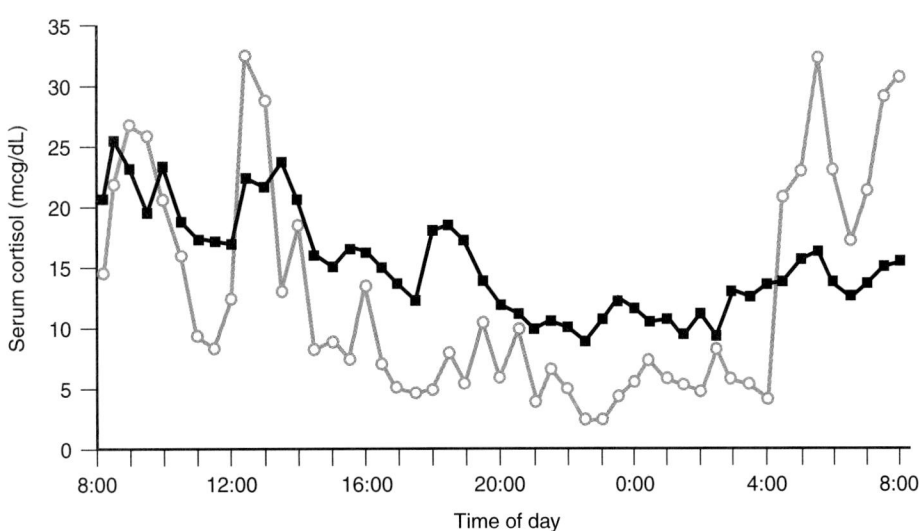

FIGURE 2. Diurnal rhythm of cortisol secretion is lost in Cushing's syndrome. Serum cortisol levels were measured every 30 minutes over 24 hours in a patient with proven Cushing's syndrome *(closed squares)* and a patient with pseudo-Cushing's syndrome *(open circles)*. Urine free cortisol (UFC) was mildly elevated in both patients (Cushing's syndrome, 75 µg/day; pseudo-Cushing's syndrome, 76 µg/day). Loss of diurnal variation in cortisol secretion is seen in the patient with Cushing's syndrome, whereas the patient with pseudo-Cushing's syndrome demonstrated normal diurnal variation with low serum cortisol levels (2.2 µg/dL) at midnight. (Data courtesy of Dr. Mary H. Samuels.)

pituitary corticotroph adenoma as the source of ACTH. A number of biochemical tests exist to distinguish pituitary from ectopic sources, the most accurate of which is the high-dose dexamethasone suppression test. This test involves comparison of a baseline 24-hour UFC with one collected during the second day of dexamethasone (Decadron) 2 mg by mouth every 6 hours for eight doses. Although failure to suppress more than 90% from the baseline UFC has been reported to have 100% specificity for identifying ectopic tumors, the sensitivity of this test is poor, and there have been subsequent reports of lower specificity. Because of this, we do not rely on biochemical testing. Rather, once ACTH-dependent disease is confirmed, we perform magnetic resonance imaging (MRI) of the pituitary gland. In approximately one half of patients, a definite tumor is identified, and we then proceed with transsphenoidal adenomectomy. However, another reasonable strategy is to proceed with pituitary surgery only if both MRI and high-dose dexamethasone testing suggests a pituitary tumor.

If a tumor is not definitely identified, inferior petrosal or cavernous sinus sampling with oCRH stimulation is required to localize the ACTH source. Finding a central (cavernous sinus or petrosal sinus) to peripheral ratio of more than 2.0 before oCRH or greater than 3.0 after oCRH is highly accurate for identifying a pituitary source of ACTH. In addition, a pre-oCRH lateralization (right to left or left to right) ratio more than 1.4 suggests the intrapituitary location of the tumor. Sampling must be performed by experienced personnel, and the accuracy of the test is highly dependent on oCRH administration, symmetric catheter placement, symmetric flow through the venous sinuses, and hypercortisolemia at the time of testing. In addition, it is critical that the diagnosis of Cushing's syndrome and ACTH-dependence be confirmed before proceeding with sampling. Normal individuals and patients with pseudo-Cushing's syndrome have inferior petrosal sinus sampling (IPSS) results that falsely suggest a pituitary tumor. Patients with ACTH-independent disease (primary adrenal disease) with low but measurable ACTH levels can have IPSS results that falsely suggest either a pituitary tumor or the ectopic ACTH syndrome.

Recently, internal jugular venous sampling has been evaluated as a less invasive alternative to petrosal sinus sampling. A jugular to peripheral ratio of greater than 1.7 before oCRH or more than 2.5 after oCRH indicate a pituitary source with high accuracy. Nondiagnostic ratios are unreliable and should be further evaluated with inferior petrosal or cavernous sinus sampling.

If sampling suggests an ectopic source of ACTH, imaging is then performed to locate the tumor, starting with high resolution CT or MRI of the chest. If those areas are unrevealing, neck, abdomen, and pelvis CT are performed. Octreotide scanning may be helpful but only rarely identifies an abnormality not already seen on anatomic imaging. Often, the culprit lesion is not seen at initial imaging, but becomes apparent on serial studies performed every 6 to 12 months.

Although IPSS is highly accurate, occasional false-negative and rare false-positive results have been reported. In situations where IPSS ratios indicate the ectopic ACTH syndrome but no ectopic tumor can be found, distinguishing a truly occult ectopic ACTH-producing tumor from a false-negative IPSS is extremely difficult. Review of the response of peripheral ACTH levels to oCRH stimulation should be done, because pituitary adenomas have significantly more robust responses than ectopic tumors. Repeat IPSS and consideration of pituitary exploration are appropriate, particularly if the ACTH response to oCRH, biochemical testing, and/or MRI are consistent with a pituitary adenoma.

Therapeutic Interventions

EXOGENOUS GLUCOCORTICOID USE

Once identified, the treatment for iatrogenic Cushing's syndrome is straightforward but often difficult because of the therapeutic benefit of pharmacologic glucocorticoids. Tapering the steroid needs to occur gradually, with close monitoring of the underlying disease process and optimization of nonsteroid therapeutics. Alternate-day dosing regimens may assist in HPA axis recovery but may be limited by the underlying disease process. Patients should wear Medic Alert identification until the taper is completed and normal HPA function is demonstrated.

ENDOGENOUS CUSHING'S SYNDROME

The therapeutic intervention in essentially all etiologies of endogenous Cushing's syndrome is surgical resection of the autonomous tumor or tissue, except for the case of lung carcinomas causing the ectopic ACTH syndrome, where therapy is tailored to the stage of the cancer. Postoperatively, all patients are treated with stress doses of glucocorticoids, tapering quickly to doses approximately twice physiologic replacement, usually hydrocortisone (Cortef)[1] 20 mg by mouth twice or three times daily. Further slow taper is done over the next several months as tolerated by cortisol withdrawal symptoms and recovery of the HPA axis. A morning serum cortisol level less than 2 µg/dL on the second postoperative day is highly predictive of surgical cure; patients with low but detectable serum cortisol levels, such as less than 5 µg/dL, have varying cure rates. Periodic morning cortisol levels and cosyntropin (Cortrosyn)[1] stimulation testing assess recovery of the HPA axis during and after the glucocorticoid taper.

Cushing's Disease

Transsphenoidal adenomectomy is recommended for the vast majority of patients with pituitary tumors, except where extensive cavernous sinus involvement indicates a transfrontal approach. Intraoperative ultrasound or MRI can assist in the localization of tumors. If a tumor is not identified at surgery, hemihypophysectomy based

---

[1]Not FDA approved for this indication.

Rakel and Bope: *Conn's Current Therapy 2006.*

on preoperative MRI and/or IPSS or CSS lateralization ratios may result in cure. Often, tumors are not identified on pathology, because they are semiliquid and "lost" during suctioning.

Mortality and morbidity are generally low in experienced centers, but complications can include cerebrospinal fluid leaks, meningitis, visual impairment, hypopituitarism, hemorrhage, venous thromboembolism, and death. Careful monitoring for abnormalities in vasopressin secretion postoperatively is required, both for diabetes insipidus and the syndrome of inappropriate antidiuretic-hormone secretion. Testing of pituitary function including free T4, IGF-1 with possible growth hormone stimulation testing and testosterone levels or menstrual history is performed at 6 weeks postoperatively.

Even in experienced hands, long-term cure of hypercortisolemia is difficult, with initial success rates reported from 68.5% to 91% and relapse rates of up to 15% over a 10-year period. Cure rates are worse for macroadenomas or invasive tumors and second surgeries, reported at 40% to 55%. Even with biochemical cure and improvement in symptoms, studies show persistent compromise in quality of life.

Primary Adrenal Disease

The laparoscopic approach has essentially replaced open surgery with similar mortality, morbidity, and operative times; and shorter postoperative recovery, hospital stays, and decreased acute and chronic pain. The laparoscopic approach is not used in cases of adrenocortical carcinoma or patients with coagulopathy, previous surgery or trauma. Lesion size was previously a limitation, but with increasing experience appears to no longer be a significant factor. Unilateral adrenalectomy is indicated for adrenal adenomas and adrenocortical carcinomas; the rare nodular hyperplasias are treated with bilateral surgery. Adrenalectomy is curative for adrenal adenomas and hyperplasia, but carcinomas are often advanced at presentation and generally have a poor prognosis. Adrenolytic therapy with mitotane (Lysodren) may be necessary to control hypercortisolemia and tumor growth in carcinomas postoperatively.

9

TABLE 2 Drugs Used in the Medical Therapy of Cushing's Syndrome

Medication	Mechanism of Action	Typical Dosage	Reported Efficacy	Common Toxicities
Steroid Biosynthesis Inhibitors				
Ketoconazole (Nizoral)[1]	Blocks multiple steps in cortisol synthesis	200-1200 mg/d	70%	Hepatotoxicity, gynecomastia, nausea, edema, rash
Metyrapone (Metopirone)[1]	Blocks 11β-hydroxylase	500-6000 mg/d	85%	Hirsutism, acne, lethargy, dizziness, ataxia, edema, nausea, rash
Aminoglutethimide (Cytadren)	Blocks cholesterol to pregnenolone conversion	750-2000 mg/d	>60% Useful additive to metyrapone	Lethargy, somnolence, dizziness, rash, fever, nausea, anorexia, hyopthyroidism
Mitotane (o,p'-DDD, Lysodren)[1*]	Blocks side-chain cleavage Adrenolytic	500-12,000 mg/d	83%	Gastrointestinal, impaired mentation, dizziness, hyperlipidemia, gynecomastia, transient rash, hepatotoxicity
ACTH Release Inhibitors				
Cyproheptadine (Periactin)[1]	Impairs ACTH secretion	24 mg/d	30%-50%	Somnolence, hyperphagia, weight gain
Bromocriptine (Parlodel)[1]	Impairs ACTH secretion	3.75-30 mg/d	25%-42%	Nausea, dry mouth, postural hypotension
Octreotide (Sandostatin)[1]	Inhibits ACTH release	100-600 μg/d	Limited experience, additive to ketoconazole	Diarrhea, gallstones
Valproic acid (Depakene)[1]	Potentiate GABA inhibition of CRH and ACTH release	1-2 g/d	Limited experience, additive to metyrapone	Sedation, nausea, hepatotoxicity, pancreatitis
Glucocorticoid Receptor Antagonist				
Mifepristone (RU-486, Mifeprex)[1]	Glucocorticoid receptor antagonist	10-25 mg/kg/d	Limited experience	Nausea, vomiting, irregular menses

[1]Not FDA approved for this indication.
*FDA approved for treatment of adrenocortical carcinoma.
Abbreviations: ACTH = adrenocorticotropic hormone; CRH = corticotropin-releasing hormone; GABA = gamma-aminobutyric acid.

Rakel and Bope: *Conn's Current Therapy 2006.*

Secondary Therapy for Failed Pituitary Surgery or Occult Ectopic Tumors

If transsphenoidal surgery fails to resolve the hypercortisolemia, patients can be offered pituitary irradiation. If a lesion can be targeted, stereotactic radiosurgery with a linear accelerator (LINAC) system, gamma-knife system, or proton beam system offers lower radiation exposure to surrounding normal tissue and theoretically more effective higher doses to the residual tumor than conventional fractionated radiation therapy. Time to control of hypercortisolemia is variable, reported from 6 to 36 months, requiring interim control of hypercortisolemia by either medical therapy or adrenalectomy. Complications of radiation therapy include hypopituitarism, rare optic neuropathy, and rare (and debated) induction of second tumors and brain necrosis. The risk of Nelson's syndrome (rapid and aggressive growth of corticotroph tumors after adrenalectomy) may be lessened with radiation therapy.

Alternatively, and in the cases of ectopic tumors remaining occult, bilateral adrenalectomy can be performed offering immediate control of hypercortisolemia. Both glucocorticoid and mineralocorticoid (fludrocortisone [Florinef] 0.1 mg by mouth once or twice daily) replacement are generally required. Glucocorticoids are tapered as described above to physiologic doses of hydrocortisone (Cortef)[1] 20 to 30 mg by mouth daily in single or divided doses. Continued surveillance with imaging is required, because of the risk of development of Nelson's syndrome and the occasional, locally invasive, and rarely metastatic potential of ectopic tumors.

Medical Management of Hypercortisolemia

Medical management of hypercortisolemia has an inadequate efficacy and side-effect profile for primary or long-term use. However, it has a very important role in temporizing the pathologic effects of long-standing Cushing's syndrome in preparation for surgical treatment and while awaiting definitive cure from radiation therapy. Strategies include medications (Table 2) that block glucocorticoid synthesis, inhibit pituitary ACTH secretion, or block glucocorticoid action. None of the agents that inhibit ACTH release is very effective but might be useful in combination therapy. The most effective medications are those that block glucocorticoid synthesis including ketoconazole[1] (Nizoral), metyrapone[1] (Metopirone), and mitotane[1*] (o,p'DDD, Lysodren).

---

[1]Not FDA approved for this indication.
*FDA approved only for adrenocortical carcinoma.

CURRENT DIAGNOSIS

- The clinical presentation of Cushing's syndrome is nonspecific and overlaps that of other more common diseases such as polycystic ovary syndrome, the metabolic syndrome, and depression.
- Signs and symptoms more specific for Cushing's syndrome include unexplained osteoporosis, muscle weakness, spontaneous ecchymoses, hypokalemia, central obesity, and plethora. Children present with growth failure, generalized obesity, and menstrual irregularities.
- A stepwise approach to the diagnosis helps avoid pitfalls in the interpretation of diagnostic tests. The first step is to confirm the diagnosis of Cushing's syndrome. The second step is to determine if the patient has ACTH-dependent or ACTH-independent disease. The final step is to determine if the ACTH source is eutopic (from the pituitary gland) or ectopic (the ectopic ACTH syndrome).
- The 1 mg ON dex test is easy to perform and has good sensitivity for diagnosing Cushing's syndrome. However, because of its poor specificity, confirmatory testing with measurement of urine free cortisol, midnight serum or salivary cortisol or the dex-CRH test is required.
- Random or CRH-stimulated ACTH levels greater than 10 pg/mL indicate ACTH-dependent disease.
- Biochemical testing is inadequate for distinguishing pituitary tumors from the ectopic ACTH syndrome. Jugular venous sampling has a high positive predictive value, but if negative, inferior petrosal or cavernous sinus sampling with CRH stimulation is required.
- Pituitary MRI is positive in only approximately one half of patients with corticotroph adenomas.

Abbreviations: ACTH = adrenocorticotropic hormone; CRH = corticotrophin-releasing hormone; dex = dexamethasone; MRI = magnetic resonance imaging; 1 mg ON dex test = 1 mg overnight dexamethasone suppression test.

CURRENT THERAPY

- Treatment for Cushing's syndrome is primarily surgical and targeted to the pathologic lesion.
- Transsphenoidal adenomectomy is recommended for pituitary-dependent Cushing's disease, but has a long-term success rate of only 60% to 80%.
- Laparoscopic adrenalectomy has replaced open approaches in the management of primary adrenal lesions except for adrenocortical carcinoma, and for second-line treatment after failed pituitary surgery or failure to localize an occult ectopic tumor.
- Definitive secondary treatments for failed pituitary surgery include pituitary irradiation and bilateral adrenalectomy.
- Medical therapy for Cushing's syndrome is difficult, and reserved for surgical failures awaiting benefit from radiation therapy or in preparation for surgical therapy.

Rakel and Bope: *Conn's Current Therapy 2006.*

These are usually dosed to partially block cortisol production, suppressing it into the normal range. Alternatively, complete adrenal blockade with replacement hydrocortisone can be attempted. Finally, very limited experience with blockade of the glucocorticoid receptor with mifepristone (Mifeprex)[1] has shown clinical efficacy. Because glucocorticoids levels are unaffected, titration of this medication must be done on clinical grounds.

REFERENCES

Bochicchio D, Losa M, Buchfelder M: Factors influencing the immediate and late outcome of Cushing's disease treated by transsphenoidal surgery: A retrospective study by the European Cushing's disease survey group. J Clin Endocrinol Metab 1995;80:3114-3120.

Hammer GD, Tyrrell JB, Lamborn KR, et al: Transsphenoidal microsurgery for Cushing's disease: Initial outcome and long-term results. J Clin Endocrinol Metab 2004;89:6348-6357.

Ilias I, Chang R, Pacak K, et al: Jugular venous sampling: An alternative to petrosal sinus sampling for the diagnostic evaluation of adrenocorticotropic hormone-dependent Cushing's syndrome. J Clin Endocrinol Metab 2004;89:3795-3800.

Leinung MC, Zimmerman D: Cushing's disease in children. Endocrinol Metab Clin North Am 1994;23:629-39.

Mahmoud-Ahmed AS, Suh JH: Radiation therapy for Cushing's disease: A review. Pituitary 2002;5:175-180.

Nieman LK: Medical therapy of Cushing's disease. Pituitary 2002; 5:77-82.

Oldfield E, Doppman J, Nieman L, et al: Petrosal sinus sampling with and without corticotropin-releasing hormone for the differential diagnosis of Cushing's syndrome. N Engl J Med 1991;325:897-905.

Papanicolaou DA, Mullen N, Kyrou I, Nieman LK: Nighttime salivary cortisol: A useful test for the diagnosis of Cushing's syndrome. J Clin Endocrinol Metab 2002;87:4515-4521

Reincke M: Subclinical Cushing's syndrome. Endocrinol Metab Clin North Am 2000;29:43-56.

Yanovski J, Cutler G, Chrousos G, Nieman L: Corticotropin-releasing hormone stimulation following low-dose dexamethasone (Decadron) administration. JAMA 1993;269:2232-2238.

[1]Not FDA approved for this indication.

Diabetes Insipidus

Method of
Alan G. Robinson, MD

Diabetes insipidus literally means excretion of tasteless urine and is a disorder caused by different diseases that affect the ability of the kidney to produce concentrated urine because of lack of the hormone vasopressin or lack of response to the hormone. The excretion of a large volume of urine, polyuria, must be distinguished at the outset from frequency, urgency, and urinary symptoms that do not connote a large urine volume. In considering therapy for this disorder, one must have determined the cause among the major differential types of diabetes insipidus: hypothalamic neurohypophyseal diabetes insipidus caused by an inability to secrete (and usually synthesize) vasopressin; nephrogenic diabetes insipidus caused by an inappropriate response to vasopressin at the level of the kidney; transient diabetes insipidus of pregnancy in which there is excessive metabolism of vasopressin; and primary polydipsia in which there is no abnormality of vasopressin but only an inappropriate ingestion of water. It is assumed here that the pathologic cause of the diabetes insipidus has been determined (infiltrated disease, tumor, trauma, idiopathic, renal disease with nephrogenic, etc.) and that the underlying disease has been appropriately treated. It should also be noted that children with diabetes insipidus require special attention and should be seen by a pediatric endocrinologist. The recommendations and dosages described here are for adult patients.

If sufficient water is taken in, lack of vasopressin alone and inability to concentrate the urine do not usually cause any biochemical abnormality in the body. It is, however, inconvenient for the patient to be constantly in need of a large volume of water to drink and to continuously excrete a large volume of urine. A major goal of therapy is to reduce the urine volume and the inconvenience of the patient to a minimum. This assumes that the patient is conscious and able to sense thirst. Patients who are unable to sense thirst constitute a special therapeutic challenge (which is discussed) and patients who are unconscious are at risk for severe dehydration and medical complications from dehydration. It is suggested that patients with diabetes insipidus carry a card or medical alert bracelet indicating the diagnosis and including the name of a physician knowledgeable about the disorder, so in an emergency diabetes insipidus is not confused with diabetes mellitus.

Central Neurohypophyseal Diabetes Insipidus

Box 1 lists the agents available to treat diabetes insipidus.

In the past much was made of distinguishing complete severe hypothalamic diabetes insipidus from partial hypothalamic diabetes insipidus. In fact, whether there is no vasopressin secreted or a small amount of vasopressin secreted that is inadequate to the need has little influence on the recommended therapy. In both cases replacement of vasopressin with desmopressin (DDAVP) is the preferred therapy. Desmopressin (1-[3-mercaptopropanoic acid]-8-D-arginine vasopressin) is

---

BOX 1 Therapeutic Agents to Treat Diabetes Insipidus

- Water
- Water-retaining agents
  - Arginine vasopressin (Pitressin)
  - Desmopressin (DDAVP)
  - Chlorpropamide (Diabinese)[1]
  - Indomethacin (Indocin)[1]
- Natriuretic agents
  - Thiazide diuretics
  - Amiloride (Midamor)[1]

[1]Not FDA approved for this indication.

a synthetic analogue of arginine vasopressin in which D-arginine is substituted in position 8 and the terminal amine is eliminated. These two changes produce an agent that is nearly 2000 times more specific for antidiuresis than vasopressin. There is considerable variability among patients in response to desmopressin, and it is useful in initiating therapy to determine the duration of a dose by asking the patient to keep a diary recording the volume and time of each voided urine. The patient is allowed ad lib fluid, and when the flow equals that equivalent to what would produce approximately 4 L per day, a dose of desmopressin can be given. Desmopressin reaches a maximum action in 1 to 2 hours and will, in most patients, persist for 6 to 12 hours or longer, depending on the dose and delivery of desmopressin. Once a total duration of action is determined, a dosage schedule can be devised to produce minimum antidiuresis, especially during the important part of the patient's day (e.g., work and/or sleep).

Most patients prefer to begin with the desmopressin tablets available in 0.1- and 0.2-mg tablets. Therapy is begun with a low dose, 0.1 mg or one half of that tablet, and increased as necessary. It is important to note that stepwise doubling of the dose often produces only a modest increase in the duration of the dose of a few hours and no increase in the maximum urinary concentration. Usually a dose is found that can be given two or three times per day and that maintains the patient in an asymptomatic state. An occasional early dose or extra dose may be necessary to assure antidiuresis for a specific event.

Desmopressin is also available as an intranasally administered spray (Minirin) or as a liquid that is given with a rhinal catheter. The spray has the disadvantage of less flexibility because it is fixed at 10 μg in a 100-μL spray, and the rhinal catheter has the disadvantage of an inconvenient form of administration. However, the rhinal catheter does allow more variability in the dose that is administered and, for some patients, may be more reliable than the oral medication. Patients should be trained in the appropriate use of the rhinal catheter and it should be noted that the liquid form of desmopressin requires refrigeration for storage.

Parenterally administered desmopressin is available in various sized vials or ampules at a concentration of 4 μg/mL. This is rarely used for routine management of ambulatory patients, but can be administered in a dose of 0.5 to 2 μg total dose given either subcutaneously, intramuscularly, or intravenously in a patient hospitalized for another condition or when there is some other reason that the patient cannot receive desmopressin orally or intranasally. If used for maintenance therapy, a much smaller dose given subcutaneously with an insulin syringe will often suffice.

The complication that must be considered when using desmopressin therapy is hyponatremia, which will occur if a patient drinks excessive amounts of fluid while antidiuretic because of the pharmacologic therapy. This must be considered when allowing the patient to follow a flexible dosage schedule. In addition to checking the patient's symptoms of polyuria and polydipsia, one should regularly check serum sodium to be certain

this it is maintained within a normal range. When starting therapy, serum sodium should be checked more regularly (i.e., daily). When diabetes insipidus is adequately treated, absence of thirst provides protection against drinking excessively. One can avoid the possibility of hyponatremia by occasionally delaying a dose of desmopressin and allowing the patient to excrete any excess fluid that might have been retained.

Although not approved as an antidiuretic agent, chlorpropamide (Diabinese)[1] increases the action of vasopressin and has been used to treat diabetes insipidus. It must be noted in the record that permission was obtained from the patient to use this agent off-label. Therapy can be initiated with 100 mg per day and increased every 4 days until satisfactory diuresis is maintained. The usual dose is 250 to 500 mg per day. Chlorpropamide is not recommended for children and care must be taken to prevent hypoglycemia especially in patients who are panhypopituitary. Maintenance of regular food intake and routine testing of the blood sugar are required.

There are several clinical situations in which there are special considerations regarding therapy of hypothalamic diabetes insipidus.

HYPOTHALAMIC DIABETES INSIPIDUS AFTER INTRACRANIAL SURGERY

It is important to recognize that after any surgical procedure, if large amounts of fluid are administered, large amounts of urine will be excreted. Consequently, it should always be determined that polyuria persists without administration of large volumes of fluid and in spite of an elevation of serum sodium. If the patient is alert and able to respond to thirst, the usual guidelines for treatment with desmopressin can be instituted and the patient's thirst will be a guide to appropriate therapy. However, if fluids are being administered intravenously, one must check the serum sodium regularly and exercise caution to avoid precipitating hyponatremia. It should also be noted that after pituitary surgery the diabetes insipidus may be transient, and after 5 to 7 days, followed by a phase of uncontrolled release of vasopressin from damaged posterior pituitary neurons. The released vasopressin can produce an antidiuresis and the syndrome of inappropriate secretion of antidiuretic hormone (SIADH) with hyponatremia for several days, which might then be followed by return of diabetes insipidus. The hyponatremia may present quite precipitously with vomiting or seizures and require therapy and fluid restriction to raise the Na$^+$. Some recent studies report using a continuous intravenous infusion of dilute arginine vasopressin (Pitressin) to control diabetes insipidus postoperatively. Infusions of 0.25 to 2.7 mU/kg per hour have been used with the advantage touted that the short half-life of vasopressin (10 to 20 minutes) is an advantage of this form of therapy. The author has no personal experience with this form of therapy, but it is obvious that serum sodium and urine output should be monitored closely.

---

[1]Not FDA approved for this indication.

TRAUMATIC DIABETES INSIPIDUS

Traumatic diabetes insipidus may occur with injury to the head, usually from a motor vehicle accident with injury to the skull and damage or section of the pituitary stalk. The symptoms and course are similar to those of diabetes insipidus after hypothalamic surgery. The risk is that the diabetes insipidus will not be diagnosed in the emergency situation. It is essential also in these situations to consider loss of anterior pituitary function and to treat with appropriate doses of hydrocortisone.

DIABETES INSIPIDUS WITH INADEQUATE THIRST

This produces a difficult management problem. There are reports that chlorpropamide[1] might increase thirst in some of these patients; consequently, a therapeutic trial might be considered to treat both the diabetes insipidus and lack of thirst. There is a special form of partial diabetes insipidus with inadequate thirst in which there is no response of the osmoreceptor to sense thirst or to stimulate secretion of vasopressin, yet the volume/baroreceptors are intact. These patients left to their own devices become hypernatremic but then stabilize at a constant level of hypernatremia because when dehydrated, the stimulation of the baroreceptors stimulate enough vasopressin release to maintain low urine volume. Polyuria may only return when sufficient fluid is given to replace the volume deficit.

In these cases, the most advantageous therapy is to select a dose of antidiuretic agent (usually desmopressin [DDAVP]) that produces chronic antidiuresis and then to vary the amount of liquid given to maintain the patient in a normal sodium balance. A rigid regimen of administered antidiuresis and water intake prescribed every 6 to 8 hours to maintain the required 24-hour intake must be maintained. These patients require frequent measure of serum sodium to insure adequate therapy.

DIABETES INSIPIDUS IN PREGNANCY

Diabetes insipidus in pregnancy may be caused by the action of the normally occurring cysteine aminopeptidase (oxytocinase) that is produced by the placenta and also destroys vasopressin. Normal levels of cysteine aminopeptidase may produce symptomatic diabetes insipidus in patients with otherwise asymptomatic diabetes insipidus (e.g., there is limited ability to concentrate the urine, but a urine volume of 3 to 4 L/day is acceptable to the patient). A rare syndrome of markedly excessive oxytocinase will produce diabetes insipidus in otherwise normal women. Desmopressin is the recommended therapeutic agent, because in the doses used to treat diabetes insipidus desmopressin has minimal oxytocic action on the uterus. It is important that the physician be aware of the expansion of extracellular fluid and the decrease in serum sodium that is normal during pregnancy, and that therapy be sufficient to maintain the normal decrease in serum sodium. As with

any patient receiving desmopressin, care should be taken with fluid administration during delivery to avoid producing hyponatremia. With the decrease in oxytocinase after delivery, diabetes insipidus may disappear or the patient may become asymptomatic with an acceptable urine volume.

Nephrogenic Diabetes Insipidus

Potential offending agents (e.g., lithium or other drugs) should be discontinued if possible. Potential contributing clinical situations (e.g., hypercalcemia or hypokalemia) should be corrected. Adequate water intake should always be maintained and may be lifesaving in congenital nephrogenic diabetes insipidus. Because these patients will not respond to administered desmopressin, therapy is aimed at reducing urine volume by causing volume contraction. This can be done by reducing total body sodium with diet and a thiazide diuretic. The major action is to decrease the glomerular filtration rate (GFR) and increase proximal sodium and water reabsorption, thus decreasing delivery of fluid to the distal diluting segment. Potassium replacement or co-administration of a potassium-sparing antidiuretic may be useful. Amiloride (Midamor)[1] is a preferred agent and is especially useful in lithium-induced nephrogenic diabetes insipidus because it decreases lithium entry into cells in the distal tubule. Co-administration of indomethacin (Indocin)[1] may be of benefit in these patients, but the possibility of inducing duodenal ulcer and gastrointestinal (GI) hemorrhage requires that this be administered with caution.

Primary Polydipsia

There is no specific treatment for primary polydipsia, but any disorder of the hypothalamus that can cause diabetes insipidus may cause disordered thirst and induce primary polydipsia. In these cases the possible coexistence of diabetes insipidus must be considered and treated if present. The disadvantage of using an antidiuretic agent such as desmopressin in a patient of primary polydipsia is the potential to produce SIADH and hyponatremia. If the disorder is a result of a psychiatric syndrome, treating that syndrome may be helpful. Often there is a habitual lifetime pattern of excessive drinking that is refractory to attempts to restrict fluid.

Managing Diabetes Insipidus in Association With Other Therapy

DIABETES INSIPIDUS WITH PANHYPOPITUITARISM

In diabetes insipidus with panhypopituitarism, remember that patients with hypoadrenalism and hypothyroidism have an inability to excrete water. Therefore, when

---

[1]Not FDA approved for this indication.

---

[1]Not FDA approved for this indication.

these deficiencies coexist with diabetes insipidus and are not treated, there may be no polyuria. If a patient with hypothyroidism and hypoadrenalism is replaced with thyroid hormone and hydrocortisone, diabetes insipidus may become manifest. It is important, therefore, for patients with combined anterior and posterior pituitary deficiencies to maintain uninterrupted and full replacement for all anterior pituitary deficiencies, as well as treatment of diabetes insipidus.

SURGICAL PROCEDURES

Routine surgical procedures are often sufficiently limited in time that the patient can have their normal dose of desmopressin and then limit the fluid administered during the procedure to maintain normal serum sodium. The anesthesiologist and endocrinologist should confer prior to the procedure.

SALINE DIURESIS

Promoting a saline diuresis is necessary for some medical treatments (e.g., chemotherapy) and when a large amount of normal saline is given to a patient taking desmopressin, the fluid may induce natriuresis and hyponatremia (SIADH). Withholding desmopressin to allow return of diabetes insipidus and replacing the urine volume with normal saline will lead to hypernatremia. Continuous ultra low-dose vasopressin (e.g., 0.08 to 0.1 mU/kg/hour) is reported to control diuresis while allowing administration of normal saline. Fluid input/output and serum sodium must be monitored carefully.

HYPERTONIC ENCEPHALOPATHY

Hypertonic encephalopathy may occur in the treatment of diabetes insipidus. Usually diabetes insipidus and hypernatremia are known to be acute and treatment with desmopressin and water can be used to bring the sodium back to normal. When the duration of hypernatremia is unknown and is believed to be chronic, the brain may have accommodated to the hypernatremia with production of "idiogenic osmols." Overly rapid normalization of the serum sodium may produce cerebral edema and worsening of the neurologic condition. In such cases, the degree of correction of hypernatremia should not exceed 0.5 mEq/L per hour, and the patient should be continuously checked for signs of cerebral edema.

ORGAN DONORS

Organ donors may have diabetes insipidus because diabetes insipidus commonly occurs when a patient becomes brain dead. If the patient is a candidate for organ donation, it is reasonable to consider treatment of the diabetes insipidus with desmopressin to maintain normal sodium. This is another situation in which continuous administration of low-dose vasopressin intravenously, as described above, may be an appropriate therapy.

Hyperparathyroidism and Hypoparathyroidism

Method of
Jeffrey A. Jackson, MD

Hyperparathyroidism

PRIMARY HYPERPARATHYROIDISM

Primary hyperparathyroidism (PHPT) is a generalized disorder of calcium and phosphate metabolism resulting from an increased production of parathyroid hormone (PTH) caused by an intrinsic abnormality of the parathyroid glands. It is the most common cause of hypercalcemia in nonhospitalized patients. The incidence of PHPT has been declining over recent decades for unclear reasons: from 91 per 100,000 of the general population in 1979; to about 21 per 100,000 during the period 1983-1992; to 4 per 100,000 in 1992 (in Rochester, Minnesota). Women are more affected than men (3:2 ratio) except in the inherited conditions associated with PHPT; the incidence of PHPT rises with age, especially in postmenopausal women. Over time, the clinical profile of PHPT has shifted from a symptomatic disease with overt bone disease, nephrolithiasis, renal failure and severe hypercalcemia toward an asymptomatic one.

Etiology

Box 1 lists the causes of hyperparathyroidism: 80% to 85% of cases are caused by single adenomas (mostly

---

> **BOX 1   Causes of Hyperparathyroidism**
>
> **Primary HPT**
> - Single and multiple adenomas
> - Multigland hyperplasia-sporadic, familial HPT ± jaw tumors, MEN-1, MEN-2A
> - Parathyroid carcinoma
> - Familial benign hypocalciuric hypercalcemia
> - Neonatal primary HPT
> - Drug-related (chronic lithium)
>
> **Secondary HPT**
> - Vitamin D deficiency—nutritional, postgastric surgery, malabsorption syndromes, hepatobiliary disease, drugs (anticonvulsants, sun blockers, and others)
> - Chronic renal insufficiency
> - Vitamin D dependency—defective renal 1-hydroxylase, defective calcitriol receptor, X-linked hypophosphatemic rickets/bone disease, other causes of prolonged hypophosphatemia or phosphate supplementation
>
> **Tertiary HPT**
> - Renal osteodystrophy
>
> ---
> *Abbreviations*: HPT = hyperparathyroidism; MEN-1 = multiple endocrine neoplasia type 1; MEN-2A = multiple endocrine neoplasia type 2A.

monoclonal tumors). Multigland hyperplasia may be sporadic but often indicates a hereditary cause (multiple endocrine neoplasia [MEN] syndromes or hereditary PHPT with or without jaw tumors). MEN-1 includes parathyroid hyperplasia and pituitary and pancreatic islet cell tumors, and has been mapped to the MEN-1 tumor-suppressor gene locus (11q13). MEN-2A includes parathyroid hyperplasia, bilateral C-cell hyperplasia and medullary thyroid carcinoma, and bilateral adreno-medullary hyperplasia and pheochromocytomas, and is associated with mutations in the RET proto-oncogene (chromosome 10q). Parathyroid carcinoma is more common in the familial syndromes and accounts for less than 1% of PHPT. It is associated with HRPT2 (hyper-parathyroidism 2) gene mutations (chromosome 1q, the same gene associated with hereditary hyperpara-thyroidism [HPT] and jaw tumors).

Sporadic PHPT may be associated with prior external head/neck irradiation and chronic lithium therapy. PHPT may often be brought out by the hypocalciuric effects of thiazide diuretics. Familial benign hypocalci-uric hypercalcemia (FBHH) should always be distin-guished from other causes of PHPT because surgical intervention is unnecessary in these patients.

Clinical Features

Classic symptoms of PHPT (skeletal-osteitis fibrosa cystica or "brown" tumors; renal-nephrocalcinosis and azotemia; gastrointestinal-peptic ulcer disease or pancre-atitis [the latter no longer clearly associated with PHPT])

BOX 2 Nonparathyroid Causes of Hypercalcemia
Malignant Disease
• Parathyroid hormone-related peptide excess (carcinomas of the lung, breast, head and neck, T-cell lymphomas, and others)
• Multiple myeloma
• Cancers metastatic to bone
• 1,25-dihydroxyvitamin D excess (rare; lymphomas)
Endocrinopathies/Metabolic Disorders
• Hyperthyroidism
• Adrenal insufficiency
• Milk-alkali syndrome
• Hypophosphatemia
Granulomatous Disease (1α-Hydroxylase [Vitamin D] Mediated)
• Sarcoidosis
• Other: tuberculosis, chronic berylliosis, fungal diseases, etc.
Drug-Induced
• Vitamins A and D
• Thiazides
• Lithium
• Aluminum intoxication, etc.
Other
• Immobilization with high bone turnover (children, Paget's disease)
• Acute and chronic renal failure

Rakel and Bope: *Conn's Current Therapy 2006.*

---

are now rare. These "bones, stones, and abdominal groans" have been replaced by subtle neuromuscular symptoms (muscle weakness or aching) or central nervous system symptoms (depression or reduced sense of well-being)—"psychic moans and fatigue overtones"—although pres-entation with renal lithiasis is not uncommon. Physical findings are usually sparse; band keratopathy is uncom-mon. Palpable neck masses are usually of thyroid origin (rarely giant parathyroid adenomas or carcinomas).

Diagnosis

The biochemical hallmarks of PHPT are hypercalcemia and elevated or inappropriate levels of PTH. Measurement of ionized calcium may be useful in the occasional "nor-mocalcemic" patient with mild PHPT. These patients typ-ically have high-normal total serum calcium levels with clinical suspicion of PHPT (history of kidney stones, unexplained osteopenia or hypercalciuria—especially premenopausal women or postmenopausal women on estrogen). Ionized calcium assays may be helpful in hypoalbuminemic or hypoproteinemic patients in whom the formula for "corrected" serum calcium (add 0.8 mg/dL for every 1 g/dL fall in serum albumin) is often inaccurate. Spurious hypercalcemia may occur postprandially or with prolonged tourniquet application during venesection.

Most commercial assays for PTH now measure intact hormone (two-site immunoradiometric assays typically). These assays have no cross-reactivity for PTH-related peptide (PTHrP) and are not affected by renal insuffi-ciency (in which PTH fragments interfere with older assays). The concept of "inappropriate normality" is a crucial one in endocrinology: inappropriately normal PTH levels are seen in 25% to 30% of patients with PHPT, especially in hereditary causes including FBHH. Box 2 lists the nonparathyroid causes of hypercalcemia.

Serum phosphorus tends to be in the lower range of normal, except in azotemic patients. A small increase in serum chloride and decrease in the serum bicarbonate level reflect the renal acid-base effects of PTH. Serum alkaline phosphatase (of osteoblast origin) may be a marker for skeletal involvement. Urinary calcium is typically elevated (>250 mg per 24 hours in women; >300 mg per 24 hours in men) in PHPT. Low levels (<80 to 100 mg per 24 hours) may be the tip-off for FBHH (confirmed by calculating calcium-to-creatinine clearance ratio [<0.01] from spot urine/serum calcium and creatinine). Very high levels (>550 to 600 mg per 24 hours) may indicate coexisting occult nonpara-thyroid disease or renal hypercalciuria. Circulating 1,25-dihydroxyvitamin D levels are typically normal or elevated in patients with PHPT, in contrast to those with PTHrP excess. Newer bone turnover markers (serum osteocalcin, urinary N-telopeptides, etc.) are typ-ically high in PHPT and seldom clinically necessary.

In patients with confirmed PHPT, measurement of bone mineral density (BMD) is useful. Patients with PHPT typically have preferential loss of cortical bone (proximal forearm and hip) with sparing of cancellous bone (spine). Dual-energy x-ray absorptiometry (DEXA) of the spine and hip is the most common technique used, although peripheral DEXA or radiogrammetry of the forearm are occasionally obtained. Nephrotomography or ultrasonography may be useful in PHPT patients without stone history to detect silent stones, which may serve as a surgical indication.

Patients with vitamin D deficiency may have masked hypercalcemia and severe PHPT manifestations, particularly bone disease. Patients on thiazide diuretics or lithium may present major diagnostic uncertainty. They usually present with less severe hypercalcemia (usually <13 mg/dL) and low urine calcium, but their PTH levels may be inappropriate or frankly elevated. If there is no clinical urgency, stopping the drugs for several months and retesting will usually clarify the diagnosis.

Treatment

The only cure for PHPT is surgical excision of abnormal parathyroid glands. It is clear that surgery is indicated for all patients with symptomatic PHPT. However, the role of surgical intervention in asymptomatic patients is controversial. The National Institutes of Health (NIH) Workshop on Asymptomatic PHPT in 2002, revised the prior 1990 guidelines for surgical intervention of these patients (Box 3). Surgery is also indicated for any patient in whom surveillance is not desired or possible. With these guidelines, less than 50% of patients will be managed without surgery. For these patients, appropriate long-term surveillance is needed: biannual serum calcium and annual serum creatinine and bone mass measurements. Approximately 15% to 25% of patients followed without surgery will develop evidence of progressive PHPT and require surgery.

Conventional neck surgery for PHPT has involved either bilateral or unilateral explorations usually under general anesthesia by an experienced surgeon (expected cure rate >95%). Recently, minimally invasive parathyroidectomy (MIP) has been developed using preoperative localization techniques—primarily technetium-99m-sestamibi radioisotope scanning plus neck ultrasonography—to limit the operative field. The use of an intraoperative gamma probe further minimizes parathyroid surgery in patients in whom preoperative sestamibi scanning detects the parathyroid adenoma. Comprehensive cost analysis and comparative studies of MIP techniques are in process. For patients with multiglandular disease, total parathyroidectomy with a remnant left in situ or autotransplanted in the nondominant forearm is required.

BOX 3 **Indications for Surgery in Asymptomatic Primary Hyperparathyroidism**

- Serum calcium ≥1.0 mg/dL above assay upper limit of normal
- 24-hour urinary calcium >400 mg
- Reductions in age- and gender-matched creatinine clearance by ≥30%
- Bone mineral density: T score <2.5 at any site
- Age <50 years

Patients with unsuccessful initial surgery may require extensive localization studies. Radioisotope scanning and ultrasound are followed by computed tomography and magnetic resonance imaging. Invasive localization by arteriography or selective venous sampling for PTH may be required if the noninvasive studies are not definitive.

Postoperatively, PHPT patients may have transient hypocalcemia while the normal previously suppressed parathyroid glands regain calcium sensitivity. "Hungry bone" syndrome with rapid deposition of calcium and phosphate into bone may cause prolonged postoperative hypocalcemia and is still occasionally seen in patients with severe hyperparathyroid bone disease. Postoperative hypoparathyroidism is more commonly seen in patients with prior neck exploration or those undergoing parathyroidectomy with autotransplantation for multiglandular disease. Recurrent laryngeal nerve injuries with vocal cord paralysis are now uncommon complications of parathyroid surgery.

Patients with PHPT who either refuse surgery or cannot have surgery performed because of operative risk (a shrinking population as a result of MIP techniques under local anesthesia) may be considered for medical management. Oral phosphate therapy may reduce serum calcium levels, but PTH levels rise and metastatic calcification may occur if the calcium-phosphorus ion product exceeds 65 to 75. Estrogen[1] may reduce serum and urinary calcium levels and antagonize PTH bone effects, although the findings of the Women's Health Initiative Study (2002) have resulted in patient and physician discomfort with the use of hormone therapy. Progestin-only therapy may attenuate calcium levels. Bisphosphonate therapy—orally with alendronate (Fosamax)[1] 10 mg daily or 70 mg weekly, ibandronate (Boniva) 2.5 mg daily or 150 mg monthly, or 70 mg weekly, risedronate (Actonel)[1] 5 mg daily or 35 mg weekly, or parenterally with pamidronate (Aredia)[1] 60 to 90 mg intravenously every 1 to 3 months, or zoledronic acid (Zometa)[1] 1 to 4 mg intravenously every 3 to 12 months—may improve BMD and stabilize calcium levels. Thiazide diuretics may reduce hypercalciuria and stone risk but potentially may cause worsened hypercalcemia and traditionally are avoided in PHPT patients. New calcimimetic agents with action at the level of the extracellular calcium-sensing receptor may prove to be safe and effective in the future in PHPT (as well as secondary/tertiary HPT).

Hypercalcemic crisis in PHPT is generally a surgical emergency, although aggressive forced saline diuresis along with the use of intravenous bisphosphonates, or less commonly, gallium nitrate or mithramycin (plicamycin [Mithracin]),[1] may be temporarily effective in reducing serum calcium levels.

SECONDARY HYPERPARATHYROIDISM

Secondary HPT is characterized by low or normal serum calcium and elevated serum PTH. It is caused most frequently by chronic renal failure with impaired

---

[1]Not FDA approved for this indication.

1α-hydroxylation of 25-hydroxyvitamin D or gastrointestinal malabsorption of vitamin D (as indicated by low 25-hydroxyvitamin D level); other causes are shown in Box 1. Treatment involves control of serum phosphate by nonaluminum phosphate binders, low-phosphorus diets, and aggressive calcium and calcitriol or vitamin D analogue therapy in renal failure patients; vitamin D sterols are used in patients with vitamin D malabsorption. Secondary HPT is an important cause of irreversible bone loss; the subgroup without severe renal impairment may also often require treatment for osteoporosis with oral bisphosphonates-alendronate (Fosamax) or risedronate (Actonel) or teriparatide (Forteo) once PTH levels have normalized.

TERTIARY HYPERPARATHYROIDISM

Hypercalcemia caused by autonomous secretion of PTH may develop in any patient with prolonged severe secondary HPT over time. It is most commonly seen in chronic renal disease patients (see Box 1) and can be associated with metastatic calcification and calciphylaxis. Total parathyroidectomy with autotransplantation may be necessary in these patients if hypercalcemia and associated symptoms are severe or response to potent vitamin D sterols or analogues (intravenous calcitriol [Calcijex], 1α-hydroxyvitamin D_2 [doxercalciferol-Hectorol], or 19-nor-1α-hydroxyvitamin D [paricalcitol-Zemplar]) is inadequate.

Hypoparathyroidism

Hypoparathyroidism is an uncommon and heterogeneous clinical disorder that is caused by inadequate PTH secretion for the maintenance of normal extracellular fluid calcium levels or from impaired PTH action in target tissues.

ETIOLOGY

Box 4 lists the causes of hypoparathyroidism. The most common cause is postsurgical following thyroidectomy, parathyroidectomy, or radical surgery for head and neck cancers.

CLINICAL FEATURES

Increased neuromuscular irritability caused by hypocalcemia is responsible for the symptoms and signs of hypoparathyroidism: circumoral and acral paraesthesias; muscle cramps; tetany-carpopedal spasm and laryngeal stridor; impaired consciousness; and convulsions. Symptoms usually occur when the serum calcium is below 7.5 mg/dL. The acute symptoms may be precipitated by pregnancy or lactation, the menstrual cycle, intercurrent illness, exercise, or states of alkalosis. Chronic hypocalcemia may be associated with basal ganglia calcification and occasionally with extrapyramidal

---

BOX 4 **Causes of Hypoparathyroidism**

Parathyroid Gland Destruction
- Surgical
- Polyglandular autoimmune
- Radiation
- Infiltration (iron or copper overload, malignancy, granulomatous disease)

Altered PTH Production or Secretion
- Primary: calcium sensing receptor mutations, PTH mutations
- Secondary: hypomagnesemia, maternal HPT

Impaired PTH Action
- Hypomagnesemia
- Pseudohypoparathyroidism (with or without Albright's hereditary osteodystrophy)
- Drugs: bisphosphonates, calcitonin, mithramycin

Abnormal Parathyroid Gland Development
- Isolated hypoparathyroidism
- DiGeorge syndrome
- Complex genetic syndromes

Abbreviations: HPT = hyperparathyroidism; PTH = parathyroid hormone.

9

manifestations, subcapsular cataracts, eczematous dermatitis, brittle hair and nails, alopecia, and abnormal dentition. Clinical signs can include Chvostek and Trousseau signs and pseudopapilledema. Prolonged QT interval may be present on electrocardiography. Occasionally, hypoparathyroidism may be diagnosed only after the finding of low serum calcium on routine laboratory testing. Polyglandular autoimmune deficiency syndrome (type 1) may also include mucocutaneous candidiasis, Addison's disease, type 1 diabetes, alopecia, steatorrhea, thyroid and gonadal failure, hepatitis, pernicious anemia, and vitiligo. Pseudohypoparathyroidism may present with or without Albright's hereditary osteodystrophy and G-subunit α deficiency (short stature, brachydactyly, subcutaneous ossification, round facies, and dental hypoplasia). Pseudohypoparathyroid patients may also develop primary thyroid and gonadal failure.

DIAGNOSIS

The biochemical hallmarks of hypoparathyroidism are low serum calcium and elevated serum phosphorus in the presence of normal renal function. Measurement of ionized calcium may be useful in hypoproteinemic patients. PTH levels are low or undetectable except in patients with impaired PTH action (hypomagnesemia or pseudohypoparathyroidism) in whom 25-hydroxyvitamin D levels should be normal. Urinary calcium is low reflecting reduced filtered calcium load. Alkaline phosphatase levels are usually normal.

TREATMENT

Correction of hypocalcemia in hypoparathyroidism of any etiology includes oral calcium supplementation (elemental 1 to 3 g daily in divided doses, avoiding calcium phosphate preparations) and vitamin D, except in mild

---

[1]Not FDA approved for this indication.

Rakel and Bope: *Conn's Current Therapy 2006.*

cases, particularly following parathyroid adenomectomy, which may just require temporary calcium supplementation alone. Vitamin D preparations include vitamin D_2 (ergocalciferol [Drisdol]) or D_3 (cholecalciferol [Delta D]) 25,000 to 100,000 units daily; 1α-hydroxyvitamin D_2 (Hectorol) 0.5 to 2.0 μg daily; or calcitriol (1,25-dihydroxyvitamin D_3) 0.25 to 1.0 μg daily. Vitamins D_2 and D_3 are less expensive but have slow onset of action and long duration (because of fat solubility), which can result in prolonged toxicity. This makes the other preparations advantageous and preferable. Requirements for vitamin D are generally lower in pseudohypoparathyroid patients with intact distal renal tubular function than in PTH-deficient patients.

Significant hypercalciuria and risk of nephrolithiasis and nephrocalcinosis may occur with therapy if calcium levels are even brought into the mid-normal (or higher) range as a result of deficient hypocalciuric PTH effect on the kidney. Low-normal serum calcium is generally an appropriate target unless the hypoparathyroid patient is also treated with thiazide diuretics. Thiazides (hydrochlorothiazide 25 to 100 mg daily or potassium-sparing agents) with a low-sodium diet are frequently used to control serum and urinary calcium levels with a cost-effective vitamin D-sparing effect. Phosphate-binding antacids may be required if serum phosphorus levels rise to >6 mg/dL. Once stabilization occurs, serum calcium may be followed at 6- to 12-month intervals, with periodic urinary calcium monitoring, if the patient is not treated with thiazide diuretics.

For acute hypocalcemic tetany, bolus intravenous calcium (dosage 2 mg/kg elemental; 90 mg per 10 mL as 10% calcium gluconate) followed by an infusion of 15 mg/kg over 6 to 12 hours is appropriate. Careful observation and monitoring are essential for these patients. Serum magnesium should always be checked in symptomatic hypocalcemic patients. Hypomagnesemia can occur in hypoparathyroid patients, and parenteral magnesium replacement (2 g [16 mEq] $MgSO_4$ infusion every 8 hours) is also appropriate in these patients.

Primary Aldosteronism

Method of
William F. Young, Jr., MD

Hypertension, hypokalemia, suppressed plasma renin activity (PRA), and increased aldosterone excretion characterize the syndrome of primary aldosteronism (PA), which was first described in 1955. Bilateral idiopathic hyperaldosteronism (IHA) and aldosterone-producing adenoma (APA) are the most common subtypes of PA (Box 1). A much less common form, unilateral or primary adrenal hyperplasia (PAH), is caused by zona glomerulosa hyperplasia of predominantly one adrenal gland.

BOX 1 Forms of Primary Aldosteronism

- Aldosterone-producing adenoma (APA)
- Bilateral idiopathic hyperaldosteronism (IHA)
- Primary (unilateral) adrenal hyperplasia (PAH)
- Aldosterone-producing adrenocortical carcinoma
- Familial hyperaldosteronism (FH)
  - Glucocorticoid-remediable aldosteronism (FH type I or GRA)
  - FH type II (APA or IHA)

Two forms of familial hyperaldosteronism (FH) are described: FH type I and FH type II. FH type I, or glucocorticoid-remediable aldosteronism (GRA), is autosomal dominant in inheritance and associated with varying degrees of hyperaldosteronism, high levels of hybrid steroids (e.g., 18-hydroxycortisol and 18-oxocortisol), and suppressibility with exogenous glucocorticoids. FH type II refers to the familial occurrence of APA or IHA or both.

Diagnosis

SCREENING

In the past, clinicians did not consider the diagnosis of PA unless the patient presented with spontaneous hypokalemia, and then the diagnostic evaluation required discontinuing antihypertensive medications for 2 weeks. The "spontaneous hypokalemia/no antihypertensive drug" diagnostic approach resulted in predicted PA prevalence rates of <0.5% of hypertensive patients. Today it is recognized that most patients with PA are not hypokalemic and present with asymptomatic hypertension, which may be mild or severe. When hypokalemia does occur, it may be associated with nocturia, polyuria, muscle cramps, or palpitations. Screening can be completed with a simple morning (8-10 AM) blood test (plasma aldosterone concentration [PAC] to plasma renin activity [PRA] ratio) in a seated ambulant patient. The patient may take any antihypertensive drugs except aldosterone-receptor blockers (spironolactone [Aldactone] and eplerenone [Inspra]). Hypokalemia is associated with false-negative ratios, and any potassium deficit should be corrected before testing. Although there is some uncertainty about test characteristics and lack of standardization, the PAC-to-PRA ratio is widely accepted as the screening test of choice for PA. Spironolactone (Aldactone) and eplerenone (Inspra) should be discontinued 4 to 6 weeks before testing for PA.

CONFIRMING THE DIAGNOSIS

The use of the PAC-to-PRA ratio as a screening test followed by aldosterone suppression confirmatory testing has resulted in much higher prevalence estimates (5% to 13% of all hypertensives) for PA. The prevalence of PA approaches 20% in patients with resistant hypertension. Patients with hypertension and hypokalemia, regardless of presumed cause (e.g., diuretic treatment),

WHEN TO CONSIDER SCREENING FOR PRIMARY ALDOSTERONISM:

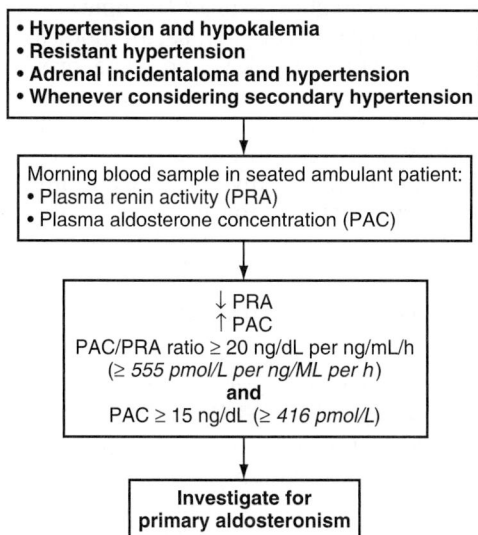

FIGURE 1. In patients with suspected primary aldosteronism, screening can be accomplished by measuring a morning (preferably 8 AM) ambulatory paired random plasma aldosterone concentration and plasma renin activity. This test may be performed while the patient is taking antihypertensive medications and without posture stimulation. Spironolactone (Aldactone) and eplerenone (Inspra) are the only medications that absolutely interfere with interpretation of the ratio.

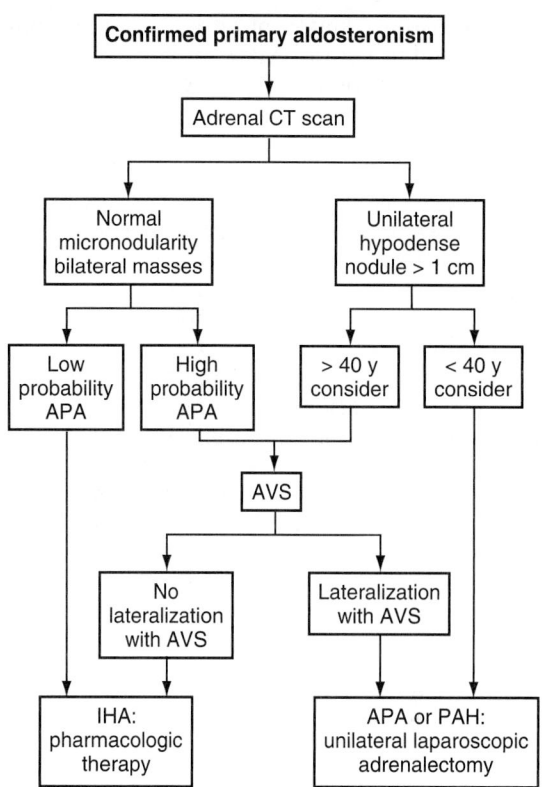

FIGURE 2. Subtype evaluation of primary aldosteronism. See text for details. APA = aldosterone-producing adenoma; AVS = adrenal venous sampling; CT = computed tomography; GRA = glucocorticoid-remediable aldosteronism; IHA = idiopathic hyperaldosteronism; PAH = primary adrenal hyperplasia. (Modified and adapted from Young WF Jr, Hogan MJ: Renin-independent hypermineralocorticoidism. Trends Endocrinol Metab 1994;5:97-106.)

and most patients with treatment-resistant hypertension should undergo screening for PA with a PAC-to-PRA ratio (cutoff is laboratory dependent) (Figure 1). A high PAC-to-PRA ratio is a positive screening test result, a finding that warrants confirmatory testing, which is completed with sodium suppression testing (oral sodium loading, saline suppression test, or fludrocortisone [Florinef] suppression testing; see references for details on these testing protocols). At the Mayo Clinic, we prefer the high-sodium diet for 3 to 4 days with 24-hour urine collection (day 3 to 4) for aldosterone, sodium, and creatinine. When the 24-hour urinary sodium is >200 mEq (confirming adequate sodium loading), patients with PA demonstrate autonomous aldosterone production with urinary aldosterone levels >12 µg/24 hour. During the oral sodium loading it is important to monitor serum electrolytes and blood pressure daily and increase potassium supplementation and antihypertensive medications as indicated.

SUBTYPE EVALUATION

Unilateral adrenalectomy in patients with APA or PAH results in normalization of hypokalemia in all; hypertension is improved in all and cured in approximately 30% to 60% of these patients. In IHA, unilateral or bilateral adrenalectomy seldom corrects the hypertension. IHA and GRA should be treated medically. For those patients who want to pursue a surgical cure, therefore, the accurate distinction among the subtypes of PA is a critical step (Figure 2). The subtype evaluation may require one or more tests, the first of which is imaging the adrenal

glands with computed tomography (CT) (see Figure 2). When a solitary unilateral macroadenoma (>1 cm) and normal contralateral adrenal morphology are found on CT in a patient younger than age 40 years with PA, unilateral adrenalectomy is a reasonable therapeutic option. In many cases, however, CT may show normal-appearing adrenals, minimal unilateral adrenal limb thickening, unilateral microadenomas (<1 cm), or bilateral macroadenomas. Of 203 patients who were evaluated with both CT and adrenal vein sampling, we found that CT accurately distinguished APA from IHA in only 53%. Small APAs may be labeled incorrectly as IHA on the basis of CT findings of bilateral nodularity or normal-appearing adrenals. Also, apparent adrenal microadenomas may represent areas of hyperplasia, and unilateral adrenalectomy would be inappropriate. In addition, nonfunctioning unilateral adrenal macroadenomas are not uncommon, especially in patients older than age 40 years.

Patients with APAs have more severe hypertension, more frequent hypokalemia, higher plasma (>25 ng/dL; >694 nmol/L) and urinary (>30 µg/24 h; >83 µmol/L per day) levels of aldosterone, and are younger (younger than age 50 years) than those with IHA. Patients fitting these descriptors are considered to have a "high probability of APA" (see Figure 2). These factors are not absolute predictors of unilateral versus bilateral adrenal disease, however. With the addition of adrenal venous sampling (AVS), we found unilateral APAs in 36% of patients with clinically "high-probability" APA who had normal findings or unilateral adrenal limb thickening on CT. Several studies have found that CT contributes to lateralization in the minority of patients with PA and that AVS is essential to direct appropriate therapy in patients with PA who want to pursue a surgical treatment option.

AVS is a difficult procedure because the right adrenal vein is both small and difficult to cannulate; the success rate depends on the proficiency of the angiographer. According to a review of 47 reports, the success rate for cannulating the right adrenal vein in 384 patients was 74%. With experience, the success rate approximates 90% to 96%. Some centers perform AVS in all patients diagnosed with PA. A more practical approach is the selective use of AVS outlined in Figure 2. Using this approach for the subtype evaluation of 120 PA patients in 1999 at the Mayo Clinic, 7% of patients had an adrenalectomy based on CT findings alone and 21% had AVS to guide therapy.

Treatment Principles

The treatment goal is to prevent the morbidity and mortality associated with hypertension, hypokalemia, and cardiovascular damage. The cause of the PA helps determine the appropriate treatment. Normalization of blood pressure should not be the only goal in managing the patient with PA. In addition to the kidney and colon, mineralocorticoid receptors are present in the heart, brain, and blood vessels. Excessive secretion of aldosterone is associated with increased cardiovascular morbidity. Therefore, normalization of circulating aldosterone or aldosterone receptor blockade should be part of the management plan for all patients with PA.

SURGERY

Unilateral laparoscopic adrenalectomy is an excellent treatment option for patients with APA or unilateral hyperplasia. Although blood pressure control improves in nearly 100% of patients postoperatively, average long-term cure rates of hypertension after unilateral adrenalectomy for APA range from 30% to 60%. Persistent hypertension following adrenalectomy correlates directly with having more than one first-degree relative with hypertension, using more than two antihypertensive agents preoperatively, older age, increased serum creatinine, and duration of hypertension, and it is most likely because of coexistent primary hypertension.

Laparoscopic adrenalectomy is the preferred surgical approach and is associated with shorter hospital stays and less long-term morbidity than the conventional open approach. The blood pressure response to spironolactone (Aldactone) preoperatively often predicts the blood pressure response to unilateral adrenalectomy in patients with APA. To decrease the surgical risk, hypokalemia should be corrected with spironolactone (Aldactone) preoperatively; treatment with this drug should be discontinued postoperatively.

Aldosterone concentrations in blood or urine should be measured shortly after the operation. For the first few weeks postoperatively, serum potassium levels should be monitored weekly and a generous sodium diet followed to avoid the hyperkalemia of hypoaldosteronism that may occur because of the chronic suppression of the renin-angiotensin-aldosterone axis. The hypertension typically resolves in 1 to 3 months postoperatively. Adrenalectomy for APA is significantly less expensive than long-term medical therapy alone.

PHARMACOLOGIC TREATMENT

IHA and GRA should be treated medically. In addition, APA patients may be treated medically if the treatment includes mineralocorticoid receptor blockade. A sodium-restricted diet (<100 mEq of sodium per day), maintenance of ideal body weight, tobacco avoidance, and regular aerobic exercise contribute significantly to the success of pharmacologic treatment. No placebo-controlled randomized trials have evaluated the relative efficacy of drugs in the treatment of PA. Spironolactone (Aldactone) has been the drug of choice to treat PA for more than three decades. It is available in 25-, 50-, and 100-mg tablets. The dosage is 25 mg per day initially, which is increased to 400 mg per day if necessary to achieve normokalemia without the aid of oral potassium chloride supplementation. Hypokalemia responds promptly, but hypertension may take as long as 4 to 8 weeks to correct. After several months of therapy, this dosage often can be decreased to as little as 25 to 50 mg per day; dosage titration is based on a goal serum potassium level in the high-normal range. Serum potassium should be monitored frequently during the first 4 to 6 weeks of therapy (especially in patients with renal insufficiency or diabetes mellitus). Spironolactone (Aldactone) increases the half-life of digoxin. Patients taking digoxin may need their dosages adjusted when they begin treatment with spironolactone (Aldactone). Concomitant therapy with salicylates should be avoided because they interfere with the tubular secretion of an active metabolite and decrease the effectiveness of spironolactone (Aldactone). Unfortunately, spironolactone (Aldactone) is not selective for the aldosterone receptor. For example, antagonism at the testosterone receptor may result in painful gynecomastia, impotence, and menstrual irregularity. The incidence of gynecomastia in 699 patients treated with spironolactone (Aldactone) was dose dependent (6.9% at doses of <50 mg per day and 52% at daily doses of >150 mg).

The FDA approved eplerenone (Inspra),[1] a new steroid-based antimineralocorticoid that acts as a competitive and selective aldosterone receptor antagonist, for the treatment of uncomplicated essential hypertension in late 2003. The 9,11-epoxide group in eplerenone (Inspra) results in a significant reduction of the molecule's progestational and antiandrogenic actions compared with spironolactone (Aldactone); eplerenone (Inspra) has 0.1% of the binding affinity to androgen

---

[1]Not FDA approved for this indication.

Rakel and Bope: *Conn's Current Therapy 2006.*

CURRENT DIAGNOSIS

- Most patients with primary aldosteronism are not hypokalemic and typically present with asymptomatic hypertension, which may be mild or severe.
- Screening can be completed with a simple morning (8-10 AM) blood test (plasma aldosterone concentration [PAC] to plasma renin activity [PRA] ratio) in a seated ambulant patient.
- A high PAC:PRA ratio is a positive screening test result, a finding that warrants confirmatory testing.
- The subtype evaluation may require one or more tests, the first of which is imaging the adrenal glands with computed tomography.
- Adrenal vein sampling is essential to direct appropriate therapy in patients with primary aldosteronism who want to pursue a surgical treatment option.

CURRENT THERAPY

- Because of aldosterone-related cardiovascular toxicity, normalization of circulating aldosterone or aldosterone receptor blockade should be part of the management plan for all patients with primary aldosteronism.
- Unilateral laparoscopic adrenalectomy is an excellent treatment option for patients with aldosterone-producing adenoma or unilateral hyperplasia.
- Patients with bilateral idiopathic hyperaldosteronism and glucocorticoid-remediable aldosteronism should be treated medically with an aldosterone-receptor antagonist (e.g., spironolactone [Aldactone] or eplerenone [Inspra]).

receptors and <1% of the binding affinity to progesterone receptors compared with spironolactone (Aldactone). Treatment trials comparing the efficacy of eplerenone (Inspra) versus spironolactone (Aldactone) for the treatment of PA are not published. Eplerenone (Inspra) presumably will prove the superior drug if it is shown to be as effective as spironolactone (Aldactone) for the treatment of mineralocorticoid-dependent hypertension and if it lacks the limiting antiandrogen side effects of spironolactone (Aldactone).

Patients with IHA frequently require a second antihypertensive agent to achieve good blood pressure control. Hypervolemia is a major reason for resistance to drug therapy, and low doses of a thiazide (e.g., 12.5 to 50 mg of hydrochlorothiazide daily) or a related sulfonamide diuretic are effective in combination with the aldosterone-receptor antagonist. Because these agents often lead to further hypokalemia, serum potassium levels should be monitored.

Special Treatment Indications

GLUCOCORTICOID-REMEDIABLE ALDOSTERONISM

Before initiating treatment, GRA should be confirmed with either genetic testing or a measurement of 24-hour urinary excretion of 18-hydroxycortisol. We perform these tests in patients with a family history of primary aldosteronism or of strokes at a young age (<50 yrs) or an onset of primary aldosteronism at a young age (<20 yrs). In the patient with GRA, chronic treatment with physiologic doses of a glucocorticoid normalizes blood pressure and corrects hypokalemia. Treatment with spironolactone (Aldactone) in these patients is just as effective, however, and avoids the potential disruption

of the hypothalamic-pituitary-adrenal axis and risk of iatrogenic side effects.

ALDOSTERONE-PRODUCING ADRENAL MALIGNANCIES

It is difficult to make the diagnosis of adrenal malignancy on the basis of microscopic examination. The only absolute criteria are local invasion or metastatic lesions. Surgical excision is the treatment of choice. Mitotane (Lysodren, *o,p'*-DDD [1-(*o*-chlorophenyl)-1-(*p*-chlorophenyl)-2,2-dichloroethane]) or cisplatin (Platinol)[1] is used in patients with a persistent tumor. Associated excessive glucocorticoid and mineralocorticoid overproduction may be controlled with ketoconazole (Nizoral).[1]

REFERENCES

Lim PO, Young WF, MacDonald TM: A review of the medical treatment of primary aldosteronism. J Hypertens 2001;19:353-361.
Montori VM, Young WF Jr: Use of plasma aldosterone concentration-to-plasma renin activity ratio as a screening test for primary aldosteronism: A systematic review of the literature. Endocrinol Metab Clin North Am 2002;31:619-632.
Mulatero P, Stowasser M, Loh K-C, Fardella CE, et al: Increased diagnosis of primary aldosteronism, including surgically correctable forms, in centers from five continents. J Clin Endocrinol Metab 2004;89:1045-1050.
Sawka AM, Young WF Jr, Thompson GB, Grant CS, et al: Primary aldosteronism: Factors associated with normalization of blood pressure after surgery. Ann Intern Med 2001;135:258-261.
Sywak M, Pasieka JL: Long-term follow-up and cost benefit of adrenalectomy in patients with primary hyperaldosteronism. Br J Surg 2002;89:1587-1593.
Young WF Jr: Primary aldosteronism: Management issues. Ann N Y Acad Sci 2002;970:61-76.
Young WF Jr: Mini-review: Primary aldosteronism-changing concepts in diagnosis and treatment. Endocrinology 2003;144:2208-2213.
Young WF Jr, Hogan, MJ: Renin-independent hypermineralocorticoidism. Trends Endocrinol Metab 1994;5:97-106.
Young WF Jr, Klee GG: Primary aldosteronism: Diagnostic evaluation. Endocrinol Metab Clin North Am 1988;17:367-395.
Young WF Jr, Stanson AW, Thompson GB, Grant CS, et al: Role for adrenal venous sampling in primary aldosteronism. Surgery 2004;136:1227-1235.

---

[1]Not FDA approved for this indication.

Rakel and Bope: *Conn's Current Therapy 2006.*

---

[1]Not FDA approved for this indication.

Hypopituitarism

Method of
Andjela Drincic, MD,
and Robert J. Anderson, MD

Hypopituitarism implies the loss of one or more of the clinically important pituitary hormones. These include growth hormone (somatropin-GH), adrenocorticotropic hormone (ACTH), thyroid-stimulating hormone (TSH), follicle-stimulating hormone (FSH), luteinizing hormone (LH), prolactin (PRL), and antidiuretic hormone (ADH). The picture of hypopituitarism is often one of a gradual cumulative loss of hormones (starting with GH and usually followed in sequence by LH, FSH, TSH, and ACTH), but the presentation can be widely varying and is influenced by the etiology. In patients with pituitary tumors, the mass effect of the tumor (leading to headache and visual disturbance) and hormonal hypersecretion may further complicate the picture. A man may have an inexorable onset of fatigue, weakness, decreased libido, erectile dysfunction, and finally, pressure symptoms of headache and visual disturbance associated with an expanding pituitary tumor. Soft, pale, waxy skin with fine facial wrinkles and female body habitus may suggest the diagnosis. Premenopausal women are usually diagnosed early because they present with amenorrhea and infertility. Progression may be rapid and dramatic in pituitary apoplexy or after head trauma. Isolated loss of a hormone occurs less frequently. If it is found care should be exercised to avoid missing progression to a multihormone deficiency. Common causes of hypopituitarism are pituitary adenoma, craniopharyngioma, traumatic injury, pituitary surgery, irradiation, ischemic necrosis, infiltrative disease, and autoimmune disease (see Current Diagnosis Box). Loss of posterior pituitary ADH is less frequent and suggests pituitary stalk or hypothalamic disease (refer to the article "Diabetes Insipidus").

There are several guidelines for the treatment of hypopituitarism. Hormone deficiency should be documented by baseline testing and further stimulation testing if necessary. The picture is usually one of an endocrine-target gland deficiency (for example, low thyroxine T$_4$) without the corresponding increase in the pituitary tropic hormone (a *normal* or low TSH). Except for GH and ADH, hormone replacement is with the target hormones—such as L-thyroxine (Synthroid, Levoxyl, Levothroid)—because they are less expensive, can be given orally or transdermally rather than parenterally, and are not immunogenic. Finally, even though the replacement schedules are frequently the same as treatments for primary endocrine deficiencies, follow-up monitoring is less ideal because the feedback response of the pituitary is lost. This article details specific treatments. Stimulation test protocols are available in endocrinology textbooks.

---

[1]Not FDA approved for this indication.

Growth Hormone Deficiency

DIAGNOSIS

Only GH deficiency in the adult patient is discussed here. Random measurement of GH cannot be used as a diagnostic tool because of the pulsatile nature of GH release. Insulin-like growth factor-1 (IGF-1) provides an average indication of GH presence but cannot be used as the sole diagnostic test because it may be in the normal range in some GH-deficient patients. The insulin tolerance test (ITT), with the demonstration of a failure of GH to respond to hypoglycemia, is still considered the gold standard test to document GH deficiency. However, ITT is cumbersome to perform and is contraindicated in patients with coronary artery disease, seizure disorders, or cerebrovascular insufficiency. Hypothalamic GH-releasing hormone (GHRH) sermorelin acetate (Geref) given intravenously in conjunction with (intravenous) IV arginine has been useful as an accurate and less stressful method for detection of GH response. In addition, patients with an appropriate clinical history, and either the presence of three or more pituitary hormone deficiencies or a serum IGF-1 less than 84 mg/L, do not require GH-stimulation testing for the diagnosis of growth-hormone deficiency (GHD).

TREATMENT

Current practice is to replace GH in adults with documented GH deficiency. In aging adults with low IGF-1 levels because of decreased GH secretion, but without clear hypopituitarism, replacement of GH is investigational. Hypopituitary patients experience premature mortality because of cardiovascular disease. Metabolic sequelae associated with the lack of GH may contribute. Subjects treated with GH have an improved sense of well-being and quality of life, increased muscle strength, decreased body fat, and increased lean body mass and bone density. GH replacement in recent studies appeared to provide protection from myocardial infarction. Because of the expense of the recombinant GH preparations, the deficiency must be documented. Baseline lipids, prostate-specific antigen (PSA), glucose, and bone mineral density are helpful for monitoring therapy. GH somatropin (Humatrope, Nutropin, Genotropin) is given as a single subcutaneous daily dose. Individualized dose titration regimens were found to have similar efficacy and better tolerability than a fixed body weight–based dosing regimens. Therefore, we recommend that therapy with GH should be initiated at a dose of 200 μg/d and titrated by 200 μg/d at 2-month intervals based on a clinical and serum IGF-1 response (with an IGF-1 level goal at the mid- to normal range for age and gender). Women taking oral (but not transdermal) estrogens may need slightly higher doses of GH to reach the same IGF-1 goals because of relative GH resistance. Patients must be monitored for the more common side effects of peripheral edema, musculoskeletal pain, or aggravation of hypertension. The prostate gland should be monitored with a digital rectal examination and prostate-specific antigen (PSA) at least yearly in men older than 50 years of age. Potential growth of persistent but stable pituitary tumors is under study. Use in the presence of any active cancer is contraindicated.

Adrenocorticotropic Hormone Deficiency

DIAGNOSIS

The diagnosis of secondary adrenal insufficiency is important because this condition is life-threatening. Exogenous glucocorticoid suppression of the hypothalamic-pituitary-adrenal axis is the most common cause of secondary adrenal insufficiency. A careful history will detect exogenous glucocorticoid administration and subsequent unnoticed or inadvertent interruption of treatment. The patient may present in an acute crisis with cardiovascular collapse. More commonly, a patient presents with chronic symptoms such as general malaise, fatigue, and lack of skin pigmentation. Women lose pubic and axillary hair because of the loss of adrenal androgens. Pale skin, lack of hyperkalemia, and low or *normal* ACTH levels help differentiate secondary from primary adrenal insufficiency. Baseline hormonal measurements may be within normal ranges, but an early morning cortisol less than 3 µg/dL is diagnostic of adrenal insufficiency and an early morning cortisol greater than 18 µg/dL makes it very unlikely. Chronic secondary adrenal insufficiency leads to adrenal atrophy. Therefore a rapid adrenocortical screen with the synthetic ACTH cosyntropin (Cortrosyn) usually shows a less-than-adequate response (cortisol <18 µg/dL at 30 minutes). A normal response does not exclude secondary (pituitary) adrenal insufficiency. Insulin-induced hypoglycemia (still considered the *gold standard*) or metyrapone testing will evaluate the complete pituitary-adrenal axis. However, these tests are often unnecessary and may be dangerous because of precipitation of a hypoadrenal crisis if unmonitored. If the patient has already been treated with glucocorticoids and the picture is unclear, the use of a 1- to 3-day IV ACTH infusion will document the presence of adrenal function.

TREATMENT

The major goal in treatment is to restore normalcy by attempting to reproduce the diurnal rhythm of cortisol production with a glucocorticoid preparation, not with ACTH. Our previous efforts at replacement often have used higher average doses, which increased the risk for accelerated bone resorption. We prefer hydrocortisone at a dose of 10 mg in the morning, 5 to 10 mg at noon, and 5 mg in the late afternoon. The dose has to be individualized. Occasionally patients will become cushingoid on the estimated doses and require a smaller twice-daily dose or a daily dose. We avoid prednisone and other longer-acting preparations such as dexamethasone because of the inability to monitor dosing and the higher occurrence of exogenous Cushing's syndrome. A mineralocorticoid preparation is not required in most cases because the renin-angiotensin system should be intact. How do we know how much is enough? The 24-hour urine-free cortisol and a 9 AM cortisol should be in the normal range to avoid overtreatment. The blood pressure, serum electrolytes, and the clinical examination and history should be followed. Glucocorticoids replacement may unmask underlying mild diabetes insipidus in some patients. We make certain that the patient understands the need to increase the dose during sick days. Each patient receives a detailed sheet that lists how to adjust the medicine. They double the dose during the 1 to 3 days of a moderate illness such as the flu with a low-grade fever (>37.7°C [<100°F]) and triple the dose if fever (<37.7°C [100°F]) is present. They are given injectable hydrocortisone sodium succinate (Solu-Cortef), in a ready-to-mix vial containing a 100-mg dose of hydrocortisone, or injectable dexamethasone (Decadron Phosphate), in a dose of 4 mg/mL in a 1-mL vial, to use if they are vomiting and cannot get immediate medical care. They give the contents of one vial intramuscularly (IM) and repeat, if necessary, every 8 to 12 hours before arriving at the hospital. The patients must get a medical information bracelet or necklace that details their need for cortisol (Medic Alert, P.O. Box 1009, Turlock, California, 95381-1009; telephone 800-625-3788).

Glucocorticoid coverage for surgery and stressful procedures is essentially the same for primary and secondary adrenal insufficiency. We give a depot of 100 mg hydrocortisone sodium-succinate (Solu-Cortef) IM on call to surgery and then 50 to 100 mg hydrocortisone intravenously every 6 hours (starting in surgery) the first 24 hours. The dose is decreased by 50% each day as indicated by patient progress until the oral glucocorticoid can be resumed. Treatment of acute adrenal insufficiency requires IV glucocorticoid (Solu-Cortef) 50 to 100 mg every 6 hours, dextrose and saline IV fluids, and an aggressive review to define the precipitating event (refer to the article "Adrenocortical Insufficiency").

Despite adequate glucocorticoid replacement, women sometimes continue to complain of fatigue, depression, and impaired quality of life. In those cases low-dose dehydroepiandrosterone (DHEA) (20-30 mg daily) may be considered because this therapy may have positive effects on behavior in early clinical trials. However, because there are no FDA-approved DHEA supplements, patients should be closely followed. Clinical effects on hair and skin should be monitored, and the DHEA dose should be adjusted to achieve normalization of morning serum levels of dehydroepiandro-sterone sulfate (DHEAS).

Thyroid Stimulating Hormone

DIAGNOSIS

Patients are clinically hypothyroid but often not as severely myxedematous as patients with primary hypothyroidism. Clinical hypothyroidism with the finding of a low free and/or total thyroxine (T$_4$) and

9

a low or *normal* TSH gives the diagnosis of secondary (central) hypothyroidism (for our purposes this includes hypothalamic hypothyroidism). An absent or blunted response of TSH to IV thyrotropin releasing hormone (TRH, protirelin [Relefact]) is of limited usefulness because it occurs in only 21% of patients with central hypothyroidism.

TREATMENT

The great advances that have occurred in titrating thyroid hormone replacement doses with more sensitive TSH assays are lost in hypopituitary patients. In replacement therapy of primary hypothyroidism, our goal is to keep the TSH within the normal range. With this measurement lost in hypopituitary patients, it is best to follow the free T_4 to maintain it within the normal range and to adjust the dose carefully based on symptoms. We use synthetic L-thyroxine (Synthroid, Levoxyl, Levothroid) for replacement. Triiodothyronine (Cytomel) is not desirable for chronic replacement because of its short half-life. A general estimate for T_4 replacement is 1.6 to 1.8 µg/kg per day. Variations in requirements occur and individualization of the dose is necessary. In patients younger than 60 years of age, in good health, and with a short duration of hypothyroidism, we usually start at 50 to 75 µg per day and increase by 25 µg increments every 6 to 8 weeks to normalize the free T_4. Such patients may be given the full estimated daily dose without adverse effects. Patients older than 60 years of age with prolonged hypothyroidism (greater than 6 months), and those with known ischemic heart disease, start with 25 µg per day to avoid aggravation of cardiac disease. We increase the dose by 25 µg in 4 weeks if there are no adverse symptoms, and then increase by 25 µg increments every 6 to 8 weeks until the free T_4 is normal. The patient is then followed every 6 to 12 months to maintain a normal level. Chronic over-replacement should be avoided to prevent potential accelerated bone loss in a patient who may already have several problems that could contribute to loss of bone (GH and gonadal steroid deficiency and potential over-replacement with glucocorticoids). Care is taken to replace cortisol beforehand or concomitantly to avoid precipitating an adrenal crisis with increased metabolic demands of thyroid hormone replacement.

Gonadotropin Deficiency

DIAGNOSIS

Because both LH and FSH are secreted from the gonadotrope, these glycoproteins are usually lost in tandem. The classic presentation in the adult is hypogonadotropic hypogonadism (secondary hypogonadism) with low or *normal* LH and FSH and low gonadal steroid levels (testosterone in men, estradiol in women). Both men and women experience loss of libido, decline in secondary sex characteristics, and decreased bone density. Women are amenorrheic. Men will be impotent. Testing with doses of IV gonadotropin releasing hormone (GnRH)

gonadorelin (Factrel) has not provided the discrimination needed to diagnose a central lesion or to define pituitary LH/FSH reserve. A magnetic resonance image (MRI) of the sella usually is necessary once biochemical evidence of secondary hypogonadism is documented. In men and postmenopausal women, the loss of LH and FSH may be sequential after the loss of GH, and it may be clinically silent until a pituitary adenoma expands to cause symptomatic defects and compression.

TREATMENT

Women

Replacement therapy with the gonadal steroid is required in premenopausal women. Premenopausal women with a uterus are given a full schedule to allow menstruation. We use oral conjugated estrogens (Premarin, Menest) at 0.3 to 1.25 mg per day on days 1 to 25 with medroxyprogesterone (Provera) 5 to 10 mg per day added from days 13 to 25. For menses, 5 to 6 days are allowed. Alternative treatments include an oral micronized estradiol (Estrace) 1 to 2 mg/per day or a transdermal system with which 0.05 to 0.1 mg patches are applied once (Climara) or two times weekly (Alora, Vivelle) on days 1 to 25, in conjunction with medroxyprogesterone as noted on days 13 to 25. Pregnancy can be attained after induction of ovulation with human menopausal gonadotropins (menotropins [Pergonal]) followed by human chorionic gonadotropin (hCG). The procedure is beyond the scope of this article. The addition of small doses of intramuscular testosterone (enanthate or cypionate, 25-50 mg each month) can be considered if libido remains decreased because of loss of adrenal androgen production stimulated by ACTH. Lower dose testosterone patches and oral testosterone that does not affect liver function may be available options in the future. Side effects of acne, hirsutism, and virilization should be avoided. In hypopituitary postmenopausal woman, the same considerations apply to the decision for gonadal steroid replacement as apply in a postmenopausal woman with normal pituitary function.

Men

Replacement therapy is given to men to attempt to normalize sexual function, increase the sense of well-being, maintain secondary sex characteristics, increase lean body mass, decrease fat mass, and prevent bone resorption. It is important to tell the patient that treatment will lead to progressive testicular atrophy if the hypopituitarism has not caused it already. In addition, it should be pointed out that fertility is usually lost. Treatment with pulsatile GnRH (if the defect is hypothalamic) or with hCG, and human menopausal gonadotropin (hMG) can be attempted to recover fertility in appropriate cases. The usual therapy is chronic testosterone replacement in those who do not desire fertility. Oral, intramuscular, transdermal, and buccal treatments are available in the United States. We avoid oral methyltestosterone preparations (Virilon, Testred) because of the potential for hepatotoxicity presenting as cholestatic hepatitis, jaundice, peliosis hepatis, or hepatoma. The dose and frequency of testosterone are based primarily on the patient evaluation of improved strength, energy, libido and sexual function, and the goal of mid- to normal-range testosterone levels. Monitoring of testosterone replacement in secondary hypogonadism is less than ideal because adequate LH or FSH levels often are unavailable to allow an estimate of feedback response. Some patients prefer testosterone enanthate (Delatestry) or testosterone cypionate (DEPO-Testosterone) IM every two weeks. This interval avoids the wide fluctuations in levels that can occur with 3- to 4-week intervals, but variations still occur. A family member or the patient can give the injections to avoid additional cost. We start with 50 to 100 mg for the severely hypogonadal individual and 100 to 200 mg every 2 weeks for most other patients. Men older than 60 years of age may require the lower doses. Testosterone levels are measured 7 days after injection for an estimate of the mid- to normal-range value and at 2 weeks to determine the nadir. We prefer the transdermal testosterone delivery systems because they mimic the diurnal pattern of testosterone secretion, and they avoid the fluctuations inherent in intramuscular delivery. Nonscrotal testosterone patches (Androderm 2.5 and 5 mg) and testosterone gels (AndroGel 1%, 2.5g and 5g packets Testim 1%) are the available transdermal systems. The gels are applied to nongenital skin each morning. The testosterone patches (Androderm) is applied each evening. Testosterone levels can be monitored 6 to 8 hours after application of the patches to maintain a mid to normal range. The testosterone patch (Androderm) are associated with more frequent and more severe skin reactions. Those reactions have been minimized with the use of testosterone gel preparation (AndroGel), but patients need to be warned about a possibility of transdermal testosterone transfer during a close contact with another person. With the testosterone buccal system (Striant), a 30-mg, sustained-release mucoadhesive tablet is applied to the buccal mucosa (just above the incisor tooth) twice daily. It achieves physiologic

9

TABLE 1 Treatment of Hypopituitarism

	Hormone lost		Treatment	Monitor
1.	GH (somatropin)	Men and women on transdermal estrogen	200 µg/d to start, ↑100-200 µg/d q8wk as indicated by IGF-1	IGF-1 Lipids
		Women on oral estrogens	400 µg/d to start, ↑100-200 µg/d q8wk as indicated by IGF-1	PSA Bone mineral density Body composition Blood pressure
2.	ACTH	Hydrocortisone	10 mg PO AM 5-10 mg PO Noon 5 mg PO PM	Sense of well-being, strength Avoid cushingoid changes 24 h urine-free cortisol, 9 AM cortisol BP, electrolytes
3.	TSH	L-Thyroxine	1.6-1.8 µg/kg/d Target dose by age: <60: 100-125 µg/d >60: 75-100 µg/d (may be lower with increased patient age)	Free T_4 T_4-sensitive proteins (ACE, SHBG) if needed Avoid hyperthyroid + hypothyroid signs and symptoms
4.	LH	Women:		Menstrual cycle
5.	FSH	Conjugated estrogens day 1-25 or Estradiol or Estrogen patch and	0.3-1.25 mg/d 1-2 mg/d 0.05mg-0.1mg (see text)	Libido Estrogen-sensitive tissue Libido
		Medroxyprogesterone Day 13-25	5-10 mg/d	Sense of well-being Strength, endurance
		Men: IM testosterone Ester Or gels Or nonscrotal patch	100-200 mg q2wk 2.5-5 g/d 2.5-5 mg/d	Sexual function Testosterone levels, PSA Hemoglobin, hematocrit
6.	Prolactin	None		Lactation
7.	ADH	DDAVP	Intranasal, oral, or subcutaneous (refer to "Diabetes Insipidus" article)	Thirst Intake and output Weight Serum sodium, urine osmolality

Abbreviations: ACE = angiotensin-converting enzyme; ACTH = adrenocorticotropic hormone; ADH = antidiuretic hormone; DDAVP = desmopressin acetate; FSH = follicle-stimulating hormone; GH = growth hormone; IGF-1 = insulin-like growth factor-1; IM = intramuscular; LH = luteinizing hormone; PSA = prostate-specific antigen; SHBG = sex hormone-binding globulin; T_4 = thyroxine; TSH = thyroid-stimulating hormone.

Rakel and Bope: *Conn's Current Therapy 2006.*

testosterone replacement but can cause severe gum irritation. All transdermal systems are more expensive than the intramuscular injections, but frequent visits to the physician's office for injections are inconvenient and costs can approach the daily transdermal treatment. Problems with acceleration of benign prostatic hyperplasia, occult prostate cancer, polycythemia or sleep apnea are uncommon in our experience with carefully monitored replacement doses. Baseline digital rectal examination, PSA, and hemoglobin should be done and followed yearly in men older than the age of 50 years and as needed in younger men. Patients should be warned about the possible occurrence of acne, oily skin, and breast tenderness.

Prolactin

DIAGNOSIS

A well-known clinical setting of PRL loss is postpartum pituitary necrosis and resultant failure of lactation (Sheehan's syndrome). Gradual progression to multi-hormone deficiency usually ensues. Any female with hypopituitarism can have failure of PRL production if pregnancy is attained. Hyperprolactinemia occurs in men but it is detected less often. The diagnosis is made by documenting a low baseline PRL in the absence of any suppressing agent, and the lack of PRL response to TRH. There is no clear clinical syndrome known in men without PRL. The hormone may have an effect on sexual behavior and fluid balance, but the effect is not completely clear. PRL is not replaced.

ANTIDIURETIC HORMONE DEFICIENCY

Replacement of ADH in diabetes insipidus is usually required to maintain normal water balance. The vasopressin analogue desmopressin (DDAVP) is used most frequently as nasal, oral, and subcutaneous preparations. Details are given in the article "Diabetes Insipidus."

Documentation of pituitary hormone loss is essential prior to treatment. Select stimulation tests (ACTH, corticotropin-releasing hormone [CRH], ITT, GHRH) can be done when appropriate. Glucocorticoids must be replaced first to avoid life-threatening deterioration. Cortisol is given before or with thyroid hormone to avoid precipitation of a hypoadrenal crisis. Gonadal steroids and GH can be replaced once contraindications are excluded. Periodic monitoring of replacement therapy is essential. Patients can live well with total replacement, but they will be inconvenienced. A patient with panhypopituitarism may need cortisol, L-thyroxine gonadal steroids, GH, and DDAVP[1] (Table 1), all of which can enhance the quality of life and potentially decrease long-term morbidity and mortality. The dose of cortisol must be adjusted during illness. The ability to fine tune the treatment to the best levels for each individual is not optimal because the feedback centers are lost. Research into sensitive tissue indicators of adequate

CURRENT DIAGNOSIS

Etiology of Hypopituitarism
- Tumors
  Pituitary adenomas—functioning + nonfunctioning
  Craniopharyngioma
- Pituitary surgery
- Traumatic injury
- Infarction/vascular
  Ischemic necrosis—(Sheehan's-postpartum, diabetes mellitus, sickle-cell disease)
  Pituitary apoplexy—necrosis of tumor
- Radiation of pituitary—usually gradual + progressive
- Infiltrative and infectious diseases
  Sarcoidosis
  Hemochromatosis
  Meningitis
  Tuberculosis
- Autoimmune—lymphocytic hypophysitis
- Genetic diseases—Gene mutations: prop-1 (deficiency of LH, FSH, GH, TSH, or PRL); pit-1 (deficiency of GH, PRL, variable TSH)
- Idiopathic
- Iatrogenic—Discontinuation of exogenous glucocorticoid treatment or inadequate glucocorticoid coverage during stress in patients on chronic or intermittent glucocorticoids by any route.
- Hypothalamic diseases—Craniopharyngioma. Any hypothalamic tumor, injury, radiation, infarction, infiltrative, or infectious diseases also can affect hypothalamic hormone secretion.

Abbreviations: FSH = follicle-stimulating hormone; LH = luteinizing hormone; GH = growth hormone; PRL = prolactin; TSH = thyroid-stimulating hormone.

replacement will enhance our treatment of this important group of patients.

REFERENCES
Alexopoulou O, Beguin CL, De Nayer PH, Maiter D: Clinical and hormonal characteristics of central hypothyroidism at diagnosis and during follow-up in adult patients. Eur J Endocrinol 2004; 150:1-8.

American Association of Clinical Endocrinologists: Medical guidelines for clinical practice for growth hormone use in adults and children—2003 update. Endocr Pract 2003;9(No.1)65-76.

Arlt W, Allolio B: Adrenal insufficiency. Lancet 2003;361:1881-1893.

Bengtsson B, Karlsson FA: Low dose dehydroepiandrosterone affects behaviour in hypopituitary androgen-deficient women: A placebo-controlled trial. J Clin Endocrinol Metab 2002;87:2046-2052.

Biller, BMK, Samuels MH, Zagar A, et al: Sensitivity and specificity of six tests for the diagnosis of adult GH defciency. J Clin Endocrinol Metab 2002;87:2067-2079.

Cameron DR, Braunstein GD: Androgen replacement therapy in women. Fertil Steril 2004;82:273-289.

Hartman ML, Crowe BJ, Biller BMK, et al: Which patients do not require a GH stimulation test for the diagnosis of adult GH deficiency? J Clin Endocrinol Metab 2002;87:477-485.

Hoffman AR, Strasburger CJ, Zagar A, et al: Efficacy and tolerability of an individualized dosing regimen for adult growth hormone replacement therapy in comparison with fixed body weight-based dosing. J Clin Endocrinol Metab 2004;89:3224-3233.

Johannsson G, Burman P, Wiren L, et al: Low dose dehydroepiandrosterone affects behavior in hypopituitary androgen-deficient women: A placebo-controlled trial. J Clin Endocrinol Metab 2002;87: 2046-2052.

Rhoden EL, Morgentaler A: Risk of testosterone-replacement therapy and recommendations for monitoring. N Engl J Med 2004;350: 482-492.

Hyperprolactinemia

Method of
Jeremy A. King, MD,
and Howard A. Zacur, MD, PhD

Prolactin is a polypeptide hormone secreted primarily by lactotrophs in the anterior pituitary gland. In humans, it has lactogenic, steroidogenic, and immunoregulatory functions. Hyperprolactinemia, defined simply as circulating plasma prolactin concentrations exceeding the upper limit of normal, may be caused by a variety of physiologic, iatrogenic, or pathologic conditions. An understanding of the physiology and regulation of prolactin is required to distinguish pathologic conditions from physiologic responses.

Regulation of prolactin production and secretion is multifactorial. The primary regulatory mechanism is chronic inhibition by dopamine. Dopamine secreted by neurons in the hypothalamus reaches the anterior pituitary via the portal circulation. The result of dopaminergic stimulation of lactotrophs is diminished prolactin production and release. Prolactin may also inhibit its own release by providing negative feedback at the level of the lactotroph or by stimulating the release of hypothalamic dopamine. Several substances are known to stimulate prolactin secretion. These include epidermal growth factor (EGF), vasoactive intestinal peptide (VIP), thyrotropin-releasing hormone (TRH), gonadotropin-releasing hormone (GnRH), and estrogens.

Signs and Symptoms

Premenopausal women with hyperprolactinemia may present with menstrual disturbances, infertility, and/or galactorrhea. When galactorrhea is identified in women with regular menstrual cycles, prolactin levels will be normal in at least 80% of cases. When both galactorrhea and amenorrhea are experienced, however, the incidence of hyperprolactinemia is 90%.

Hyperprolactinemia accounts for 10% to 38% of secondary amenorrhea. GnRH secretion is suppressed by prolactin acting at the hypothalamus thereby lowering release of gonadotropins. The resulting hypogonadism can cause hot flashes, vaginal dryness, and decreased bone mineral density caused by decreased levels of circulating estradiol. In males hyperprolactinemia causes impotence and decreased libido caused by lowered testosterone levels. Large prolactin-secreting pituitary lesions can cause neurologic symptoms such as severe headaches or visual impairment.

Causes of Hyperprolactinemia

Excess prolactin secretion can be caused by a variety of physiologic, iatrogenic, or pathologic conditions (Box 1). Elevation of prolactin levels to as high as 600 ng/mL may occur during a normal pregnancy. Stimulation or irritation of the chest wall from herpes zoster or local trauma may cause prolactin levels to rise. Conflicting data exist regarding the impact of clinical breast examination on prolactin levels. Sleep, physical or emotional stress, and food ingestion at lunch or dinner (but not breakfast) are all associated with a transient rise in prolactin values. Any pharmacologic agent that prevents the release of or blocks the action of dopamine can elevate prolactin levels. Common examples include many antipsychotics and antidepressants, H_2 receptor blockers, methyldopa, verapamil, reserpine, and metoclopramide.

BOX 1   Causes of Hyperprolactinemia

Physiologic
- Stress
- Sleep
- Lunch or dinner
- Chest wall stimulation
- Pregnancy

Pharmacologic
- Neuroleptics
- SSRIs
- H_2 receptor blockers
- Methyldopa
- Verapamil
- Reserpine
- Metoclopramide
- Protease inhibitors

Pathologic
- Prolactinoma
- Nonfunctioning pituitary tumors
- Empty sella syndrome
- Infiltrative disorders or CNS masses
- Hypothyroidism
- Renal failure

Idiopathic

Abbreviations: CNS = central nervous system; SSRI = selective serotonin reuptake inhibitor.

Pathologic hyperprolactinemia may be caused by lactotroph adenomas, decreased inhibition of prolactin secretion, or underlying medical conditions. Pituitary adenomas are found in at least 40% of hyperprolactinemic patients. They are almost always benign. Any abnormal process within the hypothalamus and/or pituitary that interrupts the normal secretion of dopamine to the portal circulation can cause hyperprolactinemia. Examples include tumors such as craniopharyngiomas, infiltrative diseases such as sarcoidosis, or trauma. Primary hypothyroidism is associated with hyperprolactinemia because TRH is a stimulator of prolactin release.

Evaluation

Diagnosis of pathologic hyperprolactinemia is made only after physiologic or iatrogenic causes have been excluded. More than one blood sample should be used to verify the diagnosis. Pregnancy must be ruled out. When an elevation of serum prolactin levels has been confirmed and careful history has excluded other known causes of hyperprolactinemia, proper evaluation consists of measuring serum thyroid-stimulating hormone (TSH) to rule out primary hypothyroidism and imaging of the pituitary gland.

We prefer to image the pituitary whenever the circulating prolactin level is above the normal range rather than waiting until levels exceed a given cutoff value. Many hyperprolactinemic patients will have a detectable pituitary abnormality (regardless of the magnitude of prolactin elevation). Magnetic resonance imaging (MRI) is the most sensitive diagnostic modality. Prolactinomas less than 10 mm in diameter are classified as microadenomas. Lesions 1 cm or larger are termed macroadenomas.

Pituitary lesions are capable of secreting any pituitary hormone. Adenomas of any cell origin are capable of causing lactotrophs to secrete excess prolactin. Therefore, when pituitary lesions are identified in the hyperprolactinemic patient, screening tests should be performed to rule out the secretion of other pituitary hormones before a diagnosis of a prolactinoma is made. Measurements of the following should be checked:

- Serum insulin-like growth factor I (IGF)-I (to exclude acromegaly)
- Follicle-stimulating hormone (FSH) and luteinizing hormone (LH) (to exclude gonadotroph tumors)
- TSH levels (to rule out thyrotroph tumors)
- 24-hour urine-free cortisol level (to exclude Cushing's syndrome)

Management

Management options include observation, medication, and surgery. Selection of the most appropriate option depends on the findings of pituitary imaging and the patient's fertility desires (Figure 1).

NO ADENOMA, PREGNANCY NOT DESIRED

Two therapeutic choices are available for the patient without a detectable pituitary abnormality who does not desire pregnancy. These are observation or dopamine agonist therapy. One third of the time, an elevated prolactin level in the absence of a detectable adenoma will normalize spontaneously within 5 years. Extended observation of the hyperprolactinemic patient with amenorrhea may be inadvisable because osteopenia or osteoporosis may result from prolonged hypoestrogenism. In addition to pituitary imaging, patients not receiving therapy should undergo periodic bone density monitoring.

Medical therapy is best achieved with dopamine agonists. Agonist therapy will successfully normalize prolactin levels and restore menstruation in up to 90% of women with nontumoral hyperprolactinemia. Medical therapy is directed at stimulating dopamine receptors, which inhibit prolactin production and secretion. Drugs that accomplish this effect include the ergot-derived bromocriptine (Parlodel), cabergoline (Dostinex), and pergolide (Permax),[1] and the apomorphine-derived quinagolide (Norprolac).[2]

Bromocriptine (Parlodel) and cabergoline (Dostinex) are currently approved by the FDA for the treatment of primary hyperprolactinemia. Bromocriptine (Parlodel) has been used for more than 30 years. Its efficacy and safety are well established. Cabergoline (Dostinex), approved for treatment of hyperprolactinemia in 1996, has the advantages of being slightly more efficacious, better tolerated, and can be taken at a much longer dosing interval. Both drugs cause side effects such as nausea, vomiting, postural hypotension, dizziness, syncope, and nasal congestion. Up to 12% of patients will not tolerate bromocriptine (Parlodel), whereas only 3% are intolerant to cabergoline (Dostinex).

We generally initiate bromocriptine (Parlodel) treatment with one half of a 2.5-mg tablet at night. The dose is then increased every few days as needed to normalize the serum prolactin concentration to a maximum of 2.5 mg three times a day. The graduated dose increase helps minimize adverse effects. Vaginal administration (with 2.5 to 5 mg/d) is also effective and is often better tolerated. Oral dosing with cabergoline (Dostinex) begins at 0.25 mg twice a week or 0.5 mg weekly. This dose is often therapeutic but can be increased if needed. Prolactin level monitoring can be performed within a few days of initiating or modifying medical therapy.

Pergolide (Permax)[1] is currently FDA approved for the treatment of parkinsonism but has been used successfully to treat hyperprolactinemia. It is the least expensive dopamine agonist available. Quinagolide (Norprolac)[2] is also effective but is currently available only in Europe. Both drugs are administered once daily.

If contraception is desired, the patient's choice of options need not be restricted by hyperprolactinemia. Although estrogen is known to stimulate pituitary prolactin secretion, oral contraceptive users rarely

---

[1]Not FDA approved for this indication.
[2]Not available in the United States.

The Endocrine System

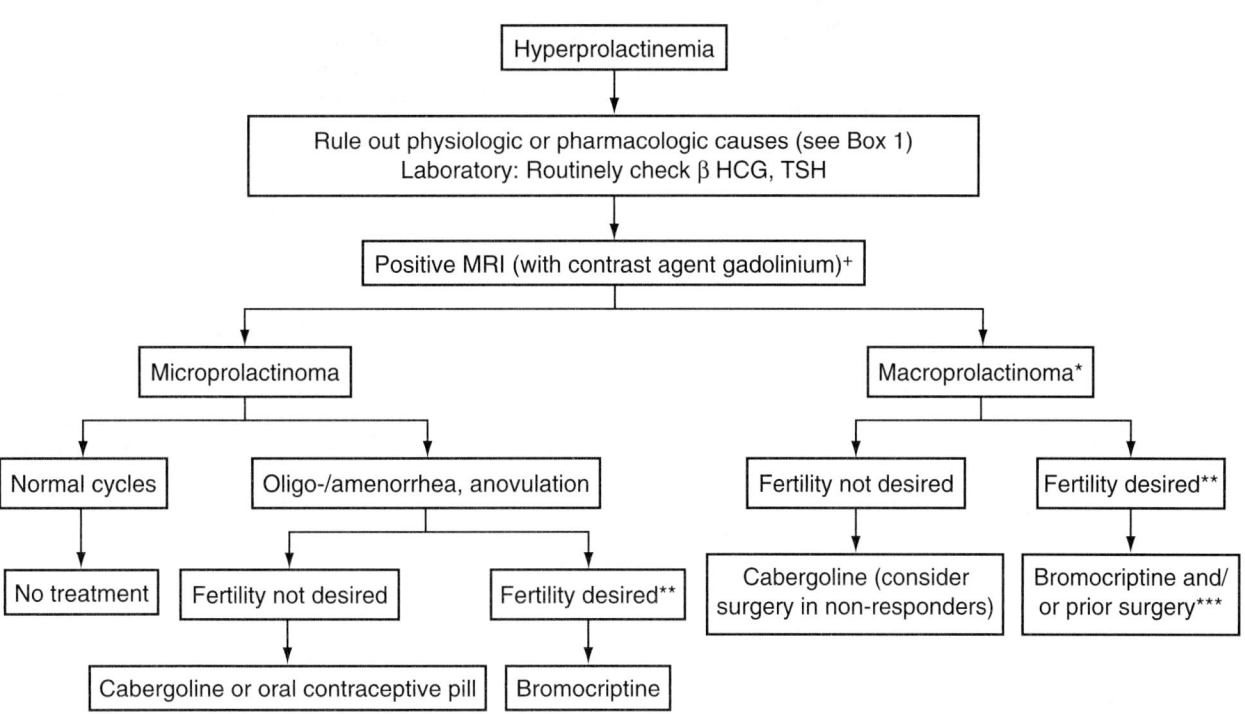

+ Patients who have a normal MRI are diagnosed with idiopathic hyperprolactinemia; they are medically managed in the same way as patients with microprolactinomas.
* In macroprolactinomas, prolactin levels are usually > 200 ug/L.
** When fertility is desired, bromocriptine (Parlodel) is preferred given a greater safety experience with this agent.
*** Patients with macroprolactinomas require medical treatment to reduce tumor volume or surgical treatment to excise the adenoma prior to attempting to conceive.

FIGURE 1. Management of hyperprolactinemia.

experience rising prolactin levels or formation of pituitary adenomas. Because tumor growth has been reported in some cases, however, pituitary imaging should be ordered if headaches or rising prolactin levels are observed.

ADENOMA PRESENT, PREGNANCY NOT DESIRED

As mentioned previously, it is important to exclude other hormone-producing adenomas when a pituitary lesion is visualized. Once other lesions are excluded, treatment for hyperprolactinemia may be considered. For patients with microadenomas, observation may be an appropriate option. Ninety percent to 95% of microadenomas remain stable or shrink over time. Dopamine agonist therapy will achieve normal prolactin levels and reduce adenoma size in 70% to 90% of patients (depending on lesion size). Medical therapy is indicated for any patient with a macroadenoma or with neurologic signs or symptoms. Periodic monitoring by MRI is recommended with more frequent monitoring if a macroadenoma is present.

Surgery, which is usually accomplished as a transsphenoidal partial hypophysectomy, is another option. Unfortunately, surgical therapy fails to cure

hyperprolactinemia approximately one third of the time. Roughly 20% of patients experience adenoma recurrence. Complication rates can be high. These include pituitary insufficiency, diabetes insipidus, cerebral spinal fluid fistulas, carotid artery injury, loss of vision, and meningitis. The incidence of malignancy in prolactinomas is rare. Current data do not support surgery for the purpose of excluding malignancy. Surgery is indicated for patients with pituitary apoplexy or with lesions that grow despite agonist therapy. Patients who are intolerant or unwilling to use long-term medical therapy may also consider surgical resection.

Treatment of hyperprolactinemia will result in increased fertility. Women desiring estrogen-containing contraceptives should be aware that rare case reports have documented an association of such agents with an increase in adenoma size. However, several larger series have failed to demonstrate any association with increases in lesion size or prolactin levels.

NO ADENOMA, PREGNANCY DESIRED

Infertility associated with hyperprolactinemia is the result of chronic hypogonadism. When pregnancy is desired, bromocriptine (Parlodel) is the first line

CURRENT DIAGNOSIS

- Repeat serum prolactin measurements.
- Exclude known physiologic and iatrogenic causes.
- Measure serum TSH.
- Image pituitary (preferably MRI with contrast).
- Check serum IGF-I, FSH, LH, TSH, and 24-hour urine free cortisol level if a pituitary lesion is identified.

Abbreviations: FSH = follicle-stimulating hormone; IGF = insulin-like growth factor; LH = luteinizing hormone; MRI = magnetic resonance imaging; TSH = thyroid-stimulating hormone.

of therapy. Normalization of prolactin levels and resumption of menses typically occur within 8 weeks of therapy. The drug is discontinued when pregnancy is diagnosed. Discontinuation does not increase the chance of pregnancy loss. Children conceived during bromocriptine (Parlodel) administration are not at increased risk for congenital malformation. Cabergoline (Dostinex) also restores normal gonadotropic activity effectively. However, there are insufficient data about the impact of this drug on early pregnancy. Some hyperprolactinemic, anovulatory patients fail to respond to dopamine agonists or cannot tolerate the side effects. In such cases clomiphene citrate or gonadotropins are used for ovulation induction. Because of the normal elevation and variation of prolactin levels in pregnancy there is no clinical usefulness in measuring serum values.

ADENOMA PRESENT, PREGNANCY DESIRED

Identification of pituitary hormone secretion other than prolactin from pituitary lesions is essential. Next the patient is managed in a manner similar to that described for the hyperprolactinemic patient without a lesion. Dopamine agonists or ovulation induction agents may be used. Patients should be counseled about the risks of pregnancy. Gland and adenoma enlargement often

CURRENT THERAPY

- Management of hyperprolactinemia depends on the presence and size of an adenoma and the patient's desire for fertility.
- Dopamine agonists are highly effective for treating hyperprolactinemia with or without adenomas present.
- Although all agonists are effective, cabergoline is often more effective and better tolerated.
- Because more data are available for bromocriptine use during pregnancy, bromocriptine (Parlodel) should be the drug of choice when pregnancy is desired.
- In general, surgical resection of prolactinomas should be a last resort.

occurs under the influence of elevated estrogen levels. The chance of developing headaches or visual changes is only 1% to 5% for women with microadenomas, but it can be as high as 36% when a macroadenoma is present.

When pregnancy is achieved dopamine agonists are discontinued by tapering the daily dose to avoid adenoma infarction. Visual field testing and pituitary imaging with MRI are performed if symptoms occur. Measurement of prolactin levels during pregnancy is not useful for detecting adenoma enlargement. Dopamine agonist therapy may be restarted if optic nerve compromise occurs.

Breast-feeding is not contraindicated. Dopamine agonists can be administered during lactation if neurologic symptoms occur. Occasionally spontaneous infarction of an adenoma occurs postpartum. This can result in lowered prolactin levels and resumption of normal menses.

REFERENCES

Bankowski BJ, Zacur HA: Dopamine agonist therapy for hyperprolactinemia. Clin Obstet Gynecol 2003;46(2):349-362.
Bevan JS, Webster J, Burke CW, Scanlon MF: Dopamine agonists and pituitary tumor shrinkage. Endocr Rev 1992;13(2):220-240.
Biller BM, Luciano A, Crosignani PG, et al: Guidelines for the diagnosis and treatment of hyperprolactinemia. J Reprod Med 1999;44(Suppl 12):1075-1084.
Corenblum B, Donovan L: The safety of physiological estrogen plus progestin replacement therapy and with oral contraceptive therapy in women with pathological hyperprolactinemia. Fertil Steril 1993;59(3):671-673.
Kleinberg DL, Noel GL, Frantz AG: Galactorrhea: A study of 235 cases, including 48 with pituitary tumors. N Engl J Med 1977;296(11):589-600.
Losa M, Mortini P, Barzaghi R, et al: Surgical treatment of prolactin-secreting pituitary adenomas: Early results and long-term outcome. J Clin Endocrinol Metab 2002;87(7):3180-3186.
Molitch M: Prolactinoma. In Melmed S (ed): The Pituitary, 2nd ed. Malden, Mass, Blackwell Publishing, 2002, pp 455-495.
Schlechte J, Dolan K, Sherman B, et al: The natural history of untreated hyperprolactinemia: A prospective analysis. J Clin Endocrinol Metab 1989;68:412-418.
Webster J, Piscitelli G, Polli A, et al: A comparison of cabergoline and bromocriptine in the treatment of hyperprolactinemic amenorrhea. Cabergoline Comparative Study Group. N Engl J Med 1994;331(14):904-909.

Hypothyroidism

Method of
Peter A. Singer, MD

Hypothyroidism is probably the most common thyroid disorder encountered in clinical practice. It is estimated that approximately 15 million persons living in the United States have hypothyroidism, or roughly 2% of the population. Hypothyroidism increases in prevalence with increasing age; approximately 10% of 65-year-old women are hypothyroid, and perhaps 15% of 75-year-old women are hypothyroid. Women are affected much more often than men, in a ratio of 8 to 1 or 9 to 1. Approximately 95% of hypothyroidism in the United States is from primary thyroid failure, either from chronic autoimmune (Hashimoto's) thyroiditis or surgical or radioiodine ablation. There are numerous other causes of hypothyroidism, including transient forms of the disorder associated with either subacute painful thyroiditis, or with postpartum thyroiditis. In addition, certain drugs, including the antiarrhythmic agent amiodarone and the cytokines interferon (IFN)-alpha and interleukin (IL)-2, may cause transient hypothyroidism by causing thyroiditis. Amiodarone, which is heavily iodinated, may cause hypothyroidism by inhibiting thyroid hormone secretion, as may the antidepressant lithium carbonate. Much less common causes of hypothyroidism include congenital hypothyroidism, affecting approximately 1 to 3500 live births in the United States, and certain rare chronic inflammatory or infiltrative disorders including hemochromatosis, cystinosis, and Riedel's struma. In geographic areas of iodine deficiency, lack of iodine is the principle cause of hypothyroidism; there are no known areas of iodine deficiency in the United States. All the aforementioned causes of hypothyroidism are termed primary *hypothyroidism* because of the thyroid gland's deficiency in secreting thyroid hormone. *Secondary hypothyroidism*, on the other hand, occurs when there is a deficiency of thyroid-stimulating hormone (TSH) secretion because of an abnormality of the hypothalamic-pituitary axis, usually from pituitary tumors or craniopharyngiomas, although other disorders may cause deficient TSH secretion. Table 1 lists the different etiologies of hypothyroidism.

Symptoms and Signs

The symptoms and signs of hypothyroidism are typically multiple and varied, nonspecific, and often suggestive of other clinical conditions. Symptoms depend on the patient's age, the severity of the hypothyroidism, and its duration. Young patients typically have fewer symptoms, whereas older individuals are less able to tolerate thyroid hormone deficiency. Typical symptoms of hypothyroidism include fatigue, dry skin and hair, increased need for sleep, cold intolerance, constipation, weight gain, and slowing of intellectual functioning. Increased menstrual flow may also be present. A common misconception among patients (and even many physicians) is that significant weight gain is associated with hypothyroidism; even with overt hypothyroidism patients gain no more than 10% to 15% over baseline weights, because hypothyroidism is associated with a decreased appetite.

Signs of hypothyroidism may include bradycardia, mild diastolic hypertension, a waxy and pale complexion, puffiness of the eyelids, slowing or even slurring of speech, goiter, muffled heart tones, and delayed deep tendon reflexes. As with symptoms, signs depend on the degree of thyroid hormone deficiency, duration of the disorder, and patient age.

Rakel and Bope: *Conn's Current Therapy 2006.*

TABLE 1 Etiologies of Hypothyroidism

Primary Hypothyroidism
Permanent Hypothyroidism
Chronic autoimmune (Hashimoto's) thyroiditis (most common cause in industrialized countries)
Thyroid ablation (radioactive iodine therapy for hyperthyroidism; thyroidectomy)
External radiotherapy (for head and neck cancers, lymphoma)
Congenital (~1 per 3500 live births in the United States; caused by thyroid agenesis)
Infiltrative disorders (hemochromatosis, amyloidosis, Riedel's thyroiditis, cystinosis, scleroderma, leukemia—all are infrequent to rare)
Iodine deficiency (principally in Asia, Africa, and areas of Latin America)
Iodine excess—rom iodine containing medications, such as amiodarone, SSKI (occurs in patients with underlying autoimmune thyroid disease)
Transient Hypothyroidism
Subacute painful (viral) thyroiditis
Subacute painless thyroiditis—most frequently postpartum
Drug induced
• IF-alfa; IL-2; amiodarone (the drugs induce a thyroiditis-like response)
• Exogenous iodides, including amiodarone (euthyroidism returns after drug withdrawal)
• Antithyroid drugs—methimazole, propylthiouracil (resolves after medication withdrawal)
• Lithium carbonate (resolves after medication withdrawal; occurs only in patients with underlying autoimmune thyroid disease)
Secondary (Central) Hypothyroidism
Pituitary adenoma, craniopharyngioma
Pituitary apoplexy, Sheehan's syndrome
Lymphocytic hypophysitis
Pituitary irradiation
Cranial radiation
Pituitary stalk section; other major head trauma
Congenital hypopituitarism (rare)
Infiltrative disorders (Langerhans histiocytosis, hemochromatosis)
Granulomatous disorders (sarcoidosis)

Abbreviations: IF = interferon; IL = interleukin; SSKI = saturated solution of potassium iodide.

Laboratory Diagnosis

The serum thyrotropin is the cornerstone in the biochemical diagnosis of primary hypothyroidism, and it should be the first test employed in screening for hypothyroidism. If the serum TSH is elevated, a serum-free thyroxine (FT_4) or its estimate should be obtained to assess the degree of thyroid deficiency. Mild TSH elevation (i.e., greater than 5 mIU/L and less than 20 mIU/L) associated with a normal FT_4 is termed *subclinical hypothyroidism, mild hypothyroidism,* or *mild thyroid failure,* whereas a low FT_4 associated with an elevation in serum TSH is termed *overt hypothyroidism.* A normal- or low-serum TSH is associated with a low FT_4 and suggests secondary hypothyroidism. In such cases pituitary imaging with magnetic resonance imaging (MRI) is indicated.

Whether to measure thyroid antibodies in patients with elevated TSH levels is a matter of debate. Because most patients with spontaneous hypothyroidism have chronic autoimmune thyroiditis, antimicrosomal (thyroperoxidase [TPO]) antibodies will usually be elevated. Thus, if there is clinical and biochemical evidence of hypothyroidism, measurement of antibodies may be superfluous in terms of treatment, because their presence or absence will not influence the decision to treat. If the TSH is mildly elevated and the FT_4 is normal, measurement of TPO antibodies may help to determine whether there is spurious (transient) TSH elevation; in such cases, TPO antibodies will be negative, and the clinician may wish to defer therapy until persistent TSH elevation has been documented.

It should be noted that there are pitfalls in the interpretation of serum TSH levels. It is most reliable when measured in ambulatory individuals. In hospitalized euthyroid patients, however, the TSH may be either high or low, depending on the severity of the nonthyroidal illness. Thus, a serum TSH that is mildly abnormal in an ill patient should be repeated following recovery. Serum TSH values may also become mildly elevated with the use of certain drugs, especially dopamine antagonists such as metoclopramide or domperidone; the degree of TSH elevation with such agents tends to be mild. Elevated serum TSH levels occur in thyrotoxic patients, such as those with TSH-secreting pituitary adenomas; such patients are clinically and biochemically thyrotoxic and should not be confused with patients with suspected hypothyroidism. Finally, mild TSH elevations, even in healthy ambulatory individuals, may be transient, and before initiating therapy for hypothyroidism the serum TSH should be repeated.

Treatment

There is virtual unanimity of opinion among endocrinologists that levothyroxine (LT_4) is the drug of choice for the treatment of hypothyroidism. Approximately 80% of LT_4 is absorbed from the gastrointestinal tract, and the T_4 half-life of 1 week ensures that a constant level of thyroid hormone in serum is easily achieved. LT_4 is administered in a daily oral dose, and the goal of therapy is to achieve a normal serum TSH level; although laboratory reference ranges of TSH may be fairly broad, practicing endocrinologists prefer that the TSH be maintained in the range of approximately 0.5 to 2 mIU/L.

The average LT_4 dose for healthy adults is approximately 1.6 μg/kg per day; patients younger than 50 or 55 years of age may be started on full-replacement therapy, whereas older patients are generally started on doses of between 25 and 50 μg per day. Those with underlying coronary disease, or other significant comorbidity, such as diabetes mellitus, hypertension, and hyperlipidemia (metabolic syndrome), should be started on doses no greater than 25 μg per day.

After therapy has been initiated, patients should be reevaluated in approximately 6 to 8 weeks, with a clinical examination and measurement of serum TSH level. There is little usefulness in checking the TSH sooner

because serum T_4 and TSH levels take approximately 6 weeks to equilibrate. If the serum TSH continues to be elevated, the dose of LT_4 should be increased by 25 μg per day, and the patients reevaluated in another 6 to 8 weeks, and every 2 to 3 months thereafter, with 25 μg dose adjustments, until the TSH normalizes. If the TSH level is suppressed, the dose should be decreased, and further adjustments made every few months until normalization of the serum TSH concentration is achieved. Once patients are on a stable dose of LT_4, they may be reevaluated yearly, or more often as the clinical situation dictates.

Patients should be instructed to take LT_4 on an empty stomach, and to refrain from eating for an hour, as food appears to inhibit LT_4 absorption, albeit slightly. In addition, patients should be instructed to avoid taking iron and/or calcium supplements at the same time as LT_4, because the supplements have a mild inhibitory effect on LT_4 absorption; spacing should be at least 2 hours apart. In addition to interfering with absorption of LT_4, a number of conditions and drugs alter LT_4 dose requirements (Table 2).

OTHER CONSIDERATIONS

Pregnancy

Pregnancy increases LT_4 requirements by as much as 40%. The need for the dose increase is multifactorial, in part related to increased T_4 clearance, as well as increased transfer of T_4 to the fetus. The estrogen-mediated increase in thyroxine-binding globulin (TBG) appears to increase T_4 requirements also. It is essential for normal fetal growth and intellectual development that the hypothyroid mother be euthyroid during pregnancy; therefore, once pregnancy is confirmed, a maternal serum TSH should be obtained within 4 weeks. A rise in TSH warrants an immediate increase in LT_4 dose, usually by 25 μg per day. The serum TSH should be checked once each trimester, and the LT_4 dose

---

TABLE 2 Factors Affecting Levothyroxine Dose

Increased LT_4 Dose Requirement
Increase in TBG—pregnancy, estrogen therapy
Weight gain
Impaired gastrointestinal absorption of LT_4
- Inflammatory small bowel disease, celiac disease
- Vitamins and supplements containing iron, calcium carbonate; aluminum hydroxide gels
- Sucralfate; bile acid-binding sequestrants (cholestyramine, colestipol)
- Diet high in soy
Drugs increasing LT_4 metabolism—phenytoin, carbamazepine, phenobarbital, rifampin
Smoking
Decreased LT_4 Dose Requirement
Decrease in TBG—androgen therapy; nephrotic syndrome
Aging (old age)
Significant weight loss

Abbreviations: LT_4 = levothyroxine; TBG = thyroxine-binding globulin.

Rakel and Bope: *Conn's Current Therapy 2006.*

should be adjusted accordingly. An alternative method would be to empirically increase the LT_4 dose by approximately 40% once pregnancy is confirmed, rather than wait for an increase in TSH. In my experience the *40% rule* is inconsistent, and I prefer waiting until a need for increased dose is demonstrated. Following delivery, the prepregnant dose of LT_4 may be resumed without hesitation.

Subclinical Hypothyroidism

The issue of whether to treat patients with mild TSH elevations and normal FT_4 concentrations is still controversial. Some clinicians use a serum TSH of 10 mIU/L as the lowest cutoff to initiate treatment with LT_4, whereas others suggest treating any patient with an elevated TSH, regardless of the level. I advocate obtaining TPO antibodies in patients with elevated TSHs, and if the antibodies are positive, I encourage LT_4 therapy (usually with a starting dose of 25 to 50 µg per day), because individuals with positive antibodies and TSH levels above the normal range are likely to develop overt hypothyroidism at a rate of approximately 5% per year. Thus, early initiation of treatment in such patients will avoid the inadvertent development of overt hypothyroidism.

Levothyroxine Product Switching

A common scenario nowadays is product switching by pharmacists, driven by insurance companies' desire to

---

CURRENT THERAPY

- Healthy patients younger than 50 years of age: L-thyroxine 1.6 µg/kg body weight per day (full replacement)
- Older healthy patients: L-thyroxine 25 to 50 µg per day
- Older patients with coronary disease, or otherwise unwell: L-thyroxine 12.5 to 25 µg per day

---

reduce costs. Therefore, the least expensive preparation is frequently substituted for the product the physician has prescribed. Most endocrinologists strongly urge that patients take a *branded* preparation, and if the product is switched when the prescription is refilled, that the patient be reevaluated with a serum TSH, no sooner than 6 weeks, because not all products are bioequivalent.

Other Thyroid Hormone Preparations

In addition to LT_4, there are other thyroid hormone preparations available, including desiccated thyroid, combinations of T_4 and T_3, and T_3 (Cytomel) alone. Some patients have strong preferences for such preparations, and for various reasons, a common one being that they know that T_3 (Cytomel) is the biologically active form of thyroid hormone. Because T_4 is converted to T_3 (Cytomel) in peripheral tissues, there clearly is no advantage to the use of T_3 (Cytomel)-containing preparations. Moreover, there may be disadvantages to their use, including inconsistent bioavailability, and the supranormal increases in serum T_3 (Cytomel) levels that may occur within a few hours after taking them. In patients with underlying heart disease, a significant increase in T_3 (Cytomel) concentration may result in angina or arrhythmia. Despite the caveats provided to patients, some are insistent and believe that they will feel better by taking T_3 (Cytomel) alone, or in combinations with T_4. My solution to situations such as this, if my explanation regarding the advantages of LT_4 therapy is insufficient, is to prescribe one of the preparations in a dose tailored to mimic the LT_4 dose. I carefully explain that suppression of TSH must be avoided, and that they may not feel better. It is preferable to ensure some measure of compliance, than to have the patient go untreated.

TREATMENT OF SECONDARY HYPOTHYROIDISM

Patients with secondary hypothyroidism usually have other pituitary hormone deficiencies, and before thyroid hormone therapy is initiated it is imperative that the remainder of pituitary status be evaluated; it is essential that LT_4 not be prescribed unless patients with adrenocorticotropic hormone (ACTH)-cortisol

---

CURRENT DIAGNOSIS

Common Symptoms
- Fatigue
- Increased need for sleep
- Cold intolerance
- Dry skin and hair
- Weight gain (mild)
- Constipation
- Intellectual slowing

Common Signs
- Slowed pulse
- Slowed speech
- Dry, flaky skin
- Pallor (with overt hypothyroidism)
- Goiter
- Periorbital edema
- Distant heart tones (with marked hypothyroidism)
- Delayed deep tendon reflexes

Biochemical Diagnosis
- Elevated serum TSH
- Low free T_4
- Elevated serum TSH, and normal free T_4 (with subclinical hypothyroidism)
- Normal or low serum TSH, and low free T_4 (with secondary hypothyroidism)

Abbreviations: TSH = thyroid-stimulating hormone.

Rakel and Bope: *Conn's Current Therapy 2006.*

deficiency are on glucocorticoid therapy as well. LT$_4$ therapy alone could precipitate adrenal crisis. Because the serum TSH cannot be used as an endpoint of therapy, the clinician must rely on the serum FT$_4$ (or estimate) concentration, which should be kept in the upper half of the normal range.

REFERENCES

Alexander EK, Margusee E, Lawrence J, et al: Timing and magnitude of increases in levothyroxine requirements during pregnancy in women with hypothyroidism. N Engl J Med 2004;351:241-249.

Canaris GJ, Manowitz NR, Mayor G, Ridgway EC: The Colorado thyroid disease prevalence study. Arch Intern Med 2000;160: 526-534.

Cooper DS: Clinical practice: Subclinical hypothyroidism. N Engl J Med 2001;345:260-265.

Ladenson PW, Singer PA, Ain KB, et al: American Thyroid Association guidelines for detection of thyroid dysfunction. Arch Intern Med 2000;160:1573-1575.

Oppenheimer JH, Braverman LE, Toft A, et al: A therapeutic controversy. Thyroid hormone treatment: When and what? J Clin Endocrinol Metab 1995;80:2873-2883.

Singer PA, Cooper DS, Levy EG, et al: Treatment guidelines for patients with hyperthyroidism and hypothyroidism. JAMA 1995;273-808-812.

Surks MI, Ortiz E, Daniels GH, et al: Subclinical thyroid disease: Scientific review and guidelines for diagnosing and management. JAMA 2004;291:228-238.

Vanderpump MP, Tunbridge WM, French JM, et al: The incidence of thyroid disorders in the community: A twenty-year follow up of the Whickham Survey. Clin Endocrinol (Oxf) 1995;43:55-68.

Hyperthyroidism

Method of
Kenneth D. Burman, MD

Hyperthyroidism is a condition resulting from overproduction of L-thyroxine (T$_4$) and/or L-triiodothyronine (T$_3$) (Box 1). The clinical diagnosis should always be confirmed with thyroid function tests and sometimes by radioisotope studies. Treatment of hyperthyroidism should preferably be conducted in consultation with an endocrinologist.

Diagnosis

HISTORY AND PHYSICAL EXAMINATION

Classically, by history and/or examination, the patient usually has one or more of the following: nervousness; weight loss; increased appetite; palpitations; tachycardia; generalized pruritus; hand tremor; hyperdefecation; diaphoresis; irritability; insomnia and muscle weakness; widened pulse pressure with systolic hypertension; hyperreflexia; lid lag; warm, moist skin; irritability; and

---

BOX 1   Causes of Endogenous Hyperthyroidism
Common
• Graves' disease
• Toxic adenoma
• Multinodular goiter
• Thyroiditis (subacute, postpartum)
• Amiodarone
Uncommon
• TSH-secreting pituitary adenoma
• Metastatic differentiated thyroid cancer
• Struma ovarii
Abbreviations: TSH = thyroid-stimulating hormone.

---

inability to concentrate. However, a given patient may exhibit these findings to a varying extent. Elderly patients in particular may present in a more subtle fashion, perhaps demonstrating only weight loss, weakness, depression, or atrial fibrillation. Commonly, patients have an enlarged thyroid gland. In Graves' disease the thyroid gland is enlarged and smooth possibly with an overlying bruit. Patients with Graves' disease may demonstrate extrathyroidal findings such as diplopia, burning or itching eyes, lid lag or retraction, extraocular muscle involvement, proptosis, or even, on rare occasions, decreased vision. Pretibial myxedema, onycholysis, and acropachy may occur. The thyroid gland is nodular in patients with a multinodular goiter or solitary autonomous nodule. Patients with granulomatous (de Quervain's thyroiditis) subacute thyroiditis may have a history of recent viral infection, neck pain that can radiate to the jaw or chest, and a tender goiter. Patients with postpartum thyroiditis present within 6 to 12 months of gestation. Subacute, postpartum, and silent thyroiditis tend to evolve through various stages of hyperthyroidism and hypothyroidism before usually returning to the euthyroid state. Patients with exogenous thyrotoxicosis may have no goiter. Those with iodine-induced thyrotoxicosis have a history of recent exposure to iodinated contrast agents (e.g., computed tomography [CT] scan, angiogram). Rarer causes of hyperthyroidism are a thyroid-stimulating hormone (TSH)-secreting pituitary tumor and human chorionic gonadotropin (hCG)-mediated disease. Metastatic follicular cancer and struma ovarii are usually evident by history and physical examination.

LABORATORY EVALUATION

The diagnosis is established by having an undetectable TSH (<0.01 mU/L) and elevated T$_4$ and/or T$_3$. TSH assays vary in their sensitivity, and in some assays a TSH less than 0.05 mU/L is also consistent with the diagnosis. Free T$_4$ (FT$_4$) hormone determinations are preferable to total T$_4$. Total T$_3$ is still more easily obtained than Free T$_3$ (FT$_3$). Binding protein abnormalities such as elevated thyroxine-binding globulin (TBG) induced by pregnancy and estrogen administration interfere with total hormone assays. However, a variety of circumstances such as systemic illness and medications may

---

BOX 2   Radioactive Iodine Thyroid Uptake and Hyperthyroidism

High uptake
- Graves' disease
- Multinodular goiter
- Toxic adenoma

Low uptake
- Thyroiditis (subacute, postpartum)
- Amiodarone (Cordarone)[1]
- Exogenous levothyroxine (Synthroid) over administration
- Struma ovarii

---

[1]Not FDA approved for this indication.

---

interfere with TSH and FT_4 and FT_3 assays. Secondary hypothyroidism, nonthyroidal illness, Amiodarone (Cordarone),[1] glucocorticoid therapy, and excess exogenous thyroid hormone administration may cause discordant thyroid hormone tests results, usually with relatively decreased T_3 concentrations. It is always prudent to interpret the thyroid function tests carefully with consideration of the clinical condition.

A radioactive iodine uptake (RAIU) and scan may be helpful (Box 2). Patients can be divided into high uptake hyperthyroidism (Graves' disease, multinodular goiter, toxic adenoma) and low uptake hyperthyroidism (subacute, silent, postpartum thyroiditis, Amiodarone (Cordarone)[1]-induced disease, and exogenous thyroid hormone administration). Patients taking thyroid hormones for replacement therapy may have subclinical or overt hyperthyroidism because of overtreatment. Thyrotoxicosis may also occur when patients unwittingly take over-the-counter *nutraceuticals* containing thyroid hormone extracts or analogues or when they surreptitiously take thyroid hormone for weight loss or other purposes. In both cases, patients usually do not have a goiter and the thyroid uptake is low (<3%; normal 24-hour 131-I uptake is 8% to 30%). Measurement of a serum thyroglobulin level (not antibody) may be helpful in discriminating different causes of low uptake hyperthyroidism. If a patient is taking exogenous L-thyroxine, the serum thyroglobulin level is low (e.g., <5 ng/mL) because there is no intrathyroidal synthesis and secretion of iodothyronines. If the patient has destructive thyroiditis (e.g., subacute, silent, postpartum), however, the serum thyroglobulin level is elevated (usually greater than 20 ng/mL) because there is release of hormones into the circulation.

Except for over-replacement with exogenous L-thyroxine administration, in all age groups, Graves' disease is the most common cause of hyperthyroidism. Graves' disease is an autoimmune disease in which thyrotropin receptor-stimulating antibodies stimulate thyroid gland growth, thyroid hormone synthesis, and release. The most important differential diagnosis is with thyroiditis (through disruption of the thyroid follicles and release of preformed thyroid hormones) and toxic nodular disease (multinodular goiter or toxic adenoma). Graves' disease is associated with increased

thyroid hormone production and is associated with high-normal (in spite of suppressed TSH levels) or more typically increased 131-I uptake. Although TSH receptor antibodies are present in almost all patients with Graves' disease, I measure them only in specific circumstances (e.g., diagnosis in doubt, pregnancy with hyperthyroidism).

Thyroiditis may be indistinguishable from Graves' disease in the absence of extrathyroidal manifestations of the latter. In contrast to Graves' disease, thyroiditis is associated with low 131-I uptake (<3%). Additionally, patients with granulomatous (subacute) thyroiditis may have anterior neck pain, elevated sedimentation rate, and elevated white blood count. Patients with transient lymphocytic thyroiditis may have a painless goiter, family history of autoimmune disease, and antithyroperoxidase (anti-TPO) antibodies. Postpartum thyroiditis occurs within approximately 6 months of delivery and also occurs more frequently in patients with thyroid antibodies.

Toxic multinodular goiters (Plummer's disease) are more frequent in the elderly and may be difficult to diagnose. Patients usually present with large multinodular glands, but in some patients the goiter could be substernal and, therefore, not palpable in the neck. Elderly patients may present with cardiac arrhythmias, weight loss, and fatigue. Patients with multinodular goiter are especially prone to developing thyrotoxicosis after iodine exposure (e.g., following radiocontrast injection). A patient with a toxic solitary adenoma has a *hot* nodule on thyroid isotope scan.

Therapy

GRAVES' DISEASE WITH HYPERTHYROIDISM

The first goal of therapy is to render the patient euthyroid with an antithyroid agent and to treat hyperadrenergic activity with a β-blocker. Thionamides are antithyroid drugs that inhibit the synthesis of thyroid hormones with gradual decreases in the concentrations of T_3 and T_4 over several weeks of treatment. I start propylthiouracil (PTU) at doses of 50 to 100 mg orally every 8 hours for mild or moderate disease and 200 mg every 8 hours for more severe disease. Alternatively, methimazole (Tapazole) at doses of 10 to 20 mg (once daily) are used for mild to moderate disease and 20 to 40 mg (once daily) for more severe disease. In men and postmenopausal women I prefer methimazole (Tapazole), rather than PTU, because it can be administered once daily. The frequency of possible complications (skin rash, arthralgias, liver toxicity, and bone marrow suppression) is probably comparable with these two medications. Methimazole (Tapazole) has been associated with a congenital defect called *aplasia cutis*. It is preferable to use PTU in child bearing aged women who may become pregnant or breast-feed as PTU binds more strongly to serum proteins (as compared with methimazole [Tapazole]), and only a small amount of PTU crosses the placenta or gets into breast milk. PTU inhibits T_4 to

T_3 conversion, but this effect probably is of minimal clinical effect. It generally takes approximately 2 to 8 weeks of antithyroid drug (ATD) treatment for the thyroid function tests to normalize. At this point, the conversations regarding definitive therapy should become more intense. Occasionally, the serum TSH concentration remains suppressed for a long time, regardless of the serum T_4 and T_3 levels. Accordingly, serum T_4 and T_3 levels and the clinical condition must be interpreted in the context of the serum TSH level to assess when a patient is euthyroid. In some instances, I administer definitive therapy initially when the patient originally presents with hyperthyroidism. This approach is also reasonable but in the majority of cases I prefer to render the patient euthyroid first. The reasons for this approach include the observation that occasionally 131-I therapy may exacerbate hyperthyroidism but, most importantly, hyperthyroid patients may have difficulty concentrating and making rational, well considered decisions. Treatment with ATDs for several weeks prior to definitive therapy allows the patient (and family) to carefully consider the options and make the best individual decision.

Definitive treatment options include ATDs, 131-I therapy, or surgery (Box 3). ATDs may be used for an arbitrary time period (usually a year) in an effort to induce a *permanent* remission. The likelihood that a persistent remission will occur is relatively unusual and appears to correlate with the multiple factors. Favorable factors at initial presentation include mild hyperthyroidism, small goiter, and negligible or undetectable titers of thyrotrophin receptor stimulating antibodies. The ATD dose is modulated on a frequent basis for the year of treatment to maintain a normal FT_4 and T_3. TSH should not be used as the sole indicator of thyroid function. To monitor for possible adverse effects of ATD, I suggest measuring CBC with differential, liver function tests and thyroid function tests every 4 to 6 weeks while taking an ATD. The long-term remission rate after ATD is discontinued is probably in the 10% to 20% range. Relevant articles in the literature are difficult to apply to a given patient population because of varying degree of initial hyperthyroidism

and varying follow-up intervals after putative remission. If someone has or is suspected of having a major side effect, the patient is asked to immediately discontinue the offending agent and to contact their primary care doctor or the emergency room if they develop a sore throat or any significant febrile illness. It is appropriate to see these patients expeditiously and obtain appropriate laboratory studies. Patients receiving ATDs require close monitoring of thyroid function during initiation, maintenance, and discontinuation to ascertain recurrence of hyperthyroidism. In my practice, few patients opt for this approach and often prefer other forms of therapy.

If the patient has a recurrence (usually 3 to 6 months after ATD discontinuation), radioactive iodine (RAI) or surgery is then recommended. RAI therapy has been used for more than 60 years and is very effective and safe. The goal of 131-I therapy is permanent hypothyroid. Hypothyroidism typically develops approximately 2 to 3 months after 131-I administration. Patients require close follow-up during this time period and frequently require ATD for 1 to 2 months after 131-I therapy. As the FT_4 and total T_3 (TT_3) return to the normal range, the dose of ATD is gradually decreased and then discontinued. When the FT_4 decreases to the lower portion of the normal range or to below it, I start L-thyroxine therapy. Frequently the TSH rises to above the normal range, but some patients have persistent suppression of this axis even despite the development of hypothyroidism. Few patients require a second dose of 131-I, which would not be given until at least 6 months after the initial dose.

The 131-I dose is estimated from goiter size and RAI uptake using the following formula:

$$100 - 200 \text{ µCi} \times \text{thyroid gland weight [g]} \text{ divided by 24 RAIU [\%]}$$

The usual dose is 10 to 20 mCi. In adult women of childbearing potential a negative pregnancy (and appropriate clinical history) is required within 2 to 3 days of the 131-I therapy. Patients are informed of the recommended radiation precautions. Some patients may experience a short-lived exacerbation of thyroid symptoms or anterior neck pain following 131-I treatment. Serum FT_4/FT_3 and TSH are checked roughly every 4 weeks after treatment. When the TSH rises above the normal range and/or the FT_4 starts to fall into the lower portion of the normal range or below the normal range, I start levothyroxine (Synthroid) (1.7 µg/kg per day) with the goal to achieve a TSH between 0.5 to 3.0 mU/L (and FT_4/T_3 within the upper part of the normal range). This therapy is continued for life with yearly monitoring. Patients with significant ophthalmopathy may have an exacerbation of their eye problems following 131-I treatment. Smoking is also considered a risk factor for ophthalmopathy. Patients with significant ophthalmopathy are given prednisone 0.5 mg/kg per day starting several days prior to 131-I therapy and continued for approximately 2 weeks with tapering over the following 1 to 2 weeks.

Near-total or bilateral subtotal thyroidectomy represents an effective treatment that resolves the

---

BOX 3   Treatment Options

- Short term
    Thionamide (PTU or methimazole [Tapazole])
    β-blocker
- Rare
    SSKI or Lugol's[1] solution
    Lithium
    Potassium perchlorate[1]
- Definitive therapy
    Thionamide
    131-I
    Thyroidectomy

[1]Not FDA approved for this indication.
Abbreviations: PTU = propylthiouracil; 131-I = radioactive iodine;
    SSKI = saturated solution of potassium iodide.

---

thyrotoxic symptoms, usually resulting in postoperative hypothyroidism requiring lifelong levothyroxine (Synthroid) replacement. Thyroidectomy is an effective option for patients who require immediate relief of their thyrotoxic symptoms, with large goiters (especially with compressive symptoms), with suspicious or malignant nodules, with contraindications to 131-I (pregnancy) or ATDs, and preferring definitive treatment without radiation. Surgical morbidity is lower in centers with more surgical experience. As a result, permanent hypoparathyroidism, vocal cord dysfunction because of recurrent laryngeal nerve injury, infection, and hematoma are rare complications.

When any thyrotoxic patient requires control of β-adrenergic symptoms, I tend to use either once daily long-acting propranolol (Inderal LA)[1] 80 mg per day, or atenolol (Tenormin),[1] 50 mg per day. Occasionally, propranolol (Inderal) [1] 20 mg twice a day may be used. β-blockers[1] provide faster relief than ATDs and are particularly useful in the preoperative period. The goal is to maintain a pulse rate below 100 beats per minute (bpm). β-Blockers[1] do not directly affect thyroid gland secretion. Stable iodine (see Box 3) decreases the release of glandular hormones and is effective for approximately 7 to 14 days. Lugol's solution (8 mg iodide per drop) given as 5 drops three times per day or saturated solution of potassium iodide (SSKI, 40 mg iodide per drop) given as 1 to 2 drops three times per day can be beneficial as adjunctive therapy in the preparation of patients for surgery (in combination with β-blockers and ATD). In atypical additional circumstances Lugol's solution or SSKI can be used as adjunctive therapy to lower thyroid hormone levels in patients who require rapid restoration of thyroid hormone levels to normal. However, stable iodine should be given cautiously because iodine-containing preparations may actually exacerbate hyperthyroidism when given to unblocked patients, especially when used for more than 10 to 14 days. Stable iodine preparations abrogate the ability of the thyroid gland to concentrate 131-I probably for at least several weeks or longer.

SPECIAL SITUATIONS

Toxic Multinodular Goiter (Plummer's Disease)

131-I therapy or thyroidectomy represent effective treatment choices for patients with a toxic multinodular goiter. If the RAIU is sufficiently elevated, a relatively high dose (30 mCi) of 131-I can be administered with follow-up measurements of TSH, FT_4 and TT_3 levels. 131-I can also be considered in patients who are poor surgical candidates, assuming the RAIU is sufficiently elevated. 131-I therapy is associated with approximately a 20% chance of recurrence, in which case patients can receive a second dose of 131-I or opt for thyroidectomy.

Toxic Adenoma

For young patients and patients with a small (less than 4 cm) toxic nodule, either radioactive iodine therapy or surgery can be used. A single dose of 20 to 30 mCi 131-I results in resolution of the hyperthyroidism with hypothyroidism occurring in approximately 28% of patients at 5 years of age and in approximately 60% at 20 years of age. The thyroid nodule may decrease its function but remain as a structural entity in approximately 50% of cases. Patients with larger nodules are generally recommended to have surgery. Although there is a scant likelihood of malignancy, I typically recommend a fine-needle aspiration.

Subacute Thyroiditis

For patients with subacute thyroiditis, treatment is supportive with β-blockers and analgesics. Patients with moderate to severe pain, usually who also have an elevated white blood count and sedimentation rate, prednisone therapy (40 mg per day for 7 to 10 days with tapering over 1 to 2 weeks) may provide immediate relief of the neck pain but is not believed to affect the natural evolution of the thyroid hormones.

Amiodarone (Cordarone)[1]

Amiodarone (Cordarone)[1]-associated hyperthyroidism may be related to iodine excess (type 1) or to a toxic effect of the molecule on the thyroid gland, resulting in thyroiditis (type 2). Type 1 disease is treated with ATD and rarely with potassium perchlorate,[1] which inhibits the ability of the thyroid gland to trap iodine, but this medication may be associated with agranulocytosis in rare circumstances. When use of potassium perchlorate[1] is necessary, it should be only for a short time. Type 2 disease can be treated with prednisone (40 mg per day for 7 to 10 days with tapering over 1 to 2 weeks). In patients with mild to moderate amiodarone (Cordarone)[1]-associated hyperthyroidism, I use β-blockers[1] and ATD. If this does not control the disease or if the original presentation is severe, the additional use of prednisone and/or perchlorate may be indicated. Most patients do not have a pure presentation of either type 1 or type 2 disease. Because 131-I therapy can not be used because of the iodine contained in amiodarone (Cordarone),[1] thyroidectomy must be considered in some patients when the medical modalities fail. Thyroidectomy in these patients is inherently fraught with difficulty: The patients may not be euthyroid and they obviously have underlying cardiac disease. The adverse thyroid effects can persist or become manifest as long as 6 to 12 months after amiodarone (Cordarone)[1] is discontinued. Amiodarone (Cordarone)[1] associated thyrotoxicosis may be very complex, and it is preferable an experienced team treats these patients.

---

[1]Not FDA approved for this indication.

[1]Not FDA approved for this indication.

Subclinical Hyperthyroidism

Subclinical hyperthyroidism is defined as subnormal TSH in the context of normal T_4 and T_3. Subclinical hyperthyroidism represents part a continuum of disease, and in general the signs and symptoms are less pronounced than in patients with overt hyperthyroidism (elevated T_4 and T_3 with decreased TSH). Patients with subclinical hyperthyroidism are at increased risk for atrial fibrillation and enhanced bone loss, especially if they are older than 60 years of age. Thyroid function tests should be repeated several times over several weeks or months to ensure the persistence of disease. The intervals of assessing repeat thyroid function tests depend on the severity of clinical disease. Because patients may even be asymptomatic, they are less willing, perhaps appropriately, to accept definitive therapy such as 131-I therapy or surgery. I prefer to offer this group of patients ATD for 6 to 12 months in an effort to induce a remission. In contrast to overt symptomatic Graves' disease, patients with subclinical hyperthyroidism may have a higher chance of persistent remission following discontinuation of ATD. Nonetheless, the pathophysiology of the subclinical hyperthyroidism is not well studied, and the likelihood of inducing a remission is also unclear. TSH values that apply to this patient group are less than 0.1 mU/L and most frequently less than 0.01 mU/L. Patients who have a TSH of 0.1 to 0.45 mU/mL may not require therapy and could be monitored, although this is a case-by-case decision.

Pregnancy

Thyrotoxicosis during pregnancy is almost always caused by Graves' disease and tends to improve as the pregnancy proceeds. PTU is the ATD of choice with the goal of keeping serum FT_4 levels in the upper part of the normal range. FT_3 is preferable to follow as compared with total T_3. FT_3 levels should be maintained in the middle portion of the normal range. TSH receptor antibodies should be measured in the second or

CURRENT DIAGNOSIS

- Use the history and physical examination, in conjunction with the thyroid function tests, to assess the degree and severity of hyperthyroidism.
- Graves' disease may be associated with extrathyroidal manifestations.
- Assessment of RAIU (low versus high) may help determine the etiology.
- TSH should be undetectable for patients with hyperthyroidism.
- Be alert for unusual or unexpected complications or special circumstances, such as thyroid nodules that may harbor malignancy, adverse effects of medications, worsening disease, or pregnancy.
- Discuss therapeutic options with the patient.

Abbreviations: RAIU = radioactive iodine uptake; TSH = thyroid-stimulating hormone.

CURRENT THERAPY

- All patients should have thorough history and physical examinations as well as complete laboratory evaluations.
- Assess clinical status; more severely ill patients should be monitored closely and treated more aggressively.
- Close monitoring with frequent analysis of clinical status and laboratory studies are important.
- In most circumstances restore moderate or severely hyperthyroid patients to the euthyroid state prior to giving definitive therapy.

third trimester because this helps predict the development of neonatal hyperthyroidism. Close cooperation is required with the obstetrician. Maternal thyroid function tests should be monitored frequently, and it may be helpful for the obstetrician to monitor fetal thyroid gland size. Mothers may experience an exacerbation of thyrotoxicosis after delivery. All infants of mothers with Graves' disease should have thyroid function tests within the first few days of life and should be seen by a neonatologist.

A separate cause of hyperthyroidism in pregnancy is because of hCG elevations. During the first trimester, in some women hCG elevations bind to the thyroidal TSH receptor and induce thyroid gland secretion with an elevation of T_4/T_3 and resultant TSH inhibition. This cause of hyperthyroidism is usually mild and may be associated with hCG-induced hyperemesis. This type of hCG-induced hyperthyroidism is usually temporary and does not typically require treatment, except in extremely unusual circumstances. In contrast to Graves' disease patients, patients with hCG-induced elevations of thyroid secretion do not have a significantly enlarged thyroid gland, TSH receptor antibodies are negative, there is no ophthalmopathy, and in general the degree of elevations of FT_4 and T_3 is minimal.

REFERENCES

Burman KD, Cooper DS: The diagnostic evaluation and management of hyperthyroidism due to Graves' disease, toxic nodules and toxic multinodular goiter. In Cooper DS (ed): Medical Management of Thyroid Disease. New York, Marcel Dekker, 2001, pp 33-92.

Burman KD, Wartofsky L: Iodine effects on the thyroid gland: Biochemical and clinical aspects. Rev Endocr Metab Disord 2000;1:19-25.

Burman KD: Graves' disease in women: Proper therapy depends on an accurate diagnosis. Women's Health in Primary Care. 2001; 4:306-308

Ceccarelli C, Bencivelli W, Vitti P, et al: Outcome of radioiodine-131 therapy in hyperfunctioning thyroid nodules: A 20 years' retrospective study. Clin Endocrinol (Oxf) 2005;62:331.

Cooper DS: Antithyroid drugs in the management of patients with Graves' disease: An evidence-based approach to therapeutic controversies. J Clin Endocrinol Metab 2003;88:3474.

Cooper DS: Antithyroid Drugs. N Engl J Med 2005;352:905.

Kazlauskaite R, Weintraub BD, Burman KD: Evaluation of thyroid function tests. In Humes HD (ed): Kelley's Textbook of Internal

Medicine, Fourth Edition. New York, Lippincott Williams and Wilkins, 2000, pp 2821-2829.

Martino E, Bartalena L, Bogazzi F, Braverman LE: Amiodarone and the thyroid. Endocr Rev 2001;22:240.

Reinwein D, Benker G, Lazarus JH, Alexander WD: A prospective randomized trial of antithyroid drug dose in Graves' disease therapy: European multicenter study group on antithyroid drug treatment. J Clin Endocrinol Metab 1993;76:1516.

Surks MI, Ortiz E, Daniels GH, et al: Subclinical thyroid disease: Scientific review and guidelines for diagnosis and management. JAMA 2004;291:228.

Torring O, Tallstedt L, Wallin G, et al: Graves' hyperthyroidism: Treatment with antithyroid drugs, surgery, or radioiodine. A prospective, randomized study. Thyroid study group. J Clin Endocrinol Metab 1996;81:2986.

Weetman AP: Graves' disease. N Engl J Med 2000;343:1236.

Thyroid Cancer

Method of
Christopher R. McHenry, MD

Thyroid cancer accounts for 1.5% of all cancers in the United States, excluding skin cancer. The incidence of thyroid cancer is steadily increasing. In 2003, the American Cancer Society estimated 22,000 new cases of thyroid cancer and 1400 deaths per year from it. Thyroid cancer is the most common endocrine malignancy, accounting for more than 95% of all cancers affecting the endocrine organs. The true incidence of thyroid cancer may actually be higher than the actual clinical incidence. Population-based autopsy studies find occult papillary microcarcinomas in 2% to 13% of thyroid glands examined. Seventy-four percent of the cases of thyroid cancer occur in women.

Histologic Classification

Most thyroid cancers are of follicular cell origin and well differentiated. The median age at the time of diagnosis of differentiated thyroid cancer is 40 to 50 years. Papillary thyroid cancer is the most common, accounting for 75% to 80% of all thyroid malignancies. It includes multiple variants: pure papillary, follicular, tall-cell, columnar-cell, oxyphilic, diffuse-sclerosing, encapsulated, and occult microcarcinomas. The tall-cell variant is notable for a higher incidence of extrathyroidal tumor spread, distant metastases, and mortality as well as a loss of radioiodine uptake. Papillary carcinoma is characterized by multicentric disease in 25% to 50%, cervical lymph node metastases in 30% to 50%, and systemic metastases in 2% of patients at the time of presentation. It accounts for 90% of radiation-induced thyroid cancer and is familial in 3% of patients. The 20-year survival rate for patients with treated papillary carcinoma is greater than 90%.

Rakel and Bope: *Conn's Current Therapy 2006*.

Follicular thyroid cancer accounts for 10% to 15% of all thyroid malignancies. It is typically solitary, often occurring in association with benign thyroid disease, and more common in areas of iodine deficiency. It is known for its propensity to spread hematogenously, most often to the lungs and bone. Lymph node metastases are present in only 10% of patients. Invasive follicular carcinoma is defined by the presence of major capsular invasion and angioinvasion. This is in distinction to minimally invasive follicular cancer, which is almost indistinguishable from a benign follicular adenoma except for the presence of minor capsular invasion. Patients with minimally invasive follicular carcinoma have a very indolent course with a near-normal life expectancy. The 10-year survival rate for treated invasive follicular carcinoma is approximately 86%.

Hürthle cell carcinoma is characterized by the presence of encapsulated collections of Hürthle cells. Hürthle cells are identified on the basis of their granular eosinophilic cytoplasm, which corresponds to abundant mitochondria. Hürthle cell carcinomas, which account for approximately 2.5% of all thyroid cancers, have a greater tendency to spread to cervical lymph nodes than follicular carcinomas and a higher incidence of distant metastases. Less than 10% of Hürthle cell cancers concentrate radioiodine, compared with 80% to 90% of patients with papillary or follicular carcinoma. Hürthle cell carcinoma has a higher recurrence rate and a higher 10-year morality rate (21%) than papillary or follicular carcinoma.

Anaplastic thyroid cancer accounts for approximately 2% of all thyroid malignancies. It typically occurs in patients older than 60 years of age who have a history of a long-standing goiter that suddenly increases in size. Anaplastic transformation may occur in patients with a preexisting differentiated carcinoma. It is an extremely aggressive cancer with an overall 5-year survival rate of approximately 3% and a median survival time of only 4 to 6 months. Systemic metastases occur in approximately 75% of patients, but the cause of death is usually from airway obstruction secondary to extensive local disease.

Medullary thyroid cancer arises from the parafollicular, or so-called C cells, of the thyroid gland. It accounts for 5% of all thyroid cancers and is usually more aggressive than differentiated thyroid cancer. Medullary thyroid carcinoma does not concentrate radioiodine. Approximately 20% to 30% of medullary carcinomas are familial, occurring as a separate entity or as part of the multiple endocrine neoplasia (MEN) type 2 syndromes (Table 1). MEN-type syndromes occur as a result of a germ line mutation in the RET proto-oncogene, which encodes for a tyrosine kinase receptor. All familial medullary carcinomas are autosomal-dominant disorders and typically characterized by multifocal and bilateral disease and associated C-cell hyperplasia. Some 25% to 63% of patients with medullary carcinoma have lymph node metastases that most commonly involve the central compartment of the neck. Lymphatic spread also occurs to the lateral neck and mediastinum. Familial and sporadic medullary thyroid carcinomas are multicentric in 90% and 20% of cases, respectively.

TABLE 1   Familial Medullary Thyroid Carcinoma

Familial Non–Multiple Endocrine Neoplasia (MEN) Medullary Thyroid Carcinoma
Multiple Endocrine Neoplasia Type 2A
Medullary thyroid carcinoma
Hyperparathyroidism
Pheochromocytoma
Lichen planus amyloidosis
Hirschsprung's disease
Multiple Endocrine Neoplasia Type 2B
Medullary thyroid carcinoma
Pheochromocytoma
Marfanoid body habitus
Mucosal neuromas
Ganglioneuromatosis of the gastrointestinal tract

Thyroid lymphoma is rare, accounting for less than 1% of all thyroid malignancies. It is usually a non-Hodgkin's lymphoma, B-cell type. Diffuse large cell lymphoma accounts for more than 50% of all lymphomas. Most lymphomas of the thyroid gland are of intermediate or high grade and arise from mucosa-associated lymphoid tissue lymphoma. They are more common in women and usually occur during the seventh decade of life. Patients with Hashimoto's thyroiditis are known to have a 70 to 80 times higher risk for developing thyroid lymphoma compared with the normal population. Patients usually present with a rapidly enlarging goiter that causes compressive symptoms.

Clinical Presentation

Most patients with thyroid carcinoma present with a palpable thyroid nodule. Less often, they present with an abnormal cervical lymph node, a rapidly enlarging goiter with dysphagia, dyspnea, or hoarseness, an incidentally discovered thyroid nodule on an imaging study of the neck, or as a result of genetic testing in a family with MEN-2. A family history of thyroid cancer may also be present in patients with familial non-medullary thyroid cancer, which accounts for 5% of all thyroid cancers. In a patient with a thyroid nodule, associated clinical features suggestive of carcinoma include a prior history of low-dose head or neck irradiation as a child or adolescent, the presence of a firm, fixed nodule, a nodule present in association with cervical lymphadenopathy, and vocal cord paralysis as documented by laryngoscopy. A patient with a dominant thyroid nodule and a prior history of head or neck irradiation has an approximate 40% incidence of carcinoma.

Thyroid nodules are common, occurring in 4% to 7% of the population, but only an approximate 5% of thyroid nodules are malignant. The evaluation of a patient with a thyroid nodule consists of a routine fine-needle aspiration biopsy (FNAB) and a routine serum thyrotropin-stimulating hormone (TSH) level. FNAB is the mainstay in the diagnosis of thyroid cancer. It has a false-positive rate of 1% to 2% and a false-negative rate of 2% to 5%. Cytologic analysis of FNAB specimens

can be classified into one of five categories: malignant (5%), suspicious for papillary cancer (5%), consistent with follicular or Hürthle cell neoplasm (20%), benign (60%), or nondiagnostic (10%). In patients with a FNAB that is malignant, suspicious for papillary cancer, consistent with a Hürthle cell neoplasm, or consistent with a follicular neoplasm or persistently nondiagnostic when the serum TSH level is normal or high, surgical therapy is recommended without any additional testing. In patients with a FNAB that is consistent with a follicular neoplasm or persistently nondiagnostic and a low serum TSH level, an iodine-123 thyroid scan is obtained to distinguish a hyperfunctioning nodule, which is malignant in less than 1% of cases, from a hypofunctioning nodule, which is malignant in 10% to 30% of cases. As a result, patients with a hyperfunctioning nodule and a FNAB that is consistent with a follicular neoplasm or persistently nondiagnostic may be observed or offered nonsurgical or surgical therapeutic options, whereas thyroidectomy is recommended for patients with a hypofunctioning nodule. Finally, patients with a benign FNAB are followed clinically.

Ultrasound may be of value in guiding FNAB for nonpalpable nodules or when repeated palpation-guided FNAB is persistently nondiagnostic. It may also be of value in patients with a FNAB that is malignant or suspicious for papillary cancer to evaluate for associated cervical lymph node disease prior to operation because physical examination is often inadequate to detect cervical lymph node metastases. When cytologic analysis of a FNAB specimen suggests medullary thyroid cancer, immunohistochemical stains for carcinoembryonic antigen (CEA) and calcitonin should be performed to arrive at a definitive diagnosis. A serum calcitonin and CEA level should also be obtained. In addition, a 24-hour urine test for vanilmandelic acid, metanephrine, and normetanephrine and a serum calcium level should be obtained to screen for pheochromocytoma and hyperparathyroidism, respectively. Pheochromocytoma occurs in 50% of patients with MEN-2A and MEN-2B, and hyperparathyroidism occurs in 10% to 20% of patients with MEN-2A.

Familial medullary thyroid cancer may be diagnosed prior to becoming clinically evident by: recognition of a marfanoid habitus or mucosal neuromas suggestive of MEN-2B, genetic testing for the RET proto-oncogene in a patient with family members known to be affected by MEN-2, or after diagnosis of other endocrinopathies associated with the MEN-2 syndromes (see Table 1).

Treatment

Certain prognostic factors are associated with a higher recurrence rate and mortality. Factors that predict a worse prognosis in patients with differentiated thyroid carcinoma include age greater than 40 years in a man, age greater than 50 years in a woman, tumor size greater than 4 cm, a high-grade tumor, the presence of extrathyroidal tumor spread, lymph node metastases in an adult patient, systemic metastases, and an incomplete resection. Intraoperatively, patients may be divided

TABLE 2 Low- and High-Risk Groups for Recurrence and Mortality From Papillary and Follicular Thyroid Cancers

Low Risk
Women <50 y
Men <40 y
Well or moderately well-differentiated tumors
Tumors <4 cm in diameter
Tumor confined to the thyroid gland
No distant metastases

High Risk
Women ≥50 y
Men =40 y
Poorly differentiated tumors, tall-cell, columnar-cell,
    or oxyphilic variants of papillary carcinoma
Tumor >4 cm
Local invasion
Distant metastases

into low-risk or high-risk groups based on the presence or absence of various risk factors (Table 2). The recurrence rate and mortality from differentiated thyroid carcinoma in low-risk patients are 5% to 11% and 0.7% to 5%, respectively, compared with 48% and 48%, respectively, in high-risk patients. Risk group definition may be used to determine the extent of thyroidectomy for patients with differentiated thyroid cancer.

Age is the most important prognostic factor for predicting mortality from differentiated thyroid cancer. In patients younger than 45 years of age, the mortality rate from differentiated thyroid cancer is 1% to 2%. In a review of more than 1500 patients with papillary thyroid carcinoma treated at the Mayo Clinic, the mortality rates was less than 1% in patients less than 50 years of age, 7% for patients 50 to 59 years of age, 20% for patients 60 to 69 years of age, and 46% for patients older than 70 years of age. The presence of extrathyroidal tumor spread is the most important prognostic factor for predicting local recurrence. Completeness of resection is also an important prognostic factor for local recurrence and long-term cancer control. Patients with differentiated thyroid cancer and distant metastases have 10-year survival rates of 25% to 40%.

No randomized prospective studies have evaluated the appropriate extent of thyroidectomy, the necessity of radioiodine, or the management of cervical lymph nodes metastases in patients with differentiated thyroid cancer. Most experts agree that a thyroid lobectomy and isthmusectomy is appropriate therapy for a papillary microcarcinoma (smaller than 1 cm) and minimally invasive follicular cancer. Most experts also agree that a total thyroidectomy is the appropriate treatment for patients with high-risk differentiated thyroid cancer. But the treatment of patients with low-risk differentiated thyroid cancer is quite controversial. It is appropriate to treat these patients with a thyroid lobectomy and isthmusectomy. In experienced hands, however, it may be preferable to treat these patients with a total thyroidectomy, which is associated with the lowest incidence of local recurrence. It also allows for the most

effective use of radioactive iodine postoperatively for detection and treatment of metastatic disease. Furthermore, serum thyroglobulin is most effectively used as a marker to detect recurrent cancer following total thyroidectomy. Finally, total thyroidectomy is important in eliminating multicentric disease as well as a 1% risk of anaplastic dedifferentiation.

Enlarged lymph nodes in the central compartment of the neck are removed and submitted for frozen section examination. For documented metastases in the paratracheal lymph nodes, a complete central neck dissection should be performed, removing all lymphatic and fibrofatty tissue between the right and left common carotid arteries from the level of the hyoid bone superiorly to the sternal notch inferiorly. Patients with metastases in the lateral neck nodes that are palpable or identified by ultrasonography are treated with a modified (functional) neck dissection. This involves removal of all lymph nodes and fibrofatty tissue anterior and posterior to the internal jugular vein from the mastoid process to the clavicle and lateral to the spinoaccessory nerve. The internal jugular vein, sternocleidomastoid muscle, and the spinoaccessory nerve are all preserved. A modified neck dissection is preferable to the so-called berry-picking procedure because of a lower incidence of recurrent nodal metastases.

All patients with medullary thyroid cancer are treated with total thyroidectomy and a routine central neck dissection. Up to 80% of patients have lymph node metastases in the central compartment of the neck. Routine central neck dissection is demonstrated to reduce recurrence and improve survival rates when compared when the removal of lymph nodes only when they are grossly enlarged. An ipsilateral modified neck dissection is performed in all patients with: tumors greater than 2 cm, palpable or microscopic metastases in the central compartment of the neck, or palpable adenopathy in the lateral neck. Some authorities advocate routine bilateral modified neck dissection in all patients with tumors greater than 2 cm. Ipsilateral nodal involvement is reported in up to 80% and contralateral nodal involvement in up to 40% of patients with palpable intrathyroidal primaries. Prior to the surgical treatment of medullary thyroid cancer, all patients should undergo appropriate screening to exclude the possibility of a coexisting pheochromocytoma, which should be treated prior to thyroidectomy.

For patients with anaplastic carcinoma or lymphoma, the role of surgical intervention is primarily to establish a diagnosis. Most patients present with locally advanced disease, which precludes resection for cure. A tracheostomy may be necessary for patients with impending airway obstruction. Anaplastic thyroid cancer does not produce thyroglobulin; nor does it concentrate radioiodine. Most patients with anaplastic thyroid cancer are treated with hyperfractionated radiation in combination with adriamycin with or without cisplatin, which are used as radiosensitizers. Rarely, patients may present early with disease limited to the thyroid gland, and surgical resection for cure is possible. It is one of the most aggressive of all cancers. Most patients die rapidly from tumor invasion into the

Rakel and Bope: *Conn's Current Therapy 2006*.

aerodigestive tract and less commonly from metastatic disease.

Although a diagnosis of lymphoma can be made by FNAB, an open surgical biopsy is often required for specific immunohistochemical studies and definitive classification of a lymphoma. This has important implications in the choice of chemotherapeutic agents used. Once a diagnosis of lymphoma is established, staging is completed to delineate the extent of disease. Most patients are treated with chemotherapy in combination with radiation therapy. The overall 5-year survival rate in patients with lymphoma ranges from 50% to 70%.

Postoperative Management and Follow-Up

The postoperative management of patients with differentiated thyroid cancer consists of: administration of thyroid hormone; iodine-131 whole-body scanning for residual normal thyroid tissue and/or metastatic disease; the use of iodine-131 for ablation of residual normal thyroid tissue and/or treatment of metastatic disease; and follow-up physical examination, serum thyroglobulin levels, and iodine-131 whole-body scans for detection of recurrent disease. The use of recombinant human thyrotropin-stimulating hormone (rhTSH) for diagnostic purposes in patients with thyroid cancer in lieu of thyroid hormone withdrawal is a recent development that avoids hypothyroidism prior to iodine-131 whole-body scans and thyroglobulin monitoring.

TSH promotes the growth of differentiated thyroid cancer cells. As a result, patients with differentiated thyroid cancer are treated with thyroid hormone in dosages that suppress TSH levels. This reduces the recurrence rate and improves survival. L-Thyroxine is started at a dose of 2 µg per kg, and a serum TSH level is measured 6 weeks following initiation of therapy. In patients without evidence of metastatic disease, the TSH level is maintained just below the lower limit of the normal range, between 0.1 and 0.4 µIU/mL. In patients with metastatic disease, dosages of L-thyroxine are increased to maintain serum TSH levels less than 0.1 µIU/mL.

Postoperative iodine-131 whole-body scanning is recommended for all patients with a papillary thyroid cancer greater than 1 cm, a papillary carcinoma of any size with lymph node metastases, invasive follicular carcinoma, and Hürthle cell carcinoma. Patients with residual iodine uptake in the thyroid bed are treated with radioiodine ablation using a 30-mCi dose of iodine-131 as an outpatient. Total ablation of residual thyroid tissue is achieved in 80% of patients following a 30-mCi dose of iodine-131. If a 30-mCi dose is unsuccessful in ablating all of the residual thyroid tissue, a second 30-mCi dose may be given 6 to 12 months later. It is well recognized that only approximately 10% of Hürthle cell carcinomas concentrate radioiodine, but most produce thyroglobulin. As a result, radioiodine ablation of residual normal thyroid tissue is important for effective monitoring of serum thyroglobulin levels for early detection of recurrence.

Differentiated thyroid cancer recurs in 20% to 40% of patients. The incidence of recurrence is greatest within the first 2 years of surgery. But it is not unusual for recurrence to occur 25 to 30 years after surgery, emphasizing the importance of lifelong monitoring. Patients with differentiated thyroid carcinoma are followed at 3- to 6-month intervals with physical examination and a serum thyroglobulin, an antithyroglobulin antibody titer, and TSH levels for the first 2 years and then yearly thereafter. In order for iodine-131 whole-body scanning and serum thyroglobulin monitoring to be useful for detection of metastatic disease, all normal thyroid tissue must be gone. This may be accomplished by a total or near-total thyroidectomy and iodine-131 ablation.

For optimal sensitivity of radioiodine whole-body scanning and thyroglobulin measurement, the serum TSH level should be more than 30 µIU/mL to stimulate the residual normal or metastatic thyroid tissue to take up the iodine. Because of the residual circulating thyroid hormone secreted prior to the removal of the thyroid gland, the necessary TSH elevation usually does not occur for at least 4 to 6 weeks after surgery. To minimize the symptoms of hypothyroidism, patients are started on triiodothyronine (T_3) 25 µg twice a day, immediately after surgery. T_3 has a half-life of 24 hours compared to 7 days for L-thyroxine. The shorter half-life of T_3 is advantageous because it reduces the time the patient is hypothyroid prior to iodine-131 whole-body scanning. Two weeks prior to radioiodine scanning, patients are placed on a low-iodine diet and T_3 is discontinued. A serum thyroglobulin level and diagnostic whole-body scan are obtained when the serum TSH level is confirmed to be more than 30 µIU/mL.

Metastatic disease, usually involving the lung or bone, occurs in 10% to 15% of patients with differentiated thyroid cancer. Patients diagnosed with metastatic disease are admitted to the hospital, treated with doses of iodine-131 varying from 150 to 200 mCi, and kept in isolation for 3 days. A follow-up whole-body scan is routinely performed 7 to 10 days after an ablative or therapeutic dose of iodine-131 to evaluate for previously undetected metastases. Approximately 35% to 60% of all metastatic lesions concentrate iodine-131.

In the absence of normal thyroid tissue, serum thyroglobulin is a sensitive and specific marker for thyroid cancer. A serum thyroglobulin level less than 3 mg/dL while on thyroid hormone rules out carcinoma with an approximate 94% sensitivity. However, it has been well documented that a patient with metastatic disease may have an undetectable serum thyroglobulin level while on thyroid hormone, emphasizing the importance of periodic measurement of TSH-stimulated thyroglobulin levels. A serum thyroglobulin level more than 10 mg/dL after withdrawal of thyroid hormone warrants repeating an iodine-131 whole-body scan. RhTSH may be used as an alternative to thyroid hormone withdrawal to stimulate iodine-131 uptake and thyroglobulin release in euthyroid patients, avoiding hypothyroidism. Multiple studies have verified its safety and efficacy in administration prior to radioactive iodine scanning and for measurement of TSH-stimulated thyroglobulin levels. Recently, data suggest that in patients with a TSH-stimulated thyroglobulin level of less than 10 mg/dL (either by withdrawal of thyroid hormone or with the use rhTSH), an iodine-131 whole-body scan is unnecessary.

Patients with medullary thyroid cancer are followed postoperatively with serum calcitonin and CEA levels every 3 to 6 months for the first 2 years and then yearly thereafter. A routine physical examination of the neck is performed and patients are evaluated for local recurrence or regional recurrence in the cervical or supraclavicular lymph nodes. Cervical lymph node recurrence is reported to occur in approximately 45% of patients. Systemic metastases, most commonly involving the liver, lungs, and bone, may be very indolent with little change over several years. Patients with MEN-2 undergo yearly testing for a pheochromocytoma consisting of a 24-hour urine collection for vanillylmandelic acid, metanephrine, and normetanephrine. In addition, patients with MEN-2 also undergo a yearly serum calcium level to screen for the development of primary hyperparathyroidism.

Medullary thyroid cancer, because it arises from the parafollicular cells or C cells of the thyroid gland, does not take up radioiodine. As a result, there is no role for iodine-131 whole-body scanning, ablation, or treatment of metastases. Medullary thyroid cancer also does not produce thyroglobulin, nor does TSH affect its growth. As a result, measurement of serum thyroglobulin is not indicated; nor is the use of TSH-suppressive doses of thyroid hormone. Patients are started on a normal replacement dose of L-thyroxine, 1.6 µg/kg, postoperatively. Some experts propose that serum testing for the RET proto-oncogene mutations associated with the MEN-2 syndromes be obtained postoperatively in all patients diagnosed with medullary thyroid cancer. The rationale for this is that up to 30% of patients believed to have sporadic medullary thyroid cancer turn out to have new germ line mutations and are index cases for a new kindred of familial cancer. If a patient has an identified RET mutation, all family members should also be tested for the mutation. The overall 5-year survival rate for all patients with medullary thyroid cancer, including sporadic and familial forms, is 78% to 92%, and the 10-year survival rate is between 61% and 75%. Five-year survival rates based on the stage of disease are 100% for stage I, 90% for stage II, 86% for stage III, and 56% for stage IV.

The most important predictor of outcome in patients with medullary carcinoma is the stage of the disease at presentation (Table 3). In addition to increasing tumor size, lymph node metastases and systemic metastases, increasing age is also a negative prognostic factor. Older patients have a higher incidence of lymph node metastases. Male gender, nondiploid DNA tumor ploidy, and decreased calcitonin immunoreactivity are also cited as factors associated with a worse outcome in patients with medullary thyroid cancer. Among the subtypes of medullary thyroid cancer, familial non-MEN medullary thyroid cancer has the best prognosis, MEN-2B has the worst prognosis, and sporadic and MEN-2A medullary thyroid cancer have similar prognoses that are intermediate between the other two subtypes.

CURRENT DIAGNOSIS

- History
    Radiation exposure
    Family history of thyroid cancer
- Examination
    Firm, fixed nodule
    Lymphadenopathy
    Vocal cord paralysis
- Laboratories
    Serum TSH
    MTC: serum calcitonin, CEA
    24-hour urine for VMA, metanephrines
    Genetic testing
- Fine-needle aspiration biopsy (FNAB)
    Immunohistochemical staining for calcitonin
        and CEA (MTC)
    Flow cytometry (lymphoma)
- Imaging
    Selective iodine-123 thyroid scintigraphy
    Ultrasound to guide FNAB and evaluate for
        lymph node metastases

Abbreviations: CEA = carcinoembryonic antigen; FNAB=fine-needle aspiration biopsy; MTC=medullary thyroid cancer; TSH=thyroid-stimulating hormone; VMA=vanillylmandelic acid.

Rakel and Bope: *Conn's Current Therapy 2006.*

TABLE 3 Staging of Thyroid Cancer

Definitions

Primary tumor (T)
T_0 = no evidence of primary tumor
T_1 = tumor ≤1 cm
T_2 = tumor >1 cm but ≤ 4 cm
T_3 = tumor >4 cm
T_4 = tumor extending beyond the thyroid capsule

Nodal diseases (N)
N_0 = no regional lymph node metastases
N_1 = regional lymph node metastases

Systemic metastases (M)
M_0 = no distant metastases
M_1 = distant metastases

American Joint Committee on Cancer Stage Grouping

	Age <45 y	Age ≥45 y
Papillary, Follicular, and Hürthle Cell Cancers		
Stage I	Any T, any N, M_0	$T_1N_0M_0$
Stage II	Any T, any N, M_1	T_2 or $T_3N_0M_0$
Stage III		T_4 or N_1M_0
Stage IV		Any T, any N, M_1
Medullary Thyroid Cancer		
Stage I	$T_1N_0M_0$	
Stage II	T_2,T_3,T_4,N_0,M_0	
Stage III	Any T, N_1,M_0	
Stage IV	Any T, any N,M_1	
Anaplastic Thyroid Cancer (all cases are classified as stage IV)		
Stage IV	Any T, any N, any M	

CURRENT THERAPY

Differentiated Thyroid Cancer
- Low risk: lobectomy or total thyroidectomy (preferable)
- High risk: total thyroidectomy
- Enlarged lymph nodes removed and FSE
- Central lymph node metastases: CND
- Lateral lymph node metastases: MND
- Postoperative:
    I-131 ablation
    TSH-suppressive doses of thyroid hormone
    Thyroglobulin monitoring with rhTSH stimulation

Medullary Thyroid Cancer
- Total thyroidectomy and CND with or without ipsilateral/bilateral MND

Anaplastic Thyroid Cancer
- Chemotherapy and radiotherapy

Lymphoma
- Chemotherapy

Abbreviations: CND = central neck dissection; FSE = frozen section examination; MND = modified neck dissection; rhTSH = recombinant human thyrotropin-stimulating hormone; TSH = thyroid-stimulating hormone.

REFERENCES

AACE/AAES medical/surgical guidelines for clinical practice: Management of thyroid carcinoma. Endocr Pract 2001;7:203-220.

Chi DD, Moley JF: Medullary thyroid cancer: Genetic advances, treatment recommendations and the approach to the patient with persistent hypercalcitoninemia. Surg Clin North Am 1998;7(4):681-706.

Kebebew E, Clark OH: Differentiated thyroid cancer: "Complete" rational approach. World J Surg 2000;24:942-951.

Konovarakii MA, Shapiro SE, Forage BD, et al: Role of perioperative ultrasonography in surgical management of patients with thyroid cancer. Surgery 2003;134:946-955.

Mazzaferri EL, Jhiang SM: Long-term impact of initial surgical and medical therapy in papillary and follicular thyroid cancer. Am J Med 1994;97:418-428.

Mazzaferri EL, Robbins RJ, Spencer CA, et al: A consensus report of the role of serum thyroglobulin as a monitoring method for low-risk patients with papillary thyroid carcinoma. J Clin Endocrinol Metab 2003;88(4):1433-1441.

McHenry CR, Slusarczyk S, Ascari AT, et al: Refined use of scintigraphy in the evaluation of nodular thyroid disease. Surgery 1998;124:656-662.

Mittendorf EA, Tamarkin S, McHenry CR: The results of ultrasound-guided fine needle aspiration biopsy for evaluation of nodular thyroid disease. Surgery 2002;132:648-654.

Pheochromocytoma

Method of
William F. Young, Jr., MD

Pheochromocytoma is a tumor frequently sought and rarely found. It is associated with spectacular cardiovascular disturbances, and when correctly diagnosed and properly treated it is curable; when undiagnosed or improperly treated it can be fatal. Catecholamine-producing tumors that arise from chromaffin cells of the adrenal medulla and sympathetic ganglia are termed *pheochromocytomas* and *paragangliomas*, respectively. However, pheochromocytoma has become the generic name for all catecholamine-producing tumors and will be used in this article to refer to both adrenal pheochromocytomas and catecholamine-secreting paragangliomas.

Presentation

Prevalence estimates for pheochromocytoma vary from 0.01% to 0.1% of the hypertensive population with an incidence of 2 to 8 cases per million people per year. These tumors occur equally in men and women, primarily in the 3rd through 5th decades. Patients harboring these tumors may be asymptomatic; however, symptoms usually are present and are caused by the pharmacologic effects of excess circulating catecholamines. Episodic symptoms include abrupt onset of throbbing headaches, generalized diaphoresis, palpitations, anxiety, chest pain, and abdominal pain. These spells can be extremely varying in their presentation and may be spontaneous or precipitated by postural changes, anxiety, exercise, or maneuvers that increase intra-abdominal pressure. The pheochromocytoma spell may last 10 to 60 minutes and may occur daily to monthly. The clinical signs include hypertension (paroxysmal in 50% of the patients and sustained in the other 50%), orthostatic hypotension, pallor, grade I to IV retinopathy, tremor, and fever. Pheochromocytoma of the urinary bladder is associated with painless hematuria and paroxysmal attacks induced by micturition or bladder distension. Frequently patients are diagnosed with possible pheochromocytoma before they are symptomatic because of genetic screening for hereditary endocrine syndromes or incidental discovery of adrenal masses on computerized abdominal imaging. These patients may harbor catecholamine-synthesizing neoplasms that are detected months or years before the onset of periodic hypersecretory states. From 1978 to 1995 10% of the benign sporadic adrenal pheochromocytoma patients who were diagnosed at the Mayo Clinic presented as adrenal incidentalomas; this proportion of incidentally discovered pheochromocytomas is expected to increase as computerized imaging is increasingly used. In addition, in five separate reports and a total of 1488 patients with adrenal incidentalomas, the *clinically silent* adrenal pheochromocytomas comprised an average of 2.6% of patients studied.

Rakel and Bope: *Conn's Current Therapy 2006.*

Diagnosis

The diagnostic approach to catecholamine-producing tumors is divided into two series of studies (Figure 1). First, the diagnosis of a catecholamine-producing tumor must be suspected, and then confirmed biochemically by the presence of increased urine or plasma concentrations of catecholamines or their metabolites. Suppression testing with clonidine[1] or provocative testing with glucagon,[1] histamine,[1] or metoclopramide (Reglan)[1] is rarely needed. Box 1 summarizes the differential diagnoses of pheochromocytoma.

The next step is to localize the catecholamine-producing tumor to guide the surgical approach.

---

[1]Not FDA approved for this indication.

Computer-assisted adrenal and abdominal imaging (magnetic resonance imaging [MRI] or computed tomography [CT]) is the first localization test. Approximately 90% of these tumors are found in the adrenals, and 98% are in the abdomen. If the abdominal imaging is negative, then scintigraphic localization with ^{123}I-meta-iodobenzylguanidine (^{123}I-MIBG) is indicated. This radiopharmaceutical accumulates preferentially in catecholamine-producing tumors; however, this procedure is less sensitive as initially hoped (sensitivity 85%; specificity 99%). Computer-assisted chest, neck, and head imaging are additional localizing procedures that can be used, but are rarely required. Positron emission tomography (PET)-scanning with ^{18}F-fluorodeoxyglucose or ^{11}C-hydroxyephedrine or 6-[^{18}F]fluorodopamine may be helpful in identifying sites of metastatic disease.

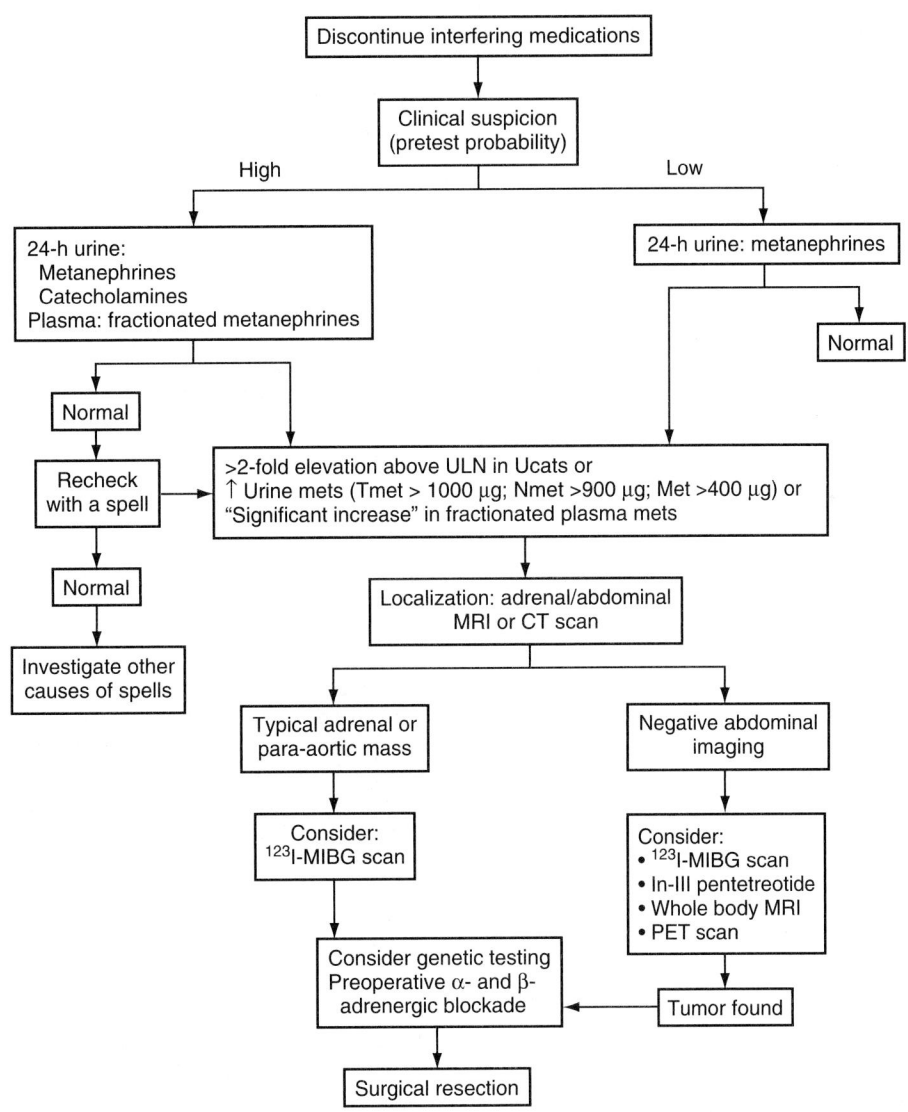

FIGURE 1. Evaluation and treatment of catecholamine-producing tumors. Clinical suspicion is triggered by the following: paroxysmal symptoms (especially hypertension); hypertension that is intermittent, unusually labile, or resistant to treatment; family history of pheochromocytoma or associated conditions; past history of pheochromocytoma; or incidentally discovered adrenal mass. The details are discussed in the text. cats = catecholamines; CT = computed tomography; mets = metanephrines; nmet = normetanephrine; MRI = magnetic resonance imaging; ^{123}I-MIBG = ^{123}I-meta-iodobenzylguanidine; ULN = upper limit of normal; U = urine. (Modified from Young WF Jr, Pheochromocytoma: 1926-1993, Trends in endocrinology and metabolism, vol 4. Elsevier Science Inc., 1993, p 122.)

Thorough discussions of the diagnostic investigation of catecholamine-producing tumors are found elsewhere.

Special Clinical Situations

HEREDITARY FORMS OF PHEOCHROMOCYTOMA AND PARAGANGLIOMA

Approximately 10% to 20% of patients with catecholamine-secreting tumors have associated germline mutations (inherited mutations present in all cells of the body) in genes known to cause genetic disease. Catecholamine-secreting paragangliomas may be associated with familial paraganglioma, neurofibromatosis type 1 (NF1), von Hippel-Lindau (VHL) disease, Carney's triad, and rarely multiple endocrine neoplasia type 2 (MEN 2). Adrenal pheochromocytoma may be associated with MEN 2, VHL disease, and NF1. Genetic testing is available for nearly all of these disorders; genetic counseling should be considered prior to performing genetic testing.

Treatment Principles

The treatment of choice for pheochromocytoma is surgical resection. Most of these tumors are benign and can be totally excised. However, prior to the operation, the chronic and acute effects of excess circulating catecholamines must be reversed.

PREOPERATIVE MANAGEMENT

Combined α- and β-adrenergic blockades are required preoperatively to control blood pressure (BP) and to prevent intraoperative hypertensive crises. α-Adrenergic blockade should be started at least 7 days preoperatively to allow for expansion of the contracted blood volume. A liberal salt diet is advised during the preoperative period. Once adequate α-adrenergic blockade is achieved, β-adrenergic blockade is initiated (e.g., 3 days preoperatively). With this approach, only 7% of patients undergoing pheochromocytoma resection at the Mayo Clinic have needed postoperative hemodynamic management.

α-Adrenergic Blockade

Phenoxybenzamine (Dibenzyline) is an irreversible, long-acting, α-adrenergic blocking agent (Table 1). Approximately 25% of an oral dose of phenoxybenzamine (Dibenzyline) is absorbed. Phenoxybenzamine (Dibenzyline) is available in 10-mg capsules. The initial dosage is 10 mg orally once or twice daily; the dosage is increased by 10 to 20 mg every 2 to 3 days as needed to control the BP and spells. The effects of daily administration are cumulative for nearly a week. The average dosage is 20 to 100 mg per day. Side effects include postural hypotension, tachycardia, miosis, nasal congestion, inhibition of ejaculation, diarrhea, and fatigue. Prazosin (Minipress),[1] terazosin (Hytrin),[1] and doxazosin (Cardura)[1] are selective α_1-adrenergic blocking agents; because of the more favorable side-effect profiles, these agents may be preferable to phenoxybenzamine (Dibenzyline) when long-term pharmacologic treatment is indicated (e.g., for metastatic pheochromocytoma). However, phenoxybenzamine (Dibenzyline) is the preferred drug for preoperative preparation because it provides α-adrenergic blockade of long duration. Effective α-adrenergic blockade permits expansion of blood volume, which usually is severely decreased as a result of excessive adrenergic vasoconstriction.

---

[1]Not FDA approved for this indication.

TABLE 1 Orally Administered Drugs Used to Treat Patients With Pheochromocytoma

Generic drug name (trade name)	Dosage (mg/d)* initial-maximum	Side effects
α-Adrenergic blocking agents		
Phenoxybenzamine (Dibenzyline)	20-100[†]	Postural hypotension, tachycardia, miosis, nasal congestion, diarrhea, inhibition of ejaculation, fatigue
Prazosin (Minipress)	1-20[‡]	First-dose effect, dizziness, drowsiness, headache, fatigue, palpitations, nausea
Terazosin (Hytrin)	1-20[†]	First-dose effect, asthenia, blurred vision, dizziness, nasal congestion, nausea, peripheral edema, palpitations, somnolence
Doxazosin (Cardura)	1-20	First-dose effect, orthostasis, peripheral edema, fatigue, somnolence
Combined α- and β-adrenergic blocking agent		
Labetalol (Normodyne, Trandate)	200-1200[†]	Dizziness, fatigue, nausea, nasal congestion, impotence
Catecholamine synthesis inhibitor		
α-Methyl-p-L-tyrosine (Demser)	1000-4000[‡]	Sedation, diarrhea, anxiety, nightmares, crystalluria, galactorrhea, extrapyramidal symptoms

*Given once daily unless otherwise indicated.
[†]Given as two doses daily.
[‡]Given in three or four doses daily.

9

β-Adrenergic Blockade

The β-adrenergic antagonist should be administered only after α-adrenergic blockade is effective because β-adrenergic blockade alone may result in more severe hypertension because of the unopposed α-adrenergic stimulation. Preoperative β-adrenergic blockade is indicated to control the tachycardia associated with both the high-circulating catecholamine concentrations and the α-adrenergic blockade. Caution is indicated if the patient is asthmatic or has congestive heart failure. Chronic catecholamine excess can produce a myocardiopathy, and β-adrenergic blockade can result in acute pulmonary edema. Noncardioselective β-adrenergic blockers such as propranolol (Inderal and Inderal LA) or cardioselective β-adrenergic blockers such as atenolol (Tenormin)[1] and metoprolol (Lopressor)[1] may be used. (Mechanisms of action, routes of metabolism, dosages and side effects are discussed elsewhere in this text.) When administration of the β-adrenergic blocker begins, the drug should be used cautiously and at a low dose. For example, propranolol (Inderal and Inderal LA) is usually initiated at 10 mg orally every 6 hours at least 1 week after the initiation of α-adrenergic blockade. The dose is then increased and converted to a long-acting preparation as necessary to control the tachycardia.

Labetalol (Normodyne, Trandate)[1] exhibits both selective α_1-adrenergic and nonselective β-adrenergic blocking activities in a ratio of approximately 1:3 (see Table 1). Some instances of paradoxical hypertensive responses in patients with pheochromocytoma treated with labetalol (Normodyne, Trandate)[1] have been reported, presumably because of incomplete α-adrenergic blockade. Therefore its safety as primary therapy is controversial. Its role in the therapy of pheochromocytoma may be in the chronic pharmacologic management of patients with metastatic disease.

Catecholamine Synthesis Inhibitor

α-Methyl-p-L-tyrosine (metyrosine; Demser) inhibits the synthesis of catecholamines by blocking the enzyme tyrosine hydroxylase. It is rapidly absorbed from the gastrointestinal (GI) tract, and most of it is excreted in the urine unchanged. Metyrosine is available in 250-mg capsules (see Table 1). The initial dosage is 250 mg orally four times daily. The dosage may be increased by 500 mg per day every day to a maximum of 4 g per day (1 g four times per day) as needed for BP control. Side effects include sedation, depression, diarrhea, anxiety, nightmares, crystalluria and urolithiasis, galactorrhea, and extrapyramidal manifestations. Therefore, this agent should be used with caution and only when other agents have been ineffective or are contraindicated. The extrapyramidal effects of phenothiazines or haloperidol (Haldol) may be potentiated; avoid use concomitantly with metyrosine. High fluid intake to avoid crystalluria is suggested for any patient taking more than 2 g daily. Although some centers have used this agent preoperatively, we have reserved it primarily for patients who, for cardiopulmonary reasons, cannot be treated with combined α- and β-adrenergic blockade.

Potential Alternative Agents and Approaches

An alternative approach that has been advocated includes the use of calcium channel antagonists for control of hypertension and expansion of intravascular

---
[1]Not FDA approved for this indication.

volume with 2 U of whole blood 12 hours before the operation. In view of our experience with combined α- and β-adrenergic blockade and its high degree of efficacy, we have not seen the need to pursue alternative strategies.

ACUTE HYPERTENSIVE CRISES

Acute hypertensive crises may occur before or during operation and should be treated with nitroprusside (Nipride) or phentolamine (Regitine) administered intravenously (IV). Because of more widespread use, nitroprusside (Nipride) is the favored agent in this setting and is discussed below.

ANESTHESIA AND SURGERY

Extirpating a pheochromocytoma is a high-risk surgical procedure, and an experienced surgeon/anesthesiologist team is required. The last oral doses of α- and β-adrenergic blockers can be administered early in the morning on the day of operation. Cardiovascular and hemodynamic variables must be monitored closely. Continuous measurements of intra-arterial pressure and heart rhythm are required. In the setting of congestive heart failure or decreased cardiac reserve, monitoring of pulmonary capillary wedge pressure is indicated. Premedication includes minor tranquilizers and barbiturates. Fentanyl/droperidol (Innovar), droperidol (Inapsine), and morphine should not be used because of the potential for stimulating catecholamine release from the pheochromocytoma. In addition, parasympathetic nervous system blockade with atropine should be avoided because of the associated tachycardia. Induction usually is accomplished with thiopental (Pentothal), and general anesthesia is maintained with a halogenated ether such as enflurane (Ethrane) or isoflurane (Forane). Hypertensive episodes should be treated with phentolamine (Regitine) (2 to 5 mg IV) or nitroprusside (Nipride) intravenous infusion (0.5 to 5.0 µg/kg/minute; maximum dose should not exceed 800 µg per minute). Lidocaine (50 to 100 mg IV) or esmolol (Brevibloc) (50 to 200 µg/kg/minute IV) is used for cardiac arrhythmia. Adverse perioperative events or complications occurred in 32% of 143 patients operated on at the Mayo Clinic between 1983 and 1996. The most common adverse event was sustained hypertension (36 patients). There were no perioperative deaths, myocardial infarctions, or cerebrovascular events. Preoperative factors univariately associated with adverse perioperative events included larger tumor size ($P = 0.007$), prolonged duration of anesthesia ($P = 0.015$), and increased levels of preoperative urinary catecholamines and catecholamine metabolites: total metanephrines ($P = 0.004$), norepinephrine ($P = 0.014$), and epinephrine ($P = 0.004$). Despite premedication of most patients with phenoxybenzamine (Dibenzyline) and a β-adrenergic blocker, varying degrees of intraoperative hemodynamic lability occurred.

In the past, an anterior midline abdominal surgical approach was usually used for adrenal pheochromocytoma. However, laparoscopic adrenalectomy is the procedure of choice in patients with solitary adrenal pheochromocytomas that are less than 8 cm in diameter. Laparoscopic adrenalectomy is one of the most significant advances in the past 20 years for the treatment of adrenal disorders. This minimally invasive approach to the adrenal gland has been used for most nonmalignant adrenal disorders that require surgery. The postoperative recovery time and long-term morbidity associated with laparoscopic adrenalectomy are significantly reduced when compared with open adrenalectomy.

If the pheochromocytoma is in the adrenal gland, the entire gland should be removed. If the tumor is malignant, as much tumor as possible should be removed. If a bilateral adrenalectomy is planned preoperatively, the patient should receive glucocorticoid stress coverage while awaiting transfer to the operating room. Glucocorticoid coverage should be initiated in the operating room if unexpected bilateral adrenalectomy is necessary. Paragangliomas of the neck, chest, and urinary bladder require specialized approaches.

POSTOPERATIVE CARE AND FOLLOW-UP

Hypotension may occur after surgical resection of the pheochromocytoma and should be treated with fluids and colloids. Postoperative hypotension is less frequent in patients who have had adequate α-adrenergic blockade preoperatively. If both adrenal glands had been manipulated, adrenocortical insufficiency can be a potential cause of postoperative hypotension. Hypoglycemia can occur in the immediate postoperative period, and therefore blood glucose levels should be monitored and the IV-administered fluid should contain 5% dextrose.

BP usually is normal by the time of dismissal from the hospital. Some patients remain hypertensive for up to 8 weeks postoperatively. Long-standing, persistent hypertension does occur and may be related to accidental ligation of a polar renal artery, resetting of baroreceptors, established hemodynamic changes, structural changes of the blood vessels, altered sensitivity of the vessels to pressor substances, renal functional or structural changes, or coincident primary hypertension.

Approximately 2 weeks postoperatively, a 24-hour urine sample should be obtained for measurement of catecholamines and metanephrines. If the levels are normal, the resection of the pheochromocytoma can be considered to have been complete. The 24-hour urinary excretion of catecholamines should be checked annually for life as surveillance for recurrence in the adrenal bed, metastatic pheochromocytoma, or delayed appearance of multiple primary tumors.

The patient should be screened for MEN-2, VHL disease, and familial pheochromocytoma either preoperatively or during the first postoperative visit. Studies to be considered include RET proto-oncogene, VHL gene mutation testing, SDH gene mutation testing, ophthalmology consult, head MRI scan, and 24-hour urinary metanephrines and catecholamines on all immediate family members.

CURRENT DIGNOSIS

- Clinical signs include hypertension (paroxysmal in 50% of the patients and sustained in the other 50%), orthostatic hypotension, pallor, grades I to IV retinopathy, tremor, and fever.
- Frequently, patients are diagnosed with possible pheochromocytoma before they are symptomatic because of genetic screening for hereditary endocrine syndromes or incidental discovery of adrenal masses (adrenal incidentaloma) on computerized abdominal imaging.
- The diagnosis of a catecholamine-producing tumor must be suspected and then confirmed biochemically by the presence of increased urine or plasma concentrations of catecholamines or their metabolites.
- Computer-assisted adrenal and abdominal imaging (MRI or CT) is the first localization test. Approximately 90% of these tumors are found in the adrenals, and 98% are in the abdomen.
- Approximately 10% to 20% of patients with catecholamine-secreting tumors have associated germ line mutations (inherited mutations present in all cells of the body) in genes known to cause genetic disease.

Abbreviations: CT = computed tomography; MRI = magnetic resonance imaging.

Special Treatment Indications

PHEOCHROMOCYTOMA IN PREGNANCY

Pheochromocytoma in pregnancy can cause the deaths of both the fetus and the mother. The treatment of hypertensive crises is the same as for nonpregnant patients. Although there is some controversy regarding the most appropriate management, pheochromocytomas should be removed immediately if diagnosed during the first two trimesters of pregnancy. Preoperative preparation is the same as for the nonpregnant patient. If medical therapy is chosen or if the patient is in the third trimester, cesarean section and removal of the pheochromocytoma in the same operation is indicated. Spontaneous labor and delivery should be avoided.

MALIGNANT PHEOCHROMOCYTOMA

The distinction between benign and malignant catecholamine-producing tumors cannot be made on clinical, biochemical, or histopathologic characteristics. Malignancy occurs in 10% to 15% of patients (with increased prevalence in paraganglioma patients) and is based on finding direct local invasion or disease metastatic to sites that do not have chromaffin tissue, such as lymph nodes, bone, lung, and liver. Although the 5-year survival rate is less than 50%, many of these patients have prolonged survival and minimal morbidity. Metastatic lesions should be resected if possible. Painful skeletal metastatic lesions can be treated with

CURRENT THERAPY

- A combined α- and β-adrenergic blockade is required preoperatively to control BP and to prevent intraoperative hypertensive crises.
- Acute hypertensive crises may occur before or during operation and should be treated with IV-administered nitroprusside (Nipride) or phentolamine (Regitine).
- Extirpating a pheochromocytoma is a high-risk surgical procedure requiring an experienced surgeon/anesthesiologist team.
- The 24-hour urinary excretion of catecholamines should be checked annually for life as surveillance for recurrence in the adrenal bed, metastatic pheochromocytoma, or delayed appearance of multiple primary tumors.

Abbreviations: BP = blood pressure; IV = intravenously.

external radiation therapy. In initial studies, local tumor irradiation with ^{131}I-MIBG has proved to be of limited therapeutic value. Radiofrequency ablation and cryoablation of hepatic and bone metastases may be very effective in select patients. If the tumor is aggressive and the affecting the quality of life, then combination chemotherapy may be considered. A chemotherapy program consisting of cyclophosphamide (Cytoxan, Neosar), vincristine (Oncovin, Vincasar), and dacarbazine (DTIC-Dome) given cyclically every 21 to 28 days has proved beneficial but not curative in these patients. Hypertension and spells can be controlled with a combined α- and β-adrenergic blockade.

REFERENCES

Assalia A, Gagner M: Laparoscopic adrenalectomy. Br J Surg 2004; 91:1259-1274.

Erickson D, Kudva YC, Ebersold MJ, et al: Benign paragangliomas: Clinical presentation and treatment outcomes in 236 patients. J Clin Endocrinol Metab 2001;86:5210-5216.

Kinney MAO, Warner ME, vanHeerden JA, et al: Perianesthetic risks and outcomes of pheochromocytoma and paraganglioma resection. Anesth Analg 2000;91:1118-1123.

Kudva YC, Sawka AM, Young WF Jr: Clinical review 164: The laboratory diagnosis of adrenal pheochromocytoma: The Mayo Clinic experience. J Clin Endocrinol Metab 2003;88:4533-4539.

Kudva YC, Young WF Jr, Thompson GB, et al: Adrenal incidentaloma: An important component of the clinical presentation spectrum of benign sporadic adrenal pheochromocytoma. The Endocrinologist 1999;9:77-80.

Neumann HP, Bausch B, McWhinney SR, et al: Germ-line mutations in nonsyndromic pheochromocytoma. N Engl J Med 2002;346: 1459-1466.

Sawka AM, Jaeschke R, Singh RJ, Young WF Jr: A comparison of biochemical tests for pheochromocytoma: Measurement of fractionated plasma metanephrines compared with the combination of 24-hour urinary metanephrines and catecholamines. J Clin Endocrinol Metab 2003;88:553-558.

Young, WF Jr: Pheochromocytoma: 1926 to 1993. Trends Endocrinol Metab 1993;4:122-127.

Young WF Jr: Management approaches to adrenal incidentalomas: A view from Rochester, Minnesota. Endocrinol Metab Clin North Am 2000;29:159-185.

9

Thyroiditis

Method of
Vahab Fatourechi, MD

Inflammatory conditions of the thyroid can be caused by an autoimmune process and by viral, bacterial, or other infectious agents. Inflammation can be induced by medications, cytokine therapy, or by radiation. Graves' disease and Hashimoto's thyroiditis are examples of autoimmune thyroiditis. Lymphocytic infiltration is more common in Hashimoto's thyroiditis than in Graves' disease. Fibrosis, common in Hashimoto's thyroiditis, is not usually seen in Graves' hyperthyroidism. These two conditions often overlap. Management of these two varieties of autoimmune thyroiditis has been discussed in detail in other sections of the book.

Autoimmune Thyroiditis

CHRONIC LYMPHOCYTIC THYROIDITIS (HASHIMOTO'S THYROIDITIS)

Hashimoto's thyroiditis is the most common cause of goiter and hypothyroidism in adults in the United States. Antithyroid antibodies are the hallmark of this condition and include thyroperoxidase antibodies (TPO antibodies) and antithymoglobulin antibodies. These antibodies are also commonly positive in Graves' disease. Some studies show that 10% of the population has elevated thyroid-stimulating hormone (TSH), indicating mild thyroid failure because of autoimmune thyroiditis. For patients with serum TSH above 10, even if peripheral thyroid hormones are still within normal range, thyroxine therapy is recommended. Seventy-five percent of patients with elevated serum TSH have levels between 5 and 10 mIU/L. Thyroxine therapy for this group of patients with mild thyroid failure is controversial and, in my opinion, should be individualized. Clinical conditions such as the presence of antithyroid antibodies, patient preference, and the presence of symptoms, pregnancy, or anticipation of pregnancy would favor therapy. For patients with overt hypothyroidism who have elevated TSH and abnormally low serum-free thyroxine levels, replacement therapy with L-thyroxine is recommended. The usual daily adult dose varies between 88 µg and 137 µg. For subclinical hypothyroidism, I use 50 to 75 µg of L-thyroxine.

POSTPARTUM THYROIDITIS

Postpartum autoimmune transient thyroiditis occurs 2 to 10 months after childbirth with a frequency of 7%. Women with type 1 diabetes and with positive antithyroid antibodies are at higher risk of developing postpartum thyroiditis (25%). It usually recurs in subsequent pregnancies. The thyroid is painless. A brief period of mild hyperthyroidism lasting 1 to 3 months may be followed by transient hypothyroidism, usually at 6 months (between 2 and 12 months). The most common presentation is hypothyroidism (43%), followed by hyperthyroidism (32%), and, less commonly, hyperthyroidism followed by hypothyroidism (25%). In some patients, postpartum depression may be associated with thyroiditis. In the hyperthyroid phase, thyroidal uptake of radioactive iodine (RAI) is minimal, TSH is suppressed, and peripheral thyroid hormone levels are mildly increased. The thyroid is only moderately enlarged, and sedimentation rate is usually normal. The condition resolves within 1 year. Persistent hypothyroidism after 12 months is usually permanent. In patients who have very high levels of antithyroid antibodies, TSH above 30 mIU/L, and large goiters, permanent hyperthyroidism is more likely. It should be noted that Graves' disease is ameliorated in the third trimester of pregnancy and may recur 3 months after childbirth. Initial presentation of Graves' disease is not uncommon after childbirth. For breast-feeding patients, TSH-receptor antibodies and severity and persistence of the condition are helpful in the differential diagnosis. For the symptomatic transient hyperthyroid phase, I administer β-blockers (long-acting propranolol 40 to 80 mg, Inderal-LA)[1] until the hyperthyroidism subsides. Antithyroid medications are not indicated for destructive low-uptake thyroiditis. For patients who are not breast-feeding, a high RAI uptake is diagnostic of Graves' hyperthyroidism. For the hypothyroid phase, if mild, no therapy is needed because of the transient nature of the condition. In symptomatic patients and in female patients planning pregnancy and for a TSH level above 10, thyroxine therapy is needed (50 to 75 µg of L-thyroxine/day). Therapy should be tapered after 12 months to see if recovery has occurred. The dose can be cut in half and TSH checked after 6 weeks. I suggest the option of continuing therapy until 1 year after completion of the family.

SILENT THYROIDITIS (SUBACUTE LYMPHOCYTIC THYROIDITIS)

Silent painless thyroiditis is similar to postpartum thyroiditis occurring unrelated to pregnancy. Silent thyroiditis can also occur in men. Some cases of glaucomatous thyroiditis, presumably of viral origin, may occur without pain. In this group of patients, a low RAI hyperthyroidism and elevation of sedimentation rate are more likely, and fine needle aspiration (FNA) may be helpful in diagnosis. Diagnosis of silent thyroiditis is made by the absence of a history of iodine ingestion and thyroid hormone products. For a definitive diagnosis, measurement of urinary iodine and serum thymoglobulin may be needed. Thymoglobulin is low in excess exogenous thyroid hormone intake and high in thyroiditis. Management of the hyper- and hypothyroid phases is similar to that described for postpartum thyroiditis.

---

[1] Not FDA approved for this indication.

Rakel and Bope: *Conn's Current Therapy 2006.*

RIEDEL'S, OR FIBROUS, STRUMA

Riedel's, or fibrous, thyroiditis is rare; in our tertiary referral center we see only one case per year. There is severe fibrotic process of the thyroid that involves other tissues in the neck. It is commonly associated with other systemic fibrotic processes such as mediastinal fibrosis, retroperitoneal fibrosis, and sclerosing cholangitis. Diagnosis is made when fibrosis is present outside of the thyroid capsule. Differential diagnosis is with fibrotic Hashimoto's thyroiditis that is limited to the thyroid and has more lymphocytic infiltration and less fibrosis. Because of the invasive nature of Riedel's thyroiditis, differentiation from thyroid cancer should be made with open biopsy. The process commonly is self-limited. Therapy is a high dose of a corticosteroid or surgical resection.

Drug-Induced Thyroiditis

CYTOKINE-INDUCED THYROIDITIS

Interferon-α and interleukin-2 therapies can cause an autoimmune thyroiditis that manifests either as hyperthyroidism or hypothyroidism. Graves' disease occasionally can be initiated by these therapies. Patients with positive thyroid antibodies are at a higher risk of developing thyroid dysfunction with these therapies. Normalization of thyroid function occurs in the majority of these cases. Also, an inflammatory low RAI uptake can occur with transient hyperthyroidism that may require β-blocker[1] therapy.

AMIODARONE-INDUCED THYROIDITIS

Amiodarone (Cordarone) is used in therapy for serious cardiac arrhythmias. It is a highly iodinated compound and remains in the body for several months. Iodine can cause hypothyroidism because of the pharmacologic inhibitory effect on organification and release of thyroid hormones. In iodine-deficient areas or in the presence of preexisting nodular goiter, it also can cause iodine-induced hyperthyroidism (type I hyperthyroidism). In this form, discontinuation of amiodarone, if possible, and therapy with antithyroid medications (40 to 60 mg of methimazole [Tapazole] per day) is effective. Type II amiodarone-induced thyroiditis is a destructive thyroiditis as a result of the toxic effect of amiodarone on the thyroid. Antithyroid medications are not effective in this type, and corticosteroid therapy is effective. Differentiation of type I from type II hyperthyroidism is difficult, and sometimes triple therapy with corticosteroids (40 mg of prednisone/day) plus antithyroid drugs (40 to 60 mg /day of methimazole) and perchlorate[1] (400 mg three times daily) may be needed. Rapid response is in favor of thyroiditis. In severely hyperthyroid patients, and in those whom continuation of amiodarone therapy is unavoidable, thyroidectomy in experienced hands is necessary. Therapy of amiodarone-induced

hyperthyroidism is complex, and an endocrinologist should be consulted.

LITHIUM-INDUCED THYROIDITIS

Preexisting thyroid autoimmunity can be activated by long-term use of lithium. Hypothyroidism and less commonly hyperthyroidism may occur. With the direct toxic effect of lithium on the thyroid, painless sporadic thyroiditis with low-uptake hyperthyroidism is also a possibility. Management of hypothyroidism and goiter will be with thyroxine therapy. High-uptake hyperthyroidism is treated similarly to Graves' disease.

RADIATION-INDUCED THYROIDITIS

External radiation administered for therapeutic purposes and RAI therapy can cause radiation-induced thyroiditis manifested by thyroid pain and, because of the release of thyroid hormones, transient hyperthyroidism. Treatment includes short-term corticosteroid therapy (prednisone 40 mg/day with taper in 2 to 3 weeks) and β-blockers[1] for hyperthyroid symptoms. Subsequent hypothyroidism usually occurs and should be managed by long-term thyroxine therapy.

Subacute Viral Thyroiditis

GRANULOMATOUS THYROIDITIS AND SUBACUTE THYROIDITIS

Granulomatous thyroiditis subacute thyroiditis, also called de Quervain's thyroiditis, is of possible viral origin because it may have a seasonal occurrence and viral elements have been isolated from thyroids of affected patients. It often follows viral upper respiratory infections and is associated with systemic febrile symptoms. The thyroid is hard and exquisitely tender on palpation, the patient has dysphagia and pain radiating to the ears, and the sedimentation rate is elevated. The combination of thyroid pain, hyperthyroidism with serum TSH, and low thyroid RAI uptake is sufficient for diagnosis. FNA is rarely needed, but, if done in questionable cases, will show multinuclear giant cells. Once the diagnosis is made, patients should be reassured because the dramatic symptoms typically make them apprehensive. Hyperthyroid symptoms should be managed with β-blockers[1] as outlined previously. Management of pain and fever in mild cases is with nonsteroidal anti-inflammatory medications (NSAIDs). One half of the patients have significant symptoms requiring corticosteroid therapy. I usually start 40 mg of prednisone daily for 2 to 4 weeks and then taper off over 2 to 3 weeks. There is usually dramatic response to corticosteroid therapy and all symptoms subside within 48 hours. If there is no response to steroids, the diagnosis should be questioned and FNA may be performed. If the symptoms return with corticosteroid taper, longer therapy may be needed. For mild symptoms after withdrawal of

---

[1] Not FDA approved for this indication.

[1] Not FDA approved for this indication.

CURRENT DIAGNOSIS

- Graves' disease: hyperthyroidism, TSH receptor antibodies, ophthalmopathy
- Hashimoto's thyroiditis: hypothyroidism, TPO antibodies, goiterous, or atrophic
- Postpartum thyroiditis: mild hyperthyroidism, transient hypothyroidism, low RAI uptake
- Silent thyroiditis: both genders, mild hyperthyroidism, transient hypothyroidism, low RAI uptake
- Riedel's thyroiditis: very rare, normal thyroid functions, fibrosis, extrathyroid extension

Drug-Induced Thyroiditis
- Lithium induced: autoimmune thyroiditis, silent thyroiditis type
- Amiodarone induced, type I: usually goiter in endemic areas, hypervascular on ultrasound
- Amiodarone induced, type II: smaller thyroid, shorter duration response to corticosteroids
- Cytokine induced: destructive thyroiditis, autoimmune hyperthyroidism or hypothyroidism

Viral or Infectious Thyroiditis
- Subacute (granulomatous): pain, high sedimentation rate, low RAI uptake
- Suppurative thyroiditis: fever, pain, high white blood count and erythrocyte sedimentation rate, abscess, Gram stain and culture

Abbreviations: RAI = radioactive iodine; TPO = thyroperoxidase; TSH = thyroid-stimulating hormone.

CURRENT THERAPY

- Graves' disease: antithyroid, RAI, surgery
- Hashimoto's thyroiditis: thyroxine therapy, if hypothyroid
- Postpartum thyroiditis: β-blockers in hyperthyroid phase, short-course thyroxine therapy for hypothyroid phase
- Silent thyroiditis: β-blockers, short-course thyroxine therapy
- Riedel's thyroiditis: corticosteroids, surgical debulking

Drug-Induced Thyroiditis
- Lithium induced: depends on type and thyroid function
- Amiodarone induced, type I: antithyroids, perchlorate, surgery
- Amiodarone induced, type II: corticosteroid therapy
- Cytokine induced: therapy depends on type and thyroid function

Viral or Infectious Thyroiditis
- Subacute (granulomatous): β-blockers, NSAIDs, corticosteroids
- Suppurative thyroiditis: drainage, specific antibiotic or antifungal

Abbreviations: NSAIDs = nonsteroidal anti-inflammatory drugs; RAI = radioactive iodine.

corticosteroid therapy, NSAIDs are sufficient. The usual course of the hyperthyroid phase is 4 to 8 weeks and very rarely may persist beyond 6 months. Approximately one third of patients develop a transient hypothyroid phase, which may not require therapy. Permanent hypothyroidism, defined as the persistence of the hypothyroid phase beyond 1 year, can occur in 10% to 15% of the patients. Recurrence can occur in 4% of the patients after several years when the immunity from the first episode is lost.

SUPPURATIVE THYROIDITIS

In general, the thyroid is resistant to infection. Suppurative thyroiditis is usually bacterial. Other infections, such as fungal, mycobacterial, and parasitic, rarely occur. In the pediatric age group, frequent bacterial infections can occur because of a patent piriform sinus. Other predisposing factors include immune deficiency and preexisting thyroid disease and systemic infection. Presentation is usually with painful thyroid mass, abscess formation, elevated erythrocyte sedimentation rate, and normal thyroid function. Diagnosis is by FNA and direct examination and culture. Therapy should include drainage and specific anti-infection therapy.

REFERENCES

Dang AH, Hershman JM: Lithium-associated thyroiditis. Endocr Pract 2002;8(3):232-236.
Feldt-Rasmussen U, Krogh Rasmussen A: Thyroiditis. In Rakel RE, Bope ET (eds): Conn's Current Therapy 2004, 56th ed. Philadelphia, Elsevier Science, 2004, pp 705-708.
Lazarus JH, Parkes AB, Premawardhana LD: Postpartum thyroiditis. Autoimmunity 2002;35(3):169-173.
Pearce EN, Farwell AP, Braverman LE: Thyroiditis. N Engl J Med 2003;348(26):2646-2655.
Slatosky J, Shipton B, Wahba H: Thyroiditis: Differential diagnosis and management. Am Fam Physician 2000;61(4):1047-1052, 1054.
Sniezek JC, Francis TB: Inflammatory thyroid disorders. Otolaryngol Clin North Am 2003;36(1):55-71.
Stagnaro-Green A: Clinical review 152: Postpartum thyroiditis. J Clin Endocrinol Metab 2002;87(9):4042-4047.

The Urogenital Tract

Bacterial Infections of the Urinary Tract in Males

Method of
John N. Krieger, MD

Urinary tract infections (UTIs) include a spectrum of clinical conditions whose common denominator is colonization and invasion of the urinary tract organs and tissues. Any portion of the urinary tract can be involved, from the renal cortex to the urethral meatus. Infection may occur predominantly at a single site, such as the bladder (cystitis), prostate (prostatitis), kidney (pyelonephritis), or perinephric space (perinephric abscess). The entire urinary tract is at risk for invasion by bacteria when any of its parts becomes infected.

Most infections occur by the ascending route, meaning that bacteria from the fecal flora colonize the perineum; then ascend via the urethra, bladder, and ureter to involve the kidney. On occasion, hematogenous dissemination of bacteria can result in seeding of the urinary tract. Classic examples of hematogenous infection are genitourinary tuberculosis and staphylococcal infection of a renal cyst ("renal carbuncle"). On rare occasions, the urinary tract may be involved by infection from contiguous structures, as may occur in patients with diverticulitis or appendicitis that involves the urinary tract.

Distinguishing Complicated from Uncomplicated Infections

The key issue for therapy is to distinguish *uncomplicated (medical)* infections from *complicated (surgical)* infections. An uncomplicated infection occurs in the absence of underlying structural or neurologic disorders of the urinary tract. These infections usually respond well to antimicrobial therapy. Thorough anatomic evaluation and imaging studies are seldom indicated in patients with uncomplicated UTIs. In contrast, complicated infections occur when the urinary tract is repeatedly invaded by bacteria, leaving residual inflammation, or, in cases accompanied by obstruction, stones, foreign bodies, or neurologic conditions that interfere with urinary drainage. Antimicrobial therapy alone is markedly less effective in complicated UTIs. Managing patients with complicated UTIs often requires thorough anatomic evaluation and imaging studies. An important differential point is that patients with complicated infections tend to have persistence of bacteria within the urinary tract in the face of antimicrobial agents to which the bacteria appear to be sensitive in laboratory tests. Often, it is necessary to correct an underlying obstructive lesion or voiding problem to clear the infection. The goal of therapy for any patient with a UTI should be total elimination of the infecting organism from the urinary tract.

Natural History

In neonates, the incidence of symptomatic UTIs is higher in males than in females. In part, this is related to circumcision status. It appears that bacteria can adhere to the prepuce of uncircumcised male infants and then gain access to the urinary tract. Neonatal circumcision appears to reduce the rate of urinary tract infections in male infants by approximately 90%. After the neonatal period, symptomatic infections in male children and adults are distinctly uncommon until middle age. This is in marked contrast with the situation in females, who experience increasing rates of both symptomatic and asymptomatic infections with a marked increase following initiation of sexual activity and then a continued gradual rise with age. Asymptomatic bacteriuria is also distinctly unusual in males when compared with females.

Well-documented UTIs in male children mandate thorough urologic investigation because of the high prevalence of structural genitourinary tract abnormalities in such patients. Often, UTI represents the key diagnostic manifestation for major abnormalities of the urinary tract. For example, vesicoureteral reflux of urine, posterior urethral valves, and other major structural abnormalities often manifest initially with a bacterial urinary tract infection. Early diagnosis and appropriate therapy offer the best chance for preservation of maximal renal function, although renal scarring may be progressive despite appropriate treatment.

Structural urinary tract abnormalities remain a major cause of renal failure in children. Morbidity can be minimized by appropriate evaluation and therapy. Our choice for evaluation of a male child with a UTI is the combination of renal ultrasound to evaluate the upper urinary tract plus a voiding cystourethrogram to evaluate the lower urinary tract. Voiding cystourethrography should be obtained after resolution of the initial infection because dilation of the upper urinary tract can be exaggerated in the face of recent infection.

Because UTIs are unusual in young men, there are few well-done natural history studies in this population. In patients without obvious neurologic or structural abnormalities, sexual intercourse can be a risk factor, particularly among homosexual men and heterosexual men who practice insertive anal intercourse. The overall contribution of these practices to bacterial UTIs in adult men is uncertain. Standard urologic teaching is to do a thorough evaluation for structural abnormalities in such patients, including radiographic studies and cystourethroscopy. However, our published experience suggests that previously healthy college-age males with well-documented urinary tract infections have low rates of structural genitourinary tract abnormalities. An excretory urogram with a postvoid film and a uroflow study are adequate to screen for structural abnormalities in this population. We reserve cystoscopy for those patients who are determined to be at risk for significant abnormalities on the basis of these screening studies and a thorough physical examination. The other major risk factors for UTIs in men are instrumentation of the urinary tract and bacterial prostatitis.

Diagnosis and Localization

Because accurate diagnosis is a prerequisite for appropriate therapy, we recommend culture and sensitivity testing of urine specimens from any male with symptoms or signs suggesting urinary infection. In patients who do not have obstructive lesions, stasis, stones, or foreign bodies, recurrent and persistent urinary tract infections are often related to bacterial prostatitis. Segmented localization cultures can be used to differentiate cystitis and urethritis from bacterial prostatitis. The procedure should be carried out at a time when the patient does not have bacteriuria.

Our procedure for lower urinary tract localization is outlined briefly. After cleaning the glans with sterile water, the first-void urine (the initial 5 to 10 mL of voided urine) is collected in a sterile container. Next, a midstream specimen is obtained. The patient is asked to stop voiding. Prostatic fluid is expressed by digital prostate massage. The postvoid urine (the next 5 to 10 mL after the massage) is then collected. Culture and sensitivity testing are then carried out. It is critical to make certain that the laboratory is aware of the purpose of these studies so that the laboratory will evaluate small numbers of uropathogens.

Diagnosis of chronic bacterial prostatitis can be made if the post-massage urine specimen or the expressed prostatic secretion contains a tenfold or greater increase in the concentration of the uropathogen when compared with that in the first-void urine specimen. In patients with well-documented bacterial prostatitis, the causative organism is identical to the one causing recurrent episodes of bacteriuria.

Only a small minority of males presenting with symptoms of prostatitis fit into the acute or chronic bacterial prostatitis categories. The great majority of patients with symptoms are classified in the chronic prostatitis/chronic pelvic pain category. In contrast with the recognized benefit of appropriate antimicrobial therapy for patients with acute and chronic bacterial prostatitis, the roles of antimicrobial therapy and other treatments have not been defined for patients with chronic prostatitis/chronic pelvic pain syndrome.

Basic Principles in Therapy

There are three keys to successful therapy for UTIs. First, eliminate or control predisposing factors. For example, we are often asked to manage "resistant urinary infections" in long-term care patients with indwelling catheters. One approach is to change their bladder management from a chronic, indwelling catheter to an intermittent self- (or assisted) catheterization program. Other examples include the removal of obstructing lesions, stones, or strictures of improved drainage of the lower urinary tract. These measures may be successful in eliminating the focus of infection, even with no antimicrobial therapy. Second, eradicate the infection as soon as possible to prevent colonization of the prostate and other structures. Third, ensure that the infection has been eliminated by obtaining cultures during or immediately after therapy and at follow-up at 1 to 2 months following therapy.

UNCOMPLICATED INFECTIONS

Uncomplicated infections generally manifest with symptoms of bacterial cystitis, with a combination of urinary frequency, urgency, dysuria, nocturia, suprapubic discomfort, low back pain, or hematuria. Systemic symptoms of fever, chills, and rigor are absent. Urine culture confirms the diagnosis, with *Escherichia coli* being the most common pathogen. Uncomplicated infections, including those introduced by a single or short course of indwelling urethral catheterization, generally respond promptly to a short course of antimicrobial therapy. The infection may persist and become difficult to eradicate if the prostate becomes colonized or if the patient has a stone or structural abnormality of the urinary tract. Thus, an effort should be made to eliminate predisposing factors while routine therapy is guided by in vitro susceptibility tests.

I prefer oral therapy with one of the agents listed in Table 1. In our geographic area, bacteria-causing UTIs have developed substantial resistance to trimethoprim-sulfamethoxazole (Bactrim). Therefore, we usually initiate empirical therapy with a quinolone. Nitrofurantoin (Macrodantin) remains highly effective and is an attractive alternative drug. In general, we recommend that

TABLE 1 Oral Antimicrobial Agents Prescribed for Urinary Tract Infections in Adult Males

Antimicrobial class	Agent	Dosage frequency
Fluoroquinolone	Ciprofloxacin (Cipro)	250-500 mg bid
	Ciprofloxacin (Cipro XR)	500-1000 mg qd
	Gatifloxacin (Tequin)	200-400 mg qd
	Levofloxacin (Levaquin)	250-500 mg qd
	Norfloxacin (Noroxin)	400 mg bid
	Ofloxacin (Floxin)	200-400 mg bid[3]
Combination agents	Trimethoprim-sulfamethoxazole (Bactrim, Bactrim DS, Septra, Septra DS)	160 mg trimethoprim + 800 mg sulfamethoxazole bid
Vn	Amoxicillin-clavulanic acid (Augmentin)	500-875 mg amoxicillin + 125 mg clavulanate bid
Cephalosporin	Cefaclor (Ceclor)	250-500 mg tid[3]
	Loracarbef (Lorabid)	200-400 mg bid[3]
Other antimicrobials	Nitrofurantoin (Macrobid)	50-100 mg qd or bid
	Nitrofurantoin (Macrodantin)	50-100 mg qid

[3]Exceeds dosage recommended by the manufacturer.
Abbreviations: bid = twice daily; qd = every day; qid = four times per day; tid = three times per day.

the duration of therapy be at least 2 weeks, although only limited data address this point in males.

COMPLICATED INFECTIONS

Patients with systemic signs or those with a history of structural or neurologic abnormalities merit thorough anatomic investigation of the urinary tract. It is important to do this early in the course of therapy because antimicrobial therapy alone may fail to cure infection and urosepsis may develop unless there is specific management of the underlying problem. Our initial choice for evaluation of these patients is either a computed tomography (CT) scan with contrast or an excretory urogram with postvoid film. If an abscess in the retroperitoneal space or the prostate is suspected, CT scanning is superior to the other modalities for diagnosis.

Prolonged courses of therapy are indicated for patients with persistent infections. I often use 3 to 4 months of therapy in this situation. In patients with chronic bacterial prostatitis, elderly patients, or those in nursing homes, continuous therapy may be necessary to suppress bacteriuria, even though eradication may prove impossible. Thus, for patients with recurrent or complicated infections, I recommend an attempt to eradicate the focus of infection, following thorough evaluation of the urinary tract. The therapy is usually with the same drugs listed in Table 1. My first choice for curative therapy is usually a quinolone. For patients with persistent or frequently relapsing infections, I consider long-term therapy (months or years) using low dosages of antimicrobial drugs for prophylaxis or suppression with periodic monitoring by culture to be sure that the agent continues to be effective.

PROSTATITIS

Acute and chronic bacterial prostatitis can manifest with local urinary tract symptoms characteristic of bacterial cystitis or with systemic signs and symptoms.

Acute bacterial prostatitis is usually manifest with the sudden onset of chills, fever, malaise, and low back and perineal pain, as well as difficulty with urination. On rectal examination, the prostate is tense and exquisitely tender. Excessive palpation can induce septicemia. For patients who require hospitalization, my initial choice is the combination of a β-lactam drug and an aminoglycoside until the results of antimicrobial sensitivity testing are available. Following parenteral therapy, the patient is managed with continued antimicrobial therapy for at least 4 weeks, usually employing a quinolone. Patients with acute bacterial prostatitis usually respond well to a variety of antimicrobial agents that penetrate an acutely inflamed prostate. Many of these agents are not effective in chronic bacterial prostatitis.

In contrast with acute bacterial prostatitis, chronic bacterial prostatitis is often insidious in onset. Patients usually have recurrent UTIs and sometimes have recurrent episodes of acute prostatitis. Between symptomatic episodes, patients might be totally asymptomatic. Diagnosis depends on the localization cultures described earlier. Treatment must be prolonged because diffusion of antimicrobial agents into the prostates is poor. My initial choice is usually a quinolone, with trimethoprim-sulfamethoxazole (Septra, Bactrim) as a second choice agent. Carbenicillin indanyl sodium (Geocillin) is also approved for this indication, but has not been particularly effective in my experience. It is important not to confuse bacterial prostatitis with chronic prostatitis/chronic pelvic pain syndrome. Chronic prostatitis is the most common cause of symptomatic prostatitis, but these patients do not have bacteriuria.

LONG-TERM CARE PATIENTS

Long-term care patients, including those with incontinence and indwelling urinary catheters or other devices and chronic asymptomatic bacterial colonization, should not be treated. It is impossible to sterilize the urine permanently in such cases. Furthermore, resistant

Rakel and Bope: *Conn's Current Therapy 2006.*

10

CURRENT DIAGNOSIS

- Urinary tract infections include a wide clinical spectrum.
- Infection at any site in the urinary tract places the entire system at risk.
- The critical clinical issue is to distinguish uncomplicated (medical) from complicated (surgical) infections.
- Anatomic evaluation and imaging studies are seldom indicated for patients with uncomplicated infections.
- Well-documented UTIs in male children require thorough urologic investigation because of the high prevalence of structural urinary tract abnormalities.
- We recommend culture and sensitivity testing of urine specimens for any male with symptoms or signs suggesting a UTI.
- In contrast, we discourage routine screening urine cultures in long-term care patients who have no signs or symptoms suggesting a UTI.

Abbreviation: UTI = urinary tract infection.

organisms are likely to emerge, making subsequent therapy difficult. I treat such patients only if they develop acute symptoms referable to the urinary tract or prior to genitourinary tract procedures. We strongly recommend against obtaining screening cultures in such patients because these cultures often lead to unnecessary therapy that selects resistant bacterial flora. Furthermore, there is evidence that bacterial colonization with relatively benign strains can inhibit the establishment of symptomatic infections caused by more virulent bacteria.

CURRENT THERAPY

- Antimicrobial therapy alone is markedly less effective for patients with complicated UTIs than for patients with uncomplicated UTIs.
- Managing patients with complicated UTIs often requires anatomic evaluation and imaging studies.
- The goal of therapy is elimination of the infecting organism from the urinary tract.
- For patients with complicated UTIs it is often necessary to eliminate or control predisposing factors.
- Rapid eradication of the infection may limit the potential for infection of adjacent structures.
- Ensure elimination of the infection by repeating urine cultures.
- A prolonged course of antimicrobial therapy may prove necessary for patients with persistent infections.

Abbreviations: UTIs = urinary tract infections.

REFERENCES

Abarbanel J, Engelstein D, Lask D, Livne PM: Urinary tract infection in men younger than 45 years of age: Is there a need for urologic investigation? Urology 2003;62:27-29.
Andrews S, Brooks PT, Hanbury DC, et al: Ultrasonography and abdominal radiography versus intravenous urography in investigation of urinary tract infection in men: Prospective incident cohort study. BMJ 2002;324:454-456.
Bjerklund Johansen TE: Diagnosis and imaging in urinary tract infections. Curr Opin Urol 2002;12:39-43.
Bonacorsi S, Lefevre S, Clermont O, et al: *Escherichia coli* strains causing urinary tract infection in uncircumcised infants resemble urosepsis-like adult strains. J Urol 2005;173:195-197.
Hummers-Pradier E, Ohse AM, Koch M, et al: Urinary tract infection in men. Int J Clin Pharmacol Ther 2004;42:360-366.
Koyle MA, Barqawi A, Wild J, et al: Pediatric urinary tract infections: The role of fluoroquinolones. Pediatr Infect Dis J 2003;22:1133-1137.
Krieger JN, Ross SO, Simonsen JM: Urinary tract infections in healthy university men. J Urol 1993;149:1046-1048.
Naber KG: Levofloxacin in the treatment of urinary tract infections and prostatitis. J Chemother 2004;16(Suppl 2):18-21.
Talan DA, Klimberg IW, Nicolle LE, et al: Once daily, extended release ciprofloxacin for complicated urinary tract infections and acute uncomplicated pyelonephritis. J Urol 2004;171:734-739.
Ulleryd P, Zackrisson B, Aus G, et al: Selective urological evaluation in men with febrile urinary tract infection. BJU Int 2001;88:15-20.

Urinary Tract Infections in Women

Method of
Burke A. Cunha, MD

General Concepts

Urinary tract infections (UTIs) are common in adult women. The two major clinical manifestations of UTIs in adult women are cystitis or pyelonephritis. Young adult women may also present with so-called dysuria pyuria syndrome (abacteriuric cystitis), previously known as acute urethral syndrome, as outpatients. Hospitalized compromised female hosts with cystitis may be complicated by bacteremia or ascending infection. Renal abscess may complicate pyelonephritis in normal or compromised female hosts.

Cystitis Versus Pneumonias

The therapeutic approach to UTIs in adult women depends on accurate localization of the site of infection in the urinary tract. The most common clinical problem is differentiating cystitis from pyelonephritis. Patients with acute bacterial cystitis present with dysuria and frequency, which may or may not be accompanied by suprapubic discomfort or lower back pain. The fever accompanying cystitis is $\leq$ to 38.9°C (102°F) and is not usually associated with chills. The clinical manifestation of cystitis is confirmed by finding pyuria and significant bacteriuria, (i.e., $\geq 10^6$ CFU/mL) in such patients. The urinalysis in acute cystitis is not usually accompanied by microscopic hematuria.

Staphylococcus saprophyticus is the only uropathogen in the ambulatory setting that is responsible for the majority of cases of UTIs accompanied by microscopic hematuria. Microscopic hematuria in a urinalysis in a patient with an apparent UTI should be carefully observed and should disappear after therapy of the UTI. If the microscopic hematuria disappears, then the physician can safely assume it was related to the UTI. Particularly in elderly patients, if the microscopic hematuria persists after eradication of the UTI, then the patient should be investigated for a bladder or renal source of the microscopic hematuria.

Dysuria-Pyuria Syndrome

There are three other types of UTIs that mimic or resemble cystitis. In sexually active young women, the dysuria-pyuria syndrome manifests with the symptoms of cystitis but with negative urine cultures, or if organisms are cultured, they are present in low numbers ($\leq 10^3$ CFU/mL). Most cases of dysuria-pyuria syndrome are caused by *Chlamydia trachomatis*. In patients with dysuria-pyuria syndrome, if the urine is cultured for *Chlamydia*, cultures are frequently positive.

Catheter-Associated Bacteriuria (CAB)

Hospitalized patients with indwelling Foley catheters often acquire bacteriuria as a function of time that the Foley catheter is in place. Pyuria is often in the urine of patients with indwelling Foleys because the catheter elicits inflammation of the urinary tract. The presence of pyuria and bacteriuria in a patient with an indwelling Foley suggests either UTI or CAB. The majority of such patients are asymptomatic and afebrile. More than 95% of the time these patients have colonization of the urinary tract without infection. The urinalysis in patients with indwelling Foley catheters is helpful if either bacteria without pyuria or pyuria without bacteria is demonstrated. Bacteriuria without pyuria signifies colonization of the urinary tract, whereas pyuria without bacteriuria indicates inflammation of the urinary tract. In non–Foley catheter patients, the presence of pyuria plus significant bacteriuria is diagnostic of a UTI. This is not the case with CAB. As mentioned in the setting of the Foley catheter, bacteriuria plus pyuria almost always represents colonization and not a UTI.

Benign Bacteriuria of the Elderly

In elderly female patients, varying degrees of relaxation of the pelvic musculature are common. Patients often have varying degrees of cystocele of rectocele, which changes anatomic relationship and the angularity of the urethra as it enters the bladder and predisposes to colonization of the bladder urine by the introital flora, such as coliform flora derived from the colon. For this reason, elderly female patients often have bacteriuria with few or no symptoms of a UTI. The presence of bacteriuria/pyuria is often discovered on a routine urinalysis obtained as part of either admission laboratory work or an outpatient workup/screening test battery. The presence of bacteriuria/pyuria in an elderly female patient without underlying genitourinary (GU) disease or impaired host defenses has been appropriately termed *benign bacteriuria of the elderly*; it has been shown that these patients do not go on to have symptomatic UTIs, ascending infection (e.g., pyelonephritis/ renal abscess), or bacteremia from the urinary tract.

Recurrent Urinary Tract Infections: Reinfection Versus Relapse

Most UTIs in women are acute. CAB is often incorrectly considered a chronic UTI because in most cases it represents colonization rather than infection. Recurrent UTIs are chronic in the sense that they persist over a long period of time, but are really episodic infections. However, the approach to recurrent UTIs is based on determining whether the recurrence is on the basis of reinfection or relapse. The reinfection variety of recurrent UTIs is defined as a recurrent UTI because of different organisms being cultured during each UTI episode. The relapse form of recurrent UTIs is defined as demonstrating the same organism during repeated bouts of UTIs. The reinfection form of recurrent UTIs is usually because of rapid colonization of the vaginal introitus/entry into the urethra, usually following sexual intercourse. The relapse variety of recurrent UTI by the same organism recovered during each episode suggests an underlying structural abnormality of the GU tract. The correct diagnostic approach to recurrent UTIs because of relapse is a thorough investigation of the GU tract from the urethra to the kidneys, which determines a possible source for the focus for the organisms to periodically reappear as a relapsing UTI. Relapse UTIs cannot be successfully approached therapeutically without correcting the underlying condition predisposing to relapse (i.e., bladder calculi, kinked ureters, renal stones, renal abscesses).

Acute Pyelonephritis

Acute pyelonephritis is most common in pregnancy and as a complication of an ascending infection from cystitis/GU instrumentation. An acute episode of

10

pyelonephritis may occur in patients who have chronic pyelonephritis; the acute episode is superimposed on the chronic condition. Renal abscess may complicate acute and chronic pyelonephritis. Renal cortical abscesses are often caused by gram-positive cocci (e.g., staphylococci acquired hematogenously), whereas medullary abscesses are usually caused by aerobic gram-negative bacilli (e.g., coliforms or enterococci).

Acute pyelonephritis may be differentiated from cystitis by the presence of unilateral costovertebral angle (CVA) tenderness (otherwise unexplainable) and a temperature of ≥ 38.9°C (102°F). Bilateral pyelonephritis is unusual, and the presence of bilateral CVA tenderness should suggest an alternative diagnosis. Pyelonephritis is often bilateral pathologically, but clinically it is almost always unilateral in its presentation with CVA tenderness. The urinalysis in pyelonephritis is the same as in cystitis, for example with significant pyuria/bacteriuria in addition to the findings suggestive of pyelonephritis. The clinical presentation of renal abscess may resemble pyelonephritis if CVA tenderness is present, but this is not an invariable finding. The urinalysis in renal abscess may reveal pyuria and bacteria if the abscess is medullary but only pyuria if the renal abscess is cortical. Renal imaging studies are usually unnecessary in cystitis or pyelonephritis. If there is confusion regarding the presence or absence of chronic pyelonephritis, then a computed tomography/magnetic resonance imaging (CT/MRI) scan of the abdomen or renal ultrasound is appropriate.

Chronic Pyelonephritis

Chronic pyelonephritis results in shrunken and distorted kidneys with a distorted collecting system. If the patient presents with *chronic pyelonephritis* and has kidneys of normal or large size, then an alternate explanation should be sought. The only way to diagnose a renal abscess with certainty is with renal imaging studies. For this purpose, the CT/MRI of the kidneys is vastly superior in picking up small lesions than is the renal ultrasound. For the purposes of excluding a renal abscess, a negative renal ultrasound should never be used to rule out the diagnosis. A negative renal ultrasound should always be followed with a renal CT/MRI of the kidneys if a renal abscess is in the differential diagnosis.

Therapeutic Considerations

ACUTE CYSTITIS

The initial episode of acute complicated cystitis in a normal host without GU abnormalities/preexisting renal disease need not be treated with antimicrobial therapy. Usually treatment with phenazopyridine (Pyridium), which has no antibacterial effect, is sufficient to relieve bladder spasm and the relative urine obstruction because of the bladder spasm, and the bacteria will spontaneously clear itself without antimicrobial therapy.

Repeated episodes of acute cystitis should have appropriate diagnostic studies, for example a urinalysis and urinary culture with sensitivities with each episode to differentiate reinfection from relapse. If cystitis occurs in a nonleukopenic compromised host (e.g., with diabetes mellitus, systemic lupus erythematosus, multiple myeloma, cirrhosis, etc.), then a seven-day course of therapy is recommended with an oral agent such as nitrofurantoin (Macrodantin), trimethoprim-sulfamethoxazole (TMP-SMX) (Bactrim), or amoxicillin (Amoxil). Ampicillin should be avoided because of its resistance potential with coliform bacteria.

DYSURIA-PYURIA SYNDROME

The dysuria-pyuria syndrome because of *Chlamydia* should be treated with a two-week course of doxycycline (Vibramycin). Patients unable to tolerate doxycycline (Vibramycin) may be treated with a macrolide for the same period of time. A grossly hemorrhagic cystitis suggests a viral etiology for which no specific therapy is available. Patients with cystitis and microscopic hematuria are often infected with *S. saprophyticus*.

Fortunately, *S. saprophyticus* is susceptible to a wide range of antibiotics and virtually any agent selected to treat a UTI will be effective. Antimicrobial resistance has not been a problem in *S. saprophyticus* UTIs. Chronic interstitial cystitis is not an infectious disorder and therefore antimicrobial therapy is unnecessary.

CATHETER-ASSOCIATED BACTERIURIA

CAB in hospitalized patients who are normal hosts without structural abnormalities need not be treated, because virtually all of these patients are colonized and not infected. CAB in nonleukopenic compromised hosts (with diabetes mellitus, systemic lupus erythematosus, multiple myeloma, cirrhosis, and so forth), should be treated to prevent ascending infection/bacteremia from the lower urinary tract. Such individuals should be treated with an oral agent such as amoxicillin (Amoxil), nitrofurantoin (Macrodantin), or TMP-SMX (Bactrim) for 1 to 2 weeks.

Nonleukopenic compromised hosts with enterococci CAB are best treated with oral nitrofurantoin (Macrodantin), which is effective against enterococcal strains such as *S. faecalis* (non-vancomycin-resistant *Enterococcus* [non-VRE]) as well as *E. faecium* [VRE]). *Enterococcus faecalis* strains may also be treated with oral amoxicillin (Amoxil). These instances represent prophylaxis/early therapy because the majority of patients who are nonleukopenic-compromised hosts will have colonization of the urinary tract prior to catheterization or rapidly develop it soon thereafter. Therefore, prevention of ascending infection/bacteremia is the primary aim of therapy in patients with CAB who are compromised on the basis of their host defenses or GU tract abnormalities (e.g., ureteral stents).

ACUTE PYELONEPHRITIS

Acute pyelonephritis may be caused by aerobic gram-negative bacilli, such as coliforms or enterococci (almost always *E. faecalis*). The empirical treatment of pyelonephritis is based on a Gram stain of the urine, which, if the diagnosis is pyelonephritis, will show significant pyuria and a single predominant organism. In a patient with presumed pyelonephritis, the absence of bacteria in the Gram stain of the urine in an acutely ill patient essentially eliminates the diagnosis of pyelonephritis from further consideration, and an alternate explanation for the patient's fever and CVA tenderness should be sought (e.g., renal imaging studies).

Because acute pyelonephritis is often accompanied by bacteremia (urosepsis), parenteral agents may be used initially followed by oral agents; or in mild-to-moderate cases, oral agents may be used for the entire course of therapy. The parenteral agents useful in the treatment of acute pyelonephritis because of aerobic

---

 CURRENT DIAGNOSIS

- Acute uncomplicated cystitis is the most common type of UTI in adult women.
- The initial peak incidence of cystitis occurs with sexual intercourse and gradually increases through adulthood.
- Cystitis may occur as a single event or may be recurrent because of reinfection or relapse.
- Cystitis is usually caused by coliform or enterococci from the fecal flora or by *Staphylococcus saprophyticus* from the skin flora.
- Clinically, cystitis is marked by low-grade fever (≤38.9°C [102°F]) with lower abdominal/suprapubic discomfort, and/or dysuria.
- *Staphylococcus aureus*, *Streptococcus pneumoniae*, groups A, C, G streptococci, and *Bacteroides fragilis* are not uropathogens in cystitis.
- In elderly women, *cystitis* manifests as pyuria and bacterluria without fever or dysuria, which is termed *benign bacteriuria of the elderly*.
- A variant of cystitis, the so-called *dysuria/pyuria syndrome* is also known as *abacteriuric cystitis*.
- Dysuria/pyuria syndrome, most common in young adult women, manifests as cystitis, but urine cultures are negative for bacteria or uropathogens such as *Escherichia coli* are present in low numbers. *Chlamydia trachomatis* is frequently isolated if the urine is cultured for *Chlamydia*.
- Pyelonephritis in women may occur as an uncommon complication of cystitis or during pregnancy.
- It is not possible to predict the uropathogen of cystitis from clinical features except for *S. saprophyticus*.
- *S. saprophyticus* cystitis is characterized by a fishy urine odor, microscopic hematuria, and an alkaline urinary pH.
- Cystitis with alkaline urine suggests infection secondary to *S. saprophyticus*, *Ureaplasma urealyticum*, or a struvite stone with associated infection caused by a urea-splitting organism such as *Proteus*.
- Microscopic hematuria is common with *S. saprophyticus* cystitis but is uncommon with other uropathogens. If a patient with cystitis and microscopic hematuria fails to promptly resolve with antimicrobial therapy, work up the patient for a bladder/renal neoplasm or renal TB.
- The diagnosis of cystitis in women is made by demonstrating pyuria and significant bacteriuria (≥ 10^6 col/mL) in the setting of cystitis symptoms.
- Cystitis symptoms with gross hematuria should suggest a viral hemorrhagic cystitis or a renal lesion.
- Pyuria without bacteriuria indicates urinary tract inflammation. Persistent pyuria without bacteriuria should suggest interstitial cystitis or renal TB.
- With cystitis, the specific gravity of the urine is not decreased in contrast to pyelonephritis where the specific gravity is decreased.
- Urinary concentration returns to normal with treatment in pyelonephritis.
- Pyelonephritis may be differentiated from cystitis by the presence of fever ≥38.9°C (102°F) and otherwise unexplained unilateral CVA tenderness.
- The urine analysis/culture findings in pyelonephritis and cystitis are the same. Bacteremia frequently occurs with pyelonephritis but is not a feature of cystitis in normal hosts.
- Nonleukopenic compromised hosts, such as diabetes mellitus, systemic lupus erythematosus, multiple myeloma, cirrhosis, and so on, with cystitis may be complicated by pyelonephritis or bacteremia.
- Pyelonephritis is caused by the same uropathogens that cause cystitis; however, *S. saprophyticus* occurs only in cystitis.
- Acute pyelonephritis clinically improves unless complicated by renal abscess.
- Clinically, pyelonephritis is almost always unilateral, but pathophysical findings may be bilateral.
- Bilateral CVA tenderness should suggest an alternate diagnosis.
- In pyelonephritis, radiologic studies typically show unilateral renal involvement characterized by cortical scarring, medullary abnormalities, and renal shrinkage.
- Bilateral, normal-sized, or enlarged kidneys should suggest an alternate diagnosis to pyelonephritis.

Abbreviations: CVA = costovertebral angle; TB = tuberculosis; UTI = urinary tract infection.

Rakel and Bope: *Conn's Current Therapy 2006.*

gram-negative bacilli include aminoglycosides, aztreonam (Azactam), antipseudomonal penicillin (e.g., ticarcillin [Ticar]), piperacillin (Pipracil), or a renally excreted respiratory quinolone. Patients presenting with acute pyelonephritis, who have streptococci in the Gram stain of the urine indicating enterococci, may be treated empirically with ampicillin and antipseudomonal penicillin, ticarcillin (Ticar), piperacillin (Pipracil), or meropenem (Merrem). In the rare instance where there is enterococcal urosepsis complicating acute pyelonephritis because of VRE, then linezolid (Zyvox), quinupristin-dalfopristin (Synercid), or daptomycin (Cubicin) may be used. In patients presenting with acute pyelonephritis where a Gram stain is unobtainable or unavailable, then empirical coverage for both aerobic gram-negative bacilli and enterococci (*E. faecalis*), may be achieved with antipseudomonal penicillins, nonrenally eliminated respiratory quinolones, or meropenem (Merrem). After the organism responsible for the pyelonephritis is subsequently identified by urine/blood culture, then the patient may be switched to one of the agents mentioned. Similarly, if the patient is shown to have enterococci as the cause of their urosepsis, it may be treated initially as non-VRE, as indicated previously in the article. Patients with pyelonephritis are usually treated for 1 to 2 weeks.

Particularly in critically ill patients, initial therapy is often started parenterally. Patients may be switched to an oral agent as soon as the patient clinically defervesces or treated entirely by an oral agent for the duration of therapy. The ideal oral antibiotic has the same spectrum as its parenteral counterpart and has excellent bioavailability; blood/tissue levels are approximately the same after intravenous/oral (IV/PO) administration. For example, by giving 1 g of amoxicillin (Amoxil) every 8 hours, the same blood/tissue levels are achieved as by giving ampicillin by intramuscular injection (IM). Nonrenally eliminated respiratory quinolones, such as levofloxacin (Levaquin) and gatifloxacin

 CURRENT THERAPY

- Virtually all cases of initial uncomplicated cystitis will resolve spontaneously with or without treatment. No urine analysis/culture is needed with the initial episode of cystitis.
- For the dysuria of cystitis, phenazopyridine (Pyridium), which has no antibacterial properties but relieves pain and relative urinary obstruction from muscle spasm, may be used. Relief of spasm promptly clears the bacteriuria.
- Recurrent cystitis of the reinfection variety is because of different uropathogens with each episode that the urine is cultured. Reinfection is related to vaginal introital colonization following sexual intercourse and may be treated with a postcoital/HS of an appropriate antibiotic.
- Although the initial attack of cystitis resolves in virtually all patients without treatment, those who prefer to treat may use single-dose therapy with nitrofurantoin (Macrodantin), TMP-SMX (Bactrim), or amoxicillin (Amoxil).
- Cystitis in a nonleukopenic compromised host (discussed previously) should be treated for 1 to 2 weeks to prevent bacteremia/ascending infection, such as pyelonephritis/renal abscess.
- Ampicillin should be avoided because of its high resistance potential. Amoxicillin should be used instead, which has not been associated with resistance and is effective against the common coliforms and enterococci (*Enterococcus faecalis*).
- Nitrofurantoin has no resistance potential, is effective against all common uropathogens and all enterococci, such as *E. faecalis* (non-VRE) and *Enterococcus faecium* (VRE). Nitrofurantoin

(Macrodantin) is useful in cystitis or catheter-associated bacteremia but is not to be used in pyelonephritis/bacteremia.
- Recurrent UTI of the relapse variety is caused by the same uropathogen with each occurrence. The problem in relapse UTIs is not therapeutic but diagnostic. Relapsing UTIs have an underlying structural abnormality or ureteral shunts that do not permit antimicrobial therapy to be effective.
- The treatment of pyelonephritis is with IV or PO antibiotics, depending on the severity of the clinical manifestation. Treatment is for 2 to 4 weeks with an effective antibiotic.
- For pyelonephritis, parenteral agents useful against coliforms are cephalosporins, aztreonam (Azactam), aminoglycosides, TMP-SMZ (Bactrim), or renally eliminated quinolones. Against enterococci (most of which are non-VRE), parenteral ampicillin, antipseudomonal penicillins, and meropenem (Merrem) are useful.
- Oral antibiotics useful against coliform causes of pyelonephritis include renally eliminated quinolones, amoxicillin (Amoxil), antipseudomonal penicillins, or TMP-SMZ (Bactrim).
- Linezolid (Zyvox) may be used for pyelonephritis caused by enterococci (non-VRE), amoxicillin (Amoxil), or for VRE.
- Patients with acute pyelonephritis become afebrile/nearly afebrile within 72 hours with or without treatment. Persistence of high fevers for greater than 72 hours should be considered as representing a renal abscess until proved otherwise.

Abbreviations: HD = half dose; IM = intramuscular; IV = intravenous; TMP-SMZ = trimethoprim-sulfamethoxazole; UTI = urinary tract infection; VRE = vancomycin-resistant *Enterococcus.*

Rakel and Bope: *Conn's Current Therapy 2006.*

(Tequin), achieve the same blood and tissue levels when given either by the IV or PO route. This permits completion of therapy at home and does not require 2 to 4 weeks of inpatient hospitalization for intravenous drug therapy. There is some rationale for treating acute pyelonephritis for an extended period, such as 2 to 4 weeks, to prevent chronic pyelonephritis.

CHRONIC PYELONEPHRITIS

Patients with chronic pyelonephritis are a therapeutic challenge because of the distorted intrarenal architecture and decreased blood supply to the kidney, which limits access of white blood cells (WBCs), impairs host defenses, and limits penetration of the antibiotic into the infected/diseased areas of the kidney. Treatment of chronic pyelonephritis should be based on susceptibility testing of the isolates that are present in the urine. In chronic pyelonephritis, bacteriuria is intermittent but is present over a long period of time and will persist after short or inadequate treatment. The antibiotic selected should be effective against the isolate recovered from the urine in patients with chronic pyelonephritis and possess the ability to penetrate into diseased kidneys. The ideal oral agents for therapy are TMP-SMX (Bactrim), doxycycline (Vibramycin), or a nonrenally eliminated respiratory quinolone.

RENAL ABSCESS

Acute pyelonephritis treated appropriately results in a rapid defervescence of temperature and decrease in CVA tenderness within 72 hours. If the temperature does not decrease after 72 hours of appropriate therapy, suggest a renal abscess until proved otherwise. Renal abscesses should be treated for the presumed organism based on the location of the abscess by renal imaging studies. If sensitivities from an isolate available from the urine or percutaneous aspiration of the abscess are unavailable, then empirical treatment directed against aerobic gram-negative bacilli for medullary abscesses is indicated. Treatment is the same as for pyelonephritis except is more prolonged and should be given until the abscess is drained or it resolves. For cortical abscesses in the absence of culture and sensitivity data, antibiotic therapy should be directed against *Staphylococcus aureus* and *E. faecalis*, and treated in the same manner as pyelonephritis but for an extended period of time. Acute pyelonephritis with or without acteremia is usually treated for 7 days.

RECURRENT UTIs

Reinfection may be treated with nitrofurantoin (Macrodantin), TMP-SMX (Bactrim), or amoxicillin (Amoxil) as a single postcoital dose. Therapeutic approach to relapse is to remove the underlying condition responsible for perpetuating the bacteriuria. Antimicrobial therapy may be selected based on the susceptibility of the organism, but antimicrobial therapy alone will not eradicate the relapsing form of recurrent UTI.

Rakel and Bope: *Conn's Current Therapy 2006.*

REFERENCES

Cunha BA: Clinical concepts in the treatment of urinary tract infections. Antibiotics for the Clinician 1999;3:88-93.
Cunha BA: Nosocomial catheter-associated urinary tract infections. Hosp Physician 1986;22:13-16.
Cunha BA: *Staphylococcus saprophyticus* urinary tract infections. Intern Med 1985;6:82-89.
Cunha BA: Single-dose therapy of urinary tract infections. Hosp Physician 1983;19:35-37.
Cunha BA. Urinary tract infections: Pathophysiology/diagnosis. Postgrad Med 1981;70:141-145.
Cunha BA: Urinary tract infections: Therapy. Postgrad Med 1981;70:149-157.
Cunha BA, Comer JB: Pharmacokinetic considerations in the treatment of urinary tract infections. Conn Med 1979;43:347-353.
Gupta K, Hooton TM, Roberts PL, Stamm WE: Patient-initiated treatment of uncomplicated recurrent urinary tract infections in young women. Ann Intern Med 2001;135:9.
Hooton TM: The current management strategies for community-acquired urinary tract infection. Infect Dis Clin North Am 2003;17:303-332.
Kahan E, Kahan NR, Chinitz DP: Urinary tract infection in women—Physician's preferences for treatment and adherence to guidelines: A national drug utilization study in a managed care setting. Eur J Clin Pharmacol 2003;59:663-668.
Kraft JK, Stamey TA: The natural history of symptomatic recurrent bacteriuria in women. Medicine (Baltimore) 1977;56:55.
Meiland R, Geerlings SE, Hoepelman LI: Management of bacterial urinary tract infections in adult patients with diabetes mellitus. Drugs 2002;62:1859-1868.
Miller LG, Tang AW: Treatment of uncomplicated urinary tract infections in an era of increasing antimicrobial resistance. Mayo Clin Proc 2004;79:1048-1053.
Nicolle LE: Urinary tract infection: Traditional pharmacologic therapies. Am J Med 2002;113(Suppl 1A):35S-44S.
Nicolle LE, Ronald AR: Recurrent urinary tract infection in adult women: Diagnosis and treatment. Infect Dis Clin North Am 1987;1;793.
Ronald AR, Conway B: An approach to urinary tract infection in women. Infection 1992;20(Suppl 3):S203.
Schaeffer AJ, Stuppy BA: Efficacy and safety of self-start therapy in women with recurrent urinary tract infections. J Urol 1999;161:207.
Wong ES, McKevitt M, Running K, et al: Management of recurrent urinary tract infections with patient administered single-dose therapy. Ann Intern Med 1985;102:302.

10

Bacterial Infections of the Urinary Tract in Girls

Method of
Candice E. Johnson, MD, PhD

Urinary tract infections (UTIs) are bacterial infections of any mucosal surface of the urinary tract including the urethra, the bladder, the ureters, and the renal calyces, as well as the renal parenchyma (Box 1). The best indicator for differentiating clinical pyelonephritis from cystitis is fever higher than 38.5°C (101.3°F). The classification of UTIs by anatomic location is complicated by the ascending nature of virtually all these infections. Thus, a girl with pyelonephritis usually has cystitis and urethritis simultaneously. Box 2 gives the

---

BOX 1 Classification of Urinary Tract Infections

- **Urethritis:** Dysuria, frequency or enuresis, accompanied by pyuria, but colony count of 10^3/mL of urine or less.
- **Cystitis:** Afebrile UTI. Dysuria, frequency or enuresis with colony count of at least 10^4/mL of urine. Hematuria may be present, but casts, flank pain, temperature more than 38.5°C (101.3°F) and systemic toxicity are absent.
- **Clinical pyelonephritis:** Febrile UTI (≥38°C [100.4°F]), usually accompanied by flank and abdominal pain. The colony count is usually greater than or equal to 10^5/mL of urine except with *Staphylococcus saprophyticus* or enterococci. Cystitis symptoms may also be present.
- **Proved pyelonephritis:** Shows evidence of acute inflammation on radiologic evaluation by CT, ultrasound, or radionuclide scan.

Abbreviations: CT = computed tomography; UTI = urinary tract infection.

---

colony count criteria generally accepted for clinical use, although research studies are usually more stringent.

Epidemiology and Pathogenesis

Approximately 2.2% of girls will have a UTI in the first 24 months of life. In the first year of life, most UTIs in females are febrile and may be hard to diagnose. Because of this difficulty, girls younger than 36 months with no source of fever should have a urine culture and urinalysis obtained. Unfortunately, the sensitivity of a standard urinalysis is only 82%, although it is 92% specific. For unknown reasons, the prevalence of UTI is much higher in white compared with African American girls, with Hispanics having a rate between the two groups.

Risk factors for UTI include:

- A history of recurrent UTI in the mother
- Family history of vesicoureteral reflux (VUR)
- Dysfunctional voiding patterns
- Constipation

Cleanliness and methods of wiping with toilet paper are not risk factors. In girls, an "unstable bladder" is the main cause of dysfunctional voiding. An unstable bladder has strong contractions at volumes 50% to 75% of capacity. These contractions cause both frequency

---

BOX 2 Colony Count Criteria for Urinary Tract Infection in Children

- If suprapubic aspiration is performed any growth is significant for UTI
- If catheterization of female is performed greater than 1000 CFU/mL is significant for UTI
- If clean-void urine is performed greater than 10,000 CFU/mL in pure culture is suggestive; >100,000 CFU/mL is highly likely.
- Growth of two or more species suggests contamination, but does not exclude true infection. Repeat the culture.

BOX 3 Antibiotic Choices for the Treatment of Urinary Tract Infections

Oral

- Trimethoprim (Primsol oral solution)—8-12 mg/kg/day divided every 12 hours (max dose 320 mg).
- Trimethoprim-sulfamethoxazole (TMP/SMX) (Bactrim, Septra)—8-12 mg of TMP component divided every 12 hours (max dose 320 mg).
- Amoxicillin (Amoxil)—children <40 kg: 40 mg/kg/day divided every 12 hours; children >40 kg: 875 mg every 12 hours.
- Cephalosporins:
  Cefprozil (Cefzil)[1]—30 mg/kg/day divided every 12 hours (max dose 1 g/day).
  Cefixime (generic only)—infants and children: 8 mg/kg/day divided every 12 hours; adolescents and adults: 400 mg/day divided every 12-24 hours.
  Cefdinir (Omnicef)[1]—Infants and children (older than 6 months to 12 years): 14 mg/kg/day divided every 12 hours (max dose 600 mg/day).
  Cephalexin (Keflex)—25-50 mg/kg/day divided every 6 to 8 hours (max dose 4 g/day).
- Nitrofurantoin (Macrodantin) for afebrile infections only—5-7 mg/kg/day divided every 6 hours; children older than 12 years and adults, 300 mg every 12 hours or 600 mg every 24 hours.

Parenteral

- Gentamicin (Garamycin)—5-6 mg/kg/day divided every 8 hours or 5 mg/kg as a single dose every 24 hours (with measured levels after third dose).
- Trimethoprim sulfamethoxazole (Bactrim, Septra) at 8 mg/kg/day of the TMP component, divided every 12 hours.
- Cephalosporins:
  Ceftriaxone (Rocephin)—50 mg/kg/day once every 24 hours.
  Ceftazidime (Fortaz)—100-150 mg/kg/day divided every 8 hours; (max dose : 600 mg)
  Cefotaxime (Claforan)—50-150 mg/kg/day divided every 6-8 hours. (max dose: 12 grams/day)
- Fluoroquinolones are not approved for under age 18 years, but may be required for resistant organisms.

[1]Not FDA approved for this indication.

---

and incontinence, and girls may sit on their feet to attempt to prevent voiding (Vincent's curtsy). In the most severe cases the girl tightens the external sphincter during bladder contraction, and this leads to high bladder pressure. A thickened and trabeculated bladder often occurs as well as VUR.

Diagnosis

A high index of suspicion is needed to diagnose all UTIs, especially those in infants and toddlers. In addition to fever, manifesting symptoms include anorexia and emesis, abdominal pain, fussiness, neonatal jaundice, poor weight gain, enuresis, and hematuria.

Urine should be collected only by catheter or suprapubic aspiration until the child is toilet trained, because urine bags have contamination rates of up to 50%.

Rakel and Bope: *Conn's Current Therapy 2006.*

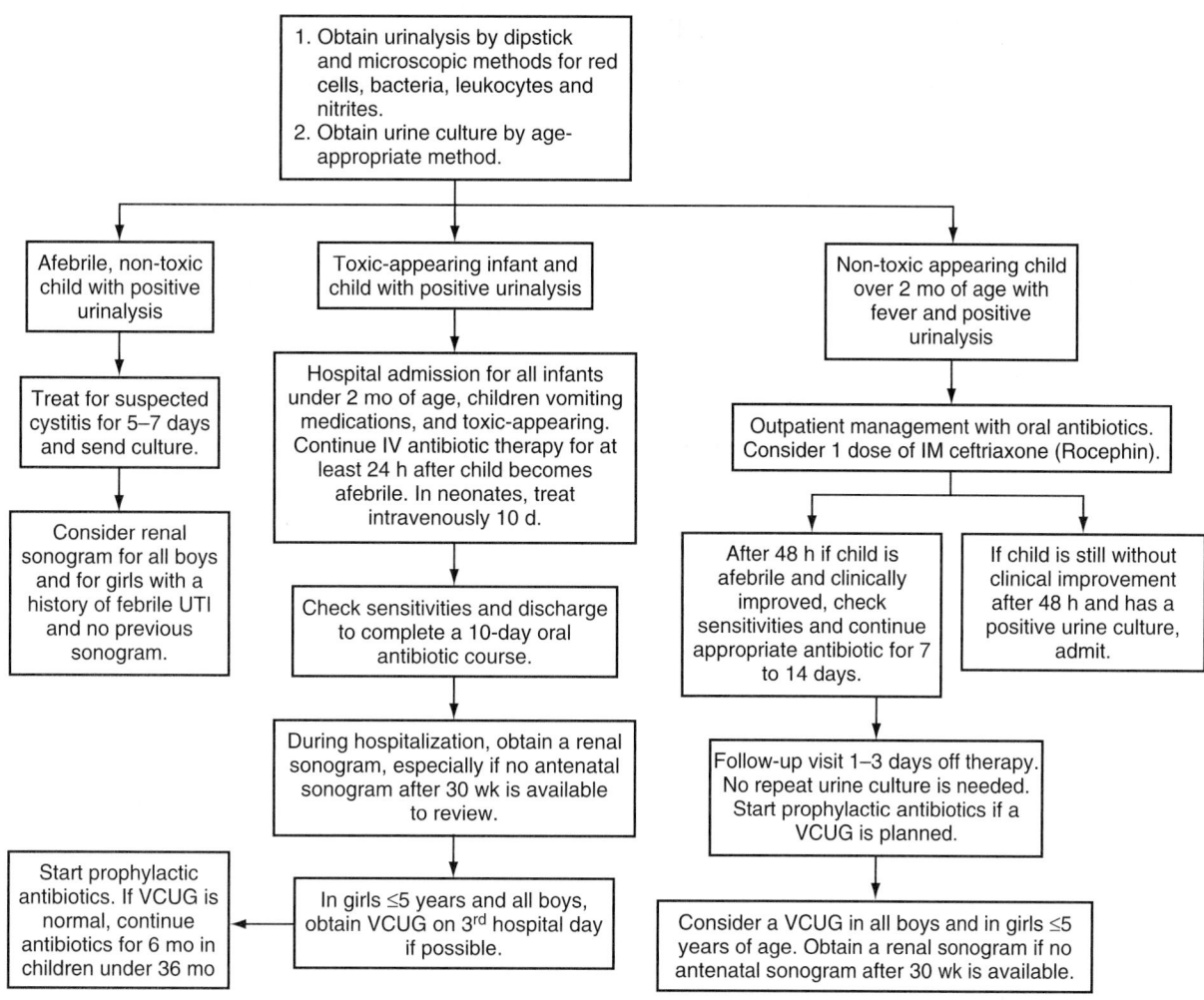

FIGURE 1. Treatment of suspected urinary tract infection in children younger than 13 years old.

Box 2 shows the colony counts that best differentiate real UTIs from contamination.

Urinalysis continues to be performed in most laboratories by a dipstick combined with spun urine sediment. This continues despite studies since 1983 showing that unspun urine counted in a hemocytometer is more sensitive and specific. In a private office, the dipstick results for leukocyte esterase, nitrites, and hematuria are sufficient to decide on empirical treatment of girls. Urine cultures should still be sent, even with a negative dipstick, because, unlike adult women, radiologic workups may be needed for confirmed UTIs in girls.

Treatment of Afebrile Urinary Tract Infection

Treatment of a girl with an afebrile UTI (cystitis or lower tract) is straightforward, requiring only a knowledge of national and local antibiotic resistance rates. *Escherichia coli* causes more than 90% of cystitis in girls, with other Enterobacteriaceae and *Staphylococcus saprophyticus* comprising the remainder. *E. coli* is

resistant to amoxicillin (Amoxil) more than 50% of the time, so this is not appropriate initial therapy. Rates of resistance to trimethoprim (Proloprim) and sulfonamides are highest in the Pacific Coast states, and rates of first-generation cephalosporin resistance vary widely. Drugs that retain high sensitivity rates are the second- and third-generation cephalosporins and nitrofurantoin (Macrodantin). Box 3 provides doses of commonly used drugs, and amoxicillin is preferred if the organism is sensitive.

Treatment of Febrile Urinary Tract Infection

Unlike the majority of viral and bacterial infections, a single kidney infection may cause permanent damage (i.e., renal scarring) if not treated rapidly and with effective antibiotics. In 1999, outpatient management of febrile UTIs was demonstrated to be effective in a study of 306 children under 24 months of age. A 2004 study in Montreal of 291 patients who were 3 months to 5 years of age showed that at least 75% of febrile children with

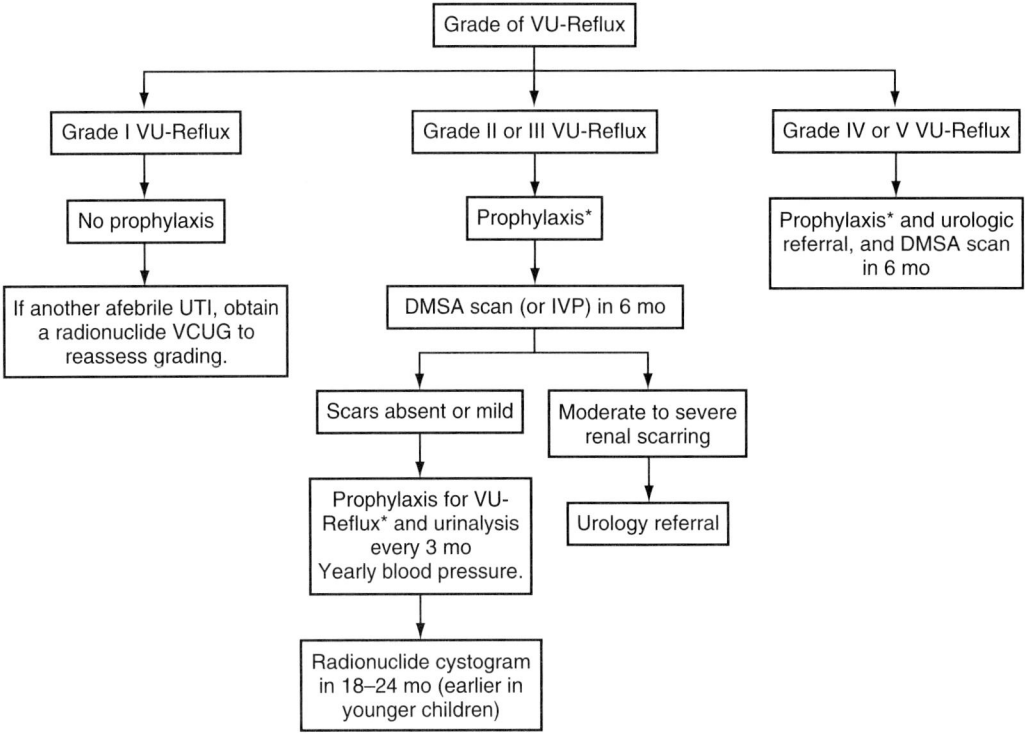

*Trimethoprim (Primsol) (1–2 mg/kg/d at bedtime) or nitrofurantoin (Macrodantin) (same dosage)

FIGURE 2. Radiologic management of a child with vesicoureteral reflux.

UTI could be managed in a day treatment center (DTC). These children had a mean of 3.5 visits to the DTC for intravenous gentamicin (Garamycin), followed by an oral antibiotic to complete 10 days of treatment.

BOX 4 Proposed Criteria for Hospitalization of Children With Febrile Urinary Tract Infection

- Sufficient emesis is present to prevent oral therapy.
- Family is judged likely to be noncompliant with antibiotics or follow-up appointments.
- Toxic or ill-appearing child which is suggestive of sepsis.
- Age is younger than 2 months.
- Prolonged duration of symptoms exists (>5 days).
- Renal scarring or impaired renal function is known to be present.
- Diabetes, AIDS, sickle cell, or other serious chronic disease is present.

Successful treatment was seen in 97% of the UTI episodes, and all first UTIs were evaluated by renal sonography and cystography at the DTC.

Because the DTC concept is not widely available for children in the United States, Figure 1 shows a suggested decision tree that does not use a DTC. Inpatient management is recommended for infants younger than 8 weeks as they do not absorb oral antibiotics predictably. Box 4 lists other variables to consider in deciding on inpatient versus outpatient treatment. Antibiotic choices are given in Box 3. Duration of symptoms before presentation is very important, because renal scarring was seen in British studies after as few as 5 days of delayed diagnosis.

Once on antibiotic therapy, defervescence may be expected in approximately 68% of children younger than 2 years by 24 hours and in 89% by 48 hours. The 11% who remain febrile at 48 hours were no more likely to have renal abscesses or hydronephrosis than the others, and they may be discharged after sensitivities

---

TABLE 1 Prophylactic Antibiotics for Childhood Urinary Tract Infections

Drug	Dose	Timing	Side effects
Trimethoprim-sulfamethoxazole (TMP-SMX) (Bactrim)	2 mg/kg of TMP component (up to 40 mg)	Bedtime	Rash in ~6%
Nitrofurantoin (Macrodantin capsules 25, 50, or 100 mg preferred over oral suspension)	1-2 mg/kg/d up to 100 mg	Bedtime	Vomiting, abdominal pain
Trimethoprim (Primsol oral solution 50 mg/mL or 100 mg tablets)	2 mg/kg up to 40 mg	Bedtime	Rash in ~1%

Rakel and Bope: *Conn's Current Therapy 2006*.

are known. It is convenient to the family to perform the cystogram, if indicated, during hospitalization and it greatly improves compliance.

Prophylaxis

There is expert agreement that further prospective studies of antibiotic prophylaxis for childhood UTI are needed. In adult women, the cost-to-benefit ratio favors prophylaxis with three or more UTIs per year. In children, because young age is the major risk for renal scarring, studies are lacking, but expert opinion favors 6 months of prophylaxis after a febrile UTI, with or without VUR. Guidelines from the American Urological Association also suggest prophylaxis for all children with VUR, but the Swedish experts suggest stopping at age 24 months in boys and 5 years in girls. Table 1 lists suggested agents. Unfortunately, the choice of antibiotic is becoming limited as trimethoprim (Proloprim) resistance rates rise.

Radiologic Evaluation

No area of childhood UTI evaluation is as controversial as determining which children merit sonography, radionuclide scans, and cystograms. Two recent studies have helped clarify these issues, and several professional academies have agreed on guidelines for febrile children younger than 2 years of age (Pediatrics, Family Practice, Emergency Physicians, Urological, and College of Radiology). These associations recommend a renal sonogram and a voiding cystogram soon after the first febrile UTI. Figure 2 indicates that the initial cystogram should be a standard fluoroscopic examination to permit accurate grading of VUR. Follow-up cystograms may be radionuclide studies, which carry less risk of gonadal radiation.

CURRENT DIAGNOSIS

- A high level of suspicion is required in all febrile infants.
- Boys outnumber girls 10:1 in the neonatal period.
- Girls are at highest risk for UTI when younger than 12 months of age and again at 3 to 5 years of age.
- Urine for culture should not be obtained with a bag, but requires a catheterization or suprapubic aspiration, if the child is not toilet trained.
- The colony count cutoff to define a UTI differs with the method used for collection.
- With a negative urinalysis, febrile UTI becomes much less likely, but an afebrile UTI cannot be ruled out.

Abbreviations: UTI = urinary tract infection.

Rakel and Bope: *Conn's Current Therapy 2006.*

CURRENT THERAPY

- Outpatient therapy of febrile UTIs is usually appropriate in infants older than 2 months of age.
- A single dose of intramuscular ceftriaxone (Rocephin) will cover the first 24 hours after diagnosis when emesis is most likely to occur and antibiotic sensitivities are unknown.
- Febrile girls should be seen between 36 and 48 hours after diagnosis to assess clinical improvements and check urine culture results.
- A voiding cystogram remains essential for febrile girls younger than 5 years of age and all boys.

Abbreviations: UTI = urinary tract infection.

Hoberman and colleagues also question the value of the initial renal sonogram. In a cohort of 309 febrile children who had paired dimercaptosuccinic acid (DMSA) radionuclide renal scans and sonography performed within 48 hours of diagnosis, neither study changed management. All had had an antenatal sonogram after 30 weeks of gestation, and anomalies were presumably corrected before UTI could occur. The argument in favor of doing this painless and medically safe study is that children with "dilating reflux" (i.e., grades III-V) would be identified, and the doctor could track down these children if they fail to keep an appointment for a cystogram. In other words, in the absence of a cystogram, a sonogram with hydronephrosis or pelvic caliectasis *will* change management. In the patient with no health insurance who cannot afford both studies, the more important study is the voiding cystogram, not the sonogram.

REFERENCES

Abelson Storby K, Osterlund A, Kahlmeter G: Antimicrobial resistance in *Escherichia coli* in urine samples from children and adults: A 12 year analysis. Acta Paediatr 2004;93:487-491.

Bollgren I: Antibacterial prophylaxis in children with urinary tract infection. Acta Paediatr 1999;(Suppl 431):48-52.

Gauthier M, Chevalie I, Sterescu A, et al: Treatment of urinary tract infections among febrile young children with daily intravenous antibiotic therapy at a day treatment center. Pediatrics 2004;114:469-476.

Hellerstein S: Urinary tract infections in children. Infections in Medicine 2002;19:554-560.

Hoberman A, Charros M, Hickey RW, et al: Imaging studies after a first febrile urinary tract infection in young children. N Engl J Med 2003;348(3):195-202.

Hoberman A, Wald ER, Hickey RW, et al: Oral versus initial intravenous therapy for urinary tract infections in young febrile children. Pediatrics 1999;104(1)79-86.

Jakobsson B, Esbjorner E, Hansson S: Minimum incidence and diagnostic rate of first urinary tract infection. Pediatrics 1999;104(2 Pt):222-226.

Johnson CE: Dysuria. In: Kliegman RM, Greebaum LA, Lye PS, (eds): Practical Strategies in Pediatric Diagnosis and Therapy, 2nd ed. Philadelphia, WB Saunders, 2004, pp 397-411.

Lin D-S, Huang F-Y, Chiu N-C, et al: Comparison of hemocytometer leukocyte counts and standard urinalysis for predicting urinary tract infections in febrile infants. Pediatr Infect Dis J 2000;19:223-227.

Lowe LH, Patel MN, Gatti JM, and Alon US: Utility of follow-up renal sonography in children with vesicoureteral reflux and normal initial sonogram. Pediatr 2004;113:548-550.

Roberts KB: A synopsis of the American Academy of Pediatrics' practice parameter on the diagnosis, treatment, and evaluation of the initial urinary tract infection in febrile infants and young children. Pediatr Rev 1999;20(10):1-4.

Rushton HG: Urinary tract infections in children: Epidemiology, evaluation, and management. Pediatr Clin North Am 1997;44(5):1133-1169.

Childhood Enuresis

Method of
Frank Cernigliar, MD

In general, *enuresis* is associated with purely nighttime wetting. The term, however, means involuntary wetting (day or night) beyond the age of anticipated control. Childhood enuresis includes both day (diurnal) and night (nocturnal) wetting. The latter is further subdivided into primary and secondary nocturnal enuresis. Enuresis is one of the most common problems seen by the pediatric primary care physician and is referred to the pediatric urologist.

The problem, which dates back to as early as 1500 BC, has been the subject of many dissertations on diagnosis, causes, and remedies. Childhood wetting problems, or voiding dysfunctions, affect 5% to 10% of school-aged children and can be a profound source of distress for the child and family as a whole. The number of potential causes for abnormal voiding include anatomic, neuropathic, and functional disorders. Most children who present with day and/or nighttime wetting have a non-neurologic functional voiding abnormality requiring no complex evaluation or invasive study.

Development of Bladder Control

Urinary continence develops in an ordered process of sequenced maturation that requires no teaching. To attain continence, one needs a low-pressure storage vessel surrounded by smooth muscle to "squeeze" out the urine from the bladder, an "involuntary" internal sphincter, and a complex external sphincteric mechanism with intertwined smooth and skeletal muscle that is under voluntary control. These three mechanisms work in accord to accomplish bladder emptying. The neonate voids by reflex through the sacral spinal cord. The bladder reaches a functional capacity stretch point, and afferent signals are sent to the spinal cord to activate sympathetic outflow to the bladder and urethra. The result is relaxation of the external sphincter and contraction of the detrusor; bladder emptying ensues.

Urinary frequency, incontinence, and nocturnal enuresis are all normal occurrences in the very young child. Infants are asleep approximately 60% of the time with 40% of their voiding episodes occurring during sleep. In year 1 of life, the child voids approximately 20 times per day. During the next 2 years, voiding frequency decreases by as much as 50% while the voided volumes (and bladder capacity) increase by as much as three to four times. Beginning at age 2 years, conscious sensation of bladder fullness develops, although control is not yet mastered. By 4 years, most children have achieved an adult pattern of voiding in which micturition can occur at less than total bladder capacity or be postponed until absolute functional bladder capacity is reached. For the transition to this pattern, three separate events must occur:

1. Capacity of bladder must increase so it can function as a reservoir.
2. The child must gain control over the external sphincter so urination can be allowed or terminated at will.
3. Direct voluntary control over the voiding reflex must develop to allow the child to initiate or inhibit bladder contraction voluntarily.

Simply put, urinary control is obtained when the bladder fills under low pressure to an adequate capacity and then can be emptied, with a detrusor contraction coordinated with complete relaxation of the external sphincter. However, one needs to understand this happens on a continuum. Nocturnal bowel control occurs first, followed by daytime bowel control, daytime urine control, and finally nighttime dryness. Most, but not all, children achieve these functions by the 4th year.

Evaluation

Pure voiding dysfunction is urinary incontinence without any underlying structural or obvious neurologic abnormality. On the whole, patients with an anatomic abnormality usually have leaked their entire lives, unable to gain continence at any point. The incontinence, instead of being diurnal or nocturnal only, is a combination of both. Children with suspected anatomic defects should be evaluated with imaging of both the kidneys and bladder by ultrasound and voiding cystogram with or without a fluoroscopic urodynamics study. Children with voiding dysfunction are able to gain continence for a varying period of time followed by incontinence.

It is important during history taking to ask the child's primary caregiver for valuable insight into the general aspects of the child's voiding habits. One should ask precise questions, understandable to the child, in order to get accurate answers. This information can be augmented with a voiding diary because many parents may not be totally aware of the specifics and finer points of the child's voiding habits.

ONSET

At what age was the child toilet trained? If the child was trained, at what point did he or she start wetting? Were there any occurrences in the child's life coinciding with the onset of wetting? Has the child ever been able to be toilet trained? Is the wetting new over the last few days, weeks, or months?

Rakel and Bope: *Conn's Current Therapy 2006.*

FREQUENCY

Voiding diaries can be very helpful in diagnosing and treating voiding abnormalities. They can be kept over a 3- to 4-day period and include voiding times, volumes, wet versus dry, and any associated symptoms. Appropriate volumes can be calculated as age (in years) plus 2 oz. One should determine if the volumes are less than expected. Does the child void infrequently with larger-than-anticipated amounts? How many voids per day? How many accidents per week? Does the child wet multiple times during the day or only at night?

CHARACTER OF VOIDING

Does the male child compress his urethra while or after voiding? Does he sit or stand to void? Can the parent hear him voiding (good forceful stream) or does he dribble? Does the little girl void with her legs tightly closed? Does she sit back on the toilet or perch on the edge of the seat to help maintain balance (causing pelvic contraction)? Is the child in a rush? Does he or she delay voiding? Is there posturing (squatting, crossing legs)?

DEGREE

Does the child wet enough to require clothes to be changed, or does the wetting consist of only spotting in the underwear? Is the wetting before voiding (unstable bladder) or after voiding (vaginal pooling)?

Two other important aspects of the history are bowel habits and family history of wetting. Any bowel dysfunction must be corrected before one can treat any wetting abnormality successfully. One should obtain a family history because it is now evident that a genetic component is linked to conditions such as primary nocturnal enuresis. One should also ask about other associated urologic, neurologic, or nephrologic conditions (valves, reflux, renal insufficiency) or any previous surgeries.

Physical Examination

Once the history is taken, the physical examination should be performed, taking into account not only vitals (height, weight, blood pressure), as a basic starting point, but the general appearance of the child. Uncleanliness, poor hygiene, or poor dentition may suggest neglect or abuse. An abdominal examination should seek to identify masses, a palpable bladder, or stool in the colon. Careful inspection of the child's back for occult spinal dysraphisms includes looking for lipomas, scoliosis, hair patches, cutaneous lesions, sacral or coccygeal defects, or gluteal asymmetry. A basic neurologic examination is essential and should include such points as gait, reflexes, and brief examination room maneuvers to substantiate that no nerve deficits are contributing to the incontinence. Examination of the rectal area is important, but often passed over, and should incorporate assessing sphincter tone, ruling out pelvic masses, and looking for signs of fecal soiling. Additionally, one should inspect the external genitalia to diagnose labial adhesions in young girls,

female epispadias (causing total incontinence), and signs of vaginal pooling (butterfly "rash" and irritation of the labia and perineal and perianal areas). In boys, one should look for narrowing or inflammation of the meatus, unretractable foreskin, hypospadias, or epispadias. If the physician can observe the child void, valuable information can be gained about the quality and pattern of the urinary stream.

Laboratory/Radiograph Examination

A urinalysis should be performed to check for infection, glucosuria, and proteinuria. A specific gravity test can exclude polyuria as a cause for incontinence and indicates if the kidneys concentrate properly. If indicated, a urine culture should be done. If all of the tests just mentioned are normal, no further testing is needed at this initial stage. After the history, physical examination, and urinalysis, the abnormality is classified as anatomic, functional, or neurogenic. When an anatomic problem is suspected, imaging of the upper tract as well as the bladder is needed. Usually a renal ultrasound and voiding cystourethrogram is performed. The same is required if the urine is infected, a neurologic disorder is diagnosed, or there is history of either. More complex testing (magnetic resonance imaging [MRI] or computed tomography [CT] scan) may need to be done if abnormal physical findings of the lower spine or sacrum are found. Although urodynamics testing may be invasive and is not done routinely as a screen, it may be valuable in those select patients with severe symptoms refractory to standard treatment or in the child with a neurologic lesion.

Diurnal Enuresis

Daytime wetting, or diurnal enuresis, is much more troubling to the school-aged child and adolescent because it is often obvious to family, friends, and peers as well as being socially unacceptable and a source of embarrassment and ridicule. Children who are wet during the day generally experience urge and urge incontinence and may be wet at night as well. They may posture, and when the urine volume is measured, a small bladder capacity may be found. Children generally outgrow daytime wetting as they mature, but until that time treatment can be offered, which parents generally expect. Initial treatment measures are usually directed toward placing the child on a timed voiding schedule (every 2 to 3 hours to empty the bladder before the child has an uninhibited bladder contraction), practicing good hygiene, and, of utmost importance, correcting constipation with stool softeners and a high-fiber diet.

The next step commonly is pharmacologic treatment of the voiding dysfunction. This must be tailored to the type of abnormality and whether there is associated infection or vesicoureteral reflux. For many years, the drug of choice has been oxybutynin (Ditropan) because the mainstay of treatment has been long-term anticholinergic use. Once the underlying bladder overactivity or instability is quashed and the overactivity of the external sphincter lessened, the result is diminished or eliminated elevated intravesical pressure. Another preparation used recently is tolterodine (Detrol).[1] Both of these drugs are now available in once-a-day long-acting formulations (Ditropan XL, Detrol LA). Both have been reported to have side effects in varying degrees such as facial flushing, dry mouth, diminished sweating, occasional blurred vision, and constipation. Other drugs, which have been used with varying levels of success, include hyoscyamine sulfate (Levsin),[1] propantheline (Pro-Banthine),[1] and dicyclomine hydrochloride (Bentyl).[1]

The child who fails initial treatment may need a further workup with fluoroscopic urodynamics studies to assess bladder function, filling pressure, and sphincter coordination with voiding.

Nocturnal Enuresis

Nocturnal enuresis (NE) has been described in early literature dating back to the Ebers papyrus with various documented causes and remedies across the centuries. It continues to be a very common problem affecting 15% to 20% of school-aged children. The prevalence falls to 5% at 10 years old and affects 1% of 15-year-old teenagers. Fifteen percent of children with monosymptomatic primary nocturnal enuresis experience spontaneous resolution each year. NE can have a serious impact on the child, leading to shame, guilt, and diminished self-esteem. Only about one third of parents seek medical attention; about the same number punish the child for wetting, mistakenly thinking laziness or purposeful behavior has caused the problem. It is therefore incumbent on anyone who treats young children to screen for bed-wetting, educate the parents, and offer treatment if appropriate.

There is no one isolated cause for bed-wetting. It has been attributed to a multifactorial maturational delay in arousal to a full bladder, a delay in maturation of the bladder resulting in a diminished nocturnal bladder capacity, and a diminished circadian rhythm of antidiuretic hormone production. Even a genetic component is implicated because bed-wetting has been shown to run in families.

Although bed-wetting is considered benign from a physical standpoint, because of the previously described negative impact, treatment options should be offered to the child age 6 years and older. The focus of the physician treating NE should be to ensure the child has no physical abnormality causing the bed-wetting. The child who has pure monosymptomatic nocturnal enuresis needs no further evaluation than a good history and physical examination and a urinalysis.

Treatment should be first directed at treating constipation or any daytime frequency or wetting component,

which can be a benign association in 15% to 25% of cases. Treatment measures should include patient education because once the child (and parents) have an understanding of the mechanisms behind bed-wetting, compliance and success of treatment often improve. Initial therapy should also center on evening fluid restriction, avoidance of caffeine and artificial dyes (particularly red number 40), and motivational therapy with rewards and praise for dry nights. The child has no control over wet nights and should never be punished for a wet bed.

If the parents decide treatment is desirable, they can choose between pharmacologic and nonpharmacologic options. For those wishing to avoid medication, conditioning therapy with a moisture-sensitive alarm is an option. Several enuresis alarms are available on the market, all with the goal of awakening the child at or shortly after the time of micturition. The first drops of urine complete a circuit, activating a buzzer designed to awaken the child. It is important for a family member to be involved in the process to ensure the child wakes up and completes the voiding process in the toilet. Over time a conditioned response develops, and the child awakens voluntarily to a full bladder without help from the alarm. This process can take weeks to months, therefore requiring a patient and dedicated family and child to achieve success. The overall success rate has been stated as 50%, but with family involvement and proper use it can be as high as 70% to 90%.

Additional nonpharmacologic treatments offered include motivational therapy, bladder training exercises, hypnotherapy, bladder training, night wakening, and fluid restriction and diet therapy. All except motivational therapy have shown disappointing results.

The alternative to the alarm is pharmacologic treatment. The most commonly used drug now is desmopressin acetate (DDAVP) in tablet form and less commonly nasal spray. Desmopressin acetate is a synthetic analogue of vasopressin, a potent antidiuretic hormone produced by the pituitary gland. Desmopressin acetate tablets are dosed starting at 0.2 mg 1 hour before bed (food and drink should be withheld 1 hour before dosing) and increased by one tablet per week up to 0.6 mg or until dryness is achieved at a lower dose. Success rates increase with higher doses and can be as high as 60% to 70%. Side effects are rare even at the higher doses. If a child responds, that dose is continued for 3 to 6 months before structured weaning by one less tablet a night per week. The drug can also be used

---

 CURRENT THERAPY

- Treatment of constipation is the initial measure.
- Children should not be punished for wet nights.
- For the bed-wetting alarms to be effective, family involvement is critical.
- Patience and understanding of the process are important for compliance with therapy and attaining success.

---

[1]Not FDA approved for this indication.

CURRENT DIAGNOSIS

- Obtain a good voiding history, including family history of wetting, history of all elimination habits, and dietary history.
- Do a thorough physical examination, including neurologic and rectal if appropriate and indicated.
- Educate the family and debunk any myths about wetting.
- Give the family multiple treatment options, both pharmacologic and nonpharmacologic, including observation.

long term without reservation. Another advantage is its ability to be used intermittently in situations like nightly or weekend sleepovers at a friend's house or overnight trips.

Another acceptable alternative is imipramine (Tofranil), a tricyclic antidepressant that has generalized effects on the bladder including weak α-adrenergic and anticholinergic effects. It weakly increases arousal and additionally may have some antidiuretic properties. Dosage begins at 25 mg at bedtime and is increased if necessary to 50 mg at bedtime in preadolescents and 75 mg per night in adolescents. There has been some hesitancy recently using imipramine because of certain profound side effects that have been observed. These include insomnia, weight loss, extrapyramidal symptoms, anxiety, and personality changes. Fatal cardiac dysrhythmias have been reported with overdosage. If dosed properly, imipramine can be an effective and safe drug. If effective, medicine is dosed for 6 months before attempts to wean.

REFERENCES

Cendron M: Primary nocturnal enuresis: Current concepts. Is Fam Physician 1999;59:1295-1213.
Hinsl KK, Hurwitz RS: Urol Clin North Am 1991;18(2):283-293.
Roth DR: Enuresis. In Rakel RE, Bope ET (eds): Conn's Current Therapy 2003, 55th ed. Philadelphia, Elsevier Science, 2003.
Rushton HG: Wetting and functional voiding disorders. Urol Clin North Am 1995;22(1):75-93.
Rushton HG, Belman AB: Enuresis and voiding dysfunction: A national kidney foundation guide to the child who wets. Washington, DC, Children's National Medical Center, 1999.

Urinary Incontinence

Method of
Niall T.M. Galloway, MD

Key Points

- Incontinence is a very common condition and patterns of problems run in families.
- There are many contributing causes and most are readily treated.
- Simple treatments are effective, but results are best when the treatment starts early.
- Surgery should be reserved for those with moderate or severe symptoms who have failed conservative therapy.

Definition

The unwanted or involuntary loss of urine that is objectively demonstrable and is a social or hygienic problem.

10

Significance

- More than 25 million Americans suffer from bladder control problems.
- Incontinence is more common in women than men, but all ages may be affected.
- Incontinence may occur after childbirth or after pelvic surgery (e.g., hysterectomy or prostatectomy).
- Prevalence is greater in the elderly (3% of women ages 20 to 29 years, 32% of women >80 years old).

Cost of incontinence can be measured in personal, social, and economic terms.

- Personal issues—loss of confidence, reduced quality of life, negative impact on employment, restriction of activities
- Social—isolation, unable to do sports or exercise, and later not able to go out are often the key factors that push the elderly out of their homes and into residential care
- Economic—$27.8 billion a year estimated to be spent on continence treatments and care for those older than 65 years of age in the United States; more feminine protection products are used to control incontinence problems than for menstrual loss

The Agency for Health Care Policy and Research (AHCPR) developed a *Clinical Practice Guideline for Urinary Incontinence* in 1996, which was published by the U.S. Department of Health and Human Services. This guideline has been accepted widely, for the evaluation and management of urinary incontinence, as a standard for care by medical and nursing practitioners.

Causes

Incontinence can be caused by many factors.

Stress incontinence is used to describe leakage that occurs with coughing, sneezing, or lifting. Stress incontinence implies weakness of the closure mechanism (urethral sphincter muscle). Elements include anatomic displacement of the bladder base, incompetence of the bladder neck, and/or intrinsic urethral sphincter weakness.

Urge incontinence describes leakage that occurs with a strong feeling of needing to go, but the patient is not able to hold on without leaking. Urge leakage is usually more difficult for the patient, because it is unpredictable and often sudden. When urge leakage does occur, it may be a flood (large volume of loss) rather than drops. Urge may be a result of inappropriate contractions of the bladder (overactive bladder) or unwanted relaxation of the pelvic floor and sphincter muscles. Stroke, spinal cord injury, MS (multiple sclerosis), and other nervous system problems can be associated factors.

Overflow incontinence implies that the bladder fails to empty properly. The overfull bladder will spill over as the pressure within exceeds the closure pressure of the urethra. Overflow leakage will occur with any activity by day and at night. Failure to empty the bladder may lead to increased bladder pressures, which will offer resistance to drainage of urine from the kidneys and can lead to kidney damage.

Extraurethral leakage implies that the urine is not leaking from the natural opening of the urethra, but from an abnormal opening. Extraurethral leakage is rare and is usually the result of previous surgery. In adults, there may be a fistula (abnormal opening) from the bladder into the vagina after hysterectomy.

In addition, unwanted urinary leakage can be provoked by other factors that are not related to bladder and urethral function. Epileptic seizures are classically associated with urinary leakage. Coma or excessive sedation can provoke overfilling of the urinary bladder and lead to incontinence. Excessive or inappropriate medications can provoke or exacerbate problems of urinary incontinence. Diuretics can provoke increased urine volume, antihypertensive agents can relax the smooth muscle of the bladder neck and worsen leakage problems. Anti-inflammatory medications and analgesics can provoke incontinence and worsen leakage. Review of medications is always helpful.

There are physical factors in the pelvis that will predispose to incontinence. The bladder shares space in the pelvis with the other pelvic organs, including the colon and rectum, and in women, the uterus and cervix. Enlargement of the uterus during pregnancy will compress the bladder and leave little or no space in the bladder to hold urine. In the final weeks of a pregnancy, urinary symptoms may include increased frequency, nocturia, or urgency, and urinary leakage is a common complaint. The enlarged uterus, crowded with fibroid tumors, can provoke incontinence in the same way. The constipated bowel, loaded with stool, can provoke unwanted urinary leakage at any age, but it is a particularly common cause in the elderly.

Stress and urge incontinence account for at least 80% of urinary incontinence. Extra urethral incontinence is treated by surgical repair of the abnormal opening. Overflow incontinence is treated by intermittent drainage using clean catheterization. If there is an anatomic obstruction that is preventing the flow, such as an enlarged prostate, surgical relief of the obstruction may restore normal voiding and resolve the urinary incontinence.

Signs and Symptoms

A typical patient with stress urinary incontinence is a 57-year-old mother of three with a 7-year history of urinary leakage. At first the episodes of leakage were infrequent and provoked only by vigorous coughing or sneezing, but in the last 2 years, leakage occurs every day and she must wear two or three pads a day for protection. Leakage problems have caused her to stop playing tennis and to avoid vigorous activity. There is a family history of problems—the patient's mother and aunt also experienced bladder control problems.

The symptom is unwanted urinary leakage that occurs with coughing or lifting. Other symptoms may be present, such as skin irritation and dermatitis, or episodes of urinary tract infection. Urinary symptoms of increased urinary frequency and urgency may be prominent. There may be prolapse of the pelvic organs, which may result in an awareness of "something coming down" in the vagina. The patient may see or feel a bulge in the vagina and might complain that the bladder has "dropped down" or "fallen."

Incontinence is not only a complaint and a condition, it is also a clinical sign. When we examine the patient, we should look at the clothing and underwear for signs of wetting or urinary staining. The demonstration of urinary leakage can occur without provocation as the patient moves or turns during clinical examination. If incontinence is less severe, it will be necessary to use some provocation, such as coughing or straining, to provoke urinary leakage. It is important to examine the patient with a full or at least partly full bladder. If incontinence is severe, leakage may be demonstrated with the first cough in the supine position, but if there is no leak in the supine position, you must examine the patient standing. Ideally, the patient should be examined standing on a towel, with one foot raised on a standing stool and one foot on the floor.

Leakage may be provoked by asking the patient to cough gently. For less severe problems, it is necessary to use more vigorous and repeated coughing or straining (Valsalva maneuver) to demonstrate urinary loss. The physician should kneel beside the patient and observe the urethral meatus and vaginal introitus during the efforts to provoke leakage. If leakage occurs, the examining fingers can be used to support the anterior vaginal wall and prevent downward movement of the bladder neck. Repeated provocation will help to determine whether the urinary leakage is or is not controlled by supporting the bladder neck (Marshall test).

Other physical signs and features are commonly associated with incontinence. Recognition of these features will help the physician to develop a management plan to resolve the bladder control problem.

Abdominal distention is very common in incontinence and can be recognized by inspection of the abdomen in the supine position. The patient should be able to push out the anterior abdominal wall and to draw it inward. If there is significant distention, the patient cannot draw the abdominal wall inward from the resting position. This would imply that the abdominal cavity is "full," like a suitcase that is packed too tightly, leaving no space inside. There are five usual causes of distention: fat, fetus, fluid, flatus, and feces. In practice, the most common causes are flatus and feces. Fat is distributed uniformly throughout the body. If the arms, shoulders, and breasts are not heavy with fat, abdominal distention is most unlikely to be a result of fat.

The physician should palpate the abdomen and examine the left and right lower quadrants. The cecum is like the stomach in that it should contain fluid mulch and not solids. The cecum is never palpable in health. If the abdomen is distended and the right colon is palpable, this would imply at least some element of constipation or bowel inertia. Fluid is dull to percussion, and the dullness may be demonstrated to shift when the patient is rolled to one side. Percussion of the abdomen will distinguish the characteristic shifting dullness that suggests the presence of abnormal fluid, such as ascites. Percussion should include the epigastric and suprapubic areas to reveal the presence of a distended bladder.

Hypothyroidism is common in perimenopausal and postmenopausal women. Slowing of the thyroid will contribute to constipation, abdominal distention, and symptoms of urinary incontinence. *Hyperthyroidism* might be found in younger patients. Overactivity of the thyroid is associated with urinary frequency, urgency, and urge incontinence.

The state of hydration is important. Excessive fluid and salt intake can drive urinary symptoms and contribute to problems of polyuria and peripheral edema. Ankle swelling and pitting edema that are evident by day will contribute to excessive fluid mobilization at night when the lower limbs are elevated. This will lead to excessive urine production at night and the need to empty the bladder more often at night (nocturia). In the elderly, this pattern will contribute to problems of nocturnal bed-wetting. New onset of bed-wetting in adults or the elderly is an important sign and it should prompt the physician to examine the patient to exclude chronic urinary retention, urinary tract infection, renal failure, or fecal impaction.

The patient who is troubled by urinary frequency or incontinence will often try to avoid fluids, which will lead to clinical features of dehydration. The tongue and mucous membranes may be dry, the eyes dark and deeper in the orbits, skin turgor will be increased, and the pulse may be thin and rapid. Examination of the voided urine will reveal small volumes of dark, concentrated, amber-colored urine. The specific gravity will be increased (>1.020). Patients complain of fatigue, headache, and abdominal discomfort. When the body is deprived of adequate fluids, extra water is reabsorbed from the colon and the stool becomes more dry and stiff and difficult to evacuate. As the bowel becomes more slow and loaded with stool, so there is more crowding of the bladder, which will worsen symptoms of pelvic pressure, urinary frequency, and incontinence.

Physical characteristics are associated with problems of urinary incontinence. The distended abdomen has been mentioned, but aspects of obesity, gait, posture, and lower extremities are also important. The nerves that are responsible for the activity of the muscles of the pelvic floor are located in the most distal segments of the spinal cord (S2, S3, S4, and S5). These nerves are more caudal in the spinal cord than the nerves for the muscles of the feet and toes (S2 and S3). There may be a history of back or neck problems, including disc disease or spinal stenosis. Examination should include inspection of the back and buttocks. The gluteal form and folds will also reflect the relative strength of the pelvic floor structures.

Inspection of the feet and buttocks is important, because they offer a mirror that will reflect the condition of the muscles of the pelvic floor. The patient who has severe urinary incontinence because of muscle weakness will often have a corresponding pattern of weakness in the intrinsic muscles of the feet. A typical pattern would be flat feet with loss of intrinsic muscles in the lateral toes. This would be marked by an inability to abduct the toes (spread the toes apart in the line of the toes). In health, the toes should lie flat on the floor, like the fingers of a hand palm down on a tabletop. The patient with intrinsic muscle weakness of the sacral segments may have clawing of the toes—hyperextension of the metatarsophalangeal joints and flexion of the interphalangeal joints-so that the toe nails are pointing downward in a vertical direction, instead of horizontal. Lateral deviation of the great toe (hallux valgus) is often present and the lateral toes may be hypoplastic.

Sensory deficits may be recognized by simple clinical examination of the sacral dermatomes. Examine the patient in a lateral position with the knees drawn up. Use two orange sticks held with the tips 4 cm apart to assess two-point discrimination in the perianal and postanal dermatomes. The sensory deficits are typically less marked than the motor deficits.

The physician should complete an examination of the perineum, including inspection with a speculum and bimanual examination. Leakage may be demonstrated by cough in the supine position. Repeated coughing or abdominal straining may be needed to demonstrate leakage if incontinence is not severe. When leakage is not demonstrated in the supine position, examine the patient in a standing position with a full, or at least partly full, bladder. Stand the patient on a towel, with one foot elevated on a low stool. Coughing in this position will usually provoke leakage in the patient with moderate or severe stress urinary incontinence.

Screening and Diagnosis

Prevalence of incontinence is high and many patients will accept symptoms as if incontinence is a normal consequence of childbirth or an expected part of aging, but it is not. Many patients are embarrassed and reluctant to seek help. Many physicians are also embarrassed and reluctant to inquire about these problems, because they may lack interest or awareness about these problems. Some physicians may not have had much training about the assessment and treatments for incontinence. The interest of the physician is often directed to other aspects of health care, and it is easy to miss the opportunity to recognize and resolve urinary leakage problems.

Urinary incontinence is a condition and its symptoms will vary from day to day until the problem becomes severe. Screening may be done as a part of the clinical interview at routine annual visits for cervical smear or other clinical examinations. We must remember that patients are often embarrassed about bladder control problems and may be reluctant to ask their doctor for help. There may be clues in the form of odor, or the presence of pads in the underclothes or urine staining on clothing, bedding, or furniture. The physician must be willing to ask about the problem, but don't ask, "Are you incontinent?" Instead ask, "How much trouble are you having with bladder control?"

When the problem of involuntary leakage has been recognized, it is necessary to distinguish whether the leakage is transient or chronic. Transient leakage will resolve when the provoking factors have been resolved. If incontinence is chronic, the type of incontinence can usually be distinguished by history taking, physical examination, and simple testing to determine whether the bladder is able to empty or not. The physician should consider the reversible factors that might provoke or sustain incontinence. Initial treatment should be directed to resolve the reversible factors.

Prevention and Treatment

It is appropriate to consider how to preserve continence and pelvic health, in the same way that we might modify behaviors, lifestyle, and diet to preserve a healthy heart. Little attention has been paid to strategies that might prevent problems of urinary incontinence in the United States, but other countries do take a more active approach. In France, for example, there is a national program that provides pelvic floor therapy to restore muscle strength after childbirth. The rate of hysterectomy in the women of France is dramatically less than in the United States (1:9).

It has been usual for patients to wait far too long to address the problems of urinary incontinence. Patients may be too embarrassed or mild symptoms may not warrant attention. There may be a fear of surgical treatment and some may not realize that nonsurgical treatments are available and effective. On average, the typical patient will tolerate symptoms of urinary leakage for more than 7 years, before seeking medical attention.

Modification of the diet is appropriate for many patients. Some foods are bladder irritants and will worsen symptoms of urinary frequency urgency and incontinence. These include spicy foods, acidic or citrus fruits, and beverages, including caffeine and alcohol. Patients should be encouraged to drink more water (four to six 8-oz glasses a day) to dilute the urine and improve bowel function. There are no adequate randomized controlled trials to study the impact of these primary management strategies.

The most common cause for incontinence is weakness of the muscles of the pelvic floor. We are not all blessed with the same structures and there are wide differences in pelvic floor muscle strength between one patient and another. There is a tendency for similar structures to be found in members of the same family, and similar symptoms and bladder control problems are shared as a result. It may be easy to dismiss bladder problems as "normal" if several members of the family share the same symptoms.

Pelvic floor muscles can be weakened or damaged by vaginal delivery. As the baby's head passes through the birth canal, the perineum will be stretched and pelvic floor muscles and the pelvic support structures can be torn away from their normal attachments within the pelvis. For some women, the risk of vaginal delivery may be sufficient to warrant cesarean section.

In addition, violent forces on the pelvic floor such as those associated with exceptional stresses of power lifting, gymnastics, or parachute jumping can result in damage to the pelvic floor muscles and the internal attachments of the pelvic support anatomy and pelvic organs. Less dramatic forces are associated with chronic coughing, morbid obesity, and abdominal straining. These activities can also contribute to pelvic floor muscle weakness. We should encourage avoidance of these exceptional and chronic forces in individuals at risk for incontinence problems.

Like other muscles, the pelvic floor muscles can be strengthened by exercise. Kegel exercises are repetitive gripping and tightening contractions of the pelvic floor. These exercises are easy to learn when the pelvic floor is strong, but not so easy when the muscles are weak. These exercises are the time-honored way of treating urinary incontinence by pelvic floor muscle strengthening. Verbal or written instructions alone do not prepare patients adequately. When a trained nurse or therapist provides instruction and coaching with Kegel exercises results are improved.

Postnatal pelvic floor muscle exercises are effective for treating postpartum incontinence. In a randomized controlled trial of 8000 women surveyed 3 months after delivery, 749 reported persistent incontinence and were randomized to instructed pelvic floor muscle exercises and bladder retraining or routine postnatal exercises. At 12 months postpartum, the treatment group showed a significant reduction in stress urinary incontinence.

Biofeedback techniques can be used to help patients to generate more effective contractions and to guide their efforts to target the contractions in the pelvic floor. It is a paradox that the patient with the strongest pelvic muscles (and no symptoms) will master Kegel contractions easily, but those with weaker muscles will find them more difficult to do.

Weighted vaginal cones can be used to help build pelvic floor muscle strength and endurance. This is a classic method of treatment (sometimes referred to as "Chinese eggs"). The patient is taught to insert a graded vaginal weight, starting with a light one and progressing to heavier weights through a range as muscle strength and endurance improve.

Stimulated contractions can be used to strengthen the pelvic floor muscles. If the patient is unable to localize the pelvic floor muscles and cannot generate any useful contraction, electrical stimulation can be used. These treatments use electrodes mounted on a probe that is placed in the vagina or anus or skin patches that are applied to the pelvic floor for stimulation with low-energy direct current. These treatments are widely available in Europe and have an established place in the clinical management of urinary incontinence. The results of electrical stimulation therapy vary from center to center, according to treatment protocols and patient selection. Success with electrical stimulation requires a skilled staff and a motivated patient, but in the best hands, the clinical results are excellent.

Studies have compared electrical stimulation with sham treatment and with pelvic floor exercises alone. Electrical stimulation was associated with improved outcomes for number of leakage episodes, pelvic floor muscle strength, and leakage on pad weight testing. Patients will not always accept electrical stimulation as a treatment option. Some are reluctant to use a probe in the vagina or anus. Some complain of discomfort or irritation with a probe. Even the use of patches on the skin may cause local irritation and skin problems for some patients.

Extracorporeal magnetic innervation is a new technology that uses a pulsed magnetic field flux to induce contractions of the muscles, but without the need for probes or patches and without the need to undress for treatments. The therapy head consists of a magnetic field generator (similar to magnetic resonance imaging) that is built into the seat of a special chair (NeoControl). For treatment the patient sits comfortably, fully clothed, on the chair, and the changing magnetic field will induce effective contractions of the pelvic floor muscles. Treatment is painless and the rate of contractions can be much faster than with conventional Kegels. NeoControl treatments are usually used for 20 minutes twice a week for 8 weeks. (See www.neotonus.com for more information).

VAGINAL PESSARY

A formed support can be worn in the vagina to correct prolapse or incontinence. The type and form of the pessary are selected based on the nature of the problem and the shape, internal dimensions, and the size of the vaginal opening. Pessaries for incontinence treatment may include a ring-shaped design with a thickened area that should be positioned beneath the urethra to restore the anterior vaginal wall and bladder neck to a more normal position and to help close the bladder outlet.

Some pessaries include the hormone estrogen, which can be absorbed directly with contact to nourish and restore the vaginal mucosa.

Occlusive devices have been developed that offer a physical barrier, which may be a patch over the urethral opening or a plug that can be worn inside the natural opening of the urethra. There is a place for these in select patients.

Collection and containment systems have a role in managing the problem of leakage until effective treatments are complete or for those who may not be candidates for definitive therapy. External collection systems are to be preferred over internal catheters, which may be associated with problems of urinary infections, stone formation bleeding, and other complications.

MEDICATIONS

There is an important role for medication, particularly in the treatment of urge incontinence. Overactive detrusor contractions can be reduced or eliminated by anticholinergic drugs such as hyoscyamine (Levsin, Levbid),[1] oxybutynin (Ditropan), and imipramine (Tofranil).[1] The side-effect profile of the traditional anticholinergic medications includes dry mouth and constipation, which may limit the therapeutic benefit. Newer preparations include sustained-release forms (Ditropan XL), which have an improved profile, and newer agents such as tolterodine (Detrol). This is also available as a once-a-day formulation (Detrol LA).

α-Adrenergic agonist medication (phenylpropanolamine)[2] has been used in the treatment of stress urinary incontinence. A randomized controlled trial has compared medication with pelvic floor muscle exercise and revealed no significant benefit of medication over exercise.

SURGICAL TREATMENTS

Bulking agents have an established role in the treatment of stress urinary incontinence. Collagen can be injected at the bladder neck to help close the bladder outlet to prevent unwanted leakage. This is an outpatient treatment that includes cystoscopy to guide the placement of the injections. Collagen treatments can be done without the need for a general anesthetic. Repeat injections may be needed to obtain the best results and further injections may be needed in the future to improve the closure, if the cushions of collagen reduce in size over time. Newer materials have been proposed for use as bulking agents.

NEEDLE-SUSPENSION PROCEDURES AND THE BURCH PROCEDURE

Early surgical procedures were designed to elevate and fix the bladder neck and urethra in an effort to prevent stress urinary leakage. There is less enthusiasm for

---

[1]Not FDA approved for this indication.
[2]Not available in the United States.

these procedures because long-term results are disappointing. New symptoms of voiding difficulty, frequency, urgency, urge leakage, and pain are common after these surgeries. Longer follow-up reveals significant problems with pelvic organ prolapse.

Surgeries can be done using access and exposure that can be from the abdomen, from the vagina, or from both. The development of minimally invasive techniques has led to minimal access procedures that may replace traditional open surgeries. Laparoscopic, vaginal, and endoscopic procedures offer surgical choices for the patient and the surgeon.

Modern techniques reflect a more complete understanding of the mechanisms of pelvic prolapse and incontinence. These techniques recognize that the support structure of the pelvic floor extends to include all of the boundaries of the pelvic floor. If the urethra is not in the correct position, the anterior vaginal wall has lost some of its normal attachments. To correct displacement of the urethra, it is critical to include reattachment of the vaginal wall to its normal attachments within the pelvis. Repair of a lateral detachment of the vagina is called a *paravaginal repair*.

Modern techniques recognize that problems of vaginal prolapse (or bulging from the vagina) rarely include only a single support defect. It is common to find multiple support defects and our surgical repairs should recognize and correct all of the problems in a single procedure. There are patterns of support defect that occur together and can be readily corrected by the appropriate site-specific surgical repairs.

There is fashion in surgery, as in all things, and there is a rush to adopt the newest methods and to be up to date. At the same time, we must remember that the results of our surgical procedures are best judged not early at 2 months or 6 months, but after years. Patients should expect a surgical repair to last and the best repairs should last for years. Any new techniques must be adopted with caution until there is adequate follow-up and long-term outcomes are known. There are significant differences in practice between the urologist and the gynecologist. The urologist tends to favor endoscopic or open surgical procedures, whereas the gynecologist tends to favor vaginal or laparoscopic procedures. There are limited data from randomized comparative studies.

Colposuspension is a surgical procedure that will fix the anterior vaginal wall (adjacent to the bladder neck) to the pelvic bones at Cooper's ligament. This procedure is used by both urologists and gynecologists. Colposuspension has been compared with anterior colporrhaphy (plication of the anterior vaginal wall) and with needle-suspension procedures. After 1 year, results favor colposuspension and the results reveal a stronger difference at 3 years (88% versus 57%) and 14 years (74% versus 42%).

Surgical methods that are currently popular include sling procedures that may use the patient's tissue (autologous fascia), or banked tissue (cadaveric fascia), or animal-derived materials (xenograft), or nonbiologic artificial materials (prosthetic sling). Prosthetic slings are associated with unacceptable complications, including erosion and infection. Natural materials are preferred over artificial for sling procedures.

Results of sling procedures may be better when combined with surgical repairs of the associated pelvic support defects, such as paravaginal detachments or vaginal vault prolapse. There is a trend toward minimally invasive surgical procedures, including the use of laparoscopic access for colposuspension and other continence procedures. There are few prospective randomized studies to compare traditional with minimally invasive surgeries. The limited study, that has compared results after 1 and 3 years, suggests that traditional open surgery was significantly more effective.

Clinical Indicators

- Number of leak episodes
  The patient should be asked to keep a record of the number of leak episodes and the factors that provoked leak episodes (examples: coughing, sneezing, lifting, a feeling of urgency or leakage without awareness).
- Severity of leakage
  The severity of leakage refers to the volume of urine loss (drops, moderate, or a flood of leakage).
- Pad use
  The number of pads used per day and the type of pads or protective garment is a useful measure.
- Bladder chart (bladder diary or log)
  Patients are given a measuring cup (like an inverted hat that can be placed in the commode) to measure the volume of every void for an interval of 24 hours. Analysis of the chart will reveal the largest voided volume (called the functional bladder capacity) and the number of voids by day and at night. Addition of all of the voided volumes will reveal the total urine output in 24 hours. This volume should be in the order of 1.5 to 2 L per day. Patients with urinary frequency and incontinence may have volumes of more than 8 L per day. Dehydrated patients may be oliguric with voided volumes of less than 600 mL per day.
- Incontinence-specific quality-of-life measures (e.g., I-QOL short survey)
  Quality-of-life measures are useful indicators of the impact of urinary incontinence on our patients. There are validated surveys—both long and short forms—that may be used.

Prognosis

Cure is a reasonable goal for most patients. If incontinence is mild to moderate, leakage can usually be resolved without surgery. Effective nonsurgical treatments include fluid and bowel management, timed or prompted voiding, and pelvic floor muscle strengthening exercises (Kegel). If pelvic floor muscles are weak and the patient is unable to grip effectively with the exercises, biofeedback techniques can be used to improve muscle contraction strength and duration.

Rakel and Bope: Conn's Current Therapy 2006.

Electrical stimulation of the pelvic floor muscles can be used if the patient is unable to generate effective contractions. Electrical stimulation involves the use of patches that are placed on the skin of the perineum or probes that are introduced into the vagina or anus. This method involves repeated intervals of stimulation, but when used on a regular treatment regimen, it can be effective. Extracorporeal magnetic innervation is a new technology that uses a pulsed magnetic field flux to induce contractions of the muscles without the need for probes.

Surgery is considered when symptoms have failed to resolve with conservative therapies. Symptoms should be moderate or severe to warrant surgical treatment. There are always risks associated with any type of surgical procedure and the patient and surgeon should weigh the risks and benefits of surgery before electing to proceed. If anatomic defects are responsible, then surgery can be used to correct the defects. Before proceeding with surgery, it is appropriate to consider the role of urodynamic testing. Urodynamic testing is used to define the specific causes of the urinary incontinence and to plan the choice of surgical procedures. There is no single procedure that will be appropriate for all patients, but the principles of effective surgical correction are to define the anatomic defects and to restore normal anatomy by site-specific surgical repairs. Procedures that create compensatory abnormalities (such as sling procedures) should be reserved for those patients with severe defects that cannot be corrected by restoring the normal anatomic relations.

If incontinence is chronic and severe, complete resolution is less likely because of confounding factors such as immobility and irreversible neurologic deficits. For the most frail of our elderly patients, cure may not be possible because of the confounding factors and the goal should be to make the problem a manageable one. If incontinence is to be managed, the goal is to reduce the severity of leakage. We need to aim to avoid the complications of incontinence such as urinary infection, dermatitis, and ulceration of the skin. It is important to define the objectives of the management plan with the patient and caregivers. Try to define what is the worst aspect of the problem for the patient. This should be the first target for change in the plan.

Alternative/Complementary Medicine

Bowel management is an important element of pelvic health. The urinary bladder shares space in the pelvis with the bowel (and the uterus) and when the lower bowel is empty, the bladder capacity is optimal and bladder control will be better. There are many complementary and alternative strategies for bowel management. A high-fiber diet is helpful for maintaining stool volume, form, and regularity. The addition of specific foods, such as warm prune juice, prunes, figs, or rhubarb, can act as natural stimulants for the bowel. Natural lubricants, such as olive oil, can improve the bowel pattern. Other oils are more palatable in the

form of capsules such as flaxseed oil,[*,1] fish oil,[*,1] or aloe products.[*,1] Use of appropriate laxatives, such as herbal remedies, oriental green tea,[*,1] and similar preparations, is indicated if the simpler measures are insufficient. Suppositories, enemas, or colon cleansing do have a place in bowel management, but the simpler measures are preferred. Physical methods of abdominal palpation and kneading can be helpful to stimulate bowel transit. No randomized controlled trial data are available to compare the outcomes of alternative strategies.

Research Frontiers

SURGICAL TREATMENTS

There is great interest in efforts to make surgical treatments for incontinence less invasive and easier for the patient and the surgeon. The simpler forms of outpatient surgery use some form of fixation staples or screws to attach the soft tissues of the anterior vaginal wall to the bones of the pelvis. These techniques include influence and vesica procedures.

The transvaginal tape (TVT) procedure is a new form of sling procedure that involves the passage of two long needles from a small wound in the anterior vaginal wall beneath the urethra to the abdominal wall. Each needle is attached to the end of a tape of artificial material and as the needles are passed upward, the tape is carried into position. The needles and excess tape are trimmed and the small wounds are closed. This technique is simple to perform and early results are encouraging, but it is too early to predict what the long-term results might be.

Bulking agents have an established role in the treatment of stress urinary incontinence. Collagen was the preferred material to inject at the level of the bladder neck and urethra to help prevent leakage, but newer agents are in development and some are now available. These include artificial substances such as carbon particles and silicone suspension (Macroplastique). Some investigators are using cultured cartilage cells (taken from the back of the patient's own ear) as a bulking material. The cells are grown in tissue culture and then injected in suspension. This technique offers the advantage of using living cells that may be able to remain in place without significant change for years. Long-term results are awaited.

REFERENCES

Abrams P, Blaivas JG, Stanton SL, et al: Standardization of terminology of lower urinary tract function. Scand J Urol Nephrol 1988;114(Suppl):5-19.

Berghmans LCM, Hendricks HJM, Bo K, et al: Conservative treatment of stress urinary incontinence in women: A systematic review of randomized controlled trials. Br J Urol 1998;82:181-191.

Black NA, Downs SH: The effectiveness of surgery for stress incontinence in women: A systematic review. Br J Urol 1996;78: 497-510.

---

[*]Available as a dietary supplement.
[1]Not FDA approved for this indication.

Bo K, Hagen RM, Kvarstein B, et al: Pelvic floor muscle exercises for the treatment of female stress incontinence. III. Effects of two different degrees of pelvic floor muscle exercises. Neurourol Urodyn 1990;9(5):489-502.

Bump RC, Hurt WG, Fantl A, Wyman JF: Assessment of Kegel pelvic muscle performance after brief verbal instruction. Am J Obstet Gynecol 1991;165:322-329.

Burton G: A three year prospective randomized urodynamics study comparing open and laparoscopic colposuspension. Neurourol Urodyn 2997;16:353-354.

Cammu H, Van Nylen J, Derde MP, et al: Pelvic physiotherapy in genuine stress incontinence. Urology 1991;38(4):332-337.

Colombo M, Vitobello D, Proietti F, et al: Randomized comparison of Burch colposuspension versus anterior colporrhaphy in women with stress urinary incontinence and anterior vaginal wall prolapse. Br J Obstet Gynaecol 2000;107:544-551.

Gladzener CMA, Lang G, Wilson PD, et al: Postnatal incontinence: A multicenter controlled trial of conservative treatment. Br J Obstet Gynaecol 1998;105(Suppl 117):47.

Leach GE, Dmochowski RR, Appell RA, et al: Female stress urinary incontinence clinical guidelines panel: Summary report on surgical management of female stress urinary incontinence. J Urol 1997;158:875-880.

Simeonova Z, Milsom I, Kullendorf AE, et al: The prevalence of urinary incontinence and its influence on quality of life in women from an urban Swedish population. Acta Obstet Gynecol Scand 1999;78:546-551.

Wagner TH, Hu TW: Economic costs of incontinence in 1995. Urology 1998;51(3):355-361.

Epididymitis

Method of
Michael Thomas Gambla, MD,
and Darrew Chapman, MD

Epididymitis refers to inflammation or infection of the epididymis. *Acute epididymitis* is defined by a duration of symptoms of less than 6 weeks, typically with pain and swelling. *Chronic epididymitis* refers to a longer duration of pain, usually not accompanied by swelling.

Epidemiology

Acute epididymitis is a major cause of urologic morbidity. In a survey published by Collins and colleagues of almost 60,000 ambulatory office visits of all medical specialties, epididymitis accounted for 1 in 345 (0.29%), making it the fifth most common urologic cause of an office visit, behind prostatitis, urinary tract infection (UTI), kidney stones, and sexually transmitted diseases (STDs) in men ages 18 to 50 years. In a review of 121 patients, Kaver and Matzkin found it most commonly occurs in patients ages 16 to 30 and 51 to 70 years. Mittemeyer and colleagues' data on 610 U.S. Army soldiers also demonstrated a peak incidence in the 20- to 29-year-old age range. There is no predilection for laterality, and up to 9% of cases can be bilateral. There is no racial bias.

Pathophysiology

Before Berger published his landmark paper in 1979, reflux of urine into the vas deferens was considered the cause of epididymitis. Using cultures and epididymal aspirates, however, Berger proved that most cases of epididymitis are caused by bacterial infection. The causative organisms vary according to the age of the patient. *Neisseria gonorrhoeae* and *Chlamydia trachomatis* are the common isolates in men younger than 35 years; *Escherichia coli* is usually found in men older than 35 years. Thus in younger, sexually active men, it is the common causes of sexually transmitted urethritis that cause epididymitis, whereas in the older age groups, it is the common urinary pathogens. Note that in men who practice anal intercourse, coliform bacteria are the common causative organisms. Less common pathogens include the sexually transmitted *Ureaplasma urealyticum,* as well as the common urinary pathogens *Proteus* species, *Klebsiella pneumoniae, Pseudomonas aeruginosa,* and *Haemophilus influenzae. Mycobacterium tuberculosis* is a rare cause of epididymitis but must be considered in patients at risk for this disease. One fifth of men with mumps develop acute epididymo-orchitis because of the virus. Cytomegalovirus (CMV) is another viral cause of epididymitis, but it is associated with HIV-positive patients. Noninfectious causes are the vasculitides as well as the antiarrhythmic amiodarone (Cordarone).

Presentation and Evaluation

The most comprehensive review of the presentation of epididymitis was published by Kaver and Matzkin. In their evaluation, 90% of patients presented with a duration of symptoms of 1 week or less. Dysuria was present in one third, and 75% had a temperature higher than 37.5°C (99.5°F), but only 20% reported chills. Orchitis, an infection of the testicle, was present in 58%. Scrotal skin erythema was present in 62%. Peripheral leukocytosis occurred in 64%. Hematuria was present in 53%, and pyuria in 79%.

The Centers for Disease Control and Prevention (CDC) has made recommendations for the evaluation of patients with epididymitis. An intraurethral swab or Gram stain as well as a culture of the urethral exudate should be obtained. Patients with a gonoccocal infection should be identified. If the urethral Gram stain is negative, a urinalysis, urine Gram stain, and urine culture should be obtained. Syphilis serology and HIV testing should also be performed.

Differential Diagnosis

The most important differentiation that must be made is between acute epididymitis and torsion of the testicle. Physical findings can be helpful in that torsion manifests with a high transversely oriented testicle, whereas the testicle is in its normal anatomic position in epididymitis. A swollen, tender epididymus often can be palpated in the patient with acute epididymitis. Prehn's sign, or relief of pain with elevation of the testicle, may be present in epididymitis, whereas elevating a torsed testicle generally induces more pain. The physical examination may be difficult in a patient with an inflamed hemiscrotum and a reactive hydrocele. Testicular ultrasound is a reliable noninvasive test that can distinguish between epididymitis and testicular torsion. If the diagnosis is in question, immediate surgical exploration is warranted because time is critical in the treatment of torsion. Testicular cancer, although less commonly misdiagnosed as epididymitis, should also be considered. An ultrasound is helpful in making this distinction as well. If this diagnosis is considered, tumor markers (α-fetoprotein, β-human chorionic gonadotropin [β-hCG], and lactic dehydrogenase [LDH]) should be sent.

Management

Patients should be treated with empirical antibiotic therapy. For patients with presumptive gonococcal or chlamydial infections, a single dose of ceftriaxone (Rocephin) 250 mg intramuscularly and doxycycline (Vibramycin) 100 mg orally twice a day for 10 days is the regimen recommended by the CDC. An oral dose of 1 g of azithromycin (Zithromax) may be substituted for doxycyline if compliance is an issue. In patients whose epididymitis is caused by coliform bacteria, or in those who are allergic to cephalosporins and/or tetracyclines, a 10-day course of ofloxacin (Floxin), 300 mg orally twice a day, should be prescribed. For symptomatic improvement, a 2-week course of anti-inflammatories begun at the time of antibiotics has proved very effective in reducing both pain and swelling. Patients should adhere to a regimen of decreased activity and scrotal elevation. Those who do not improve within 3 to 5 days should be reevaluated. Patients who are systemically ill, or those with a scrotal abscess or pyocele, should be hospitalized and treated with intravenous antibiotics. Surgical therapy is usually reserved for the most severe cases.

Prognosis

Acute epididymitis caused by a sexually transmitted infection usually resolves quickly with appropriate therapy. Complications are more common in cases

 CURRENT THERAPY

Age Younger Than 35 Years
- Ceftriaxone (Rocephin) 250 mg IM × 1
  and either
- Doxycycline (Vibramycin) 100 mg PO bid × 10 days
  or
- Azithromycin (Zithromax) 1 g PO × 1

Age Older Than 35 Years
- Ofloxacin (Floxin) 300 mg PO bid × 10 days

All Patients
- Anti-inflammatories
- Decreased activity
- Scrotal elevation
- Pain control

Abbreviations: bid = twice a day; IM = intramuscular; PO = by mouth.

caused by coliforms and include testicular abscess, testicular infarction, and testicular atrophy. Reduced spermatogenesis and subfertility may also occur. Chronic pain is uncommon but is a clinical and therapeutic dilemma.

REFERENCES

Berger RE, Alexander ER, Harnisch JP, et al: Etiology, manifestations and therapy of acute epididymitis: Prospective study of 50 cases. J Urol 1979;121:750-754.
Berger RE, Lee JC. Sexually transmitted diseases: The classic diseases. In Walsh PC, Retik AB, Vaughan ED, et al. (eds): Campbell's Urology, 8th ed. Philadelphia, WB Saunders, 2002, pp 671-691.
Centers for Disease Control and Prevention. Sexually transmitted diseases treatment guidelines. MMWR 1998;47:1-118.
Collins MM, Stafford RS, O'Leary MP, et al: How common is prostatitis? A national survey of physician visits. J Urol 1998;159:1224-1228.
Kaver I, Matzkin H: Epididymo-orchitis: A retrospective study of 121 patients. J Fam Pract 1990;30:548-552.
Luzzi GA, O'Brien TS: Acute epididymitis. BJU Int 2001;87:747-755.
Mittemeyer BT, Lennox KW, Borski AA: Epididymitis: A review of 610 cases. J Urol 1966;95:390-392.

 CURRENT DIAGNOSIS

- Onset greater than or equal to 1 week
- Pain on palpation of epididymis
- Scrotal skin erythema
- Leukocytosis
- Elevated temperature
- Pyuria
- Association with gonorrhea, chlamydia, or *Escherichia coli* infection
- Scrotal ultrasound to differentiate epididymitis, testicular torsion, and tumor

Rakel and Bope: *Conn's Current Therapy 2006.*

Primary Glomerular Disease

Method of
Daniel Catteran, MD,
and Penny Turner, MD

Primary, or idiopathic, glomerular diseases encompasses a wide variety of clinical scenarios and management. They vary from the treatment of asymptomatic urinary abnormalities to the complexity of renal replacement therapy. This article focuses on their clinicopathologic correlations and management.

Clinical Presentation

The most common presentations and their histologies are described in the following text and summarized in Table 1.

• Acute nephritic syndrome (ANS): This is defined by the presence of hypertension, active urine sediment, and usually some degree of renal insufficiency. Active sediment implies that dysmorphic (misshapen) red blood cells (RBCs) and RBC casts are in the urine. Rapidly progressive glomerulonephritis (RPGN) is the most extreme example of this syndrome. Renal function declines rapidly over weeks and months, often to the point of requiring dialysis.
• Nephrotic syndrome: This is defined by the presence of edema, hypoalbuminemia, hypercholesterolemia, and proteinuria greater than 3.5 g per day (>50 mg/m^2 in children). Renal function is usually normal.
• Asymptomatic microhematuria and/or proteinuria: This state is defined by the findings of a positive urine dipstick test for blood and/or protein in a completely asymptomatic individual.
• Gross hematuria: This is characterized by redness in the urine that can be seen by the naked eye.
• Uremic syndrome: This state is accompanied by symptoms of chronic renal failure, including decreased appetite, weight loss, pruritus, decreased energy, and other symptoms of chronic kidney failure.

Approach to Diagnosis

All patients with suspected primary glomerular disease have serum creatinine, urinalysis, and a quantitative estimate (24-hour urine collection or aliquot for protein-to-creatinine ratio) of proteinuria if positive on dipstick. The urine dipstick is a sensitive test for microhematuria and proteinuria, often the two earliest signs of glomerular disease. If the dipstick results are positive, perform a urine microscopic examination to identify other signs of glomerular disease such as dysmorphic RBCs, RBC casts, granular casts, and oval fat bodies.

Patients with signs or symptoms suggesting glomerular disease, such as persistent proteinuria and/or impaired renal function, should be considered for renal biopsy. This is the best way to classify the primary glomerular diseases for prognosis and treatment. The risk of biopsy is low. The only major hazard is significant bleeding, and in expert hands it occurs in fewer than 1% of procedures.

Secondary glomerular renal disease can occur as a consequence of a systemic process, often closely mimics primary glomerular disease, and can only be excluded after close clinical and laboratory evaluations (Table 2). Their treatment is targeted at the underlying causative factor and is often different from primary glomerular disease.

TABLE 1 Primary Glomerular Diseases and their Common Presentations

Primary glomerular disease	Presentation
Minimal Change Disease	Nephrotic syndrome
FSGS	Nephrotic syndrome, +/– reduced renal function, +/– hypertension in up to 50%
Membranous Glomerulopathy	Nephrotic syndrome, usually normal renal function
MPGN	Nephritic (10-30%), Nephrotic syndrome (40-50%), Asymptomatic proteinuria (20-40%)
Diffuse Proliferative GN	Acute nephritic syndrome
IgA Nephropathy	Asymptomatic hematuria +/– proteinuria (40-70%), Nephrotic syndrome (2-30%), Acute nephritic syndrome (10-20%)
Crescentic GN	Acute nephritic syndrome

TABLE 2 Secondary Glomerular Diseases Pathology and their Common Causes

Pathology type	Causative factor
Minimal Change Disease	Medications Malignancy
Focal Segmental Glomerulosclerosis	HIV Obesity Reflux nephropathy
Membranous Nephropathy	Hepatitis B Systemic lupus erythematosis Malignancy Medications
MPGN Type 1	Hepatitis C Systemic lupus erythematosis
Diffuse Proliferative GN	Bacterial infection
IgA Nephropathy	Liver disease
Type 1 Crescentic GN	Anti-glomerular basement Membrane antibodies
Type 2 Crescentic GN	Systemic lupus erythematosis Bacterial infection
Type 3 Crescentic GN	Systemic vasculitis

Rakel and Bope: *Conn's Current Therapy 2006.*

Treatment

TARGETS OF THERAPY

The therapy goals are to:

- Slow or prevent loss of renal function
- Complete reversal of proteinuria
- Reduce proteinuria

The management of primary glomerular diseases can be divided into conservative and specific therapies.

CONSERVATIVE THERAPY

Conservative therapy is aimed at slowing the progression of the underlying glomerular disease. Blood pressure (BP) targets are substantially lower than in the past; 130/80 mm Hg or lower (e.g., 125/75 mm Hg in patients with ≥1 g/day of proteinuria) is recommended. The initial agent should be an angiotensin-converting enzyme inhibitor (ACEI) because it not only lowers BP but also has an independent renal protective benefit. The latter is reflected in greater reductions in proteinuria compared with other classes of antihypertensive agents per mm Hg BP decrease. Angiotensin receptor blockers (ARBs) also have a similar additive benefit. ACEI used in combination with ARBs are synergistic in regard to their benefit in proteinuria and renal function preservation. The serum creatinine may initially rise 5% to 10% with the initiation of an ACEI or ARB, but this is hemodynamic rather than nephrotoxic and will stabilize after 2 to 3 months. An important caveat with single or combined ACEI/ARB therapy is the careful monitoring of the serum potassium level because hyperkalemia is a risk, especially if renal function is 50% of normal or less.

Diuretics like furosemide (Lasix) are used as necessary to control symptoms secondary to volume overload and work well if used in conjunction with a low-sodium diet. Spironolactone (Aldactone) is often a useful addition, especially if the nephrotic syndrome is severe. Again, watch for hyperkalemia if ACEI/ARB plus spironolactone (Aldactone) is used.

Metolazone (Zaroxolyn), a powerful thiazide diuretic, may need to be added in cases of refractory edema and/or if renal insufficiency is severe. Care must be taken to maintain euvolemia. Excessive intravascular volume depletion not only increases the risk of decreased renal perfusion and acute renal failure, but it may also increase the thrombotic tendency in the severely nephrotic patient and accentuate muscle cramping.

Cholesterol is usually elevated with either nephrotic range proteinuria and/or with chronic kidney impairment. The hyperlipidemia is an independent cardiovascular risk factor and lipid-lowering therapy, most commonly with beta-hydroxy-β-methylglutaryl-coenzyme A (HMG-CoA) reductase inhibitors such as atorvastatin (Lipitor) 20 to 40 mg daily to achieve a low-density lipoprotein (LDL) cholesterol of less than 100 mg/dL is recommended.

Rakel and Bope: *Conn's Current Therapy 2006.*

TABLE 3 Immunosuppressive Treatment of Primary Glomerular Disease

Primary glomerular disease	Specific therapy
Minimal Change Disease	First Line: prednisone Second Line: cyclosporine[A] (Neoral) or cytotoxics
FSGS	First Line: prednisone Second Line: cyclosporine[A]
Membranous Glomerulopathy	First Line: cyclosporine[A] or cytotoxis/corticosteroids Second Line: mycophenolate mofetil[A] (CellCept)
MPGN	Alternate day low dose prednisone for children
Diffuse Proliferative GN	Supportive therapy only, unless crescents
IgA Nephropathy	ACE inhibitors and/or ARBs, fish oil supplements,[A] corticosteroids[A] +/– cyclophosphamide[A] (Cytoxan)
Crescentic GN	Corticosteroids, cyclophosphamide[A] +/– azathioprine[A] (Imuran) +/– plasmapheresis

[A]Not FDA approved for this indication.

SPECIFIC THERAPY

The *specific* therapy of primary glomerular diseases, based on their underlying renal pathology, is discussed in the following text; and Table 3 summarizes it as well.

MINIMAL CHANGE DISEASE

Pathology

Minimal change disease (MCD) is named for the absence of any abnormalities on light and immunofluorescence microscopy. The identifying characteristic of this disease is diffuse effacement of the epithelial foot processes with loss of slit diaphragms on electron microscopy.

Treatment

MCD remains the most common cause of the idiopathic nephrotic syndrome in children. Treatment for children is prednisone at 60 mg/m^2 per day (up to 80 mg/day) for 4 weeks, and then 40 mg/m^2 on alternate days for 4 to 8 weeks, slowly tapering off over 4 to 6 weeks. Remission is achieved in more than 90% of cases within 8 weeks. Up to 75% of children will have at least one relapse, and 50% will have a frequently relapsing course, defined by two or more relapses within a 6-month period. Initially, most relapses are retreated with prednisone alone. Renal biopsy in this age group is usually only performed after at least 4 weeks of therapy, if the patient is unresponsive, or if the response is incomplete. Approximately 10% of children will have steroid-resistant disease and most will subsequently have focal and segmental glomerulosclerosis on biopsy.

MCD is an uncommon cause of the nephrotic syndrome in adults, but its presentation is similar. In contrast to children, however, there may be age-related renal insufficiency and/or hypertension. Treatment with prednisone in doses of 1 mg/kg per day up to a maximum of 80 mg per day is often required, but for a longer period (12 to 16 weeks) before a complete remission is induced. In addition, there is a lower rate (approximately 75%) of success than in children.

Steroid-resistant and steroid-dependent patients (especially if maintenance is >10 mg/day and/or drug toxicities are accumulating with prednisone) will require treatment with an immunosuppressive agent such as cyclophosphamide (Cytoxan)[1] or cyclosporine (Neoral).[1] Cyclophosphamide (Cytoxan)[1] in doses of 1.5 to 2 mg/kg per day for 12 weeks in combination with low-dose prednisone is an effective regimen. Careful monitoring for cytopenias and infections is essential. If cyclosporine (Neoral)[1] is selected, it is initiated at 3 to 4 mg/kg in two divided doses and adjusted to maintain a 12-hour trough level of 100 to 175 ng/mL. This drug is also often used in combination with low-dose prednisone. Therapy with cyclosporine (Neoral),[1] if the patient responds, should be continued for up to 12 months before tapering, always with careful monitoring of renal function to minimize nephrotoxicity. If one of these routines is unsuccessful, considering using the other, often after a drug-free holiday (off all immunosuppressive agents for 2 to 4 months). Any patient on prolonged high-dose steroids and/or an immunosuppressive agent should be on *Pneumocystis carinii* pneumonia (PCP) prophylaxis with trimethoprim-sulfamethoxazole (Bactrim or Septra) 80 mg/400 mg daily, barring sulfa drug allergy. In addition, bisphosphonate therapy should be considered if prolonged oral corticosteroids are used to minimize osteoporosis.

FOCAL AND SEGMENTAL GLOMERULOSCLEROSIS

Pathology

In focal and segmental glomerulosclerosis (FSGS), focal (some glomeruli) and segmental (parts of individual glomeruli) scarring of the glomerular tuft at the vascular pole, with or without adhesions to Bowman's capsule, and mesangial collapse in these areas are the classic lesions on light microscopy. Immunofluorescence may show nonspecific IgM and C1 trapping in these areas, and electron microscopy demonstrates diffuse epithelial foot process effacement.

Treatment

Treatment of primary FSGS should begin with prednisone in a dose of 1 mg/kg per day up to 80 mg maximum per day for up to 16 weeks before steroid

resistance can be declared. If a patient is at risk of steroid toxicity (e.g., the patient is older than age 60 years, obese, or has a family history of diabetes) and/or if a 50% reduction in proteinuria is not seen by 8 weeks, the addition of a second agent is recommended with an associated taper of steroids to more acceptable levels (10 to 20 mg/day) to minimize complications.

Cyclosporine (Neoral)[1] therapy is effective in the treatment of steroid-resistant or steroid-dependent FSGS. The initial dose and management are the same as in steroid-resistant MCD. If there is no significant change in proteinuria (a minimum 50% decrease) by 6 months, and/or there is a sustained rise in serum creatinine (30% or more) unimproved by a reduction in cyclosporine (Neoral)[1] dosage, it should be discontinued. If the patient is responsive to cyclosporine (Neoral),[1] it should be continued at the lowest possible dose for at least 1 year before slowly tapering it off.

There is insufficient evidence from retrospective reviews to support prolonged cytotoxic therapy with an agent such as cyclophosphamide (Cytoxan)[1] in steroid-resistant FSGS.

MEMBRANOUS NEPHROPATHY

Pathology

Glomeruli look normal on light microscopy at the earliest phase of disease, but as the immune complexes continue to be deposited, there is glomerular basement membrane (GBM) matrix increase and the capillary loops begin to look rigid and diffusely thickened. On silver stain, spikes of matrix may be visible on the epithelial side of the capillary wall, representing new GBM enclosing the immune complex deposits. Subepithelial immune complexes are confirmed by electron microscopy, positive granular staining along the GBM for IgG, and complement on immunofluorescence.

TREATMENT

The prognosis in idiopathic membranous glomerulonephritis (MGN) follows the rule of thirds: one third will progress slowly to end-stage renal disease (ESRD), one third will have persistent low- to medium-grade proteinuria with preserved renal function over many years, and one third will have a spontaneous remission. Demographic markers of a poor outcome at onset include male gender, older age, hypertension, interstitial fibrosis and tubular atrophy on renal pathology, and reduced renal function and high-grade proteinuria (>8 g/day) on laboratory examination. These factors should all be considered before deciding how to manage the patient. Conservative therapy should be initiated immediately, but an observation period of up to 6 months is recommended before deciding if immunosuppressive treatment is warranted. A semiquantitative assessment that can categorize the patients in terms of their risk of progression has been constructed and validated.

---

[1]Not FDA approved for this indication.

[1]Not FDA approved for this indication.

Rakel and Bope: *Conn's Current Therapy 2006.*

Its application can substantially help in assessing the risk benefit of immunosuppressive therapy for both the physician and the patient. If proteinuria remains less than 4 g per day for 6 months, continued conservative treatment is recommended; seriously consider immunosuppressives if proteinuria will not decrease lower than 4 to 8 g per day; and if more than 8 g per day and/or progressive deterioration in renal function ensues, immunosuppressives therapy should be initiated even prior to the completion of 6 months of observation. Options include corticosteroids with cytotoxics or cyclosporine (Neoral).[1] Prednisone as monotherapy is not sufficient treatment. A 6-month course of alternating monthly prednisone, 0.5 mg/kg per day, with a month of either chlorambucil (Leukeran),[1] 0.2 mg/kg per day, or cyclophosphamide (Cytoxan),[1] 2.5 mg/kg per day orally, is effective. Cyclosporine (Neoral)[1] therapy initiated at 3 to 4 mg/kg in two divided doses targeting a 12-hour trough level of 100 to 175 ng/mL for a minimum of 6 months has also been proved effective in a randomized controlled trial.

Mycophenolate mofetil (CellCept),[1] 500 to 2000 mg daily, in an open-label pilot study significantly reduced and stabilized renal function in approximately 30% of a group of MGN patients resistant to other forms of therapy and can be considered if all else fails. Rituximab (Rituxan),[1] a monoclonal antibody against B-cell marker CD20, has also had positive results in a pilot study.

MEMBRANOPROLIFERATIVE GLOMERULONEPHRITIS

Pathology

There is mesangial hypercellularity, increased mesangial matrix, and capillary-wall thickening on light microscopy in both subtypes of membranoproliferative glomerulonephritis (MPGN). Immunofluorescence is varied and nondiagnostic. On electron microscopy there are subendothelial immune complex deposits in type I MPGN, and ribbon-like, dense deposits within the GBM in MPGN type II.

Treatment

C3 complement levels are reduced in both types I and II MPGN, and the C4 complement component is low in type I, but usually normal in type II. Treatment of idiopathic MPGN is challenging, and few treatments have demonstrated a significant benefit over conservative therapy alone. Alternate day, prolonged (>2 years), low-dose prednisone in children has the best evidence, but even it is limited to retrospective albeit long-term analyses. Cyclophosphamide (Cytoxan)[1] has been reported to be of benefit in a small study, but was associated with significant toxicity, and based on current evidence cannot be recommended. Initially, aspirin[1] and dipyridamole (Persantine)[1] were felt to have a favorable

effect on proteinuria, but later results from these studies have suggested no long-term benefits on either proteinuria or renal survival.

DIFFUSE PROLIFERATIVE GLOMERULONEPHRITIS

Pathology

In diffuse proliferative glomerulonephritis (DPGN), light microscopy shows proliferative glomerular lesions with increases in both mesangial and endothelial cells, often with an associated intracapillary inflammatory infiltrate of polymorphs. Immunofluorescence shows varying amounts of complement and Ig deposition, and on electron microscopy the characteristic subepithelial *humps* or deposits along the GBM are evident. In severe cases epithelial crescent formation may be found.

Treatment

The most common known causal factor in DPGN is infection. Poststreptococcal glomerulonephritis (PSGN) is less prevalent in the developed world with antibiotic use, but it can still occur. Other bacteria commonly associated with subtle chronic infections such as endocarditis, infected atrioventricular shunts, skin infections, and visceral abscesses can also be associated with proliferative glomerulonephritis (PGN).

Hypocomplementemia is often found in the acute phase. The symptoms and signs of DPGN usually spontaneously resolve within 4 to 8 weeks. Conservative therapy includes BP control, diuretics, and sodium restriction. Dialysis support may be necessary during the acute phase. The underlying infection should be treated if it has not resolved spontaneously. In children the prognosis is excellent with little long-term sequelae, and more than 80% of adults will have no residual renal dysfunction. If crescent formation is present, these patients should be treated as outlined in the idiopathic crescentic GN section later in this article.

IMMUNOGLOBULIN A NEPHROPATHY

Pathology

IgA nephropathy has mesangial hypercellularity and matrix expansion on light microscopy. Crescents are rarely present and are usually segmental in nature. Immunofluorescence shows mesangial IgA (± IgG) and complement deposits and their location is confirmed on electron microscopy.

Treatment

Management depends on the clinical features, the degree of proteinuria, and the severity of renal insufficiency. Patients with only microhematuria, no proteinuria, and normal renal function with no hypertension need only be followed at regular intervals. If proteinuria is less than 1 g per day and the patient has a

---

[1]Not FDA approved for this indication.

normal serum creatinine, treatment should include ACEI and/or ARBs therapy, even in the absence of hypertension, to reduce proteinuria to the lowest level possible. If proteinuria is greater than 1 g per day with normal renal function, ACEI and/or ARBs should be instituted and proteinuria and BP normalization targeted. Fish oil supplements[1] at a dose of 1.8 g per day of eicosapentaenoic acid (EPA) and 1.2-g per day doses of docosahexaenoic acid (DHA) daily should be considered. Although results from trials have been varied, the risk of this treatment is negligible. If renal function is deteriorating or proteinuria persists at doses of ≥1 g per day despite maximum conservative therapy after 6 months, immunosuppressive therapy should be considered. In the group with persistent proteinuria but stable, well-preserved renal function, pulse methylprednisolone (Solu-Medrol) doses of 1 g per day for 3 days in the beginning of months 1, 3, and 5 with low-dose prednisone (0.5 mg/kg/day) on alternate days for 6 months has been shown to be effective. In the group with persistent proteinuria and rising serum creatinine, cytotoxic therapy should be considered in addition to prednisone. Prednisone doses of 40 mg per day, tapering to 10 mg per day within 2 years, combined with cyclophosphamide (Cytoxan)[1] orally for 3 months followed by azathioprine (Imuran)[1] for a minimum of 2 years, both at 1.5 mg/kg per day, has been studied in this type of patient in a RCT with good results. A recent RCT using mycophenolate mofetil (CellCept)[1] as a single agent showed no benefit on either proteinuria or renal survival if initial serum creatinine was 3 mg/dL or more. This would support the futility of using immunosuppressive therapy once severe chronic renal insufficiency (creatinine clearance ≤35 mL/minute) has been reached.

CRESCENTIC GLOMERULONEPHRITIS

Pathology

Light microscopy will show varying degrees of cellular or fibrocellular crescent formation in Bowman's space, surrounding, and in some cases obliterating, the glomerular tuft. Immunofluorescence staining helps distinguish between the three main types: Type 1, or anti-GBM disease, has linear IgG staining of the GBM;

CURRENT DIAGNOSIS

- All persistent hematuria and proteinuria above 150 mg per day need to be investigated.
- Secondary causes of glomerular disease must be excluded.
- Renal biopsy is often necessary for proper classification, prognosis, and therapy.

CURRENT THERAPY

- Blood pressure (BP) should be controlled below 130/80 mm Hg or less than 125/75 mm Hg if significant proteinuria is present (>0.5 g/d).
- Angiotensin-converting enzyme inhibitors and angiotensin receptor blockers provide renal protection independent of their effect on BP control.
- Specific immunosuppressive therapy in primary glomerular disease depends on careful assessment of the likelihood of progression/complication of the disease and the risks of therapy.
- Treatment is directed at the underlying cause in secondary glomerular diseases.

type 2, or immune complex disease, has diffuse granular staining along the GBM; and type 3, or pauci-immune, has little or no staining in the glomeruli.

Treatment

Rapid institution of treatment is critically important to reverse or stabilize renal function. The overall renal survival rate in crescentic GN is 75% to 85% and patient survival rate is 85% to 90%. Therapy should be focused first on induction and then on maintenance treatment. Induction should be with methylprednisolone (Solu-Medrol) at 5 to 15 mg/kg per day for 3 days, then prednisone at 1 mg/kg per day. Additional immunosuppressive therapy includes cyclophosphamide (Cytoxan),[1] 1.5 to 2.5 mg/kg per day orally. The dose of cyclophosphamide (Cytoxan)[1] should be reduced in elderly patients in proportion to their degree of renal failure aiming to maintain a neutrophil count above 2.5 cu[3]. Cyclophosphamide (Cytoxan)[1] is not always required in the induction phase. It is not recommended, for instance, in idiopathic type-2 crescentic GN of postinfectious origin. When pulmonary hemorrhage is present in anti-GBM disease (and also associated with vasculitis), plasma exchange is added for up to 10 exchanges, or until anti-GBM antibodies are negative, using 4-L exchanges with albumin (or fresh-frozen plasma if bleeding risk is high). In the vasculitis type, maintenance consists of cyclophosphamide (Cytoxan)[1] for 3 months, then azathioprine (Imuran) maintenance therapy is substituted at 1 to 2 mg/kg per day if the disease is quiescent. Long-term maintenance therapy is unnecessary in anti-GBM crescentic GN, and all therapy can usually be discontinued after 6 to 9 months.

REFERENCES

Bakris GL, Weir MR: Angiotensin-converting enzyme inhibitor-associated elevations in serum creatinine: Is this a cause for concern? Arch Intern Med 2000;160:685-693.

---

[1]Not FDA approved for this indication.

---

[1]Not FDA approved for this indication.

Ballardie FW, Roberts ISD: Controlled prospective trial of prednisolone with cytotoxics in progressive IgA nephropathy. J Am Soc Nephrol 2002;13:142-148.

Cattran DC, Appel GB, Hebert LA, et al: A randomized trial of cyclosporine in patients with steroid-resistant focal segmental glomerulosclerosis. Kidney Int 1999;56:2220-2226.

Cattran DC, Appel GB, Hebert LA, et al: Cyclosporine in patients with steroid-resistant membranous nephropathy: A randomized trial. Kidney Int 2001;59:1484-1490.

Cattran DC, Pei Y, Greenwood CM, et al: Validation of a predictive model of idiopathic membranous nephropathy: Its clinical and research implications. Kidney Int 1997;51:901-907.

ISEN Group (Gruppo Italiano di Studi Epidemiologici in Nefrologia): Randomised placebo-controlled trial of effect of ramipril on decline in glomerular filtration rate and risk of terminal renal failure in proteinuric, non-diabetic nephropathy. Lancet 1997;349:1857-1863.

Jayne D, Rasmussen N, Andrassy K, et al: A randomized trial of maintenance therapy for vasculitis associated with antineutrophil cytoplasmic autoantibodies. N Engl J Med 2003;349:36-44.

Klahr S, Levey AS, Beck GJ, et al: The effects of dietary protein restriction and blood-pressure control on the progression of chronic renal disease. N Engl J Med 1994;330:877-884.

Miller G, Zimmerman R, Radhakrishnan J, Appel G: Use of mycophenolate mofetil in resistant membranous nephropathy. Am J Kidney Dis 2000;36:250-256.

Nakao N, Yoshimura A, Morita H, at al: Combination treatment of angiotensin-II receptor blocker and angiotensin-converting-enzyme inhibitor in non-diabetic renal disease (COOPERATE): A randomised controlled trial. Lancet 2003;361:117-124.

Pei Y, Cattran D, Delmore T, et al: Evidence suggesting under-treatment in adults with idiopathic focal segmental glomerulosclerosis. Am J Med 1987;82:938-944.

Ponticelli C, Altieri P, Scolari F, et al: A randomized study comparing methylprednisolone plus chlorambucil versus methylprednisolone plus cyclophosphamide (Cytoxan) in idiopathic membranous nephropathy. J Am Soc Nephrol 1998;9:444-450.

Praga M, Gutierrez E, Gonzalez E, et al: Treatment of IgA nephropathy with ACE inhibitors: A randomized and controlled trial. J Am Soc Nephrol 2003;14:1578-1583.

Acute Pyelonephritis

Method of
Kurt A. McCammon, MD,
and Carol F. McCammon, MD

Acute pyelonephritis results from infection and inflammation of the renal parenchyma and renal pelvis. Most infections ascend to the kidney from the lower urinary tract (LUT), and many patients relate a history of recent dysuria, frequency, or urgency. Patients in general present ill-appearing, febrile, and complain typically of unilateral flank pain often associated with nausea and vomiting.

Physical findings include fever, costovertebral angle (CVA) tenderness, and sometimes mild abdominal discomfort on examination. Although the majority of patients may be treated as outpatients successfully, remember that inadequate or delayed eradication of infection can result in serious sequelae including hypertension, renal scarring, and end-stage renal disease (ESRD).

Rakel and Bope: Conn's Current Therapy 2006.

Fortunately, timely diagnosis and appropriate treatment can greatly reduce the risk of these complications.

Etiology

The most common pathogens causing acute pyelonephritis are aerobic gram-negative bacteria. Most cases result from ascending lower urinary tract infections (LUTIs); therefore, the etiologic agents parallel. Nearly 85% of community-acquired cases of acute pyelonephritis result from the *Escherichia coli.* Other less-common pathogens include *Proteus, Klebsiella, Enterococcus,* and *Staphylococcus saprophyticus.* Nosocomial infections are predominantly caused by *E. coli* (approximately 50%); other pathogens include (in order of frequency) *Enterococcus, Klebsiella, Enterobacter, Citrobacter, Serratia, Pseudomonas aeruginosa,* and *Staphylococcus epidermidis.* Urine cultures usually produce single bacterium because pyelonephritis is rarely polymicrobial.

Pathology

The susceptible host frequently develops acute pyelonephritis from the LUT. Colonization of the perineum by the intruding organism may be the initial event. If untreated at the LUT level, the organism may further ascend the urinary tract (UT) via the ureters to the renal pelvis and renal parenchyma, resulting in the clinical manifestations of acute pyelonephritis. This retrograde progression may result from the presence of fimbriae on the surface of many bacteria that invade the UT. Culture-proved fimbriated organisms occur in 8% of cases of acute pyelonephritis.

Hematogenous seeding of the renal parenchyma from a remote site of infection causes pyelonephritis in approximately 5% of cases. Patients will more frequently exhibit bilateral flank pain, and CVA tenderness and sources other than the UT must be sought and appropriately treated. Individuals at risk include patients on immunosuppressive therapy or a history of intravenous (IV) drug use. A gram-positive bacterial urine culture is nearly always a result of blood-borne, distant infection.

Epidemiology

There are 250,000 cases of acute pyelonephritis each year in the United States. Women are most frequently affected by acute pyelonephritis with a 50% chance of developing a LUTI. Only 2% of these LUTIs are found to ascend. Pregnancy adds a significant risk, particularly in the second and third trimesters when ureteral compression and urinary stasis from the enlarging uterus play anatomic roles in establishing urinary infection. Thus, treatment of asymptomatic bacteriuria is recommended in pregnant women. In children, vesicoureteral reflux and anatomic anomalies are most often associated with the development of pyelonephritis.

Differential Diagnosis

Any disease process that causes fever and flank or abdominal pain must be considered in the differential diagnosis of acute pyelonephritis. Generally, diverticular disease, appendicitis, cholecystitis, hepatitis, and pancreatitis should be considered. Renal colic from calculi or other obstructing lesions may manifest similarly. In women, consider pelvic inflammatory disease, Fitz-Hugh-Curtis syndrome, and when pregnant, hemolysis, elevated liver enzymes, and low platelet (HELLP) syndrome. Men should also be evaluated for prostatitis, epididymitis, and orchitis as well, and their presence may be a preceding factor in the cause of acute pyelonephritis. Overall, the patient's history, physical examination, and appropriate ancillary testing will help distinguish between these numerous possibilities in differential diagnosis.

Ancillary Testing

Urinalysis and urine culture are indicated preferably before institution of antibiotic therapy when appropriate because pyelonephritis, by definition, is a complicated UTI. Urinalysis and urine culture require adequate clean urine; in females, a catheterized specimen is recommended. The urinalysis frequently shows pyuria, bacteria, esterase, and nitrites. It should not contain epithelial cells, which indicate contamination and renders the specimen inadequate for culture.

White blood cell (WBC) casts are often seen in the setting of acute pyelonephritis. Taking blood for complete blood cell count and culture should also be considered because the WBC count can be followed for signs of response to treatment along with clinical progress. The blood culture is useful in the treatment of particularly ill-appearing patients, and 20% to 30% of patients will have a positive blood culture. Renal function should also be ascertained because acute pyelonephritis may cause renal dysfunction in severely affected patients, those with co-morbid conditions, or those with a single kidney. Antibiotic choice and further radiographic evaluation may be altered in the patient with a disturbance in renal function. Empirical treatment should promptly begin while awaiting culture results.

Patients with significant co-morbid conditions and those who do not respond well to initial antimicrobial therapy, prepubescents, and the elderly should be considered for radiographic evaluation. Indications include pyelonephritis in pregnancy, history of urolithiasis, prior genitourinary surgery, recurrent pyelonephritis, and fever for more than 5 to 7 days without appropriate medical evaluation.

Intravenous pyelogram (IVP) is the initial study of choice in nonpregnant patients with adequate renal function. IVP will demonstrate segmental or global renal enlargement, delay in nephrograms, anatomic anomalies, and/or UT obstruction. However, 75% of studies prove normal.

Alternatively, computed tomography (CT) may be useful (without contrast) to quickly evaluate for obstructing stones. Other abnormalities may also be suggested by the CT, which could help in patient management. Ultrasound (US) is less invasive, safe in pregnancy, and will not disturb renal function; however, it may not provide as much information as IVP. It is sensitive in identifying the presence of perinephric or intrarenal abscess, segmental renal abnormalities, and hydronephrosis and may detect larger renal calculi.

Management

First, it must be determined whether the patient has a complicated or uncomplicated case of acute pyelonephritis. Patients with uncomplicated cases of acute pyelonephritis are generally treated as outpatients (Figure 1). After an adequate urinalysis and culture are obtained, the patient can be started on oral antibiotics, most often a fluoroquinolone or other antibiotic with similar coverage (Box 1). Antipyretics, analgesia, and fluids are recommended. The patient should be re-evaluated in 72 hours and, if the patient is appropriately improving, may continue outpatient treatment for 14 to 21 days. At the end of treatment, the patient should return for repeat urinalysis and culture to prove complete adequate treatment. If this culture is positive, retreatment with an appropriately targeted antibiotic should be started and radiographic evaluation of the UT considered. Nonsteroidal anti-inflammatory drugs[1] and vitamins A[1] and E may potentially decrease renal scarring even if there is a delay in initial antibiotic treatment.

Patients with complicated cases of acute pyelonephritis should be strongly considered for inpatient treatment with at least 3 days of IV antibiotics (Box 2 and Figure 2). These patients are at risk for serious sequelae in the face of treatment failure and should be monitored closely. After adequate urinalysis and culture,

---

[1]Not FDA approved for this indication.

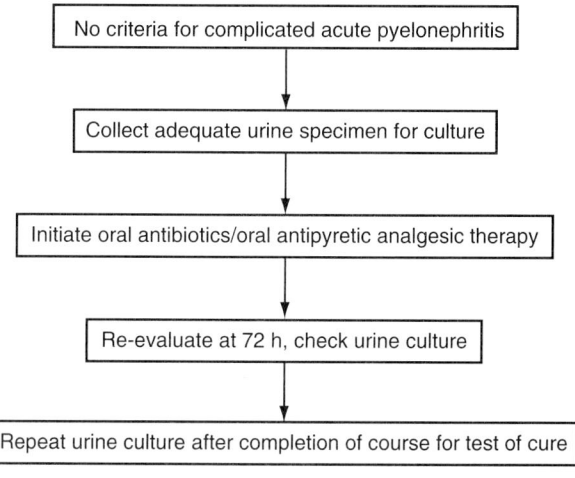

FIGURE 1. Treatment algorithm for uncomplicated acute pyelonephritis.

Rakel and Bope: *Conn's Current Therapy 2006.*

BOX 1 Oral Antibiotic Regimens for Outpatient Treatment*

Primary
Ciprofloxacin (Cipro)[1] 500 mg bid
Ofloxacin (Floxin)[1] 200-400 mg PO q12h
Levofloxacin (Levaquin) 250-500 mg qd

Alternative
Amoxicillin/clavulanate (Augmentin)[1] 875 mg bid
Cephalexin (Keflex)[1] 500 mg tid-qid
Cefadroxil (Duricef)[1] 1-2 g divided bid
Cefaclor (Ceclor)[1] 250-500 mg tid
Cefprozil (Cefzil)[1] 250-500 mg bid
Cefdinir (Omnicef)[1] 600 mg qd
Cefpodoxime (Vantin)[1] 100-400 mg bid
Ceftibuten (Cedax)[1] 400 mg qd
Trimethoprim/sulfamethoxazole DS PO bid

---

*Check antibiotic resistance patterns in your region to guide empirical therapy.
[1]Not FDA approved for this indication.
Abbreviations: bid = twice daily; PO = orally; qd = every day; qid = four times daily; tid = three times daily.

BOX 2 Criteria for Complicated Pyelonephritis[1]

- Anatomic or functional urinary tract abnormalities
- Immunocompromised host
- Prepubertal age
- Male gender
- Sepsis
- Nausea and vomiting
- Significant co-morbid conditions

Consider Admission[1]

BOX 3 Intravenous Antibiotic Regimens for Inpatient Treatment* of Adults with Normal Renal Function

Primary
Ciprofloxacin[1†] 400 mg q12h
Levofloxacin (Levaquin) 250-500 mg q24h
Ofloxacin (Floxin)[1†] 200-400 mg q12h
Ampicillin 1-2 g q4-6h plus gentamicin 3-5 mg/kg/day divided q8h[2]
Ceftriaxone (Rocephin)[1†] 1 g q24h
Ceftizoxime (Cefizox)[1†] 1-2 g q8-12h
Ceftazidime (Fortaz)[1†] 1-2 g q8-12h
Cefotaxime (Claforan)[1†] 1-2 g q6-8h

Alternative
Ticarcillin/clavulanate (Timentin)[1†] 3.1 g q4-6h
Ampicillin/sulbactam (Unasyn)[1†] 1.5-3 g q6h
Piperacillin/tazobactam (Zosyn)[1] 3.375-4.5 g q6h
Ertapenem (Invanz)[1] 1.0 g IV qd

---

*Check antibiotic resistance patterns in your region to guide empirical therapy.
[1]Not FDA approved for this indication.
[2]Follow peak/trough levels during treatment.
[†]For gram-positive organisms, consider adding vancomycin 1 g q12h.

the patient should promptly be started on an IV broad-spectrum antibiotic regimen (Box 3). The patient should have a complete blood cell count, blood culture, and creatinine level drawn. Supportive measures of IV fluids, antipyretics, analgesia, and antiemetics should be administered. Radiographic evaluation in the hemodynamically stable patient should be considered early in

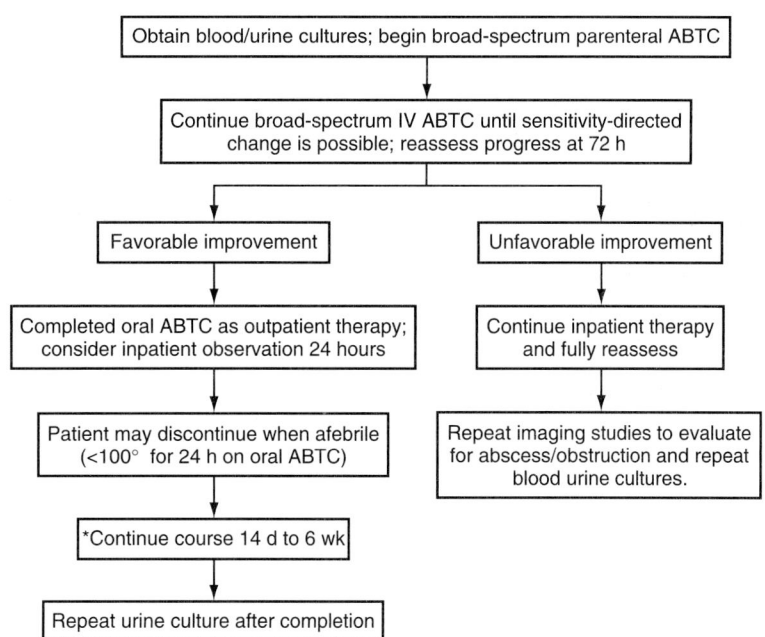

CRITERIA FOR COMPLICATED ACUTE PYELONEPHRITIS

* Prolonged courses are typical for patients with underlying prostatitis, with indwelling foreign body, and after genitourinary surgical procedure. *Abbreviation*: ABTC = antibiotic.

FIGURE 2. Treatment algorithm for complicated acute pyelonephritis. ABTC = antibiotic; IV = intravenous.

Rakel and Bope: *Conn's Current Therapy 2006.*

the course of treatment. If fever abates and there is clinical improvement within 72 hours, the patient may be switched to a tailored oral regimen. Another day of observation is recommended to make certain the patient remains afebrile. If the patient does not improve within 72 hours, review cultures and sensitivity and perform studies to rule out renal abscess, perinephric abscess, UT obstruction, or other abnormality. If any are present, appropriate management by an urologist is indicated.

Management in Pregnancy

Obstetric/gynecologic (OB/GYN) consultation in these patients is appropriate in management of acute pyelonephritis. Antibiotic regimens that are category B or C are acceptable under most circumstances, provided the patient has no allergies. Nearly all of these patients should have IV antibiotics and initial inpatient management because preterm labor and miscarriage are risks of persistent infection. Avoid sulfa during the third trimester because newborns may develop kernicterus. Tetracycline discolors teeth in the fetus and therefore is also contraindicated in all trimesters. Fluoroquinolones have been shown to cause cartilaginous disorders in fetal animals and are not recommended.

Special Pediatric Considerations

Pediatric patients with acute pyelonephritis are likely to have UT anomalies. These patients must have radiographic evaluation to include renal US and voiding cystourethrography to further evaluate the anatomy of the UT. Once initial infection is eradicated, the patient with an anatomic abnormality should be maintained on daily antibiotic suppressive therapy until it is deemed unnecessary by the urologist or the abnormality is appropriately corrected.

Neurologic Impairment

Patients with spinal cord injury above the level of renal innervation (T11 or higher) can have a delayed presentation and much more vague symptomatology. Similarly, patients with multiple sclerosis (MS) and other neurologic diseases can have an atypical presentation because of sensory loss. They may be unable to identify dysuria, flank pain, and other classic symptoms of pyelonephritis; additionally, many of these patients have indwelling or intermittent catheterization, which can interfere with interpretation of urinalysis. The presence of fever and pyuria/bacteriuria with absence of other foci of infection may be the only clinical indicators of the presence of pyelonephritis. These patients should undergo radiographic imaging to rule out upper-urinary obstruction in addition to management in the complicated pyelonephritis pathway.

Complications

Aggressive early treatment of acute pyelonephritis prevents most complications of the disease. However, patients who are inadequately treated or who present late in a fulminant process can suffer significant complications, including sepsis and death. Emphysematous pyelonephritis is a rare form and occurs primarily in diabetics. It is a fulminant, necrotizing infection, commonly caused by *E. coli*. An examination of the kidney, ureter, and bladder may show air in the nephric shadow. The involved kidney functions poorly; therefore, an IVP is not helpful in confirming the diagnosis. Emphysematous pyelonephritis is an indication for emergency nephrectomy. Percutaneous drainage helps in the appropriate clinical setting. Renal and perinephric abscess should be evaluated by a urologist and may respond to antibiotics alone. Some may require percutaneous or surgical drainage or possibly nephrectomy. Chronic renal scarring may lead to hypertension. Recurrent episodes can cause enough scar formation to contribute to chronic renal failure.

Trauma to the Genitourinary Tract

Method of
Sean P. Elliott, MD

Urologic trauma spans the spectrum from renal hilar injuries, which require expedient operative intervention to avoid rapid exsanguination, to urethral injuries, which may necessitate only urinary diversion in the acute setting. Several principles should guide the evaluation and management of the urologic trauma patient. First, understand the context of the urologic injury in the setting of the patient's associated injuries, which may be more life-threatening. Second, know the indications for imaging and accurately interpret the subtle findings. Third, formulate a management plan ranging from acute repair to temporization. Finally and most importantly, know which intervention to pursue based on the patient's overall status.

Renal Trauma

Renal injuries account for 1.4% to 3.25% of all traumas. Most renal injuries are the result of blunt trauma—from motor vehicle accidents or falling from a height—with penetrating trauma accounting for less than 20% of all renal injuries. Blunt impact causes direct trauma to the kidney or disruption of the kidney from its attachments at the renal vessels or the ureteropelvic junction. A low-velocity, penetrating wound causes a renal laceration along the path of the knife or bullet, whereas a high-velocity firearm can also cause extensive surrounding tissue necrosis from blast effect. The kidneys are protected by perinephric fat, surrounding vertebral bodies, back muscles, and bowel; therefore, the renal injury rarely occurs in isolation because the force necessary to injure the kidney usually damages the surrounding structures.

A renal injury should be suspected in the trauma patient when any of the following scenarios are present:

- Penetrating injury with gross or microscopic (>2 red blood cells [RBCs]/high-power field [HPF]) hematuria
- Blunt injury with gross hematuria
- Blunt injury with microscopic hematuria and shock (systolic blood pressure [BP] <90 mm Hg)

Hypotension is a less reliable indicator of injury in children. Hematuria should be evaluated from the first aliquot of urine, with either a urine dipstick or microscopic analysis. In the absence of hematuria, a renal injury is still possible in the patient sustaining a rapid deceleration injury or a blunt or penetrating wound to the flank or upper abdomen, as well as in the patient with multiple associated injuries. In the stable patient, evaluation should consist of a computerized tomography (CT) scan with contrast and delayed views. Contrast images enable evaluation of the renal vasculature and renal parenchyma (Figure 1), whereas delayed views demonstrate any urinary extravasation along the course of the collecting system from the renal calyces to the distal ureter. If the patient is brought immediately to the operating room (OR) for abdominal exploration, the kidneys should be explored only if there is an expanding or pulsatile retroperitoneal hematoma. Most children with blunt trauma and fewer than 50 RBCs/HPF will have a minor renal injury. Therefore, it may be possible to eliminate the CT scan in hemodynamically stable children with fewer than 50 RBCs/HPF; whereas unstable children should go immediately for abdominal exploration.

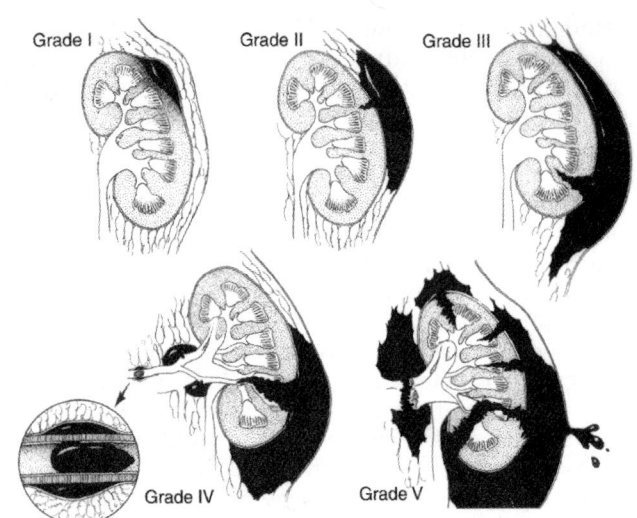

FIGURE 2. The AAST grading system for traumatic renal injuries. Grade I: renal contusion and subcapsular hematoma; grade II: cortical laceration and perirenal hematoma; grade III: laceration into medulla or segmental renal artery thrombosis without a parenchymal injury; grade IV: laceration involving the collecting system, with or without a devascularized segment and contained vascular injury; grade V: renal artery thrombosis, avulsion of the renal pedicle, and shattered kidney. AAST = Association for the Surgery of Trauma. (From McAninch JW [ed.]: Traumatic and reconstructive urology. Philadelphia, WB Saunders, 1996.)

Renal injuries are classified by a validated grading system developed by the American Association for the Surgery of Trauma (AAST) (Figure 2). Most renal injuries are graded on a scale of I to V and can be managed nonoperatively with bed rest and frequent BP and hematocrit measurements. The patient can walk when the hematocrit and BP are stable and any gross hematuria has cleared. Absolute indications for renal exploration include renal hilar avulsion, expanding or pulsatile hematoma, or persistent life-threatening hemorrhage believed to stem from renal injury. Relative indications for exploration include coexistent intra-abdominal injuries requiring exploration, a large laceration of the renal pelvis or ureteropelvic junction, a devitalized renal segment with associated urine leak, complete renal artery thrombosis of both kidneys or a solitary kidney, renal vascular injuries that have failed angiographic management, and renovascular hypertension. Operative management includes repair of the injured kidney if possible and nephrectomy if there is main renal artery injury, main renal vein avulsion, or hemodynamic instability.

Ureteral Trauma

Ureteral injuries from external trauma are uncommon. Gunshot wounds (GSWs) cause 60% to 95% of ureteral injuries, but the ureter is involved in only 2% to 3% of abdominal GSWs. As in renal trauma, the ureters are well protected in the retroperitoneum and the bony pelvis; thus ureteral injury from external violent trauma requires significant blunt impact or penetrating injury with frequent injury to surrounding organs.

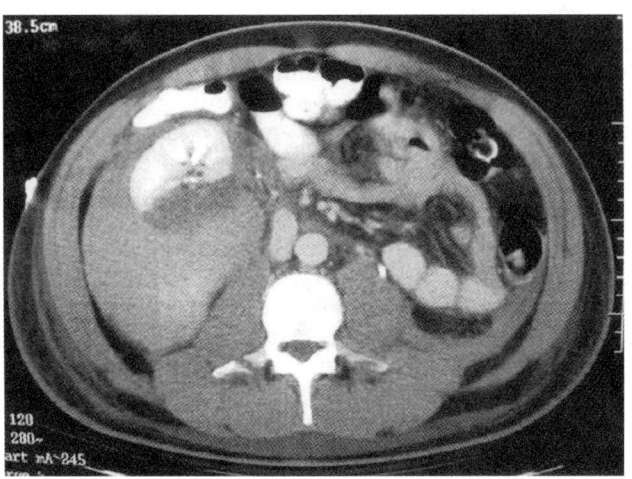

FIGURE 1. Computed tomography scan demonstrating large, right perirenal hematoma and thrombosed posterior segmental artery. Classified as a grade IV renal injury.

Rakel and Bope: *Conn's Current Therapy 2006.*

Hematuria is present in 75% of cases, and hypotension occurs in approximately 50%. Imaging indications and techniques are the same as those for renal injury. Additionally, patients with rapid deceleration injuries or penetrating injury to the flank should be imaged. Findings indicative of injury include urinary contrast extravasation, ureteral narrowing, and delayed peristalsis (Figure 3).

Although a small extravasation of urinary contrast in the intrarenal collecting system in the setting of a renal injury can often be observed, any ureteral injury should be stented and/or repaired immediately. Delay in diagnosis or delay in therapy leads to increased complications from urinary leakage, including infected urinoma and urosepsis. In the stable patient with a minor ureteral injury and no associated injuries requiring laparotomy, consider cystoscopy with ureteral stenting—re-epithelialization often occurs within days and complete healing by 6 weeks. The vast majority of ureteral injuries occur in association with other intra-abdominal injuries, however, in which case the ureter should be surgically repaired. The type of repair depends on the location and the length of the injury, with options

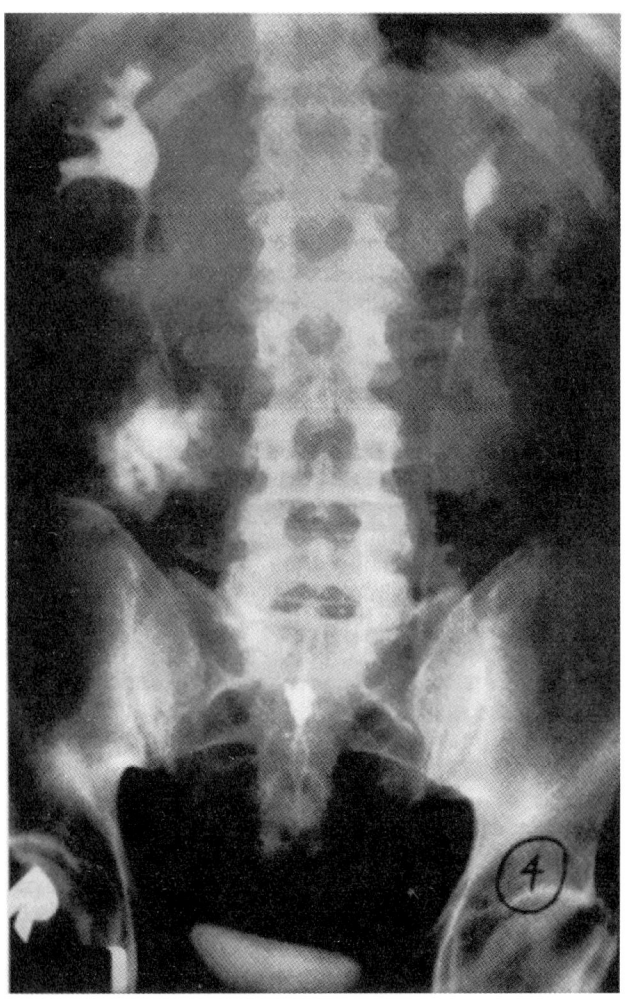

FIGURE 3. Intravenous pyelogram demonstrating extravasation of urine from the right midureter.

including ureteroureterostomy, transureteroureterostomy, or ureteroneocystostomy with or without a psoas hitch, Boari flap, ileal ureter, or autotransplantation. In the unstable patient, the ureter may be ligated and a percutaneous nephrostomy tube placed 2 to 3 days postoperatively. All repairs should be performed over a stent, which is removed in 6 weeks.

Bladder Trauma

Etiology of bladder rupture is blunt trauma in 71% to 88% and penetrating trauma in 12% to 29%. Gross hematuria is universally present. As in renal and ureteral injuries, bladder trauma is frequently associated with other injuries. Of patients with bladder rupture attributable to blunt trauma, approximately 90% have an associated pelvic fracture, whereas only 10% of all patients with pelvic fractures have an associated bladder rupture. Bladder rupture is classified as intraperitoneal (36%), extraperitoneal (56%), or both (8%). Pathogenesis of intraperitoneal bladder rupture caused by blunt trauma is a sharp rise in bladder pressure followed by perforation of the bladder at the dome where the muscular support is the weakest. However, extraperitoneal bladder injuries are usually along the anterolateral bladder wall near the bladder base and are caused by the shear force induced by bony pelvic ring disruption.

If a bladder injury is suspected based on mechanism and gross hematuria, then a cystogram should be performed. Either a plain film cystogram or a CT cystogram is appropriate. Generally the patient requires evaluation of other intra-abdominal organs or pelvic fracture, so a CT cystogram is preferred. If a plain film cystogram is to be performed, it should be preceded by a plain abdomen and pelvis film. The bladder should then be filled retrograde with 300 to 400 mL (in children use 60 mL plus 30 mL per year of age up to 300 mL) of contrast solution and films taken both in the anteroposterior view and oblique. The bladder is then drained and another anteroposterior film taken. If a CT cystogram is preferred, then the bladder should be filled retrograde with a 1 to 6 dilution of contrast solution. It is inadequate to clamp the urethral catheter and wait for previously injected IV contrast to drain down from the kidneys to fill the bladder. A single CT series may be done with the bladder distended; it is unnecessary to obtain prefilling and drainage scans.

Intraperitoneal rupture is characterized on plain films and CT cystography by contrast outlining loops of bowel (Figure 4). All intraperitoneal bladder ruptures should be repaired immediately to avoid the complication of urine peritonitis and to speed the healing time of the frequently long lacerations. The abdomen is explored and the bladder closed in layers with absorbable suture. The bladder is drained with a urethral catheter for 7 to 10 days. A suprapubic catheter may be added if there is significant hematuria.

Extraperitoneal bladder ruptures, on the other hand, are characterized on plain film cystography by a flame-like distribution of contrast either limited to the perivesical space or extending up the retroperitoneum.

Rakel and Bope: *Conn's Current Therapy 2006.*

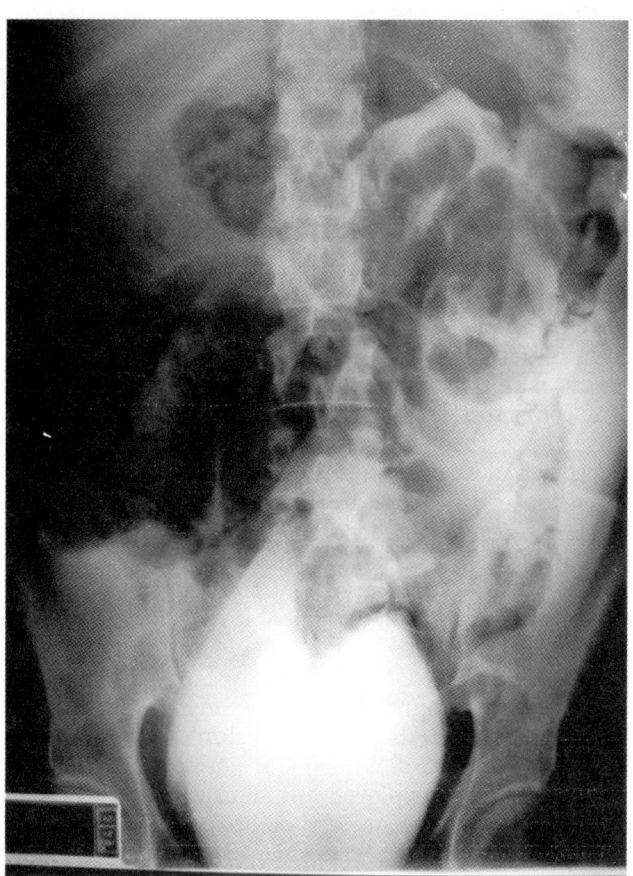

FIGURE 4. Intraperitoneal bladder rupture is demonstrated. Note contrast extravasating from the dome of the bladder and outlining the small intestine and left colon.

On a CT cystogram, contrast is limited to the extraperitoneal potential space (Figure 5), which can generally be managed nonoperatively. Bladder drainage is optimized with a urethral catheter, and the bladder laceration heals in 7 to 10 days. Indications for operative repair of extraperitoneal bladder rupture include excessive

hematuria requiring placement of a suprapubic tube, laparotomy for repair of other injuries, bladder-neck injury, and foreign body in the bladder such as bone.

Urethral Trauma

Male urethral injuries are characterized according to whether they occur in the posterior urethra or the anterior urethra, each with a different pathogenesis and management. Female urethral injuries are rare because of the short course of the urethra.

Approximately 90% of all urethral injuries occur as a result of blunt trauma. Posterior urethral injuries occur at the membranous urethra as a result of the stretching and shear forces that occur in an unstable pelvic fracture. This type of injury, combined with the large pelvic hematoma that often results, may cause significant urethral distraction. Anterior urethral injuries from blunt trauma are most common in the bulbar urethra and result from straddle injuries in which the urethra is crushed between the foreign object and the pubic arch under which the bulbar urethra passes. Anterior urethral injuries in the pendulous urethra are more often the result of a penile fracture or penetrating trauma. Female urethral injuries can be complicated because of involvement of the sphincter, bladder neck, and/or a concomitant vaginal laceration.

Urethral injury should be suspected in any patient with blood at the urethral meatus, especially when the mechanism, inability to void, or associated pelvic fracture would suggest urethral injury. A retrograde urethrogram should be performed before any attempts at passage of a urethral catheter. This is done in the oblique position. With the penis on stretch, 20 to 40 mL of contrast solution should be injected retrograde from the meatus (Figure 6).

Along with treatment of life-threatening associated injuries, the primary goal in treatment of urethral injuries should be to obtain adequate urinary drainage. This minimizes the risk of potential complications

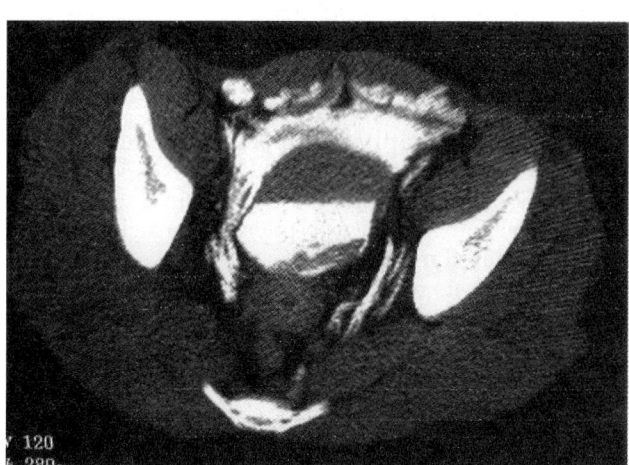

FIGURE 5. Extraperitoneal bladder rupture seen on computed tomography cystogram.

Rakel and Bope: *Conn's Current Therapy 2006.*

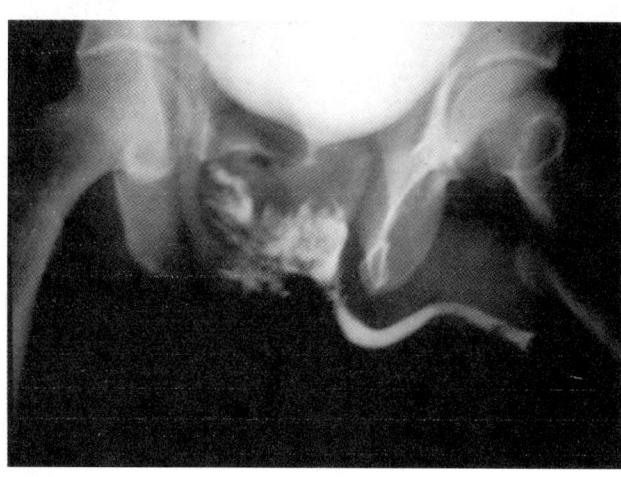

FIGURE 6. Retrograde urethrogram diagnostic of partial bulbar urethral transection resulting from straddle injury.

including urinary retention, urinary fistula, infected urinoma, and Fournier's gangrene. Operative repair of urethral injuries requires debridement of nonviable tissue with primary urethral anastomosis, use of local skin flaps, or placement of grafts. Because hematoma and crush injury make such repairs difficult at the time of injury, acute operative exploration of urethral injuries should be done only in cases of penetrating anterior urethral injury or in cases of urethral injury associated with penile fracture. In these select cases, the possibility of concomitant corporal cavernosal injury and urethral injury argues for exploration to avoid the potential complication of urethra-corporal fistula. However, such injuries are infrequent as blunt traumatic urethral injury. If there is a partial disruption after blunt injury, then one attempt at passage of a urethral catheter is permitted. The management is more controversial in cases of complete disruption or if urethral catheter insertion is unsuccessful. A suprapubic tube may be placed to divert the urine away from the injury. Almost 100% of patients will develop a stricture, which then will be repaired with an open operation in a delayed fashion. In the stable patient, others advocate primary realignment using cystourethroscopy followed by catheter placement over a wire. This may avoid stricture and delayed repair in approximately one third of patients, but it may cause additional harm during cystourethroscopy.

External Genitalia

Of all testicular injuries, 85% are from blunt trauma. Most injuries are sustained during athletic activities; patients present with acute onset of testicular pain. A heterogeneous echo pattern in the testicular parenchyma on ultrasound suggests testicular injury (sensitivity 64%, specificity 75%); whereas visualization of a tear in the tunica albuginea is rare (Figure 7). All testicular injuries

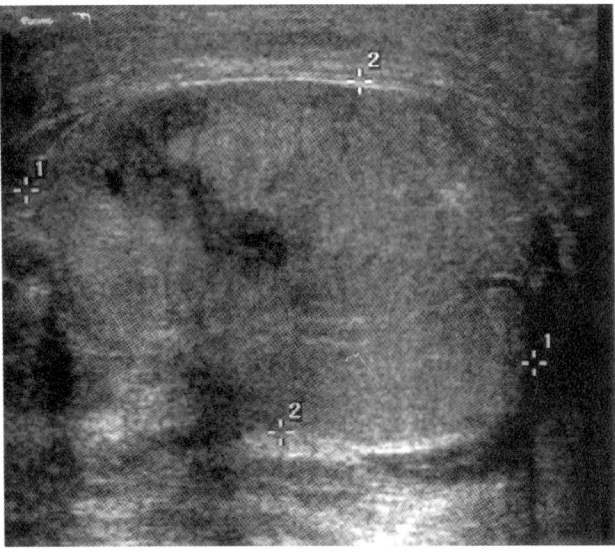

FIGURE 7. Testis ultrasound demonstrating heterogeneous architecture characteristic of testicular rupture.

should be explored. Extruded seminiferous tubules are debrided and the testicle closed. Testicular salvage rate is 90% when explored acutely but drops to 45% when exploration is delayed more than 72 hours.

A traumatic tear in the tunica albuginea of the corpora cavernosa is commonly referred to as a penile *fracture*. Intercourse is described as the cause in 33% to 58% of injuries and is the result of the penis slipping out of the vagina and thrusting against the pubic bone resulting in an acute angulation of the erect penis. Patients report hearing a *crack* or *pop* followed by intense penile pain and rapid detumescence. Buck's fascia usually remains intact, limiting the resulting hematoma to the penis. In some cases hematoma may extend into the scrotum indicating that Buck's fascia was torn. All cases of penile fracture should be explored to evacuate the hematoma and close the tunical tear. The incidence of concomitant urethral injury is approximately 20%. Blood at the meatus, inability to void, and hematuria are suggestive, but not diagnostic, of urethral injury; so one must have a high degree of suspicion. Routine urethrography to rule out urethral injury is advised.

Penetrating injuries to the external genitalia and injuries with extensive genital skin loss (i.e., burns, large abrasions, and avulsions from motor vehicle accidents) should be explored and debrided in an effort to stage the injury and prevent complications such as urinoma and Fournier's gangrene. Skin grafting can be delayed.

 CURRENT DIAGNOSIS

- Indications of GU for CT scan with IV contrast and delayed images:
  Penetrating abdominal trauma with microscopic (>2 RBCs/HPF) or gross hematuria
  Blunt abdominal trauma with gross hematuria
  Blunt abdominal trauma with microscopic hematuria and hypotension (systolic BP <90 mm Hg)
  Rapid deceleration injuries
  Flank trauma
- Indications for cystogram
  Absolute
  Gross hematuria with pelvic fracture
  Relative
  Gross hematuria without pelvic fracture
  Pelvic fracture with microhematuria
  Isolated microhematuria
- Indications for retrograde urethrogram
  Blood at the urethral meatus
  Inability to void
  Pelvic fracture with displacement of the pubic ramus
- Indications for scrotal ultrasound
  Any blunt or penetrating trauma to the scrotum

Abbreviations: BP = blood pressure; CT = computed tomography; GU = genitourinary; HPF = high-power field; IV = intravenous; RBC = red blood cell.

CURRENT THERAPY

Renal Trauma
- Management of grades I to III (or IV) renal trauma in the hemodynamically stable patient
  Bed rest
  Serial hematocrits and transfuse as needed
  Walk when urine is clear and hematocrit stable
- Indications for renal exploration with repair versus nephrectomy
  Absolute
    Renal hilar avulsion
    Expanding or pulsatile hematoma
    Persistent life-threatening hemorrhage believed to stem from renal injury
  Relative
    Coexistent intra-abdominal injuries requiring exploration
    Large laceration of the renal pelvis or ureteropelvic junction
    Devitalized renal segment with associated urine leak
    Complete renal artery thrombosis of both kidneys or of a solitary kidney
    Renal vascular injuries that have failed angiographic management
    Renovascular hypertension

Bladder
- Intraperitoneal rupture: abdominal exploration and closure
- Extraperitoneal: urethral catheter drainage for 7 to 10 days

Urethra
- If partial disruption, then one attempt at urethral catheter placement
- If unsuccessful or if complete urethral disruption, then cystoscopy with primary realignment for suprapubic tube placement with delayed repair

Testis
- Exploration and repair
- Extraperitoneal bladder rupture seen on computed tomography cystogram

Traumatic penile amputation occurs rarely and is usually the result of assault, but it can also be self-inflicted and related to unresolved gender or psychosexual issues, usually in the setting of intoxication. If the penis is brought to the hospital, it should be stored in saline-soaked gauze pads on ice. Reconstruction should be performed within 24 hours.

The care of the urologic trauma patient is challenging in that it requires the efficiency and fortitude to repair complex injuries in the acutely ill patient as well as the wisdom to recognize when to delay repair of non–life–threatening injuries in the unstable patient.

Rakel and Bope: *Conn's Current Therapy 2006.*

REFERENCES

Brandes S, Coburn M, Armenakas N, McAninch JW: Diagnosis and management of ureteric injury: An evidence-based analysis. BJU Int 2004;94(3):277-289.
Chapple C, Barbagli G, Jordan G, et al: Consensus statement on urethral trauma. BJU Int 2004;93(9):1195-1202.
Elliott SP, McAninch JW: Ureteral injuries from external violence: The 25-year experience at San Francisco General Hospital. J Urol 2003;170(4 Pt 1):1213-1216.
Gomez RG, Ceballos L, Coburn M, et al: Consensus statement on bladder injuries. BJU Int 2004;94(1): 27-32.
Morey AF, Metro MJ, Carney KJ, et al: Consensus on genitourinary trauma: External genitalia. BJU Int 2004;94(4):507-515.
Santucci RA, Wessells H, Bartsch G, et al: Evaluation and management of renal injuries: Consensus statement of the renal trauma subcommittee. BJU Int 2004;93(7):937-954.
Wessells H, Suh D, Porter JR, et al: Renal injury and operative management in the United States: Results of a population-based study. J Trauma 2003;54:423-430.

Prostatitis

Method of
Michel A. Pontari, MD

Prostatitis, one of the most commonly seen urologic conditions in both primary care and urology offices, accounts for an estimated 2 million visits per year to physicians in the United States. The term *prostatitis* refers to a wide array of clinical syndromes, from true bacterial infection to symptoms of chronic pelvic pain with no identifiable infection, as well as to histologic evidence of prostatic inflammation in the absence of symptoms. The National Institutes of Health (NIH) classification of prostatitis reflects this diversity (Box 1).

Category I: Acute Bacterial Prostatitis

Acute prostatitis, characterized by the sudden onset of fever and dysuria, represents a true acute infection of the prostate, caused by bacteria including *Escherichia coli, Klebsiella, Enterobacter,* and *Pseudomonas.* Voiding symptoms, in addition to burning with urination, can include frequency, urgency, and hesitancy. On physical examination, the prostate should be palpated

BOX 1	National Institutes of Health Classification of Prostatitis
Category I	Acute bacterial prostatitis
Category II	Chronic bacterial prostatitis
Category III	Chronic pelvic pain syndrome
Category IIIA	Inflammatory
Category IIIB	Noninflammatory
Category IV	Asymptomatic inflammatory prostatitis

with caution because vigorous massage or repeat examinations theoretically could produce bacteremia and precipitate urosepsis. The postvoid residual urine should be measured, preferably by ultrasound, to avoid catheterization. Laboratory studies should include both urine and blood cultures and a white blood cell (WBC) count.

TREATMENT

Patients are generally admitted to the hospital because they are acutely ill on presentation. Intravenous (IV) fluids are started as well as IV antibiotics. Traditionally, an aminoglycoside and ampicillin are started. An IV fluoroquinolone is also acceptable. If the patient has a significantly elevated postvoid residual, a suprapubic tube is recommended to avoid a urethral catheter that could exacerbate the infection. If the patient is in retention, an α-blocker[1] helps with urination once the inflammation subsides. Nonsteroidal anti-inflammatory agents reduce prostate inflammation and help with discomfort. The IV antibiotics are continued until the patient is afebrile for 24 hours or as per indicated by the blood culture results. Oral antibiotic therapy is then started as per the culture and sensitivity and continued for 4 weeks to try to prevent bacterial colonization and chronic bacterial prostatitis. Usually fluoroquinolones are used as the oral agent. If a patient has persistent symptoms and fever, a computed tomography (CT) scan should be performed to rule out a prostatic abscess. If an abscess is present, it should be drained transurethrally.

Category II: Chronic Bacterial Prostatitis

Chronic bacterial prostatitis is characterized by relapsing episodes of urinary tract infections, usually with the same organism seen on urine cultures. These patients are usually asymptomatic between infections. True chronic bacterial prostatitis is relatively uncommon. The manifestation is that of a urinary tract infection, with dysuria, frequency, and low back pain. Patients usually do not have the elevated temperature or toxic appearance of patients with acute bacterial prostatitis. Evaluation includes prostate examination, determination of postvoid residual urine, and a urine culture. If the patient has multiple recurrent infections, an ultrasound of the kidneys and a cystoscopy can rule out other causes of recurrent urinary tract infection (UTI).

TREATMENT

Antibiotics are prescribed based on the result of the urine culture. While waiting for the results of the culture, empirical therapy is started with either sulfa-based antibiotics or a fluoroquinolone. Treatment should be

for 2 to 4 weeks. For cases of more frequent repeat episodes in the absence of an anatomic cause, such as urinary retention, prophylaxis with daily antibiotics can be used for 3 to 6 months.

Category III: Chronic Prostatitis/ Chronic Pelvic Pain Syndrome

Patients with category III, chronic prostatitis/chronic pelvic pain syndrome (CP/CPPS), have chronic pelvic pain that can be relapsing and remitting. Sites of discomfort include the penis, suprapubic area, testes, and perineum, as well as dysuria and pain after ejaculation. The term *chronic pelvic pain* indicates that not all the discomfort in these men comes from the prostate, and it may include the bladder, rectum, penis, or even central nervous system (CNS) as sources of discomfort. Associated systemic symptoms such as fatigue are common, as is erectile dysfunction. Category IIIA is inflammatory CPPS with WBC present in either semen, expressed prostatic secretions (EPS), or post-prostate massage urine (VB3 [voided bladder 3]). Category IIIB includes individuals without WBC in any of these fluids. No significant differences exist clinically between categories IIIA and IIIB, so it is not necessary to measure WBC in these specimens. But a midstream urine culture should be obtained to rule out a UTI as the source of pelvic pain. Fractionated cultures of VB1 (voided bladder 1) (first 10 mL), VB3, and EPS are not indicated because recent studies show that asymptomatic men have as many localizing bacteria in the prostate as do men with CPPS.

The main tenet of evaluation of men with CPPS is to identify treatable causes of pelvic pain. Unfortunately, in the vast majority of men, a clear cause is not found. In addition to a urine culture, the evaluation should include a thorough history and physical examination. An assessment of symptoms is facilitated by using the NIH-Chronic Prostatitis Symptom Index (NIH-CPSI), a self-administered validated symptom index. Originally designed as an outcome measure for use in treatment trials, it also is very helpful for symptom assessment in the office and now available in a Spanish translation. The history should also include history of infections, trauma, or any neurologic disease, including vertebral disc problems. The physical examination should search for extraprostatic causes of pain, including penile

---

 CURRENT DIAGNOSIS

- Urinalysis for hematuria indicative of cancer
- Urine culture to exclude ongoing infection
- Urinary retention excluded
- Neurologic abnormalities identified
- Scrotal ultrasound for orchalgia
- Computerized tomography scan for concomitant abdominal pain

---

[1]Not FDA approved for this indication.

Rakel and Bope: *Conn's Current Therapy 2006.*

CURRENT THERAPY

- First line: 4 to 6 weeks of antibiotics; repeat courses only for documented urinary tract infection
- α-Blockers
- Anti-inflammatory medications
- Second line: Medications for pain: tricyclic antidepressants, anticonvulsants
- Medications for urinary frequency: anticholinergics
- Pelvic floor physical therapy

---

lesions, testicular masses, and perirectal processes. In addition to a urine culture, a urinalysis looking for hematuria is mandatory. Men with irritative voiding symptoms should have a urine cytology to rule out carcinoma in situ of the bladder. Another recommended investigation is determining postvoid residual urine, which is especially important in men older than 50 years of age, given their greater risk of retention from benign prostatic hypertrophy (BPH) than in younger men with CP/CPPS. Imaging studies should be determined by specific findings, such as looking for midline cysts in men with pain on ejaculation. CT scan should be considered in patients who present with concomitant abdominal pain in addition to the pelvic pain. Urodynamics may be helpful in patients with voiding symptoms or elevated residual. Prostate-specific antigen (PSA) is not a part of the standard evaluation of men with CPPS, and an elevated PSA should not a priori be ascribed to prostate inflammation but be further evaluated for the possibility of prostate cancer as it would be in any asymptomatic man.

TREATMENT

Men with chronic pelvic pain and symptoms similar to those of a prostate infection are treated with one initial 4-week course of antibiotics, even with a negative urine culture. If they respond, antibiotics are continued for another 2 to 4 weeks. Repeated courses of antibiotics after this initial treatment are not used unless there is a positive urine culture. Second-line therapies in men with persistent symptoms include α-adrenergic blockers[1] and nonsteroidal anti-inflammatory medications. For men with persistent pain, tricyclic antidepressants[1] can be beneficial because of their effect on neuropathic pain. Other pain medications include antiseizure medications[1] and newer non-narcotic analgesics. Urinary frequency and irritative symptoms may be helped by anticholinergic agents and medications used to treat interstitial cystitis, such as antihistamines[1] and synthetic heparinoids (Pentosan, Elmiron). Pelvic floor physical therapy may be helpful. For refractory cases, sacral neuromodulation is an option. Surgery on the

---

[1]Not FDA approved for this indication.

Rakel and Bope: *Conn's Current Therapy 2006.*

prostate either transurethrally or to remove the prostate is not recommended.

Category IV: Asymptomatic Inflammatory Prostatitis

Prostatic inflammation is found on many prostate biopsies and specimens from transurethral resections. Patients with asymptomatic histologic prostate inflammation require no further evaluation or specific treatment.

Benign Prostatic Hyperplasia

Method of
Gopal H. Badlani, MD,
and Matthew E. Karlovsky, MD

10

Epidemiology

Bladder outlet obstruction (BOO) secondary to benign prostatic hyperplasia (BPH) is one of the most common medical conditions in older men and represents up to a 40% clinical risk for urinary retention in a man's lifetime. It is the most prevalent condition in the aging male, affecting 14 million men in the United States, with an annual cost of $4 billion to treat. Age and normal androgenic function are two of the better established risk factors. Whereas BPH is rare before the age of 40, the prevalence of histologic BPH at autopsy is 50% by 60 years of age and 90% by 85 years of age. Approximately 40% of males 70 years of age or older have lower urinary tract symptoms (LUTS) secondary to BPH, and with age, the prevalence increases. Symptomatically, approximately 25% of 55-year-old men experience decreased urinary flow rate and other symptoms of BPH. By 75 years of age, the appearance of this symptom increases to 50%. Age, however, is not a causative factor of BOO. Although the risk for developing symptoms from BPH doubles for each decade of life between 60 and 90 years of age, clinical symptoms of the individual patient do not necessarily progress with age. BPH is more commonly diagnosed because of increased life expectancy and a greater tendency today to seek medical advice at an earlier disease stage.

Normal androgenic function is required for development of BPH. Both androgenic and estrogenic hormonal stimulation can induce prostatic hypertrophy. Other factors, such as race, sexual activity, smoking, socioeconomic status, vasectomy, alcohol intake, and diet, have been implicated in BPH development. Identifying men at clinical risk for BPH and its progression has clinical usefulness in selecting the appropriate intervention when necessary.

Pathophysiology

The pathophysiology of BPH is poorly understood because no direct correlation can be made between prostatic glandular enlargement and the symptomatology of BPH. Because the condition is rare in those younger than 40 years of age and does not develop in castrated men, it is accepted that BPH development requires aging and functional testes for androgen production. BPH is believed to originate in the transitional zone of the prostate, which surrounds the prostatic urethra between the bladder neck and the verumontanum, and is progressive.

Both a static and a dynamic component are involved in BPH development. The static component relates to epithelial and stromal cell proliferation in the prostatic transitional zone (TZ); enlargement is evident as median or lateral lobe hypertrophy. Proliferation is induced by testosterone and its biologically active conversion product, dihydrotestosterone. Conversion of testosterone to dihydrotestosterone occurs via the enzyme 5α-reductase. Two forms of this enzyme have been described, type 1 and type 2. Type 1 is present in liver, skin, and other organs. Type 2 is present in urogenital tissues. Individuals lacking 5α-reductase type 2 do not develop genitalia and prostates.

Conversely, the dynamic component relates to prostatic smooth muscle. High concentrations of α_1-adrenergic receptors occur in the prostatic capsule and bladder neck. An increase in smooth muscle tone is responsible for increased urethral resistance and pressure. Pharmacologic blockade with α_1 antagonists blocks prostatic smooth muscle contraction and decreases urethral resistance and pressure, subsequently relaxing the dynamic component of BPH.

Symptoms

The diagnosis of BPH is presumptive, based on symptoms. These symptoms, commonly referred to as lower urinary tract symptoms (LUTS), are not specific for BPH. LUTS include frequency, retention, intermittency, decreased force of stream (FOS), straining, urgency, and nocturia. Individuals with LUTS should be carefully assessed to determine the cause, to confirm diagnosis of BPH, and to exclude other bladder and prostate processes. Normal prostate size on digital rectal examination (DRE) does not rule out a diagnosis of BPH because palpable prostate size does not correlate with degree of obstruction or severity of LUTS. However, the odds of having moderate to severe symptoms are five times higher for men with enlarged prostates compared with those with normal prostates. Symptoms of BPH are difficult to assess and quantify, yet they are the keys to proper diagnosis and treatment. Because the vast majority of procedures performed for BPH are to provide symptomatic relief, it is necessary to quantify the level of interference in the quality of life of the patient. Assessment of interference on quality of life can be reliably accomplished using the well-validated International Prostate Symptom Score (IPSS) (Figure 1).

Symptoms based on overall score are classified as mild (0 to 7), moderate (8 to 19), and severe (20 to 35). The subjective impact of these symptoms on overall quality of life must also be taken into account. The patient with a severe-range IPSS may feel the symptoms are less bothersome than a patient with a lower IPSS, and this subjective impact on quality of life can direct therapeutic options.

Diagnosis

Diagnosis of BPH relies on an accurate medical history eliciting the specific voiding complaints, as well as quantification of these symptoms using the IPSS. Other possible causes of LUTS also must be ruled out, including urinary tract infection (UTI), urolithiasis, diabetes, urethral stricture, overactive or neurogenic bladder, prostate/bladder cancer, or congestive heart failure. Medications that can exacerbate obstructive symptoms include tricyclic antidepressants, anticholinergic agents, diuretics, narcotics, and first-generation antihistamines and decongestants. Physical examination should include DRE for prostatic abnormalities, such as palpable nodules, induration or irregularities of malignancy, or infection. On DRE, the posterior lobes, not the transition zone, are palpable. Abdominal examination may detect a suprapubic or low abdominal mass in a patient with BPH-induced retention. The American Urological Association and the American Cancer Society recommend all men older than age 50 receive an annual prostate-specific antigen (PSA) serum level to screen for prostate cancer. In black men or men with a family history of prostate cancer in a first-degree relative, PSA screening should begin at 40 years of age or younger. The normal range for PSA is up to 4.0 μg/mL. Other valuable laboratory data include urinalysis to rule out infection or hematuria, a serum creatinine level to determine renal function, and urine cytologic studies if irritative voiding symptoms are present. More sophisticated studies, such as urinary flow rate, postvoid residual, and pressure flow urodynamic studies, are appropriate for evaluation of men with more severe symptoms (IPSS >8) or with more complex comorbidities. These tests are often used to determine baseline function prior to initiation of therapy or to determine subsequent response to therapy. In patients who fail medical therapy, urodynamic pressure-flow studies and cystoscopy may be appropriate to evaluate the need for operative intervention and to rule out other urologic pathologies. Cystoscopy is also reserved for situations in which invasive treatment is strongly considered. If watchful waiting or noninvasive therapies are appropriate, invasive diagnostic tests are usually not necessary. The variables of importance of disease progression in an artificial neural network analysis were PSA, obstructive symptom score, and transitional zone volume. The Olmstead County study showed risk progression of acute urinary retention (AUR) with age. Overall, a 60-year-old man has a 23% chance of AUR if he survives the next 20 years. The average annual change in prostate volume was 1.6% for all ages. The annual increase was

Rakel and Bope: *Conn's Current Therapy 2006.*

Name: Date:

	Not at all	Less than 1 time in 5	Less than half the time	About half the time	More than half the time	Almost always	Your score
Incomplete emptying Over the past month, how often have you had a sensation of not emptying your bladder completely after you finish urinating?	0	1	2	3	4	5	
Frequency Over the past month, how often have you had to urinate again less than two hours after you finished urinating?	0	1	2	3	4	5	
Intermittency Over the past month, how often have you found you stopped and started again several times when you urinated?	0	1	2	3	4	5	
Urgency Over the past month, how difficult have you found it to postpone urination?	0	1	2	3	4	5	
Weak stream Over the past month, how often have you had a weak urinary stream?	0	1	2	3	4	5	
Straining Over the past month, how often have you had to push or strain to begin urination?	0	1	2	3	4	5	

	None	1 time	2 times	3 times	4 times	5 times or more	Your score
Nocturia Over the past month, how many times did you most typically get up to urinate from the time you went to bed until the time you got up in the morning?	0	1	2	3	4	5	

Total IPSS score							

Quality of life due to urinary symptoms	Delighted	Pleased	Mostly satisfied	Mixed— about equally satisfied and dissatisfied	Mostly dissatisfied	Unhappy	Terrible
If you were to spend the rest of your life with your urinary condition the way it is now, how would you feel about that?	0	1	2	3	4	5	6

FIGURE 1. International prostate symptom score (IPSS).

not significantly related to baseline age but was significantly related to baseline prostate volume.

Treatment

WATCHFUL WAITING

Indications for treatment of BPH rely, in large part, on the subjective nature of the symptoms. For the majority of patients with BPH, symptoms are not severe or bothersome enough to warrant long-term medical or surgical intervention. Men with an IPSS of less than 8 are usually treated with expectant management. Advising the patient toward lifestyle modifications, such as minimizing evening fluid intake, avoiding caffeine, and avoiding decongestants, anticholinergics, and other medications that impair voiding, often provides an effective resolution of symptoms. In a study of 556 men with moderate symptoms of BPH comparing outcomes following transurethral resection of the prostate (TURP) with watchful waiting for more than 3 years, 8% of men randomized to TURP and 17% of men with watchful waiting failed treatment. Treatment failure with watchful waiting was mostly because of high postvoid residuals and significant increases in IPSS symptoms. Patients who respond poorly to watchful waiting have multiple medical and surgical options for treatment of BPH.

α₁-ADRENERGIC BLOCKING AGENTS

The α_1-adrenergic antagonists have been shown in numerous randomized placebo-controlled trials to be safe and effective in the treatment of BPH. The most commonly prescribed α_1-adrenergic blockers appear to have similar safety profiles and clinical efficacy and are the common first approach for urologists. Terazosin (Hytrin) and doxazosin (Cardura) were the first α antagonists available for treatment of BPH; however, orthostatic hypotension was a significant concern, requiring careful dose titration. Tamsulosin (Flomax), a highly selective α-blocker, does not induce orthostatic hypotension and so does not require dose titration. Overall, the most common side effects include headaches, dizziness, asthenia, and drowsiness. Sexual side effects are limited to retrograde ejaculation. Alfuzosin (Uroxatral), a newer nonspecific α-blocker, has minimal vasoactive or retrograde ejaculation side effects. Table 1 provides a list for medication dosing and schedules.

5α-REDUCTASE INHIBITION

Finasteride (Proscar) and dutasteride (Avodart) are 5α-reductase inhibitors (type 1 and type 1/2, respectively) that block conversion of testosterone to dihydrotestosterone, the androgen involved in development of BPH. These medications represent the paradigm for androgen suppression of BPH. They have their greatest therapeutic effect in men with prostates greater than 40 g, and treatment for 6 months or more is usually required for a clinical response. The first randomized, multicenter, double-blind, placebo-controlled trial investigating the efficacy of finasteride demonstrated significant improvements in maximum flow rate and decreased prostatic volume. Since then, further studies have confirmed a reduced risk of acute urinary retention and surgical intervention with finasteride use. Finasteride can reduce BPH-associated hematuria. It is effective as adjuvant therapy, following other treatments, and as neoadjuvant therapy prior to minimally invasive therapy.

Adverse effects include decreased libido, ejaculatory dysfunction, and gynecomastia. In the patient being monitored for prostate cancer with PSA testing, finasteride therapy must be taken into account when interpreting PSA values; finasteride decreases PSA values by 50%, leading to a false-negative result.

Efficacy of Medical Therapy

The Medical Therapy of Prostate Symptoms (MTOPS) study evaluated the efficacy of doxazosin and finasteride to determine if medical therapy delays or prevents disease progression. At 4 years, combination therapy was most effective for reducing risk of clinical progression (AUR) and improving symptom score and urinary flow rate. Finasteride and combination therapy significantly reduced the risk of AUR and invasive therapy over 4 years. Monotherapy with either medication reduced symptom score and improved flow significantly, but to a lesser degree than combination therapy. Doxazosin delayed time to progression of AUR and invasive therapy but not the risk. Without treatment, the risk of BPH progression was 20% more during the trial. Risk factors for progression include baseline prostate volume (>40 g) and higher serum PSA value (>2 μg/mL).

Phytotherapy

Saw palmetto (*Serenoa repens*)[1,2] extract is the most popular phytotherapeutic agent. Its likely mechanism is inhibition of 5α-reductase. A recent meta-analysis of numerous randomized trials using saw palmetto described a mild to moderate improvement in flow and LUTS; however, because of small study sample, varying products, short treatment times, and varying outcomes, these study conclusions are difficult to interpret. Other popular preparations are African plum (*Pygeum africanum*)[1,2] and South African star grass (*Cynodon nlemfuënsis*).[1,2] The former has been shown to have several in vitro effects, such as antiestrogen effects, leukotriene blockade, and inhibition of fibroblast

---

[1]Not FDA approved for this indication.
[2]Available as a dietary supplement.

TABLE 1   Common Medications for Benign Prostatic Hyperplasia

Medication	Class	Dose	Schedule
Alfuzosin (Uroxatral)	α-1 Blocker	10 mg	Once daily
Doxazosin (Cardura)	α-1 Blocker	1-8 mg, titrated	Once daily at bedtime
Tamsulosin (Flomax)	α-1a Blocker	0.4 mg	Once daily
Terazosin (Hytrin)	α-1 Blocker	1-10 mg, titrated	Once daily at bedtime
Dutasteride (Avodart)	5-α Reductase inhibitor	0.5 mg	Once daily
Finasteride (Proscar)	5-α Reductase inhibitor	5 mg	Once daily

growth factors. The latter has been shown in vitro to increase plasminogen activators, as well as to stimulate release of transforming growth factor-β, an inducer of apoptosis, yet these in vitro effects have not been shown to occur in vivo. A meta-analysis of four clinical trials of South African star grass extract, β-sitosterol, concluded that β-sitosterol improved urologic symptoms and flow rates in men.

There is no standard of care for management of patients using phytotherapy. Nor have the long-term safety effects been established. Patients should be cautioned that doses, efficacy, side effects, and drug interactions with phytotherapy are unknown. For the patient refusing medical therapy of α-blockers and 5α-reductase inhibitors, phytotherapy may be attempted as long as the patient understands the limitations of these agents. If retention, UTI, calculi, or decreased renal function occurs, phytotherapy should be discouraged and more aggressive medical and surgical management undertaken.

Minimally Invasive Therapies

The most commonly employed surgical procedure, and the gold standard for BPH, is transurethral resection of the prostate (TURP), involving endoscopic resection of the obstructive component of the prostate. TURP is highly effective, improving symptoms in up to 95% of patients. Common complications include inability to void postoperatively, clot retention, incontinence, impotence, and retrograde ejaculation. A number of new minimally invasive therapies have been developed to reduce the complications associated with TURP, as well as provide alternatives for the unfavorable surgical candidate. Most minimally invasive therapies use energy, such as radio waves, laser, ultrasound, microwaves, or electrical current.

Transurethral incision of the prostate (TUIP) involves endoscopic placement of one to two incisions into the prostate and capsule to reduce urethral constriction. This procedure is highly effective on prostate glands less than 30 g and is well documented and safe, with efficacy comparable with TURP. TUIP is associated with a 78% to 83% improvement of symptoms. Because TUIP is associated with fewer retrograde ejaculations, less morbidity, and a reoperation rate of less than 1% in 10 years, this procedure is the treatment of choice for small gland BPH in men concerned with fertility and ejaculation.

In transurethral needle ablation (TUNA), low-level energy is transferred by radio frequency to the prostate, creating a well-defined necrotic lesion within the prostatic parenchyma while preserving the urethral mucosa. A cystoscope-like instrument with two needles set at 90 degrees from each other ablates tissue in 3 to 5 minutes when needles reach temperatures of 27° to 38°C (80° to 100°F). Urethral and rectal temperatures are also vigorously monitored as the device adjusts. Preliminary studies show an increase in peak flow and a decrease in symptom score following TUNA, with no major complications. Transient urinary retention is reported in 10% to 40% of patients. In a prospective study, TURP was superior to TUNA in increasing flow rates but demonstrated comparable improved symptoms at 1 year postoperatively. Transurethral microwave thermotherapy (TUMT) heats prostatic transitional zone tissue to between 60° and 80°C (140° to 176°F), inducing tissue damage. Thermotherapy preferentially destroys smooth muscle by coagulative necrosis while water-conductive cooling of the urethral mucosa preserves periurethral tissues. Although prospective studies indicate that TURP produces more pronounced urinary improvements versus TUMT, thermotherapy consistently improves symptom scores by 75% and increases peak flow rates by 75%. Furthermore, TUMT is a procedure done under local anesthesia. Retrograde ejaculation and urinary retention with prolonged catheterization occurs in greater than one third of patients.

Ultimately, therapeutic decisions depend in large part on symptom scores. Men with low symptom scores without bother are appropriately managed through watchful waiting. As scores increase, or if progression with clinical morbidity develops, more aggressive management is appropriate.

REFERENCES

Bhargava S, Canda AE, Chapple CR: A rational approach to benign hyperplasia evaluation: Recent advances. Curr Opin Urol 2004;14:1-6.
Djavan B, Waldert M, Ghawidel C, Marberger M: Benign prostatic hyperplasia progression and its impact on treatment. Curr Opin Urol 2004;14:45-50.
Fong YK, Milani S, Djavan B: Role of phytotherapy in men with lower urinary tract symptoms. Curr Opin Urol 2005;15:45-48.
Hoffman RM, MacDonald R, Monga M, Wilt TJ: Transurethral microwave thermotherapy vs. transurethral resection for treating benign prostatic hyperplasia: A systematic review. BJU Int 2004;94:1031-1036.
Walsh, PC, Retik A, Vaughan D (eds): Campbell's Urology, 8th ed. Philadelphia, Saunders Elsevier Science, 2002.

10

Erectile Dysfunction

Method of
Luciano Kolodny, MD

The term *erectile dysfunction* (ED) is relatively new, having replaced *impotence* approximately a decade ago. ED is defined as the "inability of the male to attain or maintain an erection sufficient for satisfactory sexual intercourse." ED affects millions of men worldwide with implications that go far beyond sexual activity alone. ED is now recognized as a sentinel event in cardiovascular disease, diabetes mellitus (DM), and depression. It can also be damaging to interpersonal relationships and self-esteem.

Epidemiology

The Massachusetts Male Aging Study is one of the pivotal studies on the prevalence of ED. Between 1987 and 1989, men between the ages of 40 and 70 years received questionnaires inquiring about several aspects of their sexual health. Of the 1790 men who received the questionnaires, 1290 responded. They revealed that 52% of them had some degree of dysfunction, 17% with minimal, 25% with moderate, and almost 10% with complete absence of erectile function. It also showed the extremely detrimental link between coronary artery disease (CAD), DM, and ED. A few years later another group used the same patient database and followed up on these subjects. The risk of ED was 26 cases per 1000 men annually, which increased with age, lower education, DM, heart disease, and hypertension.

Physiology of Erection

The penile erection requires intact vascular, neuronal, and hormonal systems. The intricate details of this process are beyond the scope of this article, but in summary, after any sensorial stimulation, which can be visual, tactile, auditory, or olfactory, nitric oxide (NO) and other neurotransmitters are released at the cavernous nerve terminals. The endothelial cells then release vasoactive relaxing factors, which lead to vasodilatation of the penile blood vessels and increased blood flow. As blood flow increases, compression of the subtunical venular plexuses will substantially decrease venous outflow and finally cause the penis to change from flaccid to erect (Figure 1).

NO is the principal neurotransmitter involved in penile erection, but other vasoactive substances such as vasoactive intestinal peptide, neuropeptide Y, calcitonin gene-related peptide (CGRP), substance P, and serotonin also play roles. High levels of intrapenile NO facilitate the relaxation of intracavernosal trabeculae, thereby maximizing blood flow and penile erection. Nonadrenergic, noncholinergic neurons have been found to release NO, leading to increased production of cyclic guanosine monophosphate (cGMP). Through a series of reactions, cGMP will lead to relaxation of the smooth muscle, directly impacting the ability to go from a flaccid to an erect penile state. The return from erect to flaccid requires the hydrolysis of cGMP to guanosine monophosphate (GMP) by phosphodiesterase 5 (PDE5) (see Figure 1).

Testosterone and Erectile Function

Testosterone provides intrapenile nitrous oxide synthase (NOS), which has an important role in enhancing the production of NO, subsequent local vasodilatation, and penile erection. There is no correlation between serum testosterone levels and the degree of ED. However, hypogonadal men may experience significantly reduced libido. Hypogonadism is associated with decreased self-esteem, depression, osteoporosis, insulin resistance, increased fat mass, decreased lean body mass, and cognitive dysfunction.

Pathophysiology of Erectile Dysfunction

ED can be classified as psychogenic, organic (hormonal, vascular, drug-induced, or neurogenic), or mixed psychogenic and organic. Up to 80% of ED cases have

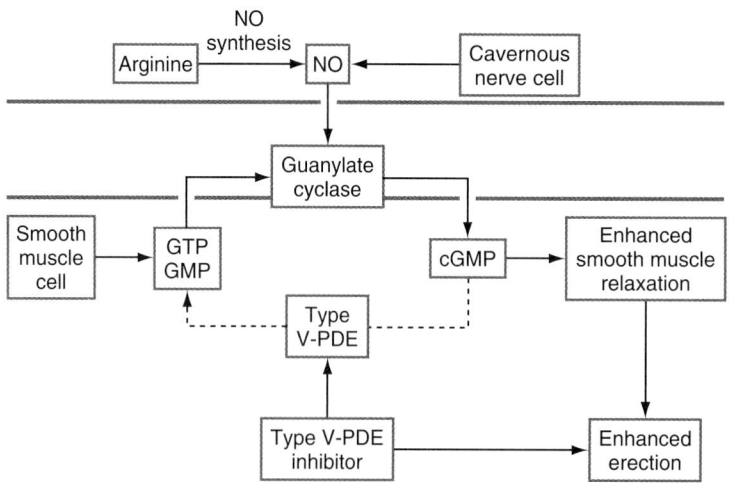

FIGURE 1. The biochemical process involved in erections and the mechanism of action of sildenafil citrate (Viagra). The cavernous nerves (S2-S4) innervate the penis and release NO. NO stimulates the production of cGMP in the smooth muscle cells of the penis. cGMP is directly responsible for increasing smooth muscle relaxation, which leads to increased arterial inflow and an erection. When cGMP is metabolized by PDE5, the penis undergoes detumescence. Sildenafil citrate (Viagra) inhibits PDE5 and increases the available cGMP, thereby leading to an enhanced erection. cGMP = cyclic guanosine monophosphate; NO = nitric oxide; PDE5 = phosphodiesterase 5. (From Kim ED: Erectile dysfunction. In Rakel RE, Bope ET [eds]: Conn's Current Therapy 2004, 56th ed. Philadelphia, 2004, WB Saunders. Used with permission.)

BOX 1   **Classification of Erectile Dysfunction**

Endocrine
- Hypogonadism
- Hyperprolactinemia

Drug Induced
- β-Blockers
- Calcium channel blockers
- Alcohol
- Nicotine
- Antiandrogens
- Cocaine
- Heroine
- Marijuana
- Cimetidine
- Metoclopramide
- Antidepressant medications
- Antipsychotic medications

Vascular
- Coronary artery disease
- Peripheral vascular disease
- Hypertension
- Diabetes mellitus

Psychogenic
- Depression
- Performance anxiety

Neurogenic
- Spinal cord injury
- Neuropathy (diabetic, hypertensive)
- Cerebrovascular disease
- Radical prostatectomy
- Pelvic surgery

Multifactorial
- Aging
- End-stage renal disease
- Pelvic trauma (neurogenic and vasculogenic)
- Diabetes mellitus (neurogenic, vasculogenic, drug induced)

---

an organic origin. The most common cause of ED is vascular disease (Box 1).

Atherosclerosis is the most common cause of vasculogenic ED, wheras endothelial damage is the most common mechanism. Aging is a well-known risk factor for ED, and it is hypothesized that there are alterations in the levels of NO that occur as a consequence of the aging endothelium. Additionally, chronic illness, depression, and lack of a sexual partner are all prevalent in this age population.

Chronic tobacco use is a major risk factor for the development of vasculogenic ED because of its effects on the vascular endothelium. Additionally, blood nicotine levels rise after smoking, which increases sympathetic tone in the penis and leads to nicotine-induced, smooth-muscle contraction in the cavernosal body. Chronic smoking also leads to decreased penile NOS activity and neuronal NOS content.

DM is a major risk factor for ED. In the Massachusetts Male Aging Study, the diabetic subset had a threefold increased prevalence of ED compared with nondiabetic subjects (28% versus 9.6%). In the same study, the overall incidence rate of ED was 26 cases per 1000 man-years

in nondiabetics and 50 cases per 1000 man-years in the diabetic population. The pathogenesis of ED in the diabetic patient is related to accelerated atherosclerosis, alterations in the corporal erectile tissue, and neuropathy.

Hypertension is another major risk factor for ED. Whether ED in patients with hypertension is related to the disease itself or to the use of antihypertensive medications has been debated for years. In a study looking at 104 subjects, the differences in incidence or severity of ED were minor between distinct types of antihypertensive medications or the number of agents being used simultaneously. This favors the concept that antihypertensive agents as well as the disease itself contribute to the appearance of ED. There are, however, classes of antihypertensive medications that are notorious for their negative impact on erectile function such as thiazides and β-blockers. The only β-blocker not associated with significant incidence of ED is carvedilol (Coreg).

Hyperlipidemia is another etiologic factor for ED. It is believed to contribute to ED by its relationship to endothelial dysfunction. One study showed that decreasing total cholesterol to less than 200 mg/dL by using atorvastatin (Lipitor) led to significant improvement of ED as measured by the International Index of Erectile Function (IIEF).

ED may be a sentinel manifestation of vascular disorders. In a study of 980 subjects seeking ED advice, 18% were suffering from undiagnosed hypertension, 16% had DM, 5% had ischemic heart disease, 15% had benign prostatic hyperplasia, 4% had prostate cancer, and 1% had depression. ED can itself be an independent marker for CAD. In addition, the extent of CAD correlates with the prevalence of ED.

Quantification of the Severity of Erectile Disfunction and Improvement

There are several tools designed to assess the severity of ED, as well as to measure the efficacy of different treatments. We discuss three different measures, the IIEF, the Sexual Encounter Profile (SEP), and the Global Assessment Question (GAQ) (Box 2).

PATIENT HISTORY

When assessing sexual dysfunction, it is important to inquire about a number of issues:

1. Differentiate between decreased libido and ED: assess whether the patient has one or both
2. Tobacco use: type, amount, duration
3. Alcohol intake
4. History of depression or anxiety disorder
5. Presence of social/relationship stressors
6. Ability to have erections while masturbating versus when with partner
7. List of all prescription, over-the-counter, and herbal medications

Rakel and Bope: *Conn's Current Therapy 2006.*

Tools used in the quantification of the severity of erectile dysfunction (ED) include the International Index of Erectile Function (IIEF), the Sexual Encounter Profile (SEP), and the Global Assessment Question (GAQ).

International Index of Erectile Function

The IIEF is a standardized questionnaire designed to measure ED and detect treatment-related changes. It is a 15-item questionnaire addressing five different domains: erectile function, orgasmic function, sexual desire, intercourse satisfaction, and overall satisfaction. The IIEF is the most frequently used efficacy measurement employed in ED drug trials. Using a scale from 1 (never/almost never) to 5 (almost always/always), men grade each domain. It is very sensitive and specific, and has been validated in 20 languages to assess treatment-related changes in sexual function. The questions 1-5 and 15 are used to quantify erectile dysfunction severity and are as follows:

1. How often were you able to get an erection during sexual activity?
2. When you had erections with sexual stimulation, how often were your erections hard enough for penetration?
3. When you attempted sexual intercourse, how often were you able to penetrate (enter) your partner?
4. During sexual intercourse, how often were you able to maintain your erection after you had penetrated (entered) your partner?
5. During sexual intercourse, how difficult was it to maintain your erection to completion of intercourse?
15. How do you rate your confidence that you could get and keep an erection?

And it is scored as follows:

26-30	Normal ED
22-25	Mild ED
17-21	Mild to moderate ED
11-16	Moderate ED
≤10	Severe ED

Sexual Encounter Profile

SEP is a five-question survey provided to patients with ED in clinical studies of oral therapies. The survey is completed after each sexual attempt. The questions are as follows:

1. Were you able to achieve at least some erection?
2. Were you able to insert your penis into your partner's vagina?
3. Did your erection last long enough to have successful intercourse?
4. Were you satisfied with the hardness of your erection?
5. Were you satisfied with the overall sexual experience?

Answers to questions 2 and 3 are the ones most often used in the literature.

Global Assessment Questions

GAQ is usually administered at the end of the treatment period during efficacy studies.
Question 1: Has the treatment taken during the study improved your erections?
Question 2: If yes, has the treatment improved your ability to engage in sexual activity?
This is very subjective, and its responses tend to be valued less than SEP and IIEF.

8. Knowledge of whether nocturnal erections are present
9. History of drug use: marijuana, cocaine, other recreational drugs
10. History of genitourinary trauma
11. History of prostatic disease, or possible related symptoms
12. History of hypertension, hyperlipidemia, CAD, peripheral vascular disease, cerebrovascular disease
13. History of DM
14. History of spinal cord injury
15. History of penile plaques: possible Peyronie's disease
16. Frequency of intercourse or attempted intercourse
17. Ability to ejaculate

PHYSICAL EXAMINATION

The physical examination should include a careful testicular examination to assess testicular size, asymmetries, presence of hernias, or varicoceles. Additionally, a digital rectal examination to assess the prostatic size, consistency, and presence of nodules is warranted. Penile inspection and palpation should be performed, with special attention to possible fibrotic plaques. Palpation and auscultation of femoral arteries for possible bruits is another important part of the examination.

LABORATORY STUDIES

Laboratory workup on a patient with ED should include total and bioavailable testosterone levels drawn in the morning, prolactin, prostate-specific antigen, fasting glucose, and fasting lipid panel. Further studies may be warranted depending on the results of the aforementioned.

Management of Erectile Dysfunction

The landscape of ED was revolutionized with the introduction of sildenafil citrate (Viagra), the first oral medication for the treatment of this condition. Since then, oral agents have become the preferred mode of treatments by patients in surveys worldwide. There are three oral agents that inhibit PDE5 currently on the market:

1. Sildenafil citrate (Viagra)
2. Vardenafil (Levitra)
3. Tadalafil (Cialis)

All three drugs work by inhibiting PDE5, which maintains intracavernosal levels of cGMP, subsequently producing vasodilatation and penile erection (see Figure 1).

SILDENAFIL CITRATE (VIAGRA)

Sildenafil citrate (Viagra) is an orally active, potent, and selective inhibitor of cGMP-specific PDE5. The predominant phosphodiesterase isoform in the penile tissue is type 5. The selectivity of sildenafil citrate (Viagra) for PDE5 is approximately 4000-fold greater than its selectivity for phosphodiesterase 3 (PDE3), the isoform involved in the control of cardiac contractility. Sildenafil citrate (Viagra) is absorbed rapidly after oral administration, with an absolute bioavailability of 40%. The time of maximal (T-max) plasma after oral dosing in the fasting state is between 30 and 120 minutes. A high-fat meal increases the time to peak plasma concentration by 60 minutes and reduces the peak plasma concentration by 29%. The half-life of the drug is from 3 to 5 hours. Sildenafil citrate (Viagra) is metabolized by hepatic microsomal cytochrome P450 isoenzyme 3A4 for the most part. Cytochrome P450 3A4 inhibitors, cimetidine (Tagamet), erythromycin, ketoconazole (Nizoral), and protease inhibitors may retard the metabolism of sildenafil citrate (Viagra).

The recommended dose is from 25 to 100 mg as needed approximately 1 hour before sexual activity. In some individuals, the onset of activity may be seen as early as 11 to 19 minutes, but this is not the norm. The usual starting dose is 50 mg.

The maximum recommended dose is 100 mg, and the maximum dosing frequency is once daily. A starting dose of 25 mg can be considered for patients older than age 65 years as well as for patients with severe hepatic cirrhosis or severe renal impairment.

There are more than two-dozen, randomized, double-blind, placebo-controlled studies involving this agent. It produces positive results regardless of the etiology of ED. It has been studied in patients with DM, CAD, postcoronary artery bypass graft (post-CABG), spinal cord injury, depression, hypertension, prostate cancer post-prostatectomy, benign prostate enlargement post-transurethral resection of the prostate (TURP), patients on hemodialysis, as well as recipients of renal transplants. Results vary according to underlying condition causing ED in the first place, ranging from 50% to 85%.

The most common side effects of sildenafil citrate (Viagra) include vasodilatory effects such as headaches, flushing, and nasal congestion caused by hyperemia of the nasal mucosa, as well as dyspepsia. Up to 30% of patients may get at least one side effect. Another side effect that presents on occasion is blurred or blue-green vision because of inhibition of phosphodiesterase 6 (PDE6) in the retina. It is absolutely contraindicated in men taking long-acting or short-acting nitrate drugs, and men taking any form of nitrates should be informed about the dangerous interaction.

Do not prescribe sildenafil citrate (Viagra) to patients with unstable CAD who need nitrates. Assess the need for ordering treadmill testing in select patients. Initial monitoring of blood pressure (BP) after the administration of sildenafil citrate (Viagra) may be indicated in men with complicated congestive heart failure (CHF). α-Blockers should not be used in combination with sildenafil citrate (Viagra) because of possible orthostatic hypotension.

VARDENAFIL (LEVITRA)

Vardenafil (Levitra) is a highly potent inhibitor of PDE5. It was approved for use in the United States in late 2003. It is a more selective PDE5 inhibitor than sildenafil citrate (Viagra). The absorption of vardenafil (Levitra) is delayed by a fatty content of more than 30% in a meal. However, that does not seem to affect its effectiveness in different trials. The half-life of vardenafil (Levitra) is 4.4 to 4.8 hours, and the clinical effectiveness may be as long as 12 hours. The time for maximum plasma concentration is between 42 and 54 minutes. The first trial using the agent included 580 patients, excluding patients with spinal cord injury, radical prostatectomy, hypogonadism, thyrotoxicosis, or DM.

The successful rates of intercourse were 71% to 75% on patients taking 5 or 10 mg at a time. Those taking 20 mg had a success rate of 80%. The placebo groups had an average success rate of 30%.

Vardenafil (Levitra) has been tested in patients with type 2 DM; 452 patients were enrolled in a double-blind, placebo-controlled trial. The success rate in the vardenafil (Levitra) group ranged from 57% to 72%.

In a different study involving 736 subjects including men with DM and stable CAD, the success rates were 28% for the placebo group, 65% for those taking 5 mg, 80% for those taking 10 mg, and 85% for the 20-mg group.

Patients who were unresponsive to sildenafil citrate (Viagra) at a dose of 100 mg on several attempts were given vardenafil (Levitra) in doses of 10 and 20 mg (proved in trial). Vardenafil (Levitra) produced statistically and clinically significant results compared with placebo in men who were historically unresponsive to sildenafil citrate (Viagra). The dose that offers the best clinical results is 20 mg. It should not be taken more than once every 24 hours. Safety studies have shown no deleterious effects with long-term daily use of this drug for up to 12 months.

The most common side effects include headaches (10% to 21%), flushing (5% to 13%), rhinitis (9% to 17%), and dyspepsia (1% to 6%) because vardenafil (Levitra) does not inhibit PDE6. Unlike sildenafil citrate (Viagra), it does not produce problems of blurred vision or blue-green visual disturbances. The same warning regarding the use of nitrates as sildenafil citrate (Viagra) applies to vardenafil (Levitra). Patients taking vardenafil (Levitra) may use α-blocking agents with caution.

TADALAFIL (CIALIS)

The third oral agent of this class is tadalafil (Cialis). It has a half-life of 17.5 hours, with two thirds of patients experiencing clinical benefits of this drug up to 36 hours after its use. The clinical onset of action occurs in less than 1 hour. There is no interaction between food and alcohol on the absorption of the drug.

There have been numerous phase II and III studies in Europe, Canada, and the United States using doses of 2, 5, 10, and 25 mg of the drug in comparison with placebo. The average success rates on these studies averaged 17% for placebo, 51% for the 2-mg dose, and 80% for the other doses, as well as up to 88% on the 25-mg dose in one study. In one study looking at

10

216 subjects with type 2 DM, improved erections were reported in 56% to 64% of the patients.

A recent article looking at all the previously published patient data showed that among 2102 men studied in 11 randomized placebo-controlled trials lasting 12 weeks, each mean improvement in IIEF at 20 mg of tadalafil (Cialis) was 8.6. Mean positive Sexual Encounter Profile Diary Question 3 (SEP3) response was 68% versus 31% in placebo groups. Mean GAQ was 84% versus 33% in placebo group.

In a multicenter, randomized, double-blind, crossover study looking at 181 men who received either sildenafil citrate (Viagra) or tadalafil (Cialis), 73% (132) preferred tadalafil (Cialis) at 20 mg instead of sildenafil citrate (Viagra) at 50 or 100 mg.

The most clinically effective dose of tadalafil (Cialis) is 20 mg. It should be taken at least 30 minutes before intercourse. It may be used with caution in patients using α-blocking agents. Nitrates are absolutely contraindicated for use in patients taking tadalafil (Cialis). The most common side effects include headaches, dyspepsia, back pain, rhinitis, and flushing. There are no visual side effects reported.

APOMORPHINE (UPRIMA)[1]

Apomorphine (Uprima)[1] is a potent emetic that acts on central dopaminergic receptors. The stimulation of central dopaminergic receptors transmits excitatory signals down the spinal cord to the sacral parasympathetic nucleus, stimulating activity of the sacral nerves supplying the penis. It has been used successfully in up to 67% of patients when administered through a sublingual preparation. Subcutaneous injections[2] of apomorphine (Uprima)[1] produce almost a 100% erectile response, but nausea and vomiting are limiting factors to this mode of administration.

The most common side effects are headache, nausea, and dizziness. Rare syncopal episodes have been reported.

PHENTOLAMINE (REGITINE)

Phentolamine (Regitine) is an α_1- and α_2-adrenergic receptor antagonist.

The sympathetic system via the release of noradrenaline (NA) is the primary determinant of cavernosal smooth muscle contraction and detumescence. A relative predominance of NA-induced contraction over NO-induced smooth muscle relaxation may contribute to ED.

In large phase III studies, 55% to 59% of patients receiving 40 and 80 mg were able to achieve vaginal penetration. Adverse effects include nasal congestion (10%), headaches (3% to 5%), dizziness (3% to 5%), tachycardia (3%), and nausea.

TRAZODONE (DESYREL)[1]

Trazodone (Desyrel)[1] is a serotonin reuptake inhibiting agent. Its action in ED is believed to be the result of central serotonergic and peripheral α-adrenolytic activity. The efficacy of trazodone is poorly demonstrated; however, it may have a place in those with performance anxiety. Side effects include drowsiness, insomnia, headaches, and weight loss.

DIETARY SUPPLEMENTS AND ERECTILE DYSFUNCTION

Yohimbine[1] is an α_2-adrenoreceptor antagonist with short duration of action. It is administered orally, and it is believed to have a central effect at adrenergic receptors in brain centers associated with libido and penile erection. A meta-analysis of seven studies established that it is superior to placebo, although results can be very erratic. Side effects include palpitations, tremors, and anxiety. Yohimbine should *not* be recommended as part of the management of ED.

A study with 60 patients who had failed papaverine[1] injections (50 mg or less) were treated with an extract of *Ginkgo biloba,* 60 mg for 12 to 18 months. After 6 months, 50% of the patients reported improvement in erectile function. A placebo-controlled randomized trial using 240 mg of *Ginkgo biloba* extract daily for 24 weeks in patients with vasculogenic ED did not demonstrate significant differences between the groups.

L-Arginine[1] is an amino acid that is the precursor to NO. Three small studies are looking at this drug. There are encouraging results in one study.

Zinc is found in high concentrations in seminal fluid. Anecdotal reports of improvement in ED.

ALPROSTADIL (PROSTAGLANDIN E1, CAVERJECT, MEDICATED URETHRAL SYSTEM FOR ERECTION)

Prostaglandin E1 (PGE_1) exerts a number of pharmacologic effects including systemic vasodilatation, inhibitory actions on platelet aggregation, and relaxation of smooth muscle. PGE_1 binds to PGE receptors and causes a relaxation response mediated by cyclic adenosine monophosphate (cAMP). It can be administered intracavernosally or intraurethrally.

It has been used in combination with papaverine,[1] and the combination was superior to PGE_1 alone. The intracavernosal administration seems to be more effective than transurethral (medicated urethral system for erection [MUSE]). MUSE should be administered in 1-mg doses, applied intraurethrally. Responses to intracavernosal injections (Caverject) as high as 80% may be expected in patients with organic ED with a dose of 20 μg, and much lower to MUSE (35% to 43%). Injections are given with 27- to 30-gauge needles. The administration of PGE_1 is usually relegated as an alternative in patients who have contraindications to the use of phosphodiesterase 5 (PDE5) inhibitors. The possible side effects include penile fibrosis, priapism, urethral bleeding, hypotension, or syncopal episodes.

---

[1]Not FDA approved for this indication.
[2]Not available in the United States.

---

[1]Not FDA approved for this indication.

Papaverine[1] is a nonspecific phosphodiesterase inhibitor that increases cAMP and cGMP levels in penile erectile tissue. It produces smooth muscle relaxation and vasodilatation. It decreases the resistance to arterial inflow and increases the resistance to venous outflow. It is highly effective in psychogenic and neurogenic ED but not vasculogenic. It has been commonly used in combination with phentolamine (Regitine). Major side effects include priapism, corporeal fibrosis, and possible elevation of liver transaminases.

Moxisylyte chlorohydrate[2] is an α-blocking agent. In a study where 156 subjects received either alprostadil or moxisylyte in a dose-escalating fashion, alprostadil had much better success rates (46% versus 81%).

Chlorpromazine (Thorazine)[1] is useful when given in combination with alprostadil or papaverine. It has α-blocking properties, and it is cheaper than phentolamine (Regitine).

Decreased concentration of vasoactive intestinal polypeptide (VIP)* has been reported in the penile tissue of men with ED. VIP is believed to play a role in the erectile process. It is ineffective when administered alone but can be quite effective in combination with phentolamine (Regitine). In a small study of 52 subjects with organic ED, 100% of them achieved an erection sufficient for intercourse. Further studies into the effectiveness of VIP may be needed.

PENILE PROSTHESES

This surgical approach used to be quite common before the advent of oral agents. The use of prostheses is still a suitable alternative for those who are unresponsive to less invasive treatments. Prostheses can be classified as rod, one-piece inflatable, two-piece inflatable, and three-piece inflatable. Postsurgical infections and malfunctions are the most common complications. Patients are usually satisfied with the results of prosthetic placement.

Vacuum Constrictive Device

Vacuum constrictive device is a plastic cylinder that is placed over the penis and connected to a pump that creates a partial vacuum. After achieving penile rigidity, a band is placed around the base of the penis to maintain the erection. This is a safe, noninvasive, and effective method of treating ED. It requires an understanding partner and the quality of the erection is not ideal; but patients are usually satisfied.

Testosterone

Patients who have low testosterone levels may benefit substantially from replacement. Men may expect significant improvements in libido, self-esteem, and overall energy levels. Additionally, testosterone is necessary for NO generation in the penile tissue.

---

[1]Not FDA approved for this indication.
[2]Not available in the United States.
*Investigational drug in the United States.

Rakel and Bope: *Conn's Current Therapy 2006.*

CURRENT DIAGNOSIS

- The risk factors for ED include tobacco, alcohol, and drug use, as well as DM, hypertension, hyperlipidemia, and prostate disease.
- ED is widely prevalent, and incidence sharply increases with age.
- ED is a cardiovascular sentinel event, and its occurrence warrants a cardiac workup.
- The workup of ED should include checking testosterone levels, prolactin, glucose, and lipid levels.
- First-line therapies include the use of PDE5 inhibitors such as sildenafil citrate (Viagra), vardenafil (Levitra), and tadalafil (Cialis).

Abbreviations: DM = diabetes mellitus; ED = erectile dysfunction; PDE5 = phosphodiesterase 5.

The different testosterone preparations include injections such as testosterone enanthate (Delatestryl), cypionate (Depo-Testosterone) given as an intramuscular (IM) injection in doses of 100 to 200 mg, every 2 weeks on average. They also include transdermal testosterone patches (Androderm and Testoderm, 5 mg/d) or transdermal gel (AndroGel 5-g packets, one daily; or Testim 1% testosterone gel, one packet daily). Testosterone gel preparations provide physiologic replacement of testosterone and are preferred more than depot IM injections.

Future Trends

In the next few years we will see a sharp rise in the use of combination drugs, such as PDE5 inhibitors and apomorphine (Uprima),[1] PDE5 inhibitors and phentolamine (Regitine), and combinations of PDE5 inhibitors and intraurethral and intracavernosal agents. ED will

---

[1]Not FDA approved for this indication.

CURRENT THERAPY

- PDE5 Inhibitors
  Sildenafil citrate (Viagra) 25-100 mg
  Vardenafil (Levitra) 10-20 mg
  Tadalafil (Cialis) 10-20 mg
- Alprostadil (PGE₁)
  Intracavernosal injections (Caverject) 20 μg
  Intraurethral application (MUSE) 1-mg pellet
- Papaverine injections[1] 30-60 mg
- Agents not yet approved for use by the FDA:
  Apomorphine (Uprima)[1] 3, 4, 6 mg
  Phentolamine (oral)[1] 40, 60, 80 mg

[1]Not FDA approved for this indication.

Abbreviations: MUSE = medicated urethral system for erection; PDE5 = phosphodiesterase 5; PGE₁ = prostaglandin E1.

be recognized universally as a cardiovascular sentinel event and also as a risk factor for vascular disease in general.

REFERENCES

Archer SL: Potassium channels and erectile dysfunction. Vascul Pharmacol 2002;38:61-71.
Burchardt M, Burchardt T, Baer L, et al: Hypertension is associated with severe erectile dysfunction. J Urol 2000;164(10):1188-1191.
Carson CC, Rajfer J, Eardley I, et al: The efficacy and safety of tadalafil: An update. BJU Int 2004;93:1276-1281.
Crowe SM, Streetman DS: Vardenafil treatment for erectile dysfunction. Ann Pharmacother 2004;38:77-85.
Feldman HA, Goldstein I, Hatzichristou DG, et al: Impotence and its medical and psychosocial correlates: Results of the Massachusetts Male Aging Study. J Urol 1994;151(1):54-61.
Jackson G, Betteridge J, Dean J, et al: A systematic approach to erectile dysfunction in the cardiovascular patient: A consensus statement—Update 2002. Int J Clin Pract 2002;56(9):663-671.
Jaynat D, Shepherd MD: Evaluation and treatment of erectile dysfunction in men with diabetes mellitus. Mayo Clin Proc 2002; 77(3):276-282.
Johannes CB, Araujo AB, Feldman HA, et al: Incidence of erectile dysfunction in men ages 40 to 69 years old: Longitudinal results from the Massachusetts Male Aging Study. J Urol 2000;163(2): 460-463.
Kirby M, Jackson G, Betteridge J, et al: Is erectile dysfunction a marker for cardiovascular disease? Int J Clin Pract 2002;55(9): 614-618.
Lue TF: Drug therapy: Erectile dysfunction. N Engl J Med 2000; 342(24):1802-1813.
Michelakis E, Tymchak W, Archer S: Sildenafil: From the bench to the bedside. CMAJ 2000;163(9):1171-1175.
NIH Consensus Development Panel on Impotence: Impotence (NIH Consensus Conference). JAMA 1993;270(1):83-90.
Padma-Nathan H: Intra-urethral and topical agents in the management of erectile dysfunction. In Carson CC III, Kirby RS, Goldstein I (eds): Textbook of Erectile Dysfunction. Oxford, Isis Medical Media, 1999, pp 323-326.
Rhoden EL, Teloken C, Mafessoni R, et al: Is there any relation between serum levels of testosterone and the severity of erectile dysfunction? Int J Impot Res 2002;14:167-171.
Shokeir AA, Alserafi MA, Mutabagani H: Intracavernosal versus intraurethral alprostadil: A prospective randomized study. BJU Int 1999;83:812-815.
Spahn M, Manning M, Juenemann KP: Intracavernosal therapy. In Carson CC III, Kirby RS, Goldstein I (eds): Textbook of Erectile Dysfunction. Oxford, Isis Medical Media, 1999, pp 345-353.
Sullivan ME, Thompson CS, Dashwood MR, et al: Nitric oxide and penile erection: Is erectile dysfunction another manifestation of vascular disease? Cardiovasc Res 1999;43:658-665.

Acute Renal Failure

Method of
John J. Friedewald, MD and Hamid Rabb, MD

Epidemiology, Cause, and Course of Acute Renal Failure

Acute renal failure (ARF), also known as acute kidney injury (AKI), is a common condition that must be recognized and treated promptly. The frequency among hospitalized patients is 1% at admission, 2% to 5% during hospitalization, 4% to 15% following cardiopulmonary bypass, and in 30% to 50% of deceased donor kidney transplants. There are multiple definitions of ARF, but generally accepted guidelines include an increase in serum creatinine of 0.5 mg per dL or more over the baseline value, a reduction in the calculated creatinine clearance of 50%, or a decrease in renal function that results in the need for dialysis. Approximately 30% of patients with ARF require dialysis at some point.

ARF can be divided into three categories: *prerenal* failure, *intrinsic* renal (or *intrarenal* failure), and *postrenal* failure. A careful history and physical examination should help focus the differential diagnosis (Table 1). Special attention should be paid to recent medications. The course of patients with ARF is highly varied, often depending on the cause and other co-morbid conditions (Table 2).

Prerenal Azotemia

Prerenal ARF stems from inadequate maintenance of glomerular filtration because of decreased perfusion pressure, most commonly because of reduced intravascular volume. Hemorrhage, overdiuresis, poor fluid intake, vomiting, and diarrhea can lead to a true depletion of the circulating intravascular volume. Other conditions can lower the *effective* circulating intravascular volume, including congestive heart failure, cirrhosis or hepatorenal syndrome, and the nephrotic syndrome. Finally, conditions can arise that limit the glomerular filtration rate (GFR) despite a normal intravascular volume. Renal artery stenosis and the vasoactive mechanisms of various agents, including angiotensin-converting enzyme (ACE) inhibitors, nonsteroidal anti-inflammatory drugs (NSAIDs), radiocontrast agents, and immunosuppressive calcineurin inhibitors, can all lead to prerenal azotemia.

The diagnosis of prerenal azotemia is often made by history and physical examination (consistent with volume depletion), but it can be suggested by certain laboratory abnormalities. A plasma blood urea nitrogen (BUN)-to-creatinine (Cr) ratio should be calculated. A ratio greater than 20 favors a prerenal cause, whereas ratios between 10 and 20 favor intrinsic or postrenal failure. The urine sediment should be examined by light microscopy. With prerenal ARF, a bland urinary sediment is the norm with trace or no proteinuria and perhaps a few hyaline casts. The fractional excretion of sodium (FENa – $[P_{Cr}/U_{Cr}]/[P_{Na}/U_{Na}]$) should be calculated on all patients with oliguria. A FENa less than 1% is common in euvolemic subjects in Na^+ balance with normal renal function and moderate salt intake. Clinically, a high FENa (>1%) is most often caused by acute tubular necrosis (ATN) (discussed later) but may also be seen in volume depletion (up to 10% of the time) or in volume depletion with ongoing diuretic therapy (causing salt wasting). Conversely, a low FENa (<1%) is more commonly associated with prerenal causes of ARF. In the instance of ongoing diuretic therapy,

TABLE 1 Differential Diagnosis of Acute Renal Failure

Types and underlying problems	Possible causes
Prerenal Acute Renal Failure	
True intravascular depletion	Hemorrhage, overdiuresis, poor fluid intake, vomiting, diarrhea
Decreased effective circulating volume to the kidneys	Congestive heart failure, cirrhosis or hepatorenal syndrome, nephrotic syndrome
Impaired renal blood flow caused by exogenous agents	ACE inhibitors, NSAIDs, calcineurin inhibitors
Intrinsic Acute Renal Failure	
Acute tubular necrosis	Ischemia
Toxins: drugs (e.g., aminoglycosides), contrast agents, pigments (myoglobin or hemoglobin)	
Sepsis	
Glomerular disease	*Rapidly progressive glomerulonephritis:* systemic lupus erythematosus, small-vessel vasculitis (Wegener's granulomatosis or microscopic polyangiitis), Henoch-Schönlein purpura (immunoglobulin A nephropathy), Goodpasture's syndrome *Acute proliferative glomerulonephritis:* endocarditis, poststreptococcal infection, postpneumococcal infection
Vascular disease	*Microvascular disease:* atheroembolic disease (cholesterol-plaque microembolism), thrombotic thrombocytopenic purpura, hemolytic uremic syndrome, HELLP syndrome, or postpartum acute renal failure *Macrovascular disease:* renal artery occlusion, severe abdominal aortic disease (aneurysm)
Interstitial disease	Allergic reaction to drugs, autoimmune disease (systemic lupus erythematosus or mixed connective tissue disease), pyelonephritis, infiltrative disease (lymphoma or leukemia)
Postrenal acute renal failure	Benign prostatic hypertrophy, prostate cancer, cervical cancer, retroperitoneal fibrosis, intratubular obstruction (crystals or myeloma light chains), pelvic mass or invasive pelvic malignancy, intraluminal bladder mass (clot, tumor, or fungus ball), neurogenic bladder, urethral strictures

Abbreviations: ACE = angiotensin-converting enzyme; HELLP = hemolysis, elevated liver enzymes, low platelets; NSAIDs = nonsteroidal anti-inflammatory drugs.
Adapted from Agrawal M, Swartz R: Acute renal failure. Am Fam Phys 2000;61(7):2077-2088.

evaluating the fractional excretion of urea (FE_{urea}) may be useful (by using the same FENa equation and substituting urea concentration for sodium). The FE_{urea} is normally 50% to 65% and usually below 35% in prerenal states.

Once identified, any known causes of prerenal ARF should be discontinued or eliminated if possible, especially in the case of medications. Volume-depleted states should be treated with infusions of saline or oral rehydration. However, some patients with total body volume overload despite low effective circulating blood volume (as with cirrhosis, congestive heart failure, or nephrotic syndrome) can present with oliguria or anuria. In this instance, efforts should be made to correct the underlying disorder (such as using positive inotropic agents for the treatment of decreased cardiac output, etc.). It is usually the case that prerenal ARF resolves rapidly (hours to days) with prompt restoration of renal plasma flow. It is also common to see partial rapid recovery of renal function in response to intravascular volume expansion when varying degrees of prerenal and ischemic acute tubular necrosis coexist because of their shared pathophysiology.

Rakel and Bope: *Conn's Current Therapy 2006.*

TABLE 2 Causes of Hospital-Acquired Acute Renal Failure: Associated Frequency and Mortality

Cause	Frequency	Mortality
Decreased renal perfusion	39%	13.6%
Medications	16%	15%
Radiographic contrast media	11%	14%
Postoperative	9%	2.8%
Sepsis	6.5%	76%
Post–liver transplant	<5%	28.6%
Post–heart transplant	<5%	35%
Obstruction	<5%	28.6%
Hepatorenal	<1%	71.4%
Rhabdomyolysis, artifact, glomerulonephritis, nephrectomy, atheroemboli, hypercalcemia, unknown	<1%	

Adapted from Nash OK, Hafeez A, Hou S: Hospital-acquired renal insufficiency. Am J Kidney Dis 2002;39(5):930-936.

Intrarenal Acute Renal Failure

The differential diagnosis for causes of intrarenal, or intrinsic, ARF is extensive (see Table 1). The most common cause of intrarenal ARF is acute tubular necrosis (ATN), either from an ischemic insult or toxic substances, usually medication (Table 3). The diagnosis of underlying causes of intrarenal ARF relies more heavily on microscopic and laboratory analyses of the urine, as well as blood tests (Figure 1).

TUBULAR DISEASE

Acute tubular injury (also called acute tubular necrosis or ATN) is the most common cause of ARF in hospitalized patients, comprising nearly 50% of cases. The causes of ATN are divided into ischemic and toxic. As previously mentioned, the pathophysiology of ischemic ATN is shared with prerenal azotemia. A decrease in renal perfusion leads to anoxic injury and apoptosis in tubular epithelial cells. Microvascular inflammation and decreased perfusion perpetuate the initial injury. The injured epithelium loses polarity, which results in abnormal solute trafficking, especially in the proximal tubules. The subsequent increase in sodium chloride delivery to the distal nephron leads to a further decrease in GFR through tubuloglomerular feedback. The epithelial cells detach from the basement membrane and slough into the urinary space, forming granular casts that are often visible in the urine sediment. ATN is associated with an increased FENa (more than 2%) and elevated urine sodium (usually greater than 40 mEq/L). A usual hallmark of ATN is the inability to concentrate urine, with urine osmolality less than 450 mOsm/kg. Patients may be oliguric or nonoliguric.

In the setting of oligoanuria, volume overload can be problematic. Furosemide or other loop diuretics should initially be used to treat hypervolemia. A dose between 20 and 100 mg of furosemide should be administered, and if an inadequate response is not achieved in the first hour, the dose should be doubled. If the volume overload is life-threatening and not adequately treated with medication, ultrafiltration via dialysis may be necessary (discussed later).

Toxic ATN results from direct or indirect tubular damage from a variety of substances, usually medications. Aminoglycoside antibiotics, cisplatin, radiocontrast agents, heavy metals, NSAIDs, amphotericin, hemoglobin (with hemolysis), myoglobin (with rhabdomyolysis), and uric acid (from tumor lysis syndrome) are all examples of commonly encountered causes of toxic ATN. The course of ATN, regardless of the cause, depends highly on the removal of the offending stimulus. This includes cessation of medications and restoration of renal plasma flow. With removal of the offending agent, renal recovery is likely, with a usual course of 7 to 21 days. Recovery is usually heralded by a rise in urine output, followed by improvements in renal function parameters. Although transient dialysis support may be required to manage uremia or volume overload in hospitalized patients that develop ATN, with removal of the ischemia or nephrotoxins most patients recover adequate renal function to discontinue dialysis.

Although many strategies are employed to alter the course of ATN, no effective, approved treatments are available to date. Some drugs, including loop diuretics and low-dose infusions of dopamine, are known to increase urine output during ATN, but they do not improve the speed or incidence of recovery from ATN. No trials to date suggest the effectiveness of diuretics in

---

TABLE 3 Drugs Associated with Acute Renal Failure

Mechanism	Drug
Reduction in renal perfusion through alteration of intrarenal hemodynamics	NSAIDs, ACE inhibitors, cyclosporine, tacrolimus (FK-506), radiocontrast agents, amphotericin B, interleukin (IL)-2*
Direct tubular toxicity	Aminoglycosides, radiocontrast agents, cisplatin, cyclosporine, tacrolimus, amphotericin B, methotrexate, foscarnet, pentamidine, organic solvents, heavy metals, IV immunoglobulin (IG)†
Heme pigment–induced tubular toxicity (rhabdo myolysis)	Cocaine, ethanol, lovastatin‡
Intratubular obstruction by precipitation of the agent	Acyclovir, sulfonamides, ethylene glycol,§ chemotherapeutic agents,‖ methotrexate
Allergic interstitial nephritis	Penicillins, cephalosporins, sulfonamides, rifampin, ciprofloxacin, NSAIDs, thiazide diuretics, furosemide, cimetidine, phenytoin, allopurinol¶
Hemolytic-uremic syndrome	Cyclosporine, tacrolimus, mitomycin, cocaine, quinine, conjugated estrogens

Abbreviations: ACE = angiotensin-converting enzyme; AIN = acute tubular necrosis; IV = intravenous; NSAIDs = nonsteroidal anti-inflammatory drugs.
*IL-2 produces a capillary leak syndrome with volume contraction.
†Mechanism unclear, may be caused by additives.
‡ARF most likely to occur when lovastatin is given in combination with cyclosporine.
§Ethylene glycol–induced toxicity can cause calcium oxalate crystals.
‖Uric acid crystals may form as a result of tumor lysis.
¶Many other drugs in addition to those listed here cause AIN.
Adapted from Thadhani, et al: Acute renal failure. N Engl J Med 1996;334:1448.

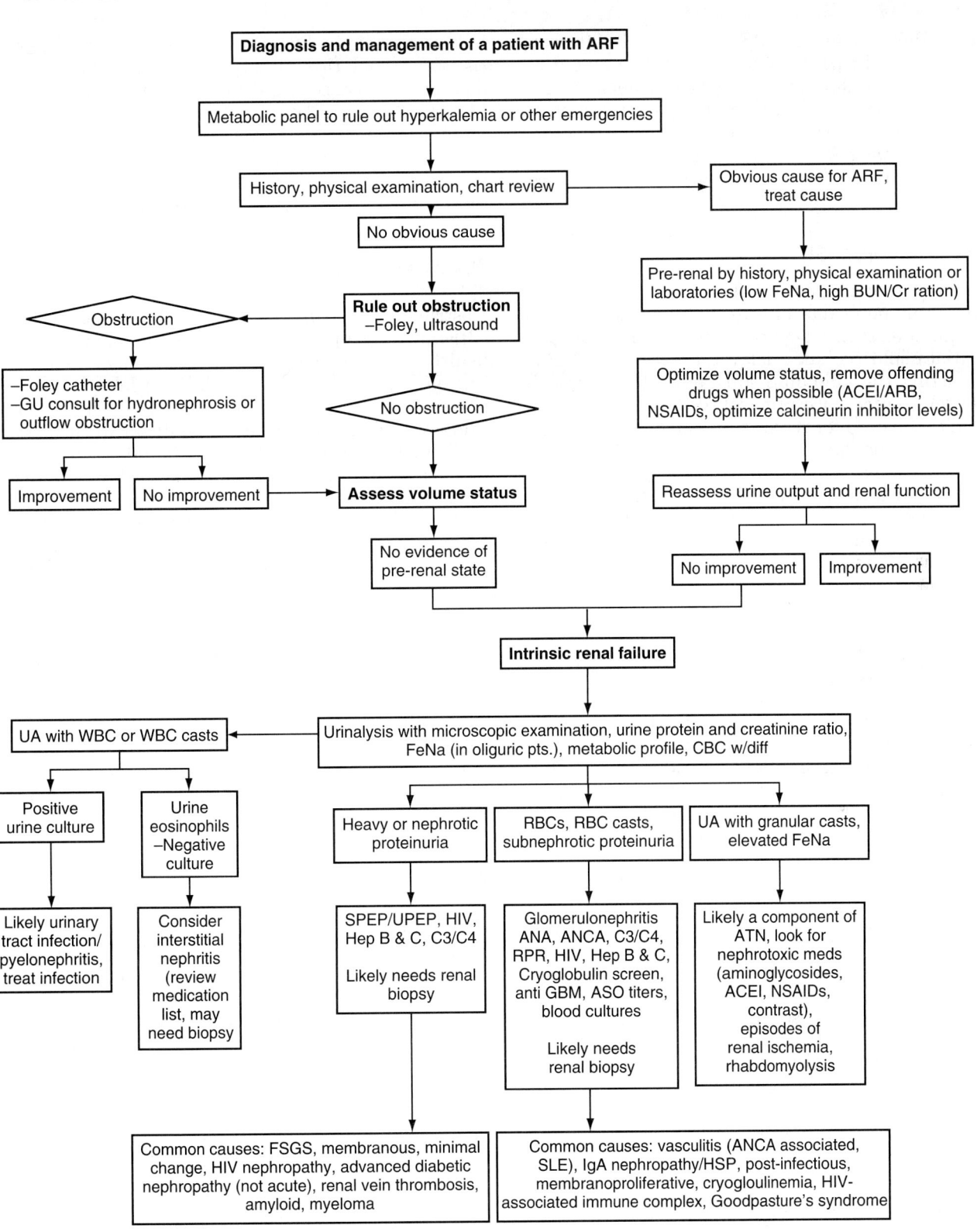

FIGURE 1. Diagnosis and management of a patient with Acute Renal Failure.

Rakel and Bope: *Conn's Current Therapy 2006.*

changing the course of ARF when solely used to change from an oliguric to nonoliguric state. Prevention (see section on radiocontrast nephropathy) and supportive care continue to be the mainstays of therapy. As more is discovered about the underlying inflammatory nature of ischemic ARF, there is growing interest in anti-inflammatory therapy to modify the disease course.

INTERSTITIAL DISEASE

Disorders of the tubulointerstitium can lead to ARF. The most common cause of acute interstitial nephritis is allergic interstitial nephritis (AIN). Most allergic interstitial nephritis has a delayed onset, up to 7 days after starting the offending substance. The course is usually self-limited with removal of the agent but can progress to the need for renal replacement therapy. The gold standard for diagnosis of AIN is visualization of interstitial edema and infiltrating lymphocytes and eosinophils on a renal biopsy. However, the diagnosis can be suggested in a less invasive manner by identifying peripheral blood eosinophilia or eosinophiluria (using a Hansel stain). The positive predictive value for eosinophilia is around 50%, but the negative predictive value (other than in NSAID-associated AIN) is greater than 90%. The laboratory evidence is accompanied by clinical findings of fever or rash in up to one third of patients. The most common offending agents for AIN include β-lactam antibiotics, especially methicillin, sulfonamides, rifampin, and quinolone antibiotics. Severe courses of AIN that do not improve in 3 to 5 days following discontinuation of the offending drug often respond to a course of immunosuppressive therapy. If the diagnosis of AIN is fairly certain, especially following renal biopsy, an initial 2- to 3-week course of prednisone, 1 mg/kg orally every day or 2 mg/kg orally every other day, can be initiated, and if effective tapered over a 2- to 3-month period. Other therapies can be considered if steroid resistance occurs in biopsy-proved cases of AIN, such as cytotoxic therapy or immunosuppressive therapy with mycophenolate mofetil.

Another cause of interstitial disease that can lead to ARF is pyelonephritis. In addition to pyuria, hematuria, and a positive urine culture, the urine sediment may contain WBC casts, suggesting the diagnosis of pyelonephritis. *Escherichia coli* causes 70% to 95% of cases of pyelonephritis with staphylococcus saprophyticus responsible for 5% to 20%.

GLOMERULAR DISEASE

Diseases affecting the glomerulus comprise 10% to 15% of cases of ARF. This diagnosis is suggested by characteristic changes in the urinary sediment as well as by frequent association with systemic disease symptoms (see Table 1 and Figure 1). Examination of the urine sediment frequently reveals red blood cells or red cell casts, proteinuria, and granular casts. In the instance of suspected glomerulonephritis, a renal biopsy is usually indicated to aid in diagnosis. An acute glomerulonephritis with rapid rise in serum creatinine is a medical emergency because of the mortality and morbidity from kidney and extrarenal manifestations and also because many can be effectively treated if diagnosed promptly. Therapy for glomerular disease often involves immunosuppressive or cytotoxic therapy that should be guided by renal pathology and clinical presentation.

Postrenal

Obstruction of urinary flow is an infrequent cause of ARF, making up less than 5% of cases. Because one healthy kidney can excrete the body's generated nitrogenous waste adequately, unilateral ureteral obstruction does not usually manifest itself with ARF. The level of obstruction must be distal to the bladder neck or, if proximal, it must be found in conjunction with a solitary functioning kidney or be bilateral to produce clinical ARF. The most frequent site of obstruction is at the bladder neck and usually results from prostate pathology (hypertrophy or malignancy). Bladder dysfunction, either from anticholinergic medication or autonomic insufficiency (as with advanced diabetes), can also cause postrenal ARF (see Figure 1). The diagnosis of postrenal ARF is usually made by demonstrating hydronephrosis on an ultrasound of the kidneys. Placement of a Foley bladder catheter is the most effective method for diagnosing and treating obstruction of the urethral tract. Despite the relative infrequency of postrenal ARF, because of the reversibility of obstruction, all patients with newly discovered ARF should undergo renal imaging and/or temporary bladder catheterization.

Special Situations

Hyperkalemia can complicate ARF and requires prompt therapy. An electrocardiogram (ECG) should be performed to assess for myocardial irritability. Hyperkalemia can be associated with sinus bradycardia, sinus arrest, slow idioventricular rhythms, ventricular tachycardia, and ventricular fibrillation. More commonly, there can be peaked T waves, lowering of P-wave amplitude, prolongation of the PR interval, second-degree atrioventricular (AV) block, intraventricular conduction defects, and finally a widened "sine-wave" QRS that can precede asystole. The sequence of ECG changes is not orderly, and potentially lethal ventricular arrhythmias and asystole may occur at any time. When present, severe ECG changes should be rapidly antagonized with calcium in the form of calcium gluconate (one to two ampules) or calcium chloride (one half to one ampule) given intravenously. The patient should be in a cardiac-monitored setting. The effects of calcium last 30 to 60 minutes, and definitive methods of lowering serum potassium should be undertaken. The most reliable agent for promoting a transcellular shift of potassium is insulin. It should be given 10 U intravenously

The Urogenital Tract

with 50 mL of 50% dextrose solution with careful monitoring for hypoglycemia. Other options include sodium bicarbonate in the setting of acidemia and β_2-agonists in the form of nebulized albuterol. The exchange resin sodium polystyrene sulfonate (Kayexalate) with 70% sorbitol (50 to 70 mL) can help eliminate potassium from the gut and thereby lower serum concentrations by up to 1 mEq/L (following a 60-g oral dose). Kayexalate should be avoided in patients with known gastrointestinal dysmotility or recent bowel surgery. Generally, with ECG changes and serum potassium more than 6.5 mEq/L, the definitive method for correcting hyperkalemia is hemodialysis.

Metabolic acidosis, if severe (bicarbonate level less than 12 mEq/L or pH less than 7.2), can be treated with sodium bicarbonate in either oral or intravenous forms. The base deficit can be calculated to determine how much bicarbonate is needed:

$$Bicarbonate\ deficit\ (mEq/L) = 0.5 \times weight\ (kg) \\ \times (24 - measured\ serum\ HCO_3)$$

This formula is a conservative estimate of bicarbonate deficit and may underestimate the true deficit with serum bicarbonate less than 10 mEq/L. Using sodium bicarbonate in patients with lactic acidosis is controversial, especially in the intensive care unit (ICU) setting, with some authors questioning its ability to reverse myocardial depression induced by acidemia.

CONTRAST NEPHROPATHY

Use of radiocontrast agents often leads to acute reductions in renal function, especially in patients with preexisting renal dysfunction, diabetic nephropathy, hypovolemia, or those on drugs that affect renal blood flow (i.e., ACE inhibitors). Several therapeutic interventions are employed to prevent ARF with varied success. The best evidence still supports hydration with isotonic saline before and after radiocontrast exposure and the use of nonionic, iso-osmolar contrast agents. Recent evidence suggests that the addition of sodium bicarbonate to standard saline hydration could further reduce ARF: 150 mEq of sodium bicarbonate can be added to a liter of D5W (5% dextrose in water) and 3 mL/kg of body weight should be infused over the hour prior to the radiocontrast administration, followed by 1 mL/kg/hour for the 6 hours following the contrast exposure. Prophylaxis with the antioxidant acetylcysteine (Mucomyst, 600 mg orally twice daily before and after the procedure) can prevent reductions in renal function in patients with preexisting renal insufficiency (patients had a mean serum creatinine of 2.4 mg/dL). Although the effectiveness of Mucomyst is questioned, a meta-analysis of randomized clinical trials supports its use. Debate about it continues, but it is a relatively innocuous medication and therefore should be considered in all patients with the risk factors described earlier for ARF from radiocontrast agents. Other putative renoprotective agents like fenoldopam are being evaluated but still lack significant proof of effect. Given cost and side-effect issues, hydration, acetylcysteine, and bicarbonate are the most reasonable preventive strategies at this point.

ACUTE RENAL FAILURE FOLLOWING RENAL TRANSPLANTATION

ARF following renal transplantation is referred to as delayed graft function (DGF). DGF is usually a result of ischemia-reperfusion injury-induced ATN. DGF is usually defined as the need for renal replacement therapy in the first week post-transplant. Many patients have "slow graft function" with significant ischemic ATN that does not require dialysis. Depending on the induction immunosuppressive regimen, most centers perform protocol allograft biopsies in the first 1 to 2 weeks post-transplant to rule out acute allograft rejection or drug toxicity. Limited studies have determined that the type of dialysis membrane (biocompatible versus less biocompatible) used does not have a significant influence on the duration of DGF. Most clinicians agree that patients should be maintained at or slightly above their dry weight to avoid hypoperfusion of the allograft. The use of antilymphocyte antibody induction therapy can allow for delayed initiation of calcineurin-inhibitor medications, which have known acute ischemic nephrotoxic effects. In addition, antilymphocyte antibodies could decrease ARF by directly reducing inflammation and T-cell function during ischemia. Agents like sirolimus (Rapamycin) and mycophenolate mofetil (CellCept) may potentially delay recovery from ARF and at least sirolimus should be avoided until DGF is improving.

RENAL REPLACEMENT THERAPY

The need for renal replacement therapy in the setting of ARF should be decided individually in consultation with a nephrologist. The optimal modality also depends on the clinical scenario. Standard intermittent hemodialysis is feasible for most patients in need of acute dialysis. Patients with hypotension (either with or without vasopressor therapy), ongoing highly catabolic state with abundant generation of metabolic toxins (as with severe rhabdomyolysis or tumor lysis syndrome), or large daily volume intake (usually more than 3 L per day) may benefit from continuous venovenous hemodialysis (CVVHD) therapy. Local practices dictate the type of continuous therapy, either hemofiltration or hemodiafiltration.

Several studies address the optimal timing and frequency of dialysis in the setting of ARF, mainly in the ICU. One study shows that in a group of trauma patients in the ICU, there are advantages both in survival and length of stay when dialysis is started while the BUN is less than 60 mg/dL (early start). Another controversial study looked at daily (high-dose) versus every-other-day (standard-dose) dialysis in ICU patients. There was an apparent advantage in the high-dose dialysis group. Another single-center study shows a benefit to 23 mL/kg/hour CVVH as compared with 20 mL/kg/hour. A large randomized clinical trial currently is readdressing the question of dialysis dose in ICU patients with ARF.

General Management of Patients With Acute Renal Failure

Aside from the maneuvers just described to diagnose and treat ARF, there are some general principles of patient management. All medications should be reviewed and proper dose adjusted to account for possible increased serum concentrations with the reduction in GFR. It is generally advisable to keep a patient in the hospital until the course of ARF is improving or at least stabilized, given the excessive associated morbidity and mortality. Elective and semielective surgical procedures should be postponed when possible until ARF resolves and the serum creatinine is near baseline. Nutrition should be adequate and low-potassium regimens should be administered in most cases. Consultation with a nephrologist should be sought early when a patient presents with ARF, even before dialysis is indicated.

REFERENCES

Alonso A, Lau J, Jaber BL, et al: Prevention of radiocontrast nephropathy with N-acetylcysteine in patients with chronic kidney disease: A meta-analysis of randomized, controlled trials. Am J Kidney Dis 2004;43(1):1-9.
Bellomo R, Ronco C, Kellum JA, et al: Acute renal failure—definition, outcome measures, animal models, fluid therapy and information technology needs: The Second International Consensus Conference of the Acute Dialysis Quality Initiative (ADQI) Group. Crit Care 2004;8(4):R204-R212.
Clarkeson M, Lieberthal W, Brady HR: Acute renal failure. In Brenner B (ed): Brenner & Rector's The Kidney. Philadelphia, WB Saunders, 2004.
Forsythe SM, Schmidt GA: Sodium bicarbonate for the treatment of lactic acidosis. Chest 2000;117(1):260-267.
Friedewald JJ, Rabb H: Inflammatory cells in ischemic acute renal failure. Kidney Int 2004;66(2):486-491.
Merten GJ, Burgess WP, Gray LV, et al: Prevention of contrast-induced nephropathy with sodium bicarbonate: A randomized controlled trial. JAMA 2004;291(19):2328-2334.
Nash OK, Hafeez A, Hou S: Hospital-acquired renal insufficiency. Am J Kidney Dis 2002;39(5):930-936.
Tepel M, van der Giet M, Schwarzfeld C, et al: Prevention of radiographic-contrast-agent-induced reductions in renal function by acetylcysteine. N Engl J Med 2000;343(3):180-184.

Chronic Renal Failure

Method of
Jeffrey A. Kraut, MD

Chronic renal failure is defined as a reduction in glomerular filtration rate (GFR) below the normal values of approximately 120 to 130 mL/minute developing over months to years. Its incidence has increased significantly over the last several years, but this probably reflects more accurate estimations of GFR. However, there is an increased prevalence of type II diabetes mellitus, a frequent cause of renal disease, in Western societies that could contribute to a higher incidence of chronic renal failure. When renal failure is severe (GFR <10 mL/minute), renal replacement therapy, either dialysis or renal transplantation, is required to preserve life. However, even before several renal failure ensues, the presence of chronic renal failure has an important impact on organ function and can contribute to the development of significant electrolyte derangements, important hormonal abnormalities, and anemia. Also, its presence can alter the metabolism and therefore the blood concentrations and tissue concentrations of drugs administered for the treatment of various diseases. Moreover, a reduced GFR is associated with an increased risk of death, increased incidence of cardiovascular events, and hospitalizations independent of known risk factors or a history of cardiovascular diseases. Finally, the mortality of several surgical procedures is substantially increased by the presence of chronic renal failure. Therefore, detecting and treating patients with chronic renal failure is extremely important.

Causes of Chronic Renal Failure

Many disorders can cause chronic renal failure. However, epidemiologic studies indicate that diabetes mellitus and hypertension account for the majority of cases (>60%). Chronic glomerulonephritis, polycystic kidney disease, obstructive uropathy, and ischemic nephropathy caused by atherosclerotic renal artery stenosis are less common, but important causes of renal impairment. The latter disorder is postulated to be more frequent than previously believed and is an important undiagnosed cause of chronic renal impairment.

Recent studies have indicated that a reduction in GFR occurs with aging in the absence of factors known to produce renal injury such as hypertension or diabetes. Indeed, the average GFR of subjects in the 8th decade of life in one large study was 40 to 50 mL/minute. Pathologic examination of these individuals, when available, may reveal only benign nephrosclerosis.

Importantly, because a majority of individuals older than 60 years of age have lower muscle mass, the reduced GFR is not accompanied by a rise in serum creatinine concentration. Therefore, renal failure is not detected unless the physician considers other variables such as the patient's age and muscle mass in assessing GFR (see the following section).

Approach to the Diagnosis of Chronic Renal Failure

The first step in the diagnosis of chronic renal failure is, of course, to detect a reduction in GFR. In the past, estimations of GFR were based on the measurement of serum creatinine concentration alone. In adults, the

The Urogenital Tract

  ## CURRENT DIAGNOSIS

The following lists the optimal care of patients with chronic kidney disease:

- Test for albuminuria and estimate glomerular filtration rate using MDRD formula yearly for early diagnosis and stratification of CKD.
- If possible, determine cause of kidney disease.
- Initiate treatment to delay to prevent progression of disease including use of converting enzyme inhibitors and/or angiotensin receptor blockers to reduce BP to less than 138/80 and urine protein excretion to less than 1 g/24 hours.
- Control or prevent biochemical or clinical abnormalities including those of serum potassium, serum bicarbonate, serum phosphorus, parathyroid hormone, and hemoglobin.
- Evaluate patients for presence of and treat important co-morbid conditions, particularly heart disease.
- If the GFR is less than 30 mL/min, consider referral to a nephrologist.

Abbreviations: BP = blood pressure; CKD = care of patients with chronic kidney disease; GFR = glomerular filtration rate; MDRD = modification of diet in renal disease.

normal serum creatinine ranges between 0.6 and 1.3 mg/dL. Individuals with values greater than this are said to have renal failure. However, there is a wide range of normal values. Also, creatinine production, which is dependent on muscle mass, is a critical variable affecting serum creatinine concentration. Thus, a large group of individuals with reduced muscle mass can have serum creatinine values within the normal range, but a decreased GFR. The most common situation in which this paradox is encountered is in the elderly and in individuals with malignancy or chronic liver disease.

Precise measurement of GFR is accomplished by calculating the clearance of creatinine in a timed urine collection, generally 24 hours in duration:

$$\text{Creatinine clearance (mL/minute)} = \text{Ucr (mg/dL)} \times \text{volume (mL)/ Scr(mg/dL)/1440.}$$

where Ucr = urine creatinine concentration

Scr = plasma creatinine concentration

However, timed urine collections are often inaccurate because of errors in collection. Moreover, as renal function progresses and serum creatinine rises, or in the presence of nephrotic range proteinuria, GFR tends to be overestimated by creatinine clearance. Most recently, formulas derived from studies of large groups of patients—such as those by Cockroft and Gault and the Modification of Diet in Renal Disease (MDRD) in which GFR was correlated with other factors (e.g., body

weight, age, and serum albumin)—are sufficiently accurate to use for clinical purposes:

$$\text{Cockroft-Gault: CrCl (mL/minute)} = \{(140 - \text{age}) \times \text{wt} \times [1 - (0.15 \times \text{gender})]\}/(0.814 \times \text{Scr})$$

$$\text{MDRD: GFR} = 170 \times [\text{PCr}]^{-0.999} \times [\text{Age}]^{-0.176} \times [0.762 \text{ female}] \times [1.180 \text{ if patient is black}] \times [\text{SUN}]^{-0.170} \times [\text{Alb}]^{+0.318}$$

Once renal function is depressed, the physician determines whether this represents acute or chronic renal failure, When previous measurements of GFR are available, it is relatively easy to determine if the renal failure is chronic in nature. However, if these studies are not available, demonstration that the kidneys are small in size (less than 8 to 9 cm when they are normally approximately 10 to 12 cm) by renal ultrasound will confirm the chronicity of the disease. Evidence of increased echogenicity reflecting augmented fibrous deposits is also suggestive of chronic disease. However, several disorders associated with chronic renal failure have normal kidney size such as diabetes mellitus, polycystic kidney disease, and amyloidosis. Therefore, normal kidney size does not exclude chronic renal failure. If individuals have normal kidney size, the presence of anemia and/or certain abnormalities of divalent ion metabolism can also suggest the disease is chronic in nature.

Once impaired renal function is recognized, measurements of blood urea nitrogen (BUN), sodium, potassium, chloride, bicarbonate, hemoglobin and hematocrit, and calcium and phosphorus are obtained. A urinalysis is obtained looking for increased excretion of protein, presence of blood in the urine, and abnormal cellular elements. In patients with diabetes, studies to find microalbuminuria (albumin urine concentrations less than 300 mg per day) are important to detect the early stages of renal disease. A 24-hour or spot urine protein and creatinine determination to assess the urine's protein-to-creatinine ratio is obtained to quantitate the amount of protein being excreted. Urine protein excretion in excess of 3.5 g daily indicates the presence of glomerular pathology, whereas interstitial disease is characterized by values below 2 g. However, urine protein excretion can vary with glomerular disease so values below 3.5 g are still consistent with this diagnosis. Assessment of urine protein excretion is important for diagnostic purposes, but also because urine protein excretion is often followed to assess effectiveness of therapy.

Obstruction uropathy, an important cause of chronic renal failure and exacerbation of renal failure, can be excluded in the majority of cases by ultrasound of the kidneys. Doppler ultrasound of the renal arteries performed at the same time is helpful in excluding obstruction of the renal arteries. The necessity of obtaining other diagnostic studies such as measurement of serum complement, blood and urine eosinophils, serum and urine and protein electrophoresis, antiglomerular basement membrane antibodies, anti–double-stranded DNA (dsDNA) antibodies, hepatitis B and C antibodies, sedimentation rate, and HIV studies depends on the context of the renal failure.

10

Finally, a renal biopsy may be required in certain situations to make a definitive diagnosis. Because treatment of specific diseases can vary, making a precise pathologic diagnosis can be extremely important for proper management. Unfortunately, once the renal failure is moderate to severe in nature, renal pathologic examination may not always be helpful in determining the cause.

Clinical and Laboratory Abnormalities in Chronic Renal Failure

Because the kidney plays a critical role in the regulation of the serum concentrations of sodium, potassium, bicarbonate, chloride, calcium, and phosphorus as well as the levels of hemoglobin and hematocrit, blood pressure and extracellular volume, chronic renal injury can lead to derangements in these parameters as summarized in Table 1.

HYPONATREMIA AND HYPERNATREMIA

The kidney plays an essential role in excreting water by producing a dilute urine (less than 1/6 plasma osmolality) or retaining water by producing a concentrated urine (three to four times plasma osmolality). The ability to concentrate or dilute the urine in the majority of cases is usually retained until GFR falls to less than 30% of normal, and therefore hyponatremia or hypernatremia are uncommon until that time. If the disease is primarily interstitial in nature, alterations in urine concentrating ability can appear prior to significant reductions in GFR. However, even with higher levels of GFR the patient can be at risk for either of these electrolyte abnormalities should they ingest large quantities of fluid or be deprived of appropriate fluid intake.

TABLE 1 Clinical and Electrolyte Abnormalities Noted With Chronic Renal Failure

Clinical or laboratory disorder	GFR or Stage of Renal Failure*
Hypertension	GFR <60 mL/min (stage 2)
Hyponatremia or Hypernatremia	GFR <30 mL/min (stage 3)
Hyperkalemia*	GFR <30 mL/min (stage 3)
Hyperphosphatemia*	GFR <30 mL/min (stage 3)
Metabolic acidosis	GFR <30 mL/min (stage 3)
Anemia	GFR <60 mL/min (stage 2)
Uremic symptoms Nausea, vomiting, disturbances in sleep	GFR <15 mL/min (stage 5)

*Descriptions of the various stages are presented in the text. These electrolyte abnormalities can be seen at higher levels of GFR.
Abbreviations: GFR = glomerular filtration rate.

HYPERKALEMIA

The kidney plays the most critical role in the regulation of potassium balance. Adaptive changes in renal tubular function and possible colonic function enable the kidney to maintain serum potassium within the normal range until GFR falls below 20% to 25% of normal (serum creatinine of 4 mg/dL or greater). Recent studies indicate a tendency for elevations in serum potassium to appear at even modest reductions in GFR (<60 mL/min). When disease of the kidney involves the medullary portion or hormonal derangements such as hyporeninemic hypoaldosterinism are present, hyperkalemia can be observed prior to significant declines in GFR. In addition, patients with even moderate renal failure have a reduced reserve to eliminated potassium and therefore can develop hyperkalemia if potassium load is increased dramatically.

METABOLIC ACIDOSIS

A fall in plasma bicarbonate concentration in association with a reduced blood pH (metabolic acidosis) is frequently observed when GFR falls below 20% to 25% of normal. The acidosis results from acid excretion falling below acid production leading to positive proton balance. Recent studies have documented that a tendency to the development of metabolic acidosis can be seen with mild reductions in GFR (<60 mL/min).

The electrolyte pattern seen with the metabolic acidosis of renal failure is often of the high anion gap variety, but frequently a hyperchloremic (normal anion gap) or combined anion gap and hyperchloremic pattern can be observed. The degree of acidosis is usually mild to moderate with plasma bicarbonate concentration ranging from 12 to 22 mEq/L. Of interest, at any given level of GFR, the acidosis is often not progressive, but plasma bicarbonate concentration remains stable unless renal function declines further or there is an increment in acid production.

ABNORMAL DIVALENT IN METABOLISM

Serum phosphorus is regulated by the kidney but in most cases remains within the normal range until GFR falls below 20% to 25% of normal. This stabilization of serum phosphorus is attributed to increased tubular excretion of phosphorus as a result of increased parathyroid hormone secretion. As with potassium and bicarbonate, recent studies demonstrate a tendency for elevation in serum phosphorus can be observed with mild renal failure (<50 to 60 mL/min). Serum calcium is usually in the normal range, but varies receiprocally with serum phosphorus. Because of derangements in divalent ion metabolism bone disease with increased tendency to fractures and disordered soft tissue structures can be observed.

Hyperparathyoridism is a common occurrence in patients with renal failure, the values usually being higher with a greater degree of renal impairment. The elevated PTH values are usually induced by hypocalcemia, although increased serum phosphorus concentrations independent of serum calcium values can also play a role. The increased parathyroid hormone levels can induce damage to bone and soft tissue structures, but also may affect other functions such as cardiac function and the production of red blood cells.

ANEMIA

The kidney is the source of erythropoietin, the hormone that regulates bone marrow production of red blood cells. Thus, with the development of renal impairment, there is a fall in red blood cell production. A fall in red cell survival also contributes to development of anemia. Anemia generally appears when GFR falls below 60 mL/minute. There is a rough correlation between the severity of renal failure and the degree of anemia: the more severe the renal failure the greater the degree of anemia. However, this relationship is not invariable, and many patients have only mild reductions in hemoglobin and hematocrit.

Anemia initially was believed to contribute only to changes in oxygen delivery. However, recent studies show that anemia can contribute to the genesis of left ventricular hypertrophy and other cardiomyopathies noted with chronic renal failure and can raise mortality in patients with chronic renal failure.

HYPERTENSION

Recent studies emphasize the importance of the kidneys in the regulation of blood pressure, and the bulk of patients with diabetes or other glomerular disease will develop hypertension in the course of their renal failure. In many instances, hypertension does not develop until GFR is below 40% to 50% of normal. The type of renal disease underlying chronic renal failure appears to be important, as hypertension is less common with pyelonephritis. Hypertension might be observed earlier in the course of renal failure, however, in patients with polycystic kidney disease or ischemic nephropathy. Because hypertension is one of the most critical factors in the genesis of cardiovascular disease and can accelerate the progression of renal failure, careful attention of control of hypertension is important.

VOLUME OVERLOAD

Salt retention often accompanies chronic renal failure even when GFR is not severely compromised. The degree of salt retention can be profound if significant albuminuria with resultant hypoalbuminemia is seen and is more severe as GFR falls below 20% to 25% of normal. Salt retention is a critical factor in the development of hypertension and can promote congestive heart failure.

Symptoms and Signs of Renal Failure

Patients with chronic renal failure are often asymptomatic with little evidence of disease other than laboratory abnormalities until late in the course of renal failure.

Rakel and Bope: *Conn's Current Therapy 2006.*

If anemia is present, patients may complain of fatigue; and if significant elevations in parathyroid hormone levels are noted, bone pain, ruptured tendons or other disorders of soft tissue structures can be noted. Once moderate to severe renal failure appears, symptoms of the electrolyte abnormalities can be observed. Hyperkalemia, if severe, can lead to arrythmias or heart block and muscle weakness. Metabolic acidosis can contribute to fatigue. Anemia can contribute to fatigue and changes in mentation and physical stamina. Weight loss related to metabolic acidosis and or retention of various uremic toxins may occur. Sexual dysfunction characterized by reduced libido and reduced fertility are common with moderate to severe renal failure.

Once severe renal failure develops (stage 4 or 5), the uremic syndrome can be observed characterized by a decreased appetite, nausea, vomiting, and subtle changes in mental status including changes in sleep patterns. However, even with severe renal failure many patients feel surprisingly well.

Management of Chronic Renal Failure

STAGING OF CHRONIC RENAL FAILURE

As noted earlier, within the last several years, a great deal of effort has been expended into developing guidelines for the evaluation, monitoring, and treatment of patients with chronic renal failure. To this end, experts working with the National Kidney Foundation have divided chronic renal failure into different states based on measurements or estimations of GFR. The value of staging to the physician is that the studies necessary to monitor patients and the complications of chronic renal failure are often different depending on the stage of renal failure.

Stage 0 (GFR Greater Than 90 mL/minute With Risk Factors for Renal Disease)

Patients at stage 0 have increased risk for development of chronic renal failure, such as those with diabetes or hypertension but who have GFR greater than 90 mL/minute in the absence of proteinuria or urinary sedimentary abnormalities. These patients should have their blood pressure and diabetes controlled. Estimates of GFR should be obtained approximately every 6 months from measurement of serum creatinine, and qualitative tests for urine protein excretion should be obtained. In diabetics measurement of microalbumin should also be obtained. Because control of disease may forestall progression glycosylated hemoglobin (HbA1C) values should also be obtained.

Stage 1 (GFR Greater Than 90 mL/minute With Albuminuria)

Once evidence of renal damage is obtained, as reflected by microalbuminuria or proteinuria, but GFR is either normal or increased, patients are said to be in stage 1. These individuals should be monitored more closely and strict attention must be given to maintain blood pressure below 130/80. Furthermore, angiotensin converting enzyme inhibitor (ACEI) or angiotensin receptor blocker (ARB) should be given to prevent evolution of microalbuminuria to full blown proteinuria (see the following). No clinical or laboratory abnormalities are observed at this stage.

Stage 2: Mild Renal Failure (GFR 60 to 90 mL/minute)

When GFR is mildly reduced to values from 60 to 90 mL/minute, patients are in stage 2. These patients should also be carefully monitored and blood pressure tightly controlled. If diabetes is present, strict attention to maintaining HbA1C within recommended guidelines should be given. Again, it is rare at this stage for any significant clinical abnormalities other than hypertension to be present.

Stage 3: Moderate Renal Failure (GFR 30 to 59 mL/minute)

When GFR ranges between 30 to 59 mL/minute, patients are in stage 3. At this point hypertension may appear, mild abnormalities in serum phosphorus might be observed, and anemia can be seen. Also in some patients an elevation in serum potassium can be noted, particularly if they are ingesting a relatively high potassium diet. These patients need to be followed more closely, and it is recommended that patients at this stage be monitored by a nephrologist.

Stage 4: Moderate to Severe (GFR from 15 to 29 mL/minute)

Once GFR falls to values from 15 to 29 mL/minute, patients have severe renal failure, or stage 4 disease. At this level of GFR, significant electrolyte abnormalities such as metabolic acidosis, hyperkalemia, and hyperphosphatemia are frequent. Anemia is common and the patient may begin to note reductions in appetite and have a fall in muscle mass. However, there is great variability in the appearance of symptoms or laboratory derangements.

Stage 5: Severe (GFR Less Than 15 to 29 mL/minute)

When GFR falls below 15 mL/minute, severe electrolyte abnormalities are often present, anemia is common. Clinical symptoms can develop. Renal replacement therapy, either dislysis or transplantation, is usually required at this stage.

Recommendations for treatment of patients are summarized below. The frequency of patient visits, of course, largely depends on the complications of renal disease present and co-morbid conditions. Therefore, these are only general recommendations for frequency of examination.

When patients are in stage 0, they should be seen once per year for renal evaluation. When GFR remains normal or elevated, but proteinuria is present, renal evaluation should be performed every 6 months. When stage 3 develops, we usually repeat renal evaluation every 3 months. Patients in stage 4 are seen more frequently, usually at the minimum of once per month. Patients with end-stage disease require renal replacement therapy.

GENERAL APPROACH TO TREATMENT OF CHRONIC RENAL FAILURE

Treatment of chronic renal failure can be divided into the modalities that are specific to the underlying disorder and those that are used to treat all patients with chronic renal failure. Thus, patients with systemic lupus erythematosus or other immune-mediated or inflammatory disease may benefit from treatment with steroids and immunosuppressive agents. Treatments specific for individual disorders are beyond the scope of this article.

The physician treating the patient with renal failure has two goals: preventing or delaying progression of renal failure, and alleviating the electrolyte and hormonal abnormalities that can lead to symptoms or complications of the disease. Understanding the methods to accomplish the former requires knowledge of those factors that are integral to progression of the disease.

FACTORS CAUSING PROGRESSION OF CHRONIC RENAL FAILURE

It has been recognized for several years that once renal failure has developed, renal function can decline at a predictable rate in the absence of further insults to the kidney. Essential to the optimal approach used to treat chronic renal failure, therefore, is an understanding of those factors that can cause progression of renal failure, including:

- Systemic and intraglomerular hypertension
- Glomerular hypertrophy
- Intrarenal precipitation of calcium and phosphorus
- Hyperlipidemia
- Altered metabolism of prostanoids
- Metabolic acidosis
- Anemia
- Tubulointerstitial disease
- Proteinuria

Intraglomerular Hypertension and Glomerular Hypertrophy

As nephrons are lost, changes are induced in the kidney to preserve GFR such as renal vasodilatation, an increase in glomerular capillary pressure, and an increment in size of individual glomeruli raising wall stress. These adaptive mechanisms probably induce damage by causing endothelial cell damage with detachment of epithelial cells allowing enhanced flux of water and solutes that might cause narrowing of capillary lumens. Also, strain on mesangial cells causes them to produce cytokines and extracellular matrix with resultant expansion of the mesangium and glomerular sclerosis.

Proteinuria

Although proteinuria has traditionally been a marker of glomerular injury, with greater amounts of urinary protein excretion being associated with more severe injury, recent studies indicate that proteinuria, can induce mesangial and tubular damage. Therefore, treatments to reduce proteinuria, may be beneficial in limiting further renal damage.

Tubulointerstitial Disease

Some component of tubulointerstitial disease is generally found in individuals with chronic renal failure even when the primary process affects the glomerulus. It has been postulated that the tubulointerstitial disease can produce atrophy of tubules or obstruction destroying individual nephrons. Even when tubular inflammation is treated, progressive scarring can continue unabated. Thus, treatments designed to reduce interstitial fibrosis may be important for preventing progression of disease. At present, only experimental drugs not available for human use have been examined for this purpose.

Hyperlipidemia

Hyperlipidemia is frequently observed in disorders associated with nephrotic range proteinuria, but is also noted in a large percentage of the general population without renal disease. Experimental evidence obtained from animal studies shows hyperlipidemia can promote progression of renal failure. Thus, loading with cholesterol augments renal injury and treatment with cholesterol-lowering drugs slows the rate of progression. This effect is synergistic to that achieved by lowering blood pressure.

The mechanisms underlying the effects of lipids are not well understood, but possible explanations include mesangial lipid deposition leading to glomerular injury or tubular injury. A few studies performed in human subjects have demonstrated benefit from lipid lowering on the progression of renal injury, although they are not conclusive. Because patients with chronic renal failure have a high prevalence of cardiovascular disease, it is reasonable to inititate therapy with statin drugs to lower serum cholesterol and lipid levels.

Calcium-Phosphate Deposition

A rise in serum phosphorus, usually seen at the later stages of renal failure, can lead to precipitation of calcium phosphate in the renal interstitium. The deposits can then induce an inflammatory response producing interstitial fibrosis and tubular atrophy. Some have indicated that the deposits may form prior to detectable elevations in serum phosphorus concentrations.

Increased Glomerular Prostaglandin Production

An increment in glomerular prostaglandin production has been found in several studies of chronic renal failure.

The increased prostanoids produce renal vasodilatation and a rise in intraglomerular pressure, factors that augment progression of disease.

METABOLIC ACIDOSIS

Metabolic acidosis commonly develops in the course of chronic renal failure. In response to the acidosis, ammonia production per residual functioning nephron is augmented. It has been postulated that the increased local production of ammonia in some way induces tubulointerstitial damage. This issue remains controversial, as some studies do not support this possibility.

SPECIFIC TREATMENT MEASURES

Treatment of patients with chronic renal failure should be designed to ameliorate those factors that can cause progression of renal injury, treat or prevent important

---

 CURRENT THERAPY

The recommendations for the treatment of patients with renal failure is as follows:

Recommendation	Goal
Control BP	130/80
Reduce proteinuria by administering angiotensin converting enzyme inhibitors or angiotensin receptor blockers. In some cases both agents may have to be given concomitantly.	Decrease urine protein excretion to less than 1 g per day by gradual titration of dose.
Control phosphate concentrations with phosphate binders with noncalcium containing binders when possible.	Serum phosphate <4.5 mg/dL
Prevent hyperparathyroidism with vitamin D or calcimimetics.	Maintain PTH <150 pg/mL
Correct anemia with erythropoietin and iron replacement as needed.	Maintain Hg between 11 and 12 mg/dL
Administer diuretics to control hypertension and volume overload.	Maintain euvolemia when possible
Control serum potassium with dietary restriction, diuretics, and/or potassium exchange resin as necessary.	Maintain serum potassium <5.0 mEq/L
Keep protein intake at 0.6 to 0.8 g/kg body weight per day.	Slow progression of renal disease to prevent protein depletion
Control metabolic acidosis with administration of sodium citrate (Citra pH).	Maintain serum HCO$_3$ >20 mEq/L

Abbreviations: BP = blood pressure; HCO$_3$ = bicarbonate; Hg = mercury; PTH = parathyroid hormone.

10

complications, and normalize important laboratory abnormalities that contribute to symptoms of the disease.

Measures Designed to Reduce the Rate of Progression of Renal Failure

CONTROL OF SYSTEMIC AND INTRAGLOMERULAR HYPERTENSION

Experimental and human studies demonstrate that control of systemic hypertension can slow the rate of progression of renal disease substantially. Recent evidence indicates that target blood pressure levels should be lower than recommended for the general population (<130/80). Control of hypertension with the use of myriad agents can benefit the patient with renal failure. However, as indicated previously, reduction in intraglomerular hypertension may be the most important factor underlying the benefits from blood pressure control. Therefore, when possible, treatment with ACEIs, ARBs, or the combination of these agents should be first-line antihypertensive therapy in these patients. Patients who do not tolerate these drugs might benefit from administration of non-dihydropyridine calcium channel blockers. In patients with proteinuria, even if blood pressure is controlled or they are normotensive, the doses of ACEIs or ARBs should be raised to levels even greater than recommended to reduce urine protein excretion to levels less than 500 mg. This reduction in proteinuria is the most optimal in protecting the kidney.

Potentially serious complications with ACEIs or ARBs include acute reduction in GFR and hyperkalemia. If these complications occur, a reduction in dose or even discontinuation of these agents might be required. It is recommended that these agents be continued less than 20 mL/minute. Given the potential severity of these complications, patients should be monitored closely.

PROTEIN RESTRICTION

The benefits of protein restriction in preventing progression are unclear, but it has suggested that reducing protein intake to 0.8 to 1.0 g/kg body weight of high biologic value is beneficial. Others have indicated that 0.6 g/kg body weight should be used. In patients with substantial proteinuria, the quantity of protein recommended will have to be adjusted to prevent hypoalbuminemia. Once patients reached later stage 4, protein restriction may be useful to prevent expression of uremic symptoms. Reducing protein intake will have the added benefit of decreasing acid, potassium, and phosphate production.

CONTROL OF LIPIDS

Control of cholesterol with statins may help prevent progression and should reduce the burden of cardiovascular disease, which remains the most lethal disorder for patients with chronic renal failure. Adherence to the newly proposed aggressive recommendation appears reasonable.

Measures Designed to Treat Significant Laboratory Abnormalities

ANEMIA

Patients with renal anemia should be treated with erythropoietin (Procrit). Although this requires subcutaneous injection once per week, newer, long-lasting forms (darbepoetin [Aranesp]) enable patients to be treated every 3 weeks. Because iron stores need to be repleted for anemia to be successfully treated, these should be monitored and iron given. Because of the vagaries of ferritin measurements, we use serum iron and iron binding capacity with the goal of maintaining saturation above 20% and near 30%. At present, the target hemoglobin and hematocrit varies between 11 mg/dL and 12 mg/dL 33 and 36, respectively.

METABOLIC ACIDOSIS

Controversy exists as to the target value of bicarbonate for patients with chronic renal failure. Some experts recommend raising plasma bicarbonate to levels above 20 mEq/L, whereas others recommend complete normalization of plasma bicarbonate. To properly raise plasma bicarbonate concentration, the deficit should be calculated from the formula:

Desired − prevailing level of plasma bicarbonate
$\times 50\%$ body weight = Total bicarbonate deficit.

The deficit should be corrected slowly over several days.

Because patients experience gas when the base is given as bicarbonate, the base is usually administered as Shohl's solution sodium citrate,* the citrate being metabolized to bicarbonate in the liver. Each milliliter of Shohl's solution represents 1 mEq of the base.

DIVALENT ION METABOLISM

Serum phosphorus is controlled by administration of phosphate binders usually starting with calcium citrate (Citracal) or acetate (PhosLo). If these are not successful or if patients have elevated calcium levels, then sevelomer (Renagel) can be used either alone or in combination with calcium binders. Physicians should aim to maintain serum phosphorus levels below 5 mg/dL and keep serum calcium phosphorus product below 60.

Parathyroid hormone (PTH) levels should be maintained slightly below 150 pg/mL, values that have been associated with proper bone remodeling but not to values observed in patients without kidney disease.

---

*May be compounded by pharmacists.

Suppression of parathyroid hormone secretion can be achieved by administration of various vitamin D analogues. The recent recognition of the calcium-sensing receptor and development of calcimimetic drugs that are extremely effective in lowering PTH secretion may make using vitamin D compounds obsolete in the future.

HYPERKALEMIA

As this is the most serious electrolyte disorder encountered, patients should be monitored closely. Serum potassium concentrations should be maintained below 5 mEq/L. If hyperkalemia develops during treatment with ACEIs or ARBs, the doses of these agents should be reduced or discontinued. Diuretic administration, often given for control of hypertension, can help control hyperkalemia, but if it should develop, particularly when GFR falls below 20% of normal, it can be treated with the potassium exchange resin, sodium polystyrene sulfonate (Kayexalate).

ELEVATED BLOOD UREA NITROGEN CONCENTRATION

The precise solutes that are retained, which are important for the pathogenesis of the uremic syndrome, are not clear. However, BUN is a marker for other retained solutes and is roughly correlated with development of uremic symptoms. When the BUN is greater than 100 mg/dL and serum creatinine concentration is greater than 8 mg/dL uremic symptoms may develop. These symptoms will often abate merely with protein restriction and reduced production of these compounds. Protein restriction is usually not instituted until GFR is less than 15% to 20% of normal. Prior to that time, it is important to maintain protein intake to keep serum albumin within the normal range.

VOLUME OVERLOAD

Because salt retention is an essential component of the development of hypertension and underlies volume overload, diuretic administration is usually necessary in the treatment of chronic renal failure. Thiazides frequently used in the treatment of hypertension or volume overload in subjects with normal renal function may not be efficacious once GFR is less than or equal to 33% of normal. Therefore, loop diuretics, such as furosemide (Lasix) or a combined loop and proximal tubule diuretic such as metolozone (Zaroxolyn), are generally indicated. Because the effectiveness of both agents requires access to the tubule lumen, the effective dose is often higher than in those with normal renal function. Once patients are in stage 4 renal failure, use of diuretics is hampered by worsening of renal failure and often must be used cautiously.

REFERENCES

Beco JA, Bansal VK: Medical nutrition therapy in chronic kidney failure: Integrating clinical practice guidelines. J Am Diet Assoc 2004;104:404-409.

Rakel and Bope: *Conn's Current Therapy 2006.*

Clase CM, Garg AX, Kiberd BA: Prevalence of low glomerular filtration rate in nondiabetic Americans: Third National Health and Nutrition Examination Survey (NHANES III). J Am Soc Nephrol 2002;13.
Cleveland DR, Jindal KK, Hirsch DJ, et al: Quality of pre-referral care in patients with chronic renal insufficiency. Am J Kidney Dis 2002;40:30-36.
Curtin RB, Becker B, Kimmel PL, Schatell D: An integrated approach to care for patients with chronic kidney disease. Semin Dial 2003;16:399-402.
Djamali A, Kendziorski C, Brazy PC, Becker BN: Disease progression and outcomes in chronic kidney disease and renal transplantation. Kidney Int 2003;64:1800-1807.
Kopple JD: National Kidney Foundation K/DOQI clinical practice guidelines for nutrition in chronic renal failure. Am J Kidney Dis 2001;37:S66-S70.
Maschio G, Alberti D, Janin G, et al: Effect of the angiotensin-convering-enzyme inhibitor benazepril on the progression of chronic renal insufficiency. N Engl J Med 1996;334:939-945
Tonelli M, Gill J, Pandeya S, et al: Slowing the progression of chronic renal insufficiency. Can Med Assoc J 2002;166:906-907.

Malignant Tumors of the Urogenital Tract

Method of
Brett S. Carver, MD, Guido Dalbagni, MD, and Joel Sheinfeld, MD

Genitourinary malignancies account for approximately 42% of all cancers in men and 5% of all cancers in women. In this article, the four most common genitourinary malignancies—prostate, bladder, renal, and testicular cancers—are reviewed, with a concise description of the epidemiologies, clinical diagnoses, treatment paradigms, and recent advances in their management.

Prostate Cancer

Prostate cancer is the most commonly diagnosed cancer in men in the United States and the second most common cause of male cancer deaths. An estimated 230,000 new cases and 29,000 deaths related to prostate cancer will occur in 2004. Its incidence increases with advancing age, and the median age of diagnosis is 70 years. With the widespread implementation of serum prostate-specific antigen (PSA) screening initiated in the early 1990s, a stage migration has occurred with approximately 40% of cases diagnosed by an elevated serum PSA alone. The current American Cancer Society prostate cancer screening recommendations include an annual serum PSA and digital rectal examination starting at 50 years of age, or at age 40 years for African American men or those with a family history of the disease. With the high prevalence of prostate cancer, several investigators are evaluating the role of chemoprevention. In a recent randomized prospective trial, finasteride (Proscar)[1] taken daily was shown to decrease the prevalence of prostate cancer by 24.8% compared with placebo. Unfortunately, a higher incidence of high-grade (Gleason score >7) prostate cancer observed in the finasteride group was associated with this finding. Clinical trials are currently under way to evaluate the role of vitamin E[1] and selenium[1] for the chemoprevention of prostate cancer.

Transrectal ultrasound-guided prostate biopsy is the method of choice for diagnosing men with prostate cancer. Currently, a nuclear medicine bone scan is recommended for men with high-grade tumors and serum PSA levels greater than 10 µg/dL, and a computerized tomography (CT) scan of the pelvis is recommended to evaluate for lymphadenopathy if serum PSA levels are greater than 20 µg/dL. Table 1 shows the staging system for prostate cancer. Patients diagnosed with clinically localized prostate cancer face a daunting variety of management choices including expectant management, radical prostatectomy, or radiation therapy.

EXPECTANT MANAGEMENT

Although the lifetime risk of developing an autopsy-detectable prostate cancer is approximately 42%, the lifetime risk of dying of prostate cancer is only approximately 3%. The high prevalence of prostate cancer in the male population and the fact that some cancers would not affect an individual's life expectancy has led to the treatment paradigm of expectant management ("watchful waiting"). Expectant management is based on close surveillance of patients deemed to be at low risk for prostate cancer progression using a combination of serum PSA testing, digital rectal examination, and additional prostate biopsies while not

---

[1]Not FDA approved for this indication.

TABLE 1   1997 American Joint Committee on Cancer TNM Staging Classification for Prostate Cancer

Stage	Definition
T1a	Tumor in <5% of transurethrally resected specimen
T1b	Tumor in >5% of transurethrally resected specimen
T1c	Tumor identified by an elevated prostate-specific antigen serum alone
T2a	Tumor confined to one lobe
T2b	Tumor confined to both lobes
T3a	Extracapsular extension
T3b	Seminal vesicle invasion
T4	Invasion of bladder or rectum
N0	No regional lymph node metastasis
N1	Regional lymph node metastasis
M0	No distant metastasis
M1	Distant metastasis

compromising the potential opportunity for curative therapy. Although the selection criteria for men entering an expectant management program are not well standardized, the consensus is that expectant management should be reserved for men with well-differentiated (Gleason score 6 or less) low-volume (organ-confined, small percentage of biopsy cores positive) prostate cancer, and those with a life expectancy of less than 10 years. Although a recent prospective randomized trial comparing radical prostatectomy with watchful waiting demonstrates a disease-specific survival advantage for the group of men undergoing radical prostatectomy (4.6% versus 8.9%), this study has limitations because the majority of men entering the study had a higher grade and stage than would be considered for watchful waiting in the United States. Several series demonstrate that expectant management is a viable treatment option for select men with prostate cancer and that curative therapy is not compromised. Further studies incorporating both clinical and molecular biologic markers are needed to better characterize the selection criteria for men who would benefit from an expectant management program.

RADICAL PROSTATECTOMY

With improved knowledge of the pelvic anatomy, neurovascular bundles, and urethral sphincter mechanism, the surgical technique of the radical prostatectomy has evolved over recent years. Radical prostatectomy provides excellent long-term cancer control with a 10-year disease-specific survival of approximately 85% for patients with clinically organ-confined tumors. For patients undergoing radical prostatectomy, predictors for disease recurrence include Gleason score (histologic grade), pathologic stage, and serum PSA level. When disease is pathologically confined to the prostate, 90% of patients remain free from disease recurrence at 10 years following radical prostatectomy. Pathologic extension of prostate cancer beyond the prostatic capsule and invasion into the seminal vesicles decreases the 10-year probability of freedom from progression to 75% and 45%, respectively. Lymph node metastases occur in 3% to 6% of all patients undergoing radical prostatectomy. Secondary to the benefit of local tumor control following radical prostatectomy, it is recommended that radical prostatectomy be completed even in the face of micrometastatic lymph node disease.

The risk of incontinence following radical prostatectomy varies from 5% to 30%. Urinary incontinence tends to improve with time, and the majority of patients achieve continence by 3 to 6 months after the surgery. With an appropriately performed nerve-sparing radical prostatectomy, recovery of erection occurs in approximately 70% of patients. The probability of erectile function recovery is related to patient age, preexisting erectile function, and surgical technique.

Laparoscopic radical prostatectomy is being performed with increasing frequency, and reports have shown disease-free survival rates similar to open radical prostatectomy. This procedure is technically challenging with a steep learning curve. Laparoscopic radical prostatectomy results in better cosmesis, reduced hospital stay, reduced need for blood transfusion, and a quicker postoperative recovery time. Little is reported in the literature regarding recovery of continence or potency.

RADIATION THERAPY

Radiation therapy in the treatment of prostate cancer encompasses external beam radiation therapy, brachytherapy, and a combination of the two modalities. With the improvement in technology, radiation therapy continues to evolve with higher therapeutic doses being delivered over recent times. In general, outcomes following external beam radiation therapy for clinically organ-confined prostate cancer are reportedly similar to those obtained with radical prostatectomy. The criteria used to define disease recurrence vary widely between external beam radiotherapy and radical prostatectomy, however, and to date no comparative trials have been conducted. The administration of hormonal therapy concomitantly with radiation therapy has been shown previously in several large trials to improve freedom from recurrence and disease-specific survival. However, current trials are under way to evaluate if hormonal therapy still adds benefit to the higher doses of radiation provided by intensity-modulated radiation therapy (IMRT). In patients with clinically organ-confined prostate cancer, 10-year disease-specific survival rates are approximately 85%. For patients with locally advanced prostate cancer, results are less favorable with a 10-year disease-specific survival of approximately 50%.

With the improved techniques in the delivery of external beam radiotherapy, the radiation oncologist has been able to deliver increasing doses of therapeutic radiation while at the same time reducing the incidence and severity of associated complications. Common side effects following radiation therapy are generally short lived and include irritative voiding symptoms, diarrhea, and occasional rectal bleeding, which occurs to varying degrees in approximately one third of patients. Erectile function tends to diminish over time, rendering only 50% of patients potent following treatment with external beam radiation therapy.

Interstitial brachytherapy is a treatment option typically reserved for patients with clinically organ-confined disease, well-differentiated tumors, and a serum PSA less than 10. In this select cohort of men, results are similar to those of radical prostatectomy. Interstitial brachytherapy is well tolerated with mild side effects, predominantly urinary urgency and frequency and occasional proctitis.

METASTATIC PROSTATE CANCER

The most common sites of prostate cancer metastasis are the axial skeletal system, lungs, and pelvic lymph nodes. Symptoms secondary to metastatic prostate cancer are typically related to bony metastases and include pain, anemia, pathologic fractures, and epidural spinal cord compression. The majority of prostate cancers depend on androgens for tumor proliferation, and

the initial mainstay of treatment for metastatic prostate cancer is androgen ablation. Several techniques are available to achieve androgen deprivation, including surgical castration, medical castration, and androgen receptor blockade. Long-acting gonadotropin-releasing hormone (GnRH) agonist-antagonists, goserelin acetate (Zoladex), and leuprolide acetate (Lupron), act by down-regulating the secretion of luteinizing hormone (LH) and follicle-stimulating hormone (FSH), resulting in a brief rise and subsequent fall in testosterone to castration levels. Because of the initial flare in testosterone, GnRH analogues alone are contraindicated in patients with spinal metastases and imminent cord compression. This flare can be prevented by pretreatment with an antiandrogen (bicalutamide [Casodex], flutamide [Eulexin]) prior to administration of a GnRH analogue.

For patients who progress to androgen-independent prostate cancer, the median survival is approximately 18 months. This group of patients has been generally treated with the addition of an antiandrogen and subsequent antiandrogen withdrawal for progressive hormone refractory disease. A multicenter clinical trial recently demonstrated the benefit of chemotherapy based on docetaxel (Taxotere) in patients with hormone-refractory metastatic prostate cancer. In this study, median survival was significantly improved in men receiving chemotherapy. Future trials are currently being developed to evaluate the efficacy of tumor vaccines[4] and targeted therapy in the management of hormone refractory prostate cancer.

Bladder Cancer

Urothelial malignancies encompass tumors arising from the urothelial lining of the urinary tract, with the bladder the most common site of disease. In men, bladder cancer is the fourth most common malignancy, accounting for 6% of all cancer cases; in women, it is the eighth most common, accounting for 2% of all cases. The incidence of bladder cancer increases with age, and factors reported to be associated with the development of bladder cancer include cigarette smoking, occupational exposure to chemical carcinogens, infections and chronic bladder inflammation, and bladder calculi. Cigarette smoking is clearly the most important single cause of bladder cancer, attributed to more than 50% of cases in men. The relative risk varies from two- to tenfold, in a dose-dependent relationship, and the risk may persist for 10 years or longer after smoking cessation.

Transitional cell carcinoma is the most prevalent histologic subtype, representing approximately 90% of bladder tumors in the United States. Although squamous cell carcinoma represents only 5% of bladder tumors in the United States, it is an important cause of bladder cancer worldwide and prevalent in countries where exposure to *Schistosoma haematobium* (bilharziasis) is common.

10

Rakel and Bope: *Conn's Current Therapy 2006.*

[4]Not yet approved for use in the United States.

Painless gross hematuria is the most common presenting symptom, occurring in greater than 90% of patients with bladder tumors. Irritative voiding symptoms such as urinary frequency, urgency, or dysuria are less frequent symptoms of an urothelial malignancy, but their presence should not be overlooked and are more commonly seen with carcinoma in situ (CIS) of the bladder. Evaluations of patients with documented gross or microscopic hematuria should include an intravenous pyelogram or computerized tomography (CT) urogram to evaluate the kidneys, ureters, and bladder; a urine specimen for culture and sensitivity to rule out an infectious cause; a urine specimen for cytology; and a cystoscopy to examine the bladder thoroughly. Patients presenting with irritative symptoms alone should be evaluated with a urinary cytology and cystoscopy when indicated to rule out bladder CIS. Other noninvasive urine tests such as nuclear matrix protein (NMP-22) and bladder tumor antigen (BTA) have been evaluated in the diagnosis of bladder cancer and have a potential role in the workup and monitoring of patients with bladder cancer when urinary cytology is not readily available, but they should not be used to replace cystoscopy.

Transurethral resection of the bladder tumor (TURBT) is both a diagnostic and therapeutic procedure. An accurate pathologic assessment of the bladder tumor specimen provides information regarding histologic grade, pathologic stage, and the presence of concomitant CIS, all of which are important in subsequent management decisions. A bimanual examination performed under anesthesia and a CT scan or magnetic resonance imaging (MRI) of the abdomen and pelvis are important in staging the extravesical extent of the tumor.

In general, bladder cancer can be divided into superficial disease, muscle-invasive disease, and metastatic disease. Approximately 75% of patients have superficial bladder tumors at presentation, and 25% present with muscle-invasive disease. The management of patients with bladder cancer is determined by tumor stage (Table 2) as well as histologic grade.

MANAGEMENT OF SUPERFICIAL BLADDER CANCER

Superficial bladder cancer encompasses tumors with pathologic stages Ta, T1, and Tis, each of which may have varying behaviors with regard to tumor recurrence and progression. Approximately 70% of superficial bladder tumors are stage Ta, and 30% are T1. In situ carcinoma (Tis) occurs in approximately 10% of bladder cancers, often coexisting with papillary bladder tumors. Following TURBT, which is curative for the majority of superficial bladder tumors, further management is directed according to the risk of tumor recurrence and progression. Although patients with low-grade superficial bladder tumors have recurrence rates of 50% to 60%, the risk of progression to muscle-invasive disease is low (2% to 10%), and patients are usually managed with TURBT alone with adjuvant intravesical chemotherapy (mitomycin C [Mutamycin])[1] reserved to prevent disease recurrence in patients with a history of multiple tumor recurrences. Patients with solitary high-grade superficial bladder tumors have recurrence rates of up to 80%, and approximately 20% to 50% of patients have progression to muscle-invasive disease if TURBT alone is performed. Therefore, for patients with high-grade solitary T1 tumors or diffuse CIS, intravesicle immunotherapy with bacille Calmette-Guérin (BCG) is recommended following TURBT. Intravesicle BCG has been proved to treat CIS effectively and to decrease tumor recurrence and progression. Patients with BCG-refractory CIS or T1 tumors should be considered candidates for radical cystectomy because progression to muscle-invasive disease occurs in up to 80% of these patients. For patients with unresectable T1 tumors and multifocal high-grade T1 tumors, radical cystectomy should be considered because 30% to 50% of these patients will have underlying muscle-invasive disease.

MANAGEMENT OF MUSCLE-INVASIVE BLADDER CANCER

Radical cystectomy with an extended pelvic lymph node dissection and urinary diversion remains the standard of care for patients with muscle-invasive bladder cancer. A recent multicenter randomized prospective trial found that neoadjuvant chemotherapy prior to radical cystectomy provided a 5-year survival advantage of 14% compared with radical cystectomy alone (57% versus 43%, respectively). Therefore, neoadjuvant chemotherapy should be discussed with and offered to patients with muscle-invasive bladder cancer prior to radical cystectomy. Survival following radical cystectomy is related to tumor stage and the presence of lymph node metastasis, with a probability of survival at 5 years of 70% for organ-confined tumors, 50% for tumors with extravesicle extension, and 35% for lymph node metastases. The options for urinary diversion following radical cystectomy include an ileal conduit, a continent cutaneous pouch, and an orthotopic neobladder.

TABLE 2 1997 American Joint Committee on Cancer TNM Staging Classification for Bladder Cancer

Stage	Definition
Ta	Noninvasive papillary tumor
Tis	In situ carcinoma
T1	Tumor invades lamina propria
T2	Tumor invades muscularis propria
T3	Tumor invades perivesicle tissue
T4	Tumor invades adjacent structures (prostate, vagina, rectum, pelvic wall)
N0	No regional lymph node metastasis
N1	Metastasis in a single lymph node <2 cm
N2	Metastasis in multiple lymph nodes or a single lymph node >2 cm
M0	No distant metastasis
M1	Distant metastasis

---

[1]Not FDA approved for this indication.

Rakel and Bope: *Conn's Current Therapy 2006.*

The only absolute contraindication to performing an orthotopic neobladder is a positive urethral margin. Thus, a urethral margin frozen section should be performed prior to orthotopic urinary diversion. Studies show that patients undergoing an orthotopic neobladder have complication rates similar to the other forms of urinary diversion and may provide patients with a better quality of life after radical cystectomy.

METASTATIC BLADDER CANCER

Despite the recognized chemosensitivity of transitional cell carcinoma of the bladder, more than 10,000 deaths per year in the United States are attributable to this disease. At initial presentation, approximately 18% of patients have metastatic disease involving the regional lymph nodes and 3% have distant metastases. In addition, 20% to 40% of patients recur with metastatic disease following radical cystectomy. A number of single chemotherapeutic agents have demonstrated efficacy in the treatment of metastatic bladder cancer, but because the majority of these responses are incomplete and of short duration, multidrug regimens are preferred. The traditional MVAC (methotrexate, vinblastine [Velban], doxorubicin [Adriamycin], and cisplatin [Platinol]) chemotherapy regimen has recently been supplanted by other regimens, which have shown similar response rates with a significant reduction in side effects. Long-term survival may be obtained in 10% to 15% of patients with metastatic disease.

Renal Cancer

Renal cell carcinoma (RCC) accounts for 3% of all adult malignancies, and approximately 12,000 patients die of the disease annually. Although the majority of cases are sporadic, several familial syndromes are associated with renal cell carcinoma, including von Hippel-Lindau (VHL) disease, tuberous sclerosis, and congenital polycystic kidney disease. The VHL gene is a tumor suppressor gene located on chromosome 3. Approximately 28% to 45% of patients with germ line mutations in the VHL gene develop RCC. In patients with sporadic RCC, approximately 60% to 80% demonstrate mutations or loss of heterozygosity of the VHL locus. Other risk factors associated with RCC include cigarette smoking, obesity, and acquired renal cystic disease in end-stage renal failure patients.

Renal cell carcinoma includes a variety of histologic subtypes with varying biologic behavior. The Heidelberg classification system for renal cortical tumors defines major histologic categories including clear cell carcinoma, papillary carcinoma, and chromophobe carcinoma. These different histologic subtypes display distinct cytogenetic abnormalities and differing propensities for metastasis. Benign renal cortical lesions such as oncocytoma are often clinically indistinguishable from renal cell carcinoma.

The classic triad of flank pain, hematuria, and flank mass occurs in fewer than 10% of patients diagnosed with RCC, and when it does, the disease is often metastatic.

Rakel and Bope: *Conn's Current Therapy 2006.*

TABLE 3 TNM Staging Classification for Renal Cancer

Stage	Definition
T1	Tumor confined to kidney <7 cm
T2	Tumor confined to kidney >7 cm
T3a	Tumor invades adrenal gland
T3b	Tumor extends into renal vein or infradiaphragmatic IVC
T3c	Tumor extends into supradiaphragmatic IVC
T4	Tumor invades beyond Gerota's fascia
N0	No regional lymph node metastasis
N1	A single regional lymph node metastasis
M0	No distant metastasis
M1	Distant metastasis

Abbreviation: IVC = inferior vena cava.

The majority of patients (60%) with RCC are diagnosed incidentally during an abdominal ultrasound or CT scan performed for another medical purpose. With the increase in the number of incidentally detected renal tumors, a stage migration has occurred, resulting in the detection of a larger number of smaller renal lesions. Table 3 shows the staging system for renal cancer. The evaluation of patients with suspected RCC includes a triphasic CT scan of the abdomen and pelvis to evaluate the primary renal tumor, regional lymph nodes, and visceral organs for metastasis. A chest roentogram should also be performed to evaluate for pulmonary metastasis, with a CT scan of the chest reserved for patients with suspicious lesions on chest radiograph. An MRI is indicated for patients with suspected renal vein or inferior vena cava (IVC) tumor thrombus to delineate its cephalad and caudad extent.

SURGICAL MANAGEMENT

With the evolving stage migration and the reduction in tumor size as more renal tumors were detected incidentally, the standard treatment for RCC has evolved over the years. Radical nephrectomy remains the standard of care for patients with larger (>4 cm) renal tumors. Partial nephrectomy, previously reserved for patients with bilateral renal tumors or tumors in a solitary kidney, however, has emerged as a viable treatment option if not approaching standard of care for patients with renal tumors smaller than 4 cm. For patients undergoing partial nephrectomy, local recurrence rates are less than 5%, and overall survival is comparable with patients undergoing radical nephrectomy. Concomitant adrenalectomy is indicated in patients undergoing nephrectomy for larger lesions involving the upper pole of the kidney. Although the role of regional lymphadenectomy in the treatment of RCC is not yet established definitively, a large multi-institutional trial is ongoing to evaluate patients undergoing radical nephrectomy with or without regional lymphadenectomy. Thus far, no difference in disease progression has been noted, 5.2% versus 6.7%, respectively, and regional lymphadenectomy is not routinely recommended for patients undergoing radical nephrectomy. Inferior vena cava tumor thrombus is reported to occur in 5% of patients with RCC. Renal vein or IVC tumor thrombus associated with an organ-confined renal tumor does not portend a poor prognosis, and radical nephrectomy with tumor thrombectomy results in an overall 5-year survival rate of 56% to 72%.

With the advancements in laparoscopy, laparoscopic radical and partial nephrectomies are being performed with increasing frequency. Laparoscopic radical nephrectomy offers a reduced postoperative recovery time, improved cosmesis, decreased requirement for postoperative analgesics, and a shorter hospital stay without compromising cancer control and cure. Although laparoscopic partial nephrectomy appears feasible for small exophytic lesions, tumors centrally located or involving the renal collecting system are reported to have a higher complication rate compared with open partial nephrectomy.

METASTATIC RENAL CELL CARCINOMA

Approximately 30% of patients with renal cell carcinoma present with metastatic disease at the time of diagnosis. The prognosis of metastatic RCC is poor, with a median survival of 6 to 10 months and a probability of survival at 5 years of 1% to 2%. Previous attempts to treat locally advanced or metastatic RCC with chemotherapy, hormonal therapy, or radiation therapy have been unsuccessful. Currently immunotherapy with or without radical nephrectomy is the standard of care for the initial treatment of metastatic RCC. Several large clinical trials have evaluated the use of peginterferon alfa-2a (PEG-Intron, Intron A)[1] and high-dose interleukin-2 (Proleukin) for the management of metastatic RCC. The overall response to these regimens is approximately 15%, and patients with a good performance status, solitary pulmonary metastasis, and those undergoing a cytoreductive nephrectomy are most likely to benefit from these regimens. Currently, several multicenter clinical trials are being performed to address the roles of vaccine therapy, gene therapy, and targeted therapy in patients with metastatic RCC.

Testicular Cancer

Testicular cancer is the most common malignancy in men 20 to 35 years of age. With the combination of surgery and chemotherapy for the management of testicular cancer, overall survival rates for all stages currently exceed 95%. Cryptorchidism has been the most consistently associated risk factor for the development of testis cancer. Approximately 8.5% of patients diagnosed with testicular cancer have a history of cryptorchidism. A prior history of infertility is found in approximately 3% of patients with testicular cancer, and therefore

testicular cancer should be ruled out in men undergoing evaluation for infertility.

The most common symptom at the time of diagnosis is painless swelling or enlargement of the testis. Symptoms manifesting secondary to metastatic disease include a mass in the left neck, pulmonary complaints such as hemoptysis or dyspnea, abdominal mass, or back pain that can often be disabling. In approximately 3% of patients, tenderness of the breast is reported. A delay in diagnosis has been reported in the literature ranging from 2.5 to 4.4 months and is associated with a more advanced clinical stage at the time of diagnosis. Reasons for the delay in diagnosis are multifactorial but include both a physician and patient component. Previous reports have shown that approximately 18% to 33% of patients with testicular cancer were initially treated for epididymitis by their physician. Testicular ultrasonography is the initial imaging modality of choice with a high sensitivity and specificity in detecting testicular tumors. The serum tumor markers α-fetoprotein (AFP) and human chorionic gonadotropin (hCG) have established a clear role in both the diagnosis and clinical management of testicular germ cell tumors. Elevation of one or both markers occurs in 80% of metastatic germ cell tumors of the testis.

Whenever an intratesticular mass is diagnosed, an inguinal radical orchiectomy should be performed for primary tumor control and pathologic diagnosis. Although scrotal violation does not compromise overall survival, the practice of transscrotal orchiectomy or testicular biopsy should be discouraged because it has the potential to alter metastatic pathways and increase the burden of therapy on the patient.

Germ cell tumors of the testis are categorically divided into seminomatous and nonseminomatous tumors based on the pathologic assessment of the orchiectomy specimen and the serum tumor marker (animal protein factor [APF], hCG) levels. Nonseminomatous germ cell tumors (NSGCTs) include embryonal carcinoma, choriocarcinoma, yolk sac tumor, and/or teratoma. Serum tumor markers are frequently elevated in patients with NSGCT. Seminomatous germ cell tumors include only pure seminoma and demonstrate no elevation of serum AFP, but hCG may be elevated in approximately 10% to 15% of cases. Seminomatous tumors found in combination with nonseminomatous tumors or those with elevated serum AFP are appropriately categorized and managed as nonseminomas. The initial staging evaluation should include a CT scan of the chest, abdomen, and pelvis, as well as serum tumor marker levels both pre- and postorchiectomy. The clinical staging system for germ cell tumors (Table 4) is the only staging system of the urologic malignancies to incorporate serum tumor markers. Treatment paradigms are described based on tumor pathology, clinical staging, and risk stratification.

NONSEMINOMA

Following radical orchiectomy the majority of patients with clinical stage I disease are cured. Approximately 20% to 30% of patients are understaged by CT scan, however, and either relapse systemically or in

---

[1]Not FDA approved for this indication.

TABLE 4 Clinical Staging System for Testicular Germ Cell Tumors

Stage	Definition
I	Tumor confined to the testis
IS	Tumor confined to the testis with elevated serum tumor markers
IIa	Regional lymph node metastasis <2 cm
IIb	Regional lymph node metastasis 2-5 cm
IIc	Regional lymph node metastasis >5 cm
III	Distant metastasis

the retroperitoneum. Surveillance protocols have been developed that include periodic physical examinations, serum tumor marker evaluation, and frequent chest radiographs and CT scans. The cornerstone to a surveillance program is patient compliance, and noncompliant patients should never be offered surveillance as a treatment option. Primary retroperitoneal lymph node dissection (RPLND) is both a diagnostic and therapeutic procedure. Patients at high risk for relapse in the retroperitoneum, that is, predominant embryonal carcinoma, vascular invasion, or extension into the tunica or scrotum, should undergo primary RPLND if serum tumor markers have normalized. A nerve-sparing procedure should be performed with successful preservation of ejaculatory function in approximately 95% of men.

BOX 1 International Germ Cell Cancer Consensus Group Classification System

Good Prognosis
- Nonseminoma
- Testis or retroperitoneal primary
- No nonpulmonary visceral metastases
- AFP <1000 µg/mL, hCG <5000 IU/L, and LDH <1.5 times normal
- Seminoma
- Any primary tumor site
- No nonpulmonary visceral metastases
- Normal AFP, any hCG or LDH level

Intermediate Prognosis
- Nonseminoma
- AFP 1000-10,000 µg/mL, hCG 5,000-50,000 IU/L
- LDH 1.5-10 times normal
- Seminoma
- Nonpulmonary visceral metastases

Poor Prognosis
- Nonseminoma
- Any of the following:
  Mediastinal primary
  Nonpulmonary visceral metastases
  AFP >10,000 µg/mL, hCG >50,000 IU/L, or LDH >10 times normal

Abbreviations: AFP = α-fetoprotein; hCG = human chorionic gonadotropin; LDH = lactate dehydrogenase.

Rakel and Bope: *Conn's Current Therapy 2006.*

 CURRENT DIAGNOSIS

Prostate Cancer
- Screening guidelines include an annual serum PSA and DRE starting at 50 years of age (high-risk groups should initiate screening at 40 years of age).
- An elevated serum PSA or abnormal DRE should be evaluated with a TRUS-guided prostate biopsy.

Bladder Cancer
- Hematuria (gross or microscopic) should be evaluated with a urine cytology, urine culture, CT urogram or IVP, and a cystoscopy.
- TURBT should be performed because it is both diagnostic and therapeutic.

Renal Cancer
- The vast majority of renal carcinomas are currently detected incidentally by abdominal imaging (CT scan, MRI, ultrasound) during a nonrelated medical evaluation.
- Patients with a palpable flank mass or hematuria should have a triphasic CT scan of the abdomen to evaluate for a renal cortical mass.

Testicular Cancer
- All palpable testicular masses should be evaluated with a bilateral testicular ultrasound.
- Radical inguinal orchiectomy is both a diagnostic and therapeutic procedure and should be performed promptly following confirmation of an intratesticular lesion.

Abbreviations: CT = computerized tomography; DRE = digital rectal examination; IVP = intravenous pyelogram; MRI = magnetic resonance imaging; PSA = prostate-specific antigen; TRUS = transrectal ultrasound; TURBT = transurethral resection of the bladder tumor.

Approximately 20% of patients with clinical stage I NSGCT have retroperitoneal metastases at the time of RPLND, of whom the vast majority do not require adjuvant chemotherapy. With either approach overall survival exceeds 98%, although patients suffering a relapse after surveillance may have a higher treatment burden. Patients with clinical stage IIa NSGCT (nodes <2 cm) and normal serum tumor markers are managed with primary RPLND with adjuvant chemotherapy reserved for patients at an increased risk of systemic relapse following surgery.

SEMINOMA

Radical orchiectomy followed by retroperitoneal external beam radiation therapy cures approximately 98% of patients with stage I seminomas. Because of the minimal morbidity of radiation therapy to this region and the risk of late relapse of patients on surveillance protocols, surveillance is generally not recommended in the United States. Patients with clinical stage IIa seminoma are also treated with retroperitoneal radiation therapy with an excellent overall survival.

CURRENT THERAPY

Prostate Cancer
- Clinically localized disease (>10 years life expectancy): Radical prostatectomy and external beam or interstitial radiotherapy provide excellent tumor control, and curative rates are fairly similar.
- Clinically localized disease (<10 years life expectancy): The curative treatment options still remain; however, strong consideration should be given to expectant management.
- Metastatic disease: Initial therapy includes androgen ablation, with chemotherapeutic and alternative options for men with progressive androgen-independent disease.

Bladder Cancer
- Superficial disease: TURBT followed by surveillance cystoscopy, with intravesical therapy reserved for patients at a high risk for recurrence or progression.
- Muscle-invasive disease: Radical cystectomy remains the main form of treatment, and neoadjuvant cisplatin-based chemotherapy should be offered because it improves overall survival.
- Metastatic disease: Chemotherapy is the current mainstay of therapy, although overall survival is poor.

Renal Cancer
- Clinically localized disease: Radical nephrectomy or partial nephrectomy (for tumors <4 cm) is the current recommended treatment.
- Metastatic disease: Immunotherapy with or without radical nephrectomy benefits patients with metastatic disease. Patients who have a good performance status and a solitary pulmonary site of disease have the best outcome and should be considered for surgical resection.

Testicular Cancer
- Seminoma (I, IIA): Adjuvant or therapeutic radiation therapy to the retroperitoneum offers cure rates in excess of 98%.
- Seminoma (IS, IIB-III): Cisplatin-based chemotherapy should be given based on IGCCCG risk classification. Postchemotherapy surgery is reserved for patients with residual masses greater than 3 cm and a positive PET scan.
- Nonseminoma (I, IIA): For patients at a high risk for retroperitoneal disease (or recurrence), a primary retroperitoneal lymph node dissection should be performed.
- Nonseminoma (IS, IIB-III): Cisplatin-based chemotherapy should be given based on IGCCCG risk classification. Postchemotherapy RPLND should be performed with resection of other sites limited to those with residual masses.

Abbreviations: IGCCCG = International Germ Cell Cancer Consensus Group; PET = positron emission tomography; RPLND = primary retroperitoneal lymph node dissection; TURBT = transurethral resection of the bladder tumor.

ADVANCED GERM CELL TUMORS

Regardless of histology, patients with advanced germ cell tumors (cIs, cIIb, cIIc, and cIII) and those with persistently elevated tumor markers following radical orchiectomy are treated initially with platinum-based chemotherapy according to the International Germ Cell Cancer Consensus Group (IGCCCG) risk stratification (Box 1). Patients are generally treated with three cycles of bleomycin (Blenoxane), etoposide (VePesid), and cisplatin (Platinol) or four cycles of etoposide and cisplatin for good-risk disease. Patients with intermediate-risk or high-risk disease traditionally receive four cycles of bleomycin, etoposide, and cisplatin. Postchemotherapy RPLND is an integral component in the management of advanced NSGCT. Following induction chemotherapy, approximately 40% of patients undergoing RPLND have a teratoma in their retroperitoneum, and an additional 10% to 15% have a viable germ cell tumor. Teratoma is chemorefractory and has an unpredictable biologic potential with the possibility of devastating late relapse if not completely resected. For patients with residual masses following chemotherapy for seminoma, postchemotherapy RPLND has traditionally been reserved for patients with a residual mass greater than 3 cm. A recent report demonstrates the usefulness of a positron emission tomography (PET) scan in evaluating postchemotherapy residual masses in patients with seminoma. In this study, the PET scan demonstrated a specificity of 100% and a sensitivity of 80% in patients with residual masses greater than 3 cm. Therefore, current recommendations for performing postchemotherapy surgery in men with seminoma include a residual mass greater than 3 cm and a positive PET scan.

REFERENCES

De Santis M, Becherer A, Bokemeyer C, et al: 2-[18]fluro-deoxy-D-glucose positron emission tomography is a reliable predictor for viable tumor in postchemotherapy seminoma: An update of the prospective multicentric SEMPET trial. J Clin Oncol 2004;22(6):1034-1039.

Gillenwater, JY, Grayhack JT, Howards SS, et al: Adult and Pediatric Urology, 4th ed. Philadelphia, Lippincott Williams and Wilkins, 2002.

Grossman HB, Natale RB, Tangen CM, et al: Neoadjuvant chemotherapy plus cystectomy compared with cystectomy alone for locally advanced bladder cancer. N Engl J Med 2003;349(9): 859-866.

Holmberg L, Bill-Axelson A, Helgeson F, et al: A randomized trial comparing radical prostatectomy with watchful waiting in early prostate cancer. N Engl J Med 2002;347(11):781-789.

Thompson IM, Goodman PJ, Tangen CM, et al: The influence of finasteride on the development of prostate cancer. N Engl J Med 2003;349(3):215-224.

Vogelzang NJ, Scardino PT, Shipley WU, et al. (eds): Comprehensive Textbook of Genitourinary Oncology, 2nd ed. Philadelphia, Lippincott Williams and Wilkins, 2000.

Walsh, PC, Retik AB, Vaughn ED, et al. (eds): Campbell's Urology, 8th ed. Philadelphia, Saunders Elsevier Science, 2002.

Urethral Stricture

Method of
Stephen Boorjian, MD,
and Mark Horowitz, MD

Anatomy and Etiology

Urethral stricture disease generally refers to a scarring process that results in narrowing or obliteration of the urethral lumen. Anatomically, urethral strictures are generally classified as either posterior urethral strictures, referring to strictures of the membranous or prostatic urethra, or anterior urethral strictures, referring to processes in the penile and bulbar urethra. The membranous urethra refers to the urethral segment, which is surrounded by the striated external sphincter; the anterior urethra lies within the corpus spongiosum of the penis.

Importantly, the urethra has a dual blood supply, consisting of the bulbourethral artery and the dorsal artery of the penis. Both arise from the common penile artery, which is the terminal branch of the internal pudendal artery. This dual blood supply is relevant clinically because it allows the urethra to be detached at either end during repair without compromise.

The etiology of urethral stricture disease was predominantly linked historically to gonococcal urethritis. However, with improved antibiotic therapy, gonococcal infections now infrequently progress to urethral stricture formation. A role for other infectious agents, such as *Chlamydia* and *Ureaplasma urealyticum,* in the formation of urethral strictures has been suspected but is less well defined. Balanitis xerotica obliterans (BXO), an inflammatory process of uncertain etiology, however, remains an important cause of urethral strictures, particularly of the penile urethra. Often considered an advanced stage of the chronic dermatitis condition lichen sclerosis et atrophicus, BXO appears as a whitish plaque and is characterized histologically by hyperkeratosis. It usually begins clinically on the foreskin and glans, and it may initially cause contraction of the prepuce onto the glans, then progress to meatal stenosis, and ultimately result in stricturing of the anterior urethra.

Currently, however, most strictures of both the anterior and posterior urethra result from trauma. The majority of traumatic anterior urethral strictures occurs following straddle injuries and may go unrecognized for a period of time after the injury, often until obstructive voiding symptoms develop. Traumatic posterior urethral strictures, meanwhile, are usually observed in the setting of pelvic fractures. Indeed, the prostatomembranous urethra is injured in approximately 10% of patients sustaining a pelvic fracture. The posterior urethral distraction injury often heals with considerable surrounding fibrosis, thus resulting in stricture formation.

In addition to external trauma, iatrogenic injuries to the urethra may result in the development of a stricture as well. Anterior urethral strictures may result from repeated, aggressive urethral instrumentation or catheterization; posterior urethral strictures may occur following radical prostatectomy or transurethral resection of the prostate. Postoperative stricturing of the posterior urethra may occur in isolation at the bladder neck and in such cases is termed *bladder neck contracture.*

Other, less common causes of urethral strictures include urethral ischemia, which can occur during cardiopulmonary bypass surgery, and urethral carcinoma, which must be suspected in the setting of a urethral stricture or fistula manifesting in a man over age 50. A final category of urethral strictures, although rare, is congenital strictures. These strictures, primarily found in children, may be classified as congenital in the absence of a history of trauma, instrumentation, infection, or other known predisposing factors as previously described. Of note, strictures in the pediatric population, as in adults, may be classified as either congenital or acquired. Acquired strictures in children usually occur in the setting of external urethral trauma or develop following hypospadias repair.

Diagnosis and Evaluation

The presentation of patients with urethral stricture disease most often consists of obstructive voiding symptoms, which include a weakened urinary stream, straining to void, hesitancy, and postvoid dribbling. Uncommonly, the first presentation of a urethral stricture may be complete urinary retention. Patients may also report frequency, dysuria, and, because of the increased voiding pressure needed to facilitate emptying across a strictured urethra, gross hematuria. As mentioned, in cases of traumatic urethral strictures, these symptoms may manifest at a considerable delay from the inciting injury. Alternatively, patients may present with urinary tract infections, epididymitis, or prostatitis, caused in part by stasis of urine from incomplete emptying across a strictured urethra.

Given the various etiologies of urethral stricture disease discussed in the previous section, a complete medical and surgical history should be obtained, including any history of pelvic/perineal/penile trauma, urinary tract infections, sexually transmitted diseases, and previous urethral instrumentation/catheter placement. The physical examination of a patient with urethral stricture disease may qualitatively suggest the extent of the scarring process and the depth of fibrosis in the surrounding corpus spongiosum. In patients with BXO, moreover, physical examination often reveals a thickened, whitish foreskin and meatal stenosis.

Initial evaluation of a suspected urethral stricture, particularly for the patient presenting with urinary retention, may involve an attempt at urethral catheter placement. For patients in whom initial attempts at catheterization are unsuccessful, catheter placement is often performed under direct visualization, using a flexible cystoscope, with insertion of a guidewire through the scope, across the stricture, and into the bladder, and subsequent placement of a Councill-tip Foley catheter (which has a terminal hole allowing guidewire placement) over the guidewire into the bladder. In fact, serially larger Councill-tip catheters may be inserted and removed over the guidewire, dilating the stricture. Given the ready availability of flexible endoscopy today, blind dilation of a suspected urethral stricture using filiform and followers or urethral sounds should not be common practice. In cases where catheter placement is unsuccessful, even with the assistance of direct vision, suprapubic cystostomy catheter placement is indicated.

Once the diagnosis of urethral stricture has been raised based on history, physical examination, and/or attempted catheter placement, the extent, location, and density of the stricture should be investigated to devise an appropriate treatment plan. Characterization of the stricture may be performed with a combination of radiographic assessment, ultrasonography, and urethroscopy. Retrograde urethrography has been the long-standing initial diagnostic study for patients with urethral strictures, and it may be performed either with static images or dynamic fluoroscopy. In either case, it is important to obtain images in more than one projection to ensure complete visualization of the stricture. Retrograde urethrography may be combined with an antegrade radiographic assessment of the urethra proximal to the stricture, either via voiding cystourethrogram for patients with a suprapubic tube or for patients in whom catheter placement is possible, or double-contrast intravenous pyelogram for patients without access to the proximal urethra.

More recently, ultrasonography is being used in the workup of patients with urethral strictures, specifically to evaluate the depth and density of the fibrosis associated with the stricture. Endoscopic examination of the urethra also plays a role in the assessment of patients with a urethral stricture, both to determine the degree of elasticity of the spongy tissue and to visualize the urethra proximal and distal to the stricture and thus define the limits of the urethral segment involved in the stricture.

Treatment

The primary goal of treatment, regardless of cause, is restoration of a functional urethra. A variety of treatment options exists for the management of urethral stricture disease, including dilation, endoscopic incision, and open reconstruction. The optimal approach must be tailored to the individual patient based on the nature, location, and extent of the stricture, as well as the patient's goals regarding the treatment outcome.

Urethral dilation is the most widely employed treatment modality for stricture disease and may be used for either anterior or posterior strictures. Serial dilations to gradually achieve a larger urethral lumen are repeated over time and may be performed by the patient at home. Balloon-dilating catheters have been used to achieve the same goal. Urethral dilation is a particularly effective form of treatment for strictures without underlying spongiofibrosis. The goal of dilation

is to stretch the scar without tearing the stricture and incurring further trauma.

In contrast, internal urethrotomy enlarges the urethral diameter by incising the stricture under direct vision. Healing is then by secondary intention. Internal urethrotomy may also be performed in both the anterior and posterior urethra. Generally, this procedure involves incising the urethra at the 12-o'clock position, although an argument has been made for incisions at the 3- and 9-o'clock positions instead because the corpus spongiosum covering the urethra is thinnest over the anterior urethra. Incisions that penetrate through the spongiosum may injure the adjacent corpus cavernosum, potentially resulting in significant hemorrhage and/or erectile dysfunction. An indwelling urethral catheter is usually left in place after internal urethrotomy for 3 to 5 days, during the initial healing phase.

Internal urethrotomy is particularly successful for strictures of the bulbar urethra that are less than 1.5 cm in length and without associated deep spongiofibrosis. The most common complication from this procedure is stricture recurrence. Importantly, repeat internal urethrotomy procedures do not increase the success rates, and therefore patients should be referred for consideration of open reconstruction after a failed internal urethrotomy. Attempts to prevent stricture recurrence following internal urethrotomy, including prolonged catheterization and self-dilation, have consistently failed to demonstrate improved patency rates.

On a final note regarding internal urethrotomy, various types of lasers, including carbon dioxide, argon, potassium titanyl phosphate (KTP), Nd:YAG, holmium:YAG, and excimer, have recently been employed for endoscopic incision and/or vaporization. Long-term data on the efficacy of these new treatment modalities, however, are lacking.

Urethral stent placement either may be used as a primary treatment for urethral strictures or employed in association with internal urethrotomy. Urethral stents are available in both removable and permanently implantable forms. The permanently implantable UroLume stent is FDA approved and is best used for short strictures in the bulbar urethra. These stents should not be used in patients who have undergone prior substitution urethral reconstruction (see later) or those with deep spongiofibrosis associated with the stricture. In addition to stricture recurrence, potential complications of urethral stents are related to the site of placement. Patients with stents placed in the anterior urethra may complain of pain with sitting or with intercourse; those with stents in the membranous or prostatic urethra may experience urinary incontinence and bladder stone formation.

For patients in whom urethral dilation and/or endoscopic management has failed or is not feasible, open surgical urethral reconstruction (urethroplasty) is necessary. Broadly, the types of urethral reconstruction can be classified as either anastomotic repairs or substitution urethroplasties. The choice of repair should be tailored to the characteristics, including location, length, and depth of the particular stricture. Anastomotic repair consists of excising the strictured urethral segment and area of fibrosis and then creating a tension-free, spatulated anastomosis of the proximal and distal urethral ends. This technique, which involves mobilization of the corpus spongiosum, is used primarily for bulbar and membranous urethral strictures. The use of anastomotic repairs in the anterior urethra has been limited by the subsequent development of ventral penile curvature. Anastomotic repair has been readily employed for strictures of 1 to 2 cm in length, as well for strictures up to 4 cm. The success rate of anastomotic repairs is reportedly in excess of 95%.

When the strictured segment is too long for primary reanastomosis, substitution urethroplasty may be employed. Substitution repairs use either a tissue flap or graft to bridge the urethral defect. Flap repairs use an area of redundant hairless skin on either the scrotum or (particularly in uncircumcised men) the penis. Skin flaps include the underlying dartos fascia and are mobilized on a vascular pedicle to bridge the urethral defect. Graft repairs, meanwhile, have generally involved the use of one of four urethral substitutes: full-thickness skin grafts, split-thickness skin grafts, bladder epithelial grafts, and, more recently, buccal mucosal grafts. Buccal grafts may be harvested from either the inner check or lip and have demonstrated excellent, albeit short-term, results.

The most common complication of substitution urethroplasty is restricturing the urethra at the site of repair. In particular, tubularized, as opposed to onlay, repairs should be avoided whenever possible because of the associated high recurrence rate. Excision with primary anastomosis remains the procedure of choice for urethroplasty; however, because not all strictures are amenable to anastomotic repair, the reconstructive surgeon must be comfortable with the principles of tissue transfer.

Future Directions

Current research in urethral stricture disease misdirected toward improving both diagnostic and treatment options. Advancements in the definition of ultrasonography have led to further exploration of the role of

CURRENT DIAGNOSIS

- Strictures are anatomically classified as either anterior or posterior urethral strictures.
- Most urethral strictures today result from either external trauma or iatrogenic injury.
- Urethral strictures usually manifest with obstructive voiding symptoms.
- Catheter placement in the patient with a urethral stricture may be performed under direct vision using a flexible cystoscope.
- Characterization of the stricture includes a combination of retrograde urethrography, ultrasound, and endoscopic visualization.

CURRENT THERAPY

- Urethral dilation is the most widely employed treatment technique for urethral strictures and may be used for both anterior and posterior defects.
- Internal urethrotomy involves incising the urethral stricture under direct endoscopic vision.
- Repeat internal urethrotomy does not increase the success rate after a failed previous internal urethrotomy.
- Open urethral reconstruction consists of anastomotic repair or substitution urethroplasty.
- Substitution urethroplasty may use either a tissue flap or graft to bridge the strictured segment.
- Tissue flaps use either penile or scrotal skin; grafts include full-thickness skin grafts, split-thickness skin grafts, bladder epithelial grafts, and buccal mucosal grafts.

ultrasound in the evaluation of the patient with a suspected urethral stricture. In addition, three-dimensional spiral computed tomography (CT) is being used as a diagnostic tool to investigate potential urethral defects. Static and dynamic CT images are taken with contrast cystourethrography to define the anatomy of the stricture.

Regarding the treatment of urethral strictures, although efforts continue with tissue engineering to develop better options for urethral substitution, recent reports have suggested the use of *botulinum toxin* (Botox)[1] as an alternative treatment approach.

REFERENCES

Barbagli G, Palminteri E, Rizzo M: Dorsal onlay graft urethroplasty using penile skin or buccal mucosa in adult bulbourethral strictures. J Urol 1998;160:1307-1309.

Baskin LS, Duckett JW: Changing concepts in the management of pediatric urethral strictures. AUA Update Series, vol 13, lesson 33, 1994.

Choudhary S, Singh P, Sundar E, et al: A comparison of sonourethrography and retrograde urethrography in evaluation of anterior urethral strictures. Clin Radiol 2004;59(8):736-742.

El-Kassaby AW, Osman, T., Abdel-Aal A, et al: Dynamic three-dimensional spiral computed tomographic cysto-urethrography: A novel technique for evaluating post-traumatic posterior urethral defects. BJU Int 2003;92(9):993-996.

Jordan GH: Complications of interventional techniques of urethral stricture disease: Direct visual internal urethrotomy, stents, and laser. In Carson C (ed): Topics in clinical urology: Complications of interventional techniques. New York, Igaku-Shoin, 1996.

Jordan GH (Guest editor): Reconstruction for urethral stricture. In Atlas of Urologic Clinics of North America. Philadelphia, WB Saunders, 1997.

Jordan GH, Schlossberg SM: Surgery of the penis and urethra. In Walsh PC, Retik AB, Vaughan ED Jr., Wein AJ (eds): Campbell's Urology, 8th ed. Philadelphia, WB Saunders, 2002.

[1]Not FDA approved for this indication.

Khera M, Boone TB, Smith CP: Botulinum toxin type A: A novel approach to the treatment of recurrent urethral strictures. J Urol 2004;172(2):574-575.

Milroy E: Treatment of sphincter strictures using permanent UroLume stent. J Urol 1993;150:1729-1733.

Morey AF, McAninch JW: Ultrasound evaluation of the male urethra for assessment of urethral stricture. J Clin Ultrasound 1996;24:473-478.

Venn SN, Mundy AR: Urethroplasty for balanitis xerotica obliterans. Br J Urol 1998;81:735-737.

Webster GD, Venn SN: Strictures of the male urethra. In Gillenwater JY, Grayhack JT, Howards DD, Mitchell ME (eds): Adult and Pediatric Urology, 4th ed. Philadelphia, Lippincott Williams & Wilkins, 2002.

Renal Calculi

Method of
Nicholas J. Hegarty, MD,
and Stevan B. Streem, MD

Urolithiasis affects 5% to 15% of adults and the incidence of stone disease appears to be increasing. Calcium stones are the most frequent, and they present most often between the 3rd and 5th decades of life. They are two to three times more common in males than females. Incidence is threefold higher in whites than African Americans with people of Asian or Hispanic background having an intermediate incidence. More than one half of those presenting with their first stone episode will suffer a second stone event within 10 years. Thus, there are two important considerations in approaching patients with stone disease: the management of the initial stone episode and the prevention of further stone formation.

Presentation and Initial Management

The most common presenting symptom is acute onset flank pain. This is generally described as severe and colicky in nature, but may be mild. Pain may radiate anteriorly, to the groin and ipsilateral testis or labia. Associated symptoms may include nausea and diaphoresis. Patients are often restless, moving about in an attempt to obtain relief. Other than indicating the side of the stone, pain location does not correlate well with the position of the stone in the ureter. The onset of irritative bladder symptoms, however, suggests progression of the stone to the ureterovesical junction. The presence of fever or systemic symptoms is worrisome as they suggest the coexistence of a urinary tract infection and the need for urgent treatment (Figure 1). Physical examination may reveal upper quadrant or renal angle tenderness, but no guarding nor rebound, which indicates peritonitis. Basic investigations include urinalysis and microscopy, which usually, but not invariably, show the presence of red blood cells. A pregnancy test is

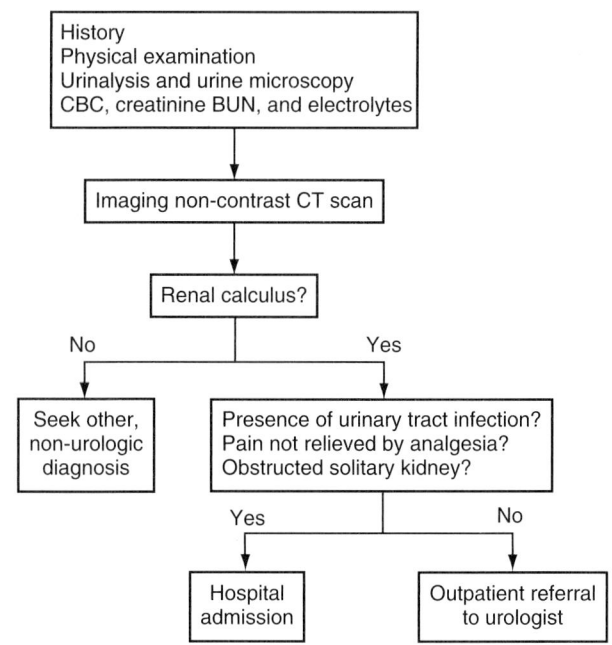

FIGURE 1. Acute stone episode algorithm.

performed in women of childbearing age prior to abdominal imaging, and blood urea nitrogen (BUN) creatinine, and electrolytes are performed prior to the administration of contrast, in order to give an indication of renal function. Pain relief should not be delayed and requires a nonsteroidal anti-inflammatory drug (NSAID) such as ketorolac (Toradol), 30 mg every 6 hours, or opiates such as morphine sulfate or meperidine (Demerol), 1mg/kg every 8 hours, or a combination of these.

Imaging

Radiologic imaging is performed to confirm the diagnosis and determine stone size, location, and degree of obstruction. Other findings that may influence treatment are urinary tract anatomy and ipsilateral and overall renal function. Local availability and the clinical setting influence the choice and combination of imaging technique(s). Abdominal plain radiograph will reveal more than 90% of calcium-containing stones, but small stones or those composed of uric acid or cystine are difficult to visualize. Renal ultrasound can demonstrate shadowing of renal stones and hydronephrosis, but is limited in showing ureteral calculi. Intravenous pyelogram (IVP) is the traditional urologic investigation of choice, as it identifies the location of stones in the collecting system. It offers some functional detail and demonstrates the presence or absence of obstruction and any renal or ureteral anomalies. However, it does require exposure to radiographs and intravenous iodine-based contrast. It can also be quite time-consuming, particularly if there is delayed excretion secondary to obstruction. In most centers, noncontrast computed tomography (CT) has superseded IVP. It has greater sensitivity and specificity comparable with that of IVP. All stones, other than certain drug-related crystals, are visualized by this method. Thin-cut spiral CT can be performed in one breath hold and can also provide details of nonurologic causes of abdominal pain. Magnetic resonance urography has little role in stone disease, but may be considered in pregnancy or a patient who has a complex genitourinary anatomy. In some chronic and complicated cases, radionuclide studies are performed to assess remaining function in a compromised kidney, prior to deciding between stone removal and nephrectomy.

Indications for Intervention

The presence of ureteral calculus and urinary tract infection constitutes a surgical emergency that requires prompt intervention. Impaired function in the obstructed kidney mandates an increase in antimicrobial dosage (intravenous administration is usually required). Drainage, either by percutaneous nephrostomy or retrograde stent placement, further assists the resolution of infection prior to considering definitive management. Similarly, an obstructing calculus in an anatomically or functionally solitary kidney may result in anuria and acute renal failure. In general, there is less urgency associated with the treatment of stones and many can be treated expectantly if pain control is sufficient. Stone size is the single most important determinant of the likelihood of spontaneous stone passage. The majority of stones less than 5 mm can be expected to pass, whereas almost all stones greater than 8 mm will require intervention. Along with analgesia, hydration and activity are recommended (although there is, in fact, little evidence to suggest these measures result in an improved outcome). Studies of ureteral physiology have proposed a number of strategies including calcium channel blockers,[1] steroids,[1] and phosphodiesterase inhibitors.[1] Perhaps the most promising of these are the α-adrenergic blocking agents.[1] The vesicoureteral junction is rich in α-adrenergic receptors. Oral administration of $α_1$-blockers in the acute stone episode reduces analgesic requirements and results in more rapid and higher overall rates of spontaneous stone passage. Experience with their use in benign prostatic hyperplasia has shown their safety, tolerability, and freedom from interaction with other drug groups (other than phosphodiesterase inhibitors). How long to wait is a question that remains unanswered. With complete obstruction, renal damage is evident at 2 weeks and irreversible damage at 6 weeks, although truly "complete" obstruction rarely develops from ureteral calculi. Longer periods of partial or intermittent obstruction can be tolerated, and many studies show few untoward effects in the follow-up of nonobstructing distal ureteral calculi after 1 year. Nevertheless, we feel that failure to progress at 4 to 6 weeks probably corresponds to a high probability that the stone is unlikely to progress with

further observation. We generally recommend intervention at this stage if there has been no caudal stone movement.

Interventional Options

SHOCK WAVE LITHOTRIPSY

Shock wave lithotripsy (SWL) is a noninvasive technique whereby shock waves from an external source bring about stone fragmentation. Radiograph fluoroscopy, ultrasound, or dual imaging is used to bring the stone to the focal point of the shock wave generator. Typical treatments are comprised of 3000 shock waves, and, in most cases, the procedure is performed as an outpatient. It is an option for patients with relatively small renal and ureteral stones—although the need for re-treatment is higher than some other minimally invasive alternatives. SWL is less invasive than ureteroscopy or percutaneous management, and its side-effect profile is less. Cystine and calcium oxalate monohydrate stones are resistant to fragmentation by SWL, and radiolucent uric acid stones may pose difficulty with focusing. Obesity may also give rise to difficulty with stone visualization, and dissipation of shock wave energy by excessive interposed adipose tissue can reduce treatment efficacy. Reduced power settings are recommended in children to protect the growing kidney. Use can be extended to stones larger than 1 cm in children, but ureteral stenting is often required to prevent obstruction as fragments are passing. The presence of distal ureteral obstruction is a contraindication to SWL, and certain abnormalities of collecting system anatomy, particularly in dependent lower poles, may preclude drainage of stone debris, despite successful fragmentation.

URETEROSCOPY

Ureteroscopy or ureterorenoscopy can be performed with rigid, semirigid, or flexible scopes. It provides direct visualization of stones during manipulation and extraction. Early series reported a 2% to 6% rate of ureteral injury or perforation. We recommend the use of a floppy-tipped safety wire in all cases, as this allows placement of a ureteral stent if injury occurs, or in the rare instance that an impacted stone cannot be removed. Two wires are required for flexible ureteroscopy—a working wire, for introducing a ureteral access sheath or guiding the flexible scope into the ureter, and a safety wire. Large stones require fragmentation prior to extraction. A number of modalities are available, the most frequently used being holmium laser lithotripsy. Laser fibers allow stone break up with little propulsion of fragments. The holmium laser is capable of fragmenting all stone types, but care must be taken to avoid ureteral damage. Laser fibers are suitable for use in rigid, semirigid, and flexible ureteroscopes, and most centers now use a holmium laser almost exclusively as the fragmentation modality of choice.

---

[1]Not FDA approved for this indication.

PERCUTANEOUS EXTRACTION

This is recommended for renal stones greater than 1 to 1.5 cm and stones refractory to SWL. Fragmentation can be accomplished with an ultrasound wand or, more recently, a single device combining both ultrasound and pneumatic lithotripsy. Laser fragmentation is considerably slower but can be used with a flexible scope to access difficult calyces or the ureter in an antegrade manner. Fragments inaccessible to percutaneous management can be treated by SWL to achieve greater stone clearance rates. Percutaneous surgery also allows correction of coexisting infundibular stenosis or ureteropelvic junction (UPJ) obstruction. The indications for open or laparoscopic surgery are progressively fewer, and today such management is applied to less than 1% of stone patients requiring intervention. Nephrectomy is an option for a stone-bearing kidney with irreversible loss of function (with a differential function less than 10% to 15% on radionuclide scanning).

Stone Prevention

General recommendations can be given to reduce the incidence of further stones. These include maintaining adequate hydration and reducing intake of dietary purines, oxalates, and vitamin supplements (Box 1). Opinions differ on which patients should undergo metabolic evaluation, when they should be tested, and how extensive testing should be. A comparable incidence of finding a treatable abnormality is found in those presenting with their first stone as compared with subsequent stones. However, full investigation of all stone formers would incur considerable expense and inconvenience for such a large patient group. This has prompted some units to propose an abbreviated investigation for the majority of patients, with full investigation for a small minority. In our unit, we recommend complete investigation for those who are likely to require medical treatment (Box 2). Serum studies include electrolytes, creatinine, BUN, calcium, phosphorous, and uric acid. The need for more detailed investigations with further tests such as parathyroid studies should be assessed based on initial results. A single, 24-hour urinary collection is taken, with the patient on a normal diet. Urinary volume, creatinine, calcium, citrate, oxalate, uric acid, and sodium are all measured. A creatinine value of 1 to 2 g per day is an

---

BOX 1 General Recommendations for All Calcium Stone Formers

General dietary measures include the following:
• Fluid intake >2 liters per day
• Low sodium (<4 g NaCl per day)
• Normal calcium intake
• Oxalate restriction
• Moderate protein restriction
• Low fat, high fiber diet
• Avoidance of vitamin C and D supplements

BOX 2 Metabolic Evaluation

Serum
• Blood urea nitrogen
• Creatinine
• Sodium
• Potassium
• Chloride
• Calcium
• Phosphorous
• Uric acid
• Parathormone*

24-Hour Urine
• Volume
• Creatinine
• Calcium
• Citrate
• Oxalate
• Uric acid
• Sodium
• Cystine†

Stone Analysis
• Calcium oxalate
• Calcium phosphate
• Uric acid
• Struvite
• Cystine

*Parathormone levels performed if calcium elevated or phosphorous low.
†Test for urinary cystine if cystine stone on stone analysis or family history of cystine stones.

---

important indicator of a properly collected specimen. The most frequently detected abnormalities are hypercalciuria, hyperuricosuria, hypocitraturia, hyperoxaluria, and a combination of these.

HYPERCALCIURIA

In the absence of hypercalcemia, hypercalciuria is termed idiopathic. It may be considered absorptive or "renal leak," but we do not differentiate between them as both represent an increased sensitivity to vitamin D and respond to thiazide diuretics (hydrochlorothiazide, 25 to 50 mg per day).[1] Thiazides reduce the urine calcium load by increasing its tubular absorption and increasing calcium availability to the bones. Calcium supplements are restricted to 600 mg daily, but we do not restrict dietary calcium because longitudinal studies show that dietary calcium restriction may promote stone formation, and because creating a negative calcium balance promotes bone resorption and osteoporosis. We routinely recommend dietary sodium restriction, as a high sodium intake increases urinary calcium, especially in hypercalciuric patients.

HYPERURICOSURIA

Hyperuricosuria may be primary or secondary to high dietary purine intake. If it persists with dietary restriction,

---

[1]Not FDA approved for this indication.

allopurinol (Zyloprim), 300 mg daily, should be commenced. Persistent acid urine and elevated serum uric acid suggest gout. Treatment is aimed at alkalinization of the urine with potassium citrate (Urocit K), 10 to 20 mEq three or four times per day, or sodium bicarbonate.

HYPOCITRATURIA

Acidosis inhibits citrate production causing hypocitraturia. Most often, it is associated with alkaline loss from inflammatory bowel disease (IBD) or hypokalemia connected with thiazide use. IBD may also cause malabsorption of citrate. Treatment is aimed at correcting the underlying condition and citrate replacement (typically Urocit K, 30 to 60 mEq per day). Marked hypocitraturia may suggest the presence of renal tubular acidosis. Usually, there will be an associated hyperchloremic, hypokalemic acidosis. Where electrolytes are normal, an acid load test may be considered to confirm the diagnosis.

HYPEROXALURIA

Hyperoxaluria may result from endogenous, or, more frequently, exogenous sources. Endogenous causes include congenital deficiencies of glyoxylate transamination or oxidation, excess vitamin C ingestion, or pyridoxine deficiency. Hydration, vitamin C restriction, and dietary oxalate restriction are recommended initially. In those with persistent hyperoxaluria, vitamin B_6 (pyridoxine),[1] starting at 200 mg daily, may be effective. Exogenous causes include malabsorption from previous gastrointestinal surgery or inflammatory bowel disease. Malabsorption promotes saponification of calcium. There is less calcium available to bind oxalate in the gut, which is then absorbed in greater quantities. Treatment is the same as for endogenous causes, along with treatment of the underlying condition.

---

[1]Not FDA approved for this indication.

CURRENT DIAGNOSIS

■ General
  Consider and rule out life-threatening causes of acute abdominal pain (e.g., abdominal aortic aneurysm rupture).
  Rule out concurrent urinary tract infection.
■ Imaging
  Computed tomography stone protocol provides greatest sensitivity and specificity.
■ Metabolic
  Full metabolic workup is indicated in those likely to require medical treatment.
  Serum studies, stone analysis, and a single 24-hour urine usually provide sufficient information to guide treatment.

Calcium citrate may reverse metabolic acidosis and increase oxalate binding in the gut. In those with stones from jejunoileal bypass, bypass reversal may be required if stones cannot otherwise be controlled.

Cystine Stones

Cystinuria is an autosomal recessive condition characterized by abnormal intestinal and renal absorption of dibasic amino acids (cystine, ornithine, lysine, and arginine). Excess urinary cystine leads to stone formation in a minority of patients. Initial treatment is aimed at increasing the solubility of cystine by increasing fluid intake to 2 to 3 L per day and alkalinization with citrate or bicarbonate. If this fails, D-penicillamine (Cuprimine) 1.5 to 2 mg per day or α-mercaptopropionylglycine (Thiola), 800 to 1200 mg per day, should be commenced.

CURRENT THERAPY

Acute Stone Event
- Pain relief to be instituted and diagnosis established.
- Choice of treatment influenced by position and size of stone, patient comorbidity and preference, and available treatment modalities.
- α-Adrenergic blockade[1] may facilitate spontaneous stone passage.
- Presence of urinary tract infection, persistent pain, obstruction in a solitary kidney, and patient social circumstances may mandate prompt intervention.

Intervention
- Minimally invasive techniques have all but replaced open stone surgery.
- Shock wave lithotripsy is suitable first-line treatment for small ureteral and renal calculi.
- Ureteroscopy has higher treatment success rates, but is more invasive than SWL.
- In an otherwise healthy patient, staghorn calculi, even when asymptomatic, should be treated.
- Percutaneous extraction is the first-line treatment for most patients with large stones, and certainly for staghorn calculi.

Stone Prevention
- Hydration and general stone preventive measures should be recommended to all stone formers.
- Medical treatment is tailored to the individual patient, based on lifestyle and metabolic findings.
- Metabolic abnormalities frequently coexist.

---

[1]Not FDA approved for this indication.

10

Staghorn Calculi

Typically these are infective (struvite) in nature, but may also be composed of uric acid, cystine, or calcium oxalate. Infection-related stones form only in the setting of urease-producing organisms, and patients typically have a high urinary pH. Untreated, these tend to result in chronic pyelonephritis with atrophy of the kidney or life-threatening pyonephrosis. Unless the patient's condition precludes treatment, it is generally recommended that staghorn calculi be treated, that is, removed. Infection remains within the stone matrix and is probably impossible to completely eradicate in the presence of the stone. Percutaneous extraction is the treatment of choice for most staghorn calculi. The position and number of access tracts will be determined by the stone morphology and anatomy of the collecting system. Repeat procedures may be required or SWL may be used to treat remaining or inaccessible fragments. Entire stone clearance is usually required for eradication of infection and to prevent further stone formation. Where there is little useful function remaining in a kidney with a staghorn calculus, nephrectomy is a reasonable option.

REFERENCES

Dellabella M, Milanese G, Muzzonigro G: Efficacy of tamsulosin in the medical management of juxtavesical ureteral stones. J Urol 2003;170(6):2202-2205.

Fielding JR, Steele G, Fox LA, et al: Spiral computerized tomography in the evaluation of acute flank pain: A replacement for excretory urography. J Urol 1997;157(6):2071-2073.

Klein LT, Frager D, Subramanium A, Lowe FC: Use of magnetic resonance urography. Urology 1998;52(4):602-608.

Pak CY, Peterson R, Poindextrer JR: Adequacy of a single stone risk analysis in the medical evaluation of urolithiasis. J Urol 2001;165(2):378-391.

Segura JW, Preminger GM, Assimos DG, et al: Ureteral Stones Clinical Guidelines Panel summary report on the management of ureteral calculi: The American Urological Association. J Urol 1997;158(5):1915-1921.

Segura JW, Preminger GM, Assimos DG, et al: Nephrolithiasis Clinical Guidelines Panel summary report on the management of staghorn calculi: The American Urological Association Clinical Guidelines Panel. J Urol 1994;151(6):1648-1651.

Stamatelou KK, Francis ME, Jones CA, et al: Time trends in reported prevalence of kidney stones in the United States: 1976-1994. Kidney Int 2003;63(5):1817-1823.

Sexually Transmitted Diseases

Chancroid

Method of
George P. Schmid, MD, MSc

Haemophilus ducreyi, a small gram-negative bacillus, causes chancroid, one of the three sexually transmitted diseases (STDs) characterized by genital ulceration (genital herpes and syphilis are the other two). A common STD in the United States before World War II, cases decreased markedly with the introduction of penicillin. In the latter 1980s, however, chancroid resurged with the introduction of crack cocaine and an attendant high-risk sex-for-drugs trade. Since a peak of 4986 cases in 1989, case numbers have diminished for unclear reasons, and in 2003 only 54 cases were reported. In sub-Saharan Africa and parts of Asia, chancroid remains common and is responsible for facilitating transmission of many cases of the HIV epidemic; nevertheless, in sub-Saharan Africa, chancroid is declining in frequency for uncertain reasons.

Chancroid should be suspected if a patient has one or a few very painful genital ulcers; in approximately half the cases, painful inguinal adenopathy occurs. The ulcers are raw and often deep, accompanied by bleeding. Definitive diagnosis is difficult because special culture media required to grow *H. ducreyi* are not often available; polymerase chain reaction (PCR) testing may be available from referral laboratories.

Treatment

Several therapies are equally effective: azithromycin (Zithromax), 1 g orally, once; ceftriaxone (Rocephin), 250 mg intramuscularly, once; ciprofloxacin (Cipro), 500 mg orally twice a day for 3 days; and erythromycin base, 500 mg orally three times a day for 7 days. Antimicrobial resistance to these drugs has rarely, if ever, occurred.

Successfully treated patients report subjective improvement within 48 to 72 hours, and objective improvement is apparent within 3 to 7 days. If there is no clinical improvement by 7 days, the clinician should consider whether patients took their medication, antimicrobial resistance may exist, there is coinfection with *Treponema pallidum* or herpes simplex virus (seen in approximately 10% of patients), or the diagnosis is wrong. Patients should be followed until the ulcer completely heals.

Patients with fluctuant buboes benefit from drainage to prevent spontaneous rupture and fistula formation. Drainage may be accomplished either by needle aspiration or by incision and drainage with packing of the node. The former approach may require subsequent reaspiration; the latter approach is more invasive. Despite successful therapy, nodes not fluctuant enough for drainage when patients are seen initially may become fluctuant later and require drainage.

Patients who are uncircumcised or who have HIV infection do not respond as well as circumcised patients or those without HIV infection; some experts prefer multiple-dose regimens for these patients. All patients with suspected chancroid should have an HIV test initially and, if negative, again 3 months later (because HIV seroconversion rates are high among those who are initially HIV negative). It is prudent to schedule a follow-up visit several days after initial diagnosis to check for evidence of healing and for counseling about the results of the initial HIV test.

Sex partners within the 10 days before the appearance of the ulcer should be notified, examined, and treated. Asymptomatic ulcers occasionally occur in the vagina or on the cervix. Asymptomatic carriage of *H. ducreyi* in cervical secretions has been described but

CURRENT DIAGNOSIS

- Chancroid is rare in the United States.
- Ulcers are invariably painful.
- Diagnostic tests may not be available.

CURRENT THERAPY

- Short courses of antimicrobials are highly effective.
- Buboes often require drainage.

is rare. Suspected cases should be reported to the local health department.

REFERENCES

Centers for Disease Control and Prevention: Sexually transmitted diseases treatment guidelines 2002. MMWR 2002:51(No. RR-6).

Ernst AA, Marvez-Valls E, Martin DH: Incision and drainage versus aspiration of fluctuant buboes in the emergency department during an epidemic of chancroid. Sex Transm Dis 1995;11:217-220.

Mertz KJ, Weiss JB, Webb RM, et al: An investigation of genital ulcers in Jackson, Mississippi, with use of a multiplex polymerase chain reaction assay: High prevalence of chancroid and human immunodeficiency virus infection. J Infect Dis 1998;168:1060-1066.

Schmid GP: Treatment of chancroid, 1997. Clin Infect Dis 1999; Suppl 1:S14-S20.

Steen R: Eradicating chancroid. Bull World Health Organ 2001; 79:818-826.

Gonorrhea

Method of
George P. Schmid, MD, MSc

Gonorrhea, caused by *Neisseria gonorrhoeae*, is a sexually transmitted disease (STD) that is globally the most important cause of urethritis in men and pelvic inflammatory disease (and its consequences of infertility and ectopic pregnancy) in women. Most cases, however, are asymptomatic or associated with symptoms that are so mild that persons do not recognize they have a sexually transmitted infection (STI). Efforts to create a vaccine against *N. gonorrhoeae* have been unsuccessful, and control depends upon enhancing safer sex behaviors to prevent acquisition of infection, screening to detect those who are asymptomatically infected, and appropriate management of detected cases.

Epidemiology

More than 300,000 cases of gonorrhea are reported annually to state health authorities, and *N. gonorrhoeae* is second in frequency only to *Chlamydia trachomatis* among reported communicable infections. Frequency of infection is highest in young persons, 15 to 24 years old, and approximately equal numbers of reported cases occur in men and women. Before the AIDS epidemic, gonorrhea was extremely common in men who have sex with men (MSM). With the adoption of safer sex practices

by MSM, rates plunged. In the past several years, however, the number of cases of gonorrhea in MSM has risen markedly as adherence to safer sex practices has declined. Other groups at risk for gonorrhea include sex workers, those who abuse drugs, and minorities; geographically, gonorrhea is concentrated in large cities and the southeastern United States.

Gonorrhea is efficiently spread. The risk of a woman acquiring *N. gonorrhoeae* from a single act of sex with an infected male is approximately 50%; the risk of a man acquiring *N. gonorrhoeae* from a single act of sex with an infected woman is approximately 20%.

Microbiology and Diagnosis

N. gonorrhoeae is an aerobic, gram-negative bacterium that occurs in pairs (a diplococcus), with adjacent, flattened sides. Culture is accomplished using a special medium (traditionally, the Thayer-Martin medium) incubated at 35°C to 36°C (95°F to 96.8°F) in an atmosphere enriched by 3% to 5% carbon dioxide (CO_2). Recovery rates from infected individuals are highest if specimens, particularly those from women (who have fewer organisms than symptomatic men), are plated directly onto media rather than placed into transport media.

Nonculture diagnostic techniques are replacing culture because of ease of transport and, with some tests, the ability to use noninvasively collected specimens such as urine. The initial nonculture test for gonorrhea was an enzyme-linked immunosorbent assay (ELISA). This test has been supplanted by the more sensitive nucleic acid hybridization and nucleic acid amplification tests, which detect either chromosomal or plasmid DNA, or ribosomal RNA. The sensitivity of these tests on cervical or urethral secretions appears to approach that of culture, and they are highly (>99%) specific. A considerable advantage of the nucleic acid amplification tests is that they can be used on a broad range of specimens, in particular, urine, making the necessity of an intraurethral swab in men or an endocervical swab in women unnecessary—this is particularly beneficial in screening situations. Sensitivity of the tests on urine specimens is, however, less than on endocervical or urethral secretions.

In symptomatic men, a Gram stain of urethral secretions remains highly useful, and sensitivity of the detection of intracellular diplococci is 95% to 99% specific. For women, a Gram stain of endocervical secretions is only approximately 50% sensitive, and other cervical flora can be confused with *N. gonorrhoeae*, decreasing specificity.

In some instances, only culture should be used, such as in cases of medicolegal importance—to definitively identify *N. gonorrhoeae* and to retain the organism as evidence—and if testing for antimicrobial resistance is desired.

Clinical Characteristics

Infection may occur at whatever anatomic site sex occurs. The most common sites of infection are the urethra in men and the cervix in women. In MSM, rectal infection occurs in approximately 25% of men with an infection at any site. Nearly 35% to 50% of women with an endocervical infection will also have rectal infection caused by contamination of the anus by secretions from the vagina. Among persons with infection at any site, pharyngeal infection occurs in approximately 5% of heterosexual men, 15% of heterosexual women, and 15% of MSM.

The incubation period of gonorrhea is best characterized in men, with a typical incubation period of 3 to 5 days. Women who become symptomatic develop more vague, local symptoms, and the initial symptoms may be caused by pelvic inflammatory disease (PID). In both genders, symptoms may be scant or nonexistent at any site that is infected, and most women and probably most men are asymptomatic. Alternately, they may have symptoms that are so mild that they are overlooked.

Symptoms of urethral infection in men are dysuria and discharge. The discharge is classically purulent (yellow or green), as opposed to the white or clear discharge of nongonococcal urethritis, although testing is required to distinguish the two. Rectal infection (proctitis) in MSM, when symptomatic, results in anal discharge, discomfort, and tenesmus; few women with rectal infection have symptoms. Most pharyngeal infections are asymptomatic, although occasionally pharyngitis of mild to moderate severity occurs.

Complications of infection occur in individuals who are untreated. Disseminated gonococcal infection (DGI), also called the arthritis-dermatitis syndrome, occurs in 1% to 2% of infected individuals and is the most common cause of septic arthritis in young people. It occurs as a result of bacteremia in individuals typically without genital tract symptoms and is characterized by moderate fever, tenosynovitis, arthritis, and skin lesions (a small number of pustules with a red base on the periphery of the arms and legs). Gram stain of the lesions or joint fluid typically yields the initial diagnosis, and culture of these sites (if affected) and blood should be done. PID occurs in 20% to 40% of untreated women, most commonly during the first few menstrual cycles following infection.

Therapy

UNCOMPLICATED GENITAL TRACT OR RECTAL INFECTION

Uncomplicated infection is effectively treated by a single dose of an antimicrobial (Box 1). Quinolone resistance is common in the developing world, particularly Asia, and has appeared in the United States, initially in Hawaii and then in California. In these states and for infections acquired in many countries outside the United States (including England and Wales), quinolones are not recommended. Because quinolone resistance has been particularly prevalent among MSM, quinolones are not recommended for treatment of MSM with gonorrhea. Resistance to cephalosporins has only rarely been reported.

Rakel and Bope: *Conn's Current Therapy 2006.*

> **BOX 1** Uncomplicated Infection of the Urethra, Cervix, or Rectum*
>
> - Ceftriaxone (Rocephin), 125 mg IM once; or
> - Ciprofloxacin (Cipro), 500 mg PO once; or
> - Ofloxacin (Floxin), 400 mg PO once; or
> - Levofloxacin (Levaquin), 250 mg PO once;
> - Each of the previously listed medications along with (unless chlamydial infection is excluded): Azithromycin (Zithromax), 1 g PO once; or Doxycycline (Vibramycin), 100 mg PO twice a day for 7 days.
>
> *Cefixime, 400 mg, PO, can be used but the distribution of cefixime in the United States has been discontinued by the manufacturer.
> *Abbreviations:* IM = intramuscularly; PO = orally.

Alternate cephalosporin or quinolone regimens can be used but offer either no advantage over the drugs in Box 1 or have lesser therapeutic experience. Spectinomycin (Trobicin), 2 g intermuscularly (IM), is highly effective against genital and rectal infection and can be used if cephalosporins or quinolones cannot.

Co-infection by *C. trachomatis* of individuals with gonorrhea occurs in 10% to 30% of cases. Unless testing for *C. trachomatis* infection is performed, all patients with gonorrhea should be treated for a possible co-existing chlamydial infection with either azithromycin (Zithromax) or doxycycline (Vibramycin).

Patients should be serologically tested for syphilis and offered testing for HIV infection. All cases of gonorrhea confirmed by laboratory testing should be reported promptly to health authorities.

Patients should be counseled about the need to adhere to therapy, the possible side effects of medication, the need to return if symptoms do not abate, the need to refrain from sex until they complete therapy (as do any sex partners), and the need to refer sex partners. Because the onset of symptoms is not always clear and a reliable incubation period is difficult to establish, referral of sex partners within the past 60 days is recommended. Partners should be evaluated, tested, and routinely treated. If there has been no sex partner in the last 60 days, the most recent sex partner should be examined.

The effectiveness of recommended regimens is so high (>98%) that patients do not need to return for follow-up but should if symptoms persist. If they do persist, the clinician should consider other causes of symptoms, antibiotic resistance of *N. gonorrhoeae*, and whether the patient adhered to therapy.

PREGNANCY

Pregnant women should not be treated with quinolones or tetracyclines. A cephalosporin or spectinomycin should be used, and possible co-infection with *C. trachomatis* should be treated with erythromycin or amoxicillin.

PHARYNGEAL INFECTION

Pharyngeal infection is more difficult to cure than anogenital infections. Ceftriaxone (Rocephin) or ciprofloxacin (Cipro) can be used, but cure rates may not exceed 90%. Pharyngeal infection by *C. trachomatis* is uncommon, but co-treatment for *C. trachomatis*, whether an oral or asymptomatic genital infection, is recommended.

DISSEMINATED GONOCOCCAL INFECTION

Initial hospitalization is advisable for patients with disseminated gonococcal infection, particularly those with septic arthritis or other significant illness—a questionable diagnosis—or who may not comply with outpatient therapy. Ceftriaxone (Rocephin), 1 g IM or intravenously (IV) every 24 hours, is recommended. Alternately, cefotaxime (Claforan, 1 g IV every 8 hours), ceftizoxime (Cefizox, 1 g IV every 8 hours), ciprofloxacin (Cipro, 400 mg IV every 12 hours), ofloxacin (Floxin, 400 mg IV every 12 hours), levofloxacin (Levaquin, 250 mg IV daily), or spectinomycin (Trobicin, 2 g IM every 12 hours), may be used. Once clinical response has occurred, therapy may be continued orally with ciprofloxacin (Cipro), 500 mg twice daily, or ofloxacin (Floxin), 400 mg orally (PO) twice daily.

PELVIC INFLAMMATORY DISEASE

Article 270, "Pelvic Inflammatory Disease," describes the treatment of PID caused by *N. gonorrhoeae*.

COMPLICATIONS

Infection rarely causes severe invasive disease (e.g., endocarditis or meningitis) or local disease (e.g., ophthalmitis). If these types of complications occur, other sources should be consulted.

INFECTION OF NEONATES AND CHILDREN

All neonates should receive ocular prophylaxis against gonococcal ophthalmia with 1% silver nitrate or an appropriate topical antimicrobial. Infants born to mothers with cervical infection are at risk of gonococcal ophthalmia or disseminated gonococcal infection and should be evaluated and treated with ceftriaxone (Rocephin), 25 to 50 mg/kg IV or IM, not to exceed 125 mg, once. Infection in older children should prompt an investigation of child abuse. Quinolones are not recommended for children younger than 18 years of age,

and ceftriaxone (Rocephin) is preferred (125 mg IM unless the child weighs >45 kg, in which case an adult dose is used).

REFERENCES

Centers for Disease Control and Prevention: Increases in fluoroquinolone-resistant *Neisseria gonorrhoeae* among men who have sex with men—United States, 2003, and revised treatment recommendations for gonorrhea treatment, 2004. MMWR Morb Mortal Wkly Rep 2004;43:335-338.

Centers for Disease Control and Prevention: Screening tests to detect *Chlamydia trachomatis* and *Neisseria gonorrhoeae* infections—2002. MMWR Recomm Rep 2002;51(RR15):1-27.

Centers for Disease Control and Prevention: Sexually transmitted diseases treatment guidelines 2002. MMWR 2002: 51(No. RR-6).

Golden MR, Whittington WL, Handsfield HH, et al: Effect of expedited treatment of sex partners on recurrent or persistent gonorrhea or chlamydial infection. N Engl J Med 2005;17:676-685.

Monroe KW, Weiss HL, Jones M, Hook EW 3rd: Acceptability of urine screening for *Neisseria gonorrhoeae* and *Chlamydia trachomatis* in adolescents at an urban emergency department. Sex Transm Dis 2003;30:850-853.

Shain RN, Piper JM, Holden AE, et al: Prevention of gonorrhea and chlamydia through behavioral intervention: Results of a two-year controlled randomized trial in minority women. Sex Transm Dis 2004;31:401-408.

Nongonococcal Urethritis

Method of
*Heidi M. Bauer, MD, MS, MPH, and
Kimberly Workowski, MD*

Nongonococcal urethritis (NGU) is estimated to affect more than 4 million men in the United States every year. This syndrome is characterized by urethral inflammation that may be asymptomatic in 30% to 50% of cases. Symptoms of urethritis include urethral discharge, dysuria, or meatal pruritus. The majority of infectious cases are sexually transmitted. Because of its well-defined role in the development of upper tract disease and infertility in women, *Chlamydia trachomatis* remains the most important pathogen, accounting for 15% to 40% of cases of NGU. Other etiologies include *Mycoplasma genitalium, Trichomonas vaginalis,* and herpes simplex virus. The role of *Ureaplasma urealyticum,* enteric bacteria, anaerobes, and *Candida* species is less well defined. Complications of untreated NGU include epididymitis in less than 3% of cases and, rarely, Reiter syndrome. Although NGU can be caused by chemical, allergic, or autoimmune processes, the syndrome should be presumed infectious. Evaluation and treatment for both gonorrhea and chlamydia is warranted. Furthermore, clinical evaluation and treatment of sex partners is critical for preventing complications and interrupting sexual transmission. Pathogens responsible for NGU are associated with cervicitis, pelvic inflammatory disease (PID), and tubal infertility.

Diagnosis

Although the clinical presentation varies, the incubation of NGU averages 7 to 14 days with gradual onset of mild dysuria and mucoid discharge. In some high-risk populations, up to 50% of infections are asymptomatic.

Because of its high sensitivity and specificity, the Gram stain is the preferred rapid diagnostic test for evaluating urethritis. Gonococcal infection can be established by documenting the presence of white blood cells (WBCs) containing intracellular gram-negative diplococci. The presence of gram-negative rods should raise the suspicion for enteric bacteria. Confirmatory tests are important for identifying a specific etiology, which may improve compliance and facilitate partner management. *Neisseria gonorrhoeae* and *C. trachomatis* can be detected using culture, DNA hybridization tests on a urethral specimen, or nucleic acid amplification tests (NAATs) on a urethral or urine specimen. Because of their increased sensitivity, NAATs are recommended for chlamydia testing. For urine-based NAATs, 10 to 15 mL of first-catch urine is collected.

Diagnostic tests for mycoplasmas are available in research settings; however, these are not available for routine clinical use. Although culture is available for *T. vaginalis,* specific medium is necessary for isolation; both urethral and urine specimens are recommended.

CURRENT DIAGNOSIS

The diagnosis of urethritis is confirmed by documenting evidence of inflammation on a urethral smear or in the urine:

- Urethral discharge that is mucoid or purulent
- Gram stain of urethral exudate demonstrating five or more white blood cells (WBCs) per oil immersion field (×1000)
- Positive leukocyte esterase test on first-void urine or microscopic examination of first-void urine sediment demonstrating 10 or more WBCs per high power field (×400)

Treatment

If gonorrhea cannot be ruled out with a stat test (i.e., Gram stain of urethral exudate), patients should be treated for both gonorrhea and chlamydia. Both azithromycin (Zithromax) and doxycycline (Vibramycin) are highly effective in treating chlamydial NGU. Azithromycin provides convenient dosing and the opportunity for directly observed therapy. Doxycycline is inexpensive but requires a twice-daily dosing for a full week. Alternatives include erythromycin (E-Mycin) and fluoroquinolones.

Among patients with erratic health care seeking behavior in whom poor compliance is anticipated, azithromycin offers the easiest administration. Further, *M. genitalium* appears to respond better to macrolides compared with tetracyclines. Patients should be advised to abstain from sex until therapy is completed, symptoms have resolved, and sex partners have been treated. Patients should return for evaluation and treatment if their symptoms persist or recur after completion of therapy. Patients should refer all sex partners in the past 60 days for evaluation and treatment. Sexual contacts of patients with NGU should be offered evaluation and treatment.

Persistent or Recurrent Urethritis

Chronic urethritis is defined as persistent or recurrent urethritis within 6 weeks following treatment. An estimated 20% to 40% of NGU cases do not respond to first-line therapy. Although up to 20% of men with chlamydial NGU have recurrence, up to 50% of men with nonchlamydial NGU have recurrence. Noncompliance and reinfection are important considerations. Other causes include organisms that do not respond to the standard treatment regimens, such as trichomoniasis, tetracycline-resistant *Ureaplasma,* viral etiologies, and other bacteria. Up to 30% of NGU has no identifiable infectious etiology. These cases may involve allergy and postinfectious immunologic response. Before administering therapy, the presence of urethral inflammation

---

CURRENT THERAPY

Recommended Regimens

- Azithromycin(Zithromax), 1 g PO in a single dose
- Doxycycline (Vibramycin), 100 mg PO bid × 7 days

Alternative Regimens

- Erythromycin base (E-Mycin, ERYC, E-Base), 500 mg PO qid × 7 days
- Erythromycin ethylsuccinate (EES), 800 mg PO qid × 7 days
- Ofloxacin (Floxin), 300 mg PO bid × 7 days
- Levofloxacin (Levaquin), 500 mg PO qd × 7 days

Abbreviations: bid = two times a day; PO = by mouth; qd = once daily; qid = four times a day.

should be documented. Patients with persistent or recurrent urethritis who did not comply with therapy or who had exposure to an untreated sex partner should be retreated with the initial drug regimen. Otherwise, recommended treatment regimens include metronidazole (Flagyl), 2 g orally in a single dose, plus either erythromycin base (E-Base), 500 mg orally four times a day for 7 days, or erythromycin ethylsuccinate (EES), 800 mg orally four times a day for 7 days.

REFERENCES

Centers for Disease Control and Prevention: Sexually transmitted diseases treatment guidelines 2002. MMWR Morb Mortal Wkly Rep 2002;51(RR-6):30-42.
Centers for Disease Control and Prevention: Screening tests to detect *Chlamydia trachomatis* and *Neisseria gonorrhoeae* infections—2002. Morb Mortal Wkly Rep 2002;51(RR-15):3-19.
Jensen JS: *Mycoplasma genitalium:* The aetiological agent of urethritis and other sexually transmitted diseases. J Eur Acad Dermatol Venereol 2004;18(1):1-11.
Kodner C: Sexually transmitted infections in men. Prim Care 2003; 30:173-191.

Granuloma Inguinale (Donovanosis) and Lymphogranuloma Venereum

Method of
A.A. Hoosen, MSc, MB, ChB, MMed, FC Path

The initial clinical presentation of granuloma inguinale (GI) (or donovanosis) and lymphogranuloma venereum (LGV) is genital ulceration, and these conditions are considered in the differential diagnosis of genital ulcer disease (GUD) or genital ulcer syndrome (GUS).

In view of the difficulty in making an accurate clinical diagnosis of the exact etiology of GUD and also because more than one sexually transmitted pathogen may cause an infection concurrently in high-risk populations, syndromic management of sexually transmitted infections (STIs) is promoted. The World Health Organization (WHO) has published guidelines for syndromic management, which are being followed in many countries; however, other countries have modified these according to the local prevalence of STIs. Antimicrobial agents shown to be efficacious for the eradication of GI (donovanosis) and LGV are always included in the protocols for the management of genital ulcer disease.

Management is important with these diseases not only, for public health reasons, to curtail their spread among the population but also because these diseases enhance the spread of HIV.

Granuloma Inguinale

Granuloma inguinale (GI)/Donovanosis is a chronic, progressive ulcerative condition of the genitalia caused by an encapsulated bacterium called *Calymmatobacterium granulomatis*. A recent proposal is that this organism be reclassified as *Klebsiella granulomatis*. The infection occurs in selected foci worldwide including southeast India, Papua New Guinea, the Caribbean, Brazil, eastern South Africa, Zimbabwe, Zambia, and Australia.

The primary lesion begins as a small, painless papule that ulcerates to form an exuberant, beefy red granulomatous ulcer with rolled edges. The lesions are painless and bleed easily on contact. Healing may be accompanied by scar formation and, in severe cases, lymphedema with resultant elephantiasis and deformities. In men, the lesions usually appear on the penile shaft, coronal sulcus, and prepuce; in women they occur commonly on the labia and fourchette. Intravaginal and cervical lesions mimic carcinoma of the cervix clinically and may result in complications such as hydronephrosis.

In large characteristic beefy lesions, the diagnosis is usually made clinically. However, for smaller lesions and where mixed infections are suspected, tests to exclude other causes of GUD need to be undertaken. The mainstay of laboratory diagnosis for GI is visualization of characteristic intracellular Donovan bodies in monocytes in tissue smears stained by Giemsa and Wright stains. Donovan bodies are encapsulated, short rods showing a characteristic bipolar staining. Specimens are collected by taking scrapings or swab specimens from the edge of lesions. Tissue biopsy lesions taken from the edge of the lesions assist in excluding malignancy, and these are stained with Giemsa and silver stains for ease of diagnosis. The causative organism has been successfully cultured in monocytes and in HEp-2 cells, but this requires elaborate laboratory facilities and expertise, which are not readily available in many routine diagnostic laboratories. Molecular diagnostic assays are not available commercially and have only been used in a few research studies.

A number of antimicrobial agents provide successful therapy for GI. The recommended duration of therapy is until lesions re-epithelize. Our recommendation for patients with severe lesions is hospitalization and administration of an aminoglycoside (e.g., gentamicin at 4.5 to 5 mg/kg per day or amikacin 15 mg/kg per day intravenously in a single daily dose for 10 to 14 days) together with a macrolide agent (e.g., erythromycin at 500 mg four times per day until resolution of lesions). Tetracycline, 500 mg four times per day; doxycycline, 100 mg twice daily; and trimethoprim/sulfamethoxazole, 80/400 mg twice daily, are also reported to be effective by various centers. There is no difference in clinical outcome for HIV co-infected individuals.

Lymphogranuloma Inguinale

Lymphogranuloma venereum (LGV) is caused by serovars L1, L2, and L3 of *Chlamydia trachomatis*.

CURRENT DIAGNOSIS

Clinical

- Characteristic signs are large beefy, exuberant, painless lesions that bleed easily on contact.
- A transient papular ulcer is followed by regional lymphadenopathy that develops into a bubo and may suppurate.

Laboratory

- Mainstay of diagnosis is the demonstration of a characteristic bipolar staining of Donovan bodies in monocytes, which appear in Giemsa-stained tissue smears.
- Serology most widely used is biopsied tissue stained with Giemsa and silver stains.
- Current test of choice is the microimmunofluorescence (MIF) test.

CURRENT THERAPY

- For large lesions, use combination therapy with intravenous aminoglycoside plus oral erythromycin followed by oral erythromycin until lesions re-epithelize.
- Antimicrobials such as tetracycline, ceftriaxone, azithromycin, chloramphenicol, and co-trimoxazole are used with good success; the most widely used agent is doxycycline, 100 mg twice daily for 2 to 3 weeks.
- Alternative agents include erythromycin and sulfisoxazole.
- Fluctuant buboes must be aspirated before they rupture.

The initial clinical presentation is a small transient papular lesion; the characteristic regional lymphadenopathy occurs later. The disease is endemic in Africa, India, Southeast Asia, South America, and the Caribbean.

Classic LGV disease has three distinct stages. The first stage is the formation of the primary lesion, usually on the genitalia, which is a papular ulcer and is usually asymptomatic. The lesion appears approximately 3 days to 3 weeks after acquisition of infection and heals without scar formation. The secondary stage is characterized by regional lymphadenopathy and manifestation of systemic symptoms. In men, the inguinal area is usually affected, and in the majority of cases it is a unilateral lymphadenopathy. In women vulval lesions lead to inguinal and femoral lymphadenopathy, and for upper vaginal or cervical lesions the iliac nodes are affected. The simultaneous enlargement of the femoral and inguinal lymph nodes gives an appearance of a groove and this "groove sign" is said to be characteristic of LGV. The lymph nodes coalesce and form a bubo that may rupture spontaneously and lead to fistulae and sinus tracts. In the third stage, there is chronic granulomatous enlargement with ulceration of the external genitalia. These changes may lead to lymphatic obstruction resulting in elephantiasis.

Diagnosis of a chlamydial infection is usually made either by demonstrating the causative agent in stained smears, by antigen detection, by culture, by serologic tests, or by molecular tests such as the polymerase chain reaction (PCR). For the diagnosis of LGV, Giemsa-stained smears of ulcerative lesions are not helpful because of the presence of competing genital flora. Antigen detection by monoclonal immununofluoresence assays has been used; culture in HEp-2, HeLa, and McCoy cell lines have shown yields of up to 30%; and molecular tests are not currently commercially available. Diagnosis is usually made by serologic assays. The classic complement fixation test is rarely used nowadays; the current test of choice is the microimmunofluorescence test (MIF or micro IF) as it allows for discrimination between the serovars of *C. trachomatis*.

A number of antibacterial agents such as tetracycline, doxycycline, minocycline, chloramphenicol, and erythromycin have been used for successful therapy. The recommended duration of therapy is at least 14 days in view of the unique intracellular life cycle of this pathogen. The Centers for Disease Control and Prevention (CDC) recommends the use of doxycycline, 100 mg twice daily for 21 days, with erythromycin and sulfisoxazole as alternative agents. The use of the azalide azithromycin (1 g orally) allows for a single-dose regimen for the management of chlamydial infections, and this may allow for better compliance of therapy.

It is extremely important to aspirate fluctuant buboes to prevent complications of rupture and sinus tract formation.

REFERENCES

Carter J, Hutton S, Sriprakash KS, et al: Culture of the causative organism of donovanosis (*Calymmatobacterium granulomatis*) in Hep-2 cells. J Clin Microbiol 1997;35:2915-2917.

Carter JS, Bowden FJ, Bastian I, et al : Phylogenetic evidence for reclassification of *Calymmatobacterium granulomatis* as *Klebsiella granulomatis* comb. Nov. Int J Syst Bacteriol 1999;49:1695-1700.

Centers for Disease Control and Prevention: Sexually transmitted diseases: Treatment guidelines, 2002. MMWR Morb Mortal Wkly Rep 2002;51(RR6):1-80.

Hoosen AA, Draper G, Moodley J, Cooper K: Granuloma inguinale of the cervix: A carcinoma look-alike. Genitourin Med 1990;66:380-382.

Hoosen AA, Mphatsoe M, Kharsany ABM, et al: Granuloma inguinale in association with pregnancy and HIV infection. Int J Gynaecol Obstet 1996;53:133-138.

Kharsany ABM, Hoosen AA, Kiepiela P, et al: Growth and cultural characteristics of *Calymmatobacterium granulomatis*—the aetiological agent of granuloma inguinale (donovanosis). J Med Microbiol 1997;46:579-585.

Mahony JB, Coombes BK, Chernesky MA: *Chlamydia* and Chlamydophila. In: Murphy PR, et al (eds): Manual of Clinical Microbiology. Washington, DC, American Society of Microbiology, 2003, pp 991-1004.

O'Farrell N, Hoosen AA, Coetzee K, van der Ende J: A rapid stain for the diagnosis of granuloma inguinale. Genitourin Med 1990;66:200-201.

Richens J: The diagnosis and treatment of donovanosis (granuloma inguinale). Genitourin Med 1991:67:441-452.

Stamm WE, Jones RB, Balteiger BE: *Chlamydia trachomatis*. In: Mandell GL, Bennett JE, Dolin R (eds):. Principles and Practice of

Infectious Diseases. New York, Churchill Livingstone, 2005, pp 2239-2255.

Wasserheit JN: Effect of changes in human ecology and behaviour on patterns of sexually transmitted diseases, including human immunodeficiency virus infection. Proc Natl Acad Sci U S A 1994;91:2430-2435.

World Health Organization. Guidelines for the management of sexually transmitted infections. World Health Organization, 2003, pp 1-91.

Syphilis

Method of
Mrunal Shah, MD

One of the oldest infections known, syphilis dates back more than 500 years. It was known as "The Great Pox" because of its skin manifestations; in contrast to the "small pox" seen around the same time. Studies were done before the use of antibiotics, which is where most of our natural history information comes from. The most recent epidemic occurred in 1990 (20.3 cases per 100,000 population) and has fallen steadily each year since. In the year 2000, the rate was at an all time low of 2.2 cases per 100,000 population. This was a 9.6% drop since 1999. The Centers for Disease Control and Prevention (CDC) hopes to eradicate the disease completely by 2005, but this may be difficult.

Peak ages are 30 to 39 years of age in men and 20 to 24 years of age in women. African Americans have always had higher incidences than whites. In the 1990s, it was 60:1, but the incidence has since declined to 30:1.

Microbiology

Treponema pallidum is the bacterium responsible for causing syphilis. It is very small and cannot be detected by ordinary microscopy, a feature that complicates diagnosis. The organism can be seen with darkfield microscopy, a technique that uses a special condenser to cast an oblique light. This allows visualization of a corkscrew-shaped organism with tightly wound spirals. This organism is extremely sensitive to penicillin, as is discussed later in the article. It has a very slow doubling rate, therefore requiring longer courses of treatment.

Pathophysiology

T. pallidum initiates infection when it gains access to subcutaneous tissues through microabrasions that can occur during sexual intercourse. Even though it has a slow doubling time (30 hours), it escapes host immune defenses and leads to the initial ulcerative lesion, the chancre. These can be seen anywhere around the genitalia including the cervix, perianal and rectal areas, and the oral mucosa. Regional lymphadenopathy also can be seen. As the host immune system fights the initial infection, *T. pallidum* is disseminated throughout the host. This is known as latency, as the patient will have no symptoms. There is also vertical spread in utero or during delivery, which is why prenatal panels include screening tests for syphilis.

Clinical Manifestations

The initial clinical manifestation is also called *primary* syphilis. This usually consists of a painless chancre at the site of inoculation. Primary syphilis represents a local infection, but it quickly becomes systemic with widespread dissemination of the spirochete. Because it is painless, most people do not seek medical attention. Even without treatment, the chancre will resolve in 4 to 6 weeks. It is this painlessness that helps separate it from herpes simplex virus (genital herpes) and *Haemophilus ducrey*i (chancroid).

In approximately weeks to months after the resolution of the chancre, patients will develop *secondary* syphilis, which includes systemic symptoms of rash, fever, headache, malaise, anorexia, and diffuse lymphadenopathy. The rash typically involves the palms and soles but can also include mucosal surfaces. Many patients do not realize that they had these lesions. These symptoms usually resolve spontaneously but can relapse for up to 5 years.

After symptoms resolve, and for up to many years later, the disease goes into *latent* syphilis, which is characterized by a lack of symptoms but seropositive test results. This can be separated into early and late latent phases based on being potentially infectious in the early phase. This is defined by the United States Public Health Service (USPHS) as infection of 1 year's duration or less. Anything longer is late latent.

Finally, for the next 1 to 30 years, untreated patients have a 25% to 40% risk of developing *late* or *tertiary* syphilis. It may involve many tissue types, so the spectrum of disease can be very confusing. Moreover, patients need not have had symptoms of primary or secondary syphilis prior to developing late syphilis. Tissues involved include cutaneous (gumma formation), cardiovascular (aortic disease), and central nervous system (CNS) (tabes dorsalis, meningitis, neurosyphilis) diseases (Table 1).

Diagnosis

The quickest, most direct method of diagnosing primary and secondary syphilis is direct visualization of the spirochete of moist lesions by means of darkfield microscopy. This is difficult and requires using laboratories that perform a high volume of sexually transmitted disease analyses. In general, a moist lesion should be cleaned with saline (not iodine because of bacteriocidal effect). Then, using gauze, the lesion should be unroofed. Any serosanguineous material should be collected on a dry slide for examination.

Rakel and Bope: *Conn's Current Therapy 2006*.

TABLE 1 Clinical Manifestations and Treatment of Syphilis

Stage	Clinical manifestation	Treatment
Primary	Painless ulcer (chancre), adenopathy	Benzathine penicillin G (Bicillin LA), 2.4 million U IM × 1
Secondary (weeks to months)	Rash, mucocutaneous lesions, adenopathy, hepatitis, arthritis, glomerulonephritis, condyloma lata	Benzathine penicillin G, 2.4 million U IM × 1
Latent	Asymptomatic	
Early (<1 year)		Benzathine penicillin G, 2.4 million U IM × 1
Late		Benzathine penicillin G, 2.4 million U IM weekly × 3
Tertiary (late) 1-30 years		
Cutaneous	Gummatous lesions	Benzathine penicillin G, 2.4 million U IM weekly × 3
Cardiovascular	Aortic aneurysm, aortic insufficiency	Benzathine penicillin G, 2.4 million U IM weekly × 3
CNS	Neurosyphilis, tabes dorsalis, Argyll-Robertson pupils, paresis, seizures, subtle psychiatric manifestations, dementia; may be asymptomatic	Aqueous crystalline penicillin G, 18-24 million U/d given as 3-4 million units IV q4h for 10-14 days or Procaine penicillin (Wycillin), 2.4 million U qd with probenecid 500 mg PO qid for 10-14 days

Abbreviations: CNS = central nervous system; IM = intramuscularly; IV = intravenously; PO = orally; qd = daily; qid = 4 times per day.
Adapted from the CDC: Guidelines for the treatment of STDs. MMWR Morb Mortal Wkly Rep 2002;51(RR-06):1-80.

11

More common is serologic testing that can be done in most laboratories. The two most common screening tests are rapid plasma reagin (RPR) and the Venereal Disease Research Laboratory (VDRL) test. These tests are designed to test for IgM and IgG antibodies against a cardiolipin-cholesterol-lecithin antigen. Positive tests are reported as a dilutional titer. False positives are less than 1:4, whereas higher titers (1:16 to 1:128) are found in secondary and early latent syphilis. This titer is important as a benchmark to follow treatment. Lack of expected decreases in titer indicate inadequate treatment, false-positive result, re-infection, or late-stage therapy.

Before treatment, a positive screening test needs to be confirmed with specific *T. pallidum* antigen testing, such as the fluorescent treponemal antibody absorption test (FTA-ABS). These tests are expensive and have a high false-positive rate, making them unsuitable as screening tests. They also remain positive for life in most people.

Newer molecular tests include the use of polymerase chain reaction (PCR), which can be used to detect multiple organisms. It has high sensitivity and specificity and can distinguish among *H. ducreyi*, herpes simplex virus, and *T. pallidum*. This test is very expensive and is likely to be available only in specialized laboratories, for now.

The most significant morbidity of syphilis occurs during the tertiary phase and includes neurosyphilis. *T. pallidum* can be found in the cerebrospinal fluid (CSF) during primary and secondary phases, but it usually resolves on its own. Those patients who have an abnormal CSF during the latent phase are at higher risk for symptomatic neurosyphilis, making it helpful to distinguish asymptomatic neurosyphilis. The CDC recommends that CSF testing be done whenever there is clinical evidence of neurosyphilis or vision changes, active tertiary syphilis, treatment failure, or HIV infection. CSF-VDRL is highly specific, but, unfortunately, very insensitive (as low as 30%) and therefore can rule in but cannot exclude neurosyphilis.

Although the HIV epidemic showed a resurgence of syphilis, it is controversial as to what diagnostic changes occurred in testing. Several studies show contradictory information; one shows that there was an increase in the false-positive rates, whereas a second study showed a decrease in true-positive rates, and a third study showed higher false negatives. In any case, testing should still be performed as in non-HIV patients and followed accordingly.

Pregnancy poses only increased risk, including perinatal death, premature delivery, low birth weight, congenital anomalies, and active congenital syphilis of the neonate. Physical examination and serologic testing should be performed in any female considering pregnancy or during initial antepartum testing at least. Treatment, discussed below, should be given as if the patient is not pregnant.

Treatment

In all stages, the main reason for treatment is to prevent progression and spread of the disease. Historic treatments included mercury, salvarsan (an arsenic derivative), fever therapy, and malarial injection. Today's treatment has been in use since 1943, since the introduction of penicillin. Because there has been no reported resistance, penicillin remains the treatment of choice, so much so that penicillin-allergic patients have undergone desensitization therapy in order to receive it. Although penicillin G, given parenterally, is the preferred drug, the preparation used (benzathine, procaine, crystalline), dosage, and duration of therapy depend on stage and clinical manifestations (see Table 1). Oral penicillin is not considered appropriate for treatment. Alternative treatments could include doxycycline (Vibramycin), tetracycline, erythromycin, or ceftriaxone (Rocephin).[1]

---

[1]Not FDA approved for this indication.

Once treatment is started, physicians should be aware of a potential complication called the Jarisch-Herxheimer reaction. It is an acute, febrile reaction accompanied by headache and myalgias, which represents treponemal cell death and release of toxins. It peaks within 2 hours and subsides within 24 hours, and is most common in primary and secondary disease.

Follow-up of Treated Patients

Any patient with syphilis diagnosed at any stage should get testing for HIV and should be retested in 3 to 6 months if a member of a high-risk population. After treatment, repeat serologic testing should be done at 6 and 12 months and titers at 24 months. If there is not at least a fourfold decrease in 6 months, there is likely treatment failure. A lumbar puncture should be done to rule out neurosyphilis, and retreatment with three weekly injections of 2.4 million units of benzathine penicillin (Bicillin LA) is recommended unless there is evidence of neurosyphilis.

Partners of patients with syphilis should also be notified and treated. In primary disease, any partner within the previous 3 months should be identified. Empiric treatment is recommended unless there is good follow-up and serologic surveillance.

Rakel and Bope: *Conn's Current Therapy 2006.*

Diseases of Allergy

Anaphylaxis and Serum Sickness

Method of
Marcia Torres Lima, MD, and
Gailen D. Marshall, Jr., MD, PhD

Anaphylaxis

In 1902, Portier and Richet described the experimental induction of hypersensitivity in dogs immunized with the venom from coelenterate invertebrates (sea anemones) while attempting to confer sting prophylaxis. The dogs were sensitized to the venom unexpectedly and had fatal reactions to previously nonlethal doses of the venom. To describe this phenomenon, Portier and Richet proposed the term anaphylaxis, which was derived from Greek words ana- (*against*) and phylaxis (*immunity, protection*). Anaphylaxis is an acute, potentially life-threatening clinical condition that is most often caused by a systemic allergic reaction. The term *anaphylaxis* should be reserved only for IgE-mediated systemic reactions as a consequence of release of inflammatory mediators, and *anaphylactoid* should be used to describe systemic reactions from non–IgE-mediated mechanisms that induce mast cell and basophil activation. They are otherwise clinically indistinguishable. The distinction becomes important in therapeutic considerations (discussed later).

Mast cells are located primarily near mucous membranes and around blood vessels. The skin, conjunctiva, gastrointestinal tract, and upper and lower respiratory systems are the organs that most frequently come in contact with a foreign antigen. Because of their relatively high concentration of mast cells, they are the initial sites of degranulation. IgE is bound to the surface of mast cells by its high-affinity Fc receptor (FcERI). Once antigens cross-link the Fab component, a series of cytoplasmic events takes place. Unlike mast cells, basophils commonly circulate in peripheral blood. However, they also have IgE bound to the Fc receptor and can be activated by antigen binding or other physical/chemical factors.

Biochemical mediators and chemotactic substances are released during degranulation of mast cells and basophils. These include preformed granule-associated substances, such as histamine, tryptase, chymase, and heparin; histamine-releasing factor and other cytokines; and newly generated lipid-derived mediators, such as prostaglandin D_2 (PGD_2), platelet-activating factor, leukotriene B_4 (LTB_4), and the cysteinyl leukotrienes (LTC_4, LTD_4, and LTE_4). Eosinophils may play either a direct toxic role (release of cytotoxic granule-associated proteins) or a proinflammatory role (metabolism of vasoactive mediators) to increase vascular permeability, decrease systemic vascular resistance, etc.).

Histamine activates H_1 and H_2 receptors. Pruritus, rhinorrhea, tachycardia, and bronchospasm are caused by activation of the H_1 receptors, whereas both H_1 and H_2 receptors mediate headache, flushing, and hypotension. Serum histamine levels correlate with the severity and persistence of cardiopulmonary manifestations but not with formation of urticaria. Gastrointestinal signs and symptoms (abdominal cramping, nausea, vomiting) are associated with histamine more than tryptase levels.

Tryptase is the only protein that is concentrated selectively in the secretory granules of human mast cells. Tryptase levels correlate with clinical severity of anaphylaxis. Postmortem measurements of serum tryptase may be useful in establishing anaphylaxis as the cause of death in subjects experiencing sudden death of uncertain cause.

INCITING ETIOLOGIC AGENTS

In fact, any agent capable of activating mast cells or basophils might potentially cause anaphylaxis or an anaphylactoid reaction. However, as previously reported, multiple mechanisms can be involved in some cases of anaphylaxis. The most common definable causes of anaphylaxis are foods, medications, and insect stings.

The list of foods implicated in anaphylactic reactions is extensive. However, the same few foods, such as peanuts, tree nuts, shellfish, milk, and eggs, are reported to provoke the majority of anaphylactic reactions. In westernized countries, peanuts and tree nuts, fish (cod and whitefish), and shellfish (shrimp, lobster, crab, scallops, oyster) are most often implicated in fatal or near-fatal reactions. These foods also tend to induce a "persistent sensitivity" in the vast majority of patients, in contrast to other foods, such as milk, eggs, and soybeans, which are frequently associated with milder reactions that can usually be "outgrown" by avoidance for 2 to 3 years.

Risk of drug-induced anaphylaxis increases with age, peaking in the elderly, probably as a consequence of the higher proportion of older people who regularly use one or more drugs. In hospital settings, anesthetic agents are commonly used. Muscle relaxants are responsible for the majority of intraoperative anaphylaxis episodes. However, latex also accounts for a significant number of these reactions, and its incidence is actually increasing. There are specific subpopulations who are at increased risk for anaphylaxis to latex: atopic individuals, individuals with increased previous exposure to latex, health care workers who are exposed to latex mainly by inhalation (from glove powder), and possibly patients who have undergone multiple surgical procedures (particularly intra-abdominal) and therefore have been repeatedly exposed to latex intravascularly and/or via genitourinary tract by catheterization. Peptide hormones such as insulin and antidiuretic hormone (desmopressin, DDAVP) and enzymes such as streptokinase (Streptase) can induce anaphylaxis. Colloids, opioids, and radiocontrast material can also induce anaphylactoid reactions. Penicillin is a relatively common cause of anaphylaxis; reactions may also be triggered by penicillin derivatives. Up to 10% of those with documented penicillin allergy will also be allergic to cephalosporins (particularly first- generation cephalosporins). The risk of anaphylactoid reactions in those using aspirin and nonsteroidal anti-inflammatory drugs should be considered in general practice. However, the physiopathology of those agents is not completely understood.

Venoms from the stings of bees and wasps are an important cause of anaphylaxis and differentiating between the two is important because immunotherapy is an effective treatment approach in this group. This is accomplished with venom-specific allergen skin test or radioallergosorbent test (RAST).

DIAGNOSIS AND DIFFERENTIAL DIAGNOSIS

It is essential for effective management that a rapid and accurate diagnosis be made and that those who are at greatest risk of reaction be rapidly identified. The most important systems involved are respiratory and cardiovascular. Early signs of anaphylaxis can include flushing and systemic urticaria. However, the clinical manifestations of intraoperative reactions often differ from those of anaphylactic reactions outside of anesthesia. Cutaneous manifestations are less common and cardiovascular collapse may be more common during anesthesia. The diagnosis can be more difficult because patients cannot express symptoms. Anaphylaxis typically begins within 5 to 60 minutes of exposure to the inciting agent. The more rapid the onset of symptoms after exposure, the more severe the clinical reaction is likely to be. Latex-induced anaphylaxis is, however, known to develop more slowly, normally over a period of about 30 to 90 minutes. Box 1 summarizes the main clinical findings. The clinician must be aware of several

BOX 1 Clinical Findings of Anaphylaxis

- Cardiovascular: Feeling of faintness, syncope, and hypotension
- Cutaneous: Pruritus, flushing, urticaria, and angioedema
- Gastrointestinal: Nausea, vomiting, diarrhea, and abdominal pain
- Neurologic: Anxiety, feeling of "impending doom," and loss of consciousness
- Oral: Pruritus of lips, tongue, and palate, edema of lips and tongue
- Respiratory: Rhinitis, sneezing, "a lump in the throat," dysphagia, dysphonia, hoarseness, stridor, cough, chest tightness, dyspnea, and wheezing

diseases that may mimic an anaphylaxis reaction (Box 2). Recurrent or biphasic anaphylaxis occurs 8 to 12 hours after the initial attack in up to 20% of subjects who experienced anaphylaxis. Pre-event use of calcium channel blockers, β-adrenergic antagonists, or angiotensin-converting enzyme inhibitors may increase risk of recurrent anaphylaxis.

If the diagnosis remains uncertain, or if the patient is stabilized before the physical examination, laboratory testing can be done to confirm the diagnosis. Levels of histamine and tryptase change with an anaphylactic event. The concentration of serum histamine rises 5 to 10 minutes after the trigger event and remains elevated for 30 to 60 minutes. Urinary histamine may remain elevated for several hours after a reaction. Serum tryptase peaks 1 to 1.5 hours after anaphylaxis, and can still be detected as long as 3 to 6 hours later.

TREATMENT

Anaphylaxis is a medical emergency that requires immediate treatment. Rapid assessment and stabilization of the airway, breathing, and circulation are of the greatest importance. The cornerstone of pharmacologic treatment is the administration of epinephrine. The dosage for adults is 0.3 to 0.5 mL of a 1:1000 dilution, and recent research has established the intramuscular route to be superior to the subcutaneous route, and the lateral aspect of the thigh is the site of choice. The dosage for children is 0.01 mL/kg, up to a maximum of 0.3 mL of a 1:1000 dilution. Epinephrine can be reinjected at 10-minute intervals, until improvement occurs. Intravenous epinephrine (1:10,000 dilution) should be administered only in severe hypotensive shock.

BOX 2 Differential Diagnosis of Anaphylaxis

- Acute or chronic urticaria
- Carcinoid syndrome
- Globus hystericus
- Hereditary angioedema
- Mastocytosis
- Serum sickness
- Vasovagal reaction

Continuous hemodynamic monitoring is essential to monitor possible induction of cardiac arrhythmias.

Additional therapy for anaphylaxis includes the use of H_1 antihistamines, diphenhydramine (Benadryl), 1 to 2 mg/kg to a maximal dose of 50 mg, and H_2 antihistamine, ranitidine (Zantac),[1] 0.5 to 1.5 mg/kg to a maximal dose of 150 mg, each given parenterally. Inhaled β_2-agonists (e.g., albuterol [Proventil]) are useful when bronchospasm is present. Early use of corticosteroids such as intravenous methylprednisolone (Solu-Medrol), 1 to 2 mg/kg, may help to prevent or minimize late-phase reactions. Patients who use β-blockers may not respond completely to epinephrine, in which case glucagon should be administered at a dose of 5 to 15 µg/min intravenously.

Anaphylaxis resulting from allergen immunotherapy injections or venom should also be treated by placement of a tourniquet proximal to the injection site or the site of sting.

After appropriate treatment, prevention is of the greatest importance. The first essential step for prevention of anaphylaxis is identification of the inciting agent. Referral of all patients who experienced a generalized reaction to a qualified allergy specialist is the key step to ensuring that patients are appropriately investigated and advised on ways to minimize or prevent future reactions. In case of drug or food allergy, not only must the offending agent be avoided, but the potential for crossreactivity must also be recognized. Allergen immunotherapy should be considered in those with history of venom-induced anaphylaxis.

Patients should be prescribed, and be instructed in the use of, self-injectable epinephrine (EpiPen or EpiPen Jr) and told to keep it with them all the time. They should also wear a Medic Alert bracelet or necklace.

Serum Sickness

Serum sickness was first described in humans by von Pirquet and Schick in 1905, as a syndrome resulting from the repeat administration of heterologous serum (usually equine) as an antitoxin. Hyperimmune antiserum was the major therapeutic option in the pre-antibiotic era for infectious and toxin-related diseases. It was observed that a significant number of patients developed rash, fever, lymphadenopathy, and arthralgia 7 to 10 days after receiving this treatment for at least the second time. The term *serum sickness* was coined to describe the clinical syndrome. Serum sickness may also occur in response to the administration of foreign proteins such as streptokinase (Streptase), antithymocyte and antilymphocyte globulins (Atgam), vaccines, and hymenoptera venoms.

The incidence of iatrogenic serum sickness has decreased as a result of the general decline in the need for foreign antisera with the advent of effective immunization procedures, antimicrobial therapy, and the development of specific human immune serum globulins.

However, a serum sickness–like reaction that is clinically similar to classic serum sickness may result from the administration of a number of nonprotein drugs.

The immunopathology of serum sickness results from antigen-antibody complex formation in relative antigen excess with foreign protein as the antigen. If the complexes are of an appropriate size and sufficient quantity, they can deposit in endothelial surfaces at a number of tissue sites. Antigen can also combine with specific IgE on mast cells and basophils, leading to the release of platelet-activating factor. Subsequent platelet aggregation triggers its histamine and serotonin release. These substances increase vascular permeability and thus facilitate the deposition of immune complexes into vascular endothelium. Complement activation by immune complexes results in formation of C3a and C5a, which are potent anaphylatoxins. These substances stimulate macrophages, neutrophils, and lymphocytes to release inflammatory toxins. In classic serum sickness reaction, symptoms typically begin 6 to 21 days after drug administration; in previously immunized patients, the reaction may begin as early as 2 to 4 days after initiation of the inciting agent.

The diagnosis is made from the patient's history and by interpreting the appropriate laboratory findings associated with symptoms of rash (urticaria or vasculitis), arthritis, myalgia, and lymphadenopathy. No specific laboratory finding is universally present in serum sickness. However, an elevated sedimentation rate, eosinophilia, and depleted complement levels are often observed. Urinalysis may reveal microscopic hematuria or mild proteinuria. Also, the creatinine and liver transaminases may be transiently elevated.

The removal of the offending agent is the key for the treatment of serum sickness. Mild symptoms can be controlled with an oral antihistamine and nonsteroidal anti-inflammatory agents, whereas severe symptoms often require a course of systemic corticosteroids. Several preparations can be used, such as methylprednisolone (Medrol) 1 to 2 mg/kg per day given orally in twice-daily dosing. Steroids should be given for 3 to 5 days in the majority of cases, although in severe cases, patients may need to be weaned over a 2-week period. Because the cutaneous symptoms of serum sickness may last for several weeks, treatment with antihistamine is recommended for 6 weeks or longer. Hydroxyzine (Atarax), 2 mg/kg per day divided into four doses in children, or 25 mg four times daily in adults, may be used; or diphenhydramine (Benadryl) or the new generation of nonsedating antihistamines—fexofenadine (Allegra), 180 mg per day; loratadine (Claritin), 10 mg per day; or cetirizine (Zyrtec), 10 mg per day—can be used.

12

---

[1]Not FDA approved for this indication.

Asthma in Adolescents and Adults

Method of
Louis-Philippe Boulet, MD

Asthma is one of the most common respiratory diseases in adults and children, and its prevalence is increasing worldwide. This rise is mostly attributed to an increase in allergic diseases, probably of multifactorial origin. With the recent improvements in our understanding of the disease and the availability of various therapeutic options, it should have a minimal impact in most asthma sufferers. But the human and socioeconomic burden of asthma is unfortunately still high.

Definition and Pathophysiology: Targets for Therapy

Asthma is defined as a condition characterized by paroxysmal or persistent symptoms such as wheezing, chest tightness, phlegm production, and cough, associated with variable airway obstruction and hyperresponsiveness to various stimuli. These changes are mostly caused by underlying airway inflammation and structural changes (remodeling). The asthmatic airway inflammatory process, in which eosinophils, mast cells, and lymphocytes are abundant compared to normal subjects, is caused by the influence of TH_2 cells, producing mediators such as interleukin (IL)-3, IL-4, IL-5, IL-13, and granulocyte-macrophage colony-stimulating factor (GM-CSF). Some of these mediators (IL-4) activate B lymphocytes to produce immunoglobulin E (IgE) or perpetuate eosinophilic airway inflammation (IL-3, IL5, GM-CSF). Changes in airway structure in asthma include epithelial damage, subepithelial fibrosis, increased airway vasculature, changes in proteoglycans, and increased smooth-muscle mass, among many others.

The etiology of asthma is unknown, but its development likely results from environmental exposures in individuals genetically predisposed to develop this condition. Many genes determine the susceptibility to develop asthma, and the number of polymorphisms associated with asthma is still increasing. In regard to environmental exposures, allergen sensitization plays a major role. According to the hygiene hypothesis, the increase in allergic diseases observed in the last two decades may be related to a change in the immune system in favor of a TH_2-type lymphocyte response, mostly programmed at producing antibodies against environmental allergens, to the detriment of the mostly anti-infectious TH_1-type response; this may be the result of reduced exposure to infectious agents and therefore endotoxins, in the context of an expanding so-called Western lifestyle. In regard to ambient or outdoor pollutants, their influence on asthma is complex, but they may contribute to its development. The increasing prevalence of

various sensitizers at the workplace may also be involved.

Diagnosis

Although typical symptoms of asthma may suggest its diagnosis, the disease should be confirmed by objective measures that demonstrate either variable airway obstruction or hyperresponsiveness because various conditions may mimic asthma. Box 1 lists the diagnostic criteria. Ideally, spirometry should be done to measure expiratory flows; otherwise, a peak expiratory flow (PEF) may be measured with a portable device. A bronchoprovocation test may reveal airway hyperresponsiveness, a classic hallmark of symptomatic asthma. Physical examination is often normal unless the patient is seen during an asthma exacerbation. Chest radiograph is usually normal except in the presence of an associated condition or complication.

Triggers and Inducers

Box 2 categorizes exposures causing or increasing airway inflammation (inducers) and noninflammatory stimuli that provoke symptoms (triggers). Indoors allergens such as animal danders and house dust mites are recognized as more "asthmogenic" than outdoor ones. Various sensitizers may be present at the workplace, divided into high- (e.g., flour) or low-molecular-weight (e.g., isocyanates) substances. Potential environmental exposures and their relationship to symptoms should be documented. Allergy skin prick tests help determine if IgE antibodies are produced against the common airborne allergens. Upper and lower respiratory infections, particularly of viral origin, may lead to asthma exacerbations and could be involved in the development of asthma in predisposed individuals. Finally, exposure to respiratory irritants, cold air, or emotional stress can result in bronchoconstriction, depending on the degree

---

BOX 1   Diagnostic Criteria of Asthma

Variable airway obstruction
- Improvement of FEV_1
  >12% postbronchodilator, ideally 15% (minimum 180 mL for adults)
  >20% over time or after corticosteroid treatment (minimum 250 mL for adults)
- Improvement in PEF
  20% postbronchodilator or over time

Airway hyperresponsiveness
- Positive bronchial provocation test (e.g., with methacholine)

Abbreviations: FEV_1 = forced expiratory flow in 1 second; PEF = peak expiratory flow.
Adapted from Boulet LP, Becker A, Bérubé D, et al., on behalf of the Canadian Asthma Consensus Group: Canadian asthma consensus report. Can Med Assoc J 1999;30;161(11 Suppl):S1-S61.

BOX 2 Triggers and Inducers of Asthma

Inducers of airway inflammation
- Allergens indoors: domestic animals, house dust mites, cockroaches, molds, etc.
- Allergens outdoors: pollen, molds, foods (more rarely)
- Workplace sensitizers:
  Animal origin: laboratory animals, seafood processing, etc.
  Vegetable origin: flour, wood dust, etc.
  Chemical: isocyanates, phthalic anhydrides
  Biologic agents: *Bacillus subtilis*
  Metals: nickel, platinum salts
- Viral respiratory infections

Factors that can increase or modify the type of airway inflammation:
- Environmental pollutants (SO_2, NO_2, ozone)
- Tobacco smoke

Other potential triggers of asthma in most asthmatic patients:
- Exercise, cold air, temperature changes, humidity
- Strong odors, respiratory irritants
- β-Blockers
- Emotional stress

Other potential triggers of asthma in selected subgroups of with asthma:
- Aspirin and nonsteroidal anti-inflammatory agents
- Food additives (sulfites, benzoates, monosodium glutamate)
- Premenstrual increase in asthma
- Gastroesophageal reflux

TABLE 1 General Management of Asthma Differential

Confirm the diagnosis and assess initial severity.	Evaluate symptoms and measure expiratory flows ± airway responsiveness.
Determine possible triggers and inducers.	Questionnaire, allergy tests, other tests (assess environment, workplace, etc.)
Initiate treatment.	Prescribe medication required to achieve asthma control and treat associated conditions.
Initiate education.	Provide basic elements and refer to an asthma educator.
Determine the best results achievable.	Check asthma control criteria (symptoms, activities, "rescue" medication needs, expiratory flows).*
Determine the minimum medication needed.	Once asthma is well controlled, reduce medication while keeping control.
Devise an action plan.	Write and discuss with the patient a plan for management of exacerbations.
Ensure regular follow-up.	Check control criteria, including expiratory flows.*

*And maybe in the near future from noninvasive measures of airway inflammation.
Adapted from Boulet et al., 2001.

12

of airway responsiveness. Tobacco smoke can trigger asthma and when tobacco is used regularly it may reduce the efficacy of treatment. Gastroesophageal reflux is common in asthma, and its contribution to asthma symptomatology should be assessed. Exercise may induce asthma symptoms but could be prevented by taking a short-acting bronchodilator beforehand. Increasing bronchoconstrictive response to exertion suggests a loss of control of the asthma.

Management and Treatment

Table 1 summarizes the global management of asthma, and Figure 1 shows the therapeutic scheme of asthma treatment. According to the international guidelines "Global Initiative on Asthma (GINA) (http://www.ginasthma.com), asthma management includes the following suggestions:

- Educate patient to develop a partnership in asthma management.
- Assess and monitor asthma severity with symptom reports and, when possible, measurement of lung function.
- Avoid exposure to risk factors.
- Establish an individual medication plan for long-term management.
- Establish an individual plan for managing exacerbations.
- Provide regular follow-up care.

GOALS OF TREATMENT

The goals of asthma treatment are to promote a normal active life, including adequate exercise tolerance, no or minimal asthma symptoms, optimal pulmonary function; to prevent exacerbations, to reduce asthma severity or the potential for irreversible airflow limitation, and to minimize asthma-related morbidity and mortality while experiencing no significant side effects from treatment.

These goals could be achieved by obtaining rapid and long-term optimal control of asthma, including optimal pulmonary function, from avoidance of triggers, particularly those inducing airway inflammation. The minimal medication allowing optimal control of symptoms should be determined and reevaluated regularly (Table 2). The patient with asthma must fully understand the disease and its treatment and know how to avoid triggers and exposures that could induce symptoms but, more importantly, those that could increase airway inflammation.

ASSESSMENT OF CONTROL AND SEVERITY

Treatment needs are based on achievement of control criteria, which means minimal symptoms and rescue medication needs and optimal pulmonary function.

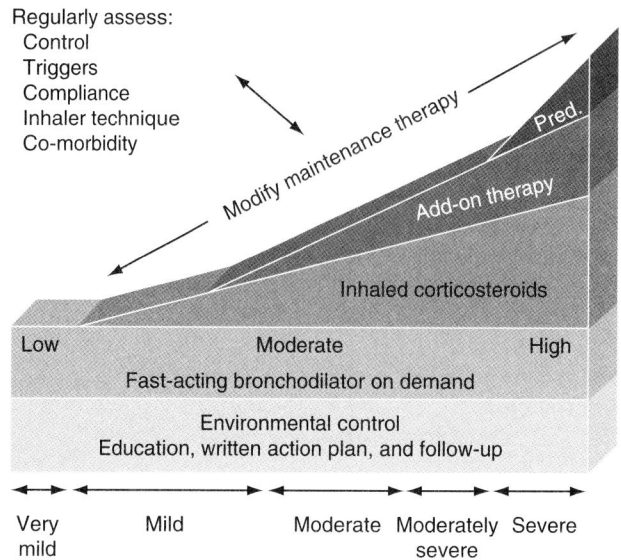

Regularly assess:
Control
Triggers
Compliance
Inhaler technique
Co-morbidity

Modify maintenance therapy

Pred.

Add-on therapy

Inhaled corticosteroids

Low   Moderate   High
Fast-acting bronchodilator on demand

Environmental control
Education, written action plan, and follow-up

Very   Mild   Moderate Moderately Severe
mild   severe

FIGURE 1. Therapeutic Scheme of Asthma. The Canadian Guidelines suggest that asthma management be considered as a continuum: Inhaled corticosteroids (ICS) are introduced as initial maintenance treatment, even with symptoms less than three times a week. LTRAs are a second-choice alternative, particularly for patients who cannot or will not use ICS agents. If control is inadequate on low-dose inhaled corticosteroids, the reasons for poor control are researched, and if needed, additional therapy with long-acting β_2 agonists, LTRAs (leukotriene receptor antagonists), or theophylline, as a third therapeutic option, is offered. The dose of inhaled corticosteroid is adapted to the severity of asthma. Severe asthma may require additional systemic steroids. Asthma control, compliance, and maintenance therapy must be regularly reassessed. See stepwise Approach for Managing Asthma in Adults and Children Older Than 5 Years of Age (p. 132). Available online at http://www.nhlbi.nih.gov/guidelines/asthma/ execsumm.pdf

Additional measures of control have been suggested, such as airway responsiveness, airway eosinophilia from induced sputum analysis, and NO measurement in expired air, but they are not currently recommended in most guidelines. Severity is best defined by the minimum medication needed to achieve asthma control (Table 3).

TABLE 2 Asthma Control Criteria

Parameters	Frequency or value
Daytime symptoms	<4 days/week
Nighttime symptoms	<1 night/week
Physical activity	Normal
Exacerbations	Mild, infrequent
Absenteeism from work or school because of asthma	None
Need for β2-agonist as needed	<4 doses/week*
FEV₁ or PEF	90% or more of personal best
PEF diurnal variation	<0% to 15% diurnal variation

*May use one dose per day before exercise.
Abbreviations: FEV$_1$ = forced expiratory flow in 1 second; PEF = peak expiratory flow.
Adapted from Boulet LP, Becker A, Bérubé D, et al, on behalf of the Canadian Asthma Consensus Group: Canadian asthma consensus report. Can Med Assoc J 1999;30;161(11 Suppl):S1–S61; and Lemiere C, Bai T, Balter M, et al: Adult Asthma Consensus Guidelines Update 2003. Can Respir J 2004;11(Suppl A):9A–18A.

ASTHMA EDUCATION

Education of asthmatic patients and their families is mandatory to achieve adequate asthma control and optimize treatment compliance and self-management, particularly at the onset of asthma exacerbations. A written individualized action plan should indicate how to manage these exacerbations. Various programs and networks offer asthma education. The educational intervention initiated in the physician's office is ideally completed by an asthma educator. Education should result in an improvement in the patient's health behaviors and self-management abilities. Asthma-control criteria must be explained and instructions provided on preventive measures and ways to adjust the treatment rapidly in case of exacerbation. Meta-analyses show that asthma education, including a written action plan and regular review, could lead to a reduction of asthma-related morbidity. Asthma education should especially be offered to patients with high asthma-related morbidity or severe asthma. Good communication between the patient and the physician/educator is essential, and the patient's feedback should be obtained to address any barrier to an adequate control of the disease.

ENVIRONMENTAL CONTROL AND AVOIDANCE OF TRIGGERS

Environmental control is another important aspect of asthma management. Contacts with respiratory irritants, particularly with allergens to which patients are sensitized, should be avoided. Although preventive measures

Diseases of Allergy

TABLE 3 Asthma Severity According to Long-Term Treatment Needs

Severity*	Symptoms	Treatment required
Very mild	Mild/infrequent	None, or inhaled β_2 agonist, rarely
Mild	Well controlled	β_2 agonist occasionally + low-dose ICS
Moderate	Well controlled	β_2 agonist + low/moderate doses ICS ± additional therapy
Severe	Well controlled	β_2 agonist + high doses ICS + additional therapy
Very severe	Not well controlled	β_2 agonist + high doses ICS + well-controlled additional therapy + oral glucocorticosteroid

*The primary measure of asthma severity in the treated patient should be the minimum therapy required to achieve acceptable control.
Abbreviation: ICS = inhaled corticosteroid.
Reproduced from Boulet LP, Becker A, Bérubé D, et al., on behalf of the Canadian Asthma Consensus Group: Canadian asthma consensus report. Can Med Assoc J 1999;30;161(11 Suppl):S1-S61.

are usually implemented for house dust mites, they are more rarely done for domestic animal avoidance. However, control of indoor exposures in sensitized subjects is key to asthma control (Box 3). The best measure for an allergy to domestic animals is to stop exposure to the animal, although secondary measures may be applied if the patient is unwilling in this regard. Asthmatic patients who smoke have an accelerated decline in lung function, respond less to treatment, and suffer an increased asthma-related morbidity. All of these patients should be offered participation in a smoking cessation program when available.

Asthmatic patients with nasal polyps are often intolerant of aspirin and nonsteroidal anti-inflammatory agents (e.g., for arthritis) and should avoid them. β-Blockers are contraindicated in asthma because they can trigger severe bronchospasm. Regular exercise is recommended and is associated with improved asthma control.

PHARMACOTHERAPY

Asthma medications are usually categorized as *relievers* for acute intermittent symptoms and as *controllers* for long-term maintenance treatment and prevention of the manifestations of asthma (Box 4). Therapeutic plans are suggested by current guidelines, either in the form of a continuum of treatment or using a stepwise approach (see Figure 1). Basically, that medication should be adapted to the severity of the disease, and the minimum amount of drugs and dosage required to keep asthma controlled is a good index of its severity.

Relievers

Fast-acting β_2 agonists, such as the short-acting agents salbutamol, fenoterol, and terbutaline or the long-acting formoterol (in certain patients already using this medication and an inhaled corticosteroid), are used for treating intermittent asthma symptoms. For this purpose, however, they should be used on demand at the least frequent dose possible. A frequent or increasing need for these drugs reveals a loss of asthma control

---

BOX 3 Environmental Measures

- Avoid respiratory irritants, particularly tobacco smoke.
- Minimize exposure to relevant allergens, particularly indoor allergens:
  House dust mites
  - Maintain relative humidity below 50%.
  - Encase mattress and box spring (and possibly pillows) in mite- and mite allergen–impermeable covers.
  - Launder bed linen in hot (55°C [131°F]) water.
  - Remove carpeting whenever possible.
  [*Note*: Air filters do not affect reservoir levels of house dust mite allergens.]
  Pet allergens:
  - Removal of the pet from the home is the most effective approach.
  - Where removal is not possible, the following may decrease airborne pet allergens:
  - Pet exclusion from the bedroom
  - HEPA (high-efficiency particulate air [filter]) room air cleaner
  - Mattress and pillow covers
  - Removal of carpeting
  - Frequent vacuuming of upholstered furniture with a HEPA-filtered vacuum
  - Washing the pet may temporarily reduce allergen load but the allergic individual must not do the washing

Adapted from Boulet et al., 2001. Regular exercise is recommended and is associated with improved asthma control.

BOX 4 Categories of Asthma Medications

Relievers
- Short-acting β_2 agonists
- Formoterol (usually if already used with an inhaled corticosteroid)
- Anticholinergics (if intolerance to β_2 agonists)*

Controllers
- Anti-inflammatory medications
  Corticosteroids: inhaled and systemic
  Nonsteroidal agents: Leukotriene receptor antagonists:
  Omalizumab (Anti-IgE)*
  Cromoglycate and nedocromil (antiallergics)
  Methotrexate, ketotifen*
- Bronchodilators
  Long-acting β_2 agonists
  Theophyllines*

*Rarely prescribed.

12

and/or abuse of the medication and is associated with increased incidence of severe asthma events.

Controllers

Inhaled Corticosteroids

Inhaled corticosteroids (ICSs) are the mainstay of long-term asthma treatment and act at numerous sites of the inflammatory cascade. They should be prescribed for all patients with more than very mild asthma. They help obtain and maintain asthma control by reducing symptoms and improving lung function, decreasing airway responsiveness, preventing asthma exacerbations, and reducing the morbidity and mortality associated with asthma. Most of the benefit is obtained at low to moderate doses. Depending on asthma severity, the dose-response of the therapeutic effect of ICS agents plateaus at moderate to high doses. Table 4 shows the comparative potency of the available agents.

Too much phobia still exists about using corticosteroids. The side effects of low to moderate doses in adolescents and adults are minimal, mostly in the form of occasional dysphonia or oropharyngeal candidiasis, reduced by rinsing the mouth after intake or the use of a spacer. At high doses, they may slightly increase bone loss and possibly, in predisposed groups of patients, produce ecchymosis or promote the development of glaucoma or cataracts. Osteoporosis prophylaxis is not recommended for patients on ICS agents unless they regularly use high doses, particularly with intermittent or regular oral corticosteroids.

Recent studies suggest that introducing an ICS early in the course of the disease may be beneficial because it may reduce asthma-related events; whether this could influence the course of the disease remains to be documented. An ICS cannot be stopped in most asthmatic patients without recurrence of symptoms and reduction in pulmonary function, indicating that the ICS may control the disease but does not induce a long-term remission. A reduction of doses to the minimum that keeps asthma under control is warranted, and if doses higher than low (to sometimes moderate) are needed, there are benefits to adding another controller.

Long-acting β_2 Agonists

The long-acting β_2 agonists (LABAs) salmeterol (Serevent) and formoterol (Oxeze) are now introduced earlier in the asthma treatment plan than before and are an excellent choice as add-on treatment when low to moderate doses of an ICS alone are insufficient to control asthma. Because LABAs have little or no effect on airway inflammation, they should always be taken with a corticosteroid. As monotherapy, they are associated with an increased incidence of severe asthma events. Unlike with short-acting β_2 agonists, their regular use with an ICS leads to improved asthma control in a large number of patients. They improve airway caliber for 12 hours or more and therefore are usually prescribed twice daily. Although they seem to add little to an ICS in mild corticosteroid-naïve patients compared to an ICS alone, in patients already on this last type of medication, even on low doses, they provide an added benefit, even compared to doubling the dose of ICS. A possible synergy with ICS is suggested at the molecular level, but its clinical relevance is not confirmed. Formoterol has a rapid onset of action and could also act as a reliever in patients on ICS already using this medication. The prescription of a combination of ICS and LABA in the same inhaler (combination therapy) may simplify the treatment, improve compliance, and prevent the need for LABA monotherapy. Such formulations may include budesonide and formoterol (Symbicort) or fluticasone and salmeterol (Advair).

Leukotriene Receptor Antagonists

Leukotriene receptor antagonists (LTRAs), such as montelukast (Singulair) and zafirlukast (Accolate), block the effects of leukotrienes, acting as receptor antagonists. Most guidelines consider LTRAs the second best choice for anti-inflammatory treatment of asthma, and they may be useful in those who cannot or will not use inhaled corticosteroids. They may possibly act even better at earlier stages of asthma, and their proposed role in the treatment of rhinitis may improve asthma as well and possibly influence its natural history, although we need more studies to determine if that is the case.

LTRAs may also be prescribed as an add-on therapy to corticosteroids when asthma is not sufficiently controlled. Some patients may like the fact that they are used in an oral form. They are considered very safe. Most of their therapeutic effect is usually seen within the first 2 weeks of treatment. Zafirlukast is given twice daily, should not be taken with food, and interacts with warfarin. Montelukast does not have these limitations and is taken once daily.

Other Medications

So-called antiallergic drugs, such as cromolyn (Intal) and nedocromil (Tilade), are now infrequently prescribed

TABLE 4 Inhaled Corticosteroid Equivalences

Product	Dose, µg/d		
	Low	**Medium**	**High**
BDP pMDI and spacer (CFC)	≤500	501-1000	>1000
BUD Turbuhaler*	≤400	401-800	>800
FP pMDI and spacer	≤250	251-500	>500
FP Diskus†	≤250	251-500	>500
BDP pMDI (HFA)‡	≤250	251-500	>500
BUD wet nebulization§	≤1000	1001-2000	>2000

Note: For children, the consensus group defines low dose as <400 µg of BDP delivered via a pMDI attached to a spacer.
*Budesonide Turbuhaler.
†Fluticasone propionate Diskus.
‡In solution with alcohol (QVAR); other HFA inhalers may provide dose equivalencies similar to BDP delivered with a traditional pMDI.
§Budesonide solution for wet nebulization.
Abbreviations: BDP = beclomethasone dipropionate; BUD = budesonide; FP = fluticasone propionate; HFA = hydrofluoroalkane (propellant); pMDI = pressurized metered-dose inhaler.
Adapted from Boulet LP, Becker A, Bérubé D, et al., on behalf of the Canadian Asthma Consensus Group: Canadian asthma consensus report. Can Med Assoc J 1999;30;161(11 Suppl):S1-S61.

because low doses of ICS agents or LTRAs have replaced them. Furthermore, they have to be taken four times a day. They may still have an adjunct role in the prevention of exercise-induced asthma.

Theophylline has immunomodulatory properties and is suggested as a third choice add-on treatment because it is less effective than LABAs and has a narrow therapeutic window. Ipratropium (Atrovent) and tiotropium (Spiriva) are rarely used for the long-term treatment of asthma unless there is an associated component of chronic obstructive pulmonary disease (COPD). Ipratropium is used in acute asthma and as a reliever in patients intolerant to β_2 agonists.

Omalizumab (Xolair) is a monoclonal antibody that is now available. Although asthma guidelines have not yet evaluated its role in asthma treatment, it could be particularly useful for the treatment of severe allergic asthma. Its cost and the need to be administered subcutaneously may be considered limitations, however.

Oral corticosteroids are required in very few patients today for long-term treatment of severe asthma. Their need should be carefully assessed, dosage kept at the minimum required, and compliance to the other treatments and environmental measures checked. Prophylaxis for osteoporosis is required in these patients. Some immunosuppressive drugs, such as methotrexate, gold salts, and cyclosporine, may reduce oral steroids needs, but their benefits are sometimes small compared to their potential side effects. If considered, they should be used only in specialized centers after extensive evaluation.

Immunotherapy is used variably from one country to another. It is generally reserved for patients in whom environmental measures and medication are insufficient to control the disease adequately. It is more beneficial in allergic rhinitis. Its benefits should be weighed against the possible occurrence of complications (transient increase in asthma, local allergic responses, etc.), its cost, time involvement, and the possibility of achieving control by other means.

Other Measures

An increased prevalence of asthma or asthma-like symptoms is described in the obese patient. Weight loss is associated with an improvement of asthma.

Vaccination for influenza is recommended in asthmatic subjects.

Although some studies suggest the asthmatic's diet should include sufficient antioxidants to help reduce inflammatory responses and that omega 3 (e.g., in fish oil) may have some beneficial effects, no specific dietary measures—other than those dictated by general health principles—are currently recommended, in the absence of a food allergy, which is rare.

Yoga and stress reduction techniques may sometimes improve asthma, but their effect is small.

Controlling Asthma

Asthma control should be assessed regularly and the treatment adjusted accordingly. Box 5 summarizes some

---

BOX 5   Possible Causes of Uncontrolled Asthma
• Wrong diagnosis • Current smoking • Noncompliance with medication • Environmental exposures • Untreated co-morbidities • Chronic obstructive pulmonary disease (COPD) component • Inadequate inhaler technique • Steroid resistance • Severe asthma

of the reasons asthma control may not be achieved. If the cause of this lack of adequate control is uncertain or if asthma is severe, the patient benefits from a referral to an asthma specialist.

FOLLOW-UP

Asthma is a chronic condition and remissions are rare. Regular medical and educational follow-up should be ensured to adjust treatment and repeat the essential information needed to obtain an effective self-management of the disease. Box 6 outlines the ideal elements for follow-up visits.

MANAGEMENT OF EXACERBATIONS

Asthma exacerbations are an important cause of morbidity and health-care costs. Patients should be educated about how to modify their medication according to control criteria, and these guidelines should be summarized in a written action plan. Basically, corticosteroid treatment should be rapidly stepped up (dose more than doubled) until symptoms and expiratory flows improve. If exacerbation is severe, systemic (usually oral) corticosteroids should be prescribed.

BOX 6   Follow-Up Visits
When asthmatic patients are seen at follow-up or unscheduled visits, the following elements should be checked: • Control criteria (symptoms, expiratory flows) • Current treatment: understanding and compliance • Untoward reactions to the medication • Exacerbations, emergency department visits, or hospital admissions • Current exposure to triggers (particularly cigarette smoke, relevant allergens, workplace exposures) • Inhaler technique • Co-morbidities (e.g., rhinitis, GOR) (additional investigation required?) • Possible reassessment of treatment and educational needs • Understanding and use of an action plan to manage exacerbations • New prescriptions; follow-up visit scheduled

Rakel and Bope: *Conn's Current Therapy 2006*.

CURRENT DIAGNOSIS

- The diagnosis of asthma should be confirmed by the objective measures of variable airflow limitation or airway hyperresponsiveness.
- Control of asthma is the main parameter to adjust the treatment and should be assessed regularly according to current guideline criteria, including symptoms and expiratory flows.
- Triggers (particularly relevant allergen exposure, workplace sensitizers, smoking) and co-morbidities (e.g., rhinitis, gastroesophageal reflux) of asthma should be identified.

THE FUTURE OF ASTHMA MANAGEMENT

Asthma in most patients can be well controlled with the available therapies, and most often, insufficient asthma control is because of inadequate treatment and insufficient self-management skills. We should nevertheless improve modes of delivery of asthma care and better integrate evidence-based asthma guidelines into current practice. Asthma education is still not integrated into care enough, and self-management skills should be acquired by those suffering from asthma, including adequate assessment of asthma control from symptoms and ideally occasional measurement of expiratory flows. Goals of treatment should be understood by the patient, and information and advice provided by caregivers should be consistent and their interventions well articulated.

CURRENT THERAPY

- Asthma education, environmental control, and smoking cessation are mandatory for optimal treatment.
- A fast-acting bronchodilator should be available for occasional symptoms and used at the minimal frequency and dosing.
- If asthma symptoms become regular (e.g., every week or more), an anti-inflammatory agent (first choice: inhaled corticosteroid) should be introduced.
- If an inhaled corticosteroid at low to moderate doses is not sufficient to control asthma, after compliance, environmental, inhaler technique, and co-morbidities are checked, an add-on therapy such as an inhaled long-acting β_2 agonist or a leukotriene antagonist should be introduced.
- If asthma is severe or difficult to control, it should be reassessed by an asthma specialist.
- Compliance with therapy and environmental measures, as well as inhaler techniques, should be verified regularly.
- Regular medical and educational follow-up should be ensured.

New medications and procedures are developing that could be useful in the future treatment of asthma. Phosphodiesterase 4 (PDE4) inhibitors are proposed as a means to reduce airway inflammation. Cytokine inhibitors, such as anti–IL-5 and anti–IL-4, are being tested, but results are not conclusive. Other potential therapies include inhaled modulation of the TH_1/TH_2 balance through vaccines or oligonucleotides, as well as more targeted immunotherapy and inhibition of various adhesion molecules, chemokines, and mediators. Bronchothermoplasty is an intriguing new procedure for the treatment of asthma currently in the experimental stage. Finally, progress is being made in the field of gene therapy that may lead to the identification of individuals at risk of developing asthma or better targeting of treatments.

REFERENCES

Abramson MJ, Puy RM, Weiner JM: Allergen immunotherapy for asthma. Cochrane Database Syst Rev 2000;(2):CD001186.
Boulet LP: Asthma guidelines and outcomes. In Adkinson NF, Adkinson Jr NF, Yunginger JW, Busse WW, et al: (eds): Middleton's Allergy Principles and Practice, 6th ed. St. Louis, Mo, Mosby, 2003, pp 1283-1301.
Boulet LP, Becker A, Bérubé D, et al., on behalf of the Canadian Asthma Consensus Group: Canadian asthma consensus report. Can Med Assoc J 1999;30;161(11 Suppl):S1-S61.
Gibson PG, Powell H, Coughlan J, et al: Self-management education and regular practitioner review for adults with asthma (Cochrane Review). Cochrane Database Syst Rev 2003;(1):CD001117.
Global Initiative on Asthma. Available 2005 online at http://www.ginasthma.com
Lemiere C, Bai T, Balter M, et al: Adult Asthma Consensus Guidelines Update 2003. Can Respir J 2004;11(Suppl A):9A-18A.
Masoli M, Fabian D, Holt S, Beasley R: Global Initiative for Asthma (GINA) Program. The global burden of asthma: Executive summary of the GINA Dissemination Committee report. Allergy 2004; 59:469-478.
National Expert Report Guidelines for the Diagnosis and Management of Asthma: Update on selected topics 2002. National Asthma Education and Prevention Program (NAEPP). Available online at http://www.nhlbi.nih.gov/guidelines/asthma/execsumm.pdf
Partridge MR, Hill SR: Enhancing care for people with asthma: The role of communication, education, training and self-management. 1998 World Asthma Meeting Education and Delivery of Care Working Group. Eur Respir J 2000;16:333-348.
Tattersfield AE, Knox AJ, Britton JR, Hall IP: Asthma. Lancet 2002;360:1313-1322.

Asthma in Children

Method of
Jonathan M. Spergel, MD, PhD, and
Matthew I. Fogg, MD

Asthma is the most common childhood chronic disease. However, because there is no specific immunologic, biologic, or physiologic marker for asthma, clinicians must base their diagnosis on a variety of factors, including family history, symptom patterns, risk factors, diagnostic tests, and responses to therapeutic interventions.

"Wheezing" in children is not diagnostic of asthma as infants can wheeze from other causes: structural, cardiac, or viral. Approximately 20% of children younger than age 2 years develop wheezing secondary to viral infections and small airways. As their airways enlarge, a majority of children will stop wheezing, with 15% continuing to wheeze into adolescence with the most severe asthma phenotype. Even though many children "outgrow" their wheezing, approximately 30% of children with asthma develop symptoms within their first year of life, 50% by age 2 years, and 80% by the time they start school. Certain risk factors (discussed below) place the early wheezing infant at risk for continued wheezing or asthma.

Epidemiology and Morbidity

Asthma affects 4.8 million (6.9% prevalence) children younger than age 18 years. There is significant morbidity as a result of asthma. The National Health Interview Survey of 17,000 families found that asthmatic children had 10.1 million missed school days, as well as 200,000 hospitalizations, resulting in 1.9 million days of inpatient care. The prevalence of asthma worldwide, like all allergic diseases, has increased over the last 30 to 50 years. The reasons for this increase in prevalence may relate to increased urban living, proximity to coastal regions, changes in native bacteria flora, exposure to endotoxin, and obesity.

Hospitalization and Mortality

Hospitalization rates for children with asthma gradually increased from 1980 to 1996 and leveled off from 1996 to 1999, with greatest increase in rates occurring in children up to 4 years of age and among black children. Male children 5 to 14 years of age were 1.3 times more likely to be hospitalized than were female children of the same age. Similarly, asthma-related deaths increased from 1980 to 1999, peaking in 1996. Higher mortality rates are found in adolescents and black, non-Hispanic children. The individual risk factors for fatal asthma are similar in children and adults (Box 1).

Risk Factors for Developing Asthma

There is no one cause for asthma. Asthma is a classic multifactorial disease with both genetic and environmental factors. Atopy, perinatal, environmental, genetic, and viral factors are all thought to play a role in development of asthma.

ATOPY

Atopy or allergies are a major risk factor for asthma. Eighty percent to 90% of children with asthma have allergies. Fifty percent of children with atopic dermatitis or eczema (allergies of the skin) develop asthma. Additionally, a family history of allergies, including hay

---

BOX 1   Risk Factors for Fatal Asthma

- Prior intensive care unit, hospitalization, or emergency care visit(s) for asthma in the past year
- Noncompliance
- Previous near-fatal episodes
- Current use of systemic corticosteroids
- Poor access to health care
- Low socioeconomic status
- Psychiatric disease or psychosocial problems
- Passive smoke exposure

---

fever (allergic rhinitis), is a risk factor for asthma in the child.

PERINATAL FACTORS

Prenatal and perinatal risk factors for the development of asthma in inner-city children include lower birth weight and gestational age, oxygen supplementation, and positive-pressure ventilation in the neonatal period. Other risk factors include maternal smoking and no prenatal care.

ALLERGENS

Exposure to high levels of house dust mite allergen in the first year of life increases the risk of developing asthma by the time the child is 5 years of age by threefold. But exposure to animals as a risk factor for asthma is unclear. Studies have found exposure to several cats, dogs or farm animals may decrease the risk for asthma. Nevertheless, once a child is sensitized to animals, exposure to animals is a risk factor for more severe disease and symptoms. These findings indicate that the timing and amount of allergen exposure, as well as the allergen itself, may significantly influence allergic sensitization and possibly asthma as well.

VIRAL INFECTIONS

In infants and children, viruses are the predominant cause of infection-induced wheezing. Lower respiratory tract infections in the first 3 years of life increase the risk of a child's developing asthma when evaluated prospectively at both 6 and 11 years of age, with most infections caused by viruses. However, daycare children have an increased number of lower respiratory illnesses and wheezing but a lower rate of asthma later in childhood. Furthermore, respiratory syncytial virus, the most common cause of bronchiolitis in infancy, was found to be a risk factor for asthma in some studies but not in others. At the current time, it is unclear whether viral infections are a true risk factor for asthma. Again, the exposure and quantity of virus, similar to allergens, have a complex role in the development of asthma.

GENETIC

Family history of asthma or atopy is a marked risk factor for asthma. There is no one individual genetic defect that is responsible for asthma. However, regions have been identified in several genomic screens. The most common identified regions are the cytokine gene cluster of interleukin (IL)-4, IL-13, IL-5, CD14, and granulocyte-macrophage colony-stimulating factor on 5q; major histocompatibility complex (MHC) region on 6p; the high-affinity IgE receptor on 11q13, and chromosomes 12q and 13q. Additionally, genetic polymorphisms in the alpha subunit of the IL-4 receptor, the β-adrenergic receptor, *ADAM33* gene, and the major cell surface receptor for endotoxin (CD14) may further influence disease expression and responses.

SOCIOECONOMIC FACTORS

Poverty itself, independent of coexistent factors such as urban living, is not a risk factor for developing asthma. Children living in poverty are more likely to use an emergency department as a primary care source than are children from higher socioeconomic environments. However, sensitization to cockroach allergen, which is more prevalent in inner-city children, is associated with symptomatic asthma.

ENVIRONMENTAL FACTORS

Exposure to cigarette smoke during pregnancy or second-hand smoke during childhood increased the risk of developing asthma by at least twofold. Exposure to pollution (particulate matter, NO_2, and ozone) from living near a busy highway increased individual asthma symptoms, hospital admissions, and incidence of asthma by at least twofold in several studies in the United States, Europe, and Asia.

The Rise of Asthma and the Hygiene Theory

The increasing prevalence of asthma in westernized cultures, coupled with evidence that factors such as childhood infections, daycare attendance, and microbe exposure may be protective, led to the initial development and later expansion of the "hygiene hypothesis." The theory is that a decrease in exposure to "good dirt and bacteria" leads to lower expression of cytokines designed to fight these infections (Th1 cytokines) with a concomitant increase in Th2 cytokines that promote allergies. Exposure to these bacteria and their endotoxin induce a switch from the native fetal Th2 milieu to a Th1 environment. Other factors that support the "hygiene hypothesis" include (a) decreased asthma rates in individuals with infection from enteric pathogens; (b) decreased asthma rates in children with a greater number of older siblings or who attended daycare during the first 6 months of life with a subsequent increased number of infections; (c) decreased asthma rates with increased environmental endotoxin exposure from farm animals or pets; (d) certain genetic polymorphisms for the major endotoxin receptor CD14 that are associated with decreased asthma rates; and (e) frequent oral antibiotic administration with subsequent alterations in gastrointestinal flora that is associated with increased asthma rates. However, it is not a straightforward change of Th1 cytokines (IL-2 and interferon [IFN]-γ; proinflammatory) to Th2 cytokines (IL-4, IL-5, and IL-13; proallergic) because proinflammatory diseases, such as diabetes and inflammatory bowel disease, are also on the rise. The latest theory is a loss of function of T regulatory cells, which down-regulate both Th1 and Th2 cellular function, leading to an increase of cytokines promoting both types of diseases.

Pathophysiology

The basic finding in asthma is reversible airflow obstruction with airway inflammation. This occurs even in patients with mild asthma and in children. The pathologic changes seen in adult and severe asthma, including connective tissue deposition, intraluminal obstruction, thickened subepithelial collagen, loss of cilia, lymphocyte accumulation, and evidence of mast cell degranulation, have been noted in children as young as 5 years of age.

Additional changes can be seen at the start of persistent symptoms, as bronchoalveolar lavage found increased number of total cells, most significantly lymphocytes, in wheezy infants compared with normal children.

The start of asthma may be in utero; all patients at birth have a Th2 phenotype because of placental factors. Furthermore, studies have found a decreased ability to produce IFN-γ in patients who develop asthma. The decrease in IFN-γ production may shift the lungs toward a Th2 phenotype, resulting in asthma. This process is further propagated in children with atopic dermatitis. In children with atopy and later asthma, the first sign of atopy is often atopic dermatitis. Patients with atopic dermatitis have a Th2 cytokine profile in the skin, as well as systemically. Therefore, patients susceptible to asthma have a Th2 cytokine profile in the lung prior to allergen or viral exposure. The body generates a Th2 response to the allergen or viral stimuli, causing eosinophilia and lymphocyte accumulation. This accumulation along with interaction of the native lung smooth-muscle cells generates the airway obstruction noted in asthma.

Differential Diagnosis

The differential diagnosis of asthma depends on the age of the child. Eighty percent to 90% of asthma patients are atopic and have either allergic rhinitis, atopic dermatitis, food allergy, or a family history of atopy. If a child does not, other diagnoses should be considered. The differential diagnosis for young infants and toddlers includes foreign-body aspiration, gastroesophageal reflux secondary to vagal nerve bronchospasm, viral-induced bronchiolitis, and bronchopulmonary dysplasia. Other rare causes include vascular rings or laryngeal webs, laryngotracheomalacia, tracheal stenosis, bronchostenosis, and enlarged lymph nodes or tumor. Children of any age with frequent lower respiratory infections and wheezing should also be ruled out for cystic fibrosis, dysmotile cilia syndrome, α_1-antitrypsin deficiency, and immunodeficiencies. Vocal cord dysfunction and psychogenic cough should be considered in school-age children or adults with cough who are not responding to therapy.

Diagnosis

HISTORY

A thorough clinical history is extremely important when evaluating a child for the presence of asthma. The patient's baseline level of asthma symptoms is an important factor to consider when making the diagnosis. Specifically, the physician should ascertain the frequency and nature of the symptoms the child is experiencing. (Box 2 lists some important questions to ask.) Families often may ascribe asthma symptoms to other diseases, such as bronchitis or colds. It is important to ask specifically about cough, wheezing, shortness of breath, chest tightness, and sputum/mucus production. The seasonal pattern of symptoms is important in understanding a patient's disease. A patient whose asthma flares in the early spring may be experiencing allergic reactivity to tree pollens as an asthma trigger, while a patient who gets sicker in the winter may be suffering from recurrent rhinovirus-induced flares or flares induced by an indoor aeroallergen.

When evaluating a child for asthma, it is essential to ascertain what factors cause exacerbations of the child's disease. Precipitating factors that should be asked about include respiratory viruses, indoor and outdoor environmental allergens, changes in environment (i.e., new home or daycare), exercise, irritants (tobacco smoke, perfumes, etc.), changes in weather, foods, medications, and strong emotion. It is also important to ascertain the patient's history of disease. The age of onset of respiratory symptoms, history of emergency visits and hospitalizations, intensive care unit admissions, endotracheal intubations, number of steroid courses, and other respiratory conditions are important factors that help the physician to ascertain the severity of the child's disease.

BOX 2   Key Questions in the Diagnosis of Asthma

- Does your child cough, wheeze (a whistling sound when breathing), or have chest tightness or shortness of breath?
- Does your child cough or wheeze with exercise, play, and laughter or during temper tantrums?
- Does your child cough or wheeze after exposure to pets, dust, or other allergens?
- Do colds go right to your child's chest and last longer than 1 week?
- Is your child sick all winter with a cold?
- Is there a family history of asthma or allergies?
- What triggers your child's symptoms—colds, allergens (like the family pet), or exercise?
- Is coughing or wheezing keeping you and your child up at night?

The physician should also attempt to understand the impact of the disease on the life of both the child and the family in terms of missed school for the child or missed work for the caregivers.

The patient's past medical history should be examined, with particular emphasis on symptoms of sinus disease, gastroesophageal reflux, cystic fibrosis, and other allergic diseases, such as rhinitis, conjunctivitis, and atopic dermatitis. As with any medical history, it is important to ascertain a complete family history focusing on atopic diseases in close relatives. A social and environmental history of pets and exposure to cigarette smoke is also important to assess for other asthma risk factors. Finally, the physician should attempt to ascertain the patient's and family's perception of the disease.

PHYSICAL EXAMINATION

A complete and thorough physical examination is essential when evaluating a child for asthma. Attention should be focused on the upper and lower respiratory tracts, as well as on potential allergic disease of other organ systems. Examination of the eyes for conjunctival erythema, cobblestoning, and allergic shiners should be undertaken, as should examination of the nose for mucosal edema, discharge, and an allergic crease, because allergic rhinitis and conjunctivitis are frequent co-morbid conditions with asthma. A purulent nasal discharge and malodorous breath may signify the presence of sinusitis, a condition that may exacerbate asthma. The chest exam should document the patient's respiratory rate, work of breathing, air entry, adventitious breath sounds (wheezes, rales, rhonchi, etc.), symmetry, inspiratory-to-expiratory ratio, and abnormalities of chest configuration (i.e., pectus deformity). An increased anteroposterior diameter of the chest may signify air trapping from asthma. The patient's digits should also be examined for clubbing, which may be seen in a variety of cardiac and pulmonary conditions. The skin should be closely examined for the presence of coexisting atopic dermatitis.

PULMONARY FUNCTION TESTS

While the clinical history and physical exam are extremely important in the diagnosis of asthma, pulmonary function tests, when practical, are extremely important in confirming or excluding the presence of asthma. Pulmonary function tests provide objective data, which can be compared to population normals. The tests take little time, are inexpensive to perform, and can be easily performed in the outpatient setting in children older than 5 years of age. These tests are particularly useful because some families may over- or understate a child's asthma symptoms. Thus, a family who is alarmed that their child is sick and wheezing "all the time" can be comforted by normal spirometry. Conversely, abnormal spirometry documenting the presence of asthma can help a family accept the diagnosis and begin a necessary course of treatment.

Spirometry is an accurate, reproducible way to measure several important pulmonary function parameters. FEV_1 is the forced expiratory volume in 1 second.

A postbronchodilator increase of 12% in FEV_1 confirms the diagnosis of asthma. Additionally, spirometry measures the forced expiratory flow from 25% to 75% of forced vital capacity (FVC). This value is known as $FEF_{25\%-75\%}$. A postbronchodilator increase of 25% in $FEF_{25\%-75\%}$ also confirms the diagnosis of asthma. Spirometry also measures the peak expiratory flow rate (PEFR), which some patients can monitor on an outpatient basis. The PEFR is a notoriously effort-dependent and inconsistent value, however. Consequently, patients must be well trained and know a personal-best reference before using peak flows for home monitoring. Spirometry also measures the FVC, which, in conjunction with FEV_1, can be used to distinguish restrictive from obstructive lung disease.

Other measurements of pulmonary function that can be performed include flow-volume loops, plethysmography (which measures lung volumes and airway mechanics), infant pulmonary function tests, and bronchial provocation tests to methacholine (Provocholine), exercise, cold air, or histamine, which tests are available at asthma specialists or children's medical centers. A detailed description of these methods is beyond the scope of this article.

TESTS FOR ALLERGEN-SPECIFIC IgE

Tests for allergen-specific IgE should be performed on all asthmatic children whose disease level is classified as persistent because 80% to 90% of children with asthma have allergies. Tests for allergen-specific IgE can be performed with a skin-prick test by a practicing allergist. In vitro tests, such as the radioallergosorbent test (RAST), are also available but are less sensitive and specific than skin-prick tests for aeroallergens.

All patients with persistent asthma should be screened for the presence of allergen-specific IgE because exposure to both perennial indoor aeroallergens (e.g., dust mites, cockroaches, cats, dogs, and molds) and outdoor seasonal aeroallergens (e.g., trees, grasses, and weeds) may cause asthma symptoms. Importantly, removing the offending allergen from the patient's environment may significantly improve asthma symptoms and progression of disease. Some allergens, such as pollens, are ubiquitous during certain seasons. Complete avoidance of these pollens may not be possible, but immunotherapy to these allergens often significantly reduces asthma symptoms during pollen seasons. Immunotherapy is also possible for some perennial indoor allergens if avoidance measures are unsuccessful.

OTHER LABORATORY TESTS

Routine chest radiography is rarely necessary for the outpatient management of chronic asthma. Additionally, chest radiography should be reserved in acute asthma for situations where complications such as pneumonia, pneumothorax, or pneumomediastinum are suspected. A sweat test for cystic fibrosis should be performed if the patient has atypical symptoms (e.g., failure to thrive, gastrointestinal [GI] malabsorption, pancreatic insufficiency, recurrent pneumonia, or sinusitis) or physical examination findings (e.g., digital clubbing, failure to thrive, nasal polyps) suggestive of cystic fibrosis. Tests for polymorphisms in the β_2-adrenergic receptor are available in some specialized centers. These polymorphisms may be associated with asthma severity and responses to β-agonist medications such as albuterol (Proventil).

Acute and chronic sinusitis may exacerbate or mimic asthma symptoms. Patients who have congestion and a purulent nasal discharge for greater than 10 days should have a sinus computed tomography (CT) scan performed to evaluate for sinusitis. Additionally, some asthmatics may have chronic sinus disease, which makes controlling their asthma difficult. A sinus CT should also be considered for chronic asthmatics who experience a deterioration in symptoms that does not respond well to aggressive asthma therapy. Another condition that frequently complicates asthma care in children is gastroesophageal reflux disease (GERD). Patients with chronic asthma that fails to respond to therapy, young children and infants with postprandial symptoms, and children with predominantly nocturnal symptoms should be screened for reflux with a barium esophagram and esophageal pH monitoring. Alternatively, some specialists choose to empirically treat for reflux rather than perform diagnostic testing.

Management of Chronic Asthma

The management of chronic asthma requires a proper classification of the patient into a disease severity category. This is best done with the National Asthma Education and Prevention Program (NAEPP) *Guidelines for the Diagnosis and Management of Asthma*. These guidelines classify a patient's asthma by the presence and frequency of day and night symptoms. For children older than age 5 years and adults, spirometry and symptoms are also used to classify the disease. Patients with daytime symptoms more often than twice a week or nocturnal symptoms more frequently than twice a month require low-dose inhaled corticosteroids (ICSs) to control the disease. In addition, a child 5 years or younger with more than three episodes of wheezing in 1 year lasting more than 1 day, and that affects sleep, is classified as mild persistent. In addition, a young child with severe exacerbations less than 6 weeks apart is also considered mild persistent by the NAEPP classifications. Table 1 (and www.nhlbi.nih.gov/guidelines/asthma, appendix A-1) lists the NAEPP guidelines for the management of chronic asthma.

The optimal choice of ICS is a matter of great debate. The choice of ICS is based on a variety of factors including ease of use, bioavailability, potency, and lipophilicity (see www.nhlbi.nih.gov/guidelines/asthma, appendix A-2). The available ICSs (as of January 2004) include beclomethasone (Vanceril), budesonide (Pulmicort), flunisolide (AeroBid), fluticasone (Flovent), and triamcinolone acetate (Azmacort).

Other preventive medications for the treatment of asthma include leukotriene modifiers (montelukast [Singulair], zafirlukast [Accolate], and zileuton [Zyflo]), theophylline (Theo-Dur, Uniphyl), cromolyn (Intal), salmeterol (Serevent), formoterol (Foradil), and

TABLE 1 National Heart, Lung, and Blood Institute Asthma Severity Guidelines

Classify severity before treatment or adequate control	*Symptoms day* symptoms night	PEF$_1$ or FEV$_1$ % of predicted	Daily medications
Step 4: Severe persistent	*Continual* Frequent	<60%	High-dose inhaled corticosteroid (ICS) and long-acting β agonists
Step 3: Moderate persistent	Daily >1 night/wk	60%-80%	Low- to medium-dose ICS and long-acting β agonists Alternatives: High-dose ICS, low- to medium-dose ICS with theophylline (Theo-Dur) or leukotriene modifiers
Step 2: Mild persistent	>2×/wk >2 nights/mo	>80%	Low-dose ICS Alternatives: Leukotriene modifiers, theophylline, cromolyn (Intal), or nedocromil (Tilade)
Step 1: Mild intermittent	<2 *days/wk* <2 nights/mo	>80%	None

nedocromil (Tilade). Salmeterol, leukotriene modifiers, and theophylline have synergistic or additive effects with ICSs without increasing ICS adverse events. Because of these factors and ease of use, the combination of fluticasone and salmeterol (Advair) is the preferred therapy in patients with persistent asthma symptoms per the current guidelines. However, salmeterol and formoterol cannot be used as a monotherapy as they have no anti-inflammatory properties as a monotherapy, whereas the remaining medications can be used as monotherapies. ICSs are more effective than any other preventive medications for the treatment of asthma.

MONITORING PATIENTS ON INHALED CORTICOSTEROIDS

The biggest concern regarding chronic use of ICSs for asthma is the linear growth of children. However, the best studies of this issue show that whereas prepubertal children may experience a transient decrease in growth velocity in the first year of therapy on some ICSs, *children on chronic ICS therapy successfully attain predicted adult height*. Furthermore, it should be emphasized that children with chronic asthma may experience impairment in growth based on their chronic disease process. The physician should chart the child's growth at all visits.

Another concern that has been raised regarding ICSs is the effect on bone mineral density (BMD) in growing children. A large study showed that moderate doses of ICSs did not alter BMD in children 5 to 12 years of age with mild to moderate asthma. ICS-induced clinically relevant hypothalamic-pituitary-adrenal (HPA) axis suppression in children on ICSs is exceedingly rare, as ICS therapy does not alter HPA function in a clinically relevant manner in most children. Finally, the available evidence suggests that ICSs *do not* cause cataracts in children.

There is much fear among parents and some physicians regarding the use of ICSs in childhood asthma. Fortunately, the available evidence supports the safety of ICSs for childhood asthma with regard to long-term growth, HPA axis suppression, BMD, and cataract formation. Parental fears regarding these side effects

should be alleviated by the data in favor of therapy with the most effective medicine for persistent asthma.

Additionally, support of ICSs is the comparison of daily inhaled versus burst of oral corticosteroids (CSs). The dose of 1 year of low-dose ICSs is one fifteenth of the dose of one course of oral steroids (Box 3). We note that there is a difference between short-burst and chronic medications. However, studies show that as few as four short bursts of oral steroids a year increases fracture rate, so short bursts of corticosteroid are not benign. ICSs show a dramatic decrease in the number of asthma exacerbations, which are typically treated with oral steroids. Therefore, for patients requiring oral steroids more often than once a year, daily preventive ICSs are preferred.

OMALIZUMAB

Omalizumab (Xolair) is the newest therapy for the treatment of asthma. It is a recombinant DNA-derived humanized IgG monoclonal antibody to IgE. The subcutaneously injected monoclonal anti-IgE binds circulating free IgE, thereby blocking IgE binding to the high-affinity receptor FcεR$_1$. Randomized, placebo-controlled trials of omalizumab for chronic asthma in patients 12 to 76 years old showed that omalizumab reduced asthma exacerbations even with the use of lower doses of ICSs. In addition, omalizumab significantly improved peak flow rates and forced expiratory volume at 1 second (FEV$_1$), although the increase in the latter was small.

BOX 3 Daily Inhaled Versus Oral Burst Steroids

- Typical 5-day course of oral steroids in a 20-kg child
  2 mg/kg/day for 5 days:
  $2 \times 20 \times 5 = 200$ mg
  Total dose: 200 mg
- One-year course of low-dose ICS
  Assumption: 20% bioavailability of inhaled dose
  Fluticasone 44 µg 2 puffs 2 × per day for 365 days
  $44 \times 2 \times 365 \times 0.2 = 12.8$ mg
- 200 mg/12.8 mg = 15.6 years of daily ICS use

Omalizumab is indicated for patients older than age 12 years with moderate to severe persistent asthma (step 3 or 4) who have a positive skin test or in vitro reactivity to a perennial aeroallergen and whose symptoms are inadequately controlled on ICSs. The patient's pretreatment IgE level should be between 100 and 700 for omalizumab to be considered. Dosing is based on weight and IgE level.

Omalizumab is generally well tolerated and no drug-related serious adverse effects have been reported. Anaphylaxis has occurred within 2 hours of omalizumab administration in less than 0.1% of treated patients. Additionally, malignant neoplasms of different organ systems were observed in 0.5% of patients in the omalizumab group, as compared to 0.2% in the control population. However, the rate of malignancy with omalizumab treatment was no greater than in the general population.

ENVIRONMENTAL CONTROL

Another major treatment for patients with asthma and demonstrable aeroallergen-specific IgE is environmental control. This is particularly important for perennial indoor aeroallergens such as dust mite, cat, dog, cockroach, mouse, and some molds. There is significant evidence that reducing exposure to these allergens in sensitized children will reduce asthma symptoms and improve disease control. Exposure to dust mite allergens can be significantly reduced by using allergy covers for mattresses, box springs, and pillows, with frequent washing of all bedding including blankets. If a patient still has significant symptoms after attempts to reduce dust mite exposure, allergen immunotherapy may reduce or eliminate allergic sensitivity to dust mite and alleviate asthma symptoms.

Household pets frequently are a major cause of asthmatic lung inflammation. At a minimum, patients who are sensitized to a pet should never have the pet in their bedroom. Additionally, efforts should be made to limit the animal's exposure to areas where the child plays and areas with carpeting that may act as a reservoir for animal dander. The only proven method to eliminate exposure to pet dander is removal of the pet from the home. Allergen immunotherapy for household pets

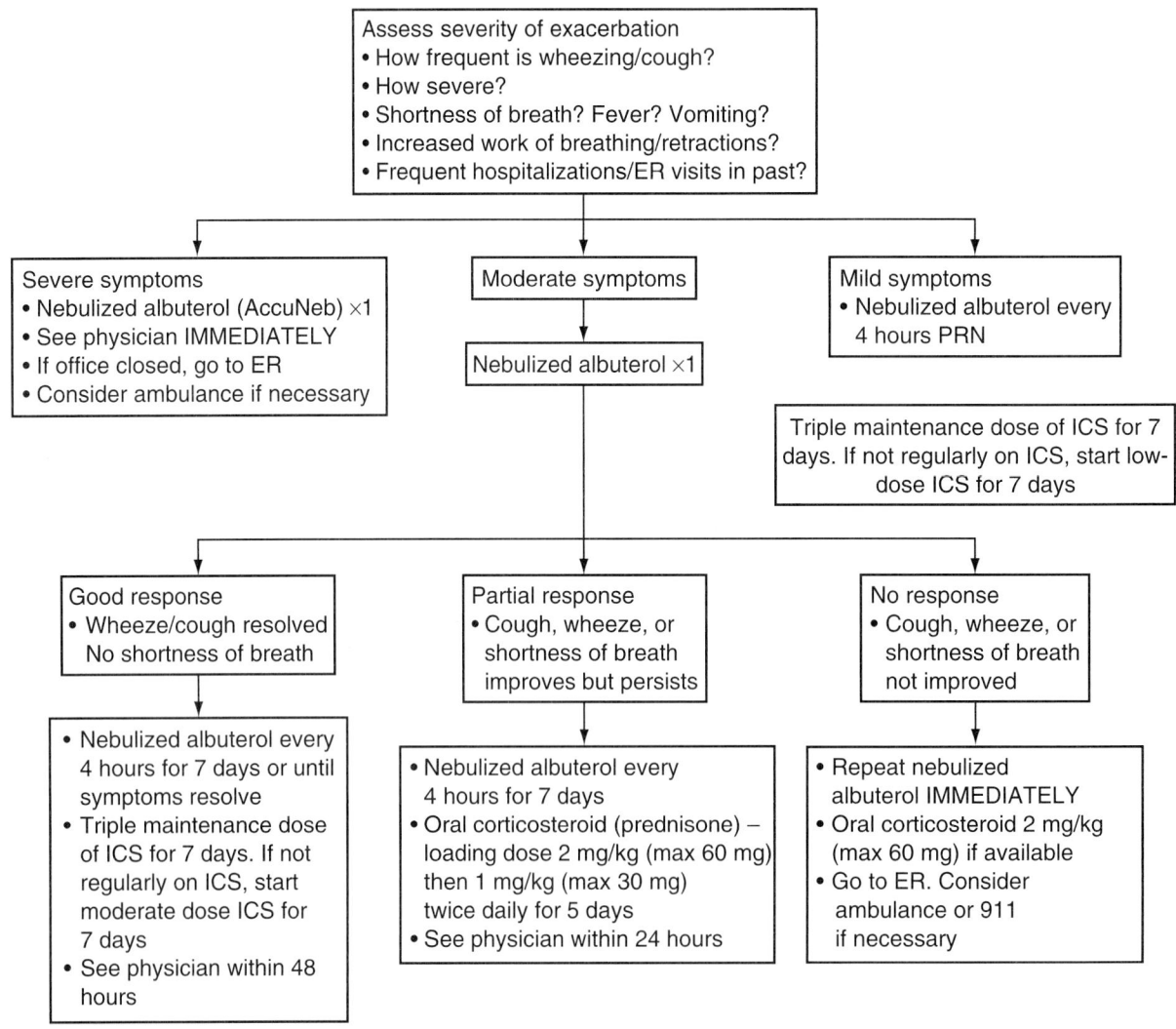

FIGURE 1. Acute asthma exacerbation guidelines for home management based on the current National Asthma Education and Prevention Program of the National Heart, Lung, and Blood Institute. ER=emergency department; ICS=inhaled corticosteroids; PRN=as needed.

Rakel and Bope: *Conn's Current Therapy 2006.*

is controversial. Extermination efforts to reduce exposure to household pests such as cockroaches or mice should be undertaken in all households with children sensitized to these allergens. However, families should be warned not to purchase a cat to eliminate mice, as a child sensitized to mouse will likely become sensitized to cats as well.

Environmental tobacco smoke has been proven to increase the incidence of asthma and otitis media as well as induce airway hyperreactivity, exacerbate lung function, and increase asthma symptoms. Simply stated, children with asthma should never be exposed to tobacco smoke.

IMMUNOTHERAPY

Allergen immunotherapy has been shown to be extremely effective for allergic rhinitis. Its role in asthma care is less clear. A recent meta-analysis performed by the Cochrane group concluded that there is strong evidence that allergen-specific immunotherapy significantly reduces asthma symptoms, rescue medication use, and

airway hyperreactivity. However, the review suggested that these benefits should be weighed against the risks of immunotherapy (anaphylaxis). Given the low risk of anaphylaxis from immunotherapy, it should be considered for patients with documented allergen-specific IgE whose asthma is not well controlled using medications and avoidance measures. It should be strongly considered for asthmatics with significant allergic rhinitis.

EDUCATION

Asthma education for both child and family is an extremely important component of asthma care. Education should address several key issues regarding asthma including: the pathophysiology of disease, symptoms of acute and chronic asthma, the importance of proper medication use and compliance, reduction of allergic and irritant triggers, and when to contact the provider. Patients may not have familiarity with using respiratory devices such as spacers, discus devices, and nebulizers. Effective medicine delivery depends on the

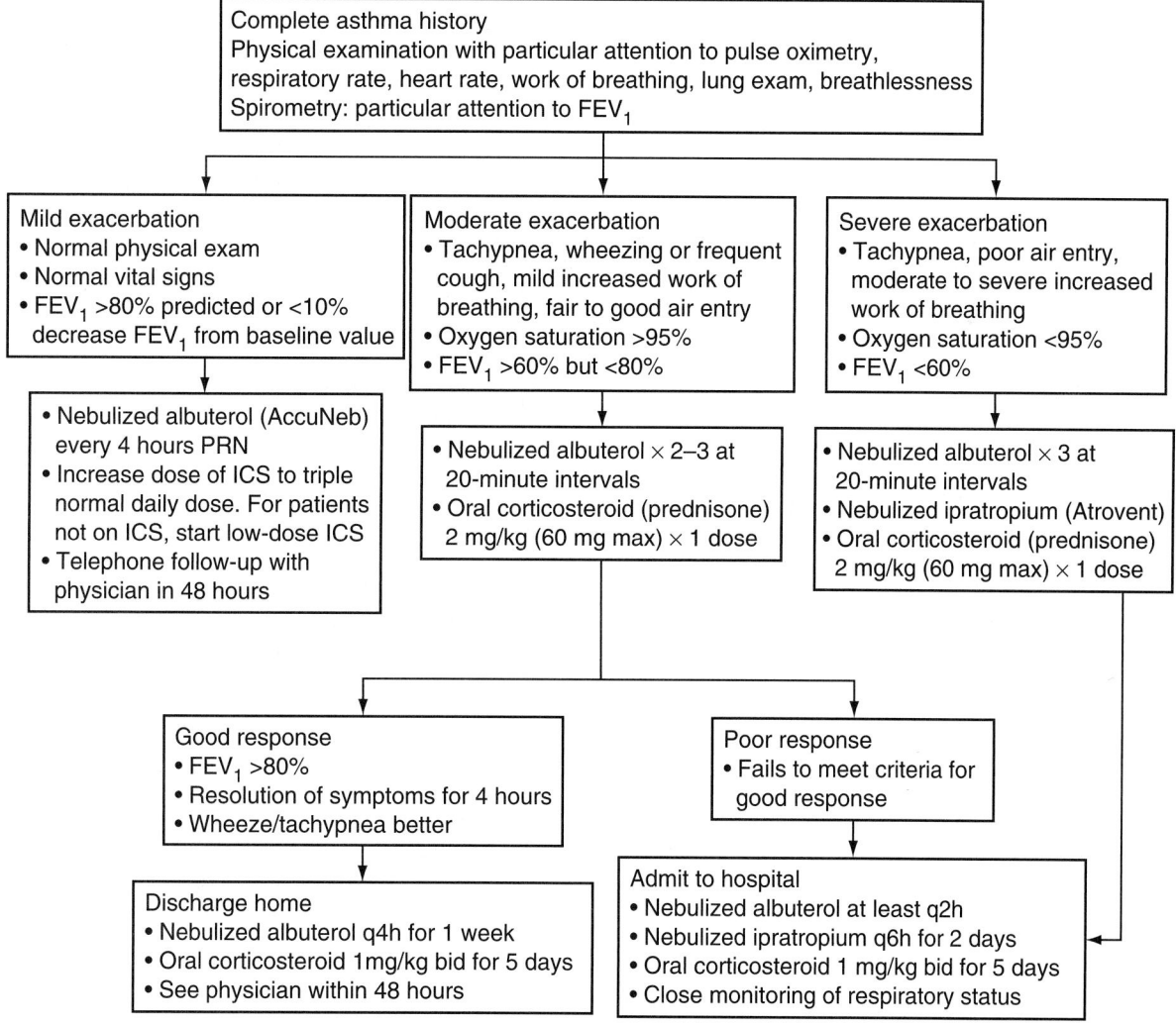

FIGURE 2. Acute asthma exacerbation guidelines for physician office management based on the current National Asthma Education and Prevention Program of the National Heart, Lung, and Blood Institute. FEV$_1$=forced expiratory volume in 1 second; ICS=inhaled corticosteroid; PRN=as needed.

Rakel and Bope: *Conn's Current Therapy 2006.*

technique of medication administration. Teaching families to recognize early symptoms of an acute exacerbation is also important because early recognition of an asthma flare allows a family to intensify asthma treatment before the exacerbation has become severe. Families should also be taught that, under optimal control, asthma should not cause symptoms and should not limit the child's activities or life in any way.

Most patients with asthma should have a written asthma management plan that includes medicines the child should be using every day (if any) as well as how to manage an acute exacerbation. These asthma "action plans" help families treat their children at the onset of an exacerbation. Although there is not a lot of literature in support of the practice, the use of written asthma management plans is very common among asthma specialists and is becoming increasingly common among primary care physicians.

Management of Acute Exacerbations

HOME MANAGEMENT

Home management of asthma exacerbations via telephone is often extremely difficult. Some families are excellent at judging the severity of symptoms with telephone guidance. Others may under- or overestimate the severity of symptoms. For these patients daily peak flow monitoring is helpful. Figure 1 provides a childhood asthma home management algorithm. It should be stressed that if the parents are uncomfortable about their child's respiratory status, they should see a physician immediately.

OFFICE MANAGEMENT

Most providers are more comfortable with office management of acute exacerbations because the physician can examine the child and perform spirometry. Figure 2 shows a childhood asthma office/emergency department management algorithm. Antibiotics are not recommended for acute management of asthma exacerbations in the absence of signs or symptoms of pneumonia.

Asthma is the most common chronic disease of childhood. It is responsible for an enormous amount of health care costs, hospitalizations, emergency department visits, outpatient visits, and mortality. In addition, many children live with poorly controlled or uncontrolled asthma symptoms without access to or treatment with inhaled corticosteroids. Aggressive, early treatment with ICSs of any child with daytime asthma symptoms that occur more often than twice a week, or with nocturnal symptoms that occur more often than twice a month, should be undertaken to improve asthma symptoms and lung function, as well as to reduce the need for acute care and hospitalizations. In addition, allergic triggers and other irritants such as environmental tobacco smoke should be removed from the asthmatic child's home. With good asthma care, the asthmatic child should be able to lead a normal life.

Allergic Rhinitis

Method of
Michael Wein, MD

Rhinitis, an inflammatory disorder of the mucous membranes of the nose and related structures, can be allergic, nonallergic, or both. Rhinitis affects almost 20% of the U.S. population, and the annual economic impact is enormous—billions of dollars spent on prescriptions, office visits, missed work, and lost productivity. Although not associated with hospitalization or surgery, allergic rhinitis significantly impacts quality of life. The increase in allergic diseases has been explained by the *hygiene hypothesis*: A decline in the prevalence of childhood infections and a cleaner home environment results in a shift of T-helper lymphocytes away from expressing the Th1 set of cytokines, which enhance antimicrobial activity, in favor of a second, or Th2, set of cytokines, which up-regulate allergic responses.

Pathogenesis

Sensitization by allergen induces production of allergen-specific IgE by B cells. IgE binds to mast cells in the nasal mucosa. Further allergen exposure triggers the *early-phase* response with release of histamine, chymase, and tryptase, and initiates a *late-phase* response with production of leukotrienes, prostaglandins, cytokines, bradykinin, platelet-activating factor, and other mediators. These mediators produce itching, sneezing, nasal discharge, sinus pressure, and nasal congestion, as well as systemic symptoms of fatigue, irritability, and reduced concentration.

Once the immune system is *primed,* a magnified response may be seen on subsequent exposure with the same amount of allergen. Nonspecific hyperreactivity to a wide range of allergic and nonallergic triggers may also result, which explains the reaction to strong odors, smoke, spicy foods, alcohol, or changes in temperature and relative humidity seen in allergic individuals.

Evaluation of Rhinitis

Most patients present to the physician after antihistamines have failed. At this point a careful and complete history should include the nature of symptoms and their severity pattern of symptom progression, duration, seasonality, exacerbating and alleviating factors, response to self-treatment, co-morbid conditions, occupational and avocational exposures, medication history, family history, and identification of other notable environmental factors. Published questionnaires can help the physician more rapidly acquire the large amount of data needed to optimally treat rhinitis patients.

The history should include impact on daily activities and effect of treatment on various symptoms (Box 1).

BOX 1 Symptoms of Allergic Rhinitis

Primary
- Itching of the nose (and eyes, ears, throat)
- Sneezing
- Rhinorrhea
- Nasal congestion

Secondary
- Mouth breathing
- Headache
- Sore throat
- Postnasal drip
- Cough
- Anosmia or hyposmia
- Eustachian tube dysfunction
- Sleep apnea or sleep disturbance
- Fatigue
- Halitosis

Include questions about anosmia, snoring, sleep problems, fatigue, and cough. The differential diagnosis includes acute infections, structural problems, hormonal factors, and side effects from medications (Box 2).

When history suggests outdoor symptoms, the physician should suspect pollen and mold. Although there is great variability across regions, tree pollen is released during the spring, grass pollen peaks in early summer, and weed pollen peaks in late summer or early fall. Some species are entomophilous (pollinated by insects and not by wind), so they do not contribute significantly. Pollen levels are tracked by the National Allergy Bureau (http://aaaai.org/nab/index.cfm?p=pollen/). Mold or fungi are also found outdoors almost year-round, and counts are affected by temperature, humidity, wind, and precipitation. In dry weather *Alternaria* and *Cladosporium* may predominate outdoors; in wet weather *Fusarium*, *Phoma*, and *Cephalosporium* may increase.

BOX 2 Selected Causes of Nasal Symptoms

Allergic sensitivity
  Pollen: trees, grasses, weeds
  Mold: indoor and outdoor
  Dust mites
  Animal dander
  Cockroaches
  Occupational allergens
- Infection (viral, bacterial, fungal)
- Hormonal (e.g., hypothyroidism, pregnancy, contraceptives)
- Anatomic (e.g., septal deviation, concha bullosa, foreign body)
- Granulomatous (e.g., Wegener's, midline granuloma, sarcoidosis)
- Vasomotor (e.g., temperature, humidity)
- Pharmacologic (e.g., antihypertensives, aspirin, rhinitis medicamentosa)
- Trauma (e.g., cerebrospinal fluid rhinorrhea)
- Neoplastic (e.g., inverted papilloma, squamous carcinoma)
- Other (ciliary dysmotility, nonallergic rhinitis with eosinophilia)

When symptoms predominate indoors, mold, pets, or dust mites may be responsible. The growth of indoor mold such as *Penicillium* and *Aspergillus* is influenced by many factors, but relative humidity is of primary concern. All warm-blooded animals are capable of producing allergen, including birds and farm animals, but cat allergen is especially ubiquitous, can remain airborne for prolonged periods, and is inadvertently transported to sites without cats, leading to significant levels even in hospital corridors, schools, and shopping malls. The major source of allergen in house dust is the fecal residue of dust mites, which tends to be highest in the bedroom, especially in carpets, bedding, and upholstery. Particles carrying dust mite allergens are relatively heavy and remain airborne for roughly 30 minutes and should be suspected if symptoms worsen shortly after a disturbance such as vacuuming.

Recent Allergic Rhinitis and its Impact on Asthma (ARIA) guidelines discourage the classification of seasonality and distinguish intermittent from persistent rhinitis, with the latter indicating symptoms more than 4 days per week and more than 4 weeks per year (Box 3). This change reflects the concept of a minimal persistent mucosal inflammation in patients who are continuously exposed to relevant allergens. In such patients, even a slight additional swelling of the nasal mucosa might lead to complete obstruction, whereas the same degree of additional swelling might go unnoticed by patients without baseline edema. Both intermittent and persistent rhinitis can be mild or moderate to severe, with the latter indicating symptoms that interfere with work, school, leisure, or sleep. The temporal nature, severity of rhinitis, and impairment of daily activities are important historical points and should guide therapy. In particular, the physician should consider the impact of disease on quality of life by inquiring about changes in work habits, limitations in recreational activity, social functioning, energy level, mood, ability to concentrate, and sense of well-being.

BOX 3 ARIA Symptom Classification*

Frequency	
Intermittent	**Persistent**
<4 days per week *or* <4 weeks per year	>4 days per week *and* >4 weeks per year
Severity	
Mild	**Moderate/Severe**
Normal sleep	Abnormal sleep
Normal daily activities	Impaired activities
	• sports/leisure
	• work/school problems
No troublesome symptoms	Troublesome symptoms

*Classification is based on untreated patients and adapted from World Health Organization guidelines on Allergic Rhinitis and its Impact on Asthma.

A history of other allergic diseases, especially asthma, is helpful and relates to the concept of inflammation throughout the airway representing a single allergic disease process. Roughly 50% to 80% of patients with asthma have rhinitis, and 25% of patients with rhinitis have asthma. Exacerbations of rhinitis often trigger asthma, whereas treatment of rhinitis frequently leads to improved control of asthma.

Physical Examination

Physical findings may be nonspecific. Nasal mucosa often appears swollen, with a blue tinge and enlarged turbinates. Other findings include conjunctival injection, chemosis, lacrimation, infraorbital creases (Dennie-Morgan lines), infraorbital edema (allergic shiners), middle ear effusion, and a transverse nasal crease from excessive rubbing. Chronic mouth breathing may result in the typical allergic face with a high arched palate, narrow maxillary arch, and greater anterior facial height. Other findings may include nasal polyps and giant papillae or cobblestone appearance of the tarsal conjunctiva.

Diagnostic Testing

Skin testing to detect cell-bound allergen-specific IgE is the best evidence of an allergic basis. Skin testing is accurate, cost-effective, and safe and provides immediate results to guide treatment. Testing can be done with plastic devices rather than needles, rendering the test almost painless. Less accurate and more expensive blood tests to detect circulating IgE are available if the patient has extensive skin disease. Except for children under age 4, most patients with allergic rhinitis will be found to react to multiple inhalant allergens. Testing blood for total IgE is unhelpful because up to 50% of patients with allergic rhinitis have normal IgE levels, and up to 20% of nonallergic patients have elevated total IgE. Blood testing for allergen-specific IgG or IgG_4 antibodies has no value in the diagnosis of allergic rhinitis.

THERAPY

Therapy for rhinitis includes environmental control, pharmacotherapy, and immunotherapy (Box 4). Allergen avoidance should be stressed because it is safe and relatively inexpensive. Reducing exposure to outdoor allergens such as pollen and mold is often impractical, but patients may find improvement if they decrease the time outdoors, especially in the morning or on windy days with low humidity. Physicians should focus on the indoor environment because it is more easily altered. Americans spend a greater portion of time indoors, and the exposure is year-round and at high allergen levels. In addition, reduction of exposure to indoor allergens may reduce reactivity even to outdoor allergens by limiting nonspecific hyperreactivity.

BOX 4   Management Options for Allergic Rhinitis

- Avoidance
- Immunotherapy (desensitization with allergy vaccine)
- Pharmacotherapy
  Intranasal anticholinergics (ipratropium [Atrovent 0.03%])
  Intranasal antihistamines
  Intranasal cromolyn (NasalCrom)
  Intranasal decongestants
  Intranasal glucocorticoids
  Intranasal saline
  Oral antihistamine–decongestant combinations
  Oral antihistamines
  Oral antileukotrienes
  Oral decongestants
  Oral glucocorticoids

Avoidance

Emphasis should be placed first on the removal of allergen sources, next on the elimination of reservoirs, and only as a last resort on removal of the free allergen itself. This makes sense because houses usually contain, in total, many milligrams of pure allergens, of which only a few nanograms (i.e., <0.001%) may be airborne at any one time. Allergen is thus replaced even if all the airborne allergen is removed from the air, just as the water is replaced if it is pumped out of a leaking boat.

Indoor mite allergen levels are reduced if relative humidity is kept below 50%. Encasing pillows and mattresses with allergen-impermeable covers, removing carpeting, and laundering with water temperature at least 55°C (130°F) may also decrease mite allergen levels (Box 5). Although mean mite allergen concentrations of 20 to 40 µg/g of dust are often observed, meticulous allergen control to levels below 2 µg/g of dust may result in dust mite skin tests becoming negative over a period of 2 to 3 years.

Many interventions to reduce mite allergens are destined for futility. Washing in 37°C (98.6°F) water with detergent and bleach kills only a portion of dust mites, which can recolonize. Reliance on chemical intervention is not recommended; although benzyl benzoate

---

BOX 5   Strategies for Avoidance of Indoor Dust Mite Allergens

- Decrease ambient humidity below 50%, using a dehumidifier and hygrometer
- Encase pillow and mattress in mite-impermeable covers
- Remove carpeting
- Remove ceiling fans
- Remove feather pillows and stuffed animals
- Remove upholstered furniture and drapery from bedrooms
- Use vacuum and consider HEPA filter attachment
- Wash bedding weekly in hot water (at least 130°F [55°C])

Abbreviations: HEPA = high-efficiency particulate air.

(Acarosan)[1] kills dust mites, the allergen remains present. Tannic acid denatures mite allergen, but the mites are not killed and can produce more allergen. Neither residential air-cleaning devices nor ozone generators have clinical efficacy.

Among pets cat allergen has been the most intensively studied. Production of allergen varies widely between animals and over time. There are no allergen-free breeds of cats or dogs, but a cat genetically deficient in the major cat allergen has been experimentally designed and bred. Cat shedding of allergen is not reduced by washings, Allerpet-C spray, or acepromazine (PromAce).* Studies demonstrate that using a new high-efficiency particulate air (HEPA) filter vacuum cleaner actually increased inhaled allergen, probably by recruiting allergen from the carpet acting as a reservoir. Even high-quality air filtration is less effective in the presence of carpets. Cat allergen from saliva, urine, and dander is associated with small particles (<5 μm), remains airborne for days, and can be reduced by a combination of a HEPA room air filter, carpet removal, and cat exclusion from the bedroom.

Air conditioners and dehumidifiers may inhibit the growth of indoor mold, such as *Aspergillus* and *Penicillium*. Fungal studies found inconsistencies and inadequacies in exposure and outcome measures, and mold abatement efforts may yield mixed results. Fungicidal agents are commercially available, and as with most allergens, emphasis should be placed on reducing or eliminating the source—eliminate moisture or fungal contamination whenever possible.

Air-treatment devices, especially ionizers and ozone generators, have not shown clinical benefit in well-controlled studies; nevertheless, these products are heavily advertised. Reliance on clean air delivery rate (CADR) is insufficient. Furthermore, air filters that hang around the neck barely reduce particle concentration in the surrounding air.

Pharmacotherapy

Most patients have already self-medicated with over-the-counter first-generation antihistamines to reduce itching, sneezing, and rhinorrhea with minimal effect on congestion. Although histamine may increase vascular permeability, vasodilation, mucosal blood flow, and goblet cell secretion, histamine is only one of many mediators involved, and it is not surprising that symptoms often persist despite antihistamine use. Antihistamines tend to be less effective if taken after exposure to the relevant allergen, and they are also less effective for nonallergic rhinitis. Although many studies show differences in antihistamine-induced wheal suppression, receptor binding affinity, and onset of action, many of these parameters are only weakly associated with

clinical efficacy. For example, one pill of astemizole (Hismanal)[2] may eliminate the skin-test wheal response for days with virtually no parallel reduction of symptoms. Studies show that patients are often unaware of cognitive and performance impairment with first-generation antihistamines, leading many to drive cars with reaction times equivalent to someone who is legally drunk. In addition to visual–motor impairment, multiple studies show that first-generation antihistamines impair children's learning and academic performance. It is noteworthy that the time to onset of clinically important relief with nonsedating antihistamines has a median of 60 to 148 minutes, depending on the agent used, quite a bit longer than the first-generation.

Safety, side-effect profile, and dosing interval lead physicians to choose second- instead of first-generation antihistamines. Second-generation antihistamines also lack many drug interactions and cause no significant anticholinergic effects. Clinical studies show only minimal improvement when the FDA-recommended dose is exceeded, so there is little reason to ingest more than the recommended dose. Tachyphylaxis generally does not occur, and the peak effect of most occurs at approximately 5 to 7 hours after a single oral dose. Those with known risk of cardiac arrhythmia have already been withdrawn from the U.S. market. Each has a unique profile; for example, cetirizine (Zyrtec) is technically a second-generation antihistamine despite sedation in 15% of patients, tends to be excreted in the urine rather than metabolized in the liver, and has some interesting anti-inflammatory properties, especially at higher doses (Table 1).

Intranasal antihistamines are at least as effective as oral antihistamines, and may have a somewhat faster onset of action, but 11.5% report somnolence with azelastine (Astelin), the only FDA-approved antihistamine for intranasal use. Third-generation antihistamines such as desloratadine (Clarinex) and tecastemizole (Soltara)[2] may show some mild improvement of congestion, but the latter is not yet FDA approved. Other antihistamines in the pharmaceutical pipeline include levocetirizine (Xyzal),* oral ketotifen (Zaditor), oxatomide (Tinset),* levocabastine nasal spray,* and mizolastine (Mizollen).* Mizolastine (Mizollen)* is approved for use in Europe, shows significant benefit on congestion, and inhibits the production of leukotrienes.

Oral decongestants reduce congestion, but insomnia and nervousness limit their utility. Phenyl-propanolamine was withdrawn from the market because of an association with stroke in women, and pseudoephedrine (Sudafed) and phenylephrine (AH-chew D) must be used with caution in patients with hypertension, glaucoma, or thyroid or cardiac disease. The latter medication has extremely poor oral bioavailability.

Nasal decongestants can lead to rapid rebound nasal congestion and tachyphylaxis and should generally be avoided. Nasal cromolyn (NasalCrom) is extremely safe but only minimally effective and must be used four to

---

[1]Not FDA approved for this indication.
*Not yet approved for human use in the United States. For animals only.

*Investigational drug in the United States.
[2]Not available in the United States.

Rakel and Bope: *Conn's Current Therapy 2006.*

TABLE 1   Second-Generation Antihistamines

Generic (trade)*	Minimum age indication	Usual adult dose	Pregnancy category	Dose in renal Impairment	Dose in hepatic impairment	Incidence of somnolence[†]	Onset of action	Pediatric dose
Cetirizine (Zyrtec)	6 mo	10 mg qd	B	5 mg qd	5 mg qd	13.7% (6.3%)	<1 h	2-5, 0.5 tsp
Fexofenadine (Allegra)	6 y	60 mg bid or 180 mg qd	C	60 mg qd	NC	1.3% (0.9%)	1 h	(2, 5 mg) qd Under 12, 30 mg bid
Loratadine (Claritin)	2 y	10 mg qd	B	10 mg qod	10 mg qod	8% (6%)	1-3 h	Under 6, 1 tsp (5mg) qd
Azelastine (Astelin)	5 y	2 sprays bid	C	NC	NC	11.5% (5.4%)	2-3 h	
Desloratadine (Clarinex)	12 y	5 mg qd	C	5 mg qod	5 mg qod	2.1% (1.8%)	<1 h	

*Levocetirizine (Xyzal) and tecastemizole (Soltara) are not yet FDA approved and are not included in the table.
[†]Somnolence data in parentheses is for placebo.
Abbreviations: bid = twice daily; NC = no change; qd = daily; qod = every other day.

six times daily. In addition, it is only effective if used before allergen exposure. Nasal ipratropium bromide (Atrovent 0.03%) is effective for the treatment of rhinorrhea but has no effect on other symptoms.

Leukotriene receptor antagonists are significantly less effective than intranasal corticosteroids for allergic rhinitis, even in combination with antihistamines. Studies show that montelukast (Singulair) is roughly as effective as second-generation antihistamines. Combination of montelukast (Singulair) with antihistamines is less effective than nasal corticosteroids alone, and it is not effective in perennial allergic rhinitis. Although it might seem plausible to use antileukotrienes to treat rhinitis when asthma is also present, standard treatment of rhinitis with many other medications has already been shown to improve asthma control and reduce emergency department visits for asthma in a dose-dependent manner.

Intranasal steroids are the cornerstone of pharmacologic management for allergic rhinitis, but they are less effective for ocular symptoms. One study showed that 78% of patients obtain at least moderate relief with nasal corticosteroids, compared with 58% for second-generation antihistamines. In vitro, budesonide (Rhinocort) and fluticasone (Flonase) have the highest pharmacologic potency based on receptor-binding affinity studies and topical vasoconstrictor potency, but this does not correlate directly with clinical efficacy. Mometasone (Nasonex) has the lowest age indication, down to age 2 years, and has extremely low systemic bioavailability. All require prolonged use over weeks to achieve optimal effectiveness, but some studies do show benefit with initial use, suggesting a very limited role for as-needed use. Choosing among the various intranasal steroids also requires a consideration of patient preference as well as characteristics of the preparation itself (Table 2). The dose-response curve for intranasal steroids plateaus, and if a low dose is ineffective, then further increases are likely to increase side effects such as epistaxis without any significant clinical benefit. If one nasal steroid is

TABLE 2   Nasal Corticosteroid Formulations

Generic (trade)	Minimum age	Usual adult dose per nostril spray	Dose frequency	Intranasal bioavailability (%)*	Pediatric dose
Beclomethasone dipropionate (Vancenase AQ 42)	6 y	1 or 2	bid	44	(<12 y, 1 spray bid)
Fluticasone (Flonase)	4 y	1 or 2	qd	0.5-2.0	(4-12 y, 1 spray qd)
Triamcinolone (Nasacort AQ)	6 y	2	qd	46	(6-12 y, 1 spray qd)
Flunisolide (Nasalide, Nasarel)	6 y	2	bid/tid	49	(6-14 y, 1 spray tid)
Mometasone (Nasonex)	2 y	2	qd	0.1	(3-12 y, 1 spray qd)
Budesonide AQ (Rhinocort Aqua)	6 y	1 or 2	qd	34	(Over 6 y no change)

Note that higher doses occur along the plateau of the dose–response curve. As a result, higher-than-recommended doses tend to cause increasing side effects without much improved therapeutic benefit.
Patients should taper to the lowest effective maintenance dosage to minimize systemic effects. All are pregnancy category C, but budesonide nasal spray is category B. Ciclesonide has not yet been approved by the FDA.
*Bioavailability studies were not based on direct comparison in a single study; data are not to be interpreted otherwise.
Abbreviations: bid = twice daily; qd = daily; tid = three times per day.

ineffective, it is unlikely that another will yield significantly better results for the same patient.

The FDA requires all nasal steroids to carry a warning regarding growth suppression. Except for intranasal dexamethasone (Decadron Turbinaire),[2] the risk of significant systemic side effects with nasal corticosteroids is minimal, although testing of corticotrophin-releasing hormone can reveal subtle changes in the hypothalamic-pituitary axis. Other demonstrations of systemic side effects with nasal steroids are linear growth suppression in children 6 to 9 years old with intranasal beclomethasone (Vancenase) taken for 1 year, decreased overnight urinary cortisol levels in healthy volunteers with a 4-day course of fluticasone (Flonase) 200 mg per day, and a slight increase in the prevalence of cataracts with high cumulative lifetime doses (>2000 µg) of inhaled corticosteroids. The physician must watch for rare cases of septal perforation. High doses of inhaled corticosteroid therapy used to treat asthma are another reason to use the lowest effective dose and titrate down whenever possible.

Prolonged use of oral steroids is not a viable option because of the risk of cataracts, osteoporosis, glaucoma, hypertension, glucose intolerance, and aseptic necrosis. Rare individuals may be more susceptible even to intranasal steroids.

Allergen Vaccines (Desensitization)

Allergen immunotherapy is the injection of a vaccine against relevant allergens and is a safe and highly effective treatment to relieve or eliminate allergic rhinitis, is the only treatment able to alter the natural course of the disease, and may even prevent the onset of asthma in some cases. It is usually reserved for patients with persistent symptoms, at least moderate in severity, who have failed other treatment options (Box 6). At the cellular level, allergen vaccination blocks the seasonal rise in IgE, decreases histamine release, prevents recruitment of inflammatory cells, reduces the number of mast cells in tissue, and reduces cytokine production. Clinically, allergen vaccination can improve allergic symptoms, reduce medication use, and increase pulmonary function. Although effective in 85% to 90% of patients, if a clinical response is not seen within the

---

[2]Not available in the United States.

BOX 6 **Considerations for Allergen Immunotherapy**
• Desire for long-lasting relief without medication • Excessive medication use • Inadequate control with allergen avoidance and pharmacotherapy • Intolerable medication side effects • Unavoidable exposure

first 12 months, then immunotherapy is usually stopped. Immunotherapy should generally not be administered to children under age 5 years, to patients using β-blockers, or to those experiencing an acute asthma exacerbation because of the risk of anaphylaxis. Effectiveness requires experienced practitioners exercising careful attention to allergen selection, dosing, and administration. It may be safely continued during pregnancy but should not be initiated in pregnant patients. Data based on Medicare's Resource-Based Relative Value Scale indicate that allergen immunotherapy is cost-effective. After a maintenance level is reached, the frequency of injections can be reduced to one injection every 1 to 3 weeks. A course of 3 to 5 years is usually sufficient to induce a remission that can persist for years, even after injections are discontinued.

Pregnancy

Pregnant patients with rhinitis represent a special challenge, especially because uncontrolled rhinitis may exacerbate asthma and affect pregnancy outcome. Although intranasal cromolyn (NasalCrom) is first-line therapy in this situation, most patients will require additional treatment, either with an antihistamine from pregnancy category B (e.g., chlorpheniramine [Chlor-Trimeton], loratadine [Claritin], cetirizine [Zyrtec]) or an intranasal corticosteroid. The most desirable corticosteroids would be either beclomethasone (Vancenase), because of its long record of use, or budesonide (Rhinocort), which was suggested for use in pregnancy by the American College of Obstetrics and Gynecology. Ipratropium (Atrovent nasal spray), lodoxamide (Alomide ophthalmic solution), and montelukast (Singulair) are also pregnancy category B but are not widely used in this situation because of limited clinical experience in pregnancy and less utility than the other options noted previously. Avoidance becomes more important in this situation, and as noted patients should not increase or initiate immunotherapy while pregnant.

Future Therapy

The FDA has approved a monoclonal antibody, anti-IgE injection (omalizumab [Xolair]),[1] which can reduce asthma exacerbations by more than 40% in patients already treated optimally with inhaled steroids for asthma. Anti-IgE similarly reduces symptoms in patients with rhinitis already treated optimally with allergen immunotherapy. At the time of this writing, it is not expected to be approved for use in allergic rhinitis, and I would not recommend off-label use. Perhaps the most exciting rhinitis research involves vaccines using allergen genes, antisense single-stranded DNA, or synthetic CpG deoxynucleotides that mimic microbial DNA and are able to down-regulate Th2 responses through toll-like receptor 9. Future approaches to block the recruitment

---

[1]Not FDA approved for this indication.

KEY TREATMENT ALGORITHM

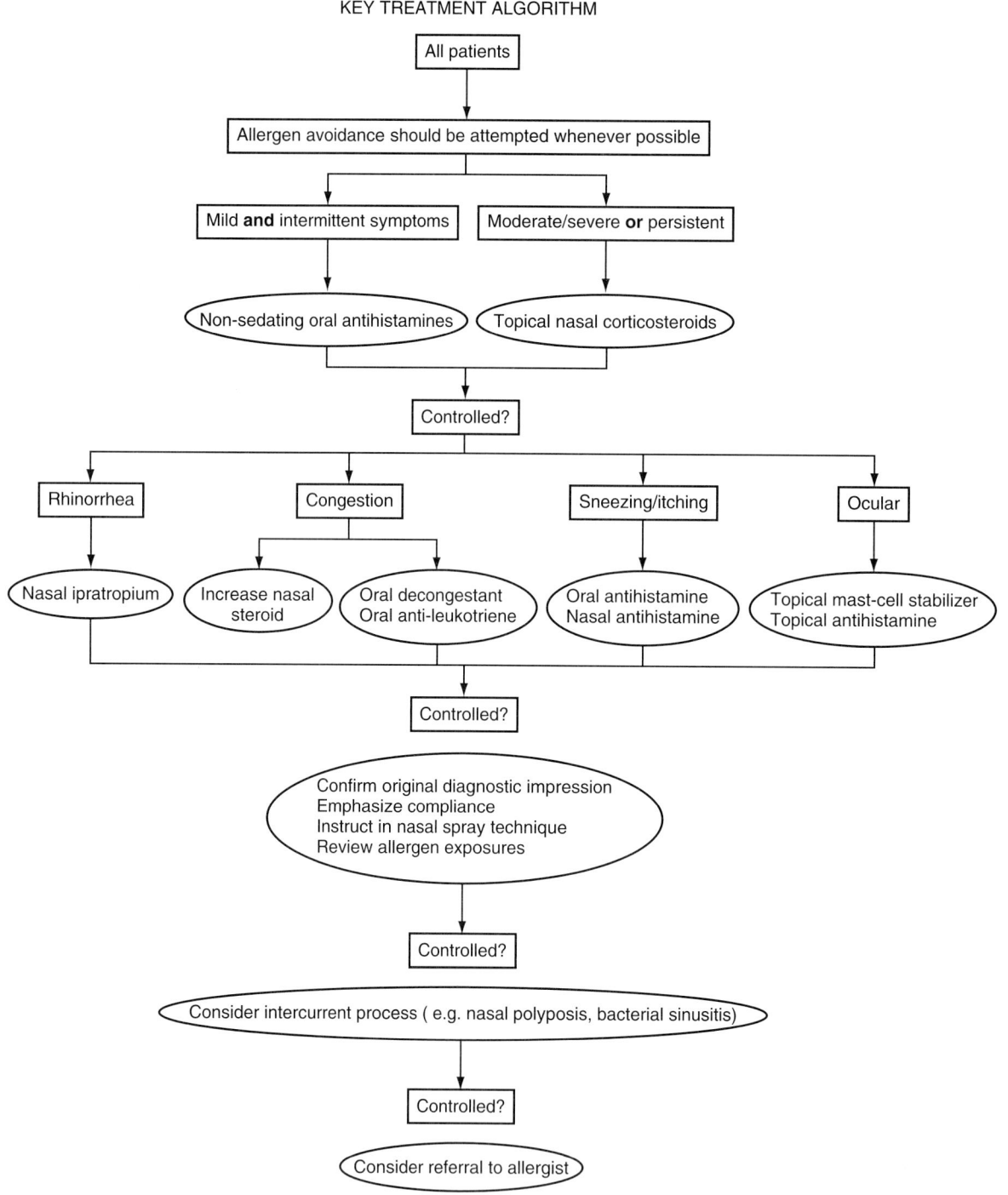

FIGURE 1. Key treatment for allergic rhinitis.

of inflammatory cells involve monoclonal antibodies directed against chemokines, adhesion molecule antagonists, or interleukins (ILs) as well as soluble cytokine receptors. One example is the compound R112, an intranasal inhibitor of the tyrosine kinase called Syk. Syk phosphorylates many intracellular signaling proteins and leads to the release of inflammatory mediators. The compound R112 is already in clinical trials and looks promising.

Patients with allergic rhinitis experience systemic as well as local symptoms, and the primary complaint is usually either congestion or fatigue. The disease involves multiple mediators and responds best to an approach targeted to reducing inflammation, rather than blocking a single mediator. Even though some nonsedating antihistamines may be available over-the-counter, intranasal steroids are more effective except for ocular symptoms. Leukotriene antagonists are not more effective

Rakel and Bope: *Conn's Current Therapy 2006.*

CURRENT DIAGNOSIS

- Allergic rhinitis is a serious disease affecting millions of people, costing billions of dollars, and significantly impairing quality of life.
- Allergic rhinitis should be characterized by duration as intermittent or persistent and by severity as either mild/moderate or severe.
- Allergic rhinitis is frequently associated with asthma and other atopic disorders.
- Nonspecific hyper-reactivity to a wide range of nonallergic triggers may also occur and often leads to a delayed diagnosis.
- A complete history should include questions about the upper and lower airway and also the effect on work, social activities, energy level, impact on the patient's quality of life, impairment of school/work performance, interference with leisure activities, and sleep disturbances.
- Skin testing is the best evidence of allergic sensitization and provides immediate, accurate, and cost-effective results to guide treatment.

 CURRENT THERAPY

- Allergen avoidance should be the first line of treatment whenever possible. It is the safest, least expensive, and most effective intervention whenever feasible. For most patients air-treatment and air-filtration devices, while heavily advertised, are clinically ineffective.
- Second-generation antihistamines are especially useful because of their excellent side-effect profile and long dosing interval. Patients are often unaware of cognitive and performance impairments with first-generation antihistamines.
- Adjunctive agents, such as eye drops and nasal anticholinergic medications, should always be considered if symptoms warrant their use.
- Intranasal steroids are the cornerstone of pharmacologic management, but they are less effective for ocular symptoms.
- Allergen immunotherapy is the only treatment currently available that is able to alter the natural course of the disease and may even prevent the development of asthma in some patients.
- Referral to a board-certified allergist should be considered, especially if medications lead to inadequate control or intolerable side-effects.

than antihistamines, and they are less effective than nasal steroids.

If avoidance has failed to provide adequate relief, the patient can (a) use daily nonsedating antihistamine in the morning, (b) add the lowest possible dose of inhaled steroid sufficient to provide relief, and (c) avoid known or suspected triggers. Common reasons for lack of a clinical response to treatment are incorrect diagnosis, medication noncompliance, persistent exposure to allergens (e.g., incomplete patient education), and improper selection of medication (e.g., nasal steroids for ocular symptoms). Common reasons for referral to an allergist are (a) pharmacotherapy and avoidance yield poor control or undesirable side effects; (b) co-morbid conditions such as asthma, nasal polyposis, or sinusitis recur; and (c) quality-of-life issues prompt consideration of more intensive treatment, including avoidance or immunotherapy.

REFERENCES

Bousquet J, van Cauwenberge P, Khaltaev N: Allergic rhinitis and its impact on asthma: ARIA workshop report. J Allergy Clin Immunol 2001;108:S147-334.

Creticos PS, Chen YH, Schroeder JT: New approaches in immunotherapy: Allergen vaccination with immunostimulatory DNA. Immunol Allergy Clin North Am 2004;24(4):569-581, v. Review.

Durham SR, Walker SM, Varga EM, et al: Long-term clinical efficacy of grass-pollen immunotherapy. N Engl J Med 1999;341(7):468-475.

Dykewicz MS, Fineman S, Skoner DP, et al: Diagnosis and management of rhinitis: Complete guidelines of the Joint Task Force on Practice Parameters in Allergy, Asthma and Immunology. American Academy of Allergy, Asthma, and Immunology. Ann Allergy Asthma Immunol 1998;81(5 Pt 2):478-518.

Halken S: Prevention of allergic disease in childhood: Clinical and epidemiological aspects of primary and secondary allergy prevention. Pediatr Allergy Immunol 2004;15(Suppl 16):4-5, 9-32.

Joint Task Force on Practice Parameters: Allergen immunotherapy: A practice parameter. American Academy of Allergy, Asthma and Immunology. American College of Allergy, Asthma and Immunology. Ann Allergy Asthma Immunol. 2003;90(1 Suppl 1):1-40.

Ross RN, Nelson HS, Finegold I: Effectiveness of specific immunotherapy in the treatment of allergic rhinitis: An analysis of randomized, prospective, single- or double-blind, placebo-controlled studies. Clin Ther 2000;22:342-350.

Skoner D, Rachelefsky G, Meltzer E, et al: Detection of growth suppression in children during treatment with intranasal beclomethasone dipropionate. Pediatrics 2000;105:E23.

Ten RM, Klein JS, Frigas E: Allergy skin testing. Mayo Clin Proc 1995;70(8):783-784.

12

Allergic Reactions to Drugs

Method of
Donald McNeil, MD

Drug allergic reactions fall under the broader category of adverse drug reactions (ADRs), which also include toxic drug effects, drug interactions, drug intolerance, and, finally, allergic (or immunologic) drug reactions.

Adverse drug reactions are common and often result in only trivial consequences. Some may be severe and life-threatening, and may result from both allergic and nonallergic causes.

The incidence of adverse drug effects is unknown but estimates of 20% of hospital admissions are not unreasonable. A skin rash is the most common manifestation; more importantly, however, severe life-threatening reactions occur, of which only a small portion have an allergic etiology. Most drug reactions are the result of unknown mechanisms. Drug intolerance, drug overdose, and side effects of drugs, as well as drug interactions, all play a significant role. These reactions should be considered both common and predictable.

Although allergic drug reactions are potentially severe, they are also the least common and least predictable. Allergic drug reactions are given particular attention because of the unpredictable, costly, and severe consequences that occasionally arise.

Several mechanisms may play a role in the underlying etiology of immunologic drug reactions. Immediate IgE-mediated reactions represent the classic allergic reaction. This is well characterized and the best understood, but other mechanisms also exist, for example, a cytotoxic reaction in which drug-induced antibodies result in hemolytic anemia. Another example is immune complex formation resulting in organ damage. This is commonly referred to as a "serum sickness" reaction and is characterized by fever, rash, and arthralgia beginning 2 to 4 weeks after initiation of drug. Finally, a delayed-type hypersensitivity reaction occurs when drug-specific T-lymphocytes react. This completes the picture of the four types of immunologic-mediated drug reactions according to the original Gell and Coombs classification. These are referred to as Type I, II, III, or IV reactions, respectively.

Cutaneous reactions comprise the most frequent type of allergic drug reaction. Approximately 94% cause a morbilliform rash and only 5% cause an urticarial reaction. Idiosyncratic reactions are still the most likely cause for a rash and occur much more frequently than a true drug-induced allergic reaction. Ampicillins in conjunction with a viral hepatitis or sulfa drugs taken in the AIDS population are common examples.

Both allergic and nonallergic reactions are known to be associated with severe reactions, including fatalities. Contrast media agents, allergic extracts, anesthetics, and antibiotics are the most commonly implicated drugs. Penicillin remains the most common cause of fatal drug reactions and accounts for up to 75% of these severe drug reactions in the United States.

An allergy to penicillin is the most frequently reported, but as many as 90% of patients labeled "penicillin allergic" are able to tolerate penicillin. This allergy is often mislabeled because of underlying illness or interaction between antibiotic and illness. Unfortunately one third to half of vancomycin (Vancocin) prescriptions in hospitals are given because of a history of "penicillin allergy." This raises the incidence of drug-resistant bacteria because of broad-spectrum antibiotic overuse. The economic impact of treating antibiotic-resistant infections is roughly $4 billion annually.

Pathophysiology

Some drugs are capable of reacting in the body without further alteration in chemical structure, whereas others must first be metabolized to become immunogenic. Many drugs are too small to be immunogenic alone and are incapable of eliciting an immune allergic response. These drugs require binding to a high-molecular-weight protein followed by antigen processing and presentation by the macrophage in the presence of major histocompatibility complex (MHC)-specific antigen to appropriate T-cell receptors.

Penicillin is capable of inducing an allergic reaction in more than one manner. Benzylpenicilloyl, the major penicillin determinant, is able to produce a strong antigenic response. A commercially available product, benzylpenicilloyl-polylysine (PPL) (Pre-Pen), provides the means to reproduce the same allergic response by simple skin testing. Minor determinants are metabolic derivatives of penicillin that may also produce an immune response. The diagnostic capabilities of a penicillin allergy are strengthened by including some measure of the allergic response to the minor determinants when skin testing is conducted for penicillin (Figure 1).

Patients with a history of penicillin allergy but negative skin testing to PPL and the minor determinants rarely experience allergic reactions on re-exposure. If they should occur, these are not fatal, but rather mild and self-limited.

PPL alone will potentially miss a significant percentage of allergic reactions to penicillin. Allergy testing with fresh benzylpenicillin G, aged penicillin (reconstituted more than 24 hours) as well as skin testing with the specific penicillin in question will greatly enhance the likelihood of uncovering of penicillin allergy in a patient with a positive history.

Cephalosporins do not provide the same degree of certainty with respect to an allergic evaluation. Cross-reactivity with penicillin allergy patients is known to exist, and although uncommon, it is also unpredictable. To err on the side of safety, a patient with a known penicillin allergy should not be treated with a cephalosporin. A patient with a previous cephalosporin reaction with a negative penicillin skin test cannot safely receive penicillin or another cephalosporin unless further diagnostic measures are taken. This patient may be allergic to a side chain on the cephalosporin that has not been identified by penicillin skin testing. Others recommend a graded oral challenge using a cephalosporin with a different side chain. The latter should be done realizing that standardized procedures have not been developed for this and therefore false negative results may occur.

Successful desensitization to penicillin has permitted a similar approach with other drugs. If the drug in question is required, either intravenous or oral drug administration is possible by incremental doses given usually every 15 minutes. A 10,000-fold dilution of the initial dose is usually sufficient to begin, followed by higher doses, 2-fold or greater. The vital signs are monitored throughout the procedure with timely medical intervention if problems arise.

Rakel and Bope: *Conn's Current Therapy 2006*.

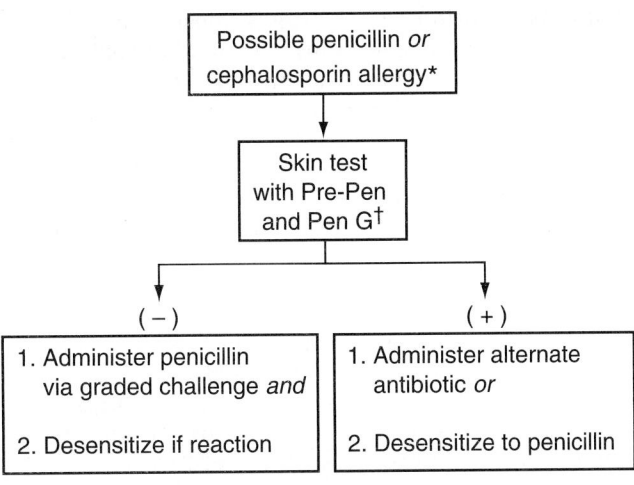

*Only 10%–20% of patients who report a penicillin allergy are actually allergic.
†Benzylpenicilloyl polylysine (Pre-Pen) and penicillin G (Pen G) will not include all potential penicillin derivatives. The additional benefit of testing with the minor determinant mixture is impractical and usually not available.

FIGURE 1. Penicillin allergy evaluation.

Sulfonamides typically cause cutaneous reactions, infrequently in healthy individuals but extremely common in AIDS patients. Reactions may be relatively benign in nature such as urticaria or fixed-drug eruption, but may also cause more serious reactions (Stevens-Johnson syndrome, toxic epidermal necrolysis). A variety of mechanisms may exist, alone or in combination, using IgE antibody response, T-lymphocytes, and inflammatory cytokines. Because of our inadequate understanding of these mechanisms, there are no universally acceptable means of evaluating sulfonamide hypersensitivity. Unless there has been previously severe reaction, a graded challenge with the drug in question is considered a reasonable alternative (Box 1). Although a theoretical risk exists between sulfonamides and drugs with sulfonamide derivatives (diuretics, COX-2 inhibitors), little data show this is actually true.

Radiographic contrast media (RCM) produce an anaphylactoid reaction by an unknown mechanism. Conventional RCM is hypertonic. The newer nonionic RCM with lower osmolarity are associated with fewer anaphylactoid or allergic-like reactions. Complement system activation, which is capable of causing histamine release, is thought to be the method by which this reaction occurs.

In the continuum of adverse drug effects with suspected hypersensitivity, exposure to *aspirin* and other nonsteroidal anti-inflammatory drugs (NSAIDs) rarely exhibits features that are IgE mediated and allergic in nature, and are more often nonimmunologic mediated. A non–IgE-mediated event must still be approached with caution because the consequences are potentially life-threatening.

More commonly, NSAIDs are associated with the asthma triad syndrome associated with nasal polyps or rhinitis, and severe asthma. This is not an allergic drug reaction, but it represents a largely unrecognized subpopulation of asthmatics who will benefit by avoiding the use of NSAIDs.

The antibiotic *vancomycin* (Vancocin) causes a reaction referred to as *red man syndrome*. Histamine and other mast cell mediators are released, but not through vancomycin-induced IgE antibody (rare cases have been reported). Most, but not all, cases of the red man syndrome are related to the rate of the infusion, and most will subside once the medication is stopped. A graded challenge with the drug or a full course of desensitization usually permits resumption of treatment.

Angiotensin-converting enzyme (ACE) inhibitors are well known to be associated with cough and angioedema, but like NSAIDs, the mechanism is unknown. Newer ACE inhibitors have been described to cause similar reactions but at a much lower incidence. The symptoms of cough and angioedema may continue to recur for several months and up to a year after the discontinuation of the drug.

As seen from the discussion above, IgE-mediated allergic drug reactions represent only a portion of immune-mediated drug reactions. To assist in the diagnosis, a 7- to 10-day delay in the appearance of the drug reaction

---

BOX 1 Graded Challenge

1. Cautious administration of medications to patient not likely allergic to drug.
2. Not to be considered equivalent to desensitization.
3. Used when insufficient evidence available to exclude drug allergy.
4. Medication administered in incremental doses beginning at 1:100 dilution of final dose.
5. Adequate medical resources exist to treat allergic reaction.

after initial treatment or immediate reactivation on re-exposure suggests an immunologic etiology. Oftentimes, only the history will provide this index of suspicion. Confirmation by positive skin testing with the drug in question is highly predictive of IgE-mediated hypersensitivity.

Attempts to label reactions as either IgE- or non–IgE-mediated may prove to be costly, time-consuming, and of no immediate benefit. Non-IgE reactions are capable of eliciting changes in vital signs, pulmonary function, and cutaneous effects similar to anaphylaxis and are referred to as anaphylactoid. These need to be regarded with the same degree of caution as IgE-mediated reactions. Narcotics, radiographic contrast media, and chemotherapeutic agents may directly affect mast cell mediator release with the consequences listed above. Antihistamines and corticosteroids given prior to administration of these drugs are usually sufficient to prevent a reoccurrence, or at least to minimize these reactions.

Drug desensitization is indicated for those patients with positive skin tests who must receive the drug, but should not be assumed to be universally safe or protective. Some chemotherapeutic agents, such as etoposide (VePesid) and teniposide (Vumon), have a much higher incidence of anaphylactoid reactions. Readministration of these drugs in the face of a previous reaction and in spite of prophylactic measures often leads to disappointing results.

Current biologic response modifier agents, as well as others soon to arrive, are associated with adverse reactions. Monoclonal antibodies, T- and B-cell inactivators, and others may prove to have adverse immunologic effects that will only become more apparent with the experience of increased use.

Evaluation of Drug Allergy in Practice

The importance of a reliable history in a medical evaluation is never more evident than during the initial workup of a suspected drug allergy. The timing of exposure, with the first allergic reaction occurring within days of the priming dose or immediately upon re-exposure, strongly points to an allergic etiology. Multiple exposures to the same drug on previous occasions do not preclude an allergic reaction de novo. Similarly, a previous history of an allergic drug reaction does not by itself predict a reoccurrence on re-exposure. The allergic diathesis may wane over time for drugs just as it may occur for other allergens.

Armed with this suggestive drug history and clinical findings such as a rash, fever, bronchospasm, or anaphylaxis, the evaluation becomes more straightforward. In the appropriate clinical setting, eosinophilia will also support a drug-allergic reaction.

Avoiding the implicated drug may be the simplest approach because confirmation of the diagnosis with appropriate skin testing is often unavailable. (Standardized skin testing exists only for penicillin, but even this does not provide 100% reliability.) Skin testing with the drug is questionable, but using both a positive and negative control of histamine and saline may still provide useful information. A positive skin test would certainly discourage use of this drug unless adequate precautions were taken.

If a non–life-threatening history of a reaction exists and the drug cannot be appropriately substituted, the option exists for a graded oral challenge to confirm the diagnosis. This should not be considered to be the same as desensitization because it involves higher doses and exposure over a shorter period of time than would be considered safe in a truly allergic individual. A challenge such as this should be conducted in suitable medical facilities under close medical supervision.

If the drug in question has been shown to cause an allergic reaction but still must be used, then a carefully monitored drug desensitization program should be considered. Under medical supervision, the drug should be administered orally or intravenously beginning with doses that are tenfold more dilute than the final strength. Incrementally higher doses of the drug should be administered every 15 minutes, increasing the dose twofold each time.

Drug-induced skin reactions are common and warrant particular attention. Early recognition is necessary to avoid an incorrect diagnosis and to institute appropriate interventional measures as soon as possible.

The following points will assist the physician in arriving at a correct diagnosis. The *timing of the onset* of the reaction in relation to the time the drug was given provides an important clue. Often signs and symptoms develop 1 to 2 weeks after time of initial drug exposure. Symptoms may develop rapidly on repeat exposure. *Pruritic urticarial lesions* strongly suggest an adverse drug reaction. A *symmetrical or truncal distribution* or a rash that occurs only in sun-exposed areas (polymorphous light eruption) also supports an ADR finding. The morphology of the reaction is helpful, although many types occur (lichenoid, morbilliform, eczematous). The histopathology of the lesion on skin biopsy may reveal eosinophils, which may also be detected in the peripheral blood.

Drugs that commonly cause ADRs tend to be antibiotics. The most common is the morbilliform rash when ampicillin is given in the presence of a viral infection such as infectious mononucleosis or cytomegalovirus. Rarely is this IgE mediated and it should not be regarded as a basis for a history of penicillin allergy. It should also be noted that not all ADRs are caused by prescription medications. A patient may fail to disclose over-the-counter medications that might be responsible (e.g., St. John's wort).

The *response to treatment* may aid in the recognition of an ADR. An incomplete response to topical steroids is typical of an ADR and systemic steroids may turn out to be the therapy of choice. Finally, the *response to withdrawal* of drug may range from a rapid recovery to slow clearing over many weeks, but a favorable response nonetheless.

Table 1 lists several drugs used to treat AIDS/HIV that are worthy of mention. Not all should be considered to be an allergic cause of ADR.

Rakel and Bope: *Conn's Current Therapy 2006.*

TABLE 1 Drugs Used to Treat AIDS/HIV

Drug	Reaction
Zidovudine, AZT (Retrovir)	Hyperpigmentation
Zalcitabine, ddC (Hivid)	Oral ulcers
Abacavir (Ziagen)	Severe rash/anaphylaxis
Nevirapine (Viramune)	Toxic epidermal necrolysis
Foscarnet	Urethral ulceration
Trimethoprim-sulfamethoxazole (TMP-SMX) (Bactrim)	Morbilliform rash or erythema multiforme

A careful and systematic approach to the patient with a suspected drug allergy will provide valuable information for both the immediate and the long-term management of the patient. A suspected drug allergy that is disproved will facilitate good medical care because unnecessary expense and the risk of further sensitizing the patient to a new medication will be spared if the patient is not allergic. On the other hand, a positive screen for a suspected drug allergy will result in a safe alternative. It should be emphasized, however, that neither a family history of a drug allergy nor a patient requesting a "test" for a possible drug allergy without other reason is an indication for further drug allergy evaluation because of the risk of false-negative results.

Allergic Reactions to Insect Stings

Method of
Mark S. Dykewicz, MD, and
J. Keith Lemmon, MD

Types of Reactions

The normal reaction to an insect sting consists of pain, erythema, and swelling around the sting site lasting 1 to 2 hours. Allergic reactions to insect stings, in contrast, can occur locally or systemically and vary in their time courses. The two main reaction types are the large local reaction and the systemic reaction. A third type of reaction, the unusual delayed reaction, can also occur.

Large local reactions develop 12 to 24 hours following a sting and usually represent a late-phase IgE-dependent inflammatory mechanism. Symptoms include painful swelling beginning at the sting site and extending at least 10 cm in diameter; the edema and overlying inflammation occasionally can involve an entire limb. Symptoms typically peak at 48 hours and last for 5 to 10 days. Local reactions are generally not dangerous and do not indicate significant risk for future systemic reactions. If the oropharynx is stung, however, resultant swelling can mimic laryngeal edema.

Systemic reactions produce symptoms distant from the sting site, generally occur within 30 to 60 minutes of the sting, and represent an IgE-mediated immediate hypersensitivity reaction. Systemic reactions vary but include manifestations of anaphylaxis such as generalized urticaria and/or angioedema (in >80% of cases), laryngeal edema, bronchospasm, and hypotension.

Unusual delayed-type reactions are reported and include cases of Guillain-Barré syndrome, glomerulonephritis, late-onset urticaria, and serum sickness–like reactions following an insect sting. Many of these illnesses develop several days to weeks after the stinging incident. An exact immunologic mechanism has yet to be fully elucidated for this reaction type.

Epidemiology

The stinging insects responsible for causing allergic reactions belong to the Hymenoptera order, of which three families sting most frequently: Apids (honeybees, bumblebees), vespids (yellow jackets, hornets, wasps), and formicids (fire ants). Large local reactions occur in an estimated 10% of adults. The prevalence of systemic reactions following an insect sting is almost 1% in children and approximately 3% in adults. At least 50 deaths per year in the United States are attributable to insect stings. Data regarding the prevalence of insect sting allergic reactions likely underestimate the actual frequency of reactions and associated fatalities.

Although systemic reactions occur more frequently in children, adults suffer more fatal outcomes to insect stings. Nearly 50% of deaths related to insect stings are in patients without prior history of allergic reactions to stings. Risk factors for a poor outcome to anaphylaxis include the presence of cardiovascular disease and certain medications such as β-blockers or angiotensin-converting enzyme (ACE) inhibitors.

Studies in both adults and children show that symptoms upon re-sting are typically no more severe than those of the initial systemic reaction. In children with a history of systemic reaction limited to cutaneous manifestations (e.g., urticaria, angioedema), the risk of another systemic reaction is 10%, with only 1% of cases increasing in severity (e.g., the addition of laryngeal edema or respiratory or cardiovascular symptoms). In adults the incidence of developing another systemic reaction upon re-sting is roughly 50%.

Diagnosis

A careful history should elicit the reaction's symptoms and time course and the degree of its severity, and should clarify whether a local or systemic process occurred. Further testing is not necessary in patients who suffer large local reactions, but patients who suffer a systemic reaction should be referred to an allergist/immunologist.

To confirm the diagnosis of stinging insect hypersensitivity, the presence of specific IgE antibodies to Hymenoptera venom must be established in patients with a history of systemic reaction. The preferred and

Rakel and Bope: *Conn's Current Therapy 2006.*

more sensitive diagnostic procedure is skin testing using dilute concentrations of honeybee, yellow jacket, white-faced hornet, yellow hornet, and wasp venoms, or, in the case of fire ants, whole body extract. Skin testing should not take place until 4 to 6 weeks following a sting reaction because a transient refractory period can produce false-negative results.

Skin testing is reserved for patients with a history of systemic reaction because asymptomatic venom sensitization in the general population is roughly 25%; hence the predictive value of skin testing in patients without a history of systemic reaction is low. If a patient with a history of systemic reaction has negative skin test results, measurement of venom-specific IgE antibodies using in vitro testing should be considered.

Therapy

ACUTE TREATMENT OF INSECT STINGS
(see Fig. 1)

Large local reactions are treated with a combination of oral H_1 antagonists, ice packs, and elevation of the affected area. If swelling is particularly massive or affects the head and neck region, a short course of oral corticosteroids may be beneficial. Intense erythema and lymphangitic streaking can often overlie the edema, giving an appearance of cellulitis. If this finding occurs within 2 days of the sting, however, it usually does not indicate cellulitis.

Primary treatment for systemic reactions in adults is aqueous epinephrine 1:1000 (weight/volume) dilution administered intramuscularly at doses of 0.2 to 0.5 mL.

CURRENT DIAGNOSIS

Large Local Reactions
- Represent late-phase IgE dependent reaction.
- Reactions can consist of painful edema with overlying erythema and lymphangitic streaking.
- Symptoms develop within 12 to 24 hours following insect sting and can persist for 5 to 10 days.
- No diagnostic testing is required.

Systemic Reactions
- Represent immediate IgE-mediated hypersensitivity reaction.
- Sting produces symptoms distant from sting site, usually within 30 to 60 minutes.
- Reactions vary but include manifestations of anaphylaxis such as generalized urticaria and/or angioedema (in more than 80% of cases), laryngeal edema, bronchospasm, and hypotension.
- Diagnostic testing for specific IgE antibodies to Hymenoptera venom is indicated using skin testing; in certain cases, in vitro testing may be useful.

Unusual Delayed-Type Reactions
- Exact immunologic mechanism unknown.
- May develop days to weeks after a sting.
- Cases of Guillain-Barré syndrome, glomerulonephritis, late-onset urticaria, and serum-like sickness are reported.

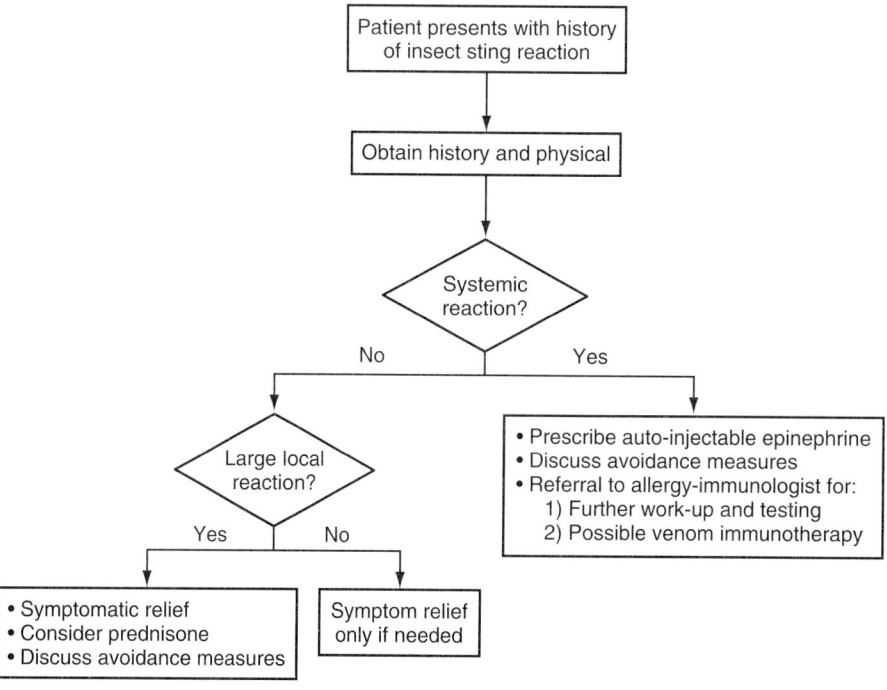

FIGURE 1. Treatment algorithm. (Modified from Moffitt JE, Golden DB, Reisman RE, et al: Stinging insect hypersensitivity: A practice parameter update. J Allergy Clin Immunol 2004;114(4):869-886.)

This may be repeated every 10 to 15 minutes as needed up to a maximum of 1 mg per dose. In children, the dose is 10 µg (0.01 mg) per kg body weight up to a maximum of 500 µg (0.5 mg) per dose or 0.5 mL of 1:1000 (weight/volume). The epinephrine dose can be repeated every 15 minutes for two doses and then every 4 hours as needed. If the patient responds poorly to several doses of intramuscular epinephrine, intravenous epinephrine might be considered (see later for dosing). Depending on the reaction severity, patients may require oxygen and inhaled β-agonist medications such as aerosolized albuterol. Because laryngeal edema can obstruct the airway, treating physicians must assess the need for intubation vigilantly. Large volumes of intravenous fluids and vasopressors may be needed to compensate for hypotension. Patients taking β-adrenergic blocking agents may be refractory to epinephrine, in which case glucagon, 1 to 5 mg (20 to 30 µg per kg [maximum 1 mg] in children) administered intravenously over 5 minutes and followed by an infusion of 5 to 15 µg per minute, should be considered. Antihistamines (e.g., diphenhydramine 1 to 2 mg per kg or 25 to 50 mg per dose given parenterally) can be given to attenuate urticaria and associated pruritis. Additionally, the use of H_2 antihistamines combined with H_1 antihistamine blockade may be useful in reversing refractory hypotension. Anaphylaxis can have a biphasic temporal course, and patients should be monitored for at least 6 hours. Corticosteroids (e.g., 200 mg of intravenous hydrocortisone) may be used in an effort to diminish the potential for late-phase responses.

PREVENTIVE MEASURES

Avoidance precautions should be discussed with patients. Recommendations include wearing shoes when outside to minimize the risk of stings on the foot. Patients must exercise care when eating and drinking outdoors and

---

 CURRENT THERAPY

Large Local Reactions

- Cold compresses and elevation of affected limb.
- Oral H_1 receptor antagonists (e.g., diphenhydramine 25 to 50 mg orally every 4 to 6 hours as needed for adults; in children ages 2 to 6 years, the dose is 6.25 mg orally every 4 to 6 hours as needed; in children ages 6 to 12 years, the dose is 12.5 to 25 mg orally every 4 to 6 hours as needed).
- Analgesics (e.g., acetaminophen, 325 to 650 mg orally every 4 to 6 hours, as needed for adults; 10 to 15 mg per kg orally every 4 to 6 hours, as needed for children).
- Short course of oral corticosteroids.
- Antibiotics generally not indicated for associated erythema and lymphangitic streaking if occurring within 2 days of the sting.

Systemic Reactions

- Cardiopulmonary resuscitation (CPR) should be performed if loss of circulation or respiration occurs. The airway should be closely monitored and maintained via intubation if necessary.
- *Epinephrine* is the immediate drug of choice:
  In the field, auto-injector kits (e.g., EpiPen, 0.3 mg, for adults or EpiPen Jr., 0.15 mg, for children) should be given intramuscularly immediately following a sting.
  In a monitored setting, the initial adult dose is 0.2 mL to 0.5 mL of a 1:1000 (weight/volume) dilution given intramuscularly every 10 to 15 minutes as needed up to a maximum of 1 mg per dose. For children, the dose is 10 µg (0.01 mg) per kg body weight up to a maximum 500 µg (0.5 mg) per dose or 0.5 mL of 1:1000 (weight/volume). This dose can be repeated every 15 minutes for two doses and then every 4 hours as needed.

  If refractory shock occurs, intravenous epinephrine should be administered in adults using a formulation of 1:10,000 (0.1 mg per mL) epinephrine or by first diluting a 1:1000 (1 mg per mL) dilution (weight/volume) of epinephrine to a 1:10,000 dilution. Either preparation can then be initially infused starting at 1 µg per minute and then increasingly titrated to 2 to 10 µg per minute. In children, the initial intravenous epinephrine dose is 10 µg (0.01 mg) per kg body weight or 0.10 mL of 1:10,000 (weight/volume) dilution. Subsequent doses are 100 µg per kilogram (1 mL of 1:10,000) (weight/volume) every 3 to 5 minutes, and if the shock is still refractory, the dose may be increased to 200 µg per kg.
- Vasopressors and large amounts of intravenous fluids/colloids may be necessary to compensate for peripheral vasodilation and intravascular third spacing.
- H_1 antihistamines should be given (e.g., diphenhydramine, 1 to 2 mg per kg or 25 to 50 mg per dose parenterally). H_2 antihistamines combined with H_1 antihistamine blockade may be useful in reversing refractory hypotension.
- Inhaled nebulized bronchodilators may be administered for bronchospasm (e.g., albuterol, 2.5 to 5 mg nebulized as needed every 1 to 4 hours).
- Corticosteroids may be used in an effort to attenuate possible late-phase responses (e.g., 200 mg intravenous hydrocortisone).
- Patients taking β-adrenergic blocking agents may be refractory to epinephrine, in which case glucagon, 1 to 5 mg (20 to 30 µg per kg [maximum 1 mg] in children) administered intravenously over 5 minutes and followed by an infusion of 5 to 15 µg per minute, should be considered.

Rakel and Bope: *Conn's Current Therapy 2006.*

should avoid garbage cans where stinging insects scavenge. They should minimize wearing bright colors and floral prints as well as scented soaps or fragrances.

Self-treatment injectable epinephrine kits should be prescribed to patients at risk for anaphylactic reactions; such kits include the EpiPen, 0.3 mg, and the EpiPen Jr., 0.15 mg. Physicians should review and demonstrate the indications and technique for injectable epinephrine with their patients.

VENOM IMMUNOTHERAPY

Venom immunotherapy (VIT) is 95% to 97% effective in preventing systemic reactions in venom-sensitized patients; this protective effect can persist for 10 to 20 years after completing VIT. VIT is indicated for adult patients with a history of systemic reaction who demonstrate venom-specific IgE hypersensitivity via positive skin tests or in vitro testing methods. In children (younger than 16 years of age), VIT is limited to venom-sensitized patients whose systemic reaction included respiratory and/or cardiovascular manifestations. VIT is not indicated in venom-sensitized children with systemic reactions limited to cutaneous signs and symptoms because their risk for developing severe anaphylaxis upon re-sting is 1%. VIT is not indicated for large local reactions.

VIT is administered via subcutaneous injections of increasing doses of specific venoms (although fire ant immunotherapy uses whole body extract). VIT is administered weekly until a maintenance dose is achieved and then injections are spaced to every 4 weeks for 1 year. During the remaining years of therapy, the interval for VIT injections can increase to 6 weeks. Adverse reactions include large local reactions in roughly 50% of patients and systemic symptoms in 5% to 15% of patients. There are no known negative long-term sequelae from VIT. The duration of VIT is generally 3 to 5 years, although specific guidelines are evolving regarding the cessation of therapy. Patients with particularly severe reactions may benefit from lifelong VIT.

REFERENCES

Freeman TM: Clinical practice. Hypersensitivity to hymenoptera stings. N Engl J Med 2004;351(19):1978-1984.
Lieberman P, Kemp SF, Opperheimer J, et al: The diagnosis and management of anaphylaxis: An updated practice parameter. J Allergy Clin Immunol 2005; 115(3):S483-S523.
Moffitt JE, Golden DB, Reisman RE, et al: Stinging insect hypersensitivity: A practice parameter update. J Allergy Clin Immunol 2004;114(4):869-886.
Portnoy JM, Moffitt JE, Golden DB, et al: Stinging insect hypersensitivity: A practice parameter. J Allergy Clin Immunol 1999;103 (5 Pt 1):963-980.

Diseases of the Skin

Acne and Rosacea

Method of
Guy F. Webster, MD, PhD

Acne

Acne vulgaris is an extremely common disease. To some degree, signs of the disease can be found in nearly all adolescents, and regardless of severity, acne is often of greater psychological effect than cutaneous. Most patients overestimate the severity of their disease, whereas most doctors underestimate the impact of acne on their patients. Studies show that those with severe acne as teens are less employable as adults, and self-esteem in acne patients is low. These facts, combined with routine adolescent tensions, make acne a difficult disease to treat.

PATHOGENESIS

The pathogenesis of acne is multifactorial with disturbances of keratinization, hormonal secretion, and immunity. The central defect involves the formation of the comedo, a plug in the follicle that results from aberrant desquamation of the follicular wall. Comedones are described clinically as *open* if the pore is visible and *closed* if it is not. The black tip of an open comedo results from the oxidation of sebaceous lipid and melanin, and it is not dirt (contrary to worldwide maternal advice). The cause of comedo formation is not known but may relate to bacterial stimulation of aberrant keratinization within the sebaceous duct. Comedones do not result from poor hygiene or diet or use of name-brand cosmetics (big companies have a reputation to lose and test for acnegenicity).

The acne of many patients remains in this first non-inflamed stage, but it may progress to inflammatory lesions of varying severity. The target of inflammation is *Propionibacterium acnes*, an aerotolerant anaerobic member of the normal flora in sebaceous regions of the skin. *P. acnes* lives in the follicle and metabolizes sebaceous triglycerides into fatty acids and glycerol. It consumes the glycerol and casts off the fatty acids.

In years past it was believed the fatty acids in sebum were the cause of acne inflammation, but it is now clear the organism itself is the target.

P. acnes is a highly inflammatory, activating complement, secreting neutrophil and monocyte chemotactic factors, activating toll-like receptors and lymphocytes, and inducing lysosomal enzyme release. In addition, the organism is degraded only very slowly, resulting in a persistent follicular inflammatory response.

Because all individuals have significant levels of *P. acnes* and some degree of follicular plugging, it is curious that everyone does not have active acne. The explanation lies in the level of the immune response to the organism. Patients with excessive humoral and cellular immunity to *P. acnes* mount a more destructive inflammatory response that produces clinical lesions. This response represents a true hypersensitivity to *P. acnes*, in that the organism is a beneficial commensal and of minimal infectious potential.

A minority of women have an endocrine aspect to their acne. Although not necessarily severe, their acne may become very refractory. Such patients may give a history of irregular menses, be overweight, or have increased facial hair or androgenetic alopecia. Measurement of serum androgen levels and subsequent corrective therapy usually improves their acne as well. Although only two contraceptives are currently approved for marketing as acne therapy, probably all oral contraceptives are of some benefit.

There are many acne grading systems. Those that involve pimple counting are useful for clinical trials but too cumbersome for office use. A gestalt system is more useful, in which the physician and patient reach some consensus on the degree of the acne by combining severity of actual lesions with the impact of the disease on the patient. Inflammatory acne lesions range from superficial pustules to deep scarring nodules. Patients generally have a mixture of lesion types, and their acne should be graded based on the most severe lesions present (i.e., a patient with 3 scarring nodules has more severe acne than one with 50 superficial pustules). The presence of acne on the chest or back also connotes more severe and hard-to-treat disease.

The terms *inverse acne, triad acne,* and *hidradenitis suppurativa* all describe a follicular process that results in comedo formation and inflammation in the scalp, axilla, and groin. In the past, this was believed to be an apocrine disease, but recent work describes it as a disease of the hair follicle, like acne. Unlike acne, *P. acnes* plays little or no role in this acne of nonsebaceous regions. Various bacteria, enterics, pseudomonads, and streptococci colonize these lesions and provoke inflammation and scarring. Sinus tract formation is common and results in disease that is often best treated surgically.

TREATMENT

The first step in treatment of patients with acne is to be certain they (and their parents) have not fallen prey to the numerous myths about the disease. Acne is not caused by dirt, diet, or impure thoughts. Patients commonly believe one particular food, usually a greasy or sweet one (never asparagus), worsens their acne. Trying to correct this misconception is fruitless; it is better to focus on the proper use of medicine. Hair on the forehead does not make pimples, and the disease cannot be treated effectively with soap and water. Although satisfying, popping pimples is bad; it promotes scarring and prolongs the life of many lesions. Stress may play a role in acne, but it is a small one, and most patients' acne does not benefit from tranquilizers.

Patients and doctors need to communicate particularly well during the treatment of acne. During the first visit, patients should be given realistic expectations and disabused (if possible) of incorrect ideas. Teens, in particular, expect quick results. They must understand that 3 to 6 weeks (although an eternity) is the quickest that acne can be expected to improve. Bigger lesions may take longer, as do open comedones. To most patients, so-called scarring is any mark on the face after a pimple is gone; they need to learn to distinguish between true scars and transient postinflammatory pigment changes.

Acne regimens vary widely among dermatologists. Some use one or two drugs in each patient; others use five or six. In general, one or two properly chosen drugs do better and are easier to comply with than a more complex regimen.

The central lesion in acne is the microcomedo in both comedonal and inflammatory acne types. Thus most effective regimens include a retinoid such as adapalene, tretinoin or tazarotene. Indeed, with sufficient patience, topical retinoids are excellent monotherapy for all but the most severe acne. But because topical retinoid monotherapy takes several months to really clear inflammatory acne, it is sensible to add a drug that reduces inflammation by reducing *P. acnes* populations. Purely noninflammatory (comedonal) acne is the mildest form of disease but can be the hardest to treat. Comedones are usually firmly ensconced in the follicle and, untreated, they cannot be easily expressed. Tretinoin (vitamin A acid) cream is the standard against which all other anticomedonal agents are compared. It inhibits comedo formation and eliminates comedonal acne in a few months. The only significant side effect is the irritation that is greatest after a few weeks. It usually does not require intervention, but if desired, a moisturizing lotion may be prescribed. Because their skin is inherently irritable, patients with atopic diseases may not tolerate topical retinoids even with moisturization.

Other drugs are also useful for noninflammatory acne. Adapalene is a naphthoic acid derivative that binds to nuclear retinoid receptors and has retinoid effects. It is effective for comedonal acne and also has a measure of anti-inflammatory activity. Adapalene is roughly equivalent to topical tretinoin but with somewhat less irritation. Tazarotene is a potent anticomedonal retinoid cream that is only slightly more irritating than tretinoin.

In the past 15 years, most dermatologists have observed a reduced efficacy of topical erythromycin and clindamycin. When first introduced the drugs were quite effective, but they have become of little use because of a dramatic increase in the resistance of *P. acnes* to the drugs. Fortunately, this resistance does not translate into hard-to-treat infections, just in hard-to-treat acne. The solution to the problem is to use the two drugs along with benzoyl peroxide, which effectively prevents the acquisition of resistance.

Oral antibiotics that are effective in acne include erythromycins, tetracyclines, trimethoprim-sulfamethoxazole, and ciprofloxacin. Because of concerns about generating resistant gastrointestinal (GI) flora, the latter two drugs should be reserved for problematic patients. Tetracyclines have the significant advantage of additional anti-inflammatory activity in acne and are the most widely prescribed. Doxycycline and minocycline have the greatest effect on acne and are well tolerated and generally safe.

Because of the clear link to androgens, acne is often perceived as a hormonal disease, but it is unusual for a hormonal drug to be effective as monotherapy. Adding a hormonal therapy to acne regimens in women is occasionally helpful. Two types of drug may be used: oral contraceptives and spironolactone. As stated earlier, although only two oral contraceptives are currently approved for marketing as an acne treatment, it is likely that most are helpful in acne to a degree.

In treating acne during pregnancy, tetracyclines may cause staining of teeth and bones and are contraindicated. Although commonly thought to be a teratogen, topical tretinoin does not raise circulating vitamin A levels or result in fetal deformity when used. Nevertheless, many patients and doctors are concerned and do not use the drug during pregnancy. Benzoyl peroxide, azelaic acid, and oral erythromycin are generally agreed to be safe for use during pregnancy; however, because nausea and heartburn often accompany pregnancy, avoiding erythromycin and treating acne topically is recommended.

Although occasionally helpful, topical steroids actually cause acne and invariably cause atrophy of facial skin if used for any length of time. They should be avoided. Intralesional triamcinolone acetonide is useful to calm big nodules but can cause pitting and hypopigmentation, both of which eventually resolve (0.05 mL of a 2 mg per mL dosage is commonly used).

Nodular scarring acne that resists oral antibiotics and topical retinoids is usually treated with oral isotretinoin, a potent and effective therapy for severe acne. After 4 to 6 months, most patients have little or no disease. Eighty percent have a complete long-term remission (possible cure) of their acne if treated with

1 mg/kg per day for 4 to 6 months. The duration of benefit after therapy is linked to dosage; lower dosages minimize side effects but increase the relapse rate.

Unfortunately, isotretinoin has significant side effects. There is an initial flare of acne in many patients that can be blunted by beginning at a low dose (e.g., 20 mg) and then increasing to around 1 mg/kg after 1 month. Patients with truncal acne may have a particularly severe flare of disease known as acne fulminans. This is a vicious scarring process that must be avoided. These patients are usually started on 20 mg of isotretinoin along with 20 mg of prednisone for the first month. The drug also produces dry skin and mucosae, elevated triglycerides in approximately 30% of patients, and occasional muscle or joint aches. Transaminases are occasionally elevated, but investigation usually determines they are muscle derived rather than of hepatic origin. Patients who exercise vigorously are at greater risk for muscle enzyme leakage.

Much public concern focuses on depression caused by isotretinoin, but both personal experience and large studies fail to show a correlation between the drug and mental illness. Unfortunately, disproving a negative can be nearly impossible. Discussing the issue with patients and parents and agreeing to bring up any problems that arise is beneficial.

The major issue with isotretinoin is teratogenicity. The drug produces a tremendous rate of miscarriage and deformed babies, and pregnancy must be rigorously prevented while patients are undergoing treatment. Fortunately, isotretinoin is rapidly eliminated, and patients may conceive safely one full menstrual period after stopping the drug. Perhaps surprisingly, the patient most likely to become pregnant while taking isotretinoin is in her 20s or 30s. All female patients taking the drug must be either surgically sterile or use two means of contraception; one hormonal and one barrier method. A negative pregnancy test must be obtained monthly.

Rosacea

Although usually considered along with acne, rosacea is a distinct disease. Comedo formation, the hallmark of acne, is absent. Rather, the predisposing factor seems to be vascular hyperreactivity. Patients who blush, especially the fair skinned, often develop some degree of rosacea, although the condition is not limited to the very pale and can be seen in all races if closely observed.

The mildest form of disease is the permanent malar blush. Telangiectasia may follow as may inflammatory papules and nodules. Some patients develop sebaceous overgrowth, particularly on the nose. Termed *rhinophyma,* this process is disfiguring and stigmatizing because people believe it is a sign of alcoholism.

Approximately 50% of rosacea patients also have ocular involvement. Styes, blepharitis, and corneal surface disease may result. The severity of ocular rosacea bears no relation to the severity of facial disease, and all patients should be questioned about symptoms and have their conjunctivae examined.

The pathogenesis of rosacea is a matter of great debate, and few hard facts are available. Vasodilation clearly plays a role, but what it does to promote the process is unclear. The resulting edema fluid is suggested as the cause of inflammation. Any food or medication that induces blushing worsens rosacea, but probably no one's rosacea has ever been treated effectively by diet alone. *P. acnes* probably plays a role in some patients' inflammatory disease, but drugs that reduce the organism without anti-inflammatory activity are not very effective. *Demodex* mites and gastrointestinal *Helicobacter* were suggested for years as having a role in rosacea, but no convincing studies exist.

No medication adequately treats the vascular phase of rosacea. The temptation to use topical corticosteroids must be avoided; it always makes the condition worse in the long run.

Inflammatory rosacea may be treated topically with azelaic acid or metronidazole creams. Benzoyl peroxide is sometimes helpful. Because vasodilation worsens disease, creams should be used that are not irritating to the patient. Oral therapy with tetracyclines, especially doxycycline and minocycline, is best for refractory, severe, or ocular rosacea. In extreme cases, isotretinoin is an appropriate last resort.

CURRENT DIAGNOSIS

- Determine severity of acne: comedonal, papular, nodular.
- Evaluate possibility of endocrinopathy.
- Evaluate rosacea patients for ocular involvement.

CURRENT THERAPY

- Topical retinoids are the cornerstone of acne therapy.
- Mild disease is well treated with topical therapy (e.g., retinoid plus benzoyl peroxide or clindamycin).
- More severe inflammatory acne usually requires oral doxycycline or minocycline.
- Resistant nodular acne may be treated with isotretinoin.
- Ocular rosacea is best treated with doxycycline.

REFERENCES

Webster GF: Acne vulgaris. BMJ 2002;325:475-479.

Leyden JJ: A review of the use of combination therapy for the treatment of acne vulgaris. J Am Acad Dermatol 2003;49:S200-S210.

Diseases of the Hair

Method of
Azim J. Khan, MD, Dwight Scarborough, MD, and Emil Bisaccia, MD

Like any other disease entity, diseases of the hair require a thorough history, good physical examination, and sometimes the pertinent laboratory examinations to reach the correct diagnosis. History should always include the duration of onset, the location and the extent of hair loss, family history of similar hair loss, any drug intake, systemic illness, any endocrine abnormality, and history of pulling at the hairs (including compulsive or incidental pulling caused by hair styling and use of hair styling techniques). The examination should include:

- Careful examination of the hair-bearing areas to evaluate the hair density, caliber, and quality
- Examination of the scalp to look for any sign of inflammation and/or scarring
- Examination of the thyroid gland to rule out any thyromegaly
- Examination of the nails

Visual examination of the hair density is usually not very accurate. Approximately 50% of the hairs are generally lost before any hair loss is visually apparent. Parting the hairs at different scalp sites and then comparing the width of the part is more accurate in determining the hair density. Hair density is higher during childhood and decreases with age in both sexes. Crown hair density is usually less than the density at the sides of the scalp.

The history may guide the physician to perform a more detailed examination, including the performing of any pertinent laboratory workup. For example, a case of nonscarring, generalized hair thinning can be a sign of thyroid abnormality, thus necessitating a thyroid-stimulating hormone (TSH) level determination. Similarly a patient with irregular menstruation, acne, and hair loss may require a workup to rule out any androgen excess by performing testosterone and dehydroepiandrosterone sulfate (DHEAS) level tests. A patient with anemia and nonscarring alopecia should be checked for ferritin levels, which is an exceedingly important cause to rule out in most female patients with nonscarring alopecia. In patients with low levels of ferritin (<20 µg/L), generalized thinning of the hair is noted much earlier than the development of anemia. Usually a ferritin level of greater than 40 µg/L is required for the normal growth and development of healthy hairs. Most diseases of the hair can be easily understood and diagnosed by comprehending two vital concepts. The first is the concept of normal hair cycling, and the second involves the clinical classifications of alopecias.

Normal Hair Growth Cycle

On average, a normal scalp contains 100,000 hair follicles. Every hair follicle goes through three phases in its growth cycle:

1. Anagen is the growing phase (lasting an average of 3 years).
2. Telogen is the resting phase (lasting approximately 3 months).
3. Catagen is the destructive phase (lasting approximately 3 weeks).

Approximately 90% of hair follicles on a healthy scalp are in the anagen phase, approximately 10% are in the telogen phase, and less than 1% of hair follicles are in the catagen phase at any given time. It is of note that telogen or catagen hairs are the hairs that fall out spontaneously on a daily basis, and their number usually ranges from 100 to 150 hairs in a normal individual. This is important to know, as many patients may perceive this much hair shedding, which is normal, as pathogenic.

Classifications of Alopecia

Many classifications of alopecia are proposed, but one of the more useful classifications involves dividing the alopecias into scarring and nonscarring categories. On a close visual examination of any area of alopecia, one should be able to discern the presence or absence of hair follicle ostia even if the area is devoid of terminal hairs. If the follicular ostia are present, one of the nonscarring alopecias should be considered in the differential diagnosis. On the other hand, the scarring alopecias are diagnosed by the presence of scar tissue without any follicular ostia visible in it. This distinction is clinically important not only in the diagnosis but also in determining the prognosis of the disease, as most of the scarring alopecias result from severe inflammation of the hair follicle resulting in irreversible damage to the follicle and poor prognosis. Many of the nonscarring alopecias, however, are reversible.

The most common causes of hair loss include androgenetic alopecia (male and female pattern baldness), alopecia areata, trichotillomania secondary to compulsive or incidental hair pulling and traction, telogen effluvium, infections, hair shaft abnormalities, and hereditary and congenital dermatosis, among others. Following are brief descriptions and treatment options for some of the most commonly encountered hair disorders.

NONSCARRING ALOPECIA

Androgenetic Alopecia

Androgenetic alopecia (AGA) is characterized by receding hairline in the frontotemporal fashion in males and generalized thinning of hair in the central scalp in women without any hairline recession. Nonscarring, diffuse, low-density, and thinner caliber hairs, without any distinct patchy hair loss, can easily differentiate AGA from other types of alopecias. Family history on the maternal or paternal side is usually an indicator for AGA. The disease affects at least 50% of men by age 50 and probably a similar percentage of women as well. It can begin at any age after puberty. Testosterone is converted into dihydrotestosterone, which in turn is believed to cause the miniaturization of the susceptible hair follicles in the frontoparietal scalp. The conversion of testosterone into dihydrotestosterone is brought about by enzymatic action of 5α-reductase type II found in hair follicles and prostate glands. Finasteride (Propecia), a 5α-reductase inhibitor, at a dose of 1 mg orally every day, is the most effective FDA-approved treatment for AGA in men that is available today.

In placebo-controlled studies, 100% of men noted hair loss in the placebo group whereas 65% in Propecia group had no further hair loss and 35% had retained greater hair density compared to the placebo group. Thus, at the minimum, Propecia can halt or slow the further progression of the hair loss in men. Because finasteride lowers the prostate-specific antigen (PSA) level, a baseline PSA level should be obtained, in case there is a need to follow them in the future. This can be valuable, especially in the middle-aged-to-elderly population who are being monitored for serial PSA levels because of prostatic pathology.

The use of Propecia, however, should not mask the detection of prostate cancer. Some suggest doubling the value of PSA in patients on Propecia for interpretation purposes. Propecia is usually a well-tolerated medication, as it does not affect spermatogenesis or semen production. Sexual side effects encountered in less than 2% of patients are almost always reversible on discontinuation of therapy and resolve in approximately 50% of patients who continue therapy. The benefit of the therapy can be maintained as long as the therapy is continued. Propecia is not recommended for use in females. Pregnant women should not even handle the pills because of possible transcutaneous absorption and possible feminization of the male fetus.

In females, AGA manifests as generalized thinning rather than hairline recession and frank baldness. A strong family history of female pattern baldness may predispose patients to this condition at an early age; otherwise this pattern of hair loss is generally seen in perimenopausal patients. If seen in a younger patient, a workup to rule out androgen excess is warranted, especially if other signs of hyperandrogenism (acne, hirsutism) are co-existent. This is done by testing testosterone and DHEAS levels.

Adrenal hyperplasia and polycystic ovary disease are more likely to be encountered in a young patient with AGA as compared to a woman over 65 years of age. Also, female patients thought to have AGA should be ruled out for other systemic causes, such as thyroid abnormality and decreased ferritin level, as generalized hair thinning in female patients is often multifactorial. As opposed to males, multiple therapy options to counteract androgen excess exist for female patients. Most of them, however, are not FDA approved for AGA

in particular. Either increasing the estrogen levels or decreasing the androgen levels can be effective. Estrogen-dominant oral contraceptives like Premarin[1] alone or in combination with progesterone (Provera)[1] can be used for estrogen replacement therapy. An antiandrogen like spironolactone (Aldactone),[1] 50 to 200 mg per day, is an effective antiandrogen. Some physicians like to monitor serum K^+ levels, especially if Aldactone is given in higher doses. Dexamethasone,[1] 0.125 to 0.25 mg orally at night, can effectively suppress adrenal-based androgen excess. Although effective, none of these treatments is FDA approved for AGA in females.

Telogen Effluvium

Telogen effluvium is a very common nonscarring, generalized alopecia that is caused by a variety of physical or emotional traumas. Usually pregnancy, crash dieting, and intense physical or emotional stress, including major surgeries, are the most frequent causes of telogen effluvium. The diagnosis is usually made clinically on careful history depicting some form of trauma within a few months (6 weeks to 4 months) before the onset of the hair loss. The diagnosis of telogen effluvium can be further strengthened by performing a *hair-pluck* trichogram, a painful procedure that is falling out of favor because of the discomfort it poses to the patient. The test is performed by firmly plucking approximately 50 hairs using a hemostat whose jaws are covered with tape to afford a firm grip on the hair. The analysis of the roots of these hairs is easily performed by sandwiching them between two glass slides under a low-power microscope. If the telogen club-shaped hairs are found in more than 10% of the hair sample, it usually indicates telogen effluvium. The plucked anagen hairs are broomstick-shaped and covered with glistening inner and outer hair root sheaths; the plucked telogen hairs are smooth and club shaped at the base. This information is usually helpful in determining the percentage of hairs that are in the anagen versus the telogen phase.

Anagen Effluvium

Most commonly caused by cancer-treating chemotherapeutic agents, anagen effluvium is clinically characterized by marked thinning of the scalp hair, which begins shedding after 1 to 2 weeks of chemotherapy treatment—or other insults like radiation therapy or protein calorie malnutrition—and becomes most evident within 1 to 2 months. Broken hairs show a progressive narrowing of the hair shaft proximally caused by the arrest in keratinization and impaired DNA synthesis, which makes the hair shaft narrow and fragile. A tourniquet band or pressure cuff applied around the scalp during the chemotherapy session is effective in preventing hair loss secondary to chemotherapy. After the cessation of the chemotherapy, hair growth almost always returns to normal.

---

[1]Not FDA approved for this indication.

Alopecia Areata

Alopecia areata (AA) is a cell-mediated, autoimmune disease that manifests as patchy round or oval nonscarring hair loss of scalp or any other hair-bearing area. In a small number of patients, a positive family history for alopecia areata can be elicited. Quite often patients give a history of some emotional trauma or stress prior to its onset. The most commonly affected areas include scalp, beard area, eyebrows, eyelashes, and, less commonly, other hair-bearing body areas. If the whole scalp is involved, it is termed *alopecia totalis;* if the whole body is involved, the disease is termed *alopecia universalis.* The diagnosis is usually clinical except in rare, difficult situations requiring a punch biopsy of the scalp. On close clinical examination, smooth noninflammatory nonscarring patch(es), sometimes containing a few short proximally tapered hairs (exclamation point hairs), are seen. One helpful clue is the presence of nail pitting, which is seen in many patients with alopecia areata. Some related abnormalities include Hashimoto's thyroiditis, vitiligo, and other autoimmune diseases. Many physicians routinely perform a TSH hormone level test to rule out any related thyroid abnormality. Others suggest antithyroid antibody determination to screen patients who may be at risk for hypothyroidism in the future. Mostly, however, alopecia areata occurs without any associated disease.

Spontaneous recovery is seen in most patients within a few months even without any treatment. Treatment, however, seems to promote the regrowth of the alopecia patches sooner than spontaneous recovery, and thus is recommended in most cases. If the areas involved are small and few in number, then a potent topical steroid like clobetasol (Temovate Gel),[1] 0.1% gel twice daily, or intralesional triamcinolone acetonide,[1] 5 to 10 mg/mL repeated every 6 weeks, can be effective. In resistant cases, or in rapidly spreading larger areas, a short course of oral steroids in tapering doses followed by topical or intralesional steroids can be effective. Small, localized patches in postpubertal patients are usually a good prognostic sign. Poor prognostic signs include prepubertal onset, widespread involvement, alopecia totalis or universalis, involvement of the occipital hairline (ophiasis pattern), and disease process of more than 5-year duration.

The challenging nonrespondent cases may require prolonged use of oral steroids, but caution is advised because of the side-effect risks. Other agents shown to be of some benefit in resistant cases include topical sensitizers such as topical 1% anthralin[1] used for 10 to 20 minutes a day and then washed off to produce a local-controlled inflammatory response. Similarly diphencyprone,[1] squaric acid dibutylester,[1] and dinitrochlorobenzene[1] are some of the local sensitizers that can be considered in resistant cases. Most of these agents, however, are not FDA approved for AA therapy. Also, concern regarding the use of low-level, chronic inflammation-causing sensitizers, reactive lymphoid hyperplasia, and possible mutagenic potential has kept many from using these sensitizing agents. Oral psoralen plus ultraviolet light of A wavelength (PUVA)[1] has also been used in resistant cases with some success.

Whether spontaneous or secondary to treatment, the regrowth is initially fuzzy hairs, usually grey in color, which gradually become thicker and regain the pigment slowly. Many patients with complete recovery may experience recurrences at other areas down the road and should be educated about this possibility. The National Alopecia Areata Foundation is a useful education and support group resource for patients, especially those with severe disease.

Trichotillomania

Trichotillomania is obsessive, compulsive, or habitual picking or plucking of hairs causing traumatic breakage of hair shafts at different lengths. It is usually associated with anxiety, depression, or obsessive-compulsive disorders. If performed repeatedly, it can cause permanent damage to the hair follicle and lead to scarring alopecia. The diagnosis is usually clinical but can be quite difficult in certain cases. Some suggest asking the patient *catch questions* like, "How do you pluck hairs," rather than asking, "Do you pluck hairs," as most of the patients deny that they are plucking the hairs at all. Another helpful technique is to shave a small affected area and then watch for the normal hair regrowth as the patient cannot pluck the newly regrowing tiny hairs. A 4-mm punch biopsy can usually confirm the diagnosis in most difficult situations. The characteristic findings include pigmented casts and hemorrhage in the hair follicles, usually without inflammatory changes. Psychotherapy or psychopharmacologic medications are the treatment of choice for this condition. A psychiatric referral can be beneficial in most cases.

CICATRICIAL (SCARRING) ALOPECIA

Cicatricial or scarring alopecia results from the inflammatory destruction of the hair stem cells that reside in the bulge portion of the hair follicle. If this portion is irreversibly destroyed, it can lead to irreversible hair loss and scarring. The end stage in many inflammatory cicatricial alopecias results in a clinical picture termed *pseudopelade of Brocq,* which refers to the resultant scarring rather than the etiology that caused scarring in the first place. Major causes of cicatricial alopecia are infections (e.g., bacteria-like folliculitis decalvans, viral or fungal), physical injuries (e.g., burns, trauma), congenital defects (e.g., aplasia cutis), neoplasms (e.g., cutaneous T-cell lymphoma), and many inflammatory dermatoses of the scalp (e.g., lupus, lichen planopilaris). To determine the cause of the inflammation that is causing the localized scarring, a culture sensitivity of any suspicious infection for the suspected agent (bacterial, viral, or fungal), as well as a 4-mm punch biopsy, can be extremely helpful. This is especially true if biopsy is obtained early in the course of the disease rather than from an end-stage scar, which is usually nondiagnostic.

---

[1]Not FDA approved for this indication.

[1]Not FDA approved for this indication.

If diagnosed early, with the appropriate treatment of the underlying cause, the scarring process can usually be halted.

Folliculitis Decalvans

Folliculitis decalvans is characterized by a progressive destruction of the hair follicles secondary to folliculitis. The exact etiology is not known; however, *Staphylococcus aureus* is a common pathogen in many cases. The clinical picture varies according to the extent of the disease but often involves the follicular-based papules and pustules that result in confluent, erythematous plaques sometimes with tufted folliculitis with *doll-like* hairs. In cases with bacterial etiology, long-term antibiotic therapy may halt the process.

Lichen Planopilaris

Also termed *follicular lichen planus,* lichen planopilaris is a variant of lichen planus. Approximately 50% of lichen planopilaris patients also have typical cutaneous or oral lichen planus lesions concurrently or prior to the onset of lichen planopilaris. The disease is four times more common in females ages 30 to 70 years old, and it usually involves the scalp and eyebrows only. Typical clinical presentations involve the follicular erythema, follicular hyperkeratosis, and, eventually, scarring alopecia if not treated early on. Treatments usually include potent topical steroids or intralesional steroids.

Discoid Lupus Erythematosus

Discoid lupus erythematosus (DLE) is mostly confined to the skin (approximately 95%) without any systemic involvement. In rare instances a larger area, especially below the neck, is also involved; in this case a systemic involvement is more likely. The characteristic erythematous, indurated hypo- or hyperpigmented patches, or plaques with atrophic centers and follicular plugging, are usually seen on the scalp, nose bridge, malar surfaces, and the ears. Scarring alopecia is a common sequela of scalp DLE. Clinical diagnosis can be easily confirmed on biopsy, and treatment with local or intralesional steroids usually suffices. In more resistant cases and in systemic involvement, an antimalarial agent may be helpful.

Hair Shaft Abnormalities

Increased fragility that results from most hair shaft abnormalities is the main cause of alopecia seen in these disorders. A number of inherited hair shaft disorders have been described in many different syndromes involving many systemic complaints. Trichorrhexis nodosa is the most commonly acquired hair shaft abnormality and is caused by chemical or physical damage to the hair shaft. Chronic bending of the weakened hair shaft produces the broomstick appearance that characterizes trichorrhexis nodosa. The diagnosis can be easily performed with light microscopic examination of the hair shaft. Treatment involves avoiding the physical or chemical substances that caused damage to the hair shaft along with gentle handling and aggressive use of gentle hair conditioners. The inherited form of trichorrhexis nodosa is an autosomal dominant condition that is usually found in argininosuccinicaciduria.

Cancer of the Skin

Method of
Richard F. Wagner, Jr., MD

Ultraviolet light (UVL) skin damage plays an important etiologic role in most basal cell carcinoma (BCC) and squamous cell carcinoma (SCC). UVL interacts with a variety of factors, including host genotype, Fitzpatrick skin type, and immunocompetence, that determine whether acute (sunburn) and chronic cumulative UVL injury will cause skin cancer. Less frequent causes of skin cancer in the United States are ionizing radiation exposure, arsenic ingestion, traumatic skin injury, tobacco (SCC of lip), and chemical carcinogen. Many genetic disorders predispose patients to skin cancer through a variety of mechanisms, such as albinism, basal cell nevus syndrome, xeroderma pigmentosum, and epidermolysis bullosa. Genital SCC is almost always associated with human papilloma virus (HPV), often identified as HPV-16 or -18. HPV interacts with sunlight to result in life-threatening SCC in a rare skin disease, epidermodysplasia verruciformis.

Clinical Features

Nodular BCC is the most common subtype of BCC (80%), and it classically manifests as a shiny papule with visible telangiectasia. Nodular BCC may be pigmented and can be confused with nodular melanoma. Superficial BCC (15%) usually appears as an erythematous thin plaque on the trunk, with a subtle threadlike raised border. The most difficult type of primary BCC to recognize clinically is the morpheaform or sclerotic type, appearing much like a scar. Neglected BCC, although usually painless, may ulcerate ("rodent ulcer") and bleed, have a foul odor, and reach enormous size.

SCC may be difficult to distinguish clinically from BCC. The presence of keratotic scale and the absence of classic BCC morphology are the best clinical indicators for SCC. Organ transplant patients on immunosuppressive therapy are more likely to have SCC than BCC. SCC remains the most common malignancy of the mucosal lip. Bowen's disease, or SCC in situ (SCCIS), may resemble superficial BCC. When SCCIS arises on the uncircumcised mucosal penis (erythroplasia of Queyrat), it is typically moist and bright red with sharp clinical margins. SCCIS may develop into invasive SCC, and invasive SCC may also arise from actinic keratoses. Invasive SCC

13

classically manifests as a red papule or nodule with scale. The keratoacanthoma is regarded by many dermatopathologists as a subtype of well-differentiated invasive SCC, often having a history of sudden rapid growth and a central keratotic crater. Large (2-cm diameter or greater) invasive SCC are more likely to have perineural invasion, especially if the tumor is recurrent.

Regional lymph nodes should be examined for patients with BCC and SCC, and a bimanual examination of the mouth is recommended for patients with SCC of the mucosal lip. Pathologic lymph nodes should be referred to a specialist for fine-needle aspiration (FNA) and imaging studies to exclude metastatic skin cancer to lymph nodes, the most frequent site of metastasis.

Treatment Cryosurgery

Cryosurgery with liquid nitrogen, an effective treatment for BCC and SCC, relies on the destructive effect of the freeze-thaw cycle on living cells. It should be performed under the guidance of a thermocouple to ensure an adequate depth of freeze. Cold sensitivity disorders such as cryoglobulinemia are contraindications.

Electrodesiccation and Curettage

Electrodesiccation and curettage (EDC) remains the most frequently used treatment modality for BCC and SCC in the United States. It is highly effective in selected tumors, and although variability is reported among physicians using the technique, 95% cure rates are cited for small primary BCC and SCC. It is often the fastest and least expensive treatment, and it is very effective for small BCC and SCC (5 mm or less) that arise on areas of skin that are not high tumor recurrence zones, such as on the arms, legs, and trunk. It can also be effective for superficial BCC and SCCIS, as long as the tumor does not extend down the hair follicle. EDC treatment sites heal by second intention and are usually flat and hypopigmented. In one private dermatology practice setting, there was no statistical difference in recurrence rates for primary BCC and SCC treated with either EDC or excision, although previous studies from academic centers favored excision.

Other Destructive Options

Surgical lasers such as the carbon dioxide and the erbium:yttrium-aluminum-garnet (Er:YAG) are also used to ablate small or superficial BCC and SCCIS.

Standard Surgical Excision

For primary BCC less than 2 cm in diameter, excision with a 4-mm margin yields a 95% cure rate. Margins for primary SCC of the same size should be 4 to 6 mm, adjusted for specific tumor characteristics. If excision is initially attempted and the surgical margin is

subsequently reported positive, Mohs' micrographic surgery (MMS) or adjuvant radiation therapy should be considered.

Mohs' Micrographic Surgery

Mohs' micrographic surgery fully integrates the roles of dermasurgeon and dermatopathologist, and it achieves the highest statistical cure rates for BCC and SCC with maximal conservation of uninvolved tissue. MMS has a wide range of indications, including BCC and SCC arising in areas of high recurrence (nose, lip, eyelid, ear, etc.) or areas where maximal tissue sparing is needed and for tumors that are recurrent, have specific histologic subtypes, show perineural invasion, have poorly defined clinical margins, or have a diameter greater than 1 cm on the face or 2 cm elsewhere.

Photodynamic Therapy

The basis of photodynamic therapy (PDT) is the activation of selectively absorbed photosensitizers by skin cancer and subsequent destruction of these cells by visible light. Superficial BCC and SCCIS are successfully treated with topically applied photosensitizers, but currently this method is not widely available in the United States.

Radiation Therapy

Fractionated radiation therapy (typical total of 4000 to 6000 cGy) is an effective but costly treatment for primary and recurrent BCC and SCC, with reported 90% cure rates. It is especially useful for treating tumors in patients with co-morbid medical conditions that put them at high risk for surgical complications or when surgical treatment would result in extensive morbidity. Because of the lower statistical cure rate than MMS and the risk for late local cutaneous complications, including the rare risk of another primary tumor in the radiation portal (SCC is most common), primary radiation therapy for BCC and SCC is not widely employed in healthy patients younger than 50 years in the United States. For surgically treated SCC with perineural invasion and unusually aggressive BCC and SCC, adjuvant radiation therapy is offered at many medical centers to decrease the risk of tumor recurrence. It is relatively contraindicated for patients with basal cell nevus syndrome, xeroderma pigmentosum, and epidermodysplasia verruciformis.

Topical Medicines

Topical 5-fluorouracil (Efudex) is used successfully to treat superficial BCC, but patients frequently cannot complete the recommended treatment course because of brisk local inflammation (pregnancy category X). Imiquimod (Aldara) cream, a biologic response modifier,

Diseases of the Skin

CURRENT DIAGNOSIS

- BCC and SCC can arise anywhere on the skin, but sun-exposed surfaces are the most likely.
- Clinical distinction between BCC and SCC is possible (shiny papule with telangiectasia for the most frequent type of BCC and the presence of keratotic scale in SCC), but a skin biopsy is necessary for a definitive diagnosis.

Abbreviations: BCC = basal cell carcinoma; SCC = squamous cell carcinoma.

recently gained FDA approval for nonfacial superficial BCC that are less than 2.0 cm in diameter in immunocompetent adults and are not located in the hands, feet, or anogenital skin, when surgery is less appropriate and patient follow-up is likely (pregnancy category C).

CURRENT THERAPY

- Electrodesiccation and curettage is an excellent treatment for small BCC and SCC with distinct clinical margins (diameter 5 mm or less) that are not on high recurrence risk areas and do not demonstrate high recurrence risk histopathology or perineural invasion.
- Standard surgical excision is a good treatment option for facial BCC and SCC that have distinct clinical margins and are 1.0 cm or less in diameter when the tumors are not in high-risk areas for tumor recurrence or show histopathology associated with aggressive biologic behavior. It is also a good option for primary BCC and SCC elsewhere that have distinct clinical margins and are 2.0 cm in diameter or less and do not have high recurrence risk histopathology or perineural invasion. If surgical pathology reveals marginal tumor involvement, referral for Mohs' micrographic surgery should be considered because such tumors are often larger than the initial clinical impression.
- Mohs' micrographic surgery has the highest statistical chance for cure for BCC and SCC. It should be a consideration for primary BCC and SCC arising in high recurrence risk areas (nose, ears, eyelids, lips, etc.), tumors that are greater than 1.0 cm diameter anywhere on the face or greater than 2 cm elsewhere on the body, and for recurrent BCC and SCC or those with specific histopathologic patterns or findings such as morpheaform, micronodular, and perineural invasion.
- Radiation therapy is usually reserved for patients who are 50 years of age or older and not good surgical candidates because of uncontrolled medical co-morbidity or extensive morbidity associated with surgical treatment options.

Abbreviations: BCC = basal cell carcinoma; SCC = squamous cell carcinoma.

Rakel and Bope: *Conn's Current Therapy 2006.*

Systemic and Topical Chemoprophylaxis

No FDA-approved prescription medications for skin cancer prevention are currently available.

Patient Follow-up and Aftercare

Scheduled follow-up visits every 6 months in the case of primary BCC and every 3 months for recurrent BCC and primary or recurrent SCC are recommended to check for tumor recurrence. Patients presenting with a BCC skin cancer have approximately a 36% risk for additional primary BCC.

Patients with a history of nonmelanoma skin cancer should be advised to reduce their UVL exposure. It is reasonable to advise these patients to take daily oral supplemental vitamin D every day (200 IU to age 50, 400 IU from age 51 to 70, and 600 IU at age 71 and older) to compensate for decreased sunlight exposure. Immunosuppressed patients may be vitamin D deficient because of sun avoidance and other factors, and they may require specialized protocols and monitoring to normalize and maintain their vitamin D levels.

REFERENCES

Brodland DG, Zitelli JA: Surgical margins for excision of primary cutaneous squamous cell carcinoma. J Am Acad Dermatol 1992;27(2 Pt 1):241-248.
Robinson JK: Risk of developing another basal cell carcinoma. A 5-year prospective study. Cancer 1987;60(1):118-120.
Shriner D, McCoy DK, Goldberg DJ, Wagner RF Jr: Mohs micrographic surgery. J Am Acad Dermatol 1998;39(1):79-97.
Taub AF: Photodynamic therapy in dermatology: History and horizons. J Drugs Dermatol 2004;3(1 Suppl):S8-S25.
Werlinger KD, Upton G, Moore AY: Recurrence rates of primary nonmelanoma skin cancers treated by surgical excision compared to electrodesiccation-curettage in private dermatological practice. Dermatol Surg 2002;28(12):1138-1142.
Wolf DJ, Zitelli JA: Surgical margins for basal cell carcinoma. J Am Acad Dermatol 1987;123(3):340-344.

Cutaneous T-cell Lymphomas (Mycosis Fungoides and Sézary's Syndrome)

Method of
Christiane Querfeld, MD, Steven T. Rosen, MD, and Timothy M. Kuzel, MD

Cutaneous T-cell lymphomas (CTCLs) represent clinically and biologically a heterogeneous group of non-Hodgkin's lymphomas (NHLs) with clonal proliferation of skin-homing malignant T lymphocytes. CTCLs are characterized by a prolonged clinical course with a different

13

clinical behavior and outcome compared to their systemic counterpart. But disease progression may involve lymph nodes, peripheral blood, and visceral organs with a less favorable prognosis. Features of the different types of CTCL are recognized in the new revised European Organization for Research and Treatment of Cancer (EORTC) and World Health Organization (WHO) classification for primary cutaneous lymphomas, which distinguishes indolent types such as mycosis fungoides (MF) from aggressive types such as Sézary syndrome (SS).

The most common types of CTCL, MF and SS, represent monoclonal T helper memory lymphomas. MF/SS is predominantly a disease of older patients, with a median age of onset of 55 years, a male predominance of approximately 2:1, and an age-adjusted ratio of African Americans to whites of 1:7. It has an annual incidence of approximately 0.36 cases per 100,000 people that overall represents 2.2% of all NHLs.

Cutaneous lymphomas include other entities such as the adult T-cell leukemia/lymphoma (ATLL), which is etiologically associated with human T-cell leukemia virus 1 (HTLV-1). The chronic smoldering form is frequently associated with skin lesions often resembling MF. Lymphomatoid papulosis (LyP) and anaplastic large T-cell lymphoma (ALCL) belong to the CD30+ lymphoproliferative disorders. Their common phenotypic hallmark is the CD30+ T lymphocyte that resembles Reed-Sternberg cells morphologically. Cutaneous ALCL rarely carries the t(2;5) translocation and is usually large cell anaplastic lymphoma kinase (ALK) negative. Both appear to have a favorable clinical course. Subcutaneous panniculitis-like T-cell lymphoma is a cytotoxic T-cell lymphoma that involves the subcutaneous tissue, mimicking panniculitis. The heterogeneous group of peripheral T-cell lymphoma includes provisional entities such as cutaneous aggressive CD8+ cytotoxic T-cell lymphoma, cutaneous γ/δ T-cell lymphoma, and cutaneous CD4+ small/medium-sized pleomorphic T-cell lymphoma. Other hematologic neoplasms, such as the EBV(Epstein-Barr virus)-associated extranodal NK/T-cell lymphoma, nasal type, and the EBV-negative blastic NK-cell lymphoma, frequently occur in the skin with or without concurrent extracutaneous manifestations.

Clinical and Pathologic Features

MF has numerous clinical and histologic variants. Besides the classical Alibert-Bazin type of MF, three major variants are recognized in the new EORTC-WHO classification, including granulomatous slack skin, folliculocentric MF, and pagetoid reticulosis. MF is typified by the development of patches, plaques, or tumors (Table 1). Most patients remain in clinical stages limited to the skin; however, a small percentage progress to the tumor or erythrodermic stages, and their estimated 5-year survival rate is only 40%. SS is the erythrodermic and aggressive variant of CTCL with a leukemic component, characterized by circulating, atypical, malignant T lymphocytes with cerebriform nuclei (Sézary cells), the presence of erythroderma, and often lymphadenopathy. Severe pruritus, ectropion, alopecia, and palmoplantar

TABLE 1 Stage Classification for Mycosis Fungoides/Sézary Syndrome

Stage	T	N	NP	M
IA	1	0	0	0
IB	2	0	0	0
IIA	1/2	1	0	0
IIB	3	0/1	0	0
III	4	0/1	0	0
IVA	1-4	0/1	1	0
IVB	1-4	0/1	0/1	1

Abbreviations: M = metastases; N = node; NP = performed lymph node biopsy; T = tumor.

keratoderma are common associated features. Patients with SS have an unfavorable prognosis with an estimated 5-year survival rate of 15%.

Several histologic features are useful in establishing a diagnosis of MF/SS. In most cases, it consists of an upper-dermal bandlike lymphocytic infiltrate with atypical lymphocytes, variable findings of inflammatory cells, and epidermal involvement with solitary cells or small clusters of malignant lymphocytes (Pautrier's microabscesses). Tumor lesions express more diffuse and deep infiltrates with diminished epidermotropism. Biopsies from erythrodermic MF or SS are often lacking these features; thus the presence of a dominant T-cell clone is an important diagnostic criterion. Procedures based on polymerase chain reaction (PCR) are the most sensitive to detect clonality and represent an important adjuvant procedure, in association with histopathology and immunophenotyping, to support the clinical diagnosis.

In cases of classical MF/SS, the neoplastic lymphocytes bear a T-helper/memory antigenic profile (CD2+, CD3+, CD4+, CD5+, CD7+, CD8-, CD26-, CD45RO+) with frequent loss of the CD5 and/or CD7 antigen in advanced stages. Recently, CD158k, a major histocompatibility complex (MHC) class I antigen receptor, was found selectively expressed on circulating and cutaneous malignant T cells from SS patients, which might represent a new phenotypic marker. Patients with advanced-stage MF/SS show a helper T-cell type 1 and 2 (T_h1/T_h2) imbalance with a predominant type 2 immune response characterized by increased cytokine production of interleukin-4 (IL-4), IL-6, and IL-10 and decreased interferon-γ (IFN-γ) and IL-2 resulting in an impaired cell-mediated immunity. In advanced stages, the number of reactive cytotoxic CD8+ T cells and dendritic cells, which are characteristic in early patch stage cutaneous lesions, tend to decrease with an increase of neoplastic CD4+ T cells.

Etiology, Molecular Biology, and Molecular Genetics

Many factors are implicated in the etiology of CTCL, including microbiologic, environmental, or occupational theories, but none are yet verified. Previous studies on the pathogenesis reveal acquired oncogene abnormalities

Rakel and Bope: *Conn's Current Therapy 2006.*

such as diminished expression of the tumor suppressor genes TGF-β receptor II, Fas, p15, p16, and overexpression of JUNB on peripheral malignant CD4+ T lymphocytes, suggesting they may be crucial in the pathogenesis of CTCL. Comparative analyses of clonal lymphocytes derived from SS patients revealed aberrations in signaling pathways by the signal transducer and activator of transcription (STAT) family and by impaired CD40/CD40L interaction. cDNA microarray analysis, a novel technique for genomic analysis in tumors, is used to screen rapidly for genomic imbalances and to show oncogene changes globally in MF and SS. A recent study shows that the antiapoptotic T-cell oncogene *Twist* and the growth-promoting tyrosine kinase receptor EpH4 are among the highly and selectively expressed genes in malignant T lymphocytes. CTCL is characterized by the accumulation of genetic mutations during disease progression. Molecular cytogenetic studies identify common regions of chromosomal deletion and amplification, involving structural rearrangements of chromosomes 1, 2, 6, 9, 14, and 16 and numerical abnormalities of 6, 8, 10, 11, 13, 17, and 21. Microsatellite instability, consistent with deficits in DNA repair, was found in a large number of biopsies from patients with MF with a higher prevalence in higher tumor stages. Promoter hypermethylation leading to tumor suppressor gene inactivation appears associated with disease progression.

Staging and Prognostic Factors

The recommended staging system is the TNMB (tumor, node, metastasis, blood), which considers the extent of skin involvement, presence of lymph node or visceral disease, and detection of Sézary cells in the peripheral blood (Box 1 and Table 1). Routine evaluation should include complete physical examination, complete blood count with differential, and Sézary cell assessment, chemistry panel with lactate dehydrogenase (LDH), skin biopsy for histology, immunophenotyping and gene rearrangement studies, and lymph node biopsies in cases with enlarged nodes at presentation. Diagnosis in early stages of MF is improved because of advances in TCR gene rearrangement techniques with increased sensitivity and specificity. Imaging studies should be reserved for patients with clinical and laboratory findings suggestive of systemic disease or prominent lymphadenopathy. Patients with T1 disease have a normal life expectancy, whereas patients with increased tumor burden have a significantly decreased survival. The median survival time of patients who develop extracutaneous disease is approximately 25 months.

Several studies attempt to identify clinical, biologic, histopathologic, or immunophenotypic characteristics that can predict outcome. So far, the main prognostic factors identified in MF/SS are the type and extent of skin involvement, extracutaneous manifestation of the disease, initial response to treatment, histologic large cell transformation, high serum level of lactate dehydrogenase (LDH), and the detection of a cutaneous or peripheral blood T-cell clone. A high Sézary cell count, loss of T-cell markers, blood eosinophilia, chromosomal

---

> **BOX 1   TNMB Classification for Mycosis Fungoides/Sézary Syndrome**
>
> **T (skin)**
>   T1 limited patch/plaque (<10% of BSA)
>   T2 generalized patch/plaque(>10% of BSA)
>   T3 tumors
>   T4 generalized erythroderma
> **N (nodes); LN (lymph nodes)**
>   N0 no clinically abnormal peripheral lymph nodes
>   N1 clinically abnormal peripheral lymph nodes
>   NP0 biopsy performed, not CTCL
>   NP1 biopsy performed, CTCL
>   LN0 uninvolved
>   LN1 reactive lymph node
>   LN2 dermatopathic node, small clusters of convoluted cells (<6 cells per cluster)
>   LN3* dermatopathic node, small clusters of convoluted cells (>6 cells per cluster)
>   LN4* lymph node effacement
> **M (viscera)**
>   M0 no visceral metastasis
>   M1 visceral metastasis
> **B (blood)**
>   B0 atypical circulating cells not present (<5%)
>   B1 atypical circulating cells present (>5%)
>
> *Abbreviations:* BSA = body surface area; CTCL = cutaneous T cell lymphoma; TNMB = tumor, node, metastasis, blood.
> *Pathologically involved lymph nodes.

13

---

abnormalities in T cells, and high serum concentration of soluble alpha chain of the interleukin-2 receptor (sIL-2R) are also independently associated with a poor outcome. The presence of cytotoxic CD8+ T lymphocytes in the dermal infiltrate, as well as the density of epidermal Langerhans cells greater than 90 cells/mm^2, is associated with a better prognosis.

Treatment: Early-Stage Disease

The treatment of MF/SS is stage dependent and regarded as palliative because no definitive curative treatment strategies are available at present. Patients with early-stage CTCL are ideally treated with topical agents such as nitrogen mustard, carmustine, retinoids, rexinoids, narrowband-ultraviolet light B (NB-UVB), photochemotherapy with psoralens and ultraviolet light A (UVA) (psoralen plus ultraviolet light of A wavelength [PUVA]), and total skin electron-beam irradiation. Multiagent chemotherapy regimens, used early in the course, demonstrate no survival benefit. Two recent retrospective studies support this approach. Kim and colleagues reported on 203 patients with MF/SS clinical stages I through III treated with topical nitrogen mustard. Relapse-free rates in T1 at 2 and 5 years were 74% and 54%, respectively, and in T2, 54% and 29%, respectively. Most relapses occurred within 2 years. Querfeld and colleagues reported on long-term remissions of patients with early-stage disease treated with PUVA. Depending on T stage, 30% to 50% of patients remain disease free after 10 years, but based on the occurrence of late relapses a permanent cure is not suggested. Our current approach for early-stage patients is the use of a topical monotherapy. If patients fail to respond, we switch to a different topical therapy. Our first-line treatment for early-stage patients is PUVA or NB-UVB therapy. In cases of refractory early stages, however, we consider combination therapy such as PUVA or NB-UVB with low-dose systemic bexarotene or IFN-α-2a (Roferon-A).

PHOTOTHERAPY

Since 1974 PUVA therapy has been widely used in treating psoriasis, vitiligo, and other skin disorders. 8-Methoxypsoralen (8-MOP), after oral ingestion, becomes activated when exposed to UVA light. UVA (320 to 400 µm), with its peak emission wavelength between 330 and 340 µm, penetrates the skin approximately 1 to 2 mm into the mid-dermis. The combination is thought to act at the nuclear level of cells, inhibiting DNA and RNA synthesis through formation of mono- or bifunctional thymine products, induction of gene mutations, or sister chromatid exchanges. Initial exposure times of patients are limited to the phototype according to the Fitzpatrick grading system, the ability to tan, and the patient's history of sunburns. The initial UVA dosage is approximately 0.5 J/cm^2 and increased per treatment as tolerated or up to the minimal erythema dose. Therapy is typically given three times a week until complete remission is achieved. Additional maintenance therapy can be administered while gradually reducing PUVA from once per week to once every 4 to 6 weeks, to maintain longer remission times.

Phototherapy is extremely effective at clearing patch and plaque disease with successfully reapplied courses in relapsed patients. Several studies confirm the efficacy of this treatment, with reported complete remissions (CRs) in up to 71.4% of patients. Long-term remissions of more then 8 years are reported in patients with early-stage MF. Disease-free survival rates for stage IA at 5 and 10 years were 56% and 30%, respectively, and for stage IB/IIA, 74% and 50%. The most common reported acute side effects are erythema, pruritus, and nausea, which are usually mild at presentation and generally manageable with dose adjustments of UVA or psoralens or dose interruptions. Long-term exposure is associated with an increased risk for developing chronic photodamage and skin cancer.

NB-UVB is considered less carcinogenic and may be an alternative treatment option in early-stage MF. In three small retrospective analyses, patients with clinical stage IA/IB and parapsoriasis treated with NB-UVB showed CR rates between 54.2% and 83%. Remission times were short, however, and a maintenance schedule was difficult to establish.

TOPICAL NITROGEN MUSTARD

Many investigators demonstrate the efficacy of topical nitrogen mustard (Mustargen) in early-stage MF with occasional long-term remissions of more then 8 years. Updates on 203 patients with MF treated with topical nitrogen mustard demonstrated its efficacy with reported CR rates of 76% to 80% for patients with stage IA and 35% to 68% for those with stage IB disease. The median duration of remission was short at 12 months, although less than 10% of patients developed progression to a higher stage disease. Topical nitrogen mustard is equally effective when used after disease relapses. The most common adverse effects are irritant contact dermatitis.

TOPICAL RETINOIDS

Application of topical retinoids may be an effective approach in early-stage MF. They exert their effects through two basic types of nuclear receptors: the retinoic acid (RAR) and rexinoid (RXR) receptor family. No comparison of different retinoids exists. Bexarotene 1% gel (Targretin gel), a new rexinoid, was approved by the Food and Drug Administration (FDA) as a therapy for stages IA through IIA MF. In a dose-escalating trial of bexarotene from 0.1% to 1.0%, the CR rate was 21%, with a 63% overall response rate. The median duration of remission was 24 months. A multinational phase III study of patients with refractory and/or persistent early-stage MF, treated with 1% bexarotene gel in a dose frequency escalating fashion, demonstrated an overall response rate of 54% and CR in 10%. The median duration was less favorable at 7 months. Reported events were mostly localized skin irritation.

TOTAL SKIN ELECTRON BEAM TREATMENT

In total skin electron beam treatment (TSEBT), ionizing radiation is administered to the entire skin surface, penetrating at least 4 mm into the dermis. The standard total dose is 36 Gy delivered with electrons of at least 4 MeV energy and fractionated over 8 to 10 weeks. Techniques, including dynamic rotation, 6-field, or regional patch treatments, are used to administer the electron beam. Published data of therapeutic efficacy of total skin electron beam therapy (TSEBT) from centers with extensive experience show 40% to 98% CR rates among patients from stage IA to IB, with approximately 50% of patients with clinical stage IA and 25% of patients with clinical stage IB remaining in long-term remission. TSEBT in early stages remains controversial because of its potential toxicity. Side effects can be significant and consist of erythema, edema, scaling, ulceration, and irreversible loss of skin adnexae. TSEBT may be repeated for palliative effects although at reduced doses. Adjuvant therapy, including PUVA, photopheresis, and INF-α, may improve the duration of response.

Treatment:
Advanced-Stage Disease

Treatment goals in advanced stages should be to reduce tumor burden, relieve symptoms, delay disease progression, and preserve quality of life. In particular, SS is refractory to most therapies, and historically no demonstrated treatment modifies significantly its natural course. Approaches for advanced disease treatment include spot radiation for single or localized skin tumors, mono- or polychemotherapy, extracorporeal photopheresis, interferon-α, oral retinoids, monoclonal antibodies, recombinant toxins, combination approaches of those just described, and high-dose chemotherapy with allogeneic bone marrow transplant. Nonrandomized clinical trials do not suggest any one treatment is preferable. Treatment choice should be made with the patient's preference and practitioner's skill in mind. The toxicity of treatment should not outweigh the cosmetic and functional disability of the disease.

SYSTEMIC CHEMOTHERAPY

Single-agent and combination chemotherapies in advanced/refractory MF/SS are associated with high response rates but are short lived. Their use is limited to palliation of symptoms. Options include single-agent or multiagent chemotherapy, including steroids, methotrexate, chlorambucil (Leukeran), vincristine (Oncovin), doxorubicin (Adriamycin), cyclophosphamide (Cytoxan), etoposide (VePesid), and alkylators. Combination regimens, including cyclophosphamide, doxorubicin, vincristine, and prednisone (CHOP) or CHOP-like therapy, achieve higher response rates of approximately 70% to 80%, compared to 25% to 35% for monotherapy.

Among single-agent chemotherapies, liposomal doxorubicin (Doxil), pentostatin (Nipent), and gemcitabine (Gemzar) are reportedly particularly effective. Pegylated liposomal doxorubicin tested empirically in MF/SS patients showed an overall response rate of 80% with CR in 6 of 10 patients (60%). More recent published multicenter data of pegylated doxorubicin in 34 patients with recurrent or recalcitrant CTCL reveals a response rate of 88.2%. Twenty-seven patients (79.4%) achieved CR with a median duration of 12 months ranging from 9.5 to 44 months. Adverse effects were generally mild compared with other chemotherapy regimens.

Gemcitabine, a pyrimidine antimetabolite with a low-toxicity profile, was evaluated in a phase II study for advanced and relapsed patients with MF or peripheral T-cell lymphoma. The compound was administered intravenously on days 1, 8, and 15 of a 28-day schedule at a dose of 1200 mg/m^2 for a total of three cycles. The reported overall response rate for 21 patients with MF/SS was 70%, with CR in 10% of patients and only mild hematologic toxicities observed.

Treatment with temozolomide (Temodal), an oral alkylating agent, appears effective in patients with MF and SS. Patients with MF/SS have low levels of the DNA repair enzyme O^6 alkylguanine DNA alkyltransferase (AGT), which inhibits the drug activity. Preliminary data reported a response in 5 of 19 patients with MF/SS (26%) with a median duration of 4 months. Response rate correlated with low levels of AGT. Patients with high AGT expression did not respond to treatment.

BIOLOGIC THERAPIES

Increased understanding of the pathophysiology of the disease has led to attempts to develop agents that may augment the host antitumor response to target the malignant cells selectively.

Retinoids

Retinoids have been used therapeutically since the early 1980s, and the benefits of some derivatives such as isotretinoin, etretinate, and acitretin were confirmed in several small monotherapy studies. Response rates ranged from 44% to 67%, with CR rates from 21% to 35% and median response duration around 8 months. Common side effects consisted of skin and mucous membrane dryness. The FDA has approved oral bexarotene (Targretin), a novel synthetic rexinoid, for the treatment of refractory or relapsed CTCL. In two multicenter phase II-III clinical trials in early and advanced stages of CTCL patients, reported response rates in early stages were between 45% and 54%. An overall response rate in 94 patients with advanced disease was with only 4% complete responders and a median duration of 10 months. The recommended dose of 300 mg/m^2 daily is associated with significant side effects, such as hyperlipidemia, hypothyroidism, and cytopenias. Retrospective comparison data suggest little difference in efficacy between bexarotene and agents such as all-*trans*-retinoic acid (RAR-specific retinoid), but clear differences in toxicity exist. New insights into the immunomodulatory function of retinoids with potential augmentation or reconstitution of T-helper cell type 1 response suggest opportunities for combined treatment with IFN-α, denileukin diftitox, or phototherapy.

Interferon-α

IFN-α (Roferon) is the most effective agent in the treatment of CTCL. It is initiated at low doses between 1 and 3 million IU (MU) three times weekly, with gradual escalation to 9 to 12 MU daily or as tolerated. T_h1 cytokines support cytotoxic T-cell–mediated immunity, and it is speculated that IFN-α maintains or enhances a T_h1 cell population balance for an effective cell-mediated response to malignant T lymphocytes. Bunn and colleagues first reported in 1984 the treatment of advanced and heavily pretreated patients with MF/SS with IFN-α. There was an overall response rate of 45%. Papa and colleagues achieved response rates between 70% for advanced-stage disease and 80% for early-stage disease. Olsen and colleagues tested 3 versus 36 MU daily of IFN-α-2a in 22 patients with clinical stage I to IV MF/SS; an overall response rate of 38% was observed in patients treated with low doses compared to 79% treated with high doses. Side effects are dose related and most commonly flulike symptoms. With chronic administration, depression, cytopenias, or impaired liver function tests occur. The development of neutralizing antibodies is associated with IFN-α therapy with variable impact on response rates. Combination therapy with IFN-α and PUVA results in higher response rates and shows superiority to other interferon combinations. Kuzel and colleagues reported on 39 patients with progressive disease treated with combined IFN-α/PUVA with an overall response rate of 92% and CR in 62% of patients and a median duration of 28 months. The combination abrogated the development of neutralizing antibodies.

Extracorporeal Photochemotherapy

Extracorporeal photochemotherapy (or photopheresis) (ECP) was originally designed as a modified PUVA treatment. It is a leukapheresis-based method for patients, in which after 8-MOP ingestion, circulating mononuclear cells are exposed to 1 to 2 J UVA in the machine and returned to the patient. It is performed on two consecutive days every 14 to 28 days. A suggested mechanism of action is induction of apoptosis of malignant circulating T lymphocytes with subsequent release of tumor antigens leading to a systemic antitumor response against the malignant T-cell clone. Reported response rates are 36% to 64% for patients with advanced disease, especially erythrodermic diseases with circulating neoplastic T cells. Optimal candidates for ECP are patients with SS with modest tumor burden and circulating neoplastic cells and almost normal counts of circulating $CD8^+$ T lymphocytes. Treatment of patients with plaques and tumors is not as effective.

TARGETED MODALITIES

Denileukin Diftitox (DAB389-IL-2, Ontak)

Recombinant toxins are genetically engineered proteins consisting of a toxin fused to a ligand that binds selectively to a target cell. The recombinant fusion protein denileukin diftitox, composed of diphtheria toxin coupled to human interleukin-2 (IL-2), is FDA approved for use in advanced and refractory CTCL. It targets the intermediate- and high-affinity IL-2 receptor (IL-2R) on malignant T lymphocytes. Once bound to the IL-2R, it is internalized by endocytosis with subsequent inhibition of ADP-ribosyltransferase and subsequent inhibition of protein synthesis with induction of apoptosis. Response rates to denileukin diftitox in patients with relapsed and refractory MF/SS range from 30% to 37%. Response correlates with improved quality of life. Adverse effects include acute infusion-related events, such as fever, rash, chills, dyspnea, and hypotension, and later effects, such as myalgias, elevated serum transaminases, and vascular leak syndrome (VLS). VLS occurred in 27% of patients and may be diminished by premedication with steroids. Bexarotene is known to up-regulate the expression of the high-affinity form of IL-2R in malignant lymphocytes and thus enhance the susceptibility of leukemia cells to denileukin diftitox.

MONOCLONAL ANTIBODIES

The developments of T-lymphocyte-specific monoclonal antibodies (MoAb) may add to the treatment of MF/SS. MoAb can mediate antitumor effects through three major mechanisms: intrinsic cytotoxic activity, antibody-dependent cellular cytotoxicity, and activation of complement-dependent cytolysis.

Alemtuzumab (Campath-1H)

Alemtuzumab is a humanized monoclonal IgG_1 antibody that targets the CD52 antigen abundantly expressed on normal and malignant B and T lymphocytes but not on hematopoietic stem cells. It is FDA approved for the treatment of chronic lymphocytic leukemia. A multicenter European study on alemtuzumab in low-grade NHL included 8 patients with heavily pretreated relapsed/refractory MF/SS with reported overall response rate (RR) of 50% and CR in 2 patients (25%). A recently published phase II trial of alemtuzumab in 22 patients with advanced MF/SS demonstrated a clinical response in 55% of cases and 32% CRs, with most impressive results demonstrated in SS patients. Median response duration was 12 months. Alemtuzumab was administered at a dose of 30 mg three times per week after using an initial dose escalating regimen. The compound is associated with significant hematologic toxicities and infectious complications consisting of reactivation of cytomegalovirus, herpes zoster, miliary tuberculosis, and pulmonary aspergillosis. Cytopenias and prolonged immunosuppression require both prophylactic antibiotic, antiviral, and antifungal treatment and potential support with granulocyte colony-stimulating factor (G-CSF).

PERIPHERAL STEM CELL TRANSPLANTATION

Autologous stem cell transplantation after high-dose chemotherapy yields disappointing results. Despite reported CRs in the majority of patients treated, relapses occurred rapidly. Allogeneic transplants are known to achieve much more durable complete remissions, most likely because of an immune-mediated graft-versus-lymphoma (GVL) effect. Response durations as far as 6 years post transplant are reported, suggesting it may be a curative option. It does carry a higher risk of treatment-related mortality, however, including life-threatening infections and graft-versus-host disease (GVHD). Reduced-intensity (mini) allogeneic transplants potentially offer a GVL effect with lesser toxicities related to the conditioning regimen.

INVESTIGATIONAL APPROACHES

CD4 Antibodies

Therapeutic effects of a chimeric (mouse/human) anti-CD4 antibody were observed as an active agent in MF/SS as early as 1991. Two phase I trials reported clinical improvement in patients with refractory MF. The reported overall response rate of patients was 88% (7 of 8 patients) with a median disease-free period of 25 weeks. The treatment was well tolerated without evidence of immunosuppression.

HuMax-CD4 is a fully human anti-CD4 ($IgG_1\kappa$) MoAb that targets the CD4 receptor expressed on T-helper/memory cells. Two ongoing phase II trials show promising results with an acceptable toxicity rate. Clinical improvement according to the Physician's Global Assessment was reported in 36% to 55% of early-stage patients and in 30% to 38% of advanced-stage patients treated for 16 weeks. Higher response rates were achieved with greater doses in early and advanced stages.

Histone Deacetylase Inhibitors

Hyperacetylation of tumor suppressor genes is frequently observed in CTCL. These genes are silenced by histone deacetylases, which remove acetyl groups from histones and then form complexes with DNA (nucleosome). Histone deacetylase (HDAC) inhibitors may restore the expression of tumor suppressor and/or cell cycle regulatory genes by increasing the acetylation of histones. Depsipeptide and suberoylanilide hydroxamic acid (SAHA), potent HDAC inhibitors, are shown in vitro and in vivo cytotoxic activity against various tumors. In recently conducted phase I trials, depsipeptide and SAHA were active in both MF and peripheral T-cell lymphoma.

Immunomodulators

Cytosine-phosphorothiolated guanine-containing oligodeoxynucleotides (CpG ODN) represent a new immune-modulating class of compounds being tested because host immune function appears to play an integral role in mediating responses in MF. Trials investigating the effects of a synthetic ODN with CpG motifs (CpG 7909) are under way. This drug activates dendritic cells following binding to toll-like receptor 9 (TLR9). Preliminary results demonstrate that the cytotoxic $CD8^+$ T-cell population increased within tumor infiltrates after systemic administration.

CURRENT DIAGNOSIS

- Clinical
    Early stage: persistent patches/plaques in non-sun-exposed areas
    Advanced stage: generalized erythroderma
- Lymphadenopathy
- Histopathological
    Epidermotropism
    Bandlike infiltrate
    Pautrier's microabscesses
    Atypical lymphocytes
- Immunophenotypic
    Early stage: $CD4^+$, $CD8^-$ phenotype (skin); $CD4^+$, $CD8^-$ phenotype (blood)
    Advanced stage: loss of $CD5^-$ and/or $CD7^-$
- Molecular
    Clonal T cell receptor gene rearrangement (skin)
    Clonal T cell receptor gene rearrangement (blood)
- Laboratory
    Sézary cells
    Elevated lactate dehydrogenase (LDH)

Vaccine Therapy

Therapeutic vaccination against MF/SS requires the characterization of tumor-specific epitopes, activation of dendritic cells for tumor antigen processing, and generation of a cytotoxic $CD8^+$ T-cell response. One strategy uses the T cell receptor (TCR) as a target to develop a TCR idiotype vaccine, but this is complicated by the variability of TCR-α and TCR-β chains. Berger and colleagues observed that extracorporeal photopheresis induces apoptosis in malignant T cells and maturation of immature dendritic cells with presentation of tumor-specific antigens, leading to a cytotoxic $CD8^+$ T-cell response. These findings led to the development of so-called transimmunization, which induces transfer of tumor-specific antigens to dendritic cells, initiating an immunization against the malignant T cells. Vaccines based on dendritic cells show efficacy in animal models. CpG ODN, added as an immunoadjuvant in DC (dendritic cell)-based vaccinations, may enhance tumor-specific immune responses.

CURRENT THERAPY

- Topical
    Topical steroids
    Phototherapy
    Nitrogen mustard
    Retinoids
- Radiation
- Systemic chemotherapy
    Single agent
        Pegylated doxorubicin
        Nucleoside analogues (pentostatin)
        Gemcitabine
        Temozolomide
    Multiagent
        CHOP and CHOP-like
- Biologic therapy
    IFN-α
    Retinoids
    ECP
    Denileukin diftitox
- Stem cell transplant
    Allogeneic transplant
    Mini allogeneic transplant
- Combined therapy
    Bexarotene and phototherapy
    IFN-α and bexarotene
    IFN-α and phototherapy
    ECP and IFN-α
    ECP and bexarotene
- Investigational therapy
    Antibodies (Alemtuzumab, HuMax)
    Histone deacetylase inhibitors
    Immunomodulators (CpG ODN)
    Cytokines (IL-2, IL-12)
    Vaccination strategies

Abbreviations: CHOP = cyclophosphamide, doxorubicin, vincristine, and prednisone; CpG ODN = cytosine-phosphorothiolated guanine-containing oligodeoxynucleotides; ECP = extracorporeal photochemotherapy (or photopheresis); IFN = interferon.

At present, there is no cure for this disease, and stage-dependent therapy remains the best approach. Treatment goals are disease palliation, improvement of survival, and improvement of quality of life. Given the nature of the disease and despite initial responses to standard therapy, all patients eventually relapse. Immunomodulatory regimens in patients should be used initially in patients with all stages of MF/SS to reduce the need for cytotoxic therapies with more damaging side effects. Investigational strategies continue to be developed to improve outcomes.

REFERENCES

Grange F, Bagot M: Prognosis of primary cutaneous lymphomas. Ann Dermatol Venereol 2002;129:30-40.

Kuzel TM: Systemic chemotherapy for the treatment of mycosis fungoides and Sézary syndrome. Dermatol Ther 2003;16:355-361.

Kuzel TM, Roenigk HH, Samuelson E, et al: Effectiveness of interferon alfa-2a combined with photochemotherapy for mycosis fungoides and Sézary syndrome. J Clin Oncol 1995;13:257-263

Oyama Y, Guitart J, Kuzel TM, et al: Long-term remission after allogeneic hematopoietic stem cell transplantation for refractory cutaneous T-cell lymphoma. Hematol Oncol Clin North Am 2003; 17:1475-1483.

Querfeld C, Rosen ST, Kuzel TM, et al: Long-term follow-up of patients with early stage cutaneous T-cell lymphoma who achieved complete remission on PUVA monotherapy. Arch Dermatol 2005; 141:1-7.

Querfeld C, Rosen ST, Guitart J, et al: Comparison of selective RAR and RXR retinoid mediated efficacy, tolerance, and survival in refractory cutaneous T-cell lymphoma. J Am Acad Dermatol 2004; 51:25-32.

Querfeld C, Guitart J, Kuzel TM, Rosen ST: Primary cutaneous lymphomas: A review with current treatment options. Blood Rev 2003;17:131-142.

Rook AH, Lessin SR, Jaworsky C, et al: Immunopathogenesis of cutaneous T-cell lymphoma. Abnormal cytokine production by Sézary cells. Arch Dermatol 1993;129:486-489.

Rosen ST, Foss FM: Chemotherapy for Mycosis fungoides and the Sézary syndrome. Hematol Oncol Clin North Am 1995;9:1109-1116.

Willemze R, Jaffe E, Burg G, et al: WHO-EORTC classification for cutaneous lymphomas. Blood 2005;105:3768-3785.

Papulosquamous Eruptions

Method of
Dana Kazlow Stern, MD, and
Mark G. Lebwohl, MD

Papulosquamous eruptions are a varied group of cutaneous disorders characterized by a common morphologic feature: papules covered with scale. A description of the more common papulosquamous eruptions encountered in clinical practice is provided in this article. Table 1 lists papulosquamous eruptions.

TABLE 1 Papulosquamous Eruptions

Psoriasis	Tinea corporis*
Lichen planus	Secondary syphilis
Pityriasis rosea	Lupus erythematosus
Pityriasis rubra pilaris	Lichen striatus
Seborrheic dermatitis	Lichen nitidus
	Parapsoriasis

*Items listed in this column are not discussed in this article.

Psoriasis

Psoriasis is a common, chronic, immunologically mediated, relapsing, inflammatory, papulosquamous cutaneous disorder that affects 2% to 3% of the U.S. population and occurs with equal frequency in both sexes. The precise etiology is unknown, but multifactorial inheritance is believed to be of central significance. The average age of onset is 28 years; however, the natural history of psoriasis can vary tremendously. It is characterized clinically by round, well-circumscribed erythematous plaques covered with a grayish silvery white scale. Symptoms, including pruritus, burning, and pain, coupled with the psychological impact of the disease can severely impact patient quality of life. The scalp, extensor surface of the limbs (elbows, knees), and the umbilical and sacral regions are typical areas of involvement. Nail findings can include pitting, onycholysis (detachment of the nail plate from the nail bed), subungual hyperkeratosis, discoloration of the nail bed, and splinter hemorrhage. Between 5% and 42% of psoriasis patients develop psoriatic arthritis. Medications known to exacerbate psoriasis include lithium, antimalarials, angiotensin-converting enzyme (ACE) inhibitors, β-blockers, and withdrawal from systemic steroids. In addition, psoriasis can be exacerbated by emotional stress, and physical trauma can result in the Koebner phenomenon whereby new psoriatic lesions occur at sites of trauma. In addition to classic plaque-type psoriasis, several variants exist including guttate, inverse, pustular, and erythrodermic.

GUTTATE PSORIASIS

The word *guttate* is derived from gutta, the Latin word for drop. Guttate psoriasis is characterized by small, droplike, scaling papules that typically erupt abruptly following an upper respiratory infection in patients younger than 30 years of age. A streptococcal infection should be sought when this occurs. Guttate psoriasis responds particularly well to phototherapy with ultraviolet B (UVB), which may be preferable to topical therapy because of the extensive body surface area involvement associated with this form of psoriasis.

INVERSE PSORIASIS

Inverse psoriasis has a characteristic distribution in skin folds and typically affects the axillae, groin, inframammary folds, intergluteal crease, and umbilicus. The skin appears red and inflamed and lacks the scaling seen with plaque-type psoriasis. Treatment includes topical corticosteroids, calcipotriene (Dovonex), tars, and anthralin (Psoriatec). Because of the self-occluding anatomic nature of the intertriginous regions, caution should be taken when treating inverse psoriasis with corticosteroids because these areas are particularly sensitive to steroid side effects such as atrophy and formation of striae.

PUSTULAR PSORIASIS

Pustular psoriasis is a rare form of psoriasis that occurs in either an acute, generalized distribution (von Zumbusch's psoriasis), or as a localized eruption. The variant of von Zumbusch's psoriasis, which can be life-threatening, is characterized by tender, painful skin that develops widespread areas of erythema with pustules that are described as lakes of pus that appear in a generalized pattern. Constitutional signs and symptoms such as fever, chills, malaise, anorexia, and nausea accompany these cutaneous manifestations. Patients require supportive care, usually in a hospital setting where they can be treated for infection, fluid loss, and electrolyte imbalance. The localized pattern, in contrast, tends to be more subacute and does not manifest systemically. The most common cause of pustular psoriasis is withdrawal of systemic corticosteroids. However, many drugs including iodine, lithium, salicylates, tar, anthralin (Psoriatec), antimalarials, and minocycline are some of the reported causes.

ERYTHRODERMIC PSORIASIS

Erythrodermic psoriasis is an inflammatory form of psoriasis that appears as fiery erythema and scaling that can affect the entire cutaneous surface and ultimately becomes exfoliative. Just as in generalized pustular psoriasis, the protective barrier function of the skin becomes compromised, predisposing the patient to infection, electrolyte imbalance, severe dehydration, and an inability to control temperature. It is essentially the same mechanism as a burn injury, and supportive care in a hospital is often required because these complications can be life-threatening. Withdrawal of systemic corticosteroids is the most common precipitator.

TREATMENT

Topical Therapies

Initial treatment of plaque-type psoriasis, for patients with less than 10% body surface involvement, usually involves topical therapies such as corticosteroids, vitamin D analogues, tazarotene (Tazorac), coal tar (DHS tar, Neutrogena T/Gel, Polytar), anthralin (Psoriatec), and salicylic acid. The topical immunomodulators, tacrolimus (Protopic)[1] 0.1% ointment and pimecrolimus (Elidel)[1] 1% cream are also used off-label to treat facial and intertriginous psoriasis.

Topical corticosteroids, available in creams, lotions, ointments, foams, gels, sprays, and occlusive tapes, are the most common therapeutic agents used to treat psoriasis. Steroids are ranked in groups, from I (super potency) to VII (low potency). Choosing the potency compound to use depends on disease location and severity. In general, group I superpotent steroids should be used to treat thick plaques on the trunk and extremities and should be avoided on the face, genitalia, or intertriginous areas. Treatment regimens are usually once or twice daily, limited to 2-week treatment intervals. Ideally, group I corticosteroids should be avoided in children if possible. Ointments, although greasy and messy to apply, tend to be more occlusive and are, therefore, generally more potent than creams and lotions. For especially resistant plaques, occlusion with Saran Wrap or other dressings may be used for a maximum of a few days. Lotions, foams, and gels tend to be particularly effective for scalp psoriasis. For psoriasis of the face and intertriginous areas, although nonsteroidal agents like the topical immunomodulators are preferred, low-potency topical steroids should be used once or twice daily. Side effects of topical corticosteroids include atrophy, telangiectasia, striae, folliculitis, perioral dermatitis, and tachyphylaxis. Pulse therapy, sometimes called *weekend therapy* because a superpotent corticosteroid is only applied on weekends, is a popular treatment method used to minimize side effects and prolong psoriasis remissions. Clinically significant hypothalamic-pituitary-adrenal axis suppression is rarely associated with topical application of steroids.

The vitamin D–derived analogue calcipotriene (Dovonex) is a nonsteroidal topical therapy that induces epidermal differentiation and inhibits keratinocyte proliferation. Calcipotriene is effective for the treatment of mild to moderate plaque-type and scalp psoriasis without producing any of the side effects associated with corticosteroids. Calcipotriene can be used as monotherapy or in conjunction with topical corticosteroids as sequential therapy, in which potent agents (high-potency topical corticosteroids, for example) are used to initiate disease clearance, and safer, less effective agents are used to maintain disease remission. Calcipotriene can also be used to treat the face and intertriginous areas—sites that are particularly vulnerable to the side effects of topical corticosteroids. Local irritation is the only cutaneous side effect associated with this form of therapy and can be avoided by diluting the medication with petrolatum.

Tazarotene (Tazorac), a topical retinoid (vitamin A derivative), acts by binding to specific retinoic acid receptors, resulting in normalization of the differentiation and proliferation of the epidermis. Tazarotene is available as a topical gel or cream in 0.05% and 0.1% strengths for the treatment of mild to moderate plaque psoriasis. Applied once daily, usually at bedtime, it can be used to treat most parts of the body, including the face and scalp. The most limiting side effect is local irritation. Treatment in combination with a topical corticosteroid is proven to not only minimize side effects but also to be more effective than tazarotene (Tazorac) alone. Retinoids are photosensitizers, so caution should

---

[1]Not FDA approved for this indication.

be taken with sun exposure. Because of the teratogenic potential of retinoids, female patients of childbearing potential must use adequate contraception, and pregnancy should be excluded before treatment begins.

Tar and tar-containing products have been used for more than a century for the treatment of psoriasis. Tars are effective, have few side effects, and are considered extremely safe. They are valuable alternatives to corticosteroids for treating intertriginous areas, the face, and scalp disease. It is believed that the more pungent, dark, and cosmetically unacceptable the tar, the more effective the treatment. However, the staining property, odors, and extended treatment times needed to induce a favorable clinical response have made them an unpopular treatment option for patients. Tar products* are available in gels, creams, emollient creams, ointments, and as emulsions that are added to the bath. Coal tars (DHS tar, Neutrogena T/Gel, Polytar) are more commonly used for the treatment of psoriasis than other tar types, and tar shampoos are probably the most commonly used tar products. Shampoos are effective for treating scalp psoriasis but cause discoloration and have an unpleasant odor.

Anthralin (Psoriatec), a hydoxyanthracene derivative, has been used for many years for the treatment of psoriasis but had until recently fallen out of favor because of the unwanted side effects of local irritation and staining associated with it. However, recent novel treatment methods such as short-duration therapy and innovative treatment vehicles have simplified treatment regimens and minimized these side effects. A new formulation of 1% anthralin, which is packaged in a semicrystalline vehicle, releases the anthralin content at skin surface temperatures, resulting in less prohibitive staining. Anthralin can also be used with corticosteroids or calcipotriene as combination therapy.

Combinations of salicylic acid and topical corticosteroids, tar, and anthralin are successfully used to treat thick, scaly plaques associated with psoriasis. It is a particularly useful agent when used in combination with corticosteroids because its keratolytic effect allows greater absorption of other topical therapies. When combined with steroids, the mixture must be compounded by a pharmacist because premixed combinations are currently unavailable. Caution should be taken when treating young children and patients with renal/hepatic impairment because of the potential for elevated serum salicylate levels. When considering using salicylic acid as part of a dual treatment regimen, be aware that salicylic acid blocks ultraviolet (UV) light and inactivates calcipotriene when applied concurrently.

Phototherapy/Photochemotherapy

UVB therapy, narrowband B therapy, and psoralen plus ultraviolet light of A wavelength (PUVA) therapy are the three main types of light therapy used for the treatment of psoriasis. These treatment modalities are ideal for patients with psoriasis who have either widespread disease that is too impractical to treat with topical therapy or psoriasis that is unresponsive to topical treatments.

UVB phototherapy, or broadband, delivers light in the range 290 to 320 nm. A history of improvement with sun exposure is a useful indication that this form of therapy will be appropriate. Prior application with petrolatum or mineral oil improves treatment efficacy. Treatment is generally three times per week. In addition, combination therapies with a variety of topical and systemic agents have shown additional benefit. For example, topical agents, calcipotriene and tazarotene are proven to enhance therapeutic efficacy when combined with UVB. Calcipotriene is inactivated by UVA and should, therefore, be applied after phototherapy. When used with UVB oral retinoids[1] and methotrexate (Trexall)[1] result in increased efficacy and reduce the total dose of systemic agent required. Sunburn is the major potential adverse event associated with UVB therapy.

Narrowband UVB phototherapy (311 nm) is a relatively new phototherapeutic modality that is proven to be superior to broadband and is useful for patients who have not responded sufficiently to broadband. Narrowband light bulbs deliver monochromatic light within the 305 to 315 nm range, exactly the spectrum that is most effective for treating psoriasis. Although narrowband treatment has demonstrated clinical disease resolution that is superior to broadband, the long-term safety data are not as well known at this time. Narrowband is considered to be safer than PUVA, but it is less clinically effective.

PUVA is a type of photochemotherapy whereby the patient ingests a photosensitizing medication (8-methoxypsoralen)[1] and is subsequently exposed to UVA light (320 to 400 nm). 8-Methoxypsoralen is dosed at 0.4 to 0.6 mg/kg body weight and should be taken 1.5 to 2 hours before UVA phototherapy, depending on the formulation. Treatments are given two or three times per week. Side effects include burning, sun sensitivity, nausea, and vomiting. Nausea can be minimized by late-day dosing or dividing doses with food; if nausea is severe, bath PUVA is available at some centers. It is well known that chronic exposure to PUVA can lead to the development of cutaneous malignancies. Recent evidence also supports an increased incidence of malignant melanoma in patients who had received more than 250 PUVA treatments. As a result of these findings, many dermatologists are advocating PUVA as a combination agent to minimize cumulative doses of PUVA. Combining PUVA with oral retinoids,[1] often referred to as Re-PUVA, is a method that is viewed as PUVA sparing. In fact, there is some evidence to support that retinoids may be protective against the development of PUVA- and cyclosporine (Neoral)-induced cancers. Contraindications to PUVA therapy include severe hepatic and renal function impairment, and light-aggravated and -induced diseases such as lupus erythematosus, porphyria, and xeroderma pigmentosum. PUVA is contraindicated during pregnancy.

---

*May be compounded by pharmacists.

[1]Not FDA approved for this indication.

Rakel and Bope: *Conn's Current Therapy 2006.*

The excimer laser is a relatively new technology that is approved for the treatment of psoriasis. The light emitted from this light source is in the UVB range at 308 nm. Because the laser beam can be selectively focused on lesional skin, this treatment modality is able to spare surrounding normal skin from unnecessary light exposure. This advantage, coupled with the need for fewer treatments than with other forms of phototherapy and photochemotherapy, has made the excimer laser a valuable treatment option for treating plaques of limited size.

Systemic Agents

The systemic agents acitretin (Soriatane), methotrexate (Trexall), and cyclosporine (Neoral) are used for moderate to severe plaque-type psoriasis. These agents are particularly effective for the treatment of pustular and erythrodermic psoriasis. Systemic therapies may be associated with varying degrees of long-term toxicity and, therefore, may be inappropriate for long-term monotherapy. To minimize long-term toxicity, these therapies are frequently rotated with UVB and/or PUVA at various clinically appropriate intervals.

Acitretin, a metabolite of etretinate, is a systemic retinoid that has replaced etretinate for the treatment of psoriasis because of its significantly shorter half-life and similar treatment efficacy. Because acitretin is completely undetectable in serum 3 weeks after treatment is terminated, women are theoretically able to conceive significantly sooner after therapy than they were with the defunct etretinate. However, women must completely avoid all alcohol, including even the most minute amounts found in cough syrups and food, because in the presence of alcohol acitretin is esterified to etretinate, its active metabolite. Therefore it is recommended that pregnancy be avoided for 3 years after treatment with acitretin.

The oral retinoids—acitretin, started at 25 mg daily, and isotretinoin (Accutane),[1] started at 1.5 to 2.0 mg/kg per day—are particularly effective as monotherapy for both pustular and erythrodermic psoriasis. Acitretin is modestly effective as monotherapy for the treatment of plaque-type psoriasis in relatively high doses of 50 and 75 mg[3] daily. However, when acitretin is used in combination with UVB or PUVA, clearance of plaque-type psoriasis is expedited and both lower ultraviolet and acitretin doses are needed. Side effects include cheilitis, alopecia, xerosis, hyperostosis, elevation of serum lipids (particularly triglycerides), and elevation of liver function tests. Hypercholesterolemia and hypertriglyceridemia can be treated with atorvastatin (Lipitor). Caution must always be taken when treating women of childbearing potential, because all retinoids are potent teratogens.

Methotrexate is used to treat moderate to severe recalcitrant plaque-type psoriasis; erythrodermic, acute, localized pustular psoriasis; and moderate to severe psoriatic arthritis. Doses are given as a single weekly oral dose of 7.5 mg to 30 mg per week, or the dose is divided into thirds and given at three 12-hour intervals. Hepatotoxicity and bone marrow suppression are the two most significant side effects. Therefore before initiation of therapy, a thorough history and physical exam should be done to rule out preexisting risk factors for liver disease. Additionally, lab work should be performed to exclude severe anemia, leukopenia, thrombocytopenia, renal function abnormalities, and significant liver function abnormalities (including hepatitis A, B, and C). Compete blood count (CBC) with platelet differential and count, renal function tests, and liver chemistries should be monitored throughout the treatment course.

Relative contraindications to methotrexate include active infectious disease, excessive alcohol consumption, hepatitis, and cirrhosis. Pregnancy and nursing are absolute contraindications to treatment with methotrexate. Monitoring hepatotoxicity by performing periodic liver biopsies is advocated for psoriasis patients treated with methotrexate. Rheumatologists do not obtain liver biopsies in rheumatoid arthritis patients treated with methotrexate, but it is clear that hepatic fibrosis occurs more commonly in psoriasis. Even with normal liver chemistries, liver biopsy is advocated at approximately 1.0 to 1.5 g of cumulative methotrexate and repeated with every additional 1.5 g. There is some evidence supporting the concomitant administration of folic acid (1 to 5 mg per day) to reduce nausea and megaloblastic anemia. The two leading causes of methotrexate overdosage are impaired renal function and concomitant treatment with trimethoprim-sulfamethoxazole (TMP-SMZ) (Bactrim). An immediate parenteral or oral dose of leucovorin calcium is the only antidote.

Cyclosporine is an extremely effective immunosuppressive agent approved for the treatment of psoriasis in doses up to 4 mg/kg daily but prescribed up to 5 mg/kg daily.[3] Cyclosporine is an effective agent for plaque-type, erythrodermic, and pustular psoriasis and is particularly useful for treating acute psoriatic flares because it results in rapid clinical improvement. Because of the concerning side effects of decreased renal function and hypertension, treatment should be initiated only after first trying less toxic therapies, and short-term therapy is ideal when possible.

Before initiation of cyclosporine therapy, baseline monitoring should include a history including a medication history, physical exam, two separate serum creatinine values, chemistry panel including lipid profile, liver function tests, electrolytes, magnesium, and uric acid. Laboratory values should be measured every 2 weeks for at least the month of therapy and monthly thereafter. Patients should be examined for side effects including malaise, nausea, headaches, tremors, sensitivity to extremes of temperature, hypertrichosis, and gingival hyperplasia. The associated hypertension can be effectively treated with a calcium channel–blocking agent. Kidney biopsies and drug level monitoring are not routinely performed. Absolute contraindications to cyclosporine include renal disease, poorly controlled

---

[1]Not FDA approved for this indication.
[3]Exceeds dosage recommended by the manufacturer.

---

[3]Exceeds dosage recommended by the manufacturer.

hypertension, and severe infections. Long-term treatment with cyclosporine is associated with cyclosporine-induced nephropathy. Therefore treatment periods should be limited and cyclosporine should be used as part of a rotational therapy regimen.

Biologic Agents

Recent advances in the understanding of how T cells play a paramount role in both the development and maintenance of psoriatic plaques has led to an explosive research effort toward the creation and development of biologic agents for the treatment of psoriasis. Psoriasis is now recognized to be a Th$_1$-mediated T-cell disorder. By selectively targeting specific steps in this T-cell-mediated inflammatory cascade, biologic agents can theoretically control disease with minimal impairment of immune function and few side effects.

Like systemic agents, biologics are generally used to treat psoriasis patients who have moderate to severe disease and have not responded to other treatment measures. However, unlike the systemic agents currently in use, biologic agents are neither hepatotoxic nor nephrotoxic. Thus, these new agents represent a significant addition to our current psoriasis therapy armamentarium.

Three types of biologic agents are used for the treatment of psoriasis and psoriatic arthritis:

1. Recombinant human cytokines or growth factors
2. Monoclonal antibodies
3. Fusion proteins

Table 2 shows examples of the latter two kinds of biologics, which are in various stages of approval for psoriasis.

At the time of this publication, alefacept (Amevive), a novel fusion protein, efalizumab (Raptiva), a monoclonal antibody, and etanercept (Enbrel), a dimeric fusion protein are currently the only biologic agents that are FDA approved for the treatment of moderate to severe plaque-type psoriasis in adult patients who are candidates for systemic therapy or phototherapy. Alefacept, efalizumab, and etanercept are safe, tolerable, and effective treatments for psoriasis.

Alefacept is administered as a 15 mg intramuscular (IM) weekly dose for 12 weeks. Safety and tolerability profiles were similar to placebo for one or two 12-week courses of alefacept IM. After a 12-week rest period off-drug, a second 12-week course can be administered. Before starting treatment, patients should have a history and physical, as well as laboratory examination of blood including CBC with total lymphocyte and CD4+ T-cell counts. Lymphocyte and CD4+ T-cell counts should be within normal limits before initiating therapy. Current recommendations are to monitor weekly CD4+ counts and to hold therapy if CD4+ counts fall below 250/μL.

Data from four randomized, placebo-controlled, phase III studies show efalizumab to be a safe and effective therapy for the treatment of moderate to severe plaque psoriasis in doses of 1.0 mg/kg per week to 2.0 mg/kg per week. Clinical response was observed as early as 2 weeks after treatment initiation. Additional new and ongoing trials are being conducted to define optimal dosing schedules, determine optimal strategies for withdrawal of therapy, and further support efalizumab as a potential long-term therapy. Adverse events that occurred at least 2% more frequently in efalizumab patients than in the placebo group include infection (mostly upper respiratory), headache, chills, nausea, pain, myalgia, flu syndrome, fever, back pain, and acne. For the third and subsequent doses, the incidence of adverse events was similar to placebo.

TABLE 2 Some of the Well-Known Biologic Agents for the Treatment of Psoriasis and Psoriatic Arthritis

	Type of agent	Mechanism of action	Administration method	Status
Alefacept (Amevive)	Fusion protein	Blocks T-cell activation; selective reduction of memory effector T cells	IM	Psoriasis—FDA approved for chronic moderate to severe plaque-type psoriasis, January 2003; psoriatic arthritis—phase I
Efalizumab (Raptiva)	Monoclonal antibody	Anti-CD11a; blocks T-cell activation; reduces trafficking of T cells to inflamed skin	SC	Psoriasis—FDA approved for chronic, moderate to severe plaque-type psoriasis, October 2003; psoriatic arthritis—phase II
Etanercept (Enbrel)	Fusion protein	TNF-α inhibitor	SC	Psoriasis—FDA approved for chronic, moderate to severe plaque-type psoriasis, April 2004; psoriatic arthritis—FDA approved, January 2002
Infliximab (Remicade)	Monoclonal antibody	TNF-α inhibitor	IV	Psoriasis—phase III[1]; psoriatic arthritis
Adalimumab (Humira)	Monoclonal antibody	TNF-α inhibitor	SC	Psoriasis—phase III[1]; psoriatic arthritis—phase III[1]

[1]Not FDA approved for this indication.
Abbreviations: IM = intramuscular; IV = intravenous; SC = subcutaneous; TNF = tumor necrosis factor.

Rakel and Bope: *Conn's Current Therapy 2006.*

Etanercept is indicated for the treatment of moderate to severe plaque-type psoriasis in the dose of 50 mg subcutaneously (SC) twice weekly for three months followed by a reduction to a maintenance dose of 50 mg per week. It is also indicated for the treatment of psoriatic arthritis. More than 130,000 patient years of treatment experience (mostly in the rheumatoid arthritis population) have demonstrated etanercept to be safe and effective. Laboratory monitoring is not required during treatment with etanercept. Injection site reactions were the only adverse events that occurred significantly more often in etanercept-treated patients than in placebo-treated patients in controlled clinical trials.

It should be noted that alefacept, efalizumab, and etanercept are fairly new agents without a long history of use, thus limiting our knowledge of the potential long-term side effects of these treatments.

Lichen Planus

Lichen planus is a common papulosquamous disorder of unknown etiology, characterized by small, violaceous, flat-topped, polygonal papules that are extremely pruritic. Lichen planus occurs equally among males and females, and without predisposition to race. Although more than 33% of patients are between 30 and 60 years of age, it does occur, albeit uncommonly, in children. Close examination of individual papules reveals a superficial fine scale that is crossed with gray-white streaks known as Wickham's striae. The eruption tends to occur at the flexor aspects of the upper extremities (especially the wrist), trunk, thighs, shins, buccal mucosa, and glans penis. Scalp involvement can occur as well. Oral involvement occurs on the buccal mucosa or tongue as either an atrophic or ulcerative pattern. Oral disease may occur with or without concomitant cutaneous involvement. Lichen planus can also affect the nails with characteristic nail plate longitudinal grooving and ridging. If nail involvement is severe, the matrix can be destroyed, resulting in pterygium formation. There are several clinical variants of lichen planus including linear, annular, follicular, hypertrophic, atrophic, bullous, and ulcerative forms. (A detailed description of these entities is beyond the scope of this article.)

The pathogenesis of lichen planus is a T-cell-mediated immune response of unknown cause. Although the disease course is highly variable, cutaneous disease tends to resolve in less than 1 year—in contrast to mucous membrane involvement, which tends to be chronic and is reported to have a mean duration of 5 years. Because ulcerated lichen planus of the oral mucosa, vulva, and anus is associated with an increased risk of malignant transformation to squamous cell carcinoma, suspicious, erosive, or ulcerated lesions should be biopsied.

There is a well-known association between lichen planus and hepatitis C infection. Because the cutaneous presentation is the same in patients regardless of underlying disease status, hepatitis C should be sought at initial presentation. In addition, many drugs are associated with lichenoid eruptions; therefore,

a thorough drug history should be taken to rule out drug-induced lichen planus (Table 3).

First-line therapies include class I or II topical corticosteroids, intralesional corticosteroid injections, and antihistamines. Topical corticosteroids should be applied twice daily for 2 to 4 weeks, and concomitant treatment with occlusive dressings is proven to improve efficacy. Intralesional corticosteroid injections are more ideal for limited, recalcitrant, discrete lesions. Oral lesions can be treated with mixtures of high-potency corticosteroids and benzocaine (Orabase), or intralesional injections can be used for unresponsive oral regions. Treatment with high-potency corticosteroids should be limited to prevent unwanted side effects. Pruritus can be quelled with antihistamines such as hydroxyzine (Atarax) in doses of 25 to 100 mg by mouth every 4 to 6 hours.

Second-line therapies—systemic corticosteroids, oral retinoids, and PUVA—are more ideal for widespread disease. Oral prednisone in doses of 30 to 60 mg daily for 2 to 6 weeks is an effective therapy and should be followed by a long taper (2 to 6 weeks) to prevent relapse. Acitretin,[1] in doses of 30 mg daily, also is proven effective for the treatment of cutaneous lichen planus. Isotretinoin (Accutane),[1] in doses of 10 mg orally twice daily for 2 months, shows efficacy for both oral and cutaneous lichen planus with fewer mucocutaneous side effects than with high-dose acitretin.[1] Lastly, there is limited evidence supporting bath PUVA with methoxsalen[1] at 1 mg/L as an effective therapy for lichen planus.

Cyclosporine,[1] tacrolimus (Protopic) (FK506),[1] metronidazole (Flagyl),[1] TMP-SMZ,[1] griseofulvin, itraconazole,[1] levamisole,[1] photodynamic therapy, azathioprine, interferon, and mycophenolate mofetil are some of the many therapies that can be considered third-line therapies for

---

[1]Not FDA approved for this indication.

TABLE 3 Medications Associated With Induction of a Lichenoid Eruption

β-Blockers
Methyldopa
Penicillamine (Cuprimine)
Quinidine
Quinine
Nonsteroidal anti-inflammatory drugs (NSAIDs)
Allopurinol (Zyloprim)
Tetracyclines
Furosemide (Lasix)
Hydrochlorothiazide (Esidrix)
Isoniazid (Nydrazid)
Phenytoin (Dilantin)
Hepatitis B vaccination
Angiotensin-converting enzyme inhibitors
Chlorpropamide
Carbamazepine (Tegretol)
Gold
Lithium

13

the treatment of lichen planus. These therapies tend to either have limited evidence-based data to support their efficacy or are more likely to have potentially severe associated toxicities. Cyclosporine,[1] for example, is extremely effective for the treatment of severe lichen planus; however, because of the nephrotoxicity associated with it, this therapy should be reserved for severe, recalcitrant cases.

Pityriasis Rosea

Pityriasis rosea is a self-limited, inflammatory papulosquamous disorder of unknown etiology, characterized by oval, salmon-colored macular and papular lesions that are covered in fine scale. The lesions are distributed with the long axis of the macule parallel to the lines of cleavage, a pattern that is classically described as having a *Christmas tree distribution*. Although it can affect any age group, it most commonly occurs in children and young adults; women are more frequently affected. In the United States it is most prevalent in the spring and fall.

The outbreak usually begins with the appearance of a solitary pink herald patch followed in 1 to 2 weeks by a generalized eruption primarily on the trunk, sparing sun-exposed areas. Patients may experience mild constitutional symptoms before the onset, and pruritus tends to occur in most patients. Resolution usually occurs after approximately 6 weeks. Atypical presentations are common in approximately 20% of patients. It is, therefore, important to differentiate pityriasis rosea from a number of other disorders that it resembles such as lichen planus, nummular dermatitis, pityriasis lichenoides, erythema dyschromicum perstans, guttate psoriasis, seborrheic dermatitis, syphilis, tinea versicolor, and tinea corporis. Mycologic examination of skin scrapings and syphilis serology may be warranted to rule out dermatophyte infections and syphilis, respectively.

To date, the etiology of pityriasis rosea remains unknown. It is believed to be caused by a viral infection, but no single causal agent has been identified. In addition, there are reports of medication-induced pityriasis rosea–like eruptions with certain drugs such as captopril (Capoten), metronidazole (Flagyl), ketotifen (Zaditor), arsenicals, gold, bismuth, clonidine (Catapres), and barbiturates. However, there is no evidence to support that pityriasis rosea is drug induced.

Pityriasis rosea is self-limiting. Therefore, treatment is only indicated to relieve pruritus, or as an attempt to expedite disease resolution. First-line therapies include medium potency topical corticosteroids applied twice daily, emollients, and oral antihistamines such as hydroxyzine (Atarax) in doses of 25 mg every 4 to 6 hours. For patients with significant pruritus and extensive disease, UVB phototherapy administered daily for 5 to 10 treatments is proven to ameliorate symptoms and reduce disease severity.

Pityriasis Rubra Pilaris

Pityriasis rubra pilaris (PRP) is a papulosquamous disorder with a clinically distinct presentation characterized by keratotic follicular papules, palmoplantar hyperkeratosis, and generalized red-orange scaling. Follicular papules are topped by a central horny plug and initially distributed on the dorsum of the proximal phalanges, wrists, neck, and trunk. These characteristic papules are described as looking like goose flesh or as nutmeg grater papules. Eventually the eruption can become diffuse, and any body area may be affected including the nails, mucous membranes, and eyes; however, small areas of well-circumscribed uninvolved skin remain spared. As PRP progresses, palmoplantar keratoderma can become severely fissured and painful. In addition, nails can become discolored, thickened, and brittle. Unlike in psoriasis, however, pitting is extremely unusual. In severe cases, a generalized erythroderma may develop, compromising the protective barrier of the skin and predisposing patients to infection, inability to control temperature, and electrolyte imbalances.

The etiology of PRP is unknown. It is classified into several subtypes. The classic adult type is the most common form of PRP. This form manifests acutely in adulthood, has the classic aforementioned clinical features, and carries the best prognosis, with 80% of patients going into remission within 3 years. A familial form of the disease with an autosomal-dominant inheritance pattern tends to present in childhood. More recently, there are reports of an HIV-associated form, which is characterized by HIV infection, cutaneous lesions of PRP, nodulocystic and pustular acneiform lesions, hidradenitis suppurativa, and lichen spinulosus.

PRP has a variable clinical response to therapy. Treatment can be challenging and therapeutic response somewhat unpredictable. Medium potency topical corticosteroids applied with bland emollients can help to relieve pruritus. Both retinoids and methotrexate (Trexall)[1] are considered first-line therapies for the treatment of PRP. Isotretinoin (Accutane)[1] in doses of 1.0 to 1.5 mg/kg per day for 3 to 6 months is proven to be a particularly effective treatment. There are also reports of successful treatment with acitretin (Soriatane)[1] combined with UVA phototherapy. As previously mentioned, potential side effects of retinoids include elevation of serum lipids and liver function tests as well as cheilitis, alopecia, xerosis, hyperostosis, and teratogenicity. Methotrexate (Trexall), in doses of 7.5 to 25 mg weekly for 3 to 4 months, is also an effective treatment option. Hepatotoxicity and bone marrow suppression are important side effects to be aware of with this type of therapy. Marked clinical improvement can be achieved with azathioprine (Imuran)[1] in doses of 150 to 200 mg daily. Azathioprine can be considered a second-line therapy. Potentially significant side effects associated with azathioprine include myelosuppression, increased malignancy rates, nausea and vomiting, hypersensitivity reactions, and increased susceptibility

---

[1]Not FDA approved for this indication.

[1]Not FDA approved for this indication.

Rakel and Bope: *Conn's Current Therapy 2006.*

Diseases of the Skin

to opportunistic infections. Clinical responses to cyclosporine (Neoral)[1] are inconsistent. Patients with HIV-associated PRP, while resistant to standard therapies, respond to triple antiretroviral therapy with zidovudine (AZT) (Retrovir),[1] in doses of 250 mg twice daily, lamivudine (3TC [Epivir]),[1] in doses of 150 mg twice daily, and saquinavir (Invirase, Fortovase)[1] in doses of 600 mg three times daily. Clinical response is directly related to fall in viral load.

Seborrheic Dermatitis

Seborrheic dermatitis is a common, chronic, papulosquamous disorder characterized by sharply demarcated, greasy, flaky, yellowish, crusted patches overlying red, inflamed skin. It tends to affect sebum-rich areas, with a predilection for the scalp, eyebrows, eyelids, nasolabial folds, beard, postauricular regions, external auditory canal, sternum, axillae, and groin. It can occur in any age group, manifesting, for example, on the scalp as cradle cap in infants and as pityriasis sicca, or

---

[1]Not FDA approved for this indication.

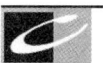

CURRENT DIAGNOSIS

- Psoriasis is a chronic inflammatory cutaneous disorder that can have a major psychologic impact on patient quality of life.
- In addition to the classic plaque-type psoriasis, other variants include guttate, inverse, pustular, and erythrodermic.
- Many psoriasis patients also suffer from psoriatic arthritis.
- A streptococcal infection should be sought in patients with guttate psoriasis. The most common cause of pustular and erythrodermic psoriasis is withdrawal of systemic corticosteroids.
- Lichen planus is characterized by small, violaceous, flat-topped, polygonal papules that are intensely pruritic. Oral involvement also occurs.
- There is a possible association between lichen planus and hepatitis C infection.
- Pityriasis rosea classically begins with the appearance of a solitary pink herald patch, followed in 1 to 2 weeks by a generalized eruption described as having a *Christmas tree distribution*.
- Pityriasis rubra pilaris (PRP) is characterized by keratotic follicular papules, palmoplantar hyperkeratosis, and generalized red-orange scaling.
- Seborrheic dermatitis is characterized by sharply demarcated, greasy, flaky, yellowish-crusted patches overlying inflamed sebum-rich skin.
- Seborrheic dermatitis is associated with Parkinson's and HIV infection.

dandruff, in adults. It is associated with and may be exacerbated in patients with Parkinson's disease, particularly those with neuroleptic-induced disease, and in patients with HIV.

Although the exact etiology is controversial, seborrheic dermatitis is believed to be associated with the lipophilic yeast *Pityrosporum ovale* (*Malassezia furfur*); however, the mechanism of the disease process remains unresolved. Some argue that *P. ovale* is present in abundance in skin lesions of seborrheic dermatitis patients and, therefore, believe that this yeast is the culprit. Others have challenged this cause-and-effect relationship by showing that *P. ovale* may be present in profuse levels in patients who have no clinical evidence of seborrheic dermatitis. Some studies demonstrate that it is the higher concentrations of skin lipids in patients with seborrheic dermatitis that result in promotion of growth of the organism and, ultimately, the disease. Yet others believe that seborrheic dermatitis is associated with normal levels of the yeast, and that it is the host's inadequate immune response that is causative.

Seborrheic dermatitis of the scalp responds well to treatment at least two or three times per week with medicated shampoos such as ciclopirox (Loprox), ketoconazole (Nizoral), selenium sulfide (Selsun or Exsel), pyrithione zinc (DHS Zinc or Head & Shoulders), propylene glycol, and coal tar (DHS tar, Neutrogena

13

CURRENT THERAPY

- First-line therapy for psoriasis patients with less than 10% body surface involvement is topical therapy. Other management options include phototherapy/photochemotherapy, systemic agents, and the newer biologic agents.
- In general, when treating papulosquamous disorders, group I superpotent steroids should be avoided on the face, genitalia, and intertriginous areas. Treatment regimens are usually twice daily, limited to 2-week treatment intervals.
- Side effects of topical corticosteroids include atrophy, telangiectasia, striae, folliculitis, perioral dermatitis, and tachyphylaxis.
- First-line therapy for lichen planus includes high potency topical corticosteroids, intralesional corticosteroid injections, and antihistamines. Systemic corticosteroids, oral retinoids, and PUVA are more ideal for widespread disease.
- Pityriasis rosea is self-limiting, so treatment is only indicated to relieve pruritus.
- Treatment of PRP can be challenging. Retinoids and methotrexate are considered first-line therapies.
- Seborrheic dermatitis of the scalp responds well to treatment with medicated shampoos. Shampoo should be massaged into a rich lather on the scalp and allowed to remain for 5 minutes before rinsing.

Abbreviations: PRP = pityriasis rubra pilaris; PUVA = psoralen plus ultraviolet light of A wavelength.

T/Gel, Polytar). Shampoo should be massaged into a rich lather on the scalp and allowed to remain for 5 minutes before rinsing. A keratolytic agent such as salicylic acid can be of added benefit, by allowing greater penetration of other medications. For treating seborrheic dermatitis of the face, scalp, trunk, and extremities, low potency topical corticosteroids such as hydrocortisone applied once daily for a minimum of 3 weeks, and antimicrobial preparations such as ketoconazole or ciclopirox gel 0.77% can be helpful. These agents can be used alone or in combination. Ketoconazole, the most commonly prescribed azole, is available as a 2% cream, an oil-in-water emulsion, a foaming gel or, as previously mentioned, as a shampoo. Caution should be taken when treating seborrheic blepharitis with corticosteroids because steroids in this area may induce glaucoma and cataracts. Instead, the eyelashes should be cleansed with baby shampoo on a cotton-tipped applicator. For severe or refractory seborrheic dermatitis, oral therapies may be more efficacious. Oral ketoconazole[1] in doses of 200 mg daily for 1 month is proven to be effective for widespread disease. A number of new potential therapies have recently gained attention including the azoles, fluconazole (Diflucan),[1] metronidazole (Flagyl),[1] ciclopirox, tacrolimus (Protopic),[1] and pimecrolimus (Elidel).[1] Lithium succinate ointment (Efalith)[1] is proven to be effective for facial involvement and particularly for the treatment of AIDS-related seborrheic dermatitis.

REFERENCES

Allen RA, Janniger CK, Schwartz RA: Pityriasis rosea. Cutis 1995;56(4):198-202.

Callen JP, Krueger GG, Lebwohl M, et al: AAD consensus statement on psoriasis therapies. J Am Acad Dermatol 2003;49(5):897-899.

Cohen PR, Prystowsky JH: Pityriasis rubra pilaris: A review of diagnosis and treatment. J Am Acad Dermatol 1989;20(5 Pt 1):801-807.

Fox BJ, Odom RB: Papulosquamous diseases: A review. J Am Acad Dermatol 1985;12(4):597-624.

Gottlieb AB, Evans R, Li S, et al: Infliximab induction therapy for patients with severe plaque-type psoriasis: A randomized, double-blind, placebo-controlled trial. J Am Acad Dermatol 2004;51(4):534-542.

Gupta AK, Madzia Se, Batra R: Etiology and management of seborrheic dermatitis. Dermatology 2004;208(2):89-93.

Lebwohl M, Tyring SK, Hamilton TK, et al: A novel targeted T-cell modulator, efalizumab, for plaque psoriasis. N Engl J Med 2003;349(21):2004-2013.

Leonardi CL, Powers JL, Matheson RT, et al: Etanercept as monotherapy in patients with psoriasis. N Engl J Med 2003;349(21):2014-2022.

---

[1]Not FDA approved for this indication.

Connective Tissue Disorders

Method of
*John Varga, MD, Susan M. Manzi, MD, MPH,
and Gabriella Lakos, MD, PhD*

Systemic lupus erythematosus (SLE), scleroderma (or systemic sclerosis), and the inflammatory myopathies are distinct but related idiopathic autoimmune connective tissue diseases. Each of these diseases is associated with significant morbidity and mortality. Each is characterized by considerable clinical heterogeneity and a chronic and unpredictable clinical course, often with remissions and relapses. Each is more common in women than men and associated with progressive damage to multiple organs. Prominent target organs include the skin, the cardiovascular system, the lungs, and the musculoskeletal system; in SLE, the brain and the kidneys are also affected. At the tissue level, inflammation and progressive scarring are prominent. Furthermore, each of these diseases is associated with high levels of autoantibodies in the circulation. Autoimmunity, a hallmark of connective tissue diseases, reflects a fundamental breakdown in immunologic self-tolerance. Although the connective tissue diseases have no cure, many effective treatment options are currently available. Because of their clinical heterogeneity, protean multiorgan systemic manifestations, and chronic and unpredictable course, the evaluation and management of patients with connective tissue diseases present unique challenges.

Systemic Lupus Erythematosus

Chronic inflammation and immune dysregulation characterize SLE. The precise etiology is unknown but likely results from a combination of genetic, hormonal, and environmental factors. The spectrum of manifestations in SLE is quite broad and the time course extremely variable. Some patients develop life-threatening irreversible organ damage, whereas the most incapacitating condition in others may be fatigue. Therapy should be tailored to the individual patient and designed not only to suppress disease activity but also to alleviate symptoms as well. Patients with SLE are optimally managed by a team of specialists that may include, in addition to the rheumatologist, a dermatologist, nephrologist, cardiologist, psychiatrist, psychologist, pulmonologist, gastroenterologist, orthopedic surgeon, and physical therapist.

Although a definitive cure for SLE remains elusive, recent advances, both nonpharmacologic and pharmacologic, have significantly improved survival and quality of life. According to Manzi, established treatments fall into four main categories: nonsteroidal anti-inflammatory drugs, antimalarial agents, corticosteroids, and cytotoxic and immunosuppressive agents.

Choosing an appropriate treatment regimen requires careful thought in light of the complexity and marked clinical heterogeneity of the disease and the potential long-term side effects of the drugs used. Consultation with a rheumatologist or other subspecialist with expertise in lupus is recommended.

GENERAL PRINCIPLES OF THERAPY

As patients become more information savvy, the role of health professionals in patient education becomes crucial. Physicians and their staff should assist patients in evaluating the flow of information available through modern technology such as the Internet. A patient may be alarmed by hearing or reading about worst-case scenarios. Reassurance that the manifestations and course of disease vary considerably may ease this anxiety. Providing information about support groups may also be helpful. Moreover, physicians should recognize and address the psychological impact that a diagnosis of a chronic, potentially serious disease may have on a previously healthy individual.

Although not life-threatening, fatigue is a challenge for many SLE patients. Physicians should search for contributing factors such as hypothyroidism, fibromyalgia, or depression and must emphasize the importance of adequate rest. Overexposure to ultraviolet (UV) radiation may cause systemic disease flares in addition to skin rashes. Photosensitive patients should avoid excessive exposure to sunlight and wear protective clothing and sunscreen (SPF [sun protection factor] of 35) routinely. Certain prescription drugs, including sulfa drugs and other antibiotics, can exacerbate photosensitivity as well as other lupus disease activity.

Unexplained fever should not be ignored because lupus patients are susceptible to infections. To minimize this risk, physicians should exercise caution when prescribing immunosuppressive agents and corticosteroids and consider influenza and pneumococcal immunizations. Because a disease flare during pregnancy poses risk to the fetus, pregnancies in women with lupus are considered high risk. High-dose estrogen contraceptives should generally be avoided, particularly in patients with increased risk of blood clots; low-dose estrogen, progesterone-only pills, or other effective means of contraception should be considered. Planning pregnancies during periods of disease remission and careful monitoring of both the mother and fetus can improve the chances for healthy outcomes.

Other considerations in the general management of patients with SLE include their increased risk of cardiovascular disease and osteoporosis. Patients should be screened for these conditions and be advised to adopt a cardioprotective lifestyle and take measures to ensure their bone health. These actions include smoking cessation, moderate intake of alcohol, heart-healthy diet, adequate intake of dietary calcium and vitamin D, and regular weight-bearing exercise. Although no definitive link is established between SLE and malignancy, routine gynecologic testing and breast examinations should be performed.

NONSTEROIDAL ANTI-INFLAMMATORY DRUGS

Although nonsteroidal anti-inflammatory drugs (NSAIDs) do not have disease-modifying properties in SLE, they are used to treat fever, pleuritis, pericarditis, and musculoskeletal complaints (Figure 1). Because SLE patients may take NSAIDs for long periods of time, consideration should be given to gastroprotective agents. Furthermore, the potential adverse effects of these drugs on the kidney, liver, and central nervous system may be confused with worsening disease activity. Table 1 lists the general recommendations for monitoring NSAIDs and other commonly used agents in SLE.

ANTIMALARIAL AGENTS

Antimalarial agents are frequently prescribed in the treatment of SLE. The most commonly used are hydroxychloroquine (Plaquenil)[1] and chloroquine (Aralen).[1] Antimalarials are regularly used in the management of cutaneous and musculoskeletal manifestations, constitutional symptoms, and in some cases serositis. Antimalarials may be used in combination when one agent by itself is ineffective because their actions can be synergistic. A particular benefit of antimalarial agents is their steroid-sparing effect. Hydroxychloroquine[1] (200 to 400 mg daily) is generally well tolerated, but it may take 6 to 8 weeks for the benefit to become apparent. Because of potential ophthalmologic toxicity, patients should have an ophthalmologic examination when they begin treatment and every 6 to 12 months thereafter. Although it is unclear whether antimalarials prevent major organ disease, they do have lipid-lowering and possible antiplatelet activities.

CORTICOSTEROIDS

Corticosteroids are used to treat a broad spectrum of lupus manifestations. Oral administration of 5 to 30 mg of prednisone daily in single or divided doses is effective in treating constitutional symptoms, cutaneous disease, arthritis, and serositis. Once immediate relief is achieved, their dose is often tapered while slower-acting agents such as antimalarials or immunomodulatory therapy are added. For more serious organ involvement, such as nephritis, central nervous system or hematologic abnormalities, or systemic vasculitis, prednisone at higher doses (1 to 2 mg/kg) daily or parenteral corticosteroid preparations in equivalent doses are given. Pulses of methylprednisolone (1000 mg) can be given for 3 consecutive days in severe situations. According to Ionnaou and Isenberg, the infusion should be given over several hours to minimize the risk of reactions such as joint pain, flushing, headache, or tachycardia. Although high-dose corticosteroids may be required to preserve major organ function, patients who require such aggressive treatment over extended periods are subjected to highly unfavorable side effects, including emotional lability, weight gain,

[1]Not FDA approved for this indication.

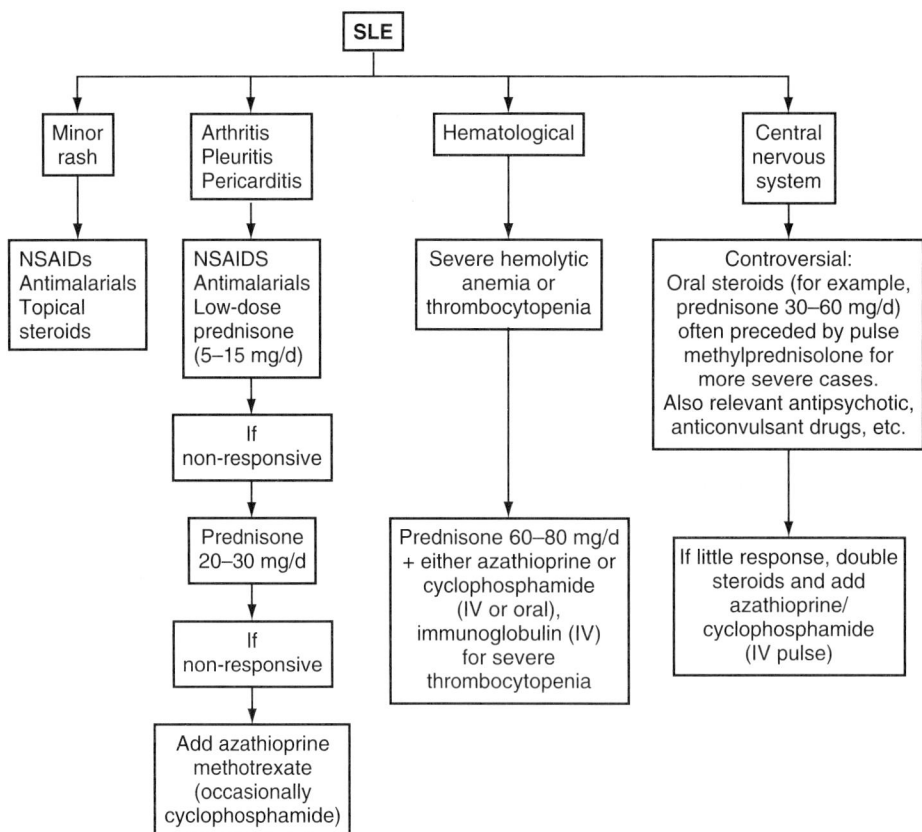

FIGURE 1. Management of nonrenal lupus. (Adapted from Ioannou Y, Isenberg DA: Current concepts for the management of systemic lupus erythematosus in adults: A therapeutic challenge. Postgrad Med J 2002;78:599-606.)

hypertension, hyperlipidemia, diabetes, glaucoma, risk of infection, avascular necrosis of bone, and osteoporosis. It is recommended that treating physicians attempt to taper corticosteroids to discontinuation or to a minimal dose administered daily or on alternate days once disease activity is controlled.

CYTOTOXIC AGENTS

Aggressive therapy with cytotoxic agents is required for patients with severe disease involving major organs. In general, such therapy should be administered by specialists aware of the potential dangers involved. Cyclophosphamide (Cytoxan)[1] and azathioprine (Imuran),[1] are the agents most commonly prescribed. Methotrexate (Rheumatrex),[1] mycophenolate mofetil (CellCept),[1] and intravenous immunoglobulin (IVIG)[1] also show promising results.

Cyclophosphamide

According to Ortmann and Klippel, cyclophosphamide[1] is the drug of choice for treating most forms of lupus nephritis (Figure 2). Glucocorticoids in combination with intravenous bolus regimens of cyclophosphamide (0.5 to 1.0 g/m^2) is more effective than glucocorticoids alone in preserving renal function. Cyclophosphamide[1]

appears to be most effective in diffuse proliferative lupus nephritis, although it may also be useful in membranous nephropathy. Less severe forms of lupus nephritis are commonly treated with corticosteroids alone; however, physicians should be prepared to administer immunosuppressive agents if more severe nephritis develops or if patients develop unacceptable side effects from corticosteroids. Renal biopsy is helpful in determining the therapy of choice. Regardless of the type of immunosuppressant used, it is necessary to control blood pressure effectively to prevent irreversible organ damage. Cyclophosphamide[1] is also effective in nonrenal manifestations of SLE, such as cytopenia, central nervous system disease, pulmonary hemorrhage, and vasculitis.

Cyclophosphamide[1] has numerous undesirable side effects. Nausea, vomiting, hair loss, infertility, and bone marrow suppression are the most common. Gastrointestinal toxicity can be minimized with the administration of antiemetics, and hair loss is normally reversible when treatment is discontinued. Older age and cumulative dose appear to be the major risk factors for infertility. Adjusting the dose of cyclophosphamide[1] can often regulate leukopenia, which typically peaks 8 to 12 days after intravenous administration. Patients on cyclophosphamide[1] are also at increased risk for infections, particularly herpes zoster. Bladder carcinoma can develop even years after cyclophosphamide[1] therapy has stopped;

---

[1]Not FDA approved for this indication.

[1]Not FDA approved for this indication.

TABLE 1 Standard Drug Therapies in Systemic Lupus Erythematosus and Recommended Monitoring Strategies

Drug	Toxicities requiring monitoring	Baseline evaluation	Monitoring	
			System review	Laboratory
Salicylates, nonsteroidal anti-inflammatory drugs	Gastrointestinal bleeding, hepatic toxicity, hypertension	CBC, creatinine, urinalysis, AST, ALT	Dark/black stool, dyspepsia, nausea/vomiting, abdominal pain, shortness of breath, edema	CBC yearly, creatinine yearly
Hydroxychloroquine	Macular damage	None unless patient is over 40 y of age or has previous eye disease	Visual changes	Funduscopic and visual fields q 6-12 mo
Glucocorticoids	Hypertension, hyperglycemia, hyperlipidemia, hypokalemia, osteoporosis, avascular necrosis, cataract, weight gain, infections, fluid retention	BP, bone densitometry, glucose, potassium, cholesterol, triglycerides (HDL, LDL)	Polyuria, polydipsia, edema, shortness of breath, BP at each visit, visual changes, bone pain	Urinary dipstick for glucose q 3-6 mo, total cholesterol yearly, bone densitometry yearly to assess osteoporosis
Azathioprine	Myelosuppression, hepatotoxicity, lymphoproliferative disorders	CBC, platelet count, creatinine, AST or ALT	Symptoms of myelosuppression	CBC and platelet count q 1-2 wk with changes in dose (q 1-3 mo thereafter), AST yearly, PAP test at regular intervals
Cyclophosphamide	Myelosuppression, myeloproliferative disorders, malignancy, immunosuppression, hemorrhagic cystitis, secondary infertility	CBC and differential and platelet count, urinalysis	Symptoms of myelosuppression, hematuria, infertility	CBC and urinalysis monthly; urine cytology and PAP test yearly for life
Methotrexate	Myelosuppression, hepatic fibrosis, cirrhosis, pulmonary infiltrates, fibrosis	CBC, chest radiograph within past year, hepatitis B, C serology in high-risk patients, AST, albumin, bilirubin, creatinine	Symptoms of myelosuppression, shortness of breath, nausea/vomiting, oral ulcer	CBC and platelet count, AST or ALT, and albumin q 4-8 wk, serum creatinine, urinalysis
Mycophenolate mofetil	Myelosuppression, gastrointestinal	CBC and differential and platelet count, creatinine, AST, ALT	Symptoms of myelosuppression, nausea, diarrhea	CBC and platelet count q1-2 wk with changes in dose (q 1-3 mo thereafter), AST, ALT, creatinine q 1-3 mo.

Abbreviations: ALT = alanine transaminase; AST = aspartate transaminase; BP = blood pressure; CBC = complete blood count; HDL = high-density lipoprotein; LDL = low-density lipoprotein.
Adapted from Manzi S: Treatment of systemic lupus erythematosus. In Klippel JH, Stone J, Weyand C, Crofford LJ (eds): Primer on the Rheumatic Diseases. Atlanta, Arthritis Foundation, 2001, pp 346-352.

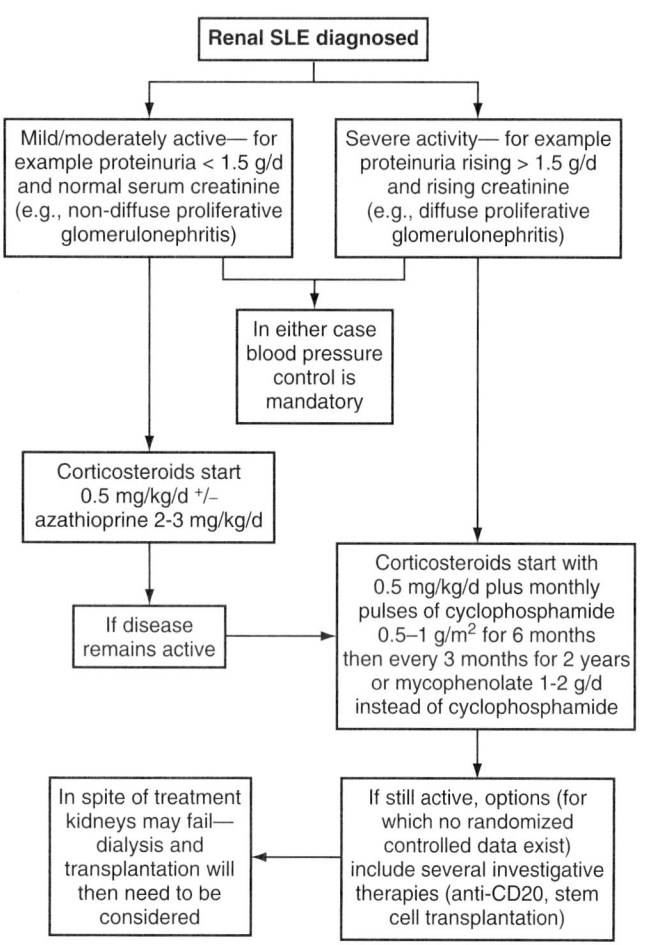

FIGURE 2. Management of renal lupus. (Adapted from Ioannou Y, Isenberg DA: Current concepts for the management of systemic lupus erythematosus in adults: A therapeutic challenge. Postgrad Med J 2002;78:599-606.)

thus urinalysis, urine cytology, and cystoscopy are indicated in patients with hematuria.

Azathioprine (Imuran)

Azathioprine[1] can be used for lupus nephritis, as a steroid-sparing agent in patients with nonrenal manifestations, and in patients at low risk for progressive renal failure. Azathioprine[1] is generally started at 50 mg daily and increased by 25 mg per week to a maintenance dose of 2 to 3 mg/kg daily. Azathioprine[1] is generally better tolerated than cyclophosphamide[1]; however, bone marrow, hepatic, and gastrointestinal toxicity are common.

Methotrexate (Rheumatrex)

Much evidence supports the effectiveness of methotrexate in rheumatoid arthritis, but very few controlled studies have been conducted in SLE. Evidence suggests that methotrexate at 15 to 20 mg per week is effective in controlling cutaneous and articular manifestations.

[1]Not FDA approved for this indication.

Because side effects are common at high doses, methotrexate[1] is currently used primarily as a steroid-sparing agent in milder SLE.

Mycophenolate Mofetil (CellCept)

Mycophenolate mofetil[1] (500 to 1000 mg twice daily) appears to be effective for lupus nephritis. In one small study, it is effective in reducing proteinuria and improving serum creatinine in severe lupus nephritis refractory to cyclophosphamide. In a larger study, mycophenolate mofetil in combination with prednisone appeared to be as effective as combination cyclophosphamide[1]/prednisolone in lupus nephritis and produced fewer side effects.

Intravenous Immunoglobulin

Intravenous immunoglobulin (IVIG)[1] is used most commonly for the treatment of refractory thrombocytopenia. Platelet counts rise rapidly following initiation of treatment at 400 mg/kg daily. Similar doses have produced improvements in arthritis, nephritis, fever, mucocutaneous manifestations, and immunologic parameters. Patients with SLE-associated IgA deficiency should be treated with alternative therapies.

Scleroderma/Systemic Sclerosis

Scleroderma, or systemic sclerosis (SSc), is a chronic connective tissue disease characterized by evidence of widespread vascular injury, autoimmunity, fibroproliferative process, and variable clinical course. Localized sclerodermas (morphea and linear scleroderma) are distinct from SSc, occur more frequently in children, and are not associated with internal organ involvement. According to Mayes and colleagues, median survival in SSc is 11 years. Survival is determined by the extent of internal organ involvement. Prominent target organs include the skin, lungs, heart, kidneys, and gastrointestinal tract (Box 1). SSc has substantial clinical heterogeneity. Based on the constellation of clinical and laboratory findings present, patients are subclassified

[1]Not FDA approved for this indication.

BOX 1   Prominent Organ Involvement in Systemic Sclerosis (SSc)

- Skin (inflammation, induration and tethering; hyper- and hypopigmentation, calcinosis)
- Lungs (alveolitis and pulmonary fibrosis; pulmonary arterial hypertension)
- Heart (restrictive cardiomyopathy, pericarditis)
- Peripheral vascular (mucocutaneous telangiectasia, Raynaud's phenomenon, digital ulcers and infarction, watermelon stomach, male erectile dysfunction)
- Gastrointestinal tract (see Box 4)
- Muscle (myositis)
- Joints (contractures, arthralgia, tendon friction rubs)

as "limited cutaneous SSc" or "diffuse cutaneous SSc" (Box 2). These two subtypes predict distinct patterns of organ involvement, clinical course, and survival. Some patients with SSc show features of overlap with other autoimmune diseases and manifest sicca syndrome, arthritis, myositis, or thyroiditis.

GENERAL PRINCIPLES OF THERAPY

In light of the clinical heterogeneity of SSc and its variable course, treatment must be individualized according to the unique needs of each patient; some need early aggressive intervention, whereas others need a conservative symptom-based approach with close monitoring. According to Bryan and colleagues, predictors of poor outcome include older age onset (>60 years of age), anemia, evidence of significant cardiac or pulmonary involvement, tendon friction rubs, and the presence of antitopoisomerase antibodies. In general, therapies fall into two groups: those that target the underlying pathophysiologic process, and those that alleviate or reverse target organ complications. Because major internal organ involvement develops early, disease-modifying interventions should be considered before tissue damage becomes established. Because SSc is invariably a multisystem disease, a coordinated approach to evaluation and management by an integrated multidisciplinary team including a rheumatologist, pulmonologist, cardiologist, gastroenterologist, vascular or orthopedic surgeon, and physical therapist is desirable. Patients should also be given the opportunity to participate in controlled clinical trials on novel therapeutic agents.

DISEASE-MODIFYING THERAPIES

To date, no therapy is shown conclusively to be disease modifying in SSc. Nonetheless, based on historical or anecdotal evidence or empirical considerations, many agents are used widely in an attempt to reverse or halt the progression of the immunologic, vascular, and fibrotic damage (Box 3). In light of the potential toxicities associated with these therapies and their lack of proven benefit, decisions regarding their use must be

---

> **BOX 2**   **Clinical Features of Systemic Sclerosis (SSc) Subsets**
>
> - Limited cutaneous SSc
>   - Limited extent of skin induration (distal extremities and face); no truncal skin involvement; slowly progressive
>   - Prominent vascular involvement (cutaneous telangiectasia, Raynaud's phenomenon, digital ulcers; pulmonary hypertension)
>   - Calcinosis cutis
>   - Antibodies to centromere
> - Diffuse cutaneous SSc
>   - Progressive and diffuse skin induration; truncal involvement frequent
>   - Pulmonary fibrosis
>   - Scleroderma renal crisis
>   - Antibodies to topoisomerase-I

> **BOX 3**   **Potentially Disease-Modifying Interventions for Systemic Sclerosis (SSc)**
>
> - Immunomodulatory
>   - Methotrexate*
>   - Cyclophosphamide*
>   - Mycophenolate mofetil*
>   - Antithymocyte globulin
>   - Autologous stem cell therapy (with or without immune oblation)
> - Antifibrotic
>   - D-Penicillamine*
>   - Interferon γ
>
> ---
> *Although commonly used, to date these interventions have not been demonstrated in controlled clinical trials to be of unequivocal benefit in the treatment of SSc.

---

considered carefully. In patients with limited SSc and stable disease, organ-based treatments directed toward specific complications of the disease (see later) are generally more appropriate than these generalized disease-modifying treatment strategies.

ORGAN-BASED TREATMENT APPROACHES

Therapy for Skin Involvement

Skin induration can be progressive and widespread in diffuse cutaneous SSc, whereas it is generally not prominent in limited cutaneous form. Extensive skin involvement often, but not invariably, predicts severe internal organ involvement. In diffuse SSc, skin induration generally peaks in the first 2 to 4 years of SSc, after which it regresses with spontaneous softening. In early disease, inflammation of the skin dominates, with edema, erythema, and pruritus. Patients at this stage benefit form antihistamines such as hydroxyzine (Atarax),[1] 25 mg at bedtime. Low-dose glucocorticoids such as prednisone,[1] 5 mg daily, provide substantial symptomatic relief for inflammation in early SSc but should be used with caution in light of the increased risk of scleroderma renal crisis (see later); patients taking low-dose prednisone[1] should be instructed to monitor their blood pressure daily. Digital ulcers can be managed using Duoderm[1] application to promote healing and topical povidone-iodine (Betadine)[1] solution for cleansing.

Therapy for Vascular Involvement

Raynaud's Phenomenon and Its Complications

Widespread damage of small and medium-sized peripheral blood vessels is virtually universal in SSc. Endothelial cell injury is associated with release of vasoconstrictors such as thromboxane and endothelin 1 (ET1), impaired production of vasodilators such as nitric oxide and prostacyclin, and platelet aggregation and thrombosis. What starts out as a reversible dysfunction of vascular smooth muscle often progresses to irreversible structural

---

[1]Not FDA approved for this indication.

alterations characterized by intimal layer proliferation, medial hypertrophy, and adventitial fibrosis. Reduced blood flow and repeated episodes of ischemic reperfusion in the digits, kidneys, lungs, heart, and other involved organs cause tissue ischemia, progressive vascular damage, and fibrosis.

Cold-induced Raynaud's phenomenon is the most common presenting problem in SSc and may precede other manifestations of the disease by years. Repeated and increasingly severe Raynaud's episodes lead to digital ischemia, resulting in painful ulcers and nonhealing pitting scars and, in extreme cases, digital infarction and gangrene. Patients should be counseled to stop smoking and to avoid cold exposure, which triggers vasoconstriction; not only the hands but the whole body should also be kept warm. Mild Raynaud's phenomenon can be effectively treated with orally active vasodilators (Table 2) and treatment is most commonly started with calcium channel blockers. Infection complicating digital ulcers should be treated aggressively with antibiotics; such ulcers may take months to heal and may progress to osteomyelitis. The ET1 receptor blocker bosentan (Tracleer),[1] 125 mg twice daily, is effective in preventing digital ulcers. Patients with impending digital infarction may respond to intravenous epoprostenol (Flolan),[1] 0.5 to 6 μg/kg body weight per minute for 6 to 24 hours, or nonpharmacologic interventions such as sympathetic ganglion blockade and surgical digital sympathectomy. The role of statin drugs, antioxidants such as tocopherol (vitamin E)[1] (400 IU daily), and diets rich in fish oils in preventing vascular damage in Raynaud's phenomenon are not yet adequately studied.

Pulmonary Arterial Hypertension

Pulmonary arterial hypertension (PAH), which occurs in at least 15% of SSc patients, has a major impact on survival. PAH may complicate interstitial pulmonary fibrosis or may occur in the absence of parenchymal lung disease; the latter is indistinguishable from primary (idiopathic) and familial pulmonary hypertension. Because PAH may be asymptomatic until advanced, it was historically underdiagnosed in SSc. Moderately severe PAH is associated with exertional dyspnea, chest pain, and syncope; right-sided heart failure is seen in late-stage disease. Emphasis must be placed on early preclinical recognition of PAH. A combination of pulmonary function testing and Doppler echocardiography is appropriate for screening and should be performed yearly. Right heart catheterization is the gold standard for determining pulmonary arterial pressures and cardiac index and for excluding pulmonary embolism.

Several new classes of agents provide at least short-term symptomatic and hemodynamic improvement in PAH. Patients with New York Heart Association functional class III or IV symptoms (ordinary activity causing dyspnea, chest pain, or near syncope) should start an orally active ET1 receptor blocker such as bosentan (Tracleer). In addition, warfarin anticoagulation (to achieve an INR [international normalized ratio] of 1.5 to 2.0), low-flow oxygen therapy, diuretics, and digitalization are generally indicated. Patients who fail to respond to ET1 antagonists may benefit from parenteral prostacyclin analogues such as inhaled iloprost (Ventavis), every 2 hours up to 45 μg daily, or continuous infusions of subcutaneous treprostinil (Remodulin) 1.25 μg/kg per minute, or intravenous epoprostenol (Flolan), 2 to 10 μg/kg per minute. A major limitation of these therapies is their cost, now exceeding $30,000 per year. Furthermore, because of their short half-lives, prostacyclin analogues must be administered by continuous infusion or frequent inhalations. Epoprostenol requires long-term ambulatory central venous catheterization, which may be complicated by line sepsis and pump failure with potentially catastrophic consequences. Combinations of a prostacyclin analogue together with an ET1 antagonist or a phosphodiesterase type 5 inhibitor such as sildenafil (Viagra),[1] up to 50 mg three times daily, appear to be well tolerated and provide added benefit. Surgical options for patients unresponsive to pharmacologic therapies include atrial septostomy and lung transplantation. In light of the complexity involved, the evaluation and management of PAH in SSc patients should be coordinated by specialized centers having appropriate expertise.

---

[1]Not FDA approved for this indication.

TABLE 2 Oral Vasodilator Therapy for Raynaud's Phenomenon in Systemic Sclerosis

Agent	Dose
Calcium Channel Blockers	
Nifedipine (Procardia)	10-30 mg three times daily
Diltiazem (Cardizem)	30-120 mg three times daily
Amlodipine (Norvasc)	5-20 mg daily
Felodipine (Plendil)	2.5-10 mg daily
Angiotensin II Receptor Antagonists	
Losartan (Cozaar)	25-100 mg daily
Valsartan (Diovan)	80-320 mg daily
Sympatholytic Agents	
Prazosin (Minipress)	1-5 mg daily
Doxazosin (Cardura)	1-16 mg daily
Nitroglycerin	2% ointment topically once daily

Adapted from Wigley FM: Raynaud's phenomenon. N Engl J Med 2002;347(13):1001-1008.

Therapy for Interstitial Lung Disease

Some degree of interstitial lung disease is present in most patients with SSc and is a leading cause of death. The extent and progression of pulmonary fibrosis are major determinants of outcome. Combined with pulmonary function testing, high-resolution computed tomography (HRCT) scan of the chest is more sensitive for interstitial lung disease screening than chest radiography. A ground-glass appearance generally correlates with active inflammation (alveolitis). Patients with

---

[1]Not FDA approved for this indication.

alveolitis may benefit from cyclophosphamide (Cytoxan)[1] (orally up to 50 mg daily, or intravenously as pulse therapy up to 1000 mg/m[2] monthly) to stabilize lung function. Low-dose prednisone[1] (up to 20 mg daily) is often used in combination with cyclophosphamide. The optimal duration of cyclophosphamide[1] treatment is uncertain, but some experts recommend at least a year. General supportive measures include pneumococcal vaccination and yearly influenza immunization, avoidance of smoking, prevention of gastroesophageal reflux, nasal oxygen supplementation, and bronchodilators. Respiratory tract infections should be treated with empirical antibiotics. For selected patients with progressive respiratory decline, lung transplantation remains an option.

Therapy for Gastrointestinal Tract Involvement

Gastrointestinal involvement is common, can be extensive, and significantly contributes to the morbidity of SSc. Gastroesophageal reflux may be associated with dyspepsia, dysphagia, and regurgitation and can lead to chronic esophagitis and its complications (Box 4). Reflux should be managed by elevating the head of the bed, eliminating triggers such as chocolates, alcohol, and tobacco, and restricting food intake before going to sleep. Most patients require long-term treatment with proton pump inhibitors such as omeprazole (Prilosec)[1] in doses sufficient to suppress reflux symptoms (up to 160 mg daily). Prokinetic agents such as metoclopramide (Reglan)[1] (10 mg four times daily) or erythromycin[1] (250 mg three times daily) may be effective for gastroparesis. Chronic diarrhea and malabsorption caused by small bowel bacterial overgrowth can be treated with periodic courses of tetracycline[1] (500 mg four times daily) or metronidazole (Flagyl)[1] (500 mg three times daily). Some patients benefit from subcutaneous octreotide injections (Sandostatin,)[1] (50 μg one to four times daily). Nutritional assessment and support are important aspects of management. Gastric vascular ectasia (watermelon stomach) is frequent in SSc and causes recurrent occult gastrointestinal bleeding. It can be effectively treated with laser argon ablation.

---

[1]Not FDA approved for this indication.

> **BOX 4   Gastrointestinal Tract Complications of Systemic Sclerosis (SSc)**
>
> - Esophageal dysmotility leading to dysphagia and chronic gastroesophageal reflux; dyspepsia, esophagitis, strictures, ulcers, pulmonary aspiration; Barrett's esophagus and esophageal adenocarcinoma
> - Watermelon stomach with upper gastrointestinal bleeding
> - Gastroparesis and small bowel hypomotility
> - Blind loop syndrome with malabsorption, weight loss, diarrhea
> - Large bowel pseudo-obstruction
> - Colonic perforation
> - Pneumatosis cystoides intestinalis

Rakel and Bope: *Conn's Current Therapy 2006.*

Therapy for Renal Involvement

Scleroderma renal crisis, which develops in up to 15% of patients with SSc, was uniformly fatal in the pre–angiotensin-converting enzyme (ACE)[1] inhibitor era. Risk factors include progressive skin induration, male sex, and glucocorticoid use. Renal crisis characteristically manifests with an abrupt rise in blood pressure, frequently associated with retinal hemorrhages, and occasionally with seizures and pulmonary hemorrhage, microangiopathic hemolysis, and rapidly progressive oliguric renal insufficiency. The key to controlling this dreaded complication of SSc is early recognition. Accordingly, high-risk patients should monitor their blood pressure daily, and if there is a rise in blood pressure, a new onset of proteinuria, or a rise in creatinine, patients should be hospitalized for close monitoring and aggressive management. Some patients (<10%) develop scleroderma renal crisis in the absence of hypertension. Treatment with increasing doses of ACE inhibitors such as captopril (Capoten)[1] (up to 200 mg daily) should be started immediately. The creatinine may continue to rise even on ACE inhibitor therapy[1] and with adequate blood pressure control. Despite aggressive treatment, progressive renal insufficiency may ensue, necessitating dialysis. Nevertheless, up to 40% of patients may ultimately recover adequate renal function to discontinue dialysis. There is insufficient evidence to support prophylactic use of ACE inhibitors[1] in SSc.

Polymyositis/Dermatomyositis

Idiopathic inflammatory myopathies (IIM) include adult and childhood dermatomyositis (DM), polymyositis (PM), myositis associated with malignancy or other connective tissue diseases, and inclusion body myositis (IBM) (Table 3). Although the etiology of IIM is unknown, the presence of cellular infiltrates in the muscle provides strong evidence for an immune mechanism of muscle damage. In DM, the main immune effector response appears to be humoral and directed against the microvasculature, whereas in both PM and IBM, cytotoxic CD8[+] T cells and macrophages invade and destroy muscle fibers. Inflammatory myopathies are characterized by progressive symmetric weakness of the proximal muscles, causing difficulty walking, standing, and lifting objects. In DM, a characteristic erythematous rash on the face, eyelids, neck, upper chest, and back is seen. Muscle biopsy is helpful in differentiating PM/DM from drug-induced myopathies and from endocrine and metabolic myopathies. Myositis-specific antibodies may be of prognostic value; patients with Jo-1 or other anti–aminoacyl-tRNA autoantibodies are at high risk for interstitial lung disease (ILD) and show poor response to therapy. The levels of serum creatine kinase (CK) are useful in assessing disease activity. Involvement of the gastrointestinal muscles can lead to dysphagia. Patients with new myositis and especially adults with dermatomyositis, should be carefully screened for malignancy.

---

[1]Not FDA approved for this indication.

13

TABLE 3 Clinical Characteristics of Idiopathic Inflammatory Myopathies

Dermatomyositis	Polymyositis	Inclusion	Body myositis
Female to male	2:1	1:1	1:3
Age (y)	10-80	30-60	50-70
Muscle atrophy	Frequent	Rare	Frequent
Skin rash	Yes	No	No
Lung disease	Frequent	Frequent	
Dysphagia	Frequent	Rare	Rare
Arthralgia	Frequent	Rare	No
Malignancy	5%-17%	Rare	No

GENERAL PRINCIPLES OF THERAPY

Immunosuppressive therapies are the primary treatment for the IIM. Early intervention is crucial to prevent irreversible muscle damage. Because long-term administration of high doses of corticosteroids is associated with significant morbidity, a second-line agent such as methotrexate[1] or azathioprine[1] should be introduced early. Intravenous Ig therapy,[1] cyclophosphamide (Cytoxan),[1] and cyclosporine (Neoral)[1] are also used with some benefit. Rehabilitative and physical therapeutic interventions are essential to complement pharmacologic therapy. Although PM and DM can usually be controlled by immunosuppressive agents, the treatment of IBM remains unsatisfactory.

Corticosteroids

Prednisone[1] (1 mg/kg daily) is effective as initial therapy in the majority of the cases. In patients with rapidly progressive myositis or extramuscular manifestation such as ILD, intravenous pulse methylprednisolone[1] (1 g daily for 3 days) may be used. Both muscle strength and functional status and serum levels of CK should be checked regularly. Clinical improvement usually follows a fall in CK levels. Prednisone at 10 mg daily may be needed for 6 to 12 months. Progressive weakness in the face of declining CK levels suggests steroid myopathy.

[1]Not FDA approved for this indication.

Other Immunosuppressive Agents

In patients who fail to respond to corticosteroids, azathioprine[1] (2 mg/kg daily) or methotrexate[1] (20 mg weekly) may be used. Box 5 shows the indications for using second-line agents. Blood cell counts and liver functions should be closely monitored. Intermittent bolus IVIG (up to 2 g/kg infused every 4 to 8 weeks) may also be effective in some steroid-resistant DM patients and for severe esophageal involvement.

Treatment of Extramuscular Manifestations

Alveolitis and ILD are frequent complications. Some experts recommend high-dose daily corticosteroids in combination with a second-line immunosuppressive agent (cyclophosphamide,[1] azathioprine,[1] or cyclosporine[1]) early in the treatment. Skin rash can be effectively treated with hydroxychloroquine (Plaquenil)[1] (200 to 400 mg daily). Patients with severe proximal dysphagia may need a feeding tube to prevent aspiration and malnutrition.

Rehabilitative Measures

The goal of physical therapy is to preserve existing muscle function and to prevent muscle atrophy and joint contractures. Bedridden patients should receive passive exercise, stretching, and massage. As muscle strength improves, resistive exercise followed by an active aerobic conditioning regimen can be introduced. Proximal oropharyngeal dysphagia should be managed by speech therapy.

[1]Not FDA approved for this indication.

BOX 5 Rationale for Using a Second-Line Immunosuppressive Agent in Idiopathic Inflammatory Myopathy (IIM)

- Increased risk of corticosteroid-related side effects (diabetes mellitus, osteoporosis)
- Disease relapse after corticosteroid tapering attempts jeopardy
- Corticosteroid complications (myopathy)
- Severe or progressive myositis
- Serious extramuscular manifestations
- Lack of efficiency of corticosteroid as a single agent

 CURRENT DIAGNOSIS

- Protean manifestations in multiple organs
- Marked clinical heterogeneity
- Unpredictable, often remitting-relapsing clinical course
- Diagnosis based on characteristic constellations of clinical and laboratory features (criteria)
- Accurate diagnosis, specific subset, and stage of disease must be established

CURRENT THERAPY

- Prompt diagnosis and early intervention are desirable.
- Treatment strategies must be individualized.
- Treatment plan must consider both short-term symptom control and long-term strategies.
- Both organ-based and disease-modification approaches are used.
- Immunosuppression is often complicated by side effects.
- Management by a multispeciality team of experts is desirable.

REFERENCES

Bryan C, Knight C, Black CM, Silman AJ: Prediction of five-year survival following presentation with scleroderma: Development of a simple model using three disease factors at first visit. Arthritis Rheum 1999;42(12):2660-2665.

Dalakas MC: High-dose intravenous immunoglobulin in inflammatory myopathies: Experience based on controlled clinical trials. Neurol Sci 2003;24(Suppl 4):S256-S259.

Ionnaou Y, Isenberg DA: Current concepts for the management of systemic lupus erythematosus in adults: A therapeutic approach. Postgrad Med J 2002;78:599-606.

Isenberg DA, Allen E, Farewell V, et al: International consensus outcome measures for patients with idiopathic inflammatory myopathies. Development and initial validation of myositis activity and damage indices in patients with adult onset disease. Rheumatology (Oxford) 2004;43(1):49-54.

Manzi S: Treatment of systemic lupus erythematosus. In Klippel JH, Stone J, Weyand C, Crofford LJ (eds): Primer on the Rheumatic Diseases. Atlanta, Arthritis Foundation, 2001, pp 346-352.

Mayes MD, Lacey JV Jr, Beebe-Dimmer J, et al: Prevalence, incidence, survival, and disease characteristics of systemic sclerosis in a large US population. Arthritis Rheum 2003;48(8):2246-2255.

Oddis CV: Idiopathic inflammatory myopathies: A treatment update. Curr Rheumatol Rep 2003;5(6):431-436.

Ortmann RA, Klippel JH: Update on cyclophosphamide for systemic lupus erythematosus. Rheum Dis Clin North Am 2000;26:363-375.

Ramirez A, Varga J: Pulmonary arterial hypertension in systemic sclerosis: Clinical manifestations, pathophysiology, evaluation, and management. Treat Respir Med 2004;3(6):339-352.

Wigley FM: Raynaud's phenomenon. N Engl J Med 2002;347(13):1001-1008.

Cutaneous Vasculitis

Method of
*Thomas M. Bush, MD, and
Matthew H. Kanzler, MD*

Cutaneous vasculitis is a form of systemic vasculitis that typically involves the venules, capillaries, and arterioles of the skin. In more severe cases, the kidneys, gastrointestinal (GI) tract, or peripheral nerves may be involved. The hallmark of the disease is palpable purpura, a rash consisting of slightly raised nonblanching papules that usually appear first in the lower extremities (Figure 1).

Rakel and Bope: *Conn's Current Therapy 2006.*

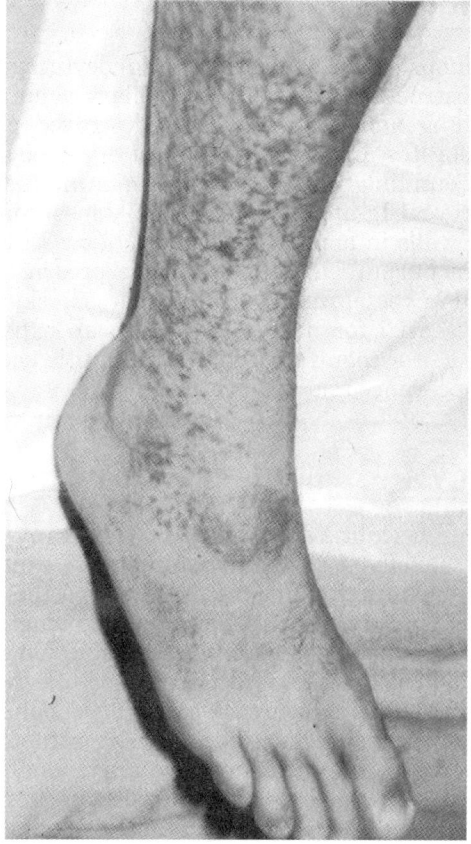

FIGURE 1. Right calf of a patient with palpable purpura.

Clinical Presentation

Cutaneous vasculitis typically manifests with a crop of lesions in dependent areas, most commonly the lower extremities. The lesions are usually raised, red to light purple, and nonblanchable. The papules range from 1 mm to several centimeters and may occasionally be vesicular, ulcerated, or urticarial. They are asymptomatic, mildly pruritic, and occasionally associated with pain or a burning sensation. Although the lesions usually begin on the lower extremities, subsequent crops of eruptions may involve the trunk and arms. Individual lesions fade over a period of several weeks, sometimes leaving residual hyperpigmentation.

Typically 50% of patients with cutaneous vasculitis experience an acute or transient course, 30% develop chronic disease, and 20% experience relapsing disease. Approximately 50% of patients with cutaneous vasculitis have multisystemic involvement. Polyarthritis often manifests with tender and swollen joints with painful range of motion. The knees, wrists, and ankles are commonly involved. Nephritis may evolve into chronic renal failure, the most serious long-term sequelae of cutaneous vasculitis. An additional serious complication of cutaneous vasculitis is GI disease. Symptoms may range from mild colicky abdominal pain to rare cases of hemorrhage or intussusception. Unusual complications include peripheral neuropathies or pulmonary hemorrhage.

Pathology

A skin biopsy may demonstrate leukocytoclastic vasculitis destruction of small postcapillary venules, with surrounding nuclear debris from destroyed polymorphonucleocytes and extravasation of erythrocytes into the surrounding dermis. Direct immunofluorescent studies reveal Ig and/or complement deposition in the vascular walls in approximately 85% of cases. Henoch-Schönlein purpura is notable for the presence of IgA deposited in vessel walls. In typical cases, a skin biopsy is not essential for diagnosis because an experienced clinician can recognize cutaneous vasculitis accurately by its appearance and distribution.

Etiology

Cutaneous vasculitis is considered an aberrant immune response usually triggered by an infection, exposure to a drug, or an autoimmune disease. The specific etiology of palpable purpura is identified in approximately 50% of cases. Infectious agents are responsible for approximately 20% of cases. A wide variety of infections are linked to palpable purpura. Bacterial infections associated with cutaneous vasculitis include streptococcus, staphylococcus, and gram-negative organisms. Several viral agents can trigger palpable purpura, including HIV, hepatitis B, and hepatitis C. Twenty percent of cases are possibly triggered by an exposure to a drug. Many drugs are reported to cause palpable purpura, most commonly antibiotics (penicillins, sulfonamides), anticonvulsants, isoniazid (Laniazid), and cardiac medications. Less than 5% of cases are associated with an underlying connective tissue disease such as systemic lupus erythematosus, rheumatoid arthritis, Sjögren's syndrome, and Wegener's granulomatosis. Rarely are cases of palpable purpura reported in patients with malignancies, including Hodgkin's disease, mycosis fungoides, and adult T-cell lymphoma.

The most likely cause of transient vasculitis in patients in whom the workup fails to pinpoint an etiology is an undetected viral infection or overlooked medication or chemical ingestion. Chronic vasculitis (months to years) suggests a primary autoimmune disorder if cryoglobulinemia and chronic hepatitis C infection are ruled out.

Differential Diagnosis

The differential diagnosis of purpuric skin lesions includes trauma, pigmented purpuric eruptions (Schamberg's disease), coagulopathies, thrombocytopenia, and embolic or thrombotic disorders. Pigmented purpuric eruptions are benign disorders most commonly appearing on the lower legs as chronic yellow-brown irregular patches with superimposed pinpoint red macules. These disorders are usually distinctive clinically, and pathology is limited to mild capillaritis of the skin. Purpuras caused by coagulopathies are generally nonpalpable and retiform, branching, or stellate. Associated livedo reticularis and

necrosis are common. Thrombocytopenia manifests with petechial lesions that are nonpalpable and usually smaller than palpable purpura lesions, in the range of 1 to 5 mm. Coagulopathy panels and platelet counts promptly distinguish these different conditions. It may be more difficult to readily diagnose embolic or thrombotic disorders. Cholesterol emboli may appear with a showering of purpuric lesions in the lower extremities. This condition typically follows an invasive vascular procedure and frequently is associated with hypereosinophilia. A skin biopsy may be necessary for establishing a diagnosis based on typical cholesterol clefts. Bacterial sepsis or endocarditis may also manifest with septic emboli that resemble palpable purpura. Patients with this condition are generally systemically ill and exhibit positive blood cultures.

Henoch-Schönlein Purpura

Henoch-Schönlein purpura (HSP) deserves specific mention because of its history and frequency. Heberden described the first case in a 4-year-old boy in 1801. Schönlein in 1837 and Henoch in 1874 reported additional cases in children. This condition classically appears in children between 5 and 15 years of age with palpable purpura, arthritis, nephritis, and colicky abdominal pain. Thirty percent of cases follow an upper respiratory infection, and 10% are associated with the use of β-lactam antibiotics. The clinical outcome is excellent in more than 90% of cases without treatment. A small percentage of patients develop persistent renal or gastroenterologic manifestations and may require immunosuppressive therapy. Direct immunofluorescence of skin biopsies demonstrates perivascular IgA deposits.

Cryoglobulinemia

Another important subtype of cutaneous vasculitis is related to hepatitis C and cryoglobulins. Cryoglobulinemia is a trigger for palpable purpura. It was considered an idiopathic condition until 1990 when Pascual described a link between hepatitis C and essential mixed cryoglobulinemia. It is now well recognized that 40% of patients with chronic hepatitis C infection produce cryoglobulins, which is a type of rheumatoid factor (antibodies that react with the Fc portion of other antibodies) that precipitates in the cold. Ten percent of patients with cryoglobulinemia develop cutaneous vasculitis with palpable purpura, Raynaud's phenomenon, nephritis, and peripheral neuropathy. It is important to recognize patients who have palpable purpura caused by hepatitis C because the key to their treatment is antiviral therapy.

Treatment

Cutaneous vasculitis is usually a relatively benign condition. The most important intervention is often the recognition and removal of an underlying trigger, such as a medication or infection. Symptomatic improvement may be achieved with leg elevation, nonsteroidal anti-inflammatory drugs, and antihistamines. Persistent palpable purpura without significant internal organ complications may respond to treatment with colchicine[1] (0.6 mg given twice daily), hydroxychloroquine (Plaquenil)[1] (200 mg given at a dose of 6.25 mg/kg per day), or dapsone[1] (100 to 200 mg per day).

Repeated clinical evaluation of patients for indication of renal, GI, or neurologic manifestations is essential. Physical examination and urine analysis for microscopic hematuria and proteinuria should be conducted periodically until the patient stabilizes. Development of internal organ involvement usually indicates a need for systemic corticosteroid therapy. Prednisone[1] can be started at a moderate dose (0.5 to 1 mg/kg per day), gradually tapering once the patient's symptoms stabilize. Unfortunately, no prospective randomized trials of immunosuppressant medications are available to guide treatment of these patients. If patients develop severe renal disease, more potent immunosuppressive medications, such as azathioprine (Imuran)[1] (2 mg/kg per day), methotrexate[1] (7.5 to 15 mg once per week), or cyclophosphamide (Cytoxan)[1] (2 mg/kg per day), may be indicated. Patients with cryoglobulinemia secondary to hepatitis C should be treated with antiviral agents, such as interferon-α[1] (3 MU three times per week) and

[1]Not FDA approved for this indication.

CURRENT DIAGNOSIS

History
- Acute versus chronic?
- Antecedent illness, exposure to new drugs?
- Symptoms indicating systemic involvement?
- Symptoms indicating connective tissue diseases?
- Symptoms indicating underlying malignancy?

Physical Exam
- Small vessel vasculitis: palpable purpura, pinpoint papules, vesicles, petechiae splinter hemorrhages, pustules, and urticaria
- Arthritis: tender, swollen joints

Laboratory Evaluation
- Biopsy: not always necessary in classic presentation of small vessel disease
- Urinalysis: most cost-effective screen for systemic involvement
- Sedimentation rate: not helpful in diagnosis; only useful for monitoring disease activity
- Further laboratory workup typically reserved for patients with chronic vasculitis or systemic symptoms: CBC, LFTs, HBV/HCV, stool guaiac, CXR, cryoglobulins, and complement levels
- Other tests ordered at direction of history and physical exam (e.g., ANA, RF if connective tissue symptomatology)

Abbreviations: ANA = antinuclear antibody; CBC = complete blood count; CXR = chest radiograph; LFTs = liver function tests; HBV/HCV = hepatitis B virus/hepatitis C virus; RF = rheumatoid factor.

Rakel and Bope: *Conn's Current Therapy 2006.*

CURRENT THERAPY

Initial Therapy
- Removal of underlying trigger
- Leg elevation
- Nonsteroidal anti-inflammatory drugs
- Antihistamines
- Colchicine
- Hydroxychloroquine
- Dapsone

If Internal Organ Involvement
- Prednisone
- Azathioprine
- Methotrexate
- Cyclophosphamide

ribavirin[1] (1000 mg per day). In life-threatening cases, prednisone, cyclophosphamide, and plasmapheresis may be indicated.

Cutaneous vasculitis is a relatively common and benign form of vasculitis. It usually presents with palpable purpura but may occasionally progress to involve the joints, kidneys, bowel, or peripheral nerves. The most important step in treating these patients is often the correct identification and treatment of an underlying drug, infection, or connective tissue disease that has triggered the vasculitis. In the majority of patients, the vasculitis resolves spontaneously and they do not need immunosuppressive therapy. If patients develop internal organ complications, a course of prednisone or other immunosuppressive medication may be indicated.

REFERENCES

Blanco R, Martinez Taboada VM, Rodriguez-Valverde V, Garcia-Fuentes M: Cutaneous vasculitis in children and adults: Associated diseases and etiologic factors in 303 patients. Medicine 1998; 77:403-418.
Jeannette JC, Falk RJ: Medical progress: Small-vessel vasculitis. N Engl J Med 1997;337:1512-1523.
Lotti T, Ghersetich I, Comacchi C, Jorizzo JL: Cutaneous small-vessel vasculitis. J Am Acad Dermatol 1998;39:667-687.
Sais G, Vidaller A, Jucgla A, et al: Prognostic factors in leukocytoclastic vasculitis: A clinicopathologic study of 160 patients. Arch Dermatol 1998;134:309-315.
Stone JH, Nousari HC: "Essential" cutaneous vasculitis: What every rheumatologist should know about vasculitis of the skin. Curr Opin Rheum 2001;13:23-34.

[1]Not FDA approved for this indication.

13

Diseases of the Nails

Method of
Robert Baran, MD

Dermatitis

Allergic or irritant contact dermatitis involving the digits may interfere with nail plate formation and produce transverse grooves and pitting. Associated onycholysis is more frequent than subungual hyperkeratosis. Paraben-free topical corticosteroids, applied two to three times daily to surrounding soft tissues, are effective, observing thorough protection of hands (cotton gloves beneath vinyl gloves).

Epidermoid Carcinoma

The best treatment for epidermoid carcinoma is Mohs' micrographic surgery, allowing adequate excision with maximal preservation of normal tissue and function. It can be performed with routine instrumentation as well as with the carbon dioxide laser in a focused beam incisional mode. This technique avoids bleeding and ensures minimal postoperative discomfort for the patient.

Excisional surgery may be used for limited lesions or for complete removal of the nail apparatus, with healing by secondary intention or grafting and supplemented by repair with a bridge flap. Electrosurgery is a therapeutic alternative in a few selected cases. Liquid nitrogen may give good results. Bone involvement requires amputation of the distal phalanx. Besides local 5-fluorouracil (Adrucil),[1] imiquimod cream (Aldara) and photodynamic therapy are recent treatments that require the test of time.

Exostosis and Osteochondroma

The treatment of exostosis and osteochondroma consists of local curettage or excision of the excess bone under aseptic conditions. If the tumor is located in the nail bed, the nail plate is partially removed and a longitudinal incision made in the subungual tissue.

Whenever possible, removal of tumor by an L-shaped or a fish-mouth incision is performed to avoid nail plate avulsion. The osseous growth with its cartilaginous cap is carefully dissected using fine skin hooks to avoid damage to the fragile nail bed, and the tumor is removed with a fine chisel.

Fibrokeratoma and Koenen's Tumors

Fibrokeratoma and Koenen's tumors are cured by simple excision. Tumors growing out from under the proximal

nail fold are removed after reflecting the fold back by making lateral incisions down each margin in the axis of the lateral nail grooves. Subungual fibroma are removed after avulsion of the corresponding part of the nail plate.

Glomus Tumor

When the bluish-red spot of a glomus tumor involves the middle of the nail bed, a 6- to 8-mm punch removes a disk of keratin and enables a longitudinal incision. The caviar-like material is dissected from the surrounding tissue. The disk of keratin is then placed back. In the matrix area, horizontal incision should be performed. Tumors in a lateral position are removed by an L-shaped incision of the tip of the digit, allowing dissection of the nail bed from the bone until the tumor is reached.

Green Nails

Green nails are usually caused by infection with *Pseudomonas* that grows in a wet pocket under the posterior fold or under the nail plate. Drying out the pocket and using alcohol or an alcohol-based antibiotic such as clindamycin[1] kills the organism, but discoloration persists until the nail grows out. The green stain can be removed by sodium hypochlorite (Dakin's solution), one drop twice daily around the nail. It is also possible to cover the nail with dark polish until the green hue disappears. Cotton gloves beneath vinyl gloves for any wet work prevents recurrence.

Habit-Tic Nail Deformity

Onychophagia and onychotillomania are nervous habits. Periungual warts are a complication common in nail biters. Use of distasteful preparations may discourage nail biting and chewing. Oral fluoxetine hydrochloride[1] (Prozac), 20 mg per day, is suggested.

The longitudinal split known as Heller's median nail dystrophy is probably caused by repeated pressure on the base of the nail, the proximal nail fold kept intact. It usually affects the thumbs and must be differentiated from the washboard nail appearing with transverse ridging crossed by a longitudinal depression. This condition results from pushing back the cuticle. Micropore tape, changed daily and maintained for 6 months, may deter the patient's habit.

Hematoma

Hematoma occurs shortly after a single trauma involving the nail apparatus. In partial hematoma of the proximal area of the nail apparatus, drainage of the hematoma with a fine-pointed scalpel blade gives prompt relief from pain.

[1]Not FDA approved for this indication.

[1]Not FDA approved for this indication.

A hematoma involving more than 25% of the nail is observed when there is an injury to the nail bed. The possibility of an underlying fracture must be considered and a radiograph performed. After the nail plate is removed, the hematoma is evacuated, the wound repaired, and the nail replaced.

Hallopeau's Acrodermatitis

For systemic treatment of Hallopeau's acrodermatitis, etretinate,[2] 0.5 mg/kg per day, or acitretin (Soriatane)[1] is used. Nimesulide,[2] 200 mg per day, has been suggested. For topical treatment, calcipotriene (Dovonex),[1] topical steroids, or both (Daivobet) are helpful.

Hangnails

Hangnails that may become infected should be removed with sharp-pointed scissors. Mupirocin ointment (Bactroban) prevents or clears low-grade infection.

Ingrown Nails

Regardless of the initial cause, an ingrown nail ultimately has a nail bed that is too narrow for its nail plate.

DISTAL NAIL EMBEDDING

Sculptured artificial nails can be used to override and lower the distal nail wall. When this procedure fails, a crescent wedge-shaped tissue excision is carried out around the entire distal phalanx, and the defect is closed with a 5-0 monofilament suture.

JUVENILE INGROWING TOENAIL

Treatment of the early stage (pain and erythema) of juvenile ingrowing toenail is conservative. The distal-lateral nail spicule is removed under local anesthesia, and a wisp of cotton wool, kept moist with a disinfectant, is placed beneath the nail and between its lateral edge and the lateral nail groove.

In the advanced stage (edema, granulation tissue, purulent drainage), the aim of the treatment is to narrow the nail. A lateral strip of the offending nail is removed. After protection of the surrounding skin with petroleum jelly, a saturated solution of phenol is applied in a bloodless field to the matrix horn on a small cotton pack for 3 minutes. Infection may be prevented by soaking the foot twice daily in a quart of warm water containing three capsules[2] of povidone-iodine (Betadine).

HYPERTROPHIC LATERAL NAIL LIP

Hypertrophic lateral nail lip results from long-standing ingrown nails. An elliptic wedge of tissue, taken from the lateral nail wall of the toe to the bone, pulls away the lateral nail fold from the offending lateral nail margin. Associated phenol cautery of the matrix horn prevents recurrences.

PINCER NAIL

The nail brace technique, using a stainless steel wire fitted to the nail, is useful for correcting a pincer nail, a mild inward distortion. In advanced cases, phenol cautery of the lateral horns of the matrix gives excellent results.

Lichen Planus

Treatment of lichen planus prevents severe and sometimes permanent lesions, such as pterygium and onychatrophy. An intralesional long-acting steroid should be used in the same manner as for treating psoriatic nails. If more than two digits are affected and there is no medical contraindication, triamcinolone acetonide (Kenalog-10)[1] is injected intramuscularly (80 mg the first month, then 40 mg monthly for 6 months). The frequency of the injections should be adjusted to the patient's response. Treatment may last for 18 months to 2 years.

Etretinate[2] or acitretin[1] is effective before the scarring stage. Azathioprine (Imuran),[1] 100 mg per day, is suggested.

Longitudinal Melanonychia

In adults with fair complexions, complete excisional biopsy may be recommended for both diagnosis and treatment of longitudinal melanonychia with an irregular dermoscopy pattern. The appropriate technique depends on the width of the band, the matrix melanin production site, and the anatomic location of the band of the nail. Longitudinal melanonychia with periungual pigmentation, nail dystrophy, ulceration, or a bleeding mass should be treated as a malignant melanoma.

Myxoid Pseudocyst

Liquid nitrogen can produce up to an 86% cure rate for myxoid pseudocyst. The field treated includes the cyst and the adjacent proximal area to the transverse skin creases overlying the terminal joint. Two freeze/thaw cycles are carried out, each freeze time 30 seconds after the ice field forms; the intervening thaw times are at least 4 minutes. Nail fold excision for cysts involving the distal portion of the posterior fold is advocated.

The careful extirpation of the lesion is often recommended. A drop of methylene blue solution, mixed with fresh hydrogen peroxide, is injected into the distal interphalangeal joint at the volar joint crease. The joint accepts only 0.1 to 0.2 mL of dye. This clearly identifies

---

[1]Not FDA approved for this indication.
[2]Not available in the United States.

[2]Not available in the United States.
[1]Not FDA approved for this indication.

the pedicle connecting the joint to the cyst and the cyst itself.

High success rates are found with osteophytectomy, even without removal of the cystic lesion. Complications following resection of myxoid pseudocysts are mainly joint stiffness, loss of residual motion, persistent swelling, pain, deviation of the distal interphalangeal joint, and infection.

Injection of a sclerosing agent, such as 1% sodium tetradecyl sulfate (Sotradecol),[1] into myxoid pseudocysts is effective. After the cyst has been pierced and its jellylike material expressed, 0.10 to 0.20 mL is injected. One single procedure is rarely enough. A second or a third one can be performed at 6-week intervals. Adverse reactions such as permanent nail dystrophy are reported.

Nail Fragility Syndrome

In the nail fragility syndrome, nails may split lengthwise or laterally into layers. It occurs mostly in persons who have an occupation involving exposure to moisture. The following procedures are helpful:

- Repeated immersions in soap and water should be avoided.
- Each hydration should be followed by application of an ointment (e.g., containing phospholipids, urea hyaluronic acid [Restylane],[2] α-hydroxy acids, etc.) to retain the moisture in the nail plate.
- Applications of dimethyl urea 2%[1] can be applied as a base coat preparation (Toughen Up).[1]
- Cetaphil can be used as an alternative to excessive exposure to water.
- The nails should be kept short.
- Oral iron[1] for 6 months, even in the absence of overt anemia, may be helpful, as well as biotin[2] (10 mg/day) and/or cystine.[2]
- Nail polish is protective; oily removers should be used.
- Nail wrapping limited to the distal portion of the nail may afford protection.

Onychogryphosis

The nail is thickened and distorted in onychogryphosis, often resembling a ram's horn in those over 65 years of age. Conservative treatment is indicated using rotating grinders at regular intervals. Should radical treatment be needed, matricectomy and nail bed ablation are obtained with 88% phenol cautery.

Onycholysis

In onycholysis, separation of the nail plate starts distally and spreads toward the proximal edge. Whatever the cause, thorough clipping away of as much detached nail as possible is helpful, repeated at 1- or 2-week intervals.

[1]Not FDA approved for this indication.
[2]Not available in the United States.

Gentle brushing with plain soap and water once daily should be followed by careful rinsing and drying.

Depending on the cause of the complaint (e.g., fungal organisms, psoriasis, impaired peripheral circulation), appropriate local treatment, systemic therapy, or both are prescribed. In all cases, dryness of the onycholytic areas should be maintained.

Onychomycosis

Before initiating treatment of onychomycosis, potassium hydroxide examination and mycologic culture are essential. Sometimes isolation of fungi is difficult (proximal white subungual onychomycosis) because the patient has already received antifungal treatment. A washout period should be considered. In difficult cases, nail samples should be sent to the pathologist.

Providing the distal half of the nail plate is spared, it may be possible to achieve a cure using topical therapy alone, with ciclopirox (Penlac) or amorolfine.[1] The success rates can be increased by associating a nail lacquer with a systemic treatment.

Other treatments are as follows:

- Terbinafine (Lamisil), 250 mg daily for 6 weeks, for fingernail onychomycosis, and 3 to 6 months for toenails
- Intermittent therapy of itraconazole (Sporanox), 400 mg daily for 1 week a month (two pulses for fingernail onychomycosis and three or four for toenails)
- Fluconazole (Diflucan),[1] 300 mg once weekly for 9 to 12 months

Results may be improved further using an adjunct of 40% urea paste applied under an occlusive dressing.

Partial surgical nail avulsion for onychomycosis of limited extent reduces the time needed for systemic therapy by 50%. Partial surgical avulsion is also advisable in mold paronychia and *Candida* paronychia with secondary nail invasion. Nail abrasion of pathologic keratin is an alternative. Recurrences may be prevented by the regular application of topical antifungals on the previously affected nails, soles, and toe webs, and application of an antifungal nail lacquer every 2 weeks.

Parakeratosis Pustulosa

The lesions of parakeratosis pustulosa are usually limited to one digit in a child and improve spontaneously with time. Topical steroids may be used for limited periods.

Paronychia

ACUTE PARONYCHIA

If very superficial, pus may be released with a sharp-pointed scalpel without anesthesia. Any whitlow can extend more deeply into the tissue to give rise to a felon

[1]Not FDA approved for this indication.

Rakel and Bope: *Conn's Current Therapy 2006.*

that connects to the tendon sheath or extends under the nail plate.

If deeper infection does not respond within 48 hours to penicillinase-fast antibiotics associated with dressings moistened with alcoholic solution under occlusion, it should be treated surgically by removing the base of the nail plate, whose proximal third is cut transversally with a nail splitter. When pus forms below the nail plate, probing determines the most painful area and provides an indication for the site of fenestration of the nail plate.

CHRONIC PARONYCHIA

Chronic paronychia represents an inflammatory reaction of the proximal nail fold to irritants or allergens. Secondary colonization with *Candida albicans* and/or bacteria occurs in most cases. Patients should follow the same rules described for nail fragility.

In patients nonallergic to neomycin, Mycolog ointment should be applied twice daily until the cuticle has regrown. Intralesional injection of triamcinolone[1] acetonide suspension (2.5 mg/mL) into the affected nail fold facilitates quick resolution of the paronychia.

Methylprednisone,[1] 20 mg per day for 1 week, can be prescribed in severe polydactylous cases. Antifungals are usually unnecessary.

Chronic paronychia that does not respond to medical therapy is usually associated with a foreign body. Such cases should be treated by excising a crescent-shaped full-thickness segment of the proximal nail fold, including its swollen portion.

Psoriasis

Nail polish may be used to hide discrete nail changes. Potent topical corticosteroids are helpful in treating the dorsal aspect of the proximal fold. Although the efficacy of topical corticosteroids can be enhanced by overnight occlusion, this technique should be used only for limited periods. Tazarotene gel (Tazorac) or calcipotriol (Dovonex), combined with clobetasol (Temovate), are useful after the nail bed is exposed, using 40% urea as in chemical avulsion or after clipping away as much detached nail as possible.

Depending on the location of the affected structures, an intralesional long-acting steroid is injected into the proximal nail fold to treat the proximal matrix or into the subungual area through the lateral aspect of the nail walls, using triamcinolone acetonide (Kenalog-10), diluted to 2.5 mg/mL, at a dose of 0.2 to 0.5 mL per nail.

A 30-gauge needle with fine volume gradations is locked to the syringe and injections should be repeated monthly for 6 months, then every 6 weeks for the next 6 months, and finally every 2 months for 6 to 12 months. A digital block is useful to make the treatment less painful, especially in nail bed psoriasis, but when several digits are involved, a wrist block may be the appropriate anesthesia.

The standard steroid of triamcinolone acetonide, 10 mg/mL, may be used as an alternative because weaker solutions may not be a test of efficacy. An injection of 0.05 to 0.1 mL is inserted on both sides of the distal digit, in each of four sites depending on whether the nail matrix or bed requires treatment. Benefit should appear in 2 to 3 months. This treatment may be followed by repeated injections of weaker strengths.

With the exception of acropustulosis, in which the treatment is consistently effective, good response to etretinate[2] or acitretin (Soriatane) is found in hyperkeratotic nail psoriasis. All female subjects of childbearing potential must undergo a pregnancy test and agree to use adequate birth control. Pregnancy continues to be contraindicated for 3 years after cessation of therapy.

Pyogenic Granuloma

Under local anesthesia, pyogenic granuloma, a vascular post-traumatic tumor, is easily removed by surgical shaving (for the pathologist to examine). Hemostasis is achieved with aluminium chloride solution.

Twenty-Nail Dystrophy

Twenty-nail dystrophy, usually observed in children, is characterized by nail roughness and excessive ridging. It can be idiopathic or associated with alopecia areata, lichen planus, and, less often, psoriasis. The nail changes usually regress spontaneously within a few years. No treatment is required. Nevertheless, biotin oral administration for 6 months is advocated.

Warts

Recurrences of warts are frequent. A spontaneous or so-called magic cure is by no means unusual. Liquid nitrogen is often used despite a throbbing pain. Under local anesthesia, a multiple puncture technique with a bifurcated vaccination needle introducing bleomycin sulfate (Blenoxane)[1] (1 µg/mL) sterile saline solution into warts is the best treatment.

Periungual and subungual warts respond well to carbon dioxide laser treatment. Imiquimod (Aldara)[1] may be effective.

Yellow Nail Syndrome

Fluconazole (Diflucan),[1] 300 mg once a week combined with vitamin E, 1000 to 1200 IU daily, produces a positive effect on nail growth in yellow nail syndrome (YNS). Total resolution of yellow nails and lymphedema may be observed following oral zinc supplementation for 2 years. Topical vitamin E solution in dimethylsulfoxide[2] applied twice a day is successful.

---

[1]Not FDA approved for this indication.

[1]Not FDA approved for this indication.
[2]Not available in the United States.

Monthly repeated intradermal triamcinolone acetonide[1] suspension injections into the proximal nail matrix are effective.

REFERENCES

Baran R: Nail fungal infections and treatment. Hand Clin 2002;18: 625-628.

Baran R: The new oral antifungal drugs in the treatment of the yellow nail syndrome. Br J Dermatol 2002;147:189-191.

Baran R, Haneke E, Richert B: Pincer nails: Definition and surgical treatment. Dermatol Surg 2001;27:261-266.

Baran R, Perrin C, Thomas L, Braun RP: Melanocytic system of the nail and its disorders. In Nordlung JJ, Boissy RE, Hearing VJ, et al (eds): The Pigmentary System: Physiology and Pathophysiology, 2nd ed, Oxford, Blackwell Publishing (in press).

De Berker D: Diagnosis and management of nail psoriasis. Dermatol Ther 2002;15:165-172.

Haneke E, Baran R: Longitudinal melanonychia. Dermatol Surg 2001;27:580-584.

---

[1]Not FDA approved for this indication.

Keloids

Method of
Woraphong Manuskiatti, MD

Keloids are a frequent reason for dermatologic consultation requests. Clinically, keloids appear as firm, bulbous nodules or markedly elevated plaques following the healing process of a skin injury that extends beyond the confines of the original wound. They do not regress spontaneously and tend to recur after excision. Histologically, keloids are characterized by foci of markedly thickened, brightly eosinophilic-staining collagen bundles arranged randomly that appear within the mass of fibrillary collagen. The presence of a keloid is often cosmetically unacceptable to the affected individuals. In addition, it may be painful or pruritic, and it may restrict range of motion. Keloids represent abnormal wound healing in response to cutaneous surgery, physical trauma, or inflammatory responses. Keloids occur in all races, with a preponderance in individuals with darker pigmentation.

Pathogenesis

The exact mechanisms of keloid pathogenesis are yet to be determined and may be multifactorial. Studies have demonstrated both overproduction of collagen and increased procollagen levels, as well as decreased levels of collagenase in keloidal tissue. Proposed mechanisms for the cause of keloid formation include tension and vessel occlusion, as well as genetic, hormonal, and immune-mediated mechanisms. Much of the current research is concentrated on the immunoregulation of collagen production and deposition.

Treatment

Prevention should be the first rule of keloid therapy. Nonessential surgical and cosmetic procedures should not be performed on patients with histories of forming keloids or in anatomical regions prone to keloid formation, including the midchest, shoulder, back, and posterior neck. All postoperative and cutaneous trauma sites should be treated with appropriate antibiotics to prevent infection. All surgical wounds should be closed with normal tension. If possible, incision should not cross joint spaces, and skin excisions should be horizontal ellipses in the same direction as the skin tension lines.

Several forms of treatment are used with varying degrees of success. No single therapy is superior. Use of multiple modalities is often necessary to treat the lesions successfully. The selection of therapeutic techniques typically depends on size, location, depth, patient age, past responses to treatment, and the economic status of individuals (Table 1).

Medical Therapies

CORTICOSTEROID INJECTIONS

Intralesional corticosteroid injections are the mainstay therapy for treatment of keloids. Corticosteroids decrease excessive scarring by reducing synthesis of collagen and glycosaminoglycans and by reducing inflammatory mediators and fibroblast proliferation during the wound healing process. The most commonly used corticosteroid is triamcinolone acetonide (Kenalog-10),[1] 10 to 40 mg/mL, administered intralesionally at 2- to 4-week intervals over the course of months to years. Response rates vary from 50% to 100%, with a recurrence of 9% to 50%. Results are improved when corticosteroids are combined with other therapies such as excision and cryosurgery. Complications of repeated corticosteroid injections include atrophy, telangiectasia, and hypopigmentation at and around the injection sites (Figure 1).

INTERFERON

Interferon (IFN)[1] causes a decrease in collagen I and III synthesis by reducing cellular messenger ribonucleic acid. Intralesional IFN-γ injection administered twice weekly for 4 weeks shows improved to complete resolution of keloids. But injections tend to be exceedingly painful and complicated by flulike symptoms.

5-FLUOROURACIL[1]

Treatment of keloids with intralesional 5-fluorouracil (5-FU) (Adrucil)[1] injection combined with corticosteroids

---

[1]Not FDA approved for this indication.

TABLE 1 Common Therapeutic Regimens for Keloids

Treatment modality	Regimen	Treatment interval
IL corticosteroids	TAC (10-40 mg/mL)	q 2-4 wk
IL 5-FU plus TAC	5-FU (45 mg/mL) mixed with TAC (1 mg/mL)	q 1-2 wk
Excision	Scalpel or CO_2 laser excision	Should be followed by another treatment modality
Cryosurgery	Two to three freeze-thaw cycles of 10 to 30 sec	q 3-4 wk
Pressure therapy	Pressure maintained between 24 and 30 mm Hg, 18 to 24 hr per day	At least 6-12 mo
Pulsed-dye laser	7-mm spot, 5-7 J/cm^2	q 2-4 wk
Silicone gel sheeting	Apply for at least 12 h per day	At least 3 mo

Abbreviations: CO_2 = carbon dioxide; 5-FU = 5-fluorouracil; IL = intralesional; q = every; TAC = triamcinolone acetonide.

is as effective as intralesional corticosteroids alone, but the latter is much more likely to cause adverse effects. 5-FU[1] appears to work by decreasing keloid fibroblast proliferation. Injections are given once a week at the beginning and then adjusted up or down according to the therapeutic response. Side effects of intralesional 5-FU include spots of purpura, pain during injection, and localized superficial tissue slough.

IMIQUIMOD[1]

A study on the effect of postoperative application of imiquimod (Aldara)[1] 5% cream on the surgically excised keloids for a period of 8 weeks noted a lower recurrence rate than that of excision alone. Theoretically, imiquimod induces production of IFN, thus down-regulating collagen synthesis. Reported side effects include local skin irritation and mild hyperpigmentation.

[1]Not FDA approved for this indication.

Surgical Therapies

EXCISION

Surgical excision of keloids without adjunctive therapy yields a high rate of recurrence (45% to 100%). Decreased recurrence rates are consistently reported with excision in combination with other postoperative treatment modalities, such as intralesional corticosteroids, radiation, pressure therapy, silicone gel sheeting (SGS), or imiquimod cream. Surgical techniques to minimize tissue trauma, closing with minimal tension and using buried sutures when necessary for layered closure, are recommended to decrease the possibility of recurrence.

CRYOSURGERY

Freezing keloids with cryogen such as liquid nitrogen affects the microvasculature and causes cell damage. This occurs via intracellular crystallization leading to tissue anoxia with subsequent tissue necrosis and sloughing, followed by tissue flattening. Cryosurgery

13

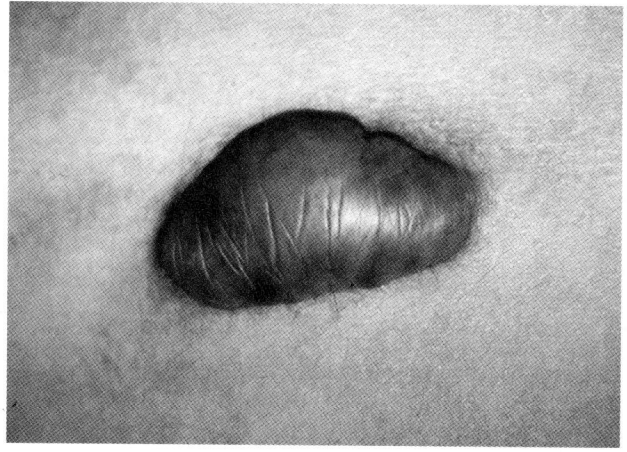
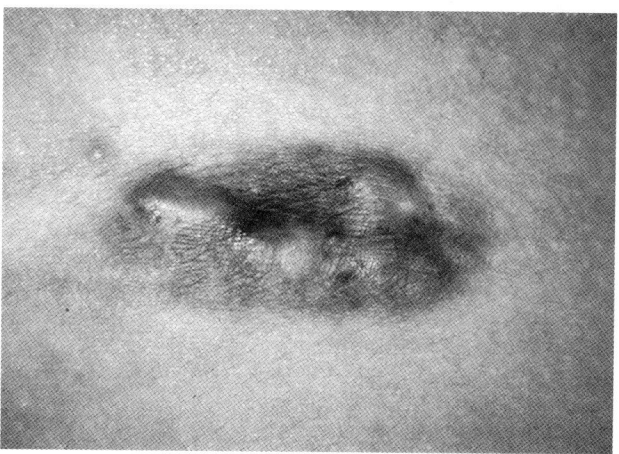

A   B

FIGURE 1. A keloid on the back before **(A)** and after **(B)** four intralesional corticosteroid (10 mg/mL) injections. Note side effects of skin atrophy, telangiectasia, and hypopigmentation. (Adapted from Manuskiatti W: Guidelines for the treatment and management of keloids and hypertrophic scars. Siriraj Hosp Gazette 2003;55:251.)

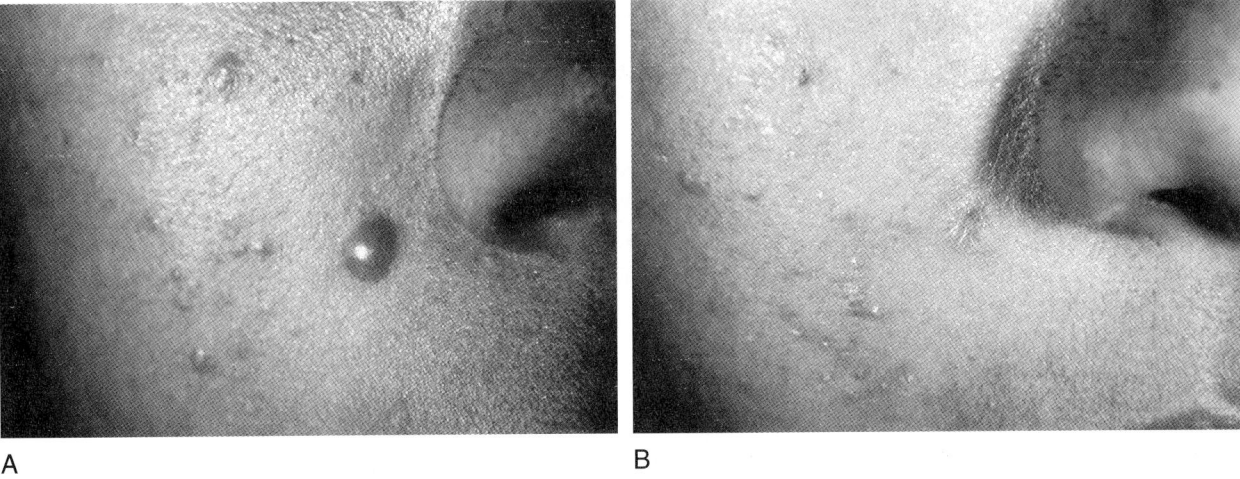

A   B

FIGURE 2. A keloid developing after acne on the cheek before **(A)** and after **(B)** two pulsed-dye laser treatments, combined with two intralesional corticosteroids plus 5-fluorouracil injections.

alone causes complete flattening in more than half of patients after two or more sessions performed at 3- to 4-week intervals. Limitations to this treatment include postoperative pain, slow healing, and hypopigmentation (especially in patients with darker skin).

Radiation Therapy

Radiation may be used as a monotherapy or combined with surgery to prevent recurrence of keloids following excision. Radiation therapy theoretically works by inhibiting fibroblast proliferation and neoangiogenesis in wound healing. When used as a monotherapy, radiation is not very effective, with a high recurrence rate of 50% to 100%. The risks of carcinogenicity associated with radiotherapy are controversial. Caution is advised when treating young children or when treating areas around the breasts and thyroid because of the increased radiosensitivities of these tissues.

Physical Modalities

PRESSURE THERAPY

The mechanism involved in how pressure therapy reduces keloid formation is unknown, but it is hypothesized that pressure induces tissue hypoxia, resulting in fibroblast degeneration and subsequent collagen degradation. It is generally recommended that the pressure be maintained between 24 and 30 mm Hg, 18 to 24 hours a day for at least 6 to 12 months, for this therapy to be effective. Pressure therapy is commonly used in combination with other modalities such as SGS and postsurgical excision. Patient compliance is the limiting factor, given the need for long-term pressure application for therapeutic success.

LASER THERAPY

At present, the common use of lasers to treat keloids is based on two different approaches. One technique is an

application of a carbon dioxide (CO_2) laser for nonspecific destruction of keloids. Keloid vaporization or excision by CO_2 laser alone results in high (40% to 90%) recurrence rate and provides no distinct advantage over scalpel excision. The CO_2 laser is now reserved for debulking large keloids, prior to the initiation of other treatment modalities. Another method used is 585-nm pulsed-dye laser (PDL) for selectively damaging the microvasculature of the keloids (Figure 2). Multiple (more than two) PDL treatment sessions decrease scar height and erythema and improve scar texture and dysesthesia.

SILICONE GEL SHEETING

The mode of action of SGS is unknown but thought to occur through an increased scar hydration effect provided by the sheet, leading to anti-keloidal effects. To be effective, the sheets must be applied for at least 12 hours daily. SGS may be especially useful in children and others who cannot tolerate the pain associated with other treatment modalities.

Miscellaneous Therapies

Although additional novel therapies are available, many treatments are anecdotal and require confirmation of efficacy and safety through formal studies. Some of these

 CURRENT DIAGNOSIS

- Clinical characteristic: A raised, firm scar, possibly painful or pruritic, extending beyond wound borders
- Histologic characteristics: Thick bundles of hyalinized collagen arranged in dense swirls or nodules

CURRENT THERAPY

Medical Therapies
- Corticosteroid injections[1] (Kenalog-10)
- Interferon (IFN)[1]
- 5-Flourouracil (5-FU) (Adrucil)[1]
- Imiquimod (Aldara)[1]

Surgical Therapies
- Primary excision
- Cryosurgery

Radiation Therapy

Physical Modalities
- Pressure therapy
- Laser therapy
- Silicone gel sheeting (SGS)

Miscellaneous Therapies
- Topical vitamin E,[1] onion extract cream (Mederma),[1] topical retinoic acid (Retin-A),[1] IL verapamil,[1] colchicines,[1] ultraviolet A1 phototherapy

[1]Not FDA approved for this indication.

therapies include topical vitamin E,[1] onion extract cream (Mederma),[1] topical retinoic acid (Retin-A),[1] intralesional verapamil,[1] colchicines,[1] and ultraviolet A1 phototherapy.

In conclusion, therapeutic management of keloids remains a challenge because of their high rate of recurrence and lack of curative treatment. Treatment approaches to keloids depend not only on the size of the lesion but also on the age and location. Use of several approaches in combination or sequentially, based on the patient's individual requirements and responses, is recommended to maximize the therapeutic outcome.

REFERENCES

Alster TS, Handrick C: Laser treatment of hypertrophic scars, keloids, and striae. Semin Cutan Med Surg 2000;19:287-292.

Berman B, Flores F: The treatment of hypertrophic scars and keloids. Eur J Dermatol 1998;8:591-596.

Manuskiatti W, Fitzpatrick RE: Treatment response of keloidal and hypertrophic sternotomy scars: Comparison among intralesional corticosteroid, 5-fluorouracil, and 585-nm flashlamp-pumped pulsed-dye laser treatments. Arch Dermatol 2002;138:1149-1155.

Murray JC: Keloids and hypertrophic scars. Clin Dermatol 1994; 12:27-37.

Mustoe TA, Cooter RD, Gold MH, et al: International clinical recommendations on scar management. Plast Reconstr Surg 2002;110: 560-571.

Niessen FB, Spauwen PH, Schalkwijk J, Kon M: On the nature of hypertrophic scars and keloids: A review. Plast Reconstr Surg 1999;104:1435-1458.

Urioste SS, Arndt KA, Dover JS: Keloids and hypertrophic scars: Review and treatment strategies. Semin Cutan Med Surg 1999;18:159-171.

[1]Not FDA approved for this indication.

Warts (Verrucae)

Method of
Tamara Salam Housman, MD, and
Phillip M. Williford, MD

Viral warts afflict approximately 10% of the population and are caused by human papillomavirus (HPV). HPV, a nonenveloped, double-stranded DNA virus, is of the papovavirus class and invades both mucous and squamous epithelium. At least 130 known types of HPV have been identified. HPV causes both clinical and subclinical infection and plays a role in certain cutaneous carcinomas, including squamous cell carcinoma (SCCa) of the anogenital area and nail unit. HPV is found in the basal layer of the epidermis but replicates only in the superficial, well-differentiated layer. The subsequent cellular proliferation gives rise to thick, hyperkeratotic lesions generally known as warts.

Cutaneous warts are mainly divided into common warts, plantar warts, flat warts, and genital warts. Common warts account for 70% of all cutaneous warts and are probably associated with HPV types 1, 2, and 4. Two thirds of untreated common warts spontaneously regress within 2 years, but these previously infected individuals have a higher rate of developing new warts than those who were never infected. Treatment of warts with salicylic acid and/or cryotherapy has demonstrated a 60% to 80% cure rate.

Transmission is via skin-to-skin contact, including sexual, and is seen with greater frequency where groups of people are in close contact, including in school-age children, with a frequency of 20% for common warts. Extent of infection is determined by the immune response, and immunocompromised hosts are at increased risk. Symptoms may include pain and bleeding, and warts may interfere with daily functioning, especially if located on the palms, soles, or digits. Warts can be professionally and socially stigmatizing, especially if located on the hands or fingers of patients who must touch others on a daily basis.

Types of Warts

Verrucae vulgares (common warts) are flesh-colored, hyperkeratotic, verrucous, fissured, firm papules that disrupt normal skin lines on fingers and toes. They may be distinguished from calluses and corns by paring down of the stratum corneum (the uppermost horny layer of skin) to reveal thrombosed/ bleeding capillaries seen as brown/black dots. A subtype is a butcher's wart, which is seen on the hands of butchers and fish and meat handlers/packers, and appears as large, cauliflower plaques. Differential diagnoses (DDx) include seborrheic keratosis, molluscum contagiosum, keratoacanthoma, amelanotic melanoma, SCCa in situ, and invasive SCCa. Verrucae vulgares warts are associated with HPV subtypes 1, 2, 4.

13

TABLE 1 Treatment of Verrucae

	Available Preparations	Mechanism of Action	Application	Dosage	Disadvantages Therapy Adverse Effects
Salicylic acid keratolytic) (Compound W)	Solution Gel/lotion/cream Plaster Pad 10%–60%	Destruction of infected epidermis; irritation leads to stimulation of immune response.	Patient applied. Adjunct to other treatment modalities. May pare down/shave wart then apply keratolytic to increase penetration.	qhs until clear, usually weeks to months.	Irritation
Cryosurgery	Liquid nitrogen (–196°C [–320.8°F]): cryospray or cotton-tipped applicator	Destruction of infected epidermis; induces inflammation leading to stimulation of immune response.	Physician applied. Paring of thick lesions liquid nitrogen freeze for 30–60 sec to include a 1–2 mm rim around wart → let thaw → repeat × 2 cycles total.	May repeat q 3–4 wk.	Pain Erythema Vesicle/bullae Crusting Possible infection Hypopigmentation Scarring (if freeze too deep) Onychodystrophy (if not careful with periungual warts)
Cantharidin[1,2]	Colloidal solution, 0.7%	Destruction of epidermis and leads to blister formation; extract of blister beetle.	Adjunct to other treatment modalities. Careful with periungual warts, overlying tendons, and on lower extremities. Physician applied. Paring of thick lesions. Apply using very fine applicator only to wart then patient is to wash off in 6–8 h. Painless—good for children.	May repeat q 2–4 wk.	Vesicle/bullae Crusting Avoid face or near eyes
Surgical excision Curettage Electrocautery	N/A	Destruction by surgical removal of wart.	Physician applied. Surgical excision of wart or surgical removal by curetting wart then cauterizing the base.	Usually only performed once but may repeat if wart recurs.	Painful (minimal if use local anesthesia but some postoperative pain) Scarring
Trichloroacetic acid (Tri-Chlor) Bichloroacetic acid	Solution, up to 50% concentration	Destruction of infected epidermis.	Physician applied.	Most useful for mucosal warts.	Painful reactions
Lasers: Carbon dioxide Pulsed-dye Erbium:YAG	N/A	Destruction of infected epidermis.	Physician applied.	May repeat q 4–6 wk.	Expensive Risk of viral spread via laser plume Not superior to conventional therapy
Imiquimod	Cream, 5%	Immunomodulator: indirect in vivo anti-tumor and antiviral effects mediated by induction of cytokines—IFN-α, TNF-α, IL-1, -6, -8, and others.	Patient applied. On nonmucosal skin, including plantar/palmar warts, apply keratolytic, followed by occlusion in PM, followed by imiquimod in AM; may also occlude imiquimod if not getting any erythema. If irritation is severe, stop regimen for few days then resume, if possible. May initiate therapy with cryosurgery followed by keratolytic-imiquimod combination therapy for 6 wks then repeat if necessary.	3 times/wk on mucosal skin; 5–7 times/wk on keratinized skin.	Irritation Erythema Pruritus Burning Crusting Infection Scarring

Rakel and Bope: *Conn's Current Therapy 2006.*

Drug	Preparation	Mechanism	Notes/Application	Dose	Side Effects/Comments
Cimetidine (Tagamet)[1]	Tablets: 200 mg, 300 mg, 400 mg, 800 mg; liquid: 300 mg/5 mL	Immunomodulator: at high doses may enhance immune response.	Patient initiated.	25 to 40 mg/kg daily, divided bid to qid.	True efficacy unclear
DPC[1] SADBE[1] DNCB[1]	Acetone solution, 0.001-2% Acetone solution, 0.01-1%	Immunomodulator: inducing a delayed hypersensitivity reaction thus leading to stimulation of immune response.	Physician applied. Sensitize patient by applying 2%-3% solution of SADBE/DPC to 1 cm area on inner arm → may need to resensitize every 10-14 d until get local reaction (erythema/vesicle).	After sensitization, apply to wart using 0.03%-2% solution once per wk until clear.	DNCB—possibly mutagenic May be unable to sensitize some patients Irritation Erythema Vesicle/bullae
Retinoids	Acitretin (Soriatane),[1] 10 mg or 25 mg tabs Isotretinoin (Accutane),[1] 10 mg, 20 mg, 40 mg tabs Topical tretinoin (Retin-A),[1] cream/microgel	Antimitotic: interferes with epidermal differentiation and proliferation.	Patient applied/initiated. Good prevention for immunosuppressed/immunocompromised patients with multiple warts or EDV. Topical retinoids for flat warts.	Systemic: least effective qd or qod dose. Topical: apply qhs to warts only.	Topical: local irritation, erythema, and dryness Systemic: mucocutaneous dryness, abnormal liver function tests, elevated triglycerides,
Bleomycin (Blenoxane)[1]	Aqueous solution, 0.1% (1 mg/mL)	Antimitotic.	Physician applied. Intralesional.	Single dose of 0.1 mL of 1 unit/mL in 0.1% solution with normal saline (unclear if repeat q 2-3 wk).	Pain (use with local anesthesia) Tissue necrosis Scarring Loss of nail Raynaud's at local site Possible significant systemic absorption
5-Fluorouracil (Adrucil)	Cream, 5%	Antimitotic: inhibition of DNA and RNA synthesis leading to keratinocyte death.	Patient applied. May be combined with topical tretinoin therapy	Once per wk.	Irritation Erythema Edema

[1]Not FDA approved for this indication.
[2]Not available in the United States.
Abbreviations: bid = twice daily; DNCB = dinitrochlorobenzene; DPC = diphencyclopropenone; EDV = epidermodysplasia verruciformis; q = every; qd = every day; qhs = at bedtime; qid = four times daily; qod = every other day; SADBE = squaric acid dibutylester; YAG = yttrium-aluminum-garnet.

Rakel and Bope: *Conn's Current Therapy 2006.*

Verrucae plantares (plantar warts) are flesh-colored, hyperkeratotic, endophytic papules or plaques located on the soles of the feet that also disrupt normal skin lines and may have thrombosed capillaries manifested as brown/black dots. These can be quite painful and interfere with mobility and daily functioning, especially if located on sites of pressure. A mosaic wart occurs if multiple plantar warts coalesce into a plaque. DDx include callus, corns, exostosis, and acral melanoma. Verrucae plantares warts are associated with HPV subtypes 1, 2, 4, 27, 57.

Verrucae planae (flat warts) are tan- to flesh-colored, flat, sharply demarcated papules located on the dorsum of hands, distal lower extremities, and face; and are often in a linear arrangement after trauma. DDx include molluscum contagiosum, epidermodysplasia verruciformis, and benign syringomas on the face. Verrucae planae warts are associated with HPV subtypes 3, 10.

Epidermodysplasia verruciformis (EDV) is a rare, autosomal recessive, hereditary disorder manifesting with extensive, flesh-colored to pink to tan, round, flat papules on the trunk, hands, upper and lower extremities, and face. These do have malignant potential, especially on the face on sun-exposed areas. Patients with EDV are usually infected with multiple types of HPV. DDx include seborrheic keratosis, actinic keratosis, basal cell carcinoma, SCCa in situ, or invasive SCCa. EDV warts are classified into more than 30 associated HPV subtypes, including types 3, 5, 8, 9, 12, 14, 15, 17, 19-25, 36-38, 47, 49, 50.

Verrucous carcinoma is a slow-growing variant of SCCa arising in three sites:

1. Oral mucosa (oral florid papillomatosis)
2. Anogenital region (giant condyloma of Buschke and Löwenstein)
3. Plantar foot (epithelioma cuniculatum)

Verrucous carcinoma warts are associated with HPV subtypes 6, 11.

Diagnosis

Diagnosis is mainly based on clinical findings. In immunocompromised or immunosuppressed patients, biopsy should be performed in large or suspicious lesions to rule out SCCa.

Therapy

It is well accepted that the treatment of warts must be individualized and that usually more than one therapeutic modality is required to achieve complete resolution (Table 1). Conventional destructive treatments include repeated application of topical chemotherapy (i.e., salicylic acid [Compound W], cantharidin,[2] podophyllin [Podofin], 5-fluorouracil [Adrucil], etc.), cryosurgery, surgical excision, curettage and/or electrosurgery, and laser therapy. Other approaches include immunotherapy

---

[2]Not available in the United States.

(i.e., intralesional interferon [IFN] [Alferon N], diphencyprone[2]), tape occlusion, and observation. In 20% of immunocompetent individuals, the warts will spontaneously resolve within 3 months. Cure rates for common and plantar verrucae with salicylic acid vary from 60% to 80%. Also, overall cure rates with cryosurgery range from 60% to 80%; and with carbon dioxide and pulsed-dye laser, they range from 45% to 90%. However, these methods are usually painful and expensive. Nonetheless, with most methods, recurrence is common, and repeat visits to the physician are costly.

Intralesional IFN-α, although promising with a 36% to 62% clearance rate of anogenital warts, requires multiple injections in the physician's office, is expensive, and may cause systemic adverse effects. Imiquimod (Aldara),[1] a self-applied topical agent that induces interferon production at the site of application, is reported to have a 50% eradication rate in the treatment of genital warts. Other treatments include:

- Hyperthermia with hot water (113°F [45°C]) immersion
- Intralesional injection of *Candida*[1]/mumps[1] antigen
- Photodynamic therapy with aminolevulinic acid (Levulan Kerastick)[1] followed by red light irradiation
- Hypnosis
- Duct tape occlusion

Special attention should be paid to immunosuppressed or immunocompromised patients in whom there is a higher rate of malignant transformation of warts and in whom warts tend to be more resistant and more numerous and thus may require systemic retinoids as a maintenance regimen.

---

[2]Not available in the United States.
[1]Not FDA approved for this indication.

Condyloma Accuminata (Genital Warts)

Method of
Karl R. Beutner, MD, PhD, and Alice N. Do, DO

Genital warts are the most common manifestation of infection of the genital area with the human papilloma virus (HPV). Genital HPV infection is the most common viral sexually transmitted disease. Approximately 1% of the general population has genital warts at any time.

Proliferation of HIV-infected keratinocytes results in a genital wart. More than 100 genotypes of HPV exist. Low-risk HPV types 6 and 11 cause genital warts. High-risk HPV, most often types 16 and 18, are commonly associated with squamous cell carcinoma (SCC) in situ, also known as bowenoid papulosis or vulvar intraepithelial neoplasia of the external genital area, as well as abnormal Papanicoulaou (Pap) smears including in situ and invasive SCC of the cervix. In immunocompetent hosts,

Rakel and Bope: *Conn's Current Therapy 2006.*

in situ SCC of the skin rarely, if ever, evolves into invasive SCC. Genital skin appears not to be as susceptible to the oncogenic potential of HPV as are the transformation zones of the uterine cervix and the anal canal.

Diagnosis is clinical, so identification of various presentations of genital warts involves understanding the different genital skin types that influence wart morphology. Three types of genital skin are fully keratinized hair-bearing, fully keratinized non–hair-bearing, and partially keratinized non–hair-bearing. The later appears moist and is often mistakenly referred to as mucous membranes. However, there are no mucus glands, and it appears moist because it is partially keratinized.

Treatment can be directed by skin type and wart morphology. The four morphologic types of genital warts are:

1. Cauliflower-type, or condyloma acuminatum
2. Smooth papular type, which are skin-colored, dome-shaped, 1 to 4 mm papules
3. Keratotic type, which may mimic seborrheic keratoses or common warts
4. Flat type, which are slightly raised.

Condyloma acuminatum occurs most commonly on moist, partially keratinized skin, whereas the smooth papular and keratotic types are seen most frequently on fully keratinized areas; the flat type is seen on all types of genital skin.

Genital warts may appear on the penile shaft, scrotum, perineum or perianal areas, labia, vulva, or pubic area, or in the crural folds. They can also be found in the urethra or bladder or in the oral cavity. The oral cavity should also be examined in patients being evaluated for genital warts.

Biopsy is usually unnecessary to confirm a clinical diagnosis of external genital warts. However, a biopsy should be considered when lesions are atypical, pigmented, ulcerated, indurated, or fixed to underlying tissue; fail to respond to treatment or worsen during treatment; frequently recur; exhibit individual (noncoalescent) warts larger than 1 cm in diameter; or are suspicious for malignancy. Biopsy should also be considered when diagnosis is unclear.

Acetowhitening to aid in diagnosis of external genital warts is no longer recommended because it lacks adequate specificity and sensitivity.

Differential diagnosis includes lichen planus, skin tags, seborrheic keratoses, molluscum contagiosum, condyloma latum, pearly penile papules, sebaceous glands, lichen nitidus, Crohn's disease, and SCC in situ.

Treatment

Genital warts may spontaneously resolve or persist. Discuss expectations of therapy with patients. The goal is to eliminate symptoms, namely visible wart lesions, rather than to address HPV infection. Rather than a treatment, a course of therapy is required to achieve a wart-free state. It is unknown whether wart elimination will decrease or eliminate the patient's infectivity to current or future sexual partners. Even after proper treatment, recurrence is due to latent HPV in the surrounding normal tissue, and not necessarily due to reinfection. Once two individuals are infected with the same HPV type, they will not continue to reinfect one another. Any given treatment carries a 40% to 75% change of clearing and a 25% to 50% chance of recurrence. Recurrence is responsible for a prolonged course for the patient. Treatment failure is commonly caused by improper selection or use of a therapeutic modality. At the present time, all treatments are comparable in effectiveness.

Choice of Treatment

Selection of treatment is influenced by wart morphology, anatomic site, total wart area, wart count, clinician's experience, and patient preference. Not all patients respond equally well to all modalities. Proper matching of patient with modality will usually shorten treatment duration. Pregnancy and immunosuppression are associated with larger and more numerous genital wart lesions. Certain treatment modalities are more appropriate in pregnancy. Immunosuppressed patients do not respond as well to therapy and have a high recurrence rate. These patients have a higher incidence of SCC. Have a plan or set protocol, particularly when a limited number of modalities are available. In general, if after three to four treatments with a given therapy a clinically significant response is not seen, or if after six treatments no clearance is achieved, the treatment modality should be changed and the diagnosis should be re-evaluated.

TREATMENT MODALITIES

Current treatments are divided into provider-administered and patient-applied therapies. Provider-administered therapies include cryotherapy, podophyllin resin (Podocon-25), trichloroacetic acid (Tri-Chlor)[1], and surgery. Patient-applied therapies allow the patient greater control and include podofilox (Condylox) and imiquimod (Aldara). However, these require good compliance and that the patient be able to view and reach the warts.

PROVIDER-ADMINISTERED THERAPIES

Cryotherapy

Cryotherapy works well for small, flat, few warts in dry or moist areas. It can be used on the penile shaft and vulva with little scarring. It can be used during pregnancy. It is not recommended for large wart areas, which can be quite painful and cause wound-care issues. A small, tightly wound cotton swab (Q-tip) that holds inadequate amounts of liquid nitrogen cannot effectively freeze a wart. Apply liquid nitrogen with a large, loosely wound piece of cotton on a wooden stick or with a cryoprobe.

A few small warts can be frozen without an anesthetic. Patients with more warts should be offered local anesthesia, with either injection of 1% lidocaine[1] or topical application of a eutectic mixture of 2.5% lidocaine and 2.5% prilocaine (EMLA cream).[1] Freeze the wart and 1- to 2-mm surrounding border. For larger warts, two freeze-thaw cycles are effective. How *hard* to freeze the warts can be learned with experience.

Cryotherapy requires proper training. Complications are rare but inexperienced clinicians often underfreeze areas, reducing efficacy. Overfreezing increases pain and the probability of scarring and other complications. Warn patients about post-treatment pain and blistering.

Podophyllin Resin

Podophyllin resin (Podofin, Podocon-25, Podofilm) is from the plant species *Podophyllum peltatum* or *Podophyllum emodii*. This resin contains podofilox (podophyllotoxin), 4-dimethylpodophyllotoxin, α-peltatum, and β-peltatum, which cause cellular mitotic arrest and lead to tissue necrosis. It is a good choice for moist warts and up to a 10 cm^2 surface area. It is ineffective in dry areas, such as the scrotum, penile shaft, and labia majora.

Podophyllin resin lacks a standardized preparation, but it is commonly used as a 10% to 25% solution in tincture of benzoin. Use a cotton tip and apply a thin layer directly to the wart and allow to air dry before the patient assumes a normal anatomic position. Traditionally, patients were advised to wash off podophyllin 2 to 4 hours after application, but benzoin is water insoluble and cannot be removed simply with soap and water. Another ill-advised but not uncommon practice is to create a *barrier* around the wart with Vaseline or K-Y jelly, and apply podophyllin resin to the central wart. Body temperature thins the barrier, which mixes with the podophyllin resin, and spreads over the entire area, creating an impressive irritant reaction. I advise patients to leave the podophyllin resin on overnight and avoid washing, bathing, or sexual contact until the next day. Local side effects include erythema, pain, and irritation. Systemic side effects are caused by increased toxic absorption and are associated with large treatment area (>10 cm^2) or allowing the resin to absorb for an extended time. Avoid podophyllin resin in pregnancy.

Trichloroacetic Acid (Tri-Chlor)[1]

Trichloroacetic acid ([TCA] Tri-Chlor)[1] chemically coagulates warts and adjacent skin. Use for small, few, moist warts. TCA[1] can be used during pregnancy. Although 30% to 70% solutions are employed, the optimal

concentration is undetermined. Use extreme caution with the higher concentrations, which can be highly caustic. Apply sparingly to lesions, being careful not to let the solution run onto normal skin. Treatment can be repeated weekly, or every other week, as needed. TCA[1] can be neutralized, if needed, with soap and sodium bicarbonate.

Surgery

Surgery renders the patient wart free with a single visit. It is a good choice for limited or large treatment areas. There is no clearly superior surgical modality. Selection of a surgical approach depends on clinician experience and availability of equipment. Good results can be achieved with superficial tangential scissors, electrodessication, hot cautery, curettage, or CO_2 laser.

PATIENT-APPLIED THERAPIES

Podofilox

The major active lignin in podophyllin resin is podofilox, available as a 0.5% solution or gel (Condylox). Apply to warts twice daily for 3 days followed by a treatment-free period of 4 days. Repeat this cycle four to six times to achieve wart clearance. A maximum of 10 cm^2 should be treated, and podofilox should be avoided in pregnancy.

Imiquimod

Imiquimod (Aldara) is a 5% cream, applied three times weekly at bedtime to moist wart areas. Dry and nonintertriginous areas may respond better to daily application. It can be used for up to 16 weeks. As imiquimod stimulates an inflammatory response, however, local irritation, burning, and ulceration are expected side effects and are similar to those seen with other modalities.

5-Fluorouracil

5-Fluorouracil creams (Carac, Effudex),[1] used previously for genital warts, are no longer recommended because of side effects, uproven efficacy, and the availability of other treatments.

----

[1]Not FDA approved for this indication.

[1]Not FDA approved for this indication.

 CURRENT DIAGNOSIS

Diagonis of genital warts requires their identification on physical exam. The clinician should become adept at recognizing the various morphologies of genital warts, which are influenced by the overlying genital skin type.

External wart morphology	Description	Skin type
Condyloma accuminatum	Coalescent cauliflower-like plaques	Moist/partially keratinized
Smooth papular	Skin-colored, dome shaped, 1 to 4 mm papules	Fully keratinized
Keratotic	Discrete, warty papules	Fully keratinized
Flat type	Slightly raised, flat-topped papules	Moist/partially keratinized or fully keratinized

Rakel and Bope: *Conn's Current Therapy 2006.*

CURRENT THERAPY

Treatment modalities can be divided into either provider-administered or patient-applied therapies. The choice of therapy will depend on skin type, wart quantity, and location.

Treatment	Mechanism	Good choice for	Poor choice for	Procedure
Provider administered				
Cryotherapy	Direct tissue destruction	• Small, flat, few warts • Dry or moist warts • Pregnancy OK	• Large wart areas (> 10 cm²)	• Liquid nitrogen applied on a large, loosely wound piece of cotton on a wooden stick; or with a cryoprobe, by the spray technique • Freeze the wart and 1 to 2-mm surrounding border
Podophyllin resin	Arrest in mitosis leading to tissue necrosis	• Moist warts	• Dry wart areas • Do not exceed 10 cm² treatment area • Not for pregnancy	• Use a cotton tip and apply a thin layer to wart and allow to air day before the patient assumes a normal anatomic position • Leave on overnight and avoid washing, bathing, and sexual contact • Repeat treatment 1 week later, as needed
TCA (Tri-Chlor)[1]	Chemical coagulation of wart proteins	• Small, moist, few warts • Pregnancy OK	• Large wart areas (> 10 cm²) • Dry warts	• Apply sparingly to the lesion, being careful not to let the solution run onto normal skin • Repeat weekly or every other week, as needed
Surgery	Direct removal of lesions	• Large or small treatment areas • Rectal lesions OK • Pregnancy OK	• Bleeding disorders	• Superficial tangential scissor excision, electrodessication, hot cautery, curettage, or CO_2 laser may be used
Patient applied				
Podofilox (Condylox)	Arrest in mitosis → tissue necrosis	• Moist warts	• Do not exceed 10 cm² treatment area • Not for pregnancy • Poor compliance	• Apply bid for 3 days following by a 4-day treatment-free period • Repeat weekly cycles four to six times, as needed
Imiquimod (Aldara)	Immunomodulator	• Moist warts	• Large wart areas (> 10 cm²) • Dry warts • Poor compliance	• Apply every other night on moist warts or intertriginous areas, or every night on dry warts • May be used for up to 16 weeks, as tolerated

[1]Not FDA approved for this indication.
Abbreviations: TCA = trichloroacetic acid.

Transmission and Prevention

HPV is a sexually transmitted disease (STD). Educate patients to tell sexual partners that they have this infection. Condoms may decrease transmission but do not completely prevent infection. Asymptomatic partners can harbor a subclinical infection, and examination for genital warts is appropriate if lesions are suspected. It is unknown whether treatment of genital wart lesions eliminates infectivity. Discuss the oncogenic potential of HPV types associated with bowenoid papulosis. Women with external genital warts or whose male partners have lesions should have a Pap smear and remain in the system for monitoring for cervical cancer. Investigations for other STDs should be done if suspected.

Acquiring an STD carries a negative social stigma and emotional trauma. Patients often fear discovery and rejection and feel guilty and victimized. They view themselves as less sexually desirable, enjoy sex less, and have concerns about transmission. Teaching and educational materials are available from the American Social Health Association (1-919-361-8422).

REFERENCES

Beutner KR, Richwald GA, Wiley DJ, et al: External genital warts: Report of the American Medical Association consensus conference. Clin Infect Dis 1998;27:796-806.
Beutner KR, Wiley DJ, Douglas JM, et al: Genital warts and their treatment. Clin Infect Dis 1999;28(Suppl 1):S37-S56.

[1]Not FDA approved for this indication.

Habif TP: Sexually transmitted viral infections. In Hodgson S, Cook L (eds): Clinial Dermatology, A Color Guide to Diagnosis and Therapy, 4th ed. Philadelphia, Mosby 2004, pp 336-342.

Odom RB, James WD, Berger TG: Viral diseases. In Fathman EM, Geisel EB, Salmo A, (eds): Andrew's Diseases of the Skin, Clinical Dermatology, 9th ed. Philadelphia, WB Saunders, 2000; pp 541-519.

Nevi

Method of
Scott C. Wickless, DO, and Joan Guitart, MD

Nevi (singular, nevus) are considered benign proliferations of normal skin constituents. Although the term *nevi* describes an assortment of nonmelanocytic and melanocytic entities of the skin, the scope of this discussion is limited to congenital and common acquired types of melanocytic nevi, also known as nevocellular nevi or moles.

Epidemiology

Melanocytic nevi commonly appear in childhood and adolescence (*acquired*). Less commonly, nevi may also be present at birth (*congenital*). The incidence of melanocytic nevi increases during the first 3 decades of life. The prevalence of nevi is related to race and age. Genetic factors and sun exposure may encourage their development as well. Individuals with a fair complexion (Fitzpatrick types I and II) are more likely to have higher counts of acquired nevi, especially if they have extensive sun exposure. Furthermore, an increased risk of melanoma is associated with high counts of nevi with or without dysplastic features. Broad-spectrum sunscreens may decrease the development of melanocytic nevi when used in children. The highest counts of melanocytic nevi are seen in the fourth and fifth decades of life, and the incidence with each successive decade decreases. In contrast, congenital melanocytic nevi are best regarded as an error in the development and migration of neuroectodermal elements. They present at birth or soon thereafter, although some small congenital nevi remain inconspicuous until years later.

Clinical Presentations

Nevi may appear as macules (flat), papules (raised), or even nodules with varying degrees of pigmentation. Common acquired nevi are usually symmetrical and smaller than 0.5 cm. Infrequently, they may be grouped. Nevi are characterized histologically by their nested collections of pigment-producing cells present in the dermis and/or epidermis. Melanocytes present only in the dermoepidermal junction are referred to as *junctional nevi*, often occurring on the acral surfaces as pigmented macules. Melanocytes present in the dermoepidermal junction and the dermis are referred to as *compound nevi*. These are often raised and may be papillomatous. Melanocytes present exclusively in the dermis are referred to as *dermal nevi*. These are typically flesh colored. Each has a typical clinical presentation, although considerable overlap of features is seen (Table 1). Lesions larger than 0.5 cm are often *dysplastic nevi* or *congenital nevi*.

Congenital nevi are present at birth and have the specific histologic characteristics of nevus cells occurring deep around skin structures. They are divided into small (<1.5 cm), medium (1.5 to 20 cm), and large (>20 cm) (Table 2). Small congenital nevi have a low risk for melanoma development, whereas large congenital melanocytic nevi have a substantially higher risk of cutaneous or even leptomeningeal melanoma. Because the melanocytes occur deep in the subcutaneous fat and even fascia, excision can be quite disfiguring.

Many variants of melanocytic nevi exist. *Halo nevi* (Sutton's nevi) are pigmented nevi surrounded by a well-circumscribed white halo caused by the cytotoxic effect of infiltrating T lymphocytes. Halo nevi are more common in adolescents than in adults. Patients beyond age 40 years with halo nevi, especially if multiple lesions are present, should be evaluated for the presence of melanoma elsewhere on the body or in the lesion.

Blue nevi are typically heavily pigmented lesions and usually located on the dorsal hands and feet, as well as the scalp and sacral region. They are believed to arise from dermal melanocytes that failed to complete migration to the epidermis during gestation. It is important to note that not all blue nevi appear blue and the color varies depending on the light source. Dark brown, black, or even gray hues are often noted. Although color variation exists, blue nevi have a hard consistency and are typically small and symmetric.

Nevus spilus (speckled lentiginous nevus) most commonly affects the trunk and extremities. They are characterized by a tan patch (flat) ranging from 1 to 4 cm with

TABLE 1 Clinical and Histologic Features of Common Acquired Melanocytic Nevi

Feature	Junctional	Compound	Dermal
Size	<5 mm	<5mm	<10 mm
Color	Tan to brown	Brown	Flesh colored to tan or pink
Primary lesion	Macule (flat)	Papule (raised)	Papule (raised)
Clinical location	Head, neck, trunk, upper extremities	Head, neck, trunk	Face, head, neck, trunk, upper/lower extremities
Histologic location	Dermoepidermal junction	Dermoepidermal junction and dermis	Dermis

TABLE 2 Clinical Features of Small, Medium, and Large Congenital Nevi

Feature	Small and medium	Large
Size	<1.5 cm (small) 1.5-20 cm (medium)	>20 cm
Color	Tan to brown with follicular accentuation	Brown to black
Primary lesion	Plaquelike, pebbled	Plaquelike, furrowed
Clinical location	Anywhere, especially head, neck	Anywhere, including involvement of major anatomic region

a tan background and a dark brown specked pattern. Microscopically, the epidermis contains increased single melanocytes at the dermoepidermal junction. Meanwhile, the 1 to 6 mm smaller interspersed multiple speckles of dark brown macules or papules may demonstrate increased single melanocytes or melanocytic nesting with or without dermal involvement (compound or junctional nevus).

Spitz nevi or *epithelioid and spindle cell nevus* were formerly known as benign juvenile melanoma because of their cellular composition resembling melanoma cells. They are single flesh-colored or slightly pigmented papules or nodules commonly seen on children and young adults that can mimic melanoma histologically. Rarely, they occur with multiple lesions grouped together. This form is known as agminated Spitz nevus. The head and neck region is the most common site, although they may be present on the trunk or extremities. Clinically, Spitz nevi are often difficult to distinguish from conventional nevi. Some Spitz nevi can be heavily pigmented and demonstrate hemangioma-like features, but in general they are less pigmented than common nevi, appearing as tan-colored dome-shaped papules.

Dysplastic or *atypical melanocytic nevi* (Clark's nevus, nevus with architectural disorder) are pigmented lesions with irregular borders in a haphazard variety of colors ranging from pink, brown, and dark brown to black. Erythema may be present around the nevus as a perilesional halo or within the lesion. These may be flat or raised and in general are larger than common acquired nevi. Lesions most commonly involve the trunk but can be identified in any skin location, and the number can range from one to hundreds of lesions. Atypical isolated lesions have a low risk of melanoma, whereas patients with a strong family history of melanoma and patients with multiple larger lesions are at an increased risk for the development of melanoma.

Recurrent nevi (pseudomelanoma) result from incompletely removed nevi, especially after shave removal. The lesion is usually macular and demonstrates irregular borders and coloration within or adjacent to the previous surgical scar (Box 1). Loss of pigment and stippling and mottling may be present. More than half of recurrent nevi are noted to occur within 6 months after the procedure.

Treatment

SHAVE BIOPSY/EXCISION

The shave biopsy is a quick method performed with a scalpel (usually a number 15 blade). A straight razor blade allows for easily controlling depth by increasing or decreasing the convexity of the blade. This technique requires little training, and sutures are not required for closure. A small depressed scar is expected at the biopsy site. Shave biopsy/excision is not generally used for pigmented lesions because an unanticipated melanoma cannot be properly staged if only the superficial portion is removed. Shave biopsies are preferred for lesions with less suspicious pathology confined to the epidermis, such as actinic keratoses, skin tags, and superficial basal cell carcinomas (Box 2).

The saucerization technique involves deeper removal of the lesion by taking 1- to 2-mm margins of normal skin surrounding the lesion. The blade is first directed downward at a 45-degree angle to the skin as the blade approaches the deep dermis and then directed upward at the same angle. This technique provides significantly more tissue for histologic evaluation of depth. Prolonged healing time and increasing scar size may result.

PUNCH BIOPSY/EXCISION

The punch biopsy uses a round cutting instrument ranging in diameter from 2 to 10 mm. The punch is an ideal procedure for diagnostic skin biopsy because it provides full-thickness evaluation while providing a better cosmetic result than a shave biopsy. Punch biopsies are quick and easily performed, with a low incidence of significant scarring. The size of the punch biopsy instrument should be slightly larger than the biggest dimension of the lesion. Ideally, the entire lesion should be removed for proper evaluation. If smaller than 3 mm, wounds may heal satisfactorily by secondary intention. Punches greater than 3 mm may heal best when closed with one or two sutures. Sutures are removed after 5 to 7 days on the face and 12 to 14 days elsewhere.

BOX 1 The ABCD Approach to the Clinical Evaluation of Suspicious-Appearing Lesions

- Asymmetry in shape
- Border irregularities
- Color variation
- Diameter more than 6 mm

13

BOX 2   Indications for Biopsy/Excision

- Atypical clinical appearance suspicious for melanoma
- Changing lesion
- Repeated irritation (including bleeding, ulceration, pruritus, pain)
- Recurrence of old lesion
- Presence of new lesion
- Cosmetic reasons

ELLIPTICAL EXCISION

Elliptical excision removes the pigmented lesion with a variable amount of clinically normal skin. It is indicated for any lesion that is suspicious for malignancy, especially when lesions cannot be removed with a punch because of depth, location, or size. The ellipse is created with a length-to-width ratio of 3:1, with the depth extending into the fat. This type of excision provides plentiful

 CURRENT DIAGNOSIS

- The diagnosis of a nevus is based on the clinical presentation. If the clinician suspects a possible melanoma, the diagnosis is confirmed by histologic examination.
- A thorough physical examination of patients with lesions should be performed in adequate lighting that involves careful inspection of the lesion in question, as well as a recommended total skin examination. This includes the scalp, palms, soles, genitalia, buttocks, axillae, and between digits.
- Nevi must be distinguished from melanoma.
- Suspicious lesions are usually larger than 0.6 cm.
- Irregular borders, asymmetry, and variable pigmentation also suggest melanoma (see Box 1).
- Patient education regarding clinical signs of melanoma is imperative, and sun protection should be encouraged.
- Any patient history with persistent change in a long-lasting pigmented lesion or the development of a new pigmented lesion warrants careful inspection.
- Appropriate documentation of the lesion should include the location, color, and size of the lesion. A simple drawing or chart may be beneficial. A magnifying lens may also be useful in visualizing lesions.
- Dermoscopy (epiluminescence microscopy, dermatoscopy) in the hands of an experienced clinician may provide further diagnostic accuracy, by using a handheld magnifier (×10) with or without polarization and oil interface.
- Photographic documentation of lesions is helpful for people with multiple lesions who require comparative examinations in the future.

 CURRENT THERAPY

- Although most melanocytic nevi are static and benign in appearance, some require a biopsy with complete histologic examination to exclude the possibility of melanoma.
- Indications for biopsy and treatment include typical clinical appearance suspicious for melanoma (see Box 1); changing lesion; repeated irritation (including bleeding, ulceration, pruritus, pain); incomplete removal or recurrence of an old lesion; presence of a new lesion; or cosmetic reasons (see Box 2).
- Patients should be informed of the potential for scarring if the indication is purely cosmetic.
- Although multiple biopsy/treatment methods for nevi are available, certain variables may help to determine which procedure is most appropriate: convenience, amount of healing time, adequacy of specimen for histologic examination, and cosmetic result.
- Pigmented melanocytic lesions should never be destroyed by cryosurgery because it impairs the ability to diagnose the lesion properly. Treatment may include biopsy and/or excision.

tissue for histologic interpretation and provides a good cosmetic result with rapid healing. The major disadvantages include the need for greater amount of expertise and time, as well as an increased length of scar.

REFERENCES

Barnhill RL: Textbook of Dermatopathology, 2nd ed. New York, McGraw-Hill, 2004.
Bolognia JL, Jorizzo JL, Rapini RP, et al: Dermatology. St Louis, Mosby, 2003.
Crowson AN, Magro CM, Mihm MC: The Melanocytic Proliferations: A Comprehensive Textbook of Pigmented Lesions. New York, Wiley-Liss, 2001.
Elder D, Elenitsas R, Jaworsky C: Lever's Histopathology of the Skin. Philadelphia, Lippincott Williams & Wilkins, 1997.
Freedburg IM, Eisen AZ, Wolff K, et al: Fitzpatrick's Dermatology in General Medicine. New York, McGraw-Hill, 2003.
Weedon D: Skin Pathology. New York, Churchill Livingstone, 2002.

Malignant Melanoma

Method of
Douglas Tyler, MD, and Hilliard Seigler, MD

Malignant melanoma is the ninth most common cancer and the leading cause of death from cutaneous malignancy. Melanoma ranks second only to adult leukemias in potential lives lost. The incidence of melanoma is rising faster than any other malignancy, with the number of new cases doubling over the last 35 years. It is currently projected that 1 in 82 women and 1 in 58 men will develop melanoma in the course of their lifetime. Thus in the United States in 2005, more than 55,000 new cases of melanoma will be diagnosed, and approximately 7600 individuals will die from this disease.

Diagnosis

Melanoma has a variety of appearances and can be located anywhere on the body. Common clinical features include an asymmetric lesion, a diameter greater than 6 mm, color variation within the lesion, and border irregularity. Any change in a preexisting or new nevus is also suggestive of melanoma. The physician generally should have a low threshold to evaluate skin lesions diagnostically if melanoma is suspected. The skin lesion in question should be completely removed with an excisional biopsy. The biopsy needs to include full thickness of the skin into the subcutaneous tissue to allow an accurate measurement of the tumor's thickness. Punch biopsy is a good technique for small lesions, whereas elliptical excision may be necessary for larger ones. Shave biopsies should not be done because of the risk of transecting the melanoma, preventing accurate assessment of its depth.

Pathology

Melanoma traditionally is broken down into four subtypes based on pathology and growth pattern: superficial spreading melanoma (SSM), acral lentiginous melanoma (ALM), lentigo maligna melanoma (LMM), and nodular melanoma. SSM accounts for approximately 70% of melanomas, typically arises from a preexisting nevus, and has a radial growth phase before becoming invasive. ALM accounts for 10% of melanomas and usually arises on the soles, palms, and mucous membranes, and subungually. ALM also has a radial growth phase, but it is frequently misdiagnosed early on because of the nonsuspicious locations where it develops. LMM accounts for 5% of melanomas and most frequently arises in the head and neck region. LMM has a slow radial growth pattern and usually develops in older patients from a lentigo maligna precursor lesion. Nodular melanoma, the second most common type of melanoma (15% to 20%), is unlike the other types just described because it is associated with no radial growth phase. Nodular melanomas more commonly arise de novo, and a history of rapid onset over several months is not uncommon.

Histologic evaluation of the primary melanoma provides important information for determining prognosis and clinical treatment. The Breslow thickness and Clark level are measurements of tumor thickness and histologic depth, respectively. Breslow depth and, to a lesser degree, Clark level are directly associated with prognosis. Other factors that also appear important include ulceration, regression, evidence of lymphatic or vascular invasion, and satellitosis. Each of these is associated

with a more aggressive form of melanoma that should be factored into clinical decision making.

Staging

The American Joint Commission on Cancer (AJCC) revised its staging system for melanoma in 2002 (Table 1). The modifications incorporated into the new staging system include subclassification using Breslow categories based on whole numbers. In addition, the new system takes into account tumor ulceration, which is an independent predictor of survival. It is also becoming clearer that the number of positive lymph nodes, not the size of the largest lymph node, is the most important factor for nodal staging. The presence of satellitosis is also incorporated into the AJCC staging system.

For patients with melanomas less than 4 mm deep, the initial staging workup consists of a baseline lactate dehydrogenase (LDH) and chest radiograph. For patients with melanomas greater than 4 mm, a more extensive staging workup is performed using chest, abdomen, and pelvic computed tomography (CT) scans or a dual PET (positron emission tomography)/CT scan. Intraoperative lymphatic mapping and sentinel lymph node biopsy for the evaluation of lymph node status in melanoma patients is a widely accepted staging tool for patients with melanomas greater than 1 mm. It is used in patients with greater than 4 mm melanomas if their imaging workup is negative as well as in patients with thin melanomas that are less than 1 mm but carry poor prognostic features such as a discordant Clark level, ulceration, regression, or depth between 0.75 and 1 mm. Although it is clear that melanoma does spread in an orderly and predictable fashion through regional lymphatics, most people believe that when tumor cells metastasize from the primary site, they can also shed directly into the bloodstream either bypassing the lymphatics or floating through them at the same time.

Extensive histologic examination of the sentinel lymph node demonstrates that routine histologic examination of the sentinel lymph node can identify 1 tumor cell in 10,000 lymphocytes. Application of serial sectioning and immunohistochemistry for melanoma-specific markers (HMB-45 or S100) can improve tumor detection to 1 tumor cell in 100,000 lymphocytes. Molecular biology techniques using reverse transcriptase polymerase chain reaction (RT-PCR) for detection of mRNA for melanoma-associated gene products (such as tyrosinase, gp [gene product] 100, MAGE [melanoma-associated gene] 3, or MART-1 [melanoma antigen recognized by T cells]) have the capability of detecting 1 tumor cell in 1,000,000 lymphocytes. Recent studies demonstrate that patients who have a histologically negative, RT-PCR-positive sentinel lymph node have a statistically significant shorter disease-free survival than patients with histologically negative, RT-PCR-negative sentinel lymph nodes. Overall, sentinel lymph node biopsy is emerging as an important staging tool that ensures accurate prognostic and staging information on each patient as well as identifying a group of patients who may benefit from adjuvant therapy.

TABLE 1 American Joint Commission on Cancer Staging System for Cutaneous Melanoma

Pathologic stage	TNM	Thickness (mm)	Ulceration	Number of positive lymph nodes	Nodal size	Distant metastasis
IA	T1a	≤1	No	0	—	—
IB	T1b	≤1	Yes or Clark IV, V	0	—	—
	T2a	1.01-2.0	No	0	—	—
IIA	T2b	1.02-2.0	Yes	0	—	—
	T3a	2.01-4.0	No	0	—	—
IIB	T3b	2.01-4.0	Yes	0	—	—
	T4a	>4.0	No	0	—	—
IIC	T4b	>4.0	Yes	0	—	—
IIIA	N1a	Any	No	1	Micro	—
	N2a	Any	No	2-3	Micro	—
IIIB	N1a	Any	Yes	1	Micro	—
	N2a	Any	Yes	2-3	Micro	—
	N1b	Any	No	1	Macro	—
	N2b	Any	No	2-3	Macro	—
	N2c	Any	Any	0, satellite, or in transit present		
IIIC	N1b	Any	Yes	1	Macro	—
	N2b	Any	Yes	2-3	Macro	—
	N3	Any	Any	4, or satellite, or in transit with any node	Micro or macro	—
IV	M1a	Any	Any	Any	Any	Skin, SC
	M1b	Any	Any	Any	Any	Lung
	M1c	Any	Any	Any	Any	Other visceral

Abbreviations: SC = subcutaneous; TNM = tumor, node, metastasis.

Treatment: Primary Lesion and Regional Lymph Nodes

Once the diagnosis of melanoma is made, treatment focuses on appropriate management of the primary lesion to prevent recurrence and address the status of the lymph nodes in patients thought to be at risk of harboring metastatic disease. The current recommendations for re-excision of primary melanomas are as follows. Melanoma in situ should be re-excised with a 5-mm margin. Thin melanomas with a Breslow thickness less than 1 mm should be re-excised with a 1-cm margin. Intermediate-thickness melanomas with a Breslow thickness between 1 and 4 mm should undergo a 2-cm-wide local excision. Although some controversy exists regarding the size of the re-excision margin for thick melanomas carrying a Breslow thickness greater than 4 mm, recent consensus suggests a 2-cm-wide local excision should be adequate. A recently published study that compares 1- versus 3-cm-wide local excision margins from England fails to provide significant data to change these recommendations.

Evaluation of nodal status is based on the Breslow thickness, which helps determine the likelihood that the regional lymphatics are involved.

MELANOMAS LESS THAN 1 MM

Although the prognosis for patients with thin melanoma is excellent, approximately 10% of these patients go on to die of their disease. Several studies try to determine the characteristics of thin lesions that are more likely to metastasize. Features of regression, vertical growth phase, high mitotic index, ulceration, and/or discordant Clark level of IV or V are generally associated with a worse prognosis in this subgroup of patients. Intraoperative lymphatic mapping may be another way to evaluate patients further with thin melanomas whose primary tumors have poor prognostic features. Although currently no data suggest this group of patients receive a survival benefit from a therapeutic lymph node dissection based on a positive sentinel lymph node, they are candidates for adjuvant therapies either in the form of interferon or immunotherapy trials.

MELANOMAS BETWEEN 1 AND 4 MM

Much controversy surrounds the appropriate management of patients with intermediate-thickness melanomas with regard to lymph nodes. Some believe patients in this group have a higher probability of regional nodal disease (15% to 60%) as compared to distant metastatic disease (8% to 15%), and as such they may benefit theoretically from removal of regional lymph nodes. When intraoperative lymphatic mapping and sentinel lymph node biopsy was first described, only a few retrospective studies demonstrated a survival advantage to removing the regional lymph nodes prophylactically or electively. In addition to a few large retrospective studies that show no benefit to elective removal of the regional lymph node in this patient population, three prospective randomized clinical trials fail to show any benefit from early lymph node removal.

To address many of the concerns raised by the initial randomized prospective clinical trials, the Intergroup Surgical Trial was initiated and accrued 781 patients between 1983 and 1991. This study stratified patients by tumor thickness, ulceration, and site. At the most recent analysis it has greater than 5-year follow-up in all patients and a mean follow-up of 10 years. Although no overall survival advantage to elective lymph node dissection was discerned when the entire group of patients was examined, there did appear to be some groups of patients who did benefit from lymph node dissection as identified by subgroup analysis. The analysis of prospectively stratified groups demonstrated significant reductions in mortality for patients with nonulcerated lesions (29%), extremity lesions (27%), and lesions with Breslow thickness between 1 and 2 mm (35%). In addition, although not stratified prospectively, age appeared to be an important factor because patients younger than 60 years showed improved survival from elective lymph node dissection.

Although the Intergroup trial demonstrates some survival advantages to certain subgroups of patients with intermediate-thickness melanoma, the majority of these patients (70% to 80%) do not have micrometastatic disease and thus would not benefit from lymph node dissection. Because lymph node dissection is not without morbidity, many surgeons hesitate to perform elective lymph node dissection on all patients potentially to benefit a few. A recent study from the John Wayne Cancer Institute matches more than 500 patients and compares elective lymph node dissection to selective lymph node dissection (a lymph node dissection is performed only if the sentinel lymph node is positive). This study suggests the two procedures are therapeutically equivalent because no differences in the incidence of tumor positive dissections, tumor recurrence, or survival are found. Most centers now offer patients with intermediate-thickness melanomas a selective lymph node dissection based on the status of the sentinel lymph node because this provides not only important prognostic information, but also allows patients to be candidates for adjuvant therapy trials and may provide a survival advantage in certain groups in whom a selective lymph node dissection is performed.

Two large clinical trials examining the role of intraoperative lymphatic mapping and sentinel lymph node biopsy in patients with intermediate-thickness melanoma have closed. The Multicenter Selective Lymphadenectomy Trial-I (MSLT-I) randomized patients to wide local excision (WLE) alone versus WLE plus intraoperative lymphatic mapping and sentinel lymph node biopsy and closed to accrual in March 2002. If the sentinel lymph node biopsy was positive, patients underwent a completion lymph node dissection. The Sunbelt Melanoma Trial enrolled patients with melanomas greater than 1 mm in depth and incorporated molecular pathologic staging (RT-PCR) in an attempt to determine whether early intervention with lymphadenectomy and/or interferon

alfa-2b will improve survival. This trial closed at the end of 2003. All patients underwent intraoperative lymphatic mapping and sentinel lymph node biopsy. The sentinel lymph node had a small piece removed for RT-PCR analysis, and the rest of the lymph node was examined with serial sectioning and immunohistochemistry. Patients with a histologically positive sentinel lymph node underwent completion nodal dissection. If the sentinel lymph node was the only positive lymph node, the patient was randomized to observation or adjuvant high-dose interferon for 1 month. If the sentinel lymph node was histologically negative, RT-PCR analysis was performed. If the node was positive, patients were randomized to observation, completion lymphadenectomy, or completion lymphadenectomy plus 1 month of high-dose interferon. Preliminary findings from this study suggest that approximately 30% of patients had a histologically positive sentinel lymph node and approximately 55% of patients had an RT-PCR–positive sentinel lymph node. The results of the MSLT-I and Sunbelt trials will not be available for several years until the data are more mature.

Two current large sentinel lymph node trials accruing patients with intermediate-thickness melanomas focus on examining the need for completion lymph node dissection in patients with a positive sentinel lymph node. The Multicenter Selective Lymphadenectomy Trial-II (MSLT-II) randomizes patients to observation versus completion lymph node dissection but allows patients to receive any adjuvant therapy, whereas the Florida Melanoma Trial-II randomizes patients to observation versus completion lymph node dissection, but all patients receive 1 year of high-dose interferon. Both of these studies are in their early stages of patient accrual.

MELANOMA LESIONS GREATER THAN 4 MM

Most studies suggest that the patient population with melanoma lesions greater than 4 mm has a very high chance of harboring distant metastatic disease, and as a result no survival benefit is ever demonstrated for patients undergoing elective regional lymph node dissection. Our approach to this patient population is to perform a staging workup consisting of chest, abdomen, and pelvic CT scan or obtain a dual PET/CT scan. If no metastatic disease is identified, we offer intraoperative lymphatic mapping and sentinel lymph node biopsy to these patients if they are interested in participating in an adjuvant therapy trial should their sentinel lymph node be positive. The additional benefit of performing a sentinel lymph node biopsy in this patient population is that individuals who have a negative sentinel lymph node have an excellent prognosis, much better than would be expected for the group of patients with thick melanomas as a whole.

Treatment: Adjuvant Therapy

Because patients with metastatic nodal disease have a greater than 50% chance of developing recurrent disease, a tremendous effort is being made to identify an effective adjuvant therapy for patients after lymph node resection. Only one therapy, high-dose interferon alfa-2b (Intron A), is shown to have potential benefit in preventing recurrent disease in high-risk melanoma. The Eastern Cooperative Oncology Group (ECOG) 1684 trial, which randomized patients to either high-dose interferon or observation after resection of positive lymph nodes, demonstrated a statistically significant improvement in 5-year disease-free survival from 26% to 37% and overall survival from 37% to 46%. The follow-up ECOG trial 1690, which randomized patients to high-dose interferon, low-dose interferon, or observation after resection found on interim analysis (52-month follow-up) that high-dose interferon leads to a reproducible improvement in 5-year disease-free survival. Interestingly, there was no improvement in overall 5-year survival between any of the study arms because the observation group did significantly better in terms of survival in the 1690 trial as compared to the 1684 trial. The reasons for this improvement are still being investigated, but the fact that many patients who recurred in the observation arm were subsequently treated with interferon alfa-2b is a major confounding factor. A more recent trial, ECOG 1694, randomized patients to 1 year of high-dose interferon or 2 years of a ganglioside GM2 vaccine. This trial was stopped early because during an interim analysis, the high-dose interferon was associated with significantly improved relapse-free and overall survival. A review of all the interferon data suggests that although it clearly improves relapse-free survival, most studies if followed long enough fail to demonstrate a sustained overall survival difference.

Although approved by the FDA for the adjuvant treatment of metastatic melanoma ever since ECOG 1684 was published, high-dose interferon is associated with significant side effects that when taken in conjunction with its controversial survival benefit leads many physicians to suggest other adjuvant alternatives to patients, such as vaccine trials. Vaccine therapies appeal to patients because they usually have few side effects and are frequently viewed as a way potentially to help the immune system. Although a number of different vaccine strategies have been tried, the observation of an immune response induced by the vaccine has not translated into a survival advantage. Current approaches[4] include:

- Whole-cell vaccines using either allogeneic or autologous irradiated cell lines
- Lysate vaccines
- Vaccinia melanoma cell lysate vaccines
- Shed antigen vaccines
- Ganglioside vaccines using purified gangliosides such as GM2 alone or conjugated to the carrier protein keyhole limpet hemocyanin (KLH) and the adjuvant QS21
- Peptide vaccines
- Dendritic cell vaccines
- DNA vaccines

To date, only one of these trials, a small phase III clinical trial of stage III AJCC patients using a shed

[4]Not yet approved for use in the United States.

antigen vaccine, demonstrates a survival advantage in the range of 11 months for patients receiving vaccine therapy. Two large phase III randomized trials involving the Canvaxin vaccine, a form of active immunotherapy, in the postsurgical adjuvant setting are currently in progress. The trial for patients treated in the stage III adjuvant setting has just completed accrual, whereas the trial for patients treated in the stage IV setting is still open for accrual.

Treatment: Metastatic Disease

Treatment options for patients who develop metastatic disease depend on the pattern of disease. When patients present with metastatic disease they should undergo an extensive staging workup. This workup traditionally consists of chest, abdomen, and pelvis CT scans along with either a magnetic resonance imaging (MRI) or CT scan of the brain. More recently, PET scans are proving a more useful tool for staging this patient population. Patients with metastatic disease should initially be considered for surgical resection. Involvement of regional lymph nodes should be treated with surgical resection because long-term survival occurs in 20% to 25%. A similar observation is seen in patients who undergo pulmonary resection of solitary melanoma metastasis. Patients with solitary lesions in other areas should also be considered surgical candidates because between 5% and 10% achieve long-term survival.

Patients with regionally advanced disease in the form of local recurrence or in-transit disease confined to an extremity should be considered for hyperthermic isolated limb perfusion (HILP). HILP with melphalan (Alkeran) is the standard treatment for this group of patients and associated with response rates of 50% to 80%. Several studies suggest the addition of tumor necrosis factor (TNF) to melphalan could improve response rates in patients with large tumors and/or large tumor burdens (greater than 10 nodules). Recently, however, the American College of Surgeons Oncology Group closed its randomized prospective trial comparing HILP with melphalan to HILP with melphalan and TNF in an attempt to better define which subgroups of patients, if any, benefit from the addition of TNF to HILP with melphalan. The interim analysis suggests no difference between the two arms of this study. Another regional treatment, called isolated limb infusion (ILI), is popular in Australia. In contrast to HILP, ILI consists of a 30-minute infusion in an acidotic, hypoxic extremity

 CURRENT DIAGNOSIS

- Asymmetric lesion
- Lesion diameter greater than 6 mm
- Color variation within the lesion
- Border irregularity of the lesion
- Change in preexisting pigmented lesion
- Rapid growth of new lesion

CURRENT THERAPY

- Full-thickness biopsy
- Wide local excision of primary lesion
  - Melanoma in situ: 5-mm margin
  - Invasive melanoma up to 1 mm in depth: 1-cm margin
  - Invasive melanoma 1 mm to 4 mm in depth: 2-cm margin
  - Invasive melanoma greater than 4 mm in depth: 2- to 3-cm margin
- Intraoperative lymphatic mapping and sentinel lymph node biopsy
  - Melanoma in situ: not recommended
  - Invasive melanoma up to 1 mm in depth: Lesions with poor prognostic features such as ulceration, vertical growth phase, discordant Clark level (IV, V), regression, or high mitotic index should be considered
  - Invasive melanoma 1 mm to 4 mm in depth: Recommended
  - Invasive melanoma greater than 4 mm in depth: Recommended after staging patient with PET/CT scan

Abbreviations: CT = computerized tomography; PET = positron emission tomography.

using melphalan and dactinomycin (Cosmegen).[1] Although the response rate at the Sydney melanoma unit is approximately 85% (41% complete response [CR] and 44% partial response [PR]), this technique is only currently performed in a few centers in the United States.

For patients with widely metastatic disease, the prognosis is poor, with mean survivals measured in the range of 6 to 9 months. A number of treatment options are used, including chemotherapy, biologic response modifiers, and a combination of both. Single-agent therapies, the most effective of which are dacarbazine (DTIC) and temozolomide (Temodar),[1] have response rates in the 10% to 20% range. With multiagent therapy, most notably the Dartmouth regimen (cisplatin,[1] DTIC, BCNU [carmustine], and tamoxifen[1]) or CVD (cisplatin,[1] vinblastine, and DTIC), response rates are improved somewhat, but no significant changes in overall survival are observed. Combinations of biologic response modifiers with combination chemotherapy result in slightly higher response rates but at the price of higher toxicity. Interleukin-2 alone can produce very durable long-term complete responses in approximately 5% of treated patients. In general, therapy of advanced disease is mainly palliative, with younger patients usually receiving a cisplatin-based combination therapy protocol and older patients, who usually tolerate cisplatin poorly, receiving single-agent therapy.

REFERENCES

Balch CM, Buzaid AC, Soong, SJ, et al: Final version of the AJCC staging system for cutaneous melanoma. J Clin Oncol 2001:19:3635-3648.

[1]Not FDA approved for this indication.

Rakel and Bope: *Conn's Current Therapy 2006.*

Balch CM, Soong SJ, Bartolucci AA, et al: Efficacy of an elective regional lymph node dissection of 1 to 4 mm thick melanomas for patients 60 years of age and younger. Ann Surg 1996;224:255-266.

Balch CM, Soong, SJ, Gershenwald JE, et al: Prognostic factor analysis of 17,600 melanoma patients: Validation of the new AJCC melanoma staging system. J Clin Oncol 2001;19:3622-3634.

Gershenwald JE, Thompson W, Mansfield PF, et al: Multi-institutional melanoma lymphatic mapping experience. The prognostic value of sentinel lymph node status in 612 stage I or II melanoma patients. J Clin Oncol 1999;17:976-983.

Kirkwood JM, Ibrahim JG, Sosman JA, et al: High-dose interferon alfa-2b significantly prolongs relapse-free and overall survival compared with the GM2-KLH/QS-21 vaccine in patients with resected stage IIb-III melanoma: Results of intergroup trial E1694/S9512/C509801. J Clin Oncol 2001;19:2370-2380.

McMasters KM, Reintgen DS, Ross MI, et al: Sentinel lymph node biopsy for melanoma: How many radioactive nodes should be removed? Ann Surg Oncol 2001;8:192-197.

Morton DL, Thompson JF, Essner R, et al: Validation of the accuracy of intraoperative lymphatic mapping and sentinel lymphadenectomy for early-stage melanoma-a multicenter trial. Multicenter Selective Lymphadenectomy Trial Group. Ann Surg 1999;230:453-463.

Morton DL, Wen DR, Wong JH, et al: Technical details of intraoperative lymphatic mapping for early stage melanoma. Arch Surg 1992:127:392-329.

Tsao H, Atkins MB, Sober AJ: Management of cutaneous melanoma. N Engl J Med 2004;351:998-1012.

13

Premalignant Lesions

Method of
Forrest C. Brown, MD

The most common malignant lesions of the skin are basal cell carcinoma (BCC), squamous cell carcinoma (SCC), and malignant melanoma (MM). Less common tumors are dermatofibrosarcoma protuberans, microcystic adnexal carcinoma, malignant fibrohistiocytoma, and Merkel cell carcinoma. The premalignant expressions of BCC, SCC, and MM skin cancers are discussed in this article; there are no commonly accepted definitions for the premalignant lesions of the less common tumors mentioned above. Additionally, several conditions are not premalignant in themselves, but they seem to set the stage for conversion of benign-to-malignant growths.

Nonmelanoma skin cancer is the most commonly occurring group of cancers worldwide. The cost to health care systems has never been accurately quantified, but it is obviously extremely high. Mortality figures for nonmelanoma skin cancer are notoriously flawed, because the recorded lethal event may actually be cardiac arrest or sepsis caused by the debilitated condition and treatment of the skin cancer. With the increasing occurrence rate of nonmelanoma and melanoma skin cancers throughout most of the world—because of increasing carcinogenic exposure of the sun and immune suppression of various causes, both environmental and iatrogenic—these cancers represent an enormous public health problem.

Skin cancers are even more significant because they are so readily curable by early diagnosis and treatment if the mind and eye are schooled to recognize the early and premalignant forms of the tumors. Recognition of an individual likely to have a skin cancer and recognition of premalignant lesions, along with their treatment, are the thrust of this article.

Typically, it is the fair-skinned person with sun exposure who is a likely candidate for both melanoma and nonmelanoma skin cancer. As one moves toward the equator the rate of skin cancer rises significantly in the indigenous population as the intensity of actinic radiation rises. Newer evidence, however, seems to indicate that it is the number of painful sunburns before the age of 20 years that correlates well with nonmelanoma skin cancer, whereas in melanoma, it may be the total sun exposure, but that is not clear.

Burn scars, long-standing skin ulcers, chronic skin sinuses and infections, as well as areas of chronic edema, are sites where skin cancer frequently develops and may be regarded as occasionally premalignant because of the possibility that these are sites of localized, lowered, or compromised immunity.

Given all these factors, the index of suspicion is highest in a fair-skinned person who has signs of significant sun exposure such as weathered thin skin, increased telangiectasia, rough patches, and pigment irregularities, or in an individual with signs or history of immune depression.

Actinic Keratosis

Actinic keratoses (AK) are separated into two significant but artificial divisions. The first is a very small papular lesion commonly classified as a clinically detectable keratosis, and the second is a larger lesion classified as clinically visible keratosis. This is a significant separation because sun damage in skin may manifest as multiple micro foci of abnormal keratinization that may or may not progress; whereas larger, visible keratoses are more likely to progress on their own to cancer.

The clinically detectable actinic keratosis may be perceived only by touch as a roughness in sun-damaged skin. Often, it is in an area that has received the most sun, such as ears, cheekbones, nose, and upper forehead. Magnified vision reveals surface irregularities and a few small, dilated red vessels. These lesions progress with summer sun exposure, fall dormant in the winter, then grow larger the following summer if sun protection is not provided.

The clinically visible actinic keratosis should be considered a likely precursor for SCC and BCC. Removal with close follow-up is necessary on all lesions, especially on body areas that receive routine sun exposure such as the face, hands, ears, and back of the neck. Any actinic keratosis that demonstrates increasing thickness or width and/or redness should be removed, as there is evidence that the conversion of a premalignant to a malignant lesion is accompanied by erythema.

Two special forms of actinic keratosis should be recognized, hypertrophic actinic keratosis and proliferative actinic keratosis. Hypertrophic actinic keratosis is a very thick, crusting nodule of approximately 1 cm (or more) that generally occurs on the dorsum of the hands and arms. Nodules of this type are in active transition to malignancy, with approximately 50% showing active foci of either BCC or SCC. Proliferative actinic keratosis is an active, enlarging lesion that is often superficially ulcerated and shows deep proliferation and rapid progression to SCC. Both of these forms require significantly aggressive therapy including wide excision or, alternatively, deep shave excision that encompasses 3 mm of normal skin followed by intense liquid nitrogen spray, which creates an ice front approximately 3 mm beyond the excised margin.

With the exception of hypertrophic actinic keratosis and proliferative actinic keratosis, I have, for many years, treated most actinic keratosis lesions with liquid nitrogen cryospray. It is effective, rapid, and simple. However, this simplicity has led many to undertreat, resulting in treatment failures and recurrences. Liquid nitrogen is not without problems; it may result in significant blistering, scarring, and very noticeable post-treatment hypopigmentation. However, in trained hands it remains very popular for treating a few isolated lesions where hypopigmentation is not a significant consideration.

When treating the face, especially in younger individuals, cosmetic result and treatment morbidity are very important considerations. Even the slightest possibility of a scar or perceived disfigurement is to be avoided, if possible, in the treatment of these epidermal lesions. The nonsteroidal anti-inflammatory agent diclofenac (Solaraze), a recently introduced form of topical therapy, may be used with little or no perceived evidence of treatment except for lesion clearing; however, the treatment regimen requires 3 months.

Topical treatments with either low- or standard-strength 5-fluorouracil (5-FU) (Efudex) usually require a relatively short treatment time (a few weeks), but redness may last significantly longer.

With all self-administered therapies for these premalignant lesions, some very important ground rules must be kept in mind:

- Treat for the full time recommended unless the reaction makes it impossible.
- Never allow these medications to be used ad lib.
- Always biopsy an area that is slow to heal or recurs after treatment.

Physicians should never have a cavalier attitude toward these medications. Numerous reports have been published regarding their improper use; for example, only the tops of unrecognized cancers may be removed by treatment, and large, dangerous subsurface tumors later develop at the lesion sites.

A new treatment that eliminates the dangers of self-directed therapy recently received FDA approval. This treatment, aminolevulinic acid (ALA) (Levulan Kerastick), is a topical photodynamic therapy. Protoporphyrin IX is created in the cells of the actinic keratosis following exposure to topical ALA after a few hours of incubation. The area is then exposed to coherent light (laser) or noncoherent light (ordinary) for a short time. The photoreaction that occurs destroys very specifically the metabolically active cells of the actinic keratosis. Although there is discomfort during the light exposure, the procedure is popular with many patients because it eliminates the time required to build up to the maximum effect with 5-FU.

The decision to treat actinic keratosis is sometimes questioned. I believe treatment should be given when:

- Lesions are located on areas of the body that continue to receive sun exposure.
- Lesions are showing signs of activity such as thickening or widening.
- Lesions show development of erythema.

DISSEMINATED SUPERFICIAL ACTINIC POROKERATOSIS

Disseminated superficial actinic porokeratosis (DSAP) is an actinic keratosis with a familial history; it probably represents a combination of sun exposure and clones of slightly atypical cells. These lesions appear in individuals after the age of 40 years (primarily in women) on the sun-exposed portions of the extremities. Diagnosis is by pathologic examination, but the lesions are clinically detected by their very definite palpable border and by their erythematous bases. Conversion to squamous cell carcinoma is well documented. Treatment is by liquid nitrogen or by topical treatment; with either, the treatment must be more intense and carried out for a longer period of time than when treating the usual actinic keratosis. Post-treatment erythema may last for many months.

Cutaneous Horn

Cutaneous horn is diagnosed clinically by observing what is at the base of the lesion. Warts, inflamed seborrheic keratoses, mollusca, hypertrophic actinic keratoses, keratoacanthomas, and squamous cell carcinomas are all possible causes. The treatment is deep shave or excision for diagnosis and appropriate follow-up therapy depending on the microscopic diagnosis.

Nevus Sebaceus

Nevus sebaceus is a congenital lesion occurring primarily on the head and neck that thickens and becomes nodular after puberty. Thereafter, patients should be followed closely, because some percentage develop either BCC or SCC during their lifetime. Excision of the lesion in its entirety is the preferred treatment, but if that is not possible, then any suspicious area should be biopsied.

Premalignant Fibroepithelioma

Premalignant fibroepithelioma is a term coined many years ago by a dermatopathologist for a particular microscopic pattern. It is an unfortunate designation

for it is neither premalignant nor a fibroepithelioma; it is a BCC and should be treated accordingly.

Bowen's Disease

Bowen's disease is SCC that has not yet progressed to invasion (SCC in situ). The lesion should be considered malignant and removed. It is tempting to perform only superficial removal because of the intraepithelial nature of the tumor; however, migration down hair follicles is common, and recurrence after such treatments is the usual course. If the lesion is not too large, excision is the best treatment. For larger lesions, destructive therapy followed by excision of any recurrences may be an option. Photodynamic therapy is successful according to some reports. Removal by Mohs micrographic surgery is indicated in areas where tissue conservation is important, such as the face.

Leukokeratosis of the Lip

Leukokeratosis, or leukoplakia, of the lip is the mucosal expression of an actinic keratosis. The entire lip should be considered suspect, because new areas or continuations develop after localized treatment of individual lesions. Carbon dioxide laser ablation of the mucosal surface with healing by second intention is a very effective treatment. Intense liquid nitrogen treatment of the lip usually offers a good result. It is a popular treatment and should be considered before excision and mucosal advancement surgery.

Bowenoid Papulosis

Bowenoid papulosis is multiple papules of histologic Bowen's disease (SCC in situ) that occur in the genital area although a few cases are reported on distant sites. Human papilloma virus has been identified in some cases. Some lesions resolve spontaneously. They should, however, be considered at least premalignant and removed in a simple manner, such as with liquid nitrogen or curettage and desiccation. Recently, excellent response has been reported with the topical immune response modifier imiquimod cream (Aldara).

Special Considerations

The problems of premalignant lesions are very troublesome for the healthy patient, but they take on extreme importance in immunosuppressed individuals. In these patients, the biology of a premalignant lesion is so altered that every lesion should be considered as a developing malignant lesion, *not* a premalignant lesion. Therapy as well as the decision to institute therapy should be aggressive to prevent damage by an immunologically unrestrained cancer.

Bacterial Diseases of the Skin

Method of
Michael G. Wilkerson, MD

Bacterial diseases of the skin (Table 1) range from trivial annoyances to life-threatening emergencies affecting not only sick patients but also otherwise healthy individuals. Normal skin flora includes staphylococci, streptococci, diphtheroids, and *Propionibacterium* and gram-negative bacteria below the waist. Knowledge of common bacterial flora, their sensitivities to common antibiotics, and initial empirical treatment is essential. Even when bacteria grow quickly on laboratory medium, cultures and sensitivities require a minimum of 48 to 72 hours.

The traditional paradigm of empirical treatment with cultures reserved for nonresponsive cases is rapidly changing because of the emergence of bacterial resistance. The overuse and incomplete treatment of infections, use of bacteriostatic rather than bacteriocidal antibiotics, and other adaptive factors that are not well understood may well be fueling the current resistance crisis. The most important resistance at this time is methicillin-resistant *Staphylococcus aureus* (MRSA) in the institutional setting and now community-acquired methicillin-resistant *S. aureus* (CA-MRSA) in the community. Vancomycin-resistant *S. aureus* (VRSA) is now reported with increasing frequency.

Although treatment of skin infections remains empirical, bacterial cultures are almost becoming mandatory. In nonresponsive cases, mycobacterium and fungal cultures in healthy patients should be obtained. The recent outbreak of atypical mycobacterium lower extremity infections associated with nail salon foot baths in otherwise healthy patients resembling *S. aureus* folliculitis and abscesses illustrates the need to expand our differential diagnosis in nonresponsive cases. Bioterrorism with infectious agents including anthrax are now a potential concern.

Impetigo and Ecthyma

Impetigo is a well-known disease of school-age children that is easily transmitted. In past years it was thought that much of impetigo was secondary to group A β-hemolytic streptococci; most cases now involve *S. aureus*. Occasionally mixed infections of streptococci and *S. aureus* are seen. Impetigo has a predilection for areas of traumatized skin such as contact dermatitis or eczema. Warm moist environments, poor living conditions, and close living conditions aggravate impetigo.

Impetigo is classified as bullous or nonbullous. The nonbullous form is much more common (approximately 70%) of cases. Bullous impetigo is often linked to *S. aureus* group II phage. The bullae usually appear on the trunk, buttocks, perineum, or face. A toxin produced by this particular type of *S. aureus* is thought to induce the bullae. Complications of impetigo include glomerulonephritis, septicemia, pneumonia, septic arthritis, osteomyelitis, and necrotizing fasciitis.

TABLE 1 Bacterial Skin Infections

Infection	Primary organisms	Recommended treatments
Impetigo	Group A streptococcus or *Staphylococcus aureus*	Bacterial culture. If mild, topical mupirocin (Bactroban) twice daily × I wk. More difficult cases, dicloxacillin (Dynapen), cephalexin (Keflex), erythromycin, or clarithromycin (Biaxin).
Folliculitis	*S. aureus* (most common); *Klebsiella, Enterobacter* (long-term acne antibiotics); *Pseudomonas* (hot tub exposure); atypical mycobacterium (nail salon foot bath)	Bacterial culture. Superficial: topical mupirocin, erythromycin, clindamycin, and personal hygiene measures. More severe cases: dicloxacillin, cephalexin, amoxicillin-clavulanate (Augmentin), cefdinir (Omnicef), and clarithromycin. Fungal and mycobacterium cultures for recalcitrant cases. Hot tub folliculitis may require ciprofloxacin (Cipro) if recalcitrant.
Cellulitis	β-Hemolytic streptococci; *S. aureus; Haemophilus influenzae* (young children); gram negatives "below the waist," especially in immunocompromised patients	Culture by needle aspiration or tissue biopsy. Localized, nontoxic presentation: dicloxacillin, amoxicillin-clavulanate, cephalexin, and clarithromycin. Progressive, toxic, or immunocompromised: β-lactamase-resistant intravenous antibiotics. Newer antibiotics should be considered.
Staphylococcal scaled skin syndrome	*S. aureus* phage group II	β-Lactamase-resistant antibiotics. Mupirocin for nares.
Necrotizing fasciitis	Polymicrobial infections with aerobic and anaerobic organisms	Surgical consultation. Should not delay waiting on imaging studies, early débridement, broad-spectrum intravenous antibiotics for aerobic and anaerobic bacteria.
Anthrax	*Bacillus anthracis*	Skin biopsy for cultures and immunohistochemical stains; lab director, pathologist, dermatologist, and public health officials should be consulted. Ciprofloxacin or doxycycline (Vibramycin) depending on patient's age and condition.

Nephritogenic strains of streptococcus may produce postinfectious glomerulonephritis after 18 to 21 days, particularly in young children 3 to 7 years of age. Antibiotic treatment does not appear to prevent this complication in susceptible individuals.

Ecthyma is a clinical variant of impetigo that affects mainly immunocompromised patients with diabetes, HIV infection, and neutropenic states from cancer chemotherapy and other immunosuppressants. The same causative organisms as impetigo are found. The lesions are more punched out and painful than impetigo lesions and not responsive to topical therapy.

TREATMENT

Limited superficial impetigo can be treated with topical therapy such as mupirocin (Bactroban) ointment or cream. This product must be applied two to three times a day for 2 to 3 weeks. Treatment of the anterior nares with mupirocin ointment (Bactroban Nasal) is helpful because they are a harbor for chronic carriage. In limited disease this treatment is helpful and avoids the use of systemic antibiotics. All known isolates of group A β-hemolytic streptococcus are sensitive to mupirocin; however, some isolates of *S. aureus* appear to be becoming resistant as longtime use of mupirocin occurs. Some authorities now recommend not treating the anterior nares for more than 4 to 6 weeks. More extensive cases of impetigo and ecthyma should be treated with systemic antibiotics that are β-lactamase resistant, such as dicloxacillin (Dynapen), cephalexin (Keflex), amoxicillin-clavulanate potassium (Augmentin), cefdinir (Omnicef), erythromycin (E-mycin), and clarithromycin (Biaxin). Macrolides such as erythromycin and clarithromycin may be used for limited disease in low-risk individuals who are sensitive to penicillin and/or cephalosporin.

Basic hygiene should be enforced, along with warm compresses to help remove crust followed by application of mupirocin ointment or cream. In cases of underlying dermatitis, control of the dermatitis is also helpful.

Folliculitis

Folliculitis is a common infection involving the hair follicle or pilosebaceous unit. It usually manifests as follicular-based yellow pustules. Sometimes the patient has excoriated or shaved them away, which may make the diagnosis less obvious. Spreading with scratching or shaving is a helpful clue. Patients who shave, work, or exercise in sweaty environments are particularly predisposed.

TREATMENT

Superficial folliculitis frequently responds to changes in local environment, use of topical antibacterial soaps, changes in razors, less frequent shaving, and use of adequate shaving cream or lubricants. Most cases are caused by *S. aureus* and can be treated with topical antibiotics such as mupirocin (Bactroban), erythromycin 2% (A/T/S), or clindamycin 1% (Cleocin T). More severe recalcitrant cases may require systemic

β-lactamase-resistant antibiotics. Cultures are now recommended in view of CA-MRSA and nosocomial-acquired MRSA and VRSA. Fungal cultures are also recommended in recalcitrant cases, particularly in patients with tinea pedis, tinea cruris, tinea corporis, and tinea capitis, because these infections mimic bacterial disease. Atypical mycobacterium should also be cultured for in recalcitrant cases. Less common causes include gram-negative bacteria such as *Klebsiella* or *Enterobacter* that may be seen as a consequence of antibiotic therapy for acne vulgaris. *Pseudomonas aeruginosa* and *Pseudomonas cepacia* are associated with hot tub exposure ("hot tub folliculitis"). Low disinfectant levels in hot tubs need to be addressed prior to patients reentering the hot tub. Hot tub folliculitis is usually self-limited and resolves in 7 to 10 days. *Proteus* is occasionally seen as a deeper, more nodular type of lesion.

Furuncles and Carbuncles

Furuncles are more involved infections of the pilosebaceous unit resulting in indurated, red painful nodules. Carbuncles are further extensions of this process to include multiple lesions that are interconnected to form multiloculated abscesses. The most common organism is *S. aureus*. Environmental factors, including sweating, friction, oils and grease, poor hygiene, preexisting dermatoses, nutritional factors, and immune status, are all-important contributors. The most common areas of involvement include the face, buttocks, thighs, perineum, breast, and axillae. Carbuncles involve the neck more commonly because of the thickness of the skin in this area.

TREATMENT

Bacterial cultures, good hygiene, and warm compresses along with appropriate empirical systemic antibiotic therapy clear most cases. Mupirocin ointment may be applied to the anterior nares, axillae, groin, gluteal cleft, and folds of the neck in patients with recurrent disease to attempt to reduce the carrier state. Use of antiseptic soaps in these patients is discouraged because of lack of efficacy and the potential for developing additional resistance patterns. Large abscesses may require incision and drainage. Bacterial cultures should be obtained if possible prior to institution of therapy and in recalcitrant cases.

Hidradenitis suppurativa is a condition that at first may resemble chronic furunculosis. Primary involvement is seen in the axillae, nape of the neck, inframammary folds, and perineum. These patients form large abscesses, which are usually subcutaneous without evidence of follicular origin. Hidradenitis is treated with incision and drainage, antibiotics, and, in severe cases, extirpation with grafting of the involved skin.

Cellulitis and Erysipelas

Cellulitis is a more invasive infection of the skin and associated soft tissues. Erysipelas is a more superficial form of cellulitis and occurs predominantly on the face and legs. Because of the acute onset and fiery red appearance, it is sometimes called "St. Anthony's fire."

Cellulitis is frequently preceded by some type of superficial injury to the skin. Tinea pedis, dermatitis, varicella, or traumatic injuries are common precipitators. *S. aureus* and β-hemolytic streptococci are the most common causes. *Haemophilus influenzae* (less common since the *Haemophilus influenzae* type b [Hib] vaccine), group B streptococci in newborns, and pneumonococcal cellulitis in immunocompromised patients also occurs. Less common causes include atypical mycobacterium, *Vibrio vulnificus* (exposure to sea water), and gram-negative bacteria such as *Pseudomonas* and *Klebsiella*.

Localized skin abscesses with necrosis, gangrene, septicemia, ascending lymphangitis, and thrombophlebitis, may occur. Anaerobic infections with clostridium originating from soil and bacteroides from fecal material are also seen. Many of these infections are polymicrobial and can be quite aggressive, dissecting along fascial planes.

TREATMENT

Treatment of cellulitis begins with a choice of systemic antibiotics on an empirical basis bearing in mind the wound, immune status of the patient, and observed toxic state of the patient. Localized disease may be treated in an otherwise nontoxic healthy individual with oral antibiotics and outpatient follow-up. More aggressive infections in immunocompromised patients require intravenous antibiotic therapy along with incision and drainage and/or débridement if abscesses or necrotic tissue are present. Simpler infections require antibiotics that cover *S. aureus* and streptococci. In children, *H. influenzae* must be considered because it is best treated with amoxicillin/clavulanate (Augmentin) or other effective antibiotics. Needle aspiration and tissue cultures are helpful in some cases, but yield from such procedures is typically less than 10% to 20% recovery of causative organisms. In infections that do not appear to respond or progress despite adequate therapy, the clinician should consider the possibility of resistant organisms, atypical organisms, and necrotizing fasciitis.

Staphylococcal Scalded Skin Syndrome

Staphylococcal scalded skin syndrome (SSSS) is a toxin-mediated manifestation of infection with staphylococci, usually phage group II. It occurs mainly in children and manifests with acute fever, skin tenderness, and a scarlatiniform erythema. Flaccid bullae and erosions develop in 1 to 2 days followed by desquamation.

TREATMENT

Treatment is directed at the *S. aureus* with β-lactamase-resistant antibiotics. Sicker children and adults should be admitted for initial stabilization and then may be discharged on oral antibiotics once stable. Most cases heal without significant scarring, although darker individuals may have variation of pigmentation that can persist for some time.

Necrotizing Fasciitis

Necrotizing fasciitis is a deep infection of subcutaneous soft tissue involving fascia and fat. It is classified in two categories: type I and type II. Immunocompromised individuals including diabetics, patients with peripheral vascular disease, young children, and those over 65 years of age are at increased risk. The frequency is increasing in normal individuals, however, including athletes or following minor injuries, varicella, and trauma.

Type I necrotizing fasciitis occurs most commonly after surgical procedures, in patients with diabetes, and in patients with peripheral vascular diseases. It is a mixed infection with both aerobic and anaerobic bacteria including *S. aureus, Escherichia coli,* group A *Streptococcus* (GAS), *Peptostreptococcus* species, *Prevotella* and *Porphyromonas* species, *Clostridium* species, and *Bacteroides fragilis.*

Type II necrotizing fasciitis is caused by GAS and shares clinical features with spontaneous gangrenous myositis. Many of the patients are not as chronically ill as those in type I disease and present from the community following varicella, injection drug use, lacerations, childbirth, surgical procedures, blunt trauma, and exposure to other patients.

Initial presentation of necrotizing fasciitis is not always dramatic. It may only involve localized swelling of an extremity, followed by a dusky purple nonblanching skin, and localized tenderness to underlying muscle groups. Patients may be relatively asymptomatic, particularly those who are chronically ill, until sepsis and hypotension develop. Laboratory values including leukocytosis and hyperglycemia are usually nonspecific, and a high index of suspicion is necessary to suspect the diagnosis. Most cases progress rapidly to frank septicemia, hypotension, and necrosis. Despite adequate intervention with systemic antibiotics and surgical débridement, mortality may approach 40% to 50%, particularly in patients with multiple underlying medical conditions.

If necrotizing fasciitis is considered in the diagnosis, prompt surgical consult with a surgeon experienced in management of these patients may be lifesaving. Imaging studies may be helpful in some cases but could delay diagnostic and therapeutic surgical intervention.

Newer Antimicrobial Agents

Several novel agents are available in the war against resistant *S. aureus*. These include linezolid (Zyvox), daptomycin (Cubicin), and quinupristin/dalfopristin (Synercid). The use of these antibiotics should be limited to those patients in whom traditional therapies are contraindicated. Clinicians should familiarize themselves with all prescribing information and side effects prior to use of the agents in the absence of appropriate consultation.

Rakel and Bope: *Conn's Current Therapy 2006.*

Linezolid (Zyvox) is a novel compound of the oxazolidinone class intended for treatment of nosocomial and community-acquired pneumonias and skin infections caused by staphylococcus and streptococcus. It is effective against MRSA; however, it should be noted that is a bacteriostatic antibiotic. Dosing is based on severity of the infection. For uncomplicated infection the suggested dose is 400 mg orally twice daily. An intravenous dose of 600 mg twice daily is recommended for complicated infections.

Quinupristin and dalfopristin (Synercid) is a synergistic combination of two semisynthetic pristinamycin derivatives of the streptogramin class. The drug is administered parentally and indicated for complicated skin and skin structure infections caused by MRSA and *Staphylococcus pyogenes*. Normal intravenous dosing is 7.5 mg/kg every 12 hours for 7 days, increased to every 8 hours for bacteremic patients.

Daptomycin (Cubicin) is a cyclic lipopeptide indicated for complicated skin infections caused by MRSA and MSSA. Its use is potentially limited because of the potential of skeletal muscle toxicity. It is administered parentally at 4 mg/kg/24 hours for 7 to 14 days. The dosage should be decreased in patients with a creatinine clearance of less than 30 mL/minute (see package insert for further details).

Anthrax

Anthrax infections of the skin were considered rare until bioterrorism events of the last few years. Ability to recognize cutaneous infection requires good diagnostic skills, index of suspicion, and appropriate laboratory evaluation. Early recognition of an outbreak can lead to appropriate lifesaving treatment of the patient involved, as well as treatment of asymptomatic exposed individuals with appropriate antibiotic prophylaxis.

Cutaneous anthrax, caused by *Bacillus anthracis*, is a gram-positive, spore-forming bacillus. *Anthrax* is derived from *anthrakos,* the Greek word for coal or charcoal. The bacillus has two plasmids. One of these codes is for a glutamic acid capsule that prevents phagocytosis. The other codes for toxin subunits.

Cutaneous anthrax results from direct inoculation of spores into the skin, usually from minor abrasions to the skin. After a latency period of approximately 5 days (range is 1 to 12 days), a nontender pruritic macule or papule is noted. Within 24 to 48 hours the lesion progresses to a vesicle or bulla that enlarges up to 2 cm. It ruptures, forms an ulcer, and develops a hemorrhagic crust. Edema and satellite vesicles also ensue. Regional adenopathy, low-grade fever, and malaise may occur. The overlying crust develops into a dark, painless ester. Differential diagnosis includes brown recluse spider bite and ulceroglandular tularemia. In anthrax, the edema and painlessness are important differentiating signs. Diagnosis is confirmed by use of cultures and skin biopsy prior to institution of antibiotic therapy. In suspected cases, consultation with laboratory directors, a pathologist, and a dermatologist should be obtained to ensure that an adequate sample is obtained and proper handling

 CURRENT DIAGNOSIS

- Cultures and sensitivities are becoming essential prior to treatment.
- Empirical treatment may be started while awaiting culture results.
- Fungal and mycobacterium cultures should be obtained in recalcitrant cases or in immunocompromised patients.
- Unusual presentation or clustering of atypical infections should be immediately reported to local health authorities.

of specimens results in confirmation of diagnosis. Public health officials should be alerted in all suspected cases because they will coordinate public health response and treatment of other potentially exposed patients.

TREATMENT

Once material is obtained by biopsy, treatment of the infection can begin with ciprofloxacin or doxycycline. Ciprofloxacin (Cipro) is favored in young children, pregnant women, and breast-feeding mothers. Initial therapy in normal adults is ciprofloxacin, 500 mg orally twice daily, or doxycycline (Vibramycin), 100 mg orally twice daily. Therapy for children is ciprofloxacin, 15 mg/kg every 12 hours (not to exceed 1 g/day); doxycycline 100 mg every 12 hours in children older than 8 years and weight greater than 45 kg; in smaller children, 2.2 mg/kg every 12 hours if medically indicated rather than ciprofloxacin. Pregnant women may be treated with the normal adult dose of ciprofloxacin. Doxycycline is favored in pregnant women only if susceptibilities are known. Immunocompromised patients are treated at the same dose levels as normal adults. Duration of treatment in all confirmed/suspected cases is 100 days.

 CURRENT THERAPY

- β-Lactamase-resistant antibiotics should be used as empirical treatment in most skin infections. Full course of therapy and use of mupirocin ointment to treat carrier state is suggested.
- Use of newer agents approved for MRSA should be used only when clinically appropriate. Documented resistance, complicated infections, immunocompromised patients, and toxic patients may be candidates for such drugs.
- Incision and drainage and débridement are important adjuncts in complicated infections and abscesses.
- Imaging studies and appropriate surgical and infectious disease consultation should be sought in complex cases if available. Transfer of patient should be considered if services are not available.

13

REFERENCES

Eady EA, Cove JH: Staphylococcal resistance revisited: Community-acquired methicillin resistant *Staphylococcus aureus*-an emerging problem for the management of skin and soft tissue infections. Curr Opin Infect Dis 2003;16:103-124.

Iyer S, Jones DH: Community-acquired methicillin-resistant *Staphylococcus aureus* skin infection: A retrospective analysis of clinical presentation and treatment of local outbreak. J Am Acad Dermatol 2004;50:854-858.

Martin SJ, Zeigler DG: The use of fluoroquinolones in the treatment of skin infections. Expert Opin Pharmacother 2004;5:237-246.

Raghavan M, Linden PK: Newer treatment options for skin and soft tissue infections. Drugs 2004;64:1621-1642.

Schweiger ES, Weinberg JM: Novel antibacterial agents for skin and skin structure infections. J Am Acad Dermatol 2004;50(3):331-340; quiz: 341-342.

Sniezek PJ, Graham BS, Lederman ER, et al: Rapidly growing mycobacterial infections after pedicures. Arch Dermatol 203;139(5):629-634.

Viral Diseases of the Skin

Method of
Sylvia L. Brice, MD

Herpes Simplex Virus Types 1 and 2

Herpes simplex virus types 1 and 2 (HSV-1 and HSV-2) are the most closely related members of the human herpesvirus family (Table 1), and the skin lesions they produce are clinically indistinguishable. Clusters of tense blisters on an erythematous base often quickly evolve into erosions or ulcerations with associated crusting. Lesions may develop at any mucocutaneous site but are typically found in the perioral or anogenital regions. Both HSV-1 and HSV-2 are transmitted by direct mucocutaneous contact with an infected host. Following viral replication in the skin or mucosa, intact viral nucleocapsids travel via sensory neurons to the corresponding dorsal root ganglia to establish latency. Later, a variety of stimuli may trigger reactivation. The virus travels back along the sensory neurons to the mucocutaneous surface to replicate and induce active or subclinical infection. In the case of subclinical infection, no active skin lesions are evident, but infectious particles are present, a state known as asymptomatic shedding. Although the viral titer is much lower than during clinically active disease, asymptomatic shedding of the virus in oral and genital secretions is thought to be responsible for the majority of cases of HSV transmission.

Primary, initial nonprimary (or *first episode*), and *recurrent* are terms used to further define the nature of the HSV infection. A primary infection refers to a patient's first infection with either type of HSV at any site. These patients are seronegative initially but subsequently develop HSV type-specific antibodies. A patient who is already infected with one HSV type and then develops an infection with the alternate type will experience what is known as an initial nonprimary or first-episode infection (e.g., the first episode of genital herpes in a patient with a prior history of orofacial herpes). These patients are seropositive for one type-specific HSV antibody (e.g., HSV-1) and later develop antibodies specific for the alternate HSV type (e.g., HSV-2). Finally, a recurrent infection is that which occurs at a site of prior infection. These patients are seropositive for HSV-1 or HSV-2, or both. Because most primary infections, whether oral or genital, are asymptomatic, the first evidence of disease often represents a recurrent or initial nonprimary infection.

OROFACIAL HERPES SIMPLEX VIRUS

Orofacial HSV, also known as herpes labialis, fever blisters, or cold sores, is commonly acquired during childhood or adolescence. Symptomatic primary disease

TABLE 1 The Human Herpesviruses

Human Herpesvirus	Alternate Name	Associated Clinical Infection
Human herpesvirus-1 (HHV-1)	Herpes simplex virus type 1	Orofacial herpes, genital herpes, herpetic whitlow, eczema herpeticum
Human herpesvirus-2 (HHV-2)	Herpes simplex virus type 2	Genital herpes, herpetic whitlow, eczema herpeticum, orofacial herpes
Human herpesvirus-3 (HHV-3)	Varicella-zoster virus	Varicella (chickenpox), herpes zoster (shingles)
Human herpesvirus-4 (HHV-4)	Epstein-Barr virus	Infectious mononucleosis, oral hairy leukoplakia
Human herpesvirus-5 (HHV-5)	Cytomegalovirus	Viral exanthem, *blueberry muffin* baby, chronic perianal ulceration in HIV
Human herpesvirus-6 (HHV-6)	None	Roseola infantum (also known as exanthem subitum, sixth disease)
Human herpesvirus-7 (HHV-7)	None	
Human herpesvirus-8 (HHV-8)	Kaposi's sarcoma–associated herpesvirus	Kaposi's sarcoma

usually takes the form of gingivostomatitis with or without additional lesions on the cutaneous perioral surfaces. Fever, malaise, and tender lymphadenopathy may also be present. In recurrent episodes, clusters of blisters erupt along the vermillion border of the lips with subsequent erosions and crusting persisting for several days up to 2 weeks. Lesions may develop anywhere in the perioral area, especially on the cheeks. In men, a viral folliculitis of the beard area (herpetic sycosis) may be mistaken for a bacterial process because it is often pustular in nature. The presence of a prodrome and recurrence in the same site are clues to the correct diagnosis. Although recurrent intraoral lesions of HSV may occur, they are uncommon in immunocompetent individuals. Exposure to ultraviolet light is a common trigger factor for herpes labialis as is fever or intercurrent infection.

GENITAL HERPES SIMPLEX VIRUS

When symptomatic, primary genital herpes often involves bilaterally distributed lesions in the anogenital area with associated fever, inguinal adenopathy, and dysuria or urinary retention. Aseptic meningitis may also occur. The lesions often persist for 2 to 3 weeks or longer. Nonprimary infections are usually less severe with fewer constitutional symptoms. Recurrent episodes tend to be milder and shorter in duration. Often, there is a prodrome of tingling or burning followed by the development of localized vesicles that may quickly rupture, leaving nonspecific erosions or ulcerations. The lesions may be anywhere within the anogenital region but tend to recur close to the same area in subsequent episodes. The time between exposure and development of primary disease is estimated to be from 3 to 14 days. However, more often the first clinical indication of disease is a recurrence, which may occur weeks to years after the initial infection. Prior infection with HSV-1 provides some protection against acquisition of HSV-2.

Based on seroepidemiologic evidence, it is estimated that at least 22% of the population in the United States 12 years of age and older is infected with HSV-2. Most of these individuals have not been officially diagnosed with this disease and are unaware that they are infected. Nevertheless, they experience asymptomatic shedding and unknowingly transmit the disease to sexual partners. Interrupting this cycle of transmission has become a major focus among health care givers who work with these patients. A combination of patient education and appropriate use of systemic antiviral agents may gradually have some impact on this epidemic. Recommendations for patients with genital herpes include avoidance of sex with uninfected partners when active lesions or prodromal symptoms are present, and the routine use of latex condoms to minimize transmission during periods of asymptomatic shedding. Chronic suppressive doses of oral antiviral agents (Table 2), including acyclovir (Zovirax), valacyclovir (Valtrex),

TABLE 2 Recommendations for Systemic Antiviral Treatment of Mucocutaneous Herpes Simplex Virus (HSV) Infection

Genital HSV		
Primary/first episode	Acyclovir (Zovirax)	400 mg PO tid or 200 mg PO 5 × per d × 10d (mild to moderate) 5 mg/kg IV q8h × 5d (severe)
	Valacyclovir (Valtrex)	1 g PO bid × 10d
	Famciclovir (Famvir)	250 mg PO tid × 10d
Recurrent episode	Acyclovir	400 mg PO tid or 200 mg PO 5 × per d × 5d
	Valacyclovir	500 mg PO bid × 3d
	Famciclovir	125 mg PO bid × 5d
Chronic suppressive therapy	Acyclovir	400 mg PO bid or 200 mg PO tid; adjust up or down according to response (>6 outbreaks per year)
	Valacyclovir	500 mg PO qd (<10 outbreaks per year) 1 g PO qd (10 or more outbreaks per year)
	Famciclovir	250 mg PO bid (6 or more outbreaks per year)
Orofacial HSV		
Recurrent	Acyclovir	400 mg PO 5 × per d for 5d; start at prodrome
	Valacyclovir	2 g PO bid × 1d; start at prodrome
	Famciclovir	500 mg PO tid × 5d; minimally more effective than 250 mg PO tid; start at prodrome
Chronic suppressive therapy	Acyclovir	400 mg PO tid (adjust up or down according to response)
	Valacyclovir	500 mg-1 g PO qd
	Famciclovir	250 mg PO bid
Orolabial or Genital HSV in Immunosuppressed Patients		
Recurrent/suppressive	Acyclovir	400 mg PO 5 × per d or 5-10 mg/kg IV q8h
	Valacyclovir	500 mg PO bid
	Famciclovir	500 mg PO bid

Abbreviations: bid = twice daily; IV = intravenous; PO = by mouth; qd = daily; tid = three times a day.

Rakel and Bope: *Conn's Current Therapy 2006.*

and famciclovir (Famvir), significantly reduce the frequency of clinical recurrences as well as the rate of asymptomatic shedding and may be recommended together with these other practices to reduce the risk of transmission.

Although HSV-2 is the etiologic agent in a majority of cases of genital herpes infections, an increasing number of genital herpes infections are caused by HSV-1. Symptomatic recurrences and asymptomatic shedding are less frequent with genital HSV-1 infection than with genital HSV-2 infection, and this distinction becomes important for patient counseling and prognosis.

OTHER MUCOCUTANEOUS HERPES SIMPLEX VIRUS INFECTIONS

Eczema herpeticum, also known as Kaposi's varicelliform eruption, represents a cutaneous dissemination of HSV usually seen in patients with atopic dermatitis or other underlying skin disease. Herpetic vesicles develop over an extensive mucocutaneous surface, most often the face, neck, and upper trunk, presumably spreading from a recurrent oral HSV infection or asymptomatic shedding from the oral mucosa. Eczema herpeticum may also develop in the presence of genital HSV. As with other HSV infections, eczema herpeticum may be recurrent. In addition, patients may develop localized, recurrent HSV in previously involved areas. Because of the extensive and inflammatory nature of the process and the possible secondary bacterial infection, the underlying viral etiology may be obscured. A history of eczema and recurrent HSV in the patient and careful observation for the grouped vesicles or erosions can be key to the correct diagnosis.

Herpetic whitlow refers to HSV infection of the hand, usually one or more distal digits. Previously thought to be limited to health care professionals with exposure to oral secretions of their patients, it is now recognized that autoinoculation from orolabial or genital HSV contributes to a significant number of cases.

Herpes gladiatorum is a problem seen most commonly in athletes who participate in close contact sports such as wrestling. Typically transmitted from active herpes labialis or asymptomatic shedding in oral secretions of an infected opponent, herpes gladiatorum often affects the head, neck, or shoulders and may be recurrent.

Varicella-Zoster Virus (Herpes Zoster)

Varicella-zoster virus (VZV), another member of the human herpesvirus family (see Table 1), produces two specific patterns of disease in the skin. The primary infection results in varicella, also known as chickenpox, a widespread vesicular eruption usually seen in the pediatric population (see Section 2 of this book). Following the primary infection, VZV establishes latency in the dorsal root ganglia until some later point in time when reactivation may occur. The ensuing unilateral

dermatomal distribution of blisters, often preceded by neuralgic pain, is known as *herpes zoster* or *shingles*. Herpes zoster is especially common in patients older than 50 years of age, but it may be seen at any age. It is also seen more frequently in the immunocompromised patient population such as organ-transplant recipients or individuals infected with HIV. Herpes zoster is no longer considered a marker for underlying cancer, and evaluation for occult malignancy in an otherwise asymptomatic individual is not indicated. A single recurrence of herpes zoster, usually in the same dermatome, may occur in up to 4% of zoster patients. Additional recurrences, however, suggest a dermatomal form of HSV, and laboratory assessment for this possibility should be performed.

The most common dermatomes involved with herpes zoster are in the thoracolumbar (T3-L2) and trigeminal (V1) regions. Skin lesions typically evolve from papules to vesicles and pustules, and then crusted erosions, before healing approximately 2 to 4 weeks after onset. The associated neuropathic pain commonly persists after the lesions have healed. If pain continues for more than 1 month after resolution of the skin lesions, it is referred to as *postherpetic neuralgia,* one of the most common and debilitating complications of this infection.

Several clinical presentations of herpes zoster deserve additional attention. Ophthalmic zoster, with lesions along the tip, side, or base of the nose indicating involvement of the nasociliary branch of the trigeminal nerve (Hutchinson's sign), may be associated with increased risk for ocular complications. Prompt initiation of a systemic antiviral agent (see Table 1) and evaluation by an ophthalmologist are recommended. Disseminated zoster, with more than a few lesions outside the primary and immediately adjacent dermatomes, can be indicative of visceral involvement and its associated complications. The term *zoster sine herpete* is used to describe patients with neuropathic pain resembling zoster but without any skin lesions. The diagnosis can be supported by demonstration of increased IgG antibody titers between the acute and convalescent phases. Chronic zoster is seen predominantly in HIV-infected individuals. Single or multiple warty growths may persist for weeks or months in areas of skin previously involved by typical lesions of varicella or herpes zoster. Chronic zoster is often acyclovir (Zovirax) resistant. Both tissue biopsy and viral cultures, with further testing for antiviral resistance, may aid in assessment.

Diagnosis

HERPES SIMPLEX VIRUS

Viral culture remains the preferred method for diagnosis of HSV infection. This method is sensitive when specimens are obtained from lesions that have not yet become too dry or crusted, usually during the first 2 to 3 days after onset. An adequate sample, obtained by unroofing the blister and swabbing the base, increases the likelihood of an accurate result. Antigen detection tests may remain positive even after lesions have dried, as long as the specimen includes epithelial cells and not just debris. For this method, a scraping from the lesion is usually smeared on a glass slide to be sent to the laboratory. Not all antigen detection methods are designed to distinguish HSV-1 from HSV-2. The Tzanck smear (cytologic detection) is both insensitive and nonspecific but may be of use in some clinical settings. It does not differentiate HSV types or HSV from VZV. Polymerase chain reaction (PCR) is highly sensitive but not routinely used for diagnosis of mucocutaneous HSV infections.

Serologic testing for HSV was previously of limited use because it could not reliably differentiate HSV-1 from HSV-2. Because they share significant genetic homology, HSV-1 and HSV-2 code for a number of common proteins that are not antigenically distinct. However, they also code for type-specific proteins that can be used to differentiate them. Current tests based on detection of type-specific viral glycoprotein G (gG-based, type-specific assays) are accurate and should be requested for this purpose. A positive HSV-2 serology may be useful in confirming the diagnosis of genital herpes in a patient with a negative viral culture or with unrecognized or asymptomatic disease. Alternatively, a negative serology may exclude the diagnosis of HSV in a patient with chronic, nonspecific oral or genital symptoms.

HERPES ZOSTER

Diagnosis of herpes zoster is often made on clinical grounds alone. A Tzanck smear may provide additional support of the viral etiology. With atypical presentations, however, the diagnosis is best confirmed by either an antigen detection method or viral culture. Both will differentiate VZV from HSV. Samples submitted for viral culture should be obtained from vesicular fluid because dried or crusted lesions are unlikely to

---

BOX 1 Recommendations for Systemic Antiviral Treatment of Herpes Zoster

Immunocompetent Patients
Acyclovir (Zovirax) 800 mg PO 5 × per d × 7-10d
Valacyclovir (Valtrex) 1 g PO tid × 7d
Famciclovir (Famvir) 500 mg PO tid × 7d
Immunosuppressed Patients
Acyclovir 800 mg PO 5 × per d for 10d*
    10 mg/kg/dose IV q8h × 7-10d*
Valacyclovir 1 g PO tid × 10d*
Famciclovir 500 mg PO tid × 10d*

*Continue until there are no new lesions for 48 hours.
Abbreviations: IV = intravenous; PO = by mouth; tid = three times a day.

---

yield positive results. Viral cultures are required if there is a need to assess possible antiviral resistance. PCR can be useful for detection of VZV in bodily fluids such as cerebrospinal fluid. VZV serology is rarely useful for diagnosis, because a majority of the population is seropositive.

13

Treatment

There are three systemic antiviral agents routinely used for the treatment of HSV and VZV infections: acyclovir (Zovirax), valacyclovir (Valtrex), and famciclovir (Famvir). All three are highly effective and generally well tolerated. Because they inhibit only actively replicating viral DNA, they have no impact on latent infection. Recommendations for antiviral treatment of mucocutaneous HSV infections and herpes zoster, localized topical measures, and available formulations are outlined in Box 1 and Tables 2, 3, and 4. Optimal antiviral dosage schedules for less common HSV infections,

---

TABLE 3 Topical Treatment Options for Mucocutaneous Herpes Simplex Virus (HSV) and Varicella-Zoster Virus (VZV) Infections

Topical Treatment	Comment
Cool, moist compresses using tap water or aluminum acetate 1:20 to 1:40 (Burow's solution, Domeboro, Bluboro)	Good for moist, oozing lesions to accelerate drying. Apply wet dressing to involved skin and cover with dry cloth to allow evaporation.
Calamine lotion or similar shake lotion containing alcohol, menthol, and/or phenol; Aveeno colloidal oatmeal	Useful as drying and antipruritic agent. May be applied after wet dressing.
Bacitracin[1], Polysporin, mupirocin1 (Bactroban)	Use if there is concern for localized secondary bacterial infection.
2% Viscous lidocaine, compounded* suspensions (e.g., Kaopectate or Maalox, diphenhydramine, lidocaine)	Useful for temporary pain relief of oral or genital mucosal involvement.
Acyclovir (Zovirax) ointment	Used together with systemic antiviral agents, may be of benefit to immunocompromised individuals for localized HSV.
Penciclovir (Denavir) cream	May decrease the duration of lesions in herpes labialis by half a day if applied every 2h while awake for 4 days beginning at the first sign of disease.

[1]Not FDA approved for this indication.
*May be compounded by pharmacies.

TABLE 4 Formulations of Acyclovir, Valacyclovir, and Famciclovir

Drug	Oral	Topical	Intravenous
Acyclovir (Zovirax)	200, 400, 800 mg 200 mg/5 mL suspension	5% Ointment (3 g, 15 g tube)	Yes
Valacyclovir (Valtrex)	500 mg, 1 g	No	No
Famciclovir (Famvir)	125, 250, 500 mg	No	No
Penciclovir (Denavir)	No	1% Cream (1.5 g tube)	No

such as herpetic whitlow, have not been determined. The doses outlined in Table 2 for either episodic or chronic suppressive therapy can be used as a guideline in these cases.

Acyclovir (Zovirax) became available more than 20 years ago and continues to be widely used. Inside an infected host cell, acyclovir must be phosphorylated—first by a virally encoded enzyme (thymidine kinase) and then by host-cell enzymes—to the active form of the drug, acyclovir triphosphate. As a nucleotide analogue, acyclovir triphosphate is incorporated into replicating viral DNA, abruptly terminating further synthesis of that viral DNA chain. Acyclovir triphosphate also interferes with viral DNA replication by directly inhibiting viral DNA polymerase. Valacyclovir (Valtrex) is an oral prodrug of acyclovir and has a much higher bioavailability. After ingestion, valacyclovir is rapidly metabolized to acyclovir and the subsequent mechanism of action is as just described. Famciclovir (Famvir) is an oral prodrug of penciclovir, designed for greater bioavailability. Similar to acyclovir, penciclovir must first be phosphorylated by viral thymidine kinase and then by cellular enzymes to penciclovir triphosphate.

In this active form, penciclovir-triphosphate interferes with viral DNA synthesis and replication by inhibiting viral DNA polymerase. Famciclovir has both greater bioavailability and a longer intracellular half-life than acyclovir. For all three agents, the required activation by viral thymidine kinase and the preferential inhibition of viral DNA synthesis contribute to the highly specific antiviral activity.

If taken as recommended, acyclovir, valacyclovir, and famciclovir are generally comparable in their safety and effectiveness. Valacyclovir and famciclovir offer the convenience of less frequent dosing. Dosing for all three should be adjusted in the presence of renal insufficiency (Table 5).

Although antiviral therapy does not decrease the incidence of postherpetic neuralgia, all three agents decrease the time for lesion healing and shorten the overall duration of pain if initiated within 48 to 72 hours after the onset of herpes zoster. Valacyclovir and famciclovir appear to be more effective than acyclovir for this purpose. An otherwise healthy individual younger than 50 years of age with discrete involvement on the trunk and mild to moderate pain may benefit minimally or

TABLE 5 Recommended Antiviral Dose Modification in Patients with Impaired Renal Function

Initial Genital HSV		Recurrent Genital HSV	Genital HSV—Chronic Suppression	Herpes Zoster
Acyclovir (Zovirax)				
CrCl >25	200 mg 5 × per d	200 mg 5 × per d	400 mg q12h	800 mg 5 × per d
CrCl 10-24	200 mg 5 × per d	200 mg 5 × per d	400 mg q12h	800 mg q8h
CrCl <10	200 mg q12h	200 mg q12h	200 mg q12h	800 mg q12h
Valacyclovir (Valtrex)				
CrCl >50	1 g q12h	500 mg q12h	500 mg-1 g q24h	1 g q8h
CrCl 30-49	1 g q12h	500 mg q12h	500 mg-1 g q24h	1 g q12h
CrCl 10-29	1 g q24h	500 mg q24h	500 mg q24-48h	1 g q24h
CrCl <10	500 mg q24h	500 mg q24h	500 mg q24-48h	500 mg q24h
Famciclovir (Famvir)				
CrCl >60		125 mg q12h	250 mg q12h	500 mg q8h
CrCl 40-59		125 mg q12h	250 mg q12h	500 mg q12h
CrCl 20-39		125 mg q24h	125 mg q12h	500 mg q24h
CrCl <20		125 mg q24h	125 mg q24h	250 mg q24h

Abbreviation: CrCl = creatinine clearance.

not at all from this intervention, especially if it is initiated after 72 hours of lesion onset. However, patients who are older than 50 years of age, are immunosuppressed, have involvement in the ophthalmic distribution, or have more extensive lesions or severe pain should receive systemic antiviral therapy, even if the 72-hour deadline has expired. Adequate pain control, often requiring opiates, is also important. The addition of systemic corticosteroids to the antiviral regimen remains controversial. There is evidence to suggest this can lessen the severity of the acute episode but does not decrease the incidence or duration of postherpetic neuralgia. Corticosteroids should not be used without concomitant antiviral therapy.

Despite widespread use of these antiviral agents, antiviral resistance is rarely a problem in the immunocompetent population. However, it does arise in the setting of immunosuppression. The basis for the resistance is most commonly a mutation in the gene coding for thymidine kinase. Less often there is a mutation in the viral DNA polymerase. In either case, all three standard drugs become ineffective. Alternative antiviral agents available for treatment of acyclovir-resistant HSV and VZV infections include foscarnet (Foscavir)[1] and cidofovir (Vistide).[1]

Hand-Foot-and-Mouth Disease

Hand-foot-and-mouth disease is typically a disease of childhood. The etiologic agent is an enterovirus, and transmission is via the oral-oral or fecal-oral route. It is highly contagious. Several days after exposure, a prodrome of low-grade fever, malaise, abdominal pain, or respiratory symptoms may develop, followed by the appearance of papulovesicles on the palate, tongue, or buccal mucosa. Similar lesions may subsequently develop on the feet and hands. The eruption persists for 7 to 10 days and then resolves. Treatment is symptomatic.

Parvovirus B19

Cutaneous manifestations of parvovirus B19 infection include the childhood exanthem known as erythema infectiosum (fifth disease) and, less commonly, petechial or purpuric eruptions. The virus is transmitted primarily via respiratory secretions and, to a much lesser extent, through blood or blood products. The host cells for viral replication are erythroid progenitor cells, which subsequently undergo cell lysis.

A child with erythema infectiosum typically develops a low-grade fever and nonspecific upper respiratory symptoms approximately 2 days before the onset of rash. The rash has been described as having a *slapped cheeks* appearance with prominent redness over the malar eminences. This is followed by a pink-to-red lacy

or reticular eruption over the trunk and extensor surfaces of the arms and legs. The rash usually lasts a week to 10 days but may transiently recur over months in response to precipitating factors such as sunlight, exercise, and bathing. Diagnosis of erythema infectiosum is usually made on clinical grounds, and treatment is symptomatic. By the time the rash appears and the diagnosis has been made, the child is no longer infectious.

Infection with parvovirus B19 in older adolescents and adults often manifests with arthralgias or arthritis rather than a rash. In certain patient populations, parvovirus B19 infections may be associated with complications including transient aplastic crisis, chronic anemia, and hydrops fetalis. In these less typical presentations, serology (anti-B19 IgM or documented seroconversion) may be needed for diagnosis. Intravenous immunoglobulin (IVIG [Gamimune N][1]) is used successfully for treatment of chronic/persistent infection in immunosuppressed individuals.

---

[1]Not FDA approved for this indication.

CURRENT DIAGNOSIS

HSV-1 and HSV-2
- Grouped vesicles or erosions, especially in perioral or anogenital location
- Tzanck smear, viral culture, antigen detection, gG-based type-specific serology

VZV
- Papules, pustules, vesicles in diffuse (varicella) or dermatomal (herpes zoster) distribution
- Tzanck smear, antigen detection, viral culture

Hand-Foot-and-Mouth Disease
- Papulovesicles on oral mucosa, hands, feet following fever, constitutional symptoms
- Viral culture, PCR, serology

Parvovirus B19
- "Slapped cheeks" reticular erythema on trunk or extremities following fever, constitutional symptoms; arthralgias, arthritis, purpuric eruptions; transient aplastic crisis, fetal hydrops
- B19 specific IgM serology, nucleic acid amplification testing

Molluscum Contagiosum
- Few to multiple 1- to 4-mm umbilicated flesh-colored papules
- Histopathology if clinical appearance atypical

Orf
- One to several solid to vesicular nodules on hands, forearms; history of exposure to sheep, goats, cattle
- Histopathology if clinical appearance atypical

Abbreviations: gG = glycoprotein G; HSV = herpes simplex virus; IGIV = immunoglobulin intravenous; PCR = polymerase chain reaction.

---

[1]Not FDA approved for this indication.

13

Poxviruses

MOLLUSCUM CONTAGIOSUM

Molluscum contagiosum are benign umbilicated papules caused by infection with the Molluscipoxvirus, a member of the poxvirus family. Lesions are limited to the mucocutaneous surface and typically appear in clusters on the face, trunk, and skin fold areas in children versus thighs, lower abdomen, and suprapubic areas in sexually active adults. Large numbers of lesions in an extensive distribution may be seen in the immunosuppressed population. Transmission routinely occurs by skin-to-skin contact with an infected host, but transmission from contaminated fomites has been reported. Autoinoculation commonly occurs. Diagnosis is usually based on clinical exam, but histopathology of atypical lesions may be used for confirmation. Because molluscum contagiosum tend to be self-limited, treatment is not always required, but it may reduce the risk of autoinoculation and transmission to others. Treatment modalities are primarily aimed at lesion destruction, similar to those used for verruca vulgaris (Table 6). In the case of sexual transmission, evaluation for other sexually transmitted diseases may be indicated.

ORF AND MILKER'S NODULES

Orf (also known as ecthyma contagiosum) and milker's nodules are caused by the closely related Parapoxvirus, a member of the poxvirus family. The virus responsible for orf is widespread in sheep and goats, whereas the virus causing milker's nodules is found in cattle. Transmission to humans is by direct contact with infected animals and is usually seen several days up to 2 weeks after exposure. Orf and milker's nodules most commonly appear as one to several nodules on the dorsal aspect of the hands or forearms. Lesions evolve through several clinical stages over a period of 3 to 5 weeks ranging from solid red nodules to vesicular, exudative, or wartlike tumors. As with other poxvirus infections,

CURRENT THERAPY

HSV-1 and HSV-2
- Acyclovir (Zovirax), valacyclovir (Valtrex), famciclovir (Famvir)
- For acyclovir resistance: foscarnet (Foscavir),[1] cidofovir (Vistide)[1]

VZV
- Acyclovir, valacyclovir, famciclovir (Famvir)
- For Acyclovir resistance: foscarnet,[1] cidofovir (Vistide)[1]

Hand-Foot-and-Mouth
- Supportive care

Parvovirus B19
- Supportive care, IVIG

Molluscum contagiosum
- Surgical or chemical methods of destruction
- Immunomodulators (imiquimod, cimetidine)

Orf
- Self-limited

[1]Not FDA approved for this indication.
Abbreviations: HSV = herpes simplex virus; IVIG = intravenous immunoglobulin.

lesions of orf often demonstrate central umbilication. Regional lymphadenopathy and lymphangitis are commonly seen. Diagnosis is based on a history of exposure and clinical exam. Tissue biopsy for histopathology or electron microscopy may also be used. The lesions are self-limited and treatment is not routinely required.

REFERENCES

American College of Obstetricians and Gynecologists: Clinical management guidelines for obstetrician-gynecologists, number 57, November 2004. Gynecologic herpes simplex virus infections. Obstet Gynecol 2004;104:1111-1118.
Bikowski JB Jr: Molluscum contagiosum: The need for physician intervention and new treatment options. Cutis 2004;73:202-206.
Corey L, Wald A, Patel R, et al: Once daily valacyclovir to reduce the risk of transmission of genital herpes. N Engl J Med 2004;350:11-20.

TABLE 6 Treatment Options for Molluscum Contagiosum

Treatment	Comment
Cryotherapy (liquid nitrogen)	Freeze individual lesions for 5-10 seconds. Repeat PRN in 2-3 weeks.
Curettage	Entire lesion may be removed using a curette. This results in bleeding. Removal of central core with toothpick or other pointed instrument is also effective.
Cantharidin (Cantharone)[1]	Blister-inducing agent. Apply to lesion with toothpick, air dry. Cover with tape or adhesive bandage. Patient to wash area after 24 hours (or sooner if significant pain).
Podophyllin (25% in tincture of benzoin)[1]	Cytotoxic agent. Apply to lesion with toothpick. Patient to wash off after 4-6 hours. Contraindicated in pregnancy.
Podofilox (Condylox 0.5% gel or solution)[1]	Done by patient. Apply bid for 3 consecutive days per week for 2-4 weeks. Contraindicated in pregnancy.
Salicylic acid/lactic acid (Occlusal, Duofilm)	Done by patient. Apply daily.
Imiquimod (Aldara) 5% cream[1]	Done by patient. Apply daily 5 consecutive days per week. Leave on overnight. Continue for 8-12 weeks.
Cimetidine (Tagamet)[1]	30 mg/kg/d PO for 6-12 weeks. May boost cell-mediated immunity.

[1]Not FDA approved for this indication.
Abbreviations: PO = by mouth; PRN = as needed.

Gnann JW, Whitley RJ: Herpes zoster. N Engl J Med 2002;347: 340-346.

Kimberlin DW, Rouse DJ: Genital herpes. N Engl J Med 2004; 350:1970-1977.

Schillinger JA, Xu F, Sternberg MR, et al: National seroprevalence and trends in herpes simplex virus type 1 in the United States, 1976-1994. Sex Transm Dis 2004;31:753-760.

Scott LA, Stone MS: Viral exanthems. Dermatol Online J 2003;9(3):4.

Vander Straten M, Carrasco D, Lee P, Tyring SK: Reduction of postherpetic neuralgia in herpes zoster. J Cutan Med Surg 2001; 5:409-416.

Parasitic Diseases of the Skin

Method of
Philip D. Shenefelt, MD, MS

Parasitic afflictions of the skin are caused by protozoa, helminths, and arthropods. Table 1 lists cutaneous parasites, geographic distribution, and parasitic diseases and their treatment. Although a number of cutaneous parasites occur geographically in the tropics, world travel exposes increasing numbers of people from temperate climates to these pathogens. Travel history and recreational/occupational history are important when cutaneous findings indicate that parasitic skin disease is in the differential diagnosis spectrum.

Protozoa

AMEBIASIS

Cutaneous amebiasis caused by *Entamoeba histolytica* is rare and occurs by direct inoculation from feces or an abscess. The lesion typically is an irregular painful ulcer on the perineum, buttock, or abdomen. Trophozoites may be found in the ulcer or stool. Metronidazole (Flagyl), 750 mg orally every 8 hours for 5 to 10 days, is recommended, followed by iodoquinol (Yodoxin), 650 mg three times daily for 20 days, to eliminate the intestinal source.

LEISHMANIASIS

Cutaneous leishmaniasis is transmitted by the bite of an infected sandfly, with several *Leishmania* species involved. The lesion is an ulcer with elevated border and central crater. Sodium stibogluconate (Pentostam)[1] is available from the Centers for Disease Control and Prevention (CDC) Drug Service. The dose is 20 mg/kg per day pentavalent antimony (0.2 mL Pentostam) intravenous or intramuscularly for 21 to 28 days.

TRYPANOSOMIASIS

Chagas' disease caused by *Trypanosoma cruzi* often is clinically inapparent on the skin but may manifest as Romaña's sign (unilateral eyelid edema and conjunctivitis) or a chagoma (an erythematous indurated subcutaneous nodule). This occurs at the bite site from an infected reduviid bug. Early treatment is important to prevent late sequelae of cardiomyopathy or gastrointestinal involvement. Nifurtimox (Lampit)[1] is available through the CDC Drug Service and is given 8 to 10 mg/kg per day orally in four divided doses for 120 days.

African sleeping sickness is transmitted by the bite of the tzetze fly infected with a *Trypanosoma brucei* variant, *gambiense* or *rhodesiense*. Approximately half of patients develop an initial 2- to 5-cm erythematous nodule surrounded by a white halo at the bite site 5 to 15 days after the bite. An evanescent macular eruption may occur weeks to months later. Early treatment is very important to prevent central nervous system involvement. For *Trypanosoma brucei* variant *gambiense*, eflornithine (Ornidyl),[1] available from the World Health Organization, is given at 400 mg/kg orally in four divided doses for 2 weeks, followed by 300 mg/kg per day orally for 3 to 4 weeks. Suramin sodium (Antrypol), available from the CDC Drug Service, can be used to treat either *Trypanosoma brucei* variant (*gambiense* or *rhodesiense*). The dosage is a 100-mg test dose followed by 20 mg/kg to a maximum of 1 g intravenously on days 1, 3, 7, 14, and 21.

Helminths

CREEPING ERUPTION (CUTANEOUS LARVA MIGRANS)

Cutaneous larval migrans, or creeping eruption, occurs when the larvae of the cat and dog hookworm, *Ancylostoma braziliense*, penetrate skin in contact with the ground. The infestation usually occurs in warm, moist, sandy areas such as the beach, playgrounds, sandboxes, and under houses. Within a few hours of contact, an erythematous papule appears at the site of skin penetration. In a day or two, pruritic erythematous serpiginous tracks develop. They usually progress at 1 to 2 cm per day. The larvae are accidental intruders and usually die within a few weeks, although some may persist for up to a year with cycles of remission and exacerbation.

Small numbers of lesions can be treated with ethyl chloride or liquid nitrogen freezing. Larger numbers can be treated topically with a thiabendazole (Mintezol) 10% to 15% suspension applied three times a day until the lesions have resolved. Oral thiabendazole, 25 to 50 mg/kg per day in two divided doses up to a maximum of 1.5 g per day for patients who weigh more than 70 kg, may be given for 2 consecutive days after weighing the benefits with the potential adverse reactions. Oral ivermectin (Stromectol), 200 µg/kg orally in a single dose, is a good alternative.

---

[1]Not FDA approved for this indication.

Rakel and Bope: *Conn's Current Therapy 2006.*

---

[1]Not FDA approved for this indication.

TABLE 1 Cutaneous Parasites, Parasitic Diseases, and Their Treatment

Class	Causative organism	Geographic distribution	Cutaneous manifestations	Recommended treatment
Protozoa	*Entamoeba histolytica*	Worldwide	Amebiasis cutis	Metronidazole (Flagyl) 750 mg PO q8h for 5-10 d
	Leishmania species	Africa, Asia, Middle East, Central and South America	Cutaneous leishmaniasis	Sodium stibogluconate (Pentostam)* 20 mg/kg/d IV or IM for 21-28 d
	Trypanosoma cruzi	Central and South America	Chagas' disease	Nifurtimox (Lampit)* 8-10 mg/kg/d in 4 doses for 120 d
	Trypanosoma brucei	Africa	Chancre or macular eruption	Trypanosomal eflornithine* (Ornidyl) or suramin*
Helminths	*Ancylostoma braziliense*	Worldwide	Cutaneous larva migrans	Topical 10-15% thiabendazole* suspension (Mintezol) bid for 2d; ivermectin[†] (Stromectol) 200 µg/kg
	Ancylostoma duodenale, Necator americanus	Africa, Asia, Mediterranean, Central and South America, southeastern North America	Ground itch, dew itch	Mebendazole (Vermox) 100 mg PO q12h for 3 days
	Dracunculus medinensis	Asia, Africa, Middle East,	Guinea worm	Surgical removal
	Loa loa	Africa	Calabar swellings	Diethylcarbamazine (Hetrazan)* 6 mg/kg/d PO for 21 d
	Onchocerca volvulus	Africa, Central and South America	Onchodermatitis, river blindness	Ivermectin[†](Stromectol) 150 µg/kg q 6-12 mo
	Schistosoma species	Africa, Asia, Middle East, Caribbean, South America	Schistosomiasis, cercarial dermatitis, swimmer's itch	Praziquantel (Biltricide) 20 mg/kg bid or tid for 1 d
Strongyloides	*Stercoralis urticaria*	Worldwide	Larva currens	Ivermectin[†] (Stromectol) 200 µg/kg PO
	Wuchereria bancrofti, Brugia species	Asia, Africa, Caribbean, South America	Lymphatic filariasis, elephantiasis	Diethylcarbamazine (Hetrazan) 6 mg/kg/d PO for 6-12 d
Arthropoda	*Dermatobia hominis,*	Worldwide	Myiasis, botflies	Surgical removal
	Pediculus humanus	Worldwide	Head lice, body lice	1% permethrin (Nix Creme Rinse) for 10 min, repeat in 1 wk
	Phthirus pubis	Worldwide	Pubic lice	5% permethrin cream for 10 min
	Sarcoptes scabiei	Wordwide	Scabies	5% permethrin cream or ivermectin[†]
	Tunga penetrans	Central and South America, Africa	Tungiasis	Surgical removal

*Only available from the Centers for Disease Control and Prevention.
[†]Ivermectin is officially indicated only for onchocerciasis and gastrointestinal strongyloidiasis.
Abbreviations: bid = two times per day; IM = intramuscular; IV = intravenously; PO = by mouth; q = every; tid = three times per day.

Patients should be instructed in preventive measures. Minimizing contact with the ground, covering sandboxes when not in use, and draping the ground with plastic prior to performing work in areas frequented by domestic animals help prevent further exposure.

DRACUNCULIASIS

Dracunculiasis occurs when the larvae are swallowed inside infected water fleas. *Dracunculus medinensis*, the Guinea worm, can be extracted by winding it around a small stick as it emerges from the subcutaneous tissues. Metronidazole,[1] 250 mg orally three times daily for

[1]Not FDA approved for this indication.

10 days, reduces inflammation and facilitates removal of the worm.

LOIASIS

Migratory angioedema, called Calabar swellings, and worms visible in the scleral conjunctiva typify the cutaneous manifestation of *Loa loa*. Transmission is by infected tabanid fly bite. Treatment is with diethylcarbamazine (Hetrazan), 8 mg/kg per day orally in three divided doses for 21 days.

LYMPHATIC FILARIASIS

Elephantiasis occurs as a late sequela of lymphatic channel obstruction by *Wuchereria bancrofti* or *Brugia*

species, which are transmitted by bites from infected mosquitos. Microfilariae may be visible in blood samples viewed under the microscope. Treatment is with diethylcarbamazine (Hetrazan), 6 mg/kg per day orally in three divided doses for 6 to 12 days.

ONCHODERMATITIS

Pruritic dermatitis and subcutaneous nodules are characteristic of *Onchocerca volvulus* infections. Transmission is by blackflies. It tends to occur adjacent to the rivers where the blackfly larvae develop, hence the name *river blindness* for the ocular manifestations. Microfilariae may be visible in blood samples viewed under the microscope. Treatment with ivermectin (Stromectol), 150 µg/kg orally every 6 to 12 months, keeps the microfilaria under control. The adult worms are resistant to this treatment, hence the need for ongoing suppression of the microfilariae.

SCHISTOSOMIASIS

Skin exposure to contaminated water is the cause of schistosomiasis. The duck/snail schistosome causes cercarial dermatitis, or swimmer's itch, with pruritic erythematous papules that last 5 to 7 days. Infection with the nonhuman species of *Schistosoma* is self-limited, not requiring treatment. Human/snail schistosomiasis can be treated with praziquantel (Biltricide), 20 mg/kg two or three times in a single day.

LARVA CURRENS

Strongyloides stercoralis often causes a serpiginous eruption similar to cutaneous larval migrans, but migration is much more rapid, up to 10 cm per day. It is often accompanied by diarrhea and proximal bowel infection. Ivermectin (Stromectol),[1] 150 to 200 µg/kg orally as a single dose, is very effective for both the bowel and cutaneous involvement.

UNCINARIAL DERMATITIS

The human hookworms *Ancylostoma duodenale* and *Necator americanus* cause dew itch or ground itch similar to cutaneous larval migrans, but the larvae penetrate venules, exit into the lungs, ascend the trachea, are swallowed, attach to the small intestine, and mature. Treatment is with mebendazole (Vermox), 100 mg orally every 12 hours for 3 days.

Arthropods

MYIASIS

Human myiasis may occur with *Dermatobia hominis* or one of several other species of botfly, screwworm fly, or flesh fly. These Diptera deposit eggs on the skin and the larva burrow into the skin, creating an erythematous

pruritic papule with a central punctum within which the tip of the larval abdomen periodically appears. Occlusion of the central punctum with petroleum jelly may force the larva to emerge to avoid suffocation. Otherwise diagnosis and treatment is accomplished by surgical extirpation.

PEDICULOSIS

Human lice are of three types. *Phthirus pubis*, the pubic louse or crab louse, prefers the pubic hair but can be found on body and axillary hair, eyebrows, eyelashes, and occasionally the occipital scalp. *Pediculus humanus* variant *capitis*, the head louse, and variant *corporis*, the body louse, are elongated and fast moving. The head louse prefers the scalp, whereas the body louse hides in seams in clothing. The eggs or nits of the pubic and head louse are cemented to the bases of hairs, whereas those of the body louse are laid on clothing. Nits remain viable for up to a month. They hatch and evolve into adults within 2 or 3 weeks. Spread occurs from one person to another by close contact or sharing a bed or clothing. The louse bite results in a red pruritic macule with a central hemorrhagic center.

Pediculosis Pubis

Crab lice are identified by their characteristic shape and slow movement. They are difficult to see. The nits also can be seen attached to the bases of hairs. In addition to the pubic hair, the body hair, axillary hair, eyebrows, eyelashes, and occipital scalp should also be examined. Pruritus and excoriations are common, and secondary impetiginization may supervene. Scattered bite sites may be seen on the skin near hairs.

Permethrin 5% cream (Elimite)[1] should be applied to the affected areas as a lotion for 10 minutes, then showered off. Alternatively, lindane (Kwell, Gamene) shampoo should be applied to the affected areas for 5 to 10 minutes, then showered off. A fine-toothed nit comb may be used to remove nits by combing the hairs. The treatment may be repeated once in 5 to 7 days. Eyelash infestations may be treated with careful mechanical removal of nits and lice using a fine forceps. Alternatively, petrolatum[1] may be applied in a thick layer twice a day for a week. Clothing and bedding should be laundered in hot soapy water and mechanically dried for at least 20 minutes. Close contacts should be treated if infested.

Pediculosis Capitis

Head lice move quickly, so one must be alert for sudden movement when parting the hair. The nits are easier to find. The areas of heaviest nit involvement typically are at the occipital scalp. Nits are attached at the bases of hairs. Pruritus with excoriations is usually present. Secondary impetiginization may occur. Because head lice are highly contagious in children, all closely associated children should be treated.

[1]Not FDA approved for this indication.

Rakel and Bope: *Conn's Current Therapy 2006.*

[1]Not FDA approved for this indication.

Permethrin (Nix) is effective as a single-dose treatment. It is applied after shampooing and toweling dry. After 10 minutes it is rinsed out with water. A nit comb is used to remove nits.

Pyrethrin piperonyl butoxide liquid (Rid) is applied to dry hair and then shampooed out after 10 minutes. Because it is less effective as an ovicide, treatment should be repeated once in a week. Nits should be removed using a nit comb.

Lindane (Kwell, Gamene) shampoo has poor ovicidal activity. It is applied in contact with the scalp and hair for 4 minutes, then removed by shampooing. Nit combing must be thorough. Repeat treatments may be necessary.

Pediculosis Corporis

Body lice are most commonly found on vagabonds or in wartime. Because the louse lives in the seams of clothing, it is not often observed on the skin. Typical feeding sites are on the trunk and buttocks. The resulting red papules are often extensively excoriated. Secondary impetiginization is common. Nits and lice should be sought in the seams of clothing for diagnosis.

Laundering or dry cleaning the clothes and bedding kills the lice and nits. After cleansing the skin with soap and water, pruritus may be treated with topical corticosteroid creams and oral antihistamines.

SCABIES

Scabies is a skin infestation by the mite *Sarcoptes scabiei*. The mite lives and breeds in the stratum corneum. Usually the human host does not notice the initial exposure infestation until several weeks have passed. Sensitization to the mite or its scybala (fecal droppings) then results in intense pruritus, accentuated at night. Reinfestation results in pruritus, usually within a day. Because of the asymptomatic initial phase of infestation, close contacts of a scabies patient should be treated even if not symptomatic. A successfully treated patient may continue to experience pruritus for a few weeks after treatment.

The distribution of scabies on the body typically involves the finger webs, wrists, ankles, elbows, axilla, waistline, under the breasts and on the nipples in women, umbilicus, genitalia, and buttocks. Typically, lesions are small red papules, often excoriated. Secondary impetiginization may supervene. Uncommonly, nodules may appear on the genitalia, groin, or axilla. Vesicles can occur, especially in children. A pathognomonic lesion, the burrow, can sometimes be identified as a tiny line on a finger web or lateral finger. Lesions do not ordinarily occur above the neck except in infants and toddlers. If the reaction to scabies has been partially suppressed by topical or systemic corticosteroids, scabies incognito may occur and be difficult to recognize. At the other extreme, a mentally retarded or debilitated or immunocompromised patient may have thick crusted areas and thousands of mites, even burrowing into the fingernails. This condition is known as Norwegian or crusted scabies.

A presumptive diagnosis of scabies can be made from the clinical presentation just described. To confirm the

CURRENT DIAGNOSIS

- Obtain careful travel and exposure histories.
- Consider parasitosis if blood eosinophils are elevated.
- Suspect scabies if skin eruption is highly pruritic.
- Screen for intestinal parasites with stool ova and parasites three times.

diagnosis, using a number 15 scalpel blade dipped in mineral oil, several lesions are scraped down almost to the point of pinpoint bleeding and the scrapings are transferred to a drop of mineral oil on a clean glass slide. After placing a cover slip over the specimen, the slide is examined under a microscope using the 10× or 40× objective. Finding the mite, its eggs, or its scybala (droppings) clinches the diagnosis. Treatment of scabies is generally quite effective. To prevent reinfestation, asymptomatic close contacts should be treated simultaneously. Bed sheets and all clothing worn in the past 3 days should be laundered in hot soapy water or dry cleaned.

Permethrin 5% cream is applied from the neck down and left on overnight for 8 to 12 hours. Reapplication after 5 days is often advisable. If used on infants and toddlers, it should be applied to the head and scalp also.

Lindane 1% lotion is applied from the neck down and left on overnight for 8 to 12 hours. Reapplication after 5 days is often advisable. Lindane should usually be avoided in infants, pregnant women, and epileptics because of its neurotoxicity. Up to 40% of scabies mites may be resistant to lindane.

Precipitated sulfur 6% in petrolatum[1] is applied daily for 3 consecutive days without removal or bathing during the 3-day time interval. Treatment of infants and toddlers should include the face and scalp. This agent is preferred for infants, toddlers, and pregnant women because of its minimal toxicity. Oral ivermectin, 200 µg/kg orally in a single dose, may be useful for crusted scabies or scabies in an immunocompromised host.

TUNGIASIS

The burrowing female flea, *Tunga penetrans*, typically manifests as an erythematous papule with a central

CURRENT THERAPY

- Educate patient how to minimize/avoid future exposure risks.
- Check for patient compliance/reexposure if recommended treatment (see Table 1) failed to obtain cure.
- With resistant or crusted scabies, consider oral ivermectin.
- With recurrent head lice, check for adequate nit removal.

black spot. Location is usually on the foot. Diagnosis is confirmed and treatment is accomplished by surgical removal of the embedded flea.

REFERENCES

Hunter GW, Strickland GT, Magill AJ: Hunter's Tropical Medicine and Emerging Infectious Diseases, 8th ed. Philadelphia, WB Saunders, 1997.
Goddard J: Physician's Guide to Arthropods of Medical Importance, 4th ed. Boca Raton, Fla, CRC Press, 2002.

Fungal Diseases of the Skin

Method of
Adelaide A. Hebert, MD

Fungal infections are caused by organisms that infect keratin-containing tissues such as skin, nails, and hair shafts. The most common organism involved in these processes is a group known as the dermatophytes (*Trichophyton, Microsporum, Epidermophyton*), often referred to as tinea infections, but fungal infections can also be caused by nondermatophytes such as yeast (*Candida*) or *Malassezia* species.

The spores and hyphae of dermatophytes rarely invade growing tissues, confining themselves to the soft keratin composing the skin of the trunk, arms, and ventral feet and hands. For this reason, topical therapeutics can penetrate and cure these cutaneous infections, which include tinea corporis, tinea manuum, tinea faciei, and tinea cruris.

Hair and nails are composed of hard keratin, which topical medications cannot penetrate. Oral therapy must be used for hair and nail involvement, as well as for more chronic or extensive skin involvement.

Diagnosis

Diagnosis is often clinically based, but 20% potassium hydroxide (KOH) preparations for microscopic visualization of hyphae can confirm the diagnosis. In skin and scalp infections, a sample can be obtained by lightly scraping the scaly area with a #15 blade. Nail samples must be acquired by curetting the affected surface of the nail plate, scraping under the nail bed, or taking nail clippings, depending on the region of the nail involved. Fungal cultures are still useful to verify the causative organism, particularly in scalp or nail infections where oral therapy will be required for successful infection control.

TINEA PEDIS

Tinea pedis is the most common fungal infection of the skin in the United States, popularly known as athlete's foot. Most commonly caused by *Trichophyton rubrum*, this infection commonly appears as maceration between the toes with fissuring. Tinea pedis can also involve more diffuse erythema and scaling favoring the plantar surface of the foot (moccasin-type). Differential diagnosis includes contact dermatitis, dyshidrotic eczema, and cellulitis.

TINEA CRURIS

Tinea cruris, or jock itch, affects men more than women, occurring in the groin where there is increased sweating and friction. This condition more often occurs in warm, humid environments or in the summer months; causal organisms include *T. rubrum, Trichophyton mentagrophytes*, or *Epidermophyton floccosum*. The pruritic plaques are well demarcated in the inner thighs, usually sparing the scrotum. This sparing is in contrast to a candidal infection in the groin, which can involve the scrotum. The differential must include psoriasis, seborrheic dermatitis, erythrasma, and candidiasis.

TINEA CORPORIS

Fungal infections can occur on the trunk or extremities and are commonly caused by *T. rubrum*. Characteristic findings include circular lesions with central clearing, but follicular pustules can also be seen. Differential diagnosis includes nummular eczema and pityriasis rosea. Watch for secondary bacterial infections in these cases.

Important note: Cutaneous fungal infections that have been misdiagnosed and treated with topical steroids can have unusual features caused by the reduced inflammation with a loss of defined borders and scale. This condition is known as tinea incognito. In such cases discontinue the use of topical steroids and treat with topical antifungals or appropriate oral therapy if progression is extensive.

TINEA MANUUM

Some patients with tinea pedis may also have involvement of the hands with a diffuse erythema along with fairly well-demarcated scaling. Dry, peeling skin can be slowly progressive and mildly pruritic. Tinea manuum is most often unilateral, and in more acute presentations it may be related to animal or soil contacts. Hand involvement can also mimic eczema, dyshidrosis, keratolysis exfoliativa, or the palmoplantar pustulosis type of psoriasis.

TINEA CAPITIS

Trichophyton tonsurans is the common culprit in scalp fungal infections in the majority of the United States. Tinea capitis is most often seen in children, causing patchy hair loss with scaling and possibly a boggy scalp with tender plaques (kerion). Cervical lymphadenopathy is common in this condition. The differential includes alopecia areata, which has no scale, and seborrheic dermatitis, which may have scaling with minimal to no hair loss. In black-dot tinea capitis, the hair shaft is

CURRENT THERAPY

Treatment of Cutaneous Fungal Infections

	Preferred treatment	Alternatives	Comments or considerations
Dermatophytes			
Tinea pedis	**Systemic:** terbinafine (Lamisil) 250mg/day for 2 wk; itraconazole (Sporanox) 200 mg bid for 2 wk **Topical:** butenafine (Mentax) 1-2 times daily for 2-4 wk	**Systemic:** fluconazole (Diflucan) 150 mg/wk for 4 wk	Topicals can be used concurrently with oral therapy. Prevent recurrence with moisture-absorbing foot powder, wide-toe shoes, and frequent changes of socks and shoes.
Tinea cruris	**Topical:** miconazole, bid, 4 wk clotrimazole, bid, 4 wk econazole, bid, 4 wk	Systemic therapy for resistant cases: **Oral:** griseofulvin ultramicrosized 333 to 500 mg/day for 2 wk; terbinafine 250 mg/day for 2 wk; fluconazole 150 mg once a week for 2-4 wk	Inflamed lesions: butenafine (Mentax) qd for 4 wk.
Tinea corporis	**Topical:** clotrimazole or terbinafine bid for 2 wk **Systemic** (for extensive involvement): itraconazole 200 mg/d 2 wk	**Topical:** miconazole bid, 2 wk **Oral:** terbinafine 250 mg/d 2 wk **Oral:** fluconazole 150 mg once a week for 4 wk	Watch for secondary bacterial infections in these cases.
Tinea capitis	**Systemic:** griseofulvin liquid microsized 20-25 mg/kg/d for 8 wk; griseofulvin pill ultramicrosized 15-20 mg/kg/d for 8 wk	**Systemic:** terbinafine 5mg/kg/d for 4-8 wk	Concurrent topical use of 2% ketoconazole or 1% selenium sulfide shampoo helps kill spores on the hair, decreasing transmission. Topicals should not be used as monotherapy, as systemic therapy is required.
Tinea barbae	**Systemic:** griseofulvin ultramicrosized 500 mg or 330 mg 1-2/d	**Systemic:** itraconazole 200 mg/d for 2-4 wk terbinafine 250 mg/d for 2-4 wk	
Tinea unguium (Onychomycosis)	**Systemic:** terbinafine 250 mg/d for 6 wk (fingernails), 12 wk (toenails)	**Systemic:** itraconazole 400 mg bid for 1 wk, repeat in next 1 to 2 mo fluconazole 300 mg once a week for 6-9 mo	Nails will not look clear after 12 wk; patients must be reassured. Onychomycosis can be caused by Candida alone or in combination with dermatophytes; treat accordingly
Nondermatophytes			
Tinea versicolor	**Topical:** miconazole, clotrimazole, econazole bid for up to 4 wk Selenium sulfide 2.5% lotion; use an antiseborrheic shampoo 2/wk **Systemic:** itraconazole 200 mg/d for 1 wk or ketoconazole (Nizoral) 400 mg once	ketoconazole (Nizoral) be used for 3 d Salicylic acid soap, terbinafine spray	Oral therapy reserved for nonresponsive, extensive involvement Recurrence rates are high Pityrosporum folliculitis, also caused by same *Pityrosporum orbiculare* is treated with similar drugs and dosing

CURRENT THERAPY—cont'd

Treatment of Candidiasis

	Preferred treatment	Alternative	Other considerations
Onychomycosis	**Systemic:** itraconazole 200 mg/d for 3-5 mo	Fluconazole 150-300 mg/wk for 6-12 mo	May have concurrent dermatophyte infection.
Intertriginous candidiasis	**Topical:** miconazole bid for 2 wk nystatin 2-3/d	Clotrimazole bid, 2 wk ketoconazole bid, 2 wk	Water compresses with Burrow's solution to affected areas. Moisture-absorbing powders applied to body folds to prevent recurrence.
Diaper candidiasis, Candidial balanitis	**Topical:** miconazole apply bid 2 wk nystatin (Mycostatin) 2-3/d	Clotrimazole ketoconazole	For concurrent bacterial infections: mupirocin cream or ointment 2% tid for 8 d. For inflammation use 1% hydrocortisone cream.
Vaginal candidiasis	**Systemic:** fluconazole 150 mg once **Topical:** clotrimazole miconazole	Itraconazole 400 mg once	**Topical forms:** creams, ointments and suppositories; depending on patient preference.
Mucocutaneous candidiasis	**Systemic:** fluconazole 150 mg/wk for 4 wk	Clotrimazole lozenges nystatin suspension swish and swallow	

13

brittle and breaks off at the level of the scalp. Differential diagnosis includes seborrheic dermatitis, psoriasis, eczema, poor hygiene, or adherent scalp products such as styling gels.

TINEA BARBAE

In men's beard and mustache areas, a fungal infection is typically unilateral and spares the upper lip. In contrast to the other main differential diagnosis, bacterial folliculitis, tinea barbae is more insidious. The causal organisms include *T. mentagrophytes* and, more rarely, *Trichophyton verrucosum*. Secondary bacterial infection is common and can cause regional lymphadenopathy.

TINEA UNGUIUM (ONYCHOMYCOSIS)

Fungal infections of the nail are more common in adults (affecting approximately 2% of the U.S. population) and can be caused by dermatophyte species (tinea unguium), other fungal species, or yeasts. The most common dermatophytic presentation is the distal lateral subungual type, involving thickened nails with dystrophic edges and yellow to brown discoloration. White superficial onychomycosis produces a dry, soft surface on the nail. Differential diagnosis includes psoriasis, leukonychia, trachyonychia, and onycholysis.

Important note: Onychomycosis can also be caused by various other fungal organisms, including *Candida* species. Concurrent bacterial infection is also a consideration.

OTHER FUNGAL INFECTIONS

Tinea Versicolor

Pityrosporum orbiculare is a normal inhabitant of human skin, but overzealous colonization defines tinea versicolor. Tinea versicolor is common during adolescence and in humid, tropical regions. Generally asymptomatic, the lesions manifest acutely as circular, pink, or hypopigmented scaling macules on the trunk. Chronically, these lesions can become greyish-tan and confluent. Differential diagnosis includes vitiligo, pityriasis alba, pityriasis rosea, and guttate psoriasis. Diagnosis is confirmed with a KOH examination of the scale, which will reveal a characteristic *spaghetti and meatballs* appearance of the hyphae and spores.

Pityrosporum Folliculitis

This is an infection of the hair follicle caused by the yeast *Pityrosporum orbiculare*. The condition causes an itchy, diffuse papulopustular eruption of the upper trunk and shoulders. Differential diagnosis includes acne, bacterial folliculitis, and scabies.

CANDIDIASIS

Most cutaneous candidiasis is caused by the yeast *Candida albicans* infecting skin and mucous membranes. This species is part of normal human flora, growing best in moist, warm areas or where skin touches skin. Pregnancy, diabetes, immunosuppression, and the use of birth control pills, topical steroids, and antibiotics can all predispose to these skin infections. The presentation usually includes pustules with a red, glistening border. A KOH preparation is helpful but not always diagnostic in differentiating these pseudohyphae from dermatophytes.

Intertriginous candidiasis involves skin folds such as the axillae, submammary folds, groin, and perineum areas. Obese and diabetic patients are at particular risk, with moisture, heat, and friction predisposing the skin to these infections.

Diaper dermatitis, diaper rash, appears as erythematous small pustules with similar satellite lesions involving the genitalia, buttocks, and perineum, but characteristically sparing the genitocrural folds. Bacterial superinfection and/or concurrent contact diaper dermatitis can occur. Pseudohyphae can be seen on KOH prep. *Candida*-induced diaper dermatitis must be differentiated from staphylococcus impetigo, atopic dermatitis, or contact diaper dermatitis.

Candidal balanitis involves erythema and vesiculopustules on the glans penis and is especially prevalent in the uncircumcised penis or in cases of poor hygiene. Vulvovaginal candidiasis involves pruritus, burning, and dyspareunia with a creamy white discharge. This vulvovaginitis is common in women taking antibiotics, those in late pregnancy, or those who are diabetic with low vaginal pH.

Oral thrush is a candidal infection in the oropharynx. Dryness or burning of the mouth and/or dysphagia may or may not be present. Thrush is most often associated with immunocompromised states such as HIV infection but may also occur in healthy infants.

Treatment

Griseofulvin and ketoconazole (Nizoral) are the oldest treatments for dermatophyte infections but are becoming less popular because of longer treatment courses with lower cure rates. Despite these drawbacks, griseofulvin, which is fungistatic, is still the drug of choice for tinea capitis. Fat aids in the absorption of griseofulvin, so this medication should be taken with meals or dairy foods.

Ketoconazole (Nizoral) is effective against dermatophyte, *Malassezia,* and *Candida* species and comes in cream, shampoo, and oral tablets. This drug is reserved for recalcitrant cutaneous infections and those unresponsive to topical therapies or oral griseofulvin. Hepatotoxicity is a rare but possible side effect, and liver function should be monitored regularly.

The development of imidazole derivatives has ushered in broad spectrum efficacy. The triazole antifungal itraconazole (Sporanox) is active against dermatophytes, *Candida,* and even some molds. Reversible hepatitis is a risk, and liver function should be monitored in patients with liver problems. Other problems include cardiac side effects (such as congestive heart failure) and multiple drug interactions. Fluconazole (Diflucan) has high oral absorbability and may become a favored alternative for infections previously treated with griseofulvin.

Side effects are usually mild and include nausea and headaches.

Allylamines make up another newer class of antifungals and include naftifine (Naftin) and terbinafine (Lamisil). Some patients taking these medications report taste changes that persist for a period after therapy is concluded. The benzylamine drug butenafine (Mentax) is another option with the added benefit of an anti-inflammatory effect. Mentax is useful for dermatophyte infections with marked inflammatory reactions in the infected tissue.

Ciclopiroxolamine (Loprox) comes in a lotion, cream, or shampoo form for *Candida* and dermatophyte infections of the skin. Ciclopirox 8% (Penlac Nail Lacquer) is the only topical nail treatment approved for infections not involving the lunula, but it must be applied daily for up to a year with only limited cure rates being reported.

Nystatin (Mycostatin) is a polyene available in both oral and topical versions and is only effective for *Candida* infections. *Candida* can also be treated with both topical and oral imidazole derivatives, such as ketoconazole (Nizoral). Ciclopiroxolamine and allylamines such as terbinafine are also effective options.

The key to successful management of dermatophyte, tinea versicolor, and *Candida* infections is to correctly identify the diagnosis prior to initiating therapy. Simple techniques such as KOH examinations and cultures can support clinical findings and validate a diagnosis in most cases. Therapy should be directed at the causative agent with consideration given to the patient's other medical conditions, treatments, and ability to comply with the outlined regimen.

REFERENCES

Aly R, Forney R, Bayles C: Treatments for common superficial fungal infections Dermatol Nurs 2001;12(2):91-94.
Boucher HW, Groll AH, Chiou C, Walsh T: Newer systemic antifungal agents: Pharmacokinetics, safety and efficacy. Drugs, 2004;64(18): 1997-2000.
Chan YC, Freidlander SF: New treatments for tinea capitis. Curr Opin Infect Dis 2004;17:97-103.
Cribier BJ, Bakshi R: Terbinafine in the treatment of onychomycosis: A review of its efficacy in high-risk populations and in patients with nondermatophyte infections. Br J Dermatol 2004;150:414-420.
Foster KW, Ghannoum M, Elewski B: Epidemiologic surveillance of cutaneous fungal infection in the United States from 1999 to 2002. J Am Acad Dermatol 2004;50(5):748-752.
Greenburg HL, Shwayder TA, Bieszk N, Fivenson DP: Clotrimazole/ betamethasone dipropionate: A review of costs and complications in the treatment of common cutaneous fungal infections. Pediatr Dermatol 2002;19(1);78-81.
Grin C: Tinea: Diagnostic clues, treatment keys. Consultant 2004; 44(2):14.
Gupta AK: Systemic antifungal agents. In Wolverton SE (ed): Comprehensive Dermatologic Drug Therapy. Philadelphia, WB Saunders, 2001, pp 55-70.
Gupta AK, Bluhm R: Ciclopirox (Loprox) gel for superficial fungal infections. Skin Therapy Lett 2004;9(7):4-5.
Gupta AK, Chaudhry M, Elewski B: Tinea corporis, tinea cruris, tinea nigra, and piedra. Dermatol Clin 2003;21(3):395-400.
Gupta AK, Ryder J, Summerbell RC: Comparison of efficacy criteria across onychomycosis trials: need for standardization. Int J Dermatol 2003;42;312-315.
Habif et al: Skin disease: Diagnosis and treatment, St. Louis, Mosby, 2001, pp 206-209.
Loeffler J, Stevens DA: Antifungal drug resistance. Clin Infect Dis 2003;36(2):S31.

Rakel and Bope: *Conn's Current Therapy 2006.*

Piraccini BM, Tosti A: White superficial onychomycosis: Epidemiological, clinical and pathological study of 79 patients. Arch Dermatol 2004; 140:696-701.

Vander Straten MR, Hossain MA, Ghannoum MA: Cutaneous infections dermatophytosis, onychomycosis, and tinea versicolor. Infect Dis Clin North Am 2003;17(1):87-112.

Weinstein A, Berman B: Topical treatment of common superficial tinea infections. Am Fam Physician 2002;65(10):2095-2102.

Diseases of the Mouth

Method of
Carl M. Allen, DDS, MSD

A wide variety of disease processes other than dental caries and periodontal disease affect the oral region. These diseases may be classified based on the etiopathogenesis of the disease (e.g., viral, neoplastic); the clinical form of the lesions (e.g., plaque, vesicle, ulcer); or the anatomic region affected (e.g., lips, buccal mucosa). The clinical form and anatomic region are particularly useful for the clinician confronted by an unknown lesion. An accurate diagnosis is the most important aspect of patient management because treatment is predicated on diagnosis. The lesions that tend to affect certain oral mucosal sites preferentially are listed here according to their frequency; space limitations prohibit discussion of rare entities.

Generalized Oral Involvement

Xerostomia is the subjective feeling of a dry mouth. In most instances, it is caused by any of a variety of medications (antihypertensives, antihistamines, psychoactive drugs), and withdrawal or substitution of the medication may be helpful. A smaller number of patients may have xerostomia secondary to autoimmune destruction of the salivary gland tissue (Sjögren's syndrome) or caused by radiation therapy of the head and neck region. Such patients may develop a number of problems. The mucosa is not as well lubricated and becomes susceptible to traumatic ulceration. The dry environment predisposes the individual to the erythematous or angular cheilitis forms of oral candidiasis. If the patient has natural teeth, a marked increase in dental caries is noted.

A number of over-the-counter artificial saliva substitutes, in both liquid and gel form, are available to help manage the symptoms of dryness. Oral ulcerations should be managed conservatively using a protective hydroxypropylcellulose medication (Zilactin),[1] applied as often as necessary. Oral candidiasis can be treated with any of several antifungal medications, although

those with high sucrose content, such as nystatin pastilles (Mycostatin Oral Pastilles), should probably be avoided in dentulous patients because these agents could contribute to caries activity. A prescription-strength topical fluoride preparation, such as 1.1% neutral sodium fluoride gel (PreviDent), should be used daily by patients who have natural teeth to prevent dental decay. Application of the topical fluoride is best performed at night after brushing the teeth and before retiring. Several drops of the fluoride gel should be placed on the toothbrush and gently massaged onto the surfaces of the teeth next to the gum tissue.

Lips

COMMON CONDITIONS

Fordyce's Granules

Fordyce's granules, a variation of normal anatomy, are heterotopic sebaceous glands seen in more than 80% of adults. They occur as 1-mm yellow-white submucosal dots distributed on the lateral upper lip and the buccal mucosa. No treatment is indicated because of the completely benign nature of the condition.

Angular Cheilitis

Angular cheilitis is characterized by inflammation of the corners of the mouth, accompanied by fissuring and sometimes scaling. This condition was thought to be caused by B vitamin deficiency, but the vast majority of these lesions are now thought to be caused by a low-grade infection of *Candida albicans*, with or without *Staphylococcus aureus*.

These lesions can be easily treated with a topical antifungal agent such as nystatin-triamcinolone cream (Mycolog-II Cream). Another alternative is iodoquinol-hydrocortisone cream (Vytone Cream),[1] which is both antifungal and antibacterial but must be used externally. Either medication should be applied three to four times daily for at least 1 week. With recurrence, a careful search for an intraoral source of infection may be indicated, and the possibility of HIV infection may need to be ruled out. Angular cheilitis with associated intraoral candidiasis requires treatment. Topical agents include clotrimazole troches (Mycelex Oral Troches) and nystatin pastilles, each dissolved in the mouth four to five times daily for 7 to 10 days. Systemic therapy with fluconazole (Diflucan) may be more convenient for some patients because it is given orally, 200 mg the first day, followed by 100 mg daily for the next 6 days.

Herpes Labialis

Recurrent herpes labialis affects approximately 25% of the population. Reactivation of the virus is usually triggered by sun (ultraviolet light) exposure, with many patients experiencing an itching or tingling sensation in the prodromal phase. A cluster of vesicles then develops

[1]Not FDA approved for this indication.

13

on the vermilion zone of the lip or on perioral skin, rupturing within 1 to 3 days and leaving a crusted area that resolves after a few more days.

No curative therapy exists for this condition, and treatment results may be difficult to interpret because of the strong placebo effect in some instances. High sun protection factor (SPF) sun-blocking agents significantly reduce the frequency of episodes triggered by exposure to ultraviolet light. Low-dose acyclovir (Zovirax)[1] or valacyclovir (Valtrex)[1] may prevent attacks if it is taken continuously (400 mg twice daily; 1 g per day, respectively), but attacks resume as usual once the medication is stopped. Systemic valacyclovir, 2-g doses 12 hours apart given during the prodromal phase, reduces lesion formation in a subset of individuals affected by this condition. Topical acyclovir ointment shows no benefit in double-blind, placebo-controlled trials in immunocompetent patients, whereas topical penciclovir cream (Denavir) has only a modest effect on the course of the lesions.

Melanotic Macule

Melanotic macule, a solitary lesion, usually develops on the vermilion zone of the lips, but it may be seen intraorally. The lesion occurs as a 1- to 5-mm macule that exhibits a uniform, well-demarcated brown to black color.

If the patient indicates the lesion has been present for several years and has not observed any change in size or color, no treatment is indicated unless the patient is concerned about cosmetic appearance. If changes in the lesion are recent, excisional biopsy is indicated to rule out the possibility of an early melanoma.

Actinic Keratosis (Cheilitis)

Actinic keratosis is a premalignant process affecting the lower vermilion zone of the lip of fair-skinned adults with a history of chronic sun exposure. The lesions have a scaly texture and ill-defined margins.

Excision, by either scalpel or laser, or cryosurgery is indicated for treatment. Excision is often accomplished by vermilionectomy, in which the entire vermilion zone is removed as a strip for histopathologic examination. The labial mucosa is then advanced over the resulting defect. When topical chemotherapy with fluorouracil (Efudex) is used, dysplastic epithelial cells persist histologically. All patients with sun-damaged lips should be advised to use a sunscreen with high SPF, applied particularly to the lower lip when sun exposure is anticipated.

UNCOMMON CONDITIONS

Squamous Cell Carcinoma

The malignancy of squamous cell carcinoma affects the lower vermilion zone, typically arising in a preexisting actinic keratosis. Such lesions usually have a relatively slow, steady growth, with a roughened or ulcerated surface. The diagnosis should be established by biopsy.

[1]Not FDA approved for this indication.

Wide surgical excision, obtaining at least a 1-cm margin of normal tissue, is usually adequate treatment because these lesions are rather indolent and do not metastasize until relatively late in their course.

Reactive Cheilitis

Patients may present occasionally with a complaint of fissured, painful lips. Evaluation of the problem should include a history of onset, duration, and use of medications and cosmetics. Lipstick and artificially flavored cinnamon products may produce a contact cheilitis. Isotretinoin (Accutane) often causes exfoliative cheilitis. Solitary chronic lip fissures, which usually occur in the winter months, may respond to topical antibiotic preparations, with surgical excision reserved for resistant lesions. Many cases of reactive cheilitis appear to be factitial, although patients may be reluctant to admit their habit of licking and nibbling at the vermilion zone. Constant moistening of the lips also predisposes the individual to a superimposed candidal infection, which exacerbates the inflammatory symptoms, and petrolatum-based lip balms may contribute to the problem by trapping moisture and thereby promoting the growth of yeast.

Telangiectasias

Superficial dilated blood vessels may occur on the vermilion zone of the lips as an isolated finding or, if multiple, as a component of either hereditary hemorrhagic telangiectasia or CREST (calcinosis, Raynaud's phenomenon, esophageal dysfunction, sclerodactyly, and telangiectasias) syndrome. Patients should be evaluated to distinguish between these two entities because their prognoses are different. Treatment of the telangiectatic lesions can be performed by laser excision, cryotherapy, or electrodesiccation.

Labial Mucosa

COMMON CONDITIONS

Mucocele

The mucocele represents a collection of extravasated mucin within the submucosal connective tissue caused by the disruption of a minor salivary gland duct by minor trauma. Most mucoceles develop on the lower labial mucosa, appearing suddenly as a painless, soft, bluish, circumscribed swelling. A cycle of swelling, breaking, and swelling again is typical. Surgical excision of the mucous deposit and the associated gland usually is necessary for resolution of the problem.

Varix

The varix, similar to varicose veins of the leg, is seen on the labial mucosa, lips, buccal mucosa, and tongue of patients older than 50 years. Patients usually describe the gradual onset of a painless purplish or bluish nodule.

Generally, no treatment is indicated. If the lesion is a cosmetic problem or if it occurs in areas likely to be traumatized, the varix may be treated by surgical excision or cryotherapy.

Aphthous Ulcer (Canker Sore)

The aphthous ulcer is perhaps one of the most misdiagnosed, mismanaged, and misunderstood of all oral diseases. Most authorities believe that aphthous ulcers are immunologically induced. No convincing scientific data link the process to viral infection. Furthermore, studies suggesting the lesions are associated with certain foods or vitamin deficiencies have not been duplicated. Several mechanisms may initiate the abnormal immune response leading to focal destruction of the oral mucosa. The lesions are typically recurrent, ranging from 1 to 24 episodes per year. The most common form of aphthous ulcer is the minor aphthous ulcer, manifesting as a 1- to 10-mm ulceration with an erythematous periphery and smooth borders. From one to five ulcers may develop simultaneously. Aphthous ulcers are located on movable mucosa, not mucosa bound to periosteum, a situation directly opposite to recurrent intraoral herpes. The patient typically reports pain that seems out of proportion to the size of the lesion. With no treatment, minor aphthae heal within 5 to 10 days. Patients with frequent attacks should be questioned regarding ocular complaints or genital ulcerations to rule out Behçet's syndrome. Infrequently, aphthous-like oral ulcerations may be a manifestation of Crohn's disease as well.

Topical application of a relatively strong corticosteroid, such as fluocinonide (Lidex Gel),[1] betamethasone dipropionate (Diprolene Gel),[1] or clobetasol (Temovate Gel),[1] is most effective in controlling the lesions. For optimum response, small amounts of the medication should be applied as a thin film often (four to five times daily) and as early in the course of the lesion as possible.

UNCOMMON CONDITIONS

Major Aphthous Ulcers

Major aphthae are debilitating oral lesions that resemble minor aphthae, except they are much larger (ranging up to 3 cm), and they persist for periods of up to 6 weeks before healing. Topical application of fluocinonide,[1] betamethasone dipropionate,[1] or clobetasol[1] usually controls this process. If the lesions are in the posterior segments of the mouth, betamethasone syrup (Celestone Syrup),[1] used as a mouth rinse and swallowed (10 mL after meals and at bedtime for 7 to 10 days), often provides relief.

Herpetiform Aphthous Ulcers

Herpetiform aphthous ulcers resemble primary herpetic gingivostomatitis, and they can be distinguished from that condition by their history of recurrence. Herpetiform aphthae are most effectively treated with one of the topical corticosteroid preparations or rinses described earlier.

---

[1]Not FDA approved for this indication.

Rakel and Bope: *Conn's Current Therapy 2006.*

Angioedema

Angioedema is thought to occur because of localized release of histamine from mast cells. Most cases are sporadic and harmless. The lips are most frequently affected, followed by the tongue. A tingling sensation usually precedes the sudden onset of rather dramatic, nontender swelling. The overlying skin appears normal, and the patient is otherwise asymptomatic; these features should help distinguish this condition from cellulitis associated with a dentoalveolar abscess. With no treatment, the condition resolves in 24 to 48 hours; however, oral antihistamine therapy seems to speed resolution. Attacks are commonly recurrent, and the precipitating factor is often difficult to identify. A rare hereditary form, caused by a deficiency of C1 esterase inhibitor, can be life-threatening if the laryngeal tissues are involved. With persistent swelling, biopsy may be indicated to rule out relatively rare conditions such as orofacial granulomatosis (cheilitis granulomatosa, Melkersson-Rosenthal syndrome).

Buccal Mucosa

COMMON CONDITIONS

Linea Alba

The oral linea alba merely represents a mild thickening of the epithelium along the plane of occlusion in dentate patients. The extent to which it is evident varies tremendously from patient to patient. No treatment is indicated for this completely benign condition.

Leukoedema

Leukoedema is considered a variation of normal. Clinically, it has a whitish, filmy, almost opalescent appearance, usually affecting the buccal mucosa. Stretching the mucosa causes the white appearance to diminish greatly or disappear completely. The surface epithelial cells histologically are edematous but otherwise normal, and no treatment is necessary for this benign condition.

Cheek-Chewing

Cheek-chewing is a harmless chronic habit. Although the anterior buccal mucosa is the most common site, the labial mucosa and lateral tongue may also be affected. A white, ragged alteration of the mucosa is seen clinically. Actual ulceration is uncommon because only the outer layers of the epithelium (which have no nerve fibers) are nibbled. The patient usually admits to the habit if questioned. This habit is completely benign and requires no further management once it is identified.

Fibroma (Irritation Fibroma, Focal Fibrous Hyperplasia)

The fibroma represents an accumulation of dense collagenous connective tissue at a site of irritation.

13

For this reason, most of these lesions are found on the buccal mucosa. The lesion appears clinically as a sessile, dome-shaped, smooth-surfaced nodule. Patients may complain because they bite the lesion inadvertently.

Because this lesion cannot be definitively differentiated clinically from a wide array of other neoplasms, excisional biopsy is generally indicated. Recurrence is uncommon.

Lichen Planus

Lichen planus is an immunologically mediated condition of unknown cause that affects adults. The oral lesions manifest in two patterns: reticular and erosive. The reticular pattern is more common and usually seen bilaterally on the posterior buccal mucosa, occurring as white fine interlacing lines or papules. The gingivae and the tongue may also be affected. The erosive form of the condition is symptomatic because of the presence of ulcerations. These ulcerations usually have a central yellow-white area of fibrin surrounded by an erythematous halo and radiating white striae.

Reticular lichen planus requires no treatment. In 20% of cases, candidiasis is present, which should be treated with an antifungal agent. Erosive lichen planus can usually be managed effectively with the more potent topical corticosteroids such as fluocinonide,[1] betamethasone dipropionate,[1] or clobetasol.[1] Application of a thin film of medication to the lesional areas, four to five times daily, often resolves the ulcers within a few days. Other conditions, such as epithelial dysplasia, lichenoid amalgam reactions, contact stomatitis, lichenoid drug reactions, and systemic lupus erythematosus, may mimic lichen planus clinically; biopsy is thus warranted if classic clinical features are not present. Malignant transformation of reticular lichen planus is not thought likely, although erosive lichen planus could possibly be premalignant. Affected patients should be reevaluated periodically for evidence of significant mucosal change, with rebiopsy performed if necessary.

UNCOMMON CONDITIONS

Verrucous Carcinoma

Verrucous carcinoma is a relatively low-grade malignancy of surface epithelial origin. It appears as a diffuse, white, rough-surfaced, spreading plaquelike lesion affecting the buccal mucosa, palate, or alveolar process in patients over 65 years of age.

Treatment is complete surgical excision, via scalpel or laser, with evaluation of the lesional tissue histopathologically because 25% of verrucous carcinomas may contain foci of routine squamous cell carcinoma. The prognosis is generally good because this lesion does not metastasize.

---

[1]Not FDA approved for this indication.

Oral Mucosal Cinnamon Reaction

The oral mucosal cinnamon reaction affects the buccal mucosa, the lateral tongue, and gingivae. The lesions appear as diffuse areas of mucosal erythema with varying degrees of superimposed white plaques and, less commonly, ulceration. Such lesions may be mistaken clinically for lichen planus, candidiasis, leukoplakia, or erythroplakia. Discontinuing the artificially flavored cinnamon product (usually chewing gum) resolves the lesions within 1 week. The diagnosis can be confirmed by challenging the oral mucosa with the offending agent, although patients are often reluctant to do so after their lesions clear.

Hard Palate

COMMON CONDITIONS

Torus

Palatal tori are common developmental lesions representing a benign accumulation of dense bone in the midline posterior hard palate region. The diagnosis can be made clinically because no other condition manifests as a bony hard midline palatal mass. No treatment is necessary for this benign process, although denture construction may be hampered. Removal of the torus by an oral surgeon is recommended in that situation.

Denture Stomatitis

Denture stomatitis is almost invariably associated with a maxillary removable denture worn 24 hours per day. The palatal mucosa directly beneath the denture appears red, although it is asymptomatic. The redness is confined to the denture-bearing mucosa.

In many cases, simply having the patient remove the denture at night may resolve the palatal erythema. If the patient has a complete upper denture, it can be soaked in a mild sodium hypochlorite solution (Clorox) (1 teaspoon in 8 ounces of water) each night for a week to disinfect it. (Note: Chrome-cobalt metal denture frameworks should not be soaked in Clorox; severe corrosion will result and ruin the denture.) Because denture stomatitis is a benign and asymptomatic condition, treatment need not be a top priority.

Inflammatory Papillary Hyperplasia

Inflammatory papillary hyperplasia (IPH) (denture papillomatosis) is seen almost exclusively in patients who wear ill-fitting complete upper dentures. The lesions appear as multiple, erythematous 1- to 2-mm papules typically confined to the palatal vault area. These papules are composed of dense fibrous connective tissue that has accumulated secondary to chronic irritation in the superficial mucosa.

Treatment of this benign process is somewhat controversial. Some prosthodontists prefer to have these lesions surgically removed prior to constructing a new denture, although this procedure may not be necessary in every case.

UNCOMMON CONDITIONS

Recurrent Intraoral Herpes

Recurrent intraoral herpes is much less common than aphthous ulcerations, a condition with which it is frequently confused. Recurrent intraoral herpes affects only the hard palate and the attached gingiva (the paler firm gum tissue directly adjacent to the teeth). Most patients experience mild symptoms and may give a history of recurrent episodes. Lesions appear as a cluster of 1- to 2-mm shallow ulcerations that heal within 1 week. Generally no treatment is necessary, although the patient should be cautioned that virus is being shed from the lesion.

Salivary Gland Tumors

The posterior hard palate/anterior soft palate region is the most common site for the development of intraoral salivary gland neoplasia. This type of lesion presents as a slowly growing, rubbery firm, nontender mass that may or may not be ulcerated. The clinical appearance does not distinguish benign form malignant tumors, so a biopsy should be obtained that includes a margin of normal adjacent tissue. Approximately 50% of these tumors are pleomorphic adenomas, whereas the remainder represent mucoepidermoid carcinoma, polymorphous low-grade adenocarcinoma, adenoid cystic carcinoma, or acinic cell carcinoma. Complete excision is recommended for the pleomorphic adenoma, including overlying mucosa and underlying periosteum. The malignancies should be treated with a much more aggressive surgical approach, depending on the histologic type, the extent of bone involvement, and the size of the lesion. Adjunctive radiation therapy may be indicated for adenoid cystic carcinoma and high-grade mucoepidermoid carcinoma.

Soft Palate/Tonsillar Pillars

COMMON CONDITIONS

Papilloma

The squamous papilloma is the most common benign epithelial neoplasm that affects the oral mucosa, typically occurring as a solitary exophytic growth with numerous finger-like or frondlike projections on its surface. The soft palate/tonsillar pillar region is the most common site for the papilloma, and its color may range from pink to white.

Excisional biopsy, including the base of the lesion, should be performed. For those lesions of the posterior soft palate, periodic observation may be appropriate, particularly if the patient is experiencing no symptoms and the lesion is clinically characteristic.

UNCOMMON CONDITIONS

Pemphigus Vulgaris

Pemphigus vulgaris is an immunologically mediated condition characterized by the formation of vesicles and bullae secondary to attack of desmosomal complexes of the surface epithelium by autoantibodies. The condition usually is first seen intraorally, with painful, erosive lesions distributed diffusely on the oral mucosa. The soft palate is a primary site of involvement. Diagnosis should be established by light microscopy with direct and indirect immunofluorescence studies. Systemic immunosuppressive therapy is necessary to control this condition addressed in other areas of the text.

Tongue

COMMON CONDITIONS

Coated and Hairy Tongue

Coated and hairy tongue represents the accumulation of excess keratin on the filiform papillae of the dorsal tongue, resulting in the formation of elongated filamentous strands that superficially resemble hairs. Contrary to the description in numerous textbooks, this condition is not caused by an overgrowth of yeast.

No treatment is required, but if the patient is concerned about the appearance of the tongue, gentle daily débridement with a tongue scraper or the edge of a spoon assists in removing the accumulations of dead keratinized cells.

Fissured Tongue

Fissured tongue is essentially a variation of normal that usually develops sometime after the first decade of life. The patient may be concerned about the appearance of the tongue, but no symptoms are associated with the condition. The extent and pattern of fissuring can vary, and no treatment is indicated.

Benign Migratory Glossitis (Erythema Migrans, Geographic Tongue)

Benign migratory glossitis, a condition of unknown etiology, is seen in approximately 2% of the population. Most patients are asymptomatic, with lesions detected on routine examination. The dorsal tongue exhibits one or more well-demarcated zones of papillary atrophy that are surrounded, at least partially, by yellow-white slightly raised linear serpentine borders. The lesions typically resolve in one area and move to another, appearing in various stages of resolution and activity concurrently.

Because this is a benign condition, treatment is usually unnecessary. Approximately 5% of patients complain of sensitivity to hot or spicy foods when their lesions are active, but usually they do not require treatment. With severe symptoms, topical fluocinonide

(Lidex Gel)[1] or one of the other stronger topical corticosteroids, applied as a thin film to the lesions several times daily, seems to reduce the discomfort.

Traumatic Ulcer

The traumatic ulcer occurs most frequently on the lateral tongue, buccal mucosa, and overlying bony prominences such as tori and exostoses. Most of these lesions are associated with relatively little pain. The traumatic ulcer manifests clinically as a defect covered by creamy white fibrin. Although most of these lesions heal within a week or so, some tend to persist, developing a rolled margin and peripheral induration.

Often no treatment is required because of the minimal degree of discomfort and the rapid healing time. If the patient complains of tenderness when eating salty or acidic foods, a protective medication (Zilactin) can be applied as needed. Topical corticosteroids should probably not be used because they may delay healing in this situation. If an ulcer is present for longer than 2 weeks, with or without previous treatment, a biopsy is mandatory to rule out malignancy. A possible exception to this rule might be those ulcers overlying tori because they are notoriously difficult to resolve.

Burning Tongue Syndrome (Idiopathic Glossopyrosis)

The burning tongue syndrome seems to affect postmenopausal women predominantly. The patient often reports the rather sudden onset of a sensation that feels like the tongue was scalded. Symptoms are usually localized to the anterior tongue, although the labial mucosa and anterior hard palate may also be affected. Clinically, the mucosa appears normal. If mucosal erythema is identified, a variety of conditions should be ruled out, including candidiasis, anemia, local trauma, and erythema migrans. A culture for *Candida albicans* should be performed. If the workup shows no evidence of these conditions, a diagnosis of burning tongue syndrome can be made. Because there is no medically proven therapy, no specific treatment exists. The numerous suggested treatments in the literature have generally not been examined in controlled trials, and their efficacy is typically no more than that of the placebo effect. Reassuring patients this is a harmless condition, nothing more than a nuisance, and that the condition often resolves spontaneously after a period of months or years is usually sufficient.

UNCOMMON CONDITIONS

Squamous Cell Carcinoma

The lateral/ventral tongue is one of the most common sites for squamous cell carcinoma. In the early stages, the lesion is relatively asymptomatic, which underscores the importance of a regular and thorough oral mucosal examination. Slight thickening or nodularity within a white or red plaque frequently heralds the onset of invasion. As the lesion grows, the surface becomes ulcerated and symptoms of pain and tenderness develop. On palpation, squamous cell carcinomas are usually firm and show infiltrative borders. Biopsy is mandatory because other chronic ulcerative processes, such as chronic traumatic ulcer, deep fungal infections, mycobacterial infections, Wegener's granulomatosis, and other malignancies, may have a similar clinical presentation.

Treatment consists of wide surgical resection or radical radiation therapy, or both, depending on a number of factors. Prognosis is directly related to the tumor stage, although, in general, these patients do poorly because their lesions are not diagnosed until the later stages.

Hairy Leukoplakia

Hairy leukoplakia is an HIV-related lesion, significant because it often heralds a rapid decline in the patient's immune status. The lesion affects the lateral borders of the tongue, usually bilaterally, appearing as white plaques with vertical streaks. Sometimes the degree of keratinization may be great enough to produce hairlike projections, hence the name. Because this is otherwise a benign condition, no treatment is necessary. Hairy leukoplakia is caused by Epstein-Barr virus, thus medications used against other herpes viruses, such as acyclovir (Zovirax),[1] valacyclovir (Valtrex),[1] and dihydroxypropoxymethyl guanine (DHPG) (ganciclovir [Cytovene]),[1] may produce transient resolution.

Herpes in the Immunocompromised Host

With an immunocompromised host, the normal rules governing the location of the lesions of recurrent herpes are not applicable. The virus is not contained by the host, as in the normal individual, and the result is the formation of large, shallow, painful ulcerations with slightly elevated serpentine or scalloped margins. The diagnosis should be established by exfoliative cytology or viral culture, and treatment should be instituted immediately with systemic acyclovir, orally or intravenously, depending on the severity of the clinical infection.

Macroglossia

Macroglossia is the term used to describe enlargement of the tongue. Among the more frequent causes of macroglossia are hemangiomas and lymphangiomas. Hemangiomas are usually present at birth or develop shortly thereafter, with the tongue the most common site. These lesions are typically red or purple in color. If no compromise in function of the involved tissue is seen, treatment should be delayed until the child is older than 6 years of age because many of these lesions regress spontaneously. For those lesions that do not regress, argon laser excision is the optimal therapy. Other methods of management include cryotherapy and sclerosing agents.

---

[1]Not FDA approved for this indication.

[1]Not FDA approved for this indication.

Lymphangiomas affecting the oral tissues often exhibit a characteristic so-called frog-egg or tapioca-pudding surface morphology because of the dilated lymphatic vessels that are close to the surface. Treatment is surgical excision, although the decision to treat may depend on the size and site of the lesion. Recurrence rates as high as 40% are reported in some series of cases.

Other causes of macroglossia are much less common and include amyloidosis as well as benign and malignant tumors. Biopsy would be indicated to establish a diagnosis prior to treatment planning.

Floor of the Mouth

COMMON CONDITIONS

Leukoplakia

Leukoplakia is a clinical term that should be applied only to those white patches of the oral mucosa that cannot be wiped off and cannot be diagnosed as any other condition clinically. Leukoplakia is considered a premalignant condition and usually diagnosed in the sixth and seventh decades of life. Clinically, the condition appears as a well-defined white plaque that may show varying degrees of redness. The most worrisome sites of involvement include areas prone to cancer development, such as the lateral tongue, floor of the mouth, and the tonsillar pillar region.

Ideally, treatment is complete removal with microscopic evaluation of the excised specimen. Cryotherapy and laser excision may be used, but tissue may be rendered unsuitable for histopathologic examination. More concern should be given to leukoplakias found in nonsmokers, in high-risk areas for oral cancer, in lesions with a red component, in multifocal lesions, or those found in patients 20 to 50 years of age. If complete excision is accomplished, 30% of leukoplakias still recur, so careful follow-up with rebiopsy is indicated.

Sialolithiasis

Sialolithiasis (salivary duct stones) may appear with symptoms or be discovered on routine examination. The classic presentation is sudden painful unilateral swelling of the involved salivary gland occurring at mealtime. Most stones involve the submandibular gland, and these can be palpated as a hard submucosal mass in the floor of the mouth. Treatment usually involves surgical removal of the stone with repositioning of the salivary duct opening proximally. Sialography should then be performed to assess the function of the gland, and if it appears abnormal, it should probably be removed to prevent subsequent episodes of chronic recurrent sialadenitis.

UNCOMMON CONDITIONS

Erythroplakia

The premalignant lesion of erythroplakia represents the nonkeratinized version of leukoplakia. Erythroplakia appears as a well-demarcated, velvety red plaque that is

typically asymptomatic. Dysplastic changes are likely, and treatment should consist of complete removal by the most expedient means.

Squamous Cell Carcinoma

The clinical appearance of squamous cell carcinoma at this site is similar to that of the lateral tongue, as is the treatment.

Alveolar Process/Gingiva

COMMON CONDITIONS

Mandibular Tori/Exostoses

Mandibular tori/exostoses are benign developmental lesions that consist of dense, viable bone. Mandibular tori are located on the lingual surface of the mandible in the premolar region, whereas exostoses occur on the alveolar process in other sites. Radiographic evaluation of any asymmetric bony swelling is indicated, and the exostosis should appear as a well-defined radiopacity. Generally, no treatment is necessary unless the bony outgrowths interfere with denture construction, in which case surgical removal is indicated.

Amalgam Tattoo

The amalgam tattoo is produced by the iatrogenic implantation of dental amalgam into the oral soft tissues. Amalgam tattoos are usually macular and range in color from gray to blue to black or brown. Periapical radiographs often show the fine radiopaque metallic particles.

No treatment is necessary if the diagnosis can be made definitively from the radiograph. If no radiopacity is seen, biopsy is generally indicated to rule out a relatively rare oral melanocytic process such as a nevus or melanoma.

Dental Sinus Tract (Parulis)

The lesion of the dental sinus tract (parulis) represents a proliferation of granulation tissue at the drainage site of a sinus tract originating form the apical root portion of a nonvital tooth. Clinically, the parulis appears as an erythematous papule on the alveolar mucosa. Symptoms of pain may wax and wane. Treatment consists of either extraction or endodontic therapy for the offending tooth, and the prognosis is good.

Acute Necrotizing Ulcerative Gingivitis (Trench Mouth, Vincent's Infection)

Acute necrotizing ulcerative gingivitis is a disease produced by bacteria that are normal inhabitants of the oral microflora. The condition, which occurs in the third or fourth decade of life, is associated with poor oral hygiene, poor diet, and stress. College students are especially vulnerable during final examinations, and the condition may be seen in HIV-positive patients as well. Patients invariably present with a complaint of painful, foul-smelling gingivae. Examination shows punched-out ulceration of the interdental papillae. Acute necrotizing ulcerative gingivitis is frequently confused with primary herpes, which also is associated with pain and ulceration, but the punched-out interdental papillae are not seen in herpes infection.

Débridement, often requiring topical or local anesthesia, or both, is very important. This should be combined with systemic antibiotic therapy, such as tetracycline,[1] 250 mg every 6 hours, or potassium penicillin V, 500 mg every 6 hours. HIV-infected patients should also use chlorhexidine (Peridex) mouth rinse twice daily to prevent recurrence of acute necrotizing ulcerative gingivitis. For non-HIV patients, the prognosis is reasonably good, assuming they improve their diet and oral hygiene status.

Primary Herpetic Gingivostomatitis

Primary herpetic gingivostomatitis is caused by the initial exposure of the patient to herpes simplex virus, usually type I. Most of these infections occur during childhood, but occasionally an individual escapes contact with the virus until adulthood. Patients present with fever, cervical lymphadenopathy, malaise, and oropharyngeal pain. Examination of the oral mucosa reveals multiple shallow ulcerations distributed diffusely throughout the mouth, although the gingivae are often markedly affected. The gingival involvement is different from that of acute necrotizing ulcerative gingivitis, in that the interdental papillae do not show the punched-out ulcerations with the herpetic infection.

Patients should be managed symptomatically with analgesics, antipyretics, and topical anesthetics as indicated. Dehydration is sometimes a problem if oral pain prevents intake of fluids. Having the patient rinse with 5 mL of viscous lidocaine (Xylocaine Viscous) or dyclonine HCl (Dyclone) prior to meals provides temporary relief. Systemic acyclovir (Zovirax)[1] or valacyclovir (Valtrex)[1] may have a significant impact on the course of this disease if given during the first few days of the infection.

Inflammatory Fibrous Hyperplasia (Denture Epulis, Epulis Fissuratum, Denture Fibroma)

Inflammatory fibrous hyperplasia is caused by low-grade irritation from an ill-fitting denture. Clinically, the lesions are seen as smooth-surfaced sessile masses that appear to arise from the mucosa of the alveolar process or vestibule. Sometimes a groove or fissure runs lengthwise across the lesion, corresponding to the denture flange. Ulceration of the surface may be seen.

Surgical excision of the lesion is indicated prior to construction of new dentures. If the lesion is removed and the patient continues to wear the old denture, inflammatory fibrous hyperplasia recurs, but it is a completely benign process that does not undergo malignant transformation.

---

[1]Not FDA approved for this indication.

UNCOMMON CONDITIONS

Pyogenic Granuloma, Peripheral Giant Cell Granuloma, and Peripheral Ossifying Fibroma

Pyogenic granuloma, peripheral giant cell granuloma, and peripheral ossifying fibroma are benign gingival lesions probably initiated by chronic irritation in most instances. Although they are histologically distinctive, their clinical appearance and biologic behavior are similar. All of these lesions appear as sessile, dome-shaped masses that develop mainly on the gingiva (although pyogenic granuloma may be seen on any surface). They range from pink to reddish purple in color and are often ulcerated. Excisional biopsy is recommended to rule out the less likely possibility of metastatic neoplasm, which may clinically appear very similar. A recurrence rate of 15% can be expected for each of these lesions.

Generalized Gingival Hyperplasia

Generalized gingival hyperplasia usually develops as a side effect of medication: phenytoin (Dilantin), calcium channel blocking agents, or cyclosporine (Sandimmune). Only 30% to 50% of patients receiving one of these drugs show the diffuse gingival enlargement, which is usually related to the level of oral hygiene of the patient. If the drug cannot be discontinued or substituted, periodic periodontal surgery with reinforcement of oral hygiene instruction can usually control the problem. Rarely such enlargement may be associated with any of several genetic syndromes. These patients typically require periodic surgical reduction of the gingival tissues by a periodontist. Generalized gingival hyperplasia may also be a manifestation of myelomonocytic leukemia, although these patients usually complain of other signs and symptoms related to their leukemic state. Biopsy and appropriate hematologic evaluation are necessary to establish a diagnosis.

Desquamative Gingivitis

Desquamative gingivitis is a descriptive term for a reaction pattern that affects the gingival tissues of adults. Patients complain of red, tender gingival mucosa that has a tendency to slough with minor manipulation. Vesicles may sometimes be reported. This condition must be biopsied for light microscopic evaluation as well as direct immunofluorescence studies because it invariably represents one of several distinct entities: erosive lichen planus, cicatricial pemphigoid, linear IgA disease, pemphigus vulgaris, or chronic ulcerative stomatitis. Once the definitive diagnosis is established, the patient can be managed appropriately.

REFERENCES

Neville BW, Damm DD, Allen CM, Bouquot JE: Oral and Maxillofacial Pathology, 2nd ed. Philadelphia, Elsevier Science, 2002.
Neville BW, Day TA: Oral cancer and precancerous lesions. CA Cancer J Clin 2002;52:195-215.
Regezi JA, Sciubba JJ, Jordan RCK: Oral Pathology. Clinical Pathologic Correlations, 4th ed. Philadelphia, Elsevier Science, 2003.

Sapp JP, Eversole LR, Wysocki GP: Contemporary Oral and Maxillofacial Pathology, 2nd ed. Philadelphia, Elsevier Science, 2004.

Scully C, Gorsky M, Lozada-Nur F: The diagnosis and management of recurrent aphthous stomatitis: A consensus approach. J Am Dent Assoc 2003;134:200-207.

Venous Ulcers

Method of
Markéta Límová, MD

Leg ulcers caused by venous insufficiency present a significant problem worldwide. Although the exact prevalence is unknown, in some studies it is reported to affect up to 1% of the general population. In the United States, the estimates range from 600,000 to 2.5 million patients. Although the differential diagnosis of leg ulcers is rather lengthy, the overwhelming majority of these ulcers are caused by venous insufficiency (70% to 90%). Box 1 lists arterial insufficiency (10% to 20%), neuropathy (5% to 10%), and other less common causes. Many patients have more than one contributing factor and the etiologies overlap. In many cases, one condition leads to the development of ulceration (trauma, surgery, vasculitis, etc.), but the underlying venous insufficiency keeps the wound from healing.

The exact mechanism by which venous insufficiency or, more correctly, venous hypertension, leads to ulceration is not clear, but research shows that a certain cascade of events contributes to its development. Increased pressure of the deep venous system because of vein valve incompetence, outflow obstruction, or calf muscle pump failure leads to distention of vessel walls, increased capillary permeability, and activation of white blood cells (CBCs). Extravasation of fibrinogen and various macromolecules leads to the development of so-called fibrin cuff, which is thought to bind various growth factors, making them unavailable in the tissue. Activated white blood cells release a number of enzymes that contribute to further tissue damage.

Evaluation

Evaluation of a patient with a lower leg ulcer consists of a thorough history and physical examination as well

13

BOX 1 Differential Diagnoses of Venous Ulcers

- Venous disease
  - Primary (congenital)
  - Secondary (trauma, thrombosis)
- Arterial disease
  - Atherosclerosis
  - Cholesterol embolism
  - Thromboangiitis obliterans
- Neuropathic
  - Spina bifida
  - Secondary (diabetes, syphilis, leprosy, etc.)
- Lymphedema
  - Congenital
  - Secondary following surgery, radiation, infection
- Malignancy
  - Primary cutaneous (squamous and basal cell carcinoma, melanoma, others)
  - Secondary (metastatic)
  - Sarcoma
- Trauma
  - Burns (thermal, chemical)
  - Pressure
  - Radiation dermatitis
  - Cold injury (frostbite, pernio)
  - Factitial
- Vasculitis
  - Hypersensitivity vasculitis
  - Rheumatoid arthritis
  - Polyarteritis nodosa
  - Wegener's granulomatosis
  - Systemic lupus erythematosus
  - Scleroderma
  - Drug-induced vasculitis
- Metabolic disease
  - Diabetes
  - Necrobiosis lipoidica diabeticorum
  - Gout
  - Porphyria cutanea tarda
  - Pancreatic disease
  - Gaucher's disease
- Hematologic disease
  - Hypercoagulable disease (protein C, S deficiency, lupus anticoagulant, antithrombin III deficiency, cryofibrinogen)
  - Sickle cell anemia
  - Thalassemia
  - Leukemia
  - Lymphoma
  - Macroglobulinemia
  - Hereditary spherocytosis
  - Polycythemia vera
- Drugs
  - Halogens
  - Ergotamine (ergotism)
  - Anticoagulant necrosis (warfarin, heparin)
- Infection
  - Bacterial
  - Mycobacterial
  - Fungal
  - Spirochetal
  - Viral
- Other
  - Insect bites (brown recluse spider)
  - Sweet's syndrome
  - Pyoderma gangrenosum
  - Lichen planus (ulcerative)
  - Bullous diseases
  - Panniculitis
  - Other

Rakel and Bope: *Conn's Current Therapy 2006.*

as some basic vascular testing. Typical venous ulcers are located in the malleolar ("gaiter") area, although they can be located anywhere from the dorsum of the foot to just below the knee with single or multiple ulcers present. Generally, they are irregular shaped, relatively shallow, and may be covered with a fibrinous slough (Figure 1). The surrounding tissue may show varying degrees of erythema, scaling, hemosiderin deposition (stasis dermatitis), induration, and fibrosis (lipodermatosclerosis). Varicose veins and dependent edema of the leg may be clinically evident, and patients may complain of leg heaviness and aching. Atrophic white scars as evidence of previous ulcerations may also be present (Figure 2).

A basic vascular evaluation is indicated in most patients with lower extremity ulceration because compression is an important component of venous ulcer therapy, but it must be used with caution in patients with arterial disease. Venous insufficiency diagnosis can be made definitively by duplex ultrasound or plethysmography, which are both noninvasive tests of the venous system. Photoplethysmography is a functional test of the venous refill time and has the advantage that it is quick, noninvasive, and easy to do during the office visit. Ankle-brachial index (ABI) is a screening test for arterial disease. It is a ratio of systolic pressures in the ankle and the arm. A normal ABI is around 1.0; a ratio of less than 0.85 indicates some degree of arterial compromise. An ABI of 0.5 is associated with severe occlusive disease, and patients frequently complain of claudications on exertion and resting pain with leg elevation. The ABI may be artificially high in patients with calcified noncompressible vessels, such as in the elderly (usually > 80 years old) or in patients with diabetes. All patients with an abnormal ABI need further evaluation because

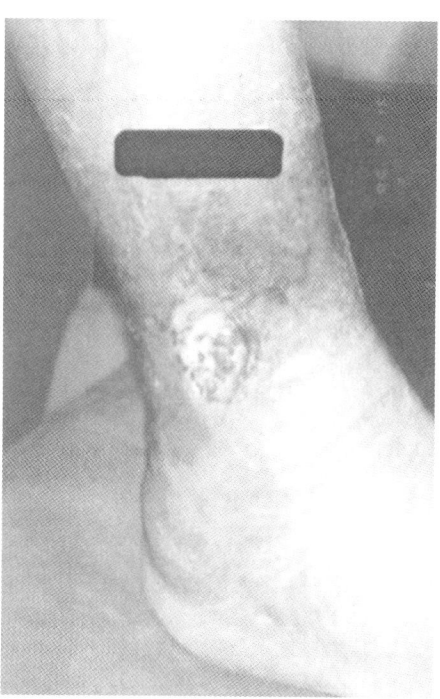

FIGURE 1. Typical venous ulcer in the malleolar area surrounded by dermatitis and hemosiderin pigmentation.

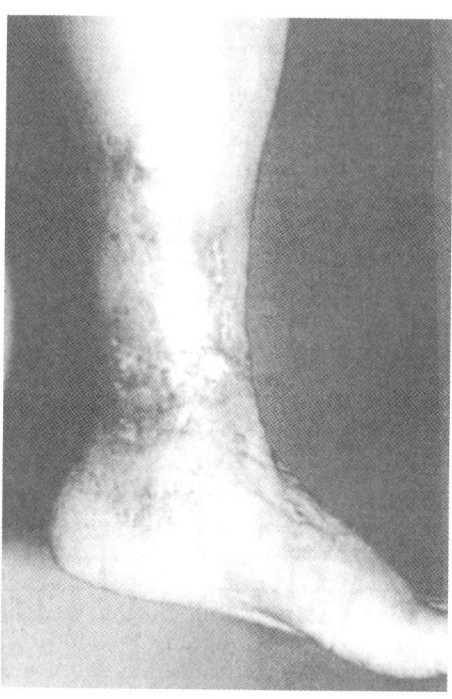

FIGURE 2. Patient with long-standing venous disease showing an irregular ulcer with an area of lipodermatosclerosis and multiple atrophic scars from previous ulcers.

it is also a predictor of coronary and cerebrovascular disease.

Additional tests for patients with a chronic leg ulcer may include laboratory evaluation (CBC, glucose, ANA [acetylneuraminic acid], RA [rheumatoid agglutinin], lupus anticoagulant, cryoglobulin, cryofibrinogen, protein C and S deficiency, antithrombin III, homocysteine, and others) and a skin biopsy for culture and histopathology to help confirm or establish a diagnosis. Generally, a 4- to 6-mm punch biopsy from the wound edge yields enough tissue and can be performed with local anesthetic on an outpatient basis. When possible, histopathology should be interpreted by a dermatopathologist for highest diagnostic accuracy because findings may be complex and need interpretation within the clinical context.

Treatment

The goals of therapy of venous ulcers are not only the healing of the cutaneous wound but also improvement of dermatitis and fibrosis, relief of edema and pain, improvement of hemodynamics, and prevention of reulceration. Care of any particular ulcer should be based on good wound care principles, which include cleaning, débridement, and choosing an appropriate dressing. In cases of venous ulcers, a compression bandage must be applied to the extremity because without correcting the underlying venous hypertension the ulcer is unlikely to heal. All venous ulcers have some degree of exudate, frequently copious until edema is controlled and compression applied. Varying degrees of contamination, colonization, or infection may be present. These issues

TABLE 1 Common Wound Dressing Classes

Dressing class	Composition	Characteristics	Brand names (alphabetical)
Films	Polyurethane or polyethylene membranes	Adhesive Waterproof Vapor permeable Nonabsorbent	Bioclusive Op-site Tegaderm
Hydrogels	Polyethylene oxide, polyacrylonitrile or methacrylate and variable amount of water sheet or gel	Maintains moisture Comfortable Nontraumatic on removal Lightly absorbent	Aquasorb IntraSite Tegagel Vigilon
Hydrocolloids	Polymer with hydrophilic colloidal particles bound to polyurethane foam or paste	Adhesive (sheet form) Waterproof Speeds autolytic débridement Absorbs exudate	Comfeel RepliCare DuoDERM CGF Tegasorb
Alginates and hydrofibers	Calcium Alginate Carboxymethyl cellulose	Nonadherent/very absorbent Maintains moisture Nonocclusive: needs secondary dressing	Kaltostat Sorbsan Tegagen Aquacel
Foams and sponges	Polyurethane or collagen May be film coated	Highly absorbent Conforms to contours/cushion Occlusive or permeable Adhesive or nonadhesive	Allevyn Hydrasorb Lyofoam Comfeel foam
Antimicrobial dressings	Any of above dressing compositions with silver, povidone iodine, gentian violet (or other) incorporated into dressing	Moisture delivery to lightly absorptive depending on composition Controls bacterial overgrowth and infection	Acticoat Contreet SilvaSorb Hydrofera blue Iodoflex

13

must be taken into account to select the most appropriate treatment regimen.

Cleaning may be done with saline or various wound-cleansing agents that are not harmful to the wound tissue. Antiseptics such as chlorhexidine, sodium hypochlorite (Dakin's solution), or povidone iodine (Betadine) are generally not recommended because they are cytotoxic and can impair wound healing. Topical medications, such as antibiotic ointments, also need to be used with caution because up to 20% of chronic ulcer patients develop an allergic contact dermatitis to one of the components (bacitracin, neomycin, lanolin, preservatives, etc.). Débridement of fibrinous and necrotic tissue decreases infection and facilitates granulation tissue formation and epithelialization. This can be done mechanically (wet to dry scrubbing) or surgically, although both of these methods may be painful and nonspecific, may require use of local anesthetic agents, and can damage surrounding tissue. Autolytic débridement can be facilitated with some occlusive dressings and further enhanced with enzymatic débriding agents (collagenase [Santyl] or papain urea [Accuzyme]). Biologic débridement (medical maggots) is also being used more frequently because it is extremely efficient, specific, and relatively painless. Table 1 summarizes the wide variety of wound dressings available. The choice of a particular dressing depends on wound characteristics, such as size, amount of exudate, presence of necrotic material, and condition of surrounding skin, which indicate a specific one based on its properties of conformability,

absorption, and ease of use, as well as availability. The goal generally is to choose a dressing that helps provide a moist environment, manages exudate, and can remain in place for several days at a time to help minimize wound trauma at the time of dressing changes.

One of the important aspects of venous ulcer treatment is compression therapy. Without external compression of 30 to 40 mm Hg, the extremity hemodynamics are not normalized and the ulcer will not heal or will heal very slowly. Compression can be achieved in several ways. The most common compression methods are paste bandages (Unna's boot), four-layer compression, and compression stockings. Paste bandages consist of gauze impregnated with zinc oxide paste and a second layer of elastic wrap. This bandage provides graduated pulsatile compression with ambulation and it exerts

CURRENT DIAGNOSIS

- Extremity warm, edematous
- Ulcer below knee, malleolar region most common
- Irregular shape, relatively shallow, exudative
- Surrounding skin with stasis dermatitis, hemosiderin pigmentation, and lipodermatosclerosis
- Results of duplex ultrasound, plethysmography, and ankle-brachial index supportive of diagnosis

Rakel and Bope: *Conn's Current Therapy 2006.*

CURRENT THERAPY

- Cleaning: noncytotoxic agents
- Débridement: autolytic/mechanical/surgical
- Dressing: absorbs exudates while maintaining a moist wound environment
- Compression: critical component of therapy; corrects venous hypertension
- Infection: treated when culture positive or clinical signs of infection present

relatively low compression when the patient is at rest, making it suitable for patients with some degree of arterial insufficiency. Four-layer bandages provide a sustained high degree of compression and are effective at reducing edema, but they cannot be used in patients with arterial insufficiency. Compression stockings provide graduated compression and are convenient, although they can be difficult to get on and must be fitted to the patient. Other options include nonelastic orthotics (CircAid), which are relatively easy to apply but bulky, and pneumatic compression pumps, which provide intermittent sequential compression and are comfortable and very effective but require immobility for a few hours per day to use.

Approximately two thirds of venous ulcers heal with a proper wound care regimen and compression. For those that do not, a number of biologically active materials are available that increase wound healing and epithelialization. These include topical growth factors (becaplermin [Regranex]),[1] granulocyte-macrophage colony stimulating factor (Leukine),[1] dressings to decrease metalloprotease activity (Promogran), biologically active membranes (small intestinal submucosa [Oasis]), and bioengineered skin substitutes (OrCel Apligraf Dermagraft[1]). Systemic therapy that improves healing along with compression is pentoxifylline (Trental)[1] as well as aspirin.[1]

Patient education during the treatment process is of utmost importance. Because these patients are at high risk for recurrence, especially individuals with previous deep venous thrombosis or a history of orthopedic surgery of the leg, consistent long-term use of compression stockings (30 to 40 mm Hg) or other compression devices is extremely important.

REFERENCES

Belcaro G, Cesarone MR, Nicolaides AN, et al: Treatment of venous ulcers with pentoxifylline: A 6-month randomized, double-blind, placebo controlled trial. Arch Med Res 2002;33(3):281-289.

Choucair M, Phillips T: Compression therapy. Dermatol Surg 1998; 24:141-148.

Eisenbud D, Huang NF, Luke S, Silberklang M: Skin substitutes and wound healing: Current status and challenges. Wounds 2004; 16(1):2-17.

Harding KG, Morris HI, Patel GK: Healing chronic wounds. BMJ 2002;324:160-163.

Límová M: Dressings for chronic wounds. In Maibach HI, Bashir SJ, McKibbon A (eds): Evidence-Based Dermatology. Hamilton, Ontario, Canada, BC Decker, 2002, Chapter 13.

---

[1]Not FDA approved for this indication.

Lin P, Phillips T: Ulcers. In Bolognia JL, Jorizzo JL, Rapini RP (eds): Dermatology. Toronto, Ontario, Canada, Mosby, 2003, Chapter 106.

Margolis DJ, Berlin JA, Strom BL: Risk factors associated with the failure of a venous ulcer to heal. Arch Dermatol 1999;135:920-926.

Mostow EN: Wound healing: A multidisciplinary approach for dermatologists. Dermatol Clin 2003;21:371-387.

Valencia IC, Falabella A, Kirsner RS, Eaglstein WH: Chronic venous insufficiency and venous leg ulceration. J Am Acad Dermatol 2001;44:401-421.

Pressure Ulcers

Method of
David R. Thomas, MD

A pressure ulcer is the visible evidence of pathologic changes in blood supply to the dermal and underlying tissues, usually because of compression of the tissue over a bony prominence.

A differential diagnosis of ulcer type is critical to treatment. Chronic ulcers of the skin include arterial ulcers, venous stasis ulcers, diabetic ulcers, and pressure ulcers. Pressure ulcers generally appear in soft tissue over a bony prominence. A classic presentation aids the diagnosis. For example, arterial ulcers occur in the distal digits or over a bony prominence, diabetic ulcers occur in regions of callous formation, and venous stasis ulcers occur on the lateral aspect of the lower leg. Atypical presentations may occasionally obscure the etiology. The treatment of these various etiologies differs considerably. This discussion is limited to the treatment of pressure ulcers and should not be used to treat other types of ulcers.

Seven principles of management guide treatment of pressure ulcers. The chief cause of these ulcers is pressure applied to the tissues, which compromises blood flow. Thus the first treatment principle is to relieve pressure. Pressure relief can be obtained by positioning the patient frequently and at a fixed interval to relieve pressure over the compromised area. Turning and positioning may be difficult to achieve because of a patient's self-positioning or medical treatments that interfere with the ability to position the patient. A number of medical devices, classified as static or dynamic, are designed to relieve pressure. Static devices include air-, gel-, or water-filled containers that reduce the tissue-to-surface interface. Dynamic devices use a power source to fill compartments with air that support the patient's weight or alternate the pressure on different areas of the body. A static device works when the patient has good bed mobility, and a dynamic device is useful when the patient cannot self-position in bed.

Results of reported clinical trials do not favor one device over another. The choice should be based on durability, ease of use, and patient comfort. A simple check for bottoming out should be done for all devices. The hand should be inserted palm upward under the patient's sacrum between the device and the bed surface.

If no air column is apparent between the patient and the bed surface, the device is ineffective and should be changed. No device is effective in reducing heel pressure, the second most common site for pressure ulcers. Bridging with pillows is effective in reducing heel pressure in immobile patients; patients with high bed mobility may require boot devices to elevate the heel off the bed surface. Patients who fail to improve or who have multiple pressure ulcers should be considered for a dynamic-type device, such as a low-air-loss bed or air-fluidized bed.

The second principle of pressure ulcer therapy is to assess pain. Pressure ulcers do not always result in pain, particularly in insensate patients, but those that do should be treated aggressively. Oral or parenteral pain medications should be used to control symptoms.

The third principle of ulcer therapy is to assess nutrition and hydration. Pressure ulcers occur in sicker individuals in whom nutrient intake may be reduced by coexisting illness. Increased intake of protein (1.2 to 1.5 g/kg/day) is associated with higher healing rates. Achievement of high protein intake may be difficult because of anorexia of aging or anorexia associated with coexisting diseases. Adequate calories, adjusted for stress (30 to 35 kcal/kg/day), should be prescribed. Adequate dietary intake should provide adequate vitamins and minerals. No difference in healing rates is associated with supertherapeutic doses of vitamin C or zinc. If adequate dietary intake is compromised, a supplemental vitamin/mineral prescription at recommended daily allowance (RDA) doses should be considered. Adequate hydration can be maintained by 30 mL/kg per day of water. The decision to institute enteral feeding in patients with pressure ulcers who are unable to maintain adequate oral intake should not be undertaken lightly. The patient's wishes, overall goal of care, and complications of enteral feeding must be considered. In several studies, the long-term result of enteral feeding is associated with poorer outcomes in patients with pressure ulcers.

The fourth principle of pressure ulcer management requires removing necrotic debris. Phagocytosis removes necrotic debris naturally. Accelerating the rate of removal may shorten healing time. Options include sharp surgical débridement, mechanical débridement with gauze dressings, application of exogenous enzymes, or autolytic débridement under occlusive dressings. Surgical débridement is indicated if the ulcer is infected. It is the fastest method but may remove some viable tissue and cause discomfort, and it is the most expensive method, especially if performed in an operating room. Applying moist gauze that is allowed to adhere to the ulcer bed by drying is a form of débridement. When the dry dressing is removed, nonselective tissue removal occurs. This method is associated with discomfort and may delay healing while débridement is in progress. It is often defeated when the dressing is remoistened prior to removal. Enzymatic débridement can digest necrotic material. Three enzymatic preparations available in the United States are collagenase, papain/urea, and papain/urea combined with chlorophyll. Enzyme preparations are nonselective, possibly resulting in some damage to fibroblasts, epithelial cells, or granulation tissue. Enzymatic débridement is

slower, is associated with discomfort, and should be limited in duration until a clean wound bed is obtained. Autolytic débridement is achieved by allowing autolysis under an occlusive dressing. Both enzymatic and autolytic débridement may require 2 to 6 weeks to achieve a clean wound bed. Unless clinically infected, heel ulcers are better left undébrided because they occur in poorly vascularized tissues.

The fifth principle of pressure ulcer management is to maintain a moist wound environment, associated with more rapid healing rates compared to dressings that are allowed to dry. Continuously moist saline gauze is the historical standard dressing for stage II through IV pressure ulcers. Care must be taken to change the gauze frequently to prevent drying, which may delay healing. Newer wound dressings provide a low moisture vapor transmission rate (MVTR), a measure of how quickly the dressing allows drying. A MVTR of less than 35 g of water vapor per square meter per hour is required to maintain a moist wound environment. Woven gauze has a MVTR of 68 g/m^2/hour; impregnated gauze has a MVTR of 57 g/m^2 per hour. By comparison, hydrocolloid dressings have a MVTR of 8 g/m^2 per hour. Dressings with low MVTR provide a healing environment that encourages granulation tissue formation and epithelialization.

The use of occlusive-type dressings is more cost effective than gauze dressings, primarily because of a decrease in nursing time for dressing changes. Occlusive dressings can be divided into broad categories of polymer films, polymer foams, hydrogels, hydrocolloids, alginates, and biomembranes. Each has advantages and disadvantages. No single agent is perfect. The choice of a particular agent depends on the clinical circumstances. Nonpermeable polymers can be macerating to normal skin. Polymer films are not absorptive and may leak, particularly when the wound is highly exudative. Most films have an adhesive backing that may remove epithelial cells when the dressing is changed. Hydrogels, hydrophilic polymers that are insoluble in water but absorb aqueous solutions, are available in amorphous gels or sheet dressings. They are poor bacterial barriers and nonadherent to the wound. Because of their high specific heat, these dressings are cooling to the skin, aiding in pain control and reducing inflammation. Most of these dressings require a secondary dressing to secure them to the wound. Hydrocolloid dressings are complex dressings similar to ostomy barrier products. They are impermeable to moisture and bacteria and highly adherent to the skin. Hydrocolloid dressings have an accelerated healing of 40% compared to moist gauze dressings. They are particularly suited for areas subject to urinary and fecal incontinence. Their adhesiveness to surrounding skin is higher than some surgical tapes, but they are nonadherent to wound tissue and do not damage epithelial tissue in the wound. The adhesive barrier is frequently overcome in highly exudative wounds. Hydrocolloid dressings cannot be used over tendons or on wounds with eschar formation. Alginates are complex polysaccharide dressings that are highly absorbent in exudative wounds. This high absorbency is particularly suited to exudative wounds. Alginates are nonadherent to the wound, but if the wound is allowed to dry,

CURRENT DIAGNOSIS

- Differentiate among pressure, diabetic, venous stasis, and arterial ulcers.

CURRENT THERAPY

The seven principles of pressure ulcer therapy are as follows:
1. Relieve pressure.
2. Assess pain.
3. Assess nutrition and hydration.
4. Remove necrotic debris.
5. Maintain a moist wound environment.
6. Encourage granulation and epithelial tissue formation.
7. Control infection.quality of life.

damage to the epithelial tissue may occur with removal. Alginates may be used under other dressings to absorb exudate. The biomembranes are very expensive and not readily available.

Stages I and II pressure ulcers can be managed with a polymer film or hydrocolloid dressing. Stages III and IV dressings may require a wound filler, such as a calcium alginate or an amorphus hydrogel, to obliterate dead space and decrease anaerobic colonization.

Electrotherapy has been used for stages III and IV pressure ulcers unresponsive to conventional therapy. Several clinical trials suggest that electrotherapy is likely to be effective. Hyperbaric oxygen, ultrasound, infrared, ultraviolet, and low-energy laser irradiation have insufficient data to recommend their use currently. Data do not support the use of a systemic vasodilator, hemorrheologics, serotonin inhibitors, or fibrolytic agents in the treatment of pressure ulcers. Topical agents such as zinc, phenytoin,[1] aluminum hydroxide,[1] honey, sugar, yeast, aloe vera gel, or gold[1] have not been effective in clinical trials.

Because the theory of augmenting ulcer healing under the newer dressings suggests that wound fluid contains favorable healing factors, the dressings should not be changed too frequently. Unless the wound fluid seeps from under the dressing, it should not be changed more often than every 3 to 7 days.

The sixth principle of pressure ulcer treatment is to encourage granulation tissue formation and promote re-epithelialization. Growth factors show promising early results, but the data do not suggest accelerated healing of pressure ulcers. It is important not to affect granulation and epithelial tissue negatively. A number of wound cleaners and antiseptics are toxic to fibroblasts and epithelial tissues, including benzalkonium chloride,[1] povidone iodine solution (Betadine),[1] Dakin's solution,[1] hydrogen peroxide, Granulex, Hibiclens, and pHisoHex. The use of these agents in a pressure ulcer should be restricted to infected ulcers and strictly limited in duration.

The seventh principle of pressure ulcer management is to control infection. Quantitative microbiology alone is a poor predictor of clinical infection in chronic wounds. All pressure ulcers are colonized with bacteria, usually from skin or fecal flora. The presence of microorganisms alone (colonization) does not indicate an infection in pressure ulcers. The diagnosis of infection in chronic wounds must be based on clinical signs—erythema, warmth, pain, edema, odor, fever, or purulent exudate. In the presence of clinical signs of infection, enteral or parenteral antibiotics should be used. In ulcers that

are not progressing toward healing, an empirical trial of topical antimicrobial may be considered, although the data are inconclusive.

REFERENCES

Thomas DR: The role of nutrition in prevention and healing of pressure ulcers. Geriatr Clin North Am 1997;13:497-512.

Thomas DR: Are all pressure ulcers avoidable? J Am Med Dir Assoc 2001;2:297-301.

Thomas DR: Improving the outcome of pressure ulcers with nutritional intervention: A review of the evidence. Nutrition 2001;17:121-125.

Thomas DR: Issues and dilemmas in managing pressure ulcers. J Gerontol Med Sci 2001;56:M238-M340.

Thomas DR: Prevention and management of pressure ulcers. Rev Clin Gerontol 2001;11:115-130.

Thomas DR: The promise of topical nerve growth factors in the healing of pressure ulcers. Ann Intern Med 2003;139:694-695.

Thomas DR: Management of pressure ulcers. J Am Med Dir Assoc (in press).

Atopic Dermatitis

Method of
Asad Salim, MD, and
Lawrence F. Eichenfield, MD

Atopic dermatitis, also called atopic eczema, is the most common of the chronic eczematous eruptions in childhood. The current prevalence is approximately 17% to 20% of children and 2% or greater of adults in the United States.

Eczema is a morphologic term used to describe the lesions in a variety of different dermatoses that manifest with similar morphologic findings and histologic findings of edema between keratinocytes, termed *spongiosis*. An acute eczematous rash consists of erythema, scaling, and crusts. Additional changes such as lichenification and pigmentary changes are seen as eczema becomes chronic.

---

[1]Not FDA approved for this indication.

Diagnosis

Atopic dermatitis is a syndrome with the following clinical features.

I. Essential features (may be present)
   A. Pruritus
   B. Eczematous dermatitis (acute, subacute, or chronic)
      1. Typical morphology and age-specific patterns
      2. Chronic or relapsing history
II. Important features (seen in most cases, adding support to the diagnosis)
   A. Early age of onset
   B. Atopy
      1. Personal and/or family history
      2. Immunoglobulin E (IgE) reactivity
   C. Xerosis

Treatment

Atopic dermatitis has a significant impact on the quality of life of patients and families. Treatment of this chronic condition involves addressing psychosocial aspects and basic skin care.

Basic skin care of atopic dermatitis encompasses education, avoidance of irritants, hydration with moisturizers, use of topical steroids and topical calcineurin inhibitors, and, in a minority of cases, avoidance of specific allergens or foods.

PSYCHOSOCIAL ASPECTS

Addressing the psychosocial aspects is as important as prescribing medicine because this chronic condition can have a significant impact on personal and family life. Important issues are sleep deprivation, school and work absenteeism, and learned behavior perpetuating the itch–scratch cycle. Specific measures such as counseling aimed at behavior modification, relaxation therapy, and biofeedback methods may all be helpful.

EDUCATION

Understanding the chronic, relapsing nature of atopic dermatitis and the exacerbating factors is very important. Clinicians should also provide verbal and written instructions, which include general disease information along with detailed skin care recommendations.

HYDRATION

Patients with atopic dermatitis have enhanced transepidermal water loss associated with impaired function of the water permeability barrier. Keeping the skin hydrated is a fundamental part of atopic dermatitis skin care. Authors advocate a "soak and seal" approach that involves application of a moisturizer within minutes of bathing or showering.

MOISTURIZERS

Regular moisturizer therapy can help reestablish and preserve the stratum corneum barrier. Liberal use of moisturizers in large quantities with frequent application should be encouraged.

AVOIDANCE OF IRRITANTS

Patients with atopic dermatitis have a lowered threshold of responsiveness to irritants. Current recommendations include use of cleansers that are perfume and dye free with minimal defatting activity and a neutral pH. Alcohol-containing agents and astringents in skin care products and irritating chemicals or detergents should be avoided.

AVOIDANCE OF ALLERGENS

Some atopic dermatitis patients develop allergies to specific foods or aeroallergens, which may require evaluation with specific tests. These allergies may cause contact urticaria, gastrointestinal symptoms, and urticaria, and only a subset result in eczematous dermatitis. Allergens proven clinically relevant should be avoided.

TOPICAL STEROIDS

Topical steroids remain the mainstay of treatment for atopic dermatitis as they have for more than 50 years. Several large placebo-controlled studies and systematic reviews show the effectiveness of topical steroids in reducing inflammation and pruritus. In addition, topical steroids reduce *Staphylococcus aureus* skin colonization by reducing skin inflammation. Topical steroids are formulated in potencies ranging from extremely high (group 1) to low (group 7). The vehicle can alter the potency of the corticosteroid (e.g., ointments containing the same molecule are more potent than the cream preparations). Treatment with topical corticosteroids is typically twice daily. Ointments are preferred to creams because of their occlusive nature and greasiness, but in warm environments creams may be preferred. Adverse effects include local effects, such as skin atrophy, striae, telangiectasia, perioral dermatitis, and acneiform eruptions. Less frequently systemic effects, such as suppression of the hypothalamic-pituitary-adrenal axis or cataracts, can occur. Strong topical corticosteroid preparations should not be applied to the face, groin, or axillae because they can cause skin atrophy.

CALCINEURIN INHIBITORS

Calcineurin inhibitors act through steroid-receptor independent pathways and do not cause cutaneous atrophy or telangiectases the way the topical steroids may, even after chronic use. Several large studies lasting up to 12 months show them to be effective when compared with placebo with no evidence of tachyphylaxis or increase in skin infections. Side effects noted are burning and stinging at the site of application. The long-term risks

13

of using calcineurin inhibitors, such as nonmelanoma skin cancer, are not known, and patients are advised to use sunscreens. Concerns have been raised about possible carcinogenic effects based on animal studies with high systemic exposures, though effects have not been observed with topical use.

Tacrolimus ointment, marketed by Fujiwara Healthcare, Inc. as Protopic 0.03% for children 2 to 15 years of age and 0.03% and 0.1% for adults, is approved by the FDA for short-term and intermittent long-term use for moderate to severe eczema.

Pimecrolimus is an ascomycin derivative similar to tacrolimus. It is effective in mild to moderate eczema against vehicle creams but not as effective as strong topical corticosteroids. Pimecrolimus (Elidel) cream 1% is approved by the FDA for mild to moderate eczema for children older than 2 years of age. Calcineurin inhibitors have minimal local side effects and may be applied to all skin surfaces (e.g., periorbital areas).

ANTIHISTAMINES AND ANXIOLYTIC THERAPY

Pruritus is one of the major features of atopic dermatitis with the associated scratching leading to excoriations, lichenification, and induction of papulonodular changes. In addition, pruritus can cause significant sleep deprivation with a negative impact on the patient's and caregivers' quality of life. Systemic antihistamines and anxiolytics can be effective in relieving itch, primarily through their sedating effect.

Diphenhydramine (Benadryl) and hydroxyzine (Atarax) are most commonly used. Doxepin (Sinequan), a tricyclic antidepressant with a long half-life, may be used at a dose between 10 and 50 mg.

ANTI-INFECTIVE THERAPY

Atopic dermatitis skin is commonly colonized and may become clinically infected with *S. aureus*. Infected eczema may be treated with systemic antibiotics. Where possible,

CURRENT DIAGNOSIS

- Eczematous dermatitis
- Pruritus
- Dryness
- Dennie-Morgan folds (accentuated lines or grooves below the margin of lower eyelids)
- Allergic shiners (darkening beneath the eyes)
- Facial pallor
- Pityriasis alba
- Keratosis pilaris
- Ichthyosis vulgaris
- Hyperlinearity of palms and soles
- White dermographism
- Keratoconus
- Anterior subcapsular cataracts
- Elevated serum immunoglobulin E (IgE)
- Immediate skin test reactivity

bacterial cultures should be obtained prior to treatment. Cephalosporins such as cephalexin (Keflex), 25 to 50 mg/kg per day, are usually used, although the changing spectrum of staphylococcus resistance patterns may require different antibiotic selection for appropriate coverage. Long-term maintenance antibiotic therapy should be avoided because it may predispose to colonization by methicillin-resistant organisms. Localized areas of infection can be treated with a topical antibiotic such as mupirocin (Bactroban, Centany), applied three times a day for 7 to 10 days. Eczema herpeticum in children is treated with systemic antiviral agents and may require hospital admission.

[4]Not yet approved for used in the United States.

CURRENT THERAPY

Mild Atopic Dermatitis
Step 1
- Emollient bid
Step 2
- Emollient bid
- Intermittent low-potency TS for flares; TCI alternative; ± antihistamines
Step 3
- Emollient bid
- Mid-potency TS for flares or TCI alternative; ± antihistamines
Moderate Atopic Dermatitis
Step 1
- Emollient bid
- Intermittent low-potency TS for flares or TCI alternative; ± antihistamines
Step 2
- Emollient bid
- Mid to higher potency TS for flares or TCI long-term/intermittent; ± antihistamines
- Antibiotic if clinical infection
Step 3
- Emollient bid
- High-potency TS for flare control
- TCI long-term/intermittent antihistamines
- Antibiotics if clinical infection
Severe Atopic Dermatitis
Step 1
- Emollient bid
- Moderate to higher potency TS for flares
- TCI long-term/intermittent; ± antihistamines
Step 2
- Mid to higher potency TS for flares
- TCI long-term/intermittent; ± antihistamines
Step 3
- Phototherapy *or*
- Systemic treatment (e.g., cyclosporine, prednisone)
- TCI long-term/intermittent; ± antihistamines
- Antibiotics if clinical infection

Abbreviations: bid = twice daily; TCI = topical calcineurin inhibitors; TS = topical steroids.

Rakel and Bope: *Conn's Current Therapy 2006.*

SYSTEMIC THERAPY

Severe or refractory atopic dermatitis may require phototherapy or systemic therapy with oral corticosteroids in short courses. Immunosuppressants such as cyclosporine (Sandimmune)[1] at a dose of 2 to 4 mg/kg may be useful for several-month courses for severe disease.

REFERENCES

Ehlers A, Stangier U, Gieler U: Treatment of atopic dermatitis: A comparison of psychological and dermatological approaches to relapse prevention. J Consult Clin Psychol 1995;63:624-635.

Eichenfield LF: Consensus guidelines in diagnosis and treatment of atopic dermatitis. Allergy 2004: 59(Suppl 78):86-92.

Eichenfield LF, Hanifin JM, Luger TA, et al: Consensus conference on pediatric atopic dermatitis. J Am Acad Dermatol 2003;49:1088-1095.

Eichenfield LF, Lucky AW, Boguniewicz M, et al: Safety and efficacy of pimecrolimus (ASM 981) cream 1% in the treatment of mild and moderate atopic dermatitis in children and adolescents. J Am Acad Dermatol 2002;46:495-504.

Hanfin JM, Ling MR, Langley R, et al: Tacrolimus ointment for the treatment of atopic dermatitis in adult patients: I. Efficacy. J Am Acad Dermatol 2001;44:S28-S38.

Hoare C, Li Wan Po A, Williams H: Systemic review of treatments of atopic eczema. Health Technol Assess 2000;4:1-191.

Luger T, Van Leent EJ, Graeber M, et al: SDZ ASM 981: An emerging safe and effective treatment for atopic dermatitis. Br J Dermatol 2001;144:788-794.

Paller A, Eichenfield LF, Leung DY, et al: A 12-week study of tacrolimus ointment for the treatment of atopic dermatitis in pediatric patients. J Am Acad Dermatol 2001;44:S47-S57.

---

[1]Not FDA approved for this indication.

Erythema Multiforme, Stevens-Johnson Syndrome, and Toxic Epidermal Necrolysis

Method of
Marcia G. Tonnesen, MD

Historically, erythema multiforme (EM), Stevens-Johnson syndrome (SJS), and toxic epidermal necrolysis (TEN) were considered a disease spectrum, and therefore they are addressed together here. Current evidence, however, supports a clear distinction between EM, with characteristic acrally distributed target lesions and an etiologic link to herpes simplex virus (HSV) infection, and SJS/TEN, with focal to widespread skin and mucous membrane involvement, characterized by epidermal destruction, and an etiologic link to adverse drug reactions. EM is typically mild and self-limited and requires only symptomatic care. In contrast, because of the degree and extent of epidermal and mucosal involvement that occurs in SJS and TEN, careful monitoring is critical and hospitalization for supportive care often required. Thus early diagnosis is critical. Elimination of any identified or presumed precipitating factors is of prime importance. Therapy should combine symptomatic and supportive measures with observation for and treatment of associated complications, depending on the clinical characteristics and severity of the episode. Optimal therapeutic intervention is hindered because specific pathogenic mechanisms of tissue injury are not yet completely defined. In addition, few controlled studies have evaluated the effectiveness of proposed therapeutic agents. Nevertheless, recent advances elucidating unique morphologic features and novel mechanisms of epidermal necrosis enhance the likelihood of successful therapeutic intervention.

Erythema Multiforme

EM is an acute, self-limited, but frequently recurrent, inflammatory cutaneous disorder, characterized by the sudden onset of a symmetric erythematous eruption with primarily an acral distribution. Skin lesions begin as fixed (lasting longer than 24 hours) erythematous flat macules, rapidly progress to erythematous raised papules, and then develop a pale or dusky central zone because of edema or bulla formation. This characteristic morphology is now termed *raised atypical target*. Some further evolve to form distinctive raised target lesions with at least three zones of color (dusky/bullous center, pale edematous halo, erythematous border), termed *typical target*. Individual lesions occasionally sting or itch, appear in successive crops for 24 to 72 hours, and spontaneously resolve within 1 to 4 weeks. Mucosal involvement, when present, is usually limited to the lips, buccal mucosa, and tongue.

Most recurrent EM cases are associated with herpes simplex virus (HSV) type I or II infection and typically occur 3 to 14 days after the appearance of a recurrent HSV lesion (oral, genital, or other location). Subclinical episodes of herpes can also induce EM. HSV DNA is detected in EM lesions. Herpes-associated erythema multiforme is currently believed to result from the HSV-specific host immune response.

THERAPEUTIC APPROACH

Elimination of Etiologic Factor

In recurrent herpes-associated EM, a course of acyclovir (Zovirax), 200 mg orally five times daily for 5 days, should be initiated at the first symptom of HSV infection. Acyclovir therapy is not effective if initiated after the development of HSV or EM lesions.

Symptomatic Measures

For pruritic or painful skin lesions, systemic antihistamines or analgesics may provide symptomatic relief. Topical acyclovir and topical corticosteroids are not beneficial. Care for skin and mouth erosions is addressed in the following section.

Rakel and Bope: *Conn's Current Therapy 2006.*

Preventive Measures

Because of the common etiologic association between recurrent HSV infections and EM, measures that attempt to prevent recurrences of HSV may lessen the frequency of subsequent episodes. Avoidance of sun exposure by using sunscreens (SPF [sun protection factor] 15 or higher), sun sticks (sunscreen-containing lip balm), and UV (ultraviolet)-protective clothing and by minimizing sun exposure from 10 AM to 3 PM (the peak period for ultraviolet B [UVB]) may reduce ultraviolet light–induced HSV recurrences. Attempts should be made to minimize stress, a well-known precipitating factor of HSV. Topical antiviral preparations do not prevent or abort recurrent HSV infections.

Prophylactic administration of acyclovir abolishes recurrent HSV infections and ensuing episodes of EM. In patients with frequently recurring, debilitating, herpes-associated EM, the treatment of choice is daily oral acyclovir for a period of 6 months or longer. The recommended adult starting dose is 400 mg orally twice daily, with tapering of the dose after the disease is brought under control. Because asymptomatic subclinical HSV episodes can also trigger EM, patients with so-called idiopathic recurrent EM often benefit from prophylactic antiviral therapy. If acyclovir fails to prevent recurrences of HSV, newer antiviral agents with enhanced bioavailability, such as valacyclovir (Valtrex) or famciclovir (Famvir), should be tried. Because of the known occurrence of acyclovir resistance and the unknown long-term side effects of chronic acyclovir therapy, the drug should be stopped periodically and the need for its continuance reassessed.

Patient Education

Patients should be reassured regarding the usual benign, self-limited course, educated regarding the frequent association of EM with recurrent HSV infections, and advised regarding preventive measures.

Stevens-Johnson Syndrome and Toxic Epidermal Necrolysis

SJS is a severe mucocutaneous illness characterized by an extensive blistering eruption with a primarily facial and truncal distribution and extensive mucosal erosions, typically involving the mouth and conjunctivae. A prodrome with constitutional symptoms and fever usually heralds the onset of the eruption. Skin lesions begin as erythematous flat macules, frequently develop dusky central vesiculation, and may progress to bullae formation with epidermal necrosis. The current morphologic terms for these characteristic lesions are *macule with or without blister* if only one color and *flat atypical target* if two concentric zones of color are present. Epidermal detachment may involve up to 10% body surface area (BSA). Painful mucosal erosions result in characteristic hemorrhagic-crusted lips, foul-smelling mouth, and decreased oral intake. Ocular involvement with photophobia and painful conjunctival erosions may lead to residual scarring, lacrimal abnormalities, and permanent visual impairment. Disease duration is 4 to 6 weeks. Recurrences are infrequent. SJS is now recognized as strongly related to adverse drug reactions and linked to some infections, particularly *Mycoplasma pneumoniae*, but never to herpes virus infection.

TEN is characterized by widespread sheetlike necrosis and sloughing of the epidermis, involving greater than 30% of the BSA. (Epidermal detachment between 10% and 30% of the BSA is classified as SJS/TEN overlap.) Following a 1- to 3-day prodrome of fever and flulike symptoms, the cutaneous eruption characteristically begins symmetrically on the face and upper body. Initial painful erythema rapidly progresses within hours to days to widespread bulla formation. Sheetlike areas of epidermal necrosis with extensive denudation involve significant or total BSA. Alternatively, TEN may begin as erythematous or violaceous macules that then develop bullae and coalesce. Involvement of multiple mucosal surfaces is present in nearly all patients. The order of frequency is oropharynx (in severe cases extending to larynx and tracheobronchial tree), eyes, genitalia, and anus. TEN is considered a manifestation of "acute skin failure" with abnormal barrier function resulting in fluid, electrolyte, and protein loss, increased susceptibility to infection, impaired thermoregulation, altered immune status, and increased energy expenditure. Morbidity is significant, and the mortality rate is 25% to 40%. The leading cause of death is sepsis.

Adverse drug reactions are the only well-documented cause of TEN. The most common offenders (Box 1) include antibiotics, particularly sulfonamides, anticonvulsants, nonsteroidal anti-inflammatory agents (NSAIDs), and more recently antiretroviral agents, although more than 100 drugs are implicated. The greatest risk for antibiotics occurs during the initial weeks of use; for most anticonvulsants, the risk is highest during the

---

BOX 1   Drugs With Highest Risk of Stevens-Johnson Syndrome/ Toxic Epidermal Necrolysis

Antibiotics
- Sulfonamides
- Cephalosporins
- Quinolones
- Tetracycline
- Aminopenicillins
- Imidazole antifungals

Anticonvulsants/Antianxiety
- Carbamazepine
- Chlormezanone[2]
- Phenytoin
- Phenobarbital
- Valproic acid
- Lamotrigine
- Nonsteroidal anti-inflammatory drugs, particularly oxicams
- Allopurinol
- Antiretroviral agents

[2]Not available in the United States.

first 2 months. Although the specific pathogenic mechanism is not fully elucidated for SJS/TEN, the characteristic epidermal necrosis is now believed to be a result of keratinocyte apoptosis. Current evidence supports important roles in the induction of keratinocyte death for Fas/Fas ligand–mediated apoptosis, cytokines such as tumor necrosis factor-α (TNF-α), and cytotoxic T lymphocytes, as well as specific genetic defects in detoxification of reactive drug metabolites. Recent novel attempts at therapeutic intervention are based on these proposed mechanisms of epidermal necrosis.

THERAPEUTIC APPROACH

Elimination of Etiologic Factors

Immediate withdrawal of any suspected or potential causative drug(s) is critical because cessation of the offending agent no later than the stage of early blister formation may decrease mortality. For SJS, *Mycoplasma pneumoniae* and other infections, if diagnosed, should be appropriately treated.

Intervention with Systemic Therapy to Stop Progression

Indication for the use of systemic therapy in SJS/TEN is highly controversial because no randomized, controlled trials document efficacy of any systemic intervention. Because widespread epidermal necrosis is associated with a high mortality rate, however, early administration of systemic therapy in the progressive phase of the disease process is advocated to attempt to limit the extent of tissue damage. Use of systemic glucocorticosteroids has proved particularly controversial. There is no evidence-based documentation of their efficacy, and some retrospective studies indicate that patients treated with systemic steroids have an increased incidence of morbidity, prolonged hospitalization, and mortality. Thus other agents are currently being assessed and advocated. Case studies or uncontrolled trials involving small numbers of patients report benefit from a variety of systemic agents. Immunosuppressive therapy with oral cyclosporine (Sandimmune)[1] or high-dose intravenous cyclophosphamide (Cytoxan)[1] is claimed to help several patients. Plasmapheresis may be of some benefit. Innovative treatment is not without risk, however. For example, a double-blind, placebo-controlled trial of thalidomide, which suppresses production of TNF-α, had to be aborted because of a dramatic increase in thalidomide-related mortality.

Currently the most promising and widely advocated systemic therapy is the early administration of high-dose intravenous immunoglobulin (IVIG)[1] to inhibit epidermal apoptosis mediated by the Fas/Fas ligand death receptor. An initial landmark pilot study by Viand and colleagues of 10 TEN patients treated with IVIG demonstrates rapid cessation of disease progression and 100% survival. Subsequently, numerous case reports, retrospective analyses, and uncontrolled prospective studies

support the overall safety as well as the efficacy of IVIG to decrease mortality, with only a few dissenting. Improved survival appears to depend on use of high-dose IVIG (1 g/kg/day given more than 3 to 4 days for a total dose of 3 to 4 g/kg) because increased risk of mortality occurs at lower total doses (2 g/kg/day or less). A randomized placebo-controlled trial of IVIG for TEN has not yet been done and will be challenging to accomplish, given the rarity of the disease and the high mortality rate.

In the absence of documented efficacy, use of systemic therapy to limit disease progression in a specific patient remains at the discretion of the physician. However, it is now clear that if systemic intervention is administered, once disease progression ceases and the wound healing process begins, or if no response is noted within 3 to 6 days, treatment should be abruptly discontinued to minimize risk of associated complications.

Supportive Care

Because of the extensive epidermal and mucosal necrosis and detachment that can occur in SJS and TEN, careful monitoring is critical and hospitalization is often required. Early referral of severe cases to an intensive care or burn unit decreases mortality. Poor outcome can be predicted by a TEN-specific severity of illness score and correlates with the number of specific independent risk factors for mortality present within the first 24 hours after admission to an intensive care unit (Box 2).

Skin Care

For crusted erosive discrete skin lesions, mild drying, gentle débridement, and cleansing as well as a soothing antipruritic effect is achieved with open wet to damp compresses of tepid water applied for 20 minutes three or four times per day. Lesions should be observed for signs of secondary infection, cultured when indicated, and treatment initiated with the appropriate systemic antibiotic. Topical corticosteroids are not beneficial. For pruritic or painful skin lesions, systemic antihistamines or analgesics provide symptomatic relief.

If extensive, advanced tissue necrosis occurs or is already evident (10% to 20% total BSA involvement),

---

BOX 2	SCORTEN: A Severity-of-Illness Score Predictive of Mortality in Toxic Epidermal Necrolysis

- Age >40 y
- Presence of malignancy
- Initial epidermal detachment >10% BSA
- BUN >28 mg/dL
- Glucose >252 mg/dL
- HCO_3 <20 mEq/L
- Heart rate >120 beats/min

Abbreviations: BSA = body surface area; BUN = blood urea nitrogen; HCO_3 = bicarbonate.

---

[1]Not FDA approved for this indication.

immediate transfer of the patient to an intensive care or burn unit under the care of an experienced dermatologist and skilled nurses is strongly advocated. Therapeutic protocols consist of the following:

- Measures to guard against iatrogenic infection, including withdrawal from systemic steroids; avoidance of indwelling lines and catheters whenever possible; limitation of antibiotic use to specific culture-proven infections; daily cultures of denuded skin, eyes, mouth, sputum, and urine; and aggressive treatment of sepsis if it occurs.
- Supportive care consisting of use of an air-fluidized bed, intravenous fluid therapy to restore fluid and electrolyte balance, tube feedings to ensure adequate caloric intake, adequate pain relief, respiratory and physical therapy as needed and tolerated, and continuing eye care by an ophthalmologist.
- Avoidance of all unnecessary medications, particularly those that are known etiologic factors of SJS/TEN, such as sulfonamides (including sulfa-containing eye preparations and topical dressings).

- Skin care with emphasis on wound dressings to protect the denuded dermis from desiccation and secondary infection and to facilitate rapid re-epithelialization. Reduced mortality and faster healing result from the use of synthetic dressings, biologic dressings, silver nitrate dressings, allografts, or porcine xenografts.

Mouth Care

When extensive painful mouth lesions are present, good oral hygiene is critical to minimize infection and discomfort. Hydrogen peroxide (1.5%) or sterile normal saline mouthwash every 2 hours provides cleansing and gentle débridement. Topical anesthetics, such as dyclonine, viscous lidocaine, or a 1:1 mixture of Kaopectate[1] and elixir of diphenhydramine (Benadryl), used as a mouthwash, often provides pain relief. A liquid or soft diet, usually better tolerated, contributes to the

---

[1]Not FDA approved for this indication.

 CURRENT DIAGNOSIS

Erythema Multiforme
- Symmetric erythematous acral eruption with target lesions
- Acute: Onset over 24 to 72 hours
- Unique clinical morphology: key to diagnosis
  Raised atypical target lesions
- Palpable round red with central edema/bulla
- Two concentric zones of color
  Typical target lesions
- Palpable round red with pale halo and dusky center
- Three concentric zones of color
- Mucosal involvement variable, oral only
- Self-limited: Spontaneous resolution within 1 to 4 weeks
- Recurrent EM
  Associated with HSV type I or II
  Occurs 3 to 14 days after HSV lesion

Stevens-Johnson Syndrome
- Severe mucocutaneous disease
  Extensive symmetrical blistering eruption
  Mucosal erosions: mouth, conjunctivae, then oropharynx, genitalia
- Characteristic erosions with hemorrhagic crust on lips
- Initial prodrome with fever and flulike symptoms
- Skin lesions: Erythematous/violaceous macules
  Often with central vesicles/bullae
  May progress to epidermal necrosis (<10% BSA)
- Unique clinical morphology: key to diagnosis
  Macules with or without blisters
- Flat nonpalpable (except central blister)

- Red or dusky
- May become confluent face/trunk
  Flat atypical target lesions
- Flat nonpalpable (except central blister)
- Round red/dusky or pale central blister
- Two concentric zones of color
- Duration 4 to 6 weeks; infrequent to no recurrences
- Severe adverse reaction to drug
  Or if infection: *Mycoplasma pneumoniae,* never HSV

Toxic Epidermal Necrolysis
- Severe adverse drug reaction
- Initial 1- to 3-day prodrome of fever, flulike symptoms
- Initial painful erythema of the face and upper trunk
- Rapid progression of skin involvement:
  Central, then acral
  Dusky red flat macules to flaccid blisters to large sheets of epidermal necrosis
- Unique clinical morphology: key to diagnosis
  Macules with or without blisters
- Flat nonpalpable (except central blister)
- Red or dusky
- Become confluent
  Flat atypical target lesions
- Flat nonpalpable (except central blister)
- Round red/dusky or pale central blister
- Two concentric zones of color
  Extensive areas of confluent epidermal denudation
- > 30% BSA (may involve >90% BSA)
- Involvement of multiple mucosal surfaces usual
- High morbidity; mortality rate: 25% to 40%

Abbreviations: BSA = body surface area; EM = erythema multiforme; HSV = herpes simplex virus.

Rakel and Bope: *Conn's Current Therapy 2006.*

maintenance of hydration and nutrition. More aggressive nutritional support is usually required for severe oral involvement.

Eye Care

Because of the potential for long-term sequelae resulting in loss of vision, careful monitoring of eye involvement is mandatory, and early consultation and daily continuing care by an ophthalmologist is strongly recommended. Suggested therapeutic measures might include sterile irrigation and compresses to cleanse the eye, lysis of adhesions, and instillation of topical antibiotics.

Preventive Measures

In drug-associated SJS or TEN, future avoidance of the causative drug or chemically related agents is mandatory.

Patient Education

For SJS and TEN, patients should be advised the course is self-limited but potentially severe and life-threatening, educated regarding the association with adverse drug reactions, and warned to avoid future use of the implicated medication(s).

 CURRENT THERAPY

Erythema Multiforme

- Eliminate/prevent etiologic factor by initiating acyclovir (Zovirax), 200 mg orally five times daily, for 5 days at the first symptom of HSV recurrence but not after HSV or EM lesions appear.
- Reduce UV-induced HSV recurrences.
    Apply sunscreens (SPF 15 or higher).
    Use sunscreen-containing lip balm.
    Wear UV-protective clothing and minimize sun exposure from 10 AM to 3 PM.
- Consider prophylactic acyclovir if frequent severe recurrences.
    Prescribe 400 mg orally twice daily for at least 6 months.
    Taper dose after disease under control.
    Stop periodically to reassess need.

Stevens-Johnson Syndrome/Toxic Epidermal Necrolysis

- Eliminate/prevent etiologic factor:
    Immediately stop suspected drug(s).
    Avoid exposure to causative drug and chemically related agents.
    Treat *Mycoplasma pneumoniae* if present.
- Stop progression of epidermal necrosis:
    Administer high-dose IVIG[1]
    Give total dose of 3 to 4 g/kg over 3 to 4 consecutive days, 1g/kg/day for 3 to 4 days; if renal insufficiency: lower daily dose, and lengthen the duration.
    Initiate as early as possible.
    Discontinue once disease progression ceases, or if no response in 3 to 6 days, to minimize complications.

Supportive Care

Skin care

For crusted, erosive discrete skin lesions:
- Apply open wet-to-damp compresses of sterile water for 20 minutes three to four times per day to cleanse and soothe.

- Observe for secondary infection; culture and treat with appropriate systemic antibiotic.
- Use systemic antihistamines or analgesics for discomfort.

For extensive epidermal detachment (10% to 20% BSA):
- Transfer immediately to intensive care or burn unit.
- Guard against iatrogenic infection:
    Stop all systemic steroids.
    Avoid indwelling lines and catheters.
    Limit antibiotic use to specific culture-proven infections.
    Perform daily surveillance cultures of denuded skin, eyes, mouth, sputum, and urine.
    Treat sepsis aggressively if it occurs.
- Provide supportive care:
    Try an air-fluidized bed.
    Give intravenous fluid therapy.
    Provide tube feedings.
    Provide pain relief.
    Give respiratory and physical therapy.
    Provide eye care by an ophthalmologist.
    Avoid all unnecessary medications.
    Apply wound dressings—synthetic, biologic, or silver nitrate, or use allografts/porcine xenografts.

Mouth care

- Use hygienic mouthwash such as hydrogen peroxide (1.5%) or sterile normal saline every 2 hours.
- Use a pain-relief mouthwash such as viscous lidocaine or a 1:1 mixture of Kaopectate[1] and elixir of diphenhydramine (Benadryl).
- Provide a liquid/soft diet or tube feedings.

Eye care

- Provide daily continuing care by an ophthalmologist:
    Use sterile irrigation and compresses.
    Perform lysis of adhesions.
    Provide instillation of topical antibiotics.

---

[1]Not FDA approved for this indication.

Abbreviations: BSA = body surface area; EM = erythema multiforme; HSV= herpes simplex virus; IVIG = intravenous immunoglobulin; SPF = sun protection factor; UV = ultraviolet.

Rakel and Bope: *Conn's Current Therapy 2006.*

REFERENCES

Bachot N, Revuz J, Roujeau J-C: Intravenous immunoglobulin treatment for Stevens-Johnson syndrome and toxic epidermal necrolysis: A prospective noncomparative study showing no benefit on mortality or progression. Arch Dermatol 2003:139:33-36.

Bastuji-Garin S, Rzany B, Stern RS, et al: Clinical classification of cases of toxic epidermal necrolysis, Stevens-Johnson syndrome, and erythema multiforme. Arch Dermatol 1993;129:92-96.

Green JA, Spruance SL, Wenerstrom G, Piepkorn MW: Post-herpetic erythema multiforme prevented with prophylactic oral acyclovir. Ann Int Med 1985;102:632-633.

Halebian PH, Madden MR, Finklestein JL, et al: Improved burn center survival of patients with toxic epidermal necrolysis managed without corticosteroids. Ann Surg 1986;204:503-512.

Kelemen JJ, Cioffi WG, McManus WF, et al: Burn center care for patients with toxic epidermal necrolysis. J Am Coll Surg 1995; 180:273-278.

Lehrer-Bell KA, Kirsner RS, Tallman PG, Kerdel FA: Treatment of the cutaneous involvement in Stevens-Johnson syndrome and toxic epidermal necrolysis with silver nitrate–impregnated dressings. Arch Dermatol 1998;134:877-879.

Prins C, Kerdel FA, Padilla S, et al: Treatment of toxic epidermal necrolysis with high-dose intravenous immunoglobulins: Multicenter retrospective analysis of 48 consecutive cases. Arch Dermatol 2003;139:26-32.

Roujeau J-C, Kelly JP, Naldi L, et al: Medication use and the risk of Stevens-Johnson syndrome or toxic epidermal necrolysis. N Eng J Med 1995;333:1600-1607.

Tatnall FM, Schofield JK, Leigh IM. A double-blind, placebo-controlled trial of continuous acyclovir therapy in recurrent erythema multiforme. Br J Dermatol 1995;132:267-270.

Trent JT, Kirsner RS, Romanelli P, Kerdel FA: Analysis of intravenous immunoglobulin for the treatment of toxic epidermal necrolysis using SCORTEN. Arch Dermatol 2003;139:39-43.

Viard I, Wehrli P, Bullani R, et al: Inhibition of toxic epidermal necrolysis by blockade of CD95 with human intravenous immunoglobulin. Science 1998;282:490-493.

Wolkenstein P, Latarjet J, Roujeau J-C, et al: Randomized comparison of thalidomide versus placebo in toxic epidermal necrolysis. Lancet 1998;352:1586-1589.

Bullous Diseases

Method of
Diya F. Mutasim, MD

Autoimmune bullous diseases result from an immune response to molecular components of desmosomes or the basement membrane zone (BMZ). The various types of pemphigus are caused by antibodies to desmosomal proteins. There is strong evidence that antibodies in pemphigus vulgaris (PV), pemphigus foliaceus (PF), and paraneoplastic pemphigus (PNP) cause acantholysis and blister formation by directly interfering with desmosomal function. However, the subepidermal autoimmune bullous diseases result from antibodies against components of the BMZ. In general, subepidermal vesicles result from activation of complement resulting in a cellular inflammatory infiltrate.

The discussion on drug use in this article is for off-label use. The drugs are neither approved nor evaluated by double-blind, placebo-controlled studies for bullous diseases. The quality of evidence-based practice guidelines in bullous diseases is variable but generally low. The reasons for the lack of controlled studies include the rarity of bullous diseases, the severe morbidity associated with most cases, and the ethical dilemma of giving placebo to a patient with a serious disorder. Most data are derived from case reports and case series. In addition, the experience of the author is expressed in proposed algorithms for the treatment of each disease.

Pemphigus Vulgaris

The aim of therapy in the management of patients with PV is to prevent the appearance of new lesions and produce healing of existing lesions. Successful therapy suppresses the production of pathogenic autoantibodies; therefore, immunosuppressive drugs are used. A positive clinical response is associated with a decrease in or absence of circulating autoantibodies in the serum and then absence of bound autoantibodies in the skin. There has been a dramatic decrease in the mortality of PV because of the increasing availability of immunosuppressive drugs and glucocorticoids in addition to earlier diagnosis and treatment.

The choice of therapy depends to some degree on the severity of the disease at presentation. Other factors that play a role in choosing therapy are patient related (age, general health, and associated medical illnesses such as diabetes, hypertension, or tuberculosis) and drug related (onset of action, efficacy, adverse effects, and cost). Unless there is an absolute contraindication, the initial therapy of PV is systemic glucocorticoid.

Prednisone or methylprednisone may be used. The starting dose of prednisone is 1 mg/kg per day divided into 2 to 3 doses. Most patients obtain remission within 4 to 12 weeks. The dose is then maintained for 6 to 10 weeks and then decreased by 10 to 20 mg every 2 to 4 weeks. The dose may be increased if there is slow response. When the dose is 40 mg daily, the patient is changed to an every-other-day schedule. This is accomplished by keeping the first day's dose at 40 mg and decreasing the second day's dose by 5 to 10 mg every 2 to 4 weeks. When the patient is taking 40 mg every other day, the dose is tapered by 5 mg every 2 to 4 weeks. If there is no recurrence, the patient is maintained on 5 mg daily or every other day for several years. Methylprednisolone (Solu-Medrol), administered intravenously (IV) as 1 g per day over a period of 1 to 3 hours for 3 consecutive days, is referred to as *pulse steroid therapy*. The goal of this approach is to quickly achieve the immunosuppressive effects of glucocorticoids while avoiding the long-term side effects. Side effects are rare and may include electrolyte imbalance, hypertension, pancreatitis, seizures, and cardiac arrhythmias. Patients with severe PV who do not respond to oral glucocorticoids may respond well to pulse steroid therapy.

If prednisone fails to induce a remission, or if the patient develops serious adverse effects, adjuvant immunosuppressive drugs are instituted. The preferred method involves treatment initiated with adjuvant therapy concomitant with steroid therapy to decrease the total dose of glucocorticoid needed. The glucocorticoid is tapered rapidly, and the patient is maintained on the steroid-sparing agent for 18 to 24 months. The most commonly used steroid-sparing immunosuppressive drugs are azathioprine (Imuran),[1] mycophenolate mofetil (MMF) (CellCept),[1] and cyclophosphamide (Cytoxan).[1] Cyclophosphamide[1] is used at a dose of 1 to 3 mg/kg per day, azathioprine[1] at a dose of 2 to 4 mg/kg per day, and MMF[1] at a dose of 2 to 3 g daily. The addition of cyclophosphamide[1] to prednisone often results in rapid disease control and permits a reduction in the prednisone dose.

Azathioprine[1] is less effective than cyclophosphamide[1] but is more widely used. It is less toxic and therefore requires less monitoring than cyclophosphamide.[1] Because of its relatively lower toxicity, lower risk of sterility, and lower lifetime risk of malignancy, it is indicated in younger individuals. MMF[1] is a generally safe glucocorticoid-sparing agent. It was first used for PV in 1997. Later, its use was reported in a study of 12 patients with PV who had failed combination therapy with prednisone and azathioprine[1]. These patients were given prednisone and MMF[1] (2 g per day). Of 12 patients, 11 improved without relapse during the 9- to 12-month follow-up period, even with steroid tapering. Although methotrexate (Rheumatrex)[1] is also used as a steroid-sparing agent in PV, it is generally less effective than other agents. The response of PV to cyclosporine (Neoral)[1] is controversial. The literature suggests that cyclosporine[1] is ineffective as a single agent but may be beneficial when used as adjuvant to

glucocorticoid treatment in long-term maintenance therapy of PV.

High-dose intravenous immunoglobulin (IVIG) (Gamimune N)[1] has a rapid onset of action and appears most effective when used as adjuvant to conventional therapy, especially as a steroid-sparing agent. The mechanism of action of IVIG[1] is unclear. Plasmapheresis has been used in the treatment of severe PV, especially when the disease is refractory to treatment with prednisone and immunosuppressive agents, but its effectiveness is controversial. When used in combination with prednisone, it is superior to prednisone alone. In that study, no concomitant immunosuppressive drugs were used. Other studies found it effective at reducing serum levels of autoantibodies and controlling disease activity. To avoid the rebound phenomenon (increased production of autoantibodies), immune suppression (usually with cyclophosphamide[1]) is used concomitantly with plasmapheresis.

For resistant cases of PV consider:

- Experimental therapy with extracorporeal photochemotherapy
- Rituximab (Rituxan)[1] (a mouse and human chimeric monoclonal antibody that is directed against the CD20 antigen on the surface of pre-B cells, B cells, and malignant B cells)
- High-dose intravenous cyclophosphamide[1] (50 mg/kg per day for 4 days) without stem-cell rescue
- Immunophoresis

Figure 1 is a proposed algorithm for the treatment of PV.

13

---

[1]Not FDA approved for this indication.

[1]Not FDA approved for this indication.

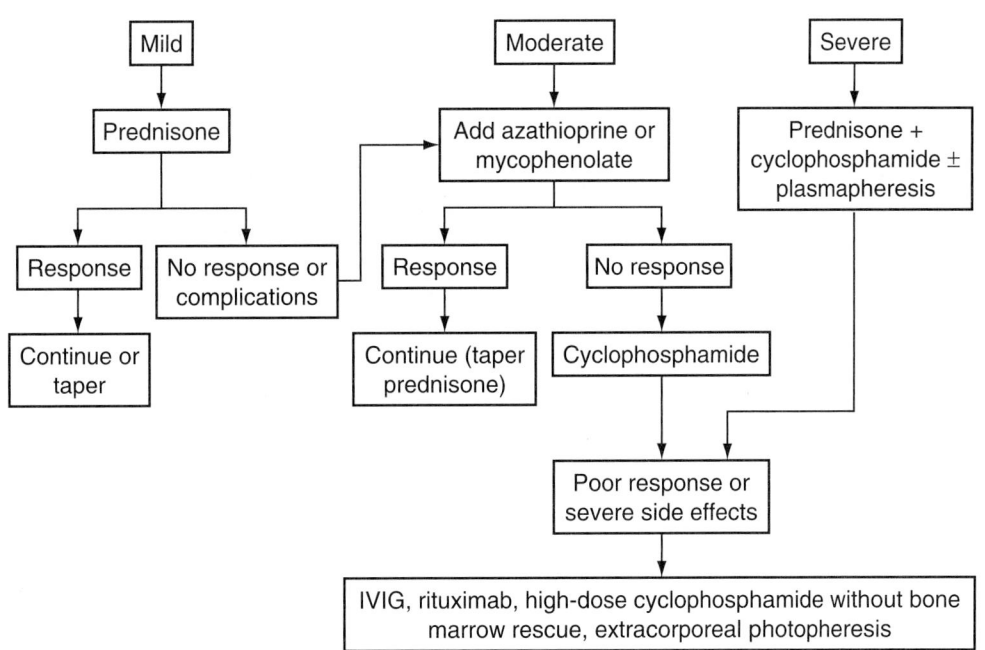

FIGURE 1. Proposed algorithm for the treatment of pemphigus.

Rakel and Bope: *Conn's Current Therapy 2006.*

Pemphigus Foliaceus

The principles and practice of managing PF are similar to those for PV. The aim of therapy is suppression of the production of pathogenic antibodies, cessation of new lesions, and healing of old lesions. This is usually accomplished with the use of systemic glucocorticoids with or without steroid-sparing agents. In addition, dapsone,[1] gold,[1] and hydroxychloroquine (Plaquenil)[1] have been used with variable success.

Paraneoplastic Pemphigus

The management of PNP consists of the treatment of the underlying neoplasm as well as immune suppression. Surgical excision of benign neoplasms, such as thymoma and Castleman disease, results in clinical and serologic improvement and remission. In patients with malignant neoplasms (B-cell lymphoma, chronic lymphocytic leukemia [CLL]), treatment of the associated neoplasm may not result in remission. Generally, skin lesions respond more rapidly than mucosal lesions. Systemic glucocorticoids are frequently used as the first-line agent in a dose of 1 to 2 mg/kg per day. Patients usually have a partial response; rarely, there is a complete resolution of lesions. Other immunosuppressive drugs are used with variable success. These include MMF,[1] azathioprine,[1] and cyclosporine.[1]

High-dose cyclophosphamide[1] without stem-cell rescue has been reported in a patient with PNP associated with chronic lymphocytic leukemia. The patient received cyclophosphamide[1] doses of 50 mg/kg per day IV on 4 consecutive days. After 2 months there was a significant improvement of the mucosal disease. Rituximab[1] was effective in a case of PNP associated with CD20[+] follicular lymphoma and in a case of PNP associated with follicular non-Hodgkin's lymphoma. The standard dose is 375 mg/m[2] weekly. Immunophoresis is a procedure that is similar to plasmapheresis in which sheep antihuman IgG bead-formed agarose gel is used to selectively immunoabsorb and remove patients' circulating IgG autoantibodies. Clinical and serologic improvement is reported in a patient after failing systemic glucocorticoid therapy.

Bullous Pemphigoid

Bullous pemphigoid (BP) is a disease that results from an autoimmune response (autoantibodies) and has prominent inflammatory features (cellular infiltrate). Unlike treating PV, successful treatment of BP may be accomplished with anti-inflammatory agents. The goal of therapy is to heal the existing lesions and prevent the appearance of new lesions.

Potent topical steroids[1] such as fluocinonide (Lidex)[1] or clobetasol (Temovate)[1] should be considered in the management of patients with localized or limited disease. Most patients with generalized BP require systemic therapy. The most commonly used systemic agents are the glucocorticoids. Prednisone is the most commonly used glucocorticoid and is sufficient as the only therapy in the majority of cases in a dose is 0.5 to 0.75 mg/kg per day. Unlike in PV, higher doses of prednisone are rarely needed. A clinical response is usually obtained within 1 to 3 weeks. The prednisone dose is then gradually decreased by relatively large portions (10 mg) initially and smaller portions (2.5 to 5 mg) later. When the daily dose is 30 to 40 mg, shifting to every other day is attempted to decrease the potential for well-known, long-term glucocorticoid side effects. In many patients, prednisone may be completely discontinued after 6 months of therapy. Some patients require longer duration of therapy. Steroid pulse therapy with methylprednisolone, IV 0.5 to 1 g daily for 3 consecutive days, may help control severe disease. Unlike in patients with PV, this therapy is rarely needed.

Immunosuppressive drug therapy is indicated for patients who require a high-maintenance dose of glucocorticoid, develop glucocorticoid side effects, or do not respond completely to glucocorticoid therapy. The most commonly used immunosuppressive agents are azathioprine,[1] MMF,[1] and methotrexate.[1] Azathioprine[1] is commonly used in a dose of 1 to 3 mg/kg per day, which may be adjusted based on clinical response and side effects. MMF[1] is used in a dose of 30 to 35 mg/kg per day or 1 gm twice daily. MMF (CellCept)[1] and azathioprine[1] are effective as sole agents or in combination with glucocorticoids. Methotrexate (Rheumatrex)[1] is effective in small doses (up to 12.5 mg per week) and may be used as sole therapy.

Tetracyclines[1] or erythromycin,[1] with or without niacinamide,[1] have been used effectively. These agents are known to have anti-inflammatory properties. Initial case reports suggest a moderate beneficial effect of tetracycline with or without niacinamide. A study that compares the effectiveness of the combination of tetracycline and niacinamide versus that of prednisone in the treatment of generalized BP finds that the combination of the two medications is equally effective as prednisone. Tetracycline[1] is given in a dose of 500 mg four times daily and niacinamide[1] in a dose of 500 mg three times daily. Minocycline (Minocin),[1] 100 mg, or doxycycline (Vibramycin),[1] 100 mg twice daily, may be used instead of tetracycline. The use of tetracycline and niacinamide[1] may be indicated in two situations. In mild cases, the combination alone may lead to a clinical remission without use of corticosteroids. In more extensive cases, the addition of this combination of drugs to prednisone may have a steroid-sparing effect.

Dapsone[1] (or a sulfapyridine[1,2]) has been used with mild to moderate response. Dapsone[1] is usually started at 50 mg daily and increased by 50 mg increments every week until a beneficial effect is obtained. The mechanism of action of dapsone[1] in BP is unclear.

---

[1]Not FDA approved for this indication.

[1]Not FDA approved for this indication.
[2]Not available in the United States.

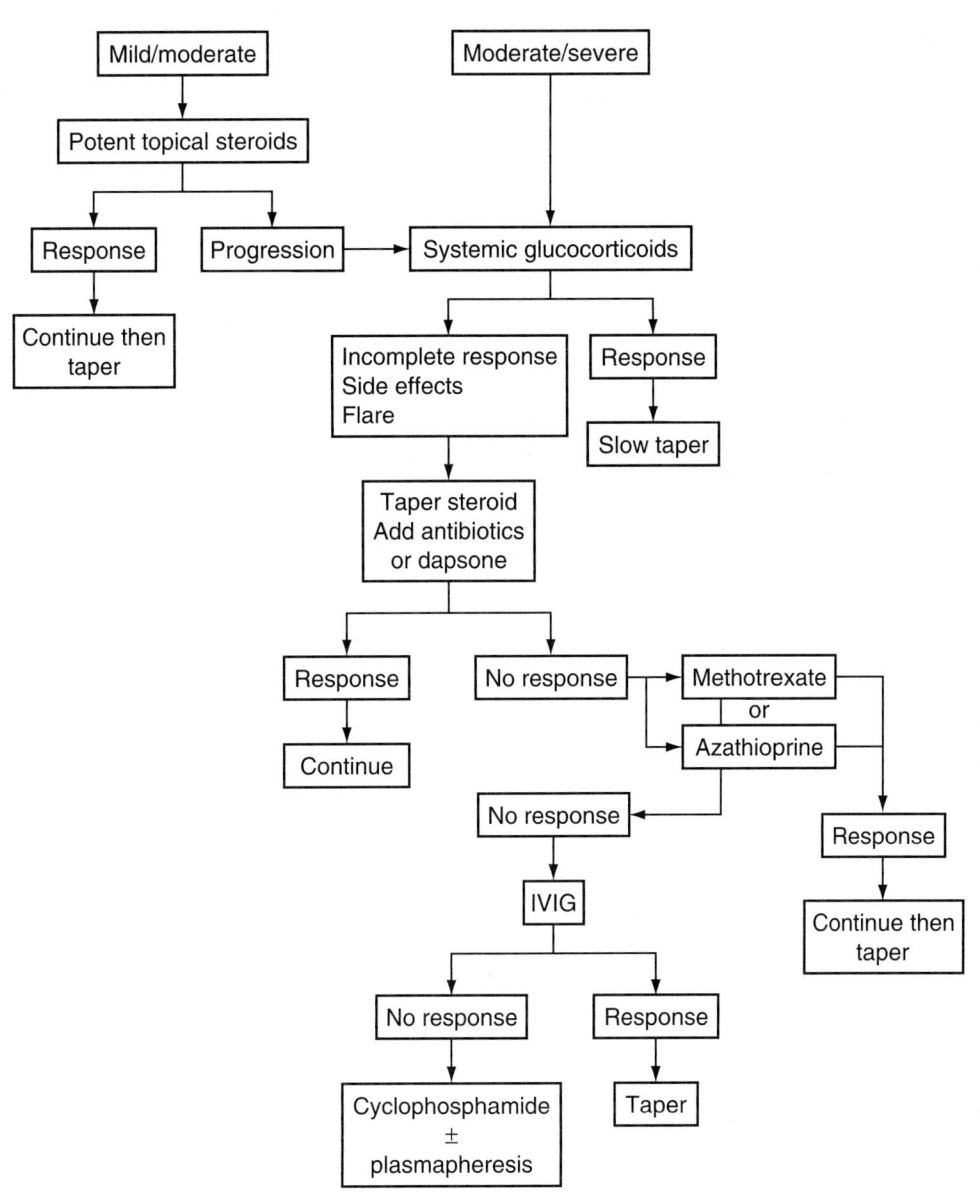

FIGURE 2. Treatment of bullous pemphigoid.

High-dose IVIG[1] is highly effective for selected cases. It is given in a dose of 2 g/kg in a cycle divided over 4 to 5 days. Patients usually receive two to four cycles (once every 3 to 4 weeks) initially and one to two cycles if their disease recurs. This therapy is extremely expensive and should be reserved for resistant cases. Plasmapheresis is used in severe cases. The procedure should be used in conjunction with immunosuppressive/cytotoxic therapy (e.g., cyclophosphamide[1]) to avoid the rebound phenomenon. Plasmapheresis is costly and time consuming and produces only temporary benefits.

A recent report reviews the literature and discusses the evidence for treating BP from six randomized,

controlled trials comprising 293 patients. No strong recommendations can be made based on the available evidence. In the proposed guidelines, systemic glucocorticoids are the best established treatment. Consideration should be given to potent topical steroids for localized disease. For mild to moderate disease, tetracyclines[1] and niacinamide[1] should be considered. Immunosuppressive agents should not be routinely used and should be considered if the glucocorticoid dose cannot be reduced to an acceptable level. Azathioprine[1] is the best established agent, followed by methotrexate.[1] Figure 2 is a proposed algorithm for the treatment of BP.

[1]Not FDA approved for this indication.

[1]Not FDA approved for this indication.

Rakel and Bope: *Conn's Current Therapy 2006.*

Mucosal Pemphigoid

Therapy of mucosal pemphigoid (MP) varies with the sites of involvement, extent, and severity. In limited oral disease, local therapy with topical anesthetic agents and topical glucocorticoids in addition to oral hygiene may suffice. The steroid may be applied under occlusion with a prosthetic device or injected intralesionally. Patients with extensive oral involvement may require systemic therapy. Dapsone[1] is effective in some patients. Oral lesions respond faster than ocular lesions, which may not respond. The drug is started at 50 mg daily and increased gradually.

Tetracyclines,[1] with or without niacinamide,[1] are effective according to some reports. In severe oral disease as well as patients with ocular, pharyngeal, or laryngeal involvement, systemic glucocorticoids, in combination with cyclophosphamide,[1] are indicated. Most of the patients have an excellent response with a prolonged remission after being treated with the combination of prednisone (1 mg/kg per day) and cyclophosphamide[1] (1 to 2 mg/kg per day). Prednisone is used for approximately 6 months, whereas cyclophosphamide[1] is used for 18 to 24 months. Azathioprine[1] and MMF[1] are generally less effective but may be used if there are contraindications to steroid or cyclophosphamide use.

High-dose IVIG[1] is sometimes successful in the treatment of patients with MP who are refractory to other therapy. The use of IVIG[1] therapy results in a faster reduction in the level of autoantibody titers. High-dose IVIG[1] results in the induction and maintenance of a sustained clinical and serologic remission. Cases with severe ocular scarring may benefit from cryotherapy ablation of eyelashes. Ocular surgery is contraindicated when the disease is active. Surgical intervention may cause severe flares of the disease. Figure 3 is a proposed algorithm for the treatment of MP.

Epidermolysis Bullosa Acquisita

Unlike other subepidermal autoimmune bullous diseases, epidermolysis bullosa acquisita (EBA) is generally resistant to therapy. The disease waxes and wanes with periods of remission and exacerbation. Trauma is known to contribute to blister formation, especially in the classical form of EBA. The inflammatory form of EBA responds more easily to therapy than the classical form. Because of the neutrophil predominance in the inflammatory form, many patients respond to dapsone.[1] The drug is started at a dose of 50 mg daily and increased by 50 mg every week until clinical remission (usually 100 to 250 mg). The dose is maintained for several months. If the patient remains in remission, the dose may be decreased slowly and ultimately discontinued. Colchicine[1] is reported to be variably effective in a few cases. Patients who do not tolerate or do not respond to

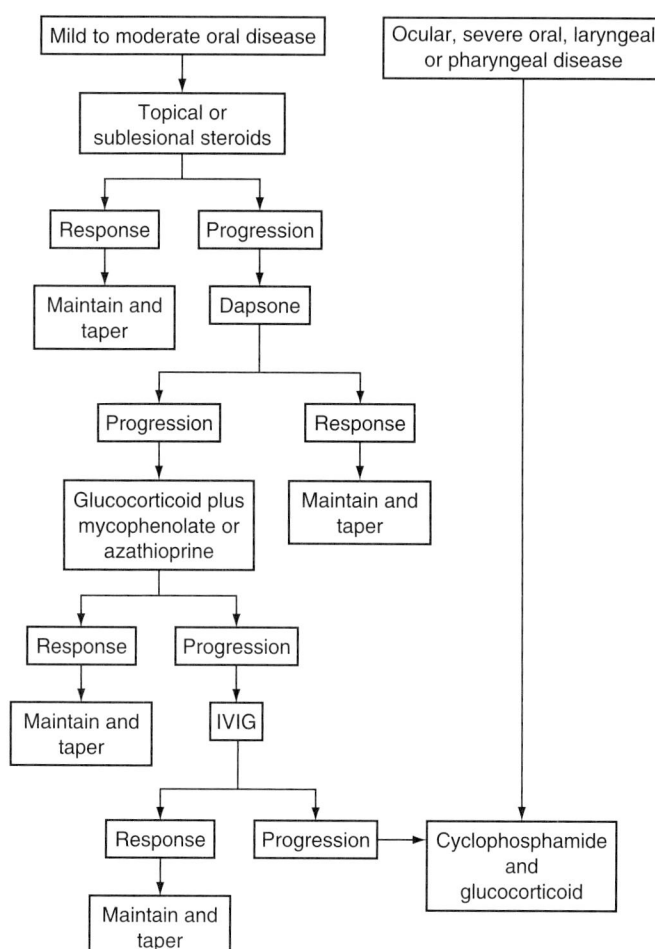

FIGURE 3. Treatment of mucosal pemphigoid.
Abbreviation: IVIG = intravenous immunoglobulin.

colchicine[1] and dapsone[1] may be treated with oral glucocorticoids such as prednisone in a dose of 0.5 to 1 mg/kg per day in divided doses.

If there is no response to glucocorticoids or if the patient develops severe adverse effects, cyclosporine[1] (4 to 6 mg/kg/day) may be initiated and is usually associated with a rapid response. Once disease activity is controlled, the dose is decreased. Decrements of 1 mg/kg per day every other week can be instituted until stabilization. Another regimen is to initiate therapy at 2.5 to 3 mg/kg per day and increase the dose by 0.5 to 1.0 mg/kg per day every 2 weeks if needed. Cyclosporine[1] should be discontinued if there is no response within a few weeks.

The same agents that are used for the inflammatory form of EBA may be used for the classical form. The latter is generally more resistant to treatment. Patients who fail to respond may be treated with immunosuppressive agents such as azathioprine[1] or cyclophosphamide[1] in a manner similar to PV, BP, and MP. Patients who

---

[1]Not FDA approved for this indication.

[1]Not FDA approved for this indication.

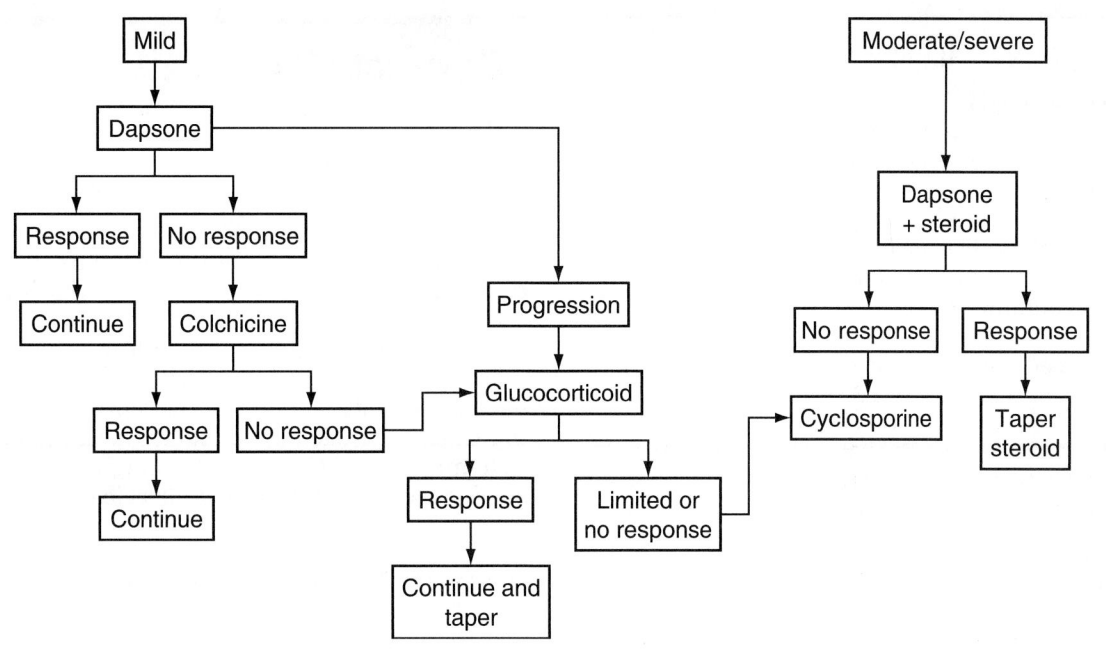

FIGURE 4. Treatment of epidermolysis bullosa acquisita.

are resistant to these agents may be treated with IVIG[1] alone or in conjunction with plasmapheresis. The advantages of IVIG[1] over plasmapheresis are the rapid onset of action and the lesser degree of invasiveness. Extracorporeal photochemotherapy was effective in four reported cases with refractory EBA. Figure 4 is a proposed algorithm for the treatment of EBA.

Linear Immunoglobulin A Disease

Linear IgA disease (LAD) is mediated by neutrophils. Dapsone[1] is the first-line agent for the treatment of LAD. The drug may be started at 50 mg daily and increased by 50-mg increments every 1 to 2 weeks until an effective dose is reached. Sulfapyridine[1,2] is an alternative agent for patients who cannot tolerate dapsone. The starting dose is 500 mg twice daily and may be increased by 1000 mg every 1 to 2 weeks until it adequately controls the disease. Colchicine[1] in doses of 0.6 mg 2 to 3 times daily may be considered. Glucocorticoids may be added if patients do not respond completely to dapsone or sulfapyridine.[1,2] Tetracyclines[1] in combination with niacinamide[1] are reported to be effective. The dose of tetracycline is 500 mg four times daily. Alternatively, doxycycline or minocycline, 100 mg twice daily, may be used. The dose of niacinamide is 500 mg three times daily. Cyclosporine[1] or high-dose IVIG[1] may be used in resistant cases.

---

[1]Not FDA approved for this indication.
[2]Not available in the United States.

Rakel and Bope: *Conn's Current Therapy 2006.*

Dermatitis Herpetiformis

Dermatitis herpetiformis (DH) results from an immune response to gluten. A gluten-free diet is extremely helpful in the management of patients with DH and is often associated with a marked decrease in the requirement for pharmacologic therapy with drugs such as dapsone.[1] A strict gluten-free diet may result in complete remission of the disease without requiring dapsone therapy. Reinstitution of a gluten-containing diet results in recurrence of the disease within a few months. The support of a dietician and disease support groups is often helpful. Many patients find a strict gluten-free diet too restrictive and choose pharmacologic therapy. The drug of choice for patients with DH is dapsone. Treatment is initiated with dapsone at 50 mg daily and is increased by 25 mg every week as needed and as tolerated. The average daily maintenance dose is 100 mg. Some patients require slowly increasing doses several years later,

---

[1]Not FDA approved for this indication.

  CURRENT DIAGNOSIS

- Histopathology
    Intraepidermal: pemphigus
    Subepidermal: pemphigoid, epidermolysis
      bullous acquisita, LAD
- Direct immunofluorescence
    Epidermal cell surface: pemphigus
    Basement membrane: subepidermal diseases

Abbreviations: LAD = linear IgA disease.

CURRENT THERAPY

- Glucocorticoids
- Nonsteroidal immunosuppressive drugs
- Purine analogs: Azathioprine (Imuran),[1] MMF (CellCept)[1]
- Calcineurin inhibitors: Cyclosporine (Neoral)[1]
- Folate antagonist: methotrexate (Rheumatrex)[1]
- Cytotoxic: cyclophosphamide (Cytoxan)[1]
- IVIG (Gamimune N)[1]
- Plasmapheresis
- Anti-B cell antibodies: Rituximab (Rituxan)[1]

[1]Not FDA approved for this indication.
Abbreviations: IVIG = intravenous immunoglobulin; MMF = mycophenolate mofetil.

which is likely secondary to increased deposition of IgA in the skin that results in increased disease activity.

In patients who are intolerant or allergic to dapsone, therapy with sulfapyridine[1,2] may be considered. The initial dose is 500 mg three times daily and may be increased slowly to 2 g three times daily. The response to sulfapyridine[1,2] is not as predictable as that to dapsone. Patients who are allergic to dapsone often tolerate sulfapyridine.[1,2] Patients who are intolerant or allergic to both dapsone and sulfapyridine[1,2] may be treated with colchicine,[1] cholestyramine,[1] heparin,[1] tetracycline,[1] and nicotinamide.[1] These agents are much less effective than dapsone and sulfapyridine.[1,2] Topical steroids are only minimally effective.

The effective management of patients with autoimmune bullous diseases requires knowledge of the pharmacologic effects of the agents used, an accurate diagnosis, knowledge of the pathophysiology of the disease process, and understanding of patient expectations.

REFERENCES

Bystryn J-C, Steinman NM: The adjuvant therapy of pemphigus. Arch Dermatol 1996;132:203-212.
Mutasim DF: Laboratory diagnosis of autoimmune bullous diseases. G Ital Dermatol Venereol 2002;137:383-393.
Mutasim DF: Management of autoimmune bullous diseases: Pharmacology and therapeutics. J Am Acad Derm 2004; 51(6): 859-880.
Mutasim DF, Anhalt GJ: Bullous diseases in the elderly. In Gilchrest BA (ed): Clinics in Geriatric Medicine, Philadelphia, WB Saunders, 2002, pp 43-58.
Nousari HC, Sragovich A, Kimyai-Asadi A, et al: Mycophenolate mofetil in autoimmune and inflammatory skin disorders. J Am Acad Dermatol 1999; 40:265-268.

[1]Not FDA approved for this indication.
[2]Not available in the United States.

Contact Dermatitis

Method of
Denis Sasseville, MD

Contact dermatitis is an exogenous inflammatory disorder of the skin resulting from the interaction of the integument with a chemical or biologic aggressor. Although it can sometimes manifest as urticaria, lichen planus, or erythema multiforme, approximately 95% of cases exhibit an eczematous morphology, with varying degrees of edema, vesiculation, desquamation, and lichenification. Contact dermatitis is traditionally subdivided into irritant and allergic dermatitis.

Irritant Contact Dermatitis

Irritant contact dermatitis accounts for 75% to 80% of all cases. It results from the direct cytotoxic effect of the offending agent on the cells of the skin. Strong irritants such as concentrated acids or alkalis cause an acute contact dermatitis, manifested by a painful burn accompanied by erythema, edema, blistering, or necrosis.

Mild irritants such as water, detergents, solvents, and dilute solutions of alkalis or acids require repeated exposure to induce visible changes. The threshold for irritation varies from one individual to another, and atopics are much more susceptible to irritation. The interval between exposure and onset of dermatitis may vary from a few days to many years. Patients complain of pain rather than itch, and the clinical picture is a subacute or chronic eczema, characterized by desquamation, crusting, fissuring, and a grayish thickening of the epidermis known as *lichenification*. The prototype of chronic irritant contact dermatitis is housewives' eczema, caused by repeated contact with water and cleaning products.

Allergic Contact Dermatitis

Allergic contact dermatitis occurs in a minority of individuals who develop an immunologic reaction to a foreign substance deposited on the skin. This delayed lymphocyte-mediated event is similar to the rejection of a graft. The epidermis contains a network of antigen-presenting cells called Langerhans cells that capture incomplete antigens, or haptens. These haptens are internalized, combined with proteins to become complete antigens, and presented to naïve T cells that undergo clonal expansion and divide into memory and cytotoxic T cells. This initial, or sensitization, phase lasts approximately 3 weeks and is usually asymptomatic. The elicitation phase is triggered when already primed T lymphocytes are once again presented with the allergen and release proinflammatory cytokines that generate visible lesions. This second phase usually begins after 24 to 48 hours and may last between 2 and 8 weeks after a single exposure.

Rakel and Bope: *Conn's Current Therapy 2006.*

The usual clinical presentation is an acute or subacute eczema. A classic example of acute allergic contact dermatitis is the intensely itchy, vesiculobullous dermatitis, often distributed in linear streaks, that follows contact with *Toxicodendron* species (poison ivy/poison oak). At times, however, allergic contact dermatitis manifests as chronic eczema, especially after repeated exposure to a low-grade unrecognized allergen. Examples include the painful, keratotic, and fissured dermatitis of the fingertips seen in dental assistants sensitized to acrylates in composite restorative materials or florists allergic to tulip bulbs and *Alstroemeria* ("tulip fingers").

Relying solely on the symptoms, morphology, and distribution of the lesions is often insufficient to distinguish between irritant and allergic contact dermatitis. More than 3700 chemicals are potential allergens, and many are both irritants and allergens. They range from metals to glues and resins, preservatives in cosmetics, paints, and metalworking fluids, rubber additives, textile dyes, and topical medications. The gold standard technique for detecting contact allergens is patch testing. Standardized allergens (Thin-Layer Rapid Use Epicutaneous [TRUE] Test and others) are applied on the patient's back and read after 48 and 96 hours in a fashion similar to a tuberculin test. According to the North American Contact Dermatitis Group, the 10 most common sensitizers are nickel, balsam of Peru, neomycin, fragrance mix, thimerosal, gold, formaldehyde, quaternium-15, bacitracin, and cobalt.

Treatment

Treatment of acute irritant contact dermatitis is the same as for a thermal burn, with the extra step of copious lavage with water to remove the offending chemical. Alkali burns are more extensive than acid burns and require more prolonged irrigation and mechanical scrubbing. Analgesia and standard wound care with nonadherent dressings and surgical débridement constitute the essential of subsequent care.

Management of iterative, subacute, or chronic contact dermatitis starts with recognition and avoidance of the aggressor. Withdrawal from work may be necessary and should be long enough to allow restoration of the epidermal barrier, which may require 4 to 6 weeks after visible lesions have cleared. Mid-strength to potent corticosteroids, such as triamcinolone acetonide (Kenalog), betamethasone valerate (Valisone), betamethasone dipropionate (Diprosone), or halcinonide (Halog), are used, preferably in their ointment formulations. The addition of 3% to 5% salicylic acid helps reduce lichenification. Liberal use of moisturizers is encouraged, and in most circumstances, the greasiest are best. Petroleum jelly or thick water-in-oil emulsions are effective emollients against water-soluble irritants, whereas oil-in-water preparations work best with solvents or oils. These emollients act passively by seeping between corneocytes to replace lost natural lipids. Newer moisturizers, based on cholesterol, free fatty acids, and ceramide, may behave in a more active fashion because their components are internalized by living keratinocytes to

regenerate the disrupted lipid barrier. When frequent hand washing cannot be avoided, mild synthetic detergents (Dove, Aveeno Bar) should be substituted for harsh soaps and abrasive cleansers.

Recognition and removal of the offending agent is also the crucial initial step in the management of allergic contact dermatitis. In the acute stage, treatment is directed at alleviation of symptoms and suppression of inflammation. Thin wet dressings saturated with tap water, saline, or Burow's solution (Domeboro), applied for 20 to 30 minutes three or four times per day, dry up oozy lesions. Sedating antihistamines such as hydroxyzine (Atarax), 25 to 100 mg/day, or diphenhydramine (Benadryl), 50 to 200 mg per day, bring some relief from pruritus but produce considerable drowsiness. Nonsedating antihistamines are devoid of side effects but ineffective as antipruritics in allergic contact dermatitis. Glucocorticosteroids are the mainstay of treatment in acute cases of allergic contact dermatitis. When lesions are limited in extent and severity, topical formulations in creams, gels, or lotions usually suffice. Because the duration of treatment is expected to be short, superpotent agents such as clobetasol propionate (Temovate) or halobetasol propionate (Ultravate) can be used, even on the face or genitalia. For more extensive or severe lesions, systemic corticosteroids are warranted. Oral prednisone is prescribed at an initial dose of 1 mg/kg per day for 6 to 10 days, decreased to 0.5 mg/kg per day for an additional 6 to 10 days, and then stopped. Intramuscular triamcinolone acetonide (Kenalog) is an alternative that is administered as a single dose of 40 to 60 mg. When corticosteroids are contraindicated, oral cyclosporine (Neoral)[1] can be used at a dose of 5 mg/kg per day.

Chronic allergic contact dermatitis is usually treated with topical glucocorticosteroids. Selection of the preparation should be guided by the location of the dermatitis and by the presumed duration of therapy. The least potent effective formulation should be chosen to avoid side effects of atrophy, acneiform eruptions, and tachyphylaxis. Tacrolimus (Protopic ointment)[1] and pimecrolimus (Elidel cream)[1] are newer immunomodulators devoid of atrophogenic potential and safe to use on delicate skin. They are expensive and may not be potent enough to replace stronger corticosteroids on difficult-to-treat areas such as the hands and feet.

Patients who fail to improve with topical treatment often respond to psoralen plus ultraviolet A (PUVA)[1] phototherapy. This treatment consists of topical or oral

---

[1]Not FDA approved for this indication.

 CURRENT DIAGNOSIS

- Eczematous morphology occurs in most cases.
- Irritant contact dermatitis manifests as painful chemical burn or subacute/chronic eczema.
- Allergic contact dermatitis manifests as pruritic, acute/subacute dermatitis.
- Patch testing is helpful in finding the cause of allergic contact dermatitis.

13

CURRENT THERAPY

- Exposure to the offending agent must be stopped.
- Wet dressings and corticosteroid creams, gels, or lotions are used in acute dermatitis.
- Short courses of systemic prednisone or cyclosporine[1] are used for severe or extensive lesions.
- Chronic dermatitis is treated with corticosteroid ointments and emollients.
- Psoralen ultraviolet A (PUVA) phototherapy[1] or grenz rays are alternatives for localized refractory dermatitis.
- Systemic immunosuppressants may at times be needed.

[1]Not FDA approved for this indication.

administration of photosensitizing psoralens followed by precisely dosed incremental exposures to ultraviolet A light, usually given three times per week. Superficial radio therapy (grenz rays) is a less frequently used but an effective modality of treatment for refractory hand or foot eczema. Systemic immunosuppressants may occasionally be necessary. Methotrexate,[1] 10 to 25 mg per week, is given in divided doses on 2 consecutive days. Azathioprine (Imuran)[1] is also used with success in doses ranging from 100 to 150 mg per day. Cyclosporine[1] is often effective when administered 3 to 5 mg/kg per day, but nephrotoxicity may preclude long-term use. The newer drug is mycophenolate mofetil (CellCept),[1] given orally in doses that range from 1500 to 2500 mg per day. Toxicity is low and consists of mild myelosuppression, nausea, and diarrhea.

REFERENCES

Belsito DV: Allergic contact dermatitis: Immunological aspects. In Adams RM (ed): Occupational Skin Disease, 3rd ed. Philadelphia, WB Saunders, 1999, pp 28-34.

Brandt CP, Fratianne RB: Diagnosis and management of common industrial burns. Dermatol Clin 1994;12:469-475.

De Groot AC. Patch Testing. Test Concentrations and Vehicles for 3700 Chemicals, 2nd ed. Amsterdam, Elsevier, 1994.

Elsner P. Irritant dermatitis in the workplace. Dermatol Clin 1994; 12:461-467.

Mao-Qiang M, Brown BE, Wu-Pong S, et al: Exogenous nonphysiologic vs. physiologic lipids. Arch Dermatol 1995;131:809-816.

Marks JG Jr, Belsito DV, DeLeo VA, et al: North American Contact Dermatitis Group patch test results, 1998 to 2000. Am J Contact Dermat 2003;2:59-62.

Rietschel RL, Fowler JF Jr: Noneczematous contact dermatitis. In Rietschel RL, Fowler JF (eds) Fisher's Contact Dermatitis, 5th ed. Philadelphia, Lippincott William & Wilkins, 2001, pp 71-88.

Warshaw E, Lee G, Storrs FJ: Hand dermatitis: A review of clinical features, therapeutic options, and long-term outcomes. Am J Contact Dermat 2003;14:119-137.

[1]Not FDA approved for this indication.

Pruritus Ani and Vulvae

Method of
Libby Edwards, MD

Anogenital pruritus, or itching, is a symptom, not a diagnosis. The word *itching* encompasses a number of sensations, including irritation, prickling, and crawling sensations as well as a sensation of needing to scratch. Specifically excluded are burning, soreness, and other pain adjectives.

Unlike medication for pain, no nonspecific anti-itch medications are available. Thus the management of anogenital pruritus begins with an evaluation to diagnose the underlying cause, followed by specific therapy for that etiology (Box 1). The usual causes of itching are infection, dermatosis, neuropathy, or anxiety/depression. Several factors may play a role.

Acute itching is most often related to infection, especially *Candida albicans*. Herpes simplex virus infection, trichomoniasis, *Staphylococcus aureus,* and scabies are less common causes of itching. The most common dermatosis to produce sudden-onset itching is allergic or irritant contact dermatitis, in which something touching the skin (overcleaning, stool retained in skin folds, topical medications, etc.) causes itching.

Chronic itching is most often caused by skin disease, often with exacerbating factors such as secondary infection or irritation from topical medications. The most common dermatoses to cause chronic itching are eczema/ lichen simplex chronicus (LSC) and lichen sclerosus (LS). Less common pruritic dermatoses that can affect anogenital skin include psoriasis and nonerosive lichen planus (LP). Although infection is almost never the primary cause of chronic anogenital itching, infection can complicate and perpetuate itching from dermatoses. Some patients exhibit chronic itching despite a normal

---

BOX 1   Causes of Anogenital Itching

Acute Itching
Infection
- *Candida albicans*
- Pinworms
- Trichomoniasis
- Herpes simplex virus infection
- Mollusca contagiosa
- Genital warts, bacterial vaginosis, group B streptococcus

Dermatoses
- Irritant or allergic contact dermatoses
- Eczema, lichen sclerosus, psoriasis, lichen planus

Chronic Itching (Often Multifactorial)
- Dermatoses: Lichen simplex chronicus/eczema, lichen sclerosus, psoriasis, lichen planus
- Neuropathy
- Anxiety/depression
- Infection: Usually only a complicating factor in the face of underlying dermatosis

---

physical examination and negative cultures. Most often these patients have subtle eczema, but itching on the basis of neuropathy or anxiety/depression can occur. These diagnoses are made by excluding infection and skin disease and by response to therapy.

Management

The first step in management is a very careful examination of the anogenital area, including vulvar and perianal skin folds and the vaginal epithelium (Box 2). Severe symptoms sometimes are produced by subtle signs. Cultures of vaginal secretions and scrapings of scaling skin to evaluate for infection are indicated.

Acute itching on the basis of an infection can generally be cleared rapidly and definitively by treatment of

---

BOX 2 Treatment of Anogenital Itching

Nonspecific Measures
- Patient education and reassurance
- Careful evaluation for infection and dermatoses
- Elimination of irritants: Overwashing, infection, nighttime scratching, unnecessary topical medications and lubricants, infections
- Topical anesthetics: Topical lidocaine (Xylocaine) jelly 2%/ointment 5%, as needed; pramoxine (Summer's Eve Anti-itch Gel) as needed; topical benzocaine (Vagisil) and diphenhydramine (Benadryl) should be avoided
- Nighttime sedation
- Cool soaks/ice (frostbite avoided by wrapping ice in a towel)

Specific Measures
- Itching because of infection
    Acute itching: Treatment with standard therapy.
    Chronic itching: Evaluation for concomitant dermatosis; infection treated and suppressed long enough for skin to heal and itching to respond to therapy for concomitant process.
- Itching because of dermatoses
    Lichen sclerosus: Clobetasol propionate (Temovate) ointment two times per day until skin texture is normal, then three times per week for life (prepubertal girls occasionally experience remission at puberty; boys remit after circumcision). Or chronic tacrolimus (Protopic) 0.1%, two times per day.
    Eczema/lichen simplex chronicus (LSC): Clobetasol propionate ointment two times per day until skin is normal and itching controlled, then frequency tapered to three times weekly, twice weekly, once weekly, then discontinued; restarted when flares occur. Or tacrolimus (Protopic) or pimecrolimus (Elidel), two times per day.
- Itching without objective abnormalities
    Treated as for eczema/lichen simplex chronicus with clobetasol propionate for presumed subtle eczema/LSC.
    Amitriptyline (Elavil) (tapered up as high as 150 mg at bedtime), venlafaxine (Effexor) (tapered up as high as 150 mg extended release per day), gabapentin (Neurontin) (up to 3600 mg per day) for neuropathic pain
    Anxiety/depression addressed

Rakel and Bope: *Conn's Current Therapy 2006.*

the infection. All dermatoses, whether producing acute or chronic itching, can be treated with an ultrapotent topical corticosteroid ointment (e.g., clobetasol propionate [Temovate]). Ointments are less irritating than creams or gels. Although potent corticosteroids can produce atrophy, striae, and steroid dermatitis when used chronically without supervision, short-term twice-daily use produces safe and rapid control of symptoms. The frequency of application can be tapered when itching is controlled, or a lower potency medication can be substituted. Some dermatoses (LS, psoriasis) require long-term or lifetime thrice-weekly dosing of a corticosteroid to maintain control, whereas others (LSC) usually achieve remission, and medication can be discontinued, at least for prolonged times. Tacrolimus (Protopic) is beneficial for LSC, LS, and LP, although it is slow in onset and produces burning with application. Itchy anogenital skin without evidence of an infection or a visible dermatosis should be treated with a potent topical corticosteroid. If unresponsive to a steroid, the addition of medication for neuropathy (amitriptyline [Elavil], gabapentin [Neurontin], venlafaxine [Effexor]) or attention to anxiety/depression should be considered.

Whatever the cause, certain nonspecific measures can improve itching and contribute to a more rapid response to specific therapy, including the following:

- Avoidance of irritants, such as overwashing and unnecessary topical medications.
- Topical anesthetics (lidocaine [Xylocaine] jelly 2% or ointment 5%) that can temporarily improve itching and minimize ongoing irritation from scratching (but topical benzocaine [Vagisil] and diphenhydramine [Benadryl], which can be irritating and allergenic, should be avoided).
- Nighttime sedation, which can both provide well-needed respite from sleepless itchy nights and protect the skin from irritating scratching during nighttime hours. Tricyclic medications such as amitriptyline and doxepin (Sinequan) produce deeper sleep and less scratching than diphenhydramine and hydroxyzine (Atarax).

Although many clinicians use antihistamines for all itching, this class of medication has no intrinsic anti-itch properties and is generally useful only for the histamine-mediated itch of urticaria, usually a generalized rather than anogenital process.

Other, less potent measures that can be used in patients with recalcitrant symptoms include topical doxepin (Zonalon), tacrolimus (Protopic 0.1%), or pimecrolimus (Elidel). These medications are beneficial primarily in patients with mild to moderate eczema/LSC.

 CURRENT DIAGNOSIS

- Examination for skin disease
- Microscopic examinations and cultures for infection
- History of contactants and irritants

CURRENT THERAPY

- Careful evaluation for underlying etiologies
- Specific therapies for all appropriate underlying etiologies
- Specific therapy continued long enough for the skin to heal and the itch-scratch cycle to cease
- Patient education regarding the chronic/recurrent nature of itching and the role of irritants
- Consideration of neuropathy and anxiety/depression in patients without observable disease who are resistant to topical corticosteroid therapy

Patients should be advised that all causes of itching can be chronic or recurrent. Thus recurrence of itching does not necessarily reflect a failure of diagnosis or therapy but rather a need for recurrent or chronic therapy that is sufficiently prolonged for the skin to heal completely and for the itch-scratch cycle to be broken.

REFERENCES

Bauer A, Deier J, Elsner P: Allergic contact dermatitis in patients with anogenital complaints. J Reprod Med 2000;45:649-654.
Bohm M, Frieling U, Luger TA, et al: Successful treatment of anogenital lichen sclerosus with topical tacrolimus. Arch Dermatol 2003; 48:444-448.
Bornstein J, Heifetz S, Kellner Y, et al: Clobetasol dipropionate 0.05% versus testosterone propionate 2% topical application for severe vulvar lichen sclerosus. Am J Obstet Gynecol 1998;178(1, Pt 1): 80-84.
Cohen AD, Masalha R, Medvedovsky E, Vardy DA: Brachioradial pruritus: A symptom of neuropathy. J Am Acad Dermatol 2003; 48(6):825-828.
Kirtschig G, Van Der Meulen AJ, Ion Lipan JW, et al: Successful treatment of erosive vulvovaginal lichen planus with topical tacrolimus. Br J Dermatol 2002;147:625-626.
Reitamo S, Rustin M, Ruzicka T, et al: Efficacy and safety of tacrolimus ointment compared with that of hydrocortisone butyrate ointment in adult patients with atopic dermatitis. J Allergy Clin Immunol 2002;109:547-555.
Stellon A: Neurogenic pruritus: An unrecognized problem? A retrospective case series of treatment by acupuncture. Acupunct Med 2002;20(4):186-190.

Urticaria and Angioedema

Method of
Eugene W. Monroe, MD

Urticaria (hives) is a skin reaction pattern characterized by transient, pruritic, edematous, lightly erythematous papules or wheals, frequently with central clearing. *Angioedema* describes swellings of the deep dermis or subcutaneous tissue involving mucous membranes and loose tissues around the eyes, lips, or genitalia. Urticaria is extremely common. Approximately 15% to 20% of the general population have at least one episode of urticaria, angioedema, or both during their lives. The potential causes of urticaria are numerous, including drugs, food, infections, internal diseases, inhalants, bites/stings, contactants, immunologic processes, psychogenic factors, genetic abnormalities, and physical agents (dermographism and pressure, cholinergic, cold, solar, and heat urticaria).

Classification

Urticaria is classified as acute or chronic, depending on the duration of the condition. Most cases of urticaria are classified as acute because they persist for only a few days to a few weeks. The incidence of acute urticaria is between 10% and 20% of the population. The etiology is usually detected, often an allergic reaction to a food or medication, or related to an acute infection. Many cases of urticaria are never seen by a physician. The initial aspect of therapy is the elimination of any suspected cause. Drug therapy should begin with the use of a so-called nonsedating H_1 antihistamine. In severe urticarial reactions or in cases associated with asthma or laryngeal edema, stronger medical management is required, including the use of subcutaneous injection of epinephrine or systemic corticosteroids.

When urticaria persists longer than 6 weeks, it is classified as chronic urticaria. The incidence of this form is between 0.1% and 3% of the population. The course is variable, from months to years, with 20% lasting longer than 20 years. Approximately 40% of the cases are associated with angioedema. Unfortunately, the etiology is not found in 60% to 95% of these cases, with most either idiopathic or autoimmune in nature. Treatment programs for chronic urticaria focus on measures that provide symptomatic relief.

Diagnosis

The clinical diagnosis of urticaria is reasonably easy. Finding an underlying cause, especially for chronic urticaria, however, is usually extremely frustrating for the patient and the physician.

The most important diagnostic test in the evaluation of a patient with urticaria is a detailed history, which should include the location of lesions, morphology of lesions, pattern of attacks, precipitating factors, review of medical systems, and review of potential etiologies of urticaria. Diagnostic tests are selected on the basis of suspicions elicited by a meticulous history and physical examination. Potential minimal baseline tests might include a complete blood count with differential, a chemistry panel, and a sedimentation rate. Other possible tests based on the history might include thyroid autoantibodies, physical urticaria challenge tests, autologous serum skin testing, and so on.

Treatment

The ideal treatment for urticaria is identification and removal of its cause. If that is not possible, the reduction of various triggering factors should be attempted, especially in cases of physical urticaria. The drug management of urticaria centers around four theoretical treatment approaches: blocking the effects of already released histamine on the receptor sites of cutaneous blood vessels; blocking the release of histamine and other mediators from mast cells; blocking mediators other than histamine that can cause hives; and modulating the inflammatory, cellular, and immunologic components of the urticarial process.

H_1 antihistamines remain the first line of therapy for urticaria. First-generation antihistamines such as hydroxyzine (Atarax), diphenhydramine (Benadryl), and chlorpheniramine (Chlor-Trimeton) are moderately effective in treating urticaria. The usefulness of these agents is sometimes limited by undesirable side effects, however, especially central nervous system (CNS) effects such as daytime sedation and anticholinergic effects. Because of these problems, a new class of peripherally acting second-generation antihistamines, most of which are labeled "nonsedating," are now available.

Four second-generation antihistamines are currently available on the market in the United States. In order of their FDA approval, these are loratadine (Claritin), cetirizine (Zyrtec), fexofenadine (Allegra), and desloratadine (Clarinex). Table 1 compares these agents in terms of dosing, potency, and side effects.

In clinical studies of chronic urticaria, the efficacy of the second-generation antihistamines is statistically superior to placebo and clinically comparable to the strongest of the first-generation agents such as hydroxyzine. The few clinical studies comparing the second-generation agents with each other in chronic urticaria show no statistically significant differences in efficacy.

The second-generation H_1 antihistamines are a heterogeneous group of compounds with lesser sedation than the first generation. Loratadine, desloratadine, and fexofenadine are nonsedating at the recommended dosage. Cetirizine is sedating at recommended dosage, but less than the first-generation agents. Only fexofenadine is totally nonsedating at any dosage above recommended levels.

What if monotherapy with a second-generation H_1 antihistamine does not adequately control the signs and symptoms of urticaria? Figure 1 summarizes a practical treatment algorithm for patients with chronic urticaria. The next step is to add another H_1 antihistamine to the original second-generation antihistamine, either an additional second-generation agent or a first-generation agent at night. The next option is to add an agent that blocks the H_2 receptors, either a tricyclic antidepressant such as doxepin (Sinequan) or an H_2 receptor antagonist.

The use of H_2 receptor antagonists is supported by the evidence that the cutaneous blood vessels possess H_2 receptors as well as the commonly recognized H_1 receptors, and these receptors are involved in the mediation of cutaneous vasodilatation and vascular permeability. Tricyclic antidepressants such as doxepin are potent H_1 and H_2 antihistaminic antagonists. Studies show doxepin to have comparable efficacy and side effects to hydroxyzine in the treatment of chronic urticaria. The usual initial dosage is 10 to 25 mg at night, which can be increased to two or three times daily if necessary. Several clinical studies show that the combination of an H_1 antihistamine and an H_2 antihistamine in both chronic urticaria and dermographism has added benefit compared to the use of an H_1 antihistamine alone. The dosage of the H_2 antihistamine is similar to that used for gastrointestinal disease—cimetidine (Tagamet), 300 mg four times daily, or ranitidine (Zantac), 150 mg twice daily.

Several mediators other than histamine can increase vascular permeability and thus cause hives. A few recent studies show that leukotriene receptor antagonists, such as montelukast (Singulair, 10 mg once daily) and zafirlukast (Accolate, 20 mg twice daily), may be beneficial in some cases of chronic urticaria.

Systemic corticosteroids are sometimes indicated for the management of moderate to severe acute urticaria, pressure urticaria, or urticarial vasculitis. They have no place in extended therapy of chronic urticaria, although they may occasionally be used as a short course of therapy to break the cycle of a resistant case. A common routine

TABLE 1 Comparison of Second-Generation H_1 Antihistamines

Drug	Recommended dosage	Efficacy in urticaria	Side effects at recommended dosage	Side effects at higher than recommended dosage
Loratadine (Claritin)	10 mg qd	+++	None	Mild sedation
Cetirizine (Zyrtec)	10 mg qd	+++	Mild sedation	Dose-related increases in sedation
Fexofenadine (Allegra)	60 mg bid or 180 mg qd	+++	None	None
Desloratadine (Clarinex)	5 mg qd	+++	None	Mild sedation

Abbreviations: bid = twice per day; qd = every day.

Rakel and Bope: *Conn's Current Therapy 2006.*

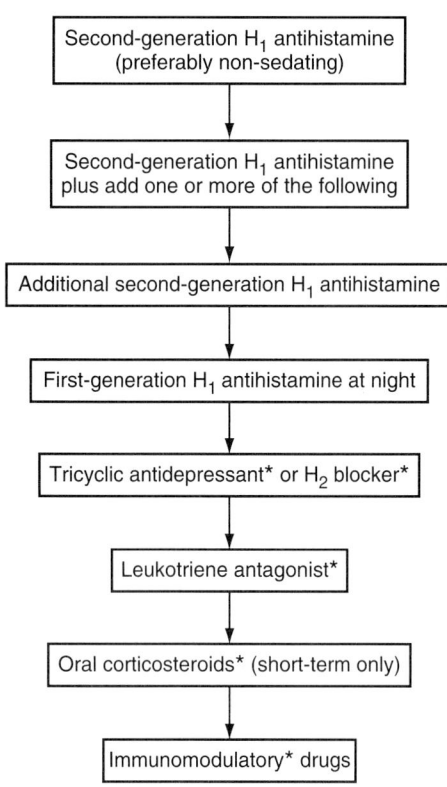

* Not FDA approved in this indication.

FIGURE 1. Treatment algorithm for patients with chronic urticaria.

is the use of prednisone beginning at 30 to 40 mg daily, tapered over 2 to 4 weeks. Systemic corticosteroids should be discontinued as soon as possible or at most maintained on an alternate-day basis.

In refractory cases of severe chronic urticaria or cases of "steroid-dependent" urticaria, other medications might be considered. Cyclosporine (Neoral, Sandimmune) in doses of 4 mg/kg per day is shown in some controlled studies to be effective in severe refractory cases of chronic urticaria or autoimmune urticaria.

In urticarial vasculitis, patients present clinically with urticaria that by skin biopsy is shown to be leukocytoclastic vasculitis. Treatment of this condition is often unsatisfactory. In addition to the use of antihistamines, other occasionally beneficial agents include nonsteroidal anti-inflammatory drugs such as indomethacin

 CURRENT DIAGNOSIS

The key clinical features of urticaria are the following:
- Erythematous, edematous papules or wheals, often with central clearing
- Pruritus (usually without signs of excoriation) and transient nature of individual lesions, which last 1 to 12 hours but definitely less than 24 to 48 hours.

 CURRENT THERAPY

- H_1 antihistamines remain the first choice of therapy for urticaria, both acute and chronic.
- The second-generation, so-called nonsedating antihistamines are the treatment of choice for many patients with urticaria because of their comparable efficacy and better safety profile compared to the first-generation antihistamines.
- Several other agents demonstrate additive value when monotherapy with H_1 antihistamines is not sufficient to control the refractory cases of chronic urticaria.

(Indocin), 25 to 50 mg three times daily; colchicine, 0.6 mg twice daily; dapsone, 50 to 300 mg daily; or hydroxychloroquine (Plaquenil), 200 to 400 mg per day. Systemic corticosteroids are also sometimes effective.

REFERENCES

Finn AF, Kaplan AP, Fretwell R, et al: A double-blind, placebo-controlled trial of fexofenadine HCl in the treatment of chronic idiopathic urticaria. J Allergy Clin Immunol 1999;103:1071-1078.
Grattan CEH, Sabroe RA, Greaves MW: Chronic urticaria. J Am Acad Dermatol 2002;46:645-657.
Greaves M: Chronic urticaria. J Allergy Clin Immunol 2000;105:664-672.
Kaplan AP: Chronic urticaria and angioedema. N Engl J Med 2002;346:175-179.
Kaplan AP: Chronic urticaria: Pathogenesis and treatment. J Allergy Clin Immunol 2004;114:465-474.
Lee EE, Maibach HI: Treatment of urticaria. An evidence-based evaluation of antihistamines. Am J Clin Dermatol 2001;2:151-158.
Monroe EW: Urticaria. Curr Probl Dermatol 1993;V:113-140.
Monroe E, Finn A, Patel P, et al: Efficacy and safety of desloratadine 5 mg once daily in the treatment of chronic idiopathic urticaria: A double-blind, randomized, placebo controlled trial. J Am Acad Dermatol 2003;48:535-541.
Zuberbier T. Urticaria. Allergy 2003;58:1224-1234.

Pigmentary Disorders

Method of
Kowichi Jimbow, MD, PhD and
Hiroyuki Hara, MD, PhD

Of the various factors responsible for human skin color, melanin is the major determinant, primarily reflecting the color brown and occasionally the color blue. Melanin pigment is produced within the melanosomal compartment of the melanocyte. Increased melanin pigmentation of the skin is primarily related to the size, shape, type, and color of melanosomes and their distribution patterns in melanocytes and keratinocytes. In contrast, hypomelanosis is related to the absence (amelanosis) or decreased function of the melanocyte, which may result in the altered size, shape, and color of melanosomes as well as their transfer from the melanocyte to surrounding keratinocytes and their distribution and degradation there. The partnership of a melanocyte and a neighboring group of keratinocytes is called an *epidermal melanin unit.* Thus abnormal pigmentation (hypermelanosis or hypomelanosis including amelanosis) reflects the alteration of the epidermal melanin unit. Hypermelanosis, however, also derives from the abnormal accumulation of melanosomes within the dermis that reflects the presence of abnormal melanocytes in the dermis (dermal melanocytosis) or incontinence (dropping off) of epidermal melanosomes in the dermis.

Box 1 presents the classification for hypermelanosis and hypomelanosis. It is often possible to distinguish

epidermal hypomelanosis from dermal after clinical examination and inspection with a Wood's lamp. Epidermal pigmentation is usually dark brown or black and accentuated under a Wood's lamp examination. In contrast, dermal pigmentation is often slate gray or blue and becomes less prominent under a Wood's lamp examination. Hypopigmentation can also be grouped into two components: decreased or absent melanin pigmentation. Again, the distinction of these two clinical forms can be differentiated by a Wood's lamp examination. Distinguishing hyperpigmentation and hypopigmentation has therapeutic implications in choosing the most effective treatment modalities based on the location of abnormal pigmentation in the skin. For example, most of the topical treatments are best suited for epidermal causes of hyperpigmentation, whereas surgical options

---

BOX 1 Major Pigmentary Disorders

Hyperpigmentation
Epidermal/Brown
CONGENITAL
POEMS syndrome
Albright syndrome
Café au lait macules
Becker's melanosis
Nevus spilus
Lentigenes syndrome (e.g., Peutz-Jeghers syndrome, centrofacial lentiginosis, Moynahan's syndrome, LAMB syndrome)
Urticaria pigmentosa
Cronkhite-Canada syndrome
Acanthosis nigricans (benign familial)
Dyschromatosis (universalis/simmetrica)
Acropigmentatio reticularis
ACQUIRED
Suntan melasma
Freckles
Solar lentigo
Lentigo malgna
Postinflammatory (porphyria cutanea tarda, lichen planus, tinea versicolor, atopic dermatitis, arsenic ingestion, lupus erythematosus, pellagra, etc.)
Macular amyloidosis
Drugs (e.g., phenytoin, contraceptives, estrogens, bleomycin, psoralen, tar, cyclophosphamide)
Systemic diseases (hyperthyroidism, renal insufficiency, billary cirrhosis)
Addison's disease
Hemochromatosis
Acanthosis nigricans (malignant)
Dermal/Blue, Slate Gray
CONGENITAL
Nevus of Ota
Extrasaccral mongolian spots
Incontinentia pigmenti
Franceschetti-Jadassohn syndrome
ACQUIRED
Riehl's melanosis
Melasma
Fixed drug eruption
Ochronosis
Erythema dyschromicum perstans
Chronic nutritional insufficiency

Metastatic melanoma with melanogenuria
Tattoos
Drugs (e.g., minocycline, amiodarone, phenothiazine, antimelarials, chlorpromazine)
Heavy metals (e.g., bismuth, chrysiasis, argyria)
Hemosiderin
Alkaptonuria
Erythema abigne
Hypopigmentation
Epidermal/White
CONGENITAL
Plebaldism
Tuberous sclerosis
Albinism
Phenylketonuria
Nevus depigmentosus
Ataxia telangiectasia
Nevus anemics
Nevus if Ito (incontinentia pigmenti achromians)
Waardenburg's syndrome
Ziprowski-Margolis syndrome
Woolf syndrome
Idiopathic guttate hypomelanosis
Menke's steely hair disease
Hemocystinuria
ACQUIRED
Vitiligo
Postinflammatory (e.g., lupus erythematosus, eczema, psoriasis)
Chemicals (e.g., arsenicals, chloroquine, hydroquinone, glucocorticoids, retinoids)
Pityriasis alba
Leprosy
Sarcoidosis
Syphillis
Tinea versicolor
Burns
Scleroderma
Systemic diseases (e.g., Addison's disease, hypopituitarism, hypothyroidism)
Epidermal/White
CONGENITAL
None
ACQUIRED
None

Rakel and Bope: *Conn's Current Therapy 2006.*

(e.g., laser surgery) are effective for both epidermal and dermal types of hyperpigmentation.

The history of onset and evolution of the pigmentary changes are also important: Are the lesions congenital, as in piebaldism or hypomelanosis of Ito, or are they acquired, as in vitiligo? Not all congenital pigmentary disorders, particularly hypomelanosis, are obvious at the outset. In a fair-skinned child not exposed to sunlight in the first year or early years of life, congenital hypopigmented lesions may be mislabeled as acquired. A white infant born in the late fall may not tan; hence the hypomelanosis may be invisible until the child goes outside to play and tans after sun exposure in the following year.

Common Diseases of Hyperpigmentation

MELASMA

Melasma is a common patchy, irregular, tanned brown pigmentation usually located on the face of women. It occurs in one of three, usually symmetric, facial patterns. The most common is a centrofacial pattern involving cheeks, forehead, upper lip, nose, and chin. Less common is the malar pattern, involving cheeks and nose, and the mandibular pattern, involving the ramus of mandible. Melasma occurs exclusively in sun-exposed areas and is more apparent during and after periods of solar exposure and less obvious during the winter. Multiple factors affect the degree of melasma pigmentation: pregnancy, oral contraceptives, endocrine dysfunction, genetic factors, medication, nutritional deficiency, and hepatic dysfunction. It is commonly seen during several pregnancies. Often melasma becomes apparent followed childbirth or upon continuation of oral contraceptives.

Hydroquinone is a common topical approach to melasma. Treatment modalities include the application of hydroalcoholic lotion of hydroquinone at concentrations of 2% to 5%. Decreasing skin color is observed after 4 weeks of therapy, and optimal depigmentation is achieved after 6 to 10 weeks of therapy. The effectiveness of hydroquinone is enhanced by concomitant daily use of an effective broad-spectrum sunscreen cream. However, the daily and prolonged use of hydroquinone with high concentrations (4% to 5%) produces a high incidence of primary irritant reactions. Treatment of melasma with monobenzyl ether of hydroquinone may result in irreversible chemical depigmentation or may incite vitiligo in a predisposed individual. Thus the use of monobenzyl ether of hydroquinone is contraindicated.

Good results can be obtained with the combination of retinoic acid (0.1%), hydroquinone (4.0%), and triamcinolone acetonide (0.025%). Formulations containing 1% and 0.05% or 0.1% retinoic acid can also lighten melasma skin. A high concentration of retinoic acid (more than 1.5%) may irritate the skin. Patients with macules of dermal melasma do not respond satisfactorily to hydroquinone therapy.

Azelaic acid is a dicarboxylic acid originally isolated from *Pityrosporum ovale*, the organism responsible for pityriasis versicolor. It is a competitive inhibitor of tyrosinase in vitro and used successfully to treat melasma. Azelaic acid is associated with few side effects, which suggests it may be beneficial if prolonged treatment is necessary. Kojic acid is a fungal metabolite produced by many species of *Aspergillus* and *Penicillium*. It is structurally related to maltol. Like maltol, it is a good chelator of transition metal ions and inhibits tyrosinase activity. Kojic acid inhibits tyrosinase isolated from black-and-gold-colored fish and suppresses melanogenesis in cultured pigment cells. When fed the coat color of black goldfish, they become almost yellow-brown.

Phenolic thioethers such as 4-S-cysteaminylphenol (*N*-acetyl or *N*-propionyl) represent a new family of depigmenting compound related to phenols. These melanocytotoxic agents are derived from sulfur homologues of phenols. In a preliminary clinical study using a 4% preparation of *N*-acetyl 4-S-cysteaminylphenol conducted on patients with melasma, marked to moderate improvement is seen. The compound appears less irritating to the skin than hydroquinone. Side effects are minimal. The depigmentation is associated with a decreased number of both functioning melanocytes and melanosomes transferred to keratinocytes. Both *N*-acetyl and *N*-propionyl 4-S-cysteaminylphenols are the tyrosinase substrate, and, upon exposure to tyrosinase, they form melanin-like pigments. An in vivo study indicates that *N*-acetyl and *N*-propionyl 4-S-cysteaminylphenols have both cytostatic and cytocidal effects on melanocytes.

Although hydroquinone is still considered the gold standard for the treatment of melasma, using chemical peels, also referred to as chemexfoliation, is an established technique for improving or treating hyperpigmentation disorders and now also a popular method for treating facial melasma. Superficial, medium-depth, and deep chemical peels are often used to treat melasma, in combination with chemical agents.

Topical application of glycolic acid in the form of chemical peels is a safe and effective method for treating hyperpigmentation disorders. The effectiveness of peels is enhanced by the use of 10% to 15% glycolic acid lotion plus hydroquinone (2%). Resorcinol, an isomer of catechol, was one of the earliest chemical peels. At the concentration of 50%, resorcinol results in medium-depth peels and is useful in treating patients with melasma as well as freckles and solar lentigines. Kojic acid chemical peels, which consist of kojic acid at 2% concentration, can be performed if hyperpigmentation of melasma persists after initial kojic acid gel treatment. They may be less drying to the skin than glycolic acid chemical peels. Both glycolic acid/kojic acid and glycolic acid/hydroquinone are highly effective in reducing the hyperpigmentation of melasma patients. The kojic acid preparation, however, is more irritating than hydroquinone. It has a high sensitizing potential and a comparatively high frequency of contact sensitivity. Its use as a topical agent is prohibited in Japan. Salicylic acid chemical peels, at a concentration of 20% to 30%, are also used for hyperpigmentation of melasma patients. Moderate to significant improvement is observed in patients suffering from postinflammatory hyperpigmentation. Trichloroacetic acid can be used when treatment with kojic acid peels is unsatisfactory. These medium-depth peels work as an adjuvant to treat the persistent diffuse hyperpigmentation of melasma lesions.

SOLAR LENTIGINES

Solar, or senile, lentigines are dark brown macules, usually 1 to 3 cm in diameter, that appear on the chronically sun-exposed skin of senior individuals (>60 years of age). They must be carefully distinguished histopathologically from lentigo maligna. Solar lentigines show elongated epidermal rete ridges with club-shaped or budlike extensions, frequent branching and fusing, a thinned or atrophic epidermis between rete ridges, and an increased number of epidermal melanocytes without formation of nesting. Scant to moderate perivascular mononuclear cell infiltrates appear in the upper dermis, usually associated with melanin-laden macrophages (melanophages). In contrast, lentigo maligna is a type of malignant melanoma in situ with a prolonged radial (horizontal) growth that is a precursor of invasive melanoma. Histopathologically, lentigo maligna is characterized by an atrophic epidermis with thinning and loss of rete ridges and increased numbers of atypical basilar melanocytes. These melanocytes vary in appearance, size, and shape, and they have nuclei of different sizes. A mononuclear cell infiltrate is characteristically seen in the superficial lesions of papillary dermis below the proliferated melanocytes.

Topical depigmenting agents listed for the treatment of melasma with or without chemical peels are used with various degrees of success. 4-Hydroxyanisole with or without tretinoin is reported effective. Solar lentigines can also be treated by other methods, such as gentle freezing with liquid nitrogen. Melanocytes are particularly susceptible to this treatment, but the production of skin necrosis must be avoided. Dark-skinned patients should not have lesions frozen except in special circumstances because of the risk of permanent depigmentation.

Solar lentigines respond well to a variety of pulsed and continuous wave (CW) lasers. The most commonly used pulsed lasers are the frequency-doubled Q-switched Nd:YAG (neodymium:yttrium=aluminum=garnet) laser at 532 μm, the Q-switched ruby laser (694 μm), the Alexandrite laser, and the pulsed-dye green laser (510 μm). All these lasers work well, with the exception of the green wave-length laser. The Alexandrite laser appears the most effective for the treatment of solar lentigines. Intense pulsed light, a broad-band visible flash light from noncoherence, is also well tolerated and may be a modality for treating solar lentigines.

FRECKLES (EPHELIDES)

Freckles are small, usually less than 0.5 cm in diameter, discrete brown macules that appear on the sun-exposed skin, especially on the face. In freckled skin, the number of functioning melanocytes is not increased, but they are highly dendritic, strongly DOPA (3,4-dihydroxyphenylalanine) positive, and have many

stage IV mature melanosomes. The treatment of freckles is primarily the same as that of solar lentigines. The laser treatment described earlier is effective. Liquid nitrogen treatment is efficacious too but often leaves some marginal pigmentation and may cause permanent depigmentation in dark-skinned people.

POSTINFLAMMATORY HYPERPIGMENTATION

Hyperpigmentation in many cases follows the resolution of specific eruptions. Certain rashes, such as those deriving from contact dermatitis to poison ivy, are particularly likely to result in postinflammatory hyperpigmentation. These pigmentary changes, which are characteristically discrete macules with hazy, feathered margins, correspond exactly with a primary eruption and may persist for months. The pathophysiology of postinflammatory hyperpigmentation is primarily related to either an increased production of melanin pigments or an alteration of the distribution pattern of melanin pigments within the epidermis, but not primarily because of the increased number of melanocytes. In some cases, postinflammatory hyperpigmentation is blue or slightly gray, deriving from incontinence of melanin pigments from the epidermis to the dermis.

The epidermal form of hyperpigmentation may respond well to bleaching depigmenting agents. Dermal hyperpigmentation does not respond to any medical treatment except for lasers. Major postinflammatory hyperpigmentation derives from the interaction of cytokines and/or growth factors released from dermal inflammatory cells or epidermal keratinocytes. The principle of the treatment, therefore, is to reduce and settle the inflammatory changes. Optimal management of the primary underlying skin problem is thus essential for the treatment and prevention of further hyperpigmentation.

SUNTAN

Tanning reactions after exposure to sunlight result from two different mechanisms. Long-wave ultraviolet light (ultraviolet A [UVA], 320 to 400 μm) and visible light cause an immediate tanning reaction of pigments (previously called immediate pigment darkening). This occurs within a few minutes after exposure to the UVA and visible light and disappears spontaneously within hours. It is caused by the oxidization of preexisting melanin pigments as well as the alteration in the distribution patterns of melanin pigments (melanosomes) within the epidermis. It is not associated with the activation or an increased population of epidermal melanocytes.

Short-wave ultraviolet light (ultraviolet B [UVB], 290 to 320 μm), which produces a delayed tanning reaction, is often associated with sunburn. The delayed tanning reaction is associated with an increased population of epidermal melanocytes as the result of the proliferation and even replication of melanocytes as well as the increased production of melanin pigments that derives from increased synthesis and the activation of tyrosinase and tyrosinase-related proteins. It generally takes 4 to 7 days to develop and lasts for many weeks.

13

Both long-wave and short-wave UV light contribute to the enhancement or augmentation of the aging process (photoaging), and both increase the risk of developing skin cancers. UVB is primarily responsible for this process and UVA may not be directly responsible for this skin cancer development, but will accommodate with UVB for this process. Patients must recognize that sun-induced pigmentation can be reversed only by protecting the skin from sun exposure and all forms of UV light. Many physical sunblocks are available that reflect UV light and protect the skin. Tightly woven outerwear and a hat provide excellent protection. Physical sunblocks, such as zinc oxide, calamine, talc, titanium dioxide, and kaolin, are opaque, and they scatter and reflect the sunlight. For those individuals who are especially sensitive to sunlight and also enjoy outdoor activities, the application of sunblock is essential.

Chemical sunscreens function in a different way and absorb UV light in the UVB and, to some extent, the UVA ranges. Para-aminobenzoic acid (PABA) (and its derivatives), salicylates, and cinnamates absorb sunlight radiation in the UVB range. Benzophenone derivatives absorb sunlight radiation mainly in the range of UVA. The ideal broad-spectrum sunscreen contains an agent that absorbs UVB and an agent that absorbs UVA. Two factors should be considered when choosing a sunscreen: the sun protection factor (SPF) and its ability to withstand perspiration and immersion in water.

SYSTEMIC CAUSES OF HYPERPIGMENTATION

Generalized hyperpigmentation is associated with many systemic disorders. Usually the color is caused by melanin pigments, as seen in Addison's disease. Metabolic, nutritional, or endocrine disorders should be considered in patients with widespread or diffuse hyperpigmentation. Drugs or heavy metals also can cause generalized hyperpigmentation. Treatment is directed at correcting underlying diseases or discontinuing the medication.

CAFÉ-AU-LAIT MACULES

Café-au-lait macules are macular pigmented lesions with a uniformly pale brown color, serrated or irregular margins, and variable sizes. They are present in 10% of the normal population and seen in association with neurocutaneous syndromes such as neurofibromatosis, Albright's syndrome, tuberous sclerosis, Silver-Russell syndrome, Westerhof's syndrome, Watson's syndrome, and Bloom syndrome. Multiple lesions are especially common in the neurofibromatosis (NF) of Recklinghausen's disease (NF type 1). Café-au-lait macules can be good candidates for treatment with Q-switched lasers because submicrosecond laser pulses interact selectively with melanosomes in melanocytes and in keratinocytes of the epidermis. However, treatment of Q-switched lasers may not consistently yield successful results. Complete and partial clearance followed by recurrence appears in approximately half of the cases. Nonetheless, Q-switched ruby or Q-switched

Nd:YAG laser is the treatment of choice for the café-au-lait macules present on exposed areas.

BECKER'S NEVUS

Becker's nevus may vary in color from tan to dark brown and is well demarcated from the normal skin. Following the onset, a Becker nevus is likely to grow slowly for a few years producing black terminal hairs; hence the patient often presents two complaints: hyperpigmentation and hypertrichosis. Hyperpigmentation lesions can be treated with Q-switched lasers. However, satisfactory results are not always obtained. Decreased hair growth is seen after Q-switched laser treatment, but the effect appears brief. The long-pulse ruby laser (3 ms, 40 to 60 g/cm^2) is the correct choice for hypertrichosis.

NEVUS SPILUS

Nevus spilus is a circumscribed tan-colored macule containing smaller darkly pigmented macules or small papules. Nevus spilus can be treated as a combined disease of café-au-lait macules with junctional nevi. The treatment of choice is Q-switched laser. Successful treatment of nevus spilus is also reported with intense pulsed light source emitting a wavelength of 500 to 1200 μm. However, careful follow-up is necessary because melanoma can occur in nevus spilus after incomplete laser treatment.

OTA NEVUS (OCULODERMAL MELANOCYTOSIS)

Ota nevus, nevus fuscoceruleus ophthalmomaxillaris, is usually congenital but may appear in childhood or in the teenage years. It is characterized by unilateral blue-black or slate-gray macules intermingled with small brown flat spots, occurring most characteristically in the skin innervated by the first and second branches of the trigeminal nerve. Mucosae, conjunctivae, and tympanic membranes may be involved. The skin lesions may sometimes be bilateral. Ota nevus does not improve with time.

The Q-switched ruby laser is a safe and effective treatment. Multiple treatments, five to six courses, generally increase the response, resulting an excellent lightening (70% or more). Satisfactory results can be also obtained with Q-switched ruby laser, Q-switched 1064-μm Nd:YAG laser, and Q-switched 755-μm Alexandrite laser with a range from 5 to 6 g/cm^2.

Common Diseases of Hypopigmentation

VITILIGO

Vitiligo is a common, idiopathic, acquired disease with a loss of normal melanin pigments and functioning melanocytes from otherwise healthy-looking skin. Clinically, vitiligo can be grouped into several unique subtypes. The localized type includes focal and segmental vitiligo. Generalized ones are vitiligo vulgaris, acrofacial, and universal vitiligo. Although it is acquired, a genetic predisposition is considered. The leukoderma of vitiligo does not contain any functioning melanocytes.

At present, no universally effective medical or surgical modality is available for vitiligo therapy. A number of active therapeutic approaches are effective, such as oral or topical application of psoralen followed by exposure to long-wave UVA (PUVA). It is the most popular therapy for vitiligo, and hence the detailed guideline of PUVA is well described. Although the use of Oxsoralen is the standard of the treatment, the new Oxsoralen-Ultra (a preparation containing ultramicronized 8-MOP) is an option. It has faster bioavailability and drug absorption time was less before PUVA than that of traditional Oxsoralen. Vitiligo is also treated successfully with narrow-band UVB phototherapy. Intradermal and topical corticosteroids are used to treat vitiligo with mixed results. Recently, successful treatment of vitiligo depigmentation was reported with topical application of pseudo-catalase and calcium followed by short-term UVB light exposure. This treatment appears to rely on the presence of tyrosinase activity in the depigmented epidermis of patients with vitiligo. It is also known that calcipotriene may act in vitiligo either by 1,25-dihydroxyvitamin D_3 receptors on melanocytes or by modifying defecting calcium homeostasis in the epidermal unit. The combination of calcipotriene and PUVA or calcipotriene plus narrow-band UVB achieves earlier pigmentation.

Furthermore, surgical graft of autologous epidermal sheet or cultured melanocytes (often combined with keratinocyte co-cultures) can repigment the depigmented areas where PUVA is ineffective. PUVA therapy after autologous skin graft can enhance the repigmenting efficiency. Although PUVA with or without surgical procedure represents a useful tool in vitiligo treatment, the degree of psychological impairment caused by the vitiligo should be assessed. In addition, normal skin of vitiligo can be totally depigmented by monobenzyl ether of hydroquinone to match the skin color in certain patients with generalized vitiligo.

The 308-μm excimer laser shows promise for the treatment of vitiligo. Unlike narrow-band UVB phototherapy and PUVA, the 308-μm excimer laser modality can selectively treat single vitiliginous patches and spare nonaffected areas. Furthermore, the combination treatment of topical tacrolimus plus the 308-μm excimer laser is superior to 308-μm excimer laser monotherapy.

ALBINISM

Albinism refers to genetic abnormalities of melanin synthesis associated with a normal number and structure of melanocytes. Reduced melanin synthesis in the melanocyte of the skin, hair, and eyes is termed *oculocutaneous albinism* (OCA), and hypopigmentation primarily involving the retinal pigment epithelium of the eye is termed *ocular albinism* (OA). The precise definition of albinism includes specific changes in the

TABLE 1. Classification of Albinism

Type	Subtypes	Gene Locus	Includes	Mechanism(s)
OCA1	OCA1A	Tyrosinase	Tyrosinase-negative OCA	Inactive/missing enzyme due to tyrosinase gene mutation
	OCA1B	Tyrosinase	Minimal pigment OCA	Partially active enzyme due to tyrosinase gene mutation
			Platinum OCA	
			Yellow OCA	
			Temperature-sensitive OCA	
			Autosomal recessive OCA	
OCA2	P		Tyrosinase-positive OCA impaired tyrosinase transport?	Partially active enzyme due to tyrosinase gene mutation
			Brown OCA	
			Autosomal recessive OCA (some)	
OCA3	TYRP1		Rufous OCA	Partially active enzyme to *TYRP1* gene mutation
			Red OCA	OA1
OA1	OA1		X-linked OA	Partially active enzyme due to tyrosinase gene mutation
Unrelated to Mutations of Tyrosinase Family Genes				
HPS	HPS		Hermansky-Pudlak syndrome	Mutation of *AP-3*, leading to impaired vesicular transport
CHS	CHS		Chediak-Higashi syndrome	Mutation of *LYST*, leading to impaired vesicular transport

Abbreviations: AP = adaptor protein; OA = ocular albinism; OCA = oculocutaneous albinism; TYRP1 = tyrosinase-related protein 1.

Rakel and Bope: *Conn's Current Therapy 2006.*

development and function of the eye and optic nerves, and ocular changes are necessary to make the diagnosis. The ocular system changes in albinism include reduction of iris pigments, reduction of retinal pigments, foveal hypoplasia, misrouting of the optic fibers at the chiasm, nystagmus, and alternating strabismus. Any child or adult with cutaneous hypopigmentation must have these ocular changes to make the diagnosis of albinism. Once it is established the individual has albinism, the determination of the specific type is made with a family history and clinical examination. A family history of affected men related through unaffected women indicates an X-linked inheritance pattern consistent with OCA1.

For OCA, the family history is usually negative or there is an affected sibling of either sex, indicative of autosomal recessive inheritance.

All individuals with albinism should be under the care of an ophthalmologist and have annual examinations until adulthood. Most are hyperopic or myopic and may have significant astigmatism. Protection from UV radiation of the sun is necessary for individuals with OCA who have little or no skin and hair pigment. This care is the same as that for individuals without albinism who have type I or II skin and includes the use of sunscreens, hat, long sleeves, and sun avoidance (Table 1).

 CURRENT DIAGNOSIS

Melasma
- Patchy irregular brown pigmentation of the face with three basic patterns: centrofacial, malar, and mandibular.
- Degree of pigmentation is affected by multiple factors: pregnancy, oral contraceptives, endocrine dysfunction, genetic factors, nutritional deficiency, and hepatic dysfunction.

Solar Lentigines
- Dark brown macules, 1 to 3 mm in diameter, on the chronically sun-exposed skin of elderly individuals (>60 years of age).
- Must be carefully distinguished from lentigo maligna (a type of malignant melanoma in situ).

Freckles
- Small, discrete brown macules, usually less than 0.5 mm in diameter, on the sun-exposed skin of the face.

Postinflammatory Hyperpigmentation
- The three major patterns of hyperpigmentation are epidermal, dermal, or a combination of the epidermal and dermal type.
- Epidermal hyperpigmentation results from increased production of melanin pigments and/or alterations in the distribution pattern of melanin pigments in the epidermis.
- Dermal hyperpigmentation, although less common than the epidermal type, derives from incontinence of melanin pigments from the epidermis to the dermis.

Suntan
- Two forms of suntan occur after exposure to the sunlight: immediate tan (previously called immediate pigment darkening) and delayed tan.
- Immediate tan derives from exposure to UVA (320 to 400 μm) and visible light, occurring within a few minutes and disappearing within hours spontaneously.
- Delayed tan occurs after exposure to UVB (290 to 320 μm) and often is associated with sunburn. It takes 4 to 7 days to develop and lasts for many weeks.

Systemic Causes of Hyperpigmentation
- Generalized hyperpigmentation is caused by many systemic disorders.
- Treatment should be directed at corresponding underlying diseases or discontinuing the medication.

Café-Au-Lait Macules
- Multiple numerous lesions of café-au-lait macules are seen in the neurofibromatosis of Recklinghausen's disease.
- Multiple café-au-lait lesions are seen in other neurocutaneous diseases, such as Albright's syndrome, tuberous sclerosis, Silver-Russell syndrome, and Bloom syndrome.

Becker's Nevus
- Becker's nevus is hyperpigmented tan to dark brown plaque associated with hypertrichosis.

Nevus Spilus
- Nevus spilus is a tan-colored macule resembling a café-au-lait macule and associated with smaller darkly pigmented spots or papules of junctional nevi.

Ota Nevus
- Ota nevus is a blue-black macular lesion of the skin and mucosa occurring most commonly on the first and second branches of the trigeminal nerve.

Vitiligo
- Vitiligo is an acquired depigmenting disease with loss or death of functioning melanocytes in the skin.
- Depigmented chalk- or milk-white macules are best seen under Wood's light examination.

Albinism
- The two major forms of albinism are oculocutaneous albinism (OCA), with hypopigmentation (including amelanosis) of skin, hair, and eyes, and ocular albinism (OA), with hypopigmentation of skin and eyes.
- The diagnosis of albinism should include careful evaluation of ocular changes that include reduction of iris pigments, reduction of retinal pigments, foveal hypoplasia, misrouting of the optic fibers at the chiasm, nystagmus, and alternating strabismus.

Abbreviations: UVA = ultraviolet A; UVB = ultraviolet B.

CURRENT THERAPY

Melasma

- Currently hydroquinone is most commonly used.
- Hydroquinone combined with other topical agents, such as retinoic acid (0.1%) and triamcinolone acetonide (0.025%), can also result in good depigmenting effect.
- Other topical agents include kojic acid and phenolic thioether amines.
- Chemical peels with or without the combination of the topical agents just cited are also popular.

Solar Lentigines

- Topical depigmenting agents with or without chemical peels are effective.
- 4-Hydroxyanisole with or without tretinoin is also effective.
- Gentle freezing with liquid nitrogen is effective, but care must be taken in treating dark-skinned people because it can cause permanent depigmentation.
- A variety of pulsed and continuous wave (CW) lasers are now widely used.

Freckles

- Treatment of freckles is basically the same as that of solar lentigines.
- Laser and liquid nitrogen treatment is effective.

Postinflammatory Hyperpigmentation

- The principle of treatment is to reduce and settle the inflammatory changes of the skin, which derives from the interaction of cytokines and growth factors released from dermal inflammatory cells or epidermal keratinocytes.

Suntan

- Chemical sunscreens absorb UV light in the range of UVB and, to some extent, UVA.
- PABA (and its derivatives), salicylates, and cinnamates absorb sunlight in the UVB range, whereas benzophenone derivatives absorb sunlight in the range of UVA.
- When choosing a sunscreen, the sun protection factor (SPF) and the ability to withstand perspiration and water immersion are important criteria.

Systemic Causes of Hyperpigmentation

- Generalized hyperpigmentation is caused by many systemic disorders.
- Treatment should be directed at corresponding underlying diseases or discontinuing the medication.

Café-Au-Lait Macules

- Café-au-lait macules are well treated by Q-switched lasers (ruby or Nd:YAG).
- Although complete or partial clearance is achieved with Q-switched laser treatment, recurrence may occur in approximately half of the cases.

Becker's Nevus

- Hyperpigmentation is best treated with Q-switched laser, and hypertrichosis can be treated with long-pulse ruby laser.

Nevus Spilus

- The treatment of choice is Q-switched laser.

Ota Nevus

- Five to six courses of Q-switched lasers (ruby, Nd:YAG, and Alexandrite types) are the best choice of treatment.

Vitiligo

- No universally effective medical or surgical modality is available for vitiligo therapy.
- PUVA is the most popular therapy. Narrow-band UVB phototherapy is a recent successful treatment.
- Successful treatment of vitiligo depigmentation is noted with topical application of pseudo-catalase and calcium followed by UVB exposure.
- Autologous skin graft or cultured melanocyte graft followed by PUVA is introduced to repigment the depigmented areas where PUVA is ineffective.

Albinism

- All albinism patients should have annual eye examinations until adulthood.
- Protection from UV radiation of the sun is necessary for patients with oculocutaneous albinism.

Abbreviations: PABA = para-aminobenzoic acid; UVA = ultraviolet A; UVB = ultraviolet B; PUVA = psoralen plus long-wave ultraviolet A.

REFERENCES

Balkrishnan R, Kelly AP, McMichael A, Torok H: Improved quality of life with effective treatment of facial melasma: The pigment trial. J Drugs Dermatol 2004;3(49):377-381.

Chen YF, Yang PY, Hu DN, et al: Treatment of vitiligo by transplantation of cultured pure melanocyte suspension: Analysis of 120 cases. J Am Acad Dermatol 2004;51:68-74.

Espinal-Perez LE, Moncada B, Castanedo-Cazares JP: A double-blind randomized trial of 5% ascorbic acid vs. 4% hydroquinone in melasma. Inter J Dermatol 2004;43:604-607.

Jimbow K: N-Acetyl-4-S-cysteaminylphenol as a new type of depigmenting agent for the melanoderma of melanoma patients. Arch Dermatol 1991;127:1528-1534.

Kawada A, Shiraishi H, Asai M, et al: Clinical improvement of solar lentigines and ephelides with a intense pulsed light source. Dermatol Surg 2004;28:504-508.

Kawaler AZ, Spencer JM, Phelps RG: Combined excimer laser and topical tacrolimus for the treatment of vitiligo: A pilot study. Dermatol Surg 2004;30:130-135.

Khunger N, Sarkar R, Jain RK: Tretinoin peels versus glycolic acid peels in the treatment of melasma in dark-skinned patients. Dermatol Surg 2004;30:756-760.

Moreno-Arias GA, Bulla F, Vilata-Corell JJ, Camps-Fresneda A: Treatment of widespread segmental nevus spilus by Q-switched Alexandrite laser (755 µm, 100 nsec). Dermatol Surg 2001;27:841-843.

Parsad D, Saini R, Verma N: Combination of PUVAsol and topical calcipotriol in vitiligo. Dermatology 1998;197:167-170.

Zouboulis CC, Rosenberger AD, Adler Y, Orfanos CE: Treatment of solar lentigo with cryosurgery. Acta Derm Venereol 2004;79:489-490.

Sunburn

Method of
K. Wade Foster, MD, PhD and Craig A Elmets, MD

Diagnosis

Sunburn is the visible short-term effect of overexposure of the skin to ultraviolet (UV) light emanating from the sun or artificial light sources. It is typified by erythema caused by cutaneous vasodilatation and may be followed by blister formation and/or desquamation. The erythema peaks at 12 to 24 hours after exposure and is accompanied by noticeable tenderness. In severe cases, confluent blistering with concomitant malaise, edema, chills, fever, nausea, and tachycardia may be present with symptoms lasting up to 1 week. Long-term effects of overexposure to UV radiation include photoaging of the skin, non-melanoma skin cancers (including squamous cell and basal cell carcinomas), melanoma, and a subtle form of immunosuppression.

UV light is artificially subdivided into categories of varying wavelengths: UVA (320 to 400 μm), UVB (290 to 320 μm), and UVC (200 to 290 μm). Nearly all UVC radiation is absorbed by the ozone contained in Earth's atmosphere, so natural UV light with wavelengths of less than 290 μm is virtually undetectable on Earth's surface. The major artificial sources that emit UVC are germicidal lamps. Consequently, UVA and UVB have the greatest relevance to human disease. In normal human skin, the ability to induce sunburn is inversely related to wavelength. Thus UVB light is responsible for most sunburns. In fact, it takes approximately 1000 times the amount of UVA radiation to produce a sunburn as it does UVB. In contrast, UVA is much more effective at producing a suntan than UVB. The depth of penetration of UV light is wavelength dependent, with longer UVA wavelengths penetrating more deeply than UVB. Cutaneous absorption of UV light results in DNA damage, the formation of cytotoxic reactive oxygen intermediates, and the generation of inflammatory mediators. Evidence supports a role for prostaglandin E_2, histamine, kinins, interleukins (IL-1, -6, -8, -10, -12), tumor necrosis factor-α (TNF-α), Substance P, calcitonin gene-related peptide, and nitric oxide in the erythematous response, vasodilatation, and inflammation present in sunburned skin.

Once the signs and symptoms of sunburn are present, no form of treatment is unequivocally effective. Hence prevention of sunburn is of utmost importance. The best means of preventing sunburn is sun avoidance between 10 AM and 4 PM when UVB intensity is at its peak. The amount of UV radiation reaching Earth's surface is affected by regional ozone depletion, seasonal changes, and day-to-day variations in the weather. An online UV index predictor is available from the National Weather Service and U.S. Environmental Protection Agency. Using a zip code or city and state, the predictor analyzes regional factors and provides a forecast of the following day's UV radiation levels. This tool can be found online at http://www.epa.gov/sunwise/uvindex.html.

Barrier protection with hats and clothing is also an important means of sunburn prevention. Most articles of clothing, however, only afford moderate photoprotection, and it is possible to receive sufficient amounts of UV radiation to develop a sunburn through clothing, especially wet clothing. For patients who are very photosensitive, manufacturers make special sun-protective clothing that is effective at preventing excessive exposure of the skin to both UVA and UVB.

Sunscreen agents are another important form of barrier protection. They should be used regularly, including on cloudy days, because 80% of the sun's UV rays pass through the clouds. Sunscreens work by absorbing, reflecting, or scattering the sun's rays as they strike the skin, and they are traditionally divided into two groups: chemical and physical. Chemical sunscreens absorb high-energy UV waves, and physical sunscreens are broad-spectrum UV blockers that reflect or scatter UV light. Table 1 lists several recommended sunscreens, and a more comprehensive catalog of agents available in the United States and Canada can be found online at http://www.uspdqi.org/pubs/monographs/index1.html.

All sunscreens are labeled with an SPF (sun protection factor) rating that indicates the level of protection from UVB–induced erythema. Higher SPF sunscreens offer greater protection from sunburn, whereas lower SPF sunscreens afford less protection. The SPF rating of a sunscreen is calculated by comparing the amount of time needed to produce a mild sunburn response (i.e., erythema) on sunscreen-protected skin to that of unprotected skin. For example, a sunscreen with an SPF of 15 allows one to multiply the original burning time by a factor of 15. It is important to remember that SPF values are calculated in a laboratory setting in which unusually large amounts of sunscreen are applied to the skin. Patients generally apply only approximately 25% of the amount required to achieve the full SPF value indicated by a product's label. Consequently, in practice, the SPF value is an overestimate of the true degree to which sunscreen users are actually protected. For these reasons, most dermatologists recommend that patients evenly apply a sunscreen with an SPF value of at least 15 to dry skin 15 to 30 minutes before going outdoors and reapply it at 2-hour intervals. A good rule of thumb is that anyone going out in the sun for more than 20 minutes needs a sunscreen. Lips should also be protected with a lip balm with an SPF rating of 15 or higher.

Part of evaluating a sunburn when it does occur is determining whether it is a typical sunburn caused by overexposure to UVB light, a phototoxic reaction to a medication, or a photosensitivity disease masquerading as a sunburn. Box 1 lists some common photosensitizing agents that can increase sensitivity to UV light. Although UVA radiation plays only a minor role in typical sunburns, it is very important in phototoxic reactions. For this reason, individuals taking potentially phototoxic medications should select a sunscreen with UVB and broad UVA coverage when sun exposure cannot be avoided. Suspicion of a phototoxic response

TABLE 1 Recommended Sunscreen Agents

Brand name	Form	Composition	Sun protection factor (SPF)	Waterproof (WP), water-resistant (WR)	Coverage
PreSun	Lotion	Aminobenzoic acid Padimate O Oxybenzone	15	-	UVA/UVB
PreSun Sunscreen	Cream	Avobenzone Octyl methoxycinnamate Octyl salicylate Oxybenzone	30	WP	UVA/UVB
PreSun Sunscreen for Kids	Cream	Avobenzone Octyl methoxycinnamate Octyl salicylate Oxybenzone	30	WP	UVA/UVB
Shade UVA Guard	Lotion	Avobenzone Octyl methoxycinnamate Oxybenzone	15	WR	UVA/UVB
Ombrelle Sunscreen	Lotion	Avobenzone Octyl methoxycinnamate Oxybenzone	15	WP	UVA/UVB
Coppertone Waterproof Sunblock	Lotion	Homosalate Octocrylene Octyl methoxycinnamate Oxybenzone	30	WP	UVA/UVB
Coppertone All Day Protection	Lotion	Homosalate Octyl methoxycinnamate Octyl salicylate Oxybenzone	30	WP	UVA/UVB
Neutrogena No Stick Sunscreen	Lotion	Homosalate Octyl methoxycinnamate Octyl salicylate Oxybenzone	30	WP	UVA/UVB
Total Eclipse Oily and Acne Prone Skin Sunscreen	Lotion	Lisadimate Oxybenzone Padimate O	15	—	UVA/UVB
Neutrogena Sunblock	Cream	Menthyl anthranilate Octocrylene Octyl methoxycinnamate	30	WP	UVA/UVB
Coppertone All Day Protection	Lotion	Octocrylene Octyl methoxycinnamate Octyl salicylate Oxybenzone	45	WP	UVA/UVB
Shade Sunblock	Lotion	Octocrylene Octyl methoxycinnamate Octyl salicylate Oxybenzone	45	WP	UVA/UVB
Bullfrog Sport	Lotion	Octocrylene Octyl methoxycinnamate Octyl salicylate Oxybenzone Titanium dioxide	18	WP	UVA/UVB
SolBar PF Ultra	Cream	Octocrylene Octyl methoxycinnamate Oxybenzone	50	WP	UVA/UVB
Bullfrog Body	Lotion	Octocrylene Octyl methoxycinnamate Oxybenzone	18, 36	WP	UVA/UVB
Banana Boat Faces Sensitive Skin Sunblock	Cream	Octyl methoxycinnamate Octyl salicylate Oxybenzone	15, 23	WP	UVA/UVB
PreSun Active Clear	Gel	Octyl methoxycinnamate Octyl salicylate Oxybenzone	15, 30	WP	UVA/UVB

Continued

Rakel and Bope: *Conn's Current Therapy 2006.*

13

TABLE 1 Recommended Sunscreen Agents—cont'd

Brand name	Form	Composition	Sun protection factor (SPF)	Waterproof (WP), water-resistant (WR)	Coverage
Banana Boat Active Kids Sunblock	Lotion	Octyl methoxycinnamate Octyl salicylate Oxybenzone	30+	WP	UVA/UVB
Sundown Sunblock	Lotion	Octyl methoxycinnamate Octyl salicylate Oxybenzone Titanium dioxide	15, 30	WP	UVA/UVB
Total Eclipse Moisturizing Skin	Lotion	Octyl salicylate Padimate O	15	—	UVB
Neutrogena Chemical-Free Sunblocker	Lotion	Titanium dioxide	17	WR	UVA/UVB
Vaseline Intensive Care Baby Moisturizing Sunblock	Lotion	Titanium dioxide	15	WP	UVA/UVB

Abbreviations: UVA = ultraviolet A; UVB = ultraviolet B.

should be high if a patient complains of a sunburn reaction from a tanning bed. The lights used in tanning beds emit large amounts of UVA radiation. Thus patients given photosensitizing medications should be counseled to avoid tanning beds. Another clue to suggest a phototoxic reaction caused by a drug rather than a typical sunburn is that the erythema response can be elicited through window glass. Window glass filters out virtually all UVB but only a small fraction of UVA radiation.

A number of photosensitizing diseases can masquerade as a sunburn. Patients with these conditions may report a sunburn that occurs with lower than expected doses of sun exposure, a burning sensation perceived by the patient concomitant with sun exposure, or complaints of a sunburn with an unusual time course, either earlier or later than would otherwise be expected. The differential diagnosis of photosensitivity is large and includes a diverse group of genetic and metabolic diseases. Of these, polymorphic light eruption (PMLE), known by the general public as "sun poisoning," is the most common. Typical characteristics of PMLE are nonscarring pruritic, erythematous papules, plaques, or vesicles on sun-exposed skin occurring mainly in the V area of the neck, arms, and face that develop 30 minutes to several hours after sun exposure. The eruption of PMLE may persist for a few hours to as long as 2 weeks. The condition has a female predominance and tends to affect fair-skinned individuals. Lupus erythematosus (LE) is also typified by a photosensitive rash affecting sun-exposed parts of the body. The rash in systemic LE is characteristically confluent erythema, edema, and erythematous macules and papules occurring on the malar eminence and the nasal bridge, although bullae are sometimes present in severely affected individuals. Of particular interest in understanding the relationship of photosensitivity and LE is subacute cutaneous lupus erythematosus. This LE variant routinely manifests with photosensitivity, and

serologically most affected individuals have Ro (SS-A) antibodies, thought to be a marker for photosensitivity. The antinuclear antibody (ANA) titer may be negative in these patients even though they are Ro (SS-A) antibody positive. Erythropoietic protoporphyria is another photosensitive condition that can also be confused with sunburn. This disease usually first manifests in childhood, and clinical features include subjective complaints of a burning pain within minutes to hours after exposure to the sun. These complaints may or may not be accompanied by skin lesions, which are present on exposed areas and disappear when the sun is avoided. Patients with suspected photosensitivity disorders should be referred for evaluation and management to a dermatologist specializing in photosensitivity diseases.

Treatment

No consensus exists on an algorithm for the treatment of sunburn, and most studies demonstrate little if any efficacy of corticosteroids, nonsteroidal anti-inflammatory medications (NSAIDs), antioxidants, antihistamines, or emollients in decreasing recovery time. Symptomatic treatment of UV light–induced symptoms, including erythema, pain, and pruritus, remains the most effective and practical approach to acute sunburn. Mildly sunburned skin does not require any specific treatment, but may benefit from emollients (e.g., Cetaphil or Eucerin Cream or Lotion) to help rehydrate the affected area. Moderately sunburned skin may benefit from cool tap water compresses, cool baking soda baths, or cool dilute acetic acid compresses. NSAID medications such as naproxen (Naprosyn) or ibuprofen (Motrin) are effective in controlling the inflammatory response and pain associated with sunburn. Patients with pruritus may benefit from antihistamines such as hydroxyzine (Atarax), and a moderate potency topical corticosteroid

BOX 1 Common Photosensitizing Agents

Antiarrhythmics
Amiodarone (Cordarone)
Diltiazem (Cardizem)
Antidiabetics
Glipizide (Glucotrol)
Glyburide (DiaBeta)
Diuretics
Furosemide (Lasix)
Chlorothiazide (Diuril)
Hydrochlorothiazide (HydroDIURIL)
NSAIDs
Piroxicam (Feldene)
Naproxen (Aleve)
Nabumetone (Relafen)
Phenothiazines
Chlorpromazine (Thorazine)
Prochlorperazine (Compazine)
Psoralens
8-Methoxypsoralen
Quinolones
Lomefloxacin (Maxaquin)
Nalidixic acid (NegGram)
Sparfloxacin (Zagam)
Ciprofloxacin (Cipro)
Retinoids
Topical (e.g., Retin-A, Tretinoin)
Oral (e.g., Accutane, Isotretinoin)
Tetracyclines
Demeclocycline (Declomycin)
Doxycycline (Adoxa)
Topical photosensitizers
5-Aminolevulinic acid (Levulan)

Abbreviation: NSAIDs = nonsteroidal anti-inflammatory drugs.

CURRENT THERAPY

Mild Sunburn
- No treatment
- Emollients (Cetaphil, Eucerin Cream or Lotion) to rehydrate the affected area

Moderate Sunburn
- Emollients (Cetaphil, Eucerin Cream or Lotion)
- Cool tap water compresses, cool baking soda baths (1 cup per tub of cool tap water), or cool dilute acetic acid compresses (1:20 vinegar to cool tap water)
- Atarax, 10 to 25 mg every 6 hours, as needed for pruritus
- Nonsteroidal anti-inflammatory drugs (e.g., Motrin tabs or liquid) for pain relief
- Topical triamcinolone 0.1% cream, twice daily, to affected areas
- Oral prednisone (Sterapred), 40 to 60 mg per day for 10 to 14 days

Severe Sunburn
- Same as for moderate sunburn
- Discontinuation of the offending medication in presence of phototoxic drug reaction
- Admission to the hospital for individuals with significant loss of skin barrier function and/or unstable vital signs

REFERENCES

Elmets CA, Anderson CY: Sunscreens and photocarcinogenesis: An objective assessment. Photochem Photobiol 1996;63:435-440.
Gould JW, Mercurio MG, Elmets CA: Cutaneous photosensitivity diseases induced by exogenous agents. J Amer Acad Dermatol 1995;33:551-573, 574-576.
Hönigsmann, H: Erythema and pigmentation. Photodermatol Photoimmunol Photomed 2002;18:75-81.
Odom RB, James WD, Berger TG: Andrews' Diseases of the Skin, Clinical Dermatology, 9th ed. 2000, pp 21-48.
Roelandts, R: The diagnosis of photosensitivity. Arch Dermatol 2000;136:1152-1157.
Scheinfeld N, Deleo VA: Photosensitivity in lupus erythematosus. Photodermatol Photoimmunol Photomed 2004;20:272-279.
Tutrone WD, Spann CT, Scheinfeld N, Deleo VA: Polymorphic light eruption. Dermatol Ther 2003;16:28-39.

13

such as triamcinolone 0.1% cream can provide some relief of irritation, pruritus, and erythema. In moderate to severe cases, patients may benefit from a tapering course of oral prednisone (Sterapred), beginning at 40 to 60 mg per day for 10 to 14 days. Rarely, in severe cases with confluent blistering, changes in vital signs, severe pain, edema, chills, fever, and significant skin barrier disruption, hospitalization may be warranted.

CURRENT DIAGNOSIS

- Mild sunburn is characterized by cutaneous erythema with accompanying tenderness that peaks 12 to 24 hours after sun exposure.
- Patients with severe cases of sunburn may have cutaneous erythema with confluent blistering, marked discomfort, malaise, edema, chills, fever, nausea, and tachycardia.
- Symptoms may last for up to 7 days and are often followed by desquamation.
- A medical history should be obtained, including current oral and topically applied medications used by the patient that could potentiate a phototoxic reaction.

The Nervous System

Alzheimer's Disease

Method of
Jody Corey-Bloom, MD, PhD

Alzheimer's disease (AD) is the most frequent type of dementia in the United States and Europe, comprising approximately 50% to 80% of elderly subjects presenting with dementing disorders (Table 1). An estimated 4 million individuals in the United States currently have AD, and that number is projected to increase to at least 14 million by the year 2050. AD is a major cause of disability and mortality, and its impact on health care costs, including direct and indirect medical and social service costs, is estimated as greater than $100 billion per year.

Pathology

The brain of a patient with AD often shows marked atrophy, with widened sulci and shrinkage of the gyri. Microscopically, there is significant loss of neurons, in addition to shrinkage of large cortical neurons. Loss of synapses is believed to be the critical pathologic substrate. The neuropathologic hallmarks of AD are neuritic plaques (NPs) and neurofibrillary tangles (NFTs),

although these lesions are by no means unique to AD and occur in a variety of other neurodegenerative disorders. Classic NPs are spherical structures consisting of a central core of fibrous protein (amyloid) that is surrounded by degenerating nerve endings (neurites). NFTs are found inside neurons and composed of paired helical filaments of hyperphosphorylated microtubule-associated tau protein. NP and NFT are not distributed evenly across the brain in AD but concentrated in vulnerable neural systems. Other pathologic alterations commonly seen in the brains of patients with AD include neuropil threads, granulovacuolar degeneration, and amyloid angiopathy.

Pathologic criteria for the diagnosis of AD at autopsy require the demonstration of a sufficient number of NP and NFT on microscopic examination. The most consistent neurochemical change associated with AD is the well-documented decline in cholinergic activity that has inspired many attempts to treat AD with cholinergic drugs. Additional deficiencies in glutamate, norepinephrine, serotonin, somatostatin, and corticotropin-releasing factors are also described.

Epidemiology

Our understanding of the epidemiology of AD has advanced rapidly during the past decade with the emergence of various demographic, genetic, and exposure-related risk factors for its development. Table 2 lists the most important clinical risk factors for the development of AD.

Age is clearly the major risk factor for AD; the overall prevalence of AD after the age of 65 years is approximately 10%. Overall prevalence is, however, much less

TABLE 1 Common Causes of the Dementia Syndrome

Alzheimer's disease (AD)	50%-80%
Lewy body dementia	20%
AD and vascular dementia (mixed dementia)	10%
Depression	5%-10%
Vascular dementia	5%
Metabolic disorders	<5%
Drug intoxication	<5%
Infections	<5%
Structural lesions	<5%
Dementia secondary to alcohol	<5%
Hydrocephalus	<5%
Parkinson's disease	<5%
Pick's and other frontal dementias	<1%

TABLE 2 Risk Factors for Alzheimer's Disease

Age*
Genetic influences*
Apolipoprotein E status*
Female gender
Lack of education
Head trauma
Myocardial infarction

*Most important.

TABLE 3 Alzheimer's Disease: Genetic Loci

Chromosome	Gene	% of AD	Age at onset (y)
21	APP	<1	45-60
14	PS-1	1-5	30-60
1	PS-2	<1	50-65
19	Apo E	50-60	60+

Abbreviations: AD = Alzheimer's disease; APP = amyloid precursor protein; PS-1 = presenilin-1; PS-2 = presenilin-2; Apo E = apolipoprotein E.

meaningful than age-specific prevalence. From ages 65 to 85 years, the prevalence of AD doubles approximately every 5 years. Prevalence rises from approximately 2% in the age range 65 to 69 years to 4% in ages 70 to 74 years, 8% in ages 75 to 79 years, 16% in ages 80 to 85 years, and approximately 35% to 40% in those older than age 85 years.

In addition, genetic influences are important in AD, but their mechanism of action and whether they are operative in all cases of AD remain to be elucidated. In some cases, AD is inherited (familial AD) in an autosomal fashion with the gene linked to markers on three separate chromosomes (1, 14, and 21) (Table 3). Familial AD families are those with multiply affected individuals in which the disease segregates in a manner consistent with fully penetrant autosomal dominant inheritance. Disease onset is usually early in familial AD. Although these cases probably comprise less than 5% of all cases with AD, they are a source for significant advances in understanding its molecular basis.

The importance of an individual's apolipoprotein E (Apo E) gene status is receiving significant attention as an important genetic susceptibility risk factor for the development of the more typical or "sporadic" AD. Apo E is a protein involved in cholesterol transport with three possible alleles: ε2 (rare), ε3 (most frequent), and ε4.

Individuals who are homozygous and carry two Apo E ε4 alleles have an increased probability (more than 90%) of developing AD by age 85 years and do so approximately 10 years earlier than individuals carrying the ε2 or ε3 allelic variants. The exact mechanism by which this occurs remains unsettled; because up to 50% of late-onset AD patients do not possess an ε4 allele, Apo E genotyping for diagnostic purposes is currently not recommended.

Epidemiologic studies show a higher prevalence of family history of AD even in patients with sporadic AD. A family history of AD in a first-degree relative increases the risk of developing dementia by approximately fourfold. Other demographic factors, including gender (women may be more susceptible to AD than men) and lack of education, are also emerging as putative risk factors for AD. Head trauma, either a single episode leading to unconsciousness or repeated head injuries as in the case of boxers, appears to be a risk factor for AD. Whether exposure to nonsteroidal anti-inflammatory drugs or estrogen *reduces* the risk of developing AD remains unclear.

Clinical Features

The diverse spectrum of symptoms of AD reflects dysfunction of widespread regions of the cerebral cortex. Symptoms begin insidiously and progression is generally gradual and inexorable with occasional pauses. Memory loss is the cardinal and commonly presenting complaint in AD. Initially the patient has difficulty recalling new information, such as names or details of conversation, whereas remote memories are relatively preserved. With progression, the memory loss worsens to include remote memory (Table 4). Language is frequently normal early in AD, although reduced conversational output may be noted. As dementia progresses, more difficulty with naming and increased loss of

TABLE 4 Common Clinical Features of Alzheimer's Disease by Stage

	Early	Intermediate	Late
Cognitive memory	Poor recall of new information Remote memories relatively preserved	Remote memories affected	Untestable
Language	Dysnomia Mild loss of fluency	Nonfluent, paraphasias Poor comprehension Impaired repetition	Near-mutism
Visuospatial	Misplacing objects Difficulty driving	Getting lost Difficulty copying figures	Untestable
Behavioral	Delusions Depression Insomnia	Delusions Depression Agitation Insomnia	Agitation Wandering
Neurologic	Abnormal face-hand test Agraphesthesia Frontal release signs	Abnormal face-hand test Agraphesthesia Frontal release signs	Muteness Incontinence Frontal release signs Rigidity Loss of gait ± myoclonus

fluency may be noted. Later, language becomes obviously nonfluent until, terminally, the patient may be reduced to a state of near-mutism. Visuospatial impairment in AD results in symptoms such as misplacing objects or getting lost, difficulty with recognizing and drawing complex figures, and impaired driving. Difficulty with calculation (affecting skills such as handling money), apraxia, and agnosia are further problems that develop in AD. Early in AD, deficits in problem solving, abstraction, reasoning, decision making, and judgment may become apparent, suggesting executive dysfunction as a result of involvement of the frontal lobes. Patients may have difficulty organizing complex tasks such as a vacation trip, large family meal, or financial and other business deals. Impaired judgment may lead to unusual susceptibility to requests or solicitations and difficulty driving. Social comportment and interpersonal skills are often strikingly preserved in AD, however, and they may remain relatively intact long after memory and insight are lost.

Behavioral or psychiatric symptoms occur frequently in AD. Although major depression is uncommon, depressive symptoms occur in as many as 50% of patients. Delusions are common in AD, although they are rarely as systematized as in schizophrenia. They often have a paranoid flavor, with fears of personal harm, theft of personal property, and marital infidelity. "Phantom boarder" delusions, in which the patient believes that unwelcome individuals are living in the home, and misidentification syndromes also occur. Television characters are believed real or patients commonly fail to recognize their own reflection in a mirror. Hallucinations, primarily visual, are much less common than delusions, occurring in up to 20% of patients with AD. In addition to depression and psychotic symptoms, patients with AD show a wide range of behavioral abnormalities including agitation, wandering, sleep disturbances, and disinhibition. These often impose a significant burden on caregivers and may precipitate nursing home placement. In contrast to psychotic symptoms, behavioral disturbances are more clearly associated with the degree of dementia.

As neuronal degeneration progresses in AD, all of the symptoms just described worsen, and eventually patients become uncommunicative and unable to care for themselves, walk, or maintain continence. They require total care, including feeding, and are often institutionalized. In end-stage AD, death usually results from the complications of being bed bound, such as aspiration pneumonia, urinary tract infections, sepsis, or pulmonary embolism. Although mean survival after symptom onset is highly variable, ranging from 2 to more than 16 years, an excess mortality is consistently reported. Median duration of survival in most studies ranges from 5.3 to 5.9 years.

Diagnostic Evaluation

Several criteria are available to diagnose AD. The two most widely used are those of the *Diagnostic and Statistical Manual of Mental Disorders, Fourth Edition*

(*DSM-IV*) and those formulated by the National Institute of Neurological and Communicative Disorders and Stroke and the Alzheimer's Disease and Related Disorders Association (NINCDS-ADRDA) joint task force in 1984. According to the *DSM-IV*, primary degenerative dementia of the Alzheimer type requires an insidious onset, a generally progressive deteriorating course, and exclusion of all other specific causes of dementia. The more detailed NINCDS-ADRDA criteria classify AD into definite, probable, and possible levels of diagnostic certainty. Using NINCDS-ADRDA or other criteria with suitable laboratory and diagnostic studies, at least 85% to 90% accuracy in the clinical diagnosis of AD is achieved.

No single element of the clinical picture is unique to AD, but a skillfully taken history may reveal a change from a prior level of performance in several areas of intellectual function (e.g., difficulty recalling details of recent events, diminished attention, language difficulties, visuospatial problems, and impaired judgment). For most patients, an informant should substantiate this information. In taking a history, changes in functional abilities are helpful in confirming the presence of new impairment. Finally, the tempo of cognitive decline is extremely important in the evaluation of the patient with dementia. Acute or subacute onset of disability, a more rapid course, or episodic changes along the course suggest possibilities of dementia etiology other than AD.

Cognitive testing can be conducted according to the preference of the individual physician but should include assessment of attention, orientation, recent and remote memory, language, praxis, visuospatial abilities, calculations, and judgment. Brief mental status screening instruments that neurologists find useful and may enhance clinical judgment include the Mini Mental State Examination (MMSE). It should be emphasized, however, that age, education, ethnicity, and language of the respondent can influence responses to mental status test items, and the clinician must make allowances for each of these in assessing patients with cognitive difficulties. Recommended cutoff points are by no means definitive, and patients who are mildly demented may score in the normal range. Test scores do not, of themselves, make a diagnosis of dementia, nor do they determine the etiology of the dementing illness. Although not a routine part of the clinical evaluation, neuropsychological testing may be helpful in specific instances, for example, in high-functioning individuals whose history and initial evaluation are borderline or suspicious or in distinguishing depression from dementia.

The physical neurologic examination is often normal, especially early in AD. A thorough examination may reveal significant or lateralizing abnormalities, however, such as a visual field cut or hemiparesis that may suggest diagnoses other than AD. In intermediate or advanced stages of AD, patients often develop variable features, including extrapyramidal signs (rigidity and bradykinesia), nonspecific gait disturbances leading to an increased risk of falls, and myoclonus.

14

TABLE 5 Laboratory Evaluation of Patients with Dementia

Routine	When indicated
Complete blood count	Erythrocyte sedimentation rate
Chemistry panel	Urinalysis
Thyroid function tests	Toxicology
Vitamin B$_{12}$ level	Chest radiography
Computed tomography/	Heavy metal screen
magnetic resonance	HIV testing
imaging	Syphilis serology
	Cerebrospinal fluid examination
	Electroencephalography
	Positron emission tomography/
	single-photon emission
	computed tomography

No laboratory test currently can confirm AD during life or permit identification of individuals at risk for the disease. Several promising avenues—genotyping, imaging, other biomarkers—are actively being pursued, and ideally one or several will emerge with the sensitivity and specificity necessary for a diagnostic test. Thus the primary goal of laboratory testing at present is to exclude other etiologies of mental status impairment. Testing should be designed to evaluate treatable disorders systematically and include the studies cited in Table 5. Other tests, although not recommended as routine studies, may be helpful in certain circumstances.

Treatment

SPECIFIC THERAPIES FOR ALZHEIMER'S DISEASE

Although currently no treatment can either cure or permanently arrest AD, presently available AD-specific therapies are of two types: symptomatic approaches based on enhancement of neurotransmitter systems and neuroprotective strategies using antioxidant compounds. The most successful cholinergic strategy to date comprises the class of compounds known as cholinesterase inhibitors (Table 6). These agents reduce the metabolism of acetylcholine, thereby prolonging its action at cholinergic synapses in the brain. Three cholinesterase inhibitors are currently marketed for the treatment of mild to moderate AD: donepezil (Aricept), galantamine (Reminyl), and rivastigmine (Exelon). As a class, these agents demonstrate measurable, albeit modest, effects on cognition, behavior, activities of daily living, and global measures of functioning versus placebo in clinical trials. Cholinergic treatment probably does not alter the progression of neurodegeneration in the brain; however, possible long-term benefits of cholinergic therapy may include delayed institutionalization, possible decreased mortality, and economic savings in the cost of patient care. The primary side effects associated with treatment are gastrointestinal (e.g., nausea, vomiting, diarrhea, anorexia, weight loss); not surprisingly, better tolerability accompanies dosing that occurs on a full stomach. Insomnia, vivid dreams, and leg cramps are also reported side effects of treatment. In the absence of head-to-head comparisons of the cholinesterase inhibitors, the main differences appear to be their side effect profiles, titration schedules, and dosing regimens. Donepezil is administered once daily, either at bedtime or, alternatively, in the morning if insomnia or nightmares should occur. The initial dose is 5 mg and patients may be increased to 10 mg after 4 to 6 weeks. Both galantamine and rivastigmine require twice-daily dosing and should be slowly titrated to maximal dosing as tolerated. The recent American Academy of Neurology (AAN) practice parameter on the management of dementia concludes that cholinesterase inhibitors should be considered in patients with mild-to-moderate AD. This same parameter describes a potential benefit of neuroprotective agents such as α-tocopherol (vitamin E) and possibly selegiline because these compounds are shown to reduce functional loss and slow the progression to major milestones in AD. Furthermore, it notes that prospective data do not support the use of anti-inflammatory agents, prednisone, or estrogen to treat AD.

The FDA recently approved an *N*-methyl-D-aspartate (NMDA) receptor antagonist, memantine (Namenda), for the treatment of moderate-to-severe AD. This compound was very well tolerated in clinical trials. It is recommended that dosing be initiated at 5 mg once daily and increased in 5-mg increments to 10 mg twice daily (with a minimum interval of 1 week between dose increases).

TABLE 6 Features of Cholinesterase Inhibitors Currently Marketed for Alzheimer's Disease

Name (trade name)	Class	Selectivity	Time to maximum serum concentration	Metabolism	Daily dose (mg)
Donepezil (Aricept)	Piperidine	Acetylcholinesterase	3-5 h	CYP2D6 CYP3A4	5-10
Galantamine (Reminy)	Phenanthrene alkaloid	Acetylcholinesterase Allosteric nicotinic modulator	30-60 min	CYP2D6 CYP3A4	8-24
Rivastigmine (Exelon)	Carbamate	Acetylcholinesterase Butyrylcholinesterase	30-120 min	Nonhepatic	3-12

Rakel and Bope: *Conn's Current Therapy 2006.*

TABLE 7 Pharmacologic Treatment of Depression

Drug	Recommended dosage	Potential side effects
SSRIs		
Citalopram (Celexa)	10 to 40 mg/d	Nausea, insomnia, headache, tremor, restlessness,
Escitalopram (Lexapro)	10 to 20 mg/d	GI disturbances, sexual dysfunction. Paroxetine
Fluoxetine (Prozac)	10 to 40 mg/d	more anti cholinergic than other SSRIs.
Paroxetine (Paxil)	10 to 40 mg/d	
Sertraline (Zoloft)	25 to 100 mg/d	
Tricyclics		
Nortriptyline (Pamelor)	10 to 100 mg/d	Drowsiness, dizziness, dry mouth, tachycardia
Desipramine (Norpramin)	10 to 100 mg/d	
Other		
Venlafaxine (Effexor)	37.5 to 150 mg/d	Headache, nausea, anorexia

Abbreviations: GI = gastrointestinal; SSRI = selective serotonin reuptake inhibitor.

ADJUNCTIVE THERAPIES FOR THE BEHAVIORAL SYMPTOMS OF ALZHEIMER'S DISEASE

Because behavioral disturbances impair patients' function, increase their need for supervision, and often influence the decision to institutionalize them, their control is a priority in managing patients with AD. The principal treatable behavioral disturbances in AD are agitation, psychosis, depression, anxiety, and insomnia. Treating behavioral symptoms in AD is probably more of an art than a science. For virtually every group of symptoms, older and newer classes of medications are available, with proven efficacy in patients who are not demented and less clear results in those with AD. Until the appropriate trials are conducted in patients with AD, including comparative studies of different agents, it is recommended that clinicians choose a few medications, know their pharmacokinetic and half-life profiles in depth, and follow the general principles that apply to using any medication in older adult patients. For example, it is important to target therapy clearly by defining the most offending behaviors or symptoms. Precipitating causes of behavioral symptoms (e.g., physical illness or medication side effects) should be treated when present. Environmental modification and nonpharmacologic

strategies should be employed whenever possible. For example, mild degrees of pacing or wandering can be channeled into physical activity by simplifying surroundings and providing an enclosed yard to walk in. Drugs should be initiated at very low doses and increased slowly, monitoring carefully for common and less frequent side effects. As much as possible, dose schedules should be simplified with day-by-day pill dispensers, and caregivers should be enlisted to supervise medication compliance. Withdrawal of a drug that produces symptomatic improvement should always be considered, especially if the targeted symptom is known to be stage specific.

Treatment of depressive symptoms in AD commonly uses selective serotonin reuptake inhibitors, such as citalopram (Celexa), escitalopram (Lexapro), fluoxetine (Prozac), paroxetine (Paxil), or sertraline (Zoloft) (Table 7). Alternatively, tricyclic antidepressants with low anticholinergic side effects (such as desipramine [Norpramin] or nortriptyline [Aventyl HCl, Pamelor]) or the combined noradrenergic and serotonergic reuptake inhibitor venlafaxine (Effexor) can be tried.

Classes of agents used to treat agitation in AD include antipsychotics, mood-stabilizing anticonvulsants, trazodone (Desyrel), and anxiolytics (Table 8). Although many consider antipsychotics a mainstay in managing

14

TABLE 8 Pharmacologic Treatment of Psychosis and Agitation

Drug	Recommended dosage	Potential side effects
Neuroleptics		
Haloperidol (Haldol)	0.5 to 3.0 mg/d	Parkinsonism
Atypical Neuroleptics		
Risperidone (Risperdal)	0.25 to 3.0 mg/d	Orthostatic hypotension, nausea
Olanzapine (Zyprexa)	2.5 to 10.0 mg/d	Weight gain, elevated liver tests
Quetiapine (Seroquel)	12.5 to 200.0 mg/d	Sedation
Benzodiazepines		
Lorazepam (Ativan)	0.5 to 2.0 mg/d	Lethargy, confusion, dependence
Oxazepam (Serax)	10 to 30 mg/d	Ataxia

TABLE 9 Pharmacologic Treatment of Anxiety and Insomnia

Drug	Recommended dosage	Potential adverse effects
Tricyclics		
Nortriptyline (Pamelor)	10 to 75 mg qhs; 10 to 20 mg bid	Drowsiness, dizziness, dry mouth, tachycardia
Benzodiazepines		
Lorazepam (Ativan)	0.5 to 1 mg qhs	Lethargy, confusion, dependence
Oxazepam (Serax)	10 to 20 mg qhs	Ataxia
Other		
Trazodone (Desyrel)	12.5 to 75 mg qhs	Orthostatic hypotension
Buspirone (BuSpar)	2.5 to 10 mg bid or tid	Dizziness, headache, insomnia

Abbreviations: bid = twice a day; qhs = each bedtime, every night; tid = three times a day.

agitation, others reserve their use for psychosis because these agents may produce serious side effects, including parkinsonism, tardive dyskinesia, confusion, and falls. Parkinsonism and tardive dyskinesia may persist for weeks to months after cessation of antipsychotics and, for some, may never remit. Extrapyramidal side effects are more common with typical than with atypical antipsychotics, which appear to be better tolerated than traditional agents. Atypical antipsychotics are the treatment of choice for patients with psychotic symptoms. Sedation is the most common side effect reported in patients receiving these agents. The initial antipsychotic dose in AD subjects should be low, approximately one quarter of that used in young adults, and the total daily dose should be gradually increased as needed, titrating against side effects such as cognitive deterioration, low blood pressure, and parkinsonism.

Most patients with anxiety do not require pharmacologic treatment. For those needing it, however, benzodiazepines should be avoided if at all possible, given their potential deleterious effects on cognition (Table 9). Nonbenzodiazepine anxiolytics such as buspirone (BuSpar) are preferred. For insomnia, it is worthwhile to try nonpharmacologic sleep hygiene measures, including sleep restriction and keeping patients awake during the day as an adjunct to pharmacologic management. If medications are necessary, sedating antidepressants such as trazodone (Desyrel) may be effective choices for promoting sleep in AD, but anticholinergic hypnotics should be avoided.

CURRENT DIAGNOSIS

- Memory loss is the cardinal and commonly presenting complaint in Alzheimer's disease (AD).
- Social comportment and interpersonal skills are often strikingly preserved in AD, and they may remain relatively intact long after memory and insight are lost.
- The two most widely used criteria for the diagnosis of AD are those of the *DSM-IV* and those formulated by the NINCDS-ADRDA joint task force in 1984.
- AD cannot be diagnosed when consciousness is impaired by delirium or if conditions exist (such as decreased visual or auditory acuity) that prevent adequate evaluation of mental status.
- In taking a history, changes in functional abilities, such as preparing a balanced meal, playing games of skill, pursuing previously enjoyed hobbies, filling out business forms, handling financial records, and shopping alone, are helpful in confirming the presence of new impairment.
- AD characteristically has an insidious onset with slowly progressive worsening; thus acute or subacute onset of disability, a rapid course, or episodic changes along the course suggest possibilities of dementia etiology other than AD.
- Cognitive testing can be done according to the preference of the individual physician but should include assessment of attention, orientation, recent and remote memory, language, praxis, visuospatial relations, calculations, and judgment.
- Test scores do not, of themselves, make a diagnosis of dementia, nor do they determine the etiology of the dementing illness.
- No laboratory test currently confirms AD during life or permits identification of individuals at risk for the disease.
- Although neuroimaging is especially useful for excluding treatable causes of dementia, its use in making a positive diagnosis of AD is limited because the most prominent features—cortical atrophy and ventricular enlargement—are neither sensitive nor specific markers of AD, and they often accompany normal aging.
- Among patients who meet criteria for dementia, approximately 10% to 20% have a specific treatable or reversible etiology for their dementing syndrome.

Abbreviations: DSM-IV = Diagnostic and Statistical Manual of Mental Disorders, Fourth Edition; NINCDS-ADRDA = National Institute of Neurological and Communicative Disorders and Stroke and the Alzheimer's Disease and Related Disorders Association.

CURRENT THERAPY

- Presently available specific therapies for Alzheimer's disease (AD) include symptomatic approaches based on enhancement of the cholinergic and glutamatergic systems.
- The most successful cholinergic strategy to date—cholinesterase inhibitors—have modest effects on cognitive, behavioral, functional, and global measures in AD patients.
- In the absence of head-to-head comparisons of the efficacies of cholinesterase inhibitors, the main differences appear to be their side effect profiles, titration schedules, and dosing regimens.
- Because behavioral disturbances impair patients' function, increase their need for supervision, and often influence the decision to institutionalize them, their control is a priority in managing patients with AD.
- The principal treatable behavioral disturbances in AD are agitation, psychosis, depression, anxiety, and insomnia.
- Environmental modification and nonpharmacologic strategies should be used whenever possible, recognizing that some behavioral symptoms in AD may be transient and stage specific.
- Although often considered a mainstay in managing agitation, antipsychotics should be reserved for psychosis because these agents may produce serious side effects, including parkinsonism, tardive dyskinesia, confusion, and falls.
- Atypical antipsychotics are the treatment of choice for AD patients with psychotic symptoms.

REFERENCES

Chung JA, Cummings JL: Neurobehavioral and neuropsychiatric symptoms in Alzheimer's disease: Characteristics and treatment. Neurol Clin 2000;18:829-846.
Consensus recommendations for the postmortem diagnosis of Alzheimer's disease: The National Institute on Aging, and Reagan Institute Working Group on Diagnostic Criteria for the Neuropathological Assessment of Alzheimer's Disease. Neurobiol Aging 1997;18(Suppl 4):S1-S2.
Corey-Bloom J, Thal LJ, Galasko D, et al: Diagnosis and evaluation of dementia. Neurology 1995;45,211-218.
Cummings J, Vinters H, Cole G, Khachaturian Z: Alzheimer's disease: Etiologies, pathophysiology, cognitive reserve, and treatment opportunities. Neurology 1998;51(Suppl 1):S2-S17.
Doody RS, Stevens JC, Beck C, et al: Practice parameter: Management of dementia (an evidence-based review). Report of the Quality Standards Subcommittee of the American Academy of Neurology. Neurology 2001;56:1154-1166.
Jorm AF, Jolley D. The incidence of dementia: A meta-analysis. Neurology 1998;51:728-733.
Klatka L, Schiffer R, Powers J, Kazee A: Incorrect diagnosis of Alzheimer's disease. A clinicopathologic study. Arch Neurology 1996;53:35-42.
Knopman DS, DeKosky ST, Cummings JL, et al: Practice parameter: Diagnosis of dementia (an evidence-based review). Report of the

Quality Standards Subcommittee of the American Academy of Neurology. Neurology 2001;56:1143-1153.
Morris JC: Clinical presentation and course of Alzheimer disease. In Terry RD, Katzman R, Bick KL, Sisodia SS (eds): Alzheimer Disease, 5th ed. Philadelphia, Lippincott Williams & Wilkins, 1999, pp 11-24.
Selkoe DJ: Translating cell biology into therapeutic advances in Alzheimer's disease. Nature 1999;399:A23-A31.
Terry R, Masliah E, Hansen L: The neuropathology of Alzheimer disease and the structural basis of its cognitive alterations. In Terry RD, Katzman R, Bick KL, Sisodia SS (eds): Alzheimer Disease, 2nd ed. Philadelphia, Lippincott Williams & Wilkins, 1999, pp 187-206.

Sleep Disorders Except Insomnia and Sleep Apnea

Method of
Mary B. O'Malley, MD, PhD

14

Sleep complaints are common in primary care. Although the most common sleep problem in westernized nations is simply insufficient sleep, many millions of adults suffer from the effects of underlying primary sleep disorders. The route to diagnosis and appropriate treatment is complicated by several factors. First, symptoms of sleepiness and insomnia are underreported to physicians, and patients instead turn to over-the-counter treatments. Second, when patients do seek medical attention, even physicians who manage obstructive sleep apnea and insomnia effectively may lack knowledge or confidence in dealing with the many other intrinsic sleep disorders that may be just as common. The fact that patients' presenting complaints are often vague also does not help identify a solution. The clinician armed with some specific guides for evaluation, however, is prepared to discern probable causes and can use appropriate treatments for a range of common sleep disorders.

Taking a Sleep History

Sleep disorders are classified into three broad groups:

1. Disorders of the sleep process, or dyssomnias
2. Disorders of arousal and disruptions in the transition between sleep and wake, or parasomnias
3. Sleep disturbances that arise from an underlying medical or psychiatric illness

A targeted sleep history can often identify the presence of a sleep disorder and suggest solutions to some as well. Box 1 provides a sample of a structured sleep history, much of which the patient could answer on a questionnaire prior to an office visit. The patient's sleep schedule, including work hours, and the patient's habits relative to sleep are the core of a sleep history. Having patients use sleep diaries to illustrate graphically the pattern of sleep over several days is often invaluable.

Sleep Timing
- "How many hours of sleep do you need to feel rested? When did you last feel that way?"
- "What is your bedtime and usual wake time?" "Any evening or night shift work?"
- "How regular is your sleep period (weekday versus weekend)?"
- "Any difficulty falling asleep?"
- "Do you have a creepy, crawly, tingly, or restless feeling in your legs?
- "Ever feel a need to move, pace, or stretch?"
- How much do you worry about not sleeping well?"

Snoring
- "Has your snoring been loud enough to bother others? Has anyone witnessed apneas?"

Awakenings
- "Are you having difficulty sleeping through the night?"
- "Ever awaken with heartburn, choking, anxiety, pain, or hot flashes?"
- "How often do you awaken to urinate? Ever find you've urinated in bed?"
- "Once awake, how long before sleep returns?"
- "What keeps you from falling back asleep?"
- "How do you feel upon awakening for the day: rested? headache, dry mouth, congested?"

Daytime Symptoms
Excessive sleepiness versus fatigue:
- "How often do you feel drowsy when reading, watching TV, or at work?"
- "Do you take naps? Are they ever unintentional (e.g., at work, in the evening at home)?"
- "Ever drowsy at the wheel? Accidents or near-misses because of drowsiness?"
- "How often do you feel fatigued (tired, but not sleepy)?"
- "Do you have any trouble doing what you'd like to do because of fatigue?"

For reference, it is helpful to discover when, if ever, patients feel they sleep well, how much sleep is usual for them per night, and their state of health at that time. Everyone has a hard-wired circadian rhythm that defines preferred sleep timing relative to exposure to morning sunlight. For instance, a man who presents with complaints of excessive sleepiness and great difficulty waking up for work at 9 AM, but who reports that during college he felt fine when operating on an extreme night-owl schedule, may be diagnosed with a circadian rhythm misalignment.

Despite most people's perceptions that they "can get by with less sleep," chronic partial sleep restriction (e.g., sleeping 6 hours rather than 8 hours per night for most adults) leads to an insidious rise in sleepiness and an impairment in higher cognitive functioning. Consequently, knowing a patient is not overtly sleep deprived but is manifesting symptoms of excessive sleepiness helps identify a high likelihood of an underlying primary sleep disorder. Evaluating daytime functioning in low-stimulus conditions—reading quietly, driving while stopped in traffic—should be included in even the briefest of sleep assessments to identify problem sleepiness. Patients should be asked whether they have had accidents or near-misses caused by drowsiness

while driving. Falling-asleep-at-the-wheel accidents are often fatal and can be prevented if patients and their doctors identify chronic sleepiness.

The Presentation and Management of Common Sleep Disorders

PARASOMNIAS

Parasomnias are a broad array of disruptive behaviors that occur in or around sleep. These sleep disorders are often easy to identify because patients complain of unwanted events or experiences (e.g., nightmares, sleeptalking) that interfere with a good night's sleep. Daytime fatigue or sleepiness may be present as a consequence, but these are usually a secondary concern compared with the behavior itself. Parasomnias are caused by incomplete arousals from sleep. Many parasomnias are common during childhood because the brain is maturing and becoming more facile with the transitions between sleep and wake. In contrast, adulthood parasomnias often signal an underlying illness, medication effect, or marked psychological stress.

Parasomnia symptoms depend on the type of sleep stage at the time of the arousal. The timing of symptoms relative to the onset of sleep, the extent of mentation, memory for the event, and movement involved can often identify the type of parasomnia (Table 1). During normal rapid eye movement (REM) sleep, a flaccid paralysis is evoked of all skeletal muscles except the diaphragm and extraocular muscles. Thus dream activity is not able to be acted out. If a sleeper emerges rapidly from REM sleep, wakefulness may be experienced before the paralysis has lifted, leaving the sleeper immobile, but awake and aware, and often frightened about the situation. This condition, *sleep paralysis*, can occur in normal sleepers, but frequent bouts are not normal and may indicate an underlying diagnosis of narcolepsy. In contrast, people who do not maintain sufficient paralysis during dreaming (REM) sleep may act out their dreams, often with injury to self or bed partner. This uncommon condition, *REM sleep behavior disorder*, is a somewhat ominous diagnosis because it often heralds the development of a neurodegenerative disease such as parkinsonism. Some medications (e.g., venlafaxine) may infrequently induce reversible symptoms of REM sleep behavior disorder, however, so reviewing any coincident changes in medications or substance use is essential in patients manifesting these symptoms.

During REM sleep, mentation is richly detailed and recalled as dreams upon wakening. During non-REM sleep, mentation is usually vague and movement is not suppressed. Incomplete arousals from deep non-REM sleep may manifest as *sleepwalking, sleeptalking, confusional states*, or *night terrors*. Sleepwalking (somnambulism) is prevalent during childhood (up to 17% affected), and more common in adults than generally acknowledged (2.5%). Occasionally, sleepwalking episodes include behaviors such as binge eating or eating non-nutritive substances (e.g., drinking ketchup). Embarrassment over

TABLE 1 Parasomnias

Parasomnia type	Arousing from sleep stage	Usually normal?	Suggested treatment
Nightmare	REM	Not if chronic	Dream scripting* Medications†
Sleep paralysis	REM	Yes if infrequent	Education
		No if frequent	Evaluation for narcolepsy, OSA
REM behavior disorder	REM	No	Medications‡
Hypnagogia	NREM	Yes	Education
Somnambulism (sleepwalking)	NREM	Yes in children No in adults	Safety, education Safety, medications
Night terrors	NREM	In children usually	Parent education about adequate sleep
		No in adults	Screening for severe stress Medication changes§ Stress management Screening for PTSD
Enuresis	All	Not if chronic	Fluid management, interval awakenings screening for OSA and urologic disorders Medications¶
Bruxism	NREM	No	Protective mouth guard Medications‡

*As described in Germain A, Nielsen T: Behav Sleep Med 2003;1(3):140-154.
†Prazosin (Minipress), 1.0 mg at bedtime titrated up slowly by 0.5 mg increased every 3 nights to a maximum of 9.5 mg, or topiramate (Topamax), 25 to 100 mg at bedtime, or gabapentin (Neurontin), 300 to 1200 mg at bedtime.
‡Clonazepam (Klonopin), 0.5 to 2.0 mg at bedtime.
§Eliminate alcohol, nonbenzodiazepine hypnotics.
¶Nasal DDAVP (desmopressin acetate) or imipramine (Tofranil), 25 to 75 mg every day at bedtime.
Abbreviations: NREM = non–rapid eye movement; OSA = obstructive sleep apnea; PTST = post-traumatic stress disorder; REM = rapid eye movement.

14

evidence of nighttime eating activities or resultant weight gain may prompt desire for treatment. Patients with sleep-related eating disorders have variable levels of recall of the event, but amnesia is typical for sleep-walking events, and attempts to waken the individual may fail.

Night terrors are the most dramatic disorder of arousal. An episode is often initiated with a bloodcurdling scream, followed by a display of panic or terror, and often attempts to run around, striking out aimlessly. The sufferer may appear awake but not responsive to attempts to communicate. Children with night terrors are inconsolable during often prolonged (15- to 45-minute) episodes of crying, screaming, and panic-stricken confusion, which is later lost on the sleeper but not by the shaken parents. Anxious dreams or *nightmares*, in contrast, are recalled in frightened detail. Chronic nightmares may accompany depressive or anxiety disorders, especially post-traumatic stress disorder (PTSD).

Both adults and children may develop night terrors in response to trauma, as part of a larger PTSD. Patients with this type of night terror may have other features of an anxiety disorder. Sometimes night terrors are the only signal that severe emotional distress is present. This is true especially in patients who are in intolerable situations, but in which they have no control (e.g., in the case of severe child abuse), or in those who fear the expression of anger.

Enuresis (bed-wetting) is a disorder of sleep arousal. Common in children, enuresis has three main pathogenic factors: detrusor muscle hyperactivity, polyuria, and a high-arousal threshold during sleep. Children with persistent enuresis have evidence of very deep non-REM sleep, so the usual sensory input of a full bladder does not prompt awakening. The bladder dysfunction, and/or polyuria, also lowers the threshold for urination, so when combined with the child's very deep, imperturbable sleep, it prompts urination without awakening. Enuresis may occur as part of a sleep-related seizure or from obstructive sleep apnea, especially in adults, because the effort to overcome a blocked upper airway during obstructive events can generate a very powerful Valsalva maneuver that can trigger bladder emptying.

Sleep-related teeth grinding, or *bruxism*, is less often a serious disruption to sleep. Although the noise may bother the bed partner, treatment is more often motivated by the development of morning jaw pain, headaches, or damaged teeth. Bruxism may be secondary to medications such as antidepressants, a malocclusion, or stress-related muscle tension.

Testing for Parasomnias

Patients with parasomnias may present with resulting injuries, but otherwise no signs of these disorders are apparent on physical examination. Although often not necessary for the diagnosis, nocturnal polysomnograms may be able to confirm physiologic changes that predispose the patient to parasomnia behavior. Sleep studies are also helpful to rule out underlying seizure

Rakel and Bope: *Conn's Current Therapy 2006*.

disorders or secondary sleep disorders that contribute to the development of parasomnias or occasionally mimic symptoms of parasomnias.

Treatment of Parasomnias

Before searching for the cause, patients with any unintended sleep behavior should be advised to make the environment safe. Especially for sleepwalkers, routes out of the home—windows and doors—should be locked, blocked, or rigged with motion sensor alarms to prevent the inadvertent wandering into harm's way. The bedroom and adjacent areas should also be safety-proofed to protect from falls and sharps. Educating the patient and the bed partner or family is important to allay fears, increase safety, and help avoid the conditions that increase the likelihood of sleepwalking: sleep deprivation, stress, alcohol, and nonbenzodiazepine short-acting hypnotics. Most patients need no further intervention than these educational and preventative measures. Emphasizing the need to address ongoing stress and referral for psychological support is often an effective direction for patients who see their symptoms as scary and unmanageable.

In adult patients with sleepwalking or night terrors, a careful review of their medications and substance use may yield a culprit. Referral to a sleep center is advised for any patients with injurious behavior or in whom a second underlying sleep disorder is suspected. Clues to underlying severe distress or psychiatric illness must be picked up. Referral for psychiatric evaluation should be strongly considered in patients with repetitive night terrors, especially if no other precipitant can be identified.

Medications are a necessary adjunct to the behavioral management strategies of parasomnias if the episodes are hazardous. Benzodiazepines decrease slow-wave sleep as well as REM sleep, and so they are useful to treat both REM sleep behavior disorders as well as the non-REM parasomnias of sleepwalking and night terrors (clonazepam [Klonopin], 0.5 to 2.0 mg every day at bedtime). For persistent nightmares in patients with PTSD, bedtime doses of prazosin (Minipress, titrated up to a maximum dose of 9.5 mg at bedtime) may be effective. Alternatively, some anticonvulsants show benefits for reducing nightmares in some PTSD sufferers (gabapentin [Neurontin], 300 to 1500 mg; tiagabine [Gabitril], 4 to 12 mg every day at bedtime; or topiramate [Topamax], 25 to 100 mg).

Primary enuresis ends when nocturnal self-wakening can occur readily. Enuresis alarms may be used for any child older than age 6 years who elects to use one. These alarms teach the skill of nocturnal self-wakening, and combined with fluid management they have the highest cure rate of any intervention. When the alarm alone is unsuccessful, adding medications is usually effective (bedtime doses of imipramine [Tofranil], 25 to 75 mg a half-hour before bedtime, or desmopressin [DDAVP] nasal spray, 5 to 10 µg at bedtime). If enuresis is a persistent problem or recurs in a child after a period of dryness (secondary enuresis), the clinician should evaluate new contributing factors such as excess fluid or caffeine intake, sleep deprivation (increases sleep depth), development of sleep apnea, or medication side

effects. Occasionally, urologic disorders may be at fault, so referral is helpful if symptoms continue.

For bruxism, dental examination are advised to assess for occlusal problems, and mouth guards may be made to protect teeth. Unfortunately, mouth guards do not stop the grinding. If bruxism causes significant sleep disruption, or daytime sequelae, bedtime doses of muscle relaxants or benzodiazepines, diazepam (Valium), 10 mg, clonazepam (Klonopin), 0.5 mg, or other muscle relaxants are usually effective.

RESTLESS LEGS SYNDROME AND PERIODIC LIMB MOVEMENT DISORDER

Restless legs syndrome (RLS) is a common sleep disorder, estimated to affect 9% of the U.S. adult population. The disorder is characterized by painful or creepy-crawly sensations in the limbs at rest, with an irresistible desire to move, which alleviates the discomfort. The symptoms have a circadian rhythm, increasing as evening turns into night, postponing sleep onset by the need to pace or stretch the limbs. Once asleep, RLS may disrupt sleep throughout the night, prompting awakenings with the recurrent need to move until the sensations subside around dawn. The condition may frequently cause significant discomfort that is present even during the day. With milder symptoms, patients accommodate the need to move and may only notice they cannot fall asleep. The symptoms of RLS are similar to the medication-induced movement disorder akathisia, but akathisia does not follow a circadian pattern. Medications such as antidepressants, antihistamines, and caffeine may aggravate RLS. In children, RLS is often misdiagnosed as "growing pains."

The underlying etiology of RLS appears related to defective iron transport and storage that causes iron deficiency within the central nervous system (CNS). Because iron is a necessary cofactor for dopamine synthesis, this leads to a deficiency of dopamine and hypoactivity in dopaminergic motor areas. Idiopathic RLS follows an autosomal dominant inheritance pattern with variable expression of symptoms. Secondary RLS is associated with pregnancy, iron deficiency anemia (Ekbom syndrome), and neuropathy of chronic disorders (uremia, cryoglobulinemia, diabetes mellitus, infections). The clinical course is chronic, waxing and waning over the time, in relation to co-morbid illness or aggravating factors. Signs of RLS are not evident on neurologic examination.

Many patients with RLS also have a second sleep movement disorder, *periodic limb movement disorder* (PLMD), repetitive small myoclonic twitches of the legs or arms that literally kick a sleeper awake for a few seconds but go unobserved because the movements are small. When these events are frequent, sleep is severely disrupted, and sleepers complain of fatigue, sleepiness, or even insomnia because they find themselves awake occasionally. Jerking movements of the limbs, especially the legs, may be reported prior to sleep onset as well. Both RLS and PLMD account for a significant amount of the insomnia seen in patients older than age 60 years.

Rakel and Bope: *Conn's Current Therapy 2006.*

Testing for Restless Legs Syndrome and Periodic Limb Movement Disorder

A history alone easily diagnoses RLS. Any history of discomfort, accompanied by the need to move, that the patient observes to be worse as evening progresses is characteristic of the disorder. Anxiety symptoms may be reported as "restlessness," but the patient upon further questioning can distinguish the feeling is not a physical need to move so much as a desire to keep busy. A diagnosis of PLMD must be confirmed by polysomnography. A serum ferritin level should be determined in patients with these disorders; results below 50 μg/mL indicate that iron supplementation may be helpful in reducing symptoms, even if other signs of iron deficiency (e.g., microcytic anemia) are not present.

Treatment of Restless Legs Syndrome and Periodic Limb Movement Disorder

First the patient should be helped to eliminate offending factors: caffeine, chocolate, alcohol, nicotine, antidepressants, and antihistamines. Iron supplements, if indicated, begin the treatment. Mild to moderate RLS symptoms may respond to oral iron (65 mg elemental iron equivalent [Feosol; Slow Fe] twice daily, with 250 mg of vitamin C to enhance iron absorption). Initial studies indicate that severe RLS symptoms may respond rapidly to intravenous iron therapy (600 to 1000 mg ferrous gluconate [Ferrlecit] in divided doses), especially in patients with end-stage renal disease.

Many pharmacologic therapies are recommended to treat RLS and PLMD (Table 2). For medication to be most effective, dosing should begin in the evening or afternoon, before restlessness starts, with supplemental doses prior to bedtime. For patients with PLMD, dosing at bedtime is sufficient. Dopaminergic agents reduce the motor movements of PLMD and the motor restlessness of RLS. These agents are useful for many patients; however, side effects of nausea or daytime somnolence may be limiting. For many patients, unfortunately, the use of dopaminergic medications prompts a rebound of increased RLS symptoms the following day. This phenomenon, known as augmentation, may begin within a few months of treatment, and it may require discontinuing dopaminergic medications. Another widely used approach is the off-label use of anticonvulsants; these agents decrease the activity at night and ameliorate RLS sensations. Benzodiazepines may be useful to diminish the arousals from sleep, but they do not reduce the leg movements or alleviate the RLS sensations completely. Although commonly used, clonazepam (Klonopin) and others can cause residual daytime sedation, and tolerance may occur. Finally, although less appealing to many prescribers, opiate medications can often be very effective for even severe symptoms of RLS. Extended-release preparations such as oxycodone (OxyContin) or methadone (Dolophine; Methadose) may prevent the need for repeat dosing during the night.

NARCOLEPSY

Narcolepsy is a neurologic disorder of disrupted sleep-wake regulation. It is characterized clinically by pathologic sleepiness despite what appears to be adequate quality and quantity of nighttime sleep. People with narcolepsy develop such overwhelming sleepiness that they experience episodes of uncontrollable need for sleep, or so-called sleep attacks. This extreme sleepiness is in fact so characteristic of narcolepsy that clinicians often mistakenly use the term *narcolepsy* to refer to sleepiness itself. Other sleep disorders, and even total sleep deprivation, can produce an equivalent degree of extreme sleepiness. What distinguishes narcolepsy from

TABLE 2 Medications for Restless Legs Syndrome and Periodic Limb Movement Disorder

Agent	Initial and maximum doses	Side effects
Ferrous sulfate	65 mg (or equivalent) elemental iron*	Constipation, stool darkened
Ferrous gluconate (Ferrlecit)	125 mg intravenous in normal saline infused over an hour*	Hypotension, edema, nausea/vomiting, rare anaphylaxis
Carbidopa/levodopa (Sinemet)	25/100 to 100/400 SR-mg†	Insomnia, hallucination
Pergolide (Permax)	0.025 to 0.5 mg‡,§	Orthostasis, augmentation nausea/ vomiting, and sedation
Pramipexole (Mirapex)	0.125 to 1.5 mg‡,§	
Ropinirole (Requip)	0.125 to 1.5 mg‡,§	
Gabapentin (Neurontin)	300 to 3600 mg§	Dizziness, ataxia, sedation
Hydrocodone	5 to 20-30 mg‡,§	Constipation, dependence, euphoria, and sedation
Codeine	30 to 180 mg‡,§	
Oxycodone XR (OxyContin)	10 to 20-30 mg‡,§	
Methadone (Methadose)	2.5 to 20 mg‡	
Morphine sulfate XR (MS Contin)	15 to 30-45 mg‡,§	

*In patients with serum ferritin below 50 μg/mL.
†Single evening or bedtime dose.
‡Total daily dose, divided two times per day.
§Total daily dose, divided three times per day.

Rakel and Bope: *Conn's Current Therapy 2006.*

other sleep disorders is the absence of overt causes of sleepiness and the predisposition to slip in and out of REM sleep especially. The clinical features of narcolepsy are excessive sleepiness; disrupted nighttime sleep; frequent REM-related parasomnias (vivid dreams, sleep paralysis, hypnagogic hallucinations), and cataplexy (brief loss of muscle control triggered by strong emotions).

The pathophysiology of narcolepsy is linked to a loss of functional Orexin/hypocretin peptide in a cell group of the hypothalamus that regulates wakefulness and sleep onset. This is a suggested autoimmune-mediated process; people carrying the HLA DQB1 0602 gene are more likely to develop the disorder. People with narcolepsy typically develop symptoms during their teen years, with an unremitting course throughout their life. The symptoms of cataplexy may be dramatic—such as knees buckling after hearing a funny joke—or as mild as slurred speech. Cataplexy episodes last only seconds to a few minutes, and consciousness is maintained, although patients may be unresponsive. Unfortunately, cataplexy is often mistaken as syncope or seizure. For this and other reasons, proper diagnosis and treatment of people with narcolepsy often comes years after the initial onset of symptoms.

Testing for Narcolepsy

No specific signs of narcolepsy are evident on physical examination. Cataplexy symptoms may be observed in affected patients if they become emotional. A diagnosis of narcolepsy usually relies on polysomnographic testing: nighttime testing to rule out other sleep disorders, and the following day, during opportunities to nap, sleep onset is rapid with repeated transitions into REM sleep. HLA testing may be helpful in confirming the likelihood of the disorder in ambiguous cases but is not required for the diagnosis.

Treatment of Narcolepsy

Behavioral management strategies such as napping can be helpful, but the pathologic sleepiness associated with narcolepsy is debilitating and also necessitates the use of alerting medications. The current first-line alerting agent is modafinil (Provigil; 100 to 600 mg daily as single or divided doses) because of its more selective wake-promoting effects, tolerability, and lack of abuse potential. Traditional stimulants have been used for years to control sleepiness in these patients, and they remain effective for many patients. Table 3 lists the typical doses of the alerting agents necessary to treat narcolepsy. Antidepressant medications are effective in suppressing intrusive REM phenomena such as cataplexy. Any of the selective serotonin reuptake inhibitors (at doses comparable to that used to treat depressive disorders) or the nonsedating tricyclics such as protriptyline (Vivactil, 5 mg twice a day) can be effective as anticataplectics. For patients with severe cataplexy symptoms, sodium oxybate (Xyrem), 4.5 to 9.0 g at bedtime in divided doses, can be extraordinarily effective, usually used in combination with their alerting medications. In many patients, Xyrem may also significantly improve their alertness over time, lessening the need for other wake-promoting medications.

CIRCADIAN RHYTHM DISORDERS

Sleep timing relative to our 24-hour day is set by a hard-wired internal clock in the suprachiasmatic nucleus, our circadian rhythm. The clock's timing is set by the exposure to morning sunlight and triggers a drive for wakefulness until the fall of darkness, which prompts the secretion of melatonin. The drive for wakefulness then dissipates to allow sleep to occur. In this way, people's rhythms are regularly synchronized with the extrinsic day-night schedule, and most find that sleep is best between 11 PM and 7 AM. Individuals with circadian rhythm disorders, however, have an internal clock that is set differently, so normal sleep occurs at the "wrong time" relative to the usual hours for work and school.

Circadian rhythm disorders have a familial component. Families affected with advanced sleep phase syndrome are known, but because their sleep timing—in bed by 7 PM, up at 3 AM—still accommodates the 9-to-5 work world, these people often do not present for treatment. In contrast, those whose sleep timing is naturally at the other extreme—delayed sleep phase syndrome

---

TABLE 3 Medications for Excessive Sleepiness Because of Narcolepsy

Agent	Daily dose range	Side effects
Modafinil (Provigil)	100 mg every morning to 600 mg in divided doses	Headache, dry mouth, rare anxiety/dysphoria
Methylphenidate (Ritalin)	Up to 80 mg in divided doses Occasionally as high as 300 mg Up to 40-60 mg in children	Anxiety, euphoria Tachycardia, anorexia Growth retardation, insomnia
Dextroamphetamine (Dexedrine) Amphetamine salts (Adderall)	Up to 60 mg	Dependence
Methamphetamine Desoxyn	5-30 mg in divided doses Occasionally as high as 100 mg	Dependence Psychosis
Pemoline (Cylert)	37.5 to 150 mg	Anxiety; rare but fulminant liver failure
Sodium oxybate (Xyrem)	2.0-4.5 g taken just prior to sleep and repeated again 2.5-4 later during the night (total dose, 4.5-9.0 g/night)	Nausea, vomiting, enuresis, lethargy, confusion

Rakel and Bope: *Conn's Current Therapy 2006.*

(DSPS)—often need help to manage their sleep because it conflicts with school and work schedules. Patients with this disorder have a lifelong tendency to fall asleep quite late, evident when sleep timing is first organized in childhood. Typically parents do not seek treatment for their children until their problems falling asleep before 2 to 4 AM wreak havoc with the demands for early rising times for middle and high school. Of course, like other teens, those affected with this disorder often are accused of trying to avoid daytime responsibilities or staying up at night deliberately. Compounding the problem, the need for sleep increases during puberty to 9 hours a night, so the teens with this circadian disorder really suffer from enormous difficulty arising in time for school. The differential diagnosis of this disorder includes mood disorders, problems with limit setting, and other sleep disorders such as RLS. A telltale sign of this intrinsic circadian rhythm disturbance is consistent difficulty waking at early times, even for pleasurable events such as a vacation.

A more common circadian-dependent sleep disorder is shift work sleep disorder (SWSD). Although it is common for night or evening shift workers to report intermittent problems remaining awake during work and /or sleeping during the day after work, some individuals have extreme difficulty functioning on these schedules. These workers appear to have a biologic failure to adapt to the imposed schedule that produces debilitating sleepiness at night and/or insomnia during the day. This condition affects approximately 10% to 15% of all evening- and night-shift workers and causes persistent sleepiness as extreme as seen in people with narcolepsy. In reviewing their sleep history, people develop these symptoms only in relation to their non-standard work hours.

Sleepiness is a leading cause of industrial and motor vehicle accidents, and this minority of workers may contribute a disproportionate amount of accidents caused by untreated sleepiness. Diagnosis of SWSD is made by history alone. People with this sleep disorder are typically morning types and more sensitive to sleep deprivation. Telltale signs of SWSD are excessive sleepiness in any sedentary conditions, but especially at night while at work and on their drive home. Despite attempts to optimize their sleep, they may experience sleeplessness during the day. The patient may continue to have persistent sleep complaints even after returning to a day-shift job if this is possible. Of course, most shift workers are not able to change their work schedule. For people with SWSD, the pathologic sleepiness necessitates a multilevel treatment approach to optimize both sleep and wakefulness.

Testing for Circadian Rhythm Disorders

There are no physical signs of circadian rhythm disorders. Sleep logs are useful to chart sleep-wake patterns to see evidence of chronic difficulty getting sufficient sleep when desired, unless the schedule allows internally preferred sleep times. Reports of excessive sleepiness are evident, especially at the times their clock favors sleep (e.g., morning classes for DSPS, at

night during work for SWSD). Referral to a sleep center is not necessary to make these diagnoses, but it is often helpful to rule out secondary sleep disorders.

Treatment of Circadian Rhythm Disorders

Overall, a goal for any patients with a circadian rhythm disorder is eventually to find a lifestyle that can allow them to sleep when their body sleeps best, although this is not always possible. In the meantime, patients should start behavioral management strategies first: develop realistic sleep schedules (e.g., 6 hours and a nap, rather than a straight 8 hours), optimize the sleep environment, and avoid excess caffeine, nicotine, and alcohol. For young people with DSPS, exposure to therapeutic bright lights (5000 to 10,000 lux) for 30 minutes upon waking can help facilitate setting their clock to the desired time. Evening melatonin supplements (1 to 3 mg taken 3 hours before sleep is desired) may also help initiate sleep. Short-acting hypnotics may be helpful, but benzodiazepine hypnotics should be avoided.

For those with SWSD, the alerting medication modafinil (Provigil) is approved to treat excessive sleepiness on the job at night. Dosing modafinil (200 mg) approximately an hour before the night shift improves alertness for most SWSD patients studied. Based on

14

 CURRENT DIAGNOSIS

- Patients should complete a sleep inventory at each office visit. The interval development of sleep disorders may be evident from a historical review of specific sleep items.
- Any patient who describes regular drowsiness in low-stimulus conditions has potentially dangerous sleepiness. If sleep deprivation and medication effect are ruled out, an underlying sleep disorder is suspected.
- Sleepwalking in adults is most often prompted by medications or alcohol.
- Children or adults with frequent sleepwalking or night terrors episodes may be getting insufficient sleep, which predisposes the parasomnia to occur. Their history should be reviewed for evidence that episodes are less frequent after a few nights of extra sleep. If this correlation is not apparent, other factors should be considered, including an underlying anxiety disorder.
- RLS and PLMD account for a significant amount of the insomnia seen in patients older than age 60 years. If RLS symptoms are present, check the serum ferritin level.
- In narcolepsy patients, cataplexy may be mild or frequent. Ask about sudden muscle weakness associated with any strong emotion (laughter, anger, and surprise are most frequent) that lasts only a minute or so. Consciousness is preserved even if eyes are closed and there are no associated symptoms or sequelae.

Abbreviations: PLMD = periodic limb movement disorder; RLS = restless legs syndrome.

CURRENT THERAPY

- Any patient with drowsy driving should be assessed fully and told to stop or limit driving until the sleepiness is resolved. Sleepiness blunts insight into the danger involved while driving.
- Patients with symptoms of restless legs who have a serum ferritin level below 50 µg/mL should begin oral iron supplements (65 mg elemental iron twice daily) to help alleviate symptoms. Additional pharmacologic treatment may be needed, but the iron supplements may need to be continued.
- Any parasomnia behavior has the potential for injury. The sleeper should be provided with safety-proofing instructions. Bed partners may need to be advised to sleep separately until the behavior resolves.
- Narcolepsy patients need chronic medication for alertness, often at high doses. The misuse or abuse of medications is rare in these patients. The aim is to maintain their alertness throughout the day and allow them flexibility in dosing to achieve this goal.

experience with other chronically sleepy people, higher doses may be necessary in some people (e.g., 400 mg in one or divided doses during the work period). The goal is for alertness throughout the wake period, including the drive home. Modafinil does not interfere with sleep later, but these patients may benefit from a short-acting hypnotic or melatonin (or both) to facilitate better sleep during the day. Attention to their total sleep time, sleep environment, and any demands on them that interfere with sleep is important at all follow-up visits.

Sleep disorders are varied in their presentation and effects on patient health. Many sleep disorders can be effectively managed by primary care practitioners in the office setting. Clinicians need to become comfortable integrating a standardized sleep history in their clinical practice to identify patients with treatable sleep disorders. The range of available safe treatment options is increasing for symptoms such as sleepiness, giving clinicians a new opportunity to manage debilitating symptoms successfully in their patients. As the evidence grows that poor sleep creates specific health problems, the addition of sleep medicine to primary care practice represents a necessary step toward better health for all.

REFERENCES

Allen RP, Picchetti D, Hening WA, et al: Restless legs syndrome. Diagnostic criteria, special considerations, and epidemiology: A report from the restless legs syndrome diagnosis and epidemiology workshop at the National Institutes of Health. Sleep Med 2003;4:101-119.
Black JE, Brooks SN, Nishino S: Narcolepsy and syndromes of primary excessive daytime somnolence. Semin Neurol 2004;24(3):271-282.
Drake CL, Roehrs T, Richardson G, et al: Shift work sleep disorder: Prevalence and consequences beyond that of symptomatic day workers. Sleep 2004;27(8):1453-1462.
Krakow B, Hollifield M, Johnston L, et al: Imagery rehearsal therapy for chronic nightmares in sexual assault survivors with posttraumatic stress disorder: A randomized controlled trial. JAMA 2001;286(5):537-545.
Mahowald MW, Bornemann MC, Schenck CH: Parasomnias. Semin Neurol 2004;24(3):283-292.
Montplaisir J: Abnormal motor behavior during sleep. Sleep Med 2004;5(Suppl 1):S31-S34.
Raskind MA, Peskind ER, Kanter ED, et al: Reduction of nightmares and other PTSD symptoms in combat veterans by prazosin: A placebo-controlled study. Am J Psychiatry 2003;160(2):371-373.
Schmitt BD: Nocturnal enuresis. Pediatr Rev 1997;18(6):183-190.
Schwartz JR, Nelson MT, Schwartz ER, Hughes RJ: Effects of modafinil on wakefulness and executive function in patients with narcolepsy experiencing late-day sleepiness. Clin Neuropharmacol 2004;27(3):152.
Thorpy MJ: Approach to the patient with a sleep complaint. Semin Neurol 2004;24(3):225-235.
Van Dongen HPA, Maislin G, Mullington JM, Dinges DF: The cumulative cost of additional wakefulness: Dose response effects

Intracerebral Hemorrhage

Method of
James M. Gebel Jr, MD

Parenchymal intracerebral hemorrhage (ICH) represents approximately 10% of all strokes and two thirds of hemorrhagic strokes in the United States. Despite advances in ICH diagnosis and improved understanding of its natural history and prognosis, mortality is unchanged over the past 30 years.

Epidemiology

The incidence of ICH is more than twice that of subarachnoid hemorrhage and kills more than 20,000 Americans annually. An estimated 67,000 cases of ICH occurred in the United States in 2002. The incidence of ICH fell in the 1960s and 1970s with the increasing prevalence of antihypertensive therapy but then has leveled off over the past 30 years.

The risk of ICH increases dramatically with age. Ethnicity is a second important nonmodifiable ICH risk factor. A recent population-based study estimates the annual incidence of ICH at 18 per 100,000 for whites and 37 per 100,000 per year for blacks. Rates of ICH in blacks ages 55 or younger are especially disproportionately higher as compared to whites, with up to a fivefold relative risk. Persons of Asian and, to a lesser extent, Hispanic ethnicity are also at increased risk of ICH.

Risk Factors and Causes

HYPERTENSION

Hypertension is the single most significant and prevalent modifiable risk factor for so-called spontaneous, primary, or hypertensive ICH, and it accounts for the

TABLE 1 Annual Incidence of Intracerebral Hemorrhage as Related to Initial Systolic Blood Pressure in Hiroshima and Nagasaki, Japan

Initial systolic blood pressure (mm Hg)	Subsequent annual incidence per 100,000 persons
Less than 110	0
110-139	30
140-179	113
180 or greater	252

vast majority of preventable attributable risks for ICH. Merely treating hypertension in those in whom it is suboptimally controlled would eliminate an estimated 17% to 28% of all ICHs. As expected, a dose-response curve exists between hypertension severity and subsequent ICH risk. Table 1 reviews this dramatic risk relationship.

CEREBRAL AMYLOID ANGIOPATHY

Cerebral amyloid angiopathy is a common cause of lobar ICH in the elderly (age 65 years or older). Distinct from generalized amyloidosis, the amyloid protein is selectively deposited in the subcortical arterioles of the brain. Dementia and recurrent lobar ICH are its primary clinical manifestations. Its prevalence dramatically increases with age, observed in approximately 5% to 8% of persons in their 60s versus 55% to 60% of those 90 years of age or older. Magnetic resonance imaging (MRI), specifically with gradient echo sequencing that detects previous microscopic hemorrhages, should be employed in anyone with suspected cerebral amyloid angiopathy.

COAGULOPATHY

Coagulopathy is implicated in up to 7.8% of cases with ICH and most often caused by warfarin therapy, which increases relative ICH risk by 6- to 11-fold overall, with risk paralleling the degree of anticoagulation. Absolute risk of ICH from warfarin therapy ranges from 0.3% to 1.7% per year, depending on the reason for anticoagulation.

STRUCTURAL LESIONS

Vascular malformations, which are often treatable, account for a progressively larger fraction of ICH etiologies with decreasing age. They should be strongly considered in any patient with ICH under age 45 years, including those with hypertension, and represent a significant ICH fraction (4% to 5%) in some series. Up to 10% of aneurysmal ruptures result in parenchymal ICH. Angiography and brain MRI are recommended in all patients with ICH under age 45 years, and in older patients who lack traditional risk factors for ICH.

Rakel and Bope: *Conn's Current Therapy 2006.*

DRUG-RELATED CASES

Drug abuse is a final important consideration in non-traumatic ICH, representing approximately 0.5% of overall ICH, but a much higher percentage in adolescents and young adults. Cocaine and amphetamine abuse, in particular, represent important identifiable and potentially modifiable etiologies for ICH. A toxicology screen should generally be performed in any young patient with ICH. Finally, alcohol, the most common abused drug in American society, is associated with increased ICH risk.

Diagnosis

With the advent of computerized tomography (CT) scanning, ICH diagnosis is greatly facilitated. Patients classically present with headache, depressed or diminishing level of consciousness, and gradually evolving, rather than sudden maximal-at-onset, focal neurologic deficits, which often fail to conform to a specific vascular territory. Many patients with ICH fail to conform to this classic presentation, however, so CT scanning is mandatory to differentiate ischemic from hemorrhagic stroke.

Special mention should be given to the presenting signs of cerebellar hemorrhage, namely headache, nausea and vomiting, nystagmus, and dysmetria or ataxia. Unless thin 3-mm or 5-mm posterior fossa cuts are ordered, it is possible to miss a cerebellar hematoma by routine 10-mm-thickness CT scanning. Because cerebellar hemorrhage is readily treatable by surgical decompression, which is often both life and disability saving, it is important to maintain a high level of suspicion for patients with the appropriate clinical presentation, as well as to walk the patient to detect truncal ataxia, which is often the only clinically apparent examination finding (if any).

Treatment

INITIAL MEDICAL THERAPY

Medical therapy begins with the ABCs (airway, breathing, circulation). Airway protection in patients whose level of consciousness or gag reflex is markedly diminished is mandatory. Extremes of blood pressure should be promptly treated.

BLOOD PRESSURE MANAGEMENT

Controversy exists over how aggressively and quickly blood pressure should be lowered. A large clinical trial funded by the National Institutes of Health (NIH) is investigating whether or not aggressive lowering of blood pressure in patients with acute ICH reduces the frequency of hematoma growth during the first 24 hours post-ICH, which is as high as 38%. Studies of perihematomal cerebral blood flow by both MRI and xenon CT suggest that in the vast majority of patients, unlike

14

ischemic stroke, little or no penumbra is present. Overly aggressive use of potent vasodilating antihypertensive medications, however, can precipitate herniation in those with large hematomas by increasing intravascular volume. Current American Heart Association practice guidelines recommend lowering mean arterial pressure (MAP) to below 130 mm Hg in those with a prior history of hypertension. In patients with elevated increased intracranial pressure (ICP), cerebral perfusion pressure should be kept above 70 mm Hg. Pressors are recommended in those patients whose *systolic* blood pressure drops below 90 mm Hg.

TREATMENT OF INCREASED INTRACRANIAL PRESSURE

Intubation and hyperventilation are often the fastest way to lower ICP. Osmotic diuretics such as intravenous mannitol or glycerin are also used. Neither is shown to improve overall mortality or functional outcome in patients, although clinical trials employ arbitrary, regularly scheduled, fixed dosing of such agents, which does not mirror their use in clinical practice. Corticosteroids are *not* shown to benefit overall outcome of these patients. In fact, infection and hyperglycemic complication rates are much higher in dexamethasone-treated patients in clinical trials employing steroid use.

SURGICAL TREATMENT

Data are available from eight randomized controlled trials of surgical versus conservative therapy for ICH (Table 2). Early trials were greatly limited by no imaging confirmation and/or small size. Auer and colleagues demonstrated a lower mortality rate for endoscopically surgically treated patients with deep ICHs with a trend toward better survival in patients whose ICH volume was less than 50 mL, despite not demonstrating an overall statistically significant benefit.

The most significant clinical trial of surgical therapy for ICH is the recently completed 1024-patient International Surgical Trial of ICH (ISTICH), which evaluated the efficacy of early craniotomy (within 24 hours of admission) versus a conservative therapy group, which underwent craniotomy only when signs of impending

herniation were evident, in patients presenting within 72 hours of ICH onset. No difference was discerned in the rate of favorable outcome in the early surgery group (26.1%) and the conservative management group (23.8%), nor in mortality rates. A trend did favor early surgery for lobar ICH.

TREATMENT OF COAGULOPATHY-RELATED INTRACEREBRAL HEMORRHAGE

Warfarin-related ICH should be treated immediately with recombinant factor VIIa where available, which is now FDA-indicated for life-threatening warfarin-related bleeding. It can reverse warfarin in 5 minutes or less. Fresh-frozen plasma and vitamin K should also be administered because factor VIIa has only a 3-hour half-life.

MEDICAL COMPLICATIONS

Much of ICH mortality is caused ultimately by medical complications such as aspiration pneumonia. As with any patient with an impaired level of consciousness or stroke, swallowing function should be carefully assessed and aspiration risk-monitored and treated as necessary with aspiration-reducing strategies including early tracheostomy and gastrostomy in patients who are likely to have sustained aspiration risk. Deep venous thrombosis prophylaxis with pneumatic air stockings in paretic or paraplegic legs can begin immediately. Decubitus prophylaxis should be tailored to individual patient risk as ascertained by Braden score or other comparable risk assessment tool. Fall risk assessment should be performed in potentially ambulatory patients. Adequate hydration and nutrition, especially protein, should be maintained while considering aspiration risk.

Secondary Prevention

Only one large clinical trial indirectly addresses the issue of pharmacologic means of recurrent ICH prevention above and beyond reduction of modifiable risk factors. The perindopril protection against recurrent stroke study (PROGRESS) trial reported a 75% relative

TABLE 2 Summary of All Prospective, Randomized Placebo-Controlled Trials for the Treatment of Intracerebral Hemorrhage in the Post–Computerized Tomography Era

Study/year	Number of patients	Intervention	Benefit
ISTICH/2003	1024	Early (<24 h) surgery	None
Yu/1992	216	Glycerol	None
Batjer/1990	21	Surgery	None
Auer/1989	100	Endoscopic surgery	Yes*
Juvela/1989	52	Surgery	None
Italian/1988	164	Hemodilution	None
Poungvarin/1987	93	Dexamethasone	None
Tellez/1973	40	Dexamethasone	None

*Decreased mortality in surgically treated (30%) versus medically treated (70%) patients (*P* < .05); increased proportion of neurologically intact patients in surgically treated arm (*P* < .01).

CURRENT DIAGNOSIS

- Obtain an emergency noncontrast CT scan of the brain upon arrival.
- Determine whether the patient is on anticoagulant therapy.
- Ascertain antecedent hypertension history and control.
- Order MRI/MRA and/or angiography for underlying cause in patients younger than 45 years of age or for lobar ICH.

Abbreviations: CT = computed tomography; ICH = intracerebral hemorrhage; MRI/MRA = magnetic resonance imaging/magnetic resonance arteriography.

CURRENT THERAPY

- Remember the ABCs (airway/breathing/circulation).
- Reverse warfarin coagulopathy immediately with recombinant factor VII, vitamin K, and fresh-frozen plasma.
- Lower extreme hypertension aggressively upon presentation.
- Monitor for rebleeding within the first 24 hours.
- Do not use corticosteroids.

risk reduction in recurrent hemorrhagic stroke in patients treated with a combination of perindopril and indapamide as compared to placebo. The effect of these medications appears not to be explained simply by their blood pressure reduction effect, suggesting that additional effects (such as on the endothelium of cerebral arterioles) may be responsible for part or all of the treatment effect.

Outcome

Overall outcome in ICH is poor. Mortality rates for so-called spontaneous ICH generally remain in the 30% to 50% range. A simple bedside prognostic scale, the ICH score, is used in clinical practice to determine mortality risk in patients with ICH, and incorporates factors most strongly correlated to ICH mortality risk, such as age, hematoma volume, hydrocephalus, and intraventricular extension (Table 3).

Emerging Therapies

Recently completed and ongoing studies are evaluating the efficacy of ultra-early hemostatic medications such

as recombinant factor VIIa, neuroprotective drugs such as NXY-059, aggressive versus conservative blood pressure reduction, and aggressive versus conventional management of hyperglycemia.

ICH represents a significant fraction of all strokes and causes a disproportionate amount of stroke-related morbidity and mortality, especially in blacks age 55 years or younger. Treatment of hypertension is the single most important means of preventing ICH. Although diagnosis is greatly improved in the CT/MRI era, morbidity and mortality remain essentially unchanged. A high level of suspicion for cerebellar hemorrhage must be maintained. A toxicology screen, MRI, and angiography should be strongly considered in all patients with ICH under age 45 years. Patients presenting with hyperacute ICH need to be closely monitored because there is a 38% risk of rebleeding within the first 24 hours post-ICH onset. Patients with warfarin-related ICH should be immediately treated with recombinant factor VII infusion. Corticosteroids are of no value in ICH treatment and may increase risk of hyperglycemia and infection. Mortality risk can be predicted by the ICH score, a useful bedside prognostic scale.

14

TABLE 3 The Intracerebral Hemorrhage (ICH) Score

Variable	ICH score points
Glasgow Coma Score 3-4	2
Glasgow Coma Score 5-12	1
Glasgow Coma Score 13-16	0
ICH volume 30 mL or greater	1
ICH volume < 30 mL	0
Intraventricular extension present	1
Intraventricular extension absent	0
Infratentorial ICH	1
Supratentorial ICH	0
Age ≥ 60 y: check	1
Age < 60 y	0

Note: Mortality rate for score of 0 = 0%; 1 = 13%; 2 = 26%; 3 = 72%; 4 = 97%; 5 or 6 = 100%.

REFERENCES

Broderick JP, Adams HP Jr, Barsan W, et al: Guidelines for the management of spontaneous intracerebral hemorrhage. Stroke 1999;30:905-915.

Broderick JP, Brott T, Tomsick T, et al: ICH is more than twice as common as subarachnoid hemorrhage. J Neurosurg 1993;78:188-191.

Brott TG, Broderick JP, Kothari R, et al: Early hemorrhage growth in patients with ICH. Stroke 1997;28:1-5.

DelZoppo GJ, Mori E: Hematologic causes of ICH and their treatment. Neurosurg Clin North Am 1992;3:637-658.

Hemphill JC, Bonovich DC, Besmertis L, et al: The ICH Score: A simple, reliable grading scale for ICH. Stroke 2001;32:891-897.

Kissela B, Schneider A, Kleindorfer D, et al: Stroke in a biracial population: The excess burden of stroke among blacks. Stroke 2004;35:426-431.

Mendelow AD, Gregson BA, Fernandes HM, et al: Early surgery versus initial conservative treatment in patients with spontaneous supratentorial intracerebral haematomas in the International Surgical Trial in Intracerebral Haemorrhage (STICH): a randomised trial. Lancet 2005;365(9457):387-397.

Poungvarin N, Bhoopat W, Viriyavejakul A, et al: Effects of dexamethasone in primary supratentorial ICH. N Engl J Med 1987;316:1229-1233.

PROGRESS Collaborative Group. Randomised trial of a perindopril-based blood-pressure lowering-regimen among 6,105 individuals with previous stroke or transient ischaemic attack. Lancet 2001;358(9287):1033-1041.

Woo D, Haverbusch M, Sekar P, et al: The effect of untreated hypertension on hemorrhagic stroke. Stroke 2004; 35:1703-1708.

Zhu XL, Chan MSY, Poon WS: Spontaneous ICH: Which patients need diagnostic cerebral angiography? A prospective study of 206 cases and a review of the literature. Stroke 1997;28:1406-1409.

Ischemic Cerebrovascular Disease

Method of
Enrique C. Leira, MD,
and Harold P. Adams Jr, MD

Stroke is the third most common cause of death and a leading cause of disability in the United States. Approximately 3 million stroke survivors are living in the United States, many of whom are disabled. Stroke is a disease that primarily affects the elderly. Given the aging of the American population, the economic and social burden from cerebrovascular diseases is expected to grow considerably during the next 50 years. In the United States, the majority (80%) of strokes are ischemic. Acute stroke is an emergency and needs to be treated accordingly. Physicians should educate patients with vascular risk factors about the warning signs of stroke, including the advice to call 911 in case of suspected stroke to minimize extrahospital and intrahospital delays. The goal for emergent acute ischemic stroke management is to prevent neurologic deficit and death, achieved by promoting flow to the area of underperfused brain tissue around the core of the infarction, known as the ischemic penumbra, and preventing and treating early neurologic and systemic complications. Acute management should avoid delays and follow the suggested steps outlined here.

Initial Management and Stabilization

As in any other emergency, the management of acute stroke starts with assessment of the airway, breathing, and circulation (ABCs). Following stroke, most patients do not require intubation. The decision whether to intubate a stroke patient should be clinical and based on the likelihood of aspiration or obstruction developing given the neurologic deficit and findings. High-risk patients are those with either a depressed level of consciousness or bulbar dysfunction. Following strokes, oxygenation parameters are usually normal initially.

Arrhythmias and concomitant acute myocardial ischemia can follow a cerebral infarction. In addition, stroke is a potential consequence of heart disease, including acute myocardial ischemia. Consequently, assessment of the circulatory status should include an electrocardiogram and blood pressure monitoring. Blood pressure management is crucial. Some patients have elevations in blood pressure aimed to maintain cerebral perfusion in ischemic brain areas with impaired autoregulation. Such a compensatory blood pressure elevation should be treated conservatively. Current guidelines recommend that lowering the blood pressure be avoided, unless the mean is above 130 mm Hg or the systolic is above 220 mm Hg. Exceptions to this rule are those situations when the blood pressure needs to be treated more aggressively, such as strokes with concomitant myocardial infarction, aortic dissection, or evidence of hypertensive end-organ damage. Another exception is the administration of thrombolytic therapy in which, to minimize secondary hemorrhagic complications, the blood pressure is treated if above 185 mm Hg systolic or 110 mm Hg diastolic. A sustained elevation in blood pressure greater than the parameters just cited is a contraindication to treatment with thrombolytic therapy. A potential mistake is to administer sublingual nifedipine to an acute stroke patient with moderate blood pressure elevation. A sudden, profound, or sustained drop in perfusion pressure can result and the neurologic deficit may worsen. If blood pressure needs to be treated, intravenous short-acting β-blocking agents are preferred given their predictable response and minimal vasodilatory effect that could potentially worsen intracranial pressure.

Patients should not take food or liquid by mouth until a swallowing evaluation can be performed. Because many patients are dehydrated and the ischemic penumbra around the infarct may benefit from additional perfusion pressure, generous intravenous fluids should be started barring a major contraindication, such as congestive heart failure. Because fluids containing dextrose can potentially exacerbate the ischemic cerebral damage, normal saline is the fluid of choice. Peripheral intravenous access is preferred because central lines constitute a relative contraindication for thrombolytic therapy. The patient should be kept initially at bed rest to avoid worsening cerebral ischemia from positional-induced decline in flow in perfusion-dependent areas. An evaluation to address the differential diagnosis of stroke should be performed as soon as the person is stabilized to proceed with specific acute therapies (Table 1).

TABLE 1 Differential Diagnosis of Acute Ischemic Stroke

Intracerebral or subarachnoid hemorrhage
Subdural/epidural hematoma
Hypoglycemia
Postseizure (Todd's) paralysis
Complicated migraine
Brain tumors/metastasis
Brain abscess
Encephalitis (e.g., herpes simplex)
Multiple sclerosis
Metabolic/septic encephalopathy (exacerbating a previous neurologic deficit)
Psychogenic

Rakel and Bope: *Conn's Current Therapy 2006.*

Evaluation for Specific Therapies

Reperfusion therapy with intravenous recombinant tissue-type plasminogen activator (rt-PA) is currently the only approved pharmacologic treatment for acute ischemic stroke in the United States. Two randomized double-blinded clinical trials in acute ischemic stroke show the odds ratio for a favorable outcome at 3 months in intravenous rt-PA treated patients compared with placebo is 1.7 (95% confidence interval [CI] 1.2-2.6). That translates into a 32% relative increase in so-called favorable outcomes with rt-PA. Unfortunately, the therapy is not risk free. These trials also showed a 10-fold increase in the risk of symptomatic intracerebral hemorrhage with rt-PA treatment (0.64% versus 6.4%), and half of these hemorrhages were lethal. Table 2 shows eligibility for intravenous thrombolysis with rt-PA, and Table 3 describes the protocol. The minimal recommended requirements for administering rt-PA include familiarity with the NIH Stroke Scale, availability of emergent interpretation of brain computerized tomography (CT) scans, urgent laboratory blood tests (cell count and coagulation), and capacity to handle intracranial bleeding complications. Intra-arterial thrombolysis was beneficial in one study testing angiographically proven middle cerebral artery occlusions less than 6 hours old and is a promising alternative or complement to intravenous rt-PA, but it is considered experimental at this point. Mechanical thrombolysis with a cerebral embolus retrieval device is FDA approved for acute stroke. No neuroprotective agent is effective. Early full anticoagulation does not improve neurologic outcomes and has a risk of hemorrhagic transformation, so current guidelines do not recommend heparin in the treatment of most patients with stroke.

General Acute Medical Care

The use of specialized acute stroke units with dedicated medical, nursing, and rehabilitation personnel also improves outcome after stroke independently of any other therapy. In addition, stroke unit care can be given to a broader population of patients with stroke than rt-PA. Specialized stroke units should be promoted as an intervention that improves outcome. Although the reason for such benefit is uncertain, it is probably multifactorial and related to differences in ancillary care. Given that benefit, physicians should manage patients in the same way that stroke units do. Table 4 shows

14

TABLE 3 Protocol for Intravenous Recombinant Tissue-Type Plasminogen Activator (rt-PA) in Acute Ischemic Stroke

Total dose 0.9 mg/kg. (max dose 90 mg)
10% bolus, rest over 1 hour
Avoid central arterial lines for 24 hour
Avoid aspirin or anticoagulants for 24 hour
Admit to neurologic intensive care unit or stroke unit
Frequent blood pressure monitoring
Treat BP > 185/110 mm Hg with intravenous labetalol
Neurology checks every hour

Abbreviations: rt-PA = recombinant tissue-type plasminogen activator.

TABLE 2 Eligibility for Intravenous Recombinant Tissue-Type Plasminogen Activator (rt-PA) in Acute Ischemic Stroke

Eligible
Time of onset < 3 hours*
Significant measurable neurologic deficit
Symptoms attributed to cerebral ischemia (see Table 1)
Patient and family consent

Ineligible
Minor neurologic deficit (NIHSS 1-2 points)
NIHSS > 22 points
Patient comatose
Deficit rapidly self-improving
Blood pressure > 185/110 mm Hg
Seizure at onset of stroke
Abnormal CT of the brain (including "soft signs" of early ischemia)
Prolonged PT or PTT
Patient anticoagulated
Thrombocytopenia
Recent surgery, myocardial infarction, stroke, hemorrhage

*If patient wakes up with a deficit, the last time he or she was seen normal is counted as time of onset.
Abbreviations: CT = computerized tomography; NIHSS = National Institutes of Health Stroke Scale; PT = prothrombin time; PTT = partial thromboplastin time; rt-PA = recombinant tissue-type plasminogen activator.

TABLE 4 Typical Admission Orders for an Ischemic Stroke Patient

Activity: bed rest initially.
Telemetry monitored bed.
Neurology checks q 1-2 hours.
Notify physician if change in level of consciousness or neurologic deficit.
Blood pressure q 15-30 minutes.
Diet: nothing orally (until swallowing evaluated; then as appropriate).
Fluids: normal saline 70-100 mL/hour.
Pneumatic leg compression devices
Medications: hold all taken at home antihypertensives initially.
Aspirin 325 mg/day.*
Subcutaneous low-dose heparin or low-molecular-weight heparin.*
Sliding-scale insulin.
Labetalol, 5-10 mg IV, if blood pressure exceeds 220 mm Hg systolic or 130 diastolic (185/110 mm Hg if rt-PA was given).
Physical, speech, and occupational therapy consultations.

*None for 24 hours if rt-PA was given.
Abbreviations: IV = intravenous; q = every; rt-PA = recombinant tissue-type plasminogen activator.

suggested admission orders. An early neurologic complication of stroke is hemorrhagic transformation of the
infarction, more commonly seen after large cardioembolic
strokes or with the use of anticoagulants or thrombolytic agents. Measures to treat this complication include
aggressive blood pressure control. In some cases, surgical evacuation of a large symptomatic hematoma may
be needed. Another potentially life-threatening complication is brain edema, which is typically noticeable 3 to
5 days after large hemispheric infarctions or in the first
48 hours in cerebellar strokes. Prophylaxis includes
measures to maintain oxygenation, lower temperature,
and modest dehydration. Symptomatic brain edema
is usually managed initially with osmotic agents (e.g.,
mannitol), head elevation, or hyperventilation. In some
instances, surgical interventions (ventriculostomy or
hemicraniectomy) are required. Such procedures are
life-saving, but the risk of serious residual morbidity is
considerable. Aspiration pneumonia and urinary tract
infections are common complications that should be
addressed with antibiotic therapy to prevent sepsis and
neurologic deterioration. Deep venous thrombosis and
pulmonary embolism are prevented by pneumatic compression devices and subcutaneous low-dose anticoagulation and treated if necessary with full anticoagulation.
Patients should be monitored under telemetry to address
the potential cardiac arrhythmias and myocardial infarction that could follow stroke. Rehabilitation and mobilization should be promoted soon after a stroke while
preserving safety with fall precautions.

Early Secondary Stroke Prevention

Patients who have an ischemic stroke are at high risk
for subsequent events. Secondary prevention should
be initiated as soon as possible during hospitalization.
The control of modifiable risk factors (blood pressure,
hypercholesterolemia, diabetes, and smoking) is appropriate for every ischemic patient. Other strategies for
secondary prevention are not universal. To choose the
most appropriate strategy, the subtype of the ischemic
stroke (Table 5) needs to be first determined following
an algorithm employing clinical and ancillary test data
(Table 6). Cardioembolic strokes are best prevented by

TABLE 5 Acute Ischemic Stroke Subtypes (TOAST Classification)

Atherothrombotic (large-artery atherosclerosis)
Lacunar (small-vessel atherosclerosis)
Cardioembolic
Other etiology:
   Nonatherosclerotic arteriopathies (e.g., dissection,
     vasculitis)
   Procoagulant state
   Undetermined cause (unclear after complete workup or
     multiple mechanisms present)

Abbreviations: TOAST = Trial of Org 10172 in Acute Stroke Treatment.

TABLE 6 Investigations Required in Patients With Acute Stroke

All Patients
Unenhanced CT or brain MRI
Serum glucose, PT, PTT, electrolytes, cell and platelet
  blood count, cardiac enzymes
Electrocardiography
Pulse oximetry or arterial blood gas
Echocardiography (TTE or TEE)
Carotid ultrasound or neck MRA

Selected Patients
Intracranial MRA
Cerebral angiography
Lumbar puncture
Blood cultures
Electroencephalography
Hypercoagulability workup

Abbreviations: CT = computed tomography; MRA = magnetic resonance
arteriography; MRI = magnetic resonance imaging; PT = prothrombin
time; PTT = partial thromboplastin time; TEE = transesophageal
echocardiography; TTE = transthoracic echocardiography.

the long-term use of oral anticoagulants. If a major
contraindication exists, or the patient is at high risk
for bleeding, aspirin may be an option. Conversely,
non–cardioembolic strokes (atherothrombotic, lacunar,
or strokes of undetermined etiology) are best prevented
with antiplatelet agents. Warfarin is a second-line alternative for non–cardioembolic strokes because it does
not provide additional benefits over aspirin and has the
potential for serious hemorrhagic complications. Available
antiplatelets are aspirin, aspirin and dipyridamole, and
clopidogrel. Ticlopidine is another option but it is now
considered a second-line therapy because of the risks
of neutropenia and thrombotic thrombocytopenic purpura. All the newer antiplatelet agents show a modest
benefit over aspirin but are more expensive.

 CURRENT THERAPY

- The two proven effective interventions for acute
  stroke are intravenous recombinant tissue-type
  plasminogen activator (rt-PA) for selected cases
  less than 3 hours old and organized ancillary
  care in a dedicated stroke unit.
- Stroke prevention is achieved by controlling
  modifiable risk factors, such as hypertension,
  hypercholesterolemia, diabetes, obesity, and
  smoking.
- In addition, antiplatelet agents are effective in
  preventing recurrent noncardioembolic stroke.
  Anticoagulants are the agent of choice to prevent
  recurrent cardioembolism.
- Endarterectomy and angioplasty/stenting can
  further reduce the risk of recurrence for certain
  strokes caused by large artery atherosclerosis.

In addition to antiplatelet agents, some patients with large-artery disease can benefit from surgery or endovascular procedures. Endarterectomy is of proven value for those patients with more than 50% stenosis of the ipsilateral carotid artery if the angiographic and surgical procedural complications of death and disabling stroke can be kept below 2%. Therefore, this approach may not be effective for high-risk medical patients or institutions without the adequate experience. Angioplasty and stenting is becoming an alternative to endarterectomy for patients with symptomatic carotid disease.

Patients with stroke because of other causes may benefit from different specific secondary prevention interventions. For example, strokes caused by antiphospholipid antibodies may be best prevented with anticoagulants. Similarly, strokes caused by isolated angiitis (vasculitis) of the nervous system may be best prevented with immunosuppressants, whereas syphilitic strokes are best prevented with antibiotics.

REFERENCES

Adams HP Jr, Bendixen BH, Kappelle LJ, et al: Classification of subtype of acute ischemic stroke. Definitions for use in a multicenter clinical trial. TOAST. Trial of Org 10172 in Acute Stroke Treatment. Stroke 1993;24(1):35-41.
Adams HP Jr, Brott TG, Crowell RM, et al: Guidelines for the management of patients with acute ischemic stroke. A statement for healthcare professionals from a special writing group of the Stroke Council, American Heart Association. Circulation 1994;90(3):1588-1601.
Adams HP Jr, Brott TG, Furlan AJ, et al: Guidelines for Thrombolytic Therapy for Acute Stroke: A Supplement to the Guidelines for the Management of Patients with Acute Ischemic Stroke. A statement for healthcare professionals from a Special Writing Group of the Stroke Council, American Heart Association. Stroke 1996;27(9):1711-1718.
Albers GW, Amarenco P, Easton JD, et al: Antithrombotic and thrombolytic therapy for ischemic stroke. Chest 2001;119(1 Suppl):300S-320S.
American Heart Association: Heart and Stroke Facts. Dallas, Author, 2002.
Barnett HJ, Taylor DW, Eliasziw M, et al: Benefit of carotid endarterectomy in patients with symptomatic moderate or severe stenosis. North American Symptomatic Carotid Endarterectomy Trial Collaborators. N Engl J Med 1998;339(20):1415-1425.
Endovascular versus surgical treatment in patients with carotid stenosis in the Carotid and Vertebral Artery Transluminal Angioplasty Study (CAVATAS): A randomised trial. Lancet 2001;357(9270):1729-1737.
Evans A, Perez I, Harraf F, et al: Can differences in management processes explain different outcomes between stroke unit and stroke-team care? Lancet 2001;358(9293):1586-1592.
Furlan A, Higashida R, Wechsler L, et al: Intra-arterial prourokinase for acute ischemic stroke. The PROACT II study: A randomized controlled trial. Prolyse in Acute Cerebral Thromboembolism. JAMA 1999;282(21):2003-2011.
Mohr JP, Thompson JL, Lazar RM, et al: A comparison of warfarin and aspirin for the prevention of recurrent ischemic stroke. N Engl J Med 2001;345(20):1444-1451.
Stroke Unit Trialists' Collaboration: Organised inpatient (stroke unit) care for stroke. Cochrane Database Syst Rev 2000;(2):CD000197.
The National Institute of Neurological Disorders and Stroke rt-PA Stroke Study Group: Tissue plasminogen activator for acute ischemic stroke. N Engl J Med 1995;333(24):1581-1587.

Rehabilitation of the Stroke Patient

Method of
Karl J. Sandin, MD

Of the approximately 700,000 Americans who will have a stroke this year, an estimated half of them will need some sort of rehabilitation effort to maximize function. Whether because of thromboembolic disease, subarachnoid hemorrhage, or intracerebral hemorrhage, stroke is the third leading cause of disability in the United States. Although typically ineffective or unnecessary for either the minimally affected or tremendously impaired stroke survivor, for the large middle cohort of individuals with mild, moderate, or severe disability after stroke, rehabilitation programs provide improvements in outcome over natural recovery alone.

Rehabilitation is a coordinated program that provides reliable, conscientious, patient-centered restorative care to minimize impairment, disability, and handicap caused by a particular set of medical conditions. *Impairment* is any loss or abnormality of psychological, physical, or anatomic structure or function. *Disability* is any restriction to perform an activity in the manner within the range considered normal for a human being. *Handicap* is a social disadvantage that results from impairment or disability that limits fulfillment of a normal role. After stroke, a patient may have hemiparesis (impairment) that limits ambulation (disability), subsequently affecting ability to work (handicap). Some authors prefer to emphasize functions that remain after stroke, so they speak of ability and participation instead of disability and handicap. When rehabilitation is delivered by a well-functioning team, it provides a level of service excellence greater than the sum of its parts.

Rehabilitation settings include acute-care hospitals, acute rehabilitation hospitals and units, skilled nursing facilities, outpatient facilities and departments, the community (including the home, licensed residential care facilities, and assisted living centers), and transitional living facilities. Typically a patient with stroke is admitted through the emergency department to the hospital, preferably to a dedicated stroke unit. Use of these specialized service areas decreases morbidity and mortality after stroke and sets the stage for maximal recovery. From there patients with a substantial level of disability, yet good endurance for rehabilitation efforts and a reasonable prognosis to achieve a functional level that will allow them to live in a community setting, are referred to acute comprehensive stroke rehabilitation. Patients with less endurance or community discharge uncertainty are often referred to skilled nursing facilities for a less intensive program of rehabilitation. Some patients with less disability are referred directly from hospital care to outpatient or home health programs. Patients move from setting to setting as their medical condition and rehabilitation needs demand; services should continue in the least restrictive setting possible until the patient reaches a plateau. Younger stroke survivors, for whom community and vocational reentry is paramount, benefit greatly from transitional living center care. Gresham and colleagues in *Post-Stroke Rehabilitation* (in Chapter 5) effectively summarize decision trees to help choose a rehabilitation setting.

Apart from the patient and family, rehabilitation team clinical members include physicians (especially physiatrists—medical doctors specializing in physical medicine and rehabilitation—internists, and neurologists), nursing personnel of all levels, therapists (physical, occupational, recreational), speech/language pathologists, counselors (vocational, psychological), case/program managers, and others (dietitians, pharmacists, chaplains, etc.). The degree of involvement of each team member depends primarily on the setting and the stroke survivor's rehabilitation needs. In general, doctors are very involved in stroke rehabilitation as primary physician and team captain in acute rehabilitation settings but less so in community-based programs. Therapists are often more peripheral in intensive care unit settings but integral in home- and community-based treatment.

The antiquated term *cerebral vascular accident* (CVA) should never be used to describe a stroke. Accidents happen without warning or foreknowledge, whereas definable, manageable risk factors for stroke include homocystinemia, cardiac rhythm disturbances such as atrial fibrillation, obesity, dyslipidemia, nicotine dependence/tobacco use, stress, cocaine use, hypertension, diabetes, and autoimmune disease. Although nonmodifiable risk factors for stroke exist such as age (the older the person the higher the risk), gender (women die more of stroke than men, but men have more strokes), ethnicity (even controlled for other risk factors, people of color have more strokes than whites), and family history, primary and secondary stroke risk can be managed. Using the best medical care, family counseling, and education, stroke rehabilitation efforts should always seek to prevent future stroke. Secondary prevention of stroke through diet, exercise, cessation of smoking, and compliance with medical regimens remains a primary rehabilitation concern.

Prevention and early recognition of medical complications of stroke maximize neurologic and functional recovery. Thromboembolic disease, respiratory complications, cardiac problems, neurologic change, bowel and bladder dysfunction, skin breakdown, and pain can particularly affect stroke rehabilitation. All rehabilitation providers have the opportunity to recognize the signs and symptoms of these obstacles to improvement. Prompt recognition and diagnosis of medical problems improve patient care and outcome.

After stroke, deep venous thrombosis (DVT) and pulmonary embolism (PE) occur 40% to 50% and 9% to 15% of the time, respectively. These phenomena are the fourth most common cause of death in the first 30 days after stroke. Risk factors for their development include venous stasis, hypercoagulability, and endothelial injury. The first two are typically present in the stroke survivor because of immobility and acute-phase reaction. Primary prevention of these complications is critical. Stroke survivors not on systemic anticoagulation need either heparin or inferior vena caval filter placement. Because of lower morbidity compared with standard heparin, most stroke patients (including those with CNS [central nervous system] hemorrhage not requiring neurosurgical evacuation) receive low-molecular-weight fractionated heparin (enoxaparin sodium [Lovenox], 40 mg every day). Heparin prophylaxis continues until thromboembolic risk is minimized, typically defined as walking without physical assistance for 200 feet at a time. Pragmatically, prophylaxis is often stopped at institutional discharge but should be continued for at least 3 weeks after stroke. Intermittent pneumatic compression has little relevance in rehabilitation programs because patients are spending considerable time out of bed; elastic stockings provide no DVT/PE prevention. Recognition of failure of prevention requires clinical vigilance and forethought because 50% of DVT cases are clinically silent. A low threshold to check for DVT using Doppler ultrasound or other noninvasive testing or for PE using spiral chest computed tomography (CT) should inform the physician caring for the stroke survivor.

Pneumonia is the third major cause of death in the first 30 days after stroke. An estimated 32% of all stroke survivors develop pneumonia, especially after subarachnoid hemorrhage and in patients with coma because of stroke. Common risk factors include aspiration of oral contents, including saliva, liquids, and food, decreased chest wall compliance, poor expiratory muscle strength, decreased immune response after stroke, and general debility. Although pneumonia classically presents with shaking chills, hemoptysis, and pleuritic pain, in the stroke survivor the only symptom(s) may be low-grade fever, lethargy, loss of neurologic or functional status, or malaise. Prevention of pneumonia requires early assessment for and treatment of dysphagia, strict oral hygiene, such as sterilizing the mouth with an oral antiseptic (chlorhexidine gluconate [Peridex] on a foam-tipped mouth brush every 8 hours, preventive respiratory care including frequent incentive spirometry and inspiratory muscle training, and supervised posturally appropriate eating. Treatment of pneumonia includes rest, antibiotics, and tracheobronchial hygiene and may interrupt the stroke rehabilitation program.

At least 75% of patients with stroke have cardiac disease, which may have caused the stroke (e.g., atrial fibrillation) and may affect stroke recovery (e.g., cardiomyopathy). Cardiac disease is the second leading cause of early mortality and the leading cause of late mortality after stroke. Of stroke patients, 66% have coronary artery disease, 50% have dysrhythmias, and 20% have congestive heart failure (CHF). Effective management of CHF improves function after stroke. Cardiovascular and neurovascular disease commonly exist together, so stroke rehabilitation providers should assume all stroke survivors younger than 70 years have at least latent heart disease. Regardless of rehabilitation setting, patients should be monitored for vital signs and for signs and symptoms of well-being at the inception of the exercise components of stroke rehabilitation (and to some degree throughout).

Neurologic conditions may change or appear after stroke. Seizures complicate less than 10% of strokes;

half occur in the first few days after stroke. Patients who seize after stroke typically have more brain damage and therefore a worse prognosis. Many patients with large bland infarcts or intracerebral and subarachnoid hemorrhage are placed on antiseizure agents as a prophylaxis against seizures. This controversial practice may impair the function of surviving normal brain and is discouraged in rehabilitation settings. A short (1-week) course of seizure prophylaxis is warranted after craniotomy. Bland infarcts may hemorrhagically transform, often presenting with changes in neurologic or functional status. A low threshold for repeat neurologic imaging (especially brain CT) should uncover this phenomenon and enable transfer, as is typically required, to a higher level of medical care. Change in neurologic status because of new stroke or intolerance of medications is not unusual during rehabilitation.

Neuromuscular conditions aggravate and facilitate stroke rehabilitation. After stroke, many survivors are initially hypotonic. As a result, their joints are poorly protected, so normal assistance moving in bed can result, for example, in shoulder trauma and pain. In the first few months after stroke, flaccidity is typically replaced with spasticity, a symptom complex of resistance to passive stretch, brisk reflexes, and hypertonicity because of loss of descending inhibition of spinal interneurons. Although spasticity can have its benefits, such as causing lower extremity rigidity that provides knee and ankle stiffness and allows a stable circumducted gait, it also can cause pain, contracture, and loss of function. Physical exercises, medications (dantrolene sodium [Dantrium], up to 100 mg four times daily), chemodenervation (botulinum toxin A [Botox]), and neuro destructive techniques seek to preserve some level of tone, thereby allowing maximal motor control. Yet much of the disability after stroke is caused by underlying weakness or sensory disturbances, losses not impacted by spasticity control.

Most stroke survivors have bowel and bladder dysfunction. Bladder problems include infection, incontinence, retention, and preexisting genitourinary disease, and they are often complicated by impairments in cognition, language, and mobility in the stroke patient. Continence, a complex feat of awareness, control, mobility, and dexterity, is vulnerable at many points to the direct and indirect effects of stroke. Cortical lesions can cause symptoms of urinary urgency at low urine volumes because of an unstable detrusor, the most common finding on urodynamic testing of stroke survivors with persistent incontinence. Brainstem strokes can cause detrusor sphincter dyssynergia. Patients with large strokes that cause aphasia, alteration in consciousness, or high levels of physical disability are typically bladder incontinent during initial stroke care. Patients with postvoid urinary retention (demonstrated by ultrasound postvoid measurement of bladder volume) have higher rates of incontinence and infection. Urinary tract infection occurs in almost all stroke survivors and responds well to targeted antibiotic therapy. Incontinence rates drop in the first 3 months after stroke. Stroke survivors often require bladder retraining with timed voiding every 2 to 3 hours around the clock, elimination of

medications with anticholinergic side effects that cause increased sphincter tone, and voiding trials in upright rather than recumbent positions to regain continence. Bowel dysfunction is common after stroke because of physical inactivity, inadequate fluid and/or dietary fiber, direct effect of a neurologic lesion of central defecation centers, side effects of medication, or impaction because of prolonged constipation. Conversely, some patients have diarrhea after stroke because of antibiotic side effects including *Clostridium difficile* infection, overstimulation of the colon with laxative, or obstipation. To normalize bowel function, stroke survivors require proper fluid, nutrition, fiber, and opportunity to eliminate in an upright position on their normal schedule. Often patients require a stimulant laxative (senna [Senokot], 2 to 4 tablets) followed 8 hours later by a postprandial rectal suppository (bisacodyl [Dulcolax]). Excessive use of bulk-forming agents does not help restore bowel regularity in the stroke survivor with altered mobility.

Neuropathic and nociceptive pain are common after stroke. Most worrisome is shoulder-hand syndrome (reflex sympathetic dystrophy, CPRS [Complex Regional Pain Syndrome, type 1]) that presents with pain in the eponymous parts, edema, dystrophic skin, and vasomotor instability. Triple-phase radionuclide bone scanning complemented by diagnostic and therapeutic blockade confirm the diagnosis. Additional therapies include transdermal clonidine, contrast baths, and axial loading extremity exercises. Most shoulder pain after stroke is caused by contracture, glenohumeral subluxation, rotator cuff disease, or bicipital tendonitis. Many stroke survivors have co-morbid conditions, such as osteoarthritis, which flare symptomatically with restorative efforts. True neuropathic pain because of stroke (central poststroke pain) is rare and difficult to treat.

Impairments after stroke include weakness (hemiparesis), loss of coordination (ataxia), hemisensory loss, visual deficits, agnosia, apraxia, disorders of language, and cognitive losses. After stroke, weak extremities often swell, usually because of flaccidity, loss of muscle control, or clot. If a thrombus is ruled out, extremity swelling requires elevation, such as for the upper extremity on a hemilap tray, or an external pressure gradient such as a 25 to 35 mm Hg below-knee compression stocking. Stroke survivors may have loss of light touch, pinprick, temperature, proprioception, kinesthetic, or vibratory sense, singularly or in combination. Even with normal strength, the patient with sensory loss may be very disabled. Visual deficits after stroke include field cuts, disregard, and disorders of perception. Anecdotal reports of improvement in visual functioning through behavioral optometry are not supported by well-designed studies. Agnosia (a deficit in afferent processing or inability to interpret or recognize information in one sensory modality when the end-organ is intact) particularly involves vision, touch, and hearing. Apraxia (a deficit in efferent processing or the inability to perform purposefully despite normal coordination and motor function) can involve language, dressing, or construction. Language problems include aphasia (impairment of the capacity to interpret and formulate multimodal language symbols), dysarthria (imprecise or poorly coordinated speech production with decreased articulation and intelligibility without problems in word retrieval or comprehension), and speech apraxia (a verbal or oral impairment of voluntary execution of complex speech-motor activities). Cognitive sequelae of stroke are inattention, memory loss, and loss of insight and judgment, which in combination may result in inability to initiate, plan, and complete (executive functioning) daily tasks. Various rehabilitation techniques such as transfer of training, neurodevelopmental technique (NDT) of Bobath, cutaneous stimulation of Rood, proprioceptive neuromuscular facilitation (PNF) of Voss and Knott, and motor relearning have particular disciples and adherents, although most rehabilitation therapists use a combination of various theories to improve function.

Strict attention to patient safety vis-à-vis falls and swallowing limits morbidity after stroke. Stroke survivors, regardless of location, have high fall rates. Falls can be prevented by placing the patient near the nurse's station, using bed movement alarms and mobility monitors, eliminating wet or uneven surfaces, providing one-to-one supervision, and avoiding polypharmacy, especially with cognitively impairing medications. Approximately 50% of stroke survivors have dysphagia because of deficits in oral, pharyngeal, or esophageal stages of swallowing. Of those, one third aspirate (some silently), defined as entrance of material into the airway below the level of the true vocal folds. Although the history and physical offer some tools to identify and treat swallowing problems, most rehabilitation therapists use functional endoscopic or videofluoroscopic swallowing studies to determine swallowing ability and guide management of dysphagia. Stroke survivors with dysphagia should eat only in highly structured, distraction-free environments using techniques such as double swallow and chin tuck to mitigate risk of aspiration. At time of advancement to more difficult diet textures or consistencies, strokes survivors should receive special attention to ensure a safe transition.

In the past, stroke rehabilitation paradigms focused almost exclusively on disability limitation. Today, changes in medical and societal perspective and improved neuroscience understanding are leading to newer techniques of care that seek to first improve physical function, automatically lessening disability. Examples of such efforts in stroke rehabilitation include partial weight-bearing treadmill training, constraint-induced movement therapy, and residential aphasia training. Although there is some overlap with disability treatment, a primary goal of these interventions is to avoid or eliminate learned nonuse, demanding maximal performance of the CNS for the physical or cognitive task at hand. At a cellular level, stroke rehabilitation improves outcome in two major ways: synaptogenesis and uncovering of dormant or vestigial CNS pathways.

Neuropharmacology augments the stroke rehabilitation process. Deficits in attention can be decreased by stimulants (methylphenidate [Ritalin], up to 10 mg twice daily). The addition of dextroamphetamine (Dextrostat) biweekly to speech/language pathologist language retraining improves aphasia and verbal apraxia compared to therapy alone. Although no controlled studies exist, many practitioners use acetylcholinesterase inhibitors designed to treat dementia (donepezil [Aricept], 5 to 10 mg every day) for cognitive disorders after stroke. Selective serotonin reuptake inhibitor (SSRI) and serotonin-norepinephrine reuptake inhibitor (SNRI) antidepressants effectively treat poststroke depression and may directly improve neural recovery after stroke.

Regardless of setting, stroke rehabilitation affects outcome beneficially. Major outcome measurement tools include the National Institutes of Health (NIH) stroke scale, a 14-item assessment scoring various impairments. Functional (disability) scales are the bedrock of analysis of stroke rehabilitation success and include, most prominently, the Barthel index and the Functional Independence Measure (FIM). Few scales assess participation, although arguably ability to return to active community living best reflects stroke rehabilitation success. Using diagnostic and demographic data and FIM scores, stroke survivors undergoing acute comprehensive rehabilitation paid by Medicare are assigned to a case-mix group (CMG) from which prospective payment derives. Payment for stroke rehabilitation is a controversial topic because rehabilitation hospitals, skilled nursing facilities, outpatient departments, and home health agencies all believe current funding schemes under-reimburse their services.

Perhaps the biggest burden after stroke is psychosocial. Depression and anxiety are common after stroke, with an incidence of approximately 40% each at 6 months. Many standard tests for these psychological conditions require normal cognitive and language function, so they have limited usefulness in the stroke survivor. Emotionalism (emotional lability) is present up to 1 year after stroke in 21% of patients. Social problems after stroke include economic strain (46%), social isolation (53%), decreased community involvement (43%), disruption of family function (52%), poor motivation, dependency, and loss of control. Social isolation is more common in women and those with higher educational achievement. Families are often called on to provide care for stroke survivors, but they may have neither the emotional nor physical ability to do so. As a result, caregivers burn out, culminating in severe situations with neglect

---

CURRENT THERAPY

- Stroke rehabilitation improves outcome over natural recovery alone.
- Stroke rehabilitation is most effective when team members work together on shared functional goals.
- Reduction of future stroke risk is a primary stroke rehabilitation concern.
- Most common medical problems after stroke include DVT/PE, pneumonia, UTI, and CHF, conditions that can usually be prevented, and if they occur must be managed well to secure stroke rehabilitation success.

Abbreviations: CHF = congestive heart failure; DVT/PE = deep venous thrombosis/pulmonary embolism; UTI = urinary tract infection.

Rakel and Bope: *Conn's Current Therapy 2006*.

or abuse. The incidence of depression in spouses of stroke patients is three times that of controls. To maximize the chances of a satisfying life for stroke survivors and their families, liberal use of community services within the entire first year after stroke should be encouraged. If the challenges of resuming a meaningful life are not met, patients and their families may respond with illness and maladaptive behaviors (Current Therapy Box).

REFERENCES

Bode RK, Heinemann AW, Semik P, Mallinson T: Patterns of therapy activities across length of stay and impairment levels: Peering inside the "black box" of inpatient stroke rehabilitation. Arch Phys Med Rehabil 2004;85(12):1901-1908

Bogey RA, Geis CC, Phillip R, et al: Stroke and neurodegenerative disorders: III. Stroke: Rehabilitation management. Arch Phys Med Rehabil 2004;(Suppl 1)85(3):15-20

Da Cunha IT Jr, Lim PA, Qureshy H, et al: Gait outcomes after acute stroke rehabilitation with supported treadmill ambulation training: A randomized controlled pilot study. Arch Phys Med Rehabil 2002;83:1258-1265.

Dettmers C, Teske U, Hamzei F, et al: Distributed form of constraint-induced movement therapy improves functional outcome and quality of life after stroke. Arch Phys Med Rehabil 2005;86(2):204-209.

Gresham GE, Duncan PW, Stason WB, et al: Post-Stroke Rehabilitation. Clinical Practice Guideline, No. 16. Rockville, Md, U.S. Department of Health and Human Services. Public Health Service, Agency for Health Care Policy and Research. AHCPR Pub. No. 95-0662. May 1995.

McLean DE: Medical complications experienced by a cohort of stroke survivors during inpatient, tertiary-level stroke rehabilitation. Arch Phys Med Rehabil 2004;85:466-469.

Sandin KJ, Mason KD: Manual of Stroke Rehabilitation. Boston, Butterworth-Heinemann, 1996.

Seizures and Epilepsy in Adolescents and Adults

Method of
Annemarei Ranta, MD,
and Nathan B. Fountain, MD

Seizures and epilepsy were long misunderstood by physicians, but a logical framework for the approach to seizures is finally emerging. This is especially important today because eight new antiepileptic drugs (AEDs), developed since 1993, are now approved in the United States, and their proper use depends on a systematic approach.

This article follows the systematic analysis that should accompany the approach to treating patients with seizures and epilepsy by dividing the process into five steps. Step 1 confirms the paroxysmal symptom of concern is a seizure. Step 2 determines the specific type of seizure present, classifying it as focal or generalized in onset. Step 3 determines the neuroanatomic site of seizure onset to direct investigations toward identifying pathology at that site. Step 4 identifies the etiology or

determines the epilepsy syndrome if the etiology is not identifiable. Step 5 selects the appropriate therapy.

Some terms used to describe seizures and epilepsy have definitions unique to the study of epilepsy. *Seizures,* behavioral changes that result from abnormal paroxysmal neuronal discharges, are a symptom of an underlying brain problem. A seizure may result from a transient perturbation of neuronal physiology such as during acute head trauma, alcohol withdrawal, or hypocalcemia, or a seizure may result from an enduring tendency to seizures, commonly referred to as epilepsy. *Epilepsy,* therefore, is not a single disease but rather any disease characterized by the spontaneous recurrence of seizures. Epilepsy syndromes are characterized exclusively or primarily by the occurrence of seizures with few other systemic or neurologic symptoms. When the etiology of seizures is definitely known—for example, when caused by a brain tumor or penetrating brain injury—then classification into an epilepsy syndrome is less important. But when the etiology is unknown because it is not identifiable or the evaluation is incomplete, classification becomes useful. Patients grouped into a specific epilepsy syndrome are presumed to share a similar pathophysiology and therefore a similar natural history and response to therapy.

Diagnosis

DIFFERENTIAL DIAGNOSIS OF PAROXYSMAL SYMPTOMS

Several entities present with symptoms similar to seizures. Syncope is commonly accompanied by motor movements, especially clonic or brief tonic arm movements. An electroencephalogram (EEG) recording during such "convulsive syncope" or "syncopal seizure" shows profound suppression of brain activity because of cerebral anoxia; it does not show seizure discharges, and thus convulsive syncope is not an epileptic seizure. Syncope is distinguished from a true seizure by the presence of presyncopal symptoms (nausea, flushing, and lightheadedness), brief loss of consciousness, and the return of normal cognition within a few seconds after arousal. Migraine headaches may occasionally be accompanied by complex visual phenomena or sensorimotor symptoms that could be confused with seizures. Postictal headaches may be confused with migraine. Complicated migraine with hemiparesis may be mistaken for a postictal paralysis. A history of migraine headaches and preservation of normal consciousness help identify the spells as migraine. Rarely, basilar migraines may be accompanied by loss of consciousness. Transient ischemic attacks (TIAs) should almost never be mistaken for seizures because TIAs cause focal negative phenomena, such as weakness, numbness, aphasia, or ataxia, whereas seizures usually cause positive phenomena, such as jerking, tingling, automatisms, or movements. Some movement disorders, sleep disorders, and hypoglycemia may also mimic seizures.

Psychiatric disease can present with symptoms nearly identical to seizures. Anxiety attacks can be characterized by anxiety, palpitation, facial flushing, and incoherence, as can seizure auras. Seizure auras usually progress to complex partial seizures at some point in the evolution of epilepsy, and auras are usually more stereotyped than anxiety attacks. Pseudoseizures, also termed *psychogenic nonepileptic seizures,* may be identical to seizures in their presentation, but pseudoseizures are more likely to be long in duration, involve bizarre or unusual symptoms and movements, have pelvic thrusting or thrashing, be precipitated by psychologically stressful events, and persist despite AED therapy. Unfortunately, epileptic seizures may also have these characteristics, and video/EEG monitoring may be the only way to distinguish seizures definitively from pseudoseizures. Surprisingly, as many as 30% of the patients admitted to inpatient epilepsy units for the diagnosis of spells end up with a diagnosis of pseudoseizures.

SEIZURE CLASSIFICATION

The International League Against Epilepsy (ILAE) developed a classification of seizures based on the site of seizure origin to facilitate communication (Figure 1). Seizures are divided into partial (or focal) and generalized classes. Consciousness is preserved in partial seizures because only a small region of the brain is affected. Consciousness is lost in generalized seizures because the entire cortex is affected. Partial seizures may secondarily generalize. "Primary" generalized seizures involve the whole brain from the onset.

Partial seizures are subdivided into simple partial and complex partial subtypes. Simple partial seizures arise in a small region of the cortex and produce discrete symptoms, depending on the area from which they arise, without altering consciousness. For example, seizures arising in the primary motor cortex in the frontal lobe cause clonic jerking of the contralateral limb, usually the hand. The most common simple partial seizures are indescribable auras arising in the temporal lobe and causing autonomic symptoms. Complex partial seizures (CPS) are characterized by staring with a fixed gaze and lack of distractibility to examiners. Automatisms are common, especially picking or pulling at clothing, lip smacking, and swallowing.

Generalized seizures are classified based on the predominant motor activity. Generalized tonic–clonic (GTC) seizures begin with sudden tonic extension of the extremities, often with an expiratory scream, followed by clonic rhythmic jerking of the extremities. Postictally, patients are always unresponsive for at least a brief period and usually sleep for minutes to hours. Tonic seizures contain only the tonic phase; clonic seizures contain only the clonic phase. Myoclonic seizures are a brief lightning-like jerk, most commonly of the arms. Atonic seizures consist of sudden unprotected falling with loss of muscle tone. Absence seizures are associated with nondistractible staring, similar to complex partial seizures, but they are very brief, frequent, occur primarily in children, and are associated with a generalized 3-Hz spike-and-wave pattern on EEG. Atypical absence seizures are similar but more prolonged and often accompanied by brief myoclonic jerks or loss of tone, and the EEG shows a slow or atypical generalized spike-and-wave pattern.

ETIOLOGY AND EPILEPSY SYNDROME CLASSIFICATION

The underlying pathology or etiology of seizures ultimately determines the natural history and, to some degree, the response to therapy. The ILAE established a systematic approach to epilepsy classification to help the clinician make appropriate decisions regarding the evaluation and treatment of patients with epilepsy (Table 1).

The most important division of epilepsy syndromes is into *focal epilepsies* (or localization related), in which pathology is localized to one region of the brain, and *generalized epilepsies,* in which the pathology is expressed throughout the whole brain. Focal epilepsies generally present with simple partial, complex partial, or secondary GTC seizures. Generalized epilepsies typically present with primary generalized seizures such as absence, primary GTC, atonic, or myoclonic seizures.

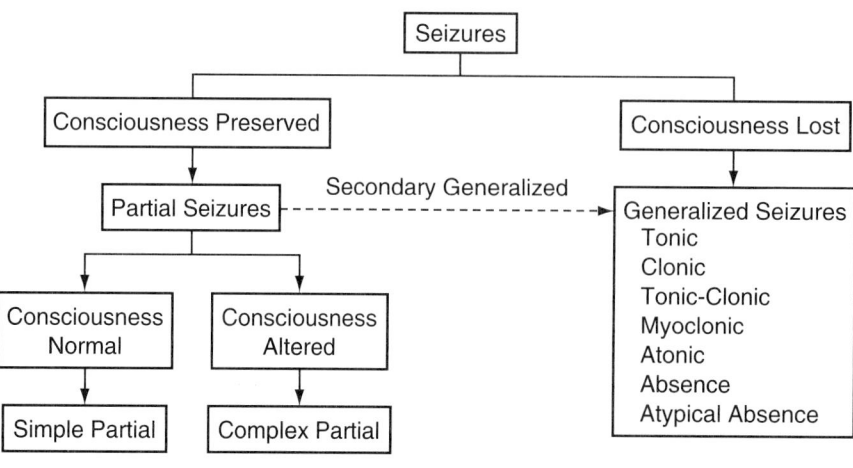

FIGURE 1. Algorithm for seizure classification.

Rakel and Bope: *Conn's Current Therapy 2006.*

TABLE 1 Examples of Epilepsy Syndromes in Adolescents and Adults

	Focal (localization-related)	Generalized
Idiopathic	Benign childhood epilepsy with centrotemporal spikes	Childhood absence epilepsy
		Juvenile absence epilepsy
	Benign occipital epilepsy	Juvenile myoclonic epilepsy
	Autosomal dominant nocturnal frontal lobe epilepsy	Epilepsy with generalized tonic–clonic seizures on awakening
		Cortical malformations
Symptomatic	Temporal lobe	Cortical dysplasias
	Frontal lobe	Metabolic abnormalities
	Parietal lobe	West's syndrome
	Occipital lobe	Lennox-Gastaut syndrome
		West's syndrome (unidentified pathology)
Cryptogenic	Any occurrence of partial seizures without obvious pathology	Lennox-Gastaut syndrome (unidentified pathology)

The epilepsies can be further subdivided into three categories:

1. Those that are symptomatic of an identified underlying brain lesion
2. Cryptogenic, in which an anatomic lesion is suspected but cannot be identified with current technology
3. Idiopathic, in which an identifiable lesion is neither identified nor suspected

The idiopathic syndromes are possibly caused by inherited abnormalities of neurotransmission without corresponding anatomic lesions. The importance of the latter distinction is that an aggressive search for underlying pathology is not necessary or indicated for idiopathic epilepsies, but it is necessary for cryptogenic cases.

Temporal lobe epilepsy (TLE), one of the most common types of epilepsy encountered in adults, is characterized by refractory complex partial seizures with occasional secondary generalization, originating in the temporal lobe. If neuroimaging is normal, the patient's condition is described as "cryptogenic focal epilepsy," the most common type of epilepsy in adults. Quite frequently, however, magnetic resonance imaging (MRI) demonstrates atrophy and gliosis of the hippocampus in the temporal lobe. Histopathologically, this neuronal loss and gliosis of the hippocampus and several mesial temporal structures gives rise to the term *mesial temporal sclerosis*. Mass lesions in the temporal lobe may present in a similar manner and include malformations and tumors, such as astrocytomas and dysembryoplastic neuroepithelial tumors (DNETs). Patients with such abnormalities on MRI suffer from symptomatic focal epilepsy. TLE is an important syndrome to recognize because temporal lobectomy renders more than 60% of patients essentially seizure free.

Juvenile myoclonic epilepsy (JME) is an example of a common adulthood idiopathic epilepsy. It is named for the characteristic onset in adolescence of brief myoclonic arm jerks and GTC seizures. JME is associated with a characteristic EEG pattern of generalized "polyspike and waves" in between seizures. Imaging studies are

normal, as is the case for all idiopathic generalized epilepsies. The etiology is undoubtedly an abnormality of neurotransmission and localized to at least two separate chromosomal loci, but the pathophysiology is still unknown. Many other epilepsies are encountered in adults, including those that begin in childhood (discussed in the article titled, "Epilepsy in Infancy and Childhood"), those caused by lesions in areas other than the temporal lobe, and other less commonly encountered adult-onset, idiopathic, generalized epilepsies.

DIAGNOSTIC EVALUATION

The evaluation of new-onset seizures is aimed at finding acute transient causes such as metabolic abnormalities and excluding acute life-threatening etiologies, such as infection, neoplasm, or hemorrhage. Most patients seek emergency care after the first seizure. At that time, it is usually impossible to determine whether the seizure represents epilepsy or an acute medical illness. Consequently, simple screening laboratory tests may be indicated, including electrolytes, complete blood count, liver enzymes, and urine drug screen. If central nervous system (CNS) infection is suspected, a lumbar puncture should be performed. An EEG is key because it may reveal interictal epileptiform discharges of the type present in patients with epilepsy, but it is not needed acutely. Neuroimaging is always indicated in the evaluation of a partial-onset seizure to exclude acute or serious focal pathology. The imaging technique of choice is an MRI scan, but if unavailable, a noncontrasted head computed tomography (CT) can be substituted in the acute setting.

The evaluation of established epilepsy is aimed at defining the underlying cause of the epilepsy syndrome, which is usually more subtle. An EEG is always indicated because it may reveal focal epileptiform discharges and assist in classifying the seizure type and epilepsy syndrome, but a normal EEG does not exclude epilepsy. The first EEG is abnormal in only approximately 40% of patients with clinically definite localization-related epilepsy. The EEG remains normal in approximately 20% of these patients, even after as many as seven EEGs.

Rakel and Bope: *Conn's Current Therapy 2006.*

14

The diagnostic evaluation of intractable epilepsy is intertwined with the presurgical evaluation and discussed later.

Antiepileptic Drug Therapy

PHARMACOKINETIC PRINCIPLES

No logical system exists to classify AEDs. One convenient method is to divide them into conventional, new, unconventional, and experimental categories. *Conventional AEDs* are those that were available before 1993. Of the several conventional AEDs, only phenytoin (Dilantin), carbamazepine (Tegretol), valproate (Depakote), phenobarbital, and primidone (Mysoline) are widely used today. *New AEDs* are those that have been approved since 1993. *Unconventional AEDs* are either outdated, used only in specific circumstances, or primarily used for non–epilepsy-related purposes. This review focuses on the conventional and new AEDs.

Conventional AEDs are frequently accompanied by side effects that often depend on the pharmacokinetics of the drug (Table 2). The half-life of these drugs is important because it determines the dosing interval and is often affected by concomitant AEDs. Infrequent dosing is key to improve compliance, so long half-life drugs are desirable. Some AEDs have a narrow therapeutic window so at the peak of the serum level patients may experience side effects. More frequent dosing of smaller amounts may avoid peak dose side effects.

New AEDs have few drug interactions; however, among conventional AEDs, phenobarbital, carbamazepine, and phenytoin are enzyme inducers that can decrease levels of one another and valproate (Table 3). All AEDs necessarily affect the brain, so pharmacodynamic interactions make CNS side effects of lethargy, ataxia, and blurry vision more common when more than one AED is taken at a time. Even as monotherapy, all AEDs cause CNS side effects at high doses.

Several principles to guide dosing help avoid problems. When initiating therapy, it is best to "start low and go slow." Most side effects are experienced at the initiation of therapy and can be avoided by starting with a low enough dose and increasing more slowly than recommended by the manufacturer. Table 4 provides general target doses that are usually therapeutic, but the maintenance doses given cover a wide range because there is no set final dose for any of the AEDs. The only way to know a given dose is "therapeutic" is to observe a decreased frequency of seizures. Serum drug levels are available for conventional and essentially all new AEDs, keeping in mind that oxcarbazepine (Trileptal) and tiagabine (Gabitril) levels are of very limited use because of their pharmacokinetic properties. In some instances, drug levels can provide a general guide, but many patients are on a so-called therapeutic dose while their blood level is below the usual normal range. Blood levels can help guide dose increases, however, by warning that toxic side effects may occur with further increases when the blood level is at the upper limit of the established therapeutic range. Nonetheless, it is important to increase each drug to the maximum tolerated dose before labeling it ineffective. This strategy usually requires increasing the drug until side effects occur and then reducing the dose by one step. Patients must be informed of how this works or they may refuse to take the drug, even at a lower dose. If neither seizure control improves nor side effects set in, despite high doses of a given AED, checking a serum level can help uncover noncompliance, a problem especially frequent among adolescents.

When substituting one AED for another, it is important to start the second drug and determine it is effective before gradually withdrawing the first drug. This system affords at least some protection from seizures at all times. After a 2-year seizure-free period, a trial of

---

TABLE 2   Conventional, New, Unconventional, and Experimental Antiepileptic Drugs

Conventional	New	Unconventional	Experimental
Carbamazepine (CBZ) (Tegretol)	Felbamate (FBM) (Felbatol)	Adrenocorticotropic hormone (ACTH)[1]	Clobazam (Frisium)*,‡
Ethosuximide (ESM) (Zarontin)	Gabapentin (GBP) (Neurontin)		Eterobarb‡
Phenobarbital (PB)	Lamotrigine (LMT) (Lamictal)	Acetazolamide (Diamox)	Ganaxolone‡
Phenytoin (PHT) (Dilantin)	Levetiracetam (LEV) (Keppra)	Amantadine (Symmetrel)[1]	Losigamone‡
Primidone (PRM) (Mysoline)	Oxcarbazepine (OXC) (Trileptal)	Bromides[1,†]	Nitrazepam (Mogadon)*,‡
Valproic acid (VPA) (Depakene)	Tiagabine (TGB) (Gabitril)	Clomiphene (Clomid)[1]	Piracetam (Nootropil)‡
	Topiramate (TPM) (Topamax)	Ethotoin (Peganone)	Pregabalin‡
	Zonisamide (ZNS) (Zonegran)	Mephenytoin (Mesantoin)	Progabide‡
		Mephobarbital (Mebaral)	Remacemide‡
		Methsuximide (Celontin)	Rotigotine‡
		Trimethadione (Tridione)	Retinamide‡
			SPM927 (Harkoseride)‡
			Stiripentol‡
			Vigabatrin (Sabril)*,‡

[1]Not FDA approved for this indication.
*Approved in other countries.
†May be compounded by pharmacists.
‡Investigational drug in the United States.

Rakel and Bope: *Conn's Current Therapy 2006.*

TABLE 3 Pharmacokinetics of Conventional and New Antiepileptic Drugs

Drug	Metabolized by inducible enzymes (mechanism)	Induces hepatic enzymes	Half-life (hours)	Protein bound (%)
Carbamazepine (Tegretol)	Yes (oxidized)	Yes	12-17	76
Ethosuximide (Zarontin)	Yes (oxidized)	No	30-60 (30 in child)	0
Felbamate (Felbatol)	Yes (multiple mechanisms)	No	20-23	25
Gabapentin (Neurontin)	No	No	5-7	<3
Lamotrigine (Lamictal)	Yes (glucuronidated)	No	25 alone or with both 60 with valproate 12 with enzyme inducer	55
Levetiracetam (Keppra)	No	No	6-8	<10
Oxcarbazepine (Trileptal)	Yes (converted to MHD, glucuronidated)	Mixed	9-11 (for MHD)	67
Phenobarbital	Yes (hydroxylated, glucuronidated)	Yes	80-100	45
Phenytoin (Dilantin)	Yes (hydroxylated, glucuronidated)	Yes	22	90
Primidone (Mysoline)	Yes (similar to phenobarbital)	Yes	8-15 (shorter with EI)	20
Tiagabine (Gabitril)	Yes (glucuronidation, oxidation)	No	7-9 (alone) 4-7 (with EI)	96
Topiramate (Topamax)	Yes (hydroxylated, hydrolyzed, glucuronidated)	No	20-24	13-17
Valproic acid (Depakene)	Yes (glucuronidated, oxidized)	No	9-16 (shorter with EI)	70-90 (varies with level)
Zonisamide (Zonegran)	Yes (acetylated, reduced)	No	63	40

Abbreviations: EI = enzyme inducer; MHD = monohydroxy derivative.

drug withdrawal should be considered in patients who do not have a known continued tendency for seizures. The risk of seizure recurrence after drug withdrawal is lowest in patients who have a normal MRI and EEG and are not diagnosed with an adult-onset idiopathic epilepsy.

CONVENTIONAL ANTIEPILEPTIC DRUGS

Phenytoin (Dilantin) is probably the most widely used and familiar AED, despite having the most problematic side effects. The metabolism of phenytoin is saturable, which means it shows zero-order kinetics at high blood levels. Very steep elevations in the blood level may occur with even small dosage increases when the level is near

TABLE 4 Antiepileptic Drug Interactions That Influence Serum Concentrations*,†

Drug added	CBZ	ESM	FBM	GBP	LMT	LEV	OXC	PB	PHT	TGB	TPM	VPA	ZNS
CBZ	→	→	→	–	→→	–	→	–	→	→→	→→	→	→
ESM	?	–	?	?	–	?	?	?_	?__	?	?	?__	?
FBM	→ epox	?	–	?	–	?	?			?	?		?
GBP	–	?	?	–	?	–	?	–	–	?	?	–	?
LMT	–	–	–	?	–	–	?			?	?	→	?
LEV	–	?	?	–	–	–	?	–	–	?	?	–	?
OXC	–	?	?	?	→	?	–			?	?	–	?
PB	→	→	→	–	→→	–	→	–		→→	→	→	→
PHT	→	→	→	–	→→	–	→	–		→→	→→	→	→
TGB	–	?	?	?	?	?	?	?		–	?	→	?
TPM	–	?_	?	?	?__	?	?			?	–	→	?
VPA	→ epox	→	–	–	–	?	–	–	–	–	–		–
ZNS	–	–	?	?	?	?	?			?	?	–	–

Abbreviations: CBZ = carbamazepine; ESM = ethosuximide; FBM = felbamate; GBP = gabapentin; LEV = levetiracetam; LMT = lamotrigine; OXC = oxcarbazepine; PB = phenobarbital; PHT = phenytoin; TGB = tiagabine; TPM = topiramate; VPA = valproic acid; ZNS = zonisamide.
*Effect of adding the drug listed in the first column on the blood concentration of the drugs listed in the other columns.
†Clinically significant effects are double arrows; other effects (single arrows) are not usually clinically relevant. Question marks indicate unknown interactions.

Rakel and Bope: *Conn's Current Therapy 2006.*

The Nervous System

14

20 µg/mL, despite the occurrence of a linear increase in the blood level with dose increases when blood levels are below 20 µg/mL. For example, the blood level may be 10 µg/mL with 200 mg per day, then increase to 15 µg/mL with 300 mg per day, and then increase to 20 µg/mL with 400 mg per day, but with an increase to 500 mg per day, the level may skyrocket to more than 30 µg/mL if the metabolism is saturated. Phenytoin's idiosyncratic side effects of hepatitis and blood dyscrasias are rare. One benefit of phenytoin is the availability of Dilantin Kapseals and other slow-release preparations so it can be dosed once per day, unlike other phenytoin preparations, such as the suspension or the Infatab, which must be dosed at least twice a day. Cumulative side effects of phenytoin, which occur over many years, include gum hypertrophy, hirsutism, coarsening of features, ataxia (as a consequence of cerebellar atrophy), osteoporosis, and peripheral neuropathy.

Intravenous (IV) phenytoin solution is very basic (pH 11), which frequently causes venous irritation, and occasionally "purple glove syndrome" and severe acute necrosis leading to amputation. IV phenytoin is mixed in polyethylene glycol, causing bradycardia and hypotension, which limits the rate of infusion to less than 50 mg per minute. This can be a significant problem in the treatment of status epilepticus or frequent seizures. Fosphenytoin (Cerebyx) is a phenytoin prodrug in which the phosphate group is rapidly cleaved off upon entering the bloodstream, yielding phenytoin. It is mixed in an aqueous solution and has a more neutral pH. Thus it is much better tolerated and can be given as fast as 150 mg per minute.

Carbamazepine (Tegretol), like phenytoin, is metabolized by the liver and induces hepatic metabolism. It also undergoes autoinduction, inducing its own metabolism for up to 3 weeks after initiating it, so steady-state blood levels are not achieved for several weeks. Carbamazepine has a relatively narrow therapeutic window, with usual therapeutic blood levels of between only 7 and 12 µg/mL. It commonly causes acute toxicity (ataxia, diplopia, and lethargy) with only a small increase in the dose. Carbamazepine does not have cumulative side effects and rarely causes serious idiosyncratic side effects, including blood dyscrasias, hepatitis, and hyponatremia. Mild leukopenia is common and does not require intervention unless the white blood cell count falls below 3000 cells/mm^3. Extended-release preparations (Tegretol XR and Carbatrol) that can be dosed twice daily are now available.

Valproic acid (or valproate) is very useful because it is effective for both partial and generalized seizures (see later). It is available as valproic acid (Depakene), sodium divalproex (Depakote), and an extended-release form (Depakote ER). Valproic acid (Depakene) frequently causes dyspepsia and other gastrointestinal side effects. Sodium divalproex (Depakote) is immediately cleaved to valproate in the stomach, but this preparation is tolerated much better. Valproate is usually dosed three times per day because of its relatively short half-life. Depakote ER was recently approved for once-per-day dosing, but it is actually released over less than 24 hours, so twice-daily dosing may be more useful for the treatment of epilepsy.

Valproate is now available as an IV preparation (Depacon), dosed identically to the oral forms.

Valproate is usually well tolerated, but it occasionally causes weight gain, alopecia, tremor, and thrombocytopenia. It can cause potentially fatal hepatitis and pancreatitis. Hepatitis occurs in only 1 in 40,000 adult patient exposures, but it is much more common in children (as much as 1 in 500) who are on multiple AEDs and with mental retardation, possibly because they have an undiagnosed metabolic abnormality. Carnitine[1] supplementation may reduce the risk of hepatitis. Although not proved, it is prudent for children with unknown causes of mental retardation on valproate to take carnitine. The overall incidence of birth defects associated with valproate is greater than with other AEDs, and it is more often associated with neural tube defects, which are more serious. Folic acid supplementation at 1 to 5 mg per day can reduce this risk. All women of childbearing potential on valproate should practice an effective method of birth control and take folic acid.

Phenobarbital fell out of favor as an AED because it occasionally induces lethargy, depression, and learning difficulties. However, it is usually well tolerated in adults, is effective for partial-onset and primary generalized tonic–clonic seizures, is inexpensive, and can be given IV. It can be dosed once per day and has a very long half-life, which is an advantage in poorly compliant patients. Primidone (Mysoline) is a prodrug of phenobarbital that also has its own antiseizure effects but less often causes lethargy.

Ethosuximide (Zarontin) is unique because it is the only AED that is effective exclusively for absence seizures with no efficacy for other types of seizures. It is usually well tolerated but occasionally causes nausea, anorexia, headache, and blood dyscrasias. It can be dosed once per day because of its very long half-life but is usually better tolerated twice daily.

NEW ANTIEPILEPTIC DRUGS

Felbamate (Felbatol) was approved in 1993 as the first new AED since valproate in 1978. It held great promise because it was highly effective for the most intractable epilepsies, such as the Lennox-Gastaut syndrome, as well as for partial-onset seizures, despite frequent side effects of anorexia, insomnia, and agitation, and the occurrence of frequent AED interactions. However, in 1994, after approximately 100,000 prescriptions were dispensed, 35 cases of aplastic anemia and 18 cases of fulminant hepatitis were reported. This led to a sudden change in practice and labeling so the drug is now only indicated for intractable epilepsy, in cases where the potential benefit outweighs the risk of potentially fatal side effects. Some clinicians obtain written consent from patients prior to prescribing. Its use should probably be limited to epilepsy centers.

Gabapentin (Neurontin) is very well tolerated and has no pharmacokinetic interactions because it is renally excreted unchanged. It has engendered an unwarranted

---

[1]Not FDA approved for this indication.

Rakel and Bope: *Conn's Current Therapy 2006.*

poor reputation as an AED because some believe it is ineffective. Clinical studies examined doses that statistically reduced the frequency of seizures with minimal side effects but were not high enough to determine the maximum tolerated dose; thus gabapentin was approved and initially used at relatively low doses of 900 to 1800 mg per day. Clinical experience suggests that doses as high as 3600 mg per day may be required for effectiveness in most patients, but high doses may not increase blood levels because drug absorption may be saturated at doses above 4000 mg per day.

Lamotrigine (Lamictal) is particularly useful because it is effective for both partial and generalized seizures. It is severely affected by other AEDs, so its dosing is drastically different depending on concomitant AEDs (Table 5). When taken alone (or with a combination of an enzyme inducer and inhibitor), the half-life of lamotrigine is approximately 25 hours, but reduced to 12 hours when taken with enzyme inducers (such as phenytoin, phenobarbital, carbamazepine), and prolonged to as much as 60 hours when taken with valproate (an enzyme inhibitor). Thus the anticipated maintenance dose and dose escalation rate are different depending on the concomitant AED. The only potentially serious side effect of lamotrigine is rash, whose occurrence also depends on concomitant AEDs. Mild rash is common and was present in as many as 1 in 50 children and 1 in 1000 adults during initial clinical studies. The rash can be life-threatening in the form of Stevens-Johnson syndrome or toxic epidermal necrolysis, but the incidence of the serious rash is only approximately 1 in 40,000. The rash is most likely to occur after the first 3 weeks of therapy but can happen at any time, and it is more common with high initial doses and titration rates and when taken with valproate. The titration rates in Table 5 were accompanied by a very low incidence of rash, probably because the titration rate is so slow—so slow that patients are unlikely to see an effect for many weeks or months and may require encouragement from the physician. When a rash is reported, the patient must be examined immediately and serious consideration given to stopping the drug.

Levetiracetam (Keppra) is approved as add-on therapy for partial seizures in adults, and studies in children are ongoing. It is very well tolerated and not associated with serious side effects. It can be titrated relatively rapidly so its effectiveness in a patient can be determined in a few months. It is primarily excreted unchanged with only 24% hydrolyzed before excretion, so it is unlikely to have significant drug interactions.

Oxcarbazepine (Trileptal) is a derivative of carbamazepine. The primary CNS side effects of carbamazepine are caused by epoxide 10,11-carbamazepine, a metabolite produced by oxidation. Oxcarbazepine cannot undergo this conversion and thus does not produce this metabolite, so it is better tolerated than carbamazepine and much less likely to cause diplopia and ataxia. The incidence of blood dyscrasias also appears lower than with carbamazepine. It is associated with hyponatremia. It does not induce AED-metabolizing liver enzymes (although it does induce other liver enzymes) or undergo autoinduction. Carbamazepine can be converted to oxcarbazepine, but the ratio is not 1:1 and responses are not 100% predictable. It is effective as monotherapy, so in the future oxcarbazepine probably will replace carbamazepine entirely.

Tiagabine (Gabitril) is approved as add-on therapy of partial-onset seizures. It is the only AED designed for a specific mechanism of action; it inhibits the reuptake of γ-aminobutyric acid (GABA) in the synaptic cleft. It has a very short serum half-life, but it affects the GABA transporter for at least 12 hours so it can be dosed twice daily. Some patients may require more frequent dosing. It is not associated with any end-organ toxicity, but it can precipitate nonconvulsive status epilepticus in those who are predisposed, usually patients with generalized epilepsy.

Topiramate (Topamax) is effective for partial seizures and some types of generalized seizures, especially the Lennox-Gastaut syndrome. It has an unwarranted reputation for causing cognitive side effects, probably because clinical studies appropriately determined the maximum tolerated dose by finding the dose at which an unacceptable frequency of side effects occur. Considering all topiramate clinical studies together, the incidence of subject dropout in those treated with more than 400 mg per day was twice that of the group taking less than 400 mg per day, which was approximately equal to placebo. This indicates that the average maximum tolerated dose is approximately 400 mg per day. Topiramate is a weak carbonic anhydrase inhibitor and can cause kidney stones, metabolic acidosis, and oligohidrosis; the use of other carbonic anhydrase inhibitors is relatively contraindicated. Acute narrow-angle glaucoma is reported in a few cases and requires immediate discontinuation. End-organ toxicities are not reported with topiramate.

Zonisamide (Zonegran) is the most recently released AED, although it was available for many years in Japan. It appears to be effective for both focal and some generalized epilepsies. Its pharmacology is not well described, but it is metabolized by multiple mechanisms and has a very long half-life, which may allow it to be dosed once per day. It rarely causes kidney stones. It also may cause oligohidrosis (reduced sweating) and rarely is associated with blood dyscrasias.

CHOOSING AN ANTIEPILEPTIC DRUG

Drugs of Choice by Seizure Type and Epilepsy Syndrome

AEDs should be selected based on the epilepsy syndrome or seizure type if the syndrome is not known. All types of partial-onset seizures respond to the same medications, so they can be considered together. The available data suggest that all AEDs, except for ethosuximide (Zarontin), are equally effective. Therefore, to select among them, consideration must be given to the relative importance of the side-effect profile, dosing interval, pharmacokinetics, and cost for each patient. In general, the new AEDs have less frequent side effects, daily or twice-daily dosing, and simple pharmacokinetics, which suggest they are more desirable than conventional AEDs. But conventional AEDs are familiar, have

TABLE 5 Titration Guidelines for Conventional and New Antiepileptic Drugs

Generic name	Common brand name	Dosing schedule	Initial dose	Adult increment (mg)	Maintenance (mg/day)	Child's initial dose (mg/kg/day)	Maintenance (mg/kg/day)
Carbamazepine	Tegretol, Tegretol XR, Carbatrol	tid-qid bid	200 bid	200 q wk	600-1800	10 qd	10-35 (for age <6 yr)
Ethosuximide	Zarontin	qd-bid	250 qd	250 q3-7d	750	15	15-40
Felbamate	Felbatol	tid	600-1200 qd	600-1200 q1-2wk	2400-3600	15	15-45
Gabapentin	Neurontin	tid	300 qd	300 q3-7d	1200-3600	10	25-50
Lamotrigine	Lamictal	bid	25 qd	25 q2wk	100 with VPA 400 alone; 600 with EI	0.15-0.5	0.5-5 with VPA; 5 alone; 5-15 with EI
Levetiracetam	Keppra	bid	500 bid	500 q wk	2000-4000	20	40-100
Oxcarbazepine	Trileptal	bid	300 qd	300 q wk	900-2400	8-10	30-46
Phenobarbital	(Generic)	qd-bid	30-60 qd	30 q1-2wk	60-120	3	3-6
Phenytoin	Dilantin, Kapseals liquid, Infatab	qd, bid-tid	200 qd	100 q5-7d	200-300	4	4-8
Primidone	Mysoline	tid	125-250 qd	250 q1-2wk	500-750	10	10-25
Tiagabine	Gabitril	bid-qid	4 qd	4-8 q wk	16-32	0.1	0.4 without EI; 0.7 with EI
Topiramate	Topamax	bid	25 qd	25 q1-2wk	100-400	3	3-9
Valproic acid	Depakene, Depakote, Depakote ER	tid-qid, bid	250 qd	250 q3-7d	750-3000	15	15-45
Zonisamide	Zonegran	bid	100 qd	100 q2wk	200-400	4	4-12

Abbreviations: bid = twice a day; EI = enzyme inducer; qd = every day; qid = four times a day; tid = three times a day; VPA = valproic acid.

Rakel and Bope: *Conn's Current Therapy 2006.*

a proven track record, can often be administered intravenously, and are inexpensive. Most neurologists still prefer to start therapy with a conventional AED, but they move quickly to a new AED if necessary. New AEDs are gradually starting to replace conventional AEDs for the initial treatment of partial seizures.

Each type of generalized seizure must be considered individually. GTC seizures, tonic seizures, and clonic seizures seem to respond to the same AEDs as partial-onset seizures, but this may be because historically little distinction was made between primary generalized and secondary generalized seizures during drug development. All conventional AEDs, except ethosuximide, seem to be effective. Few published studies of the efficacy of new AEDs are available, but lamotrigine (Lamictal), felbamate (Felbatol), topiramate (Topamax), and zonisamide (Zonegran) seem to be effective, and the others are unknown. Absence seizures respond to valproate (Depakote), ethosuximide (Zarontin), and lamotrigine but not to carbamazepine (Tegretol), gabapentin (Neurontin), or tiagabine (Gabitril). The efficacy of other new AEDs is not yet demonstrated. Myoclonic seizures respond to valproate and lamotrigine, and occasionally to benzodiazepines.

A few epilepsy syndromes in adults and adolescents respond particularly well to specific AEDs. Myoclonic and GTC seizures occurring in juvenile myoclonic epilepsy respond very well to valproate or lamotrigine. Atonic, tonic, and atypical absence seizures occurring as part of the Lennox-Gastaut syndrome respond very well to valproate, lamotrigine, and topiramate. This is one case in which the potential benefit of felbamate usually outweighs the risk. Approximately 30% of patients with childhood absence epilepsy have seizures that persist into adulthood, and valproate or lamotrigine is usually a better alternative than ethosuximide when they have GTC seizures in addition to absence seizures.

Special Considerations

Children represent a special population because their seizure types, epilepsy syndromes, etiologies, and pharmacokinetic responses are different from adults. This leads to important dosing differences, such as dosing based on body weight rather than absolute amounts (see Table 5). Long-term cosmetic cumulative side effects of phenytoin (Dilantin) make it a poor choice for the chronic treatment of children, especially girls. Children are addressed in the article titled, "Epilepsy in Infancy and Childhood," but it is important to recognize that many childhood epilepsies persist into adulthood and may evolve.

The elderly deserve special consideration because they are more likely to have side effects, take multiple medications, and have hepatic and renal impairment. Seizures beginning in late adult life are always partial seizures from acquired etiologies, especially stroke. Phenytoin is particularly poorly tolerated in the elderly, and in addition, may have a prolonged half-life, so levels are unexpectedly high. Some new AEDs are better tolerated and less likely to cause drug interactions. Gabapentin (Neurontin) is particularly desirable

because it has no drug interactions. Oxcarbazepine (Trileptal) and levetiracetam (Keppra) are also usually well tolerated.

Women pose several potential difficulties when selecting an AED. Women with epilepsy have increased rates of infertility as a consequence of intrinsic hormone changes, anovulatory cycles, irregular menstrual cycles, and altered sexuality. The effects of AEDs can compound these situations, especially valproate (Depakote), associated with polycystic ovarian disease. Hysterectomy with bilateral oophorectomy may seem like a reasonable treatment for seizures clustering around the menstrual period, but it is usually ineffective and deprives patients of the protective effects of estrogen. Osteopenia is common in postmenopausal women and augmented by chronic phenytoin use.

Potential teratogenicity is an important consideration for women of childbearing potential, but data in humans are only available for the conventional AEDs. The incidence of birth defects in women taking an AED is approximately 5% to 6%, compared to 1% to 2% in the general population. The rate of birth defects appears the same for all conventional AEDs. Most birth defects associated with phenytoin (Dilantin), carbamazepine (Tegretol), and phenobarbital are considered mild or cosmetic, but valproate frequently causes neural tube defects. Folic acid, 1 to 5 mg per day, reduces the rate of teratogenicity, especially neural tube defects. It is indicated for women on valproate and is good practice for all women of childbearing potential. Some new AEDs are teratogenic in animal models, but the effects in humans are unknown. Blood levels should be monitored regularly during and immediately after pregnancy because of significant changes in blood volume and metabolism. AEDs are transmitted to infants via breast milk, but the benefits of breast-feeding are probably greater than any potential harm from AED exposure.

Hepatic disease may impair the ability to clear hepatically metabolized drugs (see Table 3), a particular problem for conventional AEDs, which are all hepatically metabolized. Among the new AEDs, gabapentin (Neurontin) and levetiracetam (Keppra) are not hepatically metabolized at all and not affected even by severe liver disease, and even the other new AEDs are not affected until liver disease is severe. The dose reduction of hepatically metabolized AEDs in hepatically impaired patients is determined by the prolongation of clearance, which is different in each patient. Therefore, no standard dosing recommendations can be made.

Renal disease may impair clearance of AEDs, which are normally eliminated unchanged by the kidneys. All conventional AEDs are primarily deactivated by hepatic metabolism before urinary elimination of inactive metabolites. Therefore, they are not significantly affected by renal disease until the end stage, in which case the small amount normally excreted unchanged may build up. Some newer AEDs, such as gabapentin (Neurontin), levetiracetam (Keppra), oxcarbazepine (Trileptal), and topiramate (Topamax), have a significant portion excreted unchanged by the kidneys and therefore require empirical or calculated dose reduction with renal impairment.

A more significant problem in the treatment of renally impaired patients is the removal of free drug during hemodialysis. The amount of drug removed depends on the free fraction, duration and volume of dialysis, and other factors, so a predictable change in blood levels cannot be determined. After each hemodialysis session, the blood level and effectiveness must be ascertained to decide how much drug must be given until a steady state of postdialysis dosing is reached. Phenytoin (Dilantin) is not significantly affected by hemodialysis because only 10% exists in the free dialyzable form, but free levels should be monitored. A mild to moderate amount of phenobarbital is removed during dialysis, but if the level falls significantly after dialysis, a bolus can be given. Changes in valproate (Depakote) dosing are usually not necessary because although 20% is removed by dialysis, the half-life increases by 20%, which compensates. Among newer AEDs, gabapentin (Neurontin) is the most severely affected; 60% is removed by hemodialysis, but the half-life becomes nearly infinite so only very small doses are required once the patient becomes anuric, such as only 300 mg after each dialysis.

Refractory Epilepsy

EVALUATION OF INTRACTABLE SEIZURES

The definition of refractory epilepsy is evolving. In statistical terms, patients who continue to have seizures after trying therapeutic doses of two AEDs are very unlikely to respond to additional AEDs, although some do. The definition is becoming increasingly important because refractory patients should be referred to an epilepsy center for diagnosis and consideration of the many therapeutic options now available, including epilepsy surgery to resect the seizure focus, palliative surgery to reduce the severity of some seizure types, unconventional AEDs, and experimental AEDs.

The evaluation of intractable seizures depends on a careful history and physical examination directed at elucidating the seizure type, neuroanatomic site of seizure origin, and the epilepsy syndrome or etiology. The most important diagnostic test is prolonged (24 hours per day) simultaneous video and EEG monitoring to capture seizures. Video/EEG is vitally important to determine that the spells in question are indeed seizures, to define the seizure type, and to localize the site of origin. Video/EEG may need to continue for days or weeks to capture enough spells to make a correct diagnosis. MRI of the brain using special acquisition protocols to define fine brain anatomy often reveals abnormalities that are not obvious on routine MRI, especially in the temporal lobe where seizures often arise. Positron emission tomography (PET) may reveal focal hypometabolism in the region of seizure onset. Interictal single-photon emission computed tomography (SPECT) occasionally reveals focal hypoperfusion at the focus. To perform an ictal SPECT scan, the radiotracer is injected within 90 seconds of seizure onset, and subsequent scanning often reveals focal hyperperfusion in the region of seizure onset. Magnetic resonance spectroscopy is primarily a research

tool but can reveal focal changes in the region of the seizure focus. Neuropsychological testing may demonstrate lateralized or localized deficits.

EPILEPSY SURGERY

Surgery to resect the epilepsy focus is the only method of curing epilepsy available today. Successful surgery depends heavily on correctly localizing the seizure focus. Presurgical evaluation is usually carried out in three phases. Phase 1 consists of extracranial monitoring and the noninvasive tests just noted. If the findings yield a general area from which the seizures arise but do not pinpoint the exact site of onset, the patient may proceed to phase 2, which is intracranial EEG monitoring through electrodes placed on or into the brain. Phase 3 is the removal of the seizure focus. Fortunately, most patients do not require intracranial monitoring now because neuroimaging often identifies an anatomic abnormality to corroborate the EEG findings.

Any area of the brain is a candidate for resection, but in reality a vast majority of patients have temporal lobe epilepsy (TLE) and undergo anterior temporal lobectomy (ATL) to remove the anterior 4 to 5 cm of the temporal lobe containing the hippocampus and amygdala. Approximately 70% of patients are essentially seizure free after ATL, and the risk of stroke or other serious complications is less than 1%. Extratemporal resections are more complicated. The seizure focus must be more precisely localized, and electrical brain mapping or other methods must be used to ensure that important brain functions will not be removed during surgery. This usually requires intracranial monitoring. Approximately 50% of patients are rendered essentially seizure free. The risk of complications, such as a motor deficit, is only slightly higher than with ATL. More drastic surgeries,

---

 CURRENT DIAGNOSIS

- Consider Non-epileptic origin for paroxysmal event
  - Syncope, migraine, TIA, sleep disorder, Movement disorder, hypoglycemia, Psychiatric disease
- Exclude general medical etiology
  - Laboratory Tests: complete blood count, electrolytes, glucose, liver enzymes, urine drug screen
  - Perform LP, if CNS infection is considered
  - Neuroimaging, preferable MRI. CT is acceptable in the acute setting to rule out hemorrhage (neoplasms may be missed by head CT)
- Characterize seizure type and etiology or epilepsy syndrome
  - High-resolution MRI
  - Routine EEG. If unrevealing consider sleep deprived EEG
  - Consider inpatient video/EEG monitoring to capture and event if seizures occur at least once per week.

CURRENT THERAPY

- Select an AED by seizure type and epilepsy syndrome
- Consider side effect profile, dosing schedule, drug interactions, and cost
- "Start low and go slow" in starting AED therapy
- Increase dose to maximum tolerated dose (toxicity) before changing
- Substitute one drug at a time in an attempt to achieve montherapy
- Refer to an epilepsy center for consideration of surgery if seizures are refractory to two AEDs
- After a seizure-free period of at least 2 years withdrawal of AEDs may be considered
- Risk of seizure recurrence is lowest if MRI and follow-up EEG are both normal

such as hemispherectomy or corpus callosotomy, are indicated in special circumstances.

Vagus nerve stimulation is a recently developed novel approach to seizure control. A small generator is placed subcutaneously in the left chest wall and wire electrodes are led to the left vagus nerve. The generator supplies a few seconds of current every few minutes at predetermined settings. Its efficacy in blinded controlled trials is approximately the same as a new AED; it reduces the frequency of seizures by 50% in approximately half of the subjects.

The treatment of epilepsy is rapidly changing and more complex than in previous years because physicians now have 14 AEDs from which to choose, technologic advances make diagnostic tests more useful, and epilepsy surgery is safer and more readily available. A systematic approach yields some basic guidelines for therapy.

REFERENCES

Commission of Classification and Terminology of the International League Against Epilepsy: Proposal for revised classification of epilepsies and epileptic syndromes. Epilepsia 1989;30:389-399.

Dreifuss FE, Bancaud J, Henriksen O, et al: Proposal for the revised clinical and electroencephalographic classification of epileptic seizures. Epilepsia 1981;22:489-501.

Engel J Jr, Wiebe S, French J, et al: Practice parameter: Temporal lobe and localized neocortical resections for epilepsy: Report of the Quality Standards Subcommittee of the American Academy of Neurology, in association with the American Epilepsy Society and the American Association of Neurological Surgeons. Neurology 2003;60(4):538-547.

Farhat G, Yamout B, Mikati MA, et al: Effect of antiepileptic drugs on bone density in ambulatory patients. Neurology 2002;58(9):1348-1353.

French JA, Kanner AM, Bautista J, et al: Efficacy and tolerability of the new antiepileptic drugs: I. Treatment of new onset epilepsy. Neurology 2004;62:1252-1260.

French JA, Kanner AM, Bautista J, et al: Efficacy and tolerability of the new antiepileptic drugs: II. Treatment of refractory epilepsy. Neurology 2004;62:1261-1273.

Hauser WA, Rich SS, Annegers JF, Anderson VE: Seizure recurrence after a first unprovoked seizure: An extended follow-up. Neurology 1990;40;1163-1170.

Kwan P, Brodie MJ: Early identification of refractory epilepsy. N Engl J Med 2000;342:314-319.

Marson AG, Kadir ZA, Hutton JL, Chadwick DW: The new antiepileptic drugs: A systematic review of their efficacy and tolerability. Epilepsia 1997;38(8):859-880.

Mattson RH, Cramer JA, Collins JF, et al: Comparison of carbamazepine, phenobarbital, phenytoin, and primidone in partial and secondarily generalized tonic clonic seizures. N Engl J Med 1985;313(3):145-151.

Mattson RH, Cramer JA, Collins JF, et al: A comparison of valproate with carbamazepine for the treatment of complex partial seizures and secondarily generalized tonic-clonic seizures in adults. The Department of Veterans Affairs Epilepsy Cooperative Study No. 264 Group. N Engl J Med 1992;327:765-771.

Weibe S, Blume WT, Girvin JP, et al: A randomized, controlled trial of surgery for temporal-lobe epilepsy. N Engl J Med 2001;345:311-318.

Epilepsy in Infancy and Childhood

Method of
Raj D. Sheth, MD

14

Definition

Seizures are a sudden self-limited clinical event that results from abnormal and excessive firing of cortical neurons. Paroxysmal events that are not cerebral in origin may mimic seizures, and in infants these commonly include breath-holding spells, vasovagal syncope, or cardiac arrhythmias.

Classification

Seizures can be classified based on their onset as either *partial* (starting in a focal area of the brain), *partial with secondary generalization* (starting as a partial seizure but then secondarily spreading to other areas of the brain, usually involving both cerebral hemispheres), or *primary generalized* (involving all of the brain from the onset of the seizure) (Box 1). Partial seizures may be either simple partial, if consciousness is preserved during the seizures, or complex partial, if impairment of consciousness or confusion occurs during the seizure. Partial seizures typically present with brief motor movement, sensation, or autonomic symptoms.

Such a classification scheme, which works well in a child older than 7 years, may be difficult to apply to a younger child or infant. This feature adds considerable difficulty in determining if an event is an epileptic seizure or simply a behavioral phenomenon. For example, a young child with staring spells might simply be daydreaming or might be having an epileptic seizure such as an absence seizure or a complex partial seizure. Useful features to distinguish these events are that seizures may occur in both active and passive modes, whereas behavioral staring events are typically only seen in a passive mode (e.g., while watching television).

Generalized seizures include absence seizures, myoclonic seizures, or primary generalized tonic-clonic seizures.

Provoking Factors

Seizures may be acutely provoked by a fever (febrile seizures) or be symptomatic of an underlying acute cerebral insult such as a severe head injury, central nervous system infection, electrolyte imbalance, or metabolic derangement. In these patients, treatment is directed at the underlying cause of the seizure. Patients with acute symptomatic seizures may require temporary seizure medication to control seizures but may not need long-term treatment with seizure medication.

Idiopathic and Symptomatic Epilepsy

Epilepsy is the occurrence of two or more unprovoked seizures and indicates an underlying tendency toward seizures. Epilepsy that does not appear to be caused by an underlying cerebral abnormality (normal neurologic examination and cognitive function and a normal cranial magnetic resonance imaging [MRI] scan) is referred to as idiopathic epilepsy. Approximately 50% of childhood cases are idiopathic. The prognosis for idiopathic epilepsy is usually good for either spontaneous remittance of seizures or for their control. Idiopathic epilepsy is frequently related to a genetic multifactorial tendency toward the disorder. When it is a symptom of underlying remote cranial trauma, congenital cerebral malformations, tumors, or vascular anomalies, it is referred to as symptomatic epilepsy. Approximately two thirds of these patients have difficult to control seizures. When a cause cannot be identified but cognitive impairment is present, epilepsy is called cryptogenic. Patients with cryptogenic epilepsy have a similar prognosis as those with symptomatic epilepsy.

Epidemiology

Approximately 3% to 5% of all children experience a single seizure, with febrile seizures the most frequent. The incidence of seizures is highest in the first year of life, particularly in the neonatal period (first 4 weeks of life). Approximately 1% of these children have unprovoked seizures, and half of those have two or more seizures and are said to have epilepsy. Of those with epilepsy, approximately half have generalized seizures. Half of all children have epilepsy that is symptomatic of an underlying brain lesion, with the remainder having idiopathic epilepsy indicative of a genetic tendency.

Diagnosis

The first priority is to determine if the event the patient experienced was a seizure or a nonepileptic paroxysmal event. Nonepileptic events in children include breath-holding spells, temper tantrums, vasovagal syncope, night terrors, hyperventilation, and panic attacks. The history is often sufficient to differentiate these events from seizures.

Evaluation of seizures requires a careful history, with particular attention given to the onset of the seizure (eye deviation, fear) and any focal weakness following the seizure to determine if the seizure was partial. The neurologic examination is very useful. When a child exhibits neurologic deficits, it strongly suggests the seizure resulted from a focal brain lesion and warrants a cranial MRI.

ELECTROENCEPHALOGRAM

The electroencephalogram (EEG) is central to the evaluation of seizures and should be obtained in all patients who had a seizure other than those with a simple febrile seizure. The EEG can help diagnosis and guide treatment by helping classify seizures, and it also offers some indication about prognosis. Generally, two features on the EEG are helpful in the evaluation: the background EEG activity and the epileptiform discharges. Background activity may be in either the normal or slow range. Normal background activity typically suggests idiopathic epilepsy, whereas background slowing is more indicative of seizures that are symptomatic of an underlying cerebral abnormality. Epileptiform discharges can occur even when the patient is not acutely seizing and are seen in approximately two thirds of patients known to have epilepsy. They are also seen in approximately 1% of children who have never experienced a seizure. Importantly, epileptiform discharges can help differentiate between partial and generalized seizures, thereby guiding treatment. Focal epileptiform discharges are present in one part of the brain and indicate partial epilepsy. Generalized epileptiform discharges occur throughout the brain. Specific generalized seizures can be diagnosed: 3-Hz generalized spike-and-wave activity (indicative of absence seizures) or polyspike-and-wave activity (indicative of myoclonic or tonic–clonic seizures) are suggestive of generalized epilepsy. Severe forms of epilepsy, including infantile spasms, are associated with hypsarrhythmia, and the Lennox-Gastaut syndrome, associated with slow spike-and-wave activity, can be diagnosed with the EEG.

CRANIAL IMAGING

In an acute situation, a cranial computed tomography (CT) can help evaluate urgently for intracranial blood or trauma, although a comprehensive evaluation requires an MRI scan in most patients. New-onset seizures may require evaluation with gadolinium enhancement to exclude a brain tumor. Patients with temporal lobe epilepsy require specific studies, which include a temporal lobe protocol to determine if there is mesial temporal sclerosis.

DIFFERENTIAL DIAGNOSIS

Movement in the neonatal period can be difficult to differentiate from seizures. In an intensive care unit (ICU) setting, approximately 90% of events thought to be epileptic seizures turn out to be nonepileptic. Jitteriness can be separated from seizures because seizures can be stopped by changing the position of the limb. Clonic movements are the most specific for epileptic seizures. An EEG is very helpful at this point. A consistent precipitant suggests nonepileptic events. Breath holding can be associated with brief nonepileptic convulsive activity. Importantly, seizures are stereotypic. Parental home videos of the events can be helpful in better characterization.

In children older than age 5 years and adolescents, complicated migraine, sleep disorders, and syncope may be difficult to separate from seizures. Hyperventilation and panic events should also be considered. When there is doubt about the diagnosis, an EEG may be very helpful, with approximately 70% of patients showing epileptiform discharges between seizures.

Epilepsy Syndromes

FEBRILE SEIZURES

Febrile seizures occur between ages 6 months and 5 years, with the majority presenting by age 3 years. Simple febrile seizures last less than 15 minutes, with a single seizure within a 24-hour period, and they are not associated with Todd's paralysis. All other seizures are complex and may require further evaluation. Antipyretic measures and therapy are often recommended, although no evidence indicates this strategy prevents recurrence. Approximately one third of patients experience a recurrence. Rectally administered diazepam (Diastat) may help reduce the length of a seizure and is typically recommended for seizures that last longer than 5 minutes. Phenobarbital and valproate (Depakene) are effective in preventing recurrence of febrile seizures, although given the adverse effect of chronic therapy they are rarely indicated. Patients with prior febrile seizures who subsequently experience a seizure without fever should be evaluated for epilepsy.

INFANTILE SPASMS AND LENNOX-GASTAUT SYNDROME

Infantile spasms and Lennox-Gastaut syndrome, although uncommon, are severe epilepsies and should be evaluated promptly. Infantile spasms occur between ages 3 and 18 months, and Lennox-Gastaut syndrome is typically diagnosed after that. Untreated infantile spasms often transition into Lennox-Gastaut syndrome.

Spasms are typically brief, lasting 1 to 5 seconds, with symmetric contraction of the trunk, extension of the arms, and tonic extension of the legs. Spasms, which occur in clusters, are associated with irritability and often seen as the child awakens or transitions to sleep. The EEG is hypsarrhythmic, showing a markedly abnormal and chaotic background with multifocal epileptiform discharges. The triad of infantile spasms, hypsarrhythmia, and developmental regression is referred to as West's syndrome. An underlying etiology is present in 80% of infants and usually associated with a poorer outcome than those in whom an etiology is not found. Corticotropin (ACTH)[1] treatment frequently results in control of spasm, improvement in EEG background, and an improvement in development. Vigabatrin (Sabril)[*] is an oral agent that can control infantile spasms, particularly those associated with tuberous sclerosis.

Lennox-Gastaut syndrome develops in 50% of children with infantile spasms. The EEG shows a diffuse slow spike-and-wave pattern. Patients have a combination of tonic, myoclonic, and atypical absence seizures. Seizures are intractable to medical treatment and the outcome is poor, with mental retardation seen in up to 90% of patients.

ABSENCE EPILEPSY

Absence seizures resemble staring spells, although they may occur in both an active or passive state. Fifty seizures a day are typical, with subtle behavioral arrest that may be associated with eyelid twitching. The EEG shows 3-Hz generalized spike and waves. Absence seizures occur in childhood absence, juvenile absence, and juvenile myoclonic epilepsy.

Childhood absence epilepsy develops between 4 and 10 years of age and remits in most patients by 10 years of age. Seizures are easily treated with ethosuximide (Zarontin), although valproate (Depakote) and lamotrigine (Lamictal) can also be used.

Juvenile absence epilepsy develops between ages 6 and 10 years and usually does not remit. Unlike the childhood form, seizures do not remit and may be associated with tonic–clonic seizures. Ethosuximide is usually not effective for the tonic–clonic seizures, and valproate or lamotrigine are usually considered.

Juvenile myoclonic epilepsy, the most common epilepsy syndrome seen in children of normal intellect, has a similar age of onset as juvenile absence epilepsy and does

---

[1]Not FDA approved for this indication.
[*]Investigational drug in the United States.

not remit. The EEG shows generalized polyspike-and-wave discharges. Valproate is an effective medication for this epilepsy, although lamotrigine can also be considered. The latter is not as effective as valproate in controlling myoclonic seizures, although it has a better side-effect profile compared to valproate.

BENIGN PARTIAL EPILEPSY WITH CENTROTEMPORAL SPIKE

Benign partial epilepsy with centrotemporal spike (BECTS) accounts for approximately 15% of epilepsy in childhood. Seizures are partial, with face twitching, of which the child is usually aware. Generalized tonic–clonic seizures may occur at night. The EEG shows a normal background with epileptiform spikes in the centrotemporal regions. If the child is only experiencing simple partial seizures, treatment may be withheld. Seizures remit in the vast majority of children. Control of seizures is seen with low-dose medication, and carbamazepine (Tegretol) or oxcarbazepine (Trileptal) are both effective treatment options.

Treatment

After a careful diagnosis of epileptic seizures, treatment decisions are made to reduce the risk of seizure-associated injury, prevent the risk of prolonged seizures (status epilepticus), reduce the adverse cognitive effects of frequent seizures, and deal with social factors, such as driving. Decisions should be discussed with the child and family, weighing the benefits with the risks of treatment. Factors that help guide treatment include seizure type, etiology, frequency, duration, and impact on the patient's life, along with age and level of activity.

The goal of treatment is prevention of seizures; therefore, assessment of the recurrence risk should be made. Following a first unprovoked seizure, there is a 50% risk of a second seizure. With the second seizure, the risk of the third increases to 80%. A normal neurologic examination, MRI, and EEG are all factors that lower the risk to 25% to 33%, whereas abnormalities found in these tests and a family history of epilepsy increase the recurrence risk to 75%. An EEG that shows 3-Hz generalized spike wave discharges seen in absence of seizures, however, increases that risk to virtually 100%. Treatment is often suggested after a patient has a second unprovoked seizure.

The underlying principles guiding treatment are that the patient should be free from both seizures and the adverse effects of medications (Table 1). Choosing among the different medications requires an understanding of adverse effects and efficacy. Seizures that respond well to treatment include the benign syndromes discussed earlier. In these patients, the lowest dose of recommended medication should be tried and gradually titrated depending on response (Table 2).

Medications should be titrated slowly to minimize adverse effects. Medication serum levels can help guide treatment, but medications should be titrated to response. Serum levels can be helpful in deciding if breakthrough seizures are a result of noncompliance or lack of efficacy. Some patients require more than one

TABLE 1 Commonly Used Antiepileptic Medications

Agent	Pediatric dose (mg/kg/d)	Half-life (h)*	Dosing schedule	Side effects
Carbamazepine (Tegretol)	10-35	25-65 (initial) 12-17 (chronic)	bid-qid	r, hep, bd, s, n dip, hypn, ost
Clonazepam (Klonopin)	0.01-0.2	18-50	bid-tid	s, a, h, b
Ethosuximide (Zarontin)	10-15 (initial) 15-40 (maint)	30-40	qd-tid	gi, n, an, s, d, b, r, bd
Gabapentin (Neurontin)	30-60	5-7	tid-qid	s, d, a, ny, wg
Lamotrigine (Lamictal)				
Off valproate:	0.6 (initial) 5-15 (maint)	7	bid	r, hep, d, a, s, n
On valproate	0.15 (initial) 1-5 (maint)	45	qd-bid	
Levetiracetam (Keppra)†	20-60	6-8	bid	s, d, ha, b
Oxcarbazepine (Trileptal)	8-10 (initial) 20-50 (maint)	8-10	bid	r, hep, s, diz, n dip, a, ha, hypn
Topiramate (Topamax)	1-3 (initial) 5-9 (maint)	18-30	bid	s, an, ks, ps, wl
Valproic acid (Depakote)	15-60	9-20	bid-qid	hep, bd, n, s, d, wg, hl, r, gi
Zonisamid (Zonegran)†	2-4 (initial) 4-8 (maint)	50-70	qd-bid	r, bd, hep, s, diz, an, n, ha, wl, ks

*Half-life is based on monotherapy and assumes normal renal function.
†Not FDA approved for this indication in children.
Abbreviations: a, ataxia; an, anorexia; b, behavioral difficulties; bd, blood dyscrasia; d, dizziness; dip, diplopia; gi, gastrointestinal distress; h, hyperactivity; ha, headache; hep, hepatotoxicity; hl, hair loss; hypn, hyponatremia; ks, kidney stones; maint, maintenance; n, nausea; ny, nystagmus; ost, osteomalacia; ps, psychomotor slowing; r, rash; s, sedation; wg, weight gain; wl, weight loss.

TABLE 2 Which Medications for Which Seizure Types?

Seizure Type	First-Line Therapy	Second-Line Therapy	Third-Line Therapy
Partial (all types)	CBZ, OXC	LTG, VPA, GBP, TPM, PHT	TGB, LEV,[A] ZNS,[A] PB
Generalized			
Tonic-clonic	VPA	LTG, TPM, PHT	PB, ZNS[A]
Myoclonic	VPA	LTG, CZP	PB, ZNS[A]
Tonic	VPA	LTG	CZP, TPM, ZNS[A]
Absence (before age 10)	ESM*	VPA, LTG	ZNS, TPM
(after age 10)	VPA	LTG	ESM, TPM, ZNS[A]
Epilepsy syndromes			
CAE	ESM	VPA, LTG	ZNS, TPM
JAE	VPA	LTG	ESM, TPM, ZNS[A]
JME	VPA, LTG	TPM, ZNS[A]	CZP, PHT
Lennox-Gastaut	VPA	LTG, TPM	CZP, ZNS,[A] FBM
Infantile spasms	ACTH, VGB[†]	VPA, TPM, TGB, CZP	FBM, ZNS[A]
BECTS	CBZ, OXC	VPA, PHT, CBZ	LTG, TPM

*Assuming no convulsive seizures.
Abbreviations: ACTH, adrenocorticotropic hormone; BECTS, benign epilepsy of childhood with centrotemporal spikes; CAE, childhood absence epilepsy; CBZ, carbamazepine (Tegretol); CZP, clonazepam (Klonopin); ESM, ethosuximide (Zarontin); FBM, felbamate (Felbatol); GBP, gabapentin (Neurontin); JAE, juvenile absence epilepsy; JME, juvenile myoclonic epilepsy; LEV, levetiracetam (Keppra); LTG, lamotrigine (Lamictal); OXC, oxcarbazepine (Trileptal); PB, phenobarbital; PHT, phenytoin (Dilantin); TGB, tiagabine (Gabitril); VGB, vigabatrin (Sabril); ZNS, zonisamide (Zonegran).
[A]Not FDA approved for this indication in children.
[†]Investigational drug in the United States.

14

medication to control seizures. Unfortunately, many patients, despite multiple medications, continue to have seizures.

WHEN MEDICATIONS FAIL TO CONTROL SEIZURES

Approximately 33% of patients' seizures are not controlled by medication, and alternative approaches can be considered. Options include the vagus nerve stimulator, the ketogenic diet, and epilepsy surgery. The first two measures typically reduce but do not abolish seizures. These decisions are best made using a multidisciplinary approach and require referral to a comprehensive epilepsy center. Patients who do not respond to a first medication choice should be referred for consultation.

STOPPING MEDICATIONS

Discontinuing medications depends on the type of seizures and epilepsy. Generally, when a patient is seizure free for 2 years, discontinuing medication can be considered. With this strategy, 60% to 75% of patients remain seizure free. However, a higher relapse rate is seen in remote symptomatic epilepsy, epileptiform discharges on EEG, and structural cerebral lesions on MRI. Recurrences usually occur in the first year, but late recurrence is also seen. Discontinuing medications should be considered before adolescents start driving because once patients are driving the decision to stop medication becomes much more complicated.

Attention Deficit Hyperactivity Disorder (ADHD)

Method of
Anouk Scheres, PhD,
and F. Xavier Castellanos, MD

Attention deficit hyperactivity disorder (ADHD), as defined in the *Diagnostic and Statistical Manual of Mental Disorders, Fourth Edition (DSM-IV)* of the American Psychiatric Association, is differentiated into three subtypes, predominantly inattentive, predominantly hyperactive/impulsive, and a combination of the two. The diagnosis relies on subjective reports of developmentally inappropriate behavior in the domains of inattention, hyperactivity, and/or impulsiveness that have been present for at least 6 months, and in more than one setting, such as school and home. At least some of the symptoms must be associated with impairment before the age of 7 years, and symptoms must clearly interfere with social, academic, or occupational functioning. The diagnosis does not apply if the symptoms can be better accounted for by a pervasive developmental disorder, schizophrenia, or other psychotic disorders, or by any other specific mental disorder.

The prevalence of ADHD in school-age children is at least 3% to 5%, although some estimates exceed 10%. ADHD is diagnosed more frequently in males than females, with ratios ranging between 2:1 and 9:1

depending on the mode of ascertainment. The diagnosis of ADHD is reached with more difficulty at the extremes of the age distribution. For example, the behavior of preschool-age children is more variable than that of older children, and attention demands on younger children are not as high, which makes it hard to discern attention deficits in very young children. Numerous studies demonstrate that ADHD persists into adulthood, although estimates vary from 4% to 80%. Applying the diagnosis of ADHD to adults is problematic, as the criteria were developed for and field tested with children and adolescents 6 to 14 years of age. Furthermore, retrospective reports of symptoms are unreliable. In practice, many adults are diagnosed after their own children have been determined to have ADHD.

Children are occasionally diagnosed only with ADHD, but 60% to 80% are found to have another disorder as well. The possible co-morbid conditions generally include oppositional defiant disorder, conduct disorder, learning disabilities, and tic disorders. Anxiety or mood disorders may also be present.

In some cases, juvenile bipolar (manic-depressive) disorder may initially present as severe ADHD. ADHD also represents a risk for later drug and alcohol abuse, particularly when conduct disorder is also present.

Assessment

There is no objective test for diagnosing ADHD. Rather, the diagnosis is based exclusively on the history of symptoms, derived optimally from more than one informant, such as a parent and a teacher. Children with ADHD are rarely aware of the full impact of their symptoms and their direct assessment is mainly aimed at ruling out alternative diagnoses, such as pervasive developmental disorders or psychotic disorders, and determining whether or not tic disorders or obsessive-compulsive disorder might be present. Standardized parent and teacher rating scales are commonly used to provide a rapid screen for the symptoms associated with ADHD.

The most frequently used questionnaires include:

- The *Child Behavior Checklist*
- The *Teacher Report Form*
- The *Revised Conners Parent and Teacher Rating Scales*
- The *Swanson, Nolan and Pelham (SNAP) Teacher and Parent Rating Scales* (may be downloaded from http://www.adhd.net)

The *Child Behavior Checklist* and *Teacher Report Form* differ from the others in that they are designed to stratify "externalizing behaviors," such as hyperactivity and aggression, and "internalizing behaviors" that are related to anxiety and mood concerns along a continuum from normal to abnormal, and they are not linked to specific psychiatric diagnoses. They are in wide use around the world and serve as an effective screening tool as well as a tool to assist researchers comparing samples crossculturally. Conners, SNAP, and similar scales are linked to the *DSM-IV* criteria for ADHD–oppositional defiant disorder and conduct disorder. Raters are asked

to indicate how each symptom applies to a child on a four-point scale, ranging from "not at all" to "very much."

While rating scales are an economical and efficient manner of measuring the severity of behavioral symptoms, at least as rated by observers, they do not suffice for a diagnostic evaluation. The most comprehensive evaluations, such as those performed in research clinics, also use structured or semistructured psychiatric interviews. In structured interviews the interviewer does not interpret the informant's response. In semistructured interviews, interpretation by a clinically astute interviewer is required. Highly structured interviews are more reliable but may be less valid, and semistructured interviews tend to be more valid but less reliable. Structured or semistructured interviews are rarely used in clinical practice, but the goals of reviewing the full range of disruptive behavior disorders, and assessing for the presence of co-morbid learning disorders (mood and anxiety disorders, substance use and abuse, high-risk behaviors), and excluding pervasive developmental disorders and psychotic disorders should be met. Formal psychoeducational evaluation alerts the clinician to the presence of co-morbid learning disorders, which are found in 25% to 40% of children with ADHD, and their extent. Such evaluations should also highlight the individual's cognitive strengths, as those may be easily overlooked. In-person evaluation of the child cannot either confirm or refute a diagnosis of ADHD. However, such examination is generally necessary to assess for the presence of tic disorders, to confirm the social dexterity of the child and thus exclude pervasive developmental disorders, and to probe for the presence of anxiety and mood disorders, including depression and obsessive-compulsive disorder. It also serves crucially to initiate the therapeutic alliance.

Treatment

Treatment of ADHD can be divided into two categories, pharmacologic (with psychostimulant drugs being the first choice) and psychosocial/behavioral treatments. Neither type of treatment seems to carry over; when treatment stops, the effects on symptoms also stop. The Multimodal Treatment Study of ADHD (MTA) in 579 children with combined-type ADHD compared:

- The effect of medication treatment (mainly psychostimulants, with methylphenidate [Ritalin] being the drug of first choice)
- Intensive behavioral treatments
- The combination of the two
- Community care (which consisted mostly of medication treatment provided by community mental health providers chosen by the parents)

Children in all groups showed reduction of core ADHD symptoms; although medication treatment and combined treatment were equally effective, both were more effective than behavioral treatment alone or community care.

These data suggest that for most children with combined-type ADHD, carefully conducted medication

TABLE 1 Immediate-Release Stimulants for Treatment of Attention Deficit Hyperactivity Disorder

Drug	Doses (mg)	Typical duration	Schedule
MPH (Ritalin, Metadate, generic)	5, 10, 20	3-4 h	bid-tid
d-MPH (Focalin)	2.5, 5, 10	3-4 h	bid-tid
d-Amphetamine (Dexedrine, generic)	5, 10	4-8 h	qd-bid
d-l-Amphetamine (Adderall, generic)	5, 7.5, 10, 12.5, 15, 20, 30	4-8 h	qd-bid

Abbreviations: bid = two times per day; MPH = methylphenidate; qd = every day; tid = three times per day.

management is likely to be the most cost-effective manner of reducing ADHD symptoms as rated by parents and teachers. The study also demonstrates that medication management in typical community settings produces suboptimal benefits, perhaps because of underdosing, insufficient monitoring, and lack of regular feedback from teachers.

Perhaps not surprisingly, the MTA data continue to provide support for a range of approaches to treatment selection. For many children, psychosocial interventions provided appreciable benefit, and were rated as more acceptable than medication by parents, even when medication produced greater quantitative benefits. Children with a greater burden of risk factors or higher rates of co-morbidity tended to respond best to the combination of optimal medication management and state of the art psychosocial interventions. Unfortunately, such interventions are still mostly unavailable outside the rarefied context of research studies. Thus the challenge to clinicians is how to approximate the effectiveness of optimally delivered treatment within the constraints of usual practice settings. The absence of definitive guidelines regarding optimal treatment means that the parents, along with their child, depending on the child's age, are the ones who select treatment regimens. It is the clinician's task to provide the parents (and preadolescents or adolescents) with relevant information about the known effects of treatments, along with an informed perspective, which can form the basis for collaborative decisions.

PHARMACOLOGIC TREATMENT

The three primary types of medications used to treat ADHD are the psychostimulants, nonstimulant or adrenergic reuptake blockers, and α-agonist antihypertensive agents. Although the specific molecular mechanisms of action differ, all the stimulants increase synaptic levels of dopamine and norepinephrine. Nonstimulants include the tricyclic antidepressants[1], which are now rarely prescribed because of concerns of cardiac toxicity, and the new noradrenergic reuptake inhibitor atomoxetine (Strattera). The antihypertensive agents clonidine (Catapres)[1] and guanfacine (Tenex)[1] also affect noradrenergic neurotransmission via a different mechanism. Methylphenidate (MPH) (Ritalin, Concerta, Metadate CD, Ritalin LA) remains the most common pharmacologic treatment for children with ADHD (Tables 1 and 2). Therapeutic doses of methylphenidate block the dopamine and norepinephrine transporters and result in an increase of synaptic dopamine and norepinephrine. Other psychostimulants used are dextroamphetamine (Dexedrine and Dexedrine Spansules), a mixture of amphetamine salts (Adderall and Adderall XR), and pemoline (Cylert) (see Tables 1 to 3). These psychostimulants are equally efficacious in group comparisons, although not all individuals respond equally to the different types of stimulants. On average, more than 70% of individuals with ADHD are classified as partial or full responders when treated with methylphenidate or one of the amphetamines. When the other type of stimulant is administered, the total response rate increases to more than 90%. Pemoline is now rarely prescribed because of the potential for fatal hepatotoxicity. Placebo response rates vary by study, but are generally between 10% and 20%. A positive response to a stimulant does not confirm the diagnosis of ADHD, as children and adults without ADHD have been shown to also demonstrate improvements in attention and decreases in locomotor activity.

The most notable development over the past several years has been the marketing of long-acting formulations of methylphenidate (Concerta, Metadate CD, and Ritalin LA) and amphetamine (Dexedrine Spansules

---

[1]Not FDA approved for this indication.

14

TABLE 2 Extended-Release Methylphenidate for Treatment of Attention Deficit Hyperactivity Disorder

Drug	Method	Immediate release	Extended release	Typical duration
Ritalin SR (20 mg) Metadate SR (10-20 mg)	100% wax matrix	Minimal	More sustained than immediate release	<5 h
Concerta ER (18, 27, 36, 54 mg)	Osmotic system	22% overcoat	78%	10-12 h
Metadate CD (20 mg)	Beads; can sprinkle	30%	70%	8 h
Ritalin LA (20, 30, 40 mg)	Beads; can sprinkle	≈50%	≈50%	8 h

TABLE 3 **Extended-Release Amphetamines for Treatment of Attention Deficit Hyperactivity Disorder**

Drug	Method	Immediate release	Extended release	Typical duration	Comments
Dexedrine Spansules (5,10,15 mg)	Beads	≈1/3	≈2/3	8-13	Excretion $t_{1/2} > 10$ h for all amphetamines
Adderall XR (5, 10, 15, 20, 25, 30 mg)	Beads	≈50%	≈50%	12+	Absorption delayed by high-fat breakfast

and Adderall XR). These once-daily formulations use a variety of different drug delivery systems to extend their effects. Concerta uses an osmotic release system that pumps drug out of the capsule over 10 hours to achieve up to 12 hours of efficacy. The remaining long-acting compounds all use beads that dissolve at different rates once swallowed. Two of the methylphenidate formulations (Metadate CD and Ritalin LA) are designed to provide approximately 8 hours of efficacy. Thus these forms may require a second dose for late afternoon coverage. The long-acting amphetamines are generally only given once per day because their plasma half-lives are up to three times longer than that of methylphenidate. For these reasons, long-acting amphetamines are the most likely compounds to produce substantial suppression of appetite and decreased ability to fall asleep. Finally, the manufacturer of Ritalin has also marketed the d-isomer under the brand name Focalin (dexmethylphenidate). The chief advantage seems to be that the dosages administered are half those of the racemic parent compound.

Despite the large number of options, many clinicians continue to begin treatment with one of the methylphenidate formulations. The immediate-release methylphenidate formulation is bioequivalent, but many physicians are starting with one of the branded long-acting formulations such as Concerta, Metadate CD, or Ritalin LA. The first of these lasts the longest, providing up to 12 hours of benefit compared to double-blind placebo. However, it comes as a rigid capsule in a limited range of doses (18, 27, 36, or 54 mg). Although higher doses are not yet FDA approved, many adolescents or adults require 72 mg per day. Besides differing in duration of effect, the three formulations differ somewhat in the proportion, of methylphenidate that is available for immediate release once swallowed. Concerta has the lowest proportion, at 22% of the total dose. By contrast, Metadate CD provides 30% immediately released, and 70% released 4 hours later; and Ritalin LA is designed to release 50% immediately and 50% 4 hours later.

The mixture of d- and l-amphetamine known as Adderall XR is one of the most commonly prescribed stimulants. It and the long-acting Dexedrine Spansules tend to last much longer than the methylphenidates, and they also tend to have stronger effects on the noradrenergic system.

One of the most interesting developments is the introduction of atomoxetine (Strattera). This selective noradrenergic reuptake inhibitor is significantly more effective than placebo for the treatment of ADHD in children, adolescents, and adults, and it is the first drug

approved by the FDA for treating ADHD in adults. Because the drug does not affect striatal dopamine levels, it does not have the same potential to produce substance abuse as the stimulants, and it is not controlled by the Drug Enforcement Administration, as are all the stimulants. Studies by the pharmaceutical company have reported equivalent efficacy to methylphenidate, but this does not seem to match the perception of clinicians in practice. However, Strattera is unquestionably now the first choice for anyone with ADHD and a history of substance abuse. It is also worth considering for individuals with ADHD and a tic disorder such as Tourette's disorder. Because of the potential for gastrointestinal adverse effects, which are generally mild and transient, atomoxetine should be titrated upward more slowly than the stimulants. Interestingly, despite a plasma half-life of less than 6 hours, many individuals seem to be able to take Strattera only once a day. Dosages should be started at no more than 0.5 mg/kg per day for up to 1 week, and increased at weekly intervals until effects are obtained or to a maximum of 1.4 mg/kg per day in children, or to a maximum of 80 mg per day in those who weigh more than 70 kg. Benefits have been reported for both inattention and hyperactivity/impulsivity symptoms. Additionally, Strattera appears to be effective for improving frustration tolerance and decreasing irritability.

Clonidine (Catapres)[1] and guanfacine (Tenex)[1] are α_2 agonists that are also occasionally used for the treatment of ADHD, although rarely as monotherapy. Clonidine is strongly sedating, and is useful for individuals who have difficulty going to sleep, although care must be taken to monitor potential rebound effects when only bedtime dosing regimens are used. Physicians need to remember that clonidine tablets are 0.1 mg each; usual total daily doses are below 0.25 mg per day. Guanfacine is more selective and consequently much less sedating in low doses (<2 mg per day). Some individuals seem to benefit from even lower doses (as little as 0.5 mg per day) when supplementing a stimulant, although there are no controlled trials to guide such adjunctive treatment.

Some physicians use a range of other options for treating ADHD including bupropion (Wellbutrin)[A] and venlafaxine (Effexor XR).[1] However, given the wide range of other options, there is much less reason to use these off-label approaches.

---

[1]Not FDA approved for this indication.

Rakel and Bope: *Conn's Current Therapy 2006.*

Once a drug and a dose are proven to be efficacious in a child, it is important to re-evaluate the effect of the drug regularly (at least once per year). Is the drug still having a positive effect on the child's behavior, and is medication treatment still needed, or does the dose need to be changed? Especially in adolescents with ADHD, some of the symptoms could decrease naturally without drug use, and therefore a period without medication is recommended in order to reassess the need for medication management. It is also an important means of maintaining the therapeutic alliance with adolescents.

BEHAVIORAL TREATMENT

In addition to medication treatment, behavioral treatment should always be considered. Parents find behavioral treatments intrinsically more satisfying than medications, even though the benefits may not be as large. Although most ADHD can be ascribed to neurobiologic causes, parents and teachers can play an important role in managing the behaviors, or in making them worse. Clinics that specialize in ADHD typically offer parent education classes or groups, which may also be available through parent support groups such as Children and Adults with Attention Deficit Disorder (CHADD).

Child-Focused Behavioral Treatment

Cognitive training and social skills training have been extensively tried in children with ADHD with little meaningful effect on social behaviors or academic achievement. Intensive summer treatment programs are sometimes available and combine intensive behavioral management techniques with the socialization of summer camps. In general, the short-term improvements in summer treatment programs can be large, but evidence is lacking regarding their long-term benefits, as is the case for all interventions for ADHD.

Parent Training

Some degree of parent training is important, regardless of whether the primary treatment is through medications or through behavioral techniques. Typically, parent training programs involve 10 or so group sessions that focus on teaching parents how to manage the behavior of their children. These techniques include setting up school and home daily report cards, rewarding and ignoring the child's behavior, learning how to give effective commands to children, learning how to encourage compliance with instructions, and learning how to use token economies and time-out as a consequence of negative behavior. One of the most important goals of parent training is to help parents to not take their child's ADHD behaviors as personal affronts, and to recalibrate their expectations based on the slower maturation rate of most ADHD children. Such reframing can decrease critical or negative expressed emotion on the part of parents about their children, which seems to mediate many of the poor outcomes of ADHD.

Rakel and Bope: *Conn's Current Therapy 2006.*

 CURRENT DIAGNOSIS

Criteria

- HD-inattentive type: At least six symptoms of inattention are specified in the *DSM-IV.*
- ADHD hyperactive/impulsive type: At least six symptoms of hyperactivity/impulsivity should be present for a diagnosis.
- ADHD-combined type: Both of the above must be present for a diagnosis.
- Symptoms need to have been present for at least 6 months, in more than one setting.
- Some of the symptoms must have been associated with impairment before age 7 years.
- Symptoms must clearly interfere with social, academic, or occupational functioning.
- The diagnosis does not apply if the symptoms can be better accounted for by a pervasive developmental disorder, schizophrenia, or other psychotic disorders, or by any other specific mental disorder.

Co-morbidity

- In 60% to 80% of children with a diagnosis of ADHD there is another disorder as well.
- Common co-morbidities include oppositional defiant disorder, conduct disorder, learning disabilities, tic disorders, anxiety or mood disorders.
- In some cases, juvenile bipolar (manic-depressive) disorder may initially present as severe ADHD.

Assessment

- Diagnosis is based on history of symptoms, derived from informants such as parents and teachers.
- Frequently used questionnaires (note that questionnaires do not suffice for a diagnostic evaluation) are:
  Child Behavior Checklist
  Teacher Report Form
  Revised Conners Parent and Teacher Rating Scales
  Swanson, Nolan and Pelham (SNAP) Teacher and Parent Rating Scales
  Structured or semistructured psychiatric interviews
  Diagnostic Interview Schedule for Children (DISC)
  Schedule for Affective Disorders and Schizophrenia for School-Age Children (K-SADS)

Abbreviations: ADHD = attention deficit hyperactivity disorder; *DSM-IV = Diagnostic and Statistical Manual of Mental Disorders, Fourth Edition.*

Teacher Consultation

Problem behaviors and situations should be discussed with the child's teacher. Teachers are the most effective observers of the symptoms of ADHD, and of the improvement in symptoms with treatment. They can also notice adverse effects that may be missed by parents and clinicians. Unfortunately, the availability of long-acting medications has made it possible for parents to avoid

14

CURRENT THERAPY

Pharmacological Treatment

- Psychostimulants
- Methylphenidate (Ritalin, Concerta, Metadate CD, Ritalin LA)
- Dextroamphetamine (Dexedrine and Dexedrine Spansules)
- A mixture of amphetamine sales (Adderall and Adderall XR)
- Pemoline (Cylert). Note that pemoline is now rarely prescribed because of the potential for fatal hepatotoxicity
- Long-acting formulations of methylphenidate
- Concerta
- Metadate CD
- Ritalin LA
- Long-acting formulations of amphetamine
- Dexedrine Spansules
- Adderall XR
- Nonstimulant noradrenergic reuptake blockers
- Tricyclic antidepressants are now rarely prescribed because of concerns of cardiac toxicity
- Atomoxetine (Strattera)
- α-Agonist anti-hypertensive agents
- Clonidine (Catapres) and Guanfacine (Tenex)

Psychosocial/Behavioral Treatment

- Parent training
- Teaching parents how to manage the behavior of their child
- Teacher consultation
- Child-focused behavioral treatments
  Cognitive training
  Social skills training

informing the school and their child's teacher about the diagnosis of ADHD and its treatment. While protection of the child's confidentiality is important, much can be lost when the perspective and insights of an experienced teacher are not available.

When a good working relationship is established amongst parents, teachers, and clinicians, behavioral control can be greatly supported by using a daily report card coupled with home-based rewards, or by the use of a token system in order to reinforce desired behavior within the classroom. During teacher consultation, teachers are advised about several issues such as classroom structure and rules, task demands, clear commands, rewarding and ignoring behavior, individualizing task instructions, token economies, time-out, and others.

ADHD is a common behavioral disorder that needs careful diagnostic assessment, including the use of validated questionnaires and thorough interviews to determine the current and past behavior of the child. Information should always be obtained from multiple sources, including parent, child, and teacher reports. ADHD frequently co-occurs with other conduct disorders, (anxiety, learning disorders), and these possible co-morbid conditions also require attention by the clinician. Treatment for ADHD should involve a combination of

carefully evaluating the efficacy of pharmacologic treatment (long-acting psychostimulant drugs being the first choice), and behavioral intervention (parent training and teacher consultation), depending on the individual child.

Gilles de la Tourette Syndrome

Method of
Roger D. Freeman, MD

Tourette's syndrome (TS), otherwise known as Gilles de la Tourette syndrome or Tourette's disorder, is characterized by waxing and waning motor and vocal tics over a period of at least 1 year. For historic and arbitrary reasons, at least one vocal tic is required to fulfill all criteria, although lists of tics often confuse the issue by incorrectly including sniffing as "vocal." (There seems to be no valid reason to privilege a vocal tic in the definition.) A child with multiple changing tics (not necessarily simultaneous) almost certainly fulfills criteria for TS later, even if only a few weeks have passed; the 12-month rule is again arbitrary. The media loves to portray coprolalia, the involuntary emission of expletives or unacceptable words, noises, or phrases, but it occurs in only approximately 5% to 15% of cases as a significant problem and may be transient. Tics, like other neurodevelopmental disorders, are highly familial and probably influenced by multiple genetic and environmental factors.

Clinical Features and Course

Tics are very common, occurring in up to 20% of boys in any one school year. Most of these are single tics that may resolve with further development and never come to a physician's attention. It is now generally accepted that the current criteria for TS is satisfied by approximately 0.5% to 1% of the child population, with boys outnumbering girls by approximately four to one and a mean age at onset of 6 to 7 years. These two stable findings around the world indicate that the underlying process is neurodevelopmental and may be influenced by gender-specific factors, but it is unlikely that diet, environmental toxins, allergies, or infections is a major cause. Psychological factors are not sufficient to cause tics but may sometimes influence their severity or form. "Automatic suppression" of tics in the presence of strangers may mean the physician sees many fewer symptoms than the parents do, and the teacher sees less than at home. The experience of having obvious tics is the result of a complex mixture of biologic, psychological (learning, meanings), family, and sociocultural factors in which information, attitudes, talent, time, and support have important roles to play. Tics are at their most severe and unstable prior to puberty (approximately age 10 to 12 years) and usually diminish gradually and become more stable in or after adolescence. Follow-up studies and clinical experience agree that no matter how severe the tics in childhood, substantial improvement is likely. The quality of life is then determined not by the cross-sectional severity or impairment, but by how childhood is endured with the tics and the kind of individual who emerges into adulthood.

Co-Occurring Conditions and Problems

Depending on whether subsyndromal obsessive-compulsive symptoms are included as a disorder, approximately 12% to 20% of clinical cases simply have tics (TS-Only); the remainder, varying by clinic from almost all to approximately 60%, have (on average) two co-occurring disorders (TS+) by our current classification system and may therefore present with (or develop) a wide variety of problems; often the tics are the least of these. Attention deficit hyperactivity disorder (ADHD) and obsessive-compulsive disorder (OCD) are the most common co-occurring conditions, and the trio is well known by all clinicians in the field, typically starting with ADHD, tics developing around age 6 to 8 years, and OCD often somewhat later. Those patients with this complex picture are also at risk for learning disabilities; anxiety disorders, oppositional-defiant disorder, and mood disorders. Families need to understand the evolution of a complex clinical picture with multiple diagnoses does not mean that separate diseases are acquired, but that the complexity of the underlying problem and its adaptive manifestations has changed and will likely evolve further. All disorders or problem behaviors cannot be treated simultaneously or rigidly; assessment of all areas of functioning, strengths as well as weaknesses, is required to determine the need for treatment. Patients with TS-Only that persists for a few years without the development of co-morbid disorders are unlikely to have problem behaviors, self-injurious behavior (SIB), sleep disorders, or a learning disability.

Assuming the diagnosis is made correctly, the goals in the management of TS are:

- The development of tolerance for tics, which minimizes the need for long-term medication and the burden of suffering.
- The development of ways of thinking conducive to a balanced view of the child.
- Suppression of tics in some cases at some times.
- Treatment of co-occurring disorders or problems

THE DEVELOPMENT OF TIC TOLERANCE

Parents do not like to see their child acting strangely or others looking askance at them. They may hesitate to take their child to the movies or to church where their tics will be noticeable or hear their child complaining of

sore muscles or teasing. Many actions can be taken to reduce the impact for most children:

- Ensure that both parents have a basic understanding of key information. Other important family members may need the same information, especially absent fathers and involved grandparents.
- Seek school support with understanding by staff and schoolmates, advocacy where necessary, and monitoring of teasing and bullying. Teachers may need explanations tailored to the individual child if tics are prominent, causing misunderstanding/rejection or interfering with attention, writing, or peer relationships.
- Offer the child explanations at his or her level and the opportunity to develop brief, simple explanations of symptoms for peers and others.
- Find ways to work around certain tics like ßeyerolling, which results in a loss of focus on the line while reading.
- Manage muscle soreness conservatively (heat, massage, analgesics), especially with a frequent new tic.
- Optimize family functioning and activities to promote positive experiences.
- Ensure the continued accessibility of the clinician for questions about new symptoms and for reassessment as needed. This works best in the context of a continuing relationship.
- Learn not to attribute all problems to tics. Ask, "Could the same or a similar problem occur without tics?" Often the answer is "yes." Resist trying obsessively to find causes for new symptoms or distinguish a tic from compulsions and all other behaviors.
- Find support groups after the situation is stabilized that share tips and reduce a sense of negative uniqueness. Note: Support groups may create problems if attended primarily by persons with worse difficulties or with an idiosyncratic agenda.

A BALANCED VIEW

At first, many parents react as if the tics and associated symptoms override all other characteristics of their child. In cases in which the child has good social skills, interests, and talents, these important qualities need to be gradually restored to their rightful place in the parental repertoire of reactions and meanings. An exploration of the individual significance of that child and his or her success in life or apparent suffering for being different may be helpful and is sometimes necessary when a balanced view cannot be restored. The continuing influence of spouses and relatives must also be taken into account, and sometimes it is necessary to help them with their understanding.

TIC SUPPRESSION

Except in extreme instances, the need for a tic suppressant is not determined by the tics themselves, but by their specific effects and meanings at a particular stage of development of the child and family and in an individual context. If a rapid response is needed, a neuroleptic is the first choice (pimozide, haloperidol, or risperidone), followed by tetrabenazine (available in Canada and probably soon in the United States). The general principle is to start very low and increase dosages slowly. If that rule is followed, concurrent usage of antiparkinsonian agents is usually unnecessary, and acute extrapyramidal (dystonic) reactions are very rare. The dosage-related onset of school or work avoidance as a new problem is reason to suspect the "neuroleptic separation anxiety syndrome" and to test its relationship to neuroleptic dosage. Tardive dyskinesia is fortunately a very rare occurrence but may not always be reversible, so the need for medication must be very clear. Information about the long-range side effects of the atypical neuroleptics is still emerging (prolactin effects, weight gain, increased risk of diabetes or cardiovascular disease), so their advantage over the typical neuroleptics may not be great. If a slower response is tolerable, clonidine or guanfacine may be tried. Refractory cases should be treated by (or in consultation with) a TS expert. Finally, there are three important rules:

1. Complete tic suppression is undesirable. It leads to excessive drug dosages and obscures the continuing need for medication.
2. Because tics wax and wane spontaneously, there should be a delay in responding to an upsurge, and because of confusion caused by rebound, medication dosage should be tapered rather than suddenly stopped.
3. A baseline electrocardiogram and close monitoring are essential to minimize complications, especially when a new drug is initiated and dosages are changed.

CO-OCCURRING DISORDERS OR PROBLEMS

Co-occurring ADHD, with all of its ramifications, is diagnosed in approximately 60% of clinical TS cases. Because ADHD is itself highly familial, other family members with such problems may need consideration in comprehensive management. The use of stimulant medications is usually quite successful without causing tic exacerbations beyond that which could occur by chance with any medication. Experience with the non-stimulant atomoxetine (Strattera) is just beginning but looks promising.

In approximately 25% of TS cases, OCD is diagnosed. Subthreshold but significant symptoms appear in another 35%. Treatment with selective serotonin reuptake inhibitors (SSRIs) or clomipramine is the usual approach, with low-dosage pimozide augmentation for some refractory cases with tics. Cognitive behavior therapy (with or without medication) is also useful for fixed symptom patterns in cooperative patients and may have longer lasting effects than medication.

Sleep disorders (25%) are highly associated with ADHD, not tics, although new or complex tics may make it difficult to fall asleep. When sleep initiation difficulty fails to respond to modifications in sleep hygiene, timing of stimulant medication, or treatment

of obsessive-compulsive symptoms, 0.1 mg of clonidine[1] or 3 to 9 mg of melatonin* are effective for many children.

Anger control problems, sometimes referred to as "rage," are uncommon in TS-Only but common in TS+ cases (40% or more). Co-occurring obsessive-compulsive features or mood lability may serve as triggers, but problems occurring in school may also have a learning problem (often unrecognized) as a factor. It is important to try to identify target symptoms that may be contributing to these problems.

Self-injurious behavior (SIB) is reported in 15%. SIB is not uncommon in the general population and in many of the childhood neuropsychiatric disorders. It is much more common in TS+OCD than in TS-Only, and it may take bizarre forms. It may or may not respond to neuroleptic and/or antiobsessional treatment.

Anxiety disorders are diagnosed in 15% to 20%. Many of the same measures used in childhood anxiety without tics can be equally useful, but SSRI medications have more unpredictable effects than in adults and may have paradoxical effects.

Mood disorders are diagnosed in 20%. In practice, formal mood disorders seem less common than complaints about "moodiness," high reactivity, or a negative approach to problems and frustrations. The distinction between juvenile bipolar disorder and ADHD may be difficult in some cases.

Pervasive developmental disorders (PDD) are diagnosed in approximately 5%. Several epidemiologic studies show a high rate of tics and TS in children with Asperger's syndrome and autism; as those children age, obsessive-compulsive symptoms and severe sleep disorders may become very troublesome. These cases typically require consultation or management by a specialist.

Management of the Typical Case of Tourette's Syndrome-Only

Children with TS are now brought to physicians significantly earlier than in the past. The child is usually not the one worried about the tics. The parents may already have done research, perhaps with resulting confusion and likely with considerable anxiety. Almost certainly they have heard something about TS and require remedial learning. They often fear social rejection (especially because of coprolalia, a dire prognosis from cases shown on television) and the use of potentially dangerous drugs. They may have guilt over blaming the child for deliberate behavior rather than involuntary symptoms, disagreeing with each other over the nature of the tics and fruitless attempts at diagnosis and treatment. If the child has friends, reasonable intelligence, hobbies and interests, and at least average school achievement, reassurance and education are usually all that is needed. Parents can learn that these positive features are the

---

[1]Not FDA approved for this indication.
*Based on open-label experience; randomized clinical trials are complete and the results are expected to be published soon.

Rakel and Bope: *Conn's Current Therapy 2006.*

TABLE 1 Medications for Tics

Drug	Starting dose	Maintenance dose	Side effects	Comments
Haloperidol (Haldol)	0.25 mg every morning	0.5-3 mg/d	Cognitive blunting at higher dosages; extrapyramidal symptoms	Drops available
Pimozide (Orap)	0.5 mg every morning or evening	2-6 mg/d	Tremor, akinesia, extrapyramidal symptoms	May be used bid
Risperidone (Risperdal)	0.25 mg/d	0.5-4 mg/d	Extrapyramidal symptoms, weight gain, diabetes	Oral solution available
Clonidine (Catapres)	0.025 bid-tid	0.1 mg tid	Somnolence, dry mouth	
Guanfacine (Tenex)	1 mg every morning	1-2 mg/d	Somnolence, dry mouth	
Olanzapine (Zyprexa)	2.5 mg	5-10 mg/d	Extrapyramidal symptoms, weight gain, diabetes	
Quetiapine (Seroquel)	25 mg bid	100-300 mg/d	Diabetes, extrapyramidal symptoms	Not well established yet for TS
Ziprasidone (Geodon)	20 mg/d	40-120 mg/d	Increased QT_c interval, possibly less weight gain	Not yet well evaluated for tics

Abbreviations: bid = two times per day; QT_c = corrected for heart rate; tid = three times per day; TS = Tourette's syndrome.

14

most important. Even with competent diagnosis and information, however, the next few upsurges often require support before tolerance of tics develops. The school may need confirmation of the diagnosis or explanation of its significance. As development proceeds, monitoring school progress, social development, and any new symptoms that may indicate the presence of a co-morbid disorder is important, and parents need to know whom to contact in that event. If parental anxiety does not diminish, more work to uncover its current or remote sources may be necessary.

Management of the More Complex Case (Tourette's Syndrome Plus)

Complexity in management is not always correlated with the number of co-morbid disorders. Some TS-Only cases can be more difficult to manage than cases with three or more diagnostic labels, but ongoing management of difficult cases is really the province of the specialist with extensive experience. Additional consultation with colleagues may be indicated. Psychological testing is often helpful, especially when there are school problems, either academic or behavioral. When medications are needed for tics, they need to be started at very low dosages and raised and lowered slowly (Table 1).

Management of Adults

Many of the same considerations as previously outlined apply to adults with TS. The original assessment may be inadequate by current standards, however, and a fresh look therefore needs to be taken. The delay between onset of tics and the diagnosis may be quite long.

Discussion of etiology years ago may have centered on psychogenic factors. The consequences of misunderstanding the nature of the condition and the effects on family relationships may be severe and enduring. Education or re-education of the patient and important family members must be considered.

A knowledgeable and interested clinician can manage many cases of TS-Only, and—with the advice of a specialist—some co-morbid TS+ cases. In spite of tics and other symptoms, patients and families who can develop a well-balanced perspective may experience a good quality of life.

REFERENCES

Chowdhury U, Heyman I: Tourette's syndrome in children. British Med J 2004;329:1357-1358.

Cohen AJ, Leckman JF: Sensory phenomena associated with Gilles de la Tourette's syndrome. J Clin Psychiatry 1992;53:319-323.

Freeman RD, Fast DK, Burd L, et al: An international perspective on Tourette syndrome: Selected findings from 3500 individuals in 22 countries. Dev Med Child Neurol 2000;42:436-447.

Gadow KD, Nolan EE, Sprakin J, et al: Tics and psychiatric comorbidity in children and adolescents. Dev Med Child Neurol 2002;44:330-338.

Goetz CG, Leurgans S, Chmura TA: Home alone: Methods to maximize tic expression for objective videotape assessments in Gilles de la Tourette syndrome. Mov Disord 2001;16:693-697.

Grados MA, Riddle MA, Samuels JF, et al: The familial phenotype of obsessive-compulsive disorder in relation to tic disorders: The Hopkins OCD family study. Biol Psychiatry 2001;50:559-565.

Hoekstra PJ, Steenhuis MP, Kallenberg CG: Association of small life events with self reports of tic severity in pediatric and adult tic disorder patients: A prospective longitudinal study. J Clin Psychiatry 2004;65:426-431.

Hoekstra PJ, Steenhuis MP, Troost PW, et al: Relative contribution of attention-deficit hyperactivity disorder, obsessive-compulsive disorder, and tic severity to social and behavioral problems in tic disorders. J Dev Behav Pediatr 2004;25:272-279.

Kadesjö B, Gillberg C: Tourette's disorder: Epidemiology and comorbidity in primary school children. J Am Acad Child Adolesc Psychiatry 2000;39:548-555.

Kurlan R: Tourette's syndrome: Are stimulants safe? Curr Neurol Neurosci Rep 2003;3:285-288.

Kurlan R, Como PG, Miller B, et al: The behavioral spectrum of tic disorders: A community-based study. Neurology 2002;59:414-420.

Kushner HI: A Cursing Brain? The Histories of Tourette Syndrome. Cambridge, Mass, Harvard University Press, 1999.

Leckman JF: Tourette's syndrome. Lancet 2002;360:1577-1586.

Leckman JF, Cohen DJ (eds): Tourette's Syndrome—Tics, Obsessions, Compulsions: Developmental Psychopathology and Clinical Care. New York, John Wiley, 1999.

Leckman JF, Zhang H, Vitale A, et al: Course of tic severity in Tourette syndrome: The first two decades. Pediatrics 1998;102:14-19.

Mantel BJ, Meyers A, Tran QY: Nutritional supplements and complementary/alternative medicine in Tourette syndrome. J Child Adolesc Psychopharmacol 2004;14:582-589.

Singer HS, Giuliano JD, Zimmerman AM, et al: Infection: A stimulus for tic disorders. Pediatr Neurol 2000;22:380-383.

Snider LA, Seligman LD, Ketchen BR, et al: Tics and problem behaviors in schoolchildren: Prevalence, characterization, and associations. Pediatrics 2002;110:331-336.

Headache

Method of
R. Michael Gallagher, DO

Headache is a disturbing and sometimes fearsome affliction that has plagued humankind throughout recorded history. It often is debilitating and particularly disturbing to the sufferer because the pain is located in the head, the very center of the body's cognitive and control functions. With its accompanying pain and debilitating symptoms, stress can mount and the headache can become all consuming.

Headache is experienced by all age groups from young children to the elderly. It is more common than asthma, diabetes, mental illness, or rheumatoid arthritis. In fact, the World Health Organization identifies severe migraine, along with psychosis and quadriplegia, as "one of the most debilitating chronic conditions." Although the majority of Americans experience tension-type headaches at some time in their lives, approximately 30 million experience migraine headache—13% of women and 6% of men, predominantly in their most productive years between the ages of 13 and 55 years. Prepubescent boys and girls suffer equally, whereas boys often outgrow their migraine attacks as they mature and are less subjected to hormonal influences. Smaller percentages of people, by comparison, suffer with other chronic headaches such as cluster headache or chronic daily headache.

No sure diagnostic tests are available to differentiate headache types. The headache condition can progress over time in frequency, severity, and debilitation. Each sufferer can be different and may require a detailed evaluation and individualized treatment plan; the more frequent or prolonged attacks often necessitate a more comprehensive treatment plan. Thus the headache

problem can be a challenge for both the sufferer and the clinician.

During the 20th century, dramatic advancements were made in medicine. Longevity and quality of life improved for many. Unfortunately, for headache sufferers, most of these advances were for maladies that killed or maimed rather than the non–life-threatening conditions. It was not until the 1960s that even a reasonable preventive medication, propranolol (Inderal), was introduced, and by the 1980s only a handful of medications were available for wide use. Physicians had to improvise with medications and treatments that were originally designated for other medical conditions.

In the late 1980s and 1990s, epidemiologic, psychosocial, and pharmacologic research resulted in an increase in available headache information and treatment possibilities. The development of the triptans, serotonin agonists, brought a new awareness to both physicians and sufferers. Today, seven triptans and two relatively new preventive medications are available. In spite of this, a minority of migraine sufferers use these options and more than 50% continue to self-treat without benefit of professional care.

In the past, patients wanted the physician to believe their headache problem was real. They hoped to be taken seriously and that a sincere attempt would be made to help them. The headache patient has changed. The headache sufferer who seeks treatment today is more knowledgeable and interested in rapid relief and tolerability of medication.

Evaluation and Diagnosis

An accurate diagnosis is essential for the effective management of patients with the more commonly encountered headaches. Because no biologic markers or diagnostic tests exist to determine headache type, the history is the single most important element in the headache patient evaluation. Various headache types sometimes have similar initial presentation, or patients may suffer with more than one type of headache (e.g., migraine and tension-type headache), which can be confusing at first, but the careful history usually differentiates the headache type. In general, little is needed in the way of diagnostic testing unless a physical cause is suspected. Some physicians prefer to perform simple laboratory tests to establish a baseline for medication toleration and monitoring as necessary.

The headache complaint can on occasion be a sign of a more serious medical condition such as a tumor, infection, or aneurysm. For this reason, the clinician always must be cautious and diligent in establishing an accurate and timely diagnosis. Certain so-called red flags in the history require immediate attention. These include any complex of symptoms or history that does not fit a typical headache type; report of a significant neurologic deficit; late-onset migraine (older than age 30 years); sudden onset of a new head pain without history of similar headaches; changes in headache character; headache associated with elevated temperature; or completely unresponsive attacks in the absence of analgesic or caffeine overuse. When any of these symptoms are present or there are significant findings on physical examination, further diagnostic evaluation with imaging studies and consultation is imperative.

The appropriate headache patient evaluation includes a thorough history, physical examination with special attention to the head, neurologic, cardiovascular, and musculoskeletal systems, and diagnostic tests when appropriate. The history should include headache onset, location, pain character (e.g., pressure, throb), frequency, duration, associated symptoms, aura or prodrome, triggers, previous treatment, and family history. Certain clues in the history may lean toward migraine, such as motion sickness, absence of headache during pregnancy, and headache relationship to menses, sun glare, oversleep, fatigue, fasting, foods, or alcohol.

Various diagnostic screening questionnaires and tools were developed over the years to assist busy clinicians in establishing the diagnosis of migraine. Most are long and cumbersome and do not easily become a part of routine patient evaluation. A simple three-question screener for migraine is helpful for generalist clinicians. A "yes" answer to all of these three questions indicates a strong possibility of the migraine diagnosis:

1. Do you experience headaches severe enough to see a physician?
2. Are your headaches accompanied by other symptoms?
3. Are your headaches intermittent (i.e., nondaily)?

Note: This screener should not be substituted for a complete history and used only for screening purposes.

TENSION-TYPE HEADACHE

Tension type headache (TTHA) is the most common of headaches and first was believed to be caused by sustained muscle contraction of the neck, jaw, scalp, or facial muscles. However, it is now thought the sustained muscle contraction can, in fact, be an epiphenomenon to possible central disturbances rather than a primary process. Evidence suggests that altered levels of serotonin, substance P, and neuropeptide Y in the serum or platelets of patients with TTHA may be responsible.

TTHA is characterized by intermittent or persisting bilateral pain, usually described as a squeezing pressure or a bandlike sensation around the head. Most patients experience their symptoms in the frontal, temporal, or occipital areas of the head. Location frequently varies with the attack, and tightness of the neck and shoulders is common. Intensity varies greatly, and attacks can last from hours to days, and in some extreme cases they may last for months. Aura, nausea, photophobia and phonophobia, and incapacitation are not typically associated with TTHA.

Many TTHA sufferers easily recognize the origin of their attacks. TTHA typically results from emotional upset, periods of stress, and major life changes. Anxiousness, poor adaptation skills, and anxiety and depression often are present. Physical causes such as degenerative joint disease, trauma to the head or neck, poor posture, or temporomandibular joint dysfunction

also can precipitate attacks. Those over 50 years of age are prone to excessive muscle contraction because of arthritis of the neck and jaw, poor posture, or stress. TTHAs that are consistently precipitated by the neck frequently are referred to as cervicogenic headache. In contrast to migraine headache, TTHA is more likely to begin in later life.

MIGRAINE HEADACHE

Migraine headache is a familial disease characterized by unilateral or bilateral paroxysmal headache lasting hours to days. Adult women experience attacks more than men 3:1, whereas children and the elderly experience migraine equally. Attacks occur from as infrequently as one or two per year to several times weekly. Associated symptoms usually occur and frequently include throbbing, nausea, vomiting, photophobia, phonophobia, fluid retention, or mood changes.

There are two basic types of migraine headache: *migraine with aura* (previously called classic migraine) and *migraine without aura* (previously called common migraine). Migraine with aura is preceded by an aura, a transient neurologic symptom that usually is visual, such as scotoma, teichopsia, tunnel vision, or visual field deficit, lasting 10 to 30 minutes. Migraine without aura is more commonly experienced and comes on gradually or is present on awakening from sleep. In some, these headaches are associated with a nonspecific prolonged prodrome such as mood changes, food cravings, or fluid retention hours before the pain.

The underlying cause of migraine headache is not clearly established and various theories are proposed. It appears that migraine is of genetic origin and an inflammatory disease, which causes disturbances in serotonin (5-HT) use and activity. Strong evidence indicates the migrainous attack originates in the central nervous system by stimulation of the locus ceruleus and dorsal raphe nuclei. Resultant changes alter cerebral and extracranial blood flow, activate the trigeminovascular system, and cause vascular dilation, neurogenic inflammation, and pain. Various precipitants are known, and many sufferers report that migraine attacks frequently are associated with menstruation or triggered by foods containing vasoactive amines, strong odors, too much or too little sleep, sun glare, stress, altitude, weather changes, exertion, or fasting (Boxes 1 and 2).

Some physicians classify migraine according to its precipitant or description (e.g., menstrual migraine, exertional migraine, coital migraine, cervicogenic migraine, cyclic migraine, acephalic migraine). Regardless, the fundamentals of evaluation and treatment remain the same.

CLUSTER HEADACHE

The cause of cluster headache is unknown and little credible research is available. Various possibilities or theories are suggested and include, but are not limited to, disturbances in histamine production or use; hypothalmic biorhythm dysfunction; or serotonin and neurotransmitter mechanisms similar to migraine.

1120   Headache

BOX 1 Migraine Dietary Triggers

- Dairy: ripened cheese (cheddar, brie, camembert, half-cup limit of sour cream)
- Meats: processed lunch meats, hot dogs, sausage, bologna, salami, chicken liver
- Fish: pickled or dried herring
- Grains: sourdough bread
- Fruits: bananas, raisins, figs, avocado, half-cup limit of citrus
- Vegetables: broad and fava beans, onions, snow peas
- Other: chocolate, nuts, peanut butter, pickled foods, Chinese food with MSG
- Beverages: most wine and alcohol, 200 mg daily limit of caffeine
- Additives: monosodium glutamate (MSG), soy sauce, meat tenderizers, aspartame, sulfites, garlic

---

Some authorities consider cluster headache one of the most severe pain conditions known to humankind.

Cluster headache predominantly affects men, with a male-to-female ratio of 6:1, and occurs in well under 0.5% of the population. Later life onset, after the age of 30 years, is common, and patients sometimes report head injury or a traumatic event months before onset. Attacks occur on a daily or near-daily basis for weeks or months at a time and mysteriously disappear for months to years regardless of treatment, only to recur and cycle again. Although nonspecialist physicians only occasionally encounter the patient with cluster headaches, it is important to consider cluster headaches in the differential diagnosis.

The typical patient with a cluster headache experiences relatively brief attacks (45 to 90 minutes) of horrible unilateral head pain associated with ipsilateral lacrimation, scleral injection, rhinorrhea, or eyelid droop. The hallmark of the syndrome is its associated symptoms and its severe and intense pain. During attacks, most cluster patients move about, trying unsuccessfully to get more comfortable, similar to renal colic, in contrast to migraine sufferers who prefer to lie quietly in a dark quiet room. Few triggers are identified and alcohol almost always precipitates an attack during a cluster

---

BOX 2 Migraine Triggers

- Altitude
- Alcohol
- Caffeine withdrawal
- Fluorescent or flickering lights
- Sun glare
- Weather changes
- Stress, stress letdown
- Foods
- Skipping meals
- Smoky environment
- Noisy environment
- Strong odors
- Lack of sleep, oversleep
- Exertion
- Hormonal changes

"on" cycle. A rare form of cluster headache does not cycle and continues on a daily or near-daily basis without cessation.

Treatment

The doctor-patient relationship frequently is the key to treatment success in the headache patient. Although to some, this statement would seem an obvious truism, its importance cannot be overemphasized. Patients who experience frequent, near-daily, or daily headaches invariably require a comprehensive treatment program that necessitates good communication. Anxious patients sometimes do not comprehend medical explanations or instructions; busy doctors sometimes do not have or take the time to ensure that the patient understands.

There are two elements of headache treatment: *abortive treatment,* directed at attacks once they have begun, and *prophylactic treatment,* directed at preventing or reducing the frequency of attacks. In general, the abortive approach is for patients who suffer infrequent attacks and for those who experience breakthrough attacks while on prophylactic therapy. Prophylactic therapy should be instituted when headaches are frequent, unresponsive to abortive medication, or when there are contraindications to abortives.

Headache treatment can include nonpharmacologic measures such as physical exercise, stretching, stress avoidance, relaxation exercises, biofeedback, manipulation, massage, or cold/warm packs. Pharmacologic therapies can include a vast array of medicaments from over-the-counter (OTC) drugs to prescription drugs such as triptans, other vasoconstrictors, β-blockers, antiepileptic agents, antidepressants, nonsteroidal anti-inflammatory drugs (NSAIDs), analgesics, muscle relaxants, anxiolytics, and others.

Whether prophylactic or abortive, treatment should follow a definite plan incorporating the clinician and patient into a team focused on reducing the headache frequency, severity, and disability. As mentioned earlier, impressions and physical findings should be explained to the patient and as detailed as necessary, for a complete understanding. The complexity of the headache condition needs to be explained emphasizing its chronicity, rather than its curability, and that the treatment goal is to control the disease.

The degree of comprehensiveness of the patient's treatment plan depends on the frequency of their attacks. The more frequent and severe the attacks, the more detailed plan may be necessary. Patients experiencing infrequent attacks (e.g., once or twice monthly) may require only an abortive medication and little else. Patients with more frequent attacks may benefit from dietary restrictions, psychosocial intervention, biofeedback relaxation training, manipulation, and physical modality intervention, in addition to medication.

TENSION-TYPE HEADACHE TREATMENT

Tension-type headache often is associated with emotional stress and muscle strain or tension of the shoulders and neck. Simple self-administered measures such as stress avoidance, stretching, warm packs, or relaxation techniques can be helpful in reducing or relieving attacks. More comprehensive professional intervention such as manipulation, physical therapy, local injections, or biofeedback training are considerations for the more frequent or severe cases.

Prophylactically, the use of OTC or prescription medications can be considered in addition to nonmedicinal measures to reduce the frequency and duration of attacks. NSAIDs, muscle relaxants, or antidepressants (TCA [tricyclic antidepressant], SSRI [selective serotonin reuptake inhibitor]), at the lowest effective doses, are more commonly used.

The daily use of the longer acting NSAIDs, such as naproxen (Naprosyn)[1] or celecoxib (Celebrex),[1] in the appropriately screened patient, over a 2- to 3-week period, can be an effective preventative. Tricyclic antidepressants (TCAs), such as nortriptyline (Pamelor)[1] or amitriptyline (Elavil),[1] in low doses at night over 1 to 3 months, is frequently effective, especially in patients with anxiety or mild depression. The SSRI drugs, such as fluoxetine (Prozac)[1] or sertraline (Zoloft),[1] similarly can be useful. The muscle relaxant cyclobenzaprine (Flexeril),[1] at low doses, with similar mechanisms to the TCAs, can be administered at night for limited periods. Other muscle relaxants occasionally can be effective. Potential side effects can limit the use of NSAIDs (GI [gastrointestinal] irritation) and the TCAs (tiredness and weight gain).

The *abortive* or *symptomatic treatment* of TTHA can include simple OTC medications (e.g., aspirin or acetaminophen), NSAIDs (short acting), muscle relaxants, combination analgesics, and in some cases opioid or opioid-like drugs. Caution should be exercised in prescribing potentially habituating drugs. The daily or nearly daily use of analgesics can lead to analgesic rebound headache, which can compound the patient's headache problem.

Botulism toxin (Botox)[1] is reported to be helpful in treatment of tension-type and migraine headache. Although controlled studies are limited, a diluted solution of botulism toxin is injected into various muscles of the face, scalp, neck, or shoulders. Because this treatment frequently is used in headache specialty and pain centers, simultaneous comprehensive measures and medication may contribute to positive results. Side effects from Botox are low when injected properly.

MIGRAINE TREATMENT

Migraineurs are unique individuals, and the effectiveness and tolerance of medications can vary from patient to patient. Medication changes, combinations of medications, and trial and error may be necessary in the early stages of treatment.

Nonmedicinal measures for migraine sufferers include biofeedback stress reduction, caffeine and dietary restrictions, regimentation of meals and sleep, rest, exercise, stretching, and the avoidance of work or activity overload. Limiting caffeine to less than 200 mg per day is important to avoid the caffeine headache (rebound headache). Eliminating vasoactive foods such as chocolate, aged cheese, or processed meats and the avoidance of fasting for more than 4 hours can be helpful for those with more frequent attacks (Table 1). Regular exercise and stretching, planned relaxation, regular sleep schedules, and following a healthy lifestyle are frequently included in a comprehensive treatment regimen. In some patients, especially children and adolescents, biofeedback stress reduction or psychotherapeutic intervention may be necessary.

The more commonly used medications for prophylaxis are β-blockers, calcium channel blockers, antiepileptics (neurostabilizers), and the antidepressants. Treatment should be continued for a 4- to 8-week trial before discontinuation for ineffectiveness. The determination of which medication to use depends on co-morbidities, interactions with concomitant medications, and tolerability.

β-Blockers such as propranolol (Inderal) and timolol (Blocadren) are nonselective and carry FDA approvals for migraine prevention. Other β-blockers, nadolol (Corgard),[1] metoprolol (Lopressor),[1] and atenolol (Tenormin),[1] also can be effective. The mechanism of action in migraine is not wholly understood, but it is thought to involve anxiolytic effects as well as vascular changes and stabilization. The usual dosage is recommended (e.g., timolol, 10 to 30 mg per day, propranolol, 120 to 160 mg per day), and many consider the nighttime dose the more significant.

---

[1]Not FDA approved for this indication.

[1]Not FDA approved for this indication.

TABLE 1 Triptans

Medication	Brand name	Half-life	Form/strength
Sumatriptan	Imitrex	1.5 h	Oral: 25, 50, 100 mg; NS: 20 mg; injection: 6 mg
Naratriptan	Amerge	6 h	Oral: 2.5 mg
Zolmitriptan	Zomig	3 h	Oral: 2.5, 5 mg; Melt: 2.5, 5 mg; NS: 5 mg
Rizatriptan	Maxalt	2-3 h	Oral: 5, 10 mg; Melt: 10 mg
Almotriptan	Axert	3-4 h	Oral: 6.25, 12.5 mg
Frovatriptan	Frova	25 h	Oral: 5 mg
Eletriptan	Relpax	4 h	Oral: 20, 40 mg

Abbreviations: Melt = oral disintegrating; NS = nasal steroid.

Rakel and Bope: *Conn's Current Therapy 2006.*

Calcium channel antagonists are well tolerated in general and can be as effective as the β-blockers. They are believed to alter serotonin release and inhibit platelet serotonin uptake and release within the brain. Verapamil (Calan)[1] is considered the more effective and is commonly recommended to patients. Dosage can vary from 120 mg to 480 mg per day. Nimodipine (Nimotop)[1] is equally effective, but because of its high cost in the United States it is rarely used.

Antiepileptic medications such as phenytoin (Dilantin)[1] and carbamazepine (Tegretol)[1] were prescribed for migraine prevention over the years with mixed results. However, with the advent of newer, more easily tolerated agents, such as divalproex sodium (Depakote) and topiramate (Topamax), their use is now limited.

Divalproex sodium is effective in migraine attack reduction and particularly useful in patients with coexisting head injury, seizure disorders, and bipolar disorders. It is thought to improve inhibitory and excitatory amino acid imbalance in the brain. It is best to start with a lower dose and gradually increase as needed and tolerated. The dosage of 500 to 1000 mg per day is more frequently prescribed. A commonly experienced side effect is sedation, which can sometimes be used to the patient's advantage when anxiolytic effects are needed.

Topiramate is the most recent preventive medication approved by the FDA for migraine prophylaxis. It has multiple mechanisms of action, but its exact mechanism in migraine headache is yet unknown. Its effectiveness is believed to involve sodium ion channel stabilization, calcium ion channels, GABA (γ-aminobutyric acid) receptors, and neuronal membrane stabilization. The average daily dose is variable and ranges from 30 mg to 100 mg per day. A most unusual side effect of weight loss or appetite suppression can be used to the patient's advantage in preventing weight gain, which frequently accompanies migraine prophylactic medications.

The TCAs can be useful in patients who experience frequent attacks and in those who experience anxiety and depression. The TCAs inhibit synaptic reuptake of serotonin, thereby reducing neuron firing and release of neurotransmitters. Starting with a low dose in the evening and titrating up to efficacy and tolerability is recommended. Significant anticholinergic and sedation effects sometimes limit their use. The SSRIs[1] are reported helpful in some patients, but their use in migraine prevention is limited.

In general, prophylactic medications should be taken for 6 to 8 weeks to determine efficacy. If effective, a course of 4 to 6 months is recommended before an attempt is made to discontinue medication.

A variety of abortive treatment options are available for migraine sufferers. The triptans have generated much interest, and although frequently prescribed, other medications continue to be used by clinicians, including ergotamine and its derivatives, isometheptene, and NSAIDs. Many of the abortive medications do carry significant prescribing limitations that must be taken into consideration before prescribing.

Vasoconstrictor medications are contraindicated in those with cardiovascular or peripheral vascular disease. NSAIDs should not be used in those with GI or bleeding disorders. As with all medications, the clinician must consider appropriate prescribing, contraindication, and side-effect information.

The vasoconstrictor ergotamine is available in oral, rectal, and sublingual forms (Ergomar). Ergotamine has a relatively long half-life and duration of action (up to 3 days) and should be used no more frequently than every 4 to 5 days to avoid ergotamine rebound headache. The ergot derivative dihydroergotamine (DHE-45, Migranal NS) is available for intramuscular (IM), subcutaneous (SC), intravenous (IV), and intranasal use. IV dihydroergotamine (DHE-45) sometimes is used for intractable migraine (status migrainosis) in emergency departments and in-patient settings. The intranasal form (Migranal) is an effective treatment when administered correctly by the patient. Unfortunately, dihydroergotamine is not absorbed by the GI tract, and unlike other abortive nasal sprays, any swallowed medication will be wasted. Dihydroergotamine has a low headache recurrence rate of approximately 12%. All forms of ergotamine and dihydroergotamine are more effective when taken early in attacks.

Isometheptene is found in combination with dichloralphenazone and acetaminophen (Midrin, Duradrin). It is slow acting and more effective when taken early in attacks and for those attacks preceded or accompanied by stress and muscle tension of the neck. Although isometheptene is considered less potent than ergotamine and triptans, it is preferred by many patients whose headaches have features of both migraine and TTHA.

At the present time, seven serotonin agonists (triptans) are approved in the United States for abortive migraine treatment (see Table 1). As a category, the triptans are approximately 65% to 70% effective in published clinical trials. Their similarities are greater than their differences, but each triptan is not necessarily effective across all patients, and familiarity with their differences can be helpful to the treating physician. Half-life, onset and duration of action, adverse events, tolerability, recurrence of headache, and routes of administration may vary and allow the physician to match the medication to the individual patient. For example, a slower onset of action and longer lasting triptan may be appropriate for slow-onset, longer lasting migraine attacks.

Like other treatments, oral tablets of triptans are more effective in the early phases of migraines. It is thought that peripheral sensitization, allodynia, is a sign of later phase migraine, and treating before this phenomenon occurs is important. When there is a delay in treatment or the patient awakens with severe migraine, the injection, nasal spray, or rapidly acting triptans may be more beneficial. As a group, although very effective, recurrence of headache, after initial relief, requiring retreatment is common and can be as high as 40%. The recurrence rate tends to be less in triptans with a longer half-life.

The ergots and triptans are contraindicated in patients with ischemic heart disease, uncontrolled hypertension, and cerebrovascular disease. Physicians initially were

---

[1]Not FDA approved for this indication.

extremely cautious in recommending triptans for patients when they first were introduced in the United States. However, significant human exposure to the triptans reveal that catastrophic myocardial infarction or serious ischemia is rare. Chest pain following triptan use affects a small percentage of patients, and, although its significance is not always clear, refraining from future use is recommended.

Sumatriptan (Imitrex), the first triptan approved in the United States, is available in nasal spray (20 mg), SC (6 mg), and oral formulations (25, 50, 100 mg). The half-life is approximately 1.5 hours, and its duration of action is less than 4 hours. The injectable form produces rapid relief in 70% to 80% of patients and appears to be the most effective of all the available triptan forms. Conversely, it also appears to cause the most side effects, and for this reason, it should be used for the more severe attacks only. The oral forms are more favorable regarding adverse effects (AEs) and their effectiveness is similar to other triptans (approximately 65%). Because of sumatriptan's short half-life and duration of action, recurrence of headache is common, necessitating repeat dosing.

Zolmitriptan (Zomig) is available in 2.5- and 5-mg oral and oral disintegrating tablets (ZMT), and a 5-mg nasal spray. The efficacy of oral zolmitriptan is approximately 65% and 70% in the nasal form. Its half-life is 3 hours and its duration of action is longer, improving on the need to remedicate. The nasal spray form has a biphasic absorption curve, which accounts for a favorable AE profile over the 5-mg oral tablet.

Naratriptan (Amerge) was the first of the gradual onset, longer acting triptans. It is available in oral 2.5-mg tablets and has a half-life of 6 hours. Naratriptan is well tolerated by patients and often is used in patients with slow-onset migraine. Some specialists prescribe naratriptan daily for limited periods of time for menstrual or intractable migraine attacks.

Rizatriptan (Maxalt) is available orally in 5- and 10-mg tablets and an oral disintegrating form (MLT). It has a relatively rapid onset of action and a favorable one-dose 2-hour response rate. Patients who are simultaneously being treated with propranolol should take the lesser 5-mg dose because of a resultant increased rizatriptan plasma level.

Almotriptan (Axert) is available in 6.25- and 12.5-mg tablets. It has a half-life of 3.5 hours and, because of a broad T_{max} (time of maximal concentration) range of 1.4 to 3.8 hours, a relatively rapid onset of action. Almotriptan has a favorable adverse effect and headache recurrence profile. Chest pain symptoms after its use are similar to placebo in clinical trials.

Frovatriptan (Frova) is a long-acting triptan available in 2.5-mg oral tablets. It has the longest half-life of 25 hours and a favorable recurrence rate. Frovatriptan is frequently used in the treatment of menstrual migraine and in those who suffer attacks of longer duration. Some specialists use frovatriptan on a daily basis for a limited period of time for menstrual and prolonged migraine attacks.

Eletriptan (Relpax) is the most recently approved triptan. It is available in 20- and 40-mg oral tablets and has a half-life of nearly 5 hours. Eletriptan has a relatively rapid onset but a longer duration of action and a favorable recurrence rate. In studies, some patients respond to eletriptan when unresponsive to other triptans.

Various attempts were made to compare triptans. There have been head-to-head trials, but most involved one triptan compared to sumatriptan. A meta-analysis of 53 clinical trials was published in 2001 comparing efficacy, recurrence, duration of action, and tolerability of all available triptans. Almotriptan and eletriptan were rated favorably across the major parameters of onset of action, efficacy, adverse events, and recurrence. In spite of efforts to adjust for variations in protocols and placebo response, there is no clear consensus among specialists as to their validity or value.

NSAIDs frequently are recommended for acute migraine and can be effective when taken early. Their effects on the physiology of pain, inflammation, and platelets are believed to be the mechanisms involved. Various agents are used, and significant efficacy superiority does not appear to exist among the rapid-acting NSAIDs. The OTC ibuprofen (Motrin) and aspirin, in combination with caffeine and acetaminophen (Excedrin Migraine), carry migraine indications by the FDA.

The symptomatic treatment of pain may be necessary in patients who do not respond to recommended abortive treatment. Any effective analgesic can be appropriate, provided its use is infrequent and does not approach daily or near-daily frequency. In general, the more effective analgesics are those containing anti-inflammatory and sedative properties.

CLUSTER HEADACHE TREATMENT

Cluster headache is one of the more unusual pain conditions occasionally encountered by physicians. The pain onset is rapid and the duration of the attack is brief. For this reason, prophylactic treatment usually is the most practical. Abortive prescriptions frequently are given, but for most, by the time medication is absorbed, the cluster attack is resolving.

Nonmedicinal prophylactic measures are extremely limited. The reduction of cigarette smoking, the addressing of individual stress and hostility issues when appropriate, and complete cessation of alcohol during cluster periods should be a part of any treatment program. Prophylactic medications include the calcium channel blockers verapamil (Calan)[1] and nimodipine (Nimotop),[1] the neurostabilizers valproate (Depakote)[1] and topiramate (Topamax),[1] various NSAIDs, ergotamine (Ergomar),[1] lithium (Eskalith),[1] and, in extreme cases, steroids.[1] These medications are used in average therapeutic doses, and combinations of medications are commonly needed (Table 2). The preventatives should be used during the cluster cycle and discontinued during off-cycle periods.

Abortive treatment is less preferred for cluster headache, as already noted. However, inhalation oxygen via facial mask at 6 L terminates cluster attacks in 75%

[1]Not FDA approved for this indication.

TABLE 2 Cluster Headache Prophylactic Medications

Medication	Brand	Average daily dose
Verapamil[1]	Calan, Isoptin, Verelan	240-420 mg
Divalproex[1]	Depakote	500-1500 mg
Topiramate[1]	Topamax	50-200 mg
Indomethacin[1]	Indocin	100-150 mg
Naproxen[1]	Naprosyn	1000-1500 mg
Lithium[1]	Lithobid	600-1200 mg*
Ergotamine[1]	Bellergal[1]	1 tablet bid[†]
Prednisone[1]	—	100 mg, decrease to 0

[1]Not FDA approved for this indication.
*With serum level monitoring.
[†]0.6 mg ergotamine with phenobarbital 40 mg and 0.2 mg *l*-alkaloids of belladonna.

to 80% of sufferers within 12 minutes. Other possibilities include sumatriptans (Imitrex) SC or nasal spray,[1] zolmitriptan (Zomig) nasal spray,[1] or dihydroergotamine injection (DHE-45) or nasal spray (Migranal).[1] The occasional patient reports relief with the oral triptans or analgesics. When triptans, ergotamine, or analgesics are used, appropriate prescribing and frequency guidelines should be followed. In general, with the exception of oxygen, daily as-needed medications should be avoided.

Headache continues to present a challenging problem for clinicians as well as the suffering patient. In spite of recent treatment advances and more public awareness, millions continue to needlessly endure pain and debilitation. At first glance, the headache problem appears complex and difficult when in actuality, most sufferers experience straightforward, easily diagnosed headaches. The interested generalist or specialist who takes the time to elicit a careful history can establish the headache diagnosis and be able to direct a simple treatment plan that can make a tremendous difference in the headache sufferer's life.

REFERENCES

Astin JA, Ernst E: The effectiveness of spinal manipulation for the treatment of headache disorders: A systematic review of randomized clinical trials. Cephalalgia 2002;22:617-623.

Diamond and Dalessio's The Practicing Physician's Approach to Headache, 5th ed. Philadelphia, WB Saunders, 1999.

Ferrari MD, Roon KI, Lipton RB, et al: Oral triptans (serotonin 5HT-IB/ID-agonists) in acute migraine treatment: A meta-analysis of 53 trials. Lancet 2001;358:1668-1675.

Gallagher RM, Kunkel R: Migraine medication attributes important for patient compliance: Concerns about side effects may delay treatment. Headache: J Head Face Pain 2003;43(1):36-43.

Goadsby PJ, Lipton RB, Ferreri MD: Migraine current understanding and treatment. N Engl J Med 2002;346(4):257-270.

Vernon H, McDermaid C, Hagino C: Systematic review of randomized clinical trials of complementary/alternative therapies in the treatment of tension-type and cervicogenic headache. Complement Ther Med 1999;7:142-155.

Wolff's Headache and Other Head Pain, 7th ed. New York, Oxford University Press, 2001.

---

[1]Not FDA approved for this indication.

Viral Meningitis and Encephalitis

Method of
Bruce A. Cohen, MD

Viruses are the most common cause of central nervous system (CNS) infections in the United States. Most of the neurotropic viruses responsible for CNS infections may cause either meningitis or encephalitis in a given individual, and in some instances the features of both are combined as a meningoencephalitis. Susceptibility to particular agents and presentations may vary in hosts with immune deficiencies. In approaching a patient suspected to have a viral CNS infection, the physician must consider the clinical presentation, including extraneurologic findings, the season of the year, travel history, any potential environmental exposures, and the status of the patient's immune system.

Clinical Features

Viral meningitis typically presents with fever and headache associated with signs of meningeal irritation. Meningismus may be absent in immunosuppressed patients. Fatigue, malaise, photophobia, and myalgias are common. Features of a respiratory or gastrointestinal (GI) infection may precede or accompany the neurologic symptoms, including cough, chills, dyspnea, nausea, vomiting, or diarrhea. Irritability is common in infants and small children, and dehydration may lead to lethargy. In older children, adolescents, and adults, the sensorium is normal. Clues to specific agents may lie in the associated signs and symptoms of other organ system involvement, such as rash and cardiac or hepatic disease.

Viral encephalitis is a febrile illness associated with evidence of brain parenchymal dysfunction, typically including neurologic deficits such as weakness or sensory impairments, changes in sensorium and behavior, seizures, and ataxia in varying combinations. Some viral infections may be associated with a postinfectious encephalitis attributed to an immune response directed against the pathogen that cross-reacts to normal CNS proteins.

Etiologies

Enteroviruses (Picornaviridae), which include the echoviruses, coxsackieviruses, numbered enteroviruses, and the polioviruses, are the most common agents causing viral meningitis, accounting for more than 80% of cases. Human-to-human transmission usually occurs through fecal-oral contamination, although some strains may be acquired by inhalation of respiratory droplets. In the United States, the peak incidence for enterovirus infections is in the summer and early autumn. Epidemics may occur, and school-age children constitute the majority of cases, although all age groups are affected. Enterovirus 71 is seen in the Asian Pacific region where it causes hand, foot, and mouth disease and brainstem encephalitis.

Primary infection with enteroviruses occurs in the GI tract. Seeding of the CNS and other organs results from a viremia. A biphasic fever pattern may occur with initial constitutional symptoms followed by a period of improvement and then recurrent fever with the onset of neurologic symptoms. A variety of exanthems may be associated. Coxsackieviruses may cause concurrent myocarditis, pericarditis, pleurodynia, and conjunctivitis. Individuals with hypogammaglobulinemia may develop a chronic, recurrent meningoencephalitis, which may be associated with a dermatomyositis-like rheumatologic syndrome.

The most common cause of viral encephalitis is herpes simplex virus type 1 (HSV-1). A prodromal syndrome of behavior or personality change may evolve over days into fever, seizures, and cognitive and focal neurologic deficits with depressed sensorium. The disease occurs sporadically and has a predilection for the temporal lobes. Herpes simplex virus type 2 (HSV-2) most often causes meningitis, usually in the setting of concurrent genital infection. When associated with primary genital infection, urinary retention may occur. Both HSV-1 and HSV-2 are also associated with recurrent (Mollaret's) meningitis. Encephalitis caused by varicella-zoster virus (VZV) may be seen in association with primary infection (chickenpox) and in older individuals or those with compromised cell-mediated immunity. Reactivation of VZV infection in patients with impaired cell-mediated immunity may be associated with meningitis, meningomyelitis, or meningoencephalitis, which may occur in the absence of the typical dermatomal rash. Human herpesvirus 6 (HHV-6) causes exanthem subitum in infants and can cause meningitis and meningoencephalitis with associated febrile seizures. Other herpesviruses are less frequent causes of encephalitis in normal individuals, but they may cause meningitis or encephalitis in patients with AIDS, immunosuppression following organ or bone marrow transplantation, or treatment with myelosuppressive medications. Cytomegalovirus (CMV) in immunosuppressed patients may produce meningitis, meningomyeloradiculitis, or encephalitis and affect the retina, GI tract, lungs, and adrenal glands. Epstein-Barr virus (EBV) in AIDS patients is associated with primary CNS lymphoma and may be a cause of encephalitis or lymphoproliferative syndrome in immunosuppressed individuals. HSV-2, HHV-6, and HHV-7 are also reported as causes of encephalitis in transplant and AIDS patients.

Arboviruses comprise a variety of pathogens transmitted by arthropod vectors and therefore occur most frequently in summer and fall. The West Nile virus (WNV), a flavivirus with worldwide distribution carried by birds and spread to humans by mosquitoes, is the most prominent arbovirus in the United States. Transmission by blood transfusion and organ transplantation is also reported. Infants and individuals older than 50 years of age are at increased risk of encephalitis. A poliomyelitis that produces severe flaccid weakness

also occurs. Additional CNS syndromes are still being identified. Prodromal fever, headache, anorexia, nausea, vomiting, lymphadenopathy, myalgia, and a maculopapular or roseolar rash on the face and trunk may precede CNS disease.

St. Louis encephalitis (SLE), also a flavivirus, is found particularly in the central and western states but also occurs throughout North and South America. Encephalitis occurs in about half of infected patients and occurs more commonly in those over the age of 60. Neurologic symptoms may be preceded by a prodrome including malaise, fever, headache, myalgias, conjunctivitis, and upper respiratory tract symptoms. Powassan virus is a tick-borne flavivirus reported to cause occasional cases of encephalitis in New York and New England. Eastern equine encephalitis (EEE), a togavirus, is most prevalent in the Atlantic and Gulf of Mexico coastal regions of the United States. Prodromal symptoms include fever, headache, myalgia, lethargy, vomiting, and abdominal pain. Seizures are common and hyponatremia may be seen. Reported mortality is high, with neurologic sequelae in many survivors. Western equine encephalitis (WEE) is found in the western United States and Canada and is currently an infrequent cause of encephalitis. The La Crosse virus (LACV) is found in the midwestern and mid-Atlantic states and typically affects children and adolescents. Seizures occur in half the cases, and focal findings may be present with changes on electroencephalogram (EEG) resembling those found in HSV-1 encephalitis. Japanese encephalitis virus (JEV) is one of the most important pathogens causing encephalitis worldwide. Currently it is primarily found in southern and east Asia with occasional cases in the Philippines and Pacific Islands. Clinical features include headaches, nausea, vomiting, behavioral changes, altered sensorium, and seizures. Tremor, choreoathetosis, rigidity, and flaccid paralysis may also be seen. The disease strikes healthy children and young adults, with mortality rates of up to 33% of cases and significant neurologic sequelae in a high proportion of survivors. Nipah virus (NV) occurs in pigs and recently caused epidemic encephalitis in pig farmers in Malaysia. Cerebellar and brainstem signs and segmental myoclonus are described.

Mumps, a paramyxovirus, is infrequently seen in the United States today; however, meningitis is the most frequent neurologic manifestation. Infection results from inhalation of respiratory droplets and spreads hematogenously. Parotitis is typical, but myocarditis, orchitis, oophoritis, and pancreatitis may also be associated.

Lymphocytic choriomeningitis virus (LCMV) is an arenavirus transmitted by rodents and may infect field mice, rats, and hamsters. Transmission to humans may occur by exposure to rodent urine through contaminated food or open wounds, and it may affect individuals living in less hygienic impoverished conditions or who own or work with rodents. The peak incidence occurs in winter. Myocarditis, pericarditis, orchitis, or arthritis may be associated.

A reovirus, which causes Colorado tick fever, is transmitted by a wood tick found in mountainous areas in the western United States. Meningitis is associated with retro-orbital pain and, in some cases, a macular rash. Leukopenia and thrombocytopenia are common, and bleeding complications may result.

Acute infection with HIV may be associated with meningitis as part of a mononucleosis syndrome. JC virus (JCV) infects oligodendrocytes and causes progressive multifocal leukoencephalopathy in immunosuppressed individuals, most commonly in AIDS. Rarely, influenza types A and B may cause encephalitis. Influenza A is associated with particularly aggressive necrotizing encephalitis. Rabies is rare in the United States where isolated cases of encephalitis are linked to bat bites.

Postinfectious encephalomyelitis is an acute demyelinating disease that may follow infection with an enterovirus, influenza virus, measles virus, or herpesvirus. It may also be seen following vaccination. Multifocal neurologic symptoms and signs, headache, seizures, or depressed sensorium appear within weeks of the preceding infection or vaccination. The illness is monophasic and may resolve with or without neurologic sequelae.

Diagnosis

A variety of conditions that may mimic viral meningitis or encephalitis need to be excluded in the diagnostic evaluation (Boxes 1 and 2).

Magnetic resonance imaging (MRI) is the imaging study of choice. In viral meningitis, MRI is usually normal, although nonspecific enhancement of meninges is seen following gadolinium contrast infusion. In HSV-1

encephalitis, MRI reveals a lesion with increased signal on T2 sequences and enhancement following gadolinium contrast infusion on T1 sequences, usually in the medial and inferior temporal lobe. In WNV and CMV encephalitis, enhancement of meninges or ventricular ependyma and, in some cases of WNV, lesions in the basal ganglia and thalami may be seen. White matter lesions are found with VZV, JCV, and NV.

Cerebrospinal fluid (CSF) is the most useful examination in evaluating patients with meningitis and encephalitis, and it is important both to exclude alternative conditions and attempt to establish a specific etiologic diagnosis. CSF typically reveals a lymphocytic pleocytosis with less than 1000 cells/mm^3, although higher cell counts are seen with some arboviruses. An early polymorphonuclear response may be found in the first 24 hours, and CMV is associated with a persistent polymorphonuclear pleocytosis in immunosuppressed individuals. Protein is usually elevated but may be normal in some patients with meningitis. Glucose levels are generally normal but may be depressed with LCMV, mumps, and the herpesviruses. The most sensitive and specific technique for viral diagnosis is detection of genetic material using polymerase chain reaction (PCR) amplification techniques. For RNA viruses, reverse transcriptase PCR (RT-PCR) is used. In HSV-1 encephalitis, PCR eliminates the need for brain biopsy in most cases.

Demonstration of virus-specific IgM responses in blood or CSF or of fourfold elevations of specific IgG in convalescent serum samples, compared to acute, are alternative ways of establishing an etiologic diagnosis. Diagnosis of WNV is established by finding specific IgM in CSF, which appears by the end of the first week. WNV RNA can also be detected by RT-PCR. IgM antibodies to WNV may persist in serum for up to 6 months. IgG antibodies to WNV appear after a week and rise in

---

BOX 1 Differential Diagnosis of Viral Meningitis

Bacterial meningitis
Parameningeal infections
  Sinusitis
  Paravertebral abscess
Fungal meningitis
Mycobacterium tuberculosis meningitis
Lymphomatous and carcinomatous meningitis
Syphilis
Lyme disease
Leptospirosis
Parasitic meningoencephalitis
Subarachnoid hemorrhage
Dural sinus thrombosis
Noninfectious inflammatory diseases
  Sarcoidosis
  Systemic lupus erythematosus
  Behçet's disease
  Vasculitis
Drug-induced meningitis
  Nonsteroidal anti-inflammatory agents
  Muromonab-CD3 (OKT-3)
  Sulfonamides
  Intravenous immunoglobulin
  Carbamazepine (Tegretol)
  COX-2 inhibitors
  Metronidazole (Flagyl)

BOX 2 Differential Diagnosis of Viral Encephalitis

Bacterial abscesses
Subdural empyema
Brain tumors
Mycobacterium tuberculosis
Fungal infection
Parasitic infections
Rickettsia
Drug intoxication
Delirium tremens
Malignant hyperthermia
Metabolic diseases
  Thyroid disease
  Electrolyte disorders
  Hyperglycemia, hypoglycemia
  Hypoxia
Vasculitis
Subdural hematoma
Multiple cerebral infarctions
Syphilis
Sarcoidosis
Paraneoplastic encephalitis
Acute psychosis

---

serum but may cross-react with SLE or JEV. Thus they must be confirmed with a more specific test such as a plaque neutralization assay. Diagnosis of other arbovirus infections is based on findings of virus-specific IgM antibody in CSF, a fourfold rise in titer of specific viral antibodies in serum, or isolation of the pathogen. Antibodies are less useful for herpesvirus infections; in HSV-1 they are not found in the CSF until 10 to 14 days following onset of infection. Enteroviruses may be isolated from stool or throat cultures; however, because viral shedding may persist for weeks after active infection, recovery from these sites is inconclusive unless virus is also recovered from blood or CSF. PCR testing is available for enteroviruses. It has been advocated, despite the benign natural history of enterovirus meningitis in most cases, as cost-effective in reducing duration of hospitalization and antibiotic therapy.

In patients with postinfectious encephalitis, CSF reveals a lymphocytic pleocytosis, normal glucose, elevated protein, and myelin basic protein, sometimes with oligoclonal bands.

Electroencephalography may reveal periodic lateralized epileptiform discharges in patients with HSV-1 or LACV, but it is most commonly nonspecific. Brain biopsy

is less often pursued because of the availability of PCR; however, when a lesion is identified and no specific diagnosis established, tissue sampling may still be required. Boxes 3 and 4 list diagnostic studies.

Treatment

In the immunocompetent individual, most episodes of viral meningitis are self-limited and benign in their outcome. Coverage with a third-generation cephalosporin such as ceftriaxone (Rocephin), 2 g every 12 hours, or cefotaxime (Claforan), 2 g every 6 hours, and vancomycin, 500 to 750 mg every 6 hours, should be initiated until bacterial meningitis is excluded. Ampicillin may be added if *Listeria monocytogenes* is of concern. Treatment is supported by administering analgesics and antipyretics,

---

BOX 3 Evaluation of Suspected Viral Meningitis

Cerebrospinal fluid studies
 Opening pressure
 Cell count and differential
 Glucose with matching serum glucose
 VDRL or FTA-ABS
 Gram stain and bacterial culture
 Acid-fast culture and smear, PCR for *Mycobacterium tuberculosis*
 Fungal culture and India ink
 Cryptococcal antigen
 Cytology
 PCR for HSV-1, HSV-2, EBV, VZV, CMV
 RT-PCR for enteroviruses and West Nile virus
Blood studies
 Cultures
 CBC
 Sedimentation rate
 Electrolytes
 Glucose
 Thyroid-stimulating hormone
 Hepatic and renal chemistries
 HIV-1 serology
 Antinuclear antibodies
 VDRL or FTA-ABS
 Protein electrophoresis
 Acute and convalescent serologies for arboviruses and enteroviruses
 Serology for borella burdorferi (Lyme disease)
Urine drug screen
MRI if indicated to exclude a parameningeal focus, dural venous thrombosis

Abbreviations: CBC = complete blood count; CMV = Cytomegalovirus; EBV = Epstein-Barr virus; FTA-ABS = fluorescent treponemal antibody absorption (test); HSV = herpes simplex virus; MRI = magnetic resonance imaging; PCR = polymerase chain reaction; RT-PRC = reverse transcriptase polymerase chain reaction; VDRL = Venereal Disease Research Laboratory (test); VZV = varicella-zoster virus.

BOX 4 Evaluation of Suspected Viral Encephalitis

Brain MRI
 Cerebrospinal fluid
 Cell count and differential
 Glucose with matching serum glucose
 Protein
 Mycobacterium tuberculosis culture, smear, and PCR
 Fungal culture and antigen studies
 Gram stain and bacterial studies
 VDRL
 Cytology
 PCR studies for HSV-1, CMV, VZV, EBV, HHV-6, HSV-2, JCV
 RT-PCR for West Nile virus, enteroviruses as indicated
 Antibody studies for arboviruses
 Borrelia burgdorferi antibodies (Lyme disease)
 If suspected postinfectious encephalitis: IgG index and oligoclonal bands with matching serum samples
Blood studies
 Serologies for arboviruses, *Toxoplasma gondii,* HIV-1
 Cultures
 CBC
 Sedimentation rate
 Hepatic and renal chemistries
 Electrolytes
 Thyroid-stimulating hormones
 VDRL or FTA-ABS
 Antinuclear antibodies
 Angiotensin-converting enzyme
 Protein electrophoresis
 Paraneoplastic antibody panel
Chest radiograph
Urine toxicology screen
EEG
Imaging of other symptomatic organ systems as indicated
In selected instances, brain biopsy

Abbreviations: CBC = complete blood count; CMV = Cytomegalovirus; EBV = Epstein-Barr virus; EEG = electroencephalogram; FTA-ABS = fluorescent treponemal antibody absorption (test); HHV = human herpesvirus; HSV = herpes simplex virus; JCV = JC virus; MRI = magnetic resonance imaging; PCR = polymerase chain reaction; VDRL = Venereal Disease Research Laboratory (test); VZV = varicella-zoster virus.

14

CURRENT DIAGNOSIS

- Viral meningitis is a syndrome of headache and fever usually with accompanying neck stiffness.
- Viral encephalitis may present with combinations of fever, headache, seizures, confusion or obtundation, and focal neurologic deficits.
- Herpes encephalitis may begin with behavioral or personality changes followed by fever and neurologic symptoms.
- Clues to the specific diagnosis of viral meningitis and encephalitis may reside in the history of environmental exposures through residence, seasonal occurrence, or travel.
- Accompanying symptoms indicating extraneurologic organ system involvement may also provide clues to the etiologic diagnosis.
- Postinfectious encephalitis typically follows a prodromal infection within weeks.
- In patients who are immunosuppressed, diagnosis may be more difficult because of the absence of common features related to the inflammatory response.
- The most sensitive imaging test for patients with encephalitis is magnetic resonance imaging.
- The most used test for specific etiologic diagnosis is sampling of cerebrospinal fluid, including polymerase chain reaction amplification assays for viral genetic material.

CURRENT THERAPY

- Specific antiviral therapy is currently limited to agents from the herpesvirus family.
- Acyclovir is the treatment of choice for HSV-1 and HSV-2 and is usually effective also for herpes zoster.
- CMV, HSV-6, and acyclovir-resistant herpes zoster is treated with ganciclovir, foscarnet, or cidofovir, sometimes in combination for immunosuppressed patients with encephalitis.
- Patients with postinfectious encephalitis are typically treated with high-dose steroids.
- Supportive therapy includes treatment for seizures, respiratory compromise, increased intracranial pressure (when required), prophylaxis for deep vein thrombophlebitis, protection against decubitus ulceration, and management of fluids, nutrition, and electrolyte balance.
- Early initiation of passive and, when possible, active physical and occupational therapy may mitigate risk of later contractures.

Abbreviations: CMV = cytomegalovirus; HSV = herpes simplex virus (types 1, 2, 6).

and, particularly in infants and young children, monitoring fluid and electrolyte balance. Pain may be treated with nonsteroidal anti-inflammatory drugs (NSAIDs) and amitriptyline (Elavil) or other tricyclic agents. Although not FDA approved for this use, many physicians combine anticonvulsant agents such as gabapentin (Neurontin), carbamazepine (Tegretol), or lamotrigine (Lamictal) with tricyclics or NSAIDS. In cases of severe pain, short-term use of opiates such as hydrocodone (Norco, Vicodin) may be required. Antiviral therapy is available for the herpesviruses, and acyclovir (Zovirax), 200 mg five times daily, or valacyclovir (Valtrex), 1000 mg twice daily, may be given to immunocompetent patients with HSV-2 meningitis complicating genital infection. In immunocompromised patients, HSV-2 meningitis should be treated with high-dose intravenous acyclovir, as described later for HSV-1 encephalitis.

Acyclovir (Zovirax) is specific therapy for HSV-1 encephalitis in doses of 10 mg/kg intravenously every 8 hours for 14 to 21 days. A similar course of therapy can be used for VZV encephalitis. CMV or HHV-6 meningoencephalitis in immunosuppressed individuals who are not responsive to acyclovir can be treated initially in individuals with normal renal function using ganciclovir (Cytovene), 5 mg/kg every 12 hours; foscarnet (Foscavir), 90 mg/kg every 12 hours; or for CMV, once-weekly cidofovir (Vistide), 5 mg/kg given over 1 hour intravenously in conjunction with 2 g probenecid 3 hours before, and 1 g of probenecid 2 and 8 hours following

the infusion. Following successful induction, doses are lowered for maintenance therapy. Careful monitoring of hepatic and renal function is required for all of these agents. Individuals taking cidofovir must have regular monitoring of ocular pressure to prevent blindness related to hypotony. Although no controlled trials are available, some authors recommend initial combined therapy with both ganciclovir and foscarnet in AIDS patients with CMV encephalitis.

Pleconaril is an antiviral agent with efficacy against enteroviruses. Although not currently released for use in the United States, it has efficacy for life-threatening enteroviral infections. Ribavirin inhibits WNV and LACV in vitro and is being investigated for therapeutic use. No specific treatment is currently available for other viral encephalitides.

Most neurologists treat patients with postinfectious encephalomyelitis with intravenous methylprednisolone (Solu-Medrol) in typical doses of 1000 mg daily for 5 days, followed by an oral tapering dose, although no controlled trial as yet supports efficacy.

Supportive measures include anticonvulsants to control seizures, control of increased intracranial pressure when required using mannitol, 0.25 to 0.5 g/kg every 3 to 4 hours (adjusting the dose to maintain serum osmolality to between 300 and 320 mOsm/L), management of fluid and electrolyte balance, assisted ventilation as required, prophylaxis for deep vein thrombophlebitis, nutritional support, early initiation of physical therapy to prevent contracture formation, prophylaxis for decubitus, and hygienic measures to limit complicating secondary infections. When the patient is sufficiently stable, more aggressive cognitive and physical rehabilitation measures are initiated.

REFERENCES

Cinque P, Bossolasco S, Lundkvist A: Molecular analysis of cerebrospinal fluid in viral diseases of the central nervous system. J Clin Virol 2003;26:1-28.

Debiasi RL, Tyler KL: Molecular methods for diagnosis of viral encephalitis. Clin Microbiol Rev 2004;17:903-925.

Johnson RT: Emerging viral infections of the nervous system. J Neurovirol 2004;9:140-147.

Kennedy PG: Viral encephalitis: Causes, differential diagnosis, and management. J Neurol Neurosurg Psychiatry 2004;75(Suppl 1): i10-i15.

Romero JR, Newland JG: Viral meningitis and encephalitis: Traditional and emerging viral agents. Semin Pediatr Infect Dis 2003;14:72-82.

Tyler K: Herpes simplex virus infections of the central nervous system: Encephalitis and meningitis, including Mollaret's. Herpes 2004;11(Suppl 2):57A-64A.

Multiple Sclerosis

Method of
Randall T. Schapiro, MD

Multiple sclerosis (MS) has been called a primary demyelinating disease of the central nervous system, but that is somewhat inaccurate. Charcot's description of MS included damage to the axon, which has been especially emphasized in the past decade. Today MS is described not only as a disease of myelin, but also of the cell that makes myelin (oligodendrocyte) and also the axon. All these are primary targets in the destructive process that appears to be directed by the immune system, and thus MS is more properly called an immune-mediated disorder. The immune system can cause direct destruction and inflammation. It also can program the targets (cells, axons) to self-destruct over time (apoptosis).

The pathology of MS has been elucidated more thoroughly in the past several years thanks to international projects that began with descriptions of biopsied specimens from brain lesions of patients with the disease. Some individuals had a high involvement of the immune system; a minority had less. Four different varieties are separable. These types (I through IV) provide a way to separate the disease potentially into different categories. This combination of possibilities puts MS into both the inflammatory and degenerative categories. Much work is left to do in this area, but in the next decade treatments may be dictated by the variety of pathologic processes occurring as the disease changes over time.

While describing MS at a microscopic level, it is easy to lose sight of the fact that, at a global level, it is a disease of people with all of their complexities. The person with MS is typically diagnosed early in the third decade of life and has a family, work, and responsibilities in the community, making this potentially disabling disease one of the most important acquired, nontraumatic neurologic diseases in the world.

Rakel and Bope: *Conn's Current Therapy 2006.*

Relative to the past, MS today is a disease with very active treatment strategies aimed in three general directions. The ideal goal is to slow or stop the disease itself. Disease management is now routine, with five Federal Drug Administration (FDA)-approved medications available to slow MS. Symptom management remains one of the principal directions of treatment in MS. Superimposed on these two very obvious directions is the psychological support necessary to keep people with neurologic dysfunction performing at their highest level. The psychological area is often ignored in the office but is of equal importance in offering a quality of life for those with the disease.

Etiology

The cause of multiple sclerosis remains unknown. Despite numerous advances, the discussion of MS causation has changed little in the past decade. No simple explanation is available for why MS occurs. For more than 40 years, a population gradient to MS has been understood. As one moves away from the equator north and south, the number of MS cases increases. Much of that may be because of the ethnic origin of the people in those areas. They tend to be northern European and Scandinavian, but migration studies demonstrate that the disease spreads beyond ethnic backgrounds when generations remain in the targeted geographic regions. Studies in the Faeroe and Shetland/Orkney islands off the coast of Scotland and other regions give credence to the possibility of a viral or other infectious influence. Despite decades of modern viral isolation techniques, no virus has stood the test of time in MS. Each decade has produced its own target virus. In the 1970s, it was the measles virus, in the 1980s, the herpesvirus, and in the 1990s, the retroviruses of tropical spastic paraparesis. Then, one after another, the human herpesvirus type 6 and the chlamydia bacteria were implicated. None appeared conclusive, although many continue under investigation.

What does seem clear is the involvement of the immune system in MS. The understanding of the influence of the immune system continues to evolve as newer and better techniques to explore this complex area develop. MS is now described as an immune-mediated disease to distinguish it from a classic autoimmune disease. The immune system clearly is more active toward a central nervous system antigen. Just what that antigen is remains mysterious, but several candidates have emerged, including myelin and it components, the oligodendrocyte, the axon, and other surrounding tissues and cells. For the immune system to attack the nervous system, something must trigger it. That is likely the environmental influence, and after it is programmed to attack a nervous system element, it must make its way through the blood–brain barrier to find the target. It is the very complexity of the process that may make it susceptible to intervention. Strategies are being or have been developed to interfere with the initial reaction of the antigen-presenting cell (macrophage) to the antigen, the passage through the blood-brain barrier, and the reaction once in the central nervous system.

14

The immune system appears to be the genetic link in MS. Although MS is said to be nonhereditary, it clearly has a genetic component. The likelihood of getting MS with no one in the family having it is approximately 0.2%. If a parent has the disease and the child is a girl, the risk jumps to 3% to 4%. If the child is a boy, the risk is 2%. If an identical twin has MS, the risk to the sibling is 30%. But if MS were wholly a hereditary disease, it would be 100%.

Thus the cause of MS is unknown, but it must be a multifactorial process. It takes a susceptible individual who has an immune system capable of being genetically stimulated by an exogenous factor, and all these factors must be at the right time in the right place.

Course of the Disease

The disease has numerous presentations. Virtually any symptom that can result from an irritated central nervous system may be present in MS. Fatigue is the single most common symptom, but numbness, tingling, dizziness, visual distortion, weakness, clumsiness, pain, urinary, bowel, sexual, and psychological effects are often present as well. The course of MS is also very unpredictable and variable. Today MS is divided into four broad categories. Approximately 80% of MS begins with a fluctuating course with relapses of neurologic deficit followed by periods of relative quiet, termed *relapsing-remitting MS.*

Over time, half of those untreated with relapsing-remitting MS stop fluctuating and slowly get worse. This is called *secondary progressive MS.* If the course of secondary progressive MS fluctuates, it is called *secondary progressive with relapses.* The common feature of the progressive variety is that it progresses between relapses if relapses are present.

Approximately 10% of MS gets worse from the beginning, which is called *primary progressive,* and approximately 5% begins progressive and then has a relapse or two and is labeled *progressive-relapsing.*

Even though MS is divided into categories, it remains MS, which is especially true of the relapsing-remitting and secondary progressive types that are almost certainly the same process. Primary progressive and progressive-relapsing may be variants, but the two of them are also almost certainly the same process.

Approximately 20% of people with MS do fairly well, with their disease accumulating little disability over time, even untreated. The exact number is controversial, but even autopsy studies demonstrate repeatedly that MS appears without clinical evidence much more than would be expected. Those autopsied died from other causes and did not even recognize they had MS.

Many experts believe MS is a spectrum of diseases that appear clinically similar. Little actual data support the theory, but in the past few years when researchers at the Mayo Clinic, together with many others around the world, looked at biopsied specimens of lesions that turned out to be MS, they saw great variability among them. This discovery has prompted a new classification based on the pathology that divides MS into four broad categories. At one end is a very immunologically based pathology, at the other end is a very degenerative pathology, and in between are two that blend between the extremes. Thus MS is highly diverse, both clinically and pathologically, and yet there is also much similarity.

Diagnosis

Under normal circumstances, MS typically is not difficult to diagnose when following simple clinical dictums. There are three criteria in the clinical diagnosis of MS:

1. The person should be relatively young, between the ages of 15 and 55 years.
2. She or he should have neurologic symptoms that fluctuate.
3. The neurologic examination should demonstrate multiple abnormalities within the central nervous system, hence the name *multiple* sclerosis.

Other obvious reasons for the clinical picture should be ruled out, and then the diagnosis of MS can be made very accurately. Schumacher codified these criteria in the 1970s before the days of elaborate testing. When evoked potentials and spinal fluid tests became more accurate, Poser and his committee added the use of those modalities to allow for a diagnosis when a clinical piece is missing. Magnetic resonance imaging (MRI) advanced the cause rapidly, allowing for more precision in diagnosis, and recently the McDonald committee added its use to speed the diagnostic process. The MRI scan has to show significant specific abnormalities to be substituted for a clinical loss, and to be effective, all these criteria still depend on the initial clinical presentation.

Despite the emphasis on the clinical picture in diagnosing MS, laboratory testing continues to play a role in confirming the diagnosis. Evoked potentials are electrical potentials stimulated within the brain by a stimulus (visual, auditory, or somatosensory). They can be measured via electrodes placed on the scalp. With the aid of computerized signal averaging, normal transmission can be separated from abnormal, thus extending the neurologic examination to find more subtle abnormalities of the sensory system. The spinal fluid can be analyzed in a very sophisticated way for immune abnormalities. Detection of unique oligoclonal banding in the IgG spectrum is characteristic of MS. Increased production of IgG and the presence of myelin basic protein are also common.

Blood (and sometimes cerebrospinal fluid) should be analyzed to eliminate mimicking diseases such as lupus, Sjögren's, sarcoid, B_{12} deficiency, Lyme disease, vasculitis, and other autoimmune processes.

Management

The complexity and variability of multiple sclerosis make it a classic example of a disease best managed by a team approach. The team may require participation from physicians, nurses, rehabilitation professionals, psychologists, and social workers. The extent of participation should be determined by the complexity of the individual situation. It is not necessary or appropriate for all professionals to be involved with all patients, but an educated team makes the management of complicated patients much more effective.

With the advent of immune-modulating medication, treatment has expanded greatly. These medications have revolutionized the medical approach toward the disease, but their expense and their lack of total efficacy must be taken into consideration when determining their use.

It is abundantly clear that patients cannot get back what is lost in the destruction of the central nervous system. Thus the goal of management is to prevent loss and maintain function. In MS the immune system becomes programmed to attack the myelin, oligodendrocyte, or other nerve component. Whether that programming antigen is a virus or other stimulus does not change the fact that an antigen-presenting cell (usually a macrophage) engulfs the antigen and presents it. This causes a stimulation of T-helper cells, which separate into the highly inflammatory Th1 and the anti-inflammatory Th2 cells. In MS there is a shift of the balance, with increased Th1 allowing for increased destruction. The programmed cells then cross the blood–brain barrier looking for the part of the nervous system that resembles their programming. Stopping this from occurring has become the principal treatment strategy. The interferons appear to keep the flow of Th1 cells from crossing the blood–brain barrier, thus decreasing their likelihood of destruction. Glatiramer acetate appears to cross the barrier and stimulate increased Th2 production, changing the balance of immune regulation toward a more modulating course. Another agent awaiting approval (Natalizumab, Antegren) works to shore up the blood–brain barrier by preventing it transport across via inhibition of adhesion molecule movement.

Keeping an activated immune system from getting to the myelinated central fibers appears to slow the process of demyelination in MS. Therefore the principle of treatment in MS today revolves around immune modulation. Over the past dozen years more scientifically proven treatments for MS have evolved than in all other years combined. Today five FDA-approved medications are available.

Interferons are proteins that the body makes in response to a foreign stimulation. Thus with a viral infection the body makes interferons that modulate the immune system. The three main categories of interferon are alfa (α), beta (β), and gamma (γ). Interferon γ stimulates the immune system and makes MS worse, whereas interferon β calms the system down and decreases attack rates, increases the time between attacks, and decreases the damage seen on MRI scans.

Studies done in various ways show approximately one third of the attacks in an actively affected MS population can be diminished during the first 2 years. The preponderance of information leads to the conclusion that the higher the dose of interferon, the more potent the response. Many studies show that in the appropriate person, with the appropriate dose, interferons change the course of the disease. The potent anti-inflammatory effects of interferons have a dramatic effect on the MRI, with a decrease in T2 and T1 contrast-enhancing lesions.

These human gene interferons come in two formulations: interferon beta-1a (Avonex, Rebif) made in a hamster and interferon beta-1b (Betaseron) made in bacteria. The recommended doses of Rebif and Betaseron appear to be equivalent (three to four times per week); that of Avonex is significantly lower (once per week).

Glatiramer acetate is a polypeptide that appears to fool the immune system. As noted earlier, it shifts the Th1-Th2 balance toward the Th2. Appearing to mimic myelin, it may also decrease the attack by blocking the cells headed toward myelin and preventing damage. It, too, appears to decrease attack rates by approximately a third in the first 2 years of use.

All of these medications are administered parentally. They all have side effects and are all costly. The β-interferons may be toxic to the blood and liver and can exaggerate depression in a susceptible individual that is generally mild but should be monitored. Glatiramer acetate has less toxicity but can cause a systemic reaction that mimics a heart attack, although it is not, and clears in 20 minutes. Although rare, this reaction can be frightening. All of the drugs can produce skin reactions except for the intermuscular interferon beta-1a (Avonex).

All of these agents were studied in the relapsing forms of MS. Although this does not preclude effectiveness in more progressive forms, there is a paucity of data for that use. Clinical experience, together with evidence-based data, gives a picture of the high-dose interferons having the most potent effect, followed by glatiramer acetate, and then low-dose interferon.

Based on the aggressiveness of the MS and the lifestyle of the patient, the physician should select the agent. The goal must include maintaining the person on the medication and preventing noncompliance. Although patients must be included in the decision making, they should not be given the choice without a recommendation from the health professional. Many neurologists tend to abdicate the decision making to patients, who are not prepared to make such a decision.

Knowing that approximately 20% of patients do well without treatment and many more do well for a significant period of time without treatment begs the question of how early to treat. As stated earlier, it is impossible to retrieve damaged neurons consistently. The issue is whether to treat 100% of patients with MS immediately at the time of diagnosis if only 80% will need to be treated eventually. If the drugs were curative, time limited, or inexpensive, all would agree on treating all patients. Given the fact they are not, who should be treated and when is an issue.

All experts agree that early treatment is necessary, but the question is how to define "early." Much controversy surrounds the question of whether it is advisable to wait and see into what group an individual falls. Studies on so-called pre-MS, what is called the "clinically isolated syndrome," do not answer the question. The clinically isolated syndrome is a first attack, usually accompanied by an abnormal MRI. Two attacks are required for diagnosis. Studies clearly show that the second attack, leading to the diagnostic label, can be delayed by treatment, but that says nothing about long-term disability. This dilemma is especially pertinent because often the disease quiets after diagnosis and can go decades or more before reactivating. Attempts to look at that issue scientifically have come up short. The CHAMPS (Controlled High Risk Avonex Multiple Sclerosis) study looked at people with a first attack who did not meet the criteria for clinically definite MS. The study showed that the immune treatment (interferon beta-1a [Avonex]) did delay the second attack, but it says nothing about whether such early treatment changes disability later in life, a very important question that remains unanswered. A European study (ETOMS [Early Treatment of MS] with interferon beta-1a [Rebif]) leaves the same question.

Prognostic indicators can help predict whether a more aggressive course is impending. A large burden of disease on initial MRI scanning and the presence of weakness, ataxia, cognitive problems, frequent attacks, and spinal cord symptoms all point to a worse prognosis and should lead to earlier treatment. Numbness, tingling, blurred vision, dizziness, pain, and fatigue do not usually evolve into the more aggressive forms of MS, and immediate treatment may not be as necessary. All experts agree with the National Multiple Sclerosis Society's practice guideline, which states that if the disease is *active,* treatment should be instituted with one of the four agents.

Thus prevention is the key, but despite best efforts, breakthrough attacks do occur. People, treated or untreated, may develop new symptomatology, which is deemed a relapse. The use of the potent anti-inflammatory cortisone agents has been used to settle attacks for many decades. There are many regimens that individual experts use depending on the severity of the attack. If the attack is relatively minor and not encroaching on function, a hand-holding approach with no steroids is recommended. If the attack is slightly more severe, two dose packs of methylprednisolone may be given simultaneously. If the attack is even more severe with increased disability, 1000 mg of methylprednisolone may be administered each day for 3 to 5 days. If the attack is such that aggressive inpatient rehabilitation is warranted, a dose of dexamethasone beginning at 64 mg with a taper over 1 week is given. After either the outpatient high-dose or the inpatient high-dose steroid plan, a 1-month taper of oral methylprednisolone is included. All of these are based on experience rather than evidence-based data.

Once the decision is made that the person has active disease, requiring ongoing immunomodulation, a decision about which agent to use becomes paramount. If the disease is highly inflammatory with aggressive relapses and/or MRI evidence of blood–brain barrier breakdown (contrast-enhancing lesions), a high-dose β-interferon is used. If the person's lifestyle cannot tolerate that, an adjustment of medication to a less anti-inflammatory agent (glatiramer acetate or interferon beta-1a, at a lower dose) is suggested. If the disease is less aggressive but the patient is experiencing much depression, glatiramer is preferred. The use of medication is not random but represents the best fit of the drug to the situation. This is with the understanding that high-dose interferon β (Betaseron, Rebif) is the most potent, with glatiramer acetate (Copaxone) following and low-dose interferon beta-1a (Avonex) next.

If the disease cannot be controlled with the four immunomodulating medications, as seen by ongoing progression of disability with continued relapses, immunosuppression with mitoxantrone (Novantrone) is administered. The MRI scan can be of some help in the decision making but correlates poorly with the clinical picture. Thus it should not be the most important factor in decision making. Mitoxantrone is administered intravenously in a regimen of 12 mg/m². There is a total lifetime dose of 140 mg/m² before heart damage becomes a major concern. Examination of the heart at appropriate levels for ejection fraction and function is necessary. A typical course is 1 year of therapy and then continued evaluations without further mitoxantrone until (or if) progression resumes.

The use of oral immune suppressants including azathioprine (Imuron) and methotrexate (Rheumotrex) were more popular before the newer agents became available. They are still used as adjunct therapy in difficult cases of progressive disease.

Natalizumab (Tysabri, previously called Antegren) is a monoclonal antibody that prevents immune cells from moving from the blood to the central nervous system by blocking integrin, the adhesion molecule. It was originally approved by the FDA on the basis of impressive data obtained in the first year of a 2-year study. There is a dramatic lowering of relapse rate and a significant decrease in MRI activity. This treatment is a once-monthly intravenous infusion. Two large studies were conducted. One was Tysabri versus placebo and the second was Tysabri plus Avonex versus placebo plus Avonex. Unfortunately, shortly after release of the treatment by the FDA, two cases of progressive multifocal leukoencephalopathy (PML) were recognized in the Avonex plus Tysabri group, and these people died. As a result, the distribution of Tysabri was halted pending further evaluation.

Studies on intense immunosuppression with bone marrow transplantation (autologous and stem cell) continue but are not positive enough to recommend its use.

Despite the time, effort, and success given to slow the disease, the bulk of a clinician's time with multiple sclerosis is devoted to symptomatic management. The tools available include pharmacologic, rehabilitative, and psychological approaches. Fatigue is the single most common and most disabling symptom seen in MS. Five different "fatigues" are apparent in MS: normal, neuromuscular, deconditioning, fatigue of depression, and lassitude (MS-related fatigue). Normal fatigue is the same that occurs in everyone who tires after working hard. Neuromuscular fatigue is the tiring of muscles when they are required for activities such as walking. The fatigue of deconditioning is the result of a lack of sufficient activity to maintain endurance. Depression can result in poor sleep and ongoing fatigue. The most common fatigue is a tiredness that occurs without significant activity. It comes on spontaneously and is likely the result of a neurochemical imbalance in the brain. Neurochemically active drugs including amantadine and modafinil are helpful in its management.

Occupational therapy can teach energy conservation and improve activities of daily living to increase efficiency and decrease fatigue. In managing fatigue the health professional must rule out a sleep disturbance or other contributing confounding problem and then develop a plan based on the specific fatigue present.

Spasticity is managed with a multicentered approach. Noxious stimuli are minimized initially because they can increase muscle tone. An exercise program emphasizing stretching and range of motion is instituted. If more management is necessary, baclofen, tizanidine, benzodiazepines, and gabapentin may be added to appropriate doses. Failing all of the preceding, intrathecal administration of baclofen via a pump or selected muscle weakening with botulinum toxin is effective.

The bladder and bowel are often involved with MS. Bladders may become hypertonic, small, and fail to store or they may become hypotonic, large, and fail to empty. Sometimes the bladder and the sphincter become dyssynergic. Anticholinergic medication often helps the small bladder and controls the bladder spasms. Catheterization techniques may help the large bladder (self, intermittent, and indwelling). Combinations of therapy can aid the dyssynergic bladder including α-adrenergic blocking agents. A bowel program can lead to improved independence by scheduling the bowel movement rather than allowing it to be entirely spontaneous. Taking advantage of the gastrocolic reflex, attempting evacuation following a meal with the judicious use of bulking agents, stool softeners, and suppositories is the start to taking charge.

Sexual function may require attention. Erectile dysfunction in men is managed with Viagra, Levitra, or Cialis. Injection of prostaglandin (Caverject) is clearly more potent than the oral agents but requires the ability to directly inject the penis. Prostaglandin suppository (Muse) places the medication within the urethral orifice but is less potent than the injection. Women often experience decreased libido, decreased sensation, decreased lubrication, or sometimes pain. The use of various vibrators along with external water-soluble lubricants with the gentle application of cold can be helpful. Many of the commonly used antidepressant medications can decrease sexual desire and may need adjustment.

Neuropathic type pain is surprisingly common in MS (50%). The newer anticonvulsants, including gabapentin, Trileptal, Topamax, and Lamictal, are commonly dosed sufficiently to decrease the pain. Amitriptyline can be helpful, especially at night.

Cognitive problems likewise occur in approximately 50% of those with MS. Watching for depression and the contribution of other medications to the problem is essential. Keeping people in society and not allowing them to withdraw may decrease the secondary exaggeration of the symptom.

Ataxia, tremor, and balance problems often go together and are very difficult to manage. Although a number of medications can help any one person, none are consistent. Bracing across a joint can be helpful. Compensatory training for balance sometimes helps that symptom.

A number of paroxysmal symptoms relatively unique to MS are managed with anticonvulsant medications. These include spasms of an extremity. Sensory aberrations rapidly coming and going may include the pain of trigeminal neuralgia or fluctuating pain in an extremity. Paroxysmal visual blurring or speech slurring can be seen. These fluctuations may occur many times a minute, only to settle down for hours.

Ambulation can be affected through many mechanisms including weakness and ataxia. Ambulatory support through the appropriate use of devices (canes, crutches, walkers, and ankle-foot orthoses) is recommended to enhance mobility. If ambulation becomes too difficult, other mobility devices should be used freely. One of the major answers to disability is maintaining mobility.

Progressive resistive exercises must take into account the strength of innervation of the specific muscle. Fatigue results from the overzealous use of strengthening exercises. If a muscle is not used, however, atrophy results. Thus an intelligent strengthening program can be helpful if not overdone.

The role of aerobic exercise has evolved significantly over the past 2 decades, and an appropriate training program can benefit an individual if tailored to his or her deficits. The program must emphasize the slow buildup of intensity of the exercise over as much time as it takes to prevent fatigue from becoming overwhelming with each session.

Because of the individuality of the disease for each person, generalizations are hard to make. What is clear is that simply having the diagnosis causes a ripple effect even in the patients with the mildest symptoms. The family experiences the problems of their loved ones and thus this becomes a family disease like few others. The age of the patient influences vocational planning. It also influences family roles and child rearing. Thus counseling may be a very necessary component of a well-rounded approach. The complexity of all of this has made MS centers a popular choice for many who have issues surrounding the MS. These allow for experienced therapists to communicate with the medical professionals

CURRENT DIAGNOSIS

- Clinical history of fluctuating neurologic symptoms (exacerbations and remissions)
- Multiple abnormalities seen on neurologic examination
- Absence of other systemic disorder (e.g., lupus, Lyme, other autoimmune processes)
- Confirmatory laboratory studies of benefit: MRI (using McDonald criteria); CSF, looking for increased immune activity including oligoclonal IgG banding, increased IgG synthesis, and index; abnormal evoked potentials indicating multiple abnormalities potentially not found on routine neurologic examination

Abbreviations: CSF = cerebrospinal fluid; MRI = magnetic resonance imaging.

Rakel and Bope: *Conn's Current Therapy 2006.*

CURRENT THERAPY

- Education and psychological support
- Symptomatic management of appropriate symptoms
- Immune modulation with interferon beta-1a, interferon beta-1b, or glatiramer acetate early in the active disease course and ongoing
- Regular follow-up with clinical examination and magnetic resonance imaging if additional information is needed

and the patients to develop a comprehensive management strategy.

The diagnosis and management of MS has drastically evolved over the past 2 decades. It has gone from a disease characterized by the late Labe Scheinberg, MD, as "diagnose and adios" to one in which physicians are arguing about how early and how aggressively treatment strategies should be applied. We have come a long way but still have far to go to find the cause and eventual cure to this very difficult problem.

REFERENCES

Jacobs LD, Cookfair DL, Rudick RA, et al: Intramuscular interferon beta-1a for disease progression in relapsing multiple sclerosis. Ann Neurol 1996, 39(3):285-294.
Johnson KP, Brooks BR, Cohen JA, et al: Copolymer 1 reduces relapse and improves disability in relapsing-remitting multiple sclerosis: Results of a phase III multi-center, double-blind, placebo-controlled trial. Neurology 1995;45:1268-1276.
Petajan JH, White AT: Recommendations for physical activity in multiple sclerosis. Sports Med 1999;27(3):179-191.
PRISMS Study Group and University of British Columbia MS MRI Analysis Group: PRISMS-4: Long-term efficacy of interferon-beta 1a in relapsing MS. Neurology 2001;56:1628-1636.
Rao S, Leo GT, Bernardin L, Unverzagt F: Cognitive dysfunction in multiple sclerosis: I. Frequency, pattern and predictors. Neurology 1991;41(5):685-691.
Sadovnik AD, Remick RA, Allen J, et al: Depression and multiple sclerosis. Neurology 1996;46:628-632.
Schapiro RT: The Management of MS Symptoms. New York, Demos Medical Publishing, 2003.
The IFNB Multiple Sclerosis Group, University of British Columbia MS/MRI Analysis Group: Interferon beta-1b in the treatment of multiple sclerosis: Final outcome of the randomized controlled trial. Neurology 1995;45:1277-1285.

Myasthenia Gravis and Related Disorders

Method of
Robert M. Pascuzzi, MD

Myasthenia gravis (MG) is an autoimmune disorder of neuromuscular transmission involving the production of autoantibodies directed against the nicotinic acetylcholine receptor. Acetylcholine receptor antibodies are detectable in the serum of 80% to 90% of patients with MG. The prevalence of MG is approximately 1 in 10,000 to 20,000 people. Women are affected approximately twice as often as men. Symptoms may begin at virtually any age with a peak in women in the second and third decades, while the peak in men occurs in the fifth and sixth decades. Associated autoimmune diseases such as rheumatoid arthritis, lupus, and pernicious anemia are present in approximately 5% of patients. Thyroid disease occurs in approximately 10%, often in association with antithyroid antibodies. Approximately 10% to 15% of MG patients have a thymoma, while thymic lymphoid hyperplasia with proliferation of germinal centers occurs in 50% to 70% of cases. In most patients the cause of autoimmune MG is unknown. However, there are three iatrogenic causes for autoimmune MG. D-Penicillamine (Cuprimine) (used in the treatment of Wilson's disease and rheumatoid arthritis) and alfa-interferon therapy are both capable of inducing MG. In addition, bone marrow transplantation is associated with the development of MG as part of the chronic graft-versus-host disease.

Clinical Features

The hallmark of MG is fluctuating or fatigable weakness. The presenting symptoms are ocular in 50% of all patients (25% of patients initially present with diplopia, 25% with ptosis), and by 1 month into the course of illness, 80% of patients have some degree of ocular involvement. Presenting symptoms are bulbar (dysarthria or dysphagia) in 10%, leg weakness (impaired walking) in 10%, and generalized weakness in 10%. Respiratory failure is the presenting symptom in 1% of cases. Patients usually complain of symptoms from focal muscle dysfunction such as diplopia, ptosis, dysarthria, dysphagia, inability to work with arms raised over the head, or disturbance of gait. In contrast, patients with MG tend not to complain of generalized weakness, generalized fatigue, sleepiness, or muscle pain. In the classic case, fluctuating weakness is worse with exercise and improved with rest. Symptoms tend to progress later in the day. Many different factors can precipitate or aggravate weakness, such as physical stress, emotional stress, infection, or exposure to medications that impair neuromuscular transmission (perioperative succinylcholine

[Anectine], aminoglycoside antibiotics, quinine, quinidine, botulinum toxin [Botox]).

Diagnosis

The diagnosis is based on a history of fluctuating weakness with corroborating findings on examination. There are several different ways to validate or confirm the clinical diagnosis.

EDROPHONIUM (TENSILON) TEST

The most immediate and readily accessible confirmatory study is the edrophonium (Tensilon) test. To perform the test, choose one or two weak muscles to judge. Ptosis, dysconjugate gaze, and other cranial deficits provide the most reliable endpoints. Use a setting where hypotension, syncope, or respiratory failure can be managed as patients occasionally decompensate during the test. If the patient has severe dyspnea, defer the test until the airway is secure. Start an IV. Have intravenous atropine, 0.4 mg, readily available in case bradycardia or extreme gastrointestinal (GI) side effects occur. Edrophonium, 10 mg (1 mL), is drawn up in a syringe; 1 mg (0.1 mL) should be given as a test dose while checking the patient's heart rate (to ensure the patient is not supersensitive to the drug). If no untoward side effects occur after 1 minute, another 3 mg is given. Many MG patients will show improved power within 30 to 60 seconds of giving the initial 4 mg, at which point the test can be stopped. If after 1 minute there is no improvement, give an additional 3 mg; if there is still no response, 1 minute later give the final 3 mg. If the patient develops muscarinic symptoms or signs at any time during the test (sweating, salivation, GI symptoms), one can assume that enough edrophonium has been given to see improvement in strength and the test can be stopped. When a placebo effect or examiner bias is of concern, the test is performed in a double-blind, placebo-control fashion. The 1 mL control syringe contains saline, 0.4 mg atropine, or nicotinic acid,* 10 mg. Improved strength from edrophonium lasts for just a few minutes. When improvement is clear-cut, then the test is positive.

If the improvement is borderline, it is best to consider the test negative. The test can be repeated several times. Sensitivity of the edrophonium test is approximately 90%. The specificity is difficult to determine, as improvement following IV edrophonium has been reported in other neuromuscular diseases including Lambert-Eaton syndrome, botulism, Guillain-Barré syndrome, motor neuron disease, and lesions of the brainstem and cavernous sinus.

Neostigmine† has a longer duration of effect and, in selected patients, may be an alternative cholinesterase inhibitor (CEI) for diagnostic testing, especially in children. For performance of a neostigmine test, 0.04 mg/kg is given intramuscularly or 0.02 mg/kg intravenously (one time only).

ACETYLCHOLINE RECEPTOR ANTIBODIES

The standard assay for receptor binding antibodies is an immunoprecipitation assay using human limb muscle for acetylcholine receptor antigen. In addition, assays for receptor-modulating and receptor-blocking antibodies are available. Binding antibodies are present in approximately 80% of all myasthenia patients (50% of patients with pure ocular MG, 80% of those with mild generalized MG, 90% of patients with moderate to severe generalized MG, and 70% of those in clinical remission). By also testing for modulating and blocking antibodies, the sensitivity improves to 90% overall. Specificity is outstanding with false-positives exceeding rare in reliable labs. If blood is sent to a reference laboratory, the test results are usually available within 1 week.

MUSCLE-SPECIFIC KINASE ANTIBODIES

More recently, data show that 25% to 47% of patients who are seronegative for acetylcholine receptor antibodies have muscle-specific kinase (MuSK) antibodies. MuSK antibodies can now be measured by a commercially available immunoprecipitation assay. The clinical features of MuSK-positive patients may differ from non-MuSK MG patients. Such patients, who tend to be younger women (younger than age 40 years), have lower likelihood of abnormal repetitive stimulation and edrophonium test results. Bulbar symptoms are significantly more common at onset of disease in MuSK antibody–positive patients. MuSK antibodies may also be more commonly associated with patients having weakness of neck extensor, shoulders, or respiratory muscles.

ELECTROPHYSIOLOGIC TESTING

Repetitive stimulation electrophysiology (EMG) testing is widely available and has variable sensitivity, depending on number and selection of muscles studied and various provocative maneuvers. However, in most laboratories this technique has a sensitivity of approximately 50% in all patients with MG (lower in patients with mild or pure ocular disease). In general, the yield from repetitive stimulation is higher when testing muscle groups that have clinically significant weakness. Single-fiber EMG (SFEMG) is a highly specialized technique, usually available in major academic centers, with a sensitivity of approximately 90%. Abnormal single-fiber results are common in other neuromuscular diseases, and, therefore, the test must be used in the correct clinical context. The specificity of single-fiber EMG is an important issue because mild abnormalities can clearly be present with a variety of other diseases of the motor unit, including motor neuron disease, peripheral neuropathy, and myopathy. Disorders of neuromuscular transmission other than MG can have substantial abnormalities on SFEMG. In contrast, acetylcholine receptor antibodies (and MuSK antibodies) are not found in non-MG patients. In summary, the two highly sensitive laboratory studies are single-fiber EMG and acetylcholine receptor antibodies; nonetheless, neither test is 100% sensitive.

---

*Not available in the United States in parenteral form.
†FDA indicated for treatment but not diagnosis.

Rakel and Bope: *Conn's Current Therapy 2006.*

Prognosis

Appropriate management of the patient with autoimmune MG requires understanding of the natural course of the disease. The long-term natural course of MG is not clearly established other than that it is highly variable. Several generalizations can be made. Approximately 50% of MG patients present with ocular symptoms, and by 1 month 80% have eye findings. The presenting weakness is bulbar in 10%, limb in 10%, generalized in 10%, and respiratory in 1%. By 1 month symptoms remain purely ocular in 40%, generalized in 40%, limited to the limbs in 10%, and limited to bulbar muscles in 10%. Weakness remains restricted to the ocular muscles on a long-term basis in approximately 15% to 20% (pure ocular MG). Most patients with initial ocular involvement tend to develop generalized weakness within the first year of the disease (90% of those who generalize do so within the initial 12 months). Maximal weakness occurs within the initial 3 years in 70% of patients. In the modern era, death from MG is rare. Spontaneous long-lasting remission occurs in approximately 10% to 15%, usually in the first year or two of the disease. Most MG patients develop progression of clinical symptoms during the initial 2 to 3 years. However, progression is not uniform, as illustrated by 15% to 20% of patients whose symptoms remain purely ocular and those who have spontaneous remission.

Treatment

FIRST-LINE THERAPY: PYRIDOSTIGMINE BROMIDE

Cholinesterase inhibitors (CEIs) are safe, effective, and first-line therapy in all patients. Inhibition of acetylcholinesterase (AChE) reduces the hydrolysis of acetylcholine (ACh), increasing the accumulation of ACh at the nicotinic postsynaptic membrane. The CEIs used in MG bind reversibly (as opposed to organophosphate CEIs, which bind irreversibly) to AChE. These drugs cross the blood–brain barrier poorly and tend not to cause central nervous system (CNS) side effects. Absorption from the gastrointestinal (GI) tract tends to be inefficient and variable, with oral bioavailability of approximately 10%. Muscarinic autonomic side effects of GI cramping, diarrhea, salivation, lacrimation, diaphoresis, and, when severe, bradycardia may occur with all of the CEI preparations. A feared potential complication of excessive CEI use is skeletal muscle weakness (cholinergic weakness). Patients receiving parenteral CEI are at the greatest risk to have cholinergic weakness. It is uncommon for patients receiving oral CEI to develop significant cholinergic weakness even while experiencing muscarinic cholinergic side effects. Table 1 summarizes the commonly available CEIs.

Pyridostigmine (Mestinon) is the most widely used CEI for long-term oral therapy. Onset of effect is within 15 to 30 minutes of an oral dose, with peak effect within 1 to 2 hours, and wearing off gradually at 3 to 4 hours postdose. The starting dose is 30 to 60 mg three to four times per day, depending on symptoms. Optimal benefit usually occurs with a dose of 60 mg every 4 hours. Muscarinic cholinergic side effects are common with larger doses. Occasional patients require and tolerate more than 1000 mg per day, dosing as frequently as every 2 to 3 hours. Patients with significant bulbar weakness will often time their dose approximately 1 hour before meals in order to maximize chewing and swallowing. Of all the CEI preparations, pyridostigmine has the least muscarinic side effects. Pyridostigmine may be used in a number of alternative forms to the 60-mg tablet. The syrup may be necessary for children or for patients with difficulty swallowing pills. Sustained-release

TABLE 1 Commonly Available Cholinesterase Inhibitors

Cholinesterase inhibitors	Unit dose	Average dose (adult)	Children's dose
Pyridostigmine bromide tablet (Mestinon)	60-mg tablet	30-60 mg every 4-6 h	Tablet: 1 mg/kg every 4-6 h
Pyridostigmine bromide syrup	12 mg/mL	30-60 mg every 4-6 h	Syrup: 60 mg/5 mL
Pyridostigmine bromide sustained-release (Mestinon Timespan)	180-mg tablet	1 tablet twice daily	
Pyridostigmine bromide (parenteral)	5 mg/mL ampules	1-2 mg every 3-4 h (1/30 of oral dose)	
Neostigmine bromide (Prostigmin)	15-mg tablet	7.5-15 mg every 3-4 h	
Neostigmine methylsulfate (parenteral)	0.25-1.0 mg/mL every 2-3 h	0.5 mg IM, IV, or SC ampules	For treatment: 0.01-0.04 mg/kg dose, IM, IV, or SC every 2-3 h as needed For diagnosis*: 0.1 mg/kg IM or SC once, or 0.05 mg/kg IV once
Edrophonium (Tensilon)	For diagnosis only See text, page 1067		For diagnosis: 0.1 mg/kg IV, (or 0.15 mg/kg IM or SC, which prolongs the effect), preceded by a test dose of 0.01 mg/kg

*FDA indicated for treatment, but not for diagnosis.
Abbreviations: IM = intramuscular; IV = intravenous; SC = subcutaneous.

pyridostigmine, 180 mg (Mestinon Timespan), is sometimes preferred for nighttime use. Unpredictable release and absorption limit its use. Patients with severe dysphagia or those undergoing surgical procedures may need parenteral CEI. Intravenous pyridostigmine should be given at approximately 1/30 of the oral dose. Neostigmine (Prostigmin) has a slightly shorter duration of action and slightly greater muscarinic side effects.

For patients with intolerable muscarinic side effects at CEI doses required for optimal power, a concomitant anticholinergic drug such as atropine sulfate (0.4 to 0.5 mg orally) or glycopyrrolate (Robinul) (1 to 2 mg orally) on an as-needed basis or with each dose of CEI may be helpful. Patients with mild disease can often be managed adequately with CEIs. However, patients with moderate, severe, or progressive disease usually require more effective therapy.

THYMECTOMY: FOR WHOM, WHAT TYPE, AND WHAT TO TELL THE PATIENT TO EXPECT

Association of the thymus gland with MG was first noted around 1900, and thymectomy has become standard therapy for more than 50 years. Prospective, controlled trials have not been performed for thymectomy (although such a trial is currently in the planning stage). Nonetheless, thymectomy is generally recommended for patients with moderate to severe MG, especially those who are inadequately controlled on CEI, and those younger than 55 years of age. All patients with suspected thymoma undergo surgery. Approximately 75% of MG patients appear to benefit from thymectomy. Patients may improve or simply stabilize. For unclear reasons the onset of improvement tends to be delayed by 1 or 2 years in most patients (some patients do not seem to improve until 5 to 10 years after surgery). The majority of centers use the transsternal approach for thymectomy with the goal of complete removal of the gland. The limited transcervical approach has been largely abandoned because of the likelihood of incomplete gland removal. Many centers perform a maximal thymectomy in order to ensure complete removal. The procedure involves a combined transsternal–transcervical exposure with en bloc removal of the thymus. If thymectomy is to be performed, choose an experienced surgeon, anesthesiologist, and center with a good track record and insist that the entire gland is removed.

Which patients do not undergo thymectomy? Patients with very mild or trivial symptoms do not have surgery. Most patients with pure ocular MG do not undergo thymectomy even though there has been some reported benefit in selected patients. Thymectomy is often avoided in children because of the theoretical possibility of impairing the developing immune system. However, reports of thymectomy in children as young as 2 to 3 years of age have shown favorable results without adverse effects on the immune system. Thymectomy has been largely discouraged in patients older than 55 years of age because of expected increased morbidity, latency of clinical benefit, and frequent observation of an atrophic, involuted gland. Nonetheless there are older patients reported to benefit from thymectomy. Major complications from thymectomy are uncommon so long as the surgery is performed at an experienced center with anesthesiologists and neurologists familiar with the disease and perioperative management of MG patents.

Common, although less serious, aspects of thymectomy include postoperative chest pain (which may last several weeks), a 4- to 6-week convalescence period, and a cosmetically displeasing incisional scar.

CORTICOSTEROIDS

There are no controlled trials documenting the benefit of corticosteroids in MG. However, nearly all authorities have personal experience attesting to the virtues (and complications) of corticosteroid use in MG patients. In general, corticosteroids are used in patients with moderate to severe, disabling symptoms that are refractory to CEI. Patients are commonly hospitalized to initiate therapy because of the risk of early exacerbation. Opinions differ regarding the best method of administration. For patients with severe MG, it is best to begin with high-dose daily therapy of prednisone,[1] 60 to 80 mg per day orally. Early exacerbation occurs in approximately 50% of patients, usually within the first few days of therapy and typically lasting 3 or 4 days. In 10% of cases the exacerbation is severe, requiring mechanical ventilation or a feeding tube (thus the need to initiate therapy in the hospital). Overall, approximately 80% of patients show a favorable response to steroids with 30% attaining remission and 50% marked improvement. Mild to moderate improvement occurs in 15% of patients, and 5% have no response. Improvement begins as early as 12 hours and as late as 60 days after beginning prednisone, but usually the patient begins to improve within 1 or 2 weeks. Improvement is gradual, with marked improvement occurring at a mean of 3 months, and maximal improvement at a mean of 9 months. Of patients having a favorable response, most maintain their improvement with gradual dosage reduction at a rate of 10 mg every 1 to 2 months. More rapid reduction is usually associated with a flare-up of the disease. While many patients can eventually be weaned off of steroids and maintain their response, the majority cannot. They require a minimum dose (5 to 30 mg on alternate days) to maintain their improvement. Complications of long-term high-dose prednisone therapy are substantial, including cushingoid appearance, hypertension, osteoporosis, cataracts, aseptic necrosis, and other well-known complications of chronic steroid therapy. Older patients tend to respond more favorably to prednisone.

An alternative prednisone regimen involves a low-dose, alternate-day, gradually increasing schedule in an attempt to avoid the early exacerbation. Patients receive prednisone, 25 mg on alternate days with increases of 12.5 mg every third dose (approximately every fifth day), to a maximum dose of 100 mg every other day or until sufficient improvement occurs. Clinical improvement usually begins within 1 month of treatment.

[1]Not FDA approved for this indication.

The frequency and severity of early exacerbation are less than are those associated with high-dose daily regimens. High-dose intravenous methylprednisolone (Solu-Medrol)[1] (1000 mg intravenously daily for 3 to 5 days) can provide improvement within 1 to 2 weeks, but the clinical improvement is temporary.

Alternative Immunosuppressive Drug Therapy

MYCOPHENOLATE MOFETIL

Mycophenolate mofetil (CellCept)[1] is a purine inhibitor widely used in recent years for the treatment of MG. While prospective, controlled trials are underway, the anecdotal uncontrolled experience suggests that approximately 75% of MG patients benefit from the drug with the typical onset of improvement within 2 to 3 months. The drug is, in general, well tolerated. Typically the drug regimen begins with 250 to 500 mg orally twice daily, and over 2 to 4 weeks the dose is increased to 1000 mg orally twice daily.

Azathioprine

Azathioprine (Imuran)[1] is a cytotoxic purine analogue with extensive use in MG (but largely uncontrolled and retrospective). The starting dose is 50 mg orally daily, with complete blood count (CBC) and liver function tests weekly in the beginning. If the drug is tolerated and if the blood work is stable, the dose is increased by 50 mg every 1 to 2 weeks, aiming for a total daily dose of approximately 2 to 3 mg/kg per day (approximately 150 mg per day in the average-size adult). When azathioprine is first started, approximately 15% of patients will have intolerable GI side effects (nausea, anorexia, abdominal discomfort) that are sometimes associated with fever, leading to discontinuation. Bone marrow suppression with relative leukopenia (white blood cell count [WBC] 2500 to 4000 cells/mm^3) occurs in 25% of patients but is usually not significant. If the WBC drops below 2500 cells/mm^3, or the absolute granulocyte count goes below 1000 cells/mm^3, the drug is stopped (and the abnormalities usually resolve). Macrocytosis is common and of unclear clinical significance. Liver enzymes elevate in 5% to 10% of patients but this is usually reversible, and severe hepatic toxicity occurs in only approximately 1%; infection occurs in approximately 5%. There is a theoretical risk of malignancy (based on observations in organ transplant patients), but this increased risk has not been clearly established in the MG patient population. Approximately 50% of MG patients improve on azathioprine with onset approximately 4 to 8 months into treatment. Maximal improvement takes approximately 12 months. Relapse after discontinuation of azathioprine occurs in more than 50% of patients, usually within 1 year.

Cyclosporine

Cyclosporine (Sandimmune)[1] is used in patients with severe MG who cannot be adequately managed with corticosteroids or azathioprine. The starting dose is 3 to 5 mg/kg per day given in two divided doses. Cyclosporine blood levels should be measured monthly (aiming for a level of 200 to 300 mg) along with electrolytes, magnesium, and renal function (in general, serum creatinine should not be 1.5 times more than the pretreatment level). Blood should be sampled before the morning dose is taken. More than 50% of patients improve on cyclosporine. The onset of clinical improvement occurs approximately 1 to 2 months after beginning therapy and maximal improvement occurs at approximately 3 to 4 months. Side effects include renal toxicity and hypertension. Nonsteroidal anti-inflammatory drugs (NSAIDs) and potassium-sparing diuretics are among the list of drugs that should be avoided while on cyclosporine. In patients on corticosteroids, the addition of cyclosporine can lead to a reduction in steroid dosage (although it is usually not possible to discontinue prednisone).

PLASMA EXCHANGE

Plasma exchange (plasmapheresis) removes acetylcholine receptor antibodies and results in rapid clinical improvement. The standard course involves removal of 2 to 3 L of plasma every other day or three times per week until the patient improves (usually a total of three to five exchanges). Improvement begins after the first few exchanges and reaches maximum within 2 to 3 weeks. The improvement is moderate to marked in nearly all patients, but usually wears off after 4 to 8 weeks because of the reaccumulation of pathogenic antibodies. Vascular access may require placement of a central line. Complications include hypotension, bradycardia, electrolyte imbalance, hemolysis, infection, and access problems (such as pneumothorax from placement of a central line). Indications for plasma exchange include any patient in whom a rapid temporary clinical improvement is needed.

HIGH-DOSE INTRAVENOUS IMMUNOGLOBULIN

High-dose intravenous immunoglobulin (IVIG)[1] administration is associated with rapid improvement in MG symptoms in a time frame similar to plasma exchange. The mechanism is unclear but may relate to downregulation of acetylcholine receptor antibody production or to the effect of anti-idiotype antibodies. The usual protocol is 2 g/kg spread over 5 consecutive days (0.4 g/kg per day). Different IVIG preparations are administered IV at different rates (contact the pharmacy for guidelines). The majority of MG patients improve, usually within 1 week of starting IVIG. The degree of response is variable, and the duration of response is limited, like plasma exchange, to approximately 4 to 8 weeks. Complications include fever, chills, and headache,

---

[1]Not FDA approved for this indication.

[1]Not FDA approved for this indication.

which respond to slowing down the rate of the infusion and giving diphenhydramine. Occasional cases of aseptic meningitis, renal failure, nephrotic syndrome, and stroke have been reported. Also, patients with selective IgA deficiency can have anaphylaxis, which can be avoided by screening for IgA deficiency ahead of time. The treatment is relatively expensive, comparable to plasma exchange.

GENERAL GUIDELINES FOR MANAGEMENT

1. Be certain of the diagnosis.
2. Conduct patient education. Provide the patient with information about the natural course of the disease (including the variable and somewhat unpredictable course). Briefly review the treatment options pointing out effectiveness, time course of improvement, duration of response, and complications. Provide the patient with educational pamphlets prepared by the Myasthenia Gravis Foundation of America or the Muscular Dystrophy Association.
3. Determine when hospitalization is necessary. Patients with severe MG can deteriorate rapidly over a period of hours. Therefore, those having dyspnea should be hospitalized immediately in a constant observation or intensive care setting. Patients with moderate or severe dysphagia, weight loss, as well as those with rapidly progressive or severe weakness should be admitted urgently. This will allow close monitoring and early intervention in case of respiratory failure, and will also expedite the diagnostic workup and initiation of therapy.
4. Be aware that myasthenic crisis (Box 1) is a medical emergency characterized by respiratory failure from diaphragm weakness or severe oropharyngeal weakness leading to aspiration. Crisis can occur in the setting of surgery (postoperative), acute infection, or following rapid withdrawal of corticosteroids (although some patients have no precipitating factors). Patients should be placed in an intensive care unit (ICU) setting and have forced vital capacity (FVC) checked every 2 hours. Changes in arterial blood gases occur relatively late in neuromuscular respiratory failure. There should be a low threshold for intubation and mechanical ventilation. Criteria for intubation include a drop in the FVC below 15 mL/kg (or below 1 L in an average-size adult), severe aspiration from oropharyngeal weakness, or labored breathing regardless of the measurements. If the diagnosis is not clear-cut it is advisable to secure the airway with intubation, stabilize ventilation, and only then address the question of the underlying diagnosis. If the patient has been taking CEI, the drug should be temporarily discontinued in order to rule out the possibility of cholinergic crisis.
5. Screen for and correct any underlying medical problems such as systemic infection, metabolic problems (like diabetes), and thyroid disease (hypo- or hyperthyroidism can exacerbate MG).
6. Be aware of drugs to avoid in MG. Avoid using D-penicillamine (Cuprimine), interferon alfa, chloroquine (Aralen), quinine, quinidine, procainamide, and botulinum toxin (Botox). Aminoglycoside antibiotics should be avoided unless needed for a life-threatening infection. Neuromuscular blocking drugs such as pancuronium (Pavulon) and D-tubocurarine can produce marked and prolonged paralysis in MG patients. Depolarizing drugs such as succinylcholine (Anectine) can also have a prolonged effect and should be used by a skilled anesthesiologist who is well aware of the patient's MG.

GUIDELINES FOR SPECIFIC THERAPIES (Box 2)

Treatment must be individualized. Mild diplopia and ptosis may not be disabling for some patients, but for a pilot or neurosurgeon, for example, mild, intermittent diplopia may be critical. In similar fashion, some patients may tolerate side effects better than others.

1. Mild or trivial weakness, either localized or generalized should be managed with a CEI (pyridostigmine).
2. Moderate to marked weakness, localized or generalized, should initially be managed with CEI. Even if symptoms are adequately controlled, patients younger than 55 years of age undergo thymectomy early in the course of the disease (within the first year). In older patients, thymectomy is usually not performed unless the patient is thought to have a thymoma. Thymectomy is performed at an experienced center with the clear intent of complete removal of the gland. All patients with suspected thymoma (by chest scan) should have thymectomy, even if their myasthenic symptoms are mild. Unless a thymoma is suspected, patients with pure ocular disease are usually not treated with thymectomy.
3. If symptoms are inadequately controlled on CEI, immunosuppression is used. High-dose corticosteroid

---

14

> **BOX 1   The Acutely Deteriorating Myasthenic Patient**
>
> **Myasthenic Crisis**
> - Respiratory distress
> - Respiratory arrest
> - Cyanosis
> - Increased pulse and blood pressure
> - Diaphoresis
> - Poor cough
> - Inability to handle oral secretions
> - Dysphagia
> - Weakness
> - Improvement with edrophonium
>
> **Cholinergic Crisis**
> - Abdominal cramps
> - Diarrhea
> - Nausea and vomiting
> - Excessive secretions
> - Miosis
> - Fasciculations
> - Diaphoresis
> - Weakness
> - Worsening with edrophonium

Rakel and Bope: *Conn's Current Therapy 2006.*

BOX 2   Treatment of Myasthenia Gravis

1. Mild weakness: cholinesterase inhibitors
2. Moderate-marked localized or generalized weakness:
   a. Cholinesterase inhibitors, and
   b. Thymectomy for patients under age 55 (complete removal)
3. If symptoms are uncontrolled on cholinesterase inhibitors, use immunosuppression
   a. Prednisone if severe or urgent
   b. Mycophenolate mofetil (CellCept)[1] or azathioprine (Imuran)[1]
      Prednisone contraindicated
      Prednisone failure
      Excessive prednisone side effects
4. Plasma exchange or IVIG[1]
   a. Impending crisis, crisis
   b. Preoperative boost (if needed)
   c. Chronic disease refractory to drug therapy
5. If the above fails:
   a. Search for residual thymus tissue
   b. Cyclosporine (Sandimmune)[1]
   c. Long-term high-dose IVIG or PE
   d. Referral to neuromuscular specialty group

[1]Not FDA approved for this indication.
Abbreviations: IVIG = intravenous immunoglobulin; PE = plasma exchange.

---

therapy is the most predictable and effective long-term option. If patients have severe, rapidly progressive, or life-threatening symptoms the decision to start corticosteroids is clear-cut. Patients with disabling but stable symptoms may instead receive mycophenolate mofetil (CellCept),[1] especially if there are particular concerns about using corticosteroids (i.e., the patient is already overweight, diabetic, or has cosmetic concerns). Patients who respond poorly or have unacceptable complications on steroids are started on mycophenolate.

4. Plasma exchange or IVIG are indicated in:
   a. Rapidly progressive, life-threatening, impending myasthenic crisis, or actual crisis, particularly if prolonged intubation with mechanical ventilation is judged hazardous.
   b. Preoperative stabilization of MG (such as before thymectomy or other elective surgery) in poorly controlled patients.
   c. Disabling MG refractory to other therapies.
5. If these options fail, azathioprine (Imuran)[1] or cyclosporine (Sandimmune)[1] are used.
6. If the patient remains poorly controlled despite use of the above treatments, then a repeat chest CT scan looking for residual thymus should be obtained. Some patients improve after repeat thymectomy. There may be other medical problems (diabetes, thyroid disease, infection, and coexisting autoimmune diseases).

7. Referral to a neurologist or center that specializes in neuromuscular disease is advised for all patients with suspected MG and can be particularly important for complicated or refractory patients.

Other Issues

TRANSIENT NEONATAL MYASTHENIA

Transient neonatal myasthenia occurs in 10% to 15% of babies born to mothers with autoimmune MG. Within the first few days after delivery the baby has a weak cry or suck, appears floppy, and occasionally requires mechanical ventilation. The condition is caused by maternal antibodies that cross the placenta late in pregnancy. As these maternal antibodies are replaced by the baby's own antibodies the symptoms gradually disappear, usually within a few weeks, and the baby is normal thereafter. Infants with severe weakness are treated with oral pyridostigmine, 1 to 2 mg/kg every 4 hours.

CONGENITAL MYASTHENIA

Congenital myasthenia represents a group of rare hereditary disorders of the neuromuscular junction. The patients tend to have lifelong relatively stable symptoms of generalized fatigable weakness. These disorders are nonimmunologic, without acetylcholine receptor antibodies, and, therefore, patients do not respond to immune therapy (steroids, thymectomy, and plasma exchange). Most of these patients improve on CEI. There are many established subtypes of congenital myasthenia, and several are worth noting partly because of specific therapeutic implications.

The fast-channel congenital myasthenic syndrome tends to be static or slowly progressive, but it is usually very responsive to combination therapy with 3,4-diaminopyridine[1] (which enhances release of acetylcholine) and pyridostigmine (Mestinon) (which reduces metabolism of acetylcholine).

Congenital slow-channel myasthenic syndrome typically worsens over years as the end plate myopathy progresses. Although cholinesterase inhibitors typically worsen symptoms, quinidine[1] and fluoxetine (Prozac),[1] which reduce the duration of acetylcholine receptor channel openings, are both effective treatments for slow-channel syndrome.

The congenital myasthenic syndrome associated with acetylcholine receptor deficiency tends to be relatively nonprogressive and may even improve slightly as the patient ages. The disorder typically responds to symptomatic therapy with pyridostigmine and/or 3,4-diaminopyridine. Ephedrine[1] produces benefit in some cases.

Patients with end plate acetylcholinesterase deficiency usually present in infancy or early childhood with generalized weakness, underdevelopment of muscles, slowed pupillary responses to light, and either no

---

[1]Not FDA approved for this indication.

[1]Not FDA approved for this indication.

response or worsening response with cholinesterase inhibitors. No effective long-term treatment has been described for congenital end plate acetylcholinesterase deficiency.

LAMBERT-EATON SYNDROME

Lambert-Eaton syndrome (LES) (the myasthenic syndrome) is a presynaptic disease characterized by chronic fluctuating weakness of proximal limb muscles. Symptoms (Box 3) include difficulty walking, climbing stairs, or rising from a chair. In LES there may be some improvement in power with sustained or repeated exercise. In contrast to myasthenia gravis, ptosis, diplopia, dysphagia, and respiratory failure are far less common. In addition, LES patients often complain of myalgias, muscle stiffness of the back and legs, distal paresthesias, metallic taste, dry mouth, impotence, and other autonomic symptoms of muscarinic cholinergic insufficiency. LES is rare compared to myasthenia gravis, which is approximately 100 times more common. Approximately 50% of LES patients have an underlying malignancy that is usually small cell carcinoma of the lung. In patients without malignancy, LES is an autoimmune disease and can be associated with other autoimmune phenomena. In general, patients older than 40 years of age are more likely to be men and have an associated malignancy, whereas younger patients are more likely to be women and have no associated neoplasm. LES symptoms can precede detection of the malignancy by 1 to 2 years.

The examination typically shows proximal lower extremity weakness (although the objective bedside assessment may suggest mild weakness relative to the patient's history). The muscle stretch reflexes are absent. On testing sustained maximal grip, there is a gradual increase in power over the initial 2 to 3 seconds (Lambert's sign).

The diagnosis is confirmed with EMG studies, which typically show low amplitude of the compound muscle action potentials and a decrement to slow rates or repetitive stimulation. Following brief exercise, there is marked facilitation of the compound muscle action potential (CMAP) amplitude. At high rates of repetitive stimulation, there may be an incremental response. Single-fiber EMG is markedly abnormal in virtually all patients with LES. The pathogenesis involves autoantibodies directed against voltage-gated calcium channels at cholinergic nerve terminals. These IgG antibodies also inhibit cholinergic synapses of the autonomic nervous system. More than 75% of LES patients demonstrate these antibodies to voltage-gated calcium channels in serum, providing another useful diagnostic test. In patients with associated malignancy, successful treatment of the tumor can lead to improvement in the LES symptoms. Symptomatic improvement in neuromuscular transmission may occur with the use of cholinesterase inhibitors such as pyridostigmine. 3,4-Diaminopyridine (DAP) increases ACh release by blocking voltage-dependent potassium conductance and thereby prolonging depolarization at the nerve terminal and enhancing the voltage-dependent calcium influx. 3,4-DAP is clearly for most patients with LES, with relatively mild toxicity, and is becoming increasingly available, such that it represents first-line symptomatic therapy for LES. The typical beginning dose is 10 mg every 4 to 6 hours, with gradual increases, as needed, up to a maximum of 100 mg per day.

Immunosuppressive therapy is used in patients with disabling symptoms. Long-term high-dose corticosteroids, plasma exchange, and IVIG have all been used with moderate success. In general, the use of these therapies should be tailored to the severity of patient's symptoms.

14

BOX 3 **Lambert-Eaton Syndrome (LES)**
Symptoms
• Proximal limb weakness
Legs > arms
• Fatigue or fluctuating symptoms
• Difficulty rising from a sitting position, climbing stairs
• Metallic taste in mouth
• Autonomic dysfunction
Dry mouth
Constipation
Blurred vision
Impaired sweating
Signs
• Proximal limb weakness
Legs > arms
• Weakness on examination is less compared to patient's level of disability
• Hypoactive or absent muscle stretch reflexes
• Lambert's sign (grip becomes more powerful over several seconds)

Rakel and Bope: *Conn's Current Therapy 2006.*

Trigeminal Neuralgia

Method of
Alexander Mauskop, MD

Trigeminal neuralgia (TN), or tic douloureux, is associated with one of the most severe types of pain. Fortunately, the majority of these patients are helped by pharmacologic or surgical means.

The prevalence of TN is anywhere between 43 and 155 cases per 1,000,000 population, and it is higher for women than for men. An estimated 15,000 new cases are diagnosed each year. TN occurs mostly in the elderly. TN in young adults can be caused by multiple sclerosis. Hypertension is another confirmed risk factor. Spontaneous remissions often occur, and the average duration of TN is between a few months and 7 years.

Clinical Features

The definition of TN according to the classification by the International Headache Society (IHS) is provided later (Current Diagnosis). The typical pain of TN is lancinating, like an electric shock, extremely intense but very brief, lasting no longer than a few seconds. Several studies indicate that patients with atypical trigeminal neuralgia (not as intense, with aching and longer lasting pain) are less responsive to treatment than those with typical features. These atypical patients often have symptomatic trigeminal neuralgia because of other treatable causes (Box 1). Conditions that most commonly mimic the pain of TN include posterior fossa tumors, aneurysms, and arteriovenous malformations. On surgical exploration of posterior fossa in patients with TN, tumors are found in up to 2% to 3% of cases.

Many patients with TN grimace each time they experience the intense lightning-like pain. Others are able to maintain their composure and may not appear to be in severe pain. Some patients can continue to function despite the pain, whereas others become disabled, malnourished, and depressed.

In addition to the usual triggers, which include chewing, talking, brushing teeth, and touching the face, some patients have attacks provoked by vigorous physical activity, by lowering their head with blood rushing into the face, and even by wind blowing at their face. Trigger areas are most commonly situated around the mouth and nose.

The right side is affected more frequently than the left. When a single branch of the trigeminal nerve is affected, most frequently it is the second branch (44%); the third is involved in 36% and the first in 20%. Approximately a third of all patients with TN have involvement of both the second and third divisions. In 3% to 5% of patients, pain occurs bilaterally and should raise the suspicion of demyelinating disease.

Pathophysiology

Vascular compression of the trigeminal nerve root is seen in many patients who undergo posterior fossa surgery. The high efficacy of microvascular decompression suggests that a peripheral lesion causes TN. Some features of TN, however, indicate a central mechanism: triggering of pain by a stimulus outside the area of pain, latent period between the triggering event and pain, as well as a refractory period after the pain when another paroxysm of pain cannot be provoked. It is thought that a peripheral anatomic lesion leads to segmental demyelination of the nerve with development of ephaptic transmission, or cross-talk, which eventually leads to secondary changes in the spinal trigeminal nucleus. These changes include reduction in the mechanism of surround inhibition with activation of a larger than normal number of wide dynamic range neurons that leads to perception of pain from a tactile stimulus. Carbamazepine is thought to relieve pain of TN by facilitating inhibition in the spinal trigeminal nucleus.

BOX 1   Causes of Facial Pain

Dental
- Acute pulpitis
- Acute periodontitis
- Periodontal abscess
- Cracked tooth syndrome
- Denture trauma
- Temporomandibular joint (TMJ) disorder
- Atypical odontalgia

Diseases of the Jaw
- Acute osteomyelitis
- Fractures
- Infected cysts
- Malignant tumors

Diseases of the Salivary Glands
- Salivary calculi
- Acute infection

Sjögren's Syndrome
- Tumors

Sinus Disease
- Sinusitis
- Viral
- Bacterial
- Fungal
- Mucocele
- Malignant tumors
- Carcinoma
- Sarcoma
- Lymphoma

Ear Pain
- Injury
- Squamous cell carcinoma
- Infections
- Otitis
- Mastoiditis
- Cellulites
- Perichondritis
- Chondritis
- Herpes simplex
- Herpes zoster

Ophthalmic
- Glaucoma
- Optic neuritis
- Iritis and uveitis
- Orbital pseudotumor
- Orbital tumor

Intracranial
- Glossopharyngeal neuralgia
- Trigeminal neuralgia
- Cluster headache
- Ice pick pain
- Inflammation
- Infections
- Aneurysm
- Stroke
- Tumor

Rakel and Bope: *Conn's Current Therapy 2006.*

Medical Therapy

FIRST-LINE DRUGS

Carbamazepine (CBZ) (Tegretol) is the drug of first choice for the treatment of TN. The medication is started at a low dose of 100 mg twice per day to avoid nausea and somnolence that can be intolerable at a higher starting dose. The dose is increased by 100 mg every day to the point of pain relief or development of unacceptable side effects. The daily dose, which is usually 300 to 1600 mg per day, is divided into three or four doses, although long-acting forms of CBZ (Tegretol XR, Carbatrol), which can be given twice a day, are available. Monitoring blood levels is necessary when malabsorption, noncompliance, or toxicity is suspected. Correlation between the blood level and the analgesic effect in TN is established. It is not unusual to see a decline in the efficacy of CBZ on a steady dose, often caused by the phenomenon of autoinduction of metabolism of CBZ. By increasing the dose of CBZ and bringing the drug level up again, pain control can be regained. Unfortunately, patients often develop tolerance, and pain may recur even with a high therapeutic blood level. The much feared blood dyscrasias because of CBZ are less common than originally believed. They are also thought to be idiosyncratic reactions, and monitoring the blood cell count may not always prevent them. Some decline in the white cell count is common after the initiation of carbamazepine therapy. Various schedules of blood monitoring can be found in the literature. It is reasonable to check a blood cell count prior to initiating treatment and then 2 weeks, 1 month, and 3 months afterward. Hepatic functions may be checked at the same time because of potential hepatotoxicity, although it is very rare. It is more important to warn the patient to contact a physician if a fever, sore throat, bruises, stomatitis, or other symptoms develop.

Oxcarbazepine (Trileptal) is a drug similar to CBZ but somewhat better tolerated with a lower incidence of serious side effects. Blood monitoring is not required when prescribing oxcarbazepine, but it is reported to cause hyponatremia. Its efficacy in TN is less proven, however.

Patients who do not respond to CBZ can be given baclofen (Lioresal). It had 74% effectiveness in a double-blind study of 50 patients. This drug is an analogue of γ-aminobutyric acid (GABA), an inhibitory neurotransmitter. It is used for the treatment of spasticity in multiple sclerosis and spinal cord injuries. The usual starting dose is 5 mg, three times per day, with a gradual increase up to 20 mg, four times a day. Although 80 mg is the highest recommended dose, higher doses are sometimes used. The most common side effects are transient drowsiness, dizziness, and fatigue. The effectiveness of baclofen, like that of CBZ, can decline with time. In such patients, the combination of baclofen with carbamazepine can be synergistic and provide better relief than either of these drugs alone.

The first reports of phenytoin efficacy in TN appeared soon after its introduction as an anticonvulsant. Phenytoin (Dilantin) is somewhat less effective than CBZ, but it has certain advantages. As with CBZ, general principles of phenytoin use as an anticonvulsant apply to its use for TN. Titration of the daily dose is necessary in many cases, but there is no need to start with a low dose. The usual daily amount of 300 mg can be given in a single daily dose. Phenytoin has the advantage of being available parenterally for patients who are in a crisis or unable to take medications by mouth. Side effects of phenytoin include drowsiness, nausea, and (with long-term use) gingival hyperplasia and hirsutism. Dose-related side effects include nystagmus, slurred speech, ataxia, and confusion.

Less frequently used drugs include clonazepam (Klonopin), divalproex sodium (Depakote), topiramate (Topamax), pimozide (Orap), corticosteroids, oral local anesthetics, and opioid analgesics.

Clonazepam is reported effective in two thirds of patients with TN. Clonazepam is a benzodiazepine with a potential for addiction, although in patients with a typical trigeminal neuralgia it is rarely a concern. The most common side effect of clonazepam is sedation, but gradual escalation of the dose allows time for the development of tolerance to this side effect. The usual starting dose is 0.5 mg, three times daily. The maximum recommended daily dose is 20 mg.

Divalproex sodium is another anticonvulsant that can be used with some success. The same principles used for the treatment of seizures apply when treating TN. The initial dose is 125 to 250 mg twice a day with escalation sometimes much higher, depending on the response, side effects, and blood levels. The average therapeutic level of 50 to 100 μg/mL can be exceeded if the patient tolerates it. Common side effects include nausea, sedation, and tremor. Transient hair loss and weight gain occasionally occur.

Topiramate is an anticonvulsant that has the advantage of weight loss as a side effect. Cognitive side effects often limit its usefulness.

In a double-blind crossover study comparing pimozide with CBZ, all 48 patients with TN improved on pimozide, whereas only 56% improved on CBZ. Pimozide is a neuroleptic drug approved as a second-line drug for treatment of tics in patients with Tourette's disorder. Because of the potential for serious side effects such as tardive dyskinesia and cardiac arrhythmia, this drug should be reserved for patients who failed other medical approaches and are not willing to undergo surgery.

A large intravenous bolus of corticosteroids (e.g., 20 to 40 mg dexamethasone) can be tried in a patient who is in a crisis with an attack of very frequent and severe tics. Corticosteroids should not be used for any length of time because of their potential for serious side effects and low efficacy.

Opioid analgesics are rarely effective without producing sedation and should be also reserved for unusually severe and refractory cases when a short period of sedation is desirable.

Surgical Approaches

PERIPHERAL PROCEDURES

A variety of procedures involving the peripheral branches of the trigeminal nerve have been attempted. This is a logical first step after the failure of medical therapy.

CURRENT DIAGNOSIS

Diagnostic criteria according to the International Headache Society's classification are as follows:

1. Paroxysmal attacks of facial or frontal pain that last a few seconds to less than 2 minutes occur.
2. Pain has at least four of the following characteristics:
   - Distribution along one or more divisions of the trigeminal nerve
   - Sudden, intense, sharp, superficial, stabbing, or burning in quality
   - Pain intensity severe
   - Precipitation from trigger areas, or by certain daily activities such as eating, talking, washing the face, or cleaning the teeth
   - Between paroxysms, patient, entirely asymptomatic
3. No neurologic deficit occurs.
4. Attacks are stereotyped in the individual patient.
5. Other causes of facial pain are excluded by history, physical examination, and special investigations when necessary.

CURRENT THERAPY

Pharmacologic
- Carbamazepine
- Lioresal
- Phenytoin
- Clonazepam
- Topiramate

Nonpharmacologic
- Percutaneous radiofrequency gangliolysis
- Microvascular decompression

The relief is usually not sustained, but many patients prefer to repeat these procedures rather than undergo more risky gangliolysis or microvascular decompression. A block of the trigger zones is usually done using local anesthetics. If this procedure provides some temporary relief, alcohol injection or cryotherapy can produce a remission that lasts for 3 to 6 months in some patients. Some surgeons perform nerve avulsion, but the rate and duration of success of this procedure are not known.

RADIOFREQUENCY GANGLIOLYSIS

Percutaneous radiofrequency lesioning of the gasserian ganglion is probably the most popular surgical procedure, with more than 14,000 cases published in 33 reports. Although a selective destruction by graded heating of A-δ and C fibers is assumed, the evidence for this selectivity in humans is not convincing. Initial pain relief occurs in 88% to 99% of patients, but the recurrence rate is 20% to 30%. The electrode is introduced into the ganglion under fluoroscopic guidance as in all percutaneous procedures. Mild stimulation is used to position the electrode. When this stimulation produces paresthesias in the affected branch of the nerve, the current is turned up. Surgeons are cautioned to undertreat to reduce the chance of anesthesia dolorosa and sensory loss. Such undertreatment by reducing the temperature and duration of thermocoagulation produces a lower success rate, but the treatment can be repeated.

MICROVASCULAR DECOMPRESSION

Proponents of microvascular decompression claim to address the etiology of TN, which they assume to be compression of the trigeminal nerve by a blood vessel. Large numbers of patients treated by this method were found to have various blood vessels compressing the trigeminal nerve, but the role of such compression in producing TN remains unclear. The major disadvantage of this approach is the need for craniotomy. The long-term response rate is approximately 80%. Major complications in the most experienced hands include death in less than 1%, hematoma or infarction (1%), pneumonia, and meningitis. As with any other surgical procedure, less experienced surgeons have a much higher incidence of complications.

REFERENCES

Fromm GH: Medical treatment of patients with trigeminal neuralgia. In Fromm GH, Sessle BJ (eds): Trigeminal Neuralgia. Boston, Butterworth-Heinemann, 1991, pp 131-144.

Janetta PJ: Surgical treatment: Microvascular decompression. In Fromm GH, Sessle BJ (eds): Trigeminal Neuralgia. Boston, Butterworth-Heinemann, 1991, pp 145-157.

Katusic S, Beard CM, Bergstralh E, Kurland LT: Incidence and clinical features of trigeminal neuralgia. Rochester, Minnesota, 1945-1984. Ann Neurol 1990;27:89-95.

Lunsford LD: Percutaneous retrogasserian glycerol rhizotomy. In Rovit RL, Murali R, Jannetta PJ (eds): Trigeminal Neuralgia. Baltimore, Williams & Wilkins, 1990, pp 145-164.

Mullan S: Percutaneous microcompression of the trigeminal ganglion. In Rovit RL, Murali R, Jannetta PJ (eds): Trigeminal Neuralgia. Baltimore, Williams & Wilkins, 1990, pp 137-144.

Murali R: Peripheral nerve injections and avulsions in the treatment of trigeminal neuralgia. In Rovit RL, Murali R, Jannetta PJ (eds): Trigeminal Neuralgia. Baltimore, Williams & Wilkins, 1990, pp 95-108.

Penman J: Trigeminal neuralgia. In Vinken PJ, Bruyn GW (eds): Handbook of Clinical Neurology, vol 5. Amsterdam, Elsevier/North Holland, 1968, pp 296-322.

Sweet WH: The treatment of trigeminal neuralgia (tic douloureux). N Engl J Med 1986;315:174-177.

Acute Facial Paralysis (Bell's Palsy)

Method of
Bruce J. Gantz, MD, Ted A. Meyer, MD, PhD, and Peter C. Weber, MD

Bell's palsy and *idiopathic facial paralysis* are synonymous terms for acute facial paralysis of unknown etiology. McCormick first postulated that Bell's palsy was caused by herpesvirus in 1972. More recently, Murakami and coworkers (1996) further substantiated this claim when they identified DNA fragments of herpes simplex virus type 1 (HSV-1) in the perineurial fluid of 11 of 14 subjects undergoing facial nerve decompression during the acute phase of the illness. Burgess and colleagues (1994) found HSV-1 DNA in a temporal bone section in the region of the geniculate ganglion in a patient who had died of other causes 6 days after the onset of Bell's palsy. These two independent pieces of evidence strongly support the concept that the facial paralysis known as Bell's palsy is caused by a viral infection that induces inflammatory edema within the facial nerve. The nerve lies within the bony fallopian canal as it traverses the temporal bone. The labyrinthine segment, which has a diameter of approximately 0.6 mm, lies just medial to the geniculate ganglion. As the facial nerve swells, it is constricted to the greatest extent in the labyrinthine segment, and the ensuing neural conduction block causes paralysis of the voluntary facial musculature seen in Bell's palsy. An animal model of Bell's palsy has also been developed by inoculating the auricles and tongues of mice with herpes simplex virus, providing further evidence that a viral infection is an important cause in this disease. Together, this information provides more than circumstantial support for a herpes simplex viral etiology of Bell's palsy. This article highlights the epidemiology, clinical manifestations, evaluation, and treatment of Bell's palsy, taking into account the new information regarding etiology.

Epidemiology

The incidence of Bell's palsy is approximately 30 cases per 100,000 individuals per year, thus making it the most common cause of unilateral facial paralysis. Approximately 40,000 cases occur in the United States each year. There appears to be no gender predilection, and the ages range from infancy to elderly, with manifestation in the fifth and sixth decades of life most common. Right- and left-sided facial palsies occur equally. Recurrence may be unilateral or contralateral in up to 10% of patients, but the physician should be alerted to perform a rigorous examination to rule out other causes. Pregnancy triples the risk, whereas hypertension and diabetes mellitus are associated with only a small increase in incidence. Roughly 10% have a familial orientation, and 70% of patients relate an upper respiratory tract infection preceding the onset.

Recovery begins within 3 weeks for 85% of the patients, with full recovery occurring in 6 months. Approximately 10% to 15% of patients are troubled with asymmetric movement, mass movement of all branches, or movement of the mouth when closing the eye (synkinesis). Only 4% to 6% of patients, however, experience severe deformity with minimal return of facial movement. Some of these patients are completely unable to close the eye. Identification of this poor recovery group using electrophysiologic testing must be accomplished within 2 weeks of the onset of complete paralysis. Delay beyond 2 weeks renders approximately 50% of this group with residual facial dysfunction for the rest of their lives.

Evaluation

A detailed history is mandatory for any patient with facial paralysis. Date of onset, duration of associated symptoms, and other precipitating factors are important to document. Many patients report an antecedent viral illness 7 to 10 days before the onset of paralysis. A description of otalgia associated with skin and auricular blebs or blisters is not Bell's palsy but rather herpes zoster oticus (Ramsay Hunt syndrome), which is best treated with antiviral agents (valacyclovir [Valtrex])[1]. The facial paralysis in Bell's palsy may be abrupt or worsen over 2 to 3 days. It is not slowly progressive over weeks to months. Patients with Bell's palsy do not complain of facial twitching, decreased hearing, otorrhea, severe otalgia, or balance dysfunction. It is equally important to rule out recent trauma, tick bites (Lyme disease), or current ear infections.

Physical examination should confirm a facial paralysis of all branches. If the forehead is intact, a central etiology is of concern, whereas involvement of a single branch indicates a parotid tumor or trauma. The middle ear, tympanic membrane, and external canal should be normal. No aural or oral vesicular lesions should be seen. The parotid gland is palpated bimanually to ensure against a deep lobe tumor. All other cranial nerves should function normally, including cranial nerve V, even though patients may complain of vague facial numbness.

Audiometric evaluation is necessary for every patient. Unilateral hearing loss or acoustic reflex decay is suggestive of a cerebellopontine angle tumor and an indication for further retrocochlear evaluation. If vestibular complaints are present, an electronystagmogram (ENG) is obtained.

Although radiographic studies are important in patients with facial paralysis, it is not necessary to image all patients with acute facial paralysis immediately, especially patients with classic symptoms of Bell's palsy. Imaging studies are obtained immediately if the signs and symptoms are not compatible with Bell's palsy or if no return of facial motion is observed at 6 months. Both high-resolution computed tomography (HRCT) and magnetic resonance imaging (MRI) with gadolinium are useful. Computed tomography (CT) allows better visualization of the fallopian canal and associated temporal

---

[1]Not FDA approved for this indication.

bone structures. Magnetic resonance imaging can demonstrate inflammatory changes associated with Bell's palsy as well as tumors.

Electrodiagnosis

Electroneurography (ENog) and voluntary electromyography (EMG) are the two electrical diagnostic tests used most often to assess facial paralysis. ENog can estimate the amount of severe nerve fiber degeneration from an injury or conduction block, such as neurapraxia. It takes approximately 3 days for wallerian degeneration to occur after severe injury; therefore, ENog is not performed until more than 3 days after total paralysis. Electrical testing is not employed if a patient exhibits paresis, because the presence of even minimal voluntary motion after 3 days indicates minor injury, with full recovery to be expected.

ENog uses an electrical stimulus to activate the facial nerve as it exits the temporal bone at the stylomastoid foramen. Resulting facial movement generates a compound muscle action potential (CMAP) that is measured with surface electrodes. The amplitude of the CMAP biphasic response correlates with the number of remaining stimulatable fibers. The CMAP from the paralyzed side can be compared with the CMAP of the normal side. The percentage of functioning or degenerated nerve fibers can then be calculated. Degeneration of 90% or more of the fibers indicates poor recovery in more than 50% of patients. Conversely, if 90% of degeneration is not obtained by 2 weeks, a good prognosis is indicated. In addition to the percentage of degeneration, the time course of the degeneration is important. Patients reaching 90% degeneration within 5 days have a far worse prognosis than those who exhibit 90% degeneration in 2 to 3 weeks.

If the ENog demonstrates 100% degeneration and no CMAP is discernible, then voluntary EMG testing is performed, which measures voluntary motor activity: The patient is asked to make forceful facial muscle contractions, and the single motor unit action potentials are recorded. Because all nerve fibers must synchronously depolarize to generate a CMAP, no response may be seen on ENog, even when polyphasic potentials (a sign of regenerating nerve fibers) are noted on EMG. ENog is also not of benefit in long-standing facial paralysis (>3 weeks) because of polyphasic potentials when degeneration and regeneration are occurring. For similar reasons, ENog is not a useful diagnostic test for facial paralysis caused by tumors.

Treatment Protocols

The management of patients with idiopathic facial paralysis depends on a number of variables. An overview of our treatment protocol is shown in the flow chart in Figure 1. This chart is a general guide. Alterations may be made on an individual basis depending on specific circumstances.

Patients with paresis (partial paralysis) seen within the initial 2 days of onset are treated with oral corticosteroids and antiviral medication. Electrodiagnostic evaluation is not performed until at least 3 days of total paralysis. Prednisone[1] is usually prescribed at 60 to 80 mg per day for 7 days without tapering, and the recommended dosage of valacyclovir (Valtrex)[1] is 500 mg three times per day for 7 days. Patients are re-evaluated within 5 days to assess the progress of the disease. If during the course of treatment complete flaccid paralysis ensues, the patient is managed according to the acute paralysis protocol (see Figure 1). Patients coming to medical attention more than 14 days after onset are followed with only intermittent examinations.

Patients with complete paralysis seen within the first 14 days are started on oral prednisone,[1] 60 to 80 mg per day, and valacyclovir (Valtrex),[1] 500 mg three times a day. ENog is performed no sooner than the third day after the onset of paralysis. If degeneration is less than 90%, medical management is continued for a full 7 days. ENog testing is repeated based on the percentage of degeneration until 2 weeks have elapsed from the date of onset of total paralysis. If more than 90% neural degeneration occurs within the 2-week period after complete paralysis, then surgical decompression of the internal auditory canal, labyrinthine segment, and tympanic portion of the facial nerve through a middle cranial fossa approach is recommended.

Surgical decompression of the facial nerve in Bell's palsy has been controversial since it was reported in 1932. Decompression of the mastoid segment of the nerve provides no benefit to severely degenerated facial nerves compared with the natural history of the disease. Decompression of the nerve medial to the geniculate ganglion, including the meatal foramen, through a middle cranial fossa craniotomy, improves facial nerve return in cases of severe degeneration. We have reported a series of patients with severely degenerated facial nerves that were decompressed through the middle fossa approach (Gantz and colleagues, 1999). Ninety-one percent of decompressed patients exhibited normal or near-normal return of facial function 6 months after the onset of their paralysis. A group of control patients electing not to undergo decompression exhibited normal or near-normal facial function in only 42% of the cases. This study demonstrates that surgical decompression of the meatal foramen and labyrinthine segment of the facial nerve in severely degenerated cases of Bell's palsy provides significantly improved return of facial function compared to those with similar neural degeneration not decompressed ($P = .0002$). Surgical decompression through the middle fossa more than 2 weeks after the onset of paralysis provided results similar to the control group and did not result in improved facial function. If ENog demonstrates 100% degeneration, voluntary EMG is performed to confirm that complete wallerian degeneration has occurred. EMG testing is also performed if patients come to medical attention more

---

[1]Not FDA approved for this indication.

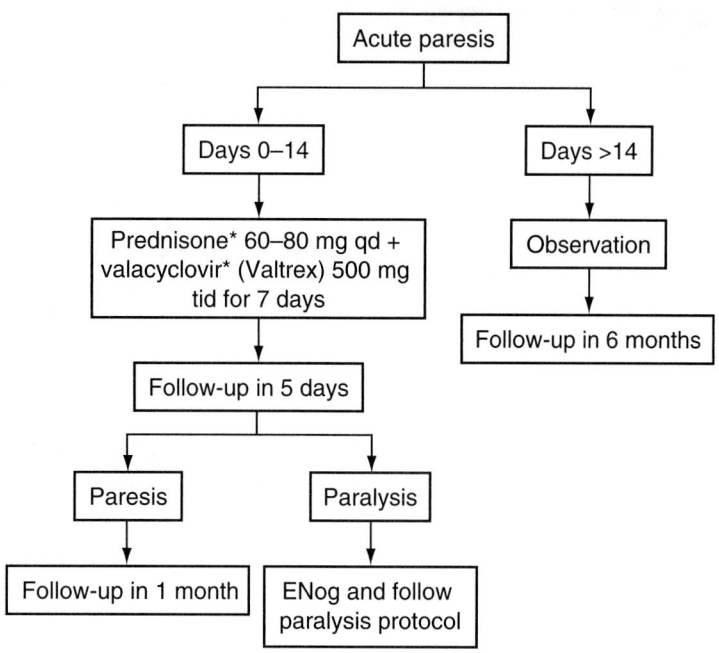

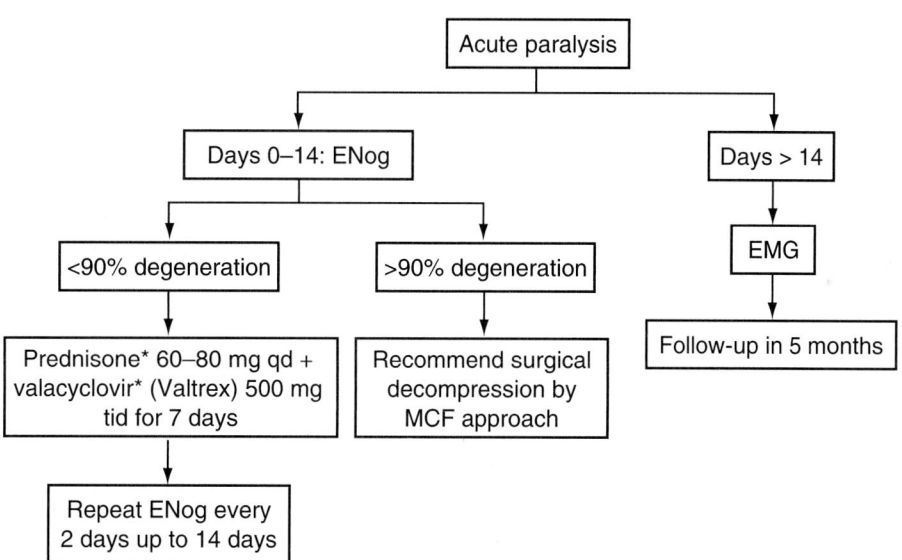

*Not FDA approved for this indication.

FIGURE 1. Acute facial paralysis flow chart. *Abbreviations*: EMG = electromyography; ENog = electroneurography; MCF = middle cranial fossa.

than 3 weeks after the onset of paralysis. EMG testing will demonstrate nerve regeneration with polyphasic potentials.

Preventive eye care is mandatory for all patients with Bell's palsy. Failure to keep the eye moist (with drops during the day and ointment/moisture chamber at night) may result in corneal abrasions and ulcers.

Any problems that develop with the eye should be managed by an ophthalmologist. Bell's palsy invariably demonstrates some improvement by 6 months. If no movement is identified 6 months after the onset of paralysis, the original diagnosis of Bell's palsy should be questioned and imaging studies, to rule out a neoplastic process, must be performed.

Rakel and Bope: *Conn's Current Therapy 2006.*

Parkinsonism

Method of
Dee E. Silver, MD

Idiopathic Parkinson's disease (IPD) is a chronic and progressive neurodegenerative disease that may be at least in part a protein deposition disease not unlike Alzheimer's disease and prion diseases. It is best understood and clinically recognized as a syndrome. IPD has a quartet of clinical signs and symptoms, usually with an asymmetric clinical presentation. Resting tremor is present in 80% of patients. Postural tremor may also be seen in some cases. Thus tremor, bradykinesia/akinesia, rigidity, and, later in the clinical journey, postural instability make up the four clinical features.

The prevalence of IPD depends on age because age is the syndrome's greatest risk factor. The term *juvenile parkinsonism* is used in the rare patients who are younger than 20 years. Early onset of IPD (ages 20 to 50 years) is less common, and the average age of onset is 60 years. In older age groups (65 years of age and older), it is as common as 1 in 100. There are approximately 1 million IPD patients in North America. IPD is probably significantly underdiagnosed because it may have an insidious onset and mild clinical features in the early stages; hence it may be undetectable for many months. Approximately 10% to 20% of patients with IPD have a positive family history. Genetics and also environmental factors play a significant role. Hence etiology is said to have a double-hit phenomenon. Chromosome 4 is associated with autosomal-dominant IPD and with mutations for α-synuclein and the ubiquitin-proteasome system. Clinically, it is a Parkinson's syndrome different from classic IPD. The gene mutations, many probably not yet known, probably lower the threshold for multiple gene interactions and/or for environmental factors to bring about clinical parkinsonism (Table 1). *N-Methyl*-4-phenyl-1,2,3,6-tetrahydropyridine (MPTP), as an exogenous toxin associated with parkinsonism in humans and animals, solidifies the environmental association with IPD. Now rotenone in animal models also supports this environmental role in etiology and clarifies the possible mechanisms of cell death. Rural living, consumption of well water, proximity to wood pulp factories, exposure to herbicides and pesticides, and welding are all environmental factors possibly associated with the development of IPD. Smoking is associated with a reduced incidence of developing IPD, as is coffee drinking, in some Asian populations.

Pathophysiology

The underlying pathophysiology of IPD is not definitely known, but greater understanding is certainly occurring. Initially there is a striatal nigral dopamine-producing cell degeneration, primarily in the substantia nigra (SN). Later there is downstream degeneration in other cells.

In areas of cell death there is the presence of α-synuclein-containing Lewy bodies, mainly in the substantia nigra but also in the cortex and spinal cord. Because the striatal nigral neurons terminate in the caudate and putamen (striatum), there is a deficiency of dopamine in the caudate and putamen. Hence normal physiologic continuous dopamine stimulation (CDS) at the postsynaptic receptor sites is altered and results in abnormal pulsatile stimulation (PS). The degenerating SN with loss of dopamine cells can no longer manage the levodopa physiologically because of loss of presynaptic neuronal capacity. The levodopa can no longer be buffered, and hence other cells take up levodopa and release it in a nonphysiologic manner. Then instead of CDS occurring, there is PS. This PS is associated with at least two downstream consequences: gene changes, which can be measured by microarray analysis in cells downstream, and glutamate excitotoxicity.

This abnormal excitotoxicity is associated with altered intracellular signaling in cells of the medium spiny neurons in the striatum. Genes dictate protein formation; altered or mutated abnormal genes may give abnormal proteins, which, in turn, cannot be appropriately broken down into amino acids by an abnormally functioning ubiquitin proteasome system. Therefore, there may be an abnormal protein deposition. The protein deposition may be part of the process of cell death. The deposition of α-synuclein results in Lewy bodies. The exact mechanism of developing motor fluctuations and dyskinesias is not known, but current thought is that downstream ramifications of PS play a significant role. The downstream changes related to glutamate toxicity are associated with the development of motor complications, motor fluctuations, and dyskinesias. It is also known that with SN degeneration and dopamine deficiency, an excessive activity or output from the globus pallidus interna (GPi) and the subthalamic nucleus (STN) develops. This excessive output inhibits thalamic-to-cortical activity, resulting in some parkinsonian features. The etiology of cell death is unknown and may well be multifactorial. However, mitochondrial dysfunction (complex I deficiency), excitotoxicity, free radicals and oxidative stress, and ubiquitin-proteasome dysfunction with consequent protein deposition may play some role either in an interactive cascade or as a multifactorial mechanism with varying influences.

Differential Diagnosis

The diagnosis of IPD, unless there is a stereotypical asymmetric presentation, occurs often as a diagnosis by exclusion, and other parkinsonian syndromes must be considered. Essential tremor (ET) is often confused with IPD or vice versa. ET usually starts at a younger age, has a strong positive family history in 70% of the cases, and is usually a postural or kinetic tremor that involves the hands, arms, head, and voice and less likely the chin and lower extremities. The patient usually has a long history of tremor and little or no rigidity or akinesia. Wilson's disease, often with a family history, must be ruled out in those younger than 65 years of age by appropriate laboratory testing. Serum copper and ceruloplasmin levels should be ordered, and liver function tests should be obtained.

Dementia with Lewy bodies (DLB) has a clinical picture of fluctuating levels of somnolence and attention robust visual hallucinations, dementia, and basal ganglia disease. The clinical course is much shorter than that of IPD, and dementia and behavioral changes become the predominant clinical feature. Frontal temporal dementia, prion disease, normal-pressure hydrocephalus, and mass lesions, such as subdurals and frontal or deep tumors, must be considered in the differential diagnoses in atypical cases of parkinsonism.

Metabolic, infectious, and other neurodegenerative diseases must also be considered. Magnetic resonance imaging (MRI) may be required to help rule out other diseases that mimic parkinsonism. Atypical Parkinson's disease (APD) or Parkinson-plus syndromes, such as multisystem atrophy (MSA) and progressive supranuclear palsy (PSP), are differential diagnoses with IPD but are usually separated later in the disease's journey by historical and physical findings. APD often has symmetric rigidity and bradykinesia and, less likely, has resting tremor. It also sometimes has postural tremor and myoclonus. Early presentation of gait disturbance; falling, speech, and swallowing difficulty; and a rapidly progressive course over 5 to 6 years are more likely for APD than IPD. Supranuclear gaze palsy is seen with PSP and involves the vertical and then horizontal gaze palsy, usually somewhat early. Dysautonomia—primarily orthostatic hypotension, bladder symptoms, and impotence—are seen in MSA.

Corticobasal degeneration is an APD associated with cortical symptoms and dementia and noted classically to have an alien limb. Dementia occurs robustly in DLB, but also in PSP, and less commonly, if at all, in MSA. However, 30% of patients with IPD have dementia later in the disease, usually occurring after 10 years unless dementia of the Alzheimer's type (DAT) or DLB is the etiology. APD cases may have a mild, somewhat transient therapeutic response to dopamine agonists (DAs) or levodopa (Sinemet), unlike in IPD where there is a robust clinical response that is sustained. Approximately 10% to 20% of patients with cirrhosis of the liver have a spectrum of symmetric parkinsonism. These patients have mild symmetric rigidity and akinesia with infrequently resting tremor. It is important to detect this parkinsonism in cirrhosis patients because many have a significant therapeutic response to levodopa. Drug-induced parkinsonism may be difficult to distinguish from IPD. Drugs such as metoclopramide, reserpine, antipsychotics, and antiemetics are most likely to cause this drug-induced syndrome. Atypical neuroleptics, such as quetiapine (Seroquel), are less likely associated with drug-induced parkinsonism and tardive dyskinesia.

Treatment

Nonpharmacologic therapy for IPD revolves around education for the patient, spouse, and caregiver, allowing for better clinical communication, understanding, and compliance. This results in more effective, efficient

medical care, better quality of life for the patient, and more cost-effective care. With education there is greater knowledge and understanding of end-dose failure, wearing off, motor fluctuations, and dyskinesias. The patient and caregiver can communicate needed and important information to the physician so the treatment can be individualized and tailored to the patient. Exercise for the patient, regardless of the stage of the disease, is crucial, not only for rigidity, akinesia, gait, and safety, but also for mental well-being. Clinical experience and studies document the significance of the ongoing benefits of regular exercise. Adequate nutrition is also paramount. Support groups are closely related to education and also help caregivers' mental well-being. The caregiver role is difficult, and any help is appreciated and needed. Treatment of known or impending co-morbidity in IPD is finally being recognized as important. Aging patients have morbidity and mortality from various diseases related to stroke and central nervous system (CNS) white matter disease, referred to as subacute atherosclerotic encephalopathy (SAE). These two diseases and other vascular diseases are related to diabetes, hypertension, smoking, obesity, hyperlipidemia, and elevated homocysteine levels. Hence, because in the aging patient with IPD the accumulation of co-morbidity adds to the pathology and disability, it is important to diagnose and treat the co-morbid diseases aggressively (Figure 1).

Pharmacologic therapy can start with any number of drugs, usually depending on the degree of impairment, age, co-morbidity, and state of cognition (see Tables 2 and 3). Anticholinergic drugs show efficacy in IPD, more so for resting tremor than rigidity and akinesia. Trihexyphenidyl (Artane) is started at 0.5 mg twice daily and then slowly and carefully increased up to 2 mg three times per day or until it is of benefit. Benztropine (Cogentin) is used at the same dosage. Biperiden (Akineton) is also available. Neuropsychiatric dysfunction (NPD), often heralded by vivid dreams and later associated with agitation, hallucinations, and paranoid ideation, is a contraindication, as is cognitive impairment in the elderly and those that have significant co-morbidity. Adverse events that may occur are confusion, hallucinations, memory impairment, dry mouth, constipation, urinary retention, blurred vision, and tachycardia. Patients with benign prostatic hypertrophy (BPH) and closed-angle glaucoma should be given anticholinergics with caution. Cognitive changes, NPD, or confusion warrant gradual withdrawal of the anticholinergic. Amantadine (Symmetrel), now known as a glutamate antagonist, was first known to reduce presynaptic dopamine uptake and to increase dopamine release. It improves rigidity, akinesia, and, less so, tremor in approximately 60% of patients. It also reduces the severity and presence of dyskinesias, probably through its glutamate antagonism. The elderly and patients with cognitive impairment and NPD have more adverse events, which are vivid dreams, hallucinations, confusion, and insomnia. A benign ankle edema and livedo reticularis can occur. Amantadine is often introduced in younger patients to give theoretical neuroprotection and as monotherapy to delay the use of levodopa (Sinemet). It is also added to levodopa to reduce dyskinesias

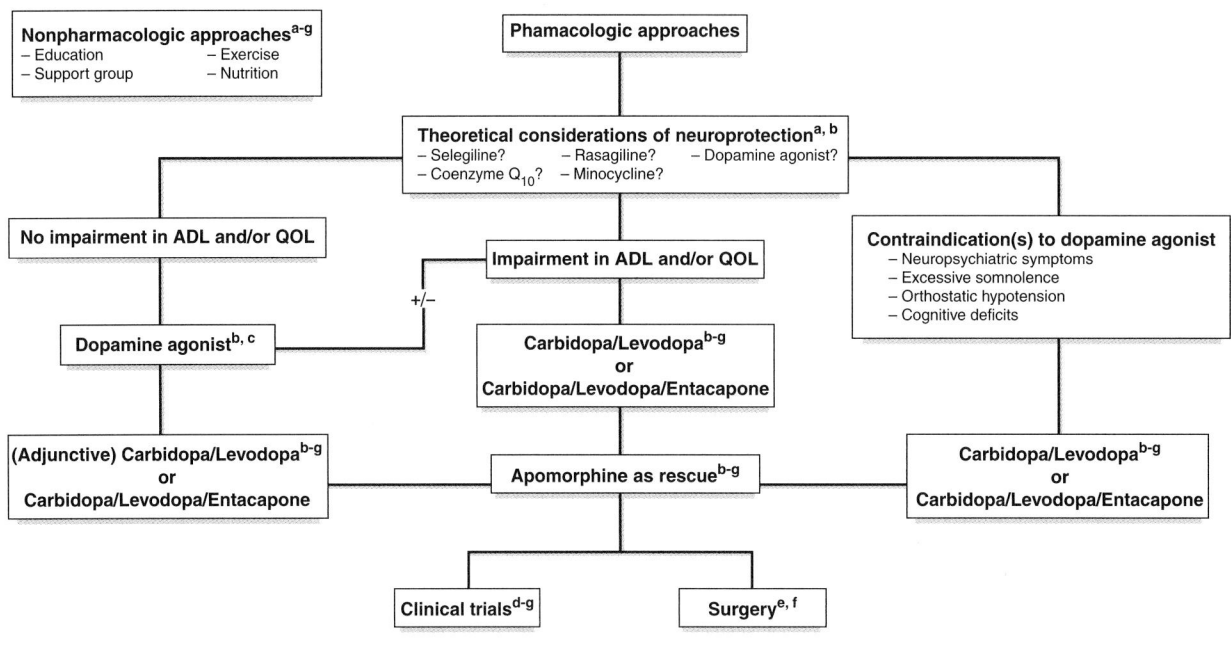

FIGURE 1 Treatment algorithm for elderly patients with PD. ADL, activities of daily living; QOL, quality of life.

in approximately 50% to 70% of patients with IPD. Amantadine also improves activities of daily living (ADLs). Amantadine should be slowly withdrawn from patients with adverse events because often the rigidity, akinesia, and ADLs worsen. It is used at 100 mg once daily, increasing slowly up to 100 mg three times per day; but usually the dose is twice daily, in the morning and at noon.

DAs act directly on the dopamine receptors and were initially used as adjunctive therapy with levodopa. Studies show their clinical benefits with and without levodopa and the ability to reduce the levodopa dose or delay the need of levodopa. DAs bypass the degenerating SN dopamine neurons and do not require metabolic conversion to an active neurotransmitter. They act directly on the postsynaptic or presynaptic receptor. They also have longer half-lives than levodopa's 90-minute half-life. A shorter drug half-life allows for less CDS and hence more PS. Dopamine agonists are without interference from amino acids at the gastrointestinal (GI) or brain transport sites, so they can be taken with food or protein without affecting transport, unlike with levodopa. Bromocriptine (Parlodel), with a half-life of approximately 5 hours, is a D_2 and D_3 agonist with dosing that ranges from 5 to 30 mg, starting at 0.25 mg three times per day. Pergolide (Permax) is a D_1 and D_2 agonist whose half-life is 10 to 18 hours. Usually the starting dose is 0.05 mg three times per day, and it is increased to a total dose of 3 to 5 mg per day. The latter two dopamine agonists are ergots. Ropinirole (Requip) and pramipexole (Mirapex) are nonergot derivatives that are primarily D_2 and D_3 receptor agonists. These drugs in adjunctive studies show improvement in the amount of off time in levodopa-treated patients and allow levodopa dose reduction. Also, dopamine agonists show superior antiparkinson effect compared to placebo in

levodopa-treated patients. Later studies comparing placebo and DAs in newly diagnosed, untreated IPD patients show DAs give robust clinical benefit. DA monotherapy is now the trend in newly diagnosed IPD patients, sparing and delaying the need for levodopa.

Three placebo-controlled, double-blind trials compare the agonist pramipexole with levodopa against the motor complications of Parkinson's disease (CALM-PD [Comparison of the Agonist pramipexole with Levodopa on Motor development in Parkinson's Disease]) study (Mirapex) and the O56 (Requip) study. Several key results are noted in both of these studies. Approximately 30% of patients could maintain DA monotherapy for 4 to 5 years. Only a small percentage of DA-only treated patients developed dyskinesias at 4 to 5 years (7% to 10%), whereas 50% or more of the patients on levodopa/ carbidopa alone developed dyskinesias. Approximately the same percentage was true for motor fluctuations, wearing off, and on-off times. However, levodopa gave a slightly more robust clinical benefit with most noticeably better Unified Parkinson's Disease Rating Scale (UPDRS) motor scores. When additional levodopa was added to a DA as compared to the levodopa/carbidopa-only group, the DA group with added levodopa had less chance of developing dyskinesias compared to the supplemented levodopa group, approximately 25% compared to 50%. Also, the DA group had significantly less disabling dyskinesias compared to the levodopa group. Hence the studies support using a DA first as monotherapy to allow delaying the need for levodopa and to delay motor fluctuations and dyskinesias. Imaging tests were also done on patients in these two studies. Positron emission tomography (PET) scans for ropinirole and a 2β-carbomethoxy-3β-(4-iodophenyl) tropane single-photon emission computed tomography (β-CIT SPECT) study for pramipexole both measured different

Rakel and Bope: *Conn's Current Therapy 2006.*

biochemical aspects. The results show 35% (PET scan) and 37% (β-CIT SPECT) relative differences in reduction in loss of uptake for the DA group. This loss of reduction uptake could represent a reduction in the SN neuronal loss when using a DA as compared to levodopa. However, some feel the reason for the reduction in loss of uptake is uncertain or may be a pharmacologic effect. Hence neuroprotection by a DA cannot be stated with certainty. Further clinical studies are needed.

Ropinirole can be started at 0.25 mg three times per day and increased slowly up to 16 to 20 mg a day. Pramipexole is started at 0.125 mg three times per day and increased to 1.5 to 3 mg per day. Sumanirole,* a new D_2-D_3 agonist, is in clinical trials and looks very promising for efficacy for improving symptoms and disability and delaying the need for levodopa. It appears to have the same adverse event profile as the other DAs, which are also seen in dopaminergic medications, most noticeably nausea, vomiting, somnolence, excessive daytime sleepiness (EDS), hallucinations, and postural hypotension. Going low and slow with the dose and titrating carefully helps reduce some of the adverse events. Cognitively impaired and NPD patients have a higher incidence of hallucinations. Rarely, erythromelalgia, ankle edema, and valvular, pulmonary, and retroperitoneal fibrosis are seen (maybe more so with the ergot DA). Recent case reports show valvular fibrosis occurs with pergolide; however, the frequency is uncertain. This may well be a class effect and needs to be carefully monitored in all patients on DAs.

Apomorphine is used in Europe and has been released in the United States. Apomorphine is a strong D_1-D_2 agonist used subcutaneously with an autoinject pen. Injected subcutaneously, it has clinical benefit in 10 minutes and lasts 20 to 60 minutes. It is a rescue drug used when the patient is having wearing off or just going off. It cannot be used if the patient is allergic to sulfides. Adverse effects seen with apomorphine are somnolence, yawning, rhinorrhea, nausea, dizziness, chest pressure or discomfort, skin nodules, and dyskinesias. Apomorphine may be a drug that enables some IPD patients to avoid or delay surgery. It may also prove useful in patients where other drugs are not possible because of NPD or cognitive changes. Apomorphine is also being studied as a skin patch and as a nasal spray.

Rotigotine* is a DA skin patch being studied that shows clinical benefit. A_2A antagonists have a different mechanism of action but are not yet available for the treatment of IPD. So far studies are promising and demonstrate clinical benefit. It is yet uncertain what effect this class of drugs has on dyskinesias—probably little or no reduction and in some patients slightly worse.

Levodopa/carbidopa (Sinemet) is the most commonly used form of levodopa. However, it is associated with motor complications, mainly motor fluctuations seen as wearing off, on-off, never on or delayed, or on and freezing. Dyskinesia, another motor complication, occurs frequently with levodopa and in the young and advanced patient is the most difficult adverse event to treat and manage. Obviously some development of the motor fluctuations and the dyskinesias is also related to the progressive loss of the dopamine neurons in the SN. The short 90-minute plasma half-life also is a factor for allowing PS rather than CDS.

Levodopa with carbidopa comes in immediate-release (IR) and continuous-release (CR) (Sinemet) forms. Clinical studies show some clinical and probably minor advantages. Sinemet CR was developed to give a more continuous release of the levodopa and allow for a smoother levodopa plasma level, hence more CDS and less PS. There are concerns of variable or unpredictable absorption with Sinemet CR. At 5 years, 25% of the IR and CR patients had dyskinesia, but the clinical study may have had some design flaws. The starting dose should be low and then increased slowly. In the IR levodopa, half a tablet made up of 25 mg carbidopa and 100 mg levodopa may be started once a day and gradually increased to three times per day, then to four or five times per day. Doses of more than 600 to 800 mg should be used infrequently and cautiously, and combination therapy is the ideal therapeutic goal (Tables 1 to 3).

_____

*Investigational drug in the United States.

TABLE 1 Chromosomes, Loci, Gene, and Inheritance Patterns in Parkinson's Disease

Name	Chromosome	Locus	Gene	Inheritance
Park1	Ch4	4q21-23	α-synuclein	AD
	Ch4	4q21-23	duple/triple	AD
Park2	Ch6	6q23-27	Parkin	AR
Park3	Ch2	2q13	?	AD
Park4	Ch4	4p15	?	AD
Park5	Ch4	4q14-15	UCHL-1	AD
Park6	Ch1	1p35	PINK-1	AR
Park7	Ch1	1p36	DJ1	AR
Park8	Ch1	12p11	Dordain	AR
	Ch12	12p11.2-q13.1	LRRK2	AD
Park9	Ch1	1p36	?	AR
Park10	Ch1	1p32	?	S
Park11	Ch2	2q36-37	?	NM

Abbreviations: AD = autosomal dominant; AR = autosomal recessive; NM = nonmendelian; S = susceptibility.

Rakel and Bope: _Conn's Current Therapy 2006._

14

TABLE 2 Medications for the Treatment of Parkinson's Disease

Generic name	Dosage unit (mg)	Daily dose	Mechanism of action
FDA Approved			
Selegiline	5	10	MAO-B inhibitor
Trihexyphenidyl	2 and 5	4-6	Anticholinergic
Benztropine	0.5, 1.0, 2.0	0.5-8.0	Anticholinergic
Amantadine	100	100-300	Release of dopamine, dopamine reuptake inhibitor anticholinergic, NMDA antagonist
Carbidopa/levodopa	10/100 and 25/250	100-1600	Dopa decarboxylase inhibitor/dopamine precursor
Carbidopa/levodopa CR	25/100 and 50/200	50/200-250/2,000	Dopa decarboxylase inhibitor/dopamine precursor
Carbidopa/levodopa disintegrating	10/100 and 25/100	100-1600	Dopa decarboxylase inhibitor/dopamine precursor
Carbidopa/levodopa/entacapone	50/100/150	50-1600	Dopamine decarboxylase inhibitor/dopamine precursor/COMT inhibitor
Bromocriptine	2.5 and 5.0	7.5-40	Dopamine agonist/ergot
Pergolide	0.05, 0.25 and 1	0.5-4.0	Dopamine agonist/ergot
Ropinirole	0.25, 0.5, 1, 2, and 5	0.025-24	Dopamine agonist/nonergot
Pramipexole	0.125, 0.25, 1 and 1.5	0.125-4	Dopamine agonist/nonergot
Lisuride	0.2	0.2-0.6	Dopamine agonist/ergot
Cabergoline	0.5	0.5-10	Dopamine agonist/ergot
Apomorphine	0.1 mL/1 mg subcutaneous autoinjector	2-10 as needed for rescue	Dopamine agonist/nonergot
Entacapone	200	200-1600	COMT inhibitor
Tolcapone	100 and 200	200-1600	COMT inhibitor
In Phase III Testing			
Zydis sublingual selegiline	1.25 or 2.5	1.25 or 2.5	MAO-B inhibitor
Rasagiline	0.5 and 1.0	0.5-1.0	MAO-B inhibitor
Rotigotine	Patch	Patch	Dopamine agonist/nonergot
Rivastigmine (for PD dementia)	1.5, 3.0, 4.5, 6.0	3.0-12.0	Acetylcholinesterase inhibitor

Abbreviations: COMT = catechol *O*-methyltransferase; MAO-B = monoamine oxidase type B; NMDA = N-Methyl-D-aspartate; PD = Parkinson's disease.

Combination therapy is comprised of a DA, levodopa, and perhaps an anticholinergic and a monoamine oxidase type B (MAO-B) inhibitor. It is considered ideal to increase the DA to the highest effective yet tolerated dose before maximizing the levodopa dose or, if levodopa was started first, a DA can be added. As the DA is increased, the levodopa can be gradually reduced. The CR formulation has reduced absorption and hence

TABLE 3 Effects of Selected Dopamine Agonists Used as Adjunctive Therapy In Reducing Awake "Off" Time

Medication	Mean reduction in "off" time (hours)
Zydis selegiline	1.75
Rasagiline mesylate (0.5 mg)	0.49
Rasagiline mesylate (1.0 mg)	0.94
Pergolide	1.6
Ropinirole	1.5
Pramipexole	2.0
Tolcapone	1.8
Entacapone	1.2

needs 25% to 30% more levodopa dose to be equivalent to the IR dose. Adverse events with all medications containing levodopa may be nausea, vomiting, hypotension, somnolence, hallucinations, dyskinesia, and motor fluctuations.

Catechol *O*-methyltransferase (COMT) inhibitors, which should only be used (and only provide benefit) in combination with levodopa, have therapeutic efficacy in IPD. Although tolcapone (Tasmar) improves on time by approximately 2 hours, it can cause drug-induced hepatitis, and the FDA has restricted its use significantly. Tolcapone is still available, however, but it must be used cautiously and weekly laboratory tests are required.

Entacapone (Comtan), like tolcapone, inhibits one pathway of levodopa metabolism by COMT inhibition in the plasma and hence reduces the formation of 3-*O*-methyldopa (3-OMD). This gives more available levodopa to the brain and may reduce peripheral dopamine-adverse events. Entacapone improves on time by approximately 1.5 hours in fluctuating patients. The plasma levodopa half-life with entacapone COMT inhibition is increased by 75%, area under curve (AUC) is increased by 48%, and there is no change in maximal concentration (C-max); however, the plasma levels gradually increase throughout the day. Hence entacapone allows for a smoother plasma level, increases the availability of levodopa to the brain, and enhances CDS. This theoretically and ideally reduces the development of motor fluctuations and dyskinesias. Robust evidence of clinical improvement in UPDRS motor scores and ADLs, as well as a reduction in levodopa dose requirement, is present for fluctuating patients when entacapone is added to levodopa.

Nonfluctuating patients are patients that do not have wearing off, end-dose failure, or dyskinesias. There appear to be more than just the theoretical reasons to use entacapone in nonfluctuating patients, which is supported by some early studies that show improvement in ADLs and other quality-of-life measures. (Even more theoretical would be its use at the time of initiating levodopa therapy in levodopa-naïve patients. This might be done to try to maximize CDS and reduce PS as soon and as much as possible.) The positive study results with entacapone led to the development of Stalevo, a triple pill that contains entacapone, carbidopa, and levodopa. Stalevo allows all the pharmacologic advantages of entacapone with levodopa and carbidopa, along with the ease, convenience, and compliance advantage that one pill obviously offers. Antidotal experience and initial studies with Stalevo show efficacy and patient acceptance and preference with Stalevo. It may become the first-line drug when initiating levodopa in levodopa-naïve patients.

Entacapone and Stalevo are easy to use and generally well tolerated. However, some adverse events may slightly limit their use in levodopa-naïve patients, mainly diarrhea. Entacapone is associated with a 5% incidence of diarrhea, sometimes transient, yet at times requiring the discontinuance of the drug. Bismuth subsalicylate (Pepto-Bismol) or other antidiarrheal medicines can be used to reduce the initial diarrhea until it dissipates. Also, a benign brownish-yellowish urine discoloration may occur with entacapone and Stalevo. The patient must be warned about this side effect. For the use of entacapone alone when adding to levodopa, dyskinesias are the most common adverse events because of increased central dopaminergic effect. Occurrence is usually when dyskinesias are already present and/or when the threshold for developing them is low. When switching patients on levodopa to Stalevo, care must be taken to observe for dyskinesia development. Dyskinesias can then be reduced by reducing the levodopa dose by 25%. Entacapone comes in 200-mg tablets and can be cut in half, allowing for either a 100- or 200-mg dose to be given with each levodopa dose. A maximum of 1600 mg can be given a day. Only one tablet should be given with each dose of levodopa. Stalevo is formulated as carbidopa/levodopa/entacapone in the following combinations:

- 50 (12.5/50/200 mg)
- 100 (25/100/200 mg)
- 150 (37.5/150/200 mg)

The Stalevo pill should never be crushed or cut, and only one Stalevo pill should be given with each dose. No more than eight total Stalevo pills per day should be given.

Rakel and Bope: *Conn's Current Therapy 2006.*

Neuroprotection

Neuroprotection (NP) is a theoretical consideration at the present time. Vitamin E* is suggested as neuroprotective although this is not confirmed by the Deprenyl and Tocopherol Antioxidative Therapy Of Parkinsonism (DATATOP) study. It is probably not easily absorbed into the brain. Coenzyme Q10* was investigated in a small, double-blind, placebo-controlled study at three doses, 300, 600, and 1200 mg. There was a trend to show improvement with coenzyme Q10; however, longer and larger studies are needed, and one multiple-drug NP study is ongoing. Selegiline (Eldepryl), a MAO-B inhibitor, certainly was considered a potential neuroprotector. The DATATOP study's comparison of vitamin E, selegiline (Eldepryl), and placebo shows symptomatic benefits with selegiline (Eldepryl) but could not, in most opinions, document neuroprotection. It is started at 5 mg a day in the morning and usually increased to two 5-mg doses taken in the morning and at noon. It is used mostly for symptomatic improvement, but many use it as theoretical NP. Several new drugs being studied are MAO-B inhibitors, such as rasagiline. It is being studied as monotherapy and for NP. Rasagiline is effective in improving symptoms and is also safe and tolerable.

Surgical therapy for IPD (not APD) began in 1940 when Meyers at the University of Iowa investigated its use. We now have a better understanding of its limitations, indications, and efficacy. Thalamotomy for essential tremor and pallidotomy for IPD gained acceptance in the 1980s and 1990s. Pallidotomy showed efficacy in IPD, especially for dyskinesias but also somewhat for akinesia, rigidity, and tremor contralaterally. However, when this ablative procedure was done bilaterally, despite robust benefit for dyskinesias, cognitive changes, dysphagia, and dysarthria were more common; this has significantly limited the use of bilateral pallidotomy. Ablation of the STN may have some investigative use and is being used clinically on a limited investigational basis.

Deep brain stimulation (DBS) in the GPi and the STN are the most frequently performed surgical procedures for IPD now. Both sites are efficacious. However, DBS in the STN may be slightly more beneficial. Tremor, rigidity, akinesia, dyskinesia, and maybe gait can be improved, and there is an improvement in UPDRS motor scores and dyskinesia scores. Levodopa doses can often be reduced by 50%. Adverse events are not uncommon, and intracerebral hemorrhage can occur in 0.5% of cases. Infection can be as frequent as 2% to 5%, and electrode and connective wires can be fractured. Batteries eventually need to be replaced. Also, cognitive changes can occur as well as NPD. Before a patient should be considered a candidate for pallidotomy or DBS, he or she should have frequent attempts at optimal pharmacologic management, optimal pharmacologic alteration, and individualized tailoring of all medicines. Older patients with significant co-morbidity, cognitive changes, and NPD are generally likely to have significant adverse events and so are not candidates for

14

---

*Available as dietary supplement, and not FDA approved for this indication.

DBS. Patients must be screened for dementia and depression before decisions regarding surgery are made. Most of the clinical series for DBS are done in patients younger than age 70 years. Vivid dreams and hallucinations make it difficult to consider DBS because these often worsen after the surgery. A poor therapeutic response to levodopa indicates a poor surgical response. Patients at best will probably be only as good after the DBS surgery as they were when they were maximally improved on their dopamine agonist and levodopa.

Dementia

Cognitive impairment occurs in 30% of patients with IPD, and the first treatment is to taper off antiparkinson medicines slowly and sequentially that may be associated with adverse events such as cognition and NPD. Patients who have IPD and other neurologic diseases must be screened for dementia. The physician must be aware of the patients who are at risk for dementia such as those older than 65 years of age, those with IPD, and those with other neurologic diseases. Age is the greatest risk factor for dementia just as it is for IPD. Patients at risk for dementia must be screened for dementia, and the Mini Mental State Examination (MMSE), although not ideal, is easy and quick to use. If antiparkinson or UPD drugs must be tapered because of cognitive impairment, they are usually discontinued in the following order:

1. Anticholinergics—amantadine (Symmetrel) and selegiline (Eldepryl)
2. Dopamine agonists
3. Levodopa

In place of these medications, a trial of acetylcholinesterase inhibitors (AChEIs) should first be considered. These are donepezil (Aricept),[1] rivastigmine (Exelon),[1] and galantamine (Reminyl).[1] These are given not only for cognitive improvement but also for behavior issues. Memantine (Namenda),[1] a glutamate antagonist, may also be considered for improving cognition and behavior in IPD. Memantine can be used in combination with the AChEI; it is uncertain if the combination adds cognitive benefit, but it may allow the AChEI to be better tolerated. Hallucinations and delusions need the same scrutinizing for the tapering off of likely drug offenders, as already mentioned.

AChEI can be used for NPD but they do not help, atypical neuroleptics such as quetiapine (Seroquel)[1] or clozapine (Clozaril)[1] may be used. Olanzapine (Zyprexa),[1] risperidone (Risperdal),[1] haloperidol (Haldol),[1] perphenazine (Trilafon),[1] and chlorpromazine (Thorazine)[1] all make the rigidity and akinesia of parkinsonism more pronounced and may well affect the ADLs of the patient. Clozapine needs careful weekly laboratory monitoring. The FDA has added black box warnings to all atypical neuroleptics, stating an increase in rate of death.

Depression occurs in 30% to 40% of patients with IPD, often closely associated with cognitive impairment.

As with dementia, patients suspected of depression must be screened. The Bender Depression Index is easy to use and clinically helpful. Evaluation for other causes of depression must be carefully considered. Education and counseling are important in the treatment of depression, but usually the tricyclics or selective serotonin reuptake inhibitors (SSRIs) are needed to obtain some relief. Constant awareness of changing and developing symptoms of dementia and depression in a progressive, chronic disease journey brings the realization that repetitive screening is needed.

Constipation is treated with eight glasses of water a day and a third to half a cup of oat bran in the morning. These two are the foundation for resolving constipation. If this does not bring relief, stool softeners should be added. Lactulose (Cephulac), starting at 1 tablespoon once or twice per day and increasing up to 5 to 6 tablespoons per day, may be needed. Exercise is important also.

Sleep disorders in IPD are common, and EDS is present in 70% to 80% of IPD patients. A careful workup is needed, including screening with the Epworth Sleepiness Scale (ESS). Insomnia or sleep fragmentation is very common. Good sleep hygiene must be established. To help promote sleep, clonazepam (Klonopin),[1] at low doses of 0.25 or 0.5 mg at night, is of transient benefit. Also, quetiapine (Seroquel)[1] is helpful in refractory insomnia cases. EDS is common in IPD and APD and associated with reduced ADLs and quality of life (QOL). The ESS is of some benefit in detection of EDS, but it is probably of limited benefit for diagnosis of sudden sleep events (SSEs). These SSEs can occur at any time but are most concerning when they occur with driving. The patient with IPD, with or without dopaminergic medications, must be warned about sleep disorders and especially SSEs. They are more likely to occur in IPD patients on dopaminergic medications, most noticeably the DAs. Not only the patient, but the spouse and other caregivers must be questioned about sleep disorders, especially SSEs. For EDS and SSEs, modafinil (Provigil)[1] may be considered if caffeine or maybe amantadine (Symmetrel)[1] does not work. Rapid eye movement (REM) behavior disorder (RBD) is an amnestic state in which the patient is asleep and where there is acting out of dreams by violent motor activity that may be harmful to the patient or the caregiver. RBD is seen not only in IPD but also DLB. Clearly, RBD can precede the onset of IPD. If a diagnosis is made without any clinical features of IPD, the patient must be carefully followed for the development of a neurologic disease. The treatment is clonazepam (Klonopin),[1] 0.5 mg at night, and can be cautiously increased.

Restless legs syndrome (RLS) is sometimes seen in IPD, but it is a separate disorder and often associated with a number of diseases. The symptoms are usually present in the evening or at night but also sometimes after sitting for a long time. The symptoms manifest as an uncomfortable feeling associated with aching, burning, cramping, or dysesthesias. There is an uncontrollable

---

[1]Not FDA approved for this indication.

---

[1]Not FDA approved for this indication.

desire to move the legs, and with the movement there is some relief of the discomfort. Diagnosis is often delayed and late, but treatment should be as early as possible. The first drugs to use for the treatment of RLS are the DAs. They are given before bedtime or in the early evening. Compared to other medications, the DAs are less likely to cause augmentation, which is an increasingly earlier appearance of the symptoms during the day. Levodopa/carbidopa (Sinemet),[1] gabapentin (Neurontin),[1] opiates, or clonazepam (Klonopin) can be tried if DAs fail to treat the symptoms.

Bladder symptoms need to be diagnosed and treated. Nocturia is the most common and earliest urinary symptom. Detrusor hyperactivity is the most common etiology of urinary symptoms in IPD. Awareness of residual bladder volume is important, and if it is more than 200 mL, bladder retention may be indicated. Reducing evening and late afternoon fluids is the first step toward improving nocturia and reducing evening urgency and frequency. Regular voiding throughout the day is also very helpful. Oxybutynin (Ditropan), 5 to 10 mg at bedtime or three times per day, can be tried. Tolterodine (Detrol), 4 mg at bedtime, can also be used. Both of these peripherally acting anticholinergics are now in long-acting formulations.

Orthostatic hypotension is not uncommon in IPD and needs to be diagnosed and managed. Patients examined in the office must be checked for orthostatic hypotension. It usually occurs asymptomatically first and then becomes symptomatic with dizziness and lightheadedness when standing and falling when getting up. It may also be associated with loss of consciousness when getting up from a reclining position. An overview of the patient's medications is the first step in addressing this problem. Any antihypertensive medication that is not needed should be eliminated. Behavior modification and education are very important for the patient and the caregiver. Next, increasing fluid and salt intake is important. Elevation of the bed by 15 to 30 degrees is also helpful. Fludrocortisone (Florinef)[1] can be initiated at very low doses if orthostatic hypotension is not controlled. The dose is started at 0.1 mg per day and can be carefully and slowly increased up to 0.5 mg per day,[3] which is a high dose. Midodrine (ProAmatine), a selective α_1-agonist, can be used starting in the morning with 2.5 mg and increasing up to 5 or 10 mg three times per day. It is used mainly in the morning and at noon to avoid evening supine hypertension. Recently, pyridostigmine has been used to treat orthostatic hypotension with and without midodrine.

There is a great interest in premorbid personality in IPD and a great deal of uncertainty whether one truly exists. However, it is definitely known that many IPD patients have an impulsive-obsessive personality. Often this does not interfere with their daily lives. The anecdotal case reports of sexual misbehavior or excessive sexual appetite and, most recently, excessive gambling may well be an example of the inability to control the intrusive abnormal impulsive-obsessive behavior.

---

[1]Not FDA approved for this indication.
[3]Exceeds dosage recommended by the manufacturer.

Rakel and Bope: *Conn's Current Therapy 2006.*

What the norm is for the same age groups is uncertain for these two behaviors, and more studies need to be done.

The treatment of IPD is rapidly advancing, and the pathophysiology is now better understood than ever before. Combination therapy using different medications with different mechanisms of action will be the rule.

Peripheral Neuropathies

Method of
Marina Grandis, MD, and Michael Shy, MD

Anatomy

Peripheral neuropathy is the common term for disorders affecting the peripheral nervous system (PNS). The PNS consists of motor, sensory, and autonomic neurons that extend outside the central nervous system (CNS) and are associated with Schwann cells or ganglionic satellite cells. The PNS includes the dorsal and ventral spinal roots, spinal and cranial nerves, sensory and motor terminals, and the bulk of the autonomic nervous system. Motor neurons extend from their cell body in the ventral horn of the spinal cord to the neuromuscular junctions at the muscle they innervate. The cell bodies of primary sensory neurons lie outside the spinal cord in the dorsal root ganglia (DRG) where they extend peripherally to specialized sensory end-organs including nociceptors, thermoreceptors, and mechanoreceptors. Central projections from the DRG enter the spinal cord through the dorsal roots. At each spinal segment the ventral roots, carrying motor axons, and the dorsal roots, carrying sensory axons, join to form mixed sensorimotor nerves. In the cervical, brachial, and lumbosacral areas, the mixed spinal nerves form plexuses from which the major anatomically defined limb nerves emanate. Each mixed nerve is composed of large numbers of myelinated and nonmyelinated nerves of varying diameters. The large myelinated axons include motor neurons and large fiber sensory nerves that subserve position and vibration senses. Small thinly myelinated or nonmyelinated axons primarily subserve nociception and autonomic modalities. Preganglionic sympathetic autonomic fibers begin in the intermediolateral column of the spinal cord and synapse in the sympathetic trunk with sympathetic ganglia. Preganglionic parasympathetic fibers travel long distances from their cell bodies in the brainstem or sacral spinal cord to reach terminal ganglia that are near the organs the parasympathetic fibers innervate. The sympathetic and parasympathetic divisions work synergistically to mediate motivational and emotional states as well to monitor the body's basic physiology.

14

An Approach to the Patient With Peripheral Neuropathy

The use of a systematic approach is essential to evaluate a patient with peripheral nerve disease. A multitude of laboratory abnormalities, toxins, and hereditary and acquired disorders can cause peripheral neuropathy. A so-called shotgun approach in which every conceivable cause of neuropathy is excluded is expensive, may not identify the cause of the neuropathy, and is therefore not in the patient's best interests. It is better to use the history and physical examination to demonstrate peripheral nerve disease, use neurophysiologic testing to characterize the demyelinating or axonal nature of the process, and then order the relevant tests to diagnose the neuropathy.

SYMPTOMATOLOGY

Peripheral neuropathies are characterized by negative symptoms, caused by a loss of function of motor, sensory, or autonomic nerve fibers, and positive symptoms, mainly caused by abnormal electrical activities in damaged peripheral nerves.

Motor Symptoms

Weakness and loss of muscle bulk are the main motor symptoms associated with peripheral neuropathies. Weakness is usually length dependent, so the lower extremities are more involved than upper extremities. Furthermore weakness is often most accentuated in muscles providing foot dorsiflexion and eversion (anterior tibialis, peroneus brevis, and longus) and in intrinsic hand muscles (first dorsal interosseus, adductor digiti minimi, and abductor pollicis brevis). Loss of muscle bulk (atrophy) can occur with either demyelinating or axonal neuropathies (see later) because even demyelinating neuropathies develop axonal loss and denervation secondary to the demyelination.

Positive motor symptoms include cramps, fasciculations, and myokymia. Cramps are painful spontaneous contractions of a muscle and frequently occur with chronic denervation. Fasciculations, defined as the spontaneous electric discharge of a motor unit (motor neuron, its axon, and the muscle fibers it innervates), appear as irregular twitches of a muscle. Although fasciculations are most characteristic of motor neuron disorders, they can occur in peripheral neuropathies, particularly in the case of conduction blocks. Finally, myokymia is a continuous rippling contraction of the muscles and can be localized or generalized in a disorder such as Isaacs' syndrome.

Sensory Symptoms

Sensory symptoms are separable into those involving small thinly myelinated or unmyelinated fibers and those affecting large myelinated fibers. Small-fiber symptoms involve pain and temperature; large-fiber symptoms involve proprioception, or position sense. Common complaints in small-fiber neuropathy include feeling like one's feet are "walking on pebbles" or difficulties determining bath water temperature with one's feet. Large-fiber symptoms usually involve an unsteady gait, particularly at night or in crowds where it is more difficult to use vision as a way to compensate for the neuropathy.

Positive sensory symptoms can either occur spontaneously or in response to stimulation; they include *paresthesias*, such as tingling and prickling feelings, and painful *dysesthesias,* such as burning, cutting pain, or the feeling of being stuck with pins. Paresthesias and dysesthesias are associated with small-fiber abnormalities, and, like weakness and sensory loss, they tend to be length dependent.

Autonomic Symptoms

Autonomic symptoms are particularly frequent in certain neuropathies such as those associated with diabetes and amyloidosis. They include urinary retention or incontinence, abnormalities of sweating, constipation alternating with diarrhea, and lightheadedness when changing position. Impotence is a frequent component of autonomic neuropathies.

FINDINGS ON NEUROLOGIC EXAMINATION

Muscle Weakness

Muscle weakness is usually distal and expressed as an abnormality of gait or clumsiness in running. Some increased instability at the ankle, a tendency to varus deformity of the foot, and steppage gait are typically observed. In steppage gait, the knees have to be raised higher than normal to lift the feet off the ground. Muscle weakness and atrophy typically begin insidiously in the foot and leg muscles and especially affect intrinsic foot and peroneal muscles. Calf and intrinsic hand muscles are affected later. Occasionally, in more severe cases, proximal thigh muscles become affected. The atrophy tends to affect the distal part of the gastrocnemius, soleus, and distal quadriceps muscles, leaving only a small mass of muscle at the proximal end. Muscle tendon reflex loss, particularly at the Achilles tendon is frequent, *although not invariable.*

Sensory Findings

Sensory loss is usually found in a stocking-glove distribution for both large- and small-fiber neuropathy. Cold, erythematous, or bluish discolored feet suggest a loss of small-fiber function, although other factors may also contribute. Large-fiber sensory loss, or "sensory ataxia," in the upper extremities is often detected by the inability of the patient to localize the thumb with the opposite index finger accurately while eyes are closed or by the presence of a characteristic irregular tremor (pseudoathetosis) of the fingers. The sensory examination should include vibration, position, and light touch as well as pain and temperature. A determination of the degree and the extent of sensory loss as well as the pattern of the deficits (symmetric or asymmetric; distal or

TABLE 1 Predominantly Motor Neuropathies

Immune Mediated
- Guillain-Barré syndrome
- Chronic inflammatory demyelinating polyneuropathy (CIDP)
- Multifocal motor neuropathy (MMN) (often with conduction block)

Toxic
- Lead
- Dapsone

Paraneoplastic
- Motor neuropathy associated with lymphoma

Hereditary
- Distal hereditary motor neuropathies (HMNs)
- Porphyria
- Hexosaminidase A deficiency

TABLE 3 Neuropathies With Autonomic Features

Associated With Systemic Disease
- Diabetes mellitus
- Amyloidosis

Toxins
- Vacor

Hereditary
- Riley-Day syndrome
- Shy-Drager syndrome
- Hereditary sensory and autonomic neuropathies (HSANs)

generalized; focal, multifocal, or diffuse) in both upper and lower extremities is important.

Most peripheral neuropathies involve motor and sensory abnormalities. Occasional forms involve primarily motor or sensory findings (Tables 1 and 2). In addition, autonomic abnormalities are particularly frequent in neuropathies (Table 3).

LABORATORY EVALUATION

Determining when to order particular tests is one of the major challenges in caring for patients with neuropathy. There are literally hundreds of different causes of neuropathy, tests can be expensive, and neuropathies with different etiologies can present similarly. Certain laboratory tests are routinely ordered on most patients

TABLE 2 Predominantly Sensory Neuropathies

Large-Fiber Neuropathies
Immune mediated
- Sensory neuropathy associated with Sjögren's syndrome

Toxic/metabolic
- Cisplatin

Vitamin E deficiency
Vitamin B$_{12}$ deficiency
Excess vitamin B$_6$
Paraneoplastic
- Sensory neuropathy with "anti-Hu" antibodies

Hereditary
- Hereditary sensory neuropathy
- Abetalipoproteinemia

Small-Fiber Neuropathies
Associated with systemic disease
Diabetes mellitus
Amyloidosis
HIV

Toxic metabolic
Alcoholic neuropathy
- *Nucleoside reverse transcriptase inhibitors (NRTIs)*
Vincristine

Hereditary
Hereditary sensory neuropathy
Fabry's disease
Tangier disease

when they are first evaluated. For example, it is usually necessary to obtain a blood sugar, as well as a set of electrolytes, to evaluate renal function and a complete blood count (CBC) to evaluate hemoglobin levels and red blood cell morphology (for macrocytosis). In the absence of an obvious cause of neuropathy, many also order vitamin B$_{12}$ levels, HIV, rapid plasma reagent (RPR), and serum immunofixation electrophoresis (IFE) early in the evaluation of a patient. This test for monoclonal gammopathy is more sensitive and specific than serum protein electrophoresis (SPEP) or routine immunoelectrophoresis (IPEP). It is at this point that neurophysiologic testing should be obtained.

Specifically, testing is not advisable at this time for the presence of specific antibodies or for genetic causes of neuropathy without an electromyelogram (EMG), even if there is a family history of neuropathy. Interpreting the significance of antibodies reacting with ganglioside G$_{M1}$ or myelin-associated glycoprotein (MAG) should be done in the context of the patient's clinical presentation and physiology. Similarly, genetic testing is most effective when candidate genes are selected based on the patient's nerve conduction studies, inheritance pattern, and clinical presentation. Testing for the presence of specific antibodies or genes is expensive, not always useful, and is most helpful when ordered based on characteristic presentations with characteristic neurophysiology.

Unless the history suggests specific toxin ingestion or deficiency states, testing for these substances without an EMG should not be considered because different toxins or deficiency states present with different nerve conduction abnormalities. Finally, diabetic neuropathies, acquired demyelinating neuropathies, infectious neuropathies, and vasculitic neuropathies all have characteristic patterns of EMG abnormalities.

NEUROPHYSIOLOGY

The use of EMG, including nerve conduction studies (NCS), suggests whether a neuropathy is primarily demyelinating or axonal and whether the process is symmetrical or asymmetrical. If the neuropathy is demyelinating, NCS can determine whether the disorder is purely motor (as seen in multifocal motor neuropathy), distally accentuated (as seen in anti-MAG neuropathies), or uniformly slow (as seen in many genetic neuropathies). If the neuropathy is axonal, the EMG can help distinguish between symmetric axonal neuropathies or the asymmetric mononeuritis multiplex.

Rakel and Bope: *Conn's Current Therapy 2006.*

14

It can also help identify whether the neuropathy is chronic. These distinctions are important because they identify potentially treatable neuropathies. Acquired demyelinating neuropathies or mononeuritis multiplex may respond to specific treatments. But interpretation of EMG findings works best when the study is used as an extension of the neurologic examination. When EMG studies are performed in the absence of quality clinical information, the testing is much less useful. Box 1 lists common laboratory tests useful in evaluating neuropathies.

Classification and Approach to Peripheral Neuropathies

ACQUIRED NEUROPATHIES

Neuropathies Associated With Metabolic Disorders

Diabetes mellitus (DM) is the most frequent cause of neuropathy in the Western world. The estimated prevalence of peripheral nervous system impairment in diabetic patients varies in different studies from 30% to 60% as a result of differences in the measures used for assessment. Although diabetes is associated with a broad spectrum of peripheral nervous system complications, the most typical is the diabetic polyneuropathy (DPN).

Clinical features of DPN include a length-dependent, distal, symmetric, predominantly sensory nerve disorder that may occur in both type I and type II DM patients. DPN tends to develop after several years of metabolic impairment and is associated with other diabetic complications such as nephropathy and retinopathy.

The pathogenesis of diabetic neuropathy is probably multifactorial, involving both microvascular and metabolic abnormalities. The Diabetes Control and Complication Trial (DCCT), performed in 1983, confirmed a definitive causal link between increased blood glucose level and the development and progression of diabetic neuropathy.

In particular, the study evaluated conventional therapy versus intensive treatment and demonstrated a 60% reduction in the intensively treated patients compared with conventionally treated ones. A strict control of diabetes remains the only established therapy for diabetic neuropathy. The mechanisms by which hyperglycemia causes nerve dysfunction are probably multiple and still not completely elucidated.

Current pathogenic mechanisms thought to cause DPN include activation of the polyol pathway, extensive glycation, altered diacylglycerol (DAG)/protein kinase activity (PKC), and oxidative stress. All these factors are targeted by new therapeutic approaches, and many clinical trials are under way. Additionally, a large body of evidence, mainly derived from animal model studies, suggests a role for neurotrophic factors, in particular nerve growth factor (NGF), which selectively supports small fiber sensory and sympathetic neurons, in future treatments of DPN. Specific treatments for diabetic neuropathy are still not available, however, and the current therapy is based on the control of hyperglycemia, the management of symptoms, and foot care. Nonetheless, an increasing understanding of the pathogenic mechanisms may lead to truly effective treatment.

Diabetic patients may also develop acute mononeuropathies, including mononeuropathy multiplex, although the incidence is much less than with the symmetrical sensory neuropathy. The basis for these mononeuropathies is probably nerve infarction. Typical clinical presentations of these focal neuropathies are ophthalmoplegia (third, fourth, or sixth nerve palsies), proximal leg weakness (femoral neuropathy or "diabetic amyotrophy"), and thoracic pseudoradiculopathy (intercostal neuropathies). The mononeuropathies usually present with pain followed by loss of function of the nerve involved. Thus symptoms may be motor or sensory depending on the nerve. Gradual recovery of function may occur over a period of months. Finally, patients with diabetes also are more likely to develop compression neuropathies such as carpal tunnel syndrome, tarsal tunnel syndrome, or ulnar neuropathy.

Polyneuropathies Associated With Other Metabolic Disorders

A peripheral neuropathy may complicate severe renal failure, but these are now less common, in part because of better care for renal disease such as dialysis. Hypothyroidism may be associated with PNS impairment, particularly in the form of entrapment syndromes such as carpal tunnel syndrome.

Toxic and Deficiency Neuropathies

In Western countries, toxic neuropathies are more frequently side effects of medications rather than a result of environmental exposures. In most cases iatrogenic neuropathy presents as length-dependent or dying-back axonal neuropathies. The treatment involves a correct diagnosis and the discontinuation of the drug, but improvement is often slow and may take several months.

Rakel and Bope: *Conn's Current Therapy 2006.*

Neuropathies Associated With Antineoplastic Agents

Vincristine is a vinca alkaloid, used for solid tumors, lymphoma, and leukemia, which acts by blocking tubulin polymerization into microtubules, thus arresting the cell cycle. The neuropathy manifests as a distal, painful, sensory-predominant axonal polyneuropathy. Occasionally vincristine is administered to patients with subclinical hereditary neuropathy, causing an acute and severe PNS impairment.

Paclitaxel (Taxol) is a taxoid mainly administered for ovarian and breast cancers. Similar to vincristine, paclitaxel blocks the polymerization of tubulin and causes a painful axonal polyneuropathy. A recent randomized trial with vitamin E demonstrated promising results in preventing the neuropathy.

Cisplatin is a platinum-derived compound, generally used for ovarian and small cell lung tumors. Cisplatin treatment is limited by a dose-dependent sensory neuronopathy because of toxicity on DRG. Many studies address the role of possible neuroprotectant agents, including NGF, acetyl-L-carnitine, BNP7787, and its derived molecule mesna, to prevent the neuropathy, but data are not conclusive.

Suramin is an old medication that recently demonstrated anticancer properties. It may be associated with both a dose-dependent axonal neuropathy and a more severe, acute, demyelinating neuropathy, similar to Guillain-Barré syndrome.

Thalidomide recently demonstrated anticancer properties and is used against brain tumors and multiple myeloma. Similarly to cisplatin, it causes a sensory neuronopathy by inducing DRG degeneration.

Neuropathies Associated With Antimicrobials

A peripheral neuropathy is described in association with several antibiotic molecules, including chloramphenicol, chloroquine, dapsone, isoniazid, metronidazole, and nitrofurantoin. In most cases the peripheral neuropathy is a prevalent sensory polyneuropathy, with the exception of dapsone, a basic drug for leprosy, which produces a predominantly motor neuropathy.

Isoniazid-induced neuropathy is caused by a vitamin B_6 deficiency and may be prevented by pyridoxine administration (100 mg per day).

Nucleoside reverse transcriptase inhibitors (NRTIs), including zidovudine, zalcitabine, didanosine, stavudine, and lamivudine, are associated with a distal painful sensory axonopathy that is difficult to distinguish from a sensory neuropathy caused by HIV. If the neuropathy is caused by the medications, it usually begins near the onset of the therapy and may ameliorate after its suspension.

Neuropathies Associated With Cardiac Medications

Different medications commonly used for cardiac disease may determine a peripheral neuropathy. Amiodarone, an antiarrhythmic drug, and perhexiline, commonly used for angina pectoris, may bind to Schwann cell lysosomes and cause a demyelinating sensorimotor neuropathy. *Hydralazine* is an antihypertensive drug that, similarly to isoniazid, may cause a polyneuropathy related to a vitamin B_6 deficiency.

Neuropathies Associated With Other Medications

Colchicine, used for gout, may, like vincristine and paclitaxel, prevent tubulin polymerization into microtubules. *FK 506* (tacrolimus) is an immunosuppressant associated with a CIDP (chronic inflammatory demyelinating polyneuropathy)-like neuropathy, usually responding to plasma exchange (PE) or intravenous immunoglobulin (IVIG). *Gold salts,* used for rheumatoid arthritis, can cause both a subacute, mainly demyelinating polyneuropathy and a chronic axonal disease with myokymia. *Phenytoin,* an anticonvulsant drug, may be rarely responsible for a mild polyneuropathy. *Disulfiram* (Antabuse), employed in alcohol abuse discontinuation, may cause peripheral nerve damage. *Pyridoxine* (vitamin B_6) in doses greater than 200 mg per day causes a degeneration of DRG, leading to a severe sensory polyneuropathy.

Neuropathies Associated With Heavy Metals

Several heavy metals are associated with peripheral neurotoxicity, but the observation of related neuropathies is becoming less frequent because of better public control on health hazards. The treatment remains the removal of the source of contamination, eventually associated with chelating agents in case of severe poisoning.

Lead, no longer used in water containers and pipes, is still used as a component for solder and batteries and may cause a prevalent motor neuropathy typically affecting the wrist extensors and the dorsal tibialis.

Today the intoxication of *arsenic* mainly derives from homicide or suicide attempts, but, rarely, intoxication may derive from by-products of copper and lead smelting or from pesticides that may contaminate the soil and water. In case of severe intoxication, systemic symptoms prevail; if the dosage is not life-threatening, however, a painful sensory neuropathy may occur.

Organic *mercury* may be concentrated in fish and shellfish, whereas inorganic mercury is widely used in scientific instruments such as thermometers and barometers, potentially causing a poisoning in subjects working in the production of such instruments, but also in research institutions where such instruments are used extensively. Concerns regarding the safety of silver-mercury amalgam fillings continue to be raised but are unfounded.

Thallium is used in pesticides and rodenticides. A sensory painful neuropathy may accompany hair loss, which is the main clinical manifestation.

Neuropathies Associated With Chemical Compounds

The monomeric form of *acrylamide,* used in plastic and grouting industries, may cause a sensory ataxic neuropathy, particularly through skin contact.

Carbon disulfide is employed in the manufacture of rayon and cellophane and may be responsible for a sensory neuropathy. The intoxication is rare, however, because of the continuous monitoring of workers exposed to this substance.

Ethylene glycol is the main compound in automobile antifreeze and may be ingested accidentally or following a suicide or homicide attempt. It causes a prevalent renal failure associated with a polyradiculopathy with cranial nerve involvement.

The *hex carbons* n-hexane and methyl-n-butyl ketone are proven neurotoxic agents. They enter the composition of glue and solvents, and the inhalation may occur in workers exposed to those products or may be intentional (glue sniffing). The chronic exposure causes a slowly progressive sensory neuropathy characterized by giant axonal swellings observed on pathologic examination, whereas acute exposure may cause a subacute, prevalently motor neuropathy, mimicking Guillain-Barré syndrome (GBS).

Organophosphate esters, molecules used in the plastic industry and as insecticides in agriculture, are acetylcholinesterase inhibitors, which may give rise to an acute intoxication because of a direct anticholinesterase effect. As a result of a chronic low-dose exposure, particularly to triorthocresyl phosphate, a slowly progressive predominantly motor neuropathy, associated with pyramidal signs, may occur, secondary to the inhibition of a specific neuropathy target esterase.

Vacor, a rodenticide usually ingested for suicidal purposes, results in diabetes and severe autonomic neuropathy. Early niacinamide may be successful in preventing these episodes.

Deficiency Neuropathies

In Western countries a severe *vitamin B₁ deficiency* is usually secondary to severe ethanol consumption, even if an additive direct toxic effect of ethanol is likely.

Vitamin B₁₂ deficiency may cause a mild chronic sensorimotor polyneuropathy, but the prominent signs are caused by the spinal cord impairment.

Vitamin E deficiency may be genetically determined and is associated with ataxia (AVED [ataxia with vitamin E deficiency]) or, more frequently, occurs secondary to disorders affecting vitamin E absorption such as liver disease or disorders of fat metabolism (abetalipoproteinemia).

Infectious Neuropathies

The peripheral nervous system may be involved in all phases of HIV infection. The most common peripheral neuropathy is a distal, painful, sensory polyneuropathy, which is very similar to the toxic neuropathy caused by NRTIs; as already mentioned, a temporal criteria may help in the differential diagnosis, but in several cases both factors overlap. When a mainly iatrogenic neuropathy is suspected, the removal of NRTIs may improve the symptoms, whereas a direct HIV-related neuropathy may stabilize or ameliorate with a specific antiretroviral scheme. In the initial phases of HIV infection,

inflammatory neuropathies prevail and may present as either acute or chronic inflammatory demyelinating neuropathies. Differently from idiopathic inflammatory neuropathies, the cytoalbuminemic dissociation usually present in the cerebrospinal fluid (CSF) is less evident in HIV patients because of a mild mononuclear pleocytosis. The response of those neuropathies to plasma exchange or IVIG is generally good. In the late stages, cytomegalovirus (CMV) may cause both an acute lumbosacral polyradiculopathy because of the direct invasion of nerve roots or a mononeuritis multiplex through a vasculitic mechanism. CMV complications are usually treated with ganciclovir.

Varicella-zoster virus (VZV) tends to remain latent in cranial or spinal ganglia after the resolution of a systemic infection. Reactivation tends to occur in elderly persons or immunocompromised patients and determines a vesicular skin eruption, associated with pruritus and dysesthesias. Herpes zoster normally undergoes a spontaneous resolution but is frequently followed by a severe postherpetic neuralgia, which is defined as a pain persisting for more than 6 weeks after the rash appearance. Early treatment with oral acyclovir (800 mg, five times daily for 7 days) may reduce both the duration of the acute phase and the chances of developing a postherpetic neuralgia, which is usually treated with symptomatic drugs for neuropathic pain (see later).

Neuropathy Associated With Lyme Disease

Borrelia burgdorferi causes a disease in which three stages may be recognized. Shortly after a tick bite, in the same area, a nonpruritic rash develops (erythema migrans) and spontaneously disappears after a few weeks. The second phase is frequently associated with neurologic complications such as lymphocytic meningitis, focal and multifocal peripheral and cranial neuropathies, in particular unilateral or bilateral facial palsy, and radiculitis. The third stage is associated with severe neurologic complications, including encephalopathy, encephalomyelitis, and mainly sensory axonal polyneuropathy. A lymphocytic pleocytosis on the CSF analysis associated with a serologic demonstration of *B. burgdorferi* infection on serum or CSF are the main laboratory findings. Whereas early stages are treated with a 3-week course of oral antibiotics (doxycycline, 100 mg twice daily, or amoxicillin, 500 mg three times daily), intravenous penicillin or cephalosporins should be given in late stages.

Neuropathy Associated With Leprosy

Leprosy is the main cause of peripheral neuropathy in developing countries, although it is infrequent in the Western world. Leprosy may manifest in different forms, depending on the host's immune system. Patients with a normal cell-mediated immunity are more likely to have a tuberculoid form characterized by hypopigmented skin lesions associated with hypoesthesia, whereas patients with inefficient immune responses may develop a lepromatous form, which is a more severe disease leading to large disfiguring lesions. A multineuropathic pattern with a prominent superficial sensory loss is the more typical clinical presentation of leprosy. A long-term multiple-drug regimen (daily dose of dapsone, 100 mg, associated with rifampicin, 600 mg, and clofazimine, 50 mg) is normally applied.

Neuropathy Associated With Diphtheria

Although infrequent in the Western world because of intensive vaccination, diphtheria is still an important cause of subacute neuropathy in developing countries. Some strains of *Corynebacterium diphtheriae* produce a potent neurotoxin that causes a palatal weakness, accommodation deficit, and extraocular palsies, followed by an ascending paralysis because of a demyelinating neuropathy that shares many clinical features with GBS. The treatment is based on horse serum antitoxin, as early as possible, and erythromycin or penicillin to eradicate the infection and stop the toxin production.

Immune-Inflammatory Neuropathies

Immune-mediated neuropathies are frequent disorders and potentially treatable conditions. Because many treatments are proposed in the literature, the focus here is mainly on the more common forms.

Guillain-Barré Syndrome

Also defined as acute inflammatory demyelinating polyneuropathy (AIDN), GBS is a rapidly evolving sensorimotor polyneuropathy characterized by prevalent motor deficits, usually with an ascending pattern involving initially the distal parts of the limbs and gradually spreading to the proximal segments. Typically, a progressive phase develops in a few days or weeks (up to 4) followed by stabilization and finally by a slow spontaneous recovery lasting weeks or months. Most of the patients undergo either a complete recovery or are left with minor problems; approximately 20% report a persistent significant disability, and 5% to 8% die from complications of the disease.

GBS frequently is preceded by a respiratory tract infection (cytomegalovirus, Epstein-Barr virus) or gastroenteritis (*Campylobacter jejuni*) that is thought to trigger an autoimmune response directed against myelin antigens of the PNS, probably because of a molecular similarity (molecular mimicry) between a viral or bacterial antigen and myelin proteins epitopes.

Examination of the CSF reveals an increase of protein content with a normal or only moderately elevated (less than 10) cell count (myoalbumin dissociation). Electrodiagnostic studies are characterized by slow nerve conductions and partial or complete conduction blocks.

Recent evidence suggests the clinical presentation of GBS may be more heterogeneous than previously thought. Acute motor axonal neuropathy (AMAN) and acute motor sensory axonal neuropathy (AMSAN) define two variants of GBS characterized by a prominent axonal damage, frequently preceded by *C. jejuni* gastroenteritis.

Miller Fisher syndrome is another variant of GBS with specific clinical features, including ophthalmoplegia, ataxia, and areflexia, and associated with distinct antibodies recognizing the GQ1b ganglioside that appears to be particularly expressed in the paranodal region of oculomotor nerves.

A main point in the management of GBS, particularly for nonambulant patients, is careful medical and nursing care, including proper positioning and frequent turning to avoid cutaneous pressure sores, urinary catheterization to prevent urinary infections, and subcutaneous heparin and support stockings to avoid venous thromboembolism. Patients should be strictly monitored to select those who will require intensive care measures. In the presence of a rapid disease progression, bulbar dysfunction, bilateral facial weakness, dysautonomic signs, and rapid decrease in vital capacity, patients should be admitted to intensive care units and eventually intubated to start mechanical ventilation.

Therapies directed at nonspecifically modulating the immune system are proving effective in many of these disorders. PE was the first treatment to prove superior to supportive measures alone and is therefore considered the gold standard therapy. The usual PE regimen involves four exchanges of 1.5 L of plasma, each spread over a 10-day period. Two PE are sufficient in mild cases, whereas six exchanges are not superior to four in severely affected patients. The therapy should be administered preferentially within the first 2 weeks and not later than 4 weeks from clinical onset.

IVIG therapy, given at a dose of 2 g per kg divided over 2 to 5 days, is equally effective as PE. The shorter scheme acts more rapidly but is associated with higher rates of adverse effects. The effects of IVIG are ascertained if the therapy is administered within the first 2 weeks. Because both PE and IVIG are equally effective, at least in the first 2 weeks, IVIG is often preferred because of the technical convenience of this treatment compared with PE, unless there are contraindications such as low serum immunoglobulin A (IgA) levels, renal failure, severe hypertension, or hyperosmolar state.

Ten percent of GBS patients experience a secondary worsening of their neurologic condition after successful PE or IVIG, but they usually respond to a second cycle of the previously effective treatment. A combined treatment of PE followed by IVIG does not significantly change the prognosis and is therefore not recommended.

A recent examination of the use of corticosteroids in different forms (intravenous methylprednisolone, oral prednisolone or prednisone, intramuscular ACTH [adrenocorticotropic hormone]) by a Cochrane systematic review did not find them beneficial. A recent Dutch trial examined the effects of intravenous methylprednisolone (500 mg per day for 5 days) in association with IVIG compared with IVIG alone, showing a slight initial advantage for the combination regimen, without significant differences in disability at long-term evaluation.

Chronic Inflammatory Demyelinating Polyneuropathy

Considered a closely related disorder to GBS, CIDP shares an autoimmune pathogenesis and a demyelinating

14

damage of motor and sensory peripheral nerves. The clinical course develops insidiously over weeks to months (minimum 8 weeks) or years, however, and may be slowly progressive or relapsing-remitting. Unlike GBS, an antecedent infection is rare, and although considered treatable, the prognosis of CIDP overall is less favorable compared to monophasic GBS. Laboratory features include an increase of CSF protein levels, with a normal or only mildly elevated cell count, and slow conduction velocities. Laboratory tests to evaluate diabetes and monoclonal gammopathy should always be performed because those conditions may be associated with CIDP and influence the clinical course of the disease; in particular, the association of CIDP with IgM monoclonal gammopathy of unknown significance predicts a worse prognosis.

Corticosteroids are the traditional therapy for CIDP and are proven effective. A standard approach is to use oral prednisone (1 mg/kg/day) for 6 to 8 weeks, followed by very slow tapering over several months. To prevent serious side effects, H_2-receptor antagonists; osteoporosis prophylaxis; and sodium-restricted, low-carbohydrate, and a protein-rich diet should be prescribed. Long-term corticosteroids therapy leads always to weight gain, however, and it frequently causes diabetes and hypertension. Particularly because improvement with prednisone may take several months to occur, PE and IVIG are at the moment the usually preferred initial therapies.

Different immunosuppressive drugs (azathioprine, cyclosporine A, cyclophosphamide, methotrexate, mycophenolate mofetil, rituximab, and interferons α and β) are administered to patients who are refractory to conventional therapies, but no definitive evidence proves the efficacy of these drugs.

Multifocal Motor Neuropathy

Multifocal motor neuropathy (MMN), originally considered related to CIDP, is now described as a distinct neuropathy characterized by progressive, predominantly distal, asymmetric limb weakness, mainly affecting the upper limbs. Mild sensory symptoms may be present, but a definitive sensory deficit is usually absent. Electrophysiologic features include the presence of conduction blocks in motor nerves outside the normal sites of nerve compression, prolonged distal motor and F wave latencies, and normal sensory conduction parameters. The CSF examination is often normal, but in some cases a mild increase of protein content may be observed. Anti-G_{M1} IgM antibodies are reported by ELISA (enzyme-linked immunosorbent assay) in 30% to 80% of MMN patients and, even if their pathogenetic role has never been proven, they may be helpful in differentiating MMN from other lower motor neuron syndromes.

Unlike in CIDP, MMN patients usually do not respond to corticosteroids and PE and may even experience a clinical worsening of neurologic deficits following both kinds of treatments. The large majority of patients rapidly improve after an IVIG cycle (2 g/kg over 2 to 5 days), but in most cases the effect is short lasting and the treatment must be repeated every 3 to 4 weeks to

---

TABLE 4   Immune-Inflammatory Neuropathies

Guillain-Barré syndrome: rapid onset
CIDP: subacute to chronic onset
Associated with plasma cell dyscrasia: chronic onset
IgM anti-MAG: subacute to chronic onset
IgG with POEMS: subacute to chronic onset
MMN with conduction block: subacute to chronic onset

Abbreviations: CIDP = chronic inflammatory demyelinating polyneuropathy; IgG anti-MAG= immunoglobulin G anti-myelin-associated glycoprotein; IgM = immunoglobulin M; MMN = multifocal motor neuropathy; POEMS = polyneuropathy, organomegaly, endocrinopathy, monoclonal protein, and skin changes.

---

prevent neurologic deterioration. Because of the high costs of this therapy, immunosuppressive drugs have been tried to reduce or eliminate the dependency of MMN patients on IVIG. Cyclophosphamide, azathioprine, mycophenolate mofetil, and interferon beta-1a have been used, but controlled studies are not available for these therapies. Table 4 lists some of the more common immune-inflammatory neuropathies.

Neuropathy Associated With Vasculitis

Vasculitic neuropathy may be associated with primary or secondary systemic vasculitides or, less frequently, may be restricted to the PNS. Primary systemic vasculitides include polyarteritis nodosa, Wegener's granulomatosis, Churg-Strauss syndrome, and microscopic polyangiitis. In secondary systemic vasculitides, blood vessel inflammation occurs in the context of the following conditions:

- Connective tissue diseases: rheumatoid vasculitis, Sjögren's syndrome, systemic lupus erythematosus, sarcoidosis, systemic scleroderma
- Systemic infections: HIV, hepatitis B and C viruses (HBV and HCV), with or without mixed cryoglobulinemia, cytomegalovirus, human T cell leukemia/lymphoma virus, Epstein-Barr virus, tuberculosis, Lyme disease
- Vaccinations
- Tumors: paraneoplastic vasculitis (described in the paraneoplastic neuropathies)
- Drug reactions: carbimazole, amiodarone, naproxen, allopurinol, hydralazine, sulfasalazine

The clinical appearance reflects multifocal ischemic nerve damage, presenting as mononeuritis multiplex or asymmetric polyneuropathy with subacute evolving burning pain and sensory loss, whereas motor deficits are less frequent and appear later. If the neurologic evaluation is made late in the disorder, mononeuritis multiplex may be mistaken for a symmetric process because of multiple nerve involvement.

If a vasculitic neuropathy is suspected, beyond a complete blood count and a metabolic panel, serum should be checked for:

- ESR (erythrocyte sedimentation rate)
- ANA (antinuclear antibody)
- ENA (extractable nuclear antigen)

- Rheumatoid factor
- p-ANCA (perinuclear antineutrophil cytoplasmic antibody)
- c-ANCA (cytoplasmic antineutrophil cytoplasmic antibody)
- Complement and circulating immunocomplex levels
- Cryoglobulins
- HBV, HCV, and HIV
- Angiotensin-converting enzyme level

In case of a PNS-restricted vasculitis, these examinations are usually normal. Nerve conduction studies may confirm a multifocal axonal neuropathy. Protein content of CSF is usually normal or mildly elevated, except in paraneoplastic neuropathy, in which proteins may be markedly increased. A sural nerve biopsy may show fibrinoid necrosis, obstruction of epineural arteries lumen, perivascular inflammation, and hemosiderin deposits.

In the case of systemic vasculitides, treatment usually requires a high dosage of glucocorticosteroids (prednisone, 1 mg/kg/day, or intravenous methylprednisolone, 1000 mg/day for 3 to 5 days followed by oral prednisone), eventually associated with an immunosuppressant drug like cyclophosphamide, for very acute multisystemic diseases, or methotrexate and azathioprine, for milder forms. In the case of a PNS-restricted vasculitis, a less aggressive approach is applied, including oral prednisone, azathioprine, or weekly methotrexate.

Neuropathy Associated With Paraproteinemia

Paraproteinemia includes different disorders such as monoclonal gammopathy of undetermined significance (MGUS), multiple myeloma, solitary plasmocytoma, osteosclerotic myeloma, Waldenström's macroglobulinemia, primary amyloidosis, and cryoglobulinemia, all characterized by a monoclonal antibody produced by a single clone of abnormally proliferating plasma cells. A monoclonal protein may be found in approximately 5% of all patients with polyneuropathy, in approximately 10% of patients with idiopathic neuropathies, but also in 3% of the general population over the age of 50 years. The presence of a monoclonal antibody therefore does not necessarily mean it is causing a neuropathy. The neuropathy frequently is the main clinical manifestation of an underlying hematologic disorder. Even if in some cases the monoclonal protein may react against nerve antigens, in most cases the causal link between the monoclonal protein and the neuropathy is not clear.

Neuropathy Associated With Monoclonal Gammopathy of Undetermined Significance

MGUS refers to an asymptomatic and often benign condition that may rarely evolve into a malignant form (1% per year). The neuropathy, frequently the only sign of the disease, is more common with IgM-MGUS compared with IgG- or IgA-MGUS. In approximately half of the patients with neuropathy associated with IgM-MGUS, the monoclonal protein reacts against the MAG, a protein mainly localized in the paranodal region

of myelinated fibers, suggesting a direct role of anti-MAG monoclonal protein.

The clinical features of this neuropathy, affecting mainly the elderly, are well defined and include predominant sensory impairment presenting with hypoesthesia, paresthesia, dysesthesia, and unsteadiness of gait. Distal weakness tends to develop in the course of the disease, whereas a postural tremor in the upper limbs may occur in the early phases. The clinical evolution tends to be slowly progressive, but approximately 50% of the patients report a significant disability after 15 years.

Electrophysiologic studies show demyelinating features with extremely prolonged distal latencies. Sural nerve biopsy demonstrates a demyelinating neuropathy with a typical enlargement of myelin lamellae at the electron microscopy and, in most cases, deposits of IgM and complement can be seen around myelin sheaths.

Different forms of neuropathies are also associated with IgG- or IgA-MGUS, but the causal link between the hematologic disorder and the neuropathy is not at all definite.

Based on the likely hypothesis that anti-MAG involves pathogenetic factors, patients are treated with both immunomodulatory and immunosuppressive therapies, including steroids, plasma exchange, cyclophosphamide, chlorambucil, IVIG, fludarabine, interferon alfa with partial responses in open studies, although the effects were never confirmed by randomized trials. Because those patients are usually elderly and all the cited treatments may have important chronic side effects, some caution should be used before starting an aggressive regimen. The anti-B lymphocyte (CD20) humanized monoclonal antibody (rituximab) is being studied in open pilot trials with promising results, and a randomized controlled trial is currently under way.

Neuropathy Associated With Multiple Myeloma

Neuropathy, although not very frequent, may be the presenting sign or may be found along with fatigue, bone pain, anemia, hypocalcemia, and increased erythrocyte sedimentation rate. The clinical presentation of the neuropathy is heterogeneous, probably reflecting different pathogenetic mechanisms, including nerve root compression because of lytic bone lesions, metabolic and toxic effects of both myeloma and the chemotherapeutic drugs, and rarely amyloidosis deriving from light chain deposition. Treatment of the myeloma is only rarely associated with the improvement of the neuropathy.

Neuropathy Associated With Osteosclerotic Myeloma

Although osteosclerotic myeloma is a rare disease, peripheral neuropathy may occur in approximately 50% of the patients and is often the presenting sign. Osteosclerotic myeloma is frequently associated with a complex syndrome called POEMS (polyneuropathy, organomegaly, endocrinopathy, monoclonal protein, and skin changes). The neuropathy is a mainly distal sensorimotor polyneuropathy associated with electrophysiologic demyelinating features and increased CSF protein content. Local radiation or surgical excision of the sclerotic lesions may improve the PNS impairment, especially in the case of a single lesion. Patients with multiple bone lesions are treated with alkylates, prednisone, PE, and tamoxifen.

Neuropathy Associated With Waldenström's Macroglobulinemia

Waldenström's macroglobulinemia (WM) is a monoclonal IgM gammopathy (with κ light chain in most cases), clinically characterized by fatigue, weight loss, bleeding, organomegaly, and hyperviscosity syndrome (dizziness, numbness, visual disturbances, hearing problems, epistaxis, and congestive heart failure). A peripheral neuropathy may occur in more than 10% of cases, and in 30% to 40% of the patients it is associated with an anti-MAG immunoreactivity of the monoclonal protein, sharing the same pathogenetic and clinical features of the neuropathy described in association with IgM-MGUS. In most patients, neuropathy presents as a sensorimotor polyneuropathy that may derive from different mechanisms, including cryoglobulinemia or amyloidosis. Plasma exchange, prednisone, melphalan, chlorambucil, the nucleoside analogues fludarabine or cladribine, rituximab, and allogeneic bone marrow transplantation have been tried, but definitive conclusions cannot be drawn.

Neuropathy Associated With Primary Amyloidosis

Primary systemic amyloidosis includes rare hereditary forms caused by mutations in the transthyretin gene and acquired lymphoproliferative disorders associated with a monoclonal paraprotein, usually IgG or IgM. Congo red–stained deposits, in the majority of cases, of amyloid are found in different organs and consist of fragments from the variable region of the immunoglobulin light chains or the light chains themselves and misfolded transthyretin in the hereditary ones. The neuropathy is a painful, distal, sensory polyneuropathy with prominent autonomic involvement (orthostatic hypotension and impotence), frequently associated with bilateral carpal tunnel syndrome. Liver transplantation is the only therapy for familial amyloidosis, whereas hematologic disorders may be treated with prednisone and melphalan to slow the progression of renal and cardiac involvement and prolong survival. It is rare, however, to see improvement in the neuropathy.

Neuropathy Associated With Cryoglobulinemia

Cryoglobulins are immunoglobulins that undergo reversible precipitation at low temperatures and may damage peripheral nerves through immune complex deposition and consequent vasculitis. Cryoglobulins are usually divided into three groups:

1. Type I (monoclonal) associated with lymphoproliferative disorders and mixed cryoglobulinemia
2. Type II (monoclonal and polyclonal)
3. Type III (polyclonal) associated with autoimmune disorders or chronic infections, particularly HCV infection

Peripheral nerve involvement is a common complication and may manifest as a multiple mononeuropathy or, more frequently, as a distal sensorimotor polyneuropathy. The therapy is based on corticosteroids, cyclophosphamide, and plasma exchange. In case of HCV infection, the treatment is based on interferon-alfa, alone or associated with ribavirin.

Paraneoplastic Neuropathies

The peripheral nervous system is frequently involved in paraneoplastic neurologic syndromes. The pathogenetic link between the tumor and the neurologic impairment is probably represented by a host immune response to cancer antigens cross-reacting with neural epitopes. The tumors more likely related to paraneoplastic peripheral neuropathies include small cell carcinoma of the lung (SCLC) followed by carcinoma of the stomach, breast, colon, rectum, ovary and prostate, lymphoma and Hodgkin's disease.

Subacute Sensory Neuronopathy

The best clinically characterized paraneoplastic neuropathy is the subacute sensory neuronopathy (Denny-Brown syndrome), presenting with neuropathic pain and progressive sensory loss leading to numbness and ataxic gait. The clinical course is generally rapidly evolving, but a slowly progressive evolution may be possible. In most cases it is associated with SCLC, and frequently the neuropathy is the first clinical sign of the underlying disease. Laboratory findings include the demonstration of serum anti-Hu (ANNA-1 [anti-neuronal nuclear antibody) antibodies by immunohistochemical reaction against the Purkinje cells on rat cerebellar section, a normal or mildly elevated CSF protein content, and a marked decrease or absence of sensory nerve action potential (SNAPs).

The detection and treatment of the tumor may stabilize the neuropathy, although a remission is infrequent, whereas immunomodulant treatments (corticosteroids, PE, and IVIG) are usually unhelpful.

Other Paraneoplastic Neuropathies

A sensorimotor polyneuropathy may occur in a variable percentage of neoplastic patients (5% to 50%), without a specific association to a particular histotype, but the causal association between the neoplasm and the neuropathy is always very difficult to prove and therefore the best treatment remains undetermined.

A prevalent motor neuropathy may be associated with non-Hodgkin's lymphoma. A few cases of paraneoplastic neuropathies presenting with prominent dysautonomic features also have been described recently. Finally, different types of neoplasms (SCLC, lymphoma, renal, stomach, and prostate cancers) are associated with a paraneoplastic vasculitis of peripheral nerves presenting

TABLE 5 Axonal Causes of Mononeuritis Multiplex

Diabetes mellitus
Vasculitis
- Polyneuritis nodosa (PAN)
- Wegener's granulomatosis
- Allergic granulomatous angiitis (Churg-Strauss syndrome)
- Rheumatoid arthritis
Chronic Inflammatory Diseases
- Sarcoidosis
Infectious
- HIV (cytomegalovirus)
- Leprosy
- Cryoglobulinemia
Amphetamine abuse
Tumors (myeloma, neurofibromatosis)

as an asymmetric painful neuropathy with increased protein content. This neuropathy usually responds to the treatment of the cancer associated with steroids and cyclophosphamide.

Because many of the neuropathies described in the preceding few sections can present as mononeuritis multiplex, Table 5 presents a brief list of neuropathies presenting in this manner.

Inherited Neuropathies

Charcot-Marie-Tooth (CMT) disease, a class of heritable peripheral neuropathies, is among the most frequent of the genetic neuromuscular disorders with a prevalence of approximately 1:2500. In recent years, more than 30 different genes causing CMT have been identified, and loci are known for at least another 10 causes (http://www.molgen.ua.ac.be/CMTMutations/default.cfm). Despite a marked genetic heterogeneity, some prevalent clinical features may provide clues to the etiology. Patients with CMT tend to be slow runners in childhood, develop foot problems in their teenage years because of high arches and hammertoes, and often require orthotics for ankle support as adults. Sensory loss is variable and affects both large- and small-fiber modalities. Although the combination of weak ankles and decreased proprioception often leads to problems with balance, the vast majority of patients remain ambulatory throughout their life, which is not shortened by their disease. The most frequent form, CMT1A, is caused by a duplication on chromosome 17, containing the gene-encoding peripheral myelin protein 22 (PMP22), leading to an overexpression of PMP22 and producing a demyelinating polyneuropathy. Although no cures are available for CMT, rehabilitation and orthopedic surgery may improve the quality of life and help preserve independence.

NEUROPATHIC PAIN

Pain is a major problem in many peripheral neuropathies, significantly affecting the quality of life of patients. This section reviews the main medications used to control neuropathic pain.

Rakel and Bope: *Conn's Current Therapy 2006.*

Topical Agents

Topical anesthetic creams may provide a local relief without systemic toxicity and are therefore indicated in case of localized neuropathic pain. *Capsaicin cream* acts by depleting P substance from unmyelinated fibers and may be beneficial for some patients. When the treatment is started it may cause a temporary worsening of the burning sensation, which then decreases with repeated use. *Lidocaine* and *prilocaine emulsion* are also used topically for the treatment of postherpetic neuralgia.

The tricyclic antidepressants *amitriptyline, nortriptyline,* and *desipramine* are low-cost efficacious medications. Amitriptyline is the most frequently administered drug in this category. The dosage required for pain control may be significantly lower compared with the doses normally used for antidepressive purpose. Patients should begin at 10 mg, 2 hours before bedtime, and slowly increase in increments of 5 to 10 mg every 3 to 5 days until reaching a significant improvement. The usual dosage is included between 50 and 200 mg daily, but some patients respond to lower ranges. The main side effects include orthostatic hypotension, dry mouth, urinary retention, confusion, and somnolence. They may also increase the risk of cardiac arrhythmias.

Antiepileptic Drugs

The anticonvulsant *gabapentin* is recently approved by the FDA for the treatment of neuropathic pain. The mechanism of action of this molecule is not completely clear, but it was designed as a precursor of GABA and shown to increase the GABA content in brain synapses. It is also supposed to decrease the influx of calcium ions into neurons. The standard dosage for neuropathic pain is between 1200 to 3600 mg per day, divided in three doses. The initial dose is 300 mg, taken 2 hours before bedtime, with a gradual increase of 300 mg per day every 3 days. A slow increase is associated with a reduced risk of dizziness and gait problems, thus improving the compliance, especially in elderly patients. The main side effects—dizziness, gait problems, and somnolence— usually disappear after 10 days of treatment and may be minimized by slow increases in dosage. The only contraindication is renal failure.

Lamotrigine acts through the inhibition of voltage-gated sodium-channels and is efficacious in the painful neuropathy associated with HIV. The usual dose is 200 to 500 mg per day divided in two doses. The starting dose is 50 mg, which should be incremented by 50 mg every 2 weeks. The reason for slow increments is to prevent hypersensitivity. Side effects include dizziness, ataxia, and nausea. If a skin rash appears, the drug should be discontinued because more serious allergic reactions may develop. Multiorgan failure or blood dyscrasias rarely occur.

Carbamazepine is mainly used for trigeminal neuralgia but also is proposed for other painful neuropathies. The dosage is 200 to 1200 mg, divided in two doses daily. The most common side effects, dizziness, ataxia, and dyspepsia, may be prevented by advancing the dose

14

by slow increments. A complete blood count should be carefully monitored to detect blood dyscrasias, including agranulocytosis and aplastic anemia, which may occur as a result of idiosyncrasy.

Oxycarbazepine, a second-generation antiepileptic drug, has proven to be as efficacious as carbamazepine in reducing neuropathic pain, but with significantly fewer side effects. The usual starting dose is 300 mg, twice daily. Most patients respond to a daily dose ranging from 600 to 1200 mg, but occasionally it may require 2400 mg/day.

Management of Head Injuries

Method of
Todd W. Vitaz, MD

Traumatic brain injury (TBI) most commonly results from motor vehicle crashes (MVC) and typically affects males in the 2nd through 4th decades of life. These sudden random acts can have long-lasting effects on the patient and family, but these events also impact society as a whole when a young, viable working-age individual becomes suddenly disabled and dependent on the care of others. TBI has no regard for age or gender, however, and can be seen in infants as a result of nonaccidental trauma as well as in geriatric patients following falls. The management of these patients can become extremely complicated and often requires the close interaction of numerous different health care providers ranging from trauma, orthopedic, and neurologic surgeons to nurses, social workers, speech, occupational, and physical therapists. Unfortunately, current interventions are still limited to the avoidance or minimization of secondary injury and rehabilitative intervention. However, when these patients are managed with aggressive, comprehensive, multidisciplinary approaches, the outcomes at times can be rewarding.

TBI can be categorized based on numerous factors. Most commonly it is differentiated based on mechanism and injury type (closed versus penetrating), whether it has occurred with or without systemic injuries (isolated versus multisystem), and the severity (mild, moderate, severe).

The Glasgow Coma Scale (GCS) (Table 1), which was initially developed as a prognostic indicator following closed head injury, has become the principal triage tool for evaluating these patients. Patients are scored based on their best response in each of the three categories (eye opening, verbal responses, and motor score) and then subdivided into mild (13 to 15), moderate (9 to 12), and severe (3 to 8). One caveat to this assessment tool is that it can be affected by numerous alterations: hypoxia, hypotension, hypothermia, intoxication, infection, and other metabolic derangements, which are commonly seen in the trauma population.

Pathology

Another common classification system following TBI is based on pathophysiologic findings. Concussion commonly occurs following mild or moderate TBI as the result of transient (typically seconds to minutes) neurologic dysfunction in the setting of a normal computed tomography (CT) scan. Brief loss of consciousness, commonly with amnesia regarding the event, is not uncommon and is often associated with nausea, vomiting, headache, dizziness, and transient visual obscuration. These symptoms may persist for several hours to weeks as part of the *postconcussive syndrome* and, in rare instances, especially following repetitive injury, these alterations may become long-lasting. As a result of these persistent problems, in addition to a better understanding of the neurocognitive effects following this type of injury, there has been an enormous emphasis placed on their prevention (see text following).

Skull fractures may occur in isolation or be associated with other types of brain injuries. They are commonly classified based on whether they are open (overlying laceration) or closed, linear or comminuted, nondepressed or depressed. Skull fractures occur either as the result of a large force directed to a small area (i.e., depressed skull fracture following a blow to the head with a golf club) or when larger forces are dissipated throughout the skull resulting in fracture through the weakest area (linear fractures through frontal skull base, petrous, or squamous temporal bone). Linear fractures are commonly associated with raccoon eyes (frontal skull base fractures), Battle's sign (posterior skull base fracture), cerebrospinal fluid leak (otorrhea or rhinorrhea) or olfactory, facial or acoustic nerve injury (amnesia, facial palsy, sensorineuronal deafness).

TABLE 1 Glasgow Coma Scale

Best motor score	Best verbal response	Best eye opening
6 Obeys commands	5 Normal speech	4 Spontaneous
5 Localizes to pain	4 Confused	3 To voice
4 Withdraws to pain	3 Inappropriate words	2 To pain
3 Flexor posturing	2 Incomprehensible sounds	1 No eye opening
2 Extensor posturing	1 No verbal response	
1 No motor reponse	Intubated patients receive a 1 with the suffix T added to score	

In addition, temporal bone fractures may also be associated with epidural hematomas (EDHs). These extra-axial blood clots are most commonly caused by laceration of the middle meningeal artery and result in accumulation of *high-pressure arterial bleeding* in the potential space between the dura and skull. EDHs are more commonly seen in younger individuals probably because of the decreased skull thickness and lack of adhesions between the skull and dura mater in this population. Commonly, these lesions appear on CT scan as lens-shaped, extra-axial hematomas most often in the temporal region and can be rapidly expansive secondary to the high-pressure arterial bleeding. The clinical course in these patients is classically described by a brief loss of consciousness from the initial concussion, followed by a "lucid interval" in which the patient may be awake and alert, which then gives way to another episode of decreased mental status that may be rapidly progressive and associated with signs of brain stem compression (flexor or extensor posturing, dilated nonreactive pupil). EDHs are usually treated surgically unless they are extremely small and constitute one of the few true neurosurgical emergencies where mere minutes may make an enormous difference in the patient's outcome.

Unlike EDHs, subdural hematomas (SDHs) are often associated with other types of brain injury and thus typically involve an altered level of consciousness (LOC) from the onset. SDHs are typically caused by bleeding from bridging veins that get torn when the brain moves within its cerebrospinal fluid (CSF) buffer while the veins remain tethered at their dural insertions; however, other causes such as venous or arterial hemorrhage from a brain laceration also exist. CT scanning reveals that these lesions commonly appear more crescent-shaped but never cross the dural boundaries (falx or tentorium). Unlike the high-pressure EDHs, SDHs typically expand at a slower rate but still cause devastating neurologic dysfunction from compression of the underlying brain. In addition mortality rates tend to be higher with worse outcome for SDH as a result of the common underlying brain injury. Once again these extra-axial clots frequently require surgical evacuation unless they are small and fail to have substantial compression on the underlying brain, where they are managed with serial imaging and close neurologic observation. In patients for whom a small SDH is not treated surgically, the physician must remain cognizant of the fact that a small proportion of these will increase in size between 1 and 4 weeks following the trauma and can be a cause of delayed deterioration or increased headache and new neurologic findings.

Intraparenchymal hematomas occur quite commonly following TBI and can be either hemorrhagic or nonhemorrhagic. These lesions range in size from 1 to 2 mm, up to several centimeters, and can cause a full range of symptoms and neurologic findings based on their location, size, and degree of compression on surrounding structures. Just like extra-axial hematomas, these lesions may increase in size and commonly coalesce or mature and *blossom* during the first 12 to 24 hours following the trauma. In addition, larger hematomas incite an inflammatory reaction in the surrounding brain resulting in increased edema around the lesion, which may result in increases in the intracranial pressure (ICP) (commonly seen on postinjury days [PIDs] 3 to 7). Management of these lesions depends on their size, location, and associated findings and ranges from serial observation and repeat imaging, surgical evacuation of the hematoma, or decompressive craniectomy with or without lobectomy.

The final category of pathologic abnormalities following TBI occurs as the result of shear injury to the axons themselves, called diffuse axonal injury (DAI). This is caused by either acceleration and deceleration or rotational forces to the axons resulting in micro- or macroscopic areas of injury and axonal transection. Most commonly this is encountered in the setting where a patient clinically has signs of a severe TBI, often with a GCS score less than 6; however, the CT scan is either unimpressive or shows only small areas of petechial hemorrhage. In addition ICP recording typically shows normal or only slightly elevated values. Magnetic resonance imaging (MRI) is commonly used in this subset of patients and can be used as a predictive indicator for determining the severity of injury, especially if CT is negative. MRI commonly shows areas of increased intensity on fluid attenuation inversion recovery (FLAIR) and T2-weighted sequences in the brainstem, diencephalon, deep white matter tracts, or corpus callosum. Recovery following this type of injury is variable and depends more on the injury location (reticular activating system of brainstem versus supratentorial white matter tracts) rather than the injury volume.

In addition to these abnormalities, patients with TBI are also at risk for damage to the spinal cord and vertebral and carotid arteries. Thus, patients with altered LOC should be assumed to have spinal instability and possible spinal cord injury (SCI); they should remain immobilized until the absence of these can be confirmed. The incidence of carotid and vertebral artery injury associated with severe TBI is unknown, but patients with facial or cervical fractures and those with soft tissue neck or chest injury (seat belt sign) have been found to be at higher risk. The appropriate screening for and treatment of these injuries have become a topic of intense debate in recent years but should be suspected in a patient with focal neurologic findings without identifiable cause on other imaging.

INTRACRANIAL PRESSURE AND THE MONROE-KELLIE DOCTRINE

Regardless of the pathophysiologic type of injury, the end result commonly is the generation of increases in the ICP, which can then lead to secondary brain injury. ICP dynamics are easily understood if one considers the principles of the volume pressure relationships outlined by the Monroe-Kellie doctrine. The basis of this principle resides on the fact that the skull is a fixed and rigid volume; because of this any changes to the volume of its contents will directly affect the pressure within this rigid space. In simplest terms the intracranial cavity contains blood, water, and tissue. Blood may be intravascular (IV) or extravascular (EV) in the case of extra-axial blood clots; water includes not only cerebrospinal fluid, which may build up in cases of hydrocephalus, but also edema following traumatic injuries; brain parenchyma typically compromises the tissue component but in select instances tumors or cysts may also fall into this category.

As increases in any or all three of these categories occur, the pressure inside the cranial cavity increases proportionally. At first compensatory changes occur, which accommodate for these increases, resulting in only mild pressure changes; however, eventually a critical volume is reached where the compensatory mechanisms are saturated, resulting in rapid and dramatic pressure changes. The following scenario illustrates these principles. A patient is involved in a motor vehicle crash and suffers a head injury with a small epidural hematoma. Initially he is awake and alert without any focal neurologic findings. The epidural hematoma creates an increase in the EV blood component of the Monroe-Kellie doctrine; however, compensatory changes in intracranial CSF volume result in decreases in the water component, thus preventing significant changes in ICP. However, the hematoma continues to enlarge, causing increases in ICP exhibited clinically by slow deterioration in the patient's level of consciousness. The patient is now intubated and mildly hyperventilated causing vasoconstriction, therefore decreasing the intravascular blood component and reducing ICP with an improvement in the patient's neurologic condition. Unfortunately, as the operating room (OR) is being prepared, the patient suffers a rapid decrease in his level of conscious, becoming unresponsive with flexor posturing and a nonreactive pupil. Although the hematoma has expanded at a constant rate over time, the rapid change in the patient's condition is the result of him reaching the critical point where all compensatory mechanisms have been exhausted, thus causing profound rapid changes in the patient's ICP.

Treatment of Elevated Intracranial Pressure

Acute changes in ICP result in altered LOC, and at times other localizing neurologic findings such as *blown* (dilated, nonreactive) pupils and flexor or extensor posturing, and such findings may be the sign of impending herniation and death without immediate intervention. In a patient without a ventricular drain already in place, hyperventilation is the most rapid mechanism for acutely lowering elevated ICP. Currently, aggressive hyperventilation (Pco$_2$ < 30) is recommended only for short durations in cases of impending cerebral herniation while patients are being stabilized. As stated previously, hyperventilation causes vasoconstriction, which reduces intravascular blood within the cranial vault and almost instantaneously lowering ICP. However, several studies have now shown that the routine use of aggressive hyperventilation in the management of patients with severe closed head injury (CHI) results in decreased outcomes because of hypoxic injury and possible stroke caused by the sustained hyperventilation. Our current practice is to maintain Pco$_2$ values between 35 and 38 with controlled ventilation in all patients with

severe CHI; because of this we leave all these patients intubated and mechanically ventilated until their ICPs normalize and all other therapies are withdrawn.

Adequate sedation and pain control are also important elements of ICP control. Patients who are restless and agitated will have higher ICPs than similar patients who are resting quietly in bed. Another important point is the prevention of venous congestion. This occasionally is evident in cervical collars, which are fastened too tight or with the use of trach ties that are wrapped too tightly around the neck to hold the endotracheal tube in place.

Several medications are available for the treatment of elevated ICP with the most common one being mannitol. Although this agent acts as an osmotic diuretic and helps pull excess interstitial fluid into the vascular space and thus lower ICP, there are several other hypothetical mechanisms that probably also increase its efficacy such as increasing RBC flexibility, decreasing RBC and platelet clumping in small arterioles and capillaries, and increasing intravascular volume, thus improving cardiac function. Other diuretics such as furosemide (Lasix)[1] or urea (Ureaphil) may also be used but have less dramatic effects on ICP. Hypertonic saline (NaCl 3% to 5%)[1] has also been used more recently by some physicians and has been shown to have many of the same effects as mannitol.

CSF diversion is one of the simplest, quickest acting methods for decreasing ICP especially if a ventricular drain is already in place. The emergent surgical evacuation of mass lesions such as large epidural, subdural, or intraparenchymal hematomas is also extremely effective for controlling ICP, and in many instances it is also life-saving. However, in some instances, underlying brain injury or stroke from prolonged brain compression may be exhibited as massive intraoperative brain swelling and in these instances may necessitate that the bone flap be left off (craniectomy).

Management of Severe Closed Head Injury

The current recommendations of the Brain Trauma Foundation Guidelines for the management of closed head injuries call for the placement of ICP monitors in all patients who fall into the severe category (GCS score < 9). At our institution we routinely place combination intraventricular monitors and drains in all patients with a postresuscitation GCS score of less than 7. Monitors are inserted into patients with a GCS score of 7 to 9 on an individual basis depending on whether there are distracting reasons, such as intoxication, to cause the altered LOC. If patients are intubated and not following commands but are purposeful in their movements, we will sometimes elect not to place a ventriculostomy and follow the patient's clinical course over several hours. Other factors include CT findings and the need to go to the operating room during the acute period for the

---

[1]Not FDA approved for this indication.

Rakel and Bope: *Conn's Current Therapy 2006.*

treatment of other life-threatening injuries, age, or for heavy sedation secondary to other injuries or pulmonary problems. At times patients in this GCS range will be given 6 to 12 hours and treated medically to see whether or not they improve prior to placement of an ICP monitor.

Once an ICP monitor and drain have been placed elevations in ICP are treated in a systematic order. Target values include attempts to keep ICP less than 15 to 20 and cerebral perfusion pressure (CPP) greater than 60. Low CPP (CPP = mean arterial blood pressure [MAP] – ICP) is caused by either elevated ICP or low MAP. For patients with low MAP or uncontrolled ICP, vasopressors may be used to increase blood pressure (BP) and central venous pressure. At the University of Louisville, dopamine (Intropin) is used as a first line agent, followed by phenylephrine (Neo-Synephrine) and norepinephrine (Levophed) in refractory cases. ICP elevations are initially treated with adequate sedation and pain control, such as midazolam (Versed),[1] propofol (Diprivan), and/or morphine (Lioresal),[1] to prevent agitation and elevated airway pressures, which can further increase ICP and intermittent CSF diversion. In cases where this fails to control ICP, mannitol is then added to the treatment protocol along with more continuous CSF diversion and finally chemical paralysis. Mannitol is administered as a bolus infusion in doses ranging from 0.25 to 1.0 mg/kg body weight every 4 to 8 hours with the endpoints being either ICP control or measured serum osmolarity greater than 315 mOsmL.

Patients who continue to have sustained increases in their ICP despite these interventions are considered to have refractory ICP and at our facility are considered for one of two potential salvage treatments. Pentobarbital (Nembutal)[1] coma has been used successfully on occasion in young patients without mass lesions to decrease the metabolic demands of the brain during these periods of sustained ICP. Patients need to be chosen wisely for this therapy because it carries enormous risks in addition to the possibility of preserving the patient in a long-term, nonfunctional, persistent vegetative state. Initiation of pentobarbital (Nembutal)[1] coma causes severe hypotension, and patients almost always require the use of pressors in addition to volume expansion. At our facility we also place all of these patients on a Rotorest bed in an attempt to minimize the pulmonary complications that frequently occur with the use of this technique.

The second salvage therapy is decompressive craniectomy. This procedure involves the removal of a significant area of skull, typically almost an entire hemisphere or both frontal regions with opening of the dura. This permits the injured swollen brain to herniate through the opening and is the only intervention that increases the volume of the intracranial compartment, thereby reducing pressure. In addition this technique allows for the evacuation of large hemorrhagic contusions, or in cases of extreme ICP elevations it can be coupled with either frontal or temporal lobectomy. Once again,

patients must be selected carefully for this intervention. Decompressive craniectomy is used much more frequently than pentobarbital (Nembutal)[1] coma at our institution. We use this strategy for patients with elevated ICP—more than 30 to 40 for more than 30 minutes—or a significant change in neurologic condition that is nonresponsive to all other interventions. In order for either of these two salvage approaches to be effective, they must be used at the first signs of refractory ICP prior to the occurrence of complications such as ischemic infarcts or brainstem compression or hemorrhage.

Patients treated with decompressive craniectomies are at risk for significant alterations in CSF dynamics that may result in delayed deterioration. Signs of hydrocephalus either in the form of ventriculomegaly or extra-axial or interhemispheric CSF fluid collections will be evident in 50% to 80% of these patients. When necessary these patients will be treated with external ventricular or subdural drains followed by early cranioplasty (replacement of the bone plate). In many instances these changes will resolve following cranioplasty and therefore avoid the need for ventriculoperitoneal shunting, with its associated risks and complications.

All patients with abnormal head CT scans (regardless of GCS score) are treated with close neurologic observation most commonly in an intensive care unit (ICU) setting, serial CT scans (4 to 6 hours later and on PID 1), and placed on 7 days of phenytoin (Dilantin). Temkin and colleagues showed that patients with post-traumatic intracranial hemorrhage were at increased risk of suffering seizures in the acute period; treatment with antiepileptics beyond 7 days did not decrease the risk of these patients from developing epilepsy or delayed seizures but there were increased risks associated with side effects from medication administration. Patients who experience a seizure following CHI (with the exception of acute post-traumatic seizures) should be maintained on antiepileptics for at least 3 to 6 months and possible indefinitely depending on their clinical condition and EEG results. Patients with acute post-traumatic seizures (within the first several minutes following the event) are not felt to be at increased risk for developing further seizures and receive the routine 7-day treatment. At the University of Louisville we have found that changing phenytoin dosing to a weight-based schedule (15 mg/kg load, 2 mg/kg every 8 hours unless elderly [≥70 years old], then 2 mg/kg every 12 hours) increases the chance of achieving a therapeutic dose earlier in the treatment course and lowers the costs of monitoring these agents.

Finally, the treatment of these patients requires a tight-knit group of specialists and ancillary service providers with open communication channels. We have found that the use of a time-independent phased outcome clinical pathway helps maximize the level of patient care and maintain cost-effectiveness. By using such an approach all routine interactions are initiated at the time of admission and each care provider has a clear role and responsibility; one of the most important aspects of this system is the creation of a clinical coordinator whose

[1]Not FDA approved for this indication.

[1]Not FDA approved for this indication.

Rakel and Bope: *Conn's Current Therapy 2006.*

responsibility includes ensuring that all aspects of patient care and family education are completed at the appropriate intervals. We believe another key component of this is our philosophy toward early feeding (prior to PID 3) and early tracheotomy and percutaneous endoscopic gastrostomy (PEG) feeding tube placement in a majority of these individuals (PID 4). We have shown that such an aggressive approach to these issues helps reduce infectious complications and minimizes length of ICU stay.

Treatment of Mild and Moderate Traumatic Brain Injury

In many circumstances patients with moderate TBI are treated almost as though they had severe TBI, with the exception of invasive ICP monitoring. Many patients will be intubated at the time of admission and require sedation and adequate pain management. This can be difficult because it is of utmost importance to maintain the ability to perform serial neurologic examinations. Therefore, we commonly use a combination of propofol (Diprivan) infusions and intermittent morphine (Lioresal)[1] injections in these patients, thereby allowing hourly assessment of neurologic function. We have found that a subset of patients (older than age 45 years, multisystem trauma, presence of early pneumonia) with moderate TBI requires more aggressive treatment with early tracheostomy and PEG tube placement and at times ICP monitors.

The subset of patients with moderate TBI who are not intubated at the time of admission are also watched closely in the ICU. Once again, close monitoring of neurologic function and vigorous pulmonary toilet is of key importance because some patients may be lethargic and are at risk of pulmonary decompensation. We have found ipratropium (Atrovent)[1] and albuterol (Proventil)[1] nebulizers and early mobilization minimize pulmonary problems. Patients with progressive lethargy, worsening neurologic function, hypoxia, hypercapnia, or the inability to protect their airways are intubated and placed on mechanical ventilation. Once again, patients unable to tolerate a diet by PID 3 have a nasogastric feeding tube placed to allow for early enteral nutritional support; however, PEG tubes are not placed until later in the hospital course in the predischarge phase because many patients in this category will improve throughout their hospitalization and be able to tolerate an oral diet by the time of discharge.

Patients with mild TBI are treated over a much wider continuum, ranging from discharge from the emergency room (ER) with appropriate adult supervision to observation in the ICU to immediate surgical treatment of surgical mass lesions. The two most important factors in determining treatment algorithms for these patients are presence or absence of abnormal CT findings and neurologic function, with associated symptoms such as nausea, vomiting, dizziness, or visual problems. Headache is a common complaint in all of

these patients and must be taken in context with other complaints and imaging results. Patients with severe headaches, dizziness, and vomiting (postconcussive syndrome) may commonly require a brief hospital stay to allow for delayed imaging and at least partial resolution of some of the complaints.

Early and Delayed Neurologic Changes

Any patient suffering a significant neurologic injury requires close neurologic monitoring. Although most patients remain unchanged or show gradual improvement in the early phases, a small percentage will show signs of neurologic deterioration. At first these signs may be subtle (agitation, mild increase in lethargy, protracted vomiting); but eventually they may become more profound and can be precursors to impending neurologic demise and death. When these changes are the result of either expanding mass lesions or increases in ICP, treatment instituted in the early phases is more likely to be more successful compared to instances when interventions are performed under conditions associated with cerebral herniation syndromes. Thus any patient showing persistent signs of neurologic decline should be promptly evaluated by a physician and many may also require repeat CT scanning.

However, not all neurologic changes are the result of changes in ICP or expansion of mass lesions, and such irregularities may be caused by a long list of other metabolic or neurologic conditions. Some of the more common causes are seizures, strokes (especially from carotid or vertebral dissections), electrolyte imbalances, hypoxia, hypercarbia, fever, excess sedation, or drug and/or alcohol withdrawal.

Concussions and Sports-Related Injuries: Return to Play Guidelines

Over the past 2 decades, the knowledge regarding the detrimental effects of repetitive mild head injuries has led to intense public debate concerning whether athletes should be allowed to return to play following such injuries. Concussions are not uncommon among participants of competitive sports including football, hockey, baseball, and soccer. Concerns regarding the full negative impact of repetitive, almost innocuous injury have led many youth soccer leagues to ban or modify rules regarding *heading* of the ball. In addition, other concerns exist following more severe concussions such as development of other life-threatening neurologic injuries such as subdural or epidural hematomas, development of the double-impact syndrome (rapid uncontrolled increases in ICP following sequential minor traumas), and the long-term neuropsychological impact of these injuries. As a result of these concerns, the guidelines concerning when and if an athlete should be allowed to return to play have undergone modification

---

[1]Not FDA approved for this indication.

CURRENT DIAGNOSIS

Classification of Head injuries
- Closed versus Penetrating
- Isolated versus multisystem injuries
- Severity
  - Mild (GCS 13-15)
  - Moderate (GCS 9-12)
  - Severe (GCS 3-8)

Pathologic Findings with Closed Head Injuries
- Skull fractures
- Epidural hematomas
- Subdural hematomas
- Parenchymal contusions
- Intraparenchymal hematomas
- Diffuse axonal injury

CURRENT THERAPY

Management of Elevated Intracranial Pressure
- Prevention of venous engorgement
- CO_2 control (mild hyperventilation)
- Sedation and pain control
- Cerebrospinal fluid drainage
- Mannitol
- Lasix
- Hypertonic saline
- Decompressive craniectomy
- Pentobarbital coma

since development of the earlier criteria. Because of these frequent changes, readers are encouraged to check with their local medical agencies or recent publications and Internet sources if faced with these issues. In short, if a player loses consciousness or has persistent symptoms (>15 to 20 minutes), they should not be allowed to return to play on that day or even not for 1 to 2 weeks following the complete resolution of all symptoms. It should also be stressed that an individual may have a concussion without loss of consciousness and that concussion is defined as any transient change in mental status. To this end many organizations including the National Football League have developed a sideline neuropsychological screening test that can often help illustrate these deficits even when the athlete appears normal.

Restorative Therapies

Patients suffering any type of TBI can have long-lasting cognitive, psychological, and emotional dysfunction in addition to their functional and neurologic deficits. Although most people assume that the resolution of decreased alertness and consciousness symbolizes resolution of the overall neurologic injury, this is not the case in most patients. In our series of patients with moderate TBI, we found that almost 50% of patients at median follow-up of 27 months complained of persistent emotional or cognitive problems that interfered with their lifestyle despite the fact that they all were discharged from the hospital with a GCS score of 14 to 15. Long-term speech and cognitive therapies as well as individual, group, and family counseling will be helpful for many of these patients.

In the late hospital and early rehabilitative stages, numerous pharmacologic agents may be helpful to overcome some of the neurologic side effects following TBI. Patients with autonomic storms (intermittent episodes of diaphoresis, tachycardia, fever, agitation) may respond

to adrenergic antagonists such as clonidine (Catapres)[1] or propanolol (Inderal),[1] in addition to volume resuscitation, morphine (Lioresal),[1] baclofen,[1] and bromocriptine (Parlodel).[1] Patients with hypoarousal are treated with amantadine[1] (Symmetrel), 100 mg at 8 AM and 12 PM, and bromocriptine,[1] 5 to 15 mg every day. Trazodone (Desyrel), 50 to 100 mg at bedtime, may be helpful in restoring sleep-wake cycles, whereas risperidone (Risperdal),[1] olanzapine (Zyprexa),[1] and quetiapine (Seroquel)[1] may be helpful to control agitation and combativeness during the subacute recovery phases.

Future Considerations

The previously mentioned treatment strategies include what is considered common practice at the University of Louisville; however, newer, more aggressive treatments and monitoring capabilities are always being developed. Some of the newer monitoring systems under development include cerebral oximetry measurements (frequently through invasive indwelling catheters) or cerebral microdialysis systems, in which continuous assessments are performed to determine the concentrations of critical markers such as lactate in the brain or CSF. Both of these methods provide physiologic feedback for the metabolic environment of the brain, are sensitive enough to predict changes in regional oxygenation, and have been found to be correlated with outcomes in small nonrandomized studies.

REFERENCES

Brain Trauma Foundation: Management and Prognosis of Severe Traumatic Brain Injury. New York, Brain Trauma Foundation, 2000.

Mcilvoy L, Spain DA, Raque G, et al: Successful incorporation of the Severe Head Injury Guidelines into a phased-outcome clinical pathway. J Neurosci Nurs 2001;33(2):72-78, 82.

Miller PR, Fabian TC, Bee TK, et al: Blunt cerebrovascular injuries: Diagnosis and treatment. J Trauma 2001;51(2):279-286.

Temkin NR, Dikmen SS, Wilensky AJ, et al: A randomized, double-blind study of phenytoin for the prevention of post-traumatic seizures. N Engl J Med 1990;323:497-502.

Vitaz TW, McIlvoy L, Raque GH, et al: Development and implementation of a clinical pathway for severe traumatic brain injury. J Trauma 2001;51(2):369-375.

[1]Not FDA approved for this indication.

14

Vitaz TW, McIlvoy L, Raque GH, et al: Development and implementation of a clinical pathway for spinal cord injuries. J Spinal Disord 2001;14(3):271-276.

Vitaz TW, Jenks J, Raque GH, Shields CB: Outcome following moderate traumatic brain injury. Surg Neurol 2003;60(4):285-291.

Traumatic Brain Injury in Children

Method of
Stephen R. Deputy, MD

Traumatic brain injury (TBI) is one of the leading causes of death and disability among children, adolescents, and young adults. An estimated 185 per 100,000 children (ages 0 to 14 years) and 550 per 100,000 adolescents (ages 15 to 19 years) are hospitalized each year for TBI. The etiology of TBI varies depending on the age of the patient, with younger children more likely to be injured from falls and pedestrian injuries, and adolescents more often injured in motor vehicle accidents and assaults. Inflicted TBI (shaking-impact syndrome of infancy) is the leading cause of injury-related deaths in children younger than 4 years of age and accounts for 80% of deaths from head trauma in children younger than 2 years of age.

Types And Severity of Head Injury

Closed head injury is the most common type of TBI seen in children. Forces from rapid deceleration are applied diffusely throughout the brain and consciousness is frequently impaired. *Open head injuries*, in which the dura is breached, are caused by focal penetrating forces, and the risk of post-traumatic epilepsy is relatively high.

Primary brain injury is caused by the mechanical forces of the trauma itself. Diffuse axonal injury is an example of primary brain injury. During rapid deceleration, angular forces applied to the head cause the brain to rotate about its center of gravity. Shifting regions of differing densities within the brain itself result in shearing along planes such as the gray-white junction, corpus callosum, and brainstem. The shearing of axons effectively serves to "disconnect" the cortex from the brainstem and consciousness becomes impaired. Translational (straight-line) forces applied to the head produce impact-loading contact phenomena, resulting in focal injuries to the scalp, skull, and brain, such as lacerations, skull fractures, cerebral contusions, and epidural hematomas. *Subdural hematomas* may occur because of tearing of fragile dural bridging veins during rapid decelerations.

Secondary brain injury follows and is the consequence of primary injury. Examples include hypoxic-ischemic injury (secondary to low cerebral perfusion pressure or anoxia), disrupted cerebral autoregulation, seizures or status epilepticus, diffuse cerebral edema, hydrocephalus, and raised intracranial pressure. The goal of treatment for TBI is to reduce or prevent secondary brain injury from occurring because the primary brain injury has already happened at the time of trauma and cannot be altered.

The severity of TBI can be broken down into mild, moderate, and severe. *Mild* TBI is defined as head trauma with an initial Glasgow Coma Scale (GCS) score of 13 to 15. *Moderate* TBI occurs with an initial GCS score of 9 to 12. *Severe* TBI occurs with an initial GCS score of 8 or less. The GCS is modified for use in infants under the age of 36 months (Table 1).

Special attention should be given to those infants with TBI who do not show evidence of external facial or head trauma and who may not be presented by their caregivers as having a history of head injury. The *shaking-impact syndrome* is usually found in infants younger than 3 years of age with a peak incidence in infants younger than 1 year of age. Presenting symptoms include irritability, lethargy, or coma, apnea or

TABLE 1 Glasgow Coma Scale for Children

Score	Eyes open	Best verbal response	Best verbal response	Best motor response (<36 mo)	Best motor response (<36 mo)
6	—	—	—	Follows commands	Normal spontaneous movements
5	—	Oriented and converses	Coos and babbles	Localizes pain	Withdraws to touch
4	Spontaneously	Confused	Irritable to pain	Withdraws to pain	Withdraws to pain
3	To verbal commands	Inappropriate words	Cries to pain	Flexor posturing	Flexor posturing
2	To painful stimuli	Nonspecific sounds	Moans to pain	Extensor posturing	Extensor posturing
1	None	None	None	No response	No response

breathing irregularities, and seizures. Retinal hemorrhages may be found in from 65% to 95% of these patients and should be actively looked for with a dilated funduscopic examination in any case where head trauma is suspected. Computed tomography (CT) imaging most commonly shows evidence of acute or remote subdural hematomas with or without evidence of cerebral infarction. Workup should include a skeletal survey to look for evidence of skull, posterior rib, or long bone fractures of different healing stages. Infants may be more susceptible to shaking-impact syndrome given their relatively large head size compared to their underdeveloped neck musculature. Infants also have thinner skulls, and translational forces may cause more severe contusions. Relatively longer subdural veins that bridge the infant's enlarged subarachnoid spaces can be easily lacerated from angular forces, resulting in subdural hematomas.

Management of Traumatic Brain Injury in Children

MILD TRAUMATIC BRAIN INJURY

Mild TBI accounts for more than 90% of all pediatric admissions for TBI. Children in this category should have a GCS score of 15 upon arrival to the emergency room, no focal neurologic deficits, and no signs of increased intracranial pressure (ICP). These children may have had a brief loss of consciousness (less than 1 minute), amnesia for the event, an immediate impact seizure, vomiting, or lethargy (as long as the GCS score is 15 during the evaluation). Children without loss of consciousness or amnesia may be observed or sent home with competent caregivers without performing neuroimaging studies. Vigilance for any change in the child's neurologic status should be maintained for up to 72 hours after the injury. If there has been a brief loss of consciousness or amnesia for the event, the risk of intracranial hemorrhage is still relatively low, and it is up to the discretion of the treating physician whether CT imaging is warranted.

Clinical predictors of intracranial hemorrhage are less reliable for children under the age of 2 years, and nonaccidental trauma also comes into consideration in this age group. Therefore, most children under the age of 2 years with TBI should undergo CT imaging followed by careful observation.

MODERATE TRAUMATIC BRAIN INJURY

Patients who fall within the moderate category generally need more intensive monitoring and medical management to avoid secondary brain injuries. As with all critical illness, attention should first be paid to following the ABCs (airway, breathing, circulation).

Airway

Patients with a GCS score of 9 or greater usually do not require endotracheal intubation for airway protection, although they should be kept NPO (nothing by mouth) in case of clinical deterioration.

Breathing

Hypoxemia and hypoventilation may increase ICP, so supplemental oxygen by nasal cannula may be helpful.

Circulation

It is important to avoid hypotension to maintain adequate cerebral perfusion pressure (CPP). Isotonic intravenous fluids should be provided with care to avoid fluid overload, hypoglycemia, or hyperglycemia. Careful attention should be paid to fluid and sodium balance because these patients may be at risk for developing diabetes insipidus. Likewise, the head of the bed should be raised to 30 degrees and the patient's head kept midline to optimize venous return from the cranium to the right side of the heart. Sedation with short-acting sedatives (propofol [Diprivan] or midazolam [Versed]) or opioids may be necessary to avoid agitation, which can also reduce venous return to the heart.

Early post-traumatic seizures are fairly rare in children with moderate TBI. The need for empirical anticonvulsant therapy in this group remains controversial and should be reserved for those patients in whom raised intracranial pressure is of concern. Likewise, empirical use of mannitol has little clinical support for this group.

SEVERE TRAUMATIC BRAIN INJURY

Patients in the severe group are at the highest risk for secondary brain injuries. The following additional interventions are recommended.

Airway

By definition, these patients have a GCS score of 8 or lower and require endotracheal intubation for airway protection.

Breathing

Hyperventilation with a goal P_{CO_2} of 26 to 30 mm Hg should be performed only if there is impending brainstem herniation or to bridge the gap until more definitive neurosurgical intervention can be performed to lower intracranial pressure. The benefit of hyperventilation is generally short lived (1 to 24 hours) and may worsen local ischemia following trauma or acute stroke.

Circulation

In the setting of suspected raised intracranial pressure, the goal of fluid and blood pressure management should be to maintain the cerebral perfusion pressure greater than 50 to 70 mm Hg. Recall that CPP equals MAP (mean arterial blood pressure) minus ICP. Because children generally have a lower MAP than adults, it is not always necessary to provide vasopressor therapy to keep the CPP above 70 mm Hg unless there is evidence of raised ICP. Invasive intracranial pressure monitoring should be considered if the GCS score is lower than 8 or in the setting of elevated ICP to optimize CPP.

Rakel and Bope: *Conn's Current Therapy 2006.*

CURRENT DIAGNOSIS

- Children under the age of 2 years with traumatic brain injury (TBI) may require neuroimaging because clinical predictors of intracranial hemorrhage are less reliable in this age group.
- Children under the age of 1 year presenting with lethargy, irritability, apnea, or seizures should be evaluated with computed tomography (CT) imaging and a dilated funduscopic examination to rule out shaking-impact syndrome.

Other Techniques to Lower Intracranial Pressure

NEUROSURGICAL

Obvious mass lesions, such as hydrocephalus, subdural and epidural hematomas, and contused cortical tissue should be surgically evacuated whenever feasible. CT scanning is able to identify most of these surgical lesions. Decompressive craniectomy is now used more frequently to relieve pressure when multifocal contusions or diffuse cerebral edema is present. As mentioned earlier, ICP monitoring is usually warranted for all severe TBI patients.

OSMOTHERAPY

Mannitol (20% solution) may be given as an initial bolus of 0.5 to 1 g/kg. Repeat doses of 0.25 to 0.5 g/kg are given every 6 to 8 hours as needed to maintain the serum osmolality and sodium levels to less than or equal to 320 mOsmL and 150 mEq, respectively. Osmotic diuretics should be used with caution in patients with renal insufficiency. The beneficial effects occur within minutes, peak at 1 hour, and last 4 to 24 hours. Potential disadvantages include worsening of focal cerebral edema in areas where the blood-brain barrier is disrupted.

BARBITURATES

Sedating agents may lower ICP by reducing pain as well as by making the brain metabolically less active. Pentobarbital is given as a loading dose of 5 to 20 mg/kg, followed by a continuous infusion of 1 to 4 mg/kg per hour. Continuous EEG monitoring to maintain a burst suppression pattern is warranted with this therapy. Potential disadvantages include systemic hypotension and a long half-life that may interfere with the declaration of brain death.

ANTICONVULSANT THERAPY

Children with severe TBI are at a high risk for early post-traumatic seizures, which can further elevate the ICP. It is generally recommended empirically to load these children with 20 mg/kg of intravenous phenytoin (Cerebyx). Maintenance therapy can be achieved with

CURRENT THERAPY

- Children with mild TBI and a GCS score of 15 at presentation can usually be observed clinically without the need for neuroimaging.
- The goal of treatment for TBI is to minimize *secondary* brain injury.
- In the setting of raised ICP, it is important to maintain CPP above 50 to 70 mm Hg.
- Early post-traumatic seizures are relatively frequent in open head injury and in severe TBI. They should be empirically treated in any patient in whom raised ICP is a concern.
- Direct intracranial pressure monitoring should be considered in any TBI patient with a GCS score of 8 or less.

Abbreviations: CPP = cerebral perfusion pressure; ICP = intracranial pressure; GCS = Glasgow Coma Scale; TBI = traumatic brain injury.

5 mg/kg per day divided every 8 hours with target blood levels of 10 to 20 mg/dL.

HYPOTHERMIA

More centers are including hypothermia as an option for patients with elevated ICP not responsive to medical or surgical management. The best method of cooling (i.e., whole body versus head only) and the optimal core temperature are not established for children.

Of note, apart from neurosurgical interventions, none of the techniques just described are shown definitively to reduce morbidity or mortality in children with severe TBI.

REFERENCES

Annegers JF, Grabow JD, Grover RV, et al: Seizures after head trauma: A population study. Neurology 1980;30:683-689.
Bruce DA, Zimmerman RA: Shaken impact syndrome. Pediatr Ann 1989;18:482-494.
Committee on Quality Improvement, American Academy of Pediatrics: The management of minor closed head injury in children. Pediatrics 1999;104(6):1407-1415.
Deputy SR: Shaking-impact syndrome of infancy. Semin Pediatr Neurol 2003;10(2):112-119.
Kraus JF, Nourjah P: The epidemiology of uncomplicated brain injury. J Trauma 1988;28:1637-1643.
Schutzman SA, Barnes P, et al: Evaluation and management of children younger than two years old with apparently minor head trauma: Proposed guidelines. Pediatrics 2001;107:983-993.

Brain Tumors

Method of
Ashwatha Narayana, MD

Primary brain tumors accounted for an estimated 18,400 new cases diagnosed and 12,690 deaths in the year 2004 in the United States. Several histopathologically different tumors arise in the brain, reflecting the diversity of phenotypically distinct cells within the central nervous system (CNS) that have a capacity for neoplastic transformation. Gliomas, the most common tumors, are considered first in this article, followed by a description of many of the principles of brain tumor management. Then less common tumors are briefly presented, and the article closes with a discussion about managing metastatic brain tumors.

Gliomas

INCIDENCE

Malignant gliomas make up 35% to 45% of primary brain tumors, and of these, nearly 85% are glioblastoma multiforme. The incidence of anaplastic astrocytoma peaks in children younger than 10 years of age and then remains constant in each subsequent decade of life. In contrast, the incidence of glioblastoma multiforme increases dramatically after the age of 40 years. Low-grade astrocytomas make up 5% to 15% of primary brain tumors and 67% of low-grade gliomas. The remainder of low-grade gliomas are mixed oligoastrocytomas (19%) and oligodendrogliomas (13%). Unlike their malignant counterparts, low-grade gliomas are most common between the ages of 20 and 40 years and rarely occur after the age of 50 years.

GENETICS AND ETIOLOGY

Genetic abnormalities are demonstrated for 50% to 75% of adult astrocytomas. It is hypothesized that p53 gene mutations are associated with the transition to grade II tumors. Malignant progression to anaplastic astrocytoma is associated with loss of heterozygosity (LOH) for chromosomes 9p, 13q, or 19q and CDK4 gene amplification. Subsequent LOH on chromosome 10 and amplification of the epidermal growth factor receptor genes characterize further progression to glioblastoma multiforme. A second, p53-independent, pathway that leads more directly to glioblastoma multiforme development is also described.

Losses of genetic information from chromosomes 1p and 19q are commonly seen in oligodendroglioma specimens, whereas losses on 17p and p53 gene mutations are notably less frequent, suggesting that early events in their oncogenesis are distinct from those associated with astrocytic tumors.

Although some environmental factors are linked with brain tumor development, they do not appear responsible for most brain tumors. Radiation-induced gliomas are reported, mainly in children with acute leukemia who received prophylactic cranial irradiation and chemotherapy. The hereditary syndromes associated with an increased risk of brain tumors include neurofibromatosis type 1 and neurofibromatosis type 2, tuberous sclerosis, Li-Fraumeni syndrome, familial polyposis, Turcot's syndrome, Gardner's syndrome, and von Hippel-Lindau disease.

PATHOLOGY

CNS tumors are generally classified as follows (Table 1):

- Gliomas
- Neuronal/glioneuronal neoplasms
- Embryonal neoplasms
- Meningeal neoplasms
- Miscellaneous nonglial neoplasms

Reliance on a pathologic classification of brain tumors is a requisite for treatment. Indeed, histopathology is more important than anatomic staging in determining the clinical behavior and prognosis of these tumors. Neuropathologists do not all agree on a uniform classification system for astrocytic gliomas. The World Health Organization system, which divides astrocytic tumors into four grades—from grade I, corresponding to pilocytic astrocytomas, to grade IV, corresponding to the glioblastoma multiforme—is used more often.

Low-grade astrocytomas are well-differentiated tumors that display increased cellularity compared with normal brain tissue and have mild to moderate nuclear pleomorphism (Figure 1). The cytoplasmic processes that extend from the astrocytes contain a characteristic filamentous protein, glial fibrillary acidic protein (GFAP), which provides an immunohistochemical marker for these tumors. Over time, at least 50% of these tumors transform into more anaplastic lesions. The characteristic histopathologic features of anaplastic astrocytomas include moderate hypercellularity, moderate cellular and nuclear pleomorphism, variable mitotic activity, and microvascular proliferation. The presence of tumor necrosis is the hallmark that distinguishes anaplastic astrocytoma from glioblastoma multiforme (Figure 2).

Oligodendrogliomas, in contrast, are composed of small uniform cells with round central nuclei and distinct cytoplasmic borders. Formalin fixation causes a perinuclear halo that produces a "fried egg" or "honeycomb" appearance. The cells lack fibrillary cytoplasmic processes. Calcification is a frequent feature.

CLINICAL PRESENTATION

The presenting symptoms and signs of brain tumors include those associated with a mass effect and increased intracranial pressure and those that are focal. The most common presenting symptom with gliomas is headache. Approximately two thirds of adult patients

TABLE 1 Histopathology of Brain Tumors

Major classification	Variants	WHO grade
Gliomas		
Astrocytic: circumscribed	Pilocytic astrocytoma	I
	Subependymal giant cell astrocytoma (SEGA)	I
	Pleomorphic xanthoastrocytoma (PXA)	II
Astrocytic: diffuse	Astrocytoma	II
	Anaplastic astrocytoma	III
	Glioblastoma multiforme	IV
Oligodendroglial	Oligodendroglioma	II
	Anaplastic oligodendroglioma	III
Mixed gliomas	Oligoastrocytoma	II
	Anaplastic oligoastrocytoma	III
Ependymal	Subependymoma	I
	Myxopapillary ependymoma	I
	Ependymoma	II
	Anaplastic ependymoma*	III
Choroid plexus	Choroid plexus papilloma	I
	Choroid plexus carcinoma*	III
Cranial and peripheral nervetumors	Schwannoma	I
Neuronal and glioneuronal tumors	Gangliocytoma/ganglioglioma	I–III
	Desmoplastic infantile ganglioma (DIG)	I
	Dysplastic cerebellar gangliocytoma	I
	Central neurocytoma	I
	Dysembryoplastic neuroepithelial tumor	I
	Paraganglioma	I
Pineal parenchymal tumors (PPTs)	Pineocytoma	II
	PPT with intermediate differentiation	III
	Pineoblastoma	IV
Embryonal tumors	Medulloepithelioma*	IV
	Primitive neuroectodermal tumor (PNET),* including medulloblastoma and variants*	IV
	Atypical teratoid/rhabdoid tumor (AT/RT)	IV
	Cerebral neuroblastoma/ganglioneuroblastoma	IV
	Ependymoblastoma*	IV
	Olfactory neuroblastoma (esthesioneuroblastoma)	IV
Meningeal tumors	Meningioma	I
	Atypical meningioma	II
	Anaplastic (malignant) meningioma	III
Germ cell tumors	Hemangiopericytoma†	II–III
	Germinoma	NA
	Mature teratoma	NA
	Nongerminomatous germ cell tumors	NA
Tumors of the sellar region	Craniopharyngioma: adamantinomatous	I
	Craniopharyngioma: papillary	I
Hemopoietic neoplasms	Primary central nervous system lymphoma (PCNSL)	NA
	Secondary lymphoma/leukemia	NA
	Histiocytic tumors and histiocytoses	NA
Secondary tumors/metastases	Carcinomas and sarcomas	NA

*Indicates those tumors with a tendency to disseminate throughout the central nervous system (CNS).
†The origin of hemangiopericytoma is uncertain.
Abbreviations: WHO = World Health Organization; NA = not applicable.

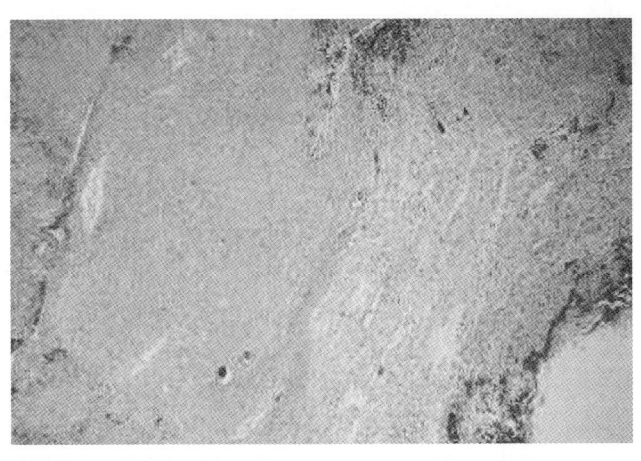

FIGURE 1. Low-grade astrocytoma showing mildly increased cellularity with uniform cells and nuclei.

with low-grade astrocytomas and 20% of patients with malignant tumors present with seizures but are otherwise neurologically intact. Others exhibit a slowly progressive neurologic syndrome consisting of headache, vomiting, motor deficit, visual or sensory loss, language disturbance, or personality change. Symptoms may be present for months or years before the diagnosis is made.

ROUTES OF SPREAD

The most common route of spread for gliomas is through local extension. As they enlarge, malignant gliomas extend directly into adjacent lobes and disseminate along anatomically defined nerve fiber pathways. Multicentric gliomas are found in less than 5% of patients. Dissemination by seeding through the CPF pathways occurs in approximately 10% of cases but is usually a late event. Metastases rarely arise outside the CNS.

DIAGNOSTIC STUDIES

Computed tomography (CT) and magnetic resonance imaging (MRI) play indispensable roles in the management of brain tumors. CT is a reliable screening and

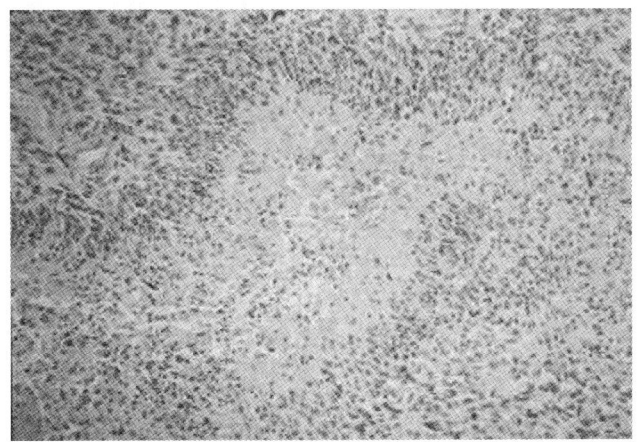

FIGURE 2. Glioblastoma multiforme with the hallmark features of necrosis with peripheral pseudopalisading of neoplastic nuclei.

Rakel and Bope: *Conn's Current Therapy 2006.*

diagnostic method for suspected supratentorial brain tumor lesions. MRI, now more frequently used in patients with malignant brain tumors, is the screening procedure of choice for diagnosing and localizing tumors in the brainstem, posterior fossa, and spinal cord. Ordinary astrocytomas appear as diffuse, poorly defined, low-density, nonenhancing lesions. Approximately 40% of ordinary astrocytomas enhance, and calcification is found in 10% of cases. Although the majority of malignant gliomas enhance with contrast media, as many as 30% of anaplastic astrocytomas present as nonenhancing lesions. In both low-grade and malignant gliomas, parenchymal infiltration by isolated tumor cells may be present in regions of T2-weighted abnormality that appear normal on CT (Figures 3 and 4). Positron emission tomography (PET), single-photon emission computed tomography (SPECT) with thallium-201 (^{201}Tl), and magnetic resonance spectroscopy (MRS) are other imaging approaches used in brain tumor management.

STAGING

No accepted staging system exists for primary brain tumors. The American Joint Committee on Cancer proposed a staging scheme for primary brain tumors based on tumor size and metastases as well as tumor grade. Because this system was not generally adapted to clinical use, it was subsequently removed.

PROGNOSTIC FACTORS

Age, histologic appearance, Karnofsky performance score (KPS), mental status, duration of symptoms, neurologic functional class, extent of surgery, and radiation dose are identified as significant partitioning covariates in clinical trials. This information is important for correctly interpreting the results of studies comparing different treatment regimens and for assessing the potential of new therapeutic methodologies.

STANDARD THERAPEUTIC APPROACHES FOR GLIOMAS

Surgery

The combination of surgery, radiation therapy, and chemotherapy represents the standard approach to the treatment of gliomas. The goals of surgery are to provide a histologic diagnosis, to alleviate intracranial hypertension and focal neurologic deficits because of a mass effect, and to permit rapid corticosteroid dose tapering. Pilocytic astrocytomas are relatively well circumscribed, and 60% to 80% are amenable to total removal. Resection of the more common diffuse astrocytomas is limited by the lack of clear demarcation between the infiltrating tumor and normal brain tissue. Evidence suggests that patients with more complete resections live longer and have an improved functional status compared with those who undergo a biopsy or partial resection only. Advances in neurosurgery, including diagnostic ultrasound, lasers, ultrasonic tissue aspirators, cortical mapping, functional imaging, and computer-assisted stereotactic laser techniques, have improved the ability of neurosurgeons to radically remove intracranial tumors.

Radiation Therapy

Limited radiation fields are used for the treatment of gliomas. Three-dimensionally designed complex treatment plans with multiple fields are used whenever appropriate to limit the high-dose volume and to minimize the risk of long-term radiation sequelae. Doses of 50.4 to 54 Gy are usually recommended for low-grade gliomas and 59.4 to 60 Gy for high-grade gliomas. Rapid fractionation schemes (such as 30 to 36 Gy) may be appropriate for some elderly or poor performance status patients with glioblastoma multiforme who have relatively short survival expectancies.

In low-grade gliomas, the role of radiation therapy is debatable. Although it improves disease-free survival, overall survival is not altered, indicating that deferring postoperative therapy is an option for selected group of patients. Evidence also indicates that lower doses of radiation therapy are probably as effective as higher doses of radiation for low-grade gliomas.

Randomized trials provide seminal evidence that external beam irradiation favorably affects the outcome of malignant gliomas. These trials demonstrate both a significant survival advantage and ability to maintain a full or partial working capacity for irradiated patients.

Chemotherapy

Chemotherapy has little established role in adult low-grade astrocytomas, but adjuvant chemotherapy is part of the standard therapeutic regimen for malignant gliomas. The addition of chemotherapy to radiation therapy improves the 1-year survival by 10% and the 2-year survival by 8.6%. The nitrosoureas, especially BCNU (*N,N′*-bis(2-chloroethyl)-*N*-nitrosourea, carmustine), are the most active single agents. No benefit of chemotherapeutical agents such as tirapazamine, topotecan (Hycamtin), paclitaxel (Taxol), B-IFN (Avonex), and thalidomide (Thalomid) is noted when used with standard radiation in clinical trials. Temozolomide (Temodar) is an alkylating agent that demonstrates an improvement in survival by an additional 2 to 3 months when given concurrently with radiation in high-grade gliomas. Anaplastic oligodendrogliomas are chemosensitive tumors. PCV (procarbazine, lomustine [CCNU], and vincristine) chemotherapy regimens produce response rates of 50% to 75% in both recurrent and newly diagnosed anaplastic oligodendrogliomas. Unfortunately, improved response to chemotherapy does not translate into improved survival for these tumors.

Some of the newer biologic agents explored today in gliomas include tyrosine kinase inhibitors, matrix metalloproteinase inhibitors, and antitenascin antibodies.

Outcome

The 5-year recurrence-free survival rates of patients with low-grade astrocytomas or mixed oligoastrocytomas

who undergo total or radical subtotal tumor resection range from 52% to 95%. The median survival times for high-grade gliomas using conventional radiation therapy alone or with chemotherapy consistently range from 9 to 14 months. The median survival for patients with glioblastoma multiforme is 10 to 12 months, whereas the 3-year survival rate is only 6% to 8%. The median survival for patients with anaplastic astrocytoma is 36 months, and the 3-year survival rate is approximately 50%.

Uncommon Primary Brain Tumors

PRIMARY CENTRAL NERVOUS SYSTEM LYMPHOMA

Primary CNS lymphomas (PCNSLs) represent approximately 2% to 5% of all intracranial neoplasms. During the last 2 decades, the incidence has increased in both the AIDS and immunocompetent general population. PCNSLs most frequently arise in the supratentorial paraventricular region of the brain. Multifocal tumors are present at diagnosis in 25% to 50% of immunocompetent patients and in 60% to 80% of AIDS patients. Cytologic examination of CPF reveals malignant cells in up to two thirds of immunocompetent patients and in nearly all AIDS patients. The neoplastic cells are similar to those of non-Hodgkin's lymphoma arising in extranodal sites. Single or multiple uniformly contrast-enhancing lesions in the paraventricular regions, basal ganglia, thalamus, or corpus callosum on MRI are characteristic findings.

The role of surgery is to establish a tissue diagnosis only. Primary CNS lymphomas respond dramatically to corticosteroid therapy. At least 90% of patients improve clinically, whereas 40% of lesions shrink considerably. Whole-brain irradiation with corticosteroids is the standard treatment for PCNSL. Recommended doses range from 36 to 45 Gy. Several reports document improved survival when chemotherapy is added to radiation therapy. The outcome is better with high-dose methotrexate-based regimens, often combined with intrathecal chemotherapy.

Survival times for primary CNS lymphoma with no treatment or steroids alone are approximately 1 to 4 months. The median survival for radiotherapy alone varies from 12 to 20 months. Median survival times for treatment programs that include high-dose methotrexate-based chemotherapy range from 33 to 42 months.

EPENDYMOMA

Ependymomas represent approximately 5% of all intracranial gliomas. The incidence peaks at 5 years and again at 34 years of age. Approximately 60% to 70% of ependymomas arise in the infratentorial brain. Ependymomas are separated into low-grade and high-grade lesions. The 5-year survival for low-grade tumors ranges from 60% to 80%, whereas it varies from 10% to

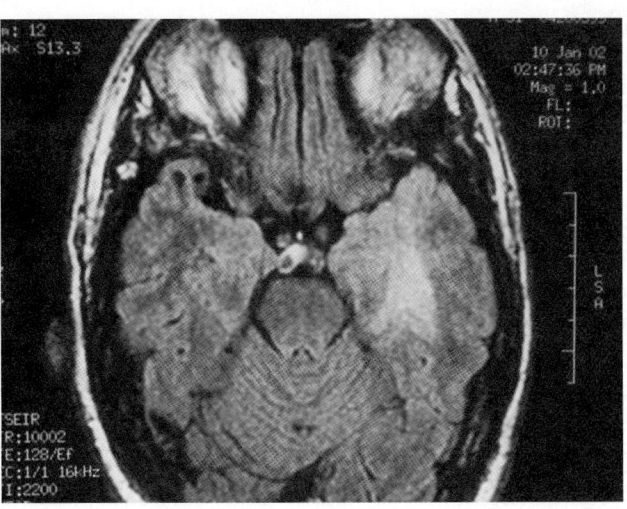

FIGURE 3. Axial magnetic resonance imaging scan of low-grade astrocytoma of left temporal lobe.

47% for high-grade tumors. Supratentorial ependymomas generally have a poorer prognosis than their infratentorial counterparts.

Most ependymomas cannot be completely excised because of their location and growth characteristics. Postoperative irradiation improves local tumor control and survival and is an accepted part of the standard treatment for these tumors. Although most ependymomas are slow growing, others are more aggressive and may disseminate throughout the CSF pathways. Current therapy for high-grade ependymomas after surgical debulking is with local fields to a dose of 59.4 Gy. The value of chemotherapy in adults with ependymomas and anaplastic ependymomas is not well defined.

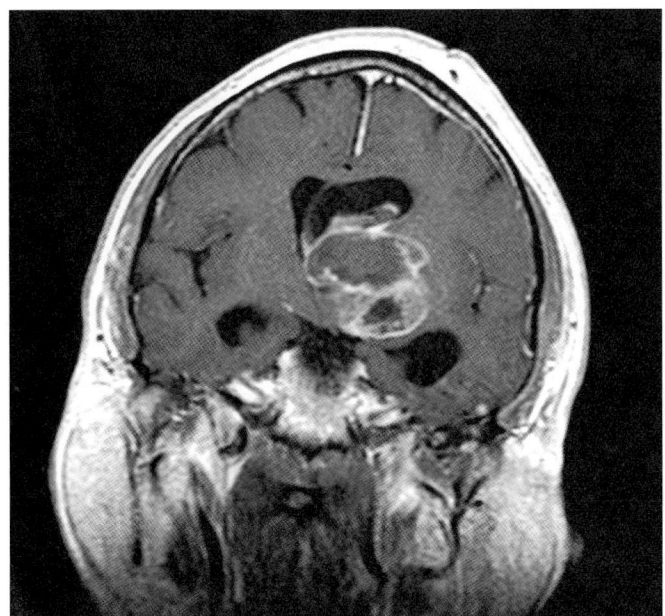

FIGURE 4. Coronal magnetic resonance imaging scan of high-grade astrocytoma of left internal capsule and brainstem region.

Rakel and Bope: *Conn's Current Therapy 2006.*

BRAINSTEM GLIOMA

Brainstem gliomas account for less than 2% of brain tumors. Children constitute approximately two thirds of the reported cases. Diagnostic imaging is sufficient for the majority of the cases. The role of surgery is minimal and limited to biopsy only if there are questions about the diagnosis. Radiation therapy alone by conventional fractionation to 54 Gy in symptomatic or large brainstem lesions is recommended. Chemotherapy does not show any benefit in the management of brainstem gliomas. The median survival time is 9 to 12 months.

MEDULLOBLASTOMA

Medulloblastoma accounts for a third of pediatric brain tumors and is the most common tumor arising in the posterior fossa in children. It arises from the roof of the fourth ventricle or from the vermis. The presenting symptoms include headache, vomiting, and imbalance. On microscopic examination, small blue undifferentiated cells are noted consistent with primitive neuroectodermal tumor. CSF involvement is noted in 25% to 40% of the patients. Five-year survival rates range from 50% to 80%, and 10-year rates vary from 40% to 55%.

Surgery involves maximal resection of the tumor. Radiation therapy to the entire craniospinal axis is essential. The dose to the craniospinal axis is 23.4 to 36 Gy. A boost of 18 to 31.4 Gy is given to the posterior fossa to bring the total to 54 Gy. The role of chemotherapy is to decrease the craniospinal radiation dose and to improve the survival in poor-risk patients. Combinations of vincristine, CCNU, and *cis*-platinum are used.

Brain Metastases

EPIDEMIOLOGY

Metastases to the brain occur in as many as 30% of patients with systemic cancer and represent the most common type of intracranial tumor. Brain metastases exert a profound effect on the quality and length of survival, and despite the best current management, they represent the direct cause of death in 25% to 30% of affected patients. Melanoma and carcinomas of the lung, breast, and colorectum have a higher propensity to metastasize to the brain. Approximately 50% of patients present with a solitary lesion. Most brain metastases, particularly those that arise from primary sites other than the lung, occur at a late stage when metastatic dissemination is present elsewhere in the body.

STANDARD TREATMENT APPROACHES

Because the majority of patients with metastatic brain lesions have or will soon develop widely disseminated disease, treatment is dictated by the need to achieve immediate short-term palliation and the desire for durable symptom-free remission. The median survival of patients with symptomatic brain metastases is approximately 1 month without treatment and 2 months with corticosteroid administration. Survival is longer and the quality of life better if brain metastases are treated.

Corticosteroids

Corticosteroids rapidly ameliorate many symptoms of brain metastasis and should be used at the onset for all symptomatic patients. Symptomatic but stable patients can begin with approximately 16 mg of dexamethasone daily in two to four divided doses. Patients who are receiving whole-brain irradiation should receive steroids for at least 48 hours before treatment. Steroid tapering may begin during week 2 of radiotherapy. For patients receiving 16 mg of dexamethasone, the drug should be tapered by 2 to 4 mg every fifth day.

Surgery

Surgery establishes the diagnosis of metastatic brain disease when it is uncertain and serves as a treatment for single metastases. Surgery can provide better local control and immediate relief of neurologic signs and symptoms because of a mass effect. Surgically treated patients also live longer, have fewer recurrences of cancer in the brain, and enjoy a better quality of life compared with those treated by radiotherapy alone. Only 10% of patients are ideal candidates for surgical extirpation, however.

Whole-Brain Radiation Therapy

Radiotherapy is the appropriate treatment for most patients with brain metastases, including those with multiple lesions and those with single metastases who are not candidates for surgery. The standard approach is to treat the whole brain to 30 Gy in 10 daily fractions over 2 weeks. Depending on the symptom, the response rate varies from 70% to 90%. Neurologic function is improved overall in 50% of patients. The median survival with radiation therapy is 4 to 6 months. Overall, 75 to 80% of remaining life is spent in an improved or stable neurologic state.

Stereotactic Radiosurgery

Stereotactic radiosurgery (SRS) is an excellent alternative to surgical extirpation of solitary and multiple brain metastases. The procedure involves the delivery of a single large dose of radiation to a small volume of the brain region under stereotactic frame guidance. Recently, data from a large randomized trial show that addition of SRS to whole-brain radiation therapy improves both the survival and the quality of life in patients with limited brain metastases. Although surgery and SRS have never been compared directly in a clinical trial, local control, survival, and quality of life in selected patients seem comparable in retrospective trials.

Chemotherapy

Chemotherapy can be considered in selected patients who progress locally after whole-brain irradiation. Systemic chemotherapy shows a response rate of 25% to 50%. Temozolomide shows promise both as an adjuvant to whole-brain radiation therapy and in patients who fail radiation therapy.

REFERENCES

Andrews DW, Scott CB, Sperduto PW, et al: Whole brain radiation therapy with or without stereotactic radiosurgery boost for patients with one to three brain metastases: Phase III results of the RTOG 9508 randomised trial. Lancet 2004;363:1665-1672.

Deangelis LM, Hormigo A: Treatment of primary central nervous system lymphoma. Semin Oncol 2004;31:684-692.

Henson JW, Gaviani P, Gonzalez RG: MRI in treatment of adult gliomas. Lancet Oncol 2005;6:167-175.

Jemal A, Tiwari RC, Murray T, et al: Cancer statistics, 2004. CA Cancer J Clin 2004;54:8-29.

Kleihues P, Cavenee WK: Pathology and Genetics: Tumours of the Nervous System, 2nd ed. Lyon, France, IARC Press, 2000, pp 6-7.

Narayana A, Leibel SA: Primary and metastatic brain tumors in adults. In Leibel SA, Philips TL (eds): Textbook of Radiation Oncology, 2nd ed. Philadelphia, WB Saunders, 2004, pp 463-496.

Patchell RA, Tibbs PA, Regine WF, et al: Postoperative radiotherapy in the treatment of single metastases to the brain: A randomized trial. JAMA 1998;280:1485-1490.

Reifenberger G, Collins VP: Pathology and molecular genetics of astrocytic gliomas. J Mol Med 2004;82:656-670.

The Locomotor System

Rheumatoid Arthritis

Method of
Joseph C. Shanahan, MD, and
E. William St. Clair, MD

Rheumatoid arthritis (RA) is a chronic disease characterized mainly by a polyarthritis, with frequent progression to articular cartilage and bone damage, physical dysfunction, and work disability. Most patients with RA have circulating autoantibodies such as rheumatoid factor (RF) and anticyclic citrullinated peptide (anti-CCP) reflecting the autoimmune features of this disease. RA is a common illness, with an estimated worldwide prevalence of 1% to 2%. It typically develops in the fourth to sixth decades, with predominance among women of approximately 2.5:1. RA may be associated with extra-articular inflammatory features, including fatigue, subcutaneous nodules, pleuritis and pericarditis, interstitial lung disease, vasculitis, and Sjögren's syndrome. Patients with RA have excess mortality, but the most frequent cause of death appears to be complications of atherosclerotic cardiovascular disease. The increased risk of cardiovascular disease in this population occurs independently of traditional cardiovascular risk factors and corticosteroid therapy and may be related to the systemic inflammatory process.

The natural history of RA is a steady decline in joint function caused by progressive cartilage damage, bone erosions, and tendon rupture. As a result, work disability rates among patients with RA are more than 50% within 10 years of disease onset. Early rheumatoid arthritis is characterized by bone erosions detectable within 2 years of disease onset in as many as 70% of patients. In some patients RA progresses rapidly, leading to early work disability if effective therapy is not started to control the inflammatory response and joint damage.

Most patients with RA are initially treated with a combination of nonsteroidal anti-inflammatory agents and corticosteroids to provide sufficient time to confirm the persistence of joint inflammation and complete the diagnostic workup. Shortly thereafter, disease-modifying antirheumatic drugs (DMARDs) are added because they can afford long-term protection from joint damage and disability. DMARDs (Box 1) are defined by the ability to reduce the signs and symptoms as well as slow the progression of joint damage, as measured by radiographic changes in the amount of bone erosions and joint space narrowing.

Over the past 20 years there has been an evolution in the treatment paradigm for RA. These advances derive from early initiation of DMARD therapy and the expanded availability of effective DMARDs. Moreover, clinical trials examining the effect of multi-DMARD treatment for early RA have shown a long-lasting and improved benefit in terms of both disease control and improved health-associated quality of life compared with single DMARD therapy. As a result, the present treatment paradigm for RA incorporates the following three goals:

1. Early diagnosis and intervention
2. First-line therapy with DMARDs that reduces progressive joint damage followed by adding more DMARDs if disease activity persists
3. Management of co-morbidities such as disease- and treatment-related osteoporosis

Traditional DMARDs notable for their excessive toxicity, such as gold and penicillamine, are no longer in widespread use. However, the availability of safer DMARDs that can be used effectively in combination has expanded RA treatment options. In particular, a major advance has been the development of tumor necrosis factor-α (TNF-α) blocking agents that include etanercept (Enbrel), infliximab (Remicade), and adalimumab (Humira). Encouraging results from phase II clinical trials involving B-cell–directed therapies and other novel biologic immune response modifiers suggest that better RA control and possibly remission-inducing treatments are on the horizon. For now, RA remains a chronic illness usually managed with lifelong, anti-inflammatory, and immunomodulating treatment aimed at abrogating joint damage and minimizing disability.

Diagnosis

In the absence of a definitive diagnostic test, the diagnosis of RA is based on clinical features and supportive laboratory tests. Established in 1987, the American College of Rheumatology (ACR) criteria require at least

BOX 1 Drugs Used for Treatment of Rheumatoid Arthritis

Traditional DMARDs
- MTX
- Leflunomide (Arava)
- Sulfasalazine (Azulfidine)
- Gold (intramuscular or oral) (Myochrysine, Solganal, Auranofin)
- Azathioprine (Imuran)
- Cyclosporine (Neoral)
- Corticosteroids

Biologic Agents
- Anti-TNF monoclonal antibodies
- Infliximab (Remicade)
- Adalimumab (Humira)
- Soluble TNF receptor
- Etanercept (Enbrel)
- IL-1ra
- Anakinra (Kineret)

Abbreviations: DMARD = disease-modifying antirheumatic drug; IL-1ra = interleukin-1 receptor antagonist; MTX = methotrexate; TNF = tumor necrosis factor.

TABLE 1 American College of Rheumatology Criteria for Rheumatoid Arthritis Diagnosis*

Criterion	Definition
Morning stiffness	In and around joints lasting at least 1 h before maximal improvement
Arthritis in at least three joint areas†	Simultaneously involved by soft tissue swelling or fluid observed by a physician
Arthritis of hand joints	At least one area swollen: wrist, MCP, PIP
Symmetric arthritis	Simultaneous involvement of the same joint areas on both sides of the body (bilateral involvement of PIPs, MCPs, or MTPs acceptable without absolute symmetry)
Rheumatoid nodules	Subcutaneous nodules over bony prominences, extensor surfaces, or in extra-articular regions observed by a physician
Serum rheumatoid factor	Abnormal amounts by any method for which the result has been positive in <5% of normal control subjects
Radiographic changes	Typical of RA on posteroanterior hand and wrist radiographs, which must include erosions or unequivocal bony decalcification localized or most obvious adjacent to involved joints (osteoarthritis changes alone do not qualify)

*Patient must satisfy four of the seven criteria listed. Criteria 1 through 4 must be present at least 6 weeks.
†Joint areas (14 total) include: right or left PIP, MCP, wrist, elbow, knee, ankle, and MTP joints.
Abbreviations: MTP = medial tibial plateau; MCP = metacarpophalangeal; PIP = proximal interphalangeal; RA = rheumatoid arthritis.

four of seven features be present for longer than 6 weeks to make the diagnosis (Table 1). These criteria were not originally designed for use in the clinic; they were to classify subjects diagnosed with RA for the purpose of clinical research. As a result, the ACR criteria are highly sensitive (95%) but only modestly specific (75% to 89%) for making the clinical diagnosis of RA in patients with established disease. In studies of early inflammatory arthritis, the ACR criteria are poorly sensitive in the first 2 years following disease onset, but improve thereafter. Although characteristic radiographic lesions, particularly marginal joint erosions, strongly support the diagnosis of RA, such lesions are only present in up to 70% of patients within the first 2 years of disease. Recently, both musculoskeletal ultrasound (US) and magnetic resonance imaging (MRI) have been shown to detect erosive lesions early in the disease course, and in many cases, before they are evident on plain radiographs. However, the impact of these imaging techniques on diagnostic accuracy in early RA remains uncertain. Another recent diagnostic advance is the measurement of anti-CCP antibodies. In studies of stored sera, these autoantibodies are detectable as long as 10 years before the clinical diagnosis of RA. Anti-CCP antibodies are more specific, but less sensitive, for the diagnosis of RA than serum RF. RF such as IgM or IgG antibodies with binding specificity for the Fc portion of γ-globulin are detectable in approximately 70% of patients with RA. The presence of either RF or anti-CCP increases the diagnostic sensitivity for RA to more than 80%.

Primary care providers play an important role in the diagnosis of RA. Recognition of inflammatory arthritis and rapid referral to rheumatologists leads to early initiation of effective, joint protective therapies. Early inflammatory polyarthritis may not always meet diagnostic criteria for RA; however, approximately 30% of these cases of undifferentiated arthritis will ultimately evolve into RA.

The importance of early, accurate diagnosis of RA has grown with evidence that early, intensive therapy, using multiple DMARDs, can alter the natural history of the disease. In one study subjects with early RA (less than 2 years of disease duration) were randomized to intensive, multidrug therapy consisting of high-dose corticosteroids, methotrexate (MTX), and sulfasalazine or monotherapy with sulfasalazine alone. The combination therapy was gradually withdrawn over 6 months until all subjects were taking sulfasalazine alone. At 1 year, no differences in disease activity were noted between the groups; however, long-term radiographic follow-up showed at 5 years that progression of joint damage was slower in the group originally treated with multiple DMARDs, even after controlling for DMARD treatment after the initial year of the study. Several other studies supporting the outcomes of the Combinatietherapie Bij Reumatoide Artritis (COBRA) trial have shown that early introduction of combination therapy using a variety of different DMARDs with and without corticosteroids benefits long-term radiographic outcomes.

Whether this translates into corresponding reductions in work disability is still under investigation.

Therapeutic Goals

Successful treatment of RA is predicated on reduction in symptomatic joint pain and swelling, relief of joint stiffness, return of lost function, and prevention of joint damage (Figure 1). Clinically, response to therapy may be determined by examining joints for tenderness and swelling, obtaining laboratory measures of inflammation (erythrocyte sedimentation rate [ESR] and C-reactive protein [CRP]), and assessing patient-reported outcomes using questionnaires, such as the Health Assessment Questionnaire (HAQ), or visual analogue scales. Long-term therapy goals include reducing missed work days, delaying disability, and decreasing early mortality. Frequent surrogates for long-term outcomes are

radiographic changes indicative of joint damage (e.g., joint erosions and joint space narrowing). In clinical trials radiographic outcomes are quantified using the van der Heijde modification of the Sharp score, a validated scoring system in which the extent of joint space narrowing and erosions are quantified on standard radiographs of the hands, wrists, and feet.

Both short- and long-term goals may be reached using DMARDs that reduce joint inflammation as well as retard the development of radiographic joint damage. The most commonly used DMARD, MTX, has a long track record of efficacy and acceptable toxicity and is often the treatment against which other agents or regimens are compared. Other DMARDs used previously for the treatment of RA, such as gold salts, penicillamine, azathioprine, and cyclophosphamide, are rarely used today because of either relatively poor efficacy or excessive toxicity, or both. A generation of novel DMARDs that inhibit inflammatory cytokines, termed *biologic response modifiers*, have essentially taken their place.

Methotrexate

A purine antimetabolite, MTX reduces symptoms of joint inflammation and decreases radiographic joint damage in patients with RA. Evidence of clinical efficacy has been shown in many studies. MTX is generally well tolerated; the majority of patients still use the drug after 5 years of treatment. Side effects may be divided into so-called nuisance toxicities, including nausea, diarrhea, mucosal ulcerations, and alopecia, and serious complications such as hepatotoxicity, bone marrow suppression, and pneumonitis (Table 2). Nuisance toxicities are an infrequent cause of MTX discontinuance and can often be managed with folic acid supplementation or by switching from oral to parenteral administration. Hepatotoxicity is typically characterized by fibrosis and cirrhosis, which occur rarely with frequent monitoring for possible toxicity. The ACR guidelines recommend monitoring hepatic transaminases and serum albumin at 4- to 8-week intervals and reserving liver biopsy for an otherwise unexplained decrease in albumin or persistent or recurrent elevation of transaminases. A rare complication, MTX-induced pneumonitis typically develops early after initiation and is characterized by cough, dyspnea, and fever. Chest radiographs reveal diffuse interstitial changes. The development of pneumonitis after MTX initiation should be managed with immediate drug discontinuation, and consideration of corticosteroid treatment in severe cases. Pneumonitis recurs frequently with rechallenge; therefore, patients experiencing this complication should be treated with an alternative DMARD. MTX is contraindicated in patients with impaired renal function because delayed clearance increases drug levels, and hence, the risk of side effects.

MTX is administered in once-weekly doses. It is important to maximize the beneficial effects of MTX by titrating to 20 to 25 mg per week because lower doses are often less effective. There has been little additional benefit observed in patients treated with doses greater

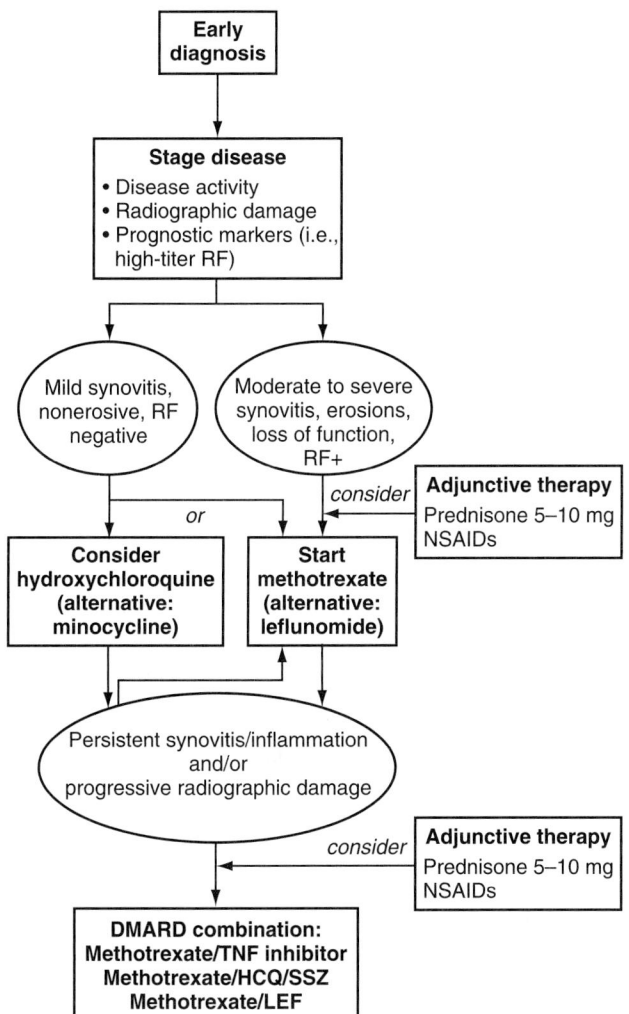

FIGURE 1. This flow diagram illustrates key decision points for RA therapy, based on the recommendations of the ACR. RA = rheumatoid arthritis. (American College of Rheumatology Subcommittee on Rheumatoid Arthritis Guidelines: Guidelines for the management of rheumatoid arthritis: 2002 update. Arthritis Rheum 2002;46:328-323.)

TABLE 2 Disease-Modifying Antirheumatic Drug monitoring

DMARD	Tests	Interval
Methotrexate (MTX)	Hepatic transaminases, serum creatinine, CBC, albumin	Baseline and q 4-8 wk
	CXR, HBV and HCV serology, β-HCG	Baseline
Leflunomide (Arava)	Hepatic transaminases, serum creatinine, CBC, albumin, HBV and HCC serology, β-HCG	Baseline
	ALT	q mo for 6 mo, then q 6-8 wk
	Hepatic transaminases, serum creatinine, CBC, albumin	q 6-8 wk
TNF inhibitors (etanercept, infliximab, adalimumab [Humira])	PPD, CXR (if positive PPD, emigration from TB endemic country, or TB exposure history), CBC	Baseline
	CBC	q 6-8 wk
Sulfasalazine (Azulfidine)	CBC, hepatic transaminases, creatinine	Baseline and q 2 wk for 3 mo, then q 4 wk for 3 mo, then q 12 wk
	G6PD screen	Baseline
Hydroxychloroquine	Serum creatinine and G6PD deficiency screen	Baseline
	Ophthalmologic evaluation: visual acuity and retinal function tests	Baseline and q 6 mo
Cyclosporine (Neoral)	Serum creatinine, hepatic transaminases, CBC, potassium, blood pressure	Baseline and q 2 wk until dosage is stable, then q mo
Azathioprine (Imuran)	CBC, hepatic transaminases, creatinine	Baseline and then q 2 wk for 3 mo, then q mo for 3 mo, then q 2-3 mo
Anakinra (Kineret)	CBC	Baseline and then q 4-8 wk

Abbreviations: ALT = alanine aminotransferase; CBC = complete blood count; CXR = chest radiograph; DMARD = disease-modifying antirheumatic drug; G6PD = glucose-6-phosphatase deficiency; HBV = hepatitis B virus; HCC = hepatitis contagiosa canis; HCV = hepatitis C virus; q = every; TB = tuberculin.

than 25 mg per week; however, toxicities become more common at these higher doses.

Inhibitors of Tumor Necrosis Factor-α

TNF-α is a pleiotropic cytokine expressed by activated T lymphocytes and macrophages and acts in an autocrine and paracrine fashion to upregulate production of other proinflammatory cytokines, including interleukin (IL)-1 and IL-6, matrix metalloproteinases, and reactive oxygen intermediates that provoke inflammation and injure articular cartilage and bone. In addition, TNF-α promotes receptor activation of nuclear factor-κB ligand (RANK ligand) expression that leads to differentiation and activation of osteoclasts. In RA, osteoclasts are responsible for articular bone loss characterized by erosions and osteopenia. In addition, TNF-α drives the differentiation of synoviocytes into a fibroblastic phenotype that confers invasive, tumor-like qualities on these cells. Fibroblast-like synoviocytes form the synovial pannus, a tumor-like mass unique to rheumatoid joints that invades and damages cartilage.

Clinical studies of several TNF-inhibiting agents have demonstrated the therapeutic benefits of TNF blockade on RA disease activity and joint damage. The three TNF-inhibiting drugs approved for the treatment of RA—etanercept (Enbrel), infliximab (Remicade), and adalimumab (Humira)—appear similarly efficacious for the treatment of this disease, but they have not been

directly compared in clinical trials. Many clinical trials have compared treatment using TNF inhibitors with placebo controls in patients with active RA despite taking MTX. In these studies, 40% to 60% of patients met American College of Rheumatology (ACR) criteria for improvement at week 20 (Box 2). Approximately 10% to 20% of patients improved even more, reaching ACR 70 criteria. The add-on design of these trials simulates current practice patterns in which a second DMARD is added to MTX in patients with persistent synovitis. Long-term follow-up of subjects

---

BOX 2 American College of Rheumatology 20 Criteria for Improvement in Rheumatoid Arthritis

Requires 20% improvement in each of the first two domains and in three of the following seven domains:
1. Tender joint count (68 joints)
2. Swollen joint count (66 joints)
3. Patient assessment of pain (10 cm visual analogue scale)
4. Patient assessment of disease activity (10 cm visual analogue scale)
5. Physician global assessment of disease activity (10 cm visual analogue scale)
6. Patient assessment of physical function (HAQ score)
7. Serum CRP or erythrocyte sedimentation rate

Abbreviations: ACR = American College of Rheumatology; CRP = C-reactive protein; HAQ = Health Assessment Questionnaire; RA = rheumatoid arthritis.

enrolled in these trials has shown clinically important improvement in quality-of-life measures and reduction of disability.

The TNF-blocking agents are generally well tolerated. However, an increased risk for reactivation of latent tuberculosis has led to the recommendation in the United States and certain other countries that, prior to use of a TNF inhibitor, a purified protein derivative (PPD) skin test should be performed. A chest radiograph should be obtained in patients with a history of tuberculosis exposure, positive PPD, or emigration from countries where tuberculosis is endemic. Clinical trials of TNF inhibitors in patients with advanced congestive heart failure and multiple sclerosis suggest that these conditions may be exacerbated by these drugs. Demyelinating syndromes have been reported rarely in association with therapeutic TNF blockade. TNF inhibitors have been associated in trials with a slight increase in minor infections (primarily upper respiratory). Postmarketing surveillance suggests that infections with organisms that promote granulomatous inflammatory responses, such as histoplasmosis, coccidioidomycosis, and listeriosis may occur more frequently in patients treated with TNF inhibitors. There have been rare reports of lupus-like syndromes characterized by rash, serositis, and antinuclear and anti–double-stranded DNA autoantibodies.

A total of three TNF-inhibiting agents are commercially available. Etanercept (Enbrel) is a soluble TNF-receptor type II (p75)-to-Fc fusion protein. Infliximab (Remicade) is a chimeric human-to-mouse monoclonal anti-TNF antibody, whereas adalimumab (Humira) is a fully human anti-TNF monoclonal antibody. Etanercept (Enbrel) is administered by subcutaneous injection at a dose of 25 mg twice weekly or 50 mg once weekly. Adalimumab (Humira) is administered subcutaneously at a dose of 40 mg every 1 or 2 weeks. Infliximab (Remicade) is given as an intravenous infusion. Standard initial dosing for infliximab (Remicade) calls for 3 mg/kg to be given at 0, 2, and 6 weeks followed by regular infusions at 8-week intervals. The dosage may vary among patients from 3 to 10 mg/kg, and the interval may be adjusted between 4 and 8 weeks, depending on the individual's clinical response. Although TNF inhibitors may be used as monotherapy, more commonly they are added to MTX or other DMARD therapy to improve disease control. However, clinical trials in early RA suggest that combining MTX with a TNF inhibitor may be more effective than either therapy alone.

Other DMARDs

Other DMARDs may be used alone or in combination to treat RA. Some traditional DMARDs such as gold and D-penicillamine are now rarely used because of toxicity concerns. In some cases of mild RA, agents such as hydroxychloroquine or minocycline may be useful, particularly in early disease. Hydroxychloroquine is an antimalarial drug that may be used by itself in early and mild RA, or as part of a combination regimen. It is typically prescribed at doses of 5 to 7.5 mg/kg per day.

The primary serious side effect is retinal toxicity, so routine ophthalmologic evaluation is suggested. Gastrointestinal side effects and skin rashes may also occur with hydroxychloroquine use.

Leflunomide is a pyrimidine antimetabolite that has been shown in clinical trials to be as efficacious as MTX. The recommended starting dose is 20 mg per day. The dose may be reduced to 10 mg per day when used in combination with MTX or if the starting dose is not tolerated. Leflunomide side effects are typically observed 2 to 4 weeks after starting treatment. The most important serious toxicities are hepatotoxicity and cytopenias. Therefore, laboratory monitoring of hepatic transaminases and a complete blood count should be performed at 4- to 8-week intervals. Leflunomide is an alternative to MTX as a first-line DMARD in patients intolerant of MTX or with renal insufficiency. Leflunomide may be used in combination with MTX. Because both drugs cause hepatotoxicity, however, hepatic transaminases and serum albumin should be monitored carefully. The safety data for combining leflunomide with TNF-α blockers are limited to open-label studies with infliximab (Remicade), but suggest that leflunomide may be used safely in combination with TNF inhibition.

Other DMARDs include sulfasalazine and cyclosporine. With respect to efficacy, these agents compare similarly with MTX as monotherapy, and also improve control of synovitis when combined with MTX. Sulfasalazine treatment is started at 500 mg twice daily and may be titrated gradually to 4.5 g per day, given in two or three divided doses. Gastrointestinal toxicity may limit the dose. Interval monitoring for hepatotoxicity and cytopenias is also required. Cyclosporin is started at 2.0 to 2.5 mg/kg per day in two divided doses. It may be titrated to 4.5-5 mg/kg per day, but the dose may be limited by hypertension or renal toxicity. Long-term side effects such as nephrotoxicity and hirsutism make it difficult for most patients to maintain therapy with cyclosporin for long periods. Gold salts administered parenterally provide significant clinical improvement in up to 30% of patients with RA and prolonged complete remissions have been observed. Unfortunately, many patients are forced to discontinue gold because of side effects that include cytopenia, nephropathy, and cutaneous hypersensitivity.

Anakinra (Kineret), a recombinant IL-1 receptor antagonist (IL-1ra), is a biologic agent that blocks the proinflammatory activities of IL-1. IL-1 shares many of the proinflammatory abilities of TNF-α in promoting the symptoms of arthritis and joint damage in RA. IL-1ra is a naturally occurring anti-inflammatory molecule that competes with soluble IL-1β for binding to cells expressing the IL-1 receptor type I. IL-1ra binding does not induce signaling through the IL-1 receptor, resulting in IL-1 inhibition. Anakinra modestly reduces joint pain and swelling when administered in combination with MTX to patients with RA that is refractory to MTX monotherapy. Anakinra use has been limited by cost and aversion to daily subcutaneous administration (100 mg/day). Many patients develop local injection site reactions, but these are self-limited and usually subside over time.

Rakel and Bope: *Conn's Current Therapy 2006*.

Azathioprine and cyclophosphamide, traditional cytotoxic agents, have shown efficacy in RA, but their use is limited by toxicity. These drugs are usually reserved for use in life-threatening extra-articular manifestations of RA such as interstitial lung disease or vasculitis.

Corticosteroids

Corticosteroids are potent anti-inflammatory agents used for controlling signs and symptoms of synovitis. The use of corticosteroids in RA is limited by the side effects associated with long-term therapy. For short periods, high doses (0.25 to 0.5 mg/kg/day) may be used to control severe flare-ups of arthritis. However, corticosteroids are most commonly used in low daily doses (5 to 10 mg/day) as bridge treatment while a DMARD takes effect or as adjuvant therapy to control persistent symptoms in patients with DMARD-refractory disease. In clinical studies, low-dose corticosteroids can reduce the number of radiographic erosions that develop early after disease onset. These doses are rarely sufficient to completely control synovitis, and are therefore most commonly used in conjunction with traditional DMARDs or biologic agents. Low-dose corticosteroids are generally well-tolerated, but careful monitoring for complications, particularly osteoporosis, should be performed. An alternative to systemic corticosteroids is intra-articular injection of triamcinolone (Kenalog, Aristocort), betamethasone (Celestone), or methylprednisolone (Depo-Medrol), particularly for disproportionately inflamed joints or joints responding slowly to systemic therapies. Clinicians should be careful not to assume a disproportionately swollen joint is because of RA. In such cases, synovial fluid aspiration is performed first to exclude infection because RA is a leading risk factor for joint sepsis.

Combination Therapy

Although many patients' disease appears to be well controlled using a single DMARD, persistent synovitis or progressive radiographic joint damage is common with such an approach. The current treatment paradigm favors a rapid *step-up* strategy, which calls for the addition of a second or third DMARD if synovitis persists despite adequate dosing with a single DMARD. There are several possible approaches. One approach is that inadequate responders to MTX can add a TNF inhibitor. Another approach is to convert to *triple therapy,* which consists of sulfasalazine and hydroxychloroquine in addition to MTX. Triple therapy reduces disease activity in patients with an inadequate response to MTX. An alternative combination regimen, adding leflunomide to MTX, reduces joint inflammation in otherwise refractory disease states. Available data suggest that combination therapy improves radiographic and functional outcomes for patients with RA inadequately controlled with a single DMARD. In subjects with RA refractory to combination therapy, alternative DMARDs may be used, either singly or in combination;

but such patients, albeit in the minority, represent a small group that may be difficult to treat with currently approved agents.

Nonsteroidal Anti-Inflammatory Drugs

Nonsteroidal anti-inflammatory drugs (NSAIDs) are used widely to reduce pain, swelling, and stiffness in joints affected by RA. Although NSAIDs are useful adjunctive agents, they are not considered disease-modifying drugs. Traditional NSAIDs inhibit cyclooxygenase (COX) enzymes and therefore block the conversion of arachidonic acid into prostaglandins, molecules that may stimulate inflammation. Two forms of COX enzymes exist, COX-1 and COX-2. COX-1 is expressed constitutively in the gastric mucosa, where it functions to protect the stomach from luminal acid secretion, and in the kidney, where it serves to maintain renal perfusion. COX-2 is expressed at sites of inflammation and is also expressed constitutively in the kidney. Traditional NSAIDs, which block the function of both COX-1 and COX-2, have anti-inflammatory effects, but they also produce gastrointestinal toxicity that may manifest as gastritis, peptic ulcers and hemorrhage, or enteritis. NSAIDs that specifically antagonize COX-2 activity, termed *coxibs* (celecoxib [Celebrex]), have similar anti-inflammatory efficacy as the nonselective NSAIDs; but they cause significantly less gastrointestinal toxicity. Some evidence suggests that the gastrointestinal benefits of coxibs may be reduced by the concurrent use of aspirin. In addition, rofecoxib (Vioxx) and valdecoxib (Bextra) have been associated with an increased risk of cardiovascular and cerebrovascular events and have been withdrawn from the market.

Emerging Biologic Therapies

Novel biologic agents are being developed that target various inflammatory pathways or mediators deemed to be important in the pathogenesis of RA. T-cell activation, for example, is believed to be a central mechanism that initially triggers RA. The activation of T cells requires two interactions between cell surface receptor-ligand pairs. The first interaction occurs between the T-cell receptor (TCR) and an antigen complexed with an HLA molecule on the surface of an antigen-presenting cell (APC). On their surface, T cells also express CD28, which provides a second activating signal to the T cell when it associates with its ligands B7-1 or B7-2 (CD80/86), which are expressed on the APC. Failure of inducing a second signal through CD28 may result in anergy, which is a process that silences T cells. Cytotoxic T-lymphocyte antigen-4 (CTLA4, CD152) is also expressed on T-cell surfaces and competes with CD28 for binding to B7-1 and B7-2. CTLA-4 does not send an activating signal after binding to B7 molecules; however, it appears to downregulate T-cell activation. Abatacept, a fusion protein consisting of CTLA4 and the Fc portion of IgG, is presently under development for treatment of RA. It binds to B7-1 and B7-2 (CD80/86) and thereby blocks the costimulatory signal for T cells and inhibits T-cell activation. Studies show that abatacept can reduce disease activity in RA.

Recently, B cells have emerged to play an important role in the pathogenesis of RA. This belief is supported by the recognition that rituximab, an anti-CD20 monoclonal antibody that depletes B cells, can improve the signs and symptoms of RA. Rituximab is currently approved for the treatment of certain types of lymphoma and is under development as a possible treatment for RA.

Other biologic therapies that block the function of proinflammatory cytokines include anti–IL-6 receptor antibody, anti–IL-12, and anti–IL-15 have also shown efficacy for treating RA. These agents are at earlier stages of clinical development.

Overview of RA Treatment Strategies

The effectiveness of RA treatment has improved dramatically with recent advances in early diagnosis, the development of less toxic and more effective disease-modifying treatments, and more intensive DMARD regimens that control persistent synovitis and progressive radiographic damage. Furthermore, recognition of the impact of associated disorders including osteoporosis and atherosclerotic disease, in addition to appropriate therapeutic intervention for these disorders, will likely result in improved morbidity and mortality among patients with RA. Figure 1 depicts the most commonly employed strategy in use today, and the strategy favored by the authors. Effective treatment begins with early initiation of effective DMARDs before substantial joint damage has occurred. Careful follow-up, particularly

CURRENT DIAGNOSIS

- Synovitis—palpable swelling or effusions are present.
- Symmetry—similar joints are involved on both sides of the body.
- RA-specific joints—MCP and wrist involvement is present with DIP sparing.
- Persistence—synovitis lasting longer than 6 weeks excludes most reactive arthritis.
- Synovial fluid—joint aspiration is favored to exclude crystal-induced polyarthritis.
- Imaging—erosions in the hands or feet are commonly found early in disease; periarticular osteopenia reflects intra-articular inflammation.
- Laboratory features include:
  Inflammation—elevated ESR or CRP
  Autoimmunity—rheumatoid factor and/or
      anti-CCP antibodies

Abbreviations: CRP = C-reactive protein; DIP = distal interphalangeal; ESR = erythrocyte sedimentation rate; MCP = metacarpophalangeal; RA = rheumatoid arthritis.

CURRENT THERAPY

- Early initiation of DMARD
- Regular reassessment of disease progression
- MTX (or leflunomide if MTX contraindicated or poorly tolerated) as first-line DMARD
- Step up to combination therapy
- NSAIDs as tolerated for improved symptom control
- Low-dose corticosteroids to reduce synovitis and damage early after diagnosis
- Regular monitoring for associated diseases that contribute to morbidity
- Regular BP monitoring
- Annual fasting lipid profile
- Annual assessment of glucose tolerance (HbA_{1c} or fasting glucose)
- DEXA scan

Abbreviations: BP = blood pressure; DEXA = dual-energy radiograph absorptiometry; DMARD = disease-modifying antirheumatic drug; HbA_{1c} = glycosylated hemoglobin; MTX = methotrexate; NSAID = nonsteroidal anti-inflammatory drug.

15

using objective measures that account for physical findings, patient disease assessment, and laboratory measures of systemic inflammation, should guide clinicians about the need for combination therapy, in which new DMARDs are added to existing ones, with special attention to suppressing joint inflammation as much as possible. Most patients today are able to live productively with RA because of the advent of new drugs and more intensive early treatment. The future likely holds an expanded therapeutic armamentarium, which promises to afford even better disease control and less disability.

REFERENCES

Arnett FC, Edworthy SM, Bloch DA, et al: The American Rheumatism Association 1987 revised criteria for the classification of rheumatoid arthritis. Arthritis Rheum 1988;31:315-324.

Hansen KE, Cush J, Singhal A, et al: The safety and efficacy of leflunomide in combination with infliximab in rheumatoid arthritis. Arthritis Rheum 2004;51:228-232.

Kirwan JR: Effects of glucocorticoids on joint destruction in rheumatoid arthritis. N Engl J Med 1995;333:142-146.

Kremer JM, Alarcon GS, Lightfoot RW Jr, et al: Methotrexate for rheumatoid arthritis. Suggested guidelines for monitoring liver toxicity. American College of Rheumatology. Arthritis Rheum 1994;37:316-328.

Kremer JM, Genovese MC, Cannon GW, et al: Concomitant leflunomide therapy in patients with active rheumatoid arthritis despite stable doses of methotrexate. A randomized, double-blind, placebo-controlled trial. Ann Intern Med 2002;137:726-733.

Landewe RB, Boers M, Verhoeven AC, et al: COBRA combination therapy in patients with early rheumatoid arthritis: Long-term structural benefits of a brief intervention. Arthritis Rheum 2002;46:347-356.

Lee DM, Schur PH: Clinical utility of the anti-CCP assay in patients with rheumatic diseases. Ann Rheum Dis 2003;62:870-874.

O'Dell JR, Haire CE, Erikson N, et al: Treatment of rheumatoid arthritis with methotrexate alone, sulfasalazine and hydroxychloroquine, or a combination of all three medications. N Engl J Med 1996;334:1287-1291.

St. Clair EW, Wagner CL, Fasanmade AA, et al: The relationship of serum infliximab concentrations to clinical improvement in rheumatoid arthritis: Results from ATTRACT, a multicenter, randomized, double-blind, placebo-controlled trial. Arthritis Rheum 2002;46:1451-1459.

van der Heijde DM: Plain x-rays in rheumatoid arthritis: Overview of scoring methods, their reliability and applicability. Baillieres Clin Rheumatol 1996;10:435-453.

van Everdingen AA, Jacobs JW, Siewertsz Van Reesema DR, Bijlsma JW: Low-dose prednisone therapy for patients with early active rheumatoid arthritis: Clinical efficacy, disease-modifying properties, and side effects: A randomized, double-blind, placebo-controlled clinical trial. Ann Intern Med 2002;136:1-12.

Treatment Update on Juvenile Arthritis

Method of
Andreas Otto Reiff, MD

Overview of Juvenile Arthritis

Juvenile arthritis (JA) is the most common rheumatic condition in childhood with an estimated annual incidence of 0.8 to 22 per 100,000 children and a prevalence of approximately 7 to 400 per 100,000 children. The wide range can be explained to some extent by significant geographic and ethnic variability and the use of different classification systems. The American College of Rheumatology (ACR) diagnostic criteria for JA require age at onset before 16 years, inflammation of one or more joints for at least 6 weeks, and exclusion of other causes of arthritis.

The pathogenesis of JA remains unknown. Associations between JA subtypes and specific human leukocyte antigen (HLA) loci suggest a genetic predisposition. Box 1 reviews the extensive differential diagnosis of JA, which encompasses other rheumatic and musculoskeletal conditions, diseases, infectious processes, and malignancies.

Because of different nomenclatures for JA in Europe (JCA or JIA) and the United States (JRA), the International League of Associations of Rheumatologists (ILAR) proposed a reclassification of childhood arthritis based on the identification of more clinically homogeneous arthritis groups. In addition to the three traditional subtypes—oligoarticular-, polyarticular- and systemic-onset JIA—the ILAR criteria also recognize psoriatic arthritis, enthesitis-related arthritis, and nonclassifiable forms of childhood arthritis. These new criteria continue to evolve, however, and the American College of Rheumatology has not yet implemented them. Although the term JRA is still commonly used, many pediatric rheumatologists use the ILAR criteria as the current classification (Table 1).

Juvenile Arthritis Subtypes

Because of space constraints, this article focuses on the three major genetically distinct JA subtypes (*pauciarticular,* or *oligoarticular onset; polyarticular onset;* and

BOX 1 Differential Diagnostic Considerations in Juvenile Rheumatoid Arthritis

Inflammatory
- Acute rheumatic fever
- Systemic lupus erythematosus
- Dermatomyositis
- Scleroderma
- Mixed connective tissue disease
- Kawasaki disease
- Reiter disease
- Psoriatic arthritis
- Sjögren's syndrome
- Transient synovitis of the hip
- Inflammatory bowel disease

Musculoskeletal
- Hypermobility syndrome
- Chondromalacia patellae
- Trauma and overuse syndrome
- Fibromyalgia syndrome
- Growing pains
- Legg-Calvé-Perthes disease
- Osgood-Schlatter disease
- Reflex sympathetic dystrophy

Infectious
- Septic arthritis
- Viral-associated arthritis
- Lyme disease
- Postinfection arthritis secondary to *Yersinia* or *Shigella*

Other
- Immunodeficiency (congenital and acquired)
- Sarcoidosis
- Sickle cell disease
- Pigmented villonodular synovitis
- Histiocytosis
- Bleeding diathesis (hemophilia with hemarthrosis)
- Neoplasm (neuroblastoma, acute leukemia, hematologic malignancy)

Data from Siegel (1993).

systemic onset), which are based on the initial clinical presentation, including number of inflamed joints and presence of fever, rash, and other systemic manifestations during the first 6 months of the disease course (Table 2). Table 1 summarizes the key characteristics of JA subtypes.

Approximately 50% of all children with JA present with pauciarticular or oligoarticular onset, involving one to four joints during the first 6 months after disease onset. This subtype particularly affects large joints in an asymmetric pattern and is usually not accompanied by significant extra-articular symptoms.

Two subgroups of pauciarticular disease are recognized: the early childhood–onset subgroup, with persistent arthritis in four or fewer joints, and the extended oligoarticular form, affecting cumulatively five or more joints after the first 6 months of disease, frequently representing a challenging patient group.

Children with early childhood–onset pauciarticular JA who are ANA (acetylneuraminic acid) positive (75% to 85%) have approximately a 30% risk for developing

TABLE 1 Classification of Juvenile Arthritis

ACR (JRA) (Cassidy, 1986)	EULAR (JCA) (EULAR, 1977)	ILAR (JIA) (Petty, 1997)	ILAR definition	%	RF	ANA	Peak onset (y)	M:F	Articular characteristics	Extra-articular features
Systemic arthritis	Systemic arthritis	Systemic arthritis	Arthritis w/or preceded by fever of 2 wk plus one of the following: rash, lymphadenopathy, serositis, hepato/ splenomegaly,	10-20	–	– (0-10%)	No peak	1:1	Multiple joint involvement; myalgia, arthralgia, or transient arthritis	Fever, rash, serositis, lymphadenopathy, hepatosplenomegaly, other systemic features
Polyarticular arthritis	Polyarticular arthritis RF negative	Polyarticular arthritis RF negative	Arthritis of ≥5 joints during first 6 mo; RF negative on two occasions (at least 3 mo apart)	20-30	–	+ (25%)	2	1:3		Mild or absent systemic symptoms
	RF positive	RF positive	Arthritis of ≥ five joints during first 6 mo; RF positive on two occasions (at least 3 mo apart)	5-10	+	+ (75%)	>8	1:6	Symmetric involvement of large and small joints plus cervical spine	Systemic symptoms generally mild, rheumatoid nodules in some
Pauciarticular arthritis	Oligoarthritis	Oligoarthritis	Arthritis of one to four joints during first 6 mo	30-40	–	+ (50%)	1-2 (early onset)	1:5	Asymmetric large joint involvement	Systemic symptoms usually absent, high risk of chronic uveitis (ANA positive)
		Persistent	Affecting only four joints during disease course							
		Extended	Affecting five or more joints after 6 mo							

Continued

15

Rakel and Bope: *Conn's Current Therapy 2006.*

TABLE 1 Classification of Juvenile Arthritis—cont'd

ACR (JRA) (Cassidy, 1986)	EULAR (JCA) (EULAR, 1977)	ILAR (JIA) (Petty, 1997)	ILAR definition	%	RF	ANA	Peak onset (y)	M:F	Articular characteristics	Extra-articular features
Spondylo-arthritis		Enthesitis-related arthritis	Arthritis and/or enthesitis with at least two of: sacroiliac tenderness and/or inflammatory spinal pain, HLA B27+; first- or second-degree relative with history of HLA B27–associated disease	10-15	–	–	>8 (late onset)	10:1	Asymmetric large joint involvement, especially hips and sacroiliac joints	Acute uveitis, occasional fever, anemia (HLA-B27+)
		Psoriatic arthritis	Arthritis and psoriasis, or arthritis and at least two of: dactylitis, nail abnormalities, first-degree relative with history of psoriasis	~3	–	–	7-11	0.95:1	Scattered asymmetric oligoarthritis of large and small joints	~3
		Non-classifiable arthritis	All forms of arthritis that do not meet criteria for other categories	~10	–	?	?	?	NA	~10

JRA = juvenile rheumatoid arthritis; JCA = juvenile chronic arthritis; JIA = juvenile idiopathic arthritis.

TABLE 2 Laboratory Studies in Juvenile Rheumatoid Arthritis

	Systemic onset	Polyarticular	Pauciarticular
WBC count	↑↑	↑	N
Hemoglobin/ hematocrit	↓↓	N	N
Platelets	↑↑	N	N
ESR	↑↑	↑↑	N,↑
CRP	↑↑	↑↑,↑	N,↑
ANA	N	N,↑	↑↑
RF	N	↑	N

WBC, white blood cell; ESR, erythrocyte sedimentation rate; CRP, C-reactive protein; ANA, antinuclear antibody; RF, rheumatoid factor; ↑, mild to moderately elevated; ↑↑, extremely elevated; N, normal or absent; ↓, mild to moderately decreased; and ↓↓, extremely decreased. Adapted from Siegel (1993), with permission.

chronic uveitis, which can result in significant loss of vision or blindness.

Approximately 40% of children with JA present with polyarticular-onset disease, involving five or more joints. This subtype of JA is more commonly observed in girls and generally characterized by symmetric arthritis of either small or large joints. Systemic manifestations are variable, and the risk of uveitis in this subgroup is approximately 5%.

Polyarticular-onset JA is further divided into two major subgroups on the basis of the rheumatoid factor (RF) status. The more common RF-negative polyarticular-onset JA affects younger patients and is less likely to involve the small joints. Usually 25% of these children are ANA positive. Conversely, RF-positive polyarthritis, associated with HLA-DR4, is seldom seen in children younger than 8 years of age and bears striking resemblance to adult-onset RA. Most of the children in this subgroup are also ANA positive, and rheumatoid nodules may be present. Early erosions are more common in RF-positive children than in those with the RF-negative subtype.

The remaining 10% to 20% of children present with systemic-onset juvenile arthritis (SOJA). Although SOJA can occur at any age, it usually affects younger children. Systemic symptoms may precede the development of arthritis by weeks or even years. The diagnosis of SOJA requires a history of arthritis in any number of joints and at least 2 weeks of daily monophasic or biphasic fever accompanied by at least one of the following:

- Salmon-pink rash on the trunk or overlying the joints
- Hepatosplenomegaly
- Lymphadenopathy
- Serositis (pericarditis)

Other rare manifestations include central nervous system (CNS) involvement. Approximately 80% of these children develop severe treatment-resistant polyarticular-course arthritis. Children with systemic JA have an increased risk of mortality and account for the majority

of children with JA who suffer from long-term disability when compared to other forms of JA.

Juvenile Arthritis Prognosis

If not treated early and aggressively enough, JA can have potentially devastating, lifelong consequences. Abnormalities include arrested or asymmetric development, retarded linear growth, and persistence of infantile proportions. Localized growth disturbances can lead to considerable deformities. Delays in gross and fine motor skills are common. Other possible sequelae include osteopenia, pericarditis, and chronic eye disease.

The once prevalent view that children typically grow out of JA is challenged by several recent epidemiologic studies. In summary, these studies describe 984 children with JA (approximately 60% with pauciarticular-onset, 30% with polyarticular-onset, and 10% with systemic-onset JA), with a mean age at onset of 7.5 years, followed over a mean of 20.5 years. Approximately 47% of these patients still had active arthritis at a mean age of 30 years, 46% reported significant difficulty in daily life, and 22% had undergone JA-related surgery. Additionally, statistically significant differences are noted for disability, pain, fatigue, physical functioning, and level of employment in patients with JA when compared to a healthy control population. Increased rates of depression and academic as well as psychosocial difficulties have also been reported in children with JA, depending on their degree of disability. Systemic-onset, polyarticular-course, and polyarticular-onset JA, particularly in girls, appear to have the worst prognosis of the three subtypes.

Juvenile Arthritis Management

Notably, long-term damage in children with JA rarely arises from overly aggressive therapy but rather from an overly conservative and cautious approach in the early stages of the disease. In addition to pharmacotherapy, early aggressive physical and occupational therapy remain one of the cornerstones of JA treatment. High-risk patients such as children with systemic-onset polyarticular course or early erosive RF-positive disease should be identified near the beginning and receive disease-modifying antirheumatic drug (DMARD) therapy within the first 3 months after disease onset.

JUVENILE ARTHRITIS PHARMACOTHERAPY
Nonsteroidal Anti-Inflammatory Drugs

Nonsteroidal anti-inflammatory drugs (NSAIDs) are commonly used as first-line agents. Ibuprofen, naproxen, and tolmetin are currently the only FDA-approved NSAIDs for JA. NSAIDs with a longer half-life and less frequent dosing such as naproxen are often preferred by children and are available in suspension form. Cyclooxygenase-2 inhibitors, such as celecoxib, are now available as a treatment alternative. A recent 12-week multinational trial in 310 children with pauci- and polyarticular-onset JA demonstrated that particularly the higher dose of rofecoxib (0.6 mg/kg/day) was safe and equally effective as naproxen in achieving JRA 30 response rates (30% improvement in a composite score of Parent/Patient's Assessment of Overall Well-Being, Investigator's Global Assessment of Disease Activity; Functional Ability [from the Children's Health Assessment Questionnaire (CHAQ)], number of joints with active arthritis and with limited range of motion; and erythrocyte sedimentation rate). Interestingly there was no difference in the gastrointestinal tolerability profile when compared to naproxen. Unfortunately, this drug was withdrawn from the market because of cardiovascular-adverse events in adult clinical trials. Celecoxib may be an alternative, but efficacy and safety data from the clinical trial in JA are not yet published.

Corticosteroids

For some JA subtypes, especially in children with monoarticular disease, treatment may be initiated with intra-articular injections of triamcinolone hexacetonide, which can result in dramatic symptomatic improvement and even remission.

Systemic steroids may still be required for treating difficult JA, especially in children with systemic-onset disease. Long-term use should be avoided, however, because of numerous well-recognized adverse effects (e.g., growth arrest secondary to premature epiphyseal closure, avascular necrosis, osteoporosis, Cushing's syndrome).

Methotrexate (Rheumatrex)

Methotrexate (MTX) is still considered the gold standard for most cases of JA and is frequently used in combination with other DMARDs. A survey of studies of MTX in JA demonstrated, however, that only 60% of children respond to a standard dose of 0.5 mg/kg once weekly, and clinical remission is achieved in merely 50% of children after a year of therapy. Relapse rates after discontinuation of MTX are high. The systemic-onset subtype appears to be even less responsive to MTX than the other subtypes. MTX is equally safe and effective whether administered orally or by intramuscular (IM) or subcutaneous (SC) injection, and it is usually given in conjunction with weekly folinic or daily folic acid supplementation. Hepatic and pulmonary toxicity, although rare in children, require regular patient monitoring.

Cyclosporine (Neoral)[1]

Cyclosporine is effective in the treatment of refractory JA and can be useful in children with systemic-onset disease, but renal toxicity and secondary infections remain a concern. In an open prospective study of 34 patients with JA, 66% withdrew from therapy because of inefficacy or side effects. In general, the benefit of cyclosporine is limited to a steroid-sparing effect and controlling fever. Effects on joints, laboratory

parameters, and uveitis are less clear. Combination therapy of MTX with cyclosporine may be superior to monotherapy with either agent alone.

Cyclophosphamide (Cytoxan)[1]

Although frequently used in pediatric systemic lupus erythematosus (SLE), only one study of four children with systemic JA has been published. After 12 to 20 pulses of intravenous (IV) cyclophosphamide (500 to 1000 mg/m²), three children achieved remission and all four patients were able to discontinue concomitant corticosteroids with subsequent increase in their linear growth.

Leflunomide (Arava)[1]

Leflunomide (LEF), a selective pyrimidine synthesis inhibitor, is comparable in efficacy to sulfasalazine and MTX in RA. In a recent 16-week, double-blind controlled pediatric trial, the safety and efficacy of leflunomide was compared to MTX. Enrolled were 94 children (47 per arm) with active polyarticular-course JA between the ages of 3 and 17 years. Both LEF and MTX were highly effective and well tolerated. Efficacy favored MTX, which was statistically superior to LEF in achieving JRA 30 response rates (see earlier). A JRA 70 response (similar to remission) was seen in 54.5% of the patients on LEF and in 65.7% of the patients on MTX. These results could not only be sustained but also slightly improved through the week 48 observation period. The most frequently observed side effects for both drugs included nausea, diarrhea, abdominal pain, headache, nasopharyngitis, and alopecia. Elevations of liver enzymes were more commonly reported in children treated with MTX than LEF, and six children (five MTX, one LEF) withdrew from the study because of serious adverse events. LEF is an effective and well-tolerated alternative to MTX in children who have failed or cannot tolerate MTX. Because of its long half-life and potential teratogenic effects, LEF should be used cautiously in girls of childbearing potential, and treatment with cholestyramine is recommended prior to pregnancy.

BIOLOGIC RESPONSE MODIFIERS (BRMS)

Etanercept (Enbrel)

Etanercept is composed of two human-soluble tumor necrosis factor-α (TNF) receptors (p75), a naturally occurring TNF-neutralizing protein, fused to the Fc portion of human immunoglobulin G1. Etanercept binds and inhibits both TNF and LT-α, formerly known as TNF-β, both of which are implicated in the pathogenesis of JA.

In a two-part open-label study in 69 children with polyarticular course JA who were refractory or intolerant to MTX, 0.4 mg per kg of etanercept injected subcutaneously twice weekly (maximum 25 mg per dose) resulted in significant improvement in the JRA 30 response rates (see earlier). At the end of 90 days of etanercept therapy (part 1 of the study), 51 children (74%) had a 30% improvement, 44 children (64%) had a 50% improvement,

---

[1]Not FDA approved for this indication.

[1]Not FDA approved for this indication.

and 25 children (36%) had a 70% improvement relative to baseline. Efficacy was sustained for up to 2 years during the extension of the trial, with no increase in rates of adverse events. Etanercept is well tolerated with injection site reactions the most frequently reported adverse event. The FDA has approved etanercept for patients with moderate to severe JA. In addition, etanercept is also used successfully in the treatment of pediatric refractory uveitis and juvenile ankylosing spondylitis.

Adalimumab

Adalimumab is a fully human monoclonal antibody against TNF, which is used successfully in adults with rheumatoid arthritis, demonstrating a rapid reduction in clinical symptoms and preventing radiographic progression. The drug is administered subcutaneously every other week. In a recent multicenter, randomized, double-blind, placebo-controlled study, adalimumab at a dose of 24 mg/m^2 body surface area (BSA) subcutaneously every other week was studied in 171 children with polyarticular course juvenile idiopathic arthritis between the age of 4 and 17 years. Eligible patients had to have a minimum of five swollen joints and three joints with limitation of motion (LOM). Patients were allowed to continue on concomitant MTX and NSAIDs. Efficacy assessments again included the JRA core set criteria for outcome (see earlier), the CHAQ, and C-reactive protein (CRP).

Eighty percent (80%) of the subjects were girls with a mean age of 11.4 years, and approximately half of them were treated with concomitant MTX. Ninety percent (155 of 171) of the children enrolled completed the 16-week open-label lead-in period. Similar to the adults, the clinical response in these 155 patients was rapid, with 67% and 77% of subjects achieving an ACR 30 Ped. 001 response after 2 and 4 weeks of treatment, respectively. At week 16, 82% of the patients on concomitant MTX and 59% of the patients on adalimumab monotherapy achieved an ACR 70 response that is close to clinical remission and were eligible to enroll in the blinded portion of the study, which is continuing to date.

The most common adverse events observed during the study were injection site reactions that were usually mild followed by infections such as mild upper respiratory infections. Three children experienced serious adverse events including pneumonia, genital herpes, and acute gastritis. No tuberculosis or opportunistic infections were reported.

Infliximab (Remicade)[1]

Infliximab, a chimeric (mouse/human) monoclonal TNF antibody, is administered intravenously usually every other month and requires concomitant MTX to suppress antibody formation. Encouraging results in several small uncontrolled trials in JA are reported. Serious infections, especially early clusters of tuberculosis, remain a concern and limit the use of this drug. In addition, occurrence of neutralizing anti-infliximab antibodies, SLE-type autoimmune features, and severe infusion reactions in response to the drug have been observed.

A multinational trial with infliximab in JA is currently under way.

Anakinra (Kineret)[1]

In addition to TNF, interleukin-1 (IL-1) plays a central role in the pathogenesis of arthritis. In a recent international multicenter, open-label study, 82 children with polyarticular course JA were treated with anakinra at 1 mg/kg per day subcutaneously for 12 weeks. Of the 82 children enrolled, 72 (88%) completed the 12-week open-label phase and 46 (58%) showed signs of clinical improvement in JRA 30 response rates when compared to baseline. Interestingly, children with systemic-onset JA showed a more favorable response than children with polyarticular- or oligoarticular-onset JA (79% versus 67% versus 52%). No difference in outcome was noted in children with or without concomitant MTX. The most common adverse events were injection site reactions (70%). In two children, isolated neutrophil counts less than 1.5 with no clinical sequelae were observed. No deaths, malignancies, opportunistic infections, or treatment-associated laboratory abnormalities were seen. Since the publication of these results, many small case series about the value of anakinra, especially for children with treatment-resistant systemic arthritis, have been published.

Anti–IL-6 Receptor Antibody

Recent studies suggest that IL-6 and IL-18 are pivotal cytokines in the pathogenesis of systemic arthritis, unlike in oligoarticular or polyarticular JA, where TNF appears to be the predominant proinflammatory cytokine. This is supported by the observation that less than 50% of children with acute systemic JA respond to TNF antagonists. In a recent phase II dose escalation trial with an anti–IL-6-receptor antibody (MRA), 11 children with treatment-resistant systemic JA were treated with up to 8 mg/kg of MRA given intravenously every other week. A dramatic treatment response with a 70% improvement in the JRA core set criteria was observed in 7 of 11 children after 2 weeks. It appeared that 8 mg/kg was the most efficacious dose. None of the children experienced a disease flare during the study and none withdrew because of adverse events. Future trials with this promising agent are currently under way.

AUTOLOGOUS BONE MARROW TRANSPLANTATION

Recent data from several small studies support autologous bone marrow transplantation as a treatment option for children with severe treatment-refractory JA. The concept is to achieve immunologic tolerance through the aggressive elimination of autoreactive B- and T-cell clones, with subsequent infusion of the patient's own purged bone marrow containing immunologically naïve stem cells. Applying slightly differing treatment regimens, approximately 45 children with refractory, predominantly systemic, JA, have been transplanted to date.

---

[1]Not FDA approved for this indication.

---

[1]Not FDA approved for this indication.

The largest series reported 31 children with treatment-refractory JA (25 with systemic onset and 6 with polyarticular onset) who had progressive disease despite treatment with NSAIDs, MTX, prednisone, cyclosporine, or IV cyclophosphamide. Treatment included antithymocyte globulin (ATG), high-dose cyclophosphamide, and whole-body irradiation (4G single fraction). After a mean follow-up of 33 months (range: 8 to 60 months), 17 children (55%) were considered in drug-free remission, and 7 children (22.5%) relapsed. Four children (13%) never responded to therapy. Three children died because of overwhelming infections or macrophage activation syndrome (MAS). These findings suggest that autologous bone marrow transplantation may be a viable option for patients with refractory JA, but with a mortality risk of approximately 10% and an expected response rate of approximately 50%, this method should be reserved for children with most severe disease.

Conclusion

With the availability of new JA outcome data, childhood arthritis is no longer considered a benign disease. Early aggressive pharmacologic intervention is a critical component of optimal disease management to prevent further disease progression, restore range of motion in the joints, and promote normal growth and development. Physicians treating children with JA need to recognize that children are not small adults and often respond less favorably to conventional RA therapy. Notably, agents used for adult RA, such as D-penicillamine, gold, and hydroxychloroquine as monotherapy, fail to demonstrate any greater benefit than placebo in children with JA.

Although the diverse nature of JA precludes a one-treatment-fits-all approach, children at risk for poor disease outcome should be identified early and receive DMARDs within the first 3 months of disease onset. High-risk patients include those with severe, erosive polyarticular disease, systemic-onset, polyarticular course disease, and extended pauciarticular disease.

New agents that may have potential in the treatment of JA are rapidly becoming available, but for most of them, data are sparse in pediatric populations. Although MTX is still considered the gold standard for most cases of JA, biologic agents such as etanercept and adalimumab have considerably raised the treatment standard and may therefore offer a significant improvement in prognosis. In contrast to adults, the effect of biologic response modifiers on radiographic progression in children is yet undetermined. To date, etanercept is the only new agent to receive FDA approval for the treatment of JA.

In addition to the agents previously discussed, other new therapeutic strategies are currently in early phases of clinical trials. These include combination therapies of biologic agents (anti-TNF/anti–IL-6), selective inhibitors of intracellular inflammatory pathways (p38 MAP kinase inhibitors), and anti–B-cell therapy (anti–CD-20, Rituximab).

REFERENCES

Arthritis Foundation: Arthritis in children, teens and young adults. Arthritis Foundation Web site. Available online at http://www. arthritis.org/communities/juvenile_arthritis/children_young_adults. asp (accessed February 24, 2004).
Giannini EH, Cassidy JT, Brewer EJ, et al: Comparative efficacy and safety of advanced drug therapy in children with juvenile rheumatoid arthritis. Semin Arthritis Rheum 1993;23(1):34-46.
Jacobs JC: Juvenile rheumatoid arthritis. In Pediatric Rheumatology for the Practitioner. New York, Springer-Verlag, 1993, pp 231-359.
Kimura Y, Pinho P, Higgins G, et al: Treatment of systemic onset juvenile rheumatoid arthritis (SOJRA) with etanercept (Abstract 1275). Arthritis Rheum 2002;46(Suppl 9):S481.
Lahdenne P, Vähäsalo P, Honkanen V: Infliximab or etanercept in the treatment of children with refractory juvenile idiopathic arthritis: An open label study. Ann Rheum Dis 2003;62(3):245-247.
Lovell DJ, Giannini EH, Reiff A, et al, for the Pediatric Rheumatology Collaborative Study Group: Etanercept in children with polyarticular juvenile rheumatoid arthritis. N Engl J Med 2000;342(11):763-769.
Manners PJ, Bower C: Worldwide prevalence of juvenile arthritis: Why does it vary so much? J Rheumatol 2002;29(7):1520-1530.
Packham JC, Hall MA: Long-term follow-up of 246 adults with juvenile idiopathic arthritis: Functional outcome. Rheumatology (Oxford) 2002;41(12):1428-1435.
Petty RE, Southwood TR, Baum J, et al: Revision of the proposed classification criteria for juvenile idiopathic arthritis: Durban, 1997. J Rheumatol 1998;25(10):1991-1994.
Wulffraat NM, Brinkman D, Ferster A, et al: Long-term follow-up of autologous stem cell transplantation for refractory juvenile idiopathic arthritis. Bone Marrow Transplant 2003;32(Suppl 1):S61-S64.

Ankylosing Spondylitis

Method of
Maxime Breban, MD, PhD

Ankylosing spondylitis (AS) is the prototypical form of a group of inflammatory rheumatic disorders, referred to as the spondyloarthropathies (SpAs). The prevalence and burden of SpA are very similar to those of rheumatoid arthritis (RA). Until recently, however, few therapeutic options were available to treat SpA. This situation changed dramatically with the arrival of the very efficacious anti–tumor necrosis factor-α (TNF-α) biologic therapies. The clinical manifestations of SpA usually begin early in adulthood (average age at onset is 22 to 23 years). The evolution tends to be chronic, with fluctuations, including the possibility of remissions and relapses. Male predominance is well established, albeit this characteristic was overrated in the past, and female cases are frequent and sometimes serious. Genetic predisposition is strong, with a trend to familial aggregation, which is partially accounted for by the striking association with the human leucocyte antigen (HLA)-B27.

Birth and Rise of the Spondyloarthropathy Concept

Recognition and even definition of SpA bear some difficulties, which relate to the nature of the disease:

- Presentation of SpA is variable from patient to patient.
- Some of the key manifestations tend to remit.

Rakel and Bope: *Conn's Current Therapy 2006.*

- Clinical manifestations lack specificity.
- Morphologic and biologic investigations are poorly contributive.
- Pathophysiology remains largely unexplained.

The different entities that make up the SpAs were originally identified on the basis of their most striking presentation features. Accordingly, AS refers to the following: an axial disorder predominantly affecting the spinal and the pelvic skeleton; psoriatic arthritis as defined by the concomitance of arthritis and psoriasis; arthritis of inflammatory bowel disease (IBD), by the combination of arthritis with Crohn's disease or ulcerative colitis; reactive arthritis, as the onset of sterile arthritis following an infection of the gastrointestinal or the urethral mucosa by invasive bacteria.

Frequent overlap of manifestations between these different entities in the same patient (simultaneously, or consecutively) and within multicase families is indicative of shared genetic background. Part of this genetic predisposition was explained by the identification of HLA-B27 as a genetic factor shared by the different entities. Classification criteria were then developed to distinguish SpAs from other unrelated rheumatic disease conditions. However, only recently was it shown in the context of familial disease that different SpA subtypes correspond to variations of the same disease, rather than to distinct entities. This assumption is consistent with the description of enthesitis (i.e., inflammation at the sites of attachment of tendons, ligaments, and capsules to bone) as a unifying target lesion shared by all SpA subtypes, as opposed to RA.

Key Manifestations of Spondyloarthropathies

AXIAL SKELETON

The most frequent manifestation of the spondyloarthropathies is back pain, which is typically persistent (i.e., 3 months) and inflammatory (responsible for nocturnal awakening and morning stiffness, improved by exercise). Symptoms usually begin in the lumbar region and diffuse upward, affecting the thoracic and less frequently the cervical spine. The sacroiliac joint is also an early affected site, manifesting as buttock pain, irradiating posteriorly to the thigh. Another frequent symptom is pain in the anterior chest wall, impairing breathing. When such symptoms occur in a young adult, 15 to 35 years of age, without alternative explanation, such as disk herniation or another mechanical spinal condition, a diagnosis of SpA must be seriously considered, even if physical examination is poor. Clear-cut improvement of the pain by nonsteroidal anti-inflammatory drugs (NSAIDs) is also indicative of the inflammatory nature of the disease. Other symptoms must then be carefully retrieved from past medical history because they are frequently absent at the time of examination.

PERIPHERAL SKELETON

Peripheral arthritis typically presents as an asymmetric oligoarthritis predominating in the large joints of lower limbs, as opposed to arthritis because of RA or other connective tissue diseases. It frequently runs an acute remitting course. It may be destructive, however, particularly in the hip and shoulder. Enthesitis most typically affects insertions of the Achilles tendon or the plantar fascia, on the calcaneus, revealing as posterior or subtalar pain, but it may affect a variety of sites, such as knee, elbow, hip, and shoulder. The physical examination is frequently poorly contributive. Dactylitis (sausage-like digit or toe) is less frequent but most typical of SpA.

EXTRA-ARTICULAR MANIFESTATIONS

The most frequent extra-articular manifestation is acute anterior uveitis, which happens at least once in 40% of the patients over 20 years of disease duration. Psoriatic skin or nail lesions are very common (15% to 20% in SpA versus 2% in the general population). Overt inflammatory bowel disease (IBD) occurs in 5% of the patients, but occult IBD could be detected more frequently by performing systematic ileocolonic investigations, including biopsies and microscopic examination. Other less frequent extra-articular manifestations are valvular insufficiency and heart conduction block.

Diagnosis

Validated classification criteria require the presence of advanced radiographic sacroiliitis for the diagnosis of AS. A major issue with this criteria is its dependency on evolution time and its inadequacy for an early diagnosis.

Biologic alterations such as raised erythrocyte sedimentation rate (ESR) or C-reactive protein (CRP) level in the serum are inconstant and not specific. The HLA-B27 allele confers a 100-fold increase in the risk of developing SpA. Thus the detection of this antigen is helpful in case of doubt. However, HLA-B27 positivity is neither mandatory nor sufficient for the diagnosis (i.e., 10% of SpA patients lack this antigen and less than 3% of HLA-B27–positive individuals ever develop SpA).

Amor and colleagues' (1990) classification criteria recapitulate all major findings typical of SpA and attribute to each of them a weight proportional to their specificity (Table 1). Although not developed for this purpose, they are frequently used as a diagnostic tool because their specificity and sensitivity are quite good, even in early disease.

To face the need for more reliable early diagnosis instrument, the most recent imaging modalities, such as magnetic resonance imaging (MRI) and ultrasonography (US), coupled with pulsed-wave Doppler (PwD), bear some hope. Both techniques may demonstrate early inflammatory changes adjacent to the affected sites (i.e., the spine, the sacroiliac or the peripheral joints, and the enthesis). Their diagnostic performance has yet to be studied systematically. However, the sensitivity of sacroiliac or spinal MRI changes seems rather poor in early SpA. In contrast, US PwD could offer greater sensitivity by showing vascularized peripheral enthesitis in most SpA patients, a very specific finding as it appears.

Rakel and Bope: *Conn's Current Therapy 2006.*

TABLE 1 Classification Criteria
for Spondyloarthropathy*

Clinical symptoms or past history	Scoring
Lumbar or dorsal pain at night or morning stiffness of lumbar or dorsal pain	1
Asymmetric oligoarthritis	2
Buttock pain	1
or	
If alternate buttock pain	2
Sausage-like toe or digit	2
Heel pain or other well-defined enthesitis	2
Iritis	1
Nongonococcal ureteritis or cervicitis within 1 mo before the onset of arthritis	1
Acute diarrhea within 1 mo before the onset of arthritis	1
Psoriasis, balanitis, or IBD (i.e., ulcerative colitis or Crohn's disease)	2
Radiologic findings	
Sacroiliitis (bilateral grade 2 or unilateral grade 3)	3
Genetic background	
Presence of HLA-B27 and/or family history of ankylosing spondylitis, reactive arthritis, uveitis, psoriasis or IBD	2
Response to treatment	
Clear-cut improvement within 48 hours after NSAIDs intake or rapid relapse of the pain after their discontinuation	2

*A patient is considered suffering from a spondylarthropathy if the score is greater than or equal to 6.
Abbreviations: HLA = human leucocyte antigen; IBD = inflammatory bowel disease, NSAIDs = nonsteroidal anti-inflammatory drugs.
From Amor et al. (1990).

Treatment

NONSTEROIDAL ANTI-INFLAMMATORY DRUGS

NSAIDs remain the cornerstone of the pharmacologic treatment of SpA. Molecules of this class can be efficacious on all osteoarticular manifestations. Selection of the molecule must be adapted to individual cases because of the high variability of response and tolerance from patient to patient. The half-life of the molecule must be considered and time of intake (bedtime is the most useful) must be adapted to obtain the greatest relief of inflammation during the second half of the night. A great proportion of patients can be satisfactorily treated with NSAIDs alone, but high dosages are required to control the most severe cases and may even be inefficacious in some cases.

CORTICOSTEROIDS

Oral or even parenteral corticosteroids are usually ineffective for skeletal manifestations. In contrast, local injections of slow-acting corticosteroids at the site of inflammation are very efficacious. Most extra-articular manifestations, such as psoriatic lesions and acute anterior uveitis, also benefit from corticosteroids.

DISEASE-MODIFYING ANTIRHEUMATIC DRUGS

Efficacy of the classic disease-modifying antirheumatic drugs (DMARDs) used to treat RA, such as gold salts or methotrexate (Rheumatrex),[1] is rarely achieved in SpA and not supported by any convincing study. Trials show some efficacy of sulfasalazine (Azulfidine),[1] 1 g two or three times daily, on peripheral manifestations but not on axial disease. These drugs were used routinely in the past to treat the most severe patients, with limited success.

In contrast, the anti–TNF-α biologic therapies in several controlled study are very efficacious in treating even the most seriously affected patients. Both the anti–TNF-α antibody infliximab (Remicade)[1] and the TNF p75-soluble receptor etanercept (Enbrel)[1] are approved to treat NSAID-resistant AS. As many as 50% of the patients enrolled in a controlled study experienced a sustained decrease of disease activity, including normalization of ESR and CRP. Patients receiving anti–TNF-α for SpA can usually decrease and frequently discontinue NSAIDs. Remicade is administered intravenously, starting with a loading regimen of three infusions (5 mg/kg per infusion) within a 6-week interval (weeks 0, 2, and 6), followed by retreatment every other 6 to 8 weeks. Enbrel is administered subcutaneously, twice weekly (25 mg per injection). Both treatments must be given permanently because relapse predictably happens upon discontinuation. The most serious adverse effects are infections, which should be minimized by a careful investigation for latent tuberculosis before treatment initiation, including a chest radiograph and a purified protein derivative (PPD) test. A 9-month prophylactic course of isoniazid should be undertaken in patients having a suspicion of untreated latent tuberculosis.

PHYSICAL THERAPY

Whenever possible, physical exercises are recommended, and physical readaptation is an important aspect of AS treatment. One to three physical therapy

---

[1]Not FDA approved for this indication.

 CURRENT DIAGNOSIS

- Retrieve relevant skeletal (axial/peripheral) and extra-articular symptoms from medical history (personal and familial).
- Search evidence for inflammation, both clinically and biologically.
- Search for clinical spinal stiffness, joint alterations, and psoriasis.
- Screen for human leucocyte antigen (HLA)-B27 positivity in case of doubt.
- Use imaging modalities as needed: pelvic radiography, tomodensitometry, magnetic resonance imaging, bone scan.

CURRENT THERAPY

- Use nonsteroidal anti-inflammatory drugs (NSAIDs) as first-line therapy.
- Add physical therapy.
- Consider local corticosteroid injections.
- Consider second-line therapy for patients with a Bath Ankylosing Spondylitis Disease Activity Index (BASDAI) of 4 out of 10 despite NSAIDs.

sessions per week are recommended, especially in patients with severe stiffness and deformities. The aim of exercises is to relax muscle stiffness, to avoid posture deformities, and to maintain muscle strength.

Follow-Up And Evaluation

Adjustment of the treatment may require a number of visits. Clinical variables to be monitored systematically are a disease activity self-assessment index, such as the Bath Ankylosing Spondylitis Disease Activity Index (BASDAI), a functional self-assessment index, such as the Bath Ankylosing Spondylitis Functional Index (BASFI), and several metrologic parameters, reflecting spinal deformity (height, occiput to wall distance, C7 spinous process to wall distance, Schober index). Other variables such as synovitis and enthesitis counts are appropriate for patients with peripheral manifestations.

The course of disease is variable during a lifetime for all patients, who must be taught how to adapt their medications. For instance, intake of NSAIDs may need to be increased during a flare, whereas discontinuation of the drug can be achieved in the case of complete remission. In the absence of clinical manifestation, including pain, swelling, stiffness, and fatigue, there is no absolute need for active treatment. Only periodic examination will then be required to check for the lack of evolution. There is no need to treat isolated biologic findings, such as elevated ESR or CRP.

REFERENCES

Amor B, Dougados M, Mijiyawa M: Critère diagnostique des spondylarthropathies. Rev Rhum Mal Ostéoartic 1990;57:85-89.

Braun J, Sieper J: Biological therapies in the spondyloarthritides—the current state. Rheumatology (Oxford) 2004;43(9):1072-1084.

Breban M, Said-Nahal R, Hugot JP, Miceli-Richard C: Familial and genetic aspects of spondyloarthropathy. Rheum Dis Clin North Am 2003;29(3):575-594.

Collantes E, Veroz R, Escudero A, et al: Can some cases of 'possible' spondyloarthropathy be classified as 'definite' or 'undifferentiated' spondyloarthropathy? Value of criteria for spondyloarthropathies. Spanish Spondyloarthropathy Study Group. Joint Bone Spine 2000;67(6):516-520.

D'Agostino MA, Said-Nahal R, Hacquard-Bouder C, et al: Assessment of peripheral enthesitis in the spondylarthropathies by ultrasonography combined with power Doppler: A cross-sectional study. Arthritis Rheum 2003;48:523-533.

Dougados M, van der Heijde D: Ankylosing spondylitis: How should the disease be assessed? Best Pract Res Clin Rheumatol 2002;16(4):605-618.

Dougados M, Van der Linden S, Juhlin R, et al: The European Spondylarthropathy Study Group preliminary criteria for the classification of spondylarthropathy. Arthritis Rheum 1991;34:1218-1227.

Maksymowych WP, Breban M, Braun J: Ankylosing spondylitis and current disease-controlling agents: Do they work? Best Pract Res Clin Rheumatol 2002;16(4):619-630.

McGonagle D: Diagnosis and treatment of enthesitis. Rheum Dis Clin North Am 2003;29(3):549-560.

van der Linden S, Valkenburg HA, Cats A: Evaluation of diagnostic criteria for ankylosing spondylitis. A proposal for modification of the New York criteria. Arthritis Rheum 1984;27:361-368.

Temporomandibular Disorders

Method of
Per-Olof Eriksson, DDS, PhD, and Hamayun Zafar, PT, PhD

Anatomic structures are more diverse in the orofacial region than in any other region. No other location expresses so many systemic and local diseases as does the oral cavity. It serves as a focal point of interest to more medical and dental specialties than any other single part of the body. Intraoral and dental diseases are the most common cause of jaw–face pain, but a number of possible etiologic factors have to be considered in patients seeking care for pain and functional impairment in the jaw–face–head region. Jaw–face pain and dysfunction may originate from dental, neurologic, otolaryngologic, vascular, cervical spine, metaplastic, infectious, or systematic diseases. Outside the dental profession, it is less known that long-standing pain and disturbed function in the jaw–face are often caused by musculoskeletal disorders, which in fact are as prevalent as the two other major dental diseases, caries and periodontitis, and therefore constitute a significant health problem. Thus the dental profession is responsible for three major so-called dental diseases that can explain jaw–face pain and dysfunction. The human jaw–face muscles show unique fiber types and contractile proteins, both for the extrafusal and the intrafusal (muscle spindles) fibers, and changes with aging in fiber type and myosin composition are opposite those of limb muscles.

Development and Maturation of Structure and Function of the Jaw–Face Region

It is generally agreed that there is an orderly development and maturation of motor control, including postural control, in a cephalocaudal direction. First comes the ability to stabilize the head, followed by stabilization of the shoulder, trunk, and hips, to allow control of the lower limbs. Similarly, development is directed proximal-distal, which means the child first learns to control proximal body segments, such as the trunk, shoulders, and hips, and hand movements after that.

The orofacial muscles are the first to develop in the body, in keeping with the cephalocaudal sequence of fetal development, and facial premuscle masses are formed between the gestational ages of 8 and 9 weeks. Muscular response to a stimulus first develops in the perioral region and is elicited at 7.5 weeks' gestational age, as a result of tactile cutaneous stimuli applied to the lips, indicating that the trigeminal nerve is the first cranial nerve to become active. Stroking the face of the 7.5-week-old embryo produces a reflex bending of the head and upper trunk away from the stimulus, an avoiding reaction, as a total neuromuscular response. Stimulation of the lips at 8.5 weeks' gestational age results in incomplete but active reflex opening of the mouth. Swallowing begins at 12 weeks' gestational age in association with extension reflexes and occurs when the fetus drinks the amniotic fluid in which it is bathed. Tongue movements may begin at 12.5 weeks' gestational age and lip movements at 14.5 weeks' gestational age. The earliest functional movements include oral actions, such as suckling and swallowing, and full swallowing and suckling permitting survival occur at only 32 to 36 weeks of fetal age. Head movements remain strongly associated with mouth movements even into the postnatal period, whereby perioral stimulation leads to ipsilateral head rotation, which in the infant is associated with suckling. Respiratory movements may be elicited by stimulation as early as 13 weeks, but spontaneous rhythmic respiration necessary for survival does not occur until much later. Increasingly complex muscle movements, producing mastication and speech, depend on development of the appropriate reflex proprioceptive mechanisms. All of the complex interrelated orofacial movements of suckling, swallowing, and breathing are reflex in origin, rather than learned, and they constitute unconditioned congenital reflexes necessary for survival. Conditioned acquired reflexes develop with maturation of the neuromuscular system and are generally learned habits. The conversion of infantile swallowing, using predominantly facial nerve muscles, into mature swallowing when molar teeth have erupted and the trigeminal nerve muscles come into action, infantile suckling into mastication, and infantile crying into speech are all examples of the substitution of conditioned reflexes acquired with maturation for the unconditioned congenital reflexes of the neonate. Superimposed on these reflex movements are voluntary activities under conscious control that are acquired by learning and experience.

Pain and Dysfunction in the Jaw–Face Region

A number of diseases may give rise to similar symptoms and signs of pain and dysfunction in the jaw–face region. Assessment, management, and treatment outcome are therefore related to the profession of the care provider. Thus pain experienced in the ear may be of muscular origin, referred to the ear region from adjacent painful jaw muscles. If such pain is interpreted as caused by infection instead of dysfunction, treatment will fail instead of being beneficial and cost-effective for the patient and society.

Symptoms and signs of musculoskeletal disorders in the jaw–face region originate preferentially in the temporomandibular joint (TMJ) and the jaw–face–head muscles. They typically include feelings of fatigue and stiffness in the jaw and face; pain in the jaw, face, ear, head, and neck regions; sounds in the TMJ; limitation of mandibular movements; and tenderness to palpation above the TMJ and jaw muscles. Pain is aggravated during jaw movements. These joint and muscle problems hamper unrestrained motor control with regard to amplitude, speed, force, coordination, direction, and endurance of movement, and they may result in difficulties in gaping, biting, chewing, and swallowing (i.e., eating behavior, yawning, and speech).

Terminology, Epidemiology, and Sex Differences

Musculoskeletal disorders in the jaw–face region are generally termed a *craniomandibular disorder* (CMD) or a *temporomandibular disorder* (TMD). Epidemiologic studies report a high prevalence of signs and symptoms of CMDs, although prevalence rates vary. Recent data, including mild symptoms and signs, reveal average values for perceived and clinically assessed CMDs to be 30% and 44%, respectively. Severe pain and dysfunction, which need treatment, are estimated to occur in about 5% to 10% of the adult population. A strong female preponderance among patients seeking care for CMDs is observed, and symptoms and signs of CMDs are more frequent, severe, and long-lasting in women than in men. No conclusive explanation for gender differences in CMD is as yet reported, in accordance with what is known for musculoskeletal disorders in other body regions.

Etiology and Treatment of Craniomandibular Disorders

Knowledge about mechanisms behind musculoskeletal disorders is in general limited. Consequently, treatment and preventive care are hampered. This is the case also for musculoskeletal disorders in the jaw–face region. Generally, it is a matter of load and capacity, and both central and peripheral factors seem important. Central factors include lifestyle-related psychogenic muscular tension and stress-induced clenching of the jaws. Peripheral factors include the stability of the bite (i.e., the relation between the lower jaw, mandibular teeth and the upper jaw, skull, or "head–neck" teeth at rest and during jaw movements). Psychogenic tension and jaw clenching in a bite that lacks stability may to various degrees give rise to an overload of dental and musculoskeletal components and accordingly result in pain and dysfunction.

Rakel and Bope: *Conn's Current Therapy 2006.*

Studies on treatment outcome involve both dental and nondental therapies, and between 65% and 95% of CMD patients who seek care for the first time are reported to improve. Treatment usually includes the following:

- Counseling
- Jaw exercises for tension relief and to regain movement skills
- A decrease of load on dental, muscle, and joint tissues by improving bite stability, which can be fulfilled by using reversible methods (e.g., intraoral appliances, bite splints) and irreversible methods (e.g., dental fillings and selective grinding of teeth)
- Drugs for relief of pain and tension
- TMJ surgery when pain and dysfunction are caused by internal derangement

Functional Coupling Between the Jaw and the Neck Regions

Evidence from neuroanatomic and neurophysiologic studies in animals demonstrates close connections between the trigeminal and the neck neuromuscular systems. In humans, a functional coupling between the craniomandibular and the cervical spine regions is suggested by intimate anatomic and biomechanical relationships, by findings of reflex activities in the neck muscles following electrical stimulation of trigeminal nerve branches, and from observations of simultaneous activation of jaw and neck–shoulder muscles during mandibular movements. The earliest reflex found in the human embryo is the trigeminal neck reflex, which consists of contraction of neck muscles elicited by light touch of the perioral region. Thus previous studies in animals and humans indicate a close functional linkage between the jaw and the neck regions. Systematic studies of integrated mandibular and head–neck behavior during natural jaw function, however, are lacking.

A series of studies in humans, using optoelectronic wireless technique for three-dimensional movement recording and electromyography, showed concomitant and well-coordinated mandibular and head–neck movements during both single and rhythmic jaw opening-and-closing tasks (Figure 1). Such movements are invariant in nature. The findings led to a new concept for natural jaw function. In this concept, functional jaw movements are the result of jointly activated jaw as well as neck muscles, leading to simultaneous movements in the temporomandibular, atlanto-occipital, and cervical spine joints. These jaw and head–neck movements have neural commands in common and are preprogrammed. Furthermore, when combined with observations in ultrasonographic studies on human fetal yawning, findings indicate that mouth opening and closing are accompanied by head extension-flexion movements, respectively, and the functional connection between the jaw and the neck in natural jaw function is innate. Thus, based on results from studies in animals and people, "natural jaw function," by definition, includes integrative jaw–neck behavior.

Significance of Functional Coupling Between the Jaw and the Neck

Connections between the trigeminal system and neck motoneurons are important for head withdrawal reactions in all species. Any sudden or unexpected stimulus in the orofacial region leads to fast head aversion, hence parallelling the flexor reflex of the limbs. Such connections are also likely critical for coordinating jaw and head–neck motions and in timing of jaw opening and closing with head–neck movements during daily activities such as eating and communication.

Free neck movements are a prerequisite for natural maximal gaping. A reduced head extension ability may limit the three-dimensional space for the mandibular movement because of impingement of the mandible with suprahyoid and airway structures. A connection between the jaw and the neck motor systems is probably of importance to allow simultaneous mandibular and head–neck movements, aimed at optimizing both the magnitude of the gape and the positioning of the gape in space. From an evolutionary perspective, such a mechanism, to optimally direct the jaw motor system (i.e., the mouth or the gape) in basic actions such as feeding, attack, and defense behavior, is probably of great survival value (e.g., during catching of prey).

Craniomandibular Disorders and Pain and Dysfunction in the Neck

Clinical trials demonstrate an association between CMDs and neck symptoms; pain and dysfunction in the neck are often present in patients with CMD. It is also known that patients with neck problems may have signs and symptoms of CMD. In fact, randomized controlled trials show that treatment of CMD in patients who were on sick leave for neck–shoulder pain and dysfunction, but who also had CMD, provided relief of both CMD and neck–shoulder symptoms. Notably, treatment outcome was measured in terms of reduced number of days on sick leave and use of medical services. The treatment consisted of improvement of bite stability by selective grinding of the lower and upper teeth. Such adjustment of peripheral input probably influences the relation between the mandible and the head–neck biomechanically, by changing the functional load on jaw and neck components, and with regard to integrative sensorimotor control of the jaw and neck.

Craniomandibular Disorders in Whiplash-Associated Disorders

Trauma to the neck from a motor vehicle accident or some other type of head–neck trauma, generally called whiplash trauma or injury, may lead to a condition

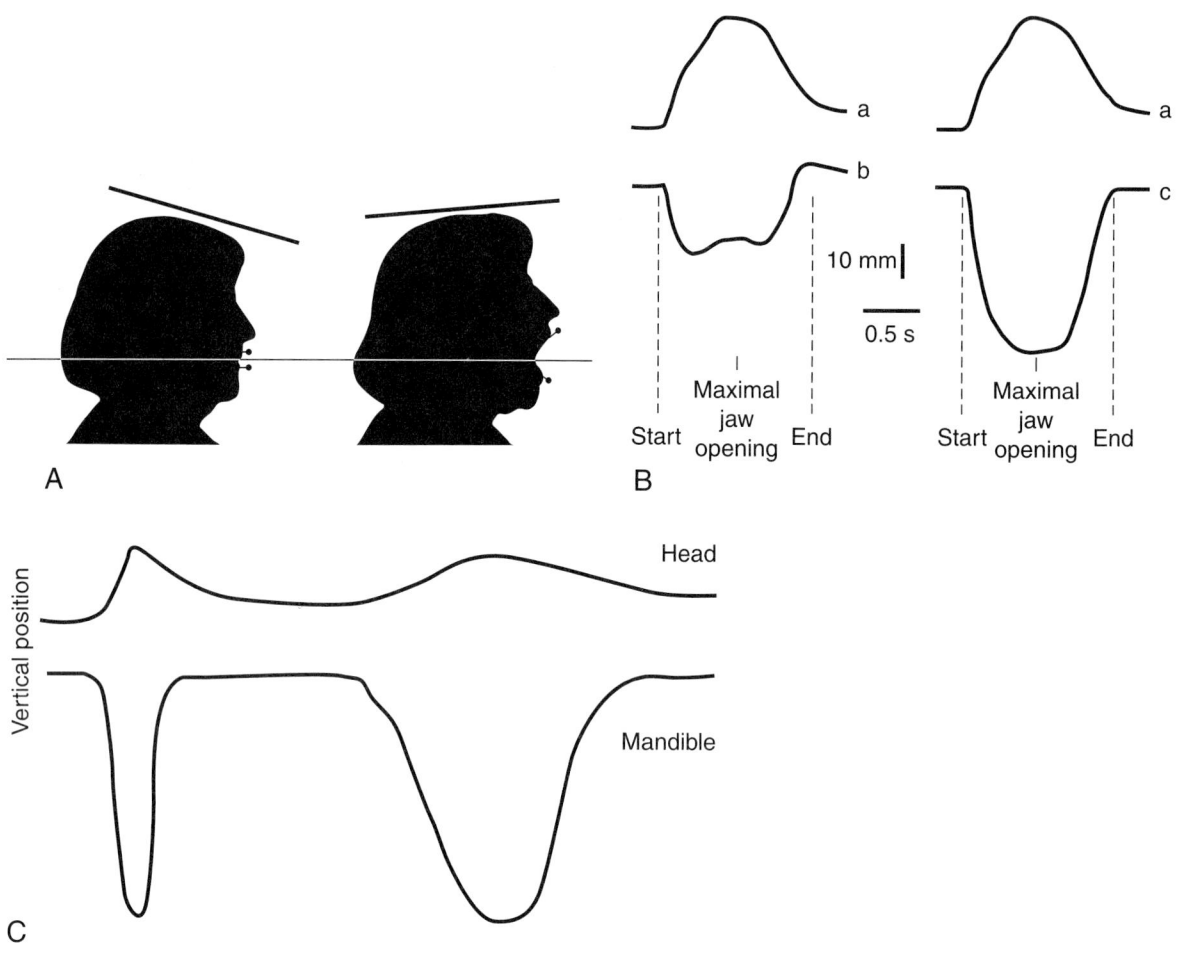

FIGURE 1. A, Head position at rest (*left*) and at maximal jaw opening (*right*). Note change in head position indicated by reference line above the head and recording markers attached to the upper and lower frontal teeth. Note also the relatively unchanged midposition of the gape at maximal jaw opening, indicated by the horizontal reference line. **B,** Movement trajectories in vertical dimension over time of the mandible (*b, c*) and the head (*a*) for a maximal jaw opening–closing movement. Start and end of movement are labeled. The *left* panel (*b*) illustrates the mandibular movement "in space," i.e., the trajectory is the result of the combined mandibular and head–neck movements. The *right* panel (*c*) shows the magnitude of the mandibular movement after mathematical compensation for head movement, i.e., in relation to the head. **C,** Movement trajectories in vertical dimension over time of head–neck and mandibular movements at fast (*left*) and slow (*right*) jaw opening–closing tasks, and after mathematical compensation for head movements. Note simultaneous start of mandibular and head movements.

comprising a number of symptoms and signs in the neck and head termed whiplash-associated disorders (WADs). Studies indicate that such head–neck trauma can result in pain and dysfunction in the jaw–face region (i.e., CMD), although the matter is under debate.

Studies on integrated jaw–neck motor control in healthy subjects and in WAD patients led to an explanatory model for the development of CMD in subjects who met with whiplash injury. Given that natural jaw actions require a healthy state with unrestricted motion of both the TMJ and the atlanto-occipital and cervical spine joints, it can be assumed that an injury to or disease of any of these three joint systems might derange natural jaw motor control. Furthermore, such a functional impairment would be reflected by disturbed jaw–neck behavior, which could be detected by recording and analyzing concomitant mandibular and head–neck movements during natural jaw actions. We recently tested this hypothesis by studying integrative

jaw–neck function in patients suffering from WADs and pain and dysfunction in the jaw–face. The results show an association between neck trauma and disturbed jaw–neck function, indicating that coordinated jaw–neck motor control during both single and rhythmic jaw opening-closing movements indeed can be disturbed following neck injury. Thus *cervicocraniomandibular disorder* (CCMD) is an appropriate term for the clinical condition comprising both jaw–face and head–neck pain and dysfunction.

Treatment Model for Improvement of Mandibular and Head–Neck Mobility

Studies on integrative jaw–neck function include measurement of magnitude, temporal coordination, speed,

Rakel and Bope: *Conn's Current Therapy 2006.*

and spatiotemporal consistency of concomitant mandibular and head–neck movements. By applying the methods we developed for analysis of healthy jaw–neck behavior in investigations of patients, we found signs of disturbed jaw–neck function in individuals suffering from WADs. Based on the findings in healthy subjects and in patients, we developed a new model for treatment of pain and dysfunction in the jaw–face and WADs. This treatment approach is aimed at improving both mandibular and head–neck mobility, thereby regaining natural jaw function. The model is based on the fact that motor control starts to develop and mature in the jaw-orofacial region (as described earlier). Data from numerous studies in animals and people suggest a close linkage between the jaw and the neck sensorimotor systems in natural jaw function. Consequently, treatment for improving jaw function should include the neck. Our studies to test this treatment model in patients with jaw–face pain and dysfunction and WADs show improvement of both jaw and neck function, results that merit further studies in randomized clinical trials.

Figure 2 shows a typical example. It is based on data from a female patient, 30 years of age, who had a car accident and developed WAD 4 years before she was referred to the department of Clinical Oral Physiology, Umeå University Hospital, Umeå, Sweden, for assessment and management of pain and dysfunction in the jaw and face. The patient had received all the care and treatment for WAD available according to routines used by the health care system. Our examination revealed severely impaired jaw and neck function and widespread pain in all body regions. The initial, pretreatment, investigation of concomitant mandibular and head–neck movements during jaw opening-and-closing tasks, using our routine protocol and optoelectronic wireless three-dimensional movement recording technique, verified the functional impairment of jaw–neck behavior. As Figure 2 illustrates, the follow-up recordings after 4 and 7 months show an increase in magnitude of movement amplitudes of both the mandibular and the head–neck movement. In addition, the speed of movement increased. The figure also shows that functional impairment, as well as change in behavior in response to treatment, can be measured and documented qualitatively and quantitatively by objective recording methods.

Treatment Regimen for Craniomandibular Disorders and Whiplash-Associated Disorders

The general aim of the treatment regimen is to regain natural jaw function by reprogramming faulty jaw–neck sensorimotor behavior. In short, this is performed in three ways:

1. Education, advice, and instructions with regard to anatomy, physiology, pathophysiology, and treatment
2. Specific jaw–neck exercises, including mandibular and head–neck movements to gain successive

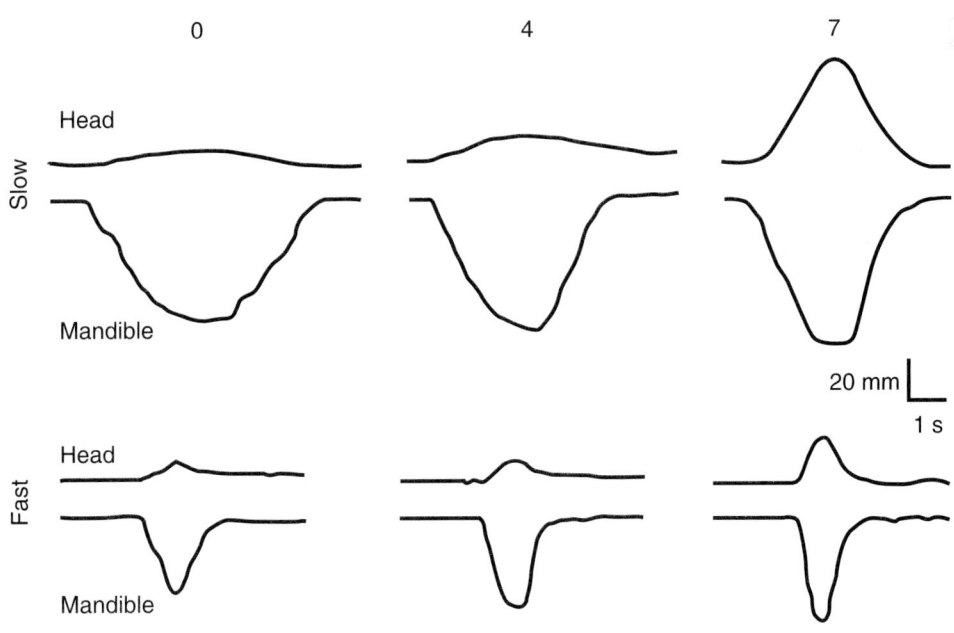

FIGURE 2. Repeated movement recordings in a female patient, 30 years old, suffering from whiplash-associated disorders and pain and dysfunction in the jaw–face. Trajectories for the vertical dimension over time of mandibular and head–neck movements at slow (*upper panel*) and fast (*lower panel*) maximal jaw opening-and-closing tasks: initial, pretreatment, recording (0), and recordings after 4 and 7 months of treatment. Note post-treatment increase in amplitude and speed for both mandibular and head–neck movements, and for both slow and fast jaw opening and closing tasks.

CURRENT DIAGNOSIS

- Because different diseases in the jaw–orofacial region may give rise to similar symptoms, proper examination and diagnosis must precede treatment.
- Musculoskeletal disorders in the jaw–face region, generally termed *craniomandibular disorders* (CMDs), are as prevalent as the two major dental diseases, caries and periodontitis, and constitute a significant health problem.
- There is a strong female preponderance among patients seeking care for CMD, and symptoms and signs are more frequent, severe, and longer lasting in women than in men.
- Between 65% and 95% of CMD patients who seek care for the first time are reported to improve.

CURRENT THERAPY

- A new concept for natural jaw function suggests that "functional jaw movements" are the result of jointly activated jaw and neck muscles, leading to simultaneous movements in the temporomandibular, atlanto-occipital, and cervical spine joints. These jaw and head–neck movements have neural commands in common, are preprogrammed, and are innate. Accordingly, natural jaw function, by definition, includes integrative jaw–neck behavior.
- A new explanatory model for the development of pain and dysfunction in the jaw–face in subjects with whiplash-associated disorders (WADs) proposes because natural jaw actions require a healthy state of the temporomandibular, atlanto-occipital, and cervical spine joints, it can be assumed that an injury to or disease of any of these three joint systems might derange natural jaw motor control.
- Based on findings of disturbed jaw–neck function in WAD, a new treatment model is suggested for patients with jaw–face pain and dysfunction and WAD. The rationale behind this approach is that intervention of jaw function by definition includes neck function. Results from implementation of this treatment model, showing improvement of magnitude and speed for both mandibular and head–neck movements, are reported.
- Finally, an appropriate term for the clinical condition comprising both jaw–face and head–neck pain and dysfunction is *cervicocraniomandibular disorders* (CCMDs).

increase in movement amplitude and speed in very minor steps (i.e., to slowly reteach the neuromuscular system to execute coordinated mandibular and head–neck movements in a cost-effective way)
3. A custom-made intraoral appliance (bite splint) attached to the upper teeth for day and night use, to change biomechanical relations (reducing detrimental load on sensitized components of the jaw–neck motor system and give pain relief) and to modulate sensorimotor settings for control of jaw–neck behavior and disturb jaw-clenching habits. In fact, ongoing studies in our laboratory indicate that this device is associated with significant changes in control mechanisms of posture and movement.

REFERENCES

Carlsson GE: Epidemiology and treatment need for temporomandibular disorders. J Orofac Pain 1999;13:232-237.

Eriksson P-O, Zafar H, Nordh E: Concomitant mandibular and head-neck movements during jaw opening-closing in man. J Oral Rehabil. 1998;25:859-870.

Eriksson P-O, Häggman-Henrikson B, Nordh E, Zafar H: Coordinated mandibular and head-neck movements during rhythmic jaw activities in man. J Dent Res. 2000;79:1378-1384.

Eriksson P-O, Zafar H, Häggman-Henrikson B: Deranged jaw-neck motor control in whiplash-associated disorders. Eur J Oral Sci. 2004;112:25-32.

Häggman-Henrikson B, Zafar H, Eriksson P-O: Disturbed jaw behavior in whiplash-associated disorders during rhythmic jaw movements. J Dent Res. 2002;81:747-751.

Häggman-Henrikson B: Neck function in rhythmic jaw activities. [Doctoral Dissertation] Umeå University, Sweden 2004; pp 1-53.

Johansson H, Windhorst U, Djupsjöbacka M, Passatore M [Eds]: Chronic work-related myalgia. Neuromuscular mechanisms behind work-related chronic muscle pain syndromes. Gävle University Press Gävle, Sweden 2003; pp 1-310.

Kirveskari P, Alanen P: Effect of occlusal treatment on sick leaves in TMJ dysfunction patients with head and neck symptoms. Community Dent Oral Epidemiol. 1984;12:78-81.

Monemi M, Kadi F, Liu JX, et al: Adverse changes in fibre type and myosin heavy chain compositions of human jaw muscle vs. limb muscle during ageing. Acta Physiol Scand. 1999;167:339-345.

Sperry GH: Craniofacial embryology. 4th ed. Wright. 1989.

Zafar H: Integrated jaw and neck function in man. Studies of mandibular and head-neck movements during jaw opening-closing tasks. [Doctoral Dissertation] Swed Dent J Suppl. 2000;(143):1-41.

Zafar H, Nordh E, Eriksson P-O: Spatiotemporal consistency of human mandibular and head-neck movement trajectories during jaw opening-closing tasks. Exp Brain Res. 2002;146:70-76.

Bursitis, Tendonitis, Myofascial Pain, and Fibromyalgia

Method of
Keith K. Colburn, MD

Soft tissue rheumatism is a term that describes musculoskeletal pain and other symptoms not caused by arthritis. Bursitis, tendonitis, myofascial pain syndrome, and fibromyalgia belong to this group of disorders. These maladies may occur in the absence of systemic disease. They are associated with persistent mild trauma and overuse of muscles, bursae, tendons, entheses, ligaments, and fascia, conditions commonly seen by primary care doctors. Localized tendonitis or bursitis is very specific and may be either self-limiting or relieved by topical or oral anti-inflammatory medications or treated with a well-placed injection. Fibromyalgia is more diffuse and may be very difficult to treat. There are no abnormal laboratory tests consistently associated with soft tissue rheumatism. Radiologic tests and scans may show abnormalities of soft tissue; it is only occasionally necessary, however, to do expensive tests to get an accurate diagnosis of these conditions. Diagnosis requires a good history and a careful physical examination of the musculoskeletal system.

Bursitis and Tendonitis

Bursitis and tendonitis may occur in any one of hundreds of locations throughout the body. A bursa is a synovial membrane-lined sac containing synovial fluid. Bursae are found in areas of potential friction, such as where tendons, ligaments, and bone rub against each other. Bursitis may occur alone or in conjunction with inflammation of a tendon in close proximity. Tendons and ligaments are fibrous cords or bands that attach muscle to other structures, usually bone. Bursitis and tendonitis are considered together here by regions of the body because diagnosis and treatment share some common principles. Treatments specific to unique locations are mentioned in the text. Otherwise, general treatment principles are listed in the Current Therapy box.

SHOULDER REGION

Shoulder pain is a common problem that increases with age. Because the shoulder has an extensive range of motion, it one of the most unstable joints in the body. Numerous ligaments, tendons, and bursae surround the shoulder joints. *Rotator cuff tendonitis,* or the *impingement syndrome,* is the most common cause of shoulder pain. *Subacromial bursitis* may be secondarily present with the impingement syndrome. Pain on active abduction and internal rotation of the glenohumeral joint and aching over the deltoid area are the main symptoms of this condition. The impingement syndrome may be acute from a recent injury or chronic

with calcific tendonitis sometimes seen on radiographs. *Rotator cuff tears* may be partial or complete, acute or chronic, exquisitely painful or hardly felt. Weakness and pain on abduction, night pain, and tenderness on palpation may indicate the presence of a torn rotator cuff. The diagnosis may be established by a shoulder arthrogram, ultrasonogram, or magnetic resonance imaging (MRI) scan. Although incomplete tears often are best treated by conservative means, over time they often become complete tears. Complete tears can often be surgically repaired, especially if they are acute and occur in younger patients. *Bicipital tendonitis* often presents as anterior shoulder pain. Sometimes the pain is diffuse, but rolling the long head of the biceps tendon under the examiner's thumb elicits localized tenderness if the tendon is inflamed. Rupture of the long head of the biceps tendon presents as an enlargement of the distal end of the biceps muscle. This complication is usually not repaired because it results in only a minor loss of strength in the biceps muscle. *Adhesive capsulitis,* or *frozen shoulder,* presents as generalized pain and tenderness of the shoulder area with a marked loss of active and passive range of motion and with muscle atrophy. Inflammatory arthritis, diabetes, immobility, low pain threshold, depression, or improper treatment of a painful shoulder can result in a frozen shoulder. Arthrography demonstrates a contracted joint capsule space. Less common painful conditions associated with the shoulder region include the *thoracic outlet syndrome, brachial plexopathy,* and *neuropathies.*

ANTERIOR CHEST WALL

Pain in the anterior chest wall is common and often needs to be differentiated from cardiac, pulmonary, or gastrointestinal pain. Point tenderness helps delineate actual chest wall pain from pain generated from an internal organ. *Costochondritis (Tietze's syndrome)* is manifested by tenderness at the costochondral junction of the anterior ribs. There is usually one distinct tender spot, although more can occur simultaneously. *Xiphodynia* is characterized by tenderness and pain over the xiphoid area.

ELBOW REGION

Olecranon bursitis occurs with repetitive mild trauma and abrasion over the elbow or with an inflammatory condition including gout, pseudogout, rheumatoid arthritis, and infection. Range of motion of the elbow is usually relatively normal and pain minimal except when infection is present. Aspiration of an uninfected bursa alone or combined with an injection of a corticosteroid is the usual treatment. Crystal identification with a polarized microscope is helpful to differentiate gout or pseudogout from infection. Antibiotic treatment, after a Gram stain and culture of purulent fluid, is indicated in a suspected infected bursa. *Lateral epicondylitis,* or tennis elbow, is a common finding in repetitive use of one's arms. Tenderness is elicited by pressing the extensor tendons 1 to 2 cm distal to the lateral epicondyle. Shaking hands or lifting a bag causes pain in the same location.

Medial epicondylitis, or golfer's elbow, is less common but diagnosed by palpating the flexor tendons attached to the medial epicondyle. A soft forearm brace may be helpful if patients would prefer not to have an injection of the tender spot. *Ulnar nerve entrapment* and *tendonitis of the musculotendinous insertion of the biceps* are conditions also found in the elbow region.

HAND AND WRIST REGION

A *ganglion* is a cyst arising from a tendon sheath or a joint, commonly located on the dorsum of the wrist. It is lined with synovium and contains a thick jelly-like liquid. *De Quervain's tenosynovitis* is inflammation and tenderness of the sheath of the abductor pollicis longus and extensor polices brevis tendons located over the radial styloid. Repetitive trauma, pregnancy, and systemic rheumatoid diseases are causes for this disorder. *Carpal tunnel syndrome* caused by the compression of the median nerve by the surrounding structures in the wrist is the most common cause of numbness and tingling in the hands. A positive Tinel or Phalen sign with a confirming nerve conduction test makes the diagnosis fairly simple. Trauma, pregnancy, and a host of metabolic or inflammatory diseases are often responsible for this condition. Treatment starts with wrist splinting at night. The use of 200 mg of vitamin B_6 daily[1] until the symptoms subside may be controversial, but in my opinion is often very helpful. If these measures are unsuccessful, a corticosteroid injection on the ulnar side of the carpal tunnel, a few millimeters away from the median nerve, usually relieves the numbness and tingling, often for months. In many patients, surgery is eventually required to release the median nerve. Other less frequent hand and wrist soft tissue problems include *pronator teres syndrome, anterior interosseous nerve syndrome, radial nerve palsy, ulnar nerve entrapment at the wrist, volar flexor tenosynovitis,* and *Dupuytren's contractures.*

HIP REGION

The trochanteric bursa lies on the posterior portion of the greater trochanter. Pain from *trochanteric bursitis* is felt in the trochanteric area and lateral thigh, and it is often thought inaccurately to be hip joint pain, which is usually felt in the groin and high in the buttock. Excessive trauma to the bursal area, such as a long hike, can precipitate trochanteric bursitis. Osteoarthritis of the lumbar spine or hip, scoliosis or leg length discrepancies, and age can contribute to trochanteric bursitis. *Iliopsoas (iliopectineal) bursitis* causes groin and anterior thigh pain, made worse on passive hyperextension and sometimes flexion of the hip with resistance. *Ischial (ischiogluteal) bursitis,* or *weaver's bottom,* is caused by trauma or sitting for a long time on hard surfaces. Pain from ischial bursitis is felt down the back of the thigh with point tenderness over the ischial tuberosity. Soft seat cushions and a corticosteroid

injection of the bursa usually help relieve the pain. *Piriformis syndrome* is not well understood. The predominant symptom is pain over the buttocks sometimes radiating down the back of the thigh and leg. Trauma is usually involved in the etiology. The diagnosis is often made on rectal or vaginal examination by detecting tenderness in the piriformis muscle. *Meralgia paresthetica* is caused by the compression of the lateral femoral cutaneous nerve (L2-L3). It causes intermittent burning pain, hyperesthesia, and numbness of the anterolateral thigh. This syndrome is seen most often in patients with obesity or diabetes, or who are pregnant.

KNEE REGION

Popliteal cysts, or Baker cysts, are associated with knee joint effusions, causing a synovial herniation into the popliteal fossa. The cyst may rupture and dissect down the calf, often to the ankle, where it may leave a purpuric "crescent sign" beneath the malleolus. A ruptured Baker cyst is acutely painful and must be differentiated from thrombophlebitis. An arthrogram or ultrasound examination of the knee may be used to diagnose a Baker cyst with or without a rupture. A venogram can exclude concomitant thrombophlebitis if necessary. An injection of a corticosteroid[1] into the cyst or the knee joint often shrinks the cyst. Surgical removal of the cyst may be necessary if the injection is ineffective. *Anserine bursitis* is diagnosed by tenderness over the medial aspect of the knee an inch or two below the joint line and occurs in predominantly obese middle-age to elderly women (35 to 80 years of age) with osteoarthritis of the knee. *Prepatellar bursitis,* or *housemaid's knee,* presents as a mildly tender swelling over the patella. It is usually caused by trauma from frequent kneeling. Aspiration of the bursa is important because occasionally septic prepatellar bursitis is present. Because the bursa does not communicate with the knee joint, treatment with oral antibiotics appropriate for the organism cultured is adequate. For sterile bursitis, an injection of a corticosteroid is helpful, as is protection of the knee from trauma. Less common painful soft tissue conditions of the knee include *patellar tendonitis, popliteal tendonitis, medial plica syndrome, rupture of the quadriceps tendon,* and *infrapatellar tendon* and *patellofemoral pain syndrome (chondromalacia patellae).*

ANKLE AND FOOT REGION

Achilles tendonitis has two predominant causes. One is trauma. The other is a group of inflammatory conditions including rheumatoid arthritis, the spondyloarthropathies, and pseudogout. Tenderness, pain, and swelling occur proximal to or at the Achilles tendon attachment to the calcaneus. Shoe corrections, heel lifts, a splint with plantar flexion, and careful stretching of the tendon constitute the safest treatment. The inflamed Achilles tendon is vulnerable to rupture, especially if a corticosteroid is injected around it. The differential

---

[1]Not FDA approved for this indication.

[1]Not FDA approved for this indication.

diagnosis of Achilles tendonitis includes *retrocalcaneal bursitis* and *subcutaneous Achilles bursitis. Plantar fasciitis* is characterized by burning, lancing or aching pain, and tenderness over the plantar surface of the heel from a variety of kinds of trauma or overuse. *Tarsal tunnel syndrome* is caused by compression of the posterior tibial nerve, posterior and inferior to the medial malleolus. A positive Tinel sign may be elicited by percussion over the entrapment site. Numbness, paresthesias, and burning pain are felt from the toes to the medial malleolus. Changing shoes and conservative therapy may help in the treatment of this condition, but surgery is often needed to decompress the nerve and provide relief. *Morton's neuroma* is an entrapment neuropathy of the interdigital nerve most commonly found between the third and fourth toes. This condition is often detected in middle-age women (35 to 60 years old) wearing high heels or tight shoes. Pain is often felt in the fourth toe as a burning, aching pain with paresthesias. Treatment consists of a metatarsal bar or a corticosteroid[1] injection in the web space of the toe where the tenderness is palpated. If these are unsuccessful, surgery to remove the neuroma may be necessary. Less common causes of nonarthritic foot pain include *posterior tibial tendonitis, hallux valgus, bunionette (tailor's bunion) of the fifth toe, hammertoes, metatarsalgia, pes planus (flat foot), pes cavus (claw foot),* and a variety of

---

[1]Not FDA approved for this indication.

 CURRENT DIAGNOSIS

Bursitis and Tendonitis

- Localized tenderness is usually palpated directly over an affected bursa or tendon.
- Most often, *active* range of motion in the affected tendon or bursa is painful, but unlike with arthritis, *passive* range of motion is frequently painless.
- With a few exceptions, blood tests and radiographs are usually normal.

Fibromyalgia

- A longer than 3-month history of chronic, widespread pain both above and below the waist and on both sides of the body in the absence of another condition to explain the pain.
- The presence of at least 11 of 18 tender points by digital palpation at previously published locations.
- Tender point sites include bilateral locations on the following locations:
  Occiput
  Anterior lower neck (C5-C7)
  Trapezius
  Supraspinatus
  Second anterior costochondral junction
  Lateral epicondyle
  Buttocks in the upper outer quadrant
  Greater trochanters
  Medial fat pad of the knees

tendon ruptures or *displacements* including the Achilles, posterior tibialis, and the peroneal tendons.

Myofascial Pain Syndrome

Myofascial pain syndromes are often referred to as localized or regional fibromyalgia. They include regional pain disorders like chronic whiplash, repetitive strain syndrome, and temporomandibular joint syndrome. Myofascial pain is characterized by the presence of trigger points, defined as localized areas of deep muscle tenderness located in a taut band in the muscle that when palpated are referred to distant zones of perceived pain. In addition to the referred pain, a local "twitch response," or muscle contraction, is seen with pressing on a trigger point. Tender points of fibromyalgia are not characterized by referred pain. Treatment includes injecting the trigger points and often adding the treatment modalities outlined in the fibromyalgia section (Current Therapy box).

Fibromyalgia Syndrome

Fibromyalgia is a chronic, diffuse pain syndrome of unknown etiology. It is characterized by widespread musculoskeletal pain of variable intensity and specific "tender points" to palpation (Current Diagnosis box). Fibromyalgia is associated with a lack of deep sleep and a relative intolerance of physical activities because of pain. Box 1 outlines the signs and symptoms associated with fibromyalgia. Many patients also complain of a history of either an emotional or physical traumatic event prior to the onset of symptoms of fibromyalgia. The incidence of fibromyalgia is estimated at 2% of the population; 90% of these cases are found in women. Primary fibromyalgia is remarkable for the lack of abnormal laboratory and radiologic tests routinely done for rheumatologic diseases. Secondary fibromyalgia, fibromyalgia linked to another disease (Box 2), may improve when the primary disease is treated. Concurrent fibromyalgia or fibromyalgia coexisting together with other conditions (see Box 2) may not respond to treatment of the other disease. The American College of Rheumatology has published diagnostic criteria for fibromyalgia (see Current Diagnosis box). Digital palpation of the tender points is done at approximately 4 kg of force, which is roughly enough pressure to blanch the thumbnail. It is extremely important that patients are made aware by the treating physician that they own this diagnosis and it requires effort on their part to get better. It then becomes the patient's responsibility to take charge of their own problem and carry out the treatment recommendations by their physicians and appropriately trained staff. Treatment with narcotics,[1] because of potential dependency problems, should be avoided if at all possible. Because there is no reliable program that eliminates all of the patient's pain, there are many

---

[1]Not FDA approved for this indication.

15

BOX 1   **Signs and Symptoms of Fibromyalgia**
• Sleep disturbance • Fatigue • Paresthesias • Stiffness • Depression • Dry eyes and mouth • Raynaud's syndrome • Headaches

treatment protocols for fibromyalgia. Self-motivated patients may find relief for a significant portion of their discomfort. My preferred method of treatment is outlined in the Current Therapy box. A compassionate, experienced physician is essential for the successful treatment of fibromyalgia. Psychological counseling may be helpful if it is presented to the patient as a modality in helping to cope with pain and not a suggestion that the patient's problems are "just" psychological. Encouraging the patient to expect small increments of improvement and not to anticipate a cure helps

---

 CURRENT THERAPY

Bursitis and Tendonitis

- Use conservative measures first in treating bursitis and tendonitis. These include rest, modifying wear-and-tear activities, heat and/or ice, physical therapy, weight loss, splinting, topical analgesics, nonsteroidal anti-inflammatory drugs (NSAIDs), and well-placed lidocaine injections with or without corticosteroids.
- There are numerous NSAID preparations, including naproxen (Naprosyn), 500 mg twice a day, ibuprofen (Motrin),[1] 400 to 800 mg every 6 to 8 hours, and the newer COX-2 selective agents, including celecoxib (Celebrex),[1] 100 to 200 mg one to two times daily. (If the patient is taking aspirin, even a baby aspirin, the COX-2 effect is eliminated. A proton pump inhibitor such as lansoprazole (Prevacid), 15 to 30 mg daily, with a traditional NSAID, gives the equivalent gastrointestinal protection of the COX-2 agents.)
- Corticosteroid injections using 0.5 to 1.0 mL of methylprednisolone acetate (Depo-Medrol) or triamcinolone acetonide (Kenalog-40) are best administered after 1 to 10 mL of lidocaine (Xylocaine) is injected with a separate syringe, leaving the needle in place while changing the syringe. This avoids the possibility of subcutaneous fat atrophy at the injection site from the corticosteroid.
- Inject around, not into, a tendon to avoid tendon rupture. For patient comfort, a number 25 or 27 needle of appropriate length should be used. (Ethyl chloride spray on the skin obscures the pain of the needle stick. Adding bicarbonate to the syringe neutralizes the stinging sensation of lidocaine.)
- Surgical solutions for bursitis and tendonitis are reserved for unresponsiveness to conservative measures.

Fibromyalgia

Initial Therapy

- See Other Tested and Possibly Helpful Therapies later in this box.

- Daily aerobic exercise, starting with as little as 5 minutes at first, progressing to between 30 to 60 minutes, is ideal. Emphasize to patients that without the progressive aerobic exercise part of treatment (i.e., walking, swimming in warm water, bicycling, jogging, etc.), they are unlikely to improve very much no matter what medications they take. It usually takes 6 to 12 months of exercise by unusually motivated patients to attain the level of fitness that is likely to diminish most or all the pain. Even some exercise is still beneficial.
- Tramadol (Ultram),[3] 50 mg, progressively up to 8 tablets daily in divided doses, for pain.
- Zolpidem (Ambien), 10 mg at bedtime (this drug is less habit forming and gives the deepest—that is, stage 3 or 4—sleep of any other sleeping medications).

Second-Line Therapy

- May be added onto or substituted for one of the first-line medications depending on drug interactions and efficacy.
- Gabapentin (Neurontin),[1] 1800 to 3600 mg daily, in progressive, divided doses, for pain.
- Amitriptyline (Elavil),[1] 10 to 200 mg, or trazodone (Desyrel),[1] 25 to 250 mg at bedtime, for sleep, depression, and mild pain relief.
- A selective serotonin reuptake inhibitor agent such as sertraline (Zoloft),[1] 50 mg daily, for depression and mild pain relief.

Other Tested and Possibly Helpful Therapies

- Muscle relaxants, such as tizanidine (Zanaflex), 4 to 8 mg three times per day, or cyclobenzaprine (Flexeril), 10 mg at bedtime, for pain and rest.
- Newer antidepressants, such as duloxetine (Cymbalta), 60 mg two times per day, for pain and, secondarily, for depression.
- Magnesium, 500 mg, combined with malic acid, 1200 to 2400 mg daily, for fatigue.
- Narcotics should be avoided.
- NSAIDs are rarely helpful.
- Prolonged bed rest and inactivity and expensive and/or dangerous alternative therapies should be avoided.

---

[1]Not FDA approved for this indication.
[3]Exceeds dosage recommended by the manufacturer.
Abbreviations: NSAID = nonsteroidal anti-inflammatory drug.

BOX 2 Conditions Associated or Concurrent with Fibromyalgia

Secondary fibromyalgia	Concurrent fibromyalgia
Hypothyroidism	Chronic fatigue syndrome
Polymyalgia rheumatica	Autoimmune diseases (systemic lupus erythematosus, rheumatoid arthritis)
Tapering off corticosteroids	Myofascial pain syndrome
Drugs (lipid-lowering and antiviral agents)	Irritable bowel syndrome
	Gulf War syndrome
Cervical stenosis?	Migraine headaches
Malignancy	Interstitial cystitis
	Viral infections (e.g., parvovirus, Lyme disease, hepatitis C)

expectations remain realistic. Patients may be referred to support groups backed by organizations like the Arthritis Foundation. Online Web sites for fibromyalgia associated with universities or reputable foundations may be very helpful to patients by providing accurate information about their condition and its treatment.

REFERENCES

Biundo JJ, Jr: Regional rheumatic pain syndromes. In: Klippel JH, Crofford LJ, Stone JH, Weyand CM (eds): Primer on the Rheumatic Diseases, 12th ed. Atlanta, Arthritis Foundation, 2001, pp 174-187.

Clauw DJ: Fibromyalgia and diffuse pain syndromes. In: Klippel JH, Crofford LJ, Stone JH, Weyand CM (eds): Primer on the Rheumatic Diseases, 12th ed. Atlanta, Arthritis Foundation, 2001, pp 188-193.

Fransen J, Russell IJ: Medical management of fibromyalgia. In Fransen J, Russell IJ (eds): The Fibromyalgia Help Book. St. Paul, Minn, Smith House Press, 1996, pp 35-58.

Goldenberg DL: Fibromyalgia and related syndromes. In: Hochberg MC, Silman AL, Smolen JS, et al (eds): Rheumatology, 3rd ed. St. Louis, Mo, Mosby, 2003, pp 701-712.

Sheon RP: Overview of soft tissue rheumatic disorders. UpToDate, online 12.3, 2004. Available online at http://www.uptodate.com.

Osteoarthritis

Method of
George E. Ehrlich, MD

In some respects, the term *osteoarthritis* is a misnomer because it refers only to a subset of joint changes—those accompanied by inflammation. An older, and still popular name in some parts of the world, is osteoarthrosis, which implies a condition of the joints without inflammation,

and perhaps this should be revived for a majority of cases, in which pain is minimal at worst. A former synonym, degenerative joint disease, has been largely discarded, as it implies a specificity that cannot be supported. The confusion arises from the fact that no adequate definition of the term exists, and osteoarthritis occurs in almost all individuals past middle life, as well as in many individuals who are younger, but symptomatic osteoarthritis afflicts only a minority of these. Part of the reason no adequate definition exists derives from the roentgenographic criteria; a narrowing of "joint space" implies loss of cartilage (there is no real space in a joint, only the distance between the bones, composed of cartilage, which is radiolucent unless it contains crystals or metabolic derivatives), but other attributes, such as marginal osteophytes, are part of the repair process, and geodes (cysts in the subchondral bone) may even be part of the pathogenesis. The pathologist's definition includes diminished cartilage, fibrillation of cartilage, cartilaginous debris, the osteophytes and geodes, eburnation (smoothing of exposed bone denuded of its cartilage), and, in many instances, angiogenesis and increased vascularity. The clinician is confronted chiefly by symptomatic osteoarthritis, although roentgenograms taken for any purpose that include diarthrodial joints may disclose joint changes that can delude one into attributing symptoms to these; this is particularly true of spinal changes at the discs and intervertebral neural foramina.

From the standpoint of therapy, only symptomatic osteoarthritis requires treatment, and even much of that remains under dispute. Prevention would obviously be best, if it could be achieved, but in such a slowly developing process as osteoarthritis, it would require a lifetime of effort and may still not be attainable. Osteoarthritis, then, is not a disease but a final common pathway for all insults, overuse, and abuse of a joint, begun by trauma, diseases of metabolism, heritable and genetic predisposition, hormonal influences, and inflammatory diseases of the joints. The initial insult may well have occurred in childhood, but the expression as osteoarthritis takes years to develop (faster when the insult is severe, as in athletic injury, slower if because of repetitive minor trauma, and slower yet if the inception was minimal). When it becomes symptomatic, however, osteoarthritis fits the definition of disease and challenges treatment paradigms.

Osteoarthritis must be viewed as a reparative process, as confirmed by its antiquity: it is found in skeletons of prehistoric animals and early hominids and afflicted all vertebrates that lived long enough. At that, it is not a manifestation of aging, only a slowly developing process that requires time and is, therefore, more common in elderly individuals. Weather changes influence symptoms but not the process itself. There is no particular geographic predilection. Although some patterns are more common in some populations (e.g., interphalangeal osteoarthritis, which, except as a consequence of trauma, is rarely found in Africans and East Asians), that applies chiefly to interphalangeal osteoarthritis in which rows of joints are involved, and not to single large joints. Obesity has been cited as a precursor, a reasonable contention for affliction of weight-bearing joints, but equally true for interphalangeal osteoarthritis, where it should theoretically play no role. Increased bone density seems to parallel osteoarthritis, but whether causal or consequential needs to be determined (similarly, osteoporosis and osteoarthritis tend to be mutually exclusive, but again cause and effect are problematic). Some investigators have looked for causes in the bone. Subchondral microfractures and bone marrow edema have been cited, but again the relationship to expression remains controversial. Box 1 lists some of the known precursors, and Box 2 lists some of the resumed risk factors. Ultimately, osteoarthritis is thought to be a disease of chondrocyte fatigue, accelerated when the weakened chondrocytes can no longer replace proteoglycans, leading to structural alterations. Chondrocalcinosis, with deposition of hydroxy apatite or calcium pyrophosphate dihydrate, commonly accompanies symptomatic osteoarthritis, but may play more of a role in causing symptoms than contributing to pathogenesis. Although some would classify osteoarthritis as primary or secondary, it probably is always secondary, even if the inception is remote in the past and long forgotten. Remember that osteoarthritis is not an acute disease, even if punctuated by acute painful episodes in approximately 15% to 20% of those in whom roentgenographic evidence of osteoarthritis exists.

BOX 1   Precursors of Osteoarthritis

- Congenital
  Slipped femoral epiphysis
  Legg-Calvé-Perthes disease
- Bone dysplasias
  ? Kashin-Beck disease
  ? Mseleni joint disease
  ? Familial
  Mediterranean fever
- Metabolic
  Ochronosis
  Hemochromatosis
  Calcium pyrophosphate deposition disease
  Gout
- Traumatic
  Acute (e.g., athletic injury)
  Chronic (repetitive trauma)
- Endocrine
  Diabetes mellitus
  Acromegaly
  ? Obesity (cofactor?)
- Idiopathic
  Rheumatoid arthritis
  Septic arthritis disease
  Joint disease
- Vascular
  Avascular necrosis
- Neurologic
  Charcot joint
  Charcot-Marie-Tooth disease
- Bone disease
  Paget's disease (osteitis deformans)

BOX 2   Risk Factors

Aging	Time duration; weak muscle control (lower extremities)
Sex	Women: interphalangeal osteoarthritis, predilection knees in valgus
Obesity	May be cofactor (interphalangeal, knees in women)
Genetics	Symmetric Heberden's nodes, Ehlers-Danlos syndrome, genetic collagen abnormalities
Endocrine	Elevated growth hormone concentrations (postmenopause?)
Diet?	
Bone density	Increased bone density; osteoporosis
Race	Site predilections that may be racially related
Occupation	Jackhammers and similar tools, habitual usage (e.g., specific finger joints in knitting shop workers, elbows in foundry workers, knees in professional football running backs, shoulders in baseball pitchers)
Avocation	Knees and hips in joggers and runners on hard surfaces (not those who continue but those who drop out)
Inflammation	Calcium pyrophosphate dihydrate, hydroxy apatite, other crystal depositions
Trauma	Acute and severe, repetitive but mild to moderate

Regional Issues

Patterns differ and give clues to pathogenesis. The knees are more frequently afflicted in women, perhaps because the broader pelvis leads to genu valgum and predisposes to knee afflictions. However, although cartilage loss on the gliding surface of the patella generally results in symptoms, even major cartilage loss in the opposing surfaces of the femur and tibia may not, and the anatomic features fail to correlate with symptomatic expression. Although proprioceptive changes were thought to play a role in the pathogenesis of knee osteoarthritis, recent studies refute this contention.

The hips tend to be more often afflicted in men. The classic FABERE maneuver (flexion, abduction, external rotation, and extension) reveals limitations of motion and elicits pain. However, in time, knee and hip osteoarthritis are nearly gender equal.

Osteoarthritis of the distal interphalangeal (DIP) joints (Heberden's nodes) and proximal interphalangeal joints (PIP), usually symmetric, occurs in white women at about the time of menopause (earlier after total hysterectomies) and implies genetic predisposition; nonsymmetric involvement of these joints is often a consequence of specific traumas or work exposure. The symmetric variety often bares erosive changes at the joint margins, and is accompanied by the traditional signs of inflammation at presentation: redness, heat, swelling, pain, and functional deficits. The joints at the bases of the thumbs (first carpometacarpal, or trapeziometacarpal joints) tend also to be involved, and even the metacarpophalangeal joints, which rarely develop osteoarthritis in other circumstances. In these women, accompanying osteoarthritis at other joints is unrelated to the hereditary familial variety, bearing a casual, not causal, relationship.

The encroachment of osteophytes on the intervertebral foramina in the movable sections of the spine (cervical and lumbar) leads to referred pain in the areas served by the appropriate nerves. The shoulders are rarely a site of osteoarthritis, but sometimes severe destructive changes (the Milwaukee shoulder) do occur. Elbows are generally spared, but "cystic" protrusions through the joint capsules of distended fluid-filled joints lead to antecubital "cysts," the corollaries of the popliteal cysts at the knees; the latter can rupture, simulating thrombophlebitis in the calves. Wrists and ankles are almost always spared, because the mosaic distribution of the small bones diffuses forces. The first metatarsophalangeal joint is subject to osteoarthritis (the bunion) but rarely other joints of the toes (thought to be spared because shoes act as splints).

Although several studies claim that jogging and running do not predispose to osteoarthritis, these studies dealt with individuals who habitually exercised and not with those who gave up exercising, so they may well not conclusively prove the advantages of exercise for the majority of patients.

I have left out the molecular biology, the catalytic enzymes and debris, and even the synovial fluid changes, as these are of greater interest to the investigator than to the clinician responsible for counseling and treating patients. They are giving us some clues to better treatments in the future, however, and a later version of this article might well give them more prominence. Of greatest importance is not necessarily to ascribe symptoms to osteoarthritis detected on imaging; false attributions can delay correct diagnoses and appropriate treatment.

Management

PREVENTION

As osteoarthritis is the culmination of all life events at the joints, it cannot really be prevented. Attempts to use bovine cartilage extracts and other substances failed to retard progression and have been largely abandoned. However, as osteoarthritis is consequent to trauma or inflammation, aggressive treatment of this initial insult might delay its onset years later, but this remains unproven. Attention must be paid to the risk factors (see Box 2), minimizing them as much as possible; weight reduction obviously decreases the load on knee and hip joints in overweight individuals. Keeping joints supple through exercising and not exposing them to shear factors (particularly in sports), jogging on soft surfaces rather than on unyielding pavement, wearing supportive footwear (spike heels may not lead to osteoarthritis per se but can lead to accidents that do,

and flat heels put excessive strain on the calf muscles and later the knees), and in general maintaining physical fitness are all helpful. Despite recently published studies that isometric exercises, especially of the quadriceps, probably cannot prevent osteoarthritis of the knees, these apply chiefly to radiographic changes and not to symptoms; it is still wise to recommend exercises that strengthen the muscles that move a joint, because function will be retained even if the anatomic changes continue. Osteoarthritis found on radiographs taken for another purpose, if asymptomatic, requires no treatment; the old dictum, "treat the patient, not the radiograph," applies. Architectural barriers should be avoided; ramps are particularly troublesome for knee and hip osteoarthritis, especially descending (that applies to stairs as well, as descent requires knee extension, which increases joint discomfort).

Symptomatic osteoarthritis occasions discomfort at times of weather changes, but the symptoms are often mild and tolerated. Many people treat themselves for these, before seeing a physician. It is important to know what they may be taking, as they often do not consider these as medicines, and potential drug interactions can occur.

COMPLEMENTARY AND ALTERNATIVE TREATMENTS

Analgesics, such as acetaminophen (Tylenol and other unbranded generics) and aspirin, and several nonsteroidal anti-inflammatory drugs are readily available on supermarket shelves and pharmacies. In these days of global travel and ethnic migrations, other approaches also are common. Ayurvedic medicine is another system, popular in Southeast Asia and spreading from there; its medicines are based on plant extracts. Ayurvedic schools are found in India and the medicines themselves are carefully prepared and tested. The most popular treatment for osteoarthritis is composed of winter cherry, Indian frankincense, turmeric, and ginger (Artrex).

Herbal medicines available chiefly in health food stores have become popular throughout the United States. These are exempted by law from testing and approval by the FDA, and their safety and efficacy remain problematic. Potential interactions with prescribed drugs have not been studied. Ginger is especially popular, but among the other preparations are boron,[1] borage oil,[1] evening primrose oil,[1] and avocado soybean saponifiables,[1] all of which are claimed to be anti-inflammatory.

Yoga is currently being studied as a potential treatment for knee osteoarthritis, and acupuncture is said to provide considerable pain relief. Chiropractic adjustment is popular, especially for back pain attributed to osteoarthritis. However, the placebo effect is very striking in most osteoarthritis; even follow-up telephone calls from the doctor's office inquiring about the health of the patient lead to improvement. Do not slight the placebo effect, though—it is, after all, an effect.

---

[1]Not FDA approved for this indication.

GENERAL PRINCIPLES

A recent symposium on osteoarthritis concluded that osteoarthritis is all about biomechanics, and normalization thereof yields better results than drug therapy (that means splints, braces, canes, shoe corrections, abolition of unsound architectural and style features). Joint damage is not the main determinant of pain, but psychosocial factors, compensation systems, and inaccurate labeling play a major role. Also, people who have osteoarthritis, because of the long duration of its inception, tend to be elderly and therefore more likely to tolerate drug therapy and surgery poorly, and because many have concurrent problems under treatment, are prone to untoward drug interactions.

As stated, only approximately 15% to 20% of individuals have sufficient pain to seek medical attention. This pain waxes and wanes, and considerable controversy addresses the best approaches to treatment. A much cited study compared acetaminophen 4 g per day with ibuprofen 1200 and 2400 μg a day during a span of 4 weeks, and concluded that there was no difference in results. However, the span is short, and proves only that analgesics are analgesic. Most patients prefer a nonsteroidal anti-inflammatory drug (NSAID), especially in anti-inflammatory dosage, as confirmed in epidemiologic and observational studies. Physical and occupational therapy can help joint-sparing mobility, ergonomic principles help at the work site, and sexual counseling, for those afflicted with hip involvement in particular, should be part of the treatment program.

For inflammatory erosive osteoarthritis of the fingers, the overnight wearing of nylon and spandex stretch gloves can inhibit nodose deformities if started early enough, before these excrescences become bony and function is compromised.

DRUG THERAPY

The severe pain of osteoarthritic joints—knees, hips, and fingers, chiefly—may be the result of secondary inflammation, caused by cartilaginous debris inciting cytokine response. A whole array of nonsteroidal anti-inflammatory drugs is available by prescription (from indomethacin [Indocin] and ibuprofen [Motrin, Advil, generics] through naproxen [Naprosyn] and diclofenac [Voltaren], with doses usually lower than those for rheumatoid arthritis), and others, not available in the United States, may be taken by patients who purchased them abroad (e.g., tiaprofenic acid[2]). These inhibit cyclooxygenase, an enzyme necessary for prostaglandin synthesis that has been found to have at least two components, COX-1, which helps protect against gastric erosion and other consequences, and COX-2, which is evoked by inflammatory mediators and may lead to adverse gastric mucosal effects (a COX-3 has been proposed as well). To avoid the latter complication, misoprostol (Cytotec) may be prescribed or incorporated into a combination formulation with diclofenac (Arthrotec), but that is not without its own complications, namely, diarrhea and cramps. To avoid the adverse effects, a series of selective (at least in

recommended dosage) COX-2 inhibitors were developed (e.g., celecoxib [Celebrex, 200 μg per day]). Lumiracoxib (Prexige),[2] 100 to 200 μg per day, was recently approved for short-term relief in osteoarthritis outside the United States. As of this writing, recommended doses may vary, so the package insert should always be consulted to determine the current appropriate dose. Gastric mucosal protection appears to be better, but there are renal consequences associated with its use and other problems are imputed. It must be stated that compounds considered safer are usually given to the patients most at risk, so the profiles do not address comparable populations. Moreover, the coxib NSAIDs are currently more expensive and not approved by all medical payment plans. Other NSAIDs, such as sulindac (Clinoril) and nabumetone (Relafen), are prodrugs, converted after absorption and hepatic biotransformation. Etodolac (Lodine) seems to work by a different mechanism; nimesulide is popular in Europe under a variety of trade names, but not available in the United States, is more COX-2 selective but less expensive, and may be brought back by travelers. Licofelone (as below) is awaiting approval in Europe. The choice of NSAIDs is relatively arbitrary; patients may respond well to one and not to another. In most instances, the most severe symptoms can be brought to a level patients will tolerate within a few days to weeks, and long-term therapy may not be necessary.

Aspirin, once the mainstay of treatment, has largely been superseded. Gastrointestinal intolerance, irreversible inhibition of platelet aggregation, and animal studies that show it to be deleterious to cartilage may be the reasons, but nonacetylated salicylates, such as salsalate (Disalcid) and choline magnesium trisalicylate (Trilisate), and simple analgesics, such as propoxyphene (Darvon)[1] and tramadol (Ultram), alone or in combination, are given alone or with NSAIDs. Narcotics are best avoided because of the potential for addiction.

Gastric mucosal erosions are found by endoscopy but usually do not translate into clinical problems. Similarly, elevation of hepatic enzymes is noncongruent with hepatotoxicity. Adverse effects on gastric mucosa are the most common; however, liver, kidney, and bone marrow complications, although uncommon, need also to be guarded against.

In most parts of the world, NSAIDs are available in creams and ointments for topical administration. The FDA is not convinced that this is more than a placebo effect so these formulations are not currently available in the United States. However, topical capsaicin, the spice in pepper plants, has been approved for use in osteoarthritis and is available under a number of trade names over the counter (a prescription no longer is necessary). During the initial period of administration, localized burning is usual. Capsaicin is also available on a patch, which is especially popular in Asia.

---

[1]Not FDA approved for this indication.
[2]Not available in the United States.

INTRA-ARTICULAR THERAPY

For nearly 50 years, cortisol derivatives have been injected into joints, usually after removal of the excess synovial fluid through arthrocentesis. When even symptomatic osteoarthritis was deemed not to be inflammatory, many clinicians cautioned that the resultant lack of pain indicated an insensitivity that could lead to further joint destruction, similar to the neuropathic Charcot joint. This fear has not been borne out and now arthrocentesis and corticosteroid instillation, preferably of a depot compound, in appropriately calibrated dosage, depending on the size of the joint, can effect long-lasting relief. However, patients should be admonished not to overuse the joint, at least for the first 3 days, as the lesions have not healed, even if the symptoms have abated. A general rule for counseling: do no more than when it hurt.

On the assumption that lubrication of the joint is impaired and corticosteroids are strictly palliative, preparations of hyaluronate have been approved for intra-articular instillation. While this procedure is called viscosupplementation, there is as yet little evidence that the instilled material is long retained in the joint or that it improves lubrication. Nevertheless, the results usually are as good as those with corticosteroids, and the duration of effect often long-lasting. The two preparations currently available are sodium hyaluronate (Hyalgan) and hylan G-F 20 (Synvisc), administered as a short series of three to five weekly injections; why they should work is problematic, and some controlled trials concluded that they were no more effective than placebo. This has been claimed for many preparations, however, because the placebo effect on pain is quite potent. Functional impairment remains, in most instances, especially at the hip, but often also at the knee. Hyaluronic acid is not indicated for interphalangeal injection, although small doses of corticosteroid into these tiny joints can sometimes lead to dramatic relief.

GLUCOSAMINE AND CHONDROITIN SULFATE

Oral glucosamine[1] is said to be as analgesic as NSAIDs and acetaminophen. Multicenter controlled trials seem to agree, but there is still much skepticism about this treatment. There is no rationale to explain why it should be analgesic, but all studies show glucosamine to be superior to placebo or reference compounds, even if not statistically in all cases. It appears to be harmless, with no untoward interactions, and the hypothesis that it might aggravate diabetes mellitus has not been borne out. Most preparations are available over the counter. The likelihood exists that any patient with symptomatic osteoarthritis is taking glucosamine, and so are many rheumatologists, empirically trusting that it has a salutary effect. Chondroitin sulfate[1] has not been shown to add anything, except in some poorly designed studies. However, the combination of glucosamine and chondroitin sulfate is marketed more frequently than either compound alone, and whole shelves in markets and pharmacies are devoted to these.

DISEASE MODIFICATION

By the time osteoarthritis becomes symptomatic and fulfills roentgenographic criteria, it is already well established. Thus, it is too late to think of "disease modification," as is now possible in rheumatoid arthritis. Nevertheless, the search for disease-modifying osteoarthritis drugs (DMOADs) goes on. All the compounds cited as possible DMOADs have been tested in animals only; no satisfactory assessment exists for studies in humans. Tetracycline derivatives, such as doxycycline,[1] seem to have merit. Drugs that work on the inner mechanisms of cells, such as chloroquine (Aralen),[1] are also under study on theoretical grounds, but have not yet proved themselves. Antioxidant vitamins, tamoxifen (Nolvadex),[1] nitric oxide inhibitors, metalloproteases, and the aforementioned nutraceuticals have all been mentioned, but no reliable protocol exists that can measure their effect on cartilage and the joint. Specialized radiography that requires positioning is too crude for the purpose; magnetic resonance imaging and ultrasound have yet to be validated and standardized for this condition.

Studies are currently underway in Europe of diacerein (Diadar)[2] and growth factors, including insulin-like growth factor β, somatomedins, fibroblast growth factor, chondrocyte growth factor, and cartilage-derived and transforming growth factors. The problem of what to study and what outcome measures to use, and the duration of the trial, also bedevil these studies. While it is true that these are experimental treatments, not currently in use, and may never come to pass, they are mentioned here to counter the argument that the neurologist diagnoses untreatable disease and the rheumatologist treats untreatable disease. If not these, other treatments deriving from our better understanding of arthritis and its pathogenesis surely are in the offing. Included among these are mesenchymal stem cells that can produce site-specific tissue, thus restoring lost cartilage and bone, but how can that be done while mechanical impediments remain? The same is true for gene manipulation, and if new cartilage and bone are created, even with no counterpressures, how will the new attach to the older remnants and what will determine that? Cartilage transplants and chondrocyte transfer and stimulation are also being investigated. A polymer of glucosamine is also available (POLY-Nag).

SURGERY

Surgery is the consequence of failure of medicine. Our inability to effect healing and repair leads to treatments

---

[1]Not FDA approved for this indication.

[1]Not FDA approved for this indication.
[2]Not available in the United States.

that would be forestalled if we could anticipate who, and under what circumstances, develops symptomatic disease and offer appropriate medical treatments. Barring that, the surgical treatment of osteoarthritis has made remarkable progress during the past 40 years. By and large, the osteotomies that were formerly performed have faded into well-deserved oblivion. Arthroscopy was hailed as a less invasive way to deal with motion-impeding osteophytes and derangements and meniscal tears, especially if combined with lavage, but the results do not materially differ from those achieved with placebos. Indeed, removal of the meniscus seems to hasten the development of the ultimate osteoarthritic lesion. The major advance was the total joint replacement, first for hips, then knees and even fingers and other small joints of the hands. These have given back life content and quality of life to myriad recipients, more than 100,000 people annually in the United States alone! While surgery is clearly not a last resort, it has successfully addressed the functional deficits and pains and permitted recipients to resume their life styles. Shut-ins are liberated. Despite the trepidation of orthopedists, travel, skiing, tennis, and golf become achievable, even with bilateral surgery. Newer materials and methods of bonding have improved the longevity of these interventions.

Osteoarthritis remains an enigma, despite the major scientific advances of the past few years. Paradoxically, we have become more effective in treating advanced osteoarthritis and symptomatic disease (because of our better understanding of inflammation and the recognition that it plays a major role in evoking symptoms) than in addressing the variety of presentations. Symptomatic relief is achievable, and restoration of function; roentgenographic and pathologic changes may fulfill the definition but do not necessarily demand treatment. The removal of infectious and other killer diseases that curtailed life expectancy in the past has paradoxically resulted in the emergence of more chronic disorders. As stated in the World Health Organization's catalogue of disabilities, the killer diseases remove the consumer shortly after the consumer ceases to be a producer; the crippling diseases leave the consumer long after the consumer ceases to be a producer. The expense and increased suffering require a humane and scientifically sound understanding.

Giant Cell Arteritis and Polymyalgia Rheumatica

Method of
John H. Stone, MD, MPH

Giant cell arteritis (GCA), the most common form of primary systemic vasculitis in adults, preferentially affects the extracranial branches of the carotid artery and also often involves the aorta and its primary branches. Polymyalgia rheumatica (PMR), an aching and stiffness of the shoulders, neck, and hip-girdle area, occurs in up to 50% of GCA cases but usually occurs alone. Age is the greatest risk factor for either GCA or PMR; essentially all patients with these conditions are older than 50 years of age. The mean age at disease onset is 72 years. PMR occurs two to four times more often than GCA. Both GCA and PMR have a predilection for individuals of northern European ancestry and occur three to four times more frequently in women than in men.

Diagnosis

The classic presenting manifestations of GCA are PMR symptoms, headache, jaw claudication, and visual disturbances (Table 1). The onset may be gradual or sudden. PMR symptoms are characterized by pain and stiffness in the neck, shoulders, and hip-girdle area that is usually much worse in the morning. Patients with PMR may report great difficulty getting out of bed, raising their arms over their heads, or rising from the commode. The most striking feature of the headache is that it is new or different from other headache patterns. Many patients describe tenderness of the scalp when brushing their hair. Some localize the tenderness to the temporal arteries, but these are enlarged or nodular in only a minority of patients. Jaw claudication—pain in the master muscles that occurs with chewing—has the highest specificity of any GCA symptom.

Approximately one third of patients present with visual symptoms, chiefly amaurosis fugax or diplopia. Blindness, which can develop abruptly, is usually preceded by episodes of blurred vision or amaurosis fugax. Visual loss results most often from infarction of the posterior ciliary artery, which supplies blood to the optic nerve head. Both eyes may be affected, sometimes in close temporal succession. Almost all patients with classic GCA features also have nonspecific manifestations such as malaise, fatigue, and anorexia. Weight loss of 2 to 10 kg is common.

Clinically overt involvement of large arteries—the aorta and its major branches—develops in at least 15% of the patients. The most commonly affected vessels include the aorta (often involving the proximal aorta, leading to valvular incompetence) and the vertebral, carotid, subclavian, and axillary arteries. Aortic involvement may lead to thoracic aortic aneurysm, the risk of which is increased 17-fold in GCA patients. Aortic aneurysm is

TABLE 1 Likelihood Ratios for Symptoms and Signs Among Patients with Suspected GCA

Symptom/sign	Likelihood ratio*
Symptoms	
Anorexia	1.2
Weight loss	1.3
Arthralgia	1.1
Diplopia	3.4
Fatigue	1.2
Fever	1.2
Temporal headache	1.5
Any headache	1.2
Jaw claudication	4.2
Myalgia	0.9
Polymyalgia rheumatica	1.0
Unilateral visual loss	0.9
Any visual symptoms	1.1
Vertigo	0.7
Signs	
Optic atrophy or ischemic optic neuropathy	1.6
Scalp tenderness	1.6
Synovitis	0.4
Beaded temporal artery	4.6
Prominent/enlarged temporal artery	4.3
Tender temporal artery	2.6
Absent temporal artery pulse	2.7

*Likelihood ratio is the probability of a positive temporal artery biopsy in a patient with a certain symptom or sign, compared to the probability of a positive biopsy in a patient without that same finding.
From Seo P, Stone JH: Large-vessel vasculitis. Arthritis Rheum 2004;51(1): 128-139.

usually a late complication of GCA, developing on average 7 years after diagnosis of the vasculitis. Abdominal aortic aneurysms, while less common, also occur in GCA.

The most common physical finding is an abnormal temporal artery, found in up to two thirds of patients. The temporal artery may be enlarged, tender, nodular, or found to have decreased pulsation. Normal temporal arteries do not exclude the diagnosis, however. Approximately 10% to 15% of patients will have axillary or subclavian disease revealed by diminished pulses, unequal arm blood pressures, or by bruits heard above or below the clavicle or along the upper arm.

The laboratory hallmarks of GCA and PMR are marked elevations of the acute phase reactants, the erythrocyte sedimentation rate (ESR), and C-reactive protein. Nearly 90% of patients with GCA present with an ESR greater than 50 mm/hour. Normochromic, normocytic anemia and thrombocytosis are also common. Approximately 20% of patients with GCA demonstrate a mildly elevated alkaline phosphatase (of liver origin). Radiologic studies such as magnetic resonance imaging (MRI) and ultrasound (US) may reveal abnormalities compatible with PMR or GCA, but the clinical uses of these tests are unclear. Neither replaces temporal artery biopsy as the gold standard for the diagnosis of GCA. Guidelines for making the

diagnosis of PMR and classifying patients with GCA have been developed. The diagnosis of PMR rests almost entirely on clinical grounds, namely symptoms of proximal limb stiffness associated with an elevated ESR and a dramatic response to prednisone.[1] Classification criteria for GCA are designed for use in the research setting, not for use as diagnostic criteria per se.

Treatment

Any patient strongly suspected of having GCA should be started on 40 to 60 mg of prednisone[1] per day and referred for temporal artery biopsy. Temporal artery

[1]Not FDA approved for this indication.

CURRENT DIAGNOSIS

Simple Diagnostic Criteria for Polymyalgia Rheumatica

- Age at onset is older than 50 years of age
- Symmetric ache/pain for at least 1 month in two of three muscle groups below, associated with morning stiffness lasting longer than 30 minutes:
  Neck or torso
  Shoulders or proximal arms
  Hips or proximal thighs
  ESR more than 40 mm per hour (Westergren method)
  Prompt, dramatic response to glucocorticoids (equivalent to prednisone[1] 20 mg once per day or less)

Criteria for the Diagnosis of Giant Cell Arteritis

- Age older than 50 years at disease onset
- New headache
- Temporal artery abnormality
- Temporal artery tenderness to palpation or decreased pulsation unrelated to arteriosclerosis of cervical arteries
- Elevated erythrocyte sedimentation rate more than 50 mm per hour
- Abnormal temporal artery biopsy
- Biopsy specimen with vasculitis characterized by a predominance of mononuclear cell infiltration or granulomatous inflammation, usually with multinucleated giant cells
- For classification purposes, a patient with vasculitis shall be said to have GCA if at least three of these seven criteria are present. The presence of any three or more criteria yields a sensitivity of 93.5% and a specificity of 91.2%.

[1]Not FDA approved for this indication.
Abbreviations: GCA = giant cell arteritis; ESR = erythrocyte sedimentation rate.
From Hunder GG, Bloch DA, Michel BA, et al: The American College of Rheumatology 1990 criteria for the classification of giant cell arteritis. Arthritis Rheum 1990;33:1122-1128.

15

CURRENT THERAPY

- No treatment other than glucocorticoids has been shown convincingly to be effective in either GCA or PMR.
- A majority of patients flare within 1 year as glucocorticoid doses are tapered.
- An appropriate strategy is to taper patients to low doses (<10 mg of prednisone/day) within several months and then to maintain 5 mg of prednisone/day for approximately 1 year. Ultimately prednisone should be tapered at the rate of only 1 mg/month.
- The usual starting dose of prednisone in GCA is 60 mg per day. The usual starting dose in PMR is 15 mg per day.

Abbreviations: GCA = giant cell arteritis; PMR = polymyalgia rheumatica.

biopsy, the only test that can secure the diagnosis of GCA, is recommended in all cases. Although it is traditional to obtain the temporal artery biopsy quickly, evidence suggests that the pathology remains intact for at least 2 weeks after the start of corticosteroid treatment. Unilateral and bilateral temporal artery biopsies are approximately 90% and 95% sensitive, respectively, at least when performed by experts in the procedure. In any setting, some patients whose histories are compelling for the diagnosis of GCA will have negative biopsies.

Patients suspected of having GCA who have experienced transient visual loss should receive high-dose intravenous methylprednisolone[1] (e.g., 1000 mg/day) for 3 days. Low-dose aspirin[1] (81 or 325 mg/day) is also prudent in patients with GCA. Patients with PMR alone are treated usually with prednisone,[1] 10 to 20 mg per day. Patients with PMR or GCA usually respond dramatically to corticosteroid treatment within 2 days or earlier. Approximately 10% of patients, however, require a week of therapy before feeling better.

Prednisone[1] tapers usually begin after 1 month. The overall goal of the prednisone taper is to discontinue the medication within 9 to 12 months. Because of the substantial toxicities of corticosteroids, one reasonable approach is to taper prednisone[1] more quickly at higher doses than at lower doses, aiming to reach 20 mg per day by 2 or 3 months after the start of treatment. Once patients with GCA reach 15 mg of prednisone[1] or PMR patients reach 10 mg, decrements of 1 mg about every 2 weeks may reduce the chance of flare. Mild to moderate ESR elevations, common during corticosteroid tapers, should not necessarily trigger increases in the prednisone[1] dose. Rather, increases in prednisone[1] should be dictated by the recurrence of clinical symptoms.

Unfortunately, 50% to 80% of patients with PMR or GCA relapse during or after the prednisone[1] taper. (Relapses at prednisone[1] doses higher than 15 mg/day are rare.) Patients who experience recurrent symptoms

---

[1]Not FDA approved for this indication.

usually respond to increasing the prednisone[1] dose 5 to 10 mg above the last dose at which the patient was asymptomatic. A substantial minority of patients require some prednisone[1]—usually in the range of 5 to 10 mg per day—for longer than 2 years. No corticosteroid-sparing agent has been proven consistently effective. Reports of the efficacy of methotrexate[1] in both PMR and GCA have been conflicting. Controlled studies of tumor necrosis factor-α inhibitors[1] are not yet available.

To prevent osteoporosis, patients starting on prednisone[1] should take 1500 to 1800 mg of calcium daily with 400 to 800 units of vitamin D. If bone density measurements indicate osteopenia or osteoporosis, bisphosphonates are usually the first-line agents for treatment.

REFERENCES

Caporali R, Cimmino MA, Ferraccioli G, et al: Methotrexate plus prednisone combined therapy in polymyalgia rheumatica. Ann Intern Med 2004;141(7):493-500.

Hoffman GS, Cid MC, Hellmann DB, et al: A multicenter, randomized, double-blind, placebo-controlled trial of adjuvant methotrexate treatment for giant cell arteritis. Arthritis Rheum 2002;46(5):1309-1318.

Hoffman GS, Stone JH. Disparate results in studies of methotrexate plus corticosteroids in the treatment of giant cell arteritis. Arthritis Rheum 2003;48(4):1160-1161.

Jover JA, Hernandez-Garcia C, Morado IC, et al: Combined treatment of giant cell arteritis with methotrexate and prednisone. A randomized, double-blind, placebo-controlled trial. Ann Intern Med 2001;134:106-14.

Salvarani C, Cantini F, Boiardi L, et al: Medical progress: Polymyalgia rheumatica and giant-cell arteritis. N Engl J Med 2002;347:261-271.

Seo P, Stone JH: Large-vessel vasculitis. Arthritis Rheum 2004;51(1):128-139.

Smetana GW, Shmerling RH: Does this patient have temporal arteritis? JAMA 2002;287:92-101.

Stone JH: Methotrexate in polymyalgia rheumatica: Kernel of truth or curse of Tantalus? Ann Intern Med 2004;141(7):568-569.

---

[1]Not FDA approved for this indication.

Osteomyelitis

Method of
Luca Lazzarini, MD

Osteomyelitis is a complex disease often associated with high morbidity and considerable health care costs. This condition can be classified by duration (acute or chronic), pathogenesis (hematogenous or contiguous spread), site, extent, and by the type of patient (infant, child, adult, or compromised host). The Waldvogel classification system subdivides osteomyelitis as being either hematogenous or secondary to a contiguous focus of infection. Contiguous focus osteomyelitis has been further subdivided into osteomyelitis with or without vascular insufficiency. An alternative to the Waldvogel classification system has been developed by Cierny and Mader. The Cierny-Mader staging system is based on the anatomy of the bone infection and the physiology of the host (Box 1). The anatomic types of osteomyelitis are medullary (stage 1), superficial (stage 2), localized (stage 3), and diffuse (stage 4). Stage 1 infection is confined to the medullary surface of the bone. Hematogenous osteomyelitis and infected intramedullary rods are examples of this anatomic type. Stage 2 is a contiguous focus infection occurring when an exposed infected necrotic surface of bone lies at the base of a soft tissue wound. Stage 3 is usually characterized by a full-thickness, cortical sequestration that can be removed surgically without compromising bony stability. Stage 4 is a through-and-through process that usually requires an intercalary resection of the bone to arrest the disease process. Further, the patient is classified as an A, B, or C host. An A host represents a patient with normal physiologic, metabolic, and immunologic capabilities. The B host is either systemically compromised, locally compromised, or both. When the morbidity of treatment is worse than that imposed by the disease itself, the patient is given the C host classification. This classification system aids in the understanding, diagnosis, and treatment of bone infections in children and adults (Table 1).

TABLE 1 Principal Antibiotics Used in the Initial Intravenous Treatment of Osteomyelitis

Staphylococci, methicillin sensitive	Nafcillin (Unipen) 2 g q4-6h (+ rifampin[Rifadin][1] 600 mg qd PO)
Staphylococci, methicillin resistant	Vancomycin (Vancocin) 1 g q12h (+ rifampin [Rifadin][1] 600 mg qd PO)
Streptococci	Penicillin[1] 2 MU q4h
Anaerobes, gram-positive	Clindamycin[1] (Cleocin) 900 mg q8h
Anaerobes, gram-negative	Metronidazole[1] (Flagyl) 500 mg q8h
Enterobacteriaceae, Pseudomonas	Ciprofloxacin (Cipro) 400 mg q12h

[1]Not FDA approved for this indication.
Abbreviations: PO = orally; q = every; qd = every day.

Etiology

In hematogenous osteomyelitis, a single pathogenic organism is almost always recovered from the bone. In infants *Staphylococcus aureus*, *Streptococcus agalactiae*, and *Escherichia coli* are most frequently isolated from blood or bones. However, in children more than 1 year of age, *S. aureus*, *Streptococcus pyogenes*, and *Haemophilus influenzae* are most commonly isolated. The incidence of *H. influenzae* infection decreases after age 4 years. However, the overall incidence of *H. influenzae* as a cause of osteomyelitis is decreasing because of the new *H. influenzae* vaccine now given to children. In adults, *S. aureus* is the most common organism isolated. Multiple organisms are usually isolated from the infected bone in contiguous focus osteomyelitis. *S. aureus* remains the most commonly isolated pathogen. However, gram-negative bacilli and anaerobic organisms are also frequently isolated. Other microorganisms, such as mycobacteria and fungi, can be involved as well.

BOX 1 The Cierny-Mader Staging System for Osteomyelitis

Anatomic Type
- Stage 1: medullary osteomyelitis
- Stage 2: superficial osteomyelitis
- Stage 3: localized osteomyelitis
- Stage 4: diffuse osteomyelitis

Physiologic Class
- A: normal host
- B: compromised host
- Bs: systemically compromised
- Bl: locally compromised
- C: treatment worse than the disease

Factors Affecting Host Status
- Systemic
  Malnutrition
  Renal and hepatic failure
  Diabetes mellitus
  Chronic hypoxia
  Immune disease
  Malignancy
  Extremes of age
  Immunosuppression
- Local
  Chronic lymphedema
  Venous stasis
  Major vessel compromise
  Arteritis
  Extensive scarring
  Radiation fibrosis
  Small-vessel disease
  Neuropathy
  Tobacco use

Clinical Manifestations

SIGNS AND SYMPTOMS

Hematogenous osteomyelitis in children may present with acute signs of infection including abrupt fever, irritability, lethargy, and local signs of inflammation. However, 50% of children present with vague complaints, including pain of the involved limb of 1 to 3 months in duration and minimal, if any, temperature elevation.

Adults with hematogenous osteomyelitis usually present with vague complaints consisting of nonspecific pain and few constitutional symptoms lasting 1 to 3 months. However, acute clinical presentations with fever, chills, swelling, and erythema over the involved bone(s) are occasionally seen. The source of bacteremia may be from a trivial skin infection or from a more serious infection such as acute or subacute bacterial endocarditis. Hematogenous osteomyelitis that involves either long bones or vertebrae is an important complication of injection drug abuse.

Patients with contiguous focus osteomyelitis often present with localized bone and joint pain, erythema, swelling, and drainage around the area of trauma, surgery, or wound infection. Signs of bacteremia such as fever, chills, and night sweats may be present in the acute phase of osteomyelitis, but not in the chronic phase.

The sedimentation rate is usually elevated, reflecting chronic inflammation, but the leukocyte count is usually normal. The chronic disease is usually either not progressive or slowly progressive. If a sinus tract becomes obstructed, the patient may present with a localized abscess and or an acute soft tissue infection. A sedimentation rate that returns to normal during the course of therapy is a favorable prognostic sign.

MICROBIOLOGY

The diagnosis and determination of the etiology of long bone osteomyelitis rests on the isolation of the pathogen(s) from the bone lesion or blood or joint culture. Except in hematogenous osteomyelitis, where positive blood or joint fluid cultures may suffice, antibiotic treatment of osteomyelitis should be based on meticulous cultures of bone taken at débridement surgery or from deep bone biopsies. If possible, cultures should be obtained before antibiotics are initiated. Sinus tract cultures are unreliable for predicting which organisms will be isolated from infected bone; however, those growing *S. aureus* show a positive correlation with bone cultures.

RADIOLOGY

In hematogenous osteomyelitis, radiographic changes usually correlate with the destructive process and are usually seen when at least 50% to 75% of the bone matrix is destroyed. This happens at least 2 weeks after the infection was initiated. The earliest radiologic changes are swelling of the soft tissue, periosteal thickening and/or elevation, and focal osteopenia. Radiographic improvement may lag behind clinical recovery, even when the patient is receiving appropriate antimicrobial therapy. In contiguous focus osteomyelitis, the radiographic changes are subtle, often found in association with other nonspecific radiographic findings, and require a careful clinical correlation to achieve diagnostic significance. Computed tomography (CT) may play a role in the diagnosis of osteomyelitis. Increased marrow density occurs early in the infection, and intramedullary gas has been reported in patients with hematogenous osteomyelitis. The CT scan can also help identify areas of necrotic bone and assess the involvement of the surrounding soft tissues. One disadvantage of this study is the scatter phenomenon, which occurs when metal is present in or near the area of bone infection. Magnetic resonance imaging (MRI) has been recognized as a useful modality for diagnosing the presence and scope of musculoskeletal infection. The resolution of MRI makes it useful in differentiating between bone and soft tissue infection, often a problem with radionuclide studies. Radionuclide scans may be obtained when the diagnosis of osteomyelitis is ambiguous or to help gauge the extent of bone and soft tissue inflammation.

Treatment

Therapy of osteomyelitis is both surgical and medical and includes adequate drainage and débridement, obliteration of dead space, soft tissue coverage, and specific antimicrobial treatment. If the patient is a compromised host, an effort is made to correct or improve the host defect.

ANTIBIOTIC TREATMENT

According to the results of animal studies, the optimal duration of antibiotic treatment is 4 to 6 weeks. The time needed for bone revascularization after débridement surgery is approximately 3 weeks. Shorter durations are probably successful when the infection is superficial (stage 2) and a complete débridement is performed and when ablative surgery (amputation above the infected region) is performed.

Antibiotic treatment for osteomyelitis is traditionally administered by the intravenous (IV) route. To reduce hospitalization and health care costs, outpatient IV therapy is currently used. This modality of administration reduces treatment cost and improves patient quality of life.

Antistaphylococcal penicillins (nafcillin [Unipen],[1] oxacillin [Prostaphlin][1]) are used for the treatment of methicillin-sensitive staphylococcal osteomyelitis. A first-generation cephalosporin, cefazolin (Ancef), is effective in the treatment of staphylococcal osteomyelitis. The glycopeptides vancomycin (Vancocin) [1] and the oxazolidinone antibiotic linezolid (Zyvox)[1] are used to treat methicillin-resistant staphylococcal osteomyelitis. Several third- and forth-generation cephalosporins, such as cefotaxime (Claforan)[1] or cefepime (Maxipime)[1] can be used to treat osteomyelitis because of gram-negative bacilli.

Oral antibiotics have also been successfully used to treat osteomyelitis. Several oral drugs, such as clindamycin (Cleocin),[1] rifampin (Rifadin),[1] cotrimoxazole (Bactrim),[1] and fluoroquinolones (e.g., ciprofloxacin [Cipro] and levofloxacin [Levaquin][1]) are currently used in the treatment of osteomyelitis. Clindamycin (Cleocin), a lincosamide antibiotic active against most gram-positive bacteria, possesses an excellent bioavailability and is currently used orally, after an initial IV treatment of 2 weeks. Oral therapy using quinolones for gram-negative organisms is used in adult patients with osteomyelitis. The current quinolones have variable *S. aureus* and *Staphylococcus epidermidis* coverage. Pediatric patients should not be given the quinolone

---

[1]Not FDA approved for this indication.

class of antibiotics because of possible damage to cartilage.

The initial treatment of most cases of osteomyelitis usually starts on an empirical basis. After cultures are obtained, a parenteral antimicrobial regimen is begun, covering the clinically suspected pathogens. Once the organism is identified, different antibiotics can be selected by appropriate sensitivity methods. If possible, antibiotics should not be initiated until the results of the bone bacterial culture and sensitivities are known.

ANTIBIOTIC TREATMENT BY CIERNY-MADER STAGE

Stage 1 osteomyelitis in children usually responds to antibiotics alone. Stage 1 osteomyelitis in adults is more refractory to therapy and is usually treated with antibiotics and surgery. The patient is treated for 4 to 6 weeks with appropriate antimicrobial therapy, dated from the initiation of therapy or after the last major débridement surgery. If after 48 hours there is no clinical improvement, surgical treatment may be needed in conjunction with another 4-week course of antibiotics.

In stage 2 osteomyelitis shorter courses of antibiotics, such as 2 weeks, are usually given. In stages 3 and 4 osteomyelitis the patient is treated with 4 to 6 weeks of antimicrobial therapy dated from the last major débridement surgery. This long treatment is needed because even when all necrotic tissue has been adequately débrided, the remaining bed of tissue must be considered contaminated with the responsible pathogen(s).

SUPPRESSIVE ANTIBIOTIC THERAPY

When surgical treatment of osteomyelitis is not feasible, a long-term antibiotic therapy is usually given to control the disease and to prevent flare-ups. Oral antibiotics are usually used. Suppressive therapy has been studied extensively in the setting of infected orthopedic implants. The efficacy of suppressive treatment in osteomyelitis without implants has not been determined. Suppressive therapy is usually administered for 6 months. If recurrence of the infection occurs after discontinuation, a new, culture-directed suppressive regimen is begun and administered indefinitely.

SURGICAL TREATMENT

Surgical treatment of osteomyelitis includes adequate drainage, extensive débridement of all necrotic tissue, obliteration of dead spaces, adequate soft tissue coverage, and restoration of an effective blood supply.

Adequate débridement may leave a large bony defect termed *dead space*. The goal of dead space management is to replace dead bone and scar tissue with vascularized tissue. Local tissue flaps or free flaps may be used to fill dead space. An alternative technique is to place cancellous bone grafts beneath local or transferred tissues where structural augmentation is necessary.

CURRENT DIAGNOSIS

- Clinical signs
- Plain radiographs
- CT, NMR, and bone scans obtained in selected cases
- Cultures from sinus tract are unreliable
- Perform bone biopsy for culture and histology whenever possible

Abbreviations: CT = computed tomography; NMR = nuclear magnetic resonance.

Antibiotic-impregnated acrylic beads may be used to sterilize and temporarily maintain dead space. The beads are usually removed within 2 to 4 weeks and replaced with a cancellous bone graft. The most commonly used antibiotics in beads are vancomycin (Vancocin),[1] tobramycin,[1] and gentamicin.[1] Because beads act as a biomaterial surface to which bacteria adhere, infection associated with the use of beads has been described.

If movement is present at the site of infection, measures must be taken to achieve permanent stability of the skeletal unit. Stability may be achieved with plates, screws, rods, and/or an external fixator. External fixation is preferred more than internal fixation because of the tendency of medullary rods to become secondarily infected and to spread the extent of the infection. The Ilizarov fixator is a type of external fixator that allows reconstruction of segmental bone defects and difficult infected nonunions. The technique is used for difficult cases of osteomyelitis when stabilization and bone lengthening is necessary.

Adequate soft tissue coverage of the bone is often necessary to arrest osteomyelitis. Small soft tissue defects may be covered with a split thickness skin graft. In the presence of a large soft tissue defect or with an inadequate soft tissue envelope, local muscle flaps and free vascularized muscle flaps may be placed in a one- or two-stage procedure. Local muscle flaps and free vascularized muscle transfers improve the local biologic environment by bringing in a blood supply important in host defense mechanisms, antibiotic delivery, and osseous and soft tissue healing.

---

[1]Not FDA approved for this indication.

CURRENT THERAPY

- Stabilization (if needed) and surgical débridement
- Antibiotic treatment of 4 to 6 weeks after surgical débridement
- Select antimicrobial according to in vitro sensitivity tests; consider toxicity, allergy, costs
- Antibiotic suppressive therapy in selected cases

REFERENCES

Cierny G, Mader JT, Pennick JJ: A clinical staging system for adult osteomyelitis. Contemp Orthop 1985;10:17-37.

Lew DP, Waldvogel FA: Osteomyelitis. Lancet 2004;364:369-379.

Shuford JA, Steckelberg JM: Role of oral antimicrobial therapy in the management of osteomyelitis. Curr Opin Infect Dis 2003;16:515-519.

Simpson AH, Deakin M, Latham JM: Chronic osteomyelitis. The effect of the extent of surgical resection on infection-free survival. J Bone Joint Surg Br 2001;83:403-407.

Common Sports Injuries

Method of
Julie J. Chuan, MD, and
Kenneth S. Taylor, MD

Sports-related injuries are commonly evaluated and treated in a physician's office. Injuries can be from acute trauma, such as a fracture or burner/stinger (see definition later), or repetitive stress, such as patellofemoral syndrome. To manage all of these injuries, the provider needs to do a focused evaluation to make the diagnosis and decide on a plan for treatment. Treatment should include rehabilitation, injury prevention, and safe return to play.

Evaluation, Diagnosis, and Treatment

When evaluating any patient with a sports injury, the date of injury and chronicity of symptoms should be determined. The mechanism of injury for all acute injuries, including when, how, and what happened after the injury, should be established. A head injury with persistent headache sustained a week ago is much more concerning for a serious concussion than one sustained an hour ago. If the patient says he or she sustained a twisting knee injury and recalls a pop followed by immediate swelling and was able to walk, an anterior cruciate ligament (ACL) injury is likely. Finally, knowing what happens after the injury can be useful. For example, weight bearing after an ankle injury makes a significant fracture much less likely.

If the injury is more chronic, a history of the sport must be obtained, including change in level or type of activity. The level of activity is important to gauge overuse injuries, including frequency, duration, and intensity. Distance runners with shin pain after increasing their distance is concerning for a stress reaction or fracture. Learning about the type of activity and evaluating for proper biomechanics can often help lead to the diagnosis. Any swimmer who complains of shoulder pain with overhead activity who recently changed from breaststroke to a freestyle stroke likely has some subacromial impingement. This is also important in rehabilitation, which should focus on correcting the biomechanics to prevent reinjury.

After the history, a focused examination of the injury, including palpation, range of motion, and neurovascular status, should be documented. Plain radiographs are useful to assess for fractures and bony alignment. Magnetic resonance imaging (MRI) is helpful to visualize soft tissues and often performed if a diagnosis is in question.

Treatment should include acute injury management, rehabilitation, and return to play. Acute injuries often respond well to rest, ice, compression, elevation, and protection/immobilization, as indicated. If pain cannot be controlled with this alone, non-narcotic analgesics can be used acutely for comfort. Rehabilitation should start as soon as the injury is stable and pain is controlled. It can range from a home exercise program to formal physical therapy. Home exercise programs can be more convenient for the patient and are most appropriate for motivated people who understand how to do the exercises properly. Physical therapists incorporate modalities such as ultrasound (phonophoresis) and electrical stimulation (iontophoresis), and they provide controlled, supervised stretching and strengthening programs that can be individualized for each patient. Finally, the decision to return to play should be addressed and be made when the injury has had adequate time to heal and rehabilitate and the patient understands how to prevent reinjury.

Specific Injuries

HEAD AND NECK INJURIES

Concussions

Concussions are traumatic brain injuries that can occur with any sport and they range in severity. Initial evaluation should include neurologic and physical examinations. Obtaining a history from the patient to assess for post-traumatic amnesia, level of awareness, concentration, and confusion, as well as history of prior concussions, can help determine the severity of injury. Friends and witnesses can be helpful to confirm the history and verify if any loss of consciousness occurred. Concussion symptoms can include but are not limited to headache, dizziness, mood lability, loss of concentration, fatigue, nausea, and vision changes. The physical examination should include pupillary response, coordination, gait, balance, and cranial nerve and strength testing. If there was minimal or no loss of consciousness and the patient is asymptomatic with a normal examination within 15 minutes after injury, the injury is mild. In the patient with prolonged loss of consciousness (more than 1 minute), prolonged or progressive symptoms (hours to days), abnormal physical examination, or severe amnesia, imaging should be strongly considered to look for more severe injury such as an intracranial bleed. Return to play should be determined based on the extent of injury and duration of symptom-free days from injury.

Rakel and Bope: *Conn's Current Therapy 2006.*

Burners and Stingers

Burners and stingers are neck injuries caused by brachial plexus traction or compression. They are common in contact sports, up to 38% in one study of 190 sports injuries. They are acute injuries usually sustained by one of three mechanisms:

1. Lateral flexion force distracting the head and neck away from the shoulder of the affected side
2. Compression injury with neck and head flexion toward the affected side
3. Direct blow to the supraclavicular region

This results in numbness, tingling, or burning down the arm into the hand, usually in the C5 or C6 distribution. Minor injuries resolve within minutes, but more severe injuries involving weakness can last hours to weeks. Athletes often do not seek treatment because symptoms resolve within a few minutes in more than 90% of injuries. If patients do complain of symptoms, evaluation should include a neck examination with palpation and range of motion, shoulder examination, and upper extremity neurologic examination. If more than one extremity is involved, the patient should be immobilized and radiographs obtained to exclude cervical spine injury. Electromyelograms (EMGs) are useful for evaluating severe injuries but may take up to 3 weeks after injury to become abnormal. Burners or stingers involving weakness for more than 72 hours have an abnormal EMG at 4 weeks. Prolonged injury can be treated with physical therapy for range of motion and strengthening. Natural history is not been well studied because permanent neurologic symptoms are rare. Return to play should not be considered until the athlete is asymptomatic with neck and shoulder range of motion and has a normal neurologic examination, including symmetric strength testing.

SHOULDER INJURIES

Acromioclavicular Separation

Shoulder pain can be from injury to the acromioclavicular (AC) joint or the glenohumeral joint. Acromioclavicular joint separations occur from a direct blow to the shoulder, an axial load from the elbow, or an axial load with an extended arm. The trauma is acute and results in swelling, bruising, pain at the AC joint, and occasionally deformity. A focused neurovascular examination should be performed because the brachial plexus is at risk of injury. Shoulder radiographs should be obtained including a true anterior-posterior, 10- to 15-degree cephalic anterior-posterior, and axillary lateral views. If the diagnosis is in question, comparison views of the contralateral side can be useful, but weighted views are not recommended because they rarely change the diagnosis and may exacerbate the injury. Separations are classified by the extent of ligamentous disruption, which is determined by examination and radiographs. Types I and II separations can be treated conservatively with a sling and early range-of-motion exercises. Type III separation treatment is not clearly defined and should be managed individually. Any type IV, V, or VI injury is unstable and usually needs surgical fixation. Treatment should be immobilization with a sling for comfort for all AC separations and referral if warranted (Table 1). Return to play in nonsurgical cases can be considered when there is no pain on palpation of the AC joint.

Shoulder Impingement

Glenohumeral joint pain in active patients without history of acute trauma is often from overuse. Repetitive overhead or throwing activities can lead to impingement or subacromial bursitis symptoms. Examination elicits pain at 70 to 120 degrees of abduction, often with positive provocative tests, such as Hawkins (passive forward flexion of the shoulder and elbow to 90 degrees with internal rotation eliciting pain) and Neer (passive forward flexion with elbow extended eliciting pain). These tests impinge the greater tuberosity against the acromion and have 75% to 90% sensitivity for bursitis and 88% sensitivity for rotator cuff pathology. Rotator cuff strength should be carefully tested for deficits suggestive of muscle or tendon tears. Radiographs are useful to assess for fractures, calcium deposits for calcific tendonitis, acromial shape for bony spurs, and alignment of the glenohumeral joint for rotator cuff or

15

TABLE 1 Acromioclavicular Separation

Acromioclavicular separation	Ligamentous disruption	Radiographs	Treatment
Type I	AC ligament sprain	Normal	Nonsurgical
Type II	AC ligament and capsule disruption	<50% AC subluxation	Nonsurgical
Type III	AC and CC ligaments disrupted; unstable joint	>25% CC separation, >50% AC separation	Nonsurgical versus surgical; controversial
Type IV	AC and CC ligaments disrupted; unstable joint	Type III with *posterior* displacement of the clavicle	Surgical
Type V	AC and CC ligaments disrupted; unstable joint	Type III with *superior* displacement of the clavicle	Surgical
Type VI	AC and CC ligaments disrupted; unstable joint	Type III with inferior displacement of the clavicle	Surgical

Abbreviations: AC = acromioclavicular; CC = coracoclavicular.

degenerative pathology. If soft tissue injury is suspected, MRI can be a useful diagnostic tool. Treatment should consist of relative rest with limited overhead activity, ice, and analgesics as needed. Strengthening the rotator cuff and focusing on kinetic chain function can help restore biomechanical motion. Subacromial injections can be used for diagnostic and therapeutic purposes. If the examination is limited by pain, a subacromial anesthetic injection usually offers significant if not complete pain relief if the source is impingement. Physical therapy is important for restoration of function, but it can be difficult for the patient to tolerate secondary to pain. A subacromial steroid injection may offer temporary pain relief that can facilitate physical therapy. If the injection does not provide any relief, consider referral for surgical decompression and débridement. This is an option for more definitive treatment and can often be performed arthroscopically to provide significant symptom relief. Return to play is contingent on the patient's level of pain. Sometimes patients can return to activity if they minimize the overhead activity that reproduces the symptoms.

KNEE INJURIES

Patellofemoral Pain

Knee injuries are a common complaint in athletes, both from overuse and acute trauma. The most common overuse injury seen in the athlete under 40 years old is patellofemoral joint pain. The pathophysiology, however, is not clear, but most accepted theories involve a combination of stress-induced cartilage defects and abnormal extensor mechanism biomechanics. The patient usually complains of anterior knee pain as well as pain after long periods with the knee held in flexion, which closes the patellofemoral joint (movie theater sign). There may be an inciting incident such as blunt trauma to the patella or simply a change in activity. Examination and treatment should focus on correction of the biomechanics of the patellofemoral joint. Femoral and tibial torsion, patellar tilt, foot hyperpronation, and varus or valgus knee malalignment can put uneven forces on the knee extensor mechanism. This is often evident by vastus medialis oblique muscle weakness or decreased muscle bulk and tightness of the lateral patellar retinaculum, rectus femoris, and/or hamstring on examination. The biomechanics can usually be improved with hamstring stretching, vastus medialis oblique strengthening, activity modification, and orthotics as needed. If symptoms are refractory to therapy, surgical intervention is an option to correct the malalignment. Return to play is contingent on the patient's level of pain and ideally should be close to pain-free prior to returning to play.

Anterior Cruciate Ligament Injury

Acute knee injuries in sports commonly result in injury to the anterior cruciate ligament (ACL). The mechanism is usually a twisting injury and/or a valgus force on the knee. The patient often reports hearing or feeling a pop followed by a significant effusion. With the high-energy force causing ACL tears, there is often associated meniscal, collateral ligament, chondral injury, or fracture. If there is an isolated ACL tear, patients are usually able to ambulate and the pain is mild. They may present chronically with complaints of instability with twisting or cutting activity because the ACL functions to provide stability for torsional forces. On examination, a Lachman test, anterior drawer, and/or pivot shift test may be positive. The Lachman test is performed with the patient lying supine and relaxed with the knee in 20 to 30 degrees of flexion. Stabilizing the femur, the examiner gently pulls the tibia forward to assess for an endpoint and anterior translation relative to the normal knee. The anterior drawer is performed in a similar fashion, except with the knee at 90 degrees of flexion; however, studies do not show it to be as sensitive as the Lachman test. The pivot shift is performed with the knee in extension, and the examiner passively internally rotates and flexes the knee while applying a valgus stress to the knee. The tibia shifts into place around 20 to 30 degrees of flexion when the ACL is torn but can only be done when the patient is completely relaxed. For the experienced clinician, the Lachman test has a high negative predictive value and the pivot shift a high positive predictive value. In acute injuries, the range of motion of the knee should be examined to ensure there is no soft tissue or bony block that may require earlier surgical intervention. If the patient is guarding or has a large knee effusion acutely and no fracture is suspected, range-of-motion bracing and/or crutches for comfort should be considered and repeat the examination a few days later when pain has decreased. Knee range of motion and strength should be optimized prior to surgery and initiated as soon as the patient's pain is controlled. Partial ACL tears can be managed conservatively with therapy and strengthening if there is no instability. Partial or complete ACL tears with clinical instability should be referred for surgical evaluation. Return to play in nonsurgical cases depends on the degree of instability and may require modification of activities.

Meniscal Injury

Meniscal injuries are a common cause of knee pain seen with acute and chronic degenerative trauma. Patients often complain of symptoms of locking, catching, giving way, and localized areas of pain. Examination of any meniscal injury should include inspecting for effusion, palpating for joint line tenderness, testing passive range of motion, and performing McMurray and Apley provocative tests. Joint line tenderness helps localize the area of injury and is a sensitive but not very specific test. The McMurray test is performed by palpating the joint line with one hand and internally and externally rotating while flexing and extending the knee. A positive test elicits a click or catch with pain at the joint line. The Apley test is performed with the patient prone and the knees flexed to 90 degrees. An axial load is placed on the knee while internally and externally rotating the tibia to load each of the menisci with a positive test reproducing the symptoms. In evaluating acute meniscal injuries, range of motion should be documented, specifically extension, to ensure there is no evidence of an extension lag suggestive of a bucket-handle meniscal tear that needs earlier surgical intervention. Because the medial and lateral menisci are much more vascular in the margins, or peripheral third areas, there is a higher chance of healing of tears in those areas. Degenerative tears occur from repetitive knee-loading activities, ranging from running to squatting (baseball catchers) or kneeling (gardening). Patients usually present with more insidious symptoms of pain in certain positions, and they rarely have locking, catching, or giving-way symptoms as in acute meniscal injuries. If meniscal symptoms are persistent, surgical intervention can repair or remove the area of damaged meniscus, depending on the area and extent of the damage. Return to play in nonsurgical cases is appropriate when the patient is symptom free, suggestive of meniscal healing, and there are no signs of meniscal injury on examination.

ANKLE INJURIES

Ankle Sprain

Ankle sprains, specifically lateral ankle sprains, are the most common sports injuries and usually occur with an inversion and plantar flexion mechanism. This usually disrupts the anterior talofibular ligament (ATFL), followed by the calcaneofibular ligament and posterior talofibular ligament. In the acute setting, swelling and pain may limit the examination and should be treated symptomatically and reevaluated to get a better examination a few days later. The examination should look for swelling, ecchymosis, areas of tenderness, and instability. Swelling, ecchymosis, and tenderness over the ATFL are suggestive of a ligament disruption. The anterior drawer test may be difficult to perform in the acute setting and should be repeated for a more accurate result approximately 5 to 7 days after injury when pain and swelling have subsided. The ankle anterior drawer test is performed with the patient seated with the foot hanging over the table. The examiner stabilizes the leg with one hand and uses the other to hold the heel and pull forward to look for anterior translation. The anterior drawer test is 73% sensitive and 97% specific. Tenderness over the ATFL with a positive anterior drawer increases sensitivity to 100% and specificity to 77%. Finally, bony tenderness suggestive of any fractures that require imaging should be checked. Box 1 lists the criteria for the Ottawa ankle rules, a useful guide to determine whether an ankle sprain requires imaging.

BOX 1 Ottawa Ankle Rules

If any of the following are positive, films are
  recommended:
- Unable to walk four steps immediately after injury and in the office
- Tenderness over the distal 6 cm of the tibia or fibula, including the malleoli
- Midfoot or navicular tenderness
- Tenderness over the proximal fifth metatarsal

 CURRENT DIAGNOSIS

- Concussions
  History of head trauma
  Loss of consciousness determined
  Neurologic examination
- Burner/stingers
  History of flexion or direct blow to the head
    or neck
  Duration of symptoms
  Neurologic deficits
- AC separations
  History of direct fall on or blow to the shoulder
  Palpation of the AC joint
  Deformity at the AC joint
- Impingement
  History of pain with overhead activity
  Neer impingement test
  Hawkins impingement test
- Patellofemoral syndrome
  History of possible increased level of activity
  Pain with prolonged sitting
- ACL injury
  History of twisting injury, instability
  Lachman test
  Pivot shift test
  Anterior drawer test
- Meniscal injury
  History of pain, clicking, locking, giving way
  McMurray test
  Apley test
- Ankle sprain
  History of injury, pain, swelling
  Anterior drawer
  Pain over the ATFL

Abbreviations: AC = acromioclavicular; ACL = accessory collateral ligament; ATFL = anterior talofibular ligament.

Swelling and pain can be treated with relative rest, ice, compression, elevation, and support (RICES). Rest may involve the use of crutches for a few days if it is difficult to bear weight, but early mobilization should be encouraged. Icing is recommended for 15- to 20-minute periods to stimulate vasoconstriction and decrease swelling. Compression acutely can be managed by an Ace wrap or pneumatic splint placing pressure on the areas of swelling to promote fluid resorption. Elevation decreases swelling because it increases venous and lymphatic drainage to the heart. Finally, supportive devices are useful in improving swelling and stability in the acute phase. Analgesics such as acetaminophen or mild narcotics can be used acutely, but a nonsteroidal anti-inflammatory drug (NSAID) should be reserved until 48 hours after injury when bruising and swelling have stabilized because it may exacerbate bleeding and swelling acutely. Finally, rehabilitation should be started when the patient is pain-free and should include range-of-motion exercises (writing the alphabet in the air), balance/proprioception exercises (balancing on the injured ankle on the floor, balance board, or

CURRENT THERAPY

- Concussions
  Monitor for resolution of symptoms
  Image for persistent symptoms, prolonged loss of consciousness, or neurologic deficit.
  Return to play when asymptomatic. If symptoms severe, may need to be asymptomatic for days to weeks prior to return to play.
- Burner/Stingers
  Monitor for resolution of symptoms.
  Consider EMG if symptoms persist.
  Return to play when asymptomatic.
- AC separations
  Provide sling for comfort.
  Refer for grade III and above injuries.
  Return to play when asymptomatic.
- Impingement
  Order physical therapy for strengthening and biomechanical retraining.
  Prescribe NSAIDs and steroid injections to improve symptoms temporarily.
  Consider referral for surgical débridement if symptoms persist.
- Patellofemoral syndrome
  Order physical therapy for strengthening.
  Correct any malalignment.
- ACL injury
  Order physical therapy for strengthening and range of motion.
  Make surgical referral for reconstruction.
- Meniscal injury
  If symptoms persist, make surgical referral for repair or débridement.
- Ankle sprain
  Prescribe RICES.
  Order physical therapy for range of motion, strengthening, and proprioception training.

Abbreviations: AC = acromioclavicular; ACL = accessory collateral ligament; EMG = electromyelogram; NSAIDs = nonsteroidal anti-inflammatory drugs; RICES = rest, ice, compression, elevation, and support.

trampoline), and strengthening exercises (controlled elastic band exercises). Return to play can be considered when the athlete gradually progresses to his or her previous level of activity, has near to full range of motion, swelling has resolved, has the ability to hop and perform sport-specific tasks without pain or instability, and has regained at least 90% of the strength of the noninjured side.

Discussion

Sports injuries are common in the active population of all ages. When evaluating any injury, understanding the patient's level of activity and goals for return to play are important in treatment. Graded return to play should be emphasized to the patient because full return to play after any injury makes reinjury likely. Physical therapists and athletic trainers are important in treating the injury, and if they are used, the clinician should monitor progress and determine the appropriate time to return to play. Finally, if the patient is not improving appropriately or the diagnosis is unclear, further imaging or referral to a specialist for evaluation should be considered.

REFERENCES

Adams WB: Treatment options in overuse injuries of the knee: Patellofemoral syndrome, iliotibial band syndrome, and degenerative meniscal tears. Curr Sports Med Rep 2004;3(5):256-260.

Bossart PJ, Joyce SM, Manaster BJ, Packer SM: Lack of efficacy of 'weighted' radiographs in diagnosing acute acromioclavicular separation. Ann Emerg Med 1988;17(1):20-24.

Cohen RS, Balcom TA: Current treatment options for ankle injuries: Lateral ankle sprain, Achilles tendonitis, and Achilles rupture. Curr Sports Med Rep 2003;2(5):251-254.

Dugan S, Weber K: Selected topics in sports medicine. Disease-A-Month. September 2002;48(9)572-616.

Ferrante MA: Brachial plexopathies: Classification, causes, and consequences. Muscle Nerve 2004;30(5):547-568.

Fithian DC: Fate of the anterior cruciate ligament-injured knee. Orthop Clin North Am 2002;33(4):621-636.

Guskiewicz KM, Bruce SL, Cantu RC, et al: National Athletic Trainers' Association Position Statement: Management of Sport-Related Concussion. J Athletic Training 2004;39(3):280-297.

Pyne SW: Diagnosis and current treatment options of shoulder impingement. Curr Sports Med Rep 2004;3(5):251-255.

Safran MR: Nerve injury about the shoulder in athletes: II. Long thoracic nerve, spinal accessory nerve, burners/stingers, thoracic outlet syndrome. Am J Sports Med 2004;32(4):1063-1076.

Tennet TD, Beach WR, Meyers JF: A review of the special tests associated with shoulder examination: I. The rotator cuff test. Am J Sports Med 2003;31(1):154-160.

Van Dijk CN: Management of the sprained ankle. Br J Sports Med 2002;36(2):83-84.

Zanda P: Shoulder pain: Involvement of the acromioclavicular joint. Am J Roentgenol Radium Ther Nucl Med 1971;112(3):493-506.

Obstetrics and Gynecology

Antepartum Care

Method of
Faith Joy Frieden, MD, and Ying Chan, MD

Pregnancy offers the health care provider a window of opportunity to influence the health of today's women and tomorrow's children. Although the cornerstone of treatment during this unique time period is antepartum care, the ideal time to begin is prior to conception.

Preconception Care

At a preconception visit, a basic history and physical examination should be performed, along with a risk assessment. Special areas of concern include preexisting maternal medical conditions, medication use, family history of birth defects, carrier screening for inherited diseases, occupational hazards, and recreational drug use, including cigarettes and alcohol. This visit provides an opportunity to determine susceptibility to infectious diseases, such as toxoplasmosis, cytomegalovirus, varicella, rubella, and HIV, and to vaccinate as appropriate. When risk factors are identified, the patient can be advised of the potential consequences. In some situations (such as uncontrolled diabetes, recent vaccination, recent viral infection, or potentially teratogenic exposure), pregnancy can be postponed until the risk factor is managed and the risk reduced.

Routine Care

INITIAL PRENATAL VISIT

At the initial prenatal visit, a thorough history is obtained, including age, menstrual history, prior obstetrical history, past medical and surgical history, family history, genetic screening, medication or drug use, and history of exposure to infections (tuberculosis, hepatitis B, genital herpes, HIV, and other sexually transmitted diseases, etc.). Any risk factors identified should be

addressed and incorporated into the plan of care for the pregnancy. Certain obstetrical conditions, such as prior preterm birth, recurrent pregnancy loss, or preeclampsia remote from term, are associated with a relatively high recurrence risk, compared with women with no such history. Medical conditions, such as diabetes, hypertension, lupus, asthma, or a seizure disorder, must be stabilized as quickly as possible. In counseling the pregnant woman with underlying medical disorders, we must consider the effects of the medical condition on a pregnancy and the effects of pregnancy on the woman's health. We also must weigh the risk of medication compared with the risks of not treating the condition. The general rule of thumb is that the best predictor of a healthy infant is a healthy mother. Many medications are available that are not known to incur any increased risk of birth defects above the background risk in the general population.

The initial physical examination should include a general physical exam as well as a pelvic exam. The prepregnancy height and weight are recorded, along with the initial vital signs. It is important to perform a thorough exam at this time because many women have not had a physical exam prior to becoming pregnant. Also, at subsequent prenatal visits, less emphasis will be placed on nonobstetric areas in the absence of complaints. The pelvic exam should include assessment of the cervix, uterine size, and adnexa, as well as a clinical impression of the adequacy of the pelvis. Table 1 lists the recommended initial and subsequent laboratory tests.

FOLLOW-UP PRENATAL VISITS

In general, prenatal visits are repeated every 4 weeks until 28 weeks, then every 2 to 3 weeks until 36 weeks, then weekly until delivery. Of course, this schedule should be individualized to the patient, and more frequent visits may be appropriate. The purpose of each prenatal visit is to assess maternal and fetal well-being. Therefore, in a systematic fashion at each visit, the patient's weight and blood pressure are recorded, along with the presence or absence of edema. A urine dipstick is performed to check for protein and glucose. The height of the uterine fundus is measured and fetal heart tones are recorded. The fetal heart rate usually can be auscultated using a Doppler device by 12 weeks.

TABLE 1 Recommended Prenatal Laboratory Screening

Preconception or First Visit	15-20 Weeks	26-28 Weeks	35-37 Weeks
Hemoglobin and hematocrit	Maternal serum screening	Diabetic screening	GBS culture
Blood type/RH factor/antibody screen		Hemoglobin and hematocrit	
Rubella titer		Antibody screen if indicated	
Hepatitis B test			
Syphilis test			
Tests for chlamydia and gonorrhea			
HIV test (offered)			
Urine analysis and culture			
Pap smear			

GBS, Group B streptococcus; HIV, human immunodeficiency virus.
Modified from Gabbe SG, Niebyl JR, Simpson JL: Obstetrics: Normal and Problem Pregnancies, 4th ed, 2002.

The patient is also asked about the perception of fetal movement, which is usually apparent by 20 weeks.

NUTRITION IN PREGNANCY

Pregnant women should increase their daily caloric intake by approximately 300 kcal. The American College of Obstetricians and Gynecologists (ACOG) recommends total weight gain for healthy women with singleton gestation to be 25 to 35 pounds. Underweight women may gain 28 to 40 pounds and overweight women 15 to 25 lb. Women carrying twins may gain 35 to 45 pounds. Pregnant women should receive 30 mg of ferrous iron supplements daily. Folic acid supplementation is advised, both on a hematologic basis and to decrease certain birth defects. The Centers for Disease Control and Prevention (CDC) recommends folic acid, 0.4 mg per day, while attempting pregnancy and during the first trimester of pregnancy for prevention of neural tube defects (NTDs). A woman with a history of a prior NTD-affected pregnancy can reduce the 3% recurrence risk of NTDs by more than 70% if she supplements her daily diet with 4 mg of folic acid for the month before conception and for the first trimester of pregnancy.

VACCINATION OF PREGNANT WOMEN

The benefits of immunization to pregnant women usually outweigh the theoretical risks to the fetus. In general, live-virus vaccines are contraindicated because of the theoretical risks of transmitting vaccine virus to the fetus. Vaccinating pregnant women with inactivated virus, bacterial vaccines, or toxoids is not contraindicated. Although the MMR (measles-mumps-rubella) vaccine is contraindicated in pregnancy, no cases of congenital mumps, measles, or rubella syndromes are identified among infants born to women who were vaccinated within 3 months prior to conception or early in pregnancy. Similarly, no adverse fetal outcomes are reported in pregnant mothers who received varicella vaccine inadvertently. In October 2001, the CDC changed the recommendations concerning the pregnancy interval after receiving rubella vaccine, reducing it from 3 months to 1 month. Influenza vaccine, tetanus-diphtheria booster,

hepatitis A vaccine, hepatitis B vaccine, rabies vaccine, and pneumococcal vaccine are safe in pregnancy and should be administered if appropriate.

HERBAL MEDICINES

Herbal medicines are increasing in popularity nowadays. Herbs were traditionally used to deal with a wide range of pregnancy complications, including morning sickness, threatened miscarriage, labor problems, and poor milk production. Some of the most commonly used herbal medicines are ginger,[1] St. John's wort,[1] and ginseng.[1] Because they originate from plants, most pregnant women perceive them as safe. But herbal medicines can potentially alter maternal hemodynamic parameters and increase bleeding complications associated with regional anesthesia and childbirth. Ginger is a potent inhibitor of thromboxane synthetase, and ginseng has an antiplatelet component. Drug-herb interactions are also described. Therefore, it is imperative that health care providers routinely ask about their use in pregnant women.

COMMON COMPLAINTS

Nausea and vomiting frequently complicate early pregnancy. Nonpharmacologic remedies include frequent small feedings and avoiding spicy foods. Several medications are used as well, including diphenhydramine (Benadryl),[1] metoclopramide (Reglan),[1] prochlorperazine (Compazine), promethazine (Phenergan), and trimethobenzamide (Tigan). One of the newer considerably successful treatment modalities is a continuous infusion of metoclopramide via subcutaneous infusion pump.

Heartburn is a frequent problem, which occurs because of relaxation of the esophageal sphincter with reflux of gastric contents into the lower esophagus. Patients should avoid spicy foods and lying completely flat. Antacids may be helpful, especially in liquid form that coats the lining of the esophagus.

---

[1]Not FDA approved for this indication.

Constipation occurs as a result of smooth muscle relaxation and delayed bowel transit time. It can usually be treated successfully with dietary modification, incorporating increased fruits, vegetables, and water. Stool softeners may also be helpful.

Environmental Hazards and Exposures

Whenever considering the teratogenic potential of an exposure, it is imperative to keep in mind the 3% background risk of major birth defects in the general obstetric population. Only a small percentage of birth defects can actually be linked to a known agent. Examples include such infectious agents as rubella virus and *Toxoplasma gondii,* drugs such as alcohol, thalidomide, and isotretinoin, physical agents such as ionizing radiation and hyperthermia, and chemicals such as lead, organic solvents, and methylmercury.

METHYLMERCURY EXPOSURE IN PREGNANCY

Fish and shellfish are an important part of a balanced diet for pregnant women. Almost all fish and shellfish contain traces of methylmercury. However, some fish contain higher levels of methylmercury that may be harmful to susceptible populations. High levels of methylmercury can impair an unborn fetus's nervous system. In April 2004, the Food and Drug Administration and Environmental Protection Agency issued a joint advisory regarding this issue. Pregnant women and women who might become pregnant should not eat shark, swordfish, tilefish, and king mackerel. They may eat up to 12 ounces, two average meals per week, of fish and shellfish that are lower in mercury: shrimp, canned light tuna, salmon, pollock, catfish.

Prenatal Diagnosis

The purpose of prenatal diagnosis is to provide information that optimizes medical care and enables the patient to make informed reproductive decisions. As health care providers, our responsibility is to assess the risks unique to each pregnancy, convey that information to the patient, and guide her through the testing process while allowing her to choose a course of action that is right for her. This nondirective approach, based on the principle of patient autonomy, is critical to the process of genetic counseling and prenatal diagnosis.

CARRIER SCREENING

Several autosomal recessive disorders occur with increased frequency in certain ethnic groups. Carrier detection should be offered whenever one or both expectant parents belong to the group at increased risk. The most frequently encountered of these conditions are Tay-Sachs disease in the Ashkenazi Jewish population, sickle cell disease in the African American population,

and the thalassemias in people of Mediterranean, African, and Asian descent. Cystic fibrosis (CF) is the most common serious autosomal recessive disorder in the caucasian population. In 2001 the American College of Obstetricians and Gynecologists and American College of Medical Genetics published clinical guidelines for CF screening. It is recommended that CF screening be offered to couples in ethnic or racial groups considered at higher risk for carrying the CF gene: caucasians, particularly those of Ashkenazi Jewish or European descent. It is also recommended that CF testing be available to those of Hispanic, African, and Asian descents, although screening in these populations is less conclusive. Screening for other genetic disorders on the basis of family history may also be indicated (e.g., fragile X syndrome for family history of mental retardation). It is important to counsel patients that a negative test result does not guarantee an unaffected pregnancy, but rather it decreases the risk.

NUCHAL TRANSLUCENCY AND BIOCHEMICAL MARKERS SCREENING

First-trimester screening, consisting of nuchal translucency, free β-human chorionic gonadotropin (hCG), and pregnancy-associated plasma protein A (PAPP-A), may be available in some centers. First-trimester screening is typically performed at 11 to 14 weeks. This allows for earlier detection and diagnosis of some fetal chromosomal and structural abnormalities. Median level of free β-hCG is higher in affected Down syndrome pregnancies. Conversely, median level of PAPP-A is lowered in affected Down syndrome pregnancies. Increased nuchal translucency is associated with chromosomal abnormalities such as trisomy 21,18, and 13, 45, X, and triploidy. It is also associated with congenital anomalies such as cardiac defects, skeletal abnormalities, and some genetic disorders. The prevalence of major cardiac defects increases with increasing nuchal translucency thickness. In fetuses with increased nuchal translucency measurement and normal chromosomes, detailed anatomic survey and fetal echocardiography are recommended.

Second-trimester maternal serum screening is offered at approximately 16 weeks' gestation. This test generally evaluates three markers, namely α-fetoprotein (AFP), hCG, and unconjugated estriol. AFP is produced by the fetus and is present in high concentrations in the amniotic fluid and, to a lesser extent, in maternal serum. Elevated levels of maternal serum AFP are associated with open neural tube defects, ventral wall defects, some renal abnormalities, multiple gestation, certain skin disorders, maternal tumors, fetal demise, placental abnormality, and otherwise unexplained adverse perinatal outcome. Low levels of maternal serum AFP are associated with Down syndrome. The addition of the other two markers enhances the detection rate, from 25% using AFP alone to approximately 60% using all three. This test is especially useful for younger women, who might not otherwise pursue prenatal diagnosis. In the event of an abnormal result, patients are offered ultrasound for confirmation of gestational age and for anatomic survey. They also have the option of amniocentesis for direct assessment of the fetal chromosomes and AFP level.

In general, first-trimester screening has comparable detection rates and positive screening rates for Down syndrome as second-trimester screening. However, integrated screening (i.e., combined first- and second-trimester screening) is believed to be the most sensitive and cost-effective test. Detection rate for fetal Down syndrome with this approach can be as high as 92%.

AMNIOCENTESIS AND CHORIONIC VILLUS SAMPLING

Genetic amniocentesis is the most commonly performed invasive prenatal diagnostic procedure. It is generally performed at 15 to 20 weeks. Although it is performed under ultrasound guidance, using sterile technique, it still carries a pregnancy loss rate attributable to the procedure of approximately 0.5%. The amniotic fluid is sent for fetal karyotyping and AFP determination, although other specific genetic testing can also be performed.

An alternative to traditional amniocentesis is chorionic villus sampling (CVS), which allows a first-trimester diagnosis. CVS can be performed at 10 to 12 weeks, using the transabdominal or transcervical approach. The pregnancy loss rate is approximately 1.3% with CVS, which is somewhat higher than with traditional amniocentesis, according to a large multicenter trial conducted by the National Institute of Child Health and Human Development. Another drawback is that AFP cannot be measured in villi. It is conceivable, therefore, that an amniocentesis might be necessary later to evaluate an elevated maternal serum AFP. Subsequent amniocentesis could also be indicated to clarify an ambiguous CVS finding, which occurs in approximately 1% of cases.

FETAL BLOOD SAMPLING

Sometimes it becomes necessary to sample fetal blood directly for rapid karyotyping, evaluating for fetal infection, or diagnosing platelet disorders prenatally. This technique, of accessing fetal blood via the umbilical cord, is known as percutaneous umbilical blood sampling (PUBS) and has an estimated fetal loss rate of 1% to 2%.

Antepartum Testing

ULTRASOUND

A variety of noninvasive techniques are available for evaluating fetal health. The most powerful tool, and perhaps the most controversial, is diagnostic ultrasound. Ultrasound technology has fundamentally altered the practice of obstetrics and refined the art of prenatal diagnosis. Its clinical utility is under constant scrutiny, analysis, and expansion. Although academics disagree about whether routine ultrasound screening is useful or cost effective in low-risk pregnancies, this tool is almost universal in the United States.

NONSTRESS TEST

The nonstress test (NST) is a simple, noninvasive method of monitoring fetal well-being by recording fetal heart rate patterns along with the maternal perception of fetal movement. It is based on the premise that the heart rate of a nonacidotic or non–neurologically depressed fetus accelerates in response to fetal movement. If two or more accelerations of 15 beats per minute, lasting for 15 seconds, are present in a 20-minute period, the test is considered "reactive," or normal. The major pitfall of this test is the high false-positive rate because "nonreactivity" is more likely associated with a fetal sleep cycle than with actual central nervous system depression.

BIOPHYSICAL PROFILE

Biophysical profile testing combines multiple biophysical parameters to assess fetal well-being, in an attempt to identify the compromised fetus more accurately. It is composed of the NST and four parameters evaluated by ultrasound, namely fetal breathing movement, fetal body movement, fetal tone, and assessment of amniotic fluid volume.

Medical Complications

DIABETES MELLITUS

Diabetes in pregnancy encompasses two very different groups of women—diabetic women who become pregnant and pregnant women who become diabetic. The former group, although smaller in number, is greater in terms of the impact on a pregnancy. Preconception counseling is most important for this group. With a two- to fourfold increase in the risk of major malformations in infants of diabetic mothers, congenital malformations are the most important cause of perinatal loss in these pregnancies. The organ systems most frequently affected are the cardiovascular, skeletal, and central nervous systems. It has been demonstrated repeatedly that excellent glycemic control at the time of conception and organogenesis can dramatically reduce this risk. Fetal overgrowth because of maternal hyperglycemia can be another complication because delivery of excessively large infants occurs up to 10 times more often in diabetic women than in the nondiabetic population. If maternal blood glucose levels are not controlled adequately, these newborns are also subject to metabolic derangements, including hypoglycemia, magnesium deficiency, and hyperbilirubinemia, as well as respiratory distress and polycythemia. When the diabetes is associated with vasculopathy, such as nephropathy or retinopathy, the fetus is at risk for intrauterine growth restriction. Therefore, it is essential that diabetic women maintain meticulous glycemic control, adhering to an appropriate diet and monitoring blood glucose levels from four to seven times daily. Target values are fasting capillary blood glucose of 60 to 90 mg/dL and 1-hour postprandial values less than 120 mg/dL. In addition, it is useful to monitor glycosylated hemoglobin levels in these women, which indicate the overall level of control for the preceding 6 weeks. Fetal well-being is assessed with ultrasound and echocardiography in the second trimester and with nonstress tests and biophysical profile exams in the third trimester. Because of the increased risk of adverse perinatal outcome in these pregnancies, delivery is usually recommended at term, as soon as fetal lung maturity is assured.

Approximately 3% of pregnant women develop carbohydrate intolerance, or gestational diabetes, during the latter part of pregnancy. Because roughly half of these women have no identifiable risk factors, it is good practice to screen all pregnant women for this condition at 28 weeks with the 1-hour 50-g oral glucose challenge test (GCT). If this result is elevated, the 3-hour 100-g OGTT is performed. In contrast to GCT, which can be performed at any time of the day, OGTT should be performed in the morning after an overnight fast of at least 8 hours and after at least 3 days of unrestricted diet (150 g carbohydrate or more per day) and physical activity. Table 2 shows the recommended cutoff values by Carpenter and Coustan. A woman who meets or exceeds two or more values is diagnosed with gestational diabetes. Approximately 15% of women with a positive GCT have a positive OGTT. The mainstay of management is diet with self-monitoring of blood glucose, in most cases four times daily (fasting and 1 hour after meals). If the target glucose values cannot be reached and maintained with this regimen, insulin therapy may be necessary. Although carbohydrate intolerance should resolve following delivery, gestational diabetic patients should know that they have a 50% chance of becoming diabetic later in life.

Surgery in Pregnancy

Whenever the physician is faced with the decision of whether to take a pregnant woman to the operating room, the risks of surgery must be weighed against the risks of conservative management, keeping in mind that the sequelae of nonintervention could actually be more severe in a pregnant patient. If surgery is performed, a general rule of thumb is to minimize uterine manipulation to minimize the risk for preterm labor. Cesarean section should be reserved for obstetric indications.

TABLE 2 Recommended Cutoff Values by Carpenter and Coustan to Diagnose Gestational Diabetes Mellitus With a 100-g Oral Glucose Tolerance Test (OGTT)

100-g OGTT	Plasma (mg/dl)
Fasting	95
1 hour	180
2 hours	155
3 hours	140

Rakel and Bope: *Conn's Current Therapy 2006.*

Appendicitis is the most common nonobstetric emergency during pregnancy. The diagnosis is complicated by the overlap of the symptoms of appendicitis with some common symptoms in pregnancy. In addition, the position of the appendix becomes higher as pregnancy advances, making it more difficult to pinpoint the source of the pain. Maternal and fetal complications are directly associated with advanced disease and delay in treatment. Therefore, once acute appendicitis is suspected in pregnancy, emergency surgery should be performed. To lower maternal and fetal morbidity, we accept a higher negative exploration rate than in the nonpregnant population.

Gallbladder disease is the second most common nonobstetric surgical condition in pregnancy, usually presenting with right upper quadrant pain, nausea, and vomiting. Medical management includes bed rest, no oral feedings, intravenous fluids for hydration, and antibiotics. When attacks are recurrent or if the patient develops an acute abdomen, cholecystectomy should be performed.

Trauma in Pregnancy

Trauma and violence are the leading causes of death in women of reproductive age. The first priority when encountering a pregnant trauma victim is treatment and stabilization of the woman. Only then should attention be directed to the fetus. Pregnancy should not alter the necessary evaluation and treatment. It cannot be overstated that necessary radiographic studies should be performed without delay, with efforts made to minimize the dose to the lower abdomen. A systematic approach to evaluation should be used, consisting of the ABCs (airway, breathing, and circulation). There are some considerations unique to pregnancy. The patient should be tilted or wedged in the left lateral position, thus deflecting the uterus off the inferior vena cava and aorta. The pregnant trauma victim requires a greater volume of blood replacement to maintain her cardiovascular integrity than a nonpregnant patient. In gestations beyond 20 weeks, electronic monitoring for uterine contractions, as well as fetal heart rate, is helpful in evaluation for placental abruption and other injury.

Motor vehicle accidents are a significant source of trauma and death, especially when the victim is ejected from the car. The three-point lap belt/shoulder harness restraint is superior to the lap belt alone in preventing maternal and fetal injury.

Perhaps the most insidious form of trauma in pregnancy is domestic violence. The actual incidence is not known, but an estimated 25% of women in the United States are abused by a current or former partner sometime in their lives. Because obstetricians are the primary care providers for many women, they are in a unique position to identify women who are victims of abuse and offer them help. If an abusive relationship is identified, the woman should be encouraged to leave the violent situation and be referred to appropriate agencies, to protect both herself and her children.

16

Obstetrical Complications

PRETERM BIRTH

Preterm birth, occurring prior to the completion of 37 weeks of gestation, complicates 9% of all births in the United States and accounts for 75% of the neonatal deaths that are not caused by congenital malformations. Despite the advent of new diagnostic and therapeutic modalities, the preterm birth rate has remained unchanged over the past 40 years. This may be largely because of the multifaceted nature of this problem. Approximately one third of such births are iatrogenic, in that they are indicated because of medical or obstetric disorders that place the mother or fetus at increased risk, such as hypertension, diabetes, hemorrhage, or intrauterine growth restriction. The remaining two thirds are attributed to preterm labor, preterm premature rupture of membranes, and cervical incompetence. Some current therapies directed at early diagnosis and treatment include home uterine activity monitoring, tocolytic therapy, ultrasonographic measurements of cervical length, and assays of fetal fibronectin levels in cervicovaginal secretions. When preterm birth is imminent, delivery in a setting with appropriate neonatal intensive care optimizes perinatal outcome.

PROLONGED PREGNANCY

A postdate or post-term pregnancy is defined as one that reaches 42 weeks after the last menstrual period. Perinatal morbidity and mortality increase dramatically after 40 weeks and especially after 42 weeks. Possible maternal complications include an increased incidence of cesarean section, hemorrhage, and trauma because of fetal macrosomia. Potential problems of these neonates include birth trauma from macrosomia and meconium aspiration. Good outcomes can be expected with accurate dating, careful fetal surveillance, and intervention when indicated.

MULTIPLE GESTATIONS

The incidence of twinning in the United States is approximately 1.2% of all pregnancies. With the increased use of assisted reproductive technologies, the incidence of higher-order multiple gestations (triplets and higher) is approximately 0.3%. These pregnancies pose special concerns for management of the mother as well as the fetuses. Increased maternal risks include an increased strain on the cardiovascular system, pulmonary edema, preeclampsia, anemia, complications related to tocolysis, and delivery complications. The greatest fetal risk is that of prematurity. In addition, when identical twin fetuses have a single placenta and a shared placental circulation, there is a significant risk for twin-twin transfusion syndrome, a potentially fatal complication of twinning. Early diagnosis of multiple gestations, frequent checkups to monitor maternal health, serial ultrasound exams to assess fetal growth and well-being, reduced maternal activity level, prompt treatment of preterm labor, close intrapartum surveillance, and appropriate neonatal personnel in the delivery room all contribute to optimizing the outcome of these pregnancies.

Infections

Certain perinatal infections, such as toxoplasmosis, cytomegalovirus, human parvovirus B19, rubella, varicella, and syphilis, have the potential for teratogenicity or fetal loss. Some infections have the potential for other adverse perinatal sequelae. For example, vertical transmission of hepatitis B has been demonstrated. Group B β-hemolytic streptococcus, although a frequent component of vaginal flora, is one of the most common and dangerous perinatal pathogens in susceptible newborns, requiring intrapartum prophylaxis. Genital herpes can colonize newborns during passage through an infected birth canal. Chorioamnionitis, or bacterial infection of the amniotic cavity and membranes, is an important cause of perinatal morbidity and mortality, best treated with intrapartum antibiotics and delivery. Increasing evidence indicates that exposure to such intrauterine infection may be associated with an increased risk of cerebral palsy.

Special attention must be paid to HIV, which is estimated to complicate 7000 pregnancies per year in the United States. HIV testing should be offered to all pregnant women, in light of the findings of the landmark study, Pediatric AIDS Clinical Trials Group 076. This study demonstrated a significant reduction in mother-to-infant transmission of the virus, from 26% in the placebo group to 8% in the group using zidovudine (ZDV, Retrovir). According to this protocol, prophylactic ZDV therapy is given to HIV-positive women starting at 14 weeks and continued throughout pregnancy, in an oral dose of 100 mg five times daily. During labor, it is given intravenously in a 1-hour loading dose of 2 mg/kg body weight, followed by a continuous infusion of 1 mg/kg body weight every hour until delivery. The neonate is then given zidovudine syrup at a dose of 2 mg/kg body weight every 6 hours for the first 6 weeks of life.

Other risk factors may affect perinatal transmission. Prolonged fetal exposure to ruptured membranes, fetal scalp sampling, fetal scalp electrodes, and any other fetal abrasions should be avoided. Breast-feeding is contraindicated in HIV-positive women because it also increases transmission.

New multiple antiretroviral regimens are available for the treatment of HIV and AIDS. Although data are limited on their use in pregnancy, they should be administered as necessary for the life and well-being of the mother and certainly should not be avoided, especially after the first trimester when organogenesis is completed.

Fetal Therapy

With improved prenatal diagnosis and the resultant opportunity for antenatal therapy, the concept of the fetus as a patient is emerging. This therapy has taken two main forms: pharmacologic manipulation of the fetal environment via maternal medication that crosses the placenta and the exciting and challenging new frontier of fetal surgery. Perhaps the most frequently used form of in utero therapy is maternal administration of betamethasone (Celestone),[1] a corticosteroid, for the purpose of accelerating fetal lung maturity when delivery is anticipated prior to 34 weeks. The recommended dosage is 12 mg given by intramuscular injection for two doses, 24 hours apart. Maternally administered antiarrhythmics, such as digoxin, are useful in treating certain fetal cardiac arrhythmias, which, if left untreated, may lead to fetal congestive heart failure. Another striking example of in utero drug therapy is the use of dexamethasone (Decadron)[1] in pregnancies at risk for

[1]Not FDA approved for this indication.

CURRENT DIAGNOSIS

- Preconceptual and initial pregnancy evaluation should include complete blood count (CBC), type and screen, rubella, syphilis, and hepatitis testing. HIV testing should also be offered.
- The following genetic disorders based on racial and ethnic background should be screened for:
    Sickle hemoglobinopathies (African American).
    B-thalassemia (Mediterranean, Southeast Asian, and African American).
    Tay-Sachs disease (Ashkenazi Jews, French Canadians, Cajuns).
    Canavan disease and familial dysautonomia (Ashkenazi Jews). Carrier screening is also available for Gaucher's disease, Niemann-Pick disease, mucolipidosis IV, Fanconi anemia, maple syrup urine disease, Bloom syndrome, glycogen-storage disease type 1a, and so on.
    Cystic fibrosis (caucaseans of European and Ashkenazi Jewish descent).
- Both first-trimester nuchal translucency/PAPP-A/free ß-hCG and second-trimester maternal serum screening may detect women at increased risk for chromosomal abnormalities.
- Total weight gain should be 25 to 35 pounds for women of normal prepregnancy weight with a singleton gestation. Underweight women may gain 28 to 40 pounds, and overweight women 15 to 25 pounds.
- All pregnant women should be screened for gestational diabetes mellitus at 26 to 28 weeks with the 1-hour 50-g oral glucose challenge test. If it is elevated, then the 3-hour 100-g oral glucose tolerance test is performed (fasting, <95 mg/dL; 1 hr, <180 mg/dL; 2 hr, <155 mg/dL; 3 hr, <140 mg/dL). A woman who meets or exceeds two or more values is diagnosed with gestational diabetes.

Abbreviations: hCG = human chorionic gonadotropin; PAPP-A = pregnancy-associated plasma protein A.

Rakel and Bope: *Conn's Current Therapy 2006.*

CURRENT THERAPY

- Although some vaccines are safe to receive during pregnancy, it is best to have all needed immunizations before becoming pregnant. Susceptible women should have MMR (measles-mumps-rubella) and varicella vaccines at least 1 month before conception. Influenza vaccine, tetanus-diphtheria booster, hepatitis A vaccine, hepatitis B vaccine, rabies, and pneumococcal vaccines are safe in pregnancy.
- The amount of folic acid found in prenatal vitamins (1 mg) is sufficient for most women. For women at increased risk for neural tube defects, the recommended dose is 4 mg of folate starting before conception and continuing through week 12 of gestation.
- Pregnant women and women who might become pregnant should not eat shark, swordfish, tilefish, and king mackerel. They may eat up to 12 ounces per week of fish and shellfish that are lower in mercury.
- In pregnant women who are HIV-positive, antepartum, intrapartum, and neonatal treatment with zidovudine (ZDV) are recommended.

congenital adrenal hyperplasia to prevent the external genital masculinization of affected female fetuses.

When fetal anemia is suspected as a cause of fetal hydrops, such as in cases of certain congenital infections or hemolytic disease because of Rh or other maternal blood group antibodies, the fetal circulation can be accessed through percutaneous umbilical blood sampling. This allows for measurement of the fetal hematocrit as well as direct intravascular fetal transfusion. A handful of fetal treatment centers in the country use fetal surgery to treat such conditions as obstructive uropathy, congenital diaphragmatic hernia, and spina bifida.

Ethical Issues

As medical technology advances, it inevitably raises new questions regarding when and how to apply it in clinical practice. Ethical principles require full disclosure of the diagnosis, prognosis, and management alternatives. The wishes of the pregnant woman, who still retains autonomy, must always be respected. An even more perplexing ethical question is how to handle feto-fetal conflicts, such as in the case of twins with competing interests, when surgery or delivery of the affected twin will jeopardize the unaffected one. Such cases are optimally managed by carefully balancing these concerns and striving for the safety of both fetuses.

Considering all the facets of antepartum care just described, it is clear why physicians who care for pregnant women play a pivotal role in guiding them through this most important time.

REFERENCES

American College of Obstetricians and Gynecologists and American College of Medical Genetics: Preconception and prenatal carrier screening for cystic fibrosis: Clinical and laboratory guidelines. Washington, DC, ACOG, October 2001.

Braun L: Herb-drug interaction guide. Aust Fam Physician 2001; 30(4):357-358.

Carpenter MW, Coustan DR: Criteria for screening tests for gestational diabetes. Am J Obstet Gynecol 1982;144(7):763-773.

Connor EM, Sperling RS, Gelber R, et al: Reduction of maternal-infant transmission of human immunodeficiency virus type 1 with zidovudine treatment. Pediatric AIDS Clinical Trials Group Protocol 076 Study Group. N Engl J Med 1994;331(18):1173-1180.

Hyett J, Perdu M, Sharland G, et al: Using fetal nuchal translucency to screen for major congenital cardiac defects at 10-14 weeks of gestation: Population based cohort study. BMJ 1999;318: 81-85.

Revised ACIP recommendation for avoiding pregnancy after receiving rubella-containing vaccine. MMWR Morb Mortal Wkly Rep 2001; 50:1117.

Wald NJ, Rodeck C, Hackshaw AK, et al: First and second trimester antenatal screening for Down's syndrome: The results of the Serum, Urine, and Ultrasound Screening Study (SURUSS). J Med Screen 2003;10(2):56-104.

Ectopic Pregnancy

Method of
Gary H. Lipscomb, MD

In the United States, the incidence of ectopic pregnancies has increased dramatically during the last several decades. Commonly cited risks include prior pelvic inflammatory disease (PID), previous tubal surgery, intrauterine device (IUD) use, previous ectopic pregnancy, ovulation induction and in vitro fertilization, progestin-containing contraceptives, smoking, previous abdominal surgery, in utero diethylstilbestrol (DES) exposure, and previous induced abortion.

A high degree of suspicion is necessary for the early diagnosis of an ectopic pregnancy. Almost all ectopic pregnancies have episodes of vaginal bleeding or lower abdominal pain prior to rupture. Such patients are appropriate candidates to evaluate for ectopic pregnancy. Figure 1 illustrates a diagnostic algorithm that is useful in efficiently coordinating and interpreting the tests used in the diagnosis of ectopic pregnancy.

Diagnosis

Serum progesterone levels are helpful as an initial screening test for ectopic pregnancy. Levels higher than 25 ng/mL are associated with ectopic pregnancy in only 1% to 2% of cases; levels less than 5 ng/mL are associated with a nonviable pregnancy (either intrauterine or ectopic) more than 99% of the time. If progesterone levels are not readily available in a timely manner, however, human chorionic gonadotropin (hCG) levels alone may be used.

Levels of hCG rise in an essentially linear fashion until after 41 days of gestation. By this gestational age, an intrauterine pregnancy (IUP) should be seen on ultrasound. In 85% of normal pregnancies, hCG doubles approximately every 2 days, rising at least 66% in 48 hours. However, 15% of normal IUPs rise less than this in 48 hours. Conversely, 15% of ectopic pregnancies rise more than 66%. But a rise of less than 50% is associated with an abnormal pregnancy 99.9% of the time.

Because the interassay variability of hCG is 15%, a change of less than this amount is considered a plateau. Plateaued levels are the most predictive of ectopic pregnancy. The use of a urine pregnancy test to rule out the possibility of phantom hCG is strongly recommended prior to surgical or medical treatment. This phenomenon, caused by heterophilic serum antibodies, produces false-positive hCG levels usually less than 1000 IU/L.

The sonographic identification of an intrauterine gestational sac essentially excludes an ectopic pregnancy. A viable IUP should always be visualized at an hCG titer of 2000 IU/L by transvaginal scan and by 6500 IU/L with transabdominal ultrasound. An adnexal mass, in a patient with a presumed ectopic pregnancy and hCG levels less than 2000 IU/L, should not automatically be assumed to be an ectopic without the presence of a yolk sac, fetal pole, or cardiac activity. Such masses are frequently corpus luteum cysts associated with an early IUP.

Except in the rare case of heterotopic pregnancy, the identification of chorionic villi in uterine contents essentially eliminates the diagnosis of ectopic pregnancy. The use of dilation and curettage (D&C) also eliminates giving methotrexate unnecessarily to a patient with a failed IUP.

A D&C is particularly important in patients with hCG titers below the discriminatory zone of ultrasound. In these patients, the appropriate use of hCG doubling times and serum progesterone levels is necessary to avoid interrupting a viable IUP. Patients with hCG titers that plateau (less than 15% change) or an hCG rise of less than 50% in 48 hours should undergo D&C to differentiate between a failed IUP and an ectopic pregnancy. Villi is absent on final histology in up to 50% of these cases. Because only the presence of villi is diagnostic, those without villi require serial hCG titers. While awaiting final histologic pathology, hCG titers are also followed. As noted in the ectopic algorithm, a serum hCG drawn after D&C is followed by a repeat level in 12 to 24 hours. Rising or inappropriately falling

---

 CURRENT DIAGNOSIS

- Screening for symptomatic patients or those with risk factors
- Diagnostic algorithm to coordinate testing
- hCG titers every 48 hours
- Ultrasound at hCG level of 2000 mIU/mL
- D&C for inappropriate hCG rise (<50% in 48 hours) below 2000 mIU/mL

Abbreviations: D&C = dilation and curettage; hCG = human chorionic gonadotropin.

Rakel and Bope: *Conn's Current Therapy 2006.*

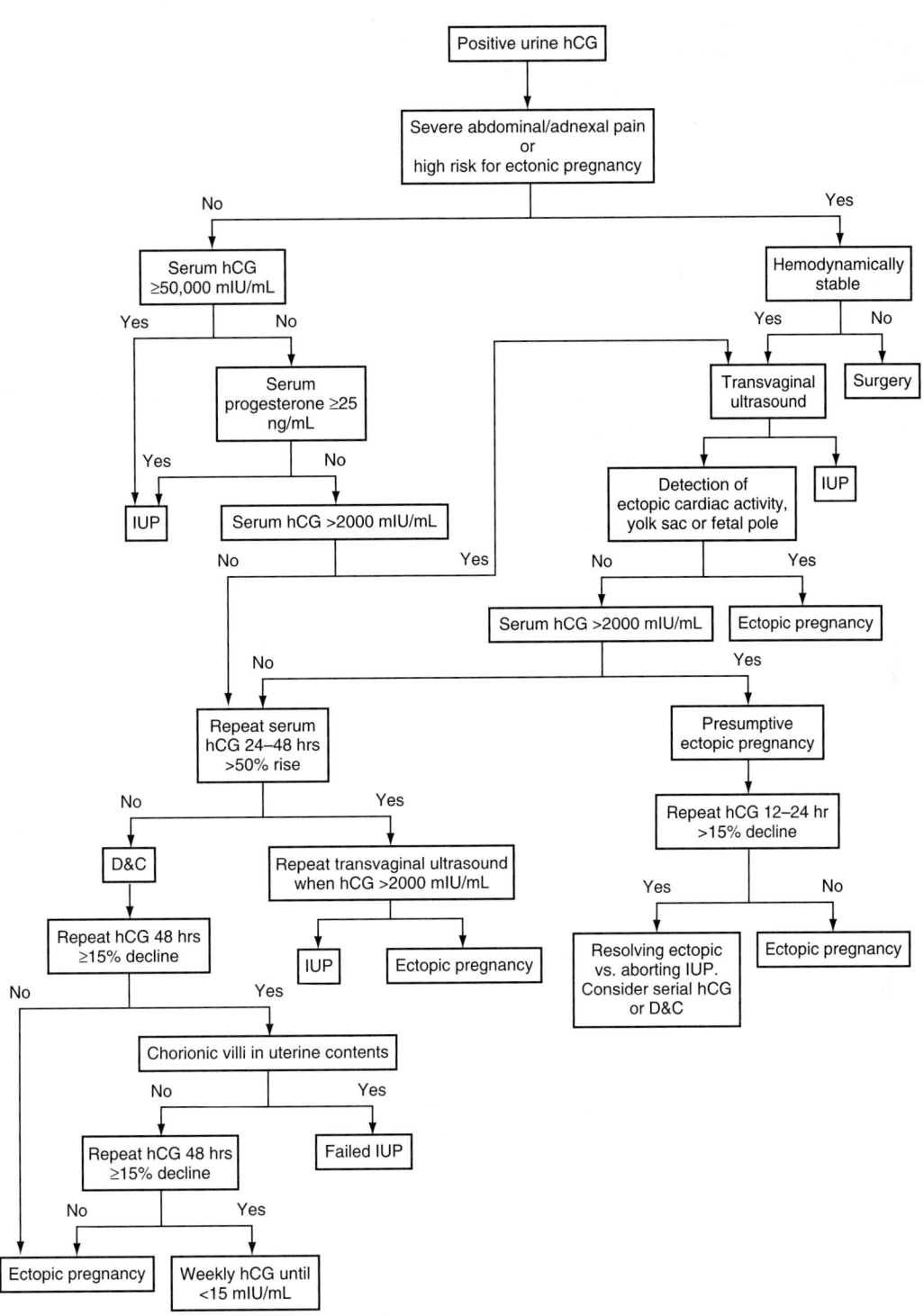

FIGURE 1. University of Tennessee Diagnostic Algorithm. D&C = dilation and curettage; hCG = human chorionic gonadotropin.

levels after D&C are considered diagnostic of an ectopic pregnancy.

Laparoscopy remains the gold standard for the diagnosis of ectopic pregnancy. It should be employed in any patient with suspected ectopic rupture, unreliable patients, or any others suspected of ectopic pregnancy for which the diagnostic algorithms are inappropriate.

Treatment

Surgery is the classic treatment for ectopic pregnancy and remains the treatment of choice in hemodynamic unstable patients, those desiring no further pregnancies, or those who are unsuitable or unwilling to risk medical therapy.

Rakel and Bope: *Conn's Current Therapy 2006.*

Medical therapy with methotrexate[1] is an acceptable option to surgical therapy. Reported success rates range from 75% to 96%, with an average of approximately 90%. Whether a multidose or single-dose methotrexate protocol is most effective remains debatable, but single-dose methotrexate is the most popular because of its ease of use and low incidence of side effects.

Contraindications to medical therapy remain ill defined, but Boxes 1 and 2 note frequently used contraindications. The hCG level is the single factor most predictive of failure. With hCG levels of 5000 to 9999, success rates fall to approximately 87%, further dropping to 82% for levels 10,000 to 14,999 and 68% if more than 15,000. These levels can be used to counsel patients about the risk of failure.

MUTLIDOSE METHOTREXATE

Intramuscular methotrexate, 1 mg/kg of actual body weight, alternating with citrovorum rescue factor (Leucovorin), 0.1 mg/kg, is given daily and continued until a 15% decline in two consecutive daily hCG titers. Human chorionic gonadotropin levels are then followed weekly. A repeat course of methotrexate/citrovorum is given if levels fall to less than 15% or rise between two consecutive hCG titers.

SINGLE-DOSE METHOTREXATE PROTOCOL

Methotrexate, 50 mg/m² based on actual body weight, is given intramuscularly. The day methotrexate is given is considered day 1. A repeat hCG is performed on days 4 and 7. If there is an appropriate decline, hCG levels are followed weekly. If the hCG level declines less than

---

[1]Not FDA approved for this indication.

 CURRENT THERAPY

- Surgery: treatment of choice for unstable patients
- Methotrexate success: correlation with hCG levels
- Multidose methotrexate: 1 mg/kg body weight IM alternate days with leucovorin 0.1 mg/kg IM until hCG declines 15%
- Multidose treatment follow-up: daily hCG until decline, then weekly
- Single-dose methotrexate: 50 mg /m² based on actual body weight
- Single-dose treatment follow-up: hCG on days 1, 4, 7, then weekly if 15% decline between days 4 and 7

Abbreviations: hCG = human chorionic gonadotropin; IM = intramuscularly.

15% between days 4 and 7, a second dose of methotrexate is given and the protocol restarted at a new day 1. Although this protocol is referred to as "single-dose methotrexate," approximately 20% of patients require more than one treatment cycle.

In conclusion, the incidence of ectopic pregnancy has reached epidemic proportions in the United States. Nevertheless, the mortality associated with this disease is steadily declining. This decline is primarily because of earlier diagnosis that allows treatment prior to rupture This earlier diagnosis is the result of improved assays for progesterone, hCG, transvaginal ultrasound, and the use of diagnostic algorithms that do not require the use of laparoscopy. Once diagnosed, numerous treatment options are now available, including the option of medical therapy. Future developments ideally will provide for an even earlier diagnosis as well as data on the optimum candidates for each form of treatment.

REFERENCES

Brenaschek G, Rudelstorfer R, Csaicsich P: Vaginal sonography versus serum human chorionic gonadotropin in early detection of pregnancy. Am J Obstet Gynecol 1988;158:608-612.
Kadar N, Freedman M, Zacher M: Further observation on the doubling time of human chorionic gonadotropin in early asymptomatic pregnancy. Fertil Steril 1980;54:783-787.
Lipscomb GH, McCord ML, Huff G, et al: Predictors of success of methotrexate treatment in women with tubal ectopic pregnancies. N Engl J Med 1999;341:1874-1878.
Lipscomb GH, Stovall TS, Ling FW: Nonsurgical treatment of ectopic pregnancy. N Engl J Med 2000;343:1325-1329.
Stovall TS, Ling FW, Buster JE: Nonsurgical diagnosis and treatment of tubal pregnancy. Fertil Steril 1990;54:537-538.
Stovall TG, Ling FW, Gray LA, et al: Methotrexate treatment of unruptured ectopic pregnancy: A report of 100 cases. Obstet Gynecol 1991;77:749-753.

Vaginal Bleeding in Late Pregnancy

Method of
Jami Star Zeltzer, MD

Vaginal bleeding in late pregnancy complicates approximately 6% of pregnancies and is associated with increased maternal and fetal morbidity and mortality. Excluding labor, the most likely causes are placenta previa and placental abruption, followed by uterine rupture and vasa previa; less common etiologies include trauma, cervical lesions, and coagulopathy. The primary focus in obstetric hemorrhage, regardless of cause, is maternal hemodynamic assessment and stabilization. Given the extraordinary blood flow to the uterus at term (600 to 800 mL/min), exsanguination can occur rapidly. Additionally, redistribution of maternal blood flow may lead to fetal hypoxia.

Early maternal signs of hemodynamic compromise include tachycardia and tachypnea; later, hypotension, weakened pulses, and oliguria ensue, along with evidence of fetal compromise. Further decompensation can ultimately result in the death of both mother and fetus. Guidelines for restoration of maternal circulating volume are approximately 3 mL of intravenous crystalloid, (i.e., normal saline or Ringer's solution) per 1 mL of blood lost (often underestimated). Laboratory evaluation includes a complete blood count, blood type, and crossmatch; in the setting of thrombocytopenia (less than 100,000 platelets), coagulation studies (prothrombin time [PT], partial thromboplastin time [PTT], fibrinogen, fibrin degradation products [FDPs]) are recommended. Packed red blood cells, fresh-frozen plasma, platelets, and/or cryoprecipitate are given to maintain maternal hemoglobin near 10 g/dL and correct coagulopathy (unlikely if whole blood is observed to clot in less than 8 minutes). Additional measures include administration of oxygen, lateral displacement of the uterus and, rarely, vasopressors. Fetal evaluation and treatment, including consideration of delivery, follow stabilization of the mother.

Placenta Previa

Placenta previa, or the implantation of the placenta adjacent to or covering the internal os, complicates approximately 0.5% of all deliveries. The degree of placenta previa may be:

- Complete (internal os covered entirely)
- Partial (portion of internal os covered)
- Marginal (placental edge at cervix or less than 2 cm away)
- Low lying (not a true previa, where the placental edge implants in the lower uterine segment but doesn't reach the cervix)

Box 1 lists the risk factors. The pathophysiology appears to involve endometrial damage, with resulting limitation of healthy uterine tissue for implantation.

The hallmark symptom is painless vaginal bleeding, presumably initiated by development of the lower uterine segment. Usually, this occurs by 29 to 30 weeks of gestation, although in approximately 33% of cases, there is no bleeding until labor. The first bleed may be self-limited, but rebleeding complicates approximately 60% of cases. The diagnosis is often made in the absence of symptoms on routine ultrasound. The incidence of placenta previa is 5% to 10% in mid-gestation; this resolves in most cases with development of the lower uterine segment (*placental migration*). When asymptomatic, expectant management is appropriate, although vaginal precautions after 28 weeks' gestation may be advised.

When a patient presents with third-trimester bleeding, speculum exams are contraindicated until placenta previa is ruled out. The most accurate method of diagnosis is transvaginal ultrasound, which is safe in experienced hands; transperineal or transabdominal ultrasound carry greater risks of false-positive and false-negative results.

Observation in the hospital is recommended following a bleed, during which time approximately 50% of patients will deliver. Steroids are indicated for enhancement of fetal lung maturation. Tocolysis can be administered if the mother and fetus are stable, preferably with magnesium sulfate to minimize cardiovascular effects. Outpatient management is acceptable if bleeding ceases, as long as the patient is compliant and has ready access to a hospital. Serial ultrasound assessment is recommended because there is an increased risk of intrauterine growth restriction. Transfusion should be offered to maintain hemoglobin greater than 10 mg/dL.

Urgent delivery by cesarean section is indicated when there is ongoing maternal hemorrhage or evidence of fetal compromise. In the stable patient, a planned cesarean section can be performed at 35 to 36 weeks, generally after an amniocentesis is performed to confirm fetal lung maturity. Vaginal delivery is preferable in the setting of fetal demise; it may be attempted if delivery is imminent, or with marginal previa, although a *double setup* for emergent cesarean section is advised.

Placenta previa predisposes to postpartum hemorrhage, either from atony of the lower uterine segment or inability to remove the placenta because of absence of the decidua basalis. The most common form of this latter condition is placenta accreta, where the trophoblast

16

BOX 1	**Risk Factors for Placenta Previa**

- Advancing maternal age
- Ethnic background (increased in Asians)
- Multiparity
- Multiple gestation
- Previous curettage
- Prior cesarean section (increases with number of sections)
- Prior placenta previa
- Smoking

adheres to the myometrium. Less common forms include placenta increta (the trophoblast invades the myometrium) and placenta percreta (trophoblast invades uterine serosa and/or adjacent organs). The primary risk factor for placenta accreta is the number of previous cesarean sections, with an incidence approaching 40% in patients with two prior cesarean sections and a placenta previa. Other risk factors include age, parity, and history of curettage. Color Doppler ultrasound and magnetic resonance imaging (MRI) are helpful but not always definitive for diagnosis. If placenta accreta is suspected, preparations can be made for scheduled delivery with trained personnel and blood products available. At delivery, the placenta should be left in place if a cleavage plane cannot be developed easily. Cesarean–hysterectomy is often required for hemostasis, although conservative management, including preoperative and intraoperative selective embolization and/or use of methotrexate, has been reported. With placenta percreta, bladder invasion may require cystoscopy and urologic repair.

Vasa Previa

Vasa previa is a rare condition (estimated 1 in 2500 deliveries) in which fetal blood vessels cross over the membranes in advance of the presenting part. This is most often associated with velamentous insertion of the umbilical cord (vessels reach the placenta after coursing through the membranes rather than by direct insertion); Box 2 lists the risk factors. Vasa previa carries a profound risk of fetal mortality from exsanguination, particularly at the time of membrane rupture (fetal blood volume at term is approximately 250 mL). Even in the absence of bleeding, vessel compression may result in compromise of the fetal circulation.

Signs include hemorrhage, as well as fetal heart rate abnormalities. A high index of suspicion is required, and advances in imaging techniques (color Doppler, transvaginal ultrasound) make prenatal diagnosis possible. If there is unexplained bleeding, an Apt test or Kleihauer-Betke test can identify fetal red blood cells. If the diagnosis of vasa previa is strongly suspected at term, or if hemorrhage is significant, prompt cesarean delivery is recommended, followed by neonatal resuscitation.

Uterine Rupture

Most often reported following prior cesarean section, uterine rupture can also occur in an unscarred uterus

---

BOX 2   **Risk Factors for Vasa Previa**

- Bilobed placenta
- In vitro fertilization
- Low-lying placenta
- Multiple pregnancy
- Succenturiate lobe
- Velamentous insertion of umbilical cord

BOX 3   **Uterine Rupture**

Risk factors
Previous cesarean section (especially classical)
Use of oxytocin, prostaglandins, or misoprostol
Multiparity
Midforceps application
Breech version/extraction
Placental abruption
Shoulder dystocia
Placenta percreta
Müllerian duct anomalies
History of pelvic radiation

Differential diagnoses
Appendicitis
Biliary colic
Pancreatitis
Peptic ulcer disease
Intestinal obstruction
Ovarian torsion
Placental abruption
Urinary tract disorders

(1 in 8000 to 1 in 15,000 deliveries). This phenomenon implies complete separation of the uterine wall (as compared to uterine dehiscence), with or without expulsion of the fetus. Box 3 lists risk factors and differential diagnoses.

Common signs and symptoms include abdominal pain/tenderness and vaginal bleeding; additional complaints include epigastric or shoulder pain, abdominal distention, and constipation. The fetal tracing may show sudden variable decelerations or abrupt and prolonged bradycardia, often accompanied by recession of the presenting part. Maternal and fetal morbidity and mortality are high, particularly with delayed diagnosis. Treatment is urgent cesarean delivery, with repair of the uterus and/or hysterectomy as needed. Repeat cesarean section is advised in the future because of the risk for recurrence.

Placental Abruption

Abruption of the placenta, or separation of the normally implanted placenta before birth, complicates 1% to 2% of pregnancies. Bleeding into the decidua basalis, with subsequent separation of varying amounts of placental tissue from the endometrium, may result in fetal compromise and/or demise. The exact pathophysiology is unclear. Box 4 lists the risk factors.

Vaginal bleeding in the second half of pregnancy is assumed to be caused by placental abruption, once placenta previa and other rare causes are ruled out. Concealed hemorrhage, present in 10% to 20% of cases, can complicate the diagnosis. Abdominal pain, back pain, uterine contractions (often described as low amplitude, high frequency), hypertonus, uterine tenderness, and/or idiopathic premature labor may be present. While ultrasound can identify placenta previa, it cannot be relied upon to definitively diagnose abruption, as clot is sonographically visible in less than 50% of cases. The differential diagnoses include uterine rupture, appendicitis, and chorioamnionitis, as well as other causes of abdominal pain.

Most commonly, bleeding is not profuse and, if the episode is self-limited, expectant management of a

---

BOX 4   Risk Factors for Placental Abruption

- Chorioamnionitis
- Cocaine use
- Ethnic background (highest in blacks)
- Hypertension
- Male fetal gender
- Multiple gestation
- Parity
- Polyhydramnios (rapid decompression at membrane rupture and/or therapeutic amniocentesis)
- Preterm premature rupture of membranes
- Previous cesarean section
- Smoking
- Trauma, including domestic violence
- Unexplained elevated second trimester alpha-fetoprotein
- Uterine anomalies/short umbilical cord

---

preterm gestation includes observation, serial fetal growth assessment, fetal well-being testing, and steroid therapy to accelerate fetal lung maturation. With ongoing significant blood loss, stabilization of the mother, fetal assessment, and laboratory evaluation are indicated. Coagulopathy is rare in the absence of fetal demise. If tocolysis is required, magnesium sulfate is preferred, as β-sympathomimetics may mask maternal cardiovascular decompensation.

Vaginal delivery is appropriate if mother and fetus are stable. Amniotomy may decrease extravasation of blood into the myometrium by head compression. Not uncommonly, effacement will precede dilatation; oxytocin (Pitocin) is acceptable for labor dysfunction. In the event of an intrauterine demise, vaginal delivery is preferred. Acute hemorrhage requires immediate cesarean delivery, with blood and coagulation factor replacement as needed.

Potential complications of abruption include hemorrhagic shock, disseminated intravascular coagulation (unlikely unless there is greater than 2000 mL blood loss and/or fetal demise), ischemic necrosis of maternal organs (especially kidney), and Couvelaire uterus (extravasation of blood into uterine muscle). Recurrence is approximately 5% to 15%, increasing with each subsequent event. There are no known preventive measures other than correcting modifiable risk factors.

Hypertensive Disorders of Pregnancy

Method of
David G. Weismiller, MD

Hypertension is the most common medical disorder during pregnancy. It occurs in 6% to 8% of pregnancies and contributes significantly to stillbirths and to neonatal morbidity and mortality. Hypertensive disorders during pregnancy are the second leading cause of maternal mortality in the United States after thromboembolism, accounting for almost 15% of such deaths. For this reason, strategies to diagnose, prevent, treat, and reduce the risk for hypertensive disorders of pregnancy receive considerable attention.

Classification of the Hypertensive Disorders of Pregnancy

The most important factor to consider in classifying disease in which blood pressure rises abnormally in pregnancy is whether the hypertensive disorder antedates the pregnancy or whether it is a potentially more ominous disease peculiar to pregnancy: preeclampsia. Elevated blood pressure is the cardinal pathophysiologic feature in chronic hypertension, whereas in preeclampsia, increased blood pressure is important primarily because it signals the underlying disorder and is a potential cause of maternal morbidity.

According to the National High Blood Pressure Education Program, increased blood pressure in pregnancy is divided into four main categories:

- Preeclampsia-eclampsia
- Chronic hypertension
- Preeclampsia superimposed on chronic hypertension
- Gestational hypertension (transient or chronic)

PREECLAMPSIA-ECLAMPSIA

Preeclampsia-eclampsia usually occurs after 20 weeks of gestation. The rate of preeclampsia ranges from 2% to 7% in healthy nulliparous women and is substantially higher in women with twin gestation (14%) and those with previous preeclampsia (18%). The disorder may occur earlier with trophoblastic diseases such as hydatidiform mole or hydrops. Preeclampsia is determined by increased blood pressure accompanied by proteinuria in a woman who is normotensive before 20 weeks (Box 1). The finding of proteinuria usually correlates with 30 mg/dL (1+ dipstick) or greater in a random urine determination with no evidence of urinary tract infection. Because of the discrepancy between random protein determinations and 24-hour urine protein

---

BOX 1 **Criteria for Diagnosis of Preeclampsia**

- Blood pressure of 140 mm Hg systolic or higher or 90 mm Hg diastolic or higher that occurs after 20 weeks of gestation in a woman with previously normal blood pressure.
- Proteinuria, defined as urinary excretion of 0.3 g protein or higher in a 24-hour urine specimen.

---

in preeclampsia (which may be either higher or lower), it is recommended that the diagnosis be based on a 24-hour urine, if at all possible, or a timed collection corrected for creatinine excretion, if a 24-hour urine is not feasible.

In the absence of proteinuria, preeclampsia is highly suspect when increased blood pressure is accompanied by the symptoms of headache, blurred vision, and abdominal pain or when it is accompanied by abnormal laboratory tests, specifically low platelet counts and abnormal liver enzymes. Diastolic blood pressure is determined by the disappearance of sound (Korotkoff 5). Gestational blood pressure elevation should be defined on the basis of at least two determinations. No randomized controlled trial evidence supports the use of ambulatory blood pressure monitoring during pregnancy.

In the past, an increase of 30 mm Hg systolic or 15 mm Hg diastolic blood pressure was used as a diagnostic criterion in preeclampsia, even when absolute values were below 140/90 mm Hg. But this diagnostic criterion is not included in the classification criteria set forth by the National High Blood Pressure Education Program. The only available evidence demonstrates that women in this group are not likely to suffer increased adverse outcomes. Still, some experts believe that women who have a rise of 30 mm Hg systolic or 15 mm Hg diastolic blood pressure warrant close observation, especially if proteinuria and hyperuricemia of 6 mg/dL or more are also present. Edema is also removed as a marker in hypertension schemes because it occurs in too many normal pregnant women to be discriminant.

Eclampsia is the occurrence of seizures that cannot be attributed to other causes in a woman with preeclampsia. Up to 40% of eclamptic seizures occur before delivery. Approximately 16% occur more than 48 hours after delivery.

Preeclampsia always presents potential danger to the mother and the fetus. As the certainty of the diagnosis of preeclampsia increases, the requirements for careful assessment and consideration for delivery also increase (Table 1).

CHRONIC HYPERTENSION

Chronic hypertension is defined as hypertension that is present and observable before week 20 of gestation, with hypertension defined as a blood pressure of 140 mm Hg systolic or 90 mm Hg diastolic or greater. Hypertension diagnosed for the first time during pregnancy that does not resolve postpartum is also classified as chronic hypertension.

TABLE 1 **Findings That Increase Certainty of Diagnosis of Preeclampsia Syndrome**

Findings	Value
Blood pressure	160 mm Hg or more systolic or 110 mm Hg or more diastolic.
Proteinuria	2.0 g or more in a 24-hour urine collection (2^+ or 3^+ g on qualitative examination). The proteinuria should occur for the first time in pregnancy and regress after delivery.
Serum creatinine	Greater than 1.2 mg/dL unless known to be previously elevated.
Platelet count	Less than 100,000 cells/mm³ and/or evidence of microangiopathic hemolytic anemia (with increased lactic acid dehydrogenase).
Hepatic enzymes	Elevated ALT or AST.
Central nervous system	Persistent headache or other cerebral or visual disturbances.
Abdomen	Persistent epigastric pain.

Abbreviations: ALT = alanine aminotransferase; AST = aspartate aminotransferase.

SUPERIMPOSED PREECLAMPSIA

Superimposed preeclampsia complicates almost 25% of pregnancies in women with chronic hypertension. The prognosis for mother and fetus is worse than with either condition alone. The incidence of superimposed preeclampsia is even higher in women who have underlying renal insufficiency, chronic hypertension that has been present 4 or more years, or who have had a hypertensive disorder complicate a previous pregnancy. Distinguishing superimposed preeclampsia from worsening chronic hypertension is a challenge (Table 2).

GESTATIONAL HYPERTENSION

Gestational hypertension refers to blood pressure elevation without proteinuria that is detected for the first time after midpregnancy. The hypertension may be accompanied by other signs of the preeclampsia syndrome, which impacts management. The final determination that the woman does not have the preeclampsia syndrome is made retrospectively postpartum. Gestational hypertension is subdivided into two types. If preeclampsia has not developed and blood pressure has returned to normal by 12 weeks postpartum, the diagnosis of transient hypertension of pregnancy is assigned. If the blood pressure elevation persists, the woman is diagnosed as having chronic hypertension.

Pathophysiology of Preeclampsia

Preeclampsia is a syndrome with well-defined maternal and fetal manifestations. The maternal disease is characterized by vasospasm, activation of the coagulation

Rakel and Bope: *Conn's Current Therapy 2006.*

TABLE 2 Findings That Increase Certainty of Diagnosis of Preeclampsia Superimposed Upon Chronic Hypertension

Finding	Value
Proteinuria	New-onset proteinuria (in women with hypertension and no proteinuria prior to 20 weeks' gestation) defined as the urinary excretion of 300 mg protein or greater in a 24-hour specimen or in women with hypertension and proteinuria before 20 weeks' gestation or sudden increase in proteinuria
Blood pressure	Sudden increase in blood pressure in a woman whose hypertension has been previously well controlled
Platelet count	Thrombocytopenia with a platelet count of less than 100,000 cells/mm^3
Hepatic enzymes	Increase in ALT or AST to abnormal levels

Abbreviations: ALT = alanine aminotransferase; AST = aspartate aminotransferase.

BOX 2   Risk Factors for Preeclampsia

Pregnancy-Associated Factors
- Chromosomal abnormalities
- Hydatidiform mole
- Hydrops fetalis
- Multifetal pregnancy
- Oocyte denotation or donor insemination
- Structural congenital abnormalities
- Urinary tract infection

Maternal-Specific Factors
- Age greater than 35 years
- Age less than 20 years
- Black race
- Family history of preeclampsia
- Nulliparity
- Preeclampsia in a previous pregnancy
- Specific medical conditions: gestational diabetes mellitus, type I diabetes, obesity, chronic hypertension, renal disease, thrombophilias
- Stress

Paternal-Specific Factors
- First-time father
- Previously fathered a preeclamptic pregnancy in another woman

16

system, and derangement in many humoral and autacoid systems that are associated with volume and blood pressure control. Oxidative stress and inflammatory-like responses may also be important in the pathophysiology of this syndrome. The pathologic changes are primarily ischemic in nature and affect the placenta, brain, liver, and kidney. Several of the so-called nonhypertensive complications can be life-threatening, even in the face of otherwise mild blood pressure elevations. Risk factors for preeclampsia are related to medical conditions, such as antiphospholipid antibody syndrome and nephropathy, or they may be related to the pregnancy itself or may be specific to the mother or father of the fetus (Box 2).

The etiology of most cases of hypertension during pregnancy, particularly preeclampsia, remains unknown. Many consider the placenta the pathogenic focus for all manifestations of preeclampsia because delivery is the only definitive cure of the disease. Much research centers on the changes in the maternal blood vessels that supply blood to the placenta. Discoveries on how alterations in the immune response at the maternal interface might lead to preeclampsia address the link between placental and maternal disease. A nonclassical human leukocyte antigen (HLA), HLA G is expressed in normal placental tissue and may play a role in modulating the maternal immune response to the immunologically foreign placenta. Additional evidence for alterations in immunity in pathogenesis includes the disease's prominence in nulliparous gestations with subsequent normal pregnancies, a decreased prevalence after heterologous blood transfusions, long cohabitation before successful conception, and observed pathologic changes in the placental vasculature in preeclampsia that resemble allograft rejection.

BLOOD PRESSURE CHANGES

Women with preeclampsia typically do not develop frank hypertension until the second half of gestation, but vasoconstrictor influences may be present earlier. Alterations in vascular reactivity may be detected by gestational week 20, and numerous surveys suggest that women destined to develop preeclampsia have slightly higher "normal" blood pressure (e.g., diastolic levels more than 70 mm Hg) as early as the second trimester, confirmed by ambulatory blood pressure monitoring techniques. Blood pressure normalizes postpartum, usually within the first few days of the puerperium, but may take as long as 2 to 4 weeks, especially in severe cases.

CARDIAC CHANGES

Typically the heart is not affected in preeclampsia. The decrements in cardiac performance represent a normally contracting ventricle against a markedly increased afterload.

RENAL CHANGES

The renal lesion characteristic of preeclampsia is termed *glomerular endotheliosis*. The glomeruli become enlarged and swollen. Both glomerular filtration rate and renal blood flow decrease in preeclampsia, leading to a decrease in filtration fraction. Because renal function normally rises 35% to 50% during pregnancy, creatinine levels in women with preeclampsia may still be below the upper limits of normal for pregnancy (0.8 mg/dL). Fractional urate clearance decreases, producing hyperuricemia. Although an elevated serum uric acid level (6.0 mg/dL) represents a useful confirmatory test for the diagnosis of preeclampsia, it has very poor predictive value among patients without preexisting hypertension. But when the patient has chronic hypertension, the serum uric acid level may be of some value. One investigator has reported that a serum uric acid level of 5.5 mg/dL or greater could identify women with an increased likelihood of having superimposed preeclampsia, which is an important marker of preeclampsia. Proteinuria may appear late in the clinical course and tends to be nonselective. Preeclampsia is associated with hypocalciuria, in contrast with the increased urinary calcium excretion observed during normal pregnancy. Even when edema is marked, plasma volume is lower than that of normal gestation, and there is evidence of hemoconcentration, believed to be caused, in part, by extravasation of albumin into the interstitium. Oliguria, commonly defined as less than 500 mL in 24 hours, also may occur, secondary to the hemoconcentration and decreased renal blood flow.

COAGULATION SYSTEM CHANGES

Thrombocytopenia is the most common hematologic abnormality in preeclampsia. Circulating fibrin degradation products occasionally may be elevated, and unless the disease is accompanied by placental abruption, plasma fibrinogen levels are unaffected. Platelet counts below 100,000 cells/mm^3 signal serious disease, and if delivery is delayed, levels may continue to fall precipitously. The cause of thrombocytopenia is unclear.

HEPATIC CHANGES

Liver damage accompanying preeclampsia may range from mild hepatocellular necrosis with serum enzyme abnormalities (aminotransferase and lactate dehydrogenase) to the ominous hemolysis, elevated liver enzymes, and low platelet count (HELLP) syndrome, with markedly elevated enzyme levels and even subcapsular bleeding or hepatic rupture. HELLP represents serious disease and is associated with significant maternal morbidity. A disproportionate elevation of lactate dehydrogenase (LDH) levels in serum may be a sign of hemolysis.

CENTRAL NERVOUS SYSTEM CHANGES

Eclampsia is the convulsive phase of preeclampsia and remains a significant cause of maternal mortality. Other central nervous system manifestations are headache and visual disturbances, including blurred vision, scotomata, and, rarely, cortical blindness. Focal neurologic signs occasionally develop, which should prompt radiologic investigation.

Clinical Considerations

Expectant mothers with hypertension are predisposed to the development of potentially lethal complications, notably abruptio placentae, disseminated intravascular coagulation, cerebral hemorrhage, hepatic failure, and acute renal failure. The clinical spectrum of preeclampsia ranges from mild to severe forms. In most women, progression through this spectrum is slow, and the disorder may never proceed beyond mild preeclampsia. In others, the disease progresses more rapidly, changing from mild to severe in days or weeks. In the most serious cases, progression may be rapid and fulminant, with mild disease progressing to severe preeclampsia or eclampsia.

DIAGNOSIS

Decisions regarding hospitalization and delivery that have significant impact on maternal and fetal health are often based on whether the patient is believed to have preeclampsia or a more benign hypertensive disorder of pregnancy, such as chronic or gestational hypertension.

The period in gestation when hypertension is first documented is helpful to consider in determining the correct diagnosis. Documentation of hypertension before conception, or before gestational week 20, favors a diagnosis of chronic hypertension (either essential or secondary). High blood pressure presenting at midpregnancy (weeks 20 to 28) may be caused by early preeclampsia (rare before 24 weeks), transient hypertension, or unrecognized chronic hypertension. Blood pressure normally falls in the initial trimesters, and this physiologic decrement may even be exaggerated in patients with essential hypertension, masking the diagnosis in pregnancy. Hypertension may be noted later in pregnancy, however, as part of the normal third trimester rise in blood pressure or when superimposed preeclampsia occurs.

LABORATORY EVALUATION

Laboratory tests recommended to diagnose or manage hypertension in pregnancy serve primarily to distinguish preeclampsia from either chronic or transient hypertension. They are also useful in assessing the severity of disease, particularly in the case of preeclampsia, which is usually associated with laboratory abnormalities that deviate significantly from those of normal pregnant women. The same measurements are usually normal in women with uncomplicated chronic or transient hypertension. Efforts to identify an ideal screening or predictive test for preeclampsia are not successful to date. At present, no single screening test is considered reliable and cost effective for predicting preeclampsia. Numerous clinical, biophysical, and biochemical tests are proposed for the prediction or early detection of preeclampsia. Most of these tests suffer from poor sensitivity and poor predictive values, although this situation may be changing. Low levels of placental growth factor (PGF) predict subsequent development of preeclampsia. Decreased urinary PGF at mid-gestation is strongly associated with subsequent early development of preeclampsia.

The laboratory evaluation of hypertensive disorders can be approached by classifying women into one of three categories:

1. High-risk patients presenting with normal blood pressure
2. Patients presenting with hypertension before gestation week 20
3. Patients presenting with hypertension after midpregnancy

High-Risk Patients Presenting With Normal Blood Pressure

Pregnant women whose gestations are considered high risk for preeclampsia benefit from a database of laboratory tests performed in early gestation. Those who are at high risk for preeclampsia include women who have a history of high blood pressure before conception or in a previous gestation (especially before week 34); women with diabetes, collagen vascular disease, underlying renal vascular disease, or renal parenchymal disease; and women with a multifetal pregnancy.

Tests that by later comparison assist in establishing an early diagnosis of preeclampsia (pure or superimposed) include hematocrit and platelet count as well as serum creatinine and uric acid levels. Observation of 1+ protein by routine urine analysis, documented by a clean-catch specimen, should be followed by a 24-hour collection for measurement of protein, as well as creatinine content, to determine accuracy of collection and to permit calculation of the creatinine clearance. High-risk patients require accurate dating and assessment of fetal growth. If circumstances are not optimal for clinical dating, sonographic dates should be established as early in the pregnancy as possible. A baseline sonogram for evaluating fetal growth should be considered at 25 to 28 weeks in these circumstances.

Patients Presenting With Hypertension Before Gestation Week 20

Most women presenting with hypertension before gestation week 20 have (or will develop) essential hypertension. Women with hypertension should be evaluated before pregnancy to define the severity of their hypertension and to plan for potential lifestyle changes that a pregnancy may require. As recommended by the Joint National Committee on Prevention, Detection, Evaluation, and Treatment of High Blood Pressure (JNC VII Report), the diagnosis should be confirmed by multiple measurements and may incorporate home or other out-of-office blood pressure readings. If hypertension is confirmed, and particularly if it is severe (stage 3, systolic pressure of 180 mm Hg or more and diastolic pressure of 110 mm Hg or more), a woman should be evaluated for potentially reversible causes.

Patients Presenting With Hypertension After Midpregnancy

Table 3 summarizes the recommended laboratory tests in the evaluation of women with hypertension after midpregnancy and the rationale for testing them

TABLE 3 Laboratory Evaluation and Rationale for Women Who Develop Hypertension After Midpregnancy

Test	Rationale
Hemoglobin or hematocrit	Hemoconcentration supports the diagnosis of preeclampsia, and it is an indicator of severity. Note that values may be decreased if hemolysis accompanies the syndrome.
Platelet count	Thrombocytopenia suggests severe preeclampsia.
Quantification of protein excretion	Gestational hypertension with proteinuria should be considered preeclampsia (pure or superimposed), until it is proved otherwise.
Serum creatinine level	Abnormal or rising serum creatinine levels, especially in association with oliguria, suggest severe preeclampsia.
Serum uric acid level	Increased serum uric acid levels suggest the diagnosis of preeclampsia (>6.0 mg/dL).
Serum transaminase levels	Rising serum transaminase values suggest severe preeclampsia with hepatic involvement.
Serum albumin, lactic acid dehydrogenase, blood smear, and coagulation profile	For women with severe disease, these values indicate the extent of endothelial leak (hypoalbuminemia), presence of hemolysis (lactic acid-dehydrogenase level increase, schizocytosis, spherocytosis), and possible coagulopathy, including thrombocytopenia.

biweekly or more often, if clinical circumstances lead to hospitalization of the patient. Such tests help distinguish preeclampsia from chronic and transient hypertension and are useful in assessing disease progression and severity. Note that in women with preeclampsia, one or more laboratory abnormalities may be present, even when blood pressure elevation is minimal.

Prevention of Preeclampsia

Preventing preeclampsia is a challenge because of the limited knowledge of its etiology. During the past two decades, numerous clinical reports and randomized trials described the use of various methods to reduce the rate and/or severity of preeclampsia. Table 4 summarizes current opinion and data on the prevention of preeclampsia. Prevention focuses on identifying women at higher risk and conducting close clinical and laboratory monitoring, to recognize the disease process in its early stages. Although these measures do not prevent preeclampsia, they may be helpful for preventing some adverse maternal and fetal sequelae.

TABLE 4 Effectiveness of Agents in Prevention of Preeclampsia

Agent	Prevention
Low-dose aspirin prophylaxis	Minimal to no reduction in the incidence of preeclampsia. The prevailing opinion is that women without risk factors do not benefit from treatment. Overall, administration of low-dose aspirin to women at risk leads to a 19% reduction in the risk of developing preeclampsia. On average, for every 69 women treated, 1 case is prevented. Starting aspirin before 12 weeks and/or using higher doses cannot be recommended for clinical practice until more information is available about safety. As the reductions in risk are small to moderate, relatively large numbers of women need to be treated to prevent a single adverse outcome.
Calcium supplementation	No data indicate that dietary supplementation with calcium prevents preeclampsia in low-risk women in the United States. Randomized trials of calcium supplementation in women considered at high risk of gestational hypertension (teenagers, previous preeclampsia, women with increased sensitivity to angiotensin II, preexisting hypertension) and in communities with low dietary calcium intake (mean intake equals 900 mg per day) demonstrate significant reductions in incidence of preeclampsia.
Magnesium supplementation	Prophylactic magnesium is not beneficial in preventing preeclampsia.
Zinc supplementation	No benefit in preventing preeclampsia.
Fish oil supplementation	No reduction in the incidence of preeclampsia.
Antioxidant therapy (vitamin C[1] and vitamin E[1])	Limited data show some promise in preventing preeclampsia.
Salt restriction	No benefit in preventing preeclampsia.
Diuretic therapy[1]	No benefit in preventing preeclampsia.

[1]Not FDA approved for the indication.

Management of Hypertensive Disorders of Pregnancy

Three factors underlie any management scheme in hypertension and pregnancy. First, delivery is always appropriate therapy for the mother but may not be for the fetus. Second, the pathophysiologic changes of severe preeclampsia indicate that poor perfusion is the major factor leading to maternal physiologic derangement and increased perinatal morbidity and mortality. Third, the pathogenic changes of preeclampsia are present long before clinical diagnostic criteria are manifest.

For maternal health, the goal of therapy is to prevent eclampsia as well as other severe complications of preeclampsia. If there is a rationale for management other than delivery, it is to palliate the maternal condition to allow fetal maturation and cervical ripening.

ANTICONVULSIVE THERAPY

Anticonvulsive therapy is usually indicated either to prevent recurrent convulsions in women with eclampsia or to prevent convulsions in women with preeclampsia. There is universal consensus that women with eclampsia should receive anticonvulsive therapy. Several randomized studies indicate that parenteral magnesium sulfate reduces the frequency of eclampsia more effectively than phenytoin (Dilantin). Parenteral magnesium sulfate is given during labor and delivery and for variable durations postpartum. There is no clear agreement concerning the use of prophylactic magnesium for women with preeclampsia. Although parenteral magnesium sulfate should be given peripartum to women with severe preeclampsia, its benefits with mild gestational hypertension or preeclampsia remain unclear.

Women with eclampsia require prompt intervention. When an eclamptic seizure occurs, the woman should be medically stabilized. First, it is important to control convulsions and prevent their recurrence with intravenous or intramuscular magnesium sulfate. One protocol is a 4- to 6-g loading dose diluted in 100 mL fluid and administered intravenously for 15 to 20 minutes, followed by 2 g per hour as a continuous intravenous infusion.

ANTIHYPERTENSIVE THERAPY

Therapy in Acute Hypertension

Antihypertensive therapy is indicated when blood pressure is dangerously high or rises suddenly in women with preeclampsia, especially intrapartum. Pharmacologic treatment with antihypertensives can be withheld as long as maternal pressure is only mildly elevated. Some experts treat persistent diastolic blood pressure of 105 mm Hg or above. Others withhold treatment until the diastolic blood pressure reaches 110 mm Hg. Table 5 summarizes the medications used to treat acute elevations in blood pressure. The goal of blood pressure reduction in emergency situations should be a gradual reduction to the normal range.

Rakel and Bope: *Conn's Current Therapy 2006.*

TABLE 5 Medications to Treat Acute Severe Hypertensive Crises in Pregnancy

	Route of dose	Pharmacologic agent	Administration notes
Arterial vasodilator (hydralazine: e.g., Apresoline)	IV or IM	5 mg over 1-2 min	After 20 min, subsequent doses are dictated by initial response; once desired response, repeat as necessary (usually 3 h)
β-Blockers (labetalol: e.g., Normodyne or Trandate)	IV	20-40 mg bolus or 1 mg/kg infusion (max 220 mg)	If effect is suboptimal to initial 20 mg IV, give 40 mg 10 min later and 80 mg every 10 min for additional two doses. Avoid in women with asthma and in those with congestive heart failure (CHF).
Calcium antagonists (nifedipine: e.g., Adalat, Procardia)	PO	10 mg PO and repeat in 30 min, if necessary	The JNC VII recommends rapidly acting nifedipine not be used for treating hypertension or hypertensive emergencies.
Sodium nitroprusside (Nipride)	IV	0.25 μg/kg/min to a maximum of 5 μg/kg/min	After failure of hydralazine, nifedipine, and labetalol. Fetal cyanide poisoning may occur if used more than 4 h.

Abbreviations: IM = intramuscularly; IV = intravenously; JNC VII = Joint National Committee on Prevention, Detection, Evaluation, and Treatment of High Blood Pressure; PO = by mouth.

Therapy in Chronic Hypertension

The role of antihypertensive therapy for pregnant women with mild to moderate chronic hypertension (stage 1 or 2 hypertension, defined as systolic blood pressure of 140 to 179 mm Hg or diastolic blood pressure of 90 to 109) is unclear. Among women with stage 1 to 2 pre-existing essential hypertension and normal renal function, most pregnancies have good maternal and neonatal outcomes. Because there is no immediate need to lower blood pressure, the rationale for treatment is that it will prevent or delay progression to more severe disease, thereby benefiting the woman and/or her infant and reducing consumption of health service resources. In addition to reducing blood pressure, these drugs are believed to reduce the risk of preterm delivery and placental abruption and improve fetal growth. A wide variety of drugs are advocated, and each group has different potential side affects and adverse effects (Table 6). More importantly, these women are candidates for nonpharmacologic therapy because to date no evidence indicates that pharmacologic treatment results in improved neonatal outcomes. Because blood pressure usually falls during the first half of pregnancy, hypertension may be easier to control with less or no medication.

The value of continued administration of antihypertensive medications to pregnant women with chronic hypertension continues to be debatable. Although it may be beneficial for the mother with hypertension to reduce her blood pressure, lower pressure may impair uteroplacental perfusion and thereby interfere with fetal development. On the basis of available data, some centers currently manage women with chronic hypertension by stopping antihypertensive medications under close observation. In patients who have had hypertension for several years, show evidence of target organ damage, or take multiple antihypertensive agents, medications may be tapered on the basis of blood pressure readings, but medications should be continued if they are needed to control blood pressure. The end point for reinstituting treatment includes exceeding threshold blood pressure levels of 150 to 160 mm Hg systolic or 100 to 110 mm Hg diastolic or the presence of target organ damage. Methyldopa (Aldomet) is preferred by most practitioners. Women who are well controlled on antihypertensive therapy before pregnancy may be kept on the same agents during pregnancy, with the exception of angiotensin-converting enzyme inhibitors and angiotensin II receptor antagonists.

For women with severe hypertension (stage 3 hypertension, usually defined as 160 to 170 mm Hg or more systolic blood pressure or 110 mm Hg or more diastolic blood pressure), there is a risk of direct arterial damage, so antihypertensive medications are indicated to lower blood pressure (see Table 6). The most effective antihypertensive drug is unclear.

Fetal Assessment

FETAL ASSESSMENT IN PREECLAMPSIA

Nonstress testing (NST), ultrasound assessment of fetal activity and amniotic fluid volume (biophysical profile [BPP]), and fetal movement counts constitute the most common fetal surveillance techniques. Although weekly to biweekly assessment usually suffices, daily testing is appropriate for women with severe preeclampsia who are being managed expectantly. If fetal surveillance (nonreactive NST, oligohydramnios, nonreassuring BPP) indicates possible fetal compromise, the decision to deliver must be significantly weighted by fetal age (Box 3).

FETAL ASSESSMENT IN CHRONIC HYPERTENSION

Much of the increased perinatal morbidity and mortality associated with chronic hypertension can be attributed to superimposed preeclampsia and/or fetal growth restriction. A plan of antepartum fetal assessment is directed by these findings. Thus efforts should be directed toward

16

TABLE 6 Antihypertensive Drug Selection

Drug	Example	Usual dose range in mg/day (daily frequency)	Notes
Central α₂-agonists	Methyldopa (e.g., Aldomet)	250-1000 (2)	First-line therapy on the basis of reports of stable uteroplacental blood flow and fetal hemodynamics
β-Blockers	Labetalol (e.g., Normodyne, Trandate)	200-800 (2)	There is a suggestion that β-blockers prescribed early in pregnancy, specifically atenolol (Tenormin), may be associated with growth restriction. None of these agents are associated to date with any consistent ill effect.
Calcium antagonists	Nifedipine long-acting (e.g., Adalat CC, Procardia XL)	30-60 (1)	Experience is limited, with most reported uses late in pregnancy.
Diuretic	Hydrochlorothiazide (e.g., HydroDIURIL)	12.5-50 mg (1)	Use is controversial; however, if their use is indicated, they are safe and efficacious agents; they can markedly potentiate the response to other antihypertensive agents, and they are not contraindicated, except in settings where uteroplacental perfusion is already reduced (preeclampsia and IUGR).
ACE inhibitors	Captopril (e.g., Capoten)	Contraindicated	Contraindicated because of association with fetal growth restriction, oligohydramnios, neonatal renal failure, and neonatal death. Fetal risks with ACE inhibitors depend on timing and dose.
Angiotensin II receptor antagonists	Losartan (e.g., Cozaar)	Contraindicated	Data are limited. Adverse effects likely to be similar to those reported with ACE inhibitors, and these agents should be avoided.

Abbreviations: ACE = angiotensin-converting enzyme; IUGR = intrauterine growth retardation.

the early detection of superimposed preeclampsia and fetal growth restriction. If these conditions are excluded, extensive fetal antepartum testing is less essential.

Most authorities recommend an initial sonographic assessment of fetal size and dating at week 18 to 20 of gestation. Fetal growth should be carefully assessed thereafter. If this assessment is not possible with usual clinical estimation of fundal height, sonographic assessment should be performed at 28 to 32 weeks and every 4 weeks until term. If growth restriction is evident, fetal well-being should be assessed by nonstress tests or biophysical profiles as usual for the growth-restricted fetus. Similarly, if preeclampsia cannot be excluded, fetal assessment as appropriate for the fetus of a woman with preeclampsia is mandatory. If the infant is normally grown and preeclampsia can be excluded, however, these studies are not indicated.

Maternal Assessment

MATERNAL ASSESSMENT IN PREECLAMPSIA

Antepartum monitoring has two goals. The first goal is to recognize preeclampsia early; the second is to observe progression of the condition, both to prevent maternal

complications by delivery and to determine whether fetal well-being can be safely monitored with the usual intermittent observations. Current clinical management of preeclampsia is directed by overt clinical signs and symptoms. Although rapid weight increase and facial edema may indicate the fluid and sodium retention of preeclampsia, they are neither universally present nor uniquely characteristic of preeclampsia. These signs are, at best, a reason to monitor blood pressure and urinary protein more closely. Early recognition of impending preeclampsia is based primarily on blood pressure increases in the late second and third trimesters. Once blood pressure starts to rise, a repeat examination within 1 to 3 days is recommended. The woman should be evaluated for symptoms suggestive of preeclampsia and undergo laboratory testing for platelet count, renal function, and liver enzymes. Quantification of a 12- to 24-hour urine sample for proteinuria is recommended. The frequency of subsequent observations is determined by the initial observations and the ensuing clinical progression. If the condition appears stable, weekly observations may be appropriate.

MATERNAL ASSESSMENT IN CHRONIC HYPERTENSION

No consensus exists as to the most appropriate fetal surveillance test(s) or interval and timing of testing in

---

BOX 3 Fetal Monitoring in Hypertensive Disorders

- Gestational hypertension—Hypertension only without proteinuria, with normal laboratory test results, and without symptoms.
    1. Perform estimation of fetal growth and amniotic fluid status at diagnosis. If results are normal, repeat testing only if a significant change occurs in maternal condition.
    2. Perform NST at diagnosis. If NST is nonreactive, perform BPP. If BPP value is 8 or if NST is reactive, repeat testing only if a significant change occurs in maternal condition.
- Mild preeclampsia—Mild hypertension plus proteinuria (300 mg or more per 24-hour period), normal platelet count, normal liver enzymes values, and no maternal symptoms.
    1. Perform estimation of fetal growth and amniotic fluid status at diagnosis. If results are normal, repeat testing every 3 weeks.
    2. Perform NST, BPP, or both at diagnosis. If NST is reactive or if BPP value is 8, repeat weekly. Repeat testing immediately if abrupt change in maternal condition occurs.
    3. If estimated fetal weight by ultrasound is less than 10th percentile for gestational age, or if there is oligohydramnios (amniotic fluid index equals or is less than 5 cm), perform testing at least twice weekly.
- Severe preeclampsia—Severe hypertension in association with abnormal proteinuria; hypertension in association with severe proteinuria (at least 5 g per 24-hour period); presence of multiorgan involvement such as pulmonary edema, seizures, oliguria (less than 500 mL per 24-hour period), thrombocytopenia (platelet count less than 100,000/mm^3), abnormal liver enzymes in association with persistent epigastric or right upper quadrant pain; persistent severe central nervous system symptoms (altered mental status, headaches, blurred vision, or blindness).
    1. Term
        Hospitalize, prevent seizures, control hypertension, and proceed with delivery.
    2. Remote from term
        Provide care in a tertiary-care setting.
        Perform laboratory evaluation and fetal surveillance (as outlined for mild preeclampsia earlier) daily depending on the severity and progression of the disorder.[1]
- Chronic hypertension—Mild hypertension (BP more than 140/90 mm Hg) or severe hypertension (BP equal or more than 180/110 mm Hg) present before the 20th week of pregnancy or hypertension present before pregnancy.
    1. Perform baseline ultrasonography at 18 to 20 weeks and repeat at 28 to 32 weeks of gestation and monthly thereafter until delivery, to monitor fetal growth.
    2. If growth restriction is detected or suspected, monitor fetal status frequently with NST or BPP.[1]
    3. If growth restriction is not present and superimposed preeclampsia is excluded, these tests are not indicated.[1]

---

[1]Not FDA approved for this indication.
Abbreviations: BPP = biophysical profile; NST = nonstress test.

---

women with chronic hypertension. Testing should be individualized, based on clinical judgment and on the severity of disease. There are no conclusive data to address either the benefits or the harms of various monitoring strategies for pregnant women with chronic hypertension. Box 3 lists the current proposed recommendations for antepartum monitoring. When chronic hypertension is complicated by intrauterine growth retardation (IUGR) or preeclampsia, fetal surveillance is warranted.

Indications for Delivery

INDICATIONS FOR DELIVERY IN PREECLAMPSIA-ECLAMPSIA

Delivery is the only definitive treatment for preeclampsia; Box 4 lists some suggested indications for delivery. All women with the diagnosis of preeclampsia should be considered for delivery at 40 weeks' gestation. Delivery may be indicated for women with mild disease and a favorable cervix at 38 weeks' gestation and should be considered in women who have severe preeclampsia beyond 32 to 34 weeks' gestation. Prolonged antepartum management with severe preeclampsia is possible in a select group of women with fetal gestational age between 23 and 32 weeks but should be attempted only at centers equipped to provide close maternal and fetal surveillance. Vaginal delivery is preferable to cesarean delivery, thus avoiding the added stress of surgery to multiple physiologic aberrations. Labor induction should be carried out aggressively once the decision for delivery is made. In a gestation that is remote from term in which delivery is indicated and fetal and maternal conditions are stable enough to permit pregnancy to be prolonged 48 hours, glucocorticoids can be safely administered to accelerate fetal pulmonary maturity.

The patient with eclampsia should be delivered in a timely fashion. Once the patient is stabilized, the method of delivery should depend, in part, on gestational age, fetal presentation, and cervical examination findings.

BOX 4 Indications for Delivery in Preeclampsia

Maternal
- Gestational age ≥38 wk
- Platelet count <100,000 cells/mm^3
- Progressive deterioration in hepatic and/or renal function
- Suspected abruption placentae
- Persistent central nervous system (CNS) manifestations: headaches or visual changes
- Persistent severe gastric pain, nausea, or vomiting

Fetal
- Severe fetal growth restriction
- Nonreassuring fetal testing results
- Oligohydramnios

16

INDICATIONS FOR DELIVERY IN CHRONIC HYPERTENSION

Pregnant women with uncomplicated chronic hypertension of a mild degree generally can be delivered vaginally at term; most have good maternal and neonatal outcomes. Cesarean delivery should be reserved for other obstetric indications. Women with mild hypertension during pregnancy and a prior adverse pregnancy outcome (e.g., stillbirth) may be candidates for earlier delivery after documentation of fetal lung maturity (as long as fetal status is reassuring). Women with severe chronic hypertension during pregnancy most often either deliver prematurely or have to be delivered prematurely for fetal or maternal indications. Delivery should be considered in all women with superimposed severe preeclampsia at or beyond 28 weeks of gestation and in women with mild superimposed preeclampsia at or beyond 37 weeks of gestation. Magnesium sulfate should be used for women with superimposed preeclampsia to prevent seizures.

Postpartum Management

Acute hypertensive changes induced by pregnancy usually dissipate rapidly, within the first several days after delivery. Resolution of hypertension is more rapid in patients with gestational hypertension and may lag in those with preeclampsia, especially those with longer duration of preeclampsia and greater extent of renal impairment. Oral antihypertensive agents may be needed after delivery (see Table 6) to help control maternal blood pressure, particularly for women who were hypertensive

 CURRENT DIAGNOSIS

- The most important factor to consider in classifying disease in which blood pressure rises abnormally in pregnancy is whether the hypertensive disorder antedates the pregnancy or arises during the pregnancy.
- Preeclampsia–eclampsia usually occurs after 20 weeks of gestation. Chronic hypertension is defined as hypertension that is present and observable before the 20th week of gestation.
- Gestational blood pressure elevation is defined as a blood pressure greater than 140 mm Hg systolic or 90 mm Hg diastolic in a woman normotensive before 20 weeks.
- Proteinuria in pregnancy is defined as the urinary excretion of 300 mg protein or greater in a 24-hour specimen.
- Laboratory tests recommended to diagnose or manage hypertension in pregnancy serve primarily to distinguish preeclampsia from either chronic or transient hypertension.
- No single screening test is considered reliable and cost effective for predicting preeclampsia.

 CURRENT THERAPY

- Prevention focuses on identifying women at higher risk and conducting close clinical and laboratory monitoring to recognize the disease process in its early stages.
- Delivery is always appropriate therapy for the mother but may not be for the fetus.
- For maternal health, the goal of therapy is to prevent eclampsia as well as severe complications of preeclampsia. Parenteral magnesium sulfate is given during labor and delivery and for variable durations postpartum to women with eclampsia and severe preeclampsia. Its benefits in mild gestational hypertension or preeclampsia remain unclear.
- Antihypertensive medications are indicated to lower blood pressure for women with severe hypertension, usually defined as 160 to 170 mm Hg or more systolic blood pressure or 110 mm Hg or more diastolic blood pressure.
- Antihypertensive therapy is indicated intrapartum when diastolic blood pressure is persistently 105 to 110 mm Hg or above.
- The goal of blood pressure reduction in emergency situations should be a gradual reduction of blood pressure to the normal range.

before pregnancy. If prepregnancy blood pressures were normal or unknown, it is reasonable to stop oral medication after 3 to 4 weeks and observe the blood pressure at 1- to 2-week intervals for 1 month, then at 3- to 6-month intervals for 1 year. If hypertension recurs, it should be treated. If the abnormalities persist, the pathology will probably be chronic.

Limited data are available on which to base our knowledge of the natural history and pathogenesis of postpartum hypertension. The women who appear to be at greatest risk for postpartum hypertension are those with antenatal preeclampsia, particularly those with higher urinary protein, serum uric acid, and blood urea nitrogen. For previously normotensive women, the risk of postpartum hypertension appears lower. Beyond the postnatal period, it is not known whether women with isolated postpartum hypertension are at increased risk of chronic hypertension.

Risk of Recurrence

Women who have had preeclampsia are more prone to hypertensive complications in subsequent pregnancies. Risk is best established for multiparas with a history of preeclampsia; the magnitude of the recurrence rate increases the earlier the disease manifested during the index pregnancy. The recurrence rate for women with one episode of HELLP is 5%. Recurrence rates are higher for those experiencing preeclampsia as multiparas compared with nulliparous women. Risk is also increased in multiparas who conceive with a new father, even when their first pregnancy was normotensive, the incidence being intermediate between that of primiparous women and monogamous multiparous women who have not had a preeclamptic pregnancy.

REFERENCES

Abalos E, Duley L, Steyn DW, Henderson-Smart DJ: Antihypertensive drug therapy for mild to moderate hypertension during pregnancy (Cochrane Review). In The Cochrane Library, Issue 4. Chichester, UK, John Wiley, 2004.

Agency for Healthcare Research and Quality: Management of chronic hypertension during pregnancy. Evidence Report/Technology assessment no. 14. AHRQ Publication No. 00-E011. Rockville, Md, Author, 2000.

American College of Obstetricians and Gynecologists: ACOG Practice Bulletin No. 29. Chronic hypertension pregnancy. Obstet Gynecol 2001;98:177-185.

Atallah AN, Hofmeyr GJ, Duley L: Calcium supplementation during pregnancy for preventing hypertensive disorders and related problems (Cochrane Review). In The Cochrane Library, Issue 4. Chichester, UK.: John Wiley, 2004.

Bergel E, Carroli G, Althabe F: Ambulatory versus conventional methods for monitoring blood pressure during pregnancy (Cochrane Review). In The Cochrane Library, Issue 4. Chichester, UK, John Wiley, 2004.

Cunningham FG, Gant NF, Leveno KJ, et al: Hypertensive disorders in pregnancy. In Cunningham FG (ed): Williams Obstetrics, 21st ed. New York, McGraw-Hill, 2001, pp 567-618.

Duley L, Henderson-Smart DJ: Drugs for treatment of very high blood pressure during pregnancy (Cochrane Review). In The Cochrane Library, Issue 4. Chichester, UK, John Wiley, 2004.

Joint National Committee: The Seventh Report of the Joint National Committee on Prevention, Detection, Evaluation, and Treatment of High Blood Pressure (JNC VII). JAMA 2003;289:2560-2571.

Levine RJ, Thadhani RT, Qian C, et al: Urinary placental growth factor and risk of preeclampsia. JAMA 2005;293:77-85.

Lim KH, Friedman SA, Ecker JL, et al: The clinical utility of serum uric acid measurements in hypertensive diseases of pregnancy. Am J Obstet Gynecol 1998;178:1067-1071.

Lucas JL, Leveno KJ, Cunningham FG: A comparison of magnesium sulfate with phenytoin for the prevention of eclampsia. N Engl J Med 1995;333:201-205.

Magee L, Sadeghi S: Prevention and treatment of postpartum hypertension (Cochrane Review). In The Cochrane Library, Issue 4. Chichester, UK, John Wiley, 2004.

Report of the National High Blood Pressure Education Program: Working group report on high blood pressure in pregnancy. Am J Obstet Gynecol 2000;183:S1-S22.

Sibai BM: Prevention of preeclampsia: A big disappointment. Am J Obstet Gynecol 1998;179:1275-1278.

Postpartum Care

Method of
Lisa R. Nash, DO

The postpartum period, or puerperium, is defined as the time needed for the anatomic and physiologic changes of pregnancy to revert to the normal state, lasting from immediately after delivery of the placenta to 6 to 8 weeks following birth.

Rakel and Bope: *Conn's Current Therapy 2006.*

The First 4 to 6 Hours

During the first few hours after delivery, blood pressure (BP), pulse, respiratory rate, temperature, vaginal bleeding, urination, and pain should be monitored every 15 minutes until the patient is stable. Complications that can occur during this time include hypotension, hemorrhage, dyspnea, fever, hypertensive disorders of pregnancy, and urinary retention. Table 1 describes the differential diagnosis and management of these disorders. Table 2 lists oxytocics used to control uterine atony.

Early skin-to-skin contact between the mother and her healthy infant should be ensured to facilitate bonding. Early breast-feeding should be encouraged. The first breast-feeding should occur prior to transfer of the healthy newborn to the nursery in facilities where rooming-in is unavailable.

The First 24 to 72 Hours

Hospitalization generally lasts 24 to 48 hours after an uncomplicated vaginal delivery and up to 72 hours after a typical cesarean delivery. During this time, the following should be addressed:

- Signs and symptoms of potential complications described in Table 1
- Transition of lochia to diminishing reddish-brown discharge
- Fundal height below umbilicus by 24 hours postpartum
- Perineal inflammation or edema and proper perineal hygiene
- Signs and symptoms suggesting deep venous thrombosis
- Resumption of normal ambulation
- Return of bowel/bladder function
- Lactation establishment
- Pain management
- Maternal mood, bonding, and family adjustment
- Contraceptive planning
- Any special requirements such as administration of $Rh_0(D)$ immune globulin (RhoGAM) or rubella vaccine

Symptoms of breast engorgement for mothers who will not breast-feed may be relieved by breast support, ice packs, and nonsteroidal anti-inflammatory medications.

Routine hospital discharge instructions should include direction to contact the physician for any of the following: heavy uterine bleeding; purulent lochia; worsening perineal pain; abdominal or breast pain; redness, warmth, tenderness, or swelling of the lower legs/calves; dysuria; fever (temperature >38°C [100°F]) and/or chills; presence of depression or problems with family adjustment. The patient should be instructed to maintain pelvic rest (nothing in the vagina) for 4 to 6 weeks, and encouraged to resume normal activities and diet.

TABLE 1 Potential Complications of the Immediate Postpartum Period Key Diagnostic and Treatment Considerations

Condition	Differential diagnosis	Management
Hypotension	Vagal response Hypovolemia Reaction to anesthesia Blood loss	Supportive—Trendelenburg position, 500-1000 mL IV crystalloid (normal saline or lactated Ringer's solution) Packed RBCs if related to blood loss
Immediate hemorrhage	Uterine atony (most common)	Table 2*
Delayed hemorrhage (>24 hours after delivery)	Retained placental tissue or blood clots Laceration or hematoma Bleeding disorders (rare) Subinvolution of former placental site Retained placental tissue or blood clots	Evacuation, oxytocics, surgical assistance as appropriate Repair Blood products Table 2* Same as for immediate hemorrhage IV crystalloids and blood products for all etiologies, as appropriate
Dyspnea	Amniotic fluid Embolism Pulmonary embolus Exacerbation of asthma	Respiratory and cardiovascular support, treatment of disseminated intravascular coagulation Antithrombolytics, anticoagulation Nebulized albuterol (Proventil)
Temperature >38°C (100°F) on any 2 d beyond first 24 h OR temperature >39°C (102.2°F) at any time	Endometritis Breast engorgement < 48 h after delivery Septic pelvic thrombophlebitis Other: abdominal wound or perineal infection, UTI, pneumonia, DVT	Clindamycin (Cleocin) 900 mg IV q8h + gentamicin (Garamycin) 100 mg (2 mg/kg) IVPB then 80 mg (1.0-1.5 mg/kg) IVPB q8h OR 2nd/3rd generation cephalosporin ± metronidazole (Flagyl) Ice packs to relieve vascular congestion (note: if >48 hours after delivery, increase breast-feeding and/or pumping) Anticoagulation with heparin
Hypertensive disorders: postpartum preeclampsia and postpartum eclampsia		Magnesium sulfate 4 g slowly IV over 15-30 min, followed by 1 to 3 g/h to keep serum magnesium levels between 4 and 7 mEq/L IV hydralazine (Apresoline) titrated to maintain blood pressure about 130/80 mm Hg
Urinary retention	Trauma of delivery Anesthesia	In-and-out bladder catheterization if spontaneous voiding does not occur within 6 h of delivery

*See Table 2 for oxytocics.
Abbreviations: DVT = deep venous thrombosis; IV = intravenous; IVPB = intravenous piggyback; RBC = red blood cell; q = every; UTI = urinary tract infection.

The 2-Week Newborn Check

The 2-week newborn check provides a good opportunity to reassess the maternal condition. Persistence of any depressive symptoms should be explored. Postpartum *blues* generally resolve by the 10th postpartum day. Although rare, postpartum psychosis generally manifests in this same time period and requires emergent intervention because of the risks of suicide and infanticide. Additional areas to assess include family

TABLE 2 Oxytocics Used for Control of Uterine Atony

Drug	Dose	Maintenance	Contraindications
Oxytocin (Pitocin)	10 U IM or infuse 10 to 40 U in 1 L of IV fluid	IV infusion maintained 1-4 h	None
Methylergonovine (Methergine)	0.2 mg IM	Repeat q 2-4 h	Hypertension, toxemia
PGF$_{2\text{-alpha}}$ carboprost; (Hemabate)	0.25 mg IM	Repeat q 15-90 min	Cardiac or pulmonary disease
PGE$_2$ (Prostin E$_2$)	20 mg suppository inserted into rectum	Repeat q 2-4 h	Hypotension (use PGF$_{2\text{-alpha}}$ instead)

Abbreviations: IM = intramuscular; IV = intravenous; PG = prostaglandin.
Reprinted and adapted from Driscoll CE: Postpartum care. In Rakel RE, Bope ET (eds):Conn's Current Therapy 2004. Copyright © 2003, with permission from Elsevier.

adjustment, breast-feeding progress or problems, urinary incontinence, anticipated time of return to sexual intimacy, and contraceptive plans. If early postpartum complications were experienced, a repeat complete blood count or urinalysis may be indicated.

The Traditional Postpartum Assessment

This assessment is generally scheduled at 6 weeks after delivery. Assessment should include vital signs and physical examination of the thyroid gland, breasts, heart, lungs, abdomen, perineum, pelvis (uterus and ovaries), and lower extremities. Papanicolaou smear should be obtained. Items listed previously for the 2-week assessment should be readdressed.

Postpartum Depression

Postpartum depression is common, occurring in approximately 20% of parturients. Postpartum thyroid dysfunction may present with similar or overlapping symptoms and should be investigated when postpartum depression is suspected. Management may be supportive and could include individual or group psychotherapy or medication. Antidepressant medications acceptable for breast-feeding mothers include sertraline (Zoloft), paroxetine (Paxil), amitriptyline (Elavil), and desipramine (Norpramin).

Family Adjustment

Many women experience transient feelings of vulnerability, inadequacy, and anxiety during the family adjustment that occurs following the addition of a new infant.

CURRENT DIAGNOSIS

- Hypo- or hypertension, tachypnea, fever, excessive vaginal bleeding, inability to void, and excessive abdominal or perineal pain are potential indicators of postpartum complications.
- Return to normal ambulation, bowel and bladder function, establishing lactation, and family adjustment and bonding are tasks for the first 24 to 72 hours postpartum.
- Persistence of depressive symptoms, family adjustment, breast-feeding progress or problems, urinary incontinence, return to sexual intimacy, and contraceptive plans should be addressed at the 2- and 6-week postpartum visits.
- Single parents, adopting parents, and parents experiencing a perinatal loss or the birth of a child with a serious illness or congenital anomaly will likely require additional/special information, services, and resources.

Feelings of attachment may vary initially but usually increase over time. Conflicting emotions elicited by increased responsibility for meeting the demands of the expanded family are common. Significant changes in lifestyle, relationships, and careers often must be made. Assessment of emotional, tangible (financial, household, childcare, etc.), and informational support can identify families who may benefit from referral to additional resources. Men typically have concerns about infant care skills, decreased personal time, changes in the marital relationship, financial security, and the health of their partner and the newborn. Common sibling responses to arrival of the new infant include behaviors that are imitating, aggressive, solicitous, or anxious. Siblings may also withdraw or become more independent. Many authorities recommend that siblings have contact with the mother during the postpartum hospitalization. Allowing siblings to assist (as age permits) in infant care and maintaining separate time for siblings to interact with parents (such as the newborn's nap time) may reduce adjustment problems. Reading children's books about new babies and discussing feelings with siblings are additional options.

Return to Sexual Activity and Contraception

The return to sexual activity and contraception should be discussed. Most couples will resume sexual activity between 6 weeks and 3 months postpartum, although some will do so sooner if perineal discomfort has resolved. The most common barriers to resumption of sexual activity include perineal pain (25%), lack of interest (more common in breast-feeding than bottle-feeding mothers), and fatigue. Anticipatory guidance is helpful for negotiating this time of transition. Breast-feeding mothers should be advised they may require a vaginal lubricant because of the hormonal changes related to breast-feeding.

Postpartum anovulatory infertility persists for 5 weeks in nonlactating women and 8 weeks or more in lactating women. The anticipated time to resume sexual activity and infant feeding plans should be considered in determining the best time to initiate contraceptive measures postpartum.

Contraceptive effects of lactational amenorrhea provide approximately 98% protection in the first 6 months if there is little or no supplemental feeding. Other options for postpartum contraception include

CURRENT THERAPY

- Specific interventions for potential complications of the immediate postpartum period are outlined in Tables 1 and 2.
- The anticipated time to resume sexual activity and infant feeding plans should be considered in the choices of contraceptive method and when to initiate contraceptive measures postpartum.

TABLE 3 Postpartum Contraception

Method	Earliest initiation	Special considerations
Lactational amenorrhea	Immediately postpartum	Additional measures required for any of the following: >6 mo postpartum, supplemental infant feeding initiation or resumption of menses
Natural family planning	Depends on return of normal menstrual cycle	
Barrier methods: condom diaphragm	3 w postpartum (coincident with earliest recommended time to resume sexual activity) 6 w postpartum	Requires full uterine involution AND refitting for patients who previously used this method
Medroxyprogesterone acetate (Depo-Provera)	Prior to hospital discharge	Does not diminish lactation Many physicians delay to 2 wk postpartum because of the potential risk for prolonged bleeding
Progesterone-only pills (Micronor)	Prior to hospital discharge	Same as medroxyprogesterone acetate (Depo-Provera)
Combination oral contraceptives	Non–breast-feeding women: 3 wk postpartum Breast-feeding women: 1 mo after lactation becomes well established	May diminish lactation
Contraceptive patch (Ortho Evra), ring (NuvaRing)	Same as combination oral contraceptives	Same as combination oral contraceptives
Intrauterine device (Mirena, ParaGard)	Within 20 min of delivery of placenta OR 6 wk postpartum	Full uterine involution must be achieved
Sterilization	After delivery/prior to hospital discharge OR 6 wk postpartum	Full uterine involution must be achieved

natural family planning, barrier methods, oral contraceptives, contraceptive patch (Ortho Evra) and ring (NuvaRing), the injectable contraceptive medroxyprogesterone acetate (Depo-Provera), intrauterine device, and sterilization (Table 3).

The usual amount of time off work allowed for employed mothers is 6 weeks.

Special Circumstances

THE SINGLE PARENT

The single parent often experiences financial and time pressures exceeding those of two-parent families. Enlisting an extended support network of family and friends in addition to a supportive and empathic physician will be helpful.

ADOPTING PARENT(S)

Adopting parent(s) usually have experienced stressful approval and unpredictable placement processes. They may have as little as a few hours' notice to make plans for the arrival of their newborn. Loss issues related to infertility may exist at various stages of resolution. Other issues may include decisions about timing and telling the adoption story to the child(ren) as well as ethnic and cultural considerations when parents and child(ren) have different backgrounds.

PERINATAL GRIEVING

Perinatal grieving occurs both for parents experiencing the death of an infant and parents of a child with a serious illness or congenital anomaly. Physicians can be helpful in this process by providing information and acknowledging when an answer is unknown. The medical team should recognize the infant as a person by using his or her name, encouraging the family's involvement in care of the infant as much as possible and providing opportunities for family members to express and discuss emotions. Parents experiencing a perinatal death should be encouraged to touch and hold their infant and photographs should be offered. Physicians should assist parents with plans for notifying siblings, friends, and relatives. Identifying available community and medical resources such as parent support groups can also be very helpful.

REFERENCES

Anderson GC, Moore E, Hepworth J, Bergman N: Early skin-to-skin contact for mothers and their healthy newborn infants. Cochrane Database Syst Rev 2003(2);CD003519.
Anonymous: Postpartum care of the mother and newborn: A practical guide. Technical Working Group, World Health Organization. Birth 1999;26(4):255-258.
Baxley E: Postpartum biomedical concerns. In Ratcliffe SD, Byrd JE, Sakornbut EL (eds): Handbook of Pregnancy and Perinatal Care in Family Practice: Science and Practice, Philadelphia, Hanley & Belfus, 1996, pp 430-446.
Driscoll CE: Postpartum Care. In Rakel RE, Bope ET (eds): Conn's Current Therapy 2004, Philadelphia, WB Saunders, 2003, pp 1076-1078.

Gabbe SG, Niebyl JR, Simpson JL (eds): Obstetrics: Normal & problem pregnancies, 4th ed. New York, Churchill Livingstone, 2002, pp 753-779.

Hatcher RA, Nelson AL, Zieman M, et al: A pocket guide to managing contraception. Tiger, Georgia, Bridging the Gap Foundation, 2003, p 27.

Killeen I, Osborn C: Postpartum care: Psychosocial concerns. In Ratcliffe SD, Byrd JE, Sakornbut EL (eds): Handbook of Pregnancy and Perinatal Care in Family Practice: Science and Practice. Philadelphia, Hanley & Belfus, 1996, pp 447-458.

Levitt C, Shaw E, Wong S, et al: Systematic review of the literature on postpartum care: Selected contraception methods, postpartum Papanicolaou test, and rubella immunization. Birth 2004; 31(3):203-212.

Montgomery, AM: Breast-feeding and postpartum maternal care. In Larimore WL (ed): Primary Care: Clinics in Office Practice. Update in Maternity Care, Vol. 27, No. 1. Philadelphia, WB Saunders, 2000, pp 237-250.

Resuscitation of the Newborn

Method of
Derek S. Wheeler, MD
and Martin J. McCaffrey, MD

Numerous and dramatic changes must occur more or less in sequential order around the time of birth, at which time the fetal cardiovascular and respiratory systems must undergo an instantaneous transition to life outside the liquid-filled uterine environment. Several events occurring prior to or at the time of delivery may interrupt this transition and lead to problems ranging from mild respiratory distress to shock, organ dysfunction, and death. Fortunately the vast majority of term newborns require no resuscitation beyond routine warming, drying, suctioning of the airway, and mild stimulation. However, rapid identification and resuscitation of those newborns experiencing a difficult transition to extrauterine life may dramatically improve outcome. Neonatal resuscitation is a team effort and requires the coordinated execution of several, simultaneous psychomotor and procedural skills. Adequate knowledge of the normal fetal, transitional, and neonatal physiology, as well as prior planning and preparation is essential to achieving the most favorable outcomes following neonatal resuscitation.

Fetal, Transitional, and Neonatal Circulations

The fetal circulation is characterized by parallel circulations, the presence of intracardiac and extracardiac shunts, a high pulmonary vascular resistance, and a relatively low systemic vascular resistance (attributed to the low-resistance placental circulation). Conversely, on delivery the right and left ventricles are in series, shunts functionally close, pulmonary vascular resistance decreases, and systemic vascular resistance increases. During intrauterine life, gas exchange occurs in the placenta; but during extrauterine life, gas exchange occurs

in the lungs. An understanding and appreciation for these differences is essential to the optimal care and resuscitation of the newborn infant.

The fetal cardiovascular anatomy differs from that of the normal newborn infant. The fetal circulation contains the two atria, two ventricles, and two great arteries but is further complemented by a foramen ovale, ductus arteriosus, and ductus venosus. In utero there exist two large anatomic shunts. One occurs between the right and left atria (the foramen ovale). The second exists between the pulmonary artery and aorta (the ductus arteriosus). The origin of blood flowing through these shunts is crucial. A streaming pattern of fetal blood flow is observed at the level of the right atrium. Less oxygenated blood from the lower body streams along the lateral wall of the inferior vena cava (IVC) crosses the tricuspid valve, and enters the right ventricle. The right ventricle also receives poorly oxygenated blood from the superior vena cava (SVC) (from the brain and upper body) and coronary sinus (from the heart). Because of the high pulmonary vascular resistance (PVR) during intrauterine life, little of the blood pumped from the right ventricle enters the pulmonary circulation. Rather, the right ventricle ejects this poorly oxygenated blood (approximately two thirds of total cardiac output) into the main pulmonary artery and into the descending aorta via the ductus arteriosus, thereby reaching the placenta (via the paired umbilical arteries) where the blood is reoxygenated. In contrast, oxygenated blood from the umbilical-placental circulation (via the single umbilical vein) bypasses the liver via the ductus venosus and travels along the medial wall of the IVC. The majority of this relatively oxygenated stream is directed across the foramen ovale into the left atrium, crosses the mitral valve, and enters the left ventricle. Although the left ventricle also receives a small percentage of poorly oxygenated blood from the lungs, the majority is relatively well oxygenated. In sum, blood in the fetal left ventricle is 20% more saturated than the blood in the right ventricle. The left ventricle ejects this blood (approximately one-third of total cardiac output) into the ascending aorta to supply the heart, brain, and upper fetal body with relatively well-oxygenated blood. A smaller percentage of left ventricular output crosses the aortic arch to the descending aorta. Therefore, the fetal right and left ventricles are functionally arranged in parallel, such that the right ventricle supplies the lower portion of the body, including the placenta, and the left ventricle supplies the upper portion of the body, including the brain. This arrangement assures that the brain receives blood with relatively higher oxygen content than does the placenta.

During birth, a number of complex events occur simultaneously. Clamping of the umbilical cord removes the low-resistance placental capillary bed from the systemic circulation, and blood flow to the placenta ceases abruptly, resulting in an increase in systemic vascular resistance (SVR). The fluid-filled lungs rapidly expand and fill with air with the first few breaths. Initiation of respirations is followed by a marked fall in PVR, and blood flow to the lungs dramatically increases. The increase in SVR results in an increase in left-sided heart pressures. The further increase in left atrial pressure resulting from increased pulmonary venous return results in closure of the foramen ovale, because left atrial pressure exceeds the right atrial pressure. Functional closure of the ductus arteriosus occurs and shunting of blood from the pulmonary artery to the aorta ceases. The fall in PVR and functional closure of the ductus arteriosus depend on several factors, the most important of which are initiation of respirations with subsequent lung inflation and increased oxygen saturation. In the majority of cases, the transition from intrauterine to extrauterine life occurs smoothly and uneventfully. However, up to 10% of all newborn infants will require some degree of intervention (e.g., positioning, suctioning, and/or stimulation to breathe) to assist with this transition. A smaller percentage will require more intensive resuscitative efforts. Certain high-risk conditions (Box 1) may preclude a smooth transition, and further resuscitation may be required to restore and support cardiopulmonary function. For example, several studies suggest that approximately 1% of newborns in the delivery room setting will require assisted ventilation.

Perinatal Asphyxia

Perinatal asphyxia occurs when oxygen delivery is insufficient to meet metabolic demands, resulting in hypoxia, hypercarbia, and metabolic acidosis. Initial compensatory

mechanisms, including tachycardia and vasoconstriction, may allow adequate oxygen delivery to the vital organs for a time. However, without resolution or treatment, these compensatory mechanisms will eventually fail, leading to a fall in heart rate and blood pressure (BP) with eventual cardiopulmonary arrest. World Health Organization (WHO) estimates from 1995 conclude that birth asphyxia is responsible for 19% of the 5 million neonatal deaths that occur annually. Intrauterine asphyxia manifests as alterations in fetal heart rate (late decelerations, bradycardia), passage of meconium (see text following), fetal gasping, and eventual apnea, termed *primary apnea*. This initial period of apnea is followed by further gasping, which gradually weakens in intensity, eventually terminating in what is termed *secondary apnea*. In the delivery room spontaneous respirations can be elicited in newborns with primary apnea by stimulation (vigorous warming and drying) or a brief trial of positive-pressure ventilation (PPV). Newborns with secondary apnea, on the other hand, have suffered a prolonged period of inadequate oxygen delivery and require aggressive resuscitation to prevent further decompensation, cardiac arrest, and death. The longer the delay in initiating resuscitation for primary apnea, the longer the time required to establish spontaneous respirations following PPV. Because there is no definitive method of differentiating between primary and secondary apnea following delivery, the neonatal resuscitation team must promptly recognize and institute proper treatment for all newborn infants with apnea and suspected perinatal asphyxia.

Neonatal Resuscitation

Neonatal resuscitation is directed toward assuring a smooth transition to extrauterine life by achieving the following goals:

- Maintaining or restoring normal body temperature
- Maintaining or establishing effective ventilation and oxygenation
- Maintaining or restoring adequate cardiac output and tissue perfusion
- Avoiding hypoglycemia

Neonatal resuscitation follows an orderly sequence known as the ABCs (airway, breathing, circulation) of resuscitation. Concurrently, the overall physiologic status of the newborn is continuously monitored via a cycle of repeated assessment and intervention (assess-intervene-assess).

Unique to newborn infants is an increased ratio of body surface area to volume; and they are at risk for significant heat loss and temperature. Temperature instability and cold stress will increase oxygen consumption and may impede an effective resuscitation. Therefore, initial efforts should be directed toward minimizing heat loss. On delivery the infant should be placed on a radiant warmer. Other heat sources, such as a heating lamp may be used if a radiant warmer is not available. Heated bags of intravenous (IV) fluid should be avoided because they may cause burns. The infant is then dried

BOX 1 Risk Factors for Neonatal Resuscitation	
Maternal factors	**Intrapartum factors**
Chronic or pregnancy-induced hypertension	Size for date discrepancy
Diabetes mellitus	Polyhydramnios or oligohydramnios
Previous fetal or neonatal death	Breech presentation
Maternal age >35 y or <18 y	Decreased fetal movement
Anemia	Prolonged labor (>24 h)
Rh isoimmunization	Prolonged rupture of membranes (>12 h)
Prematurity (<37 wk gestation)	Meconium-stained amniotic fluid
Postmaturity (>42 wk gestation)	Placental abruption
Premature rupture of the membranes	Prolapsed cord
Malnutrition or poor weight gain	Fetal distress (fetal heart rate abnormalities, fetal acidosis)
Lack of prenatal care	Emergent operative delivery
Substance abuse (including alcohol)	
Antepartum hemorrhage	
Multiple gestation	
Chronic disease (cardiovascular, rheumatologic, neurologic, etc.)	

Rakel and Bope: *Conn's Current Therapy 2006.*

vigorously with a warm, sterile towel. To minimize conductive heat losses, wet linens should be removed as soon as possible. If the newborn is otherwise stable, he or she may be placed naked against the mother's skin and covered with a clean blanket or towel.

Initial resuscitative efforts are directed toward maintaining the airway. Properly positioning the infant on his or her back, with the head and neck in a neutral, midline position will assist in opening the airway. A towel roll may be placed beneath the shoulders to assist in opening the airway. Hyperextension, which may lead to airway obstruction, should be avoided. The mouth and nose should be suctioned with a bulb syringe to remove any secretions that may contribute to airway compromise.

Drying, positioning, and suctioning usually provide sufficient stimulation to help the newborn initiate effective breathing. If respirations are adequate and cyanosis is present, supplemental oxygen should be administered, and an appropriately sized face mask should be available. Acrocyanosis (bluish discoloration of the hands and feet), on the other hand, is a normal physical finding that is often present in the first few minutes of life and does not require oxygen supplementation. Using a bag-valve-mask PPV is indicated for those infants with either absent (apnea) or slow, gasping respiratory movements. In addition, because one of the most common causes of bradycardia is lack of sufficient oxygen, PPV is indicated when the heart rate is below 100 beats per minute (bpm).

Both neonatal-sized self-inflating bags and anesthesia bags (Figure 1) are acceptable for administering PPV in the delivery room. The main advantages to using an anesthesia bag are that these devices are capable of either delivering 100% blow-by oxygen or continuous positive airway pressure (CPAP). Inspiratory pressures can be controlled and titrated with the use of an in-line manometer when using an anesthesia bag. The use of an anesthesia bag requires more expertise, however, and some centers preferentially use a self-inflating bag because of its simplicity. The main disadvantages to the self-inflating bag are that these devices require an additional oxygen reservoir attachment and inspiratory pressures cannot be closely titrated. Both devices are acceptable for use in neonatal resuscitation provided that staff is familiar with the requirements of each device.

Proper placement and sizing of the face mask is required to produce an effective seal around the mouth and nose (Figure 2). Adequate ventilation is assured using a rate of 40 to 60 breaths per minute, with a tidal volume sufficient enough to produce adequate, symmetric expansion of the chest. Initially, inspiratory pressures as high as 30 cm H_2O or more may be required for adequate lung inflation. Smaller pressures (generally 20 cm H_2O or less) are generally sufficient for subsequent breaths. An 8 or 10 F orogastric tube may be placed to decompress the stomach and improve ventilation. Ventilation via the bag-valve-mask is relatively simple to perform and can be life sustaining. Endotracheal intubation should be considered if bag-valve-mask ventilation is ineffective after attempts to optimize, if it appears that prolonged ventilation will be required or if an

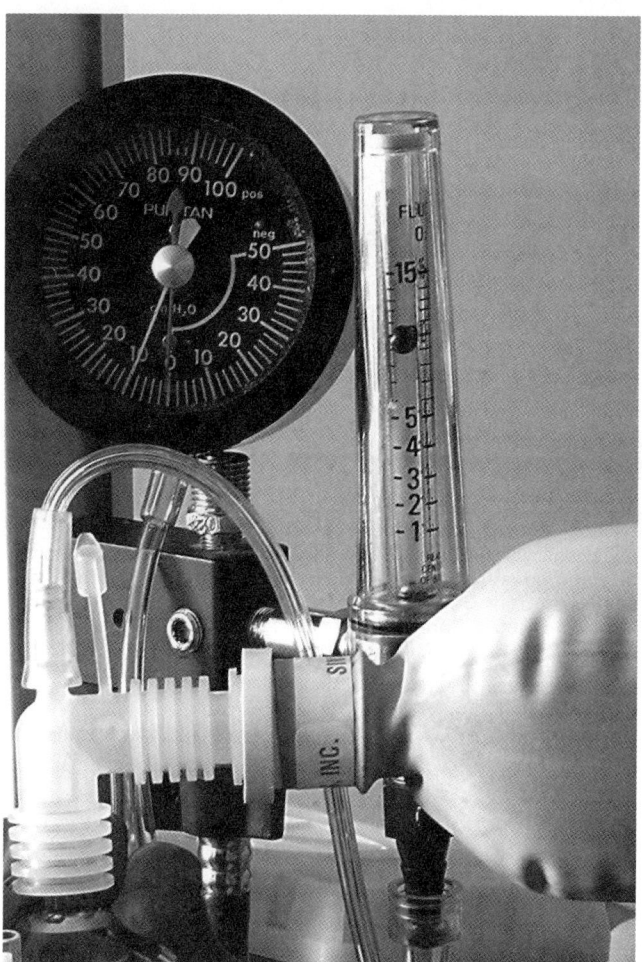

FIGURE 1. Anesthesia bag preparation. Setting the initial flow rate to 8 to 10 L/minute and the end-respiratory pressure to 8 to 10 cm H_2O allows for effective bag filling while providing positive-pressure ventilation. (Copied with permission from Golden SM: Resuscitation of the neonate. Rakel RE, Bope ET [eds]: Conn's Current Therapy, 2004. Philadelphia, WB Saunders, 2003, p 1082, Figure 1.)

intravascular route for epinephrine administration is unattainable. However, intubation should only be attempted by providers experienced with the management of the neonatal airway. Intubation of a newborn requires careful assessment to determine that the tube has been properly placed. In addition, careful ongoing assessment is required to determine that the tube remains properly positioned. Use of a disposable CO_2 indicator should be considered to confirm proper endotracheal tube placement initially and during the course of the resuscitation.

Once adequate ventilation and oxygenation are assured, attention is directed toward the circulatory system. Heart rate is assessed by palpating the brachial pulse, palpating the pulse at the base of the umbilical cord, or by auscultation of cardiac sounds with a stethoscope. The heart rate in a newborn normally ranges from 100 to 170 bpm. As mentioned previously, PPV should be initiated for infants whose heart rates are less than 100 bpm. However, chest compressions should be performed immediately if the heart rate is

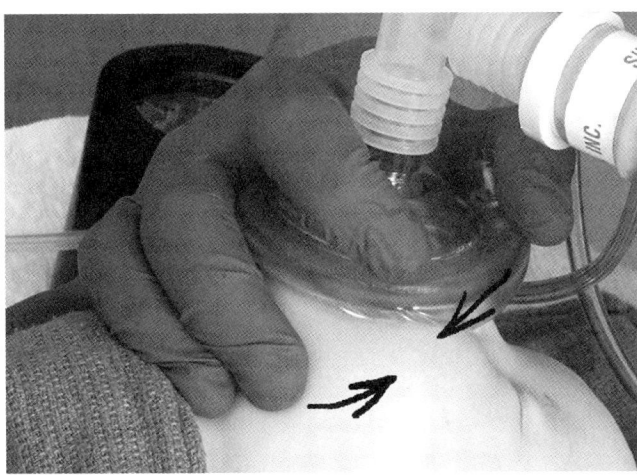

FIGURE 2. Proper placement and seal of face mask. The thumb and third finger (which is on the mandible or ramus of the mandible) are being squeezed toward each other in a *C hold.* (Copied with permission from Golden SM: Resuscitation of the neonate. Rakel RE, Bope ET [eds]: Conn's Current Therapy, 2004. Philadelphia, WB Saunders, 2003, p 1082, Figure 2.)

less than 60 bpm after 30 seconds of effective PPV with 100% oxygen (Box 2). Chest compressions are performed using either the two-thumb technique (Figure 3) or two-finger technique (Figure 4), but the two-thumb technique is thought to provide a more controlled depth of compression and better cardiac output. Team members should coordinate ventilations with chest compressions. After three compressions, a positive pressure breath with 100% oxygen should be administered (for a compression to breath ratio of 3:1). Chest compressions should be continued until the heart rate is greater than 60 bpm.

Resuscitation medications (Table 1) should be administered if the heart rate remains less than 60 bpm despite 30 seconds of chest compressions and adequate PPV. Vascular access should be established at this time, as drug, fluid and dextrose administration may be necessary, but endotracheal administration of drugs may be the most accessible route. The medication is either flushed through the endotracheal tube with 0.5 to 1 mL normal saline or pushed through a 5 F feeding tube passed to the tip of the endotracheal tube. Both methods of drug administration should be followed by several positive-pressure breaths.

Vascular access may be achieved most readily via umbilical vein cannulation. The umbilical vein is easily identified and cannulated and is therefore the preferred site of vascular access in the newborn. The umbilical vein is identified as a single, thin-walled, larger vessel compared to the small, thick-walled pair of umbilical arteries (Figure 5). A 3.5 or 5.0 F catheter is inserted until the tip of the catheter is below the skin or until blood can readily be aspirated. This should be done sterilely if possible. If not placed sterilely, however, after stabilization the catheter must be replaced to avoid potential infectious. A peripheral IV line is also perfectly acceptable but may be difficult to establish by inexperienced providers.

BOX 2   Newborn Resuscitation Equipment for the Emergency Department

Airway
- Bulb syringe
- DeLee suction catheter
- Meconium aspirator
- Laryngoscope and straight blades (sizes 0, 1)
- Endotracheal tubes, uncuffed (sizes 2.5, 3.0, 3.5, and 4.0 mm)
- Stylet
- Suction catheters (5 F, 8 F, 10 F)
- Suction source with manometer
- Nasogastric tube
- Feeding tubes (8 F, 10 F)

Breathing
- Face masks (premature, newborn, and infant sizes)
- Self-inflating ventilation bag (450 to 750 mL), with oxygen reservoir and manometer
- Oxygen source
- Chest tubes (8 and 10 F)

Circulation
- Sterile umbilical vessel catheterization tray
- Umbilical catheters (3.5 F, 5.0 F)
- Three-way stopcocks
- Syringes (tuberculin, 1, 3, 10, and 20 mL)
- Medication and fluids:
  - Epinephrine 1:10,000 concentration
  - Naloxone hydrochloride
  - Sodium bicarbonate (0.5 mEq/mL or 4.2% solution)
  - Normal saline
  - Lactated Ringer's
  - 10% Dextrose
  - 5% albumin

Miscellaneous equipment
- Radiant warmer or heat lamps
- Sterile towels
- Pulse oximeter
- Cardiorespiratory monitor with small electrocardiographic leads
- Sterile gowns, gloves
- Resuscitation chart

Epinephrine is the drug used most frequently during resuscitation of the newborn. It may be administered via the IV or endotracheal routes for either asystole or heart rate less than 60 bpm despite effective ventilations and chest compressions. Generally, the dose is 0.01 to 0.03 mg/kg (0.1 to 0.3 mL/kg of the 1:10,000 solution) administered as needed every 3 to 5 minutes. Volume expanders are also used frequently and are indicated for the treatment of hypovolemia. Generally, 10 mL/kg of either normal saline or lactated Ringer's are administered through an IV or intraosseous catheter over 5 to 10 minutes. If there is concern for significant anemia in the fetus or newborn, O-negative blood, crossmatched with the mother if possible, should be considered as a volume expander. If time does not allow, emergent-release O-negative blood should be used to initially resuscitate the severely anemic infant. Naloxone (Narcan) is administered to newborns whose mothers had narcotics within 4 hours of delivery and in whom

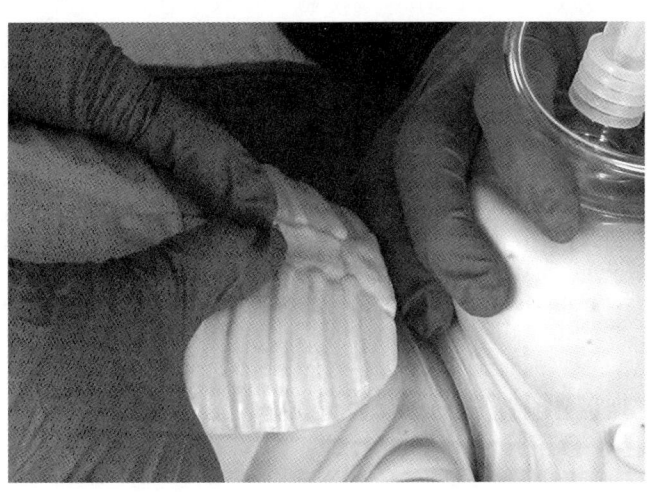

FIGURE 3. Two-thumb chest-encircling external cardiac massage technique. This is the preferred technique. Note that the thumbs are above the xyphoid process in the midsternum region. (Copied with permission from Golden SM: Resuscitation of the neonate. Rakel RE, Bope ET [eds]: Conn's Current Therapy, 2004. Philadelphia, WB Saunders, 2003, p 1083, Figure 4.)

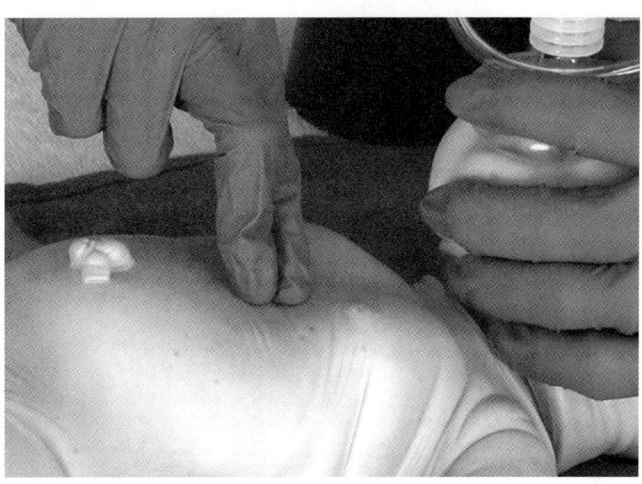

FIGURE 4. Two-finger external cardiac massage technique. Fingers are above xyphoid process; approximately one finger width beneath the nipple line. (Copied with permission from Golden SM: Resuscitation of the neonate. Rakel RE, Bope ET [eds]: Conn's Current Therapy, 2004. Philadelphia, WB Saunders, 2003, p 1083, Figure 5.)

16

heart rate and color are normal, but severe respiratory depression persists. However, naloxone (Narcan) will precipitate acute narcotic withdrawal and seizures if administered to newborns born to women with known or suspected drug abuse. IV glucose (2 mL/kg $D_{10}W$) is administered for suspected or documented hypoglycemia. Sodium bicarbonate should only be given in cases of documented severe acidosis or in prolonged resuscitations with no response to other described interventions. Finally, surfactant preparations (Survanta, Infasurf) may be administered in the

delivery room to preterm newborns with respiratory distress.

It should be emphasized that resuscitation proceeds according to the above protocols, and not according to the result of the Apgar score. The Apgar score is based on five objective signs (Table 2) and was designed to provide an easily reproducible measure of the status of a newborn shortly after birth. Scores are usually determined at 1 and 5 minutes of life. Resuscitation should *not* be delayed while awaiting the results of the 1-minute Apgar score.

TABLE 1 Drugs for Resuscitation/Stabilization

Medication	Concentration	Dosage/route	Indications	Comment
Epinephrine	1:10,000	0.1-0.3 mL/kg/dose IV or via ETT	Asystole Bradycardia that is unresponsive to PPV and chest compressions	Dilute dose with 1-3 mL normal saline for ETT. May repeat dose q 3-5 min.
Volume expanders Normal saline Lactated Ringer's		10 mL/kg IV	Hypovolemia Shock	
Glucose	10%	2 mL/kg IV	Hypoglycemia	May need to repeat.
Naloxone (Narcan)		0.1 mg/kg IV, IM, or ETT	Respiratory depression secondary to maternal narcotics	May precipitate acute life-threatening withdrawal in neonates born to drug-abusing mothers.
Sodium bicarbonate	0.5 mEq/mL	2 mL/kg IV	Documented severe metabolic acidosis or prolonged resuscitation with no response to other interventions	Administer slowly (≈2 mL/min).

Abbreviations: ETT = endotracheal tube; IM, intramuscularly; IV = intravenously; PPV = positive-pressure ventilation; q = every.

Rakel and Bope: *Conn's Current Therapy 2006.*

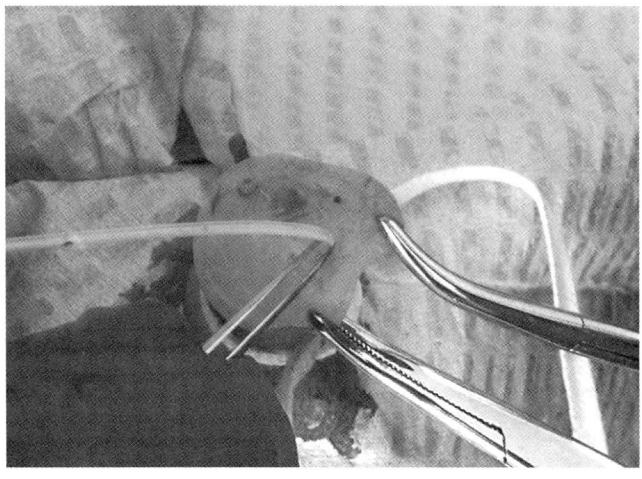

FIGURE 5. Umbilical vein catheterization. The umbilical vein is the preferred route for immediate venous access for drug medication and volume administration. (Copied with permission from Golden SM: Resuscitation of the Neonate. Rakel RE, Bope ET [eds]: Conn's Current Therapy, 2004. Philadelphia, WB Saunders, 2003, p 1084, Figure 6.)

Meconium Staining of the Amniotic Fluid

Meconium is a viscous, greenish-black substance consisting of gastrointestinal (GI) secretions, blood, bile acids, amniotic fluid, and cellular debris present in the fetal GI tract. In the majority of cases, meconium is cleared from the GI tract with the first few bowel movements. However, in approximately 10% to 15% of all deliveries, meconium is passed prior to birth, leading to meconium staining of the amniotic fluid, which increases an infant's risk of developing the meconium aspiration syndrome (MAS), a disease with serious morbidity and mortality. Current recommendations for management of meconium-stained amniotic fluid advise that as soon as the infant's head is delivered, and before the shoulders are delivered, that the mouth, nose, and pharynx should be vigorously suctioned with a specialized apparatus called a DeLee suction catheter, regardless of whether the meconium staining is thin or thick. After the infant is delivered, if the amniotic fluid contains meconium and the infant has absent or depressed respirations, decreased muscle tone, or heart rate less than 100 bpm, the infant is tracheally intubated

and the trachea is suctioned using a meconium aspirator attached directly to the endotracheal tube. Resuscitation is then performed in the usual sequence, if required. Recent studies have called into question several of the aforementioned practices, including suctioning of the mouth, nose, and pharynx prior to delivery of the shoulders and routine endotracheal intubation and suctioning of the otherwise vigorous newborn. However, until further research is available, current recommendations continue to suggest the use of the previously discussed protocol.

Newborn Resuscitation Outside the Delivery Room

Ideally, newborn resuscitation should take place in the delivery room setting. Unfortunately, many newborns are born outside the delivery room setting, such as in the home, en route to the hospital, or in the emergency department. Many mothers who deliver either outside the hospital setting or in the emergency department are more likely to represent high-risk groups (multiparous births, trauma-induced labor, lack of prenatal care, adolescent pregnancy, placental abruption, etc.). Therefore, all emergency providers should be familiar with the resuscitation of the newborn. Resuscitation of the newborn infant presents several unique challenges to emergency care providers that are infrequently found during resuscitation of either the adult or child.

In many cases, deliveries in the emergency department will occur with little prior notice. Therefore, advanced preparation and an organized approach to resuscitation are essential. In addition to a standard obstetrical tray, airway, vascular access, and other equipment unique to newborn resuscitation should be readily available (see Box 2). There is often insufficient time to obtain a complete prenatal history from the mother; however, three key pieces of information are often helpful in determining the initial priorities of resuscitation. First, if labor is premature (i.e., fewer than 37 weeks' gestation), a lengthy resuscitation with a possible need for prolonged PPV can be anticipated. Second, if twins are expected, two resuscitation teams and two sets of equipment should be available. Finally, if the membranes have ruptured, the presence of meconium will indicate the need for an additional, more specialized resuscitation sequence (see previous discussion).

Sign	0	1	2
Heart rate	Absent	Slow (less than 100 bpm)	Greater than 100 bpm
Respirations	Absent	Slow, irregular	Good, crying
Muscle tone	Limp	Some flexion	Active motion
Reflex irritability (catheter in nares)	No response	Grimace	Cough or sneeze
Color	Blue or pale	Acrocyanosis	Pink

TABLE 2 The Apgar Score*

*A score of 0, 1, or 2 is assigned in each category at 1 and 5 minutes of life.
Abbreviations: bpm = beats per minute.

CURRENT DIAGNOSIS

- Intrauterine asphyxia manifests as alterations in fetal heart rate (late decelerations, bradycardia), passage of meconium, fetal gasping, and eventual apnea, termed *primary apnea*. This initial period of apnea is followed by further gasping, which gradually weakens in intensity, eventually terminating in what is termed *secondary apnea*.
- Spontaneous respirations can be elicited in newborns with primary apnea by stimulation (vigorous warming and drying) or a brief trial of PPV. Newborns with secondary apnea, on the other hand, have suffered a prolonged period of inadequate oxygen delivery and require aggressive resuscitation to prevent further decompensation, cardiac arrest, and death.
- The longer the delay in initiating resuscitation for primary apnea, the longer the time required to establish spontaneous respirations following PPV. Because there is no definitive method of differentiating between primary and secondary apnea following delivery, the neonatal resuscitation team must promptly recognize and institute proper treatment for all newborn infants with apnea and suspected perinatal asphyxia.
- Neonatal resuscitation is directed toward assuring a smooth transition to extrauterine life by achieving the following goals:
  - Maintaining or restoring normal body temperature
  - Maintaining or establishing effective ventilation and oxygenation
  - Maintaining or restoring adequate cardiac output and tissue perfusion
  - Avoiding hypoglycemia
- Neonatal resuscitation consists of a cycle of repeated assessment and therapeutic intervention (assess-intervene-assess) until cardiorespiratory and hemodynamic stability are achieved.

Abbreviation: PPV = positive-pressure ventilation.

Ongoing Assessment

Neonatal resuscitation consists of a cycle of repeated assessment and therapeutic intervention (assess-intervene-assess) until cardiorespiratory and hemodynamic stability are achieved. The cycle of assess-intervene-assess should continue once the critically ill newborn has stabilized. During stabilization a complete blood cell count (CBC), serum electrolytes, blood urea nitrogen (BUN), creatinine, blood glucose, and an arterial blood gas to assess acid-base status should be obtained. A chest radiograph should be obtained to confirm proper placement of the endotracheal and orogastric tubes. Additional vascular access should be obtained.

Rakel and Bope: *Conn's Current Therapy 2006.*

 CURRENT THERAPY

- Initial efforts should be directed toward minimizing heat loss. On delivery, the infant should be placed on a radiant warmer. The infant is then dried vigorously with a warm, sterile towel.
- Properly positioning the infant on his or her back, with the head and neck in a neutral, midline position will assist in opening the airway. The mouth and nose should be suctioned with a bulb syringe to remove any secretions that may contribute to airway compromise.
- If respirations are adequate and cyanosis is present, supplemental oxygen should be administered.
- PPV, using a bag-valve-mask is indicated for those infants with either absent (apnea) or slow, gasping respiratory movements, and when the heart rate is below 100 bpm.
- Chest compressions should be performed immediately if the heart rate is less than 60 bpm after 30 seconds of effective PPV with 100% oxygen using either the two-thumb technique (preferred) or two-finger technique.
- Resuscitation medications should be administered if the heart rate remains less than 60 bpm despite 30 seconds of chest compressions and adequate PPV.

Abbreviations: bpm = beats per minute; PPV = positive-pressure ventilation.

In the intubated patient, further deterioration should prompt rapid, close assessment for potential endotracheal tube complications. These complications can be easily recalled at the bedside by the mnemonic *DOPE*:

*D*islodged: Has the endotracheal tube moved distally into the right or left main bronchus?
*O*bstructed: Is the endotracheal tube obstructed with inspissated secretions or blood?
*P*neumothorax: Is there a pneumothorax?
*E*sophagus: Is the endotracheal tube in the esophagus?

In conclusion, the dramatic changes in cardiovascular and respiratory physiology that occur around the time of birth pose several potential problems that could lead to an unfavorable outcome. Proper education and training in neonatal resuscitation is imperative for all health care providers working in the deliver room and nursery setting. Health care providers in these settings, as well as those physicians working in the emergency department who may also be called on to resuscitate newborn infants should have advanced knowledge and understanding of normal fetal, transitional, and neonatal physiology so that potential problems can be recognized and treated early. Only through the early recognition, resuscitation, and stabilization of the critically ill newborn will the best possible outcome be realized.

REFERENCES

Saugstad OD: Practical aspects of resuscitating newborn infants. Eur J Pediatr 1998;157(Suppl 1):S11-S15.

Palme-Kilander C: Methods of resuscitation in low-Apgar-score newborn infants: A national survey. Acta Pediatr 1992;81:739-744.

Apgar V: A proposal for a new method of evaluation of the newborn infant. Anesth Analg 1953;32:260-267.

Gelfand SL, Fanaroff JM, Walsh MC: Meconium stained fluid: Approach to the mother and the baby. Pediatr Clin North Am 2004;51: 655-667.

Vain NE, Szyld EG, Prudent LM, et al: Oropharyngeal and nasopharyngeal suctioning of meconium-stained neonates before delivery of their shoulders: multicentre, randomised controlled trial. Lancet 2004;364;597-602.

Wiswell TE, Gannon CM, Jacob J, et al: Delivery room management of the apparently vigorous meconium-stained neonate: Results of the multicenter, international collaborative trial. Pediatrics 2000; 105:1-7.

Niermeyer S, Kattwinkel J, Van Reempts P, et al: International guidelines for neonatal resuscitation: An excerpt from the Guidelines 2000 for Cardiopulmonary Resuscitation and Emergency Cardiovascular Care: International Consensus on Science. Contributors and Reviewers for the Neonatal Resuscitation Guidelines. Pediatrics 2000;106:E29.

The views presented are those of the author and do not necessarily represent the views of the Department of Defense or its components.

Care of the High-Risk Neonate

Method of
Dilcia McLenan, MD

Despite advances in prenatal care and diagnosis, the overall prematurity rate has not changed in the last two decades. The rate remains at 10% to 12% of all births in the United States. Although the overall mortality rate and the short-term morbidity rate have improved with the advances in neonatal care, premature births are still responsible for 75% to 85% of neonatal deaths. Congenital anomalies are associated with 20% to 30% of perinatal deaths. The early identification of the high-risk neonate is essential to improve outcome. The goal is to prevent the development or progression of more serious illnesses and to minimize the risk of both morbidity and mortality.

The definition of the high-risk neonate can be applied in the prenatal, perinatal or postnatal period. Approximately 75% of risk factors affecting the fetus are identified in the prenatal period. Maternal high-risk factors include age, race, socioeconomic status, nutrition and past obstetric history, current pregnancy problems, and maternal drug use. Maternal acute and chronic illness can also adversely affect the fetus. The placenta is considered fetal tissue; all conditions that affect the placenta will also affect the fetus, and vice versa. Fetal factors are limited to genetic conditions (chromosomal and nonchromosomal), and metabolic.

The prenatal diagnosis of the high-risk neonate uses many tools, such as chorionic villus sampling (CVS), amniocentesis, maternal serum screening, and cordocentesis. With the use of cytogenetics, molecular biology, and the fluorescence in situ hybridization, many genetic disorders and infectious conditions can be diagnosed. Fetal ultrasonography is another valuable tool in diagnosing high-risk conditions, including fetal growth abnormalities, which are associated with increased perinatal morbidity and mortality. The Doppler can assess blood velocity in the umbilical and fetal vessels. There is increased morbidity and mortality in fetuses with absent umbilical artery flow or with reverse end diastolic flow. The measurement of the nuchal translucency, done between 10 and 14 weeks of gestation by fetal ultrasound (US) in conjunction with the maternal serum markers, increases the detection rate of Down syndrome and other chromosomal and genetic syndromes, fetal structural malformations, and adverse pregnancy outcome.

Prenatal care facilitates the diagnosis and care of the high-risk neonate through a multidisciplinary approach. This multidisciplinary approach sets the stage for counseling, referrals, and the plan of care pre- and postnatally. When counseling the family, consider the gestational age at diagnosis, effect on maternal outcome and neonatal prognosis with or without therapy, plans for delivery, intrapartum management, and surgical intervention when applicable. General discussion with the parents during the intrapartum period regarding the preterm or high-risk neonate will include such things as anticipated birth weight and gestational age, the need for respiratory support, procedures to be expected, the need for transfusion of blood products, short- and long-term complications of each problem or condition, the need for other specialists, and morbidity and mortality. Involving the neonatologist in the counseling can aid families in making difficult decisions. One should also explain the need for transport, if delivered at a nontertiary care center, and the role the parents will have while their infant is in the neonatal intensive care unit (NICU).

The delivery management of the high-risk neonate is influenced by the factors identified in the antepartum and intrapartum period. In the intrapartum period, neonatal resuscitation facilitates the transition from the intrauterine to the extrauterine life. Approximately 5% to 10% of all newborns need help making this transition; 1% of all newborns need a more extensive intervention. The fetus is dependent on its mother and the placenta for the delivery of oxygen and nutrients as well as removal of carbon dioxide. After the umbilical cord is clamped and cut, the newborn needs to expand its lungs, establishing respirations and convert from a fetal (parallel) to an adult (in series) circulation for a successful transition, and avoid the development of asphyxia.

Resuscitation aims at facilitating the transition and reversing the process of asphyxia by clearing the airway, providing adequate oxygenation and ventilation, ensuring adequate cardiac output, and keeping oxygen consumption to the minimum. These objectives can be achieved by adhering to the four principles of neonatal resuscitation.

Rakel and Bope: *Conn's Current Therapy 2006.*

Principles of Neonatal Resuscitation

The American Heart Association (AHA) and the American Academy of Pediatrics (AAP) Neonatal Resuscitation Program (NRP) have defined the following principles of neonatal resuscitation:

- **Anticipation.** Risk factors in the antepartum and intrapartum history help identify instances that may potentially require intervention (Box 1).
- **Preparation.** In preparation of the area, equipment, and drugs should be assembled and checked.
- **Availability of qualified personnel.** At every delivery there should be at least one person skilled in neonatal resuscitation whose only responsibility is the newborn; skills include the proper use of the bag and mask. In cases of emergency or if further intervention is needed, additional competent personnel should be immediately available.

BOX 1 Antepartum/Intrapartum Factors Associated with Potential Asphyxia

Antepartum Factors

Age >35 years	Post-term gestation
Maternal diabetes	Multiple gestation
Pregnancy-induced hypertension	Size-dates discrepancy
Chronic hypertension	Drug therapy, e.g.:
Anemia or isoimmunization	Lithium carbonate
Previous fetal or neonatal death	Magnesium
Bleeding in 2nd or 3rd trimester	Adrenergic blocking drugs
Maternal infection	Maternal substance abuse
Hydramnios	Fetal malformation
Oligohydramnios	Diminished fetal activity
Premature rupture of membranes	No prenatal care

Intrapartum Factors

Emergency cesarean section	Nonreassuring fetal heart rate pattern
Breech or other abnormal presentation	Use of general anesthesia
Premature labor	Uterine tetany
Prolonged rupture of membranes >24 h before delivery	Narcotics administered to mother within 4 h of delivery
Precipitous labor	Meconium-stained amniotic fluid
Prolonged labor (>24 h)	Prolapsed cord
Prolonged second stage of labor (>2 h)	Abruptio placentae; Placenta previa

Note: Keep these factors in mind because they will alert you that depression and possibly asphyxia are potential problems.
From Bloom RS, Cropley C: The AHNAAP Neonatal Resuscitation Program Steering Committee. Textbook of Neonatal Resuscitation. Dallas, TX, 1994, Copyright American Heart Association.

- **Organized response to the emergencies—evaluation, decision, and action.** The ABCs (airway, breathing, and circulation) of resuscitation is the order in which the needed intervention will be evaluated. The evaluation assesses the breathing, heart rate, and color, then the decision or diagnosis is made followed by the action or treatment .

The initial steps of resuscitation provide the support needed to make the transition from the intrauterine to the extrauterine life (Table 1).

Shortcutting these steps prolongs the resuscitation process, increases the risk for asphyxia, and increases the likelihood of morbidity and mortality. In cases where further intervention is needed beyond the initial steps of resuscitation, a thorough evaluation should be done to diagnose conditions that might have contributed to the need for further resuscitation, such as congenital abnormalities of the airway, heart, gastrointestinal (GI) tract, genitourinary (GU) system, or secondary cardiopulmonary disorders. Infants with Apgar scores below 7 at 10 minutes should be admitted to the NICU for further observation and management.

16

Asphyxia

Asphyxia is the result of prolonged decrease of oxygen delivery to the tissues. During the event, there is redistribution of blood flow to the heart, brain, and adrenals. The continuation of the insult results in bradycardia, impaired gas exchange, and reduced tissue perfusion. These series of events can occur prenatally, intrapartum, or postnatally. In severe cases of asphyxia almost every organ of the body is affected:

- Central nervous system (CNS): hypoxic ischemic encephalopathy
- Cardiovascular: myocardial dysfunction
- Renal: renal dysfunction and or acute renal failure
- GI: liver dysfunction and increased risk of necrotizing enterocolitis
- Hematologic: coagulopathy

TABLE 1 At Birth

Initial step	Objective
Provide warmth.	Prevent heat loss, maintain oxygen consumption at a minimum, and prevent hypoglycemia.
Position, clear the airway (as necessary).	Establish an airway.
Dry stimulate and reposition.	Initiate breathing and maintain the circulation.
Give oxygen (as necessary).	Ameliorate cyanosis and provide adequate oxygen for continued circulation and adequate delivery to tissues and prevent the development of asphyxia.

- Pulmonary: activation of the mechanisms that cause persistent pulmonary hypertension of the newborn, surfactant (Survanta) deficiency, and meconium aspiration syndrome (MAS)
- Metabolic: acidosis, hypoglycemia, and hypocalcemia

After birth the normal newborn goes through a period of transition that lasts for several hours. During this period the cardiovascular, pulmonary, and sympathetic systems regulate themselves to adjust to extrauterine life. During the transition, abnormalities in color, respirations, heart rate, sleep state, motor activity, GI function, and temperature stability can be identified and will require care in the NICU. Clinical manifestations of abnormal transition include persistent tachypnea, nasal flaring, grunting, retractions, persistent cyanosis, apnea and bradycardia, pallor, temperature instability, blood pressure (BP) instability, lethargy, and other neurologic symptoms.

Postnatal Care

The postnatal care of the high-risk neonate is extremely important. There are interventions and supportive care that are common to the high-risk neonates to ensure the best possible outcome. These include thermoregulation, nutrition, developmental care, and parental involvement. Notwithstanding, individualized care that will address specific needs of each infant should always be kept in mind.

THERMOREGULATION

Thermoregulation is the balance between heat production and heat loss. It is closely linked to morbidity and mortality. In the neonate, heat loss can exceed heat production because of larger surface area to body mass ratio, decreased subcutaneous (SC) tissue or fat, increased permeability to water and small radius of curvature of exchange surfaces.

The newborn generates heat by nonshivering mechanisms—brown fat, increased muscular activity, flexion, and increased metabolic rate with increased oxygen consumption. The newborn loses heat through conduction, convection, evaporation, and radiation (Table 2).

In the neonate there is always a combination of types and mechanism of heat loss. The prevention of cold stress and hypothermia is critical for intact survival of the neonate (Figure 1).

Heat production is a result of metabolic processes that generate energy by oxidative metabolism of glucose (most efficient in the premature infant), fat, and protein. In the newborn, heat or energy production is low relative to heat or energy losses. Brown adipose tissue generates more energy than any other tissue in the body. The brown adipose tissue cells begin to differentiate by 26 to 30 weeks of gestation and continue to develop until 3 to 5 weeks after birth; it constitutes 10% of the adipose tissue in term infants.

Thermoregulation is achieved by providing the appropriate thermal environment to prevent heat loss, hypothermia, and cold stress. The neutral thermal environment (NTE) is an idealized range of ambient temperature at which the body temperature is normal, metabolic rate or oxygen consumption is minimal, and thermoregulation is achieved by basal nonevaporative physical processes. It promotes growth and stability and minimizes heat (energy) and water loss. Newborns have a narrow control range that make them vulnerable to alterations in the thermal environment. The NTE is achieved for the:

- Term infant at 32°C (89.6°F) to 33.5°C (92.3°F)
- Preterm infant greater than 1500 g at 34°C (93.2°F) to 35°C (95°F)
- Preterm infant less than 1500 g at 36.7°C (98.1°F) to 37.3°C (99.1°F)

The two common methods of supporting thermoregulation are the radiant warmer and the incubator (Table 3).

TABLE 2 Thermoregulation: Types, Mechanisms, and Management

Type/definition	Mechanism	Prevention
Conduction, transfer of heat from the body core to surface, and object in contact with body.	Cold surfaces, cold objects in contact with the body	Use rubber mattresses, warm blankets,and warm mattresses.
Convection, heat transfer from the body surface to the surrounding air.	Cool rapid air flow, cold oxygen flow	Swaddle using a cap, warm oxygen, and placing infant away from draft. Servo control air or skin incubators, warm room temperature.
Evaporation, moisture on the body surface or respiratory tract evaporates. Major source of heat loss after delivery or during bath. Inversely related to gestational age.	Wet skin, increase of activity, tachypnea, under radiant warmer and phototherapy	Dry infant immediately after birth and bath; increase humidity; use warm soaks and solutions; use polyethylene wraps, warm and humidified oxygen.
Radiation, transfer of heat from the body to surrounding cooler surfaces not in contact with the infant.	Dependent on ambient temperature, air speed and other heat loss mechanisms	Double-wall incubators, radiant warmer, and heat shield.

Rakel and Bope: Conn's Current Therapy 2006.

THERMOREGULATION

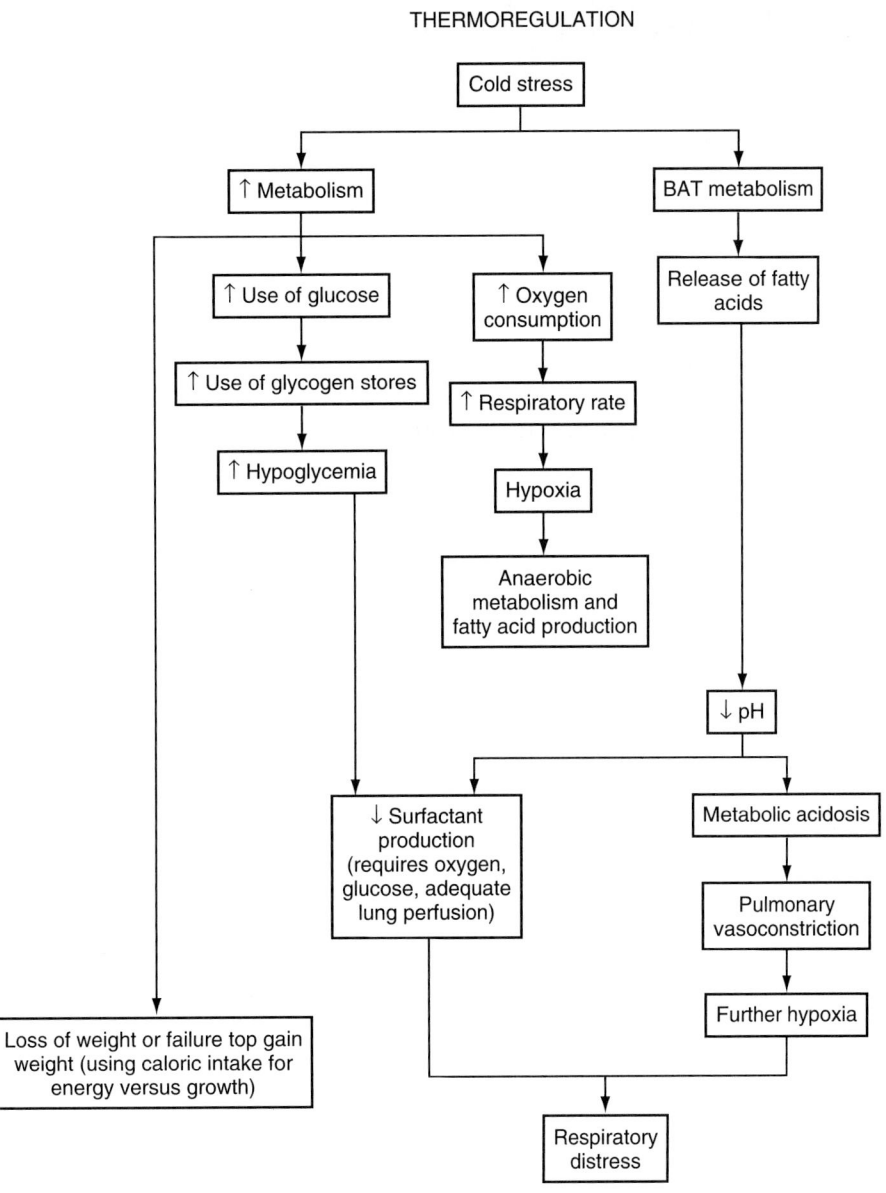

FIGURE 1. Physiologic consequences of cold stress. BAT = Brown adipose tissue.

NUTRITION

Proper nutrition is essential for adequate growth, development, and healing. Protein and lipid stores are decreased in the neonate, who has a higher baseline energy requirement compared to children and adults. The low-birth-weight (LBW) infant and the premature infant have even higher baseline requirements. The premature infant has minimal stores of fat and carbohydrates and rapidly develops nutritional deficiencies in calcium, phosphorus, iron trace elements, and vitamins. Nutritional requirements of calories and protein increase even further in the critically ill neonate with overwhelming infections, severe lung disease, and major surgical conditions. These conditions obviate the

enteral route of delivering adequate nutrition as well as the immature digestive pathways of the GI tract. In these cases parenteral nutrition is the only option. In premature infants nutritional support is aimed at achieving an intrauterine growth pattern of 15 to 30 g per day. To achieve comparable weight at term-corrected age, compared to a term infant, the daily growth rate would have to be higher to achieve catch-up growth. When there is early positive nitrogen balance, weight loss is less, there is a better rate of growth, and healing and recovery are faster.

With parenteral nutrition the fluid requirement starts at 80 mL/kg per day and increases daily up to 150 mL/kg per day. Infants with increased fluid losses, in addition to their maintenance fluid requirement,

TABLE 3 Measures to Promote Thermoregulation in Incubators and Radiant Warmers

Bed	Basis	Measures
Incubator	Decrease evaporative water and heat loss	Increase humidity
		Plastic heat shield
		Thermal blanket
		Semiocclusive dressings or emollients
	Reduce radiant and convective losses	Double-walled incubator
		Heat shield
		Thermal blanket
	Promote conductive heat gain	Heated mattress
Radiant warmer	Decrease evaporative water and heat loss	Heat shield
		Plastic wrap
		Thermal blanket
	Reduce radiant or convective losses	Heat shield
		Plastic wrap
		Thermal blanket

Modified from Sinclair, J. (1992). Management of the thermal environment. In J.C. Sinclair and M.B. Brocker (eds). Effective care of the newborn infant. Oxford: Oxford University Press.

will require replacement fluid with specific electrolytes to offset their losses. The caloric requirement varies from 80 kcal to 120 kcal/kg per day. Higher caloric needs of 20% to 30% more are required in the extremely premature infants and in the critically ill neonate. To achieve the expected postnatal growth pattern, the total nonprotein calories requirement should be at least 70 to 105 kcal/kg per day; and the protein intake should be 2.7 to 3.5 g/kg per day of protein for positive nitrogen balance, adequate nitrogen accretion, and good neurodevelopmental outcome. Protein is given in the form of an amino acid solution. These amino acids are the building blocks required for growth, preservation of skeletal muscle protein mass, tissue repair, and appropriate inflammatory response. Protein intake starts at 1 to 2 g/kg per day and increases daily, under stable conditions, up to the recommended daily intake. Critically ill neonates will also require an increase in protein intake by 10% to 20%.

Calories or energy is given through carbohydrates and fat. Glucose is the carbohydrate used in parenteral nutrition and is the preferred substrate for the brain. It provides 3.4 cal/g of glucose. Fat is given as a 20% lipid emulsion solution, and it provides 2 cal/mL. The use of the lipid emulsion will prevent essential fatty acid deficiency, improve protein use and will not increase significantly CO_2 production or metabolic rate compared to glucose. This is an important factor in infants with chronic lung disease and retention of carbon dioxide. The infusion rate of fat begins at 0.5 g/kg per day and is advanced by 0.5 g daily up to 2 to 4 g/kg per day. Close monitoring of triglycerides is required. A level above 250 mg/dL is considered high, so the rate of infusion should then be cut back. Adequate energy intake will promote or facilitate positive nitrogen balance and nitrogen accretion. Other components of parenteral nutrition are calcium, phosphorus, vitamins, and trace minerals. Sodium and potassium are added based on the serum electrolyte results.

Carnitine is added when premature infants are on prolonged parenteral nutrition.

The task of providing adequate nutrition is multidisciplinary; the neonatologist, pharmacist, and nutritionist form part of the team. Close metabolic monitoring for glucose, electrolytes, urea, lipids, and acid–base balance is an integral part of the nutritional management of their high-risk neonates. This will help assess and meet nutritional needs as well as monitor for complications such as metabolic acidosis, electrolyte imbalance, cholestatic jaundice, increased triglyceride levels, and infection. When enteral feeding is possible, human milk should be considered. Although it may not provide adequate caloric and protein intake, it has many other assets that are important in promoting healing, neurodevelopment, and protection against infection.

DEVELOPMENTAL CARE

The NICU environment plays a major role in the growth and development of the high-risk neonate and may contribute to the morbidity of these fragile infants. The amount of abnormal sensory stimulus that these fragile beings are exposed to is the source of overwhelming stress at sensitive periods of their development, and in turn will modify their brain development. The cortex of the brain is part of the sensory system, and both deprivation and overstimulation can modify its development. The sensitive period when this occurs is between 28 and 40 weeks of gestation. Therefore the NICU environment is crucial as part of the care of the sick newborn infant. These infants are subject to numerous stress factors, unpleasant procedures, continuously disrupted sleep, frequent noxious oral stimulus, noise, and bright lights. Stress causes autonomic instability, with secretion of cortisol and catecholamines. These hormones in turn interfere with tissue healing and growth.

Rakel and Bope: *Conn's Current Therapy 2006.*

When considering the NICU environment and the input or stimuli that could be beneficial to these high-risk neonates, one has to take into consideration the in utero environment and how the sensory stimulus would have been perceived in that environment, and the normal development of the sensory system for planned interventions. The hierarchal organization, maturation, and integration of the sensory system is as follows:

- Tactile
- Vestibular
- Gustatory
- Olfactory
- Auditory
- Visual

The visual sensory system is the least mature at term and maturation continues after birth. There is overlapping regarding when a sensory system maturation begins and ends, but there is clear evidence that disruption of one sensory system will affect the maturation of the system that has not yet developed. The same is true when a later sensory system is stimulated earlier than expected.

The interventions that support the development of the sensory system are as follows:

- Minimal handling
- Clustering of care
- Soft swaddling
- Stroking, rocking, and holding when appropriate
- Non-nutritive sucking
- Positioning prone or on the side
- Nesting
- Placing the infant in an infant seat; then swaddle and nest
- Soothing, soft, simple repetitive, and harmonic sounds with limited dynamic range

Limit ambient light and shield eyes and chest from bright lights. Limit the initial visual stimulus to the human face, and massage therapy. These suggested interventions should take into consideration the gestational age and the clinical acuity of the high-risk patient. The goal is to improve growth and neurodevelopmental outcome of the high-risk neonate.

PARENTAL INVOLVEMENT

When looking at specific high-risk situations, one can appreciate the scope of support needed by these high-risk neonates from various subspecialists and ancillary health care professionals. One of the things often forgotten is the major role the parents play in the healing and development of their sick infant. Parents have a sense of loss from the time their sick newborn has to be resuscitated and or is admitted to the NICU. They have a sense of loss for delivering prematurely, for not having a healthy full-term infant, loss of self-esteem, and social status as parents. Involving the parents in the care of their infant will provide some emotional, psychosocial, and spiritual support to the parents. The literature continues to support the need for and the benefits of parental

involvement in the NICU as part of the care of the high-risk neonate.

Kangaroo care, or skin-to-skin contact between the parent and the infant, provides sustained multimodal stimulation of tactile, vestibular, proprioceptive, olfactory, and auditory sensory systems. Physiologic benefits such as stable temperature; stable oxygen consumption; higher saturation levels; increased quiet sleep, which lowers cortisol levels resulting in fewer infections; and better growth have been described. It promotes non-nutritive sucking, and there is a better letdown in breast-feeding mothers. Kangaroo care acts as a behavioral organizer or facilitator, decreases motor activity, increases the quiet state in stable preterm infants, and reduces the effect of painful stimuli. These infants are also discharged sooner.

Parents can also participate in massage therapy. It has a calming effect on infants; they express fewer stress behaviors, are more alert, actively respond to face and voice, and show more organized limb movements on the Brazelton behavioral scale. Better weight gain and early discharge have been reported. At 8 months these infants continue to show better weight gain and higher scores on the Bayley Scales of Infant Development.

Conditions Associated With Abnormal Transition

A few conditions associated with abnormal transition are described in the following text.

HYALINE MEMBRANE DISEASE

Hyaline membrane disease (HMD) is the result of surfactant deficiency. Surfactant reduces the surface tension of the alveoli and prevents them from collapsing. This disorder is common to preterm infants. The clinical presentation of HMD is that of respiratory distress characterized by grunting, retractions, and flaring. Grunting is used to maintain the intra-alveoli pressure and prevent it from collapsing. The blood gas typically has hypoxemia and to a lesser degree respiratory acidosis. Radiographically the lungs have a ground glass appearance (this represents microatelectasis) and air bronchograms (the contrast of the air filled bronchi against the collapse parenchyma). These infants are managed with ventilator support and/or continuous positive airway pressure (CPAP), and surfactant (Survanta) replacement therapy. The use of antenatal steroids has decreased the incidence of HMD and the need for exogenous surfactant in the premature newborn, especially in infants who are 28 weeks gestation or more.

TRANSIENT TACHYPNEA OF THE NEWBORN

Transient tachypnea of the newborn (TTN) is described as the retention of lung fluid or transient pulmonary edema. During labor the increased level of prostaglandins causes dilation of the lymphatic vessels in the lungs

Rakel and Bope: *Conn's Current Therapy 2006.*

promoting the absorption of the pulmonary interstitial fluid. After birth, this process is further accelerated by the expansion of the lungs with air-filled alveoli and increased pulmonary circulation. Any delay in this process will result in tachypnea and occasional grunting and flaring. This is common after elective cesarean section. The arterial blood gas shows various degrees of respiratory acidosis and some hypoxemia. The typical chest radiographic findings reveal increased interstitial marking with fluid in the fissure and on occasion pleural effusion. This condition is self-limited, resolving in 1 to 2 days. These infants are managed with oxygen support by hood and rarely require ventilator support.

MECONIUM ASPIRATION SYNDROME

Meconium staining of the amniotic fluid occurs in 10% to 25% of all deliveries. It is seen in fetuses beyond 35 weeks of gestation. Passage of meconium in utero is often the result of a hypoxemic event. Meconium can be aspirated before, during, or after delivery. Once aspirated it can cause obstruction of the airway and pulmonary air leak, chemical pneumonitis and secondary bacterial infection, secondary surfactant deficiency, and pulmonary hypertension of the newborn (PPHN) if hypoxemia persists. After birth, a depressed neonate with poor or no respiratory effort should be intubated and suctioned immediately after being placed under the radiant warmer. This action will clear the airway and prevent aspiration or any further aspiration. The key in preventing meconium aspiration in neonates who did not have in utero aspiration is suctioning of the airway at the perineum by the obstetrician as soon as the head is delivered. The severity of the disease varies. The arterial blood gas pictures vary from mild respiratory acidosis with mild hypoxemia to severe respiratory failure with marked hypoxemia. The classical radiographic finding of the lungs is that of patchy infiltrates throughout the lung fields; air leak is seen in 10% to 20% of these cases. Postnatal management consists of support to minimize all factors that will perpetuate asphyxia and trigger pulmonary hypertension. Decrease energy loss and oxygen consumption by providing warmth, oxygen, and glucose. Aggressive respiratory support is needed, providing high concentration of oxygen in a hood or through the ventilator. In cases associated with severe PPHN, inhaled nitric oxide (iNO [INO$_{max}$]), and ultimately extracorporeal membrane oxygenation (ECMO) may become part of the management.

PERSISTENT PULMONARY HYPERTENSION OF THE NEWBORN

Persistent pulmonary hypertension of the newborn is the result of severe hypoxemia because of right-to-left shunting through the foramen ovale and ductus arteriosus, without associated structural heart abnormality. The pulmonary hypertension results from increased pulmonary vasoreactivity and increased muscle mass of the pulmonary arterial vessels. The increase in pulmonary smooth arterial muscle mass seen in term

infants is triggered by intrauterine stress or hypoxemia. The vasoreactive response seen after birth is caused by alteration of the balance between the circulating pulmonary vasodilator (endothelium-derived relaxing factor or endogenous nitric oxide) and pulmonary vasoconstrictors (endothelin). This vasoreactive response is seen also in preterm and term infants with primary lung disease, such as surfactant deficiency, pneumonia, or MAS. Tachypnea and cyanosis is the clinical presentation. The blood gas has severe hypoxemia and combine metabolic and respiratory acidosis. In primary PPHN, the chest radiograph is normal; in secondary PPHN, it will be characteristic of the disease in question. The diagnosis of PPHN is made with the aid of the echocardiogram, which will exclude structural heart disease, measure the pulmonary artery pressure and resistance and visualize the right-to-left shunts, and tricuspid regurgitation that is commonly present.

The management of neonates with PPHN can be challenging. The goal is to correct the hypoxemia and acidosis, both of which cause pulmonary vasoconstriction. The acidosis can be managed with hyperventilation using conventional or high-frequency ventilator (to achieve a PaCO$_2$ close to 30 mm Hg) and/or infusion of sodium bicarbonate to maintain the arterial pH around 7.40. The hypoxemia is more difficult to manage because these infants do not always respond to high concentrations of oxygen with high ventilator support. The PaO$_2$ should be maintained above 80 mm Hg. Concurrent metabolic derangement, such as hypoglycemia and hypocalcemia, and polycythemia should be corrected. The systemic arterial BP should be maintained in the high range of normal. The use of vasopressor agents (dopamine [Intropin] or dobutamine [Dobutrex]) is recommended in achieving this goal, as opposed to volume expansion. The increase in the systemic BP may decrease the right-to-left shunt through the ductus arteriosus and improve pulmonary blood flow and in turn improve the hypoxemia.

When the previously described management fails, the use of iNO at a dose of 20 ppm or less will cause selective pulmonary vasodilatation. Because many infants respond to iNO, the need for ECMO has decreased. Extracorporeal membrane oxygenation is available only in a few medical centers for those cases that fail to respond to maximum ventilator support and iNO.

The Infant with Surgical Conditions

Infants before, during, or after surgery require special consideration regarding management and support of the cardiopulmonary system, thermoregulation, fluid and electrolyte management, nutritional support, and infection control.

GASTROSCHISIS

The combined incidence of omphalocele and gastroschisis is 1:4000 live births. Of these two abdominal wall defects, gastroschisis is the more common. It is a cleft in the abdominal wall to the right of the umbilical cord with herniation of the bowel. The association of other congenital and chromosomal anomalies is rare compared with omphalocele. Common associated problems seen in gastroschisis are malrotation of the bowel, undescended testes, stenosis, and atresia of the bowel, all of which are the result of vascular injury. In 20% of the patients, necrotizing enterocolitis has been reported postoperatively.

Gastroschisis can be diagnosed in the prenatal period. This will allow for proper counseling of the family as well as the plans for intrapartum and postnatal management. The intrapartum and postnatal management consist of preventing further injury to the bowel, temperature stabilization, fluid and electrolyte management, antibiotic therapy, nutritional support, and surgical correction. The exposed bowel is at risk for further circulatory compromise. This may be avoided by having the infant lie on his or her side. Because there is a large surface area exposed to the environment, heat and fluid losses are increased. The bowel should be wrapped in cephalexin (Keflex) soaked in warm normal saline, and then covered with a plastic barrier. The prolonged exposure of the bowel to the amniotic fluid causes a severe inflammatory response that results in ileus. In addition to the increased fluid losses through the exposed bowel, there is intraluminal loss of fluid and electrolyte because of the severe ileus. In these patients 1.5 to 2 times their fluid maintenance is needed for fluid resuscitation. The bowel should be decompressed using a nasogastric or orogastric tube connected to intermittent low suction. Close monitoring of vital signs, intake and output, and serum electrolytes will give indications of the fluid and electrolyte status of these infants.

Nutritional support in infants with gastroschisis is crucial for healing and to decrease morbidity and mortality. Prior to parenteral nutrition, the mortality in these infants was very high, malnutrition and complications associated with infection being major causes. These infants may go for several weeks before enteral feedings can be attempted or tolerated. Early placement of central venous access will facilitate the long-term nutritional support and the overall management. Long-term parenteral nutrition is the key for full recovery of these infants.

The surgical approach considers two options: primary or secondary closure. Secondary closure creates an enclosed hernia, a silo with the bowel content. The bowel is then slowly returned to the abdominal cavity over several days. Antibiotics are continued until the abdominal wall is closed. Primary closure returns the bowel into the abdominal cavity in one step. It is not uncommon, especially with large defects, to have respiratory compromise requiring ventilator support. Be conscious of the need for pain management in these infants, more so in those with respiratory compromise. Other complications seen with primary closure are further bowel compromise with bloody drainage, acidosis, and infection and increased intra-abdominal pressure that causes decrease renal and or central venous perfusion.

Rakel and Bope: *Conn's Current Therapy 2006.*

CONGENITAL DIAPHRAGMATIC HERNIA

The incidence of congenital diaphragmatic hernia (CDH) is 1:2000 to 5000 live births. This condition can be diagnosed in the prenatal period. When diagnosed in the prenatal period the plan of management begins. The infant should be delivered at a tertiary care center experienced in counseling and treatment of CDH. In these patients, further workup should be done to exclude other malformations of the heart, GI tract, GU system, and CNS and chromosomal anomalies. Associated malformations should be taken into account when counseling the family and when developing the postnatal plan of management. Plans to deliver at term, and at a center where there is a pediatric surgeon, capability for iNO (INO_{max}) and ECMO is desired. Once delivered, the infant should be intubated immediately, venous access obtained in case of needed circulatory support, and a nasogastric or orogastric tube placed to decompress the bowel. Bowel distention can further compromise respiration and cardiac function.

The infant should be transferred to the NICU, an arterial line should be placed and blood obtained for blood gas and crossmatch. Obtain a chest and abdominal radiograph to confirm the diagnosis and line placement. An echocardiogram should be done to assess for structural abnormalities of the heart and to estimate the degree of pulmonary hypertension. A head US should be obtained if the infant will be placed on ECMO, because of the risk of intracranial hemorrhage in patients on ECMO.

Skilled ventilator management is important because of the coexisting pulmonary hypertension. Barotrauma should be avoided in these patients. Permissive hypercapnia is permitted once there is adequate preductal oxygenation (preductal oxygenation is measured or obtained from the right upper extremity; the preductal blood perfuses the heart and brain). The highest rates of survival result in patients in whom barotraumas are avoided and permissive hypercapnia is allowed.

A patient is considered unstable or to have failed ventilator support when the pH is <7.25, a peak inspiratory pressure of >30 cm H_2O is needed, and preductal saturation is <90% on 60% oxygen. The use of iNO (INO_{max}) may be considered in these cases, but the direct effect on pulmonary vascular resistance and right heart function need to be monitored closely. Therapy should be discontinued if no response is demonstrated. Extracorporeal membrane oxygenation is a reasonable choice for patients that have received maximum medical intervention. A venous-venous shunt is preferred unless there is significant cardiac instability.

Surgical correction is done if the infant is stable after the honeymoon period (the first 24 hours). Achievement of 90% survival is possible in a nonselect group of patients with the combination of careful ventilator management, attention to the pulmonary hypertension, delayed surgery, and aggressive early nutrition support. Survival rates are also dependent on the presence or absence of associated abnormalities and their severity. Long-term follow-up beyond the neonatal period is necessary for accurate estimation of morbidity and mortality in patients who are placed on ECMO.

TABLE 4 Common Problems and Management of the Extremely Low Birth-Weight Infant

Problems	Management
Delivery Room. It is anticipated that a complete team will be needed for resuscitation: neonatal nurse, respiratory therapist, and neonatologist.	Prevent heat loss, provide respiratory support, prevent asphyxia, and avoid trauma. Place under radiant warmer and dry well, use warm blankets and cap. Use bag and mask properly and prompt intubation when needed. Properly position the ETT; avoid high inspiratory pressure with overdistention of the lungs. Follow the ABCs of resuscitation.
NICU. The management in the delivery room and the first hours of life sets the stage for the rest of the NICU care.	In the NICU, the infant is placed under a radiant warmer for easy access and thermoregulation. Connect to all monitors, insert umbilical, venous, and arterial catheters for fluid management, BP monitoring, and to facilitate blood draw. Obtain chest and abdominal radiograph to assess the severity of lung disease and position of the ETT, venous, and arterial catheters. Cover infant with plastic wrap to decrease evaporative heat and fluid loss. Frequent weight within bed scale will estimate hydration status. There should be minimal handling and clustered care in the first week of life.
Fluid and Electrolytes. The high insensible water loss in the ELBW infant increases the risk for dehydration, hypernatremia, and hyperkalemia	Fluid requirements range from 100 to 150 mL/kg/d, given as D5W with no added electrolytes in the first 24-48 h. Monitoring of the electrolytes and strict I&O will estimate the hydration status. Monitor blood draw and replace with PRBC from a single donor, CMV negative, when 10% of blood volume is removed. Hypernatremia is caused by increased water loss and corrected with increased fluid intake. Risk of hyperkalemia is caused by water loss and is further increased if there is extravascular blood collection; this is corrected using insulin infusion with glucose, correcting acidosis with sodium bicarbonate, calcium gluconate to stabilize the myocardium, and a cation exchange resin per rectum—sodium polystyrene sulfonate (Kayexalate).
Nutrition. Long-term parenteral nutrition is required in these infants. Good nutritional support is necessary for growth and neurodevelopment.	Beginning early parenteral nutrition within the first 24 h in stable infants will provide a source of energy (glucose), protein to decrease the risk of negative nitrogen balance, calcium, vitamins, and trace minerals. Placement of percutaneous CVC should be done early in the course. Please refer to the section on nutrition in this article for further nutrition management.
CNS. There us an increased risk of developing IVH in unstable infants in the first few days of life.	To prevent IVH, stressful conditions like cold stress, hypoxemia, acidosis swing in BP, and increased intrathoracic pressure should be avoided. Initial US in the first 3 d if unstable and at the end of the first week if stable. Follow-up will depend on findings. Infants with no IVH should have a repeat at 36 weeks postmenstrual age. The use of sedation in the first week of life has not shown significant changes in the incidence of IVH.
Respiratory. HMD is the most common condition. Avoid complications associated with the disease (air leaks and pulmonary emphysema, pulmonary hemorrhage, ICH, and CLD).	Use of exogenous surfactant when indicated and rapid weaning of PIP and O_2 and close monitoring to avoid complications. Blood gas is obtained every 10-15 min after each change. Use high ventilator rate and the lowest PIP to maintain saturation 93%-95%, permissive hypercapnia ($Paco_2$ 50-60), mild acidosis (pH 7.25-7.35), and Po_2 50-70 are the goal. When stable, extubate to NCPAP. Apnea is common in these infants; they are treated with caffeine citrate (Cafcit). An initial bolus of 20 mg/kg is given followed by maintenance of 5 mg/kg every 24 h.

Continued

Rakel and Bope: *Conn's Current Therapy 2006.*

TABLE 4 Common Problems and Management of the Extremely Low-Birth-Weight Infant—cont'd

Problems	Management
Cardiovascular. PDA occurs in >50% of ELBW infants. Appearing when the lung disease is improving, clinically there is increased need for respiratory support signs including desaturation, active precordium, bounding pulses, and wide pulse pressure. The diagnosis is confirmed by echocardiogram. The ductus arteriosus of the preterm responds less to the vasoconstrictive effect of oxygen.	Medical treatment consists of fluid restriction, maintenance of hematocrit around 40%, and the use of indomethacin (Indocin IV). Complications of indomethacin (Indocin IV) are decreased GFR causing fluid retention and platelet dysfunction (contraindicated in renal failure, bleeding disorders, and low platelets). The dose is 0.2 mg/kg for four doses and a diuretic such as furosemide (Lasix) at 1 mg/kg/dose to try to prevent oliguria. If there is no response, additional dosing or courses can be given. The definitive treatment would be ligation of the ductus. Some centers use prophylactic indomethacin (Indocin IV).
Skin. Underdevelopment of the stratum corneum cause increase transepidermal water loss→dehydration→ electrolyte imbalance and evaporative heat loss. Traumatized skin is the port of entry for many infectious organisms. Acceleration of skin maturation occurs after birth over the next 10-14 d.	Use of plastic shields, increased humidity, and topical skin emollient will decrease heat and water loss and may be protective to the skin.
Glucose. Hyperglycemia is secondary to high glucose-infusion rates. When an infant becomes hyperglycemic on a stable glucose-infusion rate, consider infection and or IVH. Early hypoglycemia is common in this group of infants due to poor glycogen stores and immature hormonal adaptation of the endocrine system.	Glucose level should be >40 mg/dL in the first 48-72 h and >45 mg/dL after 72 h. When hypoglycemic, a bolus of D10W at 200 mg/kg (2 mL/kg) is given. Glucose level is obtained in 30 min, frequent monitoring is continued every 1-3 h, and further boluses are given as needed. Maintenance fluid provides 4-6 mg/kg/min of glucose infusion. This rate of infusion should be increased by 2 mg/kg/min with every need for D10W bolus. Refer to specific text for detailed management.
Calcium. The stores of calcium are limited and the reserves are rapidly depleted after birth.	Higher intake of calcium with adequate phosphorus intake is required for bone formation and growth.
Jaundice. These infants are at increased risk for brain toxicity from high bilirubin levels. High bilirubin level develops due to hepatic immaturity, shorter RBC life span, extravasation of blood, and increased enterohepatic circulation, coupled with lower serum albumin level.	The level that causes toxicity is lower in these infants. A crude method to determine the need for phototherapy at 50% the weight in kg: A 0.9 Kg infant is placed under phototherapy for a bilirubin level of 4.5 mg/dL. Exchange level is determined by the weight, in this case 9 mg/dL. The risk for toxicity increases in the unstable infant, the reason why lower levels should be used when managing. Fluid intake should be increased 15%-20% in infants under phototherapy.

Abbreviations: ABC = airway, breathing, and circulation; BP = blood pressure; CLD = chronic lung disease; CMV = cytomegalovirus; CVC = central venous catheter; ELBW = extremely low birth weight infant; ETT = endotracheal tube; GFR = glomerular filtration rate; HMD = hyaline membrane disease; I&O = intake and output; ICH = intracranial hemorrhage; IV = intravenous; IVH = intraventricular hemorrhage; NCPAP = nasal continuous positive airway pressure; NICU = neonatal intensive care unit; PDA = pulmonary disease anemia; PIP = peak inspiratory pressure; PRBC = packed red blood cells; RBC = red blood cell; US = ultrasound.

The Extremely Low Birth Weight Infant

A premature infant is a neonate who is delivered before 37 completed weeks of gestation. These infants can be further classified according to their birth weight:

- Low birth weight (LBW) if less than 2500 g
- Very low birth weight (VLBW) if less than 1500 g
- Extremely low birth weight (ELBW) if less than 1000 g

Within the ELBW infants is a subgroup called the micropremie, if birth weight is less than 750 g. The need for intrapartum and postnatal intervention and support is inversely proportional to gestational age as well as the morbidity and mortality associated with these infants. The increased risks for asphyxia, heat and water loss, intraventricular hemorrhage, and respiratory distress increase with decreasing gestational age. In the delivery room, the initial steps of resuscitation will support transition by preventing heat and water loss and asphyxia. The use of surfactant (Survanta) should be considered in ELBW infants. In infants more than 1000 g, surfactant replacement therapy should be done as soon as the neonate presents a clinical picture of surfactant deficiency (HMD). Surfactant should be given with the proper ventilator support and, it is not uncommon to require multiple doses. With delay in therapy the morbidity and mortality associated with HMD increases.

The ELBW infants are a special group within the premature infants because the advances in health care and technology seem to have had less of an impact on this group of infants. The overall morbidity and mortality

CURRENT DIAGNOSIS

- Review of risk factors: antenatal, perinatal, and postnatal
- Assessment of infants in the delivery room: airway, breathing and circulation—respiration, heart rate, and color
- Continued assessment in the nursery: respirations, heart rate, color, temperature, and CNS
- Common problems: pulmonary, circulatory, gastrointestinal, metabolic, surgical, and temperature instability

Abbreviations: CNS = central nervous system.

continue to be comparatively high in these infants and more so the micropremie or infants less than 27 weeks of gestation. Table 4 lists the common problems faced by the ELBW infant and their management.

Special Therapy

Although there are continued attempts to provide care for the ELBW infant, there are infants outside the scope of *viability*—infants with complex congenital malformations, including those labeled as *incompatible with life*, and those whose condition is irreversible and ultimately will lead to death. For such infants, we see the need for

CURRENT THERAPY

- Use functioning equipment and qualified personal in the delivery room: initial steps and ABCs of neonatal resuscitation.
- Provide neutral thermal environment. Respiratory and cardiovascular support: oxygen, mechanical ventilation vasopressor agent (dopamine).
- Infuse bolus of D10W and glucose at 6-8 mg/kg per minute or higher if needed.
- Use phototherapy for early jaundice and the bruised ELBW infant.
- Transfer to appropriate level of care when indicated.
- Monitor closely fluid and electrolytes and decreased IWL. Provide good nutritional support beginning in the first 24 hours and closely monitor for complications and tolerance.
- Provide family-centered care and appropriate environment to promote growth and development.
- Benefit special cases, especially those deemed futile, with a multidisciplinary approach.

Abbreviations: ABC = airway, breathing, and circulation; ELBW = extremely low birth weight; IWL = insensible water loss.

comfort care or palliative care. In these situations both the health care professional and parents find themselves in an awkward position. The family remains hopeful based on the perceived information that the health care professional gives, or the family goes through turmoil when interventions seem endless in a situation that they perceive as hopeless.

The decision for palliative care is made through collaboration between the health care team and the parents. The two factual considerations in making the decision for palliative care are pertinent medical facts (diagnosis, response to treatment given, potential response to other treatments, and prognosis) and the human value (what the parents anticipate, expect, and desire for their infant) and what motivates these values in the parents. The values of the health care team involved in the care of the infant are also considered.

Palliative care, as defined by the World Health Organization (WHO), is care for patients for whom cure is no longer a reasonable expectation or possibility. It is an active and comprehensive management of the entire patient, and not abandonment of care.

Practical considerations that need to be taken into account, and specific components of the palliative care that are appropriate for each individual high-risk neonate, are considered before a specific plan can be put in place. The application of palliative care in the NICU is not only possible, but necessary.

REFERENCES

Aly H: Respiratory disorders in the newborn: Identification and diagnosis. Pediatr Rev 2004;25:201-208.
Avery GB, Fletcher MA, Macdonald MG (eds): Neonatology: Pathophysiology and Management of the Newborn, 5th ed. Philadelphia, Lippincott Williams & Wilkins, 1999, pp 143-173.
Blackburn ST: Maternal, Fetal, and Neonatal Physiology: A Clinical Perspective, 2nd ed. Philadelphia, WB Saunders, 2003, pp 707-730.
Carter BS: Comfort care principles for the high-risk newborn. NeoReviews 2004;e484-e490.
Chescheir NC, Harsen WF: What's new in perinatology. Pediatr Rev 1999;20:57-63.
Downard CD, Wilson JM: Current therapy of infants with congenital diaphragmatic hernia. Semin Neonatol 2003;8:215-221.
Field TM: Stimulation of preterm infants. Pediatr Rev 2003;24:4-10.
Heird WC: Determination of nutritional requirements in preterm infants, with special reference to "catch-up" growth. Semin Neonatol 2001;6:365-375.
Klaus MH, Fanaroff MB: Care of the High-Risk Neonate, 5th ed. Philadelphia, WB Saunders, 2001, pp 195-215.
Kattwinkel J (ed): Neonatal Resuscitation Textbok, 4th ed. American Heart Association, American Academy of Pediatrics, Elk Grove Village, Ill.
Kleinman RE (ed): Pediatric Nutrition Handbook, 5th ed. American Academy of Pediatrics, Elk Grove Village, Ill, 2004, pp 23-55.
Thureen PJ, Deacon J, O'Neill P, Hernandez JA: Assessment and care of the well newborn. Philadelphia, WB Saunders, 1999, pp 83-113.
Welch KK, Malone FD: Advances in prenatal screening: Nuchal translucency ultrasonography in the first trimester. NeoReviews 2002;3:e202-e208.
Welch KK, Malone FD: Advances in prenatal screening: Maternal serum screening for Down syndrome. Neoreviews 2002;3:e209-e213.

Normal Infant Feeding

Method of
Shirley H. Huang, MD,
and Virginia A. Stallings, MD

Remarkable growth and development characterize infancy, the period from birth to 1 year of age. During this time, the goals of infant feeding are to meet nutrient requirements, provide appropriate foods in accordance with the infant's developmental stage, and establish a pattern of optimal growth and nutritional status to support lifelong normal development and health.

Important Developmental Milestones

Knowledge of the neuromuscular and digestive development of infants is vital to understand the basis for food and feeding recommendations. Neuromuscular development begins in utero as the fetus swallows amniotic fluid and exhibits the sucking reflex. The mature nutritive suck-swallow pattern is established at 33 to 34 weeks gestational age. The infant progresses from the extrusion reflex of early infancy to the ability to swallow nonliquid foods at 4 to 5 months of age. Infants lift their head and neck in prone position at 2 months, reach at 4 months, sit unsupported with good head control at 6 months, and exhibit the pincer grasp at 9 months of age. At 5 to 6 months of age, infants indicate a desire for food by opening their mouths and leaning forward, and they indicate disinterest or satiety by leaning back and turning away. These motor and communications skills aid in solid and textured food introduction with minimal risk of aspiration, help promote cup usage and finger feeding, and provide a way for the infant to indicate hunger and satiety.

Gastrointestinal (GI) processes for digestion of complex foods mature during the first year of life. Nevertheless, newborn infants are fully capable of digesting and absorbing all the constituents of human milk and infant formula in amounts needed to support growth and development. When solids are introduced at 4 to 6 months of age, the ability to digest and absorb carbohydrates, proteins, and fats is mature, and the renal concentrating ability in most infants permits the excretion of hyperosmolar loads without excessive water loss. Intestinal enzymes and bacteria efficiently metabolize lactose, the principal carbohydrate in human milk and many formulas. Glucoamylase helps digest milk at 1 month of age, and increasing levels of salivary and pancreatic amylase aid the digestion of cereals when introduced at 4 to 6 months of age. Protein digestion is relatively well developed in infancy, although trypsin and chymotrypsin activities increase during the first 4 months of life. In contrast to the digestion of protein, the digestion and absorption of fats are less well developed in early infancy.

Nonetheless, babies absorb the fat from human milk better than from cow milk. The current recommendations of the American Academy of Pediatrics (AAP) for the introducing complementary solid foods at 4 to 6 months of age are based on individual aspects of the infant's developmental progress in eating-related skills.

Nutritional Requirements

The energy and nutrient needs for rapid growth differentiate nutritional requirements in infancy from all other ages. Water requirements for infants, provided by human milk or infant formula, are much greater than for adults because of high insensible losses from the larger proportional surface area and higher percentage of body water. The healthy infant's absolute requirement for water is approximately 100 mL/kg per day after the neonatal period. A higher amount is needed during periods with water losses, increased metabolic rate, and increased susceptibility to dehydration, such as with fever, vomiting, and/or diarrhea. Energy requirements per unit of body weight are three to four times that of an adult because of the infant's relatively higher resting metabolic energy needs and rapid growth and development: 108 kcal/kg per day for 0 to 6 months of age and 98 kcal/kg per day for 6 to 12 months of age, versus 30 to 40 kcal/kg per day for an adult.

The protein requirement, including essential amino acids per unit of body weight, is also greater than that of the older child and adult. The recommended daily allowance (RDA) for protein is approximately 2.2 g/kg per day during the first 6 months of life and 1.6 g/kg per day from 6 to 12 months of age. Fat is the major source of energy for infants, providing 50% per day of energy in human milk and 40% to 50% per day in formulas. According to the recently revised Dietary Reference Intakes (DRI), the adequate intake of n-6 polyunsaturated fatty acids is 4.4 to 4.6 g per day (6% to 8% per day of total calories) and that of n-3 polyunsaturated fatty acids is 0.5 g per day (1% per day of total calories). Although the minimum requirement of the essential fatty acid linoleic acid (the parent n-6 fatty acid) in infant formulas is 2.7% per day of total calories (U.S. Food and Drug Administration [FDA], 2000), no minimum requirement exists for the essential fatty acid α-linolenic acid (the parent n-3 fatty acid). Vegetable oils that contain α-linolenic acid are used in these formulas, however. In contrast to the requirements for essential amino acids and fatty acids, there appears to be no absolute requirement for carbohydrates as long as adequate sources of fat and protein supply energy through ketones or minimal amounts of essential glucose via gluconeogenesis. The lower limit of dietary carbohydrate compatible with life or for optimal health in infants is unknown. Nonetheless, the recommended adequate intake for infants based on the average intake of carbohydrate consumed from human milk and complementary foods is 60 g per day for 0 to 6 months of age and 95 g per day for 7 to 12 months of age. Furthermore, vitamins and minerals also have recommended intake levels established in the DRI.

Rakel and Bope: *Conn's Current Therapy 2006.*

Infant Feeding

BREAST-FEEDING

The AAP recommends human milk as the preferred feeding for all infants, including premature and sick newborns, with few exceptions. National surveys in 2001 showed that the initiation of in-hospital breast-feeding in the United States reached the highest levels recorded to date at approximately 65% to 70% per day and is projected to meet the Healthy People 2010 goal of 75% per day. Continued breast-feeding at 6 months also reached highest levels at 27% to 33% per day. Significant gains are required before reaching the Healthy People 2010 goal of 50% per day, however, especially for women who are black, teenagers, primiparous, less than high school educated, or enrolled in the Supplemental Nutrition Program for Women, Infants, and Children (WIC).

The AAP recognizes human milk as the primary food source in achieving optimal infant and child health, growth, and development. Thus breast-feeding should begin as early as possible after birth and be offered to newborns every 2 to 3 hours until satiety, usually 10 to 15 minutes on each breast. Exclusive breast-feeding is recommended for the first 6 months of age. Breast-feeding should continue until 12 months of age and thereafter for as long as mutually desired.

Human milk is uniquely superior for infant feeding and exhibits many nutritional benefits. It contains hormones, immune factors, growth factors, enzymes, and viable cells, most of which cannot practically be added to infant formulas. The composition of human milk varies among individuals and with the stages of lactation. Colostrum is the breast secretion during the last part of pregnancy and for the first 4 days after delivery. It contains more protein, calcium, minerals, and immunologic factors than mature human milk. Mature milk is established by the third or fourth week postpartum and contains constituents different from cow milk. Human milk contains less protein (1.0% to 1.5% of volume) than cow milk (3.3%). Human milk protein consists of approximately 75% whey proteins, largely α-lactalbumin, and 25% casein, whereas cow milk composition is approximately reversed. Other human milk proteins, such as lactoferrin, lysozyme, and secretory immunoglobulin A, appear to protect infants against GI and upper respiratory infections. Lactose is the principal carbohydrate of both human and cow milk, with slightly higher concentrations in human milk. Human milk also contains carbohydrate polymers and glycoproteins that contribute to intestinal microbial defense. Furthermore, the fat content in human milk is higher during the latter portion of a single nursing session, which may influence the satiety of the infant. Although both human and cow milk contain mainly triglycerides, they are more readily digested in human milk. Human milk also contains long-chain metabolites of linoleic and linolenic acid, which are important fatty acid constituents in the developing retina and the nervous system. Human milk provides all of the vitamins an infant needs, with the exception of vitamin K and, potentially, vitamin D. In human milk, the calcium-to-phosphorus ratio of 2:1 (versus 1.2:1.0 in

cow milk) is favorable for calcium absorption, and iron is readily absorbed and adequate for the first 6 months.

Other compelling health benefits of breast-feeding are well documented. Strong evidence indicates that human milk decreases the incidence and/or severity of diarrhea, lower respiratory infection, otitis media, bacteremia, meningitis, urinary tract infection, and necrotizing enterocolitis. There are also possible protective effects against sudden infant death syndrome, insulin-dependent diabetes mellitus, inflammatory bowel disease, and asthma and allergic diseases (including food allergies, atopic dermatitis, and allergic rhinitis). The enhancement of cognitive development is also proposed. Moreover, the extent and duration of breast-feeding are reported to be inversely associated with the risk of obesity in later childhood. Mothers benefit as well, including less postpartum bleeding, increased weight loss, prolonged contraceptive effect, and reduced risk of ovarian and premenopausal breast cancer. Furthermore, there are also reduced health care costs and employee absenteeism for care attributable to child illness, as well as savings of at least $400 during the first year that would be spent for infant formula.

INFANT FORMULAS

Iron-fortified infant formulas are appropriate substitutes for human milk when a mother chooses not to breast-feed. The composition of formulas continues to evolve in an effort to provide health, growth, and developmental outcomes similar to those seen in a breast-fed infant. Although no infant formula has the exact composition of human milk, parents should be assured that formula-fed infants grow and develop into healthy children.

Formulas available in the United States for term infants generally can be classified into four categories based on the protein source:

1. Formulas based on cow milk
2. Formulas based on soy protein
3. Formulas based on hydrolysate
4. Formulas based on free amino acid

The Infant Formula Act of 1980, amended in 1986, establishes minimum levels for 29 nutrients and maximum levels for 9 nutrients. Average daily requirements for vitamins and minerals are met when infants are given a minimum daily intake of 25 oz of standard formula with a concentration of 20 kcal per ounce. Aside from the protein source, the carbohydrate, fat, and electrolyte components differ in various formulas. Specialized formulas are available for infants with certain medical conditions, such as metabolic disorders.

Because it is common for families to consider changing formulas with symptoms of intolerance, the AAP recommendations clarify some of the issues of allergy and formulas. Lactose intolerance is very rare in healthy term infants. Most infants with a documented IgE-mediated allergy to cow milk protein do well on soy protein or hypoallergenic (extensively hydrolyzed or free amino acid–based) formulas. Infants with documented cow milk protein-induced enteropathy or enterocolitis frequently are sensitive (cross-reactive) to soy protein

Rakel and Bope: *Conn's Current Therapy 2006.*

and should be given a hypoallergenic formula. Infants at high risk for the development of allergy, identified by a strong family history, may benefit from hypoallergenic formulas as a supplement to breast-feeding during the first year of life.

As researchers determine new components and functions of human milk, nutritional modifications of infant formulas are adjusted to approach human milk composition more closely. The importance of long-chain fatty acids is one area of recent interest. docosahexaenoic acid (DHA) and arachidonic acid (AA) are available in formulas in the United States. Infant formulas historically only contained the precursor essential fatty acids, α-linolenic acid and linoleic acid, from which formula-fed infants synthesize DHA and AA, respectively. DHA and AA are found in cell membranes, especially those of the central nervous system and retina. Studies indicate that infants fed formulas without DHA and AA have significantly less erythrocyte DHA and AA compared to those who are breast-fed. These data suggest that formulas containing only the precursor essential fatty acids are not as effective in meeting the essential fatty acid requirements as those with the DHA and AA added. Current randomized clinical trials show limited evidence for the benefit of visual or general development of term infants, however, despite increases in DHA and AA in red blood cells. The long-term effects remain to be determined through longer and larger trials.

Since 1989 an increasing number of U.S. infant formulas provide nucleotides, the nonprotein nitrogen compounds present in higher amounts in human milk than in formulas based on cow milk. Although studies report beneficial effects of nucleotide supplementation on immune function, iron absorption, lipid metabolism, and intestinal flora and function, the clinical and health benefits of nucleotides remain controversial.

Formulas try to mimic the GI flora of breast-fed infants by the addition of probiotics, such as lactobacilli, or prebiotics, such as oligosaccharides. Lactobacilli are bacteria not present in human milk. Special preparation of the formula is necessary to keep the bacteria live for administration. The addition of probiotics to infant formula decreases the incidence and severity of diarrhea. Oligosaccharides are normally found in human milk. In the prebiotic concept, the addition of oligosaccharides to formulas results in a gut flora similar to that of breast-fed infants. Limited evidence is available for health-promoting effects such as protection against invasive microorganism translocation and colonization and possible roles in immunity and allergy.

COMPLEMENTARY FOODS

Complementary foods are introduced when the infant is developmentally ready and the nutrients in human milk become growth limiting. At approximately 4 to 6 months of age, foods are introduced one at a time at weekly intervals to identify possible food intolerance. Iron-fortified foods are important initial complementary food choices, and the gradual addition of pureed individual vegetables, fruits, and meats sets the pattern for a diverse diet. At 9 months of age, the infant accepts finely chopped foods and teething biscuits. Foods such as hot dogs, nuts, grapes, raw carrots, popcorn, and round candies should never be fed to infants because of the risk of aspiration and choking. Honey should not be used to sweeten foods because of the risk of botulism. Cow milk also should not be introduced before 12 months of age because of the low concentration and bioavailability of iron, possible side effects of gastrointestinal bleeding, and the high renal solute load of cow milk protein. Fruit juice is introduced with cup feeding after 6 months of age and should be limited to 4 to 6 oz per day. Healthy infants usually require no supplemental water, except in hot weather or other conditions that promote dehydration.

SUPPLEMENTATION

Under usual circumstances, the healthy full-term infant requires little vitamin or mineral supplementation. The AAP recommends that all infants receive a single intramuscular dose of vitamin K at birth to prevent vitamin K deficiency bleeding; oral administration is questioned because of concerns about inadequate prevention of the late-onset type of vitamin K deficiency bleeding. Vitamin D should be given to breast-fed infants by 2 months of life, as well as to infants who take less than 500 mL per day of formula fortified with vitamin D. This recommendation is especially important for infants who are dark-skinned or exposed to minimal sunlight. Although iron absorption from human milk is excellent, the infant's body iron stores diminish during the first 4 months of life and the iron requirements for growth are high. Thus the breast-fed infant requires additional iron sources after 4 to 6 months of age. Moreover, vitamin B_{12} must be provided to the breast-fed infant when the mother is a vegan who consumes no animal products. Fluoride supplements are also recommended for all infants after 6 months of age when the local water supply is insufficient in fluoride.

Infant Growth

NORMAL GROWTH

Assessing the nutritional status of an infant includes the evaluation of normal growth and body composition as well as the early detection and treatment of nutritional deficiencies and excesses. Growth assessment is an essential part of pediatric care because both medical and social problems adversely affect growth. Weight, length, and head circumference should be plotted on the revised growth charts (Centers for Disease Control and Prevention, 2000), which are based on populations with a better representation of both breast- and formula-fed infants and more diverse ethnic and economic backgrounds. A newborn's weight may decrease 10% per day below birth weight in the first week of life and should regain or exceed birth weight by 2 weeks of age, gaining approximately 15 to 30 g per day during the first 9 months of life. In addition, much discussion concerns the pattern of growth in breast-fed versus bottle-fed

16

CURRENT DIAGNOSIS

- Conduct neurodevelopmental physical examination to evaluate feeding capability:
  - Suck reflex at birth
  - Lifting of head and neck in prone position at 2 months of age
  - Reaching at 4 months of age
  - Ability to swallow nonliquid foods at 4 to 5 months of age
  - Sitting unsupported with good head control at 6 months of age
  - Pincer grasp at 9 months of age
- At each well-care visit, plot weight, length, weight-for-length, and head circumference on the revised growth charts (Centers for Disease Control and Prevention, 2000).
- Carefully evaluate a child when the weight is below the third or fifth percentile or drops more than two percentile channels.
- Identify children at risk for overweight by weight-for-length (95th percentile), rate of weight gain, family history, and socioeconomic, ethnic, cultural, or environmental factors at each well-care visit.

CURRENT THERAPY

- Provide developmental evaluation and intervention if necessary for delayed milestones.
- Promote breast-feeding for at least the first 6 months of life.
- Start exclusively breast-fed babies on vitamin D supplementation during the first 2 months of life as well as iron supplementation after 4 to 6 months of age.
- Supplement fluoride for infants after 6 months of age if ingestion of fluoridated water is low.
- Limit juice intake to 4 to 6 oz per day after 6 months of age.
- Promote healthy eating patterns during infancy to prepare the child for a healthy lifestyle later in life.

infants during the first year of life. In general, exclusive breast-feeding may accelerate weight and length gain in the first few months, which then declines slowly thereafter. Some studies show no difference in weight or length by 12 months in breast-fed versus bottle-fed infants; others show that breast-fed infants tend to weigh less. Currently, it is unclear whether there are long-term consequences caused by these differences in patterns of growth over the first year of life. Nonetheless, human milk is considered the ideal food for infants.

UNDERNUTRITION

The analysis of growth patterns provides critical information for the recognition of failure to thrive (FTT) or the failure to maintain the expected rate of growth over time. Although no universal criteria define FTT, most clinicians evaluate a child carefully when weight is below the third or fifth percentile or drops more than two percentile channels. Length and head circumference are usually affected later than weight in more severe and chronic cases. Despite disagreement over the definition of FTT, all agree it describes a sign of something to evaluate further, not a diagnosis. Labeling a child with FTT has little value when the etiology is not determined and proper therapeutic efforts initiated. Categorizing the infant's condition as organic (medical) or nonorganic (nonmedical) FTT may be helpful, although the practical therapeutic distinctions often are blurred. Regardless of the cause of FTT, prompt attention to nutritional rehabilitation is essential for the infant. A multidisciplinary team approach involving the physician, nutritionist, psychologist, social worker, and other community services is often required and optimal.

OVERNUTRITION

In an era in which the prevalence of obesity is increasing in the United States, several critical periods, including early infancy, are postulated in the development of childhood- or adolescent-onset obesity. For example, high infant weight-for-age or rapid rate of weight gain during the first few months of life may be associated with obesity in childhood as well as young adulthood. At present, no known safe and effective interventions in early infancy prevent adulthood obesity. The health supervision visit (well-infant visit) is a time to identify patients at risk by virtue of family history; weight status; and socioeconomic, ethnic, cultural, and environmental factors. As evidenced by the new AAP recommendations for pediatric overweight and obesity prevention, optimal nutrition and growth during this important period by promoting healthy eating patterns to prepare the infant for a healthy lifestyle later in life is a common goal.

REFERENCES

American Academy of Pediatrics, Committee on Nutrition: Feeding the infant, In Kleinman RE (ed): Pediatric Nutrition Handbook, 5th ed. Elk Grove Village, Ill, American Academy of Pediatrics, 2004.

American Academy of Pediatrics, Committee on Nutrition: Policy statement: Soy protein–based formulas: Recommendations for use in infant feeding. Pediatrics 1998;101(1);148-153.

American Academy of Pediatrics, Work Group on Breastfeeding: Policy statement: Breastfeeding and the use of human milk. Pediatrics 1997;100(6):1035-1039.

Carver JD. Advances in nutritional modifications of infant formulas. Am J Clin Nutr 2003;77(Suppl):1550S-1554S.

Charney E, Goodman HC, McBride M, et al: Childhood antecedents of adult obesity: Do chubby infants become obese adults? N Engl J Med 1976;295:6-9.

Institute of Medicine: Dietary Reference Intakes for Energy, Carbohydrate, Fiber, Fat, Fatty Acids, Cholesterol, Protein and Amino Acids. Washington, DC, National Academy Press, 2002.

Simmer K: Long-chain polyunsaturated fatty acid supplementation in infants born at term. Review. Cochrane Database Syst Rev 2000; (2):CD000376. Update in Cochrane Database Syst Rev 2001; (4):CD000376.

Stettler N, Zemel BS, Kumanyika S, Stallings VA: Infant weight gain and childhood overweight status in a multicenter, cohort study. Pediatrics 2002;109:194-199.

Vandenplas Y: Oligosaccharides in infant formula. Br J Nutr 2002;87 (Suppl 2):S293-S296.

Zeiger RS: Food allergen avoidance in the prevention of food allergy in infants and children. Pediatrics 2003;111:1662-1671.

Diseases of the Breast

Method of
Paniti Sukumvanich, MD and
Patrick Borgen, MD

Benign Diseases of the Breast

Benign diseases of the breast historically are subdivided into proliferative and nonproliferative lesions (Table 1). In a study by Dupont and Page, patients with breast biopsies yielding nonproliferative lesions had no increased risk of subsequent breast cancer. In contrast, proliferative lesions were associated with a minimal to a fivefold increased risk of breast cancer. In clinical practice, of the proliferative lesions, only atypical epithelial lesions increase breast cancer risk significantly. Appropriate treatment and counseling of patients depends on the risk of breast cancer associated with these benign breast diseases.

Nonproliferative Lesions

Nonproliferative lesions comprise mild hyperplasia without atypia, squamous or apocrine metaplasia, duct ectasia, mastitis, and cysts. In the study of 3303 patients by Dupont and Page, only 2.2% of patients with nonproliferative lesions had breast cancer following a benign

TABLE 1 Benign Diseases of the Breast

	Increase in Breast Cancer Risk
Nonproliferative Lesions	
Mild hyperplasia without atypia	None
Squamous or apocrine metaplasia	None
Duct ectasia	None
Mastitis	None
Cysts	None
Proliferative Lesions	
Fibroadenoma	None
Moderate or florid hyperplasia	Minimal
Microglandular adenosis	Minimal
Sclerosing adenosis	Minimal
Papilloma	Minimal
Atypical ductal hyperplasia	4- to 5-fold
Atypical lobular hyperplasia	5.8-fold

Rakel and Bope: *Conn's Current Therapy 2006.*

breast biopsy with a mean follow-up time of 17 years (Figure 1).

BREAST CYSTS AND FIBROCYSTIC BREAST DISEASE

Fibrocystic breast disease is a benign process in which generalized microcystic formation with stromal proliferation leads to increased breast nodularity. Cysts within the breast are most common in perimenopausal women 50 to 59 years of age as well as premenopausal women. Postmenopausal women not on hormone replacement therapy are unlikely to develop cysts in their breasts. Benign cysts are often tender and fluctuate in size with the menstrual cycle. Cysts may be detected either on physical examination as a palpable, smooth, mobile nodule or by breast ultrasound. They may appear as a solitary nodule or in a cluster. Ultrasonographic appearance of simple benign cysts is that of an anechoic, round or oval, well-circumscribed mass with posterior enhancement. If the mass has all four criteria, the accuracy of ultrasound is close to 100% for the diagnosis of a simple benign cyst. Cysts that appear complex, with internal echoes, thick septations, and irregular walls, are suspicious for breast carcinoma and should be examined surgically or with an ultrasound-guided biopsy. Confirmation of the diagnosis can be made by fine-needle aspiration (FNA) of the cystic fluid. Bloody fluid may be an indication for a biopsy. In a study of 6782 cyst aspirates,

16

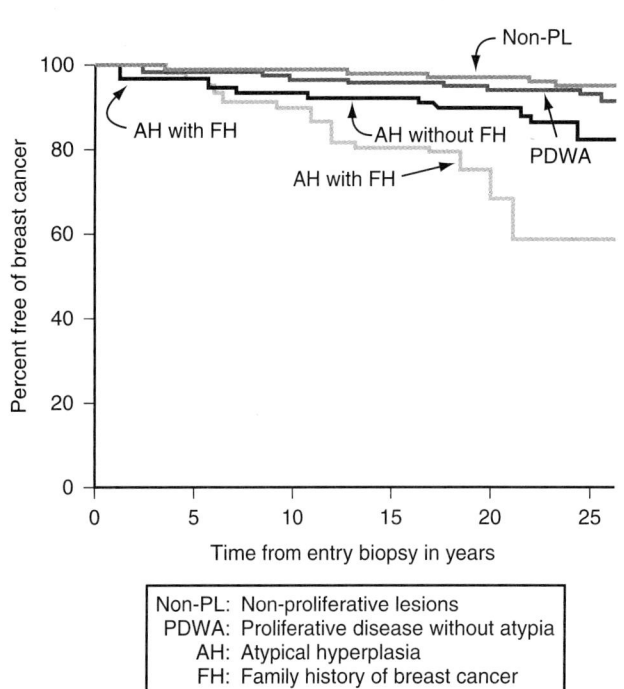

FIGURE 1. Nonproliferative lesions in breast cancer.

Ciatto and colleagues found that cytologic examination identified atypical cells in 1677 specimens. Of these specimens, only 0.3% of these cases had clinically and radiologically negative intracystic papillomas. Cytologic examination was positive in only 0.1% of these cases. Thus fluid from cyst aspirations are not sent routinely for cytologic examination. Figure 2 describes the management of suspected cysts.

MASTITIS AND DUCT ECTASIA

Mastitis is divided into lactational or nonlactational. Lactational mastitis can occur from the reflux of bacteria into the breast during breast-feeding. The causative bacteria are usually gram-positive cocci. Patients should be treated with antibiotics with the appropriate coverage and can continue to nurse or pump the breast to prevent engorgement. Nursing mothers can continue to breast-feed because the infant is not at risk for infection. Nonlactational (periductal) mastitis can be caused by duct ectasia, which occurs when the milk ducts become congested with secretions and debris, resulting in a periductal inflammation. These patients may present with greenish nipple discharge, nipple retraction, and

subareolar noncyclical pain. The treatment of nonlactational mastitis includes broad-spectrum antibiotics to cover for gram-positive cocci and skin anaerobes. Total duct excision and eversion of the nipple may be necessary to treat recurrent periductal mastitis.

Proliferative Benign Breast Diseases

Proliferative breast diseases include moderate or florid hyperplasia, microglandular and sclerosing adenosis, papilloma, fibroadenoma, and atypical ductal and lobular hyperplasia. All proliferative lesions have an increased risk of subsequent breast cancer after biopsy except for fibroadenoma. Overall, with a median follow-up of 17 years, 5.3% of patients with proliferative lesions develop breast cancer. This percentage increases to 12.9% in the presence of atypia (see Figure 1). Patients with moderate or florid hyperplasia, sclerosing adenosis, and solitary papilloma without atypia carry a minimal increase in risk of developing breast cancer over the general population. These patients are not classified as high risk. But the risk of subsequent breast cancer is

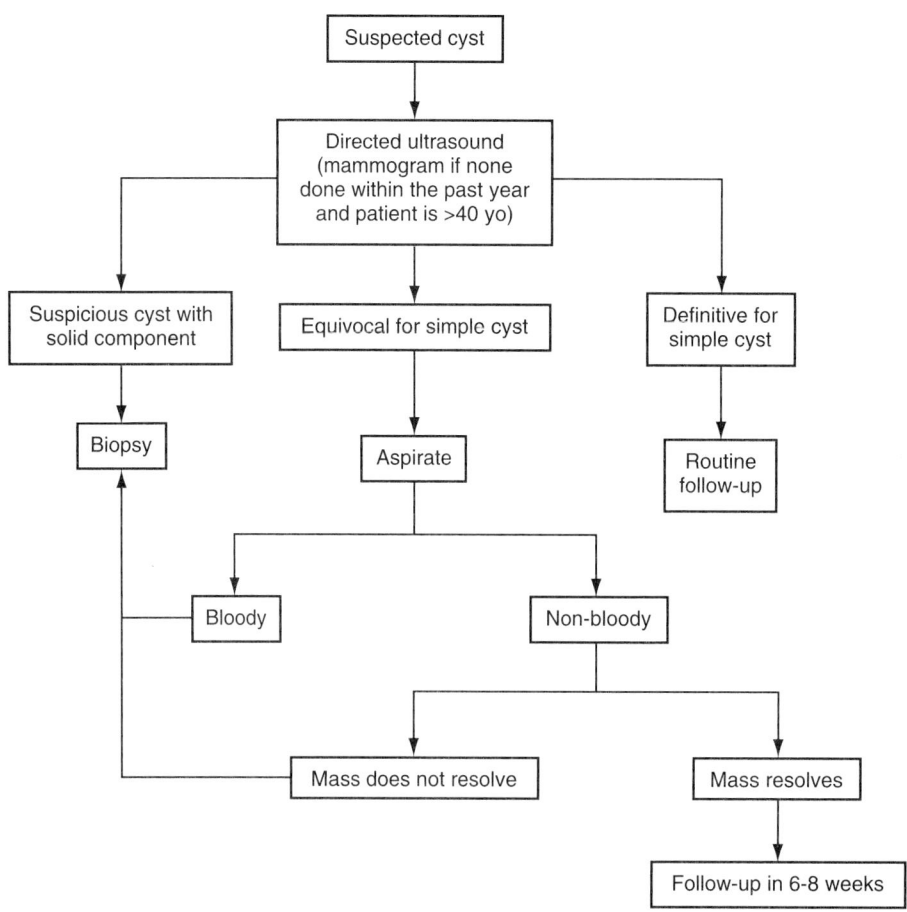

FIGURE 2. Algorithm for the management of suspected cysts.

Rakel and Bope: *Conn's Current Therapy 2006.*

increased by four- to fivefold in the presence of atypia. Atypical lobular hyperplasia carries a higher risk than atypical ductal hyperplasia, with a relative risk as high as 5.8. This increased risk applies to the contralateral breast because subsequent breast carcinomas are evenly divided between both breasts.

PROLIFERATIVE LESIONS WITH NO INCREASED RISK OF SUBSEQUENT CANCER: FIBROADENOMA

Fibroadenomas are benign tumors commonly found in young women (less than 30 years of age with a peak incidence at 21 to 25 years of age). They are characteristically detected on physical examination as well-circumscribed, rubbery, highly mobile, palpable masses. On mammograms, these lesions may appear as a well-circumscribed mass. Involution of fibroadenomas in the elderly can lead to hyalinization and dense popcorn-like calcification on mammograms. Fibroadenomas pose no increased risk of breast cancer and do not mandate surgical removal unless desired by the patient. Pregnancy can increase the size of these lesions; thus it may be reasonable to remove them prior to a planned pregnancy. Removal may facilitate follow-up, given the inability to follow breast masses adequately during pregnancy. Other types of fibroadenomas include juvenile and giant fibroadenomas. Juvenile fibroadenomas occur in adolescent women and can grow larger than 5 cm in diameter. These lesions are not malignant; given their large size, however, surgical excision may be needed to prevent asymmetry of the breasts. Giant fibroadenomas are large fibroadenomas found in the lactating breast or in the breasts of pregnant patients. These lesions may regress in size once hormonal stimulation subsides. Lesions that remain large can be excised surgically. Fibroadenomas and phyllodes tumors may be linked. Any rapidly enlarging fibroadenoma should be considered for surgical excision to rule out phyllodes tumor because it is difficult clinically to differentiate fibroadenoma from phyllodes tumor.

PROLIFERATIVE LESIONS WITH MINIMAL INCREASED RISK OF SUBSEQUENT BREAST CANCER

Multiple Peripheral Papillomas

Multiple peripheral papillomas are lesions that occur in the peripheral ducts. They most commonly present as a mass but may also present with nipple discharge. Complete excisional removal should be considered to rule out a papillary carcinoma of the breast. Approximately 10% to 33% of patients have subsequent breast cancer; thus close follow-up of these patients is warranted.

Sclerosing and Microglandular Adenosis

Sclerosing adenosis occurs as result of the proliferation of stromal tissue along with small terminal ductules. Often these lesions are picked up incidentally, but they may also present as microcalcifications on mammogram or as a mass (termed *adenosis tumor*). Sclerosing adenosis may be confused with a tubular carcinoma. Staining with immunohistochemical (IHC) markers such as actin, smooth muscle myosin heavy chain p63, or calponin may be helpful in distinguishing between the two lesions because only sclerosing adenosis contains myoepithelial cells. Microglandular adenosis is an uncommon lesion that may be mistaken for tubular carcinoma on histologic examination, and it can increase the patient's subsequent breast cancer risk. Concomitant breast cancer has been reported, so complete surgical excision should be considered for these lesions.

PROLIFERATIVE LESIONS WITH A FOUR- TO FIVEFOLD RISK OF SUBSEQUENT BREAST CANCER: ATYPICAL DUCTAL AND LOBULAR HYPERPLASIA

Atypical ductal and lobular hyperplasia are very similar to their in situ counterparts. These lesions are termed *atypical hyperplasia* because they lack some of the microscopic features of in situ disease. The distinction between atypical hyperplasia and carcinoma in situ is sometimes hard to make. In a study by Rosai, five expert breast cancer pathologists reviewed 17 cases of ductal or lobular lesions. In no case did all five agree on a diagnosis. Four out of the five were able to agree on a diagnosis in three cases (18%). In one third of the patients, the diagnosis ran the gamut from hyperplasia without atypia to carcinoma in situ. Despite such difficulty, the diagnosis of atypical hyperplasia is on the rise as mammographic screening becomes more popular. Atypical hyperplasia, which is detected secondary to microcalcifications or by serendipity, carries the highest risk of subsequent breast carcinoma among all proliferative lesions of the breast, with a four- to fivefold increased risk over the general population. Atypical lobular hyperplasia carries a higher risk than atypical ductal hyperplasia, with a relative risk as high as 5.8. This risk applies to the contralateral breast as well as the ipsilateral breast. Surgical excision of atypical hyperplasia on a core biopsy is recommended because 20% of patients are found to have breast cancer at time of surgical excision for atypical hyperplasia. It is not necessary to achieve negative margins for these lesions.

OTHER BENIGN BREAST LESIONS: FAT NECROSIS, HAMARTOMA, MONDOR'S DISEASE,RADIAL SCARS, AND PSEUDOANGIOMATOUS STROMAL HYPERPLASIA

Other benign lesions of the breast include fat necrosis, hamartoma, Mondor's disease, radial scars, and pseudoangiomatous stromal hyperplasia (PASH). Trauma to the breast may lead to fat necrosis and can be mistaken for carcinomas on clinical examination. Fat necrosis lesions present clinically as painless, irregular masses with or without associated skin changes such as skin thickening. These lesions can be normal or may have rim calcifications on mammograms. No further treatment is needed when a core biopsy definitively makes the diagnosis of fat necrosis.

Hamartomas are benign lesions that are often picked up on a mammogram. The fatty composition of the mass makes these lesions clinically occult. They can be mistaken for fibroadenomas on mammograms. Hamartomas can be left alone without histologic confirmation if diagnosed definitively on a mammogram.

Mondor's disease is a thrombophlebitis of the superficial breast veins that presents as a palpable tender cord leading to the axilla. In a study of 63 cases, 8 patients (25%) had an underlying malignancy; thus a mammogram should be done to rule out the presence of breast carcinoma.

Radial scars are benign lesions whose etiology is unknown. They are often mistaken for breast carcinoma on mammograms because of their stellate appearance. Radial scars may also mimic breast carcinoma histologically. Staining for myoepithelial cells can help distinguish between invasive carcinoma and a radial scar. Radial scars carry a 1.5-fold increase in risk of subsequent breast carcinoma, so these lesions should be considered markers of future disease.

First described in 1986, PASH is a benign proliferative lesion that may present as an incidental finding or a mobile breast mass. It can occur in all ages and also in men. On a mammogram, PASH appears as a round noncalcified mass. Histologically, PASH may be mistaken for low-grade angiosarcoma. Unlike angiosarcoma, however, there should be no evidence of mitosis or cytologic atypia in PASH specimens. The role of hormones in the pathogenesis of PASH is controversial. Although these lesions tend to occur in young patients or in elderly patients on hormone therapy, most cases tend to be negative for estrogen receptors. The treatment for PASH is complete surgical excision. Approximately 7% of cases recur despite adequate treatment.

Risk Factors for Breast Cancer

An estimated 80% of women in whom breast cancer develops have no documented risk factors or determinants. Risk factors can not be changed, whereas risk determinants can be altered to decrease a person's risk of subsequent breast cancer. Common risk factors include a familial history of breast cancer, personal breast biopsy history, menarche before 12 years of age, menopause after 55 years of age, increasing age, geographical location, and mutations of the BRCA1 or BRCA2 genes. Women known to have the BRCA1 or BRCA2 genetic mutation have an 85% lifetime risk of breast cancer as well as an increased risk of ovarian cancer. BRCA1 carriers are at a higher risk for developing ovarian cancer than BRCA2 (60% versus 20%, respectively). The risk determinants for breast cancer include reproductive factors such as nulliparity and first pregnancy after the age of 30 years and previous radiation exposure. Previous therapy for lymphoma, especially during adolescence, elevates a woman's risk of subsequent breast cancer.

Screening Techniques

Screening for breast cancer includes mammography, ultrasound, breast self-examination (BSE), and physical examination by a physician. Multiple studies such as the Göthenborg and Malmö trials show a reduction in breast cancer mortality from 30% to 40% in patients 40 to 49 years of age who undergo screening mammograms. A meta-analysis of six randomized trials indicates a 30% reduction in breast cancer mortality in patients 50 to 69 years of age. The sensitivity of mammograms depends on the patient's age and ranges from 53% to 81% in women 40 to 49 years of age to 73% to 81% in patients 50 years of age or older. An estimated 10% to 15% of breast cancer cases are not detectable on screening mammography, thus emphasizing the importance of physical breast examination by a physician and BSE that include both visual inspection and manual examination of the breast. On inspection, signs of breast malignancy include skin or nipple retraction or discoloration, nipple discharge/crusting, or peau d'orange edema of the breast. On palpation, any asymmetric mass of the breast or axilla may be regarded as a potential malignancy that deserves further evaluation.

Current recommendations are for a woman to start performing BSE at 18 years of age, have a yearly physical exam, and initiate annual mammography at 40 years of age. Little data exist on what should be the upper age limit of mammogram screening. Given that breast density decreases with age and breast cancer increases with age, mammograms should be even more sensitive and specific in the older age group. For these reasons, mammograms may be continued in very elderly patients as long as the patient is not suffering from any major comorbidities. In patients who have a very high risk of breast cancer, such as BRCA carriers, screening should start 10 years earlier than the age of onset of an affected relative or at the age of 35. Kriege screened 1909 patients (including 358 BRCA mutation carriers) who had more than a 15% lifetime risk of developing breast cancer. These patients had a biannual breast exam as well as annual mammogram and breast magnetic resonance imaging (MRI). In this population, mammograms had a sensitivity of 33% with a specificity of 95%. Breast MRI had significantly higher rates of sensitivity and specificity at 80% and 90%, respectively. Given these findings, breast MRI should be a part of the screening exam for these high-risk patients. MRI is recommended as a standard screening test in BRCA heterozygotes. Routine surveillance in high-risk patients includes a 6-month interval alternating between breast MRI and mammograms. Patients with a history of mantle radiation for lymphoma should start annual screening at 25 years of age and biannual screening 10 years after receiving radiation therapy.

Workup of a Breast Mass

DOMINANT PALPABLE MASS

The workup of a dominant palpable breast mass depends on the patient's menopausal status and the degree of suspicion. It is not unreasonable to follow a premenopausal patient with a nonsuspicious mass over one menstrual cycle and then reexamine her. Suspicious lesions present as a hard, nontender, irregular mass or as a mass in a high-risk patient. Palpable masses in postmenopausal patients may also warrant a workup. FNA should not be performed prior to diagnostic imaging because it may result in a hematoma that could obscure the image of the mass. Certain benign lesions on core biopsy should be excised, including lobular carcinoma in situ (LCIS), atypical ductal hyperplasia (ADH), radial scars, sclerosing papillary lesions, columnar cell hyperplasia with atypia, and PASH (Figure 3). Twenty percent of surgeries performed for atypical ductal hyperplasia have concurrent carcinoma in the specimen. Patients with a high-risk proliferative lesion should have close follow-up after surgery including physical examinations. Negative findings on a mammogram do not preclude the diagnosis of cancer because 10% of cancers are occult mammographically. This number drops to 3% when a lesion is occult both

mammographically and ultrasonographically. An alternative to core biopsies in younger women is the use of the triple test: a physical exam in conjunction with breast imaging (mammogram or ultrasound) and FNA. When all three components indicate the mass is benign, the negative predictive value is 100%. In a study by Morris, a triple test score assigns points to each component of the test. One point is given for benign findings, 2 points for suspicious findings, and 3 points for malignant findings. When added together, masses with scores of 4 or less are found to be benign. The triple test should only be used in women 40 years of age or younger because the incidence of breast cancer increases dramatically after that cutoff.

MASSES REVEALED ON SCREENING MAMMOGRAMS

The American College of Radiology's classification lexicon, the Breast Imaging Reporting and Data System (BI-RADS), is used in breast imaging (Table 2).

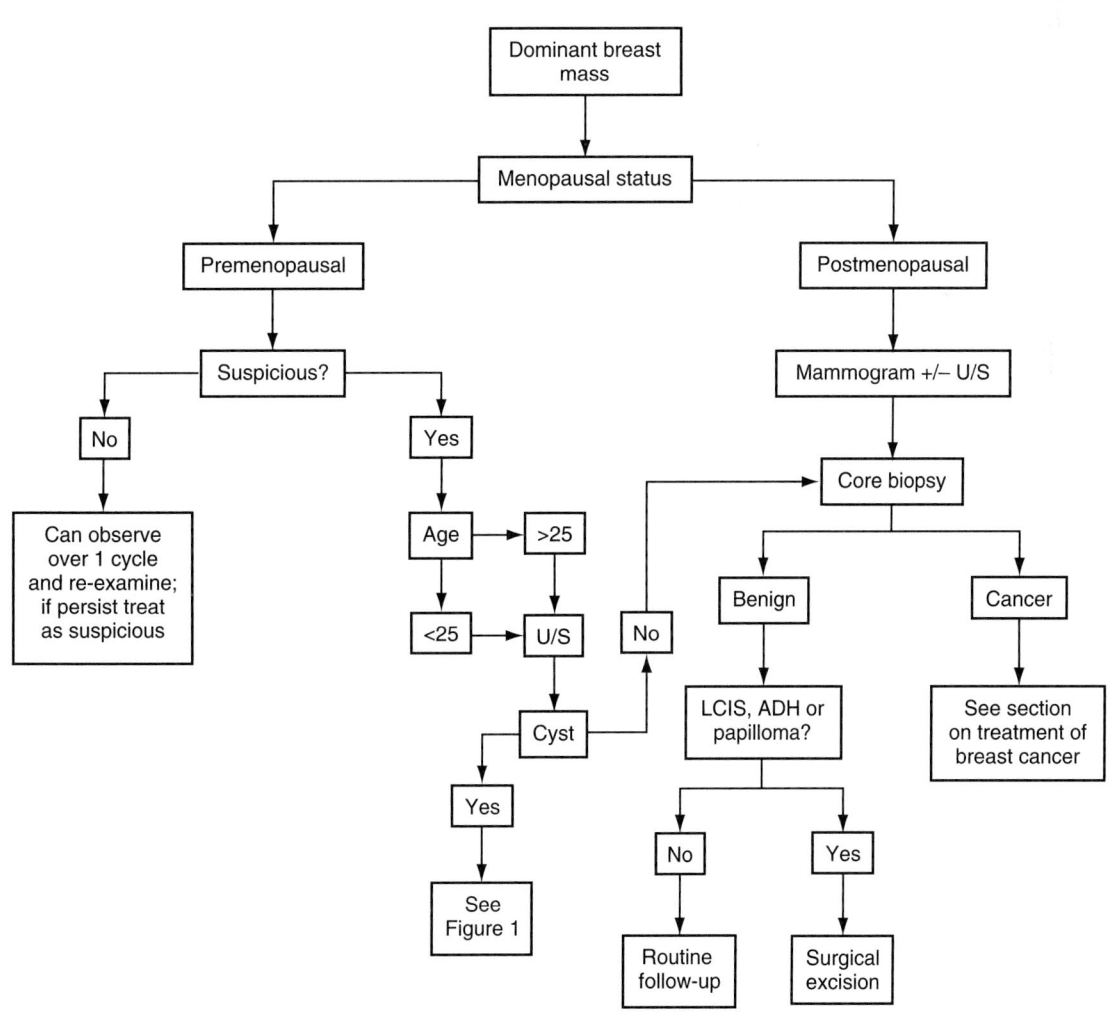

FIGURE 3. Algorithm for workup of a breast mass. ADH = atypical ductal hyperplasia; LCIS = lobular cancer in situ; U/S = ultrasound.

Rakel and Bope: *Conn's Current Therapy 2006.*

TABLE 2 BI-RADS Mammography Classification

BI-RADS category	Definition	Risk of malignancy	Recommended follow-up
0	Incomplete assessment	N/A	Further workup
1	Negative study	N/A	Repeat mammogram in 1 y
2	Benign	N/A	Repeat mammogram in 1 y
3	Probably benign	<2%	Repeat mammogram in 6 mo
4	Suspicious	20%	Biopsy should be considered
5	Highly suggestive of malignancy	90%	Appropriate action should be taken
6	Known biopsy-proven malignancy	N/A	Appropriate action should be taken

Abbreviation: BI-RADS = Breast Imaging Reporting and Data System.

BI-RADS 0 means the assessment is incomplete and more workup is needed. BI-RADS 1 indicates a normal mammogram. Mammograms with BI-RADS 2 signify benign findings. Patients with BI-RADS 3 have a 1% to 2% risk of malignancy and should have short-term follow-up with another mammogram in 6 months. BI-RADS 4 indicates the presence of suspicious lesions with a 20% to 40% probability of a malignant lesion. BI-RADS 5 is highly suggestive of cancer with a greater than 95% chance of harboring an underlying malignant lesion. BI-RADS 6, recently added as a category, indicates known malignant disease. BI-RADS 4 and 5 both indicate a biopsy.

A core biopsy via ultrasound guidance may be attempted first. A stereotactic core biopsy should be considered if this is not possible. Stereotactic biopsies may be impossible in patients with lesions that are very superficial or close to the chest wall or in patients with very small breasts that compress to less than 3 cm or who are unable to lie still for the procedure. In such situations, surgical excision with needle localization is warranted. In studies comparing surgical excision to core biopsies, the concordance rate is close to 100%. The surgeon can obviate the need for multiples surgeries in the same patient by performing a core biopsy for diagnosis. High-risk proliferative lesions, such as LCIS, atypical ductal hyperplasia, radial scars, sclerosing papillary lesions, columnar cell hyperplasia with atypia, and PASH, should be considered for an excisional biopsy if the diagnosis is made by a core biopsy.

In Situ Diseases

LOBULAR CARCINOMA IN SITU

Lobular carcinoma in situ (LCIS) should be considered a marker for future breast cancer risk and not an early noninvasive lobular cancer. This disease is most commonly seen in premenopausal women, with a peak incidence in women 40 to 50 years of age. Only 10% of LCIS occurs in postmenopausal women. Unlike ductal carcinoma in situ, LCIS is often found incidentally because typically no clinical or radiologic abnormalities are seen at time of diagnosis. In 50% of patients, LCIS is a multifocal finding. In 30% of patients, it can be found in the contralateral breast. Patients with LCIS are at

8 to 10 times the risk of the general population for subsequent breast cancer. Their overall lifetime risk is as high as 30% to 40% for the development of invasive breast cancer. In a meta-analysis, 15% of patients developed breast cancer in the ipsilateral breast, and 9.3% of patients developed cancer in the contralateral breast. The type of breast cancer can be either ductal or lobular, although the majority is ductal.

DUCTAL CARCINOMA IN SITU

Ductal carcinoma in situ (DCIS), or intraductal carcinoma, is a noninvasive breast cancer and designated stage 0. Historically, DCIS represented only approximately 5% of breast cancer cases, whereas today it constitutes 20% to 30% of all cases. This rise is predominantly attributed to the increasing use of screening mammography because DCIS is most often detected as mammographic microcalcifications. It tends to occur at a later age than LCIS and is not considered a multifocal or bilateral disease. Unlike LCIS, DCIS should be considered a true precursor lesion because if left untreated, approximately 60% to 100% of DCIS cases progress to invasive carcinoma.

TREATMENT FOR IN SITU DISEASE

Lobular Carcinoma in Situ

LCIS should be treated as a marker for increased breast cancer risk. Surgery in an attempt to achieve negative margins is not warranted for LCIS. The NSABP P-1 (the National Surgical Adjuvant Breast and Bowel Project) randomized trial examined the role of tamoxifen (Nolvadex) as a chemopreventive agent in high-risk patients, including those with LCIS. Women taking tamoxifen had a 50% reduction in the subsequent risk of breast cancer without any improvement in overall survival. The main risks of tamoxifen include increased risk of thromboembolic disease and endometrial cancer. The rate of pulmonary embolism was 3 in 1000 patients in the tamoxifen group versus 1 in 1000 in the placebo group. The rate of deep-vein thromboembolism was 5 in 1000 patients in the tamoxifen group versus 3 in 1000 in the placebo group. Endometrial cancer was seen in 9 in 1000 patients in the tamoxifen group versus 3.5 in 1000 in the placebo group. The decision to use tamoxifen as a chemopreventive agent should be made on an individual basis given these side effects. The highest reduction in breast cancer occurred in the LCIS group with a 70% reduction in risk. Despite this, no difference in survival was seen between the tamoxifen and placebo group.

Ductal Carcinoma in Situ

Treatment of DCIS has evolved from simple mastectomy to lumpectomy with radiation therapy. A simple mastectomy is associated with a 1% local recurrence rate. Thus it is still considered a viable option in patients who do not desire or are ineligible for breast conservation therapy (BCT). No difference in survival is seen in patients treated with mastectomy versus BCT. The NSABP B-17 randomized trial examined the role of lumpectomy with and without radiotherapy for the treatment of DCIS. The addition of radiotherapy decreased the recurrence rate from 16.4% to 7% with 8 years of follow-up. More importantly, it decreased the rate of invasive carcinoma from 8% to 2%. The 5-year event-free survival with lumpectomy and radiation is 84%. Limited data support excision alone in small well-differentiated DCIS with surgical margins of at least 1 cm. Silverstein showed in retrospective studies that the recurrence rate in such patients is approximately 4%. Routine axillary lymph node dissection (ALND) is not recommended for DCIS because only 1% of patients have positive axillary nodes. Recent studies, however, show that sentinel lymph node biopsy may have a role in the management of selected patients with DCIS. This is especially true in patients receiving a mastectomy as definitive treatment or if there is a question of microinvasion on the core biopsy. Patients with DCIS and microinvasion can have anywhere from a 3% to 20% incidence of nodal involvement. Indications for a sentinel node biopsy include extensive calcifications, a palpable lesion, patients undergoing mastectomy as treatment for DCIS, and lesions for which the pathology reads "can not rule out microinvasion." Tamoxifen (Nolvadex) can also be considered in cases of DCIS that are estrogen receptor positive. The NSABP B-24 randomized trial examined the utility of tamoxifen in patients treated with lumpectomy and radiotherapy. Ipsilateral tumor recurrences decreased from 13.4% without tamoxifen to 8.2% with tamoxifen. The incidence of invasive cancer was reduced by 47%. No difference in survival was observed between the placebo and the tamoxifen group. Side effects are similar to that of the NSABP P-1 trial.

Invasive Breast Cancer

INCIDENCE

An estimated 1 in 9 women living in the United States if they survive to 90 years of age will develop breast cancer. The average age at diagnosis is 64 years of age and increases along with age.

The American Joint Committee on Cancer TMN (tumor, metastasis, node) system designates breast

cancer as stage 0, I, II, III, or IV. This system categorizes breast cancer by its invasive or noninvasive character, tumor size, axillary lymph node status, and the presence of metastatic disease (see Table 2). Overall survival with breast cancer is related to stage (Table 3).

HISTOLOGY

The most common type of infiltrating carcinoma is ductal carcinoma-not otherwise specified (IFDC-NOS), which represents 85% of all invasive breast cancer. Infiltrating lobular carcinoma originates from the lobular structures of the breast and accounts for 15% of all invasive breast cancer. Other less common subtypes represent less than 10% and include tubular, medullary, mucinous, and papillary carcinoma. Additional rare subtypes of breast cancer include inflammatory carcinoma, malignant phyllodes tumor, sarcoma, lymphoma, and Paget disease.

BREAST CANCER STAGING

In 2003 the American Joint Committee on Cancer (AJCC) revised their staging system on breast cancer. This latest revision stresses the importance of nodal status as a prognostic factor by making several changes in how it is classified within the staging system. Major changes to the staging system include the following:

- Designation is made for isolated tumor cells (ITCs), which are differentiated from micrometastasis and defined as "single tumor cells or small cell clusters not greater than 0.2 mm, usually detected only by IHC (immunohistochemistry) or molecular methods, but which may be verified on H&E (hematoxylin-eosin) stains. ITCs do not usually show evidence of malignant activity, e.g., proliferation or stromal reaction." ITCs are designated as pN0 with modifiers for positive or negative IHC (i−, i+) and molecular findings (mol−, mol+).
- Internal mammary nodes (IMNs) are reclassified based on how they are detected and whether or not there is concomitant axillary lymph node metastasis.

TABLE 3 Overall Survival in Breast Cancer Patients

Stage	10-Year Overall Survival	15-Year Overall Survival
I	74%-95%	64%
II	76%	62%
IIA	81%	72%
IIB	70%	52%
III	50%	40%
IIIA	59%	49%
IIIB	36%	18%
IIIC	36%	18%
IV	18%	18%

Adapted from Rosen PP, et al: J Clin Oncol 1989;355-366; Woodward WA, Strom EA, Tucker SL, et al: Changes in the 2003 American Joint Committee on Cancer staging for breast cancer, dramatically affect stage-specific survival. J Clin Oncol 2003;3244-3248.

Detection of IMNs by sentinel node biopsy alone is classified as pN1b in the absence of positive axillary nodes or pN1c in the presence of positive axillary nodes. Internal mammary nodes detected by imaging studies (excluding lymphoscintigraphy) or by clinical exam are classified as pN2b in the absence of positive axillary nodes or pN3b in the presence of positive axillary nodes.

- Supraclavicular nodal involvement is now reclassified as N3 disease; thus a patient with supraclavicular nodal involvement does not automatically have stage IV disease.
- Infraclavicular nodal involvement is added as N3 disease.
- Axillary lymph node involvement is now classified by the number of nodes involved. Involvement of 1 to 3 axillary nodes is considered pN1 disease. Involvement of 4 to 9 axillary nodes is considered pN2 disease. Involvement of greater than 10 axillary nodes is considered pN3 disease.

Staging of breast cancer can be divided into clinical staging versus pathologic staging. Factors used for clinical staging include the size of the tumor within the breast, presence or absence of pathologically confirmed lymph nodes, and presence or absence of distant metastasis. There are five stages for breast cancer. Stage 0 is defined as the presence of in situ disease only, without evidence of nodal or distant metastasis. Stage I is considered breast cancer confined to the breast, regardless of tumor size. Exception to this general characterization includes tumors with extension to the chest wall or skin or inflammatory breast cancers. These tumors are at least stage IIIB. Stage II is considered a breast cancer of any size with pathologically positive ipsilateral mobile axillary nodes. Stage IIIA is considered a breast cancer of any size with pathologically positive ipsilateral fixed axillary nodes or clinically apparent internal mammary nodes in the absence of positive axillary nodes. Also any large tumors (bigger than 5 cm) with any type of positive axillary or internal mammary nodes are considered stage IIIA. Stage IIIB tumors are breast tumors with extension to the skin or chest wall or inflammatory breast cancer. Involvement of the pectoralis major or minor muscle does not constitute chest wall involvement. Stage IIIC tumors are breast cancers of any size with either positive infraclavicular or supraclavicular nodes or positive internal mammary nodes in the presence of positive axillary nodes. Stage IV connotes any breast cancers with distant metastasis (see Figure 3).

Pathologic staging of breast cancer is more complicated and differs from clinical staging in that the number of nodes involved as well as how nodal metastasis is detected are used in stage designation of nodal status (Figures 4 and 5).

SURGICAL TREATMENT OF THE BREAST

A significant paradigm shift in the treatment of breast cancer has occurred over the past several decades. The Halsted paradigm, popularized at the beginning of the 20th century, hypothesized that breast cancer spreads

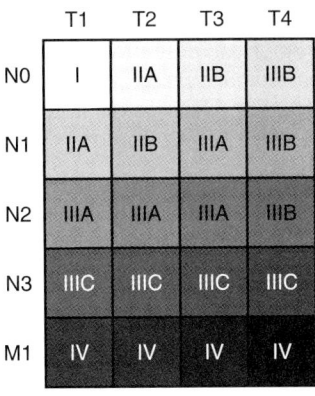

FIGURE 4. Pathologic staging of breast cancer.

in a contiguous fashion from the breast to the axillary lymph nodes and then to distant sites elsewhere in the body. The Fisher paradigm, which views breast cancer as systemic from very early in the course of the disease, modified this theory; the axillary lymph nodes act not as a barrier but as indicators of disease aggressiveness. Both paradigms are correct and incorrect. At a certain point in the evolution of a breast cancer, the disease changes from a local disease to a systemic disease. The Halsted paradigm promotes more intensive local treatment to eradicate the cancer, whereas the Fisher paradigm promotes less aggressive local treatment with the addition of systemic treatment in most women, even with relatively early disease. Because of this philosophy change and the detection of earlier disease through diligent screening techniques, surgical treatment of breast cancer is progressing toward less radical surgery and more adjuvant therapy, with equal or better outcomes. Recent mammograms of both breasts should be reviewed for any other suspicious lesions. There may be a slight increase in synchronous breast cancer in patients with invasive lobular cancer, although the rate of contralateral breast cancer is equal to that of invasive ductal carcinoma over the lifetime of the patient. The risk of distant metastasis is 25% to 50% in patients with inflammatory breast cancer.

Breast Conservation Therapy

Most small noninvasive and invasive breast cancers are treated by BCT, which consists of wide local excision with negative surgical margins and irradiation of the breast. The NSABP B-06, Milan I and Milan II, as well as other clinical trials, show no statistically significant difference in patient survival with mastectomy or BCT.

The addition of radiation treatment to wide local excision in patients with noninvasive and invasive carcinoma is currently the standard of treatment. The NSABP B-06 randomized trial evaluated local recurrence of small invasive tumors with and without irradiation after lumpectomy. It found that patients who did not

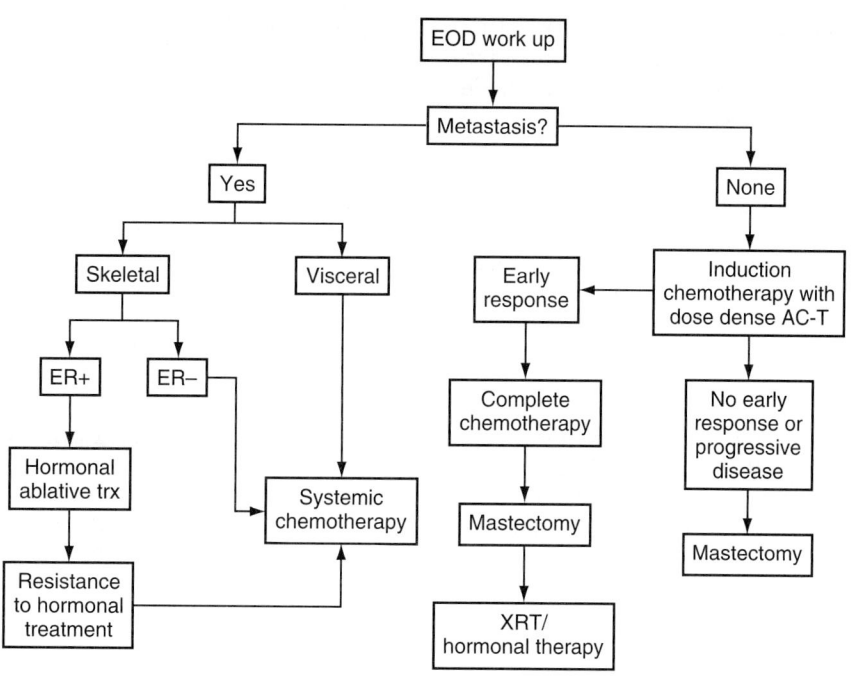

FIGURE 5. Algorithm for treatment of locally advanced breast cancer (LABC). AC-T = Adriamycin and cyclophosphamide plus Taxol; EOD = extent-of-disease; trx = treatment; XRT = x-radiation therapy.

undergo radiation therapy had significantly higher rates of local recurrence. With BCT, incidence of recurrence in the treated breast is 7% at 5 years, 14% at 10 years, and 20% at 20 years. Local recurrence rate is much lower in patients treated with mastectomy, with an overall incidence of 5% to 10%. The majority of recurrences occur in the first 3 years after surgery. Contraindications to BCT include tumor of any size that can not be adequately excised with significant deformity to the breast, multicentric disease, noncompliant patient, first- or second-trimester pregnant patient, history of significant collagen vascular disease, and history of previous radiation therapy to the chest wall. If both BCT and mastectomy are viable options, the patient's preference should also play a role in the decision to proceed with BCT versus a mastectomy.

MASTECTOMY

A patient with contraindications to breast conservation should have a mastectomy with or without immediate reconstruction. Total mastectomy surgically removes the breast parenchyma, pectoral fascia, nipple, and the areola complex. A modified radical mastectomy includes axillary dissection. A radical mastectomy, rarely done today, includes removal of the pectoralis major and minor muscles and axillary dissection.

BREAST RECONSTRUCTION

Any patient recommended to have a mastectomy should be offered the option of immediate or delayed reconstruction and referred to a plastic and reconstructive surgeon to discuss which techniques are appropriate. One commonly used method of breast reconstruction is a tissue expander breast implant. A tissue expander is placed beneath the pectoralis muscles, and expansions are performed over a period of several weeks to months to stretch the subpectoral pocket to accommodate the permanent implant. The permanent saline or silicone implant is then inserted as a secondary procedure.

Another method of breast reconstruction is the transverse rectus abdominis myocutaneous (TRAM) flap, which involves the transfer of skin, fat, and muscle from the lower part of the abdomen to create a reconstructed breast. This procedure can be performed as a free flap with the arterial and venous supply anastomosed to vessels in the axilla or as a pedicle flap with the arterial and venous supply from the superior epigastric vessels. Other types of flap reconstructions include latissimus dorsi or gluteal flaps. Reconstruction of the nipple and areola is often performed as a later procedure.

SURGICAL TREATMENT OF THE AXILLA

The status of the axilla should be assessed for metastases in any patient with invasive breast cancer for several reasons. The status of the axillary lymph nodes is important in determining the patient's stage of disease. The presence or absence of axillary lymph node metastases is predictive of the prognosis and facilitates decisions by the medical oncology team regarding adjuvant therapy. Relapse-free survival is closely related to the number of lymph nodes that are positive. In a study of 2873 patients, Hilsenbeck found that the relapse-free survival at 5 years was 80% in patients with node-negative disease. This number decreased to 70%, 60%, and 40% with 1 to 3 positive nodes, 4 to 9 positive nodes, and more than 10 positive nodes, respectively. Nodal status is now incorporated into the sixth revision of the AJCC staging system. Surgical removal of metastatic nodes in the axilla significantly decreases the possibility of axillary recurrence. ALND may improve overall survival, but this issue is debated in the medical literature.

Sentinel Lymph Node Biopsy

Axillary dissection traditionally was performed on all patients with invasive breast cancer. Today, sentinel lymphadenectomy, or sentinel lymph node (SLN) biopsy, identifies the first, or sentinel, lymph node or nodes in the axillary chain to receive drainage from the breast cancer and thus the most likely to contain metastases. The SLN biopsy is performed by injecting isosulfan blue dye and/or radioactive isotope to localize the sentinel lymph node.

The sentinel node can be identified in 95% of all cases. Multiple studies show that SLN biopsy can predict accurately the presence of axillary metastases in T1-2 breast cancer with a false-negative rate of 5% and an accuracy rate of 95%. The false-negative rate of SLN biopsy can be decreased to 1% to 3% if any palpable node is removed along with any hot or blue nodes. The SLN biopsy, a less invasive way to assess the status of the axilla, is associated with fewer complications than an axillary node dissection. Areas of controversy in SLN biopsy include T3, palpable suspicious axillary lymph nodes, and previous neoadjuvant therapy. In a study by Specht, 25% of palpable suspicious axillary lymph nodes proved benign on final pathology. Previous axillary dissection is not a strict contraindication per se because 75% of these patients can still have an identifiable sentinel node. The success rate depends on the number of nodes previously removed, with a success rate of 87% when fewer than 10 nodes are removed versus a success rate of 47% when more than 10 nodes are removed. Contraindications to SLN biopsy include T4 breast cancer and pregnancy. SLN biopsy is contraindicated in pregnancy because of the lack of data regarding fetal safety, although computer models suggest the amount of radiation exposure to the fetus is negligible.

Axillary Dissection

Patients who have metastatic cells on SLN biopsy typically undergo complete ALND. Alternatively, if a patient is not a candidate for SLN biopsy, ALND should be considered. Axillary dissection involves the removal of 10 to 30 lymph nodes from the axilla. The potential risk of axillary dissection includes the accumulation of a seroma, ipsilateral arm lymphedema, and numbness around the area of the intercostal brachial innervation if the nerve is sacrificed at the time of surgery. Because of the lifetime increased chance of arm lymphedema and possible infection, patients should avoid any trauma or procedures such as venipuncture or blood pressure measurements on the ipsilateral arm.

Adjuvant Therapy

Adjuvant therapy is used to treat patients with a demonstrable likelihood for the development of metastatic disease. Most medical oncologists consider this risk sufficient in node-negative patients with a tumor diameter of 1 cm or larger and in those with nodal metastases to justify adjuvant chemotherapy or hormonal therapy. Most commonly used cytotoxic regimens include CMF (cyclophosphamide [Cytoxan], methotrexate, and 5-FU [fluorouracil]) for 6 cycles or AC-T for 8 cycles (4 cycles of doxorubicin [Adriamycin] and cyclophosphamide followed by 4 cycles of paclitaxel [Taxol]). There appears to be a slight improvement of 3% in overall survival favoring the anthracycline-containing regimen over the CMF regimens. In the elderly population, the CMF regimen may be easier to tolerate than the AC-T regimens. In a recent study, a dose dense regimen of AC-T results in a slight improvement of disease-free and overall survival. Dose-dense regimen involves giving the chemotherapy in cycles every 2 weeks, with bone marrow support such as G-CSF (Neupogen), as opposed to the traditional cycles every 3 weeks. The improvement in survival is approximately 3%. In the Early Breast Cancer Trialists' Collaborative Group (EBCTCG) meta-analysis, adjuvant chemotherapy appears the most beneficial for women younger than 50 years of age. Combination chemotherapy resulted in the improvement of 10-year-overall survival from 71% in node-negative patients not receiving chemotherapy to 78% in those that did receive chemotherapy. This increase was even more dramatic in node-positive patients, with an improvement of overall survival from 42% to 53%. A much smaller effect was seen in patients older than 50 years of age. In this group of patients, survival was increased from 67% to 69% when node-negative patients not receiving chemotherapy were compared to those receiving chemotherapy. In node-positive elderly patients, improvement in overall survival was also minimal, with an increase of survival from 47% to 49% with chemotherapy.

Hormonal therapy, such as tamoxifen, is a commonly used adjuvant treatment in early breast cancer patients with estrogen receptor–positive tumors. The EBCTCG meta-analysis looking at the role of tamoxifen in the premenopausal patients found that tamoxifen results in an absolute improvement of 10-year overall survival of 5.6% in node-negative patients and 10.9% in node-positive patients. This effect is even greater in the postmenopausal population, with a 26% proportional reduction in 10-year mortality rates. The recommended length of treatment for node-negative patients is 5 years. Additionally, tamoxifen can be used as a chemopreventive agent to decrease the chance of an additional ipsilateral tumor developing in patients undergoing breast conservation or to decrease the possibility of contralateral breast cancer.

More recently, three large randomized trials of aromatase inhibitors, such as anastrozole (Arimidex), exemestane (Aromasin), and letrozole (Femara), was published. In the ATAC (Arimidex, Tamoxifen, Alone or in Combination) trial, patients on anastrozole had a statistically significant longer disease-free interval when compared with patients on tamoxifen alone (hazard ratio of 0.83). No difference in survival was seen between the two groups. In another large study, patients on tamoxifen for 2 to 3 years were randomized to continuing tamoxifen versus switching to exemestane for a total of 5 years of therapy. There appeared to be an improvement in disease-free survival in the aromatase inhibitor arm (hazard ratio of 0.68). No difference in survival was seen, and given the early stoppage and cross-over of patients, no survival data will be obtainable from this study. Yet another large double-blinded randomized trial involved patients who had finished a 5-year course of tamoxifen and were then randomized to receiving letrozole versus placebo. The trial was stopped at a mean follow-up of 2.4 years secondary to a significant improvement in disease-free survival in the letrozole arm (hazard ratio of 0.57). Again, no difference in survival was seen. Aromatase inhibitors are useful only in postmenopausal patients. Premenopausal patients may benefit from an aromatase inhibitor only after ovarian ablation.

Recommendations regarding tamoxifen, aromatase inhibitors, and chemotherapy depend on the clinical judgment of the treating medical oncologist. In general, if adjuvant chemotherapy is given, it should take place prior to the initiation of radiotherapy. Consideration should be given to the likelihood of systemic recurrence based on nodal status, tumor size, and tumor grade. Estrogen receptor positivity of the tumor is predictive of a response to hormonal therapy, and *HER2-neu* may determine the type of appropriate chemotherapy. Another factor is the patient's age and any co-morbid diseases that would decrease the patient's tolerance to a course of chemotherapy.

Surveillance After a Diagnosis of Breast Cancer

Surveillance should continue alter diagnosis and treatment of breast cancer to detect local recurrence or a new primary breast cancer in either the ipsilateral or contralateral breast. The National Comprehensive Cancer Network guidelines recommend that patients continue diligent monthly self-examinations and that a physician perform a physical examination at 6-month intervals to assess for evidence of local recurrence and symptoms of metastatic disease. The ipsilateral arm should be evaluated to detect early signs of lymphedema and initiate appropriate management. Bilateral mammograms should be obtained every year. Bone and computed tomographic scans and other tumor markers should be performed only on patients with symptomatic systemic disease because of the lack of evidence of improved survival with early detection of distant metastases.

Special Topics in Breast Disease

PHYLLODES TUMOR

Phyllodes tumor (cystosarcoma phyllodes) is a fibro-epithelial lesion that can be either benign or malignant. It is a rare tumor of the breast accounting for 1% of all cases. The mean age of patients is 54 years of age. These tumors often present as a breast mass on clinical and mammographic examination., and they are considered benign or malignant depending on stromal cellularity, mitotic activity, presence of necrosis, and type of borders. Treatment is complete excision without axillary node dissection. Metastases secondary to malignant phyllodes are hematogenous and primarily travel to the lungs. It is important to obtain negative margins. A mastectomy occasionally may be warranted for large lesions. Patients with malignant phyllodes have an 80% chance of 5-year survival as opposed to more than 95% for benign phyllodes.

NIPPLE DISCHARGE

Nipple discharge can occur at any age and presents as a bloody, serous, or milky discharge. Only 6% to 12% of patients with a nipple discharge are found to have an underlying malignancy. This risk is slightly elevated if the discharge is bloody. The most common cause of serous or serosanguineous nipple discharge is a benign intraductal papilloma. Numerous drugs can also cause nipple discharge, such as phenothiazine, tricyclic antidepressants, reserpine, butyrophenones, cimetidine (Tagamet), verapamil (Calan), metoclopramide (Reglan), thiazides, and hormone replacement therapy. The most common underlying malignancy is DCIS. Ductograms may be useful in locating the papilloma. When the nipple discharge is unilaterally persistent, spontaneous, or postmenopausal, further workup may be considered. Other suspicious nipple discharges are those confined to one duct or that are bloody or serous. In general, the evaluation of nipple discharge should begin with a clinical examination and a mammogram. Cytologic examination of the discharge has a low sensitivity for detection of underlying malignancy and should be not be used in the workup. Treatment consists of a major duct excision.

GYNECOMASTIA

Gynecomastia is the unilateral or bilateral benign enlargement of male breast tissue. The etiology is often related to various substances, including exogenous hormones, cimetidine (Tagamet), thiazides, digoxin, theophylline, phenothiazines, alcohol, and marijuana use; it may also be idiopathic. The main concern is to rule out the diagnosis of male breast cancer. Once breast cancer is excluded, no treatment is indicated. If medication and lifestyle etiologies are eliminated without remission of the gynecomastia, the excess breast tissue may be surgically removed for cosmetic considerations or for breast pain.

Rakel and Bope: *Conn's Current Therapy 2006.*

16

MALE BREAST CANCER

Carcinoma of the male breast represents 1% of all breast cancers. Because men are not routinely screened for breast cancer, the diagnosis is often delayed. The most common manifestation of male breast cancer is a painless, firm, subareolar breast mass. The differential diagnosis includes gynecomastia. Breast imaging with mammography and/or ultrasound may be helpful in rendering a diagnosis inasmuch as the appearance of male breast cancer is a stellate, irregular solid mass. Any suspicious breast mass in a male patient should undergo diagnostic biopsy. If a malignancy is diagnosed, standard treatment is mastectomy with assessment of the axillary nodes by SLN biopsy or ALND. Most cases of male breast cancer are estrogen receptor positive, and recommendations for adjuvant chemotherapy or hormonal therapy should be based on criteria similar to those for breast cancer in female patients.

BREAST CANCER IN PREGNANCY

Pregnancy-associated breast cancer represents less than 2% of all breast cancer diagnoses. The breast cancer frequently is diagnosed at a late stage because of the difficulty of examining the breast in pregnant women and the avoidance of mammography during pregnancy. Any suspicious lesion noted during pregnancy should be subjected to biopsy in the same fashion as in a non-gravid woman. Radiation therapy should not be administered during pregnancy, so breast conservation is generally contraindicated unless the diagnosis is made within a few weeks of delivery. Surgical treatment with mastectomy and ALND is the standard treatment of breast cancer during pregnancy. Adjuvant chemotherapy can be delivered with selective agents during the second and third trimesters. The prognosis is similar to that of nongravid women in whom breast cancer is diagnosed at a comparable stage.

INFLAMMATORY BREAST CANCER

The classic manifestation of inflammatory breast cancer is erythema, edema, peau d'orange, and color of the breast resembling an infectious process. Malignant cells within the dermal lymphatic vessels of the breast confirm the diagnosis. The usual pathology of the associated carcinoma is IFDC-NOS. Inflammatory carcinoma is a very aggressive type of breast cancer, with over 90% of patients having positive axillary lymph nodes at diagnosis. The recommended treatment is multimodality therapy, with chemotherapy preceding surgery. Surgical treatment is mastectomy followed by radiation therapy and often additional chemotherapy.

LOCALLY ADVANCED BREAST CANCER

Patients with N2 or N3 nodal status or those with four or more positive axillary nodes, T3 or T4 tumors, or involvement of the pectoralis fascia have locally advanced breast cancer (LABC). The recommended treatment for patients is neoadjuvant chemotherapy, which is administered before surgical treatment, although it has no impact on overall survival. An extent-of-disease (EOD) workup should be done in patients with LABC and includes a computed tomography (CT) of the chest, abdomen, and pelvis along with a bone scan. Figure 5 provides an algorithm for the treatment of LABC.

Endometriosis

Method of
Tommaso Falcone, MD

Endometriosis is a common benign gynecologic disorder characterized by the presence of endometrial glands and stroma in extrauterine sites. It is associated with significant morbidity that is the result of chronic pelvic pain or infertility. This disease is also responsible for a significant number of hospitalizations and surgical interventions such as laparoscopy and hysterectomy.

Epidemiology

The prevalence of endometriosis is reported in patients undergoing laparoscopy for chronic pelvic pain, infertility, or tubal sterilization. There are several obvious limitations to prevalence data based on surgical interventions that explain the wide frequency of the data reported. An estimated 35% to 50% of symptomatic patients and 6% to 10% of asymptomatic patients have endometriosis. The high prevalence in asymptomatic women implies that endometriosis diagnosed in symptomatic women may sometimes be coincidental rather than causal. Early age of menarche and shorter cycle length (less than 26 days) is associated with higher incidence. Longer duration of flow and heavier periods are also reported as potential risks for endometriosis. High parity is associated with decreased risk. Taken together, these observations point to an increase in menstrual exposure as the underlying factor that increases risk. A first-degree relative with endometriosis is associated with increased risk of disease, but no specific inheritance pattern is yet identified.

Pathophysiology

Several theories on the pathogenesis of endometriosis are proposed to explain the observations. The most commonly proposed theory is transplantation of retrograde menstruation. This theory fits with the observations of increased frequency of endometriosis in patients with heavy menstrual periods or a shortened menstrual cycle. Endometriosis is a common finding in women with obstruction to the outflow of menstrual effluent, such as with some Müllerian anomalies. It also explains the frequent finding of endometriosis in the dependent parts of the peritoneal cavity. Other theories attempt to explain the observations of endometriosis in different anatomic sites. Lymphatic spread can perhaps explain endometriosis at distant sites. Metaplasia of the coelomic epithelium is proposed to explain endometriosis of the ovary (endometriomas). Invagination of this surface epithelium can lead to ovarian cysts. Metaplasia of Müllerian rests is proposed to explain deeply infiltrating lesions of the rectovaginal septum.

Retrograde menstruation is found in most women; however, endometriosis is found in a minority of women. Thus several abnormalities are required to explain successful transplantation of the retrograde epithelium. The intraperitoneal scavenger system typically clears the menstruum. Many abnormalities of the eutopic endometrium in women with endometriosis are reported that may allow it to escape clearance. There are also abnormalities in the host immune system that seem to allow transplantation. This is within the context of genetic and environmental abnormalities that may contribute in part to the development of disease.

The immune system is involved in implantation of the ectopic endometrium and possibly the manifestations of the disease. In endometriosis, increased numbers of activated macrophages are found in the peritoneal cavity. This phenomenon is associated with increased cytokine production, especially interleukin (IL)-6 and tumor necrosis factor-α (TNF-α); angiogenic factors, such as vascular endothelial growth factor (VEGF); and growth factors. However, there is a decrease in the phagocytic activity of the macrophages as well as a decrease in natural killer (NK) cell activity. The increased secretion of these factors, along with a compromised clearance of endometriotic tissue, allows implantation to occur.

The eutopic endometrium of patients with endometriosis demonstrates aberrantly expressed genes that may allow abnormal implantation of tissue. The matrix degrading enzymes, metalloproteinases (MMPs) 7 and 11, are persistently expressed during the luteal phase and may allow endometrial tissue to invade the peritoneum. The eutopic endometrium of patients with endometriosis shows higher VEGF expression, which allows angiogenesis, an important prerequisite for successful implantation of tissue. There is also downregulation of proapoptotic genes. These are examples of alteration of the endometrium that allow implantation.

Once successful implantation of tissue occurs, the resulting lesions participate in the pathophysiology of the disease. These lesions secrete cytokines and other proinflammatory mediators, which attract activated macrophages that secrete other inflammatory mediators. The peritoneal fluid contains a large number of these cytokines. Future drug therapy may be directed toward these mediators.

The role of environmental pollutants in the development of endometriosis is unclear. Animal studies demonstrate that dioxin exposure increases the probability of disease. Two studies in Italy and Belgium, however, failed to correlate a significant impact of high dioxin exposure with the risk of endometriosis.

Rakel and Bope: *Conn's Current Therapy 2006*.

An estrogenic environment is necessary for growth of the implants. These lesions are shown to express aromatase, an enzyme that catalyzes the conversion of androgens to estrogens. Normal endometrium does not express this enzyme, but many endometriotic implants do. This local estrogen production may explain the persistence of disease after oophorectomy. In summary, endometriosis is similar to an autoimmune disease with inflammatory mediators secreted in response to endometrial cells that are abnormal.

It is unclear how endometriosis causes pain or infertility, especially in mild cases. In advanced disease with severely distorted pelvic anatomy and adhesions, infertility may be caused by a mechanical factor. In patients with mild disease, other mechanisms of infertility are proposed. For example, embryonic implantation during the luteal phase requires epithelial expression of $\alpha\beta_3$ integrins. Some women with endometriosis lack this marker and may have implantation failure. The endometriotic lesions or other peritoneal factors are thought to secrete inflammatory mediators that may have a deleterious effect on gametes or fertilization.

The precise mechanism of endometriosis that causes pain is unclear. Extent of disease does not correlate well with symptoms. The depth that these lesions infiltrate the peritoneum and subperitoneal tissues demonstrates better correlation with pain.

Several disorders associated with endometriosis may elucidate the pathophysiology further. Data support higher rates of atopic disease and other autoimmune phenomena in these patients. Fibromyalgia and chronic fatigue syndrome are often reported. Endometriosis is associated with an increased incidence of ovarian cancer, especially endometrioid and clear-cell type. There are other reports of an association with non-Hodgkin's lymphoma, dysplastic nevi, and melanoma.

Symptoms and Signs

The main symptoms of endometriosis are infertility and pain. The pain is characteristically cyclic and associated with the period (dysmenorrhea), although noncyclic chronic pelvic pain and dyspareunia are also common. These symptoms should be assessed at the first consultation. The patient should rate her pain with a 10-point severity scale (0 equals no pain, and 10 is the worst pain possible). Furthermore, the impact of these symptoms on the patient's lifestyle should be evaluated. For example, is she able to do her work or attend social events? Does the pain cause insomnia? Are there associated mood abnormalities such as depression? A psychosocial history with specific questions of potential sexual abuse should be documented. There may be associated bowel symptoms similar to irritable bowel syndrome or irritative voiding symptoms. Back pain is also quite common. The main differential diagnoses are pain syndromes associated with adhesions, irritable bowel syndrome, or interstitial cystitis. Patients may have extrapelvic endometriosis and specific symptoms associated with these different syndromes (Box 1).

16

BOX 1   Syndromes Associated With Extrapelvic Endometriosis

- Thoracic endometriosis: catamenial pneumothorax
- Diaphragmatic endometriosis: chest pain
- Sciatic nerve endometriosis: sciatica

BOX 2   Anatomic Sites Involved With Endometriosis

- Pelvic organs
- Pelvic peritoneum (broad ligament, bladder peritoneum)
- Ovaries
- Rectovaginal septum
- Rectosigmoid
- Bladder
- Ureters
- Extrapelvic organs
- Appendix
- Diaphragm
- Pleura
- Skin (umbilical, incisional)

Physical examination should be complete with a specific evaluation of other potential causes of chronic pain such as myofascial syndromes. The abdominal exam should search for abdominal hernias and myofascial or trigger point pain, as well as the standard abdominal observations. On pelvic examination, the main clinical findings suggestive of endometriosis are pelvic tenderness, mobility of the uterus, and indurations of the vagina, cul-de-sac, or adnexa. There may be an associated spasm or tenderness of the pelvic floor muscles.

Diagnostic Procedures

A delay of 8 to 9 years between the onset of pain and the diagnosis of endometriosis is common, in part because of the unavailability of an accurate nonsurgical diagnostic test. A large number of serum markers, such as CA-125, have been investigated in an attempt to arrive at a nonsurgical diagnosis, but none have sufficient sensitivity or specificity to diagnose or exclude endometriosis effectively. Imaging studies such as pelvic ultrasonography are not helpful unless an ovarian cyst is present. These imaging studies do help differentiate endometriosis from other causes of chronic pelvic pain such as adenomyosis, chronic inflammatory pelvic disease, or pelvic mass. Magnetic resonance imaging or computerized tomography is not superior to ultrasonography.

The gold standard for the diagnosis of endometriosis is a diagnostic laparoscopy. The lesions of peritoneal endometriosis demonstrate a multitude of characteristics that can lead gynecologists to diagnostic error. This error is represented by both falsely concluding that lesions do represent endometriosis as well as situations in which the diagnosis is missed. The concordance rate between the gynecologists' diagnosis and the histology is approximately 50%, depending on the phenotypic characteristic of the lesion. This underscores the importance of histologic confirmation, especially in clinical trials. The most common areas involved are the pelvic peritoneum and ovaries, but a large number of extragenital sites are identified that explain the associated symptoms (Box 2).

The extent of disease is reported as a stage similar to cancer cases. The patient is given a stage from 1 to 4 based on the extent of endometriotic implants on the ovary or peritoneum, amount of cul-de-sac disease, and the extent that adhesions are present on the ovary or fallopian tube. The extent of disease as reported by this classification does not correlate well with the severity of symptoms, although deeply infiltrating endometriosis is associated with more severe pain.

The lack of association between the extent of disease and severity of pain results in uncertainty about which lesions cause pain. For this reason a new surgical procedure called "conscious pain mapping" is reported in which a diagnostic laparoscopy is performed with the patient awake by receiving a local anesthetic and some intravenous sedation. During the procedure the surgeon touches different areas of the pelvis to evaluate if the pain is reproduced. Conscious pain mapping has not been evaluated sufficiently to recommend it routinely, however. Furthermore, the management of chronic pain is complex and uncommonly cured by the simple excision of a particularly painful lesion elicited during the procedure.

Treatment

CHRONIC PELVIC PAIN

Many patients are asymptomatic. Long-term follow-up of asymptomatic patients with endometriosis diagnosed at tubal ligation demonstrates that these patients typically do not develop symptoms. The evolution of an untreated endometriotic lesion in symptomatic patients is different. Most studies have reported progression in approximately 50% of patients and regression in approximately 30%. The main evolution of the management of chronic pelvic pain associated with endometriosis is the trend toward medical management without surgical confirmation. This empirical treatment is based on a thorough evaluation to exclude other potential causes. This treatment algorithm typically is initiated with oral contraceptives and nonsteroidal anti-inflammatory drugs (NSAIDs). Even more sophisticated drugs such as gonadotropin-releasing hormone (GnRH) agonists (leuprolide [Lupron]), however, are recommended without surgical confirmation in instances where there is a high probability of endometriosis.

Specific medical therapy for endometriosis associated with chronic pelvic pain involves the use of several drugs designed to suppress endogenous estrogen secretion and induce amenorrhea. These drugs cause regression of endometriotic lesions with symptom control, but many lesions proliferate again after resumption of ovulatory cycles. As stated, oral contraceptives and NSAIDs are used as first-line therapy for chronic pain associated with endometriosis. Continuous oral contraceptives induce amenorrhea in a large number of patients and decrease dysmenorrhea, but a recent Cochrane review concluded that there is little data to support the efficacy of oral contraceptives in these patients. Nonetheless, they are safe in reproductive-age women, have few side effects, and are therefore commonly used.

One of the earliest drugs used for endometriosis is danazol (Danocrine), a testosterone derivative. Its action is mediated through several different mechanisms including suppression of gonadotropins and direct androgenic effect on the endometrium and endometriosis implants. At the recommended dose of 800 mg daily, the drug induces amenorrhea and is quite effective at symptom control, but pain recurrence and the undesirable androgenic effects limit its use. Deaths are reported from liver failure.

Progestins such as medroxyprogesterone acetate (MPA-Provera)[1] in oral or depot form are commonly used for to treat endometriosis-associated chronic pelvic pain. Progestins given continuously and at high enough doses (typically MPA, 20 to 30 mg, or norethindrone (Aygestin), 5 to 15 mg daily) suppress the menstrual cycle and relieve pain associated with the menstrual period. Recurrence of pain is rapid after drug withdrawal. Many women dislike the side effects, such as mood abnormalities, irregular menstrual flow, weight gain, and the sensation of bloating. Patients on depot formulations may experience a prolonged delay before return of ovulatory cycles. Women interested in future fertility may not find this side effect acceptable.

The drug most commonly used as second-line therapy for the treatment of chronic pelvic pain associated with endometriosis is a GnRH agonist (Lupron, 3.75 mg monthly). The drug typically is given as an intramuscular injection for 6 months. Studies show this class of drugs is as effective as danazol, with more than 90% of patients experiencing relief. The median time to recurrence of symptoms is approximately 5 to 6 months after drug withdrawal, however.

The drug is associated with side effects such as vasomotor instability, vaginal dryness, mood changes, and osteoporosis. The decrease in bone mineral density after 6 months of GnRH agonist is slow to return to baseline and can take up to 2 years. These side effects are caused by the hypoestrogenic effects. To avoid them, an add-back therapy is recommended that consists of adding a hormone in sufficient quantities to alleviate symptoms and prevent bone loss but not enough to impede the beneficial effects on pain. A progestin (norethindrone acetate [Aygestin], 5 mg) alone or in combination with conjugated equine estrogens (Premarin,[1] 0.625 mg) is typically used. This regime effectively prevents the bone loss, and the beneficial effect is seen even if the GnRH agonist is used for 12 months of therapy. These regimens of add-back therapy with a GnRH agonist allow long-term use of the drug in select patients. Active research is looking for new drug therapies for these patients. Preliminary experience

with aromatase inhibitors such as letrozole[1] (Femara) and intrauterine devices releasing levonorgestrel[1] (Mirena) are effective in some patients with endometriosis.

A prospective double-blind randomized study in patients with stages I, II, and III endometriosis shows surgery (operative laparoscopy) to be effective in 60% of treated patients, with 23% of the control group also showing relief. The patients with the least benefit are those with early-stage disease. Using the number needed to treat (NNT) statistic provides the approximate number of operative laparoscopies that need to be performed to benefit one patient. The NNT for operative laparoscopy is 2.5. Some patients may benefit from a neurectomy performed at the same time. The uterosacral nerve resection used to be performed, but a recent Cochrane review shows no benefit. A presacral neurectomy shows benefit in two randomized clinical trials for midline pelvic pain, however. Definitive therapy for chronic pelvic pain continues to be an abdominal hysterectomy and bilateral salpingo-oophorectomy. But patients should be aware that endometriosis might recur (persist) in 5% to 10% of patients after radical therapy. Although laparoscopy and laparotomy give similar clinical outcomes, postoperative recovery is far quicker with minimally invasive surgery. Recurrence of symptoms after surgery is common: between 20% at 2 years to 40% at 5 years. Ovarian endometriomas do not respond to medical therapy and require surgical therapy.

INFERTILITY TREATMENT

Medical suppressive therapies, such as GnRH agonists, do not improve pregnancy rates. In a prospective randomized clinical trial, surgical treatment of endometriosis improved pregnancy rates. The cumulative spontaneous pregnancy rate after surgical treatment of minimal or mild endometriosis treatment is improved, but the absolute amount is open to debate. Two studies investigated this question with randomized clinical trials: a multicenter Canadian trial and an Italian trial. The Canadian trial showed improvement and the Italian trial did not. A meta-analysis of both studies showed an improvement. The NNT statistic, which gives the

---

[1]Not FDA approved for this indication.

 CURRENT DIAGNOSIS

- History
- Noncyclic chronic pelvic pain
- Dysmenorrhea
- Dyspareunia
- Physical examination
- Adnexal tenderness
- Nodularity
- Uterine mobility
- No specific serum test
- Imaging study
- Ultrasound for endometriomas

---

[1]Not FDA approved for this indication.

Rakel and Bope: *Conn's Current Therapy 2006.*

16

CURRENT THERAPY

Medical Therapy (Chronic Pelvic Pain)
- Oral contraceptives[1]
- Androgens
- Danazol (Danocrine)
- Progestins
- Norethindrone (Aygestin)
- Medroxyprogesterone acetate[1] (Provera)
- Gonadotropin-releasing hormone (GnRH) agonists with or without add-back therapy

Surgical Therapy (Infertility and Chronic Pelvic Pain)
- Ablation or excision of disease

[1]Not FDA approved for this indication.

approximate number of laparoscopies that need to be performed to achieve an extra pregnancy, is 12.

Standard infertility treatments, such as ovulation induction therapy or in vitro fertilization, result in superior outcomes to surgery. In vitro fertilization is often the final treatment option for patients with endometriosis who have failed conservative management. Although the pregnancy rates are good, recent data shows a lower pregnancy rate compared with patients without endometriosis. The odds ratio is 0.56.

Endometriosis is a chronic disease with significant morbidity. The pathophysiology involves a complex interaction of genetic aberration of the endometrium with an inflammatory host response. Diagnosis relies on history and physical examination rather than imaging techniques. Surgery and medical therapy are effective for managing chronic pelvic pain, but both have high relapse rates.

REFERENCES

Bedaiwy MA, Falcone T: Peritoneal fluid environment in endometriosis: Clinicopathological implications. Minerva Ginecol 2003;55:333-345.
Bedaiwy MA, Falcone T: Laboratory testing for endometriosis. Clin Chim Acta 2004;340(1-2):41-56.
Hornstein MD, Surrey ES, Weisberg GW, Casino L: The Lupron add-back study group. Leuprolide acetate depot and hormonal add-back in endometriosis: A 12-month study. Obstet Gynecol 1998;91:16-24.
Marcoux S, Maheux R, Berube S: Canadian Collaborative Group of Endometriosis. Laparoscopic surgery in infertile women with minimal and mild endometriosis. N Engl J Med 1997;337:217-222.
Moore J, Kennedy S, Prentice A: Modern combined oral contraceptives for pain associated with endometriosis. In the Cochrane database 2004.
Parazzini F: Ablation of lesions or no treatment in minimal-mild endometriosis in infertile women: A randomized trial. Gruppo Italiano per lo Studio dell' Endometriosisi. Hum Reprod 1999;14:1332-1334.
Sutton CJG, Ewen SP, Whitelaw N, Haines P: Prospective, randomized, double-blind trial of laser laparoscopy in the treatment of pelvic pain associated with minimal, mild, and moderate endometriosis. Fertil Steril 1994;62:696-700.

Dysfunctional Uterine Bleeding

Method of
Aydin Arici, MD, and Beth W. Rackow, MD

Abnormal uterine bleeding is a common disorder among reproductive-age women. Dysfunctional uterine bleeding, defined as bleeding that occurs with no identifiable anatomic pathology, affects 33% to 50% of women with abnormal bleeding. Normal menstrual bleeding predictably occurs at the end of an ovulatory cycle because of estrogen and progesterone withdrawal, and it lasts less than 7 days, with a cycle interval of 21 to 35 days. Any imbalance of either hormone, estrogen or progesterone, may lead to dysfunctional bleeding. Thus bleeding may occur from estrogen withdrawal because of bilateral oophorectomy or the midcycle fall in estrogen prior to ovulation; from estrogen breakthrough, such as with prolonged estrogen stimulation from chronic anovulation; from progesterone withdrawal after a short or long course of progestin therapy; and from progesterone breakthrough in the setting of a high ratio of progesterone to estrogen, such as with estrogen-progestin and progestin-based contraceptives. Dysfunctional uterine bleeding is a diagnosis of exclusion and requires eliminating other congenital and acquired abnormalities.

Evaluation of the patient with abnormal uterine bleeding must consider a broad differential diagnosis that includes a complication of pregnancy, cervical and uterine pathology (polyps, fibroids, adenomyosis, malignancies, chronic endometritis, congenital anomalies), infectious etiologies (sexually transmitted diseases, vaginitis), endocrinopathies (thyroid or androgen disorders, hyperprolactinemia), medications (exogenous hormonal therapy, anticoagulants, antibiotics, glucocorticoids, tamoxifen [Nolvadex], herbal supplements), bleeding diathesis, systemic illness (liver or renal disease), and genital trauma or foreign bodies. A thorough menstrual history is essential and should include details about past and present length of intermenstrual intervals, regularity of menses, volume and duration of bleeding during menses, onset of abnormal bleeding, factors associated with change in bleeding (postcoital, contraceptive method, postpartum, new medical diagnosis, change in weight), and associated symptoms (premenstrual symptoms, dysmenorrhea, dyspareunia, pelvic pain, hirsutism, galactorrhea). A complete medical history, list of medications, and review of systems helps identify any systemic illness or medication effect contributing to the abnormal bleeding. The physical exam should include both a careful inspection of the external genitalia, vagina, and cervix and a bimanual exam to palpate the uterus and adnexa to assess size, contour, and tenderness.

Laboratory evaluation provides further information. A pregnancy test (preferably quantitative) rules out bleeding because of a pregnancy complication. A complete blood count evaluates for anemia or thrombocytopenia and is important with prolonged or heavy bleeding. A serum progesterone timed to the luteal phase of the cycle determines if the patient is ovulatory: A level greater than 3 pg/mL is consistent with recent ovulation. Endocrine testing includes serum thyroid-stimulating hormone, prolactin, and free testosterone levels as indicated. Coagulation studies (prothrombin, partial thromboplastin, and bleeding times) should be performed in adolescents, patients with unexplained menorrhagia, and those with a personal or family history concerning a bleeding disorder. In the setting of a systemic disorder such as chronic liver or renal disease, appropriate testing should be performed.

An endometrial biopsy should be performed in patients at high risk for hyperplasia and cancer based on age (35 years and older) and duration of unopposed estrogen exposure. Young patients (less than 35 years old) with chronic anovulation, thus prolonged estrogen exposure, should also have biopsies because they can develop endometrial hyperplasia and cancer. If the biopsy (preferably done in the luteal phase) reveals secretory, not proliferative, endometrium, ovulation has occurred. A pap smear, cervical cultures, and wet mount should also be performed as indicated.

A history of regular cycles with an increasing amount or duration of bleeding, or intermenstrual bleeding, is suggestive of an anatomic cause of abnormal bleeding. Transvaginal ultrasound provides a valuable assessment of the uterus and endometrium. Pathology such as fibroids and polyps can be identified, and size and location determined. Although an endometrial biopsy may not be necessary if the endometrium is thin (less than 5 mm), clinical suspicion of endometrial pathology takes precedence. Sonohysterography involves ultrasound visualization of the uterus and endometrial cavity; whereas sterile saline distends the cavity. This test has high sensitivity and specificity for uterine and endometrial pathology and is comparable to hysteroscopy. Hysteroscopy can diagnose and treat intrauterine pathology simultaneously, but it is a more invasive procedure. Regardless, it is important to recognize when anatomic abnormalities, such as fibroids, are present but not contributing to the bleeding.

Anovulatory Dysfunctional Uterine Bleeding

A menstrual history that reveals irregular, infrequent, unpredictable bleeding, a varying amount and duration of bleeding, and no reliable symptomatology is often sufficient to diagnose anovulatory bleeding. Considered a systemic disorder, anovulatory bleeding occurs because of a variety of endocrinologic, neurochemical, and pharmacologic processes. Estrogen breakthrough is the most common scenario: Persistently high estrogen levels stimulate overgrowth of an endometrium that is fragile without the stabilizing, growth-limiting effects of progesterone, and focal areas of the endometrium breakdown, bleed, and subsequently heal because of estrogen effect. This dysfunctional bleeding is common in women with polycystic ovary syndrome or obesity, in postmenarche adolescents, and in perimenopausal women. Other conditions associated with anovulatory

states include hypothyroidism, hyperprolactinemia, androgen disorders, psychological or physical stress, eating disorders, dramatic weight changes, and insulin resistance.

Management of anovulatory bleeding involves treating both the cause of anovulation and the abnormal bleeding. Progestins are the foundation of this medical therapy. Cyclic progestins stabilize the estrogen-stimulated endometrium and result in withdrawal bleeding after the progestin course. Medications used for a 10-day course every 4 to 6 weeks include medroxyprogesterone acetate (Provera), 5 to 10 mg, and norethindrone acetate (Aygestin), 5 mg. If bleeding does not occur after progestin withdrawal, the patient may also be hypoestrogenic, and further evaluation is indicated. Estrogen-progestin contraceptives are advantageous for patients with intermittent ovulation who require contraception, and they also effectively decrease the amount of bleeding. Medroxyprogesterone acetate (Depo-Provera),[1] 150 mg intramuscularly every 3 months, can also control anovulatory bleeding, especially if patients cannot take combined contraceptives. Treatment of prolonged heavy anovulatory bleeding can be achieved with either low-dose monophasic combined contraceptives,[1] one pill twice daily for 5 to 7 days until the bleeding slows or stops, followed by routine daily use if desired, or with a higher-dose course of progestin therapy. Once the heavy bleeding is controlled, further evaluation is warranted.

Estrogen therapy is indicated for the treatment of dysfunctional bleeding with a thinned endometrium because of low estrogen levels or after prolonged bleeding. This can be accomplished with conjugated estrogens (Premarin),[1] 1.25 mg, or micronized estradiol (Estrace),[1] 2 mg daily for 7 to 10 days. Similarly, estrogen (a 7- to 10-day course) can be used to treat progesterone breakthrough bleeding in the setting of low-dose combined contraceptives or long-acting progesterone therapy (medroxyprogesterone acetate [Depo-Provera]).

Ovulatory Dysfunctional Uterine Bleeding

Heavy or prolonged bleeding may occur during ovulatory cycles, and often no specific etiology is identified. Local defects in endometrial hemostasis are implicated. A number of medical and surgical therapies are effective in this situation. Nonsteroidal anti-inflammatory drugs (NSAIDs), such as ibuprofen (Motrin),[1] naproxen (Aleve),[1] or mefenamic acid (Ponstel),[1] decrease menstrual blood loss by inhibiting prostaglandin synthesis, an important component of endometrial hemostasis. NSAIDs may decrease blood loss by 20% to 40% and should be used for 3 to 5 days upon the onset of bleeding. Similarly, oral contraceptives can reduce menstrual flow by 40% to 60%. Another option is the levonorgestrel-releasing intrauterine system (Mirena)[1]: The local progestin effect on the endometrium is profound and can reduce menstrual blood loss by 75% to 90% in women

---

[1]Not FDA approved for this indication.

16

with heavy bleeding. Although cyclic progestins are often ineffective in this setting, a course of progestin (norethindrone acetate, 5 mg three times daily) from days 5 to 26 of the cycle can suppress heavy ovulatory bleeding. Gonadotropin-releasing hormone agonists produce a hypoestrogenic state and thus cause amenorrhea as well as shrinkage of fibroids, if present. This therapy is best reserved for short-term management of heavy bleeding and severe anemia, especially prior to a surgical procedure, because of expense and significant side effects, including menopausal symptoms and bone demineralization. Less commonly employed therapies include tranexamic acid (Cyklokapron),[1] an antifibrinolytic agent used in Europe to treat menorrhagia (1 g every 6 hours for the first few days of bleeding), and danazol (Danocrine),[1] a therapy that inhibits ovulation and decreases menstrual blood loss but involves androgenic side effects (200 mg daily).

Intermenstrual bleeding can also occur during ovulatory cycles. This dysfunctional bleeding may be caused by anatomic abnormalities such as polyps or submucosal fibroids, functional ovarian cysts, pelvic infection, the preovulatory decline in estrogen, or estrogen-progestin or progestin-only contraceptive therapy. Conjugated estrogens (Premarin),[1] 1.25 mg, or micronized estradiol (Estrace), 2 mg for 2 to 3 days midcycle or 7 to 10 days for persistent breakthrough bleeding, are effective.

For patients who fail medical therapy or for those who do not desire future fertility, surgical management is appropriate. The definitive procedure is hysterectomy, but this surgery carries a significant risk of complications and involves longer recovery time. Endometrial ablation by hysteroscopic, thermal, or cryosurgical techniques is a less invasive procedure for the management of abnormal bleeding. These techniques can result in significantly reduced bleeding and even amenorrhea, as well as less dysmenorrhea, but approximately 20% of patients require additional procedures. Patients with menorrhagia attributed to uterine fibroids can be managed with myomectomy (hysteroscopic, laparoscopic, or abdominal procedures as indicated) or uterine artery embolization. Pregnancy is not recommended after the latter option because little data are available on postprocedure pregnancy outcomes.

---

[1]Not FDA approved for this indication.

 CURRENT DIAGNOSIS

- Detailed medical and menstrual history
- Thorough physical and gynecologic examination
- Pregnancy test for all reproductive-age women
- Determination of ovulatory status by history, laboratory tests
- Laboratory evaluation: complete blood count, endocrine studies, coagulation profile
- Endometrial sampling if high risk for hyperplasia or cancer
- Imaging studies to evaluate anatomy

 CURRENT THERAPY

- Progestins
  - Cyclic or intermittent use
  - Prolonged therapy
  - Progestin-releasing intrauterine device (IUD) (Mirena)[1]
- Estrogens[1]
  - Intermittent use
  - High-dose course for acute heavy bleeding
- Estrogen-progestin contraceptives[1]
  - Cyclic use
  - High-dose course with taper for heavy bleeding
- Other therapies
  - Nonsteroidal anti-inflammatory drugs[1]
  - Tranexamic acid (Cyklokapron)[1]
  - Danazol (Danocrine)[1]
  - Gonadotropin-releasing hormone agonists
- Surgical options
  - Endometrial ablation
  - Myomectomy
  - Uterine artery embolization
  - Hysterectomy

---

[1]Not FDA approved for this indication.

Uterine Hemorrhage

Acute heavy bleeding (usually with a thinned endometrium) requires high-dose estrogen therapy. Patients who need inpatient management should receive conjugated estrogens (Premarin), 25 mg intravenously every 4 hours for 24 hours or until the bleeding decreases. A Foley catheter balloon can be placed in the uterine cavity to tamponade the bleeding. Additionally, dilation and curettage is an effective way to stop acute uterine hemorrhage. If stable for outpatient management, patients can receive conjugated estrogens (Premarin),[1] 1.25 mg, or micronized estradiol (Estrace),[1] 2 mg every 4 to 6 hours for 24 hours, and when the bleeding is controlled, the dose is tapered to once daily for 7 to 10 days. Another effective regimen uses high-dose combination contraceptives[1] (3 to 4 pills daily) until the bleeding is decreased, followed by a taper to 1 pill daily for several weeks. Estrogen therapy should be followed by progestins or combined contraceptives to stabilize the estrogen-stimulated endometrium.

Because dysfunctional uterine bleeding is a diagnosis of exclusion, a thorough history and evaluation, including determination of ovulatory status, is essential. A number of medical and surgical options exist for the management of dysfunctional bleeding. However, treatment failures require further evaluation.

REFERENCES

American College of Obstetricians and Gynecologists: Management of anovulatory bleeding. ACOG Practice Bulletin, no. 14, March 2000.

---

[1]Not FDA approved for this indication.

Rakel and Bope: *Conn's Current Therapy 2006.*

Berek JS (ed): Benign diseases of the female reproductive tract. In Berek JS, ed: Novak's Gynecology. Philadelphia, Lippincott Williams & Wilkins, 2002, pp 351-373.

Munro MG: Dysfunctional uterine bleeding: Advances in diagnosis and treatment. Curr Opin Obstet Gynecol 2001;13:475-489.

Munro MG: Medical management of abnormal uterine bleeding. Obstet Gynecol Clin North Am 2000;27:287-304.

Shwayder JM: Pathophysiology of abnormal uterine bleeding. Obstet Gynecol Clin North Am 2000;27:219-234.

Speroff L, Fritz M: Dysfunctional uterine bleeding. In Clinical Gynecologic Endocrinology and Infertility. Philadelphia, Lippincott Williams & Wilkins; 2005, pp. 548-571.

Infertility

Method of
Steven R. Williams, MD

Absence of desired conception despite 12 months of unprotected intercourse generally defines infertility. Historical and physical factors allow the physician to adjust this definition to the individual patient. For example, women with longstanding amenorrhea or known distal hydrosalpinges should consider intervention before 12 months, time has elapsed. However, the couple, 22 years of age, with a negative history can be encouraged to try a bit longer than 12 months before evaluation begins. After 6 months of trying, approximately 45% of couples achieve pregnancy, and after 12 months of trying, approximately 85% will conceive. Pregnancy can occur with sex 6 days before ovulation, although one study found no pregnancies were conceived from sex the day after ovulation. Thus we recommend couples trying for a baby should plan to be active together every other day starting about 6 days before ovulation is expected (cycle day 8) until 2 to 3 days after ovulation has happened (cycle day 18). If the mood were to strike more often, that's fine with us; if the mood strikes less often, we can still be comfortable given the 6-day interval previously described. As in all of medicine, important historical points can guide the direction of the evaluation and treatment of the infertile couple.

Male-factor historical points include fathering past pregnancies or miscarriages, sexual function, urologic or hernia surgery, infections, medications, and tobacco use. Semen analysis remains the most important test for male factor evaluation. The World Health Organization (WHO) reports normal males to have more than 20 million sperm per cc with greater than 50% motility. It is probably best to advise 48 hours of abstinence before collection of the sample. A urologic exam and evaluation is indicated with abnormal counts. Modern in vitro fertilization (IVF) treatments can achieve pregnancies as long as any sperm at all can be isolated, even if that means surgical aspiration. Before pursuing assisted reproduction for severely low counts, genetic testing will be recommended because severely low counts can predict higher rates of cystic fibrosis carrier status,

balanced translocation, and perhaps microdeletions of the Y chromosome.

A women's age has a strong correlation with fertility success. Figure 1 compares the live birth rate when IVF patients used their own eggs fertilized with their partner's sperm compared to the rate when young oocyte donor's eggs are fertilized with the IVF patient's partner's sperm and the resultant embryos transferred into the IVF patient's uterus. One must conclude from these data that the majority of the decline in success is related to oocyte quality, as anyone can expect the success of a woman 25 years of age who uses the oocytes from a woman 25 years of age! Follicle-stimulating hormone (FSH) measured on day 3 of the menstrual cycle correlates well with ovarian reserve and is commonly ordered for women more than 30 years of age with infertility. In our office, day-3 FSH values lower than 9 mU/mL are reassuring with respect to ovarian reserve, whereas values greater than 20 mU/mL are rarely associated with future fertility success using that patient's eggs.

Previous full-term deliveries are reassuring, whereas recurrent abortions or preterm deliveries can predict a uterine issue. Pelvic infections, intrauterine device (IUD) use, previous abdominal surgery, dysmenorrhea, or dysparunea can predict tubal obstruction. This is explored with hysterosalpingography (HSG). After sterile preparation of the cervix, a sterile cannula is inserted, and under fluoroscopic guidance radiograph contrast is injected. The dye reveals the contour of the uterine cavity and displays uterine septa and intracavitary lesions such as fibroids or polyps. It then fills into the fallopian tubes and spills into the abdominal cavity. Most women describe the discomfort of the test as a severe menstrual cramp that lasts for several minutes. Pain is reduced by slow injection of the dye, gentle tissue handling, and pretreatment with nonsteroidal anti-inflammatory drugs (NSAIDs). Many authors suggest that the procedure itself has a fertility-enhancing effect. The American College of Obstetricians and

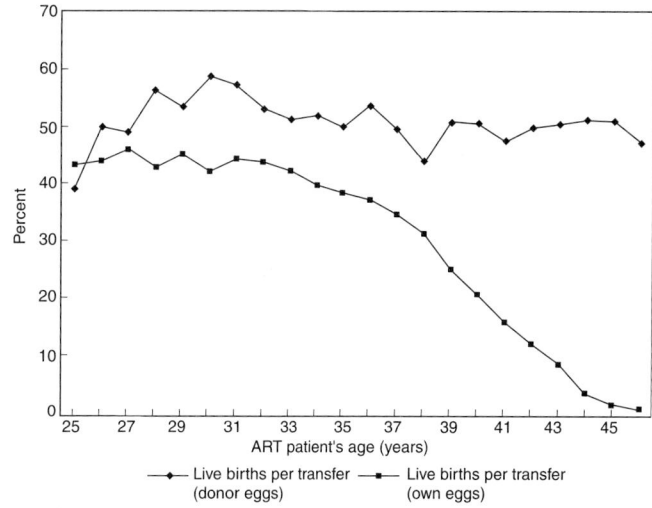

FIGURE 1. Live births per transfer for ART cycles using fresh embryos from own and donor eggs, by ART patient's age, 2002. ART = assisted reproductive technology.

Gynecologists (ACOG) suggests prophylaxis with doxycycline (Vibramycin)[1] 100 mg twice daily orally for 5 days after HSG if dilated tubes are demonstrated; no prophylaxis is indicated in a normal study. Abnormal uterine cavities can be further evaluated with saline infusion hysterograms or magnetic resonance imaging (MRI). Many uterine abnormalities can be treated completely with hysteroscopic surgery. Unilateral tubal disease noted on the HSG predicts subtle decreases in future fertility in these women compared with women with normal tubes. Bilateral tubal disease discovered on HSG predicts dramatic declines in fertility. Tubal patency established by HSG does not rule out peritubal adhesions that can affect fertility. Laparoscopy is an out-patient surgical procedure that can be used to further evaluate tubal abnormalities seen on HSG or to look for undetected peritubal adhesions. Laparoscopy also will detect endometriosis.

Endometriosis is noted in approximately 1 in 30 laparoscopies performed for tubal ligation (presumably for fertile women), although one third of women undergoing infertility evaluations will have endometriosis. Surgical treatment of minimal or mild endometriosis does appear to help with subsequent fertility somewhat. A prospective study of infertile women found to have mild or minimal endometriosis noted at laparoscopy showed a 31% preganancy rate in the next 9 months for patients randomized to treatment versus a 17% pregnancy rate in the next 9 months for women randomized to no treatment.

Irregular menstruation generally indicates irregular ovulation and diminished fertility. Even with regular menstruations, serum progesterone measurements in the luteal phase (6 to 8 days after ovulation) should be greater than 10 ng/mL for the "most fertile" of ovulations. If it is not, thyroid and prolactin studies should be ordered and induction of ovulation with clomiphene citrate (Clomid) considered. Clomiphene citrate in a 50-mg dose is taken orally for 5 days starting on menstrual day 3. Serum luteal phase progesterone is drawn 7 days after ovulation and is expected to be greater than 10 ng/dL. If it is, refills for 2 more months of treatment are written. If it is not, we recommend increasing the dose of clomiphene citrate to 100 mg daily for 5 days and repeating the luteal phase progesterone assay. If still not greater than 10 ng/dL, clomiphene citrate at 150 mg daily can be tried. If the patient is still anovulatory, referral to a gynecologist or reproductive endocrinologist is considered. For resistant patients, adjunctive treatments with the clomiphene citrate can include ultrasound monitoring with HCG injections when mature follicles are noted or adding insulin-sensitizing agents or glucocorticoids. Clomiphene ovulation induction yields approximately a 70% ovulation rate and, in young couples, approximately an 8% pregnancy rate per month. One in ten clomiphene citrate pregnancies are twins, although triplets and quadruplets are very rare on this therapy. Side effects of clomiphene citrate include hot flushes, emotional lability, mittelschmerz, headache, and sleep disturbance. Discontinue the drug

---

[1]Not FDA approved for this indication.

CURRENT DIAGNOSIS

- Medical history can guide fertility testing.
- Simple laboratory and radiograph tests can determine infertility causes.

if the patient experiences severe visual disturbance. Because the majority of clomiphene citrate pregnancies happen early in treatment, referral to reproductive specialists should be considered if the patients is not pregnant after 3 months of treatment.

Gonadotropin ovulation induction is available for women who failed to ovulate using clomiphene citrate or did not conceive on that therapy. This medication is the natural hormone used to initiate ovulation; therefore, response and pregnancy rates are better than with clomiphene citrate. Unfortunately, dramatic increases in multiple pregnancy are associated with these medications, and often they are quite expensive. One large study reviewed success and multiple pregnancy rates in patients treated with gonadotropin ovulation induction. The authors concluded the protocols employed with gonadotropin ovulation induction lead to an unacceptably high incidence of higher-order multiple pregnancies and raised the question whether that treatment could be replaced by IVF.

IVF involves induction of ovulation with gonadotropin in hopes of retrieving multiple oocytes. Ovarian response is monitored with pelvic ultrasounds and serum estradiol measurements. When the oocytes are mature, HCG is given to trigger the completion of oocyte development. Then transvaginal ultrasound is used to guide an aspirating needle through the posterior cul-de-sac and into the ovaries for aspiration of the oocytes. The procedure takes approximately 15 minutes under local anesthesia and is often performed in an office setting. Oocytes are then inseminated in the lab with the husband's sperm and cultured. In certain circumstances (vey low sperm count, surgically aspirated sperm, previous failed fertilization) the oocytes can be directly injected with the sperm via intracytoplasmic sperm injection (ICSI). The resultant embryos are then cultured for 2 to 5 days and then transferred into the uterus via a simple transcervical approach. IVF thus allows embryo development without tubal ovarial interaction, making it a great choice for patients with tubal disease or endometriosis. In fact, nothing we can find at laparoscopy that was not discovered by pelvic ultrasound and HSG will affect IVF success (Figure 2). We are developing protocols that reduce the numbers of embryos transferred for couples at high risk for multiple pregnancy to one. I believe that in the

CURRENT THERAPY

- Clomiphene citrate is a low risk treatment option when indicated.
- Assisted reproduction is delivering more and more babies with fewer multiples.

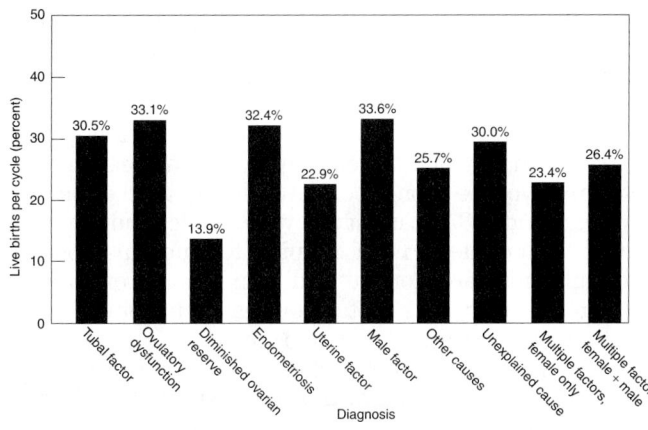

FIGURE 2. Live birth rates among women who had ART cycles using fresh nondonor eggs or embryos, by diagnosis, 2002. ART = assisted reproductive technology.

future IVF will replace both gonadotropin ovulation induction and the need for laparoscopy for treatment of infertility. The 2001 Centers for Disease Control (CDC) report on assisted reproductive technology (ART) success reported national average live birth rates in the high 30% per cycle start for women younger than 35 years of age. Some individual centers are reporting live birth rates in the 50% range. IVF is a very effective and increasingly safer alternative to older treatments for refractory infertility.

REFERENCES

American College of Obstetrics and Gynecology: Antibiotic prophylaxis for gynecologic procedures. ACOG Practice Bulletin 2003;23.

Centers of Disease Control: 2002 Assisted reproductive technology success rates, National summary and fertility clinic reports. Atlanta, Center for Disease Control, 2002.

Gleicher N, Oleske DM, Tur-Kaspa I, et al: Reducing the risk of higher order multiple pregnancy after ovarian stimulation with gonadotropins. N Engl J Med 2000;343:2-7.

Jain T, Soules MR, Collins JA: Comparison of basal follicle-stimulating hormone versus the clomiphene citrate challenge test for ovarian reserve testing. Fertil Steril 2004;82:180-185.

Jordan J, Craig K, Clifton DK, et al: Luteal phase defect: The sensitivity and specificity of diagnostic methods in common clinical use. Fertil Steril 1995;63:427-428.

Marcoux S, Maheux R, Berube S: Laparoscopic surgery in infertile women with minimal or mild endometriosis. Canadian collaborative group on endometriosis. N Engl J Med 1997;337:217-222.

Mol BW, Swart P, Bossuyt BM, et al: Is hysterosalpingography an important tool in predicting fertility outcome? Fertil Steril 1997;67:663-669.

Schwabe MG. Shapiro SS, Haning RV Jr: Hysterosalpingography with oil contrast medium enhances fertility in patients with infertility of unknown etiology. Fertil Steril 1983;40:604-606.

Trimbos JB, Trimbos-Kemper GC, Peters AA, et al: Findings in 200 consecitive asymptomatic women, having a laparoscopic sterilization. Arch Gynecol Obstet 1990;247:121-124.

Wilcox AJ, Weinberg CR, Baird DD: Timing of sexual intercourse in relation to ovulation. Effects on the probability of conception, survival of the pregnancy, and sex of the baby. N Engl J Med 1995;333:1517-1521.

Amenorrhea

Method of
Carl A. Krantz, Jr., MD

Amenorrhea occurs in approximately 5% of all reproductive-age women and is defined as one of the following:

- No menstruation by age 14 years and the absence of secondary sexual characteristics
- No menstruation by age 16 years
- The absence of periods in a previously menstruating woman, with an interval of at least three times the length of the longest cycle or 6 months of amenorrhea

Although amenorrhea is classically described as primary (never had a menses) or secondary (cessation of menses in a once-menstruating woman), the two divisions can greatly overlap. Most importantly, the workup for amenorrhea is similar in either case and always should begin with a pregnancy test, which is by far the most common etiology.

Menstrual Cycle

A clear understanding of the normal menstrual cycle is necessary to understand the complexity of the differential diagnosis of amenorrhea. Cyclic menstruation is the result of a dynamic relationship known as the hypothalamic-pituitary-ovarian axis, which stimulates follicular development with the production of estrogen. This hormonal stimulation begins the proliferation of the endometrium, which is completed with luteinizing hormone (LH) release. Ovulation occurs and secretory endometrium is produced, which prepares the uterus for implantation or results in menstruation 14 days after ovulation if fertilization does not occur. Control of the cycle begins in the hypothalamus. Pulsatile gonadotropin-releasing hormone (GnRH) is secreted by the arcuate nucleus. This pulsatile release is critical. External environmental factors as well as neurohormonal factors from higher brain centers may interfere with the pulsatile release of GnRH.

The clinical manifestation of menstruation requires an intact hypothalamic-pituitary-ovarian axis as well as a functional uterus and patent outflow tract. The workup outlined here simplifies the identification of the malfunctioning compartment of the reproductive system.

Etiology of Amenorrhea

THYROID AND PROLACTIN

Thyroid abnormalities, hyperthyroidism or, more commonly, hypothyroidism, can cause menstrual irregularities or amenorrhea. High prolactin levels inhibit

16

the pulsatile release of GnRH. Prolactin should be measured in all amenorrheic women because not all have galactorrhea as a clinical finding of hyperprolactinemia. Thyrotropine-releasing hormone stimulates both thyroid-stimulating hormone (TSH) and prolactin. In view of this relationship, those patients with an elevation in prolactin should have a TSH level drawn.

HYPOTHALAMUS

Amenorrhea associated with hypothalamic dysfunction is usually characterized by normal prolactin, low to low-normal follicle-stimulating hormone (FSH) and LH, as well as low estrogen levels. Both physical as well as psychological stress are common etiologies of hypothalamic amenorrhea. The elevation of corticotropin-releasing hormone associated with stress may inhibit GnRH pulsatility and thus cause amenorrhea. Extreme exercise may cause amenorrhea presumably because of decrease in body fat. Hormone supplementation should be considered in these patients to prevent osteoporosis and stress fractures.

Eating disorders, including bulimia and especially anorexia nervosa, are many times associated with amenorrhea. These patients are usually found to have low FSH, LH, estradiol, and 3,5,3′-triiodothyronine (T3), with normal prolactin, TSH, and cortisol.

Isolated FSH or LH deficiency is rare and probably caused by GnRH deficiency. Because of the lack of FSH and therefore estrogen production, these patients lack breast development. Hypogonadotropic hypogonadism associated with anosmia is known as Kallmann syndrome. Pseudocyesis (false pregnancy) is a rare cause of amenorrhea and can be identified when a patient has pregnancy symptoms but a negative pregnancy test.

PITUITARY

Pituitary adenomas, usually prolactinomas, cause amenorrhea. Rarely, growth hormone and adrenalotropic hormone secreting pituitary adenomas may cause amenorrhea. If prolactin levels are elevated (more than 100 µg/mL), magnetic resonance imaging (MRI) or sella tomograms are indicated. Patients with empty sella syndrome may have elevated prolactin levels and thus menstrual disturbances. Finally, Sheehan's syndrome is panhypopituitarism, caused by postpartum hypovolemic shock.

OVARY

Polycystic ovarian (PCO) syndrome is the most common ovarian disorder causing oligorrhea or amenorrhea. Many times it is associated with hyperandrogenism and insulin resistance. Patients with chromosomal abnormalities, including Turner's syndrome (45, XO), have primary amenorrhea and sexual infantilism, but Turner mosaics (46, XX/45, XO), may develop sexually and have secondary amenorrhea. These mosaic patients rarely achieve pregnancy. Deletions in the short or long arms of the X chromosome may lead to ovarian failure. Those with pure gonadal dysgenesis have primary amenorrhea and

may have a (46, XX) or (46, XY) karyotype. It is important to identify those with (46, XY) because these ovaries have a higher incidence of cancer and should be removed.

Because 50% of primary amenorrhea patients with elevated gonadotropin levels have chromosomal aberrations, a karyotype should be drawn. Many sources believe a woman under 35 years of age with an elevation of FSH should be included in karyotyping to rule out mosaics, although most are normal and simply have premature ovarian syndrome or resistant ovarian syndrome.

Androgen-secreting ovarian and, rarely, adrenal tumors may cause amenorrhea. These are associated with acne, temporal balding and hirsutism, and occasionally clitorimegaly. Adrenal tumors exhibit symptoms, including masculinization, rapidly, as compared to an androgen-secreting ovarian tumor that develops these symptoms over months. Patients with polycystic ovaries develop less significant changes over years. If the total testosterone level is greater than 200 µg/dL or DHEAS (sulfate salt of dehydroepiandrosterone) level is greater than 700 µg/dL, radiologic evaluation of ovaries and adrenals is indicated.

OUTFLOW TRACT

Complete agenesis of the müllerian ducts results in the absence of the uterus and cervix with a short blind vagina (Mayer-Rokitansky-Küster-Hauser syndrome). Cervical atresia, a transverse vaginal septum, and imperforate hymen present with amenorrhea and also with cyclic pain and sometimes endometriosis. These patients have normal ovarian function and therefore normal development of secondary sexual characteristics. Cervical stenosis may arise from cone, loop electrocautery excision procedure (LEEP), or cryosurgery and obstruct the outflow of menses from the uterus.

Uterine synechiae, resulting in obliteration of the endometrial cavity, may occur with dilation and curettage in conjunction with a recent pregnancy or missed abortion.

Testicular feminization (complete androgen insensitivity) presents with primary amenorrhea and a female phenotype. On exam, patients have a short blind vagina and scant pubic and axillary hair. The breasts are fibrous. These patients have normal male testosterone levels and one Barr body related to the (46, XY) karyotype. Because of a mutation in the androgen receptor, testosterone is rendered biologically inactive. The gonads should be removed after puberty to prevent gonadal tumors.

Diagnosis is made after a careful history and physical exam. Special attention to secondary sexual development is paramount because breasts develop with estrogen exposure. Hirsutism or more importantly, masculinization suggests androgen excess. The presence of galactorrhea suggests elevation of prolactin. A detailed pelvic exam identifies an imperforate hymen, transverse vaginal septum, cervical agenesis, or stenosis. Ultrasound identifies a uterus, cervix, and ovaries. After ruling out pregnancy, some simple

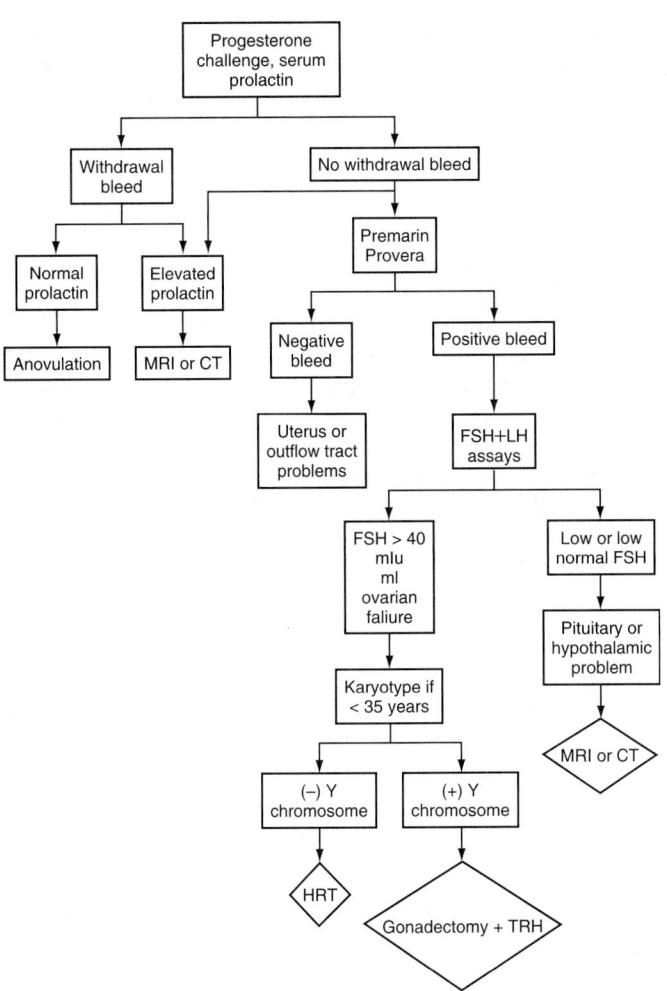

FIGURE 1. Workup for amenorrhea. CT = computerized tomography; FSH = follicle-stimulating hormone; HRT = hormone replacement therapy; LH = luteinizing hormone; MRI = magnetic resonance imaging.

 CURRENT THERAPY

- Pregnancy test
- If pregnancy test negative, thyroid-stimulating hormone (TSH), prolactin levels
- Medroxyprogesterone acetate (Provera), 10 mg for 10 days
- Algorithm as per this article

16

should be taken for 5 to 10 days. Progesterone in oil, 200 mg intramuscularly, may be substituted. Menstrual bleeding should ensue 2 to 7 days after the completion of therapy. Menstrual flow (a positive challenge test) indicates an intact outflow tract and estrogen secretion, leaving anovulation as the etiology of the amenorrhea.

- **Step III:** A negative progesterone challenge test indicates an obstructed outflow tract or a non-estrogen-primed endometrium. Once obstruction of the outflow tract is eliminated as an etiology, conjugated estrogen (Premarin, 2.5 mg) should be given orally for 21 days, and Provera, 10 mg, should be added for the last 10 days. If menstruation does not follow, the regimen should be repeated a second time. With a second negative challenge test, the uterus is the etiology of the amenorrhea. An ultrasound with hysterosonogram or hysterosalpingogram with fluoroscopy can identify both cervical stenosis and Asherman's syndrome.
- **Step IV:** A positive response to estrogen and progesterone therapy identifies a nonestrogen-primed endometrium. FSH and LH levels should be measured. Premature ovarian failure is identified if the gonadotropins are elevated, especially the FSH. If the patient is under 35 years of age, a karyotype should be considered. These patients should have hormone replacement therapy to prevent osteoporosis and pathologic stress fractures.

If the gonadotropin levels are low to low normal, a pituitary or hypothalamic problem is identified. Hypothalamic dysfunction risk factors should be sought, including stress, weight loss, extreme exercise, or eating disorders. In the absence of these, a computed tomogram or MRI of the brain should be ordered to rule out a tumor or empty sella. Here again, hormone replacement is advisable.

REFERENCES

Berek J: Novak's Gynecology, 12th ed. Philadelphia, Williams & Wilkins, 1996, pp 809-830.
Braumuald F, Hauser K, Jameson L: Harrison's Principles of Internal Medicine, 15th ed. New York, McGraw-Hill, 2001.
Copeland L: Textbook of Gynecology. Philadelphia, WB Saunders, 1993.
Speroff L, Glass R, Kase N: Clinical Gynecologic Endocrinology and Infertility, 5th ed. Philadelphia, Williams & Wilkins, 1994.

steps that will elucidate the etiology of amenorrhea are (Figure 1):

- **Step I:** The first step involves drawing a prolactin and TSH level. If the prolactin level is more than 100 µg/mL, MRI or computed tomography of the pituitary should be ordered to rule out a pituitary adenoma. Many drugs elevate prolactin levels, so a detailed medication history is a necessity.
- **Step II:** If the prolactin is normal, a progestin, medroxyprogesterone acetate (Provera), 10 mg,

 CURRENT DIAGNOSIS

- Current history; primary versus secondary amenorrhea
- Emotional, athletic, dietary history
- Weight gain or loss
- Galactorrhea?

Dysmenorrhea

Method of
Joyce Olutade, MD

Dysmenorrhea, defined as painful menstruation, affects approximately 50% of reproductive-age women and 60% to 80% of female adolescents in the United States. The result is a loss of approximately 600 million work hours annually in the United States, severely limiting school attendance and work or physical activities in approximately 10% to 45% of those affected. Dysmenorrhea is subdivided into two types: primary and secondary dysmenorrhea.

Primary Dysmenorrhea

Primary dysmenorrhea starts within 6 to 12 months of menarche when ovulatory cycles are established. The pain begins a few hours before or on the first day of menses and is most intense during the first 2 days of the menstrual period. It is a crampy, midline lower abdominal pain caused by uterine ischemia, which results from hypercontractility of the myometrium and increased uterine pressure. Prostaglandin F2α and prostaglandin E2 from secretory endometrium induce these uterine contractions. Vasopressin and leukotrienes also cause uterine contractions. Other symptoms of primary dysmenorrhea, including headaches, low back pain, diarrhea, nausea, and vomiting, are also attributable to the increased prostaglandin production. Menorrhagia is not a common feature of primary dysmenorrhea.

DIAGNOSIS

A thorough medical and gynecologic history and a pelvic examination help establish the diagnosis of primary dysmenorrhea. Age at menarche; onset of menstrual pain in relation to menarche; the duration of the menstrual cycle and menstrual period; the intensity, location, and duration of the pain; the presence of intermenstrual bleeding; the intensity of the flow; and other associated symptoms are important elements of the menstrual history. The speculum and bimanual pelvic examination are usually normal in primary dysmenorrhea.

TREATMENT

Primary dysmenorrhea is treated with nonsteroidal anti-inflammatory drugs (NSAIDs), combined oral contraceptives, or a combination of both. NSAIDs are prostaglandin synthetase inhibitors (Table 1). Cyclooxygenase-2 (COX-2) selective inhibitors are now approved for the treatment of primary dysmenorrhea (Table 2). NSAIDs (including COX-2 selective inhibitors) reduce endometrial hypercontractility through their antiprostaglandin effect. The NSAIDs, considered first-line medications for treating primary dysmenorrhea, belong to two main classes: propionic acid derivatives and fenamates. The former include ibuprofen (Motrin), ketoprofen (Orudis), and naproxen (Naprosyn). Fenamates include mefenamic acid (Ponstel), flufenamic acid,[1] and meclofenamate. Fenamates work by inhibiting prostaglandin production and by directly blocking the effect of already formed prostaglandins. One review found that naproxen, ibuprofen, mefenamic acid, and aspirin are all effective in treating primary dysmenorrhea, but ibuprofen has the best risk-to-benefit ratio. COX-2 selective inhibitors have a similar pain control profile as naproxen sodium. Other studies report fenamates to be more effective than propionic acid derivatives. NSAIDs should be started at the onset of menses. If a patient fails to respond to one class of NSAIDs, an agent from another class should be selected.

Oral contraceptives may be used as first-line medications in sexually active women who also desire contraception. NSAIDs may not be effective in approximately 30% of women. Oral contraceptives alone or in combination with NSAIDs may be beneficial in such women. If dysmenorrhea persists after a 3- to 6-month trial of second-line agents, evaluation for possible secondary dysmenorrhea should be initiated. COX-2 selective inhibitors are beneficial in women who are unable to take NSAIDs because of peptic ulcer disease. NSAIDs should always be taken with food. Adverse effects of NSAIDs include dyspepsia, gastrointestinal (GI) bleeding, hepatotoxicity, acute renal failure, and bronchospasm. COX-2 selective inhibitors have a similar adverse profile as other NSAIDs except for a lower incidence of GI bleeding and gastritis. Precautions for NSAIDs include history of GI bleeding, peptic ulcer, hypertension, congestive heart failure, renal and hepatic insufficiency, and aspirin- or NSAID-induced asthma.

By inhibiting ovulation and causing endometrial thinning, oral contraceptives reduce the production of prostaglandins and, consequently, decrease dysmenorrhea. A 2003 Cochrane review of medium-dose estrogen (35 to 50 μg) and first- or second-generation progestogens found them more effective than placebo for treating dysmenorrhea. The failure rate of the first- and second-line medications is approximately 20% to 25%.

Secondary Dysmenorrhea

Secondary dysmenorrhea is painful menstruation associated with underlying pathologic conditions. It tends to occur several years after the onset of menarche. The pain usually starts 2 to 3 days before the onset of menstruation and lasts throughout the menstrual period. It may also persist several days afterward. Excessive prostaglandin production also occurs in secondary dysmenorrhea. Menorrhagia is usually associated with secondary dysmenorrhea. Table 3 lists the major gynecologic disorders associated with secondary dysmenorrhea. Nongynecologic disorders, such as inflammatory bowel disease, psychogenic disorders, irritable bowel syndrome, and uteropelvic junction obstruction, may cause secondary dysmenorrhea.

---

[1]Not available in the United States.

Rakel and Bope: *Conn's Current Therapy 2006.*

TABLE 1 Nonsteroidal Anti-inflammatory Drugs (NSAIDs) for Treatment of Dysmenorrhea

	Formulation (mg)	Dosage
Propionic Acids		
Ibuprofen (Motrin, Advil)	200, 400, 600, 800	400 mg q4-6h; max 2400 mg/d
Ketoprofen (Orudis, Oruvail)	12.5, 25, 50, 75,100	25-50 mg PO q6-8h; max 300 mg/d
Naproxen (Naprosyn)	250, 375, 500	500 mg first dose, then 250 mg q6-8h prn; max 1250 mg/d
Naproxen sodium (Anaprox)	275, 550	550 mg PO first dose, then 275 mg PO q6-8h; max 1375 mg/d
Fenamates		
Mefenamic acid (Ponstel)	250	500 mg first dose, then 250 mg PO q6h prn; max 3 d
Meclofenamate	50, 100	100 mg PO tid; max 300 mg/d for 6 d

Abbreviations: max = maximum; PO = orally; prn = as needed; q = every; qd = once daily; tid = three times a day.

Adenomyosis has the classic features of dysmenorrhea, menorrhagia, and a uniformly enlarged uterus. The pain is limited to the menstrual period and occurs in women older than 35 years of age. The diagnosis may be confirmed by magnetic resonance imaging (MRI). A total hysterectomy is the only definitive treatment. Endometrial polyps cause irregular vaginal bleeding and dysmenorrhea and are best diagnosed by sonohysterography.

ENDOMETRIOSIS

Endometriosis is a disorder in which endometrial glands or stroma are found outside the uterine cavity and musculature. Dysmenorrhea from endometriosis may result in lower abdominal, lower back, or deep pelvic pain. The pain usually starts several years after menarche. Primary or secondary infertility, dyspareunia, menorrhagia, and shorter menstrual cycles are important clinical features. Endometriosis may occur in adolescents approximately 3 years after menarche. A bimanual examination may reveal palpably enlarged ovaries and a fixed, retroverted uterus with tender nodularity in the uterosacral ligament. MRI and pelvic ultrasonography may be helpful, but the gold standard for confirmation of endometriosis is laparoscopy.

A complete review of the treatment of endometriosis is beyond the scope of this article and discussed elsewhere in this book. Dysmenorrhea secondary to endometriosis may be treated medically or by surgery. Medical therapy includes the use of NSAIDs,[1] oral contraceptives,[1] danazol (Danocrine), gonadotropin-releasing hormone agonists, and injectable medroxyprogesterone.[1]

---

[1]Not FDA approved for this indication.

A Cochrane review found that a combination of laparoscopic laser ablation, adhesiolysis, and uterine nerve ablation relieves pelvic pain in women with minimal, mild, and moderate endometriosis. Lysis of adhesions and excision, vaporization, or coagulation of macroscopic endometriosis during laparoscopy may help relieve dysmenorrhea in 70% to 80% of treated women.

PELVIC INFLAMMATORY DISEASE

Pelvic inflammatory disease (PID) should be suspected as a cause of secondary dysmenorrhea in any sexually active woman who exhibits high-risk sexual behavior. An intrauterine contraceptive device may predispose a female to acquire PID. Chronic endometritis resulting from PID may cause intermenstrual bleeding, menorrhagia, postcoital bleeding, and dysmenorrhea. The Centers for Disease Control and Prevention's (CDC) minimum criteria for the diagnosis of PID are uterine/adnexal tenderness and/or cervical motion tenderness. A speculum examination may reveal a mucopurulent cervical or vaginal discharge or may be normal. The treatment of PID is covered in a separate article of this book. Broad-spectrum antimicrobial agents, which include *Neisseria gonorrhoeae*, *Chlamydia trachomatis*, anaerobes, gram-negative bacteria, and streptococci, are used in the treatment of PID. NSAIDs are useful for relieving the associated dysmenorrhea.

CERVICAL STENOSIS

Cervical stenosis, which may be congenital or secondary to cervical instrumentation, conization, radium

TABLE 2 Cyclooxygenase-2 (COX-2) Selective Inhibitors

Drug	Formulation (mg)	Dosage
Celecoxib (Celebrex)	100, 200, 400	400 mg PO first dose, then 200 mg PO twice per day; may take additional 200 mg on day 1
Rofecoxib	12.5, 25, 50 or 25/5 mL (suspension)	50 mg PO once per day; max 50 mg/d for 5 d
Valdecoxib	10, 20	20 mg PO bid

Abbreviations: bid = twice daily; max = maximum; PO = orally.

TABLE 3 Major Gynecologic Causes of Dysmenorrhea

Endometriosis	Endometrial polyps
Pelvic inflammatory disease	Adenomyosis
Cervical stenosis	Pelvic adhesions
Ovarian cysts	Congenital obstructive müllerian malforations

application, laser or electrical cauterization, or infection, causes severe menstrual pain in some women. The stenosis is usually at the level of the internal cervical os. Menstrual flow is impeded, causing a buildup of menstrual blood within the uterine cavity and a resulting increase in intrauterine pressure. The occurrence of hypomenorrhea and menstrual pain lasting throughout the menstrual period in a woman with a history of cervical instrumentation is highly suggestive of cervical stenosis. Some women may be amenorrheic but experience severe cyclical lower abdominal or pelvic pain. A speculum examination may reveal a scarred external cervical os. The inability to pass a cervical probe of a few millimeters' diameter through the internal cervical os is diagnostic. The diagnosis may be established using hysterosalpingography.

Cervical os dilatation relieves the resulting dysmenorrhea, but the effect is often temporary, necessitating repeated attempts to dilate the cervical os. Complete curettage of endometrial polyps, preferably during hysteroscopy, cures the majority of cases.

PSYCHOGENIC DISORDERS

Some women experience severe menstrual pain for secondary gain, a conditioned behavior for control and reward. A personality profile test helps confirm the diagnosis of conditioned behavior. Women with conditioned behavior need the help of psychologists for definitive diagnosis and behavior modification.

Stress and tension both worsen menstrual pain. Relaxation techniques, counseling, and antidepressants are useful in such cases.

Alternative Therapies for Primary and Secondary Dysmenorrhea

A Cochrane review of herbal therapies for primary and secondary dysmenorrhea shows that vitamin B_1,[1] 100 mg daily, is effective for treating dysmenorrhea. Magnesium[1] is more effective than placebo, but the effective dose is unknown. Uterine nerve ablation and presacral neurotomy are more effective in relieving primary dysmenorrhea than no treatment, but nerve interruption surgery is not recommended. Transcutaneous electrical nerve stimulation is effective for treating primary dysmenorrhea. Acupuncture may be beneficial, but spinal manipulation is not useful.

---

[1]Not FDA approved for this indication.

Premenstrual Syndrome*

Method of
Susan Thys-Jacobs, MD

Premenstrual syndrome (PMS) is a very common problem that affects approximately 40 million young women in the United States, disrupting their emotional and physical well-being. PMS is widely recognized as a recurrent, cyclical disorder related to and restricted to the latter half of the menstrual cycle, disappearing soon after the onset of menstruation. It is characterized by a complex group of signs and symptoms that may include depression, mood swings, irritability, fatigue, abdominal discomfort, and changes in appetite (Box 1). More than 150 symptoms have been described in PMS, partially explaining the difficulty of defining and studying this syndrome. The four main categories of symptoms include: negative affect, water retention, pain, and appetite changes. Although many women experience only mild symptoms, as many as 30% to 50% suffer from troublesome symptoms. Surveys indicate that approximately 5% of North American women consider their symptoms to be severe enough to have a substantially negative impact on their health and social well-being. This latter group has been referred to as severe PMS or premenstrual dysphoric disorder (PMDD).

Etiology

The pathogenesis of the cyclical mood and somatic changes in PMS is poorly understood. Numerous theories concerning the etiology of this syndrome have been proposed including hormonal imbalances such as an abnormal estrogen-progesterone ratio, progesterone

---

*This article is a modified version of a previously published article that appeared in J Am Coll Nutr 2000;19:220-227.

BOX 1   Common Symptoms of Premenstrual Syndrome

Emotional/Negative Affect
- Anger/irritability
- Depression/sadness
- Mood swings/crying spells
- Tension/nervousness

Pain
- Abdominal cramps
- Generalized aches and pains
- Headache

Bloating/Water Retention
- Abdominal bloating
- Breast swelling and tenderness

Appetite Changes
- Cravings for salt and sweets
- Increased or decreased appetite

deficiency, vitamin B_6 deficiency, and altered endogenous opiates. Most theories have been disproved, the remainder are unproven. What is known is that PMS is related to the hormonal rhythmicities of the menstrual cycle and occurs in ovulatory women, despite the unsuccessful attempts to identify differences in basal levels and pulsatility of the ovarian steroid hormones and pituitary gonadotropins between women with and women without PMS. Ovarian steroid hormones appear important in the pathogenesis of PMS and influence menstrual symptoms as well as calcium and vitamin D metabolism. Suppression or cessation of ovarian function resulting in estrogen deficiency—permanently because of menopause, temporarily because of amenorrhea, as with the administration of gonadotropin-releasing hormone agonists (Lupron),[1] or following oophorectomy—significantly diminishes and may even abolish PMS symptoms. Serotoninergic dysregulation appears to be important in the pathophysiology of the syndrome, and this is well supported by the many clinical trials demonstrating the efficacy of the serotonin reuptake inhibitors in the management of both PMS and PMDD.

Evidence now strongly suggests that PMS is associated with a calcium and vitamin D deficiency state, which is clinically unmasked during the latter half of the menstrual cycle when estradiol and progesterone predominate. The symptoms of PMS are strikingly similar to those of hypocalcemia (Box 2) and respond to calcium and vitamin D therapy. Supplemental calcium[1] alleviates symptoms such as irritability, depression, anxiety, social withdrawal, headache, and cramps. Calcium results in a beneficial clinical response in the treatment of premenstrual symptomatology in a number of studies and significantly benefits all four major categories of PMS (i.e., emotional or negative affect symptoms, bloating or water retention symptoms, food cravings, and pain symptoms), reducing overall symptoms by 50%. These clinical trials in conjunction with recent epidemiologic evidence linking lower dietary calcium and vitamin D intakes with PMS symptoms support the role of calcium in PMS and menstrual health. Calcium may ultimately affect monoamine metabolism and reverse the serotoninergic dysregulation, thus providing a

---

[1]Not FDA approved for this indication.

BOX 2 Clinical Features of Hypocalcemia

- Anxiety
- Depression
- Fatigue
- Impaired memory and intellectual capacity
- Muscle cramps
- Neuromuscular irritability
- Paresthesias
- Personality disturbances
- Tetany

Modified from Becker K (ed.): Hypocalcemia in Principles and Practices of Endocrinology and Metabolism, 3rd ed. Philadelphia, Lippincott Williams & Wilkins, 2001.

biochemical basis for the therapeutic benefit in PMS trials. In addition, variations in calcium and the calcium-regulating hormones (parathyroid hormone [PTH], 25-hydroxyvitamin D, 1,25-dihydroxyvitamin D, and ionized calcium) accompany normal ovarian steroid hormone fluctuations during the menstrual cycle. Exaggerated cyclical fluctuations of the calcium-regulating hormones across the menstrual cycle may explain many of the features of PMS. PMS may truly represent one of the most classic manifestations of a mineral deficiency syndrome.

Premenstrual Assessment and the Diagnosis of Premenstrual Syndrome

The key to diagnosis of PMS is the relationship of luteal to postmenstrual symptoms, although this relationship has been evaluated and measured differently by various authors. There is as yet no objective biochemical marker in the diagnosis of PMS, and the diagnosis depends on the menstrual pattern of symptoms cited by the woman. A prospective assessment of symptoms is recommended but not required for PMS and is strongly advised in PMDD. There is currently no uniform standard assessment of menstrual cycle symptomatology. However, the assessment can be accomplished with a menstrual calendar, daily rating scale, visual analogue scale, or symptom diary (Table 1) for at least 2 months. For PMS, current National Institute of Mental Health recommendations suggest a 30% change from luteal phase to postmenstrual phase to meet criteria of PMS. This can be measured by comparing the average symptoms scores 6 days premenstrually to scores 5 to 10 days postmenstrually. Of course, other diagnoses such as major depression, generalized anxiety, thyroid disease, and other endocrine disorders should be excluded. Of note is that the International Classification of Diseases (ICD)-10 does not require prospective confirmation or a requirement for functional impairment for the diagnosis of PMS, although it would be prudent to document the pattern of symptoms. Whether severe PMS, or PMDD, is a distinct and separate entity from PMS or is even a disease remains a controversial issue. However, a diagnosis of PMDD does require prospective symptom confirmation with specific inclusion criteria of an affective/emotional component with evidence of functional impairment (Box 3).

Current Treatments in Premenstrual Syndrome

There is no one, established therapy for PMS. A variety of treatments have been proposed over the years including lifestyle and dietary modifications, hormonal therapies, and pharmacologic interventions. The majority have proven ineffective or only temporizing, while other treatments have proven scientific efficacy. Some popular methods of treatment that have failed scientifically

TABLE 1 PMS Diary*

| Date | | | Are you presently menstruating? Yes No | | |

Rate the Average Intensity of Discomfort You Experienced During the Previous 24 Hours

PMS/Menstrual Symptoms	Absent (0)	Mild (1)	Moderate (2)	Severe (3)
1. Mood swings/crying spells				
2. Depression/sadness/feelings of hopelessness				
3. Anxiety/tension/nervousness				
4. Decreased interest in usual activities				
5. Difficulty concentrating				
6. Fatigue				
7. Increased/decreased appetite				
8. Insomnia/hypersomnia				
9. Sense of being out of control				
10. Abdominal bloating				
11. Abdominal cramps and discomfort				
12. Headache				
13. Breast tenderness/fullness				
14. Generalized aches and pains				

*Modified version of the PMS Diary. From Thys-Jacobs S, Alvir JM, Fratarcangelo P: Comparative analysis of three PMS assessment instruments—the identification of premenstrual syndrome with core symptoms. Psychopharmacol Bull 1995;31:389-396.

rigorous evaluation include progesterone therapy,[1] monamine oxidase inhibitors,[1] bromocriptine (Parlodel),[1] and evening primrose oil.[1] In general, the current approaches in the treatment of PMS include calcium supplementation,[1] the selective serotonin receptor reuptake inhibitors (SSRIs), and the gonadotropin-releasing hormone agonists.[1] Table 2 lists possible and proven treatments.

---

[1]Not FDA approved for this indication.

BOX 3 Criteria for Premenstrual Dysphoric Disorder

A. The presence of 5 or more of the following symptoms during the week before menses, with remission within the first few days after menses. One symptom must include an emotional component from items 1-4:
 1. Depression or hopelessness
 2. Anxiety or tension
 3. Mood lability or mood swings
 4. Anger or irritability
 5. Decreased interest in usual activities
 6. Difficulty in concentrating
 7. Fatigue or lack of energy
 8. Change in appetite
 9. Increase or decrease in sleep
 10. Sense of being out of control
 11. Other physical symptoms (headache, breast tenderness)
B. Evidence of functional impairment; symptoms must interfere with work or usual activities.
C. Not an exacerbation of another disorder.
D. Prospective confirmation over 2 consecutive months.

Source: The criteria are modified from the American Psychiatric Association: Diagnostic and Statistical Manual of Mental Disorders, 4th ed. Washington, DC: Author, 1994.

For some women, recommending lifestyle changes or pharmacologic interventions are not satisfactory for a natural biologic process. Herbal products are sought by many women for PMS symptom relief, as these remedies are considered more natural. However, some of the botanical therapies can be quite toxic such as blue cohosh[1] or dong quai,[1] which is considered unsafe during pregnancy. Of the herbal therapies, chasteberry,[1] also known as *Vitex agnus-castus*, appears to demonstrate some efficacy, while other data show conflicting results. It appears to diminish follicle-stimulating hormone (FSH) with decreases in estrogen synthesis and at higher doses may inhibit prolactin levels. One large clinical trial demonstrates total relief of PMS symptoms in more than 33% of the women treated. The use of chasteberry should be avoided during pregnancy and during breast-feeding.

Initially advising dietary and lifestyle modifications by increasing daily dietary calcium intake and an adequate aerobic exercise program will often alleviate PMS symptomatology. Calcium (elemental calcium)[*,1] at 1000 mg (500 mg in the form of calcium carbonate twice daily is the most convenient) and vitamin D_3–cholecalciferol[*,1] at 1000 to 2000 international units (IU) daily should be recommended to all women initially, and may be all that is required in those women with mild or even moderate symptoms. The potential for dietary supplements other than calcium to reduce PMS symptoms is less convincing. Magnesium[*,1] at a dose of 200 to 400 mg daily may alleviate PMS symptoms. Facchinetti in 1991 observed that 360 mg of magnesium reduced affective symptoms, while Walker in 1998 noted a reduction in bloated symptoms but not in mood

---

*Available as a dietary supplement.
[1]Not FDA approved for this indication.

Rakel and Bope: *Conn's Current Therapy 2006.*

TABLE 2 Current Treatments of PMS

Treatment	Dose
Chasteberry[1]	4-20 mg daily
Calcium (elemental)[1]	500 mg twice daily
Calcium carbonate (Tums)	
Calcium citrate (Citracal)	
Calcium citrate/malate	
Vitamin D[1]	
Cholecalciferol–D_3	1000-2000 IU daily
Ergocalciferol (Drisdol)–D_2	50,000 IU weekly
Calcium (elemental) and	
vitamin D combined	
Premcal Light	500 mg calcium/500 IU vitamin D_3 twice daily
Regular	500 mg calcium/750 IU vitamin D_3 twice daily
Extra strength	500 mg calcium/1000 IU vitamin D_3 twice daily
Oscal	500 mg calcium/200 IU vitamin D_3 twice daily
Magnesium (elemental)[1]	200-400 mg daily
Magnesium aspartate	
Magnesium oxide (Mag-Ox)	
Antidepressants	
Selective serotonin reuptake inhibitors	
Fluoxetine (Sarafem)	
Escitalopram (Lexapro)[1]	20 mg daily
Sertraline (Zoloft)	10-20 mg daily
Paroxetine (Paxil)[1]	25-100 mg daily
Selective serotonin and norepinephrine reuptake inhibitors	10-30 mg daily
Venlafaxine (Effexor)[1]	75-150 mg daily
Gonadotropin-releasing agonists	
Leuprolide (Lupron depot)[1]	3.75-7.5 mg monthly; 11.25 to 22.5 mg every 3 mo; 30 mg every 4 mo
Goserelin (Zoladex) implant[1]	3.6 mg every 28 d 10.8 mg every 3 mo

[1]Not FDA approved for this indication.

Side effects of the SSRIs may include anxiety, nervousness, insomnia, nausea, tremor, and somnolence.

Gonadotropin-releasing agonists (GnRH agonists) (Lupron, Zoladex) produce hypogonadotropic hypogonadism or a form of medical oophorectomy. These agents are effective, because they obliterate the normal menstrual cycle. Although they reduce PMS symptoms, the hypoestrogenic side effects and potential bone loss are of major concern. Other side effects include hot flashes, emotional lability, and insomnia. These latter drugs should be administered with great caution, and careful monitoring is highly recommended. Of all the potential remedies, GnRH agonists as well as surgical ovariectomy should be considered last. If long-term therapy is required, add-back therapy with hormone replacement is strongly recommended.

Management of Premenstrual Syndrome

It is important to document PMS symptomatology prospectively with a menstrual calendar or symptom diary for at least 2 months, particularly for severe PMS. The initial evaluation of PMS should include instruction on the use of daily diaries, and an exclusion of conditions that may compound or emulate PMS symptomatology, such as thyroid disease and depression. Laboratory evaluation consists of a baseline complete blood count (CBC), chemistries with total serum calcium, and a thyroid function panel. A calcium profile including a serum 25-hydroxyvitamin D, intact parathyroid hormone, and 24-hour urine calcium excretion should be obtained for women with moderate to severe symptoms. The acquisition of a calcium profile and urine calcium can be extremely helpful in the management of these women and often guides therapy. Hypocalciuria, when present, may indicate a malabsorption syndrome such as celiac sprue or lymphoma, and hypercalciuria may indicate that the woman has primary hyperparathyroidism or, more commonly, idiopathic hypercalciuria. Not every woman with PMS requires such an expensive laboratory evaluation. However, one can often readily treat with just the serum 25-hydroxyvitamin vitamin D concentration alone. A realistic approach is to empirically treat the woman following a 25-hydroxyvitamin D level by supplementing the diet with calcium (elemental calcium) at 1000 mg and vitamin D_3-cholecalciferol at 1000 to 2000 IU daily. Vitamin D deficiency has become more commonly recognized as a consequence of dietary deficiency and inadequate production of vitamin D by the skin. Vitamin D at 2000 IU daily in a premenopausal woman is safe. The majority of women with PMS experience a sense of well-being and relief within 1 to 2 months of treatment. For those who do not experience relief, the calcium profile along with serum 25-hydroxyvitamin D (25[OH]D), intact parathyroid hormone and 24-hour urine calcium excretion should be obtained. While a normal 25-hydroxyvitamin D concentration has been of some controversy recently, levels of 25(OH)D at 35 to 40 ng/mL appear adequate and optimal. To correct for inadequate levels of vitamin D, the following

16

symptoms. Scientific evidence on vitamins E*,[1] and B_6*,[1] is very limited. Evening primrose oil,[1] which is a rich source of γ-linolenic acid, had been suggested as a possible treatment, but two well-designed studies did not demonstrate efficacy. In a rigorous, double-blind study, progesterone therapy was not found to be better than placebo and is currently not advocated for PMS.

The antidepressants classified as SSRIs are effective, specifically in severe PMS or premenstrual dysphoric disorder. Fluoxetine (Sarafem), sertraline (Zoloft), paroxetine (Paxil), and fluvoxamine (Luvox) all appear to have similar beneficial effects. These antidepressants are usually administered daily, but intermittent therapy during the luteal phase of the cycle is efficacious.

*Available as a dietary supplement.
[1]Not FDA approved for this indication.

Rakel and Bope: *Conn's Current Therapy 2006.*

replacement regimen may be administered:

- If the 25(OH)D concentration is less than 20 ng/mL, prescribe vitamin D_3–cholecalciferol, 4000 IU daily, or ergocalciferol (Calciferol), 50,000 IU thrice weekly for 1 month. The level of 25(OH)D should be repeated in 1 and 6 months or as necessary with adjustments in dosage to achieve a 25(OH)D level of 35 to 40 ng/mL.
- If the 25(OH)D concentration is more than 21 ng/mL and less than 40 ng/mL, prescribe vitamin D_3–cholecalciferol, 2000 IU daily, or ergocalciferol, 50,000 IU weekly. The level of 25(OH)D should be repeated at 1 and 6 months or as necessary with adjustments in dosage to achieve a 25(OH)D level of 35 to 40 ng/mL.
- If the 25(OH)D concentration is more than 40 ng/ mL and normal, prescribe vitamin D at 1000 IU.
- Note that a daily maintenance dose of vitamin D may vary from 1000 IU to 4000 IU daily to achieve a 25(OH)D level of 35 to 40 ng.

Dietary modifications may be helpful as well, and adding dairy products such as yogurt or milk can reduce the total supplemental calcium while maintaining the total dietary calcium. As an example, one cup of skim milk contains 302 mg of elemental calcium, 1 ounce of Swiss cheese contains 272 mg of elemental calcium, 3 ounces of sardines contains 372 mg of elemental calcium, and 1/2 cup of cooked collards contains 168 mg of calcium. Substituting one daily yogurt and one glass of skim milk for a 500 mg calcium tablet can reduce the number of calcium supplements required while preserving total calcium intake. Increases in both dietary and supplemental calcium may cause an initial exacerbation of PMS physical symptoms, such as menstrual cramps. Women should be alerted to this initial symptom eruption, but comforted that continual treatment usually results in an overwhelming sense of balance and resolution of the majority of their symptoms within 2 to 3 months. Constipation and nausea are very common complaints that women cite with calcium supplementation. The addition of magnesium to the diet often alleviates this complaint, and ingesting the calcium supplements with meals, and not on an empty stomach, usually resolves the nausea.

In conclusion, PMS is a very common disorder among women of reproductive age, with many women experiencing emotional and physical symptoms of varying degrees. When recognized, women should be reassured that there is a probable biochemical reason for their symptoms, that this is not a psychological disorder, and that treatment for PMS is available. Evidence strongly suggests that PMS is a calcium and vitamin D deficiency syndrome. Dietary modifications with increases in total daily calcium intake may be all that is necessary. Adequate calcium and vitamin D supplementation with daily calcium intake at 1000 mg and vitamin D_3 at 1000 to 2000 IU will relieve the majority of symptoms in women with PMS. The remainder should have additional hormonal and biochemical investigations to elucidate the etiology of persistent symptoms. For women who do not adequately respond to adequate calcium and vitamin D replacement therapy, pharmacologic intervention may be required.

Menopause

Method of
Jan L. Shifren, MD, and Isaac Schiff, MD

Menopause, the permanent cessation of menstruation, occurs at a mean age of 51 years. The age at menopause appears to be genetically determined and is unaffected by race, socioeconomic status, age at menarche, or number of prior ovulations. Factors that are toxic to the ovary often result in an earlier age of menopause; women who smoke experience an earlier menopause, as do many women exposed to chemotherapy or pelvic radiation. Despite a great increase in female life expectancy, the age at menopause remains remarkably constant. A woman in the United States today will live approximately 30 years, or greater than a third of her life, beyond the menopause.

Options for caring for menopausal women have increased greatly since estrogen therapy (ET) was first introduced in the 1960s. With respect to hormone use, many choices of hormone type, dose, and method of administration are available. Not only have new forms of estrogens and progestins been introduced, but novel ways of combining the two hormones are available. In addition to hormones, selective estrogen receptor modulators (SERMs) and bisphosphonates are on the market. Women are requesting more information on complementary and alternative therapies, which are being studied more carefully.

Health Concerns After Menopause and Treatment Options

VASOMOTOR SYMPTOMS

Diagnosis

Vasomotor symptoms affect up to 75% of perimenopausal women. They last for 1 to 2 years after menopause in the majority of women, but may continue for up to 10 years. Hot flashes are the primary reason women seek care at menopause and request hormone therapy (HT). Hot flashes not only disturb women at work and interrupt daily activities, but they also disrupt sleep. Many women complain of difficulty concentrating and emotional lability during the menopausal transition. Treatment of vasomotor symptoms should improve these cognitive and mood symptoms if they are secondary to sleep disruption and resulting daytime fatigue. The incidence of thyroid disease increases as women age, so thyroid function tests should be ordered if vasomotor symptoms are atypical or resistant to therapy.

Treatment

Systemic ET is the most effective treatment available for vasomotor symptoms and associated sleep disturbance. Vasomotor symptoms appear to be the result of estrogen withdrawal, rather than simply low estrogen levels.

Abruptly stopping hormone treatment may result in a return of disruptive vasomotor symptoms. Thus, if cessation of HT is desired, the dose should be reduced slowly over several months. This recommendation is based on clinical experience because few controlled trials have examined the optimal way to cease HT use. When a woman chooses not to take estrogen or when it is contraindicated, progestin therapy alone is an option. Medroxyprogesterone acetate (Provera) and megestrol acetate (Megace) effectively treat vasomotor symptoms. Several drugs that alter central neurotransmitter pathways also are effective (Table 1). Clonidine (Catapres) may be used orally or as a weekly transdermal patch. Potential side effects include orthostatic hypotension and drowsiness.

Interestingly, selective serotonin reuptake inhibitors (SSRIs) and other antidepressants also are effective. Menopausal women experienced significant reductions in both hot flash frequency and severity in double-blind, randomized, placebo-controlled trials of paroxetine (Paxil CR) (12.5 and 25 mg per day), fluoxetine (Prozac) (20 mg per day), and venlafaxine (Effexor) (75 mg per day). The improvement in vasomotor symptoms was independent of any significant change in mood symptoms. Possible side effects include fatigue, dry mouth, nausea, and decreased libido.

Many menopausal women are interested in trying nutritional and vitamin supplements for relief of hot flashes. Many of these therapies claim to relieve hot flashes, but they are rarely studied in controlled trials. Options include dietary soy and related compounds, vitamin E (800 IU per day), black cohosh, evening primrose oil, and others. Uncontrolled studies of acupuncture, exercise, and paced respiration demonstrate an improvement in vasomotor symptoms. Lifestyle interventions, including wearing light, layered clothing, avoiding hot beverages, and the liberal use of desk fans and air conditioners, should be encouraged.

UROGENITAL ATROPHY

Diagnosis

Urogenital atrophy results in vaginal dryness and pruritus, dyspareunia, dysuria, and urinary urgency.

These are common complaints of menopausal women that respond well to therapy.

Treatment

Systemic ET is very effective for the relief of vaginal dryness, dyspareunia, and urinary symptoms. Another option for women who should not or choose not to use standard ET is topical application. Low doses of estrogen cream (Estrace, Premarin) are effective when used only one to three times weekly. An estradiol vaginal tablet (Vagifem), inserted twice weekly, is available, as is an estrogen-containing vaginal ring (Estring) placed in the vagina every 3 months. Lubricants are a nonhormonal alternative for reducing discomfort with intercourse when urogenital atrophy is present.

OSTEOPOROSIS

Diagnosis

Osteoporosis affects approximately 8 million women in the United States, with an additional 15 million women at risk for the disease. Because therapy is most likely to benefit those at highest risk, it is important to review a woman's risk factors for osteoporosis when making treatment decisions and to consider bone mineral density screening for high-risk women. Nonmodifiable risk factors include age, Asian or white race, family history, small body frame, early menopause, and prior oophorectomy. Modifiable risk factors include decreased intake of calcium and vitamin D, smoking, low body weight, excess alcohol use, and a sedentary lifestyle. Medical conditions associated with an increased risk of osteoporosis include hyperthyroidism, hyperparathyroidism, chronic renal disease, and diseases requiring systemic corticosteroid use.

Treatment

Counseling women to alter modifiable risk factors is important for both the prevention and treatment of osteoporosis. Many women have diets deficient in calcium and vitamin D and benefit from dietary changes and supplementation. Reducing the risk of osteoporosis is another of the many health benefits of smoking cessation and regular exercise. HT is very effective at both preventing and treating osteoporosis. The Women's Health Initiative (WHI) randomized controlled trial confirmed a significant 34% reduction in hip fractures in healthy women receiving HT after a mean follow-up of 5 years.

Bisphosphonates, including alendronate (Fosamax), risedronate (Actonel), and ibandronate (Boniva) specifically inhibit bone resorption and are very effective for both osteoporosis prevention and treatment. Selective estrogen receptor modulators (SERMs) are compounds that act as both estrogen agonists and antagonists, depending on the tissue. Raloxifene (Evista) is a SERM approved for both the prevention and treatment of osteoporosis. Raloxifene has estrogen-like actions on bone and lipids, without stimulating the breast

TABLE 1 Alternative Treatments for Hot Flashes

Drug*	Suggested Dose
Venlafaxine (Effexor)	37.5-75 mg XR/day
Fluoxetine (Prozac)	20 mg/day
Paroxetine (Paxil)	10-20 mg/day or 12.5-25 mg CR/day
Clonidine (Catapres)	0.1 mg/week patch
Gabapentin (Neurontin)	300-900 mg/day

*None of these medications is FDA approved for the treatment of hot flashes.
Abbreviations: CR = controlled release; XR = extended release.

or endometrium. Calcitonin nasal spray (Miacalcin) and parathyroid hormone injections (Forteo) are other therapies for osteoporosis.

CARDIOVASCULAR DISEASE

Diagnosis

Cardiovascular disease is the leading cause of death for women, accounting for approximately 45% of mortality. Nonmodifiable risk factors include age and family history. Modifiable risk factors include smoking, obesity, and a sedentary lifestyle. Medical conditions associated with an increased risk of heart disease include diabetes, hypertension, and hypercholesterolemia.

Treatment

Advising women to alter modifiable risk factors and adequately treating diabetes, hypertension, and hypercholesterolemia are important measures in reducing the risk of heart disease. In the past, prevention of heart disease was considered a potential benefit of HT use. Epidemiologic studies report an approximately 50% decrease in heart disease in women who use HT. Observational studies are prone to bias, however, and women who choose to use hormones are generally at lower risk for heart disease than those who do not.

However, the Women's Health Initiative (WHI) randomized controlled trial of combination HT versus placebo showed that not only does HT not prevent heart disease in healthy women, it actually increases its risk slightly (Table 2). This trial enrolled approximately 16,000 women nationwide between the ages of 50 and 79 years. The average age of women in the study was 63 years. The trial's major goal was to determine

---

TABLE 2 WHI & WHIMS Results: Risks per 10,000 Person-Years Attributable to Estrogen Plus Progestin

Excess Risk

Coronary heart disease	+7
Stroke	+8
Pulmonary embolism	+8
Invasive breast cancer	+8
Dementia*	+23

Reduced Risk

Colorectal cancer	−6
Hip fracture	−5

*Dementia was assessed in a subset of women from the WHI trial, ages 65 years or older. Increased risk of dementia was statistically significant when data from both estrogen plus progestin and estrogen alone trials were pooled.
Abbreviations: WHI = Women's Health Initiative; WHIMS = Women's Health Initiative Memory Study.
Adapted from: Writing Group for the Women's Health Initiative Investigators: Risks and benefits of estrogen plus progestin in healthy postmenopausal women: Principal results from the Women's Health Initiative randomized, controlled trial. JAMA 288:321-333, 2002.
Shumaker S, Legault C, Rapp S, et al: Estrogen plus progestin and the incidence of dementia and mild cognitive impairment in postmenopausal women. JAMA 289:2651-2662, 2003.

---

whether combined estrogen and progestin HT (Prempro) prevent heart disease and fractures, and whether there are associated risks. After an average of 5 years of follow-up, heart disease and stroke increased significantly in HT users by 29% and 41%, respectively. Venous thromboembolic events (VTEs) increased twofold.

Approximately 11,000 women without a uterus participated in a separate WHI study and were randomized either to estrogen alone (Premarin) or placebo. After an average follow-up of 7 years, no increased risk of heart disease was found in estrogen users. Estrogen use did have adverse vascular effects, though, increasing the risk of stroke by 39% and VTEs by 33%.

There is no role for ET in the prevention of coronary heart disease (CHD), not only in healthy women but also in women with established heart disease. The Heart and Estrogen-Progestin Replacement Study (HERS), a randomized placebo-controlled trial of HT (Prempro) for secondary prevention of heart disease, also did not demonstrate any reduction in CHD events overall. The risk of cardiovascular events actually was greater in HT users during the first year of treatment.

Of note, the WHI trials and the HERS study examined only treatment with conjugated equine estrogens and medroxyprogesterone acetate. In addition, the majority of women in the trial initiated HT many years after the menopausal transition. The outcomes after initiating HT with the onset of menopausal symptoms and the effects of other oral estrogens, transdermal estradiol, cyclic HT, or therapy with other progestins may be different. Without data from randomized controlled trials, the conservative approach is to assume that the risks of various HT regimens in menopausal women are similar.

Raloxifene (Evista) has several beneficial effects on lipids, but whether these effects translate into a reduced incidence of heart disease is currently being studied. Interestingly, in a secondary analysis of results from a randomized controlled trial of raloxifene (Evista) versus placebo in more than 7000 women with osteoporosis, no significant differences were found between groups in coronary and cerebrovascular events. Among a subset of approximately 1000 women with increased cardiovascular risk at baseline, the women who received raloxifene experienced a significant 40% reduction in cardiovascular events.

BREAST CANCER

Diagnosis

Breast cancer is the most common cancer in women and the second leading cause of cancer death. The lifetime risk of developing invasive breast cancer is 12%, so any therapies that reduce or increase this risk have a major impact on women's health. Risk factors for breast cancer include age, early menarche, late menopause, family history, and prior breast disease, including epithelial atypia and cancer. Oophorectomy and a term pregnancy before the age of 30 years are associated with reduced risk. Many of these risk factors are consistent with the hypothesis that prolonged estrogen exposure increases the risk of breast cancer.

Long-term use of HT is associated with an increased risk of breast cancer. Observational studies demonstrate a relative risk of approximately 1.3 with long-term HT use, generally defined as greater than 5 years. The WHI HT trial found a significant 26% increase in the risk of invasive breast cancer in women assigned to HT after approximately 5 years of use. Interestingly, the WHI trial of estrogen alone in women with prior hysterectomy demonstrated no increased risk of breast cancer after an average of 7 years of estrogen use.

The SERM tamoxifen (Nolvadex) is an estrogen antagonist in the breast, used in the treatment of estrogen receptor–positive breast cancer. Tamoxifen is also approved for the prevention of breast cancer in high-risk women, resulting in an approximately 50% reduction in the risk of disease. Raloxifene (Evista) also may reduce the risk of breast cancer, although it is not approved for this indication. Postmenopausal women receiving raloxifene as part of a large osteoporosis treatment trial experienced a 76% reduction in the risk of invasive breast cancer compared to placebo-treated women.

Risks are associated with SERM use. Tamoxifen and raloxifene increase the risk of VTEs approximately threefold, similar to the increased risk seen in HT users. Hot flashes are increased with raloxifene and tamoxifen use, and raloxifene is associated with leg cramps. Tamoxifen acts as an estrogen agonist in the endometrium, increasing the risk of endometrial polyps, hyperplasia, and cancer, whereas no endometrial stimulation is seen with raloxifene.

Treatment

Screening mammography annually for women over the age of 50 years is demonstrated to reduce breast cancer mortality in several large studies. Women at increased risk for breast cancer are advised not to use HT or to use it only short term. Women at high risk also may elect tamoxifen therapy.

ENDOMETRIAL CANCER

The use of unopposed estrogen is associated with an increased risk of endometrial hyperplasia and cancer. Combination estrogen-progestin therapy, therefore, is recommended for all women with a uterus. Treatment may be provided in a sequential manner, with estrogen daily and progestin for 12 to 14 days of each month or in a continuous-combined fashion with estrogen and a lower dose of progestin daily. Sequential regimens result in regular, predictable vaginal bleeding. The benefit of continuous-combined regimens is that approximately 60% to 70% of women experience amenorrhea by the end of the first year of therapy; the problem is that the bleeding that does occur is irregular and unpredictable. Several combination therapies may have a lower incidence of bleeding, including norethindrone acetate (NETA), with either ethinyl estradiol (Femhrt) or estradiol (Activella), or low-dose conjugated equine estrogens and MPA (medroxyprogesterone acetate) (Prempro 0.45/1.5 or 0.3/1.5).

Rakel and Bope: *Conn's Current Therapy 2006.*

ALZHEIMER'S DISEASE

Alzheimer's disease is the most common form of dementia. Women are at greater risk for developing the disease than men, and the number of affected Americans is expected to double to more than 8 million by 2010. Several small trials and observational studies, often of women who initiated HT early with the onset of menopausal symptoms, suggest HT use may decrease the risk of Alzheimer's disease. A randomized controlled study in women with mild to moderate Alzheimer's disease, however, demonstrated that 1 year of estrogen treatment did not slow disease progression or improve cognition. The effect of HT on cognitive function in women without dementia was studied in the WHI Memory Study (WHIMS), a randomized, double-blind, placebo-controlled trial of women aged 65 years of age or older enrolled in the WHI trial. In contrast to the findings of observational studies, women randomized to HT in WHIMS experienced a significant twofold increased risk of dementia.

Contraindications to HT use include known or suspected breast or endometrial cancer, undiagnosed abnormal genital bleeding, active thromboembolic disorders, and active liver or gallbladder disease. Relative contraindications include heart disease, migraine headaches, a history of liver or gallbladder disease, previous breast or endometrial cancer, or prior thromboembolic events.

Many options are available to address the quality of life and health concerns of menopausal women. The primary indication for HT currently is the alleviation of hot flashes and associated symptoms. Given the risks of HT, women should be advised to use the lowest dose for the shortest time that meets treatment goals. Women need to be informed of the potential benefits and risks of all therapeutic options, and care should be individualized based on a woman's needs and preferences.

  CURRENT DIAGNOSIS

Risk Factors for Osteoporosis
Nonmodifiable
- Age
- Race (white, Asian)
- Small body frame
- Early menopause
- Prior fracture
- Family history of osteoporosis

Modifiable
- Inadequate intake of calcium and vitamin D
- Smoking
- Low body weight
- Excess alcohol use
- Sedentary lifestyle

Associated Medical Conditions
- Hyperthyroidism
- Hyperparathyroidism
- Chronic renal disease
- Conditions requiring systemic corticosteroid use

CURRENT THERAPY

Treatment options for urogenital atrophy are:

- Systemic hormone therapy (if vasomotor symptoms also present)
- Vaginal estrogen cream (Estrace, Premarin): 0.5 to 1 g two to three times weekly
- Vaginal estradiol tablet (Vagifem): 1 tablet two times weekly
- Vaginal estradiol ring (Estring): 1 ring every 3 months
- Vaginal lubricants (e.g., Replens, KY Jelly): prior to intercourse as needed for dyspareunia

REFERENCES

American College of Obstetricians and Gynecologists Task Force: Hormone therapy. Obstet Gynecol 2004;104(Suppl 4):S1-S129.

Cummings S, Black D, Thompson D, et al: Effect of alendronate on risk of fracture in women with low bone density but without vertebral fractures. JAMA 1998;280:2077-2082, 2119.

Cummings S, Eckert S, Krueger K, et al: The effect of raloxifene on risk of breast cancer in postmenopausal women: Results from the MORE randomized trial. JAMA 1999;281:2189-2197.

Fisher B, Costantino JP, Wickerham DL, et al: Tamoxifen for prevention of breast cancer: Report of the national surgical adjuvant breast and bowel project P-1 study. J Natl Cancer Inst 1998; 90:1371-1388.

Laumann E, Paik A, Rosen R: Sexual dysfunction in the United States: Prevalence and predictors. JAMA 1999;281:537-544.

Shifren J, Braunstein G, Simon J, et al: Transdermal testosterone treatment in women with impaired sexual function after oophorectomy. N Engl J Med 2000;343:682-688.

Shumaker S, Legault C, Kuller L, et al: Conjugated equine estrogens and incidence of probable dementia and mild cognitive impairment in postmenopausal women: Women's Health Initiative Memory Study. JAMA 2004;291:2947-2958.

Stearns V, Beebe K, Iyengar M, Dube E: Paroxetine controlled release in the treatment of menopausal hot flashes. JAMA 2003;289: 2827-2834.

Women's Health Initiative Steering Committee: Effects of conjugated equine estrogen in postmenopausal women with hysterectomy. JAMA 2004;291:1701-1712.

Writing Group for the Women's Health Initiative Investigators: Risks and benefits of estrogen plus progestin in healthy postmenopausal women: Principal results from the Women's Health Initiative randomized controlled trial. JAMA 2002;288:321-333.

Vulvovaginitis

Method of
David A. Baker, MD

Vulvovaginitis brings large numbers of women to see their health care provider. Over the last several decades with the availability of numerous over-the-counter preparations, most patients medicate themselves to treat their symptoms. However, it is clear that the majority of patients make the wrong diagnosis. They use the wrong medications and delay bringing their symptoms and complaints to the attention of the clinician; as a result, many women will experience complications from their vaginal infection. Therefore, the clinician needs to take this condition (vulvovaginitis) seriously and view the patient as one with a significant medical, physiologic, and social problem that may lead not only to significant medical conditions and complications but also to significant interpersonal problems.

An accurate diagnosis is required to provide proper and correct treatment of this condition. Symptoms presented to the health care provider by phone can be very nonspecific and may lead to an improper diagnosis and treatment. The three major categories of vaginitis in the United States (Figure 1) are those caused predominately by candidiasis, trichomoniasis, and bacterial vaginosis (BV). Of these three abnormal symptomatic manifestations, BV is the most common in the United States. Many patients mistake BV for *Candida* infections and take over-the-counter antifungal preparations, which are costly and ineffective. Patients do not appreciate the significance of this most common condition: BV may lead to important medical complications not only during pregnancy but also when the patient is not pregnant. Of the three conditions, the only one that is considered a sexually transmitted disease (STD) is trichomoniasis. BV is associated with other STDs.

The goal of therapy is to not only treat or control the organism that is abnormally colonizing or growing in the vagina but also return the vagina to normal vaginal colonization. This objective may be difficult, and one of the major problems of recurrent vaginal infection is our inability to colonize the lower genital tract with healthy bacteria. The normal vagina has an acidic pH that is produced by a combination of normal host flora and the genus *Lactobacillus*, which produces lactic acid. The importance of *Lactobacillus* strains that produce not only lactic acid but also hydrogen peroxide cannot be overemphasized; they maintain the lower genital tract flora and act as a protective barrier to the acquisition of certain STDs, including HIV. It is therefore the goal of the treating clinician to eradicate the patient's symptoms, control the abnormal vaginal colonization, and try to propagate normal lower genital tract flora. Women with normal lower genital tract flora containing lactobacilli producing lactic acid and hydrogen peroxide were less likely to contract chlamydiosis, trichomoniasis, and symptomatic candidiasis. In addition, the prevalence of gonorrhea, chlamydiosis, and trichomoniasis was significantly lower in women who had normal vaginal *Lactobacillus* flora during pregnancy.

Bacterial Vaginosis

The term given to abnormal colonization of the lower genital tract with anaerobic bacteria is bacterial vaginosis. However, a more meaningful definition of BV may be one that includes an inflammatory component of this anaerobic bacterial overgrowth. Currently, approximately 50% of women in the United States who visit a clinician for treatment of vaginitis have BV. It is a polymicrobial infection involving an increase in anaerobic

Obstetrics and Gynecology

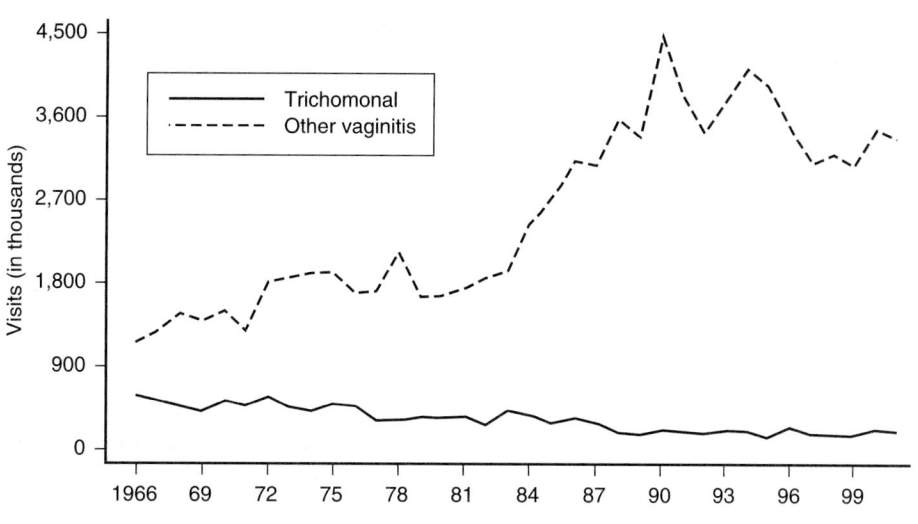

FIGURE 1. Major categories of vaginitis are candidiasis, trichomoniasis, and bacterial vaginosis.

bacteria, loss of the normal *Lactobacillus* flora, and consequently, an imbalance in the vaginal ecosystem. The absence or a decreased number of lactobacilli facilitates the overgrowth of pathogenic organism, which are predominately anaerobic bacteria.

The exact factors that trigger the overgrowth of anaerobic bacteria are still not fully understood. Douching can lead to a disturbance in the delicate balance of lower genital tract organisms. Other risk factors for BV include trichomoniasis, other STDs, early sexual experience, multiple sexual partners, and the use of an intrauterine contraceptive device.

DIAGNOSIS

Proper diagnosis is important for the treatment and eradication of BV. The diagnosis can be made during vaginal examination and does not require expensive and elaborate techniques. The current 2002 Centers for Disease Control and Prevention (CDC) STD treatment guidelines require three of the following symptoms or signs for diagnosis: a homogeneous, white, noninflammatory discharge that coats the vaginal walls smoothly; the presence of clue cells on microscopic examination; a pH of vaginal secretions of less than 4.5; and a fishy odor of the vaginal discharge before or after the addition of 10% KOH (the whiff test). Gram stain is an acceptable laboratory method for diagnosing BV. However, culture is not recommended as a diagnostic tool. In addition, cervical Papanicolaou (Pap) tests have limited clinical utility for the diagnosis of BV because of low sensitivity. Other commercially available tests add to the cost and rarely aid the clinician in diagnosing this vaginal infection.

TREATMENT

The goal of therapy is to not only control this anaerobic infection but also relieve vaginal symptoms, lessen the risk of infectious complications after procedures, and

reduce the risk of development of other infectious complications, HIV, and other STDs. All women who have symptomatic disease require treatment. Because of the increased risk of postoperative infectious complications associated with BV, it is suggested that before surgical procedures are performed on women, they be screened and treated for BV, in addition to undergoing other routine prophylactic measures.

BV during pregnancy has been associated with adverse pregnancy outcomes, including preterm labor, premature rupture of membranes, and postpartum infections. Therapy during pregnancy has the potential of reducing these potential risks, as well as reducing the risk of acquiring STDs and HIV during pregnancy. The CDC has given recommendations for the treatment of nonpregnant and pregnant women with BV (Table 1). Patients need to be informed that clindamycin (Cleocin) cream and ovules are oil-based preparations that may interfere with the efficiency of latex condoms and diaphragms. In addition, oral and topical metronidazole (Flagyl) regimens are equally efficacious. Studies of vaginal clindamycin cream appear to demonstrate that it is less efficacious than metronidazole regimens. Short-course therapy for BV in the form of metronidazole, 2 g orally in a single dose, has been proposed. The clinician must recognize that metronidazole, 2 g in a single dose, is an alternative regimen because of its lower efficacy in the treatment of BV. Unfortunately, at the current time, no preparation, either intravaginal or oral, is able to induce reversion to the normal lower genital tract vaginal flora.

BV is not considered an STD, and therefore routine treatment of sex partners is not currently recommended. When using clindamycin and metronidazole, one must differentiate between side effects and allergic reactions. Metronidazole gel (MetroGel) may be appropriate for patients who have side effects with oral metronidazole, but it should not be used in a patient allergic to metronidazole.

Rakel and Bope: *Conn's Current Therapy 2006.*

16

TABLE 1 Bacterial Vaginosis: Treatment Regimens

Recommended Regimens, Nonpregnant

Metronidazole (Flagyl), 500 mg orally twice a day for 7 d
or
Metronidazole (Metro-Gel), 0.75% gel, 1 full applicator (5 g) intravaginally once a day for 5 d
or
Clindamycin (Cleocin), 2% cream, 1 full applicator (5 g) intravaginally at bedtime for 7 d

Alternative Regimens, Nonpregnant

Metronidazole, 2 g orally in a single dose
or
Clindamycin, 300 mg orally twice a day for 7 d
or
Clindamycin ovules, 100 g intravaginally once at bedtime for 3 d

Recommended Regimens, Pregnant

Metronidazole, 250 mg orally three times a day for 7 d
or
Clindamycin, 300 mg orally twice a day for 7 d

Note: Patients should be advised to avoid consuming alcohol during treatment with metronidazole and for 24 hours thereafter. Clindamycin cream and ovules are oil based and might weaken latex condoms and diaphragms: Refer to condom product labeling for additional information.
From Centers for Disease Control and Prevention: Sexually transmitted diseases treatment guidelines 2002. MMWR Morb Mortal Wkly Rep 2002;51:42-48.

Oral regimens are recommended (see Table 1) for pregnant women. Topical clindamycin (Cleocin vaginal cream) is contraindicated in pregnancy because of the potential overgrowth of gram-negative aerobic bacteria (*Escherichia coli*) in the vagina. Patients who have BV should be offered testing for HIV and other STDs. Patients with HIV should be screened and treated for BV with the same regimens as those who are HIV negative.

Trichomoniasis

The incidence of trichomoniasis has slowly declined in the United States since the mid 1960s and has remained at a low level over the past decade. Trichomoniasis is caused by the protozoan *Trichomonas vaginalis*. Women who are infected usually have a vaginal discharge and specific symptoms, in contrast to men, who are generally asymptomatic. *T. vaginalis* is a pear-shaped flagellated protozoon that is usually identified in wet mounts by a rapid swaying motion and the presence of polymorphonuclear leukocytes. Growth is typically enhanced by anaerobic conditions and an elevated pH. The incubation period ranges from 4 to 28 days. The clinician needs to recognize that infection with this organism occurs not only in the vagina but also in the urethra, Skene's glands, and the bladder. In men, the urethra is the most common site. However, the prostate and epididymis may also be infected, and the organism may be detected in semen and urine. Trichomoniasis is an STD transmitted through sexual contact, with infection documented

in 85% of female partners of infected men. Risk factors for trichomoniasis are the presence of other STDS, an increased number of sexual partners, the presence of BV, smoking, and a vaginal pH over 4.5.

DIAGNOSIS

The patient usually has a discharge, odor, and vulvar itching with or without dysuria. The discharge is yellow-green with a frothy appearance. Further evaluation of the patient reveals that the pH of the vagina is over 4.5, the amine test may be positive, and on wet preparations, the organism and an increase in the white blood cell count (greater than 10 per high-power field) are usually found. Wet preparations and Pap smears have an approximately 50% to 60% sensitivity and greater than 90% specificity. Other techniques are in development that should better enable the clinician to diagnose this infection. Trichomoniasis in pregnant women has been associated with adverse pregnancy outcomes, specifically, preterm rupture of membranes, preterm labor, and preterm delivery. In addition, studies have shown that the presence of trichomoniasis is associated with an increased risk of acquiring HIV, so patients in whom trichomoniasis has been diagnosed should be screened for other STDs, and HIV testing should be encouraged.

TREATMENT

Current CDC treatment guidelines are presented in Table 2. The metronidazole regimen recommended has resulted in cure rates of approximately 90% to 95%. Because trichomoniasis is an STD, treatment of sexual partners is mandatory. Metronidazole gel has an efficacy of approximately 50% for the treatment of trichomoniasis. Because the organism may be found in locations other than the vagina, such treatment is less efficacious and not recommended. Women who fail oral therapy may repeat a 7-day course of therapy with topical metronidazole. Because metronidazole is currently the only approved therapy in the United States, patients with allergic reactions to metronidazole may be managed by desensitization. Tinidazole has been recently approved for the treatment of vaginal trichimoniasis. This newer medication may be of assistance in patients with the emerging problem of metronidazole-resistant trichomoniasis.

TABLE 2 Trichomoniasis: Treatment Regimens

Recommended Regimen

Metronidazole (Flagyl), 2 g orally in a single dose

Alternative Regimen

Metronidazole, 500 mg twice a day for 7 d

From Centers for Disease Control and Prevention: Sexually transmitted diseases treatment guidelines 2002. MMWR Morb Mortal Wkly Rep 2002;51:42-48.

Candidiasis

Most patients think that their symptoms are associated with a yeast infection, but in reality, studies show that 75% of patients with chronic candidiasis have another etiologic agent responsible for their problems. However, candidiasis is still one of the most common vaginal infections and is usually treated initially with over-the-counter or alternative regimens. Patients who cannot control the infection or experience recurrent symptoms generally seek medical assistance. The CDC has classified vulvovaginal candidiasis (VVC) as uncomplicated VVC or complicated VVC (Table 3). This classification is based on clinical findings, microbiology, host factors, and response to therapy. Approximately 10% to 20% of women will have complicated VVC.

DIAGNOSIS AND TREATMENT

Pruritus and an inflammatory reaction suggest the diagnosis of candidal vaginitis. A white, cheesy discharge is usually what drives the patient to buy an over-the-counter antifungal preparation. The clinician needs to use additional modalities for diagnosis, including a wet preparation with 10% KOH, Gram stain or culture, and determination of vaginal pH (less than 4.5). Because a significant number of women are colonized with *Candida*, culture in the absence of symptoms is not clinically relevant. Most patients with uncomplicated VVC have no precipitating factor; however, VVC commonly develops after antibiotic use. The CDC has recommended numerous regimens (Table 4) for the treatment of uncomplicated VVC, including 14 topical regimens and 1 single-dose oral regimen. VVC is not acquired through sexual activity, and therefore treatment of the partner is not usually recommended.

Complicated VVC is usually defined as four or more episodes of symptomatic VVC each year and should occur in only a small percentage of women. Most patients with recurrent VVC have no apparent predisposing or underlying conditions. Culture may be important in

TABLE 3 Classification of Vulvovaginal Candidiasis (VVC)

Uncomplicated	Complicated
Sporadic or infrequent VVC *or*	Recurrent VVC *or*
Mild-to-moderate VVC *or*	Severe VVC *or*
Likely to be *Candida albicans* *or*	Non-*albicans* candidiasis *or*
Nonimmunocompromised women	Women with uncontrolled diabetes, debilitation, or immunosuppression or those who are pregnant

From Centers for Disease Control and Prevention: Sexually transmitted diseases treatment guidelines 2002. MMWR Morb Mortal Wkly Rep 2002;51:42-48.

TABLE 4 Vulvovaginal Candidiasis: Recommended Treatment Regimens

Intravaginal Agents

Butoconazole (Mycelex), 2% cream, 5 g intravaginally for 3 d*
or
Butoconazole 2% cream, 5 g (butoconazole—sustained release), single intravaginal application
or
Clotrimazole (Gyne-Lotrimin), 1% cream, 5 g intravaginally for 7-14 d*
or
Clotrimazole, 100-mg vaginal tablet for 7 d
or
Clotrimazole, 100-mg vaginal tablet, 2 tablets for 3 d
or
Clotrimazole, 500-mg vaginal tablet, 1 tablet in a single application
or
Miconazole (Monistat), 2% cream, 5 g intravaginally for 7 d*
or
Miconazole, 100-mg vaginal suppository, 1 suppository for 7 d*
or
Miconazole, 200-mg vaginal suppository, 1 suppository for 3 d*
or
Nystatin, 100,000-U vaginal tablet , 1 tablet for 14 d *or*
Tioconazole (Vagistat), 6.5% ointment, 5 g intravaginally in a single application*
or
Terconazole (Terazol), 0.4% cream, 5 g intravaginally for 7 d
or
Terconazole, 0.8% cream, 5 g intravaginally for 3 d
or
Terconazole, 80-mg vaginal suppository, 1 suppository for 3 d

Oral Agent

Fluconazole (Diflucan), 150-mg oral tablet, 1 tablet in a single dose

Note: The creams and suppositories in these regimens are oil based and may weaken latex condoms and diaphragms. Refer to condom product labeling for further information.
*Preparations for intravaginal administration of butoconazole , clotrimazole, miconazole, and tioconazole are available over the counter (OTC). Self-medication with OTC preparations should be advised only for women in whom VVC has previously been diagnosed and who have a recurrence of the same symptoms. Any woman whose symptoms persist after using an OTC preparation or who has a recurrence of symptoms within 2 months should seek medical care. Unnecessary or inappropriate use of OTC preparations is common and can lead to a delay in treatment of other etiologies of vulvovaginitis that could result in adverse clinical outcomes.
From Centers for Disease Control and Prevention: Sexually transmitted disease treatment guidelines 2002. MMWR Morb Mortal Wkly Rep 2002;51:42-48.

16

determining the appropriate treatment and management of these patients. Non-*albicans* species of *Candida* are found in only 10% to 20% of patients with recurrent VVC. Different therapeutic regimens for a longer duration may be of benefit in treating recurrent VVC. The use of antifungals for maintenance therapy or in specific daily or weekly recommended regimens can be considered for up to 6 months. However, side effects and the toxicity of oral medications need to be taken into account. Once maintenance therapy is discontinued, VVC will recur in upward of 40% of women.

Nonfluconazole azole drugs are recommended as first-line therapy for non-*albicans* VVC. In this specific clinical situation, 600 mg of boric acid* by capsule intravaginally once daily for 2 weeks may be beneficial.

Specific investigation to evaluate for pregnancy, HIV infection, and systemic immunocompromising conditions such as diabetes is important in managing vulvovaginitis.

---

*Not available in the United States. May be compounded by pharmacists.

REFERENCES

Sobel JD, Nyirjesy P, Brown W: Tinidazole therapy for metronidazole-resistant vaginal trichomoniasis. Clin Infect Dis 33(8):1341-1346, 2001.

Chlamydia Trachomatis

Method of
Catherine Stevens-Simon, MD

The Scope of The Problem

Responsible for more than 3 million infections each year in the United States, *Chlamydia trachomatis* poses a public health problem of epidemic proportions. Because of the large reservoir of undiagnosed, asymptomatic infections, the number of reported cases significantly underestimates the true prevalence of this infection. Nonetheless, *C. trachomatis* is not only the most commonly reported bacterial sexually transmitted disease (STD) in the United States but also the nation's most commonly reported bacterial infection. It is difficult to give meaningful prevalence figures because the proportion of infected individuals depends on the characteristics of the population studied and how they are studied. In addition, whereas passive surveillance systems indicate that the prevalence of this infection has risen precipitously over the last decade, studies conducted at sentinel surveillance sites demonstrate a decline, which suggests that expanded screening, increased reporting, and improved test sensitivity mask a true decrease in prevalence in some sectors of American society. The epidemiologic characteristics and clinical manifestations of chlamydial infections in the United States reflect the fact that most infections are sexually transmitted and that prevalent stereotypes have an affinity for columnar epithelium. Teenage girls are most susceptible to these infections because of the following factors:

- At their age, the columnar epithelium is prominent on the ectocervix.
- Some experience a high level of unprotected, serially monogamous sexual activity with older men whose sexual risk profiles they rarely investigate.

With these two factors combined, teenage girls are at maximal biologic and social risk. Although the national prevalence of chlamydial infections in this population is unknown, school- and clinic-based studies suggest a range of 8% to 26% (compared to 3% to 5% in sociodemographically similar young adult women), with the highest age-specific prevalence reported among adolescents ages 14 to 15 years. Although readily eradicable, the economic and human costs of these infections are staggering. Annual expenditures are estimated to exceed $1.5 billion, with 75% of the cost devoted to treating sequelae of cervical infections that were initially uncomplicated. Because the majority of severe consequences of untreated infections occur in women, and as much as 66.6% of tubal factor infertility and 33.3% of ectopic pregnancies in the United States are attributed to chlamydial infections, it is estimated that every dollar spent on screening and treating asymptomatic young women and their sex partners saves approximately $12. Although this uniquely positions primary health care providers to prevent the costly sequelae of chlamydial infections, given their prevalence among teenagers, expansion of screening and treatment programs to nontraditional settings such as schools, juvenile detention centers, and drug treatment facilities is likely to be a critical component of any national strategy to control this infection.

Clinical Presentation

Chlamydial infections are an excellent example of the dependence of the clinical manifestations of disease on the intrinsic properties of the pathogen and host. In Western industrialized countries, virtually all chlamydial infections are either sexually transmitted or vertically transmitted at birth. They are caused by nonlymphogranuloma venereum stereotypes that have an affinity for columnar epithelium and can only survive by a cytotoxic, replicative cycle that evokes a variable immune response in the host. Hence, in the United States, the endocervix, urethra, rectum, and conjunctiva are preferentially affected, and clinical manifestations range from asymptomatic to florid inflammatory conditions with severe reproductive consequences. Chlamydia should be suspected in these populations:

- Women and men with dysuria and pyuria
- Women with dyspareunia; abnormal vaginal discharge; postcoital, irregular menstrual, or breakthrough contraceptive bleeding; and lower abdominal or pelvic pain
- Infants with conjunctivitis or a staccato cough

These signs and symptoms are neither a sensitive nor a specific indication of infection, however. Indeed, because nearly 90% of chlamydial infections are asymptomatic and *C. trachomatis* is isolated from less than 33.3% of women with mucopurulent cervicitis and less than 50% of men with nongonococcal urethritis, such complaints are unreliable predictors of infection. In women, the most common sign is mucopurulent cervicitis, a nonspecific clinical syndrome characterized by erythema, edema, and friability of the ectocervix and purulent endocervical exudate. Mucopurulent cervicitis, however, is also caused by other STDs and noninfectious factors (i.e., cyclical fluctuations in gonadal hormones), which increase the size of the cervical ectropion or the resident population of cervical leukocytes. Other clinical manifestations of lower genital tract chlamydial infections in women include urethritis and bartholinitis. Although pelvic inflammatory disease (PID) is a polymicrobial infection, *C. trachomatis* is also often involved, and, conversely, PID is the most common complication of chlamydial cervicitis. The estimated incidence ranges from 10% to 40% in untreated women. Young age and prolonged or recurrent infection significantly increase, whereas treatment of asymptomatic infections significantly decreases both disease severity and sequelae, such as salpingo-oophoritis, perihepatitis (Fitz-Hugh-Curtis syndrome), infertility, ectopic pregnancy, and chronic pelvic pain. Adverse outcomes associated with chlamydial infections during pregnancy include preterm labor, premature rupture of the placental membranes, low-birth-weight delivery, neonatal death, postpartum or postabortal endometritis, and vertical transmission to infants. In the infected infants, 30% to 50% develop conjunctivitis, 15% to 20% develop nasopharyngitis, and 5% to 10% develop pneumonia.

In men, the most common clinical manifestation is urethritis, the symptoms of which typically commence 1 to 3 weeks after exposure and range from mild dysuria to frank penile discharge. Other clinical syndromes in men include epididymitis, prostatitis, acute proctocolitis, and Reiter syndrome (urethritis, conjunctivitis, arthritis, and mucocutaneous lesions). These suppurative complications rarely require inpatient therapy and are far less common than those encountered in women. Nonetheless, sequelae ranging from urethral strictures to infertility do occur. Nongenital clinical manifestations, such as conjunctivitis, tenosynovitis, and arthritis, are uncommon among adults in the United States.

Diagnosis And Screening

In the United States, testing for both symptomatic and asymptomatic chlamydial infections is done with ligase chain reaction (LCR), polymerase chain reaction (PCR), and other nucleic acid amplification techniques (NAATs) because they do not require the presence of intact organisms. Urine, cervical, vaginal, or urethral fluids can be used as the analyte for these tests; specimens are stable and easy to transport; and results can be obtained within a day. This is a major advantage over the stringent collection, transport, and 3-day growth period culturing requirements associated with this fastidious organism. Although nonculture assays, non-NAATs, and rapid diagnostic tests capable of making a diagnosis within 30 minutes are available, these assays are too insensitive to be recommended for routine testing.

The signs and symptoms of chlamydial infection are nonspecific and often persist for weeks after documented eradication of the pathogen. Because of this, leukocyte, esterase-positive urine dipsticks, leukocyte-laden vaginal wet mounts, and endocervical Gram stains should

be regarded as no more than a trigger for testing. Although concerns about the consequences of underdiagnosis and undertreatment typically overshadow concerns about the consequences of overdiagnosis and overtreatment, therapeutic decisions should not be based on these poorly standardized tests. Indeed, given their low positive predictive value for chlamydial infections, the adverse psychological effects of being diagnosed with an STD, and the serious public health problems that the indiscriminate use of antibiotics creates—even in settings where the prevalence of chlamydial infections is high and patient follow-up is uncertain and in resource-poor clinics where NAATs are unavailable—enthusiasm for the practice of diagnosing chlamydial infections empirically. This must be tempered by the knowledge that to prevent one individual from suffering the sequelae of an untreated infection, hundreds will needlessly suffer the adverse psychosocial consequences of an STD diagnosis. This is true even when the diagnosis is made based on characteristic symptom complexes, suggestive leukocyte esterase urine dipsticks, and/or vaginal wet mounts. Thus, with sensitivities and specificities fluctuating approximately 98% on male urethral and urine specimens as well as on female cervical specimens, NAATs are currently the best chlamydial tests available. However, because the sensitivity of these assays for detecting infections in women is significantly lower when urine (80% to 95%) or patient- or provider-collected vaginal fluid (70% to 85%) is the analyte, endocervical specimens should be used, except in screening situations where it is impractical to perform pelvic examinations. Thus every case diagnosed on a urine or vaginal specimen is a bonus.

Despite consensus about how to screen, uncertainty continues about whom to screen and how frequently to screen them. Pregnant women and sexually active women younger than 25 years of age are the only groups for whom there is good evidence that the benefits of screening outweigh the harms. Specifically, when prevalence rates exceed 2%, testing and treating these individuals for asymptomatic chlamydial infections is a cost-effective preventive measure that:

- Averts PID and associated medical complications.
- Reduces transmission to sex partners.
- Reduces the risk of acquiring HIV.
- Lowers the prevalence of chlamydia in the community.

It is unlikely that these benefits reflect factors other than screening (i.e., increased condom use) because knowledge of sexual risk behavior adds nothing to predictive algorithms that include age and prior STD history. However, because of the highly infectious nature of this bacterium, the lack of a vaccine, and the failure of the human immune system to build up resistance to the bacteria, reinfection of effectively treated individuals tends to diminish short-term efficacy, making long-term periodic screening a prerequisite of cost efficacy.

The only other caveat is that most cost-effectiveness analyses are based on culture-proven disease and therefore may reflect a larger inoculum than infections diagnosed by NAAT assays, which can detect extremely low levels of viable and nonviable organisms. Thus further research is needed to determine if and how inoculum size affects disease presentation and to define the clinical and public health significance of NAAT-detectable infections. Specifically, studies comparing transmission rates and the clinical consequences of infections that are detected only by NAAT assay versus those that are detected by traditional assays are still needed to prove that routine, periodic, urine-based screening of asymptomatic individuals is a cost-effective way to control chlamydial infections at the population level. Moreover, because identifying infected individuals is only the first step in effective disease control, it is also important to demonstrate that once identified, the majority of these asymptomatically infected individuals and their sex partners can be contacted and treated. The randomized trial data that determine how frequently community members should be screened to lower chlamydial infections at the population level are lacking; however, observational studies consistently indicate that among sexually active teens the median time between first and repeat infections is approximately 6 months. Based on these data, biannual screening seems reasonable for women at this age (older than 25 years). Because the risk of reinfection is inversely related to age, it is unclear if this recommendation should be extended to young adults. Nevertheless, a history of prior infection predicts reinfection regardless of sexual risk behavior, and in women repeat infections are implicated in the pathogenesis of upper genital tract damage. It may be wise, therefore, to rescreen all women who were treated for chlamydial infections at 6-month intervals.

Developing selective screening criteria is a vigorously pursued public health goal. With the exception of age, however, no single demographic or behavioral risk factor or combination of risk factors consistently identifies a group of young, sexually active women who should not be screened. The utility of more selective screening is limited by the high proportion of missed infections.

Parallel evidence to support screening asymptomatic men may be lacking because before the introduction of urine screening men were not routinely tested for chlamydial infection. But because the cost of treating men is lower than the cost of treating women, a greater proportion of infected men are symptomatic than women, and the harm associated with misdiagnoses is not inconsequent, it will undoubtedly be more difficult to justify routine periodic male screening. However, false-negative test results create a reservoir of untreated disease that is likely to contribute disproportionately to the spread of *C. trachomatis*; but the psychosocial consequences of false-positive test results can range from dysphoric feelings and decreased self-esteem to the disruption of romantic relationships and domestic violence. Moreover, if treatment is initiated inappropriately, the adverse effects of drug reactions and bacterial resistance caused by antibiotic overuse must be taken into account. Thus, until more data become available, the United States Preventive Services Task Force recommends symptom-based screening for all men and for women older than 25 years of age who do not exhibit other characteristics associated with a high prevalence

of chlamydial infections (i.e., unmarried status, African American race, a history of STDs, a history of new or multiple sex partners, cervical ectopy, and inconsistent condom use).

Treatment

Recommendations for antibiotic treatment of chlamydial infections depend on the clinical syndrome. Box 1 summarizes the options for outpatient therapy of uncomplicated genital tract infections in men and women. However, because humans do not develop a natural immunity to chlamydia, treated patients remain at risk for reinfection. For this reason therapy should not be considered complete until all recent sexual contacts are treated and the patient is counseled about future disease prevention. An estimated 70% of the male partners of women with chlamydial cervicitis are infected, and, conversely, approximately 30% of the female partners of chlamydia-infected men are infected. Treatment is recommended for the most recent sex partner and all other individuals who had sexual contact with the infected person during the 60 days preceding the onset of symptoms or diagnosis. Also, partners should abstain from sexual intercourse for a week after they complete treatment.

Although patient-delivered partner treatment is as effective as partner notification, partners are more likely to be treated if informed by physicians rather than by the patients. This is because only 65% (approximately) of women with known chlamydial infections refer their sex partners for therapy, and even fewer (approximately 45%) infected men do so. Because the cure rate for single-dose azithromycin (Zithromax) therapy is close to 100% and the medication can easily be administered under medical supervision, a test of cure 3 weeks after treatment—NAATs remain positive for this long despite successful eradication of infection—is only recommended

---

   CURRENT DIAGNOSIS

- Signs and symptoms are neither a sensitive nor a specific indication of chlamydial infection and often persist for weeks after documented eradication of the pathogen.
  Most chlamydial infections are asymptomatic. *Chlamydia trachomatis* is isolated from less than half of women and men with the most common signs and symptoms (mucopurulent cervicitis and urethritis).
- Chlamydia should be suspected in:
  Women and men with dysuria and pyuria.
  Women with dyspareunia, abnormal vaginal discharge, abnormal bleeding, and lower abdominal or pelvic pain; infants with conjunctivitis or a staccato cough
- Routine periodic screening with nucleic acid amplification techniques (NAATs) is the only reliable way to diagnose this infection.

Rakel and Bope: *Conn's Current Therapy 2006.*

BOX 1 *Chlamydia Trachomatis:* Recommended Treatment Regimens by Clinical Syndrome

Asymptomatic, cervicitis, urethritis*
- First-choice regimen
- Azithromycin (Zithromax), 1 g orally in a single dose

or
- Doxycycline (Vibramycin), 100 mg orally twice a day for 7 days

Alternative Regimens (One of the Following)
- Erythromycin base (E-Mycin), 500 mg orally four times a day for 7 days
- Erythromycin ethylsuccinate (EES), 800 mg orally four times a day for 7 days
- Ofloxacin (Floxin), 300 mg orally twice a day for 7 days
- Levofloxacin (Levaquin),[1] 500 mg orally for 7 days
- Epididymitis
- Ceftriaxone (Rocephin),[1] 250 mg intramuscularly (single dose)

or
- Doxycycline,[1] 100 mg orally twice a day for 7 days

Outpatient Pelvic Inflammatory Disease
- Ofloxacin, 400 mg orally twice a day for 14 days

or
- Levofloxacin,[1] 500 mg orally for 14 days
with or without
- Metronidazole (Flagyl), 500 mg orally twice a day for 14 days

Alternative Regimens
- Ceftriaxone, 250 mg intramuscularly (single dose)

or
- Cefoxitin (Mefoxin), 2 g intramuscularly (single dose)

plus
- Probenecid, 1 g orally

plus
- Doxycycline, 100 mg orally twice a day for 14 days
with or without
- Metronidazole, 500 mg orally twice a day for 14 days

Inpatient Pelvic Inflammatory Disease†
- Cefotetan (Cefotan), 2 g intravenously every 12 hours

or
- Cefoxitin, 2 g intravenously every 6 hours

plus
- Doxycycline,[1] 100 mg orally or intravenously every 12 hours

Alternative Regimens
- Clindamycin, 900 mg intravenously every 8 hours

plus
- Gentamicin,[1] 2 g/kg of body weight loading dose, then 1.5 mg/kg of body weight every 8 hours. Treatment should be continued for 24 to 48 hours after significant clinical improvement occurs and then should consist of oral therapy with doxycycline, 100 mg orally twice a day for 14 days, or clindamycin, 450 mg orally four times a day, for a total of 14 days.

[1]Not FDA approved for this indication.
*Pregnancy: Doxycycline, erythromycin estolate (Ilosone), and ofloxacin are contraindicated, and repeat testing 3 weeks after completion of therapy is recommended because antibiotics may be less efficacious. HIV infection: Patients who have chlamydial infection and who also are infected with HIV should receive the same treatment regimen as those who are HIV-negative.
†Studies indicate that the efficacy of inpatient and outpatient treatment is comparable in terms of fertility and other long-term health outcomes (e.g., ectopic pregnancy and chronic pelvic pain). Therefore, inpatient therapy is no longer recommended except for individuals who do not respond to outpatient regimes or develop tubo-ovarian abscesses or other manifestations of severe upper genital tract disease.

Rakel and Bope: *Conn's Current Therapy 2006.*

 CURRENT THERAPY

- Antibiotic treatment is easy to summarize in tabular form but is ineffective if given in isolation of sexual network.
  - Large reservoir of asymptomatically infected partners and potential partners undermines the effectiveness of individual treatments.
  - Half of all chlamydial infections occur in previously treated persons.
- Therapy is not complete until all recent sexual contacts are treated and patient counseled about disease prevention.
- Prevalence of *Chlamydia trachomatis* in the sexual network is the best predictor of infection.
- Who an individual has sexual intercourse with puts them at higher risk for acquisition of this infection than how they do so.
- For disease prevention—condoms are plan B—plan A is choosing low-risk sexual partners.

for pregnant women (among whom antibiotic efficacy may be reduced) and when compliance is in doubt.

Approximately 50% of all chlamydial infections occur in previously treated persons. Demographic characteristics, such as age and a past history of chlamydial infection, are better predictors of infection than behavioral risk factors, such as multiple sexual partners and the failure to use condoms consistently. Being involved with a sexual network in which chlamydia is hyperendemic appears to put individuals at greater risk for infection than unsafe sexual behavior in the general population. Hence, to control the spread of *C. trachomatis,* it may be necessary to:

- Extend screening and treatment beyond recent partners to include the group of core transmitters in the infected individual's sexual network.
- Help STD patients learn to choose less risky sex partners by promoting sexual health communication within partnerships.

Although the debate about the content and duration of counseling necessary to achieve this goal is ongoing, there is a growing consensus that brief (5 minutes), personalized (provider-delivered and client-centered) counseling sessions—aimed at personal risk reduction and increasing awareness of partner risk behavior—are more effective than the conventional didactic approach to STD prevention education. They are certainly as effective as more prolonged sessions, which are difficult to conduct in busy public health clinics.

REFERENCES

Aral SO, Hughes JP, Stoner B, et al: Sexual mixing patterns in spread of gonococcal and chlamydial infections. Am J Pub Health 1999;89:825-833.
Biro F, Workowski K, Blythe MJ, Lara-Torre E: NASPAG/JPAG roundtable discussion annual clinical meeting 2003—Philadelphia, PA: Sexually transmitted diseases (STD) treatment guidelines 2002. J Pediatr Adolesc Gynecol 2004;17:143-146.

Cates W Jr: Contraception, unintended pregnancies, and sexually transmitted diseases: Why isn't a simple solution possible? Am J Epidemiol 1996;143:311-318.

Critchlow CW, Wolner-Hanssen P, Eschenbach DA, et al: Determinants of cervical ectopia and cervicitis: Age, oral contraception, specific cervical infection, smoking, and douching. Am J Obstet Gynecol 1995;173:534-543.

Duncan B, Hart G, Scoular A, Bigrigg A: Qualitative analysis of psychosocial impact of diagnosis of *Chlamydia trachomatis*: Implications for screening. BMJ 2001;322:195-199.

Ford CA, Viadro CI, Miller WC: Testing for chlamydial and gonorrheal infections outside of clinic settings. A summary of the literature. Sex Transm Dis 2004;31:38-51.

Kamb ML, Fishbein M, Douglas JM Jr, et al: Efficacy of risk-reduction counseling to prevent human immunodeficiency virus and sexually transmitted diseases: A randomized controlled trial for the Project RESPECT Study Group. JAMA 1998;280:1161-1167.

Peipert JF: Clinical practice. Genital chlamydial infections. N Engl J Med 2003;349:2424-2430.

Rietmeijer CA, Van Bemmelen R, Judson FN, Douglas JM: Incidence and repeat infection rates of *Chlamydia trachomatis* among male and female patients in an STD clinic. Sex Transm Dis 2002;29: 65-72.

U.S. Preventive Services Task Force. Screening for chlamydial infection: Recommendations and rationale. Am J Prev Med 2001;20(3S):90-94.

Pelvic Inflammatory Disease

Method of
Lydia A. Shrier, MD, MPH

Pelvic inflammatory disease (PID), which is an infection of the female upper genital tract, may include parametritis, endometritis, acute salpingitis, oophoritis, tuboovarian abscess (TOA), and pelvic peritonitis.

Risk Factors

Risk factors for PID include young age, at risk sexual behaviors (unprotected intercourse, multiple sexual partners, and intercourse during menses), smoking, and douching. Bacterial vaginosis may facilitate ascension of pathogenic organisms from the lower genital tract. Cervical ectopy, commonly seen in young women, may increase their risk of PID because pathogens readily adhere to the columnar cells exposesd on the exocervix. Cervicitis with *Neisseria gonorrhoeae* or *Chlamydia trachomatis* is clearly associated with PID. Invasive procedures, such as a therapeutic abortion or insertion of an intrauterine device within the past 30 days, increase the risk of PID. Recent studies have not found an association between the use of any hormonal contraception and PID. Scarring and impaired local barriers to infection from one episode of PID places a woman at risk for future episodes. PID is also associated with black race, low socioeconomic status, and substance abuse.

Pathophysiology

PID is a polymicrobial infection that may involve *C. trachomatis, N. gonorrhoeae, Mycoplasma hominis,* *Ureaplasma urealyticum,* nontypable *Haemophilus influenzae,* aerobes, and anaerobes (especially with TOA and with more severe PID). Lower genital tract test results do not correlate well with the presence of upper tract infection.

Infection occurs by direct canalicular spread from the endocervix along the endometrial surface to the tubal mucosa. The end of the tube may become blocked with pus, leading to pyosalpinx or TOA if the ovary is also involved. Mechanisms of ascension include direct migration transport via attachment to sperm or with refluxed menstrual blood. Chlamydial and gonococcal PID commonly occur within 7 days of the onset of menses. This is likely because of loss of the protective cervical mucus plug; sloughing of the endometrium, which produces a stickier surface for bacteria; and the presence of menstrual blood, a good culture medium.

Symptoms on Signs

Although symptoms have poor sensitivity and specificity for PID, it is useful to elicit history of:

- Lower abdominal and/or pelvic pain
- New or malodorous vaginal discharge
- Dysuria or urinary frequency
- Dyspareunia
- Onset of symptoms within 1 week of menses
- Increased or irregular menstrual flow
- Increased menstrual cramps
- A sexual partner with recent urethritis

Women with PID may also complain of fever, chills, nausea, vomiting, diarrhea, or constipation. The severity of the patient's presentation does not correlate with the severity of the pelvic infection. In fact, subclinical infection accounts for the majority of cases of PID.

Diagnosis

The diagnosis of PID is generally made on the basis of nonspecific clinical criteria. Physical examination should include vital signs, abdominal examination, and pelvic examination with visualization and a bimanual examination. Adnexal tenderness, if present, may be unilateral or bilateral. Wet preparations and pH of vaginal secretions and specimens to test for *N. gonorrhoeae* and *C. trachomatis* should be obtained. In most cases of PID, mucopurulent cervical discharge or white blood cells (WBCs) on a saline preparation of vaginal fluid is present. A pregnancy test is essential. Urinalysis and urine culture, a complete blood count with WBC differential, and erythrocyte sedimentation rate or C- reactive protein level are useful in specifying the diagnosis. However, it is important to note that all tests can be normal in a woman with PID.

Recognizing that many episodes of PID go undiagnosed, the Centers for Disease Control and Prevention (CDC) has recommended new, less stringent criteria for the diagnosis of PID (Box 1). While these new guidelines increase the sensitivity of clinical diagnosis, specificity

---

is reduced and clinicians must be sure to consider exhaustive differential diagnoses, including other gynecologic, gastrointestinal, urinary tract, orthopedic, rheumatologic/autoimmune, and psychiatric disorders. Clinicians must balance the consequences of misdiagnosing PID (e.g., cost, risk of missing other diagnoses, unnecessary exposure to antibiotics, stigma, bias toward diagnosing PID again) with the consequences of missing the diagnosis of PID and exposing the patient to undue risk of the serious complications and sequelae associated with PID.

Ultrasonography may be useful if:

• The clinician cannot adequately assess adnexae on examination
• An adnexal mass or fullness is palpated
• There is otherwise suspicion for an ovarian cyst, ectopic pregnancy, or TOA

However, a normal ultrasonographic examination does not eliminate the diagnosis of PID. Laparoscopy may be indicated if the diagnosis is very uncertain or if the patient does not respond to appropriate treatment for PID.

Management

Hospitalization and parenteral therapy is not superior to outpatient management with oral and intramuscular therapy. A woman with suspected PID should be hospitalized if:

• A surgical emergency cannot be excluded.
• She is pregnant.

Rakel and Bope: *Conn's Current Therapy 2006.*

• She has severe illness, nausea/vomiting, high fever.
• She cannot follow or tolerate an outpatient treatment regimen.
• Oral therapy has been attempted and failed to produce clinical improvement.
• TOA is present.

In addition, hospitalization may be considered for women who are less than 15 to 17 years of age, have had a gynecologic surgical procedure within the previous 14 days, have had a previous episode of PID, or have other extenuating medical or social circumstances. If a woman is to be treated as an outpatient, the clinician should assess her ability to fill prescriptions, abstain from sexual intercourse, notify her partner(s) of the need for treatment, abstain from use of illicit substances and other risk behaviors, and maintain personal safety. The patient's living situation, financial situation, and medical insurance status should also be assessed.

The recommended parenteral and oral treatment regimens are presented in Box 2. With the oral regimens,

16

some experts recommend the inclusion of metronidazole for better coverage of anaerobic organisms, although compliance may be reduced and there is the potential for more side effects. Metronidazole may also be considered if bacterial vaginosis is also diagnosed.

If the patient is treated as an outpatient, she should be reassessed within 48 to 72 hours; hospitalization should be considered if there is no clinical improvement or if she is not able to tolerate/follow the outpatient regimen. Regardless of the regimen used, if there is not substantial clinical improvement within 72 hours, the clinician should reconsider the diagnosis and evaluate for complications. Patients need to complete the full course of treatment regardless of their STD test results. HIV testing and counseling should be recommended and hepatitis B vaccination status determined. All sexual partners from at least the previous 60 days need to be treated for both *N. gonorrhoeae* and *C. trachomatis*, regardless of their symptoms or test results. The patient should be rescreened for reinfection in 4 to 6 weeks.

The complications of PID include Fitz-Hugh-Curtis perihepatitis and TOA. The patient with perihepatitis may have left upper quadrant abdominal pain or back pain, leukocytosis, an elevated erythrocyte sedimentation rate that is out of proportion with the severity of their presentation, and increased liver transaminases. The management of patients with PID and perihepatitis is no different from that of patients with PID alone. TOA requires prolonged parenteral therapy and, if it ruptures, it is a surgical emergency. Women who have had PID have an increased risk of ectopic pregnancy, infertility, chronic pelvic pain, dyspareunia, pelvic adhesions, and recurrent PID.

Primary and secondary prevention efforts are essential to reducing the burden of PID. Routine STD screening lowers the incidence of PID, and prompt recognition and treatment of PID decreases the risk of sequelae.

Uterine Leiomyomas

Method of
Tod C. Aeby, MD, and Stella Dantas, MD

Epidemiology

Uterine leiomyomas are the most common pelvic tumor in women. They affect approximately 20% of women older than 35 years of age and 40% of women older than 50 years of age, although they are found any time from puberty through menopause. Survey studies involving histologic examination of the uterus suggest they are present in more than 80% of women. Nulliparity, early menarche, and African American ethnicity increase the risk of developing leiomyomas. The incidence among women of African descent is not as high in countries other than the United States, which suggests possible dietary, environmental, and genetic influences on development. Risk is also increased in women with

a higher body mass index, presumably because of the increased estrogen production in adipocytes. Pregnancy reduces the risk of developing leiomyomas.

Pathophysiology

The etiology of uterine leiomyomas is not completely understood, but development is thought to be a multi-step process. They are benign monoclonal tumors of the smooth muscle of the myometrium that presumably derive from a normal myocyte. Estrogen and progesterone, in concert with local growth factors, lead to a somatic mutation of normal myometrium to a leiomyoma. Some growth factors that cause leiomyoma proliferation are epidermal growth factors, insulin-like growth factors, heparin-binding growth factors, and transforming growth factor-β. Leiomyomas develop during the reproductive years and increase in size during pregnancy. Growth usually ceases in menopause, and leiomyomas then decrease in volume. This supports the theory that estrogen and progesterone promote growth.

Symptoms and Signs

Most uterine leiomyomas are asymptomatic. They are categorized into subgroups based on their anatomic relationship and position in the uterus, and symptoms usually depend on those relationships. They can be subserosal, intramural, submucosal, or pedunculated. The most common symptom is abnormal uterine bleeding, usually menorrhagia, occurring in 30% of women with leiomyomas. The cause of the abnormal bleeding is not totally clear but may be the result of abnormal growth and function of the endometrium near the leiomyoma and local interference with normal physiologic mechanisms for hemostasis.

Pelvic pain and increasing pelvic pressure occur in 30% of women with leiomyomas. Other symptoms include dysmenorrhea, postcoital bleeding, and dyspareunia. Pain can be caused by leiomyomas outgrowing their blood supply and becoming necrotic. This red degeneration is common in pregnancy. Patients may have an increasing abdominal girth and pressure symptoms as a result of large fibroids. Pressure on adjacent organs such as the bladder or bowel can cause urinary frequency and urgency or constipation. Rarely, an enlarged uterus causes a palpable kidney secondary to hydronephrosis from ureteral obstruction. Patients also may be lethargic from anemia secondary to menorrhagia. Leiomyomas may also be associated with infertility, although the relationship is controversial.

A rapidly enlarging uterus should raise concern for malignant transformation. But leiomyosarcomas are extremely rare, occurring in less than 0.1% of women operated on for presumed leiomyomas.

Diagnosis

Uterine leiomyomas are typically diagnosed at pelvic exam when an enlarged and irregularly shaped uterus

TABLE 1 Comparison of Various Procedures for the Treatment of Symptomatic Uterine Leiomyoma

Therapy	Success Rate	Complication Rate	Possibility of Future Childbearing	Comments
Hysterectomy	100%	40%	No	Recovery time varies depending on the route of removal.
Myomectomy and myolysis	75%	39%	Yes	Can be associated with significant blood loss and can result in an unplanned hysterectomy. Recurrent leiomyomas are common.
Myolysis			Yes	Several methods for myolysis are available, including bipolar electrocautery, laser energy, and cryotherapy.
Uterine artery embolization	77%-91%	5%	Not currently recommended	Complication rates are low but can be severe, including infection, sepsis, and nontarget tissue necrosis. A few deaths have been reported.
Hydrothermal endometrial ablation	91%*	1%-2%	No	Hysteroscopic resection of submucosal leiomyomas, prior to endometrial ablation, improves success rates. Pregnancies have occurred after these procedures, so contraception is still required.

*Best estimate based on limited studies.

is noted. Abdominal and transvaginal ultrasound is often helpful in making the diagnosis and in differentiating leiomyomas from adnexal masses or other pelvic pathology. Serial ultrasounds also can be used to monitor their growth. During a pelvic exam, it may not be possible to palpate ovaries next to an enlarged uterus, but an adnexal tumor can be suspected if the mass moves independently of the uterus. Submucosal leiomyomas are diagnosed using saline infusion sonohysterography and hysteroscopy. Definitive diagnosis requires histologic examination.

Management

For the most part, asymptomatic leiomyoma should be managed expectantly. The approaches to the patient experiencing problems fall into the three general categories of medical management, conservative procedures, and hysterectomy. The choice should be individualized to the patient, based on the severity of her symptoms, her plans for future childbearing, and her personal interest in retaining her uterus. Other causes of abnormal bleeding should be considered.

Current medical therapy is limited to the use of gonadotropin-releasing hormone (GnRH) analogues and antagonists (i.e., leuprolide acetate [Lupron Depot], 3.75 mg monthly; nafarelin acetate [Synarel),[1] 200 μg intranasally twice a day; and goserelin acetate implant [Zoladex],[1] 3.6-mg implant monthly, cetrorelix [Cetrotide]).[1] These expensive medications are shown to decrease the uterine size by up to 65%, allowing for easier or more conservative surgical treatments. The progesterone antagonist mifepristone (Mifeprex)[1]

is also effective but not currently available for this purpose in the United States. GnRH therapy has significant side effects, mostly related to the induced hypoestrogenic state. To preserve bone density the duration of therapy must be limited. Additionally, the uterus rapidly returns to its enlarged size when the therapy is discontinued. These medications are a very effective means of inducing amenorrhea to allow for correction of an anemia prior to surgery.

Conservative procedures include myomectomy or myolysis (surgical removal or destruction of the individual fibroids while preserving the uterus), uterine artery embolization, and endometrial ablation. Each of these approaches has different risks, benefits, and complications (Table 1).

Hysterectomy remains the most common treatment for women with symptomatic leiomyoma and offers the advantage of a complete and definitive cure. The uterus can be removed through the vagina (with or without the aid of laparoscopic techniques) or through an abdominal incision. The route of removal largely depends on the size

 CURRENT DIAGNOSIS

- Abnormal uterine bleeding, postcoital spotting
- Pelvic pain, pressure, dysmenorrhea and dyspareunia
- Urinary frequency and urgency, constipation
- Lethargy
- Infertility
- Physical findings: Enlarged, irregular, and firm uterus
- Ultrasound: Diagnostic imaging modality of choice
- Saline infusion sonohysterography and/or hysteroscopy: Used to evaluate the uterine cavity

[1]Not FDA approved for this indication.

Rakel and Bope: *Conn's Current Therapy 2006.*

CURRENT THERAPY

- Only symptomatic leiomyomas require treatment.
- Medical therapy is for temporizing and making invasive procedures easier or more effective.
- Conservative procedures include myomectomy, myolysis, hydrothermal endometrial ablation, and uterine artery embolization.
- Hysterectomy is the only definitive therapy for leiomyomata.
- Choice of treatment should be made considering the severity of symptoms and respecting the patient's preferences.

of the uterus, the patient's medical and surgical history, and the experience and preference of her surgeon.

REFERENCES

Buttram VC Jr, Reiter RC: Uterine leiomyomata: Etiology, symptomatology, and management. Fertil Steril 1981;36:433-445.
Felberbaum RE, Germer U, Ludwig M, et al: Treatment of uterine fibroids with a slow-release formulation of the gonadotrophin-releasing hormone antagonist Cetrorelix. Hum Reprod 1998; 13(6):1660-1668.
Goldfarb HA: Bipolar laparoscopic needles for myoma coagulation. J Am Assoc Gynecol Laparosc 1995;2(2):175-179.
Lethaby A, Vollenhoven B, Sowter M: Pre-operative GnRH analogue therapy before hysterectomy or myomectomy for uterine fibroids. The Cochrane Database of Systematic Reviews 2001, Issue 2. Article CD000547. DOI: 10.1002/14651858.CD000547.
Parker WH, Fu YS, Berek JS: Uterine sarcoma in patients operated on for presumed leiomyoma and rapidly growing leiomyoma. Obstet Gynecol 1994;83:414.
Pron G, Bennett J, Common A, et al: Ontario Uterine Fibroid Embolization Collaboration Group. The Ontario Uterine Fibroid Embolization Trial: II. Uterine fibroid reduction and symptom relief after uterine artery embolization for fibroids. Fertil Steril 2003;79(1):120-127.
The Hydro ThermAblator system for management of menorrhagia in women with submucous myomas: 12- to 20-month follow-up. J Am Assoc Gynecol Laparosc 2003;10(4):521-527.

Ovarian Cancer

Method of
Lynne A. Eaton, MD, MS

Epithelial ovarian cancer accounts for 90% of all cases of ovarian cancer and is the leading cause of death from cancer of the female reproductive tract. Approximately 25,000 new cases and 16,000 deaths were reported in 2004 from this disease. The median age of patients with ovarian cancer is 60 years. There are few established risk factors for the disease, which include low parity, obesity, high-fat diet, and strong family history or genetic mutations. Preventative measures may include tubal ligation, hysterectomy, and breast-feeding. Oral contraceptive pills may decrease a woman's risk of developing the disease by as much as 50%, including those at highest risk for developing ovarian cancer.

Most ovarian cancers are acquired as a sporadic disease. A woman's lifetime risk of ovarian cancer increases with a family history of ovarian cancer (i.e., one first-degree relative, 4%; one-first- and one second-degree relative, 15%; and two first-degree relatives, 40%). Approximately 10% of epithelial ovarian cancers arise as a result of an inherited mutation. These cancers usually arise approximately 10 years earlier than previous generations, and most are linked to the presence of BRCA-1 or BRCA-2 gene mutation. These tumor suppressor genes have an autosomal dominant inheritance pattern and are found on chromosome 17 and 13, respectively. A woman may have up to an 80% chance of developing breast cancer and a 40% chance of developing ovarian cancer if she is BRCA-1 positive. In women who are BRCA-2 positive, their lifetime risk of developing breast and ovarian cancer is 50% to 85% and 15% to 20%, respectively. Ashkenazi Jewish women have a higher incidence of germ-line mutations in BRCA-1 or BRCA-2 genes. A second familial disorder with an increased risk of ovarian cancer is the Lynch II syndrome, or hereditary nonpolyposis colorectal cancer (HNPCC). It is caused by inherited germ-line mutations in DNA-mismatch repair genes. Women who present with a family history should be offered genetic counseling and testing for genetic mutations where appropriate. Oral contraceptives may be offered to those women who desire fertility, and oophorectomy may be considered in those who have completed their families because these measures decrease the risk of developing ovarian cancer.

Screening

Unfortunately, despite the high mortality rate of the disease, no effective screening method is available for ovarian cancer. CA-125 is an antigen found in structures derived from coelomic epithelium and in tubal, endometrial, and endocervical epithelium. The surface epithelium of the normal fetal and adult ovaries do not express CA-125, however, except in inclusion cysts, areas of metaplasia, and papillary excrescences. Serum CA-125 is quantified based on immunoradiometric assay of the monoclonal antibody OC-125. It is a serum with a low specificity and sensitivity. The elevation of the tumor marker often depends on the histology (most commonly elevated in serous histology) and can be elevated in other conditions that irritate the abdominal/pelvic cavity. These include but are not limited to endometriosis, pelvic inflammatory disease, endometrial cancer, appendicitis, liver disease, and pancreatitis. Only 50% of women with stage I disease have an elevated CA-125. Almost 80% of women with advanced disease have an elevated CA-125. This serum test is best used as a tumor marker to triage a patient with a known adnexal mass and to follow a woman postoperatively who is undergoing adjuvant chemotherapy to assess response to therapy. It can also be used as a surveillance marker, with an elevation indicating possible recurrent disease. Transvaginal ultrasonography has been examined as a screening tool. The sensitivity and specificity of this test is low in predicting ovarian cancer. Combining the two modalities may increase the screening statistical parameters. No effective screening modalities currently exist for the general population or for women at high risk of developing ovarian cancer.

Diagnosis

The symptoms of ovarian cancer are nonspecific. Many women present with abdomen pain, bloating, or fullness. They may feel their clothes are too tight or that they are gaining weight. Others complain of early satiety or dyspepsia. Some patients may present with pelvic pain because of abdominal distention from ascites or a pelvic mass. Unfortunately, at this point, 75% of women have stage III or IV disease. Diagnosis can often be made on physical examination with palpation of a mass either abdominally or on rectovaginal exam. Less frequently, the patient has a distended abdomen and a fluid wave may be present. If necessary, transvaginal ultrasound or computed tomography (CT) of the abdomen and pelvis may be performed to help establish the diagnosis. An ovarian mass that is complex in nature (i.e., having both solid and cystic components) is suspicious for ovarian cancer. This is especially true in postmenopausal women with an elevated CA-125. Women who present with a pleural effusion should also be assessed for the possibility of ovarian cancer. A CA-125 should be drawn if ovarian cancer is suspected so it may be followed postoperatively. If there is *any* suspicion a woman has an ovarian cancer, she should be referred to a gynecologic oncologist who specializes in the surgical and medical care of women with gynecologic cancers.

Management

Critical to the proper management decision in patients with ovarian cancer is the accurate staging of the disease. Comprehensive surgical staging is mandatory in this patient population. Approximately 30% to 40% of women with apparent stage I disease have occult disease outside the pelvis. Virtually every patient with ovarian cancer should undergo an exploratory laparotomy through a midline vertical incision that allows careful examination of the abdominal/peritoneal cavity. Usually a total abdominal hysterectomy with bilateral-salpingo-oophorectomy, pelvic and para-aortic lymph node dissection, and multiple peritoneal biopsies is performed. In instances of stage III or IV disease, these surgeries may additionally include rectosigmoid resections with reanastomosis, peritoneal and diaphragmatic stripping, splenectomy, and partial bladder cystectomy. The primary goal is cytoreduction of tumor nodules to less than 1.0 cm. Two large meta-analyses demonstrated that regardless of the initial tumor size, successful cytoreduction to small-volume disease increases the frequency of complete responses and enhanced survival.

Cytoreductive surgery is thought to improve survival and response rates based on the following:

- Removal of resistant clones of tumor cells decreases the likelihood of early onset of drug resistance.
- Removal of large tumor volume increases vascularity and improves drug delivery.
- More vascularized tissue has a higher growth fraction, enhancing the effect of chemotherapy.
- Smaller masses of tumor may require fewer doses of chemotherapy and decrease the possibility of acquired drug resistance.
- Removal of bulky disease may enhance the immune system.

The standard of care for adjuvant therapy in the United States today is chemotherapy using a combination of intravenous (IV) paclitaxel (Taxol) and carboplatin (Paraplatin) as an outpatient regime. This combination is a result of four large randomized trials performed through the Gynecologic Oncology Group (GOG), OV-10 (Canadian-European consortium), and AGO (Arbeitsgemeinschaft Gynakologische Onkologie; Ovarian Cancer Study Group). These trials initially compared cisplatin/cyclophospamide to cisplatin (Platinol-AQ)/paclitaxel [Cytoxan]) and found the combination of cisplatin and paclitaxel superior in regard to overall response rate, clinical complete response rate, progression-free survival, and overall survival. Efficacy trials were then performed comparing cisplatin and carboplatin, and no major therapeutic differences were found between the two drugs. Thus paclitaxel and carboplatin are defined as the gold standard for treatment of ovarian cancer. Intraperitoneal (IP) chemotherapy was evaluated in a number of randomized trials in patients with small-volume disease. These trials showed improvement in progression-free and overall survival. The IP regimens have significantly more toxicity then the IV routes of administration, however, and they are generally viewed as too toxic for routine use outside of clinical trials.

Adjuvant therapy depends on the stage and grade of the disease. In women with early-stage low-risk disease (stage IA-B, grades 1-2), no further therapy is warranted. In those women with stage IC or stage II disease, three

---

 CURRENT DIAGNOSIS

- Inherited gene mutation causes approximately 10% of ovarian cancers.
- No effective screening modalities are currently available.
- Symptoms of ovarian cancer are nonspecific.
- Physical examination and palpation of abdominal mass or fluid wave should be preformed.
- Rectovaginal exam and palpation of pelvic mass should be performed.
- Radiographic imaging demonstrates complex mass with cystic and solid components.
- Elevation of CA-125 occurs, especially in a postmenopausal woman.

CURRENT THERAPY

- Referral to gynecologic oncologist if ovarian cancer suspected based on CA-125 and/or radiographic imaging
- Adequate surgical staging of the disease by a gynecologic oncologist
- In patients with advanced disease, optimal cytoreductive surgery with tumor nodules less than 1 cm
- Adjuvant chemotherapy using paclitaxel (Taxol) and carboplatin (Paraplatin) and standard of care or enrollment in a clinical trial if available
- In patients with recurrent disease, second-line agents based on platinum sensitivity as well as consideration of convenience, toxicity, and quality of life issues

to six cycles of paclitaxel and carboplatin are given. Patients with more advanced disease generally receive six cycles of IV paclitaxel and carboplatin. They have a CA-125 drawn with each cycle of chemotherapy in hopes of a rapid downward trend. Another important option for these women is participation in clinical trials. The GOG, as well as many other cooperative groups, are leaders in the research on ovarian cancer.

Despite an initial 80% response rate to chemotherapy, 75% of patients who achieve a clinical complete response eventually relapse and die of their disease. Patients who relapse greater than 6 months from their last course of chemotherapy are considered "platinum sensitive." These women have a 30% response to second-line agents, and depending on the length of remission, they may consider retreatment with paclitaxel and carboplatin. Second-line agents include topotecan (Hycamtin), liposomal doxorubicin (Doxil), gemcitabine (Gemzar),[1] ifosfamide (Ifex),[1] and hexamethylmelamine (Hexalen), as well as other agents.

Platinum-resistant patients have a recurrence within 6 months of their last treatment. Their prognosis is considered poor because platinum-based therapy is a key factor in treatment for ovarian cancer. Treatments with second-line agents can be initiated, but response rates are low. Treatment decisions should be made based on patient convenience, toxicity, and quality of life issues. Most women with ovarian cancer ultimately die from complications related to bowel obstruction or general deterioration. When signs of an obstruction occur in a patient with end-stage ovarian cancer, it is important to initiate conversations with the patient and family regarding symptomatic care, including gastric tube placement to relieve nausea and vomiting, pain management, and hospice.

Despite the ravages of ovarian cancer, progress is being made in the treatment of the disease. Since the 1970s and the introduction of cisplatin, and more recently of paclitaxel, the median survival has progressed from

6 to 12 months to 3 to 5 years. Knowledge gained in the genetics of the disease risk-reduction procedures can be offered to those at highest risk for developing ovarian cancer. There is hope for development of new screening tools in the future. Current clinical trials are using new cytotoxic agents as well as integrating biologic agents to front-line therapy to assess their role in the armamentarium for treating ovarian cancer. It is hoped these efforts will lead to a decrease in the mortality of this disease and one day a cure for ovarian cancer.

REFERENCES

Allen DG, Heintz APM, Touw FWMM: A meta-analysis of residual disease and survival in stage III and IV carcinoma of the ovary. Eur J Gynaecol Oncol 1995;16:349-356.
Bristow RE, Tomacruz RS, Armstrong DK, et al: Survival effect of maximal cytoreductive surgery for advanced ovarian carcinoma during the platinum era: A meta-analysis. J Clin Oncol 2002;20:1248-1259.
Cannistra SA: Cancer of the ovary. N Engl J Med 2004;351:2519-2529.
Copeland LJ, Bookman M, Trimble E: Clinical trials of newer regimens for treating ovarian cancer: The rationale for Gynecologic Oncology Group Protocol GOG 182-ICON5. Gynecol Oncol 2003;90:S1-S57.
McGuire WP, Hoskins WJ, Brady MF, et al: Cyclophosphamide and cisplatin compared with paclitaxel and cisplatin in patients with stage III and stage IV ovarian disease. N Engl J Med 1996;334:1-6.
Ozols RF: Update on Gynecologic Oncology Group (GOG) trials in ovarian cancer. Cancer Invest 2004;22(Suppl 2):11-20.
Ozols RF, Bundy BN, Greer BE, et al: Phase III trial of carboplatin and paclitaxel compared with cisplatin and paclitaxel in patients with optimally resected stage III ovarian cancer: A Gynecologic Oncology Group study. J Clin Oncol 2003;21:3194-3200.
Rose PG, Nerenstone S, Brady MF, et al: Secondary surgical cytoreduction for advanced ovarian carcinoma. N Engl J Med 2004;351:2489-2497.
Thigpen T: First-line therapy for ovarian carcinoma: What's next? Cancer Invest 2004;22(Suppl 2):21-28.
Thigpen T: The if and when of surgical debulking for ovarian carcinoma. N Engl J Med 2004;351:2544-2546.

Endometrial Cancer

Method of
James J. Burke II, MD, and
Donald G. Gallup, MD

Endometrial cancer is the most common gynecologic cancer in the United States, with an estimated 40,100 new cases reported each year. Although approximately 80% of these cases are diagnosed as stage I disease, 6800 women will succumb to their disease annually.

Endometrial cancer is subdivided into two histologically and clinically separate groups. Type I endometrial cancer is directly related to an increased estrogenous state. This type of endometrial cancer is the most common and is usually found at an earlier stage, and treatment results in a more favorable outcome. Type II endometrial carcinoma is a more virulent type of carcinoma characterized by early metastasis, and it typically has a worse prognosis.

---

[1]Not FDA approved for this indication.

Rakel and Bope: *Conn's Current Therapy 2006.*

Epidemiology, Clinical Features, and Diagnosis

TYPE I ENDOMETRIAL CARCINOMA

Endometrial carcinoma is a heterogeneous mix of several histologic types with various clinical outcomes. This more common type of endometrial carcinoma represents approximately 90% of all endometrial cancers and is associated with a hyperestrogenic state. Table 1 lists risk factors associated with type I endometrial carcinoma. In the 1970s it was found that giving estrogen preparations without progestin for hormone replacement therapy led to at least a six times greater chance of endometrial carcinoma developing. Similarly, women who are obese have an increased risk of endometrial carcinoma as a result of peripheral conversion of androstenedione to estrone in peripheral adipose tissue by 5α-reductase enzyme activity. Finally, women who have untreated atypical endometrial hyperplasia, a well-known precursor to type I endometrial carcinoma, have a 29 times greater chance of endometrial carcinoma developing. Hence, intervention when this precursor is found can prevent endometrial cancer.

Although 90% of women with this type of carcinoma initially have painless, postmenopausal vaginal bleeding or some form of vaginal discharge, most postmenopausal vaginal bleeding is related to conditions other than malignancy. Nonetheless, all postmenopausal bleeding needs further evaluation. The gold standard is endometrial biopsy, usually carried out in the office with minimal patient discomfort. However, should the results of this type of in-office biopsy still be equivocal or performance of the biopsy not be possible because of cervical stenosis, formal fractional dilation and curettage should be performed. Another modality used for assessment of postmenopausal bleeding is transvaginal ultrasound (US) to measure the thickness of the endometrium. Endometrial stripes found to be thicker than 5 mm require endometrial sampling because of the higher likelihood of malignancy.

TYPE II ENDOMETRIAL CARCINOMA

Unlike type I endometrial carcinoma, type II is unrelated to an increased estrogenic state and encompasses several histologic variants that are quite aggressive. These carcinomas tend to have serous, papillary serous, or clear cell histology and typically occur in women older than age 70 years. Fortunately, carcinomas of these types account for less than 10% of all endometrial cancers; but unfortunately, they contribute the majority of deaths from endometrial cancer. Because of the aggressive nature of these cancers, most have metastasized before initial evaluation and diagnosis and spread in a fashion similar to ovarian carcinoma.

As with type I endometrial carcinoma, type II carcinomas are commonly manifested as painless, postmenopausal vaginal bleeding or vaginal discharge. However, patients may have no bleeding at all and instead have nonspecific gastrointestinal (GI) symptoms such as nausea and vomiting, constipation, early satiety, abdominal bloating, and abdominal pain. All these symptoms point to intra-abdominal metastasis, common with this type of endometrial carcinoma. In these patients, early computed tomography (CT) can aid in the diagnosis. Even when these carcinomas have not spread and are limited to the endometrium or endometrial polyps, the risk of recurrence is high.

Staging and Treatment

STAGING

Recognizing that clinical staging did not take into account pathologic or surgical prognostic information, the Gynecologic Oncology Group (GOG) conducted two large prospective surgical staging trials in the 1980s. In 1988 the Fédération Internationale de Gynécologie et d'Obstétrique (FIGO) adopted the surgical staging of endometrial cancer (Table 2). Surgical staging involves obtaining pelvic washings, extrafascial hysterectomy, bilateral salpingo-oophorectomy, and lymph node sampling from the pelvic and para-aortic regions. In addition,

16

TABLE 1 Risk Factors for the Development of Endometrial Carcinoma

Risk Factor	RR
Overweight (age 50-59 y)	
By 20-50 pounds	3
By >50 pounds	10
Nulliparity versus multiparity	5
Menopause after age 52 y	2
Diabetes	3
Unopposed estrogen replacement	6
Combination OCP	0.5

Abbreviations: OCP = oral contraceptive preparation; RR = relative risk.

TABLE 2 Fédération Internationale de Gynécologie et d'Obstétrique (FIGO) Surgical Staging Classification for Endometrial Carcinoma

Stage IA	Tumor limited to the endometrium
Stage IB	Invasion to <50% myometrium
Stage IC	Invasion to ≥50% myometrium
Stage IIA	Endocervical glandular involvement only
Stage IIB	Cervical stromal invasion
Stage IIIA	Tumor invading the serosa of the corpus uteri and/or adnexa and/or positive cytologic findings
Stage IIIB	Vaginal metastases
Stage IIIC	Metastases to the pelvic and/or paraortic lymph nodes
Stage IVA	Tumor invasion of the bladder and/or bowel mucosa
Stage IVB	Distant metastases, including intra-abdominal metastasis and/or metastasis to the inguinal lymph nodes

TABLE 3 Distribution of Endometrial Cancer by Stage	
Stage I	72.8%
Stage II	10.9%
Stage III	13.1%
Stage IV	3.2%

if high-risk histology or gross spread of disease is present at the time of surgery (common with type II endometrial cancers), removal of the omentum is recommended. Table 3 shows the typical stage distribution for endometrial carcinoma.

ADJUVANT THERAPY

Radiotherapy is currently the mainstay of adjuvant therapy for early stage endometrial carcinoma at risk for recurrence. Several trials have examined hormonal therapy or chemotherapy in an adjuvant setting for early stage disease, but none has shown any benefit in reducing recurrences.

Although 75% of endometrial carcinomas are found to be confined to the uterus after surgical staging, some patients will be at risk for recurrence and failure with surgical treatment only (Figure 1). Patients found to be at high risk for recurrence are treated with whole-pelvic radiotherapy after surgery, whereas patients who are at *intermediate* risk usually do not need radiotherapy, provided that they have been surgically staged. However, any adjuvant therapy for this group of patients remains controversial.

ADVANCED-STAGE OR RECURRENT DISEASE

A study conducted by the GOG showed that 36% of patients who were found to have metastasis to the para-aortic lymph nodes (stage IIIC) and were treated with radiotherapy were tumor free after 5 years. Similarly, if only pelvic lymph node metastasis (stage IIIC) was found and treated with radiotherapy, 72% would be alive at 5 years.

For serous or clear cell carcinomas found to have extrauterine spread at the time of surgery, *debulking* the metastasis and treating with chemotherapeutic regimens used for ovarian cancer have been shown to increase progression-free survival in several case series. Patients with gross intra-abdominal spread of endometrioid carcinoma generally have a grim prognosis and have not been shown to have prolonged survival with radiotherapy or chemotherapy. Therefore, these patients should be offered participation in clinical trials.

For most patients in whom cancer recurs, it will do so within 3 years of initial treatment. Unfortunately, if the recurrence is any place other than the pelvis (vaginal apex), the likelihood of long-term cure is poor. Depending on the location of the recurrence, radiotherapy, surgery, hormonal therapy, or chemotherapy can be used. Progestins have been studied for the treatment of recurrent disease but have demonstrated modest responses of limited duration.

FOLLOW-UP

Of the endometrial carcinomas that recur, most will do so within the first 3 years after treatment. Typically, the site of recurrence is in the pelvis, most commonly in

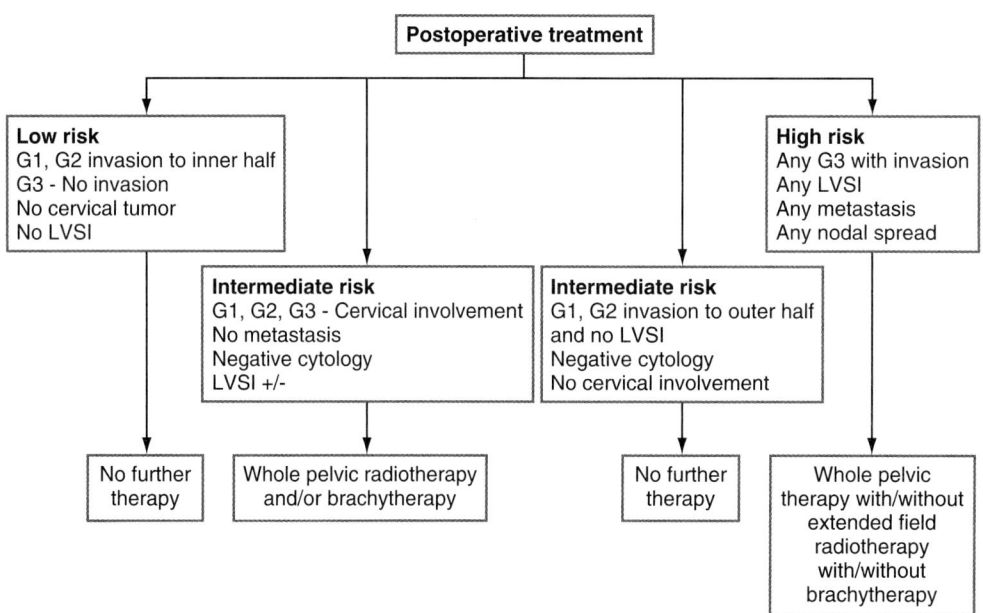

FIGURE 1. Postoperative treatment scheme at Memorial Health University Medical Center for surgical stage I endometrial carcinoma. G = grade; LVSI = lymphovascular space involvement.

Rakel and Bope: *Conn's Current Therapy 2006.*

the vaginal apex. Unfortunately a number of patients will have recurrence at distant sites such as the chest and upper part of the abdomen. Thus, patients treated for endometrial carcinoma are usually monitored closely for 5 years. At Memorial Health University Medical Center, we use an assessment program in which patients are seen every 3 months for the first year, every 4 months for the second year, and every 6 months until 5 years has elapsed since completion of treatment. In addition, a Papanicolaou (Pap) smear is performed at every visit, and chest radiographs are obtained annually for the first 2 years. Furthermore, annual mammography as well as counseling for screening colonoscopy is carried out. CT scanning is not generally used for surveillance in follow-up because of its high cost and low yield of detection. However, patients with abdominal symptoms may be assessed with CT because the likelihood of finding pathology is greater. For patients with advanced disease or high-risk histologic features, serum measurement of cancer antigen (CA) 125 may be considered. Table 4 shows 5-year survival rates of patients with endometrial carcinoma by stage.

TAMOXIFEN (NOLVADEX)

The National Surgical Adjuvant Breast and Bowel Project (NSABP) conducted a prevention trial with tamoxifen (Nolvadex), known as the P-1 trial. In this randomized, double-blind, prospective trial, women with high-risk family histories were treated with tamoxifen (Nolvadex) or placebo for 5 years. The trial demonstrated a 49% reduced risk for breast cancer, but a 2.5 times greater risk for endometrial carcinoma. Most of the endometrial carcinomas detected were stage I carcinomas, were of endometrioid histology (type I endometrial carcinoma), and were successfully treated with surgery. Additionally, other nonmalignant endometrial abnormalities were detected.

In addition to the use of tamoxifen (Nolvadex) for prevention of breast cancer, many women who have receptor-positive breast carcinomas are using tamoxifen (Nolvadex) for adjuvant treatment.

The question arises: How does one monitor patients taking tamoxifen (Nolvadex)? The consensus has been to not perform transvaginal ultrasonography or endometrial sampling in women who are asymptomatic. However, women who are taking tamoxifen (Nolvadex) and experience vaginal bleeding need to have an immediate evaluation by endometrial sampling to rule out endometrial carcinoma.

Although endometrial carcinoma remains the most common gynecologic malignancy in the United States, it is also the most curable because of its low stage at diagnosis. Surgery remains the primary treatment modality for this type of carcinoma, with adjuvant radiotherapy reserved for patients at high risk for recurrent disease after surgery. Chemotherapeutic and hormonal agents have been used to palliate advanced-stage or recurrent disease, but durable, long-term survival has not been demonstrated. Finally, women who are taking tamoxifen (Nolvadex) for prophylaxis or adjuvant treatment of breast carcinoma need no special surveillance for the development of endometrial carcinoma. However, should any postmenopausal or abnormal vaginal bleeding occur in this group of women, immediate evaluation by endometrial sampling is required.

Cancer of the Uterine Cervix

Method of
Michael P. Hopkins, MD, and Wilson Sawa, MD

Epidemiology

Invasive cancer of the cervix in the United States has decreased in morbidity and mortality significantly over the past 50 years, in large part because of mass efforts with Papanicolaou (Pap) cytologic screening. Pap smears identify many with preinvasive disease, allowing treatment prior to the development of invasive disease. In the developing world, however, cervical cancer is the third most common malignancy and accounts for significant mortality. Whereas in the United States approximately 12,000 new cases of this disease occur annually, worldwide there are approximately 500,000 new cases with 200,000 deaths. It is five to eight times more common in women affected with AIDS or HIV and represents an enormous health problem in those countries most afflicted by the virus.

The probability of a woman in the United States developing a cervical cancer is approximately 1 in 120, but this statistic is age dependent, with the highest incidence between the ages of 40 and 49 years. Invasive cervical cancer in the United States is largely reduced because of cytologic screening. Approximately 2 million abnormal Pap smears are found annually in the United States, but fortunately the vast majority are in the premalignant phase.

The risk factors for cervical cancer are closely associated with early age of intercourse, multiple sexual partners, and smoking. The unifying etiology is linked with the human papillomavirus (HPV), which is sexually transmitted. More than 90% of squamous carcinomas of the cervix have HPV DNA present, and a large percentage (more than 90%) of adenocarcinoma of the cervix

TABLE 4 Endometrial Cancer: Five-Year Survival Rate by Stage	
Stage	**5-year survival rate**
Stage IA	91%
Stage IB	88%
Stage IC	81%
Stage II	72%
Stage III	51%
Stage IV	9%

have HPV present. The high-risk HPV types include HPV-16, -18, -31, -33, and -35.

Invasive cancer is preceded by a process of cellular dysplasia that may exist for years before transitioning. The dysplastic areas termed *squamous intraepithelial lesions* also contain HPV DNA, providing strong evidence that the premalignant phase will transition into the invasive phase and the underlying etiology is also the HPV virus. Almost all the factors that increase a woman's risk of cervical cancer are associated with increased exposure to HPV. These include multiple sexual partners, early age of intercourse, contraceptive use, socioeconomic status, other venereal diseases (including herpes simplex), and cigarette smoking. Cigarette smoking may be related to cervical cancer not only because of indirect association with increased sexual activity but also because of carcinogenic cofactors found in the tobacco or possible mitigation of cervical mucosal immunologic factors that protect against HPV.

Pathophysiology

The best evidence suggests that HPV virus is the primary pathophysiologic etiology for premalignant and malignant disease of the cervix. The HPV family consists of more than 50 subtypes, classified as either low risk or high risk based on the ability to transform cells into malignancy. The high-risk cell types include HPV-16, -18, -31, -33, -35, and -51. The HPV produces an oncogenic DNA protein in E6 and E7. The epitome is incorporated into the cell that subsequently interferes with the normal cell tumor suppressor gene p53 and RB (retinoblastoma gene). This then produces a premalignant growth called squamous intraepithelial lesion or dysplasia. The cells most susceptible to infection and transformation are located in the transformation zone where the squamous epithelium is overriding the columnar epithelium, producing a metaplastic process. The dysplastic cells, especially low-grade changes, are confined to the lower level of the epithelium and may regress spontaneously in approximately 30% to 40% of patients. As transformation proceeds into a high-grade change, they are far less likely to regress spontaneously, and they eventually attain the potential to invade the basement membrane or become an invasive process. From this point on, the malignant cells invade the stroma of the cervix, eventually into the angiolymphatic spaces, and cause a local mass or ulcer through which they eventually metastasize. Hematogenous spread is less likely, but metastasis to the liver, lung, bone, and brain can occur.

Clinical Symptomatology

The symptoms of cervical cancer vary according to the extent of the disease. In the premalignant phase there are virtually no symptoms, although occasionally patients have some discharge. As a lesion begins to develop on the cervix, the hallmark symptom is postcoital bleeding, so any patient with postcoital bleeding

should be investigated. As the disease progresses, the symptoms of advanced cervical cancer are sciatica and leg edema when the disease is extending into the side wall. Physical findings are usually confined to the pelvis with advanced disease, although adenopathy in the supraclavicular or inguinal region is a possibility. The cervix either develops an ulcerative exophytic-type lesion or if it is developing in the canal, an expanding so-called barrel-shaped cervix develops with an exocervix that can appear normal. When there is a lesion on the cervix, a watery, bloody, or purulent discharge is often present. The diagnosis of cervical cancer is made by a biopsy providing a tissue diagnosis. A Pap smear is a screening test, so even though it may come back from pathology as carcinoma, a tissue biopsy must be obtained. A gross lesion of the cervix, even in the presence of a normal Pap smear, should be biopsied to avoid the misdiagnosis from a false-negative Pap smear. When an abnormal Pap smear is discovered, a colposcopy is usually performed with directed biopsies followed by further diagnostic testing. A biopsy of a grossly visible lesion with the diagnosis of invasive cancer does not mandate a cone biopsy, which should be done if there is any diagnostic question or in the presence of a biopsy that shows microinvasion. The only way to diagnose microinvasion is to have a cone biopsy with negative margins. If the colposcopy suggests invasive cancer and the biopsy does not provide the finding, a cone biopsy is necessary for diagnosis.

Pathology

The most frequent histologic subtype of cervical cancer is squamous cell cancer, accounting for approximately 80% of cases. The other main subtype, which accounts for the other 20%, is adenoma carcinoma, which can take on a variety of forms including adenosquamous, clear cell, papillary, glassy cell, mucoid type, or adenoma malignum. The percentage of adenocarcinomas is increasing because of the decreasing number of squamous cell cancers and an apparent real increase in the number of adenocarcinomas. Other rare pathologic types that can involve the cervix include melanomas, sarcomas, and small cell neuroendocrine or metastatic lesions. The literature is divided on whether the squamous cell and adenocarcinoma cell types have a similar prognosis. When corrected for tumor differentiation and stage, the survival is approximate between the cell types. The most aggressive cell type is the small cell neuroendocrine type, but fortunately these are very rare on the cervix.

Staging

Staging is one of the most critical prognostic indicators for survival, largely because of the extent of the disease and the risk for lymph node metastasis. Cervical cancer is one of the few malignancies still staged clinically, mainly because beyond stage I disease, surgery is not the treatment of choice. Rather, radiotherapy is the main

TABLE 1 International Federation of Obstetricians and Gynecologists (FIGO) Staging for Carcinoma of the Cervix (1995)

Stage 0	Carcinoma in situ, intraepithelial carcinoma
Stage I	Cancer confined to the cervix
Ia1	Microscopic invasion of stroma measuring 3 mm or less in depth and 7 mm or less in width
Ia2	Microscopic invasion of stroma measuring more than 3 mm in depth but not greater than 5 mm in depth or greater than 7 mm in width
Ib1	Lesions greater than in Ia2 but not greater than 4 cm
Ib2	Lesions greater than 4 cm
Stage II	Cancer extends beyond the cervix
IIa	Cancer involves the upper two thirds of the vagina
IIb	Obvious parametrial extension
Stage III	Extension of cancer to pelvic wall or lower vagina
IIIa	Cancer involves lower one third of vagina
IIIb	Cancer extends to pelvic wall or hydronephrosis or nonfunctioning kidney
Stage IV	
IVa	Cancer involves the bladder or rectal mucosa
IVb	Cancer metastasis to distant organs

therapy for any cervical cancer beyond stage I and also can be effective for stage I cervix cancer. The system employed for cervical cancer is the FIGO (International Federation of Obstetricians and Gynecologists) staging scheme. The stage is based on the natural route of cancer progression and the risk of lymph node metastasis. The latter relates directly to the depth of stromal invasion in stage I disease and then to the stage of disease afterward (Tables 1 and 2).

Under the FIGO system, the only acceptable diagnostic imaging studies that can be employed in addition to clinical exam are intravenous pyelogram, chest radiography, cystoscopy, and sigmoidoscopy, because in developing countries further sophisticated imaging

TABLE 2 Relationship Between Stromal Invasion or Staging and the Incidence of Lymph Node Metastasis

Invasion or Stage	Pelvic Nodes (% Positive)	Aortic Nodes (% Positive)
Less than 3 mm	0-1	
3-5 mm	2.5-5	
6-10 mm	4-8	
11-15 mm	10-25	
Ib1	15-25	5-10
Ib2	30-50	15-20
IIa	15-25	5-10
IIb	30-45	20
III	50	30

Rakel and Bope: *Conn's Current Therapy 2006.*

studies are not routinely available. In North America, sophisticated imaging studies are routinely performed for cervical cancer although not technically incorporated into the staging. These include computerized tomography (CT) and occasionally magnetic resonance imaging (MRI). In the absence of symptoms, bone scan for occult metastasis is rarely indicated. CT scans are a common pretreatment evaluation in patients with stages II to IV cancers. Their sensitivity in detecting lymph node metastasis is approximately 65%. Evaluation of suspicious lymph nodes may involve CT-guided percutaneous biopsy or retroperitoneal selective lymph node dissection. This information may alter or define treatment, but it does not change the clinical stage based on the accepted procedures. Surgical staging, employed in the past, is rarely used now except in selected institutions.

Treatment

The treatment of cervical cancer is based on the stage of disease and the patient's age and medical condition. All three modalities—chemotherapy, radiation therapy, and surgery—are used to manage invasive cervical cancer. Patients with microinvasive disease with stromal invasion less than 3 mm can be treated by conservative measures. A cone biopsy with negative margins ensures that no disease remains in the cervix. When microinvasive disease is present, expectant observation is appropriate treatment, allowing patients to preserve childbearing should they desire. In those patients for whom preservation of fertility is not an issue, a standard extrafascial hysterectomy is employed. In patients with stages Ia2, Ib1, Ib2, and in selected patients with stage IIa, radical surgery can be used. These patients can also be treated with radiation therapy. Radical hysterectomy provides an excellent overall survival for patients with early-stage cervical cancer. A radical hysterectomy is more extensive than its standard counterpart, removing lateral parametrium and a portion of the upper vagina. A lymph node dissection is also performed to identify those patients with lymph node metastasis who are at high risk of recurrence. Because cervical cancer, either adenocarcinoma or squamous cell, virtually never metastasizes to the ovaries, surgical treatment allows for preservation of ovarian function, making it the ideal operation in the patient under 40 years. Alternatively, in the population over 80 years, the vagina is quite narrowed and atrophic with the cervix flush to the fornices, so radiation treatment is often inadequate. These patients occasionally benefit from radical surgeries if their medical condition permits it. Following radical surgery patients may require radiation therapy based on high-risk features such as positive lymph nodes, positive surgical margins, and deep invasion into the cervix. In patients who are at high risk for recurrence after radical hysterectomy because of these factors, radiotherapy reduces the risk of recurrence by approximately 50%. The standard therapy for advanced disease in stages IIb to IV is with radiation therapy, both external and internal, combined with chemotherapy.

Concurrent weekly cisplatin (Platinol AQ)[1] is the usual regimen. Adjuvant chemotherapy with radiation is now routine and provides a significant improvement in survival by up to 15% to 20%. Radiation therapy typically consists of full-course external beam 45 to 50 Gy administered over 25 days by a high-energy linear accelerator, followed by intracavitary radiation with either one or two intracavitary tandem treatments or high dose after loading brachytherapy, which is now done on an outpatient basis. This provides for an additional 30 to 35 Gy to point A (a point 2 cm lateral to the internal cervical os).

Radical trachelectomy is offered as an alternative to radical abdominal or vaginal hysterectomy for patients with early-stage squamous cell cervical cancer who are interested in preserving their reproductive function. This procedure consists of removal of the cervix and the parametrium, pelvic lymph node dissection, and placement of cervical cerclage. The selected patients are in stages Ia to Ib, with most of the reported cases in stage Ib1 or lower. In addition, patients must have negative lymph nodes. The survival rates are comparable to those achieved by radical hysterectomy for similar stage and grade cervical cancer, although the number of patients treated by this new technique is limited.

Survival

Survival is related to stage and lymph node status. Table 3 shows general 5-year survival rates without concurrent chemotherapy. The survival for stage I treated by radical hysterectomy and pelvic lymphadenectomy compared to radiotherapy is equal. The survival for stage I treated with either radiotherapy or radical surgery is approximately 90% when lymph nodes are negative. This statistic drops significantly depending on the lymph node status, with survival dropping down to 60% for unilateral lymph node positivity compared to approximately 40% when lymph nodes are involved bilaterally.

Patients with normal lymph nodes but high-risk cervical factors experience a 2-year disease-free survival

---

[1]Not FDA approved for this indication.

TABLE 3 Five-Year Survival Rates for Cervical Cancer by Stage

Stage	Survival (%)
Ia1	99-100
Ia2	95
Ib1	85-90
Ib2	65-75
IIa	75-80
IIb	65
IIIa	45
IIIb	35
IV	15

of 88% when treated by postoperative pelvic radiation. In contrast, the prognosis for patients with positive nodes falls to approximately 65%. Because postoperative pelvic radiotherapy does not convincingly improve that survival, researchers are investigating postoperative chemoradiotherapy for these patients with positive pelvic nodes. This has also been reported to reduce the risk of death by 45% as an alternative. The approximate 5-year survival for locally advanced disease with a combination of chemotherapy and radiation is approximately 60%.

Surveillance

After primary treatment by either surgery or radiotherapy, patients return every 3 to 4 months for 2 years, then semiannually for an additional 3 years, followed by annual visits afterward. Physical examination and a Pap smear are routine. Annual chest radiography is optional, and CT scan should be reserved for symptomatic or high-risk patients because the yield of routine follow-up with CT scans is minimal.

Recurrent Cancer

The sites of recurrence are local recurrence in the pelvis, liver, lung, bone, lymph nodes, and brain. Although 75% are diagnosed within the first 24 months and 90% within the first 3 years, late recurrences can occur. The treatment for localized recurring cancer in the pelvis following radiation primary radiation or chemoradiation is pelvic exenteration, which consists of removal of the entire pelvic viscera, including uterus, vagina, bladder, and rectum or some combination. This operation should only be reserved if metastatic disease is not present. Preoperative and intraoperative assessment for metastatic disease excludes nearly three fourths of the patients from having this operation either initiated or completed. Patients who do undergo exenteration experience a 40% to 60% 5-year survival when margins and lymph nodes are negative.

Pelvic recurrence following primary surgical treatment usually involves the pelvic wall or the central pelvis. These patients should receive radiation, including both external radiation and intracavitary or interstitial radiotherapy. Chemotherapy can be combined with it and is a well-accepted method for treating recurrence. The use of chemotherapy with radiation for recurrence is not as well studied as for primary treatment. The treatment of distant metastasis is limited to chemotherapy, whereas radiation can be used for palliative treatment for metastatic disease to the bone or the brain. Chemotherapy consists of cisplatin (Platinol AQ) alone or in combination with topotecan (Hycamtin),[1] which has a reported response rate of approximately 30% to 40%. Although this must be viewed as palliative, if the patient is willing it should be initiated for symptomatic relief and prolongation of life.

---

[1]Not FDA approved for this indication.

REFERENCES

Keys HM, Bundy BN, Stehman FB, et al: Cisplatin, radiation, and adjuvant hysterectomy compared with radiation and adjuvant hysterectomy for bulky stage IB cervical carcinoma. N Engl J Med 1999;340(15):1154-1161.

Peters WA III, Liu PY, Barrett RJ II, et al: Concurrent chemotherapy and pelvic radiation therapy compared with pelvic radiation therapy alone as adjuvant therapy after radical surgery in high-risk early-stage cancer of the cervix. J Clin Oncol 2000;18(8):1606-1613.

Rose PG, Bundy BN, Watkins EB, et al: Concurrent cisplatin-based radiotherapy and chemotherapy for locally advanced cervical cancer. N Engl J Med 1999;340(15):1144-1153.

Neoplasms of the Vulva

Method of
Susan A. Davidson, MD

The female external genitalia includes the mons pubis, labia majora, labia minora, clitoris, perineal body, and the structures of the vaginal introitus or vestibule. Whether benign or malignant, vulvar neoplasms are uncommon, occur at all ages, and have varying characteristics. Therefore liberal use of biopsies is usually required for diagnosis and to guide treatment.

Benign Cystic Neoplasms

Benign cystic lesions of the vulva include Bartholin's duct cyst, sebaceous and epidermal inclusion cysts, mucinous cysts, Skene duct cysts, and cysts of the canal of Nuck. Bartholin's duct cyst, located in the posterior labia near the vaginal introitus, is most common. Treatment is usually not required in asymptomatic young women (<40 years). If the cyst is symptomatic or infected, however, drainage by marsupialization or use of a Word catheter, is indicated. Bartholin's gland carcinomas are rare, especially in women younger than 40 years of age. But if the mass feels firm or nodular, it should be biopsied.

Sebaceous and epidermal inclusion cysts are also common. They are prone to infection but rarely malignant. If an infection develops, they should be incised and drained. Mucinous cysts are rare and possibly arise from the minor vestibular glands. They are located anteriorly on the vulva, typically on the inner labia minora. Skene duct cysts are located next to the urethra. Excision of these cysts is necessary only if symptomatic.

Cysts of the canal of Nuck are located in the anterior portion of the labia majora at the termination of the insertion of the round ligament. These cysts represent herniation of the peritoneum through the inguinal canal and contain peritoneal fluid. If symptomatic, excision must be accompanied by closure of the fascial defect to prevent recurrence.

Rakel and Bope: Conn's Current Therapy 2006.

Benign Solid Neoplasms

The benign solid tumors of the vulva include fibromas, myomas, lipomas, hidradenomas, syringomas, myoblastomas, vestibular adenomas, and angiomas, among others. Benign pigmented lesions, such as nevi and seborrheic keratoses, may occasionally be found. Malignancy is rare, but most should be excised for diagnostic and therapeutic purposes.

CONDYLOMA ACUMINATUM

Vulvar condyloma acuminatum is a sexually transmitted verrucous lesion of the vulva caused by human papilloma virus (HPV), most frequently types 6 and 11. These lesions are warty growths that frequently cover large areas of the vulva. Smoking and immunosuppression are risk factors. Representative biopsies should be obtained to document disease and rule out malignancy. Wide local excision can be used for small lesions, although these growths are usually best treated by ablation.

Chemical ablative techniques include topical application of trichloroacetic acid (Tri-Chlor), podofilox (0.5%, Condylox), 5-fluorouracil[1] (1%, Fluoroplex or 5%, Efudex),[1] or imiquimod (5%, Aldara). Podophyllin can be applied twice daily for 3 days, repeated weekly for 4 weeks. Imiquimod can be applied three times per week for up to 16 weeks. Podophyllin and 5-fluorouracil should not be used in women who could become pregnant. Surgical ablative therapies include CO_2 laser vaporization and use of the Cavitron ultrasonic aspirator (CUSA), especially for extensive disease.

Intraepithelial Neoplasms of the Vulva

VULVAR INTRAEPITHELIAL NEOPLASIA

Vulvar intraepithelial neoplasia (VIN) is a dysplastic condition of the squamous epithelium whose incidence is increasing, especially in younger women. Risk factors are HPV types 16 and 18, smoking, and immunosuppression. Symptoms include pruritis (most common), pain, a noticeable lesion, and discoloration. Most patients with HPV-related disease have multifocal lesions including vaginal and cervical dysplasia. The most common location is in the area of the posterior fourchette and perineal body. Typical findings are raised white, gray, red, or mottled lesions; application of 4% acetic acid for several minutes can help identify faint lesions and outline abnormal vascular patterns. Diagnosis of VIN is made by punch biopsies through full thickness of the epithelium to rule out invasion, present in 20% of patients with VIN III (full-thickness dysplasia or carcinoma in situ). Of those patients with invasion, half (10% of VIN III) have invasion more than 1 mm.

Treatment of VIN can be categorized into excisional and ablative therapies. Patients at risk for microinvasion (unifocal disease, raised lesions, older age, and

_____
[1]Not FDA approved for this indication.

prior radiation) should have the lesion excised completely if possible. Skinning vulvectomy is rarely used because of psychological and sexual consequences related to scarring and disfigurement.

The ablative therapies can be divided into mechanical and chemical. The mechanical method most commonly used is the CO_2 laser, although use of the CUSA is also described. Both can ablate large or multifocal lesions successfully with an excellent cosmetic and functional outcome. The chemical method most commonly used is topical 5-fluorouracil (5%, Efudex).[1] Because of its teratogenic potential, it should not be used in women who could become pregnant. It can be applied on two consecutive nights weekly for 10 weeks. An alternative ablative therapy is use of imiquimod[1] (Aldara), as described earlier. Because of the irritation caused by these topical therapies, many patients have problems with treatment compliance. Residual disease should be excised to rule out invasion.

Patients with VIN frequently have recurrent disease, regardless of the treatment method used (Table 1). Continued smoking increases this risk, so patients should be counseled in smoking cessation. In those patients whose cancers recur and are retreated, subsequent 5-fluorouracil prophylaxis, with a single application biweekly, is used successfully to minimize further recurrences.

PAGET'S DISEASE

Paget's disease of the vulva is an uncommon condition characterized by a patchy, eczematoid lesion that frequently covers much of the vulva. Most patients are post-menopausal and present with complaints of pruritus. Although Paget's disease is an in situ disease process, 15% to 25% of patients have an underlying malignancy, usually an adenocarcinoma of the apocrine glands but occasionally an invasive Paget's. In addition, up to 30% of patients have a synchronous adenocarcinoma of the breast, colon, rectum, or upper genital tract. Screening for these cancers is therefore recommended. To assess for invasion, the lesion should be excised via wide local excision or simple vulvectomy with at least 5 mm of the adjacent subcutaneous tissue. Achieving negative margin status is frequently difficult. However, the risk of recurrence is approximately 30% whether margins are negative or positive. Thus expectant management,

[1]Not FDA approved for this indication.

TABLE 1 Recurrence of Vulvar Intraepithelial Neoplasia III

Treatment Method	% Recurrence
Chemical ablation	20-40
Mechanical ablation	20-40
Wide local excision	
Negative margin	15-25
Positive margin	30-45

TABLE 2 Incidence of Regional Node Metastases by Depth of Tumor Invasion

Depth of Invasion (mm)	% Positive Inguinal Nodes
<1	1-5
1-3	10-15
3-5	15-30
5-10	30-45
>10	>40

reserving treatment for symptomatic recurrences, is usually recommended.

Invasive Vulvar Lesions

Less than 5% of gynecologic cancers arise on the vulva. Approximately 85% are squamous cell carcinomas. The etiology of this type appears mixed. Up to 50% evolve from VIN III and are usually associated with HPV-16. These women are slightly younger (age 45-52 years). Most arise in older women (mean age 60-69 years), and suggested risk factors include immunosuppression, hypertension, diabetes mellitus, obesity, and chronic vulvar inflammation. Other histologic types are melanomas (5% to 10%), basal cell carcinomas (2% to 3%), adenocarcinomas (1%), and sarcomas (1% to 2%) Most patients present with a combination of symptoms, including pruritus, discomfort, and complaints of a mass. Examination frequently reveals a suspicious lesion, which should be biopsied for diagnosis. Vulvar cancers typically spread by local extension and lymphatic dissemination. Factors that influence dissemination include tumor size (Table 2), depth of invasion (Table 3), lymphovascular space invasion, and tumor grade. Staging is surgical and classified using the tumor, nodes, and metastasis (TNM) system (Box 1) as well as the International Federation of Gynecology and Obstetrics (FIGO) system (Box 2).

SQUAMOUS CELL CARCINOMAS AND ADENOCARCINOMAS

Surgical management of squamous cell carcinomas and adenocarcinomas depends on the size, depth of invasion, and location of the lesion. The vulvar lesion is managed

TABLE 3 Incidence of Regional Node Metastases by Tumor Diameter

Tumor Diameter (cm)	% Positive Inguinal Nodes
<1	0-15
5-20	
25-35	
35-50	
≥50	≥50

BOX 1   **TNM Classification of Vulvar Carcinoma**

T	Primary tumor
Tis	Carcinoma in situ
T1	Confined to vulva, diameter ≤2 cm
T2	Confined to vulva, diameter >2 cm
T3	Adjacent spread to urethra, vagina, perineum, or anus (any size)
T4	Infiltration of upper urethral mucosa, bladder, rectum, or bone
N	Regional lymph nodes
N0	No lymph node metastases
N1	Unilateral regional lymph node metastasis
N2	Bilateral regional lymph node metastasis
M	Distant metastases
M0	No clinical metastases
M1	Distant metastasis (including pelvic lymph node metastasis)

Abbreviation: TNM = tumor, node, metastasis.

TABLE 4   **Survival Rate by FIGO Stage for Patients With Invasive Squamous Cell Vulvar Cancer**

FIGO stage	% Surviving 5 years
I	70-90
II	50-80
III	30-50
IV	10-15

Abbreviation: FIGO = International Federation of Gynecology and Obstetrics.

chronic lymphedema. For patients with very large lesions or lesions in sensitive areas such as the clitoris, preoperative radiation, followed by less radical excision of residual disease, may minimize problems with the vulvar wound. Current investigations are ongoing in the use of sentinel lymph node dissections as a method of minimizing the groin morbidity without sacrificing survival. Positive vulvar margins or metastases to lymph nodes are managed with postoperative radiation. Survival depends on stage at diagnosis (Table 4).

MALIGNANT MELANOMA

Malignant melanoma is the second most common vulvar malignancy. Most patients have disease on the mucosal surfaces of the vulvar introitus, clitoris, and labia minora. The vulvar lesion is treated by radical excision, but management of the groins is controversial. The risk of spread is significant with a tumor thickness greater than 0.75 mm, but survival at 5 years is only approximately 10% with groin node metastases. Some argue against node dissection for this reason. However, given some long-term survivors with modern melanoma therapy, either lymphadenectomy or sentinel lymph node dissection, as is done for other cutaneous melanomas, appears indicated.

VERRUCOUS CARCINOMA

Verrucous carcinoma is a large exophytic tumor that resembles giant condyloma acuminatum. It is a variant

with a radical excision. Management of the groins is based on depth of invasion. Lesions with invasion of 1 mm have minimal risk of lymphatic spread and do not require lymphadenectomy. All others require surgical assessment of the lymph nodes. Lesions located in the midline structures require bilateral groin dissection, whereas lateral lesions are managed with ipsilateral groin dissection. This surgical approach is associated with significant morbidity including disfigurement, wound breakdown, and problems with lymphocysts and

BOX 2   **FIGO Classification (With Corresponding TNM Classification) for Vulvar Carcinoma**

Stage I (T1N0M0)	Tumor confined to vulva and/or perineum, ≤2 cm in greatest dimension; nodes are negative
Stage IA	Stromal invasion no greater than 1 mm
Stage IB	Stromal invasion >1 mm
Stage II (T2N0M0)	Tumor confined to the vulva and/or perineum, >2 cm in greatest dimension; nodes are negative
Stage III	
T3N0M0	Tumor of any size with adjacent spread to the lower urethra and/or the vagina or the anus
T3N1M0 T2N1M0	Unilateral regional lymph node metastasis
Stage IVA	
T1N2M0 T2N2M0	Tumor invades any of the following: upper urethra, bladder mucosa, rectal mucosa, pelvic bone, and/or bilateral regional node metastasis
T3N2M0 T4 any N M0	
Stage IVB	
Any T any N M1	Any distant metastasis including pelvic lymph nodes

Abbreviations: FIGO = International Federation of Gynecology and Obstetrics; TNM = tumor, node, metastasis.

 CURRENT DIAGNOSIS

- Most cystic lesions are benign. Excision is reserved for symptomatic cysts and suspicious Bartholin's gland cysts, especially in women older than 40 years of age.
- All solid lesions should be biopsied for diagnostic purposes.
- Multifocal disease requires multiple biopsies to rule out invasive disease.
- Most premalignant and malignant lesions cause pruritus, discomfort, or a noticeable lesion.
- The vagina and cervix in women with dysplastic or malignant vulvar lesions should be evaluated.

CURRENT THERAPY

- Benign solid lesions should be excised.
- After ablative treatment of vulvar intraepithelial neoplasia (VIN), excise any residual lesions to rule out occult invasive disease.
- Avoid podophyllin and 5-fluorouracil in women of reproductive potential.
- Rule out synchronous neoplasms in women with Paget's disease.
- Invasion more than 1 mm requires radical excision and lymph node evaluation.

of squamous carcinomas but has an excellent prognosis because of the lack of metastases. Verrucous carcinomas have a high tendency to recur and should be managed with radical local excision.

BASAL CELL CARCINOMA

Basal cell carcinomas typically occur in elderly white women, are commonly located on the labia majora, and have characteristics similar to basal cell carcinomas at other sites. Treatment is wide local excision only because metastases are rare. Basal cell carcinomas are prone to local recurrence, however. A malignant squamous component must be ruled out because it should be managed as a squamous cell carcinoma.

SARCOMAS

Leiomyosarcoma is the most common vulvar sarcoma and usually arises in the labia majora. Malignant fibrous histiocytoma is the second most common. Management of these lesions is radical vulvar excision.

REFERENCES

Garland SM: Imiquimod. Curr Opin Infect Dis 2003;16:85-89.
Homesley HD, Bundy BN, Sedlis A, et al: Prognostic factors for groin node metastasis in squamous cell carcinoma of the vulva (a Gynecologic Oncology Group study). Gynecol Oncol 1993;49:279-283.
Krebs HB: The use of topical 5-fluorouracil in the treatment of genital condylomas. Obstet Gynecol Clin North Am 1987;14(2):559-568.
Modesitt SC, Waters AB, Walton L, et al: Vulvar intraepithelial neoplasia III: Occult cancer and the impact of margin status on recurrence. Obstet Gynecol 1998;92(6):962-966.
Phillips GL, Bundy BN, Okagaki T, et al: Malignant melanoma of the vulva treated by radical hemivulvectomy, a prospective study of the Gynecologic Oncology Group. Cancer 1994;73:2626-2632.
Tebes S, Cardosi R, Hoffman M: Paget's disease of the vulva. Am J Obstet Gynecol 2002;187:281-284.
Trimble CL, Trimble EL, Woodruff JD: Diseases of the vulva. In Hernandez E, Atkinson BF (eds): Clinical Gynecologic Pathology. Philadelphia, WB Saunders, 1995, pp 1-90.
Wright VC, Chapman WB: Colposcopy of intraepithelial neoplasia of the vulva and adjacent sites. Obstet Gynecol Clin North Am 1993;20(1):231-255.

Contraception

Method of
Lama L. Tolaymat, MD, MPH, and
Andrew Kaunitz, MD

Each year, nearly 2% of U.S. women of reproductive age have an induced abortion. This sobering statistic underscores the importance of women and couples having access to the effective hormonal, intrauterine, and surgical methods of contraception described here.

Estrogen/Progestin Combination Oral Contraceptive Pills

Oral contraceptive (OC) use is safe for the majority of users with many noncontraceptive benefits, such as decreasing the risk of endometrial cancer, ovarian cancer, dysmenorrhea, menorrhagia, ectopic pregnancy, pelvic inflammatory disease, and acne. Although OCs represent a highly effective birth control method for correct consistent users, inconsistent or incorrect use accounts for the annual failure rate of 8% experienced overall by OC users.

OCs are usually initiated on the first day of menses or the first Sunday after menses starts. In these cases, a backup method of contraception is not needed. It is helpful to associate pill-taking with a daily routine such as tooth-brushing to improve compliance.

Conventional combination OC formulations include 21 active and 7 inactive tablets; one formulation (Mircette) includes 2 days of inactive tablets and 5 ethinyl estradiol tablets in place of the 7 inactive tablets. Some future OC formulations will likely contain 24 to 25 active tablets followed by 4 or 3 inactive tablets. The progestin component of the OCs suppresses the pituitary secretion of luteinizing hormone (LH), preventing ovulation. The estrogen component (ethinyl estradiol) suppresses secretion of follicle-stimulating hormone (FSH) and enhances cycle control (regular withdrawal bleeding with minimal unscheduled or so-called breakthrough bleeding). If 1 or 2 tablets are missed, the patient should take 1 tablet as soon as possible. Then 1 tablet should be taken twice a day until all the missed tablets are taken. Breast tenderness and nausea, common OC side effects, are related to the estrogen dose. Accordingly, if these side effects persist for more than several cycles, changing to a lower estrogen dose (e.g., switching from a 30- to 35-μg to a 20- to 25-μg) formulation may be useful. Breakthrough (unscheduled) bleeding and spotting occurs more often in women taking 20-μg estrogen OCs than in those taking 30- to 35-μg formulations. Box 1 lists medical contraindications to all estrogen-progestin contraceptives.

Progestin-Only Oral Contraceptives

Also known as minipills, progestin-only OC formulations (Micronor) contain even lower doses than

---

- Smokers: Age 35 years or older
- Hypertension: Uncontrolled or age 35 years or older
- Diabetes: Vascular disease or age 35 years or older
- Migraines: Focal neurologic symptoms or age 35 years or older
- Vascular disease: Associated with systemic lupus erythematosus
- Personal history of breast cancer or thromboembolism
- Coronary artery or cerebrovascular disease
- Acute or chronic hepatocellular disease with abnormal liver function
- Cholestatic jaundice with prior pregnancy or contraceptive use

Adapted from http://www.arhp.org/healthcareproviders/cme/onlinecme/wellwoman/TOC.cfm?ID=336.

---

combination OCs. The documented rates of failure for progestin-only pills are comparable to those of combination OCs in women who are meticulous about taking the pill at the same time every day. If one pill is taken 3 or more hours late, backup contraception is needed for 48 hours. Most commonly in the United States, minipills are used by lactating women who intrinsically have low fecundability; in this subgroup of women, contraceptive failures with progestin-only OC use are not common.

Extended-Cycle Oral Contraceptives

The first extended-cycle OC (Seasonale) to be marketed in the United States includes 84 (12 weeks) of active pills followed by 7 placebo pills, rather than the conventional 21 active tablets followed by 7 placebos. Each active pill contains 150 µg of levonorgestrel and 30 µg of ethinyl estradiol. Over time, this extended approach to OC leads to 4 rather than 13 withdrawal bleeding episodes each year. Women considering extended OC use should be counseled to expect an initially higher rate of breakthrough bleeding and spotting, which declines over time. Women with a history of menorrhagia or dysmenorrhea may be candidates for extended-cycle OC use. In the future, extended-cycle OC formulations with *no* hormone-free days may become available.

Emergency Contraception

With the manufacturer no longer making a dedicated combination emergency contraception (EC) formulation (Preven) as of summer 2004, the only dedicated EC formulation currently available is the progestin-only formulation (Plan B), which consists of two levonorgestrel 750-µg tablets.

Progestin-only EC is more effective and causes less nausea and emesis than combination EC. Package labeling for Plan B indicates that 1 tablet should be taken within 72 hours of unprotected intercourse,

followed 12 hours later by a second tablet. Taking the 2 tablets together, however, may be as effective in preventing pregnancy as dividing the dose. Furthermore, Plan B may retain its efficacy in pregnancy prevention when taken up to 5 days after unprotected intercourse.

Injectable Contraception

PROGESTIN ONLY

Depomedroxyprogesterone acetate (DMPA) (Depo-Provera) is an injectable contraceptive that provides long-acting reversible birth control, as effective as sterilization. The standard dose is 150 mg (1 mL) of DMPA intramuscularly every 3 months (or every 12 to 13 weeks). As with combination OC use, DMPA suppresses ovulation and ovarian estradiol production. In contrast with combination OC use, DMPA includes no estrogen component. Therefore, bone mineral density (BMD) declines among long-term users of DMPA. Fortunately, BMD rapidly recovers after discontinuation of DMPA, and no evidence indicates that DMPA use causes postmenopausal osteoporosis or fractures.

Although concerns regarding weight gain may discourage some women, randomized clinical trial data found that DMPA did not cause weight gain or increased appetite in short-term users. A subcutaneous DMPA formulation that should facilitate self-administration became available in 2005.

COMBINATION ESTROGEN-PROGESTIN INJECTABLE CONTRACEPTION

Lunelle was approved in 2000 as a monthly injection. This method is associated with regular bleeding episodes and a rapid return to fertility. In 2003, however, the manufacturer discontinued availability of this formulation in the United States.

Combination Patch

Ortho Evra is a once-a-week transdermal contraceptive patch applied for 3 consecutive weeks, followed by a patch-free week during which withdrawal bleeding is anticipated. The patch can be applied to the lower abdomen, upper outer arm, buttock, or upper torso (except for the breast). The patch delivers a daily systemic dose of 150 µg of norelgestromin and 20 µg of ethinyl estradiol. In a randomized clinical trial, the contraceptive efficacy of the patch was comparable to that of oral contraception. If the patch is detached for greater than 24 hours, the user should start a new patch cycle and use a backup contraceptive method (such as condoms) for 1 week.

Combination Vaginal Ring

NuvaRing is worn for 3 weeks, then removed for 1 week, during which withdrawal bleeding is anticipated.

The ring is composed of a flexible ethylene vinyl acetate copolymer, which releases approximately 120 µg of etonogestrel and 15 µg of ethinyl estradiol per day. The ring is self-inserted. In comparative clinical trials, rates of breakthrough bleeding and spotting were lower with the ring than with OCs. As with the patch, contraceptive efficacy of the ring is similar to that of combination OCs in clinical trials. Backup contraception is needed for 7 days if the ring remains outside of the vagina for more than 3 hours.

Intrauterine Devices

Intrauterine devices (IUDs) offer users convenient birth control as effective as sterilization yet completely reversible. In women in the United States, use of IUDs has declined from approximately 10% in the mid-1970s to 1% today. Concerns among clinicians and women that IUDs cause salpingitis and tubal infertility account for much of this decline. A systematic review found that if any increased risk in salpingitis is associated with IUD use, it is small and appears confined to the first month post insertion. Likewise, use of an IUD is not associated with a subsequent increased risk of tubal infertility.

The copper IUD (ParaGard) is approved for up to 10 years of use. It is appropriate for women who prefer regular cycles. Because use of the copper IUD can increase flow and cramps, it is appropriate for women who have no excess menstrual flow or cramps at baseline.

The levonorgestrel-releasing IUD (Mirena) is approved for up to 5 years of use. It releases 20 µg of levonorgestrel a day. This progestin-releasing IUD reduces menstrual flow and is therefore appropriate for women who would like their birth control method to reduce flow. Women interested in using the levonorgestrel-releasing IUD should be aware, however, that initial irregular spotting or bleeding is common after insertion of this device. Hormonal side effects, including acne and ovarian cysts, also occur in some users. Box 2 details the noncontraceptive benefits associated with use of the levonorgestrel IUD.

Progestin-Releasing Implants

Progestin-releasing contraceptive implants provide highly effective, convenient birth control. Although Norplant

---

> **BOX 2 Noncontraceptive Health Benefits of the Levonorgestrel-Releasing Intrauterine Device**
>
> - Menorrhagia because of uterine fibroids or adenomyosis and as an alternative to hysterectomy
> - Pain because of endometriosis
> - Prevention of endometrial hyperplasia in menopausal women using estrogen therapy
> - Prevention of endometrial proliferation and polyps in patients taking tamoxifen (Nolvadex)

---

and Jadelle are approved by the U.S. Food and Drug Administration (FDA), neither is currently marketed in the United States.

Norplant levonorgestrel consists of 6 capsules and provides contraception up to 5 years. The difficulty with insertion and, in particular, removal of the 6 capsules, along with frequent complaints of irregular bleeding among users, explains why U.S. clinicians, women, and

---

 CURRENT THERAPY

- Two percent of U.S. women of reproductive age have an induced abortion annually.
- Noncontraceptive benefits of oral contraceptive include decreasing the risk of endometrial cancer, ovarian cancer, ectopic pregnancy, and pelvic inflammatory disease as well as treatment of dysmenorrhea, menorrhagia, and acne.
- Combination estrogen-progestin birth control methods (pills, patch, and ring) are contraindicated in women who are smokers over 35 years old and those with a history of DVT, with cardiovascular disease, or with active liver disease.
- Progestin-only birth control methods (pills, injections, or the progestin-releasing IUD) represent appropriate contraceptive options for women who have medical problems contraindicating combination birth control methods.
- Women with menorrhagia or dysmenorrhea may benefit from extended-cycle oral contraceptive pills (Seasonale).
- Plan B, a progestin-only formulation, is the only oral formulation currently marketed for emergency contraception. Although package labeling indicates that it should be taken within 72 hours, effective postcoital contraception is provided if Plan B is taken up to 5 days following unprotected intercourse.
- Copper and progestin-releasing IUDs offer users convenient birth control as effective as sterilization yet completely reversible.
- The copper IUD (ParaGard) may increase menstrual flow and thus may not be a good method for women with menorrhagia.
- Use of the progestin (levonorgestrel)-releasing IUD (Mirena) is associated with noncontraceptive benefits including reduction in heavy menstrual flow because of fibroids or adenomyosis and decreased pain in women with endometriosis.
- Surgical tubal sterilization is associated with a 10-year cumulative failure rate of 1.8% to 3%.
- A device for occlusion of the fallopian tubes using hysteroscopy (Essure) was approved for use in the United States in 2002.
- The failure rate associated with vasectomy is 0.94% at 1 year and 1.1% at 5 years, representing pregnancy rates higher than previously reported.

Abbreviations: DVT = deep vein thrombosis; IUD = intrauterine device.

the manufacturer lost interest in this contraceptive system, which initially was in great demand when introduced in 1991.

Jadelle consists of an implant of two rods each containing 150 mg of levonorgestrel. A single-rod implant (Implanon)* is easier and quicker to insert and remove than Norplant, and its use is associated with less bleeding. The manufacturer has submitted a new drug application to the FDA; this highly effective single-rod implant system ideally will become available to patients in 2005.

Female Sterilization

Tubal sterilization involves using rings (Falope), clips (Filshie), electrocautery, or ligature/segmental excision (Pomeroy) to interrupt the patency of the fallopian tubes surgically. In the United States, approximately 700,000 tubal sterilizations are performed annually. Approximately half of them follow delivery, and half of these are performed as outpatient interval procedures. Sterilization is associated with a 10-year cumulative failure rate of 1.8% to 3%. The failure rate is higher in women younger than 28 years. Although sterilization can be reversed in some women and assisted reproductive technology can also be used to achieve pregnancy in many women following sterilization, this procedure should nonetheless be considered permanent.

Hysteroscopic tubal occlusion (Essure) is a device developed and approved for use in the United States in 2002. This device (2 mm in diameter and 4 cm long) is made of titanium, stainless steel, and nickel, and it contains Dacron fibers that induce an inflammatory reaction and fibrosis in the tubal lumen. A hysterosalpingogram is recommended following placement of the Essure device to confirm bilateral tubal occlusion.

Male Sterilization

Vasectomy involves interruption of the vas deferens, preventing passage of sperm into seminal fluid. This office-based surgical procedure does not interfere with male sexual performance. After vasectomy, couples should use backup contraception until the sperm count reaches zero. According to Jamieson, recent data indicates the failure rate following vasectomy is 9.4 per 1000 procedures at 1 year and 11.3 at 5 years, higher than the previously estimated failure rate.

---

*Investigational drug in the United States.

REFERENCES

Anderson FD, Hait H: A multicenter, randomized study of an extended cycle oral contraceptive. Contraception 2003;68:89-96.

Audet MC, Moreau M, Koltun WD, et al: Evaluation of contraceptive efficacy and cycle control of a transdermal contraceptive patch vs. an oral contraceptive: A randomized controlled trial. JAMA 2001; 285:2347-2354.

Bjarnadottir RI, Tuppurainen M, Killick SR: Comparison of cycle control with a combined contraceptive vaginal ring and oral levonorgestrel/ethinyl estradiol. Am J Obstet Gynecol 2002; 186:389-395.

Fedele L, Bianchi S, Raffaelli R, et al: Treatment of adenomyosis-associated menorrhagia with a levonorgestrel-releasing intrauterine device. Fertil Steril 1997;68:426-429.

Grigorieva V, Chen-Mok M, Tarasova M, Mikhailov A: Use of a levonorgestrel-releasing intrauterine system to treat bleeding related to uterine leiomyomas. Fertil Steril 2003;79:1194-1198.

Hubacher D, Grimes DA: Noncontraceptive health benefits of intrauterine devices: A systemic review. Obstet Gynecol Surv 2002;57:120-128.

Hubacher D, Lara-Ricalde R, Taylor DJ, et al: Use of copper intrauterine devices and the risk of infertility among nulligravid women. N Engl J Med 2001;345:561-567.

Hurskainen R, Teperi J, Rissanen P, et al: Clinical outcomes and costs with the levonorgestrel-releasing intrauterine system or hysterectomy for treatment of menorrhagia: Randomized trial 5-year follow-up. JAMA 2004;291:1456-1463.

Jain J, Jakimiuk AJ, Bode FR, et al: Contraceptive efficacy and safety of DMPA-SC. Contraception 2004;70:269-275.

Jamieson DJ, Costello C, Trussell J, et al: US Collaborative Review of Sterilization Working Group: The risk of pregnancy after vasectomy. Obstet Gynecol 2004;103:848-850.

Jones RK, Darroch JE, Henshaw SK: Contraceptive use among U.S. women having abortions in 2000-2001. Perspect Sex Reprod Health 2002;34:294-303.

Kaunitz AM. Revisiting progestin-only OCs. Contemp OB/GYN, December 1997;42:pp. 91-108.

Kaunitz AM, Garceau Rj, Cromie MA, and the LUNELLE study Group: Comparative safety, efficacy, and cycle control of LUNELLE monthly contraceptive injection (medroxyprogesterone acetate and estradiol cypionate injectable suspension) and Ortho-Novum 7/7/7 oral contraceptive (norethindrone/ethinyl estradiol triphasic). Contraception 1999;60:179-187.

Meckstroth KR, Darney PD: Implant contraception. Semin Reprod Med 2001;19:339-354.

Ubeda A, Labastida RM, Dexeus S: Essure: A new device for hysteroscopic tubal sterilization in an outpatient setting. Fertil Steril 2004;82:196-199.

Vercellini P, Frontino G, Giorgi OD, et al: Comparison of levonorgestrel-releasing intrauterine device versus expectant management after conservative surgery for symptomatic endometriosis: A pilot study. Fertil Steril 2003;80:305-309.

Westhoff C: Depot-medroxyprogesterone acetate injection (Depo-Provera): A highly effective contraceptive option with proven long-term safety. Contraception 2003 Aug 68(2): pp 75-87.

Westoff C: Emergency contraception. N Engl J Med 2003;349: 1830-1835.

Westhoff C, Davis A: Tubal sterilization: Focus on the U.S. experience. Fertil Steril 2000;73:913-922.

16

Psychiatric Disorders

Alcohol Use Disorders

Method of
Richard L. Brown, MD, MPH

Alcohol use disorders are major public health problems in the United States. Alcohol consumption is linked to 75,000 deaths per year, with 30 years of lost life per death, and substantial numbers of acute injuries, chronic diseases, hospitalizations, emergency department visits, suicides, episodes of abuse and violence, and other crimes.

Health care professionals are in ideal positions to recognize and assist patients with risky and problem drinking. Despite recommendations by the U.S. Preventive Services Task Force, the National Institute on Alcohol Abuse and Alcoholism (NIAAA), and others, few health care professionals routinely provide alcohol screening, brief intervention, and referral services. With application of the medical counseling skills commonly used to manage other chronic health conditions, health care professionals can improve health and other outcomes for many patients with alcohol use disorders.

Diagnosis

Alcohol consumption is best considered as a continuum with five major guideposts. Current recommendations on low-risk drinking do not take into account long-term cardiovascular risk. Up to two standard drinks (Box 1) per day for men and one standard drink per day for women may be beneficial in reducing cardiovascular risk; more can increase cardiovascular risk through unfavorable effects on lipids and blood pressure.

For individuals with particular health problems, such as liver disease, pancreatitis, peptic ulcer disease, cardiomyopathy, dementia, encephalopathies, neuropathies, and current or prior alcohol and drug dependencies, any use of alcohol is risky. Alcohol should also be avoided completely by pregnant women and by individuals taking medicines such as certain antibiotics, anticoagulants, anticonvulsants, antidepressants, antihistamines, anti-inflammatories, anxiolytics, H_2 blockers, hypoglycemics, muscle relaxants, and opioid analgesics.

Individuals with at-risk drinking and abuse are by definition able to control their drinking without difficulty. They can readily decrease their drinking if they wish to do so.

Alcohol dependence is synonymous with alcoholism and alcohol addiction. The primary symptom is a consistent inability, or an inconsistent ability, to control one's drinking. Alcohol dependence may occur without any physical dependence, especially in those 18 years of age or under. Dependent individuals often suffer similar and more severe negative health and social consequences than seen with alcohol abuse (Table 1).

A key neurophysiologic lesion of alcoholism and other addictions occurs in the mesolimbic dopaminergic neural pathway in the brain's ventral tegmentum. In normal individuals, this pathway provides pleasurable reinforcement when hunger or sex drives are satisfied. In addicted individuals, neuronal function in this pathway is regulated by different DNA sequences. Thus the neurophysiologic basis of the disease of addiction involves a hijacking of the mesolimbic pathway such that it drives addictive behaviors along with or instead of adaptive eating and sexual behaviors. For alcoholics, the resulting cravings and impulses to drink make it difficult to avoid alcohol.

Alcohol Screening

Alcohol screening is recommended as a component of routine preventive care for several reasons. The combined prevalence of at-risk drinking, alcohol abuse, and alcohol dependence approaches or surpasses 20% in many practice settings. Most individuals with such drinking patterns lack obvious symptoms and signs. Such drinking often responds to intervention or treatment. Early identification and management of such drinking can avert more serious and sometimes irreversible health and social consequences. Screening, followed when warranted by brief interventions, saves nearly $1000 per patient in documented costs of health care utilization, motor vehicle crashes, and criminal justice system involvement; further undocumented cost savings are likely.

In most health care settings, the best source of information for screening and more detailed assessment is the history. Physical examination reveals signs of alcohol overuse only in the relatively few patients with

BOX 1 **Standard Drinks**
• 1.5 ounces of 80-proof liquor or brandy • 2 to 3 ounces of liqueur • 3 to 4 ounces of sherry or port • 5 ounces of wine • 8 to 9 ounces of malt liquor • 12 ounces of beer or wine cooler
A standard drink is the amount of an alcoholic beverage that contains approximately 12 g of pure ethanol.

advanced alcohol dependence. Laboratory studies, such as gamma-glutamyltransferase and mean corpuscular volume, are normal in most patients with alcohol use disorders. Carbohydrate-deficient transferrin, a newer blood test that can suggest alcohol overuse, lacks sensitivity, especially for episodic heavy drinkers. Self-reports of drinking usually match or exceed reports by family members. In emergency settings, blood alcohol levels can help document alcohol-related trauma and tolerance.

Several brief batteries of yes-or-no screening questions can identify most individuals with at-risk drinking and alcohol use disorders (Box 2). Such questions can be incorporated conversationally into routine histories. The CAGE (cut down, annoyed, guilty, eye-opener) questions are used most often and are most accurate in adult men. The TWEAK questions (tolerance, worried, eye-opener, amnesia, cut down) are more accurate in women, especially pregnant women. The CRAFFT (six questions include the words *Car, Relax, Alone, Friends, Forget*, and *Trouble*) is the best validated screen for adolescents.

The SMAST-G (Short Michigan Alcoholism Screening Test–Geriatric Version) is useful for those over 65 years of age. The Two-Item Conjoint Screen (TICS) screens simultaneously for alcohol and drug problems; a conjoint screening approach has merit because one third of individuals who have substance use disorders have drug disorders.

The screens just cited are useful in identifying abuse and dependence. For patients with negative screens, questions on quantity and frequency of alcohol use can identify at-risk drinkers. Alternatively, the 10 multiple-choice questions of the AUDIT (Alcohol Use Disorders Identification Test) can be incorporated into written health history forms and can sensitively identify at-risk drinkers and patients with alcohol use disorders. An advantage of written questionnaires is they can save clinician time. A disadvantage is that they circumvent the opportunity to identify nonverbal responses to screening questions that may suggest an alcohol problem.

After Alcohol Screening

Alcohol screening provides a preliminary indication of where patients lie on the spectrum of alcohol use. Patients who abstain should be asked why. Some quit because of prior difficulties with alcohol. Others who abstain because of disillusionment about drinking by family members may be at high genetic risk for alcohol dependence. Endorsing moderate drinking for its cardioprotective benefit may be ill-advised for many abstainers, whose attempts at moderate drinking could trigger alcohol dependence.

TABLE 1 **Common Negative Consequences of Alcohol Use**

	Symptoms and Signs of Alcohol Use Disorders	
Category	**Earlier, More Reversible**	**Later, Less Reversible**
Biomedical	Gastritis, esophageal reflux, dyspepsia, peptic ulcer, hepatic inflammation, acute pancreatitis, diarrhea Hypertension Weight gain Mild traumatic injuries Sleep disturbance and fatigue Sexual dysfunction	Cirrhosis, esophageal varices, hepatic encephalopathy, chronic pancreatitis; cardiomyopathy, coronary artery disease, cardiac dysrhythmias; bone marrow and immune suppression; head, neck, and gastrointestinal cancers; cerebellar degeneration, dementia, malnutrition; major trauma-related disabilities
Psychological	Agitation, irritability, mood swings, dysphoria, anxiety disorders, depressive disorders, psychosomatic symptoms, hostility	Persistent, severe mental illness
Family	Marital and family dysfunction, childhood behavior and school problems, mental health problems in family members	Divorce, neglect, abuse, violence, estrangement
Other relationships	Alienation and loss of old friends, gravitation toward others who drink heavily	Social isolation
Work/school	Decline in performance, frequent job changes, frequent absences (especially on Mondays), requests for work excuses, initial preservation of work/school function in career-oriented individuals such as physicians	Chronic unemployment
Legal	Driving while intoxicated; various misdemeanors	Incarceration
Financial	Borrowing, debt	Insolvency, homelessness
Religious/spiritual	Shame, self-disgust, disconnection	Alienation

Rakel and Bope: *Conn's Current Therapy 2006.*

BOX 2 Alcohol Screening Instruments

CAGE Questions
1. Have you ever thought you should cut down on your drinking?
2. Have you ever felt Annoyed by others criticizing your drinking?
3. Have you ever felt bad or Guilty about your drinking?
4. Do you have a drink to help you get started in the morning (Eye-opener)?

One or more positive responses indicates the need for further assessment.

TWEAK
1. How many drinks does it take before you begin to feel the first effects of the alcohol? (Tolerance)
2. Have your friends or relatives Worried or complained about your drinking in the past year?
3. Do you sometimes take a drink in the morning when you first get up (Eye-opener)?
4. Are there times when you drink and afterward you can't remember what you said or did? (Amnesia)
5. Do you sometimes feel the need to cut (Kut) down on your drinking?

For item 1, more than two drinks scores 2 points.
For item 2, a positive response scores 2 points.
For items 3, 4, and 5, each positive response scores 1 point.
A total of 2 to 3 points indicates a possible alcohol problem.

CRAFFT
1. Have you ever ridden in a Car driven by someone (including yourself) who was high or had been using alcohol or drugs?
2. Do you ever use alcohol or drugs to Relax, feel better about yourself, or fit in?
3. Do you ever use alcohol or drugs while you are by yourself Alone?
4. Do you ever Forget things you did while using alcohol or drugs?
5. Do your Family or Friends ever tell you that you should cut down on your drinking or drug use?
6. Have you ever gotten into Trouble while you were using alcohol or drugs?

Two or more positive responses indicate the need for further assessment.

S-MAST-G
In the past year ...
1. When talking with others, do you ever underestimate how much you actually drink?
2. After a few drinks, have you sometimes not eaten or been able to skip a meal because you didn't feel hungry?
3. Does having a few drinks help decrease your shakiness or tremors?
4. Does alcohol sometimes make it hard for you to remember parts of the day or night?
5. Do you usually take a drink to relax or calm your nerves?
6. Do you drink to take your mind off your problems?
7. Have you ever increased your drinking after experiencing a loss in your life?
8. Has a doctor or nurse ever said they were worried or concerned about your drinking?
9. Have you ever made rules to manage your drinking?
10. When you feel lonely, does having a drink help?

Two or more positive responses indicate a probable alcohol problem.

Two-Item Conjoint Screen
1. In the last year, have you ever drunk or used drugs more than you meant to?
2. Have you felt you wanted or needed to cut down on your drinking or drug use in the last year?

One or two positive responses indicate the need for further assessment.

AUDIT: Alcohol Use Disorders Identification Test
Q1. How often do you consume a drink containing alcohol?
   0. Never
   1. Monthly or less
   2. 2 to 4 times a month
   3. 2 or 3 times a week
   4. 4 or more times a week
Q2. How many drinks containing alcohol do you have on a typical day when you are drinking?
   0. 1 or 2
   1. 3 or 4
   2. 5 or 6
   3. 7 to 9
   4. 10 or more
Q3. How often do you have 6 or more drinks on one occasion?
   0. Never
   1. Less than monthly
   2. Monthly
   3. Weekly
   4. Daily or almost daily
Q4. How often during the last year have you found that you were not able to stop drinking once you had started?
   0. Never
   1. Less than monthly
   2. Monthly
   3. Weekly
   4. Daily or almost daily
Q5. How often during the last year have you failed to do what was normally expected from you because of drinking?
   0. Never
   1. Less than monthly
   2. Monthly
   3. Weekly
   4. Daily or almost daily
Q6. How often during the last year have you needed a drink in the morning to get yourself going after a heavy drinking session the night before?
   0. Never
   1. Less than monthly
   2. Monthly
   3. Weekly
   4. Daily or almost daily
Q7. How often during the last year have you had a feeling of guilt or remorse after drinking?
   0. Never
   1. Less than monthly
   2. Monthly
   3. Weekly
   4. Daily or almost daily

Continued

BOX 2   Alcohol Screening Instruments—cont'd

Q8. How often during the last year have you been unable to remember what happened the night before because you had been drinking?
0. Never
1. Less than monthly
2. Monthly
3. Weekly
4. Daily or almost daily

Q9. Have you or someone else been injured as a result of your drinking?
0. No
1. Yes, but not in the last year
2. Yes, during the last year

Q10. Has a relative, a friend, or a physician or other health care worker been concerned about your drinking or suggested that you cut down?
0. No
1. Yes, but not in the last year
2. Yes, during the last year

Add up the numbers to the left of each response.
    More than 8 points: Positive for an alcohol use disorder for both men and women.
    More than 4 points: May be positive for an alcohol use disorder for women.

Alcohol Case-Finding

Case-finding involves determining whether patients who exhibit possible negative consequences of drinking (see Table 1) truly have alcohol problems. Treating the consequences of excessive drinking without addressing the root cause usually fails. Case-finding can begin with screening questions and proceed with brief alcohol assessment.

Brief Alcohol Assessment

Brief alcohol assessment identifies where individuals lie on the spectrum of alcohol use. The objectives of assessment are to discern whether patients are suffering negative consequences of drinking and additional symptoms of alcohol dependence.

The negative consequences of drinking fall into eight categories (see Table 1). Clinicians should aim to identify alcohol use disorders before later, less reversible consequences occur. Psychological consequences often occur earliest. Full-fledged mood disorders and anxiety disorders may result from or lead to alcohol use disorders, but the earliest negative consequences are often subclinical anxiety and depressive symptoms.

Alcohol-related psychological symptoms often lead to dysfunction in significant relationships. An alcohol use disorder in one family member often produces stress, anxiety, depression, and psychosomatic symptoms in others. Such symptoms should therefore prompt questions on drinking by loved ones.

Health consequences of drinking may occur early or late in the course of alcohol abuse or dependence. Alcohol can produce blood pressure elevations by a direct pressor effect on arterioles and by autonomic instability of subclinical withdrawal syndromes. Individuals who engage in episodic heavy drinking may exhibit labile hypertension. Drinking may produce fatigue by interfering with deep, restorative stages of sleep.

To assess for the loss of control seen with alcohol dependence, ask whether patients set rules about drinking and have difficulty adhering to them. To assess for preoccupying thoughts, ask whether patients sometimes have difficulty getting thoughts of drinking out of their minds. To assess for compulsive drinking, ask whether individuals have particular difficulty limiting their drinking after starting to drink. To assess for physical dependence, ask whether individuals experience shakiness hours after unusually heavy drinking. Alcohol-dependent patients may have just some of these symptoms.

Intervention

Brief interventions for alcohol problems involve counseling skills that clinicians routinely employ in managing other health problems. Recommended steps follow the FERNSS mnemonic:

- *Feedback*: Express concern that the patient's drinking may be linked with current consequences or future risks. When possible, provide authoritative medical opinion for alcohol-related health consequences. To avoid arguments, raise questions about the link between alcohol and social consequences rather than making definitive pronouncements. Emphasize risks and consequences that are important to the patient; for example, attempt to link drinking to chief complaints or to other difficulties that the patient wishes to avoid or resolve. Initially avoid alcohol-related diagnostic labels, which can elicit anger and shame. Finally, ask for the patient's point of view.
- *Education*: Explain how drinking can lead to medical or other concerns. For example, explain how alcohol can relax esophageal sphincters and cause reflux. To avoid arguments, when patients offer competing explanations for symptoms, acknowledge their possibility and affirm that alcohol is also a likely contributor.
- *Recommend*: Brief interventions are geared toward eliciting behavior change. Make a specific recommendation that the patient takes a particular action (Table 2). For patients with symptoms of alcohol dependence, initially recommend consultation with an alcohol specialist. Alternative recommendations could be a 1-month trial of abstinence to test for

TABLE 2 Recommendations to Make During Brief Interventions

Clinical Circumstances						
Alcohol Dependence Symptoms	Family History of Dependence	Health Issue or Alcohol/Medicine Incompatibility	Alcohol Abuse	At-Risk Drinking	Declined Recommendation Above	Recommendation
x						Consult with an alcohol treatment specialist or program.
					x	Attend self-help meetings.
	x	x			x	Abstain.
			x	x	x	Adhere to low-risk limits.
					x	Cut down as much as willing.

control and to assess whether possible consequences improve. Attendance at self-help meetings can help patients determine whether they have similarities to others who are committed to stop drinking. For patients with at-risk drinking or alcohol abuse and positive family histories of alcohol dependence, recommend abstinence as the safest option. As the first option for patients with alcohol abuse or at-risk drinking who have negative family histories of alcohol dependence, recommend adhering to limits for low-risk drinking.

• *Negotiate*: When patients decline recommendations, avoid arguments. Collaborate in identifying and attempting to work around barriers to adherence. Offer alternative recommendations. Express concern that continuing present drinking patterns may not allow them to attain their goals, such as more restful sleep, relief of gastric discomfort, or a better relationship. Support any commitment to decrease drinking.

• *Secure the agreement*: For patients who are willing to take action, secure concrete and specific agreement on what they will do by when. For example, for patients who are willing to set weekly and daily drinking limits, ask them to specify permissible ranges of numbers of standard drinks for each day of the week. Record the patient's agreement in writing and provide a copy for them. Written agreements are not binding but help ground discussions at follow-up visits.

• *Set follow-up*: Ask the patient to specify when follow-up contact would be useful, usually within 1 month. Provide two pieces of advice: (1) Seek immediate care for any symptoms of alcohol withdrawal, and (2) Reassure the patient that any difficulties they have implementing their plan will elicit concern and further discussion about what to do next but neither anger nor judgment.

• *At the follow-up visit*: Review the patient's progress. For patients who make positive changes, reinforce their success, and use the FERNSS approach in setting long-term plans for healthier drinking. For patients who had difficulty modifying their drinking, assess for difficulties with control; consider allowing for another try or referring for a consultation.

For patients who decline to address their risky or problem drinking, acknowledge that they are not ready to make a change. Let them know you are open to any future questions, or advise them where they can seek help if they change their minds. Although many physicians express frustration in managing alcohol use disorders, research shows that adherence to treatment recommendations on drinking is no worse than recommendations made for other chronic diseases.

Although some clinicians blame denial for patients' resistance to change, research shows that alcohol-dependent patients use denial as a defense mechanism no more frequently than non-alcohol-dependent patients. Clinicians who project warmth, empathy, respect, and partnership elicit more accurate information and adherence than those who project frustration, impatience, and judgment.

Detoxification and Withdrawal

Withdrawal from alcohol and other sedatives may be fatal. Goals are to maximize comfort, avoid oversedation and other complications, and engage patients in alcohol treatment.

Stage 1, or minor withdrawal, is characterized by tachycardia, hypertension, fever lower than 38.3°C (101°F), diaphoresis, nausea, vomiting, restlessness, agitation, and tremors. In stage 2, these symptoms and signs worsen, and hallucinations occur. Disorientation and mental clouding herald stage 3, also known as delirium tremens, or DTs. Seizures may complicate any of the three stages.

Risk factors for severe withdrawal include prior severe withdrawal, age older than 40 years, heavier and more regular drinking, higher tolerance to alcohol, poor health, and poor nutrition. Patients at low risk for severe withdrawal are best treated in supervised community settings, where favorable staffing and environmental conditions result in less need for pharmacologic treatment. Hospitalization is indicated for patients at high risk for severe withdrawal or seizures and for those with underlying medical conditions that can be aggravated by withdrawal, such as coronary artery disease or type I diabetes. Management includes ensuring appropriate hydration, restoring magnesium and other electrolyte balance, and administering thiamine and other vitamins.

Benzodiazepine loading is recommended for high-risk patients with recent and steady heavy drinking and blood alcohol levels of zero and for patients with any symptoms of withdrawal. Diazepam (Valium), 20 mg,[3] or lorazepam (Ativan),[1] 5 mg,[3] is repeated every 2 hours for a total of three doses. During loading and at any time during detoxification, sedatives should be withheld when patients become sleepy. Patients at low risk for withdrawal can be observed until symptoms begin. Long-acting benzodiazepines,[1] such as diazepam and chlordiazepoxide, provide the most comfortable detoxification. Short-acting benzodiazepines, such as lorazepam, should be reserved for patients with severe hepatic dysfunction (jaundice or elevated prothrombin times) or for patients who have already received large doses of long-acting benzodiazepines (e.g., 300 mg of diazepam). Obtain urine drug screens before administering any controlled substances.

Patients in alcohol withdrawal must be reassessed frequently. Avoid fixed, repeated doses of sedatives and imprecise "as needed" orders. Withdrawal treatment protocols that involve frequent scoring of withdrawal signs and symptoms, such as the CIWA-A (Clinical Institute Withdrawal Assessment for Alcohol), provide the most reliable guidance for continuing sedative administration.

Minor withdrawal can be treated with carbamazepine (Tegretol),[1] gabapentin (Neurontin),[1] or β-blockers. However, β-blockers can mask autonomic symptoms that herald severe withdrawal, which must be treated with a sedative. Withdrawal from alcohol or multiple sedatives can be treated with phenobarbital.[1]

Alcohol withdrawal seizures are treated with benzodiazepines and carbamazepine,[1] which should be discontinued after withdrawal. Avoid phenothiazines, which lower seizure thresholds; instead, use hydroxyzine (Atarax) for nausea and haloperidol (Haldol)[1] for agitation that does not respond to benzodiazepines.

Alcohol Treatment

According to authoritative, evidence-based reviews, treatment for alcohol dependence is effective. Although durable abstinence may elude many patients, those who receive treatment drink less, suffer fewer and less severe relapses, and exhibit better psychosocial function on average than those who do not.

A combination of professional and lay treatments is most effective. Next most effective is professionally administered treatment alone. Many patients can recover through lay-administered self-help groups, such as Alcoholics Anonymous or Rational Recovery. Physicians can facilitate referrals by arranging for

escorts by other recovering patients and by suggesting that patients try several meetings and continue at those where they feel most comfortable.

The mainstays of professionally administered alcohol treatment are nonpharmacologic. Psychoeducational, cognitive–behavioral, family, and network approaches are effective. A newer approach, motivational interviewing, is effective in changing drinking and other health-risk behaviors. Increasingly used in general medical settings, motivational interviewing can be used when brief interventions or referrals are ineffective.

Pharmacologic adjuncts can be helpful. Although disulfiram (Antabuse), an aversive agent, did not confer lasting benefit in a 1-year randomized controlled trial, it may facilitate abstinence in early recovery for patients who are prone to impulsive drinking. Naltrexone (ReVia), an opioid antagonist, reduces cravings by alcohol-dependent patients and facilitates receipt of nonpharmacologic treatment. Both medicines are safe for patients with transaminase levels less than three times normal. Approved in 2004 by the Food and Drug Administration (FDA), acamprosate (Campral) reduces cravings and bolsters abstinence for at least 12 months. Nalmefene (Revex),[1] a promising opioid antagonist, is now available in the United States. All pharmacologic treatments should supplement nonpharmacologic treatments.

---

[1]Not FDA approved for this indication.

 CURRENT DIAGNOSIS

Abstinence: No more than a few drinks per year

Low-risk drinking

- For men, no more than 14 standard drinks per week and 4 per occasion
- For women, no more than 7 to 11 drinks per week and 3 per occasion
- For elders (65 years of age or older), no more than 7 drinks per week and 1 per occasion

At-risk drinking

- Exceeding above criteria for low-risk drinking
- Any alcohol use in the presence of certain health conditions or with certain medications
- Drinking that does not qualify for abuse or dependence

Abuse

- Continued drinking despite repeated adverse health and psychosocial consequences
- Repeated alcohol use in physically hazardous situations, such as while driving
- Dependence (synonymous with alcoholism or alcohol addiction)
- Difficulty controlling drinking
- Preoccupation with obtaining or drinking alcohol
- Difficulty stopping drinking, especially once started
- Physical dependence (propensity to suffer withdrawal with sudden cessation or diminution of alcohol use)

---

[3]Exceeds dosage recommended by the manufacturer.
[1]Not FDA approved for this indication.

CURRENT THERAPY

- Intervene or refer to treatment by giving feedback and education on risks and consequences, making a recommendation, negotiating for the most behavior change, securing a concrete and specific behavioral agreement, and setting follow-up for assessing progress.
- Provide or arrange for supervised detoxification, as necessary.
- For patients who cannot abstain or maintain low-risk drinking on their own, attempt referral to specialists and/or self-help groups. Also, consider naltrexone (ReVia), disulfiram (Antabuse), and acamprosate (Campral).
- In follow-up, help patients assess progress toward their substance use and other goals, revise their plan for attaining their goals as needed, and access resources.

Diagnosis

Nearly half of patients with addictive disorders have other psychiatric disorders. A common error is to treat the concomitant psychiatric disorder without recognizing or addressing the substance use disorder. All patients with psychiatric disorders should be assessed for substance use disorders. For those with both, a best first step, if the psychiatric symptoms do not demand immediate pharmacologic treatment, is to stop the substance use. For example, sometimes stopping alcohol is effective in treating symptoms of major depression.

For patients with alcohol dependence, it is best not to prescribe potentially addictive sedatives. Insomnia is expected during the first year of recovery and best treated nonpharmacologically or with noneuphoric agents, such as trazodone (Desyrel)[1] or doxepin (Sinequan).[1] For patients with alcohol dependence and anxiety disorders, clonazepam (Klonopin)[1] and clorazepate (Tranxene), long-acting agents that generate little euphoria, are the preferred benzodiazepines for patients who do not respond to, or cannot tolerate, other classes of pharmaceuticals. Patients with alcohol dependence and chronic psychosis need regular and coordinated care by primary care, mental health, and addictions professionals; again, for patients who require benzodiazepines, long-acting agents are best.

REFERENCES

American Psychiatric Association: Diagnostic and Statistical Manual of Mental Health Disorders, 4th ed. Washington, DC, Author, 1994.
Bayard M, McIntyre J, Hill KR, Woodside J Jr: Alcohol withdrawal syndrome. Am Fam Physician 2004;69:1443-1450.
Fleming MF, Mundt MP, French MT, et al: Brief physician advice for problem drinkers: Long-term efficacy and benefit-cost analysis. Alcohol Clin Exp Res 2002;26:36-43.

[1]Not FDA approved for this indication.

Rakel and Bope: *Conn's Current Therapy 2006.*

Miller WR, Rollnick S: Motivational Interviewing: Preparing People for Change. New York, Guilford Press, 2002.
National Institute on Alcohol Abuse and Alcohol: Helping Patients With Alcohol Problems: A Health Practitioner's Guide. Rockville, Md, Author, 2004.
Sullivan JT, Sykora K, Schneiderman J, et al: Assessment of alcohol withdrawal: The revised Clinical Institute Withdrawal Assessment for Alcohol scale (CIWA-As). Br J Addict 1989;84:1353-1357.
U.S. Preventive Services Task Force: Screening and Behavioral Counseling Interventions in Primary Care to Reduce Alcohol Misuse: Recommendation Statement. Rockville, Md, April 2004. Agency for Healthcare Research and Quality on line: Available at http://www.ahrq.gov/clinic/3rduspstf/alcohol/alcomisrs.htm

Drug Abuse

Method of
Joyce A. Tinsley, MD

The U.S. Department of Health and Human Services reported that in 2001 nearly 7% of the population, or 16 million Americans age 12 and older, were actively using illegal drugs. The combination of drug and alcohol use costs taxpayers a staggering sum; an estimated $143 billion per year is spent on associated health care costs, extra law enforcement, motor vehicle accidents, crime, and lost productivity. The president's fiscal year 2003 budget included $4.4 billion for all substance abuse–related activities, with $127 million earmarked for treatment services. The abuse of legal drugs, such as prescription medications and nicotine, is also a serious problem. Nicotine dependence is responsible for more morbidity and mortality than any other abused substance and is so highly addictive that quitting eludes many who try to stop.

Many addicts in need of treatment do not get it. Reasons for this include a lack of treatment and recovery resources, the stigma surrounding drug use, and pessimism about recovery from addictions. Unfortunately, much of the clinical pessimism about addiction treatment is based on an inadequate or outdated knowledge base. At a minimum, clinicians should be familiar with the common drugs of abuse; signs of intoxication, withdrawal, and overdose; management of simple detoxification; and contemporary treatment options.

Diagnosis

In the *Diagnostic and Statistical Manual of Mental Disorders, 4th ed., Text Revision (DSM-IV-TR)*, published by the American Psychiatric Association, disorders are classified as either abuse or dependence (Box 1).

These criteria may be applied to any drug within the major classes of addictive substances. Inherent to the definition of dependence is the concept of impaired control.

17

BOX 1   *DSM IV-TR* Diagnostic Criteria

Substance Abuse
A maladaptive pattern of use leading to clinically
   significant impairment and distress in at least one of
   the following areas within a 12-month period:
1. Failure to fulfill major role obligations at work, school,
   or home
2. Use in physically hazardous situations
3. Substance-related legal problems
4. Use despite social or interpersonal problems exacerbated
   by use of the substance

Substance Dependence
A maladaptive pattern of use leading to impairment and
   distress in at least three of the following areas within a
   12-month period:
1. Tolerance—need for increasing amounts to achieve
   intoxication or desired effect or diminished effect with
   continued use of the same amount.
2. Withdrawal—development of characteristic withdrawal
   symptoms or use of the same or related substance to
   relieve or avoid withdrawal symptoms.
3. The substance is used in larger amounts or over longer
   time periods than intended.
4. Inability to cut down or control use.
5. Significant time is spent in activities related to obtaining
   the substance or recovering from its effects.
6. Social, occupational, or recreational activities are given
   up or reduced.
7. Use continues despite knowledge of harmful physical
   or psychological effects.

Adapted from: American Psychiatric Association: Diagnostic and statistical
   manual of mental disorders 4th ed., text revision (DSM-IV-TR).
   Washington, DC: Author, 2000. Used with permission.

In other words, the addict cannot predictably control when or how much of a substance he or she will use. In both abuse and dependence, the individual continues to use the substance even though it causes problems in one or more important life areas. The diagnosis is based on behaviors surrounding the drug abuse rather than the amount consumed. Substance dependence, synonymous with addiction, is the more advanced disorder.

It is often challenging to diagnose drug abuse. Patients may be hesitant to reveal illegal drug abuse or the misuse of prescription drugs. Clinicians should ask questions that are perceived to be nonjudgmental. For instance, asking, "Has anyone ever been concerned about your drug use?" is less likely to be met with resistance than initial questions that ask about quantity or frequency of use. Supplemental history from significant others and objective data from urine drug screens can help clarify the diagnosis. Some addicts readily admit their addictions. For instance, heroin users have been known to overestimate their use in order to receive a more generous opiate dose for detoxification or maintenance. Heroin and cocaine addicts with advanced dependence often acknowledge their addictions because of devastating social, legal, or physical consequences. In addition, a majority of cigarette smokers express a desire to stop smoking and attempt to get help.

Nicotine

Nicotine dependence is similar to other drug addictions in that it is best viewed as a chronic disease that requires ongoing attention. It is the addiction on which primary care clinicians may have the greatest impact. An estimated 25% of adults in the United States smoke cigarettes, and 70% of current smokers would like to quit. In view of the lethal nature of smoking, the high percentage of smokers who want to quit, and the number of individuals affected, the clinician should be prepared to encourage smoking cessation.

The nicotine withdrawal syndrome is a serious obstacle for patients who want to stop smoking. Withdrawal symptoms often begin within hours after the last cigarette, peak within 2 to 3 days, and may continue for several weeks. Nicotine cravings last much longer. Early abstinence is characterized by irritability, anxiety, restlessness, depressed mood, inattention, and insomnia. A nicotine replacement product is effective in ameliorating many of the withdrawal symptoms.

Brief counseling improves smoking cessation rates, especially when directed toward the patient's unique situation. The U.S. Public Health Service recommends easy-to-follow strategies that clinicians can use in counseling patients to quit smoking (Table 1). The "5 As" represent a strategy particularly helpful to the clinician who wants to initiate discussion about a patient's tobacco use. The "5 Rs" may be used if the patient lacks motivation to stop smoking. Finally, an action plan known by the mnemonic STAR is a guide for those ready to make a quit attempt.

TABLE 1   Office-Based Interventions for Smoking Cessation

Initial Intervention: 5 As	Motivational Intervention: 5 Rs	Action Plan: STAR
Ask about tobacco use.	Relevance: Why stop?	Set a quit date.
Advise the patient to quit.	Risks: Personalize them.	Tell others of plan.
Assess readiness to quit.	Rewards: Potential benefits.	Anticipate difficulties.
Assist in the quit attempt.	Roadblocks: Identify and address barriers.	Remove tobacco products.
Arrange follow-up.	Repetition: Repeat message at the next visit.	

Adapted from: U.S. Public Health Service: Treating tobacco use and dependence—clinician's packet. A how-to guide for implementing the public health service
   clinical practice guideline. March 2003. http://www.surgeongeneral.gov/tobacco/clinpack.html

There is solid evidence that several medications are effective in improving smokers' quit rates (Table 2). Unless there are contraindications to the use of these medications, a first-line agent, either a nicotine replacement product or bupropion (Zyban), should be recommended to patients who want to stop smoking. If initial agents are ineffective or contraindicated, the clinician should consider recommending a second-line agent, specifically clonidine (Catapres)[1] or nortriptyline (Pamelor).[1] The Public Health Service provides additional information to clinicians who want to learn more about how to help patients stop smoking on their Web site http://www.surgeongeneral.gov/tobacco.

Marijuana

Marijuana, or cannabis, is the most commonly used illegal drug in the United States. Despite purported medical uses, it is not a benign substance. Individuals who become addicted often experience impairment in multiple life areas. The active ingredient in marijuana is tetrahydrocannabinol (THC). THC is classified as a hallucinogen, which it can be in large quantities or in

---

[1]Not FDA approved for this indication.

highly sensitive individuals. More often intoxication brings relaxation, euphoria, a dreamy state, time-space distortion, and impaired attention. Perceptual disturbances may impair driving. Anxiety and paranoia are also common effects. Like other addictive substances, marijuana abuse can interfere with the assessment and treatment of psychiatric symptoms. No specific medical management is warranted for either cannabis intoxication or withdrawal.

Teenagers are among the most vulnerable users. Common signs of problematic use during adolescence include changes in sleeping and eating habits, declining school performance, changes in the adolescent's peer group, and moodiness. Physical signs include increased appetite, dry mouth, and injected conjunctiva. The University of Michigan's Monitoring the Future survey of U.S. high school students has been tracking teenage substance use for the past 25 years. In 2000, they found that by the age of 18 years, 80% of U.S. youth had used alcohol and 54% had used illicit drugs. Their drug of choice was marijuana. One in five high school seniors and nearly as many tenth graders reported marijuana use during the previous month. Treatment for marijuana abuse and dependence in adolescents or adults consists of psychotherapeutic approaches.

17

TABLE 2 Pharmacotherapy of Smoking Cessation

	Instructions	Dose	Advantages	Disadvantages
Nicotine gum/over-the-counter (Nicorette)	Chew until peppery taste, then park between cheek and gum.	2 or 4 mg per piece. Maximum 24 pieces per day. Use for up to 6 mo.	Flexibility with scheduled and/or prn doses to relieve cravings. Delivery is more rapid than the patch.	Incomplete absorption when chewed incorrectly. Cannot eat or drink while using. Caution with dental or jaw problems.
Transdermal nicotine patch/over-the-counter (Nicoderm)	Apply to skin daily. Available as 16-h or 24-h patch. Do not smoke while using.	Start 21 mg × 6 wk (14 mg if weight <100 lb or smoking <1/2 ppd). Taper to 14 mg, then 7 mg × 2-4 wk. Use for 2-3 mo total.	Easy to use. Few side effects. Releases steady dose of nicotine to reduce cravings. Can use in combination with gum.	Releases nicotine more slowly. No response for sudden cravings. Can cause skin irritation. Consider lower dosing in known cardiac disease.
Nasal spray/prescription (Nicotrol NS)	Use every 1-2 h. Take deep breath, spray into each nostril, and exhale through mouth.	From 8 to 40 times per day. Use for 3 mo with gradual taper.	Fastest delivery of nicotine. Good at reducing sudden cravings.	Nose and sinus irritation common at first. Caution with allergies or asthma.
Nasal inhaler/prescription (Nicotrol Inhaler)	Inhale nicotine by bringing inhaler to mouth when desired.	From 6 to 16 cartridges per day for first 3-6 wk. Use for 3 mo with gradual taper.	Delivers nicotine as quickly as gum. Satisfies hand-to-mouth habit. Few side effects.	May cause mouth or throat irritation. Caution with asthma or chronic lung disease.
Bupropion HCl/prescription (Zyban)	Take 1 pill in the morning, 1 in late afternoon. Start 2 wk before quit date.	150 mg SR bid. Continue for 7 to 12 weeks after quitting.	Easy to use, few side effects. May be more helpful when used with the patch.	Contraindicated in seizure, eating disorders, patients taking Wellbutrin or MAOIs, pregnancy, or breast-feeding.

Abbreviations: bid = twice daily; MAOIs = monoamine oxidase inhibitors; ppd = packs per day; prn = as needed; SR = slow release.
Adapted from: American Cancer Society: Set yourself free; deciding how to quit, a smoker's guide. 1999.

Cocaine and Other Stimulants

Cocaine is a highly addictive drug that is extracted from the coca leaf. Amphetamine, which is structurally similar to cocaine, is a synthesized product used to suppress hunger, improve energy or alertness, and improve mood. The euphoria that cocaine elicits is probably caused by increased dopamine activity. Physical effects include elevated heart rate and blood pressure, mediated by stimulation of the sympathetic nervous system. All stimulants possess these qualities, though in varying degrees and with variable risks. In overdose, these effects are intensified so that myocardial infarction, arrhythmia, stroke, and psychosis may occur. In those situations, therapeutic measures are supportive and aimed at reversing specific ill effects.

Physiologic withdrawal is not a major problem, and no medical management is indicated. However withdrawal from cocaine produces symptoms known as a *crash*. A crash may begin within hours of the last use and intensify over the next several days. During this time the addict feels extreme fatigue. Depression can be severe and carries a risk of suicidal ideation and behavior. Relapse is common during withdrawal because return to use provides quick and reliable relief.

The person who abuses cocaine may use it by snorting, injecting, or smoking. The rate at which the drug reaches the brain correlates with its addictive potential. Therefore, users with more advanced addictions commonly report a progression from snorting to intravenous use or the most rapid form of administration, smoking crack cocaine. Intravenous users are at risk for contracting hepatitis and HIV, as well as developing phlebitis and endocarditis. Treatment relies on psychotherapeutic approaches such as self-help, contingency management, and cognitive-behavioral therapy. Despite multiple medication trials, no drug effectively treats cocaine dependence.

Opiates

Among the opiates, heroin may be the most widely recognized drug of abuse. In 2000, there were an estimated 1,000,000 heroin addicts. There is concern that this number will increase because heroin has become less expensive in some parts of the country. All opiates have some abuse potential depending upon a specific drug's potency and its route of administration. Not only are illicit opiates abused, but the abuse of opiate analgesics such as methadone, hydromorphone (Dilaudid), oxycodone (OxyContin), and fentanyl (Duragesic) is also common.

Signs of intoxication include sedation, mild euphoria, pinpoint pupils, bradycardia, and low blood pressure. Overdose on drugs within the opiate class produces a reduced level of consciousness that may progress to coma and respiratory depression. When overdose is suspected, naloxone (Narcan), a synthetic opioid antagonist, can be administered to reverse the opiate's effects; the initial dose of 0.4 mg intravenously (IV) (0.01 mg/kg) can be repeated every 2 to 3 minutes as clinically indicated. Naloxone may be administered intramuscularly or subcutaneously if necessary. If the patient does not respond to a dose of 5 to 10 mg, opiate overdose is doubtful.

There is a well-defined withdrawal syndrome that occurs when an opiate is discontinued in one who is physiologically dependent (Table 3). Symptoms of withdrawal from a short-acting drug such as heroin begin within a few hours; withdrawal symptoms from a long-acting opiate such as methadone begin within 3 to 4 days. Opiate withdrawal is not a medical emergency in otherwise healthy adults. However, it is uncomfortable and may be a strong trigger for continued drug use.

There are several ways to address opiate withdrawal. In the context of a prescription medication being stopped too abruptly, the simplest approach is to restart the medication and reduce it more slowly. Planned detoxification is often accomplished by substituting methadone (Dolophine), a long-acting opioid agonist, for the shorter-acting opiate. With this method, the patient is stabilized on a methadone dose that blocks significant withdrawal. A dose of 40 mg given in divided doses during the day is adequate to block significant withdrawal symptoms in most patients. The stabilizing dose is tapered over several days. Clonidine (Catapres)[1] is a nonopiate that can be used to treat opiate withdrawal. It is a centrally acting a_2-agonist that reduces autonomic symptoms such as vomiting, diarrhea, and sweating (Table 4).

Methadone maintenance is the mainstay treatment for dependence on illicit opiates. The Food and Drug Administration (FDA) approved methadone for opioid maintenance therapy in 1972. Federal regulations placed tight restrictions on methadone programs that include special state and federal licensing. These restrictions have had an unintended effect of limiting treatment access for some opiate-addicted patients. Methadone maintenance treatment is criticized for a number of reasons:

- There is a risk that dispensed methadone will be sold on the street.
- Daily administration is inconvenient for patients.

---

[1]Not FDA approved for this indication.

TABLE 3 Symptoms of Opiate Withdrawal

	Objective	Subjective
Early	Lacrimation Rhinorrhea Diaphoresis Yawning	
Middle	Dilated pupils Piloerection	Restlessness Irritability Insomnia
Late	Tachycardia Increased blood pressure Vomiting Diarrhea Mood lability	Bone pain Nausea Abdominal cramps Depression

Rakel and Bope: *Conn's Current Therapy 2006.*

TABLE 4 Opioid Treatment Summary*

Treatment of Opioid Overdose

Drug	Administration
Naloxone (Narcan)	Initial dose 0.4 mg IV (0.01 mg/kg) Repeat every 2-3 minutes as indicated by symptoms Reevaluate diagnosis if no response to 5-10 mg Total

Sample Methadone Detoxification†

Day	Drug	Administration
Day 1	Methadone 40 mg (Dolophine)	Give initial dose of methadone 20 mg Additional doses of 10 or 20 mg may be given if withdrawal symptoms persist after 4 hours Maximum 40 mg total dose
Day 2-3	Methadone 25-30 mg	Reduce dose by 25% daily
Day 4	Methadone 20 mg	
Day 5	Methadone 10 mg	
Day 6	Methadone 5 mg	
Day 7	Discontinue	

Sample Clonidine Detoxification‡

Day	From short-acting opioid	With or without day naltrexone (ReVia) induction	From methadone
Day 1-2	0.3-0.6 mg	12.5 mg	0.3-0.6 mg
Day 3	0.3-0.8 mg	25 mg	0.4-0.6 mg
Day 4-5	0.6-1.2 mg Then reduce total daily dose by 50% each day, not to exceed 0.4 mg/d	50 mg Continue maintenance therapy	0.5-0.8 mg
Day 6-10			0.6-1.2 mg Then reduce total daily dose by 50% each day, not to exceed 0.4 mg/d

*All treatment must be individualized to meet specific patient needs and adjusted based on response to treatment.
†May be used in combination with clonidine (Catapres) or other as-needed medications. Catapres is not FDA approved for this indication.
‡Give a test dose of clonidine 0.1 mg. Continue only if blood pressure is >85/55. Clonidine 0.1-0.2 mg every 2-4 hours, hold for systolic blood pressure <85 or diastolic blood pressure <55.

- Some facilities offer inadequate adjunctive psychosocial or therapy services.

Despite concerns, methadone maintenance is effective in reducing criminal activity among heroin addicts, in decreasing the risk of HIV and hepatitis acquired through needle-sharing, and in returning some addicts to functional lifestyles.

Another synthetic opiate agonist, levomethadyl (Orlaam), is approved for maintenance therapy. This agent is also federally regulated. It has an advantage of a long half-life, allowing for less frequent dosing than methadone. However, it can prolong the QT interval, and this may account for the reluctance of some approved facilities to prescribe it.

Alternatively, an opiate antagonist may be useful for treatment of opiate addiction. Naltrexone (ReVia) blocks the euphoric effects of opiates. This medication should only be prescribed once a patient is opiate-free for 7 to 10 days, in order to avoid a precipitated withdrawal syndrome. The typical dose of naltrexone is 50 mg daily,

often initiated at 25 mg daily to reduce the risk of sedation and nausea. One group that has benefited from naltrexone maintenance is health care professionals who participate in a comprehensive recovery plan and are carefully monitored by state licensing boards.

Buprenorphine (Subutex) is a mixed opioid agonist-antagonist that was recently approved for the treatment of opiate addiction. A product (Suboxone) that combines buprenorphine with the opioid-antagonist naloxone reduces the risk of medication diversion for intravenous use. Office-based clinicians, including primary care physicians, may prescribe buprenorphine for treatment of opiate addiction after taking an approved training course and receiving a special waiver from the Drug Enforcement Agency. It is unclear to what extent approval of this newest agent will improve the care of opiate addicts. The potential advantages include greater convenience for patients, decreased risk of drug diversion, additional options for less severely addicted individuals, and fewer federal regulations for practitioners.

Rakel and Bope: *Conn's Current Therapy 2006.*

Patients at greatest risk for prescription opiate dependence include those who abuse other substances and those with a history of illicit opiate abuse. Patients with chronic pain are at risk for opiate dependence when increasing doses of medication are needed to control pain. It is advisable for clinicians who are unsure about prescribing opiates to seek the opinions of other professionals, especially when treating patients with chronic, nonmalignant pain.

Benzodiazepines

Benzodiazepines are used most often in the outpatient setting for the treatment of anxiety and insomnia. They have replaced barbiturates as the sedative-hypnotic of choice because of a greater safety profile in overdose. Benzodiazepines act on the brain's γ-aminobutyric acid (GABA) receptors, which results in relaxation and mild sedation. Signs of intoxication with benzodiazepines are similar to those experienced with alcohol, with higher doses producing greater sedation, slurred speech, and ataxia. However, benzodiazepines may be used as anesthetics, whereas alcohol is lethal in very high doses. In serious overdoses where benzodiazepines are suspected to play a role, the benzodiazepine antagonist flumazenil (Romazicon) may be administered at a dose of 0.2 mg IV over 30 seconds and repeated up to a 3-mg total dose. There is a risk of seizures in sedative-dependent individuals and in patients taking benzodiazepines as part of an antiepileptic regimen.

Benzodiazepines are effective in treating alcohol withdrawal. The symptoms of sedative withdrawal and alcohol withdrawal are similar—insomnia, anxiety, tachycardia, elevated blood pressure, and fever. In addition, seizures and delirium can be serious sequelae of an untreated alcohol- or sedative-withdrawal syndrome. Whereas opiate withdrawal is not a life-threatening condition unless it occurs in the context of medical frailty, untreated benzodiazepine withdrawal may result in death.

When a patient is addicted to a benzodiazepine and needs detoxification, it is common practice to substitute a long-acting benzodiazepine for a short-acting one. Table 5 gives an approximation of equivalent doses to ease the conversion from one medication to another. Once the patient is comfortable on the long-acting benzodiazepines, the dosage is gradually reduced and discontinued. However withdrawal does not always go smoothly and medication adjustments may be needed. The reduction schedule varies depending upon the severity of the addiction, the duration of benzodiazepine use, and the dosage used.

Hospitalized patients who are addicted to high doses of benzodiazepines often do well when converted to an equivalent dose of a long-acting agent such as clonazepam (Klonopin) or chlordiazepoxide (Librium). Then the dose may be reduced on a 10% per day schedule. In these patients it is necessary to monitor vital signs every 4 hours and have additional doses of benzodiazepine ordered for signs of withdrawal. Such signs include tremulousness, diaphoresis, blood pressure higher than

TABLE 5 Approximate Benzodiazepine Dose Equivalency

Generic Name (Trade Name)	Dose Equivalents (mg)*	Short- or Long-Acting
Alprazolam (Xanax)	1	Short
Chlordiazepoxide (Librium)	25	Long
Clonazepam (Klonopin)	0.5	Long
Diazepam (Valium)	10	Long
Flurazepam (Dalmane)	30	Long
Lorazepam (Ativan)	2	Short
Oxazepam (Serax)	30	Short
Prazepam (Centrax)	10	Long
Temazepam (Restoril)	20	Short
Triazolam (Halcion)	0.25	Short

*Doses are approximately equivalent to phenobarbital 30 mg.

150/100, and heart rate more than 100. Outpatients may require several weeks to months for detoxification. Some treatment centers use anticonvulsants, specifically valproic acid (Depakote)[1] and carbamazepine (Tegretol),[1] to prevent or minimize withdrawal symptoms.

Other Drugs of Abuse

Clinicians may deal with any number of abused substances. The popularity of particular drugs changes over time. However, there are several types of substances that come up frequently enough to warrant inclusion here. One example is the inhalants. The agents that make up this group are inexpensive and accessible in common household products such as glue, shoe polish, paint thinners, aerosols, and correction and cleaning fluids. Intoxication on these agents most resembles alcohol intoxication. Acute overdose is rare but can result in death from asphyxiation or cardiac arrhythmia. The brain, kidneys, and liver are susceptible to damage from repeated inhalant exposure. The result over the long term may be chronic delirium, psychosis, or renal failure. An estimated 15% of young adults have tried an inhalant. However, it is estimated that less than 1% are addicted to inhalant use.

Hallucinogens are another group of abusable drugs. Management of intoxication on these drugs is supportive in most cases. Lysergic acid diethylamide (LSD) is a well-known drug in this class. Like most hallucinogens it produces visual hallucinations and increases sensory awareness. Intoxication can also cause dilated pupils, facial flushing, tachycardia, and increased blood pressure. 3,4-Methylenedioxymethamphetamine (MDMA), or ecstasy, may be classified as either a hallucinogen or a stimulant because it has properties of both. It is generally considered a dangerous drug because of its potential for long-term brain damage. It may also be toxic to the heart and liver.

---

[1]Not FDA approved for this indication.

Rakel and Bope: *Conn's Current Therapy 2006.*

TABLE 6 Benzodiazepine Treatment Summary*

Treatment of Overdose

Drug	Administration
Flumazenil (Romazicon)	Initial dose 0.2 mg IV over 30 seconds. Repeat every minute up to a 3-mg total dose. Re-evaluate diagnosis if no response after 3-5 minutes.

Detoxification Guidelines

Day	Action
Day 1	Long-acting benzodiazepine until symptom control is achieved. Common upper limits are clonazepam (Klonopin), 6-8 mg per 24 hours or chlordiazepoxide (Librium), 400 mg per 24 hours.
Day 2– Completion	Taper by 25% every 1-2 days Monitor vital signs every 4 hours Have PRN doses available, i.e., clonazepam, 1 mg, chlordiazepoxide, 25 mg, for signs or symptoms of withdrawal (tremulousness, diaphoresis, systolic blood pressure >150, diastolic blood pressure >100, or heart rate >100). Consider adding anticonvulsants.

*All treatment must be individualized to meet specific patient needs and adjusted based on response to treatment.

Phencyclidine (PCP) intoxication can have a frightening presentation. The patient may become agitated and unpredictable, requiring physical and chemical restraints to ensure the safety of the patient and those around him or her. Medication may not be necessary if the patient is placed in a quiet, supportive setting. If medications are used, benzodiazepines are typically chosen first. If antipsychotics are required, agents with low anticholinergic activity are preferred. Toxic doses of PCP can produce a life-threatening condition with severe autonomic instability in which hypertension, hyperthermia, convulsions, and coma may become serious medical management problems.

Treatment

While medication management is increasingly important in the treatment of alcohol and drug dependence, nonpharmacologic approaches are the mainstay of substance abuse treatment. Alcoholics Anonymous (AA) helped many alcoholics recover before physicians had treatment techniques to offer. AA remains a proven resource, and other self-help groups are modeled after it. Narcotics Anonymous (NA) and Cocaine Anonymous (CA), similar to AA, are pivotal in the recovery of some drug abusers. The caveat is that one group may be very different from another.

There are significant problems in some self-help groups. Patients may have concerns about heavy cigarette-smoking in meetings, about attendees who actively use or sell drugs, and about criticism of prescribed psychotropic medications. Therefore, when a patient finds one group unsatisfactory for some reason, the clinician can suggest he or she try another group. Some patients object to the religious tone of traditional 12-step groups. For these individuals alternative groups such as Women for Sobriety and Rational Recovery may be more acceptable. In addition, self-help groups are free of charge, which is a factor for some patients.

Most professional addiction treatment occurs in an outpatient setting. However, higher levels of care are available in hospital, residential, or partial hospital programs if there are chaotic living situations, or pressing psychiatric or other medical needs. Social interventions are crucial for patients faced with unemployment, legal consequences, and housing dilemmas. Psychiatric disorders occur with a high frequency in drug-abusing populations, and both disorders should be treated to optimize the patient's chances for recovery. Therefore, a multidisciplinary approach to treatment often works best.

Psychiatric symptoms in patients who abuse drugs are easy to recognize. Mood lability, depression, and anxiety are common. The challenge lies in sorting out whether these symptoms are caused by the use of a mood-altering substance or represent a separate mood or anxiety disorder. Psychiatric expertise may be needed to assist in sorting out this diagnostic dilemma. Patients with schizophrenic and bipolar disorders are also at high risk for drug abuse, which can exacerbate psychoses.

The cognitive aspects of professional treatment often include educational, motivational, cognitive–behavioral, relapse prevention, and 12-step strategies. Most treatment programs try to get the patient to more fully recognize the problems associated with his or her drug use, identify reasons to change, acknowledge obstacles to sobriety, become aware of triggers to relapse, and consider ways to build a sober support network. Patients with addictive disorders do get better, and treatment of patients with drug abuse can be highly rewarding. It is important to recognize this problem as one of many chronic, relapsing conditions seen in medicine today.

Anxiety Disorders

Method of
Jacqueline Carinhas McGregor, MD

Anxiety disorders are the most common psychiatric disorders in the world among both children and adults. In the United States, 30 million people or approximately one of every four meet the criteria for an anxiety disorder in their lifetimes. It is estimated that the annual cost of anxiety disorders in 1998 dollars was more than

$63 billion. More than half of these costs were due to nonpsychiatric direct medical costs, which include undiagnosed, misdiagnosed, or inadequately treated anxiety disorders. It is clear that much of the emotional and economic burden caused by these disorders could be alleviated by improving diagnosis and treatment.

Genetics, temperament, and life stressors can all be contributors to anxiety disorders. Norepinephrine and serotonin are thought to be the major neurotransmitters involved in mediating anxiety symptoms whereas the sympathetic nervous system also plays an important role. The onset of anxiety disorders can usually be traced to childhood, adolescence, or young adulthood. With the exception of obsessive-compulsive disorder, women are more likely than men to suffer from anxiety disorders. Anxiety disorders occur across racial groups without distinction.

Anxiety is characterized by subjective feelings of worry, dread, or anticipation and can include hypervigilance, excessive negativity, and a myriad of somatic symptoms. These symptoms can include diaphoresis, palpitations, shortness of breath, dizziness, chest pain, tremulousness, gastrointestinal complaints, fatigue, dry mouth, sleep problems, hot flashes, polyuria, and restlessness. Because of the wide variety of physical complaints, underlying organic causes and disorders secondary to substances use must first be ruled out (Box 1). A detailed history of present illness, past medical history, substance history, and review of symptoms is essential. If a patient initially presents with anxiety symptoms in middle or late adulthood, has no family history of anxiety disorders, has no temporally related stressors, and does not respond to psychiatric intervention, a closer investigation of organic causes of anxiety should be undertaken.

In patients describing chest pain, cardiovascular causes such as angina, mitral valve prolapse, arrhythmias, and pulmonary embolism should be ruled out. Pulmonary ailments such as asthma, chronic obstructive pulmonary disorder, and pneumonia should be considered in patients describing shortness of breath. Hyperthyroidism, pheochromocytoma, and Cushing's

syndrome are examples of endocrine disorders that can mimic anxiety disorders. Other disorders to consider include anemia, delirium, menopause, and gastroesophogeal reflux. Medications such as stimulants (including herbal supplements and caffeine), decongestants, antipsychotics, theophylline, steroids, calcium channel blockers, and anticholenergics should all be considered. Alcohol and illicit drug use or withdrawal are other possible causes of anxiety symptoms.

The most common diagnoses of anxiety disorders include generalized anxiety disorder (GAD), panic disorder, social anxiety disorder, obsessive-compulsive disorder (OCD), posttraumatic stress disorder (PTSD), and specific phobias. Those suffering from anxiety disorders are likely to have another co-morbid psychiatric disorder such as a mood disorder or substance dependence. These patients also have a higher risk for suicidal behaviors. It is important to distinguish anxiety disorders from each other, as well as from other psychiatric disorders because the specific diagnosis may have significant impact on treatment decisions. Simple phobias, for example, are not responsive to medication and require cognitive behavioral intervention. OCD requires significantly higher doses of antidepressants than other disorders. Patients with GAD and panic disorder need lower starting doses of antidepressants to avoid iatrogenically exacerbating their symptoms. In the case of patient with comorbid bipolar disorder, special care should be used with antidepressants to prevent the induction of a manic episode.

Psychotherapeutic interventions are often considered the first line of intervention in anxiety disorders, particularly for patients with mild symptoms, those who prefer nonpharmacologic treatment, and for children. Cognitive behavior therapy (CBT) is a specific type of psychotherapy that combines behavioral therapy with cognitive therapy and has the best evidence-based research supporting its use in anxiety disorders. The behavioral component of CBT includes exposure and ritual prevention whereas the cognitive aspect includes identifying false, irrational thoughts and the automatic responses to them. It is important to find skilled therapists with specialized training in these modalities in order to facilitate helpful referrals.

The pharmacologic treatment of most anxiety disorders usually includes selective serotonin reuptake inhibitors (SSRIs) serotonin-norepinephrine reuptake inhibitors (SNRIs), and/or benzodiazepines. The SSRIs fluoxetine (Prozac) and paroxetine (Paxil) are both potent inhibitors of cytochrome P450 2D6, and significant interactions can occur with other drugs that a patient may be taking. Escitalopram (Lexapro) has the most favorable SSRI side effect profile with the least protein-binding and cytochrome-P450 interactions. The most common side effects of SSRIs are nervousness, insomnia, restlessness, nausea, and diarrhea. Venlafaxine (Effexor) has a lower risk of significant drug interactions compared to the SSRIs; however, patients prescribed venlafaxine (Effexor) should have their blood pressure monitored as it can cause or worsen existing hypertension. Benzodiazepines should be used carefully because of their addictive potential

BOX 1	Organic Causes of Anxiety Symptoms
Cardiopulmonary	Angina, mitral valve prolapse, pulmonary embolism, COPD, asthma
Endocrine	Hyperthyroidism, pheochromocytoma, Cushing's syndrome, menopause
Gastrointestinal	Gastroesophogeal reflux, irritable bowel syndrome, gastritis
Neurologic	Dementia, substance intoxication or withdrawal, seizure disorder, migraine
Medications	Stimulants, herbal supplements, decongestants, steroids, antipsychotics, theophylline, calcium channel blockers, anticholenergics

Abbreviation: COPD = chronic obstructive pulmonary disease.

and should be avoided in patients with a history of substance abuse.

As with any drug, it is important to discuss the risk and benefits of medication options with patients before coming to a treatment decision. The dosage of a medication should be carefully titrated to minimize side effects while providing adequate symptom response. The Food and Drug Administration (FDA) issued a labeling change request in October 2004 for a black box warning on antidepressant medications about the *possible* association of SSRIs with suicidality in the treatment of major depressive disorder. The antidepressant side effect of agitation has been known to trigger suicidal behavior in those with or without premorbid depression. A physician should exercise special care in using SSRI medications, especially with those younger than 18 years of age. Frequent follow-up visits are recommended to monitor side effects and treatment response. Three of the most prevalent and burdensome anxiety disorders are GAD, OCD, and panic disorder. The remainder of this article will focus on the diagnosis and treatment of GAD and OCD disorders. Panic disorder is discussed in another article.

Generalized Anxiety Disorder

DIAGNOSIS

According to the *Diagnostic and Statistical Manual of Mental Disorders IV-TR,* individuals with GAD suffer from uncontrollable, excessive anxiety and worry involving several areas of functioning on most days in a 6 month period. It must be associated with three or more of the following symptoms: restlessness, fatigue concentration difficulties, irritability, muscle tension, or sleep problems. The anxiety cannot be the result of another Axis I disorder; it must cause a significant impairment in functioning, and it cannot be due to substance abuse, a medical disorder, or occur exclusively in the context of a mood disorder, psychotic disorder, or pervasive developmental disorder.

The 12-month prevalence for GAD is 3.1%, and the lifetime prevalence is close to 5%. Women are twice as likely as men to suffer from GAD. GAD usually develops sometime during late adolescence or early adulthood, its symptoms tend to have a chronic duration, and there is a high incidence of comorbid psychiatric disorders (especially depression) associated with it.

GAD can be difficult for the physician to diagnose because patients can be reluctant to discuss their anxiety or be unable to identify it as the source of their concerns. Patient complaints of fatigue, insomnia, somatic symptoms, or chronic pain should be a signal for the physician to ask more about anxiety symptoms.

TREATMENT

Psychotherapy, pharmacotherapy, and their combination can be successfully used to treat GAD. Psychotherapy, particularly cognitive-behavior therapy and applied relaxation, are effective treatment strategies for GAD.

Rakel and Bope: *Conn's Current Therapy 2006.*

Psychotherapy can be used concomitantly with pharmacotherapy, often with better result than if either were used alone.

There are a variety of psychopharmacologic interventions that can be used for patients with GAD (Table 1). An antidepressant or the 5-HT$_{1A}$ partial agonist, buspirone (BusPar), is considered the first line of drug treatment. Paroxetine (Paxil), escitalopram (Lexapro), and venlafaxine (Effexor) are the only antidepressants that have an FDA indication for GAD, although there is evidence that both imipramine (Tofranil)[1] and sertraline (Zoloft)[1] are effective drugs in the treatment of GAD. SSRIs are usually considered the antidepressant of choice because of their safety and relatively modest side effects. Use tricyclic antidepressants such as imipramine (Tofranil) with care because of their more troublesome side-effect profile, proarrhythmic properties, and potential lethality in overdose. The most commonly noted side effects of buspirone (BusPar) are dizziness, nausea, headache, nervousness, and insomnia. Benzodiazepines can play an important role in the treatment of GAD. It is important to keep in mind the addictive potential of these medications before using them. In the first weeks of treatment with SSRIs, it can be helpful to use benzodiazepines to address acute anxiety symptoms while allowing sufficient time for the SSRI to achieve its effect. As symptoms begin to respond, the physician should consider tapering and discontinuing the benzodiazepine.

After an 8- to 10-week course of treatment with an antidepressant, if there has been an insufficient response at an adequate dose, the clinician should consider switching to or augmenting with another drug (e.g., another antidepressant, buspirone [BusPar] or a benzodiazepine). Patients need significant support and encouragement from their physician to be compliant with daily medication regimes and to continue their

---

[1]Not FDA approved for this indication.

TABLE 1 Pharmacotherapy in the Treatment of Generalized Anxiety Disorder

Drug	Starting Dose	Target Dose
SSRIs		
Paroxetine (Paxil CR)*	10 mg qd	10-60 mg qd
Escitolapram (Lexapro)*	5-10 mg qd	10-20 mg qd
Sertraline (Zoloft)	12.5-25 mg qd	50-200 mg qd
Fluoxetine (Prozac)	10 mg qd	20-40 mg qd
SNRIs		
Venlafazine (Effexor XR)*	37.5 mg qam	150-300 mg qam
OTHER		
Buspirone (BusPar)	5 mg bid-tid	10 mg bid to tid

*FDA indication for generalized anxiety disorder (GAD)
Abbreviations: bid = twice daily; qam = every morning; qd = every day; tid = three times daily.
SNRIs = serotonin-norepinephrine reuptake inhibitors; SSRIs = selective serotonin reuptake inhibitors.

medication once they begin to experience symptom relief. There is little data on the length of treatment or whether pharmacologic intervention can prevent future relapse. It is common practice to continue treatment for at least 6 to 12 months after resolution of symptoms before stopping medications. At that time a gradual tapering of the medication dose can be considered.

Obsessive Compulsive Disorder

DIAGNOSIS

The *Diagnostic and Statistical Manual of Mental Disorders IV-TR* outlines the criteria for OCD as having obsessions and/or compulsions. Obsessions are defined as recurrent, persistent thoughts, impulses, or images that are experienced as intrusive and inappropriate and cause significant distress. They cannot be excessive worries about realistic or reasonable concerns. The individual attempts to ignore the obsessions or counteract them with another thought or action and understands that the obsessions are a product of his or her own mind. Compulsions are defined as repetitive behaviors or mental acts that the individual feels compelled to perform in response to an obsession. The compulsion is aimed at reducing distress or preventing some dreaded event, but is not clearly connected to the distress or event or is clearly excessive. Except in the case of children, at some point in the course of the disorder the individual recognizes that the obsessions or compulsions are unreasonable. This last point is important in distinguishing OCD from obsessive compulsive personality disorder. The obsessions or compulsions must cause significant impairment and, if another Axis I disorder coexists, the obsessions and/or compulsions cannot be restricted only to the content of that disorder (e.g., preoccupations with food in the case of an eating disorder, hair pulling in the case of trichotillomania). As in the case of GAD, the symptoms cannot occur because of the effects of a substance or secondary to a general medical disorder.

It is not uncommon for OCD to occur with other psychiatric disorders including major depressive disorder, other anxiety disorders, eating disorders, and tic disorders. In children, streptococcal infections are associated with the development of obsessions and compulsions. Psychotic disorders can have obsessive or compulsive behaviors, but these are typically much more bizarre, and the individual has little insight into his or her behavior. It is also important to consider illnesses that can have OCD-like symptoms such as basal ganglia disorders (e.g., Huntington's disease) or tic disorders.

OCD usually appears in late adolescence or early adulthood and has a waxing and waning course. Unlike other anxiety disorders there is an equal occurrence in males and females. The lifetime prevalence rate of OCD is 2% to 3% of the population. Neuroimaging studies of OCD suggest that there are structural and functional problems in the orbitofrontal-subcortical circuitry.

People with OCD often avoid seeking treatment for their illness. Diagnosis often requires explicit questioning

 CURRENT DIAGNOSIS

Generalized anxiety disorder

- Excessive anxiety and worry about multiple concerns
- Three additional anxiety symptoms (only one in children or adolescents)
- Difficulty controlling the anxiety and worry
- Symptoms last at least 6 months

Obsessive compulsive disorder

- Obsessions and/or compulsions
- Recognition that obsessions or compulsions are excessive or unreasonable (not necessary in children or adolescents)
- Causes significant impairment

Panic disorder

- Repetitive, discrete periods of intense fear or discomfort
- At least four panic symptoms peaking within 10 minutes
- At least one panic attack followed by 1 month of anticipatory anxiety about having another panic attack

Social phobia

- Marked and persistent fear of social or performance situations in which embarrassment can occur
- Exposure to the situation provokes anxiety
- Recognition that fear is excessive or unreasonable
- Feared situation is avoided
- Avoidance causes significant impairment
- Symptoms last at least 6 months in children or adolescents

Specific phobia

- Intense fear reaction to a specific object or situation
- Level of fear in inappropriate to the situation
- Exposure to situation provokes an immediate anxiety response
- Recognition that fear is excessive or unreasonable (not necessary in children or adolescents)
- Situation is avoided or endured with significant distress

Post-traumatic stress disorder

- Follows exposure to a traumatic event
- Event is re-experienced
- Leads to avoidance behavior and increased arousal
- Symptoms last longer than 1 month

Adapted from American Psychiatric Association: Diagnostic and Statistical Manual of Mental Disorders, 4th ed, text rev. Washington, DC, American Psychiatric Association, 2000.

regarding specific behaviors such as perfectionism, rituals, washing, counting, checking, or hoarding. The physicians should also be on the lookout for excessively red or raw hands, recurring request for reassurance about medical illnesses, frequent emergency room visits, or usual repetitive behaviors observed in the examining room such as tic-like motions or tapping.

Rakel and Bope: *Conn's Current Therapy 2006*.

CURRENT THERAPY

	First intervention	Second intervention	Third intervention

GAD	CBT	SSRI OR
		   venlafaxine (Effexor) OR
		   buspirone (BusPar) OR
			Change to different antidepressant or buspirone (BusPar) OR
			Augment with a different antidepressant class, buspirone
			   (BusPar), or benzodiazepine

OCD	CBT	High dose SSRI
		   (push to maximum dose
		   in 4 to 8 weeks)
			Change to another SSRI or clomipramine (anafranil)
			OR
			Augment with atypical antipsychotic

Abbreviations: CBT = cognitive behavior therapy; GAD = generalized anxiety disorder; OCD = obsessive-compulsive disorder; SSRI = selective serotonin reuptake inhibitor.

TREATMENT

There are a variety of treatment approaches that can be used for OCD. As with GAD, psychotherapy can be utilized effectively. There is significant research that supporting cognitive behavioral therapy that incorporates exposure-response prevention is a successful treatment for obsessions and compulsions. In more severe cases of OCD, optimal treatment uses a combination of cognitive behavioral therapy and medication.

Several studies demonstrated the efficacy of SSRIs in OCD. A reasonable trial of SSRIs in OCD can be longer and requires higher doses than what would be expected in GAD or major depressive disorder. Setraline (Zoloft), fluoxetine (Prozac), paroxetine (Paxil), and fluvoxamine (Luvox) are SSRIs with FDA indications for OCD.

For those with an inadequate response to treatment with SSRIs, the clinician should consider changing SSRIs, switching to the tricyclic antidepressant, clomipramine (Anafranil), or to the SNRI, venlafaxine (Effexor).[1] The most common side effects of clomipramine (Anafranil) include dry mouth, sedation, dizziness, and weight gain, however, more serious, less common side effects include hypertension and cardiac arrhythmias.

[1]Not FDA approved for this indication.

Augmentation with a dopamine agonist such as risperidone (Risperdal)[1] or olanzapine (Zyprexa) has been shown to be an effective treatment approach as has the addition of buspirone (BusPar)[1] or benzodiazepines (Table 2).

There is some evidence to support the use of monoamine oxidase inhibitors (MAOIs) in treatment-resistant OCD, but because of the significant side effects, potential drug and food interactions, and toxicity, they are considered an option only when other medication options have proven unsuccessful. For those who fail psychotherapy and psychopharmacology and continue to have significant functional impairment, transcranial magnetic stimulation and neurosurgery are considered treatments of last resort.

Treatment of OCD can usually be accomplished on an outpatient basis; however, in severe refractory cases, inpatient treatment at a facility that specializes in OCD may be necessary. Whatever treatment strategy is employed, the physician should be mindful of the fact that the patient's family often needs to be involved in the treatment. Families often unknowingly reinforce a patient's OCD behaviors by going along with their rituals or participating in excessive reassurance.

Anxiety disorders are quite common and cause a significant burden to individuals as well as to society. The differential diagnosis of anxiety disorders is quite extensive given that anxiety symptoms are often non-specific. Anxiety disorders often go undiagnosed or are inadequately treated and are likely to occur together with other psychiatric disorders. Primary care physicians are more likely to have the opportunity to detect anxiety disorders and, in fact treat more of these disorders

[1]Not FDA approved for this indication.

TABLE 2 Pharmacotherapy in the Treatment of Obsessive-Compulsive Disorder

Drug	Starting Dose	Target Daily Dose
SSRI		
Sertraline (Zoloft)*	25-50 mg qd	100-300 mg[3]
Paroxetine (Paxil CR)*	12.5 mg qd	25-50 mg
Fluoxetine (Prozac)*	10 mg qd	20-60 mg
Fluvoxamine (Luvox)*	25-50 mg qd	100-300 mg
SNRI		
Venlafaxine (Effexor XR)	37.5 mg qam	150-300 mg
TCA		
Clomipramine* (Anafranil)	25 mg qhs	100-300 mg

*FDA indication for obsessive-compulsive disorder (OCD).
[3]Exceeds dosage recommended by the manufacturer.
Abbreviations: qam = every morning; qd = every day; qhs = at bed time.

BOX 2 Helpful Resources for Anxiety Disorders

National Alliance for the Mentally Ill	www.nami.org
National Institute of Mental Health	www.nimh.org
Anxiety Disorders Association of America	www.adaa.org
Obsessive-Compulsive Foundation	www.ocfoundation.org

than mental health care practitioners. Effective treatments for anxiety including psychotherapeutic as well as psychopharmacologic interventions are shown in Box 2.

REFERENCES

American Psychiatric Association: Diagnostic and Statistical Manual of Mental Disorders, 4th ed, text rev. Washington, DC, American Psychiatric Association, 2000.

Baer L, Rauch SK, Ballantine T, et al: *Cingulotomy for intractable obsessive-compulsive disorder*. Arch Gen Psych 1995;52:384-392.

Borkovec T, Costello E: *Efficacy of applied relaxation and cognitive-behavioral therapy in the treatment of generalized anxiety disorder*. Journal of Consulting and Clinical Psychology, 1993;61(4):611-619.

Food and Drug Administration: FDA labeling change request letter for antidepressant medications, 2004.

Greenberg BD, George MS, Martin DJ, et al: *Effect of prefrontal repetitive transcranial stimulation in obsessive-compulsive disorder: A preliminary study*. Am J Psychiatry 1997;154:867-869.

Greenberg PE, Sisitsky T, Kessler RC, et al: *The economic burden of anxiety disorders in the 1990s*. J Clin Psychiatry 1990;60:427-435.

Jenike MA, Baer L, Minichiello WE (eds): Obsessive-compulsive disorders: practical management 3rd ed. St Louis, Mosby, 1998.

Karno M, Golding JM, Sorenson SB, et al: *The epidemiology of obsessive-compulsive disorder in five US communities*. Arch Gen Psychiatry 1988;45(12):1094-1099.

Kessler RC, McGonagle KA, Zhao S: *Lifetime and 12-month prevalence of DSM-III-R psychiatric disorders in the United States*. Arch Gen Psychiatry 1994;51(1):8-19.

Kobak KA, Griest JH, Jefferson JW, et al: *Behavioral versus pharmacologic treatment of obsessive compulsive disorder: A meta-analysis*. Psychopharmacology (Berl) 1998;136:205-216.

Koran LM, Rinhold AL, Elliot MA: *Olanzapine augmentation in obsessive compulsive disorder refractory to selective serotonin reuptake inhibitors: An open label case series*. J Clin Psychiatry 2000;61:514-517.

Ladouceur R, Dugas MJ, Freeston MH, et al: *Efficacy of a cognitive behavioral treatment for generalized anxiety disorder evaluation in controlled clinical trial*. J Consult Clin Psychol 2000;68(6):957-964.

Liebowitz MR, DeMartinis NA, Weihs K, et al: *Efficacy of sertraline in severe generalized social anxiety disorder: results of a double-blind, placebo-controlled study*. J Clin Psychiatry, 2003;64(7):785-792.

McDougle CJ, Epperson CN, Pelton GH, et al: *A double blind placebo controlled study of risperidone addition in serotin reuptake inhibitor-refractory obsessive compulsive disorder*. Arch Gen Psych 2000;57:794-801.

Rickels K, Downing R, Schweizer E, et al: *Antidepressant for the treatment of generalized anxiety disorder: a placebo controlled comparison of imipramine, trazodone, and diazepam*. Arch Gen Psychiatry, 1993;50:884-895.

Rickels K, Schweizer E: *The spectrum of generalized anxiety in clinical practice: The role of short term intermittent treatment*. Br J Psychiatry 1998;173(Suppl 34):49-54.

Saxena S, Bota RG, Brody AL: Brain-behavior relationships in obsessive-compulsive disorder. Semin Clin Neuropsychiatry 2001;6(2):82-101.

Bulimia Nervosa

Method of
David B. Herzog, MD, and Kamryn T. Eddy, MD

Bulimia nervosa is a prevalent eating disorder most commonly observed in late adolescent and young adult women and often associated with psychiatric co-morbidity and medical sequelae. The course of the disorder may be chronic and relapsing, and patients may demonstrate early ambivalence regarding treatment. There is often a considerable delay between onset of symptoms and presentation for treatment that may reflect shame, control issues, and fear of change (e.g., weight gain). Currently, psychosocial treatments—particularly cognitive behavioral therapy—are considered the first-line of treatment for the disorder, having demonstrated the most successful outcomes, but psychopharmacologic interventions are also promising.

Diagnosis and Clinical Features

DIAGNOSIS

Bulimia nervosa was first recognized formally as a clinical diagnosis in 1979 by Gerald Russell. The disorder is currently defined in the *Diagnostic and Statistical Manual of Mental Disorders, Fourth Edition* (*DSM-IV*) on the basis of recurrent binge eating and compensatory behaviors and related cognitions. Binge eating is defined as the consumption of a large amount of food (typically 2000 to 4000 calories) within a discrete period of time accompanied by loss of control overeating. Loss of control overeating involves the subjective experience of being unable to control what or how much one is eating and may be characterized by eating more rapidly than usual and consuming calorie-dense foods that are typically avoided outside of binge episodes. Compensatory behaviors are designed to counteract the effects of binge eating and can be classified as purging (self-induced vomiting, misuse of laxatives, diuretics, and enemas) and nonpurging (excessive exercise, fasting). The *DSM-IV* specifies that the binge eating and compensatory behaviors occur on average at least twice weekly during a 3-month period. In addition to the behavioral components, the *DSM-IV* indicates a cognitive component of overevaluation of the importance of weight and shape on sense of self. Weight is not part of the bulimia nervosa criteria; although most patients with bulimia nervosa are within an average weight range, patients may be overweight, obese, or even underweight.

Patients with bulimia nervosa can be grouped into purging and nonpurging types based on the compensatory behaviors used. Notably, purging type appears to be predominant; less research exists on the nonpurging type.

According to the *DSM-IV* hierarchy rules, a diagnosis of bulimia nervosa is not made if the binge and compensatory behaviors occur exclusively during a period of anorexia nervosa. Similarly, a diagnosis of binge eating disorder (currently recognized in the *DSM-IV* as an eating disorder not otherwise specified) can be appropriate if recurrent binge eating is present in the absence of any compensatory behaviors.

Although the current diagnostic system is useful, limitations exist. For example, there appears to be heterogeneity within the diagnostic category of bulimia nervosa on the basis of psychosocial functioning, personality style, and co-morbidity, which may have treatment implications. Furthermore, a large subset of patients present for treatment in clinical settings with symptom profiles that closely resemble that of a patient with bulimia nervosa but do not meet all of the diagnostic criteria. For example, although a formal diagnosis of bulimia nervosa stipulates a twice-weekly binge/compensatory behaviors frequency criterion, patients often present to eating disorder clinics for the treatment of bingeing and/or purging that occurs less frequently. Thus, this treatment review derives from the literature on bulimia nervosa but can be considered applicable across patients with a spectrum of bulimic symptoms.

DIFFERENTIAL DIAGNOSIS

Consideration of a range of conditions that may be characterized by features similar to bulimia nervosa is necessary in the initial assessment. Neurologic disorders impacting appetite regulation and eating behaviors (e.g., pituitary or hypothalamic brain tumors, Kleine-Levin or Klüver-Bucy syndromes), hormonal disorders relating to malnutrition and hypometabolism (e.g., adrenal disease, diabetes mellitus, pituitary dysfunction, hyperthyroidism), and gastrointestinal (GI) disorders (e.g., malabsorption, enteritis) should be considered. Psychiatric disorders including major depression and borderline personality disorder should be considered because they may be associated with binge eating even though compensatory behaviors and cognitive features of bulimia nervosa are absent.

MEDICAL COMPLICATIONS

Patients with bulimia nervosa are generally within the normal weight range, but they may show signs of malnutrition. Medical complications secondary to bingeing and purging behaviors and malnutrition are common. Patients often present with transient facial swelling, peripheral edema, weakness and fatigue, dental problems, and abrasions on the dorsal surface of the hand (Russell's sign). Medical assessment should be based on current symptom presentation and should include complete blood count, serum electrolytes, serum blood urea nitrogen (BUN)/creatinine levels, urinalysis, and an electrocardiogram (ECG). Electrolyte and acid-based complications secondary to purging are common and may include hypochloremia, hyponatremia, and hypokalemia. Hypokalemia is related to significant cardiac problems including arrhythmias. Long-term ipecac use may lead to cardiomyopathy. Edema may be present and related to laxative and diuretic abuse. Dental complications related to chronic regurgitation of gastric contents can

include enamel erosion and caries. Swelling of the parotid glands is also common. GI difficulties ranging from constipation and bloating to esophageal disorders may also be present. Many of these symptom-related complications remit when the purging is discontinued, but additional treatment and monitoring can be warranted for some patients.

CO-MORBIDITY

Bulimia nervosa is often associated with psychiatric co-morbidity including mood, anxiety, and substance use disorders. Approximately half of patients with bulimia nervosa report a lifetime history of depression. Similarly, anxiety disorders including social phobia and obsessive-compulsive disorder are commonly reported. Although depression may precede the onset, have simultaneous onset, or follow the eating disorder onset, anxiety disorders most often precede the onset of the eating disorder. A substantial minority of patients with bulimia nervosa also reports a lifetime history of substance use disorders, with alcohol abuse being the most common.

Personality styles have received considerable attention in patients with bulimia nervosa. Research indicates that a subset of patients with bulimia can be characterized as multi-impulsive or dysregulated across multiple domains including eating, affect, interpersonal functioning, and sexuality, for example. Bulimic patients with dysregulated personality styles are more likely to present with co-morbid substance use disorders, cluster B axis II disorders, self-destructive and self-injurious behaviors, and kleptomania.

Epidemiology

Population surveys indicate a 1% to 4% lifetime prevalence rate for bulimia nervosa. However, subthreshold binge/purge symptoms and overvaluation of weight and shape are more common. Further, rates of bulimia nervosa are generally higher within given population subsets including college females, for example. Typical age of onset is in late adolescence or early adulthood and may occur during a time of transition (e.g., high school to college) or psychosocial stress. Approximately 90% of patients presenting for treatment of bulimia nervosa are female. Current research indicates that bulimia nervosa is prevalent across ethnicity and socioeconomic status. Notably, however, eating disorders are more commonly seen in industrialized nations where a thin female appearance is valued.

Etiology

A large body of research has considered the etiology of bulimia nervosa, implicating psychological, biological, and social factors. Psychological factors include general personality traits such as perfectionism and difficulty with emotion regulation, difficulty dealing with conflict, and pervasive low self-esteem. It is hypothesized that

17

these variables represent vulnerability factors that are triggered by biological and environmental variables (e.g., transition, parent eating disorder, family conflict). The biological model of bulimia nervosa is supported by the higher concordance of monozygotic than dizygotic twins, which suggests genetic factors are implicated. Further, the biological model suggests that patient-induced dietary restraint leads to binge eating. The implication of social factors is supported by the increased prevalence of bulimia nervosa in industrialized nations. The images of ideal beauty portrayed by the media are inundating in Western society, and yet they are unrealistically thin for most women; women with a childhood history of overweight and obesity may be at particular risk. This leads to internalization of a thin body ideal and associated body dissatisfaction, both of which predict bulimic symptoms. It is likely that the confluence of multiple psychological, biological, and sociocultural factors predicts the development of bulimia nervosa. Early warning signs that may be observed by family members or primary care physicians are changes in eating behaviors and weight-related concerns (e.g., not eating with the family, nighttime eating, increased body concerns in normal or underweight females), physical changes (e.g., weight loss, amenorrhea), changes in social behaviors (e.g., avoidance of activities, isolation), and mood-related changes (e.g., loss of self-esteem, depressed mood, irritability).

Treatment Options

Treatment for bulimia nervosa often involves multiple components, the most common of which are psychosocial and pharmacologic. The primary aims of treatment for bulimia nervosa are to reduce and eliminate binge/purge behaviors, modify unhealthy attitudes toward weight and shape, and encourage healthier coping styles. Most patients with bulimia nervosa can be treated on an outpatient basis; however, hospitalization may be necessary for patients who are medically unstable (e.g., because of complications secondary to bulimia nervosa or medical morbidity such as diabetes), severely depressed, or treatment-refractory.

ASSESSMENT

A comprehensive assessment is needed to determine an appropriate and individualized treatment course. Assessment should provide detailed information regarding:

- Eating disorder symptom severity (i.e., frequency, type, history)
- Medical issues and bulimia-related complications
- Developmental history
- Psychiatric history
- Treatment history
- Family history

For a subset of patients bulimia nervosa may be complicated by a concomitant medical condition; in these cases prioritizing the severity of various medical problems is necessary as a piece of the assessment.

Patients with bulimia nervosa tend to manifest shame and embarrassment about their binge/purge symptoms. There is often considerable ambivalence in these patients who, on the one hand, describe feeling out of control with their eating behaviors and perhaps wish for immediate relief and therefore may be interested in beginning a treatment that will help them regain stability over their eating. Yet, they may be hesitant to implement recommendations, demonstrating significant fears that discontinuing the binge/purge cycle will result in weight gain, which they believe would be unbearable. Determining motivation and readiness to change is an important phase of the assessment process.

Psychosocial

Several psychosocial interventions have received empirical support for the treatment of bulimia nervosa, and currently psychotherapy is regarded as the first-line of treatment for the disorder.

Cognitive behavioral therapy (CBT) is one such approach that has received the strongest empirical support. CBT has been widely studied: in clinical trials it achieves 80% reductions in bingeing and purging behavior in patients and leads to full recovery in approximately 50% of patients. CBT for bulimia nervosa works on a model in which dietary restraint leads to binge eating and subsequent compensatory behaviors; both reinforce concern about eating, weight, and shape and in turn drive the bulimic cycle. CBT aims to intervene in this cycle by targeting dietary restraint to reduce and eliminate binge eating and purging and simultaneously address dysfunctional eating, weight, and shape cognitions. Core treatment components include psychoeducation around healthy eating and the implications of disordered eating behaviors, the prescription of *regular* eating, self-monitoring (in the form of daily food logs), and cognitive restructuring around eating, weight, and shape concerns. CBT is typically short-term focused treatment comprising 15 to 20 sessions held during a 4 to 5 month period. CBT can be delivered in an individual, group, or self-help manual format. Meta-analytic review indicates that individual treatment confers an advantage over group treatment. Additionally CBT-focused self-help and guided self-help approaches have also demonstrated efficacy. Although response rates with self-help are not as high as individual CBT, advantages include the wide availability and low cost.

Interpersonal psychotherapy (IPT) has also demonstrated efficacy in the treatment of bulimia nervosa, achieving rates of improvement and recovery comparable to those of CBT but somewhat less quickly. In the treatment of bulimia nervosa, IPT was first tested as a *viable control* treatment in clinical trials of CBT for bulimia nervosa. In contrast to CBT, which directly addresses the maladaptive eating disordered behaviors and cognitions, IPT focuses on interpersonal functioning. The IPT model of bulimia nervosa hypothesizes that interpersonal difficulties lead to low self-esteem and dysphoria and that bingeing and purging are used as coping mechanisms to regulate affect. The treatment focuses on addressing interpersonal difficulties in a short-term structured treatment, which leads to improvements in bulimic symptoms that often accrue even post-treatment.

In spite of the efficacy of CBT and IPT treatments, approximately 50% of patients in clinical trials do not achieve full recovery post-treatment. Presently treatment trials are aiming to deconstruct CBT and IPT approaches to identify mechanisms of change as well as understand why treatment does not work for all patients. Integrated therapies, which incorporate elements of different treatment modalities, are often used in clinical practice and attempts to study them in controlled treatment trials are underway. One such example is an enhanced version of CBT (CBT-E), which incorporates cognitive behavioral principles, interpersonal aspects, regulation strategies taken from dialectical behavior therapy, and other techniques all in an individualized approach as they apply to the patient. Preliminary findings suggest high rates of improvement and recovery for difficult-to-treat patients.

A limitation of these clinical trials for bulimia nervosa is that patient samples are most often adult; the generalizability of these findings to adolescents with the disorder is unclear. There is some evidence to suggest that a family therapy approach to the treatment of bulimia nervosa using the Maudsley model may be helpful, particularly for younger patients who are living with their parents. Multisite family therapy trials for adolescent bulimia nervosa are currently in progress.

These empirically supported treatments are described in detail in treatment manuals available for use by treating clinicians.

Pharmacotherapy

Psychotropic medication can be helpful for patients with bulimia nervosa in reducing bingeing and purging symptoms. Controlled trials have indicated that a range of antidepressants demonstrate efficacy in reducing bulimic symptoms, with the research finding post-treatment reductions in bingeing and purging symptoms for approximately 50% of patients and post-treatment abstinence rates of 30%. Currently, the only medication that has received FDA approval in the treatment of bulimia nervosa is fluoxetine (Prozac) at a recommended dose of 60 mg every day. Studies have suggested other selective serotonin reuptake inhibitors (SSRIs) may be equally effective but controlled clinical trials and long-term follow-up data are unavailable. In particular, patients with co-morbid anxiety disorders may benefit from paroxetine (Paxil)[1] or sertraline (Zoloft).[1] Additionally, earlier studies suggested tricyclic antidepressants, particularly desipramine (Norpramin),[1] were useful in reducing bulimic symptoms, but research indicates the SSRIs may be better tolerated. Monoamine oxidase inhibitors (MAOIs) are typically avoided because they may be dangerous in patients with erratic eating patterns and nutritional instability because of bingeing and purging. Similarly, bupropion (Wellbutrin) is contraindicated in patients with bulimia nervosa because of an increased risk of seizures.

Notably, the mechanism of action in the utility of antidepressant medication in reducing bulimic behaviors is unclear. Antidepressants seem to be equally effective in patients without depressive co-morbidity, arguing against an antidepressant effect. Given the role of serotonin in appetite regulation, it has been hypothesized that certain antidepressants may act on serotonin to reduce bingeing behaviors. Additionally, several other medications have been examined in patients with bulimia nervosa demonstrating moderate efficacy, including the opiate antagonist naltrexone (ReVia),[1] and the anticonvulsant Topiramate (Topamax).[1] There is also some indication that anxiolytic and sleep medications may also be useful for patients with bulimia nervosa.

Thus psychotropic medications, particularly antidepressants, can be helpful for patients with bulimia nervosa, but they are typically less effective than cognitive behavioral therapy. Further, there is some indication that medication in combination with psychotherapy confers an advantage, but this finding is not consistent. Similar to the psychotherapy literature, however, clinical trials including adolescent patients are limited and the applicability of these findings to younger patients is unclear.

Adjunctive Treatments

A medical assessment is indicated in patients with bulimia nervosa, and ongoing medical management may be useful particularly to treat patients with complications or those discontinuing laxative and/or diuretic abuse. Nutritional counseling may also be helpful to provide additional structure, support, and education for patients who have difficulty meal planning and regulating their eating. Nutritional psychoeducation is often a component of psychotherapy (e.g., CBT), but additional

---

[1]Not FDA approved for this indication.

 CURRENT DIAGNOSIS

- *DSM-IV* defines bulimia nervosa on the basis of binge/compensatory behaviors and associated maladaptive cognitions.
- Binge eating is defined as the consumption of an objectively large amount of food within a discrete period of time accompanied by uncontrolled overeating.
- Compensatory behaviors include purging (self-induced vomiting, misuse of laxatives, diuretics, enemas) and nonpurging (excessive exercise, fasting).
- Binge/compensatory behaviors must occur on average twice weekly over a 3-month period.
- Cognitive component of overvaluation of weight and shape on sense of self.
- Differential diagnosis must consider medical and psychiatric conditions.

Abbreviations: DSM-IV = Diagnostic and Statistical Manual of Mental Disorders, Fourth Edition.

---

[1]Not FDA approved for this indication.

Rakel and Bope: *Conn's Current Therapy 2006.*

17

support may be needed for some patients. Additionally, supportive group therapy can be useful for some patients, particularly in helping them feel less isolated by interacting with that others who experience similar feelings and symptoms.

Impact of Co-Morbidity on Treatment

The role of psychiatric co-morbidity in the treatment of bulimia nervosa is unclear. Generally, improvement of bulimic symptoms is associated with an improvement in mood and anxiety, but further treatment to target co-morbidity is often warranted. Pharmacologic intervention studies indicate that antidepressants improve mood in patients with bulimia who are depressed in addition to targeting bulimic symptoms.

Course and Outcome

The longitudinal course of bulimia nervosa is variable but can be chronic and relapsing. Long-term follow-up studies suggest that 50% to 75% of patients with bulimia nervosa will achieve full recovery from their eating disorder, but approximately 33% of them will go on to relapse. A small minority of patients seem to present with chronic bulimia nervosa. It appears that a longer duration of illness, history of unsuccessful treatment attempts, co-morbid substance abuse, and cluster B personality disorders are predictive of a worse outcome for patients with bulimia nervosa.

  CURRENT THERAPY

- Goals of treatment for bulimia nervosa are to reduce and eliminate binge/compensatory behaviors, modify maladaptive eating- and body-related cognitions, and improve coping skills.
- Psychotherapy is considered first-line treatment. Psychotherapies receiving empirical support for the treatment of bulimia nervosa include CBT and IPT. Additional promising treatments include integrative psychotherapy approaches and family psychotherapy.
- Pharmacotherapy can also be helpful in targeting bulimic symptoms. Antidepressants have received the most empirical support. Fluoxetine (Prozac) at 60 mg qd is the only medication currently approved by the FDA in the treatment.
- CBT and IPT are effective in achieving reductions in binge/compensatory behaviors for the majority of patients and recovery in approximately 50% of patients. Antidepressant therapy leads to reductions in binge/compensatory behaviors for half of patients and recovery in approximately 30% of patients.
- Additional treatment research is warranted to address bulimic symptoms in the considerable subset of patients who remain ill following treatment.

Abbreviations: CBT = cognitive behavioral therapy; FDA = Food and Drug Administration; IPT = interpersonal psychotherapy.

Currently, viable psychosocial and pharmacologic treatments exist for the treatment of bulimia nervosa. Psychosocial approaches, particularly cognitive behavioral therapy, lead to substantial improvement in the majority of patients. Antidepressant therapy may also be useful for a subset of patients, but alone it does not seem to be as effective as psychotherapy. Self-help and guided self-help approaches with a cognitive behavioral focus may also be helpful for patients who have difficulty accessing care. Although these psychosocial and psychopharmacologic treatments are promising and helpful for most patients, approximately 50% of patients do not achieve full recovery even following treatment. Additional treatment research with adolescent and adults patients is needed.

REFERENCES

Agras WS, Walsh T, Fairburn CG, et al: A multicenter comparison of cognitive-behavioral therapy and interpersonal psychotherapy for bulimia nervosa. Arch Gen Psychiatry 2000;57(5):459-466.

Apple RF: Interpersonal therapy for bulimia nervosa. J Clin Psychol 1999;55:715-725.

Casper RC: How useful are pharmacological treatments in eating disorders? Psychopharmacol Bull 2002;36(2):88-104.

Fairburn CG, Cooper Z, Shafran R: Cognitive behaviour therapy for eating disorders: A "transdiagnostic" theory and treatment. Behav Res Ther 2003;41(5):509-528.

Fairburn CG, Marcus MD, Wilson GT: Cognitive-behavioral therapy for binge eating and bulimia nervosa: A comprehensive treatment manual.

Fairburn CG, Wilson GT (eds): Binge eating: Nature, assessment and treatment. New York, Guilford Press, 1993, pp 361-404.

Kotler LA, Walsh BT: Eating disorders in children and adolescents: Pharmacological therapies. Eur Child Adolesc Psychiatry 2000; 9(Suppl 1):I108-I1016.

Mitchell JE, de Zwaan M, Roerig JL: Drug therapy for patients with eating disorders. Curr Drug Targets CNS Neurol Disord 2003;2(1):17-29.

Peterson CB, Mitchell JE: Psychosocial and pharmacological treatment of eating disorders: A review of research findings. J Clin Psychol 1999;55:685-697.

Thompson-Brenner H, Westen D, Glass S: A multidimensional meta-analysis of psychotherapy for bulimia nervosa. Clin Psychol Rev 2003;10:269-287.

Wilson GT, Fairburn CC, Agras WS, et al: Cognitive-behavioral therapy for bulimia nervosa: Time course and mechanisms of change. J Consult Clin Psychol 2002;70:267-274.

Delirium

Method of
Marc E. Agronin, MD

A state of *delirium* is defined as an acute, transient, reversible brain syndrome characterized by fluctuating disturbances of consciousness, attention, perception, cognition, and neuropsychiatric function (e.g., sleep, appetite, psychomotor activity). Other common terms used for delirium include *acute confusional state, encephalitis, encephalopathy,* and *organic brain syndrome.* Delirium can present in both children and adults, but it is seen most frequently in older adults (>65 years of age) with preexisting brain disease. Although delirium is considered reversible, it can severely disrupt medical and rehabilitative recovery, unmask or even cause enduring cognitive impairment, and lead to long-standing functional decline. In addition, it is a particularly dangerous condition associated with mortality rates as high as 40% in the first year. For this reason, delirium should always be considered a medical emergency and treated aggressively.

Epidemiology

Delirium is most commonly seen in older individuals (>65 years of age), and in more women than men because of greater female-to-male ratios in late life. It is widely assumed that rates of delirium underestimate true prevalence because of delayed or missed diagnoses. Although an estimated 1% of individuals in the community suffer from delirium, prevalence rates increase dramatically in medical settings and with medical severity. Delirium is found in 10% of emergency room patients, in 10% to 30% of medical inpatients, and in up to 40% of hospitalized elderly individuals. It is seen in up to 30% of individuals after cardiac surgery, and in 30% to 40% of older individuals after hip and other orthopedic surgeries. Common factors that increase the risk of delirium across settings include the presence of multiple medical problems or medications, increased age, dementia, infection, fever, fractures, malnutrition, low albumin levels, sensory deprivation, recent surgery, alcohol or sedative dependence, physical restraints, and bladder catheters.

Clinical Presentation

Current diagnostic criteria in the *Diagnostic and Statistical Manual of Mental Disorders, Fourth Edition, Text Revision (DSM-IV-TR),* focus on three primary presenting features of delirium:

1. A disturbance in consciousness, characterized by impairment in the ability to focus, sustain, and shift one's attention to the surrounding environment
2. A change in cognition, characterized by impairment in memory, orientation, language, or perception (for example, manifested by hallucinations)
3. A development of the symptoms over a relatively short period of time (hours to days) that may fluctuate throughout the course of the day

In addition to these defining symptoms of delirium, the clinical presentation frequently involves psychomotor agitation or retardation, sleep-wake cycle disturbances, mood lability (dysphoria, anxiety, euphoria), behavioral agitation, and psychosis (hallucinations, delusions, disorganized thinking). When they occur, delusions frequently involve paranoid themes or misidentification of individuals, and they tend to be fleeting. Hallucinations can occur in all sensory modalities, although they are most commonly visual. *DSM-IV-TR* identifies four basic categories of delirium: delirium because of a general

medical condition, substance intoxication delirium, substance withdrawal delirium, and delirium because of multiple etiologies.

Delirious patients are at significant risk of harming themselves or others because their lack of insight and poor judgment impairs their ability to care for themselves independently, carry out activities of daily living, or fully cooperate with treatment. One subtype of delirium may involve psychomotor hyperactivity and agitation, leading to disruptive screaming, combativeness during caregiving, refusal to take medications or food, and pulling or picking at bandages, endotracheal tubes, or intravenous lines. Such symptoms are exacerbated by lack of sleep, overstimulating environments (such as a noisy and constantly lit intensive care unit) and lack of orientating cues to one's surroundings or time of day. Even with these symptoms, however, the delirious patient may have periods of lucidity and calm during the day.

The clinical presentation of delirium may mimic other acute psychiatric conditions such as mania, anxiety, depression, or psychosis. However, the cognitive changes that also accompany delirium are not typically seen in these conditions. Certain types of seizures or postictal states may also resemble delirium, although without ongoing symptoms beyond the day of the event. The main challenge is to distinguish delirium from dementia or to identify delirium within the setting of dementia. The diagnostic key lies in determining the individual's baseline cognition and functioning prior to the onset of more acute changes. Even though tremendous symptomatic overlap exists in terms of cognitive and neuropsychiatric impairment, the disturbance in consciousness and the fluctuating nature of symptoms that define delirium are not characteristic of most forms of dementia, with the exception of dementia with Lewy bodies. Table 1 outlines some of the main differences between dementia and delirium.

Etiology

Delirium always has a medical cause. Box 1 lists many of the medical conditions associated with delirium. Medications are the most common causes of delirium, especially when three or more medications are being administered simultaneously and one or more of them have anticholinergic, narcotic, antihistaminic, or sedative effects. Rapid discontinuation of some medications after extended use (months to years) can trigger a withdrawal delirium, particularly benzodiazepines, narcotics, stimulants, steroids, and selective serotonin reuptake inhibitor (SSRI) antidepressants. Anticholinergic medications can cause cognitive impairment or even frank delirium, and many commonly prescribed medications in the elderly have some degree of anticholinergic effects, including cimetidine, prednisolone, theophylline, digoxin, nifedipine, and furosemide. Anticholinergic delirium is the most extreme form of this impairment, caused by large doses of medications such as tricyclic antidepressants (e.g., imipramine, doxepin) or conventional antipsychotics (e.g., chlorpromazine, thioridazine).

Rakel and Bope: *Conn's Current Therapy 2006.*

TABLE 1* Clinical Differences Between Dementia and Delirium

Clinical Feature	Delirium	Dementia
Onset	Acute, over days to weeks	Chronic, over months to years
Course	Fluctuating symptoms	Stable symptoms with progressive decline
Duration	Days to weeks or months	Years until inevitable death
Awareness	Reduced	Clear
Attention	Impaired, fluctuating, distractible	Usually normal; able to focus on short, discrete tasks
Alertness	Fluctuates; lethargic or hypervigilant at times	Usually normal
Orientation	Impaired	Impaired
Memory	Immediate and recent memory impaired; remote memory intact	Recent and remote memory impaired
Perception	Hallucinations are common	Intact
Thinking	Fragmented, disorganized, with transient paranoid and other delusions	Impaired abstract thinking, vague or impoverished content; agnosia
Language	Speech slow or rapid, sometimes incoherent	Word-finding difficulty; aphasia
Psychomotor	Variable: hyper- or hypokinetic	Apraxia as dementia progresses; slowed in subcortical dementia
Sleep-wake cycle	Disrupted, reversed	Reversed or fragmented

*This table distinguishes between typical presentations of delirium and mild to moderate dementia (most consistent with Alzheimer's disease). Severe dementia is not described. Acute states of agitation and psychosis in dementia may obscure many of these clinical differences.

Acute infections are common causes of delirium across all age groups, particularly infections that affect the central nervous system (CNS). Delirium secondary to CNS infection is often referred to as an *encephalitis*. Urinary tract infections are the most common cause of delirium in nursing home residents. Delirium can also result from an array of metabolic disturbances, including various endocrine diseases, renal and hepatic failure, and rapid alterations in sodium, calcium, or glucose levels. Cerebral injury because of stroke, trauma, and neoplasm can cause delirium. The increased rates of postoperative delirium may be related to factors such as anesthesia effects, dehydration, anemia, and the use of narcotic analgesics. Older individuals undergoing orthopedic procedures and coronary artery bypass surgery are particularly susceptible.

Delirium is frequently caused by intoxication or withdrawal from substances of abuse such as alcohol and most street drugs. *Delirium tremens*, characterized by confusion, psychosis (including tactile hallucinations), agitation, and autonomic hyperactivity is a form of delirium seen in acute alcohol withdrawal, and it can be life-threatening without aggressive treatment. *Wernicke's encephalopathy* is a form of delirium resulting from thiamine deficiency. Core symptoms include confusion, nystagmus, gaze palsies, and ataxia. It is seen classically in chronic alcoholics with poor nutrition, but is less prevalent today because so many food products are vitamin fortified. *Wernicke-Korsakoff's syndrome* refers to an enduring form of learning and memory impairment that can result if the initial delirium is not treated rapidly.

It is not clear how medical problems trigger delirium, but several potential pathophysiologic mechanisms are proposed. Many conditions associated with delirium either reduce the flow of adequate blood, oxygen, or nutrients (e.g., glucose, vitamins) to the brain, increase the presence of circulating toxins in the central nervous system (either directly or indirectly by altering the blood–brain barrier), or lead to the release of endogenous mediators of infection, injury, inflammation, or stress (e.g., cytokines, cortisol). It is believed that delirium may result when one or more of these factors significantly disrupt cerebral neuronal oxidative metabolism. In addition, disruptions in several neurotransmitter systems are also implicated in delirium. Anticholinergic effects are most concerning given the central role of acetylcholine in learning, memory, and other cognitive functions. One study of hospitalized patients found a near-linear relationship between increasing serum anticholinergic activity and delirium. Dopaminergic agents can also cause delirium, and dopamine antagonists (i.e., antipsychotic medications) are used to treat delirium. Disturbances in the activity of the neurotransmitters glutamate, GABA (γ-aminobutyric acid), and serotonin are also associated with delirium.

Assessment and Treatment

Figure 1 presents a flow chart for the assessment and treatment of delirium. The first step is to identify the delirious patient, differentiating the symptoms of delirium from other psychiatric conditions that warrant attention. It is critical to obtain information from informants who have knowledge of the patient's baseline mental status prior to recent changes and who have observed the patient over time. The most salient features of delirium are the rapid change in mental status, even within the setting of advanced dementia, the disruption in the patient's attention level, and the sudden manifestation of behavioral changes, usually characterized by agitation. Sharon Inouye and colleagues developed the Confusion Assessment Method (CAM), a rating scale for delirium based on extensive research on hospitalized patients with delirium. Using this scale, a diagnosis of delirium should be considered if an acute onset

BOX 1 Etiologies of Delirium

Medications (routine use, intoxication, or withdrawal)
Antibiotics (e.g., quinolones)
Anticholinergic properties (e.g., antispasmodics, conventional antipsychotics, tricyclic antidepressants, H_2 blockers, prednisolone, theophylline)
Anticonvulsants
Antihistamines (e.g., diphenhydramine, hydroxyzine)
Antipsychotics
Cardiovascular medications (e.g., antihypertensives, calcium channel blockers, digoxin, antiarrhythmics)
Chemotherapeutic medications
Corticosteroids
Diuretics
Dopaminergic agents (e.g., levodopa, amantadine)
Immunosuppressive agents
Lithium
Muscle relaxants
Narcotics/opiates
Nonsteroidal anti-inflammatory drugs (NSAIDs)
Sedative-hypnotics (e.g., benzodiazepines, barbiturates)
Serotonergic agents (e.g., selective serotonin reuptake inhibitor [SSRI] and other antidepressants)
Stimulants/sympathomimetics
Toxins (e.g., organophosphate insecticides, carbon monoxide, organic solvents)
Infection (e.g., central nervous system [CNS] encephalitis, urosepsis, pneumonia, cellulitis)
Endocrine disease (e.g., thyroid, parathyroid, or adrenal dysfunction, hyper- or hypoglycemia)
Metabolic disturbances (e.g., hypo- or hypernatremia, hypokalemia, hypo- or hypercalcemia, dehydration, thiamine deficiency/Wernicke's encephalopathy)
Organ failure (e.g., hepatic and uremic encephalopathy)
Neurological disease (e.g., seizure disorder, transient ischemic attacks, strokes, subdural hematoma, traumatic injury, cerebral neoplasm, vasculitis)
Cardiovascular disease (e.g., arrhythmias, myocardial infarction, congestive heart failure, severe hypertension)
Pulmonary disease (e.g., chronic obstructive pulmonary disease [COPD], exacerbation, pulmonary embolism, hypoxia)
Hematologic disease (e.g., anemia, malignancies, disseminated intravascular coagulation [DIC])
Occult malignancies (especially in CNS)
Occult bone fracture
Postoperative state (e.g., anesthetic effects, hip repair, coronary artery bypass graft [CABG])
Substance abuse or withdrawal (e.g., alcohol, cocaine, phencyclidine [PCP], hallucinogens, MDMA [methylenedioxymethamphetamine]/ecstasy, heroin, amphetamines, cannabis)
Sensory impairment (e.g., severe hearing or visual loss)
Severe burns
Severe pain
Sleep deprivation

The clinician must simultaneously conduct a medical workup to identify reversible causes of delirium and make a judgment call whether disruptive behaviors require immediate treatment. This process requires intensive monitoring in a hospital or other medical setting that provides 24-hour care. The use of both chemical and physical restraints should be considered whenever there is imminent threat of self-harm or harm to others, such as from pulling out an endotracheal tube or physically fighting with staff. Although clinicians should always try to avoid the use of restraints because they can potentially worsen the delirium itself or lead to injury, they must also keep in mind that a highly agitated, delirious patient can easily extubate himself, fall out of bed and fracture a hip, or physically injure a nurse. For this same reason, a delirious patient must have 24-hour monitoring, either clearly visible from a nursing station or with a sitter. If physical restraints are needed, they must be reassessed every few hours and discontinued as soon as possible. Chemical restraints should be reevaluated daily to allow rapid titration and early discontinuation.

The medical evaluation flows from clinical suspicion but should always involve basic laboratory studies to rule out urinary tract and other infections that are common causes of delirium, as well as metabolic disturbances. A brain computed tomography (CT) or magnetic resonance imaging (MRI) scan should always be considered after any head injury or when focal neurologic symptoms are present. Such structural imaging helps identify potential causes of delirium but does not actually confirm a diagnosis. Lumbar puncture with cerebrospinal fluid (CSF) analysis and viral titers are indicated with suspected encephalitis. An electroencephalogram (EEG) is less frequently used but may help distinguish delirium from dementia or a seizure disorder. Typical EEG findings in delirium are generalized slowing across alpha, theta, and delta frequencies.

The clinician must then address the potential causes of delirium, through active treatment of a specific condition (e.g., antibiotics for an infection) or the tapering and discontinuation of potentially offending medications. Attention must be given to maintaining adequate hydration, nutrition, pain control, sensory awareness, bowel and bladder care, and treatment adherence. Medications believed to be causing delirium should be withdrawn expeditiously, although with a written taper schedule if possible, to avoid symptomatic withdrawal or rebound. Withdrawal from alcohol or benzodiazepines must be recognized and then treated with a detoxification protocol that involves close monitoring of physical symptoms of withdrawal and the administration of benzodiazepines such as lorazepam (Ativan) or oxazepam (Serax) as part of a standard taper. Narcotic analgesics can sometimes be replaced with other medications or modalities to relieve pain. In the postoperative state, potential dehydration, anemia, pain, and metabolic disturbances should be addressed.

Once the medical workup begins and the patient's safety is addressed, the next step is to consider environmental, behavioral, and pharmacologic interventions to treat the delirium. The goal is both to enhance the

and fluctuating course, inattention, and either disorganized thinking or an altered level of consciousness (rated as alert, vigilant, lethargic, stuporous, or comatose) are present. Other scales for delirium include the Delirium Rating Scale (DRS), the Delirium Symptom Interview, and the Memorial Delirium Assessment Scale (MDAS).

Rakel and Bope: *Conn's Current Therapy 2006.*

DIAGNOSE DELIRIUM
- Identify core symptoms of delirium
- Obtain observations over time, using informant reports
- Use a delirium rating scale (e.g., CAM, DRS, MDAS)

IDENTIFY AND TREAT CAUSE(S)
- Comprehensive history and physical/neurologic examination (check vital signs)
- Identify relevant medications, substances, or toxic exposures, including problematic doses or amounts, sudden cessation, or combinations (obtain tox screen if warranted)
- Evaluate for pain, sensory deprivation, dehydration, malnutrition
- Psychiatric evaluation (rule out acute mania, anxiety or panic attacks, depression)
- Rule out infection (check urinalysis and complete blood count; consider relevant cultures, chest x-ray, lumbar puncture, HIV testing, viral titers)
- Rule out metabolic disturbance (electrolytes, glucose, calcium, liver, renal, and thyroid function, and ESR)
- Rule out cerebral damage or seizure (obtain brain CT or MRI; consider EEG)
- Rule out cardiovascular source (obtain ECG; echocardiogram, Doppler studies)
- Rule out pulmonary source (check O2 sat; consider arterial blood gas, V-Q scan, etc.)

TREAT AGITATION AND PSYCHOSIS
- Identify potential threat of harm to self or others
- 24-hour observation, with sitter if necessary
- Use physical restraints only in severe situations, with close monitoring and rapid discontinuation
- Use psychotropic medications for agitation and psychosis[1]:

Antipsychotic medications[2]
Haloperidol (Haldol) 0.25–0.5 mg PO BID and Q6–8 hrs PRN
  IM haloperidol for severe agitation
  IV haloperidol in ICU setting with cardiac monitoring
  (1 mg IV, repeated with dose doubled every 30 minutes until effect)
Risperidone (Risperdal) 0.25–0.5 mg PO QD or BID and Q6–8 hrs PRN
  Elixir and orally dissolving (Risperdal M-tab) preparations available
Olanzapine (Zyprexa) 2.5–5 mg PO QHS or BID and Q6–8 hrs PRN
  IM and orally dissolving (Zyprexa Zydis) preparations available
Quetiapine (Seroquel) 25–100 mg PO QHS or BID and Q6–8 hrs PRN
Ziprasidone (Geodon) 20 mg PO BID and Q6–8 hrs PRN
  IM preparation available
Aripiprazole (Abilify) 5–10 mg PO QHS and 5 mg Q8 hrs PRN

Benzodiazepines[3]
Lorazepam (Ativan) 0.25–0.5 mg PO QD or BID and Q6–8 hrs
Oxazepam (Serax) 15–30 PO QD or BID and Q6–8 hrs PRN
  Both agents can be given IM for severe agitation or refusal to take oral medications

[1]There are no FDA-approved psychotropic medications for the treatment of delirium or its complications. Recommended medications and doses are based on standard psychiatric practice guidelines, case studies, and small prospective studies. Doses listed here may be higher in certain individuals.

[2]Electrocardiagraphic monitoring is important before and during treatment with antipsychotic agents, specifically IV haloperidol and ziprasidone. According to APA guidelines, a QTc interval >450 ms or more than 25% over the baseline value warrants dose reduction, discontinuation, and/or cardiology consultation. High doses of IV haloperidol have been associated with torsades de pointes. Also, monitor for side effects including parkinsonism (haloperidol; risperidone in doses >2 mg/day), anticholinergic effects (olanzapine > other agents), and antihistamine effects (quetiapine + others).

[3]Benzodiazepines are preferred agents with alcohol withdrawal, and then should be used according to a specific detox protocol. Otherwise, their use should be restricted to patients who cannot take or tolerate antipsychotic medications, but their efficacy will be limited to agitation and not psychosis. Monitor for excess sedation or confusion, and paradoxical effects such as increased agitation or disinhibition.

FIGURE 1. An algorithm for the assessment and treatment of delirium. APA = American psychiatric association; BID = twice daily; CAM = confusion assessment method; CT = computed tomography; DRS = delerium rating scale; ECG = electrocardiogram; EEG = electroencephalogram; ESR = erythrocyte sedimentation rate; HIV = human immunodeficiency virus; IV = intravenous; MDAS = Memorial delerium assessment scale; MRI = magnetic resonance imaging; PO = by mouth; PRN = as needed; QD = every day; QHS = at bedtime.

↓

TREAT THE DELIRIUM ITSELF
- Provide adequate hydration, nutrition, and pain control
- Employ appropriate behavioral/environmental and pharmacologic approaches:

Behavioral/environmental strategies
- Maintain a consistent, structured environment and staffing
- Provide regular orientation clues (e.g., verbal reminders, large visible clock and calendar)
- Encourage personal effects in room and visits from family and friends
- Improve sensory deprivation (e.g., hearing aides, glasses)
- Encourage sleep hygiene (structure day and night, appropriate ambient lighting, avoid excess activity, food, or caffeine before bed, warm milk or tea before bed, relaxation techniques)
- Encourage early mobilization if bed-bound or post-op state
- Avoid over- or understimulation
- Provide regular bowel and bladder care
- Minimize use of physical restraints and bladder catheters

Pharmacologic strategies[4]
Antipsychotic medications (see above for dosing)
Acetylcholinesterase inhibitors (AChEIs)
   Donepezil (Aricept) 5 mg PO QD ×4 wks, then 10 mg
   Rivastigmine (Exelon) 1.5 mg PO BID ×4 wks, then 3 mg BID
   Galantamine (Razadyne ER) 8 mg PO QD ×4 wks, then 16 mg QD
NMDA-receptor antagonist
   Memantine (Namenda) 5 mg PO QD with 5 mg weekly increments
     in BID doses to total 10 mg BID at 4 weeks

For severe insomnia, consider short-term use of zolpidem (Ambien) 5–10 mg PO QHS, zaleplon (Sonata) 5–10 mg PO QHS, or trazodone (Desyrel) 25–100 mg PO QHS. Antipsychotic medications may also improve sleep in some individuals.

[4]There are no FDA-approved medications to treat delirium. The potential benefits of antipsychotic medications, AChEIs, and NMDA-receptor antagonists to treat delirium are based on small open-label studies and case series. There are no controlled trials to support their use. Further titration of AChEIs or NMDA-receptor antagonists is dependent on either persistent symptoms or underlying dementia.

FIGURE 1, cont'd.

safety, comfort, and familiarity of the environment for the duration of the delirium and to minimize the impact of behavioral disturbances and/or psychotic and disorganized thinking. The delirious patient should be kept in a structured, familiar environment, with clear cues orienting them to person (e.g., personal photos and items), place (e.g., written sign, verbal reminders), and time (e.g., daytime lighting and nighttime darkness, visible calendar and clock, regular mealtimes, verbal reminders). Overstimulation should be avoided, although visits from family and other friendly faces can be helpful. Paranoid delusions, hallucinations, or anxiety attacks should be recognized but not given undue attention; rather, the patient should be reassured and then redirected in a warm but direct manner to more comfortable topics or simple activities. Again, family and familiar faces can play a critically supportive role here.

No FDA-approved medications for the treatment of delirium or its psychiatric complications are currently available. The acetylcholinesterase inhibitors (AChEIs) donepezil (Aricept),[1] rivastigmine (Exelon),[1] and

galantamine (Razadyne ER)[1] are used to treat delirium, with anecdotal reports and small case series suggesting benefit. Theoretically, they might benefit some patients by enhancing cholinergic activity. Similarly, the NMDA [N-methyl-D-aspartate]-receptor antagonist memantine (Namenda)[1] is used, with theoretical benefit through the modulation of glutamate-induced excitotoxicity. Figure 1 lists dosing strategies.

Antipsychotic medications are used widely to treat delirium, particularly symptoms of agitation and psychosis. Until recent years, haloperidol (Haldol)[1] was always the standard bearer, given its relatively good efficacy, versatility, and familiarity to nurses and physicians. However, the use of haloperidol carries a significant risk of extrapyramidal side effects (e.g., parkinsonism, akathisia), although interestingly enough the risk is less with intravenous (IV) preparations, even at high doses. The risk of tardive dyskinesia from extended haloperidol use is significant, with rates approaching 40% in elderly individuals after 9 months of treatment. Although ideally the use of haloperidol to treat delirium

[1]Not FDA approved for this indication.

[1]Not FDA approved for this indication.

Rakel and Bope: *Conn's Current Therapy 2006.*

is short term, on the order of days to weeks, it is common for delirious patients to be discharged to an institutional setting where the medication is continued for months or longer.

Atypical antipsychotics are being used more widely as alternatives to haloperidol because they offer excellent efficacy with significantly lower risk of both extrapyramidal side effects and tardive dyskinesia. Small studies have found improvement in cognition, agitation, and psychosis associated with delirium in up to 90% of patients treated with risperidone (Risperdal),[1] olanzapine (Zyprexa),[1] and quetiapine (Seroquel).[1] All three agents are well tolerated with minimal side effects. The atypical antipsychotics ziprasidone (Geodon)[1] and aripiprazole (Abilify)[1] may carry similar benefits. Figure 1 lists dosing strategies and potential side effects.

For individuals who have failed or cannot tolerate antipsychotic agents, and for alcohol and benzodiazepine withdrawal, low-dose and short-term use of benzodiazepines can be considered. Both short and long half-life agents should be avoided because of risks of disinhibition, sedation, dizziness, respiratory depression, confusion, and falls. Although any benzodiazepine carries a risk of these side effects, the intermediate half-life agents lorazepam (Ativan)[1] and oxazepam (Serax)[1] are preferred agents because of their simpler hepatic metabolism and lack of active metabolites. These same two benzodiazepines may be considered for short-term use in individuals with severe sleep-wake cycle disturbances; alternatively, clinicians may consider zolpidem (Ambien),[1] zaleplon (Sonata),[1] or trazodone (Desyrel).[1] Atypical antipsychotics may also improve sleep in some delirious individuals.

---

[1]Not FDA approved for this indication.

CURRENT DIAGNOSIS

- Delirium is an acute, transient brain syndrome characterized by fluctuating disturbances in consciousness, attention, cognition, perception, and behavior. Delirious patients may present with significant sleep-wake cycle disruptions, agitation, mood lability, and psychosis.
- Delirium is seen in 10% to 40% of individuals in medical settings. Key risk factors for delirium include advanced age, multiple medical problems, polypharmacy, dementia, infection, and recent surgery.
- Delirium always has a medical cause and is often multidetermined. Medications are the most common cause, followed by infection, substance intoxication or withdrawal, and metabolic disturbances.
- Delirium must be distinguished from dementia and other psychiatric disorders that involve mental status changes. Clinical history, observation over time, informant reports, and the use of a standardized instrument such as the Confusion Assessment Method can aid in diagnosis.

In general, all psychotropic medications used to treat delirium must be used cautiously and reevaluated frequently to determine if they are improving symptoms without worsening the delirium or introducing new side effects. Clinicians should consider tapering and then discontinuing these agents when symptoms abate while being vigilant for recurrence. The exception would be the use of AChEIs or memantine (Namenda)[1] in individuals with delirium and dementia; in those cases, long-term use is indicated for the treatment of the dementia itself after the delirium has abated.

Course and Prognosis

In two thirds of individuals with delirium, symptoms last from 2 days to a week. The delirium may persist for months in some individuals, and it is seen in up to 15% of sufferers after 6 months. The true efficacy of preventive strategies is unclear because several interventional studies do not demonstrate reduced rates of delirium. But one large comprehensive study of older hospitalized

---

[1]Not FDA approved for this indication.

CURRENT THERAPY

- The treatment of delirium begins with identifying and treating underlying medical causes.
- Agitation and psychosis are common manifestations of delirium and can lead to self-harm, disruption of necessary medical treatment, and harm to caregivers. Affected individuals should be monitored 24 hours, with consideration of physical and/or chemical restraints for severe behavioral disturbances.
- Antipsychotic medications, including haloperidol (Haldol), risperidone (Risperdal),[1] olanzapine (Zyprexa),[1] quetiapine (Seroquel),[1] and others, are not FDA approved for the treatment of delirium, but in small studies they have demonstrated good efficacy and relative safety for treating symptoms of delirium, particularly agitation and psychosis.
- Benzodiazepines can be used to treat alcohol or benzodiazepine withdrawal or for individuals who cannot tolerate antipsychotic medications. They treat agitation but not psychosis.
- A nonpharmacologic approach to treat delirium involves providing a familiar, structured, and consistent environment with orientation cues and appropriate but not excessive stimulation. Pharmacologic agents that may provide some benefit for delirium include antipsychotic medications, the acetylcholinesterase inhibitors donepezil (Aricept),[1] rivastigmine (Exelon),[1] and galantamine (Razadyne ER),[1] and the NMDA [N-methyl-D-aspartate]-receptor antagonist memantine (Namenda).

---

[1]Not FDA approved for this indication.

Rakel and Bope: *Conn's Current Therapy 2006.*

individuals at high risk for delirium found a lower rate, reduced duration, and fewer total episodes of delirium in individuals exposed to interventions for orientation, mobilization, sleep hygiene, sensory enhancement, and dehydration. Similar interventions that educate staff and provide adequate pain control and rapid attention to the inpatient environment and postoperative complications may help reduce both the severity and duration of delirium. Even with aggressive treatment, delirium delays functional improvement and increases the length of hospital stays, the degree of nursing care, the risk of cognitive and functional decline, and the need for home health services or nursing home placement. All of these factors are worse when there is underlying dementia and when underlying etiologies are not adequately treated. The rate of mortality ranges from 25% to 40% in the 6 to 12 months following an episode of delirium.

REFERENCES

American Psychiatric Association: Practice guideline for the treatment of patients with delirium. Am J Psychiatry 1999,156(Suppl 5):1-20.

Flacker JM, Cummings V, Mach JR Jr, et al: The association of serum anticholinergic activity with delirium in elderly medical patients. Am J Geriatr Psychiatry 1998;6:31-41.

Inouye SK. Bogardus ST Jr, Charpentier PA, et al: A multicomponent intervention to prevent delirium in hospitalized older patients. N Engl J Med 1999;340:669-676.

Inouye SK, Charpentier MP: Precipitating factors for delirium in hospitalized elderly patients. JAMA 1996;275:852-857.

Inouye SK, Rushing JT, Foreman MD, et al: Does delirium contribute to poor hospital outcome? A three-site epidemiologic study. J Gen Intern Med 1998;13:234-242.

Inouye SK, van Dyck CH, Alessi CA, et al: Clarifying confusion: The confusion assessment method: A new method for detection of delirium. Ann Intern Med 1990;113:941-948.

Liptzin B, Jacobson SA: Delirium. In BJ Sadock, VA Sadock (eds): Comprehensive Textbook of Psychiatry, 8th ed. Philadelphia, Lippincott Williams & Wilkins, 2005, pp 3693-3700.

Parellada E, Baeza I, de Pablo J, Martinez G: Risperidone in the treatment of patients with delirium. J Clin Psychiatry 2004;65(3): 348-353.

Samuels SC, Neugroschl JA: Delirium. In BJ Sadock, VA Sadock (eds): Comprehensive Textbook of Psychiatry, 8th ed. Philadelphia, Lippincott Williams & Wilkins, 2005, pp 1054-1068.

Sasaki Y, Matsuyama T, Inoure S, et al: A prospective, open-label, flexible-dose study of quetiapine in the treatment of delirium. J Clin Psychiatry 2003;64(11):1316-1321.

Skrobik YK, Bergeron N, Dumont M, Gottfried SB: Olanzapine vs haloperidol: Treating delirium in a critical care setting. Intensive Care Med 2004;30(3):444-449.

Trepacz PT: Is there a final common pathway in delirium? Focus on acetylcholine and dopamine. Semin Clin Neuropsychiatry 2000; 5:132-148.

Mood Disorders

Method of
*Michael J. Burke, MD, PhD, and
Jana Lincoln, MD*

This article reviews the diagnosis and treatment of mood disorders focusing on major depressive disorder. As a group, mood disorders represent a collection of prevalent, serious, yet highly treatable medical conditions. Untreated, mood disorders can be debilitating and cause considerable functional impairment. A potential outcome for untreated mood disorders is death by suicide, which continues to rank in the top 10 causes of death for most age groups. As an indication of the prevalence of mood disorders, in most medical settings antidepressant medications fall in the list of the top 10 most frequently prescribed drugs.

Making the Diagnosis

The several types of mood disorders are described in the *Diagnostic and Statistical Manual of Mental Disorders, Fourth Edition (DSM-IV).* Essentially when a patient presents with the complaint of "depression" or when depressive symptomatology is a focus of clinical attention, a number of diagnoses are possible (Table 1). In addition to major depressive disorder (MDD), other considerations include bipolar affective disorder and whether the depressive symptoms are a manifestation of some underlying general medical condition or are substance induced. Substance-induced mood disorders may be related to drugs of abuse (e.g., cocaine) or prescription medications (e.g., prednisone).

Mood disorders are syndromal diagnoses. In this sense, a mood disorder diagnosis represents a collection of specific signs and symptoms occurring together (Table 2). Not all patients with mood disorders display or endorse all possible signs and symptoms (e.g., diagnostic criteria) for a particular mood disorder. This is where the clinician's experience and judgment come into play in formulating a diagnosis.

The patient's age may affect how he or she presents with a mood disorder. Over the years a belief evolved that mood disorders more likely present in children and

17

TABLE 1 Differential Diagnoses for Major Mood Disorders

Major depressive disorder (single episode, recurrent)
Bipolar disorder (type I) (depressed, hypomanic, manic, or mixed episode)
Bipolar disorder (type II) (depressed, hypomanic)
Cyclothymic disorder
Dysthymic disorder
Mood disorder caused by a general medical condition
Substance-induced mood disorder

TABLE 2 Diagnostic Criteria for Depressive and Manic Episodes

Major Depressive Episode	Manic Episode
Five or more of the following symptoms present during a 2-week period: Depressed or irritable mood* Diminished interest or pleasure (anhedonia)* Disturbance in appetite Insomnia or hypersomnia Psychomotor agitation or retardation Fatigue or loss of energy Feelings of worthlessness or guilt Diminished ability to concentrate Recurrent thoughts of death, suicidal ideation, suicide attempt	**Four or five of the following symptoms present during a 1-week period or any duration if hospitalization is required:** Elevated, expansive, or irritable mood* Inflated self-esteem or grandiosity Decreased need for sleep Hyperverbal Racing thoughts, flight of ideas Distractibility Increased activity or psychomotor agitation Excessive involvement in pleasurable activities with risk for painful consequences

*For a major depressive episode diagnosis, the symptom of either depressed mood or anhedonia must be present. For a manic episode diagnosis, the altered mood symptom must be present.

adolescents as behavioral disturbances. The thought was that youths may lack the ability to express how they feel, and hence irritability and oppositional behavior may be the most prominent presenting symptoms of their mood disorder. Although it is still recognized that behavioral disturbance may bring a child with a mood disorder to clinical attention, the clinician needs to elicit additional diagnostic criteria to support a mood disorder diagnosis (see Table 2).

The elderly patient (i.e., older than 65 years of age) with a mood disorder presents another set of diagnostic challenges. On presentation, the elderly patient with a mood disorder may focus on somatic complaints, directing the clinical evaluation toward insomnia because of back pain or weight loss, and he or she may not be forthcoming with complaints of low mood, feelings of hopelessness, and suicidal thoughts. So when the clinician has a suspicion of a mood disorder in an elderly patient, the clinician must be fairly rigorous in exploring for depressive symptomatology. Regardless of the age of the patient, the approach to diagnosing a mood disorder should always include a thorough history and physical exam, with close attention to family history and medication use. The issue of substance abuse should be explored. It may be necessary to seek collateral history, particularly in the case of adolescents and children and the elderly, or when the patient is hesitant about entertaining the possibility of a mood disorder diagnosis.

Treatment of Depressive Disorders

Once the clinician makes a depressive disorder diagnosis, the next consideration is treatment. When the diagnosis is substance-induced depressive disorder or depression secondary to a general medical condition, the focus of treatment is to address the underlying cause. In the case of a substance-induced depression, suspected drugs should be discontinued, and if substance abuse is identified as

chemical dependency, treatment is indicated. For depression secondary to a general medical condition, the focus of treatment is correcting the underlying general medical condition (e.g., optimizing blood sugar regulation in a patient with diabetes). Because of the relatively low toxicity of newer antidepressant medications, the present practice supports consideration of their use while correction of the underlying causes of the mood disorder is ongoing. But this decision should be made case by case.

PHARMACOTHERAPY FOR DEPRESSIVE DISORDERS

In the last 20 years, the antidepressant armamentarium has increased dramatically. The number of antidepressant medications has increased significantly and, more importantly, the newer agents have superior safety and tolerability profiles relative to their predecessors. Approximately 20 years ago, antidepressant medications fell into two general categories: the tricyclic antidepressants (TCAs) and the monoamine oxidase inhibitors (MAOIs). These two classes of antidepressant drugs had significant safety risks and were often difficult for patients to tolerate. Today, TCAs and MAOIs are relegated to third- and fourth-line antidepressant treatment options and their use is increasingly rare. The presumed antidepressant mechanism of TCAs and MAOIs was their effects on three neurotransmitters: norepinephrine, serotonin, and dopamine. Of note, despite the improved clinical profile of newer antidepressants, their therapeutic effects are still attributed to activity on these same three neurotransmitters.

Table 3 lists currently available antidepressant medications, the recommended daily dose range for treating depressive disorders, and the presumed mechanism of antidepressant activity. The approach to conceptualizing antidepressants based on their pharmacodynamic profiles is reminiscent of how antihypertensive agents are organized and provides a basis for treatment selection. As an illustration, when a patient cannot tolerate

TABLE 3 Antidepressant Pharmacotherapy: Presumed Mechanism of Action, Dose Range, Remarks

Drug Name	Presumed Mechanism of Action	Daily Dose Range (mg/d)	Remarks
First-Line Agents			
Fluoxetine (Prozac)	SSRI	10-80	Potent inhibitor of CYP 2D6; now available in generic form
Paroxetine (Paxil)	SSRI	10-60	Potent inhibitor of CYP 2D6; most likely SSRI associated with withdrawal syndrome on abrupt discontinuation
Paroxetine (Paxil CR)	SSRI	25-62.5	Controlled-release formulation; potent inhibitor of CYP 2D6; reduced risk of SSRI withdrawal syndrome relative toimmediate-release formulation is unclear
Sertraline (Zoloft)	SSRI	25-200	
Fluvoxamine (Luvox)	SSRI	50-300	Potent inhibitor of CYP 1A2 and 2C19; only SSRI with recommended bid dosing
Citalopram (Celexa)	SSRI	20-60	
Escitalopram (Lexapro)	SSRI	10-20	S-enantiomer of citalopram
Second-Line Agents			
Venlafaxine (Effexor)	SSNRI	37.5-375	Divide daily dose as bid; associated with autonomic arousal, may cause or aggravate hypertension
Venlafaxine (Effexor XR)	SSNRI	75-225	Extended-release formulation; once-a-day dosing; associated with autonomic arousal; may cause or aggravate hypertension
Duloxetine (Cymbalta)	SSNRI	40-60	Given once a day or bid. May cause or aggravate hypertension. Also FDA approved for diabetic neuropathy
Bupropion (Wellbutrin)	NE and DA reuptake inhibitor	300-450	See PDR for strict dosing guidelines; can induce seizures; may aggravate preexisting arrhythmias; not to be used with Zyban (bupropion HCl)
Bupropion (Wellbutrin SR)	NE and DA reuptake inhibitor	150-400	Sustained-release formulation; bid for doses exceeding 150 mg; can induce seizures; may aggravate preexisting arrhythmias; not to be used with Zyban (bupropion HCl)
Bupropion (Wellbutrin XL)	NE and DA reuptake inhibitor	150-450	Alternative extended-release formulation; given as single daily dose; not to be used with Zyban (bupropion HCl)
Mirtazapine (Remeron)	SE receptor (2A, 2C, 3)	15-45	Dosed at bedtime; prominent antihistamine (H1) antagonist; effects of as α2-antagonist sedation and weight gain
Third-Line Agents			
Tricyclic agents (TCAs):	Within TCA class, each agent varies in relative potency as reuptake inhibitors of NE and SE		Cardiotoxic; lethal in overingestion. Rarely used today; titrate dose in small increments based on TDM
Amitriptyline (Elavil)		150-300	
Nortriptyline (Pamelor)		50-150	
Desipramine (Norpramin)		75-300	
Clomipramine (Anafranil)[1]		100-250	

Continued

Rakel and Bope: *Conn's Current Therapy 2006.*

TABLE 3 Antidepressant Pharmacotherapy: Presumed Mechanism of Action, Dose Range, Remarks—cont'd

Drug Name	Presumed Mechanism of Action	Daily Dose Range (mg/d)	Remarks
Monoamine oxidase inhibitors (MAOIs:)	Irreversibly inhibits enzyme that metabolizes SE, NE, DA		Rarely used today; requires restriction of diet and of other medications to avoid hypertensive crisis and hyperserotonergic syndrome
Phenelzine (Nardil)		30-90	
Tranylcypromine (Parnate)		20-60	
Trazodone (Desyrel)	SE receptor (2A) antagonist	300-600	Rarely used as an antidepressant because of sedation and orthostasis; popular in lower doses (50-100 mg) as a sleep aid; risk of priapism
Nefazodone (Serzone)	SE receptor (2A) antagonist	300-600	Bid dosing; potent inhibitor of CYP 3A4; α1 blockade may cause orthostasis; manufacturer of Serzone withdrew the drug from Canadian, European, and U.S. markets after reports of serious hepatic effects including liver failure; see June 4, 2004, FDA guidelines for use

[1]Not FDA approved for this indication.

Abbreviations: bid = twice daily; DA = dopamine; CYP = cytochrome P450 isoenzymes (inhibiting these isoenzymes is the basis for potentially serious drug interactions); MAOIs = monoamine oxidase inhibitors; NE = norepinephrine; PDR = Physicians Desk Reference; SE = serotonin; SSNRI = selective serotonin and norepinephrine reuptake inhibitor; SSRI = selective serotonin reuptake inhibitor; TDM = therapeutic drug monitoring.

a particular antidepressant or response is inadequate, the clinician selects an alternative agent that targets a different neurotransmitter or affects the same neurotransmitter through another mechanism.

Antidepressant Treatment Selection

A number of published antidepressant treatment algorithms assist with the selection of antidepressant medications in treatment-naïve patients. The tolerability and safety features of the individual antidepressants principally support these algorithms because no particular antidepressant medication or class of antidepressants has consistently superior efficacy. Hence efficacy in and of itself is not a feature that assists in treatment selection.

First-Line Antidepressants

Most published algorithms list the selective serotonin reuptake inhibitors (SSRIs) as the first-line antidepressant of choice for the treatment-naïve patient. This first-line position for the SSRIs is based in part on broad clinical experience with this group of agents over the last decade. SSRIs are well tolerated. There may be some transient gastrointestinal adverse effects during the initiation of treatment, but for most patients these tend to resolve quickly, and there is limited risk of serious adverse effects. Data support that lack of response to one SSRI does not predict lack of response to another drug in the class. Hence it is common practice for

patients to have sequential trials of more than one SSRI when the initial drug choice does not produce the desired response. For the SSRIs, sexual-adverse effects (e.g., delayed time to orgasm, anorgasmia), when they occur, may lead to drug discontinuation. This adverse effect appears to be concentration dependent and may resolve if the drug dose can be lowered. Patients who experience sexual-adverse effects with one SSRI are likely to experience them with other drugs in the class. For these patients, switching to an antidepressant medication without prominent serotonin reuptake inhibition is indicated.

Second-Line Antidepressants

In patients who do not have an optimal response or cannot tolerate SSRIs, second-line antidepressant agents include venlafaxine (Effexor), duloxetine (Cymbalta), mirtazapine (Remeron), and bupropion (Wellbutrin). In general, all of these agents are well tolerated and relatively safe, and for a given patient they might be considered first-line treatments. But each of these drugs has some at least potential disadvantages relative to SSRIs. Venlafaxine and duloxetine are potent serotonin and norepinephrine reuptake inhibitors. By virtue of targeting two neurotransmitters, these agents may carry some advantages over SSRIs. The potentiation of norepinephrine by venlafaxine and duloxetine theoretically may enhance the benefit of this medication for some patients. Some data suggest that in severely depressed patients venlafaxine may have greater efficacy than

SSRIs. But norepinephrine potentiation is also associated with potential adverse effects related to autonomic arousal, including increased blood pressure, palpitations, and diaphoresis, and severe overdose can be fatal. In the case of children and adolescents and physically healthy adult patients, the effects of norepinephrine potentiation may be tolerated without incident. But for patients who already have medical problems, such as high blood pressure or palpitations, venlafaxine and duloxetine may aggravate these conditions. Patients who experience prominent sexual-adverse effects associated with SSRIs may experience them with venlafaxine or duloxetine, which are also potent serotonin reuptake inhibitors.

Bupropion (Wellbutrin) is a relatively safe and very well-tolerated medication. It is a norepinephrine and dopamine reuptake inhibitor with little or no effect on central serotonin activity. Hence it is particularly useful for those patients who cannot tolerate the adverse effects related to serotonin potentiation (e.g., sexual dysfunction). Because of the potentiating effects on norepinephrine and dopamine, bupropion may be experienced by the patient as activating and it has the potential to cause adverse effects related to autonomic arousal. Data suggest that preexisting cardiac arrhythmias may be aggravated by bupropion. Unique to bupropion with a mechanism that is not well understood is the risk of seizures. Although the seizure risk may be reduced with the sustained-release formulations, bupropion is contraindicated in patients with seizure disorders, and its use should be scrutinized in patients with a history of head injury.

Mirtazapine (Remeron) is a unique antidepressant that is not a reuptake inhibitor but has effects on both serotonin and norepinephrine. It acts as a serotonin receptor antagonist, and it potentiates norepinephrine by blocking presynaptic α_2-adrenergic receptors. Mirtazapine has predictable sedation and weight gain associated with its use, possibly associated with the drug's potent antihistamine activity (i.e., H_1 blockade). For this reason, it is dosed at bedtime. These effects of the antidepressant may be beneficial in some patients (e.g., depressive syndrome with prominent anorexia and insomnia) but may be perceived by other patients as problematic (e.g., patients with obesity or diabetes mellitus).

Third-Line Antidepressants

At one time the cornerstones of antidepressant pharmacotherapy, TCAs and MAOIs are now relegated to a last-resort position in the antidepressant armamentarium. Their use is rare and usually confined to complicated cases in which all other treatment trials are ineffective and the patient is under the direct care of a psychiatrist. At one time considered more effective than so-called newer antidepressants, no data at present suggest that under routine circumstances TCAs or MAOIs have superior efficacy compared to other agents; hence it is difficult to justify exposing patients to the risks associated with their use.

Nefazodone (Serzone), one of the newer antidepressants from the 1990s, until recently was considered a relatively safe, well-tolerated drug with a presumed

mechanism of blocking serotonin receptors. Because of its half-life, nefazodone required twice-daily dosing, which was considered a disadvantage, but it appeared free of the sexual-adverse effects seen with SSRIs. It is a relatively potent inhibitor of the cytochrome P450 isoenzyme 3A4 and hence presented risk of interaction with other drugs requiring this enzyme for their metabolism.

Reports of adverse hepatic effects, including liver failure, led to nefazodone's removal from the Canadian and European markets in November 2003. In May 2004 Bristol-Myers Squibb pulled Serzone from the U.S. market. Generic nefazodone is currently still available in the United States. Because the serious risk of hepatic failure associated with nefazodone is now recognized, however, it anticipated use of this drug will be limited and only in rare, exceptional cases would it be initiated as antidepressant therapy. If patients are only responsive to nefazodone and stable on the drug for a period of time, the decision may be made to continue the therapy. But any use of nefazodone should require informed consent by the patient and close monitoring according to FDA guidelines. Patients with liver disease or elevated liver enzymes should not receive nefazodone.

Other Considerations in Treatment Selection

This discussion of antidepressant treatment selection so far has focused on the treatment-naïve patient. In the case of patients with recurrent mood disorders, a thorough history identifies antidepressant medications that were well tolerated and helpful to the patient in the past. In such cases, the recommendation is to resume whatever medicine was effective for the patient in treating prior mood disorder episodes. Another useful piece of history relevant to treatment selection is whether or not the patient has other family members who were treated for mood disorders and the nature of their response to particular antidepressant agents. A general belief is that if one family member has responded well to a particular antidepressant agent, the patient seeking treatment may also respond to that agent.

In addition to targeting neurotransmitters, a number of antidepressants also have effects on hepatic enzyme activity, specifically the cytochrome P450 (CYP) isoenzymes. In principle, drugs that affect a particular CYP isoenzyme activity alter the metabolism of other medications the patient may be taking that are substrates for that isoenzyme. A detailed discussion of pharmacokinetic drug interactions involving CYP isoenzymes is outside the scope of this article. Numerous references are available, and most, if not all, pharmacy departments have computer software that identifies potential pharmacokinetic drug interactions and can provide a resource as to whether or not a particular drug has an effect on CYP isoenzymes. Among currently popular antidepressant medications, fluoxetine (Prozac) and paroxetine (Paxil) are considered relatively potent inhibitors of CYP 2D6 and therefore are likely to alter the plasma concentration of other drugs the patient may be taking that require CYP 2D6 for their metabolism. As mentioned earlier, nefazodone (Serzone) is a relatively potent inhibitor of CYP 3A4. A number of other antidepressant

17

agents have mild to moderate effects on CYP isoenzymes, but their clinical significance is not clear.

An Antidepressant Treatment Trial

An antidepressant treatment trial can be conceptualized as having four principal considerations, called the four D's: diagnosis, drug, dose, and duration. For this discussion, we assume the diagnosis of a depressive disorder for which antidepressant medication is indicated. The next step is to select an antidepressant medication. As discussed, currently available antidepressants can be generally organized into first-line, second-line, and third-line agents. For a treatment-naïve patient, the clinician most likely selects a first-line antidepressant agent. Knowledge that the patient had a preferential response to a particular antidepressant in the past, or has a family member who had a preferential response to a particular antidepressant, may influence the treatment selection.

Once an antidepressant is selected, the next issue is dosing. Prior to the 1990s, antidepressant therapy often involved a lengthy process of dose titration, typically starting at very low doses to minimize toxicity and then advancing in small increments over time. In the 1990s, with the advent of better tolerated, less toxic antidepressant agents, oftentimes the starting dose was the effective dose. Perhaps the best illustration of this phenomenon is the SSRIs, where the starting doses were the effective doses for many patients. After a decade of experience with the newer antidepressant agents, it is now recognized that dose titration in and of itself is not necessarily a practice to be avoided and may offer certain advantages to patients. Several antidepressants are now available in lower-dose formulations so they can be initiated at a low dose, even if it is only for a few days or a week, to improve tolerability and positively influence treatment compliance. Some patients respond optimally to lower doses than were previously believed effective, but other patients require higher than the usually effective dose. Where a particular patient falls in this dose-response spectrum only becomes apparent during a dose titration process.

Once an antidepressant medication is initiated, the question becomes how long a treatment trial should continue before the clinician makes the decision to change the dose or switch to another antidepressant medication. The guidelines for duration of a treatment trial have shifted over the last decade. At one time, all patients were maintained for 6 to 8 weeks at the usually effective dose of a medication (e.g., fluoxetine, 20 mg per day) before considering dose titration. It was believed the antidepressant-induced biological changes in the central nervous system might take several weeks to occur. This principle has not been challenged, but data now suggest that those patients who go on to have an optimal response to an antidepressant medication are most likely to show at least a partial response by 2 to 4 weeks at the usually effective dose. Hence in current practice the response of the patient should be factored into the decision to titrate the dosage or change medication. By the 2- to 4-week

mark in a treatment trial, if the patient is in the range of the usually effective dose and showing marginal beneficial response and no adverse effects, it would be reasonable to consider advancing the medication dose. Broad variability among patients exists in the plasma drug concentrations achieved at a given antidepressant dose. Thus it is quite possible that a patient on a usually effective antidepressant dose may for a variety of reasons develop a plasma drug concentration that is much less than expected and outside the range of concentration associated with optimal response.

By the 4-week mark in a treatment trial, if the selected antidepressant agent is titrated without appreciable benefit but also without appreciable adverse effects, it is reasonable to advance the dose further. If the selected antidepressant dose is already at the recommended maximum dose or adverse effects prohibit further dose escalation, considerations include using an augmentation strategy or changing drugs. Common augmentation strategies for antidepressant medications include low-dose thyroid hormone, on the order of 25 to 50 µg per day, or low-dose lithium (Eskalith)[1] therapy, on the order of 300 or 600 mg a day. Low-dose stimulants, such as methylphenidate (Ritalin),[1] are also used as an augmentation strategy. In general, augmentation strategies should show added benefit within a relatively short period of time, on the order of 1 to 2 weeks.

Another option for the patient who has had only marginal benefit to antidepressant therapy by the 4- to 6-week mark in the treatment trial is change to a different antidepressant medication. Before switching the patient to an alternative antidepressant, the clinician should assess whether the patient had an adequate dose titration and was compliant with the treatment trial. In some cases, the clinician may decide to assay the plasma level of the antidepressant drug to assess whether the particular patient has a drug concentration much lower than would be predicted based on the antidepressant drug dose. A plasma drug level can provide the necessary data to direct either further dose titration or a drug change.

In general, 40% to 60% of patients have an optimal response to an antidepressant treatment trial. These numbers suggest that a high percentage of patients do not have an optimal response to the first treatment trial and ultimately receive sequential antidepressant treatment trials. When selecting an alternative antidepressant for a patient who has not had an optimal response during a current treatment trial, a number of options are available. Data suggest that patients who do not respond optimally to one SSRI go on to have a desired response to a second SSRI. For better or worse, it is now common practice for patients to have multiple sequential treatment trials with SSRIs. For a patient who does not respond optimally to trials of two SSRIs, although one could generate a rationale for proceeding with another SSRI treatment trial, it is reasonable to consider selecting an antidepressant with a different mechanism

---

[1]Not FDA approved for this indication.

of action. Popular non-SSRI antidepressant choices include venlafaxine (Effexor), duloxetine (Cymbalta), bupropion (Wellbutrin), and mirtazapine (Remeron).

In the primary care setting, ambulatory patients may undergo multiple sequential antidepressant treatment trials until an optimal response is achieved. Over the last several years, primary care clinicians are increasingly effective in their use of the newer antidepressant agents. That said, the time may come when it would be most appropriate to refer a patient for psychiatric specialty care. Marginal response to antidepressant treatment trials with ongoing significant functional impairment, the onset of psychotic symptoms, or when the clinician is considering the use of a third-line antidepressant medication (e.g., TCA, MAOI) are all reasons to obtain psychiatric consultation. For those patients expressing suicidal ideation or with a significant suicide risk profile (Table 4), a psychiatric referral is the appropriate strategy.

A FINAL WORD ON ANTIDEPRESSANT PHARMACOTHERAPY

In the spring of 2004, the FDA issued a public health advisory cautioning clinicians, patients, and families about the need to closely monitor all patients being treated with antidepressant drugs for the onset of suicidality. Although a causal role for antidepressants is not established, this advisory arose from ongoing concern about the potential for emerging suicidality or worsening of depressive symptoms in patients taking antidepressants. The FDA asked the makers of antidepressant drugs to add the warning for risk of emerging suicidality to the labels reflecting this advisory.

TABLE 4 SAD PERSONS Scale for Assessment of Suicide Risk

S   Sex: Males are more likely than females to kill themselves by 3:1.

A   Age: Older more than younger, especially white males.

D   Depression: A depressive episode precedes suicide in up to 70% of cases.

P   Previous attempt(s): Most people who die of suicide do so on their first or second attempt. Patients who make multiple (4+) attempts have an increased risk of future attempts.

E   Ethanol use: Recent onset of ethanol use or other sedative–hypnotic drug use increases risk.

R   Rational thinking loss: Profound cognitive slowing, psychotic depression, and preexisting brain damage.

S   Social support deficit: Social withdrawal, disconnected from family and friends, unemployed.

O   Organized plan: Person has gone beyond thinking of death and considered a plan for suicide.

N   No spouse: The absence of a spouse or significant other is a risk factor.

S   Sickness: Intercurrent medical illnesses.

Rakel and Bope: *Conn's Current Therapy 2006.*

NONPHARMACOLOGIC THERAPY FOR DEPRESSIVE DISORDERS

Psychotherapy

Although pharmacotherapy is the principal treatment intervention for patients with depressive disorders, psychotherapy should always be an option. Psychotherapy can be an adjunct to pharmacotherapy. It can be considered for those patients who prefer not to take medications, and it may be particularly suitable for patients with mild depressive symptomatology. Specifically, data support cognitive behavioral therapy (CBT) and interpersonal therapy (IT) as effective interventions for patients with milder depressive symptomatology. CBT and IT may have additive benefits for patients taking antidepressant medication. Both modalities require a practitioner who has received special training. When referring a patient for one of these particular types of psychotherapy, the clinician should inquire about the background and training of the therapist. In contrast to less well-defined psychotherapy approaches used in the past, both CBT and IT as practiced today are characterized by setting specific treatment goals and timelines for achieving those therapeutic goals.

Even in those cases where the clinician has not selected specific psychotherapies for the patient, ideally some form of generic supportive psychotherapy should be available to accompany pharmacotherapy. Elements of this generic supportive psychotherapy include psychoeducation about mood disorders and antidepressant medications, helping the patient recognize personal strengths, helping the patient prioritize what can sometimes be complex biopsychosocial problems, and in some cases offering guidance to assist with problem solving. This form of supportive psychotherapy can certainly be delegated to a therapist, but it can also be accomplished by a practiced clinician with relative efficiency.

Electroconvulsive Therapy

Perhaps the most effective treatment for depressive disorders is electroconvulsive therapy (ECT). ECT has been used for decades to treat mood disorders, and its efficacy and safety are supported by a wealth of data. Despite its effectiveness, ECT is not considered a first-line therapy for most patients with depressive disorders, principally because of the risks associated with the general anesthesia required for the treatments. ECT is indicated for patients with severe depressive symptoms, significant functional impairment, psychotic symptoms, and catatonia. There are no absolute contraindications to ECT, and it is used effectively in the frail elderly as well as in pregnant patients. In the primary care setting, the severity of depressive symptomatology or lack of response to multiple treatment trials is usually the basis for considering ECT. Whenever considering ECT, it is reasonable to obtain a psychiatric consultation first, which either offers further support for pursuing ECT or suggests alternative treatment strategies that should be implemented prior to further consideration of ECT.

17

Novel Therapies

Other nonpharmacologic interventions are either available or in development for the treatment of mood disorders. These include transcranial magnetic stimulation (TMS), vagal nerve stimulation (VNS), light therapy, and herbal/homeopathic remedies. Clinics in different parts of the country specialize in light therapy, and light sources are commercially available for patients to use in treating mood disorders. Light therapy is indicated as an adjunct to pharmacotherapy or for those patients with mild to moderate depressive symptoms who decline drug therapy. It is often used for patients who have a seasonal variation to their depressive symptoms. Further information about light therapy is available through multiple sources, including the Internet.

TMS and VNS are still considered investigational treatments for depression, and as such their use is confined to clinical trials at research centers. A multicenter trial of VNS for treatment-resistant depression (TRD) was recently completed, and the FDA is reviewing the study results

Homeopathic, herbal, and traditional medicine therapies for depression are available; however, they tend to lack rigorous scientific data to support their efficacy and safety and hence are not considered part of the standard of care of treating mood disorders.

Treatment of Bipolar Mood Disorders

Although unipolar depressive disorders are more common, no discussion of mood disorders is complete without a review of bipolar disorders. Bipolar affective disorder (BAD), formerly referred to as manic-depressive illness, can carry considerable morbidity for the patient and represents a particular challenge for the treating clinician. Clinicians in any medical setting ideally should be familiar with the various presentations of BAD (see Table 2). Increasingly, efforts are under way to manage BAD in the primary care setting.

BIPOLAR DEPRESSION

When a patient presents with a depressive episode, there may be no prior history of a bipolar diagnosis. In such cases, the clinician proceeds with antidepressant treatment as already discussed. Any antidepressant agent has the potential to induce a manic or mixed episode in a vulnerable patient (i.e., a patient with a bipolar diathesis), where *mixed* refers to a state in which the patient simultaneously meets *DSM-IV* criteria for both a depressive and manic episode. Hence part of routine management in the treatment of depression is to monitor for the possible cycling of a patient from a depressive episode into a manic or mixed episode. During the antidepressant treatment trial, if the clinician suspects the patient is cycling into mania, it is reasonable to obtain a psychiatric consultation.

Alternatively, a patient may present with a depressed episode and a prior history of BAD. This history suggests the patient is at risk for cycling into a manic or mixed state if an antidepressant medication is initiated, and hence a principal concern in treatment planning is to prevent cycling from occurring (i.e., mood stabilization). The standard approach to treating depression in the bipolar patient is to implement a mood-stabilizing medication (e.g., lithium, valproic acid,[1] carbamazepine[1]) in conjunction with an antidepressant medicine. No particular antidepressant medication carries less risk of inducing cycling to a manic or mixed episode in a vulnerable bipolar patient. Hence the guidelines discussed previously regarding antidepressant treatment selection still apply. Bupropion (Wellbutrin) may have advantages in treating depression in bipolar patients by virtue of a decreased risk of inducing cycling. But the data to support the advantages of bupropion are limited, and no consensus exists that this medication should have a particular first-line position in treating bipolar depression.

Recent industry-sponsored controlled trials suggest the atypical antipsychotic agents have mood-stabilizing properties. Olanzapine (Zyprexa), ziprasidone (Geodon), risperidone (Risperdal), quetiapine (Seroquel), and aripiprazole (Abilify) are now FDA approved for treatment of an acute manic or mixed episode of bipolar disorder. In the last few years, a number of new anticonvulsant agents were studied for mood-stabilizing properties. Of the newer anticonvulsants, only lamotrigine (Lamictal) received FDA approval as a mood stabilizer for treatment of bipolar disorder, and it is believed to have particular efficacy for bipolar depression. But the two most frequently prescribed mood stabilizers remain lithium and valproic acid (Depakote), which are considered the first-line agents for treating either bipolar depression or bipolar mania. In addition to pharmacotherapy, bipolar depression can also be treated by ECT. Because of the recognized challenge of treating bipolar depression, when this diagnosis is considered, it is reasonable to refer the patient to a psychiatrist. Once a bipolar patient is stable and euthymic, ongoing care possibly could be managed in a primary care setting.

BIPOLAR MANIA

In addition to depressive episodes, bipolar patients may present with hypomania, mania without psychosis, or mania with psychosis or in what is referred to as a *mixed state,* in which the patient exhibits symptoms of both mania and depression simultaneously. The cornerstone therapy for any one of these presentations is a mood-stabilizing agent. As discussed, first-line mood-stabilizing agents include lithium, valproic acid (Depakote), and carbamazepine (Tegretol).[1] These drugs may take days to weeks to bring about the desired clinical outcome, and often adjunctive therapy with other classes of drugs is necessary initially to help control the patient's symptoms. Patients in a manic episode may require a mood-stabilizing agent, an antipsychotic drug, and a benzodiazepine. Depending on the severity of symptoms, a second mood stabilizer may be indicated.

---

[1]Not FDA approved for this indication.

Patients identified in a manic or mixed state should be referred for psychiatry specialty care as soon as possible. Temporizing acute interventions until the patient can be seen by a psychiatrist might include benzodiazepines for insomnia and atypical antipsychotic agents for agitation. Lorazepam (Ativan),[1] 1 to 2 mg, or clonazepam (Klonopin),[1] 1 to 2 mg, are reasonable sleep aids. Olanzapine (Zyprexa), 5 mg twice daily, or risperidone (Risperdal), 1 mg twice daily, are possible acute interventions for agitation. Because of the number of variables that must be considered when instituting therapy for patients in a manic episode or mixed state, however, if the patient cannot be referred immediately, it would be reasonable to obtain a phone consultation with a psychiatrist and review the patient's particulars to formulate a treatment strategy and discuss whether hospitalization is indicated. If lithium is selected, the patient's renal function should be assessed before initiating the medication. If either valproic acid or carbamazepine[1] is selected, the patient's liver function and hematologic status should be assessed by obtaining liver function tests and a complete blood count (CBC) before initiating therapy. One advantage of the first-line mood-stabilizing agents is that they have established plasma-level ranges associated with optimal response and toxicity. A typical strategy is to initiate the mood stabilizers at low to moderate doses, allow the patient to achieve steady-state blood levels, assess the plasma concentration, and then adjust the medication accordingly.

[1]Not FDA approved for this indication.

CURRENT DIAGNOSIS

- Mood disorders are prevalent, potentially lethal, but highly treatable conditions.
- Types of mood disorders include major depressive disorder, bipolar disorder (type I and II), cyclothymic disorder, dysthymic disorder, mood disorder because of general medical condition (e.g., hypothyroidism) and substance-induced mood disorder.
- Mood disorders are syndromal diagnoses characterized by depressed or elevated mood in conjunction with vegetative signs and symptoms involving sleep, appetite, energy, libido, concentration, and psychomotor activity.
- Children and adolescents with mood disorders may present with behavioral disturbance. Elderly patients with mood disorders may present primarily with somatic complaints.
- Patients presenting with depressed or irritable mood should be evaluated and monitored for possible bipolar disorder.
- The evaluation for mood disorders must include a complete history, including medication and substance use history, a physical exam, and assessment of suicide risk (see SAD PERSONS scale, Table 4).

Mood disorders, both unipolar and bipolar, are relatively prevalent medical conditions that may occur in any clinical setting. They are serious medical conditions that can cause significant morbidity for patients and carry a significant risk of mortality either through suicide or accident. Pharmacotherapy is the principal intervention for major mood disorders. Psychotherapy is used for milder symptomatology and as an adjunct to pharmacotherapy. Mood disorders currently are being managed in the primary care setting. When patients are not responding optimally to antidepressant treatment, the symptomatology is particularly severe, the patient is at risk for suicide, or the patient presents with a manic episode or mixed state, it is advisable to obtain psychiatric consultation and refer the patient for specialty care.

CURRENT THERAPY

- The first line of treatment for depressive disorders are selective serotonin reuptake inhibitors (SSRIs) because of their tolerability and safety. The dose should be maximized as tolerated of the selected antidepressant to achieve the desired effect before switching to another antidepressant.
- Patients who do not respond to one SSRI trial may go on to have an optimal response to another agent from the same drug class.
- The second line of treatment for depressive disorders are the dual-action antidepressants, including venlafaxine, duloxetine, mirtazapine, and bupropion. They may have a higher risk of adverse effects than SSRIs but overall are also well tolerated.
- Monoamine oxidase inhibitors (MAOIs) and tricyclic antidepressants (TCAs) are third-line antidepressants. Their use is rare today and confined to complicated cases under the supervision of a psychiatrist.
- Electroconvulsive therapy (ECT) is a safe, effective treatment for mood disorders and should be considered for patients with marginal response to pharmacotherapy trials, severe symptoms, significant functional impairment, psychotic symptoms, or catatonia.
- Psychotherapy has additional benefits for patients taking antidepressant medication. It may be used as a monotherapy if the depression is mild or the patient is unwilling to try antidepressant medication.
- Treatment of bipolar disorder can be a challenge, even for an experienced psychiatrist. A mood-stabilizing agent should always be used as part of the treatment of any bipolar disorder episode to avoid cycling.
- A referral to a psychiatrist should be made if the patient is not responding to treatment, symptomatology is particularly severe, the patient is at risk for suicide, or the patient presents with manic or mixed episodes.

REFERENCES

Burt VK: Plotting the course to remission: The search for better outcomes in the treatment of depression. J Clin Psychiatry 2004; 65(Suppl 12): 20-25.

Hensley PL, Nadiga D, Uhlenhuth EH: Long-term effectiveness of cognitive therapy in major depressive disorder. Depress Anxiety 2004;20(1):1-7.

Jick H, Kaye J, Jick S: Antidepressants and the risk of suicidal behaviors. JAMA 2004;292:338-343.

Norman TR, Olver JS: New formulations of existing antidepressants: Advantages in the management of depression. CNS Drugs 2004; 18(8):505-520.

Pettinati HM: Antidepressant treatment of co-occurring depression and alcohol dependence. Biol Psychiatry 2004;56(10):785-792.

Schatzberg AF: Employing pharmacologic treatment of bipolar disorder to greatest effect. J Clin Psychiatry 2004;65(Suppl 15):15-20.

Shelton RC: The dual action hypothesis: Does pharmacology matter? J Clin Psychiatry 2004;65(Suppl 17):5-10.

Thase ME: Therapeutic alternatives for difficult to treat depression: A narrative review of the state of the evidence. CNS Spectr 2004; 9(11):808-821.

Zajecka JM, Albano D: SNRIs in the management of acute major depressive disorder. J Clin Psychiatry 2003;23(12):1668-1672.

Schizophrenia

Method of
Robert R. Conley, MD, and
Deanna L. Kelly, PharmD

Schizophrenia is one of the most challenging and complex psychiatric disorders that afflicts humans. The core symptoms of this illness are highly variable among people with schizophrenia. They include hallucinations, delusions, disorganized speech and behavior, inappropriate affect, cognitive deficits, and impaired psychosocial functioning. The onset of symptoms in most cases is insidious, usually preceded by a prodromal phase that is characterized by gradual social withdrawal, diminished interests, changes in appearance and hygiene, changes in cognition, and the onset of bizarre or odd behaviors. One percent of the population suffers from this disorder; the first presenting symptoms usually appear in late adolescence or early adulthood. Symptoms generally appear in males earlier in life than in females. Most people with the disorder require treatment with antipsychotics and comprehensive care over the course of their lives. This chapter focuses on the pharmacologic aspects of the treatment of schizophrenia. Neurobiologic and clinical aspects of these treatments are also reviewed.

Pathophysiology

The most common neuropathologic theory associated with the etiology of schizophrenia involves the dopaminergic systems. The dopamine hypothesis was formed in the late 1950s when it was discovered that antipsychotic drugs are postsynaptic dopamine antagonists. In has been observed that drugs that increase dopamine (e.g., cocaine, amphetamines) enhance or produce positive psychotic symptoms (delusions, hallucinations, suspiciousness, disorganized thinking) and drugs that decrease dopamine (e.g., antipsychotics) decrease or stop positive symptoms. There is much evidence supporting the dopamine hypothesis, particularly in areas of the brain with dopamine-2 receptors. Increased glucose metabolism in the basal ganglia and decreased metabolism in the frontal cortex may be indicative of dopaminergic hyperactivity and hypoactivity in these regions, respectively. Positron emission technology (PET) studies measuring receptor densities using dopamine-2–specific ligands such as raclopride show increased densities of dopamine-2 receptors in the basal ganglia and decreased densities in the prefrontal cortex. Other direct evidence supporting the validity of the dopamine hypothesis comes from postmortem evaluation of tissues and plasma. Investigators have measured the amount of dopamine and its metabolites, such as homovanillic acid. Brain tissue from people with schizophrenia has increased presynaptic dopamine and/or homovanillic acid levels in areas of the mesocortical and mesolimbic systems compared with levels in normal controls.

The hypothesis that the dopamine system explains symptoms of schizophrenia is far from complete, however. Recently, it has been suggested that combined dysfunction of the dopamine and glutamate transmitter systems may better explain this disorder. There has also been a great deal of speculation regarding the role of serotonin receptor antagonism with regard to antipsychotic effects. Many traditional antipsychotics are highly active at serotonin receptors, but this property does not distinguish the clinical effects of these drugs in a meaningful way. The serotonin hypothesis of psychosis actually predates the dopamine hypothesis, largely because of lysergic acid diethylamide (LSD), a drug with psychotomimetic properties, which releases serotonin. Interest in this theory was reinvigorated by the finding that clozapine, which has a 100-fold selectivity for serotonin compared with that of dopamine receptors, is highly efficacious. The other second-generation antipsychotics also have high serotonin-to-dopamine binding ratios. Serotonin receptor binding may be important to these drugs' actions, possibly by stimulating dopamine activity in mesocortical pathways. However, a compelling theory relating dopamine and serotonin receptor affinities does not yet exist.

Genetic Predisposition

The genetic component of this hypothesis is that a lesion is present at birth with the potential for *N*-methyl-D-aspartate (NMDA) receptor hypofunction, and this may not trigger psychopathologic or neuropathologic processes until late adolescence, at which time it begins to trigger schizophrenic symptoms. There is fairly strong evidence that schizophrenia is at least partially genetic in nature. For example, the risk of developing schizophrenia if a first-degree relative or both parents are diagnosed is 10% and 40%, respectively. Many genes have a weak association with the development of schizophrenia. However, there is probably no one schizophrenia gene. The possible genetic effects are either a susceptibility to schizophrenia with a certain gene or a combination of several genes that are necessary to develop the disorder. The chromosomes with the most significant evidence include 13 and 22, with some weak evidence for 6, 8, 10, 14, and 15. Environmental stimuli or triggers may contribute to the expression of symptoms.

Clinical Presentation

Schizophrenia is a chronic disorder of thought and affect and a significant disturbance in the individual's ability to function in society and develop interpersonal relationships. The clinical presentation of this disorder can be extremely varied, and despite attempts to portray a stereotype in the media, the stereotypic schizophrenic individual does not exist. In the 1970s, Strauss and others suggested that schizophrenic symptoms fell into three specific symptom complexes: positive symptoms, negative symptoms, and disorders of relating. Carpenter and others further characterized these three symptom domains into psychotic disturbances, cognitive dysfunction, and negative symptoms.

PSYCHOTIC SYMPTOMS

The acute psychotic symptoms include hallucinations (distortions or exaggeration or perception) and delusions (fixed false beliefs). Hallucinations may occur as auditory, visual, olfactory, gustatory, and tactile, but auditory hallucinations are the most common type in people with schizophrenia. Voices frequently are heard and are distinct from the person's own thoughts. The content of hallucinations is variable but is often threatening or commanding. Delusions are erroneous beliefs that usually involve a misinterpretation of perceptions or experiences and often are bizarre in nature and involve suspiciousness on the part of the patient.

COGNITIVE SYMPTOMS

Subtle disturbances in associative thinking may develop years before disorganized thinking (formal thought disorder). Inferences about thought are based primarily on the individual's speech. The schizophrenic's thinking and speech are frequently incomprehensible to others and often are illogical. Characteristics of formal thought disorder include loosening of associations, tangentiality, thought blocking, concreteness, circumstantiality, and perseveration. In addition, the average IQ of people with a schizophrenia diagnosis is 80 to 84, with the presence of prominent memory and learning difficulties.

NEGATIVE SYMPTOMS

Primary negative symptoms or deficit symptoms are quite ubiquitous in schizophrenia but are difficult to evaluate because they occur in a continuum with normality, are nonspecific, and are often due to the side effects of medication (secondary negative symptoms), mood disorder, environmental understimulation, or demoralization. The best test for establishing true negative symptoms is to examine their persistence for a considerable period of time despite efforts directed at resolving the other causes. Approximately 10% to 15% of people with schizophrenia may exhibit the majority of psychopathology as negative symptoms; these people may be referred to as having a deficit syndrome. Negative symptoms include impoverished speech and thinking, lack of social drive, flatness of emotional expression, and apathy.

PRESENTATION OF SYMPTOMS

People with a diagnosis of schizophrenia may be uncooperative, hostile, and verbally or physically aggressive owing to their misinterpretation of reality and often owing to command hallucinations. Difficulty with anxiety may be exhibited because of the presence of positive symptoms and suspiciousness. Because of negative and depressive symptoms, people with schizophrenia may have impaired self-care skills and may be dirty and unkempt. Sleep and appetite are often disturbed. People with schizophrenia often have difficulty living independently in the community and have difficulty forming close relationships with others. In addition, they have problems with initiating or maintaining employment and are often noncompliant with medications, thus increasing their risk for relapse.

Diagnosis

The commonly accepted diagnostic criteria for schizophrenia comes from the *Diagnostic and Statistical Manual of Mental Disorders, Forth Edition–Text Revision* (*DSM-IV-TR*). The essential features are a mixture of characteristic signs and symptoms as listed previously that have been present for a significant portion of time during a 1-month period (or a shorter time if successfully treated), with some signs of the disorders persisting for at least 6 months. These signs ans symptoms are associated with marked social or occupational dysfunction, are not accounted for by a mood disorder, and are not due to the direct physiologic effects of a substance or a general medical condition. Differential diagnosis of psychotic signs and symptoms may include the following: schizoaffective disorder, mood disorders, dementia, delirium, drug intoxication, pervasive developmental disorders, neurologic conditions (neoplasm, migraines, epilepsy), or medical conditions (fluid or electrolyte imbalances, metabolic conditions, autoimmune disorders).

Course and Prognosis

Although the course of schizophrenia is variable, the long-term prognosis for independent function is often poor. This illness is marked by intermittent acute psychotic episodes and a decline in psychosocial functioning. A patient may become more withdrawn, "bizarre," and nonfunctional over many years. Complete return to full premorbid functioning is not common in this disorder. Many of the more dramatic and acute symptoms disappear with time, but severe residual symptoms may persist. Family and friends may find this illness difficult to interpret and understand. Involvement with the law is fairly common for misdemeanors such as vagrancy, loitering, and disturbing the peace. The overall life expectancy is shortened primarily because of suicide, accidents, and the inability to manage self-care. The lifetime risk of suicide for persons with schizophrenia is 10% to 13%. People with schizophrenia who have fewer periods of acute psychotic episodes and those who are treated very early in their course of illness may have a better prognosis. Persistent compliance with a tolerable drug regimen also improves prognosis.

Pharmacologic and Nonpharmacologic Treatment

The cornerstone for treatment of schizophrenia is the use of both pharmacologic and nonpharmacologic therapies. Longer durations of untreated psychotic illness may lead to a poorer prognosis and functional ability later in life; thus, treatment should be initiated as soon as possible. The foundations for treatment include stabilizing therapy and preventing psychotic relapse, reducing the burden of symptoms and side effects, improving cognitive abilities, maintaining medication adherence, and rehabilitating for improvements in functional status, potential work, and/or independent living. Social skills training should be offered to patients along with rehabilitative support.

Antipsychotic drugs are used to treat nearly all forms of psychosis, including schizophrenia, schizoaffective disorder, affective disorders with psychosis, and dementias. Antipsychotic medications are the primary pharmacologic treatment of schizophrenia. Approximately 20 antipsychotic drugs are available in the United States, of which 6 are termed atypical or second-generation antipsychotics (SGAs). Adjunctive medications may be appropriate in some people and include anticholinergic medications, mood stabilizers, benzodiazepines, beta-blockers, and antidepressants. The basis for adjunctive use includes the treatment of side effects, refractory symptoms, agitation, anxiety, depression, or mood elevation.

FIRST-GENERATION ANTIPSYCHOTICS

Antipsychotics drugs have been in clinical use since the 1950s, when chlorpromazine (Thorazine) was synthesized in France. It was first used as a preanesthetic agent.

Within 2 years of use, it was found to be effective in the treatment of people with psychosis. Many other similar medications followed in the next decade. These medications were commonly referred to as neuroleptics, which meant that they caused a neurologic disorder. This name came about because of the profound extrapyramidal motor side effects they produced. Many believed the induction of motor side effects was necessary, however, for efficacy of the medications. All of the first-generation antipsychotic agents available are high-affinity D_2 receptor antagonists (e.g., haloperidol [Haldol], chlorpromazine [Thorazine]). These agents block 65% to 80% of D_2 receptors in the striatum during long-term treatment and block dopamine in the other dopamine tracts, as well. Although they differ in potency and side effect profiles, all first-generation antipsychotic agents are generally equivalent in efficacy when used in equipotent doses (300-600 CPZ units). All, however, may cause significant extrapyramidal symptoms (pseudoparkinsonism, dystonia, and akathisia) and tardive dyskinesia. The presence of extrapyramidal symptoms has a pervasive negative impact on treatment and adherence. Furthermore, worsening of negative symptoms and cognition as well as an increased risk for tardive dyskinesia has led to a new class of antipsychotic medications.

SECOND-GENERATION ANTIPSYCHOTICS

Over the past decade, six atypical or novel antipsychotics have been introduced in the United States: clozapine [Clozaril], risperidone [Risperdal], olanzapine [Zyprexa], quetiapine [Seroquel], ziprasidone [Geodon], and aripiprazole [Abilify]. What principally distinguishes these newer antipsychotic agents from the first-generation antipsychotic agents is their ability to induce an antipsychotic effect with a much lower risk of causing extrapyramidal symptoms. These agents produce a similar, if not better, effect than the first-generation antipsychotics for positive symptoms and may provide better efficacy in other domains such as negative symptoms, cognition, and mood. Thus, this class of medications should be dosed in amounts in which they are effective without causing extrapyramidal symptoms. Table 1 lists the recommended dosing in adult schizophrenia patients. Similar efficacy is observed among different antipsychotics in people with treatment-responsive schizophrenia. Clozapine, however, has superior efficacy in people who are treatment-resistant and has a response rate of approximately 30% to 60% in this population. This medication is associated with a 1% risk of causing agranulocytosis; thus, routine monitoring of white blood cells is required.

While SGAs are moving into first-line therapy in schizophrenia, it is noteworthy that treatment with this class of medications is not without side effects. Appropriate monitoring and attention should be paid to the development of side effects, and side effects should be minimized and addressed. For example, clozapine and olanzapine are associated with the greatest gains in weight and metabolic disturbances (elevations in glucose and lipids). Thus, routine weights and metabolic

TABLE 1 Dosing Recommendations for Second-Generation Antipsychotics*

Agent	Initial Target Dose	Maximal Dose Likely to Be Beneficial	Comments
Clozapine (Clozaril)	400 mg/day	500-600 mg/day	plasma level ≥ 350 ng/mL; fast-dissolving formulation available
Risperidone (Risperdal)	2-4 mg/day	6 mg/day	Long-acting injectable available for every 2-wk dosing; liquid and fast-dissolving formulations available
Olanzapine (Zyprexa)	15-20 mg/day	30-40 mg/day	> 20 mg/day is outside product labeling; fast-dissolving formulation available
Quetiapine (Seroguel)	400-600 mg/day	800-1200 mg/day	> 800 mg/day is outside product labeling
Ziprasidone (Geodon)	100-120 mg/day	160-200 mg/day	> 160 mg/day is outside product labeling; IM preparation available
Aripiprazole (Abilify)	15-30 mg/day	30 mg/day	Liquid formulation available

*Lower doses should be used in children, the elderly, persons with other diagnoses, and vulnerable populations.

parameters should be measured. Risperidone is associated with the highest risk for dose-dependent extrapyramidal symptoms and sexual dysfunction. Quetiapine is association with a high degree of early and transient sedation, ziprasidone has a tendency to prolong the QTc, and aripiprazole is associated with gastrointestinal disturbances. Side effect profiles for SGAs are listed in Table 2.

Conclusions

Although multiple treatment modalities are important in treating schizophrenia, antipsychotics remain the cornerstone of treatment. SGAs do provide advantages over first-generation antipsychotics but are much more costly. Some evidence, however, does suggest that compared with first-generation antipsychotics, SGAs

17

TABLE 2 Side Effect Profiles of Second-Generation Antipsychotics

	Clozapine	Risperidone	Olanzapine	Quetiapine	Ziprasidone	Aripiprazole	Haloperidol
Anticholinergic side effects (dry mouth, constipation, blurry vision, urinary hesitancy)	+++	∀	++ (higher doses)	∀	∀	∀	∀
EPS at clinical doses	∀	+	∀	∀	∀	∀	++
Dose-dependent EPS	0	++	+	0	+	∀	+++
Orthostatic hypotension	+++	++	+	++	+	+	+
Prolactin elevation (hormonal and sexual side effects)	0	+++	+	∀	+	0	++
QTc prolongation	+	∀	∀	∀	+	∀	∀
Sedation	+++	+	+	++	+	+	+
Seizures	++	∀	∀	∀	∀	∀	∀
Weight gain	+++	++	+++	++	+	+	∀
Glucose dysregulation	++	∀	++	∀	∀	∀	∀
Lipid abnormalities	+++	∀	+++	+	∀	∀	∀
Gastrointestinal disturbances	+	∀	∀	∀	∀	+	∀

0, absent; ∀, minimal; +, mild or low risk; ++, moderate; +++, severe; EPS, extrapyramidal symptoms.

Rakel and Bope: *Conn's Current Therapy 2006.*

CURRENT DIAGNOSIS

Characteristic symptoms: Two or more of the following, each present for a significant portion of time during a 1-month period

- Delusions
- Hallucinations
- Disorganized speech (e.g., frequent derailment or incoherence)
- Grossly disorganized or catatonic behavior
- Negative symptoms (affective flattening, alogia, avolition)

Social or occupational dysfunction in one or more of the following areas:

- Work
- Interpersonal relations
- Self-care
- Academics

Duration of symptoms and functional impairment are evident or prodromal for at least 6 months

Other disorders are ruled out such as the following:

- Schizoaffective disorder
- Bipolar disorder
- Substance abuse
- General medical condition
- Pervasive developmental disorder

are cost-effective. To maximize the benefits of SGAs, the dose of these medications should be carefully adjusted to maximize efficacy and minimize the occurrence of side effects. Proper monitoring of side effects should be implemented. Because each pharmacologic treatment has its own unique profile, clinicians should now attempt to optimize antipsychotic therapy for each patient in a highly individualized way.

CURRENT THERAPY

- Antipsychotic treatment should begin at symptom onset of schizophrenia to avoid detrimental periods of untreated psychosis
- Both pharmacologic (i.e., antipsychotics) and nonpharmacologic strategies (i.e., social skills training, psychotherapy) should be mainstays of treatment for schizophrenia
- Second-generation antipsychotics are generally recommended as first-line therapy
- Side effect liabilities vary widely among the antipsychotics, and the selection of antipsychotic agents should be tailored to individual patients
- Appropriate regular follow-up and routine monitoring for side effects is pertinent

REFERENCES

Conley RR, Kelly DL: Management of treatment resistance in schizophrenia. Biol Psychiatry 2001;50(11):898-911.

Jin H, Meyer JM, Jeste DV: Atypical antipsychotics and glucose dysregulation: A systematic review. Schizophr Res 2004;71(2-3): 195-212.

Kane JM, Leucht S, Carpenter D, Docherty JP: Expert consensus guideline series. Optimizing pharmacologic treatment of psychotic disorders. Introduction: Methods, commentary, and summary. J Clin Psychiatry 2003;64(Suppl 12):5-19.

Marder SR, Essock SM, Miller AL, et al: Physical health monitoring of patients with schizophrenia. Am J Psychiatry 2004;161(8): 1334-1349.

Marder SR, Essock SM, Miller AL, et al: The Mount Sinai conference on the pharmacotherapy of schizophrenia. Schizophr Bull 2002; 28(1):5-16.

Moller HJ: Course and long-term treatment of schizophrenic psychoses. Pharmacopsychiatry 2004;37(Suppl 2):126-135.

Seamans JK, Yang CR: The principal features and mechanisms of dopamine modulation in the prefrontal cortex. Prog Neurobiol 2004;74(1):1-58.

Wirshing DA: Schizophrenia and obesity: Impact of antipsychotic medications. J Clin Psychiatry 2004;65(Suppl 18):13-26.

Panic Disorder

Method of
*Alexander Bystritsky, MD, PhD, and
Kira Williams, MD*

Diagnosis

Panic disorder (PD) and related agoraphobia (AG) are very prevalent and disabling conditions affecting 3% to 8% of the world population. Panic disorder is characterized by sudden episodes of acute apprehension or intense fear that occur *out of the blue* without any apparent cause-panic attacks. Intense panic usually lasts no more than a few minutes, but, in rare instances, can return in *waves* for a period of up to 2 hours. During the panic itself, any of the symptoms listed in Box 1 may occur.

The attack is spontaneous, unexpected, and occurs for no apparent reason. The word *agoraphobia* means fear of open spaces; however, under many instances agoraphobia is a fear of panic attacks. Patients suffering from agoraphobia are afraid of being in situations from which escape might be difficult, or in which help might be unavailable if they suddenly had a panic attack. Many agoraphobics not only fear having panic attacks but also fear embarrassment should they be seen having a panic attack. It is common for the agoraphobic to avoid a variety of situations (Box 2). The fear usually results in travel restrictions, or a need to be accompanied by others when leaving home. They may avoid certain situations such as waiting in a line, being in crowded places (malls, theaters) and even using transportation, including driving a car. In the end, agoraphobic patients often end up completely housebound.

BOX 1 Symptoms of Panic Attack

- Dizziness, unsteadiness, or faintness
- Fear of dying
- Fear of going crazy or losing control
- Feeling of choking
- Feeling of unreality—as if you're not all there
- Heart palpitations—pounding heart or accelerated heart rate
- Hot and cold flashes
- Nausea or abdominal distress
- Numbness, pain, or tingling in hands, feet, arms, legs, fingers, toes, lips, face
- Pain or discomfort in chest, upper back, shoulder blades
- Shortness of breath or a feeling of being smothered
- Sweating
- Trembling or shaking

Impact and Cost

Panic attacks are very common events. Some studies show that lifetime prevalence of panic or panic-like episodes is somewhere from 15% to 45%. PD characterized by frequent, disturbing panic attacks accompanied by at least 1 month of persistent fear of having another attack is less frequent. Epidemiologic studies throughout the world indicate the lifetime prevalence of PD (with or without AG) ranges between 1.5% and 3.5%. Twice as many women as men suffer from panic disorder. Studies have suggested high co-morbidity, showing that 63% to 73% of PD patients have had at least one other mental health condition, including major depressive disorder, obsessive–compulsive disorder, or another anxiety disorder during their lifetime. Panic patients also tend to seek relief from their anxiety by self-medicating with alcohol and drugs (prescription and/or illicit). The professional life of a PD patient is also likely to suffer. The majority of these patients admit that the quality of their work diminished as a result of their anxiety. Those who are financially dependent and those who receive either welfare or disability benefits constitute a considerable 27% of all PD patients. Furthermore, there seems to be a lower life expectancy among PD patients because of an increased risk of developing some cardiovascular disease or because of suicidal behavior, although the evidence for this is not consistent. The actual costs of PD are difficult to evaluate because they are indirect and hidden, but it is estimated that they are quite extensive. Because of the physical nature of panic attack symptoms, most PD patients repeatedly consult their family physicians, internists or other health professionals. Current estimates of cost of these conditions in U.S. society are more than $44 billion per year, a figure comparable to the cost of cardiovascular disorders.

Differential Diagnoses

Box 3 summarizes the differential diagnoses for PD. The relationship between panic disorder and the other disorders listed in the table can be very complex, for example:

- Another disorder can mimic PD.
- Another disorder can cause or worsen PD through a variety of physiologic mechanisms.

BOX 2 Some of the More Common Situations Feared by Agoraphobics

- Being at home alone
- Crowded public places such as grocery stores, department stores, restaurants
- Enclosed or confined places such as tunnels, bridges, or the hairdresser's chair
- Public transportation such as trains, buses, subways, planes

BOX 3 Differential Diagnosis and Co-morbidity of Panic Disorder

1. Cardiac conditions
   a. Arrhythmias[a,c,d]
   b. Supraventricular tachycardia[a,c,d]
   c. Mitral valve prolapse[b,c,d]
2. Endocrine disorders
   a. Thyroid abnormality[a,b,c,d]
   b. Hyperparathyroidism[b,c,d]
   c. Pheochromocytoma[d]
   d. Hypoglycemia[a,c,d]
3. Vestibular dysfunctions[a,b,c,d]
4. Seizure disorders (temporal lobe epilepsy)[a,b,c,d]
5. Other psychiatric conditions
   a. Affective disorders
      (1) Major depression[d,e,f]
      (2) Bipolar disorder[b,d,e,f]
   b. Other anxiety disorders
      (1) Acute stress disorder[a,b,c,d,e,f]
      (2) Obsessive–compulsive disorder[a,b,c,d,e,f]
      (3) Post-traumatic stress disorder[a,b,c,d,e,f]
      (4) Social phobia[a,c,d,e,f]
      (5) Specific phobia[a,c,d,e,f]
   c. Psychotic disorders[a,d,e,f]
   d. Substance abuse and dependence
      (1) Withdrawal from central nervous system depressants[a,b,c,d,e,f]
         (a) Alcohol abuse (present in 40% of panic disorder patients)
         (b) Barbiturates
      (2) Stimulants[a,b,c,d,e,f]
         (a) Cocaine
         (b) Amphetamines
         (c) Caffeine
      (3) Cannabis[a,b,c,d,e,f]
      (4) Hallucinogens[a,b,c,d,e,f]

[a]The disorder can mimic panic disorder (PD).
[b]The disorder can cause or worsen PD through a variety of physiologic mechanisms.
[c]The disorder's symptoms could serve as triggers of panic attacks.
[d]The disorder could coexist with PD as an independent disorder.
[e]The disorder could be a co-morbid disorder with symptoms that intermingle with PD.
[f]The disorder could lead to PD or be a sequela of PD.

Rakel and Bope: *Conn's Current Therapy 2006.*

- Another disorder's symptoms could serve as triggers of panic attacks.
- Another disorder could coexist with PD as an independent disorder.
- Another disorder could be a co-morbid disorder with symptoms that intermingle with PD.
- Another disorder could lead to PD or be a sequela of PD.

One such example of this interaction is cardiac arrhythmias. Although it is uncommon, an arrhythmia can coexist with panic disorder as an independent condition, and a sudden increase of heart rate could potentially provoke panic in a patient with PD. However, arrhythmia accompanied by fear could mimic a panic attack, and patients with potentially dangerous arrhythmias may receive inappropriate treatment as the result of misdiagnosis. Another possible association is mitral valve prolapse (MVP) in patients with PD, which is a frequent finding thought to be of doubtful clinical significance. However, recent research suggested that it is possible that these two disorders in some patients are linked genetically (via chromosome 13) in a syndrome characterized by β-adrenergic hyperactivity, MVP, panic, and kidney problems. Careful initial medical and psychiatric evaluation is recommended in panic patients. However, prolonged and repetitive testing should be discouraged.

Theoretical Framework

Different theories, including cognitive-behavioral and biomedical, have been used in an attempt to describe the biologic mechanisms of panic. A brief synthesis of these theories reveals that PD is likely a combination of:

- An increase in alarm reaction
- An error in information processing (catastrophic thinking)
- Abnormal coping strategies to relieve anxiety and provide a sense of security (safety rituals and avoidance)

The disorder represents a sequential process where the symptoms start with the physical symptoms of panic and progress through the stages of abnormal thinking, rituals, and, finally, avoidance (Table 1).

These symptom clusters may be wired through different neuronal circuits and respond preferentially to different treatments. However, this theoretical frame work is incomplete, as the intricacy of the neuronal circuits and neurotransmitters is not fully understood.

Treatment Algorithm

The treatment of PD is a stepwise process that starts with treatments of proven efficacy that are capable of ameliorating symptoms and decreasing avoidance behaviors. Figure 1 provides an algorithm of the treatment steps.

Step 1 starts with a first-line medication of a selective serotonin reuptake inhibitor (SSRI) or a therapeutic approach with cognitive behavior therapy (CBT). Both treatments have demonstrated efficacy between 70% and 90% in multiple studies. The treatment choice is based on the initial patient session with the physician, in which patients usually express their preference for either medication or psychotherapy. When availability and cost of the therapy is an issue, medication is the simplest way of treating PD. If, after two trials, the SSRI is deemed unsuccessful, step 2 begins.

Step 2 should start with a discussion with the patient about his/her preference for adding another medication or switching to another treatment modality (e.g., psychotherapy).

Step 3 involves treatment with more intensive CBT or with medications or combinations of treatments that have not yet been tried. Unusual and alternative treatments may be considered at that point (an expert consultation is usually recommended).

BEHAVIORAL THERAPY

Behavior therapy can be effective in as few as four sessions and can significantly reduce a patient's distress. Box 4 gives the stages of CBT. The treatment is based on desensitizing patients to their internal sensations and external phobic situations via exposure, reduction of catastrophic thinking, and improvement in coping strategies. However, patients who have very severe anxiety accompanied by depression are frequently unable to follow the therapist's instructions and may need to be started on antidepressants early.

TABLE 1 Theory of Panic

Stages of Panic Disorder	Neuronal Circuits	Possible Treatments
Panic attacks (alarm reactions)	Periaqueductal gray amygdala, hippocampus	SSRI, SNRI, benzodiazepines, interoceptive exposure
Catastrophic thoughts (abnormal information processing)	Orbital frontal cortex, cingulum, hippocampus	SSRI, SNRI, cognitive restructuring, neuroleptics
Precaution rituals and avoidances	Prefrontal and temporal cortex	SSRI, SNRI, neuroleptics; Exposure and response prevention

Abbreviations: SNRI = serotonin-norepinephrine reuptake inhibitor; SSRI = selective serotonin reuptake inhibitor.

Step 1

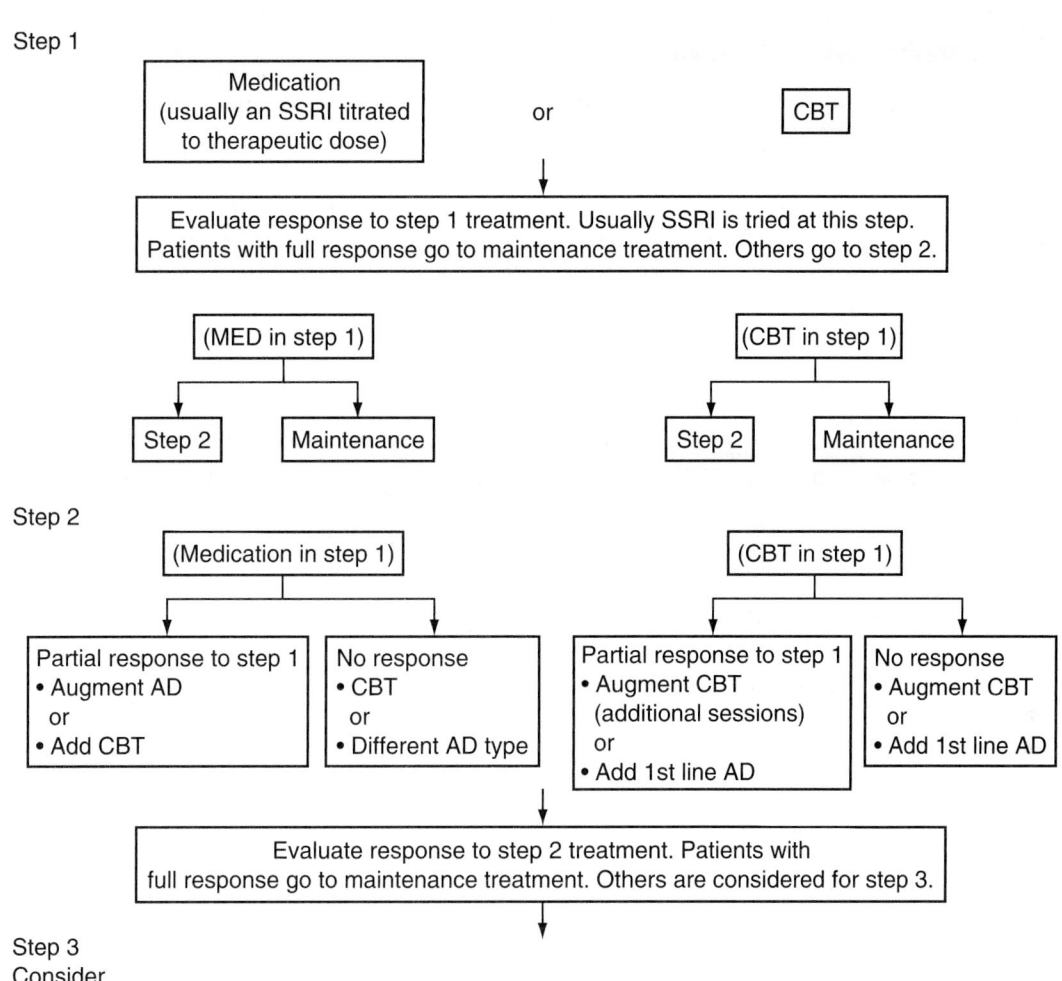

17

FIGURE 1. Treatment of panic disorder. AD = antidepressant; CBT = cognitive behavior therapy; MED = medication; PTSD = post-traumatic stress disorder; SSRI = selective serotonin reuptake inhibitor.

MEDICATION

Selection of medication depends on whether patients have received prior pharmacotherapy for the treatment of a mood or anxiety disorder, on their previous reaction to medication, and on the severity and acuity of their panic state. An SSRI is the treatment of choice for patients who have never received pharmacotherapy and have at least moderate severity of illness. In addition to treating anxiety, SSRIs will treat a co-morbid major depressive episode (MDE) and lower the risk of future MDEs. All of the SSRIs are thought to be effective in the treatment of the four major anxiety disorders (including PD, obsessive–compulsive disorder, generalized anxiety disorder, and social anxiety disorder) and have little differences except for subtle differences in side-effect profiles and differences in their effects on the cytochrome P450 liver enzyme system (Table 2). In general, selection among antidepressants should be based on the patient's anxiety symptom profile (one should avoid medications with side effects that mimic panic symptoms) and a history the side effects of medications

BOX 4   Cognitive Behavioral Therapy
• Assessment • Cognitive restructuring (de-catastrophizing thinking) • Coping enhancement • Education • Exposure and response prevention (to phobic situations) • Interceptive exposure (exposure to internal sensation) • Relapse prevention • Self-monitoring

Rakel and Bope: *Conn's Current Therapy 2006.*

TABLE 2 Antidepressants Used in Treatment of Panic

Antidepressant	Anxiolytic Efficacy*	Advantages	Disadvantages
Fluoxetine (Prozac)	Panic[†] and PTSD	Generic form Long half-life (no withdrawal)	Most stimulating Longer half-life
Fluvoxamine (Luvox)[1]	Panic, GAD, and SAD	No P450 2D6 effects	Effects on P4501A2, 2C9, and 3A4
Paroxetine (Paxil)	Panic,[†] GAD,[†] SAD,[†] PTSD[†]	Least stimulating No P4503A4 effects	Most anticholinergic Most sedating
Sertraline (Zoloft)	Panic,[†] GAD, SAD,[†] PTSD[†]	Least P450-2D6 effects Minimal P450-3A4 effects Intermediate half-life (less withdrawal)	Most diarrhea
Citalopram (Celexa)[1] Escitalopram (Lexapro)[1]	Panic	No P450 effects	Least studied

Venlafaxine ER
  (Effexor XR)[1]
	Panic, GAD,[†] SAD,[†] PTSD	No P450 effects	Short half-life
			Withdrawal with missed dose or
			  sudden discontinuation—increased
			  BP at >225 mg

Nefazodone
  (Serzone)[1]
	No controlled studies
	Open reports in panic,
	  PTSD, SAD
		Sedation, can take at
		  bedtime
			Prominent P450 3A4 effects
			Rare reports of fatal hepatotoxicity

Mirtazapine (Remeron)[1]	No controlled studies Rare open reports	Sedation	Oversedation Increased appetite and weight gain Rare agranulocytosis

Nortriptyline
  (Pamelor)[1]
	No controlled trials, but for
	  other TCAs (imipramine),
	  controlled evidence in
	  panic, GAD, PTSD
		Sedation, can take at
		  bedtime
			Too many SEs

[1]Not FDA approved for this indication.
*Data obtained from randomized clinical trials.
[†]FDA approved for this indication.
Abbreviations: BP = blood pressure; GAD = generalized anxiety disorder; PTSD = post-traumatic stress disorder; SAD = social anxiety disorder; SEs = side effects; TCAs = tricyclic antidepressants.

previously taken. Table 3 can be used as a guide. For example, in the patient with severe insomnia, one might select a sedating tricyclic, such as nortriptyline (Pamelor),[1] or perhaps mirtazapine (Remeron).[1] Paroxetine (Paxil), fluvoxamine (Luvox),[1] or citalopram (Celexa)[1] would be the SSRI of choice for patients with prominent activation. For the patient with prominent gastrointestinal (GI) side effects, one would avoid sertraline (Zoloft), and paroxetine would be the SSRI of choice. For patients with prominent palpitations and problems with weight gain, one would avoid tricyclics, paroxetine, and mirtazapine.

Benzodiazepines are not the first choice because of tolerance, dependency potential, and possible interference with CBT (especially with as-needed use). They should be reserved for emergency situations (initial panic attacks), for the reduction in extreme anxiety, or infrequent phobic situations (airplanes, elevators, etc.) before the beginning of the CBT. Finally, they can be used for maintenance of chronic patients with unremitting anxiety. If the benzodiazepines are used chronically, they should be prescribed using a pharmacokinetically appropriate schedule to minimize daily withdrawal or interdose anxiety. As-needed use of benzodiazepines should be avoided and history of alcohol and drug abuse should be assessed before beginning treatment.

TREATMENT RESISTANCE

If the patient is nonresponsive or has side effects to two prior SSRI trials, the choice is then between:

- A serotonin–norepinephrine reuptake inhibitor (SNRI)
- A newer antidepressant (e.g., venlafaxine [Effexor],[1] nefazodone [Serzone],[1] mirtazapine [Remeron][1])
- A tricyclic
- A γ-aminobutyric acid (GABA) agent (e.g., gabapentin [Neurontin][1]) (step 2)

A final consideration (step 3) involves the management of anxiety and other symptoms with a concomitant medication that would not ordinarily be a first-line treatment choice for anxiety disorders. This involves the use of sedating atypical neuroleptics such as olanzapine (Zyprexa)[1] and quetiapine (Seroquel).[1] At this point one could consider the use of monoamine oxidase inhibitors

[1]Not FDA approved for this indication.

[1]Not FDA approved for this indication.

TABLE 3 Adverse Effects of the Antidepressants*

Adverse Effect	Fluoxetine (Prozac)	Sertaline (Zoloft)	Paroxetine (Paxil)	Fluvoxamine (Luvox)	Escitalopram (Lexapro)	Citalopram (Celexa) or Nortriptyline (Pamelor)	Venlafaxine†
Headache	↑	-	-	-		↓	-
Agitation/anxiety	↑↑	↑	-	-	↑	-	↑
Tremor	↑	↑	↑	-		↑↑	↑↑
Insomnia	↑↑	↑	-	-		↓	↑↑
Drowsiness	↑	↑	↑↑	↑↑		↑↑	↑↑
Fatigue	↑	-	↑↑	-		↑↑	↑
Confusion	-	-	-	-		-	-
Dizziness	-	-	↑	-		↑	↑
Anticholinergic‡	-	-	↑	-		↑↑↑	-
Sweating	-	-	-	-		↑↑	↑↑
Weight gain	↑	↑	↑	↑		↑↑	↑
Gastrointestinal	↑	↑↑	-	↑↑		-	↑↑
Sexual	↑↑	↑↑	↑↑	↑	↑	↑	↑↑

*↑indicates the drug increases the occurrence of the adverse effect; ↓ indicates that it decreases the occurrence.
†Can increase blood pressure; must be monitored.
‡Anticholinergic side effects include dry mouth, constipation, urinary hesitancy or retention, blurred vision.

(MAOIs), which boast very impressive data supporting their efficacy. These medications require dietary restrictions and stopping concomitant antidepressants. Combining intensive CBT (several times a week) with medication augmentation strategies may also bring a desired effect. Other strategies are under development for the treatment of this resistant population, but none of them have moved past an early experimental stage.

Long-Term Management

While in some patients panic attacks stop in the course of a few months, PD is usually a chronic, waxing and waning condition. Some patients may completely recover, while others may be left with symptoms of other disorders initially masked by the panic attacks. If CBT is initiated, it is important to coordinate the medication treatment with the therapy. Completely blocking anxiety may impair patients' learning in therapy and discourage them from developing new coping techniques. Gradual reduction and stopping medication can be attempted after 2 or 3 months of complete resolution of symptoms. Approximately 20% of patients will not respond to any treatment and need to be maintained in the most comfortable state with medication or therapy or a combination thereof.

17

Physical and Chemical Injuries

Burn Treatment Guidelines

Method of
Barbara A. Latenser, MD

The initial management of the severely burned patient follows guidelines established by the American College of Surgeons (ACS). It is crucial that the patient be managed properly in the early hours after injury because the initial management of a seriously burned patient can significantly affect the long-term outcome. Optimal burn-care criteria have been established and refined by the American Burn Association (ABA) over the past 20 years.

Because of regionalization, it is common for the initial care of the seriously burned patient to occur outside the burn center. Burns are a specialized form of trauma. Therefore, the ABCs (airway, breathing, circulation) are the same as for the trauma patient: airway with cervical spine immobilization if appropriate, breathing, circulation, disability, and exposure. Also, the burn patient could be a victim of associated trauma. It is easy to be sidetracked by the obvious thermal injury. Only after the primary and secondary surveys have been performed should you evaluate the severity of the burn injury. Obtain as much information as possible regarding the incident and about the patient. An easy way to remember the information is the mnemonic AMPLE:

- Allergies
- Medications
- Past medical history
- Last meal
- Events

Universal precautions appropriate for each burn patient must be implemented by every member of the health care team.

The most commonly used guide for making an initial estimate of the second- and third-degree burns is the Rule of Nines (Figure 1). Various anatomic regions are roughly 9% of the total body surface area (TBSA) or multiples thereof. To calculate scattered burn areas, the patient's palm, including fingers, represents approximately 1% of the TBSA. A much more precise estimate of TBSA burn is provided by the Lund-Browder Classification (Figure 2). By drawing in the areas that are burned, the TBSA burn necessary for calculating resuscitation requirements can be determined. The consensus formula for the first 24 hours postburn is:

4 mL lactated Ringer's × body weight in kg × percent BSA burn

Half the calculated amount is given in the first 8 hours and the rest over the remaining 16 hours. Patients with burns on more than 20% TBSA are prone to gastric dilatation and should have a nasogastric (NG) tube. To determine hourly urine output, a urinary catheter is necessary. Intravenous (IV) morphine sulfate is indicated for control of pain associated with burns. Intramuscular (IM) or subcutaneous (SC) routes of drug administration should not be used as absorption is erratic. To calculate fluid needs, weigh the patient or estimate the preinjury weight. Reliable peripheral veins should be used to establish an IV line. Use vessels underlying burned skin if necessary. If it is impossible to establish peripheral IV access, a central line may be necessary.

The burn wound should be covered with a clean, dry sheet to prevent air currents from causing pain in partial-thickness burns and decreases fluid losses and hypothermia. Although there are many common topical antimicrobials in use, the optimal dressing prior to burn center transfer is plastic wrap such as Saran Wrap. Topical antimicrobials will just have to be washed off on arrival to the burn center, causing patient discomfort and mechanical trauma to the wound. Cold applications are appropriate only in small burns because they rapidly lead to hypothermia. Ice should never be applied because it will deepen the zone of ischemia in a thermal injury.

Escharotomies and/or fasciotomies are rarely required prior to burn center transfer, unless transfer is delayed

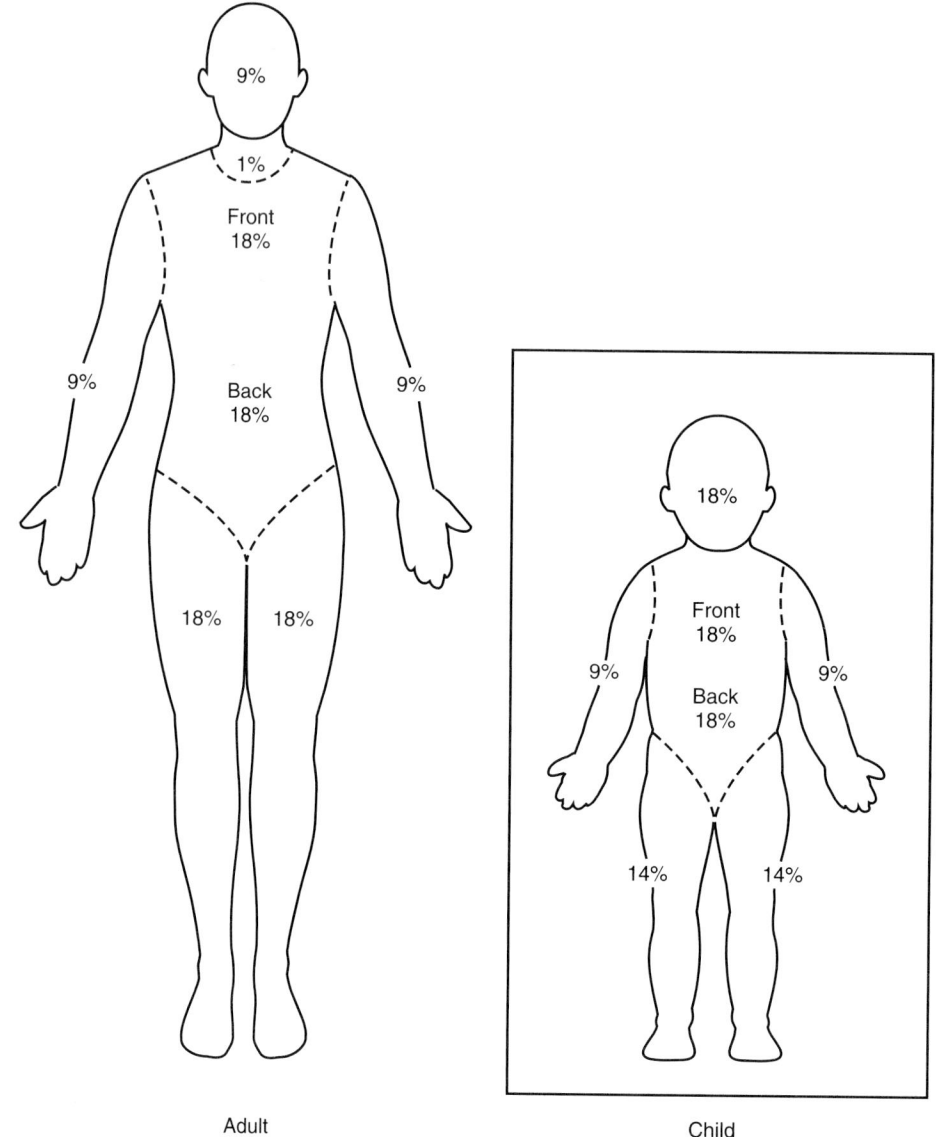

FIGURE 1. Rule of Nines.

beyond 24 hours. Patients most at risk are those with large TBSA burns, circumferential full-thickness burns, and those with electrical injury. Circumferential chest/abdominal burns may restrict ventilatory excursion. A child has a more pliable rib cage and may need an escharotomy earlier than an adult burn. If you are considering performing an escharotomy, confer with the accepting burn physician before proceeding.

So how do you know which patients should be referred to a burn center? To guide your decision making there are currently 10 burn unit referral criteria. You should have a written transfer agreement in place with a referral burn unit. The agreement should specify which patients will be referred, what stabilization is expected, who arranges transportation, and what the patient will need during transport.

Partial-Thickness Burns on More Than 10% Total Body Surface Area

Second-degree or partial-thickness burns involve a variable portion of dermis. The skin may be red, blistered, and edematous. Because sensory nerves are damaged and/or exposed, these wounds are typically extremely painful. Healing time is proportional to the depth of dermal injury. Scarring is minimal if healing occurs in 14 days or less. With closure time beyond 3 weeks, scarring will occur, the degree being greater in darker skinned individuals.

Proper fluid management is critical to the survival of patients with extensive burns. Fluid resuscitation is aimed at maintaining tissue perfusion and organ function

Rakel and Bope: *Conn's Current Therapy 2006.*

18

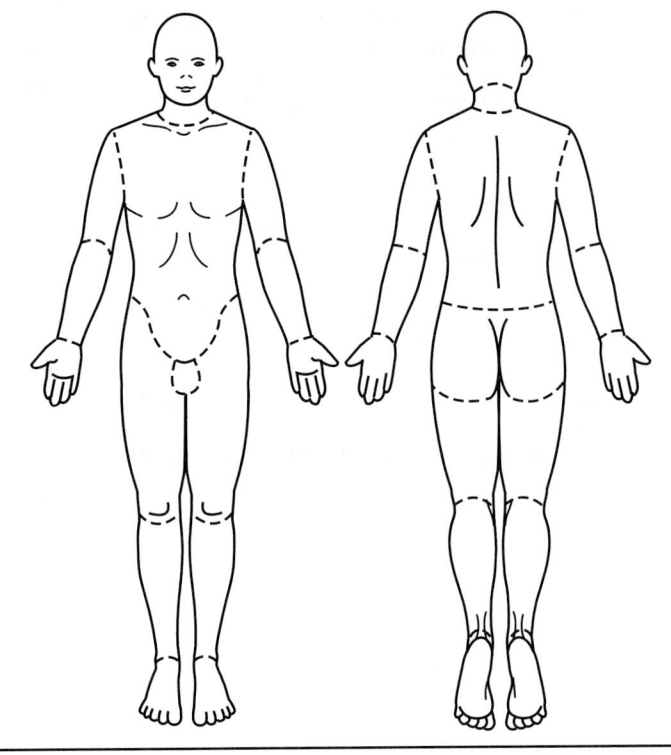

	Birth 1 yr.	1–4 yrs.	5–9 yrs.	10–14 yrs.	15 yrs.	Adult	Burn size estimate
Head	19	17	13	11	9	7	
Neck	2	2	2	2	2	2	
Anterior trunk	13	13	13	13	13	13	
Posterior trunk	13	13	13	13	13	13	
Right buttock	2.5	2.5	2.5	2.5	2.5	2.5	
Left buttock	2.5	2.5	2.5	2.5	2.5	2.5	
Genitalia	1	1	1	1	1	1	
Right upper arm	4	4	4	4	4	4	
Left upper arm	4	4	4	4	4	4	
Right lower arm	3	3	3	3	3	3	
Left lower arm	3	3	3	3	3	3	
Right hand	2.5	2.5	2.5	2.5	2.5	2.5	
Left hand	2.5	2.5	2.5	2.5	2.5	2.5	
Right thigh	5.5	6.5	8	8.5	9	9.5	
Left thigh	5.5	6.5	8	8.5	9	9.5	
Right leg	5	5	5.5	6	6.5	7	
Left leg	5	5	5.5	6	6.5	7	
Right foot	3.5	3.5	3.5	3.5	3.5	3.5	
Left foot	3.5	3.5	3.5	3.5	3.5	3.5	

Total BSAB _____

FIGURE 2. Lund-Browder Classification Burn Size and Diagram.

Rakel and Bope: *Conn's Current Therapy 2006.*

while avoiding the complications of inadequate or excessive fluid therapy. Shock and organ failure, most commonly acute renal failure, may occur as a consequence of hypovolemia in a patient with an extensive burn who is inadequately resuscitated. The increase in capillary permeability caused by the burn is greatest in the immediate postburn period and diminution in effective blood volume is most rapid at that time. A marked increase in peripheral vascular resistance accompanied by a decrease in cardiac output occurs in the first 18 to 24 hours postinjury.

In the presence of increased capillary permeability, colloid content of the resuscitation fluid exerts little influence on intravascular retention during the initial hours postburn. Crystalloid fluid is the initial resuscitation of burn patients. *Always* remember, estimates are inexact. Each patient reacts differently to burn injury and resuscitation. The actual volume of fluid infused should be varied from the calculated volume as indicated by physiologic monitoring. The patient's general condition reflects the adequacy of fluid resuscitation and should be assessed and reassessed. Mental status, anxiety, and restlessness may be signs of hypoxemia, hypovolemia, or pain.

Although urine output does not guarantee tissue perfusion, it remains the most readily available and generally reliable guide to resuscitation. Adults should produce 0.5 mL/kg per hour of urine. Children should produce 1.0 mL/kg per hour of urine, and infants 12 months or younger should produce 2.0 mL/kg per hour of urine. Oliguria is most frequently the result of inadequate fluid administration. Diuretics are contraindicated; the rate of resuscitation should be increased. During the first 24 hours, neither the hemoglobin nor the hematocrit is a reliable guide to resuscitation, and using either leads to over-resuscitation.

Measuring blood pressure (BP) by a sphygmomanometer may be misleading in a burned limb with progressive edema formation. As the swelling increases, the signal becomes diminished. If fluid infusion is increased based on this finding, edema formation may be exaggerated. Even intra-arterial monitoring may be unreliable in patients with massive burns because of peripheral vasoconstriction secondary to marked elevation of catecholamines. Heart rate is also of limited usefulness in monitoring fluid therapy. The level of tachycardia depends on the normal heart rate in each child.

Burns That Involve the Face, Hands, Feet, Genitalia, Perineum, or Major Joints

Facial burns are considered a serious injury. The possibility of respiratory tract damage must be considered. Because of the rich blood supply and loose areolar tissue of the face, facial burns are associated with extensive edema formation. To minimize this edema, keep the head of the bed elevated at 30°. Cool saline compresses on the face may also help. Careful examination of the eyes should be completed as soon as possible because the rapid onset of eyelid swelling will make this difficult. Fluorescein should be used to identify corneal injury. Chemical burns to the eyes should be rinsed with copious amounts of saline. Burns of the ears require examination of the external auditory canal and ear drum before swelling occurs.

Minor burns of the hands may result in only temporary disability and inconvenience. More extensive thermal injury may cause permanent loss of function. Monitoring the digital and palmar pulses with an ultrasonic flowmeter is the most accurate means of assessing perfusion of the tissues in the hand. The burned extremity should be elevated above the heart to minimize edema formation. Digital escharotomies are not indicated prior to transfer to a burn center. Contact the accepting burn center physician if you are concerned about the extent of the digital injury. As with burns of the upper extremity, it is important to assess the circulation and neurologic function of the feet on an hourly basis.

Third-Degree Burns in Any Age Group

A full-thickness or third-degree burn occurs with destruction of the entire epidermis and dermis, leaving no dermal elements to repopulate. A characteristic initial appearance is a waxy white color. Full-thickness injuries require emergent management. In most cases, treatment of the wound requires surgical skin grafting. Deep partial-thickness and full-thickness burns heal with severe scarring if not treated by surgical excision and skin grafting for optimal recovery. Disfigurement is common, and long-term functional problems can persist for years. There is also a high risk of infection, because an unexcised full-thickness burn behaves like an undrained abscess.

Electric Burns, Including Lightning Injury

Electrical burns can be divided into flash (typical thermal injury) and high-tension injury. The latter, caused by more than 1000 volts, produces clinically characteristic entry and exit wounds. They are usually ischemic, painless, and dry; wounds of entry may appear charred and the exit explosive. Deep-muscle injury may be present even when skin appears normal. Findings that suggest electrical injury include loss of consciousness, paralysis or mummification of an extremity, loss of peripheral pulses, flexor surface burns, myoglobinuria, serum creatine kinase (CK) more than 1000, and cardiopulmonary arrest at the scene. Electrical injuries can produce vascular thrombosis, muscle tetany causing fractures, and internal organ damage. In addition to other interventions, obtain a 12-lead electrocardiogram (ECG), cardiac enzymes, and evaluate the urine for myoglobin. If there is evidence of myoglobin from muscle damage, the urine output should be maintained at 2 mL/kg per hour until the urine grossly clears to prevent acid hematin deposition in the kidney and irreversible renal damage. Compartment pressures must be monitored. If a compartment syndrome develops, contact your burn center physician because fasciotomy may be required. The most serious immediate problem associated with electrical injuries is ventricular fibrillation, asystole, or other dysrhythmias. Life-threatening arrhythmias are treated according to advanced cardiac life support (ACLS) protocols. Survival of contact with voltage greater than 70,000 volts is uncommon.

The approximate electrical potential of a lightning bolt is 20 million volts. Lightning injury can produce an enormous spectrum of clinical symptoms and signs ranging from common (cardiac asystole, respiratory arrest, arborescent markings) to the rare (disseminated intravascular coagulation [DIC], intracerebral hemorrhage).

Rakel and Bope: *Conn's Current Therapy 2006.*

Immediate neurologic manifestations include agitation, amnesia, loss of consciousness, or motor disturbances. The eyes are particularly vulnerable to injury from electrical current, and symptoms closely correlate with the extent of the central nervous system (CNS) injury. Vitreous hemorrhage, iridocyclitis, retinal tear, macular puncture, and retinal detachment have been reported.

Lightning injuries are not usually associated with deep burns but most often with superficial injury to the skin and underlying soft tissue called *ferning*. The feathering type of burn appears as an arborescent, branching skin marking that disappears within a few days. Pathognomonic of lightning injury, they may be of great diagnostic value in a comatose patient. Often the respiratory arrest lasts longer than the cardiac arrest. Severely injured victims often present in asystole or ventricular fibrillation. Cardiac resuscitation may occasionally be successful; but direct brain trauma as well as blunt trauma, skull fracture, and intracranial injuries, are common in these patients. The prognosis for recovery in this group is usually poor.

Chemical Burns

Health care providers must wear protective clothing when caring for patients with potential chemical injury. The initial appearance of a chemical burn is usually deceptively benign. The severity of a chemical injury is related to the agent, concentration, volume, duration of contact, and mechanisms of action of the agent. Immediate irrigation decreases the concentration and duration of contact, reducing the severity of injury. If the agent is a powder, brush it off and irrigate with water. Irrigation should continue through emergency evaluation in the hospital and in general until evaluation in a burn center, especially for an alkali or if an unknown agent. Neutralizing agents are contraindicated because of the potential for heat generation, thereby giving the patient both a chemical and a thermal injury!

Acid burns are less severe than alkali burns. They are found in many household products including bathroom cleansers, drain cleaners, and swimming pool acidifiers. Tissue is damaged by coagulation necrosis and protein precipitation. Once a layer of eschar is formed, the burning process is self-limiting. The exception to this rule is hydrofluoric acid (HA), which is used to etch glass, make Teflon, and to remove rust. The pathogenesis of tissue damage in HA burns is distinct from other acids. HA readily crosses lipid membranes and has a potent diffusing capacity into the tissues. The molecule releases the freely dissociable fluoride ion, which produces extensive liquefactive necrosis of the soft tissues. Fluoride rapidly binds free calcium in the blood, and death from hypocalcemia may occur. Treatment is intra-arterial calcium gluconate[1] (or calcium chloride)[1] administered until the characteristic *pain out of proportion to the burn* has resolved.

Even small areas of contact may result in profound hypocalcemia and death. Cardiac monitoring and frequent serum calcium determinations are indicated.

Alkalis damage tissue by liquefaction necrosis and protein denaturation. Tissue pH abnormalities may persist for 12 hours postburn, allowing deeper spread of the chemical and more severe burns. Examples would include the hydroxides, caustic sodas, and ammonium compounds found in oven cleaners, fertilizer, and cement. Wet cement damages skin in three ways: allergic dermatitis as a reaction to chromate ions, abrasions caused by the gritty nature of the cement, and as an alkali with a pH of 12.5. The ability of cement to cause such injury is not well recognized, even by professional users. With the increased media interest in do-it-yourself projects, it is likely this problem will increase.

Organic compounds such as creosote and petroleum products produce contact chemical burns as well as systemic toxicity. Gasoline and diesel fuel are petroleum products that may produce a full-thickness burn that initially appears as only partial thickness. Organic compounds cause cutaneous damage by delipidation because of their fat solvent action on cell membranes. After a motor vehicle crash involving petroleum products, always look for petroleum exposure in the lower extremities, back, and buttocks. Systemic effects include elevated liver enzymes and decreased urinary output.

Inhalation Injury

Smoke inhalation injuries are the leading cause of fatalities from burn injuries, accounting for some 80% of all fire-related deaths. The major forms of inhalation injuries are carbon monoxide (CO) toxicity, injury to the upper airway, and pulmonary parenchymal damage. Each has different symptoms and signs, treatment, and prognosis. The compromised airway is protected by tracheal intubation, and respiratory failure is treated with assisted ventilation. Inhalation injury is manifested by the pathology and dysfunction that rapidly become evident in the airways, lungs, and respiratory system after inhaling the products of incomplete combustion. Patients receiving massive fluid resuscitation can develop upper airway edema with subsequent asphyxiation.

Immediate medical attention and diagnosis depend on a high index of suspicion, an appropriate history, careful examination of the upper airway, the presence of clinical symptoms, and suggestive arterial blood gases. An inhalation injury is suspected in any patient with full-thickness facial burns or with any burns combined with a history of being confined within an enclosed space. Other classic signs are soot or carbonaceous sputum, stridor or hoarseness, or blistering of the pharynx or vocal cords. Late signs include grunting, nasal flaring, retractions, wheezes, and rales. Use of prophylactic antibiotics and steroids is discouraged.

The effect of CO poisoning may be exhibited by respiratory symptoms and CNS findings such as altered level of consciousness, seizures, or coma. Cardiovascular effects include diminished cardiac output evidenced by decreased perfusion and hypotension. There is much

---

[1]Not FDA approved for this indication.

Rakel and Bope: *Conn's Current Therapy 2006.*

controversy regarding hyperbaric oxygen therapy, but there are no objective data proving the efficacy of hyperbaric oxygen in CO poisoning. At this time, hyperbaric oxygen treatment for acute CO toxicity should be restricted to randomized prospective studies. The correct treatment is administering 100% oxygen, thereby decreasing the CO half-life from 4 hours to 45 minutes.

Burn Injury in Patients with Preexisting Medical Disorders That Could Complicate Management, Prolong Recovery, or Affect Mortality

Peripheral vascular disease can lead to a decrease in wound blood flow. Diabetes, through high glucose, will impede capillary flow. Optimum control of the blood glucose is needed to optimize blood flow. A local decrease in wound-tissue oxygen tension is recognized to be a major wound-healing impediment because all phases of healing are oxygen dependent, including local infection control. Most common causes are a decrease in systemic blood volume and oxygen delivery, decrease in hemoglobin saturation, eschar on the wound surface, or infection. Treatment modalities need to focus first on correction of systemic abnormalities: correct cardiovascular and lung function, correct large vessel obstructive disease impeding wound flow, aggressive wound debridement, and eliminate tissue exudates. Patients with preexisting cardiac disease are particularly sensitive to fluids and may tolerate the necessary fluid resuscitation poorly.

Any Patient With Burns and Concomitant Trauma (Such as Fractures) in Which the Burn Injury Poses the Greatest Risk of Morbidity and Mortality

In such case, if the trauma poses the greater immediate risk, the patient may be initially stabilized in a trauma center before being transferred to a burn unit. Physician judgment will be necessary in such situations and should be in concert with the regional medical control plan and triage protocols.

Most burn-trauma publications cite a 5% frequency of burn-trauma patient. Because burn trauma is rare outside of a major conflict or disaster, most centers see only a few patients annually. By definition, child abuse falls into the burn-trauma category. It may be the burn injury that prompts relatives or neighbors to bring the child to the hospital or report the family to authority. The visibility of the injury may instigate corrective action. In a 44-month review we saw 120 cases of burns and trauma. Although motor vehicle crashes (MVCs) can result in fracture, soft tissue, and thermal injury, unique to this burn-trauma population was that the MVC injury was frequently a result of assault. With the

graying of America, elder abuse may become a larger societal problem.

Burned Children in Hospitals Without Qualified Personnel or Equipment for the Care of Children

Each year more than 2500 children die and 10,000 more sustain permanent disability from thermal injury. Children are not just little adults! They respond differently than adults to severe trauma, maintaining normal vital signs longer but decompensating rapidly. Because of the smaller cross-sectional diameter of the pediatric airway, it takes much less edema to compromise a pediatric airway. If intubation is required, the most experienced pediatric airway manager should intubate the child because repeated attempts may create sufficient airway edema as to cause obstruction. Anatomical airway differences make intubation by the inexperienced even more difficult.

The greater surface area per unit of body mass of children necessitates the administration of relatively greater amounts of resuscitation fluid. The surface area/body mass relationship of the child also defines a lesser intravascular volume per unit surface area burned. This makes the burned child more susceptible to fluid overload and hemodilution. Hypoglycemia may occur if the limited glycogen stores of the child are rapidly exhausted by the early postburn elevation of circulating levels of steroids and catecholamines. Infants should receive maintenance fluids with 5% dextrose in addition to the resuscitation fluids outlined in the consensus formula. Children younger than 2 years of age have disproportionally thin skin so that exposures that would produce only partial-thickness burns in older patients produce full-thickness injuries. Children have a relatively small muscle mass, hampering intrinsic heat generation. Children younger than 6 months of age are unable to shiver and thus are even more prone to develop hypothermia.

Stress for the burned child not only includes the body surface area (BSA) burn and the pain that is involved but also the separation from parents and loved ones. This escalates especially if the parents were also burned in the fire. Emergency management of each pediatric

---

 CURRENT DIAGNOSIS

- Maintain a high index of suspicion
- Remember the ABCs
- Rule out concomitant trauma
- Establish size and depth of burn
- Be wary of chemical and electrical burns, which may be misleading
- Establish resuscitation requirements

Abbreviations: ABC = airway with cervical spine immobilization if appropriate, breathing, circulation, disability, and exposure.

Rakel and Bope: *Conn's Current Therapy 2006.*

CURRENT THERAPY

- Communicate with your burn center early and often
- Remember the ABCs
- Cover the wound with saran wrap
- Prevent hypothermia
- Transport to the burn center

Abbreviations: ABC = airway with cervical spine immobilization if appropriate, breathing, circulation, disability, and exposure.

burn patient requires an individual care plan. Early consultation with the burn center physician is advised.

Burn Injury in Patients Who Will Require Special Social, Emotional, and/or Long-Term Rehabilitative Intervention

Failure to recognize the thermal manifestations of child abuse not only negates protection of the child but predicates potential lethal injury. Awareness of the patterns of abuse, the behavior patterns of the parents, and the physical manifestations will protect the child by early recognition and reporting. Physical child abuse victims frequently present with thermal injuries of varying degrees. The history of injury should correlate with the physical findings. The history also becomes important in identifying repetitious hospital visits for accidental injury. Not infrequently, the hospital visits will be made at different hospitals to avoid disclosure and identification.

The events leading to an injury are extremely important in the initial evaluation of an infant or child. *Always* consider the potential for child abuse. The incidence of child abuse is approximately 10% of all children presenting to an emergency department (ED), with a mortality rate less than 1%. Abused children present with a higher median Injury Severity Score, more severe injuries of the head and integument, longer hospital lengths of stay, and a high mortality rate.

A burn of any magnitude can be a serious injury. Health care providers must be able to assess the injuries rapidly and develop a priority-based plan of care. The plan of care is determined by the type, extent, and degree of burn as well as by available resources.

Burn care is complex. It involves a multisystem assessment and appropriate intervention. The first 24 hours of management are perhaps the most critical for patient survival. Burn centers provide optimal care in a cost-effective, multidisciplinary manner. Every health care provider must know how and when to contact the closest burn center. If the attending physician determines that the patient should be treated at the burn center, the extent of treatment provided at the referring hospital—and the method of transport to the burn center—should be decided in consultation with the burn center physician.

Rakel and Bope: *Conn's Current Therapy 2006.*

REFERENCES

Advanced Burn Life Support Course, American Burn Association, 625 N. Michigan Ave., Suite 1530, Chicago, IL. 60611. 2001.

American College of Surgeons Committee on Trauma: Resources for optimal care of the injured patient: 1999. Chicago, American College of Surgeons, 1999.

Andrews CJ, Cooper MA, Darveniza M, Mackerras D (eds): Lightning injuries: Electrical, medical, and legal aspects. Boca Raton, Fla, CRC Press, 1992, pp 62-63, 82-85, 88-98, 101-110.

Burd A: Hydrofluoric acid—revisited. Burns 2004;30(7):720-722.

Chang DC, Knight V, Ziegfeld S, et al: The tip of the iceberg for child abuse: The critical roles of the pediatric trauma service and its registry. J Trauma 2004;57(6):1189-1198.

Heimbach DM: Regionalization of burn care: A concept whose time has come. J Burn Care Rehabil 2003;24(3):173-174.

Latenser BA, Iteld L: Smoke inhalation injury. Seminars in Respiratory and Critical Care Medicine. 2001;22(1):13-22.

Luce EA (ed): Clinics in Plastic Surgery. An International Quarterly. Burn Care and Management. Philadelphia, WB Saunders, 2000; 27(1): 133-143.

Varghese TK, Kim AW, Kowal-Vern A, Latenser BA: Frequency of burn-trauma patients in an urban setting. Arch Surg. 2003;138:1292-1296.

High-Altitude Illness

Method of
James A. Litch, MD, DTMH

Decreased partial pressure of oxygen at high altitude results in pronounced physiologic responses that range from beneficial to pathologic. Slow ascent normally leads to acclimatization. High-altitude illness is a collective term for a cluster of acute clinical syndromes that are a direct consequence of rapid ascent to high altitude above 2500 m. The acute syndromes affecting the brain include acute mountain sickness (AMS) and high-altitude cerebral edema (HACE). The acute syndrome affecting the lung is high-altitude pulmonary edema (HAPE). All unacclimatized sojourners to high altitude are potentially at risk. The characteristic cerebral and pulmonary abnormalities are not subtle, but when unrecognized or ignored, they may progress to death. Each year millions travel to high-altitude locations on every continent, resulting in morbidity and mortality with associated economic consequences.

Normal Acclimatization

It is not uncommon for normal acclimatization of novice healthy visitors to high altitude to cause concern that they are experiencing a health problem. Normal acclimatization includes immediate hyperventilation, shortness of breath with moderate excursion, and a decreased work capacity. These are followed by diuresis, disturbed sleep (including periodic breathing), and peripheral/facial edema. It is important to recognize the signs of normal acclimatization so reassurance and education may be appropriately provided.

Incidence and Risk Factors

Determinants of whether high-altitude illness will occur are individual susceptibility, rate of ascent, altitude reached, and sleep altitude. Incidence rates of AMS reported in literature are difficult to compare because of variability in methodology and rates of ascent. Reported incident figures for AMS following ascent by hiking, vehicle, or flying range from 10% to 40% at 2700 to 3000 m, and from 40% to 95% at 3800 to 4000 m. HACE and HAPE are both far less common than mild AMS, but actual incident rates are unavailable. HAPE can occur as low as 2500 m. HACE is rare below 3600 m. Most cases of HACE and HAPE are preceded by AMS.

Risk factors for altitude illness include a history of previous high-altitude illness, residence at altitude below 1000 m, physical exertion, and preexisting cardiopulmonary conditions. Traveling in a large group presents a risk because a tight itinerary often does not allow time for acclimatization, and members are reluctant to declare symptoms for fear of being left behind. Children appear to carry the same risk for altitude illness as adults, but persons over 50 years of age seem less susceptible, possibly because of a more cautious ascent profile. There appears to be little or no gender difference for AMS, but women may be less susceptible to HAPE. Heavy physical exertion at exceedingly high altitude appears to be an important risk factor for HAPE. Rapid ascent, especially by flying or driving to altitude, places sojourners at risk for altitude illnesses.

Prevention of Altitude Illnesses

Gradual ascent to altitude over several days to allow for acclimatization reduces the likelihood of acute mountain sickness. Ascent rates of less than 300 m per day at altitudes of more than 2500 m is a common recommendation; but individuals will still experience altitude illness when abiding to this recommendation. However, the critical understanding to prevent serious life-threatening altitude illness (HAPE and HACE) is to halt further ascent until symptoms resolve.

Medications are available to help prevent the symptoms of AMS when rapid ascent (<24 hours) to altitudes more than 3000 m is anticipated, or for those with a past history of AMS with a similar ascent profile. These agents are started the evening before ascent and continued for 2 to 3 days. The most commonly used medications are acetazolamide (Diamox) (125 to 250 mg twice a day), acetaminophen[1] (325 mg four times a day), or aspirin[1] (325 mg three times a day). Acetazolamide (Diamox) is particularly useful because it actually improves oxygenation, has a positive impact on the quality of sleep at high altitude, and is effective for periodic breathing that occurs during sleep. However, these medications do not protect against the development of life threatening altitude illness: HAPE and HACE. Other medications have been suggested for use in preventing

altitude illness. Randomized double blinded placebo-controlled trails of ginkgo biloba[1] and acetazolamide (Diamox) have shown no benefit from ginkgo biloba over placebo, and reduced incidence and severity of AMS symptoms from acetazolamide (Diamox). Dexamethasone (Decadron),[1] a potent steroid, is generally best avoided as a prevention measure against AMS during ascent so it may be used, if needed, for treatment of HACE along with descent.

Nifedipine (Adalat, Procardia)[1] has been studied for use in prevention of HAPE and found to be of benefit for persons with a history of recurrent HAPE. Studies are underway to evaluate sildenafil citrate (viagra),[1] an agent that selectively lowers pulmonary artery pressure, in the prevention of HAPE. In addition, inhaled salmeterol (Serevent)[1] has been found effective for the prevention of HAPE in a small group of climbers who had previously shown susceptibility to HAPE. However, these high-risk individuals would do far better with cautious gradual ascent, rather than relying on a medication with limited effect for a life-threatening condition.

Several nonmedication measures that can prevent or ameliorate symptoms of high-altitude illness include the following:

- Begin a high-carbohydrate diet one or two days before the climb and maintain during the ascent
- Adapt plans to realistically reflect the decreased work capacity at high altitude
- Reschedule or slow the ascent should an upper respiratory or other active infection present
- Avoid overexertion during ascent by maintaining a reasonable pace and not overloading with nonessential gear
- Maintain adequate hydration on the climb to offset increased fluid loss at altitude
- Avoid nonessential medications and remedies
- Provide good ventilation for camp stoves used in confined places
- Allow for several days of altitude exposure the week prior to ascent to high altitude

Acute Mountain Sickness and High-Altitude Cerebral Edema

AMS is defined as a headache in the setting of recent altitude gain and typical symptoms which include anorexia, nausea, vomiting, insomnia, dizziness, or fatigue (Current Diagnosis box). Symptoms are nonspecific, and there is an absence of physical findings. The differential diagnosis is extensive and other conditions should be considered (Box 1). Pulse oximetry values may be high, normal, or low for the altitude and do not correlate to severity of symptoms. A careful and detailed history is essential to steer diagnostic decision making. Often in outdoor settings multiple conditions can be present such as AMS and dehydration. Rapid resolution of symptoms during treatment with oxygen

---

[1]Not FDA approved for this indication.

> ## BOX 1 Differential Diagnosis of High-Altitude Illnesses
>
> **Acute Mountain Sickness and High-Altitude Cerebral Edema**
> - Alcohol intoxication
> - Brain tumor
> - CO inhalation
> - CNS infection
> - Cerebral vascular accident
> - Dehydration
> - Diabetic ketoacidosis
> - Exhaustion
> - Hypoglycemia and insulin shock
> - Hyponatremia
> - Hypothermia
> - Migraine
> - Narcotics
> - Poisoning
> - Psychosis
> - Sedatives overdose
> - Seizures
> - Subarachnoid hemorrhage
> - Transient ischemic attack
>
> **High-Altitude Pulmonary Edema**
> - Adult respiratory distress syndrome
> - Asthma
> - Bronchitis
> - Congestive heart failure
> - Myocardial infarction
> - Pneumonia (infection or aspiration)
> - Poisoning
> - Pulmonary embolus
> - Respiratory failure
>
> *Abbreviations:* CNS = central nervous system; CO = carbon monoxide.

is very specific to AMS. Early recognition of AMS is a key principle in remote areas with limited support.

AMS is not life threatening, but ignoring it can be. Progressive neurologic deterioration may occur over hours or days as dangerous collections of fluid develop in the brain leading to HACE. HACE presents with truncal ataxia, confusion, and hallucination in the setting of recent altitude gain. The period of time from initial ataxia and confusion to onset of coma may be as little as 8 to 12 hours. If descent or oxygen supplementation is not accomplished within hours, coma and death can ensue from brain herniation. A presumptive and/or rigid diagnosis of HACE in the setting of progressive neurologic deterioration has led to tragic situations when other life-threatening conditions were actually present (see Box 1). Details of the initial presentation, response to immediate descent/supplemental oxygen, and recognition of additional signs can guide clinical decision making while maintaining a high index of suspicion for other neurologic conditions. Patients with persistent symptoms after descent require prompt evacuation and thorough evaluation. In addition, HAPE may develop concurrently with HACE resulting in shortness of breath while at rest and a further reduction of oxygen delivery to the body.

Definitive diagnosis is available using imaging studies such as CT and MRI. However, these have limited

application, because the condition should have greatly improved from oxygen/descent before the opportunity presents to obtain the study. Neuroimaging demonstrates vasogenic edema in individuals with moderate to severe AMS or HACE.

Management of AMS is directed at limiting further hypoxia by halting ascent, and providing additional oxygen should symptoms persist or progress to HACE. Acetazolamide (Diamox) is helpful for the treatment of AMS. For the management of HACE improved oxygenation is the definitive treatment. There are several methods of oxygen delivery: (1) descent, (2) supplemental oxygen via cylinder or concentrator, and/or (3) portable hyperbaric bag. These may be combined or applied in series depending on resources, location, and logistic support. Concomitant pharmacologic treatment with dexamethasone (Decadron)[1] and acetazolamide (Diamox) aid recovery. Persons with suspected HACE who do not rapidly recover during treatment or those with focal neurologic deficits should be hospitalized and undergo comprehensive neurologic evaluation including magnetic resonance imaging (MRI). The Current Therapy box summarizes management of HACE.

High-Altitude Pulmonary Edema

HAPE is defined as noncardiogenic edema resulting from hypoxia-induced changes in the pulmonary circulation. HAPE is commonly preceded by AMS, and 20% of individuals with HAPE develop HACE. Early symptoms of HAPE include decreased exercise performance beyond that expected for the altitude, often accompanied with a dry cough (see Current Diagnosis Box). Progression is rapid with even minimal continued physical activity without descent. The hallmark of progression requiring prompt action is dyspnea at rest. Rales are present at this stage. Resting pulse oximetry reveals below-normal oxygen saturation for the altitude. Tachypnea and tachycardia beyond that expected for the altitude also are present. Pink, frothy sputum develops late in the illness. Early diagnosis is important because progression of the illness further limits oxygenation and worsens the degree of hypoxemia causing the condition.

HAPE is a life-threatening emergency; immediate improvement in oxygenation is critical to arrest the progression and is the definitive treatment. In medical facilities high-flow supplemental oxygen while at rest and sitting in an upright position should be initiated immediately during the initial assessment of the patient. Response may be assessed by pulse oximetry and resting respiratory rate. Despite prompt improvement during the first few hours of treatment, maintenance of oxygenation (oxygen saturation greater than 90%) with low-flow supplemental oxygen and rest is often required for 2 to 3 days unless descent is achieved. For vacationers to high-altitude resort areas, this oxygen requirement can be maintained outside the hospital using a cylinder or concentrator as an alternative to

---

[1]Not FDA approved for this indication.

descent for informed individuals that wish to remain in the locale of family and friends. A continued requirement of high-flow oxygen of 4 to 5 L per minute or more to maintain oxygen saturation greater than 90%, or concurrent HACE, requires hospitalization. Antibiotics are indicated if infection is suspected. Endotracheal intubation and mechanical ventilation are rarely indicated. The differential diagnosis is extensive, and a high index of suspicion for other conditions should be maintained throughout the treatment course (see Box 1).

In remote areas oxygen may be administered by:

- Descent with minimal exertion
- Supplemental oxygen via cylinder or concentrator
- Portable hyperbaric bag placed on an incline to keep the head elevated

Because of a lack of equipment, immediate descent may be the only option available. In late stages more than one oxygen modality may need to be employed concurrently. These efforts place great strain on the limited resources of groups traveling in remote areas. It is common for the shared concern and cooperation among group members (tourists/staff/porters) to disintegrate or for groups to discover that they are woefully unequipped to handle HAPE. As a result fatal outcomes are common when HAPE presents in remote settings.

Pharmacologic treatment is directed at agents that reduce pulmonary artery pressure and thereby may improve oxygenation in HAPE. Medications including nifedipine (Adalat, Procardia),[1] nitric oxide (INO$_{max}$),[1] epoprostenol (Flolan),[1] and sildenafil (Viagra)[1] have been studied for use in treatment of HAPE. Current clinical experience warrants consideration of nifedipine (Adalat, Procardia) as an adjunct treatment for HAPE when immediate supplemental oxygen is unavailable or

descent is delayed. Vascular access and intravenous (IV) fluid should be immediately available if nifedipine (Adalat, Procardia) is administered because patients are often intravascularly depleted and risk a severe hypotensive event that could be devastating in the setting of concomitant HACE. Sildenafil citrate (Viagra)[1] can also selectively lower pulmonary artery pressure with less effect on systemic blood pressure, and is under study for the treatment of HAPE. Inhaled β-agonists, salmeterol

---

CURRENT THERAPY

Acute Mountain Sickness

- Halt ascent, do not exceed light activity level, oral hydration.
- Administer acetazolamide (Diamox) 250 mg PO bid.
- Administer analgesics and antiemetics.
- If readily available, administer oxygen 1 to 2 L per minute as needed to resolve symptoms.
- If no improvement after 24 hours, descend to altitude where person last slept without symptoms until fully recovered.

High-Altitude Cerebral Edema

- Administer oxygen 2 to 4 L per minute.
- In remote mountain areas, prepare for immediate descent of at least 600 m by ground or aircraft, and if oxygen unavailable, use portable hyperbaric chamber.
- Monitor at all times, and replenish/maintain hydration as needed.
- Administer dexamethasone (Decadron) 8 mg IM, IV, or PO × 1 dose, then 4 mg q6h.
- Administer acetazolamide (Diamox) 250 mg PO bid.

High-Altitude Pulmonary Edema

- Administer oxygen initially 4 to 6 L per minute, then titrate to keep arterial oxygen saturation more than 90%.
- In remote mountain areas, prepare for immediate descent of at least 600 m by ground or aircraft; and if oxygen unavailable, use portable hyperbaric chamber on incline with head end elevated.
- Sit upright at 45 degree angle, strict rest, and monitor at all times.
- Administer nifedipine (Adalat, Procardia) 10 mg PO initially, then 30 mg extended release q12h *IF* oxygen unavailable *AND* IV fluid resuscitation immediately available.
- Administer salmeterol (Serevent) inhaler, 1 puff bid *OR* albuterol (Proventil) inhaler, 4 to 6 puffs q4h.
- Administer dexamethasone (Decadron) 8 mg IM, IV or PO × 1 dose, then 4 mg q6h *IF* suspect or unsure if HACE is also present.

CURRENT DIAGNOSIS

- Acute Mountain Sickness—In the setting of a recent gain in altitude, the presence of headache and at least one of the following: GI symptoms (anorexia, nausea, or vomiting), fatigue or weakness, dizziness or lightheadedness, or difficulty sleeping
- High-Altitude Cerebral Edema—In the setting of a recent gain in altitude, the presence of a change in mental status and/or ataxia in a person with AMS, or the presence of both mental status change and ataxia in a person without AMS
- High-Altitude Pulmonary Edema—In the setting of a recent gain in altitude, the presence of at least two of the following symptoms: dyspnea at rest, cough, weakness or decreased exercise performance, chest tightness, or congestion; and two of the following signs: rales or wheezing in at least one lung field, central cyanosis, tachypnea, or tachycardia

The Lake Louise Consensus on the Definition and Quantification of Altitude Illness.
Abbreviations: AMS = acute mountain sickness; GI = gastrointestinal.

Abbreviations: bid = twice daily; IM = intramuscular; IV = intravenous; PO = orally; q = every.

(Serevent),[1] and albuterol (Proventil)[1] are currently under study for treatment of HAPE because β-agonists increase the clearance of fluid from the alveolar space and might lower pulmonary artery pressure. The Current Therapy Box summarizes the management of HAPE.

Reascent After Altitude Illness

Mild AMS is common and indicative of an ascent rate that is too rapid for a given person. Further ascent should not resume until full resolution of all symptoms. Future trips with similar ascent profiles warrant consideration of prophylaxis with acetazolamide (Diamox).

After episodes of HACE and HAPE resolve fully, reascent has been successful for many patients, some reaching exceptionally high summits. Caution is warranted, however. Persons should be advised to ascend more slowly and to recognize and act appropriately for early signs of altitude illness. Persons with multiple episodes of HAPE may benefit during subsequent ascent from prophylaxis with nifedipine (Adalat, Procardia)[1] and potentially with salmeterol (Serevent)[1] while stressing the value of cautious gradual ascent over medication. Recurrent HAPE or HAPE occurring at altitudes below 3000 m should prompt evaluation to rule out cardiac or pulmonary shunts, valvular disease, or pulmonary hypertension.

REFERENCES

Bartsch P, Merki B, Hofstetter D, et al: Treatment of acute mountain sickness by simulated descent: A randomized controlled trial. BMJ 1993;306:1098-1101.

Chow T, Browne V, Heileson HL, et al: Ginkgo biloba and acetazolamide prophylaxis for acute mountain sickness: A randomized placebo-controlled trial. Arch Intern Med 2005;165:296-301.

Consensus Group: The Lake Louise Consensus on the Definition and Quantification of Altitude Illness. In JR Sutton, G Coates, CS Houston: Hypoxia and Mountain Medicine. Burlington, Vt, Queen City Printers, 1992, 327-330.

Litch JA: Endotracheal intubation and mechanical ventilation following respiratory arrest from high altitude pulmonary edema. West J Med 1999;170(3):174-176.

Litch JA, Basnyat B, Zimmerman M: Subarachnoid hemorrhage at high altitude. West J Med 1997;167(3):180-181.

Litch JA, Bishop RA: Re-ascent following resolution of high altitude pulmonary edema (HAPE). High Alt Med Biol 2001;2(1):53-55.

Litch JA, Bishop RA: Oxygen concentrators for the delivery of supplemental oxygen in remote high altitude areas. Wilderness Environ Med 2000;11(3):189-191.

Larson EB, Roach RC, Schoene RB, Hornbein TF: Acute mountain sickness and acetazolamide—Clinical efficacy and effect on ventilation. JAMA 1982;248:328-332.

Oelz O, Maggiorini M, Ritter M, et al: Prevention and treatment of high altitude pulmonary edema by a calcium channel blocker. Int J Sports Med 1992;13(Suppl 1):S65-S68.

Pollard AJ, Niermeyer S, Barry P, et al: Children at high altitude: An international consensus statement by an ad hoc committee of the International Society of Mountain Medicine. High Alt Med Biol 2001;2(3):389-403.

Rabold MB: Dexamethasone for prophylaxis and treatment of acute mountain sickness. West J Med 1992;3:54-60.

Sartori C, Allemann Y, Duplain H, et al: Salmeterol for the prevention of high-altitude pulmonary edema. N Engl J Med 2002; 346(21): 1631-1636.

[1]Not FDA approved for this indication.

Disturbances Due To the Cold

Method of
Daniel F. Danzl, MD

Accidental Hypothermia

Accidental hypothermia occurs when the body's core temperature unintentionally drops below 35°C (95°F). At this temperature, the compensatory physiologic responses to conserve heat begin to fail. Primary hypothermia results from exposure in previously healthy patients, but the mortality is much higher when diseases or injuries result in secondary hypothermia, which is often underreported. Cold-induced tragedies continue to afflict both military and civilian populations. Urban indoor and outdoor settings produce the most cases in the United States.

PATHOPHYSIOLOGY

Humans are unable to generate sufficient heat to maintain thermoneutrality under a variety of conditions (Box 1). Significant cold exposure normally activates the preoptic anterior hypothalamus, which orchestrates thermoregulation. Physiologic responses to the cold include shivering thermogenesis as well as endocrinologic and autonomic nervous system activities. Adaptive behavioral responses include donning of more clothing and seeking a heat source. Radiation normally accounts for 55% to 65% of the heat loss. Conductive losses increase up to 5 times in wet clothing and 25 times in water. Compensatory responses to heat loss through radiation, conduction, convection, evaporation, and respiration eventually fail. As the core temperature continues to fall, the patient becomes poikilothermic and cools to the ambient temperature.

Each organ system is affected uniquely. Cerebral metabolism is depressed 6% to 7% per 1°C. Cerebrovascular autoregulation remains intact until below 25°C (77°F), which helps maintain cortical blood flow. The electroencephalographic activity is clearly not prognostic and silences around 19° to 20°C (66.2° to 68°F). Cardiovascular effects are often pronounced. After the initial tachycardia, there is progressive bradycardia. The heart rate drops to half its normal rate at 28°C (82.4°F). Hypothermia also progressively depresses the mean arterial pressure and cardiac index. Core temperature *afterdrop* refers to the continual decline in core temperature after removal from the cold. This phenomenon results from temperature equilibration and reversal of circulatory arteriovenous shunting in the extremities.

All atrial arrhythmias are commonly encountered and should have a slow ventricular response; therefore they are considered innocent. The clinical significance of ventricular arrhythmias is more difficult to assess because suppressed preexistent ectopy may reappear during rewarming. The decreased ventricular fibrillation

18

Physiologic
Decreased Heat Production
- Age extremes (infants, elderly)
- Prior cold injury
- Dehydration or malnutrition
- Overexertion
- Endocrinologic insufficiency
- Trauma (multisystem or extremity)
- Physical conditioning
- Diaphoresis or hyperhidrosis
- Hypoxia
- Insufficient fuel

Increased Heat Loss
- Vascular diseases
- Shock
- Poor acclimatization or conditioning
- Dermatologic malfunction
- Burns
- Emergency resuscitation
- Cold infusions

Impaired Thermoregulation
- Central nervous system trauma, disease
- Spinal cord injury
- Pharmacologic or toxicologic agents
- Metabolic disorders
- Sepsis

Psychological
- Mental status or attitude
- Fear or panic
- Peer pressure
- Fatigue
- Intense concentration on tasks
- Hunger
- Intoxicants

Environmental
- Heat loss (conductive, evaporative, radiative, convective)
- Ambient temperature or humidity
- Duration of exposure
- Wind chill factor
- Altitude with or without associated conditions
- Quantity of exposed surface area

Mechanical
- Inadequate insulation
- Constricting or wet clothing or boots
- Immobility or cramped positioning

threshold is a real hazard below 28°C (82.4°F). Cardiac cycle prolongation is pronounced, as reflected in the corrected QT interval on the electrocardiogram (ECG). The characteristic J wave, or Osborn hypothermic hump, may be present at the junction of the QRS complex and ST segment. Because hypothermic ECG changes are not easily computer programmable, the misdiagnosis of a current injury can result in dangerous thrombolytic therapy.

Respiratory stimulation is followed by a progressive reduction in respiratory minute volume, which reflects the metabolic depression. Carbon dioxide production falls 50% for each 8°C drop in temperature. Although renal blood flow declines, there is a large initial paradoxical diuresis.

CLINICAL PRESENTATION

Historical circumstances suggest the diagnosis when exposure is obvious. More subtle presentations predominate in urban settings. In such cases, the clinician may misfocus on a solitary diagnosis of a medical, toxicologic, neurologic, traumatic, or psychiatric emergency. Symptoms are often vague and physical findings nonspecific or deceptive. For example, if tachycardia is disproportionate for the temperature, the physician should consider a secondary cause of hypothermia, such as hypoglycemia, hypovolemia, or a drug overdose. Persistent hyperventilation suggests a central nervous system (CNS) lesion or an organic acidosis, such as lactic acidosis or diabetic ketoacidosis. A cold-induced ileus and rectus spasm can both mimic and mask an acute abdomen. When the level of consciousness is inconsistent with the temperature, an overdose or CNS trauma or infection should be suspected. Hypothermic areflexia can also obscure a spinal cord injury. Last, temporary psychiatric sequelae during hypothermia include maladaptive behavior such as paradoxical undressing, which is the inappropriate removal of clothes in response to cold stress.

Hypothermia is confirmed with a core temperature (e.g., rectal, esophageal, tympanic) measurement, preferably from two sites. Further heat loss should be gently prevented and cardiac monitoring initiated. Hypothermia adversely affects tissue oxygenation by numerous mechanisms, including the leftward shift of the oxyhemoglobin dissociation curve. Most patients are significantly dehydrated and benefit from a bolus crystalloid administration.

Routine hematologic evaluations should include arterial blood gases uncorrected for temperature. An uncorrected pH of 7.4 and Pco_2 of 40 mm Hg reflect acid-base balance at any temperature. The hematocrit also increases 2% per 1°C drop in temperature, which can mask anemia. Leukopenia does not imply the absence of infection because bone marrow suppression and white blood cell sequestration are common. Unfortunately, there is no safe predictor of the electrolyte status. For example, hyperkalemic electrocardiogram changes are obscured by hypothermia. Hypokalemia is more common in chronic hypothermia. Finally, cold induces a renal glycosuria, which as a result does not imply normoglycemia.

A full clotting screen is necessary because cold hemagglutination and coagulation are aberrant. Platelet function is impaired. Cold also directly inhibits the enzymatic reactions of the coagulation cascade. Kinetic tests of coagulation are performed in the laboratory at 37°C (98.6°F). As a result, the observed in vivo coagulopathy is not reflected by a reported deceptively normal prothrombin time, activated partial thromboplastin time, or international normalized ratio (INR).

REWARMING STRATEGIES

The key clinical decision is choosing passive versus active rewarming. Passive external rewarming is noninvasive and ideal for mild cases in previously healthy persons.

Rakel and Bope: *Conn's Current Therapy 2006.*

The patient should simply be covered with insulating materials. Active rewarming should be considered in the following situations: core temperature below 32°C (90°F), age extremes, CNS dysfunction, endocrine insufficiency, and cardiovascular instability.

Active external rewarming can be accomplished with heating blankets, radiant heat sources, and immersion. Forced-air heating blankets are the safest. There is a potential for thermal injury to vasoconstricted skin with the use of electric blankets. Limiting heat application to the trunk minimizes many of the physiologic concerns with heating the extremities. For example, heating the extremities after the occurrence of the diuresis and fluid sequestration common to chronic hypothermia causes a core temperature afterdrop.

Many techniques are available to deliver direct heat internally. Active core rewarming options include inhalation of heated humidified oxygen, heated intravenous fluids and irrigation of the peritoneum or thorax, and extracorporeal rewarming. Airway rewarming 40° to 45°C (104° to 113°F) with a mask or endotracheal tube is a valuable adjunct in all cases because the access is simple. Preoxygenation and gentle technique prevent intubation arrhythmias. The inhalation eliminates respiratory heat loss. During massive volume resuscitations, administration of heated intravenous fluid and blood is helpful. The use of countercurrent heat exchangers is the most efficient method for heating and delivering the fluid.

Peritoneal lavage is another option for severely hypothermic patients. Peritoneal dialysate at 40° to 45°C (104° to 113°F) delivered by two catheters with outflow suction transfers heat efficiently. Thoracostomy tube irrigation with warm saline is also valuable. The sterile saline is warmed to 42°C (107.6°F), infused anteriorly, and then drained from the efferent midaxillary tube. Finally, irrigation of the gastrointestinal tract is of limited value and should be reserved for use in combination with all available techniques in patients with cardiac arrest.

Extracorporeal rewarming is potentially indicated in patients with cardiac arrest, completely frozen extremities, or severe rhabdomyolysis. The standard circuit uses a mechanical pump with an oxygenator and heat exchanger. Other options are continuous arteriovenous, venovenous, and hemodialysis rewarming. Cardiopulmonary resuscitation is indicated unless:

- A do-not-resuscitate (DNR) status is documented and verified.
- Obviously lethal injuries are present.
- Chest wall depression is impossible.
- Any signs of life are present.
- Rescuers are endangered by evacuation delays or altered triage conditions.

The misdiagnosis of a cardiac arrest is a real concern. Palpation of peripheral pulses is difficult when an extreme bradycardia is coupled with peripheral vasoconstriction. The examiner should take a full minute to check for a central pulse, especially if no cardiac monitor is available. After attempts to defibrillate with 2 watt-seconds per kg, active rewarming should be continued

past 32°C (89.6°F). Successful reestablishment of flow below that temperature is rare.

Resuscitation pharmacology usually reflects standard therapeutic activity while the patient is cold, which progresses to toxicity after rewarming. Drug protein binding increases, and metabolism and excretion are impaired. Low-dosage infusions of catecholamines should be initiated in euvolemic patients who fail to rewarm and are disproportionately hypotensive. The treatment of ventricular arrhythmias is problematic. Class III agents possess direct antifibrillatory activity, but bretylium is unavailable and the safety of amiodarone (Cordarone) questionable. For severe bradydysrhythmias that do not resolve with rewarming, external noninvasive pacing with pads is preferable to transvenous pacing. The empirical use of levothyroxine (Synthroid)[1] and corticosteroids[1] is hazardous.

The clinical treatment of hypothermia should be predicated on the duration and extent of temperature depression and the severity of the predisposing factors. Outcome is difficult to predict. Indicators of a grave prognosis include evidence of cell lysis (hyperkalemia with potassium levels greater than 10 mEq per L), intravascular thrombosis (fibrinogen value below 50 mg per dL), a pH below 6.5, and a core temperature below 10° to 12°C (50° to 53.6°F). Recently, a physician was successfully resuscitated from 13.7°C (56.66°F).

Peripheral Cold Injuries

Peripheral local cold injuries include freezing and non-freezing syndromes. Frostbite is the most common freezing injury. Trench foot and immersion foot are nonfreezing injuries resulting from exposure to wet cold. Nonfreezing injury after exposure to dry cold is called chilblain (pernio). With cold stress, the core temperature is maintained via a life-versus-limb mechanism at the expense of vasospasticity and shunting, which prevent heat distribution to the extremities.

PATHOPHYSIOLOGY

A unique aspect of peripheral cold injury is the pathogenesis of the freezing injury cascade. Tissue is initially damaged by the freeze-thaw insult and subsequently by progressive dermal ischemia. Before freezing, tissue cooling increases the viscosity of the vascular contents as the microvasculature constricts.

The freeze-thaw sequence begins during extracellular fluid crystallization. Water exits the cell, causing intracellular dehydration, hyperosmolality, cellular shrinkage, and collapse. Arachidonic acid breakdown products are then released from underlying damaged tissue into the vesicle fluid. Both prostaglandin $F_{2\alpha}$ and thromboxane A_2 produce platelet aggregation, leukocyte immobilization, and vasoconstriction. Endothelial cells are quite sensitive to cold injury, and the microvasculature becomes distorted and clogged.

---

[1]Not FDA approved for this indication.

After tissue thawing, progressive edema formation continues for 48 to 72 hours. Subsequent thrombosis and early superficial necrosis develop. This tissue eventually mummifies and demarcates, often more than 60 to 90 days later—hence the surgical aphorism "Frostbite in January, amputate in July."

The incidence and severity of peripheral cold injury are determined by the duration and intensity of cutaneous cold exposure. Box 1 lists the factors predisposing to peripheral cold injuries.

CLINICAL PRESENTATION

The initial presentation of frostbite is often deceptively benign. Unlike in burns, classification of frostbite by degrees is often inaccurate prognostically and misleading therapeutically. The physical findings at 24 to 72 hours after completion of rewarming are more reliably used to classify frostbite. Superficial or mild frostbite does not entail eventual tissue loss, but deep or severe frostbite does. *Frostnip* is a superficial cold insult producing transient numbness or tingling that resolves after rewarming without tissue destruction.

All patients with frostbite have some initial sensory deficit in light touch, pain, or temperature. Acral areas and distal extremities are the usual insensate sites. Patients also complain of being clumsy or having a "chunk of wood" sensation in the extremity.

Deep frostbite may initially appear deceptively benign. Tissues remaining frozen can appear mottled, violaceous, pale yellow, or waxy. Favorable presenting signs are warmth, normal color, and some sensation. If the subcutaneous tissue is soft and pliable or the dermis can be rolled over the bony prominences, the injury may be superficial.

Rapid rewarming produces an initial hyperemia, even in severe cases. A residual violaceous hue is ominous. Early formation of clear large blebs is a more favorable sign than smaller dark, hemorrhagic blebs, which imply cold damage to the subdermal vascular plexus.

Chilblain (pernio) is a form of dry cold injury often developing after repetitive exposures. These so-called cold sores typically involve facial areas and the dorsa of the hands and feet. Young women, especially those with a history of Raynaud's phenomenon, are at risk. Persistent vasospasticity and vasculitis result in pruritus, erythema, and mild edema. Plaques, blue nodules, and ulcerations eventually develop. Treatment of perniosis is difficult; the physician should consider using nifedipine (Procardia)[1] at a dose of 20 to 60 mg daily.

Immersion (trench) foot is produced by prolonged exposure to wet cold at above-freezing temperatures. Feet often appear erythematous, edematous, or cyanotic. The bullae are indistinguishable from those seen in frostbite. This vesiculation proceeds to ulceration and liquefaction gangrene. In milder cases, hyperhidrosis, cold sensitivity, and painful ambulation persist for many years.

Warm-water immersion foot affects the soles of the feet and results from waterlogging of the thick stratum corneum. This commonly occurs in persons who lack shelter wearing wet shoes for prolonged periods.

Ancillary diagnostic adjuncts have limited value with peripheral cold injuries. Doppler ultrasonography, digital plethysmography, thermography, routine radiography, and angiography do not consistently predict tissue loss at presentation. Early scintigraphy may predict tissue loss and monitor the efficacy of treatment. Magnetic resonance angiography is emerging as a tool to predict eventual demarcation. Delayed studies may guide subsequent therapy.

Treatment

Mills popularized rapid immersion rewarming after extensive experience with severe Alaskan frostbite cases. Before thawing, frozen parts should not be exposed to dry heat sources. Tissue refreezing is also disastrous; as an extreme example, it is preferable to ambulate to safety on frozen extremities.

A circulating tank is ideal for rewarming the extremities, but a large container suffices for the hands and feet. The process starts with water at 38° to 40°C (100.4° to 104°F) and the temperature is gradually increased. Care should be taken to avoid thermal injury, which occurs if the water temperature markedly exceeds 45°C (113°F). A very common error is premature termination of rewarming because the establishment of reperfusion is quite painful and requires parenteral analgesia. Rewarming may take up to 1 hour.

Extreme caution should be exercised in treating patients with completely frozen extremities because invariably they are hypothermic. Thawing produces significant core temperature, fluid, and electrolyte fluxes. Persistent cyanosis after a complete thaw should suggest elevated fascial compartment pressures.

Management of frostbite vesicles also varies. Large clear blisters should be sterilely aspirated or débrided. The débridement of hemorrhagic vesicles, however, can extend the injury by allowing secondary desiccation of deep dermal layers. There are two strategies for inhibition of prostaglandins. Topical aloe vera ointment (Dermaide Abe)[1]* is a specific thromboxane inhibitor but it is not proven to salvage tissue. An acceptable alternative is topical antibiotic ointment. Systemically, ibuprofen is preferable to the salicylates. Ibuprofen produces fibrinolysis in addition to limiting the accumulation of inflammatory mediators. Parenteral ketorolac (Toradol) is another antiprostaglandin option.

Multiple antithrombotic and vasodilatory treatment regimens are proposed. There is no conclusive evidence of enhanced tissue salvage with administration of dextran,[1] heparin,[1] steroids,[1] nonsteroidal anti-inflammatory drugs (NSAIDs),[1] dimethylsulfoxide (DMSO),[1] nonionic detergents,[1] dipyridamole (Persantine),[1] calcium channel

CURRENT DIAGNOSIS

- Obtain core temperature measurement.
- Anticipate atypical presentations.
- Identify predisposing factors that decrease heat production; increase heat loss, or impair thermoregulation.
- Decide whether to use passive or active rewarming.

blockers,[1] or hyperbaric oxygen.[1] Pentoxifylline (Trental),[1] 400 mg given orally every 8 hours, may facilitate small-vessel perfusion.

A long-acting α-blocker, phenoxybenzamine (Dibenzyline),[1] 10 mg per day up to 60 mg per day, may decrease the refractory vasospasm that develops during the clinical course in selected patients. Aggressive hydration is essential to minimize orthostatic hypotension. Chemical sympathectomy with intra-arterial

---

[1]Not FDA approved for this indication.

CURRENT THERAPY

The following lists treatment of frostbite:

Before Thawing

- Stabilize core temperature.
- Address medical or surgical conditions.
- Protect and do not massage frozen part.
- Avoid partial thawing and refreezing.
- Extricate from environment.
- Begin rehydration.

Thaw

- Provide parenteral analgesia and hydration.
- Rapidly rewarm entire part in 38° to 40°C (100.4° to 104°F) circulating water until distal flush occurs (thermometer monitoring).
- Ask patient to spend 10 to 60 minutes moving part gently without friction massage; "partial thaw" should be avoided.

After Thawing

- For clear vesicles: aspirate if intact; débride if broken.
- For hemorrhagic vesicles: do not débride; may aspirate.
- Apply topical aloe vera (Dermaide Aloe)[1] or antibiotic ointment every 6 hours.
- Use ibuprofen, 400 mg orally every 8 hours.
- Consider tetanus diphtheria (Td) (toxoid) and streptococcal prophylaxis.
- Elevate part in protective cradle.
- Use whirlpool hydrotherapy three times daily (37°C [98.6°F]).
- Avoid vasoconstrictors, including nicotine.
- Consider phenoxybenzamine (Dibenzyline)[1] in severe cases.

---

[1]Not FDA approved for this indication.

Rakel and Bope: *Conn's Current Therapy 2006.*

reserpine was helpful but is not available. Surgical sympathectomy does not enhance tissue salvage, although a sympathetic nerve block can relieve painful and refractory vasospasm.

Sequelae

Residual neuropathic symptoms are common and result from abnormal sympathetic tone and neuronal damage. Patients with chronic symptoms should be advised to avoid nicotine and cold exposure while using nonsteroidal anti-inflammatory agents and skin lubricants. Dermatologic findings include lymphedema, ulcerations, hair and nail deformities, and epidermoid or squamous carcinomas. Occult musculoskeletal injuries are most pronounced in children. Premature epiphyseal fusion and fragmentation can occur. Amputation decisions should be deferred unless there is supervening sepsis or gangrene. The ultimate tissue salvage after a spontaneous slough usually far exceeds the most optimistic initial estimates.

REFERENCES

Centers for Disease Control and Prevention (CDC): Hypothermia-related deaths—United States, 2003. MMWR 2004;53:172.
Danzl DF: Hypothermia. Semin Respir Crit Care Med 2002;23:57.
Giesbrecht GG: Cold stress, near drowning and accidental hypothermia: A review. Aviat Space Environ Med 2000;71:733.
Hildebrand F, et al: Pathophysiologic changes and effects of hypothermia on outcome in elective surgery and trauma patients. Am J Surg 2004;187:363.
Kempainen RR, Brunette DD: The evaluation and management of accidental hypothermia. Respir Care 2004;49:192.
Kibayashi K, Shojo H: Accidental fatal hypothermia in elderly people with Alzheimer's disease. Med Sci Law 2003;43:127.
Mallet ML: Pathophysiology of accidental hypothermia. QJM 2002; 95:775.
Megarbane B, et al: Hypothermia with indoor occurrence is associated with a worse outcome. Intensive Care Med 2000;26:1843.
Muszkat M, Durst RM, Ben-Yehuda A: Factors associated with mortality among elderly patients with hypothermia. Am J Med 2002; 113:234.
Pedley DK, Paterson B, Morrison W: Hypothermia in elderly patients presenting to accident & emergency during the onset of winter. Scott Med J 2002;47:10.

18

Disturbances Caused by Heat

Method of
John F. Coyle II, MD

Heat stroke is an illness caused by failure of thermoregulation with elevation of core temperature to 40.6°C (105°F) or more, associated with central nervous system dysfunction. Heat stroke is traditionally subdivided into *exertional* and *classic* (or nonexertional) forms.

Exertional Heat Stroke

Exertional heat stroke is a sporadic illness triggered by exercise in warm environmental conditions that add to the thermal load produced by muscular contraction. It mainly strikes manual laborers, soldiers in training, and athletic competitors; indeed, it is the third leading cause of death among high school and college athletes in the United States. Exertional heat stroke may occur at moderate temperatures, especially if humidity is high, but both exertional and classic heat strokes most likely develop in conditions of high heat. The incidence of heat stroke increases exponentially when heat stress exceeds a boundary value. Appearance of the first case should sound an alarm that conditions have become dangerous, and more cases should be anticipated. The typical heat stroke victim is highly motivated, poorly conditioned, obese, and not acclimatized. Fatigue and sleep deprivation are commonly encountered, and recent or ongoing febrile or dehydrating illness increases risk. Dehydration may play a role, especially if severe. The use of certain medicines also increases risk, most notably those that decrease cardiac output (β-blockers), promote dehydration (diuretics), affect hypothalamic control (major tranquilizers, neuroleptics, alcohol), inhibit sweating (anticholinergics, tricyclic antidepressants, antihistamines), or increase thermogenicity (amphetamines, cocaine).

Prevention is the ideal treatment. Because behavior is the most powerful thermoregulatory mechanism, education and empowerment have the greatest preventive potential. To avoid exertional heat stroke, organizers should schedule vigorous exercise in the coolest hours of the day (shortly after dawn or after nightfall, in difficult seasons). Exercise level should be governed by athlete fitness, acclimatization, hydration status, and freedom from intercurrent illness. Clothing should be appropriate for exercise conditions. Medication use that might interfere with effective thermoregulation should be recognized, and medical personnel must be charged with the responsibility for stopping any participant who appears to be decompensating.

Triage of those with exertional heat stroke is highly variable. Runners who are plunged unconscious into an ice water bath at the end of a race often respond promptly to treatment, reawaken, and are sometimes sent home without hospitalization. A less-favorable response necessitates hospital admission.

Classic (Nonexertional) Heat Stroke

Classic (nonexertional) heat stroke usually occurs during heat waves that cause passive warming by exposure to unrelenting hot and humid conditions, afflicting urban dwellers who are elderly, infirm, solitary, and poor. Heat waves tend to be "silent and invisible killers of silent and invisible people." Their housing lacks air-conditioning or they do not use it because of expense or confusion. Alcoholism and chronic illness, especially mental illness, predispose people to heat stroke.

Young children are susceptible, reflecting their high surface-to-volume ratio, relatively inefficient sweat glands, and dependent status. Classic heat stroke requires preventive measures at the community level. Those with chronic illness and substance abuse history are at highest risk, and they may be the most difficult to contact. Although ventilation fans are of little help in hot and humid conditions, a few hours spent in air-conditioned rooms each day can significantly reduce the likelihood of heat stroke. Whether this is primarily a physiologic or a sociologic effect is unclear. Patients with classic heat stroke usually respond slowly to treatment and require hospital admission.

Pathophysiology

The pathophysiology of heat stroke is incompletely understood. Although a vast number of runners in a marathon may develop dehydration and a high core temperature, very few proceed to heat stroke. Excessive heat is a noxious agent that causes direct cell injury. The severity of heat stroke is related to the degree and duration of temperature elevation above 41.6°C (106.9°F). Exercise lowers the thermal threshold for heat stroke because of hormonal effects and competing demands of organ systems as blood flow is directed away from the viscera to the active muscles and the skin. Gut ischemia may result in release of bacterial polysaccharides into the blood. What happens next is a complex interplay of factors including cytokines, bacterial polysaccharides, and heat shock proteins. As endothelial abnormalities accumulate, there is precipitation of a cascade of events including activation of the coagulation system and vascular dilation, resulting in hypotension and coagulation disorders. These events in many respects mimic sepsis.

Because the brain is extremely sensitive to heat stress, the first signs of heat stroke are neurologic. Judgment is impaired, and the chance for self-diagnosis is greatly reduced. After loss of consciousness, muscular activity is markedly diminished, but temperature may remain elevated for hours. Multisystem injury may follow, with the possibility of neurologic, pulmonary, cardiac, hepatic, renal, vascular, hematologic, and immunologic damage. A high percentage of classic heat stroke patients suffer infection within 36 hours of hospital admission.

Treatment

Treatment of heat stroke can be summarized easily:

- Lower rectal temperature immediately to 39°C (102.2°F).
- Support organ systems injured by heat, hypotension, inflammation, and coagulopathy.

There is a *golden hour* after the onset of heat stroke in which therapy can be extremely effective. When treating a patient outside of the hospital, the patient should be moved to a shaded area, clothes removed, and the person covered with water and fanned. When resources become available, the simplest treatment appears to be cold-water immersion in a shallow tub, with patient head, arms, and lower legs outside the tub. The high efficiency of this method comes from two properties of water: It has 25 times the thermal conductivity of air, and it makes perfect contact with all skin surfaces. In addition, the hydrostatic properties of water tend to reduce the risk of hypotension. Other methods of cooling include skin wetting with fanning, application of total-body ice packs (24 ice packs, with special emphasis on the neck, armpits, and groin), or use of a body-cooling unit (evaporation and convection).

Assessment of the patient with presumed heat stroke should be delayed pending initiation of cooling. Determination of rectal temperature, heart rate, and blood pressure can be carried out while the patient is being cooled. Oral and tympanic membrane temperatures cannot be used because they may be misleadingly low. Rectal temperature should be measured every 5 to 10 minutes, and the patient should be removed from cooling when 39°C (102.2°F) is reached, to avoid overshoot hypothermia. Hydration with normal saline or lactated Ringer's solution should be started after initiation of cooling, and most patients require 1 L in the first hour of treatment. Further rehydration needs to be guided by estimated water losses, and in difficult cases placement of a central venous monitoring catheter may be needed. Overhydration may promote cerebral edema, pulmonary edema, and hyponatremia.

CURRENT DIAGNOSIS

- Heat stroke often occurs in the first 2 hours of exercise and may occur in so-called moderate heat stress conditions.
- Heat stroke may occur in sedentary urban dwellers during heat waves, especially in the presence of drug or alcohol use, senility, or in young children.
- Abnormal mental status (coma, delirium, agitation, confusion, combativeness) is a constant feature of heat stroke.
- Rectal temperature should be checked immediately. Axillary and aural temperatures may be misleadingly low. A rectal temperature of 40.6°C (105°F) or more is required for diagnosis of heat stroke, but delayed measurement may produce a misleadingly low temperature.
- The trap of proceeding with complex diagnostic procedures (such as computed tomographic scans) before core temperature is assessed and lowered to less than 39°C (102.2°F) should be avoided.
- After cooling measures are instituted, blood samples should be obtained to assess coagulation status, hepatic function, renal function, likelihood of infection, acid-base status, and muscle injury.

CURRENT THERAPY

- Injury because of heat stroke is related to both the magnitude and duration of core temperature elevation.
- After elevated rectal temperature is documented, treatment should not be delayed. In particular, it should not be delayed to start an intravenous line or to carry out advanced testing such as computerized tomography or other radiograph study.
- Ideal treatment for heat stroke is cold-water immersion in a low tub, such as a child's wading pool, with the patient's arms, legs, and head hanging out of the tub.
- If low tub immersion is not available, constant flowing of cold water from a tap over the patient with drainage through a slotted Gurney cart in the presence of constant high-velocity electric fanning can be effective.
- Applying ice packs to the axillae, groins, trunk, and as many other skin surfaces as possible can be useful, but this method of cooling is not as efficient as cold-water immersion or constant cold-water flow because of reduced contact surface and limited thermal gradient.
- Rectal temperature should be checked every 5 minutes during cooling. Cooling measures are discontinued when rectal temperature reaches 39°C (102.2°F) to avoid excessive cooling. Clinicians should watch for rebound temperature elevation after cooling is discontinued.
- Clinicians should be prepared to support the patient through multisystem organ failure. Hemorrhage should be treated with transfusion of red blood cells, platelets, fresh-frozen plasma, and clotting factors. Heparin has no role in treatment of this consumptive coagulopathy. Volume expansion may be needed. Prolonged ventilator support and hemodialysis may be required.
- Medications that may be needed are diazepam (Valium), 5 mg intravenously (IV), for seizures; pressors; and mannitol, 0.25 g/kg IV, and furosemide (Lasix), 0.5 to 1.0 mg/kg IV, for renal protection from rhabdomyolysis, but only after adequate volume expansion is achieved.

Seizures, which occur commonly, should be managed with diazepam (Valium), 5 mg intravenously (IV). Shivering may also be treated with diazepam. The patient must be monitored closely with use of this medication, which occasionally promotes hypotension. Hypotension should be treated with cooling and volume expansion. If blood pressure remains depressed, pressors may be needed. For patients with prolonged exertional heat stroke, mannitol, 0.25 g/kg, or furosemide (Lasix), 0.5 to 1 mg/kg, should be given after volume

Rakel and Bope: *Conn's Current Therapy 2006.*

expansion is carried out to minimize the adverse effects of rhabdomyolysis on renal function.

In patients with severe multiorgan damage, disseminated intravascular coagulation (DIC) is a common finding. Bleeding in DIC should be treated with transfusion of fresh-frozen plasma, cryoprecipitate, and platelet concentrates as needed. There is no role for heparin or thrombolytics in DIC in this setting. Adult respiratory distress syndrome tends to occur in conjunction with DIC, and prolonged ventilator support may be required. Hepatic failure in heat stroke is usually transient. Renal failure may necessitate emergency hemodialysis. No evidence supports use of anti-inflammatory agents or antipyretic agents in heat stroke. Use of strategies that are helpful in sepsis may ultimately find a role in treatment of heat stroke, but such treatments should be considered experimental at this time.

Prognosis can be estimated by time to recovery of consciousness (shorter is better) and elevation of liver enzymes (lactate dehydrogenase [LDH] at 24 hours less than three times normal is a good prognostic sign).

Heat stroke should usually be regarded as an accident, like drowning. The population at highest risk is readily defined, but because of the rarity of this ailment it is difficult to maintain a high level of preparedness for its prevention and treatment. Once encountered, heat stroke must be treated with much the same urgency as cardiac arrest because prompt cooling can sometimes make the crisis little more than an inconvenience. After the process of systemic injury becomes established, heat stroke's cascade of microvascular dysfunction can take on a life of its own, eventuating in a desperate struggle against multisystem failure and a high mortality rate.

REFERENCES

Bouchama A, Knochel JP: Heat stroke. N Engl J Med 2002;346(25):1978-1988.

Crandall CG, Vongpatanasin W, Victor RG: Mechanism of cocaine-induced hyperthermia in humans. Ann Intern Med 2002;136(11):785-791.

Dematte JE, O'Mara K, Buescher J, et al: Near-fatal heat stroke during the 1995 heat wave in Chicago. Ann Intern Med 1998;129(3):173-181.

Eichner ER: Treatment of suspected heat illness. Int J Sports Med 1998;19(Suppl 2):S150-S153.

Epstein Y, Moran DS, Shapiro Y: Exertional heatstroke in the Israeli Defence Forces. In Pandolf KB, Burr RE (eds): Medical Aspects of Harsh Environments. U.S. Defense Dept., Army, Office of the Surgeon General, 2001, pp 281-292. Available free online: http://www.bordeninstitute.army.mil/medaspofharshenvrnmnts/

Gaffin SL, Hubbard RW: Pathophysiology of heatstroke. In Pandolf KB, Burr RE (eds): Medical Aspects of Harsh Environments. U.S. Defense Dept., Army, Office of the Surgeon General, 2001, pp 161-208. Available free online: http://www.bordeninstitute.army.mil/medaspofharshenvrnmnts/

Gardner JW, Kark JA: 2001. Clinical diagnosis, management and surveillance of exertional heat illness. In Pandolf KB, Burr RE (eds): Medical Aspects of Harsh Environments. U.S. Defense Dept., Army, Office of the Surgeon General, 2001, pp 221-279. Available free online: http://www.bordeninstitute.army.mil/medaspofharshenvrnmnts/

Klinenberg E: Review of heat wave: Social autopsy of disaster in Chicago. N Engl J Med 2003;348(7):666-667.

Shephard RJ, Shek PN: Immune dysfunction as a factor in heat illness. Crit Rev Immunol 1999;19(4):285-302.

Spider Bites and Scorpion Stings

Method of
Robert L. Norris, MD

Although bites and stings by spiders and scorpions are common in the United States, the consequences are rarely severe, unlike in many other regions of the world. This article discusses the most important spider and scorpion species in the United States.

Spider Bites

Of the thousands of species of spiders in the United States, relatively few are large enough and possess fangs strong enough to allow them to bite and poison humans. The two spiders of greatest medical importance in North America are the widow spiders (*Latrodectus* species) and the brown (or violin) spiders (*Loxosceles* species).

WIDOW SPIDERS (*LATRODECTUS* SPECIES)

Widow spiders are cosmopolitan in distribution and becoming established throughout much of the United States. Only the female spider is dangerous to humans. The male is too small to bite through human skin. The best known widow spider in the United States is the black widow (*Latrodectus mactans*). The female is a large black globular-shaped spider with a red to orange hourglass-shaped marking on the ventral aspect of her abdomen. The venom possesses a potent neurotoxin, α-latrotoxin, which causes an outpouring of neurotransmitters in the victim's body. The bite is often felt as an initial "pinprick" or "sting," and the victim may bring the spider in for identification. Over approximately 1 hour, the victim develops pain at the bite site as local muscles begin to spasm. Muscle spasms may become more regionalized or even generalized over time. Circulating excess catecholamines and acetylcholine may produce tachycardia, hypertension, restlessness, diaphoresis (local or systemic), nausea, vomiting, and headache. Severity of poisoning, as with many envenomation syndromes, tends to be greater for patients at the extremes of life—the very young with less body volume to dilute circulating venom and the elderly with their co-morbidities (especially cardiovascular and chronic pulmonary diseases). Table 1 shows a grading scale for severity of widow spider bites.

Field management consists of local ice application and prompt transportation to an emergency care facility. No other measures are of any proven benefit.

Management of the patient includes establishing cardiac and pulse oximetry monitoring and starting an intravenous line. Vital signs are checked and reevaluated at frequent intervals during the early evaluation. A careful history is taken, with particular focus on any significant cardiovascular or pulmonary disease.

TABLE 1 Severity Grading for Widow Spider (*Latrodectus* Species) Bites

Grade	Symptoms/signs	Vital signs
1	Asymptomatic or local pain at the bite site.	Normal
2	Muscle spasm/pain in the bitten extremity. May extend to the abdomen if bitten in the lower extremities or to the chest if bitten in the upper extremities. Local diaphoresis at the site or the involved extremity.	Normal
3	Generalized muscle pain (back, abdomen, chest).	Abnormal
	Remote diaphoresis, nausea/vomiting, headache.	SBP >140 mm Hg; DBP >90 mm Hg; heart rate >100 bpm

Abbreviations: bpm = beats per minute; DBP = diastolic blood pressure; SBP = systolic blood pressure.
Modified from Clark RF: Clinical presentation and treatment of black widow spider envenomation: A review of 163 cases. Ann Emerg Med 1992;21(7):782-787.

The bite site is examined, although local findings are usually minimal beyond some mild local erythema.

There are no diagnostic tests of value. Standard laboratory evaluation may reflect stress-induced elevations in white blood cell count and blood glucose, and there may be mild elevations in serum creatine phosphokinase if muscle contractions are severe. Occasionally microscopic hematuria and proteinuria are seen. Patients with significant histories of cardiovascular disease and/or severely elevated blood pressures should have a chest radiograph and electrocardiogram.

Management is generally focused on treating painful muscle cramps. Although there are anecdotal reports of success with many agents, such as calcium gluconate, methocarbamol (Robaxin), narcotics, and benzodiazepines, the most effective treatment for all manifestations of widow spider bite is antivenom. All antivenoms produced for various *Latrodectus* species around the world appear effective in treating widow spider bites regardless of the offending species. The antivenom produced in the United States is Antivenin (*Latrodectus mactans*) (Merck, West Point, PA), an equine-derived whole antibody antiserum that carries with it some risk of allergic phenomena (anaphylactic/anaphylactoid reactions and serum sickness). Precise indications for use of this agent are controversial. In the rare case of severe envenomation, its use is clearly indicated. Likewise, in the envenomed pregnant patient, its use should be strongly considered because of the risk of fetal demise related to widow spider venom–induced uterine contractions. Informed consent should be obtained if possible, and a skin test for allergy, as

recommended by the manufacturer, should be done. The dose is one vial administered intramuscularly or diluted into a larger volume of normal saline and given intravenously over an hour. The attending physician must be in close attendance during antivenom administration to intervene if an acute adverse reaction occurs (see article in this text on anaphylaxis). A second dose is occasionally required for the complete resolution of symptoms.

Antivenom administration in patients suffering painful muscle spasms as their only manifestation of poisoning (which may last for many days if untreated) is controversial in North America. Deciding when to take the risk of inducing a serious adverse drug reaction to treat a painful, but generally non–life-threatening venom poisoning requires significant medical judgment, and consultation with a toxinology expert or a regional poison control center can be helpful. A trial of combined parenteral narcotic and benzodiazepine can be initiated as decisions regarding antivenom are made, which may result in adequate symptom control. In Australia, physicians treat almost all significant bites by the closely related red back spider (*Latrodectus hasseltii*) with intramuscular equine-derived antivenom (CSL Red Back Spider Antivenom, Commonwealth Serum Labs, Victoria, Australia)[1] with excellent results and rare allergic reactions.

Patients with severe presentations or with findings refractory to treatment should be admitted to the hospital. Patients who have received good symptomatic relief, whether from routine analgesics or from antivenom, and are hemodynamically stable can be discharged from the emergency department (ED) with a reliable adult. Tetanus status, of course, is updated as needed. Any patient who has received antivenom should be warned about the signs of delayed serum sickness.

Mortality from widow spider bites is extremely low, certainly far less than 1%. Complications generally involve prolonged muscle soreness and weakness. Widow spiders do not cause local wound necrosis.

BROWN/VIOLIN SPIDERS (*LOXOSCELES* SPECIES)

The taxonomy for brown spiders, also known as violin or fiddle-back spiders (*Loxosceles* species) is complicated and remains in a state of flux. The most notorious North American species is the brown recluse (*Loxosceles reclusa*). All specimens have, to greater or lesser degrees, a violin-shaped marking on the dorsum of their cephalothoraces, and both sexes are capable of biting humans. Brown spiders are most common in the central and southwestern portions of the United States. *Loxosceles* venoms are all similar and contain sphingomyelinase D, which, in concert with other venom factors and with variable autopharmacologic responses in the victim, can result in local tissue necrosis at the bite site. *Loxosceles* venom sets up a cascading tissue response, beginning with effects on the local

18

[1]Not FDA approved for this indication.

microvasculature endothelium—resulting in occlusion and ischemia. This ischemic response may progress over days to weeks, and, in severe cases, it results in lesions of impressive size. Generally, only dermal and subcutaneous tissues are involved, but skin loss can be severe. In very rare cases, systemic poisoning occurs and results in a hemolytic syndrome. This tends to happen in young children and is related to red blood cell membrane destruction by sphingomyelinase D.

The bite is generally painless and often unwitnessed. Thus the offending spider is rarely produced for identification. Patients usually become concerned about a possible spider bite after they develop a painful skin lesion of unclear origin. Field management of a presumed brown spider bite includes local ice application and follow-up with a knowledgeable physician for evaluation.

It is extremely common for patients to present to an ED complaining of "brown recluse bite," even in areas of the country where these spiders are not indigenous. Such patients should be carefully evaluated with a history and physical examination to rule out, if possible, any other cause for the lesion (other arthropod bites, local infections [e.g., methicillin-resistant *Staphylococcus aureus*], pyoderma gangrenosa, etc.). The presence of multiple lesions is very uncommon for spider bites because spiders rarely bite more than once before they are killed or flee (they bite humans out of defense or by accident; they do not feed on us). Care must be used not to overly diagnose "spider bite" or "brown recluse bite" unless clear evidence indicates this is the case. A better working diagnosis, in the absence of the specific offending organism, is "possible arthropod envenomation."

If there are any systemic findings (e.g., fever, nausea, tachycardia), it is prudent to check a complete blood count (for hemolysis or platelet consumption) and a bedside urine check (for blood or myoglobin). If these tests are abnormal, the patient should be admitted for intravenous fluids and further testing to monitor for hemolysis. Although work continues to develop a reliable test for diagnosing *Loxosceles* venom poisoning, no commercially available test exists to date.

Most patients with small necrotic lesions can be managed at home with instructions to apply ice to the site frequently throughout the day for 72 hours. Spider venoms often contain thermolabile enzymatic components (such as sphingomyelinase D) whose activities can be inhibited by therapeutic cooling. Similarly, if a local secondary infection of the lesion is suspected, it is prudent to start a short course of a broad-spectrum antibiotic (e.g., a first-generation cephalosporin) because any increase in local tissue temperatures caused by inflammation or infection could worsen tissue damage. The mainstay of therapy is good conservative wound care, and tetanus status should be updated as needed. A patient with an isolated, relatively stable-appearing necrotic lesion is followed as an outpatient with daily wound checks until it is clear the wound is improving.

The use of other modalities to treat presumed brown spider bites is highly controversial. Some recommend oral dapsone[1] therapy. As a polymorphonuclear leukocyte inhibitor, dapsone has theoretical value in reducing dermonecrosis in significant *Loxosceles* bites. It is not,

however, approved by the Food and Drug Administration (FDA) for this use. It may be considered in a patient with a probable (or confirmed) *Loxosceles* bite that is rapidly progressing or in a cosmetically important area. The dose is 50 to 100 mg, divided twice a day until the lesion completely heals. A glucose-6-phosphate dehydrogenase (G6PD) level should be obtained at the onset of therapy to evaluate the risk for drug-induced methemoglobinemia or hemolysis. Informed consent should be obtained, and it should never be used in children.

Likewise, there is significant interest in the use of hyperbaric oxygen (HBO) therapy for severe presumed brown recluse bites. The literature remains unclear on the efficacy of this modality. If HBO is readily available to the patient, it can be tried, but great effort and expense in getting a patient to a remote center is not, at this time, advisable.

Steroids, by any route, are of no value in the management of dermal lesions caused by brown spiders. They may, however, be efficacious in the rare patient who develops systemic loxoscelism (hemolysis). Administering oral prednisone,[1] 1 mg per kg per day, for a few days may enhance red cell membrane stability and reduce hemolysis. No commercially available antivenom for *Loxosceles* bites is available in the U.S. at this time.

The most feared complication of *Loxosceles* bites is severe dermonecrosis. In reality, this is an uncommon sequela. Occasionally, however, the lesion progresses to a size that requires tissue grafting. In this case, surgery should be delayed for 6 to 8 weeks to allow the dermonecrotic process to burn out and not risk losing the graft. Early surgery in an attempt to remove venom and at-risk tissue is fruitless because the ultimate tissue margins are impossible to predict. Any débridement during the initial weeks of management should be conservative and done only to remove clearly dead tissue.

Although there are rare reports in the literature of deaths caused by brown recluse spider bites in the United States, no report of actually capturing the offending spider exists. But there are documented deaths caused by the South American brown spider, *Loxosceles laeta*. Thus the mortal potential, particularly for small children, from any *Loxosceles* species must be respected.

Scorpion Stings

Although a number of scorpions are indigenous to the United States, only one is of significant medical importance, the bark scorpion (*Centruroides exilicauda*), found throughout Arizona and occasionally occurring in border regions of contiguous states. Scorpions inject venom with the telson (or sting) at the distal portion of their abdomen (the "tip of the tail"). They may also bite or pinch, but they do not envenom by these routes.

Scorpion venoms, as a group, are complex. The venom of the bark scorpion contains a neurotoxin that causes an outpouring of neurotransmitters, resulting in severe

---

[1]Not FDA approved for this indication.

CURRENT DIAGNOSIS

- Precise identification of the offending organism is preferable whenever possible to help guide subsequent therapy.
- Severe muscle spasms that begin locally and progress over a short period of time should strongly suggest the possibility of a widow spider (*Latrodectus* species) bite.
- A necrotic lesion should not be diagnosed as a "brown recluse spider bite" unless the patient produces the offending organism. When the origin of a lesion is unclear, the diagnosis should be "possible arthropod envenomation."
- Children in Arizona who present with extreme restlessness and roving eye movements and no clear history of sting should be strongly suspected of envenomation by a bark scorpion (*Centruroides exilicauda*).

CURRENT THERAPY

- The most important aspect of management of any case of venom poisoning is sound, supportive care.
- Key modalities for treating severe muscle spasms following widow spider (*Latrodectus* species) bite may include parenteral narcotics and benzodiazepines. Widow spider antivenom (Antivenin) is effective for treating pain and other effects, but its potential benefits must be weighed against the risk of a possible allergic reaction to the heterologous serum.
- Management of a presumed brown spider (*Loxosceles* species) bite involves early cooling therapy and aggressive management of any early wound infection. Dapsone[1] is not approved for use in these bites but might be considered if the lesion is in a cosmetically important area and appears severe (a G6PD [glucose-6-phosphate dehydrogenase] level should be drawn at the time of initiating such therapy). Any required skin grafts following a presumed *Loxosceles* bite should be delayed for several weeks until the progression of necrosis abates.
- Most adults with bark scorpion (*Centruroides exilicauda*) stings can be managed conservatively at home. Young children with evidence of systemic toxicity should be admitted to the hospital for further management and monitoring. Ongoing trials are evaluating the use of foreign antivenoms for stings of the bark scorpion.
- Tetanus immunization status should be updated as needed in any victim of a bite or sting.

[1]Not FDA approved for this indication.

pain, restlessness, roving eye movements, hypersalivation, respiratory distress, opisthotonic contractions, hypertension, and tachycardia. Poisoning tends to be more severe in young children, although interestingly, pain is not a prominent feature in children younger than the age of 10 years. In adults, poisoning is usually manifested only by significant pain, and most adults can be treated at home without going to the hospital. Table 2 offers a grading scale for severity of poisoning by bark scorpions. Non-neurotoxic scorpion stings in the United States cause intense, short-lived pain, mild swelling, and no necrosis. Allergic reactions are much less common following scorpion stings than following hymenoptera stings.

Field management of scorpion stings should include local ice application to reduce pain. Small children stung in Arizona should be taken to a local ED for evaluation (along with the offending organism if possible).

TABLE 2 Severity Grading Scale for Bark Scorpion (*Centruroides exilicauda*) Stings

Grade	Symptoms/signs
I	Local pain and/or paresthesias Tenderness to light tapping over the site
II	Pain and/or paresthesias remote from the sting site
III	Skeletal muscle hyperkinesis *or* Cranial nerve dysfunction (roving eye movements, dysphagia, facial paresthesias, etc.)
IV	Skeletal muscle hyperkinesis (e.g., opisthotonus) *and* Cranial nerve dysfunction (uncontrolled eye movements, drooling, choking, etc.)

Modified from Bond GR: Antivenin administration for *Centruroides* scorpion sting: Risks and benefits. Ann Emerg Med 1992;21(7): 788-791.

Adults experiencing isolated pain can usually self-treat at home with ice and mild analgesics. If systemic symptoms occur or if the pain is severe, they should contact a poison control center or their doctor or go to the hospital for evaluation.

ED management begins with trying to identify the offending organism. The bark scorpion can generally be identified by a small tubercle at the tip of its "tail," just proximal to the "sting." Children may present without a history of sting but can usually be diagnosed based on the systemic presentation (hypersalivation, roving eye movements, restlessness). Victims with systemic findings receive cardiac and pulse oximetry monitoring and an intravenous line. Parenteral benzodiazepines are used to reduce restlessness and relax the patient. Some speculate that the narcotics administered to treat pain could have synergistic effects with scorpion venom; thus using narcotics for analgesia should be done with caution.

In the past, a non-FDA approved, goat-derived antivenom produced by Arizona State University appeared effective for serious bark scorpion stings.

18

This antiserum carried some risk of allergic reactions (both acute and delayed), and because of production problems, it is no longer available. Research is currently under way, however, to evaluate the use of a high-quality equine antivenom produced in Mexico (for a closely related *Centruroides* species) for bark scorpion stings in Arizona.

Young children with serious stings should be admitted to the hospital to an intensive care setting for observation. Older children and adults can generally be discharged home if they have obtained significant symptomatic relief in the ED (with or without antivenom) and appear stable.

Management of non-neurotoxic scorpion stings consists of intermittent ice application for pain control and appropriate non-narcotic and narcotic analgesics as needed. Almost all of these patients can be treated at home. In all scorpion stings, tetanus status should be updated as needed.

Deaths because of scorpion stings are common in Mexico and in other regions of the world, but they are exceedingly rare in the United States. Complications of stings by U.S. species are quite rare because they do not cause necrosis and rarely become secondarily infected.

REFERENCES

Allen RC, Norris RL: Delayed use of antivenin in black widow spider (*Latrodectus mactans*) envenomation. J Wilderness Med 1991;2:187-192.

Bond GR: Antivenin administration for *Centruroides* scorpion sting: Risks and benefits. Ann Emerg Med 1992;21(7):788-791.

Clark RF: Clinical presentation and treatment of black widow spider envenomation: A review of 163 cases. Ann Emerg Med 1992; 21(7):782-787.

Curry SC et al: Envenomation by the scorpion *Centruroides sculpturatus*. J Toxicol Clin Toxicol 1983-1984;21(4-5):417-419.

Daly FF, Hill RE, Bogdan GM, Dart RC: Neutralization of *Latrodectus mactans* and *L. hesperus* venom by redback spider (*L. hasseltii*) antivenom. J Clin Toxicol 2001;39:119-123.

Graudins A, et al: Red-back spider (*Latrodectus hasseltii*) antivenom prevents the toxicity of widow spider venoms. Ann Emerg Med 2001;37(2):154-160.

LoVecchio F, McBride C: Scorpion envenomations in young children in central Arizona. J Toxicol Clin Toxicol 2003;41(7):937-940.

Moss HS, Binder LS: A retrospective review of black widow spider envenomation. Ann Emerg Med 1987;16(2):188-191.

Russell FE, Gertsch WJ: Letter to the editor. Toxicon 1983;21(3): 337-339.

Wasserman GS: Wound care of spider and snake envenomations. Ann Emerg Med 1988;17:1331-1335.

Woestman R, Perkin R, Van Stralen D: The black widow: Is she deadly to children? Pediatr Emerg Care 1996;12(5):360-364.

Snakebite Poisoning

Method of
Terence M. Davidson, MD

Approximately 45,000 snakebites occur every year in the United States, of which an estimated 10,000 involve venomous snakes. Approximately 10 deaths are reported annually. The majority of snakes inhabiting the United States are important ecologically to maintain a balance with the rodent population and are of little to no harm to humans. Many harmless snakes are needlessly destroyed by those who believe all snakes are bad or by those who mistake them for venomous serpents. Education about this harmful practice is encouraged.

The vast majority of venomous snakes belong to two families: the vipers, such as the Northern American rattlesnake, family Viperidae, and the elapids, family Elapidae, such as the cobra, the Australian tiger snake, and the U.S. coral snakes. Although 250 to 300 species of venomous snakes belong to these two families, the vast majority of venomous snakes and venomous snakebites in the United States involve the rattlesnake and its close relatives, the cottonmouth and the water moccasin.

Coral snakes are present both in the western and eastern United States. Only the eastern coral snake is large enough to inflict a venomous human bite. One hundred or so coral snake bites are reported annually.

A growing number of exotic snakes live in the United States; many are kept illegally in private collections. Exotic snakebites are increasingly reported. Two resources are recommended when questions arise or expertise is needed:

1. The U.S. Poison Control Centers, which maintain expertise and important networking capabilities for the evaluation and management of snakebite

2. Protocols by this author to evaluate and manage snakebite around the world, which can be accessed online at http://www.drdavidson.org, under "Snakebite Protocols," or at http://www-surgery.ucsd.edu/ent/DAVIDSON/ Snake/Index.htm

Because the rattlesnake bite is the most common venomous snakebite in the United States, this article focuses on the evaluation and management of bites from rattlesnakes, copperheads, and water moccasins. Rattlesnakes are cold-blooded animals. They hibernate in the winter, emerging in the spring and returning in the fall. They are distributed throughout the southern half of the United States, but in some regions they inhabit areas up to the Canadian border.

The majority of snakebites fall into three categories:

1. The young adult man who keeps these animals as pets. The typical scenario is that following alcohol consumption the owner attempts to handle the snake or play the game of "who is faster."

These individuals present bitten on the hand and intoxicated.

2. The second group are children, typically boys, who are bitten while attempting to catch or handle a snake. These bites are usually located on the upper extremity.
3. The third group includes hikers, outdoor workers, and others moving around in snake-inhabited country. These bites are seen on the lower extremity or on the upper extremity when someone is reaching to pick up rocks, logs, brush, or other objects.

Death from snakebite is extremely rare; however, significant tissue destruction with substantial morbidity in untreated cases is common. Therefore, proper evaluation and management are important.

First aid and field management involve the following rules:

- Do not panic.
- Remove the bitten victim from the area of the snake to avoid a second bite.
- Remove constricting jewelry such as rings and watches.
- Apply lymphatic retardant.
- Transport the bitten victim to a medical facility.

Getting away from the snake and remaining calm is important. It is of no value to kill the snake or bring it to the emergency department. Both scenarios can lead to being bitten a second time by the same or another snake. The area of the bite will swell, and if jewelry is not removed immediately, it may have to be cut off later. There is enormous debate regarding the value of constricting band/lymphatic retardants. Definitive scientific findings do not exist for U.S. rattlesnakes.

For the Elapidae bites, wrapping and immobilization delays systemic onset of symptoms in areas such as Asia, Africa, and Australia where mortality is common in the untreated bite, especially for those bites occurring in areas far away from definitive medical care. In the United States, rattlesnake bite mortality is uncommon. A band applied as a tourniquet or as a constricting band, which then tightens with swelling and becomes a tourniquet, potentially causes serious consequences. However, a lymphatic retardant/constricting band such as a 1-inch Penrose drain, as used in vena puncture, slows down venom absorption and, if properly applied, is an important adjunct to first aid.

Morbidity and mortality do not occur for hours or even days. Hence transportation to a medical facility for definitive treatment is important but not urgent. Helicopters are not generally required. Particularly with a lymphatic retardant in place, a 12- to 24-hour delay before instituting medical treatment is acceptable. The victim should be transported expeditiously, but there is no need to incur added danger by hurried evacuation.

Many myths surround the management of snakebite. Cryotherapy is contraindicated because it enhances tissue destruction. Electric shock therapy is contraindicated. Once reported by the *Lancet* to be of value,

this therapy makes no physiologic sense. Electric shock treatment fails to provide any significant improvement and has resulted in reported deaths. Incision and suction is contraindicated. The Sawyer pump extractor, developed in Europe for bee sting extraction, is touted as a first-aid treatment but is of no value. Some question the advisability of carrying antivenin in the field, but it is generally discouraged unless 10 to 20 vials are carried and the medical kit contains all of the necessary equipment for cardiopulmonary resuscitation.

Evaluation in a medical facility begins with a history confirming that snakebite occurred. Hysterical people are often mistaken about what bit them.

The initial signs and symptoms of snakebite include pain and swelling, with typical onset of both in 5 to 10 minutes. As the venom is absorbed, additional proteolytic activity is seen with bleb formation and extension of the edema up the bitten extremity. The majority of venoms are hemotoxic. They lyse fibrinogen and consume platelets. Subcutaneous hemorrhage is noted as a bluish discoloration. Blebs can be filled with serosanguineous fluid. Systemic effects of venom include third spacing of fluid with hemoconcentration, decreased serum potassium, and increased serum calcium and circumoral tingling, probably as a result of the electrolyte changes just described. If a severe bite is allowed to progress, hypotension, cardiovascular collapse, coma, and death ensue.

Neurotoxic symptoms are rarely seen except in the most severe of rattlesnake bites. Systemic effects of anticoagulation include bleeding from the gums, hemoptysis, hematuria, and bleeding from needle puncture sites.

Approximately 20% of rattlesnake bites inflict no envenomation. These are often termed *dry bites*. In such cases, no local or systemic symptoms are noted. If any symptoms are noted, laboratory evaluation is required, including a complete blood count (CBC), electrolytes, calcium, some measure of hepatic and renal function, and a coagulation profile. The most important monitor of coagulation difficulties is the quantitative platelet count. Fibrinogen and fibrin split products are often useful monitors of the progression of envenomation. Intrinsic and extrinsic bleeding measures, such as ProTime, partial thromboplastin time (PTT), and international normalized ratio (INR), are rarely abnormal unless coagulopathy is advanced. Laboratory data should be repeated periodically and sometimes are useful in monitoring the progression of envenomation and the therapy.

Mild bites are those in which signs and symptoms are restricted to the bite site, typically the distal extremity. Moderate bites are those with symptoms extending up the extremity as swelling, blebs, or fasciculations. More advanced or severe bites are those with systemic manifestations, typically coagulopathy, hypotension, and generalized muscular fasciculation. Mild bites can be observed. This is not uncommon with water moccasin and cottonmouth bites. However, once symptoms advance to involve the proximal extremity, more aggressive therapy is recommended.

The mainstay of medical therapy is the intravenous infusion of antivenom. In the majority of the world, skin testing is not used. However, skin testing is typically practiced in the United States. Assuming horse serum sensitivity is not identified, the most commonly available antivenin is the Wyeth Crotalidae Antivenin, which is effective against all North American pit vipers. The Wyeth Antivenin is an immune serum obtained from horses. It is infused intravenously, and the amount required is determined by monitoring the signs and symptoms of envenomation. An ovine (sheep) antivenin called CroFab is currently available for North American crotalid envenomation. Details of administration are similar to the Wyeth equine antivenin.

The Wyeth equine antivenin is seemingly weak. It is recommended that antivenin treatment employ 5-vial aliquots. In the mildest of bites, the initial treatment may begin with 5 vials, but in more advanced bites, treatment should begin with 10 vials. The average rattlesnake treatment in the United States requires 20 vials. If a therapeutic mistake is made, it is giving too little too slowly. Five vials of antivenin are diluted in 50 mL of diluent or normal saline. The antivenin is typically infused at a rate of 1 vial every 7 to 10 minutes. The signs and symptoms of envenomation are then monitored. The antivenin typically halts progression without reversing many of the signs and symptoms. Once the antivenin infusion is completed, the patient must be monitored for progression of the symptoms. Pain is a very sensitive symptom. Edema is an insensitive sign. Progression of edema is a sensitive sign. Muscular fasciculation is typically not sensitive. Circumoral tingling is an insensitive symptom. Quantitative platelets are a sensitive laboratory sign, as is bleeding from the gums, at the bite site, or in the urine. Antivenin infusion is continued in 5-vial aliquots. As much as 5 to 10 vials of antivenin can be delivered per hour. Once the patient is stabilized and the progression of symptoms halted, the patient is monitored in an intensive care setting. The following morning, laboratory values are repeated, the patient is evaluated, and if all is well on both accounts, the patient may be discharged to home.

Immediate allergic reactions are uncommon. Some patients may respond negatively to a rapid infusion of antivenin. In these cases, simply stopping the infusion and restarting 10 to 15 minutes later at a slower rate is beneficial. Anaphylaxis is sometimes seen. In these cases, which are often extremely difficult to manage and can be fatal, the antivenin infusion must be stopped. Steroids, vasopressors, antihistamines, and fluids should all be available and administered appropriately. Delayed cutaneous allergic reactions are common, occurring in 20% to 30 % of treated patients. Patients typically present with pruritus and urticaria 7 to 20 days following treatment. Antihistamines are theoretically the first line of treatment. A short course of systemic steroids is the most effective treatment.

A number of special circumstances and conditions can arise. If the patient has a positive skin test, the inexperienced snakebite physician is strongly encouraged to call the local poison control center and request assistance from a colleague with experience in snakebite. In these cases, antivenin can very often be administered, but it must be delivered in a diluted concentration, such as 1 vial in 100 mL of lactated Ringer's solution, administered slowly, such as 1 mL per minute for 5 minutes, wait 10 minutes, then 1 mL per minute for the remaining 95 mL. Many individuals with positive skin reactions do not demonstrate systemic reactions. However, those that do have extremely serious reactions, which can be fatal.

The next question is whether there is advantage to the equine or the ovine crotalid polyvalent antivenins. Both are expensive, with the ovine antivenin costing the most. CroFab has a distinct disadvantage of often requiring additional administration at 24 hours. The ovine antivenin has the advantage of being safe in those with horse sensitivity.

Importantly, both antivenins cause allergy, so exposure potentially affects future administration. Therefore, antivenin should never be administered if not required, and both types of antivenin should never be administered for the same bite. In other words, if antivenin therapy is initiated with one antivenin, the therapy should be completed with the same antivenin. The antivenin must not be changed unless absolutely necessary.

The principles of ovine antivenin therapy are almost identical to those of equine antivenin therapy. The details differ slightly. In mild to moderate bites, 4 to 6 vials of CroFab antivenin are diluted in 100 mL of saline. In moderate to severe bites, 6 vials are diluted in 100 mL of saline, administered intravenously over a 1-hour period. The package insert recommends administering 2 additional vials every 6 hours for 3 additional doses (6 vials total). The University of California San Diego (UCSD) Poison Control Center recommends administering additional vials on an as-needed basis. If symptoms progress, 2 vials are diluted in saline and administered over 20 to 30 minutes.

Signs, symptoms, and labs are checked periodically over the ensuing 24 hours. When the patient is stable over 24 hours, he or she can be discharged to home and followed up at 48 hours and at anytime if symptoms recur. Anaphylactic and allergic reactions are uncommon, but should they occur, they are managed identically to those resulting from other medications.

In moderate and advanced bites, extremity edema can progress to a point where arterial pulses are not palpable and may even be difficult to hear by Doppler. There is always concern that a compartment syndrome has evolved and surgical intervention is indicated.

Capillary perfusion invariably persists and is best checked at the fingernail beds. Most likely, wick measurements show the subcutaneous pressures are elevated, but the compartment pressures are not raised above 30 mm. Fasciotomy is virtually never indicated, with the possible exception of the extremely uncommon bite in which venom is delivered into the muscle compartment. This scenario is extremely uncommon in North American pit viper bites.

Excision of the bite site was once recommended as a surgical therapy. Certainly if one conducts a wide

CURRENT DIAGNOSIS

The signs and symptoms of rattlesnake bite are as follows:

- Fang marks
- Swelling and edema
- Pain
- Numbness or tingling of lips or affected part
- Ecchymosis
- Decreased blood platelets
- Decreased fibrinogen
- Increased fibrin split products
- Fasciculations
- Vesiculations/blebs
- Increased blood clotting time
- Proteinuria
- Hematuria
- Necrosis
- Unconsciousness
- Convulsions

Modified from Russell, FE: Snake Venom Poisoning. Great Neck, NY, Scholium International, 1983.

excision soon after envenomation, the need for systemic antivenin might be obviated. The resultant scar is not a reasonable trade-off. Twenty vials of antivenin are far preferable than cutting off a finger or all the skin on the dorsal hand or foot. Surgical excision is therefore not indicated.

 CURRENT THERAPY

First Aid

- Get away from the snake.
- Remove constricting jewelry.
- Apply constricting band.
- Keep calm.
- Transport to medical facility.

Medical Treatment

- Start intravenous (IV) line and hydrate.
- Draw labs: complete blood count (CBC) with differential, electrolytes, calcium, phosphorus, liver function tests (LFTs), creatinine, prothrombin time (PT), partial thromboplastin time/international normalized ratio (PTT/INR), platelets, fibrinogen, and fibrin split products.
- Assess for envenomation early symptoms and signs, pain and swelling.
- For envenomation, initiate antivenom therapy with equine or ovine antivenom (requires a skin test).
- Titrate antivenom against symptoms of envenomation (average treatment is 20 vials of Wyeth polyvalent antivenom or 6 or more vials of CroFab; observe in hospital until symptom progression free for a minimum of 12 hours).

Modified from Davidson, TM: Intravenous rattlesnake envenomation. West J Med 1988;148:45-47.

Rakel and Bope: *Conn's Current Therapy 2006.*

The 10 or so deaths per year from snakebite occur predominantly in two circumstances. In the first, an intravenous bite is inflicted and the patient succumbs within 15 to 20 minutes. In the second, a large snake inflicts a large bite with a lethal venom infusion, and the patient either fails to report for medical therapy or is so far removed from medical therapy that it cannot be provided in a timely fashion.

Intravenous (IV) infusions can be managed by early recognition and treatment with 1 g of methylprednisolone (Solu-Medrol) IV followed by 20 vials of antivenin administered IV push over 5 to 10 minutes.

Treatment of coral and exotic snakebites follows identical principles. Assuming one knows the inflicting snake, one need only know the signs and symptoms and then administer the specific antivenin in appropriate quantities. Antivenin for coral snakes is commercially available. Because exotic antivenins are not typically available in the United States, this can be problematic. Poison control centers are the best resources for these cases.

As in most fields of medicine, prevention is always wise. Individuals in areas infested by snakes should be encouraged to remain sober, dress sensibly, and watch where they are reaching and stepping. Proper clothing for snake-infested areas includes long pants and ankle-high boots for most situations. In heavily infested areas in which the individual may be required to travel through brush, a midcalf boot theoretically offers greater protection. Knee-high gaiters may provide additional protection.

18

Marine Trauma, Envenomations, and Intoxications

Method of
Charles K. Brown, MD

Our planet is 71% water. Four fifths of all organisms reside there, and many have unique methods of attack and defense. Although references date to ancient times, and some of the most potent toxins known are marine in origin, only in the last several decades have physicians approached scientifically the management of injuries and illnesses produced by marine creatures. As humans increase their encounters with the marine environment, the risk of hazardous encounters with ocean-dwelling organisms increases as well. Air travel rapidly moves both people and seafood internationally, virtually eliminating regional illnesses and intoxications. Physicians encounter patients presenting after marine injuries or intoxication and must be prepared to rapidly diagnose and treat life-threatening envenomations and intoxications.

The number of potentially hazardous organisms is enormous, yet the various syndromes may be categorized and often are treated similarly. Patients present with generally one of three encounter types: traumatic incidents, toxic ingestions, or venomous bites, stings, or skin exposures (by far the most common). Traumatic incidents require basic and advanced trauma care, and the general principles of Advanced Trauma Life Support apply. Toxic ingestions are mostly self-limited gastrointestinal illnesses requiring supportive care unless the patient has co-morbid conditions that are affected and require specific measures. Some ingestions and envenomations have life-threatening cardiovascular, respiratory, and/or neurologic symptoms. Care for these patients requires analgesia and intensive support of airway and respiratory functions unless an antidote is available. Skin exposures are usually an irritant dermatitis acutely, and local care is required.

Shark

Shark attacks are overly dramatized but uncommon; less than 100 proven shark attacks and 12 deaths have been recorded in the Unites States since 1926, with 100 to 150 reported but unproven attacks annually worldwide. Inhabiting coastal waters of North America, South Africa, and southern Australia, the sharks most often implicated in human attacks are the great white, blue, mako, bull, and gray reef sharks. Safe water conduct is paramount to prevent shark attacks. Recommendations include avoiding shark-infested waters, especially at night or dusk, avoiding turbid waters near waste outlets and deep channels; and never swimming with open wounds or in isolated areas. It is controversial whether menstruating women are at higher risk of attack. Bright, reflective swimwear and equipment are attractants. Captured fish should be tethered or stored away from divers. Chemical shark repellants are not successful, and an electrical device is being developed.

Patient management centers on basic trauma care: airway, breathing, bleeding control, and management of hypovolemic shock. Tetanus immune globulin (BayTet), 250 U intramuscularly (IM), tetanus toxoid (Td), 0.5 mL IM for patients older than 7 years of age, and prophylactic trimethoprim-sulfamethoxazole DS (TMP-SMX) (Bactrim DS), 1 tablet by mouth twice a day for 7 to 10 days, or ciprofloxacin (Cipro), 500 mg by mouth twice a day for 7 to 10 days, is suggested. Imipenem cilastin (Primaxin), 250 to 1000 mg intravenously (IV) every 6 to 8 hours, or a third-generation cephalosporin, for example, ceftriaxone (Rocephin), 1 to 2 g IM/IV every 24 hours, or ceftazidime (Fortaz), 1 to 2 g IM/IV every 8 to 12 hours, is additionally indicated for established infections. Wounds is prone to contamination with aerobes and anaerobes, including *Aeromonas*, *Vibrio*, and *Clostridia*. Wound care must include vigorous irrigation, débridement, and exploration. Wounds are usually packed open, and delayed primary closure is used.

Barracuda

The great barracuda, *Sphyraena barracuda*, is the only species implicated in human attacks. Solitary fish are the rule, but occasionally schools are involved in attacks. Their wide mouth is filled with large knifelike teeth. The Atlantic range is from Brazil to Florida, and the Indo-Pacific range is from the Red Sea to Hawaii. All attacks occur in tropical seas. An attack is swift and fierce, often occurring out of confusion and in murky waters. The large knifelike teeth produce straight or V-shaped lacerations often in rows (versus an arcuate shark bite). Barracudas are attracted to the same stimuli as sharks, and avoidance is the best means of prevention. Patients should be managed as victims of penetrating trauma, analogous to shark bites.

Moray Eel

Moray eel, powerful bottom dwellers of tropical, subtropical, and temperate waters, may reach 10 feet in length. Living under rocks or coral and in holes or crevices, they evade confrontation unless cornered. Their narrow viselike jaws and sharp fanglike teeth inflict severe lacerations through biting and holding. The moray eel may need to be beheaded or have its jaw broken to release the victim. Treatment is analogous to shark bites.

Giant Grouper

Species of the family Serranidae (sea bass, grouper) inhabit tropical and temperate seas; the giant grouper grows to 12 feet in length and can weigh 1000 pounds. These curious, pugnacious, voracious feeders are feared because of their large size, boldness, and cavernous jaws. They inhabit old wrecks and caverns and lurk behind rocks. Treatment is the same as for shark bites.

Others

Sea lions can be aggressive, particularly mating males and females with pups. Bites can result in significant wounds. Because this is a mammalian bite, rabies prophylaxis may be necessary: rabies immune globulin human (Imogam Rabies HT, BayRab), 20 U/kg with as much as possible infiltrated around the wound, and then rabies vaccine (Imovax Rabies), 1 mL IM deltoid on days 0, 3, 7, 14, and 28. The killer whale, *Orcinus orca*, inhabits all oceans and grows to 30 feet in length. Although no documented attacks are recorded, a human could easily be mistaken for a sea lion. Needlefish (family Belonidae) are slender, lightning-quick surface swimmers that resemble freshwater gar. They inhabit tropical waters and attain lengths of 6 to 7 feet, often leaping out of the water and spearing people unintentionally. Treatment is according to the nature and location of the wound.

Envenomations and Intoxications

Marine zootoxins are of three types:

1. *Oral*—bacterial products and products of decomposition
2. *Parenteral*—venoms produced in specialized glands and injected with specialized devices
3. *Crinotoxin*—venoms produced in specialized glands and administered without injection (i.e., slime)

All venoms are poisons, but all poisons are not venoms. Venoms are of large molecular weight with vasoactive compounds and proteolytic enzymes, whereas poisons are smaller protein or polypeptide metabolic byproducts of animals or plants. Both can cause widespread immunologic, cardiovascular, and neurologic dysfunction. Venoms and poisons can frustrate researchers because both lack sufficient immunogenicity to foster development of antitoxins and antivenoms.

BONEY FISH

Boney fish that cause envenomation include lionfish, scorpionfish, stonefish, weeverfish, and catfish. At least 200 species of fish envenomate victims by their spines. The boney fish generally have heat-labile, short-chain polypeptide toxins that are present in the fish up to 24 hours after its death. The family Scorpaenidae is the most dangerous, composed of 30 genera and 350 species, at least 80 of which are known to cause venomous injuries. Other vertebrate envenomations occur from stingrays and sea snakes.

SCORPIONFISH

Scorpionfish inhabit warm shallow reef waters in a worldwide distribution and public and private aquariums. Less venomous varieties are seen on the west and southeast U.S. coasts. These bottom dwellers have very effective camouflage. The scorpionfish are divided into three genera: *Scorpaena* (sculpin, bullrout, and scorpionfish); *Synanceja* (stonefish); and *Pterosis* (zebrafish, lionfish, and butterfly cod). The stonefish, inhabiting Indo-Pacific waters, are the most lethal. Stonefish venom, similar to cobra venom, can precipitate cholinergic and adrenergic discharges, acting primarily on muscle. An estimated 300 scorpionfish envenomations occur annually in the United States.

The degree of envenomation depends on the species, the number and location of stings, the amount of venom injected, and the general health of the patient. Pain is severe and immediate, radiating up the extremity. Stonefish envenomation may cause pain severe enough to produce delusions and may, rarely, persist for days. Pain peaks at 60 to 90 minutes and may last 6 to 12 hours. The site is initially ischemic and pale and then cyanotic with erythema, edema, and possible vesicle formation leading to ulceration. Many systemic autonomic and neurologic manifestations can occur. The paresthesias and numbness often persist for weeks, and the wound is often present for months. With stonefish envenomation;

dyspnea, hypotension, and cardiovascular collapse occur within 1 hour, and death usually occurs within 6 hours if not treated.

The affected limb should be immersed in hot water (45°C/113°F) for 30 to 90 minutes or until pain is relieved. The extremity may be reimmersed if pain persists. Local anesthetic infiltration or regional nerve block with 1% to 2% plain lidocaine or 0.25% plain bupivacaine (Marcaine) may be needed. Cryotherapy is contraindicated. Wounds should be copiously irrigated with warm saline and explored, with all slime and debris removed. The wound should be left open and treated with antibiotics, as discussed earlier, if deep wounds are present on the hand or foot. Stonefish equine antivenom (Commonwealth Serum Laboratories, Australia) is obtained from Sea World in San Diego and Cleveland, Sharp Cabrillo Hospital in San Diego, and the Steinhart Aquarium in San Francisco. One milliliter of antivenom should neutralize 10 mg of venom. Anaphylaxis and serum sickness are possible, and sensitivity testing using 0.02 mL of 1:10 antivenom dilution intradermally should be done. If envenomation is severe, 2 mL IM or IV should be administered, repeating as needed; one vial should handle two stings.

STINGRAYS

Stingrays are the most commonly encountered venomous fish, with approximately 2000 stings reported annually. Rays burrow in sand beneath shallow water, and when startled, they hurl their tails upward defensively, their barbs causing venom-laden lacerations and punctures. Secondary infection is common. The venom is highly unstable and very heat labile. It includes a number of toxic compounds, including phosphodiesterases and 5'-nucleotidases, that produce varying degrees of cardiovascular and neurologic disturbance in addition to severe pain. Its effects do not appear because of paralysis of neuromuscular transmission. The mechanism is unclear.

Injuries occur most commonly on the lower extremities, followed by the upper extremities, abdomen, and thorax. Abdominal and thoracic wounds may cause major organ trauma. Symptoms are immediate and may persist for several days. Initial treatment, after addressing any life threats, should include rapid irrigation of the wound with cold sterile saline or water solution to provide mild anesthesia, local vasoconstriction and removal of sheath contents left in the wound, and explorations. Other suggested treatments include superficial venous and lymphatic occlusion with a wide constriction band released for 90 seconds every 10 minutes and/or mechanical suction if immediately applied. The wound should be soaked in hot water (45°C/113°F) for 30 to 90 minutes. Pain control may be augmented with infiltration locally of 1% to 2% plain lidocaine or 0.25% plain bupivacaine (Marcaine). Cryotherapy is contraindicated. Narcotics are a useful adjunct for pain control (morphine, IM/IV 0.1 mg/kg per dose titrated to effect). The wound should be débrided and packed open. Antibiotic prophylaxis is recommended, as discussed previously. Steroids and antihistamines are without evidence of efficacy.

CATFISH

More than 1000 species of freshwater and saltwater catfish exist. *Plotosus lineatus* (oriental catfish) envenomation may cause significant systemic as well as local symptoms. The venom contains dermatonecrotic, vasoconstrictive, and other bioactive agents. Both freshwater and saltwater venoms are heat labile, unaffected by freezing and poorly antigenic; they behave and are treated similarly to mild stingray venom but cause much less severe symptoms.

An instantaneous stinging, throbbing, or burning sensation occurs and usually resolves in 30 to 60 minutes. Pain occasionally lasts 48 hours. The wound appears ischemic, and swelling can be significant. Gangrene may occur. When infection occurs there is a high incidence of *Aeromonas* species, resistant to TMP-SMX (Bactrim) and tetracycline, so antibiotics should be adjusted accordingly. There are no antidotes. The spines are radiopaque and must be sought after as foreign bodies.

WEEVERFISH

Also known as adderpike, sea dragon, sea cat, and stang, weeverfish are small (less than 46 cm) stout-bodied fish inhabiting flat sandy or muddy-bottomed bays. The victims are usually professional fishers or wading vacationers who caught the fish in a net or disturbed it. Weeverfish are the most venomous fish found in the temperate zone, inhabiting the Mediterranean Sea, east Atlantic Ocean, and European coastal waters. Generally sedentary, they strike very accurately if provoked. The spines can penetrate a leather boot and result in substantial punctures. Venom contains 5-hydroxytryptamine, two peptides, and a mucopolysaccharide, among other biogenic compounds.

The puncture results in an intense burning pain that is difficult to control. Pain is instantaneous and described as burning or crushing, quickly spreading throughout the entire limb. Pain peaks at 30 minutes and usually lasts 24 hours, but it can persist for several days and produce delirium and syncope. An initially pale and edematous puncture site develops erythema, warmth, ecchymosis, and significant edema. Total healing time may take months. A broad array of systemic symptoms may accompany envenomation, and secondary infection is common. As with stingrays, no commercial antidote is available and treatment is essentially the same. Narcotics are poorly effective. Spines occasionally are found in the wound. Prevention is primarily avoidance, wearing sufficiently protective footwear, and never handling weeverfish when alive. The fish can survive for hours out of water and should still be handled with extreme caution.

SEA SNAKES

The most dangerous sea snake is *Enhydrina schistosa*, a close relative of the cobra and krait, and all 52 species

are venomous. At least seven are implicated in fatalities. They are native to Indo-Pacific waters but also found in the Gulf of California. There are no sea snakes in the Atlantic Ocean or Caribbean. Sea snakes have a patchy, finlike tail, are generally nonaggressive, and they are encountered during summer months or when entangled in fishing nets. Sea snakes have two to four maxillary fangs, each associated with paired venom glands. The fangs are short and easily dislodged; hence most bites are without envenomation. The venom, containing neurotoxins acting at both presynaptic and postsynaptic terminals, is more potent than that in any terrestrial snake. The presynaptic toxins initially release acetylcholine, then block its resynthesis both in the peripheral and autonomic nervous systems. The postsynaptic toxins attach irreversibly to the acetylcholine receptor at the motor endplate, blocking neuromuscular transmission. Myotoxins, including phospholipase A, cause striated muscle necrosis and myoglobin release, occurring as early as 30 minutes and as late as 8 hours after the bite. Many tissue-toxic enzymes, hemotoxins, direct cardiotoxins, and vasoactive compounds are also present.

When bitten, the patient is initially asymptomatic and without pain. Symptoms can develop within 5 to 10 minutes and are usually present within 2 hours after the bite and certainly by 6 to 8 hours later. Usually 1 to 4 (but up to 20) hypodermic-like punctures are found. Painful, stiff muscle movements and myoglobinuria are the hallmarks of envenomation. Initial systemic complaints are a thick tongue, euphoria, malaise, and anxiety progressing to dysarthria, ophthalmoplegia, ptosis, trismus, and ascending flaccid or spastic paralysis. The causes of death are usually respiratory failure or aspiration (bulbar paralysis), hyperkalemia, or acute renal failure from hemoglobinuria or myoglobinuria. Early congestive heart failure and late acute renal failure are noted, and intensive supportive respiratory and circulatory care is often needed. Diagnosis of the bite is based on several factors: occurrence in the water, initial absence of pain, multiple tiny fang marks, identification of the snake, and the characteristic symptoms of painful muscle movement, lower extremity paralysis, trismus, and ptosis. If no symptoms occur by 6 to 8 hours, no envenomation has occurred.

Treatment is similar to that for elapid bites, with dependent pressure immobilization to localize the venom and minimize systemic distribution. The patient should remain quiet and warm. Incision and drainage is generally not recommended, and cryotherapy is contraindicated. An equine polyvalent antivenom obtained from *Enhydrina schistosa* and *Notechis scutatus* is available from Commonwealth Serum Laboratories (Australia) and indicated in envenomation. Administration is effective up to 24 to 36 hours after envenomation and should begin promptly. After anaphylaxis skin testing, at least 1 and up to 10 ampoules may be required. Polyvalent tiger snake antivenom[1] is an accepted alternative, beginning with one ampule and titrating the dose to

---

[1]Not FDA approved for this indication.

the clinical situation. Respiratory and renal function must be closely monitored because mechanical ventilation may be required, and hyperkalemia secondary to rhabdomyolysis is not uncommon. Hemodialysis was reported effective in two cases but is not an established mode of therapy for venom removal.

Infectious Agents

Infection is a hazard with any marine wound and should be treated appropriately. *Vibrio* species are part of coastal flora and an established source of extraintestinal infections. These are potential pathogens for severe wound infection, bacteremia, and sepsis. *Vibrio vulnificus* can cause wound infection in any patient or primary septicemia in those patients with underlying chronic disease, such as diabetes, leukemia, chronic renal failure, steroid-dependent asthma, and especially chronic liver disease. Infections with this organism are most common during the warmer months and can be caused by ingesting raw or undercooked seafood. A variety of local manifestations occur, but the more severe infections have necrotic features; a pustular bullous eruption occasionally progresses to necrotizing fasciitis. These patients appear toxic, and examination reveals extensive necrotic tissue. Wounds have intense pain, swelling, and cellulitis that can rapidly progress to bullae and massive swelling. Gangrene is reported. Treatment combines aggressive wound care, including débridement of necrotic tissue and antibiotic therapy. A combination of cefotaxime (Claforan), 1 to 2 g IM/IV every 6 to 8 hours, and minocycline (Minocin), 200 mg IV/PO initially, then 100 mg every 12 hours, is shown effective in vitro.

Primary septicemia is associated with ingestion of contaminated shellfish, especially oysters. *Vibrio* enter through the gastrointestinal mucosa, and asymptomatic carriage is possible. Clinically, findings vary from abrupt onset of fever and chills with abdominal pain, nausea, vomiting, and diarrhea to bullae, hypotension, and hypoperfusion states. Mortality approaching 50% is reported. The onset of fever and chills is abrupt. Secondary skin lesions appear within 24 hours and are associated with extreme pain. Treatment of sepsis includes antibiotics, vasopressors, and intense supportive care. More than 90% mortality is reported when hypotension occurred within the first 12 hours. Treatment combines aggressive wound care, including débridement of necrotic tissue and antibiotic therapy as noted earlier.

Aeromonas hydrophilia can cause wound infections, gastrointestinal symptoms, or septicemia. Initially cellulitic soft tissue infection can progress to fasciitis, gas-forming infection, or sepsis. Fever, chills, hypotension, or jaundice is common with septicemia. Immunosuppressed patients or those with chronic liver disease are most susceptible. A host of antibiotics are effective.

Hepatitis A has produced several large outbreaks from raw clam and oyster ingestion since the 1960s. Norwalk virus causes a self-limited although potentially severe gastroenteritis after consumption of contaminated shellfish. Nine marine species of *Vibrio* are associated with human infection, including *Vibrio cholera*. Cholera can surface virtually anywhere because of both rapid worldwide transport of raw seafood and increased world travel. Cholera produces a life-threatening enteritis that may progress to hypovolemia, acidosis, or acute renal failure. *Vibrio parahaemolyticus* causes one half of food poisonings worldwide and is associated with improperly cooked crustaceans (especially shrimp). Tetracycline (Sumycin), 250 to 500 mg four times per day taken orally, may abbreviate this illness if given within the first 48 hours. *Erysipelothrix rhusiopathiae* causes fish handler's disease, which is manifested by a characteristic ring lesion around the contaminated puncture and best treated with oral penicillin (Pen-Vee K), 250 to 500 mg four times per day, or ciprofloxacin. Botulism may result from ingestion of improperly processed fish and roe. *Campylobacter, Salmonella, Shigella*, and *Escherichia coli* are only occasionally traced to seafood. Several helminthic infections are possible, primarily from the consumption of raw fish.

Venomous Invertebrates

Humans are frequently exposed to venomous invertebrates. Coelenterates of the phylum Cnidaria are commonly encountered when swimming in salt or brackish water. Stings are the most common injury. Classes are Scyphozoa (true jellyfish), Hydrozoa (Portuguese man-of-war, blue bottle), and Anthozoa (sea anemones, soft coral). These organisms envenomate prey through nematocysts bathed in venom. Composition varies between species and has direct and indirect effects on the autonomic nervous system and end organs, particularly the heart, central nervous, skin, and vascular systems. The venom is shown experimentally in animals to produce a general destabilizing action on the cell membrane.

COELENTERATES

Both living and dead jellyfish as well as separated tentacles can cause envenomation. The sting produced is a linear painful erythematous eruption, which may blister and persist for 7 days. Jellyfish produce three grades of envenomation: mild, consisting solely of skin irritation; intermediate, producing stinging, pruritus, paresthesias, throbbing, and central radiation; and severe, with systemic symptoms involving multiple organ systems. Neurologic, cardiovascular, respiratory, musculoskeletal, gastrointestinal, and ocular reactions may occur. Chronic manifestations may include keloids, hyperpigmentation, flat atrophy, contractures, gangrene, urticaria, muscle spasm, autonomic nerve paralysis, bladder paralysis, and mononeuritis. Cutaneous lesion should be sought in cases of unexplained water-related collapse or near drowning. In these circumstances, scraping fresh skin wheals with a scalpel or the edge of a glass slide or using tape to lift off nematocysts may help make the diagnosis.

Probably the most dangerous jellyfish is the box jellyfish or sea wasp, *Chironex fleckeri*, of the south Pacific, found mainly in Australian waters off northern Queensland. A much less lethal variety is found in the Chesapeake Bay. Larger specimens can inject more than 10 mL of venom, causing cardiorespiratory death in less than a minute and an overall mortality of 15% to 20%. More than 70 documented fatalities are reported from Australia. *C. fleckeri* toxin's dominant active components are proteinaceous. An active musculotoxic agent and a vasopermeability toxin, possibly serotonin, have been isolated. Sea wasp antivenom made from sheep serum (Commonwealth Serum Laboratories, Australia) is available and should be used for all *Chironex* envenomations. It is best given IV (20,000 U [one vial] over 5 minutes), but three vials can be administered IM. The same anaphylactic precautions as with other animal-based antivenoms should be observed. Clinically, if patients have more than one half of one limb involved or loss of consciousness, immediate transport to a hospital for antivenom is indicated. The Irukandji syndrome is reported from stings of the Cuboza class of jellyfish (*Carutria barnesi*). Stings are characterized by rapidly developing pulmonary edema leading to acute respiratory failure in young healthy people. Although the pathophysiology is unclear, the symptoms are similar to unchecked catecholamine release.

All patients with suspected *Chironex* envenomation should be observed for 6 to 8 hours after treatment because rebound phenomena are reported. Pain control becomes a major hurdle once the nematocysts are removed. Narcotics are generally required and should be used as needed. Methocarbamol (Robaxin), 1 g slowly, diazepam (Valium), or other muscle relaxants can be used to alleviate cramps. A 10% calcium gluconate solution (5 to 10 mL IV) is effective in relieving muscle spasms if given acutely.

Portuguese man-of-war (*Physalia physalis*) are found in the Gulf of Mexico and off Florida from July to September. Consisting of a floating sail (up to 30 cm across) and a number of tentacles up to 30 m in length, these creatures contain up to several million nematocysts. The Pacific blue bottle (*Physalia utriculus*) is smaller, having only one tentacle up to 15 m in length. *Physalia* toxin is proteinaceous and induces histamine release and prostaglandin-induced vasodilation, and it is believed to act at the level of the sarcolemma. This action may be blocked by nonsteroidal anti-inflammatory drugs. Hemolysis, because of toxin interaction with the red blood cell membrane, can occur. Clinically, *Physalia* envenomations are similar to lesser jellyfish but carry much more likelihood of a severe reaction. Acute renal failure was reported in a patient after experiencing a severe *Physalia* sting. A severe hemolytic reaction occurred and was suspected of causing pigment-induced nephropathy. Erythema nodosum is also reported and may recur up to 4 weeks later.

Treatment of a jellyfish sting is controversial on many points and must be somewhat species specific, but all authorities seem to agree on one point: Do not immerse the area in fresh water. Initial seawater rinsing is recommended to maintain isosmolar conditions. Current recommendations to inactivate nematocysts still present on the skin include application of 5% acetic acid solution (vinegar) for 30 seconds or until pain subsides. Stingose (Hamilton Laboratories, Adelaide, Australia) (aluminum sulfate surfactant) or, as a last resort, isopropyl alcohol (40% to 70%) can be used. The wound should not be rubbed because that may discharge more nematocysts or induce skin trauma. Some argue that Stingose is ineffective. For moderate to severe or large surface area stings, a pressure immobilization technique is used after vinegar application. A cloth or gauze, approximately 6 to 8 cm by 6 to 8 cm and 3 cm thick, is applied over the sting tightly but not so tight as to occlude arterial inflow. The area of the sting is believed to become locally ischemic and venous, and lymphatic obstruction may preclude systemic absorption of the venom. The extremity and patient is immobilized and transported to medical care. For minor stings, after deactivation, to care for yourself, a baking soda or sand/mud paste or shaving cream may be applied, followed by gentle shaving to remove attached nematocysts. Tetanus prophylaxis should be current. Mild topical steroids and antihistamines may be indicated for symptomatic relief. Local or topical anesthetics may be soothing when used after removal of nematocysts, but a paradoxic reaction is reported to topical benzocaine (Americaine). There is no basis for prophylactic antibiotic administration. A popular but unproven method is application of Adolph's meat tenderizer (papain). Study of optimum methods is ongoing.

Other invertebrates causing human envenomation include the *Anthozoa* (sea anemones, corals) and *Echinodermata* (sea urchins, starfish, sea cucumbers). These are usually encountered by skin divers or tide pool scavengers. Sea anemones are flowerlike sessile creatures, ranging from a few millimeters to 0.5 m in diameter. After encountering the hell's fire anemone (*Actinodendron plumosum*), the origin of the name becomes readily apparent.

Fire coral (*Millepora* species), found on rocks, pilings, and other coral, are not true corals. They resemble a tiny brush, usually 7 to 10 cm in length, but can grow to 2 m. An initial stinging or burning pain on contact is often followed by severe pruritus and urticaria. Rubbing the area worsens envenomation. Untreated, pain resolves in 90 minutes and wheals flatten within 24 hours and resolve within 1 week. Residual hyperpigmentation may persist up to 8 weeks. Treatment for both *Anthozoa* and *Millepora* stings is analogous to jellyfish stings. Persistent rash may respond to a 2-week tapered course of prednisone.

Contact with hard corals causes lacerations contaminated by debris and abundant marine microorganisms. Wounds may heal poorly, leaving a scar or forming a granuloma. Treatment includes aggressive cleansing with saline and hydrogen peroxide, appropriate débridement, and application of a topical antibiotic to cover the marine organisms mentioned previously. The term *coral reef granuloma* is a misnomer; actually it is a tropical streptococcal or staphylococcal pyoderma with wound hyperplasia.

SPINY INVERTEBRATES

There are 6,000 species of sea urchins, of which 80 are known to be poisonous or venomous. They are covered with spines or triple-jawed pedicellariae, and either can envenomate. Most spines are solid, producing only punctures and retained foreign bodies. Some are hollow and attached to a poison sac. Pedicellariae have flexible heads containing pincers or jaws that open on contact. Penetration of the spines into the skin produces the major injury and can lead to infection by marine organisms or impalement of deeper structures, that is, nerves and joints. The hand is particularly vulnerable. Pain from the puncture is similar to an insect sting with surrounding edema and erythema. A large number of urchin toxins are identified; many mediators are histamine- or kinin-like. Some species secrete an acid mucopolysaccharide. There is no known antivenom. The wound may be stained black or purple by dye within the spines and give a false impression of a retained foreign body. Spines are radiopaque. Infrequently, systemic symptoms occur with multiple embedded or undetected spines. Local pain may persist for days. One Pacific urchin, *Tripneustes*, secretes a neurotoxin with a predilection for facial and cranial nerves. Pedicellariae envenomations are more severe; symptoms are primarily neurologic. Pain may resolve in 1 hour, whereas muscular weakness or paralysis may last for up to 6 hours. A delayed reaction may manifest 2 or more months after injury. It may consist of either localized granuloma formation or a diffuse inflammatory process, most often fusiform with swelling and discoloration. Bony destruction may occur. Local nodules are usually 2 to 5 mm in diameter, pink to cyanotic in color, centrally umbilicated, and may have a keratotic surface. Pain and suppuration are not present unless the nodules occur on a weight-bearing surface. It remains undefined whether these are local allergic reactions or granulomatous inflammation. Therapy is supportive and generally symptomatic. Treatment of sea urchin injuries consists of immediate hot water (45°C/113°F) immersion, careful removal of attached pedicellariae and embedded spines, and prevention of cellulitis or synovitis by débridement. Pedicellariae must be removed or envenomation will continue. Infection is common and antibiotic prophylaxis indicated. Analgesics may be needed for several days. If delayed nodules or cysts appear, excision is indicated because they rarely heal spontaneously. Intralesional steroids have not been studied formally but are recommended with variable success. Prevention of echinoderm-mediated injuries includes careful stepping and usage of protective footwear in shallow water.

Starfish, like sea urchins, are bottom dwellers. Only a few noxious species exist. The most studied starfish, the crown-of-thorns sea star (*Acanthaster planci*), inhabits warm waters from Polynesia to the Red Sea and is particularly venomous. Foreign body granulomata may form. Treatment of starfish envenomation includes hot water immersion to relieve pain and topical treatment of the contact dermatitis (a useful agent

is calamine lotion with 0.5% menthol)[1] and supportive symptomatic treatment for the self-limited systemic reaction. The spines are a radiopaque foreign body. Local or regional anesthetic injections may be required for pain control or substituted for narcotics.

OTHER INVERTEBRATES

Sea cucumbers are free-living, bottom-dwelling, sausage-shaped echinoderms encountered at all depths. Holothurin is extruded defensively, causing an intense dermatitis or conjunctivitis on contact. Blindness can occur if the cornea is contacted and injured. Underwater swimming near sea cucumbers may cause symptoms as a result of the high concentrations of holothurin in the water. Some cucumber species eat nematocysts and may secrete this venom as well. Ingestion of the sea cucumber can cause death because holothurin is a potent cardiac glycoside. Local care includes acetic acid or isopropyl alcohol detoxification of the venom and removal of the slime with hot soapy water. Topical steroid therapy for dermatitis is indicated. If the eye is involved, topical anesthesia, copious irrigation, fluorescein staining, and immediate ophthalmologic consultation are recommended. Severe reactions may respond to systemic corticosteroids.

At least 13 species of sponges cause irritant dermatitis on contact. A slimy surface liquid contains the crinotoxin. Identified toxins include halitoxin, okadaic acid, and subcritine. Species common to the American waters include *Tedonis ignis* (fire sponge), *Fibula nolitangere* (poison bun sponge), and *Microciona prolifera* (red sponge). The Mediterranean red sponge and the tropical Pacific Hawaiian fire sponge are particularly noteworthy. Dermatitis also may be produced from silica or calcium spicule penetration of the skin. Skin lesions can progress to bullae and desquamation over several days. Stinging may increase over the first 2 or 3 days and persist for weeks. Plaques and papules may persist for several months. Eye contact may produce iritis and corneal lesions. Erythema multiforme and anaphylaxis are most common after contact with *Fibula* species.

Removal of the foreign body spicules may be accomplished with adhesive tape, rubber cement, or a facial peel. Acetic acid or isopropyl alcohol soaks for 10 to 30 minutes should be applied three times daily. Topical steroids may help the secondary inflammation but should be applied after the initial acetic acid soak. Antihistamines and topical anesthetics are other soothing measures. Severe secondary reactions may require systemic corticosteroid administration. Tetanus immunization should be current. Infected wounds should be cultured and appropriate antibiotics administered.

Marine annelids are segmented marine worms known as bristle worms. Easily detachable projections attached to the worm's parapodia penetrate the skin. These are difficult to remove and produce an intense

---

[1]May be compounded by pharmacists.

18

inflammation with erythema, pruritus, swelling, and paresthesia. Some worms can also bite. Treatment consists of spine removal analogous to sponges. Hot water (45°C/113°F) immersion for 30 minutes may provide pain relief. Secondary infection and cellulitis are not uncommon.

Ichthyosarcotoxism

Ichthyosarcotoxism refers to a variety of conditions arising from fish flesh. Ninety-nine percent of toxins involve the viscera, skin, or mucous membranes of the organisms ingested. Rarely are the gonads or blood of the organism involved. Three classes of illness can occur: allergic, toxic, and infectious. The risk of eating seafood and becoming ill is low, with most episodes consisting of self-limited gastrointestinal illness. Although a sample of these syndromes is discussed here, other more detailed sources for definitive information on this vast topic are available. The differential diagnosis for nontraumatic marine-borne illness is extensive. This discussion centers primarily on toxins ingested from seafood and includes toxins associated with shellfish, scombroid fish, and marine animals of the *Gymnothorax* and *Tetraodon* genus as well as several other serious but less common entities.

CIGUATERA

Ciguatoxin is endemic in warm water bottom-dwelling shore and reef fish. These fish are found in the temperate zone, but worldwide accounts of toxicity exist for the majority of fish-borne illness. More than 500 species are associated with ciguatera, including barracuda, sea bass, parrot fish, red snapper, grouper, amberjack, moray eel, porgy, triggerfish, surgeonfish, and wrasse. Ciguatera is the most common type of nonbacterial food poisoning in the United States and accounts for 10% to 15% of the food poisoning cases reported to the Centers for Disease Control and Prevention. Hawaii and Florida account for more than 90% of the U.S. cases, but the Caribbean and South Pacific regions are also significant sources. Patients most commonly present during the spring and summer months.

Ciguatoxin is found in blue-green algae, protozoa, and free-living dinoflagellates, which serve as the main food source for small herbivorous fish. These fish in turn are the major food source for larger carnivorous fish, and the toxin becomes more and more concentrated in tissue as it moves up the food chain. The toxin is believed elaborated by the dinoflagellate, *Gambierdiscus toxicus*. It is now believed this toxin causes inhibition of voltage-dependent sodium cell membrane channels. Toxicity patterns may be confusing, with local variation in the same geographic area. Ciguatoxin has a low molecular weight and can cross the placenta. Children born of mothers affected late in pregnancy may manifest bizarre movements in utero, and facial palsies may be present after delivery.

Patients become ill after eating either fresh or improperly frozen fish prepared by any method. Most patients experience symptoms 2 to 6 hours after ingestion with 75% by 12 hours and 100% by 36 hours. Symptoms are acute in onset, consisting of a constellation of gastrointestinal and neurologic complaints. The neurologic symptoms are predominantly dysesthesias and paresthesias but also include a strange metallic taste, perioral and oral tingling, and numbness. Also described is an odd temperature reversal sensation. Patients state that their skin is burning but feels cold underneath, or cold food is perceived as hot and vice versa. Severe headache and a feeling of loose painful teeth are often present. Deaths are very unusual, and because of respiratory paralysis and seizures possibly hypoxic. Delayed or protracted symptoms, consisting of itching, hiccups, and dysesthesias, may last for days or weeks proportional to the amount of toxin ingested.

Laboratory testing is of no diagnostic help but can eliminate other possibilities. An immunoassay is available to test fish commercially for presence of the toxin. Treatment is primarily supportive and symptomatic. Gut emptying and decontamination with charcoal are recommended, which seems illogical in the face of nausea, vomiting (40% of patients), and diarrhea (70% of patients). Atropine is indicated for bradycardia. Intravenous mannitol[1] provided rapid relief of both gastrointestinal and neurologic symptoms within minutes in one study of 24 patients. The mechanism of mannitol efficacy is unknown, but hypotheses include competitive inhibition of the toxin's effect on the sodium channel and neutralization of the toxin. Hospital admission is indicated if the diagnosis is uncertain or if significant volume depletion is present. Gastrointestinal symptoms resolve more slowly than do the neuromuscular symptoms. Dopamine (Intropin) at appropriate dose or calcium gluconate[1] as described earlier is recommended for treatment of shock. Paresthesias may respond to a course of amitriptyline (Elavil),[1] started at 25 to 100 mg orally at bedtime, increasing to 50 to 300 mg per day. Chronic symptoms may respond to acetaminophen (Tylenol)[1] or indomethacin (Indocin),[1] 25 to 50 mg by mouth or rectum three times per day. There is no immunity.

Recurrences are common and increasingly severe. They may be prevented by intake of a high-protein, high-carbohydrate diet that avoids fish, nuts, and ethanol for 3 to 6 months after symptom resolution.

Scombroid Poisoning

Scombroid poisoning, called saurine poisoning in Japan, occurs when spoiled fish are eaten. These fish include the large dark meat yellowfin, bluefin, and albacore tuna, wahoo, bonito, mackerel, and skipjack, all of which live in temperate or tropical waters. Also frequently implicated are the nonscombroid mahi-mahi, sardine, anchovy, herring, bluefish, and amberjack. The syndrome is entirely preventable and results when bacteria proliferate on warm or improperly refrigerated

---

[1]Not FDA approved for this indication.

freshly killed fish. These organisms elaborate histidine decarboxylase, which converts histidine to histamine, saurine, and other heat-stable compounds. The extent of spoilage correlates with histamine levels. The appearance, taste, and smell of the fish generally is unremarkable, but a pungent peppery taste may be noted.

A scombroid outbreak in San Francisco in 1977 revealed an uneven distribution of histamine in the flesh of an individual fish, which may explain why a variable occurrence of disease among people eating the same fish can occur. The differential diagnosis encountered in a patient with flushing as a prominent symptom is lengthy, and coincident ethanol consumption must be taken into consideration.

Symptoms of scombroid poisoning often occur within minutes but may take several hours to develop. Very similar to allergic reactions, symptoms are histamine mediated. Treatment consists of gut decontamination and supportive symptomatic care as indicated for hypotension, bronchospasm, nausea, or vomiting. The following are used successfully, but significant improvement occurs spontaneously within a matter of hours:

- Antihistamines, including both H_1 (diphenhydramine [Benadryl]), 5 mg/kg per day PO/IV, and H_2 (famotidine: Pepcid), 20 mg IV every 12 hours or 20 mg orally twice daily
- Epinephrine, 0.01 mg/kg, with a maximum does of 0.5 mg
- Parenteral steroids (dexamethasone [Decadron]), 0.5 mg/kg every 12 hours with a maximum dose of 10 mg

Diagnosis is ordinarily clinical but can be confirmed by elevated serum and urine histamine levels.

MOLLUSKS

Some 45,000 species of mollusks exist worldwide, comprising the single largest group of potentially toxic marine invertebrates. Most intoxications result from ingestion of toxic pelecypods (oysters, clams, scallops, etc.); relatively few true envenomations occur. Toxins implicated in envenomation and intoxication by both mollusks and neurotoxic fish species are very similar and produce toxicity by inactivating the voltage-dependent sodium membrane channels. The effect is very much like curare. Neuromuscular paralysis is the result, most urgently respiratory muscle paralysis. If not treated promptly, respiratory failure and anoxia occur followed by brain damage and ultimately death. Patients are alert, mentating normally unless anoxia has occurred.

Cone shells include 300 species, 18 of which are implicated in human envenomations. Comparable in size to hymenoptera toxins, these toxins are neurotoxic. Two major types are isolated, a presynaptic ω-conotoxin, which affects calcium-mediated acetylcholine release, and μ-conotoxin, which directly modifies sodium influx channels in muscle cells, thereby abolishing action potential propagation.

The puncture may resemble a minor bee or wasp sting, but *Conus geographicus* can cause death within a few hours. The initial local symptoms of burning, local cyanosis, and numbness rapidly advance to severe neurologic symptoms including respiratory paralysis. No antivenom is available, and treatment is entirely empirical and symptomatic. Some relief may be offered by hot water immersion at 45°C (113°F). For severe envenomations, the treatment is supportive and primarily respiratory, with symptoms resolving completely in 6 to 8 hours. Prevention is by patient education.

Octopi are actually shy reclusive creatures that usually pose no threat to humans. The venomous octopi are small, less than 20 cm in diameter. The blue-ringed octopus (*Hapalochlaena maculosa*) of Australia is the most well known. Yellow brown and inconspicuous when docile, it develops brilliant iridescent blue rings when threatened. Another dangerous species is *Octopus joubini*, native to the Caribbean. All octopi less than 20 cm in diameter should be handled only with protective gloves.

The bite frequently manifests as two small puncture wounds. The patient may be totally unaware of being bitten or have a mild bee sting–like burning. The maculotoxin injected appears to block peripheral nerve transmission. The blue-ringed octopus also secretes tetrodotoxin and is the only creature known to envenomate with tetrodotoxin. The wound is numb and often blanched initially, but this is followed quickly by pain that may persist for up to 6 hours. More serious envenomations involve neurotoxic symptoms with oral and facial numbness occurring within 10 to 45 minutes. Muscle weakness is next, with death caused by respiratory failure. Treatment is supportive and based on individual symptoms because no antivenom is available. First aid is the pressure immobilization dressing. Hot water is without benefit. Symptoms begin to resolve 4 to 10 hours after the bite, and recovery may take 2 to 4 days unless anoxia has occurred. Intensive respiratory support is crucial to survival. A monoclonal rabbit serum immunoglobulin (IgG) antibody is being developed.

Tetraodon Poisoning

Tetraodon poisoning occurs after ingestion of fish of the order Tetratodontiformes, which inhabit both fresh and salt water. They have no geographic restriction but are encountered most frequently off Japan, California, Africa, Australia, and South America. More than 100 species known regionally by different names and "fugu" (a specific preparation of pufferfish considered a delicacy in Japan) are capable of producing intoxication. Other sources include ocean sunfish, blue-ringed octopus, and certain species of newts and salamanders. Tetrodotoxin is a heat-stable (except at alkaline pH), basic, water-soluble, nonprotein compound. Geographic variations in toxicity occur. Tetrodotoxin effects are similar to saxitoxin (toxic shellfish), with sodium-fast channel blockade–induced paralysis, direct chemoreceptor trigger-zone stimulation resulting in emesis,

18

and respiratory depression secondary to a direct medullary effect. Tetrodotoxin relaxes vascular smooth muscle and blocks the preganglionic cholinergic motor and sensory nerves and sympathetic nervous system. Symptoms occur within minutes and may progress to ascending paralysis and respiratory death. Toxicity is significant, with an estimated 50% to 60% mortality even when appropriate therapy is given. Complete paralysis with fixed, dilated pupils and normal mentation occurs until anoxia ensues.

Respiratory support is essential. There are two reports of successful reversal of respiratory and motor paralysis with edrophonium (Tensilon),[1] 10 mg IV after a 1-mg test dose.

Toxic Shellfish

Shellfish poisoning occurs from eating healthy mollusks from the temperate zone (clams, oysters, mussels, and scallops) that have ingested and filtered large amounts of dinoflagellates. The so-called red tide intermittently found worldwide is caused by the presence of dinoflagellate blooms. Not all red tides are toxic, and toxic dinoflagellates are not necessarily associated with red tides. These toxins are similar to tetrodotoxin and other neurotoxins. A single mussel may contain 10 mg of toxin; ingestion of fewer than six clams can be lethal. Saxitoxin, one of the best characterized, is a potent paralytic neurotoxin concentrated in the gills and digestive glands of shellfish. Saxitoxin is a heat-stable, water-soluble acetylcholinesterase inhibitor rapidly absorbed from the gastrointestinal tract, which acts on the peripheral and autonomic nervous systems. A murine bioassay is used to detect the toxin because no laboratory test to do so exists.

Paralytic Shellfish Poisoning

Symptoms occur dramatically and rapidly (30 minutes) after eating a saxitoxin-containing mollusk. They are related to the amount ingested and the method of food preparation; increased toxicity exists with raw food. Oral and perioral dysesthesias and burning progress rapidly caudally. A number of neurologic symptoms occur, and patients may describe a sensation of their body "floating." Flaccid paralysis and respiratory failure may ensue. Similar to tetraodon intoxication, the patient may remain awake. Treatment consists of gut decontamination and supportive ventilatory care. Untreated, up to 75% of victims die within 12 hours.

Neurotoxic Shellfish Poisoning

Ptychodiscus brevis toxin ingestion causes a milder form of paralytic shellfish poisoning. Onset may be delayed up to 3 hours. Neurologic symptoms resemble

CURRENT DIAGNOSIS

- Sudden cardiac arrest in ocean water: *Chironex fleckeri* envenomation
- Bite: shark, barracuda, large fish, eel whale, sea lion
- Large puncture/laceration: stingray, catfish, weeverfish
  Mild: local pain
  Moderate: regional pain
  Severe: regional pain plus autonomic symptoms and cardiovascular symptoms
  Needlefish: regional penetrating trauma
- Small puncture/unnoticed sting: scorpionfish, cone shells, sea snake (must be in water), octopus, urchins, starfish
  Pain only: all of the preceding
  Pain plus neurologic symptoms: all of the preceding
  Starfish: self-limited paresthesias, weakness
  Pain plus respiratory distress: all of the preceding
  Pain plus cardiovascular symptoms: scorpionfish
  Pain plus cranial nerve findings/rhabdomyolysis: sea snakes
- Skin lesions: jellyfish, coral, sponges
  Dendritic/serpiginous: jellyfish species
  Dendritic plus cardiovascular: *Chironex* species, Portuguese man-of-war
  Adrenergic crisis/pulmonary edema: Irukandji syndrome
  Abrasions/small lacerations: sponges, coral, starfish
  Foreign body granuloma: urchins
- Ingested: ciguatoxin, scombroid, pufferfish, mollusks, shellfish
  Ciguatoxin and scombroid: usually self-limited
  Gastrointestinal (GI) symptoms: usually not mollusks, other four possible
  GI plus neurologic: all but scombroid
  GI plus histaminergic symptoms: scombroid
  Neurologic plus respiratory distress: all but scombroid
  Fasciculations: pufferfish, mollusks
  Respiratory distress: all capable
  Respiratory distress plus cardiovascular symptoms: ciguatoxin, pufferfish, mollusks

early paralytic shellfish poisoning and ciguatera. Paralysis is rare. Only a few patients have symptoms after the first 24 hours. Treatment consists of the standard methods of gut decontamination and supportive care, particularly respiratory support. The fatality rate is 8% to 9%, with death occurring in 1 to 12 hours from respiratory failure. Patients surviving beyond 12 to 18 hours have a good prognosis for complete recovery.

Rakel and Bope: *Conn's Current Therapy 2006.*

---

[1]Not FDA approved for this indication.

CURRENT THERAPY

Bite: Advanced Trauma Life Support principles for hemorrhagic shock and limb threats

- Wound care: irrigation, débridement, exploration, pack open and delayed primary closure if desired.
- Tetanus immunization: tetanus immune globulin (BayTet), 250 U IM and tetanus toxoid (Td), 0.5 mL IM if older than 7 years.
- Antibiotics: prophylaxis with trimethoprim-sulfamethoxazole DS (TMP-SMX) (Bactrim DS), 1 tablet PO twice daily for 7 to 10 days, *or* ciprofloxacin (Cipro), 500 mg PO twice daily for 7 to 10 days.
- Established infections: imipenem cilastin (Primaxin), 250 to 1000 mg IV every 6 to 8 hours *or* ceftriaxone (Rocephin), 1 to 2 g IM/IV every 24 hours, *or* ceftazidime (Fortaz), 1 to 2 g IM/IV every 8 to 12 hours.
- Rabies prophylaxis for mammal bites (sea lion, whale): rabies immune globulin (Imogam Rabies HT, BayRab), 20 IU/kg, as much as possible around wound site, *then* rabies vaccine (Imovax rabies vaccine), 1 mL IM deltoid, on days 0, 3, 7, 14, and 28.

Large Puncture/Laceration

- Needlefish: Advanced Trauma Life Support (ATLS) principles and general wound care principles.
- Pain: immersion in water at 45°C (113°F) for 30 to 90 minutes; repeat if needed:
    Plain lidocaine 1% to 2% or bupivacaine (Marcaine), 0.25% local
    Infiltration or regional nerve block
    Morphine sulfate, IM/IV 0.1 mg/kg, if needed for severe pain
Note: Cryotherapy is contraindicated.
- Autonomic/cardiovascular symptoms:
    Benzodiazepines titrated to effect
- Stonefish antivenom: 1 mL neutralizes 10 mg venom; empirical for severe envenomation; give 2 mL IM/IV after sensitivity testing
    Available sources are Sea World, San Diego, CA, and Cleveland, OH; Sharp Cabrillo Hospital, San Diego, CA; Steinhart Aquarium, San Francisco, CA.

Small Puncture/Unnoticed

- Pain control as described earlier.
- Tetanus immunization if indicated.
- If sea snake: compression bandage, extremity in dependent position.
    Note: Cryotherapy and incision/suction contraindicated.
- Antivenom: not FDA approved.
    Equine polyvalent antivenom from *Enhydrina* species and *Notechis* species *or* polyvalent tiger snake antivenom.
    Anaphylaxis testing, then 1 to 10 ampoules as needed titrated to effect.
- Skin lesions: for nematocyst removal, do not use fresh water; do not rub with sand
    Seawater immersion.
    Deactivation with 5% acetic acid (vinegar) for 30 seconds or until pain stops.
    Apply shaving cream and shave gently.
- Pain control: morphine sulfate, 0.1 mg/kg as needed.
- Cramps: benzodiazepine (Valium), 0.01 to 0.03 mg/kg *or* methocarbamol (Robaxin), 1 g IV slowly.
    Chironex species antivenom: sheep based, 20,000 U (1 vial) IV or 3 vials IM.
    Note: All moderate to severe envenomations require 6 to 8 hours of observation.
- Ingested: atropine, 0.6 mg to 1.0 mg for three doses if needed for bradycardia.
    Intensive respiratory support may be needed for days.
    Intensive fluid and blood pressure support if needed.
- Ciguatoxin: mannitol,[1] 0.25 to 0.50 g every 8 hours if needed.
- Scombroid: antihistamines: H_1 and H_2 blockers:
    Diphenhydramine (Benadryl), 5 mg/kg day PO/IV *and* famotidine (Pepcid), 20 mg IV every 12 hours or 20 mg PO twice daily.
    Epinephrine, 0.01 mg (maximum 0.5 mg) if needed.
    Dexamethasone (Decadron), 0.5 mg/kg every 12 hours (maximum 10 mg/dose).

Mollusks/Pufferfish

- Shellfish: standard GI decontamination:
    Intensive respiratory support as needed.
    Intensive supportive care until recovery.

---

[1]Not FDA approved for this indication.
Abbreviations: IV = intravenous; PO = by mouth.

Gymnothorax Intoxication

Intoxication from *Gymnothorax* genus (moray, conger, and anguillid eels) results from a neurotoxin present in the viscera, muscles, and gonads that does not affect the fish itself. The heat-stable toxin produces a cigua-toxic-like syndrome. A toxidrome of cholinergic symptoms and hemolysis may be separate from, or coincident with, the neurotoxicity. Treatment is purely supportive, with deaths occurring from respiratory paralysis and seizures.

When humans encounter marine creatures a variety of maladies may occur, ranging from dermatitis to life-threatening trauma, allergy, envenomations, or intoxications. The physician should be prepared to recognize quickly and address appropriately the potential life threats. These are primarily neurologic, respiratory, and cardiovascular. A high degree of suspicion for these illnesses is needed. Intoxications may be especially confounding, but the supportive treatment is essentially identical.

Although most of the syndromes are self-limited and treatment supportive, time is of the essence if neuromuscular paralysis, hypotension, or respiratory compromise is present.

Much folklore exists regarding detection and prevention of these entities and should be regarded as such. The last several decades have seen a marked increase in our knowledge base regarding these fascinating envenomations and intoxications. Research in the next several decades probably will produce a variety of diagnostic and therapeutic tools that will further our understanding of and ability to specifically manage these syndromes.

REFERENCES

Auerbach PS: Marine envenomations. N Engl J Med 1991;325:486-493.

Auerbach, PS: Wilderness Medicine, 4th ed. St. Louis, Mosby, 2001.

Auerbach PS, Yajko DM, Nassos PS, et al: Bacteriology of the marine environment: Implications for clinical therapy. Ann Emerg Med 1987;16:643-649.

Brown CK, Shepherd SM: Marine trauma, envenomations and intoxications. Emerg Med Clin North Am 1992;10:385-408.

Fenner, PJ: Marine envenomation: An update—a presentation on the current status of marine envenomation; first aid and medical treatments. Emerg Med 2000;12:295-302.

Fenner PJ, Williamson JA: Worldwide deaths and severe envenomation from jellyfish stings. Med J Aust 1996;165:658-661.

Garyfallon GT, Madden JF: Lionfish envenomation. Ann Emerg Med 1996;28:456-457.

Kizer KW: Marine envenomations. J Toxicol Clin Toxicol 1984;24:527-555.

Kumamoto KS, Vukich DJ: Clinical infections of *Vibrio vulnificus*: A case report and review of the literature. J Emerg Med 1998;16:61-65.

Meyer PK: Stingray injuries. Wild Environ Med 1997;8:24-31.

Semel JD, Trenholme G: *Aeromonas hydrophilia* water-associated wound infections: A review. J Trauma 1990;30:324-327.

Shepherd S, Thomas SH, Stone CK: Catfish envenomation. J Wilderness Med 1994;5:67-71.

Williamson JA, LeRay LE, Wohlfahrt M, Fenner PJ: Acute management of serious envenomation by box-jellyfish (*Chironex fleckeri*). Med J Aust 1984;141:851-856.

Williamson JA, Fenner PJ, Burnett JW: Venomous and Poisonous Marine Animals: A Medical and Biological Handbook. Sydney, Australia, University of New South Wales Press, 1996.

Medical Toxicology: Ingestions, Inhalations, and Dermal and Ocular Absorptions

Method of
Howard C. Mofenson, MD, Thomas R. Caraccio, PharmD, Michael McGuigan, MD, and Joseph Greensher, MD

Introduction and Epidemiology

According to the national Toxic Exposure Surveillance System (TESS), almost 2.4 million potentially toxic exposures were reported last year to Poison Control Centers throughout the United States. Poisonings were responsible for almost 1100 deaths and more than 500,000 hospitalizations. Poisoning accounts for 2% to 5% of pediatric hospital admissions, 10% of adult admissions, 5% of hospital admissions in the elderly (>65 years of age), and 5% of ambulance calls. In one urban hospital, drug-related emergencies accounted for 38% of the emergency department visits. An evaluation of a medical intensive care unit and step-down unit over a 3-month period indicated that poisonings accounted for 19.7% of admissions.

The largest number of fatalities resulting from poisoning reported to the TESS are caused by analgesics. The other principal toxicologic causes of fatalities are antidepressants, sedative hypnotics/antipsychotics, stimulants/street drugs, cardiovascular agents, and alcohols. Less than 1% of overdose cases reaching the hospitals result in fatality. However, patients presenting in deep coma to medical care facilities have a fatality rate of 13% to 35%. The largest single cause of coma of inapparent etiology is drug poisoning.

Pharmaceutical preparations are involved in 40% of poisonings. The number one pharmaceutical agent involved in exposures is acetaminophen. The severity of the manifestations of acute poisoning exposures varies greatly depending on whether the poisoning was intentional or unintentional. Unintentional exposures make up 85% to 90% of all poisoning exposures. The majority of cases are acute, occurring in children younger than 5 years of age, in the home, and resulting in no or minor toxicity. Many are actually ingestions of relatively nontoxic substances that require minimal medical care. Intentional poisonings, such as suicides, constitute 10% to 15% of exposures and may require the highest standards of medical and nursing care and the use of sophisticated equipment for recovery. Intentional ingestions are often of multiple substances and frequently include ethanol, acetaminophen, and aspirin. Suicides make up 52% of the reported fatalities. About 25% of suicides are attempted with drugs. Sixty percent of patients who take a drug overdose use their own medication and 15% use drugs prescribed for close relatives. The majority of the drug-related suicide attempts involve a central nervous system (CNS) depressant, and coma management is vital to the treatment.

Assessment and Maintenance of the Vital Functions

The initial assessment of all patients in medical emergencies follows the principles of basic and advanced cardiac life support. The adequacy of the patient's airway, degree of ventilation, and circulatory status should be determined. The vital functions should be established and maintained. Vital signs should be measured frequently and should include body core temperature. The assessment of vital functions should include the rate numbers (e.g., respiratory rate) and indications of effectiveness (e.g., depth of respirations and degree of gas exchange). Table 1 gives important measurements and vital signs.

Level of consciousness should be assessed by immediate AVPU (Alert, responds to Verbal stimuli, responds to Painful stimuli, and Unconscious). If the patient is unconscious, one must assess the severity of the unconsciousness by the Glasgow Coma Scale (Table 2).

If the patient is comatose, management requires administering 100% oxygen, establishing vascular access, and obtaining blood for pertinent laboratory studies. The administration of glucose, thiamine, and naloxone, as well as intubation to protect the airway, should be considered. Pertinent laboratory studies include arterial blood gases (ABG), electrocardiography (ECG), determination of blood glucose level, electrolytes, renal and liver tests, and acetaminophen plasma concentration in all cases of intentional ingestions. Radiography of the chest and abdomen may be useful. The severity of a stimulant's effects can also be assessed and should be documented to follow the trend.

The examiner should completely expose the patient by removing clothes and other items that interfere with a full evaluation. One should look for clues to etiology in the clothes and include the hat and shoes.

Prevention of Absorption and Reduction of Local Damage

EXPOSURE

Poisoning exposure routes include ingestion (70%), dermal (8%), ophthalmologic (5%), inhalation (6%), insect bites and stings (4%), and parenteral injections (0.4%). The effect of the toxin may be local, systemic, or both.

Local effects (skin, eyes, mucosa of respiratory or gastrointestinal tract) occur where contact is made with the poisonous substance. Local effects are nonspecific chemical reactions that depend on the chemical properties (e.g., pH), concentration, contact time, and type of exposed surface.

Systemic effects occur when the poison is absorbed into the body and depend on the dose, the distribution,

and the functional reserve of the organ systems. Shock and hypoxia are part of systemic toxicity.

DELAYED TOXIC ACTION

Therapeutic doses of most pharmaceuticals are absorbed within 90 minutes. However, the patient with exposure to a potential toxin may be asymptomatic at this time because a sufficient amount has not yet been absorbed or metabolized to produce toxicity at the time the patient presents for care.

Absorption can be significantly delayed under the following circumstances:

1. Drugs with anticholinergic properties (e.g., antihistamines, belladonna alkaloids, diphenoxylate with atropine [Lomotil], phenothiazines, and tricyclic antidepressants).
2. Modified release preparations such as sustained-release, enteric-coated, and controlled-release formulations have delayed and prolonged absorption.
3. Concretions may form (e.g., salicylates, iron, glutethimide, and meprobamate [Equanil]) that can delay absorption and prolong the toxic effects. Large quantities of drugs tend to be absorbed more slowly than small quantities.

Some substances must be metabolized into a toxic metabolite (acetaminophen, acetonitrile, ethylene glycol, methanol, methylene chloride, parathion, and paraquat). In some cases, time is required to produce a toxic effect on organ systems (Amanita phalloides mushrooms, carbon tetrachloride, colchicine, digoxin [Lanoxin], heavy metals, monoamine oxidase inhibitors, and oral hypoglycemic agents).

Initial Management

1. Stabilization of airway, breathing, and circulation and protection of same.
2. Identification of specific toxin or toxic syndrome.
3. Initial treatment: D50W; consider thiamine, naloxone (Narcan), oxygen, and antidotes if needed.
4. Physical assessment.
5. Decontamination: Gastrointestinal tract, skin, eyes.

DECONTAMINATION

In the asymptomatic patient who has been exposed to a toxic substance, decontamination procedures should be considered if the patient has been exposed to potentially toxic substances in toxic amounts.

Ocular exposure should be immediately treated with water irrigation for 15 to 20 minutes with the eyelids fully retracted. One should not use neutralizing chemicals. All caustic and corrosive injuries should be evaluated with fluorescein dye and by an ophthalmologist.

Dermal exposure is treated immediately with copious water irrigation for 30 minutes, not a forceful flushing. Shampooing the hair, cleansing the fingernails, navel, and perineum, and irrigating the eyes are necessary in the case of an extensive exposure. The clothes should be specially bagged and may have to be discarded.

Rakel and Bope: *Conn's Current Therapy 2006.*

TABLE 1 Important Measurements and Vital Signs

Age	Body surface area (m²)	Weight (kg)	Height (cm)	Pulse (bpm) resting	Hypotension	Blood pressure Hypertension Significant	Severe	Respiratory rate (rpm)
Newborn	0.19	3.5	50	70-190	<60/40	>96	>106	30-60
1 mo-6 mo	0.30	4-7	50-65	80-160	<70/45	>104	>110	30-50
6 mo-1 y	0.38	7-10	65-75	80-160	<70/45	>104	>110	20-40
1-2 y	0.50-0.55	10-12	75-85	80-140	<74/47	>112/74	>118/82	20-40
3-5 y	0.54-0.68	15-20	90-108	80-120	<80/52	>116/76	>124/84	20-40
6-9 y	0.68-0.85	20-28	122-133	75-115	<90/60	>122/82	>130/86	16-25
10-12 y	1.00-1.07	30-40	138-147	70-110	<90/60	>126/82	>134/90	16-25
13-15 y	1.07-1.22	42-50	152-160	60-100	<90/60	>136/86	>144/92	16-20
16-18 y	1.30-1.60	53-60	160-170	60-100	<90/60	>142/92	>150/98	12-16
Adult	1.40-1.70	60-70	160-170	60-100	<90/60	>140/90	>210/120	10-16

Data from Nadas A: Pediatric Cardiology, 3rd ed. Philadelphia, WB Saunders, 1976; Blumer JL (ed): A Practice Guide to Pediatric Intensive Care. St Louis, Mosby, 1990; AAP and ACEP: Respiratory Distress in APLS Pediatric Emergency Medicine Course, 1993; Second Task Force: Blood pressure control in children–1987, Pediatr 79:1, 1987; Linakis JG: Hypertension. In Fliesher GR, Ludwig S (eds): Textbook of Pediatric Emergency Medicine, 3rd ed. Baltimore, Williams & Wilkins, 1993.

Rakel and Bope: *Conn's Current Therapy 2006.*

TABLE 2 Glasgow Coma Scale

Scale	Adult response	Score	Pediatric, 0-1 Years
Eye opening	Spontaneous	4	Spontaneous
	To verbal command	3	To shout
	To pain	2	To pain
	None	1	No response
Motor response			
To verbal command	Obeys	6	
To painful stimuli	Localized pain	5	Localized pain
	Flexion withdrawal	4	Flexion withdrawal
	Decorticate flexion	3	Decorticate flexion
	Decerebrate extension	2	Decerebrate flexion
	None	1	None
Verbal response: adult	Oriented and converses	5	Cries, smiles, coos
	Disoriented but converses	4	Cries or screams
	Inappropriate words	3	Inappropriate sounds
	Incomprehensible sounds	2	Grunts
	None	1	Gives no response
Verbal response: child	Oriented	5	
	Words or babbles	4	
	Vocal sounds	3	
	Cries or moans to stimuli	2	
	None	1	

Data from Teasdale G, Jennett B: Assessment of coma impaired consciousness. Lancet 2:83, 1974; Simpson D, Reilly P: Pediatric coma scale. Lancet 2:450, 1982; Seidel J: Preparing for pediatric emergencies. Pediatr Rev 16:470, 1995.

18

Physical and Chemical Injuries

Leather goods can become irreversibly contaminated and must be abandoned. Caustic (alkali) exposures can require hours of irrigation. Dermal absorption can occur with pesticides, hydrocarbons, and cyanide.

Injection exposures (e.g., snake envenomation) can be treated with venom extracts. Venom extractors can be used within minutes of envenomation, and proximal lymphatic constricting bands or elastic wraps can be used to delay lymphatic flow and immobilize the extremity. Cold packs and tourniquets should not be used and incision is generally not recommended. Substances of abuse may be injected intravenously or subcutaneously. In these cases, little decontamination can be done.

Inhalation exposure to toxic substances is managed by immediate removal of the victim from the contaminated environment by protected rescuers.

Gastrointestinal exposure is the most common route of poisoning. Gastrointestinal decontamination historically has been done by gastric emptying: induction of emesis, gastric lavage, administration of activated charcoal, and the use of cathartics or whole bowel irrigation. No procedure is routine; it should be individualized for each case. If no attempt is made to decontaminate the patient, the reason should be clearly documented on the medical record (e.g., time elapsed, past peak of action, ineffectiveness, or risk of procedure).

Gastric Emptying Procedures

The gastric emptying procedure used is influenced by the age of the patient, the effectiveness of the procedure, the time of ingestion (gastric emptying is usually ineffective after 1 hour postingestion), the patient's clinical status (time of peak effect has passed or the patient's condition is too unstable), formulation of the substance ingested (regular release versus modified release), the amount ingested, and the rapidity of onset of CNS depression or stimulation (convulsions). Most studies show that only 30% (range, 19% to 62%) of the ingested toxin is removed by gastric emptying under optimal conditions. It has not been demonstrated that the choice of procedure improved the outcome.

A mnemonic for gathering information is STATS:

S—substance
T—type of formulation
A—amount and age
T—time of ingestion
S—signs and symptoms

The examiner should attempt to obtain AMPLE information about the patient:

A—age and allergies
M—available medications
P—past medical history including pregnancy, psychiatric illnesses, substance abuse, or intentional ingestions
L—time of last meal, which may influence absorption and the onset and peak action
E—events leading to present condition

The intent of the patient should also be determined. The Regional Poison Center should be consulted for the exact ingredients of the ingested substance and the latest management. The treatment information on the labels of products and in the Physician's Desk Reference are notoriously inaccurate.

Ipecac Syrup

Syrup of ipecac–induced emesis has virtually no use in the emergency department. Although at one time it was considered most useful in young children with a recent witnessed ingestion, it is advised only within 1 hour of ingestion of known agents only when a toxic amount is involved. Current guidelines from the American Association of Poison Control Centers have significantly limited the indications for inducing emesis because the risk most often exceeds the benefit derived from this procedure. The Poison Control Center should be called before one induces emesis.

Contraindications or situations in which induction of emesis is inappropriate include the following:

- Ingestion of caustic substance
- Loss of airway protective reflexes because of ingestion of substances that can produce rapid onset of CNS depression (e.g., short-acting benzodiazepines, barbiturates, nonbarbiturate sedative-hypnotics, opioids, tricyclic antidepressants) or convulsions (e.g., camphor [Ponstel], chloroquine [Aralen], codeine, isoniazid [Nydrazid], mefenamic acid, nicotine, propoxyphene [Darvon], organophosphate insecticides, strychnine, and tricyclic antidepressants)
- Ingestion of low-viscosity petroleum distillates (e.g., gasoline, lighter fluid, kerosene)
- Significant vomiting prior to presentation or hematemesis
- Age under 6 months (no established dose, safety, or efficacy data)
- Ingestion of foreign bodies (emesis is ineffective and may lead to aspiration)
- Clinical conditions including neurologic impairment, hemodynamic instability, increased intracranial pressure, and hypertension
- Delay in presentation (more than 1 hour postingestion)

The dose of syrup of ipecac in the 6- to 9-month-old infant is 5 mL; in the 9- to 12-month-old, 10 mL; and in the 1- to 12-year-old, 15 mL. In children older than 12 years and in adults, the dose is 30 mL. The dose can be repeated once if the child does not vomit in 15 to 20 minutes. The vomitus should be inspected for remnants of pills or toxic substances, and the appearance and odor should be documented. When ipecac is not available, 30 mL of mild dishwashing soap (not dishwasher detergent) can be used, although it is less effective.

Complications are very rare but include aspiration, protracted vomiting, rarely cardiac toxicity with long-term abuse, pneumothorax, gastric rupture, diaphragmatic hernia, intracranial hemorrhage, and Mallory-Weiss tears.

Gastric Lavage

Gastric lavage should be considered only when life-threatening amounts of substances were involved, when the benefits outweigh the risks, when it can be performed within 1 hour of the ingestion, and when no contraindications exist.

The contraindications are similar to those for ipecac-induced emesis. However, gastric lavage can be accomplished after the insertion of an endotracheal tube in cases of CNS depression or controlled convulsions. The patient should be placed with the head lower than the hips in a left-lateral decubitus position. The location of the tube should be confirmed by radiography, if necessary, and suctioning equipment should be available.

Contraindications to gastric lavage include the following:

- Ingestion of caustic substances (risk of esophageal perforation)
- Uncontrolled convulsions, because of the danger of aspiration and injury during the procedure
- Ingestion of low-viscosity petroleum distillate products
- CNS depression or absent protective airway reflexes, without endotracheal protection
- Significant cardiac dysrhythmias
- Significant emesis or hematemesis prior to presentation
- Delay in presentation (more than 1 hour postingestion)

Size of Tube

The best results with gastric lavage are obtained with the largest possible orogastric tube that can be reasonably passed (nasogastric tubes are not large enough to remove solid material). In adults, a large-bore orogastric Lavacuator hose or a No. 42 French Ewald tube should be used; in young children, orogastric tubes are generally too small to remove solid material and gastric lavage is not recommended.

The amount of fluid used varies with the patient's age and size. In general, aliquots of 50 to 100 mL per lavage are used in adults. Larger amounts of fluid may force the toxin past the pylorus. Lavage fluid is 0.9% saline.

Complications are rare and may include respiratory depression, aspiration pneumonitis, cardiac dysrhythmias as a result of increased vagal tone, esophageal-gastric tears and perforation, laryngospasm, and mediastinitis.

Activated Charcoal

Oral activated charcoal adsorbs the toxin onto its surface before absorption. According to recent guidelines set forth by the American Academy of Clinical Toxicology, activated charcoal should not be used routinely. Its use is indicated only if a toxic amount of substance has been ingested and is optimally effective within 1 hour of the ingestion. Because of the slow absorption of large quantities of toxin, activated charcoal may be beneficial after 1 hour postingestion.

Activated charcoal does not effectively adsorb small molecules or molecules lacking carbon (Table 3). Activated charcoal adsorption may be diminished by milk, cocoa powder, and ice cream.

Rakel and Bope: *Conn's Current Therapy 2006.*

Physical and Chemical Injuries

TABLE 3 Substances Poorly Adsorbed by Activated Charcoal

C	Caustics and corrosives
H	Heavy metals (arsenic, iron, lead, mercury)
A	Alcohols (ethanol, methanol, isopropanol) and glycols (ethylene glycols)
R	Rapid onset of absorption (cyanide and strychnine)
C	Chlorine and iodine
O	Others insoluble in water (substances in tablet form)
A	Aliphatic hydrocarbons (petroleum distillates)
L	Laxatives (sodium, magnesium, potassium, and lithium)

There are a few relative contraindications to the use of activated charcoal:

1. Ingestion of caustics and corrosives, which may produce vomiting or cling to the mucosa and falsely appear as a burn on endoscopy.
2. Comatose patient, in whom the airway must be secured prior to activated charcoal administration.
3. Patient without presence of bowel sounds.

Note: Activated charcoal was shown not to interfere with effectiveness of *N*-acetylcysteine in cases of acetaminophen overdose, so it is no longer contraindicated as was thought in the past.

The usual initial adult dose is 60 to 100 g and the dose for children is 15 to 30 g. It is administered orally as a slurry mixed with water or by nasogastric or orogastric tube. *Caution:* Be sure the tube is in the stomach. Cathartics are not necessary.

Although repeated dosing with activated charcoal may decrease the half-life and increases the clearance of phenobarbital, dapsone, quinidine, theophylline, and carbamazepine (Tegretol), recent guidelines indicate there is insufficient evidence to support the use of multiple-dose activated charcoal unless a life-threatening amount of one of the substances mentioned is involved. At present there are no controlled studies that demonstrate that multiple-dose activated charcoal or cathartics alter the clinical course of an intoxication. The dose varies from 0.25 to 0.50 g/kg every 1 to 4 hours, and continuous nasogastric tube infusion of 0.25 to 0.5 g/kg/h has been used to decrease vomiting.

Gastrointestinal dialysis is the diffusion of the toxin from the higher concentration in the serum of the mesenteric vessels to the lower levels in the gastrointestinal tract mucosal cell and subsequently into the gastrointestinal lumen, where the concentration has been lowered by intraluminal adsorption of activated charcoal.

Complications of treatment with activated charcoal include vomiting in 50% of cases, desorption (especially with weak acids in intestine), and aspiration (at least a dozen cases of aspiration have been reported). There are many cases of unreported pulmonary aspirations and "charcoal lungs," intestinal obstruction or pseudo-obstruction (three case reports with multiple dosing, none with a single dose), empyema following esophageal perforation, and hypermagnesemia and hypernatremia, which have been associated with repeated concurrent doses of activated charcoal and saline cathartics.

Catharsis was used to hasten the elimination of any remaining toxin in the gastrointestinal tract. There are no studies to demonstrate the effectiveness of cathartics, and they are no longer recommended as a form of gastrointestinal decontamination.

Whole-Bowel Irrigation

With whole bowel irrigation, solutions of polyethylene glycol (PEG) with balanced electrolytes are used to cleanse the bowel without causing shifts in fluids and electrolytes. The procedure is not approved by the U.S. Food and Drug Administration for this purpose.

Indications

The procedure has been studied and used successfully in cases of iron overdose when abdominal radiographs reveal incomplete emptying of excess iron. There are additional indications for other types of ingestions, such as with body-packing of illicit drugs (e.g., cocaine, heroin).

The procedure is to administer the solution (GoLYTELY or Colyte), orally or by nasogastric tube, in a dose of 0.5 L per hour in children younger than 5 years of age and 2 L per hour in adolescents and adults for 5 hours. The end point is reached when the rectal effluent is clear or radiopaque materials can no longer be seen in the gastrointestinal tract on abdominal radiographs.

Contraindications

These measures should not be used if there is extensive hematemesis, ileus, or signs of bowel obstruction, perforation, or peritonitis. Animal experiments in which PEG was added to activated charcoal indicated that activated charcoal-salicylates and activated charcoal-theophylline combinations resulted in decreased adsorption and desorption of salicylate and theophylline and no therapeutic benefit over activated charcoal alone. Polyethylene solutions are bound by activated charcoal in vitro, decreasing the efficacy of activated charcoal.

Dilutional treatment is indicated for the immediate management of caustic and corrosive poisonings but is otherwise not useful. The administration of diluting fluid above 30 mL in children and 250 mL in adults may produce vomiting, reexposing the vital tissues to the effects of local damage and possible aspiration.

Neutralization is not proven to be either safe or effective.

Endoscopy and surgery have been required in the case of body-packer obstruction, intestinal ischemia produced by cocaine ingestion, and iron local caustic action.

Differential Diagnosis of Poisons on the Basis of Central Nervous System Manifestations

Neurologic parameters help to classify and assess the need for supportive treatment as well as provide diagnostic clues to the etiology. Table 4 lists the effects of

TABLE 4 Agents with Central Nervous System (CNS) Effects

Agents	General manifestations	Agents	General manifestations
CNS Depressants		**Hallucinogens**	
Alcohols and glycols (S-H)	Bradycardia	Amphetamines‡	Tachycardia and dysrhythmias
Anticonvulsants (S-H)	Bradypnea	Anticholinergics	Tachypnea
Antidysrhythmics (S-H)	Shallow respirations	Cardiac glycosides	Hypertension
Antihypertensives (S-H)	Hypotension	Cocaine	Hallucinations, usually visual
Barbiturates (S-H)	Hypothermia	Ethanol withdrawal	Disorientation
Benzodiazepines (S-H)	Flaccid coma	Hydrocarbon inhalation (abuse)	Panic reaction
Butyrophenones (Syly)	Miosis	Mescaline (peyote)	Toxic psychosis
β-Adrenergic blockers (Syly)	Hypoactive bowel sounds	Mushrooms (psilocybin)	Moist skin
Calcium channel blockers (Syly)		Phencyclidine	Mydriasis (reactive)
Digitalis (Syly)			Hyperthermia
Opioids			Flashbacks
Lithium (mixed)			
Muscle relaxants		**Anticholinergics**	
Phenothiazines (Syly)		Antihistamines	Tachycardia, dysrhythmias (rare)
Nonbarbiturate/benzodiazepine glutethimide, methaqualone, methyprylon, sedative-hypnotics (chloral hydrate,ethchlorvynol, bromide)		Antispasmodic gastrointestinal preparations	Tachypnea
Tricyclic antidepressants (late Syly)		Antiparkinsonian preparations	Hypertension (mild)
		Atropine	Hyperthermia
		Cyclobenzaprine (Flexeril)	Hallucinations ("mad as a hatter")
CNS Stimulants			
Amphetamines (Sy)	Tachycardia	Mydriatic ophthalmologic agents	Mydriasis (unreactive) ("blind as a bat")
Anticholinergics*	Tachypnea and dysrhythmias	Over-the-counter sleep agents	Flushed skin ("red as a beet")
		Plants (Datura spp)/mushrooms	Dry skin and mouth ("dry as a bone")
Cocaine (Sy)	Hypertension		Hypoactive bowel sounds
Camphor (mixed)	Convulsions	Phenothiazines (early)	Urinary retention
Ergot alkaloids (Sy)	Toxic psychosis	Scopolamine	Lilliputian hallucinations ("little people")
Isoniazid (mixed)	Mydriasis (reactive)	Tricyclic/cyclic antidepressants (early)	
Lithium (mixed)	Agitation and restlessness	**Cholinergics**	
Lysergic acid diethylamide (H)	Moist skin	Bethanechol (Urecholine)	Bradycardia (muscarinic)
Hallucinogens (H)	Tremors	Carbamate insecticides (Carbaryl)	Tachycardia (nicotinic effect)
Mescaline and synthetic analogs		Edrophonium	Miosis (muscarinic)
Metals (arsenic, lead, mercury)		Organophosphate insecticides (Malathion, parathion)	Diarrhea (muscarinic)
Methylphenidate (Ritalin) (Sy)		Parasympathetic agents (physostigmine, pyridostigmine)	
Monoamine oxidase inhibitors (Sy)		Toxic mushrooms (Clitocybe spp.)	Hypertension (variable)
Pemoline (Cylert) (Sy)			
Phencyclidine (H)†			Hyperactive bowel sounds
Salicylates (mixed)			Excess urination (muscarinic)
Strychnine (mixed)			Excess salivation (muscarinic)
Sympathomimetics (Sy) (phenylpropanolamine, theophylline, caffeine, thyroid)			Lacrimation (muscarinic)
Withdrawal from ethanol, β-adrenergic blockers, clonidine, opioids, sedative–hypnotics (W)			Bronchospasm (muscarinic)
			Muscle fasciculations (nicotinic)
			Paralysis (nicotinic)

Abbreviations: H = hallucinogen; S-H = sedative–hypnotic; Sy = sympathomimetic; Syly = Sympatholytic; W = withdrawal.
*Anticholinergics produce dry skin and mucosa and decreased bowel sounds.
†Phencyclidine may produce miosis.
‡The amphetamine hybrids are methylene dioxymethamphetamine (MDMA, ecstasy, "ADAM") and methylene dioxyamphetamine (MDA, "Eve"), which are associated with deaths.

Rakel and Bope: *Conn's Current Therapy 2006.*

CNS depressants, CNS stimulants, hallucinogens, and autonomic nervous system anticholinergics and cholinergics.

Central nervous system depressants are cholinergics, opioids, sedative-hypnotics, and sympatholytic agents. The hallmarks are lethargy, sedation, stupor, and coma. In exception to the manifestations listed in Table 4, (a) barbiturates may produce an initial tachycardia; (b) convulsions are produced by codeine, propoxyphene (Darvon), meperidine (Demerol), glutethimide, phenothiazines, methaqualone, and tricyclic and cyclic antidepressants; (c) benzodiazepines rarely produce coma that will interfere with cardiorespiratory functions; and (d) pulmonary edema is common with opioids and sedative-hypnotics.

The CNS stimulants are anticholinergic, hallucinogenic, sympathomimetic, and withdrawal agents. The hallmarks of CNS stimulants are convulsions and hyperactivity.

There is considerable overlapping of effects among the various hallucinogens, but the major hallmark manifestation is hallucinations.

Guidelines for In-hospital Disposition

Classification of patients as high risk depends on clinical judgment. Any patient who needs cardiorespiratory support or has a persistently altered mental status for 3 hours or more should be considered for intensive care.

Guidelines for admitting patients older than 14 years of age to an intensive care unit, after 2 to 3 hours in the emergency department, include the following:

1. Need for intubation
2. Seizures
3. Unresponsiveness to verbal stimuli
4. Arterial carbon dioxide pressure greater than 45 mm Hg
5. Cardiac conduction or rhythm disturbances (any rhythm except sinus arrhythmia)
6. Close monitoring of vital signs during antidotal therapy or elimination procedures
7. The need for continuous monitoring
8. QRS interval greater than 0.10 second, in cases of tricyclic antidepressant poisoning
9. Systolic blood pressure less than 80 mm Hg
10. Hypoxia, hypercarbia, acid–base imbalance, or metabolic abnormalities
11. Extremes of temperature
12. Progressive deterioration or significant underlying medical disorders

Use of Antidotes

Antidotes are available for only a relatively small number of poisons. An antidote is not a substitute for good supportive care. Table 5 summarizes the commonly used antidotes, their indications, and their methods of administration. The Regional Poison Control Center can give further information on these antidotes.

Rakel and Bope: *Conn's Current Therapy 2006.*

Enhancement of Elimination

The acceptable methods for elimination of absorbed toxic substances are dialysis, hemoperfusion, exchange transfusion, plasmapheresis, enzyme induction, and inhibition. Methods of increasing urinary excretion of toxic chemicals and drugs have been studied extensively, but the other modalities have not been well evaluated.

In general, these methods are needed in only a minority of cases and should be reserved for life-threatening circumstances when a definite benefit is anticipated.

DIALYSIS

Dialysis is the extrarenal means of removing certain substances from the body, and it can substitute for the kidney when renal failure occurs. Dialysis is not the first measure instituted; however, it may be lifesaving later in the course of a severe intoxication. It is needed in only a minority of intoxicated patients.

Peritoneal dialysis uses the peritoneum as the membrane for dialysis. It is only 1/20 as effective as hemodialysis. It is easier to use and less hazardous to the patient but also less effective in removing the toxin; thus it is rarely used except in small infants.

Hemodialysis is the most effective dialysis method but requires experience with sophisticated equipment. Blood is circulated past a semipermeable extracorporeal membrane. Substances are removed by diffusion down a concentration gradient. Anticoagulation with heparin is necessary. Flow rates of 300 to 500 mL/min can be achieved, and clearance rates may reach 200 or 300 mL/min.

Dialyzable substances easily diffuse across the dialysis membrane and have the following characteristics: (a) a molecular weight less than 500 daltons and preferably less than 350; (b) a volume of distribution less than 1 L/kg; (c) protein binding less than 50%; (d) high water solubility (low lipid solubility); and (e) high plasma concentration and a toxicity that correlates reasonably with the plasma concentration. Considerations for hemodialysis and hemoperfusion are cases of serious ingestions (the nephrologist should be notified immediately), and cases involving a compound that is ingested in a potentially lethal dose and the rapid removal of which may improve the prognosis. Examples of the latter are ethylene glycol 1.4 mL/kg 100% solution or equivalent and methanol 6 mL/kg 100% solution or equivalent. Common dialyzable substances include alcohol, bromides, lithium, and salicylates.

The patient-related criteria for dialysis are (a) anticipated prolonged coma and the likelihood of complications; (b) renal compromise (toxin excreted or metabolized by kidneys and dialyzable chelating agents in heavy metal poisoning); (c) laboratory confirmation of lethal blood concentration; (d) lethal dose poisoning with an agent with delayed toxicity or known to be metabolized into a more toxic metabolite (e.g., ethylene glycol, methanol); and (e) hepatic impairment when the agent is metabolized by the liver, and clinical deterioration despite optimal supportive medical management. Table 6 gives

18

TABLE 5 Initial Doses of Antidotes for Common Poisonings

Antidote	Use	Dose	Route	Adverse reactions/Comments
N-Acetyl cysteine (NAC, Mucomyst): Stock level to treat 70 kg adult for 24 h: 25 vials, 20%, 30 mL	Acetaminophen, carbon tetrachloride (experimental)	140/mg/kg loading, followed by 70 mg/kg every 4 h for 17 doses.	PO	Nausea, vomiting. Dilute to 5% with sweet juice or flat cola.
Atropine: Stock level to treat 70 kg adult for 24 h: 1 g (1 mg/mL in 1, 10 mL)	Organophosphate and carbamate pesticides: bradydysrhythmics, β-adrenergics, calcium channel blockers	*Child:* 0.02-0.05 mg/kg repeated q5-10 min to max of 2 mg as necessary until cessation of secretions *Adult:* 1-2 mg q5-10 min as necessary. Dilute in 1-2 mL of 0.9% saline for ET instillation. *IV infusion dose:* Place 8 mg of atropine in 100 mL D₅W or saline. Conc. = 0.08 mg/mL; dose range = 0.02-0.08 mg/kg/h or 0.25-1 mL/kg/h. Severe poisoning may require supplemental doses of IV atropine intermittently in doses of 1-5 mg until drying of secretions occurs.	IV/ET	Tachycardia, dry mouth, blurred vision, and urinary retention. Ensure adequate ventilation before administration.
Calcium chloride (10%): Stock level to treat 70 kg adult for 24 h: 10 vials 1 g (1.35 mEq/mL)	Hypocalcemia, fluoride, calcium channel blockers, β-blockers, oxalates, ethylene glycol, hypermagnesemia	0.1-0.2 mL/kg (10-20 mg/kg) slow push every 10 min up to max 10 mL (1 g). Since calcium response lasts 15 minutes, some may require continuous infusion 0.2 mL/kg/h up to maximum of 10 mL/h while monitoring for dysrhythmias and hypotension.	IV	Administer slowly with BP and ECG monitoring and have magnesium available to reverse calcium effects. Tissue irritation, hypotension, dysrhythmias from rapid injection. Contraindications: digitalis glycoside intoxication.
Calcium gluconate (10%): Stock level to treat 70 kg adult for 24 h: 20 vials 1 g (0.45 mEq/mL)	Hypocalcemia, fluoride, calcium channel blockers, hydrofluoric acid; black widow envenomation	0.3-0.4 mL/kg (30-40 mg/kg) slow push; repeat as needed up to max dose 10-20 mL (1-2 g).	IV	Same comments as calcium chloride.
Infiltration of calcium gluconate	Hydrofluoric acid skin exposure	Dose: Infiltrate each square cm of affected dermis/subcutaneous tissue with about 0.5 mL of 10% calcium gluconate using a 30-gauge needle. Repeat as needed to control pain.	Infiltrate	

Rakel and Bope: *Conn's Current Therapy 2006.*

Agent	Indication	Dose/Administration	Route	Comments
Intra-arterial calcium gluconate	Hydrofluoric acid skin exposure	Infuse 20 mL of 10% calcium gluconate (not chloride) diluted in 250 mL D$_5$W via the radial or brachial artery proximal to the injury over 3-4 hours.		Alternatively, dilute 10 mL of 10% calcium gluconate with 40-50 mL of D$_5$W.
Calcium gluconate gel Stock level: 3.5 g	Hydrofluoric acid skin exposure	2.5 g USP powder added to 100 mL water-soluble lubricating jelly, e.g., K-Y Jelly or Lubifax (or 3.5 mg into 150 mL). Some use 6 g of calcium carbonate in 100 g of lubricant. Place injured hand in surgical glove filled with gel. Apply q4h. If pain persists, calcium gluconate injection may be needed (above).	Dermal	Powder is available from Spectrum Pharmaceutical Co. in California: 800-772-8786. Commercial preparation of Ca gluconate gel is available from Pharmascience in Montreal, Quebec: 514-340-1114.
Cyanide antidote kit: Stock level to treat 70 kg adult for 24 h: 2 Lilly Cyanide Antidote kits	Cyanide Hydrogen sulfide (nitrites are given only) Do not use sodium thiosulfate for hydrogen sulfide Individual portions of the kit can be used in certain circumstances (consult PCC)	Amyl nitrite: 1 crushable ampule for 30 secs of every min. Use new amp q3min. May omit step if venous access is established.	Inhalation	If methemoglobinemia occurs, do not use methylene blue to correct this because it releases cyanide.
	Cyanide Hydrogen sulfide (nitrites are given only) Do not use sodium thiosulfate for hydrogen sulfide Individual portions of the kit can be used in certain circumstances (consult PCC)	Sodium nitrite: *Child:* 0.33 mL/kg of 3% solution if hemoglobin level is not known, otherwise based on tables with product. *Adult:* up to 300 mg (10 mL). Dilute nitrite in 100 mL 0.9% saline, administer slowly at 5 mL/min. Slow infusion if fall in BP.	IV	If methemoglobinemia occurs, do not use methylene blue to correct this because it releases cyanide.
	Do not use sodium thiosulfate for hydrogen sulfide Individual portions of the Kit can be used in certain circumstances (consult PCC)	Sodium thiosulfate: *Child:* 1.6 mL/kg of 25% solution, may be repeated every 30-60 min to a maximum of 12.5 g or 50 mL in adult. Administer over 20 min.	IV	Nausea, dizziness, headache. Tachycardia, muscle rigidity, and bronchospasm (rapid administration).
Dantrolene sodium (Dantrium): Stock level to treat 70 kg adult for 24 h: 700 mg, 35 vials (20 mg/vial)	Malignant hyperthermia	2–3 mg/kg IV rapidly. Repeat loading dose every 10 minutes, if necessary up to a maximum total dose of 10 mg/kg. When temperature and heart rate decrease, slow the infusion	IV/PO	Hepatotoxicity occurs with cumulative dose of 10 mg/kg. Thrombophlebitis (best given in central line). Available as 20 mg lyophilized dantrolene powder for

Continued

Rakel and Bope: *Conn's Current Therapy 2006.*

TABLE 5 Initial Doses of Antidotes for Common Poisonings—cont'd

Antidote	Use	Dose	Route	Adverse reactions/Comments
Deferoxamine (Desferal): Stock level to treat 70 kg adult for 24 h: 17 vials (500 mg/amp).	Iron	1-2 mg/kg every 6 hours for 24-28 h until all evidence of malignant hyperthermia syndrome has subsided. Follow with oral doses 1-2 mg/kg four times a day for 24 h as necessary.	Preferred IV: avoid therapy >24 h	reconstruction, which contains 3 g mannitol and sodium hydroxide in 70-mL vial. Mix with 60 mL sterile distilled water without a bacteriostatic agent and protect from light. Use within 6 hours after reconstituting. Hypotension (minimized by avoiding rapid infusion rates) DFO challenge test 50 mg/kg is unreliable if negative.
Diazepam (Valium) Stock level to treat 70 kg adult for 24 h: 200 mg, 5 mg/mL; 2,10 mL	Any intoxication that provokes seizures when specific therapy is not available, e.g., amphetamines, PCP, barbiturate and alcohol withdrawal. Chloroquine poisoning.	Adult, 5-10 mg IV (max 20 mg) at a rate of 5 mg/min until seizure is controlled. May be repeated 2 or 3 times. Child, 0.1-0.3 mg/kg up to 10 mg IV slowly over 2 min.	IV	Confusion, somnolence, coma, hypotension. Intramuscular absorption is erratic Establish airway and administer 100% oxygen and glucose.
Digoxin-specific Fab antibodies (Digibind): Stock level to treat 70 kg adult for 24 h: 20 vials.	Digoxin, digitoxin, oleander tea with the following: (1) Imminent cardiac arrest or shock, (2) hyperkalemia >5.0 mEq/L. (3) serum digoxin >5 ng/mL (child) at 8-12 h post ingestion in adults, (4) digitalis delirium, (5) ingestion over 10 mg in adults or 4 mg in child, (6) bradycardia or second- or third-degree heart block unresponsive to atropine, (7) life threatening digitoxin or oleander posioning.	(1) If amount ingested is known total dose × bioavailability (0.8) = body burden. The body burden + 0.6 (0.5 mg of digoxin is bound by 1 vial of 38 mg of FAB) = # vials needed. (2) If amount is unknown but the steady state serum concentration is known in ng/mL: Digoxin: ng/mL: (5.6 L/kg Vd) × (wt kg) = μg body burden. Body burden + 100 = mg body burden/0.5 = # vials needed. Digitoxin body burden = ng/mL × (0.56 L/kg Vd) × (wt kg) Body burden + 1000 = mg body burden/0.5 = # vials needed. (3) If the amount is not known, it is administered in life-threatening situations as 10 vials (400 mg) IV in saline over 30 min in adults. If cardiac arrest is imminent, administer 20 vials (adult) as a bolus.	IV	Allergic reactions (rare), return of condition being treated with digitalis glycoside. Administer by infusion over 30 min through a 0.22-μ filter. If cardiac arrest imminent, may administer by bolus. Consult PCC for more details.

Rakel and Bope: *Conn's Current Therapy 2006.*

Drug	Uses	Dose	Route	Precautions/Adverse Effects
Dimercaprol (BAL in peanut oil): Stock level to treat 70 kg adult for 24 h: 1200 mg (4 amps—100 mg/mL 10% in oil in 3 mL amp)	Chelating agent for arsenic, mercury, and lead.	3-5 mg/kg q4th usually for 5-10 d	Deep IM	Local infection site pain and sterile abscess, nausea, vomiting, fever, salivation, hypertension, and nephrotoxicity (alkalinize urine).
2,3 Dimercaptosuccinic acid (DMSA succimer): 100 mg/capsule: 20 capsules	Used as a chelating agent for lead, especially blood lead levels >45 µg/dL. May also be used for symptomatic mercury exposure	10 mg/kg 3 × daily for 5 days followed by 10 mg/kg 2 × daily for 14 days.	PO	Precautions: monitor AST/ALT; use with caution in G6PD-deficient patients. Avoid concurrent iron therapy. Relatively safe antidote, rarely severe, uncommon minor skin rashes may occur.
Diphenhydramine (Benadryl) Antiparkinsonian action. Stock level to treat a 70 kg adult for 24 h: 5 vials (10 mg/mL, 10 mL each)	Used to treat extrapyramidal symptoms and dystonia induced by phenothiazines, phencyclidine, and related drugs.	*Children:* 1-2 mg/kg IV slowly over 5 minutes up to maximum 50 mg followed by 5 mg/kg/24 h orally divided every 6 hours up to 300 mg/24h *Adults:* 50 mg IV followed by 50 mg orally four times daily for 5-7 days Note: Symptoms abate within 2-5 min after IV.	IV	Fatal dose: 20-40 mg/kg. Dry mouth, drowsiness.
Ethanol (ethyl alcohol): Stock level to treat 70 kg adult for 24 h: 3 bottles 10% (1 L each)	Methanol, ethylene glycol	10 mL/kg loading dose concurrently with 1.4 mL/kg (average) infusion of 10% ethanol (consult PCC for more details)	IV	Nausea, vomiting, sedation. Use 0.22 µm filter if preparing from bulk 100% ethanol.
Flumazenil (Romazicon): Stock level to treat 70 kg adult for 24 h: 4 vials (0.1 mg/mL, 10 mL)	Benzodiazepines (may also be beneficial in the treatment of hepatic encephalopathy)	Administer 0.2 mg (2 mL) IV over 30 sec (pediatric dose not established, 0.01 mg/kg), then wait 3 min for a response, then if desired consciousness is not achieved, administer 0.3 mg (3 mL) over 30 sec, then wait 3 min for response, then if desired consciousness is not achieved, administer 0.5 mg (5 mL) over 30 sec at 60-sec intervals up to a maximum cumulative dose of 3 mg (30 mL) (1 mg in children). Because effects last only 1-5 hours, if patient responds monitor carefully over next 6 hours for resedation. If multiple repeated doses, consider a continuous infusion of 0.2-1 mg/h.	IV	Nausea, vomiting, facial flushing, agitation, headache, dizziness, seizures, and death. It is not recommended to improve ventilation. Its role in CNS depression needs to be clarified. It should not be used routinely in comatose patients. It is **contraindicated** in cyclic antidepressant intoxications, stimulant overdose, long-term benzodiazepine use (may precipitate life-threatening withdrawal), if benzodiazepines are used to control seizures, in head trauma.

Continued

TABLE 5   Initial Doses of Antidotes for Common Poisonings—cont'd

Antidote	Use	Dose	Route	Adverse Reactions/Comments
Folic acid (Folvite): Stock level to treat 70 kg adult for 24 h: 4 100-mg vials	Methanol/ethylene glycol (investigational)	1 mg/kg up to 50 mg q4h for 6 doses.	IV	Uncommon
Fomepizole (4-MP, Antizol): Stock level to treat 70 kg adult: 4 1.5-mL vials (1 g/mL)	Ethylene glycol Methanol	Loading dose: 15 mg/kg (0.015 mL/kg) IV followed by maintenance dose of 10 mg/kg (0.01 mL/kg) every 12h for 4 doses, then 15 mg/kg every 12h until ethylene glycol levels are <20 mg/dL. Fomipazole can be given to patients undergoing hemodialysis (dose q4h).	IV	Suggested: co-administer folate 50 mg IV (child1 mg/kg), thiamine 100 mg/d (child 50 mg), and pyridoxine 50 mg IV/IM q6h until intoxication is resolved. Monitor for urinary oxalate crystals. Adverse reactions include headache, nausea, and dizziness. Antizole should be diluted in 100 mL 0.9% saline or D_5W and mixed well. Antizole should not be given undiluted. Use D_5W, not 0.9% saline, to reconstitute the glucagon (rather than diluent of Eli Lilly, which contains phenol).
Glucagon: Stock level to treat 70 kg adult for 24 h: approx 25 g (50 mL of 50% or 200 mL of 12.5%)	β-Blocker, calcium channel blocker	3-10 mg in adult, then infuse 2-5 mg/h (0.05-0.1 mg/kg in child, then infuse 0.07 mg/kg/h) Large doses up to 100 mg/24h used	IV	Vomiting precautions.
Magnesium sulfate: Stock level to treat 70 kg adult for 24 h: (10 vials, 10 units)	Torsades de pointes	*Adult:* 2 g (20 mL or 20%) over 20 min. If no response in 10 min, repeat and follow by continuous infusion 1 g/h. *Children:* 25-50 mg/kg initially and maintenance is (30-60 mg/kg/24h) (0.25-0.5 mEq/kg/24h) up to 1000 mg/24h. (Dose not studied in controlled fashion.)	IV	Use with caution if renal impairment is present.
Methylene blue: Stock level to treat 70 kg adult for 24 h: 5 amps (10 mg/10 mL)	Methemoglobinemia	0.1-0.2 mL/kg of 1% solution, slow infusion, may be repeated every 30-60 min	IV	Nausea, vomiting, headache, dizziness.
Naloxone (Narcan): Stock level to treat 70 kg adult for 24 h: 3 vials (1 mg/mL, 10 mL)	Comatose patient; decreased respirations <12; opioids	In postoperative opioid depression reversal, IV 0.1-0.5 μg/kg every 2 min as needed and may repeat up to a total dose of 1 μg/kg In **suspected overdose,** administer IV 0.1 mg/kg in a child younger than 5 years of age up to 2 mg, in older children and adults administer 2 mg every 2 min up to a total of 10-20 mg. Can also be administered into the	IV, ET	**Larger doses** of naloxone may be required for more poorly antagonized synthetic opioid drugs: buprenorphine (Buprenex), codeine, dextromethorphan, fentanyl, pentazocine (Talwin), propoxyphene (Darvon), diphenoxylate, nalbuphine (Nubain), new potent "designer" drugs, or long-acting opioids such as methadone (Dolophine). **Complications.** Although naloxone is safe and effective, there are rare reports of

Rakel and Bope: *Conn's Current Therapy 2006.*

Antidote	Indication	Route	Dose	Adverse Effects/Comments
			endotracheal tube. If no response by 10 mg, a pure opioid intoxication is unlikely. **If opioid abuse** is suspected, **restraints** should be in place before administration; **initial dose** 0.1 mg to avoid withdrawal and violent behavior. The initial dose is then doubled every minute progressively to a total of 10 mg. **A continuous infusion** has been advocated because many opioids outlast the short half-life of naloxone (30-60 min). **The naloxone infusion hourly rate** to produce a response is equal to the effective dose required (improvement in ventilation and arousal). An additional dose may be required in 15-30 min as a bolus.	complications (<1%) of pulmonary edema, seizures, hypertension, cardiac arrest, and sudden death. The infusions are titrated to avoid respiratory depression and opioid withdrawal manifestations. Tapering of infusions can be attempted after 12h and when the patient's condition is stable.
Physostigmine (Antilirium): Stock level to treat 70 kg adult for 24 h: 2-4 mg (2 mL each)	Anticholinergic agents (not routinely used, only indicated if life-threatening complications).		*Child:* 0.02 mg/kg slow push to max 2 mg q30-60 min; *Adult:* 1-2 mg q5 min to max 6 mg.	
Pralidoxime (2PAM, Protopan): Stock level to treat 70 kg adult for 24 h: 12 vials (1 g per 20 mL)	Organophosphates	IV	Child ≤12 y, 25-50 mg/kg max (4 mg/min); >12 y, 1-2 g/dose in 250 mL of 0.9% saline over 5-10 min. Max 200 mg/min. Repeat q6-12h for 24-48h. Max adult 6 g/d. Alternative: Maintenance infusion 1 g in 100 mL, of 0.9% saline at 5-20 mg/kg/h (0.5-12 mL/kg/h) up to max 500 mg/h or 50 mL/h. Titrate to desired response. End point is absence of fasciculations and return of muscle strength.	Bradycardia, asystole, seizures, bronchospasm, vomiting, headaches. Do not use for cyclic antidepressants.
		IV		Nausea, dizziness, headache; tachycardia. muscle rigidity, bronchospasm (rapid administration).
Pyridoxine (vitamin B$_6$): Stock level to treat 70 kg adult for 24 h: 100 mg/mL 10% solution. For a 70 kg patient, 10 g = 10 vials	Seizures from isoniazid or *Gyromitra* mushrooms; ethylene glycol	IV	*Isoniazid: Unknown amt ingested:* 5 g (70 mg/kg) in 50 mL D$_5$W over 5 min + diazepam 0.3 mg/kg IV at rate of 1 mg/min in child or 10 mg dose at rate up to 5 mg/min in adults. Use different site (synergism). May repeat q5-20 min until seizure controlled.	After seizure is controlled, administer remainder of pyridoxine 1 g/1 g isoniazid total 5 g as infusion over 60 min. Adverse reactions uncommon; do not administer in same bottle as sodium bicarbonate. For *Gyromitra* mushrooms, some use PO 25 mg/kg/d early when mushroom ingestion is suspected.

Continued

Rakel and Bope: *Conn's Current Therapy 2006.*

TABLE 5 Initial Doses of Antidotes for Common Poisonings—cont'd

Antidote	Use	Dose	Route	Adverse reactions/Comments
		Up to 375 mg/kg have been given (52 g). *Known amount:* 1 g for each gram isoniazid ingested over 5 min with diazepam (dose above) *Gyromitra mushroom:* Child 25 mg/kg or 2-5 g, adults IV over 15-30 min to max 20 g.		
Sodium bicarbonate (NaHCO₃): Stock level to treat 70 kg adult for 24 h; 10 ampules or syringes (500 mEq)	Tricyclic antidepressant cardiotoxicity (QRS >0.12 sec; ventricular tachycardia, severe conduction disturbances); metabolic acidosis; phenothiazine toxicity *Salicylate:* to keep blood pH 7.5-7.55 (not >7.55) and urine pH 7.5-8.0. Alkalinization recommended if salicylate conc. >40 mg/dL in acute poisoning and at lower levels if symptomatic in chronic intoxication. 2 mEq/kg will raise blood pH 0.1 unit	*Ethylene glycol:* 100 mg IV daily. 1-2 mEq/kg undiluted as a bolus. If no effect on cardiotoxicity, repeat twice a few minutes apart

Adult with clear physical signs and laboratory findings of acute moderate or severe salicylism: Bolus 1-2 mEq/kg followed by infusion of 100-150 mEq NaHCO₃ added to 1 L of 5% dextrose at rate of 200-300 mL/h *Child:* Bolus same as adult followed by 1-2 mEq/kg in infusion of 20 mL/kg/h 5% dextrose in 0.45% saline. Add potassium when patient voids. Rate and amount of the initial infusion, if patient is volume depleted: 1 h to achieve urine output of 2 mL/kg/h and urine pH 7-8. | IV | Monitor sodium, potassium, and blood pH because fatal alkalemia and hyponatremia have been reported.

Monitor both urine and blood pH. Do not use the urine pH alone to assess the need for alkalinization because of the paradoxical aciduria that may occur. Adjust the urine pH to 7.5-8 by NaHCO₃ infusion. After urine output established, add potassium 40 mEq/L. |

Rakel and Bope: *Conn's Current Therapy 2006.*

In mild cases without acidosis and urine pH >6 administer 5% dextrose in 0.9% saline with 50 mEq/L or 1 mEq/kg $NaHCO_3$ as maintenance to replace ongoing renal losses. If acidemia is present and pH <7.2, add 2 mEq/kg as loading dose followed by 2 mEq/kg q3 to 4h to keep pH at 7.5-7.55. If acidemia is present, recommend isotonic $NaHCO_3$, 3 ampules to 1 L of D_5W @ 10-15 mL/kg/h or sufficient to produce normal urine flow and a urine pH of 7.5 or higher.

Drug	Indication	Dose	Route	Notes
	Long-acting barbiturates: Phenobarbital and primidone (Mysoline) Note: Alkalinization is ineffective for the short- or intermediate-acting barbiturates	$NaHCO_3$: 2 mEq/kg during the first hour or 100 mEq in 1 L of D_5W with 40 mEq/L potassium at rate of 100 mL/h in adults. Adequate potassium is necessary to accomplish alkalinization	IV	Additional sodium bicarbonate and potassium chloride may be needed. Adjust the urine pH to 7.5-8 by $NaHCO_3$ infusion.
Thiamine 100 mg/mL, 2 vials	Thiamine deficiency, ethylene glycol poisoning, alcoholism	100 mg IV followed with 100 mg V/IM for 5-7 days in an alcoholic and followed by 100 mg/d orally.	IV/IM	
Vitamin K₁ (Aqua Mephyton) 10 mg/1-5 mL; 5 mg tablets	Warfarin anticoagulant or rodenticide toxicity	Oral 0.4 mg/kg/dose child, 10-25 mg adults. If evidence of bleeding administer vitamin K_1 SC, IV 0.6 mg/kg/dose child and up to 25-50 mg adults for 6 hours depending on severity.	PO/SC, IV	Give vitamin K daily until PT/INR are normal. Examine stools and urine for evidence of bleeding.

Abbreviations: ALT = alanine aminotransferase; amp = ampule; AST = aspartate aminotransferase; BAL = British anti-Lewisite; BP = blood pressure; Conc. = concentration; ECG = electrocardiogram; ET = endotracheal; G6PD = glucose-6-phosphate dehydrogenase; IM = intramuscular; IV = intravenous; PCC = poison control center; PO = oral; PT = Prothrombin time; SC = subcutaneous.

TABLE 6 Plasma Concentrations Above Which Removal by Extracorporeal Measures Should Be Considered

Drug	Plasma concentration	Protein binding (%)	Volume distribution (L/kg)	Method of choice
Amanitin	NA	25	1.0	HP
Ethanol	500-700 mg/dL	0	0.3	HD
Ethchlorvynol	150 µg/mL	35-50	3-4	HP
Ethylene glycol	25-50 µg/mL	0	0.6	HD
Glutethimide	100 µg/mL	50	2.7	HP
Isopropyl alcohol	400 mg/dL	0	0.7	HD
Lithium	4 mEq/L	0	0.7	HD
Meprobamate (Equanil)	100 µg/mL	0	NA	HP
Methanol	50 mg/dL	0	0.7	HD
Methaqualone	40 µg/dL	20-60	6.0	HP
Other barbiturates	50 µg/dL	50	0-1	HP
Paraquat	0.1 mg/dL	poor	2.8	HP > HD
Phenobarbital	100 µg/dL	50	0.9	HP > HD
Salicylates	80-100 mg/dL	90	0.2	HD > HP
Theophylline		0	0.5	
Chronic	40-60 µg/mL			HP
Acute	80-100 µg/mL			HP
Trichlorethanol	250 µg/mL	70	0.6	HP

Abbreviations: HD = hemodialysis; HP = hemoperfusion; HP > HD hemoperfusion preferred over hemodialysis.
Note: Cartridges for charcoal hemoperfusion are not readily available anymore in most locations, so hemodialysis may be substituted in these situations.
In mixed or chronic drug overdoses, extracorporeal measures may be considered at lower drug concentrations.
Data from Winchester JF: Active methods for detoxification. In Haddad LM, Winchester JF (eds). Clinical Management of Poisoning and Drug Overdose, 2nd ed. Philadelphia, WB Saunders, 1990; Balsam L, Cortitsidis GN, Fienfeld DA: Role of hemodialysis and hemoperfusion in the treatment of intoxications. Contemp Manage Crit Care 1:61, 1991.

plasma concentrations above which removal by extracorporeal measures should be considered.

The contraindications to hemodialysis include the following: (a) substances are not dialyzable; (b) effective antidotes are available; (c) patient is hemodynamically unstable (e.g., shock); and (d) presence of coagulopathy because heparinization is required.

Hemodialysis also has a role in correcting disturbances that are not amenable to appropriate medical management. These are easily remembered by the "vowel" mnemonic:

A—refractory acid–base disturbances
E—refractory electrolyte disturbances
I—intoxication with dialyzable substances (e.g., ethanol, ethylene glycol, isopropyl alcohol, methanol, lithium, and salicylates)
O—overhydration
U—uremia

Complications of dialysis include hemorrhage, thrombosis, air embolism, hypotension, infections, electrolyte imbalance, thrombocytopenia, and removal of therapeutic medications.

HEMOPERFUSION

Hemoperfusion is the parenteral form of oral activated charcoal. Heparinization is necessary. The patient's blood is routed extracorporeally through an outflow arterial catheter through a filter-adsorbing cartridge (charcoal or resin) and returned through a venous catheter.

Cartridges must be changed every 4 hours. The blood glucose, electrolytes, calcium, and albumin levels; complete blood cell count; platelets; and serum and urine osmolarity must be carefully monitored. This procedure has extended extracorporeal removal to a large range of substances that were formerly either poorly dialyzable or nondialyzable. It is not limited by molecular weight, water solubility, or protein binding, but it is limited by a volume distribution greater than 400 L, plasma concentration, and rate of flow through the filter. Activated charcoal cartridges are the primary type of hemoperfusion that is currently available in the United States.

The patient-related criteria for hemoperfusion are (a) anticipated prolonged coma and the likelihood of complications; (b) laboratory confirmation of lethal blood concentrations; (c) hepatic impairment when an agent is metabolized by the liver; and (d) clinical deterioration despite optimally supportive medical management.

The contraindications are similar to those for hemodialysis.

Limited data are available as to which toxins are best treated with hemoperfusion. Hemoperfusion has proved useful in treating glutethimide intoxication, phenobarbital overdose, and carbamazepine, phenytoin, and theophylline intoxication.

Complications include hemorrhage, thrombocytopenia, hypotension, infection, leukopenia, depressed phagocytic activity of granulocytes, decreased immunoglobulin levels, hypoglycemia, hypothermia, hypocalcemia, pulmonary edema, and air and charcoal embolism.

Rakel and Bope: *Conn's Current Therapy 2006.*

HEMOFILTRATION

Continuous arteriovenous or venovenous hemodia fil-tration (CAVHD or CVVHD, respectively) has been suggested as an alternative to conventional hemodialy-sis when the need for rapid removal of the drug is less urgent. These procedures, like peritoneal dialysis, are minimally invasive, have no significant impact on hemodynamics, and can be carried out continuously for many hours. Their role in the management of acute poisoning remains uncertain, however.

PLASMAPHERESIS

Plasmapheresis consists of removal of a volume of blood. All the extracted components are returned to the blood except the plasma, which is replaced with a colloid protein solution. There are limited clinical data on guidelines and efficacy in toxicology. Centrifugal and membrane separators of cellular elements are used. It can be as effective as hemodialysis or hemoperfusion for removing toxins that have high protein binding, and it may be useful for toxins not filtered by hemodialysis and hemoperfusion.

Plasmapheresis has been anecdotally used in treat-ing intoxications with the following agents: paraquat (removed 10%), propranolol (removed 30%), quinine (removed 10%), L-thyroxine (removed 30%), and salicy-late (removed 10%). It has been shown to remove less than 10% of digoxin, phenobarbital, prednisolone, and tobramycin. Complications include infection; allergic reactions including anaphylaxis; hemorrhagic dis-orders; thrombocytopenia; embolus and thrombus; hypervolemia and hypovolemia; dysrhythmias; syncope; tetany; paresthesia; pneumothorax; acute respiratory distress syndrome; and seizures.

Supportive Care, Observation, and Therapy for Complications

ALTERED MENTAL STATUS

If airway protective reflexes are absent, endotracheal intubation is indicated for a comatose patient or a patient with altered mental status. If respirations are ineffective, ventilation should be instituted, and if hypoxemia persists, supplemental oxygen is indicated. If a cyanotic patient fails to respond to oxygen, the prac-titioner should consider methemoglobinemia.

HYPOGLYCEMIA

Hypoglycemia accompanies many poisonings, including with ethanol (especially in children), clonidine (Catapres), insulin, organophosphates, salicylates, sulfonylureas, and the unripe fruit or seed of a Jamaican plant called ackee. If hypoglycemia is present or suspected, glucose should be administered immediately as an intravenous bolus. Doses are as follows: in a neonate, 10% glucose (5 mL/kg); in a child, 25% glucose 0.25 g/kg (2 mL/kg); and in an adults, 50% glucose 0.5 g/kg (1 mL/kg).

A bedside capillary test for blood glucose is performed to detect hypoglycemia, and the sample is sent to the laboratory for confirmation. If the glucose reagent strip visually reads less than 150 mg/dL, one administers glucose. Venous blood should be used rather than capillary blood for the bedside test if the patient is in shock or is hypotensive. Large amounts of glucose given rapidly to nondiabetic patients may cause a transient reactive hypoglycemia and hyperkalemia and may accentuate damage in ischemic cerebrovascular and cardiac tissue. If focal neurologic signs are present, it may be prudent to withhold glucose, because hypo-glycemia causes focal signs in less than 10% of cases.

THIAMINE DEFICIENCY ENCEPHALOPATHY

Thiamine is administered to avoid precipitating thi-amine deficiency encephalopathy (Wernicke-Korsakoff syndrome) in alcohol abusers and in malnourished patients. The overall incidence of thiamine deficiency in ethanol abusers is 12%. Thiamine 100 mg intra-venously should be administered around the time of the glucose administration but not necessarily before the glucose. The clinician should be prepared to manage the anaphylaxis that sometimes is caused by thiamine, although it is extremely rare.

OPIOID REACTIONS

Naloxone (Narcan) reverses CNS and respiratory depres-sion, miosis, bradycardia, and decreased gastrointestinal peristalsis caused by opioids acting through μ, κ, and δ receptors. It also affects endogenous opioid peptides (endorphins and enkephalins), which accounts for the variable responses reported in patients with intoxications from ethanol, benzodiazepines, clonidine (Catapres), cap-topril (Capoten), and valproic acid (Depakote) and in patients with spinal cord injuries. There is a high sensi-tivity for predicting a response if pinpoint pupils and cir-cumstantial evidence of opioid abuse (e.g., track marks) are present.

In cases of suspected overdose, naloxone 0.1 mg/kg is administered intravenously initially in a child younger than 5 years of age. The dose can be repeated in 2 min-utes, if necessary up to a total dose of 2 mg. In older children and adults, the dose is 2 mg every 2 minutes for five doses up to a total of 10 mg. Naloxone can also be administered into an endotracheal tube if intravenous access is unavailable. If there is no response after 10 mg, a pure opioid intoxication is unlikely. If opioid abuse is suspected, restraints should be in place before the administration of nalox-one, and it is recommended that the initial dose be 0.1 to 0.2 mg to avoid withdrawal and violent behavior. The initial dose is then doubled every minute prog-ressively to a total of 10 mg. Naloxone may unmask concomitant sympathomimetic intoxication as well as withdrawal.

Larger doses of naloxone may be required for more poorly antagonized synthetic opioid drugs: buprenor-phine (Buprenex), codeine, dextromethorphan, fentanyl and its derivatives, pentazocine (Talwin), propoxyphene

(Darvon), diphenoxylate, nalbuphine (Nubain), and long-acting opioids such as methadone (Dolophine).

Indications for a continuous infusion include a second dose for recurrent respiratory depression, exposure to poorly antagonized opioids, a large overdose, and decreased opioid metabolism, as with impaired liver function. A continuous infusion has been advocated because many opioids outlast the short half-life of naloxone (30 to 60 minutes). The hourly rate of naloxone infusion is equal to the effective dose required to produce a response (improvement in ventilation and arousal). An additional dose may be required in 15 to 30 minutes as a bolus. The infusions are titrated to avoid respiratory depression and opioid withdrawal manifestations. Tapering of infusions can be attempted after 12 hours and when the patient's condition has been stabilized.

Although naloxone is safe and effective, there are rare reports of complications (less than 1%) of pulmonary edema, seizures, hypertension, cardiac arrest, and sudden death.

AGENTS WHOSE ROLES ARE NOT CLARIFIED

Nalmefene (Revex), a long-acting parenteral opioid antagonist that the Food and Drug Administration has approved, is undergoing investigation, but its role in the treatment of comatose patients and patients with opioid overdose is not clear. It is 16 times more potent than naloxone, and its duration of action is up to 8 hours (half-life 10.8 hours, versus naloxone 1 hour).

Flumazenil (Romazicon) is a pure competitive benzodiazepine antagonist. It has been demonstrated to be safe and effective for reversing benzodiazepine-induced sedation. It is not recommended to improve ventilation. Its role in cases of CNS depression needs to be clarified. It should not be used routinely in comatose patients and is not an essential ingredient of the coma therapeutic regimen. It is contraindicated in cases of co-ingestion of cyclic antidepressant intoxication, stimulant overdose, and long-term benzodiazepine use (may precipitate life-threatening withdrawal) if benzodiazepines are used to control seizures. There is a concern about the potential for seizures and cardiac dysrhythmias that may occur in these settings.

Laboratory and Radiographic Studies

An electrocardiogram (ECG) should be obtained to identify dysrhythmias or conduction delays from cardiotoxic medications. If aspiration pneumonia (history of loss of consciousness, unarousable state, vomiting) or noncardiac pulmonary edema is suspected, a chest radiograph is needed. Electrolyte and glucose concentrations in the blood, the anion gap, acid–base balance, the arterial blood gas (ABG) profile (if patient has respiratory distress or altered mental status), and serum osmolality should be measured if a toxic alcohol ingestion is suspected. Table 7 lists appropriate testing on the basis of

TABLE 7 Patient Condition/Systemic Toxin and Appropriate Tests

Condition	Tests
Comatose	Toxicologic tests (acetaminophen, sedative-hypnotic, ethanol, opioids, benzodiazepine), glucose.
Respiratory toxicity	Spirometry, FEV_1, arterial blood gases, chest radiograph, monitor O_2 saturation
Cardiac toxicity	ECG 12-lead and monitoring, echocardiogram, serial cardiac enzymes (if evidence or suspicion of a myocardial infarction), hemodynamic monitoring
Hepatic toxicity	Enzymes (AST, ALT, GGT), ammonia, albumin, bilirubin, glucose, PT, PTT, amylase
Nephrotoxicity	BUN, creatinine, electrolytes (Na, F, Mg, Ca, PO_4), serum and urine osmolarity, 24-hour urine for heavy metals if suspected, creatine kinase, serum and urine myoglobin, urinalysis and urinary sodium
Bleeding	Platelets, PT, PTT, bleeding time, fibrin split products, fibrinogen, type and match

Abbreviations: ALT = alanine aminotransaminase; AST = aspartate aminotransaminase; BUN = blood urea nitrogen; ECG = electrocardiogram; FEV_1 = forced expiratory volume at 1 second; GGT = γ-glutamyltransferase; PT = prothrombin time; PTT = partial thromboplastin time.

clinical toxicologic presentation. All laboratory specimens should be carefully labeled, including time and date. For potential legal cases, a "chain of custody" must be established. Assessment of the laboratory studies may provide a clue to the etiologic agent.

ELECTROLYTE, ACID-BASE, AND OSMOLALITY DISTURBANCES

Electrolyte and acid–base disturbances should be evaluated and corrected. Metabolic acidosis (usually low or normal pH with a low or normal/high $Paco_2$ and low HCO_3) with an increased anion gap is seen with many agents in cases of overdose.

The anion gap is an estimate of those anions other than chloride and HCO_3 necessary to counterbalance the positive charge of sodium. It serves as a clue to causes, compensations, and complications. The anion gap (AG) is calculated from the standard serum electrolytes by subtracting the total CO_2 (which reflects the actual measured bicarbonate) and chloride from the sodium: $(Na - [Cl + HXO_3]) = AG$. The potassium is usually not used in the calculation because it may be hemolyzed and is an intracellular cation. The lack of anion gap does not exclude a toxic etiology.

The normal gap is usually 7 to 11 mEq/L by flame photometer. However, there has been a "lowering" of the normal anion gap to 7 ± 4 mEq/L by the newer techniques (e.g., ion selective electrodes or colorimetric titration).

Rakel and Bope: *Conn's Current Therapy 2006*.

TABLE 8 Etiologies of Metabolic Acidosis

Normal anion gap hyperchloremic	Increased anion gap normochloremic	Decreased anion gap
Acidifying agents	Methanol	Laboratory error[†]
Adrenal insufficiency	Uremia*	Intoxication—bromine, lithium
Anhydrase inhibitors	Diabetic ketoacidosis*	Protein abnormal
Fistula	Paraldehyde,* phenformin	Sodium low
Osteotomies	Isoniazid	
Obstructive uropathies	Iron	
Renal tubular acidosis	Lactic acidosis[†]	
Diarrhea, uncomplicated*	Ethanol,* ethylene glycol*	
Dilutional	Salicylates, starvation solvents	
Sulfamylon		

*Indicates hyperosmolar situation. Studies have found that the anion gap may be relatively insensitive for determining the presence of toxins.
[†]Lactic acidosis can be produced by intoxications of the following: carbon monoxide, cyanide, hydrogen sulfide, hypoxia, ibuprofen, iron, isoniazid, phenformin, salicylates, seizures, theophylline.

Some studies have found anion gaps to be relatively insensitive for determining the presence of toxins.

It is important to recognize anion gap toxins, such as salicylates, methanol, and ethylene glycol, because they have specific antidotes, and hemodialysis is effective in management of cases of overdose with these agents.

Table 8 lists the reasons for increased anion gap, decreased anion gap, or no gap. The most common cause of a decreased anion gap is laboratory error. Lactic acidosis produces the largest anion gap and can result from any poisoning that results in hypoxia, hypoglycemia, or convulsions.

Table 9 lists other blood chemistry derangements that suggest certain intoxications.

Serum osmolality is a measure of the number of molecules of solute per kilogram of solvent, or mOsm/kg water. The osmolarity is molecules of solute per liter of solution, or mOsm/L water at a specified temperature. Osmolarity is usually the calculated value and osmolality is usually a measured value. They are considered interchangeable where 1 L equals 1 kg. The normal serum osmolality is 280 to 290 mOsm/kg. The freezing point serum osmolarity measurement specimen and the serum electrolytes specimens for calculation should be drawn simultaneously.

The serum osmolal gap is defined as the difference between the measured osmolality determined by the freezing point method and the calculated osmolarity. It is determined by the following formula:

$$(Sodium \times 2) + (BUN/3) + (Glucose/20)$$

(where BUN is blood urea nitrogen).

This gap estimate is normally within 10 mOsm of the simultaneously measured serum osmolality. Ethanol, if present, may be included in the equation to eliminate its influence on the osmolal gap (the ethanol concentration divided by 4.6; Table 10).

The osmolal gap is not valid in cases of shock and postmortem state. Metabolic disorders such as hyperglycemia, uremia, and dehydration increase the osmolarity but usually do not cause gaps greater than 10 mOsm/kg. A gap greater than 10 mOsm/mL suggests

that unidentified osmolal-acting substances are present: acetone, ethanol, ethylene glycol, glycerin, isopropyl alcohol, isoniazid, ethanol, mannitol, methanol, and trichloroethane. Alcohols and glycols should be sought when the degree of obtundation exceeds that expected from the blood ethanol concentration or when other clinical conditions exist: visual loss (methanol), metabolic acidosis (methanol and ethylene glycol), or renal failure (ethylene glycol).

A falsely elevated osmolal gap can be produced by other low molecular weight un-ionized substances (dextran, diuretics, sorbitol, ketones), hyperlipidemia, and unmeasured electrolytes (e.g., magnesium).

TABLE 9 Blood Chemistry Derangements in Toxicology

Derangement	Toxin
Acetonemia without acidosis	Acetone or isopropyl alcohol
Hypomagnesemia	Ethanol, digitalis
Hypocalcemia	Ethylene glycol, oxalate, fluoride
Hyperkalemia	β-Blockers, acute digitalis, renal failure
Hypokalemia	Diuretics, salicylism, sympathomimetics, theophylline, corticosteroids, chronic digitalis
Hyperglycemia	Diazoxide, glucagon, iron, isoniazid, organophosphate insecticides, phenylurea insecticides, phenytoin (Dilantin), salicylates, sympathomimetic agents, thyroid, vasopressors
Hypoglycemia	β-Blockers, ethanol, insulin, isoniazid, oral hypoglycemic agents, salicylates
Rhabdomyolysis	Amphetamines, ethanol, cocaine, or phencyclidine, elevated creatine phosphokinase

Rakel and Bope: *Conn's Current Therapy 2006.*

TABLE 10 **Conversion Factors for Alcohols and Glycols**

Alcohols/glycols	1 mg/dL in blood raises osmolality mOsm/L	Molecular weight	Conversion factor
Ethanol	0.228	40	4.6
Methanol	0.327	32	3.2
Ethylene glycol	0.190	62	6.2
Isopropanol	0.176	60	6.0
Acetone	0.182	58	5.8
Propylene glycol	not available	72	7.2

Example: Methanol osmolality. Subtract the calculated osmolality from the measured serum osmolarity (freezing point method) = osmolar gap × 3.2 (one-tenth molecular weight) = estimated serum methanol concentration.
Note: This equation is often not considered very reliable in predicting the actual measured blood concentration of these alcohols or glycols.

Note: A normal osmolal gap may be reported in the presence of toxic alcohol or glycol poisoning, if the parent compound is already metabolized. This situation can occur when the osmolal gap is measured after a significant time has elapsed since the ingestion. In cases of alcohol and glycol intoxication, an early osmolar gap is a result of the relatively nontoxic parent drug and delayed metabolic acidosis, and an anion gap is a result of the more toxic metabolites.

The serum concentration is calculated as mg/dL = mOsm gap × MW of substance divided by 10.

RADIOGRAPHIC STUDIES

Chest and neck radiographs are useful for suspected pathologic conditions such as aspiration pneumonia, pulmonary edema, and foreign bodies and to determine the location of the endotracheal tube. Abdominal radiographs can be used to detect radiopaque substances.

The mnemonic for radiopaque substances seen on abdominal radiographs is CHIPES:

C—chlorides and chloral hydrate
H—heavy metals (arsenic, barium, iron, lead, mercury, zinc)
I—iodides
P—PlayDoh, Pepto-Bismol, phenothiazine (inconsistent)
E—enteric-coated tablets
S—sodium, potassium, and other elements in tablet form (bismuth, calcium, potassium) and solvents containing chlorides (e.g., carbon tetrachloride)

TOXICOLOGIC STUDIES

Routine blood and urine screening is of little practical value in the initial care of the poisoned patient. Specific toxicologic analyses and quantitative levels of certain drugs may be extremely helpful. One should always ask oneself the following questions: (a) How will the result of the test alter the management? and (b) Can the result of the test be returned in time to have a positive effect on therapy?

Owing to long turnaround time, lack of availability, factors contributing to unreliability, and the risk of serious morbidity without supportive clinical management, toxicology screening is estimated to affect management in less than 15% of cases of drug overdoses or poisonings. Toxicology screening may look specifically for only 40 to 50 drugs out of more than 10,000 possible drugs or toxins and more than several million chemicals. To detect many different drugs, toxic screens usually include methods with broad specificity, and sensitivity may be poor for some drugs, resulting in false-negative or false-positive findings. On the other hand, some drugs present in therapeutic amounts may be detected on the screen, even though they are causing no clinical symptoms. Because many agents are not sought or detected during a toxicologic screening, a negative result does not always rule out poisonings. The specificity of toxicologic tests is dependent on the method and the laboratory. The presence of other drugs, drug metabolites, disease states, or incorrect sampling may cause erroneous results.

For the average toxicologic laboratory, false-negative results occur at a rate of 10% to 30% and false-positives at a rate of 0% to 10%. The positive screen predictive value is approximately 90%. A negative toxicology screen does not exclude a poisoning. The negative predictive value of toxicologic screening is approximately 70%. For example, the following benzodiazepines may not be detected by some routine immunoassay benzodiazepine screening tests: alprazolam (Xanax), clonazepam (Klonopin), temazepam (Restoril), and triazolam (Halcion).

The "toxic urine screen" is generally a qualitative urine test for several common drugs, usually substances of abuse (cocaine and metabolites, opioids, amphetamines, benzodiazepines, barbiturates, and phencyclidine). Results of these tests are usually available within 2 to 6 hours. Because these tests may vary with each hospital and community, the physician should determine exactly which substances are included in the toxic urine screen of his or her laboratory. Tests for ethylene glycol, red blood cell cholinesterase, and serum cyanide are not readily available.

For cases of ingestion of certain substances, quantitative blood levels should be obtained at specific times after the ingestion to avoid spurious low values in the distribution phase, which result from incomplete absorption. The detection time for drugs is influenced by many variables, such as type of substance, formulation, amount, time since ingestion, duration of exposure, and half-life. For many drugs, the detection time is measured in days after the exposure.

Common Poisons

ACETAMINOPHEN (PARACETAMOL, *N*-ACETYL-PARAAMINOPHENOL)

Toxic Mechanism

At therapeutic doses of acetaminophen, less than 5% is metabolized by P450-2E1 to a toxic reactive oxidizing metabolite, *N*-acetyl-p-benzoquinoneimine (NAPQI). In a case of overdose, there is insufficient glutathione available to reduce the excess NAPQI into nontoxic conjugate, so it forms covalent bonds with hepatic intracellular proteins to produce centrilobular necrosis. Renal damage is caused by a similar mechanism.

Toxic Dose

The therapeutic dose of acetaminophen is 10 to 15 mg/kg, with a maximum of five doses in 24 hours for a maximum total daily dose of 4 g. An acute single toxic dose is greater than 140 mg/kg, possibly greater than 200 mg/kg in a child younger than age 5 years. Factors affecting the P450 enzymes include enzyme inducers such as barbiturates and phenytoin (Dilantin), ingestion of isoniazid, and alcoholism. Factors that decrease glutathione stores (alcoholism, malnutrition, and HIV infection) contribute to the toxicity of acetaminophen. Alcoholics ingesting 3 to 4 g/d of acetaminophen for a few days can have depleted glutathione stores and require *N*-acetylcysteine therapy at 50% below hepatotoxic blood acetaminophen levels on the nomogram.

Kinetics

Peak plasma concentration is usually reached 2 to 4 hours after an overdose. Volume distribution is 0.9 L/kg, and protein binding is less than 50% (albumin).

Route of elimination is by hepatic metabolism to an inactive nontoxic glucuronide conjugate and inactive nontoxic sulfate metabolite by two saturable pathways; less than 5% is metabolized into reactive metabolite NAPQI. In patients younger than 6 years of age, metabolic elimination occurs to a greater degree by conjugation via the sulfate pathway.

The half-life of acetaminophen is 1 to 3 hours.

Manifestations

The four phases of the intoxication's clinical course may overlap, and the absence of a phase does not exclude toxicity.

- Phase I occurs within 0.5 to 24 hours after ingestion and may consist of a few hours of malaise, diaphoresis, nausea, and vomiting or produce no symptoms. CNS depression or coma is not a feature.

- Phase II occurs 24 to 48 hours after ingestion and is a period of diminished symptoms. The liver enzymes, serum aspartate aminotransferase (AST) (earliest), and serum alanine aminotransferase (ALT) may increase as early as 4 hours or as late as 36 hours after ingestion.
- Phase III occurs at 48 to 96 hours, with peak liver function abnormalities at 72 to 96 hours. The degree of elevation of the hepatic enzymes generally correlates with outcome, but not always. Recovery starts at about 4 days unless hepatic failure develops. Less than 1% of patients with a history of overdose develop fulminant hepatotoxicity.
- Phase IV occurs at 4 to 14 days, with hepatic enzyme abnormalities resolving. If extensive liver damage has occurred, sepsis and disseminated intravascular coagulation may ensue.

Transient renal failure may develop at 5 to 7 days with or without evidence of hepatic damage. Rare cases of myocarditis and pancreatitis have been reported. Death can occur at 7 to 14 days.

Laboratory Investigations

The therapeutic reference range is 10 to 20 μg/mL. For toxic levels, see the nomogram presented in Figure 1.

Appropriate and reliable methods for analysis are radioimmunoassay, high-pressure liquid chromatography, and gas chromatography. Spectroscopic assays often give falsely elevated values: bilirubin, salicylate, salicylamide, diflunisal (Dolobid), phenols, and methyldopa (Aldomet) increase the acetaminophen level. Each 1 mg/dL increase in creatinine increases the acetaminophen plasma level 30 μg/mL.

If a toxic acetaminophen level is reached, liver profile (including AST, ALT, bilirubin, and prothrombin time), serum amylase, and blood glucose must be monitored. A complete blood cell count (CBC); platelet count; phosphate, electrolytes, and bicarbonate level measurements; ECG; and urinalysis are indicated.

Management

Gastrointestinal Decontamination

Although ipecac-induced emesis may be useful within 30 minutes of ingestion of the toxic substance, we do not advise it because it could result in vomiting of the activated charcoal. Gastric lavage is not necessary. Studies have indicated that activated charcoal is useful within 1 hour after ingestion. Activated charcoal does adsorb N-acetylcysteine (NAC) if given together, but this is not clinically important. However, if activated charcoal needs to be given along with NAC, separate the administration of activated charcoal from the administration of NAC by 1 to 2 hours to avoid vomiting.

N-Acetylcysteine (Mucomyst)

NAC (Table 11), a derivative of the amino acid cysteine, acts as a sulfhydryl donor for glutathione synthesis,

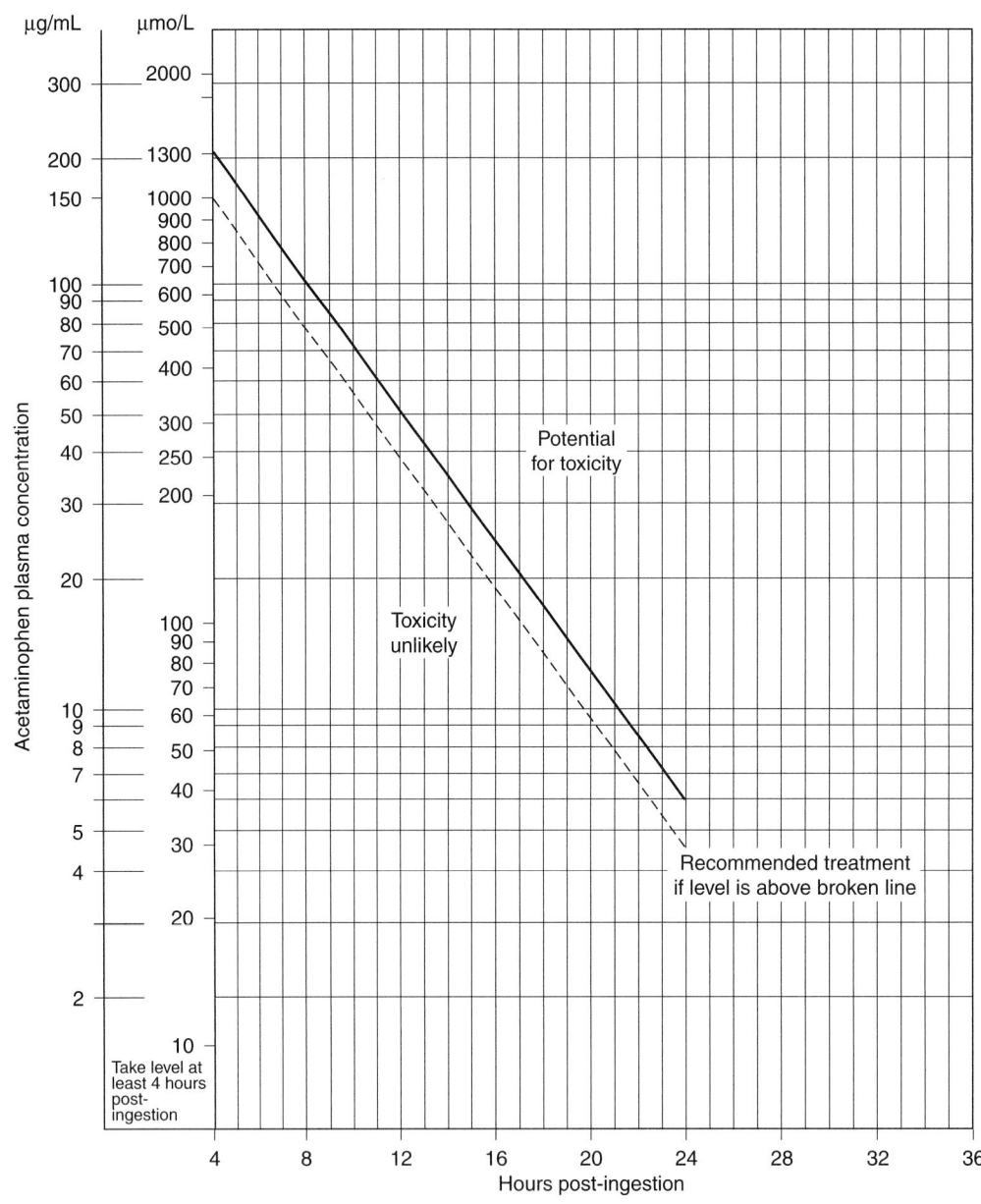

FIGURE 1. Nomogram for acetaminophen intoxication. *N*-acetylcysteine therapy is started if levels and time coordinates are above the lower line on the nomogram. Continue and complete therapy even if subsequent values fall below the toxic zone. The nomogram is useful only in cases of acute single ingestion. Levels in serum drawn before 4 hours may not represent peak levels. (From Rumack BH, Matthew H: Acetaminophen poisoning and toxicity. Pediatrics 55:871, 1975.)

TABLE 11 Protocol for *N*-Acetylcysteine Administration

Route	Loading dose	Maintenance dose	Course	FDA approval
Oral	140 mg/kg	70 mg/kg every 4 h	72 h	Yes
Intravenous	150 mg/kg over 15 min	50 mg/kg over 4 h followed by 100 mg/kg over 16h	20 h	Yes

as surrogate glutathione, and may increase the non-toxic sulfation pathway resulting in conjugation of NAPQI. Oral NAC should be administered within the first 8 hours after a toxic amount of acetaminophen has been ingested. NAC can be started while one awaits the results of the blood test for acetaminophen plasma concentration, but there is no advantage to giving it before 8 hours. If the acetaminophen concentration result after 4 hours following ingestion is above the upper line on the modified Rumack-Matthew nomogram (see Figure 1), one should continue with a maintenance course. Repeat blood specimens should be obtained 4 hours after the initial level is measured if it is greater than 20 mg/mL, which is below the therapy line, because of unexpected delays in the peak by food and co-ingestants. Intravenous NAC (see Table 11) is approved in the United States.

There have been a few cases of anaphylactoid reaction and death by the intravenous route.

Variations in Therapy

In patients with chronic alcoholism, it is recommended that NAC treatment be administered at 50% below the upper toxic line on the nomogram.

If emesis occurs within 1 hour after NAC administration, the dose should be repeated. To avoid emesis, the proper dilution from 20% to 5% NAC must be used, and it should be served in a palatable vehicle, in a covered container through a straw. If this administration is unsuccessful, a slow drip over 30 to 60 minutes through a nasogastric tube or a fluoroscopically placed naso-duodenal tube can be used. Antiemetics can be used if necessary: metoclopramide (Reglan) 10 mg per dose intravenously 30 minutes before administration of NAC (in children, 0.1 mg/kg; maximum, 0.5 mg/kg/d) or ondansetron (Zofran) 32 mg (0.15 mg/kg) by infusion over 15 minutes and repeated for three doses if necessary. The side effects of these antiemetics include anaphylaxis and increases in liver enzymes.

Some investigators recommend variable durations of NAC therapy, stopping the therapy if serial acetaminophen blood concentrations become nondetectable and the liver enzyme levels (ALT and AST) remain normal after 24 to 36 hours.

There is a loss of efficacy if NAC is initiated 8 or 10 hours postingestion, but the loss is not complete, and NAC may be initiated 36 hours or more after ingestion. Late treatment (after 24 hours) decreases the rates of morbidity and mortality in patients with fulminant liver failure caused by acetaminophen and other agents.

Extended relief formulations (*ER* embossed on caplet) contain 325 mg of acetaminophen for immediate release and 325 mg for delayed release. A single 4-hour postingestion serum acetaminophen concentration can underestimate the level because ER formulations can have secondary delayed peaks. In cases of overdose of the ER formulation, it is recommended that additional acetaminophen levels be obtained at 4-hour intervals after the initial level is measured. If any level is in the toxic zone, therapy should be initiated.

It is recommended that pregnant patients with toxic plasma concentrations of acetaminophen be treated with NAC to prevent hepatotoxicity in both fetus and mother. The available data suggest no teratogenicity to NAC or acetaminophen.

Indications for NAC therapy in cases of chronic intoxication are a history of ingestion of 3 to 4 g for several days with elevated liver enzyme levels (AST and ALT). The acetaminophen blood concentration is often low in these cases because of the extended time lapse since ingestion and should not be plotted on the Rumack-Matthew nomogram. Patients with a history of chronic alcoholism or those on chronic enzyme inducers may also present with elevated liver enzyme levels and should be considered for NAC therapy if they have a history of taking acetaminophen on a chronic basis, because they are considered to be at a greater risk for hepatotoxicity despite a low acetaminophen blood concentration.

Specific support care may be needed to treat liver failure, pancreatitis, transient renal failure, and myocarditis.

Liver transplantation has a definite but limited role in patients with acute acetaminophen overdose. A retrospective analysis determined that a continuing rise in the prothrombin time (4-day peak, 180 seconds), a pH of less than 7.3 2 days after the overdose, a serum creatinine level of greater than 3.3 mg/dL, severe hepatic encephalopathy, and disturbed coagulation factor VII/V ratio greater than 30 suggest a poor prognosis and may be indicators for hepatology consultation for consideration of liver transplantation.

Extracorporeal measures are not expected to be of benefit.

Disposition

Adults who have ingested more than 140 mg/kg and children younger than 6 years of age who have ingested more than 200 mg/kg should receive therapy within 8 hours postingestion or until the results of the 4-hour postingestion acetaminophen plasma concentration are known.

AMPHETAMINES

The amphetamines include illicit methamphetamine ("Ice"), diet pills, and formulations under various trade names. Analogues include MDMA (3,4 methylenedioxymethamphetamine, known as "ecstasy," "XTC," "Adam") and MDA (3,4-methylenedioxyamphetamine, known as "Eve"). MDA is a common hallucinogen and euphoriant "club drug" used at "raves," which are all-night dances. Use of methamphetamine and designer analogues is on the rise, especially among young people between the ages of 12 and 25 years. Other similar stimulants are phenylpropanolamine and cocaine.

Toxic Mechanism

Amphetamines have a direct CNS stimulant effect and a sympathetic nervous system effect by releasing catecholamines from α- and β-adrenergic nerve terminals but inhibiting their reuptake.

Hallucinogenic MDMA has an additional hazard of serotonin effect (refer to serotonin syndrome in the SSRI section). MDMA also affects the dopamine system in the brain. Because of its effects on 5-hydroxytryptamine, dopamine, and norepinephrine, MDMA can lead to serotonin syndrome associated with malignant hyperthermia and rhabdomyolysis, which contributes to the potentially life-threatening hyperthermia observed in several patients who have used MDMA.

Phenylpropanolamine stimulates only the β-adrenergic receptors.

Toxic Dose

In children, the toxic dose of dextroamphetamine is 1 mg/kg; in adults, the toxic dose is 5 mg/kg. The potentially fatal dose of dextroamphetamine is 12 mg/kg.

Kinetics

Amphetamine is a weak base with pKa of 8 to 10. Onset of action is 30 to 60 minutes, and peak effects are 2 to 4 hours. The volume distribution is 2 to 3 L/kg.

Through hepatic metabolism, 60% of the substance is metabolized into a hydroxylated metabolite that may be responsible for psychotic effects.

The half-life of amphetamines is pH dependent—8 to 10 hours in acid urine (pH <6.0) and 16 to 31 hours in alkaline urine (pH >7.5). Excretion is by the kidney—30% to 40% at alkaline urine pH and 50% to 70% at acid urine pH.

Manifestations

Effects are seen within 30 to 60 minutes following ingestion.

Neurologic manifestations include restlessness, irritation and agitation, tremors and hyperreflexia, and auditory and visual hallucinations. Hyperpyrexia may precede seizures, convulsions, paranoia, violence, intracranial hemorrhage, psychosis, and self-destructive behavior. Paranoid psychosis and cerebral vasculitis occur with chronic abuse.

MDMA is often adulterated with cocaine, heroin, or ketamine, or a combination of these, to create a variety of mood alterations. This possibility must be taken into consideration when one manages patients with MDMA ingestions, as the symptom complex may reflect both CNS stimulation and CNS depression.

Other manifestations include dilated but reactive pupils, cardiac dysrhythmias (supraventricular and ventricular), tachycardia, hypertension, rhabdomyolysis, and myoglobinuria.

Laboratory Investigations

The clinician should monitor ECG and cardiac readings, ABG and oxygen saturation, electrolytes, blood glucose, BUN, creatinine, creatine kinase, cardiac fraction if there is chest pain, and liver profile. Also, one should evaluate for rhabdomyolysis and check urine for myoglobin, cocaine and metabolites, and other substances of abuse. The peak plasma concentration of amphetamines is 10 to 50 ng/mL 1 to 2 hours after ingestion of 10 to 25 mg. The toxic plasma concentration is 200 ng/mL. When the rapid immunoassays are used, cross-reactions can occur with amphetamine derivatives (e.g., MDA, "ecstasy"), brompheniramine (Dimetane), chlorpromazine (Thorazine), ephedrine, phenylpropanolamine, phentermine (Adipex-P), phenmetrazine, ranitidine (Zantac), and Vicks Inhaler (L-desoxyephedrine). False-positive results may occur.

Management

Management is similar to management for cocaine intoxication. Supportive care includes blood pressure and temperature control, cardiac monitoring, and seizure precautions. Diazepam (Valium) can be administered. Gastrointestinal decontamination can be undertaken with activated charcoal administered up to 1 hour after ingestion.

Anxiety, agitation, and convulsions are treated with diazepam. If diazepam fails to control seizures, neuromuscular blockers can be used and the electroencephalogram (EEG) monitored for nonmotor seizures. One should avoid neuroleptic phenothiazines and butyrophenone, which can lower the seizure threshold.

Hypertension and tachycardia are usually transient and can be managed by titration of diazepam. Nitroprusside can be used for hypertensive crisis at a maximum infusion rate of 10 μg/kg/minute for 10 minutes followed with a lower infusion rate of 0.3 to 2 mg/kg/minute. Myocardial ischemia is managed by oxygen, vascular access, benzodiazepines, and nitroglycerin. Aspirin and thrombolytics are not routinely recommended because of the danger of intracranial hemorrhage. It is important to distinguish between angina and true ischemia. Delayed hypotension can be treated with fluids and vasopressors if needed. Life-threatening tachydysrhythmias may respond to an α-blocker such as phentolamine (Regitine) 5 mg IV for adults or 0.1 mg/kg IV for children and a short-acting β-blocker such as esmolol (Brevibloc) 500 μg/kg IV over 1 minute for adults, or 300 to 500 μg/kg over 1 minute for children. Ventricular dysrhythmias may respond to lidocaine or, in a severely hemodynamically compromised patient, immediate synchronized electrical cardioversion.

Rhabdomyolysis and myoglobinuria are treated with fluids, alkaline diuresis, and diuretics. Hyperthermia is treated with external cooling and cool 100% humidified oxygen. More extensive therapy may be needed in severe cases. If focal neurologic symptoms are present, the possibility of a cerebrovascular accident should be considered and a CT scan of the head should be obtained.

Paranoid ideation and threatening behavior should be treated with rapid tranquilization using a benzodiazepine. One should observe for suicidal depression that may follow intoxication and may require suicide precautions.

Extracorporeal measures are of no benefit.

Disposition

Symptomatic patients should be observed on a monitored unit until the symptoms resolve and then observed for a short time after resolution for relapse.

ANTICHOLINERGIC AGENTS

Drugs with anticholinergic properties include antihistamines (H$_1$ blockers), neuroleptics (phenothiazines), tricyclic antidepressants, antiparkinsonism drugs (trihexyphenidyl [Artane], benztropine [Cogentin]), ophthalmic products (atropine), and a number of common plants.

The antihistamines are divided into the sedating anticholinergic types, and the nonsedating single daily dose types. The sedating types include ethanolamines (e.g., diphenhydramine [Benadryl], dimenhydrinate [Dramamine], and clemastine [Tavist]), ethylenediamines (e.g., tripelennamine [Pyribenzamine]), alkyl amines (e.g., chlorpheniramine [Chlor-Trimeton], brompheniramine [Dimetane]), piperazines (e.g., cyclizine [Marezine], hydroxyzine [Atarax], and meclizine [Antivert]), and phenothiazine (e.g., Phenergan). The nonsedating types include astemizole (Hismanal), terfenadine (Seldane), loratadine (Claritin), fexofenadine (Allegra), and cetirizine (Zyrtec).

The anticholinergic plants include jimsonweed (*Datura stramonium*), deadly nightshade (*Atropa belladonna*), henbane (*Hyoscyamus niger*), and antispasmodic agents for the bowel (atropine derivatives).

Toxic Mechanism

By competitive inhibition, anticholinergics block the action of acetylcholine on postsynaptic cholinergic receptor sites. The toxic mechanism primarily involves the peripheral and CNS muscarinic receptors. H$_1$ sedating-type agents also depress or stimulate

the CNS, and in large overdoses some have cardiac membrane–depressant effects (e.g., diphenhydramine [Benadryl]) and α-adrenergic receptor blockade effects (e.g., promethazine [Phenergan]). Nonsedating agents produce peripheral H$_1$ blockade but do not possess anticholinergic or sedating actions. The original agents terfenadine (Seldane) and astemizole (Hismanal) were recently removed from the market because of the severe cardiac dysrhythmias associated with their use, especially when used in combination with macrolide antibiotics and certain antifungal agents such as ketoconazole (Nizoral), which inhibit hepatic metabolism or excretion. The newer nonsedating agents, including loratadine (Claritin), fexofenadine (Allegra), and cetirizine (Zyrtec), have not been reported to cause the severe drug interactions associated with terfenadine and astemizole.

Toxic Dose

The estimated toxic oral dose of atropine is 0.05 mg/kg in children and more than 2 mg in adults. The minimal estimated lethal dose of atropine is more than 10 mg in adults and more than 2 mg in children. Other synthetic anticholinergic agents are less toxic, and the fatal dose varies from 10 to 100 mg.

The estimated toxic oral dose of diphenhydramine (Benadryl) in a child is 15 mg/kg, and the potential lethal amount is 25 mg/kg. In an adult, the potential lethal amount is 2.8 g. Ingestion of five times the single dose of an antihistamine is toxic.

For the nonsedating agents, an overdose of 3360 mg of terfenadine was reported in an adult who developed ventricular tachycardia and fibrillation that responded to lidocaine and defibrillation. A 1500-mg overdose produced hypotension. Cases of delayed serious dysrhythmias (torsades de pointes) have been reported with doses of more than 200 mg of astemizole. The toxic doses of fexofenadine (Allegra), cetirizine, and loratadine (Claritin) need to be established.

Kinetics

The onset of absorption of intravenous atropine is in 2 to 4 minutes. Peak effects on salivation after intravenous or intramuscular administration are at 30 to 60 minutes.

Onset of absorption after oral ingestion is 30 to 60 minutes, peak action is 1 to 3 hours, and duration of action is 4 to 6 hours, but symptoms are prolonged in cases of overdose or with sustained-release preparations.

The onset of absorption of diphenhydramine is in 15 minutes to 1 hour, with a peak of action in 1 to 4 hours. Volume distribution is 3.3 to 6.8 L/kg, and protein binding is 75% to 80%. Ninety-eight percent of diphenhydramine is metabolized via the liver by *N*-demethylation. Interactions with erythromycin, ketoconazole (Nizoral), and derivatives produce excessive blood levels of the antihistamine and ventricular dysrhythmias.

The half-life of diphenhydramine is 3 to 10 hours.

The chemical structure of nonsedating agents prevents their entry into the CNS. Absorption begins in 1 hour, with peak effects in 4 in 6 hours. The duration of action is greater than 24 hours.

These agents are metabolized in the gastrointestinal tract and liver. Protein binding is greater than 90%. The plasma half-life is 3.5 hours. Only 1% is excreted unchanged; 60% of that is excreted in the feces and 40% in the urine.

Manifestations

Anticholinergic signs are hyperpyrexia ("hot as a hare"), mydriasis ("blind as a bat"), flushing of skin ("red as a beet"), dry mucosa and skin ("dry as a bone"), "Lilliputian type" hallucinations and delirium ("mad as a hatter"), coma, dysphagia, tachycardia, moderate hypertension, and rarely convulsions and urinary retention. Other effects include jaundice (cyproheptadine [Periactin]), dystonia (diphenhydramine [Benadryl]), rhabdomyolysis (doxylamine), and, in large doses, cardiotoxic effects (diphenhydramine).

Overdose with nonsedating agents produces headache and confusion, nausea, and dysrhythmias (e.g., torsades de pointes).

Laboratory Investigations

Monitoring of ABG (in cases of respiratory depression), electrolytes, glucose, and the ECG should be undertaken. Anticholinergic drugs and plants are not routinely included on screens for substances of abuse.

Management

For patients in respiratory failure, intubation and assisted ventilation should be instituted. Gastrointestinal decontamination can be instituted. Caution must be taken with emesis in cases of diphenhydramine (Benadryl) overdose because of the drug's rapid onset of action and risk of seizures. If bowel sounds are present for up to 1 hour after ingestion, activated charcoal can be given. Seizures can be controlled with benzodiazepines (diazepam [Valium] or lorazepam [Ativan]).

The administration of physostigmine (Antilirium) is not routine and is reserved for life-threatening anticholinergic effects that are refractory to conventional treatments. It should be administered with adequate monitoring and resuscitative equipment available. The use of physostigmine should be avoided if a tricyclic antidepressant is present because of increased toxicity. Urinary retention should be relieved by catheterization to avoid reabsorption of the drug and additional toxicity.

Supraventricular tachycardia should be treated only if the patient is hemodynamically unstable. Ventricular dysrhythmias can be controlled with lidocaine or cardioversion. Sodium bicarbonate 1 to 2 mEq/kg IV may be useful for myocardial depression and QRS prolongation. Torsades de pointes, especially when associated with terfenadine and astemizole ingestion, has been treated with magnesium sulfate 4 g or 40 mL 10% solution intravenously over 10 to 20 minutes and countershock if the patient fails to respond.

Hyperpyrexia is controlled by external cooling. Hemodialysis and hemoperfusion are not effective.

Disposition

Antihistamine H₁ Antagonists

Symptomatic patients should be observed on a monitored unit until the symptoms resolve, then observed for a short time (3 to 4 hours) after resolution for relapse.

Nonsedating Agents

All asymptomatic children who acutely ingest more than the maximum adult dose and all symptomatic children should be referred to a health care facility for a minimum of 6 hours' observation as well as cardiac monitoring. Asymptomatic adults who acutely ingest more than twice the maximum adult daily dose should be monitored for a minimum of 6 hours. All symptomatic patients should be monitored for as long as there are symptoms present.

BARBITURATES

Barbiturates have been used as sedatives, anesthetic agents, and anticonvulsants, but their use is declining as safer, more effective drugs become available.

Toxic Mechanism

Barbiturates are γ-amino butyric acid (GABA) agonists (increasing the chloride flow and inhibiting depolarization). They enhance the CNS depressant effect of GABA and depress the cardiovascular system.

Toxic Dose

The shorter-acting barbiturates (including the intermediate-acting agents) and their hypnotic doses are as follows: amobarbital (Amytal), 100 to 200 mg; aprobarbital (Alurate), 50 to 100 mg; butabarbital (Butisol), 50 to 100 mg; butalbital, 100 to 200 mg; pentobarbital (Nembutal), 100 to 200 mg; secobarbital (Seconal), 100 to 200 mg. They cause toxicity at lower doses than long-acting barbiturates and have a minimum toxic dose of 6 mg/kg; the fatal adult dose is 3 to 6 g.

The long-acting barbiturates and their doses include mephobarbital (Mebaral), 50 to 100 mg, and phenobarbital, 100 to 200 mg. Their minimum toxic dose is greater than 10 mg/kg, and the fatal adult dose is 6 to 10 g. A general rule is that an amount five times the hypnotic dose is toxic and an amount 10 times the hypnotic dose is potentially fatal. Methohexital and thiopental are ultrashort-acting parenteral preparations and are not discussed.

Kinetics

The barbiturates are enzyme inducers. Short-acting barbiturates are highly lipid-soluble, penetrate the brain readily, and have shorter elimination times. Onset of action is in 10 to 30 minutes, with a peak at 1 to 2 hours. Duration of action is 3 to 8 hours. The volume distribution of short-acting barbiturate is 0.8 to 1.5 L/kg; pKa is about 8. Mean half-life varies from 8 to 48 hours.

Long-acting agents have longer elimination times and can be used as anticonvulsants. Onset of action is in 20 to 60 minutes, with a peak at 1 to 6 hours. In cases of overdose, the peak can be at 10 hours. Usual duration of action is 8 to 12 hours. Volume distribution is 0.8 L/kg, and half-life is 11 to 120 hours. The pKa of phenobarbital is 7.2. Alkalinization of urine promotes its excretion.

Manifestations

Mild intoxication resembles alcohol intoxication and includes ataxia, slurred speech, and depressed cognition. Severe intoxication causes slow respirations, coma, and loss of reflexes (except pupillary light reflex).

Other manifestations include hypotension (vasodilation), hypothermia, hypoglycemia, and death by respiratory arrest.

Laboratory Investigations

Most barbiturates are detected on routine drug screens and can be measured in most hospital laboratories. Investigation should include barbiturate level; ABG; toxicology screen, including acetaminophen; glucose, electrolyte, BUN, creatinine, and creatine kinase levels; and urine pH. The minimum toxic plasma levels are greater than 10 µg/mL for short-acting barbiturates and greater than 40 µg/dL for long-acting agents. Fatal levels are 30 µg/mL for short-acting barbiturates and 80 to 150 µg/mL for long-acting agents. Both short-acting and long-acting agents can be detected in urine 24 to 72 hours after ingestion, and long-acting agents can be detected up to 7 days.

Management

Vital functions must be established and maintained. Intensive supportive care including intubation and assisted ventilation should dominate the management. All stuporous and comatose patients should have glucose (for hypoglycemia), thiamine (if chronically alcoholic), and naloxone (Narcan) (in case of an opioid ingestion) intravenously and should be admitted to the intensive care unit. Emesis should be avoided especially in cases of ingestion of the shorter-acting barbiturates. Activated charcoal followed by MDAC (0.5 g/kg) every 2 to 4 hours has been shown to reduce the serum half-life of phenobarbital by 50%, but its effect on clinical course is undetermined.

Fluids should be administered to correct dehydration and hypotension. Vasopressors may be necessary to correct severe hypotension, and hemodynamic monitoring may be needed. The patient must be observed carefully for fluid overload. Alkalinization (ion trapping) is used only for phenobarbital (pKa 7.2) but not for short-acting barbiturates. Sodium bicarbonate, 1 to 2 mEq/kg IV in 500 mL of 5% dextrose in adults or 10 to 15 mL/kg in children during the first hour, followed by sufficient bicarbonate to keep the urinary pH at 7.5 to 8.0, enhances excretion of phenobarbital and shortens the half-life by 50%. Diuresis is not advocated because of the danger of cerebral or pulmonary edema.

Hemodialysis shortens the half-life to 8 to 14 hours, and charcoal hemoperfusion shortens the half-life to 6 to 8 hours for long-acting barbiturates such as phenobarbital. Both procedures may be effective in patients with both long-acting and short-acting barbiturate ingestion. If the patient does not respond to supportive measures or if the phenobarbital plasma concentration is greater than 150 µg/mL, both procedures may be tried to shorten the half-life.

Bullae are treated as a local second-degree skin burn. Hypothermia should be treated.

Disposition

All comatose patients should be admitted to the intensive care unit. Awake and oriented patients with an overdose of short-acting agents should be observed for at least 6 asymptomatic hours; overdose of long-acting agents warrants observation for at least 12 asymptomatic hours because of the potential for delayed absorption. In the case of an intentional overdose, psychiatric clearance is needed before the patient can be discharged. Chronic use can lead to tolerance, physical dependency, and withdrawal and necessitates follow-up.

BENZODIAZEPINES

Benzodiazepines are used as anxiolytics, sedatives, and relaxants.

Toxic Mechanism

The GABA agonists produce CNS depression and increase chloride flow, inhibiting depolarization.

Flunitrazepam (Rohypnol; street name "roofies") is a long-acting benzodiazepine agonist sold by prescription in more than 60 countries worldwide, but it is not legally available in the United States.

Toxic Dose

The long-acting benzodiazepines (half-life >24 hours) and their maximum therapeutic doses are as follows: chlordiazepoxide (Librium), 50 mg; clorazepate (Tranxene), 30 mg; clonazepam (Klonopin), 20 mg; diazepam (Valium), 10 mg in adults or 0.2 mg/kg in children; flurazepam (Dalmane), 30 mg; and prazepam, 20 mg.

The short-acting benzodiazepines (half-life 10 to 24 hours) and their doses include the following: alprazolam (Xanax), 0.5 mg, and lorazepam (Ativan), 4 mg in adults or 0.05 mg/kg in children, which act similar to the long-acting benzodiazepines.

The ultrashort-acting benzodiazepines (half-life <10 hours) are more toxic and include temazepam

(Restoril), 30 mg; triazolam (Halcion), 0.5 mg; midazolam (Versed), 0.2 mg/kg; and oxazepam (Serax), 30 mg.

In cases of overdose of short- and long-acting agents, 10 to 20 times the therapeutic dose (>1500 mg diazepam or 2000 mg chlordiazepoxide) have been ingested with resulting mild coma but without respiratory depression. Fatalities are rare, and most patients recover within 24 to 36 hours after overdose. Asymptomatic unintentional overdoses of less than five times the therapeutic dose can be seen. Ultrashort-acting agents have produced respiratory arrest and coma within 1 hour after ingestion of 5 mg of triazolam (Halcion) and death with ingestion of as little as 10 mg. Midazolam (Versed) and diazepam (Valium) by rapid intravenous injection have produced respiratory arrest.

Kinetics

Onset of CNS depression is usually in 30 to 120 minutes; peak action usually occurs within 1 to 3 hours when ingestion is by the oral route. The volume distribution varies from 0.26 to 6 L/kg (LA, 1.1 L/kg); protein binding is 70% to 99%. For flunitrazepam, the onset of action is in 0.5 to 2 hours, oral peak is in 2 hours, and duration 8 hours or more. The half-life of flunitrazepam is 20 to 30 hours, volume distribution is 3.3 to 5.5 L/kg, and 80% is protein bound. Flunitrazepam can be identified in urine 4 to 30 days after ingestion.

Manifestations

Neurologic manifestations include ataxia, slurred speech, and CNS depression. Deep coma leading to respiratory depression suggests the presence of short-acting benzodiazepines or other CNS depressants. In elderly persons, the therapeutic doses can produce toxicity and can have an additive effect with other CNS depressants. Chronic use can lead to tolerance, physical dependency, and withdrawal.

Laboratory Investigations

Most benzodiazepines can be detected in urine drug screens. Quantitative blood levels are not useful. Some of the immunoassay urinary screens cannot detect all of the new benzodiazepines currently available. A consultation with the laboratory analyst is warranted if a specific case occurs in which the test result is negative but benzodiazepine use is suspected by the patient's history. Situations in which benzodiazepines may not be detected include ingestion of a low dose (e.g., <10 mg), rapid elimination, and a different or no metabolite. Some immunoassay methods can produce a false-positive finding for the benzodiazepines when nonsteroidal anti-inflammatory drugs (tolmetin [Tolectin], naproxen [Aleve], etodolac [Lodine], and fenoprofen [Nalfon]) are used. If this is a concern, the laboratory analyst should be consulted.

In cases in which "date rape" drugs such as flunitrazepam are suspected, a police crime or reference laboratory should be consulted for testing.

Management

Emesis and gastric lavage should be avoided. Activated charcoal can be useful only if given early before the peak time of absorption occurs. Supportive treatment should be instituted but rarely requires intubation or assisted ventilation.

Flumazenil (Romazicon) is a specific benzodiazepine receptor antagonist that blocks the chloride flow and inhibitor of GABA neurotransmitters. It reverses the sedative effects of benzodiazepines, zolpidem (Ambien), and endogenous benzodiazepines associated with hepatic encephalopathy. It is not recommended to reverse benzodiazepine-induced hypoventilation. The manufacturer advises that flumazenil be used with caution in cases of overdose with possible benzodiazepine dependency (because it can precipitate life-threatening withdrawal), if cyclic antidepressant use is suspected, or if a patient has a known seizure disorder.

Disposition

If the patient is comatose, he or she must be admitted to the intensive care unit. If the overdose was intentional, psychiatric clearance is needed before the patient can be discharged.

β-ADRENERGIC BLOCKERS (β-BLOCKER)

β-Blockers are used in the treatment of hypertension and of a number of systemic and ophthalmologic disorders. Properties of β-blockers include the factors listed in Table 12.

Lipid-soluble drugs have CNS effects, active metabolites, longer duration of action, and interactions (e.g., propranolol). Cardioselectivity is lost in overdose. Intrinsic partial agonist agents (e.g., pindolol) may initially produce tachycardia and hypertension. Cardiac membrane depressive effect (quinidine-like) occurs in cases of overdose but not at therapeutic doses (e.g., with metoprolol or sotalol). α-Blocking effect is weak (e.g., with labetalol or acebutolol).

Toxic Mechanism

β-Blockers compete with the catecholamines for receptor sites and block receptor action in the bronchi, the vascular smooth muscle, and the myocardium.

Toxic Dose

Ingestions of greater than twice the maximum recommended daily therapeutic dose are considered toxic (see Table 12). Ingestion of 1 mg/kg propranolol in a child may produce hypoglycemia. Fatalities have been reported in adults with 7.5 g of metoprolol. The most toxic agent is sotalol, and the least toxic is atenolol.

Kinetics

Regular-release formulations usually cause symptoms within 2 hours. Propranolol's onset of action is 20 to

TABLE 12 Pharmacologic and Toxic Properties of β-Blockers

Blocker	Maximum solubility	Therapeutic plasma level	Lipid solubility	Intrinsic sympathomimetic activity (Partial agonist)	Membrane stabilizing effect β-Selective β₁	β₂	Cardiac selectivity α-Selective
Acebutolol (Sectral)	800 mg	200-2000 ng/mL	Moderate	+	+	+	+
Alprenolol[2]	800 mg	50-200 ng/mL	Moderate	2+	+	–	–
Atenolol (Tenormin)	100 mg	200-500 ng/mL	Low	–	–	2+	–
Betaxolol (Kerlone)	20 mg	NA	Low	+	–	+	–
Carteolol (Cartrol)	10 mg	NA	No	+	–	–	–
Esmolol (Brevibloc) (Class II antidysrhythmic, IV only)			Low	–	–	+	–
Labetalol (Trandate)	800 mg	50-500 ng/mL	Low	+	+/–	–	+
Levobunolol (AKBeta eyedrop) (Eye drops 0.25% and 0.5%)	20 mg	NA	No	–	–	–	–
Metoprolol (Lopressor)			Moderate	–	–	2+	
Nadolol (Corgard)	320 mg	20-40 ng/mL	Low	–	–	–	–
Oxyprenolol[2]	480 mg	80-100 ng/mL	Moderate	2+	+	–	–
Pindolol (Visken)	60 mg	50-150 ng/mL	Moderate	3+	+/–	–	–
Propranolol (Inderal) (Class II antidysrhythmic)	360 mg	50-100 ng/mL	High	–	2+	–	–
Sotalol (Betapace) (Class II antidysrhythmic)	480 mg	500-4000 ng/mL	Low	–	–	–	–
Timolol (Blocadren)	60 mg	5-10 ng/mL	Low		+/–	–	–

[2]Not available in the United States.

30 minutes and peak is at 1 to 4 hours, but it may be delayed by co-ingestants. The onset of action with sustained-release preparations may be delayed to 6 hours and the peak to 12 to 16 hours. Volume distribution is 1 to 5.6 L/kg. Protein binding is variable, from 5% to 93%.

Metabolism

Atenolol (Tenormin), nadolol (Corgard), and santalol (Betapace) have enterohepatic recirculation. The duration of action for regular-acting agents is 4 to 6 hours, but in cases of overdose it may be 24 to 48 hours. The duration of action for sustained-release agents is 24 to 48 hours.

The regular preparation with the longest half-life is nadolol, at 12 to 24 hours, and the one with the shortest half-life is esmolol, at 5 to 10 minutes.

Manifestations

See "Toxic Properties" and Table 12.

Highly lipid soluble agents produce coma and seizures. Bradycardia and hypotension are the major cardiac symptoms and may lead to cardiogenic shock. Intrinsic partial agonists initially may cause tachycardia and hypertension. ECG changes include atrioventricular conduction delay or asystole. Membrane-depressant effects produce prolonged QRS and QT interval, which may result in torsades de pointes. Sotalol produces a very prolonged QT interval. Bronchospasm may occur in patients with reactive airway disease with any β-blocker because the selectivity is lost in overdose.

Other manifestations include hypoglycemia (because β-blockers block catecholamine counter-regulatory mechanisms) and hyperkalemia.

Laboratory Investigations

Measurements of blood levels are not readily available or useful. ECG and cardiac monitoring should be maintained, and blood glucose and electrolytes, BUN, and creatinine levels should be monitored, as well as ABG if there are respiratory symptoms.

Management

Vital functions must be established and maintained. Vascular access, baseline ECG, and continuous cardiac and blood pressure monitoring should be established. A pacemaker must be available. Gastrointestinal decontamination can be undertaken initially with activated charcoal up to 1 hour after ingestion. MDAC is no longer recommended, based on the latest guidelines. Whole-bowel irrigation can be considered in cases of large overdoses with sustained-release preparations, but there are no studies evaluating the efficacy of intervention.

If there are cardiovascular disturbances, a cardiac consultation should be obtained. Class IA antidysrhythmic agents (procainamide, quinidine) and III (bretylium) are not recommended. Hypotension is treated with fluids initially, although it usually does not respond. Frequently, glucagon and cardiac pacing are needed. Bradycardia in asymptomatic, hemodynamically stable patients requires no therapy. It is not predictive of the future course of the disease. If the patient is unstable (has hypotension or a high-degree atrioventricular block), atropine 0.02 mg/kg (up to 2 mg) in adults, glucagon, and a pacemaker can be used. In case of ventricular tachycardia, overdrive pacing can be used. A wide QRS interval may respond to sodium bicarbonate. Torsades de pointes (associated with sotalol) may respond to magnesium sulfate and overdrive pacing. Prophylactic magnesium for prolonged QT interval has been suggested, but there are no data. Epinephrine must not be used because an unopposed α effect may occur.

Hypotension and myocardial depression are managed by correction of dysrhythmias, Trendelenburg position, fluids, glucagon, or amrinone (Inocor), or a combination of these. Hemodynamic monitoring with a Swan-Ganz catheter or arterial line may be necessary to manage fluid therapy.

Glucagon is the initial drug of choice. It works through adenyl cyclase and bypasses catecholamine receptors; therefore, it is not affected by β-blockers. Glucagon increases cardiac contractility and heart rate. It is given as an intravenous bolus of 5 to 10 mg[C] over 1 minute and followed by a continuous infusion of 1 to 5 mg/h (in children, 0.15 mg/kg followed by 0.05 to 0.1 mg/kg/h). In large doses and in infusion therapy D_5W, sterile water, or saline should be used as a diluant to reconstitute glucagon in place of the 0.2% phenol diluent provided with some drugs. Effects are seen within minutes. It can be used with other agents such as amrinone.

Amrinone (Inocor) inhibits phosphodiesterase enzyme, which metabolizes cyclic AMP. It is administered as a bolus of 0.15 to 2 mg/kg (0.15 to 0.4 mL/kg) intravenously, followed by infusion of 5 to 10 µg/kg/min.

Hypoglycemia should be treated with intravenous glucose. Life-threatening hyperkalemia is treated with calcium (avoid if digoxin is present), bicarbonate, and glucose or insulin. Convulsions can be controlled with diazepam or phenobarbital. If bronchospasm is present, $β_2$ nebulized bronchodilators are given.

Extraordinary measures such as intra-aortic balloon pump support can be instituted. Extracorporeal measures can be undertaken. Hemodialysis for cases of atenolol, acebutolol, nadolol, and sotalol (low volume distribution, low protein binding) ingestion may be helpful, particularly when there is evidence of renal failure. Hemodialysis is not effective for propranolol, metoprolol, and timolol.

Prenalterol[A] has successfully reversed both bradycardia and hypotension but is not currently available in the United States.

Disposition

Asymptomatic patients with history of overdose require baseline ECG and continuous cardiac monitoring for at least 6 hours with regular-release preparations and for 24 hours with sustained-release preparations.

Symptomatic patients should be observed with cardiac monitoring for 24 hours. If seizures or abnormal rhythm or vital signs are present, the patient should be admitted to the intensive care unit.

CALCIUM CHANNEL BLOCKERS

Calcium channel blockers are used in the treatment of effort angina, supraventricular tachycardia, and hypertension.

Toxic Mechanism

Calcium channel blockers reduce influx of calcium through the slow channels in membranes of the myocardium, the atrioventricular nodes, and the vascular smooth muscles and result in peripheral, systemic, and coronary vasodilation, impaired cardiac conduction, and depression of cardiac contractility. All calcium channel blockers have vasodilatory action, but only bepridil, diltiazem, and verapamil depress myocardial contractility and cause atrioventricular block.

Toxic Dose

Any ingested amount greater than the maximum daily dose has the potential of severe toxicity. The maximum oral daily doses in adults and toxic doses in children of each are as follows: amlodipine (Norvasc), 10 mg for adults and more than 0.25 mg/kg for children; bepridil (Vascor), 400 mg for adults and more than 5.7 mg/kg for children; diltiazem (Cardizem), 360 mg for adults (toxic dose > 2 g) and more than 6 mg/kg for children; felodipine (Plendil), 40 mg for adults and more than 0.56 mg/kg for children; isradipine (DynaCirc), 40 mg for adults and more than 0.4 mg/kg for children; nicardipine (Cardene), 120 mg for adults and more than 0.85 mg/kg for children; nifedipine (Procardia), 120 mg for adults and more than 2 mg/kg for children; nimodipine (Nimotop), 360 mg for adults and more than 0.85 mg/kg for children; nitrendipine (Baypress)[A], 80 mg for adults and more than 1.14 mg/kg for children; and verapamil (Calan), 480 mg for adults and 15 mg/kg for children.

Kinetics

Onset of action of regular-release preparations varies: for verapamil it is 60 to 120 minutes, for nifedipine 20 minutes, and for diltiazem 15 minutes after ingestion. Peak effect for verapamil is 2 to 4 hours, for nifedipine 60 to 90 minutes, and for diltiazem 30 to 60 minutes, but the peak action may be delayed for 6 to 8 hours. Duration of action is up to 36 hours. The onset of action for sustained-release preparations is usually 4 hours but may be delayed, and peak effect is at 12 to 24 hours. In cases of massive overdose, concretions and prolonged toxicity can develop.

[A]Not available in the United States.
[C]Exceeds dosage recommended by the manufacturer.

[A]Not available in the United States.

Volume distribution varies from 3 to 7 L/kg. Hepatic elimination half-life varies from 3 to 7 hours. Patients receiving digitalis and calcium channel blockers run the risk of digitalis toxicity, because calcium channel blockers increase digitalis levels.

Manifestations

Cardiac manifestations include hypotension, bradycardia, and conduction disturbances occurring 30 minutes to 5 hours after ingestion. A prolonged PR interval is an early finding and may occur at therapeutic doses. Torsades de pointes has been reported. All degrees of blocks may occur and may be delayed up to 16 hours. Lactic acidosis may be present. Calcium channel blockers do not affect intraventricular conduction, so the QRS interval is usually not affected.

Hypocalcemia is rarely present. Hyperglycemia may be present because of interference in calcium-dependent insulin release. Mental status changes, headaches, seizures, hemiparesis, and CNS depression may occur.

Laboratory Investigations

Specific drug levels are not readily available and are not useful. Monitor blood sugar, electrolytes, calcium, ABG, pulse oximetry, creatinine, and BUN, and also use hemodynamic monitoring, ECG, and cardiac monitoring.

Management

Vital functions must be established and maintained. Baseline ECG readings should be obtained and continuous cardiac and blood pressure monitoring maintained. A pacemaker should be available. Cardiology consultation should be sought.

Gastrointestinal decontamination with activated charcoal is recommended. If a large dose of a sustained-release preparation was ingested, whole-bowel irrigation can be considered, but its effectiveness has not been investigated.

If the patient is symptomatic, immediate cardiology consult must be obtained, because a pacemaker and hemodynamic monitoring may be needed. In the case of heart block, atropine is rarely effective and isoproterenol (Isuprel) may produce vasodilation. The use of a pacemaker should be considered early.

Hypotension and bradycardia can be treated with positioning, fluids, and calcium gluconate or chloride, glucagon, amrinone (Inocor), and ventricular pacing. Calcium salts must be avoided if digoxin is present. Calcium usually reverses depressed myocardial contractility but may not reverse nodal depression or peripheral vasodilation. Calcium chloride can be given in a 10% solution, 0.1 to 0.2 mL/kg up to 10 mL in an adult, or calcium gluconate in a 10% solution 0.3 to 0.4 mL/kg up to 20 mL in an adult. Administration is intravenous, over 5 to 10 minutes. One should monitor for dysrhythmias, hypotension, and the serum ionized calcium. The aim is to increase calcium 4 mg/dL to a maximum of 13 mg/dL. The calcium response lasts 15 minutes and may require repeated doses or a continuous calcium gluconate infusion 0.2 mL/kg/h up to maximum of 10 mL/h.

If calcium fails, glucagon can be tried for its positive inotropic and chronotropic effect, or both. Amrinone (Inocor), an inotropic agent, may reverse the effects of calcium channel blockers. An effective dose is 0.15 mg to 2 mg/kg (0.15 to 0.4 mL/kg) by intravenous bolus followed by infusion of 5 to 10 µg/kg/min.

In case of hypotension, fluids, norepinephrine (Levophed), and epinephrine may be required. Amrinone and glucagon have been tried alone and in combination. Dobutamine and dopamine are often ineffective.

Extracorporeal measures (e.g., hemodialysis and charcoal hemoperfusion) are not useful, but extraordinary measures such as intra-aortic balloon pump and cardiopulmonary bypass have been used successfully.

For cases of calcium channel blocker toxicity that fail to respond to aggressive management, recent studies demonstrate that insulin and glucose have therapeutic value. The suggested dose range for insulin is to infuse regular insulin at 0.5 IU/kg/h with a simultaneous infusion of glucose 1 g/kg/h, with glucose monitoring every 30 minutes for at least the first 4 hours of administration and subsequent glucose adjustment to maintain euglycemia (70 to 100 mg/dL). Potassium levels should be monitored regularly, as they may shift in response to the insulin.

Disposition

Patients who have ingested regular-release preparations should be monitored for at least 6 hours and those who have ingested sustained-release preparations should be monitored for 24 hours after the ingestion. Intentional overdose necessitates psychiatric clearance. Symptomatic patients should be admitted to the intensive care unit.

CARBON MONOXIDE

Carbon monoxide is an odorless, colorless gas produced from incomplete combustion; it is also an in vivo metabolic breakdown product of methylene chloride used in paint removers.

Toxic Mechanism

Carbon monoxide's affinity for hemoglobin is 240 times greater than that of oxygen. It shifts the oxygen dissociation curve to the left, which impairs hemoglobin release of oxygen to tissues and inhibits the cytochrome oxidase enzymes.

Toxic Dose and Manifestations

Table 13 describes the manifestations of carbon monoxide toxicity. Exposure to 0.5% for a few minutes is lethal. Sequelae correlate with the patient's level of consciousness at presentation. ECG abnormalities may be noted. Creatine kinase is often elevated, and rhabdomyolysis and myoglobinuria may occur.

Rakel and Bope: *Conn's Current Therapy 2006.*

TABLE 13 Carbon Monoxide Exposure and Possible Manifestations

CoHB saturation (%)	Manifestations
3.5	None
5	Slight headache, decreased exercise tolerance
10	Slight headache. dyspnea on vigorous exertion, may impair driving skills
10-20	Moderate dyspnea on exertion, throbbing, temporal headache
20-30	Severe headache, syncope, dizziness, visual changes, weakness, nausea, vomiting, altered judgment
30-40	Vertigo, ataxia, blurred vision, confusion, loss of consciousness
40-50	Confusion, tachycardia, tachypnea, coma, convulsions
50-60	Cheyne-Stokes, coma, convulsions, shock, apnea
60-70	Coma, convulsions, respiratory and heart failure, death

The carboxyhemoglobin (CoHB) expresses in percentage the extent to which carbon monoxide has bound with the total hemoglobin. This may be misleadingly low in the anemic patient with less hemoglobin than normal. The patient's presentation is a more reliable indicator of severity than the CoHB level. The manifestations listed in Table 13 for each level are in addition to those listed at the level above. The CoHB may not correlate reliably with the severity of the intoxication, and linking symptoms to specific levels of CoHB frequently leads to inaccurate conclusions. A level of carbon monoxide greater than 40% is usually associated with obvious intoxication.

Kinetics

The natural metabolism of the body produces small amounts of CoHB, less than 2% for nonsmokers and 5% to 9% for smokers.

Carbon monoxide is rapidly absorbed through the lungs. The rate of absorption is directly related to alveolar ventilation. Elimination also occurs through the lungs. The half-life of CoHB in room air (21% oxygen) is 5 to 6 hours; in 100% oxygen, it is 90 minutes; in hyperbaric pressure at 3 atmospheres oxygen, it is 20 to 30 minutes.

Laboratory Investigations

An ABG reading may show metabolic acidosis and normal oxygen tension. In cases of significant poisoning, the ABG, electrolytes, blood glucose, serum creatine kinase and cardiac enzymes, renal function tests, and liver function tests should be monitored. A urinalysis and test for myoglobinuria should be obtained. Chest radiograph can be useful in cases of smoke inhalation or if the patient is being considered for

hyperbaric chamber. ECG monitoring should be maintained, especially if the patient is older than 40 years, has a history of cardiac disease, or has moderate to severe symptoms. Which toxicology studies are used is based on symptoms and circumstances. CoHB should be monitored during and at the end of therapy. The pulse oximeter has two wavelengths and overestimates oxyhemoglobin saturation in carbon monoxide poisoning. The true oxygen saturation is determined by blood gas analysis, which measures the oxygen bound to hemoglobin. The co-oximeter measures four wavelengths and separates out CoHB and the other hemoglobin binding agents from oxyhemoglobin. Fetal hemoglobin has a greater affinity for carbon monoxide than adult hemoglobin and may falsely elevate the CoHB as much as 4% in young infants.

Management

The first step is to adequately protect the rescuer. The patient must be removed from the contaminated area, and his or her vital functions must be established.

The mainstay of treatment is 100% oxygen via a nonrebreathing mask with an oxygen reservoir or endotracheal tube. All patients receive 100% oxygen until the CoHB level is 5% or less. Assisted ventilation may be necessary. ABG and CoHB should be monitored and the present CoHB level determined. *Note:* A near-normal CoHB level does not exclude significant carbon monoxide poisoning, especially if the measurement is taken several hours after termination of exposure or if oxygen has been administered prior to obtaining the sample.

The exposed pregnant woman should be kept on 100% oxygen for several hours after the CoHB level is almost 0, because carbon monoxide concentrates in the fetus and oxygen is needed longer to ensure elimination of the carbon monoxide from fetal circulation. The fetus must be monitored, because carbon monoxide and hypoxia are potentially teratogenic.

Metabolic acidosis should be treated with sodium bicarbonate only if the pH is below 7.2 after correction of hypoxia and adequate ventilation. Acidosis shifts the oxygen dissociation curve to the right and facilitates oxygen delivery to the tissues.

The decision to use the hyperbaric oxygen chamber must be made on the basis of the ability to handle other acute emergencies that may coexist in the patient and of the severity of the poisoning. The standard of care for persons exposed to carbon monoxide has yet to be determined, but most authorities recommend using the hyperbaric oxygen chamber under any of the following conditions:

- If the patient is in a coma or has a history of loss of consciousness or seizures
- If there is cardiovascular dysfunction (clinical ischemic chest pain or ECG evidence of ischemia)
- If the patient has metabolic acidosis
- If symptoms persist despite 100% oxygen therapy
- In a child, if the initial CoHB is greater than 15%
- In symptomatic patients with preexisting ischemia

Rakel and Bope: Conn's Current Therapy 2006.

- If there are signs of maternal or fetal distress regardless of CoHB level (infants and fetus are a special problem because fetal hemoglobin has greater affinity for carbon monoxide)

Although controversial, a neurologic-cognitive examination has been used to help determine which patients with low carbon monoxide levels should receive more aggressive therapy. Testing should include the following: general orientation memory testing involving address, phone number, date of birth, and present date; and cognitive testing, involving counting by 7s, digit span, and forward and backward spelling of three-letter and four-letter words. Patients with delayed neurologic sequelae or recurrent symptoms up to 3 weeks may benefit from hyperbaric oxygen chamber treatment.

Seizures and cerebral edema must be treated.

Disposition

Patients with no or mild symptoms who become asymptomatic after a few hours of oxygen therapy and have a carbon monoxide level less than 10%, and normal physical and neurologic-cognitive examination findings can be discharged, but they should be instructed to return if any signs of neurologic dysfunction appear. Patients with carbon monoxide poisoning requiring treatment need follow-up neuropsychiatric examinations.

CAUSTICS AND CORROSIVES

The terms *caustic* and *corrosive* are used interchangeably and can be divided into acids and alkalis. The U.S. Consumer Product Safety Commission Labeling Recommendations on containers for acids and alkalis indicate the potential for producing serious damage, as follows:

- Caution—weak irritant
- Warning—strong irritant
- Danger—corrosive

Some common acids with corrosive potential include acetic acid, formic acid, glycolic acid, hydrochloric acid, mercuric chloride, nitric acid, oxalic acid, phosphoric acid, sulfuric acid (battery acid), zinc chloride, and zinc sulfate. Some common alkalis with corrosive potential include ammonia, calcium carbide, calcium hydroxide (dry), calcium oxide, potassium hydroxide (lye), and sodium hydroxide (lye).

Toxic Mechanism

Acids produce mucosal coagulation necrosis and may be absorbed systemically; they do not penetrate deeply. Injury to the gastric mucosa is more likely, although specific sites of injury for acids and alkalis are not clearly defined.

Alkalis produce liquefaction necrosis and saponification and penetrate deeply. The esophageal mucosa is likely to be damaged. Oropharyngeal and esophageal damage is more frequently caused by solids than by liquids. Liquids produce superficial circumferential burns and gastric damage.

Toxic Dose

The toxicity is determined by concentration, contact time, and pH. Significant injury is more likely with a substance that has a pH of less than 2 or greater than 12, with a prolonged contact time, and with large volumes.

Manifestations

The absence of oral burns does not exclude the possibility of esophageal or gastric damage. General clinical findings are stridor; dysphagia; drooling; oropharyngeal, retrosternal, and epigastric pain; and ocular and oral burns. Alkali burns are yellow, soapy, frothy lesions. Acid burns are gray-white and later form an eschar. Abdominal tenderness and guarding may be present if perforation has happened.

Laboratory Investigations

If acid ingestion has taken place, the patient's acid–base balance and electrolyte status should be determined. If pulmonary symptoms are present, a chest radiograph, ABG measurement, and pulse oximetry are called for.

Management

It is recommended that the container be brought to the examination, as the substance must be identified and the pH of the substance, vomitus, tears, or saliva tested.

If the acid or alkali has been ingested, all gastrointestinal decontamination procedures are contraindicated except for immediate rinse, removal of substance from the mouth, and dilution with small amounts (sips) of milk or water. The examiner should check for ocular and dermal involvement. Contraindications to oral dilution are dysphagias, respiratory distress, obtundation, or shock. If there is ocular involvement one should immediately irrigate the eye with tepid water for at least 30 minutes, perform fluorescein stain of eye, and consult an ophthalmologist. If there is dermal involvement, one should immediately remove contaminated clothes and irrigate the skin with tepid water for at least 15 minutes. Consultation with a burn specialist is called for.

In cases of acid ingestion, some authorities advocate a small flexible nasogastric tube and aspiration within 30 minutes after ingestion.

Patients should receive only intravenous fluids following dilution until endoscopic consultation is obtained. Endoscopy is valuable to predict damage and risk of stricture. The indications are controversial, with some authorities recommending it in all cases of caustic ingestions regardless of symptoms, and others selectively using clinical features such as vomiting, stridor, drooling, and oral or facial lesions as criteria. We recommend endoscopy for all symptomatic patients or patients with intentional ingestions. Endoscopy may be performed immediately if the patient is symptomatic, but it is usually done 12 to 48 hours postingestion.

The use of corticosteroids is considered controversial. Some feel they may be useful for patients with second-degree circumferential burns. They recommend starting with hydrocortisone sodium succinate (Solu-Cortef) intravenously 10 to 20 mg/kg/d within 48 hours and changing to oral prednisolone 2 mg/kg/d for 3 weeks before tapering the dose. We do not usually recommend using corticosteroids because they have not been shown to be effective.

Tetanus prophylaxis should be provided if the patient requires it for wound care. Antibiotics are not useful prophylactically. Contrast studies are not useful in the first few days and may interfere with endoscopic evaluation; later, they can be used to assess the severity of damage.

Emergency medical therapy includes agents to inhibit collagen formation and intraluminal stents. Esophageal and gastric outlet dilation may be needed if there is evidence of stricture. Bougienage of the esophagus, however, has been associated with brain abscess. Interposition of the colon may be necessary if dilation fails to provide an adequate-sized passage.

Management of inhalation cases requires immediate removal from the environment, administration of humid supplemental oxygen, and observation for airway obstruction and noncardiac pulmonary edema. Radiographic and ABG evaluation should be obtained when appropriate. Intubation and respiratory support may be required.

Certain caustics produce systemic disturbances. Formaldehyde causes metabolic acidosis, hydrofluoric acid causes hypocalcemia and renal damage, oxalic acid causes hypocalcemia, phenol causes hepatic and renal damage, and picric acid causes renal injury.

Disposition

Infants and small children should be medically evaluated and observed. All symptomatic patients should be admitted. If they have severe symptoms or danger of airway compromise, they should be admitted to the intensive care unit. After endoscopy, if no damage is detected, the patient may be discharged when he or she can tolerate oral feedings. Intentional exposures require psychiatric evaluation before the patient can be discharged.

COCAINE (BENZOYLMETHYLECGONINE)

Cocaine is derived from the leaves of *Erythroxylum coca* and *Truxillo coca*. "Body packing" refers to the placement of many small packages of contraband cocaine for concealment in the gastrointestinal tract or other areas for illicit transport. "Body stuffing" refers to spontaneous ingestion of substances for the purpose of hiding evidence.

Toxic Mechanism

Cocaine directly stimulates the CNS presynaptic sympathetic neurons to release catecholamines and acetylcholine, while it blocks the presynaptic reuptake of the catecholamines; it blocks the sodium channels along neuronal membranes; and it increases platelet aggregation. Long-term use depletes the CNS of dopamine.

Toxic Dose

The maximum mucosal local anesthetic therapeutic dose of cocaine is 200 mg or 2 mL of a 10% solution. Although CNS effects can occur at relatively low local anesthetic doses (50 to 95 mg), they are more common with doses greater than 1 mg/kg; cardiac effects can occur with doses greater than 1 mg/kg. The potential fatal dose is 1200 mg intranasally, but death has occurred with 20 mg parenterally.

Kinetics

Cocaine is well absorbed by all routes, including nasal insufflation, and oral, dermal, and inhalation routes (Table 14). Protein binding is 8.7%, and volume distribution is 1.5 L/kg.

Cocaine is metabolized by plasma and liver cholinesterase to the inactive metabolites ecgonine methyl ester and benzoylecgonine. Plasma pseudocholinesterase is congenitally deficient in 3% of the population and decreased in fetuses, young infants, the elderly, pregnant people, and people with liver disease. These enzyme-deficient individuals are at increased risk for life-threatening cocaine toxicity.

Ten percent of cocaine is excreted unchanged. Cocaine and ethanol undergo liver synthesis to form cocaethylene, a metabolite with a half-life three times longer than that of cocaine. It may account for some of

TABLE 14   The Different Routes and Kinetics of Cocaine

Type	Route	Onset	Peak (min)	Half-life (min)	Duration (min)
Cocaine leaf	Oral, chewing	20-30 min	45-90	NA	240-360
Hydrochloride	Insufflation	1-3 min	5-10	78	60-90
	Ingestion	20-30 min	50-90	54	Sustained
	Intravenous	30-120 sec	5-11	36	60-90
Free base/crack	Smoking	5-10 sec	5-11	—	Up to 20
Coca paste	Smoking	Unknown	—	—	—

Rakel and Bope: *Conn's Current Therapy 2006.*

cocaine's cardiotoxicity and appears to be more lethal than cocaine or ethanol alone.

Manifestations

The CNS manifestations of cocaine ingestion are euphoria, hyperactivity, agitation, convulsions, and intracranial hemorrhage. Mydriasis and septal perforation can occur, as well as cardiac dysrhythmias, hypertension, and hypotension (with severe overdose). Chest pain is frequent, but only 5.8% of patients have true myocardial ischemia and infarction. Other manifestations include vasoconstriction, hyperthermia (because of increased metabolic rate), ischemic bowel perforation if the substance is ingested, rhabdomyolysis, myoglobinuria, and renal failure. In pregnant users, premature labor and abruptio placentae can occur.

Body cavity packing should be suspected in cases of prolonged toxicity.

Mortality can result from cerebrovascular accidents, coronary artery spasm, myocardial injury, or lethal dysrhythmias.

Laboratory Investigations

Monitoring of the ECG and cardiac rhythms, ABG, oxygen saturation, electrolytes, blood glucose, BUN, creatinine, and creatine kinase levels should be maintained. One should monitor cardiac fraction if the patient has chest pain, as well as the liver profile, and the urine for myoglobin. Intravenous drug users should have HIV and hepatitis virus testing.

Urine should be tested for cocaine and metabolites and other substances of abuse, and abdominal radiographs or ultrasonogram should be ordered for body packers. If the urine sample was collected more than 12 hours after cocaine intake, it will contain little or no cocaine. If cocaine is present, cocaine has been used within the past 12 hours. Cocaine's metabolite benzoylecgonine may be detected within 4 hours after a single nasal insufflation and for up to 114 hours. Cross-reactions with some herbal teas, lidocaine, and droperidol (Inapsine) may give false-positive results by some immunoassay methods.

Management

Supportive care includes blood pressure, cardiac, and thermal monitoring and seizure precautions. Diazepam (Valium) is the drug of choice for treatment of cocaine toxicity agitation, seizures, and dysrhythmias; doses are 10 to 30 mg intravenously at 2.5 mg per minute for adults and 0.2 to 0.5 mg/kg at 1 mg per minute up to 10 mg for a child.

Gastrointestinal decontamination should be instituted, if the cocaine was ingested, by administration of activated charcoal. MDAC may adsorb cocaine leakage in body stuffers or body packers. Whole-bowel irrigation with polyethylene glycol solution (PEG) has been used in body packers and stuffers if the contraband is in a firm container. If the packages are not visible on plain radiographs of the abdomen, a contrast study or CT scan can help to confirm successful passage. Cocaine in the nasal passage can be removed with an applicator dipped in a non–water-soluble product (lubricating jelly) if this is done within a few minutes after application.

In body packers and stuffers, venous access must be secured, and drugs must be readily available for treating life-threatening manifestations until the contraband is passed in the stool. Surgical removal may be indicated if the packet does not pass the pylorus, in an asymptomatic body packer, or in the case of intestinal obstruction.

Hypertension and tachycardia are usually transient and can be managed by careful titration of diazepam. Nitroprusside may be used for severe hypertension. Myocardial ischemia is managed by oxygen, vascular access, benzodiazepines, and nitroglycerin. Aspirin and thrombolysis are not routinely recommended because of the danger of intracranial hemorrhage.

Dysrhythmias are usually supraventricular (SVT) and do not require specific management. Adenosine is ineffective. Life-threatening tachydysrhythmias may respond to phentolamine (Regitine) 5 mg IV bolus in adults or 0.1 mg/kg in children at 5- to 10-minute intervals. Phentolamine also relieves coronary artery spasm and myocardial ischemia. Electrical synchronized cardioversion should be considered for patients with hemodynamically unstable dysrhythmias. Lidocaine is not recommended initially but may be used after 3 hours for ventricular tachycardia. Wide complex QRS ventricular tachycardia may be treated with sodium bicarbonate 2 mEq/kg as a bolus. β-Adrenergic blockers are not recommended.

Anxiety, agitation, and convulsions can be treated with diazepam. If diazepam fails to control seizures, neuromuscular blockers can be used. The EEG should be monitored for nonmotor seizure activity. For hyperthermia, external cooling and cool humidified 100% oxygen should be administered. Neuromuscular paralysis to control seizures will reduce temperature. Dantrolene and antipyretics are not recommended. Rhabdomyolysis and myoglobinuria are treated with fluids, alkaline diuresis, and diuretics.

If the patient is pregnant, the fetus must be monitored and the patient observed for spontaneous abortion.

Paranoid ideation and threatening behavior should be treated with rapid tranquilization. The patient should be observed for suicidal depression that may follow intoxication and may require suicide precautions. If focal neurologic manifestations are present, one should consider the possibility of a cerebrovascular accident and obtain a CT scan.

Extracorporeal clearance techniques are of no benefit.

Disposition

Patients with mild intoxication or a brief seizure that does not require treatment who become asymptomatic may be discharged after 6 hours with appropriate psychosocial follow-up. If cardiac or cerebral ischemic manifestations are present, the patient should be monitored in the intensive care unit. Body packers and stuffers require care in the intensive care unit until passage of the contraband.

CYANIDE

Hydrogen cyanide is a byproduct of burning plastic and wools in residential fires. Hydrocyanic acid is the liquefied form of hydrogen cyanide. Cyanide salts can be found in ore extraction. Nitriles, such as acetonitrile (artificial nail removers) are metabolized in the body to produce cyanide. Cyanogenic glycosides are present in some fruit seeds (such as amygdalin in apricots, peaches, and apples). Sodium nitroprusside, the antihypertensive vasodilator, contains five cyanide groups.

Toxic Mechanism

Cyanide blocks the cellular electron transport mechanism and cellular respiration by inhibiting the mitochondrial ferricytochrome oxidase system and other enzymes. This results in cellular hypoxia and lactic acidosis. *Note:* Citrus fruit seeds form cyanide in the presence of intestinal β-glucosidase (the seeds are harmful only if the capsule is broken).

Toxic Dose

The ingestion of 1 mg/kg or 50 mg of hydrogen cyanide can produce death within 15 minutes. The lethal dose of potassium cyanide is 200 mg. Five to 10 mL of 84% acetonitrile is lethal. Infusions of sodium nitroprusside in rates above 2 µg/kg per minute may cause cyanide to accumulate to toxic concentrations in critically ill patients.

Kinetics

Cyanide is rapidly absorbed by all routes. In the stomach, it forms hydrocyanic acid. Volume distribution is 1.5 L/kg. Protein binding is 60%. Cyanide is detoxified by metabolism in the liver via the mitochondrial thiosulfate-rhodanese pathway, which catalyzes the transfer of sulfur donor to cyanide, forming the less toxic irreversible thiocyanate that is excreted in the urine. Cyanide is also detoxified by reacting with hydroxocobalamin (vitamin B_{12a}) to form cyanocobalamin (vitamin B_{12}).

The cyanide elimination half-life from the blood is 1.2 hours. The elimination route is through the lungs.

Manifestations

Hydrogen cyanide has the distinctive odor of bitter almonds or silver polish. Manifestations of cyanide intoxication include hypertension, cardiac dysrhythmias, various ECG abnormalities, headache, hyperpnea, seizures, stupor, pulmonary edema, and flushing. Cyanosis is absent or appears late.

Laboratory Investigations

The examiner should obtain and monitor ABGs, oxygen saturation, blood lactate, hemoglobin, blood glucose, and electrolytes. Lactic acidemia, a decrease in the arterial-venous oxygen difference, and bright red venous blood occurs. If smoke inhalation is the possible source of cyanide exposure, CoHB and methemoglobin (MetHb) concentrations should be measured.

Cyanide levels in whole blood, red blood cells, or serum are not useful in the acute management because the determinations are not readily available. Specific cyanide blood levels are as follows: smokers have less than 0.5 µg/mL; a patient with flushing and tachycardia has 0.5 to 1.0 µg/mL, one with obtundation has 1.0 to 2.5 µg/mL, and one in coma or who has died has more than 2.5 µg/mL.

Management

If the cyanide was inhaled, the patient must be removed from the contaminated atmosphere. Attendants should not administer mouth-to-mouth resuscitation. Rescuers and attendants must be protected. Immediate administration of 100% oxygen is called for and oxygen should be continued during and after the administration of the antidote. The clinician must decide whether to use any or all components of the cyanide antidote kit.

The mechanism of action of the antidote kit is twofold: to produce methemoglobinemia and to provide a sulfur substrate for the detoxification of cyanide. The nitrites make methemoglobin, which has a greater affinity for cyanide than does the cytochrome oxidase enzymes. The combination of methemoglobin and cyanide forms cyanomethemoglobin. Sodium thiosulfate provides a sulfur substrate for the rhodanese enzyme, which converts cyanide into the relatively nontoxic sodium thiocyanate, which is excreted by the kidney.

The procedure for using the antidote kit is as follows:

Step 1: Amyl nitrite inhalant perles is only a temporizing measure (forms only 2% to 5% methemoglobin) and it can be omitted if venous access is established. Alternate 100% oxygen and the inhalant for 30 seconds each minute. Use a new perle every 3 minutes.

Step 2: Sodium nitrite ampule is indicated for cyanide exposures, except for cases of residential fires, smoke inhalation, and nitroprusside or acetonitrile poisonings. It is administered intravenously to produce methemoglobin of 20% to 30% at 35 to 70 minutes after administration. A dose of 10 mL of 3% solution of sodium nitrite for adults and 0.33 mL/kg of 3% solution for children is diluted to 100 mL 0.9% saline and administered slowly intravenously at 5 mL/min. If hypotension develops, the infusion should be slowed.

Step 3: Sodium thiosulfate is useful alone in cases of smoke inhalation, nitroprusside toxicity, and acetonitrile toxicity and should not be used at all in cases of hydrogen sulfide poisoning. The administration dose is 12.5 g of sodium thiosulfate or

50 mL of 25% solution for adults and 1.65 mL/kg of 25% solution for children intravenously over 10 to 20 minutes.

If cyanide symptoms recur, further treatment with nitrites or the perles is controversial. Some authorities suggest repeating the antidotes in 30 minutes at half of the initial dose, but others do not advise this for lack of efficacy. The child dosage regimen on the package insert must be carefully followed.

One hour after antidotes are administered, the methemoglobin level should be obtained and should not exceed 20%. Methylene blue should not be used to reverse excessive methemoglobin.

Gastrointestinal decontamination of oral ingestion by activated charcoal is recommended but is not very effective because of the rapidity of absorption. Seizures are treated with intravenous diazepam. Acidosis should be treated with sodium bicarbonate if it does not rapidly resolve with therapy. There is no role for hyperbaric oxygen or hemodialysis or hemoperfusion.

Other antidotes include hydroxocobalamin (vitamin B_{12a}) (Cyanokit), which has proven effective when given immediately after exposure in large doses of 4 g (50 mg/kg) or 50 times the amount of cyanide exposure with 8 g of sodium thiosulfate. Hydroxocobalamin has FDA orphan drug approval.

Disposition

Asymptomatic patients should be observed for a minimum of 3 hours. Patients who ingest nitrile compounds must be observed for 24 hours. Patients requiring antidote administration should be admitted to the intensive care unit.

DIGITALIS

Cardiac glycosides are found in cardiac medications, common plants, and the skin of the Bufo toad.

Toxic Mechanism

Cardiac glycosides inhibit the enzyme sodium/potassium-adenosine triphosphatase (NA^+, K^+, ATPase), leading to intracellular potassium loss and increased intracellular sodium, and producing phase 4 depolarization, increased automaticity, and ectopy. There is increased intracellular calcium and potentiation of contractility. Pacemaker cells are inhibited, and the refractory period is prolonged, leading to atrioventricular blocks. There is increased vagal tone.

Toxic Dose

Digoxin total digitalizing dose, the dose required to achieve therapeutic blood levels of 0.6 to 2.0 ng/mL, is 0.75 to 1.25 mg or 10 to 15 µg/kg for patients older than 10 years of age; 40 to 50 µg/kg for patients younger than 2 years of age; and 30 to 40 µg/kg for patients 2 to 10 years of age.

The acute single toxic dose is greater than 0.07 mg/kg or greater than 2 or 3 mg in an adult, but 2 mg in a child or 4 mg in an adult usually produces only mild toxicity. One to 3 mg or more may be found in a few leaves of oleander or foxglove. Serious and fatal overdoses are more than 4 mg in a child and more than 10 mg in an adult.

Acute digitoxin ingestion of 10 to 35 mg has produced severe toxicity and death. Digitoxin therapeutic steady state is 15 to 25 ng/mL. In cases of chronic or acute-on-chronic ingestions in patients with cardiac disease, more than 2 mg may produce toxicity; however, toxicity can develop within therapeutic range on chronic therapy.

Patients at greatest risk of overdose include those with cardiac disease, those with electrolyte abnormalities (low potassium, low magnesium, low T_4, high calcium), those with renal impairment, and those on amiodarone (Cordarone), quinidine, erythromycin, tetracycline, calcium channel blockers, and β-blockers.

Kinetics

Digoxin is a metabolite of digitoxin. In cases of oral overdose, the typical onset is 30 minutes, with peak effects in 3 to 12 hours. Duration is 3 to 4 days. Intravenous onset is in 5 to 30 minutes; peak level is immediate, and peak effect is at 1.5 to 3 hours.

Volume distribution is 5 to 6 L/kg. The cardiac-to-plasma ratio is 30:1. After an acute ingestion overdose, the serum concentration is not reflective of tissue concentration for at least 6 hours or more, and steady state is 12 to 16 hours after last dose.

Sixty percent to 80% of the parent compound is excreted unchanged in the urine. The elimination half-life is 30 to 50 hours.

Manifestations

Onset of manifestations is usually within 2 hours but may be delayed up to 12 hours.

Gastrointestinal effects of nausea and vomiting are frequently present in cases of acute ingestion but may also occur in cases of chronic ingestion. The "digitalis effect" on ECG is scooped ST segments and PR prolongation; in cases of overdose, any dysrhythmia or block is possible but none are characteristic. Bradycardia occurs in patients with acute overdose with healthy hearts; supraventricular tachycardia occurs in patients with existing heart disease or chronic overdose. Ventricular tachycardia is seen only in cases of severe poisoning.

The CNS effects include headaches, visual disturbances, and colored halo vision. Hyperkalemia occurs following acute overdose and correlates with digoxin level and outcome. Among patients with serum potassium levels of less than 5.0 mEq/L, all survive. If the level is 5 to 5.5, 50% survive, and if the level is greater than 5.5, all die. Hypokalemia is commonly seen with chronic intoxication. Patients with normal digitalis levels may have toxicity in the presence of hypokalemia.

Rakel and Bope: *Conn's Current Therapy 2006.*

Chronic intoxications are more likely to produce scotoma, color perception disturbances, yellow vision, halos, delirium, hallucinations or psychosis, tachycardia, and hypokalemia.

Laboratory Investigations

Continuous monitoring of ECG, pulse, and blood pressure is called for. Blood glucose, electrolytes, calcium, magnesium, BUN, and creatinine levels should also be monitored. An initial digoxin level should be measured on patient presentation and repeated thereafter. Levels should be measured more than 6 hours postingestion because earlier values do not reflect tissue distribution. Digoxin clinical toxicity is usually associated with serum digoxin levels of greater than 3.5 ng/mL in adults.

An endogenous digoxin-like substance cross-reacts in most common immunoassays (not with high-pressure liquid chromatography) and values as high as 4.1 ng/mL have been reported in newborns, patients with chronic renal failure, patients with abnormal immunoglobulins, and women in the third trimester of pregnancy.

Management

A cardiology consult should be obtained and a pacemaker should be readily available.

In undertaking gastrointestinal decontamination, excessive vagal stimulation should be avoided (e.g., emesis and gastric lavage). Activated charcoal should be administered, and if a nasogastric tube is required for the activated charcoal, pretreatment with atropine (0.02 mg/kg in children and 0.5 mg in adults) should be considered.

Digoxin-specific antibody fragments (Fab, Digibind) 38 mg binds 0.5 mg digoxin and then is excreted through the kidneys. The onset of action is within 30 minutes. Problems associated with Fab therapy are mainly from withdrawal of digoxin and worsening heart failure, hypokalemia, decrease in glucose (if the patient has low glycogen stores), and allergic reactions (very rare). Digitalis administered after Fab therapy is bound and may be inactivated for 5 to 7 days.

Absolute indications for Fab therapy include the following:

- Life-threatening malignant (hemodynamically unstable) dysrhythmias
- Ventricular dysrhythmias, unstable severe bradycardia, or second- or third-degree blocks unresponsive to atropine or rapid deterioration in clinical status
- Life-threatening digitoxin and oleander poisonings
- Relative indications for Fab therapy include the following:
- Ingestions greater than 4 mg in a child and 10 mg in an adult
- Serum potassium level greater than 5.0 mEq/L
- Serum digoxin level greater than 10 ng/mL in adults or greater than 5 ng/mL in children 6 hours after an acute ingestion
- Digitalis delirium and thrombocytopenia response

Digoxin-specific Fab fragments therapy can be administered as a bolus through a 22-μm filter if the case is a critical emergency. If the case is less urgent, then it can be administered over 30 minutes. An empiric dose is 10 vials in adults and 5 vials in a child for an unknown amount ingested in a symptomatic patient with history of a digoxin overdose.

To calculate the dose in the case of a known ingestion, the following equation is used:

$$\text{Amount (total mg)} \times (0.8) = \text{body burden}$$

If liquid capsules were taken or the substance was given intravenously the 80% bioavailability figure is not used. Instead, the body burden divided by 0.5 (0.5 mg digoxin is bound by 1 vial of 38 mg of Fab) equals the number of vials needed.

If the amount is unknown but the steady state serum concentration is known, the following equations are used:

For digoxin

$$\text{Digoxin ng/mL} \times (5.6 \text{ L/kg Vd}) \times (\text{wt kg}) = \text{mg body burden}$$

$$\text{Body burden} \div 1000 = \text{mg body burden}$$

$$\text{Body burden/0.5} = \text{number of vials needed}$$

For digitoxin

$$\text{Digitoxin ng/mL} \times (0.56 \text{ L/kg Vd}) \times (\text{wt kg}) = \text{mg body burden}$$

$$\text{Body burden} \div 1000 = \text{mg body burden}$$

$$\text{Body burden/0.5} = \text{number of vials needed}$$

Antidysrhythmic agents or a pacemaker should be used only if Fab therapy fails. For ventricular tachydysrhythmias, electrolyte disturbances should be corrected by the administration of lidocaine or phenytoin. For torsades de pointes, magnesium sulfate 20 mL 20% IV can be given slowly over 20 minutes (or 25 to 50 mg/kg in a child), titrated to control the dysrhythmia. Magnesium should be discontinued if hypotension, heart block, or decreased deep tendon reflexes are present. Magnesium is used with caution if the patient has renal impairment.

Unstable bradycardia and second-degree and third-degree atrioventricular block should be treated by Fab first. A pacemaker should be available if necessary. Isoproterenol should be avoided because it causes dysrhythmias. Cardioversion is used with caution, starting at a setting of 5 to 10 joules. The patient should be pretreated with lidocaine, if possible, because cardioversion may precipitate ventricular fibrillation or asystole.

Potassium disturbances are caused by a shift, not a change, in total body potassium. Hyperkalemia (>5.0 mEq/L) is treated with Fab only. Calcium must never be used, and insulin/glucose and sodium bicarbonate should not be used concomitantly with Fab because they may produce severe life-threatening hypokalemia. Sodium polystyrene sulfonate (Kayexalate) should not be used. Hypokalemia must be treated with caution because it may be cardioprotective. Treatment can be administered if the patient has ventricular dysrhythmias or a serum potassium level less than 3.0 mEq/L and atrioventricular block.

Extracorporeal procedures are ineffective. Hemodialysis is used for severe or refractory hyperkalemia.

One must never use antidysrhythmic types Ia (procainamide, quinidine, disopyramide [Norpace], amiodarone [Cordarone]), Ic (propafenone [Rythmol], flecainide [Tambocor]), II (β-blockers), or IV (calcium channel blockers). Class Ib drugs (lidocaine, phenytoin [Dilantin], mexiletine [Mexitil], and tocainide [Tonocard]) can be used.

Disposition

Consultation with a poison control center and a cardiologist experienced with digoxin-specific Fab fragments is warranted. All patients with significant dysrhythmias, symptoms, elevated serum digoxin concentration, or elevated serum potassium level should be admitted to the intensive care unit.

ETHANOL

Table 15 lists the features of alcohols and glycols.

Toxic Mechanism

Ethanol has CNS depressant and anesthetic effects. Ethanol stimulates the γ-aminobutyric acid (GABA) system. It promotes cutaneous vasodilation (contributes to hypothermia), stimulates secretion of gastric juice (gastritis), inhibits the secretion of the antidiuretic hormone, inhibits gluconeogenesis (hypoglycemia), and influences fat metabolism (lipidemia).

Toxic Dose

A dose of 1 mL/kg of absolute ethanol (100% ethanol, or 200 proof) gives a blood ethanol concentration of 100 mg/dL. A potentially fatal dose is 3 g/kg for children or 6 g/kg for adults. Children are more prone to developing hypoglycemia than adults.

Kinetics

Onset of action is 30 to 60 minutes after ingestion; peak action is 90 minutes on empty stomach. Volume distribution is 0.6 L/kg. The major route of elimination (>90%) is by hepatic oxidative metabolism. The first step is by the enzyme alcohol dehydrogenase, which converts ethanol to acetaldehyde. Alcohol dehydrogenase metabolizes ethanol at a constant rate of 12 to 20 mg/dL/h (12 to 15 mg/dL/h in nondrinkers, 15 to 30 mg/dL/h in social drinkers, 30 to 50 mg/dL/h in heavy drinkers, and 25 to 30 mg/dL/h in children). At very low blood ethanol concentration (<30 mg/dL), the metabolism is by first-order kinetics. In the second step, acetaldehyde is metabolized by acetaldehyde dehydrogenase to acetic acid, which is metabolized by the Krebs cycle to carbon dioxide and water. The enzyme steps are nicotinamide adenine dinucleotide–dependent, which interferes with gluconeogenesis. Less than 10% of ethanol is excreted unchanged by the kidneys. The relationship between blood ethanol concentration (BEC) and dose (amount ingested) can be calculated as follows:

$$\text{BEC (mg/dL)} = \text{amount ingested (mL)} \times$$
$$\% \text{ ethanol product} \times \text{SG (0.79)/Vd (0.6 L/kg)} \times$$
$$\text{body wt (kg)}$$

$$\text{Dose (amount ingested)} = \text{BEC (mg/dL)} \times \text{Vd (0.6)} \times$$
$$\text{body wt (kg)}/\% \text{ ethanol} \times \text{specific gravity (0.79)}$$

Manifestations

Table 16 lists the clinical signs of acute ethanol intoxication.

Chronic alcoholic patients tolerate higher blood ethanol concentration, and correlation with manifestations is not valid. Rapid interview for alcoholism is the CAGE questions:

- C—Have you felt the need to Cut down?
- A—Have others Annoyed you by criticism of your drinking?

TABLE 15 Summary of Alcohol and Glycol Features

	Methanol	Isopropanol	Ethanol	Ethylene glycol
Principal uses	Gas line antifreeze, Sterno, windshield de-icer	Solvent jewelry cleaner, rubbing alcohol	Beverage, solvent	Radiator antifreeze, windshield de-icer
Specific gravity	0.719	0.785	0.789	1.12
Fatal dose	1 mL/Kg 100%	3 mL/kg 100%	5 mL/kg 100%	1.4 mL/kg
Inebriation	±	2+	2+	1+
Metabolic change		Hyperglycemia	Hypoglycemia	Hypocalcemia
Metabolic acidosis	4+	0	1+	2+
Anion gap	4+	±	2+	4+
Ketosis	Ketobutyric	Acetone	Hydroxybutyric	None
Gastrointestinal tract	Pancreatitis	Hemorrhagic gastritis	Gastritis	
Osmolality*	0.337	0.176	0.228	0.190

*1 mL/dL of substances raises freezing point osmolality of serum. The validity of the correlation of osmolality with blood concentrations has been questioned.

Rakel and Bope: *Conn's Current Therapy 2006.*

18

TABLE 16 Clinical Signs in the Nontolerant Ethanol Drinker

Ethanol blood concentration (mg/dL)*	Manifestations
>25	Euphoria
>47	*Mild incoordination,* sensory and motor impairment
>50	Increased risk of motor vehicle accidents
>100	Ataxia (legal toxic level in many localities)
>150	*Moderate incoordination,* slow reaction time
>200	Drowsiness and confusion
>300	Severe incoordination, stupor, blurred vision
>500	*Flaccid coma,* respiratory failure, hypotension; may be fatal

*Ethanol concentrations sometimes reported in %.
Note: mg% is not equivalent to mg/dL because ethanol weighs less than water (specific gravity 0.79). A 1% ethanol concentration is 790 mg/dL and 0.1% is 79 mg/dL. There is great variation in individual behavior at different blood ethanol levels. Behavior is dependent on tolerance and other factors.

- G—Have you felt Guilty about your drinking?
- E—Have you ever had morning Eye-opening drink to steady your nerves or get rid of a hangover?

Two affirmative answers indicate probable alcoholism.

Laboratory Investigations

The blood ethanol concentration should be specifically requested and followed. Gas chromatography or a breath-analyzer test gives rapid reliable results if no belching or vomiting is present. Enzymatic methods do not differentiate between the alcohols. ABG, electrolytes, and glucose should be measured, the anion and osmolar gaps determined (measure by freezing point depression, not vapor pressure), and a check for ketosis made.

Management

The examiner should inquire about trauma and disulfiram use. The patient must be protected from aspiration and hypoxia. Vital functions must be established and maintained. The patient may require intubation and assisted ventilation.

Gastrointestinal decontamination plays no role in the management of ethanol intoxication.

If the patient is comatose, glucose should be administered intravenously, 1 mL/kg 50% glucose in adults and 2 mL/kg 25% glucose in children. Thiamine, 100 mg intravenously, is administered if the patient has a history of chronic alcoholism, malnutrition, or suspected eating disorders to prevent Wernicke-Korsakoff syndrome. Naloxone (Narcan) has produced a partial inconsistent response but is not recommended for known alcoholics.

General supportive care includes administration of fluids to correct hydration and hypotension and correction of electrolyte abnormalities and acid–base imbalance. Vasopressors and plasma expanders may be necessary to correct severe hypotension. Hypomagnesemia is frequent in chronic alcoholics. In case of hypomagnesemia, a loading dose of 2 g magnesium sulfate 10% is administered by intravenous solution over 5 minutes in the intensive care unit with blood pressure and cardiac monitoring and calcium chloride 10% on hand in case of overdose. This is followed with constant infusion of 6 g of 10% solution over 3 to 4 hours. Caution must be taken with the use of magnesium if renal failure is present.

Hypothermic patients should be warmed. See the section on disturbances caused by cold.

Hemodialysis can be used in severe cases when conventional therapy is ineffective (rarely needed).

Repeated or prolonged seizures should be treated with diazepam (Valium). The brief "rum fits" do not need long-term anticonvulsant therapy. Repeated seizures or focal neurologic findings may warrant skull radiographs, lumbar puncture, and CT scan of the head, depending on the clinical findings. Withdrawal is treated with hydration and large doses of chlordiazepoxide (Librium) 50 to 100 mg or diazepam (Valium) 2 to 10 mg intravenously; these doses may be repeated in 2 to 4 hours. Very large doses of benzodiazepines may be required for delirium tremens. Withdrawal can occur in presence of elevated blood ethanol concentration and can be fatal if left untreated.

Chest radiograph is warranted to determine whether aspiration pneumonia is present. Renal and liver function tests and bilirubin level measurement should be made.

Disposition

Clinical severity (e.g., intubation, assisted ventilation, aspiration pneumonia) should determine the level of hospital care needed. Young children with significant unintentional exposure to ethanol (calculated to reach a blood ethanol concentration of 50 mg/dL) should have blood ethanol concentration obtained and blood glucose levels monitored for hypoglycemia frequently for 4 hours after ingestion. Patients with acute ethanol intoxication seldom require admission unless a complication is present. However, intoxicated patients should not be discharged until they are fully functional (can walk, talk, and think independently), have suicide potential evaluated, have proper disposition environment, and have a sober escort.

ETHYLENE GLYCOL

Ethylene glycol is found in solvents, de-icers, radiator antifreeze (95%), and air-conditioning units. Ethylene glycol is a sweet-tasting, colorless, water-soluble liquid with a sweet aromatic fragrance.

Toxic Mechanism

Ethylene glycol is oxidized by alcohol dehydrogenase to glycolaldehyde, which is metabolized to glycolic acid and glyoxylic acid. Glyoxylic acid is metabolized to oxalic acid via a pyridoxine-dependent pathway to glycine and by thiamine and magnesium-dependent pathways to α-hydroxy-ketoadipic acid. The metabolites of ethylene glycol produce a profound metabolic acidosis, increased anion gap, hypocalcemia, and oxalate crystals, which deposit in tissues (particularly the kidney).

Toxic Dose

The ingestion of 0.1 mL/kg 100% ethylene glycol can result in a toxic serum ethylene glycol concentration of 20 mg/dL. Ingestion of 3.0 mL (less than 1 teaspoonful or swallow) of a 100% solution in a 10-kg child or 30 mL of 100% ethylene glycol in an adult produces a serum ethylene glycol concentration of 50 mg/dL, a concentration that requires hemodialysis. The fatal amount is 1.4 mL/kg of 100% solution.

Kinetics

Absorption is via dermal, inhalation, and ingestion routes. Ethylene glycol is rapidly absorbed from the gastrointestinal tract. Onset is usually in 30 minutes but may be delayed by co-ingestion of food and ethanol. The usual peak level is at 2 hours. Volume distribution is 0.65 to 0.8 L/kg.

For metabolism, see *Toxic Mechanism.*

The half-life of ethylene glycol without ethanol is 3 to 8 hours; with ethanol, it is 17 hours, and with hemodialysis it is 2.5 hours. Renal clearance is 3.2 mL/kg/minute. About 20% to 50% is excreted unchanged in the urine. The relationship between serum ethylene glycol concentration (SEGC) and dose (amount ingested) can be calculated as follows:

$$0.12 \text{ mL/kg of } 100\% = \text{SEGC } 10 \text{ mg/dL}$$

Manifestations

Phase I

The onset of manifestations is 30 minutes to several hours longer after ingestion with concomitant ethanol ingestion. The patient may be inebriated. Hypocalcemia, tetany, and calcium oxalate and hippuric acid crystals in urine can be seen within 4 to 8 hours but are not always present. Early, before metabolism of ethylene glycol, an osmolal gap may be present (see *Laboratory Investigations*). Later, the metabolites of ethylene glycol produce changes starting 4 to 12 hours following ingestion, including an anion gap, metabolic acidosis, coma, convulsions, cardiac disturbances, and pulmonary and cerebral edema. Because fluorescein is added to some antifreeze, the presence of fluorescence may be a clue to ethylene glycol exposure. However, it has been shown that fluorescent urine is not a reliable indicator of ethylene glycol ingestion and should not be used as a screen.

Phase II

After 12 to 36 hours, cardiopulmonary deterioration occurs, with pulmonary edema and congestive heart failure.

Phase III

Phase III occurs 36 to 72 hours after ingestion, with pulmonary edema and oliguric renal failure from oxalate crystal deposition and tubular necrosis predominating.

Phase IV

Neurologic sequelae may occur rarely, especially in patients who fail to receive early antidotal therapy. The onset ranges from 6 to 10 days after ingestion. Findings include facial diplegia, hearing loss, bilateral visual disturbances, elevated cerebrospinal fluid pressure with or without elevated protein levels and pleocytosis, vomiting, hyperreflexia, dysphagia, and ataxia.

Laboratory Investigations

Blood glucose and electrolytes should be monitored. Urinalysis should look for oxalate ("envelope") and monohydrate ("hemp seed") crystals. Urine fluorescence is not reliable as a screen. ABG, ethylene glycol, and ethanol levels, plasma osmolarity (using freezing point depression method), calcium, BUN, and creatinine should be measured. A serum ethylene glycol concentration of 20 mg/dL is toxic (ethylene glycol levels are very difficult to obtain). If possible, a glycolate level should be obtained. Cross-reactions with propylene glycol, a vehicle in many liquids and intravenous medications (phenytoin [Dilantin], diazepam [Valium]), other glycols, and triglycerides may produce spurious ethylene glycol levels. False-positive ethylene glycol values may occur with colorimetric or gas chromatography using an OV-17 column in the presence of propylene glycol.

The following equations can be used to calculate the osmolality, osmolal gap, and ethylene glycol level:

$$2(\text{Na+ mEq/L}) + (\text{Blood glucose mg/dL})/20 + (\text{BUN mg/dL})/3 = \text{Total calculated osmolality (mOsmL/L)}$$

$$\text{Osmolar Gap} = \text{measured osmolality (by freezing point depression method)} - \text{calculated osmolality}$$

A gap greater than 10 is abnormal. *Note:* if ethanol is involved, add ethanol level/4.6 to the calculated equation.

An increased osmolal gap is produced by the following common substances: acetone, dextran, dimethyl sulfoxide, diuretics, ethanol, ethyl ether, ethylene glycol, isopropanol, paraldehyde, mannitol, methanol, sorbitol, and trichloroethane. Table 10 gives the conversion factors for these substances.

Although a specific blood level of ethylene glycol in milligrams per deciliter can be estimated using the equation below, this is not considered to be a reliable method and should not take the place of obtaining a measured ethylene glycol blood concentration.

$$\text{osmolar gap} \times \text{conversion factor} = \text{serum concentration}$$

Caution: The accuracy of the ethylene glycol estimated decreases as the ethylene glycol levels decrease. The toxic metabolites are not osmotically active, and patients presenting late may show signs of severe toxicity without an elevated osmolar gap.

The anion gap can be calculated using the following equation:

$$Na - (Cl + HCO_3) = anion\ gap$$

The normal gap is 8 to 12. Potassium is not used because it is a small amount and may be hemolyzed. Table 8 lists factors that may account for an increased or a decreased anion gap.

Management

Vital functions should be established and maintained. The airway must be protected, and assisted ventilation can be used, if necessary. Gastrointestinal decontamination has a limited role. Only gastric aspiration can be used within 60 minutes after ingestion. Activated charcoal is not effective.

Baseline measurements of serum electrolytes and calcium, glucose, ABGs, ethanol, serum ethylene glycol concentration (may be difficult to obtain readily in some institutions), and methanol concentrations should be obtained. In the first few hours, the measured serum osmolality should be determined and compared to calculated osmolality (see osmolality equation, earlier). If seizures occur, one should measure serum calcium (preferably ionized calcium) and treat with intravenous diazepam. If the patient has hypocalcemic seizures, he or she should also be treated with 10 to 20 mL 10% calcium gluconate (0.2 to 0.3 mL/kg in children) slowly intravenously, with the dose repeated as needed. Metabolic acidosis should be corrected with intravenous sodium bicarbonate.

Ethanol therapy should be initiated immediately if fomepizole (Antizol) is unavailable (see next paragraph). Alcohol dehydrogenase has a greater affinity for ethanol than ethylene glycol. Therefore, ethanol blocks the metabolism of ethylene glycol. Ethanol therapy is called for if there is a history of ingestion of 0.1 mL/kg of 100% ethylene glycol, serum ethylene glycol concentration is greater than 20 mg/dL, there is an osmolar gap not accounted for by other alcohols or factors (e.g., hyperlipidemia), metabolic acidosis is present with an increased anion gap, or there are oxalate crystals in the urine. Ethanol should be administered intravenously (the oral route is less reliable) to produce a blood ethanol concentration of 100 to 150 mg/dL. The loading dose is 10 mL/kg of 10% ethanol intravenously, administered concomitantly with a maintenance dose of 10% ethanol of 1.0 mL/kg/h. This dose may need to be increased to 2 mL/kg/h in patients who are heavy drinkers. The blood ethanol concentration should be measured hourly and the infusion rate should be adjusted to maintain a blood ethanol concentration of 100 to 150 mg/dL.

Fomepizole (Antizol, 4-methylpyrazole) inhibits alcohol dehydrogenase more reliability than ethanol and it does not require constant monitoring of ethanol levels and adjustment of infusion rates. Fomepizole is available in 1 g/mL vials of 1.5 mL. The loading dose

is 15 mg/kg (0.015 mL/kg) IV; maintenance dose is 10 mg/kg (0.01 mL/kg) every 12 hours for four doses, then 15 mg/kg every 12 hours until the ethylene glycol levels are less than 20 mg/dL. The solution is prepared by being mixed with 100 mL of 0.9% saline or D_5W (5% dextrose in water). Fomepizole can be given to patients requiring hemodialysis but should be dosed as follows:

Dose at the beginning of hemodialysis:

- If <6 hours since last Antizol dose, do not administer dose
- If >6 hours since last dose, administer next scheduled dose

Dosing during hemodialysis:

- Dose every 4 hours

Dosing at the time hemodialysis is completed:

- If <1 hour between last dose and end of dialysis, do not administer dose at end of dialysis
- If 1 to 3 hours between last dose and end of dialysis, administer one half of next scheduled dose
- If >3 hours between last dose and end of dialysis, administer next scheduled dose

Maintenance dosing off hemodialysis:

- Give the next scheduled dose 12 hours from the last dose administered

Hemodialysis is indicated if the ingestion was potentially fatal; if the serum ethylene glycol concentration is greater than 50 mg/dL (some recommend at levels of >25 mg/dL); if severe acidosis or electrolyte abnormalities occur despite conventional therapy; or if congestive heart failure or renal failure is present. Hemodialysis reduces the ethylene glycol half-life from 17 hours on ethanol therapy to 3 hours. Therapy (fomepizole and hemodialysis) should be continued until the serum ethylene glycol concentration is less than 10 mg/dL, the glycolate level is nondetectable (not readily available), the acidosis has cleared, there are no mental disturbances, the creatinine level is normal, and the urinary output is adequate. This may require 2 to 5 days.

Adjunct therapy involving thiamine, 100 mg/d (in children, 50 mg), slowly over 5 minutes intravenously or intramuscularly and repeated every 6 hours and pyridoxine, 50 mg IV or IM every 6 hours, has been recommended until intoxication is resolved, but these agents have not been extensively studied. Folate, 50 mg IV (child 1 mg/kg), can be given every 4 hours for 6 doses.

Disposition

All patients who have ingested significant amounts of ethylene glycol (calculated level above 20 mg/dL), have a history of a toxic dose, or are symptomatic should be referred to the emergency department and admitted. If the serum ethylene glycol concentration cannot be obtained, the patient should be followed for 12 hours, with monitoring of the osmolal gap, acid–base parameters, and electrolytes to exclude development of metabolic acidosis with an anion gap. Transfer should be considered for fomepizole therapy or hemodialysis.

HYDROCARBONS

The lower the viscosity and surface tension of hydrocarbons or the greater the volatility, the greater the risk of aspiration. Volatile substance abuse has produced the "Sudden Sniffing's Death Syndrome," most likely caused by dysrhythmias.

Toxicologic Classification and Toxic Mechanism

All systemically absorbed hydrocarbons can lower the threshold of the myocardium to dysrhythmias produced by endogenous and exogenous catecholamines.

Aliphatic hydrocarbons are branched straight chain hydrocarbons. A few aspirated drops are poorly absorbed from the gastrointestinal tract and produce no systemic toxicity by this route. However, aspiration of very small amounts can produce chemical pneumonitis. Examples of aliphatic hydrocarbons are gasoline, kerosene, charcoal lighter fluid, mineral spirits (Stoddard's solvent), and petroleum naphtha. Mineral seal oil (signal oil), found in furniture polishes, is a low-viscosity and low-volatility oil with minimum absorption that never warrants gastric decontamination. It can produce severe pneumonia if aspirated.

Aromatic hydrocarbons are six carbon ring structures that are absorbed through the gastrointestinal tract. Systemic toxicity includes CNS depression and, in cases of chronic abuse, multiple organ effects such as leukemia (benzene) and renal toxicity (toluene). Examples are benzene, toluene, styrene, and xylene. The seriously toxic ingested dose is 20 to 50 mL in adults.

Halogenated hydrocarbons are aliphatic or aromatic hydrocarbons with one or more halogen substitutions (Cl, Br, Fl, or I). They are highly volatile and are abused as inhalants. They are well absorbed from the gastrointestinal tract, produce CNS depression, and have metabolites that can damage the liver and kidneys. Examples include methylene chloride (may be converted into carbon monoxide in the body), dichloroethylene (also causes a disulfiram [Antabuse] reaction known as "degreaser's flush" when associated with consumption of ethanol), and 1,1,1-trichloroethane (Glamorene Spot Remover, Scotchgard, typewriter correction fluid). An acute lethal oral dose is 0.5 to 5 mL/kg.

Dangerous additives to the hydrocarbons can be summed up with the mnemonic CHAMP: C, camphor (demothing agent); H, halogenated hydrocarbons; A, aromatic hydrocarbons; M, metals (heavy); and P, pesticides. Ingestion of these substances may warrant gastric emptying with a small-bore nasogastric tube.

Heavy hydrocarbons have high viscosity, low volatility, and minimal gastrointestinal absorption, so gastric decontamination is not necessary. Examples are asphalt (tar), machine oil, motor oil (lubricating oil, engine oil), home heating oil, and petroleum jelly (mineral oil).

Laboratory Investigations

The ECG, ABG, pulmonary function, serum electrolytes, and serial chest radiographs should be continuously monitored. Liver and renal function should be monitored in cases of inhalation of aromatic hydrocarbons.

Management

Asymptomatic patients who ingested small amounts of aliphatic petroleum distillates can be followed at home by telephone for development of signs of aspiration (cough, wheezing, tachypnea, and dyspnea) for 4 to 6 hours. Inhalation of any hydrocarbon vapors in a closed space can produce intoxication. The victim must be removed from the environment, have oxygen administered, and receive respiratory support.

Gastrointestinal decontamination is not advised in cases of hydrocarbon ingestion that usually do not cause systemic toxicity (aliphatic petroleum distillates, heavy hydrocarbons). In cases of ingestion of hydrocarbons that cause systemic toxicity in small amounts (aromatic hydrocarbons, halogenated hydrocarbons), the clinician should pass a small-bore nasogastric tube and aspirate if the ingestion was within 2 hours and if spontaneous vomiting has not occurred. Some toxicologists advocate ipecac-induced emesis under medical supervision instead of small-bore nasogastric gastric lavage; we do not.

Patients with altered mental status should have their airway protected because of concern about aspiration. The use of activated charcoal has been suggested, but there are no scientific data as to effectiveness and it may produce vomiting. Activated charcoal may, however, be useful in adsorbing toxic additives such as pesticides or co-ingestants.

The symptomatic patient who is coughing, gagging, choking, or wheezing on arrival has probably aspirated. The clinician should provide supportive respiratory care and supplemental oxygen, while monitoring pulse oximetry, ABG, chest radiograph, and ECG. The patient should be admitted to the intensive care unit. A chest radiograph for aspiration may be positive as early as 30 minutes after ingestion, and almost all are positive within 6 hours. Negative chest radiographs within 4 hours do not rule out aspiration.

Bronchospasm is treated with a nebulized β-adrenergic agonist and intravenous aminophylline if necessary. Epinephrine should be avoided because of susceptibility to dysrhythmias. Cyanosis in the presence of a normal arterial PaO_2 may be a result of methemoglobinemia that requires therapy with methylene blue. Corticosteroids and prophylactic antimicrobial agents have not been shown to be beneficial. (Fever or leukocytosis may be produced by the chemical pneumonitis itself.)

Most infiltrations resolve spontaneously in 1 week; lipoid pneumonia may last up to 6 weeks. It is not necessary to surgically treat pneumatoceles that develop because they usually resolve. Dysrhythmias may require α- and β-adrenergic antagonists or cardioversion.

There is no role for enhanced elimination procedures.

Methylene chloride is metabolized over several hours to carbon monoxide. See treatment of carbon monoxide poisoning. Halogenated hydrocarbons are hepatorenal toxins; therefore, hepatorenal function should be monitored. *N*-acetylcysteine therapy may be useful if there is evidence of hepatic damage.

Extracorporal membrane oxygenation (ECMO) has been used successfully for a few patients with life threatening respiratory failure. Surfactant used for hydrocarbon aspiration was found to be detrimental.

Disposition

Asymptomatic patients with small ingestions of petroleum distillates can be managed at home. Symptomatic patients with abnormal chest radiographic, oxygen saturation, or ABG findings should be admitted. Patients who become asymptomatic and have normal oxygenation and a normal repeat radiograph can be discharged.

IRON

There are more than 100 iron over-the-counter preparations for supplementation and treatment of iron deficiency anemia.

Toxic Mechanism

Toxicity depends on the amount of elemental iron available in various salts (gluconate 12%, sulfate 20%, fumarate 33%, lactate 19%, chloride 21% of elemental iron), not the amount of the salt. Locally, iron is corrosive and may cause fluid loss, hypovolemic shock, and perforation. Excessive free unbound iron in the blood is directly toxic to the vasculature and leads to the release of vasoactive substances, which produces vasodilation. In cases of overdose, iron deposits injure mitochondria in the liver, the kidneys, and the myocardium. The exact mechanism of cellular damage is not clear but is thought to be related to free radical formation.

Toxic Dose

The therapeutic dose is 6 mg/kg/d of elemental iron. An elemental iron dose of 20 to 40 mg/kg may produce mild self-limited gastrointestinal symptoms, 40 to 60 mg/kg produces moderate toxicity, more than 60 mg/kg produces severe toxicity and is potentially lethal, and more than 180 mg/kg is usually fatal without treatment. Children's chewable vitamins with iron have between 12 and 18 mg of elemental iron per tablet or 0.6 mL of liquid drops. These preparations rarely produce toxicity unless very large quantities are ingested and have never caused death.

Kinetics

Absorption occurs chiefly in the upper small intestine. Ferrous (+2) iron is absorbed into the mucosal cells, where it is oxidized to the ferric (+3) state and bound to ferritin. Iron is slowly released from ferritin into the plasma, where it binds to transferrin and is transported to specific tissues for production of hemoglobin (70%), myoglobin (5%), and cytochrome. About 25% of iron is stored in the liver and spleen. In cases of overdose, larger amounts of iron are absorbed because of direct mucosal corrosion. There is no mechanism for the elimination of iron (elimination is 1 to 2 mg/d) except through bile, sweat, and blood loss.

Manifestations

Serious toxicity is unlikely if the patient remains asymptomatic for 6 hours and has a negative abdominal radiograph. Iron intoxication can produce five phases of toxicity. The phases may not be distinct from one another.

Phase I

Gastrointestinal mucosal injury occurs 30 minutes to 12 hours postingestion. Vomiting starts within 30 minutes to 1 hour of ingestion and is persistent; hematemesis and bloody diarrhea may occur; abdominal cramps, fever, hyperglycemia, and leukocytosis may occur. Enteric-coated tablets may pass through the stomach without causing symptoms. Acidosis and shock can occur within 6 to 12 hours.

Phase II

A latent period of apparent improvement occurs over 8 to 12 hours postingestion.

Phase III

Systemic toxicity phase occurs 12 to 48 hours postingestion with cardiovascular collapse and severe metabolic acidosis.

Phase IV

Two to 4 days postingestion, hepatic injury associated with jaundice, elevated liver enzymes, and prolonged prothrombin time occur. Kidney injury with proteinuria and hematuria occur. Pulmonary edema, disseminated intravascular coagulation, and *Yersinia enterocolitica* sepsis can occur.

Phase V

Four to 8 weeks postingestion, pyloric outlet or intestinal stricture may cause obstruction or anemia secondary to blood loss.

Laboratory Investigations

Iron poisoning produces anion gap metabolic acidosis. Monitoring should include complete blood cell counts, blood glucose level, serum iron, stools and vomitus for occult blood, electrolytes, acid–base balance, urinalysis and urinary output, liver function tests, and BUN and creatinine levels. Blood type and match should be obtained.

Serum iron measurements taken at the proper time correlate with the clinical findings. The lavender top Vacutainer tube contains EDTA, which falsely lowers serum iron. One must obtain the serum iron measurement before administering deferoxamine. Serum iron levels of less than 350 μg/dL at 2 to 6 hours predict an asymptomatic course; levels of 350 to 500 μg/dL are usually associated with mild gastrointestinal symptoms; those greater than 500 μg/dL have a 20% risk of shock and serious iron toxicity. A follow-up serum iron measurement after 6 hours may not be elevated even in cases of severe poisoning, but a serum iron measurement taken at 8 to 12 hours is useful to exclude delayed absorption from a bezoar or sustained-release preparation. The total iron-binding capacity is not necessary.

Adult iron tablet preparations are radiopaque before they dissolve by 4 hours postingestion. A "negative" abdominal radiograph more than 4 hours postingestion does not exclude iron poisoning.

Patients who develop high fevers and signs of sepsis following iron overdose should have blood and stool cultures checked for *Yersinia enterocolitica*.

Management

Gastrointestinal decontamination should involve immediate induction of emesis in cases of ingestions of elemental iron of greater than 40 mg/kg if vomiting has not already occurred. Activated charcoal is ineffective. An abdominal radiograph should be obtained after emesis to determine the success of gastric emptying. Children's chewable vitamins and liquid iron preparations are not radiopaque. If radiopaque iron is still present, whole-bowel irrigation with polyethylene glycol solution should be considered. In extreme cases, removal by endoscopy or surgery may be necessary because coalesced iron tablets produce hemorrhagic infarction in the bowel and perforation peritonitis.

Deferoxamine (Desferal) in a dose of about 100 mg binds 8.5 to 9.35 mg of free iron in the serum. The deferoxamine infusion should not exceed 15 mg/kg/h or 6 g daily, but faster rates (up to 45 mg/kg) and larger daily amounts have been administered and tolerated in extreme cases of iron poisoning (>1000 mg/dL). The deferoxamine-iron complex is hemodialyzable if renal failure develops.

Indications for chelation therapy are any of the following:

- Very large, symptomatic ingestions
- Serious clinical intoxication (severe vomiting and diarrhea [often bloody], severe abdominal pain, metabolic acidosis, hypotension, or shock)
- Symptoms that persist or progress to more serious toxicity
- Serum iron level greater than 500 mg/dL

Chelation should be performed as early as possible within 12 to 18 hours to be effective. One should start the infusion slowly and gradually increase to avoid hypotension.

Adult respiratory distress syndrome has developed in patients with high doses of deferoxamine for several days; infusions longer than 24 hours should be avoided.

The endpoint of treatment is when the patient is asymptomatic and the urine clears if it was originally a positive "vin rosé" color.

For supportive therapy, intravenous bicarbonate may be needed to correct the metabolic acidosis. Hypotension and shock treatment may require volume expansion, vasopressors, and blood transfusions. The physician should attempt to keep the urinary output at greater than 2 mL/kg/h. Coagulation abnormalities and overt bleeding require blood products or vitamin K. Pregnant patients are treated in a fashion similar to any other patient with iron poisoning.

Hemodialysis and hemoperfusion are ineffective. Exchange transfusion has been used in single cases of massive poisonings in children.

Disposition

The asymptomatic or minimally symptomatic patient should be observed for persistence and progression of symptoms or development of toxicity signs (gastrointestinal bleeding, acidosis, shock, altered mental state). Patients with mild self-limited gastrointestinal symptoms who become asymptomatic or have no signs of toxicity for 6 hours are unlikely to have a serious intoxication and can be discharged after psychiatric clearance, if needed. Patients with moderate or severe toxicity should be admitted to the intensive care unit.

ISONIAZID

Isoniazid is a hydrazide derivative of vitamin B_3 (nicotinamide) and is used as an antituberculosis drug.

Toxic Mechanism

Isoniazid produces pyridoxine deficiency by increasing the excretion of pyridoxine (vitamin B_6) and by inhibiting pyridoxal 5-phosphate (the active form of pyridoxine) from acting with L-glutamic acid decarboxylase to form γ-aminobutyric acid (GABA), the major CNS neurotransmitter inhibitor, resulting in seizures. Isoniazid also blocks the conversion of lactate to pyruvate, resulting in profound and prolonged lactic acidosis.

Toxic Dose

The therapeutic dose is 5 to 10 mg/kg (maximum 300 mg) daily. A single acute dose of 15 mg/kg lowers the seizure threshold; 35 to 40 mg/kg produces spontaneous convulsions; more than 80 mg/kg produces severe toxicity. A fatal dose in adults is 4.5 to 15 g. The malnourished patients, those with a previous seizure disorder, alcoholic patients, and slow acetylators are more susceptible to isoniazid toxicity. In cases of chronic intoxication, 10 mg/kg/d produces hepatitis in 10% to 20% of patients but less than 2% at doses of 3 to 5 mg/kg/d.

Kinetics

Absorption from intestine occurs in 30 to 60 minutes, and onset is in 30 to 120 minutes, with peak levels of 5 to 8 µg/mL within 1 to 2 hours. Volume distribution is 0.6 L/kg, with minimal protein binding.

Elimination is by liver acetylation to a hepatotoxic metabolite, acetyl-isoniazid, which is then hydrolyzed to isonicotinic acid. In slow acetylators, isoniazid has a half-life of 140 to 460 minutes (mean 5 hours), and 10% to 15% is eliminated unchanged in the urine. Most (45% to 75%) whites and 50% of African blacks are slow acetylators, and, with chronic use (without pyridoxine supplements), they may develop peripheral neuropathy. In fast acetylators, isoniazid has a half-life of 35 to 110 minutes (mean 80 minutes), and 25% to 30% is excreted unchanged in the urine. About 90% of Asians and patients with diabetes mellitus are fast acetylators and may develop hepatitis on chronic use.

In patients with overdose and hepatic disease, the serum half-life may increase. Isoniazid inhibits the metabolism of phenytoin (Dilantin), diazepam, phenobarbital, carbamazepine (Tegretol), and prednisone. These drugs also interfere with the metabolism of isoniazid. Ethanol may decrease the half-life of isoniazid but increase its toxicity.

Manifestations

Within 30 to 60 minutes, nausea, vomiting, slurred speech, dizziness, visual disturbances, and ataxia are present. Within 30 to 120 minutes, the major clinical triad of severe overdose includes refractory convulsions (90% of overdose patients have one or more seizures), coma, and resistant severe lactic acidosis (secondary to convulsions), often with a plasma pH of 6.8.

Laboratory Investigations

Isoniazid produces anion gap metabolic acidosis. Therapeutic levels are 5 to 8 µg/mL and acute toxic levels are greater than 20 µg/mL. These levels are not readily available to assist in making decisions in acute overdose situations. One should monitor the blood glucose (often hyperglycemia), electrolytes (often hyperkalemia), bicarbonate, ABGs, liver function tests (elevations occur with chronic exposure), BUN, and creatinine.

Management

Seizures must be controlled. Pyridoxine and diazepam should be administered concomitantly through different IV sites. Pyridoxine (vitamin B_6) is given in a dose of 1 g for each gram of isoniazid ingested. If the dose ingested is unknown, at least 5 g of pyridoxine should be given intravenously. Pyridoxine is administered in 50 mL D_5W or 0.9% saline over 5 minutes intravenously. It must not be administered in the same bottle as sodium bicarbonate. Intravenous pyridoxine is repeated every 5 to 20 minutes until the seizures are controlled. Total doses of pyridoxine up to 52 g have been safely administered; however, patients given 132 and 183 g of pyridoxine have developed a persistent crippling sensory neuropathy.

Diazepam is administered concomitantly with pyridoxine but at a different site. They work synergistically. Diazepam should be administered intravenously slowly, 0.3 mg/kg at a rate of 1 mg/min in children or 10 mg at a rate of 5 mg/min in adults. After the seizures are controlled, the remainder of the pyridoxine is administered (1 g/1 g isoniazid) or a total dose of 5 g.

Phenobarbital or phenytoin is ineffective and should not be used.

In asymptomatic patients or patients without seizures, pyridoxine has been advised by some toxicologists prophylactically in gram-for-gram doses in cases of large overdoses (<80 mg/kg per dose) of isoniazid, although there are no studies to support this recommendation. In comatose patients, pyridoxine administration may result in the patient's rapid regaining of consciousness. Correction of acidosis may occur spontaneously with pyridoxine administration and correction of the seizures. Sodium bicarbonate should be administered if acidosis persists.

Hemodialysis is rarely needed because of antidotal therapy and the short half-life of isoniazid, but it may be used as an adjunct for cases of uncontrollable acidosis and seizures. Hemoperfusion has not been adequately evaluated. Diuresis is ineffective.

Disposition

Asymptomatic or mildly symptomatic patients who become asymptomatic can be observed in the emergency department for 4 to 6 hours. Larger amounts of isoniazid may warrant pyridoxine administration and longer periods of observation. Intentional ingestions necessitate psychiatric evaluation before the patient is discharged. Patients with convulsions or coma should be admitted to the intensive care unit.

ISOPROPANOL (ISOPROPYL ALCOHOL)

Isopropanol can be found in rubbing alcohol, solvents, and lacquer thinner. Coma has occurred in children sponged for fever with isopropanol. See Table 10 for ethanol features of alcohols and glycols.

Toxic Mechanism

Isopropanol is a gastric irritant. It is metabolized to acetone, a CNS and myocardial depressant. It inhibits gluconeogenesis. Normal propyl alcohol is related to isopropyl alcohol but is more toxic.

Toxic Dose

A toxic dose of 0.5 to 1 mg/kg of 70% isopropanol (1 mL/kg of 70%) produces a blood isopropanol plasma concentration of 70 mg/dL. The CNS depressant potency is twice that of ethanol.

Kinetics

Onset of action is within 30 to 60 minutes, and peak is 1 hour postingestion. Volume distribution is 0.6 kg/L. Isopropyl alcohol metabolizes to acetone. Its excretion is renal.

Note: The serum isopropyl concentration and amount ingested can be estimated using the same equation as is used in ethanol kinetics and substituting the specific gravity of 0.785 for isopropyl alcohol.

Manifestations

Ethanol-like inebriation occurs, with an acetone odor to the breath, gastritis, occasionally with hematemesis, acetonuria, and acetonemia without systemic acidosis.

Depression of the CNS occurs: lethargy at blood isopropyl alcohol levels of 50 to 100 mg/dL, coma at levels of 150 to 200 mg/dL, potentially death in adults at levels greater than 240 mg/dL.

Hypoglycemia and seizures may occur.

Laboratory Investigation

Monitoring of blood isopropyl alcohol levels (not readily available in all institutions), acetone, glucose, and ABG should be maintained. The osmolal gap increases 1 mOsm per 5.9 mg/dL of isopropyl alcohol and 1 mOsm per 5.5 mg/dL of acetone. The absence of excess acetone in the blood (normal is 0.3 to 2 mg/dL) within 30 to 60 minutes or excess acetone in the urine within 3 hours excludes the possibility of significant isopropanol exposure.

Management

The airway must be protected with intubation, and assisted ventilation administered if necessary. If the patient is hypoglycemic, glucose should be administered. Supportive treatment is similar to that for ethanol ingestions.

Gastrointestinal decontamination has no role in the treatment of isopropanol ingestion. Hemodialysis is warranted in cases of life-threatening overdose but is rarely needed. A nephrologist should be consulted if the blood isopropanol plasma concentration is greater than 250 mg/dL.

Disposition

Symptomatic patients with concentrations greater than 100 mg/dL require at least 24 hours of close observation for resolution and should be admitted. If the patient is hypoglycemic, hypotensive, or comatose, he or she should be admitted to the intensive care unit.

LEAD

Acute lead intoxication is rare and usually occurs by inhalation of lead, resulting in severe intoxication and

often death. Lead fumes can be produced by burning of lead batteries or use of a heat gun to remove lead paint. Acute lead intoxication also occurs from exposure to high concentrations of organic lead (e.g., tetraethyl lead).

Chronic lead poisoning occurs most often in children 6 months to 6 years of age who are exposed in their environment and in adults in certain occupations (Table 17). In the United States, the prevalence in children aged 1 to 5 years with a venous blood lead greater than 10 µg/dL decreased from 88.2% in a 1976-1980 survey to 8.9% in a 1988-1991 survey as a consequence of measures to reduce lead in the environment, particularly leaded gasoline. However, an estimated 1.7 million children between 1 and 5 years of age and more than 1 million workers in over 100 different occupations still have blood lead levels greater than 10 µg/dL.

Toxic Dose

In cases of chronic lead poisoning, a daily intake of more than 5 µg/kg/d in children or more than 150 µg/d in adults can give a positive lead balance. In 1991, the Centers for Disease Control and Prevention (CDC) recommended routine screening for all children younger than 6 years of age. In children a venous blood level greater than 10 µg/dL was determined to be a threshold of concern. The average venous blood level in the United States is 4 µg/dL. In cases of occupational exposure (see Table 17), a venous blood level greater than 40 µg/dL is indicative of increased lead absorption in adults.

Toxic Mechanism

Lead affects the sulfhydryl enzyme systems, the immature CNS, the enzymes of heme synthesis, vitamin D conversion, the kidneys, the bones, and growth. Lead alters the tertiary structure of cell proteins by denaturing them and causing cell death. Risk factors are mouthing behavior of infants and children and excessive oral behavior (pica), living in the inner city, a poorly maintained home, and poor nutrition (e.g., low calcium and iron).

TABLE 17 Occupations Associated with Lead Exposure

Lead production or smelting	Demolition of ships and bridges
Production of illicit whiskey	Battery manufacturing
Brass, copper, and lead foundries	Machining/grinding lead alloys
Radiator repair	Welding of old painted metals
Scrap handling	
Sanding of old paint	Thermal paint stripping of old buildings
Lead soldering	
Cable stripping	Ceramic glaze/pottery mixing
Worker or janitor at a firing range	

Modified from Rempel D: The lead-exposed worker. JAMA 262:533, 1989.

18

TABLE 18 CDC Questionnaire: Priority Groups for Lead Screening

1. Children age 6–72 months (was 12–36 months) who live in or are frequent visitors to older, deteriorated housing built before 1960.
2. Children age 6–72 months who live in housing built prior to 1960 with recent, ongoing, or planned renovation or remodeling.
3. Children age 6–72 months who are siblings, housemates, or playmates of children with known lead poisoning.
4. Children age 6–72 months whose parents or other household members participate in a lead-related industry or hobby.
5. Children age 6–72 months who live near active lead smelters, battery recycling plants, or other industries likely to result in atmospheric lead release.

TABLE 19 Sources of Lead

Product	Lead content (%) by dry weight
Paint	0.06
Solder	0.6
Plastic additives	2.0
Priming inks	2.0
Plumbing fixtures	2.0
Pesticides	0.1
Stained glass came	0.1
Wine bottle foils	0.1
Construction material	0.1
Fertilizers	0.1
Glazes, enamels	0.06
Toys/recreational games	0.1
Curtain weights	0.1
Fishing weights	0.1

The CDC questionnaire given in Table 18 is recommended at every pediatric visit. If any answers to the CDC questionnaire are "positive," a blood screening test for lead should be administered. To be more accurate, however, identifying lead exposure studies have suggested that the questionnaire will have to be modified for each individual community because it has had poor sensitivity (40%) and specificity (60%) as it stands.

Table 19 lists sources of lead. The number one source is deteriorating lead-based paint, which forms leaded dust. Lead concentrations in indoor paint were not reduced to safer (0.06%) levels until 1978. Lead can also be produced by improper interior or exterior home renovation (scraping or demolition). It is found in pre-1960 built homes. The use of leaded gasoline (limited in 1973) resulted in residue from leaded motor vehicle emissions. Lead persists in the soil near major highways and in deteriorating homes and buildings. Vegetables grown in contaminated soil may contain lead.

Oil refineries and lead-processing smelters produce lead residue. Food cans produced in Mexico contain lead

solder (95% do not in United States). Lead water pipes (until 1950) and lead solder (until 1986) deliver lead-containing drinking water (calcium deposits, however, may offer some protection). Water at a consumer's tap should contain less than 15 parts per billion (ppb) of lead (Table 20).

For occupational exposure, see Table 17. The Occupational Safety and Health Administration (OSHA) standards require employers to provide showering and clothes changing facilities for personnel working with lead; however, businesses with fewer than 25 employees are exempt from the regulation. The OSHA lead standard of 1978 set a limit of 60 µg/dL for occupational exposure to lead. At a blood lead level of 60 µg/dL, a worker should be removed from lead exposure and not allowed back until his or her lead level is below 40 µg/dL. Many authorities believe that this level should be lower. The lead residue on the clothes of the workers may represent a hazard to the family. Other occupations that are potential sources of lead exposure include plumbers, pipe fitters, lead miners,

TABLE 20 Agency Regulations and Recommendations Concerning Lead Content

Agency	Specimen	Level	Comments
CDC	Blood (child)	10 µg/dL	Investigate community
OSHA	Blood (adult)	60 µg/dL	Medical removal from work
OSHA	Air	50 µg/m³	PEL*
	Air	0.75 µg/m³	Tetraethyl or tetramethyl
ACGIH	Air	150 µg/m³	TWA†
EPA	Air	1.5 µg/m³	Three-month average
EPA	Water	15 µg/L (ppb)	5 ppb circulating
EPA	Food	100 µg/d	Advisory
FDA	Wine	300 ppm	Plan to reduce to 200 ppm
EPA	Soil/dust	50 ppm	
CPSC	Paint	600 ppm (0.06%) by dry weight	

Abbreviatons: ACGIH = American Conference of Governmental Industrial Hygienists; CDC = Centers for Disease Control and Prevention; CPSC = Consumer Product Safety Commission; EPA = Environmental Protection Agency; FDA = Food and Drug Administration; OSHA = Occupational Safety and Health Administration.
*PEL = permissible exposure limit (highest level over an 8-hour workday).
†TWA = time-weighted average (air concentration for 8-hour workday and 40 hour workweek).

Rakel and Bope: *Conn's Current Therapy 2006.*

auto repairers, shipbuilders, printers, steel welders and cutters, construction workers, and rubber product manufacturers.

Leaded pots to make molds for "kusmusha" tea represent lead exposure. Imported pottery lined with ceramic glaze can leach large amounts of lead into acids (e.g., citrus fruit juices).

Hobbies associated with lead exposure are listed in Box 1. Some "traditional" folk remedies or cosmetics that contain lead include the following:

- "Azarcon por empacho" ("Maria Louisa" 90 to 95% lead trioxide): a bright orange powder used in Hispanic culture, especially Mexican, for digestive problems and diarrhea.
- "Greta" (4% to 90% lead): a yellow powder "por empacho" ("empacho" refers to a variety of gastrointestinal symptoms), used in Hispanic cultures, especially Mexican.
- "Pay-loo-ah": an orange-red powder used for rash and fever in Southeast Asian cultures, especially among Northern Laos Hmong immigrants.
- "Alkohl" (Al-kohl, kohl, suma 5% to 92% lead): a black powder used in Middle Eastern, African, and Asian cultures as a cosmetic and an umbilical stump astringent.
- "Farouk": an orange granular powder with lead used in Saudi Arabian culture.
- "Bint Al Zahab": used to treat colic in Saudi Arabian culture.
- "Surma" (23% to 26% lead): a black powder used in India as a cosmetic and to improve eyesight.
- "Bali goli": a round black bean that is dissolved in "grippe water," used by Asian and Indian cultures to aid digestion.

Cases of substance abuse involving lead poisoning have been reported, in which the patient sniffs leaded gasoline or uses improperly synthesized amphetamines.

Kinetics

Absorption of lead is 10% to 15% of the ingested dose in adults; in children, up to 40% is absorbed, especially in cases of iron deficiency anemia. With inhalation of fumes, absorption is rapid and complete. Volume distribution in blood (0.9% of total body burden) is 95% in red blood cells. Lead passes through the placenta to the fetus and is present in breast milk.

Organic lead is metabolized in the liver to inorganic lead. Its half-life is 35 to 40 days in blood; in soft tissue, the half-life is 45 days and in bone (99% of the lead), the half-life is 28 years. The major elimination route is the stool, 80% to 90%, and then renal 10% (80 g/d) and hair, nails, sweat, and saliva. Nine percent of organic lead is excreted in the urine per day.

Manifestations

Adverse health effects are given in Table 21 and include the following.

Hematologic

Lead inhibits γ-aminolevulinic acid dehydratase (early in the synthesis of heme) and ferrochelatase (transfers iron to ferritin for incorporation of iron into protoporphyrin to produce heme). Anemia is a late finding. Decreased heme synthesis starts at >40 µg/dL. Basophilic stippling occurs in 20% of severe lead poisoning.

Neurologic

Segmental demyelination and peripheral neuropathy, usually of the motor type (wrist and ankle drop), occurs in workers. A venous blood level of lead greater than 70 µg/dL (usually >100 µg/dL), produces encephalopathy in children (symptom mnemonic "PAINT": P, persistent forceful vomiting and papilledema; A, ataxia; I, intermittent stupor and lucidity; N, neurologic coma and refractory convulsions; T, tired and lethargic). Decreased cognitive abilities have been reported with a venous blood level of lead greater than 10 µg/dL, including behavioral problems, decreased attention span, and learning disabilities. IQ scores may begin to decrease at 15 µg/dL. Encephalopathy is rare in adults.

Renal

Nephropathy as a result of damaged capillaries and glomerulus can occur at a venous blood level of lead greater than 80 µg/dL, but recent studies show renal damage and hypertension with low venous blood levels. A direct correlation between hypertension and venous blood level over 30 µg/dL has been reported. Lead reduces excretion of uric acid, and high-level exposure may be associated with hyperuricemia and "saturnine gout," Fanconi's syndrome (aminoaciduria and renal tubular acidosis), and tubular fibrosis.

Reproductive

Spontaneous abortion, transient delay in the child's development (catch up at age 5 to 6 years), decreased sperm count, and abnormal sperm morphology can occur with lead exposure. Lead crosses the placenta and

BOX 1	Hobbies Associated with Lead Exposure
Casting of ammunition	Print making and other fine arts (when lead white, flake white, chrome yellow pigments are involved)
Collecting antique pewter	
Collecting/painting lead toys (e.g., soldiers and figures)	
Ceramics or glazed pottery	Liquor distillation
Refinishing furniture	Hunting and target shooting
Making fishing weights	Painting
Home renovation	Car and boat repair
Jewelry making, lead solder	Burning/engraving lead-painted wood
Glass blowing, lead glass	Making stained leaded glass
Bronze casting	Copper enameling

TABLE 21 Summary of Lead-Induced Health Effects in Adults and Children

Blood lead level (μg/dL)	Age group	Health effect
>100	Adult	Encephalopathic signs and symptoms
>80	Adult	Anemia
	Child	Encephalopathy
		Chronic nephropathy (e.g., aminoaciduria)
>70	Adult	Clinically evident peripheral neuropathy
	Child	Colic and other gastrointestinal symptoms
>60	Adult	Female reproductive effects
		CNS disturbance symptoms (i.e., sleep disturbances, mood changes, memory and concentration problems, headaches)
>50	Adult	Decreased hemoglobin production
		Decreased performance on neurobehavioral tests
	Adult	Altered testicular function
		Gastrointestinal symptoms (i.e., abdominal pain, constipation, diarrhea, nausea, anorexia)
	Child	Peripheral neuropathy*
>40	Adult	Decreased peripheral nerve conduction
		Hypertension, age 40–59 years
		Chronic neuropathy*
>25	Adult	Elevated erythrocyte protoporphyrin in males
15-25	Adult	Elevated erythrocyte protoporphyrin in females
>10	Child	Decreased intelligence and growth
		Impaired learning
		Reduced birth weight*
		Impaired mental ability
	Fetus	Preterm delivery

*Controversial.
From Anonymous: Implementation of the Lead Contamination Control Act of 1988. MMWR Morb Mortal Wkly Rep 41:288, 1992.

fetal blood levels reach 75% to 100% of maternal blood levels. Lead is teratogenic.

Metabolic

Decreased cytochrome P450 activity alters the metabolism of medication and endogenously produced substances. Decreased activation of cortisol and decreased growth is caused by interference in vitamin conversion (25-hydroxyvitamin D to 1,25 hydroxyvitamin D) at venous blood levels of 20 to 30 μg/dL.

Other Manifestations

Abnormalities of thyroid, cardiac, and hepatic function occur in adults. Abdominal colic is seen in children at doses greater than 50 μg/dL. "Lead gum lines" at the dental border of the gingiva can occur in cases of chronic lead poisoning.

Laboratory Investigations

Serial venous blood lead measurements are taken on days 3 and 5 during treatment and 7 days after chelation therapy, then every 1 to 2 weeks for 8 weeks, and then every month for 6 months. Intravenous infusion should be stopped at least 1 hour before blood lead levels are measured. Table 22 gives a classification of blood lead concentrations in children.

One should evaluate CBC, serum ferritin, erythrocyte protoporphyrin (>35 μg/dL indicates lead poisoning as well as iron deficiency and other causes), electrolytes, serum calcium and phosphorus, urinalysis, BUN, and creatinine. Abdominal and long bone radiographs may be useful in certain circumstances to identify radiopaque material in bowel and "lead lines" in proximal tibia (which occur after prolonged exposure in association with venous blood lead levels greater than 50 μg/dL).

Neuropsychological tests are difficult to perform in young children but should be considered at the end of treatment, especially to determine auditory dysfunction.

TABLE 22 Classification of Blood Lead Concentrations in Children

Blood lead (μg/dL)	Recommended interventions
<9	None
10-14	Community intervention
	Repeat blood lead in 3 months
15-19	Individual case management
	Environmental counseling
	Nutritional counseling
	Repeat blood lead in 3 months
20-44	Medical referral
	Environmental inspection/abatement
	Nutritional counseling
	Repeat blood lead in 3 months
45-69	Environmental inspection/abatement
	Nutritional counseling
	Pharmacologic therapy
	DMSA succimer oral or CaNa$_2$EDTA parenteral
	Repeat every 2 weeks for 6-8 weeks, then monthly for 4-6 months
>70	Hospitalization in intensive care unit
	Environmental inspection/abatement
	Pharmacologic therapy
	Dimercaprol (BAL in oil) IM initial alone
	Dimercaprol IM and CaNa$_2$EDTA together
	Repeat every week

Abbreviations: BAL = British anti-Lewisite; CaNa$_2$EDTA = Edetate calcium disodium; DMS = dimercaptosuccinic acid; IM = intramuscular.

Management

The basis of treatment is removal of the source of lead. Cases of poisoning in children should be reported to local health department and cases of occupational poisoning should be reported to OSHA. The source must be identified and abated, and dust controlled by wet mopping. Cold water should be let to run for 2 minutes before being used for drinking. Planting shrubbery (not vegetables) in contaminated soil will keep children away.

Supportive care should be instituted, including measures to deal with refractory seizures (continued antidotal therapy, diazepam, and possibly neuromuscular blockers), with the hepatic and renal failure, and intravascular hemolysis in severe cases. Seizures are treated with diazepam followed by neuromuscular blockers if needed.

Lead does not bind to activated charcoal. One must not delay chelation therapy for complete gastrointestinal decontamination in severe cases. Whole-bowel irrigation has been used prior to treatment. Some authorities recommend abdominal radiographs followed by gastrointestinal decontamination if necessary before switching to oral therapy. Chelation therapy can be used for patients in whom venous blood level of lead is greater than 45 µg/dL in children and greater than 80 µg/dL in adults or in adults with lower levels who are symptomatic or who have a "positive" lead mobilization test result (not routinely performed at most centers) (Table 23).

Succimer (dimercaptosuccinic acid, DMSA, Chemet), a derivative of British anti-Lewisite (BAL), is an oral agent for chelation in children with a venous blood level of greater than 45 µg/dL. The recommended dose is 10 mg/kg every 8 hours for 5 days, then every 12 hours for 14 days. DMSA is under investigation to determine its role in children with a venous blood level less than 45 µg/dL. Although not approved for adults, it has been used in the same dosage. Monitoring should be maintained by CBC, liver transaminases, and urinalysis for adverse effects.

D-Penicillamine (Cuprimine) is another oral chelator that is given in doses of 20 to 40 mg/kg/d not to exceed 1 g/d. However, it is not FDA approved and has a 10% adverse reaction rate. Nevertheless, D-penicillamine has been used infrequently in adults and children with elevated venous blood lead levels.

Edetate calcium disodium (ethylene diaminetetraacetic acid or CaNa$_2$EDTA Versenate) is a water-soluble chelator given intramuscularly (with 0.5% procaine) or intravenously. The calcium in the compound is displaced by divalent and trivalent heavy metals, forming a soluble complex, which is stable at physiologic pH (but not at acid pH) and enhances lead clearance in the urine. EDTA usually is administered intravenously, especially in severe cases. It must not be administered until adequate urine flow is established. It may redistribute lead to the brain; therefore, BAL may be given first at a venous blood lead level of greater than 55 µg/dL in children and greater than 100 µg/dL in adults. Phlebitis occurs at a concentration greater than 0.5 mg/mL. Alkalinization of the urine may be helpful. CaNa$_2$EDTA should not be confused with sodium EDTA (disodium edetate), which is used to treat hypercalcemia; inadvertent use may produce severe hypocalcemia.

Dimercaprol (BAL) is a peanut oil–based dithiol (two sulfhydryl molecules) that combines with one atom of lead to form a heterocyclic stable ring complex. It is usually reserved for patients in whom venous blood lead is greater than 70 µg/dL, and it chelates red blood cell lead, enhancing its elimination through the urine and bile. It crosses the blood–brain barrier. Approximately 50% of patients have adverse reactions, including bad metallic taste in the mouth, pain at the injection site, sterile abscesses, and fever.

A venous blood lead level greater than 70 µg/dL or the presence of clinical symptoms suggesting encephalopathy in children is a potentially life-threatening emergency. Management should be accomplished in a medical center with a pediatric intensive care unit by a multidisciplinary team including a critical care specialist,

TABLE 23 Pharmacologic Chelation Therapy of Lead Poisoning

Drug	Route	Dose	Duration	Precautions	Monitor
Dimercaprol (BAL in oil)	IM	3-5 mg/kg q4-6h	3-5 days	G6PD deficiency Concurrent iron therapy	AST/ALT enzymes
CaNa$_2$EDTA (calcium disodium. versenate)	IM/IV	50 mg/kg per day	5 days	Inadequate fluid intake Renal impairment Penicillin allergy	Urinalysis, BUN Creatinine Urinalysis, BUN
D-Penicillamine (Cuprimine)	PO	10 mg/kg per day increase 30 mg/kg over 2 weeks	6-20 weeks	Concurrent iron therapy; lead exposure Renal impairment	Creatinine, CBC
2,3-Dimercaptosuccinic acid (DMSA; succimer)	PO	10 mg/kg per dose tid, 10mg/kg per dose bid 14 days	19 days	AST/ALT Concurrent iron therapy G6PD deficiency lead exposure	AST/ALT

Abbreviations: ALT = alanine aminotransferase; AST = aspartate transaminase; BAL = British anti-Lewisite; bid = twice daily; BUN = blood urea nitrogen; CBC = complete blood count; G6PD = glucose-6-phosphate dehydrogenase; IM = intramuscular; IV = intravenous; PO = oral; tid = three times daily.

Rakel and Bope: *Conn's Current Therapy 2006.*

a toxicologist, a neurologist, and a neurosurgeon. Careful monitoring of neurologic status, fluid status, and intracranial pressure should be undertaken if necessary. These patients need close monitoring for hemodynamic instability. Hydration should be maintained to ensure renal excretion of lead. Fluids, renal and hepatic function, and electrolyte levels should be monitored.

While waiting for adequate urine flow, therapy should be initiated with intramuscular dimercaprol (BAL) only (25 mg/kg/d divided into 6 doses). Four hours later, the second dose of BAL should be given intramuscularly, concurrently with $CaNa_2EDTA$ 50 mg/kg/d as a single dose infused over several hours or as a continuous infusion. The double therapy is continued until the venous blood level is less than 40 µg/dL.

As long as the venous blood level is greater than 40 µg/dL, therapy is continued for 72 hours and followed by two alternatives: either parenteral therapy with two drugs ($CaNa_2EDTA$ and BAL) for 5 days or continuation of therapy with $CaNa_2EDTA$ alone if a good response is achieved and the venous blood level of lead is less than 40 µg/dL. If one cannot get the venous blood lead report back, one should continue therapy with both BAL and EDTA for 5 days. In patients with lead encephalopathy, parenteral chelation should be continued with both drugs until the patient is clinically stable before changing therapy. Mannitol and dexamethasone can reduce the cerebral edema, but their role in lead encephalopathy is not clear. Surgical decompression is not recommended to reduce cerebral edema in these cases.

If BAL and $CaNa_2EDTA$ are used together, a minimum of 2 days with no treatment should elapse before another 5-day course of therapy is considered. The 5-day course is repeated with $CaNa_2EDTA$ alone if the blood lead level rebounds to greater than 40 µg/dL or in combination with BAL if the venous blood level is greater than 70 µg/dL. If a third course is required, unless there are compelling reasons, one should wait at least 5 to 7 days before administering the course.

Following chelation therapy, a period of equilibration of 10 to 14 days should be allowed and a repeat venous blood lead concentration should be obtained. If the patient is stable enough for oral intake, oral succimer 30 mg/kg/d in three divided doses for 5 days followed by 20 mg/kg/d in two divided doses for 14 days has been suggested, but there are limited data to support this recommendation. Therapy should be continued until venous blood lead level is less than 20 µg/dL in children or less than 40 µg/dL in adults.

Chelators combined with lead are hemodialyzable in the event of renal failure.

Disposition

All patients with a venous blood lead level of greater than 70 µg/dL or who are symptomatic should be admitted. If a child is hospitalized, all lead hazards must be removed from the home environment before allowing the child to return. The source must be eliminated by environmental and occupational investigations. The local health department should be involved in dealing with children who are lead poisoned, and OSHA should be involved with cases of occupational lead poisoning. Consultation with a poison control center or experienced toxicologist is necessary when chelating patients. Follow-up venous blood lead concentrations should be obtained within 1 to 2 weeks and followed every 2 weeks for 6 to 8 weeks, then monthly for 4 to 6 months if the patient required chelation therapy. All patients with venous blood level greater than 10 µg/dL should be followed at least every 3 months until two venous blood lead concentrations are 10 µg/dL or three are less than 15 µg/dL.

LITHIUM (ESKALITH, LITHANE)

Lithium is an alkali metal used primarily in the treatment of bipolar psychiatric disorders. Most intoxications are cases of chronic overdose. One gram of lithium carbonate contains 189 mg (5.1 mEq) of lithium; a regular tablet contains 300 mg (8.12 mEq) and a sustained-release preparation contains 450 mg or 12.18 mEq.

Toxic Mechanism

The brain is the primary target organ of toxicity, but the mechanism is unclear. Lithium may interfere with physiologic functions by acting as a substitute for cellular cations (sodium and potassium), depressing neural excitation and synaptic transmission.

Toxic Dose

A dose of 1 mEq/kg (40 mg/kg) of lithium will give a peak serum lithium concentration about 1.2 mEq/L. The therapeutic serum lithium concentration in cases of acute mania is 0.6 to 1.2 mEq/L, and for maintenance it is 0.5 to 0.8 mEq/L. Serum lithium concentration levels are usually obtained 12 hours after the last dose. The toxic dose is determined by clinical manifestations and serum levels after the distribution phase.

Acute ingestion of twenty 300-mg tablets (300 mg increases the serum lithium concentration by 0.2 to 0.4 mEq/L) in adults may produce serious intoxication. Chronic intoxication can be produced by conditions listed below that can decrease the elimination of lithium or increase lithium reabsorption in the kidney.

The risk factors that predispose to chronic lithium toxicity are febrile illness, impaired renal function, hyponatremia, advanced age, lithium-induced diabetes insipidus, dehydration, vomiting and diarrhea, and concomitant use of other drugs, such as thiazide and spironolactone diuretics, nonsteroidal anti-inflammatory drugs, salicylates, angiotensin-converting enzyme inhibitors (e.g., captopril), serotonin reuptake inhibitors (e.g., fluoxetine [Prozac]), and phenothiazines.

Kinetics

Gastrointestinal absorption of regular-release preparations is rapid; serum lithium concentration peaks in 2 to 4 hours and is complete by 6 to 8 hours. The onset of toxicity may occur at 1 to 4 hours after acute overdose but usually is delayed because lithium enters the brain slowly. Absorption of sustained-release preparations and the development of toxicity may be delayed 6 to 12 hours.

Volume distribution is 0.5 to 0.9 L/kg. Lithium is not protein bound. The half-life after a single dose is 9 to 13 hours; at steady state, it may be 30 to 58 hours. The renal handling of lithium is similar to that of sodium: glomerular filtration and reabsorption (80%) by the proximal renal tubule. Adequate sodium must be present to prevent lithium reabsorption. More than 90% of lithium is excreted by the kidney, 30% to 60% within 6 to 12 hours.

Manifestations

The examiner must distinguish between side effects, acute intoxication, acute or chronic toxicity, and chronic intoxications. Chronic is the most common and dangerous type of intoxication.

Side effects include fine tremor, gastrointestinal upset, hypothyroidism, polyuria and frank diabetes insipidus, dermatologic manifestations, and cardiac conduction deficits. Lithium is teratogenic.

Patients with acute poisoning may be asymptomatic, with an early high serum lithium concentration of 9 mEq/L, and deteriorate as the serum lithium concentration falls by 50% and the lithium distributes to the brain and the other tissues. Nausea and vomiting may occur within 1 to 4 hours, but the systemic manifestations are usually delayed several more hours. It may take as long as 3 to 5 days for serious symptoms to develop. Acute toxicity and acute on chronic toxicity are manifested by neurologic findings, including weakness, fasciculations, altered mental state, myoclonus, hyperreflexia, rigidity, coma, and convulsions with limbs in hypertension. Cardiovascular effects are nonspecific and occur at therapeutic doses, flat T or inverted T waves, atrioventricular block, and prolonged QT interval. Lithium is not a primary cardiotoxin. Cardiogenic shock occurs secondary to CNS toxicity. Chronic intoxication is associated with manifestations at lower serum lithium concentrations. There is some correlation with manifestations, especially at higher serum lithium concentrations. Although the levels do not always correlate with the manifestations, they are more predictive in cases of severe intoxication. A serum lithium concentration greater than 3.0 mEq/L with chronic intoxication and altered mental state indicates severe toxicity. Permanent neurologic sequelae can result from lithium intoxication.

Laboratory Investigations

Monitoring should include CBC (lithium causes significant leukocytosis), renal function, thyroid function (chronic intoxication), ECG, and electrolytes. Serum lithium concentrations should be determined every 2 to 4 hours until levels are close to therapeutic range. Cross-reactions with green-top Vacutainer specimen tubes containing heparin will spuriously elevate serum lithium concentration 6 to 8 mEq/L.

Management

Vital function must be established and maintained. Seizure precautions should be instituted and seizures, hypotension, and dysrhythmias treated. Evaluation should include examination for rigidity and hyperreflexia signs, hydration, renal function (BUN, creatinine), and electrolytes, especially sodium. The examiner should inquire about diuretic and other drug use that increase serum lithium concentration, and the patient must discontinue the drugs. If the patient is on chronic therapy, the lithium should be discontinued. Serial serum lithium concentrations should be obtained every 4 hours until serum lithium concentration peaks and there is a downward trend toward almost therapeutic range, especially in sustained-release preparations. Vital signs should be monitored, including temperature, and ECG and serial neurologic examinations should be undertaken, including mental status and urinary output. Nephrology consultation is warranted in case of a chronic and elevated serum lithium concentration (>2.5 mEq/L), a large ingestion, or altered mental state.

An intravenous line should be established and hydration and electrolyte balance restored. Serum sodium level should be determined before 0.9% saline fluid is administered in patients with chronic overdose because hypernatremia may be present from diabetes insipidus. Although current evidence supports an initial 0.9% saline infusion (200 mL/h) to enhance excretion of lithium, once hydration, urine output, and normonatremia are established, one should administer 0.45% saline and slow the infusion (100 mL/h) for all patients.

Gastric lavage is often not recommended in cases of acute ingestion because of the large size of the tablets, and it is not necessary after chronic intoxication. Activated charcoal is ineffective. For sustained-release preparations, whole-bowel irrigation may be useful but is not proven. Sodium polystyrene sulfonate (Kayexalate), an ion exchange resin, is difficult to administer and has been used only in uncontrolled studies. Its use is not recommended.

Hemodialysis is the most efficient method for removing lithium from the vascular compartment. It is the treatment of choice for patients with severe intoxication with an altered mental state, those with seizures, and anuric patients. Long runs are used until the serum lithium concentration is less than 1 mEq/L because of extensive re-equilibration. Serum lithium concentration should be monitored every 4 hours after dialysis for rebound. Repeated and prolonged hemodialysis may be necessary. A lag in neurologic recovery can be expected.

Disposition

An acute asymptomatic lithium overdose cannot be medically cleared on the basis of single lithium level. Patients should be admitted if they have any neurologic manifestations (altered mental status, hyperreflexia, stiffness, or tremor). Patients should be admitted to the intensive care unit if they are dehydrated, have renal impairment, or have a high or rising lithium level.

Rakel and Bope: *Conn's Current Therapy 2006.*

METHANOL (WOOD ALCOHOL, METHYL ALCOHOL)

The concentration of methanol in Sterno fuel is 4% and it contains ethanol, in windshield washer fluid it is 30% to 60%, and in gas-line antifreeze it is 100%.

Toxic Mechanism

Methanol is metabolized by alcohol dehydrogenase to formaldehyde, which is metabolized to formate. Formate inhibits cytochrome oxidase, producing tissue hypoxia, lactic acidosis, and optic nerve edema. Formate is converted by folate-dependent enzymes to carbon dioxide.

Toxic Dose

The minimal toxic amount is approximately 100 mg/kg. Serious toxicity in a young child can be produced by the ingestion of 2.5 to 5.0 mL of 100% methanol. Ingestion of 5-mL 100% methanol by a 10-kg child produces estimated peak blood methanol of 80 mg/dL. Ingestion of 15 mL 40% methanol was lethal for a 2-year-old child in one report. A fatal adult oral dose is 30 to 240 mL 100% (20 to 150 g). Ingestion of 6 to 10 mL 100% causes blindness in adults. The toxic blood concentration is greater than 20 mg/dL; very serious toxicity and potential fatality occur at levels greater than 50 mg/dL.

Kinetics

Onset of action can start within 1 hour but may be delayed up to 12 to 18 hours by metabolism to toxic metabolites. It may be delayed longer if ethanol is ingested concomitantly or in infants. Peak blood methanol concentration is 1 hour. Volume distribution is 0.6 L/kg (total body water).

For metabolism, see *Toxic Mechanism*.

Elimination is through metabolism. The half-life of methanol is 8 hours, with ethanol blocking it is 30 to 35 hours, and with hemodialysis 2.5 hours.

Manifestations

Metabolism creates a delay in onset for 12 to 18 hours or longer if ethanol is ingested concomitantly. Initial findings are as follows:

- 0 to 6 hours: Confusion, ataxia, inebriation, formaldehyde odor on breath, and abdominal pain can be present, but the patient may be asymptomatic. Note: Methanol produces an osmolal gap (early), and its metabolite formate produces the anion gap metabolic acidosis (see later). Absence of osmolar or anion gap does not always exclude methanol intoxication.
- 6 to 12 hours: Malaise, headache, abdominal pain, vomiting, visual symptoms, including hyperemia of optic disc, "snow vision," and blindness can be seen.
- More than 12 hours: Worsening acidosis, hyperglycemia, shock, and multiorgan failure develop,

with death from complications of intractable acidosis and cerebral edema.

Laboratory Investigation

Methanol can be detected on some chromatography drug screens if specified. Methanol and ethanol levels, electrolytes, glucose, BUN, creatinine, amylase, and ABG should be monitored every 4 hours. Formate levels correlate more closely than blood methanol concentration with severity of intoxication and should be obtained if possible.

Management

One should protect the airway by intubation to prevent aspiration and administer assisted ventilation as needed. If needed, 100% oxygen can be administered. A nephrologist should be consulted early regarding the need for hemodialysis.

Gastrointestinal decontamination procedures have no role.

Metabolic acidosis should be treated vigorously with sodium bicarbonate 2 to 3 mEq/kg intravenously. Large amounts may be needed.

Antidote therapy is initiated to inhibit metabolism if the patient has a history of ingesting more than 0.4 mL/kg of 100% with the following conditions:

- Blood methanol level is greater than 20 mg/dL
- The patient has osmolar gap not accounted for by other factors
- The patient is symptomatic or acidotic with increased anion gap and/or hyperemia of the optic disc.

The ethanol or fomepizole therapy outlined below can be used.

Ethanol Therapy

Ethanol should be initiated immediately if fomepizole is unavailable (see *Fomepizole Therapy*). Alcohol dehydrogenase has a greater affinity for ethanol than ethylene glycol. Therefore, ethanol blocks the metabolism of ethylene glycol.

Ethanol should be administered intravenously (oral administration is less reliable) to produce a blood ethanol concentration of 100 to 150 mg/dL. The loading dose is 10 mL/kg of 10% ethanol administered intravenously concomitantly with a maintenance dose of 10% ethanol at 1.0 mL/kg/h. This dose may need to be increased to 2 mL/kg/h in patients who are heavy drinkers. The blood ethanol concentration should be measured hourly and the infusion rate should be adjusted to maintain a concentration of 100 to 150 mg/dL.

Fomepizole Therapy

Fomepizole (Antizol, 4-methylpyrazole) inhibits alcohol dehydrogenase more reliably than ethanol and it does

Rakel and Bope: *Conn's Current Therapy 2006.*

not require constant monitoring of ethanol levels and adjustment of infusion rates. Fomepizole is available in 1 g/mL vials of 1.5 mL. The loading dose is 15 mg/kg (0.015 mL/kg) IV, maintenance dose is 10 mg/kg (0.01 mL/kg) every 12 hours for 4 doses, then 15 mg/kg every 12 hours until the ethylene glycol levels are less than 20 mg/dL. The solution is prepared by being mixed with 100 mL of 0.9% saline or D_5W. Fomepizole can be given to patients requiring hemodialysis but should be dosed as follows:

Dose at the beginning of hemodialysis:

- If less than 6 hours since last Antizol dose, do not administer dose
- If more than 6 hours since last dose, administer next scheduled dose

Dosing during hemodialysis:

- Dose every 4 hours

Dosing at the time hemodialysis is completed:

- If less than 1 hour between last dose and end dialysis, do not administer dose at end of dialysis
- If 1 to 3 hours between last dose and end dialysis, administer one half of next scheduled dose
- If more than 3 hours between last dose and end dialysis, administer next scheduled dose

Maintenance dosing off hemodialysis:

- Give the next scheduled dose 12 hours from the last dose administered

Hemodialysis increases the clearance of both methanol and formate 10-fold over renal clearance. A blood methanol concentration greater than 50 mg/dL has been used as an indication for hemodialysis, but recently some toxicologists from the New York City Poison Center recommended early hemodialysis in patients with blood methanol concentration greater than 25 mg/dL because it may be able to shorten the course of intoxication if started early. One should continue to monitor methanol levels and/or formate levels every 4 hours after the procedure for rebound. Other indications for early hemodialysis are significant metabolic acidosis and electrolyte abnormalities despite conventional therapy and if visual or neurologic signs or symptoms are present.

A serum formate level greater than 20 mg/dL has also been used as a criterion for hemodialysis, although this is often not readily available through many laboratories. If hemodialysis is used, the infusion rate of 10% ethanol should be increased 2.0 to 3.5 mL/kg/h. The blood ethanol concentration and glucose level should be obtained every 2 hours.

Therapy is continued with both ethanol and hemodialysis until the blood methanol level is undetectable, there is no acidosis, and the patient has no neurologic or visual disturbances. This may require several days.

Hypoglycemia is treated with intravenous glucose. Doses of folinic acid (Leucovorin) and folic acid have been used successfully in animal investigations to enhance formate metabolism to carbon dioxide and water. Leucovorin 1 mg/kg up to 50 mg IV is administered every 4 hours for several days.

An initial ophthalmologic consultation and follow-up are warranted.

Disposition

All patients who have ingested significant amounts of methanol should be referred to the emergency department for evaluation and blood methanol concentration measurement. Ophthalmologic follow-up of all patients with methanol intoxications should be arranged.

MONOAMINE OXIDASE INHIBITORS

Nonselective monoamine oxidase inhibitors (MAOIs) include the hydrazines phenelzine (Nardil) and isocarboxazid (Marplan), and the nonhydrazine tranylcypromine (Parnate). Furazolidone (Furoxone) and pargyline (Eutonyl)[2] are also considered nonselective MAOIs. Moclobemide[2], which is available in many countries but not the United States, is a selective MAO-A inhibitor. MAO-B inhibitors include selegiline (Eldepryl), an antiparksonism agent, which does not have similar toxicity to MAO-A and is not discussed. Selectivity is lost in an overdose. MAOIs are used to treat severe depression.

Toxic Mechanism

Monoamine oxidase enzymes are responsible for the oxidative deamination of both endogenous and exogenous catecholamines such as norepinephrine. MAO-A in the intestinal wall also metabolizes tyramine in food. MAOIs permanently inhibit MAO enzymes until a new enzyme is synthesized after 14 days or longer. The toxicity results from the accumulation, potentiation, and prolongation of the catecholamine action followed by profound hypotension and cardiovascular collapse.

Toxic Dose

Toxicity begins at 2 to 3 mg/kg and fatalities occur at 4 to 6 mg/kg. Death has occurred after a single dose of 170 mg of tranylcypromine in an adult.

Kinetics

Structurally, MAOIs are related to amphetamines and catecholamines. The hydrazine peak levels are at 1 to 2 hours; metabolism is hepatic acetylation; and inactive metabolites are excreted in the urine. For the nonhydrazines, peak levels occur at 1 to 4 hours, and metabolism is via the liver to active amphetamine-like metabolites.

The onset of symptoms in a case of overdose is delayed 6 to 24 hours after ingestion, peak activity is 8 to 12 hours, and duration is 72 hours or longer.

18

[2]Not available in the United States.

The peak of MAO inhibition is in 5 to 10 days and lasts as long as 5 weeks.

Manifestations

Manifestations of an acute ingestion overdose of MAO-A inhibitors are as follows:

Phase I

An adrenergic crisis occurs, with delayed onset for 6 to 24 hours, and may not reach peak until 24 hours. The crisis starts as hyperthermia, tachycardia, tachypnea, dysarthria, transient hypertension, hyperreflexia, and CNS stimulation.

Phase II

Neuromuscular excitation and sympathetic hyperactivity occur with increased temperature greater than 40°C (104°F), agitation, hyperactivity, confusion, fasciculations, twitching, tremor, masseter spasm, muscle rigidity, acidosis, and electrolyte abnormalities. Seizures and dystonic reactions may occur. The pupils are mydriatic, sometimes nonreactive with "ping-pong gaze."

Phase III

CNS depression and cardiovascular collapse occur in cases of severe overdose as the catecholamines are depleted. Symptoms usually resolve within 5 days but may last 2 weeks.

Phase IV

Secondary complications occur, including rhabdomyolysis, cardiac dysrhythmias, multiorgan failure, and coagulopathies.

Biogenic interactions usually occur while the patient is on therapeutic doses of MAOI or shortly after they are discontinued (30 to 60 minutes), before the new MAO enzyme is synthesized. The following substances have been implicated: indirect acting sympathomimetics such as amphetamines, serotonergic drugs, opioids (e.g., meperidine, dextromethorphan), tricyclic antidepressants, specific serotonin reuptake inhibitors (SSRI; e.g., fluoxetine [Prozac], sertraline [Zoloft], paroxetine [Paxil]), tyramine-containing foods (e.g., wine, beer, avocados, cheese, caviar, chocolate, chicken liver), and L-tryptophan. SSRIs should not be started for at least 5 weeks after MAOIs have been discontinued.

In mild cases, usually caused by foods, headache and hypertension develop and last for several hours. In severe cases, malignant hypertension and severe hyperthermia syndromes consisting of hypertension or hyperthermia, altered mental state, skeletal muscle rigidity, shivering (often beginning in the masseter muscle), and seizures may occur.

The serotonin syndrome, which may be a result of inhibition of serotonin metabolism, has similar clinical findings to those of malignant hyperthermia and may occur with or without hyperthermia or hypertension.

Chronic toxicity clinical findings include tremors, hyperhidrosis, agitation, hallucinations, confusion, and seizures and may be confused with withdrawal syndromes.

Laboratory Investigations

Monitoring of the ECG, cardiac monitoring, CPK, ABG, pulse oximeter, electrolytes, blood glucose, and acid–base balance should be maintained.

Management

In the case of MAOI overdose, ipecac-induced emesis should not be used. Only activated charcoal alone should be used.

If the patient is admitted to the hospital and is well enough to eat, a nontyramine diet should be ordered.

Extreme agitation and seizures can be controlled with benzodiazepines and barbiturates. Phenytoin is ineffective. Nondepolarizing neuromuscular blockers (not depolarizing succinylcholine) may be needed in severe cases of hyperthermia and rigidity. If the patient has severe hypertension (catecholamine mediated), phentolamine (Regitine), a parenteral β-blocking agent, 3 to 5 mg intravenously, or labetalol (Normodyne), a combination of an α-blocking agent and a β-blocker, 20-mg intravenous bolus, should be given. If malignant hypertension with rigidity is present, a short-acting nitroprusside and benzodiazepine can be used. Hypertension is often followed by severe hypotension, which should be managed by fluid and vasopressors. *Caution:* Vasopressor therapy should be administered at lower doses than usual because of exaggerated pharmacologic response. Norepinephrine is preferred to dopamine, which requires release of intracellular amines.

Cardiac dysrhythmias are treated with standard therapy but are often refractory, and cardioversion and pacemakers may be needed.

For malignant hyperthermia, dantrolene (Dantrium), a nonspecific peripheral skeletal relaxing agent, is administered, which inhibits the release of calcium from the sarcoplasm. Dantrolene is reconstituted with 60 mL sterile water without bacteriostatic agents. Glass equipment must not be used, and the drug must be protected from light and used within 6 hours. Loading dose is 2 to 3 mg/kg intravenously as a bolus, and the loading dose is repeated until the signs of malignant hyperthermia (tachycardia, rigidity, increased end-tidal CO_2, and temperature) are controlled. Maximum total dose is 10 mg/kg to avoid hepatotoxicity.

When malignant hyperthermia has subsided, 1 mg/kg IV is given every 6 hours for 24 to 48 hours, then orally 1 mg/kg every 6 hours for 24 hours to prevent recurrence. There is a danger of thrombophlebitis following peripheral dantrolene, and it should be administered through a central line if possible. In addition one should administer external cooling and correct metabolic acidosis and electrolyte disturbances. Benzodiazepine can be used for sedation. Dantrolene does not reverse central dopamine blockade; therefore,

Rakel and Bope: *Conn's Current Therapy 2006.*

bromocriptine mesylate (Parlodel) 2.5 to 10 mg should be given orally or through a nasogastric tube three times a day.

Rhabdomyolysis and myoglobinuria are treated with fluids. Urine alkalinization should also be treated.

Hemodialysis and hemoperfusion are of no proven value.

Biogenic amine interactions are managed symptomatically, similar to cases of overdose. For the serotonin syndrome cyproheptadine (Periactin), a serotonin blocker, 4 mg orally every hour for three doses, or methysergide (Sansert), 2 mg orally every 6 hours for three doses, should be considered. The effectiveness of these drugs has not been proven.

Disposition

All patients who have ingested more than 2 mg/kg of an MAOI should be admitted to the hospital for 24 hours of observation and monitoring in the intensive care unit because the life-threatening manifestations may be delayed. Patients with drug or dietary interactions that are mild may not require admission if symptoms subside within 4 to 6 hours and the patients remain asymptomatic. Patients with symptoms that persist or require active intervention should be admitted to the intensive care unit.

OPIOIDS (NARCOTIC OPIATES)

Opioids are used for analgesia, as antitussives, and as antidiarrheal agents and are illicit agents (heroin, opium) used in substance abuse. Tolerance, physical dependency, and withdrawal may develop.

Toxic Mechanism

At least four main opioid receptors have been identified. The μ receptor is considered the most important for central analgesia and CNS depression. The κ and δ receptors predominate in spinal analgesia. The σ receptors may mediate dysphoria. Death is a consequence of dose-dependent CNS respiratory depression or secondary to pulmonary aspiration or noncardiac pulmonary edema. The mechanism of noncardiac pulmonary edema is unknown.

Dextromethorphan can interact with MAOIs, causing severe hyperthermia, and may cause the serotonin syndrome (see *Selective Serotonin Reuptake Inhibitors*). Dextromethorphan inhibits the metabolism of norepinephrine and serotonin and blocks the reuptake of serotonin. It is found as a component of a large number of nonprescription cough and cold remedies.

Toxic Dose

The toxic dose depends on the specific drug, route of administration, and degree of tolerance. For therapeutic and toxic doses, see Table 24. In children, respiratory depression has been produced by 10 mg of morphine or methadone, 75 mg of meperidine, and 12.5 mg of diphenoxylate. Infants younger than 3 months

of age are more susceptible to respiratory depression. The dose should be reduced by 50%.

Kinetics

Oral onset of analgesic effect of morphine is 10 to 15 minutes; the action peaks in 1 hour and lasts 4 to 6 hours. With sustained-release preparations, the duration is 8 to 12 hours. Opioids are 90% metabolized in the liver by hepatic conjugation and 90% excreted in the urine as inactive compounds. Volume distribution is 1 to 4 L/kg. Protein binding is 35% to 75%. The typical plasma half-life of opiates is 2 to 5 hours, but that of methadone is 24 to 36 hours. Morphine metabolites include morphine-3- glucuronide (inactive) and morphine-6-glucuronide (active) and normorphine (active). Meperidine (Demerol) is rapidly hydrolyzed by tissue esterases into the active metabolite normeperidine, which has twice the convulsant activity of meperidine. Heroin (diacetylmorphine) is deacetylated within minutes to 6-monacetylmorphine and morphine. Propoxyphene (Darvon) has a rapid onset of action, and death has occurred within 15 to 30 minutes after a massive overdose. Propoxyphene is metabolized to norpropoxyphene, an active metabolite with convulsive, cardiac dysrhythmic, and heart block properties. Symptoms of diphenoxylate overdose appear within 1 to 4 hours. It is metabolized into the active metabolite difenoxin, which is five times more active as a regular respiratory depressant agent. Death has been reported in children after ingestion of a single tablet.

Manifestations

Initially, mild intoxication produces miosis, dull face, drowsiness, partial ptosis, and "nodding" (head drops to chest then bobs up). Larger amounts produce the classic triad of miotic pupils (exceptions below), respiratory depression, and depressed level of consciousness (flaccid coma). The blood pressure, pulse, and bowel activity are decreased.

Dilated pupils do not exclude opioid intoxication. Some exceptions to the miosis effect include dextromethorphan (paralyzes iris), fentanyl, meperidine, and diphenoxylate (rarely). Physiologic disturbances including acidosis, hypoglycemia, hypoxia, and postictal state, or a co-ingestant may also produce mydriasis.

Usually, the muscles are flaccid, but increased muscle tone can be produced by meperidine and fentanyl (chest rigidity). Seizures are rare but can occur with ingestion of codeine, meperidine, propoxyphene, and dextromethorphan. Hallucinations and agitation have been reported.

Pruritus and urticaria are caused by histamine release by some opioids or by sulfite additives.

Noncardiac pulmonary edema may occur after an overdose, especially with intravenous heroin abuse. Cardiac effects include vasodilation and hypotension. A heart murmur in an intravenous addict suggests endocarditis. Propoxyphene can produce delayed cardiac dysrhythmias.

TABLE 24 Doses and Onset and Duration of Action of Common Opioids

Drug	Adult oral dose	Child oral dose	Onset of action	Duration of action	Adult fatal dose
Camphored tincture of opium	25 mL	0.25-0.50 mL/kg (0.4 mg/mL)	15-30 min	4-5 h	NA
Codeine	30-180 mg	0.5-1 mg/kg	15-30 min	4-6 h	800 mg
	>1 mg/kg is toxic in a child, above 200 mg in adult >5 mg/kg fatal in a child				
Dextromethorphan	15 mg 10 mg/kg is toxic	0.25 mg/kg	15-30 min	3-6 h	NA
Diacetylmorphine; street heroin is less than 10% pure	60 mg	NA	15-30 min	3-4 h	100 mg
Diphenoxylate natiopine (Lomotil)	5-10 mg	NA	120-240 min	14 h	300 mg
	7.5 mg is toxic in a child, 300 mg is toxic in adult				
Fentanyl (Duragesic)	0.1-0.2 mg	0.001-0.002 mg/kg	7-8 min	Intramuscular: 1/2-2 h	1.0 mg
Hydrocodone with APAP (Lortab)	5-30 mg	0.15 mg/kg	30 min	3-4 h	100 mg
Hydromorphone (Dilaudid)	4 mg	0.1 mg/kg	15-30 min	3-4 h	100 mg
Meperidine (Demerol)	100 mg	1-1.5 mg/kg	10-45 min	3-4 h	350 mg
Methadone (Dolophine)	10 mg	0.1 mg/kg	30-60 min	4-12 h	120 mg
Morphine	10-60 mg	0.1-0.2 mg/kg	<20 min	4-6 h	200 mg
	Oral dose is 6 times parenteral dose, MS Contin sustained release prep				
Oxycodone APAP (Percocet)	5 mg	NA	15-30 min	4-5 h	NA
Pentazocine (Talwin)	50-100 mg	NA	15-30 min	3-4 h	NA
Propoxyphene (Darvon)	65-100mg	NA	30-60 min	2-4 h	700 mg

Fentanyl is 100 times more potent than morphine and can cause chest wall muscle rigidity. Some of its derivatives are 2000 times more potent than morphine.

Laboratory Investigations

For patients with overdose, one should obtain and monitor ABG, blood glucose, and electrolyte levels; chest radiographs; and ECG. For drug abusers, one should consider testing for hepatitis B, syphilis, and HIV antibody (HIV testing usually requires consent). Blood opioid concentrations are not useful. They confirm diagnosis (morphine therapeutic dose, 65 to 80 ng/mL; toxic, <200 ng/mL), but are not useful for making a therapeutic decision. Cross-reactions can occur with Vick's Formula 44, poppy seeds, and other opioids (codeine and heroin are metabolized to morphine). Naloxone 4 mg IV was not associated with a positive enzyme multiplied immunoassay technique urine screen at 60 minutes, 6 hours, or 48 hours.

Management

Supportive care should be instituted, particularly an endotracheal tube and assisted ventilation. Temporary ventilation can be provided by a bag-valve mask with 100% oxygen. The patient should be placed on a cardiac monitor, have intravenous access established, and have specimens for ABG, glucose, electrolytes, BUN, and creatinine levels, CBC, coagulation profile, liver function, toxicology screen, and urinalysis taken.

For gastrointestinal decontamination, emesis should not be induced, but activated charcoal can be administered if bowel sounds are present.

If it is suspected that the patient is an addict, he or she should be restrained first and then 0.1 mg of naloxone (Narcan) should be administered. The dose should be doubled every 2 minutes until the patient responds or 10 to 20 mg has been given. If the patient is not suspected to be an addict, then 2 mg every 2 to 3 minutes to total of 10 to 20 mg is administered.

It is essential to determine whether there is a complete response to naloxone (mydriasis, improvement in ventilation), because it is a diagnostic therapeutic test. A continuous naloxone infusion may be appropriate, using the "response dose" every hour. Repeat doses of naloxone may be necessary because the effects of many opioids can last much longer than naloxone does (30 to 60 minutes). Methadone ingestions may require a naloxone infusion for 24 to 48 hours. Half of the response dose may need to be repeated in 15 to 20 minutes, after the infusion has been started.

Acute iatrogenic withdrawal precipitated by the administration of naloxone to a dependent patient should not be treated with morphine or other opioids.

Rakel and Bope: *Conn's Current Therapy 2006*.

Naloxone's effects are limited to 30 to 60 minutes (shorter than most opioids) and withdrawal will subside in a short time.

Nalmefene (Revex), an FDA-approved long-acting (4 to 8 hours) pure opioid antagonist, is being investigated, but its role in cases of acute intoxication is unclear and it could produce prolonged withdrawal. It may have a role in place of naloxone infusion.

Noncardiac pulmonary edema does not respond to naloxone, and the patient needs intubation, assisted ventilation, positive end-expiratory pressure, and hemodynamic monitoring. Fluids should be given cautiously in patients with opioid overdose because opioids stimulate the antidiuretic hormone.

If the patient is comatose, 50% glucose (3% to 4% of comatose opioid overdose patients have hypoglycemia) and thiamine should be given prior to naloxone. If the patient has seizures that are unresponsive to naloxone, one administers diazepam and examines for metabolic (hypoglycemia, electrolyte disturbances) causes and structural disturbances.

Hypotension is rare and should direct a search for another etiology. If the patient is agitated, hypoxia and hypoglycemia must be excluded before opioid withdrawal is considered as a cause. Complications to consider include urinary retention, constipation, rhabdomyolysis, myoglobinuria, hypoglycemia, and withdrawal.

Disposition

If a patient responds to intravenous naloxone, careful observation for relapse and the development of pulmonary edema is required, with cardiac and respiratory monitoring for 6 to 12 hours. Patients requiring repeated doses of naloxone or an infusion, or those who develop pulmonary edema, require intensive care unit admission and cannot be discharged from the intensive care unit until they are symptom free for 12 hours. Intravenous overdose complications are expected to be present within 20 minutes after injection, and discharge after 4 symptom-free hours has been recommended. Adults with oral overdose have delayed onset of toxicity and require 6 hours of observation. Children with oral opioid overdose should be admitted to the hospital for observation because of delayed toxicity. Some toxicologists advise restraining a patient who attempts to sign out against medical advice after treatment with naloxone, at least until the patient receives psychiatric evaluation.

ORGANOPHOSPHATES AND CARBAMATES

Cholinergic intoxication sources are insecticides (organophosphates or carbamates), some medications, and some mushrooms. Examples of organophosphate insecticides are malathion (low toxicity, median lethal dose [LD_{50}] 2800 mg/kg), chlorpyrifos, which has been removed from market (moderate toxicity), and parathion (high toxicity, LD_{50} 2 mg/kg). Carbamate insecticides include carbaryl (low toxicity, LD_{50} 500 mg/kg), propoxur (moderate toxicity, LD_{50} 95 mg/kg),

and aldicarb (high toxicity, LD_{50} 0.9 mg/kg). Pharmaceuticals with carbamate properties include neostigmine (Prostigmin) and physostigmine (Antilirium). Cholinergic compounds also include the "G" nerve war weapons tabun (GA), sarin (GB), soman (GB), and venom X (VX).

Toxic Mechanism

Organophosphates phosphorylate the active site on red cell acetylcholinesterase and pseudocholinesterase in the serum, neuromuscular and parasympathetic neuroeffector junctions, and in the major synapses of the autonomic ganglia, causing irreversible inhibition. There are two types of organophosphate intoxication: (a) direct action by the parent compound (e.g., tetraethylpyrophosphate), or (b) indirect action by the toxic metabolite (e.g., parathoxon or malathoxon).

Carbamates (esters of carbonic acid) cause reversible carbamylation of the active site of the enzymes. When a critical amount, greater than 50%, of cholinesterase is inhibited, acetylcholine accumulates and causes transient stimulation at cholinergic synapses and sympathetic terminals (muscarinic effect), the somatic nerves, the autonomic ganglia (nicotinic effect), and CNS synapses. Stimulation of conduction is followed by inhibition of conduction.

The major differences between the carbamates and the organophosphates are as follows: (a) carbamate toxicity is less and the duration is shorter; (b) carbamates rarely produce overt CNS effects (poor CNS penetration); (c) carbamate inhibition of the acetylcholinesterase enzyme is reversible and activity returns to normal rapidly; (d) pralidoxime, the enzyme regenerator, may not be necessary in the management of mild carbamate intoxication (e.g., carbaryl).

Toxic Dose

Parathion's minimum lethal dose is 2 mg in children and 10 to 20 mg in adults. The lethal dose of malathion is greater than 1375 mg/kg and that of chlorpyrifos is 25 g; the latter compound is unlikely to cause death.

Kinetics

Absorption is by all routes. The onset of acute ingestion toxicity occurs as early as 3 hours, usually before 12 hours and always before 24 hours. Lipid-soluble agents absorbed by the dermal route (e.g., fenthion) may have a delayed onset of more than 24 hours. Inhalation toxicity occurs immediately after exposure. Massive ingestion can produce intoxication within minutes.

Metabolism is via the liver. With some pesticides (e.g., parathion, malathion), the effects are delayed because they undergo hepatic microsomal oxidative metabolism to their toxic metabolites, the -oxons (e.g., paroxon, malaoxon).

The half-life of malathion is 2.89 hours and that of parathion is 2.1 days. The metabolites are eliminated in the urine and the presence of p-nitrophenol in the urine is a clue up to 48 hours after exposure.

Rakel and Bope: *Conn's Current Therapy 2006.*

Manifestations

Many organophosphates produce a garlic odor on the breath, in the gastric contents, or in the container. Diaphoresis, excessive salivation, miosis, and muscle twitching are helpful clues to diagnosis.

Early, a cholinergic (muscarinic) crisis develops that consists of parasympathetic nervous system activity. DUMBELS is the mnemonic for defecation, cramps, and increased bowel motility; urinary incontinence; miosis (mydriasis may occur in 20%); bronchospasm and bronchorrhea; excess secretion; lacrimation; and seizures. Bradycardia, pulmonary edema, and hypotension may be present.

Later, sympathetic and nicotinic effects occur, consisting of MATCH: muscle weakness and fasciculation (eyelid twitching is often present), adrenal stimulation and hyperglycemia, tachycardia, cramps in muscles, and hypertension. Finally, paralysis of the skeletal muscles ensues.

The CNS effects are headache, blurred vision, anxiety, ataxia, delirium and toxic psychosis, convulsions, coma, and respiratory depression. Cranial nerve palsies have been noted. Delayed hallucinations may occur.

Delayed respiratory paralysis and neurologic and neurobehavioral disorders have been described following certain organophosphate ingestions or dermal exposure. The "intermediate syndrome" is paralysis of proximal and respiratory muscles developing 24 to 96 hours after the successful treatment of organophosphate poisoning. A delayed distal polyneuropathy has been described with ingestion of certain organophosphates, such as triorthocresyl phosphate, bromoleptophos, and methomidophos.

Complications include aspiration, pulmonary edema, and acute respiratory distress syndrome.

Laboratory Investigations

Monitoring should include chest radiograph, blood glucose (nonketotic hyperglycemia is frequent), ABG, pulse oximetry, ECG, blood coagulation status, liver function, hyperamylasemia (pancreatitis reported), and urinalysis for the metabolite alkyl phosphate paranitrophenol. Blood should be drawn for red blood cell cholinesterase determination before pralidoxime is given. The red blood cell cholinesterase activity roughly correlates with clinical severity. Mild poisoning is 20% to 50% of normal, moderate poisoning is 10% to 20% of normal, and severe poisoning is 10% of normal (>90% depressed). A post-exposure rise of 10% to 15% in the cholinesterase level determined at least 10 to 14 days after the exposure confirms the diagnosis.

Management

Protection of health care personnel with clothing (masks, gloves, gowns, goggles) and respiratory equipment or hazardous material suits, as necessary, is called for. General decontamination consists of isolation, bagging, and disposal of contaminated clothing and other articles. Vital functions should be established and maintained. Cardiac and oxygen saturation monitoring are needed. Intubation and assisted ventilation may be needed. Secretions should be suctioned until atropinization drying is achieved.

Dermal decontamination involves prompt removal of clothing and cleansing of all affected areas of skin, hair, and eyes. Ocular decontamination involves irrigation with copious amounts of tepid water or 0.9% saline for at least 15 minutes. Gastrointestinal decontamination, if the ingestion was recent, involves the administration of activated charcoal.

Atropine sulfate can be given as an antidote. It is both a diagnostic and a therapeutic agent. Atropine counteracts the muscarinic effects but is only partially effective for the CNS effects (seizures and coma). Preservative-free atropine (no benzyl alcohol) should be used. If the patient is symptomatic (bradycardia or bronchorrhea), a test dose should be administered, 0.02 mg/kg in children or 1 mg in adults, intravenously. If no signs of atropinization are present (tachycardia, drying of secretions, and mydriasis), atropine should be administered immediately, 0.05 mg/kg in children or 2 mg in adults, every 5 to 10 minutes as needed to dry the secretions and clear the lungs. Beneficial effects are seen within 1 to 4 minutes and maximum effect in 8 minutes. The average dose in the first 24 hours is 40 mg, but 1000 mg or more has been required in severe cases. Glycopyrrolate (Robinul) can be used if atropine is not available. The maximum dose should be maintained for 12 to 24 hours, then tapered and the patient observed for relapse. Poisoning, especially with lipophilic agents (e.g., fenthion, chlorfenthion), may require weeks of atropine therapy. An alternative is a continuous infusion of atropine 8 mg in 100 mL 0.9% saline at rate of 0.02 to 0.08 mg/kg/h (0.25 to 1.0 mL/kg/h) with additional 1 to 5 mg boluses as needed to dry the secretions.

Pralidoxime chloride (Protopam) has both antinicotinic and antimuscarinic effects and possibly also CNS effects. Successful treatment with pralidoxime chloride may allow a reduction in the dose of atropine. Pralidoxime acts to reactivate the phosphorylated cholinesterases by binding the phosphate moiety on the esteritic site and displacing it. It should be given early before "aging" of phosphate bond produces tighter binding. However, recent reports indicate that pralidoxime chloride is beneficial even several days after the poisoning. Improvement is seen within 10 to 40 minutes. The initial dose of pralidoxime chloride is 1 to 2 g in 250 mL 0.89% saline over 5 to 10 minutes, maximum 200 mg/minute, in adults or 25 to 50 mg/kg, maximum 4 mg/kg/minute, in children younger than 12 years of age. The dose can be repeated every 6 to 12 hours for several days. An alternative is a continuous infusion of 1 g in 100 mL 0.89% saline at 5 to 20 mg/kg/h (0.5 to 12 mL/g/h) up to 500 mg/h and titrated to desired response. Maximum adult daily dose is 12 g. Cardiac and blood pressure monitoring are advised during and for several hours after the infusion. The end point is absence of fasciculations and return of muscle strength.

Contraindicated drugs include morphine, aminophylline, barbiturates, opioids, phenothiazine, reserpine-like drugs, parasympathomimetics, and succinylcholine.

Noncardiac pulmonary edema may require respiratory support. Seizures may respond to atropine and pralidoxime chloride but often require anticonvulsants. Cardiac dysrhythmias may require electrical cardioversion or antidysrhythmic therapy if the patient is hemodynamically unstable. Extracorporeal procedures are of no proven value.

Disposition

Asymptomatic patients with normal examination findings after 6 to 8 hours of observation may be discharged. In cases of intentional poisoning, the patients require psychiatric clearance for discharge. Symptomatic patients should be admitted to the intensive care unit. Observation of milder cases of carbamate poisoning, even those requiring atropine, for 6 to 8 hours symptom-free may be sufficient to exclude significant toxicity. In cases of workplace exposure, OSHA should be notified.

PHENCYCLIDINE (ANGEL DUST)

Phencyclidine is an arylcyclohexylamine related to ketamine and chemically related to the phenothiazines. Originally a "dissociative" anesthetic banned in United States since 1979, it is now an illicit substance, with at least 38 analogs. It is inexpensively manufactured by "kitchen chemists" and is mislabeled as other hallucinogens. Improper phencyclidine synthesis may release cyanide when heated or smoked and can cause explosions.

Toxic Mechanism

The mechanism of phencyclidine is complex and not completely understood. It inhibits some neurotransmitters and causes a loss of pain sensation without depressing the CNS respiratory status. It stimulates α-adrenergic receptors and may act as a "false neurotransmitter." The effects are sympathomimetic, cholinergic, and cerebellar.

Toxic Dose

The usual dose of phencyclidine mixed with marijuana joints is 100 to 400 mg of phencyclidine. Joints or leaf mixtures contain 0.24% to 7.9% of PCP, 1 mg of PCP/150 leaves. Tablets contain 5 mg (the usual street dose). CNS effects at doses of 1 to 6 mg include hallucinations and euphoria, 6 to 10 mg produces toxic psychosis and sympathetic stimulation, 10 to 25 mg produces severe toxicity, and more than 100 mg has resulted in fatalities.

Kinetics

Phencyclidine is a lipophilic weak base, with a pKa of 8.5 to 9.5. It is rapidly absorbed when smoked and snorted, poorly absorbed from the acid stomach, and rapidly absorbed from the alkaline middle small intestine. It has an enterogastric secretion and is reabsorbed in the small intestine. The onset of action when smoked is 2 to 5 minutes, with a peak in 15 to 30 minutes. With oral ingestion, the onset is in 30 to 60 minutes and when taken intravenously it is immediate. Most adverse reactions in cases of overdose begin within 1 to 2 hours. Its duration of action at low doses is 4 to 6 hours and normality returns in 24 hours; in large overdoses, fluctuating coma may last 6 to 10 days.

Volume distribution is 6.2 L/kg. Phencyclidine concentrates in brain and adipose tissue. Protein binding is 70%. The route of elimination is by gastric secretion, liver metabolism, and 10% urinary excretion of conjugates and free phencyclidine. Renal excretion may be increased 50% with urinary acidification. The half-life is 1 hour (in cases of overdose, it is 11 to 89 hours).

Manifestations

The classic picture is bursts of horizontal, vertical, and rotary nystagmus, which is a clue to diagnosis (occurs in 50% of cases), miosis, hypertension, and fluctuating altered mental state. There is a wide spectrum of clinical presentations.

Mild intoxication with 1 to 6 mg produces drunken and bizarre behavior, agitation, rotary nystagmus, and blank stare. Violent behavior and sensory anesthesia make these patients insensitive to pain, self-destructive, and dangerous. Most are communicative within 1 to 2 hours, are alert and oriented in 6 to 8 hours, and recover completely in 24 to 48 hours.

Moderate intoxication with 6 to 10 mg produces excess salivation, hypertension, hyperthermia, muscle rigidity, myoclonus, and catatonia. Recovery of consciousness occurs in 24 to 48 hours and complete recovery in 1 week.

Severe intoxication with 10 to 25 mg results in opisthotonus, decerebrate rigidity, convulsions, prolonged fluctuating coma, and respiratory failure. Patients in this category have a high rate of medical complications. Recovery of consciousness occurs in 24 to 48 hours, with complete normality in a month. Medical complications include apnea, aspiration pneumonia, cardiac arrest, hypertensive encephalopathy, hyperthermia, intracerebral hemorrhage, psychosis, rhabdomyolysis and myoglobinuria, and seizures. Loss of memory and "flashbacks" last for months. Phencyclidine-induced depression and suicide have been reported.

Fatalities occur with ingestions of greater than 100 mg and with serum levels greater than 100 to 250 ng/mL.

Laboratory Investigations

Marked elevation of creatine kinase level may occur. Values greater than 20,000 units have been reported. Urinalysis should be monitored and urine tested for myoglobin. One should monitor the blood for creatine kinase, uric acid (an early clue to rhabdomyolysis), BUN, creatinine, electrolytes (hyperkalemia),

Rakel and Bope: *Conn's Current Therapy 2006.*

blood glucose (20% of patients have hypoglycemia), urinary output, liver function tests, ECG, and ABG if the patient has any respiratory manifestations. Measurement of phencyclidine in the gastric juice is called for because concentrations are 10 to 50 times higher than in blood or urine. Phencyclidine blood concentrations are not helpful. Phencyclidine may be detected in the urine of the average user for 10 days to 3 weeks after the last dose. In chronic users, it can be detected for over 1 month. The analogs of phencyclidine may not produce positive test results for phencyclidine in the urine. Cross-reactions with bleach and dextromethorphan may cause false-positive urine test results on immunoassay, and cross-reaction with doxylamine may produce a false-positive finding on gas chromatography.

Management

The patient should be observed for violent, self-destructive, bizarre behavior and paranoid schizophrenia. Patients should be placed in a low sensory environment and dangerous objects should be removed from the area.

Gastrointestinal decontamination is not effective because phencyclidine is rapidly absorbed from intestines. Overtreating the mild intoxication should be avoided. There is insufficient evidence to support the use of MDAC. In cases of severe toxicity (stupor or coma), continuous gastric suction can be tried (with protection of the airway) because the drug is secreted into the gastric juice. The value of this procedure is controversial because of limited data.

The patient must be protected from harming himself or herself or others. Physical restraints may be necessary, but they should be used sparingly and for the shortest time possible because they increase risk of rhabdomyolysis. Metal restraints such as handcuffs should be avoided. For behavioral disorders and toxic psychosis, diazepam is the agent of choice. Pharmacologic intervention includes diazepam (Valium) 10 to 30 mg orally or 2 to 5 mg intravenously initially and titrated upward to 10 mg; however, up to 30 mg may be required. "Talk down" technique is usually ineffective and dangerous. Phenothiazines and butyrophenones should be avoided in the acute phase because they lower the convulsive threshold; however, they may be needed later for psychosis. Haloperidol (Haldol) administration has been reported to produce catatonia.

Seizures and muscle spasm are managed with diazepam, from 2.5 mg up to 10 mg. Hyperthermia (>38.5°C [101.3°F]) is treated with external cooling measures. Hypertension is usually transient and does not require treatment. In the case of emergent hypertensive crisis (blood pressure >200/115 mm Hg) nitroprusside can be used in a dose of 0.3 to 2 µg/kg/min. Maximum infusion rate is 10 µg/kg/min for only 10 minutes.

Acid ion trapping diuresis is not recommended because of the danger of myoglobin precipitation in the renal tubules. Rhabdomyolysis and myoglobinuria are treated by correcting volume depletion and insuring a urinary output of greater than 2 mL/kg/h. Alkalinization is controversial because of reabsorption of phencyclidine.

Hemodialysis is beneficial if renal failure occurs; otherwise, the extracorporeal procedures are not beneficial.

Disposition

All patients with coma, delirium, catatonia, violent behavior, aspiration pneumonia, sustained hypertension greater than 200/115, and significant rhabdomyolysis should be admitted to the intensive care unit until asymptomatic for at least 24 hours. If patients with mild intoxication are mentally and neurologically stable and become asymptomatic (except for nystagmus) for 4 hours, they may be discharged in the company of a responsible adult. All patients must be assessed for suicide risk before discharge. Drug counseling and psychiatric follow-up should be arranged. Patients should be warned that episodes of disorientation and depression may continue intermittently for 4 weeks or more.

PHENOTHIAZINES AND NONPHENOTHIAZINES (NEUROLEPTICS)

Toxic Mechanism

Neuroleptics have complex mechanisms of toxicity, including (a) block of the postsynaptic dopamine receptors; (b) block of peripheral and central α-adrenergic receptors; (c) block of cholinergic muscarinic receptors; (d) quinidine-like antidysrhythmic and myocardial depressant effect in cases of large overdose; (e) lowering of the convulsive threshold; (f) effect on hypothalamic temperature regulation (Table 25).

Toxic Dose

Extrapyramidal reactions, anticholinergic effects, and orthostatic hypotension may occur at therapeutic doses. The toxic amount is not established, but the maximum daily therapeutic dose may result in significant side effects, and twice this amount may be potentially fatal. Chlorpromazine (Thorazine), the prototype, may produce serious hypotension and CNS depression at doses greater than 200 mg (17 mg/kg) in children and 3 to 5 g in an adult. Fatalities have been reported after 2.5 g of loxapine (Loxitane) and mesoridazine (Serentil) and 1.5 g of thioridazine (Mellaril).

Kinetics

These agents are lipophilic and have unpredictable gastrointestinal absorption. Peak levels occur 2 to 6 hours postingestion and have enterohepatic recirculation.

The mean serum half-life in phase 1 is 1 to 2 hours and the biphasic half-life is 20 to 40 hours. Volume distribution is 10 to 40 L/kg; protein binding is 92% to 98%. Chlorpromazine taken orally has an onset of

TABLE 25 Neuroleptics and Properties

Compound	Antipsychotic	Anticholinergic	Extrapyramidal	Hypotensive and cardiotoxic	Sedative
Phenothiazine					
Aliphatic	1+	3+	2+	2+	3+
Chlorpromazine (Thorazine)					
Promethazine (Phenergan)					
Piperazine	3+	1+	3+	1+	1+
Fluphenazine (Prolixin)					
Perphenazine (Trilafon)					
Prochlorperazine (Compazine)					
Trifluoperazine (Stelazine)					
Piperidine	1+	2+	1+	3+	3+
Mesoridazine (Serentil)					
Thioridazine (Mellaril)					
Nonphenothiazine					
Butyrophenone	3+	1+	3+	1+	1+
Haloperidol (Haldol)					
Dibenzoxazepine	3+	1+	3+	1+	2+
Loxapine (Loxitane)					
Dihydroindolone	3+	1+	3+	1+	1+
Molindone (Moban)					
Thioxanthenes	3+	1+	3+	3+	1+
Thiothixene (Navane)					
Chlorprothixene (Taractan)					

1+ = very low activity; 2+ = moderate activity; 3+ = very high activity.

18

action in 30 to 60 minutes, peak in 2 to 4 hours, and duration of 4 to 6 hours. With sustained-release preparations, the onset is in 30 to 60 minutes and duration is 6 to 12 hours.

Elimination is by hepatic metabolism, which results in multiple metabolites (some are active). Metabolites can be detected in urine months after chronic therapy. Only 1% to 3% is excreted unchanged in the urine.

Manifestations

In cases of phenothiazine overdose, anticholinergic symptoms may be present early but are not life-threatening. Miosis is usually present (80%) if the phenothiazine has strong α-adrenergic blocking effect (e.g., chlorpromazine), but anticholinergic activity mydriasis may occur. Agitation and delirium rapidly progress into coma. Major problems are cardiac toxicity and hypotension. The cardiotoxic effects are seen more commonly with thioridazine and its metabolite mesoridazine. These agents have produced the largest number of fatalities in patients with phenothiazine overdose. Cardiac conduction disturbances include prolonged PR, QRS, and QTc intervals, U- and T-wave abnormalities, and ventricular dysrhythmias, including torsades de pointes. Seizures occur mainly in patients with convulsive disorders or with administration of loxapine. Sudden death in children and adults has been reported.

Idiosyncratic dystonic reactions are most common with the piperidine group. Reactions are not dose-dependent and consist of opisthotonos, torticollis, orolingual dyskinesia, or oculogyric crisis (painful upward gaze). These reactions are more frequent in children and women. Neuroleptic malignant syndrome occurs in patients on chronic therapy and is characterized by hyperthermia, muscle rigidity, autonomic dysfunction, and altered mental state. There is one case reported with acute overdose. The loxapine syndrome consists of seizures, rhabdomyolysis, and renal failure.

Laboratory Investigations

Monitoring should include arterial blood gases, renal and hepatic function, electrolytes, blood glucose, and creatine kinase and myoglobinemia in neurol-eptic malignant syndrome. Most of these agents are detected on routine screening. Quantitative serum levels are not useful in management. Cross-reactions with enzyme multiplied immunoassay technique tests occur with cyclic antidepressants. Phenothiazines give false-negative results on pregnancy urine tests using human chorionic gonadotropin as an indicator, and give false-positive results for urine porphyrins, indirect Coombs test, urobilinogen, and amylase.

Management

Vital functions must be established and maintained. All overdose patients require venous access, 12-lead ECG (to measure intervals), cardiac and respiratory monitoring, and seizure precautions. One should monitor core temperature to detect poikilothermic effect. If the patient is comatose, intubation and assisted ventilation may be required, as well as 100% oxygen, intravenous glucose, naloxone (Narcan), and thiamine.

Emesis is not recommended. Activated charcoal can be administered if ingestion was within 1 hour. MDAC has not been proven beneficial. A radiograph of the abdomen may be useful, if the phenothiazine is radiopaque. Haloperidol (Haldol) and trifluoperazine (Stelazine) are most likely to be radiopaque. Whole-bowel irrigation may be useful when a large number of pills are visualized on radiograph or if sustained-release preparations were taken, but whole-bowel irrigation has not been evaluated in patients with phenothiazine overdose.

Convulsions are treated with diazepam or lorazepam (Ativan). Loxapine (Loxitane) overdose may result in status epilepticus. If nondepolarizing neuromuscular blockade is required, pancuronium (Pavulon) or vecuronium (Norcuron) should be used (not succinylcholine [Anectine], which may cause malignant hyperthermia), and EEG should be monitored during paralysis.

Patients with dysrhythmias should be monitored with serial ECGs. Unstable rhythms can be treated with electrical cardioversion. Class 1a antidysrhythmics (procainamide, quinidine, and disopyramide [Norpace]) must be avoided.

Hypokalemia predisposes to dysrhythmias and should be corrected aggressively. Supraventricular tachycardia with hemodynamic instability is treated with electrical cardioversion. The role of adenosine has not been defined. Calcium channel and β-blockers should be avoided.

Prolongation of the QRS interval is treated with sodium bicarbonate 1 to 2 mEq/kg by intravenous bolus over a few minutes. Torsades de pointes is treated with magnesium sulfate IV 20% solution 2 g over 2 to 3 minutes. If there is no response in 10 minutes, the dose is repeated and followed by a continuous infusion of 5 to 10 mg/min or given as an infusion of 50 mg/minute for 2 hours followed by 30 mg/minute for 90 minutes twice a day for several days, as needed. The dose in children is 25 to 50 mg/kg initially and maintenance dose is 30 to 60 mg/kg per 24 hours (0.25 to 0.50 mEq/kg per 24 hours) up to 1000 mg per 24 hours. Serum magnesium levels should be monitored.

To treat ventricular tachydysrhythmias in a stable patient, lidocaine is used. If the patient is unstable, electrical cardioversion is used. Patients with heart block with hemodynamic instability should be managed with temporary cardiac pacing.

Hypotension is treated with the Trendelenburg position and 0.9% saline. If the condition is refractory to treatment or there is a danger of fluid overload, vasopressors are administered. The vasopressor of choice is α-adrenergic agonist norepinephrine (Levophed), titrated to response. Epinephrine and dopamine should not be used because β-receptor stimulation in the presence of α-receptor blockade may provoke dysrhythmias and phenothiazines are antidopaminergic.

Hypothermia and hyperthermia are treated with external warming and cooling measures, respectively. Antipyretic drugs must not be used.

Management of the neuroleptic malignant syndrome includes the following actions:

- Immediately discontinuing the offending agent
- Hyperventilating the patient, using 100% humidified, cooled oxygen at high gas flows (at least 10 L/min) because of rapid breathing
- Administering a benzodiazepine to control convulsions and facilitate cooling measures
- Initiating appropriate mechanical cooling measures, which may include intravenous cold saline (not lactated Ringer's), ice baths, cold lavage of the stomach, bladder, and rectum, and a hypothermic blanket
- Correcting acid–base and electrolyte disturbances and treating significant hyperkalemia with hyperventilation, calcium, sodium bicarbonate, intravenous glucose, and insulin; hemodialysis may be necessary

In addition, dysrhythmias usually respond to correction of the underlying acid–base disturbances and hyperkalemia. If antidysrhythmic agents are required, calcium channel blockers must be avoided because they may precipitate hyperkalemia and cardiovascular collapse. Dantrolene sodium (Dantrium), which is a phenytoin derivative, inhibits calcium release from the sarcoplasmic reticulum and results in decreased muscle contraction. Dantrolene acts peripherally and does not reverse the rigidity or psychomotor disturbances resulting from the central dopamine blockade; it therefore is often used in combination with bromocriptine. Bromocriptine mesylate (Parlodel) acts centrally as a dopamine agonist, as does amantadine hydrochloride (Symmetrel). Bromocriptine and dantrolene have been reported to be successful in combination with cooling and good supportive measures in malignant hyperthermia.

Dosing for these agents is as follows: dantrolene sodium at 2 to 3 mg/kg IV as a bolus, then 1 mg/kg/minute to a maximum of 10 mg/kg or until the tachycardia, rigidity, increased end-tidal CO_2, and temperature elevation are controlled. *Note:* Hepatotoxicity occurs with doses greater than 10 mg/kg. To prevent symptom recurrence, 1 mg/kg should be administered every 6 hours for 24 to 48 hours after the episode. After that time, oral dantrolene can be used at a dose of 1 mg/kg every 6 hours for 24 hours as necessary. The patient should be observed for thrombophlebitis following intravenous dantrolene. It is best administered via a central line. Bromocriptine mesylate at 2.5 to 10 mg orally or via a nasogastric tube, three times a day, should be used in combination with dantrolene.

Rakel and Bope: *Conn's Current Therapy 2006.*

Idiosyncratic dystonic reaction can be treated with diphenhydramine (Benadryl) 1 to 2 mg/kg/dose intravenously over 5 minutes up to maximum of 50 mg intravenously; a response is noted within 2 to 5 minutes. This can be followed with oral doses for 4 to 6 days to prevent recurrence.

Extracorporeal measures (hemodialysis, hemoperfusion) are not effective in removing these agents.

Disposition

Asymptomatic patients should be observed for at least 6 hours after gastric decontamination. Symptomatic patients with cardiotoxicity, hypotension, and convulsions should be admitted to the intensive care unit and monitored for 48 hours.

SALICYLATES (ACETYLSALICYLIC ACID, SALICYLIC ACID)

Toxic Mechanism

The primary toxic mechanisms include (a) direct stimulation of the medullary chemoreceptor trigger zone and respiratory center; (b) uncoupling oxidative phosphorylation; (c) inhibition of the Krebs' cycle enzymes; (d) inhibition of vitamin K dependent and independent clotting factors; (e) alteration of platelet function; and (f) inhibition of prostaglandin synthesis.

Toxic Dose

Acute mild intoxication occurs at a dose of 150 to 200 mg/kg, moderate intoxication at 200 to 300 mg/kg, and severe intoxication at 300 to 500 mg/kg. Acute salicylate plasma concentration greater than 30 mg/dL (usually >40 mg/dL) may be associated with clinical toxicity. Chronic intoxication occurs at ingestions greater than 100 mg/kg/d for more than 2 days because of accumulation kinetics. Methyl salicylate (oil of wintergreen) is the most toxic form of salicylate. A dose of 1 mL of 98% contains 1.4 g of salicylate. Fatalities have occurred with ingestion of 1 teaspoonful in children and 1 ounce in adults. It is found in topical ointments and liniments (18% to 30%).

Kinetics

Acetylsalicylic acid and salicylic acid are weak acids with a pKa of 3.5 and 3.0, respectively. Acetylsalicylic acid is absorbed from the stomach, from the small bowel, and dermally. Onset of action is within 30 minutes. Methyl salicylate and effervescent tablets are absorbed more rapidly. Salicylate plasma concentration is detectable within 15 minutes after ingestion and peaks in 30 to 120 minutes. The peak may be delayed 6 to 12 hours in cases of large overdose, overdose with enteric-coated or sustained-release preparations, and development of concretions. The therapeutic duration of action is 3 to 4 hours but is markedly prolonged in cases of overdose.

Volume distribution is 0.13 L/kg for salicylic acid but increases as the salicylate plasma concentration

increases. Protein binding is greater than 90% for salicylic acid at pH 7.4 and a salicylate plasma concentration of 20 to 30 mg/dL, 75% at a salicylate plasma concentration greater than 40 mg/dL, 50% at a salicylate plasma concentration of 70 mg/dL, and 30% at a salicylate plasma concentration of 120 mg/dL.

The half-life for salicylic acid is 3 hours after a 300 mg dose, 6 hours after a 1 g overdose, and greater than 10 hours after a 10-g overdose. Elimination includes Michaelis-Menten hepatic metabolism by three saturable pathways: (a) glycine conjugation to salicyluric acid (75%); (b) glucuronyl transferase to salicyl phenol glucuronide (10%); and (c) salicyl aryl glucuronide (4%). Nonsaturable pathways are hydrolysis to gentisic acid (<1%). Ten percent is excreted unchanged.

Acidosis increases the severity of the intoxication by increasing the non-ionized salicylate that can cross membranes and enter the brain cells. In kidneys, the un-ionized salicylic acid undergoes glomerular filtration, and the ionized portion undergoes tubular secretion in proximal tubules and passive reabsorption in the distal tubules. Renal excretion of salicylate is enhanced by alkaline urine.

Manifestations

The ingestion of concentrated topical salicylic acid preparations (e.g., wart remover) can cause mucosal caustic injury to the gastrointestinal tract. Occult salicylate overdose should be considered in any patient with unexplained acid–base disturbance.

The manifestations of acute overdose of salicylates are as follows:

Minimal Symptoms

Tinnitus, dizziness, and deafness may occur at high therapeutic salicylate plasma concentrations of 20 to 30 mg/dL. Nausea and vomiting may occur immediately because of local gastric irritation.

Phase I. Mild manifestations occur at 1 to 12 hours after ingestion with a 6-hour salicylate plasma concentration of 45 to 70 mg/dL. Nausea and vomiting followed by hyperventilation are usually present within 3 to 8 hours after acute overdose. Hyperventilation, an increase in both rate (tachypnea) and depth (hyperpnea), is present but it may be subtle. It results in a mild respiratory alkalosis with a serum pH greater than 7.4 and urine pH greater than 6.0. Some patients may have lethargy, vertigo, headache, and confusion. Diaphoresis may be noted.

Phase II. Moderate manifestations occur at 12 to 24 hours after ingestion with a 6-hour salicylate plasma concentration of 70 to 90 mg/dL. Serious metabolic disturbances, including a marked respiratory alkalosis with anion gap metabolic acidosis, dehydration, and urine pH less than 6.0, may occur. Other metabolic disturbances include hypoglycemia or hyperglycemia, hypokalemia, decreased ionized calcium, and increased BUN, creatinine, and lactate. Mental disturbances (confusion, disorientation, hallucinations) may occur. Hypotension and convulsions have been reported.

Phase III. Severe intoxication occurs more than 24 hours after ingestion with a 6-hour salicylate plasma concentration of 90 to 130 mg/dL. In addition to the above clinical findings, coma and seizures develop and indicate severe intoxication. Pulmonary edema may occur. Metabolic disturbances include metabolic acidemia (pH <7.4) and aciduria (pH <6.0). In adults, alkalosis may persist until terminal respiratory failure.

In children younger than 4 years of age, a mixed metabolic acidosis and respiratory alkalosis develop earlier (within 4 to 6 hours) than in adults because children have less respiratory reserve and accumulate lactate and other organic acids. Hypoglycemia is more common in children.

Fatalities occur at 6-hour salicylate plasma concentrations greater than 130 to 150 mg/dL and result from CNS depression, cardiovascular collapse, electrolyte imbalance, and cerebral edema.

Chronic salicylism is more serious than acute intoxication and the 6-hour salicylate plasma concentration does not correlate well with the manifestations in both acute and chronic cases of intoxication. Chronic intoxication usually occurs with therapeutic errors in young children or the elderly with underlying illness, and the diagnosis is delayed because it is not recognized. Noncardiac pulmonary edema is a frequent complication in the elderly. The mortality rate is about 25%. Chronic salicylate poisoning in children may mimic Reye syndrome. It is associated with exaggerated CNS findings (hallucinations, delirium, dementia, memory loss, papilledema, bizarre behavior, agitation, encephalopathy, seizures, and coma). Hemorrhagic manifestations, renal failure, and pulmonary and cerebral edema may occur. The metabolic picture is hypoglycemia and mixed acid–base derangements. A chronic salicylate plasma concentration greater than 60 mg/dL with metabolic acidosis and an altered mental state is very serious.

Laboratory Investigations

All patients with intentional salicylate overdoses should have acetaminophen plasma level measured after 4 hours.

One should continuously monitor ECG, urine output, urine pH, and specific gravity. Every 2 to 4 hours in cases of severe intoxication, salicylate plasma concentration, glucose (in a case of salicylism, CNS hypoglycemia may be present despite normal serum glucose), electrolytes, ionized calcium, magnesium and phosphorous, anion gap, ABGs, and pulse oximeter should be monitored. Daily monitoring of BUN, creatinine, liver function tests, and prothrombin time should take place.

The therapeutic salicylate plasma concentration is less than 10 mg/dL for analgesia and 15 to 30 mg/dL for anti-inflammatory effect. Cross-reaction with diflunisal (Dolobid) will give a falsely high salicylate plasma concentration. The Done nomogram is not considered accurate in evaluating acute or chronic salicylate intoxications.

Management

Treatment is based on clinical and metabolic findings, not on salicylate levels. Continuous monitoring of the urine pH is essential for successful alkalinization treatment. One should always obtain an acetaminophen plasma level.

Vital functions must be established and maintained. If the patient is in an altered mental state, glucose, naloxone, and thiamine are administered in standard doses. Depending on the severity, the initial studies include an immediate and a 6-hour postingestion salicylate plasma concentration, ECG and cardiac monitoring, pulse oximeter, urine (analysis, pH, and specific gravity), chest radiograph, ABGs, blood glucose, electrolytes and anion gap calculation, calcium (ionized), magnesium, renal and liver profiles, and prothrombin time. Gastric contents and stool should be tested for occult blood. Bismuth and magnesium salicylate preparations may be radiopaque on radiographs. Consultation with a nephrologist is warranted in cases of moderate, severe, or chronic intoxication.

For gastrointestinal decontamination, activated charcoal is useful (each gram of activated charcoal binds 550 mg of salicylic acid) if a toxic dose was ingested up to 4 hours postingestion. MDAC is not recommended for salicylate intoxication.

Concretions may occur with massive (usually >300 mg/kg) ingestions. If blood levels fail to decline, prompt contrast radiography of the stomach may reveal concretions that have to be removed by repeated lavage, whole-bowel irrigation, endoscopy, or gastrostomy.

Fluids and electrolyte treatment of salicylate poisonings is given in Table 26. For shock, perfusion and vascular volume should be established with 5% dextrose in 0.9% saline, then the treatment can proceed with correction of dehydration and alkalinization.

For cases of acute moderate or severe salicylism (see Table 26), adults should receive a bolus of 1 to 2 mEq/kg of sodium bicarbonate ($NaHCO_3$) followed by an infusion of 100 to 150 mEq $NaHCO_3$ added to 500 to 1000 mL of 5% dextrose and administered over 60 minutes. Children should receive a bolus of 1 to 2 mEq/kg of $NaHCO_3$ followed by an infusion of 1 to 2 mEq/kg added to 20 mL/kg of 5% dextrose administered over 60 minutes. Potassium is added after the patient voids. The goal is to achieve a urine output of greater than 2 mL/kg/hr and a urine pH of greater than 8. The initial infusion is followed by subsequent infusions (two to three times normal maintenance) of 200 to 300 mL/h in adults or 10 mL/kg/h in children. If the patient is acidotic and has a serum pH of less than 7.15, an additional 1 to 2 mEq/kg of $NaHCO_3$ is given over 1 to 2 hours; persistent acidosis may require 1 to 2 mEq/kg of bicarbonate every 2 hours. The infusion rate, the amount of bicarbonate, and the electrolytes should be adjusted to correct serum abnormalities and to maintain the targeted urine output and urinary pH. Diuresis is not as important as the alkalinization. Careful monitoring for fluid overload should take place for patients at risk of pulmonary and cerebral edema (e.g., the elderly)

Rakel and Bope: *Conn's Current Therapy 2006.*

TABLE 26 Fluid and Electrolyte Treatment of Salicylate Poisoning

Type of salicylism	Metabolic disturbance	Blood pH	Urine pH	Hydrating solution	Amount of NaHCO₃ (mEq/L)	Amount of potassium (mEq/L)
Mild	Respiratory alkalosis	>7.4	>6.0	5% Dextrose, 0.45% saline	50 (adult) 1 mEq/kg (child)	20
Moderate Chronic Child <4 Years	Respiratory alkalosis Metabolic acidosis	>7.4 or <7.4	<6.0	5% Dextrose in water	100 (adult) 1-2 mEq/kg (child)	40
Severe Chronic Child <4 years	Metabolic acidosis Respiratory alkalosis	<7.4	<6.0	5% Dextrose in water	150 (adult) 2m Eq/kg (child)	60
CNS depressant co-ingestant	Respiratory acidosis	<7.4	<6.0	5% Dextrose in water	100-150*	60

*Correct hypoventilation.
Modified from Linden CH, Rumack BH: The legitimate analgesics, aspirin and acetaminophen. In Hansen W Jr (ed): Toxic Emergencies. New York, Churchill Livingstone, 1984.

and because of inappropriate secretion of the antidiuretic hormone.

In patients with mild intoxication who are not acidotic and have a urine pH greater than 6, 5% dextrose in 0.45% saline should be administered as maintenance to replace ongoing fluid loss. Some toxicologists may consider adding sodium bicarbonate 50 mEq/L or 1 mEq/kg in some cases.

To achieve alkalinization, sodium bicarbonate is administered to produce a serum pH 7.4 to 7.5 and a urine pH greater than 8. Carbonic anhydrase inhibitors (acetazolamide [Diamox]) should not be used. If the patient is acidotic, additional bicarbonate may be required. About 2 mEq/kg raises the blood pH 0.1. In children, alkalinization may be a difficult problem because of the organic acid production and hypokalemia. Hypokalemic and fluid-depleted patients cannot be adequately alkalinized. Alkalinization is usually discontinued in asymptomatic patients with a salicylate plasma concentration less than 30 to 40 mg/dL but is continued in symptomatic patients regardless of the salicylate plasma concentration. A decreased serum bicarbonate but normal or high blood pH indicates respiratory alkalosis predominating over metabolic acidosis, and the bicarbonate should be administered cautiously. An alkalemic pH of 7.40 to 7.50 is not a contraindication to bicarbonate therapy because these patients have a significant base deficit in spite of elevated blood pH.

Potassium is added, 20 to 40 mEq/L, to the infusion after the patient voids. In cases of severe, late, and chronic salicylism, 60 mEq/L of potassium may be needed. When the serum potassium is below 4.0 mEq/L, 10 mEq/L should be added over the first hour. If the patient has hypokalemia less than 3 mEq/L and flat T waves and U waves, 0.25 to 0.5 mEq/kg up to 10 mEq/h is administered. Potassium should be administered under ECG monitoring. Serum potassium is rechecked after each rapidly administered dose. A paradoxical

urine acidosis (alkaline serum pH and acid urine pH) indicates that potassium is probably needed.

Convulsions are treated with diazepam or lorazepam, but hypoglycemia, low ionized calcium, cerebral edema, and hemorrhage should first be excluded with a CT scan. If tetany develops, the NaHCO₃ therapy is discontinued and calcium gluconate 0.1 to 0.2 mL/kg 10% administered.

Pulmonary edema management consists of fluid restriction, high FIO₂, mechanical ventilation, and positive end-expiratory pressure.

Cerebral edema management consists of fluid restriction, elevation of the head, hyperventilation, osmotic diuresis, and administration of dexamethasone. Vitamin K₁ is administered parenterally to correct an increased prothrombin time (>20 seconds) and coagulation abnormalities. If the patient has active bleeding, fresh plasma and platelets are administered as needed. Hyperpyrexia is managed by external cooling measures, not antipyretics.

Hemodialysis is the choice for removal of salicylates because it corrects the acid–base, electrolyte, and fluid disturbances as well. The indications for hemodialysis include the following:

- Acute poisoning with salicylate plasma concentration greater than 100 mg/dL without improvement after 6 hours of appropriate therapy
- Chronic poisoning with cardiopulmonary disease and a salicylate plasma concentration as low as 40 mg/dL with refractory acidosis, severe CNS manifestations (coma and seizures), and progressive deterioration, especially in elderly patients
- Impairment of vital organs of elimination
- Clinical deterioration in spite of good supportive care and alkalinization
- Severe refractory acid–base or electrolyte disturbances despite appropriate corrective measures

Disposition

There are limitations of salicylate plasma levels and patients are treated on the basis of clinical and laboratory findings. Patients who are asymptomatic should be monitored for a minimum of 6 hours, and longer if enteric-coated tablets or massive overdose was taken or if there is suspicion of concretions. Those who remain asymptomatic with a salicylate plasma concentration less than 35 mg/dL may be discharged following psychiatric evaluation, if indicated. Chronic salicylate-intoxicated patients with acidosis and an altered mental state should be admitted to the intensive care unit. Patients with acute ingestion and a salicylate plasma concentration less than 60 mg/dL and mild symptoms may be able to be treated in the emergency department. Patients with moderate and severe intoxications should be admitted to the intensive care unit.

SELECTIVE SEROTONIN REUPTAKE INHIBITORS

Selective serotonin reuptake inhibitors (SSRIs) are primarily prescribed as antidepressants. SSRIs include fluoxetine (Prozac), paroxetine (Paxil), and sertraline (Zoloft).

Toxic Mechanism

The SSRIs interfere with the neuron reuptake of serotonin (5-hydroxytryptamine) at the presynaptic ganglia sites in the brain, increasing the activity of serotonin. SSRIs should not be used within 5 weeks of when a MAOI is given, nor should MAOI therapy be initiated or discontinued within 5 weeks of SSRI therapy.

Toxic Dose

The therapeutic oral dose of fluoxetine is 20 to 80 mg/d. No toxicity is seen in children with up to 3.5 mg/kg/dose orally. A fatal dose for adults is 6 g. The therapeutic dose for paroxetine is 20 to 50 mg/d. In 35 adult patients, none developed serious side effects after the ingestion of 10 to 1000 mg, and a study involving 35 children failed to demonstrate serious adverse effects at doses less than 180 mg. The therapeutic dose for sertraline is 50 mg to 200 mg/d. Patients have ingested up to 2.6 g without serious side effects. Overdose involving children who ingested less than 100 mg failed to cause adverse events.

Kinetics

Fluoxetine is well absorbed from the gastrointestinal tract, and has a peak plasma concentration at 6 to 8 hours. Volume distribution is 20 to 42 L/kg; 95% is protein bound. The half-life is 4 days (for the demethylated active metabolite norfluoxetine, the half-life is 7 to 15 days). Elimination is 80% renal. Fluoxetine and other serotonin inhibitors are inhibitors of the cytochrome P450, CYP 2D6 enzyme. Therefore interactions may occur with many other medications, such as antidysrhythmic class IC drugs (quinidine), phenytoin (Dilantin), haloperidol, lithium, tricyclic antidepressants (TCAs), β-blockers, codeine, and carbamazepine (Tegretol).

Paroxetine is almost completely absorbed from the gastrointestinal tract, with a peak in 2 to 8 hours. Protein binding is greater than 90%; volume distribution is 13 L/kg. Paroxetine undergoes extensive first-pass liver metabolism by oxidation and methylation to inactive metabolites. It inhibits the P450 system (see fluoxetine metabolism). The average half-life is 21 hours.

Sertraline peaks in 8 to 12 hours. Its volume distribution is 20 L/kg and protein binding is 98%. The average half-life of sertraline is 26 hours. It is metabolized to form a less-active metabolite, N-desmethylsertraline (half-life of 62 to 104 hours).

Manifestations

All SSRIs may cause serotonin syndrome, a potentially life-threatening reaction, if they are administered concurrently with an MAOI. Serotonin syndrome is caused by cerebral serotonergic stimulation and can cause severe hyperthermia, myoclonus, rhabdomyolysis, confusion, tremors, and a variety of psychological disturbances. In addition, cardiovascular complications and extrapyramidal side effects, including akathisia, dyskinesia, and Parkinson-like syndromes may occur. Also, increased suicidal ideation, seizures, sexual disorders, and hematologic disorders (platelet serotonin activity blockade leading to prolonged bleeding times) may develop. Inappropriate secretion of antidiuretic hormone resulting in hyponatremia may occur when SSRIs are administered to the elderly. This effect is usually seen within the first week of therapy.

Overdose effects are similar to the serotonin syndrome.

Laboratory Investigations

One should obtain a complete blood count (CBC), electrolytes, glucose levels, a coagulation profile, liver function tests, creatine kinase level, and an ECG.

Management

There is no specific antidote to SSRI intoxication.

Initial management consists of stabilizing vital functions, including thermoregulation. Supportive therapy and anticipation of potential life-threatening manifestations (hypotension, hyperthermia, seizures, coma, disseminated intravascular coagulation, ventricular tachycardia, and metabolic acidosis), are essential. Vital signs, EEG, creatine kinase, and blood chemistry should be monitored.

Benzodiazepines are administered to prevent and control muscle hyperactivity (diazepam [Valium] for seizures, clonazepam [Klonopin] for myoclonus). If benzodiazepine therapy fails to control muscle activity or seizures, anesthesia or nondepolarizing neuromuscular blockade may be necessary.

Rakel and Bope: Conn's Current Therapy 2006.

Electrolyte abnormalities and acid–base balance should be corrected. Fluids are used to maintain a urine output of greater than 2 mL/kg/h if there is a risk of myoglobinuria.

There are no data to support the use of gastrointestinal decontamination, although activated charcoal may be used if an ingestion has occurred within 1 hour. Hemodialysis and charcoal hemoperfusion are unlikely to be beneficial. Haloperidol (Haldol), phenothiazines, and other highly protein-bound drugs are to be avoided.

Benzodiazepine and cooling therapy can be used for hyperthermia. Serotonin antagonists, such as cyproheptadine (Periactin), may be useful in treating serotonin syndrome, although there are no controlled data. Dantrolene (Dantrium) and bromocriptine (Parlodel) are not recommended and may actually precipitate serotonin syndrome.

Disposition

Cases of ingestions in children up to 5 years of age of less than 180 mg of paroxetine (Paxil), less than 3.5 mg/kg of fluoxetine (Prozac), or less than 100 mg of sertraline (Zoloft) can be observed at home. Symptomatic patients should be admitted to the intensive care unit until asymptomatic for 24 hours. Asymptomatic patients should be observed for 6 hours. All patients should be assessed for risk of suicide before discharge. When taken chronically, SSRIs may increase cholesterol and triglycerides and decrease uric acid, so these test results should be followed.

THEOPHYLLINE

Theophylline (Slo-Phyllin) is a methylxanthine alkaloid similar to caffeine and theobromine. Aminophylline is 80% theophylline. Theophylline is used in the acute treatment of asthma, pulmonary edema, chronic obstructive pulmonary disease, and neonatal apnea.

Toxic Mechanism

The proposed mechanisms of action include phosphodiesterase inhibition, adenosine receptor antagonism, inhibition of prostaglandins, and increase in serum catecholamines. Theophylline stimulates the central nervous, respiratory, and emetic centers and reduces the seizure threshold. It has positive cardiac inotropic and chronotropic effects, acts as a diuretic, relaxes smooth muscle, and causes peripheral vasodilation but cerebral vasoconstriction. Gastric secretions, gastrointestinal motility, lipolysis, glycogenolysis, and gluconeogenesis are all increased.

Toxic Dose

A single dose of 1 mg/kg produces a theophylline plasma concentration of approximately 2 µg/mL. The therapeutic range usually is 10 to 20 µg/mL. An acute, single dose greater than 10 mg/kg causes mild toxicity, a dose greater than 20 mg/kg causes moderate toxicity, and a dose greater than 50 mg/kg causes serious, possibly

fatal toxicity. Fatalities occur at lower doses in patients with chronic toxicity, especially those with risk factors (see *Kinetics*).

Kinetics

The pKa is 9.5. Absorption from the stomach and upper small intestine is complete and rapid, with onset in 30 to 60 minutes. Peak theophylline plasma concentration occurs within 1 to 2 hours after ingestion of liquid preparations, 2 to 4 hours after ingestion of regular tablets, and 7 to 24 hours after ingestion of slow-release formulations. Volume distribution is 0.3 to 0.7 L/kg. Protein binding is 40% to 60% in adults, mainly to albumin (low albumin increases free active theophylline).

Elimination is 90% by hepatic metabolism to an active metabolite, 2-methyl xanthine. The half-life is 3.5 hours in a child and 4 to 6 hours in an adult. The half-life is shorter in smokers and patients taking enzyme-inducing drugs. Only 8% to 10% of the drug is excreted unchanged in the urine.

Risk factors that produce a longer half-life include age younger than 6 months or older than 60 years, use of enzyme-inhibitor drugs (calcium channel blockers, oral contraceptives, cimetidine [Tagamet], ciprofloxacin [Cipro], erythromycin, macrolide anti-biotics, isoniazid), illness (persistent fever >38.9°C [>102°F]), viral illness, liver impairment, heart failure, chronic obstructive pulmonary disease, and influenza vaccination.

Manifestations

Acute toxicity generally correlates with blood levels; chronic toxicity does not (Table 27).

In the case of an acute, single, regular-release overdose, vomiting and occasionally hematemesis occur at low theophylline plasma concentrations. CNS stimulation includes restlessness, muscle tremors, and protracted tonic–clonic seizures, but coma is rare. Convulsions are a sign of severe toxicity and usually are preceded by gastrointestinal symptoms (except with sustained-release and chronic intoxications). Cardiovascular disturbances include cardiac dysrhythmias (supraventricular tachycardia) and transient hypertension with mild overdoses, but hypotension and ventricular dysrhythmias with severe intoxications. Rhabdomyolysis and renal failure are occasionally seen. Children tolerate higher serum levels, and cardiac dysrhythmias and seizures occur at theophylline plasma concentrations greater than 100 µg/mL. Possible metabolic disturbances include hyperglycemia, pronounced hypokalemia, hypocalcemia, hypomagnesemia, hypophosphatemia, increased serum amylase, and elevation of uric acid.

Chronic intoxication, defined as multiple doses of theophylline over 24 hours, or cases in which interacting drugs or illness interfere with theophylline metabolism are more serious and difficult to treat. Cardiac dysrhythmias and convulsions may occur at theophylline plasma concentrations of 40 to 60 µg/mL and there is no correlation with TPC. The seizures occur without warning and are protracted and repetitive and

Table 27 Theophylline Blood Concentrations and Acute Toxicity

Plasma concentration (μg/mL)	Toxicity degree	Manifestations
8-10	None	Bronchodilation
10-20	Mild	Therapeutic range: nausea, vomiting, nervousness, respiratory alkalosis, tachycardia
15-25		35% have mild manifestations of toxicity
20-40	Moderate	Gastrointestinal complaints and central nervous system stimulation
		Transient hypertension, tachypnea, tachycardia; 80% will have some manifestations of toxicity
60	Severe	Convulsions, dysrhythmias
100		Hypokalemia, hyperglycemia
		Ventricular dysrhythmias, protracted convulsions, hypotension, acid–base abnormalities

Reprinted and modified from Linden CH, Rumack BH, In Toxic Emergencies (Honser W Jr [ed]): The legitimate analgesics, aspirin and acetaminophen, copyright 1984, with permission from Elsevier.

may produce status epilepticus. Vomiting and typical metabolic disturbances do not occur.

Differences with slow-release preparations are that few or no gastrointestinal symptoms occur, peak concentrations and convulsions may be delayed 12 to 24 hours postingestion, and convulsions occur without warning.

Laboratory Investigations

Monitoring includes vital signs, pulse oximeter, ABG, hemoglobin, hematocrit (for gastrointestinal hemorrhage), ECG and cardiac monitor, renal and hepatic function, electrolytes, blood glucose, acid–base balance, and serum albumin. Gastric contents and stools should be tested for occult blood. Samples for theophylline plasma concentration measurement should be drawn within 1 to 2 hours after ingestion of liquid preparations, 2 to 4 hours after ingestion of regular-release formulations, and 4 hours after ingestion of slow-release formulations. One should check the serum albumin level because a decrease in albumin levels may cause manifestations of toxicity despite normal theophylline plasma concentration. A single theophylline plasma concentration reading may be misleading; therefore,

theophylline plasma concentration measurement should be repeated every 2 to 4 hours to determine the trend until a declining trend is reached and then monitored every 4 to 6 hours until it is below 20 μg/mL.

Management

Vital functions must be established and maintained. If the patient is in a coma or has convulsions or vomiting, he or she should be intubated immediately. The theophylline plasma concentration is obtained and repeated every 2 to 4 hours to determine peak absorption, and a theophylline bezoar should be considered if the theophylline plasma concentration fails to decline. Consultation with a nephrologist about charcoal hemoperfusion is recommended.

Gastrointestinal decontamination is warranted in the case of an acute overdose, but emesis must not be induced. Activated charcoal is the choice decontamination procedure in a dose of 1 g/kg to all patients, followed with MDAC 0.5 g/kg every 2 to 4 hours until the theophylline plasma concentration is less than 20 μg/mL. MDAC is effective in treating acute, chronic, and intravenous overdoses. Activated charcoal shortens the half-life of theophylline by about 50% and may be indicated up to 24 hours following ingestion.

Whole-bowel irrigation with polyethylene-electrolyte solution has been recommended for cases of massive overdose, possible concretions, and ingestion of sustained-release preparations. If intractable vomiting occurs, the antiemetic metoclopramide (Reglan) (0.1 mg/kg adult dose), droperidol (Inapsine) (2.5 to 10 mg IV), or ondansetron (Zofran) (8 to 32 mg IV) is administered. Ondansetron, however, inhibits metabolism of theophylline after a few doses.

Convulsions are controlled with lorazepam (Ativan) or diazepam (Valium) and phenobarbital. Phenytoin (Dilantin) is ineffective. The convulsions in patients with chronic intoxication are often refractory and may require, in addition to anticonvulsants, neuromuscular paralyzing agents, sedation, assisted ventilation, and EEG monitoring.

Hypotension is treated with fluids and vasopressors, if necessary. Norepinephrine (Levophed) 0.05 μg/kg/min is preferred as the vasopressor over dopamine.

Supraventricular tachycardia with hemodynamic instability requires cardioversion. Low-dose β-blockers may be used but should not be used in patients with reactive airway disease or hypotension. Adenosine (Adenocard) is ineffective. For ventricular dysrhythmias, electrolyte disturbances should be corrected. Lidocaine is the treatment of choice but has the potential to cause seizures at toxic concentrations. Cardioversion may be needed.

Hematemesis is managed with sucralfate (Carafate) 1 g four times daily and/or Maalox TC 30 mL every 2 hours and blood replacement, if necessary. H$_2$ antihistamine blockers that are enzyme inhibitors are not used.

Fluid and metabolic disturbances should be corrected. Hyperglycemia does not require insulin therapy. Hypokalemia should be corrected cautiously, as it may be largely an intracellular shift and not total body loss. Usually adding 40 mEq potassium to a liter of fluid will suffice. The serum potassium level must be monitored closely.

Charcoal hemoperfusion is the management of choice for patients with serious intoxications. Hemoperfusion can increase the clearance twofold to threefold over hemodialysis, but hemodialysis can be used if hemoperfusion is not available. Criteria for charcoal hemoperfusion are as follows:

- Life-threatening events such as convulsions or dysrhythmias
- Intractable vomiting refractory to antiemetics
- Acute intoxications with a theophylline plasma concentration greater than 80 μg/mL or greater than 70 μg/mL 4 hours after overdose with a sustained-release formulation and greater than 40 μg/mL in the case of chronic intoxication
- Acute or chronic overdoses with a theophylline plasma concentration greater than 40 μg/mL, especially if the patient has risk factors that lengthen the half-life of the drug (see Kinetics).

Disposition

Patients with mild symptoms and a theophylline plasma concentration less than 20 μg/mL can be treated in emergency department and discharged when asymptomatic for a few hours. Any patient with acute ingestion and a theophylline plasma concentration greater than 35 μg/mL should be admitted to a monitored bed with seizure precautions and suicide precautions, if needed. If neurologic or cardiotoxic effects or a theophylline plasma concentration greater than 50 μg/mL is present, the patient should be admitted to the intensive care unit. A patient with an overdose of a sustained-release preparation, regardless of symptoms or initial theophylline plasma concentration, requires admission, monitoring, activated charcoal, and MDAC. In patients on chronic therapy, toxicity may occur at a lower theophylline plasma concentration, and these patients should not be discharged until they are asymptomatic for several hours.

TRICYCLIC AND CYCLIC ANTIDEPRESSANTS

Historically, tricyclic antidepressants are an important cause of pharmaceutical overdose fatalities. The mortality rate was reduced from 15% in the 1970s to less than 1% in the 1990s because of a better understanding of the pathophysiology of these agents and improvements in management (Table 28).

Toxic Mechanism

The major mechanisms of toxicity of the tricyclic antidepressants are (a) central and peripheral anticholinergic effects; (b) peripheral α-adrenergic blockade; (c) quinidine-like cardiac membrane stabilizing action blockade of the fast inward sodium channels; and (d) inhibition of synaptic neurotransmitter reuptake in the CNS presynaptic neurons. The tetracyclics, monocyclic aminoketones, and dibenzoxazepines possess convulsive activity

and less cardiac toxicity in overdose than the older tricyclic antidepressants. Triazolopyridine has less serious cardiac and CNS toxicity.

Toxic Dose

The therapeutic dose of imipramine (Tofranil) is 1.5 to 5 mg/kg; a dose greater than 5 mg/kg may be mildly toxic; 10 to 20 mg/kg may be life threatening, although less than 20 mg/kg has produced few fatalities; greater than 30 mg/kg carries a 30% mortality rate; and at a dose greater than 70 mg/kg, patients rarely survive. In children 375 mg and in adults as little as 500 mg have been fatal. In adults, five times the maximum daily dose is toxic and 10 times is potentially fatal. Although major overdose symptoms are associated with plasma concentrations greater than 1 μg/mL (>1000 ng/mL), plasma tricyclic levels do not correlate well with toxicity; clinical signs and symptoms should guide therapy.

The relative dosage or potency equivalents are as follows: amitriptyline (Elavil) 100 mg = amoxapine (Asendin) 125 mg = desipramine (Norpramin) 75 mg = doxepin (Sinequan) 100 mg = imipramine (Tofranil) 75 mg = maprotiline (Ludiomil) 75 mg = nortriptyline (Pamelor) 50 mg = trazodone (Desyrel) 200 mg. This allows one to determine an equivalent dosage of an agent compared with another (see Table 28).

Kinetics

The tricyclic and cyclic antidepressants are lipophilic. They are rapidly absorbed from the alkaline small intestine, but absorption may be prolonged and delayed in cases of massive overdose owing to anticholinergic action. Onset varies from less than 1 hour (30 to 40 minutes) to, rarely, 12 hours. The peak serum levels are reached in 2 to 8 hours and the peak effect is in 6 hours but may be delayed 12 hours because of erratic absorption. The clinical effects correlate poorly with plasma levels.

Cyclic antidepressants are highly protein-bound to plasma glycoproteins, 98% at a pH 7.5 and 90% at 7.0. Volume distribution is 10 to 50 L/kg. The elimination route is by hepatic metabolism. The tertiary amines are metabolized into active demethylated secondary amine metabolites. The active secondary amine metabolites undergo a 15% enterohepatic recirculation and are metabolized over a period of days into nonactive metabolites. The intestinal bacterial flora may reconstitute the metabolites, which are active.

The half-life varies from 10 hours for imipramine to 81 hours for amitriptyline and 100 hours for nortriptyline. The active metabolites have longer half-lives.

Only 3% of the ingested dose is excreted in the urine unchanged.

Manifestations

There are reports of asymptomatic patients who, upon arrival to an emergency department, suddenly have a seizure, develop hemodynamically unstable dysrhythmias,

TABLE 28 Cyclic Antidepressants, Daily Dose and Their Major Properties

Generic name	Adult daily dose (mg)	Therapeutic range (ng/mL)	Half-life (hours)	Toxicity* Antichol	Toxicity* CNS	Toxicity* Cardiac
Tertiary Amines						
Amitriptyline (Elavil)	75-300	120-250	31-46	3+	3+	3+
Imipramine (Tofranil)	75-300	125-250	9-24	3+	3+	2+
Doxepin (Sinequan)	75-300	30-150	8-24	3+	3+	2+
Trimipramine (Surmantil)	75-200	10-240	16-18	3+	3+	2+
Secondary Amines						
Nortriptyline (Pamelor)	75-150	50-150	18-93	2+	3+	3+
Desipramine (Norpramin)	75-200	75-160	14-62	1+	3+	3+
Protriptyline (Vivactil)	20-60	70-250	54-198	2+	3+	3+
Newer Cyclic Antidepressants						
Teracyclic			30-60	1+	2+	3+
Maprotiline (Ludiomil)	75-300	—	30-60	1+	2+	3+
Trizolopyridine, a noncyclic, produces less serious cardiac and CNS toxicity						
Trazodone (Desyrel)	50-600	700	4-7	1+	1+	1+
Monocyclic Aminoketone						
Bupropion (Wellbutrin)	200-400	—	8-24	1+	3+	1+
Dibenzazepine						
Clomipramine (Anafranil)	100-250	200-500	21-32	2+	2+	2+
Dibenoxazepine						
Amoxapine (Ascendin)	150-300	200-500	6-10	1+	3+	2+

*Antichol = anticholinergic effect; CNS = central nervous system effect primarily seizures; Cardiac = cardiac effect.
Other drugs with similar structures are cyclobenzaprine, a muscle relaxant (similar to amitriptyline), and carbamazepine, an anticonvulsant (similar to imipramine); however, they cause less cardiac toxicity.

and die shortly thereafter from ingestion of a tricyclic antidepressant. Most patients with severe toxicity develop symptoms within 1 to 2 hours, but symptoms may be delayed 6 hours after overdose.

Small overdoses produce early anticholinergic effects, agitation, and transient hypertension, which are not life-threatening. Large overdoses produce depression of the CNS and myocardium, convulsions, and hypotension. Death can occur within the first 2 to 6 hours following ingestion.

Some ECG screening tools for predicting cardiac or neurologic toxicity from ingestion of a tricyclic antidepressant have been developed: (a) A QRS greater than 0.10 second may produce seizures, and if greater than 0.16 second, 50% of patients may develop ventricular dysrhythmias (20% of these may be life-threatening) and seizures; (b) a terminal 40 msec of the QRS axis greater than 120 degrees in the right frontal plane may be associated with toxicity; or (c) a large R wave greater than 3 mm in ECG lead aVR may predispose the patient to toxicity. The quinidine cardiac membrane stabilizing effect produces depression of myocardium, conduction, and ECG changes. The peripheral α-adrenergic blockade produces hypotension.

The secondary amines are metabolized to inactive metabolites. The tetracyclics produce a high incidence of cardiovascular disturbances and seizures. Monocyclic aminoketones produce seizures in doses greater than 600 mg. Dibenzoxazepines produce a syndrome of convulsions, rhabdomyolysis, and renal failure.

Laboratory Investigations

If the patient has altered mental status or ECG abnormalities, ABG, ECG, chest radiograph, blood glucose, serum electrolytes, calcium, magnesium, blood urea nitrogen, and creatinine levels, liver profile, creatine kinase level, urine output, and, in severe cases, hemodynamic monitoring are indicated. Levels of the tricyclic and cyclic antidepressants less than 300 ng/mL are therapeutic; levels greater than 500 ng/mL indicate toxicity, and levels greater than 1000 ng/mL indicate serious poisoning and are associated with QRS widening.

Management

Vital functions must be established and maintained. Even if the patient is asymptomatic, intravenous access should be established, vital signs and neurologic status monitored, and baseline 12-lead ECG and continuous cardiac monitoring obtained for at least 6 hours from admission or 8 to 12 hours postingestion. QRS interval should be measured on a limb lead ECG every 15 minutes for 6 hours postingestion.

For gastrointestinal decontamination, emesis should not be induced and gastric lavage should not be used. Activated charcoal is preferable. If the patient is in an altered mental state, the airway must be protected. Activated charcoal 1 g/kg is recommended up to 1 hour postingestion. Benefit from MDAC has not been demonstrated.

Alkalinization does not control seizures; diazepam or lorazepam should be used. Status epilepticus may require high-dose barbiturates or neuromuscular blockers with intravenous diazepam. If not successful, the patient can be paralyzed with short-term nondepolarizing neuromuscular blockers such as vecuronium (Norcuron), intubation, and assisted ventilation. A bolus of sodium bicarbonate is recommended as an adjunct to correct the acidosis produced by the seizures.

Sodium bicarbonate is administered in a dose of 1 to 2 mEq/kg undiluted as a bolus and repeated twice a few minutes apart, if needed, for "sodium loading" and alkalinization, which may increase protein binding from 90% to 98%. The sodium loading overcomes the sodium channel blockage and is more important than the alkalinization. Indications include (a) a QRS complex greater than 0.12 second, (b) ventricular tachycardia, (c) severe conduction disturbances, (d) metabolic acidosis, (e) coma, and (f) seizures. A continuous infusion of sodium bicarbonate is of limited usefulness for controlling dysrhythmias. Bolus therapy should be used as needed.

Hyperventilation alone has been recommended, but the pH elevation is not as instantaneous and there is compensatory renal excretion of bicarbonate; therefore, we do not recommend it. The combination of hyperventilation and sodium bicarbonate has produced fatal alkalemia and is not recommended. One should monitor serum potassium level (the sudden increase in blood pH can aggravate or precipitate hypokalemia), serum sodium, and ionized calcium levels (hypocalcemia may occur with alkalinization) and blood pH.

Specific cardiovascular complications should be treated as follows: Hypotension is treated with norepinephrine, a predominantly α-adrenergic drug, which is preferred over dopamine. Hypertension that occurs early rarely requires treatment. Sinus tachycardia usually does not require treatment. Supraventricular tachycardia in a patient who is hemodynamically unstable requires synchronized electrical cardioversion, starting at 0.25 to 1.0 watt-second per kg, after sedation. Ventricular tachycardia that persists after alkalinization requires intravenous lidocaine or countershock if the patient is hemodynamically unstable. Ventricular fibrillation should be treated with defibrillation. Torsades de pointes is treated with magnesium sulfate IV 20% solution, 2 g over 2 to 3 minutes, followed by a continuous infusion of 1.5 mL 10% solution or 5 to 10 mg per minute. For the treatment of bradydysrhythmias, atropine is contraindicated because of the anticholinergic activity. Isoproterenol 0.1 μg/kg/minute,

used with caution, may produce hypotension. If the patient is hemodynamically unstable, a pacemaker is used.

Extraordinary measures, such as aortic balloon pump and cardiopulmonary bypass, have been successful.

Investigational treatments include FAB fragments specific for tricyclic antidepressant, which have been successful in animals. Prophylactic $NaHCO_3$ to prevent dysrhythmias is also being investigated.

Physostigmine has produced asystole, and flumazenil has produced seizures. Both are contraindicated.

Disposition

A patient with an antidepressant overdose who meets any of the following criteria should be admitted to the intensive care unit for 12 to 24 hours: (a) ECG abnormalities except sinus tachycardia, (b) altered mental state, (c) seizures, (d) respiratory depression, and (e) hypotension. Low-risk patients include those in whom the above symptoms are absent at 6 hours postingestion, those who present with minor transient manifestations such as sinus tachycardia who subsequently become and remain asymptomatic for a 6-hour period, and asymptomatic patients who remain asymptomatic for 6 hours. These patients may be discharged if the ECG remains normal, they have normal bowel sounds, and they undergo psychiatric disposition.

Even if the patient is asymptomatic upon presentation to the health care facility, intravenous access should be established, vital signs and neurologic status monitored, a baseline 12-lead ECG obtained, and cardiac monitoring continued for at least 6 hours. *Caution:* in 25% of fatal cases, the patients were initially alert and awake at presentation. However, in most cases of fatality initially deemed as sudden cardiac death, the patient, upon reexamination, actually had symptoms that were missed.

Children younger than 6 years of age with nonintentional (accidental) exposures to amitriptyline (Elavil), desipramine (Norpramin), doxepin (Sinequan), imipramine (Tofranil), or nortriptyline (Aventyl) in a dose less than 5 mg/kg, who are asymptomatic and have what are deemed reliable caregivers, can be observed at home, with close poison control follow-up for 6 hours. Parents or caregivers should be given instructions regarding signs and symptoms to be alert for. Children who are symptomatic, or who ingested greater than 5 mg/kg, should be referred to the emergency department for monitoring, observation, and activated charcoal treatment.

18

Appendices and Index

Reference Intervals for the Interpretation of Laboratory Tests

Method of
William Z. Borer, MD

Most of the tests performed in a clinical laboratory are quantitative; that is, the amount of a substance present in blood or serum is measured and reported in terms of concentration, activity (e.g., enzyme activity), or counts (e.g., blood cell counts). The laboratory must provide reference intervals to assist the clinician in the interpretation of laboratory results. These reference intervals represent the physiologic quantities of a substance (concentrations, activities, or counts) to be expected in healthy persons. Deviation above or below the reference range may be associated with a disease process, and the severity of the disease process may be associated with the magnitude of the deviation. Unfortunately, a sharp demarcation rarely exists to distinguish between physiologic and pathologic values, and the time of transition between the two is often gradual as the disease process progresses.

The terms *normal* and *abnormal* have been used to describe laboratory values that fall inside and outside the reference range, respectively. Use of these terms is inappropriate because no good definition of normality exists in the clinical sense and the term *normal* may be confused with the statistical term *gaussian*. Reference ranges are established from statistical studies in groups of healthy volunteers. These study subjects must be free of disease, but they may have lifestyles or habits that result in variations in certain laboratory values. Examples of these variables include diet, body mass, exercise, and geographic location. Age and gender may also affect reference values.

When the data from a large cohort of healthy subjects fit a gaussian distribution, the usual statistical approach is to define the reference limits as 2 standard deviations (SD) above and below the mean. By definition, the reference range excludes the 2.5% of the population with the lowest values and the 2.5% with the highest values. Nongaussian distributions are handled by different statistical methods, but the result is similar in that the reference range is defined by the central 95% of the population. In other words, the probability that a healthy person will have a laboratory result that falls outside the reference range is 1 in 20. If 12 laboratory tests are performed, the probability that at least one of the results will be outside the reference range increases to about 50%, which means that all healthy persons are likely to have a few laboratory results that are unexpected. The clinician must then integrate these data with other clinical information, such as the history and physical examination, to arrive at an appropriate clinical decision.

The reference intervals for many tests (especially enzyme and immunochemical measurements) vary with the method used. Accordingly, each laboratory must establish reference intervals that are appropriate for the methods used.

SI Units

During the 1980s, a concerted effort was made to introduce SI units (le Système International d'Unités). The rationale for conversion to SI units is sound. Laboratory data are scientifically more informative when the units are based on molar concentration rather than on mass concentration. For example, the conversion of glucose to lactate and pyruvate or the binding of a drug to albumin is more easily understood in units of molar concentration. Another example is illustrated as follows:

CONVENTIONAL UNITS

1.0 g of hemoglobin:

- Combines with 1.37 mL of oxygen
- Contains 3.4 mg of iron
- Forms 34.9 mg of bilirubin

SI UNITS

4.0 mmol of hemoglobin:

- Combines with 4.0 mmol of oxygen
- Contains 4.0 mmol of iron
- Forms 4.0 mmol of bilirubin

TABLE 1 Base SI Units

Property	Unit	Symbol
Length	Meter	m
Mass	Kilogram	kg
Amount of substance	Mole	mol
Time	Second	s
Thermodynamic temperature	Kelvin	K
Electrical current	Ampere	A
Luminous intensity	Candela	cd
Catalytic amount	Katal	kat

The use of SI units would also enhance the standardization of nomenclature to facilitate global communication of medical and scientific information. The units, symbols, and prefixes used in the international system are shown in Tables 1, 2, and 3.

Unfortunately, problems have arisen with the implementation of SI units in the United States. The introduction of this system in 1987 prompted many medical journals to report laboratory values in both SI and conventional units in anticipation of complete conversion to SI units in the early 1990s. The lack of a coordinated effort toward this goal forced a retrenchment on the issue. Physicians continue to think and practice with laboratory results expressed in conventional units, and few, if any, hospitals or clinical laboratories in the United States use SI units exclusively. Complete conversion to SI units is not likely to occur in the foreseeable future, but most medical journals will probably continue to publish both sets of units. For this reason, the values in the tables of reference ranges in this appendix are given in both conventional units and SI units.

Tables of Reference Intervals

Some of the values included in the tables that follow have been established by the Clinical Laboratories at Thomas Jefferson University Hospital in Philadelphia and have not been published elsewhere. Other values have been compiled from the sources cited in the suggested readings. These tables are provided for information and educational purposes only. Laboratory values must always be interpreted in the context of clinical data derived from other sources, including the medical history and physical examination. One must exercise individual judgment when using the information provided in this appendix.

TABLE 3 Standard Prefixes

Prefix	Multiplication Factor	Symbol
yocto	10^{-24}	y
zepto	10^{-21}	z
atto	10^{-18}	a
femto	10^{-15}	f
pico	10^{-12}	p
nano	10^{-9}	n
micro	10^{-6}	μ
milli	10^{-3}	m
centi	10^{-2}	c
deci	10^{-1}	d
deca	10^{1}	da
hecto	10^{2}	h
kilo	10^{3}	k
mega	10^{6}	M
giga	10^{9}	G
tera	10^{12}	T

SUGGESTED READINGS

Bick RL (ed): Hematology: Clinical and Laboratory Practice. St Louis, Mosby–Year Book, 1993.

Borer WZ: Selection and use of laboratory tests. In Tietz NW, Conn RB, Pruden EL (eds): Applied Laboratory Medicine. Philadelphia, WB Saunders, 1992, pp 1-5.

Campion EW: A retreat from SI units. N Engl J Med 327:49, 1992.

Drug Evaluations Annual. Chicago, American Medical Association, 1994.

Friedman RB, Young DS: Effects of Disease on Clinical Laboratory Tests, 3rd ed. Washington, DC, AACC Press, 1997.

Henry JB: Clinical Diagnosis and Management by Laboratory Methods, 19th ed. Philadelphia, WB Saunders, 1996.

Hicks JM, Young DS: DORA 97-99: Directory of Rare Analyses. Washington, DC, AACC Press, 1997.

Jacob DS, Demott WR, Grady HJ, et al (eds): Laboratory Test Handbook, 4th ed. Baltimore, Williams & Wilkins, 1996.

Kaplan LA, Pesce AJ: Clinical Chemistry: Theory, Analysis, and Correlation, 3rd ed. St Louis, Mosby-Year Book, 1996.

Kjeldsberg CR, Knight JA: Body Fluids: Laboratory Examination of Amniotic, Cerebrospinal, Seminal, Serous and Synovial Fluids, 3rd ed. Chicago, ASCP Press, 1993.

Laposata M: SI Unit Conversion Guide. Boston, NEJM Books, 1992.

Scully RE, McNeely WF, Mark EJ, McNeely BU: Normal reference laboratory values. N Engl J Med 327:718-724, 1992.

Speicher CE: The Right Test: A Physician's Guide to Laboratory Medicine, 3rd ed. Philadelphia, WB Saunders, 1998.

Tietz NW (ed): Clinical Guide to Laboratory Tests, 3rd ed. Philadelphia, WB Saunders, 1995.

Wallach J: Interpretation of Diagnostic Tests: A Synopsis of Laboratory Medicine, 6th ed. Boston, Little, Brown, 1996.

Young DS: Effects of Preanalytical Variables on Clinical Laboratory Tests, 2nd ed. Washington, DC, AACC Press, 1997.

Young DS: Effects of Drugs on Clinical Laboratory Tests, 4th ed. Washington, DC, AACC Press, 1995.

Young DS: Determination and validation of reference intervals. Arch Pathol Lab Med 116:704-709, 1992.

Young DS: Implementation of SI units for clinical laboratory data. Ann Intern Med 106:114-129, 1987.

TABLE 2 Derived SI Units and Non-SI Units Retained for Use with SI Units

Property	Unit	Symbol
Area	Square meter	m^2
Volume	Cubic meter	m^3
	Liter	L
Mass concentration	Kilogram/ cubic meter	kg/m^3
	Gram/liter	g/L
Substance concentration	Mole/cubic meter	mol/m^3
	Mole/liter	mol/L
Temperature	Degree Celsius	C = K – 273.15

Reference Intervals for Hematology

Test	Conventional Units	SI Units
Acid hemolysis (Ham test)	No hemolysis	No hemolysis
Alkaline phosphatase, leukocyte	Total score, 14-100	Total score, 14-100
Cell counts		
Erythrocytes		
Males	4.6-6.2 million/mm^3	4.6-6.2 × 10^{12}/L
Females	4.2-5.4 million/mm^3	4.2-5.4 × 10^{12}/L
Children (varies with age)	4.5-5.1 million/mm^3	4.5-5.1 × 10^{12}/L
Leukocytes, total	4500-11,000/mm^3	4.5-11.0 × 10^9/L
Leukocytes, differential counts*		
Myelocytes	0%	0/L
Band neutrophils	3-5%	150-400 × 10^6/L
Segmented neutrophils	54-62%	3000-5800 × 10^6/L
Lymphocytes	25-33%	1500-3000 × 10^6/L
Monocytes	3-7%	300-500 × 10^6/L
Eosinophils	1-3%	50-250 × 10^6/L
Basophils	0-1%	15-50 × 10^6/L
Platelets	150,000-400,000/mm^3	150-400 × 10^9/L
Reticulocytes	25,000-75,000/mm^3 (0.5-1.5% of erythrocytes)	25-75 × 10^9/L
Coagulation tests		
Bleeding time (template)	2.75-8.0 min	2.75-8.0 min
Coagulation time (glass tube)	5-15 min	5-15 min
D Dimer	<0.5 μg/mL	<0.5 mg/L
Factor VIII and other coagulation factors	50-150% of normal	0.5-1.5 of normal
Fibrin split products (Thrombo-Welco test)	<10 μg/mL	<10 mg/L
Fibrinogen	200-400 mg/dL	2.0-4.0 g/L
Partial thromboplastin time, activated (aPTT)	20-25 s	20-35 s
Prothrombin time (PT)	12.0-14.0 s	12.0-14.0 s
Coombs' test		
Direct	Negative	Negative
Indirect	Negative	Negative
Corpuscular values of erythrocytes		
Mean corpuscular hemoglobin (MCH)	26-34 pg/cell	26-34 pg/cell
Mean corpuscular volume (MCV)	80-96 μm^3	80-96 fL
Mean corpuscular hemoglobin concentration (MCHC)	32-36 g/dL	320-360 g/L
Haptoglobin	20-165 mg/dL	0.20-1.65 g/L
Hematocrit		
Males	40-54 mL/dL	0.40-0.54
Females	37-47 mL/dL	0.37-0.47
Newborns	49-54 mL/dL	0.49-0.54
Children (varies with age)	35-49 mL/dL	0.35-0.49
Hemoglobin		
Males	13.0-18.0 g/dL	8.1-11.2 mmol/L
Females	12.0-16.0 g/dL	7.4-9.9 mmol/L
Newborns	16.5-19.5 g/dL	10.2-12.1 mmol/L
Children (varies with age)	11.2-16.5 g/dL	7.0-10.2 mmol/L
Hemoglobin, fetal	<1.0% of total	<0.01 of total
Hemoglobin A$_{1C}$	3-5% of total	0.03-0.05 of total
Hemoglobin A$_2$	1.5-3.0% of total	0.015-0.03 of total
Hemoglobin, plasma	0.0-5.0 mg/dL	0.0-3.2 μmol/L
Methemoglobin	30-130 mg/dL	19-80 μmol/L
Erythrocyte sedimentation rate (ESR)		
Wintrobe:		
Males	0-5 mm/h	0-5 mm/h
Females	0-15 mm/h	0-15 mm/h
Westergren:		
Males	0-15 mm/h	0-15 mm/h
Females	0-20 mm/h	0-20 mm/h

*Conventional units are percentages; SI units are absolute cell counts.

Rakel and Bope: *Conn's Current Therapy 2006.*

Reference Intervals* for Clinical Chemistry (Blood, Serum, and Plasma)

Analyte	Conventional Units	SI Units
Acetoacetate plus acetone		
Qualitative	Negative	Negative
Quantitative	0.3–2.0 mg/dL	30-200 µmol/L
Acid phosphatase, serum (thymolphthalein monophosphate substrate)	0.1-0.6 U/L	0.1-0.6 U/L
ACTH (see Corticotropin)		
Alanine aminotransferase (ALT), serum (SGPT)	1-45 U/L	1-45 U/L
Albumin, serum	3.3-5.2 g/dL	33-52 g/L
Aldolase, serum	0.0-7.0 U/L	0.0-7.0 U/L
Aldosterone, plasma		
Standing	5-30 ng/dL	140-830 pmol/L
Recumbent	3-10 ng/dL	80-275 pmol/L
Alkaline, phosphatase (ALP), serum		
Adult	35-150 U/L	35-150 U/L
Adolescent	100-500 U/L	100-500 U/L
Child	100-350 U/L	100-350 U/L
Ammonia nitrogen, plasma	10-50 µmol/L	10-50 µmol/L
Amylase, serum	25-125 U/L	25-125 U/L
Anion gap, serum calculated	8-16 mEq/L	8-16 mmol/L
Ascorbic acid, blood	0.4-1.5 mg/dL	23-85 µmol/L
Aspartate aminotransferase (AST), serum (SGOT)	1-36 U/L	1-36 U/L
Base excess, arterial blood, calculated	0±2 mEq/L	0±2 mmol/L
Bicarbonate		
Venous plasma	23-29 mEq/L	23-29 mmol/L
Arterial blood	21-27 mEq/L	21-27 mmol/L
Bile acids, serum	0.3-3.0 mg/dL	0.8-7.6 mmol/L
Bilirubin, serum		
Conjugated	0.1-0.4 mg/dL	1.7-6.8 µmol/L
Total	0.3-1.1 mg/dL	5.1-19.0 µmol/L
Calcium, serum	8.4-10.6 mg/dL	2.10-2.65 mmol/L
Calcium, ionized, serum	4.25-5.25 mg/dL	1.05-1.30 mmol/L
Carbon dioxide, total, serum or plasma	24-31 mEq/L	24-31 mmol/L
Carbon dioxide tension (Pco_2), blood	35-45 mm Hg	35-45 mm Hg
β-Carotene, serum	60-260 µg/dL	1.1-8.6 µmol/L
Ceruloplasmin, serum	23-44 mg/dL	230-440 mg/L
Chloride, serum or plasma	96-106 mEq/L	96-106 mmol/L
Cholesterol, serum or EDTA plasma		
Desirable range	<200 mg/dL	<5.20 mmol/L
Low-density lipoprotein (LDL) cholesterol	60-180 mg/dL	1.55-4.65 mmol/L
High-density lipoprotein (HDL) cholesterol	30-80 mg/dL	0.80-2.05 mmol/L
Copper	70-140 µg/dL	11-22 µmol/L
Corticotropin (ACTH), plasma, 8 AM	10-80 pg/mL	2-18 pmol/L
Cortisol, plasma		
8:00 AM	6-23 µg/dL	170-630 µmol/L
4:00 PM	3-15 µg/dL	80-410 µmol/L
10:00 PM	<50% of 8:00 AM value	<50% of 8:00 AM value
Creatine, serum		
Males	0.2-0.5 mg/dL	15-40 µmol/L
Females	0.3-0.9 mg/dL	25-70 µmol/L
Creatine kinase (CK), serum		
Males	55-170 U/L	55-170 U/L
Females	30-135 U/L	30-135 U/L
Creatinine kinase MB isoenzyme, serum	<5% of total CK activity	<5% of total CK activity
	<5% of ng/mL by immunoassay	<5% of ng/mL by immunoassay
Creatinine, serum	0.6-1.2 mg/dL	50-110 µmol/L
Estradiol-17β, adult		
Males	10-65 pg/mL	35-240 pmol/L
Females		
Follicular	30-100 pg/mL	110-370 pmol/L
Ovulatory	200-400 pg/mL	730-1470 pmol/L
Luteal	50-140 pg/mL	180-510 pmol/L

Reference Intervals* for Clinical Chemistry (Blood, Serum, and Plasma)—cont'd

Analyte	Conventional Units	SI Units
Ferritin, serum	20-200 ng/mL	20-200 µg/L
Fibrinogen, plasma	200-400 mg/dL	2.0-4.0 g/L
Folate, serum	3-18 ng/mL	6.8-4.1 nmol/L
Erythrocytes	145-540 ng/mL	330-120 nmol/L
Follicle-stimulating hormone (FSH), plasma		
Males	4-25 mU/mL	4-25 U/L
Females, premenopausal	4-30 mU/mL	4-30 U/L
Females, postmenopausal	40-250 mU/mL	40-250 U/L
Gastrin, fasting, serum	0-100 pg/mL	0-100 mg/L
Glucose, fasting, plasma or serum	70-115 mg/dL	3.9-6.4 nmol/L
γ-Glutamyltransferase (GGT), serum	5-40 U/L	5-40 U/L
Growth hormone (hGH), plasma, adult, fasting	0-6 ng/mL	0-6 µg/L
Haptoglobin, serum	20-165 mg/dL	0.20-1.65 g/L
Immunoglobulins, serum (see table of Reference Intervals for Tests of Immunologic Function)		
Iron, serum	75-175 µg/dL	13-31 µmol/L
Iron-binding capacity, serum		
Total	250-410 µg/dL	45-73 µmol/L
Saturation	20-55%	0.20-0.55
Lactate		
Venous whole blood	5.0-20.0 mg/dL	0.6-2.2 mmol/L
Arterial whole blood	5.0-15.0 mg/dL	0.6-1.7 mmol/L
Lactate dehydrogenase (LD), serum	110-220 U/L	110-220 U/L
Lipase, serum	10-140 U/L	10-140 U/L
Lutropin (LH), serum		
Males	1-9 U/L	1-9 U/L
Females		
Follicular phase	2-10 U/L	2-10 U/L
Midcycle peak	15-65 U/L	15-65 U/L
Luteal phase	1-12 U/L	1-12 U/L
Postmenopausal	12-65 U/L	12-65 U/L
Magnesium, serum	1.3-2.1 mg/dL	0.65-1.05 mmol/L
Osmolality	275-295 mOsm/kg water	275-295 mOsm/kg water
Oxygen, blood, arterial, room air		
Partial pressure (PaO$_2$)	80-100 mm Hg	80-100 mm Hg
Saturation (SaO$_2$)	95-98%	95-98%
pH, arterial blood	7.35-7.45	7.35-7.45
Phosphate, inorganic, serum		
Adult	3.0-4.5 mg/dL	1.0-1.5 mmol/L
Child	4.0-7.0 mg/dL	1.3-2.3 mmol/L
Potassium		
Serum	3.5-5.0 mEq/L	3.5-5.0 mmol/L
Plasma	3.5-4.5 mEq/L	3.5-4.5 mmol/L
Progesterone, serum, adult		
Males	0.0-0.4 ng/mL	0.0-1.3 mmol/L
Females		
Follicular phase	0.1-1.5 ng/mL	0.3-4.8 mmol/L
Luteal phase	2.5-28.0 ng/mL	8.0-89.0 mmol/L
Prolactin, serum		
Males	1.0-15.0 ng/mL	1.0-15.0 µg/L
Females	1.0-20.0 ng/mL	1.0-20.0 µg/L
Protein, serum, electrophoresis		
Total	6.0-8.0 g/dL	60-80 g/L
Albumin	3.5-5.5 g/dL	35-55 g/L
Globulins		
α_1	0.2-0.4 g/dL	2.0-4.0 g/L
α_2	0.5-0.9 g/dL	5.0-9.0 g/L
β	0.6-1.1 g/dL	6.0-11.0 g/L
γ	0.7-1.7 g/dL	7.0-17.0 g/L
Pyruvate, blood	0.3-0.9 mg/dL	0.03-0.10 mmol/L
Rheumatoid factor	0.0-30.0 IU/mL	0.0-30.0 kIU/L
Sodium, serum or plasma	135-145 mEq/L	135-145 mmol/L

19

Continued

Rakel and Bope: *Conn's Current Therapy 2006.*

Reference Intervals* for Clinical Chemistry (Blood, Serum, and Plasma)—cont'd

Analyte	Conventional Units	SI Units
Testosterone, plasma		
Males, adult	300-1200 ng/dL	10.4-41.6 nmol/L
Females, adult	20-75 ng/dL	0.7-2.6 nmol/L
Pregnant females	40-200 ng/dL	1.4-6.9 nmol/L
Thyroglobulin	3-42 ng/mL	3-42 µg/L
Thyrotropin (hTSH), serum	0.4-4.8 µIU/mL	0.4-4.8 mIU/L
Thyrotropin-releasing hormone (TRH)	5-60 pg/mL	5-60 ng/L
Thyroxine (FT_4), free, serum	0.9-2.1 ng/dL	12-27 pmol/L
Thyroxine (T_4), serum	4.5-12.0 µg/mL	58-154 nmol/L
Thyroxine-binding globulin (TBG)	15.0-34.0 µg/mL	15.0-34.0 mg/L
Transferrin	250-430 mg/dL	2.5-4.3 g/L
Triglycerides, serum, after 12-h fast	40-150 mg/dL	0.4-1.5 g/L
Triiodothyronine (T_3), serum	70-190 ng/dL	1.1-2.9 nmol/L
Triiodothyronine uptake, resin (T_3RU)	25-38%	0.25-0.38
Urate		
Males	2.5-8.0 mg/dL	150-480 µmol/L
Females	2.2-7.0 mg/dL	130-420 µmol/L
Urea, serum or plasma	24-49 mg/dL	4.0-8.2 nmol/L
Urea, nitrogen, serum or plasma	11-23 mg/dL	8.0-16.4 nmol/L
Viscosity, serum	1.4-1.8 × water	1.4-1.8 × water
Vitamin A, serum	20-80 µg/dL	0.70-2.80 µmol/L
Vitamin B_{12}, serum	180-900 pg/mL	133-664 pmol/L

*Reference values may vary, depending on the method and sample source used.

Reference Intervals for Therapeutic Drug Monitoring (Serum or Plasma)*

Analyte	Therapeutic Range	Toxic Concentrations	Proprietary Name(s)
Analgesics			
Acetaminophen	10-40 µg/mL	>150 µg/mL	Tylenol Datril
Salicylate	100-250 µg/mL	>300 µg/mL	Aspirin Bufferin
Antibiotics			
Amikacin	20-30 µg/mL	Peak >35 µg/mL Trough >10 µg/mL	Amkin
Gentamicin	5-10 µg/mL	Peak >10 µg/mL Trough >2 µg/mL	Garamycin
Tobramycin	5-10 µg/mL	Peak >10 µg/mL Trough >2 µg/mL	Nebcin
Vancomycin	5-35 µg/mL	Peak >40 µg/mL Trough >10 µg/mL	Vancocin
Anticonvulsants			
Carbamazepine	5-12 µg/mL	>15 µg/mL	Tegretol
Ethosuximide	40-100 µg/mL	>250 µg/mL	Zarontin
Phenobarbital	15-40 µg/mL	40-100 ng/mL (varies widely)	Luminal
Phenytoin	10-20 µg/mL	>20 µg/mL	Dilantin
Primidone	5-12 µg/mL	>15 µg/mL	Mysoline
Valproic acid	50-100 µg/mL	>100 µg/mL	Depakene
Antineoplastics and Immunosuppressives			
Cyclosporine	100-300 ng/mL	>400 ng/mL	Sandimmune
Methotrexate, high-dose, 48h	Variable	>1 µmol/L, 48h after dose	
Tacrolimus (FK-506), whole blood	3-20 µg/L	>15 µg/L	Prograf

Reference Intervals for Therapeutic Drug Monitoring (Serum or Plasma)*—cont'd

Analyte	Therapeutic Range	Toxic Concentrations	Proprietary Name(s)
Bronchodilators and Respiratory Stimulants			
Caffeine	3-15 ng/mL	>30 ng/mL	Elixophyllin
Theophylline (aminophylline)	10-20 µg/mL	>30 µg/mL	Quibron
Cardiovascular Drugs			
Amiodarone (obtain specimen more than 8h after last dose)	1.0-2.0 µg/mL	>2.0 µg/mL	Cordarone
Digoxin (obtain specimen more than 6h after last dose)	0.8-2.0 ng/mL	>2.4 ng/mL	Lanoxin
Disopyramide	2-5 µg/mL	>7 µg/mL	Norpace
Flecainide	0.2-1.0 µg/mL	>1 µg/mL	Tambocor
Lidocaine	1.5-5.0 µg/mL	>6 µg/mL	Xylocaine
Mexiletine	0.7-2.0 µg/mL	>2 µg/mL	Mexitil
Procainamide	4-10 µg/mL	>12 µg/mL	Pronestyl
Procainamide plus NAPA (N-acetyl procainamide)	8-30 µg/mL	>30 µg/mL	
Propranolol	50-100 ng/mL	Variable	Inderal
Quinidine	2-5 µg/mL	>6 µg/mL	Cardioquin Quinaglute
Tocainide	4-10 ng/mL	>10 ng/mL	Tonocard
Psychopharmacologic Drugs			
Amitriptyline	120-150 ng/mL	>500 ng/mL	Elavil Triavil
Bupropion	25-100 ng/mL	Not applicable	Wellbutrin
Desipramine	150-300 ngmL	>500 ng/mL	Norpramin
Imipramine	125-250 ng/mL	>400 ng/mL	Tofranil
Lithium (obtain specimen 12h after last dose)	0.6-1.5 mEq/L	>1.5 mEq/L	Lithobid
Nortriptyline	50-150 ng/mL	>500 ng/mL	Aventyl Pamelor

*Values may vary depending on the method and sample collection device used. Always consult the reference values provided by the laboratory performing the analysis.

Reference Intervals* for Clinical Chemistry (Urine)

Analyte	Conventional Units	SI Units
Acetone and acetoacetate, qualitative	Negative	Negative
Albumin		
Qualitative	Negative	Negative
Quantitative	10-100 mg/24h	0.15-1.5 µmol/d
Aldosterone	3-20 µg/24h	8.3-55 nmol/d
δ-Aminolevulinic acid (δ-ALA)	1.3-7.0 mg/24h	10-53 µmol/d
Amylase	<17 U/h	<17 U/h
Amylase/creatinine clearance ratio	0.01-0.04	0.01-0.04
Bilirubin, qualitative	Negative	Negative
Calcium (regular diet)	<250 mg/24h	<6.3 nmol/d
Catecholamines		
Epinephine	<10 µg/24h	<55 nmol/d
Norepinephine	<100 µg/24h	<590 nmol/d
Total free catecholamines	4-126 µg/24h	24-745 nmol/d
Total metanephrines	0.1-1.6 mg/24h	0.5-8.1 µmol/d
Chloride (varies with intake)	110-250 mEq/24h	110-250 mmol/d
Copper	0-50 µg/24h	0.0-0.80 µmol/d
Cortisol, free	10-100 µg/24h	27.6-276 nmol/d

Continued

Rakel and Bope: *Conn's Current Therapy 2006.*

19

Reference Intervals* for Clinical Chemistry (Urine)—cont'd

Analyte	Conventional Units	SI Units
Creatine		
Males	0-40 mg/24h	0.0-0.30 mmol/d
Females	0-80 mg/24h	0.0-0.60 mmol/d
Creatinine	15-25 mg/kg/24h	0.13-0.22 mmol/kg/d
Creatinine clearance (endogenous)		
Males	110-150 mL/min/1.73 m^2	110-150 mL/min/1.73 m^2
Females	105-132 mL/min/1.73 m^2	105-132 mL/min/1.73 m^2
Cystine or cysteine	Negative	Negative
Dehydroepiandrosterone		
Males	0.2-2.0 mg/24h	0.7-6.9 µmol/d
Females	0.2-1.8 mg/24h	0.7-6.2 µmol/d
Estrogens, total		
Males	4-25 µg/24h	14-90 nmol/d
Females	5-100 µg/24h	18-360 nmol/d
Glucose (as reducing substance)	<250 mg/24h	<250 mg/d
Hemoglobin and myoglobin, qualitative	Negative	Negative
Hemogentisic acid, qualitative	Negative	Negative
17-Hydroxycorticosteroids		
Males	3-9 mg/24h	8.3-25 µmol/d
Females	2-8 mg/24h	5.5-22 µmol/d
5-Hydroxyindoleacetic acid		
Qualitative	Negative	Negative
Quantitative	2-6 mg/24 h	10-31 µmol/d
17-Ketogenic steroids		
Males	5-23 mg/24h	17-80 µmol/d
Females	3-15 mg/24h	10-52 µmol/d
17-Ketosteroids		
Males	8-22 mg/24h	28-76 µmol/d
Females	6-15 mg/24h	21-52 µmol/d
Magnesium	6-10 mEq/24h	3-5 mmol/d
Metanephrines	0.05-1.2 ng/mg creatinine	0.03-0.70 mmol/mmol creatinine
Osmolality	38-1400 mOsm/kg water	38-1400 mOsm/kg water
pH	4.6-8.0	4.6-8.0
Phenylpyruvic acid, qualitative	Negative	Negative
Phosphate	0.4-1.3 g/24h	13-42 mmol/d
Porphobilinogen		
Qualitative	Negative	Negative
Quantitative	<2 mg/24h	<9 µmol/d
Porphyrins		
Coproporphyrin	50-250 µg/24h	77-380 nmol/d
Uroporphyrin	10-30 µg/24h	12-36 nmol/d
Potassium	25-125 mEq/24h	25-125 mmol/d
Pregnanediol		
Males	0.0-1.9 mg/24h	0.0-6.0 µmol/d
Females		
Proliferative phase	0.0-2.6 mg/24h	0.0-8.0 µmol/d
Luteal phase	2.6-10.6 mg/24h	8-33 µmol/d
Postmenopausal	0.2-1.0 mg/24h	0.6-3.1 µmol/d
Pregnanetriol	0.0-2.5 mg/24h	0.0-7.4 µmol/d
Protein, total		
Qualitative	Negative	Negative
Quantitative	10-150 mg/24h	10-150 mg/d
Protein/creatinine ratio	<0.2	<0.2
Sodium (regular diet)	60-260 mEq/24h	60-260 mmol/d
Specific gravity		
Random specimen	1.003-1.030	1.003-1.030
24-h collection	1.015-1.025	1.015-1.025
Urate (regular diet)	250-750 mg/24h	1.5-4.4 mmol/d
Urobilinogen	0.5-4.0 mg/24h	0.6-6.8 µmol/d
Vanillylmandelic acid (VMA)	1.0-8.0 mg/24h	5-40 µmol/d

*Values may vary, depending on the method used.

Rakel and Bope: *Conn's Current Therapy 2006.*

Reference Intervals for Toxic Substances

Analyte	Conventional Units	SI Units
Arsenic, urine	<130 µg/24h	<1.7 µmol/d
Bromides, serum, inorganic	<100 mg/dL	<10 mmol/L
Toxic symptoms	140-1000 mg/dL	14-100 mmol/L
Carboxyhemoglobin, blood	Saturation, percent	
Urban environment	<5%	<0.05
Smokers	<12%	<0.12
Symptoms		
Headache	>15%	>0.15
Nausea and vomiting	>25%	>0.25
Potentially lethal	>50%	>0.50
Ethanol, blood	<0.05 mg/dL	<1.0 mmol/L
	<0.005%	
Intoxication	>100 mg/dL	>22 mmol/L
	>0.1%	
Marked intoxication	300-400 mg/dL	65-87 mmol/L
	0.3%-0.4%	
Alcoholic stupor	400-500 mg/dL	87-109 mmol/L
	0.4%-0.5%	
	>500 mg/dL	
Coma	>0.5%	>109 mmol/L
Lead, blood		
Adults	<20 µg/dL	<1.0 µmol/L
Children	<10 µg/dL	<0.5 µmol/L
Lead, urine	<80 µg/24h	<0.4 µmol/d
Mercury, urine	<10 µg/24h	<150 nmol/d

19

Reference Intervals for Tests Performed on Cerebrospinal Fluid

Test	Conventional Units	SI Units
Cells	<5 mm^3; all mononuclear	<5 × 10^6/L, all mononuclear
Protein electrophoresis	Albumin predominant	Albumin predominant
Glucose	50-75 mg/dL (20 mg/dL less than in serum)	2.8-4.2 mmol/L (1.1 mmol/L less than in serum)
IgG		
Children <14 y	<8% of total protein	<0.08 of total protein
Adults	<14% of total protein	<0.14 of total protein
IgG index		
$\left(\dfrac{\text{CSF / serum IgG ratio}}{\text{CSF / serum albumin ratio}} \right)$	0.3-0.6	0.3-0.6
Oligoclonal banding on electrophoresis	Absent	Absent
Pressure, opening	70-180 mm H_2O	70-180 mm H_2O
Protein, total	15-45 mg/dL	150-450 mg/L

Rakel and Bope: *Conn's Current Therapy 2006.*

Reference Intervals for Tests of Gastrointestinal Function

Test	Conventional Units
Bentiromide	6-h urinary arylamine excretion >57% excludes pancreatic insufficiency
β-Carotene, serum	60-250 ng/dL
Fecal fat estimation	
Qualitative	No fat globules seen by high-power microscope
Quantitative	<6 g/24h (>95% coefficient of fat absorption)
Gastric acid output	
Basal	
Males	0.0-10.5 mmol/h
Females	0.0-5.6 mmol/h
Maximum (after histamine or pentagastrin)	
Males	9.0-48.0 mmol/h
Females	6.0-31.0 mmol/h
Ratio: basal/maximum	
Males	0.0-0.31
Females	0.0-0.29
Secretin test, pancreatic fluid	
Volume	>1.8 mL/kg/h
Bicarbonate	>80 mEq/L
D-Xylose absorption test, urine	>20% of ingested dose excreted in 5h

Reference Intervals for Tests of Immunologic Function

Test	Conventional Units	SI Units
Complement, serum		
C3	85-175 mg/dL	0.85-1.75 g/L
C4	15-45 mg/dL	150-450 mg/L
Total hemolytic (CH_{50})	150-250 U/mL	150-250 U/mL
Immunoglobulins, serum, adult		
IgG	640-1350 mg/dL	6.4-13.5 g/L
IgA	70-310 mg/dL	0.70-3.1 g/L
IgM	90-350 mg/dL	0.90-3.5 g/L
IgD	0.0-6.0 mg/dL	0.0-60 mg/L
IgE	0.0-430 ng/dL	0.0-430 mg/L

Lymphocytes Subsets, Whole Blood, Heparinized

Antigen(s) Expressed	Cell Type	Percentage (%)	Absolute Cell Count
CD3	Total T cells	56-77	860-1880
CD19	Total B cells	7-17	140-370
CD3 and CD4	Helper-inducer cells	32-54	550-1190
CD3 and CD8	Suppressor-cytotoxic cells	24-37	430-1060
CD3 and DR	Activated T cells	5-14	70-310
CD2	E rosette T cells	73-87	1040-2160
CD16 and CD56	Natural killer (NK) cells	8-22	130-500

Helper/suppressor ratio: 0.8-1.8

Reference Values for Semen Analysis

Test	Conventional Units	SI Units
Volume	2-5 mL	2-5 mL
Liquefaction	Complete in 15 min	Complete in 15 min
pH	7.2-8.0	7.2-8.0
Leukocytes	Occasional or absent	Occasional or absent
Spermatozoa		
Count	$60\text{-}150 \times 10^6$ mL	$60\text{-}150 \times 10^6$ mL
Motility	>80% motile	>0.80 motile
Morphology	80-90% normal forms	>0.80-0.90 normal forms
Fructose	>150 mg/dL	>8.33 mmol/L

Rakel and Bope: *Conn's Current Therapy 2006.*

Toxic Chemical Agents Reference Chart: Symptoms and Treatment

Method of
James J. James, MD, DrPH, MHA, and
James M. Lyznicki, MS, MPH

Toxic chemical agents are poisonous vapors, aerosols, gasses, liquids, or solids that have toxic effects on people, animals, or plants. Most of these agents are liquid at room temperature and are disseminated as vapors and aerosols. They may be released as bombs, sprayed from aircraft and boats, or disseminated by other means to intentionally create a hazard to people and the environment. Some of these agents are highly toxic and persistent, features that can render a site uninhabitable and require costly and potentially hazardous decontamination and remediation. Health effects range from irritation and burning of skin and mucous membranes to rapid cardiopulmonary collapse and death.

Efficient deployment of hazardous materials (HazMat) teams is critical to control a chemical agent attack. Although all major cities and emergency medical systems have plans and equipment in place to address this situation, physicians and other health professionals must be aware of principles involved in managing a patient or multiple patients exposed to these agents. Chemical weapon agents have a high potential for secondary contamination from victims to responders. This requires that medical treatment facilities have clearly defined procedures for handling contaminated casualties, many of whom will transport themselves to the facility. Precautions must be used until thorough decontamination has been performed or the specific chemical agent is identified. Health care professionals must first protect themselves (e.g., by using protective suits, respiratory protection, and chemical-resistant gloves) because secondary contamination with even small amounts of these substances (particularly nerve agents such as VX) may be lethal.

Primary detection of exposure to chemical agents will be based on the signs and symptoms of the potential victim (Table 1). Confirmation of a chemical agent, using detection equipment or laboratory analyses, will take considerable time and will not likely contribute to the early management of mass casualty victims.

19

TABLE 1 Quick Reference Chart on Chemical Weapon Agents

Chemical Agent	Diagnostic Considerations	Treatment Considerations*
Cyanides Cyanogen chloride (CK) Hydrogen cyanide (AC)	• Symptom onset: rapid, seconds to minutes • Odor: bitter almond, musty, or chlorine-like • Nonspecific hypoxic and hypoxemic symptoms • Binds cellular cytochrome oxidase causing chemical asphyxia • Respiratory: shortness of breath, chest tightness, hyperventilation, respiratory arrest • GI: nausea, vomiting • Cardiovascular: ventricular arrhythmias, hypotension, cardiac arrest, shock • CNS: anxiety, headache drowsiness, weakness, apnea, convulsions, seizure, coma • CNS effects may be confused with carbon monoxide and hydrogen sulfide poisoning • Metabolic acidosis and increased concentration of venous oxygen (patient also may present with cyanosis) • Laboratory testing: cyanide, thiocyanate, serum lactate levels; venous and arterial partial oxygen pressure	• Immediate treatment of symptomatic patients is critical • Antidote: sodium nitrite and sodium thiosulfate; repeat one-half initial doses of both agents in 30 minutes if there is inadequate clinical response • Amyl nitrate capsules are available for first aid until intravenous access is achieved • Cyanide antidone kits are commercially available • Investigational in the United States, available in Europe: hydroxycobalamin (vitamin B_{12a}) administered with thiosulfate • Activated charcoal[A] for oral exposure • Mechanical ventilation as needed • Circulatory support with crystalloids and vasopressors • Metabolic acidosis corrected with IV sodium bicarbonate • Seizures controlled with benzodiazepines • Antidote: physostigmine salicylate (Antilirium)[A] • Support, intravenous fluids
Incapacitating Agents Agent 15 3-quinuclidinyl benzilate (BZ)	• Symptom onset: hours 0-4 h: parasympathetic blockade and mild CNS effects 4-20 h: stupor with ataxia and hyperthermia 20-96 h: full-blown delirium Resolution phase: paranoia, deep sleep, reawakening, crawling, climbing automatisms, eventual reorientation	

Continued

Rakel and Bope: *Conn's Current Therapy 2006.*

TABLE 1 Quick Reference Chart on Chemical Weapon Agents—cont'd

Chemical Agent	Diagnostic Considerations	Treatment Considerations*
Nerve Agents Cyclohexyl sarin (GF) Sarin (GB) Soman (GD) Tabun (GA) VX	• Odorless • Competitive inhibitor of acetylcholine muscarinic receptor • Mydriasis, blurred vision, dry mouth, dry skin, possible atropine-like flush, initial rise in heart rate, decreased level of consciousness, confusion, disorientation, visual hallucinations, impaired memory • Symptom onset: vapor (seconds), liquid (minutes or hours); symptom onset may be delayed up to 18 hours particularly for localized exposures • Odor: none (GB, VX), fruity (GA), camphor-like (GD) • Most toxic of known chemical agents • Irreversible acetylcholinesterase inhibitors • Eyes: excessive lacrimation, miosis may be present • Respiratory: rhinorrhea, bronchospasm, respiratory failure • GI: hypersalivation, nausea, vomiting, diarrhea • Skin: localized sweating • Cardiac: sinus bradycardia • Skeletal muscles: fasiculations followed by weakness, flaccid paralysis • CNS: loss of consciousness, convulsions, apnea, seizures • May be confused with organophosphate and carbamate pesticide poisoning • Laboratory testing: erythrocyte or serum cholinesterase activity to confirm exposure	• Rapid establishment of patent airway • Antidote: Atropine[A] and pralidoxime[A] chloride (Protopam chloride, 2-PAM); additional doses until bronchial secretions are cleared and ventilation improved • Early administration of 2-PAM is critical to minimize permanent agent inactivation of acetylcholinesterase (i.e., "aging") • Benzodiazepines to control nerve agent-induced seizures • Airway and ventilatory support as needed • Atropine,[A] pralidoxime,[A] and diazepam[A] are available in autoinjector kits through the U.S. military
Pulmonary or Choking Agents Acrolein Ammonia (NH_3) Chlorine (CL) Choloropicrin (PS) Diphosgene (DP) Nitrogen oxides (NO_x) Perflouroisobutylene (PFIB) Phosgene (CG) Sulfur dioxide (SO_2)	• Symptom onset: rapid or delayed; 1-24 h (rarely up to 72 h) • Odor (CG): freshly mown hay or grass • Easily absorbed via mucous membranes of eyes, nose, oropharynx. Degree of water solubility of the agent influences onset and severity of respiratory injury. • Eye and airway irritation, dyspnea, chest tightness, rhinorrhea, hypersalivation, cough, wheezing • High dose inhalation may produce laryngospasm, pneumonitis, and acute lung injury with delayed onset (≤48 h) of acute respiratory distress syndrome • Chest radiograph: hyperinflation, noncardiogenic pulmonary edema • May be confused with inhalation exposure to industrial chemicals (e.g., HCl, Cl_2, NH_3)	• No specific antidote • Supportive measures; specific treatment depends on the agent • IV fluids for hypotension; no diuretics • Ventilation with or without positive airway pressure • Bronchodilators for bronchospasm • Methylprednisolone[A] may be effective in preventing noncardiogenic pulmonary edema
Riot Control Agents Mace (CN) Tear gas (CS)	• Symptom onset: immediate • Odor: apple blossom (CN); pepper (CS) • Metallic taste • SN_2 alkylating agents • Burning and pain on mucosal membranes and skin • Eyes: irritation, pain, tearing, blepharospasm	• Supportive care • Irrigation as necessary • Persons with asthma, emphysema may need oxygen, inhaled bronchodilators, steroids, assisted ventilation • Lotions, such as calamine,[A] for persistent erythema

TABLE 1 Quick Reference Chart on Chemical Weapon Agents—cont'd

Chemical Agent	Diagnostic Considerations	Treatment Considerations*
Vesicant or Blister Agents	• Airways: burning in nose and mouth, respiratory discomfort, bronchospam (may be delayed 36 h) • Skin: tingling, erythema • Nausea and vomiting common • CN can cause corneal opacification • No specific laboratory tests • Symptoms onset: immediate (L, CX); delayed 2-48 h (H, HD) • Primary liquid hazard • May be confused with skin exposure to caustic irritants (e.g., sodium hydroxide, ammonia) • Intracellular enzyme and DNA alkylating agents • Clinical effects dependent on extent and route of exposure; effects may be delayed, appearing hours after exposure	• Immediate decontamination • Supportive care • Thermal burn-type treatment • Symptomatic management of lesions
Sulfur mustard (H) Distilled mustard (HD)	• Odor: garlic, horseradish, or mustard • Skin: erythema and blisters (may be delayed ≤8 h), pruritus • Eye: irritation, conjunctivitis, corneal damage, lacrimination, pain, blepharospasm • Respiratory: mild to marked acute airway damage, pneumonitis within 1-3 d, respiratory failure • GI effects (nausea, vomiting diarrhea) may be present • Bone marrow stem cell suppression leading to pancytopenia and increased susceptibility to infection • Fever, sputum production • Combination with Lewisite (called mustard-Lewisite or HL) results in rapid effects of Lewisite and delayed effects of mustard agents	• No specific antidote • Skin: silver sulfadiazine[A] • Eye: homatropine[A] ophthalmic ointment • Pulmonary: antibiotics, bronchodilators, steroids • Colony stimulating factor may be helpful for leukopenia • Systemic analgesic and antipruritics • Early use of positive-end expiratory pressure or continuous positive airway pressure • Maintain fluid and electrolyte balance (do not excessively fluid resuscitate as in thermal burns)
Lewisite (L)	• Odor: fruity or geranium • More volatile than mustard • Damages eyes, skin, and airways by direct contact • Skin: gray area of dead skin within 5 min, erythema within 30 min, blistering 2-3 h, immediate irritation or burning pain on contact, severe tissue necrosis • Eye: pain, blepharospasm, conjunctival and lid edema • Airway: pseudomembrane formation, nasal irritation • Intravascular fluid loss, hypovolemia, shock, organ congestion, leukocytosis	• Antidote: British Anti-Lewisite (BAL or Dimercaprol)
Phosgene Oxime (CX)	• Odor: freshly mown hay • Urticant, nonvesicant agent • Vapor extremely irritating; vapor and liquid cause tissue damage upon contact • Immediate burning, irritation, wheal-like skin lesions, eye and airway damage, conjunctivitis, lacrimation, lid edema, blepharospasm • No distinctive laboratory findings	• No antidote • Parenteral methylprednisolone[A] may be effective in preventing noncardiogenic pulmonary edema • Experimental: aerosolized dexamethasone[A] and theophylline[A] for pulmonary involvement

Continued

19

Rakel and Bope: *Conn's Current Therapy 2006.*

TABLE 1   Quick Reference Chart on Chemical Weapon Agents—cont'd

Chemical Agent	Diagnostic Considerations	Treatment Considerations*
Vomiting (Arsine-Based) Agents Adamsite (DM) Diphenylchlorarsine (DA) Diphenylcyanoarsine (DC)	• Symptom onset: All rapidly acting within minutes • Odor: none (DA), garlic (DC), burning fireworks (DM) • Primary route of absorption is through respiratory system • Arsine gas depletes erythrocyte glutathione and causes hemolysis • Eyes: conjunctival irritation, tearing, and blepharospasm • Airways: sneezing, mucosal lung irritation, edema, progressive cough, wheezing • Cardiac: tachypnea, tachycardia • GI: intestinal cramps, emesis, diarrhea • Skin: erythema, edema at the site of dermal contact • CNS: depression, syncope • Chest radiograph to rule out chemical pneumonitis	• Supportive care • Monitor for hemolysis • Wheezing or dyspnea; may need albuterol inhalation • Eye irrigation (water, normal saline, lactated Ringer's solution) in patients sustaining ocular exposure • Treat repetitive emesis with IV hydration and antiemetics • Blood transfusion may be required • Exchange transfusion may be required • Hemodialysis may be useful in decreasing arsenic level and treating renal failure

ᐱNot FDA approved for this indication.

*Different situations may require different treatment and dosage regimens. Please consult other references as well as a regional poison control center (1-800-222-1222), medical toxicologist, clinical pharmacologist, or other drug information specialist for definitive dosage information, especially dosages for pregnant women and children.

Abbreviations: CNS = central nervous system; GI = gastrointestinal.

Several patients presenting with the same symptoms should alert physicians and hospital staff to the possibility of a chemical attack. If a chemical attack occurs, most victims will likely arrive within a short time. This situation differentiates a chemical attack from a biological attack involving infectious microganisms. Additional diagostic clues include:

• Unusual temporal or geographic clustering of illness
• Any sudden increase in illness in previously healthy persons
• Sudden increase in non-specific syndromes (e.g., sudden unexplained weakness in previously healthy persons; dimmed or blurred vision; hypersecretion, inhalation, or burn-like syndrome)

A coordinated communication network is critical for transmitting reliable information from the incident scene to treatment facilities. Any suspicious or confirmed exposure to a chemical weapons agent should be reported to the local health department, local Federal Bureau of Investigations office, and the Centers for Disease Control and Prevention (1-770 488-7100).

Biologic Agents Reference Chart—Symptoms, Tests, and Treatment

Method of
*James J. James, MD, DrPh, MHA, and
James M. Lyznicki, MS, MPH*

Biologic weapons are devices used intentionally to cause disease or death through dissemination of microorganisms or toxins in food and water, by insect vectors, or by aerosols. Potential targets include human beings, food crops, livestock, and other resources essential for national security, economy, and defense. Unlike nuclear, chemical, and conventional weapons, the onset of a biological attack will probably be insidious. For some infectious agents, secondary and tertiary transmission may continue for weeks or months after the initial attack.

Initial detection of an unannounced biologic attack will likely occur when an astute health professional notices an unusual case or disease cluster and reports his or her concerns to local public health authorities. Physicians and other health professionals should be alert to the following:

• Unusual temporal or geographic clustering of illnesses
• Sudden increase of illness in previously healthy persons

Rakel and Bope: *Conn's Current Therapy 2006.*

- Sudden increase in non-specific illnesses (e.g., pneumonia, flulike illness; bleeding disorders; unexplained rashes, particularly in adults; neuromuscular illness; diarrhea)

To enhance detection and treatment capabilities, physicians and other health professionals in acute care settings should be familiar with the clinical manifestations, diagnostic techniques, isolation precautions, treatment, and prophylaxis for likely causative agents (e.g., smallpox, pneumonic plague, anthrax, viral hemorrhagic fevers). Table 1 provides a quick summary of diagnostic and treatment considerations for various infectious and toxic biological agents. For some of these agents, delay in medical response could result in a potentially devastating number of casualties. To mitigate such consequences, early identification and intervention are imperative. Front-line physicians must have an increased level of suspicion regarding the possible intentional use of biologic agents as well as an increased sensitivity to reporting those suspicious to public health authorities, who, in turn, must be willing to evaluate a predictable increase in false positive reports.

Medical response efforts require coordination and planning with emergency management agencies, law enforcement, health care facilities, and social services agencies. Health care agencies should ensure that physicians know whom to call with reports of suspicious cases and clusters of infectious diseases, and should work to build a good relationship with the local

TABLE 1 Quick Reference Chart on Biological Weapon Agents

Disease/Agent	Diagnostic Considerations	Treatment Considerations[1]	Prophylaxis
Bacteria			
Anthrax *Bacillus anthracis*	Incubation period: 1-5 d (perhaps ≤60 d)[2] *Cutaneous:* • Evolving skin lesion (face, neck, arms), progresses to vesicle, dispressed ulcer, and black necrotic lesions • Lethality: 20% if untreated, otherwise rarely fatal *Gastrointestinal* • Nausea, vomiting, abdominal pain, bloody diarrhea, sepsis • Lethality: approaches 100% if untreated but data are limited; rapid, aggressive treatment may reduce mortality *Inhalational* • Abrupt onset of flu-like symptoms, fever with or without chills, sweats, fatigue or malaise, non- or minimally productive cough, nausea, vomiting, dyspnea, headache, chest pain, followed in 2-5 d by severe respiratory distress, mediastinitis, hemorrhagic meningitis, sepsis, shock.[3] • Widened mediastinum on chest radiograph is characteristic for inhalational and occasionally GI anthrax.[4] • Lethality: Once respiratory distress develops, mortality rates may approach 90%; begin treatment when inhalational anthrax is suspected, do not wait for confirmatory testing.[5]	Combination therapy of ciprofloxacin (Cipro) or doxycycline (Vibramycin) plus one or two other antimicrobials should be considered with inhalational anthrax[6] Penicillin[A] should be considered if strain is susceptible and does not possess inducible β-lactamases If meningitis suspected, doxycycline (Vibramycin) may be less optimal because of poor CNS penetration Steroids may be considered for severe edema and for meningitis.	Ciprofloxacin (Cipro) or doxycycline (Vibramycin) with or without vaccination If strain is susceptible, penicillin[A] or amoxicillin[A] (Amoxil) should be considered Inactivated vaccine (licensed but not readily available); six injections and annual booster

Continued

Rakel and Bope: *Conn's Current Therapy 2006.*

TABLE 1 Quick Reference Chart on Biological Weapon Agents—cont'd

Disease/Agent	Diagnostic Considerations	Treatment Considerations[1]	Prophylaxis
	Gram stain and culture of blood, pleural fluid, cerebrospinal fluid, ascitic fluid, vesicular fluid or lesion exudate; sputum rarely positive; confirmatory serological and PCR tests available through public health laboratory network		
Brucellosis *B. abortus* *B. canis* *B. mellitensis* *B. suis*	Incubation period: 5-60 d (usually 1-2 mo) • Non-specific flu-like symptoms, fever, headache, profound weakness and fatigue, GI symptoms such as anorexia, nausea, vomiting, diarrhea, or constipation • Osteoarticular complications common • Lethality: less than 5% even if untreated; tends to incapacitate rather than kill. Blood and bone marrow culture (may require 6 wk to grow *Brucella*); confirmatory culture and serological testing available through public health laboratory network	Doxycycline (Vibramycin) plus streptomycin or rifampin[A] (Rifadin) *Alternative therapies:* Ofloxacin (Floxin)[A] plus rifampin[A] (Rifadin) Doxycycline (Vibramycin) plus gentamicin (Garamycin) TMP/SMX (Bactrim,[A] Septra) plus gentamicin (Garamycin)	Doxycycline (Vibramycin) plus streptomycin or rifampin (Rifadin) No approved human vaccine
Inhalational (pneumonic) tularemia *Francisella tularensis*	Incubation period: 3-5 d (range of 1-21 d) • Sudden onset of acute febrile illness, weakness, chills, headache, generalized body aches, elevated WBCs • Pulmonary symptoms such as dry cough, chest pain or tightness with or without objective signs of pneumonia • Progressive weakness, malaise, anorexia, and weight loss occurs, potentially leading to sepsis and organ failure • Largely clinical diagnosis • Lethality: ≈30-60% fatal if untreated Culture of blood, sputum, biopsies, pleural fluid, bronchial washings (culture is difficult and potentially dangerous); confirmatory testing available through public health laboratory network	Streptomycin or gentamicin (Garamycin) *Alternative therapies:* Ciprofloxacin (Cipro)[A] Doxycycline (Vibramycin) Chloramphenicol[A] (Chloromycetin)	Tetracycline Doxycycline (Vibramycin) Ciprofloxacin (Cipro)[A] Live attenuated vaccine (USAMRIID, IND) given by scarification; currently under FDA review; limited availability
Pneumonic plague *Yersinia pestis*	Incubation period: 1-10 d (typically 2-3 d) • Acute onset of flu-like prodrome: fever, myalgia, weakness, headache; within	Streptomycin; gentamicin (Garamycin) *Alternative therapies:* Doxycycline (Vibramycin) Tetracycline	Tetracycline Doxycycline (Vibramycin) Ciprofloxacin[A] (Cipro) Inactivated whole cell vaccine licensed but not

Rakel and Bope: *Conn's Current Therapy 2006.*

TABLE 1 Quick Reference Chart on Biological Weapon Agents—cont'd

Disease/Agent	Diagnostic Considerations	Treatment Considerations[1]	Prophylaxis
	24 h of prodrome, chest discomfort, cough with bloody sputum, and dyspnea. By day 2 to 4 illness, symptoms progressing to cyanosis, respiratory distress, and hemodynamic instability • Lethality: almost 100% if untreated; 20–60% if appropriately treated within 18-24 h of symptoms; begin treatment when diagnosis of plague is suspected; do not wait for confirmatory testing Gram stain and culture of blood, CSF, sputum, lymph node aspirates, bronchial washings; confirmatory serological and bacteriological tests available through public health laboratory network	Ciprofloxacin[A] (Cipro) Chloramphenicol[A] (Chloromycetin) is first choice for meningitis except for pregnant women	readily available; injection with boosters Vaccine not effective against aerosol exposure
Rickettsia **Q-Fever** *Coxiella burnetii*	Incubation period: 2-14 d (may be ≤40 days) • Nonspecific febrile disease, chills, cough, weakness and fatigue, pleuritic chest pain, pneumonia possible • Lethality: 1-3%. Fatalities are uncommon even if untreated but relapsing symptoms may occur Isolation of organism may be difficult; confirmatory testing via serology or PCR available through public health laboratory network	Tetracycline Doxycycline (Vibramycin)	Tetracycline Doxycycline (Vibramycin) Inactivated whole cell[B] vaccine (IND) Skin test to determine prior exposure to *C. burnetii* recommended before vaccination
Viruses **Smallpox** Variola major virus	Incubation period: 7-17 d • Prodrome of high fever, malaise, prostration, headache, vomiting, delirium followed in 2-3 d maculopapular rash uniformly progressing to pustules and scabs, mostly on extremities and face • Requires astute clinical evaluation; may be confused with chickenpox, erythema multiforme with bullae, or allergic contact dermatitis • Lethality: 30% in unvaccinated persons Pharyngeal swab, vesicular fluid, biopsies, scab material for electron microscopy and PCR testing through public health laboratory network Notify CDC Poxvirus Section at 1-404-639-2184	Supportive care Cidofovir (Vistide) shown to be effective in vitro and in experimental animals infected with surrogate orthopox virus	Live attenuated vaccinia vaccine derived from calf lymph; given by scarification (licensed, restricted supply) New vaccine being developed from tissue culture Vaccination given within 3-4 d following exposure can prevent or decrease the severity of disease

Continued

TABLE 1   Quick Reference Chart on Biological Weapon Agents—cont'd

Disease/Agent	Diagnostic Considerations	Treatment Considerations[1]	Prophylaxis
Viral Encephalitis Eastern (EEE) Western (WEE) Venezuelan (VEE)	Incubation period: 2-6 d (VEE); 7-14 d (EEE, WEE) • Systemic febrile illness, with encephalitis developing in some populations • Generalized malaise, spiking fevers, headache, myalgia • Incidence of seizures and/or focal neurologic deficits may be higher after biological attack • White blood cell count may show stricking leukopenia and lymphopenia • Clinical and epidemiologic diagnosis • Lethality: <10% (VEE); 10% (WEE); 50-75% (EEE) Confirmatory test and viral isolation available through public health laboratory network	Supportive care Analgesics, anticonvulsants as needed	Several IND vaccines, poorly immunogenic, highly reactogenic
Viral Hemorrhagic Fevers (VHFs) Arenaviruses (Lassa, Junin, and related viruses) Bunyaviruses (Hanta, Congo-Crimean, Rift Valley) Filoviruses (Ebola, Marburg) Flaviviruses (yellow fever, dengue, various tick-borne disease viruses)	Incubation period: 4-21 d • Fever with mucous membrane bleeding, petechiae, thrombocytopenia and hypotension in patients without underlying malignancies • Malaise, myalgias, headache, vomiting, diarrhea possible • Lethality: Variable depending on viral strain; 15-25% with Lassa fever to ≤ 90% with Ebola Confirmatory testing and viral isolation available through public health laboratory network Call CDC Special Pathogens Office at 1-404-639-1115	Supportive therapy Ribavirin (Virazole)[A] may be effective for Lassa fever, Rift Valley fever, Argentine hemorrhagic fever, and Congo-Crimean hemorrhagic fever	Ribavarin (Virazole)[A] is suggested for Congo-Crimean hemorrhagic fever and Lassa fever Yellow fever vaccine is the only licensed vaccine available Vaccines for some of the other VHFs exist but are for investigational use only
Biological Toxins			
Botulism *Clostridium botulinum toxin*	Symptom onset: 1-5 d (typically 12-36 h) • Blurred vision, diploplia, dry mouth, ptosis, fatigue • As disease progresses, acute bilateral descending flaccid paralysis, respiratory paralysis resulting in death • Clinical diagnosis • Lethality: 60% without ventilatory support Serum and stool should be assayed for toxin by mouse neutralization bioassay, which may require several days	Intensive and prolonged supportive care; ventilation may be necessary Trivalent equine antitoxin (serotypes A,B,E, – licensed, available from the CDC) should be administered immediately after clinical diagnosis Anaphylaxis and serum sickness are potential complications of antitoxin Aminoglycosides and clindamycin (Cleocin)[A] must not be used	Pentavalent toxoid (A-E), yearly booster (IND, CDC) Not available to the public Antitoxin may be sufficient to prevent illness following exposure but is not recommended until patient is showing symptoms
Enterotoxin B *Staphylococcus aureus*	Symptom onset: 3-12 h • Acute onset of fever, chills headache, nonproductive cough	Supportive care	No vaccine available

TABLE 1 Quick Reference Chart on Biological Weapon Agents—cont'd

Disease/Agent	Diagnostic Considerations	Treatment Considerations[1]	Prophylaxis
	• Normal chest radiograph • Clinical diagnosis • Lethality: probably low (few data available for respiratory exposure) Serology on acute and convalescent serum can confirm diagnosis		
Ricin toxin *Ricinus communis*	Symptom onset: ≤6-24 h • Weakness, nausea, chest tightness, fever, cough, pulmonary edema, respiratory failure, circulatory collapse, hypoxemia resulting in death (usually within 36-72 h) • Clinical and epidemiological diagnosis • Lethality: mortality data not available but is likely to be high with extensive exposure Confirmatory serological testing available through public health laboratory network	Supportive care Treatment for pulmonary edema Gastric decontamination if toxin ingested	No vaccine available
T-2 Mycotoxins *Fusarium* *Myrothecium* *Trichoderma* *Stachybotrys*	Symptom onset: minutes to hours • Abrupt onset of mucocutaneous and airway irritation and pain • May include skin, eyes, and GI tract; systemic toxicity may follow	Clinical support Soap and water washing within 4-6 h reduces dermal toxicity; washing within 1 h may eliminate toxicity entirely	No vaccine available
Other filamentous fungi	• Lethality: severe exposure can cause death in hours to days Consult with local health department regarding specimen collection and diagnostic testing procedures; confirmation requires testing blood, tissue, and environmental samples	No effective medications or antidotes	

[A]Not FDA approved for this indication.

[B]Not available in the United States.

[1]Different situations may require different dosage and treatment regimens. Please consult other references and an infectious disease specialist for definitive dosage information, especially dosages for pregnant women and children.

[2]Data from 22 patients infected with anthrax in October and November 2001 indicate a median incubation period of 4 d (range 4-7 d) for inhalational anthrax and a mean incubation of 5 d (range 1-10 d) for cutaneous anthrax.

[3]Limited data from the October/November 2001 anthrax infections indicate hemorrhagic pleural effusions to be strongly associated with inhalational anthrax; rhinorrhea was present in only 1/10 patients.

[4]Chest radiograph abnormalities include paratracheal and hilar fullness and may be subtle. Consider chest computed tomography if diagnosis is uncertain.

[5]Limited data from the 2001 terrorist-related anthrax infections indicate that early treatment significantly decreased the mortality rate.

[6]Other agents with in vitro activity suggested for use in conjunction with ciprofloxacin (Cipro) or doxycycline (Vibramycin) for treatment of inhalational anthrax include rifampin (Rifadin), vancomycin (Vancocin), imipenem (Primaxin), chloramphenicol (Chloromycetin), penicillin and ampicillin, clindamycin (Cleocin), and clarithromycin (Biaxin).

Abbreviations: CDC = Centers for Disease Control and Prevention; CNS = central nervous system; CSF = cerebrospinal fluid; GI = gastrointestinal; IND = investigational new drug; PCR = polymerase chain reaction; TMP-SMX = trimethoprim-sulfamethoxazole; USAMRIID, U.S. Army Medical Research Institute of Infectious Diseases; WBC = white blood cell.

Adopted for *Biological Weapons: Quick Reference Guide.* American Medical Association; 2002. Available at http://www.amaassn.org/ama1/pub/upload/mm/415/quickreference0902.pdf.

medical community. Resource integration is absolutely necessary to:

- Establish adequate capacity to initiate rapid investigation of an outbreak
- Educate the public
- Begin mass distribution of antibiotics and vaccines
- Ensure mass medical care
- Control public anger and fear

In an epidemic, overwhelming numbers of critically ill patients will require acute and follow-up medical care. Both infected persons and the *worried well* will seek medical attention, with a corresponding need for medical supplies, diagnostic tests, and hospital beds. The impact — or even the threat — of an attack can elicit widespread panic and civil disorder, overwhelm hospital resources, and disrupt social services.

Any suspicious or confirmed exposure to a biologic weapons agent should be reported immediately to the local health department, local Federal Bureau of Investigations office, and the Centers of Disease Control and Prevention (1-770-488-7100).

Some Popular Herbs and Nutritional Supplements

Method of
Miriam M. Chan, RPh, PharmD

Herb/Nutritional Supplement	Common Uses	Reasonable Adult Oral Dosage*	Precautions and Drug Interactions
Black cohosh root	Commonly used to relieve hot flashes and other menopausal symptoms Also used to treat premenstrual discomfort and dysmenorrhea	20 mg bid of rhizome extract standardized to triterpene glycosides The German guidelines do not recommend its use for >6 mo	Black cohosh may have an estrogen-like effect and should be avoided in women with breast cancer Large doses may induce miscarriage and it is contraindicated during pregnancy It may cause GI disturbances, headache, and hypotension
Bilberry fruit	Often used orally to improve visual acuity and to treat degenerative retinal conditions Also used orally to treat chronic venous insufficiency, varicose veins, and hemorrhoids Approved in Germany to use orally for acute diarrhea and topically for mild	For eye conditions and circulation, 80-160 mg tid of the extract standardized to at least 25% anthocyanosides For diarrhea, 20-60 g/d of the dried, ripe berries or as a tea preparation (5-10 g of crushed dried berries in water, brought to a boil for 10 min, then strained)	No known side effects reported with bilberry fruit and extract However, bilberry leaf taken in large quantities or with long-term use has been shown to cause wasting, anemia, jaundice, acute excitation, disturbances of tonus, and death in animals

Rakel and Bope: *Conn's Current Therapy 2006.*

Herb/Nutritional Supplement	Common Uses	Reasonable Adult Oral Dosage*	Precautions and Drug Interactions
	inflammation of the mucous membranes of mouth and throat	For external use, 10% decoction	The anthocyanidin extracts from bilberry may increase the risk of bleeding in those taking warfarin or other blood thinners
Chamomile flower	Used orally to calm nerves and treat GI spasms and inflammatory diseases of the GI tract Used topically to treat wounds, skin infections, and skin or mucous membrane inflammation	1 cup of freshly made tea three to four times daily (1 tbsp or 3 g of dried flower in 150 mL boiling water for 5-10 min)	Chamomile may cause an allergic reaction, especially in people with severe allergies to ragweed or other members of the daisy family (e.g., echinacea, feverfew, and milk thistle) It should not be taken concurrently with other sedatives, such as alcohol or benzodiazepines
Chaste tree berry (Chasteberry, Vitex)	For normalizing irregular menstrual periods and relieving premenstrual complaints For relieving menopausal symptoms For restoring fertility in women For treating acne associated with menstrual cycles Also for increasing breast milk production in lactating women	For menstrual irregularities and premenstrual complaints, 30-40 mg/d of the dried berries or an equivalent amount of aqueous-alcoholic extracts (50-70% v/v) Dried fruit extract, standardized to 0.6% agnusides, is used in doses of 175-225 mg/d For other conditions, no established dosage documented	Chaste tree berry can have uterine stimulant properties and should be avoided in pregnancy Women with hormone-dependent conditions (e.g., breast, uterine, and ovarian cancer, and endometriosis and uterine fibroids) and men with prostate cancer should avoid chaste tree berry because it contains progestins Side effects include intramenstrual bleeding, dry mouth, headache, nausea, rash, alopecia, and tachycardia High doses (≥480 mg/d extract) can paradoxically decrease lactation Chaste tree berry is thought to have dopaminergic effects and may interact with dopamine antagonists, such as antipsychotics and metoclopramide Chaste tree berry may also decrease the effects of oral contraceptives and hormone replacement therapy
Chondroitin	For osteoarthritis, commonly used in combination with glucosamine	400 mg tid; chondroitin derived from bovine cartilage may carry a potential risk of contamination with diseased animals	Occasional mild side effects include nausea, indigestion, and allergic reactions
Chromium	For diabetes For hypercholesterolemia Commonly found in weight-loss products Also promoted for body building	For diabetes, 100 µg bid for ≤4 mo or 500 µg bid for 2 mo For hypercholesterolemia, 200 µg tid or 500 µg bid for 2-4 mo For body building, 200-400 µg/d Chromium picolinate has been used in most studies, even though the chloride form is also available	Adverse effects are rare, but they may include headaches, insomnia, sleep disturbances, irritability and mood changes. Some patients may also experience cognitive, perceptual, and motor dysfunction Long-term use of high doses (600-2400 µg/day)

Continued

Rakel and Bope: *Conn's Current Therapy 2006.*

19

Herb/Nutritional Supplement	Common Uses	Reasonable Adult Oral Dosage*	Precautions and Drug Interactions
			can cause anemia, thrombocytopenia, hemolysis, hepatic dysfunction, and renal failure There have been two case reports of interstitial nephritis A few studies suggest that chromium may cause DNA damage Chromium competes with iron for binding to transferrin and can cause iron deficiency Antacids, H_2 blockers, and proton pump inhibitors can decrease the absorption of chromium
Coenzyme Q10	As adjunctive treatment for congestive heart failure, angina, and hypertension Also used for reducing cardiotoxicity associated with doxorubicin	For heart failure, 100 mg/d in two or three divided doses For angina, 50 mg tid For hypertension, 60 mg bid	Mild adverse events include gastric distress, nausea, vomiting, and hypotension Doses >300 mg/d may cause elevated liver enzymes Coenzyme Q10 may reduce the anticoagulation effects of warfarin Oral hypoglycemic agents and HMG-CoA reductase inhibitors may reduce the serum coenzyme Q10 levels
Creatine	To enhance muscle performance, especially during short-duration, high-intensity exercise	A loading dose of 20 g/d for 5-7 d followed by a maintenance dose of ≥2 g/d An alternative dosing of 3 g/d for 28 d has been suggested	Creatine can cause gastroenteritis, diarrhea, heat intolerance, muscle cramps, and elevated serum creatinine levels Creatine is contraindicated in patients taking diuretics Concurrent use with cimetidine, probenecid, or nonsteroidal anti-inflammatory drugs increases the risk of adverse renal effects Caffeine may decrease creatine's ergogenic effects
Dong quai root	Commonly used for the relief of premenstrual and menopausal symptoms Also used as a "blood tonic" and a strengthening treatment for the heart, spleen, liver, and kidneys	For premenstrual and menopausal symptoms, 3-4 g/d in three divided doses For other conditions, no established dosage documented	Dong quai should not be used in pregnant women due to its uterine stimulant and relaxant effects Women with hormone sensitive conditions (e.g., breast, uterine, and ovarian cancer, and endometriosis and uterine fibroids) should avoid dong quai because of its estrogenic effects Drinking the essential oil of dong quai is not recommended because it contains a small amount of carcinogenic constituents

Rakel and Bope: *Conn's Current Therapy 2006.*

Herb/Nutritional Supplement	Common Uses	Reasonable Adult Oral Dosage*	Precautions and Drug Interactions
			Dong quai contains psoralens that can cause photosensitivity and photodermatitis
			Dong quai also contains natural coumarin derivatives that can increase the risk of bleeding in those who are taking anticoagulant or antiplatelet drugs
Echinacea	As an immune stimulant, particularly for the prevention and treatment of the common cold and influenza Supportive therapy for lower urinary tract infections Used topically to treat skin disorders and promote wound healing	300 mg tid of *E. pallida* root or 2-3 mL tid of expressed juice of *E. purpurea* herb Do not use for >8 wk because echinacea may suppress immunity if used long term	Echinacea should not be used in transplant patients and those with autoimmune disease or liver dysfunction Allergic reactions have been reported. Adverse events are rare and may include mild GI effects It should be discontinued as far in advance of surgery as possible Echinacea may decrease effectiveness of immunosuppressants
Ephedra (ma huang)	For diseases of the respiratory tract with mild bronchospasm Commonly found in weight-loss products Also marked as a stimulant for performance enhancement	1 tsp or 2 g of dried herb (15-30 mg of ephedrine) in 240 mL boiling water for 10 min In Canada, the maximum allowable dosage is 8 mg ephedrine/dose or 32 mg ephedrine/day	Ephedra contains ephedrine, which has sympathomimetic activities; consequently, it should not be used in patients who have cardiovascular disease, diabetes, glaucoma, hypertension, hyperthyroidism, prostate enlargement, psychiatric disorders, or seizures Serious adverse effects, including seizures, arrhythmias, heart attack, stroke, and death, have been associated with the use of ephedra; as a result, the FDA has banned the sale of ephedra products in the United States Because of the cardiovascular effects of ephedrine, patients taking ephedra should discontinue use at least 24 h before surgery Concurrent use of ephedra and digitalis, guanethidine, monoamine oxidase inhibitors, or other stimulants, including caffeine, is not recommended
Evening primrose oil	For premenstrual syndrome (PMS), especially if mastalgia is present	For PMS, 2-4 g/d For atopic eczema, 6-8 g/d For rheumatoid arthritis, 2.8 g/d	Evening primrose oil may increase the risk of pregnancy complications

Continued

Rakel and Bope: *Conn's Current Therapy 2006.*

Herb/Nutritional Supplement	Common Uses	Reasonable Adult Oral Dosage*	Precautions and Drug Interactions
	Licensed in the United Kingdom for the treatment of atopic eczema Also used for other medical conditions, including rheumatoid arthritis, menopausal symptoms, Raynaud's phenomenon, Sjögren's syndrome, and diabetic neuropathy	These doses are based on products standardized to 9% γ-linolenic acid The daily dose can be given in divided doses	Side effects may include indigesion, nausea, soft stools, and headache Seizures have been reported in patients with schizophrenia who were taking phenothiazines and evening primrose oil concomitantly Evening primrose oil may interact with anesthesia and cause seizures Concomitant use of evening primrose oil with anticoagulant and antiplatelet drugs can increase the risk of bleeding
Fenugreek seed	For diabetes and hypercholesterolemia Also for constipation, dyspepsia, gastritis, and kidney ailments. Approved in Germany to use orally for loss of appetite and topically as a poultice for local inflammation	For loss of appetite, 1-2 g of the seed tip or 1 cup of tea (500 mg seed in 150 mL cold water for 3 h) several times a day Maximum 6 g/d For other conditions, no established dosage documented For topical use, 50 g powdered seed in ¼ L of hot water to form a paste	Fenugreek may cause uterine contraction and should be avoided in pregnancy Individuals who have allergies to peanuts or soybeans may also be allergic to fenugreek Fenugreek can cause diarrhea and flatulence; it may also make the urine smell like maple syrup Hypoglycemia may occur if fenugreek is taken in large amounts Repeated external applications can result in undesirable skin reactions Fenugreek contains small amounts of coumarins and may interact with anticoagulants and antiplatelet drugs The high mucilage content of fenugreek can affect the absorption of oral drugs; therefore, fenugreek should not be taken within 2 h of other drugs
Feverfew	For migraine headache prophylaxis For treatment of fever, menstrual problems, and arthritis	50-125 mg qd of the encapsulated dried leaf extract standardized to at least 0.2% parthenolide	Feverfew may induce menstrual bleeding and is contraindicated in pregnancy Fresh leaves may cause oral ulcers and GI irritation Sudden discontinuation of feverfew can precipitate rebound headache Feverfew may interact with anticoagulants and potentiate the antiplatelet effect of aspirin
Garlic	To lower blood pressure and serum cholesterol To prevent atherosclerosis	Fresh clove: 1 (4 g)/d Tablet: 300 mg bid to tid standardized to 0.6%-1.3% allicin	Intake of large quantities can lead to stomach complaints Garlic has antiplatelet effects, so patients should

Herb/Nutritional Supplement	Common Uses	Reasonable Adult Oral Dosage*	Precautions and Drug Interactions
			discontinue use of garlic at least 7 d before surgery
			Concomitant use of garlic and anticoagulants may increase the risk of bleeding
Ginger root	As an antiemetic For prevention of motion sickness	Fresh rhizome: 2-4 g/d Powdered ginger: 250 mg three to four times daily Tea: 1 cup tea tid (0.5-1 g dried root in 150 mL boiling water for 5-10 min)	Ginger should not be used in patients with gallstones because of its cholagogic effect It may inhibit platelet aggregation; cases of postoperative bleeding have been reported Large doses of ginger may increase bleeding time in patients taking anti-platelet agents
Ginkgo biloba leaf	To slow cognitive deterioration in dementia To increase peripheral blood flow in claudication To treat sexual dysfunction associated with the use of SSRIs	60-120 mg bid of extract Egb761 standarized to 24% flavonoids and 6% terpenoids	Adverse effects are rare and may include mild stomach or intestinal upset, headache, or allergic skin reaction Ginkgo can inhibit platelet aggregation; reports of spontaneous bleeding have been published Patients should discontinue ginkgo at least 36 h before surgery. Concurrent use of ginkgo and anticoagulants, antiplatelet agents, vitamin E, or garlic may increase the risk of bleeding
Ginseng root	As a tonic during times of stress, fatigue, disability, and convalescence To improve physical performance and stamina	Root: 1-2 g/d Tablet: 100 mg bid of extract standardized to 4%-7% ginsenosides A 2- to 3-week period of using ginseng followed by a 1- to 2-week "rest" period is generally recommended Ginseng is commonly adulterated, especially Siberian ginseng products	Ginseng has a mild stimulant effect and should be avoided in patients with cardiovascular disease Tachycardia and hypertension can occur Overdosages can lead to "ginseng abuse syndrome," characterized by insomnia, hypotonia, and edema Ginseng has estrogenic effects and may cause vaginal bleeding and breast tenderness Ginseng has been shown to inhibit platelets, so patients should discontinue ginseng use at least 7 d before surgery Ginseng should not be used with other stimulants Patients taking antidiabetic agents and ginseng should be monitored to avoid the hypoglycemic effects of ginseng Ginseng may interact with warfarin and cause a

Continued

Herb/Nutritional Supplement	Common Uses	Reasonable Adult Oral Dosage*	Precautions and Drug Interactions
			decreased international normalized ratio Siberian ginseng may increase digoxin levels There have been reports of a drug interaction between ginseng and phenelzine (a monoamine oxidase inhibitor) resulting in insomnia, headache, tremulousness, and manic-like symptoms
Glucosamine	For osteoarthritis	500 mg tid with meals Glucosamine is available in the form of sulfate, hydrochloride, or n-acetyl salt. Glucosamine sulfate is the form that has been used in most clinical studies	Side effects are generally limited to mild GI symptoms, including stomach upset, heartburn, diarrhea, nausea, and indigestion Glucosamine derived from marine exoskeletons may cause reactions in people allergic to shellfish Glucosamine may raise blood glucose level in patients with diabetes
Hawthorn leaf with flower	Commonly used in Germany to increase cardiac output in patients with New York Heart Association stage I and II heart failure	160-900 mg water-ethanol extract (30-169 mg procyanidins or 3.5-19.8 mg flavonoids) divided into 2-3 doses	Side effects include GI upset, palpitations, hypotension, headache, dizziness, and insomnia Concomitant use with CNS depressants may have additive CNS effects Hawthorn may potentiate effects of digoxin and vasodilators
Horse chestnut seed	To relieve symptoms of chronic venous insufficiency	250 mg bid of extract standardized to 50 mg aescin in delayed-release form It is unsafe to ingest the raw seed, which contains significant amounts of the most toxic constituent, esculin	Mild GI symptoms, headahe, dizziness, and pruritus have been reported Ingestion of high doses may cause renal, hepatic, and hematologic toxicity Concomitant use with anticoagulants may increase the risk of bleeding Horse chestnut may potentiate the effects of hypoglycemic drugs
Kava kava	As an anxiolytic for nervous anxiety, stress, and restlessness As a sedative to induce sleep	Herb and preparations equivalent to 60-120 mg kava pyrones/d Most clinical trials have used 100 mg tid of extract standardized to 70% kava pyrones for anxiety disorders	Kava should not be used by patients with depression and pregnant or nursing women Kava may affect motor reflexes and judgment, so it should not be taken while driving and/or operating heavy machinery Accommodative disturbances have been reported. Kava may exacerbate Parkinson's disease Extended use can cause a temporary yellow

Herb/Nutritional Supplement	Common Uses	Reasonable Adult Oral Dosage*	Precautions and Drug Interactions
			discoloration of skin, hair, and nails
			Reports have linked kava use to at least 25 cases of severe liver toxicity. Sale of products containing kava has been banned in Canada and several European countries
			Kava has been shown to have additive CNS depressant effects with benzodiazepines, alcohol, and herbal tranquilizers
			Kava may also potentiate the sedative effects of anesthetics and so patients taking kava should be discontinued at least 24 h before surgery
Lutein	Commonly used for preventing age-related macular degeneration (AMD) and cataracts Also used to prevent skin cancer, breast cancer, and colon cancer To protect against cardiovascular disease	For AMD and cataracts, 6-20 mg lutein/d from diet For other uses, no established dosage documented Foods containing high concentrations of lutein include kale, spinach, broccoli, and romaine lettuce It is not known if supplemental lutein is as effective as natural lutein Supplemental lutein in the form of esters may require a higher fat intake for effective absorption than purified lutein	No major adverse effects and drug interactions have been reported
Lycopene	Commonly used to prevent and treat prostate cancer Also used in cancer prevention, arthrosclerosis prevention, and reduction of asthma symptoms	For decreasing the growth of prostate cancer, 15 mg supplement bid For prostate cancer prevention, at least 6 mg/d from tomato products (or ≥10 servings/wk) For other uses, no established dosage documented Heat processing converts lycopene in fresh tomatoes from the trans to the cis-configuration. The cis isomer has better bioavailability Lycopene supplements usually do not specify the type and amount of isomers in their product labeling	Lycopene, when consumed in amounts found in foods, is generally considered to be safe Concomitant ingestion of β-carotene may increase lycopene absorption Lycopene may reduce cholesterol levels and potentiate the effects of statins
Melatonin	For jet lag, insomnia, shift-work disorder, and circadian rhythm disorders	For jet lag, 5 mg at bedtime for 2-5 d beginning the day of return	Avoid use in pregnancy because melatonin decreases serum luteinizing

Continued

Herb/Nutritional Supplement	Common Uses	Reasonable Adult Oral Dosage*	Precautions and Drug Interactions
	Also for other medical conditions, including depression, multiple sclerosis, tinnitus, headache, and cancer	For sleep disorders, 0.3-5 mg taken 2 hrs before bedtime Avoid melatonin from animal pineal gland due to possibility of contamination	hormone concentrations and increases serum prolactin levels The common adverse reactions include headache, transient depressive symptoms, daytime fatigue and drowsiness, dizziness, abdominal cramps, irritability, and reduced alertness Concomitant use of melatonin with alcohol, benzodiazepines, or other CNS depressants may cause additive sedation Melatonin can affect immune function and may interfere with immunosuppressive therapy Concomitant use with other herps that have sedative properties (e.g., chamomile, goldenseal, hop, kava, valerian) may produce additive CNS-impairing effects
Milk thistle fruit	As a hepatoprotectant and antioxidant, particularly for the treatment of hepatitis, cirrhosis, and toxic liver damage Used in Europe for the treatment of hepatotoxic mushroom poisoning from *Amanita phalloides*	Average daily dose is 12-15 g of crude drug or formulations equivalent to 200-400 mg of silymarin	Adverse effects are rare but may include diarrhea and allergic reactions Milk thistle may potentiate the hypoglycemic effect of antidiabetic agents
Red clover flower	Commonly used for conditions associated with menopause, such as hot flashes, cardiovascular health, and osteoporosis Also used for premenstrual syndrome, benign prostate hyperplasia, and cancer prevention Used topically to treat psoriasis, eczema, and other rashes	For hot flashes, 40 mg/d of the isoflavones extract (Promensil™) For other conditions, no established dosage documented	Red clover has estrogenic activity and should be avoided during pregnancy and lactation Women with hormone-dependent conditions (e.g., breast, uterine, and ovarian cancer, and endometriosis and uterine fibroids) and men with prostate cancer should also avoid taking red clover Side effects include headache, myalgia, nausea, and rash Red clover contains coumarin derivatives and may increase the risk of bleeding in those who are taking anticoagulants or antiplatelet drugs Preliminary report suggests that red clover may antagonize the effects of tamoxifen Some evidence suggests that red clover can increase levels of drugs that are

Rakel and Bope: *Conn's Current Therapy 2006.*

Herb/Nutritional Supplement	Common Uses	Reasonable Adult Oral Dosage*	Precautions and Drug Interactions
			metabolized by the cytochrome P450 3A4 isoenzyme (e.g., lovastatin, ketoconazole, itraconazole, fexofenadine, and triazolam)
SAMe (S-adenosyl-L-methionine)	For treatment of osteoarthritis, depression, fibromyalgia, and liver disease	For osteoarthritis, 200 mg tid. For depression and fibromyalgia, 800 mg bid. For liver disease, 600-800 mg bid	Common side effects include flatulence, nausea, vomiting, and diarrhea. SAMe can cause anxiety in people with depression and hypomania in people with bipolar disorder. Concurrent use of SAMe and other antidepressant may cause serotonin syndrome
Saw palmetto berry	To treat symptomatic benign prostatic hyperplasia and irritable bladder	160 mg bid of extract standardized to 8%-95% fatty acids and sterols	Adverse effects are rare but may include headache, nausea, and upset stomach. High doses can cause diarrhea
St. John's wort	Effective for the treatment of mild to moderate depression. May have anti-inflammatory and anti-infective activities	300 mg tid of hypericum extract standardized to 0.3% hypericin	St. John's wort should not be used in pregnancy. Side effects include dry mouth, GI upset, dizziness, fatigue, and constipation. St. John's wort may induce photosensitivity, especially in fair-skinned individuals. It may cause serotonin syndrome if used with other antidepressants, including SSRIs, or other serotonergic drugs. It has been shown to induce the cytochrome P450 3A4 isoenzyme and decrease blood levels of many drugs such as indinavir, nevirapine, cyclosporine, digoxin, theophylline, simvastatin, oral contraceptive pills, and warfarin. St. John's wort should be discontinued at least 5 d before surgery to avoid any potential drug interactions
Soy	Commonly used for cholesterol reduction in combination with a low fat diet. Also used for menopausal symptoms and for preventing osteoporosis and cardiovascular disease in postmenopausal women	For lowering cholesterol, 25-50 g/d of soy protein. For hot flashes, 20-60 g/d of soy protein. For osteoporosis, 40 g/d of soy protein containing 90 mg isoflavones	Soy, when consumed as whole foods (e.g., tofu or soymilk), has minimal adverse effects. Large consumption of soy may cause gastric complaints such as constipation, bloating, and nausea. Long-term use of soy tables containing isoflavones (150 mg/d × 5 y) have been shown to cause endometrial hyperplasia

Continued

Herb/Nutritional Supplement	Common Uses	Reasonable Adult Oral Dosage*	Precautions and Drug Interactions
Valerian root	Used as a mild sedative for insomnia and anxiety	2-3 g of dried root or 1-3 mL of tincture, qd to several times/d Two clinical trials have found 400-500 mg of the root extract effective for insomnia	Valerian has a bad odor and can cause morning drowsiness Long-term administration may lead to paradoxical stimulation including restlessness and palpitations Because of the risk of benzodiazepine-like withdrawal, valerian should be tapered over a period of several weeks before surgery It may potentiate the sedative effect of CNS depressants (e.g., benzodiazepines, alcohol) and other herbal tranquilizers

*All supplements are not FDA approved.
*Doses presented in the table are modified from the German Commission E Monographs and/or data from clinical trials. Products from different manufacturers vary considerably. A reliable product should have a label clearly stating the botanical name of the herb and milligram amount contained in the product. Standardized extracts should be used whenever possible and are often disclosed on the label of quality products.
CNS = central nervous system; GI = gastrointestinal; HMG-CoA = 3-hydroxy-3-methylglutaryl coenzyme A; SSRIs = selective serotonin reuptake inhibitors.

New Drugs in 2004 and Agents Pending FDA Approval

Method of
Miriam M. Chan, RPh, PharmD, and
Bella Mehta, PharmD

New Drugs Approved in 2004

Generic Name	Trade Name (Manufacturer)	Strength	Dosage Form	Normal Dosage Range	Pregnancy Rating*	FDA Approval Date	Indication	Classification
Acamprosate calcium	Campral (Forest)	333 mg	Enteric-coated tablet	666 mg tid	C	7/04	Maintenance of abstinence from alcohol in patients with alcohol dependence who are abstinent at initiation of treatment	Alcohol cessation agent
Apomorphine hydrochloride	Apokyn (Mylan Bertek)	10 mg/mL in 2 mL ampule and 3 mL cartridge	Injection	0.2 mL (2 mg) SC and titrate up to a maximum dose of 0.6 mL (6 mg)	C	4/04	For the acute, intermittent treatment of hypomobility, "off" episodes ("end-of-dose wearing off" and unpredictable "on/off" episodes) associated with advanced Parkinson's disease	Non-ergoline dopamine agonist
Azacitidine	Vidaza (Pharmion)	100 mg/vial (yields 25 mg/mL when reconstituted)	Injection	75 mg/m² SC qd for 7 d and repeat q 4 wk; dose may be increased to 100 mg/m² if no beneficial effect is observed after 2 treatment cycles	D	5/04	Treatment for myelodysplastic syndrome	Demethylating agent
Bevacizumab	Avastin (Genentech)	25 mg/4 mL in 4, 16 mL vials	Injection	5 mg/kg IV infusion over 90 min q 14 d	C	12/04	First-line treatment of patients with metastatic carcinoma of the colon or rectum, in conjunction with 5-fluorouracil	Recombinant human monoclonal IgG1 antibody

Continued

19

Rakel and Bope: *Conn's Current Therapy 2006.*

New Drugs Approved in 2004—cont'd

Generic Name	Trade Name (Manufacturer)	Strength	Dosage Form	Normal Dosage Range	Pregnancy Rating*	FDA Approval Date	Indication	Classification
Bovine hyaluronidase	Amphadase (Amphastar)	150 U/mL in 1 mL vial	Injection	For absorption and dispersion of IV drugs: add 50-300 U, most typically 150 U, to the injection solution For SC urography: 75 U SC over each scapula, followed by injection of contrast medium at the same time	C	10/04	As an adjuvant to increase absorption and dispersion of other injected drugs, for hypodermoclysis, and as an adjunct in SC urography for improving resorption of radioopaque agents	Protein enzyme injection adjuvant
Cetuximab	Erbitux (Bristol-Myers Squibb)	2 mg/mL in 50 mL vial	Injection	Loading dose: 400 mg/m^2 IV infusion over 2 h Maintenance dose: 250 mg/m^2 infused over 60 min q wk	C	6/04	Treatment of epidermal growth factor receptor-expressing, metastatic colorectal carcinoma in patients who are refractory to irinotecan-based therapy	Recombinant human/mouse chimeric monoclonal antibody
Cinacalcet hydrochloride	Sensipar (Amgen)	30, 60, 90 mg	Tablet	Parathyroid carcinoma: 30 mg bid and titrate dosage q 2-4 wk through sequential doses of 30 mg bid as necessary to normalize serum calcium levels Secondary HPT: 30 mg qd and titrate dose q 2-4 wk to target intact PTH	C	3/04	Treatment of hypercalcemia in patients with parathyroid carcinoma and for secondary hyperparathyroidism (HPT) with chronic kidney disease on daily dialysis	Calcium receptor agonist
Clofarabine	Clolar (Genzyme)	1 mg/mL in 20 mL vial	Injection	52 mg/m^2 IV infusion over 2 h daily for	D	12/04	Treatment of relapsed or refractory	Deoxyadenosine nucleoside

Generic name	Brand (Company)	Strengths	Dosage form	Dose	Pregnancy category	Date	Indication	Drug class
				5 d, repeat cycle q 2-6 wk			pediatric acute lymphoblastic leukemia after at least 2 prior regimens	antimetabolite
Darifenacin	Enablex (Novartis)	7.5, 15 mg	Extended-release tablet	7.5 mg qd, may increase to 15 mg qd as early as 2 wk after starting therapy	C	12/04	Treatment of overactive bladder with symptoms of urge urinary incontinence, urgency, and frequency	Selective muscarinic (M3) receptor antagonist
Duloxetine hydrochloride	Cymbalta (Eli Lilly)	20, 30, 60 mg	Delayed-release capsule	Major depressive disorder: 20 mg bid to 60 mg qd or 30 mg bid Diabetic neuropathy: 60 mg qd	C	8/04	Treatment of major depressive disorder and diabetic peripheral neuropathic pain	Serotonin norepinephrine reuptake inhibitor
Erlotinib hydrochloride	Tarceva (OSI Pharmaceuticals)	25, 100, 150 mg	Tablet	150 mg qd, take 1-2 h after ingestion of food	D	12/04	Treatment of locally advanced or metastatic non-small cell lung cancer after failure of at least one prior chemotherapy regimen	Antineoplastic agent – HER1/EGFR tyrosine kinase inhibitor
Eszopiclone	Lunesta (Sepracor)	1, 2, 3 mg	Film-coated tablet	2 mg immediately before bedtime; for elderly adults, start at 1 mg dose and increase to 2 mg if needed	C	12/04	For the treatment of insomnia	Non-benzodiazepine hypnotic, pyrrolopyrazine derivative of cyclopyrrolone
Gadobenate dimeglumine	Multihance (Bracco)	0.5 M (529 mg/mL)	Injection	0.1 mmol/kg (0.2 mL/kg) IV infusion at 10 mL/min	No data, not recommended	11/04	Use in MRI of the central nervous system in adults to visualize lesions	MRI paramagnetic agent
L-glutamine	NutreStore (Nutritional Restart.)	5 g/packet	Powder for oral solution	30 g/d divided in 6 doses, give with meals or snacks	C	6/04	Treatment of short bowel syndrome when use in combination with nutrition support and human growth hormone	Amino acid

Continued

19

Rakel and Bope: *Conn's Current Therapy 2006.*

New Drugs Approved in 2004—cont'd

Generic Name	Trade Name (Manufacturer)	Strength	Dosage Form	Normal Dosage Range	Pregnancy Rating*	FDA Approval Date	Indication	Classification
Human secretin	ChiRhoStim (ChiRhoClin)	16 mcg/vial	Injection	0.2 mcg/kg by IV injection over 1 min	C	4/04	For the stimulation of pancreatic secretions and gastrin to aid in the diagnosis of pancreatic exocrine dysfunction or gastrinoma and to facilitate the identification of the ampulla of vater and accessory papilla during endoscopic retrograde cholangiopancreatography	Synthetic human secretin
Icodextrin	Extraneal (Baxter Healthcare)	7.5 g/100 mL in 1.5, 2, 2.5 L bags	Intraperitoneal solution	Infuse intraperitoneally over 10-20 min at a rate comfortable to the patient with the recommended well time of 8-16 h	C	12/04	For a single dialysis exchange for the long (8-16 hours) dwell during continuous ambulatory peritoneal dialysis (CAPD) or automated peritoneal dialysis (APD) for the management of chronic renal failure	Osmotic peritoneal dialysate
Iloprost	Ventavis (CoTherix)	20 mcg/2 mL ampule	Inhalation solution	2.5 mcg initially via Prodose AAD system, then increase to the maintenance dose of 5 mcg 6-9 x/d (max 45 mcg/d)	C	12/04	Treatment of pulmonary arterial hypertension (WHO group I) in patients with NYHA Class III or IV symptoms	Synthetic analogue of prostacyclin PGI₂
Insulin glulisine	Apidra (Aventis Pharms)	100 U/mL in 10 mL vial	Injection	Give individualized dose SC within 15 minutes before a meal or within 20 minutes after starting a meal	C	4/04	For the treatment of adult patients with diabetes mellitus for the control of hyperglycemia	Rapid-acting human insulin analog

Continued

19

Generic	Brand (Manufacturer)	Strength	Form	Dosage	Pregnancy Category	Date	Indication	Class
Lanthanum carbonate	Fosrenol (Shire Pharmaceuticals)	250, 500 mg	Chewable tablet	Can be used in an external infusion pump Total daily dose 750-1500 mg/d divided and taken with meals. Titrate q 2-3 wk until serum phosphate at acceptable values Usual dosage range: 1500-300 mg	C	11/04	Treatment of hyperphosphatemia in patients with end-stage renal disease (ESRD) associated with secondary hyperparathyroidism	Phosphate binder
Lutropin alfa	Luveris (Serono Inc.)	75 IU	Injection	Female infertility: 75 IU SC qd until adequate follicular development Maximum duration of treatment: 14 days; to be used concomitantly with follitropin alfa	X	10/04	Stimulation of follicular development in infertile hypogonadotropic hypogonadal (HH) women with profound luteinizing hormone (LH) deficiency	Ovulation stimulator (gonadotropin)
Omega-3-acid ethyl esters	Omacor (Ross Labs)	1 g	Capsule	4 g/day as a single daily dose or in 2 divided doses	C	12/04	Treatment of hypertriglyceridemia (≥500 mg/dL)	Antilipemic agent
Palifermin	Kepivance (Amgen)	6.25 mg	Injection	Adults: 60 mcg/kg/day for 3 consecutive days before and after myelotoxic therapy; total of 6 doses	C	12/04	Decrease the incidence and severity of severe oral mucositis associated with hematologic malignancies in patients receiving myelotoxic therapy requiring hematopoietic stem cell support	Keratinocyte growth factor

Rakel and Bope: *Conn's Current Therapy 2006.*

New Drugs Approved in 2004—cont'd

Generic Name	Trade Name (Manufacturer)	Strength	Dosage Form	Normal Dosage Range	Pregnancy Rating*	FDA Approval Date	Indication	Classification
Pegaptanib sodium	Macugen (Eyetech)	0.3 mg/ 90 µL pre-filled syringe	Injection	0.3 mg into affected eye(s) q 6 wk	B	12/04	Treatment of neovascular (wet) age-related macular degeneration (AMD)	Ophthalmic Agent recombinant vaccine
Pemetrexed disodium	Alimta (Eli Lilly)	500 mg vial	Injection	500 mg/m² IV infusion over 10 min on day 1 of each 21 day cycle as either a single agent or in combination with cisplatin	D	2/04	In combination with Cisplatin, Alimta is indicated for treatment of malignant pleural mesothelioma for patients whose disease is unresectable or are not candidates for curative surgery. As a single use agent for patients with locally advanced or metastatic non-small cell lung cancer after prior chemotherapy	Antifolate antineoplastic agent
Pentetate calcium trisodium (Ca-DTAP)	Pentetate calcium Trisodium (Hameln Pharmaceuticals)	200 mg/mL in 5 mL	Injection	For adults and adolescents an initial therapy within 24 h of exposure: 1 g IV per day. For initial therapy of pediatrics less than 12 yo: 14 mg/kg IV (max 1 g/d) If additional chelation therapy is needed, switch to Zn-DTAP	C	8/04	For treatment of individuals with known or suspected internal contamination with plutonium, americium, or curium to increase the rate of elimination	Chelating agent
Pentetate zinc trisodium (Zn-DTAP)	Pentetate zinc trisodium (Pharma HamelnG mbH)	200 mg/mL in 5 mL	Injection	For maintenance therapy of adults and adolescents: 1 g IV/d. For maintenance therapy of	B	8/04	For treatment of individuals with known or suspected internal contamination with plutonium, americium, or	Chelating agent

Continued

curium to increase the rate of elimination.

Drug	Strengths	Form	Dosage		Date	Use	Class
Pregabalin Lyrica (Pfizer)	25, 50, 75, 100, 150, 200, 225, 300 mg	Capsule	pediatric patients (less than 12 yo): 14 mg/kg/d (max 1 g) 300-600 mg/d in divided doses	C	12/04	Management of neuropathic pain associated with diabetic peripheral neuropathy	Alpha-2 delta binder of calcium channel
Rifaximin Xifaxan (Salix)	200 mg	Tablet	200 mg tid for 3 d	C	5/04	Treatment of travelers' diarrhea in patients ≥12 years old caused by noninvasive strains of Escherichia coli	Nonsystemic antibiotic
Sodium tetradecyl sulfate Sotradecol (Bioniche Pharamaceuticals)	10, 30 mg/mL	Injection	0.5 mL IV several hours prior to administration of larger dose; 0.5-2 mL (preferred maximum: 1 mL) in each vein, maximum: 10 mL per treatment session; 3% solution reserved for large varices	C	12/04	Treatment of small, uncomplicated varicose veins of the lower extremities	Sclerosing agent
Solifenacin VESIcare (Yamanouchi)	5, 10 mg	Tablet	5 mg/d; if tolerated, may increase to 10 mg/d	C	12/04	Treatment of overactive bladder with symptoms of urinary frequency, urgency, or urge incontinence	Anticholinergic agent
Telithromycin Ketek (Aventis)	400 mg	Tablet	Chronic bronchitis, acute sinusitis: 800 mg qd for 5 d Community-acquired pneumonia: 800 mg qd for 7-10 d	C	4/04	Treatment of acute bacterial exacerbation of chronic bronchitis, acute bacterial sinusitis, and community-acquired pneumonia	Antibacterial

19

New Drugs Approved in 2004—cont'd

Generic Name	Trade Name (Manufacturer)	Strength	Dosage Form	Normal Dosage Range	Pregnancy Rating*	FDA Approval Date	Indication	Classification
Tinidazole	Tindamax (Presutti Labs)	250, 500 mg	Tablet	Trichomoniasis: A single 2 g oral dose taken with food. Giardiasis: In adults, single 2 g dose with food. In pediatrics older than 3 yo, single dose of 50 mg/kg (up to 2 g) with food Intestinal amebiasis: In adults, 2 g/d × 3 d with food. In pediatrics older than 3 yo, 50 mg/kg/d (up to 2 g) × 3 d with good Amebic liver abscess: In adults 2 g/d for 3-5 d with food. In pediatric patients 50 mg/kg/d (up to 2 g) for 3-5 d	C	5/04	Treatment of trichomoniasis caused by *T. vaginalis* in both female and male patients; treatment of giardiasis caused by *G. duodenalis* in both adults and pediatric patients older than 3 yo; treatment of intestinal amebiasis and amebic liver abscess caused by *E. histolytica* in both adults and pediatric patients older than 3 yo	Synthetic antiprotozoal agent
Tiotropium bromide	Spiriva Handihaler (Boehringer Ingelheim)	18 mcg capsules	Aerosol	Inhalation of 18 mcg qd with the HandiHaler device	C	1/4	Long-term maintenance treatment of bronchospasm associated with chronic obstructive pulmonary disease (COPD) patients, including chronic emphysema and bronchitis	Anticholinergic agent
Trospium chloride	Sanctura (Indevus Pharmaceuticals)	20 mg	Tablet	1 bid given on 1 h before meals or an empty stomach	C	5/04	Treatment of overactive bladder with symptoms of	Antticholinergic agent

urge urinary incontinence, urgency, and urinary frequency

Ziconotide	Prialt (Elan Pharmaceuticals)	100, 25 mcg/mL	Injection	2.4 mg/day, titrate ≤2.4 mcg/d (0.1 mcg/h) at intervals ≥2-3×/wk to a maximum dose of 19.2 mcg/d (0.8 mcg/h) by day 21	C	Management of severe chronic pain in patients requiring intrathecal therapy and are intolerant or refractory to other therapies	Analgesic calcium channel blocker	12/04

FDA Pregnancy Categories
A- Adequate studies in pregnant women have not demonstrated a risk to the fetus in the first trimester of pregnancy, and there is no evidence of risk in later trimesters.
B- Animal studies have shown an adverse effect, but adequate studies in pregnant women have not demonstrated a risk to the fetus during the first trimester of pregnancy, and there is no evidence of risk in later trimesters.
C- Animal studies have shown an adverse effect on the fetus, but there are no adequate studies in humans; the benefits from the use of the drug in pregnant woman may be acceptable despite its potential risks.
D- There is evidence of human fetal risk, but the potential benefits from the use of the drug in pregnant women may be acceptable despite its potential risks.
X- Adverse reaction reports indicate evidence of fetal risk; the risk of use in a pregnant woman clearly outweighs any possible benefit.
No drug should be administered during pregnancy unless it is clearly needed and potential benefit outweighs potential hazard to the fetus, regardless of the pregnancy category.

Rakel and Bope: *Conn's Current Therapy 2006.*

Agents Pending FDA Approval

Generic Name	Trade Name (Manufacturer)	Indication
Abetimus	Riquent (La Jolla Pharmaceutical)	Treatment of lupus
Anidulafungin	No brand name (Vicuron Pharmaceuticals)	Treatment of esophageal candidiasis
Ciclesonide	Alvesco (Sanofi-Aventis)	Treatment of asthma
Cilomilast	Ariflo (GlaxoSmithKline)	Treatment of patients with COPD who are poorly responsive to albuterol
Conivaptan	Vaprisol (Yamanouchi Pharma)	Treatment of hyponatremia
Estradiol/drospirenone	Angeliq (Berlex)	Treatment of menopausal symptoms
Everolimus	Certican (Novartis)	Prevention of rejection after heart and kidney transplantation
Etoricoxib	Arcoxia (Merck)	Treatment of arthritis, chronic lower back pain, acute pain, and ankylosing spondylitis
Exenatide	No brand name (Amylin Pharmaceuticals/ Eli Lilly)	Treatment of type 2 diabetes mellitus
Ferumoxtran-IO	Combidex (Advanced Magnetics/Cytogen Corporation)	Used in conjunction with magnetic resonance imaging to aid in the differentiation of cancerous from noncancerous lymph nodes
Histrelin	Vantas (Valera Pharmaceuticals)	Palliative treatment of metastatic prostate cancer
Hyaluronic acid	Orthovisc (Anika Therapeutics)	Treatment of osteroarthritis of the knee
Ibandronate sodium	Boniva (Roche)	Once monthly treatment of osteoporosis
Insulin detemir	No brand name (Novo Nordisk)	Long-acting insulin analog for the treatment of diabetes mellitus
Measles, mumps, rubella, varicella vaccine	Proquad (Merck)	Vaccine against measles, mumps, rubella, and varicella in children
Oxypurinol	Oxyprim (Cardiome)	Treatment of allopurinol-intolerant hyperuricemia
Ramelteon	Rozerem (Takeda)	Treatment of insomnia
Ranolazine	Ranexa (CV Therapeutics)	Treatment of chronic stable angina
Selegiline	Emsam Patch (Mylan Laboratories/ Waston Pharmaceuticals)	Treatment of depression

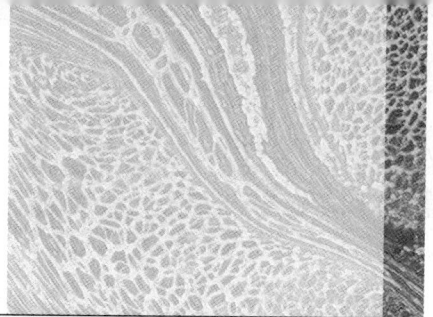

Index

Note: Page numbers followed by f, t, and b indicate figures, tables, and boxed material, respectively. Drugs are listed under the generic name.

Index

Light therapy. *See also* Phototherapy.
  for circadian rhythm disorders, 36, 37, 1083
  for depression, 1368
Lightning injury, 1384-1385
Light's criteria, for pleural effusions, 326, 326t
Limb ischemia
  in acute arterial occlusion, 450-451
  in chronic occlusive peripheral arterial disease, 448-450
Lindane
  for pediculosis, 1018t, 1019, 1020
  for scabies, 1018t, 1020
Linea alba, 1027
Linear IgA disease, 1051
Linezolid
  for bacterial meningitis, 133-134, 135t, 136t
  for staphylococcal infections, 1008, 1009
  for urinary tract infections, 832
Lip
  disorders of, 1025-1026
  herpetic lesions of, 1010-1011, 1011t, 1013-1015, 1013t, 1014t, 1025-1026
  leukokeratosis of, 1005
  melanotic macule of, 1026
  squamous cell carcinoma of, 1026
  telangiectasia of, 1026
Lipase, for steatorrhea, in chronic pancreatitis, 673
Lipid(s)
  diabetes mellitus and, 703
  malabsorption of, 655-656. *See also* Malabsorption.
Lipid-complex amphotericins, for coccidioidomycosis, 307-308, 307t
Lipid-lowering therapy, 734-737. *See also* Antilipid agents.
  for chronic renal failure, 888
  for myocardial infarction, 442
  for primary glomerular disease, 851, 851t
Lipoproteins
  metabolism of, atherogenesis and, 731-732
  target levels for, 732-733, 732t
Liposomal amphotericin B
  for coccidioidomycosis, 307-308, 308t
  for histoplasmosis, 310, 311
  for leishmaniasis, 112t, 113, 114-115
Liquid nitrogen
  for actinic keratosis, 1004
  for myxoid pseudocyst, 983-984
  for solar lentigines, 1060
Listeriosis
  food-borne, 93t, 94t, 95-96
  meningitis in, 131. *See also* Meningitis, bacterial.
Lisuride, for Parkinson's disease, 1152t
Lithium
  for antidepressant augmentation, 1366
  for bipolar disorder, 368-1369
  for cluster headaches, 1123, 1124t
  overdose of, 1468-1469
    extracorporeal therapy for, 1432t
  thyroiditis from, 823
Lithotripsy, 901
Liver. *See also under* Hepatic.
  amebiasis of, 19-22, 66-71, 690. *See also* Amebiasis.
  bacterial infections of, secondary, 605
  biopsy of, in hemochromatosis, 528
  cancer of, cirrhosis and, 604
  cirrhosis of, 601-609. *See also* Cirrhosis.
  in sarcoidosis, 338
  total parenteral nutrition complications in, 759
Liver abscess, amebic, 66-71, 690
Liver disease
  alcoholic, 606
  anticonvulsants in, 1103
  chronic, 601-609. *See also* Cirrhosis.
  drug metabolism in, 1103
  parkinsonism in, 1149
Liver dysfunction, in preeclampsia, 1238
Liver failure, total parenteral nutrition in, 755
Liver transplant
  for α₁-antitrypsin deficiency, 609
  for ascites, 603
  for esophageal varices, 612
  for hemochromatosis, 607
  for hepatocellular carcinoma, 604
  for hepatorenal syndrome, 603

Liver transplant *(Continued)*
  for portopulmonary hypertension, 605
  for primary biliary cirrhosis, 606
  for primary sclerosing cholangitis, 607
Lobectomy, for lung cancer, 299-300
Lobular carcinoma in situ, 1276-1277
Löfgren's syndrome, 338-339
Loiasis, 1018, 1018t
Lomustine, for Hodgkin's disease, 533-535
Long QT syndrome, 370, 396
Longitudinal melanonychia, 983
Loop diuretics. *See* Diuretics.
Loperamide
  for cryptosporidiosis, 692
  for malabsorption, 662
  for nausea and vomiting, in food-borne illness, 99
  for traveler's diarrhea, 100, 197
Lopinavir, for HIV infection, 52, 54t, 55t, 56t
Loracarbef, for urinary tract infections, 827t
Loratadine, 1057t
  for allergic rhinitis, 935, 936t
  for serum sickness, 917
  for urticaria, 1057, 1057t
Lorazepam
  for alcohol withdrawal, 1338
  for Alzheimer's disease, 1075, 1075t, 1076t
  for bipolar disorder, 369
  for delirium, 1358f, 1360
  for endotracheal intubation, in tetanus, 177
  for Ménière's disease, 254-255
  for nausea and vomiting, 8t, 9
Losartan
  for hypertension, 432
    in pregnancy, 1242t
  for hyperuricemia, 730
  for Raynaud's phenomenon, 976, 976t
Loteprednol, for chemical conjunctivitis, 232
Lovastatin, 734
  niacin and, 737
Low back pain, 45-47
Low-carbohydrate diets, diabetes mellitus and, 703-704
Low-molecular-weight heparin. *See also* Heparin.
  for deep venous thrombosis, 456-457
    in pregnancy, 459
  for pulmonary embolism, 333
Low-sodium diet
  for hypertension, 430
  for Ménière's disease, 254
Loxapine, properties of, 1479t
Loxosceles bites, 1399-1400
LSD, 1344
Lucio's leprosy, 117
Lumbar spinal stenosis, pseudoclaudication and, 448, 449t
Lumiracoxib, for osteoarthritis, 1210
Lund-Browder Classification, of burns, 1381, 1383f
Lung. *See also under* Pulmonary; Respiratory.
  abscess of, 316-319
  cirrhosis manifestations in, 605
Lung cancer, 296-305
  after radiotherapy, 543
  biology of, 298
  bronchoalveolar, 297-298
  carcinoid, 298
  diagnosis of, 298-299
  epidemiology of, 296-297
  histologic classification of, 297-298
  large cell, 298
  non-small cell, 300-304
  paraneoplastic syndromes in, 297, 302, 304
  preoperative assessment of, 299-300
  risk factors for, 297
  screening for, 298
  second primary, 302
  signs and symptoms of, 297
  small cell, 304-305
  squamous cell, 298
  staging of, 299
  treatment of, 300-305
Lung fluke, 699t
Lung transplant
  for COPD, 289
  gout after, 729-730
Lung volume reduction surgery, 288-289

Lupus erythematosus
  discoid, 953
  photosensitivity in, 1068
  silicosis and, 342
  systemic, 970-974
Lupus nephritis, 972-974, 974f
Luricostatic agents, 727-728, 728b
Luricosuric agents, 727, 728-729, 728b
Lutein, 1517
Luteinizing hormone, deficiency of, 796
  amenorrhea and, 1292, 1293
Lutropin alfa, 1525
Lycopene, 1517
Lyme disease, 165-169
  arthritis in, 166
  carditis in, 165-166
  chronic, 168-169
  clinical manifestations of
    in early-stage disease, 165-166
    in late-stage disease, 166-167
  peripheral neuropathy in, 1160
  prevention of, 167
  treatment of, 167-169
Lymph node biopsy
  in breast cancer, 1277, 1280
  in melanoma, 1000-1001
Lymph node dissection, retroperitoneal, for testicular cancer, 895, 896
Lymphadenitis, in cat-scratch disease, 208, 210
Lymphangiectasia, intestinal, 661
Lymphangiomas, of tongue, 1031
Lymphatic filariasis, 1018-1019, 1018t
Lymphocyte infusion, for chronic myeloid leukemia, 565
Lymphocytes, CD4+, in HIV infection, 51
Lymphocytic choriomeningitis virus, 1125
Lymphocytic thyroiditis
  chronic, 822
  subacute, 822
Lymphogranuloma venereum, 910-911
Lymphoid papulosis, 956
Lymphoma, 566-568
  gastric, 680-682, 682b
  Hodgkin's. *See* Hodgkin's disease.
  in HIV infection, 66
  primary CNS, 1178
  T-cell
    anaplastic large-cell, 956
    cutaneous, 955-962. *See also* Cutaneous T-cell lymphomas.
Lynch syndrome, 686
Lysergic acid diethylamide, 1344
Lyssaviruses, 156

M
Ma huang, 1513
Mace, 1502-1503
Macroglossia, 1030-1031
Macrolide antibiotics. *See also* Antibiotic(s).
  for bacterial pneumonia, 325, 326t
  for *H. pylori* infection, 647t
Macrosomia
  maternal diabetes and, 1228
  prolonged pregnancy and, 1228
Mad cow disease, 98
Magnesium
  deficiency of, hypoparathyroidism and, 790
  excess of, in total parenteral nutrition, 759
  supplemental
    for fibromyalgia, 1206
    for preeclampsia/eclampsia, 1240
      in postpartum period, 1246t
    for premenstrual syndrome, 1298, 1299t
    for torsades de pointes, 1428t
Magnetic innervation, for urinary incontinence, 845, 847
Magnetic resonance venography, for deep venous thrombosis, 454, 455
Malabsorption, 655-663, 656f
  causes of, 657-661, 657f
  diagnosis of, 661-662, 662b
  in primary biliary cirrhosis, 607
  of carbohydrates, 656-657

Rakel and Bope: *Conn's Current Therapy 2006.*

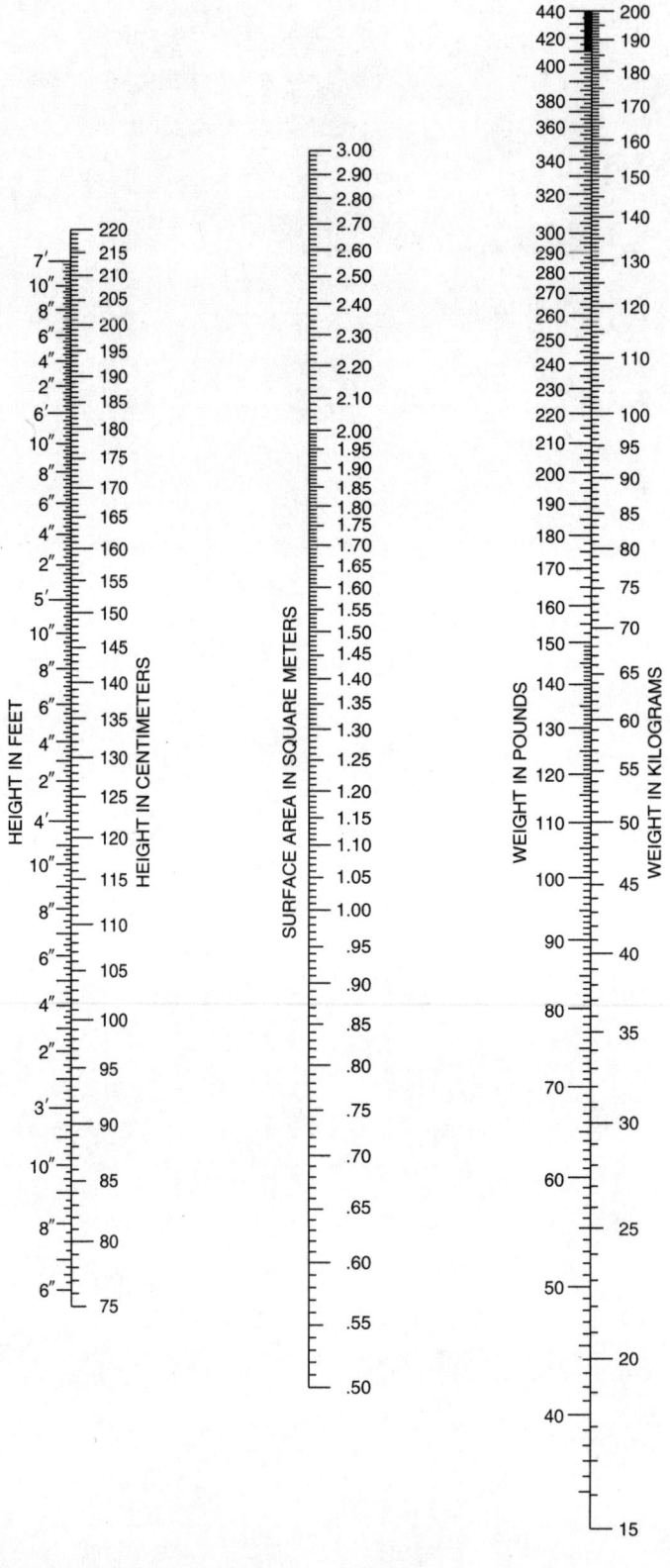